PRINCIPLES AND PRACTICE OF GYNECOLOGIC ONCOLOGY

SEVENTH EDITION

SEVENTH EDITION

PRINCIPLES AND PRACTICE OF GYNECOLOGIC ONCOLOGY

Dennis S. Chi, MD
Deputy Chief
Head of Ovarian Cancer Surgery
Gynecology Service
Department of Surgery
Memorial Sloan Kettering Cancer Center
New York, New York

Don S. Dizon, MD, FACP
Clinical Co-Director
Gynecologic Oncology
Massachusetts General Hospital Cancer Center
Associate Professor
Harvard Medical School
Boston, Massachusetts

Andrew Berchuck, MD
Director
Division of Gynecologic Oncology
Department of Obstetrics and Gynecology
Director
Gynecologic Cancer Program
Duke Cancer Institute
Duke University Medical Center
Durham, North Carolina

Catheryn Yashar, MD
Professor
Chief of Breast and Gynecologic Services
Medical Director La Jolla
University of California, San Diego
San Diego, California

Wolters Kluwer

Philadelphia • Baltimore • New York • London
Buenos Aires • Hong Kong • Sydney • Tokyo

Acquisitions Editor: Ryan Shaw
Editorial Coordinator: David Murphy
Senior *Production Project Manager:* Alicia Jackson
Design Coordinator: Holly McLaughlin
Manufacturing Coordinator: Beth Welsh
Marketing Manager: Rachel Mante Leung
Prepress Vendor: S4Carlisle Publishing Services

Seventh edition

9 8 7 6 5 4 3 2 1

Printed in China

Library of Congress Cataloging-in-Publication Data

ISBN-13: 978-1-4963-4002-3
ISBN-10: 1-4963-4002-7

Cataloging-in-Publication data available on request from the Publisher.

LWW.com

CCS0217

Dedication

This book is dedicated to our families: Hae-Young Chi and children Jessica, Stephanie, and Andrew Chi; Amy Berchuck and children Samuel, Jacob, and Benjamin Berchuck; Henry Stoll and children Isabelle, Harrison, and Sophia Dizon-Stoll; Arnold Yashar and children William, Jacob, and Drew Yashar. Their patience, good humor, encouragement, and love have inspired us throughout our careers. In this regard, they have each made significant contributions to this book.

We would also like to express our gratitude to our own esteemed professors who guided and mentored us, and to all of the colleagues we have worked alongside, learned from, and taught over the years. The Gynecologic Oncology community that the readers of this book belong to is dedicated to the advancement of knowledge in the field and its application to outstanding patient care. The considerable progress we have achieved together in the understanding, diagnosis, treatment, and prevention of these cancers is presented in this book. On behalf of the Gynecologic Oncology community, we dedicate this edition of *Principles and Practice of Gynecologic Oncology* to the brave and courageous patients we all serve, and take inspiration in the oath we all share.

HIPPOCRATIC OATH

I swear to fulfill, to the best of my ability and judgment, this covenant:

- I will respect the hard-won scientific gains of those physicians in whose steps I walk, and gladly share such knowledge as is mine with those who are to follow.
- I will apply, for the benefit of the sick, all measures which are required, avoiding those twin traps of overtreatment and therapeutic nihilism.
- I will remember that there is art to medicine as well as science, and that warmth, sympathy, and understanding may outweigh the surgeon's knife or the chemist's drug.
- I will not be ashamed to say "I know not," nor will I fail to call in my colleagues when the skills of another are needed for a patient's recovery.
- I will respect the privacy of my patients, for their problems are not disclosed to me that the world may know. Most especially must I tread with care in matters of life and death. Above all, I must not play at God.
- I will remember that I do not treat a fever chart, a cancerous growth, but a sick human being, whose illness may affect the person's family and economic stability. My responsibility includes these related problems, if I am to care adequately for the sick.
- I will prevent disease whenever I can, for prevention is preferable to cure.
- I will remember that I remain a member of society, with special obligations to all my fellow human beings, those sound of mind and body as well as the infirm.
- If I do not violate this oath, may I enjoy life and art, respected while I live and remembered with affection thereafter. May I always act so as to preserve the finest traditions of my calling and may I long experience the joy of healing those who seek my help.

International Editorial Board

Contributors

Fadi W. Abdul-Karim, MD, MEd
Department of Pathology
Vice Chair of Education
Robert J. Tomisch Pathology and Laboratory Medicine Institute
Professor of Pathology
Cleveland Clinic, Lerner College of Medicine
Cleveland, Ohio

Sunil J. Advani, MD
Associate Professor
Department of Radiation Medicine and Applied Sciences
University of California, San Diego
La Jolla, California

Ebtesam Ahmed, PharmD, MS
Associate Clinical Professor
Clinical Health Professions
St. John University
Queens, New York
Director Pharmacy Internship
MJHS Institute for Innovation in Palliative Care
New York, New York

David S. Alberts, MD
Regents Professor and Director Emeritus
University of Arizona Cancer Center
University of Arizona
Tucson, Arizona

Donald Armstrong, MD
Professor Emeritus
Memorial Sloan Kettering Cancer Center
New York, New York

Meena Bedi, MD
Assistant Professor
Department of Radiation Oncology
Medical College of Wisconsin
Milwaukee, Wisconsin

Andrew Berchuck, MD
Director
Division of Gynecologic Oncology
Department of Obstetrics and Gynecology
Director
Gynecologic Cancer Program
Duke Cancer Institute
Duke University Medical Center
Durham, North Carolina

Sushil Beriwal, MD
Associate Professor
University of Pittsburgh Cancer Institute
Department of Radiation Oncology
Magee-Womens Hospital of UPMC
Pittsburgh, Pennsylvania

Leslie Blackhall, MD
Associate Professor of Internal Medicine
Division of General Medicine, Geriatrics and Palliative Care
Department of Medicine
Palliative Care Clinic
Charlottesville, Virginia

Michael A. Bookman, MD
Director
Gynecologic Oncology Research
US Oncology and Arizona Oncology
Tucson, Arizona

David D. L. Bowtell, BVSc, PhD
Head
Cancer Genetics and Genomics and Senior Principal Research Fellow
Research Department
Peter MacCallum Cancer Centre and Garvan Institute of Medical Research
Victoria (Peter Mac) and NSW (Garvan), Australia

Mark F. Brady, PhD
Director of Statistics, GOG SDC
GOG Statistical and Data Center
Research Professor
Department of Biostatistics
Roswell Park Cancer Institute
Buffalo, New York

Donal J. Brennan, MB, MRCPI, MRCOG, PhD
Assistant Master
Department of Obstetrics and Gynecology
Rotunda Hospital
Dublin, Ireland

Louise A. Brinton, PhD
Chief
Hormonal and Reproductive Epidemiology
Division of Cancer Epidemiology and Genetics
National Cancer Institute
National Institutes of Health
Bethesda, Maryland

Robert E. Bristow, MD, MBA
Professor and Chair
Department of Obstetrics and Gynecology
University of California
Irvine, California

Jubilee Brown, MD
Professor and Associate Director
Department of Gynecologic Oncology
Levine Cancer Institute
Carolinas HealthCare System
Charlotte, North Carolina

James J. Burke II, MD
The Donald G. Gallup Scholar of Gynecologic Oncology
The Curtis and Elizabeth Anderson Cancer Institute
Memorial University Medical Center
Associate Professor and Director
Department of Gynecologic Oncology
Mercer University School of Medicine, Savannah Campus
Savannah, Georgia

Hilary Calvert, MD, FRCP
Emeritus Professor of Cancer Therapeutics
UCL Cancer Institute
Research Department of Oncology
Faculty of Medical Sciences
London, England

Susana M. Campos, MS, MD, MPH
Assistant Professor of Medicine
Medical Oncology
Harvard Medical School
Dana-Farber Cancer Institute
Boston, Massachusetts

Dennis S. Chi, MD
Deputy Chief
Head of Ovarian Cancer Surgery
Gynecology Service
Department of Surgery
Memorial Sloan Kettering Cancer Center
New York, New York

David Cibula, MD, PhD
Gynecologic Oncology Center
Department of Obstetrics and Gynecology
First Faculty of Medicine
Charles University in Prague
General University Hospital in Prague
Prague, Czech Republic

David E. Cohn, MD
Stuart M. Sloan and Larry J. Copeland Chair
Director
Division of Gynecologic Oncology
Professor
Department of Obstetrics and Gynecology
Columbus, Ohio

Mary B. Daly, MD, PhD
Chair
Department of Clinical Genetics
Fox Chase Cancer Center
Philadelphia, Pennsylvania

Robert Debernardo, MD
Director of Minimally Invasive Surgery
Gynecologic Oncology Division
Department of Obstetrics and Gynecology and Women's Health Institute
Cleveland Clinic
Cleveland, Ohio

Marcela G. del Carmen, MD
Professor
Division of Gynecologic Oncology
Harvard Medical School
Boston, Massachusetts

Don S. Dizon, MD, FACP
Clinical Co-Director
Gynecologic Oncology
Massachusetts General Hospital Cancer Center
Associate Professor
Harvard Medical School
Boston, Massachusetts

Sean C. Dowdy, MD, FACS
Professor and Chair
Division of Gynecologic Surgery Co-Leader, Women's Cancer Program
Mayo Clinic College of Medicine
Rochester, Minnesota

Linda R. Duska, MD, MPH
Professor
Department of Obstetrics and Gynecology
Fellowship Director
Division of Gynecologic Oncology
Associate Dean for Clinical Research
University of Virginia School of Medicine
Charlottesville, Virginia

David A. Edmonson, MD, FACS
Assistant Professor
Department of General Surgery
Department of Obstetrics and Gynecology
Director
Lymphedema Program, PWO
The Warren Alpert Medical School of Brown University
Program in Women's Oncology
Women and Infants' Hospital
Providence, Rhode Island

Mark H. Einstein, MD, MS
Professor and Chair
Department of Obstetrics, Gynecology, and Women's Health
Rutgers New Jersey Medical School
Newark, New Jersey

Robert E. Emerson, MD
Associate Professor
Department of Pathology and Laboratory Medicine
Indiana University School of Medicine
Indianapolis, Indiana

Beth A. Erickson, MD
Professor
Department of Radiation Oncology
Medical College of Wisconsin
Milwaukee, Wisconsin

Britt K. Erickson, MD
Assistant Professor
Gynecologic Oncologist
Department of Obstetrics and Gynecology
Division of Gynecologic Oncology
University of Minnesota
Minneapolis, Minnesota

Dariush Etemadmoghadam, PhD
Senior Research Officer
Department of Research
Peter MacCallum Cancer Centre
Victoria, Australia

Amanda N. Fader, MD
Associate Professor and Director
The Kelly Gynecologic Oncology Service
Baltimore, Maryland

Virginia L. Filiaci, PhD
Associate Director
Biostatistics and Science
GOG and NRG Oncology-Buffalo Statistics and Data Management Centers
Roswell Park Cancer Institute
Buffalo, New York

Gini F. Fleming, MD
Professor of Medicine
Director
Medical Oncology Breast Program Medical Oncology
Director
Gynecologic Oncology
The University of Chicago Medicine
Chicago, Illinois

Silvia Franceschi, MD
Group Head, Special Advisor
Infections and Cancer Epidemiology Group
International Agency for Research on Cancer
Lyon, France

Stéphanie L. Gaillard, MD, PhD
Assistant Professor
Department of Medicine/Division of Medical Oncology
Duke University Medical Center
Durham, North Carolina

Aleksandra Gentry-Maharaj, PhD
Senior Research Associate
Gynecological Cancer Research Centre
Department of Women's Cancer
Institute for Women's Health
Faculty of Population Health Sciences
UCL
London, England

David M. Gershenson, MD
Professor
Department of Gynecologic Oncology and Reproductive Medicine
The University of Texas MD Anderson Cancer Center
Houston, Texas

Charlie Gourley, BSc, MB ChB, PhD, FRCP
Professor of Medical Oncology
Nicola Murray Ovarian Cancer Research Centre
Edinburgh Cancer Research UK Centre
MRC IGMM
The University of Edinburgh
Honorary Consultant in Medical Oncology
Edinburgh Cancer Centre
Western General Hospital
United Kingdom

Laura J. Havrilesky, MD, MHSc
Professor
Division of Gynecologic Oncology
Department of Obstetrics and Gynecology
Duke University Medical Center
Durham, North Carolina

Jaroslaw T. Hepel, MD, FACRO
Assistant Professor
Department of Radiation Oncology
The Warren Alpert School of Medicine at Brown University
Rhode Island Hospital
Providence, Rhode Island

Warner K. Huh, MD
Professor and Division Director
Margaret Cameron Spain Endowed Chair in Obstetrics/Gynecology
Division of Gynecologic Oncology
University of Alabama at Birmingham
Birmingham, Alabama

Elizabeth L. Jewell, MD
Associate Professor
Department of Obstetrics and Gynecology
Weill Cornell Medical College
Associate Attending Surgeon
Department of Surgery
Memorial Sloan Kettering Cancer Center
New York, New York

Josephine Kang, MD, PhD
Assistant Professor of Clinical Radiation Oncology
Department of Radiation Oncology
New York Presbyterian/Weill Cornell Medical College
New York, New York

Noah D. Kauff, MD
Director
Clinical Cancer Genetics
Duke Cancer Institute
Duke University Health System
Durham, North Carolina

Hanan I. Khalil, MD
Assistant Professor
Department of Diagnostic Imaging
The Warren Alpert Medical School of Brown University
Rhode Island Medical Imaging
East Providence, Rhode Island

Elise C. Kohn, MD, CAPT (Ret.) USPHS
Head
Gynecologic Cancer Therapeutics
Gastroenteropancreatic Neuroendocrine Cancer Therapeutics
Lead
NCTN Core Correlative Science Committee
Clinical Investigations Branch
Cancer Therapy Evaluation Program
National Cancer Institute
Attending Physician
Women's Malignancies Branch
Medical Oncology Program
Center for Cancer Research
National Cancer Institute
Bethesda, Maryland

Shalini L. Kulasingam, MPH, PhD
Associate Professor
School of Public Health
Division of Epidemiology and Community Health
University of Minnesota, Twin Cities
Minneapolis, Minnesota

Charles A. Kunos, MD, PhD
Associate Professor
Department of Pharmaceutical Sciences
Northeast Ohio Medical Center
Rootstown, Ohio

Eric Leblanc, MD
Head
Department of Gynecological Oncology
Centre Oscar Lambret
Lille, France

Larissa J. Lee, MD
Assistant Professor
Radiation Oncology
Brigham and Women's Hospital
Dana-Farber Cancer Institute
Boston, Massachusetts

Leslie K. Lee, MD
Staff Radiologist
Department of Radiology
Brigham and Women's Hospital
Instructor of Radiology
Harvard Medical School
Boston, Massachusetts

Susanna I. Lee, MD, PhD
Associate Professor
Department of Radiology
Harvard Medical School
Staff Radiologist
Department of Radiology
Massachusetts General Hospital
Boston, Massachusetts

Carolyn Lefkowits, MD, MPH, MS
Assistant Professor
Division of Gynecologic Oncology
Department of Obstetrics and Gynecology
University of Colorado School of Medicine
Denver, Colorado

Robert D. Legare, MD
Associate Professor of Obstetrics and Gynecology (Clinical)
Associate Professor of Medicine (Clinical)
Department of Obstetrics and Gynecology
Alpert Medical School
Brown University
Providence, Rhode Island

Mario M. Leitao Jr, MD
Associate Professor
Department of Obstetrics and Gynecology
Weill Cornell Medical College
Associate Attending Surgeon
Gynecology Service
Department of Surgery
Memorial Sloan Kettering Cancer Center
New York, New York

Ernst Lengyel, MD, PhD
Chairman
Department of Obstetrics and Gynecology
Arthur L. and Lee G. Herbst Professor of Obstetrics and Gynecology
University of Chicago Medicine
Chicago, Illinois

Pauline Lesage, MD, LLM
Physician Educator
MJHS Institute for Innovation in Palliative Care
New York, New York
Associate Professor
Department of Family and Social Medicine
Albert Einstein College of Medicine
Bronx, New York

Douglas A. Levine, MD
Director
Gynecologic Oncology, Laura and Isaac Perlmutter Cancer Center
Head
Gynecology Research Laboratory
Professor
Division of Gynecologic Oncology
Department of Obstetrics and Gynecology
NYU Langone Medical Center
New York, New York

Stephanie Lheureux, MD, PhD
Associate Professor
Faculty of Medicine
University of Toronto
Staff
Department of Medical Oncology and Hematology
Princess Margaret Cancer Center
Toronto, Canada

Maria Lluria-Prevatt, PhD
Research Administrator
University of Arizona Cancer Center
University of Arizona
Tucson, Arizona

Karen H. Lu, MD
J. Taylor Wharton Distinguished Chair in Gynecologic Oncology
Department of Gynecologic Oncology and Reproductive Medicine
Division of Surgery
Chair
Department of Gynecologic Oncology and Reproductive Medicine
Division of Surgery
The University of Texas MD Anderson Cancer Center
Houston, Texas

John R. Lurain, MD
Marcia Stenn Professor of Gynecologic Oncology
Department of Obstetrics and Gynecology
Fineberg School of Medicine
Northwestern University
Chicago, Illinois

Heather MacNew, MD
Assistant Professor
Surgical Critical Care and Acute Care Surgery
Mercer University School of Medicine
Memorial University Medical Center
Savannah, Georgia

Gina M. Mantia-Smaldone, MD
Assistant Professor
Department of Surgical Oncology
Division of Gynecologic Oncology
Fox Chase Cancer Center
Philadelphia, Pennsylvania

Daniela Matei, MD
Professor
Diana Princess of Wales Professor in Cancer Research
Northwestern University Feinberg School of Medicine
Chicago, Illinois

Shaunagh McDermott, MB, BCh, BAO
Instructor
Harvard Medical School
Radiologist
Department of Thoracic Imaging
Massachusetts General Hospital
Boston, Massachusetts

D. Scott McMeekin†, MD
Virginia Cade Chair
Cancer Development Therapeutics
Deputy Director for Clinical Research
Section Chief, Gynecologic Oncology
University of Oklahoma
Oklahoma City, Oklahoma

Usha Menon, MD (RES), FRCOG
Professor of Gynaecological Cancer
Department of Women's Cancer
UCL Institute for Women's Health
London, United Kingdom

Jeffrey C. Miecznikowski, PhD
Associate Professor
Department of Biostatistics
SUNY University at Buffalo
Buffalo, New York

Bradley J. Monk, MD, FACOG, FACS
Professor
Director
Division of Gynecologic Oncology
Vice Chair
Department of Obstetrics and Gynecology
University of Arizona Cancer Center-Phoenix
Creighton University School of Medicine at
Dignity Health St. Joseph's Hospital and Medical Center
Phoenix, Arizona

John W. Moroney, MD
Associate Professor
Division of Gynecologic Oncology
Department of Obstetrics and Gynecology
University of Chicago
Chicago, Illinois

Firas Mourtada, PhD, DABR, FAAPM
Adjunct Associate Professor
Department of Radiation Oncology
Thomas Jefferson University
Philadelphia, Pennsylvania
Chief of Clinical Physics
Department of Radiation Oncology
Christiana Health Care Systems
Newark, Delaware
Associate Professor
Department of Radiation Physics
The University of Texas MD Anderson Cancer Center
Houston, Texas

Andreas Obermair, MD, FRANZCOG, CGO
Director of Research
Queensland Centre for Gynecological Cancer
Herston, Brisbane, Australia

Roisin O'Cearbhaill, MB, BCh, BAO
Assistant Professor
Department of Medicine
Weill Cornell Medical College
Assistant Attending Physician
Gynecologic Medical Oncology Service
Department of Medicine
Memorial Sloan Kettering Cancer Center
New York, New York

Kunle Odunsi, MD, PhD
Cancer Center Deputy Director
The M. Steven Piver Professor and Chair
Department of Gynecologic Oncology
Executive Director
Center for Immunotherapy
Roswell Park Cancer Institute
Buffalo, New York

Amit M. Oza, BSc, MD, MBBS, FRCP
Professor
Faculty of Medicine
University of Toronto
Co-Director
Drug Development Program
Princess Margaret Cancer Center
Toronto, Canada

Sonali V. Pandya, MD, FACS
Breast Surgeon
Department of Surgery - Clinical Instructor at Brown University
Women and Infants' Hospital
Providence, Rhode Island

Emily Penick, MD
Captain, Medical Corps, U.S. Army
Division of Gynecologic Oncology
Walter Reed National Military Medical Center
Clinical Assistant Professor
Uniformed Services University of the Health Sciences
Bethesda, Maryland

Jacobus Pfisterer, MD, PhD
Director
Gynecologic Oncology Center
Chairman
AGO Study Group
Past Chair/Member of the Executive Committee
Gynecologic Cancer Intergroup GCIG
Kiel, Germany

Russell K. Portenoy, MD
Professor
Department of Neurology
Albert Einstein College of Medicine
Executive Director
MJHS Institute for Innovation in Palliative Care
New York, New York

Scott C. Purinton, MD, PhD
Assistant Professor
Department of Obstetrics and Gynecology
Mercer University School of Medicine
Assistant Professor
Anderson Cancer Institute Surgical Associates
Anderson Cancer Institute
Memorial University Medical Center
Savannah, Georgia

Denis Querleu, MD
President-elect
European Society of Gynaecologic Oncology
Institut Bergonié Cancer Center
Bordeaux, France

Tina Rizack, MD, MPH
Medical Oncology/Hematology
Program in Women's Oncology
Women & Infants Hospital
Assistant Professor (Clinical) of Medicine and Obstetrics and Gynecology
Alpert Medical School of Brown University
Providence, Rhode Island

Kenneth Rolston, MD, FACP
Internist and Professor of Medicine
Department of Infectious Diseases, Infection Control and Employee Health
Division of Internal Medicine
The University of Texas MD Anderson Cancer Center
Houston, Texas

Paul J. Sabbatini, MD
Attending Physician
Gynecologic Medical Oncology Service
Deputy Physician-in-Chief for Clinical Research
Memorial Sloan Kettering Cancer Center
New York, New York

Amar Safdar, MD
Associate Professor of Medicine
Department of Infectious Diseases and Immunology
NYU School of Medicine
Director
Transplant Infectious Diseases
Department of Medicine
NYU Langone Medical Center
New York, New York

Vikrant V. Sahasrabuddhe, D. PH
Program Director
Division of Cancer Prevention
National Cancer Institute
Bethesda, Maryland

Mark Schattner, MD
Professor of Clinical Medicine
Department of Medicine
Weill Cornell Medical College
Attending Physician
Gastroenterology and Nutrition Service
Department of Medicine
Memorial Sloan Kettering Cancer Center
New York, New York

Julian C. Schink, MD
Professor
Department of Obstetrics and Gynecology
Michigan State University
Vice President
Clinical Integrations and Improvement
Spectrum Health
Grand Rapids, Michigan

Angeles A. Secord, MD, MHSc
Professor
Department of Obstetrics and Gynecology
Division of Gynecologic Oncology
Duke Cancer Institute
Durham, North Carolina

Jeffrey D. Seidman,* MD
Medical Officer
Office of In Vitro Diagnostics and Radiological Health
Center for Devices and Radiological Health
Food and Drug Administration
Silver Spring, Maryland

Priya Simoes, MD
Fellow
Gastroenterology and Nutrition Service
Memorial Sloan Kettering Cancer Center
New York, New York

Yukio Sonoda, MD
Professor
Department of Obstetrics and Gynecology
Weill Cornell Medical College
Attending Surgeon
Department of Surgery
Memorial Sloan Kettering Cancer Center
New York, New York

Margaret M. Steinhoff, MD FACP
Professor of Pathology and Laboratory Medicine
The Warren Alpert Medical School of Brown University
Director of Surgical Pathology
Women and Infants Hospital of Rhode Island
Providence, Rhode Island

*The opinions and assertions herein are the private views of the authors and do not purport to reflect the US FDA, Department OF HHS, or any other part of the US Government. This work was not prepared as part of Dr. Seidman's official duties in the US FDA.

Paul H. Sugarbaker, MD, FACS, FRCS
Director
Program in Peritoneal Surface Malignancy
MedStar Washington Hospital Center
Washington, DC

C. James Sung, MD
Professor of Pathology
Alpert Medical School of Brown University
Vice Chief of Pathology and Director of Clinical Pathology
Women and Infants Hospital of Rhode Island
Director of Clinical Pathology and Laboratory Informatics
Care New England Health System
Providence, Rhode Island

Carmen Tornos, MD
Professor of Pathology
Department of Pathology
Stony Brook Medical Center
Stony Brook, New York

Britton Trabert, PhD
Investigator
Division of Cancer Epidemiology and Genetics
National Cancer Institute
Bethesda, Maryland

Akila Viswanathan, MD, MPH
Associate Professor of Radiation Oncology
Harvard Medical School
Director
Gynecologic Radiation
Dana-Farber Cancer Institute
Boston, Massachusetts

Edward J. Wilkinson, MD, FACOG, FACAP
Professor and Vice Chairman
Director and Chief
Division of Anatomic Pathology
Department of Pathology and Laboratory Medicine
Adjunct Professor
Obstetrics and Gynecology
University of Florida College of Medicine
Gainesville, Florida

Aaron H. Wolfson, MD
Professor
Department of Radiation Oncology
University of Miami School of Medicine
Miami, Florida

Catheryn Yashar, MD
Professor
Chief of Breast and Gynecologic Services
Medical Director La Jolla
University of California, San Diego
San Diego, California

Anna Yemelyanova, MD
Associate Professor
Department of Pathology
The University of Texas MD Anderson Cancer Center
Houston, Texas

Robert H. Young, MD
Robert E. Scully Professor of Pathology
Harvard Medical School
Director
Gynecologic Pathology
Pathologist
Department of Pathology
Massachusetts General Hospital
Boston, Massachusetts

Dmitriy Zamarin, MD, PhD
Assistant Attending
Gynecologic Medical Oncology
Memorial Sloan Kettering Cancer Center
New York, New York

Oliver Zivanovic, MD
Assistant Professor
Department of Obstetrics and Gynecology
Weill Cornell Medical College
Assistant Attending Surgeon
Department of Surgery
Memorial Sloan Kettering Cancer Center
New York, New York

Video List

Vulva:

Video 1 Sentinel inguinofemoral lymph node identification in vulvar cancer and the use of near-infrared imaging for sentinel lymph node detection

Cervix:

Video 2 Radical abdominal trachelectomy

Video 3 Extraperitoneal lymph node dissection

Video 4 Robotic-assisted supralevator total pelvic exenteration

Video 5 Total pelvic infralevator exenteration using Ligasure

Video 6 Urinary reconstruction following cystectomy: The ileal conduit

Video 7 Urinary reconstruction after pelvic exenteration: Modified Indiana pouch

Video 8 Modified RAM flap for neovagina creation after exenteration

Uterine Corpus:

Video 9 Sentinel lymph node mapping for uterine cancer: A practical illustration of injection and mapping techniques

Video 10 Sentinel lymph node (SNL) mapping using robotic-assisted fluorescence imaging

Ovary:

Video 11 Robotic Xi infra renal aortic node dissection with lower pelvic port placement

Video 12 Retroperitoneal lymph node dissection (RPLND) for primary ovarian cancer

Video 13 Surgical vascular anatomy on the upper abdomen

Video 14 Vascular and ligamentous attachments

Video 15 How to approach suspicious lymph nodes on the upper abdomen

Video 16 Resection of tumor from the supragastric lesser sac with peritonectomy

Video 17 Morison pouch peritonectomy in cytoreductive surgery

Video 18 Diaphragm peritonectomy with resection of Glisson capsule for advanced ovarian cancer

Video 19 Diaphragm peritonectomy with full-thickness resection for advanced ovarian cancer

Video 20 Liver mobilization with diaphragm peritonectomy and liver wedge resection

Video 21 Excision of tumor along ligament venosum

Video 22 Excision of tumor along ligamentum teres

Video 23 Mobilization of right liver with wedge resection segments 6 and 7

Preface

The publication in 2017 of the 7th edition of *Principles and Practice of Gynecologic Oncology* marks the 25th anniversary of the creation of this textbook. The founding editors, William J. Hoskins, Carlos A. Perez, and Robert C. Young, represented the disciplines of Gynecologic Oncology, Radiation Oncology, and Medical Oncology. They created the first multidisciplinary textbook in the field and, in their words, "strove to produce a definitive reference written at the expert level." The focus on multidisciplinary approaches to treatment and a detailed presentation of the literature on which clinical care is based continues to be a guiding principle.

The second set of editors, Richard R. Barakat, Maurie Markman, and Marcus Randall, also represented Gynecologic, Medical, and Radiation Oncology. Over the course of several editions, they incorporated new chapters that reflected dramatic progress in the understanding and treatment of women's cancers. Simultaneously, advances in technology facilitated the use of full color throughout the book as well as increasingly user-friendly online versions that allow access to cutting-edge information at the point of care.

As the new editors of *Principles and Practice of Gynecologic Oncology*, we owe a debt of gratitude to our predecessors. We are proud to continue their tradition of bringing together multidisciplinary expertise that also includes Pathology colleagues. Given the pace of discovery and change within the field, we strove to ensure that this new edition reflects the many advances in the field. To this end, this edition includes an updated chapter on pharmacology of gynecologic cancers and a new chapter on targeted therapies. Several approaches have been developed with collaboration and support from the publisher that will enhance the value of this book for practitioners, researchers, and students.

We are increasingly becoming a single worldwide Gynecologic Oncology community. In recognition of this reality, the most significant change in the 7th edition is an enhanced global focus. This is in dramatic contrast to 25 years ago when this textbook was essentially intended to reflect the standard of care and ongoing advancement of knowledge in the developed world. Today, developed nations have embraced global efforts to eradicate health care disparities. The greatest challenge in Gynecologic Oncology globally is the lack of infrastructure for cervical cancer screening and prevention in resource-poor countries. This results in the deaths of hundreds of thousands of women annually, many of which could be prevented. Treatment of gynecologic cancers also continues to be suboptimal in many of these countries owing to lack of resources and trained personnel, and this leads to unacceptably low cure rates. In the new edition of *Principles and Practice of Gynecologic Oncology*, we invited more international experts as authors of chapters to provide their perspectives on patterns of incidence, mortality, and treatment worldwide. We also established an International Editorial Board that was charged with providing commentary on similarities and differences in management between different countries.

We have given considerable thought to the issue of how best to maintain the relevance of the book between printed editions in an era of instant access to new information on the Internet. Solutions include smartphone access to the content of the textbook with enhanced search capabilities, as well as more frequent online updates as new studies are reported. We also now include online access to a new library of surgical videos to ensure that surgical techniques are not only read, but visualized.

It is our hope that the global focus of the 7th edition will enhance the impact of this textbook by bringing a synthesis of existing knowledge and standards of practice to the entire world. All of those involved in producing this edition are united with its readers in a shared mission to cure and eradicate gynecologic cancers worldwide.

Dennis S. Chi, MD
Andrew Berchuck, MD
Catheryn Yashar, MD
Don S. Dizon, MD, FACP

Acknowledgments

The editors acknowledge the contributions of numerous individuals without whom this book would not have been possible. The talented staff of the publisher Wolters Kluwer, specifically senior product manager Emilie Moyer, editorial coordinator David Murphy, and developmental editor Martha Cushman, provided invaluable encouragement, direction, and guidance during the creative process and in technical execution. Shailaja Subramanian provided outstanding production services. From the Academic Office of the Gynecology Service, Department of Surgery, Memorial Sloan Kettering Cancer Center, we acknowledge the invaluable contributions of editors George Monemvasitis and Jenifer Levin. Their attention to detail, patience, and communication skills were of the utmost importance throughout the publication process. Our appreciation for all their efforts cannot be adequately expressed, but we hope they know how much we value their contributions.

Contents

SECTION I

Etiology, Prevention, and Molecular Biology

CHAPTER 1

Epidemiology of Gynecologic Cancers

Louise A. Brinton, Vikrant V. Sahasrabuddhe, Britton Trabert, and Silvia Franceschi

Disease-oriented texts often include a chapter on epidemiology or etiology, which is considered perfunctory if the book is used by therapists whose daily practice is rarely influenced by these considerations. This is not the case for physicians who treat patients with gynecologic cancers because these clinicians have frequent opportunities to interpret epidemiologic findings and make observations of etiologic importance. Moreover, public health measures based on epidemiologic findings influence gynecologic practice perhaps more than any other clinical discipline. In particular, epidemiologic data are critical for the prevention and treatment of cervical and uterine cancers.

From the observation 150 years ago of the rarity of cervical cancer in nuns to the most recent follow-up studies of type-specific human papillomavirus (HPV) infection, determining the cause, natural history, and prevention of this disease has focused on sexual practices and suspect infectious agents. Screening interventions based on natural history studies have fundamentally altered the usual presentation of this disease, and as more information about preceding infectious processes becomes available, even more radical changes in presentation and management are likely.

The probable estrogenic cause of uterine cancer was proposed by etiologically oriented gynecologists decades before its demonstration by epidemiologists. Unfortunately, this did not prevent the largest epidemic of iatrogenic cancer in recorded history (i.e., uterine cancer caused by menopausal estrogen therapy). The resurgent interest in menopausal hormone therapy, effects of progestins added to this regimen, and associated risk–benefit questions are certain to link the epidemiologist and the gynecologist for the foreseeable future. The iatrogenic chemoprevention of endometrial and ovarian cancer through oral contraception has similarly thrust the two disciplines together around issues ranging from basic biology to risk–benefit assessments.

The rich tradition of the mingling of epidemiology and gynecologic oncology has led to better opportunities for prevention, screening, and insights into basic mechanisms of disease than for any other subspecialty concerned with cancer. This chapter is written with the aim of clarifying how epidemiology is an integral part of the effort to reduce the morbidity and mortality from gynecologic cancers in women.

Uterine Corpus Cancer

Demographic Patterns

Uterine corpus cancer (hereafter referred to as uterine cancer) is the most common invasive gynecologic cancer and the fourth most frequently diagnosed cancer among women in the United States today. One in 40 will develop uterine cancer during their lives, and it is estimated that there were approximately 54,870 diagnoses during 2015 (1). Uterine cancers are primarily endometrial cancers, with sarcomas comprising only about 3% to 7% of all uterine malignancies, and therefore most of what is known regarding the epidemiology of uterine cancer relates to endometrial cancer. The average annual age-adjusted incidence of uterine cancer from the Surveillance, Epidemiology, and End Results (SEER) program, a cancer reporting system involving approximately 30% of US residents, was 27.5 per 100,000 women for 2012. The disease is rare before the age of 45 years, but the risk rises sharply among women in their late 40s to middle 60s (**Fig. 1.1**).

The prognosis for uterine cancers is quite good, with an age-adjusted mortality rate of 4.5 per 100,000 women and a 5-year survival rate of approximately 83.8% (2). It is estimated that approximately 10,170 women died from uterine cancer during 2015 (1).

Uterine cancer rates are highest in North America and Northern Europe, intermediate in Southern Europe and temperate South America, and low in Southern and Eastern Asia (including Japan) and in most of Africa (except southern Africa) (**Fig. 1.2**) (3). This is likely due to prevalence differences in a variety of risk factors, including reproductive patterns and obesity, although specific studies to address the impact of such differences have not been undertaken.

Over time in the United States, dramatic changes in the incidence pattern for uterine cancers have occurred. Among Whites, there was a marked increase in incidence that peaked about 1975, a trend that was later linked with the widespread use of menopausal estrogen therapy in the late 1960s and early 1970s (**Fig. 1.3**). In Blacks, there has been a progressive increase in incidence over time, eliminating the previous racial disparity that was observed for many decades. In contrast, mortality rates remain considerably higher for Blacks than for Whites.

Reproductive Risk Factors

Nulliparity is a recognized risk factor for uterine cancer. Most studies demonstrate a two- to threefold higher risk for nulliparous women than for parous women. The association of uterine cancer with nulliparity is believed to be a consequence of prolonged periods of anovulation, although both nulliparity and infertility appear to exert independent effects (4). Mechanisms that may mediate the risk associated with infertility include anovulatory menstrual cycles (i.e., prolonged exposure to estrogens without sufficient progesterone); high serum levels of androstenedione (i.e., excess androstenedione is available for conversion to estrone); low levels of serum sex hormone-binding globulin (SHBG); and the absence of monthly sloughing of the endometrial lining (i.e., residual tissue may become hyperplastic).

It has further been established that the risk of uterine cancer decreases with increasing parity, especially among premenopausal women (5). Recent attention has focused on timing of births. Several investigators have found decreased risks with shorter intervals since a last birth and have suggested that this might reflect a protective effect of mechanical clearance of initiated cells (5).

An understanding of the effects of infertility on cancer risk must also consider relationships according to different methods of birth control, including oral contraceptives (discussed later in this chapter).

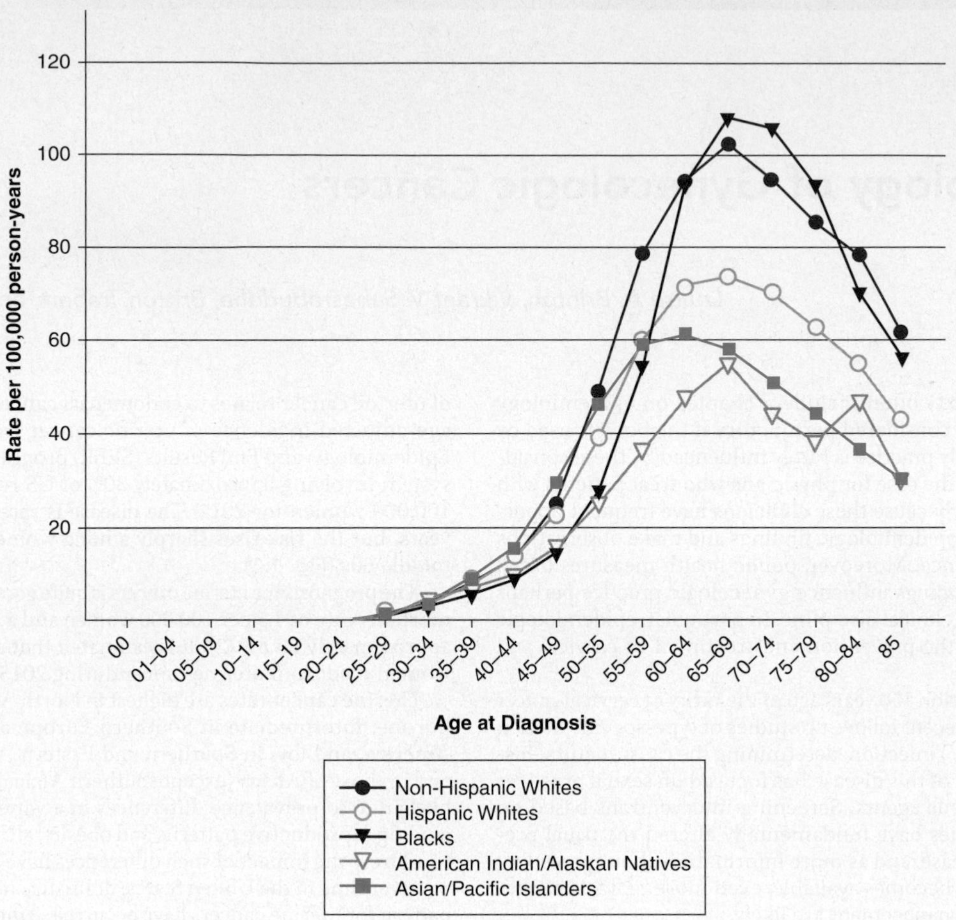

Figure 1.1. Age-specific uterine cancer incidence rates by race among US women, SEER-18, 2003 to 2012.

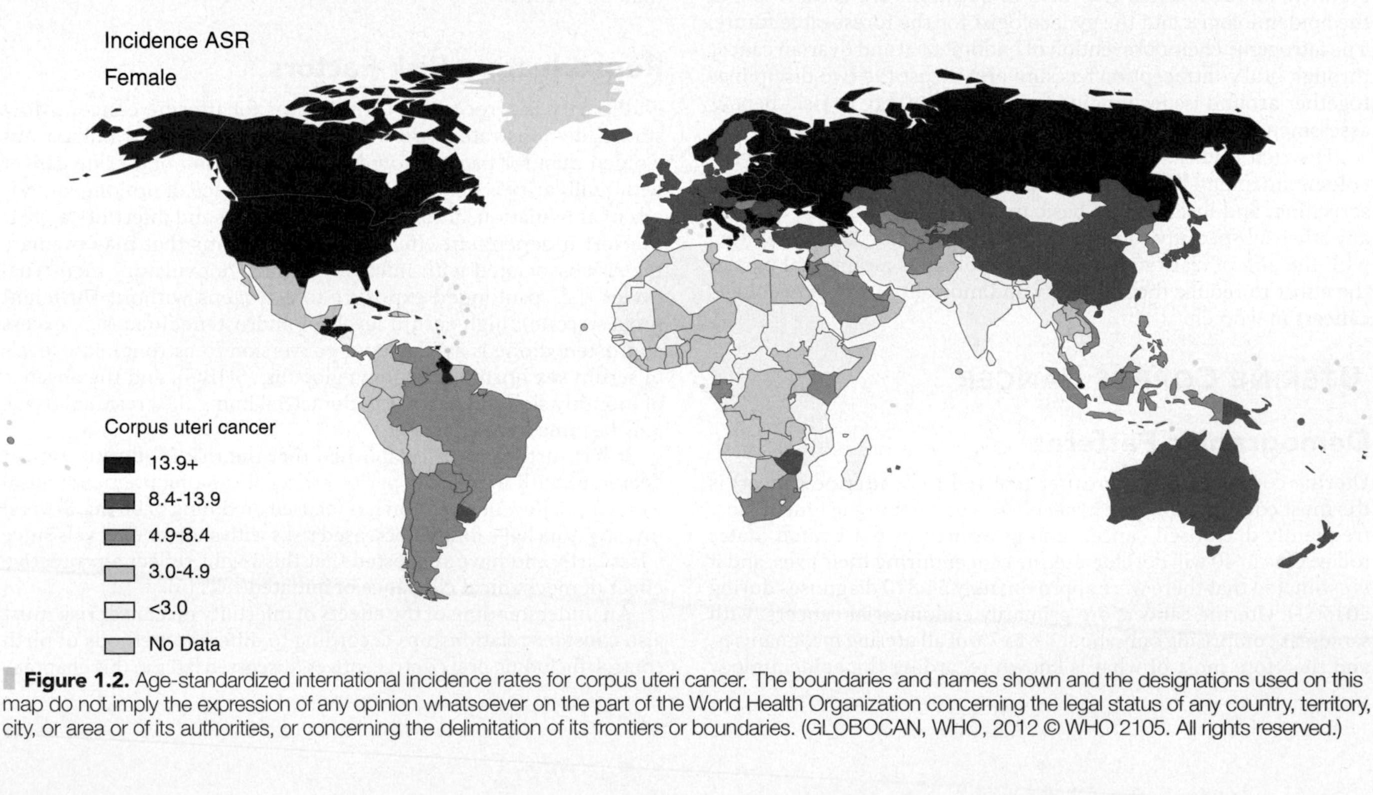

Figure 1.2. Age-standardized international incidence rates for corpus uteri cancer. The boundaries and names shown and the designations used on this map do not imply the expression of any opinion whatsoever on the part of the World Health Organization concerning the legal status of any country, territory, city, or area or of its authorities, or concerning the delimitation of its frontiers or boundaries. (GLOBOCAN, WHO, 2012 © WHO 2105. All rights reserved.)

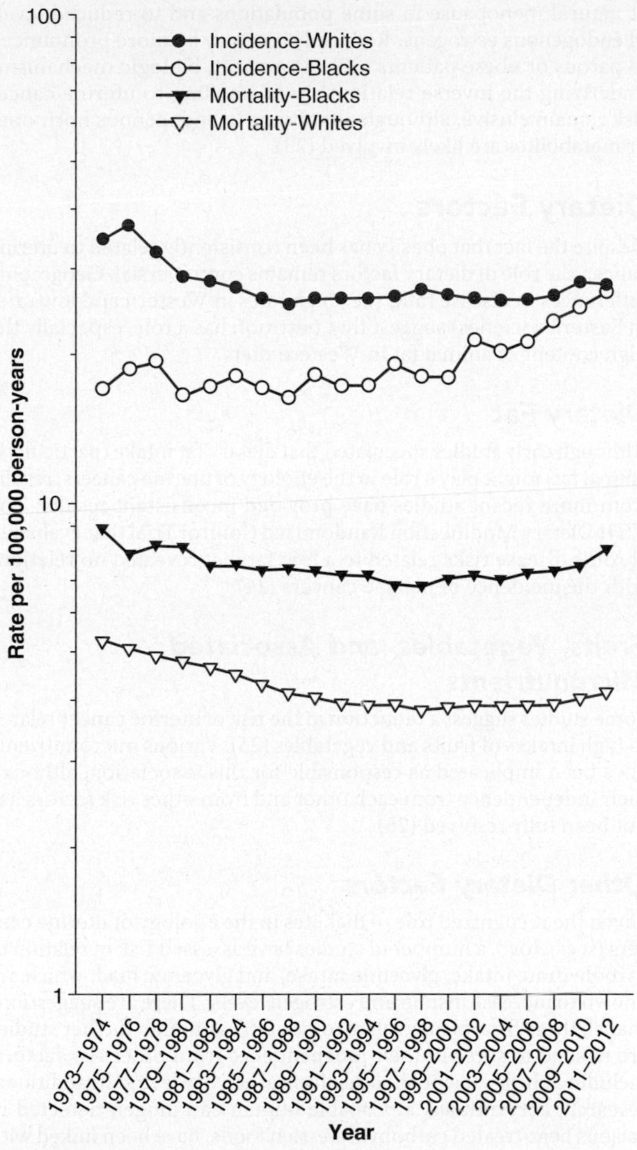

Figure 1.3. Trends in uterine incidence among US women, SEER-9, 1973 to 2012.

As elaborated in a recent pooled analysis (6), a number of investigations have noted reductions in risk among users of intrauterine devices (IUDs). The mechanisms involved with this apparent protective effect have not been elaborated, although it is possible that the devices may affect risk by causing structural or biochemical changes that alter the sensitivity of the endometrium to circulating hormones.

The use of fertility drugs has been of concern, given the structural similarity of clomiphene and tamoxifen and the fact that tamoxifen has been extensively linked with elevated risks of uterine cancers (discussed in more detail later). Although earlier studies suggested that fertility drugs might increase uterine cancer risk, the latest investigation on the topic provided no support for a relationship (7).

The potential effects of breast-feeding remain controversial. Although some studies suggest that prolonged lactation may offer protection, this has not been consistently found (5).

Menstrual Risk Factors

Early ages at menarche have generally been related to an elevated risk for uterine cancer. A large multicenter prospective cohort reported a 30% reduction in risk with later as compared with earlier ages at menarche, with the association being strongest for younger women (5). The extent to which this relationship reflects increased exposure to ovarian hormones or other correlates of early menarche (e.g., increased body weight) is unresolved.

Most studies have indicated that age at menopause is directly related to the risk of developing uterine cancer. About 70% of all women diagnosed with uterine cancer are postmenopausal. Investigations support that there is about a twofold increased risk associated with natural menopause after 52 years of age as compared with before age 49. It has been hypothesized that the effect of late age at menopause on risk may reflect prolonged exposure of the uterus to estrogen stimulation in the presence of anovulatory (progesterone-deficient) cycles. The interrelationships among menstrual factors, age, and weight are complex, and there has been substantial speculation regarding underlying biologic mechanisms.

Exogenous Hormones

Oral Contraceptives

The use of combination oral contraceptives has been shown to be associated with marked reductions in the risk of uterine cancer, with the greatest decreases seen among long-term users. In a recent meta-analysis, 5 years of use was associated with a risk ratio of 0.76 (95% confidence interval [CI], 0.73 to 0.78) (8). This reduction in risk persisted for more than 30 years, with no apparent difference in risk across calendar time periods, despite use of higher estrogen dose pills in earlier years.

Menopausal Hormones

It is well established that unopposed estrogens are associated with a 2- to 12-fold elevation in uterine cancer risk (9). In most investigations, the increased risk does not become apparent until the drugs have been used for at least 2 to 3 years, and longer use of estrogens is generally associated with higher risk. The highest relative risks (RRs) have been observed with higher drug dosages and after 10 years of use (up to 20-fold), although it is unclear whether risk increases after 15 years. Most but not all studies have found that cessation of use is associated with a relatively rapid decrease in risk, although a number of studies have found significantly elevated risks persisting for 10 or more years after last usage.

The large body of evidence linking estrogen use to increases in the risk of uterine cancers has led to estrogens being prescribed in conjunction with progestins among women who have not had a hysterectomy, given that progestins cause regression of endometrial hyperplasia, the presumed precursor of uterine cancers. In the Women's Health Initiative (WHI) clinical trial, after 5.6 years of median intervention and 13 years of follow-up, women assigned to 0.625 mg of conjugated equine estrogen plus 2.5 mg of medroxyprogesterone acetate daily had a hazard ratio (HR) of 0.65 (95% CI, 0.48 to 0.89) compared with those assigned to placebo (10). Similar results derive from a number of observational studies, including the Million Women Study in the United Kingdom, where usage of continuous combined therapy resulted in an RR of 0.71 (95% CI, 0.56 to 0.90) (9).

Although studies indicate that the excess risk of uterine cancer associated with estrogens can be significantly reduced if progestins are given for at least 10 days each month (11), some studies have shown that subjects prescribed progestins for less than 10 days per month (sequential users) experience some increase in risk, with only a slight reduction compared with estrogen-only users (12). The sharp contrast between the effects of <10 and ≥ 10 days of progestin use has led to the suggestion that the extent of uterine sloughing or of "terminal" differentiation at the completion of the progestin phase may play a critical role in determining risk. It remains questionable whether <10 days of progestin administration per month is sufficient for complete protection, particularly for long-term users. Few studies have had large numbers of long-term sequential users, but there is some evidence that this pattern of usage may result in persistent elevations in risk (13).

Studies have shown that the effects of hormonal therapy (both unopposed estrogens and combination therapy) may vary by user characteristics, most notably by a woman's body mass. Investigations have shown that the adverse effects of unopposed estrogens are greatest in nonobese women and that the beneficial effects of combined therapy are greatest in obese women (9,12).

Most data regarding the effects of hormones derive from studies of users of pills. Unresolved is whether the use of estrogen patches, creams, or injections can affect risk; given the relationship of risk with even low-dose estrogens, it is plausible that these regimens may confer some increase in risk.

Tamoxifen

A number of clinical trials have demonstrated an increased risk of uterine cancer among tamoxifen-treated breast cancer patients, with a recent meta-analysis showing a HR of 2.18 (95% CI, 1.39 to 3.42) (14). This is consistent with tamoxifen's estrogenic effects on the endometrium. Elevated risks have been observed primarily within relatively short periods after exposure and among women receiving high cumulative doses of therapy. Certain uterine cancer histologies that are normally associated with a poor prognosis may be especially elevated (15).

Anthropometry and Physical Activity

Obesity

Obesity is a well-recognized risk factor for uterine cancer and may account for up to 25% of cases (16). Very heavy women appear to have exceptionally high risks. Although studies have demonstrated significant positive trends of uterine cancer with both weight and various measures of obesity, including body mass index (BMI [weight/height^2]), height has not been consistently associated with risk. Obesity appears to affect both premenopausal and postmenopausal uterine cancer.

Although initial studies hypothesized that adolescent and long-standing obesity may be more important than adult weight, recent studies support that contemporary weight and weight gain during adulthood are the most important predictors of uterine cancer risk (17). Relationships with obesity appear stronger among women not exposed to exogenous hormones.

Recent interest has focused on determining whether the distribution of body fat predicts uterine cancer risk. A number of studies have shown that central obesity may have an effect independent of overall body size (18), although not all studies confirm this relationship (19).

Physical Activity

Investigations have suggested a potential protective effect of physical activity on uterine cancer risk independent of relationships with body weight. A potential relationship is biologically plausible given that physical activity can result in changes in the menstrual cycle, body fat distribution, and levels of endogenous hormones. One meta-analysis of prospective studies demonstrated a decreased risk of uterine cancer with moderate-to-vigorous physical activity independent of relationships with known potential confounders, namely, obesity, menopausal hormone therapy use, and parity (20). Both occupational and recreational physical activity appear to result in decreased risks.

Recent attention has focused on inadequate physical activity, specifically sedentary behavior, often measured as sitting time, which has been linked with risk increases (20). However, it is still not clear from the existing studies if the association is independent of moderate-to-vigorous physical activity or body weight (20).

Cigarette Smoking

A reduced risk of uterine cancer among smokers has been reported, with current smokers having approximately half the risk of nonsmokers (21). Cigarette smoking has been linked to an earlier age at natural menopause in some populations and to reduced levels of endogenous estrogens. Reduced risks may be more pronounced in parous or obese patients (22). At present, biologic mechanisms underlying the inverse relationship of smoking to uterine cancer risk remain elusive, although alterations in endogenous hormones or metabolites are likely involved (23).

Dietary Factors

Despite the fact that obesity has been consistently related to uterine cancer, the role of dietary factors remains controversial. Geographic differences in disease rates (i.e., high rates in Western and low rates in Eastern societies) suggest that nutrition has a role, especially the high content of animal fat in Western diets.

Dietary Fat

Although early studies speculated that dietary fat intake (particularly animal fat) might play a role in the etiology of uterine cancers, results from more recent studies have provided inconsistent results. The WHI Dietary Modification Randomized Control Trial that evaluated chronic disease risks related to a low-fat diet revealed no relations with the incidence of uterine cancers (24).

Fruits, Vegetables, and Associated Micronutrients

Some studies suggest a reduction in the risk of uterine cancer related to high intakes of fruits and vegetables (25). Various micronutrients have been implicated as responsible for this association, although their independence from each other and from other risk factors has not been fully resolved (25).

Other Dietary Factors

Given the recognized role of diabetes in the etiology of uterine cancers (see below), a number of studies have assessed risk in relation to carbohydrate intake, glycemic intake, and glycemic load, which are known to increase insulin and estrogen levels. There are suggestions that all three factors may relate to risk (26), although further studies are needed to sort out their independence from other risk factors, including obesity, diabetes, and physical activity levels. In additional research, acrylamides, a probable human carcinogen detected in various heat-treated carbohydrate-rich foods, have been linked with increases in uterine cancer risk (27), while phytoestrogens and omega-3 fatty acids (found in fatty fish) appear protective (28). However, all of these exposures warrant further research to confirm effects.

Alcohol and Caffeine

Although early studies suggested that alcohol consumption might lead to reductions in endometrial cancer risk, the findings may have reflected residual confounding by cigarette smoking. More recent studies suggest either no association or one that is increased only modestly (29).

A meta-analysis of coffee consumption and uterine cancer reported a decreased risk of cancer with one cup or more of coffee per day, with consistent findings across case–control and cohort studies (30). Additional studies are needed to determine whether there are certain subgroups that would especially benefit from increased consumption and to define biologic mechanisms for the association.

Medical Conditions

Clinical reports and several observational studies link polycystic ovarian syndrome (PCOS) with an increase in the risk of uterine cancer, with one meta-analysis showing a nearly threefold increased risk associated with the condition (31). However, the extent to which this relation is independent of obesity remains unclear.

A number of studies, and a recent meta-analysis (32), suggest a high risk of uterine cancer among diabetics, but questions remain as to the independence of this effect from that of obesity. Some studies suggest that a relationship with diabetes persists when analyses are restricted to nonobese women or are adjusted for weight. Several investigations have suggested that metformin use might reduce the risk of uterine cancer, but the latest studies on this issue have not confirmed a protective effect (33).

Studies that have shown stronger relationships of diabetes to uterine cancer risk among obese women have prompted interest in the etiologic role of selected metabolic abnormalities, including hyperinsulinemia. Recent studies have focused on effects of metabolic syndrome, with findings that this may predict risk better than merely a history of diabetes (34).

A variety of other diseases, including hypertension, arthritis, thyroid conditions, anemia, and cholecystectomy, have been suggested to predispose to uterine cancers, although without consistent findings (35). In some of these studies, positive findings may have been partially explained by the correlation of the diseases with other factors. Similar to breast cancer, patients with previous fractures have been found to have a reduced risk of uterine cancer (36), presumably reflecting the association of lowered bone density with altered endogenous hormone levels.

Given speculation that inflammatory processes might play an important role in the development of uterine cancers (37), a number of studies have assessed relationships with use of nonsteroidal anti-inflammatory drugs, with inconsistent results (38).

Host Factors

Women who have a family history of uterine cancer in a first-degree relative have been shown to be at a 1.5- to 2-fold increased risk of developing the disease themselves (39). Familial histories of colorectal cancer are also associated with increases in risk, reflective of several defined cancer syndromes. This includes Lynch syndrome or hereditary nonpolyposis colorectal cancer, a dominantly inherited syndrome associated with mutations in the DNA mismatch repair genes *MSH2*, *MLH1*, and *MSH6*; Cowden syndrome, a rare condition resulting from a mutation in the tumor suppressor gene phosphatase and tensin homolog; and a rare condition associated with the *POLD1* gene that encodes the catalytic subunit of DNA polymerase (39). Patients with Lynch syndrome have been estimated to face a 25% 10-year probability of developing subsequent uterine cancers, suggesting their need for active and early management (40).

Although numerous studies have attempted to identify genetic markers of uterine cancer risk, genome-wide association studies (GWAS) have found only one locus associated with risk, namely, a susceptibility locus close to *HNF1B* (rs4430796), which has also been positively associated with prostate cancer risk and inversely with type 2 diabetes (41). In order to determine whether rare variants may be more predictive, exome-wide association studies (EXWAS) have also been undertaken, although no variants have reached global significance, suggesting the need for greater power to detect modest associated risks (42).

Environmental and Occupational Risk Factors

Geographic variation in rates of uterine cancer, with high rates in certain industrial areas, has led to the suggestion that certain environmental agents may affect risk. Given the well-recognized influence of hormones on disease, there has been particular concern about a potential role for certain endocrine disruptors, including dichlorodiphenyltrichloroethane (DDT). Several studies have addressed this issue by comparing dichlorodiphenyldichloroethylene levels (the active metabolite of DDT) in the sera of cases and controls, finding no significant differences (43). Studies have also focused on effects of electromagnetic radiation, but results regarding associations with electric blanket or mattress covers have produced mixed results (44).

Data for occupational exposures are limited. Elevated endometrial cancer rates have been found among teachers in California (45) and individuals exposed to animal dust and sedentary work in Finland (46). The extent to which these relationships reflect the influence of social class is unknown.

Etiologic Heterogeneity

In 1983, Bokhman proposed that endometrial cancers could be divided into two broad types: Type I, the predominant form, which has a hormonally driven etiology, and Type II, which is unrelated to typical endometrial cancer risk factors, not associated with endometrial hyperplasia and generally clinically aggressive. Subsequent clinicopathologic studies led to the view that most Type I cancers correspond histologically to endometrioid adenocarcinomas, whereas Type II cancers encompass most nonendometrioid histologic types, with serous carcinoma representing the prototype. Differences in molecular markers according to histology support the notion of at least two broad classes of endometrial carcinoma.

Although it is generally now accepted that there are at least two main biological types of endometrial cancer (and possibly more), most epidemiologic studies have assessed risk factors for endometrial cancer overall—which essentially represent the risks for the predominant Type I tumors, especially in largely White populations. Registry data consistently have shown that Type II cancers occur at older ages and more often affect non-White women, consistent with etiological differences compared with Type I tumors. Recently, several epidemiologic investigations have found that Type II cancers are less strongly linked to classic Type I risk factors, such as obesity, nulliparity, and hormones (15,47), emphasizing that the disease is etiologically heterogeneous.

Biologic Mechanisms Underlying Risk Factor Associations

Many of the identified risk factors are thought to operate through alterations in various endogenous hormones. The majority of studies have found increased risks associated with higher levels of circulating estrogens among postmenopausal women that persisted after adjustment for the effects of body mass (48). There is some evidence that estrogens are less predictive of premenopausal disease, suggesting that anovulation or progesterone deficiency might be more influential.

Less well investigated is whether endogenous hormones other than estrogens are related to uterine cancer risk. It has been suggested that uterine carcinogenesis is dependent on uterine mitosis, which is increased by estrogens and reduced by progesterone, but risk associated with progesterone levels has not been well explored. Several studies have shown positive associations of uterine cancer risk with serum androstenedione and testosterone levels (48). This may reflect a role of chronic anovulation and progesterone deficiency in premenopausal women, whereas after the menopause aromatase and local conversion of estrone from androstenedione may be involved.

Obesity, which has been shown to reflect elevated estrogen levels, represents a key risk factor for both uterine carcinoma and endometrial hyperplasias, but the mechanisms mediating this are unclear. One cohort study of postmenopausal women showed that elevated serum estrogen levels appeared to account for the majority of the risk associated with obesity (49).

Conclusions

A unified theory of how risk factors for uterine cancer might operate through one common hormonal pathway has been suggested. Estrogen promotes proliferation in the endometrium, which is opposed by progesterone. Therefore, exposure to estrogen, particularly bioavailable estrogen that is weakly bound or unbound to plasma protein, is viewed as a critical carcinogen. Functional ovarian tumors, PCOS, late menopause, and administration of sequential oral contraceptives and menopausal hormone therapies produce higher levels of estrogen exposure without the antiproliferative effects of progesterone.

Obesity could also contribute in a variety of ways. Adipose tissue is the primary site for conversion of androstenedione to estrone, which is the primary source for estrogen after menopause. Obesity is associated with higher conversion rates and/or elevated plasma levels of estrogen in postmenopausal women. In addition, obesity is related to lower levels of SHBG and more frequent anovulatory menstrual cycles (i.e., less progesterone). Vegetarianism is associated with lower plasma estrogen levels, presumably on the basis of the relationship of diet composition to estrogen metabolism. The beneficial effects of combination oral contraceptives and continuous progestins added to menopausal hormone therapy presumably operate through the antiestrogenic effects of progesterone. The peculiar age incidence patterns for uterine cancer (i.e., extremely rare under age 45 years, followed by a rapid and progressive rise from ages 45 to 60 years) could also reflect the waning influence of progesterone. Nulliparity, diabetes, the absence of smoking, and race may yet be added to the unifying scheme as knowledge of endocrinologic mechanisms in endometrial tissue increases.

Although there are several identified risk factors for uterine cancer (**Table 1.1**), important gaps in knowledge currently limit a full understanding of the proposed carcinogenic process. We need to understand when in a woman's life obesity matters most and how risk is influenced by weight loss; whether the number of adipocytes, their fat composition, or other factors determine peripheral conversion of androstenedione; and the precise hormonal mechanisms associated with vegetarianism. Perhaps the most important gap is in understanding the basic mechanism of estrogen carcinogenesis. It is unclear whether estrogens are complete carcinogens, classic "promoters" that affect initiated cells, or growth stimulants for abnormal cells or carcinogens that act on vulnerable genetic material. Much of the epidemiologic data point toward estrogens acting at a relatively late stage of carcinogenesis, emphasizing the need for further attention to identify tumor initiators.

TABLE 1.1. Risk Factors for Uterine Cancer

Factors Influencing Risk	Estimated Relative Risk[a]
Older age	2.0–3.0
Residency in North America, Northern Europe	3.0–18.0
Higher levels of education or income	1.5–2.0
White race	2.0
Nulliparity	3.0
History of infertility	2.0–3.0
Menstrual irregularities	1.5
Early age at menarche	1.5–2.0
Late age at natural menopause	2.0–3.0
Use of oral contraceptives	0.3–0.5
Long-term use of menopausal estrogens	10.0–20.0
High cumulative doses of tamoxifen	3.0–7.0
Obesity	2.0–5.0
Stein–Leventhal disease or estrogen-producing tumors	>5.0
Histories of diabetes, hypertension, gallbladder disease, or thyroid disease	1.3–3.0
Moderate-to-vigorous physical activity	0.5–0.8
Cigarette smoking	0.5

[a]Relative risks depend on the study and referent group employed.

Ovarian Cancer

Demographic Patterns

Ovarian cancer accounts for 1.3% of all incident cancers in US women (2). Approximately 1 in 70 will develop ovarian cancer during their lifetime. The average annual age-adjusted incidence for all SEER areas for 2012 was 11.9 per 100,000 women (2). A total of 21,290 new cases were estimated to have been diagnosed in the United States in 2015 (1).

Diagnosis usually occurs at advanced stages; the overall 5-year survival between 2005 and 2008 was only 45.6%. The average annual age-adjusted mortality rate is 7.4 per 100,000 women (2). The estimated 14,180 deaths due to ovarian cancer in 2015 made it the fifth leading cause of cancer death among US women (1). After rising during the mid-twentieth century, age-adjusted mortality rates have been declining by 2.0% per year since 2007 among White women, but have remained stable among Blacks (1). Incidence rates have also slowly declined over the past two decades; ovarian cancer incidence rates decreased by 1.1% per year from 2003 to 2012 (2). Although there is some disparity in mortality rates between US Whites and Blacks (7.7 vs. 6.6 per 100,000 women per year, respectively), the incidence rates by race are more disparate (12.5 per 100,000 women per year among Whites vs. 10.2 among Blacks) (**Fig. 1.4**) (2).

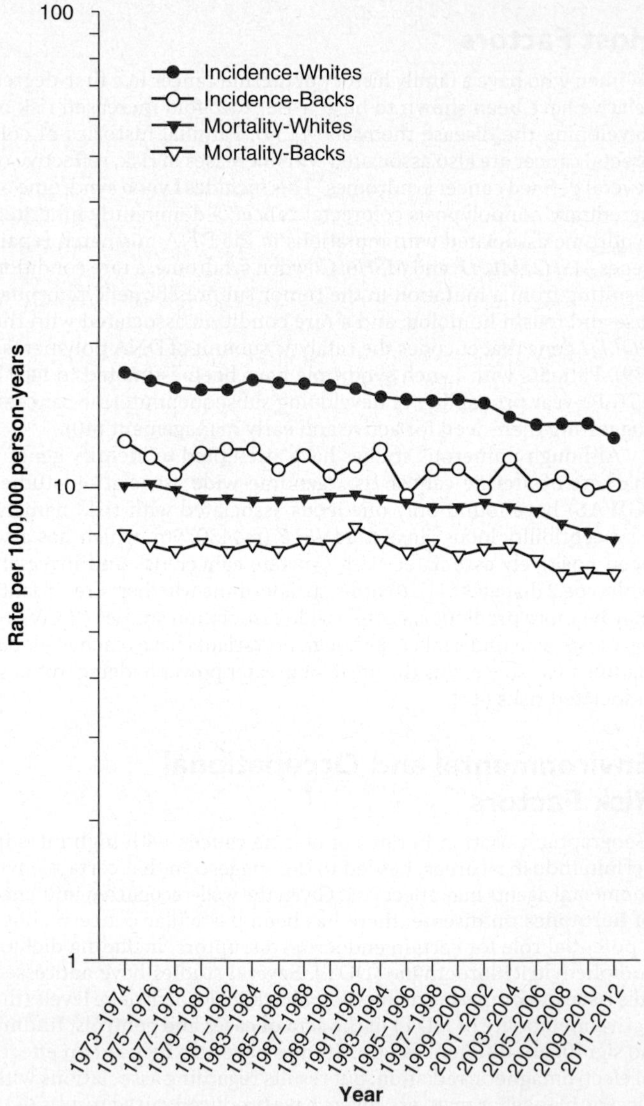

Figure 1.4. Trends in ovarian cancer incidence among US women, SEER-9, 1973 to 2012.

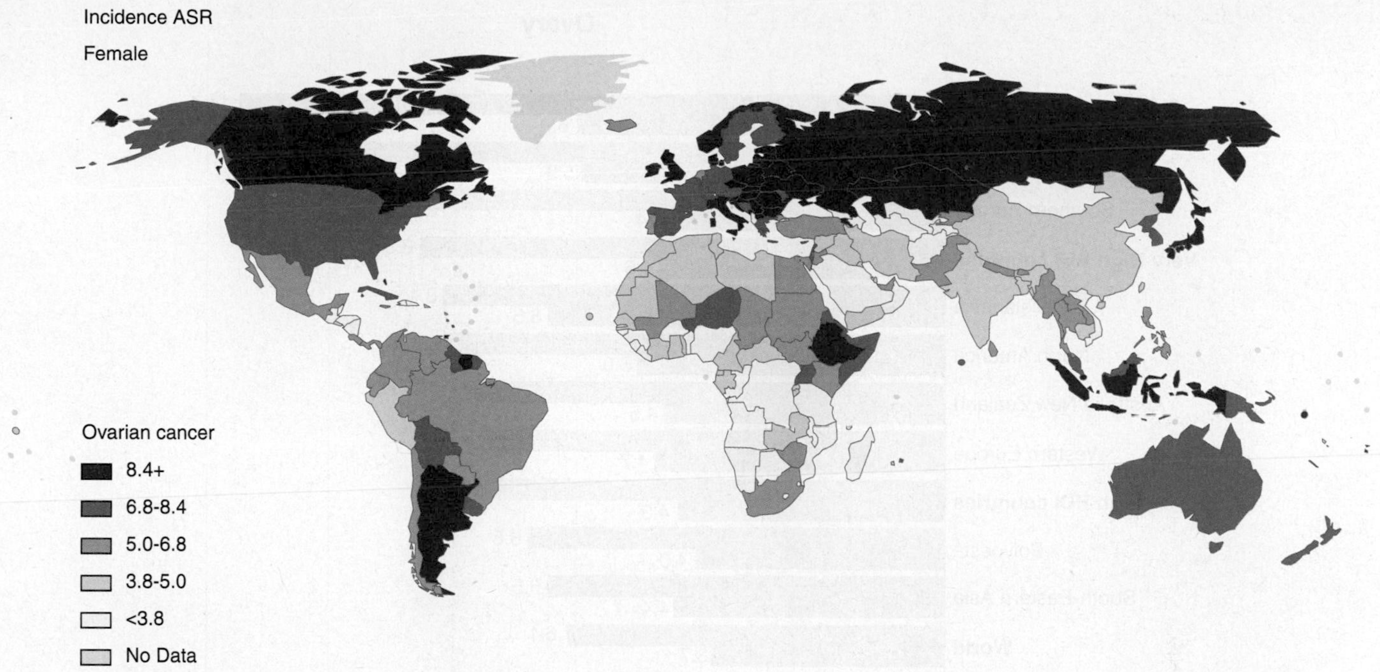

Figure 1.5. Age-standardized international incidence rates for ovarian cancer. (GLOBOCAN, WHO, 2012 © WHO 2105. All rights reserved.)

The highest incidence occurs in European, Scandinavian, and North American countries, whereas the lowest rates occur in African nations and some Eastern Asian countries, such as China (**Fig. 1.5**) (3). Age-standardized rates vary 3.7-fold across countries. Mortality data show a similar but slightly less dramatic pattern (**Fig. 1.6**). The estimated age-standardized mortality rates are 4.6 in more developed regions and range from 2.8 to 3.9 in less developed regions (3). Genetic susceptibility and differences in the prevalence of major ovarian cancer risk factors are likely to explain some of the geographic and racial/ethnic differences in rates; however, few studies have been conducted to address the influence of these factors on rate patterns.

Reproductive Risk Factors

Gravidity is consistently associated with decreased ovarian cancer risk. Compared with nulligravid women, women with a single pregnancy have an RR of 0.6 to 0.8. Each additional pregnancy decreases risk by another 10% to 15%. Although parity results in substantial reductions in risk, there is less certainty regarding the effects of incomplete pregnancies. One study (50) showed no relationship of risk with induced abortions, but an increased risk for women with multiple miscarriages, possibly reflecting a common underlying pathology. Most studies that have adjusted for parity report no residual association with age at first or last birth (51).

Although several early studies showed substantial increases in ovarian cancer risk linked to use of fertility drugs, subsequent studies have generally not confirmed an association, at least for invasive cancers (52). There are, however, lingering concerns regarding whether fertility medications might increase the risk of borderline ovarian cancers, especially given results from a recent large Dutch cohort study (53). Whether this reflects a biologic relationship or merely increased medical surveillance among infertility patients has yet to be determined.

A number of studies have found a reduced risk of ovarian cancer associated with breast-feeding, although it is unclear whether there is a dose–response relation or whether the association is independent of parity. A pooling of two large cohort studies reported an inverse trend in risk with extended breast-feeding that was independent of parity effects (54). Notably, each month of breast-feeding decreased the RR of ovarian cancer by 2%. Suppression of ovulation and decreased gonadotropin levels have been proposed as explanatory of the reduced risk, but further studies are needed to confirm this hypothesis and to clarify relations by histologic subtype.

Menstrual Factors and Gynecologic Surgery

Numerous studies have noted reduced risks among women who have had a simple hysterectomy or tubal ligation. These patients' risks were 30% to 40% lower than the risks among women who had not undergone surgery. One meta-analysis reported a 37% reduced risk of ovarian cancer with tubal ligation and evidence that the reduced risk persists 10 to 14 years after the procedure (55). It has been suggested that surgery offers an opportunity to remove abnormal-appearing ovaries, but this alone is unlikely to explain the protective effect. Partial devascularization and reduced ovarian function or partial removal of tubes, which decreases risk of tubal carcinogenesis, a precursor to serous ovarian cancer, represent possible alternative mechanisms. However, reduced exposure to potential environmental causes of inflammation resulting from tubal ligation or hysterectomy blocking the route of exposure from the outside of the body to the fallopian tube fimbria and ovaries has also been proposed.

A number of studies have linked late age at natural menopause with an increased risk of ovarian cancer, (51) although not all studies have confirmed this relationship. Most studies have not found earlier ages at menarche to increase risk (56), but some have reported weak positive associations.

Hormonal Risk Factors

Oral Contraceptives

Oral contraceptive use has been consistently associated with a lower risk of ovarian cancer. The overall estimated protection is approximately 40% for ever use and increases to more than 50% with 5 years of use or longer. A pooled analysis of 45 studies confirmed that the reduction in risk persists for 30 years beyond last use (57). The lower-dose formulations now in use seem to reduce risk at least as effectively as their higher dose predecessors; of the progestins used does not appear to differentiate risks.

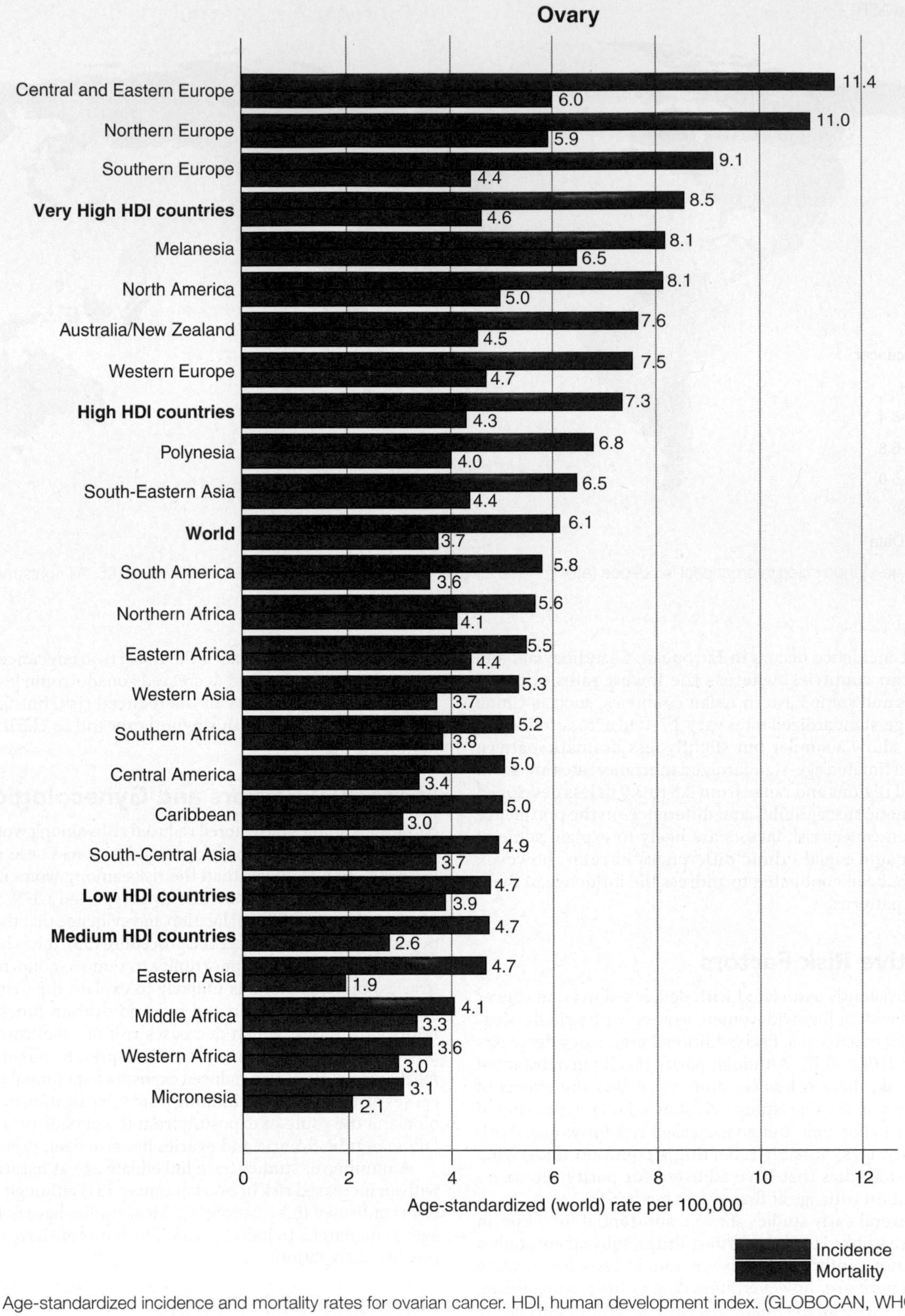

Figure 1.6. Age-standardized incidence and mortality rates for ovarian cancer. HDI, human development index. (GLOBOCAN, WHO, 2012.)

Menopausal Hormones

Unopposed estrogen menopausal hormone therapy has been consistently associated with an increased risk of ovarian cancer. Associations between estrogen plus progestin use and ovarian cancer risk have been less consistent. In the WHI clinical trial, women exposed to estrogen plus progestin therapy had an increased, albeit nonsignificant, risk of ovarian cancer compared with those receiving a placebo (RR, 2.42; 95% CI, 0.64 to 9.12) (58). However, a recent pooled analysis of 52 epidemiologic studies reported similar increased risks of ovarian cancer for both estrogen-only and estrogen plus progestin use (59). Furthermore, the Danish Sex Hormone Register study reported increased risk for both sequential and continuous estrogen plus progestin use (60), suggesting that progestins do not mitigate the increased risk associated with estrogen menopausal hormone therapy.

Endogenous Hormones

Recent interest has focused on the role of endogenous hormones in the etiology of ovarian cancer. Gonadotropins, including follicle-stimulating hormone, have been found to be inversely related to risk (61), whereas endogenous androgens have not generally shown strong risk associations (62,63). One study found some suggestion that free testosterone might play a role in early-onset ovarian cancers (64), but another investigation, which pooled data from three studies, reported null associations with estrogens, androgens, SHBG, insulin-like growth factor (IGF)-1, and associated binding proteins (62). A recent study evaluating early pregnancy hormone levels and cancer development later in life reported increased risk of invasive tumors with higher testosterone and androstenedione concentrations, while estradiol, progesterone, 17-hydroxyprogesterone, and SHBG were not substantially related to risk (65). There remains interest in further exploring the role of endogenous hormones in the etiology of ovarian cancers, especially given that they may interact with immunologic factors, which have been suggested to play an important role in ovarian carcinogenesis.

Medical Conditions and Medications

Several studies surveyed whether certain medical conditions predispose to ovarian cancer. Diabetes, hypertension, and thyroid diseases seem unrelated to risk. In line with a number of clinical studies showing simultaneous occurrences of endometriosis and ovarian cancer, epidemiologic studies have found that women with a diagnosis of endometriosis have elevated risks for developing ovarian cancer (66). In several of these studies, the relationship was shown to be especially pronounced for clear cell and endometrioid ovarian cancers, and more recently also for low-grade serous malignancies (66). As reviewed by Ness (67), the two conditions share a number of pathophysiologic processes, including estrogen excesses and progesterone deficits, immunologic responses, and inflammatory reactions. Pelvic inflammatory disease has also been found to be a possible risk factor for ovarian cancer (68), supporting the notion of a role for tubal inflammation and/or damage in ovarian carcinogenesis.

Findings have also suggested a reduced risk among women who use anti-inflammatory or other analgesic medications, and a recent pooled analysis reported a modest inverse association between aspirin use and ovarian cancer risk, with stronger risk reductions among daily aspirin users (69). However, chemoprevention via the use of these medications remains a premature concept.

Anthropometry and Physical Activity

Obesity has recently received increased scrutiny as a possible risk factor. Most individual studies fail to show an association, but pooling projects and meta-analyses are beginning to indicate increased risks associated with higher BMI (70). Some investigations have shown stronger relationships restricted to certain subgroups, including those who have never had children, premenopausal women, postmenopausal women, nonusers of menopausal estrogens, women without a family history of ovarian cancer, and physically inactive women. Furthermore, some studies have suggested that obesity is a risk factor only for certain types of tumors, with most evidence pointing to increased risks for borderline serous and invasive endometrioid and mucinous tumors (71,72).

Height has also emerged as an independent risk factor for obesity (73). Additional studies have examined effects of physical activity levels on ovarian cancer risk, with one meta-analysis reporting a 19% risk reduction associated with high levels of recreational activity; however, the association was not statistically significant when only cohort investigations were considered (74). Sedentary behavior (6+ hours of sitting per day) was recently associated with increased ovarian cancer risk (75).

Cigarette Smoking

In general, cigarette smoking is not considered a major risk factor for ovarian cancer, although it may be related to increases in risk of mucinous tumors (76). In a systematic review, smoking doubled the risk for mucinous tumors, but did not increase risk for endometrioid or clear cell tumors (77). The risk of mucinous cancers increased with amount smoked but returned to that of never smokers within 20 to 30 years of stopping smoking.

Dietary Factors

Ecologic studies of dietary factors and ovarian cancer risk led to the hypothesis that high intake of fat, milk, and eggs may be related to an increased risk of ovarian cancer, while high intake of fruits and vegetables may be related to a decreased risk. However, the majority of the observational studies targeting food classes, lactose and dairy foods, fats, vitamins/nutrients, fiber, fruits, and vegetables provide conflicting results.

Lactose Consumption

Several early studies raised concern that higher consumption of yogurt, cottage cheese, and other lactose-rich dairy products might increase ovarian cancer risk given that galactose-related enzymes can influence gonadotropin levels. Although the majority of studies fail to show increases in risk with lactose consumption or galactose metabolism, results from the Nurses' Health Study suggest that further attention may be warranted regarding effects for serous tumors (78).

Fat Intake

The WHI Dietary Modification Randomized Control Trial evaluated the effects of a low-fat dietary pattern on chronic disease incidence and reported a decreased risk of ovarian cancer associated with the intervention (a 20% reduction in total fat intake) (24). A meta-analysis of 12 cohort studies found no overall association with fat, cholesterol, or egg intakes, but some suggestion that very high levels of saturated fat intake may increase risk (79). Additional meta-analyses reported no association between red meat and inconsistent results for high intake of processed meat (80).

Fruits and Vegetables and Micronutrient Intake

Although a number of studies have suggested that ovarian cancer risk might be reduced by higher consumption of fruits and vegetables or fiber, others, including a pooling project of 12 cohort studies, fail to support such relationships (81). Some studies have shown inverse associations with particular nutrients, such as vitamins A, C, and E, β-carotene, folate, or methionine, but results have been inconsistent across studies. Meta-analyses evaluating vitamin D or the major carotenoids and ovarian cancer risk report no substantial relationships (82). Further clarification of effects may require evaluating associations according to other risk factors and within histologic subgroups.

Alcohol and Caffeine

A number of studies have examined ovarian cancer risk in relation to alcohol consumption. Most investigations, including pooling efforts (83), have not found any convincing relationships.

Caffeine and ovarian cancer risk has been evaluated in studies of coffee consumption, tea consumption, or studies of both. Although coffee consumption has been linked to an elevated risk of ovarian cancer in several studies, a recent investigation and updated meta-analysis failed to provide support for a relationship of risk with either coffee or tea consumption (84). Another meta-analysis reported reduced ovarian cancer risk with green tea consumption and no association with black tea consumption (85). Overall, there are no consistent patterns between caffeine consumption and ovarian cancer risk; however, it may be that more detailed information on type of caffeine and frequency and duration of consumption need to be evaluated.

Host Factors

A family history of ovarian cancer is the strongest risk factor identified to date. Which family member was affected is less important than the total number of affected relatives or their age at diagnosis (86). Women with two or more affected relatives or whose relative was diagnosed before 50 years of age experience the highest risks (87). Approximately 5% to 10% of ovarian cancer patients have a first-degree relative with ovarian cancer (86). Family histories of breast and colon cancer are also associated with increased ovarian cancer risk, but slightly less strongly than a family history of ovarian cancer.

Inherited mutations in two autosomal dominant genes—*BRCA1* and *BRCA2*—are strongly linked to familial ovarian cancer (and breast and other cancers) (88). Whereas the lifetime probability of developing ovarian cancer in most women is 2%, the probabilities in women with a family history or women with *BRCA1* and *BRCA2* mutations are 9.4% and 15% to 40%, respectively (89). Despite these increases, *BRCA1/2* mutations explain less than one third of the elevated risk in women with familial ovarian cancer (87). Lynch syndrome is reported to be associated with a 12% lifetime risk of ovarian cancer (90). High-penetrance genetic variation is associated with considerable disease heterogeneity; mutations in *BRCA1/2* lead to the development of serous cancers, whereas mutations of DNA mismatch repair genes are more frequently associated with mucinous and endometrioid tumors (91).

Common genetic variation and ovarian cancer risk in moderate- or low-penetrance susceptibility genes have been evaluated using candidate gene studies of single nucleotide polymorphisms (SNPs) and through GWAS. Candidate genes/SNPs have generally been selected from biologic pathways based on relevant hypotheses, and several candidate genes have been identified as possibly related to ovarian cancer risk, including *PGR, TP53,* and *CDKN2A*. GWAS have further identified susceptibility loci for ovarian cancer at 9p22.2, 8q24, 19p13, 2q31, 3q25, and 17q21 (91) and 1p36, 4q26, 9q34.2, and 17q11.2 (92). The underlying genetic basis of ovarian cancer contributes to disease heterogeneity with common low-penetrance genetic variation, with GWAS loci 9p22.2, 1p34.3, and 6p22.1 being more strongly associated with serous subtype than other subtypes (91,92). Identifying common genetic susceptibility alleles will lead to a greater understanding of disease etiology, potentially allowing the development of preventive approaches targeted toward women who have these genetic variants.

Talc

Over-the-counter talc, a silicate which chemically resembles asbestos, has been of concern with respect to ovarian cancer risk for some time. Although evaluated in many studies, results have been conflicting (93). One meta-analysis (94) indicated that exposure is associated with slight increases in risk of either all subtypes or of serous cancers, albeit with inconsistent dose–response relations. However, the WHI Observational Study reported no associations overall or by area of application, duration of use, or histologic subtype (95). Thus, it is apparent that further evaluations of this exposure are needed to fully understand potential effects.

Environmental and Occupational Risk Factors

A variety of studies have focused on effects on ovarian cancer risk of certain professions (e.g., teachers, health care workers, bookkeepers), without definitive conclusions. Specifically, there has been concern regarding potential effects of occupational exposures to either hair dyes or triazine herbicides to ovarian cancer, although no clear patterns of risk have emerged. A Monographs Working Group of the International Agency for Research on Cancer (IARC) concluded that asbestos exposure is associated with ovarian cancer, with the association confirmed in a subsequent meta-analysis of occupational cohorts (96). Until additional data address the potential for inconsistent or chance findings and the challenge of finding large populations with sufficient data on other potential confounding variables, occupational exposures beyond asbestos will likely not be considered major risk factors for ovarian cancer.

Etiologic Heterogeneity

A unified ovarian cancer progression model has not yet been established, and growing evidence demonstrates that subtypes of ovarian carcinomas have different molecular, pathological, and clinical characteristics, suggesting that there may be several distinct disease entities. Specifically, ovarian cancer subtypes appear to molecularly and morphologically resemble cancers of other sites: fallopian tube (serous), endometrium (endometrioid), gastrointestinal tract (mucinous), and unspecified glycogenated epithelium (clear cell) (97).

As previously discussed, some risk factors have been shown to have distinctive effects for certain subtypes of ovarian cancer, but there have been inconsistent findings—most likely reflecting small numbers in the studies of some of the rarer subtypes. Probably one of the more consistent findings is the propensity of endometriosis to predispose to clear cell and endometrioid tumors (66). Tubal ligation may also be more strongly related to reductions in endometrioid cancers than to other ovarian subtypes (56). Mucinous tumors also show some distinctiveness with demonstrating increased risks related to cigarette smoking (77) and decreased risks with use of menopausal hormones (72). Obesity is beginning to emerge as an especially strong predictor for certain cancers, including endometrioid cancers (71), consistent with the link of obesity to endometrial cancer (13).

It is clear that further leads regarding the etiologic heterogeneity of ovarian cancer will depend on either large studies or more likely on consortial efforts, which bring together data from multiple epidemiologic studies. Such efforts are currently underway by several groups and should provide further insights as to possibly distinct origins of some of these tumor subtypes.

Conclusions

Much of the clinical and epidemiologic evidence concerning risk factors for ovarian cancer implicates ovulatory activity (**Table 1.2**). Conditions associated with reduced ovulation (e.g., pregnancy and oral contraceptive use) consistently reduce risk. Combining these and other menstrual factors into single "ovulatory age" or "lifetime ovulatory cycles" indexes has generally produced the expected associations with ovarian cancer risk; that is, older ovulatory ages or higher cycle counts increase risk. However, the misclassification inherent in these indexes is sufficient to generate different risk estimates, and the magnitude of risk reduction for short-term oral contraceptive use or a single pregnancy exceeds the proportional decrease in ovulatory cycles that would be expected to be associated with these exposures.

The putative mechanisms behind ovulatory inhibition and the risk associated with "increased ovulation" raise additional questions. An early report suggested, based on the associations with parity and infertility, that an unidentified endocrine abnormality predisposed women to relative or absolute infertility and ovarian cancer. The protection associated with oral contraceptives seems unlikely to fit this hypothesis unless, in some improbable manner, their use induces an endocrine milieu similar to that underlying infertility.

A second popular unifying hypothesis is that ovarian cancer is the result of accumulated exposure to circulating pituitary gonadotropins. Although this is consistent with the parity, menopause, and oral contraceptive associations, there is no support for high gonadotropin levels being related to increased risk. This theory also fails to

TABLE 1.2. Risk Factors for Ovarian Cancer

Factors Influencing Risk	Estimated Relative Risk[a]
Older age	3.0
Female relative with ovarian cancer	3.0–4.0
Residency in North America, Northern Europe	2.0–5.0
Higher levels of education or income	1.5–2.0
White race	1.5
Nulliparity	2.0–3.0
History of infertility	2.0–5.0
Early age at menarche	1.5
Late age at natural menopause	1.5–2.0
History of hysterectomy or tubal ligation	0.5–0.7
Use of oral contraceptives	0.3–0.5
Long-term use of menopausal estrogens	3.0–5.0
Perineal talc exposure	1.5–2.0

[a]Relative risks depend on the study and referent group employed.

account for the risks associated with clinical infertility, and it predicts that menopausal hormone therapy use would decrease risk, because both exposures are associated with reduced gonadotropin levels.

A third explanation points to a biologic effect of ovulation on ovarian surface epithelium. Ovulation prompts a cascade of epithelial events, including minor trauma, increased local concentrations of estrogen-rich follicular fluid, and increased epithelial proliferation, followed by local inflammation and wound repair. Such proliferation, particularly near the point of ovulation, can recruit inclusions into the ovarian parenchyma. Some or all of these "incessant ovulation" events may lie on the causal path to ovarian cancer. This is consistent with most of the endocrine-related risk factors except for the risks associated with clinical infertility.

Although it has been hypothesized that epithelial inclusion cysts give rise to ovarian tumors, cancer precursors of ovarian surface epithelium remain unclear, and progress in understanding ovarian carcinogenesis, as previously mentioned, is partly limited by this lack of clarity on tissue of origin of ovarian epithelial carcinomas. Nearly all other epithelial gynecologic cancers arise via a sequence of events whereby the normal epithelium undergoes conversion to a precursor lesion that can then become an invasive neoplasia. Cervical intraepithelial neoplasia (CIN), the precursor of cervical cancer, is probably the most well-known example. More recently, increasing evidence indicates that at least a subset of high-grade serous ovarian carcinomas arise from high-grade intraepithelial serous carcinomas in the fallopian tube and spread to the ovary (97). This could help explain the inconsistent reduced risks associated with tubal ligation and hysterectomy, given that the fallopian tubes would be removed only in a subset of these procedures.

No single theory adequately incorporates the available data. A unifying hypothesis may lie in a combination of ovulation, hormones, and local effects. Additional factors, such as genetic alterations; androgens, progestins, and other hormones; inflammation; and endometriosis, also appear to be important.

Each hypothesis identifies testable possibilities. Discriminating between the roles of voluntary versus involuntary infertility could identify the mechanisms underlying the role of parity. Characterizing the specific reproductive abnormalities associated with clinical infertility could reveal new biologic mechanisms involved in ovarian carcinogenesis. Exploring the interactive contributions of the hormones along the hypothalamic–pituitary–gonadal axis could explain how specific hormones seem to influence risk at different time periods. In addition, verifying that inflammation or related conditions and pathways play an etiologic role in ovarian carcinogenesis could open new lines of inquiry.

Ovarian cancer epidemiology presents both simple and complex patterns. Rates have largely remained unchanged over the last 40 years. The highly penetrant genes account for only a small proportion (10%) of women who develop ovarian cancer, but a better understanding of the mechanisms behind those risks could introduce immediate benefits for high-risk women. A clear picture has emerged for some protective factors, such as oral contraceptives and parity, but risk associated with other important public health issues, such as smoking, obesity, and physical activity, remains uncertain. Although it is tempting to attribute the differences to histology-specific associations, such hypotheses will require substantially more epidemiologic, clinical, and genetic data before their acceptance is certain. Consistent risk factors for high-grade serous tumors, the most fatal subtype, also remain elusive. Continued attempts to account for the differences between studies should help delineate spurious associations from the etiologically relevant risk factors. Such efforts should help identify targets for improving detection, treatment, and prevention of this deadly tumor.

CERVICAL CANCER

Cervical cancer is a major source of morbidity and mortality globally. Evidence from basic biology and molecular epidemiology studies over the past three decades established the central causative role of chronic persistent infection, with carcinogenic genotypes of the HPVs in virtually all cases of cervical cancer (98). Cervical HPV infection is extremely common in all sexually active individuals, much more than the relatively rare development of precancer and the even rarer cases of cervical cancer, suggesting a role for additional etiologic factors that may modulate the HPV-induced cervical carcinogenic process. Other than intrinsic viral type-specific risk variations (HPV-16 being the most carcinogenic type, followed by HPV-18 and HPV-45 (99)) and variability in human host immunologic response, there are several cofactors, prominent among them being reproductive factors such as multiparity, hormonal influences (changes in endogenous hormonal milieu over the lifespan, as well as exogenous hormone exposures), smoking, coinfection with other infectious agents, and systemic immunosuppression.

Demographic Patterns: Global and United States

According to the latest global data from the IARC, cervical cancer is the fourth most common cancer (after breast, colorectal, and lung cancers) among women worldwide, with over 527,000 incident cases and over 265,000 deaths worldwide annually (**Fig. 1.7**) (3). The cancer burden (incidence and mortality) is disproportionately high in less developed regions of the world, which account for 85% of cases and deaths due to cervical cancer. The incidence and mortality rates are highly variable by global regions, reflective of difference in background HPV infection rates as well as disparities in access to prevention and clinical care services (**Fig. 1.8**) (3). Incidence and mortality rates of invasive cervical cancer have declined over the past six decades in a number of countries, mainly in countries that rank highly on the human development index (HDI), largely attributed to successes in screening programs for cervical cancer. However, rates remain high in most countries with low HDI, especially in countries in sub-Saharan Africa, largely reflecting lack of, or suboptimal, screening efforts, high HPV incidence, and more recent increases due to the heavy burden of human immunodeficiency virus (HIV)/acquired immune deficiency syndrome (AIDS) (100). Incidence rates are also high (over 15 per 100,000) in countries with low and medium HDI rankings, including in Latin America, Southern Asia,

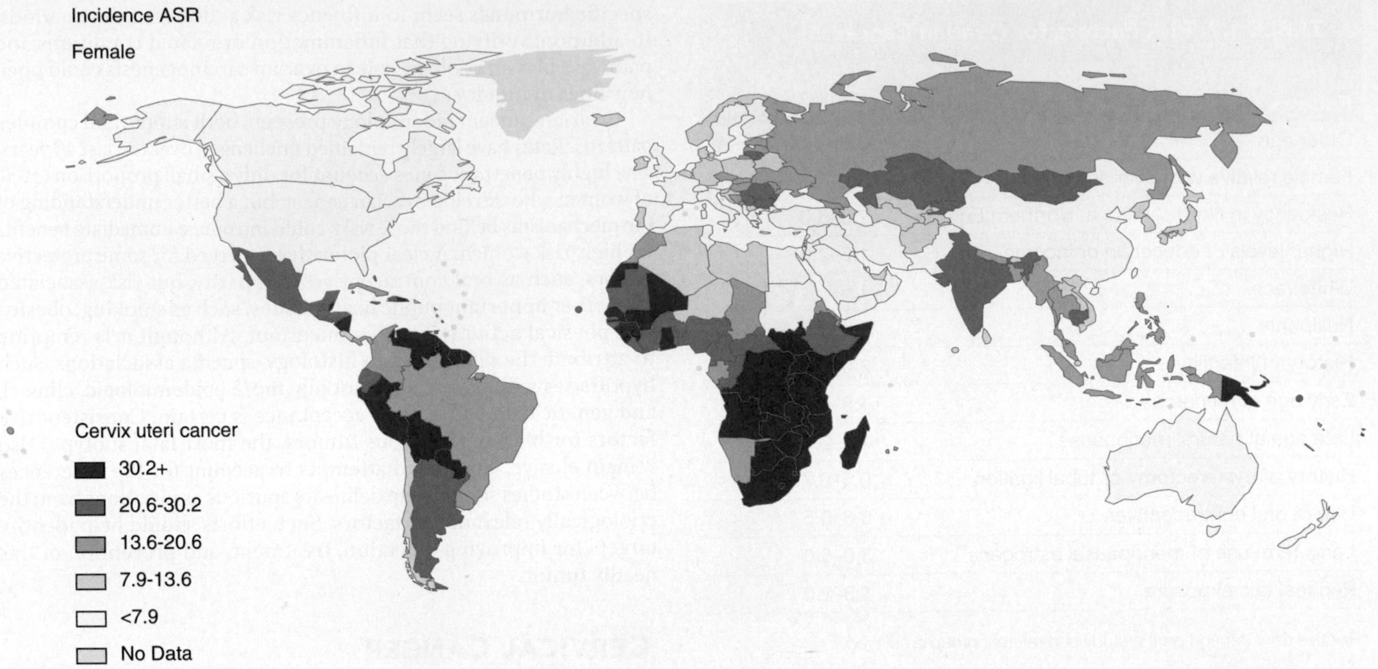

Figure 1.7. Age-standardized international incidence rates for cervical cancer. (GLOBOCAN, WHO, 2012 © WHO 2105. All rights reserved.)

and parts of Eastern Europe, also attributable to lack of widespread screening. In contrast, rates are lower in countries with medium HDI rankings including in Eastern Asia, Western Asia, and Northern Africa, despite suboptimal screening, likely attributable to lower HPV incidence.

The dramatic declines in incidence rates in countries with high HDI in the latter half of the 20th century are attributable to widespread and/or organized screening efforts (**Fig. 1.9**) (101). Despite lack of screening, several countries with medium HDI rankings have seen declines in incidence rates in the last quarter century as reflected by data from selected high-quality cancer registries in some of these countries (e.g., India, Thailand, Philippines). This is likely due to reductions in rates of multiparity, delayed ages at childbearing, and improvements in nutrition and hygiene (100). In several countries with high HDI rankings, despite general declines in incidence rates, risks by calendar period of diagnosis and birth cohorts have varied substantially, reflecting the duration and quality of screening programs over calendar time and changes in risk factors, notably sexual behaviors (e.g., earlier age at first sexual intercourse, multiple lifetime partners), over successive generations of women.

Of note, there are clear differences in incidence trends by histologic types of cervical carcinomas. While rates of squamous cell carcinomas, accounting for approximately 80% of invasive cervical cancers, have declined steadily since the introduction of Pap smear screening, adenocarcinomas (accounting for approximately 15%) have not (102). In fact, rates of cervical adenocarcinomas have risen in the past two to three decades in various countries including the United States, both relative to rates of squamous cell carcinoma and in absolute numbers.

It is estimated that 12,900 women were diagnosed with and 4,100 women died due to cervical cancer in the United States in 2015 (1). Geographic differences in incidence rates, with higher rates in underserved regions, are apparent (103). Substantial differences by race/ethnicity still persist; non-Hispanic Whites and Asian and Pacific Islanders have much lower rates compared with non-Hispanic Blacks, American Indians and Alaskan Natives, and Hispanic women.

Like other screening-preventable cancers, the age distribution of cervical cancer is affected by the availability and successes of screening. Studies prior to the introduction of screening have shown that cancer cases peak and then plateau around 45 years of age (104). It is unusual for cancer incidence rates to plateau or fall with increasing age; thus, this age structure reflects the origin and long natural history of cervical cancers from HPV infections acquired in early years of adolescence and adulthood, and is likely further influenced by several etiologic cofactors over the reproductive lifespan as well as perimenopausal hormonal changes.

Human Papillomavirus

For more than a century, epidemiologic studies have suggested an association between sexual activity and cervical cancer, but proof that HPV is the sexually transmitted agent responsible for this association was not achieved until sensitive methods for detecting HPV DNA were developed in the late 1980s. The recognition of the key etiologic role of HPV infection has profoundly altered the epidemiologic study of cervical cancer. The epidemiologic association between HPV infection and cervical cancer fulfills all of the established epidemiologic criteria for causality. As a result, HPV is now accepted to be the central, necessary causal factor for virtually all cases of cervical cancer globally (98).

Natural History of Cervical HPV Infection

Cervical HPV transmission, which is primarily sexual, is studied best at the molecular level, primarily because genotypic heterogeneity informs risk stratification. Moreover, before development of precancerous stages, most infections are not microscopically or macroscopically evident. The epidemiology of cervical cancer is most coherently understood in terms of the natural history of cervical carcinogenic HPV infection, which can be broadly categorized in the following stages: i) acquisition of HPV following sexual exposure, with clearance of infection in most cases, ii) persistence of HPV in a minority of women, with oncogenic cellular transformation progressively involving the entire thickness of the epithelium, leading to precancerous lesions, and iii) untreated precancerous lesions progressing to invasive cervical cancer. Terminologies for classifying precancerous lesions have evolved, and the most widely used CIN grading system uses increasing grades (CIN 1, CIN 2, and CIN 3) of increasing severity or extent of the squamous epithelial involvement

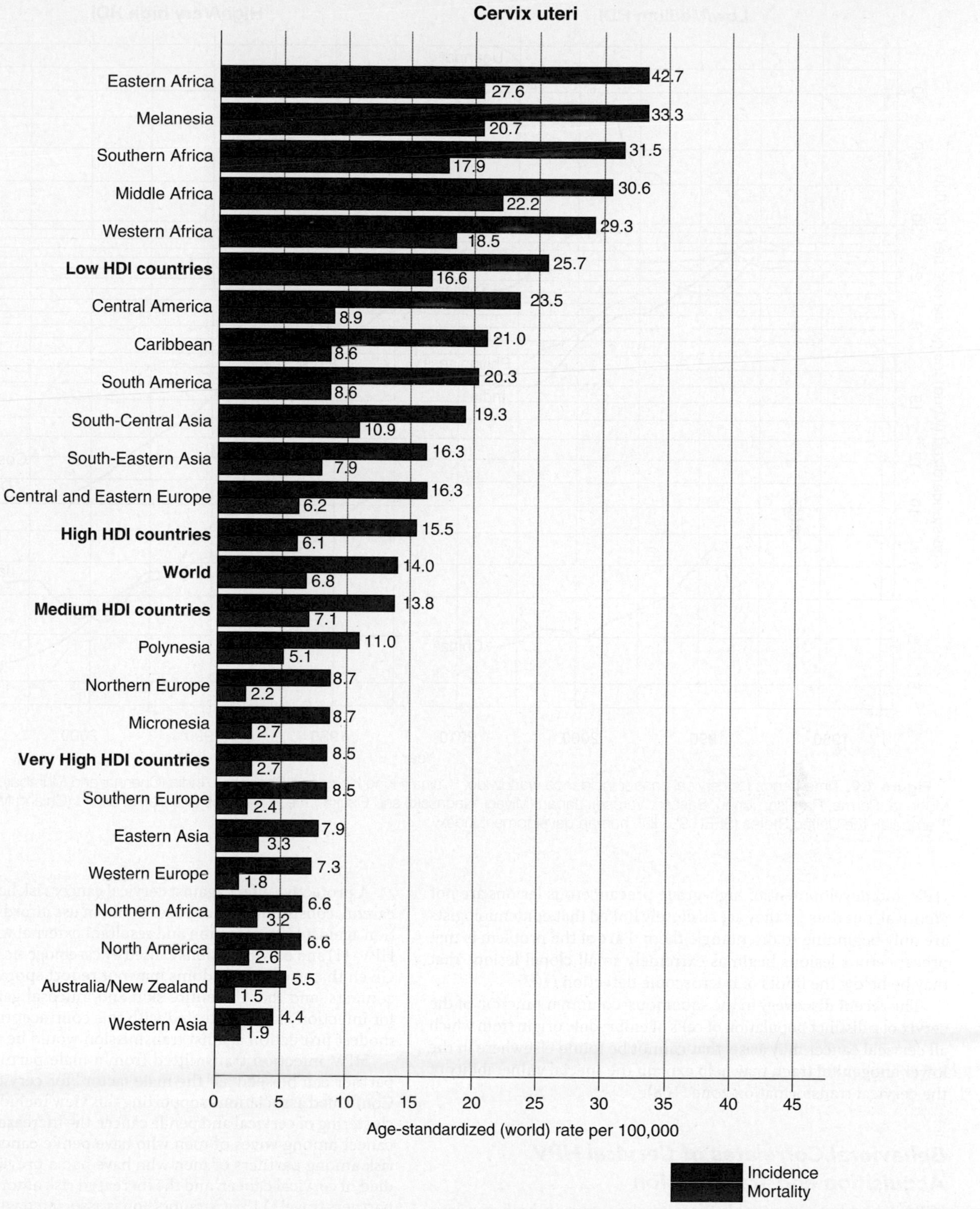

Figure 1.8. Age-standardized incidence and mortality rates for cervical cancer. HDI, human development index. (GLOBOCAN, 2012.)

on histopathology. Of note, CIN 1 is only an insensitive histopathological sign of HPV infection, CIN 2 includes a heterogeneous group of lesions which are equivocal in cancer potential, whereas CIN 3 represents the most clinically relevant lesion and is the best surrogate endpoint for efficacy against invasive cervical cancer in screening or vaccine trials (105).

As the most common sexually transmitted infection, HPV infection acquisition and transmission rates peak in the years following sexual initiation. Acquisition and clearance dynamically oppose each other, to produce the characteristic age distributions as infections are transmitted sexually when women have new partners and are then cleared (106). Transient HPV infections are ubiquitous among sexually active young women (and men), but progression to a cervical cancer precursor requires persistence of carcinogenic types. It is the overt persistence of one of the carcinogenic types that is strongly linked to precancerous lesions. Persistence of carcinogenic types of

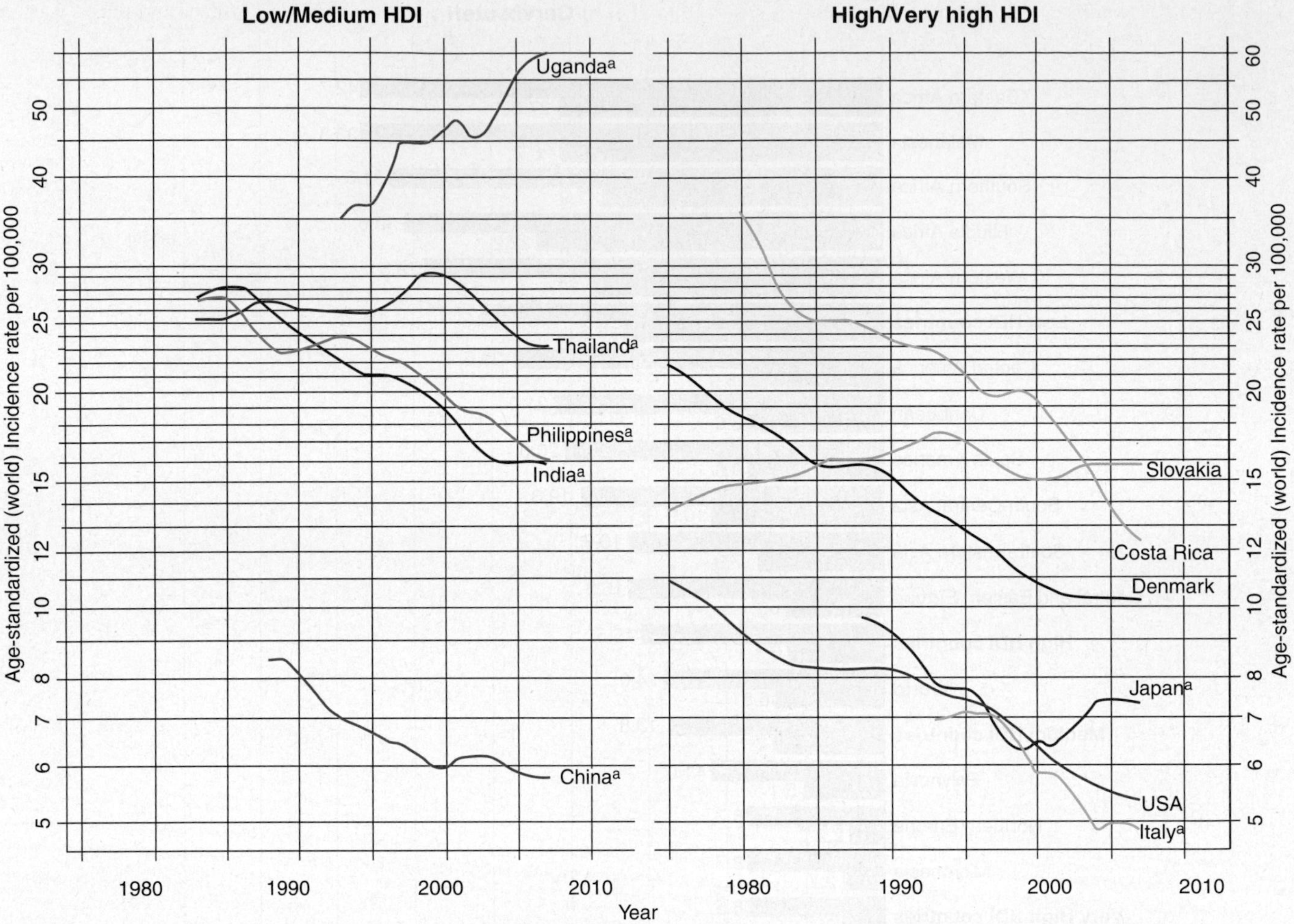

Figure 1.9. Time trends for cervical cancer incidence worldwide. [a]China (Hong Kong and Shanghai), India (Chennai and Mumbai), Italy (Ferrara, Modena, Parma, Ragusa, Torino, Sassari, Varese), Japan (Miyagi, Nagasaki, and Osaka), the Philippines (Manila), Thailand (Chiang Mai), Uganda (Kampala), the United States (SEER 9). HDI, human development index.

HPV and development of high-grade precancerous lesions are not identical, but thus far they are so closely linked that epidemiologists are only beginning to disentangle them. Part of the problem is that precancerous lesions begin as extremely small clonal lesions that may be below the limits of microscopic detection (107).

The recent discovery in the squamous-columnar junction of the cervix of a distinct population of cells of embryonic origin from which all cervical cancer may arise, that cannot be found elsewhere in the lower anogenital tract, may help explain the special vulnerability of the cervical transformation zone (108).

Behavioral Correlates of Cervical HPV Acquisition and Transmission

HPV is highly transmissible via sexual contact in both genders. Numerous epidemiologic studies have shown that markers of sexual activity, such as number of sexual partners (recent or lifetime), are among the most important correlates for HPV detection and subsequent risk of cervical precancer and cancer (109). HPV infections are easily transmitted with few acts of sexual intercourse, and therefore, sexual frequency is not a major risk factor for cervical neoplasia. The age at sexual debut serves as an apparent proxy for the time of HPV infection in nonpreviously infected women, whereas there is no evidence for a special vulnerability of the cervix close to the time of menarche (104).

A protective effect against cervical cancer risk has been noted for careful, consistent condom use. Condom use affords modest protection against HPV infection and resultant external warts (HPV-6 and HPV-11) and cervical lesions caused by carcinogenic HPV types (110). Given that users of condoms may not report sporadic unprotected contacts, and that the entire skin and mucosal genital area at risk for infection is not protected with this contraceptive method, only modest protection against transmission would be expected (111).

HPV infection transmitted from a male partner to his female partner can be seen as "the male factor" for cervical cancer (112). Confirmed associations supporting this view include the geographic clustering of cervical and penile cancer, the increased risk of cervical cancer among wives of men who have penile cancer, the increased risk among partners of men who have had a previous partner who died of cervical cancer, and the increased risk among women whose partners travel (113). Circumcision is associated with a reduced risk of HPV detection in penile samples, and wives of men with a history of multiple partners are at lower risk of cervical cancer if the men had been circumcised (113,114). Circumcision is associated with reduced prevalent male HPV infection, and randomized clinical trial evidence from Africa has now shown that voluntary adult male circumcision reduces transmission between sexual partners (114,115).

HPV Types as Determinants of Cervical Risk

HPV type greatly affects both the absolute risk of viral persistence and of progression to precancer associated with viral persistence

(116). The most common carcinogenic type, HPV-16, is also the most common type in the general population, linked to its greater propensity to persist (117). While certain noncarcinogenic types (e.g., HPV-61) can also be persistent and common, they do not cause malignant transformation (99). The average time of viral persistence that leads to diagnosable precancer is not clear. The average age at microscopic diagnosis of precancer is approximately 25 to 30 years, approximately 5 to 10 years after the average peak ages of carcinogenic HPV prevalence and associated minor cytologic abnormalities in screening populations (118). Biomarkers that predict persistence of cervical cancer and offer better discrimination of transforming versus transient HPV infections are increasingly available (119).

Noncarcinogenic HPV infections are capable of producing lesions falsely diagnosed as precancer, especially CIN 2, showing that this level of abnormality is not a perfect surrogate for cancer risk (120). Still, because of the emphasis on safety, particularly in US clinical practice, and concern over loss to follow-up, treating precancer (except as appropriate in very young women, etc.) is a valid clinical strategy to provide a margin of safety, given that it is not yet possible to know which lesions pose a threat. Eventually, better accuracy based on molecular profiling is the goal.

The distribution of HPV types in cervical cancer has been extensively studied in United States and international collaborative studies (121). The most common HPV types in descending order of frequency are HPV types 16, 18, 45, 31, 33, 52, 58, and 35, together responsible for approximately 90% of all cervical cancers worldwide. Persistent HPV-16 infection is an extremely strong risk factor for subsequent diagnoses of CIN 3 and invasive cancer, and has been classified as a Class 1 human carcinogen by IARC (89). HPV types are more predictive of risk than subtleties of minor and equivocal cytopathic effects, colposcopic findings, or behavioral cofactors such as smoking. Furthermore, intratypic sequence variants of HPV-16 and possibly other types have been associated with altered risk, although these risk modifications are weaker than the intertypic variation (122). The role of elevated viral load (i.e., HPV content in samples obtained from infected women) in predicting persistence and progression of infection is complicated and varies by HPV type and the detection of multiple infections (123). A clear trend of increasing prospective risk with increasing viral load has been demonstrated only for HPV-16, and viral load assessment is not useful clinically (124). Infection with one HPV type does not seem to influence the risk of persistence and development of precancer from another concurrent infection (116).

Host Factors Associated with HPV Persistence and Progression

Whereas humoral (antibody-mediated) immunity appears to play a central role in preventing HPV infection (leading to the prophylactic vaccines), elimination of HPV seems more closely related to mounting an effective cellular immune response. Impaired cellular immunity, attributable to HIV infection, transplantation, or immunosuppressive drugs, has been shown to increase HPV prevalence, persistence, warts, CIN, and cancer (125,126).

The immune response to HPV is an important determinant of viral clearance versus persistence and, by extension, a major determinant of cervical cancer risk (127). However, despite our growing understanding, many aspects of the interactions between HPV and the host immune system remain unknown (128). The key immune responses involved in the clearance of HPV infections are known to be cell mediated, although neutralizing antibodies are highly protective after immunization with HPV virus-like particle-based vaccines (129). A protective immune response to naturally acquired HPV infection develops in some women, but it has not been quantified adequately and is difficult to study, given the lack of site specificity and challenges in serological assay development and validation (130). Assays to measure HPV vaccine responses, on the other hand, have been extensively developed and are currently being standardized for facilitating international epidemiologic studies and future vaccine development and evaluation.

Polymorphisms in the human leukocyte antigen (HLA) genes have been implicated in the risk of HPV-associated diseases. HLAs are important determinants of the efficiency of antigen presentation to immune effector cells and, therefore, may influence the outcome of HPV infections (131). Both Class I HLA genes (those that encode HLA molecules that are present in all nucleated cells) and Class II HLA genes (those that encode HLA molecules that are present in lymphocytes and other immune-related cells) are involved in immune presentation (132). To date, HLA Class II genes have been more extensively studied than HLA Class I genes for their association with cervical cancer. A protective role for HLA DRB1*13 in cervical cancer has been consistently described in several populations. Activating combinations of HLA Class I alleles and the killer immunoglobulin-like receptor confer susceptibility to cervical cancer, whereas inhibitory combinations are associated with protection against the disease (131).

Although the biological basis is unknown, studies from nationwide tumor, twin, and other family registries in Scandinavian countries indicate that cervical cancer aggregates in families. In general, an approximate twofold increase in risk of precancer or invasive cervical cancer relative to the general population risk is observed in family members of cervical cancer patients. How much of this elevation in risk among relatives of individuals affected with cervical cancer can be attributed to shared environment versus genetic effects is not settled (133).

A major unresolved question of HPV natural history relates to the possibility of viral latency (134). In long-term studies, virtually all HPV infections become nondetectable by sensitive HPV DNA tests, usually within two years, except for those that lead to precancer. However, it is unknown if the nondetection reflects true virological clearance or a latent stage due to immunologic control that permits long-term presence (latency) below levels of detection. Indeed, the reemergence (reactivation) of viral types seen in immunocompromised individuals (e.g., immunosuppressed HIV-infected women) who have not been sexually active for a long time points to the existence of viral latency. The clinical significance of latency in terms of the fraction that can progress to precancers and cancers in immunocompetent women is unknown. In the era of HPV vaccination, many of these issues will acquire increased significance, especially with the emergence of HPV genotyping assays in clinical practice (135).

Cofactors Influencing Risk of Persistence of Carcinogenic HPV Infection and Progression of Cervical Precancer to Cancer

Since most women clear HPV spontaneously, and invasive cancer only affects a small minority of women who have persistent infection, it is very likely that cofactors influence an individual woman's risk for viral persistence, development of precancerous lesions, and finally invasion (112–114). In particular, reproductive history and hormonal influences on carcinogenic risk have been substantively explored, given the characteristic age distribution seen in unscreened populations—increasing incidence seen during the reproductive years and a perimenopausal peak (around 45 years), a feature shared with estrogen-dependent cancers (104). Some of these cofactors and the evidence supporting them are discussed below.

Multiparity

HPV-infected women who have many live births are at increased risk of cervical cancer and precancer. There is a dose-dependent increase in risk with numbers of live births, most evident among women with many full-time live births (136). Although this epidemiologic association is firmly established, the explanatory mechanism is not clear. Mechanisms underlying the association between parity and cervical neoplasia include trauma during parturition, hormonal changes associated with pregnancy, immunosuppression, and possibly altered anatomy of the transformation zone, specifically eversion. Other menstrual and reproductive factors, including miscarriages, abortions, stillbirths, ectopic pregnancies, cesarean sections, age at first pregnancy, age at menarche, and age at menopause, are not independently associated with risk (113).

Hormonal Contraceptives

Use of oral hormonal contraceptives could plausibly potentiate the carcinogenicity of HPV infection, because transcriptional regulatory regions of HPV DNA contain hormone-recognition elements and transformation of cells *in vitro* with viral DNA is enhanced by hormones (137). Pooled analyses from multicenter case–control studies found an elevated risk of invasive cervical cancer among HPV-positive women who used oral contraceptives for more than 5 years after careful adjustment for other sexual and reproductive history, duration of HPV infection, and screening history (136). Shorter durations of use or use more than 5 years prior to cancer onset were not associated with elevated risk. Evidence linking oral contraceptives to cervical abnormalities has raised concern about long-acting steroid preparations, notably depot medroxyprogesterone acetate. Although these agents are widely used in many countries, studies evaluating their effects, particularly among HPV-infected women, are limited (138).

A pooled analysis of 10 case–control studies of cervical cancer and 16 HPV prevalence surveys from four continents showed that IUD use, a common contraception option in developing countries, was associated with a decreased risk of cervical cancer, regardless of duration of use (few months up to 9 years) and after adjustment for screening status (139). This evidence contradicts a widely held assumption that IUDs may increase risk of cervical cancer and might suggest their role as protective cofactors in cervical carcinogenesis, similar to the role they play in protecting against endometrial cancer. While the precise mechanisms are subject to future investigations, it has been suggested that local cellular immunity is triggered during the process of IUD insertion or by the device itself.

The relationship between endogenous hormones and cervical cancer risk is unclear and is a topic of ongoing investigation. Recent results point to the role of circulating levels of testosterone and estradiol in modulating cervical cancer risk in premenopausal women (140). Yet, mechanistic evidence to confirm these associations and exploration of signaling pathways suggests hormone–receptor modulation in cervical cancer likely differs from other estrogen-dependent cancers (such as breast cancer) (141). The relationship between cervical cancer risk and use of menopausal hormone therapy and overweight/obesity (as determinants of circulating estrogen levels in postmenopausal women) is not well understood (142).

Socioeconomic Status

In an international meta-analysis, women defined as belonging to a low socioeconomic class were found to have twice the risk of cervical cancer compared with women defined as belonging to a high socioeconomic class (143). In the United States, a recent analysis of county-level incidence data indicated that poverty-associated infrequent screening leads to suboptimal stages at diagnosis, resulting in elevated incidence and mortality rates. Some of these affected areas included Appalachia, the southeastern Atlantic states, and the lower Mississippi Valley, as well as central counties of large metropolitan areas (103). A multicountry pooled analysis suggested that the excess of cervical cancer found in women with a low socioeconomic status in inadequately screened populations could not be explained by a concomitant excess of HPV prevalence, but rather by early events in a woman's sexually active life, that is, early sexual debut and early childbearing, that may modify the cancer-causing potential of HPV infection (144).

Cigarette Smoking

Several case–control and cohort studies, as well as collaborative pooled analyses and registry linkage studies, among groups of women infected with carcinogenic HPV have shown that smokers are at increased risk compared with infected women who do not smoke (145). Current smoking is the main risk factor, not past smoking, with no clear trend with time since stopping smoking. Among current smokers, evidence of increasing risk has been found with increasing intensity and duration (or early start) of smoking. Several investigations have attempted to define possible mechanisms by which smoking might alter the cervical epithelium (146). Some investigations have looked into measurement of tobacco-driven carcinogens such as polycyclic aromatic hydrocarbon–DNA adducts in cervical tissue of HPV-infected women (147). Tobacco-derived carcinogens are secreted into the cervix at levels higher than in serum, suggesting possible genotoxicity (147). The immunosuppressive effects of smoking may cause disturbance in the early immune responses or increase persistence through production of reactive oxygen species (148).

Nutrients

The influence of nutrient status on risk of cervical neoplasia has received substantial research attention. While dietary factors such as antioxidant micronutrient intake are likely important in cervical carcinogenesis, methodological difficulties prevent establishment of firm associations between a specific aspect of nutritional status and HPV infection or cervical cancer risk. A meta-analysis of case–control studies suggested preventive effects of micronutrients such as folic acid; vitamins B, C, and E; and β-carotene (149). However, lack of prospective studies and randomized trials preclude definitive evidence regarding the role of supplementation. The association of low folate levels and high homocysteine levels with risk of cervical cancer has led to interest in markers of one-carbon metabolism and DNA repair (119).

Infectious Agents Other Than HPV

HPV infection is known to be the central, necessary cause of cervical cancer, but other sexually transmitted agents could increase the risk of cervical cancer among HPV-infected women. Of the other agents examined, herpes simplex virus 2 was originally hypothesized to play a central role, but most attention now is focused on *Chlamydia trachomatis*. Although residual confounding by some aspect of HPV infection has not been completely ruled out, *C. trachomatis* seropositive women are at increased risk compared with seronegative women even after adjustment for HPV exposure using DNA tests and/or serology (150).

Women with HIV and AIDS have higher prevalence, incidence, and persistence of HPV infection and precancerous lesions, strongly associated with immunosuppression. It is also well established that the incidence of cervical cancer is increased severalfold in both women with HIV/AIDS and those who are iatrogenically immunosuppressed (e.g., organ transplant recipients), thus reinforcing the primary mediating role of immunosuppression in increasing this risk (151). The fraction of cancer attributable to HPV among HIV-infected women in the United States has been estimated to be 14.2%, compared with approximately 2.6% in the general female population (152). However, it is also hypothesized that interaction between HPV and HIV in the affected cervical tissue leads to the persistence of HPV infection and cervical neoplasia by various other mechanisms including depletion of Langerhans cells (153), host immune response (154), or proinflammatory cytokine expression (155). An alternative explanation is at the cellular level; HIV-specific Tat protein upregulates expression of HPV E6 and E7 oncogenes and enhances their oncogenetic transformation efficacy (156). These two mechanisms are, however, not exclusive, and joint effects most likely take place at early precancerous stages.

Risk Factors for Cervical Adenocarcinoma

While infection with a carcinogenic HPV is a necessary cause of both squamous cell carcinomas and adenocarcinomas, the distribution of carcinogenic HPV types and variants detected in these two tumor types varies (157). Multiple studies suggest that HPV-18 accounts for a relatively higher percentage of adenocarcinomas as compared with squamous cell carcinomas, although more recent evidence points to an increasingly equitable role of HPV-18 as well as HPV-16 (121).

Interpreting rates for increased cervical adenocarcinomas over time pose challenges because of gradual improvements in clinical practices (including the use of devices to obtain better endocervical sampling), stricter criteria for adequate Pap tests, development of cytologic criteria for recognizing adenocarcinoma *in situ* (AIS), and, recently, formal inclusion of the AIS category in the new Bethesda System (158). In addition, proposed but unsubstantiated explanations for these upward trends include increased rates of HPV infection without improved cytologic detection of AIS, a specific increase in rates of HPV-18 infection, and increased exposure to HPV cofactors specific to adenocarcinoma.

Although our understanding of the etiology of cervical adenocarcinoma is incomplete, a picture is emerging in which adenocarcinoma seems to share most, if not all, risk factors with cervical squamous carcinomas (acquisition of HPV through sexual contact) and others with uterine carcinoma (more related to hormones). While adenocarcinoma has most risk factors in common with squamous cell carcinoma, an important exception is smoking, which does not seem to increase the risk for adenocarcinoma. In contrast, increased weight (or related measures) appears to be related to increases in the risk of cervical adenocarcinomas (159). Oral contraceptives and menopausal hormone therapy have been linked to an increased risk for AIS or adenocarcinoma. The increased risk of cervical adenocarcinoma associated with obesity and reduced risk with smoking resemble the epidemiology of endometrial adenocarcinoma. However, the relationship between cervical adenocarcinoma and oral contraceptives is more similar to reported results for squamous carcinomas of the cervix.

Conclusions

Knowledge of the epidemiology of HPV and its causal role in cervical carcinogenesis has been successfully translated into clinical practice (107,116), particularly to reduce rates of squamous lesions. In many developed countries, newer consensus guidelines now encourage cotesting with HPV DNA and cytology to improve screening performance and reduce screening intervals, since a negative result provides strong reassurance that immediate follow-up is not required and can reduce patient anxiety and health costs (107). Screening studies are underway to develop new optimized approaches that maximize resource utilization. New low-cost and point-of-care HPV tests are in the pipeline and may improve the feasibility and quality of cervical cancer screening in low-income countries. The management of HPV-positive women, however, remains a challenge. Finally, the increasing use of prophylactic HPV vaccines is expected to impact rates of cervical precancer in the coming years (even in the lowest income countries (160)), although reductions in cancer incidence will take longer. Epidemiologic research on HPV and cervical cancer will remain integral to clinical practice recommendations and to public health strategies that improve patient management and guide and monitor successes in cervical cancer prevention and control.

VULVAR CANCER

Demographic Patterns and the Importance of Pathologic Classifications

Carcinoma of the vulva accounts for 4% of gynecological malignancies worldwide. In the United States, the average annual age-adjusted incidence in all SEER areas during 2009 to 2013 was 2.4 per 100,000 women (2). During 2015, an estimated 5,150 women developed the disease and 1,080 died as a consequence of it in the United States (1). Contrary to cervical cancer, incidence rates for vulvar cancer are similar in all ethnicities, except in Asian women, who exhibit low rates (0.9 per 100,000). Slightly lower incidence rates than in the United States have been reported from several European countries, including Denmark, the United Kingdom, and Sweden, and in Australia (1.4 to 1.7 per 100,000, world standardized) (3). In other continents, vulvar cancer rates are generally equal to or lower than 1 per 100,000, and often below 0.3. Of note, very low rates are reported by cancer registries in Africa, Latin America, and India, where cervical cancer incidence and HPV prevalence are high (see section on Cervical Cancer). This unlikely discrepancy strongly suggests a substantial underreporting of vulvar cancer in low-resource countries.

Rates of vulvar cancer have remained relatively stable over the past three decades according to SEER data (2), but previously rare vulvar invasive and *in situ* carcinomas are now more common among younger women (161). Upward incidence trends in vulvar cancer among women below 50 or 60 years of age have also been observed in other countries, for example, Denmark (162).

HPV Infection

Vulvar cancer is etiologically heterogeneous (163). The majority of cases are squamous, with two subclassifications: basaloid and warty carcinomas, which are more frequently HPV-positive (~70%) than keratinizing (differentiated) squamous tumors (~13%) (164,165). Basaloid and warty carcinomas are also substantially more frequent in young women, particularly in North American studies. Carcinomas *in situ* of the vulvar are nearly always HPV-positive (~97%) (161) and so are vulvar intraepithelial neoplasias (VIN) grade 2 and 3 (165). HPV 16, in particular, is found in 48% of vulvar cancers and 81% of *in situ* carcinomas (161). HPV-positive VINs are often detected during cervical cancer screening (165). VIN 1 is considered condyloma and should be managed conservatively (166). Non-HPV-associated vulvar cancers are poorly understood but are often associated with chronic inflammatory states such as lichen sclerosus (167).

Risk Factors

Risk factors for vulvar cancer and VIN are mainly related to those linked to an increased probability of HPV infection, for example, number of sexual partners and immunosuppression. Cancer of the vulva, therefore, occurs significantly more frequently among women with primary cancers of the cervix (168), with the two diseases often detected simultaneously (169). Although the incidence of vulvar cancer was previously thought to be related to socioeconomic class, results from one case–control study indicated that control for sexual factors eliminated this effect (170). Several studies have suggested that a history of vulvar and anogenital warts is associated with an elevated risk of vulvar cancer (171). However, HPV-6 and HPV-11, the types that cause vulvar warts, are not genetically close to the major types found in vulvar cancers (predominantly HPV-16), so the exact relationship between warts and cancer is somewhat obscure. Genetic and local inflammatory factors may also be involved in the pathogenesis of VIN and vulvar cancer (172,173). Women living with HIV (151,174) or AIDS (151) have a strongly increased risk of vulvar cancer, and VIN 2 and VIN 3. The efficacy of HPV-6/11/16/18 vaccines against VIN 2/3 in HPV-naïve women (95%) or in by-intention-to-treat analyses (79%) (175) is similar to the efficacy against CIN 2 or worse lesions. In Costa Rica, equivalent protection of the HPV-16/18 vaccine was demonstrated against prevalent HPV-16/18 infection in the vulva and cervix (176).

Conclusions

Approximately half of vulvar cancer cases worldwide and 70% in the United States are caused by HPV infection, predominantly HPV-16. Despite similar etiology, vulvar cancer is much rarer than cervical cancer. While the epithelium of the entire anogenital tract can be infected by HPV, the transformation zone of the cervix is uniquely susceptible to HPV carcinogenesis (105). The recent discovery of a distinct population of cells of embryonic origin that cannot be found elsewhere in the lower anogenital tract may help explain the special vulnerability of the transformation zone (108). A favorable role of screening in vulvar cancer prevention is not clear, but prophylactic vaccines against HPV-16 and HPV-18 may prevent an even larger fraction of VIN 2/3 and HPV-related vulvar cancer than CIN 2/3 and cervical cancer.

VAGINAL CANCER

Demographic Patterns

Cancer of the vagina is rare, with an average annual age-adjusted incidence of 0.7 per 100,000 women in the SEER areas from 2009 to 2013 (2). During 2015, it was estimated that 4,070 women developed the disease and 910 died from it in the United States (1). The majority of vaginal cancers are squamous cell carcinomas and occur in the upper part of the vagina.

Only 15% of cases are found in women younger than 40 years and almost half of cases occur in women who are 70 years or older (177). The disease is twice as common in Black as in White women. Incidence rates similar to those in the United States are found in several European countries and some parts of sub-Saharan Africa, Brazil, India, and in indigenous populations in Canada and Australia (≥1 per 100,000). Rates of 0.1 per 100,000 or lower are reported by cancer registries in parts of China and the Middle East. Underreporting of vaginal cancer is likely to occur in low-resource countries; however, the international variation of the disease somewhat differs from that of vulvar cancer, probably because the disease is less frequently detected during cervical cancer screening (108).

Risk Factors

Vaginal cancer is frequently found as a synchronous or a metachronous neoplasm with cervical cancer, pointing to the role of HPV infection (178). An international meta-analysis reported HPV detection in 70% of vaginal cancers and 94% of vaginal intraepithelial neoplasias (VAIN) (165). A large study of archival tissue samples from the United States (179) showed 75% of vaginal cancers to be HPV-positive, with 55% HPV-16/18-positive. HPV-negative cancers were more frequent in women aged 65 years or older (39% vs. 19% below age 65) (179). While a vaccine targeting HPV-16/18 potentially could prevent the majority of vaginal cancers, direct information is not available, as VIN and less frequent VAIN lesions have been combined as efficacy endpoints in the available trials (180).

Diethylstilbestrol and Vaginal Clear Cell Adenocarcinomas

In the late 1960s, cases of clear cell carcinomas of the vagina, an uncommon cancer in any age group, began to be observed with much greater frequency than expected among women between 15 and 22 years of age. Most of these cases have been linked to prenatal exposure to diethylstilbestrol (DES) use, which was stopped in the United States in 1971 (181). A registry of clear cell cancers of the vagina and cervix was established, and many more cases have been reported (182), the vagina being affected about twice as frequently as the cervix. The rate for clear cell adenocarcinoma of the vagina and cervix through 39 years of age has been estimated to be 1.6 per 1,000 DES-exposed daughters (181), and an increased risk of VAIN 3 and CIN 3 was also noted. When assessing a woman's cancer risk, whether her mother took DES in pregnancy might still be a relevant aspect of the medical history for women born during the period of DES use in pregnancy (181).

Conclusions

Less is known about risk factors for vaginal cancer than is known for vulvar cancer. It has recently been suggested that there may be two types of vaginal cancers with age-related etiology (183). In young patients, the etiology is strongly related to HPV infection, mainly HPV-16/18. HPV vaccination will therefore decrease the incidence of VAIN and vaginal cancer. The rare occurrence of vaginal adenocarcinoma in young women is distinctive in being essentially an iatrogenic disease related to *in utero* exposure to DES and other estrogens (181). A proposed mechanism involves nests of abnormal cells of Müllerian duct origin, which are stimulated by endogenous hormones during puberty and promoted into adenocarcinomas.

GESTATIONAL TROPHOBLASTIC DISEASES

Gestational trophoblastic diseases (GTDs) (which include hydatidiform moles, invasive moles, and choriocarcinoma) encompass a range of interrelated conditions characterized by abnormal growth of chorionic tissues with various propensities for local invasion and metastasis (184). Hydatidiform moles can be either complete or partial and have distinctive pathologies and etiologies. Complete moles have paternally derived nuclear DNA, but maternally derived cytoplasmic DNA. In contrast, partial moles generally have a triploid karyotype, with the extra haploid set of chromosomes being of paternal origin.

Demographic Patterns

Choriocarcinoma is a rare malignancy in the United States, with a reported incidence in all SEER areas of 0.1 per 100,000 women, or approximately 1 per 25,674 live births (185). Hydatidiform mole occurs about once in every 1,000 pregnancies, and approximately one of six occurrences results in invasive complications (either invasive mole or choriocarcinoma). Trophoblastic diseases have been reported to be more common in certain parts of the world, although some of the differences may be due to a variety of selection, detection, and reporting biases, including whether risk is expressed in relation to women at risk, conceptions, or live births. In the United States, incidence rates have declined over time, and survival has improved, but Blacks continue to have higher incidence and lower survival than women of other ethnicities.

The epidemiologic study of choriocarcinoma has been complicated by its relative infrequency. Most studies have, therefore, focused on defining risk factors for hydatidiform moles, but the extent to which these findings can be extrapolated to malignant trophoblastic disease is uncertain.

Host Factors

Trophoblastic disease rates are considerably higher in Asian and African countries, but the true extent of difference from rates in Western countries is difficult to decipher because of variations in reporting practices (184). In Europe and North America, the incidence of hydatidiform mole ranges from 0.57 to 1.1 per 1,000 pregnancies, whereas in Southeast Asia and Japan, the incidence is closer to 2.0 (186). Corresponding incidence rates in the two parts of the world for choriocarcinoma are 1 versus 9.3 per 40,000 pregnancies. These differences persist in migrants, with one study showing that the incidence of GTDs in Asians was nearly twice as high as among non-Asians (187). One survey in the United States showed that, even after adjustment for age and birth distribution effects, Blacks had a 2.1-fold greater risk and other non-White races had a 1.8-fold greater risk than Whites (188). American Indians and Alaskan natives have also been shown to have high rates of GTDs (185).

One clearly established risk factor for choriocarcinoma and hydatidiform mole is maternal age. Women with extreme maternal ages (either very early or late) have nearly twofold elevated rates, with even further age differences noted for the occurrence of complete moles (187). The recent increase in incidence of GTDs in certain European countries has been attributed in large part to increases in maternal ages (189,190).

A history of hydatidiform mole is also a strong risk factor. The risk of another molar pregnancy in a subsequent conception is about 1% (184), and the risk appears to increase to about 15% to 20% in women who have had more than one previous hydatidiform mole. This risk does not appear to be altered with a change in male partners, suggesting an influence on oocyte defects of environmental factors (191). Familial clusters of biparental complete hydatidiform moles associated with novel missense *NLRP7* gene mutations on chromosome 19q have been identified (184). Hydatidiform mole is associated with a 1,000 to 2,000 times increased risk for development of subsequent choriocarcinoma, with an even further enhancement after a complete molar pregnancy (2,500 times higher than after a live birth).

Menstrual, Reproductive, and Anthropometric Risk Factors

In several studies that have adjusted for the effects of late maternal age, parous women have remained at a substantially reduced risk of GTD compared with nulliparous women, with some evidence of further reductions in risk with multiple births (192). A number of studies have found an increased risk associated with a prior spontaneous or induced abortion, although this has not been consistently observed (192). A history of infertility has also been suggested as a risk factor for GTD, although not confirmed in all studies (192). In one study, Chinese patients reporting the use of herbal medicines during the first trimester of a previous pregnancy were at elevated risk (192).

Low body mass, unrelated to dieting or exercise, has been reported as a risk factor for choriocarcinoma in one study (193). Patients also had later onset of menarche and lighter menstrual periods than controls, possibly reflecting lower estrogen levels.

Exogenous Hormones

Several studies have found an increased risk of trophoblastic diseases associated with long-term use of oral contraceptives (194). It has also been suggested that oral contraceptives may increase the risk of malignant sequelae after mole evacuation through a tumor-stimulating effect. However, more recent studies (as demonstrated by Costa and Doyle in a systemic review published in 2006) suggest no clear evidence for such an association, prompting the suggestion that practitioners should no longer avoid use of oral contraceptives during the postmolar follow-up period.

Conclusions

Although a genetic role in the development of hydatidiform mole is now certain, little is known about genotypes that predispose to hydatidiform mole or environmental factors that may increase the risk of defective ova. Except for the possible role of oral contraceptives, few potential environmental promoters have been examined.

The trophoblast plays an active role in pregnancy, including metabolizing and detoxifying xenobiotic substances, regulating nutrient and waste product transfer, synthesizing steroid and protein hormones, and controlling the immune response of the maternofetal unit. Injury to the trophoblast can occur in pregnancy as a result of environmental exposure (e.g., heavy metals and polycyclic hydrocarbons), resulting in the breakdown of trophoblastic processes. When the trophoblast malfunctions, mutagenic, teratogenic, lethotoxic, and carcinogenic compounds gain access to the developing embryo, causing injury and death. The genotype of hydatidiform mole results in a trophoblast that malfunctions, and exposure to certain environmental agents during the molar pregnancy may promote choriocarcinoma. Before implantation, the trophoblast forms most of the embryonic tissue, which already metabolizes environmental agents. Even preimplanted moles, with their impaired metabolic capabilities, may increase the toxicity of environmental agents and promote carcinogenesis.

Recent advances in identifying genetic and molecular markers involved with partial versus complete moles (184) open a number of avenues for assessing the interaction of these markers with a variety of proposed environmental risk factors. This could include a focus on early stages in the disease process or on factors involved in the progression of molar pregnancies to more invasive complications.

SUMMARY

The goal of both medical practice and epidemiology is to reduce morbidity and mortality. For many diseases, the focus has turned to the ultimate aim of prevention. The link between identification of etiologic factors and possibilities for prevention is well illustrated for tobacco- and alcohol-related tumors and for those associated with specific pharmaceutical, radiogenic, and occupational exposures. Fortunately, for gynecologic cancers, there are a number of identified etiologic factors that are also amenable to preventive approaches.

Undoubtedly, the prospects for prevention are best for cervical cancer. For some time, secondary prevention in the form of screening for pathologic precursors of invasive disease has been the hallmark of the public health approach to this malignancy. The establishment of HPV as a central etiologic agent for the disease presents other avenues for prevention, including application of recently developed vaccines against the virus. Knowledge of when and how infection and other factors operate in the natural history of the disease has revolutionized screening strategies and shifted treatment from cell ablation to antiviral therapies. As always, combined laboratory, clinical, and epidemiologic research is needed to realize these propositions.

Many believe that more is known about the cause of endometrial carcinoma than for almost any other tumor. A unified theory of how all risk factors may operate through a final common estrogenic pathway is popular and well supported. A woman's hormonal milieu may prove to be favorable to modification at a practical level. There is substantial evidence that elimination of obesity and a reduction in fat in the diet—two interventions actively promoted for other reasons—should also reduce endometrial cancer risk. After the epidemic of endometrial cancer due to menopausal estrogen therapy, changes in the management of menopause occurred, resulting in a marked decline in the rates of endometrial cancer. More care is devoted to identifying women who truly need estrogen therapy, treatment of menopausal symptoms is for a much shorter period of time, the use of cyclic progestin in combination with estrogen is advised if indicated, and regular endometrial sampling is frequently practiced for long-term estrogen users.

Although past alterations in patient management led to a decline in endometrial cancer, current events make future patterns less clear. Previous enthusiasm for long-term treatment of large segments of the population of menopausal women with hormones to control symptoms and prevent osteoporosis and heart disease may have implications for endometrial cancer in the future. On the other hand, current patterns of use of oral contraceptives could lead to reductions in endometrial cancer rates in the general population. The impact of widespread oral contraceptive use at young ages on endometrial cancer risk at older ages is not well studied. However, if it is anywhere near the reduced risk seen at young ages, the resulting reduction in endometrial cancer overall could be substantial.

With further research, it is also possible that pharmacologic interventions aimed specifically at groups at high risk for endometrial cancer due to endogenous hormonal factors could be justified. More must be learned about the associations of risk for endometrial cancer and the quantitative levels of estrogens and other hormones and their relative proportions. Once these factors are known, women with PCOS, diabetes, morbid obesity, or other predisposing conditions could be evaluated for unfavorable hormone profiles and appropriately targeted for treatment.

Although a substantial amount has been learned about ovarian cancer risks, the prospects for meaningful preventive measures aimed at this tumor are probably worse than for the other gynecologic malignancies. Although several ovarian cancer risk factors seem to indict ovulatory activity as a common pathway to increased risk, the mechanism by which this occurs is unknown. Even if some of the hypothesized mechanisms prove to be correct (e.g., levels of circulating gonadotropins), it is unclear how reasonable any interventions may be. However, if the long-term effect of oral contraceptive use on ovarian cancer risk is similar to its short-term effect, a substantial decline in ovarian cancer rates should result from pill use patterns of the past 40 years. Another reason for the limited prospects for prevention is that for several risk factors (e.g., protection associated with hysterectomy), no credible mechanism has been suggested. The associations promising the greatest opportunities for preventive actions are several recently suggested dietary relationships, specifically, decreased risks with consumption of diets high in fruits and vegetables and certain micronutrients. However, these observations need to be replicated in additional studies. Because of the preventive implications, attempts at confirmation should have high priority.

For cervical cancer, endometrial cancer, and ovarian cancer, much is known about the risk factors. Less is known about the precise biologic mechanisms through which the known risk factors operate. There is substantial enthusiasm for current interdisciplinary studies that incorporate state-of-the-art laboratory assays into robust epidemiologic research designs focused on answering these mechanistic questions. Even among some of the more conservative etiologists, there is a belief that the gynecologic oncologist may soon be able to intervene much earlier in the natural history of these diseases and, in some instances, engage in primary prevention.

REFERENCES

1. American Cancer Society. Cancer facts & figures, 2015. http://www.cancer.org/acs/groups/content/@editorial/documents/document/acspc-044552.pdf. Accessed December 2015.
2. Howlader N, Noone AM, Krapcho M, et al. SEER cancer statistics review, 1975–2012, National Cancer Institute. Bethesda, MD: National Cancer Institute; 2015. http://seer.cancer.gov/csr/1975_2012/, based on November 2014 SEER data submission, posted to the SEER web site, April 2015. Accessed December 2015.
3. International Agency for Research on Cancer. GLOBOCAN 2012: Estimated cancer incidence, mortality and prevalence worldwide in 2012. http://globocan.iarc.fr. Accessed December 2015.
4. Yang HP, Cook LS, Weiderpass E, et al. Infertility and incident endometrial cancer risk: a pooled analysis from the epidemiology of endometrial cancer consortium (E2C2). *Br J Cancer.* 2015;112(5):925–933.
5. Dossus L, Allen N, Kaaks R, et al. Reproductive risk factors and endometrial cancer: the European Prospective Investigation into cancer and nutrition. *Int J Cancer.* 2010;127(2):442–451.
6. Felix AS, Gaudet MM, La Vecchia C, et al. Intrauterine devices and endometrial cancer risk: a pooled analysis of the Epidemiology of Endometrial Cancer Consortium. *Int J Cancer.* 2015;136(5):E410–E422.
7. Brinton LA, Westhoff CL, Scoccia B, et al. Fertility drugs and endometrial cancer risk: results from an extended follow-up of a large infertility cohort. *Hum Reprod.* 2013;28(10):2813–2821.
8. Collaborative Group on Epidemiological Studies on Endometrial Cancer. Endometrial cancer and oral contraceptives: an individual participant meta-analysis of 27 276 women with endometrial cancer from 36 epidemiological studies. *Lancet Oncol.* 2015;16(9):1061–1070.
9. Beral V, Bull D, Reeves G, et al. Endometrial cancer and hormone-replacement therapy in the Million Women Study. *Lancet.* 2005;365(9470):1543–1551.
10. Chlebowski RT, Anderson GL, Sarto GE, et al. Continuous combined estrogen plus progestin and endometrial cancer: the Women's Health Initiative Randomized Trial. *J Natl Cancer Inst.* 2016;108(3). doi: 10.1093/jnci/djv350.
11. Razavi P, Pike MC, Horn-Ross PL, et al. Long-term postmenopausal hormone therapy and endometrial cancer. *Cancer Epidemiol Biomarkers Prev.* 2010;19(2):475–483.
12. Trabert B, Wentzensen N, Yang HP, et al. Is estrogen plus progestin menopausal hormone therapy safe with respect to endometrial cancer risk? *Int J Cancer.* 2013;132(2):417–426.
13. Yang TY, Cairns BJ, Allen N, et al. Postmenopausal endometrial cancer risk and body size in early life and middle age: prospective cohort study. *Br J Cancer.* 2012;107(1):169–175.
14. Cuzick J, Sestak I, Bonanni B, et al. Selective oestrogen receptor modulators in prevention of breast cancer: an updated meta-analysis of individual participant data. *Lancet.* 2013;381(9880):1827–1834.
15. Brinton LA, Felix AS, McMeekin DS, et al. Etiologic heterogeneity in endometrial cancer: evidence from a Gynecologic Oncology Group trial. *Gynecol Oncol.* 2013;129(2):277–284.
16. Schmandt RE, Iglesias DA, Co NN, et al. Understanding obesity and endometrial cancer risk: opportunities for prevention. *Am J Obstet Gynecol.* 2011;205(6):518–525.
17. Dougan MM, Hankinson SE, Vivo ID, et al. Prospective study of body size throughout the life-course and the incidence of endometrial cancer among premenopausal and postmenopausal women. *Int J Cancer.* 2015;137(3):625–637.
18. Friedenreich C, Cust A, Lahmann PH, et al. Anthropometric factors and risk of endometrial cancer: the European prospective investigation into cancer and nutrition. *Cancer Causes Control.* 2007;18(4):399–413.
19. Ju W, Kim HJ, Hankinson SE, et al. Prospective study of body fat distribution and the risk of endometrial cancer. *Cancer Epidemiol.* 2015;39(4):567–570.
20. Moore SC, Gierach GL, Schatzkin A, et al. Physical activity, sedentary behaviours, and the prevention of endometrial cancer. *Br J Cancer.* 2010;103(7):933–938.
21. Yang HP, Brinton LA, Platz EA, et al. Active and passive cigarette smoking and the risk of endometrial cancer in Poland. *Eur J Cancer.* 2010;46(4):690–696.
22. Polesel J, Serraino D, Zucchetto A, et al. Cigarette smoking and endometrial cancer risk: the modifying effect of obesity. *Eur J Cancer Prev.* 2009;18(6):476–481.
23. Gu F, Caporaso NE, Schairer C, et al. Urinary concentrations of estrogens and estrogen metabolites and smoking in Caucasian women. *Cancer Epidemiol Biomarkers Prev.* 2013;22(1):58–68.
24. Prentice RL, Thomson CA, Caan B, et al. Low-fat dietary pattern and cancer incidence in the Women's Health Initiative Dietary Modification Randomized Controlled Trial. *J Natl Cancer Inst.* 2007;99(20):1534–1543.
25. Biel RK, Csizmadi I, Cook LS, et al. Risk of endometrial cancer in relation to individual nutrients from diet and supplements. *Public Health Nutr.* 2011;14(11):1948–1960.
26. Galeone C, Augustin LS, Filomeno M, et al. Dietary glycemic index, glycemic load, and the risk of endometrial cancer: a case-control study and meta-analysis. *Eur J Cancer Prev.* 2013;22(1):38–45.
27. Wilson KM, Mucci LA, Rosner BA, et al. A prospective study on dietary acrylamide intake and the risk for breast, endometrial, and ovarian cancers. *Cancer Epidemiol Biomarkers Prev.* 2010;19(10):2503–2515.
28. Brasky TM, Rodabough RJ, Liu J, et al. Long-chain omega-3 fatty acid intake and endometrial cancer risk in the Women's Health Initiative. *Am J Clin Nutr.* 2015;101(4):824–834.
29. Je Y, DeVivo I, Giovannucci E. Long-term alcohol intake and risk of endometrial cancer in the Nurses' Health Study, 1980–2010. *Br J Cancer.* 2014;111(1):186–194.
30. Je Y, Giovannucci E. Coffee consumption and risk of endometrial cancer: findings from a large up-to-date meta-analysis. *Int J Cancer.* 2012;131(7):1700–1710.
31. Haoula Z, Salman M, Atiomo W. Evaluating the association between endometrial cancer and polycystic ovary syndrome. *Hum Reprod.* 2012;27(5):1327–1331.
32. Liao C, Zhang D, Mungo C, et al. Is diabetes mellitus associated with increased incidence and disease-specific mortality in endometrial cancer? A systematic review and meta-analysis of cohort studies. *Gynecol Oncol.* 2014;135(1):163–171.
33. Ko EM, Sturmer T, Hong JL, et al. Metformin and the risk of endometrial cancer: a population-based cohort study. *Gynecol Oncol.* 2015;136(2):341–347.
34. Trabert B, Wentzensen N, Felix AS, et al. Metabolic syndrome and risk of endometrial cancer in the United States: a study in the SEER-medicare linked database. *Cancer Epidemiol Biomarkers Prev.* 2015;24(1):261–267.
35. Fortuny J, Sima C, Bayuga S, et al. Risk of endometrial cancer in relation to medical conditions and medication use. *Cancer Epidemiol Biomarkers Prev.* 2009;18(5):1448–1456.
36. Newcomb PA, Trentham-Dietz A, Egan KM, et al. Fracture history and risk of breast and endometrial cancer. *Am J Epidemiol.* 2001;153(11):1071–1078.
37. Modugno F, Ness RB, Chen C, et al. Inflammation and endometrial cancer: a hypothesis. *Cancer Epidemiol Biomarkers Prev.* 2005;14(12):2840–2847.
38. Brons N, Baandrup L, Dehlendorff C, et al. Use of nonsteroidal anti-inflammatory drugs and risk of endometrial cancer: a nationwide case-control study. *Cancer Causes Control.* 2015;26(7):973–981.
39. Shai A, Segev Y, Narod SA. Genetics of endometrial cancer. *Fam Cancer.* 2014;13(3):499–505.
40. Gaudet MM, Yang HP, Bosquet JG, et al. No association between FTO or HHEX and endometrial cancer risk. *Cancer Epidemiol Biomarkers Prev.* 2010;19(8):2106–2109.
41. De Vivo I, Prescott J, Setiawan VW, et al. Genome-wide association study of endometrial cancer in E2C2. *Hum Genet.* 2014;133(2):211–224.
42. Long J, Zheng W, Xiang YB, et al. Genome-wide association study identifies a possible susceptibility locus for endometrial cancer. *Cancer Epidemiol Biomarkers Prev.* 2012;21(6):980–987.
43. Weiderpass E, Adami HO, Baron JA, et al. Organochlorines and endometrial cancer risk. *Cancer Epidemiol Biomarkers Prev.* 2000;9(5):487–493.

44. Abel EL, Hendrix SL, McNeeley GS, et al. Use of electric blankets and association with prevalence of endometrial cancer. *Eur J Cancer Prev.* 2007;16(3):243–250.
45. Bernstein L, Allen M, Anton-Culver H, et al. High breast cancer incidence rates among California teachers: results from the California Teachers Study (United States). *Cancer Causes Control.* 2002;13(7):625–635.
46. Weiderpass E, Pukkala E, Vasama-Neuvonen K, et al. Occupational exposures and cancers of the endometrium and cervix uteri in Finland. *Am J Ind Med.* 2001;39(6):572–580.
47. Setiawan VW, Yang HP, Pike MC, et al. Type I and II endometrial cancers: have they different risk factors? *J Clin Oncol.* 2013;31(20):2607–2618.
48. Allen NE, Key TJ, Dossus L, et al. Endogenous sex hormones and endometrial cancer risk in women in the European Prospective Investigation into Cancer and Nutrition (EPIC). *Endocr Relat Cancer.* 2008;15(2):485–497.
49. Zeleniuch-Jacquotte A, Akhmedkhanov A, Kato I, et al. Postmenopausal endogenous oestrogens and risk of endometrial cancer: results of a prospective study. *Br J Cancer.* 2001;84(7):975–981.
50. Braem MG, Onland-Moret NC, Schouten LJ, et al. Multiple miscarriages are associated with the risk of ovarian cancer: results from the European Prospective Investigation into Cancer and Nutrition. *PLoS One.* 2012;7(5):e37141.
51. Braem MG, Onland-Moret NC, van den Brandt PA, et al. Reproductive and hormonal factors in association with ovarian cancer in The Netherlands cohort study. *Am J Epidemiol.* 2010;172(10):1181–1189.
52. Brinton LA, Sahasrabuddhe VV, Scoccia B. Fertility drugs and the risk of breast and gynecologic cancers. *Semin Reprod Med.* 2012;30(2):131–145.
53. van Leeuwen FE, Klip H, Mooij TM, et al. Risk of borderline and invasive ovarian tumours after ovarian stimulation for in vitro fertilization in a large Dutch cohort. *Hum Reprod.* 2011;26(12):3456–3465.
54. Danforth KN, Tworoger SS, Hecht JL, et al. Breastfeeding and risk of ovarian cancer in two prospective cohorts. *Cancer Causes Control.* 2007;18(5):517–523.
55. Cibula D, Widschwendter M, Majek O, et al. Tubal ligation and the risk of ovarian cancer: review and meta-analysis. *Hum Reprod Update.* 2011;17(1):55–67.
56. Merritt MA, De Pari M, Vitonis AF, et al. Reproductive characteristics in relation to ovarian cancer risk by histologic pathways. *Hum Reprod.* 2013;28(5):1406–1417.
57. Collaborative Group on Epidemiological Studies of Ovarian C, Beral V, Doll R, et al. Ovarian cancer and oral contraceptives: collaborative reanalysis of data from 45 epidemiological studies including 23,257 women with ovarian cancer and 87,303 controls. *Lancet.* 2008;371(9609):303–314.
58. Anderson GL, Judd HL, Kaunitz AM, et al. Effects of estrogen plus progestin on gynecologic cancers and associated diagnostic procedures: the Women's Health Initiative randomized trial. *JAMA.* 2003;290(13):1739–1748.
59. Collaborative Group on Epidemiological Studies of Ovarian C, Beral V, Gaitskell K, et al. Menopausal hormone use and ovarian cancer risk: individual participant meta-analysis of 52 epidemiological studies. *Lancet.* 2015;385(9980):1835–1842.
60. Morch LS, Lokkegaard E, Andreasen AH, et al. Hormone therapy and ovarian cancer. *JAMA.* 2009;302(3):298–305.
61. McSorley MA, Alberg AJ, Allen DS, et al. Prediagnostic circulating follicle stimulating hormone concentrations and ovarian cancer risk. *Int J Cancer.* 2009;125(3):674–679.
62. Lukanova A, Lundin E, Micheli A, et al. Risk of ovarian cancer in relation to prediagnostic levels of C-peptide, insulin-like growth factor binding proteins-1 and -2 (USA, Sweden, Italy). *Cancer Causes Control.* 2003;14(3):285–292.
63. Ose J, Fortner RT, Rinaldi S, et al. Endogenous androgens and risk of epithelial invasive ovarian cancer by tumor characteristics in the European Prospective Investigation into Cancer and Nutrition. *Int J Cancer.* 2015;136(2):399–410.
64. Rinaldi S, Dossus L, Lukanova A, et al. Endogenous androgens and risk of epithelial ovarian cancer: results from the European Prospective Investigation into Cancer and Nutrition (EPIC). *Cancer Epidemiol Biomarkers Prev.* 2007;16(1):23–29.
65. Schock H, Surcel HM, Zeleniuch-Jacquotte A, et al. Early pregnancy sex steroids and maternal risk of epithelial ovarian cancer. *Endocr Relat Cancer.* 2014;21(6):831–844.
66. Pearce CL, Templeman C, Rossing MA, et al. Association between endometriosis and risk of histological subtypes of ovarian cancer: a pooled analysis of case-control studies. *Lancet Oncol.* 2012;13(4):385–394.
67. Ness RB. Endometriosis and ovarian cancer: thoughts on shared pathophysiology. *Am J Obstet Gynecol.* 2003;189(1):280–294.
68. Lin HW, Tu YY, Lin SY, et al. Risk of ovarian cancer in women with pelvic inflammatory disease: a population-based study. *Lancet Oncol.* 2011;12(9):900–904.
69. Trabert B, Ness RB, Lo-Ciganic WH, et al. Aspirin, nonaspirin nonsteroidal anti-inflammatory drug, and acetaminophen use and risk of invasive epithelial ovarian cancer: a pooled analysis in the Ovarian Cancer Association Consortium. *J Natl Cancer Inst.* 2014;106(2):djt431.
70. Collaborative Group on Epidemiological Studies of Ovarian C. Ovarian cancer and body size: individual participant meta-analysis including 25,157 women with ovarian cancer from 47 epidemiological studies. *PLoS Med.* 2012;9(4):e1001200.
71. Olsen CM, Nagle CM, Whiteman DC, et al. Obesity and risk of ovarian cancer subtypes: evidence from the Ovarian Cancer Association Consortium. *Endocr Relat Cancer.* 2013;20(2):251–262.
72. Yang HP, Trabert B, Murphy MA, et al. Ovarian cancer risk factors by histologic subtypes in the NIH-AARP Diet and Health Study. *Int J Cancer.* 2012;131(4):938–948.
73. Schouten LJ, Rivera C, Hunter DJ, et al. Height, body mass index, and ovarian cancer: a pooled analysis of 12 cohort studies. *Cancer Epidemiol Biomarkers Prev.* 2008;17(4):902–912.
74. Olsen CM, Bain CJ, Jordan SJ, et al. Recreational physical activity and epithelial ovarian cancer: a case-control study, systematic review, and meta-analysis. *Cancer Epidemiol Biomarkers Prev.* 2007;16(11):2321–2330.
75. Hildebrand JS, Gapstur SM, Gaudet MM, et al. Moderate-to-vigorous physical activity and leisure-time sitting in relation to ovarian cancer risk in a large prospective US cohort. *Cancer Causes Control.* 2015;26(11):1691–1697.
76. Gram IT, Lukanova A, Brill I, et al. Cigarette smoking and risk of histological subtypes of epithelial ovarian cancer in the EPIC cohort study. *Int J Cancer.* 2012;130(9):2204–2210.
77. Jordan SJ, Whiteman DC, Purdie DM, et al. Does smoking increase risk of ovarian cancer? A systematic review. *Gynecol Oncol.* 2006;103(3):1122–1129.
78. Fairfield KM, Hunter DJ, Colditz GA, et al. A prospective study of dietary lactose and ovarian cancer. *Int J Cancer.* 2004;110(2):271–277.
79. Genkinger JM, Hunter DJ, Spiegelman D, et al. A pooled analysis of 12 cohort studies of dietary fat, cholesterol and egg intake and ovarian cancer. *Cancer Causes Control.* 2006;17(3):273–285.
80. Wallin A, Orsini N, Wolk A. Red and processed meat consumption and risk of ovarian cancer: a dose-response meta-analysis of prospective studies. *Br J Cancer.* 2011;104(7):1196–1201.
81. Koushik A, Hunter DJ, Spiegelman D, et al. Fruits and vegetables and ovarian cancer risk in a pooled analysis of 12 cohort studies. *Cancer Epidemiol Biomarkers Prev.* 2005;14(9):2160–2167.
82. Cook LS, Neilson HK, Lorenzetti DL, et al. A systematic literature review of vitamin D and ovarian cancer. *Am J Obstet Gynecol.* 2010;203(1):70 e71–78.
83. Kelemen LE, Bandera EV, Terry KL, et al. Recent alcohol consumption and risk of incident ovarian carcinoma: a pooled analysis of 5,342 cases and 10,358 controls from the Ovarian Cancer Association Consortium. *BMC Cancer.* 2013;13:28.
84. Braem MG, Onland-Moret NC, Schouten LJ, et al. Coffee and tea consumption and the risk of ovarian cancer: a prospective cohort study and updated meta-analysis. *Am J Clin Nutr.* 2012;95(5):1172–1181.
85. Butler LM, Wu AH. Green and black tea in relation to gynecologic cancers. *Mol Nutr Food Res.* 2011;55(6):931–940.
86. Hemminki K, Granstrom C. Familial invasive and borderline ovarian tumors by proband status, age and histology. *Int J Cancer.* 2003;105(5):701–705.
87. Pharoah PD, Ponder BA. The genetics of ovarian cancer. *Best Pract Res Clin Obstet Gynaecol.* 2002;16(4):449–468.
88. Venkitaraman AR. Cancer susceptibility and the functions of BRCA1 and BRCA2. *Cell.* 2002;108(2):171–182.
89. Wooster R, Weber BL. Breast and ovarian cancer. *N Engl J Med.* 2003;348(23):2339–2347.
90. Foulkes WD. Inherited susceptibility to common cancers. *N Engl J Med.* 2008;359(20):2143–2153.
91. Gayther SA, Pharoah PD. The inherited genetics of ovarian and endometrial cancer. *Curr Opin Genet Dev.* 2010;20(3):231–238.
92. Kuchenbaecker KB, Ramus SJ, Tyrer J, et al. Identification of six new susceptibility loci for invasive epithelial ovarian cancer. *Nat Genet.* 2015;47(2):164–171.
93. Cramer DW, Vitonis AF, Terry KL, et al. The association between talc use and ovarian cancer: a retrospective case-control study in two US states. *Epidemiology.* 2016;27(3):334–346.
94. Terry KL, Karageorgi S, Shvetsov YB, et al. Genital powder use and risk of ovarian cancer: a pooled analysis of 8,525 cases and 9,859 controls. *Cancer Prev Res (Phila).* 2013;6(8):811–821.
95. Houghton SC, Reeves KW, Hankinson SE, et al. Perineal powder use and risk of ovarian cancer. *J Natl Cancer Inst.* 2014;106(9). doi:10.1093/jnci/dju208.

96. Camargo MC, Stayner LT, Straif K, et al. Occupational exposure to asbestos and ovarian cancer: a meta-analysis. *Environ Health Perspect.* 2011;119(9):1211–1217.
97. Kurman RJ, Shih Ie M. Molecular pathogenesis and extraovarian origin of epithelial ovarian cancer—shifting the paradigm. *Hum Pathol.* 2011;42(7):918–931.
98. IARC Working Group on the Evaluation of Carcinogenic Risks to Humans. Meeting (2008–2009: Lyon France), International Agency for Research on Cancer, World Health Organization. *A review of human carcinogens.* Lyon, France: International Agency for Research on Cancer; 2012.
99. Guan P, Howell-Jones R, Li N, et al. Human papillomavirus types in 115,789 HPV-positive women: a meta-analysis from cervical infection to cancer. *Int J Cancer.* 2012;131(10):2349–2359.
100. Vaccarella S, Lortet-Tieulent J, Plummer M, et al. Worldwide trends in cervical cancer incidence: impact of screening against changes in disease risk factors. *Eur J Cancer.* 2013;49(15):3262–3273.
101. Gustafsson L, Ponten J, Bergstrom R, et al. International incidence rates of invasive cervical cancer before cytological screening. *Int J Cancer.* 1997;71(2):159–165.
102. Mathew A, George PS. Trends in incidence and mortality rates of squamous cell carcinoma and adenocarcinoma of cervix—worldwide. *Asian Pac J Cancer Prev.* 2009;10(4):645–650.
103. Horner MJ, Altekruse SF, Zou Z, et al. U.S. geographic distribution of prevaccine era cervical cancer screening, incidence, stage, and mortality. *Cancer Epidemiol Biomarkers Prev.* 2011;20(4):591–599.
104. Plummer M, Peto J, Franceschi S, et al. Time since first sexual intercourse and the risk of cervical cancer. *Int J Cancer.* 2012;130(11):2638–2644.
105. Schiffman M, Wentzensen N. Human papillomavirus infection and the multistage carcinogenesis of cervical cancer. *Cancer Epidemiol Biomarkers Prev.* 2013;22(4):553–560.
106. Castle PE, Schiffman M, Herrero R, et al. A prospective study of age trends in cervical human papillomavirus acquisition and persistence in Guanacaste, Costa Rica. *J Infect Dis.* 2005;191(11):1808–1816.
107. Saslow D, Solomon D, Lawson HW, et al. American Cancer Society, American Society for Colposcopy and Cervical Pathology, and American Society for Clinical Pathology screening guidelines for the prevention and early detection of cervical cancer. *CA Cancer J Clin.* 2012;62(3):147–172.
108. Herfs M, Yamamoto Y, Laury A, et al. A discrete population of squamocolumnar junction cells implicated in the pathogenesis of cervical cancer. *Proc Natl Acad Sci U S A.* 2012;109(26):10516–10521.
109. Shepherd JP, Frampton GK, Harris P. Interventions for encouraging sexual behaviours intended to prevent cervical cancer. *Cochrane Database Syst Rev.* 2011(4):CD001035.
110. Winer RL, Hughes JP, Feng Q, et al. Condom use and the risk of genital human papillomavirus infection in young women. *N Engl J Med.* 2006;354(25):2645–2654.
111. Manhart LE, Koutsky LA. Do condoms prevent genital HPV infection, external genital warts, or cervical neoplasia? A meta-analysis. *Sex Transm Dis.* 2002;29(11):725–735.
112. Burchell AN, Tellier PP, Hanley J, et al. Influence of partner's infection status on prevalent human papillomavirus among persons with a new sex partner. *Sex Transm Dis.* 2010;37(1):34–40.
113. Castellsague X, Bosch FX, Munoz N, et al. Male circumcision, penile human papillomavirus infection, and cervical cancer in female partners. *N Engl J Med.* 2002;346(15):1105–1112.
114. Auvert B, Sobngwi-Tambekou J, Cutler E, et al. Effect of male circumcision on the prevalence of high-risk human papillomavirus in young men: results of a randomized controlled trial conducted in Orange Farm, South Africa. *J Infect Dis.* 2009;199(1):14–19.
115. Wawer MJ, Tobian AA, Kigozi G, et al. Effect of circumcision of HIV-negative men on transmission of human papillomavirus to HIV-negative women: a randomised trial in Rakai, Uganda. *Lancet.* 2011;377(9761):209–218.
116. Chen HC, Schiffman M, Lin CY, et al. Persistence of type-specific human papillomavirus infection and increased long-term risk of cervical cancer. *J Natl Cancer Inst.* 2011;103(18):1387–1396.
117. Schiffman M, Glass AG, Wentzensen N, et al. A long-term prospective study of type-specific human papillomavirus infection and risk of cervical neoplasia among 20,000 women in the Portland Kaiser Cohort Study. *Cancer Epidemiol Biomarkers Prev.* 2011;20(7):1398–1409.
118. Castle PE, Fetterman B, Thomas Cox J, et al. The age-specific relationships of abnormal cytology and human papillomavirus DNA results to the risk of cervical precancer and cancer. *Obstet Gynecol.* 2010;116(1):76–84.
119. Sahasrabuddhe VV, Luhn P, Wentzensen N. Human papillomavirus and cervical cancer: biomarkers for improved prevention efforts. *Future Microbiol.* 2011;6(9):1083–1098.
120. Castle PE, Schiffman M, Wheeler CM, et al. Evidence for frequent regression of cervical intraepithelial neoplasia-grade 2. *Obstet Gynecol.* 2009;113(1):18–25.
121. Li N, Franceschi S, Howell-Jones R, et al. Human papillomavirus type distribution in 30,848 invasive cervical cancers worldwide: variation by geographical region, histological type and year of publication. *Int J Cancer.* 2011;128(4):927–935.
122. Cornet I, Gheit T, Iannacone MR, et al. HPV16 genetic variation and the development of cervical cancer worldwide. *Br J Cancer.* 2013;108(1):240–244.
123. Ramanakumar AV, Goncalves O, Richardson H, et al. Human papillomavirus (HPV) types 16, 18, 31, 45 DNA loads and HPV-16 integration in persistent and transient infections in young women. *BMC Infect Dis.* 2010;10:326.
124. Gravitt PE, Kovacic MB, Herrero R, et al. High load for most high risk human papillomavirus genotypes is associated with prevalent cervical cancer precursors but only HPV16 load predicts the development of incident disease. *Int J Cancer.* 2007;121(12):2787–2793.
125. Cohen CR, Moscicki AB, Scott ME, et al. Increased levels of immune activation in the genital tract of healthy young women from sub-Saharan Africa. *AIDS.* 2010;24(13):2069–2074.
126. Nowak RG, Gravitt PE, Morrison CS, et al. Increases in human papillomavirus detection during early HIV infection among women in Zimbabwe. *J Infect Dis.* 2011;203(8):1182–1191.
127. Wang SS, Bratti MC, Rodriguez AC, et al. Common variants in immune and DNA repair genes and risk for human papillomavirus persistence and progression to cervical cancer. *J Infect Dis.* 2009;199(1):20–30.
128. Einstein MH, Schiller JT, Viscidi RP, et al. Clinician's guide to human papillomavirus immunology: knowns and unknowns. *Lancet Infect Dis.* 2009;9(6):347–356.
129. Einstein MH. Acquired immune response to oncogenic human papillomavirus associated with prophylactic cervical cancer vaccines. *Cancer Immunol Immunother.* 2008;57(4):443–451.
130. Wentzensen N, Rodriguez AC, Viscidi R, et al. A competitive serological assay shows naturally acquired immunity to human papillomavirus infections in the Guanacaste Natural History Study. *J Infect Dis.* 2011;204(1):94–102.
131. de Araujo Souza PS, Sichero L, Maciag PC. HPV variants and HLA polymorphisms: the role of variability on the risk of cervical cancer. *Future Oncol.* 2009;5(3):359–370.
132. Hildesheim A, Wang SS. Host and viral genetics and risk of cervical cancer: a review. *Virus Res.* 2002;89(2):229–240.
133. Vink JM, van Kemenade FJ, Meijer CJ, et al. Cervix smear abnormalities: linking pathology data in female twins, their mothers and sisters. *Eur J Hum Genet.* 2011;19(1):108–111.
134. Gravitt PE. The known unknowns of HPV natural history. *J Clin Invest.* 2011;121(12):4593–4599.
135. McCredie MR, Sharples KJ, Paul C, et al. Natural history of cervical neoplasia and risk of invasive cancer in women with cervical intraepithelial neoplasia 3: a retrospective cohort study. *Lancet Oncol.* 2008;9(5):425–434.
136. International Collaboration of Epidemiological Studies of Cervical Cancer. Cervical carcinoma and reproductive factors: collaborative reanalysis of individual data on 16,563 women with cervical carcinoma and 33,542 women without cervical carcinoma from 25 epidemiological studies. *Int J Cancer.* 2006;119(5):1108–1124.
137. de Villiers EM. Relationship between steroid hormone contraceptives and HPV, cervical intraepithelial neoplasia and cervical carcinoma. *Int J Cancer.* 2003;103(6):705–708.
138. Harris TG, Miller L, Kulasingam SL, et al. Depot-medroxyprogesterone acetate and combined oral contraceptive use and cervical neoplasia among women with oncogenic human papillomavirus infection. *Am J Obstet Gynecol.* 2009;200(5):489. e481–e488.
139. Arbyn M, Castellsague X, de Sanjose S, et al. Worldwide burden of cervical cancer in 2008. *Ann Oncol.* 2011;22(12):2675–2686.
140. Rinaldi S, Plummer M, Biessy C, et al. Endogenous sex steroids and risk of cervical carcinoma: results from the EPIC study. *Cancer Epidemiol Biomarkers Prev.* 2011;20(12):2532–2540.
141. den Boon JA, Pyeon D, Wang SS, et al. Molecular transitions from papillomavirus infection to cervical precancer and cancer: role of stromal estrogen receptor signaling. *Proc Natl Acad Sci U S A.* 2015;112(25):E3255–3264.
142. Roberts JN, Kines RC, Katki HA, et al. Effect of Pap smear collection and carrageenan on cervicovaginal human papillomavirus-16 infection in a rhesus macaque model. *J Natl Cancer Inst.* 2011;103(9):737–743.
143. Parikh S, Brennan P, Boffetta P. Meta-analysis of social inequality and the risk of cervical cancer. *Int J Cancer.* 2003;105(5):687–691.
144. Franceschi S, Plummer M, Clifford G, et al. Differences in the risk of cervical cancer and human papillomavirus infection by education level. *Br J Cancer.* 2009;101(5):865–870.

145. International Collaboration of Epidemiological Studies of Cervical Cancer, Appleby P, Beral V, et al. Carcinoma of the cervix and tobacco smoking: collaborative reanalysis of individual data on 13,541 women with carcinoma of the cervix and 23,017 women without carcinoma of the cervix from 23 epidemiological studies. *Int J Cancer.* 2006;118(6):1481–1495.
146. Hellberg D, Stendahl U. The biological role of smoking, oral contraceptive use and endogenous sexual steroid hormones in invasive squamous epithelial cervical cancer. *Anticancer Res.* 2005;25(4):3041–3046.
147. Pratt MM, Sirajuddin P, Poirier MC, et al. Polycyclic aromatic hydrocarbon-DNA adducts in cervix of women infected with carcinogenic human papillomavirus types: an immunohistochemistry study. *Mutat Res.* 2007;624(1-2):114–123.
148. Siegel EM, Patel N, Lu B, et al. Biomarkers of oxidant load and type-specific clearance of prevalent oncogenic human papillomavirus infection: markers of immune response? *Int J Cancer.* 2012;131(1):219–228.
149. Myung SK, Ju W, Kim SC, et al. Vitamin or antioxidant intake (or serum level) and risk of cervical neoplasm: a meta-analysis. *BJOG.* 2011;118(11):1285–1291.
150. Madeleine MM, Anttila T, Schwartz SM, et al. Risk of cervical cancer associated with *Chlamydia trachomatis* antibodies by histology, HPV type and HPV cofactors. *Int J Cancer.* 2007;120(3):650–655.
151. Chaturvedi AK, Madeleine MM, Biggar RJ, et al. Risk of human papillomavirus-associated cancers among persons with AIDS. *J Natl Cancer Inst.* 2009;101(16):1120–1130.
152. de Martel C, Shiels MS, Franceschi S, et al. Cancers attributable to infections among adults with HIV in the United States. *AIDS.* 2015;29(16):2173–2181.
153. Walker F, Adle-Biassette H, Madelenat P, et al. Increased apoptosis in cervical intraepithelial neoplasia associated with HIV infection: implication of oncogenic human papillomavirus, caspases, and Langerhans cells. *Clin Cancer Res.* 2005;11(7):2451–2458.
154. Shrestha S, Wang C, Aissani B, et al. Interleukin-10 gene (IL10) polymorphisms and human papillomavirus clearance among immunosuppressed adolescents. *Cancer Epidemiol Biomarkers Prev.* 2007;16(8):1626–1632.
155. Behbahani H, Walther-Jallow L, Klareskog E, et al. Proinflammatory and type 1 cytokine expression in cervical mucosa during HIV-1 and human papillomavirus infection. *J Acquir Immune Defic Syndr.* 2007;45(1):9–19.
156. Syrjanen S. Human papillomavirus infection and its association with HIV. *Adv Dent Res.* 2011;23(1):84–89.
157. Scoud M, Tjalma WA, Ronsse V. Cervical adenocarcinoma: moving towards better prevention. *Vaccine.* 2011;29(49):9148–9158.
158. Solomon D, Davey D, Kurman R, et al. The 2001 Bethesda System: terminology for reporting results of cervical cytology. *JAMA.* 2002;287(16):2114–2119.
159. Lacey JV Jr, Swanson CA, Brinton LA, et al. Obesity as a potential risk factor for adenocarcinomas and squamous cell carcinomas of the uterine cervix. *Cancer.* 2003;98(4):814–821.
160. Hanson CM, Eckert L, Bloem P, et al. Gavi HPV Programs: application to Implementation. *Vaccines (Basel).* 2015;3(2):408–419.
161. Saraiya M, Watson M, Wu X, et al. Incidence of in situ and invasive vulvar cancer in the US, 1998–2003. *Cancer.* 2008;113(10, Suppl):2865–2872.
162. Baandrup L, Varbo A, Munk C, et al. In situ and invasive squamous cell carcinoma of the vulva in Denmark 1978–2007—a nationwide population-based study. *Gynecol Oncol.* 2011;122(1):45–49.
163. van der Avoort IA, Shirango H, Hoevenaars BM, et al. Vulvar squamous cell carcinoma is a multifactorial disease following two separate and independent pathways. *Int J Gynecol Pathol.* 2006;25(1):22–29.
164. de Sanjose S, Alemany L, Ordi J, et al. Worldwide human papillomavirus genotype attribution in over 2000 cases of intraepithelial and invasive lesions of the vulva. *Eur J Cancer.* 2013;49(16):3450–3461.
165. De Vuyst H, Clifford GM, Nascimento MC, et al. Prevalence and type distribution of human papillomavirus in carcinoma and intraepithelial neoplasia of the vulva, vagina and anus: a meta-analysis. *Int J Cancer.* 2009;124(7):1626–1636.
166. Darragh TM, Colgan TJ, Cox JT, et al. The Lower Anogenital Squamous Terminology Standardization Project for HPV-Associated Lesions: background and consensus recommendations from the College of American Pathologists and the American Society for Colposcopy and Cervical Pathology. *Arch Pathol Lab Med.* 2012;136(10):1266–1297.
167. van Seters M, ten Kate FJ, van Beurden M, et al. In the absence of (early) invasive carcinoma, vulvar intraepithelial neoplasia associated with lichen sclerosus is mainly of undifferentiated type: new insights in histology and aetiology. *J Clin Pathol.* 2007;60(5):504–509.
168. Judson PL, Habermann EB, Baxter NN, et al. Trends in the incidence of invasive and in situ vulvar carcinoma. *Obstet Gynecol.* 2006;107(5):1018–1022.
169. Madsen BS, Jensen HL, van den Brule AJ, et al. Risk factors for invasive squamous cell carcinoma of the vulva and vagina—population-based case-control study in Denmark. *Int J Cancer.* 2008;122(12):2827–2834.
170. Brinton LA, Nasca PC, Mallin K, et al. Case-control study of cancer of the vulva. *Obstet Gynecol.* 1990;75(5):859–866.
171. Nordenvall C, Chang ET, Adami HO, et al. Cancer risk among patients with condylomata acuminata. *Int J Cancer.* 2006;119(4):888–893.
172. Hussain SK, Sundquist J, Hemminki K. Familial clustering of cancer at human papillomavirus-associated sites according to the Swedish Family-Cancer Database. *Int J Cancer.* 2008;122(8):1873–1878.
173. Santegoets LA, van Seters M, Heijmans-Antonissen C, et al. Reduced local immunity in HPV-related VIN: expression of chemokines and involvement of immunocompetent cells. *Int J Cancer.* 2008;123(3):616–622.
174. Massad LS, Xie X, Darragh T, et al. Genital warts and vulvar intraepithelial neoplasia: natural history and effects of treatment and human immunodeficiency virus infection. *Obstet Gynecol.* 2011;118(4):831–839.
175. Munoz N, Kjaer SK, Sigurdsson K, et al. Impact of human papillomavirus (HPV)-6/11/16/18 vaccine on all HPV-associated genital diseases in young women. *J Natl Cancer Inst.* 2010;102(5):325–339.
176. Lang Kuhs KA, Gonzalez P, Rodriguez AC, et al. Reduced prevalence of vulvar HPV16/18 infection among women who received the HPV16/18 bivalent vaccine: a nested analysis within the Costa Rica Vaccine Trial. *J Infect Dis.* 2014;210(12):1890–1899.
177. Lilic V, Lilic G, Filipovic S, et al. Primary carcinoma of the vagina. *J BUON.* 2010;15(2):241–247.
178. Balamurugan A, Ahmed F, Saraiya M, et al. Potential role of human papillomavirus in the development of subsequent primary in situ and invasive cancers among cervical cancer survivors. *Cancer.* 2008;113(10, Suppl):2919–2925.
179. Saraiya M, Unger ER, Thompson TD, et al. US assessment of HPV types in cancers: implications for current and 9-valent HPV vaccines. *J Natl Cancer Inst.* 2015;107(6):djv086.
180. Madkan VK, Cook-Norris RH, Steadman MC, et al. The oncogenic potential of human papillomaviruses: a review on the role of host genetics and environmental cofactors. *Br J Dermatol.* 2007;157(2):228–241.
181. Hoover RN, Hyer M, Pfeiffer RM, et al. Adverse health outcomes in women exposed in utero to diethylstilbestrol. *N Engl J Med.* 2011;365(14):1304–1314.
182. Herbst AL, Anderson S, Hubby MM, et al. Risk factors for the development of diethylstilbestrol-associated clear cell adenocarcinoma: a case-control study. *Am J Obstet Gynecol.* 1986;154(4):814–822.
183. Troisi R, Hatch EE, Titus-Ernstoff L, et al. Cancer risk in women prenatally exposed to diethylstilbestrol. *Int J Cancer.* 2007;121(2):356–360.
184. Seckl MJ, Sebire NJ, Fisher RA, et al. Gestational trophoblastic disease: ESMO Clinical Practice Guidelines for diagnosis, treatment and follow-up. *Ann Oncol.* 2013;24 (Suppl 6):vi39–vi50.
185. Smith HO, Qualls CR, Prairie BA, et al. Trends in gestational choriocarcinoma: a 27-year perspective. *Obstet Gynecol.* 2003;102(5, pt 1):978–987.
186. Lurain JR. Gestational trophoblastic disease I: epidemiology, pathology, clinical presentation and diagnosis of gestational trophoblastic disease, and management of hydatidiform mole. *Am J Obstet Gynecol.* 2010;203(6):531–539.
187. Tham BW, Everard JE, Tidy JA, et al. Gestational trophoblastic disease in the Asian population of Northern England and North Wales. *BJOG.* 2003;110(6):555–559.
188. Brinton LA, Bracken MB, Connelly RR. Choriocarcinoma incidence in the United States. *Am J Epidemiol.* 1986;123(6):1094–1100.
189. Lybol C, Thomas CM, Bulten J, et al. Increase in the incidence of gestational trophoblastic disease in The Netherlands. *Gynecol Oncol.* 2011;121(2):334–338.
190. Salehi S, Eloranta S, Johansson AL, et al. Reporting and incidence trends of hydatidiform mole in Sweden 1973–2004. *Acta Oncol.* 2011;50(3):367–372.
191. Tuncer ZS, Bernstein MR, Wang J, et al. Repetitive hydatidiform mole with different male partners. *Gynecol Oncol.* 1999;75(2):224–226.
192. Brinton LA, Wu BZ, Wang W, et al. Gestational trophoblastic disease: a case-control study from the People's Republic of China. *Am J Obstet Gynecol.* 1989;161(1):121–127.
193. Buckley JD, Henderson BE, Morrow CP, et al. Case-control study of gestational choriocarcinoma. *Cancer Res.* 1988;48(4):1004–1010.
194. Palmer JR, Driscoll SG, Rosenberg L, et al. Oral contraceptive use and risk of gestational trophoblastic tumors. *J Natl Cancer Inst.* 1999;91(7):635–640.
195. Costa HL, Doyle P. Influence of oral contraceptives in the development of post-molar trophoblastic neoplasia—a systematic review. *Gynecol Oncol.* 2006;100(3):579–585.

CHAPTER 2

Molecular Pathogenesis of Gynecologic Cancers

Andrew Berchuck, Douglas A. Levine, Dariush Etemadmoghadam, and David D. L. Bowtell

INTRODUCTION

An overview of the molecular pathogenesis of cancer is presented in the initial sections of this chapter. A more comprehensive discussion of this topic can be found in Part I of DeVita Hellman and Rosenberg's *Cancer: Principles and Practice of Oncology* (1). Genetic alterations involved in the development of gynecologic cancers are covered in more detail in the latter sections of this chapter.

The initiating events in human cancers are diverse, but malignant transformation is invariably caused by the development of genetic and epigenetic alterations that disrupt cell growth and death (**Table 2.1**). Several classes of genetic alterations are involved in carcinogenesis, including changes in the sequence of genes (mutations), gains (amplifications) or losses (deletions) in the number of copies of genes, and rearrangement and translocation of genes from their normal chromosomal locations that sometimes create new proteins by fusing the reading frames of genes. Mutations result in activation of genes that stimulate proliferation (oncogenes), inactivation of genes that inhibit proliferation (tumor suppressor genes), and impairment of programmed cell death (apoptosis). Disruption of DNA repair systems also often occurs in the process of malignant transformation and may lead to an accelerated accumulation of genetic alterations. Because repair of genetic damage inhibits carcinogenesis, many DNA repair genes are tumor suppressors, and some of the most notable inherited cancer susceptibility genes are involved in DNA repair.

Most transforming mutations in oncogenes alter a single amino acid at specific codons that produce overactive protein products (e.g., *KRAS, BRAF*), and only one allele needs to be mutated. In contrast, inactivation of tumor suppressors (e.g., *RB1, BRCA1*) requires loss of both copies of the gene (two hits). Mutations in tumor suppressors may occur throughout the gene and are usually small insertions, deletions, or base substitutions that alter the reading frame and thereby result in truncated protein products. Loss of the second nonmutated allele generally occurs due to chromosomal deletion, leading to abrogation of tumor suppressor activity. Some tumor suppressors are inactivated by methylation of their promoters, such as *MLH1*. Cancers may have many genetic alterations, but only a small fraction of these are "driver" mutations that are responsible for malignant transformation. The majority of mutations are "passenger" events, arising through carcinogen exposure and/or genetic instability, and do not contribute to tumor growth.

Changes in gene expression due to epigenetic alterations (DNA methylation and acetylation), aberrant gene splicing, noncoding regulatory RNAs, and other mechanisms also contribute to the malignant phenotype. The histopathologic progression through hyperplasia, dysplasia, carcinoma *in situ*, and invasive carcinoma reflects the multistep, multigenic nature of malignant transformation. While some mutational changes are sequential, it is now apparent that the evolution of most cancers follows a branching pattern, akin to speciation, resulting in the generation of clonally diverse, genetically distinct populations within the patient. Cancers may arise through the accumulation of acquired (somatic) alterations or

TABLE 2.1. Molecular Alterations Involved in Cancer Pathogenesis

Genetic changes
Mutations
Mutations in oncogenes change a single amino acid and lead to gain of activity that stimulates proliferation. These mutations are dominant and not dependent on changes in the other copy of the gene
Mutations in tumor suppressor genes and DNA repair genes generally are small base insertions/deletions or single base changes that cause stop codons. These lead to truncated protein products that are nonfunctional. Loss of tumor suppressor activity is usually dependent on deletion of the other copy of the gene
Driver mutations play a critical role in the process of malignant transformation
DNA copy number changes
Deletion of one or both copies of a tumor suppressor gene due to genomic instability leads to loss of a gene product
Gain of additional copies of an oncogene leads to increased activity
Aneuploidy with gain or loss of complete chromosomes is common in many cancers
Gene rearrangements and translocations
When a gene is moved from its normal location to another chromosomal location, its expression may be increased due to proximity to a gene promoter or due to fusion of two genes
Clonal evolution
The genomic landscape of most cancers continues to evolve over time and space and the alterations observed in most cancers are often not present in all of the malignant cells
Other biologic processes
Epigenetic alterations
Hypermethylation of CpG islands in the promoter regions of tumor suppressor genes may lead to their inactivation
Loss of promoter methylation in genes that stimulate proliferation may provide an oncogenic stimulus
Changes in acetylation of histone proteins that coat DNA may play a role in carcinogenesis
Aberrant gene splicing
Alternative splice forms of genes may produce messenger RNAs and proteins with altered activity
Noncoding RNAs
Noncoding RNAs regulate gene expression, and their aberrant expression likely plays a role in the development and behavior of some cancers

through the inheritance of an alteration in the germline followed by the acquisition of additional somatic alterations. Hereditary cancers are discussed in detail in Chapter 3.

The techniques used to study genetic alterations have evolved dramatically. Advances in the 1980s and 1990s enabled the discovery of several genes that frequently play a role in the development of cancers, including the *KRAS* and HER-2/*neu* oncogenes and the *TP53* and *RB1* tumor suppressor genes. It became apparent that the spectrum of driver alterations varies considerably between cancer types, and among cancers of the same type (2). More recently, powerful new technologies have enabled comprehensive genomic studies. The Human Genome Project was completed in 2004 and provided a road map of the entire genome, including the approximately 18,000 protein-encoding genes. The HapMap project then catalogued the millions of common single nucleotide polymorphisms (SNPs) in the genome that vary at a single base in the DNA sequence between individuals. More recently, the 1000 Genomes Project has characterized rarer germline genetic variants. Large genome-wide association studies (GWAS), often involving thousands of cases and controls, have become a powerful approach for finding risk alleles that individually may have a small impact but that may interact additively or synergistically to increase an individual's genetic risk.

A road map of normal human genetic variation and the development of faster and cheaper "next generation" DNA sequencing have allowed mutational analysis of complete cancer genomes. Cancers typically have a mutation rate in the order of 1 to 10 (median of ~3) mutations per megabase (Mb), although the frequency varies over several orders of magnitude between tumor types (https://dcc.icgc.org/projects/summary). For example, mutation rates are generally high in lung cancer (median >10 mutations per Mb) and melanoma (median >60 mutations per Mb), due to exposure to tobacco smoke and UV light, respectively, whereas many pediatric tumors have few mutations (median <0.1 mutations per Mb in neuroblastoma). A small number of genes are mutated in a high fraction of cancers (e.g., *KRAS*, *TP53*), likely reflecting the strong selective advantage these alterations confer. A much larger number of genes are mutated at considerably lower frequencies. The terms "mountains" and "hills" have been used to describe genes that are commonly mutated versus rarely mutated in various types of cancers (2). Mutations in common cancers typically target multiple biological pathways, whereas some rare cancers have single dominant drivers in a majority of patients, such as ubiquitous *FOXL2* mutations in granulosa cell tumors. Several genes in a pathway may be mutated, but driver mutations in a pathway are often mutually exclusive when they involve the same pathway, as there may be little selective advantage to activating a given pathway multiple times (e.g., *KRAS* and *BRAF*).

The Cancer Genome Atlas (TCGA) Project, sponsored by the National Cancer Institute, has performed a comprehensive genomic characterization of common forms of human cancer and more recently initiated several rare tumor projects. Ovarian and endometrial cancers were among the first to be studied by TCGA and these findings have been incorporated into this chapter. The International Cancer Genome Consortium (ICGC) performed similar genomic analyses of human cancers. Both TCGA and ICGC have deposited their data online in the public domain to stimulate further research. The full spectrum and complexity of the genomic alterations in a single cancer can be best captured in a Circos plot (**Fig. 2.1**), which uses a circular ideogram layout to facilitate the display of changes across the genome.

Large-scale profiling studies provide the opportunity to perform Pan-Cancer (PANCAN) analyses to define common and distinct mutation events or patterns across cancer types (3,4). For example, analysis of base substitutions has revealed signatures associated with underlying oncogenic mutational processes. These studies have shown that the most common signature across cancer types is associated with older age at diagnosis and is characterized by a prominence of C>T substitutions at a specific trinucleotide context (NpCpG). Other signatures associated with specific mutagenic exposures (e.g., UV radiation and smoking) have also been defined (5). Integrated sequence and copy number analysis have been used to characterize cancers driven by high levels of recurrent mutations (M-class), such as renal clear cell and colorectal cancers, in contrast to those characterized predominantly by copy number alterations (C-class), including breast and high-grade serous ovarian cancers (6). PANCAN analyses are further accelerating a reclassification of cancer, from one that is based on anatomy to a molecular description. These studies are highlighting unexpected molecular similarities between anatomically distinct tumors, such as the striking similarity between high-grade serous ovarian cancer and basal-like breast cancer.

An understanding of the molecular pathogenesis of cancer provides the opportunity to better define subgroups within a given type of cancer that may differ with respect to clinical behavior and survival (7). The identification of specific mutations has facilitated the development of therapies that target these alterations. In this regard, monoclonal antibodies and small molecules targeting aberrantly expressed cellular proteins that drive malignant growth have been successful in treating some cancers (2). The evolution of Food and Drug Administration–approved targeted therapies has been accompanied by the requirement for companion diagnostic tests that demonstrate the presence of the specific alteration being targeted (e.g., HER-2/*neu* amplification/overexpression guides use of trastuzumab in breast cancer, and *BRAF* V600E mutation guides use of vemurafenib in melanoma).

Unfortunately, most metastatic gynecologic cancers have not proven amenable to targeted therapy because their growth is not driven by a single altered gene or pathway. A notable recent exception is the development of polyADP ribose polymerase (PARP) inhibitors in *BRCA1/2*-mutated ovarian cancers. Germline genetic testing of *BRCA1/2* in high-grade epithelial ovarian cancers has been driven in the past by a strong family history of breast/ovarian cancer. However, with the advent of PARP inhibitor therapy for cancers with these mutations, it may become increasingly common to perform mutational analysis in tumor tissue with reflex germline testing in cases found to have a *BRCA1/2* mutation. This allows for the detection of both somatic and germline mutations in these genes. A similar paradigm shift may occur in other cancer types in which both somatic and germline alterations may have relevance for genetic risk assessment as well as therapy.

The utility of testing for common "druggable" driver mutations is now well accepted in many tumor types. With the evolution of genomic technologies, it is now feasible to test cancers for mutations in all of the genes that are potentially targetable. In a small fraction of cases, this approach will identify actionable mutations that are not frequent in that type of cancer. However, the clinical benefit of this approach in improving survival remains uncertain and must be balanced against the high cost of targeted therapies. The value of this new paradigm is presently being explored in the context of "match" or "basket trials" in which eligibility is based on the presence of the target rather than the anatomic origin of the cancer (8). Successful therapy may therefore require the use of multiple agents that target more than one gene or pathway. A more detailed description of targeted cancer therapies is provided in Chapter 12.

Resistance to targeted therapies often occurs due to mutational heterogeneity both within the primary tumor and in metastases as clonal evolution develops over time. Cancers are continually evolving due to genetic instability and contain subclones that differ with respect to their mutational profile. Intratumoral heterogeneity can vary across metastatic sites (spatial variation) and during treatment and disease progression (temporal variation). By analogy with the shape of a tree, mutations that occur early in the development of a cancer before metastasis occurs, such as *TP53*, are called "trunk" mutations and are found across metastases. In contrast, mutations that occur late in the development of a cancer, so-called "branch" mutations, are present in a minority of tumor sites. The presence of

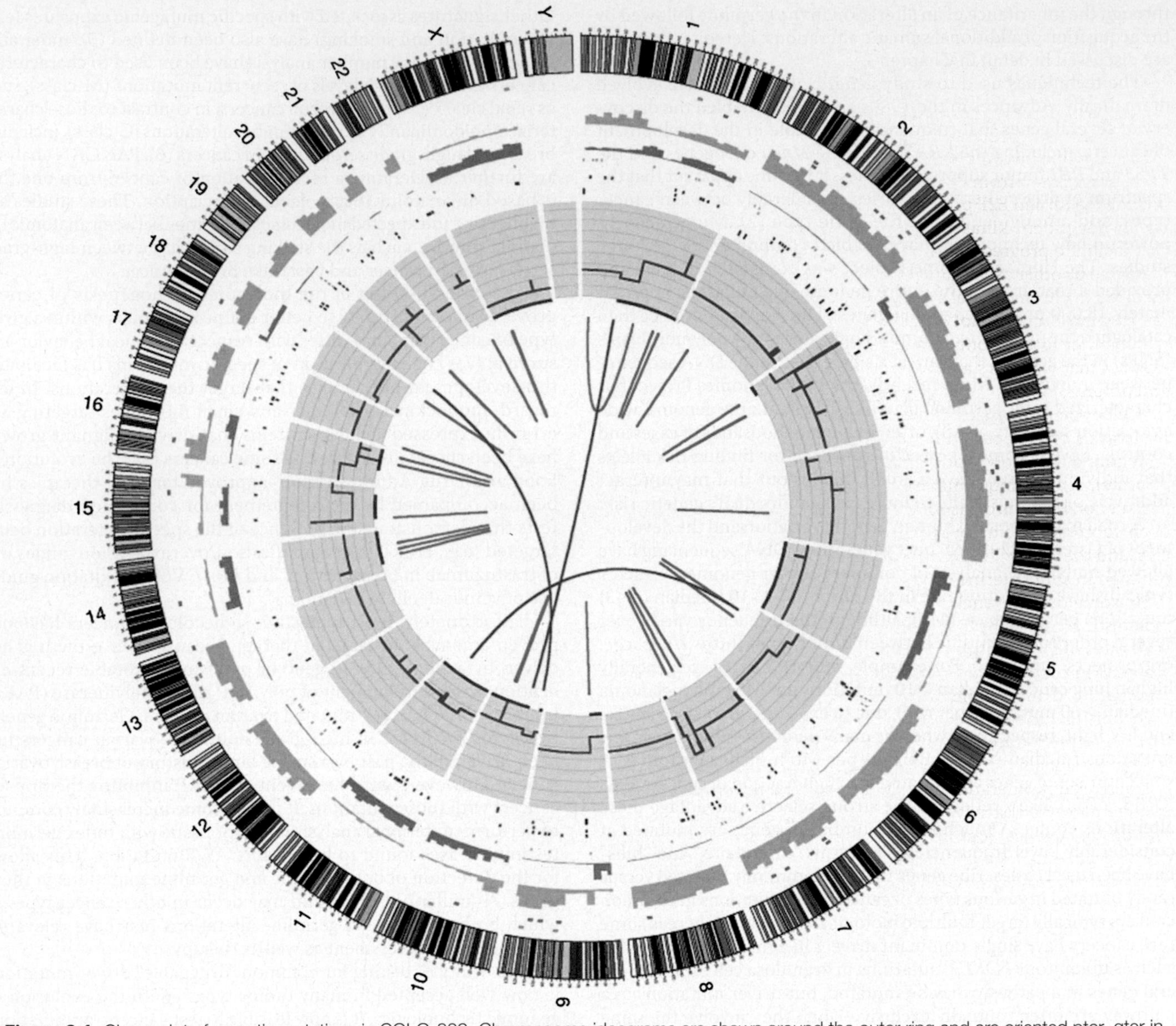

Figure 2.1. Circos plot of somatic mutations in COLO-829. Chromosome ideograms are shown around the outer ring and are oriented pter–qter in a clockwise direction with centromeres indicated in red. Other tracks contain somatic alterations (*from outside to inside*): validated insertions (*light green rectangles*); validated deletions (*dark green rectangles*); heterozygous (*light orange bars*) and homozygous (*dark orange bars*) substitutions shown by density per 10 Mb; coding substitutions (*colored squares: silent in gray, missense in purple, nonsense in red, and splice site in black*); copy number (*blue lines*); regions of loss of heterozygosity (LOH) (*red lines*); validated intrachromosomal rearrangements (*green lines*); validated interchromosomal rearrangements (*purple lines*). Reprinted by permission from Macmillan Publishers Ltd: Pleasance ED, Cheetham RK, Stephens PJ, et al. A comprehensive catalogue of somatic mutations from a human cancer genome. *Nature.* 2010;463(7278):191. [PMID: 20016485], copyright 2010.

clonal and subclonal mutations in many patients has implications for the accuracy of molecular diagnostics that rely on biopsy and evaluation of single sites in the patient. Analysis of mutations in circulating tumor cells in the blood or in DNA released into the blood from dying tumor cells may provide a more accurate representation of the molecular events present in a patient than relying on a single metastatic site (9). The presence of intratumoral heterogeneity also has implications for personalized medicine approaches that match mutational events or "actionable mutations" to specific therapeutics. Heterogeneity between clones influences sensitivity to drugs and facilitates tumor adaptation through selection and outgrowth of resistant clones, ultimately leading to treatment failure. Strategies to monitor tumor cell evolution throughout treatment would further elucidate subclonal variation, patterns of tumor evolution, and potentially improve clinical care using targeted therapies.

Finally, an increased understanding of the molecular pathogenesis of cancers provides the opportunity for early detection and prevention. This has been realized for cervical cancer with the identification of the human papillomavirus (HPV) leading to creation of a vaccine. In ovarian and endometrial cancers, identification of germline genetic alterations such as in *BRCA1* or *BRCA2* that dramatically increase risk facilitates the use of prophylactic surgery and/or screening. In addition, genetic changes that occur early in the development of cancers have the potential to serve as biomarkers for early detection and as surrogate endpoints in prevention studies. For example, it has been shown that common pathogenic mutations in endometrial and ovarian cancers can be detected in DNA from liquid Pap smears in a high fraction of cases (10). This may represent a promising step toward a broadly applicable screening methodology for the early detection of gynecologic malignancies.

CELLULAR GROWTH AND DEATH

Proliferation

The number of cells in normal tissues is tightly regulated by a balance between cellular proliferation and death. The final common pathway for cell division involves distinct molecular switches that control cell cycle progression from G1 to the S phase of DNA synthesis. These include the Rb and E2F proteins and their various regulatory cyclins, cyclin-dependent kinases (cdks), and cdk inhibitors. The events that facilitate progression from G2 to mitosis and cell division are regulated by other cyclins and cdks (**Fig. 2.2**), as well as by molecules involved in chromosomal segregation such as microtubules. When the chromosomes do not separate properly, aneuploidy may occur with gain or loss of complete chromosomes. Aneuploidy is a hallmark of many cancers and likely plays a role in their development and progression.

Cell cycle progression is also dependent on ubiquitin-mediated proteolysis of molecules involved in cell cycle arrest. Ubiquitin is a 76 amino acid polypeptide that can be linked to lysine residues of proteins, and ubiquitination marks proteins for proteolysis and destruction by the proteasome complex. Proteasome inhibitors have been successfully employed to treat some hematologic malignancies, and the *FBXW7* (*CDC4*) ubiquitin ligase has been shown to be mutated in some uterine cancers.

In some tissues—such as the bone marrow, epidermis, and gastrointestinal tract—the life span of mature cells is relatively short and high rates of proliferation are required to maintain the population, whereas in other tissues—such as liver, muscle, and brain—cells are long lived and proliferation rarely occurs. Complex molecular mechanisms have evolved to closely regulate proliferation. These involve a finely tuned balance between growth stimulatory and inhibitory signals.

Increased proliferation is one of the hallmarks of cancer. There may be increased activity of genes involved in stimulating proliferation (oncogenes) and/or loss of growth inhibitory (tumor suppressor) genes. In the past, it was thought that cancer might arise solely because of more rapid proliferation or a higher fraction of cells proliferating. It is now clear that this was an overly simplistic view. Although increased proliferation is a characteristic of many cancers, the fraction of cancer cells actively dividing and the time required to transit the cell cycle is not always strikingly increased. Altered regulation of proliferation is only one of several factors that contribute to malignant transformation.

Cell Death

In addition to being driven by increased proliferation, growth of a cancer may be attributable to cellular resistance to death. At least three distinct types of cell death pathways have been characterized, including apoptosis, autophagy, and necrosis.

Apoptosis

The term "apoptosis" derives from Greek and alludes to a process akin to leaves dying and falling off a tree. Apoptosis is an active energy-dependent process that involves cleavage of the DNA by endonucleases and proteins by proteases called caspases. Morphologically, apoptosis is characterized by condensation of chromatin, nuclear and cytoplasmic blebbing, and cellular shrinkage, which is followed by phagocytic destruction. The molecular events that effect apoptosis in response to various stimuli are complex and have only been partially elucidated, but several reliable markers of apoptosis have been discovered including annexin V, caspase-3 activation, and DNA fragmentation.

External stimuli such as tumor necrosis factor (TNF), TNF-related apoptosis-inducing ligand (TRAIL), Fas, and other death ligands that interact with cell surface receptors can induce activation of caspases and lead to apoptosis via the extrinsic pathway. The intrinsic apoptosis pathway is activated in response to a wide range of stresses including DNA damage and deprivation of growth factors. The intrinsic apoptosis pathway is regulated by a complex interaction of pro- and antiapoptotic proteins in the mitochondrial membrane that affect its permeability. Proteins that increase permeability allow release of cytochrome *c*, which activates the apoptosome complex leading to activation of caspases that effect apoptosis. Conversely, proteins that stabilize mitochondrial membranes inhibit apoptosis. The first major insight that led to the understanding of the intrinsic apoptosis pathway was the finding that an activating translocation of the *BCL-2* gene in B-cell lymphomas results in essentially complete inhibition of apoptosis. Subsequent studies demonstrated that the

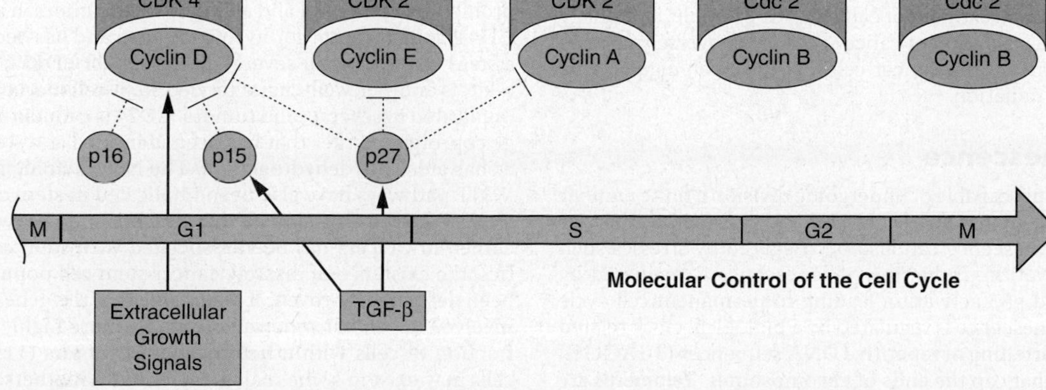

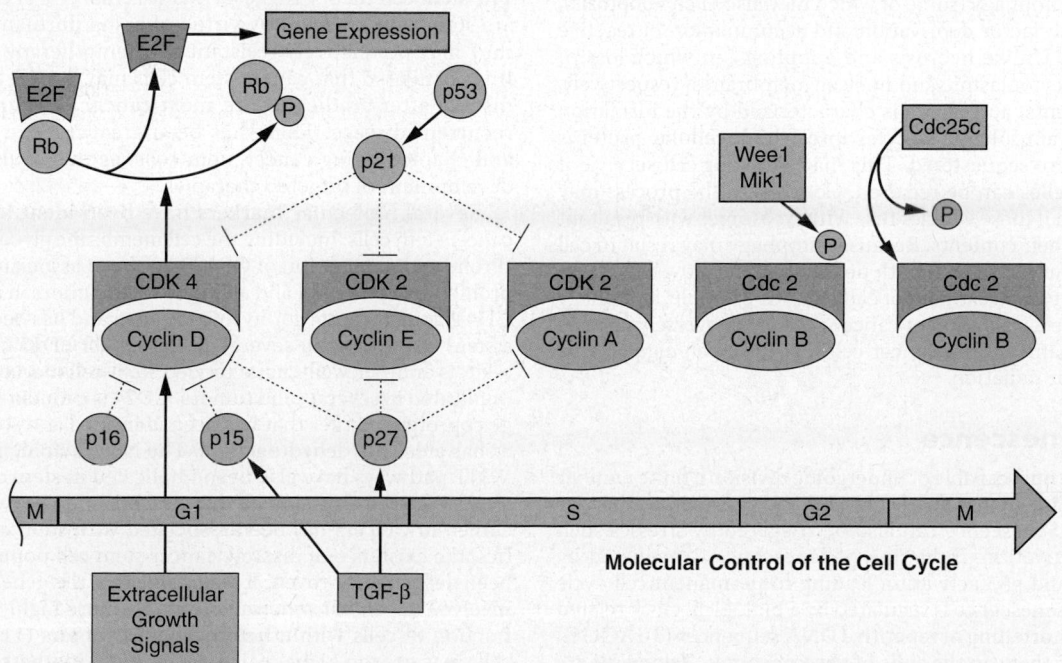

Figure 2.2. Molecular control of cell cycle progression. A linear version of the various stages of the cell cycle is shown with the various cyclin/cyclin-dependent kinase complexes corresponding to the stages that they control. CDK, cyclin-dependent kinases.

antiapoptotic effect of *BCL-2* is attributable to stabilization of the mitochondrial membrane. Additional genes related to *BCL-2*, such as *BAD*, *BCL-XL*, and others, also block apoptosis by inhibiting membrane permeability. Other genes in the *BCL* family, such as *BAX* and *BAK*, increase membrane permeability and are proapoptotic. An understanding of the complex system of checks and balances involved in regulation of apoptosis provides opportunities for the development of targeted therapies.

Apoptosis is an ongoing process to balance the birth of new cells, thereby restraining the number of cells in normal tissues. In addition, apoptosis serves an important role in preventing malignant transformation by allowing for elimination of cells that have incurred genetic damage. Following exposure of cells to mutagenic stimuli, including radiation and carcinogenic drugs, the cell cycle is arrested so that DNA damage may be repaired. If DNA repair is not sufficient, apoptosis occurs so that damaged cells do not survive. This serves as an anticancer surveillance mechanism by which mutated cells are eliminated before they proliferate or become fully transformed. The *TP53* tumor suppressor gene is a critical regulator of cell cycle arrest and apoptosis in response to DNA damage. Many of the molecules involved in apoptosis reside in the mitochondria and are encoded by mitochondrial DNA. Mutations in mitochondrial DNA have been shown to be frequent in cancer and may play a role in evasion of apoptosis.

Necrosis

Necrosis is a type of cell death that is distinct from apoptosis and is the result of bioenergetic compromise or external insult such as infection or trauma. Morphologic changes include swollen organelles and rupture of the cell membrane leading to loss of osmoregulation and cellular fragmentation. Necrosis is an unregulated process that leads to spillage of protein contents, and this may incite a brisk immune response. This is in contrast to the silent elimination of cells by apoptosis, which typically elicits a minimal immune response. There is evidence that some drugs may enhance necrotic death in tumors and this may stimulate a beneficial antitumor immune response.

Autophagy

Autophagy is a potentially reversible process in which a cell that is stressed eats itself. A wide range of stresses have been identified that may elicit autophagy (some of which may also elicit apoptosis), including growth factor deprivation and accumulation of reactive oxygen species. Unlike necrosis and apoptosis, in which loss of integrity of the cytoplasmic and nuclear membranes, respectively, are defining events, autophagy is characterized by the formation of cytoplasmic autophagic vesicles into which cellular proteins and organelles are sequestered. This may allow for cell survival if damaged organelles can be repaired. Conversely, the process may lead to cell death if these vesicles fuse with lysosomes with resultant degradation of their contents. Because autophagy may result in cell destruction or survival, it has both positive and negative effects on the development and treatment of cancers. For example, autophagy may result in the elimination of cancer cells, or conversely provide a survival mechanism for a cancer cell that has been damaged by chemotherapy or radiation.

Cellular Senescence

Normal cells are only capable of undergoing division a finite number of times before becoming senescent and this represents a barrier to immortality. Senescence can also be triggered by stresses such as oncogene activation. Induction of senescence is mediated by persistent p16 and p53 activation leading to permanent cell cycle arrest. Cellular senescence is regulated by a biological clock related to progressive shortening of repetitive DNA sequences (TTAGGG) called telomeres that cap the ends of chromosomes. Telomeres are involved in chromosome stabilization and in preventing recombination and chromosomal translocations and aneuploidy during mitosis. At birth, chromosomes have long telomeric sequences (150,000 bases) that become progressively shorter by 50 to 200 bases each time a cell divides. Telomerase is a ribonucleoprotein complex. The RNA component serves as a template for telomere extension, and the protein subunit acts to catalyze the synthesis of new telomeric repeats.

Replicative senescence serves as a defense against immortalization and malignant transformation by placing limits on proliferation of cells that have accumulated genetic damage. Reactivation of telomerase is critical to the emergence of cancers, but early in the process of malignant transformation, telomere shortening and dysfunction may promote the carcinogenic process through the generation of chromosomal rearrangements and aneuploidy. Progressive telomere shortening during adulthood may explain the association between advancing age and increased cancer risk, particularly for epithelial malignancies. Cancer risk has been mainly attributed to progressive accumulation of mutations with aging, but this theory does not explain the marked aneuploidy of most epithelial cancers.

Telomerase activity is present in a high fraction of many cancers, including ovarian, cervical, and endometrial cancers. It has been suggested that detection of telomerase might be useful for early diagnosis of cancer, but it is also found in some normal adult tissues including endometrium. Perhaps this relates to the need for a large number of lifetime cell divisions because of rapid growth and shedding of endometrial tissue each month during the reproductive years. Therapeutic approaches to inhibiting telomerase are under development that would reverse the immortalized state of cancer cells and render them susceptible again to normal replicative senescence.

Stem Cells

Stem cells in normal tissues have the capacity to undergo asymmetric division to produce daughter cells that undergo differentiation and eventually senescence and can self-renew to produce more stem cells. Stem cells have been most easily identifiable in tissues that normally are highly proliferative, such as the bone marrow, skin, and intestine, in which a constant stream of cells are being born to replace those that are differentiating and dying. It has been theorized that stem cells exist in cancers and have the capacity for self-renewal and differentiation into populations of cells that recapitulate tumor heterogeneity. Stem cells are also referred to as tumorigenic cells because of their capacity to regenerate tumors. The stem cell theory suggests that less than 1% of cells in a cancer are stem cells and that by virtue of being dormant or quiescent, they may be relatively resistant to chemotherapy and radiation. It is postulated that cancer stem cells may persist as microscopic disease after eradication of most cancer cells and give rise to recurrent disease. There has been great interest in identifying and characterizing cancer stem cells, as this could facilitate the development of targeted therapies.

Several molecular markers have been identified that define cancer stem cells, including the cell membrane glycoprotein CD133 (Prominin). Expression of CD133 has been associated with greater proliferative potential and ability to form tumors in animal models. CD44 is the receptor for hyaluronic acid and has been identified as a stem cell marker in several cancer types. CD117, also known as c-kit, is another well-characterized stem cell marker that has been implicated in several solid tumors. CD24 is a mucin-like cell surface glycoprotein marker that has been identified as a stem cell marker, as has aldehyde dehydrogenase. The Notch, Sonic Hedgehog, and WNT pathways have also been implicated in stem cell behavior.

Although expression of the markers and pathways, described earlier, in cancers has been associated with stem cell characteristics, the existence of discrete cancer stem cell populations has not been definitively proven. It is possible that the genes and pathways involved in cellular renewal are simply more highly expressed in a fraction of cells within heterogeneous tumors (11). Cancer stem cells may exist in some malignancies but not others. In this regard, demonstration of progenitor stem cells has been more robust in leukemias than in solid tumors.

ORIGINS OF GENETIC ALTERATIONS

Human cancers arise due to a series of genetic alterations that lead to disruption of normal mechanisms that govern cell growth, death, and senescence. Genetic damage may be inherited or may arise after birth due to various exposures including those related to carcinogenic substances such as tobacco and asbestos, physical factors such as ultraviolet radiation, infections such as HPV, dietary factors, obesity, and inflammation. However, much of the acquired genetic damage that causes cancer is due to endogenous mutagenic processes within the cell (**Table 2.2**). The incidence of most cancers increases with aging because the longer one is alive, the higher the likelihood of a cell acquiring sufficient damage to become fully transformed. It is thought that at least three to six alterations are required to fully transform a cell.

Inherited Cancer Susceptibility

Although most cancers arise sporadically due to acquired genetic damage, inherited mutations in cancer susceptibility genes are responsible for some familial cases. The age of cancer onset is younger in these families and it is not unusual for individuals to be affected with multiple primary cancers. Tumor suppressor genes and DNA repair genes have been implicated most frequently in hereditary cancer syndromes. The most common forms of hereditary cancer syndromes predispose to breast/ovarian (*BRCA1/2* genes) and colon/endometrial (DNA mismatch repair [MMR] genes) cancers. Although affected individuals carry the germline alteration in every cell of their bodies, paradoxically, cancer susceptibility genes are characterized by a limited repertoire of cancers. The penetrance of cancer susceptibility genes is incomplete, as all individuals who inherit a mutation do not develop cancer. The emergence of cancers is dependent on the occurrence of additional genetic alterations. Hereditary cancer syndromes are covered in detail in Chapter 3.

In addition to the high-penetrance mutations, noted earlier, that cause familial cancer syndromes, low-penetrance genetic variants may also affect cancer susceptibility, albeit less dramatically. There are over 10 million polymorphic genetic loci in the human genome. Most of these are SNPs, in which there is variation in the nucleotide at a chromosomal location (e.g., C vs. A). Many SNPs are relatively common, with the rarer of the two alleles occurring in more than 5% of individuals. GWAS have discovered over 20 SNPs that affect the risk of ovarian cancer by 10% to 50% per rare allele copy. The discovery of these common, low-penetrance-risk SNPs has been facilitated by the development of an international ovarian cancer association consortium (OCAC) that includes over 75 studies from around the world, with over 70,000 ovarian cancer cases and controls. These risk SNPs are not located within genes, but rather in regulatory regions of the genome where they are thought to play a role in regulating gene expression. A more complete understanding of the genetic factors that affect cancer susceptibility could facilitate implementation of screening and prevention approaches in subsets of the population at increased risk.

■ **TABLE 2.2. Origins of Genetic Damage in Human Cancers**

Type of Genetic Damage	Examples
Germline alterations	
High-penetrance genes	*BRCA1*, *BRCA2* (breast, ovarian cancers) *MLH1*, *MSH2* (Lynch syndrome)
Moderate-penetrance genes	*RAD51C/D*, *BRIP1* (ovarian cancer)
Low-penetrance genes	SNPs associated with various cancers
Exogenous carcinogens	
Ultraviolet radiation	*TP53* mutations in skin cancers
Tobacco	*TP53* mutations in lung cancers
Viruses	HPV inactivation of *RB* and *TP53* in cervical cancer
Endogenous DNA damage	
Cytosine methylation and deamination	*TP53* mutations in many cancer types
DNA hydrolysis	Various genes
Spontaneous errors in DNA synthesis	Various genes
Free radical production due to oxidative stress	Various genes

Acquired Genetic Damage

The etiology of acquired genetic damage in cancers has also been elucidated to some extent. For example, a strong causal link exists between cigarette smoke and cancers of the aerodigestive tract, between ultraviolet radiation and skin cancer, and between HPV and lower genital tract cancers (**Table 2.2**). For many common forms of cancer (e.g., colon, breast, prostate, endometrium, ovary), there is not a strong association with specific carcinogens. It is thought that the genetic alterations responsible for these cancers may arise mainly due to endogenous mutagenic processes. This includes methylation and deamination of cytosine residues leading to transition mutations to thymidine. In this regard, in most types of cancers that are not associated with a specific carcinogen, transition mutations from purine to purine (A/G) or pyrimidine to pyrimidine (C/T) are much more common than transversion mutations that change purine to pyrimidine (A/G to C/T) or pyrimidine to purine (C/T to A/G). An additional mechanism of endogenous damage includes spontaneous errors in DNA synthesis that frequently occur during the process of DNA replication associated with normal proliferation. Free radicals generated in response to inflammation and other cellular damage may also cause DNA damage. These endogenous processes are thought to produce mutations on an ongoing basis. Several networks of highly effective DNA damage surveillance and repair genes exist, but some mutations may elude them. The efficiency of these DNA damage response systems varies between individuals due to genetic and other factors and may affect susceptibility to cancer.

Epigenetic Changes

Epigenetics comprises heritable changes that are not due to alterations in DNA sequence. Methylation of cytosine residues that reside next to guanine residues (CpG dinucleotides) is the primary mechanism of epigenetic regulation, and this process is regulated by a family of DNA methyltransferases. CpG dinucleotides are asymmetrically distributed with about half of human genes containing CpG-rich regions termed "CpG islands" at their transcriptional start sites. Most genes are regulated without changing the methylation status of the CpG sites, but permanent silencing of genes associated with X-chromosome inactivation and genomic imprinting is due to heritable methylation of CpG islands.

Most cancers have globally reduced DNA methylation, hypomethylation, which may lead to activation of some genes. Conversely, selective hypermethylation of CpG islands in the promoter regions of tumor suppressor genes may lead to gene inactivation (e.g., *BRCA1*, *MLH1*). In addition, loss of silencing of imprinted genes that stimulate proliferation, such as *IGF2*, may provide an oncogenic stimulus. Acetylation and methylation of the histone proteins that coat DNA represent another level of epigenetic regulation that is altered in cancer. Alterations in activity of DNA methyltransferases are likely the underlying cause of epigenetic alterations in cancers.

Alterations in Signal Transduction Pathways in Malignant Transformation

Alterations in genes that stimulate cellular growth (oncogenes) can cause malignant transformation when they become overactive. Oncogenes may become overactive when affected by gain of function point mutations. In some cancers, amplification of oncogenes occurs with resultant overexpression of the corresponding protein. Instead of two copies of one of these genes, there may be many additional copies. Finally, oncogenes may be translocated from one chromosomal location to another and come under the influence of gene promoters that actuate overexpression. This latter mechanism frequently occurs as a driving event in the development of leukemias and lymphomas, but is much less frequent in gynecologic cancers. However, some other types of solid tumors may have translocations that represent significant driver events, such as those involving the *ALK* receptor gene in lung cancer. These cancers have been targeted successfully with the monoclonal antibody crizotinib.

Loss of tumor suppressor gene function also plays a role in the development of most cancers. This usually involves a two-step process in which both copies of a tumor suppressor gene are inactivated: mutation of one copy of a tumor suppressor gene and loss of the other copy due to deletion of a chromosome segment where the gene resides (e.g., *RB1*). There is also evidence that some tumor suppressor genes may be inactivated due to methylation of the promoter region of the gene (e.g., *MLH1, BRCA1*). The promoter is an area proximal to the coding sequence that binds transcription factors that regulate whether or not the gene is transcribed from DNA to RNA. When the promoter is methylated, it is resistant to activation and the gene is essentially silenced despite remaining structurally intact. This two-hit paradigm of tumor suppressor gene inactivation is relevant to both hereditary cancer syndromes, in which one mutation is inherited and the second acquired, and to sporadic cancers, in which both hits are acquired.

The sections below will review the role of oncogenes and tumor suppressor genes in signal transduction pathways that regulate cellular growth and metabolism. These pathways are complex and have considerable overlap and redundancy, and an exhaustive discussion is beyond the scope of this book. Pathways for which there is less evidence of a role in driving the development of gynecologic cancers, such as the Hedgehog, Notch, and cytokine pathways, are not covered.

Peptide Growth Factors and Receptor Tyrosine Kinases

Peptide growth factors in the extracellular space, such as those of the epidermal growth factor (EGF), platelet-derived growth factor (PDGF), and fibroblast growth factor (FGF) families, stimulate a cascade of molecular events that leads to proliferation by binding to high-affinity cell membrane receptors (**Fig. 2.3**). Growth factors are involved in normal cellular processes such as stromal–epithelial communication, tissue regeneration, and wound healing. The concept that autocrine growth stimulation might be a key strategy by which cancer cell proliferation becomes autonomous has received considerable attention. In this model, it is postulated that cancers secrete stimulatory growth factors that then interact with receptors on the same cell. Although peptide growth factors provide a growth stimulatory signal, there is little evidence to suggest that overproduction of growth factors is a precipitating event in the development of most cancers. Increased expression of peptide growth factors likely facilitates, rather than drives, malignant transformation.

Cell membrane receptors that bind peptide growth factors are composed of an extracellular ligand–binding domain, a membrane-spanning region, and a cytoplasmic tyrosine kinase domain. Binding of a growth factor to the extracellular domain results in dimerization and conformational shifts in the receptors and activation of the inner tyrosine kinase. The kinase transfers a phosphate group from ATP to specific tyrosine residues both on the growth factor receptor itself (autophosphorylation) and on molecular targets in the cell interior leading to activation of secondary signals that stimulate proliferation. Growth of some cancers is driven by overexpression of receptor tyrosine kinases. The epidermal growth factor receptor (EGFR) family of receptor tyrosine kinases plays a significant role in the development of several types of cancers and includes *ErbB-1* (EGFR), *ErbB-2* (HER-2/*neu*), *ErbB-3*, and *ErbB-4*. These receptors are activated by the binding of ligands, including EGF, transforming growth factor (TGF)-α, amphiregulin, and the neuregulins.

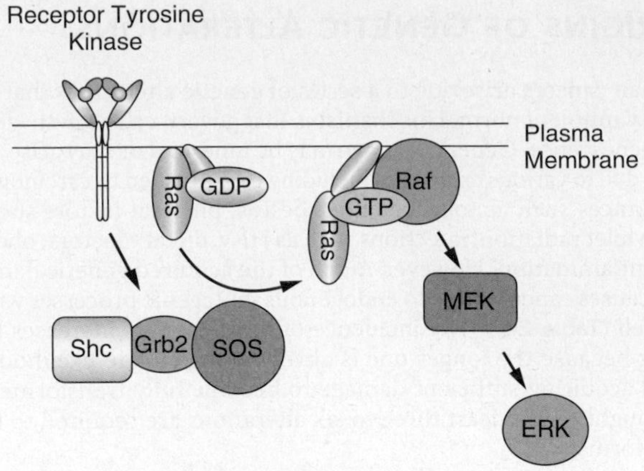

Figure 2.3. Receptor tyrosine kinase pathway. Most receptor tyrosine kinases stimulate the activity of the Ras guanine nucleotide exchange factor son of sevenless (SOS), which associates with the linker proteins Shc and Grb2. The activation of Ras by SOS stimulates a protein serine kinase cascade initiated by Raf, which stimulates MEK. MEK then activates the extracellular signaling-regulated kinases (ERKs). ERKs phosphorylate transcription factors to regulate gene expression. GDP, guanine-di-phosphate; GTP, guanine-tri-phosphate.

Because receptor tyrosine kinases are located on the cell surface, they are appealing therapeutic targets. A number of agents that target the EGFR family have been developed and translated into clinical practice. Trastuzumab is a monoclonal antibody that binds to HER-2/*neu*, blocking downstream signaling, and it is widely used in the treatment of breast cancers that overexpress this receptor (**Fig. 2.4A**). Cetuximab is a monoclonal antibody that targets the extracellular domain of EGFR, whereas gefitinib is a direct inhibitor of the EGFR tyrosine kinase (12). Lapatinib is a dual EGFR/HER-2 kinase inhibitor. Likewise, therapeutic approaches have been developed that target other receptor tyrosine kinases. Imatinib antagonizes the activity of the BCR-ABL, c-kit, and PDGF receptor tyrosine kinases and has proven highly effective in treatment of chronic myelogenous leukemias and gastrointestinal stromal tumors.

Nonreceptor Kinases and Phosphatases

Following interaction of growth factors with cell membrane receptors, secondary molecular signals are generated to transmit the growth stimulus to the nucleus. This function is served by a multitude of complex and overlapping signal transduction pathways that occur in the inner cell membrane and cytoplasm. Many of these signals involve phosphorylation of proteins by enzymes known as nonreceptor kinases. The kinases that are involved in growth regulation are of two types, those that phosphorylate tyrosine residues of target proteins, including those of the *SRC* family, and others that are specific for serine and/or threonine residues such as the *AKT* family. The activity of kinases is opposed by phosphatases such as PTEN, which act in opposition to the kinases by removing phosphates from the target proteins. The *PTEN* gene is among the most frequently mutated tumor suppressor genes in human cancers.

RAS/RAF, Mitogen-Activated Protein Kinase (*MAPK*) Pathway

Guanosine-triphosphate–binding proteins (G proteins) such as RAS represent another class of molecules involved in transmission of growth signals (**Figs. 2.4** and **2.5**). They are located on the inner aspect of the cell membrane and are positively regulated by Grb and SOS in response to receptor tyrosine kinases and other signals. They have intrinsic GTPase activity that catalyzes the exchange of GTP (guanine-tri-phosphate) for GDP (guanine-di-phosphate). In their active GTP bound form, G proteins interact with kinases that are involved in relaying the mitogenic signal, such as those of the MAP kinase family. Conversely, hydrolysis of GTP to GDP, which is stimulated by GTPase activating proteins (GAPs), leads to inactivation of G proteins. The *RAS* family of G proteins (e.g., *KRAS*) is among the most frequently mutated oncogenes in human cancers. Activation of *RAS* genes usually involves point mutations that result in constitutively activated molecules.

The *RAF* family of genes encodes serine–threonine kinases that interact with RAS proteins and propagate signaling by activating MAP kinases (MEK) which translocate to the nucleus. Mutations in the *BRAF* gene generally occur in cancers independently of *RAS* mutations (13). The mutual exclusivity of *KRAS* and *BRAF* mutations is consistent with the need to only activate one gene in a pathway. Melanomas often have mutations in codon 600 of *BRAF*. The BRAF kinase inhibitor vemurafenib has been shown to be highly active in these cancers as well as in other cancer types, including low-grade serous ovarian cancers.

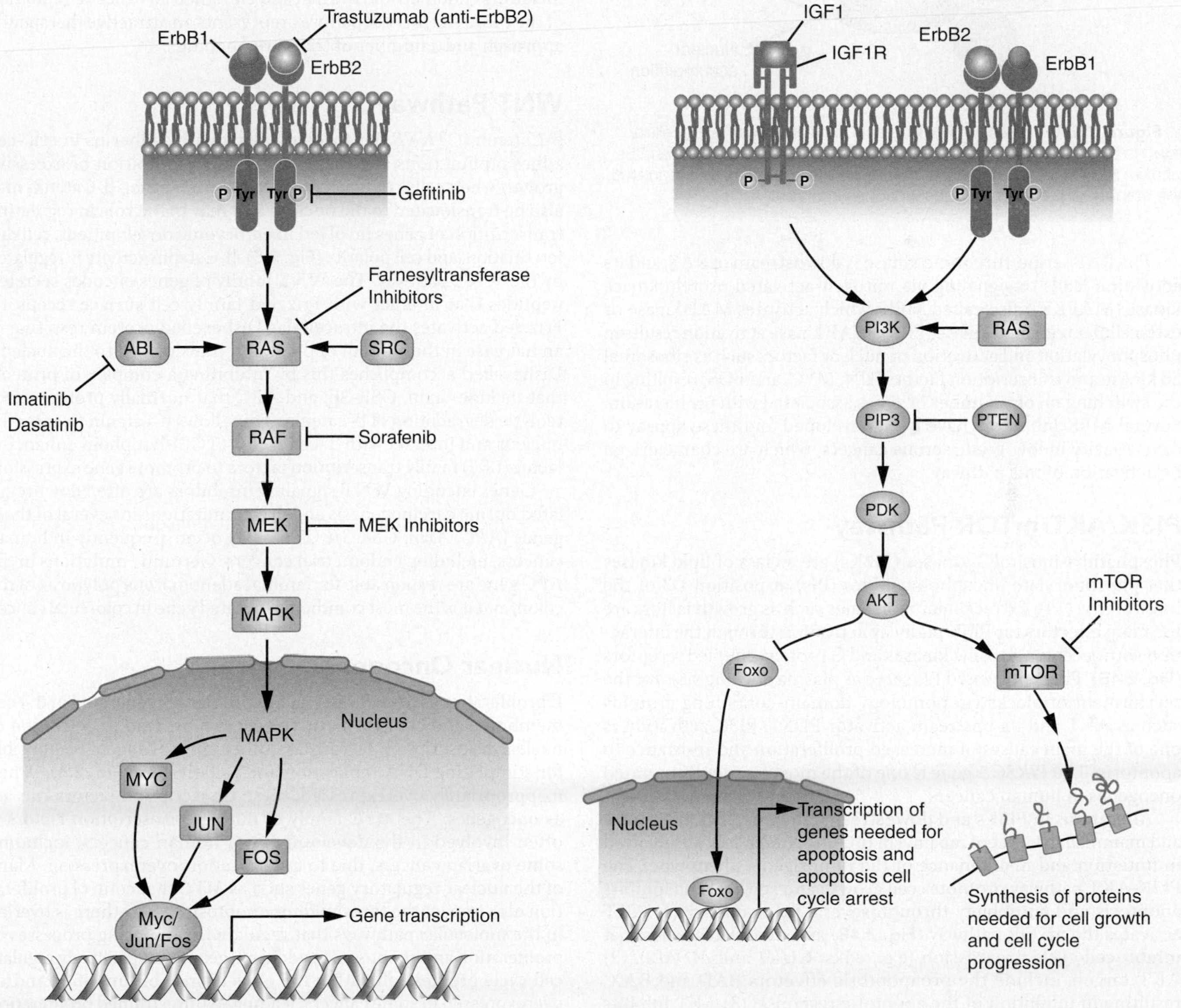

Figure 2.4. A: The ras/raf/MEK/MAPK pathway is activated by multiple growth factor receptors (here exemplified by ErbB1 and ErbB2) as well as several intracellular tyrosine kinases such as SRC and ABL. Activated RAS stimulates a sequence of phosphorylation events mediated by RAF, MEK, and ERK (MAP) kinases. Activated MAP kinase (MAPK) translocates to the nucleus and activates proteins such as MYC, JUN, and FOS that promote the transcription of numerous genes involved in tumor growth. **B:** The phosphatidylinositol 3-kinase (PI3K) pathway is activated by RAS and by a number of growth factor receptors (here exemplified by IGF1R and the ErbB1/ErbB2 heterodimer). Activated PI3K generates phosphatidylinositol-3,4,5-triphosphate (PIP3), which activates phosphoinositide-dependent kinase-1 (PDK). In turn, PDK phosphorylates AKT. PTEN is an endogenous inhibitor of AKT activation. Phosphorylated AKT transduces multiple downstream signals, including activation of the mammalian target of rapamycin (mTOR) and inhibition of the FOXO family of transcription factors. mTOR activation promotes the synthesis of proteins required for cell growth and cell cycle progression.

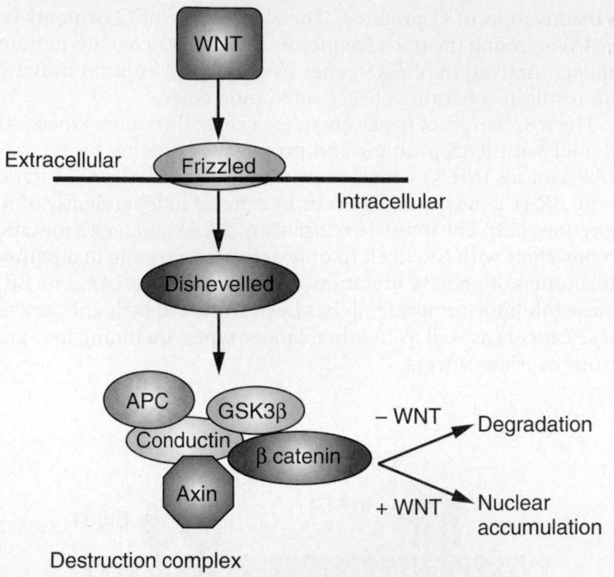

Figure 2.5. Wingless (WNT)/β-catenin signaling. WNT extracellular ligands bind Frizzled receptors and regulate the phosphorylation status of axin. Axin functions as part of the destruction complex that regulates the stability of β-catenin, a transcriptional regulator.

The RAF serine/threonine kinase is downstream of RAS, and its activation leads to signaling via mitogen-activated protein kinase kinase (MAPKK), also called MEK, which activates MAP kinase or extracellular regulated kinase (ERK). MAP kinase activation results in phosphorylation and activation of nuclear factors such as ribosomal S6 kinase and transcription factors JUN, MYC, and FOS, resulting in the switching on of a number of genes associated with proliferation. Several MEK inhibitors have been developed and these appear to have activity in low-grade serous cancers, which are characterized by activation of this pathway.

PI3K/AKT/mTOR Pathway

Phosphatidyl-inositol 3-kinases (PI3Ks) are a class of lipid kinases that phosphorylate phosphoinositides (PIs) at position D3 of the inositol ring (14). Extracellular molecules such as growth factors are the main effectors for PI3K pathway activation through the interaction with receptor tyrosine kinases and G protein-coupled receptors (**Fig. 2.4B**). Phosphorylated PIs serve as plasma docking sites for the recruitment of pleckstrin homology domain-containing proteins such as AKT and its upstream activator PDK1. PI3K activation is one of the main causes of increased proliferation and resistance to apoptosis. The *PIK3CA* gene is one of the most frequently mutated oncogenes in human cancers.

Alterations in PI3Ks and downstream effectors, including AKT and mammalian target of rapamycin (mTOR), frequently are involved in initiation and maintenance of the tumorigenic phenotype. The PI3K-AKT pathway promotes cell growth and survival and inhibits apoptosis and autophagy through several mechanisms: (1) AKT activates the mTOR pathway (**Fig. 2.4B**) and modulates genes that inhibit cell cycle progression (e.g., cdks, *CHK1* and *MDM2*). (2) AKT targets include the proapoptotic effectors BAD and BAX, resulting in inhibition of the apoptotic response. (3) AKT inhibits the expression of BH3-only proteins such as BAD and BIM through effects on transcription factors, such as Forkhead family proteins (e.g., FOXO3a) and p53. (4) AKT influences p53 activity through MDM2 phosphorylation at Ser166 and Ser186, which promotes its translocation to the nucleus with subsequent destabilization. (5) AKT can phosphorylate and activate IκB kinase-alpha, which in turn phosphorylates IκB, targeting it for degradation. This leads to nuclear translocation and activation of the transcription factor NF-κB and transcription of NF-κB–dependent prosurvival genes.

The PTEN tumor suppressor is the most important negative regulator of the PI3K signaling pathway. It is a lipid and protein phosphatase that removes phosphates in opposition to PI3K tyrosine kinases. Its ability to dephosphorylate phosphatidylinositol 3,4,5-trisphosphate (PIP3) resulting in phosphatidylinositol 4,5-bisphosphate (PIP2) inhibits oncogenic PI3K-dependent signaling. Although *PTEN* is a tumor suppressor and may be completely lost due to mutation and deletion of the two copies of the gene, mutational inactivation of one copy of the gene (haploinsufficiency) also appears to facilitate malignant transformation.

Both genetic and epigenetic alterations affect the activity of this pathway. Mutations in the *PIK3CA* gene that lead to increased activity frequently occur in human cancers, including ovarian and endometrial cancers. *PTEN* is frequently targeted by either germline or somatic mutation and is also among the most frequently mutated genes in human cancers. In addition, loss of heterozygosity (LOH) or promoter hypermethylation occurs in a broad range of cancers, including endometrioid ovarian and endometrial cancers. Inhibition of the PI3K/Akt/mTOR pathway represents an attractive therapeutic approach and a number of trials are ongoing.

WNT Pathway

β-Catenin (*CTNNB1*) is involved along with cadherins in cell–cell adhesion junctions and may play a role in inhibition of excessive growth when cells come in contact with each other. β-Catenin may also be translocated to the nucleus and may play a role in regulating transcription of genes involved in embryonic development, cell differentiation, and cell polarity (**Fig. 2.5**). β-Catenin activity is regulated by the WNT pathway. The WNT family of genes encodes secreted peptides that interact with Frizzled family cell surface receptors. Frizzled activates the intracellular Dishevelled protein resulting in an increase in the amount of β-catenin translocated to the nucleus. Dishevelled accomplishes this by inhibiting a complex of proteins that includes axin, GSK-3β, and APC that normally promote proteolytic degradation of β-catenin. This allows β-catenin to enter the nucleus and interact with T-cell factor (TCF)/lymphoid enhancing factor (LEF) family transcription factors to promote gene expression.

Genes encoding WNT signaling inhibitors are often downregulated during carcinogenesis and driver mutations in several of these genes (*APC, Axin, GSK-3β,* CTNNB1) occur frequently in human cancers, including endometrial cancers. Germline mutations in the APC gene are responsible for familial adenomatous polyposis of the colon, and it is the most commonly mutated gene in colorectal cancer.

Nuclear Oncogenes

If proliferation is to occur in response to signals generated in the cell membrane and cytoplasm, these events must lead to activation of nuclear transcription factors and other gene products responsible for stimulating DNA replication and cell division (**Fig. 2.4**). When inappropriately overexpressed, these transcription factors can act as oncogenes. The *MYC* family of nuclear transcription factors is often involved in the development of human cancers, including some ovarian cancers, due to amplification/overexpression. Many of the nuclear regulatory genes such as *MYC* that control proliferation also impact the threshold for apoptosis. Thus, there is overlap in the molecular pathways that regulate the opposing processes of proliferation and apoptosis. In addition, genes that positively regulate cell cycle progression within the nucleus may be amplified and/or overexpressed in some cancers, leading to unrestrained proliferation (e.g., cyclin D1 [*CCND1*] and cyclin E1 [*CCNE1*]).

Nuclear Tumor Suppressor Genes

The retinoblastoma gene (*RB1*) was the first tumor suppressor gene discovered and is frequently mutated in human cancers. It was named based on its discovery in the context of a rare hereditary cancer syndrome, as have many other tumor suppressor genes. The *RB1* gene plays a key role in regulation of cell cycle progression. In the G1 phase of the cell cycle, RB protein binds to the E2F family of transcription factors and prevents it from activating transcription of other genes involved in DNA replication and cell cycle progression. This serves as an important restriction point that can protect genomic integrity if DNA damage is present. G1 arrest is maintained by cdk inhibitors such as p16, p21, and p27 that prevent phosphorylation of RB. When RB is phosphorylated by cyclin/cdk complexes, E2F is released and stimulates entry into the DNA synthesis phase of the cell cycle. Other cyclins and cdks are involved in progression from G2 to mitosis. Mutations in the *RB* gene have been noted primarily in retinoblastomas and sarcomas, but less frequently in other types of cancers. By maintaining G1 arrest, the cdk inhibitors p16, p21, p27 and others act as tumor suppressor genes. Loss of p16 (*CDKN2A*) tumor suppressor function due to genomic deletion or promoter methylation occurs in some cancers. Likewise, loss of p21 and p27 has been noted in some cancers as well.

Mutation of the *TP53* tumor suppressor gene is the most frequent genetic event described thus far in human cancers and is a ubiquitous feature of some tumor types, such as high-grade serous ovarian cancers (15). The *TP53* gene encodes a 393-amino acid protein that plays a central role in the regulation of both proliferation and apoptosis. In normal cells, p53 protein resides in the nucleus and exerts its tumor suppressor activity by binding to transcriptional regulatory elements of genes, such as the cdk inhibitor p21, that act to arrest cells in G1. The *MDM2* gene product degrades p53 protein when appropriate, whereas p14ARF downregulates *MDM2* when upregulation of p53 is needed to initiate cell cycle arrest.

Many cancers have missense mutations in one copy of the *TP53* gene that result in substitution of a single amino acid, most commonly in exons 5 through 8, which encode the DNA-binding domains that are involved in regulating transcription (**Fig. 2.6**). Although these mutant *TP53* genes encode full-length proteins, they are unable to bind to DNA and regulate transcription of other genes. Mutation of one copy of the *TP53* gene often is accompanied by deletion of the other copy, leaving the cancer cell with only mutant p53 protein. If the cancer cell retains one normal copy of the *TP53* gene, mutant p53 protein can complex with wild-type p53 protein and prevent it from oligomerizing and interacting with DNA. Because inactivation of both *TP53* alleles is not required for loss of p53 function, mutant p53 is said to act in a "dominant negative" fashion. While normal cells have low levels of p53 protein because it is rapidly degraded, missense mutations encode protein products that are resistant to degradation. The resultant overaccumulation of mutant p53 protein in the nucleus can be detected immunohistochemically. A smaller fraction of cancers have mutations in the *TP53* gene that encode truncated protein products. In these cases, loss of the other allele occurs as the second event as is seen with other tumor suppressor genes.

Beyond simply inhibiting proliferation, normal p53 is thought to play a role in preventing cancer by stimulating apoptosis of cells that have undergone excessive genetic damage. In this regard, p53 has been described as the "guardian of the genome" because it delays entry into S phase until the genome has been cleansed of mutations. If DNA repair is inadequate, p53 may initiate apoptosis, thereby eliminating cells with genetic damage.

Finally, genes involved in chromatin remodeling in the context of the SWI/SNF complex in the nucleus also have been implicated as tumor suppressors (e.g., *ARID1A* in clear cell and endometrioid ovarian cancers).

TGF-β Pathway

The TGF-β family of growth factors inhibits proliferation. It is thought that TGF-β causes G1 arrest by inducing expression of cdk inhibitors such as p27. Three closely related forms of TGF-β have been discovered that are encoded by separate genes (*TGF-β1, TGF-β2, TGF-β3*). TGF-β is secreted in an inactive form bound to a portion of its precursor molecule from which it must be cleaved to release biologically active TGF-β. Active TGF-β interacts with type I and type II cell surface TGF-β receptors and initiates serine/threonine kinase activity. Prominent intracellular targets include a class of molecules called SMADs that translocate to the nucleus upon TGF-β receptor–mediated phosphorylation and act as transcriptional regulators. In the nucleus, the SMAD complex interacts with other DNA-binding transcription factors and cofactors to regulate the transcription of TGF-β target genes to initiate growth arrest. Typical events include the upregulation of cdk inhibitors (p16, p15, p21, and p27) and translation-inhibitory protein 4eBP1, as well as the downregulation of MYC. In addition to growth arrest, TGF-β also limits tumor progression through the induction of apoptosis.

Regulatory RNAs

Some RNAs that are transcribed from the genome are not translated into proteins, but rather affect various biological processes by regulating the activity of other genes. These noncoding RNAs include long noncoding RNAs (longer than 200 nucleotides) and smaller regulatory RNAs such as microRNAs (miRNAs), short interfering RNAs (siRNAs), and other species. miRNAs consist of single RNA strands of about 21 to 23 nucleotides that bind to messenger RNAs with complementary sequences and can block protein translation. Dysregulation of miRNA expression appears to play a role in the development and behavior of human cancers. miRNA production begins in the nucleus from several kilobase-long primary miRNAs (pri-miRNA). These pri-miRNAs undergo cleavage to produce short hairpin-shaped intermediates known as precursor miRNAs (pre-miRNA), which are approximately 70 nucleotides in length. Drosha, an RNAse III enzyme, processes the precursors prior to translocation to the cytoplasm. Subsequently, pre-miRNAs are cleaved by Dicer, also an RNAse III enzyme, resulting in mature miRNAs. siRNA, an approximately 21-nucleotide single-stranded sequence, is derived within the cytoplasm and does not require processing by the Drosha-DGCR8 complex. Mature miRNAs and siRNAs are then activated through the RNA-induced silencing complex, which produces host mRNA degradation and/or translational repression upon binding to the target.

Noncoding RNAs can also be used as powerful experimental tools. Exogenous constructs of either siRNAs or short hairpin RNAs (shRNA) can also be introduced into cells experimentally. shRNAs are introduced through viral vectors (transduction) to produce stable gene silencing, whereas siRNA transfection through encapsulation in lipids is transient. More recently, the CRISPR-Cas9 system has been used to engineer mutations at specific target sequences to

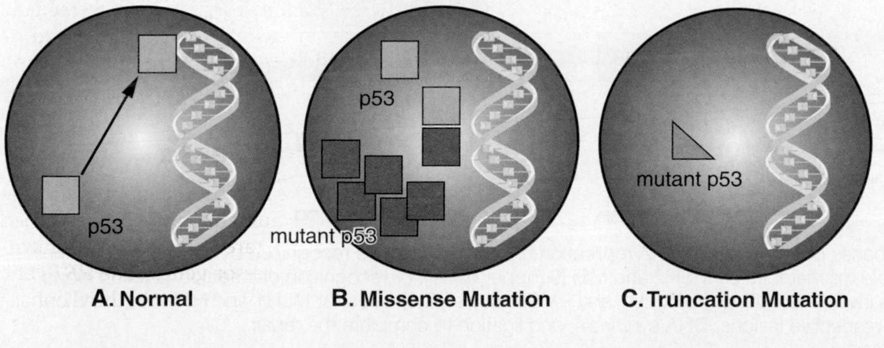

Figure 2.6. Inactivation of the p53 gene. **A:** Normal p53 protein binds to transcriptional regulatory elements in DNA. **B:** TP53 missense mutations encode proteins that no longer bind to DNA and the mutant protein complexes with and inactivates any remaining normal p53 in the nucleus. **C:** TP53 mutations that encode truncated protein products result in proteins that no longer bind to DNA, and these mutations usually are accompanied by deletion of the wild-type p53 allele.

interrogate their biological significance (16). The cas9 nuclease generates double-strand breaks guided by small RNAs that are aberrantly repaired by nonhomologous end joining (NHEJ), resulting in insertion/deletion mutations and gene disruption. Alternatively, in the presence of an introduced repair template, homology-directed repair can be utilized to induce precise mutations at the target sequence. RNA interference (RNAi) and genome editing technologies have been used as research tools to study the effect of turning off various genes and also potentially have therapeutic applications.

Energy Metabolism

Cancer cells uptake increased amounts of glucose to satisfy their metabolic demands, and this is the basis of fluorodeoxyglucose (FDG)-positron emission tomography imaging. Normal tissues generate energy using mitochondrial oxidative phosphorylation and only switch to breaking down glucose to derive energy in the absence of oxygen, which leads to the accumulation of lactate. In contrast, glycolysis of glucose to lactate occurs in cancers even in the presence of oxygen, a phenomenon called "aerobic glycolysis." This is referred to as the Warburg effect, in honor of its discoverer. Because cancers often outgrow their blood supply and become hypoxic, the ability to survive using aerobic glycolysis instead of oxidative phosphorylation may be selected for during malignant transformation. Lactate production by cancers may also promote invasion and metastasis by acidifying the microenvironment. Aerobic glycolysis also may serve the increased metabolic requirement for carbon atoms to produce the macromolecules needed to build new cancer cells. If glucose is completely broken down to carbon dioxide via the citric acid cycle, these carbon building blocks are lost.

The hypoxia-inducible transcription factor-1α (HIF-1α) plays an important role in the cellular response to decreased oxygen in the local environment. When oxygen is absent, HIF-1α accumulates and promotes transcription of proangiogenesis genes as well as those involved in glucose transport and glycolysis. HIF-1α accumulation may be a consequence of loss of the *VHL* tumor suppressor gene, providing a link between the loss of a tumor suppressor and the altered metabolic phenotype of malignant cells. Another link between glucose metabolism and cancer is the finding that isocitrate dehydrogenase (IDH), an enzyme involved in glycolysis, is frequently mutated in glioblastomas. The common amino acid-changing IDH mutations result in increased production of 2-hydroxyglutarate, which accumulates to high levels and plays a role in the development of these cancers. Activation of the PIK and RAS pathways also regulates glucose uptake and metabolism.

Differences in metabolism between normal and malignant cells represent an appealing therapeutic target. In this regard, there is a suggestion that the diabetic drug metformin may have efficacy in the treatment and prevention of cancer. This appears to be independent of blood glucose level, and the exact mechanism is unclear.

DNA Repair

It has been estimated that thousands of mutations occur in humans on a daily basis. Cells in many organs such as the skin, gastrointestinal tract, and respiratory tract that are exposed most directly to the environment constantly undergo renewal with shedding of differentiated cells that may contain mutations. Mammalian cells also have highly evolved and complex DNA repair systems to maintain the integrity of the genome. A series of cell cycle checkpoints exist that allow the opportunity to pause for successful DNA repair, or alternatively for cell death if repair cannot be accomplished. DNA damage checkpoints occur at the boundaries between G1/S and G2/M and during S phase and mitotic spindle assembly. These checkpoints serve to protect against genetic damage that can lead to malignant transformation being fixed in the genome.

There are several repair mechanisms that operate on specific types of DNA damage during these checkpoints, including MMR, nucleotide excision repair (NER), base excision repair (BER), homologous recombination (HR) repair, and NHEJ. Loss of DNA repair activity increases the likelihood of mutations being fixed in the genome, and this is a hallmark of many cancers.

DNA Mismatch Repair

MMR excises nucleotides that are incorrectly paired with the correct nucleotide on the opposite DNA strand. It involves recognition of a base pair mismatch, recruitment of repair enzymes, excision of the incorrect sequence, and resynthesis by DNA polymerase using the parental strand as a template (**Fig. 2.7**). The recognition of small loops generated by insertion or deletion of nucleotides, as well as single base mismatches, is primarily accomplished by a complex called MUTSα, which is a heterodimer of MSH2 and MSH6. MLH1 and PMS2 are recruited to the site to initiate the subsequent steps of repair, including excision, DNA synthesis, and ligation.

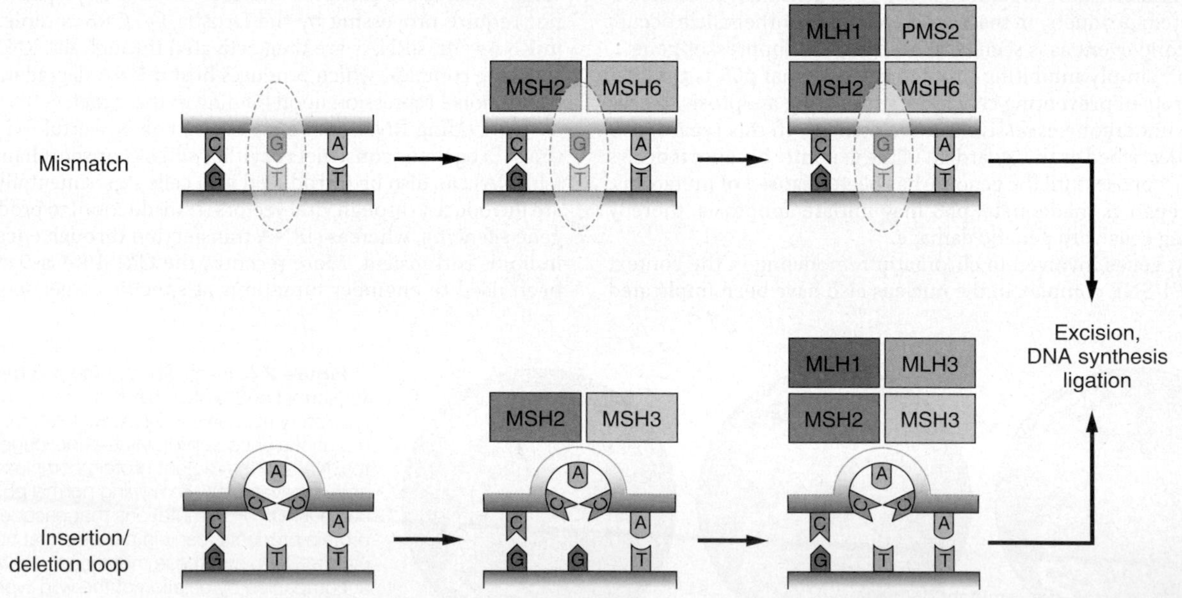

Figure 2.7. Mismatch repair pathways. Mispaired bases due to errors in DNA replication or other causes are recognized by the mismatch repair machinery. The initial step involves recognition of simple mismatches by MSH2 and MSH6 (upper panel), or recognition of insertion/deletion loops by MSH2 and MSH3 (lower panel). Subsequent steps involve recruitment of MLH1 and PMS2 to mismatch sites, or MLH1 and MLH3 to insertion/deletion loop sites. This is followed by excision of the respective lesions, DNA synthesis, and ligation to complete the repair.

Loss of MMR leads to a "mutator phenotype" in which there is accumulation of genetic mutations throughout the genome, particularly in repetitive DNA sequences called microsatellites. Examples of microsatellite sequences include mono (AAAA), di (CACACACA), and tri (CAGCAGCAGCAG) nucleotide repeats. Replication errors in these repetitive sequences are common and their inefficient repair leads to the propensity to accumulate mutations, and this is referred to as microsatellite instability (MSI). Some microsatellite sequences are in noncoding areas of the genome, whereas others are within genes. It is thought that accumulation of mutations in microsatellite sequences of tumor suppressor genes may inactivate them and accelerate the process of malignant transformation.

About 3% of endometrial cancers arise due to inherited mutations in MMR genes in the context of Lynch syndrome (17,18). Most cases are due to alterations in *MSH2* and *MLH1*, but *MSH6* and *PMS1*, *PMS2*, and *MSH3* mutations also occur. Lynch syndrome is covered in depth in Chapter 3. More frequently, the *MLH1* MMR gene is inactivated due to promoter methylation in sporadic endometrioid cancers of the endometrium leading to MSI.

Nucleotide Excision Repair/Base Excision Repair

The MMR pathway functions primarily in the recognition and repair of replication errors, while the NER and BER pathways respond to damage caused by DNA damaging agents. NER is an important DNA repair mechanism, as evidenced by severe human diseases, including xeroderma pigmentosum, that result from hereditary defects of NER proteins. The NER genes recognize and repair bulky DNA damage caused by environmental carcinogens, ultraviolet light, and chemotherapeutic agents such as platinum compounds (**Fig. 2.8**). Defects

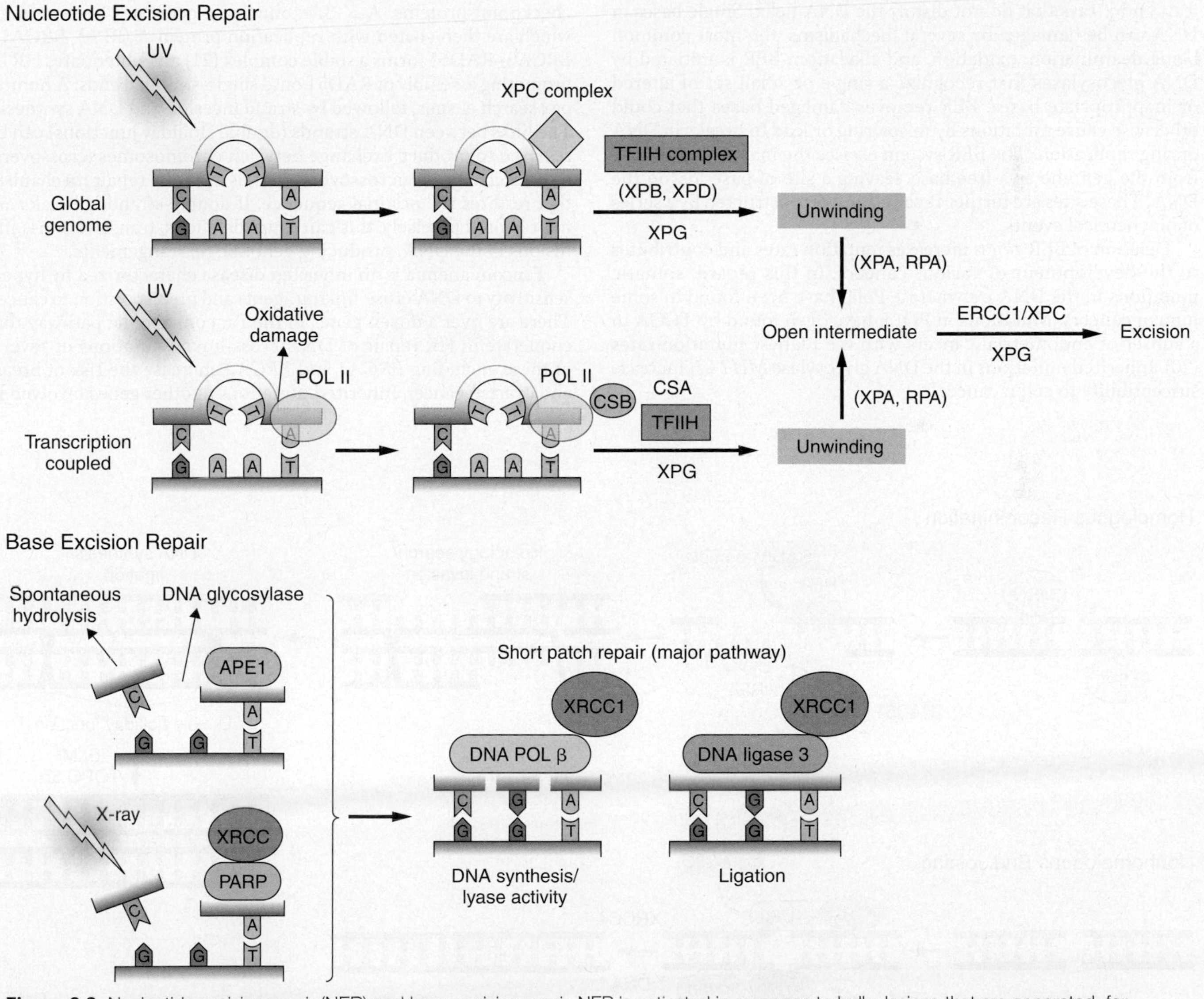

Figure 2.8. Nucleotide excision repair (NER) and base excision repair. NER is activated in response to bulky lesions that are generated, for example, by UV irradiation (upper panels). Global genome (GG) repair involves proteins identified by complementation groups in patients with xeroderma pigmentosa (XP proteins). Initial recognition of lesions occurs by a complex containing xeroderma pigmentosa C (XPC). Transcription coupled repair (TCR) also involves proteins identified by mutation in Cockayne syndrome (CS proteins) and occurs when RNA polymerase II stalls at the site of lesions. Stalled RNA polymerase II recruits Cockayne syndrome B (CSB) to the site of damage. Subsequently, DNA is locally unwound around the injured site by a TFIIH complex containing XPB and XPD. This process also involves XPG, CSA, and other proteins for TCR. Once unwound, XPA and replication protein A (RPA) contribute to stabilization of an open intermediate and recruitment of the ERCC1 and XPF endonucleases that excise the lesion. Subsequent steps involve DNA synthesis and ligation to complete the repair. In base excision repair (BER) (lower panels), abasic sites generated by spontaneous hydrolysis, action of DNA glycosylases, or x-ray–induced single-strand breaks are recognized by the APE1 endonuclease, as well as PARP and XRCC1. Subsequent repair is influenced by PARP-mediated ADP ribosylation of histones and other proteins, while XRCC1 serves as a scaffold for recruitment of DNA polymerase β and DNA ligase 3. These latter enzymes catalyze nucleotide reinsertion and ligation into the injured strand as part of the short patch repair pathway (major BER pathway).

in NER proteins predispose to various types of cancer, including skin cancer in xeroderma pigmentosum.

There are two NER pathways: one global pathway involved in scanning the entire genome and another that detects lesions that interfere with elongating RNA polymerases. The proteins required for NER assemble in an ordered stepwise fashion at sites of base damage. This assembly generates a large multiprotein complex, namely, the "repairosome." This repair complex can nick the DNA at precise distances on either side of the base damage, and these gaps are repaired using the opposite normal DNA strand as a template. There are several proteins involved in the NER process including *ERCC1, RPA, RAD23A, RAD23B XPA, XPB, XPC, XPD, XPE, XPF, XPG, CSA,* and *CSB*. *BRCA1* may also play a role in NER. *ERCC1* expression may be a marker of cisplatin resistance in cervical cancer, with low expression predicting superior 5-year disease-free survival (19).

BER is closely related to NER in that both repair lesions in DNA bases (**Fig. 2.8**). BER involves repair of small lesions due to chemicals and x-rays that do not distort the DNA helix. Single bases in DNA can be damaged by several mechanisms, the most common being deamination, oxidation, and alkylation. BER is initiated by DNA glycosylases that recognize a single or small set of altered or inappropriate bases. BER removes damaged bases that could otherwise cause mutations by mispairing or lead to breaks in DNA during replication. The BER system excises the inappropriate base from the genome as a free base, leaving a site of base loss in the DNA. These sites are further repaired and reconstructed by a series of biochemical events.

Deletion of BER genes increases mutation rates and contributes to the development of various cancers. In this regard, somatic mutations in the DNA polymerase Pol β have been found in some human cancers. Mutations in POLE have been found by TCGA in a subset of endometrial cancers with the highest mutation rates (20). Inherited mutations in the DNA glycosylase *MUTYH* increase susceptibility to colon cancer.

Double-Strand Break Repair: HR Repair, NHEJ

Double-stranded DNA damage can be caused by exogenous factors such as ionizing radiation, ultraviolet rays, alkylating agents, chemotherapeutic drugs, or by endogenous factors such as reactive oxygen species or errors in cellular DNA metabolism. Following double-stranded DNA damage, the ATM (ataxia telangiectasia mutated) and ATR kinases phosphorylate several proteins including CHK1 and CHK2 that initiate cell cycle arrest by way of p53, and this leads to DNA repair that restores genomic integrity or to apoptosis if DNA repair is inadequate.

HR is a process that provides high-fidelity, template-dependent repair of complex DNA damage such as DNA cross-links, double-strand breaks, single-strand DNA gaps, and DNA interstrand cross-links (**Fig. 2.9**). The HR pathway involves the following basic steps. Double-stranded breaks are recognized by the MRN complex and checkpoint proteins. A 5′-3, exonuclease generates 3′ overhangs, which are then coated with replication protein A (RPA). BRCA1–BRCA2–RAD51 forms a stable complex (21) and potentiates HR by promoting assembly of RAD51 onto single-stranded ends. A homology search ensues, followed by strand invasion and DNA synthesis. The links between DNA strands (double Holliday junctions) can be resolved to produce exchange between chromosomes (crossovers) or no exchange (noncrossovers). This is a precise repair mechanism that restores the original sequence. If double-stranded breaks are not repaired precisely, this can cause deletions, translocations, and fusions in the DNA, producing genomic rearrangements.

Fanconi anemia is an inherited disease characterized by hypersensitivity to DNA cross-linking agents and predisposition to cancer. There are over a dozen genes in the Fanconi anemia pathway that cooperate in HR repair of DNA cross-links. Mutations of several of these, including *BRCA1* and *BRCA2*, increase the risk of breast and ovarian cancer. Inherited mutations in other genes involved in

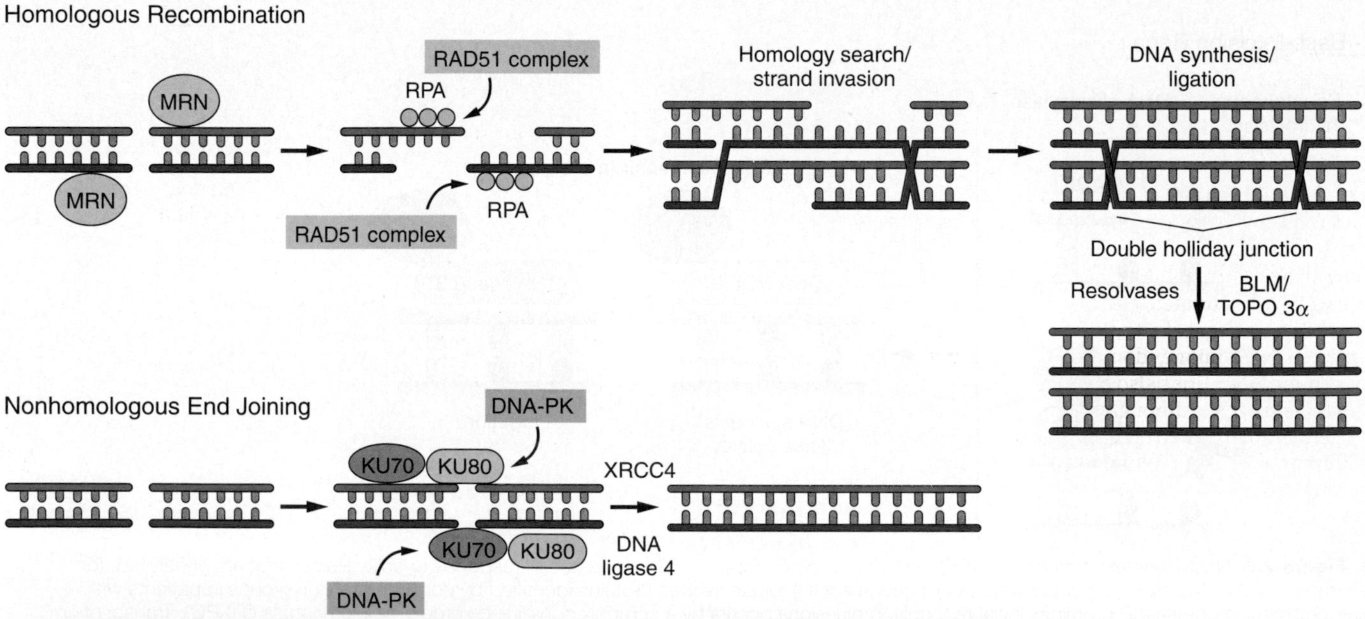

Figure 2.9. Double-strand break (DSB) repair by homologous recombination and nonhomologous end joining (NHEJ). In homologous recombination (HR), DSBs are recognized by the MRN (Mre11, Rad50 and Nbs1) complex, among other proteins. 5′-3′ exonuclease activity results in the generation of single-strand overhangs that are coated with RPA. Mediator proteins such as BRCA2 and RAD52 stimulate assembly of a RAD51 nucleoprotein filament complex that guides subsequent homology search and strand invasion into the homologous strand (e.g., the identical sister chromatid in late S/G2 phase and mitosis). Subsequent DNA synthesis and ligation result in the formation of recombination intermediates that contain double Holliday junctions. These are resolved by resolving enzymes such as the RecQ helicase BLM, in conjunction with topoisomerase 3α. The process of NHEJ involves recognition of DSB ends by the Ku70–Ku80 heterodimer, with subsequent recruitment of DNA-dependent protein kinase. DNA ends are then ligated following recruitment of XRCC4 and DNA ligase 4.

HR are associated with predisposition to these cancers, including *RAD51C* (fivefold increase) and *RAD51D* (11-fold increase) (22). *PALB2* plays a critical role in HR repair through its ability to recruit BRCA2 and RAD51 to DNA breaks. This serves as the molecular scaffold in the formation of the BRCA1–PALB2–BRCA2 complex. *PALB2* mutations confer susceptibility to breast cancer, and less likely ovarian cancer. The *BRIP1* gene is involved in the repair of DNA double-strand breaks by HR in a manner that depends on its association with BRCA1. *BRIP1* germline mutations have also been associated with ovarian cancer risk by about 11-fold (23).

DNA double-strand breaks may also be repaired through an NHEJ repair mechanism, wherein the break ends are directly ligated without the need for a homologous template (**Fig. 2.9**). Proteins associated with NHEJ include DNA-PKcs, MRE11, RAD50, XRCC4, and DNA ligase IV.

GYNECOLOGIC MALIGNANCIES

Gynecologic cancers vary with respect to grade, histology, stage, response to treatment, and survival. It is now appreciated that this clinical heterogeneity is attributable to differences in underlying molecular pathogenesis. Some cancers arise in a setting of inherited mutations in cancer susceptibility genes, but most occur sporadically in the absence of a hereditary predisposition. The spectrum of genes that are mutated varies between cancer types. For each type of cancer, there are a few genes that are frequently mutated, while a wider spectrum is altered in a small fraction of cases. There also is significant variety with respect to the spectrum of genetic changes within a given type of cancer. Cancers with a similar microscopic appearance may differ considerably at the molecular level. In some instances, molecular features may be predictive of clinical phenotypes such as stage, histologic type, and survival. An understanding of the clinical phenotypes associated with various genetic alterations in gynecologic cancers has the potential to inform prognosis and prediction of response to therapy.

ENDOMETRIAL CANCER

Etiology

Epidemiologic and clinical studies of endometrial cancer have suggested that endometrial cancer can be broadly classified into two general types. "Type I" cases are associated with unopposed estrogen stimulation and often develop in a background of endometrial hyperplasia. Obesity is the most common cause of unopposed estrogen and is often part of a metabolic syndrome that also includes insulin resistance and overexpression of insulin-like growth factors that may also play a role in carcinogenesis. Type I cancers prototypically are well-differentiated, endometrioid, early-stage lesions and have a favorable outcome. In contrast, "Type II" cancers are poorly differentiated and/or nonendometrioid and more virulent. The spectrum of genetic alterations also has been found to differ between the two types (**Table 2.3**). Although this dichotomous classification system is a useful framework to organize endometrial cancers, it lumps widely different histologic subtypes such as carcinosarcoma, clear cell, and serous into one category, leading to an oversimplification of extensive heterogeneity, and fails to account for additional heterogeneity that exists within endometrioid tumors.

Similar to other human cancers, endometrial cancers are believed to arise due to a series of genetic alterations. For Type I cancers, it has long been thought that estrogens contribute to the development of endometrial cancer by virtue of their mitogenic effect on the endometrium. A higher rate of proliferation in response to estrogens may lead to an increased frequency of spontaneous mutations. In addition, when genetic damage occurs, regardless of the cause, the presence of estrogens may facilitate clonal expansion. It also has been postulated that estrogens may act as "complete carcinogens" that both promote carcinogenesis by stimulating proliferation and act as initiating agents by virtue of their carcinogenic metabolites. Unopposed menopausal estrogen replacement therapy was found in the 1970s to increase the risk of endometrial cancer by four- to five-fold. Estrogen has been listed as a known carcinogen by the U.S. Department of Health and Human Services since 1985 and may also play a role in the development of Type II cancers. In contrast, progestins oppose the action of estrogens both by downregulating estrogen receptor levels and by decreasing proliferation and increasing apoptosis.

TABLE 2.3. Characteristics of Type 1 versus Type 2 Endometrial Adenocarcinomas

	Type 1	Type 2
Clinical features		
Risk factors	Obesity, unopposed estrogen	Older age
Precursor	Atypical endometrial hyperplasia	None or *in situ* carcinoma
Histology	Endometrioid	Serous/clear cell
Grade	1, 2	3
Stage	I/II	III/IV
Survival	Favorable	Poor
Molecular features[a]		
Ploidy	Diploid	Aneuploid
MSI	35%	Rare
Tumor suppressor genes		
TP53 mutation	15%	90%
HER-2/*neu* amplification	Rare	30%
FBXW7 mutation	10%	30%
PPP2R1A mutation	Rare	25%
ARID1A mutation	40%	10%
PTEN mutation	80%	Rare
MLH1 methylation	35%	None
POLE mutation	10%	Rare
CTCF mutation	25%	None
Oncogenes		
MYC amplification	Rare	25%
FGFR2 mutation	15%	10%
PIK3CA mutation	55%	40%
PIK3R1 mutation	40%	Rare
CTNNB1 (β-catenin) mutation	40%	None
KRAS mutation	25%	Rare

[a]Mutation frequencies obtained from TCGA data.

Lynch Syndrome and MSI

About 3% of endometrial cancers occur in women with a strong hereditary predisposition due to germline mutations in DNA MMR genes in the context of Lynch syndrome. First described by Henry

Lynch, this syndrome commonly includes malignancies of the colon, endometrium, stomach, and ovary. Less frequent malignancies that are part of this syndrome include those arising in the small bowel, upper urinary tract, brain, and biliary tract. Colorectal cancer is the most common malignancy in Lynch syndrome overall, which also is sometimes called hereditary nonpolyposis colorectal cancer syndrome. However, the risks of colorectal cancer and endometrial cancer in women are approximately equivalent (40% to 60%). Lynch syndrome is covered in more detail in Chapter 3.

Lynch syndrome is caused by inherited germline mutations in one of several DNA MMR genes—*MLH1*, *MSH2*, and, less often, *MSH6*, *MSH3*, *PMS1*, and *PMS2*. These defects lead to faulty DNA MMR. A hallmark of MMR deficiency is MSI. Microsatellites are short repetitive regions of DNA that become unstable during replication in the setting of defective MMR. In addition to germline mutations in the MMR genes, epigenetic silencing through promoter methylation, specifically in *MLH1*, is the most common mechanism of MSI in endometrial cancer (24). Methylation of *MLH1* is not a heritable condition associated with Lynch syndrome. MSI is found in up to 35% of endometrial carcinomas and is generally restricted to endometrioid cases. Methylation of the *MLH1* promoter also has been noted in endometrial hyperplasia and normal endometrium adjacent to cancers, suggesting that this is an early event in the development of some cancers (25).

The Cancer Genome Atlas Project

In 2006, The Cancer Genome Atlas (TCGA) began with studies in glioblastoma and high-grade serous ovarian cancer. The National Institutes of Health committed major resources to TCGA to collect and characterize the genomic landscape of more than 20 cancer types. A national network of research and technology teams pooled the results of their efforts to create an economy of scale and develop an infrastructure for making the data publicly accessible (http://cancergenome.nih.gov). Each cancer underwent comprehensive genomic characterization and analysis. The data generated by TCGA are available and widely used by the cancer research community through the TCGA Data Portal. The analyses included sequencing of the entire coding regions (exomes) of each cancer. Additionally, levels of gene expression, including mRNA and microRNA, were measured either through microarray-based platforms or using second-generation sequencing techniques to sequence the RNA transcriptome. Copy number alterations and methylation events were also assessed through microarray platforms. Some tumors were also hybridized to reverse-phase protein arrays when sufficient biomaterial was available.

Inherent in the design of the TCGA program are methodological aspects to be considered when interpreting the data. Only serous and endometrioid subtypes were accrued in the endometrial cancer project. Furthermore, most of the frozen tumor specimens used were previously collected and banked. Thus, larger tumors undoubtedly are overrepresented, because smaller ones are less likely to be banked. There is also an overrepresentation of serous and high-grade endometrioid cancers, with underrepresentation of the more common low-grade cancers. This was to assure adequate numbers of the former groups.

TCGA has reclassified endometrioid and serous endometrial cancers in four broad categories using comprehensive genomic approaches (**Fig. 2.10**) (20). One third of the cancers is characterized by MSI and associated hypermutation. These cancers have

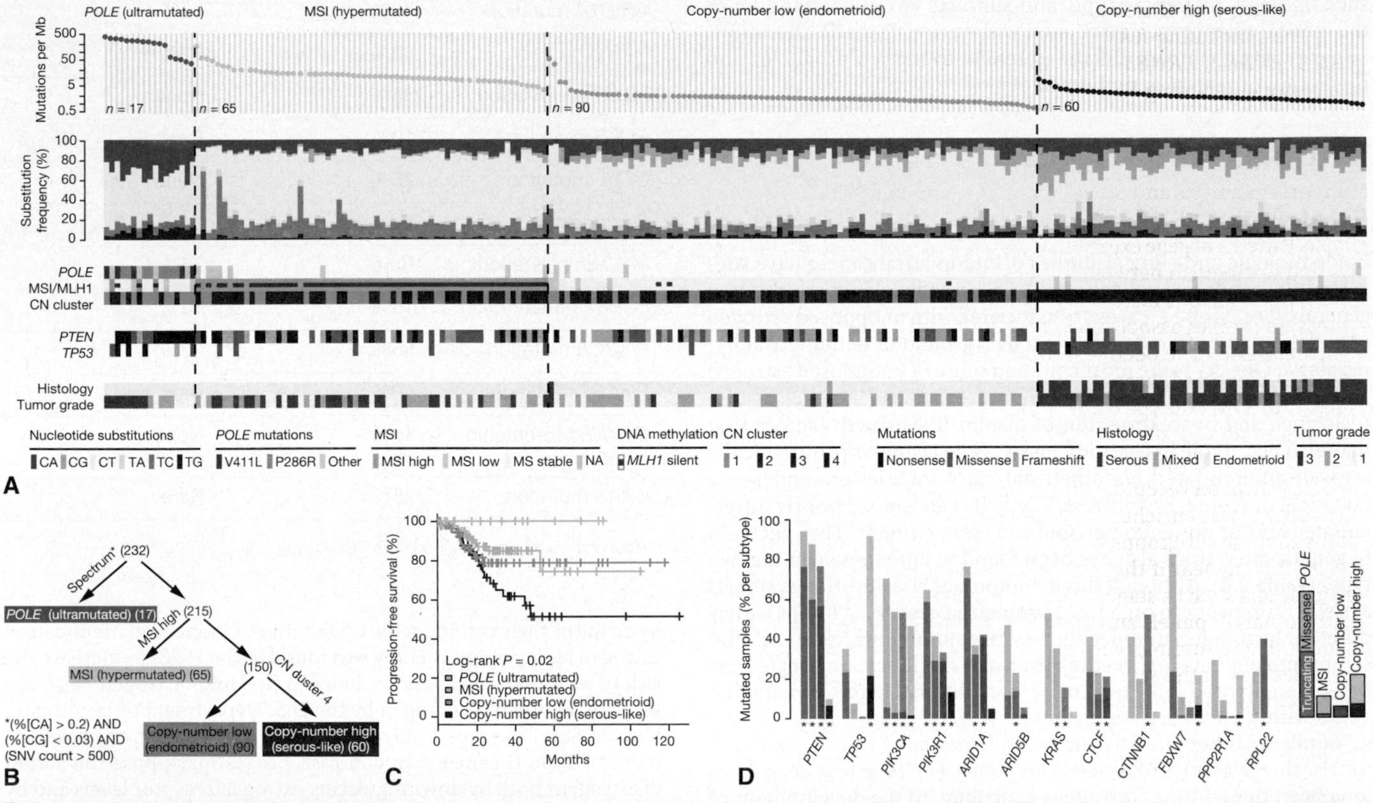

Figure 2.10. Mutation spectra across endometrial carcinomas. **A:** Mutation frequencies (vertical axis, top panel) plotted for each tumor (horizontal axis). Nucleotide substitutions are shown in the middle panel, with a high frequency of C-to-A transversions in the samples with POLE exonuclease mutations. **B:** Tumors were stratified into the four groups by (1) nucleotide substitution frequencies and patterns, (2) MSI status, and (3) copy number cluster. **C:** POLE-mutant tumors have significantly better progression-free survival, whereas copy number high tumors have the poorest outcome. **D:** Recurrently mutated genes are different between the four subgroups. Shown are the mutation frequencies of all genes that were significantly mutated in at least one of the four subgroups (MUSiC, asterisk denotes FDR < 0.05). CN, copy number; SNV, single-nucleotide variant. Reprinted by permission from Macmillan Publishers Ltd: The Cancer Genome Atlas Research Network. Integrated genomic characterization of endometrial carcinoma. *Nature* 2013;497:69; copyright 2013.

a background mutation rate (BMR) that is approximately 10-fold greater than microsatellite stable (MSS) tumors. These tumors are exclusively endometrioid and have few DNA copy number alterations. The cancers without MSI can be further separated into two groups. Serous cases with extensive DNA copy number alterations and genomic instability (similar to that seen in high-grade serous ovarian carcinoma) comprise one group, and endometrioid cases with few or only focal copy number alterations comprise the other. A smaller fourth subgroup contains samples with very high mutation rates (~100-fold or more than MSS tumors) and is characterized by mutations in the exonuclease domain of *POLE*, a DNA polymerase involved with repairing errors in transcription. Molecular features can be distinctly overlaid onto these four subclassifications and are discussed below.

DNA Copy Number

Early cytogenetic studies described gross chromosomal alterations in endometrial cancers, including changes in the number of copies of specific chromosomes. Comparative genomic hybridization (CGH) studies have also demonstrated areas of chromosomal loss and gain in endometrial cancer and atypical hyperplasia (26,27). Uterine serous carcinomas are aneuploid and have copy number alterations in nearly every chromosomal arm. Endometrioid endometrial cancers with MSI have few copy number alterations. The endometrioid cases lacking MSI have some focal copy number alterations and can be subdivided into a group with absolutely no copy number alterations and a second group with focal copy number alterations. A subset of samples also has amplification of chromosome 1q. A more global and specific approach, called GISTIC, can be used to identify recurrent focal copy number alterations. TCGA data suggest that this approach identifies approximately 81 focal copy number events, including 38 amplifications and 43 deletions (20). Amplifications occur in many oncogenes, including *KRAS, PIK3CA, PAX8, ESR1, MYC, FGFR1, FGFR3, ERBB2, ERBB3*, and *CCNE1*. Deletions occur in tumor suppressors, including *PTEN, RB1, NF1, WWOX*, and *PARK2*.

Gene Expression

Microarray analysis and other techniques have been developed that allow analysis of mRNA expression of thousands of genes in a tissue sample. Patterns of gene expression have been described using microarrays that distinguish between normal and malignant endometrium and between various histologic types of cancer (28,29). Global gene expression profiles associated with both lymph node metastasis and recurrence also have been identified in endometrial cancer.

TCGA identified three gene expression subtypes in endometrial cancer (20). One subtype contained most of the uterine serous cases and some grade 3 cases thought to be serous-like. One subtype was enriched for hormonally responsive genes and had higher expression of *ESR1* (estrogen receptor) and *PGR* (progesterone receptor). The third subtype was enriched for genes involved in immune regulation. Although these subgroups were associated with clinical outcome, at present it is unclear if they are independent of other known prognostic factors such as stage, grade, and histology. Studies to validate these biomarker panels and molecular-based prediction models are ongoing. These findings will further increase our understanding of the molecular pathogenesis of endometrial cancer and may help predict clinical phenotypes.

Tumor Suppressor Gene Alterations

TP53

Inactivation of the *TP53* tumor suppressor gene is among the most frequent genetic events in endometrial cancers. *TP53* mutation occurs in about 20% to 30% of all endometrial adenocarcinomas and is associated with several known prognostic factors, including advanced-stage, poor-grade, and nonendometrioid histology (30). *TP53* missense mutations are more common (~75%) and generally result in overexpression and accumulation of mutant p53 protein, whereas *TP53* truncating mutations (~25%; nonsense and frameshift) result in complete absence of p53 protein expression (31). Mutations in exons 5 through 8 are common and lead to loss of DNA-binding activity. Hotspots or areas of very frequent mutation exist at codons 248 and 273. Numerous studies have confirmed the strong association between p53 overexpression and poor prognostic factors and decreased survival (32). This is predominantly due to the disproportional frequency of *TP53* mutations in serous and high-grade endometrioid cancers. Most uterine serous carcinomas have *TP53* mutations as do one-quarter of high-grade endometrioid cases (20). Infrequent *TP53* mutation frequencies are found in grade 2 (~10%) and grade 1 (~5%) endometrioid cases.

PTEN

The *PTEN* tumor suppressor gene encodes a phosphatase that opposes the activity of cellular kinases that stimulate proliferation. *PTEN* is the most commonly mutated gene in endometrial carcinomas (33). Deletion of both copies of the gene had previously been thought to be a frequent event, resulting in complete loss of *PTEN* function. However, TCGA data suggest that homozygous deletion and mutation infrequently co-occur, as would be expected mechanistically, and homozygous deletion in the absence of mutation is also uncommon (20). More recent data suggest that single copy loss of *PTEN* is uncommon, and most tumors are diploid at this locus. *PTEN* mutations may be deletions, insertions, and nonsense mutations throughout the gene that lead to truncated protein products. In addition, missense mutations in the phosphatase domain can also inactivate PTEN function (**Fig. 2.11**). Loss of PTEN in endometrial cancers is associated with increased activity of the PI3 kinase, with resultant phosphorylation of its downstream substrate AKT (34). The PTEN/AKT pathway is frequently activated in many solid tumors, and endometrial cancer appears to be the tumor type with the greatest pathway activation.

Mutations in the *PTEN* gene are associated with endometrioid histology, early stage, and favorable clinical behavior (35). Well-differentiated, noninvasive cases have the highest frequency of *PTEN* mutations (>75%), which are uncommon in serous cases. In addition, *PTEN* mutations have been observed in endometrial hyperplasia, suggesting that this is an early event in the development of some endometrial cancers (36). It has been reported that loss of PTEN may occur in normal appearing endometrial glands, and it is proposed that this may represent the earliest event in endometrial carcinogenesis (37).

Other Mutated Tumor Suppressor Genes

TP53 and *PTEN* were both found to be significantly mutated genes (SMGs) in the TCGA project, as evidenced by a statistically increased mutation rate compared with an expected BMR when corrected for the size of the coding region (20). Other noteworthy SMGs in endometrial cancer include *FBXW7, ARID1A*, and *PPP2R1A*.

FBXW7 (CDC4) mediates ubiquitin-dependent proteolysis of phosphorylation-dependent ubiquitination and ubiquitin-mediated degradation of CCNE1 and other putative oncogenes. FBXW7 has also been reported to regulate mTOR signaling, and depletion of FBXW7 results in increased levels of both mTOR and phospo-mTOR. Data from TCGA and other studies suggest that *FBXW7* is mutated in a substantial fraction (~30%) of uterine serous carcinomas.

ARID1A is a large nuclear protein that participates in chromatin remodeling with downstream effects on cellular growth and other processes. It was first reported to be mutated in ovarian endometrioid and clear cell tumors and subsequently in approximately 40% of endometrioid endometrial carcinomas. Functional studies have demonstrated that *ARID1A* is a tumor suppressor gene, and more recent data suggest that it also participates in DNA repair through interaction with the checkpoint kinase ATR.

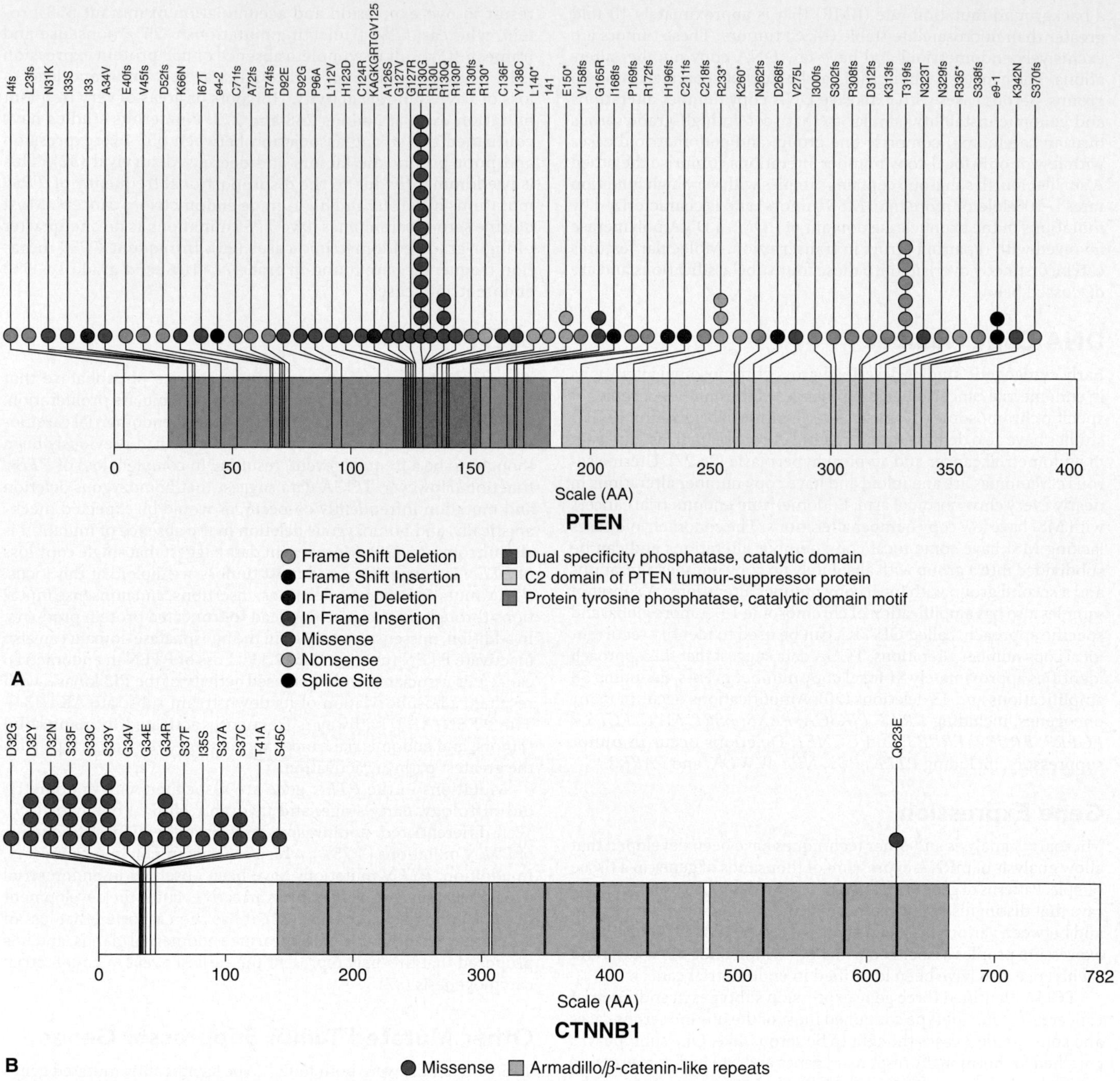

Figure 2.11. Mutational spectrum of the *PTEN* tumor suppressor gene and *CTNNB1* (β-catenin) oncogene in 68 well-differentiated nonhypermutated endometrial cancers from TCGA. **A:** Mutations in the *PTEN* tumor suppressor occur throughout the gene. **B:** Mutations in the *CTNN1B* oncogene are missense changes in critical amino acids that result in increased activity. (Figures provided by Cyriac Kandoth and Li Ding, The Genome Institute, Washington University, St. Louis, Missouri).

PPP2R1A is the constant regulatory subunit of the protein phosphatase 2A (PP2A), a serine threonine/phosphatase, and functions in control of cell growth and division. It is mutated in 20% to 30% of uterine serous carcinomas, but not in ovarian serous carcinomas. *PPP2R1A* mutations are seen in uterine endometrioid tumors at relatively low frequency.

CTCF is a transcription factor that functions as a negative regulator of both MYC and IGF2, suggesting a role as a tumor suppressor. TCGA found *CTCF* to be mutated in nearly 25% of endometrioid cancers, but mutations were not seen in serous cases. These findings suggest varied regulation of MYC with direct amplification occurring in serous tumors and loss of inhibition through *CTCF* mutation occurring in endometrioid tumors.

Oncogene Alterations

ERBB2 (HER-2/neu)

Alterations in oncogenes have been demonstrated in endometrial cancers, but occur less frequently than inactivation of tumor suppressor genes (**Table 2.3**). Increased expression of the HER-2/*neu* receptor tyrosine kinase initially was noted in 10% of endometrial cancers (38) and was associated with advanced stage and poor outcome. HER-2/*neu* overexpression is most frequently noted in serous endometrial cancers (39). TCGA data indicate that HER-2/*neu* is amplified in ~25% of uterine serous carcinomas and only ~1% of endometrioid tumors, confirming a strong association with histologic subtype (20).

Therapies that target HER-2/*neu* may have a role in the treatment of some uterine serous carcinomas. However, the levels of HER-2/*neu* overexpression in endometrial cancers are much less striking than in breast cancers. The Gynecologic Oncology Group (GOG) studied trastuzumab in advanced or recurrent HER-2/*neu*-amplified endometrial cancers. They confirmed a higher rate of overexpression in serous tumors (28%) than endometrioid tumors (7%). However, there were no major responses to therapy (40). Presently, a study of trastuzumab in combination with chemotherapy is ongoing, and PIK3CA mutations may represent a mechanism of resistance to this therapy (41).

KRAS

The *RAS* oncogenes undergo point mutations in codons 12, 13, or 61 that result in constitutively activated molecules in many types of cancers. Initial studies of endometrial adenocarcinomas in the 1990s found codon 12 of *KRAS* mutations in about 10% of American cases and 20% of Japanese cases (42,43). TCGA data indicate that *KRAS* is mutated in ~25% of endometrioid cases and rarely in serous cases (20). There is a greater frequency of *KRAS* mutations among hypermutator endometrioid cases (35%) compared with other cases (15%). *KRAS* mutations also have been identified in some endometrial hyperplasias (44), which suggests that this may be a relatively early event in the development of some Type I cancers.

PI3K

The *PTEN* tumor suppressor gene, which negatively regulates phosphatidylinositide 3-kinase (PI3K) activity, is frequently mutated in endometrioid endometrial cancers. Conversely, the *PIK3CA* gene is oncogenically activated in many cases. Activating mutations in the catalytic subunit of *PI3K* (*PIK3CA*) have been described in numerous cancer types. The p85-alpha regulatory subunit of PI3K (PIK3R1) has also been reported to be mutated and the p85-beta regulatory subunit of PI3K (PIK3R2) is mutated, although much less frequently, often in the setting of MSI.

In an initial study, *PIK3CA* mutations were seen in 36% of endometrial cancers, and 24% of cases had mutations in both *PTEN* and *PIK3CA* (45). In a subsequent study, 39% of endometrial cancers and 7% of atypical endometrial hyperplasias were found to harbor mutations in *PIK3CA* (46), implying that *PIK3CA* mutation occurs early in tumorigenesis. As in the initial study, a high fraction of cases had co-mutation in both *PTEN* and *PIK3CA*. These and other studies (47) confirm that *PIK3CA* activating mutations occur in both serous and endometrioid endometrial cancers.

TCGA identified *PIK3CA* mutations in ~50% of both serous and endometrioid tumors (20); however, *PIK3R1* mutations were generally restricted to endometrioid cases, occurring in ~40%. It has been suggested that one mechanism by which *PIK3R1* mutations are oncogenic is through the disruption of p85-alpha dimers that stabilize PTEN (48). Both inactivation of PTEN and activation of PIK3CA can lead to activation of AKT, which in turn leads to upregulation of the mTOR. Recent studies have suggested that inhibitors of the AKT/mTOR pathway such as temsirolimus may be useful in the management of endometrial cancer (49). Response to agents targeting this pathway may be enhanced by selection of patients with *PIK3CA* mutations (50).

CTNNB1 (β-catenin)

Alterations in the WNT pathway involving E-cadherin (CDH1), APC, and β-catenin (CTNNB1) have been noted in endometrial cancers. E-cadherin is a transmembrane glycoprotein involved in cell–cell adhesion, and decreased expression in cancer cells is associated with increased invasiveness and metastatic potential. E-cadherin mutations do not occur in uterine serous cancers, but occur more commonly (~7%) in endometrioid tumors with some predisposition to those cases with MSI. The cytoplasmic tail of E-cadherin exists as a macromolecular complex with the *β-catenin* and *APC* gene products, which link it to the cytoskeleton. It appears that a critical function of the *APC* tumor suppressor gene is to regulate GSK3B phosphorylation of serine and threonine residues (codons 33, 37, 41, 45) in exon 3 of β-catenin, which results in degradation of β-catenin. Mutational inactivation of APC allows accumulation of β-catenin, which translocates to the nucleus and acts as a transcription factor to induce expression of cyclin D1 and perhaps other genes involved in cell cycle progression.

Germline *APC* mutations are responsible for the adenomatous polyposis coli syndrome, and somatic mutations are common in sporadic colon cancers, but *APC* mutations have not been previously described in endometrial cancers. TCGA identified APC gene mutations, but these were mostly restricted to hypermutator cases and may be passenger rather than driver mutations. The *APC* gene may be inactivated in some endometrial cancers due to promoter methylation.

It has been shown that missense mutations in exon 3 of β-catenin lead to the same end result—namely, abrogation of the ability of APC and GSK3B to induce β-catenin degradation—which results in nuclear localization and increased transcriptional activity. β-Catenin mutations have been observed in several types of cancers, including hepatocellular, prostate, colon, and endometrial cancers. Nuclear accumulation of β-catenin protein due to mutation of the gene has been reported in about one-third of endometrioid endometrial cancers (51). Mutation of *β-catenin* has not been observed in uterine serous carcinomas. However, TCGA data indicate that the mutational frequency is ~50% in the MSS/nonhypermutator endometrioid cancers and only 15% to 20% in the MSI/hypermutator cases, suggesting that this is an important driver mutation in cases without MSI (20).

FGFR2

Mutations have also been observed in the fibroblast growth factor receptor 2 (*FGFR2*) gene in about 10% of endometrial cancers (52). In TCGA, *FGFR2* mutations were found more commonly in endometrioid cancers, with a slight predilection for MSI cases. A recent report indicates that *FGFR2* and *KRAS* mutations occur in a near mutually exclusive pattern. *FGFR2* mutations were found to be associated with a worse outcome among early-stage endometrioid tumors (53). Further studies are needed to evaluate the significance of the identified mutations, as well as the potential clinical utility of drugs targeting the receptor (54).

Other Oncogenes

Among nuclear transcription factors involved in stimulating proliferation, amplification of members of the *MYC* family have most often been implicated in the development of human cancers. It has been shown that MYC is expressed in normal endometrium with higher expression in the proliferative phase. Several studies have suggested that *MYC* may be amplified in a fraction of endometrial cancers (55). TCGA has identified a low frequency of somatic mutations in *MYC*, but 25% of uterine serous cancers have high-level amplification of the gene (20). *CTCF* is a transcription factor that functions as a negative regulator of both *MYC* and *IGF2*, suggesting a role as a tumor suppressor. TCGA found *CTCF* to be mutated in nearly 25% of endometrioid cancers, but mutations were not seen in serous cases. These findings suggest varied regulation of *MYC*, with direct amplification occurring in serous tumors and loss of inhibition through *CTCF* mutation occurring in endometrioid tumors.

Uterine Sarcomas

Although little is known regarding molecular alterations in uterine sarcomas, a number of studies are being conducted to examine uterine carcinosarcomas, leiomyosarcomas, adenosarcomas, and endometrial stromal sarcomas. The rare tumor TCGA project on uterine carcinosarcoma has identified somatic *TP53* mutations in >90% of tumors, consistent with prior reports, but distinct from uterine adenosarcomas, which only rarely harbor TP53 mutations

(56). Preliminary TCGA data from uterine leiomyosarcomas indicate that ~35% of cases have *TP53* mutations.

Endometrial stromal sarcomas are characterized by gene rearrangements that result in fusion of parts of two genes, and these are presumed to have the ability to stimulate malignant transformation. Low-grade endometrial stromal sarcomas usually present at an early stage and many have rearrangement of genes involved in chromatin binding. Most often, this is manifest in the form of t(7;17)(p15;q21), which results in a *JAZF1–SUZ12* fusion. In contrast, undifferentiated endometrial stromal sarcomas, which are more virulent and usually present at an advanced stage, frequently have t(10;17)(q22;p13) rearrangements that result in an in-frame fusion between *YWHAE* (exons 1 to 5) and one of the two highly homologous genes *FAM22A* and *FAM22B* (exons 2 to 7) (designated as *YWHAE-FAM22*) (57). Fluorescence *in situ* hybridization can be used to identify the gene fusions that differentiate low grade from undifferentiated endometrial stromal sarcomas.

OVARIAN CANCER

Etiology

About 20% of high-grade ovarian cancers arise in women who carry germline mutations in cancer susceptibility genes—predominantly *BRCA1* or *BRCA2* (58). Hereditary ovarian cancer is discussed in Chapter 3. The vast majority of ovarian cancer is sporadic and arises due to accumulation of somatic genetic damage. The causes of acquired genetic alterations remain uncertain, but exogenous carcinogens have not been strongly implicated. Cellular proliferation and oxidative stress with free radical formation with associated inflammation at the time of ovulation or in association with endometriosis or infection may also contribute to accumulation of DNA damage. Regardless of the molecular mechanisms involved, reproductive events that decrease lifetime ovulatory cycles (e.g., pregnancy and birth control pills) are protective against ovarian cancer (see Chapter 1). The action of other reproductive hormones such as estrogens, androgens, and gonadotropins may also contribute to the development of ovarian cancers.

Epithelial ovarian cancers are heterogeneous with respect to behavior (borderline vs. invasive), grade, and histologic type. It has become increasingly clear that there are striking differences in the molecular pathogenesis of various disease subsets. It has been proposed that ovarian cancers can be classified as Type I or II based on histology, grade, stage, and molecular alterations (59). Type I tumors are generally confined to an ovarian mass at diagnosis and include low-grade serous, mucinous, and most endometrioid and clear cell carcinomas. They are genetically stable and are characterized by mutations in a number of genes including *KRAS, BRAF, PTEN, CTNNB1, ARID1A*, and *PPP2R1A*. Type II cancers typically present at an advanced stage and are predominantly high-grade serous lesions, but also include high-grade endometrioid, carcinosarcoma, and undifferentiated cancers. This group of tumors has a high level of genetic instability, with frequent chromosomal gains and losses and mutation of *TP53*.

There is now strong evidence to suggest that nearly all epithelial ovarian cancers have an extraovarian origin (59). High-grade serous cancers of the ovary, fallopian tube, and peritoneum are likely derived from epithelial cells of the distal fallopian tube and fimbria (60). In this regard, most early serous cancers discovered in *BRCA1/2* carriers undergoing prophylactic surgery have been found to originate in the fallopian tube fimbria and are associated with preinvasive serous tubal intraepithelial carcinomas (STICs) that overexpress mutant *TP53*. In contrast, most endometrioid and clear cell cancers are thought to develop in deposits of endometriosis on the ovary or other pelvic structures. The origin of mucinous ovarian cancers is less clear, and some may arise from preexisting dermoid cysts (teratomas). Historically, the majority of mucinous ovarian tumors represented unrecognized metastatic gastrointestinal cancers. It has also been postulated that some mucinous and Brenner tumors arise from embryonic rests near the ovary.

As our understanding of the molecular pathogenesis of ovarian cancer continues to mature, it is likely that the various ovarian cancer subsets will increasingly be thought of as distinct entities with respect to diagnosis, treatment, and prevention (7). In view of this, each of the subtypes is discussed separately below.

High-Grade Serous Ovarian Cancer

High-grade serous ovarian cancer was the second cancer analyzed by TCGA project (58). This comprehensive genomic analysis confirmed prior findings; most notably, these cancers are characterized by a high degree of genetic instability with many copy number alterations and inactivation of *TP53* and *BRCA1/2* and other genes in the HR DNA repair pathway. Some previously unreported alterations also were discovered. This section will put the TCGA data in perspective with prior studies.

DNA Copy Number Alterations

Most high-grade serous ovarian cancers are characterized by extensive genetic instability. Initially gains and losses of various segments of the genome were demonstrated using karyotyping and later at a finer level using CGH. Likewise, LOH, indicative of deletion of specific genetic loci, was also demonstrated to occur at a high frequency on many chromosomal arms. Most recently, it has been possible using next-generation sequencing to characterize chromosomal rearrangements at the level of the actual base sequence, which facilitates analysis of their functional significance (61). Large gene deletions have been reported as well as transcriptional fusions that impact on platinum resistance.

TCGA examined DNA copy number alterations in 489 cases using a variety of high-resolution platforms (58). There were 8 chromosomal regions with recurrent gains and 22 with losses, all of which had been described previously. There were 63 recurrent focal amplifications that encoded 8 or fewer genes. The most common focal amplifications included *CCNE1* (cyclin E), *MYC*, and *MECOM*, each of which was amplified in more than 20% of cancers.

It was already known prior to the TCGA study that increased activity of transcription factors such as MYC and various cyclins might stimulate malignant transformation. Amplification of MYC had been reported to occur in some ovarian cancers (62), as had amplification and overexpression of cyclin E1 (63). In studies of advanced-stage ovarian cancers, high cyclin E1 expression was associated with poor outcome (64). Alterations of the PI3K pathway are frequent in ovarian cancer, and it also previously had been reported that the *AKT2* (65) and *PIK3CA* genes are amplified in some cases (66).

Cyclin E1 (*CCNE1*) amplification has been reported to occur independently of *BRCA1/2* mutation, and it is associated with reduced patient survival. Insensitivity of *CCNE1*-amplified tumors to platinum cross-linking agents may be partly because of an intact *BRCA1/2* pathway. These events may be mutually exclusive, because either change provides a path to tumor development, with no selective advantage to having both mutations. Using data from a genome-wide shRNA synthetic lethal screen, *BRCA1* and members of the ubiquitin pathway were shown to be selectively required in cancers that harbor *CCNE1* amplification (67). Furthermore, specific sensitivity of *CCNE1*-amplified tumor cells was shown to the proteasome inhibitor bortezomib. These findings provide an explanation for the observed mutual exclusivity of *CCNE1* amplification and *BRCA1/2* loss in high-grade serous cancers and suggest a unique therapeutic approach for treatment-resistant *CCNE1*-amplified tumors. In addition, *CDK2* was shown to be an effective therapeutic target in CCNE1-amplified cells *in vitro* (68).

TCGA identified 50 focal deletions, and the known tumor suppressor genes *PTEN, RB*, and *NF1* were deleted, albeit only in a small fraction of cases (58). The latter two genes also were targeted by mutations, consistent with the two-hit paradigm of tumor suppressor gene inactivation. Although mutations in the *RB1* tumor suppressor gene are not a common feature of ovarian cancers, evidence suggests that inactivation of *RB1* greatly enhances tumor formation in the presence of *TP53* mutations (69). A recent study identified frequent (~15%) gene breakage in *RB1* using whole-genome sequencing that had been previously overlooked through less robust sequencing approaches. A similar frequency of *NF1* loss due to gene breakage was also identified. A large number of other candidate genes are in regions that are recurrently amplified or deleted in high-grade serous ovarian cancers. Considerable effort will be required to elucidate which of these represent driver events in some cancers, as opposed to alterations of no consequence for tumorigenesis or progression.

About 30% of breast cancers express increased levels of the HER-2/*neu* (*ERBB2*) oncogene (70), usually due to gene amplification, and overexpression has been associated with poor survival. Expression of HER-2/*neu* is increased in a fraction of ovarian cancers, and overexpression has been associated with poor survival in some studies. However, ovarian cancers with HER-2/*neu* overexpression rarely have high-level gene amplification. Anti-HER-2/*neu* antibody therapy (trastuzumab) has demonstrated great efficacy in breast cancer and often is administered with chemotherapy in the context of both adjuvant therapy and treatment of metastatic disease (71). A study performed by the GOG found that only 11% of ovarian cancers exhibited significant HER-2/*neu* overexpression (72). The response rate to single-agent trastuzumab therapy was disappointingly low (7%), but there may be some benefit using it in regimens that also include cytotoxic or other biological agents.

The cdk inhibitors act as tumor suppressors by virtue of their inhibition of cell cycle progression from G1 to S phase. Expression of several cdk inhibitors appears to be decreased in some ovarian cancers. *CDKN2A* (p16) undergoes homozygous deletions in approximately 15% of ovarian cancers (73). There is evidence to suggest that *CDKN2A* (74) and *CDKN2B* (p15) (75) may be inactivated via transcriptional silencing due to promoter methylation rather than mutation and/or deletion. Likewise, decreased expression of the p21/*WAF1* cdk inhibitor has been noted in a significant fraction of ovarian cancers despite the absence of inactivating mutations (76). Loss of p27 (*CDKN1B*) also may occur and correlates with poor survival in some studies (77). It has been suggested that aberrant expression of p27 in the cytoplasm may be most associated with poor outcome (78).

Mutations

TCGA performed sequencing of the coding regions and splice sites of approximately 18,500 genes in DNA isolated initially from 316 high-grade serous ovarian cancers (58). The extent of this sequencing effort in ovarian cancer was unprecedented and would not have been possible without the recent development of massively parallel next-generation sequencing technologies. Although several genes were identified that are mutated at low frequencies, *TP53*, *BRCA1*, and *BRCA2* were confirmed to be the most frequently mutated genes in high-grade ovarian cancers.

TP53. The TCGA study validated the prior finding that mutation of the *TP53* tumor suppressor gene is the most frequent genetic event in high-grade serous ovarian cancers (**Table 2.4**). It is an early event that is found in STIC (**Fig. 2.12**) (60). About two-thirds of high-grade serous ovarian cancers have *TP53* missense mutations in the DNA-binding regions of exons 5 through 8 that result in p53 protein overexpression due to increased stability of the protein. Codons 175, 248, and 273 are mutational hot spots. These missense mutants act as dominant negative transforming genes due to their nonfunctional transcriptional activity. Loss of the other copy of the *TP53* gene is not required.

Most high-grade serous ovarian cancers that do not overexpress p53 protein have *TP53* mutations that result in truncated protein products. These are usually accompanied by loss of the other copy of the gene, consistent with the classic two-hit model of tumor suppressor gene inactivation. TCGA found *TP53* mutations in >95% of samples, suggesting that this is essentially a requisite event in the development of these cancers. Subsequent pathology review of the few cases lacking mutations found that these were probably not high-grade serous cancers (79).

BRCA1 and BRCA2. *BRCA1* and *BRCA2* germline mutations were found in 9% and 8% of high-grade serous cases, respectively, in the TCGA study, and somatic mutations in each gene occurred in an additional 3% (58). Silencing of *BRCA1* due to promoter methylation was observed in 11% of cases. Defective HR repair of double-stranded DNA damage due to loss of *BRCA1/2* was predicted in 31% of high-grade serous ovarian cancers. Other genes in the HR pathway are inactivated in some cancers, and the HR pathway may be compromised in approximately half of all cases (**Fig. 2.13**). A subsequent analysis of germline and somatic alterations in 429 TCGA ovarian carcinoma cases and 557 controls suggests that truncation variants and large deletions exist across Fanconi pathway genes in 20% of cases (80).

Patients with *BRCA1* or *BRCA2* mutations were initially noted to have increased sensitivity to platinum chemotherapy and favorable survival relative to sporadic cases (81,82). Conversely, the emergence of platinum resistance in these cancers may occur due to "revertant mutations" in which the normal *BRCA1* or *BRCA2* sequence is restored (83). More recently, studies have suggested that the initial favorable outcome seen in BRCA1/2 carriers does not persist with longer follow-up (84).

Cancers with defects in the double-stranded DNA HR repair pathway can be targeted effectively by inducing a second hit in the form of inhibition of the single-stranded DNA repair pathway. This concept of synthetic lethality—the combination of two genetic alterations, which on their own are nonlethal, but together result in a lethal phenotype—led to interest in inhibitors of enzymes such as PARP that are involved in single-stranded BER (85). Inhibition of PARP leads to the persistence of DNA lesions normally repaired by HR and makes HR-deficient cells particularly sensitive to chemotherapy-induced DNA injury. PARP inhibitors have been shown to be selective for cells with defects in the repair of double-strand DNA breaks by HR, particularly in the context of *BRCA1* or *BRCA2* mutation. While normal cells can repair the damage and survive, the BRCA-deficient cells cannot activate the HR system and therefore die (86). PARP inhibitors have demonstrated promising results in ongoing trials in ovarian cancer, and olaparib has been approved in the United States and Europe for treatment of *BRCA1/2*-mutated ovarian cancers.

TABLE 2.4. Characteristics of Common Invasive Epithelial Ovarian Carcinomas

	Mucinous	Endometrioid/Clear Cell	High-Grade Serous	Low-Grade Serous
Origin	Unclear	Endometriosis	Fallopian tube	Fallopian tube
Typical stage	Early	Early	Advanced	Advanced
Survival	Favorable	Favorable	Poor	Favorable
Commonly altered genes	*KRAS* HER-2/*neu* *TP53, CDKN2A*	*PTEN* *PIK3CA* *CTNNB1* (β-catenin) *ARID1A* *PPP2R1A*	*TP53* *BRCA1* *BRCA2*	*KRAS* *BRAF*

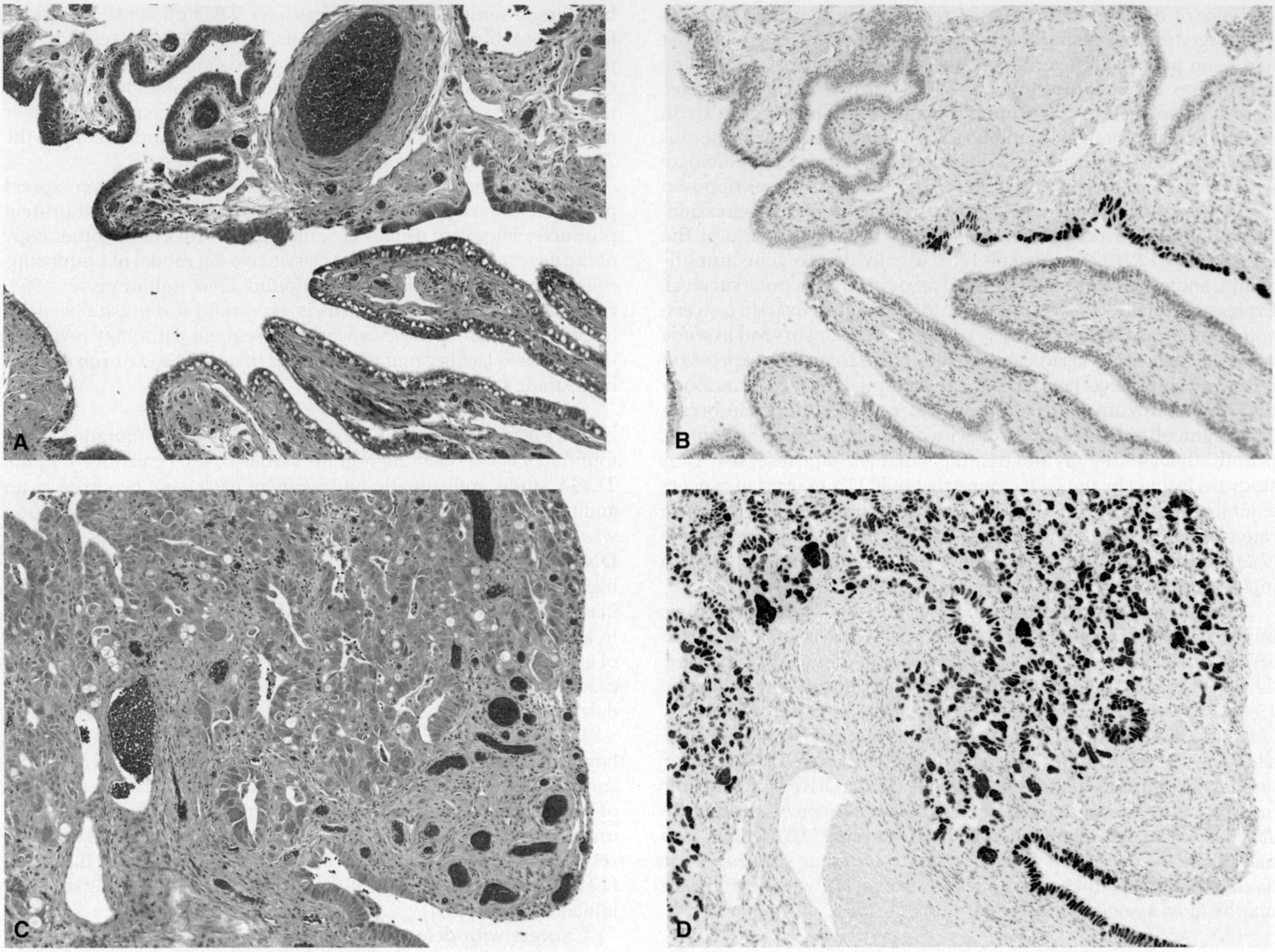

Figure 2.12. Overexpression of mutant *TP53* in serous tubal carcinoma *in situ* (**A, B**) and in high-grade serous ovarian cancer (**C, D**).

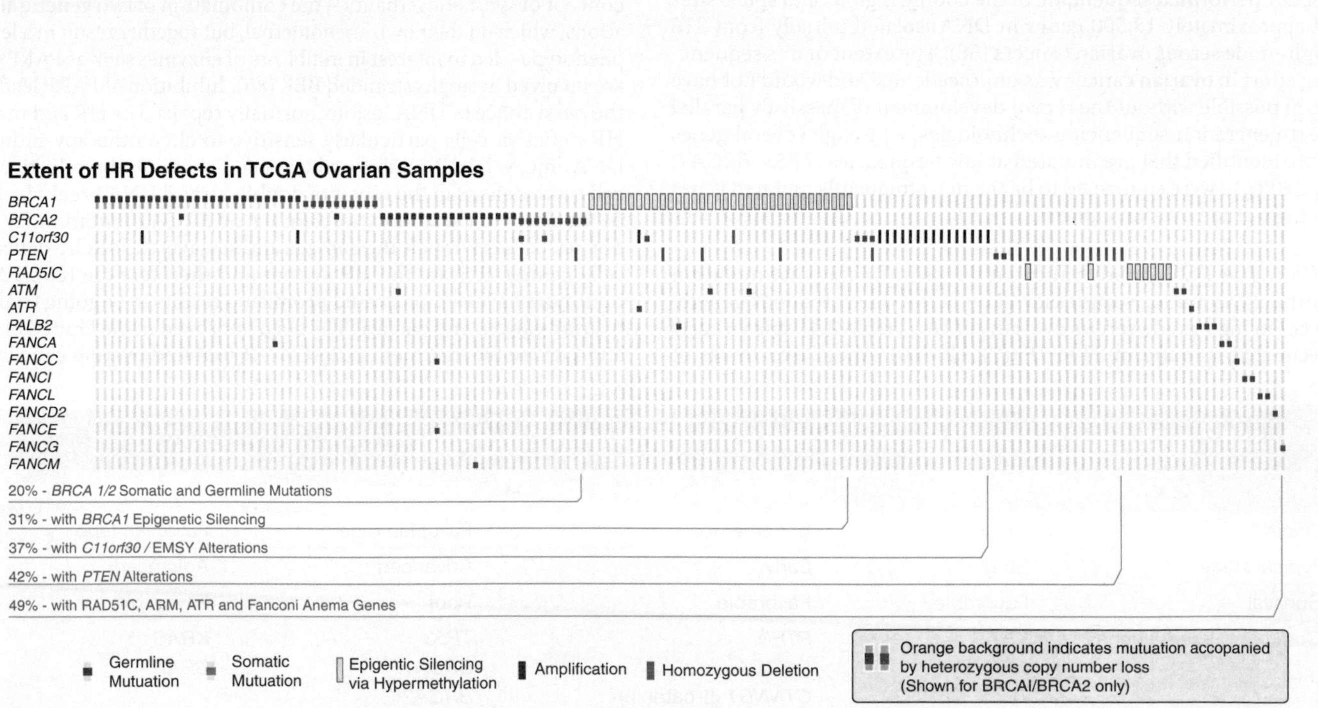

Figure 2.13. Genomic fingerprint of homologous recombination (HR) pathway alterations. Each column represents an individual case; each row represents a gene. Only cases with HR defects (N=154) are shown.

While only a minority of high-grade serous ovarian cancers have germline *BRCA1* or *BRCA2* mutations, sporadic ovarian cancers can harbor acquired genetic and epigenetic defects in *BRCA1/2* and in other HR genes and proteins, such as *RAD51C/D* and *BRIP1*, that may contribute to a "BRCAness profile" (87). Given the shared role that *BRCA1* and *BRCA2* have with other DNA repair genes, defects in these could influence response to treatment, recurrence rates, and overall survival and increase sensitivity to platinum drugs and PARP inhibitors (88). In this regard, it was shown using the TCGA data that a DNA repair pathway score was predictive of outcome in ovarian cancer (89).

More recently, investigators with the Australian Ovarian Cancer Study performed whole-genome sequencing of tumor and germline DNA from 92 patients with primary refractory, resistant, sensitive, and matched acquired resistant disease (90). It was shown that gene breakage commonly inactivates the tumor suppressors *RB1*, *NF1*, *RAD51B*, and *PTEN* and contributes to acquired chemotherapy resistance. *CCNE1* amplification was common in primary resistant and refractory disease. Several molecular events were associated with acquired resistance, including multiple independent reversions of germline *BRCA1* or *BRCA2* mutations in individual patients, loss of *BRCA1* promoter methylation, an alteration in molecular subtype, and recurrent promoter fusion associated with overexpression of the drug efflux pump *MDR1*. Clonal evolution also has the potential to affect responsiveness of high-grade serous cancers. In a genomic analysis of 31 tumor deposits from six patients, only 51.5% of mutations were present in every sample of a given case (range 10.2% to 91.4%), and *TP53* was the only mutation consistently present in all samples (91).

Other mutations. Six other genes were found to be significantly mutated by TCGA, including *RB1*, *NF1*, *FAT3*, *CSMD3*, *GABRA6*, and *CDK12*, but none was mutated in more than 6% of cancers (58). *RB1* and *NFI* are known tumor suppressor genes, while *CDK12* has also been implicated in both the regulation of RNA splicing and HR DNA repair. *FAT3* and *GABRA6* are not expressed in serous ovarian cancers or in the fallopian tube, and the significance of these mutations is unclear. A number of other known oncogenic mutations were found in *KRAS*, *NRAS*, *PIK3CA*, and *BRAF*, but at low frequencies of less than 1%. These mutations have been shown to have transforming activity and probably represent important drivers of some cancers, but may highlight cases misdiagnosed as high-grade serous.

In subsequent analysis of the TCGA whole-exome sequencing data, mutations of eight members of the ADAMTS family were noted in 10.4% of cases and were associated with a significantly higher chemotherapy sensitivity and better overall survival (58.0 vs. 41.3 months) (92). ADAMTS family members are metalloproteases that play roles in cell adhesion, migration, blood clotting, inflammation, angiogenesis, and connective tissue modeling. ADAMTS-mutated cases exhibited a distinct mutation spectrum and were significantly associated with tumors with a higher genome-wide mutation rate (median mutations per sample, 121 vs. 69).

Gene Expression

Microarray chips that contain sequences complementary to thousands of genes have been created that allow global assessment of the level of expression of each gene. Many genes have been identified that appear to be up- or downregulated in the process of malignant transformation. In addition, microarrays have demonstrated patterns of gene expression that distinguish between histologic types (93), borderline versus invasive cases (94), and between early- and advanced-stage disease (95). Molecular signatures have also been identified that are predictive of survival (96). More recently, sequencing of RNA has become technically feasible at a reasonable cost and provides a more accurate and direct representation of gene expression. RNA sequencing appears to be replacing microarrays as the preferred method for gene expression quantification.

In the TCGA ovarian cancer project, a 193-gene expression signature predictive of survival was developed and validated in several other existing data sets (**Fig. 2.14**) (58). TCGA also identified four gene expression subtypes of high-grade serous ovarian cancer that confirmed prior studies (97). These were named mesenchymal or C1, immunoreactive or C2, differentiated or C4, and proliferative or C5 subtypes based on the genes that characterized each subtype (**Fig. 2.14**). Favorable outcome is associated with the immunoreactive (C2) type, consistent with earlier studies and a worse prognosis for the mesenchymal (C1) and proliferative (C5) types (98). Alterations in gene expression may be attributable to methylation of their promoters. The TCGA examined tumor methylation using arrays that include promoters of thousands of genes. They found 168 epigenetically altered genes compared with normal fallopian tube epithelium. Further validation of genomic signatures is needed, but genomic approaches hold the potential to guide selection of therapy in the future. Patients identified as having a "poor prognosis" molecular profile might be the best candidates for investigational trials of new therapies.

With the evolving characterization of the genome, networks of molecular signals that regulate cellular proliferation and death have been identified—from receptor–ligand interactions at the cell membrane that transmit signals to the cytoplasm and then to the nucleus. The extensive genomic characterization of high-grade serous ovarian cancer by TCGA allowed for assessment of various signaling pathways. It was found that components of the RB and PI3K/RAS pathways were frequently altered, while the homologous DNA repair pathway was frequently inactivated.

Recently, 13 publicly available data sets totaling 1,525 subjects were used to develop gene expression signatures for predicting debulking status and survival in advanced-stage, serous ovarian cancer and debulking status (99). The survival signature stratified patients into high- and low-risk groups (hazard ratio = 2.19; 95% confidence interval [CI] = 1.84 to 2.61) significantly better than the TCGA signature. *POSTN*, *CXCL14*, *FAP*, *NUAK1*, *PTCH1*, and *TGFBR2* were validated by quantitative reverse transcription-polymerase chain reaction and POSTN, CXCL14, and phosphorylated Smad2/3 were validated by immunohistochemistry ($p < 0.001$) as independent predictors of debulking status. Immunohistochemistry for these three proteins classified 92.8% of samples correctly

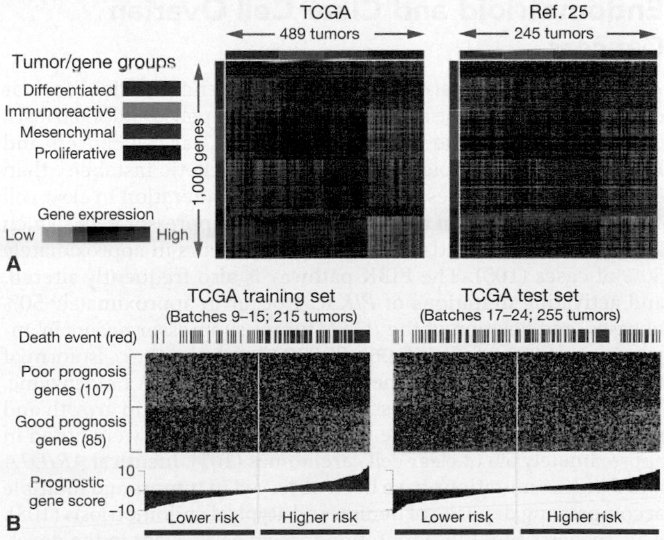

Figure 2.14. Gene expression patterns of molecular subtype and outcome prediction in high-grade serous ovarian cancers from TCGA and from reference 97. **A:** Cancers separated into four clusters on the basis of gene expression. **B:** Using a training data set, a prognostic gene signature was defined and applied to a test data set. Reprinted by permission from Macmillan Publishers Ltd: The Cancer Genome Atlas Research Network. Integrated genomic analyses of ovarian carcinoma. *Nature* 2011;474:612; copyright 2011.

for suboptimal debulking, potentially allowing for stratification of patients for primary versus secondary cytoreduction.

Borderline and Invasive Low-Grade Serous Ovarian Cancers

Similar to high-grade serous cancers, it is thought that borderline and low-grade serous cancers likely arise from fallopian tube epithelium. However, the underlying genetic alterations in borderline and low-grade tumors are different from those of high-grade cancers, suggesting that they are distinct entities rather than a single disease with varying degrees of differentiation.

Activating mutations in codons 12 and 13 of the *KRAS* oncogene are common in borderline serous ovarian tumors, occurring in about 25% to 50% of cases (100). In addition, the activating mutation V600E in the *BRAF* gene, which is a downstream effector of *KRAS*, occurs in about 20% of serous borderline tumors (101). Mutations in *KRAS* and *BRAF* have also been noted in benign epithelial cysts adjacent to serous borderline tumors, suggesting that this is an early event in their development (13). Specific inhibitors of V600E mutant BRAF protein have proven highly effective in melanomas. Mutations in these two genes are mutually exclusive and result in constitutive activation of the MAP kinase pathway.

Mutations in *KRAS*, and less frequently *BRAF*, also occur in some low-grade serous ovarian cancers (59). *KRAS* mutations are very common in recurrent cases, while *BRAF* mutations are rare (102). In another study, exome sequencing identified *BRAF, KRAS, NRAS, USP9X*, and *EIF1AX* as the most frequently mutated genes (103). *USP9X* and *EIF1AX* have both been linked to regulation of mTOR, suggesting that this pathway may be a candidate for targeted therapy trials (103), since metastatic low-grade serous and borderline cancers are generally resistant to platinum/taxane therapy. The MAP kinase pathway downstream from *KRAS/BRAF* also represents an appealing target. The MEK inhibitor trametinib and others have shown some minor activity in trials to date, but this does not correlate with *KRAS/BRAF* mutational status. In one patient who had an extraordinary response to a MEK inhibitor, genomic analysis identified a 21-base-pair deletion in the *MAP2K1* gene that encodes MEK1 (104).

Endometrioid and Clear Cell Ovarian Cancers

About 20% of epithelial ovarian cancers have endometrioid or clear cell histology, and these are thought to arise in pelvic endometriosis, on the ovary, or in the pelvic peritoneum. Clear cell cancers and low-grade endometrioid cancers have less genetic instability than high-grade serous cases. The most common alteration in clear cell cancers is mutations of the *ARID1A* tumor suppressor gene, which is involved in chromatin remodeling and occurs in approximately 50% of cases (105). The PI3K pathway is also frequently altered, and activating mutations of *PIK3CA* occur in approximately 50% of cases, and deletion of the *PTEN* tumor suppressor occurs in approximately 20% of cases (106). *PPP2R1A* encodes the α-isoform of the scaffolding subunit of the serine/threonine PP2A holoenzyme. This putative tumor suppressor complex is involved in growth and survival pathways. Missense mutations in this gene were noted in approximately 5% of clear cell carcinomas (107). Identical *ARID1A* and *PIK3CA* mutations have been observed in tumors and multiple accompanying deposits of benign and atypical endometriosis (108). This suggests that these mutations are an early event in the development of clear cell/endometrioid cancers.

Mutations of these same genes also occur in endometrioid cancers: *ARID1A* (30%), *PIK3CA* (20%) and *PTEN* (20%), *PPP2R1A* (10%) (109,110). In addition, approximately 30% of endometrioid cancers have mutations in the *CTNNB1* gene that encodes β-catenin, a nuclear transcription factor involved in the WNT pathway. These mutations occur in exon 3 at or adjacent to the serine/threonine phosphorylation sites and stabilize the protein product leading to nuclear overexpression and increased transcriptional activity. In some endometrioid ovarian cancers with abnormal nuclear accumulation of β-catenin that lack mutations in this gene, the *APC, AXIN1*, or *AXIN2* genes that regulate β-catenin activity are mutated (111). This suggests that in addition to the mutations that are also present in clear cell cancers, endometrioid cancers frequently have alterations in the WNT signaling pathway (**Table 2.4**). Mouse models in which the WNT and the PI3K/PTEN pathways are inactivated lead to the development of endometriosis and endometrioid cancers (112). Although endometrioid ovarian cancers are believed to arise from ectopic endometrium, and there is considerable overlap in pathogenic mutations, the frequency of mutations differs between endometrioid ovarian cancers and endometrioid endometrial cancers. In one comparative study (113), *PTEN* mutations were more frequent in low-grade endometrial endometrioid carcinomas (67%) compared with low-grade ovarian endometrioid carcinomas (17%). In contrast, *CTNNB1* mutations were significantly more common in low-grade ovarian endometrioid carcinomas (53%) compared with low-grade endometrial endometrioid carcinomas (28%). High-grade endometrioid ovarian cancers typically have molecular features similar to high-grade serous ovarian cancers, including genetic instability and *TP53* mutations. These tumor types may be difficult to classify by pathologists based on light microscopy.

Synchronous Endometrioid Ovarian and Endometrial Cancers

Synchronous endometrioid cancers are sometimes encountered in the endometrium and ovary that are indistinguishable microscopically. In some of these cases, identical *PTEN* mutations have been identified, suggesting that the ovarian tumor represents a metastasis from the endometrium (114). In other cases, the *PTEN* mutation seen in the endometrial cancer was not found in the ovarian tumor, suggesting that these represent two distinct primary cancers. Mutational analysis of *PTEN, CTNNB1*, and other genes frequently mutated in endometrioid cancers is helpful when a mutation is present in both cancers or in one cancer and absent in the other, but this approach may often be uninformative. It has been reported that mitochondrial DNA mutations are fairly common in endometrial cancers (115), and mitochondrial DNA sequencing has been proposed as an alternative method of determining whether synchronous endometrioid cancers of the ovary and endometrium represent separate primary cancers. Two recent papers have strongly suggested that most endometriod ovarian cancers are likely metastases from endometrial primaries and are clonally related (116,117).

Mucinous Ovarian Cancer

Historically, mucinous ovarian cancers were often misdiagnosed as metastases from the gastrointestinal tract. However, some mucinous carcinomas clearly arise from the ovary, perhaps from mucinous cystadenomas, borderline tumors, or teratomas (dermoid cysts). Similar to mucinous colorectal cancers, mucinous ovarian cancers frequently have *KRAS* mutations (59). These mutations occur in 50% to 75% of mucinous ovarian cancers and are missense changes in the hotspot codons. Identical *KRAS* mutations have been found in mucinous carcinomas and adjacent mucinous cystadenomas and borderline tumors, suggesting that the latter lesions represent premalignant precursors (59). Amplification/overexpression of HER-2/neu has been found in 19% of 154 mucinous ovarian cancers and 6% of 176 (6.2%) mucinous borderline tumors (118). Exhaustive exome sequencing analysis of these tumors revealed mutations in known drivers, such as *KRAS, BRAF*, and *CDKN2A* (119). In addition, a high percentage of mucinous ovarian carcinomas had *TP53* mutations (52%), and recurrent mutations were found in *RNF43, ELF3, GNAS, ERBB3*, and *KLF5*. Another targeted sequencing study in mucinous tumors found similar results with mutations in *KRAS, TP53, CDKN2A, PIK3CA, PTEN, BRAF, FGFR2, STK11, CTNNB1, SRC, SMAD4, GNA11*, and *ERBB2* (120). Proven and potential

RAS pathway activating changes were observed in all but one case, suggesting the potential of targeting this pathway.

Stromal Ovarian Tumors

The genetic alterations driving stromal tumors of the ovary were unknown until recently when it became possible to screen the entire genome using next-generation sequencing. Essentially all adult granulosa tumors were found to have missense mutations in codon 134 of *FOXL2*, a gene encoding a transcription factor known to be critical for granulosa cell development (121). This mutation was also found in approximately 20% of thecomas and 10% of juvenile granulosa cell tumors, but not in other types of sex cord stromal tumors.

DICER1 mutations in the RNase IIIb domain were found in approximately 30% of nonepithelial ovarian tumors, predominantly in Sertoli-Leydig cell tumors (60%) (122). These mutations were restricted to codons encoding metal-binding sites within the RNase IIIb catalytic centers, which are critical for microRNA interaction and cleavage. More recently, mutations in this part of the *DICER1* gene also have been found in approximately 2% of endometrial cancers (123). In addition, high expression of these two genes has been shown to be associated with increased survival in ovarian cancer (>11 vs. 2.7 years) (124).

CERVICAL CANCER

Etiology

Although the incidence of cervical cancer has fallen by over 80% in developed countries due to widespread implementation of cervical screening, in developing areas of the world it is still the most common cancer in women. Almost all cervical cancers are caused by sexually transmitted HPV infection, as are many vaginal and vulvar cancers. The epidemiology and biology of HPV infection and its role in screening and prevention are discussed in Chapters 1 (Epidemiology) and 7 (Preinvasive Lower Genital Tract Disease).

Unlike most other types of human cancers that occur due to mutations in oncogenes and/or tumor suppressor genes that disrupt their normal genetic sequence, cervical cancers arise as a consequence of viral inactivation of the *TP53* and *RB* tumor suppressors by the HPV E6 and E7 oncoproteins, respectively (**Fig. 2.15**). Variations in oncogenic potential between HPV subtypes may be related in part to differences in the efficiency with which E6 and E7 bind to and inactivate these tumor suppressors (125,126). In some studies, the levels of E6 and E7 in invasive cervical cancers have been found to predict outcome, whereas HPV viral load does not (127). There is also evidence that HPV E6/E7 may interact directly with other proteins such as telomerase that enhance growth and inhibit apoptosis. In addition, the cdk inhibitor p16 is strikingly upregulated in most cervical dysplasias and cancers (128). p16 detection may represent a useful adjunct to improve the positive predictive value of high-risk HPV testing for detection of cervical dysplasia.

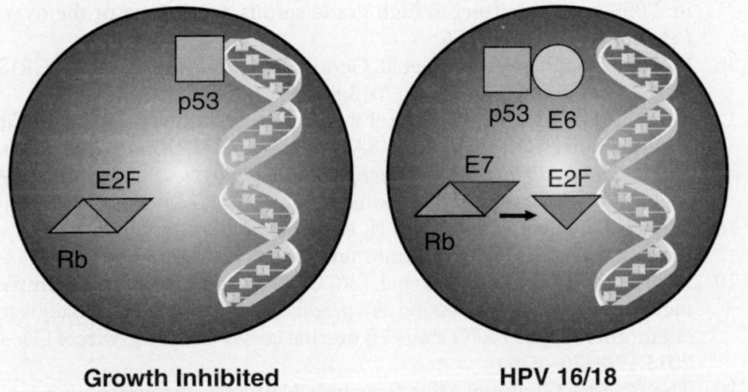

Figure 2.15. Role of *TP53* and *RB* genes in cervical carcinogenesis. The HPV-16/18 E6 and E7 proteins inactivate the *TP53* and *RB* genes, respectively.

HPV-negative cervical cancers are uncommon, but have been reported to exhibit overexpression of mutant p53 protein (129). This suggests that inactivation of *TP53* is a requisite event in cervical carcinogenesis. The biology of HPV-related transformation, including the role of E6/E7, is discussed in greater detail in Chapter 7. This chapter will focus on the secondary genetic alterations that have been observed in invasive cervical cancers.

Secondary Genomic Changes

HPV-associated cervical carcinogenesis with inactivation of the *TP53* tumor suppressor gene leads to genomic instability that results in secondary genetic alterations that play a role in the development and phenotype of these cancers. Over time, this ongoing instability leads to significant intratumoral heterogeneity as genetic damage continues to accumulate. Most cervical cancers are aneuploid, and CGH studies have shown that areas of DNA copy number gain or loss are common. A strikingly consistent finding of various studies is the high frequency of gains on chromosome 3q in both squamous cancers (130,131) and adenocarcinomas (132). Other chromosomes that exhibit frequent gains include 1q and 11q. The most common areas of chromosomal loss include chromosomes 3p, 2q and 13q (133). The frequency of gains and losses at various genomic locations may be random to a certain extent, but there are areas of the genome that are more susceptible to breakage leading to translocations or loss/gain. Abnormalities seen in invasive cancers using CGH have also been identified in high-grade dysplasias, suggesting that these are early and perhaps requisite events in cervical carcinogenesis (131,134,135).

Alterations in gene dosage due to chromosomal gains or losses have the potential to lead to changes in expression of genes involved in the regulation of processes central to malignant transformation such as growth, differentiation, and apoptosis. Cervical carcinogenesis is also accompanied by changes in DNA methylation that affect gene expression. Regardless of the cause, some changes in gene dosage likely represent collateral damage and have no effect on development and evolution of the malignant phenotype. However, it is likely that over time there is selection for clones that exhibit enhanced growth and invasive potential. It is possible that genetic instability may also enhance the emergence of resistance to radiation and chemotherapy.

A study of gene dosage in locally advanced cervical cancers using microarrays found frequent alterations, including 14 regions with recurrent gains and 14 with recurrent losses. The most common alterations were gain on 1q, 3q, 5p, 20q, and Xq and loss on 2q, 3p, 4p, 11q, and 13q, each involving 44% to 76% of the patients. Four genes on 3p (*RYBP*, *GBE1*) and 13q (*FAM48A*, *MED4*) correlated with outcome at both the gene dosage and expression level and were validated in the independent cohort. Despite circumstantial evidence provided by studies such as this, with the exception of the fragile histidine triad (*FHIT*) gene on chromosome 3p14, it has been difficult to prove that genomic gains and losses result in alterations in specific oncogenes or tumor suppressor genes that are directly involved in tumor development. The *FHIT* gene is frequently deleted in many different cancers, including cervical cancer (136). In one study, FHIT protein expression was markedly reduced or absent in 71% of invasive cancers, 52% of high-grade squamous intraepithelial lesions (HSILs) associated with invasive cancer, and 21% of HSILs without associated invasive cancer (137). In addition, reduced expression is associated with poor prognosis in advanced cervical cancers (138).

The role of several oncogenes has been examined in cervical carcinomas including most prominently the *RAS* and *MYC* genes. Mutant *RAS* genes are capable of cooperating with HPV in transforming cells *in vitro*. There is some evidence that mutations in either *KRAS* or *HRAS* may play a role in a subset of cervical cancers. *MYC* amplification and overexpression may be an early event in the development of some cervical cancers. Overexpression of *MYC* has been demonstrated in one-third of early invasive carcinomas and some cervical intraepithelial neoplasia (CIN) 3 lesions. In some studies, amplification correlated with poor prognosis in early stage cases (139).

A comprehensive genomic analysis of 115 cervical carcinomas found previously unknown somatic mutations in 79 primary squamous cell carcinomas including recurrent E322K substitutions in the *MAPK1* gene (8%), inactivating mutations in the *HLA-B* gene (9%), and mutations in *EP300* (16%), *FBXW7* (15%), *NFE2L2* (4%), *TP53* (5%), and *ERBB2* (6%) (140). Somatic mutations in *ELF3* (13%) and *CBFB* (8%) were noted in 24 adenocarcinomas. Squamous cell carcinomas have higher frequencies of somatic nucleotide substitutions occurring at cytosines preceded by thymines than adenocarcinomas. Gene expression levels at HPV integration sites were statistically significantly higher in tumors with HPV integration compared with the same genes in tumors without viral integration at the same site.

Gene silencing due to promoter hypermethylation also may play a role in cervical carcinogenesis (141). In this regard, expression of the *RASSF1A* gene on chromosome 3p21 is frequently lost in cervical cancers, particularly adenocarcinomas (142). The function of this gene is not completely understood, but is thought to be involved in *ras*-mediated signal transduction pathways. Hypermethylation of genes associated with programmed cell death (apoptosis) and tumor suppressor genes has also been described in cervical cancers.

Gestational Trophoblastic Disease

The genetic alterations that underlie gestational trophoblastic disease have been elucidated to a great extent. The most prominent feature of these tumors is an imbalance of parental chromosomes. In partial moles, this involves an extra haploid copy of one set of paternal chromosomes (XXY, XXX, or XYY). Complete moles generally are characterized by two pairs of one paternal haploid set of chromosomes (XX) and an absence of maternal chromosomes, while a minority are (XY) due to dispermy. Although the risk of repeat molar pregnancy is only about 1%, women who have had two molar pregnancies have about a 25% risk of developing another mole. Although this suggests a hereditary defect that affects gametogenesis, this remains speculative. Thus far, there is no convincing evidence that damage to specific tumor suppressor genes or oncogenes contributes to the development of gestational trophoblastic disease. However, the presence of two identical copies of each chromosome in most complete moles could facilitate transformation due to increased or decreased expression of imprinted genes involved in growth regulatory pathways. In addition, inactivation of a tumor suppressor gene on a paternal chromosome that might not normally be manifest because of the presence of a wild-type allele on the maternal chromosome could become significant in cells with two copies of the same haploid paternal genome.

The occurrence of recurrent molar pregnancy and familial aggregation in some reports suggests that genetic predisposition plays a role in some cases. Genetic mapping studies in families with multiple affected individuals identified a locus on chromosome 19q13.4, and subsequently causative mutations in the NLRP7 gene were identified (143). The mutations segregated in the studied families and each patient had two defective alleles, each inherited from one parent as expected for an autosomal recessive disease. About 42 different mutations have been described, and about 65% are truncating and 35% missense. NLRP7 and other genes in the NLRP family may also be associated with other forms of recurrent pregnancy loss in addition to molar pregnancies.

It is hypothesized that oocytes from patients with loss of NLRP7 function may be defective at several levels and are not able to sustain early embryonic development (144). Consequently, the embryos stop developing very early in these conceptions. Because these patients also have decreased cytokine secretion due to loss of NLRP7, they may fail to mount an appropriate inflammatory response to reject these arrested pregnancies as normal women would. As a result, the retention of these dead pregnancies with no embryos to later gestational stages leads to the hydropic degeneration of chorionic villi. This, combined with the potential role of NLRP7 mutations in enhancing proliferation, may lead to the three fundamental aspects of moles: aberrant human pregnancies with no embryo, abnormal excessive trophoblastic proliferation, and hydropic degeneration of CV. Discovery of NLRP7 facilitates the potential for genetic testing and counseling in patients with familial or recurrent molar pregnancies.

Microarray studies have identified several genes that are differentially expressed compared with normal villi, particularly genes associated with cellular apoptosis, immune suppression, and cell invasion (145,146). In one study in which genomic techniques were used to compare gene expression between moles that spontaneously regressed and those that subsequently developed, metastatic gestational trophoblastic neoplasia (GTN) identified 16 differentially expressed transcripts (146). Downregulation of ferritin light polypeptide (*FTL*) and insulin-like growth factor–binding protein 1 (*IGFBP1*) was confirmed in cases that subsequently developed GTN compared with those that regressed. Studies have also suggested that changes in expression of genes involved in apoptosis, such as greater expression of the antiapoptotic gene *Mcl-1*, may be involved in progression of a molar pregnancy requiring chemotherapy (147).

References

1. DeVita Jr, VT, Lawrence TS, Rosenberg SA (eds). *DeVita, Hellman, and Rosenberg's Cancer: Principles & Practice of Oncology*, 10th Ed. Philadelphia, PA: Wolters Kluwer; 2015.
2. Vogelstein B, Papadopoulos N, Velculescu VE, et al. Cancer genome landscapes. *Science*. 2013;339:1546–1558.
3. Lawrence MS, Stojanov P, Mermel CH, et al. Discovery and saturation analysis of cancer genes across 21 tumour types. *Nature*. 2014;505:495–501.
4. Hoadley KA, Yau C, Wolf DM, et al. Multiplatform analysis of 12 cancer types reveals molecular classification within and across tissues of origin. *Cell*. 2014;158:929–944.
5. Alexandrov LB, Nik-Zainal S, Wedge DC, et al. Signatures of mutational processes in human cancer. *Nature*. 2013;500:415–421.
6. Ciriello G, Miller ML, Aksoy BA, et al. Emerging landscape of oncogenic signatures across human cancers. *Nat Genet*. 2013;45:1127–1133.
7. Bowtell DD, Bohm S, Ahmed AA, et al. Rethinking ovarian cancer II: reducing mortality from high-grade serous ovarian cancer. *Nat Rev Cancer*. 2015;15:668–679.
8. Meric-Bernstam F, Brusco L, Shaw K, et al. Feasibility of large-scale genomic testing to facilitate enrollment onto genomically matched clinical trials. *J Clin Oncol*. 2015;33:2753–2762.
9. Diaz LA Jr, Bardelli A. Liquid biopsies: genotyping circulating tumor DNA. *J Clin Oncol*. 2014;32:579–586.
10. Kinde I, Bettegowda C, Wang Y, et al. Evaluation of DNA from the Papanicolaou test to detect ovarian and endometrial cancers. *Sci Transl Med*. 2013;5:167ra4.
11. Li Y, Laterra J. Cancer stem cells: distinct entities or dynamically regulated phenotypes? *Cancer Res*. 2012;72:576–580.
12. Kumar A, Petri ET, Halmos B, et al. Structure and clinical relevance of the epidermal growth factor receptor in human cancer. *J Clin Oncol*. 2008;26:1742–1751.
13. Ho CL, Kurman RJ, Dehari R, et al. Mutations of BRAF and KRAS precede the development of ovarian serous borderline tumors. *Cancer Res*. 2004;64:6915–6918.
14. Courtney KD, Corcoran RB, Engelman JA. The PI3K pathway as drug target in human cancer. *J Clin Oncol*. 2010;28:1075–1083.
15. Ahmed AA, Etemadmoghadam D, Temple J, et al. Driver mutations in TP53 are ubiquitous in high grade serous carcinoma of the ovary. *J Pathol*. 2010;221:49–56.
16. Ran FA, Hsu PD, Wright J, et al. Genome engineering using the CRISPR-Cas9 system. *Nat Protoc*. 2013;8:2281–2308.
17. Berger AH, Pandolfi PP. Cancer susceptibility syndromes. In: DeVita VT, Lawrence DK, Rosenberg SA, eds. *DeVita, Hellman, and Rosenberg's Cancer: Principles & Practice of Oncology, 9e*. Philadelphia, PA: Lippincott, Williams, and Wilkins; 2011:161–170.
18. Wijnen J, de Leeuw W, Vasen H, et al. Familial endometrial cancer in female carriers of MSH6 germline mutations. *Nat Genet*. 1999;23:142–144.
19. Park JS, Jeon EK, Chun SH, et al. ERCC1 (excision repair cross-complementation group 1) expression as a predictor for response of neoadjuvant chemotherapy for FIGO stage 2B uterine cervix cancer. *Gynecol Oncol*. 2011;120:275–279.
20. The Cancer Genome Atlas Research Network. Integrated genomic analysis of endometrial cancer. *Nature*. 2013;497:67–73.
21. Moynahan ME. The cancer connection: BRCA1 and BRCA2 tumor suppression in mice and humans. *Oncogene*. 2002;21:8994–9007.

22. Song H, Dicks E, Ramus SJ, et al. Contribution of germline mutations in the RAD51B, RAD51C, and RAD51D genes to ovarian cancer in the population. *J Clin Oncol.* 2015;33:2901–2907.
23. Ramus SJ, Song H, Dicks E, et al. Germline mutations in the BRIP1, BARD1, PALB2, and NBN genes in women with ovarian cancer. *J Natl Cancer Inst.* 2015;107(11). pii: djv214. doi:10.1093/jnci/djv214.
24. Salvesen HB, MacDonald N, Ryan A, et al. Methylation of hMLH1 in a population-based series of endometrial carcinomas. *Clin Cancer Res.* 2000;6:3607–3613.
25. Kanaya T, Kyo S, Maida Y, et al. Frequent hypermethylation of MLH1 promoter in normal endometrium of patients with endometrial cancers. *Oncogene.* 2003;22:2352–2360.
26. Baloglu H, Cannizzaro LA, Jones J, et al. Atypical endometrial hyperplasia shares genomic abnormalities with endometrioid carcinoma by comparative genomic hybridization. *Hum Pathol.* 2001;32:615–622.
27. Kiechle M, Hinrichs M, Jacobsen A, et al. Genetic imbalances in precursor lesions of endometrial cancer detected by comparative genomic hybridization. *Am J Pathol.* 2000;156:1827–1833.
28. Risinger JI, Maxwell GL, Chandramouli GV, et al. Microarray analysis reveals distinct gene expression profiles among different histologic types of endometrial cancer. *Cancer Res.* 2003;63:6–11.
29. Mutter GL, Baak JP, Fitzgerald JT, et al. Global expression changes of constitutive and hormonally regulated genes during endometrial neoplastic transformation. *Gynecol Oncol.* 2001;83:177–185.
30. Lukes AS, Kohler MF, Pieper CF, et al. Multivariable analysis of DNA ploidy, p53, and HER-2/neu as prognostic factors in endometrial cancer. *Cancer.* 1994;73:2380–2385.
31. Kohler MF, Berchuck A, Davidoff AM, et al. Overexpression and mutation of p53 in endometrial carcinoma. *Cancer Res.* 1992;52:1622–1627.
32. Hamel NW, Sebo TJ, Wilson TO, et al. Prognostic value of p53 and proliferating cell nuclear antigen expression in endometrial carcinoma. *Cancer Res.* 1996;62:192–198.
33. Tashiro H, Blazes MS, Wu R, et al. Mutations in PTEN are frequent in endometrial carcinoma but rare in other common gynecologic malignancies. *Cancer Res.* 1997;57:3935–3940.
34. Kanamori Y, Kigawa J, Itamochi H, et al. Correlation between loss of PTEN expression and Akt phosphorylation in endometrial carcinoma. *Clin Cancer Res.* 2001;7:892–895.
35. Risinger JI, Hayes K, Maxwell GL, et al. *PTEN* mutation in endometrial cancers is associated with favorable clinical and pathologic characteristics. *Clin Cancer Res.* 1998;4:3005–3010.
36. Milner J, Ponder B, Hughes-Davies L, et al. Transcriptional activation functions in BRCA2. *Nature.* 1997;386:772–773.
37. Mutter GL, Ince TA, Baak JP, et al. Molecular identification of latent precancers in histologically normal endometrium. *Cancer Res.* 2001;61:4311–4314.
38. Berchuck A, Rodriguez G, Kinney RB, et al. Overexpression of HER-2/neu in endometrial cancer is associated with advanced stage disease. *Am J Obstet Gynecol.* 1991;164:15–21.
39. Santin AD, Bellone S, Van SS, et al. Determination of HER2/neu status in uterine serous papillary carcinoma: comparative analysis of immunohistochemistry and fluorescence in situ hybridization. *Gynecol Oncol.* 2005;98:24–30.
40. Fleming GF, Sill MW, Darcy KM, et al. Phase II trial of trastuzumab in women with advanced or recurrent, HER2-positive endometrial carcinoma: a Gynecologic Oncology Group study. *Gynecol Oncol.* 2010;116:15–20.
41. Black JD, Lopez S, Cocco E, et al. PIK3CA oncogenic mutations represent a major mechanism of resistance to trastuzumab in HER2/neu overexpressing uterine serous carcinomas. *Br J Cancer.* 2015;113:1020–1026.
42. Ignar-Trowbridge D, Risinger JI, Dent GA, et al. Mutations of the Ki-*ras* oncogene in endometrial carcinoma. *Am J Obstet Gynecol.* 1992;167:227–232.
43. Enomoto T, Fujita M, Inoue M, et al. Alterations of the p53 tumor suppressor gene and its association with activation of the c-K-*ras*-2 protooncogene in premalignant and malignant lesions of the human uterine endometrium. *Cancer Res.* 1993;53:1883–1888.
44. Mutter GL, Wada H, Faquin WC, et al. K-ras mutations appear in the premalignant phase of both microsatellite stable and unstable endometrial carcinogenesis. *Mol Pathol.* 1999;52:257–262.
45. Oda K, Stokoe D, Taketani Y, et al. High frequency of coexistent mutations of PIK3CA and PTEN genes in endometrial carcinoma. *Cancer Res.* 2005;65:10669–10673.
46. Hayes MP, Wang H, Espinal-Witter R, et al. PIK3CA and PTEN mutations in uterine endometrioid carcinoma and complex atypical hyperplasia. *Clin Cancer Res.* 2006;12:5932–5935.
47. Rudd ML, Price JC, Fogoros S, et al. A unique spectrum of somatic PIK3CA (p110alpha) mutations within primary endometrial carcinomas. *Clin Cancer Res.* 2011;17:1331–1340.
48. Cheung LW, Hennessy BT, Li J, et al. High frequency of PIK3R1 and PIK3R2 mutations in endometrial cancer elucidates a novel mechanism for regulation of PTEN protein stability. *Cancer Discov.* 2011;1:170–185.
49. Oza AM, Elit L, Tsao MS, et al. Phase II study of temsirolimus in women with recurrent or metastatic endometrial cancer: a trial of the NCIC Clinical Trials Group. *J Clin Oncol.* 2011;29:3278–3285.
50. Janku F, Wheler JJ, Westin SN, et al. PI3K/AKT/mTOR inhibitors in patients with breast and gynecologic malignancies harboring PIK3CA mutations. *J Clin Oncol.* 2012;30:777–782.
51. Moreno-Bueno G, Hardisson D, Sanchez C, et al. Abnormalities of the APC/beta-catenin pathway in endometrial cancer. *Oncogene.* 2002;21:7981–7990.
52. Pollock PM, Gartside MG, Dejeza LC, et al. Frequent activating FGFR2 mutations in endometrial carcinomas parallel germline mutations associated with craniosynostosis and skeletal dysplasia syndromes. *Oncogene.* 2007;26(50):7158–7162.
53. Byron SA, Gartside M, Powell MA, et al. FGFR2 point mutations in 466 endometrioid endometrial tumors: relationship with MSI, KRAS, PIK3CA, CTNNB1 mutations and clinicopathological features. *PLoS One.* 2012;7:e30801.
54. Brooks AN, Kilgour E, Smith PD. Molecular pathways: fibroblast growth factor signaling: a new therapeutic opportunity in cancer. *Clin Cancer Res.* 2012;18:1855–1862.
55. Williams JA Jr, Wang ZR, Parrish RS, et al. Fluorescence in situ hybridization analysis of HER-2/neu, c-myc, and p53 in endometrial cancer. *Exp Mol Pathol.* 1999;67:135–143.
56. Piscuoglio S, Burke KA, Ng CK, et al. Uterine adenosarcomas are mesenchymal neoplasms. *J Pathol.* 2016;238:381–388.
57. Lee CH, Marino-Enriquez A, Ou W, et al. The clinicopathologic features of YWHAE-FAM22 endometrial stromal sarcomas: a histologically high-grade and clinically aggressive tumor. *Am J Surg Pathol.* 2012;36:641–653.
58. The Cancer Genome Atlas Research Network. Integrated genomic analyses of ovarian carcinoma. *Nature.* 2011;474:609–615.
59. Kurman RJ, Shih I. Molecular pathogenesis and extraovarian origin of epithelial ovarian cancer—shifting the paradigm. *Hum Pathol.* 2011;42:918–931.
60. Mehra K, Mehrad M, Ning G, et al. STICS, SCOUTs and p53 signatures; a new language for pelvic serous carcinogenesis. *Front Biosci (Elite Ed).* 2011;3:625–634.
61. McBride DJ, Etemadmoghadam D, Cooke SL, et al. Tandem duplication of chromosomal segments is common in ovarian and breast cancer genomes. *J Pathol.* 2012;227:446–455.
62. Tashiro H, Niyazaki K, Okamura H, et al. c-*myc* overexpression in human primary ovarian tumors: its relevance to tumor progression. *Int J Cancer.* 1992;50:828–833.
63. Etemadmoghadam D, George J, Cowin PA, et al. Amplicon-dependent CCNE1 expression is critical for clonogenic survival after cisplatin treatment and is correlated with 20q11 gain in ovarian cancer. *PLoS One.* 2010;5:e15498.
64. Rosen DG, Yang G, Deavers MT, et al. Cyclin E expression is correlated with tumor progression and predicts a poor prognosis in patients with ovarian carcinoma. *Cancer.* 2006;106:1925–1932.
65. Bellacosa A, de Feo D, Godwin AK, et al. Molecular alterations of the AKT2 oncogene in ovarian and breast carcinomas. *Int J Cancer.* 1995;64:280–285.
66. Shayesteh L, Lu Y, Kuo WL, et al. PIK3CA is implicated as an oncogene in ovarian cancer. *Nat Genet.* 1999;21:99–102.
67. Etemadmoghadam D, Weir BA, Au-Yeung G, et al. Synthetic lethality between CCNE1 amplification and loss of BRCA1. *Proc Natl Acad Sci U S A.* 2013;110:19489–19494.
68. Etemadmoghadam D, Au-Yeung G, Wall M, et al. Resistance to CDK2 inhibitors is associated with selection of polyploid cells in CCNE1-amplified ovarian cancer. *Clin Cancer Res.* 2013;19:5960–5971.
69. Flesken-Nikitin A, Choi KC, Eng JP, Shmidt EN, et al. Induction of carcinogenesis by concurrent inactivation of p53 and Rb1 in the mouse ovarian surface epithelium. *Cancer Res.* 2003;63:3459–3463.
70. Slamon DJ, Godolphin W, Jones LA, et al. Studies of HER-2/*neu* protooncogene in human breast and ovarian cancer. *Science.* 1989;244:707–712.
71. Slamon D, Eiermann W, Robert N, et al. Adjuvant trastuzumab in HER2-positive breast cancer. *N Engl J Med.* 2011;365:1273–1283.
72. Bookman MA, Darcy KM, Clarke-Pearson D, et al. Evaluation of monoclonal humanized anti-HER2 antibody, trastuzumab, in patients with recurrent or refractory ovarian or primary peritoneal carcinoma with

overexpression of HER2: a phase II trial of the Gynecologic Oncology Group. *J Clin Oncol.* 2003;21:283–290.
73. Schultz DC, Vanderveer L, Buetow KH, et al. Characterization of chromosome 9 in human ovarian neoplasia identifies frequent genetic imbalance on 9q and rare alterations involving 9p, including CDKN2. *Cancer Res.* 1995;55:2150–2157.
74. McCluskey LL, Chen C, Delgadillo E, et al. Differences in p16 gene methylation and expression in benign and malignant ovarian tumors. *Cancer Res.* 1999;72:87–92.
75. Liu Z, Wang LE, Wang L, et al. Methylation and messenger RNA expression of p15INK4b but not p16INK4a are independent risk factors for ovarian cancer. *Clin Cancer Res.* 2005;11:4968–4976.
76. Levesque MA, Katsaros D, Massobrio M, et al. Evidence for a dose-response effect between p53 (but not p21WAF1/Cip1) protein concentrations, survival, and responsiveness in patients with epithelial ovarian cancer treated with platinum-based chemotherapy. *Clin Cancer Res.* 2000;6:3260–3270.
77. Korkolopoulou P, Vassilopoulos I, Konstantinidou AE, et al. The combined evaluation of p27Kip1 and Ki-67 expression provides independent information on overall survival of ovarian carcinoma patients. *Cancer Res.* 2002;85:404–414.
78. Rosen DG, Yang G, Cai KQ, et al. Subcellular localization of p27kip1 expression predicts poor prognosis in human ovarian cancer. *Clin Cancer Res.* 2005;11:632–637.
79. Vang R, Levine DA, Soslow RA, et al. Molecular alterations of TP53 are a defining feature of ovarian high-grade serous carcinoma: a rereview of cases lacking TP53 mutations in The Cancer Genome Atlas Ovarian Study. *Int J Gynecol Pathol.* 2016;35:48–55.
80. Kanchi KL, Johnson KJ, Lu C, et al. Integrated analysis of germline and somatic variants in ovarian cancer. *Nat Commun.* 2014;5:3156.
81. Rubin SC, Benjamin I, Behbakht K, et al. Clinical and pathological features of ovarian cancer in women with germ-line mutations of BRCA1. *N Engl J Med.* 1996;335:1413–146.
82. Bolton KL, Chenevix-Trench G, Goh C, et al. Association between BRCA1 and BRCA2 mutations and survival in women with invasive epithelial ovarian cancer. *JAMA.* 2012;307:382–390.
83. Norquist B, Wurz KA, Pennil CC, et al. Secondary somatic mutations restoring BRCA1/2 predict chemotherapy resistance in hereditary ovarian carcinomas. *J Clin Oncol.* 2011;29:3008–3015.
84. Candido-dos-Reis FJ, Song H, Goode EL, et al. Germline mutation in BRCA1 or BRCA2 and ten-year survival for women diagnosed with epithelial ovarian cancer. *Clin Cancer Res.* 2015;21:652–657.
85. Scott CL, Swisher EM, Kaufmann SH. Poly (ADP-ribose) polymerase inhibitors: recent advances and future development. *J Clin Oncol.* 2015;33:1397–1406.
86. Banerjee S, Kaye SB, Ashworth A. Making the best of PARP inhibitors in ovarian cancer. *Nat Rev Clin Oncol.* 2010;7:508–519.
87. Konstantinopoulos PA, Spentzos D, Karlan BY, et al. Gene expression profile of BRCAness that correlates with responsiveness to chemotherapy and with outcome in patients with epithelial ovarian cancer. *J Clin Oncol.* 2010;28:3555–3561.
88. Pennington KP, Walsh T, Harrell MI, et al. Germline and somatic mutations in homologous recombination genes predict platinum response and survival in ovarian, fallopian tube, and peritoneal carcinomas. *Clin Cancer Res.* 2014;20:764–775.
89. Kang J, D'Andrea AD, Kozono D. A DNA repair pathway-focused score for prediction of outcomes in ovarian cancer treated with platinum-based chemotherapy. *J Natl Cancer Inst.* 2012;104:670–681.
90. Patch AM, Christie EL, Etemadmoghadam D, et al. Whole-genome characterization of chemoresistant ovarian cancer. *Nature.* 2015;521: 489–494.
91. Bashashati A, Ha G, Tone A, et al. Distinct evolutionary trajectories of primary high-grade serous ovarian cancers revealed through spatial mutational profiling. *J Pathol.* 2013;231:21–34.
92. Liu Y, Yasukawa M, Chen K, et al. Association of somatic mutations of ADAMTS genes with chemotherapy sensitivity and survival in high-grade serous ovarian carcinoma. *JAMA Oncol.* 2015;1:486–494.
93. Schwartz DR, Kardia SL, Shedden KA, et al. Gene expression in ovarian cancer reflects both morphology and biological behavior, distinguishing clear cell from other poor- prognosis ovarian carcinomas. *Cancer Res.* 2002;62:4722–4729.
94. Bonome T, Lee JY, Park DC, et al. Expression profiling of serous low malignant potential, low-grade, and high-grade tumors of the ovary. *Cancer Res.* 2005;65:10602–10612.
95. Shridhar V, Lee J, Pandita A, et al. Genetic analysis of early- versus late-stage ovarian tumors. *Cancer Res.* 2001;61:5895–5904.
96. Berchuck A, Iversen ES, Luo J, et al. Microarray analysis of early stage serous ovarian cancers shows profiles predictive of favorable outcome. *Clin Cancer Res.* 2009;15:2448–2455.
97. Tothill RW, Tinker AV, George J, et al. Novel molecular subtypes of serous and endometrioid ovarian cancer linked to clinical outcome. *Clin Cancer Res.* 2008;14:5198–5208.
98. Verhaak RG, Tamayo P, Yang JY, et al. Prognostically relevant gene signatures of high-grade serous ovarian carcinoma. *J Clin Invest.* 2013;123:517–525.
99. Riester M, Wei W, Waldron L, et al. Risk prediction for late-stage ovarian cancer by meta-analysis of 1525 patient samples. *J Natl Cancer Inst.* 2014;106. doi: 10.1093/jnci/dju048.
100. Mok SCH, Bell DA, Knapp RC, et al. Mutation of K-*ras* protooncogene in human ovarian epithelial tumors of borderline malignancy. *Cancer Res.* 1993;53:1489–1492.
101. Singer G, Oldt R III, Cohen Y, et al. Mutations in BRAF and KRAS characterize the development of low-grade ovarian serous carcinoma. *J Natl Cancer Inst.* 2003;95:484–486.
102. Tsang YT, Deavers MT, Sun CC, et al. KRAS (but not BRAF) mutations in ovarian serous borderline tumour are associated with recurrent low-grade serous carcinoma. *J Pathol.* 2013;231:449–456.
103. Hunter SM, Anglesio MS, Ryland GL, et al. Molecular profiling of low grade serous ovarian tumours identifies novel candidate driver genes. *Oncotarget.* 2015;6:37663–37677.
104. Grisham RN, Sylvester BE, Won H, et al. Extreme outlier analysis identifies occult mitogen-activated protein kinase pathway mutations in patients with low-grade serous ovarian cancer. *J Clin Oncol.* 2015;33:4099–4105.
105. Wiegand KC, Shah SP, Al-Agha OM, et al. ARID1A mutations in endometriosis-associated ovarian carcinomas. *N Engl J Med.* 2010;363:1532–1543.
106. Anglesio MS, Carey MS, Kobel M, et al. Clear cell carcinoma of the ovary: a report from the first Ovarian Clear Cell Symposium, June 24th, 2010. *Gynecol Oncol.* 2011;121:407–415.
107. Jones S, Wang TL, Shih I, et al. Frequent mutations of chromatin remodeling gene ARID1A in ovarian clear cell carcinoma. *Science.* 2010;330:228–231.
108. Anglesio MS, Bashashati A, Wang YK, et al. Multifocal endometriotic lesions associated with cancer are clonal and carry a high mutation burden. *J Pathol.* 2015;236:201–209.
109. McConechy MK, Anglesio MS, Kalloger SE, et al. Subtype-specific mutation of PPP2R1A in endometrial and ovarian carcinomas. *J Pathol.* 2011;223:567–573.
110. Obata K, Morland SJ, Watson RH, et al. Frequent PTEN/MMAC mutations in endometrioid but not serous or mucinous epithelial ovarian tumors. *Cancer Res.* 1998;58:2095–2097.
111. Wu R, Zhai Y, Fearon ER, et al. Diverse mechanisms of beta-catenin deregulation in ovarian endometrioid adenocarcinomas. *Cancer Res.* 2001;61:8247–8255.
112. Dinulescu DM, Ince TA, Quade BJ, et al. Role of K-ras and Pten in the development of mouse models of endometriosis and endometrioid ovarian cancer. *Nat Med.* 2005;11:63–70.
113. McConechy MK, Ding J, Senz J, et al. Ovarian and endometrial endometrioid carcinomas have distinct CTNNB1 and PTEN mutation profiles. *Mod Pathol.* 2014;27:128–134.
114. Lin WM, Forgacs E, Warshal DP, et al. Loss of heterozygosity and mutational analysis of the PTEN/MMAC1 gene in synchronous endometrial and ovarian carcinomas. *Clin Cancer Res.* 1998;4:2577–2583.
115. Guerra F, Kurelac I, Magini P, et al. Mitochondrial DNA genotyping reveals synchronous nature of simultaneously detected endometrial and ovarian cancers. *Gynecol Oncol.* 2011;122:457–458.
116. Schultheis AM, Ng CK, De Filippo MR, et al. Massively parallel sequencing-based clonality analysis of synchronous endometrioid endometrial and ovarian carcinomas. *J Natl Cancer Inst.* 2016;108(6):djv427. doi:10.1093/jnci/djv427.
117. Anglesio MS, Wang YK, Maassen M, et al. Synchronous endometrial and ovarian carcinomas: evidence of clonality. *J Natl Cancer Inst.* 2016;108(6):djv428. doi:10.1093/jnci/djv428.
118. Anglesio MS, Kommoss S, Tolcher MC, et al. Molecular characterization of mucinous ovarian tumours supports a stratified treatment approach with HER2 targeting in 19% of carcinomas. *J Pathol.* 2013;229:111–120.
119. Ryland GL, Hunter SM, Doyle MA, et al. Mutational landscape of mucinous ovarian carcinoma and its neoplastic precursors. *Genome Med.* 2015;7:87.
120. Mackenzie R, Kommoss S, Winterhoff BJ, et al. Targeted deep sequencing of mucinous ovarian tumors reveals multiple overlapping RAS-pathway activating mutations in borderline and cancerous neoplasms. *BMC Cancer.* 2015;15:415.

121. Shah SP, Kobel M, Senz J, et al. Mutation of FOXL2 in granulosa-cell tumors of the ovary. *N Engl J Med*. 2009;360:2719–2729.
122. Heravi-Moussavi A, Anglesio MS, Cheng SW, et al. Recurrent somatic DICER1 mutations in nonepithelial ovarian cancers. *N Engl J Med*. 2012;366:234–242.
123. Chen J, Wang Y, McMonechy MK, et al. Recurrent DICER1 hotspot mutations in endometrial tumours and their impact on microRNA biogenesis. *J Pathol*. 2015;15:415.
124. Merritt WM, Lin YG, Han LY, et al. Dicer, Drosha, and outcomes in patients with ovarian cancer. *N Engl J Med*. 2008;359:2641–2650.
125. Scheffner M, Munger K, Byrne JC, et al. The state of the p53 and retinoblastoma gene in human cervical carcinoma cell lines. *Proc Natl Acad Sci U S A*. 1991;88:5523–5527.
126. Werness BA, Levine AJ, Howley PM. Association of human papillomavirus types 16 and 18 E6 proteins with p53. *Science*. 1990;248:76–79.
127. de Boer MA, Jordanova ES, Kenter GG, et al. High human papillomavirus oncogene mRNA expression and not viral DNA load is associated with poor prognosis in cervical cancer patients. *Clin Cancer Res*. 2007;13:132–138.
128. Wang SS, Trunk M, Schiffman M, et al. Validation of p16INK4a as a marker of oncogenic human papillomavirus infection in cervical biopsies from a population-based cohort in Costa Rica. *Cancer Epidemiol Biomarkers Prev*. 2004;13:1355–1360.
129. Parker MF, Arroyo GF, Geradts J, et al. Molecular characterization of adenocarcinoma of the cervix. *Cancer Res*. 1997;64:242–251.
130. Narayan G, Pulido HA, Koul S, et al. Genetic analysis identifies putative tumor suppressor sites at 2q35-q36.1 and 2q36.3-q37.1 involved in cervical cancer progression. *Oncogene*. 2003;22:3489–3499.
131. Umayahara K, Numa F, Suehiro Y, et al. Comparative genomic hybridization detects genetic alterations during early stages of cervical cancer progression. *Genes Chromosomes Cancer*. 2002;33:98–102.
132. Yang YC, Shyong WY, Chang MS, et al. Frequent gain of copy number on the long arm of chromosome 3 in human cervical adenocarcinoma. *Cancer Genet Cytogenet*. 2001;131:48–53.
133. Lando M, Holden M, Bergersen LC, et al. Gene dosage, expression, and ontology analysis identifies driver genes in the carcinogenesis and chemoradioresistance of cervical cancer. *PLoS Genet*. 2009;5:e1000719.
134. Lin WM, Michalopulos EA, Dhurander N, et al. Allelic loss and microsatellite alterations of chromosome 3p14.2 are more frequent in recurrent cervical dysplasias. *Clin Cancer Res*. 2000;6:1410–1414.
135. Kirchhoff M, Rose H, Petersen BL, et al. Comparative genomic hybridization reveals a recurrent pattern of chromosomal aberrations in severe dysplasia/carcinoma in situ of the cervix and in advanced-stage cervical carcinoma. *Genes Chromosomes Cancer*. 1999;24:144–150.
136. Huang LW, Chao SL, Chen TJ. Reduced Fhit expression in cervical carcinoma: correlation with tumor progression and poor prognosis. *Cancer Res*. 2003;90:331–337.
137. Connolly DC, Greenspan DL, Wu R, et al. Loss of fhit expression in invasive cervical carcinomas and intraepithelial lesions associated with invasive disease. *Clin Cancer Res*. 2000;6:3505–3510.
138. Krivak TC, McBroom JW, Seidman J, et al. Abnormal fragile histidine triad (FHIT) expression in advanced cervical carcinoma: a poor prognostic factor. *Cancer Res*. 2001;61:4382–4385.
139. Bourhis J, Le MG, Barrois M, et al. Prognostic value of c-myc proto-oncogene overexpression in early invasive carcinoma of the cervix. *J Clin Oncol*. 1990;8:1789–1796.
140. Ojesina AI, Lichtenstein L, Freeman SS, et al. Landscape of genomic alterations in cervical carcinomas. *Nature*. 2014;506:371–375.
141. Dong SM, Kim HS, Rha SH, et al. Promoter hypermethylation of multiple genes in carcinoma of the uterine cervix. *Clin Cancer Res*. 2001;7:1982–1986.
142. Kuzmin I, Liu L, Dammann R, et al. Inactivation of RAS association domain family 1A gene in cervical carcinomas and the role of human papillomavirus infection. *Cancer Res*. 2003;63:1888–1893.
143. Deveault C, Qian JH, Chebaro W, et al. NLRP7 mutations in women with diploid androgenetic and triploid moles: a proposed mechanism for mole formation. *Hum Mol Genet*. 2009;18:888–897.
144. Slim R, Wallace EP. NLRP7 and the genetics of hydatidiform moles: recent advances and new challenges. *Front Immunol*. 2013;4:242.
145. Kim SJ, Lee SY, Lee C, et al. Differential expression profiling of genes in a complete hydatidiform mole using cDNA microarray analysis. *Gynecol Oncol* 2006;103:654–660.
146. Feng HC, Tsao SW, Ngan HY, et al. Differential expression of insulin-like growth factor binding protein 1 and ferritin light polypeptide in gestational trophoblastic neoplasia: combined cDNA suppression subtractive hybridization and microarray study. *Cancer*. 2005;104:2409–2416.
147. Fong PY, Xue WC, Ngan HY, et al. Mcl-1 expression in gestational trophoblastic disease correlates with clinical outcome: a differential expression study. *Cancer*. 2005;103:268–276.

CHAPTER 3

Hereditary Gynecologic Cancers

Noah D. Kauff, Andrew Berchuck, and Karen H. Lu

INTRODUCTION

Identifying a woman with gynecologic cancer as having a hereditary cancer syndrome has tremendous implications for both the patient and her family members. Hereditary breast and ovarian cancer syndrome, caused by germline mutations in *BRCA1* or *BRCA2*, and Lynch syndrome, caused by germline mutations in *MLH1, MSH2, MSH6, PMS2, or EPCAM*, are the most common high-penetrance hereditary syndromes that include gynecologic manifestations as part of their tumor spectrum. Other well-characterized high-penetrance syndromes that include gynecologic cancers are Cowden syndrome (*PTEN* germline mutation), Peutz–Jeghers syndrome (*STK11* germline mutation), and Li–Fraumeni syndrome (*TP53* germline mutation) (**Table 3.1**). These high-penetrance syndromes are generally associated with as much as a 6- to 60-fold increased risk of cancer compared to women in the general population. Recently, a number of additional genes, including *BRIP1, RAD51C, RAD51D, PALB2, ATM, CHEK2,* and *NBN,* have been associated with a moderately increased risk (generally on the order of a 2- to 6-fold increased risk) of breast, gynecologic, and in some cases other cancers.

The vast majority of both the high- and moderate-penetrance cancer susceptibility syndromes are caused by mutations in tumor suppressor genes. In order for an individual to develop a cancer associated with one of these syndromes, both the maternally and paternally inherited copy of the relevant gene must be inactivated as described by Knudson's two-hit hypothesis (1). Women with hereditary cancer syndromes have inherited, from either their mother or their father, a nonworking copy of one of the relevant genes and this defect is present in all of their cells. Therefore, in order for cancer to develop in a susceptible tissue through defects in a specific pathway, only the second working copy of the relevant gene needs to be lost. This is why the cancers occur earlier and more frequently than in the general population. This also partly explains why not all individuals with an inherited predisposition develop cancer, as it is possible that the second working copy of the relevant tumor suppressor gene is never lost in a susceptible tissue. Importantly, particularly for the moderate-penetrance cancer susceptibility genes, these genetic changes do not happen in isolation. Rather there is a genetic and environmental background which also clearly plays a role in whether or not an individual who has lost the second working copy of a relevant tumor suppressor gene in a susceptible tissue actually develops cancer.

In recent years, prognostic and therapeutic implications relevant to cancer patients with hereditary cancer syndromes have been discovered, and recommendations for prevention of hereditary cancer have been refined. Given this, there has been increasing emphasis placed on developing guidelines to assist physicians in recognizing those patients for whom genetic counseling and testing may be helpful. These developments will be reviewed in this chapter.

TABLE 3.1. Selected Hereditary Cancer Syndromes with Gynecologic Manifestations

Syndrome	Gene	Chromosome	Predominant Cancers
Hereditary breast/ovarian cancer	*BRCA1*	17q21	Breast, ovary
	BRCA2	13q12	
Lynch syndrome	*MLH1*	3p22.2	Colon, endometrium, ovary, and urinary tract
	MSH2	2p21–16	
	MSH6	2p16	
	PMS2	7p22	
	EPCAM	2p21	
Cowden syndrome	*PTEN*	10q23	Breast, thyroid, and endometrial
Li–Fraumeni syndrome	*TP53*	17p13	Breast, sarcomas, leukemias, and brain
Peutz–Jeghers syndrome	*STK11*	19p13	Colon, breast, gastric, and ovarian SCTAT
Hereditary small cell carcinoma of the ovary, hypercalcemic type	*SMARCA4*	19p13	SCCOHT

SCTAT, sex cord tumor with annular tubules; SCCOHT, small cell carcinoma of the ovary, hypercalcemic type.

HEREDITARY BREAST OVARIAN CANCER SYNDROME

Epidemiology

Of all common solid tumors, ovarian, fallopian tube, and primary peritoneal cancers have the highest proportion caused by heritable germline mutations, with mutations in *BRCA1* and *BRCA2* accounting for the vast majority. When pelvic serous cancer alone is examined, 16% to 18% of unselected patients with high-grade disease reportedly have a deleterious *BRCA1* or *BRCA2* mutation (2,3). In 2011, Zhang and colleagues reported a population-based series of 1,342 invasive ovarian cancers identified in Ontario, Canada, from 1995 to 1999 and from 2002 to 2004. In this series, 135 (18.0%) of 751 patients with serous ovarian cancer had a deleterious *BRCA1* or *BRCA2* mutation (2). Of note, 6.1% of the non-founder mutations identified in this study were large genomic rearrangements not detected on sequencing and discerned only on multiplex ligation-dependent probe amplification (MLPA) testing. Similarly, in 2012, Alsop and colleagues found 118 (16.6%) *BRCA1* and *BRCA2* mutations in 709 patients with incident pelvic serous cancers identified as part of the Australia Ovarian Cancer Study from 2002 to 2006. Notably, 62 (8.3%) of 749 patients without a significant family history had a germline *BRCA* mutation, and 44% of all the mutations identified in the study occurred in the absence of a family history (3).

Given this substantial frequency of mutations in women with pelvic serous cancer irrespective of family history, both the American College of Obstetricians and Gynecologists (ACOG) and the National Comprehensive Cancer Network (NCCN) recommend consideration of testing for *BRCA* mutations in any woman with high-grade serous ovarian cancer if it will impact the care of either the woman or her close family members (4,5).

As noted above, recently, several additional genes have recently been implicated in an inherited predisposition to breast cancer, ovarian cancer, or both. Many of these genes are in the *BRCA1*- and *BRCA2*-dependent homologous recombination (HR) repair pathway. Early studies suggest that these may be associated with as much as a 2- to 6-fold increased risk of cancer compared to women in the general population. In a series from University of Washington and the Gynecologic Oncology Group, of 1,498 patients undergoing primary therapy for high-grade serous epithelial ovarian, fallopian tube, or primary peritoneal cancer, 240 (16.0%) patients had a deleterious mutation in either *BRCA1* or *BRCA2*. Fifty-three (3.5%) patients had deleterious mutations in other tumor suppressor genes potentially associated with ovarian cancer including 22 (1.4%) in *BRIP1*, 9 (0.6%) in *PALB2*, 7 (0.5%) in *RAD51C*, 7 (0.5%) in *RAD51D*, 4 (0.3%) in *PMS2*, 3 (0.2%) in *BARD1*, and 1 (0.1%) in *MSH6*. While the authors also found mutations in a number of other genes, including *CHEK2*, *ATM*, *NBM*, *TP53*, and *RAD50*, none of these were seen to occur more frequently than in unaffected individuals genotyped as part of either the National Heart, Lung, and Blood Exome Sequencing Project or the Exome Aggregation Consortium (6). In a series of two reports evaluating frequency of non-*BRCA* mutations in 3,226 and 3,429 women with invasive epithelial ovarian, and 3,431 and 2,772 population controls, respectively, mutations in *BRIP1*, *RAD 51C*, and *RAD51D* were confirmed to be more frequent in cases than in controls. There was also a suggestion that mutations in *PALB2* were more frequent, but this did not reach statistical significance (7,8). Taken together, there is evidence that *BRIP1*, *RAD51C*, *RAD51D*, and perhaps *PALB2* may be associated with an approximately 2- to 6-fold increased risk of ovarian cancer, though wide confidence intervals for these estimates remain. Similarly, several other studies have examined breast cancer risks associated with genes in the HR repair and related pathways and have found that *ATM*, *CHEK2*, *NBN*, and *PALB2* may be associated with a 3- to 6-fold increased risk of breast cancer (9). To put these risks in perspective, *BRCA1* mutations are associated with an 18- to 36-fold increased risk of developing breast cancer prior to age 50 years and a 30- to 60-fold increased risk of developing ovarian cancer by age 70. Similarly, women with *BRCA2* mutations have a 10- to 19-fold increased risk of early-onset breast cancer and a 6- to 20-fold increased risk of ovarian cancer at any age (10). Given the generally lower relative risk of cancer associated with mutations in these genes compared to *BRCA1* and *BRCA2*, it is not yet known if risks associated with mutations in these other genes are great enough to be considered causative or if loss of function mutations in these genes act more as modifiers of cancer risk.

Pathology

BRCA1- and *BRCA2*-associated cancers appear to be preferentially associated with specific histologic subtypes of ovarian and fallopian tube cancer. In the 2011 report from Zhang et al., *BRCA* mutations were identified in 135 (18.0%) of 751 serous cancers, 26 (9.1%) of 287 endometrioid cancers, and 2 (2.2%) of 91 clear cell cancers (2). Similarly, Norquist et al. found *BRCA* mutations in 240 (16.0%) of 1,498 high-grade serous cancers, 7 (10.9%) of 64 high-grade endometrioid cancers, 4 (6.9%) of 58 clear cell cancers, and 4 (5.7%) of 70 low-grade serous cancers. No *BRCA* mutations were identified in low-grade endometrioid cancers or mucinous tumors (6).

It should be noted that the proportion of non–high-grade serous cancers associated with *BRCA* mutations may be overrepresented in these studies. Reportedly, *BRCA*-associated serous ovarian cancers frequently have a somewhat atypical histologic appearance, in some cases appearing to be "pseudo-endometrioid," or "pseudo-transitional." This can result in misclassification unless serous-specific immunohistochemical (IHC) markers are used (11). This was seen in the 2012 report from Alsop et al. In this population-based series from Australia, *BRCA1* or *BRCA2* mutations were identified in 10 (8.9%) of 119 cancers initially diagnosed as endometrioid. However, 8 of these cancers were subsequently reclassified after immunohistopathology review as serous or unspecified carcinomas, suggesting that the actual rate of *BRCA* mutations in endometrioid ovarian cancer is only 1.7%. Similarly, of the 4 (6.3%) of 63 clear cell cancers shown to have a *BRCA* mutation, 3 were reclassified as high-grade serous with focal clear cell differentiation, suggesting that the actual prevalence of *BRCA* mutations in clear cell ovarian cancer is approximately 1.6% (3).

Natural History of *BRCA*-Associated Ovarian Cancer

Over a dozen studies have reported on differences in outcome between *BRCA*-associated and sporadic ovarian and fallopian tube cancers (12). In one of the first large studies to examine this issue, Chetrit and colleagues reported on an Israeli population-based series including data from 779 Jewish women with invasive epithelial ovarian cancer genotyped for the three Ashkenazi founder mutations. In this series, *BRCA* mutation status was associated with an increase in survival from 37.9 to 53.7 months (13). More recently, investigators from The Cancer Genome Atlas (TCGA) project reported that patients with stage II to IV high-grade serous ovarian or fallopian tube cancer and germline or sporadic mutations in *BRCA1* or *BRCA2* had improved outcome compared to patients without evidence of *BRCA* deficiency (median overall survival 66.5 vs. 41.9 months, $p = 0.0003$) (14). Interestingly, in this series tumors associated with mutations in *BRCA1* or *BRCA2* also had improved outcomes compared to patients with silencing of *BRCA1* due to methylation of the *BRCA1* promoter, suggesting that the mechanism of loss of *BRCA* function may be relevant to the biology and clinical behavior of these tumors.

Until recently, most studies examining the impact of *BRCA* mutations on outcome have analyzed carriers of *BRCA1* mutations and carriers of *BRCA2* mutations together. However, mutations in *BRCA1* and *BRCA2* cause related, but distinct, cancer susceptibility syndromes. Given this, it is possible that response to therapy and clinical outcome may differ between carriers of *BRCA1* mutations and carriers of *BRCA2* mutations. In one of the first studies to examine this issue, Yang et al. reexamined data from the TCGA ovarian project. In this report, patients with *BRCA2*-associated ovarian cancer had markedly better outcome than those with *BRCA* wild-type tumors (HR = 0.33; 95% CI, 0.16 to 0.69). *BRCA1*-associated tumors also appeared to have a somewhat better outcome than *BRCA* wild-type tumors (HR = 0.76; 95% CI, 0.43 to 1.35), but this result did not reach statistical significance (15). More recently, Bolton et al. reported on a pooled series of 3,879 invasive epithelial ovarian cancers genotyped for *BRCA* mutations and found that in a model adjusted for age at diagnosis, stage, grade, and histology, both *BRCA2* (HR = 0.49; 95% CI, 0.39 to 0.61) and *BRCA1* (HR = 0.73; 95% CI, 0.64 to 0.84) had improved outcome compared to *BRCA* wild-type tumors. Tests of heterogeneity also demonstrated that hazard ratio for *BRCA2* mutation carriers was significantly different from the HR for *BRCA1* mutation carriers (16).

Similarly, ovarian cancers associated with mutations in moderate-penetrance genes in the HR pathway may be associated with different natural history depending upon the specific mutated gene. In the recent series from Norquist, ovarian cancer patients with a mutation in a non-*BRCA*-associated HR gene had an intermediate prognosis compared to *BRCA2*-associated ovarian cancers and *BRCA* wild-type ovarian cancers (6).

Given the clear differences in the outcome between *BRCA* mutated and *BRCA* wild-type tumors, several authors have recommended that, at least for participants on clinical trials, we should obtain germline *BRCA* mutation status and stratify outcomes for the presence or absence of mutations (17,18). It also makes sense to stratify outcomes depending upon whether other newly identified moderate-penetrance ovarian cancer–associated genes are also mutated.

Therapeutic Implications

BRCA1 and *BRCA2* are known to be necessary for repair of double strand DNA breaks through HR (19,20). Therefore, tumor cells from *BRCA*-associated ovarian cancers that have no working copy of either *BRCA1* or *BRCA2* are believed to be exquisitely sensitive to agents that induce double strand DNA breaks, such as platinum-based chemotherapy. While this mechanism likely explains at least some of the survival advantage seen in *BRCA*-associated ovarian cancer, until recently knowledge of this information did not provide a new therapeutic opportunity because almost all patients with serous ovarian cancer receive platinum-based chemotherapeutics as part of first-line therapy. In 2005, however, two independent groups hypothesized that the *BRCA*-dependent HR pathway could be stressed by inhibiting poly (ADP-ribose) polymerase (PARP), an enzyme necessary for the repair of single strand DNA breaks (21,22). If this enzyme (and repair of single strand DNA breaks) is inhibited during DNA replication, the advancing replication fork converts single strand DNA breaks into double strand breaks to be repaired by HR. In patients with a germline mutation in *BRCA1* or *BRCA2*, the single nonmutant allele is sufficient to allow repair in non–tumor-associated cells. However, tumor-associated cells have lost both working alleles of either *BRCA1* or *BRCA2* and therefore cannot utilize HR, forcing the cell to use error-prone nonhomologous end joining, which frequently leads to complex rearrangements and eventual apoptosis (23).

The first clinical data supporting the potential utility of PARP inhibitors in *BRCA*-associated tumors were published in 2009 (24). In this Phase I trial, 60 patients, including 22 with either a documented *BRCA1* or *BRCA2* mutation, received increasing doses of a novel PARP inhibitor, olaparib. Radiologic response or stable disease was observed in 11 (9 ovarian and 2 breast cancer) of 19 patients with heavily pretreated *BRCA*-associated ovarian, breast, or prostate cancer. Following this, a large Phase II trial of olaparib in *BRCA*-associated, platinum-resistant ovarian cancer demonstrated tumor response in 60 (31.1%) of 193 participants. Stable disease for ≥8 weeks was also noted in 78 (40%) participants (25). This data, in December 2014, led to accelerated approval in the United States of olaparib monotherapy for women with advanced ovarian cancer with a deleterious germline *BRCA* mutation who have been treated with three or more prior lines of chemotherapy. Olaparib has also been evaluated in the maintenance setting. In 2014, Ledermann et al. (26) published a preplanned analysis to examine the impact of *BRCA* mutation on the results of a randomized Phase II trial evaluating olaparib maintenance versus placebo in the setting of platinum-sensitive recurrent ovarian cancer. In this study, women with *BRCA*-associated ovarian cancer treated with olaparib maintenance after achieving clinical remission following two or more lines of platinum chemotherapy had an improved PFS compared to women treated with placebo (11.2 vs. 4.3 months; HR, 0.18; 95% CI, 0.10 to 0.31). Of note, there was a smaller but still significant difference in PFS between olaparib- and placebo- treated women who were *BRCA* wild type (7.4 vs. 5.5 months; HR, 0.54; 95% CI, 0.34 to 0.85). There was also a suggestion that *BRCA* mutant patients who received olaparib had increased overall survival, but this did not reach statistical significance (HR, 0.73; 95% CI, 0.45 to 1.17). Given the promising results of these trials, there are over half a dozen ongoing or planned Phase III trials of PARP inhibitors in *BRCA*-associated pelvic serous cancer (27). Furthermore, given the substantial frequency in pelvic serous cancer of either: (a) somatic mutations in *BRCA1* or *BRCA2*; (b) germline mutations in other genes associated with HR; or (c) epigenetic silencing of *BRCA1* through methylation of the *BRCA1* promoter (14), PARP inhibitors are also being actively investigated for treatment of ovarian cancer without germline *BRCA* mutations (28).

Genetic Counseling for Hereditary Breast and Ovarian Cancer Syndrome

Approximately 1 in 345 to 1 in 800 women have a *BRCA1* or *BRCA2* mutation associated with hereditary breast and ovarian cancer (29,30). Hereditary breast and ovarian cancer syndrome is seen in all racial and ethnic groups. However, due to the phenomenon of genetic drift, several racial and ethnic groups have experienced a marked increase in the population frequency of specific mutations, known as founder mutations. Best known of the founder mutations are the 185delAG and 5382insC mutations in *BRCA1* and the 6174delT mutation in *BRCA2* that are collectively found in 1 of 40 individuals of Eastern European Jewish (Ashkenazi) heritage. Increased incidence of *BRCA* mutations has also been seen in individuals of Icelandic, Swedish, Dutch, Polish, French Canadian, and Hungarian descent.

The vast majority of deleterious mutations in *BRCA1* and *BRCA2* are nonsense mutations that lead to a premature stop codon and a truncated protein. While the majority of protein-truncating mutations are detectable by direct sequencing of *BRCA1* and *BRCA2*, approximately 6% to 18% of deleterious mutations are caused by large genomic deletions or rearrangements that will not be identified on direct sequencing and must instead be screened for by methods such as MLPA (31–33). Additionally, depending on ethnicity, as many as 6% to 17% of individuals undergoing direct sequencing of *BRCA1* or *BRCA2* will have a missense mutation that causes a single amino acid substitution in the protein (34). These missense mutations are termed variants of uncertain significance, as it is frequently not possible to ascertain whether the protein can tolerate the resulting amino acid substitution or if the substitution will cause abrogation of protein function.

Several recent developments have fundamentally changed the manner in which genetic testing for breast and ovarian cancer is offered. The first of these developments was the Supreme Court of the United States ruling in June 2013 that: (a) segments of DNA that make up human genes were "products of nature" and not patentable under section 101 of the Patent Act; and (b) comparing a patient's isolated DNA sequence to a reference sequence was not a patentable method (35). Until this time the vast majority of commercial sequencing of *BRCA1* and *BRCA2* was performed by a single commercial lab that owned patents on both the sequence and interpretation of the genes. Within days of the Supreme Court decision, multiple molecular diagnostic companies began offering commercial testing for mutations in *BRCA1* and *BRCA2* using a variety of different methodologies and processes. However, at this time there is little standardization with respect to how individual labs assure analytic and clinical validity of sequencing results. This creates difficulties for providers in choosing labs and interpreting results (36).

The other development causing profound changes in genetic testing for hereditary breast and ovarian cancer is the advent of massively parallel sequencing technology, frequently termed next-generation sequencing. This sequencing technology allows for testing of multiple putative tumor suppressive genes at the same time that *BRCA1* and *BRCA2* are sequenced. With this development, multiple genes potentially associated with cancer risk are increasingly being added to commercial multiplex panels. While early data has suggested that some genes, including *BRIP1*, *RAD51C*, *RAD51D*, and perhaps *PALB2* may be associated with an increased risk of ovarian cancer (6–8), the actual magnitude and timing of those risks remain unclear. Furthermore, while it is hypothesized that ovarian cancer associated with non-*BRCA* HR genes may be preferentially sensitive to treatment with either platinum agents or PARP inhibitors (6), definitive studies proving or refuting this hypothesis have not yet been completed.

An additional issue with multiplex cancer susceptibility testing is that many panels include genes based on molecular pathway inference, as opposed to actual clinical data (37). However, as the cancer risks for many of these genes is uncertain, testing for them may increase the potential for false alarms and inappropriate clinical action without benefitting the patient (38). Given these issues, caution should be exercised in deciding which genes putatively associated with ovarian cancer risk should be examined in an individual undergoing genetic testing for inherited predispositions to breast and ovarian cancer.

Lastly, a number of genome-wide association studies have also identified single nucleotide polymorphisms (SNPs) that modify breast and/or gynecologic cancer risk in the setting of a *BRCA1* or *BRCA2* mutation (39). However, to date, none of these markers, either alone or in combination, have been shown to alter *BRCA*-associated cancer risk at a magnitude necessary to appreciably guide recommendations for risk-reduction strategies (40). Given the rapidly changing nature of the field, genetic counselors and other appropriately trained genetic professionals can assist in determining the most appropriate genetic tests for an individual patient. In addition, they can assist in interpreting the results in the context of the family history. Furthermore, the genetic professional can assist in identifying the most appropriate individuals for genetic testing, as in many families, it may be more informative to initiate testing in a relative of the patient, rather than in the patient herself. Importantly, genetic professionals can help identify other relatives who should be informed of a potential inherited risk (41) and can assist patients in planning such communication.

Cancer Risks Associated with a *BRCA1* or *BRCA2* Mutation

For women with mutations in *BRCA1*, lifetime risks, through age 70, of pelvic (ovarian, fallopian tube, or primary peritoneal) cancer are on the order of 39% to 46%. For women with mutations in *BRCA2*, the risk through age 70 of pelvic cancer is 12% to 20% (10,42). The average age of diagnosis of *BRCA1*-associated pelvic cancers is 53, which is approximately 10 years earlier than the average age of diagnosis of sporadic ovarian or fallopian tube cancer. Interestingly, the average age of *BRCA2*-associated pelvic cancer is 60 to 62 years, no earlier than is seen with sporadic disease (3,43). When considering the timing of approach to risk-reduction, it is also important to evaluate the risks of cancer based on the patient's approximate age of menopause. For women with *BRCA1* mutations, 10% to 21% will develop pelvic cancer by age 50, but only 2% to 3% of women with *BRCA2* mutations will develop pelvic cancer by the same age (42,44).

Breast cancer risks are also markedly elevated for women with mutations in these genes, with risks of breast cancer approaching 65% to 74% by age 70 for both carriers of *BRCA1* and *BRCA2* mutations (10,42). Breast cancer also occurs substantially earlier than is seen in the general population, with 26% to 34% of carriers of either *BRCA1* or *BRCA2* mutations developing breast cancer by age 50 (10,42,45).

For other ovarian cancer–associated genes in the HR pathway, the magnitude and timing of ovarian cancer risks are less clear. Early studies have suggested that RAD51C and RAD51D are associated with risks through age 70 of approximately 2.9% and 6.6%, respectively. BRIP1 has also been associated with a risk through age 70 of 2.5% to 6.1% (46). At present it is not clear if mutations in any of these three ovarian cancer susceptibility genes are also associated with clinically meaningful modification of breast cancer risk (9).

Guidelines for Offering Genetic Risk Assessment for Hereditary Breast and Ovarian Cancer Syndrome Caused by Mutations in *BRCA1* and *BRCA2*

Several organizations have proposed guidelines for offering genetic risk assessment for hereditary breast and ovarian cancer syndrome. For the gynecologic oncologist, the most relevant guidelines are those published by the ACOG (4), the Society of Gynecologic Oncology (SGO) (47), and the NCCN (5). Briefly, all of these guidelines state that hereditary cancer risk assessment is a process that: (a) should include assessment of risk, education, and counseling; (b) should be conducted by a physician, genetic counselor, or other provider with experience in cancer genetics; and (c) may include genetic testing after appropriate counseling and consent is obtained.

Specifically, ACOG states that it is reasonable to offer genetic risk assessment to any woman who has greater than a 5% to 10% chance of having a *BRCA1* or *BRCA2* mutation. Specific constellations of personal and family history that meet this threshold are outlined in **Table 3.2**. Given that 16% to 18% of high-grade serous ovarian and fallopian tube cancers (including 8% to 10% of patients with no significant family history) and a significant proportion of other high-grade epithelial ovarian and fallopian tube cancers segregate a *BRCA1* or *BRCA2* mutation, both SGO and NCCN recommend genetic risk assessment and testing for *BRCA1* and *BRCA2* mutation in all women with high-grade epithelial ovarian cancer, irrespective of age of diagnosis or family history. There are also several risk-prediction models, such as BRCAPRO, BOADICEA, and IBIS, that can assist in predicting the likelihood of a patient having a mutation in *BRCA1* or *BRCA2*. Each of these models, however, has unique advantages and limitations, and selecting the appropriate model is generally best done with the assistance of a genetics professional.

As noted above, the role of testing for mutations in other cancer susceptibility genes that may be associated with an inherited

TABLE 3.2. The ACOG Criteria for Offering Genetic Risk Assessment for Hereditary Breast and Ovarian Cancer Syndrome

Patients with greater than an approximate 5%–10% chance of having an inherited predisposition to breast and ovarian cancer, and for whom genetic risk assessment may be helpful:

- Women with breast cancer at age 40 y or younger
- Women with ovarian cancer, primary peritoneal cancer, or fallopian tube cancer of high-grade, serous histology at any age
- Women with bilateral breast cancer (particularly if the first case of breast cancer was diagnosed at age 50 y or younger)
- Women with breast cancer at age 50 y or younger and a close relative[a] with breast cancer at age 50 y or younger
- Women with breast cancer at age 50 y or younger and a close relative[a] with male breast cancer at any age
- Women of Ashkenazi Jewish ancestry with breast cancer at age 50 y or younger
- Women with breast cancer at any age and two or more close relatives[a] with breast cancer at any age (particularly if at least one case of breast cancer was diagnosed at age 50 y or younger)
- Unaffected women with a close relative[a] who meets one of the above criteria
- Unaffected women with a close relative[a] with a known *BRCA1* or *BRCA2* mutation

[a]Close relative is defined as a first-degree relative (mother, sister, daughter) or second-degree relative (grandmother, granddaughter, aunt, niece).

Source: Adapted from ACOG Practice Bulletin No. 103: Hereditary breast and ovarian cancer syndrome. *Obstet Gynecol*. 2009;113:957–966.

predisposition to breast and ovarian cancer is less clear. While genes such as *BRIP1*, *RAD51C*, and *RAD51D* almost certainly confer some risk of ovarian cancer, there is currently limited data to guide management of either affected or unaffected women with mutations in any of these genes. Additional tools for assessment knowledge will, however, evolve rapidly over the next several years, and physicians offering genetic risk assessment within their practice are encouraged to regularly collaborate with genetic professionals to determine the most appropriate genes to examine.

Screening and Prevention

Unaffected patients with a deleterious mutation in *BRCA1* or *BRCA2*, have several options for reducing the risk of both gynecologic and breast cancer (**Table 3.3**).

Screening

Ovarian/fallopian tube cancer. Screening for ovarian and fallopian tube cancer in the general population is not recommended. Recently, two large randomized trials of ovarian cancer screening in women not known to be at inherited risk have been reported. In 2011, the Prostate, Lung, Colorectal, and Ovarian Cancer Screening Randomized Trial reported the results of the ovarian cancer screening aim (48). In this trial, 78,216 women were randomized to either ovarian cancer screening with annual transvaginal ultrasound for 4 years and annual CA-125 determination for 6 years or usual care. After a median 12.4 years of follow-up, there was no difference in ovarian cancer mortality between the screened women and women participating in usual care (risk ratio [RR], 1.18; 95% CI, 0.82 to 1.71). Furthermore, 3,285 (8.4%) of 39,105 screened women had a false-positive result during the course of the study, with 1,080 (2.8%) undergoing surgical follow-up. In 2015, Jacobs et al. (49) reported the results of the UK Collaborative Trial of Ovarian Cancer Screening. In this trial, 202,638 women were randomized to one of three strategies: 50,640 participants were randomized to a multimodal screening strategy utilizing annual CA125 determinations analyzed by the Risk of Ovarian Cancer Algorithm (ROCA); 50,639 were randomized to annual transvaginal ultrasound; 101,299 were randomized to no screening. After a median 11.1 years of follow-up, a 15% (95% CI, –3% to 30%; $p = 0.10$) mortality reduction was seen with multimodal screening compared to no screening and an 11% (95% CI, –7% to 27%; $p = 0.21$) mortality reduction was seen with ultrasound screening compared to no screening, though neither of these reached statistical significance.

Two prospective trials specifically targeting women at familial/inherited risk have also been completed. In 2013, the results from Phase I of the UK Familial Ovarian Cancer Screening Study (UK FOCSS) were reported. In this study, 3,563 women with a greater than 10% lifetime risk of ovarian cancer were followed with annual transvaginal ultrasound and annual CA-125 blood tests (50). The results suggested a stage shift, with only 6 (26%) of 23 cancers not associated with Lynch syndrome in women screened according to protocol diagnosed at stage IIIc or higher. This was in contrast to 6 (86%) of 7 cancers being of advanced stage in women with delayed screening. This research group has now completed Phase II of the study, in which participants were followed with annual transvaginal ultrasound and every 4-month CA125 determinations, interpreted by the ROCA algorithm. Unfortunately the preliminary results, presented in abstract form, have not suggested that increasing the frequency of screening further improves the stage distribution.

The Gynecologic Oncology Group recently completed Study 0199, a prospective study of risk-reducing salpingo-oophorectomy (RRSO) and longitudinal CA-125 screening in women at increased genetic risk of ovarian cancer (51). In this study, participants at increased risk of breast and ovarian cancer elected either RRSO or surveillance with annual transvaginal ultrasound and every 3-month CA-125 interrogated with ROCA. All participants in the study were genotyped, and just under 400 of the approximately 1,600 women who elected surveillance had a *BRCA* mutation. The study has completed data collection and is currently in analysis.

Until final results are available from UK FOCSS and GOG 0199, given the lack of evidence with respect to benefit, transvaginal ultrasound and CA-125 determinations likely cannot be recommended as an alternative to RRSO in a woman with a mutation in *BRCA1* or *BRCA2* once she enters the risk period for ovarian cancer (5).

Breast cancer. For patients with a deleterious mutation in *BRCA1* or *BRCA2*, annual mammography beginning at age 30 is recommended (5,52). However, several studies have suggested that mammography alone in women with *BRCA* mutations is inadequate. In 2001, Brekelmans and colleagues (53) reported that 4 of 9 invasive breast cancers in 128 *BRCA* mutation carriers presented as palpable masses in the interval between screens. Similarly, in 2002, Scheuer et al. (54) reported that 7 of 12 invasive breast cancers diagnosed in 251 *BRCA* mutation carriers undergoing mammographic screening presented as interval cancers. Due to the relatively low sensitivity of mammography, breast MRI has been investigated as a complimentary imaging modality. Three of the largest studies to date have shown a 71% to 78% sensitivity of breast MRI for *BRCA*-associated cancers compared to a 36% to 40% sensitivity for mammography (55). Furthermore, in 2011, Warner and colleagues (56) demonstrated that the addition of annual MRI to annual mammography led to a down staging of *BRCA*-associated breast cancers (adjusted hazard ratio for the development of stage II to IV breast cancer associated with MRI screening = 0.30; 95% CI, 0.12 to 0.72). Currently, both the NCCN and the American Cancer Society recommend the combination of annual mammography and annual breast MRI, beginning by age 30, for screening in women with *BRCA* mutations (5,52).

TABLE 3.3. Risk-Reduction Recommendations for Carriers of *BRCA1* and *BRCA2* Mutations

Breast
- Annual breast MRI age 25–29 y
- Annual mammography and annual breast MRI age 30–75 y
- Breast screening considered on an individual basis for women older than 75 y
- RRSO to reduce breast cancer risk between age 35 and 40 y and when childbearing is complete. (For women with BRCA2 mutations who have already undergone bilateral mastectomy, it may be reasonable to defer RRSO until age 40–45 y.)
- Consider chemoprevention with tamoxifen, raloxifene, or an aromatase inhibitor (particularly in the setting of a *BRCA2* mutation)
- Consider RRM

Ovary/fallopian tube
- RRSO to reduce ovarian and fallopian tube cancer risk once a woman has entered the risk period for gynecologic cancers (age 35–40 y for *BRCA1*, age 40–45 y for *BRCA2*) and after childbearing is complete
- Consider chemoprevention with oral contraceptives

Source: Adapted from National Comprehensive Cancer Network: NCCN Clinical Practice Guidelines in Oncology—Genetic/Familial High-Risk Assessment: Breast and Ovarian. 2016. Version 2.2016. http://www.nccn.org

Chemoprevention

Ovarian/fallopian tube cancer. Multiple studies have suggested that use of oral contraceptives in the general population is associated with a substantial and long-lasting reduction in the risk of ovarian cancer (57). Given this, several authors have examined the impact of oral contraceptives on ovarian cancer risk in the setting of *BRCA1* or *BRCA2* mutations. In a recent meta-analysis of five case–control and retrospective cohort studies, Iodice and colleague (58) found that ever use of oral contraceptives was associated with a significant reduction in ovarian cancer risk in both *BRCA1* (summary relative risk = 0.51; 95% CI, 0.40 to 0.65) and *BRCA2* (summary relative risk = 0.52; 95% CI, 0.31 to 0.87) mutation carriers. Further, longer use was associated with a greater risk-reduction, with a 36% risk reduction seen for each 10 years of use (summary relative risk = 0.64; 95% CI, 0.53 to 0.78).

When caring for women with *BRCA1* or *BRCA2* mutations, it is important, however, to consider both breast and ovarian cancer risk, and the data regarding breast cancer risk has been somewhat more conflicting. Of five published studies addressing the impact of oral contraceptives on breast cancer risk in *BRCA1* mutation carriers, three suggested an increased risk of breast cancer with oral contraceptive use and two showed no increase in risk. Similarly, in the three studies reporting on breast cancer risk with oral contraceptive use in *BRCA2* mutation carries, two studies suggested an increased risk, and one study showed no increase in risk (58). After meta-analysis, neither *BRCA1* (summary relative risk = 1.09; 95% CI, 0.77 to 1.54) nor *BRCA2* (summary relative risk = 1.15; 95% CI, 0.61 to 2.18) mutation carriers demonstrated a statistically significant increased risk of breast cancer with oral contraceptive use. However, oral contraceptive formulations used before 1975 were associated with an increased risk of breast cancer (summary relative risk = 1.47; 95% CI, 1.06 to 2.04) (58). Given the data currently available, it likely makes sense to counsel patients that oral contraceptives may be associated with some adverse impact on breast cancer risk. This potential risk, however, needs to be balanced against the risk of unintended pregnancy and the benefit of oral contraceptives on ovarian cancer risk.

Breast cancer. The selective estrogen receptor (ER) modulators, tamoxifen and raloxifene, and to the aromatase inhibitor exemestane have been studied in the general population as chemoprevention for breast cancer. Tamoxifen is the only one of these agents that has been studied in women with *BRCA* mutations. King and colleagues (59), in a reanalysis of the NSABP P-1 trial, found a suggestion that tamoxifen was associated with protection against *BRCA2*-associated breast cancer (RR, 0.38; 95% CI, 0.06 to 1.56) but not *BRCA1*-associated breast cancer (RR, 1.67; 95% CI, 0.32 to 10.70), though neither of these results reached statistical significance. It was speculated that the reason for this possible differential effect was the different ER phenotypes of breast cancer seen between *BRCA1* and *BRCA2* mutations carriers. Sixty-five percent to 80% of *BRCA2*-associated breast cancers are ER positive, as opposed to only 10% to 25% of *BRCA1*-associated breast cancers (60,61). In 2000, Narod and colleagues examined the impact of therapeutic tamoxifen on contralateral breast cancer risk. In this study, tamoxifen appeared to be associated with a reduction of contralateral breast cancer risk in both *BRCA1* (odds ratio 0.38; 95% CI, 0.19 to 0.74) and *BRCA2* (odds ratio 0.63; 95% CI, 0.20 to 1.50) mutation carriers (62). Of potential significance, *BRCA1* mutation carriers who received tamoxifen in this study likely had ER-positive disease. Weitzel et al. (63) demonstrated that, in women with *BRCA* mutations who develop contralateral breast cancer, the ER status of the second breast cancer is highly concordant with the ER status of the first breast cancer, suggesting that women with ER-positive *BRCA1*-associated breast cancer are more likely to develop a second ER-positive cancer and therefore may be more likely to benefit from hormonal chemoprevention.

Risk-Reducing Surgery

Salpingo-Oophorectomy

Impact on ovarian cancer risk. Two of the earliest studies to examine the impact of RRSO on ovarian cancer risk were published in 2002. The first of these was a prospective cohort study from Memorial Sloan-Kettering Cancer Center. In this study, 170 women with a documented deleterious mutation in *BRCA1* or *BRCA2* elected either surveillance or RRSO. In this series, RRSO was associated with a 75% reduction in the subsequent risk of breast or *BRCA*-associated gynecologic cancer (HR = 0.25; 95% CI, 0.08 to 0.74) (64). When the impact of RRSO on gynecologic risk alone was examined, there was a an approximately 85% reduction in gynecologic cancer risk (HR = 0.15; 95% CI, 0.02 to 1.31). At the same time, a retrospective study from the University of Pennsylvania found that RRSO was associated with an approximately 96% reduction in gynecologic cancer risk (HR = 0.04; 95% CI, 0.01 to 0.16) (65). However, a commentary from Klaren et al. (66) pointed out that the retrospective study may have overestimated the conferred risk-reduction. Since that time, several other studies have suggested that RRSO is associated with a 71% to 89% reduction in gynecologic cancer risk (67), and a 2009 meta-analysis concluded that RRSO was associated with approximately 79% reduction in risk of *BRCA*-associated gynecologic cancer (HR = 0.21; 95% CI, 0.12 to 0.39) (68).

The origin of peritoneal cancers after RRSO is not entirely clear. Some of these may represent recurrence of occult ovarian or tubal malignancies that were not recognized on initial pathologic evaluation, emphasizing the need for careful pathologic evaluation of the entire ovary and fallopian tube at the time of RRSO. It has also been speculated that peritoneal cancer can arise from exfoliated tubal cells (endosalpingiosis) that implant on the peritoneum and undergo malignant transformation in that location. Lastly, some authors have suggested that peritoneal malignancies can arise exclusively in the peritoneum through Müllerian metaplasia (69). Irrespective of the origin, it is important that patients undergoing RRSO be informed of the small possibility of primary peritoneal cancer occurring after the procedure.

Impact on breast cancer risk. In the first study examining the impact of RRSO on breast cancer risk, Rebbeck and colleagues (70) found that RRSO in women with a *BRCA1* mutation was associated with a 47% reduction in *BRCA1*-associated breast cancer risk (HR = 0.53; 95% CI, 0.33 to 0.84). In a prospective study by Kauff et al. (64) reported in 2002, which examined both *BRCA1* and *BRCA2* mutation carriers, RRSO appeared to be associated with an approximately 68% reduction in breast cancer risk (HR = 0.32; 95% CI, 0.08 to 1.20). In 2008, Kauff, Rebbeck, and colleagues (71) pooled their updated prospective data and reported on 597 women with breast tissue at risk who had RRSO or surveillance and were prospectively followed for 2.8 years. When women with *BRCA1* and *BRCA2* mutations were examined together, RRSO was associated with a 47% reduction in breast cancer risk (HR = 0.53; 95% CI, 0.29 to 0.96). However, when *BRCA1* and *BRCA2* mutation carriers were examined separately, women with *BRCA2* mutations had a 72% reduction in breast cancer risk compared to women whose ovaries had been left *in situ* (HR = 0.28; 95% CI, 0.08 to 0.92). Women with *BRCA1* mutations appeared to have a 39% reduction in breast cancer risk (HR = 0.61; 95% CI, 0.30 to 1.22). However, despite this being the largest prospective study to date, these results did not reach statistical significance. An exploratory analysis examining the impact of RRSO on breast cancer stratified for ER status was also performed. In this analysis, RRSO appeared to be highly protective against ER-positive breast cancer (HR = 0.22; 95% CI, 0.05 to 1.05). However, no impact against ER-negative breast cancer was noted (HR = 1.10; 95% CI, 0.48 to 2.51).

Of note, a recent analysis from Heemskerk-Gerritsen et al. (72) has suggested that the design of several studies evaluating the impact of RRSO on breast cancer risk may have resulted in an overestimation of the risk-reduction conferred by RRSO against breast cancer. However, a reanalysis of data from Kauff et al. and Domcheck et al. according to the recommendations of Heemskerk-Gerritsen et al. suggests that, while there may be some change in the magnitude of risk-reduction conferred, the protective effect against breast cancer remains (73).

Impact on life expectancy. Domchek and colleagues (74) reported the results of a prospective cohort study concluding that RRSO in *BRCA* mutation carriers was associated with reduction in breast cancer–specific (HR = 0.44; 95% CI, 0.26 to 0.76), ovarian cancer–specific (HR = 0.21; 95% CI, 0.06 to 0.80), and all-cause mortality (HR = 0.40; 95% CI, 0.26 to 0.61). Similarly, Finch et al. (75) reported a 77% reduction in all-cause mortality (HR = 0.23;

95% CI, 0.13 to 0.39) following RRSO. While the effect of RRSO on mortality demonstrated by both Domchek et al. and Finch et al. is almost certainly present, there is a fair amount of instability in the estimates of the actual magnitude of this effect due to potential biases introduced by the respective study designs. In the Domcheck study, participants could be identified as many as 20 years prior to the identification of *BRCA1* and *BRCA2*, but in many cases only underwent genotyping (and inclusion in the final analysis) if: (a) they lived long enough for clinical testing to become available or (b) they developed a cancer of interest. Similarly, in the Finch study, participants with breast cancer, including presumably those with advanced or metastatic disease diagnosed prior to study entry, were included in the analysis of mortality. In light of this, there may have been a selective survival bias in women who ultimately elected RRSO.

Even given the limitations of the available studies evaluating the efficacy of RRSO on subsequent cancer risk and mortality, for carriers of *BRCA1* and *BRCA2* mutations, RRSO remains the best available protection against pelvic serous cancer. It should be strongly considered after childbearing is complete, once a woman has entered the risk period for *BRCA*-associated gynecologic cancer.

Technical considerations. Given that the ovaries and fallopian tubes are both at risk for malignant transformation, it is imperative that the entire ovary and distal fallopian tube are removed at the time of RRSO. To do this, it is necessary that the surgeon be able to enter the retroperitoneal space and ligate the infundibulopelvic ligament at least 2 cm from its insertion into the ovary. Malignant cells leading to upstaging of disease have also been found in peritoneal cytology specimens from a number of women undergoing RRSO (76). Given these findings, washing should probably be performed at the time of peritoneal entry in all women undergoing RRSO.

Additionally, as 2% to 10% of RRSO specimens obtained from *BRCA* mutation carriers are determined to have an occult malignancy at the time of pathologic review (77), it is essential that the entire ovary and fallopian tube be serially sectioned to minimize the possibility of a small invasive cancer going undetected (4). The fimbrial ends of the fallopian tubes are the most frequent site of occult invasive serous carcinomas (78–80), and these lesions are best visualized using the SEE-FIM (sectioning and extensively examining the fimbriated end) method (81). Briefly, SEE-FIM entails lengthwise sectioning (sagitally) of the fimbriated portion of the fallopian tube in multiple planes to maximize exposure of the tubal plicae. When this method is utilized, serous tubal intraepithelial carcinoma (STIC), a putative precursor to invasive serous carcinoma, is also identified in as many as 5% to 8% of specimens obtained at the time of RRSO in women with mutations in *BRCA1* or *BRCA2* (82,83). Patients in whom small high-grade invasive serous cancers are found incidentally at RRSO generally receive adjuvant chemotherapy. The role of adjuvant therapy in the management of STIC is less clear (76).

Recently, Wethington et al. (84) evaluated the clinical outcome of patients found to have STIC at RRSO. Of 593 patients in this study, isolated STIC was diagnosed in 12 patients (2%). Seven patients subsequently underwent hysterectomy and omentectomy, six patients had pelvic node dissections, and five patients had para-aortic node dissections. With the exception of positive peritoneal washings in one patient, no invasive or metastatic disease was identified. None of the patients received adjuvant chemotherapy. At median follow-up of 28 months (range, 16 to 44 months), no recurrences were identified. The authors concluded that the yield of surgical staging is low in patients with STICs, and short-term clinical outcomes are favorable.

Timing of procedure. For most women with mutations in either *BRCA1* or *BRCA2*, RRSO should generally be considered between age 35 and 40, and when childbearing is complete (4,5). For women with *BRCA1* mutations, this is recommended because only 2% to 3% of women with mutations in *BRCA1* gene will develop pelvic serous cancer by age 40, but 10% to 21% of *BRCA1* mutation carriers will develop pelvic serous cancer by age 50 (10,42,85). For women with *BRCA2* mutations, the risk of pelvic serous cancer by age 50 is only 2% to 3%. However, women with *BRCA2* mutations who defer RRSO until the age of natural menopause likely lose the significant protection against *BRCA2*-associated breast cancer conferred by RRSO (77). For women with *BRCA2* mutations who have already had bilateral mastectomy and ovarian ablation is not being utilized as part of adjuvant therapy for a prior breast cancer, RRSO likely can be reasonably deferred until the mid-40s.

Role of hysterectomy. While RRSO is now part of standard management for women with *BRCA1* and *BRCA2* mutations, the role of concomitant hysterectomy is controversial, as it is not clear if women with *BRCA* mutations are at increased risk of uterine cancer (4,77). Recently, Shu et al. (86) reported the results of a multicenter prospective study in which 1,083 women with deleterious *BRCA1* or *BRCA2* mutation were followed for a median 5.1 years after RRSO. Eight incident uterine cancers were observed (4.3 expected; O/E = 1.9, $p = 0.09$). Stratifying by subtype, the authors found no increased risk of endometrioid endometrial carcinoma or sarcoma. Five serous/serous-like endometrial carcinomas were observed (4 *BRCA1+*; 1 *BRCA2+*) 7.2 to 12.9 years after RRSO (*BRCA1*: 0.18 expected; O/E = 22.2, $p < 0.001$; *BRCA2*: 0.16 expected; O/E = 6.4, $p = 0.15$). Using these data, the authors estimated that a *BRCA1* mutation carrier undergoing RRSO at age 45 had a 2.6% to 4.7% risk of serous uterine cancer through age 70. They concluded that, if these results are confirmed by future studies, hysterectomy with bilateral salpingo-oophorectomy may become the preferred risk-reducing surgical approach for women with *BRCA1* mutations, unless there are strong reasons for uterine retention.

Role of salpingectomy. With evidence suggesting the distal fallopian tube epithelium is the cell of origin for pelvic serous cancer, several authors have suggested a role for risk-reducing salpingectomy with delayed oophorectomy as a bridging strategy for women with *BRCA1* and *BRCA2* mutation who are not ready to proceed with oophorectomy (87). However, caution is warranted with this approach, for several reasons (88). First, while the hypothesis that fallopian tube epithelium is the cell of origin, in at least a portion of pelvic serous cancers is compelling, it is not known what proportion of pelvic serous cancers are explained by this hypothesis. Even if the distal fallopian tube is the site of origin of the vast majority of pelvic serous cancers, it is probably not the location of neoplastic transformation in a least a fraction of pelvic serous cancers. There is no evidence of fallopian tube neoplasm in 30% to 60% of serially sectioned fallopian tubes, in the setting of a coexisting ovarian serous malignancy. Lastly, if oophorectomy is deferred until the time of natural menopause, women with *BRCA* mutation will lose the significant benefit of oophorectomy in the prevention of *BRCA*-associated breast cancer. Given this, until clear data becomes available demonstrating that salpingectomy with delayed oophorectomy reduces the risk of pelvic serous cancer, once a woman with BRCA mutation enters the risk period for gynecologic cancer RRSO remains the recommended risk-reduction strategy.

Mastectomy. Several studies have demonstrated that risk-reducing mastectomy (RRM) in women with *BRCA1* or *BRCA2* mutation is associated with at least a 90% reduction in the risk of new breast cancer (89,90). Importantly, the impact on life expectancy may be markedly less, as the majority of these cancers in women undergoing both mammography and breast MRI will be diagnosed at a curable stage. In a decision analysis by Kurian et al. (91) RRM at age 40 (in addition to RRSO at age 40 and breast screening starting at age 25) only increased the probability of survival to age 70 from 74% to 77% in carriers of *BRCA1* mutations and from 80% to 82% in carriers of *BRCA2* mutations. Given these relatively small absolute improvements in survival, intensive breast screening or RRM are likely reasonable options for a woman with a *BRCA1* or *BRCA2* mutation.

Risk-Reduction Strategies for Women with Mutations in Non-*BRCA* HR Genes

As noted above, recent advances in massively parallel sequencing have led to increased identification of individuals with germline mutations in moderate-penetrance cancer susceptibility genes that may be associated with increased risks of breast and ovarian cancer. It appears that *BRIP1*, *RAD51C*, *RAD51D*, and perhaps *PALB2* may be associated with increased risk of serous ovarian cancer. On the basis of early data from relatively small series, the lifetime risk of ovarian cancer (through age 70) associated with protein-truncating mutations in these genes is approximately 2.5% to 6.6% (46). Similarly, protein-truncating mutations in *ATM*, *NBM*, *CHEK2*, and *PALB2* may be associated with a breast cancer risk of 21% to 35% through age 70 (46). Tung et al. recently proposed a framework for counseling patients with mutations in these moderate-penetrance genes about risk-reducing strategies. Briefly, Tung et al. (46) suggested that we do not consider incremental screening or risk-reducing surgery in women with a mutation in one of these moderate-penetrance genes until the age-specific cumulative risk of cancer at least exceeds the lifetime risk of breast and gynecologic cancer in the general population. For example, the authors estimate the cumulative risk of developing ovarian cancer through age 49 in the setting of an *RAD51C* or *RAD51D* mutation is 0.6% and 1.4%, respectively. As the lifetime risk of ovarian cancer in the United States is 1.3%, the authors suggest that women with mutations in *RAD51C* or *RAD51D* do not consider RRSO until after approximately age 50. Until further data becomes available, this appears to be a reasonable starting point for discussion of risk-reduction strategies in women with mutations in moderate-penetrance cancer susceptibility genes. However, given the rapid pace of changes in our understanding of the cancer risks associated with these genes, it is recommended that patients have an ongoing discussion with clinical genetics professionals, to determine if changes in management are warranted.

Lynch Syndrome

Epidemiology

Approximately 3% to 5% of endometrial cancer cases may be attributed to an inherited predisposition (92). Lynch syndrome, or hereditary nonpolyposis colorectal cancer (HNPCC) syndrome, accounts for the majority of these cases. Individuals with Lynch syndrome have a germline mutation in one of four genes in the DNA mismatch repair family: *MLH1*, *MSH2*, *MSH6*, or *PMS2 or* a heritable deletion in the *EPCM* gene that leads to silencing of *MSH2*. While Lynch syndrome has historically been characterized by an increased risk for colorectal cancer, women with Lynch syndrome also have a substantial risk for endometrial cancer. The estimated lifetime risk for colon cancer in women is 40% to 60%, and in men as high as 80% (93,94). In women, the lifetime endometrial cancer risk is approximately 40% to 60%. In a study focusing specifically on individuals with *MSH6* mutations, risk for endometrial cancer was 26% by age 70 and as high as 44% by age 80, and lifetime risk of colon cancer was 10% by age 70 and 20% by age 80 (95). Women with Lynch syndrome also have an approximate 5% to 10% lifetime risk for developing ovarian cancer. Other cancers associated with Lynch syndrome include cancers of the stomach, small bowel, renal pelvis and ureter, and brain.

In the general population, Lynch syndrome occurs in about 1 in 600 to 1 in 3,000 individuals (96,97). In a population-based study of endometrial cancer patients, the incidence of Lynch syndrome was 2.3%, which is similar to the 2.2% incidence of Lynch syndrome among colon cancer patients (98). For women with endometrial cancer under the age of 50, the proportion with Lynch syndrome increases to 5% to 9% (99–101). The mean age of diagnosis for endometrial cancer in women with Lynch syndrome is 47 years, which is substantially lower than the mean age of diagnosis of endometrial cancer in the general population. Women with Lynch syndrome are also at increased risk of developing synchronous or metachronous cancers. In a study examining 101 women with Lynch syndrome who had developed both gastrointestinal (GI) cancer and gynecologic cancer, 51% presented first with gynecologic cancer at a median age of 44 and 49% presented with GI cancer first (102).

Pathology

Unlike the ovarian cancers associated with *BRCA1* and *BRCA2* mutations, the endometrial cancers associated with Lynch syndrome span a broader spectrum of histologies. In a study by Broaddus et al. (103), 43 of 50 (86%) endometrial cancers were endometrioid histology, with the remainder being papillary serous carcinoma, clear cell carcinoma, and malignant mixed Mullërian tumors. Interestingly, all of the non-endometrioid tumors in this study occurred in patients with *MSH2* mutations. Among all of the patients with Lynch syndrome, 78% were diagnosed at stage I, 10% at stage II, and 12% at stage III or IV. Lymphovascular space involvement was noted in 24% of the cases, and 26% had deep myometrial involvement that was defined as invasion greater than 50%. Endometrial cancers that arise in the lower uterine segment are relatively rare in the general population, but are seen more frequently in women with Lynch syndrome. In a study by Westin et al. (104), almost one-third of patients with endometrial cancers arising in the lower uterine segment were suspected to be associated with Lynch syndrome, based on tumor studies or germline testing. This characteristic phenotype is similar to the increased proportion of right-sided colon cancers seen in individuals with Lynch syndrome. Other pathologic features that have been seen more frequently in Lynch syndrome–associated colon cancers, including poor tumor differentiation and tumor-infiltrating lymphocytes, have not been seen consistently in Lynch syndrome–associated endometrial cancers.

The ovarian cancers seen in Lynch syndrome also have a different stage and histology spectrum from that seen in women with sporadic disease. In a recent series, 22 (47%) of 47 Lynch-associated epithelial ovarian cancers presented at stage I. Furthermore, serous cancers were underrepresented in this series, accounting for only 28% of tumors. Endometrioid, clear cell, and mucinous histologies were seen in 35%, 17%, and 5%, respectively (105).

Genetic Risk Assessment for Lynch Syndrome

For gynecologic oncologists, identifying Lynch syndrome in a patient with endometrial cancer has important implications for both the patient and her family members. Individuals with Lynch syndrome are at significant lifetime risk of developing a second primary malignancy. Therefore, when an endometrial cancer patient is identified as having Lynch syndrome, appropriate colon cancer screening can be initiated. Additionally, if a specific mutation in one of the DNA mismatch repair genes is identified in the endometrial cancer patient, her family members can undergo targeted predictive genetic testing for the same mutation.

Historically, guidelines to assist physicians in identifying individuals with Lynch syndrome have focused on colon cancer patients. Prior to the discovery of the genes responsible for Lynch syndrome, the Amsterdam I criteria were formulated to identify families with Lynch syndrome for research studies (106). These initial criteria only considered colon cancer as a sentinel diagnosis. The criteria were subsequently revised into the Amsterdam II criteria, to include extracolonic Lynch syndrome–associated cancers as sentinel diagnoses (107). To meet the Amsterdam II criteria, four factors must be present in a family: (a) three or more relatives have been diagnosed with Lynch syndrome–associated cancers, (b) two affected relatives are in successive generations, (c) one affected relative is a first-degree relative of the other two, and (d) one of the Lynch syndrome–associated cancers must have been diagnosed before the age of 50. While the Amsterdam criteria are quite specific, they are not sensitive enough for routine clinical use, as they only detect

13% to 36% of individuals with molecularly proven Lynch syndrome in population series (108,109).

Given the limited sensitivity of the Amsterdam I and II criteria, the Bethesda criteria were developed in 1997 and revised in 2004, to provide a more sensitive set of guidelines in order to identify patients with colorectal cancer who should be assessed further for the possibility of Lynch syndrome (110,111). However, the 2004 Bethesda criteria did not specify which patients with endometrial cancer should undergo further evaluation for Lynch syndrome. As it has become increasingly clear that female Lynch syndrome patients often present with endometrial or ovarian cancer as their first cancer, several authors have suggested modification to the 2004 Bethesda criteria to include endometrial cancer as a sentinel diagnosis (112). (**Table 3.4**)

While family history remains an important component in identifying individuals who may benefit from genetic risk assessment for Lynch syndrome, tumor testing for evidence of mismatch repair defects is increasingly being used to triage patients who may be at risk for a germline DNA mismatch repair mutation (113,114). These tumor tests include immunohistochemistry for one of the four mismatch repair proteins (MLH1, MSH2, MSH6, and PMS2) and microsatellite instability (MSI) analysis. Both of these studies can be performed on formalin-fixed, paraffin-embedded tissues and can be a first step in the evaluation of Lynch syndrome in a patient with endometrial cancer.

For immunohistochemistry-based triage, the absence of a specific mismatch repair protein in the tumor is considered abnormal. For example, a tumor may demonstrate loss of staining of the MSH2 protein, with normal staining of the MLH1, MSH6, and PMS2 proteins. The loss of staining of the MSH2 protein in the tumor indicates that both copies of the gene are nonfunctional and suggests that the woman may have an *MSH2* germline mutation.

For MSI-based triage, both tumor and normal tissues are required. MSI testing reflects the tumor phenotype of deficient DNA repair. When a tumor has deficient DNA repair capability, multiple mistakes occur in the DNA in both coding and noncoding regions. These mistakes are especially common in regions of mononucleotide and dinucleotide repeats, such as CCCCCC or CGCGCG. The National Cancer Institute has identified seven regions in the genome that can be examined for MSI testing (BAT25, BAT26, BAT40, D2S123, D5S346, D173250, and TGF-BR2). Tumors with allelic shift in two or more microsatellites in this panel are considered MSI-high. Tumors with allelic shift in only one microsatellite are considered MSI-low. Tumors with no allelic shift in all seven microsatellites are considered microsatellite-stable. For MSI-high tumors with loss of MLH1 protein expression by IHC, methylation-specific PCR for *MLH1* proximal promoter region −248 to −178 is performed to detect possible methylation of the *MLH1* promoter. When methylation is present, the patient most likely has a sporadic carcinoma rather than a Lynch syndrome–associated cancer (*MLH1* promoter methylation is discussed in more detail in Chapter 2).

Immunohistochemistry (IHC) can also direct which of the four DNA mismatch repair genes should be sequenced. This can be performed in most pathology labs, and it has become the preferred approach for initial assessment of the mismatch repair pathway in endometrial cancers. In 2014, the ACOG published a practice bulletin, including an IHC-based algorithm, for assessing the possibility of Lynch syndrome in endometrial tumors (113) (**Fig. 3.1**). Additionally, they recommend that practices taking care of women with endometrial cancer adopt one of three approaches to determine which patients should be assessed for Lynch syndrome. Briefly, they recommend that any of the following is reasonable: (a) assessing all endometrial cancer patients diagnosed prior to age 60; (b) assess all endometrial cancer patients regardless of age of diagnosis; or (c) utilize a systematic clinical screen that includes a focused personal and family medical history, to determine which endometrial cancers should be further assessed. A study from the Australian endometrial cancer study has suggested that assessing all endometrial cancer patients who present prior to age 60 with an IHC-based approach is the most cost-effective strategy for triage (115). However, local resources and limitations will clearly influence the choice of approach in individual practices.

An important limitation of IHC-based triage is that 10% to 15% of tumors with loss of either the MLH1 or PMS2 protein and 35% to 40% of tumors with loss of the MSH2 or MSH6 protein remain unexplained after comprehensive genetic evaluation, leading to counseling and management challenges. Recent data has suggested a fraction of these may be caused by biallelic somatic mutations (116), but clinical testing for this possibility is not widely available.

Given these challenges and rapid advances in next-generation sequencing technology, several authors have suggested proceeding immediately to direct germline testing of patients with a potential Lynch-associated endometrial cancer. However, while this may be a more efficient strategy in some cases, it may lead to increased genetic counseling demands due to higher rates of detection of variants of uncertain significance and potential detection of mutations in off-target genes. Furthermore, while direct germline testing may confirm the diagnosis of Lynch syndrome, only tumor testing can conclusively rule out the diagnosis.

TABLE 3.4. The 2004 Bethesda Guidelines (Modified to Include Endometrial Cancer as a Sentinel Cancer) to Identify Individuals with Colorectal or Endometrial Cancer for Whom Genetic Risk Assessment Is Recommended

- Patients with endometrial or colorectal cancer diagnosed before age 50 y
- Patient with endometrial or ovarian cancer with a synchronous or metachronous colon or other Lynch/HNPCC-associated tumor[a] at any age
- Patients with colorectal cancer with tumor-infiltrating lymphocytes, peritumoral lymphocytes, Crohn-like lymphocytic reaction, mucinous/signet-ring differentiation, or medullary growth pattern diagnosed before age 60 y
- Patients with endometrial or colorectal cancer and a first-degree relative[b] with a Lynch/HNPCC-associated tumor[a] diagnosed before age 50 y
- Patients with colorectal or endometrial cancer diagnosed at any age with two or more first-degree or second-degree relatives[b] with Lynch/HNPCC-associated tumors[a], regardless of age

HNPCC, hereditary nonpolyposis colorectal cancer.

[a]Lynch/HNPCC-related tumors include colorectal, endometrial, stomach, ovarian, pancreas, ureter and renal pelvis, biliary tract, and brain tumors (usually glioblastoma as seen in Turcot syndrome), sebaceous gland adenomas, and keratoacanthomas in Muir–Torre syndrome, and carcinoma of the small bowel.

[b]First-degree relatives are parents, siblings, and children. Second-degree relatives are aunts, uncles, nieces, nephews, grandparents, and grandchildren.

Source: Adapted from Lancaster JM, Powell CB, Kauff ND, et al. Society of Gynecologic Oncologists Education Committee statement on risk assessment for inherited gynecologic cancer predispositions. *Gynecol Oncol.* 2007;107(2):159–162.

Screening and Prevention

Screening

Guidelines for screening and prevention of Lynch syndrome–associated cancers have been published, and should be reviewed with patients when the diagnosis of Lynch syndrome is made (113,117,118) (**Table 3.5**). Colon cancer screening is recommended for individuals with Lynch syndrome every 1 to 2 years, starting at the age of 20 to 25 (or 30 years in patients with known *MSH6* mutations). This first evidence in support of this approach came from Jarvinen et al. (119), who demonstrated both a reduction in the incidence of invasive colorectal cancer from 16% to 6% ($p = 0.014$), and a relative risk of death of 0.34 (95% CI, 0.17 to 0.68) in individuals with Lynch syndrome who underwent colonoscopy or sigmoidoscopy and barium enema every 3 years, compared to those who received no routine screening. More recently, Vasen et al. (120) demonstrated an even lower risk of colorectal cancer in individuals having colonoscopy every 1 to 2 years versus every 2 to 3 years.

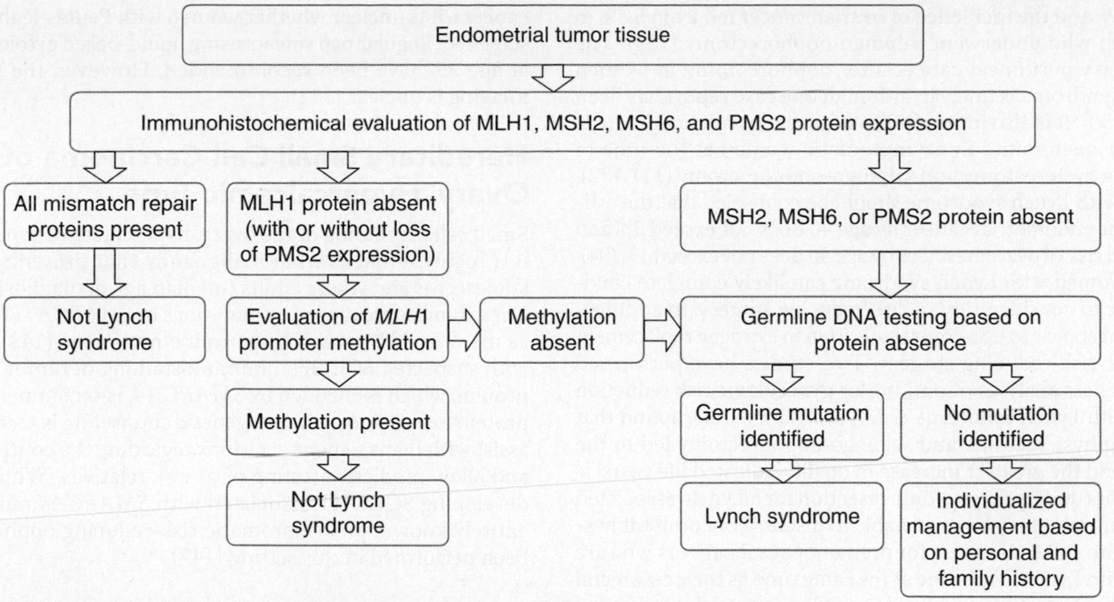

Figure 3.1. Algorithm for using IHC evaluation of mismatch repair protein expression to triage endometrial tumors for the possibility of Lynch Syndrome.

Source: Adapted from ACOG Practice Bulletin No. 147: Lynch syndrome. *Obstet Gynecol*. 2014;124:1042–1054.

TABLE 3.5. Risk-Reduction Recommendations for Women with Lynch Syndrome

GI • Colonoscopy every 1–2 y beginning at age 20–25 (or 2–5 y before the earliest colorectal cancer diagnosis in the family, whichever is earlier) • Consider esophagogastroduodenoscopy every 3–5 y beginning at age 30–35 y, if Asian descent or family history of gastric or duodenal cancer • Consider chemoprevention with aspirin (though optimal dose and duration are uncertain)
Gynecologic • Endometrial biopsy every 1–2 y beginning at age 30–35 y • Women should keep menstrual calendar, and abnormal uterine bleeding should be evaluated • Consider chemoprevention with progestin-based contraception, including oral contraceptives • Consider risk-reducing hysterectomy with bilateral salpingo-oophorectomy after completion of childbearing. In general, this procedure should be discussed with a patient by their early to mid-40s
Urologic • Consider annual urinalysis starting at age 30–35 y

Source: Adapted from ACOG Practice Bulletin No. 147: Lynch syndrome. *Obstet Gynecol*. 2014;124:1042–1054 and National Comprehensive Cancer Network: NCCN Clinical Practice Guidelines in Oncology—Genetic/Familial High-Risk Assessment: Colorectal. 2016. Version 1.2016. http://www.nccn.org

In contrast to colon cancer screening, there are no proven screening strategies for the early detection of endometrial or ovarian cancer in women with Lynch syndrome. Two European studies reported a high false-positive rate and poor efficacy of using measurement of endometrial stripe by transvaginal ultrasound as an endometrial cancer screening tool (121,122). Two more promising studies have reported identification of premalignant lesions and endometrial cancers in asymptomatic women with Lynch syndrome using office endometrial biopsy as a screening strategy (123,124). One of these studies, including 175 women with known *MLH1*, *MSH2*, or *MSH6* gene mutations, reported a stage migration, with 7% of women in the surveillance group presenting with stage III/IV disease versus 17% of women who presented symptomatically (123). The second study reported on 100 women from Lynch kindreds and demonstrated that routine endometrial sampling resulted in a significantly higher rate of malignancies and premalignancies, compared with prior historical controls in which routine endometrial sampling was not performed (6.3% vs. 1.4%, $p = 0.026$) (124). Importantly, no study to date has examined the mortality impact of routine endometrial sampling in women with Lynch syndrome. ACOG guidelines currently recommend uterine cancer surveillance with endometrial biopsy every 1 to 2 years, beginning at age 30 to 35, and keeping of a menstrual calendar, with evaluation of abnormal uterine bleeding (113). Given that endometrial biopsy is an invasive and uncomfortable procedure, a study by Huang et al. (125) demonstrated the feasibility and acceptability of performing surveillance endometrial biopsies in women with Lynch syndrome, while the patient is sedated for a screening colonoscopy. They also concluded that there was a substantial reduction in reported pain when the procedures were done concurrently under sedation.

Chemoprevention

In the general population, multiple studies have demonstrated that combination oral contraceptives reproducibly decrease endometrial and ovarian cancer risk (57,126). Progestin therapy is also effective in reversing complex atypical hyperplasia and early endometrial cancer (127). While there are no epidemiologic data that have evaluated the role of progestins or progestin-based oral contraceptives as chemoprevention in women known to have Lynch syndrome, a short-term biomarker study demonstrated a significant decrease in endometrial proliferation using either 150-mg depo medroxyprogesterone acetate or a 30-μg ethinyl estradiol/0.3 mg norgestrel oral contraceptive pill (128). An ongoing trial is examining the use of the levonorgestrel intrauterine device as a chemopreventive in women with Lynch syndrome.

Risk-Reducing Surgery

Risk-reducing hysterectomy and salpingo-oophorectomy are reasonable options for prevention of endometrial and ovarian cancer in women with Lynch syndrome. A multi-institutional retrospective study of women with Lynch syndrome demonstrated that the incidence of endometrial cancer fell from 33% to 0% in women who underwent hysterectomy, and the incidence of ovarian cancer fell from 5.4% to 0% in women who underwent salpingo-oophorectomy (129). The risk of primary peritoneal cancer after oophorectomy in women with Lynch syndrome is unclear, although one case report has been published (130). It is also important to note that occult endometrial cancers have been found in asymptomatic women at the time of risk-reducing hysterectomy and salpingo-oophorectomy (131,132).

Women with Lynch syndrome should be counseled that the estimated risk for endometrial cancer by age 40 does not exceed 2% and the estimated risk of ovarian cancer by age 40 does not exceed 1% (94). Therefore, women with Lynch syndrome can likely complete childbearing prior to consideration of risk-reducing surgery. In addition, there does not appear to be a contraindication to estrogen replacement therapy after risk-reducing surgery. Two studies have performed cost-effectiveness analyses of options for gynecologic risk reduction in women with Lynch syndrome (133,134). Both studies found that risk-reducing hysterectomy and salpingo-oophorectomy led to the lowest cost and the greatest increase in quality-adjusted life years.

For patients undergoing colonic resection for a Lynch-associated colorectal cancer, it may be reasonable to discuss concomitant hysterectomy with BSO. However, for premenopausal patients who are diagnosed with Lynch syndrome at the same time as their colorectal cancer, substantial fertility and psychosocial issues may be associated with this approach.

Other Inherited Syndromes with a Gynecologic Cancer Component

Cowden Syndrome

Cowden syndrome is caused by germline mutations in the *PTEN* gene. Individuals with Cowden syndrome are at increased risk for both benign and malignant processes. These include GI polyps, thyroid disease, and mucocutaneous lesions, as well as breast, thyroid, and endometrial cancer (135). The lifetime risk of endometrial cancer in a woman with Cowden syndrome has been estimated to be 19% to 28% (136,137). Current NCCN guidelines recommend observation for and prompt evaluation of abnormal uterine bleeding (5). Screening with endometrial biopsies and/or ultrasound measurement of the endometrial stripe is being evaluated in the context of ongoing research studies.

Li–Fraumeni Syndrome

Li–Fraumeni syndrome is caused by germline mutations in *TP53* and is characterized by early-onset breast cancer, soft tissue and bone sarcomas, adrenal cortical tumors, and brain tumors (138). Although it is not a major cancer risk in individuals with Li–Fraumeni syndrome, cases of ovarian cancer have been reported. While screening breast MRI is recommended beginning at age 20 to 25, there are no current screening recommendations for gynecologic cancers in women with Li–Fraumeni syndrome (5,139).

Peutz–Jeghers Syndrome

Peutz–Jeghers syndrome is caused by germline mutations in *STK11*. Peutz–Jeghers is generally characterized by multiple GI polyps and pigmented lesions on the lips and buccal mucosa. Women with this syndrome also have a markedly increased risk for GI and breast malignancies (140). Gynecologic cancers associated with this syndrome include sex cord–stromal tumors with annular tubules (SCTAT) of the ovary and adenoma malignum of the cervix (141). SCTATs are typically benign and bilateral. Adenoma malignum of the cervix is a rare, though aggressive, neoplasm that can also be seen in Peutz–Jeghers syndrome. It is often difficult to diagnose clinically and histologically. On imaging, the tumor appears as a multicystic endocervical mass. Histologically, the tumor appears well differentiated, but the natural history can be aggressive. Due to the rarity of both this syndrome and the associated gynecologic cancers, it is unclear whether women with Peutz–Jeghers should be screened. Regular pap smears using liquid-based cytology, beginning at age 25, have been recommended. However, the role of pelvic imaging is unclear (142).

Hereditary Small Cell Carcinoma of the Ovary, Hypercalcemic Type

Small cell carcinoma of the ovary, hypercalcemic type (SCCOHT), is a highly lethal ovarian malignancy that presents primarily in adolescents and young adults (median age of diagnosis is 25) (143). These tumors are caused by mutations in *SMARCA4* (144–146), with as many as 43% caused by germline mutations (143). For patients with suspected SCCOHT, immunostaining of tumor for the BRG1 protein, which is encoded by *SMARCA4*, is recommended. If BRG1 protein expression is absent, genetic counseling is recommended to assist with management decisions regarding the contralateral ovary and allow predictive testing of at-risk relatives. While the risk for developing SCCOHT associated with *SMARCA4* mutations is not entirely known, presymptomatic risk-reducing oophorectomy has been performed in this setting (147).

References

1. Knudson AG. Mutation and cancer: statistical study of retinoblastoma. *Proc Natl Acad Sci U S A.* 1971;68(4):820–823.
2. Zhang S, Royer R, Li S, et al. Frequencies of BRCA1 and BRCA2 mutations among 1,342 unselected patients with invasive ovarian cancer. *Gynecol Oncol.* 2011;121(2):353–357.
3. Alsop K, Fereday S, Meldrum C, et al. BRCA mutation frequency and patterns of treatment response in BRCA mutation-positive women with ovarian cancer: a report from the Australian Ovarian Cancer Study Group. *J Clin Oncol.* 2012;30(21):2654–2663.
4. American College of Obstetricians and Gynecologists; ACOG Committee on Practice Bulletins—Gynecology; ACOG Committee on Genetics; Society of Gynecologic Oncologists. ACOG Practice Bulletin No. 103: Hereditary breast and ovarian cancer syndrome. *Obstet Gynecol.* 2009;113(4):957–966.
5. National Comprehensive Cancer Network; NCCN Clinical Practice Guidelines in Oncology—Genetic/Familial High-Risk Assessment: Breast and ovarian. 2016. Version 2.2016. http://www.nccn.org.
6. Norquist BM, Harrell MI, Brady MF, et al. Inherited mutations in women with ovarian carcinoma. *JAMA Oncol.* 2016;2(4):482–490.
7. Ramus SJ, Song H, Dicks E, et al. Germline mutations in the BRIP1, BARD1, PALB2, and NBN genes in women with ovarian cancer. *J Natl Cancer Inst.* 2015;107(11).
8. Song H, Dicks E, Ramus SJ, et al. Contribution of germline mutations in the RAD51B, RAD51C, and RAD51D genes to ovarian cancer in the population. *J Clin Oncol.* 2015;33(26):2901–2907.
9. Easton DF, Pharaoh PD, Antoniou AC, et al. Gene-panel sequencing and the prediction of breast-cancer risk. *N Engl J Med.* 2015;372(23):2243–2257.
10. Antoniou A, Pharaoh PDP, Narod S, et al. Average risks of breast and ovarian cancer associated with BRCA1 or BRCA2 mutations detected in case series unselected for family history: a combined analysis of 22 studies. *Am J Hum Genet.* 2003;72(5):1117–1130.
11. Soslow RA, Han G, Park KJ, et al. Morphologic patterns associated with BRCA1 and BRCA2 genotype in ovarian carcinoma. *Mod Pathol.* 2011;25(4):625–636.
12. Zhong Q, Peng HL, Zhao X, et al. Effects of BRCA1- and BRCA2-related mutations on ovarian and breast cancer survival: a meta-analysis. *Clin Cancer Res.* 2015;21(1):211–220.
13. Chetrit A, Hirsh-Yechezkel G, Ben-David Y, et al. Effect of BRCA1/2 mutations on long-term survival of patients with invasive ovarian cancer: the national Israeli study of ovarian cancer. *J Clin Oncol.* 2008;26(1):20–25.
14. Cancer Genome Atlas Research Network. Integrated genomic analyses of ovarian carcinoma. *Nature.* 2011;474(7353):609–615.
15. Yang D, Khan S, Sun Y, et al. Association of BRCA1 and BRCA2 mutations with survival, chemotherapy sensitivity, and gene mutator phenotype in patients with ovarian cancer. *JAMA.* 2011;306(14):1557–1565.
16. Bolton KL. Association between mutations and survival in women with invasive epithelial ovarian cancer. *JAMA.* 2012;307(4):382–390.
17. Kauff ND. Is it time to stratify for BRCA mutation status in therapeutic trials in ovarian cancer? *J Clin Oncol.* 2008;26(1):9–10.

18. Hyman DM, Spriggs DR. Unwrapping the implications of BRCA1 and BRCA2 mutations in ovarian cancer. *JAMA.* 2012;307(4):408–410.
19. Husain A, He G, Venkatraman ES, Spriggs DR. BRCA1 up-regulation is associated with repair-mediated resistance to cis-diamminedichloroplatinum(II). *Cancer Res.* 1998;58(6):1120–1123.
20. Yuan SS, Lee SY, Chen G, et al. BRCA2 is required for ionizing radiation-induced assembly of Rad51 complex in vivo. *Cancer Res.* 1999;59(15):3547–3551.
21. Bryant HE, Schultz N, Thomas HD, et al. Specific killing of BRCA2-deficient tumors with inhibitors of poly(ADP-ribose) polymerase. *Nature.* 2005;434(7035):913–917.
22. Farmer H, McCabe N, Lord CJ, et al. Targeting the DNA repair defect in BRCA mutant cells as a therapeutic strategy. *Nature.* 2005;434(7035):917–921.
23. Heitz F, Harter P, Ewald-Riegler N, et al. Poly(ADP-ribosyl)ation polymerases: mechanism and new target of anticancer therapy. *Expert Rev Anticancer Ther.* 2010;10(7):1125–1136.
24. Fong PC, Boss DS, Yap TA, et al. Inhibition of Poly(ADP-Ribose) polymerase in tumors from BRCA mutation carriers. *N Engl J Med.* 2009;361(2):123–134.
25. Kaufman B, Shapira-Frommer R, Schmutzler RK, et al. Olaparib monotherapy in patients with advanced cancer and a germline BRCA1/2 mutation. *J Clin Oncol.* 2015;33(3):244–250.
26. Ledermann J, Harter P, Gourley C, et al. Olaparib maintenance therapy in patients with platinum-sensitive relapsed serous ovarian cancer: a preplanned retrospective analysis of outcomes by BRCA status in a randomized phase 2 trial. *Lancet Oncol.* 2014;15(8):852–861.
27. Drew Y. The development of PARP inhibitors in ovarian cancer: from bench to bedside. *Br J Cancer.* 2015;113(Suppl 1):S3–S9.
28. Ledermann JA, Drew Y, Kristeleit RS. Homologous recombination deficiency and ovarian cancer. *Eur J Cancer.* 2016;60:49–58.
29. Haile RW, Thomas DC, McGuire V, et al. BRCA1 and BRCA2 mutation carriers, oral contraceptive use, and breast cancer before age 50. *Cancer Epidemiol Biomarkers Prev.* 2006;15(10):1863–1870.
30. Prevalence and penetrance of BRCA1 and BRCA2 mutations in a population-based series of breast cancer cases. Anglian Breast Cancer Study Group. *Br J Cancer.* 2000;83(10):1301–1308.
31. Walsh T, Casadei S, Coats KH, et al. Spectrum of mutations in BRCA1, BRCA2, CHEK2, and TP53 in families at high risk of breast cancer. *JAMA.* 2006;295(12):1379.
32. Palma MD, Domchek SM, Stopfer J, et al. The relative contribution of point mutations and genomic rearrangements in BRCA1 and BRCA2 in high-risk breast cancer families. *Cancer Res.* 2008;68(17):7006–7014.
33. Judkins T, Rosenthal E, Arnell C, et al. Clinical significance of large rearrangements in BRCA1 and BRCA2. *Cancer.* 2012;118(21):5210–5216.
34. Hall MJ, Reid JE, Burbidge LA, et al. BRCA1 and BRCA2 mutations in women of different ethnicities undergoing testing for hereditary breast-ovarian cancer. *Cancer.* 2009;115(10):2222–2233.
35. Kesselheim AS, Cook-Deegan RM, Winickoff DE, et al. Gene patenting-the Supreme Court finally speaks. *N Engl J Med.* 2013;369(9):869–875.
36. Robson ME, Bradbury AR, Arun B, et al. American Society of Clinical Oncology policy statement update: genetic and genomic testing for cancer susceptibility. *J Clin Oncol.* 2015;33(31):3660–3667.
37. Axilbund JE. Panel testing is not a panacea. *J Clin Oncol.* 2016;34(13):1433–1435.
38. Yu PP, Vose JM, Hayes DF. Genetic cancer susceptibility testing: increased technology, increased complexity. *J Clin Oncol.* 2015;33(31):3533–3534.
39. Barnes DR, Antoniou AC. Unravelling modifiers of breast and ovarian cancer risk for BRCA1 and BRCA2 mutation carriers: update on genetic modifiers. *J Intern Med.* 2012;271(4):331–343.
40. Stadler ZK, Thom P, Robson ME, et al. Genome-wide association studies of cancer. *J Clin Oncol.* 2010;28(27):4255–4267.
41. Offit K, Groeger E, Turner S, et al. The "duty to warn" a patient's family members about hereditary disease risks. *JAMA.* 2004;292(12):1469–1473.
42. King MC. Breast and ovarian cancer risks due to inherited mutations in BRCA1 and BRCA2. *Science.* 2003;302(5645):643–646.
43. Boyd J, Sonoda Y, Federici MG, et al. Clinicopathologic features of *BRCA*-linked and sporadic ovarian cancer. *JAMA.* 2000;283(17):2260–2265.
44. Chen S, Parmigiani G. Meta-analysis of BRCA1 and BRCA2 penetrance. *J Clin Oncol.* 2007;25(11):1329–33.
45. Ford D, Easton DF, Stratton M, et al. Genetic heterogeneity and penetrance analysis of the BRCA1 and BRCA2 genes in breast cancer families. *Am J Hum Genet.* 1998;62(3):676–689.
46. Tung N, Domchek SM, Stadler Z, et al. Counseling framework for moderate-penetrance cancer-susceptibility mutations. *Nat Rev Clin Oncol.* 2016;13(9):581–588.
47. Lancaster JM, Powell CB, Chen LM, Richardson DL. Society of Gynecologic Oncology statement on risk assessment for inherited gynecologic cancer predispositions. *Gynecol Oncol.* 2015;136(1):3–7.
48. Buys SS, Partridge E, Black A, et al. Effect of screening on ovarian cancer mortality: the Prostate, Lung, Colorectal and Ovarian (PLCO) Cancer Screening Randomized Controlled Trial. *JAMA.* 2011;305(22):2295–2303.
49. Jacobs IJ, Menon U, Ryan A, et al. Ovarian cancer screening and mortality in the UK Collaborative Trial of Ovarian Cancer Screening (UKCTOCS): a randomized controlled trial. *Lancet.* 2016;387(10022):945–956.
50. Rosenthal AN, Fraser L, Manchanda R, et al. Results of annual screening in phase I of the United Kingdom familial ovarian cancer screening study highlight the need for strict adherence to screening schedule. *J Clin Oncol.* 2013;31(1):49–57.
51. Greene MH, Piedmonte M, Alberts D, et al. A prospective study of risk-reducing salpingo-oophorectomy and longitudinal CA-125 screening among women at increased genetic risk of ovarian cancer: design and baseline characteristics: a Gynecologic Oncology Group Study. *Cancer Epidemiol Biomarkers Prev.* 2008;17(3):594–604.
52. Saslow D, Boetes C, Burke W, et al. American cancer society guidelines for breast screening with MRI as an adjunct to mammography. *CA Cancer J Clin.* 2007;57(2):75–89.
53. Brekelmans CT, Seynaeve C, Bartels CC, et al. Effectiveness of breast cancer surveillance in BRCA1/2 gene mutation carriers and women with high familial risk. *J Clin Oncol.* 2001;19(4):924–930.
54. Scheuer L, Kauff N, Robson M, et al. Outcome of preventive surgery and screening for breast and ovarian cancer in BRCA mutation carriers. *J Clin Oncol.* 2002;20(5):1260–1268.
55. Leach MO, Boggis CR, Dixon AK, et al. Screening with magnetic resonance imaging and mammography of a UK population at high familial risk of breast cancer: a prospective multicentre cohort study (MARIBS). *Lancet.* 2005;365(9473):1769–1778.
56. Warner E, Hill K, Causer P, et al. Prospective study of breast cancer incidence in women with a BRCA1 or BRCA2 mutation under surveillance with and without magnetic resonance imaging. *J Clin Oncol.* 2011;29(13):1664–1669.
57. Beral V, Doll R, Hermon C, et al. Ovarian cancer and oral contraceptives: collaborative reanalysis of data from 45 epidemiological studies including 23,257 women with ovarian cancer and 87,303 controls. *Lancet.* 2008;371(9609):303–314.
58. Iodice S, Barile M, Rotmensz N, et al. Oral contraceptive use and breast or ovarian cancer risk in BRCA1/2 carriers: a meta-analysis. *Eur J Cancer.* 2010;46(12):2275–2284.
59. King MC, Wieand S, Hale K, et al. Tamoxifen and breast cancer incidence among women with inherited mutations in BRCA1 and BRCA2: National Surgical Adjuvant Breast and Bowel Project (NSABP-P1) Breast Cancer Prevention Trial. *JAMA.* 2001;286(18):2251–2256.
60. Lakhani SR. The pathology of familial breast cancer: predictive value of immunohistochemical markers estrogen receptor, progesterone receptor, HER-2, and p53 in patients with mutations in BRCA1 and BRCA2. *J Clin Oncol.* 2002;20(9):2310–2318.
61. Foulkes WD. Estrogen receptor status in BRCA1- and BRCA2-related breast cancer: the influence of age, grade, and histological type. *Clin Cancer Res.* 2004;10(6):2029–2034.
62. Narod SA, Brunet J-S, Ghadirian P, et al. Tamoxifen and risk of contralateral breast cancer in BRCA1 and BRCA2 mutation carriers: a case-control study. *Lancet.* 2000;356(9245):1876–1881.
63. Weitzel JN, Robson M, Pasini B, et al. A comparison of bilateral breast cancers in BRCA carriers. *Cancer Epidemiol Biomarkers Prev.* 2005;14(6):1534–1538.
64. Kauff ND, Satagopan JM, Robson ME, et al. Risk-reducing salpingo-oophorectomy in women with a BRCA1 or BRCA2 mutation. *N Engl J Med.* 2002;346(21):1609–1615.
65. Rebbeck TR, Lynch HT, Neuhausen SL, et al. Prophylactic oophorectomy in carriers of BRCA1 or BRCA2 mutations. *N Engl J Med.* 2002;346(21):1616–1622.
66. Klaren HM, van't Veer LJ, van Leeuwen FE, et al. Potential for bias in studies on efficacy of prophylactic surgery for BRCA1 and BRCA2 mutation. *J Natl Cancer Inst.* 2003;95(13):941–947.
67. Hartmann LC, Lindor NM. Risk-reducing surgery in hereditary breast and ovarian cancer. *N Engl J Med.* 2016;374(24):2404.
68. Rebbeck TR, Kauff ND, Domchek SM. Meta-analysis of risk reduction estimates associated with risk-reducing salpingo-oophorectomy in BRCA1 or BRCA2 mutation carriers. *J Natl Cancer Inst.* 2009;101(2):80–87.
69. Dubeau L. The cell of origin of ovarian epithelial tumors. *Lancet Oncol.* 2008;9(12):1191–1197.

70. Rebbeck TR, Levin AM, Eisen A, et al. Breast cancer risk after bilateral prophylactic oophorectomy in BRCA1 mutation carriers. *J Natl Cancer Inst.* 1999;91(17):1475–1479.
71. Kauff ND, Domchek SM, Friebel TM, et al. Risk-reducing salpingo-oophorectomy for the prevention of BRCA1- and BRCA2-associated breast and gynecologic cancer: a multicenter, prospective study. *J Clin Oncol.* 2008;26(8):1331–1337.
72. Heemskerk-Gerritsen BA, Seynaeve C, van Asperen CJ, et al. Breast cancer risk after salpingo-oophorectomy in healthy BRCA1/2 mutation carriers: revisiting the evidence for risk reduction. *J Natl Cancer Inst.* 2015;107(5).
73. Chai X, Domchek S, Kauff N, et al. RE: breast cancer risk after salpingo-oophorectomy in healthy BRCA1/2 mutation carriers: revisiting the evidence for risk reduction. *J Natl Cancer Inst.* 2015;107(9).
74. Domchek SM, Friebel TM, Singer CF, et al. Association of risk-reducing surgery in BRCA1 or BRCA2 mutation carriers with cancer risk and mortality. *JAMA.* 2010;304(9):967–975.
75. Finch AP, Lubinski J, Moller P, et al. Impact of oophorectomy on cancer incidence and mortality in women with a BRCA1 or BRCA2 mutation. *J Clin Oncol.* 2014;32(15):1547–1553.
76. Manchanda R, Drapkin R, Jacobs I, et al. The role of peritoneal cytology at risk-reducing salpingo-oophorectomy (RRSO) in women at increased risk of familial ovarian/tubal cancer. *Gynecol Oncol.* 2012;124(2):185–191.
77. Kauff ND, Barakat RR. Risk-reducing salpingo-oophorectomy in patients with germline mutations in BRCA1 or BRCA2. *J Clin Oncol.* 2007;25(20):2921–2927.
78. Powell CB, Kenley E, Chen LM, et al. Risk-reducing salpingo-oophorectomy in BRCA mutation carriers: role of serial sectioning in the detection of occult malignancy. *J Clin Oncol.* 2004;23(1):127–132.
79. Finch A, Shaw P, Rosen B, et al. Clinical and pathologic findings of prophylactic salpingo-oophorectomies in 159 BRCA1 and BRCA2 carriers. *Gynecol Oncol.* 2006;100(1):58–64.
80. Yates MS, Meyer LA, Deavers MT, et al. Microscopic and early-stage ovarian cancers in BRCA1/2 mutation carriers: building a model for early BRCA-associated tumorigenesis. *Cancer Prev Res.* 2011;4(3):463–470.
81. Medeiros F, Muto MG, Lee Y, et al. The tubal fimbria is a preferred site for early adenocarcinoma in women with familial ovarian cancer syndrome. *Am J Surg Pathol.* 2006;30(2):230–236.
82. Shaw PA, Rouzbahman M, Pizer ES, et al. Candidate serous cancer precursors in fallopian tube epithelium of BRCA1/2 mutation carriers. *Mod Pathol.* 2009;22(9):1133–1138.
83. Powell CB, Chen LM, McLennan J, et al. Risk-reducing salpingo-oophorectomy (RRSO) in BRCA mutation carriers. *Int J Gynecol Cancer.* 2011;21(5):846–851.
84. Wethington SL, Park KJ, Soslow RA, et al. Clinical outcome of isolated serous tubal intraepithelial carcinomas (STIC). *Int J Gynecol Cancer.* 2013;23(9):1603–1611.
85. Satagopan JM, Boyd J, Kauff ND, et al. Ovarian cancer risk in Ashkenazi Jewish carriers of BRCA1 and BRCA2 mutations. *Clin Cancer Res.* 2002;8(12):3776–3781.
86. Shu CA, Pike MC, Jotwani AR, et al. Uterine cancer after risk-reducing salpingo-oophorectomy without hysterectomy in women with BRCA mutations. *JAMA Oncol.* 2016;2(11):1434–40.
87. Kwon JS, Tinker A, Pansegrau G, et al. Prophylactic salpingectomy and delayed oophorectomy as an alternative for BRCA mutation carriers. *Obstet Gynecol.* 2013;121(1):14–24.
88. Hanley GE, McAlpine JN, Kwon JS, et al. Opportunistic salpingectomy for ovarian cancer prevention. *Gynecol Oncol Res Pract.* 2015;2:5.
89. Meijers-Heijboer H, van Geel B, van Putten WLJ, et al. Breast cancer after prophylactic bilateral mastectomy in women with a BRCA1 or BRCA2 mutation. *N Engl J Med.* 2001;345(3):159–164.
90. Rebbeck TR. Bilateral prophylactic mastectomy reduces breast cancer risk in BRCA1 and BRCA2 mutation carriers: the PROSE Study Group. *J Clin Oncol.* 2004;22(6):1055–1062.
91. Kurian AW, Sigal BM, Plevritis SK. Survival analysis of cancer risk reduction strategies for BRCA1/2 mutation carriers. *J Clin Oncol.* 2009;28(2):222–231.
92. Gruber SB, Thompson WD. A population-based study of endometrial cancer and familial risk in younger women. Cancer and Steroid Hormone Study Group. *Cancer Epidemiol Biomarkers Prev.* 1996;5(6):411–417.
93. Aarnio M, Sankila R, Pukkala E, et al. Cancer risk in mutation carriers of DNA-mismatch-repair genes. *Int J Cancer.* 1999;81(2):214–218.
94. Bonadona V. Cancer risks associated with germline mutations in genes in Lynch syndrome. *JAMA.* 2011;305(22):2304–2310.
95. Baglietto L, Lindor NM, Dowty JG, et al. Risks of Lynch syndrome cancers for MSH6 mutation carriers. *J Natl Cancer Inst.* 2009;102(3):193–201.
96. Dunlop MG, Farrington SM, Nicholl I, et al. Population carrier frequency of hMSH2 and hMLH1 mutations. *Br J Cancer.* 2000;83(12):1643–1645.
97. de la Chapelle A. The incidence of Lynch syndrome. *Fam Cancer.* 2005;4(3):233–237.
98. Hampel H, Frankel W, Panescu J, et al. Screening for Lynch syndrome (hereditary nonpolyposis colorectal cancer) among endometrial cancer patients. *Cancer Res.* 2006;66(15):7810–7817.
99. Lu KH, Schorge JO, Rodabaugh KJ, et al. Prospective determination of prevalence of Lynch syndrome in young women with endometrial cancer. *J Clin Oncol.* 2007;25(33):5158–5164.
100. Berends MJW. Toward new strategies to select young endometrial cancer patients for mismatch repair gene mutation analysis. *J Clin Oncol.* 2003;21(23):4364–4370.
101. Matthews KS, Estes JM, Conner MG, et al. Lynch syndrome in women less than 50 years of age with endometrial cancer. *Obstet Gynecol.* 2008;111(5):1161–1166.
102. Lu KH, Dinh M, Kohlmann W, et al. Gynecologic cancer as a "sentinel cancer" for women with hereditary nonpolyposis colorectal cancer syndrome. *Obstet Gynecol.* 2005;105(3):569–574.
103. Broaddus RR, Lynch HT, Chen LM, et al. Pathologic features of endometrial carcinoma associated with HNPCC. *Cancer.* 2006;106(1):87–94.
104. Westin SN, Lacour RA, Urbauer DL, et al. Carcinoma of the lower uterine segment: a newly described association with Lynch syndrome. *J Clin Oncol.* 2008;26(36):5965–5971.
105. Ketabi Z, Bartuma K, Bernstein I, et al. Ovarian cancer linked to Lynch syndrome typically presents as early-onset, non-serous epithelial tumors. *Gynecol Oncol.* 2011;121(3):462–465.
106. Vasen HF, Mecklin JP, Khan PM, et al. The international collaborative group on hereditary non-polyposis colorectal cancer (ICG-HNPCC). *Dis Colon Rectum.* 1991;34(5):424–425.
107. Vasen HF, Watson P, Mecklin JP, et al. New clinical criteria for hereditary nonpolyposis colorectal cancer (HNPCC, Lynch syndrome) proposed by the International Collaborative group on HNPCC. *Gastroenterology.* 1999;116(6):1453–1456.
108. Hampel H, Frankel WL, Martin E, et al. Screening for the Lynch syndrome (hereditary nonpolyposis colorectal cancer). *N Engl J Med.* 2005;352(18):1851–1860.
109. Pinol V, Castells A, Andreu M, et al. Accuracy of revised Bethesda guidelines, microsatellite instability, and immunohistochemistry for the identification of patients with hereditary nonpolyposis colorectal cancer. *JAMA.* 2005;293(16):1986–1994.
110. Rodriguez-Bigas MA, Boland CR, Hamilton SR, et al. A national cancer institute workshop on hereditary nonpolyposis colorectal cancer syndrome: meeting highlights and Bethesda guidelines. *J Natl Cancer Inst.* 1997;89(23):1758–1762.
111. Umar A, Boland CR, Terdiman JP, et al. Revised Bethesda Guidelines for hereditary nonpolyposis colorectal cancer (Lynch syndrome) and microsatellite instability. *J Natl Cancer Inst.* 2004;96(4):261–268.
112. Kauff ND. How should women with early-onset endometrial cancer be evaluated for lynch syndrome? *J Clin Oncol.* 2007;25(33):5143–5146.
113. Committee on Practice Bulletins-Gynecology; Society of Gynecologic Oncology. ACOG Practice Bulletin No. 147: Lynch syndrome. *Obstet Gynecol.* 2014;124(5):1042–1054.
114. Giardiello FM, Allen JI, Axilbund JE, et al. Guidelines on genetic evaluation and management of Lynch syndrome: a consensus statement by the US Multi-society Task Force on colorectal cancer. *Am J Gastroenterol.* 2014;109(8):1159–1179.
115. Buchanan DD, Tan YY, Walsh MD, et al. Tumor mismatch repair immunohistochemistry and DNA MLH1 methylation testing of patients with endometrial cancer diagnosed at age younger than 60 years optimizes triage for population-level germline mismatch repair gene mutation testing. *J Clin Oncol.* 2014;32(2):90–100.
116. Haraldsdottir S, Hampel H, Tomsic J, et al. Colon and endometrial cancers with mismatch repair deficiency can arise from somatic, rather than germline, mutations. *Gastroenterology.* 2014;147(6):1308–1316. e1301.
117. Lindor NM, Petersen GM, Hadley DW, et al. Recommendations for the care of individuals with an inherited predisposition to Lynch syndrome. *JAMA.* 2006;296(12):1507–1517.
118. National Comprehensive Cancer Network. *Clinical Practice Guidelines in Oncology for Genetic/Familial High-Risk Assessment: Colorectal V1.* Fort Washington, PA: National Comprehensive Cancer Network; 2016.
119. Järvinen HJ, Aarnio M, Mustonen H, et al. Controlled 15-year trial on screening for colorectal cancer in families with hereditary nonpolyposis colorectal cancer. *Gastroenterology.* 2000;118(5):829–834.

120. Vasen HF, Abdirahman M, Brohet R, et al. One to 2-year surveillance intervals reduce risk of colorectal cancer in families with Lynch syndrome. *Gastroenterology.* 2010;138(7):2300–2306.
121. Rijcken FEM, Mourits MJE, Kleibeuker JH, et al. Gynecologic screening in hereditary nonpolyposis colorectal cancer. *Gynecol Oncol.* 2003;91(1):74–80.
122. Dove-Edwin I, Boks D, Goff S, et al. The outcome of endometrial carcinoma surveillance by ultrasound scan in women at risk of hereditary nonpolyposis colorectal carcinoma and familial colorectal carcinoma. *Cancer.* 2002;94(6):1708–1712.
123. Renkonen-Sinisalo L, Bützow R, Leminen A, et al. Surveillance for endometrial cancer in hereditary nonpolyposis colorectal cancer syndrome. *Int J Cancer.* 2006;120(4):821–824.
124. Gerritzen LHM, Hoogerbrugge N, Oei ALM, et al. Improvement of endometrial biopsy over transvaginal ultrasound alone for endometrial surveillance in women with Lynch syndrome. *Fam Cancer.* 2009;8(4):391–397.
125. Huang M, Sun C, Boyd-Rogers S, et al. Prospective study of combined colon and endometrial cancer screening in women with Lynch syndrome: a patient-centered approach. *J Oncol Pract.* 2011;7(1):43–47.
126. Collaborative Group on Epidemiological Studies on Endometrial Cancer. Endometrial cancer and oral contraceptives: an individual participant meta-analysis of 27 276 women with endometrial cancer from 36 epidemiological studies. *Lancet Oncol.* 2015;16(9):1061–1070.
127. Rodolakis A, Biliatis I, Morice P, et al. European society of gynecological oncology task force for fertility preservation: clinical recommendations for fertility-sparing management in young endometrial cancer patients. *Int J Gynecol Cancer.* 2015;25(7):1258–1265.
128. Lu KH, Loose DS, Yates MS, et al. Prospective multicenter randomized intermediate biomarker study of oral contraceptive versus depo-provera for prevention of endometrial cancer in women with Lynch syndrome. *Cancer Prev Res (Phila).* 2013;6(8):774–781.
129. Schmeler KM, Lynch HT, Chen LM, et al. Prophylactic surgery to reduce the risk of gynecologic cancers in the Lynch syndrome. *N Engl J Med.* 2006;354(3):261–269.
130. Schmeler KM, Daniels MS, Soliman PT, et al. Primary peritoneal cancer after bilateral salpingo-oophorectomy in two patients with Lynch syndrome. *Obstet Gynecol.* 2010;115(Suppl):432–434.
131. Pistorius S, Kruger S, Hohl R, et al. Occult endometrial cancer and decision making for prophylactic hysterectomy in hereditary nonpolyposis colorectal cancer patients. *Gynecol Oncol.* 2006;102(2):189–194.
132. Palma L, Marcus V, Gilbert L, et al. Synchronous occult cancers of the endometrium and fallopian tube in an MSH2 mutation carrier at time of prophylactic surgery. *Gynecol Oncol.* 2008;111(3):575–578.
133. Kwon JS, Sun CC, Peterson SK, et al. Cost-effectiveness analysis of prevention strategies for gynecologic cancers in Lynch syndrome. *Cancer.* 2008;113(2):326–335.
134. Yang KY, Caughey AB, Little SE, et al. A cost-effectiveness analysis of prophylactic surgery versus gynecologic surveillance for women from hereditary non-polyposis colorectal cancer (HNPCC) Families. *Fam Cancer.* 2011;10(3):535–543.
135. Pilarski R, Burt R, Kohlman W, et al. Cowden syndrome and the PTEN hamartoma tumor syndrome: systematic review and revised diagnostic criteria. *J Natl Cancer Inst.* 2013;105(21):1607–1616.
136. Tan MH, Mester JL, Ngeow J, et al. Lifetime cancer risks in individuals with germline PTEN mutations. *Clin Cancer Res.* 2012;18(2):400–407.
137. Bubien V, Bonnet F, Brouste V, et al. High cumulative risks of cancer in patients with PTEN hamartoma tumor syndrome. *J Med Genet.* 2013;50(4):255–263.
138. McBride KA, Ballinger ML, Killick E, et al. Li–Fraumeni syndrome: cancer risk assessment and clinical management. *Nat Rev Clin Oncol.* 2014;11(5):260–271.
139. Mai PL, Malkin D, Garber JE, et al. Li–Fraumeni syndrome: report of a clinical research workshop and creation of a research consortium. *Cancer Genet.* 2012;205(10):479–487.
140. Syngal S, Brand RE, Church JM, et al. ACG clinical guideline: genetic testing and management of hereditary gastrointestinal cancer syndromes. *Am J Gastroenterol.* 2015;110(2):223–262; quiz 263.
141. Young RH, Welch WR, Dickersin GR, et al. Ovarian sex cord tumor with annular tubules. Review of 74 cases including 27 with Peutz–Jeghers syndrome and four with adenoma malignum of the cervix. *Cancer.* 1982;50(7):1384–1402.
142. Beggs AD, Latchford AR, Vasen HFA, et al. Peutz–Jeghers syndrome: a systematic review and recommendations for management. *Gut.* 2010;59(7):975–986.
143. Witkowski L, Goudie C, Ramos P, et al. The influence of clinical and genetic factors on patient outcome in small cell carcinoma of the ovary, hypercalcemic type. *Gynecol Oncol.* 2016;141(3):454–460.
144. Jelinic P, Mueller JJ, Olvera N, et al. Recurrent SMARCA4 mutations in small cell carcinoma of the ovary. *Nat Genet.* 2014;46(5):424–426.
145. Ramos P, Karnezis AN, Craig DW, et al. Small cell carcinoma of the ovary, hypercalcemic type, displays frequent inactivating germline and somatic mutations in SMARCA4. *Nat Genet.* 2014;46(5):427–429.
146. Witkowski L, Carrot-Zhang J, Albrecht S, et al. Germline and somatic SMARCA4 mutations characterize small cell carcinoma of the ovary, hypercalcemic type. *Nat Genet.* 2014;46(5):438–443.
147. Berchuck A, Witkowski L, Hasselblatt M, et al. Prophylactic oophorectomy for hereditary small cell carcinoma of the ovary, hypercalcemic type. *Gynecol Oncol Rep.* 2015;12:20–22.

CHAPTER 4

Invasion, Metastasis, and Angiogenesis

Angeles A. Secord, Charlie Gourley, and Elise C. Kohn

INTRODUCTION

Gynecologic cancers are potentially curable if diagnosed at an early stage, when the tumor remains confined to the primary organ; survival is compromised by dissemination or metastasis of the disease into, around, or adjacent to vital organs. The process of this dissemination and the result of metastasis require activation of key elements of invasive and angiogenic processes early in disease. Invasion requires activation of adhesion and deadhesion, migration, migration stimulation, and proteolytic and glycolytic events. These are activated in the early precursor cell and continue progressively along the continuum of cancer development (**Fig. 4.1**). We now know the sites of origin for all major epithelial gynecologic cancers and can map at least roughly how and when they may acquire the attributes that make them lethal cancers.

Cervical and endometrial cancers follow the classically recognized development from dysplasia/hyperplasia/metaplasia to carcinoma *in situ* to invasive cancer. Local dissemination occurs predominantly by local invasion into lymphovascular structures, allowing stepwise and generally anatomically direct progression. This permits the success of local interventions of surgery and radiotherapy that are the mainstay of treatment. The general tenet of invasion and metastasis, lymphatic and hematogenous spread to the first capillary beds, fits the common patterns of progression of these cancers. This appears to be consistent with most of the histologic types, although the process is faster for the more aggressive types of clear cell, small cell, and serous cancers, where systemic spread is rapid and necessitates systemic therapeutic intervention.

Ovarian cancer is different in several ways. As described in depth elsewhere in this text, it is now recognized that epithelial ovarian cancer comprises different types, for which there are histopathologic, demographic, and molecular differences (1). The most prevalent and most deadly is the high-grade serous and endometrioid type (HGS/epithelial ovarian cancer), generally sheets of malignant cells, with early shedding into the peritoneal cavity, causing carcinomatosis, rendering nearly all p53 dysfunctional, and initiating from fallopian tube epithelium (2,3). Clear cell and low-grade endometrioid types appear to have common endometriotic precursors, and up to 40% have somatic *ARID1a* mutations (4). Both are more frequent and have a better outcome when presenting in early-stage disease, although clear cell cancers have the highest recurrence rate of early-stage disease at ~40%. Low-grade serous cancers appear to progress from the normal surface epithelium or included surface epithelium, through serous borderline tumor, to invasive disease. They often have *RAS* and *BRAF* mutations, although data suggest that these may not be drivers of malignant or invasive behaviors (5). All types have metastatic potential and angiogenic activity and thus are potentially targetable with this broadening direction of therapeutics.

The ovary is an "inside-out" organ, where the epithelium faces the peritoneal cavity and sits on its basement membrane, the capsule of the ovary. It is a vascular organ, with further cyclical vascular changes occurring during the patient's reproductive years. This angiogenic capacity of the pelvic microenvironment makes the ovaries excellent *soil* for the *seed* of malignancy, primary or metastatic (6,7). Likewise, the fallopian tube is "inside-out," also with its epithelium facing the peritoneal cavity. This orientation facilitates shedding

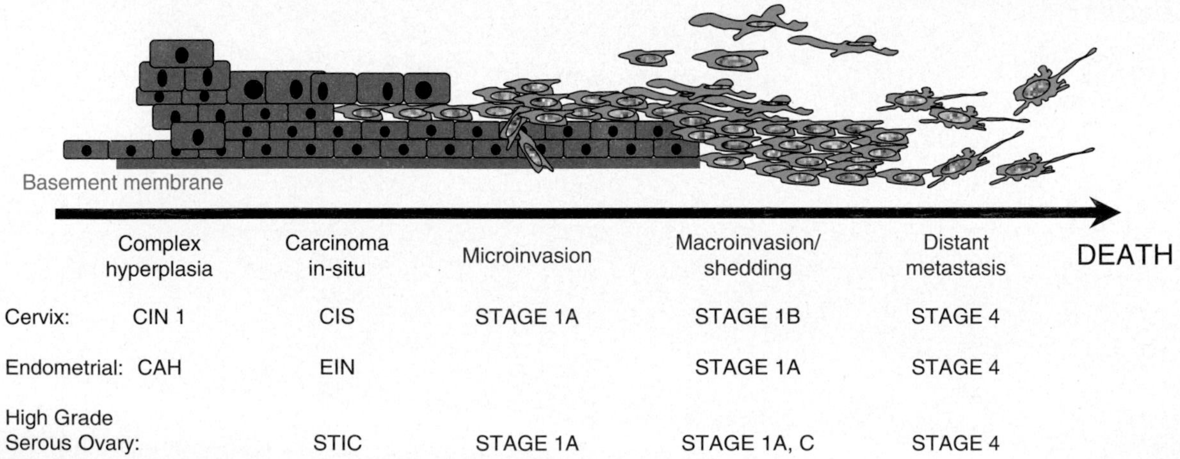

Figure 4.1. Paradigm of cancer progression. Progression from the earliest detectable event of complex hyperplasia to overt invasive and metastatic malignancy is believed to take over a decade for endometrial and cervical cancers. The tubal epithelium is now believed to be the source for type 2 high-grade serous ovarian cancer; the time frame from acquisition of p53 mutation (p53 signature) to STIC is unclear, as is the subsequent time to dissemination. Tubal epithelium can shed at an early and microscopic stage. When identified early, each of these cancers has a high cure rate and long OS. However, when identified at or beyond the stage of microinvasion, progressive disease and death from disease is common. STIC, serous tubal intra-epithelial carcinoma.

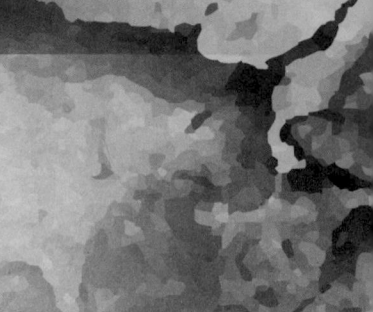

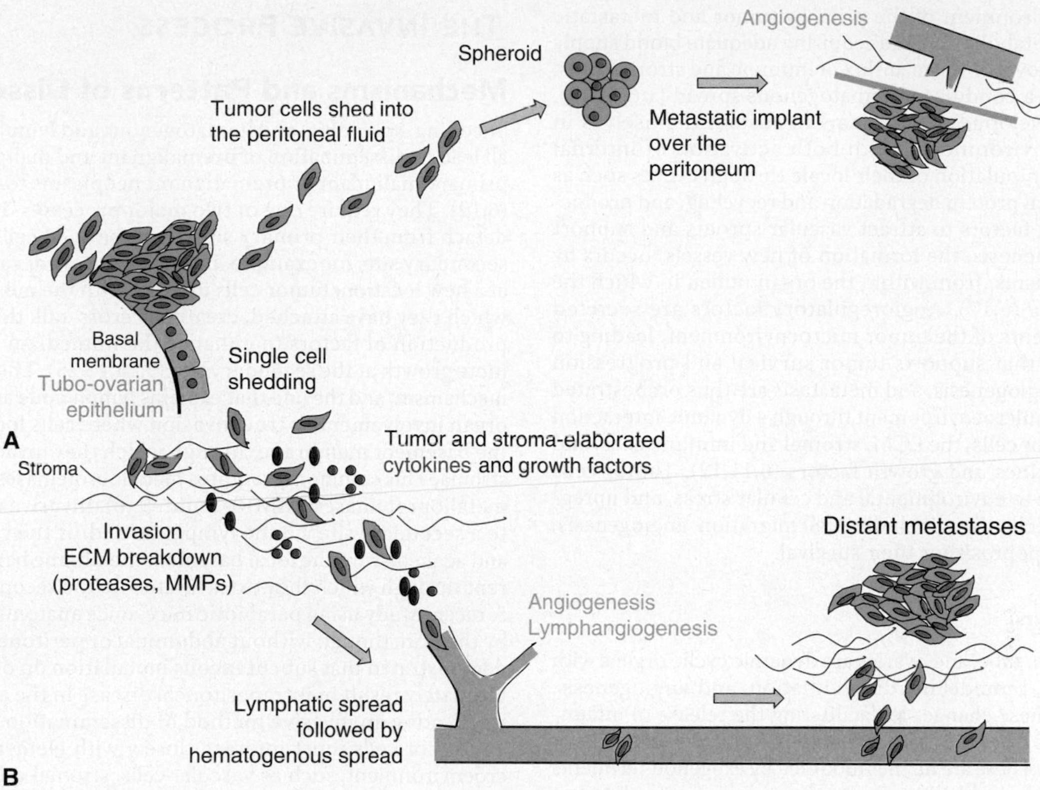

Figure 4.2. Tubo-ovarian cancer: shedding and spreading. The primary tubo-ovarian tumor metastasizes in two different ways. The first mechanism **(A)**, occurring early, is shedding of single cancer cells from the surface of the tube or ovary into the peritoneal cavity; the second mechanism **(B)**, occurring later, is invasion into surrounding and distant tissues. Cells shed in the peritoneal fluid form spheroids that have acquired mechanisms to resist anoikis. These spheroids implant on peritoneal mesothelial surfaces; cause stromal activation with desmoplasia, inflammation, and angiogenesis; and grow into metastatic deposits. ECM, extracellular matrix; MMPs, matrix metalloproteinases.

of premalignant and malignant cells, a process that can occur as early as the point of microscopic malignant disease. The first stop for such shed malignant tubal cells is the prime soil of the vascular and dynamic ovary (**Fig. 4.2**; note epithelium on the outside of the basal membrane).

The progress in understanding ovarian cancer has uncovered an unexpected migratory behavior of endometrial contents along the fallopian tubes. Here, the tubes function as retrograde conduits for endometrial materials to leave the utcrus (8). This happens during endometriosis and can result in endometrial materials enclosed in follicular cysts within the ovary and other forms of ovarian endometriosis. Such occurrences are now presumed to be precursors to clear cell and low-grade endometrioid ovarian cancers, in which *ARID1a* mutations are shared (4). The ovary is the first site reached, the most permissive and the most common site of endometriosis. The seminal processes of invasion and metastases—adhesion, migration, local microenvironmental remodeling, and angiogenesis—are pathologic processes in both benign and malignant pelvic diseases (6).

The Tumor Environment and Metastasis

The genotypic and phenotypic make-up of a tumor is a major determinant of its metastatic efficiency, and a receptive microenvironment is a prerequisite for successful tumor growth (9,10). In 1889, Sir James Paget stated that the microenvironment of each organ, *the soil*, influences the survival and growth of tumor cells, *the seed.* Multiple overlapping signal and adhesion networks cooperate to enable molecular and structural remodeling of tissues that support tumor invasion, growth, and metastatic dissemination. Cellular behavior and activation or inactivation of genes are influenced heavily by the local tumor environment. This reinforces the idea that a complex interplay of molecules and signals is needed for tumor sustainability. The tumor environment has a plasticity that allows participating elements, such as the harsh environment of hypoxia, acidosis, metabolic stress, inflammation, and cellular interactions, to vary throughout the events of cancer progression (10,11).

The tumor environment consists of its microenvironment, or proximate cellular and acellular locale, and the macroenvironment, the local perfused organ milieu. The macroenvironment changes within and between the pelvis and local region of the ovaries and the abdominal cavity and, in part, dictates the local microenvironment. The omentum, for example, has a rich background of pluripotent adipocytes and other cells that interactively promotes generation and release of enzymes and cytokines. These soluble molecules modify the local extracellular matrix (ECM), promoting invasion, proliferation, angiogenesis, and metastasis (11–14).

The microenvironment is governed by the immediate cellular and ambient regional surroundings. The ovary is the first microenvironment for tubal epithelium. The outside-in setting for the epithelium means that any growth factors, cytokines, and ECM components released by the ovarian epithelium may reach the apical or outer margin. The microenvironments of the abdominopelvic serosa, peritoneal mesothelium, and omentum are similarly favorable, though more distant, sites. The mesothelial cell, the single-cell layer of the peritoneum and outer serosal layer of organs, is a pluripotent mesenchymal cell that responds to changes in its surroundings. Such responses may be production and secretion of entities that attract and/or nurture shed tumor as well as vascular precursor cells and immune infiltrates. The omentum is a very advantageous site. Adipose tissue contains adipose stem cells that have shown the ability to differentiate into many different end cells, from bone and connective tissue cells, to vascular endothelium; this has been shown in both ovarian cancer and in endometrial cancer (13,15).

The microenvironment of the primary tumor and metastatic sites has a high metabolic demand requiring adequate blood supply for nutrients, removal of waste, influx of immune and stromal cells, and ultimately as a conduit for hematogenous spread (1,6,11,12). Tumors have developed mechanisms to sustain themselves in nutrient-poor environments, with both activation of internal pathways and manipulation of their locale through events such as autophagy, internal protein degradation and recycling, and producing and secreting factors to attract vascular sprouts and support cells (16). Angiogenesis, the formation of new vessels, occurs by multiple mechanisms, from within the organ milieu in which the tumor is growing (6,17). Angioregulatory factors are secreted into and by elements of the tumor microenvironment, leading to new vasculature that supports tumor survival and progression (11). Invasion, angiogenesis, and metastasis are thus orchestrated within the tumor microenvironment through a dynamic interaction between the tumor cells, the ECM, stromal and immune cells, and secreted chemokines and growth factors (6,11,12). Tumor cells adapt in response to environmental and cellular stress, and upregulate different mechanisms including cell migration, angiogenesis, autophagy, and apoptosis for their survival.

Inflammation

The endometrium, tube, and ovaries are dynamic cyclic organs with cycles of growth, remodeling, differentiation, and angiogenesis. Estrogen drives these changes by facilitating the release of inflammatory mediators from the epithelial, stromal, and vascular cells of the endometrium. These are further modified by exogenous elements such as pharmaceutical hormones, hormonal changes related to obesity, diet, and stress (18,19). For example, the menstrual cycle is a physiologic inflammatory process. There is a strong parallel between the immune regulation and requirements for immune tolerance in the reproductive tract and the findings that support tumor invasion and dissemination due to immune tolerance in gynecologic cancer.

Local activation of select components of the immune response promotes angiogenesis and dissemination, while others interact within the tumor microenvironment to create a potent immunosuppressive effect (20). Inflammatory mechanisms include but are not limited to the recruitment of activated CD8 T cells, production of reactive oxygen species and free radicals that directly damage DNA and proteins, and production of proinflammatory/proangiogenic molecules, such as cytokines, tumor necrosis factor-α, and interleukins (IL)-6, -8, and -10, and tumor growth factor (TGF)-β, promoting local activation and migration of proangiogenic stromal and immune components, and tumor-associated macrophages. Immunosuppressive events that may also occur in the tumor microenvironment to inhibit immune recognition of malignancy include upregulation of regulatory T cells (Tregs), T_H2 cells unable to support a cytolytic response, dysfunctional dendritic cells unable to present antigen, and M20-differentiated macrophages expressing IL-12. These events can collectively upregulate immune checkpoint inhibitors on tumor, endothelial, and immune cells, such as programmed death-1 (PD-1) and PD-ligand 1 and 2 (PDL-1 and -2) (20–23).

Cellular interactions within the tumor microenvironment are a dynamic process and can shift from an immune tolerant to an immune active antitumor mode, with changes in the local environment or with selected therapeutics (22,23). TGF-β, long recognized to be a promoter of tumorigenesis, invasion, and dissemination, also plays a role in promoting immune tolerance. Hypoxia with induction of VEGF, IL-6, and IL-8, among other cytokines and factors, promotes angiogenesis, which provides support for invasion and metastasis while also promoting recruitment and suppression of immune cell types including myeloid-derived suppressor cells, inhibitory macrophages, and Tregs (20,24). The growing understanding of the activity between immune, stromal, and tumor components is helping to guide application of novel immunotherapeutics that can modulate invasion, angiogenesis, and metastatic dissemination.

THE INVASIVE PROCESS

Mechanisms and Patterns of Dissemination

Shedding, spreading, and hematogenous and lymphatic metastasis all lead to dissemination of premalignant and malignant cells from primary malignant or premalignant neoplasms to secondary sites (6,12). They require one of two major processes. In the first, cells detach from their primary site, then the shed cells transport to a secondary site, for example, into the peritoneal cavity, and attach at a new location; tumor cells interact with the mesothelial cells to which they have attached, creating a cross-talk that results in the production of factors to enhance the immediate locale and promote growth at the secondary site (9,14,15,25). The more common mechanism, and the one that explains lymph node and parenchymal organ involvement, is true invasion where cells locally proteolyze the basement membrane through which they invade into the local stroma. This commonly requires metalloproteinases, such as matrix metalloproteinases (MMP)-2 and -9 (6). Invasive cells then travel to a secondary site via the lymphatic and/or the vascular system, and again disrupt the local basement membrane barriers to create a rent through which they extravasate into the secondary site (6,26). A recent study using parabiotic mice, mice anatomically connected by the skin, though without abdominal or peritoneal connections, demonstrated that subcutaneous inoculation on one mouse could ultimately result in intraperitoneal disease in the attached mouse, implicating an invasive method of dissemination (26).

Tumor cells must interact closely with elements in their microenvironment, such as vascular cells, stromal cells, and immune components, to achieve successful metastasis (9,12). The peritoneum, omentum, and mesenteric serosa are permissive environments to which tumor cells can attach and grow, co-opting support cells and vasculature to sustain their survival and growth. Recent preclinical studies have shown active and dynamic interactions between endometrial or ovarian cancer cells with pluripotential omental adipose cells (15,25). These data suggest that peritoneal dissemination seen in ovarian cancer may reflect the process used by endometrial and other cancers at later stages in their dissemination. Many events within the tumor cell support these outcomes.

Epithelial–Mesenchymal Transition

Epithelial–mesenchymal transition (EMT) describes a series of molecular, biochemical, and functional events that occur at a cellular level in response to local changes such as local growth factor and cytokine presence, changes, and/or exposure to the ECM (10,27). These changes progress the epithelial tumor cell along a mesenchymal-like continuum and upregulate survival and invasion signals, promoting single-cell autonomy. The tumor cells of most gynecologic cancers are epithelial in origin and nature, transforming from polarized basement membrane-bound normal cells into freely moving single cells or small groups of cells. Events occurring during EMT include downregulation of proteins that promote the homotypic cell attachment that maintains order and polarization, such as E-cadherin, and upregulation of proteins that promote heterotypic cell adhesion, such as P- and N-cadherin. These are induced by upregulation of key transcription factors, including *slug* and *snail* that inhibit transcription and expression of *CDH1*/E-cadherin, and upregulation of elements of the TGF-β pathway. Such changes occur in response to endogenous and exogenous stimuli along the EMT continuum (10,27,28). These gene expression changes were also described in the transcriptional and genomic analyses of ovarian cancers, leading to a subcategory of an aggressive subset of mesenchymal-like ovarian cancers, where patient outcome is poorest (29,30) (**Fig. 4.3**).

Anoikis is a specific apoptotic process triggered by loss of cell–cell or cell–substratum survival signals (28). It is a physiologic phenomenon that maintains cell and tissue homeostasis and is disrupted in physiologic events such as immune response and

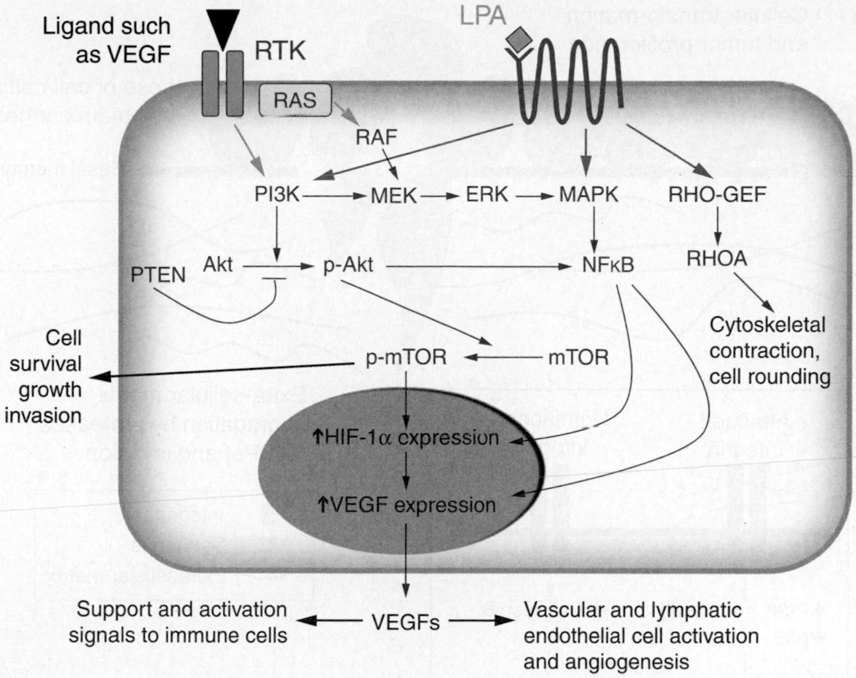

Figure 4.3. Molecular pathways. Activation of AKT is a well-recognized and potent prosurvival and proangiogenic pathway activated by LPA and growth factors and cytokines that activate RTKs. Many of these ligands are produced and secreted by gynecologic cancers, and often by mesothelial, stromal, immune, and/or vascular cells as well. LPA signals through the LPA receptor, a 7-pass transmembrane G-protein-coupled receptor. LPA promotes expression of VEGF for angiogenesis and cell survival through the PI3K/AKT, NF-κB, and MAPK signaling pathways. RTK activation also promotes cell survival, invasion, angiogenesis, and proliferation through the PI3K/AKT, NF-κB, and MAPK pathways. ERK, extracellular regulated kinase; LPA, lysophosphatidic acid; MAPK, mitogen-activated protein kinase; MEK, MAP-ERK kinase; mTOR, mammalian target of rapamycin; NF-κB, nuclear factor κB; PTEN, phosphatase and tensin homolog; Rho-GEF and RHO A are Rho family GTPases; RTK, receptor tyrosine kinases; VEGF, vascular endothelial growth factor.

pregnancy, and pathologically in cancer. Resistance to anoikis allows cancer cells to avoid apoptosis during the metastatic process, when single or small clusters of cells invade and migrate within and out of the ECM. Similarly, tumor cells require prosurvival signals when within effusions where there may be cell-bound or soluble matrix molecules, but not the classical adherent prosurvival behavior of normal epithelial cells. Anoikis resistance is thus critical in the development of carcinomatosis and ascites, creating a permissive survival signal for cancer cells shed into the peritoneal space. These viable clusters then adhere to and invade into serosal mesothelium. The mechanism by which the apoptosis of anoikis is triggered relies on the loss of prosurvival signals induced by the binding between the cell and its scaffolding. The phosphatidyl inositol-3′ kinase (PI3K)/AKT and phosphatase and tensin homolog (PTEN)/AKT pathways produce major prosurvival signals and anoikis resistance. This convergent pathway has been shown to be important in all gynecologic cancers. PI3K activation and/or PTEN loss is prevalent in endometrioid endometrial and ovarian cancers, and promotes the AKT prosurvival signaling pathway (29,31) (**Fig. 4.4**).

Extracellular Matrix

The ECM is the complex glycoproteinaceous structure surrounding and supporting cells. It comprises three major classes of biomolecules: proteoglycans, structural proteins such as collagens and elastins, and specialized matrix proteins such as fibronectin and laminins (6). The ECM serves many functions, including providing cellular scaffolding support, acting as a binding site for growth factors and cofactors, and acting as a modulator of intercellular communication. Integrins are heterodimeric transmembrane receptors that integrate microenvironment and cell signaling as mediators of bidirectional signaling, incorporating cross-talk with a variety of cell surface receptors and intracellular signaling proteins (32). The tripeptide sequence, Asp–Gly–Arg (RGD), is the important ligand recognition site for integrins. The actin cytoskeleton is connected to the cytoplasmic integrin tail through the ERM proteins, ezrin, radixin, and moesin. Ligand binding also initiates intracellular signaling cascades that provide the machinery needed for cell motility and invasion, and to support survival (28).

Adhesion

Cell attachment to other cells or to basement membrane is a requirement for normal epithelial cells. Loss of adhesion in normal epithelial cells is associated with anoikis-associated apoptosis, overruled by malignant transformation, where autologous survival stimulation occurs (10,27,28). Tumor cells interact with the local acellular microenvironment through adhesion molecules and integrins. All of these interactions can stimulate cell survival messages, or cell death messages, as may be seen in some immune interactions. There are four categories of adhesion molecules: integrins, cadherins, immunoglobulin superfamily cell adhesion molecules (CAMs), and selectins. They participate in cell–cell and/or cell–substratum binding, yielding a complexity of adherence and signaling possibilities. When expression or function of adhesion molecules becomes altered by tumor progression, new signals that can promote tumor growth, survival, and metastasis are propagated. Such adhesion interactions between tumor cells and normal cells, such as endothelial or immune cells, or fibroblasts, can result in activation of angiogenesis or the immune response, or augmentation of immune tolerance, drug resistance, and metastasis (10,11,21,26,33). Adhesion of circulating tumor cells to platelets, macrophages, or endothelial cells or matrix molecules via integrin engagement is critical to overcoming the anoikis of single-cell circulation.

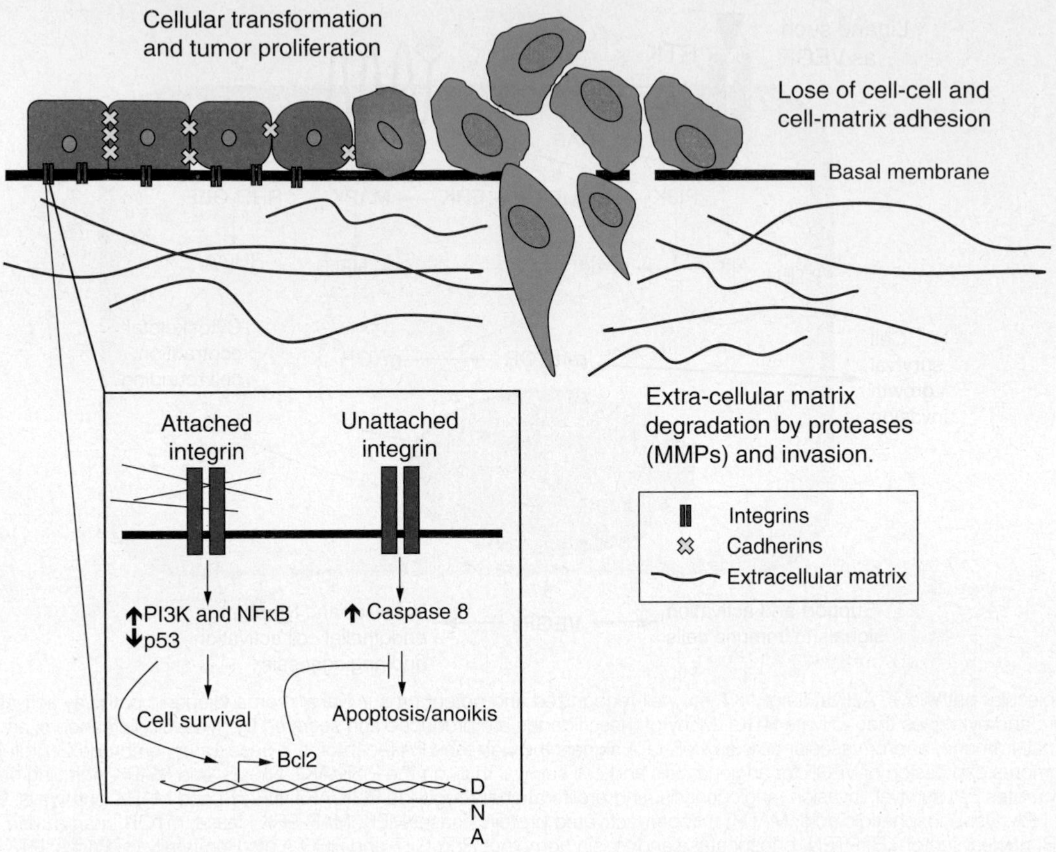

Figure 4.4. Invasion. Cancer cells lose their cell-to-cell (cadherin) and cell-to-matrix (integrin) attachment, releasing single cells and permitting cell migration. The production and secretion of proteases (MMPs, serine proteases) promotes ECM degradation forming tracks through which cancer cells migrate and invade surrounding tissues. Metastatic cancer cells have acquired mechanisms to resist anoikis. ECM, extracellular matrix; MMP, matrix metalloproteinase.

ANGIOGENESIS

All cells need a supply of nutrients and oxygen with which to sustain survival. This requires that they be located within 100 μm of a blood vessel (6,11,17). This also applies to tumor cells. They require de novo blood vessel formation to support cell cluster growth beyond 1 mm in diameter. Such new blood vessel formation is regulated by a network of pro- and antiangiogenic factors produced as a result of interaction between tumor cells, endothelial cells, and the stromal and immune macro- and microenvironments (11,17). This neovascularization occurs via a number of mechanisms, including recruitment of endothelial progenitors, vessel co-optation, vascular mimicry, sprouting angiogenesis, intussusceptive angiogenesis, and lymphangiogenesis (17).

Types of Angiogenesis

Human endothelial progenitor cells can be recruited locally or from the bone marrow in response to hypoxia or tumor-derived growth factors such as vascular endothelial growth factors (VEGFs) and fibroblast growth factors (FGFs). Response of endothelial progenitor cells to these growth factors as well as circulating ECM factors facilitates vasculogenesis by both induction of paracrine factor secretion and differentiation to form the vascular tube (34) (**Fig. 4.5**). Sprouting angiogenesis starts with the creation of a tip cell from a resting endothelial cell, and the concomitant degradation of the surrounding ECM by activated proteases. The tip cell then roams away from the parent vessel as the stalk divides under the control of the vascular endothelial growth factor receptor-2 (VEGFR-2), induction of Notch, angiopoietins (Angs), glycolysis, protein kinase A activation, and induction of the TGF-β/bone morphogenetic protein signaling pathways (35–37).

Intussusceptive angiogenesis involves the folding of the parental capillary wall into the vascular lumen, the formation of a so-called intraluminal pillar, a perforation in the core of the pillar, and subsequent splitting into two new capillaries. Factors that regulate intussusceptive angiogenesis include angiopoietins, TIE2, FGF2, and platelet-derived growth factor B (PDGFB) (38–40). It is believed that intussusceptive angiogenesis is increased in hypoxic conditions, a process that may be regulated through hypoxia-inducible factor 2α (HIF-2α) and erythropoietin.

Vascular co-option is a process whereby tumor cells grow and migrate along host blood vessels, allowing them to proliferate and metastasize without deriving their own independent blood supply. It has been proposed that this process is most frequently utilized by tumors growing in highly vascular organs such as the brain, liver, and lung (41). Information regarding the factors that specifically facilitate vascular co-option is more limited; *in vitro* models suggest that VEGF and angiopoietins are important (42). In vascular mimicry, highly dedifferentiated tumor cells, themselves, form vessel-like structures. The signaling pathways involved are well summarized (43). Key pathways include vascular-endothelial (VE)-cadherin, without which tumor cells cannot form the vascular mimicry tube. Ephrin A2, focal adhesion kinase, laminin 5γ2 chain, and HIF-2α are all additionally important in this unique process.

Lymphangiogenesis

The lymphatic system comprises the lymphatic vessels, lined by lymphatic endothelial cells, and lymphoid tissue. Two of its three primary physiologic functions are also involved in cancer progression and

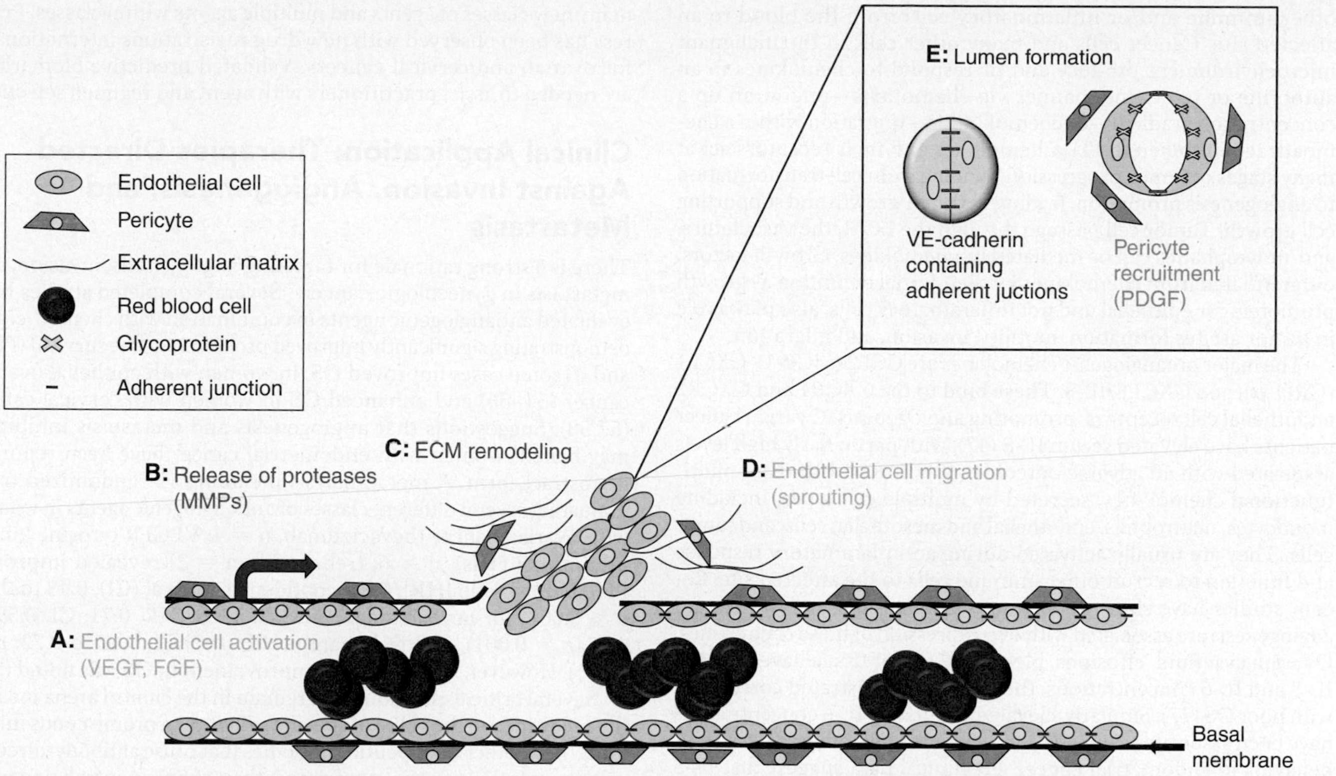

Figure 4.5. Angiogenesis sprouting. **A:** Endothelial cells are activated by multiple angiogenic factors secreted by tumor cells and cells of the tumor microenvironment. **B, C:** Proteases are released with the resulting remodeling of the ECM. **D:** Activated endothelial cells migrate into the stroma forming endothelial cords in the sprouting and other angiogenic and lymphangiogenic processes. **E:** After cellular polarization, negatively charged glycoproteins and the cytoskeleton retract, forming a vascular lumen. Pericytes are recruited for maturation of the blood vessel, mainly through the action of PDGF. ECM, extracellular matrix; FGF, fibroblast growth factors; VEGF, vascular endothelial growth factor.

metastasis: maintenance of the blood volume through reabsorption of interstitial fluid and immunological surveillance. It was previously believed that the role of lymphatic vessels in tumor metastatic spread was a passive one. It now appears that this is an active process, stimulated by the tumor, and involves both lymphangiogenesis and hyperplasia of collecting lymphatics (44). These processes are analogous to vascular angiogenesis, with recruitment and proliferation of lymphatic endothelial vessels, sprouting, and tube formation.

The signaling pathways of lymphangiogenesis remain under evaluation. They include activation of the angiogenic VEGFs/VEGFRs and of the lymphangiogenic VEGFR-3 by VEGF-C and VEGF-D (44). Lymphangiogenic VEGFs are induced by hypoxia and angiogenic signals, tumor cells, infiltrating inflammatory cells, and stromal cells. Lymph vessels are low-pressure vessels with limited basement membrane and no stromal components; they are permissive to entry and exit of tumor cells, immune cells, and pathogens; therefore, they are a ready route for metastasis. High expression of VEGF-D in epithelial ovarian tumor has been associated with higher FIGO stage, intratumoral lymphatic vessels, tumor lymphatic invasion, and lymph node metastasis. VEGF-D, intratumoral lymphatics, and lymphatic invasion have been suggested as independent prognostic factors for overall survival (OS) and disease-free survival in patients with epithelial ovarian carcinoma.

VEGFs and Receptors

It is clear from the role of vascular and lymphatic angiogenic processes that VEGFs are central factors in tumor maintenance and dissemination. VEGFs and their receptors are the focus of many of the targeted agents now being deployed for the treatment of gynecological malignancy. VEGF, first isolated from cancer xenograft ascites, was identified as a causative factor in blood vessel permeability and development (45). The VEGF family comprises seven glycoproteins, VEGF-A–E and placental growth factors-1 and -2, secreted by tumor cells, endothelial cells, stromal cells, leukocytes, and platelets. VEGF-A, the best characterized, has four in-frame isoforms determined by RNA splicing. There are three transmembrane VEGF receptor tyrosine kinases. VEGF-A, -B, and -E stimulate angiogenesis via VEGFR-1 (VEGFs-A and -B) or VEGFR2 (-A and -E). VEGFRs are predominantly found in endothelial cells and bone marrow–derived cells, though they can be expressed in other cells, including ovarian cancer cells (17,45).

Upregulation of VEGFs is mediated by many events, with tissue hypoxia, hypoglycemia, and growth factors and cytokines being the most prominent and well studied. The tumor microenvironment is hypoxic and acidic, both of which stimulate angiogenesis by induction of HIF-1α. VEGF and VEGFR-1 are under transcriptional regulation by HIF-1α, which is overexpressed in several solid tumors, including ovarian carcinomas. TGF signaling cascades, such as lysophosphatidic acid (LPA), nuclear factor (NF)-κB, and PI3K pathways, are activated by tumor and stromal-induced growth factors and can result in induction of VEGFs in gynecologic cancers. High expression of VEGF or high circulating concentrations of VEGF have been correlated with shorter OS in ovarian cancer. VEGF secreted into malignant ascites by ovarian cancer cells contributes to the increasing ascites burden and carcinomatosis through its effects on vascular permeability, modulation of the immune microenvironment, and prosurvival signals.

Soluble Factors Affecting the Tumor Microenvironment

Chemotactic cytokines, known as chemokines, are small secreted proteins or peptides that help regulate motility of a variety of cells. They are subdivided according to cysteine residue position into four groups: C, CC, CXC, and CX_3C (46). Their primary function is chemoattraction and activation of leukocytes that then recruit other immune and/or inflammatory cells from the blood to an affected site. Cancer cells and many other cells in the malignant microenvironment produce and/or respond to chemokines in an autocrine or paracrine manner via chemotaxis—migration up a concentration gradient—or chemokinesis—migration within a chemoattractant milieu (6,11). Chemokines and their receptors act at many stages of tumor progression, ranging from cell transformation to angiogenesis promotion, leading to tumor growth and supporting cell growth. Tumor cell passage through the ECM, the vasculature, and/or lymphatics can be mediated by chemokines. Growth factors, differentiated from chemokines by their initial definition as growth promoters for epithelial and not inflammatory cells, also play a role in tumor ascites formation, motility, invasion, and migration.

The major proangiogenic chemokines are CCL2 (MCP-1), CXCL1 (GRO-α), and CXCL8/IL-8. These bind to the CXCR1 and CXCR2 endothelial cell receptors, promoting angiogenesis. Ovarian cancer patients have elevated serum IL-8 (47), with particularly high levels associated with an adverse outcome (48). IL-8 and IL-6 are multifunctional chemokines, secreted by multiple cell types, including monocytes, neutrophils, endothelial and mesothelial cells, and tumor cells. They are usually activated during an inflammatory response and function to recruit other immune cells to the affected site. Recent studies have shown that tumor progression, metastasis, and angiogenesis are associated with overexpression of these chemokines. Ovarian cyst fluid, effusions, blood, and tumor tissue have elevated IL-8 and IL-6 concentrations; these have demonstrated correlation with poor OS (47). Similarly, elevated circulating IL-6 concentrations have been associated with an aggressive and chemotherapy-resistant behavior in endometrial cancer. Preclinical data suggest that IL-8 and IL-6 increase resistance to chemotherapeutic treatments in ovarian cancer cells (33). Collectively, these observations provide a rationale for targeting these chemokines therapeutically in gynecological cancers (49).

Another of the many important chemokine pairs is the receptor CXCR4 and its ligand CXCL12. Together, they activate signaling pathways that enhance proliferation, migration, angiogenesis, and invasion of gynecologic cancers. Whereas normal ovaries express very little CXCR4, in approximately 60% of ovarian cancers it is expressed with specific gene amplification in the high-grade serous histological subtype (29,50). CXCL12 is expressed in more than 90% of ovarian cancers. The CXCL12/CXCR4 pathway also controls expression of proteolytic enzymes such as urinary plasminogen activator (uPA) and MMP-9 (51) that promote local tumor and endothelial cell migration. AMD3100, a CXCR4 inhibitor, blocked CXCL12-stimulated migration of ovarian cancer cells *in vitro*. Blockade of CXCR4/CXCL12 activation led to reduced tumor growth and prolonged survival in ovarian cancer xenografts.

A fundamental requirement for successful tumorigenesis and tumor dissemination is the capacity for tumor cells to suppress host immunity (52). Ovarian cancer cells and their tumor-associated macrophages produce CCL22; CCL22 binds to CCR4 on immunosuppressive FOXP3$^+$ regulatory Tregs. This results in accumulation of Tregs at the tumor site, facilitating immune tolerance (52). Release of CXCL10 at the site of ovarian tumors causes accumulation of a second population of FOXP3$^+$ Tregs. These differ by expression of CXCR3, the CXCL10 receptor. This causes suppression of effector T-cell proliferation, again facilitating immune tolerance of the tumor (53). New data continue to emerge describing the interaction of these many types of cells in the tumor microenvironment and how, as a community, they promote tumor stability and reduce tumor susceptibility to treatment (33).

Therapeutics that Target Invasion and the Tumor Microenvironment

Development of novel agents and agent combinations to advance successful interdiction of gynecologic cancers is an ongoing need and challenge. The last decade has brought about great progress with many new classes of agents and multiple agents within classes. Progress has been observed with new drug registrations internationally for ovarian and cervical cancers. Validated predictive biomarkers are needed to assist practitioners with agent and regimen selection.

Clinical Application: Therapies Directed Against Invasion, Angiogenesis, and Metastasis

There is a strong rationale for targeting angiogenesis, invasion, and metastasis in gynecologic cancers. Several completed studies have evaluated antiangiogenic agents in combination with chemotherapy, demonstrating significantly improved progression-free survival (PFS), and in some cases improved OS, in women with epithelial ovarian cancer (54–56) and enhanced OS in women with cervical cancer (57,58). Suggestions that angiogenesis and metastasis inhibitors may benefit women with endometrial cancer have been reported in abstract form. A meta-analysis including 12 randomized trials evaluating several different classes of antiangiogenic agents in women with ovarian cancer (bevacizumab, n = 4; VEGFR tyrosine kinase inhibitors (TKIs), n = 6; trebananib, n = 2) revealed improved PFS (hazard ratio [HR], 0.61; confidence interval (CI), 0.48 to 0.79; $p < 0.001$) for bevacizumab, VEGFR TKIs (HR, 0.71; CI, 0.59 to 0.87; $p = 0.001$), and trebananib (HR, 0.67; CI, 0.62 to 0.72; $p < 0.001$). However, no significant improvement in OS was noted (59).

Several critical questions that remain in the clinical arena include the following: (a) the value of specific rather than promiscuous inhibitors; (b) whether therapeutic antibodies that cause antibody-directed cellular cytotoxicity are more active than simple neutralizing antibodies; (c) what is the best strategy for combination development with other targeted agents and/or chemotherapy; (d) whether therapy is best in treatment and/or in maintenance of response; and (e) identification of biomarkers that can accurately direct therapy. Validation and illustration of mechanism, with demonstration that the activated target is present, affected by the therapeutic, and that modulation of the target by the therapeutic is correlated with outcome, are necessary attributes of reliable biomarkers and targeted inhibitors of angiogenesis, invasion, and tumor dissemination (60,61) (**Fig. 4.6; Table 4.1**).

Inhibitors of Angiogenesis

Bevacizumab is a recombinant humanized neutralizing antihuman VEGF-A monoclonal antibody. Blocking VEGF reduces angiogenesis and related tumor growth, limits invasion and dissemination, and may alter immune function. The U.S. FDA has approved bevacizumab for use in cervical cancer and recurrent platinum-resistant ovarian cancer. Bevacizumab in combination with paclitaxel and either cisplatin or topotecan is licensed for the treatment of persistent, recurrent, or metastatic cervical cancer. It is approved in ovarian cancer in combination with paclitaxel, pegylated liposomal doxorubicin, or topotecan for the treatment of patients with platinum-resistant recurrent cancers of the ovary, fallopian tube, and primary peritoneal cancer who have received no more than two prior chemotherapy regimens. Bevacizumab has also received European Medicines Agency (EMA) approval for these gynecologic indications, as well as for the treatment of advanced newly diagnosed ovarian cancer, and (in combination with chemotherapy) for platinum-sensitive recurrent ovarian cancer.

The addition of bevacizumab to front-line chemotherapy and in maintenance therapy for epithelial ovarian cancer was evaluated in two pivotal phase III trials, GOG 218 and ICON 7. GOG 218 was a three-arm, placebo-controlled trial of front-line paclitaxel and carboplatin to which either concurrent bevacizumab or concurrent and maintenance bevacizumab were added. A PFS benefit was seen in women who received both concurrent and maintenance bevacizumab at 15 mg/kg (14.1 vs. 10.3 months; HR, 0.717; $p < 0.0001$) (55). No significant difference in OS was demonstrated (39.7 vs. 39.3 months; $p = 0.45$). ICON 7 evaluated first-line paclitaxel/

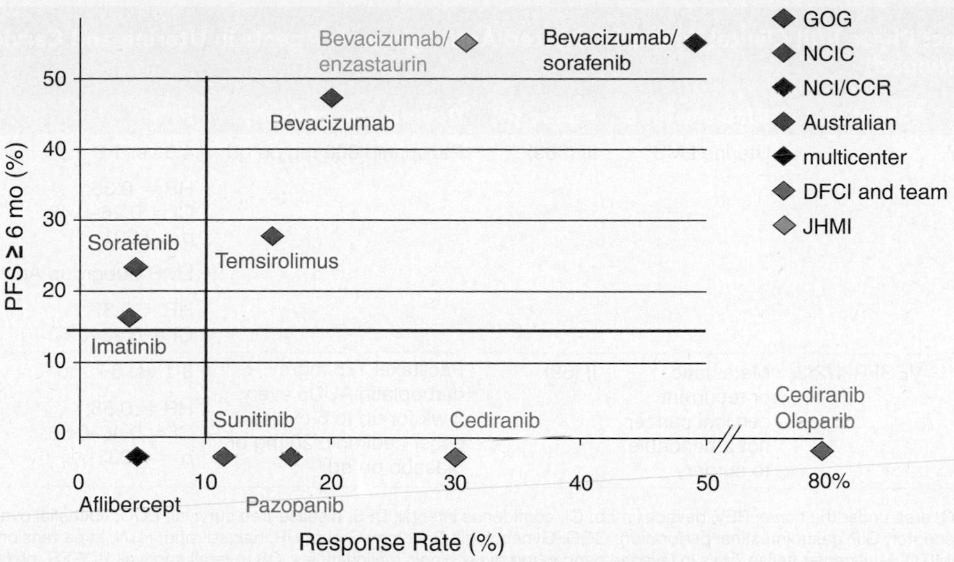

Figure 4.6. Angiogenic agents and combinations in ovarian cancer. Results of phase I–III trials of antiangiogenic agents, alone and in combinations, are plotted. Response rate and frequency of 6-month PFS are shown. PFS, progression-free survival.

TABLE 4.1. Select Phase II/III Clinical Trials of Targeted Antiangiogenic Agents in Uterine and Cervical Malignancies

Agent	Target	Disease Type	Phase (N)	Description of Study	PFS	OS
Bevacizumab GOG-0086P/NCT00977574 (ASCO 2015)	VEGF	Advanced (Stage III–IV) or Recurrent Endometrial Cancer	II (349)	A) Carboplatin AUC6 + paclitaxel 175 mg/m^2 + BEV 15 mg/kg q3 wk × 6 cycles + BEV 15 mg/kg	A) HR = 0.81; CI = 0.63–1.02	A) HR = 0.71; CI = 0.55–0.91
				B) Carboplatin AUC5 + paclitaxel 175 mg/m^2 + TEM 25 mg days 1/8 q 3 wk × 6 cycles + TEM 25 mg IV q wk days 1/8/15 q3 weeks	B) HR = 1.22; CI = 0.96–1.55	B) HR = 0.99; CI = 0.78–1.26
				C) Carboplatin AUC 6 + ixabepilone 30 mg/m^2 + BEV 15 mg/kg q 3 weeks × 6 cycles + BEV 15 mg/kg	C) HR = 0.87; CI = 0.68–1.11	C) HR = 0.97; CI = 0.77–1.23
Bevacizumab MITO END-2/ NCT01770171 (ASCO 2015)	VEGF	Advanced (Stage III–IV) or Recurrent Endometrial Cancer	II (108)	Carboplatin AUC5 + paclitaxel 175 mg/m^2 + BEV 15 mg/kg q 3 wk for 6–8 cycles + BEV 15 mg/kg	13.0 vs. 8.7 mo HR = 0.57; CI = 0.34–0.96; $p = 0.036$	
Bevacizumab GOG240/ NCT00803062 (58)	VEGF	Recurrent, persistent, or metastatic cervical cancer	III (452)	Cisplatin 50 mg/m^2 + paclitaxel 135 or 175 mg/m^2 every 3 wk or topotecan 0.75 mg/m^2 days 1–3 + paclitaxel 175 mg/m^2 every 3 wk + BEV 15 mg/kg every 3 wk	8.2 vs. 5.9 mo HR = 0.67; CI = 0.54–0.82; $p = 0.002$	17. vs. 13.3 mo HR = 0.71; CI = 0.54–0.95; $p = 0.004$
Bevacizumab RTOG0417/ NCT00369122 PMID: 24331655	VEGF	Locally advanced cervical cancer	II (49)	BEV 10 mg/kg every 2 wk × 3 cycles during chemoradiation (WPRT + brachytherapy + weekly cisplatin 40 mg/m^2)	3-year DFS: 68.7% LRF: 23.2%	3-year OS: 81.3%
Pazopanib NCT00430781 PMID:20606083	VEGFR-1/2/3, PDGFR-α/β, FGFR-1/3, and c-Kit	Stage IVb, persistent or recurrent cervical cancer	II (152)	A) Lapatinib 1500 mg po qd B) Pazopanib 800 mg po qd C) Lapatinib + pazopanib (Arm C closed for futility)	17.1 wk vs. 18.1 wk HR = 0.66; CI = 0.48–0.91; $p = 0.013$	39.1 wk vs. 50.7 wk HR = 0.67; CI = 0.46–0.99; $p = 0.045$

TABLE 4.1. Select Phase II/III Clinical Trials of Targeted Antiangiogenic Agents in Uterine and Cervical Malignancies (*continued*)

Agent	Target	Disease Type	Phase (N)	Description of Study	PFS	OS
Pazopanib PALETTE/ NCT00753688 PMID:22595799		Uterine LMS	III (369)	Pazopanib 800 mg po qd	4.6 vs. 1.6 mo HR = 0.35; CI = 0.26–0.48; $p< 0.001$ LMS Subgroup Analysis HR = 0.37 CI = 0.23–0.60	12.6 vs. 10.7 mo HR = 0.87; CI = 0.67–1.12; $p = 0{\cdot}25$ –
Cediranib CIRCCa/ NCT01229930 (62)	VEGFR-1/2/3	Metastatic or recurrent cervical cancer not amendable to surgery	II (69)	Paclitaxel 175 mg/m^2 + carboplatin AUC5 every 3 wk for up to 6 cycles + either cediranib 20 mg or placebo po qd	8·1 vs. 6·7 mo HR = 0·58; CI = 0·40–0·85; $p = 0{\cdot}032$	13.6 vs. 14.8 mo HR = 0·94; CI = 0·65–1.36; $p = 0{\cdot}42$

AEs, adverse events; AUC, area under the curve; BEV, bevacizumab; CI, confidence interval; DFS, disease-free survival; EOC, epithelial ovarian cancer; FGFR, fibroblast growth factor receptor; GIP, gastrointestinal perforation; GOG, Gynecologic Oncology Group; HR, hazard ratio; HTN, hypertension; LMS, leiomyosarcoma; LRF, locoregional failure; MITO, Multicenter Italian Trials in Ovarian cancer and gynecologic malignancies; OS, overall survival; PDGFR, platelet-derived growth factor receptor; RTOG, Radiation Therapy Oncology Group; TEM, temsirolimus; VEGF, vascular endothelial growth factor; VEGFR, vascular endothelial growth factor receptor; WPRT, whole pelvic radiation therapy.

carboplatin alone or in combination with bevacizumab followed by bevacizumab maintenance, using a 7.5 mg/kg dose (56). PFS was enhanced in the bevacizumab arm (HR, 0.81; 95% CI, 0.70 to 0.94; $p = 0.0041$), and interim analysis revealed no significant OS improvement. A post hoc exploratory subgroup analysis found an OS benefit for patients with stage IV or stage IIIC disease with >1 cm residual tumor (HR, 0.64; 95% CI, 0.48 to 0.85; $p = 0.002$). The optimal duration of bevacizumab treatment is controversial, with some advocating for continuing maintenance bevacizumab until disease progression. Two different fixed bevacizumab maintenance schedules are being evaluated in the BOOST trial (15 vs. 30 months bevacizumab; NCT01462890).

Combination chemotherapy and bevacizumab have been evaluated in women with platinum-sensitive and -resistant recurrent ovarian cancers. Two phase III trials have demonstrated survival benefit with the addition of bevacizumab to chemotherapy in women with platinum-sensitive disease. In the OCEANS trial, the bevacizumab with concurrent gemcitabine and carboplatin with maintenance bevacizumab arm showed an improved response rate (RR; 78.5% vs. 57.4%, $p < 0.0001$) and a 4-month improvement in PFS (12.4 vs. 8.4 months; HR, 0.484; $p < 0.0001$) with no difference in OS (54). GOG 213, presented as an abstract, demonstrated that bevacizumab plus platinum-based chemotherapy resulted in a 5-month improvement in OS compared with chemotherapy alone for women with first recurrence platinum-sensitive ovarian cancer (42.2 vs. 37.3 months; HR, 0.83; $p = 0.056$; abstract). The phase III AURELIA trial examined the role of the addition of bevacizumab to standard of care nonplatinum-based chemotherapy in women with recurrent platinum-resistant ovarian cancer. It reported an enhanced median PFS (6.7 vs. 3.4 months; HR, 0.48; $p < 0.001$), improved RR (27.3% vs. 11.8%; $p = 0.001$), and decreased frequency of paracentesis (17% vs. 2%) (63). Bevacizumab treatment improved patient-reported outcomes, with an increased proportion of patients achieving improvement in abdominal symptoms (21.9% vs. 9.3%; $p = 0.002$). The results of the AURELIA trial led to FDA and EMA approval of bevacizumab in women with platinum-resistant ovarian cancer.

The regulatory agencies have also approved bevacizumab for women with advanced and recurrent cervical cancer. The phase III GOG 240 trial compared taxane-based doublets (paclitaxel and cisplatin vs. paclitaxel and topotecan) in a two-by-two factorial design against use of placebo or bevacizumab with chemotherapy (58). The combination of bevacizumab and chemotherapy significantly improved RR (48% vs. 36%; $p = 0.008$), median PFS (8.2 vs. 5.9 months; HR, 0.67; $p = 0.002$), and median OS (HR, 0.71; $p = 0.004$) compared to chemotherapy alone. The addition of bevacizumab also increased toxicity, most notably demonstrating increased frequency of gastrointestinal perforations and/or genitourinary fistulas (6% vs. 0%; $p = 0.002$).

Despite suggestions of activity, no definitive role for bevacizumab has been demonstrated in endometrial cancer. Several recent studies have been presented in abstract form and await peer review. The randomized phase II GOG 86P study evaluated three experimental arms, two of which incorporated bevacizumab and one with temsirolimus, each with combination chemotherapy, in women with chemo-naïve advanced or recurrent endometrial cancer. The experimental arms were compared against historical control data. OS was statistically significantly increased with bevacizumab, paclitaxel, and carboplatin (34 vs. historical control of 22.7 months; HR, 0.71; $p < 0.039$) relative to the historical control. The randomized phase II trial, MITO END-2, compared paclitaxel and carboplatin with and without bevacizumab in women with advanced or recurrent endometrial cancer. The addition of bevacizumab significantly increased PFS (13 vs. 9.7 months; HR, 0.59; $p = 0.036$) and was associated with nonsignificant increased RR (72.7 vs. 54.3%; $p = 0.065$) and OS (23.5 vs. 18 months; $p = 0.24$).

Other Angiogenesis and Metastasis Inhibitors

Cediranib is an oral TKI that selectively targets all three VEGFRs with less potency against c-kit. Single-agent studies in recurrent ovarian cancer yielded limited RRs of 13% to 17%, with hypertension and fatigue being the most common grade 3 adverse events. Cediranib was evaluated in combination with carboplatin and paclitaxel followed by maintenance cediranib in a three-arm randomized placebo-controlled phase III trial (ICON6) in women with first recurrence platinum-sensitive disease (64). PFS was improved (8.7 vs. 11.0 months; HR, 0.56; $p < 0.001$), and preliminary OS was encouraging (17.6 vs. 20.3 months; HR, 0.70; $p = 0.04$), all favoring the concurrent/maintenance cediranib arm (NCT00532194). Adverse events were significantly more common in the cediranib maintenance arm and included hypertension, diarrhea, hypothyroidism, hoarseness, bleeding, proteinuria, and fatigue. The polyADPribose polymerase (PARP) inhibitor, olaparib, is being added to the combination for ICON9, a phase III trial under development.

Several mixed kinase inhibitors, all of which include inhibition of VEGFRs, have been examined in gynecologic cancers. *Nintedanib*/BIBF1120 inhibits VEGFRs 1, 2, and 3; PDGFR-α and -β; and FGF receptors 1 to 3. A phase III randomized placebo-controlled trial of nintedanib in combination with carboplatin and paclitaxel followed by maintenance nintedanib or placebo (AGO-OVAR12/LUME-Ovar1) in first-line treatment of ovarian cancer revealed a statistically significant PFS, but of minimal difference (17.3 vs. 16.6 months; HR, 0.84; $p = 0.0239$) (65). The most common significant adverse effects in the nintedanib arm included elevated transaminases and diarrhea. A randomized phase II trial of carboplatin and paclitaxel with or without nintedanib is ongoing in cervix cancer (NCT02009579).

Pazopanib is a kinase inhibitor that targets all three VEGFRs, both PDGFRs, and c-kit. Pazopanib is FDA approved for the treatment of patients with advanced soft tissue sarcoma who have received prior chemotherapy, including those with uterine leiomyosarcoma (LMS), based on the randomized placebo-controlled PALETTE trial (NCT00753688). Patients who received pazopanib had a statistically significant improvement in PFS compared with placebo (4.6 vs. 1.6 months; HR, 0.35; CI, 0.26 to 0.48; $p < 0.001$), with no difference in OS (66). The PazoDoble trial is currently evaluating the combination of gemcitabine and pazopanib in patients with recurrent or metastatic uterine LMS or carcinosarcoma (NCT02203760). Pazopanib also has potential value in ovarian cancer. The phase III randomized placebo-controlled maintenance trial of pazopanib 600/800 mg daily after front-line platin/taxane-based chemotherapy (AGO-OVAR16) revealed significantly longer PFS in the pazopanib group (17.9 vs. 12.3 months; HR, 0.766; CI, 0.64 to 0.91; $p = 0.002$), with no difference in OS (67). However, the benefit of pazopanib on PFS effect was not seen in East Asian women with ovarian cancer. A further exploration combined a subset of East Asian patients on the AGO-OVAR16 trial with those who participated in a separate East Asian pazopanib maintenance study. Maintenance pazopanib in this subgroup was associated with worse survival (OS HR, 1.71; CI 1.01 to 2.88; $p = 0.05$), with no identifiable factors to explain the differential findings. Weekly paclitaxel combined with pazopanib has been studied in women with recurrent platinum-resistant ovarian cancer (MITO11; NCT01644825), yielding an improved PFS (6.4 vs. 3.5 months; HR, 0.42; CI, 0·25 to 0·69; $p = 0{\cdot}0002$) and a trend toward improved OS (19.1 vs.13·7 months; HR, 0.60; CI, 0.32 to 1.13; $p = 0{\cdot}056$) (68). However, a similarly designed randomized phase II trial demonstrated conflicting results, reporting that the combination of paclitaxel and pazopanib was not superior to paclitaxel alone in women with recurrent ovarian cancer (NCT01468909; abstract).

Cabozantinib is an oral kinase inhibitor that targets c-MET, ALK, and VEGFR-2, and been shown to reduce tumor growth, invasion, and angiogenesis (69). Simultaneous targeting of the MET and VEGF signaling pathways may be a promising strategy to improve antitumor activity by blocking complementary stimulatory pathways. Cabozantinib is showing preliminary activity in a single-arm phase II trial in women with recurrent or metastatic advanced endometrioid or serous endometrial cancer and endometrial carcinosarcomas (NCT01935934). These preliminary results will be further examined in a randomized trial.

Trebananib (*AMG 386*) is a peptide-Fc fusion protein that inhibits angiogenesis by binding angiopoietin-1 and -2 and blocking their interaction with the Tie2 receptor. The phase III trial of weekly paclitaxel with trebananib or placebo for patients with recurrent ovarian cancers resulted in an improved PFS (7.2 vs. 5.4 months; HR 0.66; $p < 0.0001$), but no difference in OS (70).

Combination Therapy Opportunities Against Angiogenesis and Metastasis

Further refinement of targeted therapy is focused on the hypothesis that inhibiting biologic targets in combination may be more effective than alone. Studies have been initiated exploring the activity of targeted agents in combination with cytotoxic chemotherapy, multitargeted agent combinations, and combinations with immunomodulators. Antiangiogenic agents in combination with PARP inhibitors have been reported with promising results. It is recognized that inhibition of angiogenesis with induction of local hypoxia causes downregulation of genes involved in DNA repair (71).

Clinical successes of combination antiangiogenesis therapy, in which the microenvironmental context is synergized with other interventions, are now being reported. A randomized open-label phase II study examined the PARP inhibitor, olaparib, alone or in combination with cediranib in women with platinum-sensitive high-grade serous or endometrioid epithelial ovarian cancer or those with germline BRCA1/2 mutations (72). The median PFS was significantly longer for combination therapy compared to olaparib alone (17.7 vs. 9.0 months; $p = 0.005$). Unplanned post hoc subset analysis evaluating the interaction against deleterious germline *BRCA1* or *2* mutation carriers showed that women with no mutation or unknown status had a nearly threefold greater PFS over single-agent olaparib. Pilot biomarker studies suggest that markers indicating hypoxic injury such as induction of IL-8 and release of circulating endothelial cells may be a mechanism for synergy (73). Recent data implicate hypoxia in downregulation of BRCA1 and BRCA2 expression, creating a *BRCA*-like tumor phenotype. These findings suggest that understanding the myriad of potential pathway and microenvironmental interactions can be leveraged for clinical benefit. Success will be enhanced further by development and validation of predictive and/or patient selection biomarkers.

Biomarkers

Biomarkers are important tools with which to guide treatment and patient care decisions, in order to maximize benefit, as well as minimize cost and toxicity. It is important to differentiate predictive from prognostic markers. Predictive biomarkers differentiate patient outcome as a function of treatment intervention, such as therapy or radiation, whereas prognostic biomarkers are independent of treatment (60) (**Table 4.2**). Identification and validation of predictive biomarkers require demonstration of a treatment outcome interaction and thus cannot be evaluated on single-arm studies. Prognostic biomarkers differentiate overall outcome, such as PFS and OS, within a population and have little application to individual patients. The biology of invasion, angiogenesis, and metastasis has yielded many biomarkers of prognostic utility in gynecologic cancers, including CAMs, MMP-s, angiogenic and immune growth factors and cytokines, and their receptors.

Biomarkers can be clinical findings or measured events, such as tumor or blood factors. Ascites is known to be related to overexpression of VEGF and its associated vascular permeability (45). The presence of ascites was shown to be a positive prognostic finding in a bevacizumab trial. Several studies, reported in abstract form, have suggested that higher tumor CD31 microvessel density, higher tumor VEGF, and presence of ascites may be predictive and/or prognostic of benefit with bevacizumab treatment. In contrast, no prognostic or predictive association was seen for circulating VEGF or VEGFR-2 concentrations. Exploratory retrospective findings must be validated prospectively prior to application for patient selection or trial design as reliable predictive biomarkers.

Several promising biomarker candidates have come from retrospective exploration of serum samples. Combined serum VEGFR-3, α_1-acid glycoprotein, mesothelin, and CA125, together were denoted an as yet not validated predictive signature. The signature-positive group in the bevacizumab arm of ICON7 had improved median PFS compared with the control arm (17.9 vs. 12.4 months; $p = 0.04$) (73). The signature-negative group did not benefit from added bevacizumab. Other preliminary biomarker data suggest that serum Ang1 and Tie2 concentrations may differentiate women who may benefit or be harmed by bevacizumab. High Ang1 and low serum Tie2 levels signified benefit from bevacizumab (PFS, 23.0 vs. 16.2 months, $p = 0.006$), while both

TABLE 4.2. Biomarkers Predictive of Outcome to Antiangiogenic Therapy

Agent	Biomarker	Study	Results
Bevacizumab (ASCO 2014)	Molecularly defined proangiogenic vs. immune subgroup	ICON7	Immune subgroup had worse PFS (HR = 1.73; CI = 1.12–2.68) and OS (HR = 2.00; CI = 1.11–3.61) when treated with BEV compared to chemotherapy alone. Proangiogenic group had a nonsignificant trend to improved PFS with the addition of BEV (median 17.4 vs. 12.3 mo)
Bevacizumab (ASCO 2014)	Molecularly defined subgroups: proliferative and mesenchymal subtypes compared with immunoreactive or differentiated subtypes	ICON7	Patients with serous proliferative subtype serous ovarian cancers had greatest benefit from BEV with an improvement of median PFS of 12.8 mo ($p = 0.032$). Median PFS with BEV was not significantly greater in the differentiated, immunoreactive, and mesenchymal subtypes. Patients with mesenchymal serous cancers had improvement in median OS with BEV (HR = 0.27, CI = 0.08–0.96, $p = 0.03$)
Bevacizumab (62)	Serum VEGFR-3, α_1-acid glycoprotein, and mesothelin combined with CA125	ICON7	The signature-positive group demonstrated improved median PFS in the BEV arm compared with the control arm (17.9 vs. 12.4 mo; $p = 0.04$). The signature-negative group had an improved median PFS in the standard chemotherapy arm compared with the BEV arm (36.3 vs. 20 mo; $p = 0.006$)
Bevacizumab (74)	Serum Ang1 and Tie2	ICON7	Patients with high Ang1 and low Tie2 levels had improved PFS with BEV (23.0 vs. 16.2 mo, $p = 0.006$). Patients with high Ang1 and Tie2 levels had lower median PFS for BEV arm (12.8 vs. 28.5 mo, $p = 0.007$); patients with low Ang1 levels had no significant PFS differences associated with treatment regardless of Tie2 levels
Bevacizumab (ASCO 2015)	Tumor CD31 MVD, VEGF, VEGFR-2, NRP-1 or MET	GOG218	Higher CD31 MVD counts in BEV/BEV arm had predictive value for PFS (>Q3 MVD, HR = 0.38, CI = 0.25–0.58; ≤Q3 MVD, HR = 0.68, CI = 0.54–0.86; $p = 0.018$) and OS (>Q3 MVD, HR = 0.57, CI = 0.39–0.83; ≤Q3 MVD, HR = 1.03, CI = 0.83–1.27; $p = 0.0069$). Tumor VEGF showed potential predictive value in BEV throughout vs. control for OS (>Q3 tumor VEGF, HR = 0.62, CI = 0.43–0.91; ≤Q3 tumor VEGF, HR = 1.01, CI = 0.82–1.25; $p = 0.023$). No prognostic or predictive association was seen for plasma VEGF or VEGFR2; or tumor VEGFR-2, NRP-1, or MET
Bevacizumab (75)	Ascites	GOG218	Patients with ascites treated with BEV had improved PFS (HR = 0.72, CI = 0.63–0.83; $p < 0.001$) and OS (HR = 0.82, CI = 0.7–0.96; $p = 0.01$). Patients without ascites did not demonstrate a difference in PFS or OS
Bevacizumab (ASCO 2016)	Plasma IL-6, Ang-2, OPN, SDF-1, and VEGF-D	GOG218	IL-6 was predictive of BEV advantage for PFS and OS. Pts with high IL-6 levels treated with BEV had longer PFS (14.2 vs. 8.7 mo) and OS (39.6 vs. 33.3 mo). Both IL6 and OPN were found to be negative prognostic markers for PFS and OS

Ang, angiopoietin; BEV, bevacizumab; CI, confidence interval; GOG, Gynecologic Oncology Group; HR, hazard ratio; ICON, International Collaborative Ovarian Neoplasm; MET, MNNG HOS transforming gene also known as hepatocyte growth factor receptor; MVD, microvessel density; NRP, neuropilin; OPN, osteopontin; OS, overall survival; PFS, progression-free survival; SDF-1, stromal cell-derived factor-1; VEGF, vascular endothelial growth factor; VEGFR, vascular endothelial growth factor receptor.

high Ang1 and Tie2 levels were associated with lower median PFS with bevacizumab (12.8 vs. 28.5 months, $p = 0.007$) (74). A further study, published in abstract form only, demonstrated that a molecular subgroup characterized by high expression of immune response genes was associated with improved PFS and OS in patients treated with primary debulking and standard first-line chemotherapy. However, in a translational subgroup study of patients from the ICON7 study, patients in this immune subgroup who received bevacizumab appeared to have an inferior outcome compared to patients on the control arm. Validated predictive markers should help to optimize the use of our therapeutic opportunities to improve quality and quantity of life by predicting clinical benefit or lack thereof.

CONCLUSIONS

Continued scientific, epidemiologic, and clinical advances are critically needed until such time as successful, reproducible, and accurate early detection of gynecologic tumors becomes routine. Understanding the biology, regulation, and implications of the process of invasion and angiogenesis will continue to drive new biomarker and therapeutic target identification and intervention. The similarity between dysregulated invasion and angiogenesis and unregulated motility of metastasis allows the potential for a dual-purpose intervention. The tumor's interaction with its microenvironment becomes the focus for scientific dissection and therapeutic application. Here, the process of autocrine and paracrine regulation, signal pathway activation, and cell–cell conversation is critical. The use of the newer and high-throughput technologies to identify collections of biologic targets rather than one gene or protein at a time can make the process more streamlined and provide a broader view of the interaction of events. In addition, it is clear that there are numerous convergent and divergent angiogenic processes. New targets are emerging that may overcome angiogenesis escape, including novel endothelial cell and pericyte targets. Several new approaches including novel pathway inhibitors, immune modulators, and signaling pathway combinations are in clinical trials or presently under development. Improved understanding, study of events in the patient populations, and cooperative and collaborative progress will allow us to overcome invasion and metastasis, the major causes of morbidity and mortality in gynecologic cancers.

REFERENCES

1. Jayson GC, Kohn EC, Kitchener HC, et al. Ovarian cancer. *Lancet.* 2014;384:1376–1388.
2. Karst AM, Levanon K, Drapkin R. Modeling high-grade serous ovarian carcinogenesis from the fallopian tube. *Proc Natl Acad Sci U S A.* 2011;108:7547–7552.
3. Mehra K, Mehrad M, Ning G, et al. STICS, SCOUTs and p53 signatures; a new language for pelvic serous carcinogenesis. *Front Biosci (Elite Ed).* 2011;3:625–634.
4. Wiegand KC, Shah SP, Al-Agha OM, et al. ARID1A mutations in endometriosis-associated ovarian carcinomas. *N Engl J Med.* 2010;363:1532–1543.
5. Grisham RN, Iyer G, Garg K, et al. BRAF mutation is associated with early stage disease and improved outcome in patients with low-grade serous ovarian cancer. *Cancer.* 2013;119:548–554.
6. Liotta LA, Kohn EC. The microenvironment of the tumour-host interface. *Nature.* 2001;411:375–379.
7. Talmadge JE, Fidler IJ. AACR centennial series: the biology of cancer metastasis: historical perspective. *Cancer Res.* 2010;70:5649–5669.
8. Gadducci A, Guerrieri ME, Genazzani AR. New insights on the pathogenesis of ovarian carcinoma: molecular basis and clinical implications. *Gynecol Endocrinol.* 2012;28:582–586.
9. Friedl P, Alexander S. Cancer invasion and the microenvironment: plasticity and reciprocity. *Cell.* 2011;147:992–1009.
10. Jung HY, Fattet L, Yang J. Molecular pathways: linking tumor microenvironment to epithelial-mesenchymal transition in metastasis. *Clin Cancer Res.* 2015;21:962–968.
11. Joyce JA, Pollard JW. Microenvironmental regulation of metastasis. *Nat Rev Cancer.* 2009;9:239–252.
12. Lengyel E. Ovarian cancer development and metastasis. *Am J Pathol.* 2010;177:1053–1064.
13. Nieman KM, Kenny HA, Penicka CV, et al. Adipocytes promote ovarian cancer metastasis and provide energy for rapid tumor growth. *Nat Med.* 2011;17:1498–1503.
14. Nowicka A, Marini FC, Solley TN, et al. Human omental-derived adipose stem cells increase ovarian cancer proliferation, migration, and chemoresistance. *PLoS One.* 2013;8:e81859.
15. Klopp AH, Zhang Y, Solley T, et al. Omental adipose tissue-derived stromal cells promote vascularization and growth of endometrial tumors. *Clin Cancer Res.* 2012;18:771–782.
16. Mah LY, Ryan KM. Autophagy and cancer. *Cold Spring Harb Perspect Biol.* 2012;4:a008821.
17. Hillen F, Griffioen AW. Tumour vascularization: sprouting angiogenesis and beyond. *Cancer Metastasis Rev.* 2007;26:489–502.
18. Ibana JA, Cutay SJ, Romero M, et al. Parallel expression of enzyme inhibitors of CD8T cell activity in tumor microenvironments and secretory endometrium. *Reprod Sci.* 2016;23:289–301.
19. Weiss G, Goldsmith LT, Taylor RN, et al. Inflammation in reproductive disorders. *Reprod Sci.* 2009;16:216–229.
20. Gabrilovich DI, Ostrand-Rosenberg S, Bronte V. Coordinated regulation of myeloid cells by tumours. *Nat Rev Immunol.* 2012;12:253–268.
21. Smith HA, Kang Y. The metastasis-promoting roles of tumor-associated immune cells. *J Mol Med (Berl).* 2013;91:411–429.
22. Menderes G, Hicks C, Black JD, et al. Immune checkpoint inhibitors in gynecologic cancers with lessons learned from non-gynecologic cancers. *Expert Opin Biol Ther.* 2016;16(8):989–1004.
23. Kumar V, Patel S, Tcyganov E, et al. The nature of myeloid-derived suppressor cells in the tumor microenvironment. *Trends Immunol.* 2016;37:208–220.
24. Gutkin DW, Shurin MR. Clinical evaluation of systemic and local immune responses in cancer: time for integration. *Cancer Immunol Immunother.* 2014;63:45–57.
25. Kenny HA, Chiang CY, White EA, et al. Mesothelial cells promote early ovarian cancer metastasis through fibronectin secretion. *J Clin Invest.* 2014;124:4614–4628.
26. Pradeep S, Kim SW, Wu SY, et al. Hematogenous metastasis of ovarian cancer: rethinking mode of spread. *Cancer Cell.* 2014;26:77–91.
27. Thiery JP, Acloque H, Huang RY, et al. Epithelial-mesenchymal transitions in development and disease. *Cell.* 2009;139:871–890.
28. Frisch SM, Schaller M, Cieply B. Mechanisms that link the oncogenic epithelial-mesenchymal transition to suppression of anoikis. *J Cell Sci.* 2013;126:21–29.
29. Integrated genomic analyses of ovarian carcinoma. *Nature.* 2011;474:609–615.
30. Tothill RW, Tinker AV, George J, et al. Novel molecular subtypes of serous and endometrioid ovarian cancer linked to clinical outcome. *Clin Cancer Res.* 2008;14:5198–5208.
31. Cancer Genome Atlas Research Network, Kandoth C, Schultz N, et al. Integrated genomic characterization of endometrial carcinoma. *Nature.* 2013;497:67–73.
32. Seguin L, Desgrosellier JS, Weis SM, et al. Integrins and cancer: regulators of cancer stemness, metastasis, and drug resistance. *Trends Cell Biol.* 2015;25:234–240.
33. Wang W, Kryczek I, Dostal L, et al. Effector T cells abrogate stroma-mediated chemoresistance in ovarian cancer. *Cell.* 2016;165:1092–1105.
34. Marcola M, Rodrigues CE. Endothelial progenitor cells in tumor angiogenesis: another brick in the wall. *Stem Cells Int.* 2015;2015:832649.
35. Beets K, Huylebroeck D, Moya IM, et al. Robustness in angiogenesis: notch and BMP shaping waves. *Trends Genet.* 2013;29:140–149.
36. De Bock K, Georgiadou M, Schoors S, et al. Role of PFKFB3-driven glycolysis in vessel sprouting. *Cell.* 2013;154:651–663.
37. Larrivee B, Prahst C, Gordon E, et al. ALK1 signaling inhibits angiogenesis by cooperating with the Notch pathway. *Dev Cell.* 2012;22:489–500.
38. Makanya AN, Hlushchuk R, Baum O, et al. Microvascular endowment in the developing chicken embryo lung. *Am J Physiol Lung Cell Mol Physiol.* 2007;292:L1136–L1146.
39. Patan S. TIE1 and TIE2 receptor tyrosine kinases inversely regulate embryonic angiogenesis by the mechanism of intussusceptive microvascular growth. *Microvasc Res.* 1998;56:1–21.
40. Thurston G, Suri C, Smith K, et al. Leakage-resistant blood vessels in mice transgenically overexpressing angiopoietin-1. *Science.* 1999;286:2511–2514.
41. Donnem T, Hu J, Ferguson M, et al. Vessel co-option in primary human tumors and metastases: an obstacle to effective anti-angiogenic treatment? *Cancer Med.* 2013;2:427–436.
42. Holash J, Maisonpierre PC, Compton D, et al. Vessel cooption, regression, and growth in tumors mediated by angiopoietins and VEGF. *Science.* 1999;284:1994–1998.
43. Paulis YW, Soetekouw PM, Verheul HM, et al. Signalling pathways in vasculogenic mimicry. *Biochim Biophys Acta.* 2010;1806:18–28.
44. Stacker SA, Williams SP, Karnezis T, et al. Lymphangiogenesis and lymphatic vessel remodelling in cancer. *Nat Rev Cancer.* 2014;14:159–172.
45. Senger DR, Galli SJ, Dvorak AM, et al. Tumor cells secrete a vascular permeability factor that promotes accumulation of ascites fluid. *Science.* 1983;219:983–985.
46. Muralidhar GG, Barbolina MV. Chemokine receptors in epithelial ovarian cancer. *Int J Mol Sci.* 2014;15:361–376.
47. Lokshin AE, Winans M, Landsittel D, et al. Circulating IL-8 and anti-IL-8 autoantibody in patients with ovarian cancer. *Gynecol Oncol.* 2006;102:244–251.
48. Merritt WM, Lin YG, Spannuth WA, et al. Effect of interleukin-8 gene silencing with liposome-encapsulated small interfering RNA on ovarian cancer cell growth. *J Natl Cancer Inst.* 2008;100:359–372.
49. Coward J, Kulbe H, Chakravarty P, et al. Interleukin-6 as a therapeutic target in human ovarian cancer. *Clin Cancer Res.* 2011;17:6083–6096.
50. Archibald KM, Kulbe H, Kwong J, et al. Sequential genetic change at the TP53 and chemokine receptor CXCR4 locus during transformation of human ovarian surface epithelium. *Oncogene.* 2012;31:4987–4995.
51. Miyanishi N, Suzuki Y, Simizu S, et al. Involvement of autocrine CXCL12/CXCR4 system in the regulation of ovarian carcinoma cell invasion. *Biochem Biophys Res Commun.* 2010;403:154–159.
52. Curiel TJ, Coukos G, Zou L, et al. Specific recruitment of regulatory T cells in ovarian carcinoma fosters immune privilege and predicts reduced survival. *Nat Med.* 2004;10:942–949.
53. Redjimi N, Raffin C, Raimbaud I, et al. CXCR3+ T regulatory cells selectively accumulate in human ovarian carcinomas to limit type I immunity. *Cancer Res.* 2012;72:4351–4360.
54. Aghajanian C, Blank SV, Goff BA, et al. OCEANS: a randomized, double-blind, placebo-controlled phase III trial of chemotherapy with or without bevacizumab in patients with platinum-sensitive recurrent epithelial ovarian, primary peritoneal, or fallopian tube cancer. *J Clin Oncol.* 2012;30:2039–2045.
55. Burger RA, Brady MF, Bookman MA, et al. Incorporation of bevacizumab in the primary treatment of ovarian cancer. *N Engl J Med.* 2011;365:2473–2483.
56. Perren TJ, Swart AM, Pfisterer J, et al. A phase 3 trial of bevacizumab in ovarian cancer. *N Engl J Med.* 2011;365:2484–2496.
57. Symonds RP, Gourley C, Davidson S, et al. Cediranib combined with carboplatin and paclitaxel in patients with metastatic or recurrent cervical cancer (CIRCCa): a randomised, double-blind, placebo-controlled phase 2 trial. *Lancet Oncol.* 2015;16:1515–1524.
58. Tewari KS, Sill MW, Long HJ III, et al. Improved survival with bevacizumab in advanced cervical cancer. *N Engl J Med.* 2014;370:734–743.
59. Li X, Zhu S, Hong C, et al. Angiogenesis inhibitors for patients with ovarian cancer: a meta-analysis of 12 randomized controlled trials. *Curr Med Res Opin.* 2016;32:555–562.

60. Azad N, Yu M, Davidson B, et al. Translational predictive biomarker analysis of the phase 1b sorafenib and bevacizumab study expansion cohort. *Mol Cell Proteomics.* 2013;12:1621–1631.
61. Lee JM, Sarosy GA, Annunziata CM, et al. Combination therapy: intermittent sorafenib with bevacizumab yields activity and decreased toxicity. *Br J Cancer.* 2010;102:495–499.
62. Collinson F, Hutchinson M, Craven RA, et al. Predicting response to bevacizumab in ovarian cancer: a panel of potential biomarkers informing treatment selection. *Clin Cancer Res.* 2013;19:5227–5239.
63. Poveda AM, Selle F, Hilpert F, et al. Bevacizumab combined with weekly paclitaxel, pegylated liposomal doxorubicin, or topotecan in platinum-resistant recurrent ovarian cancer: analysis by chemotherapy cohort of the randomized phase III AURELIA trial. *J Clin Oncol.* 2015;33:3836–3838.
64. Ledermann JA, Embleton AC, Raja F, et al. Cediranib in patients with relapsed platinum-sensitive ovarian cancer (ICON6): a randomised, double-blind, placebo-controlled phase 3 trial. *Lancet.* 2016;387:1066–1074.
65. du Bois A, Kristensen G, Ray-Coquard I, et al. Standard first-line chemotherapy with or without nintedanib for advanced ovarian cancer (AGO-OVAR 12): a randomised, double-blind, placebo-controlled phase 3 trial. *Lancet Oncol.* 2016;17:78–89.
66. van der Graaf WT, Blay JY, Chawla SP, et al. Pazopanib for metastatic soft-tissue sarcoma (PALETTE): a randomised, double-blind, placebo-controlled phase 3 trial. *Lancet.* 2012;379:1879–1886.
67. du Bois A, Floquet A, Kim JW, et al. Incorporation of pazopanib in maintenance therapy of ovarian cancer. *J Clin Oncol.* 2014;32:3374–3382.
68. Pignata S, Lorusso D, Scambia G, et al. Pazopanib plus weekly paclitaxel versus weekly paclitaxel alone for platinum-resistant or platinum-refractory advanced ovarian cancer (MITO 11): a randomised, open-label, phase 2 trial. *Lancet Oncol.* 2015;16(5):561–568.
69. Yakes FM, Chen J, Tan J, et al. Cabozantinib (XL184), a novel MET and VEGFR2 inhibitor, simultaneously suppresses metastasis, angiogenesis, and tumor growth. *Mol Cancer Ther.* 2011;10(12):2298–2308.
70. Monk BJ, Poveda A, Vergote I, et al. Anti-angiopoietin therapy with trebananib for recurrent ovarian cancer (TRINOVA-1): a randomised, multicentre, double-blind, placebo-controlled phase 3 trial. *Lancet Oncol.* 2014;15:799–808.
71. Ivy SP, Liu JF, Lee JM, et al. Cediranib, a pan-VEGFR inhibitor, and olaparib, a PARP inhibitor, in combination therapy for high grade serous ovarian cancer. *Expert Opin Investig Drugs.* 2016;25(5):597–611.
72. Liu JF, Barry WT, Birrer M, et al. Combination cediranib and olaparib versus olaparib alone for women with recurrent platinum-sensitive ovarian cancer: a randomised phase 2 study. *Lancet Oncol.* 2014;15:1207–1214.
73. Lee JM, Trepel JB, Choyke P, et al. CECs and IL-8 have prognostic and predictive utility in patients with recurrent platinum-sensitive ovarian cancer: biomarker correlates from the randomized phase-2 trial of olaparib and cediranib compared with olaparib in recurrent platinum-sensitive ovarian cancer. *Front Oncol.* 2015;5:123.
74. Backen A, Renehan AG, Clamp AR, et al. The combination of circulating Ang1 and Tie2 levels predicts progression-free survival advantage in bevacizumab-treated patients with ovarian cancer. *Clin Cancer Res.* 2014;20:4549–4558.
75. Ferriss JS, Java JJ, Bookman MA, et al. Ascites predicts treatment benefit of bevacizumab in front-line therapy of advanced epithelial ovarian, fallopian tube and peritoneal cancers: an NRG Oncology/GOG study. *Gynecol Oncol.* 2015;139:17–22.

CHAPTER 5

Development and Identification of Tumor Serum Markers

Aleksandra Gentry-Maharaj and Usha Menon

Tumor markers are defined as molecules or substances produced by malignant tumors that enter the circulation in detectable amounts. They indicate the likely presence of cancer or provide information about its behavior. In the management of cancer, the most useful biochemical markers are the macromolecular tumor antigens, including enzymes, hormones, receptors, growth factors, biologic response modifiers, and glycoconjugates. A substantial number of substances have been investigated as potential tumor markers over the past decade and the list is continually growing owing to new technology employed in biomarker discovery.

Tumor markers can be used for risk stratification, screening, differential diagnosis, prognosis, predicting and monitoring response to therapy, and detecting recurrence (**Table 5.1**). The performance of a tumor marker depends on its sensitivity (percentage of patients with cancer correctly identified as a result of a positive test) and specificity (percentage of the population without cancer correctly identified as a result of a negative test) and positive predictive value (PPV, percentage of patients with positive test that have the cancer, true positives) (**Table 5.2**). An ideal tumor marker should have a 100% sensitivity, specificity, and PPV. However, in practice such a marker does not exist. As the majority of markers are tumor-associated rather than tumor-specific, and are elevated in multiple cancers, benign and physiologic conditions, they lack specificity. In addition, if sensitivity is low, a normal result may not exclude malignancy. Tumor markers discovered thus far contribute to differential diagnosis but are not themselves diagnostic. This restricts their use, with few exceptions, to monitoring therapeutic response and follow-up.

TABLE 5.1. Tumor Markers and Their Potential Uses

1. Risk stratification
Adjusting risk categorization for an individual without the disease. The marker could then be used in screening or prevention if these are proven to be effective.
2. Screening
Screening to detect cancer earlier than it would have been using clinical signs and symptoms.
3. Differential diagnosis
Use of serum and tissue tumor markers to establish the tissue of origin of a newly diagnosed cancer by differentiating between the cancer and benign conditions.
4. Prognosis
Markers used to determine prognosis in a patient, i.e., risk of invasion and metastasis in the absence of therapy.
5. Prediction
Ability of a marker to determine the likelihood of sensitivity or resistance to specific therapy.
6. Monitoring
Monitoring patients either during or after therapy to determine the status of the cancer. Patients are usually monitored during primary therapy but also during therapy for metastatic disease to determine if the patient is responding to the treatment or if an alternative therapy is needed.

TABLE 5.2. Parameters of Tumor Marker Assays

Tumor Marker Result	True Tumor Status	
	Positive	Negative
Positive	a (True positives)	b (False positives)
Negative	c (False negatives)	d (True negatives)

Sensitivity = True positives/All with tumor = a/a + c
Specificity = True negatives/All tumor-free = d/d + b
Positive predictive value (PPV) = True positives/All with positive tumor marker result = a/a + b

Tumor markers currently used in nongynecologic malignancies include:

1. Carcinoembryonic antigen (CEA), the most commonly elevated marker in colorectal cancer. Preoperative assessment is recommended by the American Society of Clinical Oncology (ASCO) as it may complement surgical staging and help in choosing the most appropriate surgical treatment. Abnormal preoperative levels may also indicate higher risk of recurrence, but there is no concrete evidence as to whether patients with colorectal cancer would benefit from adjuvant therapy based on preoperative CEA alone (1). Carcinoembryonic antigen is, however, not used in screening or early diagnosis.
2. CA15-3 measurements have been advocated (ASCO) in monitoring response to treatment in breast cancer when the disease is not measurable.
3. Prostate-specific antigen (PSA) is used in screening for prostate cancer but its use as a stand-alone marker is not recommended. Most guidelines recommend a PSA test followed by digital rectal examination, with definitive diagnosis always requiring a biopsy. PSA may have a role in detecting disease recurrence and monitoring treatment in patients with prostate cancer (2).

This chapter focuses on those markers that are clinically relevant to female genital tract malignancies.

Ovarian and Fallopian Tube Cancers

Women have approximately a 1% to 2% lifetime risk of developing ovarian cancer (OC). OC accounts for 4% of cancers diagnosed in women, with over 239,000 new cases diagnosed worldwide each year (3). Incidence rates are highest in the United States and Northern Europe and lowest in Africa and Asia. It is associated with the highest mortality rates of all female genital tract malignancies. Around 85% of cases occur over the age of 50 years and 80% to 85% are epithelial in origin. It is now widely accepted that epithelial ovarian cancer

(EOC) is a heterogeneous disease and consists of five main histologic subtypes: high-grade serous, low-grade serous, endometrioid, clear cell, and mucinous cancers, each associated with a unique origin, pathogenesis, and prognosis (4). In addition, women previously diagnosed with primary peritoneal cancers would likely be re-classified as ovarian cancers in view of the new WHO (2014) classification which states that any ovarian/tubal involvement would results in a diagnosis of ovarian cancer. The most common histologic subtype of EOC is serous OC, which usually presents at advanced stages and has the poorest outcomes (5). However, in those of reproductive age, germ cell tumors, granulosa cell/sex cord tumors, mucinous, and endometrioid tumors are more common. High-grade serous cancer which accounts for most of the OC mortality is thought to originate mainly in the fallopian tube and involve the ovaries secondarily. Given the growing evidence to support these origins as well as the notion that epithelial OC is a heterogeneous disease, it is unlikely that one marker/strategy would be equally effective in diagnosis of each subtype. Cancer antigen 125 (CA125) has been the only marker used clinically in diagnosis and management of OC. Despite decades of research to identify a better biomarker than CA125, no single marker with superior performance has been found; however, there is some encouraging data on markers that can improve the performance of CA125, and these will be discussed later in this chapter.

CA125

CA125 was first described by Bast et al. (6) in 1981. It is a 200 kD glycoprotein recognized by the OC-125 murine monoclonal antibody. CA125 carries two major antigenic domains: domain A (binds monoclonal antibody OC-125) and domain B (binds monoclonal antibody M11). The current second-generation heterologous CA125-II assay incorporates M11 and OC125 antibodies, while the original homologous assay was with OC125 alone. Currently there are a number of CA125 assays that correlate well with each other (7).

CA125 is expressed by amniotic and coelomic epithelium during fetal development. It is widely distributed in adult tissues (mesothelial cells of the pleura, pericardium, and peritoneum, tubal, endometrial, and endocervical epithelium); however, it is not expressed by the surface epithelium of normal fetal and adult ovaries with the exception of inclusion cysts, areas of metaplasia, and papillary excrescences (8). It therefore lacks complete specificity for OC.

The level of CA125 in body fluids or ovarian cysts does not correlate well with serum levels. This is probably due to the serum concentration being reflective not only of the production of the antigen by the tumor but also other factors that affect its release into the circulation. The widely adopted cutoff at 35 kU/L routinely used in clinical practice is based upon the distribution of values in 99% of 888 healthy men and women (9). However, as levels of CA125 tend to be lower in postmenopausal women or in patients who have undergone hysterectomy, levels of 20 kU/L and 26 kU/L have been suggested (10). Approximately 85% of patients with EOC have CA125 levels of >35 kU/L. Raised serum levels are found in 50% Stage I and >90% Stage II–IV cancers (11) (**Table 5.3**). CA125 levels are more frequently elevated in serous invasive compared to mucinous, clear cell, and borderline tumors (11,12). CA125 can be elevated in other malignancies (pancreas, breast, colon, and lung cancers) (**Table 5.4**), in benign conditions (**Table 5.3**), and in physiologic states such as pregnancy, endometriosis, and menstruation (11). In postmenopausal women, the diagnostic accuracy of raised CA125 is improved by absence of many of these nonmalignant conditions (**Table 5.3**). It is possible that specificity could be improved by posttranslationally modified glycosylated forms of CA125 (13).

Screening

Screening is the identification of unrecognized disease in apparently asymptomatic population by use of tests, examinations, or other procedures that allow earlier diagnosis of the disease than if it had presented clinically. The main goal of cancer screening is to reduce mortality from the disease by either preventing it (if a premalignant

TABLE 5.3. CA-125 Elevations in Benign Disorders and Ovarian Cancer

		Cutoff
Healthy women	Premenopausal[a]	35 kU/L
	Postmenopausal[b]	20 kU/L
Disease	**Condition**	**CA125 elevations over 35 kU/L (%)**
Benign ovarian disease	Overall (all benign tumors)[c]	29
	Ovarian cysts[c]	14
	Germ cell tumors (mature teratoma)[c]	21
	Sex cord stromal tumors (thecoma, fibrothecoma)[c]	52
	Cystadenoma, adenofibroma, cystadenofibroma[c]	20
	Serous epithelial tumors[c]	20
	Mucinous epithelial tumors[c]	18
	Benign, NOS[c]	27
	Benign, other (normal ovaries)[c]	22
Benign disorders of the female genital tract	Abscess/hydrosalpinx/POD[c]	37
	Fibroid (leiomyomas)[c]	26
	Acute salpingitis[d]	40.4
	Chronic salpingitis[d]	8.3
	Pelvic inflammatory disease[e]	29.4
	Endometriosis/endometrioma[c]	67
	Endometriosis (Stage I)[d]	8.0
	Endometriosis (Stage II)[d]	19.6
	Endometriosis (Stage I/II combined)[d]	11.5
	Endometriosis (Stage III)[d]	44.7
	Endometriosis (Stage IV)[d]	86.7
	Endometriosis (Stage III/IV combined)[d]	50.4
	Endometriosis (Overall)[d]	24.3
Other disorders	Cirrhosis[d]	67.1
	Cirrhosis + ascites[d]	100.0
	Acute pancreatitis[d]	32.2
	Chronic active hepatitis[d]	9.1
	Chronic pancreatitis[d]	1.9
	Renal failure[d]	14.6
	Heart failure[f]	14.7
	Diabetes[d]	0.0
Ovarian cancer[d]	**According to histology**	
	Serous	80.0
	Mucinous	69.0
	Endometrioid	75.0
	Clear cell	78.0
	Undifferentiated	88.0
	According to FIGO Stage	
	Stage I	50.0
	Stage II	90.0
	Stage III	92.1
	Stage IV	93.9
	All stages	85.1

TABLE 5.3. CA-125 Elevations in Benign Disorders and Ovarian Cancer (*continued*)

	Cutoff
According to tumor diameter	
Microscopic	21
<1 cm	38
<2 cm	46
>1 cm	79
>2 cm	70
>10 cm	100

[a]Bast RC Jr, Klug TL, St John E, et al. A radioimmunoassay using a monoclonal antibody to monitor the course of epithelial ovarian cancer. *N Engl J Med*. 1983;309(15):883–887.
[b]Bon GG, Kenemans P, Verstraeten R, et al. Serum tumor marker immunoassays in gynecologic oncology: establishment of reference values. *Am J Obstet Gynecol*. 1996;174:107–114.
[c]Moore RG, Miller MC, Steinhoff MM et al. Serum HE4 levels are less frequently elevated than CA125 in women with benign gynecologic disorders. *Am J Obstet Gynecol*. 2012;206(4):351.e351–358.
[d]Jacobs I, Bast RC Jr. The CA 125 tumour-associated antigen: a review of the literature. *Hum Reprod*. 1989;4(1):1–12.
[e]Muyldermans M, Cornillie FJ, Koninckx PR. CA125 and endometriosis. *Hum Reprod Update*. 1995;1(2):173–187.
[f]Miralles C, Orea M, España P, et al. Cancer antigen 125 associated with multiple benign and malignant pathologies. *Ann Surg Oncol*. 2003;10(2):150–154.

TABLE 5.4. CA-125 Elevations in Non-ovarian Malignancies

	Cancer	CA125 Elevations over 35 kU/L (%)
Nongynecologic malignancies	Breast[a]	17.6
	Colorectal[a]	15.1
	Pancreas[a]	52.6
	Lung[a]	29.5
	Gastric[a]	30.9
	Biliary tract[a]	45.8
	Liver[a]	49.0
	Esophageal[a]	10.5
Nonovarian gynecologic malignancies	Endometrial cancer[b,c]	21
	Endometrial cancer[d]	25
	Stage III	55
	Stage IV	86
	Cervical cancer[e]	39

[a]Jacobs I, Bast RC Jr. The CA 125 tumour-associated antigen: a review of the literature. *Hum Reprod*. 1989;4(1):1–12.
[b]Ginath S, Menczer J, Fintsi Y, et al. Tissue and serum CA125 expression in endometrial cancer. *Int J Gynecol Cancer*. 2002;12(4):372–375.
[c]Duk JM, Aalders JG, Fleuren GJ, et al. CA 125: a useful marker in endometrial carcinoma. *Am J Obstet Gynecol*. 1986;155(5):1097–1102.
[d]Bonfrer JM, Korse CM, Verstraeten RA, et al. Clinical evaluation of the Byk LIA-mat CA125 II assay: discussion of a reference value. *Clin Chem*. 1997;43(3):491–497.

condition exists) or diagnosing it earlier when treatment is more effective. Detection of the cancer of interest alone before it is symptomatic cannot justify screening.

There are cancer-specific criteria detailing which cancers could most benefit from screening that build on the WHO criteria for all diseases (**Table 5.5**) (14). To be effective and applicable to the population at large, screening must achieve high sensitivity/specificity, PPV, and negative predictive value (NPV) (**Table 5.6**), and it must

TABLE 5.5. World Health Organization Criteria for a Screening Program

1. The condition sought should be an important health problem
2. There should be accepted treatment for patients with recognized disease
3. Facilities for diagnosis and treatment should be available
4. There should be a recognizable latent or early symptomatic stage
5. There should be a suitable test or examination
6. The test should be acceptable to the population
7. The natural history of the condition, including development from latent to declared disease, should be adequately understood
8. There should be an agreed policy on whom to treat as patients
9. The cost of case finding (including diagnosis and treatment of patients diagnosed) should be economically balanced in relation to possible expenditure on medical care as a whole
10. Case finding should be a continuing process and not a "once and for all" project

From Wilson J, Jungner G. *WHO Principles and Practice of Screening for Disease.* Geneva, Switzerland: World Health Organization; 1968:66–67.

be acceptable to the populations being tested. The PPV depends on the prevalence of the disease within the population, with more false positives detected if disease prevalence is low. Well-organized national screening programmes, such as cervical cancer screening, are required to realise the true potential of screening in reducing disease-specific mortality.

In a national screening programme, issues that must be considered include: frequency of screening, age of the population to be screened, well-defined mechanisms for referral and treatment of screen-detected abnormalities, comprehensive information systems that not only send invitations at predefined intervals but also recall those with abnormalities for assessment and schedule follow-up of those treated, and quality assurance protocols to monitor and evaluate the efficacy of the screening programme. Furthermore, for a screening strategy to be successful, uptake and compliance with screening has to be high.

The established population cancer screening programmes include breast, bowel, and cervical cancer, with ongoing debates on the risks and benefits of lung and prostate cancer screening. A survey in the United Kingdom of 2,024 men and women aged 50 to 80 years demonstrated that there is a positive view of and widespread enthusiasm for cancer screening without a full appreciation of its limitations (15).

Screening for OC has been investigated in the research setting with CA125 being the only tumor marker explored in large trials. When it is interpreted using a cutoff, 2.9% of healthy postmenopausal women will have elevated CA125 levels, limiting its use as a stand-alone test (16). In the multimodal screening strategy, this is overcome by use of transvaginal ultrasound (TVS) as a second-line test in women with elevated CA125 levels, so that high specificity (99.9%) and four or fewer operations for each OC detected can be achieved (17,18). Over the last two decades, there has been a move to use CA125 profile over time rather than as a single value. A statistical algorithm (Risk of Ovarian Cancer Algorithm, ROCA), based on the age-specific risk of the disease and the behavior of CA125 over time in women with OC versus normal controls, has significantly improved both the sensitivity (19) and specificity of CA125 interpretation (19–21) for primary invasive EOC. Algorithms such as the ROCA rely on modeling the behavior of a biomarker from disease onset to clinical presentation, and use data accumulated in large trials over many years.

The first suggestion of a survival benefit with screening came from the Bart's pilot RCT of 22,000 women carried out in the 1980s, which used sequential CA125 and TVS. The trial reported

TABLE 5.6. Parameters Crucial When Evaluating Screening Tests

1. Test validity
Accuracy/Validity of the screening test is evaluated by its sensitivity and specificity. Sensitivity is the correct identification of the individuals with disease out of all with positive screening results, whereas specificity is the proportion of those with negative screening results who do not have the disease.
2. Measuring test performance
Easier to measure in research setting than in a screening program. The proportion of the population with detectable preclinical disease is an important factor in judging the effectiveness of a screening strategy. An ideal test would detect the disease early; tests that can only detect advanced disease indicate a long screening interval or poor test sensitivity.
3. PPV
Proportion of individuals with a positive screening test that will have the disease. A PPV of 10% means that only 1 out of 10 individuals investigated had the disease, the other 9 were investigated unnecessarily.
4. NPV
Proportion of individuals with a negative test result who are correctly diagnosed as not having the disease. In clinical setting, high NPV means that the test only rarely misclassifies a sick person as being healthy.
5. Test sensitivity versus program sensitivity
Test sensitivity (screening test applied once) can be different from program sensitivity (screening test applied multiple times to the same population). Program sensitivity is higher in cases where population adherence to screening is high, because if the cancer was missed in the first round of screening, it is very likely to be detected on the second round. However, if adherence to screening is poor, some cancers will be missed and diagnosed only when symptomatic.
6. Validity
RCT is the gold standard for evaluating effectiveness of a screening strategy but needs a large number of participants and takes a long time to complete (at least 15 years). Case–control studies have been used to evaluate screening tests but suffer due to potential selection bias.
7. Lead-time bias
Screening advances the time of diagnosis; therefore, the duration of time between when a cancer is detected by screening and when it would have been detected due to symptoms is referred to as lead time. However, if there is no effect on survival, i.e., the cancer is diagnosed through screening but the individual dies at the same time as if the cancer were symptomatic at the time of detection, it would appear that survival is longer in the screened population when, in fact, it is not. This is called lead-time bias.
8. Length-bias sampling
Screening tends to pick up less aggressive, slow-growing cancers and is less likely to pick up more aggressive, faster-growing cancers. Length-time bias refers to the greater likelihood of screen-detected cancers to be slow-growing—this would give the false impression of improved survival of screen-detected cancers.
9. Overdiagnosis
Screening can result in overdiagnosis, detection of the cancer that would not have been detected during that person's lifetime if not for screening. These lesions are not easy to distinguish from those that become clinically significant. There may be serious consequences for these patients, although it is unclear what proportion of them are at risk. However, any harm caused by overdiagnosis is probably miniscule when compared to the benefits of screening.
10. Selection bias
Individuals who participate in screening programs are usually more health conscious, healthier, more aware of signs and symptoms of the disease, have better access to treatment and are more likely to adhere to treatment. Hence they might have better outcomes if they develop cancer than the unscreened population. Selection bias is higher in clinical trials than in screening programs that are associated with high uptake.

NPV, Negative Predictive Value; PPV, Positive Predictive Value.

improved median survival in women with ovarian/tubal cancer in the screened (72.9 months) group when compared to control (41.8 months) group (17).

Since then, four large trials on OC screening (OCS) have reported in the general population. Aside from the Kentucky Screening Study (22), which was a single-arm annual ultrasound screening study of 25,327 women, the other three were randomized controlled trials (RCTs) and used the tumor marker CA125 together with pelvic ultrasound. The Japanese Shizuoka Cohort Study of Ovarian Cancer Screening (23) was an RCT of 82,487 low-risk postmenopausal women who were screened using an annual ultrasound and CA125 using a cutoff. Sensitivity of 77.1% and specificity of 99.9% were reported with the proportion of Stage I OCs higher in the screened group (63%) than in the control group (38%). However, it did not reach statistical significance (23) and the impact on mortality has not yet been reported.

The U.S. Prostate, Lung, Colorectal and Ovarian (PLCO) Cancer Screening Trial enrolled 78,237 women aged 55 to 74 years, with 34,202 women randomized to OCS. Women were screened using serum CA125 using a cutoff of 35 kU/L and TVS for 3 years followed by CA125 alone for a further 2 years. Evaluation and management of positive screening tests was at the discretion of participants' clinicians. The sensitivity, specificity, and PPV of this strategy for detection of primary invasive ovarian, tubal, and primary peritoneal cancers were 68.2%, 98.9%, and 7.7% (24). At a median follow-up of 12.4 years (25th to 75th centile, 10.9 to 13.0), PLCO showed no mortality benefit with OCS, with 118 and 100 deaths in the screening and control arm, respectively (mortality rate ratio of 1.18, 95% CI, 0.91 to 1.54) (**Fig. 5.1**). Moreover, excess morbidity was reported as a result of false-positive surgery with major complication rate of 15% (25).

In the UK Collaborative Trial of Ovarian Cancer Screening (UKCTOCS), 202,638 postmenopausal women aged 50 to 74 years were randomized to either control or annual screening with ultrasound (USS) or a multimodal strategy (MMS) in a 2:1:1 fashion (26,27) (**Fig. 5.2**). In the MMS group, CA125 was interpreted using the

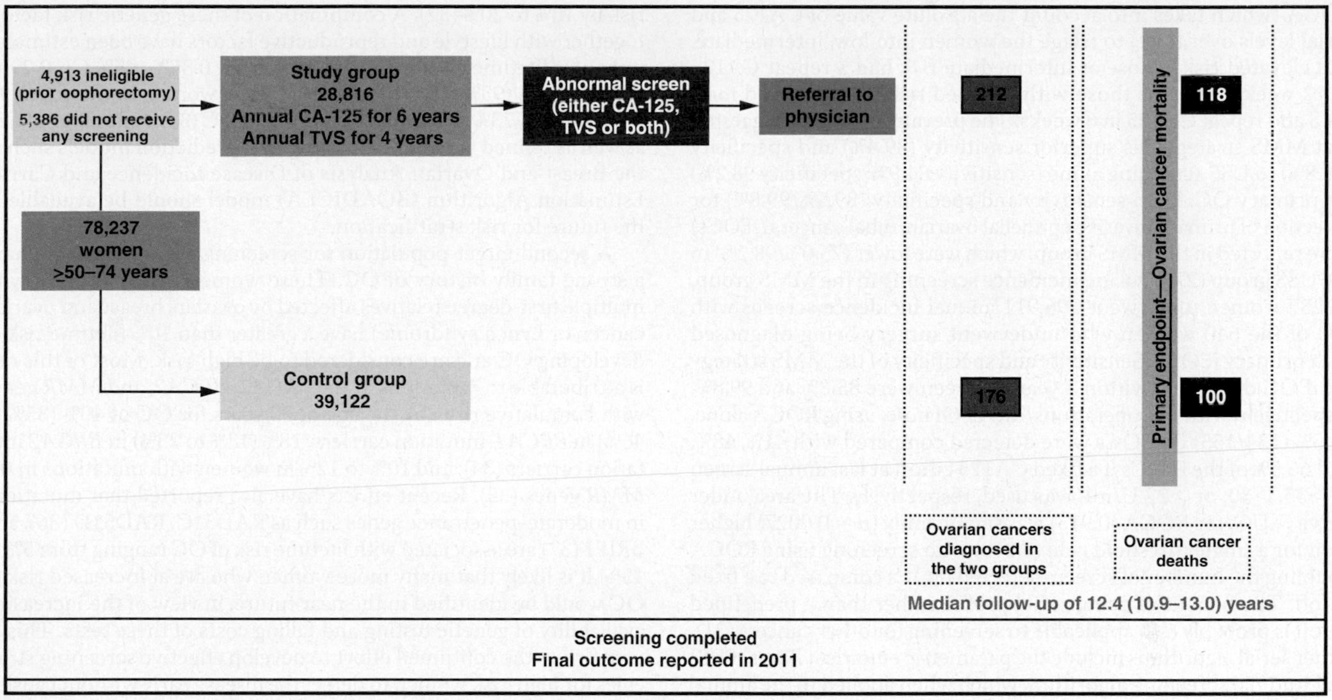

Figure 5.1. PLCO Cancer Screening Trial. Women in the trial underwent four annual screens with CA125 (interpreted using a cutoff of 35 kU/L) and TVS and two further screens with CA125 alone. If an abnormality was detected on screening, the women were referred to their physician. Final outcome (OC mortality) was reported in 2011. TVS, transvaginal ultrasound.

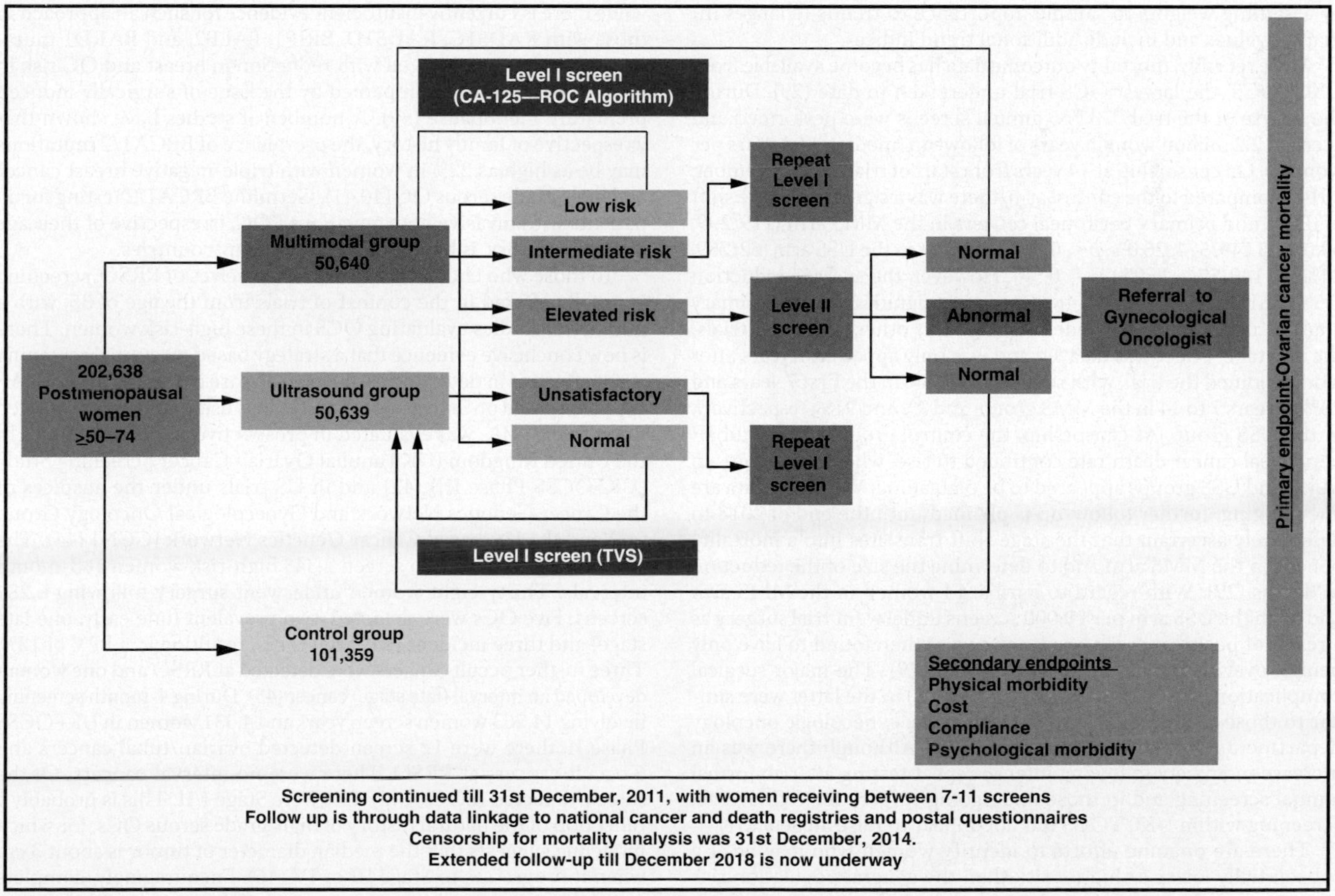

Figure 5.2. The United Kingdom Collaborative Trial of Ovarian Cancer Screening (UKCTOCS). Women in the trial, based on the Risk of Ovarian Cancer (ROC) value, are triaged into **low risk** (ROC < 1/3,500), and returned to annual screening with the next blood test in 1 year; **intermediate risk** (<1/1,000 and <1/3,500) with a repeat CA125 in 12 weeks; and **elevated risk** (>1/1,000) with Level II screen (CA125 and TVS) scheduled in 6 to 8 weeks, with earlier screens arranged if there is a high index of suspicion. Those with persistent abnormalities on Level II screen are referred to a gynecological oncologist. The screening protocol has been described in detail elsewhere. Final outcome (OC mortality) was reported in 2015. TVS, transvaginal ultrasound.

ROCA (which takes into account the absolute value of CA125 and serial levels over time) to triage the women into low, intermediate, and elevated risk. Those at intermediate risk had a repeat CA125 in 12 weeks, whereas those with elevated risk were referred for a TVS and repeat CA125 in 6 weeks. The prevalence screen suggested that MMS strategy has superior sensitivity (89.4%) and specificity (99.8%) to USS screening alone (sensitivity 84.9%; specificity 98.2%) for primary OC. High sensitivity and specificity (89.5%/99.8%) for detection of primary invasive epithelial ovarian/tubal cancers (iEOCs) were reported in the MMS group, which were lower (75.0%/98.2%) in the USS group (27). During incidence screening in the MMS group, 46,237 women underwent 296,911 annual incidence screens with 133 of the 640 women who underwent surgery being diagnosed with primary iEOCs. Sensitivity and specificity of the MMS strategy for iEOC diagnosed within 1 year of screen were 85.8% and 99.8%, respectively, with five operations/iEOC. Of note, using ROCA alone, 86.5% (134/155) of iEOCs were detected compared with 41%, 48%, and 66.5% of the iEOCs if a fixed CA125 cutoff at last annual screen of >35, >30, or >22 U/mL was used, respectively. The area under curve (AUC) for ROCA (0.915) was significantly ($p = 0.0027$) higher than for a single threshold rule (0.869) with screening using ROCA doubling the number of screen-detected iEOCs compared to a fixed cutoff. The benefit of using serial profile rather than a predefined cutoff is probably also applicable to screening for other cancers (21). Other serial algorithms include the parametric empirical Bayes (PEB) longitudinal screening algorithm, which when applied to the annual samples from 44 women who developed OC in the PLCO trial, was able to identify 20% of cases earlier than a single threshold rule ($\geq$35 kU/L) (28). A method of mean trends (MMT) algorithm has also been described that measures biomarker dynamics over time by assigning weights to sample importance to trends (changes in) marker values and include additional trend indices.

More recently, mortality outcome data has become available from UKCTOCS, the largest OCS trial undertaken to date (29). During the course of the trial 673,765 annual screens were performed and accrued 2.2 million women years of follow-up (median 11.1 years per woman). On censorship at 14 years from start of trial (31st December, 2014), compared to the control arm, there was a significant stage shift of iEOC and primary peritoneal cancers in the MMS arm (119/299, 40.0% vs. 149/574, 26.0%; $p < 0.0001$) but not in the USS arm (62/259, 24% vs. 149/574, 26.0%; $p = 0.57$). However, the average reduction (15% MMS, 11% USS) over 14 years was not significant on the primary analysis using the Cox model. As noted in other screening trials, the mortality effect was delayed and was only apparent 7 years after women joined the trial, with reductions of 8% in the first 7 years and 23% in years 7 to 14 in the MMS group, and 2% and 21%, respectively, in the USS group. At censorship, the control group ovarian/tubal/peritoneal cancer death rate continued to rise, whereas the rates in MMS and USS groups appeared to be plateauing. While the data are encouraging, further follow-up is planned until the end of 2018 to definitively ascertain that the stage shift translates into a mortality benefit in the MMS arm and to determine the size of the reduction in deaths (29). With regard to harms, 14 women in the MMS arm and 50 in the USS arm per 10,000 screens underwent trial surgery as a result of positive screen results and were then found to have only benign ovarian lesions or normal ovaries (29). The major surgical complication rate (3.1% MMS and 3.5% USS) in the latter were similar to those reported for such surgery in the gynecologic oncology departments in the United Kingdom (30). Although there was an increase in anxiety following intense repeat testing after abnormal annual screening and in those undergoing surgery for OC, overall, screening within UKCTOCS did not appear to raise anxiety (31).

There are ongoing efforts to identify women who may be at a substantially lower or higher risk than the general population risk of 1.37% based on genetic and epidemiologic factors to maximize benefit from screening. Data from the Ovarian Cancer Association Consortium (OCAC) suggests that there are currently over 30 low-penetrance single nucleotide polymorphisms (SNPs) that predispose women to OC, each individually increasing the relative risk by 10% to 20% (32). A combination of these genetic risk factors together with lifestyle and reproductive factors have been estimated to confer lifetime risk of OC ranging from 0.35% (95% CI, 0.29 to 0.42) to 8.8% (95% CI, 7.10 to 10.9). Of the women in the 4% to 9% risk category, 73% had no family history of OC (33). A number of new as well as refined versions of existing risk-prediction models such as the Breast and Ovarian Analysis of Disease Incidence and Carrier Estimation Algorithm (BOADICEA) model should be available in the future for risk stratification.

A second target population for screening are women who have a strong family history of OC. These women (from families with multiple first-degree relatives affected by ovarian, breast and ovarian cancer, or Lynch syndrome) have a greater than 10% lifetime risk of developing OC and are considered to be high-risk. Most of this risk is attributable to mutations in the *BRCA1*, *BRCA2*, and *MMR* genes with cumulative risks by the age of 70 years for OC of 40% (35% to 46%) in *BRCA1*-mutation carriers, 18% (13% to 23%) in *BRCA2* mutation carriers (34), and 10% to 12% in women with mutations in the *MMR* genes (35). Recent efforts have also reported that mutations in moderate-penetrance genes such as RAD51C, RAD51D (36), and BRIP1 (37) are associated with lifetime risk of OC ranging from 5% to 15%. It is likely that many more women who are at increased risk of OC would be identified in the near future, in view of the increasing availability of genetic testing and falling costs of these tests. This in turn drives the continued effort to develop effective screening strategies for high-risk women to detect the disease early without causing significant harm. In these women, the primary recommendation is risk-reducing salpingo-oophorectomy (RRSO) (38). In the United States, the National Comprehensive Cancer Network (NCCN) recommends RRSO in those with BRCA1, BRCA2, and Lynch syndrome, while there is currently insufficient evidence for such an approach in those with RAD51C, RAD51D, BRIP1, PALB2, and BARD1 mutations. Surgery is associated with reduction in breast and OC risk in BRCA carriers but accompanied by the issue of surgically induced premature menopause (39). A number of studies have shown that irrespective of family history, the prevalence of BRCA1/2 mutations may be as high as 22% in women with triple-negative breast cancer and high-grade serous OC (40,41). Germline BRCA1/2 testing for all patients with invasive non-mucinous EOC, irrespective of their age or family history, is being rolled out in many countries.

To those who choose not to avail themselves of RRSO, screening is usually offered in the context of trials from the age of 35, with a number of studies evaluating OCS in these high-risk women. There is now conclusive evidence that a strategy based on annual screening is not effective in detecting early-stage disease in this population. An approach based on 3- to 4-month screenings using CA125, interpreted using the ROCA, was evaluated in prospective screening studies in the United Kingdom (UK Familial Ovarian Cancer Screening Study [UKFOCSS Phase II]) (42) and in US trials under the auspices of the Cancer Genetics Network and Gynecological Oncology Group (43) and the US-based Cancer Genetics Network (CGN) (44). The latter used the ROCA to screen 2,343 high-risk women at 3-month intervals. Thirty-eight women underwent surgery following 6,284 screens. Five OCs were detected, two prevalent (one early, one late stage) and three incident (all early) cases, resulting in a PPV of 13%. Three further occult cancers were detected at RRSO and one woman developed an interval (late stage) cancer (45). During 4-month screening involving 14,263 women screen years and 4,531 women in UKFOCSS Phase II, there were 12 screen-detected ovarian/tubal cancers and 6 occult cancers at RRSO. There were no interval cancers. Of the screen-detected iEOCs, only 42% were Stage I/II. This is probably a reflection of the natural history of high-grade serous OCs, for which modeling suggests that the median diameter of tumor is about 3 cm when it progresses to Stage III or IV (46). Encouragingly, complete cytoreduction was achieved in over 90% of the women with ovarian/tubal cancers in UKFOCSS (47). Despite the intensive screening in UKFOCSS leading to women being recalled for abnormal results, only transient cancer-specific distress and no significant effect on general anxiety/depression or overall reassurance was reported (48).

The final results of the UK trial are anticipated in 2016, but this preliminary data seems to suggest that in high-risk women who decide to defer/not avail of surgery, a programme of intensive screening with ROCA and second-line TVS, together with regular discussions about RRSO, might be an option. The importance of serial monitoring of CA125 rather than using absolute cutoff is further illustrated by a case report of an asymptomatic woman seen in a familial clinic who had rising levels of CA125 within the normal range, was managed conservatively, and then went on to present with Stage IIIc OC (49).

Monitoring CA125 levels post-RRSO (although performed occasionally in high-risk women due to the small residual risk of primary peritoneal cancer [PPC]) is a contentious issue. In a recent series of 207 BRCA1/2 carriers monitored with annual CA125 between 1990 and 2008, only one woman with Stage III PPC (whose baseline CA125 before RRSO was 19.5 kU/L but 14 months after the procedure rose to 143 kU/L) was detected, supporting the majority view that CA125 monitoring post-RRSO is not effective (50).

In a 1980s biobank study, CA125 was found to be raised in 59 out of 236 (25%) stored serum samples collected from women with OC 5 years before diagnosis (51). Data from the Japanese OCS study indicate that, in serous-type OC, first elevation of CA125 to diagnosis has a shorter interval compared with those with non-serous disease (1.4 vs. 3.8 years; $p = 0.011$). Furthermore, a higher proportion (75%) of serous OCs developed following a normal CA125 (<35 kU/L) compared to 47% of non-serous OCs that developed from slightly elevated CA125 levels (35 to 65 kU/L) (52). A model of natural history of OC developed by Brown and Palmer suggests that on average it takes over 4 years for *in situ* Stage I or Stage II cancers to become clinically apparent and approximately 1 year to progress to Stage III/IV cancers (46). Serous cancers are less than 1 cm in diameter during the occult period. The model suggests that for a screening strategy to be able to detect 50% of the cancers before they progress to Stage III, an annual screen would have to detect tumors 1.3 cm in diameter, whereas to detect 80% of the cancers, the strategy would have to pick these tumors up when only 0.4 cm (53). The current tests are imprecise as they are unable to detect OCs when this small, thus the continued search for more precise markers.

Whether a raised CA125 in asymptomatic postmenopausal women is a predictor of non-gynecologic cancer is not yet clear. Data from the Bart's RCT of 22,000 postmenopausal women (17) reported that elevated serum CA125 was not a predictor of a nongynecologic malignancy on mean follow-up of 6.2 years (54). However, it was associated with significantly increased risk of death from all causes in the next 5 years (55). In contrast, data from the Norwegian OCS trial of 5,500 women showed that breast and lung cancer were overrepresented among women with elevated CA125 (56). Both trials indicate that elevated CA125 is a risk factor for death from malignant disease. This data indicates that steps should be taken to rule out other malignancies such as breast, lung, and pancreas in asymptomatic postmenopausal women with rising CA125 levels and no evidence of gynecologic malignancy.

Differential Diagnosis of an Adnexal Mass

There are certain criteria a tumor marker must fulfill to be incorporated into clinical practice (**Table 5.7**). Serum CA125 is used routinely in clinical practice in differential diagnosis of benign and malignant adnexal masses, especially in postmenopausal women. Using an upper limit of 35 kU/L, sensitivity of 78%, specificity of 95%, and PPV of 82% could be achieved for malignant disease in women with palpable adnexal masses (57). Despite further improvements in specificity being achieved by using a panel of markers (CA125 II, CA 72-4, CA 15-3, and lipid-associated sialic acid) and an artificial neural network approach to differentiate malignant from benign pelvic masses (58), these are not used in clinical practice.

The risk of malignancy index (RMI) has been the most valuable clinical tool used in the past two-and-a-half decades. It combines serum CA125 values with ultrasound findings and menopausal status. The initial study (1990) demonstrated a sensitivity of 85%

TABLE 5.7. Criteria for Incorporating Tumor Marker into Clinical Practice

1. The intended use of the tumor marker must be clearly outlined
2. The difference between "positive" and "negative" populations must be sufficient to guide change in clinical management
3. The estimate of difference must be reliable and validated
Assay must be technically stable, reproducible, and accurate
Clinical study must have been suitably designed and have sufficient power to address the utility of intended use
Statistical analysis must be rigorous

Hayes DF. Biomarkers. In: DeVita VT Jr, Lawrence TS, Rosenberg SA, DePinho RA, Weinberg RA, eds. *Cancer: Principles and Practice of Oncology.* Philadelphia, PA: Wolters Kluwer Health; Lippincott, Williams & Wilkins; 2011:694–701.

and a specificity of 97%. Patients with an elevated RMI score had on average a 42-fold increase in the background risk of OC (59). Since then, the RMI has been validated extensively. A 2009 systematic review of 109 eligible studies assessing accuracy of models for predicting malignancy in ovarian masses showed that while all models had acceptable sensitivity and specificity, RMI was the best predictor. Using a value of 200 as the cutoff, the pooled estimate for sensitivity for preoperative assessment of an adnexal mass was 78%, for a specificity of 87% (60). Varying the RMI cutoff (from 25 to 1,000) in combination with specialist ultrasound (US), magnetic resonance imaging (MRI), and radioimmunoscintigraphy (RS) can achieve a higher sensitivity (94%) and specificity (90%), thus suggesting that using this approach may improve the correct referral of cancer patients to a cancer center (61). More recently, RMI-I cutoff of 200 was shown to have a higher sensitivity (92%), but a slightly lower specificity (82%) (62). However, despite many modifications of the RMI since 1990 (by varying the cutoff levels, incorporating CA19-9), the performance between RMI-IV is comparable (63). Despite the lower accuracy of the RMI in borderline, Stage I invasive and nonepithelial OCs, the RMI is a simple, easily applicable method in the primary evaluation of patients with adnexal masses that identifies OCs more accurately than any other criterion used in diagnosis of this disease (64).

In further efforts to improve the specificity of CA125, a cancer-specific glycoform of CA125 (O-glycosylated CA125) was identified that was able to discriminate between primary iEOCs from benign ovarian neoplasms in women with moderate elevations of CA125 (30 to 500 kU/L), with a specificity of 60% and a sensitivity of 90% (13).

The International Ovarian Tumor Analysis (IOTA) group has led the effort in identifying ultrasound features that could distinguish between benign and malignant adnexal masses. Despite many studies relying on ultrasound alone, more recently, CA125 was introduced into their Assessment of Different NEoplasias in the adneXa (ADNEX) model, which achieved an AUC of 0.85 for benign versus borderline, 0.92 for benign versus Stage I cancer, 0.99 for benign versus Stage II–IV cancer, and 0.95 for benign versus secondary metastatic cancer (65), with suggestions on how this model could be applied to clinical practice (66). However, the model performed similarly to subjective assessment in predicting whether a pelvic tumor is metastatic and of non-ovarian origin (67). The latest IOTA study of 5,200 women with a pelvic mass recently reported an encouraging performance of 10 simple ultrasound rules (5 features indicative of a benign tumor and 5 indicative of malignancy) if 30% risk cutoff was used (sensitivity of 89.0%, specificity of 84.7%). The authors suggest that such an algorithm is applicable in both oncology as well as non-oncology centers and can be easily used clinically in the management of patients as well as triage to a gynecologic oncologist (68). Of all the models thus described in the literature, RMI-I and the IOTA Logistic Regression 2 (LR2) model perform best for preoperative characterization of adnexal masses in postmenopausal women. In those of reproductive age, the two best-performing models are LR2 and simple rules (63).

Prognosis

The role of CA125 (pre-, postoperative, and during treatment) in prognosis is well established (69). Single measurement of CA125 has limited value in predicting prognosis compared with a change in CA125. Preoperative serum CA125 levels are related to tumor stage, tumor volume, and histologic grade of OC and may be of value in those with localized/early-stage disease (70). Lower preoperative serum CA125 (<65 kU/L) levels indicate a significantly longer survival in those with Stage I EOC (71). These findings have been further confirmed by an international study in which those with CA125 of ≤30 kU/L (regardless of histologic subtype, substage or grade) had a good prognosis and survival and could possibly be spared from adjuvant chemotherapy (72). Additional parameters, such as cyclooxygenase-2 overexpression, in combination with preoperative CA125 <30 kU/L are independent predictors of survival (73). However, CA125 does not appear to be an independent prognostic factor in advanced OC (70).

Postoperative CA125 levels have been found to be significant prognostic factors (74). Patients with a low "CA125 prognostic score" (composed of two CA125 values, one taken preoperatively and the other taken 1 month after surgery because levels can be elevated 4 weeks post-surgery), have significantly better prognosis than patients with high scores (75). In advanced EOC, serum CA125 half-life is another way of measuring treatment response, with a half-life of 20 days most commonly used. Overall, all studies to date indicate that prolonged half-life reflects the persistent production of CA125 in OC patients and is a poor prognostic indicator (76). In patients with CA125-positive tumors, other useful prognostic indicators of survival are the serum CA125 levels prior to third course of chemotherapy (77) and the slope of the CA125 exponential regression curve. In patients treated on maintenance chemotherapy and achieving a clinically defined complete response to primary chemotherapy, with a baseline CA125 level of ≤35 kU/L, the baseline CA125 level before initiation of maintenance chemotherapy strongly predicts the risk of subsequent relapse. Patients with pre-maintenance baseline CA125 values ≤10 kU/L have a superior progression-free survival (PFS) compared to those with higher levels, even if in the normal CA125 range (78).

Serum CA125 continues to be of prognostic significance when OC recurs; patients with normal serum CA125 levels (≤35 kU/L) at relapse have a better prognosis than patients with elevated levels (79).

Monitoring Response to Treatment

It is now established that serum CA125 levels reflect progression or regression of disease in over 90% of OC patients with elevated preoperative levels (**Fig. 5.3**). Despite the widespread use of serum CA125 levels to monitor the clinical course of OC and its response to chemotherapy, CA125 should not be used as the sole criterion to determine clinical response. Studies involving second-look laparotomy have confirmed that CA125 values of <35 U/mL do not exclude active disease (80). Serial measurements are more informative than a cutoff. Rustin (81) has proposed using at least a 50% decrease in CA125 or a 75% response from pretreatment levels to define response. Response has been defined and incorporated into the RECIST criteria (82). A multicenter French study showed that pre-chemotherapy CA125, its half-life, nadir concentration, and time to nadir have a univariate prognostic value for disease-free and overall survival (OS) (83). Following first-line therapy, shorter rate of rise of CA125 (measured by CA125 doubling time) carries a worse prognosis (84). In addition to CA125 half-life, other kinetic variables have been described to assess response to therapy (85).

Detecting Recurrence

Among patients with elevated CA125 levels at diagnosis, serial monitoring following initial chemotherapy can lead to the early detection of recurrent disease. A risk of recurrence is increased in those with either a relative increase in CA125 of 100% (OR = 23.7; 95% CI, 2.9 to 192.5), or an absolute increase of 5 kU/L (OR = 8.4; 95% CI, 2.2 to 32.6) or 10 kU/L (OR = 71.2; 95% CI, 4.8 to >999.9), thus suggesting that progressive low-level increase in serum CA125 levels is strongly predictive of disease recurrence (86).

In the follow-up of OC patients, thin-section computed tomography (CT) does not aid physical examination and CA125 with ultrasound (87).

Whether to use CA125 in follow-up or wait for a symptomatic presentation of disease has been a subject of much debate. The MRC OVO5/EORTC55955 trial led by Rustin showed no benefit in CA125 monitoring in the follow-up of OC patients, as those randomized to immediate (based on CA125 levels) or delayed chemotherapy (the latter when signs and symptoms of recurrence were present) did not demonstrate a difference in survival (early arm: median 25.7 months, 95% CI, 23.0 to 27.9; delayed arm: median 27.1, 95%

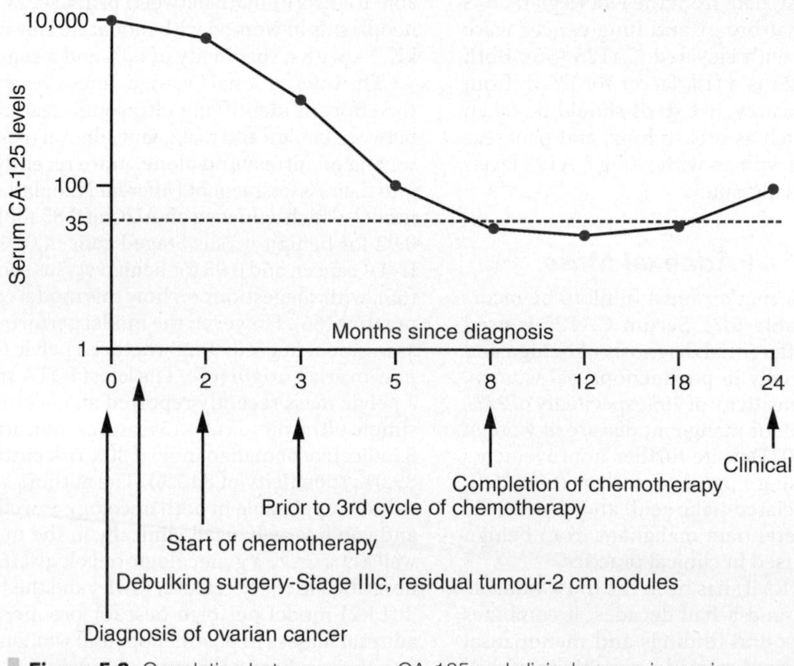

Figure 5.3. Correlation between serum CA-125 and clinical course in ovarian cancer.

CI, 22.8 to 30.9; HR 0.98, 95% CI, 0.80 to 1.20; $p = 0.85$). The trial therefore suggested that CA125 should only be measured if there is a suspicion of relapse or at patient's request (88). However, in view of the potential biases/challenges of this trial, the European Society of Gynaecological Oncology (ESGO) did not support the notion of unanimously abandoning CA125 monitoring during follow-up, as certain patient groups may benefit from such monitoring (e.g., those treated as part of a clinical trial following complete response to primary treatment, those that are not undergoing routine follow-up, those eligible for secondary surgery at recurrence, those eligible to take part in a clinical trial on second-line treatment) (89).

The usual pattern of CA125 throughout a clinical course of the disease is presented in **Figure 5.3.** CA125, remains the best-performing biomarker for OC when tumors of mucinous origin are excluded (89). However, some encouraging markers/technologies discussed below have emerged in recent years.

Human Epididymis Protein 4 (HE4)

Despite three-and-a-half decades passing since the identification of CA125, and many international efforts to find a better-performing marker or one complementing CA125, only more recently has another promising marker, Human epididymis protein 4 (HE4), been identified. HE4 is a glycoprotein in the epithelial cells of the epididymis with increased serum levels observed in OC patients.

Screening

There is as yet no clear evidence whether HE4 performs better than CA125 as a first or second-line test in screening. A case -control set (using preclinical samples collected 6 months prior to diagnosis) nested within PLCO showed that CA125 remained the single best biomarker for OC (sensitivity of 86%) followed closely by HE4 (73%) (90). Urban et al demonstrated that HE4 outperforms TVS both as a first-line (sensitivity of 35.7% vs. 28.6%) and second-line test (91). Using HE4 as a second-line test when CA125 levels are raised (>35 kU/L) was able to detect 27 out of 39 cancers (69.2%) compared with only 17 OCs detected by TVS alone (43.6%). Compared with TVS, HE4 was better at detecting Type II cancers (40% vs. 20%) than Type I cancers (18.8% vs. 56.2%). In terms of outcome, however, there is no clear advantage in diagnosing HE4-associated rather than TVS-associated tumors (91). In another nested case-control study within PLCO, none of the five predictive models, each containing six to eight biomarkers, nor a model derived from all of the 28 markers evaluated in the PLCO set, showed improvement over CA125 alone (92). A limitation of these studies was that CA125 was used in "real time" for triaging women for diagnostic workup for OC (93). There are two possibilities why studies have thus far failed to show improvement over CA125: either the current technologies are unable to identify biomarkers with greater or complementary potential for screening; or the available technologies, powerful as they are, have not yet been applied appropriately in either discovery or validation, with one of the main obstacles being use of clinical as opposed to prediagnostic/preclinical samples (94). Carotene and Retinol Efficacy Trial showed that a panel including CA125, HE4, and mesothelin may provide signal for OC 3 years before diagnosis (95) but this has not been subsequently confirmed.

Differential Diagnosis

Mean serum HE4 in patients with malignant ovarian lesions (248.7 pM) is much higher than in controls (34.1 pM) or in women with benign lesions (39.1 pM) (**Table 5.8**). HE4 levels are decreased in pregnancy (median levels of 30.5 pmol/L) (96) and levels around 50 and 60 have been demonstrated in pre- and postmenopausal women, respectively, (97) which increase with age (median 109.5 pmol/L in women over 80 years). HE4 levels are lower in many of the benign conditions that usually elevate CA125 levels (**Table 5.9**), especially in women with endometriosis.

HE4 can also be elevated in other cancers (**Table 5.10**). Initial reports stated that its specificity is superior to CA125 and of particular value for early-stage disease (98). There are conflicting reports, with some studies indicating that combining CA125 with HE4 increases sensitivity for detection of OC while maintaining high specificity (98), while others do not support this (99). An Italian multicenter study of 405 patients including 82 OCs recently demonstrated that HE4 was more specific than CA125 in ruling out patients with OCs (100).

TABLE 5.8. Mean Levels of Serum HE4 in Normal Controls, Benign and Malignant Lesions

Condition	Serum HE4 Level (Mean)
Normal Controls	34.1 pM
Benign Lesions	39.1 pM
Malignant Lesions	248.7 pM

Wang S, Dong L, Li H, et al. The application of HE4 in diagnosis of gynecological pelvic malignant tumor. *Clin Oncol Cancer Res.* 2009;6:72–74.

The performance of HE4 can be improved by being incorporated into an algorithm that includes CA125 and menopausal status (Risk of Malignancy, ROMA index). The ROMA gives a risk of OC with a value ≥13.1% predicting a high risk of EOC in premenopausal women, and a value ≥27.7% used in the postmenopausal population (101). In a single-center prospective cohort study of 432 women with a pelvic mass who were scheduled to have surgery, RMI combined with subjective ultrasound was shown to be superior to ROMA (102).

An index that uses age rather than menopausal status (as used in ROMA) has been described and evaluated in an international setting. The Copenhagen Index (CPH-I) based on serum HE4, serum CA125, and patient age was derived in a set of 809 patients with benign ovarian disease and 246 with OC. On validation in further eight international studies of 1,060 patients with benign ovarian masses and 550 patients with OC, CPH-I was able to discriminate benign from malignant ovarian disease with a sensitivity and specificity of 95.0% and 78.4%, respectively, in the training cohort, and 82.0% and 88.4% in the validation cohort (using a predefined cutoff of 0.070). It had similar AUC and specificity (at 95% sensitivity) as ROMA and RMI. Therefore, a simple index independent of US findings and menopausal status may optimize referral of women with suspected OC (103).

When evaluating new biomarkers/combinations of markers, it is important to establish the normal range in healthy individuals, especially if the marker has been shown to be very promising, such as HE4. The normal range for HE4 has been established in serum samples from 1,101 healthy women and 67 pregnant women. HE4 concentration increased with advancing age (>40 years). Median serum HE4 levels in premenopausal women (46.6 pmol/L) were significantly lower than in postmenopausal women (57.6 pmol/L; $p < 0.001$). The upper 95th percentile for HE4 levels was 89 pmol/L for premenopausal women, 128 pmol/L for postmenopausal women, and 115 pmol/L for all women. In pregnant women, median HE4 concentrations are significantly lower than their premenopausal counterparts ($p < 0.001$) (104). HE4 levels appear to be lower in the Asian population (HE4 of 33.2 pmol/L) (105). These values are important in the clinical application of the test in different populations. A recent study of 756 patients with pelvic mass (275 OCs, 53 borderline tumors, and 428 benign masses) from South China demonstrated a superior performance of HE4 and ROMA to that of CA125 in detecting borderline tumors and early-stage EOC. The authors also suggest a 70 pmol/L as the optimal cutoff in both pre- and postmenopausal women (106). Despite many studies evaluating the role of HE4 in differential diagnosis of malignant from benign adnexal masses, there is currently no consensus as to whether HE4 outperforms CA125 in this setting.

Detecting Recurrence

Schummer et al. (107) demonstrated that in patients who go on to develop a recurrence, HE4 rises earlier than CA125, with a lead

■ TABLE 5.9. Elevations of HE4 and CA125 in Women with Benign Disease and Ovarian Cancer

		HE4 > 89.1 pM (Premenopausal Women); HE4 > 128 pM (Postmenopausal Women) (%)	CA125 > 35 kU/L (%)
Benign disease[a]	Overall (all benign tumors)	8	29
	Ovarian cysts	8	14
	Germ cell tumors (mature teratoma)	1	21
	Sex cord stromal tumors (thecoma, fibrothecoma)	24	52
	Cystadenoma, adenofibroma, cystadenofibroma	20	20
	Serous epithelial tumors	8	20
	Mucinous epithelial tumors	13	18
	Benign, NOS	9	27
	Endometriosis/endometrioma	3	67
	Abscess/hydrosalpinx/POD	13	37
	Fibroid (leiomyomas)	8	26
	Benign, other (Normal ovaries)	5	22
		HE4 > 140 pmol/L (%)	CA125 > 35 kU/L (%)
Ovarian cancer[b]	Overall	75.20	80
	Stage I–II	58.3	54.2
	Stage III	78.8	86.5
	Stage IV	79.6	85.7
	Serous papillary	84.4	84.4
	Mucinous	43.8	68.8
	Other histologies	57.9	68.5

[a]Moore RG, Miller MC, Steinhoff MM, et al. Serum HE4 levels are less frequently elevated than CA125 in women with benign gynecologic disorders. *Am J Obstet Gynecol.* 2012;206:351.e351–358.
[b]Escudero JM, Auge JM, Filella X, et al. Comparison of serum human epididymis protein 4 with cancer antigen 125 as a tumor marker in patients with malignant and nonmalignant diseases. *Clin Chem.* 2011;57(11):1534–1544.

■ TABLE 5.10. Elevations of HE4 in Women with Cancers other than Ovarian

	Cancer Group	HE4 > 140 pmol/L (%)
Nongynecologic malignancies	Breast	5.6
	Digestive tract malignancy	11.3
	Lung	
	Small cell lung cancer (SCLC)	26.90
	Non-small cell lung cancer (NSCLC)	29.30
	Liver	16.3
	Melanoma	11.1
	Urologic malignancies	21.5
	Hematologic malignancies	10.0
	Mesenchymal tumors	0.0
	Non-ovarian/endometrial/NSCLC malignancies (without effusion or liver metastases)	6.5
	Non-ovarian/endometrial/NSCLC malignancies (with effusion or liver metastases)	18.5
Nonovarian gynecologic malignancies	Endometrial cancer	28
	Cervical cancer	0

Escudero JM, Auge JM, Filella X, et al. Comparison of serum human epididymis protein 4 with cancer antigen 125 as a tumor marker in patients with malignant and nonmalignant diseases. *Clin Chem.* 2011;57(11):1534–1544.

time of up to 4.5 months. It can also be elevated in patients who do not express CA125 at sufficient levels to make a clinical decision. However, as HE4 levels fail to normalize at the end of treatment, it is possible that it can be used as a marker predicting poor prognosis.

Prognosis

Elevated HE4 levels are strong and independent factors of worse prognosis in EOC patients compared to CA125 (108). High preoperative HE4 levels are poor prognostic factors, with levels over 394 pmol/L being predictors of death (HR = 1.67; 95% CI, 1.08 to 2.59) (109).

Additional Markers

In the past few years, major efforts have been made to identify either a better marker or a panel of markers that would improve the performance of CA125 in the context of screening. However, most of the studies used clinical samples (rather than preclinical samples), making their findings more relevant to differential diagnosis of benign from malignant masses, in order to avoid unnecessary operations in women with benign lesions. The latter ensures that where there is high suspicion of OC, surgery is undertaken by trained gynecologic oncologists in tertiary-care centers (110). A significant effort had been made over the years to identify other markers for OC: Interleukin-6 (IL-6), interleukin-7 (IL-7), soluble interleukin-2 receptor (sIL-2R), tumor necrosis factor (TNF), soluble receptors of TNF (sTNF-R), macrophage colony-stimulating factor (M-CSF), CA15-3, CA72-4 or TAG-72, CA19-9, OVX1, CASA/OSA, growth factors, tetranectin, tumor-associated trypsin inhibitor (TATI), galactosyltransferase associated with tumor (GAT), lipid-associated sialic acid (LASA), vascular endothelial growth factor (VEGF), immunosuppressive acid protein (IAP), lysophosphatidic acid (LPA), autoantibodies to MUC1 (111), prostasin, cadherin, shed glycans, dipeptase 1. Despite a plethora of studies, none of these markers have been shown to be useful in clinical practice. Limited sensitivities and specificities constrain their use in screening.

Apart from HE4, glycodelin is the only other marker that has shown encouraging performance (as part of multimarker panels) (112) but only improves the performance of CA125 in the screening scenario marginally (113).

Other markers such as soluble MUC1 and serum MUC1-specific antibodies have been evaluated both in early detection and as prognostic markers. Antibodies to anti-MUC1 glycopeptides are of no value in screening for OC (111) but have been shown to be prognostic for poor clinical response and reduced OS in both platinum-resistant as well as platinum-refractory OC treated with interleukin 2 (IL-2) (114).

Survivin is another marker which has shown promise as a prognostic marker for OC, as its levels positively correlated with age, advanced stage, and poor disease-free survival (DFS) (115).

Cancer-Specific Biomarkers and Novel Biospecimens

Cell-Free DNA as a Novel Biomarker

Cell-free DNA is increasingly been investigated as a potential biomarker, as it reflects the release of both normal and tumor-derived DNA (ctDNA) into the circulation through cellular necrosis and apoptosis. Cell-free DNA levels are much higher in iEOC patients (median preoperative level of 10,113 GE/mL) compared with those with benign ovarian neoplasms (median, 2,365 GE/mL; $p < 0.0001$) and controls (median, 1,912 GE/mL, $p < 0.0001$). In iEOC patients, elevated levels of cell-free DNA (>22,000 GE/mL) are associated with decreased patient survival ($p < 0.001$) and a 2.83-fold increased risk of death from disease ($p < 0.001$) (116).

The modeling of the natural history of high-grade serous OC (46) suggests that lesions would have to be detected at 1.3 cm in diameter (53) for a screening strategy to be able to detect 50% of these cancers. This suggests that early detection of low-volume rather than early-stage disease may be a more realistic target for screening in the short term, with a longer term goal of detection of the premalignant serous tubal in situ carcinoma (STIC) lesion. Over 95% of high-grade serous cancers harbor p53 mutations. A significant effort has been made to develop more sensitive assays to detect cancer-specific tumor DNA, based on mutations in TP53 and other cancer-related genes, such as *EGFR*, *BRAF*, and *KRAS*. BEAMing is one of these new technologies that is able to detect small amounts of mutant alleles in cell-free body fluids and can be quantified with unprecedented sensitivity (117). Using tagged-amplicon deep sequencing (TAm-Seq), Rosenfeld *et al.* were able to identify TP53 mutations in plasma of patients with advanced OC who had high levels of circulating tumor DNA (ctDNA). The technique was able to identify these mutations with allelic frequencies of 2% to 65%, but despite the inability of TAm-Seq to achieve a more sensitive detection limit (<2% allele frequency) so as to identify mutations in the plasma of patients with less advanced cancers, the noninvasive nature of the test holds much promise as a low-cost, high-throughput "liquid biopsy" approach for early detection of small tumors (118). This approach could also complement CA125 in women with elevated CA125 but negative imaging. A recent study of 44 ovarian/uterine cancer cases with samples collected at time of surgery demonstrated that ctDNA was detectable in women with positive CA125 and CT imaging but also in six patients with negative imaging (119).

In addition to serum and plasma, liquid cytology cervical samples provide another source of sample in which cancer-specific mutations could be detected. Using a sensitive massively parallel sequencing method to detect mutations in a panel of 12 genes, Kinde *et al.* reported that they were able to identify these expected tumor-specific mutations in 14 liquid cytology cervical samples from women with OC. These results, albeit restricted to a small study, are encouraging in that they suggest that tumor DNA could be detected in a proportion of OCs in a standard liquid-based cervical cytology specimen obtained during routine pelvic examination (120). The technique, however, needs further improvement; increasing the number of potential gene targets would increase the technical sensitivity of the test, while endometrial aspirates may help enrich the sample with cells of tubal and ovarian origin. An additional study assessing the feasibility of uterine cavity lavage in detecting shed cancer cells and its ability to provide sufficient amounts of DNA demonstrated that mutations could be identified in 80% (24/30) of patients with OC by using massive parallel sequencing and singleplex analysis (121).

In addition to its role in early detection, ctDNA holds promise as a prognostic marker in gynecologic cancers. Undetectable levels of ctDNA at 6 months following initial treatment was associated with improved progression-free and OS in a series of 44 patients with ovarian and uterine cancers (119).

DNA Methylation Profile

As changes in DNA methylation are one of the most common alterations in cancer, circulating methylated DNA may represent a new generation of tumor marker (122). Despite many studies showing hypermethylation of tumor-derived DNA in serum and plasma of cancer patients, no definitive clinically useful such marker had been described in OC patients as yet. However, encouraging data from colorectal cancer suggests that a methylated septin 9 (SEPT9) marker can increase the sensitivity of screening (to 77%) (123), and this has already been marketed as the Epi proColon commercial test.

DNA methylation profiles have been extensively studied in OC. The findings suggest that up to 21% of the CpG islands are hypomethylated, with a different panel of genes displaying hypo/hypermethylated pattern according to histologic subtype (124). Despite some encouraging data that DNA methylation profile could predict active disease (125), response to treatment (126) and OS (127), profiling is yet to be used in clinical practice.

Salivary Transcriptomes as Novel Markers

In an effort to derive tests that are not only noninvasive (such as a blood test) but would require no visit to a clinic, saliva has been proposed as a suitable alternative. Many groups are now focusing on this approach, and a strategy examining salivary transcriptomes has identified that a combination of five biomarkers (AGPAT1, B2M, BASP2, IER3, and ILI1) yielded an encouraging sensitivity (85.7%) and specificity (91.4%) for early detection of the disease (128). However, the study only included 32 OC patients, so would need validation in further studies.

Proteomics

Since the initial report by Petricoin in 2002 about the promise of proteomics in the search for OC biomarkers (129), the race has yet to abate. Surface-enhanced laser desorption ionization time-of-flight (SELDI-TOF) analysis and matrix-associated laser desorption ionization time-of-flight (MALDI-TOF) technologies have been employed over the past few years to identify patterns or changes in protein profile between those with and without cancer. However, the lack of markers identified may not be due to the issues with the technologies as much as the way the samples had been collected and processed. The biomarkers identified through the proteomics approaches include apolipoprotein A1, a truncated form of transthyretin, and elevated levels of a cleavage fragment of inter-alpha-trypsin inhibitor heavy chain H4 (ITIH4), all of which have been independently validated (130). Apolipoprotein A1, truncated transthyretin, and connective tissue–activating protein III (CTAP III) when combined with CA125 can improve the sensitivity of CA125 alone from 68% to 88% (131). A test called OVA1, which includes these markers, is marketed in the United States as part of the diagnostic workup and determination to refer to a gynecologic oncologist (132). The complexity of mass-spectrometry data requires use of algorithms to identify the most informative "common" peaks. This may be one of the reasons why despite years of proteomics biomarker discovery, a limited number of markers for OC have been identified. A proteomics study using preclinical samples from UKCTOCS identified CTAPIII and putative platelet factor 4 (PF4) as markers that could discriminate cases from controls up to 15 and 11 months before diagnosis, respectively, but, more importantly, earlier than CA125 alone (133).

In contrast, in a nested case–control study from the PLCO trial with samples collected <12 months before cancer diagnosis, a panel of markers (CA125 and apolipoprotein A1, truncated transthyretin, transferrin, hepcidin, β-2 microglobulin, connective tissue–activating protein III, and interalpha-trypsin inhibitor heavy chain 4) did not improve the sensitivity of CA125 alone (61.5%) (134).

In a case–control study nested within UKCTOCS, using isobaric tags (iTRAQ), Russell *et al.* were able to identify Protein Z as a novel early-detection biomarker, which can discriminate between Type I and Type II OC. Unlike CA125, Protein Z was significantly downregulated up to 2 years prediagnosis in Type I; whereas in Type II, it was significantly upregulated up to 4 years before diagnosis ($p = 0.01$). There was a statistically significant increase in the AUC for CA125 and CA125 combined with protein Z, from 77% to 81% for Type I and 76% to 82% for Type II. This new data suggest that Protein Z could add to CA125 and potentially ROCA in screening (135).

A more promising approach has been put forward with the use of Serial Window Acquisition of Theoretical Spectra-Mass Spectrometry (SWATH-MS), which would allow creation of a permanent OC profiling map and data mining for years to come.

Metabolite Profiling

Metabolites are the end products of cellular regulatory processes. Alterations in their levels can be regarded as response to genetic or environmental changes. In a study of 66 invasive OCs and 9 borderline ovarian tumors by gas chromatography/time-of-flight mass spectrometry (GC-TOF MS), 291 metabolites were detected, of whom 114 were already annotated compounds. Principal component analysis as well as additional supervised predictive models allowed a separation of 88% of the borderline tumors from the carcinomas. This suggests that metabolomics is a promising high-throughput, automated approach in addition to functional genomics and proteomics for analyses of molecular changes in malignant tumors (136).

Encouraging data from a U.S. study of 50 patients with serous OC and 50 with serous benign tumors indicate that plasma metabolite/lipidomics biomarkers identified by liquid chromatography–mass spectrometry could distinguish between malignant and benign serous tumors, with the performance of the top four lipid metabolites (0.85, SD = 0.07) being similar to that of CA125 alone (AUC = 0.87, SD = 0.07); however, they performed best in combination with CA125 (AUC = 0.91, SD = 0.05) (137).

MicroRNA-Based Ovarian Cancer Biomarkers

MicroRNAs (miRNAs) are small noncoding RNAs that regulate gene expression by translational inhibition or mRNA degradation. They are involved in diverse biologic processes including development, proliferation, differentiation, and apoptosis. In recent years, several unique OC miRNA signatures have been described (miR-200 family, miR-199/214 cluster, let-7 paralogs) due to their potential role as therapeutic targets in advanced disease or chemoresistant tumors. Initial studies examining tissue profiling of OCs and normal ovaries showed upregulation (miR-200a, miR-200b, miR-200c, miR-141) or downregulation (miR-199a, miR-140, miR-145 or miR-125b1) of certain miRNAs (138). One advantage of using miRNAs as biomarkers is that they are generally stable and can be detected in serum and plasma. More recently, eight miRNAs extracted from serum (e.g., miR-21, miR-141, miR-200a, miR-200b, miR-200c, miR-203, miR-205, or miR-214) were compared in exosomes isolated from sera from women with benign disease and OC, demonstrating that exosomal microRNA profile in OC patients is distinct from those with benign disease (139). Resnick et al. (140) have shown other miRNAs being up- (miR-21, miR-92, miR-93, miR-126, miR-29a) or down- (miR-155, miR-127, miR-99b) regulated, but more encouragingly, they have demonstrated upregulation of miR-21, miR-92 and miR-93 in three cancer patients with normal CA125 levels. Although miRNA signature/profile is not of established value in diagnosis, prognosis, or response to treatment, further understanding of the role of miRNAs in OC is warranted.

Carcinoembryonic Antigen (CEA)

CEA was first identified in 1965 in the serum of rabbits immunized with colon carcinoma (141). It is an oncofetal antigen which is found in small amounts in the adult colon. Elevated levels are associated with colon and pancreatic cancer but CEA levels are also raised in benign diseases of the liver, gastrointestinal tract, and lung, and in smokers. In OC, CEA is expressed by most endometrioid and Brenner tumors and in areas of intestinal differentiation in mucinous tumors. In contrast to CA125, this marker is not expressed in normal and inflammatory conditions of the adnexa. Around 25% to 50% of OC patients have elevated levels of CEA and the correlation with OC is not as well established as with the other markers (142,143).

Serum CEA is more informative in borderline ovarian tumors (Stage IB-IV) (144) and more frequently overexpressed at the tissue level (18% LMP vs. 4% OC), in which using a 30% overexpression cutoff carries a worse disease-specific survival (145). Despite an encouraging sensitivity of preoperative CEA and CA-125 serum levels of 82% to 85% (146), CEA is not routinely used in the clinic in diagnostic workup.

Alpha-Fetoprotein

Alpha-Fetoprotein (AFP) is an oncofetal protein produced by the fetal yolk sac, liver, and upper gastrointestinal tract. Elevated levels of AFP occur in pregnancy and benign liver disease. Serum levels are raised in most patients with liver tumors and in some patients with gastric, pancreatic, colon, and bronchogenic malignancies (142). AFP is rarely raised in iEOC but is elevated in patients with the rarer germ cell tumors (endodermal sinus tumors, or immature teratomas, or dysgerminomas) that present in younger women and adolescents (147). Alpha-Fetoprotein also accurately predicts the presence of yolk sac elements in mixed germ cell tumors (148).

In women with endodermal sinus tumors, AFP is a reliable marker for monitoring therapeutic response and detecting recurrence (149,150). Levels of over 1,000 ng/mL, age over 22 and histology are main prognostic factors in patients with ovarian and extragonadal germ cell tumors (151).

In postmenopausal women, yolk sac tumors are aggressive tumors (requiring adjuvant platinum-based chemotherapy) with poor outcome (152,153).

Simultaneous detection of multiple markers has not shown much promise; however, a sensitive chemiluminescence (CL) imaging immunoassay method for detection of multiple tumor markers with high throughput, easy operation, and low cost has been developed. The proof of concept study included four markers (AFP, CA125, CA-153, and CEA) to screen patients with liver, breast, or ovarian cancers. The method showed very good reproducibility, accuracy, and wide detection range, thus making it an ideal platform to study the performance of the panel in clinical and preclinical sets of samples from OC patients accumulated over the past decade (154).

Human Chorionic Gonadotropin

Human chorionic gonadotropin (hCG) is synthesized in pregnancy by the syncytiotrophoblast. It is a glycoprotein hormone made up of two dissimilar covalently linked subunits α and β, which could be released into the circulation and therefore routinely measured. hCG is elevated in virtually all cases of gestational trophoblastic disease (hydatidiform mole, invasive mole, and choriocarcinoma) and serves as an ideal tumor marker. There is a close correlation between hCG levels and tumor burden, and hCG levels are used in staging and clinical management. Serum hCG can also be detected in patients with non-trophoblastic cancers. Although gynecologic cancers are prominent in this group, the sensitivity of using hCG is lower than for other markers in current use, except in germ cell tumors with a chorionic component (155).

Elevated levels of serum hCG-β and AFP are significant predictors of OS in patients with Stage IC to IV malignant ovarian germ cell tumors; age at diagnosis is of no prognostic value (156).

In pediatric patients (mean age 12.5 years), elevated hCG-β, AFP, and CA125 are observed in over half of the cases (54%). However, the best indicators of malignancy in these young patients are complaints of a mass or precocious puberty, a mass exceeding 8 cm or a mass with solid imaging characteristics (157).

hCG levels are elevated in 67% of OCs (mainly in Stage II mucinous tumors) compared with 26.7% of benign ovarian tumors ($p = 0.000$). hCG tissue expression is positive in 68% of OCs and carries a favorable outcome (when also LH-R positive/FSH-R negative) (158) suggesting that hCG and LH-R may be useful targets in novel cancer therapies.

In gynecologic malignancies, serum-free β-subunit or its urinary degradation product β-core fragment is produced by 68% of ovarian, 51% of endometrial, and 46% of cervical cancers. The free β-subunit enhances growth and invasion in all these malignancies and is therefore associated with poor prognosis. In clinical practice, confusion arises when a patient presents with persistently low positive hCG in absence of pregnancy and no obvious malignancies (159). The first aim is to rule out a tumor in these patients, then consider a false-positive test by assaying hCG in the urine. A further possibility in women aged over 35 with oligomenorrhea, amenorrhea, or following bilateral salpingo-oophorectomy is pituitary hCG.

Inhibin and Related Peptides

Inhibin is a heterodimeric glycoprotein (composed of a common α-subunit and one of two β-subunits), resulting in either inhibin A (αβA) and inhibin B (αβB). There are other forms (α subunit not attached to the β subunit, pro-αC, and pro-αN-αC). The original Monash assay detected immunoreactive inhibin that included a range of inhibin-related peptides in addition to biologically active inhibin dimers.

Inhibin is elevated in women with granulosa cell tumors and is clinically used in differential diagnosis and surveillance of these malignancies. In the clinic, in addition to inhibin A and B, measurement of anti-Müllerian hormone (Müllerian inhibitory factor, AMH) levels is of value in the diagnosis of granulosa cell tumors. Elevated AMH and inhibin B are significantly elevated in patients with primary adult-type granulosa tumors and recurrent disease, and the combination of two markers is superior to inhibin B alone (160). The role of the inhibin peptides in EOC is less clear. Although there is encouraging data suggesting elevated serum inhibin levels in EOCs using either the original Monash assay (25% to 90%) or the total inhibin assay described in 2004 (93% of serous, 94% of mucinous tumors) (161), assays that measure inhibin A alone did not confirm this, as only 5% to 31% of patients with EOC had elevated levels (162). Use of pro-αC alone is not of use, but in combination with CA125 improves sensitivity for detection of EOC (163). Inhibin B is the main form secreted by granulosa cell tumors and reflects disease progression much better than inhibin A, and thus may be of value in the follow-up of these patients (164). As inhibin is rarely elevated in serous compared to mucinous tumors, it is used sparsely in the clinical setting.

The elevations of inhibin in patients with ovarian malignancies are presented in **Table 5.11**.

Activin is a dimer of the two β subunits of inhibin and exists as activin A (βAβA), activin B (βB βB), and activin AB (βA βB). Although serum activin A has been shown to be significantly elevated in EOC (165), with highest levels detected in undifferentiated tumors, the role of activin in OC requires further investigation. There is a suggestion that high concentrations of activin A in the peritoneal fluid of women with serous ovarian carcinoma can distinguish it from cystadenoma (166).

Kallikreins

The human kallikrein gene family currently consists of 15 members. There is accumulating evidence that in addition to prostate-specific antigen (PSA, hK3) and human glandular kallikrein (hK2) (both prostate cancer biomarkers), many other members of the human kallikrein gene family are differentially regulated in breast, ovarian, and testicular cancers. The malignant phenotype of ovarian cancer cells can be enhanced by overexpression of the human tissue kallikrein genes 4, 5, 6, and 7 (167). Potential biomarkers for OC include kallikreins 5, 6, 7, 8, 10, 11, and 14. Some kallikreins (e.g., K4) are upregulated in effusions from EOC patients (168) and may differentiate ascites between OC and non-OC patients (169). Kallikrein-related peptidase, KLK5, was found to be significantly elevated in the serum and ascitic fluid (41/41) of OC patients (42/52), with increased levels associated with poor patient outcome (170).

Of the kallikreins either expressed by ovarian cancer cells (KLKs 2 to 11 and 13 to 15) or elevated in serum (KLKs 5 to 8, 10, and 13), kallikrein-related peptidase 6 (KLK6) has been the most promising OC biomarker (171), and a specific ELISA serum assay has been developed. Kallikreins are key components of OVSCORE, an algorithm to predict surgical outcome in OC patients based on volume of ascites on ultrasound, tumor grade (laparoscopy/CT-guided biopsy), and KLK tissue expression, with KLK7 being an independent marker of OS. The hope is that OVSCORE, if independently validated, could aid in identification of patients who are unlikely to benefit from primary surgery (172). These findings are in keeping with the role of kallikrein-related peptidases in metastasis in OC (173).

Osteopontin

Despite encouraging data on the performance of osteopontin and mesothelin in OC, neither has been validated for any clinical use.

TABLE 5.11. Elevations in Inhibin or CA125 Levels in Women with Ovarian Cancer

	Cancer Group	Elevations in Inhibin[a] Levels (%)	CA125 > 35k U/L (%)	Inhibin + CA125 (%)
Malignant ovarian tumors	Serous	18	94	97
	Mucinous	84	71	94
	Endometrioid	54	91	90
	Other ovarian cancers	33–44	78–100	89–100
	Granulosa cell tumor	100	30	100
	All ovarian cancers	50	82	95

[a]Total inhibin.

Robertson DM, Pruysers E, Jobling T. Inhibin as a diagnostic marker for ovarian cancer. *Cancer Lett*. 2007;249(1):14–17.

Osteopontin is a biomarker that has been identified using gene expression profiling techniques. Its tissue expression is weak or absent in 93% of OCs compared with positive expression in 81.5% in borderline tumors and 50% in omental and lymph node implants. Its expression does not correlate with histologic type, grade, or clinical stage (174). A 2015 systematic review and meta-analysis that included 13 studies (839 OC patients and 1,439 controls) reported a sensitivity of 66% (95% CI, 51 to 78) and a specificity of 88% (95% CI, 78 to 93). Despite encouraging AUC of 0.85 (95% CI, 0.81 to 0.88), use of osteopontin is not recommended because the eligible studies were subject to selection bias (175). Osteopontin levels have been shown to correlate with the presence of ascites, bulky disease, and recurrence (176), and may be of value in detecting recurrent OC, as levels rise in 90% of these patients (177). Statins can inhibit OC proliferation by up to 50% with the effect being mediated by changes in osteopontin gene expression. Simvastatin-treated mice survive significantly longer compared to the controls. These findings need further exploration as a possible new drug therapy in OC (178).

Mesothelin

Mesothelin is a marker initially identified in mesotheliomas and OCs in 1996 (179). Serum levels are higher in OC patients when compared with women with benign ovarian tumors or healthy women. The levels increase significantly from early to advanced stages. Elevated mesothelin levels before therapy are associated with poor OS both in patients with optimal debulking surgery and in those with advanced disease (180). Mesothelin and MMP7 have both been assessed as part of multimarker panels but cannot add to the performance of CA125 and HE4 in predicting recurrence (107). Although it is possible that mesothelin may prove to be a useful tumor marker in the future, both for differential diagnosis of EOC as well as for prognosis, there is currently little data to suggest its significance.

Cytokines

Cytokines are soluble mediator substances produced by cells that exercise a specific effect on other target cells. Their importance in tumor biology has increased since it was shown that many cytokines are produced by cancer cells and can influence the malignant process in a positive or a negative manner (181). However, cytokines do not fulfill the classic criteria for tumor markers, as they may be elevated in a number of pathologic conditions, are invariably produced by nonmalignant surrounding tissue rather than the tumor itself, and are not specific for one cell type. Despite this, their measurement in malignant conditions may provide valuable clinical information regarding prognosis and response to treatment.

The role of cytokines as biomarkers in OC is limited. A majority are at an early stage of evaluation and conflicting reports are associated with some. The one studied the most, serum M-CSF (or CSF-1), was shown to have a high specificity for OC in the initial reports, with elevation being related to stage (182,183). It has been investigated in combination with other markers (CA125II, CA 72-4 and M-CSF) and was shown to have encouraging sensitivity for detecting early-stage disease compared to CA125II alone (70% vs. 45%), while maintaining high specificity (98%) (184). Elevated serum levels are associated with poor outcome (185). When combined with CA125 and HE4, M-CSF has an encouraging sensitivity for detecting serous OC, early-stage disease, and distinguishing OCs from benign lesions (186).

Interleukins have also been studied in OC. Although IL-6 is elevated in 50% of OCs, combination of IL-6 and CA125 does not improve the sensitivity of CA125 alone (187). More encouragingly, a combination of IL-7 and CA125 was found to accurately predict 69% of OC patients, without falsely classifying patients with benign pelvic mass (188).

Cytokeratins

Cytokeratins are intermediate filaments that are part of the cytoskeleton of all epithelial cells. They are specific markers of epithelial differentiation and continue to be expressed by epithelial cells following malignant transformation. Fragments of cytokeratins, in contrast to cytokeratins themselves, are soluble in serum and can be detected and measured using monoclonal antibodies. Their role as tumor markers in various malignancies has been investigated.

Tissue polypeptide-specific antigen (TPS) and CYFRA 21-1 (fragment of cytokeratin 19), although showing an encouraging sensitivity of around 50% in the original reports, have not shown further promise; some more recent studies suggest that CYFRA 21-1 is elevated in only 19.6% of OC patients (189).

Other Markers

Other serum markers have been assessed in isolation or as part of biomarker panels in women with OC, both in the context of screening and differential diagnosis, as well as in assessing prognosis, monitoring response to treatment, and detecting recurrence. **Table 5.12** details their current role in OC.

It is important to note that in women with OC, no single marker or combination of markers has emerged with a clear clinical advantage over CA125, except in specific tumor subtypes such as germ cell tumors with yolk sac and chorionic elements, and granulosa cell tumors. Few markers (TATI, CA19-9, CA 72-4, CEA combined with CA125) may be of value in non-mucinous OC (190). The results of the new approaches such as SWATH in proteomics and ctDNA are eagerly awaited. The consensus is that these new approaches are most likely to identify novel markers or marker panels that, in combination with CA125, will improve biomarker accuracy in OC.

With the ongoing efforts to detect OC using noninvasive approaches, saliva, liquid cytology, and more recently urine autofluorescence (191) may prove promising sources of novel biomarkers for OC.

ENDOMETRIAL CANCERS

A majority of women with endometrial cancer present symptomatically with abnormal vaginal bleeding, and are usually investigated using pipelle biopsy or hysteroscopy. Therefore, the role of serum markers has not been investigated with as much enthusiasm as in OC. Currently, there are no serum markers with an established role in the clinical management of endometrial cancer. Serum CA125 is elevated in 10% to 31% of patients, with elevated levels detected in 63% to 67% of patients with advanced stage compared with only 10% to 19% of those with early-stage disease (192). Preoperative assessment of serum CA125 may be useful in predicting the presence of extrauterine and metastatic disease, and to a lesser extent myometrial invasion, but it is not of benefit in the follow-up of these patients (193). Levels over 40 kU/L are correlated with higher stage, higher grade, increased depth of myometrial invasion, lymph node metastases, and the presence of lymphovascular space involvement, compared with lower levels (CA125 <40 kU/L) denoting a longer OS and recurrence-free survival (194). Despite some encouraging data on elevated CA125 and CA15-3 being poor prognostic factors, these markers are not used in the clinic.

Since the 1990s, a number of serum markers have been explored in endometrial cancer (CYFRA 21-1, urinary β-core or UGF levels, SCC and CA15-3, CA19-9, amino-terminal propeptide of type III procollagen, placental protein 4, CA72-4, OVX1 antigen, soluble interleukin-2 receptor, M-CSF, kallikrein 6, inhibinβB, matrix metalloproteinase 2 [MMP-2], survivin, p53, p21, polipoprotein A1, prealbumin, transferrin, Cathepsin-B, and serum amyloid A). However, none proved very useful, as evidenced by the lack of further publications.

Endogenous estrogens have a major role in endometrial carcinogenesis. Women with high circulating estradiol are at increased risk of endometrial cancer (RR 2.1 to 4.1) (195–197). Apart from estradiol levels, elevated estrogen metabolites (4-hydroxyestradiol (4-OHE2) may indicate risk of estrogen-induced endometrial cancer (198). Alongside estrogens and androgens, a number of other biomarkers associated with adiposity have been investigated in endometrial cancer such as

■ TABLE 5.12. Status of Current Tumor Markers in Ovarian Cancer

	Screening	Differential Diagnosis of an Adnexal Mass	Prognostic Indicator	Monitoring Response to Therapy	Monitoring Disease and Recurrence
Epithelial cancers					
Clinical practice		CA125 is the main marker—when combined with menopausal status and ultrasound features in the risk of malignancy index (RMI), a sensitivity of 71%–85% and specificity of 96%–97% is achieved. CEA	CA125 levels post surgery and during chemotherapy are independent prognostic indicators. Various criteria are used based on CA125 half-life.	Serial CA125 levels reflect clinical course in 90% of positive tumors and are used routinely for monitoring patients. HE4	CA125 detects recurrence with a sensitivity of 84%–94% and a false-positive rate of <2%. Median lead time compared with clinical diagnosis of recurrence is 60–99 days. HE4
Research	Serum CA125 being assessed in screening trials in the general (UKCTOCS and high-risk UKFOCSS and trials by GOG and CGN in USA) populations. Results from PLCO reported in 2011 and from UKCTOCS in 2015. The results from the high-risk trials are expected in 2016/17. Main emphasis on algorithms to interpret serial CA125 and transvaginal ultrasound as a second-line test.	Inhibin pro-alpha C/total inhibin, kallikreins, mesothelin, prostasin, osteopontin, M-CSF, TPS, proteomic markers (profile, transthyretin, apolipoprotein A)	Kallikrein 8, mesothelin, CYFRA 21-1, M-CSF, TATI, VEGF, CASA, tetranectin	CASA	Osteopontin, TPS
		CA-15-3, CA-72-4, CA-19-9, TATI, GAT, free serum DNA methylation, free glycans, IL-7, TNF α receptors HE4 micro RNAs metabolite profiling	HE4		CASA
Germ cell tumors					
Clinical practice		Serum AFP in tumors with endodermal sinus/yolk sac elements, serum beta hCG in tumors with chorionic elements			
Research		M-CSF especially in dysgerminomas			
Sex cord stromal tumors					
Clinical practice		Inhibin in granulosa cell tumors		Inhibin in granulosa cell tumors	

insulin, glucose, IGF-1, SHBG, adiponectin, leptin, prolactin, and TSH (199). A 2014 review suggested that a routine measurement of adiponectin in patients with lifestyle-related diseases such as endometrial cancer may be recommended (200). Circulating adiponectin levels are inversely associated with risk of endometrial cancer (independent of BMI), suggesting that insulin and estrogen pathways are working in parallel in predisposing women to endometrial cancer (201).

Proteomic markers for endometrial cancer have recently been identified in the serum (HSPA8) (202) and urine (N-glycopeptides) (203). Distinct miRNA profiles (miR-26a, let-7g, miR-21, miR-181b, mir-199c, miR-200c, miR-192, miR-215, miR-200c, and miR-205) have also been described in endometrial cancer patients. Further work in elucidating their role in these patients is warranted.

HE4 is also elevated in endometrial cancer. HE4, included as one of a panel of biomarkers, may be of use in risk stratification in endometrial cancer at an early stage in patients at high risk (204). Preoperative serum HE4 levels over 8 mfi (median fluorescence intensity units) was shown to be superior in detecting advanced stage disease compared with CA125. Median HE4 levels were significantly elevated in both Type I (>50% myometrial invasion and >2 cm tumor diameter) and Type II endometrial cancer. HE4 may therefore be of value in preoperative prediction of high-risk disease and guide the need for definitive surgical staging (205), and it may be of value in identifying high-risk patients within low-grade endometrioid endometrial cancer who may benefit from lymphadenectomy (206).

L1CAM (L1 Cell Adhesion Molecule) overexpression can identify low/intermediate risk patients with endometrial cancer at high risk of recurrence. More recently, its role in prognosis of high-risk endometrial cancer was investigated in a study of 116 endometrial cancers (86 endometrioid, 30 non-endometrioid subtype) with high-risk features (such as high tumor grade and deep myometrial invasion). Use of a much higher threshold (50% positive staining compared to 10% in lower risk groups) identified women with L1CAM and p53 expression, which in combination may be useful prognostic markers (207). As a third of high-risk endometrial cancers overexpress L1CAM, it may be a potential novel therapeutic target in this subgroup of patients.

DNA methylation profile (ADCYAP1, ASCL2, HS3ST2, HTR1B, MME, NPY, SOX1) can discriminate carcinoma from benign endometrium with an AUC of 0.93 (208).

The last 5 years have seen promise in identification of novel biomarkers for endometrial cancer for risk stratification and early detection. With rising rates of obesity across the world combined with prolonged life expectancy, it is very likely that endometrial cancer incidence will increase within the next decade. Novel biomarkers/approaches may demonstrate a clinical utility for risk stratification and early detection in the future.

Cervical Cancers

Screening for cervical cancer is one of the most prevalent and successful public health measures for cancer prevention. The screening strategy is based on exfoliative cytology, liquid-based cytology, and high-risk HPV DNA detection in cervical specimens. Currently no serologic markers have been identified that are sensitive or specific enough for screening purposes. However, a variety of serum markers have been investigated in assessing prognosis, monitoring response to treatment, and detecting recurrence.

Squamous Cell Carcinoma Antigen (SCCA)

Squamous cell carcinoma antigen (SCCA) is one of 14 subfractions of tumor antigen TA-4. Elevated levels of SCCA are found in 57% to 70% of women with primary squamous cell carcinoma (SCC) of the cervix (209). SCCA is not specific for cervical SCC; elevated levels are found in other SCCs of the head and neck, esophagus and lung, and in adenocarcinoma of the uterus, ovary, and lung. SCCA is probably a marker of cellular differentiation of squamous cells, as the incidence of elevated serum levels is higher in women with well-differentiated (78%) and moderately differentiated carcinoma (67%) than in those with poorly differentiated tumors (38%) (210). Its levels before treatment indicate poor response to chemotherapy and indicate a high risk of recurrence (211).

Similar to the other gynecologic cancers, the ability of a marker to detect the disease/recurrence early works in tandem with optimal treatment being delivered. In cervical cancer, rising levels of SCCA precede clinical detection of recurrent disease and can therefore be used in its earlier diagnosis. However, SCCA monitoring is not implemented routinely because adequate curative strategies are currently not available (212). There is no evidence that earlier detection of recurrent disease influences treatment outcome or prognosis after primary treatment.

SCCA may be of value in individualizing treatment, but no randomized trials have yet been conducted to confirm this hypothesis. There is no evidence that more aggressive treatment improves pelvic control and survival in patients with elevated SCCA levels (213).

Preliminary studies suggest that SCCA isoforms (free SCCA2, total SCCA2, total SCCA1, and total SCCA) may provide additional clinical information when compared to total SCC antigen. Roijer *et al.* evaluated specific serum immunoassays for the different isoforms of SCCA. Patients with recurrence or progressive disease have rising levels of SCCA1 and SCCA2, with elevations in SCCA2 being more prominent than that in SCCA1 (214).

In a more recent series of 138 patients with Stage I-IVA cervical cancer, SCCA was shown to be the only independent prognostic factor for DFS, with the combination of IL-6 and SCCA being prognostic for OS. In women with early-stage disease (of whom 45% recurred), VEGF was of prognostic value for DFS while IL-6 and CYFRA 21-1 was of prognostic value for OS. The findings indicate that these markers measured prior to diagnosis may be useful prognostic indicators (215).

In conclusion, SCCA may prove useful in the pretreatment identification of squamous cervical cancer patients at high risk of lymph node metastasis, and in pretreatment prediction of prognosis, monitoring response to treatment, and detecting recurrence. However, further studies are needed before clinical recommendations can be made.

CYFRA 21-1, CA125, CEA

Elevated CYFRA 21-1 levels are observed in squamous cell carcinoma (SCC) (35% Stage IB-IIA, 64% Stage IIB-IV disease) (216) and 63% of patients with cervical adenocarcinoma (217). Despite some data suggesting it has a role in follow-up and predicting residual tumor post-chemoradiation (218), the evidence available so far does not justify its routine measurements.

Serum CA125 has a limited value in cervical cancer. It is more frequently elevated in cervical adenocarcinoma compared with SCC. (219). CA125 levels rise with advancing stage of cervical cancer akin to SCCA levels (220). Falling CA125 levels are observed in those who respond to chemotherapy (221). Serum CEA alone is less useful in cervical cancers, with an overall sensitivity of 15% (at a 90% specificity) (222).

Other Markers

Methylation markers (DNA methyltransferase, tyrosine phosphatase receptor type R promoter) have been evaluated in cervical cancer and may play a role in cancer development and metastasis (223). As p16(INK4a) is overexpressed in virtually all HPV-transformed cells, it can improve the accuracy of cytology-based cancer early-detection programs (224). It is anticipated that the introduction of prophylactic HPV vaccines will reduce the incidence of cervical cancer and its malignant precursors, thus focusing effort on identifying women at high risk who would then require treatment, as well as improve the triage of the HPV-positive tests. It is believed that biomarkers will also serve an important role in the optimization of this alternative screening algorithm; therefore, the efforts continue to identify the biomarkers best-suited for this purpose.

As in OC, ctDNA has been explored as a biomarker in cervical cancer, with circulating Bmi-1 mRNA shown as an independent prognostic factor for DFS and OS (225).

Programmed death ligand 1 (PD L1) expression has been shown in many cancers and anti-PD L1 therapy has shown significant promise in recent years. In cervical cancer, PDL1 expression has not been shown in normal cervical epithelia even when adjacent to CIN or cancer but increased expression was reported in 95% of CIN and 80% of cervical squamous cell cancers suggesting a potential role for anti-PD L1 therapy in cervical cancer. In contrast, only 19% of endometrial and 13% of ovarian cancers expressed PD L1 (226).

Efforts of the past 5 years have focused on noninvasive samples that women could easily collect themselves. Cervicovaginal fluid captured on tampons is one way of testing that could, in principle, identify precancerous lesions. A multicenter randomized controlled trial of 14,041 women demonstrated that mailing of a self-collection kit to the woman's home resulted in a higher participation in a screening programme compared to a clinic visit, even in those having HPV as the primary screening test (227).

Vulvar and Vaginal Cancer

Tumors of the vulva and the vagina are rare and there are relatively few studies on circulating markers in these conditions. Few markers have been evaluated; TPS being elevated in 80% of patients with vulvar or vaginal cancer (228), SCC in 43% (229), urinary core fragment of the β-subunit of hCG in 38% (230). The latter is a poor prognostic factor (90% of patients with elevated levels die within 24 months vs. 32% of those with normal levels). Very few markers have been explored in vulvar cancer, with data from a small study suggesting that loss of Rho-associated coiled-coil-containing protein kinase 1 (ROCK1) expression at a tissue level is associated with poorer survival (231). Whether this translates into a role for circulating ROCK1 in vulvar cancer is not known.

In view of the recent advances in sequencing technology, there has been a wealth of data gathered on biomarkers for gynecologic cancers. However, it will be some time before we are able to unravel the complexities of these molecular changes in a way that translates into therapeutic benefit (232).

References

1. Sturgeon C. Practice guidelines for tumor marker use in the clinic. *Clin Chem*. 2002;48:1151–1159.
2. Sturgeon CM, Lai LC, Duffy MJ. Serum tumour markers: how to order and interpret them. *BMJ*. 2009;339:b3527.
3. Cancer Research UK. *Ovarian Cancer Statistics: Ovarian Cancer Incidence*. London, UK: Cancer Research UK; 2012.
4. Meinhold-Heerlein I, Fotopoulou C, Harter P, et al. The new WHO classification of ovarian, fallopian tube, and primary peritoneal cancer and its clinical implications. *Arch Gynecol Obstet*. 2016;293:695–700.
5. Seidman JD, Horkayne-Szakaly I, Haiba M, et al. The histologic type and stage distribution of ovarian carcinomas of surface epithelial origin. *Int J Gynecol Pathol*. 2004;23:41–44.
6. Bast RC Jr, Feeney M, Lazarus H, et al. Reactivity of a monoclonal antibody with human ovarian carcinoma. *J Clin Invest*. 1981;68:1331–1337.
7. Mongia SK, Rawlins ML, Owen WE, et al. Performance characteristics of seven automated CA 125 assays. *Am J Clin Pathol*. 2006;125:921–927.
8. Kabawat SE, Bast RC Jr, Bhan AK, et al. Tissue distribution of a coelomic-epithelium-related antigen recognized by the monoclonal antibody OC125. *Int J Gynecol Pathol*. 1983;2:275–285.
9. Bast RC Jr, Klug TL, St John E, et al. A radioimmunoassay using a monoclonal antibody to monitor the course of epithelial ovarian cancer. *N Engl J Med*. 1983;309:883–887.
10. Bon GG, Kenemans P, Verstraeten R, et al. Serum tumor marker immunoassays in gynecologic oncology: establishment of reference values. *Am J Obstet Gynecol*. 1996;174:107–114.
11. Jacobs I, Bast RC Jr. The CA 125 tumour-associated antigen: a review of the literature. *Hum Reprod*. 1989;4:1–12.
12. Fotopoulou C, Sehouli J, Ewald-Riegler N, et al. The value of serum CA125 in the diagnosis of borderline tumors of the ovary: a subanalysis of the prospective multicenter ROBOT study. *Int J Gynecol Cancer*. 2015;25:1248–1252.
13. Chen K, Gentry-Maharaj A, Burnell M, et al. Microarray Glycoprofiling of CA125 improves differential diagnosis of ovarian cancer. *J Proteome Res*. 2013;12:1408–1418.
14. Wilson JA, Jungner G. *WHO Principles and Practice of Screening for Disease*. Geneva, Switzerland: World Health Organization; 1968:66–67.
15. Waller J, Osborne K, Wardle J. Enthusiasm for cancer screening in Great Britain: a general population survey. *Br J Cancer*. 2015;112:562–566.
16. Bonfrer JM, Korse CM, Verstraeten RA, et al. Clinical evaluation of the Byk LIA-mat CA125 II assay: discussion of a reference value. *Clin Chem*. 1997;43:491–497.
17. Jacobs IJ, Skates SJ, MacDonald N, et al. Screening for ovarian cancer: a pilot randomised controlled trial. *Lancet*. 1999;353:1207–1210.
18. Jacobs I, Davies AP, Bridges J, et al. Prevalence screening for ovarian cancer in postmenopausal women by CA 125 measurement and ultrasonography. *BMJ*. 1993;306:1030–1034.
19. Menon U, Skates SJ, Lewis S, et al. Prospective study using the risk of ovarian cancer algorithm to screen for ovarian cancer. *J Clin Oncol*. 2005;23:7919–7926.
20. Lu KH, Skates S, Hernandez MA, et al. A 2-stage ovarian cancer screening strategy using the Risk of Ovarian Cancer Algorithm (ROCA) identifies early-stage incident cancers and demonstrates high positive predictive value. *Cancer*. 2013;119:3454–3461.
21. Menon U, Ryan A, Kalsi J, et al. Risk algorithm using serial biomarker measurements doubles the number of screen-detected cancers compared with a single-threshold rule in the united kingdom collaborative trial of ovarian cancer screening. *J Clin Oncol*. 2015;33:2062–2071.
22. van Nagell JR Jr, DePriest PD, Ueland FR, et al. Ovarian cancer screening with annual transvaginal sonography: findings of 25,000 women screened. *Cancer*. 2007;109:1887–1896.
23. Kobayashi H, Yamada Y, Sado T, et al. A randomized study of screening for ovarian cancer: a multicenter study in Japan. *Int J Gynecol Cancer*. 2008;18:414–420.
24. Partridge E, Kreimer AR, Greenlee RT, et al. Results from four rounds of ovarian cancer screening in a randomized trial. *Obstet Gynecol*. 2009;113:775–782.
25. Buys SS, Partridge E, Black A, et al. Effect of screening on ovarian cancer mortality: The Prostate, Lung, Colorectal and Ovarian (PLCO) Cancer Screening Randomized Controlled Trial. *JAMA*. 2011;305:2295–2303.
26. Menon U, Gentry-Maharaj A, Ryan A, et al. Recruitment to multicentre trials—lessons from UKCTOCS: descriptive study. *BMJ*. 2008;337:a2079.
27. Menon U, Gentry-Maharaj A, Hallett R, et al. Sensitivity and specificity of multimodal and ultrasound screening for ovarian cancer, and stage distribution of detected cancers: results of the prevalence screen of the UK Collaborative Trial of Ovarian Cancer Screening (UKCTOCS). *Lancet Oncol*. 2009;10:327–340.
28. Drescher CW, Shah C, Thorpe J, et al. Longitudinal screening algorithm that incorporates change over time in CA125 levels identifies ovarian cancer earlier than a single-threshold rule. *J Clin Oncol*. 2013;31:387–392.
29. Jacobs IJ, Menon U, Ryan A, et al. Ovarian cancer screening and mortality in the UK Collaborative Trial of Ovarian Cancer Screening (UKCTOCS): a randomised controlled trial. *Lancet*. 2016;387:945–956.
30. Iyer R, Gentry-Maharaj A, Nordin A, et al. Predictors of complications in gynaecological oncological surgery: a prospective multicentre study (UKGOSOC-UK gynaecological oncology surgical outcomes and complications). *Br J Cancer*. 2015;112:475–484.
31. Barrett J, Jenkins V, Farewell V, et al. Psychological morbidity associated with ovarian cancer screening: results from more than 23,000 women in the randomised trial of ovarian cancer screening (UKCTOCS). *BJOG*. 2014;121:1071–1079.
32. Sakoda LC, Jorgenson E, Witte JS. Turning of COGS moves forward findings for hormonally mediated cancers. *Nat Genet*. 2013;45:345–348.
33. Pearce CL, Stram DO, Ness RB, et al. Population distribution of lifetime risk of ovarian cancer in the United States. *Cancer Epidemiol Biomarkers Prev*. 2015;24:671–676.
34. Chen S, Parmigiani G. Meta-analysis of BRCA1 and BRCA2 penetrance. *J Clin Oncol*. 2007;25:1329–1333.
35. Aarnio M, Sankila R, Pukkala E, et al. Cancer risk in mutation carriers of DNA-mismatch-repair genes. *Int J Cancer*. 1999;81:214–218.
36. Song H, Dicks E, Ramus SJ, et al. Contribution of Germline Mutations in the RAD51B, RAD51C, and RAD51D Genes to Ovarian Cancer in the Population. *J Clin Oncol*. 2015;33:2901–2907.
37. Ramus SJ, Song H, Dicks E, et al. Germline mutations in the BRIP1, BARD1, PALB2, and NBN genes in women with ovarian cancer. *J Natl Cancer Inst*. 2015;107.
38. National Institute for Health and Clinical Excellence: Guidance. *Familial Breast Cancer: Classification, Care and Managing Breast Cancer and Related Risks in People with a Family History of Breast Cancer: Risk Reduction and Treatment Strategies*. Cardiff, UK: National Collaborating Centre for Cancer; 2016.
39. Marchetti C, De Felice F, Palaia I, et al. Risk-reducing salpingo-oophorectomy: a meta-analysis on impact on ovarian cancer risk and all cause mortality in BRCA 1 and BRCA 2 mutation carriers. *BMC Womens Health*. 2014;14:150.
40. Alsop K, Fereday S, Meldrum C, et al. BRCA mutation frequency and patterns of treatment response in BRCA mutation-positive women with ovarian cancer: a report from the Australian Ovarian Cancer Study Group. *J Clin Oncol*. 2012;30:2654–2663.
41. Hoberg-Vetti H, Bjorvatn C, Fiane BE, et al. BRCA1/2 testing in newly diagnosed breast and ovarian cancer patients without prior genetic counselling: the DNA-BONus study. *Eur J Hum Genet*. 2016;24:881–888.
42. Rosenthal AN, Fraser L, Manchanda R, et al. Results of annual screening in phase I of the United Kingdom familial ovarian cancer screening study highlight the need for strict adherence to screening schedule. *J Clin Oncol*. 2013;31:49–57.

43. Greene MH, Piedmonte M, Alberts D, et al. A prospective study of risk-reducing salpingo-oophorectomy and longitudinal CA-125 screening among women at increased genetic risk of ovarian cancer: design and baseline characteristics: a Gynecologic Oncology Group study. *Cancer Epidemiol Biomarkers Prev*. 2008;17:594–604.
44. Clinical Trial to Screen Participants Who Are at High Genetic Risk for Ovarian Cancer. 2013. Available at: www.clinicaltrials.gov. Accessed June 16, 2016.
45. Skates SJ, Drescher CW, Isaacs C, et al. *A Prospective Multi-Center Ovarian Cancer Screening Study in Women at Increased Risk*. Chicago, IL: American Society of Clinical Oncology; 2007:276s.
46. Brown PO, Palmer C. The preclinical natural history of serous ovarian cancer: defining the target for early detection. *PLoS Med*. 2009;6:e1000114.
47. Rosenthal AN, Fraser L, Philpott S, et al; on behalf of the UKFOCSS collaborators. *Results of 4-Monthly Screening in the UK Familial Ovarian Cancer Screening Study (UK FOCSS Phase 2)*. Chicago, IL: American Society of Clinical Oncology; 2013.
48. Brain KE, Lifford KJ, Fraser L, et al. Psychological outcomes of familial ovarian cancer screening: no evidence of long-term harm. *Gynecol Oncol*. 2012;127:556–563.
49. Dilley J, Manchanda R, Johnson M, et al. Importance of serial CA125 measurements over an absolute cut-off value for the detection of asymptomatic ovarian cancer in high-risk patients. *Int J Gynaecol Obstet*. 2016;133:239–240.
50. Chen Y, Bancroft E, Ashley S, et al. Baseline and post prophylactic tubal-ovarian surgery CA125 levels in BRCA1 and BRCA2 mutation carriers. *Fam Cancer*. 2014;13:197–203.
51. Zurawski VR Jr, Orjaseter H, Andersen A, et al. Elevated serum CA 125 levels prior to diagnosis of ovarian neoplasia: relevance for early detection of ovarian cancer. *Int J Cancer*. 1988;42:677–680.
52. Kobayashi H, Ooi H, Yamada Y, et al. Serum CA125 level before the development of ovarian cancer. *Int J Gynaecol Obstet*. 2007;99:95–99.
53. Hori SS, Gambhir SS. Mathematical model identifies blood biomarker-based early cancer detection strategies and limitations. *Sci Transl Med*. 2011;3:109ra116.
54. Jeyarajah AR, Ind TE, Skates S, et al. Serum CA125 elevation and risk of clinical detection of cancer in asymptomatic postmenopausal women. *Cancer*. 1999;85:2068–2072.
55. Jeyarajah AR, Ind TE, MacDonald N, et al. Increased mortality in postmenopausal women with serum CA125 elevation. *Gynecol Oncol*. 1999;73:242–246.
56. Sjovall K, Nilsson B, Einhorn N. The significance of serum CA 125 elevation in malignant and nonmalignant diseases. *Gynecol Oncol*. 2002;85:175–178.
57. Einhorn N, Bast RC Jr, Knapp RC, et al. Preoperative evaluation of serum CA 125 levels in patients with primary epithelial ovarian cancer. *Obstet Gynecol*. 1986;67:414–416.
58. Zhang Z, Barnhill SD, Zhang H, et al. Combination of multiple serum markers using an artificial neural network to improve specificity in discriminating malignant from benign pelvic masses. *Gynecol Oncol*. 1999;73:56–61.
59. Jacobs I, Oram D, Fairbanks J, et al. A risk of malignancy index incorporating CA 125, ultrasound and menopausal status for the accurate preoperative diagnosis of ovarian cancer. *Br J Obstet Gynaecol*. 1990;97:922–929.
60. Geomini P, Kruitwagen R, Bremer GL, et al. The accuracy of risk scores in predicting ovarian malignancy: a systematic review. *Obstet Gynecol*. 2009;113:384–394.
61. van Trappen PO, Rufford BD, Mills TD, et al. Differential diagnosis of adnexal masses: risk of malignancy index, ultrasonography, magnetic resonance imaging, and radioimmunoscintigraphy. *Int J Gynecol Cancer*. 2007;17:61–67.
62. Hakansson F, Hogdall EV, Nedergaard L, et al. Risk of malignancy index used as a diagnostic tool in a tertiary centre for patients with a pelvic mass. *Acta Obstet Gynecol Scand*. 2012;91:496–502.
63. Kaijser J, Sayasneh A, Van Hoorde K, et al. Presurgical diagnosis of adnexal tumours using mathematical models and scoring systems: a systematic review and meta-analysis. *Hum Reprod Update*. 2014;20:449–462.
64. Andersen ES, Knudsen A, Rix P, et al. Risk of malignancy index in the preoperative evaluation of patients with adnexal masses. *Gynecol Oncol*. 2003;90:109–112.
65. Van Calster B, Van Hoorde K, Valentin L, et al. Evaluating the risk of ovarian cancer before surgery using the ADNEX model to differentiate between benign, borderline, early and advanced stage invasive, and secondary metastatic tumours: prospective multicentre diagnostic study. *BMJ*. 2014;349:g5920.
66. Van Calster B, Van Hoorde K, Froyman W, et al. Practical guidance for applying the ADNEX model from the IOTA group to discriminate between different subtypes of adnexal tumors. *Facts Views Vis Obgyn*. 2015;7:32–41.
67. Epstein E, Van Calster B, Timmerman D, et al. Subjective ultrasound assessment, the ADNEX model and ultrasound-guided tru-cut biopsy to differentiate disseminated primary ovarian cancer from metastatic non-ovarian cancer. *Ultrasound Obstet Gynecol*. 2016;47:110–116.
68. Timmerman D, Van Calster B, Testa A, et al. Predicting the risk of malignancy in adnexal masses based on the Simple Rules from the International Ovarian Tumor Analysis group. *Am J Obstet Gynecol*. 2016;214:424–437.
69. Hogdall E. Cancer antigen 125 and prognosis. *Curr Opin Obstet Gynecol*. 2008;20:4–8.
70. Hogdall CK, Norgaard-Pedersen B, Mogensen O. The prognostic value of pre-operative serum tetranectin, CA-125 and a combined index in women with primary ovarian cancer. *Anticancer Res*. 2002;22:1765–1768.
71. Petri AL, Hogdall E, Christensen IJ, et al. Preoperative CA125 as a prognostic factor in stage I epithelial ovarian cancer. *APMIS*. 2006;114:359–363.
72. Obermair A, Fuller A, Lopez-Varela E, et al. A new prognostic model for FIGO stage 1 epithelial ovarian cancer. *Gynecol Oncol*. 2007;104:607–611.
73. Raspollini MR, Amunni G, Villanucci A, et al. COX-2 and preoperative CA-125 level are strongly correlated with survival and clinical responsiveness to chemotherapy in ovarian cancer. *Acta Obstet Gynecol Scand*. 2006;85:493–498.
74. Makar AP, Kristensen GB, Kaern J, et al. Prognostic value of pre- and postoperative serum CA 125 levels in ovarian cancer: new aspects and multivariate analysis. *Obstet Gynecol*. 1992;79:1002–1010.
75. Rosen A, Sevelda P, Klein M, et al. A CA125 score as a prognostic index in patients with ovarian cancer. *Arch Gynecol Obstet*. 1990;247:125–129.
76. Riedinger JM, Eche N, Basuyau JP, et al. Prognostic value of serum CA 125 bi-exponential decrease during first line paclitaxel/platinum chemotherapy: a French multicentric study. *Gynecol Oncol*. 2008;109:194–198.
77. Gadducci A, Zola P, Landoni F, et al. Serum half-life of CA 125 during early chemotherapy as an independent prognostic variable for patients with advanced epithelial ovarian cancer: results of a multicentric Italian study. *Gynecol Oncol*. 1995;58:42–47.
78. Markman M, Liu PY, Rothenberg ML, et al. Pretreatment CA-125 and risk of relapse in advanced ovarian cancer. *J Clin Oncol*. 2006;24:1454–1458.
79. Makar AP, Kristensen GB, Bormer OP, et al. Is serum CA 125 at the time of relapse a prognostic indicator for further survival prognosis in patients with ovarian cancer? *Gynecol Oncol*. 1993;49:3–7.
80. Gallion HH, Hunter JE, van Nagell JR, et al. The prognostic implications of low serum CA 125 levels prior to the second-look operation for stage III and IV epithelial ovarian cancer. *Gynecol Oncol*. 1992;46:29–32.
81. Rustin GJ. Use of CA-125 to assess response to new agents in ovarian cancer trials. *J Clin Oncol*. 2003;21:187s–193s.
82. Rustin GJ, Vergote I, Eisenhauer E, et al. Definitions for response and progression in ovarian cancer clinical trials incorporating RECIST 1.1 and CA 125 agreed by the Gynecological Cancer Intergroup (GCIG). *Int J Gynecol Cancer*. 2011;21:419–423.
83. Riedinger JM, Wafflart J, Ricolleau G, et al. CA 125 half-life and CA 125 nadir during induction chemotherapy are independent predictors of epithelial ovarian cancer outcome: results of a French multicentric study. *Ann Oncol*. 2006;17:1234–1238.
84. Han LY, Karavasilis V, Hagen T, et al. Doubling time of serum CA125 is an independent prognostic factor for survival in patients with ovarian cancer relapsing after first-line chemotherapy. *Eur J Cancer*. 2010;46:1359–1364.
85. Colloca G, Venturino A, Governato I. CA125-related tumor cell kinetics variables after chemotherapy in advanced ovarian cancer: a systematic review. *Clin Transl Oncol*. 2016;18(8):813–824.
86. Santillan A, Garg R, Zahurak ML, et al. Risk of epithelial ovarian cancer recurrence in patients with rising serum CA-125 levels within the normal range. *J Clin Oncol*. 2005;23:9338–9343.
87. Fehm T, Heller F, Kramer S, et al. Evaluation of CA125, physical and radiological findings in follow-up of ovarian cancer patients. *Anticancer Res*. 2005;25:1551–1554.
88. Rustin GJ, van der Burg ME, Griffin CL, et al. Early versus delayed treatment of relapsed ovarian cancer (MRC OV05/EORTC 55955): a randomised trial. *Lancet*. 2010;376:1155–1163.
89. Soletormos G, Duffy MJ, Othman Abu Hassan S, et al. Clinical use of cancer biomarkers in epithelial ovarian cancer: updated guidelines from the European group on tumor markers. *Int J Gynecol Cancer*. 2016;26:43–51.
90. Pepe MS, Feng Z, Janes H, et al. Pivotal evaluation of the accuracy of a biomarker used for classification or prediction: standards for study design. *J Natl Cancer Inst*. 2008;100:1432–1438.

91. Urban N, Thorpe JD, Bergan LA, et al. Potential role of HE4 in multimodal screening for epithelial ovarian cancer. *J Natl Cancer Inst.* 2011;103:1630–1634.
92. Zhu CS, Pinsky PF, Cramer DW, et al. A framework for evaluating biomarkers for early detection: validation of biomarker panels for ovarian cancer. *Cancer Prev Res (Phila).* 2011;4:375–383.
93. Cramer DW, Bast RC Jr, Berg CD, et al. Ovarian cancer biomarker performance in prostate, lung, colorectal, and ovarian cancer screening trial specimens. *Cancer Prev Res.* 2011;4:365–374.
94. Jacobs I, Menon U. The sine qua non of discovering novel biomarkers for early detection of ovarian cancer: carefully selected preclinical samples. *Cancer Prev Res.* 2011;4:299–302.
95. Anderson GL, McIntosh M, Wu L, et al. Assessing lead time of selected ovarian cancer biomarkers: a nested case-control study. *J Natl Cancer Inst.* 2010;102:26–38.
96. Molina R, Escudero JM, Auge JM, et al. HE4 a novel tumour marker for ovarian cancer: comparison with CA 125 and ROMA algorithm in patients with gynaecological diseases. *Tumour Biol.* 2011;32:1087–1095.
97. Moore RG, Miller MC, Steinhoff MM, et al. Serum HE4 levels are less frequently elevated than CA125 in women with benign gynecologic disorders. *Am J Obstet Gynecol.* 2012;206:351.e1–351.e8.
98. Moore RG, Brown AK, Miller MC, et al. The use of multiple novel tumor biomarkers for the detection of ovarian carcinoma in patients with a pelvic mass. *Gynecol Oncol.* 2008;108:402–408.
99. Partheen K, Kristjansdottir B, Sundfeldt K. Evaluation of ovarian cancer biomarkers HE4 and CA-125 in women presenting with a suspicious cystic ovarian mass. *J Gynecol Oncol.* 2011;22:244–252.
100. Romagnolo C, Leon AE, Fabricio AS, et al. HE4, CA125 and risk of ovarian malignancy algorithm (ROMA) as diagnostic tools for ovarian cancer in patients with a pelvic mass: an Italian multicenter study. *Gynecol Oncol.* 2016;141:303–311.
101. Fujirebio Diagnostics Inc. *CA125, HE4 and ROMA.* Malvern, PA: Fujirebio Diagnostics, Inc.; 2008.
102. Van Gorp T, Veldman J, Van Calster B, et al. Subjective assessment by ultrasound is superior to the risk of malignancy index (RMI) or the risk of ovarian malignancy algorithm (ROMA) in discriminating benign from malignant adnexal masses. *Eur J Cancer.* 2012;48(11):1649–1656.
103. Karlsen MA, Hogdall EV, Christensen IJ, et al. A novel diagnostic index combining HE4, CA125 and age may improve triage of women with suspected ovarian cancer—An international multicenter study in women with an ovarian mass. *Gynecol Oncol.* 2015;138:640–646.
104. Moore RG, Miller MC, Eklund EE, et al. Serum levels of the ovarian cancer biomarker HE4 are decreased in pregnancy and increase with age. *Am J Obstet Gynecol.* 2012;206:349.e1–349.e7.
105. Park Y, Kim Y, Lee EY, et al. Reference ranges for HE4 and CA125 in a large Asian population by automated assays and diagnostic performances for ovarian cancer. *J Int Cancer.* 2012;130:1136–1144.
106. Xu Y, Zhong R, He J, et al. Modification of cut-off values for HE4, CA125 and the ROMA algorithm for early-stage epithelial ovarian cancer detection: results from 1021 cases in South China. *Clin Biochem.* 2016;49:32–40.
107. Schummer M, Drescher C, Forrest R, et al. Evaluation of ovarian cancer remission markers HE4, MMP7 and Mesothelin by comparison to the established marker CA125. *Gynecol Oncol.* 2012;125:65–69.
108. Steffensen KD, Waldstrom M, Brandslund I, et al. Prognostic impact of prechemotherapy serum levels of HER2, CA125, and HE4 in ovarian cancer patients. *Int J Gynecol Cancer.* 2011;21:1040–1047.
109. Trudel D, Tetu B, Gregoire J, et al. Human epididymis protein 4 (HE4) and ovarian cancer prognosis. *Gynecol Oncol.* 2012;127:511–515.
110. Engelen MJ, Kos HE, Willemse PH, et al. Surgery by consultant gynecologic oncologists improves survival in patients with ovarian carcinoma. *Cancer.* 2006;106:589–598.
111. Burford B, Gentry-Maharaj A, Graham R, et al. Autoantibodies to MUC1 glycopeptides cannot be used as a screening assay for early detection of breast, ovarian, lung or pancreatic cancer. *Br J Cancer.* 2013;108:2045–2055.
112. Havrilesky LJ, Whitehead CM, Rubatt JM, et al. Evaluation of biomarker panels for early stage ovarian cancer detection and monitoring for disease recurrence. *Gynecol Oncol.* 2008;110:374–382.
113. Blyuss O, Gentry-Maharaj A, Fourkala EO, et al. Serial patterns of ovarian cancer biomarkers in a prediagnosis longitudinal dataset. *Biomed Res Int.* 2015;2015:681416.
114. Budiu RA, Mantia-Smaldone G, Elishaev E, et al. Soluble MUC1 and serum MUC1-specific antibodies are potential prognostic biomarkers for platinum-resistant ovarian cancer. *Cancer Immunol Immunother.* 2011;60:975–984.
115. No JH, Jeon YT, Kim YB, et al. Quantitative detection of serum survivin and its relationship with prognostic factors in ovarian cancer. *Gynecol Obstet Invest.* 2011;71:136–140.
116. Kamat AA, Baldwin M, Urbauer D, et al. Plasma cell-free DNA in ovarian cancer: an independent prognostic biomarker. *Cancer.* 2010;116:1918–1925.
117. Li M, Diehl F, Dressman D, et al. BEAMing up for detection and quantification of rare sequence variants. *Nat Methods.* 2006;3:95–97.
118. Forshew T, Murtaza M, Parkinson C, et al. Noninvasive identification and monitoring of cancer mutations by targeted deep sequencing of plasma DNA. *Sci Transl Med.* 2012;4:136ra168.
119. Pereira E, Camacho-Vanegas O, Anand S, et al. Personalized circulating tumor DNA biomarkers dynamically predict treatment response and survival in gynecologic cancers. *PLoS One.* 2015;10:e0145754.
120. Kinde I, Bettegowda C, Wang Y, et al. Evaluation of DNA from the Papanicolaou test to detect ovarian and endometrial cancers. *Sci Transl Med.* 2013;5:167ra164.
121. Maritschnegg E, Wang Y, Pecha N, et al. Lavage of the uterine cavity for molecular detection of mullerian duct carcinomas: a proof-of-concept study. *J Clin Oncol.* 2015;33:4293–4300.
122. Widschwendter M, Menon U. Circulating methylated DNA: a new generation of tumor markers. *Clin Cancer Res.* 2006;12:7205–7208.
123. Molnar B, Toth K, Bartak BK, et al. Plasma methylated septin 9: a colorectal cancer screening marker. *Expert Rev Mol Diagn.* 2015;15:171–184.
124. Earp MA, Cunningham JM. DNA methylation changes in epithelial ovarian cancer histotypes. *Genomics.* 2015;106:311–321.
125. Teschendorff AE, Menon U, Gentry-Maharaj A, et al. An epigenetic signature in peripheral blood predicts active ovarian cancer. *PloS One.* 2009;4:e8274.
126. Dai W, Teodoridis JM, Zeller C, et al. Systematic CpG islands methylation profiling of genes in the wnt pathway in epithelial ovarian cancer identifies biomarkers of progression-free survival. *Clin Cancer Res.* 2011;17:4052–4062.
127. Ho CM, Lai HC, Huang SH, et al. Promoter methylation of sFRP5 in patients with ovarian clear cell adenocarcinoma. *Eur J Clin Invest.* 2010;40:310–318.
128. Lee YH, Kim JH, Zhou H, et al. Salivary transcriptomic biomarkers for detection of ovarian cancer: for serous papillary adenocarcinoma. *J Mol Med.* 2012;90:427–434.
129. Petricoin EF, Ardekani AM, Hitt BA, et al. Use of proteomic patterns in serum to identify ovarian cancer. *Lancet.* 2002;359:572–577.
130. Zhang Z, Bast RC Jr, Yu Y, et al. Three biomarkers identified from serum proteomic analysis for the detection of early stage ovarian cancer. *Cancer Res.* 2004;64:5882–5890.
131. Clarke CH, Yip C, Badgwell D, et al. Proteomic biomarkers apolipoprotein A1, truncated transthyretin and connective tissue activating protein III enhance the sensitivity of CA125 for detecting early stage epithelial ovarian cancer. *Gynecol Oncol.* 2011;122:548–553.
132. Eskander RN, Carpenter BA, Wu HG, et al. The clinical utility of an elevated-risk multivariate index assay score in ovarian cancer patients. *Curr Med Res Opin.* 2016;32:1161–1165.
133. Timms JF, Menon U, Devetyarov D, et al. Early detection of ovarian cancer in samples pre-diagnosis using CA125 and MALDI-MS peaks. *Cancer Genomics Proteomics.* 2011;8:289–305.
134. Moore LE, Pfeiffer RM, Zhang Z, et al. Proteomic biomarkers in combination with CA 125 for detection of epithelial ovarian cancer using prediagnostic serum samples from the Prostate, Lung, Colorectal, and Ovarian (PLCO) Cancer Screening Trial. *Cancer.* 2012;118:91–100.
135. Russell MR, Walker MJ, Williamson AJ, et al. Protein Z: A putative novel biomarker for early detection of ovarian cancer. *Int J Cancer.* 2016;138:2984–2992.
136. Denkert C, Budczies J, Kind T, et al. Mass spectrometry-based metabolic profiling reveals different metabolite patterns in invasive ovarian carcinomas and ovarian borderline tumors. *Cancer Res.* 2006;66:10795–10804.
137. Buas MF, Gu H, Djukovic D, et al. Identification of novel candidate plasma metabolite biomarkers for distinguishing serous ovarian carcinoma and benign serous ovarian tumors. *Gynecol Oncol.* 2016;140:138–144.
138. Iorio MV, Visone R, Di Leva G, et al. MicroRNA signatures in human ovarian cancer. *Cancer Res.* 2007;67:8699–8707.
139. Taylor DD, Gercel-Taylor C. MicroRNA signatures of tumor-derived exosomes as diagnostic biomarkers of ovarian cancer. *Gynecol Oncol.* 2008;110:13–21.
140. Resnick KE, Alder H, Hagan JP, et al. The detection of differentially expressed microRNAs from the serum of ovarian cancer patients using a novel real-time PCR platform. *Gynecol Oncol.* 2009;112:55–59.

141. Gold P, Freedman SO. Specific carcinoembryonic antigens of the human digestive system. *J Exp Med*. 1965;122:467–481.
142. Onsrud M. Tumour markers in gynaecologic oncology. *Scand J Clin Lab Invest Suppl*. 1991;206:60–70.
143. Roman LD, Muderspach LI, Burnett AF, et al. Carcinoembryonic antigen in women with isolated pelvic masses. Clinical utility? *J Reprod Med*. 1998;43:403–407.
144. Nomelini RS, da Silva TM, Tavares Murta BM, et al. Parameters of blood count and tumor markers in patients with borderline ovarian tumors: a retrospective analysis and relation to staging. *ISRN Oncol*. 2012;2012:947831.
145. Hogdall EV, Christensen L, Kjaer SK, et al. Protein expression levels of carcinoembryonic antigen (CEA) in Danish ovarian cancer patients: from the Danish 'MALOVA'ovarian cancer study. *Pathology*. 2008;40:487–492.
146. Sorensen SS, Mosgaard BJ. Combination of cancer antigen 125 and carcinoembryonic antigen can improve ovarian cancer diagnosis. *Dan Med Bull*. 2011;58:A4331.
147. Kawai M, Kano T, Kikkawa F, et al. Seven tumor markers in benign and malignant germ cell tumors of the ovary. *Gynecol Oncol*. 1992;45:248–253.
148. Olt G, Berchuck A, Bast RC Jr. The role of tumor markers in gynecologic oncology. *Obstet Gynecol Surv*. 1990;45:570–577.
149. Chow SN, Yang JH, Lin YH, et al. Malignant ovarian germ cell tumors. *Int J Gynaecol Obstet*. 1996;53:151–158.
150. Zalel Y, Piura B, Elchalal U, et al. Diagnosis and management of malignant germ cell ovarian tumors in young females. *Int J Gynaecol Obstet*. 1996;55:1–10.
151. Mayordomo JI, Paz-Ares L, Rivera F, et al. Ovarian and extragonadal malignant germ-cell tumors in females: a single-institution experience with 43 patients. *Ann Oncol*. 1994;5:225–231.
152. Boussios S, Attygalle A, Hazell S, et al. Malignant ovarian germ cell tumors in postmenopausal patients: The Royal Marsden Experience and Literature Review. *Anticancer Res*. 2015;35:6713–6722.
153. Roma AA, Przybycin CG. Yolk sac tumor in postmenopausal patients: pure or associated with adenocarcinoma, a rare phenomenon. *Int J Gynecol Pathol*. 2014;33:477–482.
154. Zong C, Wu J, Wang C, et al. Chemiluminescence imaging immunoassay of multiple tumor markers for cancer screening. *Anal Chem*. 2012;84:2410–2415.
155. Mann K, Saller B, Hoermann R. Clinical use of HCG and hCG beta determinations. *Scand J Clin Lab Invest Suppl*. 1993;216:97–104.
156. Murugaesu N, Schmid P, Dancey G, et al. Malignant ovarian germ cell tumors: identification of novel prognostic markers and long-term outcome after multimodality treatment. *J Clin Oncol*. 2006;24:4862–4866.
157. Oltmann SC, Garcia N, Barber R, et al. Can we preoperatively risk stratify ovarian masses for malignancy? *J Pediatr Surg*. 2010;45:130–134.
158. Lenhard M, Tsvilina A, Schumacher L, et al. Human chorionic gonadotropin and its relation to grade, stage and patient survival in ovarian cancer. *BMC Cancer*. 2012;12:2.
159. Muller CY, Cole LA. The quagmire of hCG and hCG testing in gynecologic oncology. *Gynecol Oncol*. 2009;112:663–672.
160. Farkkila A, Koskela S, Bryk S, et al. The clinical utility of serum anti-Mullerian hormone in the follow-up of ovarian adult-type granulosa cell tumors—A comparative study with inhibin B. *Int J Cancer*. 2015;137:1661–1671.
161. Tsigkou A, Marrelli D, Reis FM, et al. Total inhibin is a potential serum marker for epithelial ovarian cancer. *J Clin Endocrinol Metab*. 2007;92(7):2526–2531.
162. Robertson DM, Pruysers E, Jobling T. Inhibin as a diagnostic marker for ovarian cancer. *Cancer Lett*. 2007;249:14–17.
163. Lambert-Messerlian GM, Steinhoff M, Zheng W, et al. Multiple immunoreactive inhibin proteins in serum from postmenopausal women with epithelial ovarian cancer. *Gynecol Oncol*. 1997;65:512–516.
164. Mom CH, Engelen MJ, Willemse PH, et al. Granulosa cell tumors of the ovary: the clinical value of serum inhibin A and B levels in a large single center cohort. *Gynecol Oncol*. 2007;105:365–372.
165. McNeilly AS. Diagnostic applications for inhibin and activins. *Mol Cell Endocrinol*. 2012;359:121–125.
166. Cobellis L, Reis FM, Luisi S, et al. High concentrations of activin A in the peritoneal fluid of women with epithelial ovarian cancer. *J Soc Gynecol Invest*. 2004;11:203–206.
167. Prezas P, Arlt MJ, Viktorov P, et al. Overexpression of the human tissue kallikrein genes KLK4, 5, 6, and 7 increases the malignant phenotype of ovarian cancer cells. *Biol Chem*. 2006;387:807–811.
168. Davidson B, Xi Z, Klokk TI, et al. Kallikrein 4 expression is up-regulated in epithelial ovarian carcinoma cells in effusions. *Am J Clin Pathol*. 2005;123:360–368.
169. Oikonomopoulou K, Scorilas A, Michael IP, et al. Kallikreins as markers of disseminated tumour cells in ovarian cancer—a pilot study. *Tumour Biol*. 2006;27:104–114.
170. Dorn J, Magdolen V, Gkazepis A, et al. Circulating biomarker tissue kallikrein-related peptidase KLK5 impacts ovarian cancer patients' survival. *Ann Oncol*. 2011;22:1783–1790.
171. Emami N, Diamandis EP. Utility of kallikrein-related peptidases (KLKs) as cancer biomarkers. *Clin Chem*. 2008;54:1600–1607.
172. Dorn J, Bronger H, Kates R, et al. OVSCORE—a validated score to identify ovarian cancer patients not suitable for primary surgery. *Oncol Lett*. 2015;9:418–424.
173. Dong Y, Loessner D, Irving-Rodgers H, et al. Metastasis of ovarian cancer is mediated by kallikrein related peptidases. *Clin Exp Metastasis*. 2014;31:135–147.
174. Tiniakos DG, Yu H, Liapis H. Osteopontin expression in ovarian carcinomas and tumors of low malignant potential (LMP). *Hum Pathol*. 1998;29:1250–1254.
175. Hu ZD, Wei TT, Yang M, et al. Diagnostic value of osteopontin in ovarian cancer: a meta-analysis and systematic review. *PLoS One*. 2015;10:e0126444.
176. Brakora KA, Lee H, Yusuf R, et al. Utility of osteopontin as a biomarker in recurrent epithelial ovarian cancer. *Gynecol Oncol*. 2004;93:361–365.
177. Schorge JO, Drake RD, Lee H, et al. Osteopontin as an adjunct to CA125 in detecting recurrent ovarian cancer. *Clin Cancer Res*. 2004;10:3474–3478.
178. Matsuura M, Suzuki T, Suzuki M, et al. Statin-mediated reduction of osteopontin expression induces apoptosis and cell growth arrest in ovarian clear cell carcinoma. *Oncol Rep*. 2011;25:41–47.
179. Chang K, Pastan I. Molecular cloning of mesothelin, a differentiation antigen present on mesothelium, mesotheliomas, and ovarian cancers. *Proc Natl Acad Sci U S A*. 1996;93:136–140.
180. Huang CY, Cheng WF, Lee CN, et al. Serum mesothelin in epithelial ovarian carcinoma: a new screening marker and prognostic factor. *Anticancer Res*. 2006;26:4721–4728.
181. Michiel DF, Oppenheim JJ. Cytokines as positive and negative regulators of tumor promotion and progression. *Semin Cancer Biol*. 1992;3:3–15.
182. Suzuki M, Ohwada M, Aida I, et al. Macrophage colony-stimulating factor as a tumor marker for epithelial ovarian cancer. *Obstet Gynecol*. 1993;82:946–950.
183. Suzuki M, Ohwada M, Sato I, et al. Serum level of macrophage colony-stimulating factor as a marker for gynecologic malignancies. *Oncology*. 1995;52:128–133.
184. Skates SJ, Horick N, Yu Y, et al. Preoperative sensitivity and specificity for early-stage ovarian cancer when combining cancer antigen CA-125II, CA 15-3, CA 72-4, and macrophage colony-stimulating factor using mixtures of multivariate normal distributions. *J Clin Oncol*. 2004;22:4059–4066.
185. Scholl SM, Bascou CH, Mosseri V, et al. Circulating levels of colony-stimulating factor 1 as a prognostic indicator in 82 patients with epithelial ovarian cancer. *Br J Cancer*. 1994;69:342–346.
186. Bedkowska GE, Lawicki S, Gacuta E, et al. M-CSF in a new biomarker panel with HE4 and CA 125 in the diagnostics of epithelial ovarian cancer patients. *J Ovarian Res*. 2015;8:27.
187. Scambia G, Testa U, Benedetti Panici P, et al. Prognostic significance of interleukin 6 serum levels in patients with ovarian cancer. *Br J Cancer*. 1995;71:354–356.
188. Lambeck AJ, Crijns AP, Leffers N, et al. Serum cytokine profiling as a diagnostic and prognostic tool in ovarian cancer: a potential role for interleukin 7. *Clin Cancer Res*. 2007;13:2385–2391.
189. Wojcik E, Rychlik U, Skotnicki P, et al. Utility of ProGRP determinations in cancer patients. *Clin Lab*. 2010;56:527–534.
190. Stenman UH, Alfthan H, Vartiainen J, et al. Markers supplementing CA 125 in ovarian cancer. *Ann Med*. 1995;27:115–120.
191. Martinicky D, Zvarik M, Sikurova L, et al. Fluorescence analysis of urine and its potential for ovarian cancer screening. *Neoplasma*. 2015;62:500–506.
192. Gadducci A, Ferdeghini M, Prontera C, et al. A comparison of pretreatment serum levels of four tumor markers in patients with endometrial and cervical carcinoma. *Eur J Gynaecol Oncol*. 1990;11:283–288.
193. Kurihara T, Mizunuma H, Obara M, et al. Determination of a normal level of serum CA125 in postmenopausal women as a tool for preoperative evaluation and postoperative surveillance of endometrial carcinoma. *Gynecol Oncol*. 1998;69:192–196.
194. Chen YL, Huang CY, Chien TY, et al. Value of pre-operative serum CA125 level for prediction of prognosis in patients with endometrial cancer. *Aust N Z J Obstet Gynaecol*. 2011;51:397–402.

195. Lukanova A, Lundin E, Micheli A, et al. Circulating levels of sex steroid hormones and risk of endometrial cancer in postmenopausal women. *Int J Cancer*. 2004;108:425–432.
196. Allen NE, Key TJ, Dossus L, et al. Endogenous sex hormones and endometrial cancer risk in women in the European Prospective Investigation into Cancer and Nutrition (EPIC). *Endocr Relat Cancer*. 2008;15:485–497.
197. Gunter MJ, Hoover DR, Yu H, et al. A prospective evaluation of insulin and insulin-like growth factor-I as risk factors for endometrial cancer. *Cancer Epidemiol Biomarkers Prev*. 2008;17:921–929.
198. Zhao H, Jiang Y, Liu Y, et al. Endogenous estrogen metabolites as biomarkers for endometrial cancer via a novel method of liquid chromatography-mass spectrometry with hollow fiber liquid-phase microextraction. *Horm Metab Res*. 2015;47:158–164.
199. Fader AN, Arriba LN, Frasure HE, et al. Endometrial cancer and obesity: epidemiology, biomarkers, prevention and survivorship. *Gynecol Oncol*. 2009;114:121–127.
200. Kishida K, Funahashi T, Shimomura I. Adiponectin as a routine clinical biomarker. *Best Pract Res Clin Endocrinol Metab*. 2014;28:119–130.
201. Dal Maso L, Augustin LS, Karalis A, et al. Circulating adiponectin and endometrial cancer risk. *J Clin Endocrinol Metab*. 2004;89:1160–1163.
202. Shan N, Zhou W, Zhang S, et al. Identification of HSPA8 as a candidate biomarker for endometrial carcinoma by using iTRAQ-based proteomic analysis. *Onco Targets Ther*. 2016;9:2169–2179.
203. Mu AK, Lim BK, Aminudin N, et al. Application of SELDI-TOF in N-glycopeptides profiling of the urine from patients with endometrial, ovarian and cervical cancer. *Arch Physiol Biochem*. 2016;122:111–116.
204. Li J, Dowdy S, Tipton T, et al. HE4 as a biomarker for ovarian and endometrial cancer management. *Expert Rev Mol Diagn*. 2009;9:555–566.
205. Kalogera E, Scholler N, Powless C, et al. Correlation of serum HE4 with tumor size and myometrial invasion in endometrial cancer. *Gynecol Oncol*. 2012;124:270–275.
206. Brennan DJ, Hackethal A, Metcalf AM, et al. Serum HE4 as a prognostic marker in endometrial cancer—a population based study. *Gynecol Oncol*. 2014;132:159–165.
207. Van Gool IC, Stelloo E, Nout RA, et al. Prognostic significance of L1CAM expression and its association with mutant p53 expression in high-risk endometrial cancer. *Mod Pathol*. 2016;29:174–181.
208. Wentzensen N, Bakkum-Gamez JN, Killian JK, et al. Discovery and validation of methylation markers for endometrial cancer. *Int J Cancer*. 2014;135:1860–1868.
209. Yoon SM, Shin KH, Kim JY, et al. The clinical values of squamous cell carcinoma antigen and carcinoembryonic antigen in patients with cervical cancer treated with concurrent chemoradiotherapy. *Int J Gynecol Cancer*. 2007;17:872–878.
210. Crombach G, Scharl A, Vierbuchen M, et al. Detection of squamous cell carcinoma antigen in normal squamous epithelia and in squamous cell carcinomas of the uterine cervix. *Cancer*. 1989;63:1337–1342.
211. Li X, Zhou J, Huang K, et al. The predictive value of serum squamous cell carcinoma antigen in patients with cervical cancer who receive neoadjuvant chemotherapy followed by radical surgery: a single-institute study. *PLoS One*. 2015;10:e0122361.
212. Salvatici M, Achilarre MT, Sandri MT, et al. Squamous cell carcinoma antigen (SCC-Ag) during follow-up of cervical cancer patients: role in the early diagnosis of recurrence. *Gynecol Oncol*. 2016;142:115–119.
213. Sturgeon CM, Duffy MJ, Hofmann BR, et al. National Academy of Clinical Biochemistry Laboratory Medicine Practice Guidelines for use of tumor markers in liver, bladder, cervical, and gastric cancers. *Clin Chem*. 2010;56:e1–e48.
214. Roijer E, de Bruijn HW, Dahlen U, et al. Squamous cell carcinoma antigen isoforms in serum from cervical cancer patients. *Tumour Biol*. 2006;27:142–152.
215. Kotowicz B, Fuksiewicz M, Jonska-Gmyrek J, et al. The assessment of the prognostic value of tumor markers and cytokines as SCCAg, CYFRA 21.1, IL-6, VEGF and sTNF receptors in patients with squamous cell cervical cancer, particularly with early stage of the disease. *Tumour Biol*. 2016;37:1271–1278.
216. Tsai SC, Kao CH, Wang SJ. Study of a new tumor marker, CYFRA 21-1, in squamous cell carcinoma of the cervix, and comparison with squamous cell carcinoma antigen. *Neoplasma*. 1996;43:27–29.
217. Ferdeghini M, Gadducci A, Annicchiarico C, et al. Serum CYFRA 21-1 assay in squamous cell carcinoma of the cervix. *Anticancer Res*. 1993;13:1841–1844.
218. Pras E, Willemse PH, Canrinus AA, et al. Serum squamous cell carcinoma antigen and CYFRA 21-1 in cervical cancer treatment. *Int J Radiat Oncol Biol Phys*. 2002;52:23–32.
219. Borras G, Molina R, Xercavins J, et al. Tumor antigens CA 19.9, CA 125, and CEA in carcinoma of the uterine cervix. *Gynecol Oncol*. 1995;57:205–211.
220. Zhi W, Ferris D, Sharma A, et al. Twelve serum proteins progressively increase with disease stage in squamous cell cervical cancer patients. *Int J Gynecol Cancer*. 2014;24:1085–1092.
221. Leminen A, Alftan H, Stenman UH, et al. Chemotherapy as initial treatment for cervical carcinoma: clinical and tumor marker response. *Acta Obstet Gynecol Scand*. 1992;71:293–297.
222. Lam CP, Yuan CC, Jeng FS, et al. Evaluation of carcinoembryonic antigen, tissue polypeptide antigen, and squamous cell carcinoma antigen in the detection of cervical cancers. *Zhonghua Yi Xue Za Zhi (Taipei)*. 1992;50:7–13.
223. Gokul G, Gautami B, Malathi S, et al. DNA methylation profile at the DNMT3L promoter: a potential biomarker for cervical cancer. *Epigenetics*. 2007;2:80–85.
224. von Knebel Doeberitz M, Reuschenbach M, Schmidt D, et al. Biomarkers for cervical cancer screening: the role of p16(INK4a) to highlight transforming HPV infections. *Expert Rev Proteomics*. 2012;9:149–163.
225. Zhang X, Wang C, Wang L, et al. Detection of circulating Bmi-1 mRNA in plasma and its potential diagnostic and prognostic value for uterine cervical cancer. *Int J Cancer*. 2012;131:165–172.
226. Mezache L, Paniccia B, Nyinawabera A, et al. Enhanced expression of PD L1 in cervical intraepithelial neoplasia and cervical cancers. *Mod Pathol*. 2015;28:1594–1602.
227. Giorgi Rossi P, Fortunato C, Barbarino P, et al. Self-sampling to increase participation in cervical cancer screening: an RCT comparing home mailing, distribution in pharmacies, and recall letter. *Br J Cancer*. 2015;112:667–675.
228. Salman T, el-Ahmady O, Sawsan MR, et al. The clinical value of serum TPS in gynecological malignancies. *Int J Biol Markers*. 1995;10:81–86.
229. Nam JH, Chang KC, Chambers JT, et al. Urinary gonadotropin fragment, a new tumor marker. III. Use in cervical and vulvar cancers. *Gynecol Oncol*. 1990;38:66–70.
230. Carter PG, Iles RK, Neven P, et al. Measurement of urinary beta core fragment of human chorionic gonadotrophin in women with vulvovaginal malignancy and its prognostic significance. *Br J Cancer*. 1995;71:350–353.
231. Akagi EM, Lavorato-Rocha AM, Maia Bde M, et al. ROCK1 as a novel prognostic marker in vulvar cancer. *BMC Cancer*. 2014;14:822.
232. Liu J, Westin SN. Rational selection of biomarker driven therapies for gynecologic cancers: the more we know, the more we know we don't know. *Gynecol Oncol*. 2016;141:65–71.

CHAPTER 6

Cancer Prevention Strategies

Mary B. Daly and Gina M. Mantia-Smaldone

INTRODUCTION

As our knowledge of the genetic, physiologic, environmental, and lifestyle factors associated with the carcinogenic process grows, the prevention of cancer is increasingly becoming a reality and being incorporated into oncology practice. Options for the primary prevention of cancer are expanding and include avoidance of carcinogens (e.g., smoking cessation, sun avoidance, removal of asbestos), diet modification, exercise and weight loss, use of cancer vaccines, prophylactic surgery, and chemoprevention. Avoidance of tobacco and sun exposure and elimination of obesity could have a major public health impact on cancer incidence, as well as other chronic conditions (1,2). Options for secondary prevention through screening for occult disease when treatment may be more effective are also becoming more sophisticated. Great strides have been made in the prevention of many of the most common cancers.

The most common risk factor for lung cancer, which is the largest cause of death from cancer for both men and women, is tobacco use. Primary prevention strategies, including tax increases on tobacco products, mass media campaigns, restrictions on smoking in public places, and the physiologic and psychological treatment of nicotine addiction, have all contributed to the reduction in smoking prevalence rates and the decrease in the incidence of lung cancer (3,4). Recently, low-dose spiral CT (LDCT) scans have been shown to detect earlier-stage lung cancer, resulting in a reduction in lung cancer mortality (5). This has led to the recommendation of LDCT screening in at-risk populations by the United States Preventive Services Task Force (6).

Nonsteroidal anti-inflammatory drugs (NSAIDs) reduce the risk of adenomatous polyps and invasive cancer among individuals with very high risks of colon cancer due to hereditary syndromes (7). Their use for primary prevention among individuals at average risk, however, is not recommended due to potential side effects. A moderate risk reduction has been seen among individuals at population risk for colorectal cancer who use long-term aspirin prophylaxis (8). There is also evidence that alteration of lifestyle factors, including adoption of a healthy diet and avoidance of obesity, smoking, and heavy alcohol use, would have a significant impact on colon cancer incidence (9). Perhaps the greatest contribution to the prevention of colorectal cancer is the increasing adoption of screening colonoscopy to identify and remove premalignant polyps (10).

Alcohol consumption and obesity in postmenopausal women are associated with an increased risk of breast cancer, suggesting that changes in dietary patterns would have a protective effect on breast cancer incidence (11). Large randomized trials have established the efficacy of both tamoxifen and raloxifene to prevent estrogen receptor–positive breast cancer (12–14). More recently, the aromatase inhibitors anastrozole and exemestane have been shown to confer a similar risk reduction in the incidence of breast cancer among high-risk women (15,16). With the demonstration of the increased risk in breast cancer associated with combined estrogen and progesterone hormone replacement therapy (HRT) by the Women's Health Initiative, the use of these products has declined significantly, and the decline is thought to be associated with a subsequent decrease in breast cancer incidence (17,18). Both prophylactic mastectomy and prophylactic oophorectomy reduce the risk of breast cancer and are considered options for women with hereditary syndromes that convey high rates of breast and ovarian cancer (19,20). There have been several advances in screening modalities for breast cancer. The recent addition of breast tomosynthesis to digital mammography has been shown to reduce the recall rate and increase cancer detection rate among women at population risk of breast cancer (21). The use of screening breast MRI in selected high-risk individuals has improved the detection of early-stage occult cancers and has led to a downstaging of disease (22,23).

A large randomized trial of finasteride, which reduces the androgenic stimulation of the prostate, produced a 30% reduction in prostate cancer incidence (24). Several other agents targeting inflammatory, antioxidant, and other pathways have been proposed as chemopreventive agents for prostate cancer, but so far none have proven efficacy (25). The role of prostate cancer screening with digital rectal examination and serum prostate-specific antigen (PSA) levels among average-risk men has recently been challenged on the basis of high rates of detection of indolent disease (26). The role of screening high-risk men, African American men, and those with a family history of this cancer is the subject of ongoing studies.

The prevention of gynecologic cancer is becoming a reality due to the recognition that the initiation and progression of gynecologic cancers is a multistep process characterized by distinct molecular genetic events that provide opportunities to intervene in the carcinogenic process at several steps and reverse its early stages. The concept of preventing gynecologic cancer is based on an understanding of causally related risk factors, their role in carcinogenesis, and opportunities for their avoidance and/or reversal of their effect. There are three distinct models that can be applied to gynecologic cancer prevention: (a) *risk avoidance and adoption of protective practices*, which includes the identification of key risk factors and the development of strategies for their avoidance. Included in risk avoidance are the avoidance of exogenous and endogenous exposures (chemical, hormonal, infectious, etc.) and the avoidance of risky health behaviors. The adoption of protective practices, such as vaccination with the human papillomavirus (HPV) vaccine, a healthy diet, and exercise, may forestall early premalignant events; (b) the use of *chemopreventive agents*, both natural and synthetic, to reverse early, premalignant changes; and (c) *surgical prophylaxis* to remove either healthy at-risk organs or tissues with premalignant changes.

In addition to establishing valid interventions for cancer prevention, it is important to identify optimal target populations for their application and to tailor the interventions to the level of risk. Interventions for use in the general population at average risk must be highly effective, safe, inexpensive, and socially acceptable. Population groups with high risks may tolerate interventions that confer more risk and higher costs. All prevention efforts are greatly enhanced by public and professional education about their use and by a health care system that values, promotes, and invests in prevention activities.

The avoidance of environmental, occupational, and lifestyle risk factors through public education and social policies has the potential to prevent a large proportion of human cancer. The epidemiologic literature has provided a wealth of information about the risks associated with cancers of the cervix, uterus, and ovary, which allows us to devise risk avoidance and risk reduction strategies. This chapter focuses on the opportunities for primary prevention of these three cancers and directions for the future.

CERVICAL CANCER

Risk Factors

Approximately 13,000 new cases of cervical cancer are diagnosed per year in the United States, and over 4,000 women die of the disease. The disease burden is not distributed equally but is overrepresented among African American, Hispanic/Latina, and American Indian women (27). However, the greatest burden of cervical cancer is in the developing countries (**Fig. 6.1**), which account for 86% of the cases and 88% of deaths (28). Traditionally, the most significant factors associated with the risk of cervical cancer have been the number of sexual partners and early onset of sexual activity. This observation has led to the discovery that the primary cause of cervical cancer, and its precursor, intraepithelial lesions, is persistent infection with HPV, which is sexually transmitted. The HPVs comprise a large (over 100 types) family of viruses that infect skin and mucosa (**Fig. 6.2**). Of the approximately 40 HPV types that infect the genital tract, about one-half are associated with anogenital warts that are nononcogenic or are considered to pose a low risk of malignancy. The other half may give rise to a range of anogenital cancers, including cancers of the cervix, vulva, and anus in women, and penis and anus in men, and are referred to as high risk or oncogenic (29). HPV types 16 and 18 alone account for >70% (**Fig. 6.3**) of all cervical cancers.

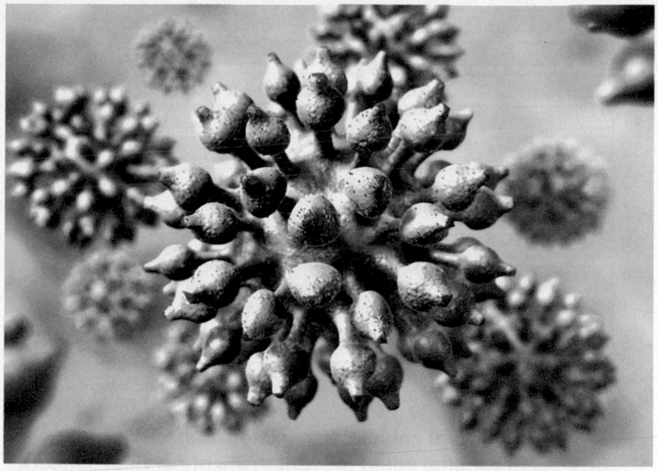

Figure 6.2. Human papillomavirus.

Source: Reprinted from Villa LL. Assessment of new technologies for cervical cancer screening. *Lancet Oncol.* 2008;9:910–911, with permission from Elsevier.

Similarly, HPV types 6 and 11 account for >90% of all anogenital warts. In the United States, where the median age of sexual debut is 17 years, close to 20% of girls are sexually active by age 15 years and close to 60% are sexually active at age 18 years. As a result, the infection rate of HPV among the general population is high, peaking in the second and third decades of life when infection rates range from 27% to 46% (30). The median length of infection is 8 to 12 months, and most individuals have cleared the virus by 2 years. A small proportion, 10% to 13%, however, develop chronic persistent HPV infection, which can lead to genital warts, cervical

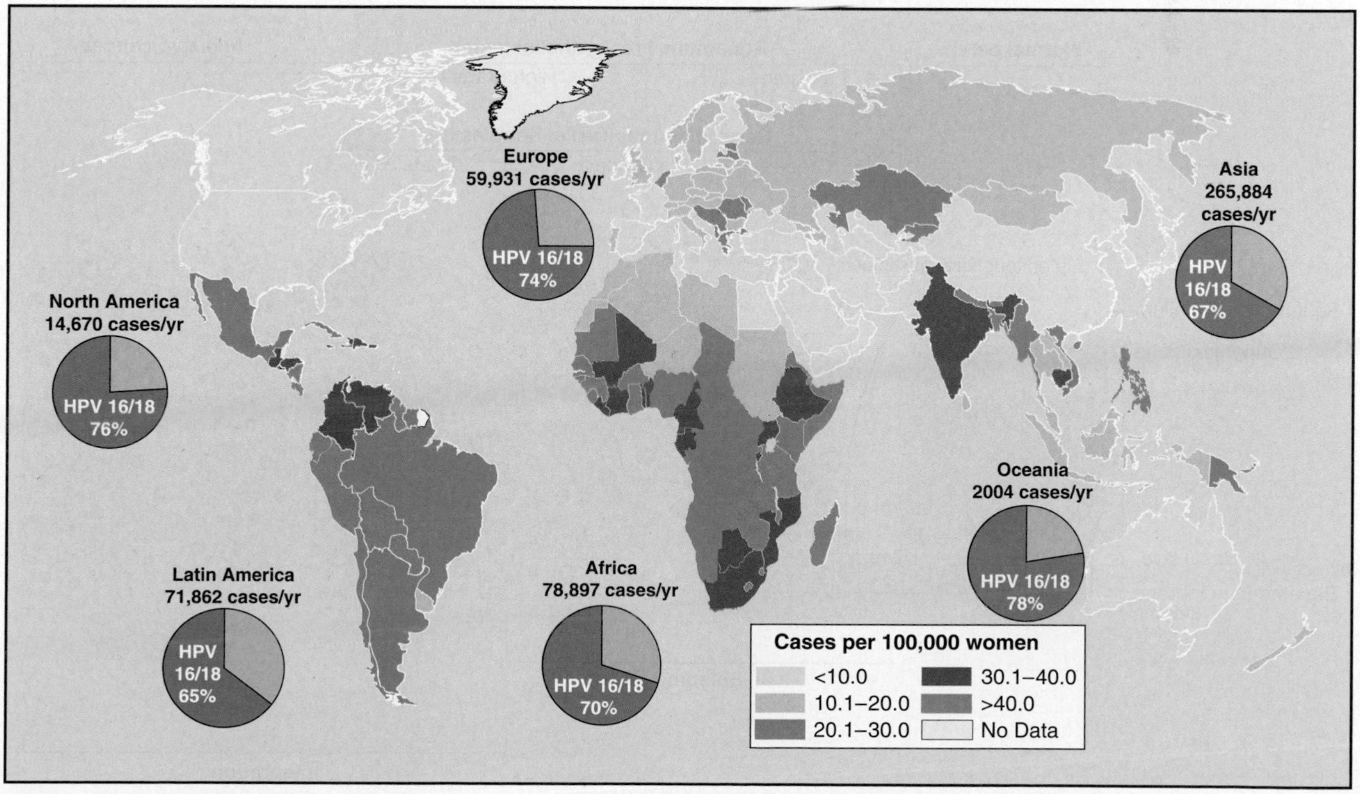

Figure 6.1. Age-standardized rates of new cases of cervical cancer per 100,000 women, 2002.

Source: Reprinted from Agosti JM, Goldie SJ. Introducing HPV vaccine in developing countries—key challenges and issues. *N Engl J Med.* 2007;356:1908–1910, with permission from the Massachusetts Medical Society.

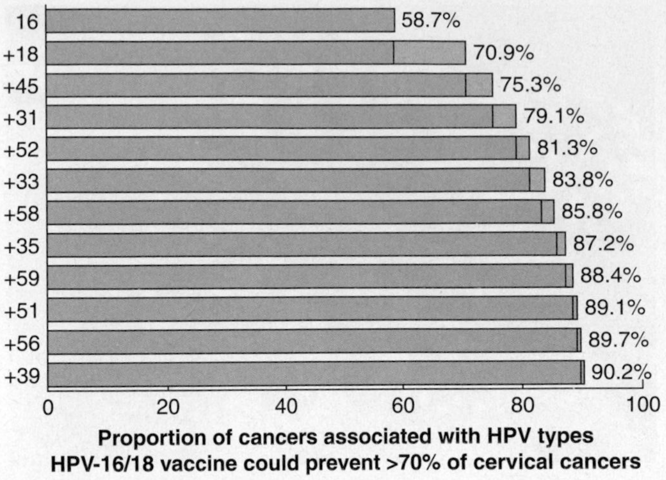

Figure 6.3. HPV types in cervical cancer.

Source: Reprinted from Monk BJ, Mahdavi A. Human papillomavirus vaccine: a new chance to prevent cervical cancer. *Recent Results Cancer Res*. 2007;174:81–90, with permission from Springer.

dysplasia, carcinoma *in situ* (CIS), and invasive cancer (**Fig. 6.4**). Persistence of HPV infection is likely to be related to modifying factors, including immune status, the use of oral contraceptives (OCPs), smoking, and infection with other sexually transmitted diseases (31). Prolonged duration of OCP use is thought to function as a promoter of HPV-related carcinogenesis, not as a facilitator of HPV infection, although the mechanisms are uncertain (32). Tobacco carcinogens have been found in cervical secretions, and it is postulated that smoking constituents may interact with HPV to induce immunologic changes leading to cervical dysplasia, or may produce genomic damage via genotoxins (33,34).

Prevention

Risk Reduction and/or Adoption of Healthy Practices

Cervical cancer prevention requires decreasing the risk of infection with oncogenic strains of HPV. Few sexual partners and the use of condoms have been associated with a reduced risk for cervical cancer (35). Avoidance of factors that enhance the persistence of HPV infection, viz. smoking and OCP use, has the potential to reduce the rate of malignant change. OCPs, however, are the most effective means of contraception, and their avoidance overall is not a wise public health strategy. Safe and effective vaccines now offer the best option for cervical cancer prevention. Early studies in animal models provided the proof of principle that neutralizing antibodies, directed to determinants on the major viral capsid protein, were generated by infection with HPV and could be detected in the serum. In the early 1990s, it was found that the L1 protein, when expressed in recombinant vectors, self-assembled into virus-like particles (VLPs), which closely resemble the antigenic characteristics of the wild-type virions. VLPs formulated on aluminum adjuvants were shown to induce a strong virus-neutralizing antibody response in nonhuman primates (36,37), leading to their development for human populations. A series of phase 1 trials in humans tested the immunogenicity and safety of monovalent VLP-based vaccines and found that they generated levels of neutralizing antibodies that far exceeded those seen in natural infections, and were sustained at long-term follow-up. The predominant antibody responses are of the immunoglobulin G1 (IgG1) subclass (29). In these early trials, vaccine efficacy against infection with HPV-16/18 and against cervical intraepithelial neoplasia (CIN) 2+ at 6.4 years of follow-up was 100% (38).

Subsequently, three vaccines have been developed for use in humans: Gardasil (Merck), a quadrivalent vaccine that includes HPV-16, -18, -6, and -11 and is formulated with aluminum adjuvant; Gardasil 9, which includes five additional oncogenic HPV types;

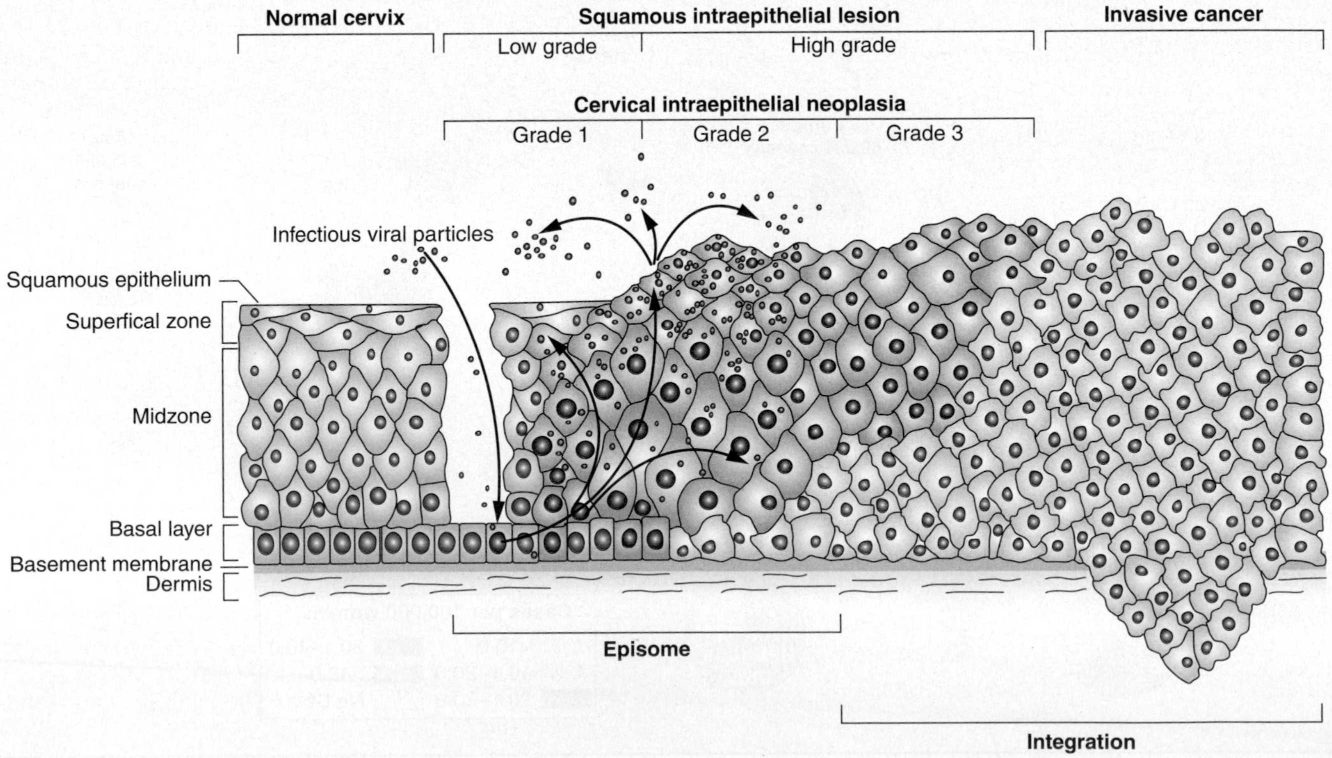

Figure 6.4. HPV-mediated progression to cervical cancer.

Source: Reprinted from Woodman BJW, Collins SI, Young LS. The natural history of cervical HPV infection: unresolved issues. *Nat Rev Cancer.* 2007;7:11–22, with permission from the Nature Publishing Group.

and a bivalent vaccine Cervarix (GlaxoSmithKline), which includes HPV-16 and -18 and is formulated with a proprietary adjuvant, AS04, which contains aluminum and a bacterial lipid. Data from several clinical trials of the quadrivalent vaccine Gardasil reported vaccine efficacy of 99% against CIN grade II–III or adenocarcinoma *in situ*. Protection remains evident 8 years after completion of a three-dose protocol (39). Combined analysis of the FUTURE I and FUTURE II randomized double-blind trials has also demonstrated protection against low-grade HPV-related lesions. At 42 months of follow-up, efficacy in the HPV naïve population was 96% for CIN grade I, 99% for condyloma, and 100% for vulvar and vaginal intraepithelial neoplasia (40).

A recent international randomized, double-blind clinical trial compared the immunogenicity, efficacy, and safety of a new nine-valent HPV vaccine, which includes the original quadrivalent HPV types and five additional oncogenic types, 31, 33, 45, 52, and 58, with the quadrivalent vaccine. The incidence of disease associated with HPV types 6, 11, 16, and 18 was similar in the two groups. There was a 96% reduction in incidence of high-grade cervical, vulvar, and vaginal lesions associated with HPV types 31, 33, 45, 52, and 58 in the nine-valent arm. Nearly 100% of women in the nine-valent arm underwent seroconversion within 1 month of vaccination. The rate of mild to moderate injection-site adverse events was higher in the nine-valent vaccine, and is attributed to an increase in the amount of HPV VLP antigens compared with the quadrivalent vaccine. As the nine types of HPV included in the new vaccine account for 90% of all cervical cancer, the introduction of this vaccine is likely to represent an important advance in the elimination of cervical cancer (41,42).

In June 2006, Gardasil received Food and Drug Administration (FDA) approval for the vaccination of females aged 9 to 26 years, followed closely by approval for its use in children and adults aged 9 to 26 years by the European Commission.

Early studies of the bivalent vaccine Cervarix established its immunogenicity, efficacy, and safety. In the large double-blind randomized trial, the Papilloma Trial against Cancer In young Adults (PATRICIA), high vaccine efficacy for Cervarix was shown among women aged 15 to 25 years against persistent infection and high-grade CIN associated with HPV-16 and -18, with some cross-reactivity with other HPV types. In the final event-driven analysis of PATRICIA, vaccine efficacy was 50%, 70%, and 87% against CIN 1+, CIN 2+, and CIN 3+, respectively, among women negative for evidence of HPV infection at baseline. Among the total vaccinated cohort, which included some women with evidence of previous or current HPV infection, the vaccine prevented 30% and 33% of CIN 2+ and CIN 3+, respectively. Immunogenicity persisted through 36 months of follow-up (43).

The demonstrated efficacy of the HPV vaccines in young women led to similar trials of vaccine efficacy in males, in whom HPV is associated with a significant proportion of anal, penile, and oropharyngeal cancers, as well as anogenital warts. In a randomized, double-blinded, placebo-controlled trial, the quadrivalent HPV vaccine resulted in seroconversion for HPV-6, 11, 16, and 18 in over 97% of vaccinated subjects. Efficacy against external genital lesions associated with these HPV types was 90.4%, and an 85.6% reduction in persistent infection was observed (44). The vaccine is currently recommended for males aged 9 through 26 years.

The Advisory Committee on Immunization Practices (ACIP) of the Centers for Disease Control and Prevention (CDC) recommends routine vaccination for HPV of girls aged 11 to 12 (range, 9 to 26 years) and has added Gardasil to its Vaccines for Children Program (45,46). Similarly, the American Academy of Pediatrics recommends that all girls should be vaccinated against HPV at age 11 to 12 years (47). The more recent data on vaccine efficacy in males have expanded the indication for HPV vaccination to include males. Currently, the CDC recommends a three-dose series of four-valent and nine-valent HPV vaccine for boys and men aged 9 to 26 years.

There are several questions remaining regarding the use of HPV vaccines. The duration of protection afforded by HPV vaccines is not fully known, although data from the large efficacy trials report continuing protection 8 years after completion of the vaccination protocol (39). The need for a booster dose and the degree of cross-reactivity are also unknown. Despite official recommendations for vaccination, and improving insurance coverage for the cost of the vaccine, uptake of at least one dose of HPV vaccine among females in the United States was only 57% in 2013 (48), and rates are even lower among males. One of the factors most strongly related to vaccine uptake is recommendation by a provider. However, surveys have found that only a minority of providers routinely recommends HPV vaccine and the recommendation is often inconsistent, behind schedule, and without urgency (49).

Much work remains to be done to educate the public about HPV and cervical cancer. Recent studies have shown that the majority of women are unaware of the link between HPV and cervical cancer. Awareness of HPV is increased among young women, more educated women, and those with more access to the health care system (50,51). Public health efforts to introduce the vaccine should clearly be accompanied by vigorous educational programs directed at both young women and their parents to increase acceptability and the success of the HPV vaccine program. Since the introduction of Gardasil into clinical care, there has been vigorous debate about the issue of compulsory HPV vaccination. Concerns raised include the lack of long-term safety data, the expense of the vaccine, and resistance to governmental coercion (52). Another concern that parents and other groups have expressed is the fear that vaccination against HPV may lead to a sense of invulnerability, would undermine abstinence-based messages, and may increase high-risk sexual behavior. There is no data, however, to suggest that fear of HPV is an important deterrent from sexual activity in young men or women. Several states have considered legislation to mandate HPV vaccination, although few have actually enacted such laws. All of the proposed laws have opt-out provisions for parents who object. However, they do not address the potential financial burdens imposed by the mandate. Mandating HPV vaccination would certainly boost vaccine coverage rates but at a price of loss of parental autonomy.

These and other vaccine-related concerns will need to be addressed by primary care providers as well as public health officials. Vaccine delivery by primary care practitioners in the United States is approximately 32% among 13- to 17-year-old girls. In contrast, rates of vaccination completion in the UK and Australia, where vaccine programs are school-based, are much higher (≥84% and ≥72%, respectively) (53).

The most significant unresolved issue pertains to the application of HPV vaccines to underdeveloped nations, where the greatest burden of disease attributable to HPV is found (**Fig. 6.5**). Contributing to this burden is a lack of understanding of the dimensions of the disease, weak infrastructures and insufficient funds for population-wide vaccination programs, and lack of political will to address the behavioral and public health issues pertinent to a sexually transmitted disease. The delivery of a new vaccine to a nonpediatric population is particularly problematic in countries with limited public health resources. Yet it is precisely in these countries that the potential benefit for a widespread vaccination program is greatest. Administering the vaccine in infancy along with other basic childhood vaccines may be the best choice, even though the duration of protection is at this time unknown. Clearly, the support of the international community will be required to make HPV vaccination a reality in the third world.

Chemoprevention

Several promising targets for the chemoprevention of cervical cancer have been identified, including topical retinoids, carotenoids, prostaglandins, indole-3-carbinol, green tea, folic acid, and immune modulators (54–56). In phase 1 and 2 trials, topical retinoids applied directly to the cervix resulted in significant complete histologic regression of CIN 2 lesions compared to placebo (57). None of the proposed agents, however, have been subject to definitive phase 3 randomized trials.

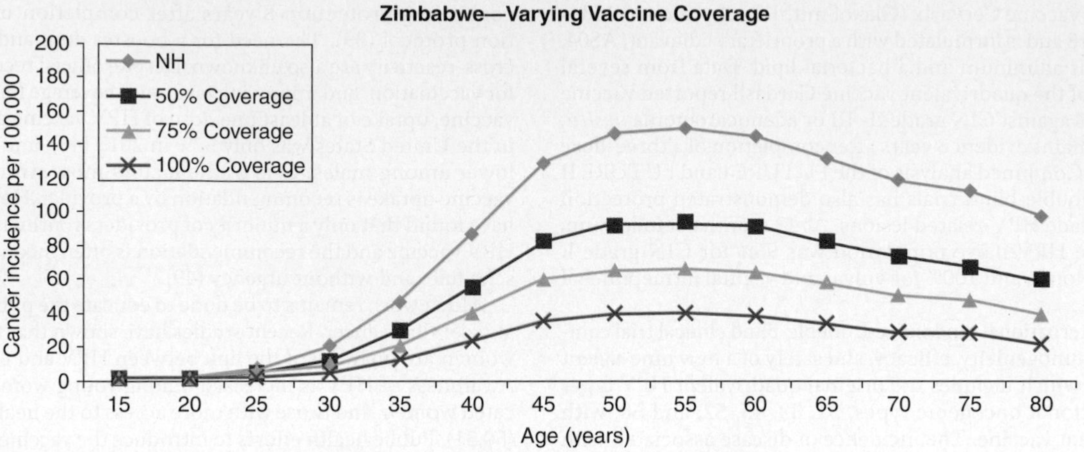

Figure 6.5. Impact of HPV-16/18 vaccines on incidence of cervical cancer.

Surgical Prophylaxis

The introduction of widespread cervical cancer screening using the Papanicolaou (Pap) smear has dramatically reduced the incidence of invasive cervical cancer through the detection of treatable, premalignant lesions, referred to as CIN. Recently, the detection and quantification of oncogenic HPV DNA in cervical epithelial cells has been added to routine Pap screening in selected situations, with demonstrated improvement in sensitivity. Co-testing with HPV DNA detects high-grade lesions earlier, thus providing a subsequent longer low-risk period. HPV screening is recommended in women with atypical squamous cells of undetermined significance (ASCUS) on cytology, co-testing with cytology in asymptomatic women aged 30 years and older, among whom a positive HPV screen is thought to represent persistent infection, and in the follow-up of treated individuals for more aggressive detection and management of persistent HPV infection (30). Its use in asymptomatic women under the age of 30 leads to overdiagnosis because of the transient nature of infection in this age group. Studies of cost-effectiveness of co-testing with HPV DNA and cytology offer a cost saving by allowing for a reduction in the frequency of screening (58). Primary high-risk HPV (hrHPV) screening is being evaluated as an alternative to cytology-based testing (59).

Transient HPV infections are associated with low-grade lesions (CIN 1). When oncogenic HPV infections persist, the viral genome is integrated into the host genome and cervical lesions progress to more advanced lesions (CIN 2 and VIN 3) (60). Because of the high rate of spontaneous regression, management of women with CIN 1 and satisfactory colposcopy (visualization of the entire squamocolumnar junction) is repeat cytology at 6 and 12 months or DNA testing for oncogenic types of HPV at 12 months. Alternatively, ablative (cryotherapy, electrocoagulation, or laser vaporization) or excisional (cold-knife conization or loop electrosurgical excision procedure [LEEP]) treatment may be offered. If the entire squamocolumnar junction cannot be visualized, an excisional procedure is the preferred approach. Treatment of CIN 2–3 lesions with satisfactory colposcopy involves excision or ablation of the entire transformation zone rather than just the colposcopically identified lesion (61). Cryotherapy, laser vaporization, and LEEP all appear to be effective modalities, although over time LEEP has become the procedure most widely chosen. When colposcopy is not satisfactory, a diagnostic excisional procedure is recommended. A variety of posttreatment surveillance protocols utilizing cervical cytology with or without colposcopy and HPV testing at frequent intervals have been proposed. Hysterectomy is reserved for recurrent or persistent biopsy-confirmed CIN 2–3, for positive margins when repeat diagnostic excision is not possible, or for women with persistent CIS who have been previously treated and who no longer desire fertility (62).

This approach to cervical cancer prevention based on large-scale cytologic screening programs is not feasible, however, in countries in the developing world, due to lack of infrastructure, funding, and public health education (**Tables 6.1** and **6.2**).

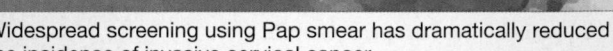

TABLE 6.1. Cervical Cancer—Major Points
Widespread screening using Pap smear has dramatically reduced the incidence of invasive cervical cancer.
Virtually all cervical cancer is related to persistent infection with HPV.
HPV infection is common, affects up to 50% of women, and peaks in the second and third decades of life.
Altered immune status, smoking, and the use of OCPs affect the rate of persistent HPV infection.
Cervical cancer is a leading cause of cancer morbidity and mortality among women in the underdeveloped world.
Three HPV vaccines have shown high efficacy in eliminating persistent HPV infection and cervical lesions in previously uninfected women.

HPV, human papillomavirus; OCPs, oral contraceptives.

TABLE 6.2. Cervical Cancer—Remaining Questions
What is the duration of protection of HPV vaccines?
What is the extent of cross-vaccination with the current HPV vaccines?
What is the sociocultural acceptability of vaccinating adolescent girls?
What is the added benefit of vaccinating males?
What is the impact of effective vaccination on subsequent screening practices and screening performance?
Which methods will best educate the public about HPV vaccines?
How should HPV vaccines be made available to underdeveloped nations?
What are the best cervical cancer screening approaches for use in underdeveloped countries?

HPV, human papillomavirus.

OVARIAN CANCER

Risk Factors

Ovarian cancer is the most common cause of death from a gynecologic cancer in the United States and accounts for approximately 14,180 deaths per year (63). Worldwide there are 238,700 new cases (64) and 157,800 deaths per year (65). Ovarian cancers are categorized as serous, endometrioid, clear cell, and mucinous. These categories are further divided into high grade and low grade. High-grade serous cancer represents the majority of epithelial ovarian cancers (66). Due to a lack of effective screening tools to identify ovarian cancer at early, highly curable stages, the majority of ovarian cancers are diagnosed at advanced stages when survival is poor. Historically, the origin of epithelial ovarian cancer was believed to be from the invagination of ovarian surface epithelium (OSE) into the ovarian stroma forming inclusion cysts, which had the potential to undergo malignant transformation (67). The recent adoption of prophylactic salpingo-oophorectomy for women with deleterious mutations in *BRCA1* and *BRCA2*, however, has challenged that theory. Careful examination of the fallopian tubes obtained at the time of prophylactic surgery has identified a high prevalence of occult primary serous carcinomas and serous tubal intraepithelial carcinomas (STIC) in the fimbrial end of the fallopian tube. Up to 15% of women with *BRCA1/2* mutations who undergo prophylactic bilateral salpingo-oophorectomy (BSO) harbor these lesions in the fallopian tubes (68,69). Both lesions are often accompanied by p53 mutations, also at the fimbriated end of the fallopian tube (70,71), suggesting that STIC is the precursor lesion for invasive ovarian carcinoma. While these changes were originally thought to be present only in women with *BRCA1* or *BRCA2* mutations, there is growing evidence pointing to the existence of these precursor lesions among women who develop sporadic serous ovarian cancer (72). Up to 60% of women with sporadic ovarian cancer may also have STICs or early invasive fallopian tube cancers identified (68). The distal fallopian tube, therefore, is increasingly being seen as the origin of tubal, ovarian, and peritoneal serous ovarian cancer. The fallopian tube is also implicated in the presentation of endometrioid and clear cell ovarian cancers, which are attributed to the passage of endometriosis tissue from the uterus through the fallopian tube to implant on the surface of the ovary or the peritoneum where it can undergo malignant transformation (73).

While our understanding of the biology of epithelial ovarian cancer is rapidly advancing, most of our current knowledge regarding risks for ovarian cancer has emerged from the epidemiologic literature. Advancing age, reproductive factors (specifically, nulliparity), and heredity are established risk factors for the disease. The majority of ovarian cancers are diagnosed after menopause. Rates are higher in nulliparous women, while parity has been found to offer protection. The risk of ovarian cancer is increased twofold in women who are infertile, and the risk appears to be independent of fertility drug treatment (74). Chronic inflammation, with its attendant increase in cell proliferation and potential for DNA disruption, has been proposed as a precursor for many cancers, including ovarian cancer. Endometriosis and pelvic inflammatory disease, both of which induce chronic inflammatory states, and possibly talc are associated with ovarian cancer (75,76).

Although the majority of cases of ovarian cancer are sporadic, up to 20% are thought to fit a hereditary pattern of autosomal dominant inheritance (77). Epidemiologic studies have estimated a two- to fourfold increase in risk among first-degree relatives of women with ovarian cancer. Recently, a number of genes have been identified that account for a large percentage of hereditary ovarian cancer and that allow more precise estimates of risk. Since the identification of *BRCA1* on chromosome 17q in 1994, and *BRCA2* on chromosome 13q in 1995, several hundred mutations in these genes have been characterized, many of which lead to premature truncation of protein transcription and, therefore, presumably defective gene products. Ovarian cancer in these families is characterized by multiple cases of ovarian and breast cancer in successive generations, earlier age of onset, and evidence of both maternal and paternal transmission (**Fig. 6.6**). The penetrance of *BRCA1/2*, that is, the likelihood that a mutation will actually result in ovarian cancer, is estimated to range anywhere from 36% to 46% for *BRCA1* mutation carriers, and from 10% to 27% for *BRCA2* mutation carriers (20). Some mutations may be more specifically related to ovarian cancer risk than others. Ovarian cancer cluster regions have been identified within the *BRCA1* gene from c.1380 to c.4062 (within exon 11) and within the *BRCA2* gene from c.3249 to c.5681 (near c.5946 dekT) and

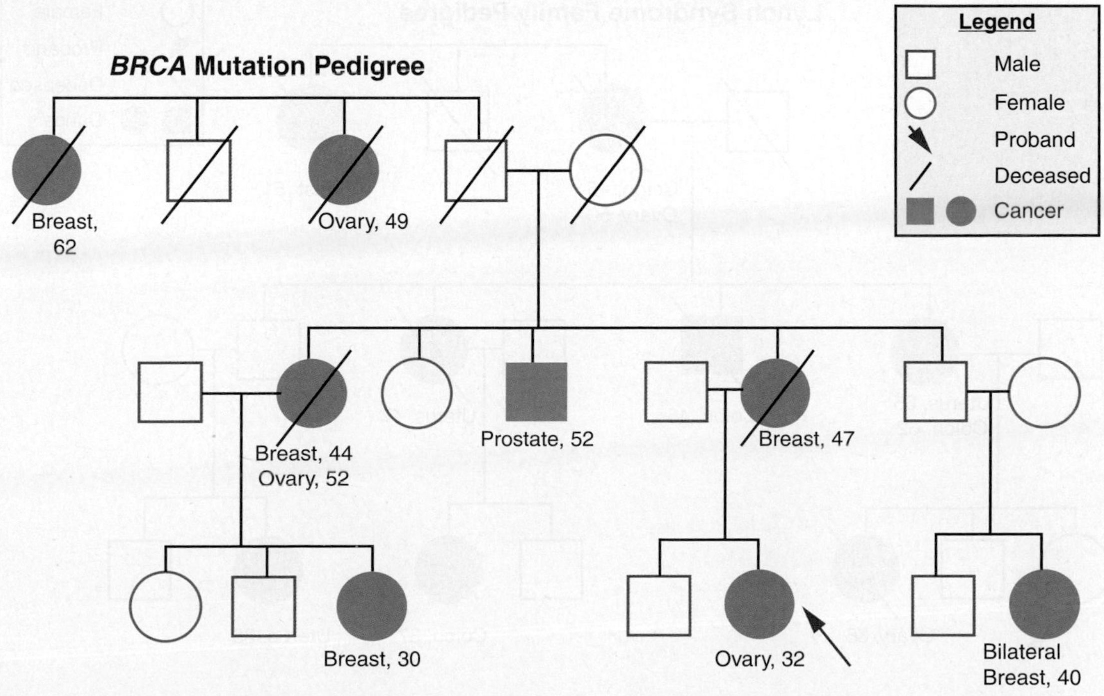

Figure 6.6. Family pedigree illustrating *BRCA* mutation.

from c.6645 to c.7471, which carry a higher risk of ovarian cancer than breast cancer (78). The wide variation in penetrance observed may also reflect the interaction of the genetic mutation with other genetic and/or environmental factors, and suggests that these genes may function as "gatekeepers" and, when lost, allow other genetic alterations to accumulate. Ovarian cancer is also included in the phenotype of the mismatch repair genes (*MSH2, MSH6, MLH1,* and *PMS1*) associated with the hereditary nonpolyposis colon cancer, or Lynch syndrome, in which the lifetime risk for ovarian cancer is estimated to be approximately 12%, and the median age at diagnosis 42.7 years (**Fig. 6.7**). The risk may be highest for women with *MLH1* or *MSH2* mutations, with up to 24% lifetime risk compared with 11% for women for *MSH6* and <10% for *PMS2* (79–81).

With the expansion of next-generation sequencing platforms and commercialization of numerous multigene panels, additional gene mutations have been identified, which may account for an increase of ovarian cancer among women who test negative for *BRCA1/2* and Lynch syndrome. Panel screening affords the opportunity to simultaneously screen for numerous genetic mutations in a single setting and may uncover mutations in less common ovarian cancer susceptibility genes, permitting use of preventive strategies for ovarian cancer. Multigene panel testing, however, may also uncover genetic variants of uncertain significance that can contribute to distress among patients and confusion among providers regarding their true pathogenic potential, and may result in inappropriate use of interventions (82).

A multigene sequencing panel for cancer risk assessment was assessed in a cohort of 198 women referred for clinical *BRCA1/2* testing in the Stanford Clinical Center Genetics program (83). Among 141 who tested negative for *BRCA1/2* mutations, pathogenic variants were identified in *ATM, BLM, CDH1, CDKN2A, MLH1, NBN, PRSS1* and *SLX4*, suggesting that selected patients may benefit from multiple-gene sequencing. Lincoln and colleagues examined a 29-gene panel in 1,105 patients and found pathogenic variants, most commonly in *ATM, PALB2, CHEK2, MLHI, MSH2, MSH6,* and *PMS2* in approximately 4% of *BRCA*-negative ovarian cancer cases (84).

Early data from studies among *BRCA1/2*-negative women suggest that upon retesting with multigene panels, approximately 3% to 5% will have a pathogenic mutation in other genes thought to be associated with breast/ovarian cancer (83,84). Mutations in genes belonging to the BRCA-Fanconi anemia pathway, including *RAD51C, RAD51D, PALB3,* and *BRIP1,* have been identified in *BRCA*-negative patients, and up to 3.5% of unselected ovarian cancers may have a loss of function mutation on one of these four genes. Similar to *BRCA1/2*, these genes are critical for DNA repair of double-stranded breaks via homologous recombination. Odds ratios for all ovarian subtypes were 5.2 (95% CI, 1.1 to 24) for *RAD51C* and 12 (95% CI, 1.5 to 90) for *RAD51D* (85).

BRIP1 mutations are associated with an eightfold increased risk of ovarian cancers and can be found in 1.4% of unselected ovarian cancer cases. The average age at diagnosis is 61.6 years in mutation carriers (86).

The identification of these additional hereditary syndromes of ovarian cancer provides new opportunities to understand the biology of the disease and to devise novel preventive strategies.

Prevention

Risk Avoidance and/or Adoption of Protective Practices

The available evidence regarding factors that lower ovarian cancer risk has been based primarily on the results of case–control studies retrospectively comparing the reproductive, hormonal, or behavioral characteristics of ovarian cancer cases with matched controls, not on prospective randomized trials. These studies have consistently shown an inverse association of ovarian cancer with increasing parity, with the first birth conferring significantly more protection (35%) than subsequent births (15%). The protective effect of pregnancy occurs regardless of fertility history and is not age-dependent (87). Pregnancy is characterized by a prolonged period of anovulation as well as high levels of circulating progesterone, which may cause terminal differentiation of premalignant cells (88,89).

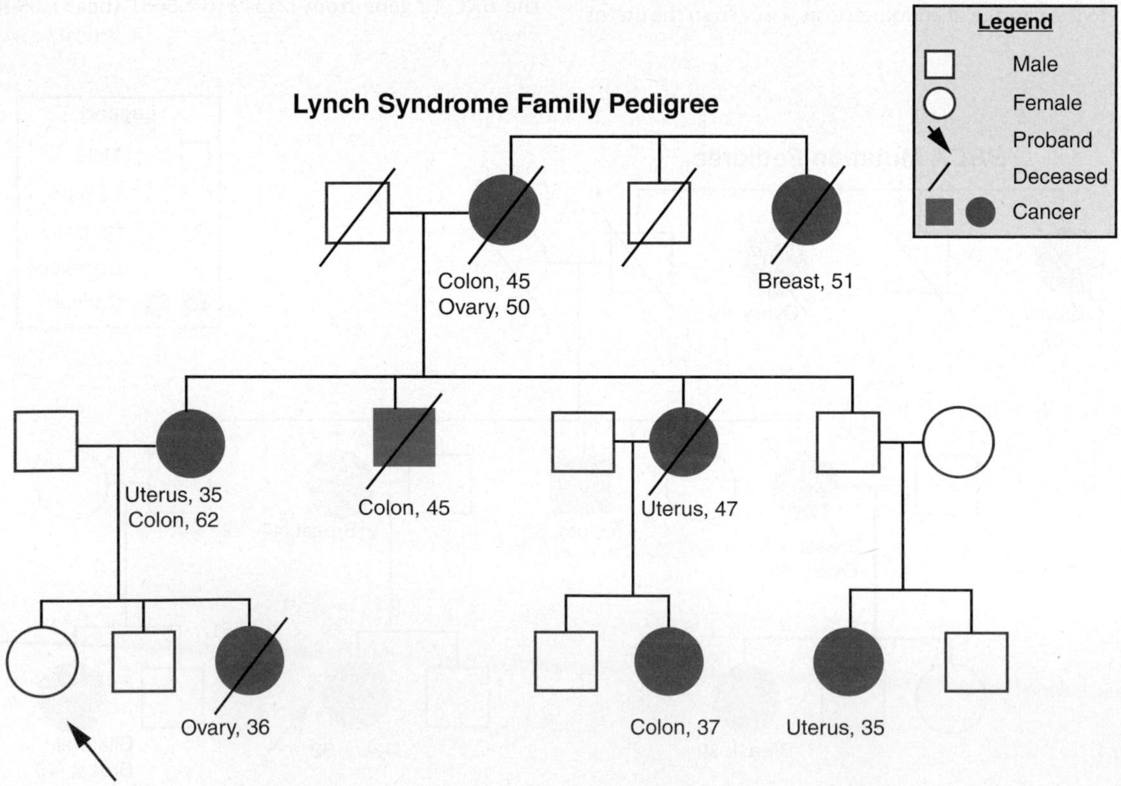

Figure 6.7. Family pedigree illustrating Lynch syndrome.

The evidence supporting a protective effect of breast-feeding against epithelial ovarian cancer risk is weak and inconsistent. Some studies suggest a 10% to 20% decrease in ovarian cancer risk associated with breast-feeding. In the studies that are positive, the impact of breast-feeding on ovarian cancer risk appears to be greatest for the first 6 months of lactation, with longer-term lactation conferring no apparent increase in protective effect (90,91).

Several studies have examined the association of HRT with ovarian cancer risk. While the majority find a modest increase in risk, most lack statistical significance. The strongest association is seen in endometrioid histologies, where relative risks range from 1.2 to 5.5 (92).

Several retrospective and prospective studies have examined associations between dietary factors and ovarian cancer risk. Modest levels of protection have been reported for fruits and vegetables in general, and for vitamin A and β-carotene in particular, although findings are inconsistent. While there is some case–control data that invasive ovarian cancer is reduced among women who report frequent high-intensity exercise, the relationship between physical activity and ovarian cancer risk is inconsistent, and may differ by histologic type (74,93–95).

Chemoprevention

The majority of theoretical models of ovarian cancer chemoprevention have been based on the assumption that the origin of ovarian cancer is the OSE. As the paradigm has shifted to identifying the epithelial surface of the fallopian tube as the site of origin, it is not clear how to interpret the previous theories. Prior research has explored the presence of receptors for most members of the steroid hormone superfamily, including receptors for progestins, retinoids, androgens, and vitamin D. Progestins, retinoids, and vitamin D have been shown to exert a broad range of common biologic effects in epithelial cells, including induction of apoptosis, upregulation of transforming growth factor-β (TGF-β), cellular differentiation, and inhibition of proliferation. In addition to hormonal agents, there is growing evidence that NSAIDs may have ovarian cancer preventive effects (96). *It is yet to be demonstrated that these agents are active in the fallopian tube epithelium.*

To date, only OCP use has been consistently shown to be protective against ovarian cancer. OCPs were first introduced in the United States in the 1960s. Most formulations include estrogen, progesterone, or a combination of the two. In addition to suppressing ovulation, OCPs also reduce pituitary secretion of gonadotropins and protect against chronic inflammation associated with pelvic inflammatory disease (97). In addition to these potential mechanisms, a 3-year study on primates demonstrated that the progestin component of an OCP had a potent effect on apoptotic and TGF-β signaling pathways in the ovarian epithelium, raising the possibility that progestin-mediated biologic effects may underlie the protective effects of OCPs (98). The use of OCPs appears to decrease a woman's risk for ovarian cancer by 30% to 60%. Risk reduction is apparent with as little as 3 months of use, increases in magnitude with increased duration of use, and persists for as long as 10 years after discontinuation of use. The risk reduction applies to nulliparous as well as parous women; to all histologic subtypes, including tumors of low malignant potential; to women with a hereditary risk for ovarian cancer; is consistent across races; and is independent of age at use or menopausal status (72,89,99). Although there has never been a randomized clinical trial to demonstrate the protective effect of OCPs on ovarian cancer risk, it is often recommended empirically to women at high risk for ovarian cancer to reduce their risk.

Epidemiologic and laboratory evidence suggest a potential role for retinoids as preventive agents for ovarian cancer (73). Retinoids are natural and synthetic derivatives of vitamin A. They have great potential for cancer prevention due to a broad range of important biologic effects on epithelial cells, including inhibition of cellular proliferation, induction of cellular differentiation, induction of apoptosis, cytostatic activity, and induction of TGF-β. The most significant evidence supporting a rationale for retinoids as chemopreventive agents for ovarian cancer is that of a chemoprevention study in Italy, which suggested an ovarian cancer preventive effect from the retinoid 4-HPR. Among women randomized to receive either 4-HPR or placebo in a trial designed to evaluate 4-HPR as a chemopreventive for breast carcinoma, significantly fewer ovarian cancer cases were noted in the 4-HPR group as compared to controls (100).

Vitamin D is a fat-soluble vitamin that is essential as a positive regulator of calcium homeostasis. The vitamin D receptor and the retinoic acid receptors share strong homology and readily dimerize, making it likely that vitamin D and retinoids have common signaling pathways in the cell (101). Vitamin D has been shown to have diverse biologic effects in epithelial cells relevant to cancer prevention, including retardation of growth, induction of cellular differentiation, induction of apoptosis, and upregulation of TGF-β (102). With regard to ovarian cancer, a recent study has correlated population-based data regarding ovarian cancer mortality in large cities across the United States with geographically based long-term sunlight data reported by the National Oceanic and Atmospheric Administration. The study demonstrated a statistically significant inverse correlation between regional sunlight exposure and ovarian mortality risk suggesting that sunlight induces production of native vitamin D in the skin (103). However, a systematic review of 20 ecologic and case–control studies failed to find consistent evidence for a relationship between vitamin D exposure and ovarian cancer incidence or mortality (104).

Epidemiologic studies have suggested that use of NSAIDs may lower ovarian cancer risk (105). Several biologic mechanisms have been proposed to account for the chemopreventive effects of NSAIDs, including inhibition of ovulation, inhibition of COX, and downregulation of prostaglandins, enhancement of the immune response, and induction of apoptosis (89,106,107). Similarly, dietary antioxidants have shown an inverse association with ovarian cancer (108). The role of β-blockers has recently been examined in ovarian cancer patients as a means to decreased adrenergic activation and thus decrease ovarian cancer growth and metastasis and has been associated with a significant improvement in overall survival (109). The role of β-blockers for chemoprevention of ovarian cancer has yet to be defined. Despite a growing body of preclinical data indicating chemopreventive effects of several agents, clinical research exploring their efficacy to reduce rates of ovarian cancer is hindered by the relatively low incidence of the disease, insufficient understanding of the preclinical course of ovarian cancer, the lack of validated preclinical biomarkers, and inadequate screening strategies.

Surgical Prophylaxis

For women with a family history of ovarian cancer, or a hereditary pattern of breast cancer, BSO has been shown to lower the risk of subsequent epithelial ovarian cancer by 80% to 95% (20,110). Prospective follow-up of a large international cohort of 2,482 *BRCA* carriers found not only a lower risk of ovarian cancer, but also a significantly lower all-cause mortality (HR 0.40; 95% CI, 0.26–0.61) and ovarian cancer–specific mortality (HR 0.21; 95% CI, 0.06–0.76). There is also a 50% reduction in rates of breast cancer in women who undergo prophylactic BSO (111). Occult invasive and *in situ* tumors have been found at the time of BSO in 2% to 10% of *BRCA1/2* mutation carriers (112), a large proportion of which occur in the fimbrial end of the fallopian tube (97,113), emphasizing the need for both deliberate removal of the fallopian tubes at the time of prophylactic surgery and of careful pathologic examination of the surgical specimen (114). The incidence of primary peritoneal cancer following BSO is reported to be approximately 2% to 5% (115). Because the median age of diagnosis of ovarian cancer among women with a hereditary risk is 50 years for *BRCA1* carriers and 60 years for *BRCA2* carriers, the recommended age for prophylactic surgery is at the completion of childbearing, or between age 35 and 40 years for *BRCA1* carriers and 40 and 45 years for *BRCA2* carriers (116). Although the incidence of premenopausal ovarian cancer is higher in *BRCA1* carriers than *BRCA2* carriers, removal of the ovaries before menopause is recommended for both groups given the added benefit of breast cancer risk reduction, which is highest for women who undergo the surgery before natural menopause (28). In addition, because there is an approximate 15% risk of ovarian cancer after age 60 years among *BRCA* carriers, BSO is also justified at older ages for women who still have intact ovaries (117). Women undergoing prophylactic hysterectomy for a deleterious mutation related to Lynch syndrome are also counseled to remove their ovaries because of the approximate 10% to 12% incidence of ovarian cancer (118).

In addition to the significant reduction in ovarian cancer incidence associated with BSO, several studies have found a significant decline in ovarian cancer worry and anxiety following the procedure (119). These potential benefits of prophylactic oophorectomy must, however, be weighed against its adverse consequences, including the short- and long-term surgical risks, the physical and psychological impact of early menopause, and the potential subsequent risks of cardiovascular disease and osteoporosis related to early estrogen/progesterone depletion (120). Although the use of combined estrogen/progesterone HRT has been associated with an increased risk for breast cancer among postmenopausal women in the general population, one study with short follow-up found no increased risk of breast cancer among *BRCA1/2* mutation carriers who took HRT following BSO (121). Also, data from the Mayo Clinic showed that there was no increase in breast cancer among women under the age of 50 years undergoing BSO (122). Women seeking information regarding prophylactic oophorectomy should be counseled about the practical short- and long-term sequelae of the surgery, the risks and benefits of postoperative HRT, and the small potential for primary peritoneal cancer.

Given the recent evidence that a majority of ovarian cancers arise in the fimbrial end of the fallopian tube, alternative surgical procedures, including radical fimbriectomy as well as bilateral salpingectomy with delayed oophorectomy have been introduced. The principle is that complete removal of both fallopian tubes will remove the source of the premalignant changes in the fallopian tube, which give rise to serous ovarian cancer. In addition, removing the tubes will prevent any endometrial tissue from reaching the ovary or peritoneal cavity. These surgical procedures have been proposed as a temporary solution which will prolong the production of ovarian hormone for *BRCA1/2* carriers, thus postponing the onset of premature menopause (123,124). Because prospective data to establish the efficacy of this approach are lacking, and because there is still a proportion of ovarian cancer that may arise out of inclusion cysts in the ovary, radical fimbriectomy or salpingectomy alone are not considered standard of care and are discouraged outside of a clinical trial by current National Comprehensive Cancer Network (NCCN) guidelines. However, salpingectomy could be considered in place of tubal ligation among those women desiring permanent sterilization or among those undergoing hysterectomy for benign indications. This is referred to as opportunistic salpingectomy by some. Tubal ligation has been associated with lower ovarian cancer risk in both case–control and cohort studies. A strong inverse association was observed between tubal ligation and ovarian cancer risk in the Nurses Health Study, with a relative risk (RR) of 0.33 (CI, 0.16–0.64) after controlling for age, OCP use, and parity (125). A recent meta-analysis of 13 case–control, retrospective, and prospective studies found that tubal ligation reduced the risk of invasive epithelial ovarian cancer by 34% (RR, 0.66; 95% CI, 0.60–0.73) (126). The International *BRCA1/2* Carrier Cohort Study found a 52% reduction in ovarian cancer among *BRCA1* carriers who had undergone tubal ligation (72). Proposed mechanisms include changes in local or circulating hormones, reduced access of carcinogens to the ovary, or a reduction in inflammatory processes. As it appears that a significant proportion of ovarian cancers arise in the fallopian tube, tubal ligation may reduce the risk by compromising the blood supply to the fimbrial end of the fallopian tube. Although the protective effect of tubal ligation appears to be substantial, the ability to perform BSO using a laparoscopic approach would seem to make this procedure a preferable choice among women with an increased risk of ovarian cancer (**Tables 6.3** and **6.4**).

TABLE 6.3. Ovarian Cancer—Major Points

Several risk factors, including age, nulliparity, and family history, have been identified for ovarian cancer.
Germ-line mutations in the *BRCA1/2* genes and the DNA mismatch repair genes associated with Lynch syndrome significantly increase the risk of ovarian cancer
The fimbrial end of the fallopian tube, not the OSE, has been identified as the source of most serous ovarian cancers.
OCPs confer significant protection from ovarian cancer, and the level of protection is related to the duration of use.
Tubal ligation also confers significant protection from ovarian cancer, although the physiologic mechanism is unknown.
Prophylactic BSO is the most effective method of preventing ovarian cancer in women with a hereditary pattern of ovarian cancer.
Radical fimbriectomy has been proposed as a temporary alternative to BSO in high-risk women to forestall surgical menopause.
Opportunistic salpingectomy has been proposed as a reasonable prophylactic measure among women undergoing tubal ligation or hysterectomy for benign conditions.

OCPs, oral contraceptives.

TABLE 6.4. Ovarian Cancer—Remaining Questions

What is the duration of latent, preclinical ovarian cancer?
Can effective screening strategies, using biomarkers and/or imaging studies, be identified?
Are there effective chemopreventive agents that will reduce the risk of ovarian cancer?
What degree of protection from ovarian cancer does radical fimbriectomy confer?

Because of the risk reduction associated with BSO among high-risk women, some have advocated the routine removal of the ovaries among all women undergoing hysterectomy for benign conditions. However, data do not support the removal of the ovaries at the time of hysterectomy for benign disease in women at average risk of ovarian cancer, among whom the negative cardiovascular and metabolic impact of early surgical menopause outweighs any potential benefit (127,128). However, opportunistic salpingectomy is reasonable in this population.

ENDOMETRIAL CANCER

Risk Factors

Endometrial cancer is the most common gynecologic cancer in the United States. Over 54,870 new cases are diagnosed each year, and there are 10,170 deaths annually (27). Unlike many other tumors, the incidence and mortality from endometrial cancer is increasing, with a lifetime risk of 2.7% and a 16% risk of death (129–131). The increasing incidence of endometrial cancer is thought by some to be related to an overall increased life expectancy and the increased prevalence of obesity (132). Globally, endometrial cancer is more common in more developed countries than less developed countries (64). The relatively low-case fatality rate is due to early detection and treatment of early-stage disease. The majority of risk factors associated with type 1 (endometrioid) endometrial cancer, increased age, nulliparity, early age at menarche, late age at menopause, obesity, long-term use of unopposed estrogen replacement therapy, polycystic ovary syndrome, and the use of tamoxifen are all thought to exert their effect through estrogen-induced endometrial proliferation leading to hyperplasia and malignant transformation. The increased risk associated with diabetes, hypertension, and thyroid disease also suggests a role for altered growth hormone pathways in addition to the steroid hormone pathways (**Fig. 6.8**). Genetic syndromes account for approximately 5% of all endometrial cancer cases. Women with germ-line mutations in the DNA repair genes associated with the HNPCC or Lynch syndrome have a 40% to 60% risk of endometrial cancer. The mean age at diagnosis in this group is approximately 50 years (81). Epigenetic silencing of the Lynch syndrome genes by hypermethylation is also thought to contribute to endometrial cancer risk (133). Recently, universal screening of endometrial cancers using immunohistochemical staining and/or microsatellite instability staining has been adopted by many centers to identify women at risk for Lynch syndrome. Endometrial cancer is also a component of Cowden syndrome, in which it is estimated that mutations in the *PTEN* gene confer a lifetime risk for endometrial cancer of approximately 19% to 28%, with the increased risk occurring mainly before the age of 50 (134). Type 2 serous endometrial cancer is uncommon and is not related to unopposed estrogen exposure.

Prevention

Risk Avoidance and Uptake of Protective Behaviors

It has been estimated that approximately 40% of endometrial cancers are attributable to excess body weight of many patients in developed countries (132) (**Fig. 6.9**). Maintenance of ideal body weight, regular physical activity, and control of diseases associated with endometrial cancer (diabetes, hypertension, and thyroid disease) are prudent approaches to reduce disease risk. Vigorous physical activity helps to control, prevent, or reverse weight gain; improve insulin sensitivity; and reduce circulating estrogen levels, thus leading to a 22% reduction in endometrial cancer (135). Tamoxifen is a proven chemotherapeutic strategy to reduce the incidence of breast cancer in women at increased risk. While acting as an estrogen antagonist in the glandular epithelium of the breast, tamoxifen acts as an agonist in the endometrium, increasing the risk of postmenopausal bleeding, endometrial hyperplasia, endometrial polyps, and endometrial cancer. Although the absolute numbers were small, the RRs for endometrial cancer in the National Surgical Adjuvant Breast and Bowel Project (NSABP) Breast Cancer Prevention Trial (BCPT) for women on the tamoxifen arm compared to placebo were 2.53 (95% CI, 1.35–4.97) for all women, and 4.01 (95% CI, 1.70–10.90) for women aged 50 years and older (136). Women considering the use of tamoxifen for breast cancer risk reduction should carefully weigh the greater-than-twofold risk of endometrial cancer with the benefits as they make their decision (137). Women experiencing abnormal uterine bleeding while taking tamoxifen for chemoprevention of breast cancer should be instructed to seek immediate gynecologic evaluation to exclude endometrial hyperplasia or malignancy.

Chemoprevention

The addition of a progestin to the estrogen component of HRT has been shown to eliminate the increased risk of endometrial cancer. Progesterone controls many pathways resulting in growth inhibition and tissue homeostasis, and reverses the estrogen effect on the endometrium, thus preventing the development of hyperplasia. The use of combined estrogen and progesterone OCP decreases the risk of endometrial cancer by 50%, although their effectiveness in obese women is not clear (138). For every 5 years of OCP use, the risk of endometrial

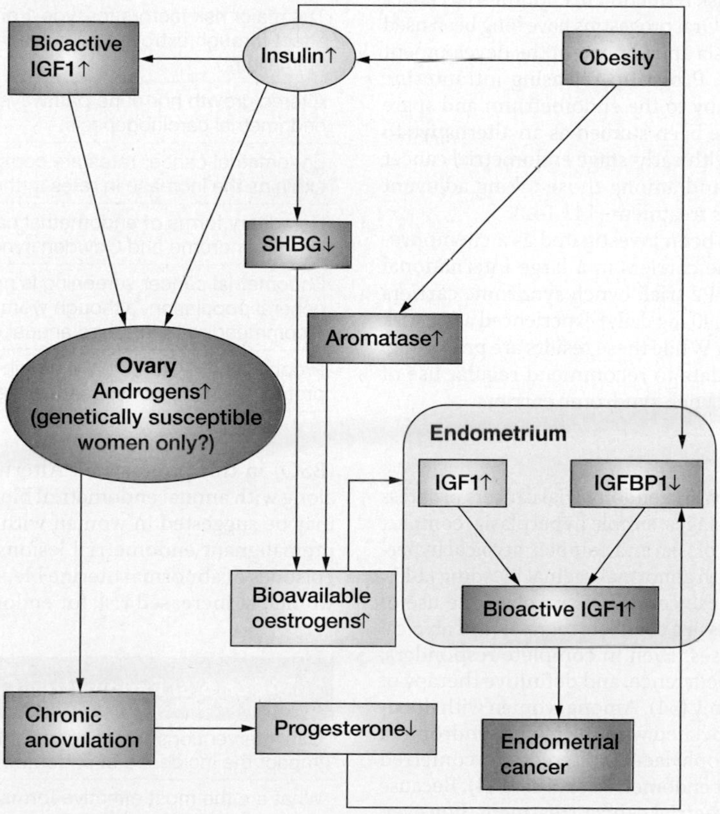

Figure 6.8. Molecular pathways involved in obesity and endometrial cancer. IGF, insulin-like growth factor; IGFBP, insulin-like growth factor-binding protein; SHBG, sex hormone-binding globulin.

Source: Reprinted from Fader AN, Arriba LN, Frasure HE, et al. Endometrial cancer and obesity: epidemiology, biomarkers, prevention and survivorship. *Gynecol Oncol.* 2009;114:121–127, with permission from Elsevier.

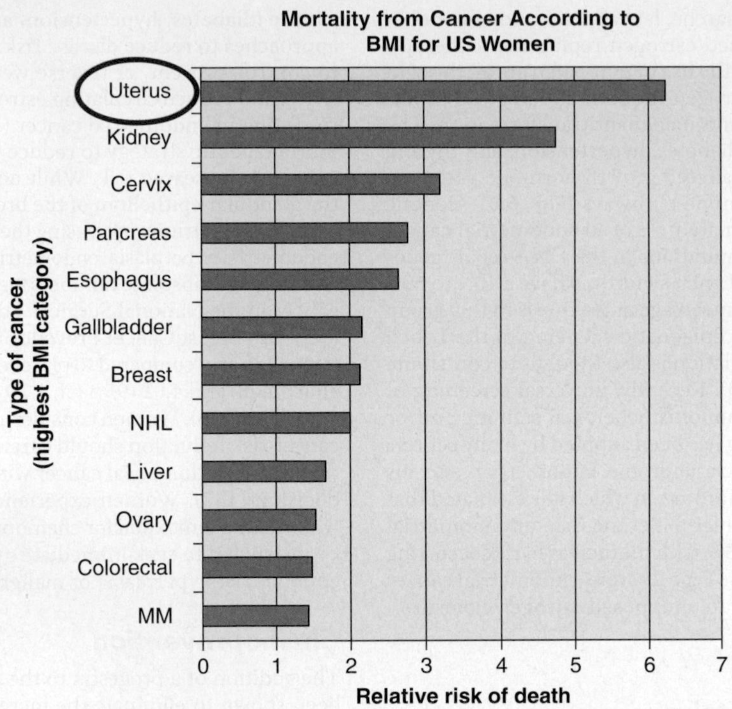

Figure 6.9. Relative risk of death among US women by body mass index (BMI). MM, multiple myeloma; NHL, non-Hodgkin lymphoma.
Source: Reprinted from Fader AN, Arriba LN, Frasure HE, et al. Endometrial cancer and obesity: epidemiology, biomarkers, prevention and survivorship. *Gynecol Oncol.* 2009;114:121–127, with permission from Elsevier.

cancer may decrease by 24%, and this risk reduction may persist for more than 30 years after OCP use (139). Women with Lynch syndrome can experience greater than 60% risk reduction in endometrial cancer with use of OCP for ≥1 year (140). Oral progestins have long been used to reverse premalignant hyperplasia and to prevent the development of endometrial carcinoma (130). Progestin-releasing intrauterine devices, which deliver local therapy to the endometrium and spare some of the systemic effects, have been studied as an alternative to oral progestins both for women with early-stage endometrial cancer who desire to preserve fertility and among those taking adjuvant tamoxifen following breast cancer treatment (141,142).

Daily aspirin use has recently been investigated as a chemopreventive agent in Lynch syndrome carriers in a large international randomized trial (7). In the CAPP2 trial, Lynch syndrome carriers who were randomized to aspirin (600 mg daily) experienced a 30% risk reduction in extracolonic tumors. While these results are promising, there is currently not sufficient data to recommend regular use of aspirin for chemoprevention in Lynch syndrome carriers.

Surgical Prophylaxis

It is thought that the majority of invasive endometrial cancers progress through a series of premalignant stages, simple hyperplasia, complex hyperplasia, simple atypical hyperplasia, and complex atypical hyperplasia, all of which may present with abnormal vaginal bleeding (143). Conservative management of these conditions involves the use of progestational agents, which results in a complete regression of atypical hyperplasia in 50% to 94% of cases. Even in complete responders, however, there is a high rate of recurrence, and definitive therapy of atypical hyperplasia is hysterectomy (54). Among women with documented germ-line mutations associated with the Lynch syndrome, a retrospective study found that prophylactic hysterectomy conferred 100% protection from subsequent endometrial cancer (144). Because of the high success rate for endometrial cancer treatment, however, it is not clear if this protection would translate into a significant survival benefit. This study also found 100% protection from ovarian cancer, which may warrant the consideration of prophylactic total abdominal hysterectomy (TAH)–bilateral salpingo-oophorectomy (BSO) in this population. Alternatively, transvaginal ultrasound along with annual endometrial biopsies starting at age 30 to 35 years may be suggested in women with Lynch syndrome to detect early, premalignant endometrial lesions (145) (**Tables 6.5** and **6.6**). Any episodes of abnormal uterine bleeding should prompt evaluation in women at increased risk for endometrial cancer.

TABLE 6.5. Endometrial Cancer—Major Points
The major risk factors for type 1 endometrial cancer exert their effect through estrogen stimulation of the endometrial surface epithelium.
Altered growth hormone pathways may also be involved in endometrial carcinogenesis.
Endometrial cancer rates are correlated with obesity, which explains the increase in rates in the United States and globally.
Hereditary forms of endometrial cancer have been associated with Lynch syndrome and Cowden syndrome.
Endometrial cancer screening is not recommended for the general population, although women with a hereditary risk are recommended to undergo annual endometrial biopsy.
Prophylactic hysterectomy in high-risk women has been shown to protect women from subsequent endometrial cancer.

TABLE 6.6. Endometrial Cancer—Remaining Questions
Can interventions targeting weight control and physical activity impact the incidence of endometrial cancer?
What are the most effective forms of progesterone-containing contraceptive preparations for reducing the incidence of endometrial cancer?
Does prophylactic hysterectomy in hereditary cases translate into a survival benefit?

FUTURE DIRECTIONS

The prevention of gynecologic malignancies involves many disciplines and requires the collaboration of basic scientists, clinicians, behavioral scientists, and policy makers. The successful development of the HPV vaccines is a major breakthrough in the prevention of cervical cancer and will likely undergo further improvements and refinements. Advances in molecular genetics, molecular pathology, and molecular imaging will contribute to the early identification of specific markers of premalignant change associated with gynecologic malignancies. The identification of safe and effective chemopreventive agents will provide additional strategies for prevention. Accompanying this progress will be the need to address the psychosocial and cultural barriers to the adoption of preventive strategies.

REFERENCES

1. Dart H, Wolin KY, Colditz GA. Commentary: eight ways to prevent cancer: a framework for effective prevention messages for the public. *Cancer Causes Control*. 2012;23(4):601–608.
2. Meyer J, Rohrmann S, Bopp M, et al. Impact of smoking and excess body weight on overall and site-specific cancer mortality risk. *Cancer Epidem Biomar*. 2015;24(10):1516–1522.
3. Bala MM, Lesniak W. Efficacy of non-pharmacological methods used for treating tobacco dependence: meta-analysis. *Pol Arch Med Wewn*. 2007;117(11–12):504–511.
4. Bala MM, Lesniak W, Strzeszynski L. Efficacy of pharmacological methods used for treating tobacco dependence: meta-analysis. *Pol Arch Med Wewn*. 2008;118(1–2):20–28.
5. Christensen JD, Chiles C. Low-dose computed tomographic screening for lung cancer. *Clin Chest Med*. 2015;36(2):147–160, vii.
6. Moyer VA, U.S. Preventive Services Task Force. Screening for lung cancer: U.S. Preventive Services Task Force recommendation statement. *Ann Intern Med*. 2014;160(5):330–338.
7. Burn J, Gerdes AM, Macrae F, et al. Long-term effect of aspirin on cancer risk in carriers of hereditary colorectal cancer: an analysis from the CAPP2 randomised controlled trial. *Lancet*. 2011;378(9809):2081–2087.
8. Chan AT, Ogino S, Fuchs CS. Aspirin use and survival after diagnosis of colorectal cancer. *JAMA*. 2009;302(6):649–659.
9. Chan AT, Giovannucci EL. Primary prevention of colorectal cancer. *Gastroenterology*. 2010;138(6):2029–2043.e10.
10. Levin B, Lieberman DA, McFarland B, et al. Screening and surveillance for the early detection of colorectal cancer and adenomatous polyps, 2008: a joint guideline from the American Cancer Society, the US Multi-Society Task Force on Colorectal Cancer, and the American College of Radiology. *CA Cancer J Clin*. 2008;58(3):130–160.
11. Advani P, Moreno-Aspitia A. Current strategies for the prevention of breast cancer. *Breast Cancer*. 2014;6:59–71.
12. Vogel VG, Costantino JP, Wickerham DL, et al. Update of the National Surgical Adjuvant Breast and Bowel Project Study of Tamoxifen and Raloxifene (STAR) P-2 trial: preventing breast cancer. *Cancer Prev Res*. 2010;3(6):696–706.
13. Fisher B, Costantino JP, Wickerham DL, et al. Tamoxifen for the prevention of breast cancer: current status of the National Surgical Adjuvant Breast and Bowel Project P-1 study. *J Natl Cancer Inst*. 2005;97(22):1652–1662.
14. Cuzick J, Sestak I, Cawthorn S, et al. Tamoxifen for prevention of breast cancer: extended long-term follow-up of the IBIS-I breast cancer prevention trial. *Lancet Oncol*. 2015;16(1):67–75.
15. Cuzick J, Sestak I, Forbes JF, et al. Anastrozole for prevention of breast cancer in high-risk postmenopausal women (IBIS-II): an international, double-blind, randomised placebo-controlled trial. *Lancet*. 2014;383(9922):1040–1048.
16. Goss PE, Ingle JN, Ales-Martinez JE, et al. Exemestane for breast-cancer prevention in postmenopausal women. *N Engl J Med*. 2011;364(25):2381–2391.
17. Chlebowski RT, Anderson GL, Gass M, et al. Estrogen plus progestin and breast cancer incidence and mortality in postmenopausal women. *JAMA*. 2010;304(15):1684–1692.
18. Majumdar SR, Almasi EA, Stafford RS. Promotion and prescribing of hormone therapy after report of harm by the Women's Health Initiative. *JAMA*. 2004;292(16):1983–1988.
19. Heemskerk-Gerritsen BA, Menke-Pluijmers MB, Jager A, et al. Substantial breast cancer risk reduction and potential survival benefit after bilateral mastectomy when compared with surveillance in healthy BRCA1 and BRCA2 mutation carriers: a prospective analysis. *Ann Oncol*. 2013;24(8):2029–2035.
20. Rebbeck TR, Kauff ND, Domchek SM. Meta-analysis of risk reduction estimates associated with risk-reducing salpingo-oophorectomy in BRCA1 or BRCA2 mutation carriers. *J Natl Cancer Inst*. 2009;101(2):80–87.
21. Friedewald SM, Rafferty EA, Rose SL, et al. Breast cancer screening using tomosynthesis in combination with digital mammography. *JAMA*. 2014;311(24):2499–2507.
22. Boetes C. Update on screening breast MRI in high-risk women. *Obstet Gynecol Clin North Am*. 2011;38(1):149–158, viii–ix.
23. Berg WA, Zhang Z, Lehrer D, et al. Detection of breast cancer with addition of annual screening ultrasound or a single screening MRI to mammography in women with elevated breast cancer risk. *JAMA*. 2012;307(13):1394–1404.
24. Thompson IM Jr., Cabang AB, Wargovich MJ. Future directions in the prevention of prostate cancer. *Nat Rev Clin Oncol*. 2014;11(1):49–60.
25. Sandhu GS, Nepple KG, Tanagho YS, et al. Prostate cancer chemoprevention. *Semin Oncol*. 2013;40(3):276–285.
26. Moyer VA, U.S. Preventive Services Task Force. Screening for prostate cancer: U.S. Preventive Services Task Force recommendation statement. *Ann Intern Med*. 2012;157(2):120–134.
27. Torre LA, Siegel RL, Ward EM, et al. Global cancer incidence and mortality rates and trends-an update. *Cancer Epidemiol Biomarkers Prev*. 2016;25(1):16–27.
28. Sahasrabuddhe VV, Parham GP, Mwanahamuntu MH, et al. Cervical cancer prevention in low- and middle-income countries: feasible, affordable, essential. *Cancer Prev Res*. 2012;5(1):11–17.
29. Stanley M. HPV vaccines. *Best Pract Res Clin Obstet Gynaecol*. 2006;20(2):279–293.
30. Saslow D, Solomon D, Lawson HW, et al. American Cancer Society, American Society Colposcopy and Cervical Pathology, and American Society for Clinical Pathology screening guideline for the prevention and early detection of cervical cancer. *CA Cancer J Clin*. 2012;62(3):147–172.
31. Garland SM, Quinn MA. How to manage and communicate with patients about HPV? *Int J Gynecol Obstet*. 2006;94:S106–S112.
32. Moreno V, Bosch FX, Munoz N, et al. Effect of oral contraceptives on risk of cervical cancer in women with human papillomavirus infection: the IARC multicentric case-control study. *Lancet*. 2002;359(9312):1085–1092.
33. McCann MF, Irwin DE, Walton LA, et al. Nicotine and cotinine in the cervical mucus of smokers, passive smokers, and nonsmokers. *Cancer Epidemiol Biomarkers Prev*. 1992;1(2):125–129.
34. McIntyre-Seltman K, Castle PE, Guido R, et al, ALTS Group. Smoking is a risk factor for cervical intraepithelial neoplasia grade 3 among oncogenic human papillomavirus DNA-positive women with equivocal or mildly abnormal cytology. *Cancer Epidemiol Biomarkers Prev*. 2005;14(5):1165–1170.
35. Bailey J, Cymet TC. Planning for the HPV vaccine and its impact on cervical cancer prevention. *Compr Ther*. 2006;32(2):102–105.
36. Lowe RS, Brown DR, Bryan JT, et al. Human papillomavirus type II (HPV-11) neutralizing antibodies in the serum and genital mucosal secretions of African green monkeys immunized with HPV-11 virus-like particles expressed in yeast. *J Infect Dis*. 1997;176(5):1141–1145.
37. Palker TJ, Monteiro JM, Martin MM, et al. Antibody, cytokine and cytotoxic T lymphocyte responses in chimpanzees immunized with human papillomavirus virus-like particles. *Vaccine*. 2001;19(27):3733–3743.
38. Romanowski B, de Borba PC, Naud PS, et al. Sustained efficacy and immunogenicity of the human papillomavirus (HPV)-16/18 AS04-adjuvanted vaccine: analysis of a randomised placebo-controlled trial up to 6.4 years. *Lancet*. 2009;374(9706):1975–1985.
39. Nicol AF, de Andrade CV, Russomano FB, et al. HPV vaccines: their pathology-based discovery, benefits, and adverse effects. *Ann Diagn Pathol*. 2015;19(6):418–422.
40. Future I/II Study Group, Dillner J, Kjaer SK, et al. Four year efficacy of prophylactic human papillomavirus quadrivalent vaccine against low grade cervical, vulvar, and vaginal intraepithelial neoplasia and anogenital warts: randomised controlled trial. *BMJ*. 2010;341:c3493.
41. Cuzick J. Gardasil 9 joins the fight against cervix cancer. *Expert Rev Vaccines*. 2015;14(8):1047–1049.
42. Joura EA, Giuliano AR, Iversen OE, et al. A 9-valent HPV vaccine against infection and intraepithelial neoplasia in women. *N Engl J Med*. 2015;372(8):711–723.
43. Apter D, Wheeler CM, Paavonen J, et al. Efficacy of human papillomavirus 16 and 18 (HPV-16/18) AS04-adjuvanted vaccine against cervical infection and precancer in young women: final event-driven analysis of the randomized, double-blind PATRICIA trial. *Clin Vaccine Immunol*. 2015;22(4):361–373.

44. Giuliano AR, Palefsky JM, Goldstone S, et al. Efficacy of quadrivalent HPV vaccine against HPV infection and disease in males. *N Engl J Med.* 2011;364(5):401–411.
45. Markowitz LE, Dunne EF, Saraiya M, et al. Quadrivalent human papillomavirus vaccine: recommendations of the Advisory Committee on Immunization Practices (ACIP). *MMWR Recomm Rep.* 2007;56(RR-2):1–24.
46. Charo RA. Politics, parents, and prophylaxis - mandating HPV vaccination in the United States. *N Engl J Med.* 2007;356(19):1905–1908.
47. Brady MT, Byington CL, Davies HD, et al. Policy statement Hpv vaccine recommendations. *Pediatrics.* 2012;129(3):602–605.
48. Henry KA, Stroup AM, Warner EL, et al. Geographic factors and human papillomavirus (HPV) vaccination initiation among adolescent girls in the United States. *Cancer Epidemiol Biomarkers Prev.* 2016;25(2):309–317.
49. Gilkey MB, Malo TL, Shah PD, et al. Quality of physician communication about human papillomavirus vaccine: findings from a national survey. *Cancer Epidemiol Biomarkers Prev.* 2015;24(11):1673–1679.
50. Moreira ED Jr., de Oliveira BG, Neves RC, et al. Assessment of knowledge and attitudes of young uninsured women toward human papillomavirus vaccination and clinical trials. *J Pediatr Adolesc Gynecol.* 2006;19(2):81–87.
51. Tiro JA, Meissner HI, Kobrin S, et al. What do women in the US know about human papillomavirus and cervical cancer? *Cancer Epidemiol Biomarkers Prev.* 2007;16(2):288–294.
52. Colgrove J, Abiola S, Mello MM. HPV vaccination mandates–lawmaking amid political and scientific controversy. *N Engl J Med.* 2010;363(8):785–791.
53. Wheeler CM. Less is more: a step in the right direction for human papillomavirus (HPV) vaccine implementation. *J Natl Cancer Inst.* 2011;103(19):1424–1476.
54. Alberts DS, Barakat RR, Daly M, et al. *Prevention of Gynecologic Malignancies.* Philadelphia, PA: Elsevier Ltd; 2004.
55. Zou C, Liu H, Feugang JM, et al. Green tea compound in chemoprevention of cervical cancer. *Int J Gynecol Cancer.* 2010;20(4):617–624.
56. Zhou X, Meng Y. Association between serum folate level and cervical cancer: a meta-analysis. *Arch Gynecol Obstet.* 2016;293:871–877.
57. Meyskens FL Jr., Surwit E, Moon TE, et al. Enhancement of regression of cervical intraepithelial neoplasia II (moderate dysplasia) with topically applied all-trans-retinoic acid: a randomized trial. *J Natl Cancer Inst.* 1994;86(7):539–543.
58. Kulasingam S, Havrilesky L. Health economics of screening for gynaecological cancers. *Best Pract Res Clin Obstet Gynaecol.* 2012;26(2):163–173.
59. Huh WK, Ault KA, Chelmow D, et al. Use of primary high-risk human papillomavirus testing for cervical cancer screening interim clinical guidance. *Obstet Gynecol.* 2015;125(2):330–337.
60. Brown AJ, Trimble CL. New technologies for cervical cancer screening. *Best Pract Res Clin Obstet Gynaecol.* 2012;26(2):233–242.
61. Spitzer M, Apgar BS, Brotzman GL. Management of histologic abnormalities of the cervix. *Am Fam Physician.* 2006;73(1):105–112.
62. Wright TC Jr., Cox JT, Massad LS, et al. 2001 Consensus guidelines for the management of women with cervical intraepithelial neoplasia. *J Low Genit Tract Dis.* 2003;7(3):154–167.
63. Siegel RL, Miller KD, Jemel A. Cancer statistics, 2016. *CA Cancer J Clin.* 2016;66(1):7–30.
64. Torre LA, Bray F, Siegel RL, et al. Global cancer statistics, 2012. *CA Cancer J Clin.* 2015;65(2):87–108.
65. Mortality GBD, Causes of Death Collaborators. Global, regional, and national age-sex specific all-cause and cause-specific mortality for 240 causes of death, 1990-2013: a systematic analysis for the Global Burden of Disease Study 2013. *Lancet.* 2015;385(9963):117–171.
66. Tone AA, Salvador S, Finlayson SJ, et al. The role of the fallopian tube in ovarian cancer. *Clin Adv Hematol Oncol.* 2012;10(5):296–306.
67. Mingels MJ, Roelofsen T, van der Laak JA, et al. Tubal epithelial lesions in salpingo-oophorectomy specimens of BRCA-mutation carriers and controls. *Gynecol Oncol.* 2012;127(1):88–93.
68. Kurman RJ, Shih Ie M. Molecular pathogenesis and extraovarian origin of epithelial ovarian cancer–shifting the paradigm. *Hum Pathol.* 2011;42(7):918–931.
69. Powell CB, Chen LM, McLennan J, et al. Risk-reducing salpingo-oophorectomy (RRSO) in BRCA mutation carriers: experience with a consecutive series of 111 patients using a standardized surgical-pathological protocol. *Int J Gynecol Cancer.* 2011;21(5):846–851.
70. Lee Y, Miron A, Drapkin R, et al. A candidate precursor to serous carcinoma that originates in the distal fallopian tube. *J Pathol.* 2007;211(1):26–35.
71. Folkins AK, Jarboe EA, Roh MH, et al. Precursors to pelvic serous carcinoma and their clinical implications. *Gynecol Oncol.* 2009;113(3):391–396.
72. Antoniou AC, Rookus M, Andrieu N, et al. Reproductive and hormonal factors, and ovarian cancer risk for BRCA1 and BRCA2 mutation carriers: results from the International BRCA1/2 Carrier Cohort Study. *Cancer Epidemiol Biomarkers Prev.* 2009;18(2):601–610.
73. Brewer MA, Johnson K, Follen M, et al. Prevention of ovarian cancer: intraepithelial neoplasia. *Clin Cancer Res.* 2003;9(1):20–30.
74. Hanna L, Adams M. Prevention of ovarian cancer. *Best Pract Res Clin Obstet Gynaecol.* 2006;20(2):339–362.
75. Nezhat F, Datta MS, Hanson V, et al. The relationship of endometriosis and ovarian malignancy: a review. *Fertil Steril.* 2008;90(5):1559–1570.
76. Cramer DW, Vitonis AF, Terry KL, et al. The association between talc use and ovarian cancer: a retrospective case-control study in two US states. *Epidemiology.* 2016;27(3):334–346.
77. Walsh T, Casadei S, Lee MK, et al. Mutations in 12 genes for inherited ovarian, fallopian tube, and peritoneal carcinoma identified by massively parallel sequencing. *Proc Natl Acad Sci U S A.* 2011;108(44):18032–18037.
78. Rebbeck TR, Mitra N, Wan F, et al. Association of type and location of BRCA1 and BRCA2 mutations with risk of breast and ovarian cancer. *JAMA.* 2015;313(13):1347–1361.
79. Bonadona V, Bonaiti B, Olschwang S, et al. Cancer risks associated with germline mutations in MLH1, MSH2, and MSH6 genes in Lynch syndrome. *JAMA.* 2011;305(22):2304–2310.
80. Senter L, Clendenning M, Sotamaa K, et al. The clinical phenotype of Lynch syndrome due to germ-line PMS2 mutations. *Gastroenterology.* 2008;135(2):419–428.
81. Celentano V, Luglio G, Antonelli G, et al. Prophylactic surgery in Lynch syndrome. *Tech Coloproctol.* 2011;15(2):129–134.
82. Norquist BM, Swisher EM. More genes, more problems? Benefits and risks of multiplex genetic testing. *Gynecol Oncol.* 2015;139(2):209–210.
83. Kurian AW, Hare EE, Mills MA, et al. Clinical evaluation of a multiple-gene sequencing panel for hereditary cancer risk assessment. *J Clin Oncol.* 2014;32(19):2001–2009.
84. Lincoln SE, Kobayashi Y, Anderson MJ, et al. A systematic comparison of traditional and multigene panel testing for hereditary breast and ovarian cancer genes in more than 1000 patients. *J Mol Diagn.* 2015;17(5):533–544.
85. Song H, Dicks E, Ramus SJ, et al. Contribution of germline mutations in the RAD51B, RAD51C, and RAD51D genes to ovarian cancer in the population. *J Clin Oncol.* 2015;33(26):2901–2907.
86. Ramus SJ, Song H, Dicks E, et al. Germline mutations in the BRIP1, BARD1, PALB2, and NBN genes in women with ovarian cancer. *J Natl Cancer Inst.* 2015;107(11):1–8.
87. Whiteman DC, Murphy MF, Cook LS, et al. Multiple births and risk of epithelial ovarian cancer. *J Natl Cancer Inst.* 2000;92(14):1172–1177.
88. Pike MC, Pearce CL, Wu AH. Prevention of cancers of the breast, endometrium and ovary. *Oncogene.* 2004;23(38):6379–6391.
89. Barnes MN, Grizzle WE, Grubbs CJ, et al. Paradigms for primary prevention of ovarian carcinoma. *CA Cancer J Clin.* 2002;52(4):216–225.
90. Risch HA, Marrett LD, Howe GR. Parity, contraception, infertility, and the risk of epithelial ovarian cancer. *Am J Epidemiology.* 1994;140(7):585–597.
91. Rosenblatt KA, Thomas DB. Lactation and the risk of epithelial ovarian cancer. The WHO Collaborative Study of Neoplasia and Steroid Contraceptives. *Int J Epidemiol.* 1993;22(2):192–197.
92. Auranen A, Hietanen S, Salmi T, et al. Hormonal treatments and epithelial ovarian cancer risk. *Int J Gynecol Cancer.* 2005;15(5):692–700.
93. Weiderpass E, Margolis KL, Sandin S, et al. Prospective study of physical activity in different periods of life and the risk of ovarian cancer. *Int JCancer.* 2006;118(12):3153–3160.
94. Rossing MA, Cushing-Haugen KL, Wicklund KG, et al. Recreational physical activity and risk of epithelial ovarian cancer. *Cancer Causes Control.* 2010;21(4):485–491.
95. Cannioto RA, Moysich KB. Epithelial ovarian cancer and recreational physical activity: A review of the epidemiological literature and implications for exercise prescription. *Gynecol Oncol.* 2015;137(3):559–573.
96. Rodriguez-Burford C, Barnes MN, Oelschlager DK, et al. Effects of nonsteroidal anti-inflammatory agents (NSAIDs) on ovarian carcinoma cell lines: preclinical evaluation of NSAIDs as chemopreventive agents. *Clin Cancer Res.* 2002;8(1):202–209.
97. Salvador S, Gilks B, Kobel M, et al. The fallopian tube: primary site of most pelvic high-grade serous carcinomas. *Int J Gynecol Cancer.* 2009;19(1):58–64.
98. Rodriguez GC, Nagarsheth NP, Lee KL, et al. Progestin-induced apoptosis in the Macaque ovarian epithelium: differential regulation of transforming growth factor-beta. *J Natl Cancer Inst.* 2002;94(1):50–60.
99. Whittemore AS, Balise RR, Pharoah PDP, et al. Oral contraceptive use and ovarian cancer risk among carriers of BRCA1 or BRCA2 mutations. *Br J Cancer.* 2004;91(11):1911–1915.
100. De Palo G, Veronesi U, Camerini T, et al. Can fenretinide protect women against ovarian cancer? *J Natl Cancer Inst.* 1995;87(2):146–147.
101. Campbell MJ, Park S, Uskokovic MR, et al. Expression of retinoic acid receptor-beta sensitizes prostate cancer cells to growth inhibition

mediated by combinations of retinoids and a 19-nor hexafluoride vitamin D3 analog. *Endocrinology*. 1998;139(4):1972–1980.
102. Studzinski GP, Moore DC. Sunlight—can it prevent as well as cause cancer? *Cancer Res*. 1995;55(18):4014–4022.
103. Lefkowitz ES, Garland CF. Sunlight, vitamin D, and ovarian cancer mortality rates in US women. *Int J Epidemiol*. 1994;23(6):1133–1136.
104. Cook LS, Neilson HK, Lorenzetti DL, et al. A systematic literature review of vitamin D and ovarian cancer. *Am J Obstet Gynecol*. 2010;203(1):70. e71–70.e78.
105. Moysich KB, Mettlin C, Piver MS, et al. Regular use of analgesic drugs and ovarian cancer risk. *Cancer Epidemiol Biomarkers Prev*. 2001;10(8):903–906.
106. Rodriguez C, Patel AV, Calle EE, et al. Estrogen replacement therapy and ovarian cancer mortality in a large prospective study of US women. *JAMA*. 2001;285(11):1460–1465.
107. Akhmedkhanov A, Toniolo P, Zeleniuch-Jacquotte A, et al. Aspirin and epithelial ovarian cancer. *Prev Med*. 2001;33(6):682–687.
108. Gates MA, Tworoger SS, Hecht JL, et al. A prospective study of dietary flavonoid intake and incidence of epithelial ovarian cancer. *Int J Cancer*. 2007;121(10):2225–2232.
109. Watkins JL, Thaker PH, Nick AM, et al. Clinical impact of selective and nonselective beta-blockers on survival in patients with ovarian cancer. *Cancer*. 2015;121(19):3444–3451.
110. Kauff ND, Domchek SM, Friebel TM, et al. Risk-reducing salpingo-oophorectomy for the prevention of BRCA1- and BRCA2-associated breast and gynecologic cancer: a multicenter, prospective study. *J Clin Oncol*. 2008;26(8):1331–1337.
111. Domchek SM, Friebel TM, Singer CF, et al. Association of risk-reducing surgery in BRCA1 or BRCA2 mutation carriers with cancer risk and mortality. *JAMA*. 2010;304(9):967–975.
112. Rabban JT, Barnes M, Chen LM, et al. Ovarian pathology in risk-reducing salpingo-oophorectomies from women with BRCA mutations, emphasizing the differential diagnosis of occult primary and metastatic carcinoma. *Am J Surg Pathol*. 2009;33(8):1125–1136.
113. Manchanda R, Abdelraheim A, Johnson M, et al. Outcome of risk-reducing salpingo-oophorectomy in BRCA carriers and women of unknown mutation status. *BJOG*. 2011;118(7):814–824.
114. Hirst JE, Gard GB, McIllroy K, et al. High rates of occult fallopian tube cancer diagnosed at prophylactic bilateral salpingo-oophorectomy. *Int J Gynecol Cancer*. 2009;19(5):826–829.
115. Finch A, Beiner M, Lubinski J, et al. Salpingo-oophorectomy and the risk of ovarian, fallopian tube, and peritoneal cancers in women with a BRCA1 or BRCA2 Mutation. *JAMA*. 2006;296(2):185–192.
116. Daly MB, Pilarski R, Axilbund JE, et al. NCCN Practice Guidelines in Oncolgy (NCCN Guidelines) Genetic/Familial High-Risk Assessment: Breast and Ovarian. *2016 National Comprehensive Cancer Network, Inc.* 2016; Version 2:2016 ©.
117. van der Kolk DM, de Bock GH, Leegte BK, et al. Penetrance of breast cancer, ovarian cancer and contralateral breast cancer in BRCA1 and BRCA2 families: high cancer incidence at older age. *Breast Cancer Res Treat*. 2010;124(3):643–651.
118. Yang KY, Caughey AB, Little SE, et al. A cost-effectiveness analysis of prophylactic surgery versus gynecologic surveillance for women from hereditary non-polyposis colorectal cancer (HNPCC) families. *Fam Cancer*. 2011;10(3):535–543.
119. Michelsen TM, Dorum A, Dahl AA. A controlled study of mental distress and somatic complaints after risk-reducing salpingo-oophorectomy in women at risk for hereditary breast ovarian cancer. *Gynecol Oncol*. 2009;113(1):128–133.
120. Finch A, Metcalfe KA, Chiang JK, et al. The impact of prophylactic salpingo-oophorectomy on menopausal symptoms and sexual function in women who carry a BRCA mutation. *Gynecol Oncol*. 2011;121(1):163–168.
121. Rebbeck TR, Friebel T, Wagner T, et al. Effect of short-term hormone replacement therapy on breast cancer risk reduction after bilateral prophylactic oophorectomy in BRCA1 and BRCA2 mutation carriers: the PROSE Study Group. *J Clin Oncol*. 2005;23(31):7804–7810.
122. Olson JE, Sellers TA, Iturria SJ, et al. Bilateral oophorectomy and breast cancer risk reduction among women with a family history. *Cancer Detect Prev*. 2004;28(5):357–360.
123. Leblanc E, Narducci F, Farre I. Radical fimbriectomy: a reasonable temporary risk-reducing surgery for selected women with a germ line mutation of BRCA1 or 2 genes? Rationale and preliminary development. *Gynecol Oncol*. 2011;121:472–476.
124. Green MH, Mai PL, Schwartz PE. Does bilateral salpingectomy with ovarian retention warrant consideration as a temporary bridge to risk-reducing bilateral oophorectomy in BRCA1/2 mutation carriers? *Am J Obstet Gynecol*. 2011;204:19.e11–e16.
125. Hankinson SE, Hunter DJ, Colditz GA, et al. Tubal ligation, hysterectomy, and risk of ovarian cancer. A prospective study. *JAMA*. 1993;270(23): 2813–2818.
126. Cibula D, Widschwendter M, Majek O, et al. Tubal ligation and the risk of ovarian cancer: review and meta-analysis. *Hum Reprod Update*. 2011;17(1):55–67.
127. Hickey M, Ambekar M, Hammond I. Should the ovaries be removed or retained at the time of hysterectomy for benign disease? *Hum Reprod Update*. 2010;16(2):131–141.
128. Berek JS, Chalas E, Edelson M, et al. Prophylactic and risk-reducing bilateral salpingo-oophorectomy: recommendations based on risk of ovarian cancer. *Obstet Gynecol*. 2010;116(3):733–743.
129. Leslie KK, Thiel KW, Yang S. Endometrial cancer: potential treatment and prevention with progestin-containing intrauterine devices. *Obstet Gynecol*. 2012;119(2 Pt 2):419–420.
130. Yang S, Thiel KW, Leslie KK. Progesterone: the ultimate endometrial tumor suppressor. *Trends Endocrinol Metab*. 2011;22(4):145–152.
131. Siegel RL, Miller KD, Jemal A. Cancer statistics, 2015. *CA Cancer J Clin*. 2015;65(1):5–29.
132. Rice LW. Hormone prevention strategies for breast, endometrial and ovarian cancers. *Gynecol Oncol*. 2010;118(2):202–207.
133. Backes FJ, Cohn DE. Lynch syndrome. *Clin Obstet Gynecol*. 2011;54(2):199–214.
134. Pilarski R, Burt R, Kohlman W, et al. Cowden syndrome and the PTEN hamartoma tumor syndrome: systematic review and revised diagnostic criteria. *J Natl Cancer Inst*. 2013;105(21):1607–1616.
135. Moore SC, Gierach GL, Schatzkin A, et al. Physical activity, sedentary behaviours, and the prevention of endometrial cancer. *Br J Cancer*. 2010;103(7):933–938.
136. Fisher B, Costantino JP, Wickerham DL, et al. Tamoxifen for prevention of breast cancer: Report of the National Surgical Adjuvant Breast and Bowel Project P-1 study. *J Natl Cancer Inst*. 1998;90(18):1371–1388.
137. Gabriel EM, Jatoi I. Breast cancer prevention. *Expert Rev Anticancer Ther*. 2012;12(2):223–228.
138. Schmandt RE, Iglesias DA, Co NN, et al. Understanding obesity and endometrial cancer risk: opportunities for prevention. *Am J Obstet Gynecol*. 2011;205(6):518–525.
139. Collaborative Group on Epidemiological Studies on Endometrial Cancer. Endometrial cancer and oral contraceptives: an individual participant meta-analysis of 27 276 women with endometrial cancer from 36 epidemiological studies. *Lancet Oncol*. 2015;16(9): 1061–1070.
140. Dashti SG, Chau R, Ouakrim DA, et al. Female hormonal factors and the risk of endometrial cancer in Lynch syndrome. *JAMA*. 2015;314(1): 61–71.
141. Brown AJ, Westin SN, Broaddus RR, et al. Progestin intrauterine device in an adolescent with grade 2 endometrial cancer. *Obstet Gynecol*. 2012;119(2 Pt 2):423–426.
142. Chin J, Konje JC, Hickey M. Levonorgestrel intrauterine system for endometrial protection in women with breast cancer on adjuvant tamoxifen. *Cochrane Database Syst Rev*. 2009;(4):CD007245.
143. Sherman ME, Sturgeon S, Brinton L, et al. Endometrial cancer chemoprevention: implications of diverse pathways of carcinogenesis. *J Cell Biochem Suppl*. 1995;23:160–164.
144. Syngal S, Brand RE, Church JM, et al. ACG clinical guideline: genetic testing and management of hereditary gastrointestinal cancer syndromes. *Am J Gastroenterol*. 2015;110(2):223–262; quiz 263.
145. Auranen A, Joutsiniemi T. A systematic review of gynecological cancer surveillance in women belonging to hereditary nonpolyposis colorectal cancer (Lynch syndrome) families. *Acta Obstet Gynecol Scand*. 2011;90(5): 437–444.

CHAPTER 7

Preinvasive Disease of the Lower Genital Tract

Britt K. Erickson, Mark H. Einstein, and Warner K. Huh

INTRODUCTION

Human papillomavirus (HPV) is central to any discussion of preinvasive and invasive lesions of the lower genital tract. Infection with HPV is necessary for the development of almost all preinvasive cervical and vaginal lesions, and it is present in roughly half of preinvasive vulvar disease. It is also highly associated with anal cancer and implicated in the development of carcinoma of the penis and oropharynx. HPV is the most commonly diagnosed sexually transmitted infection in the United States, with a point prevalence in young women of over 40% and an estimated lifetime probability of infection of almost 85% (1,2). Our knowledge surrounding HPV biology and epidemiology has increased exponentially in the past three decades, leading to improved screening modalities and strategies as well as development of prophylactic vaccination.

In this chapter, we will discuss the biology and epidemiology of HPV infections as they relate to cervical, vaginal, and vulvar carcinogenesis. Additionally, we will review the clinical and HPV-associated risk factors for the development of disease and the pathology of preinvasive lesions including cytology and histology and discuss the efficacy and impact of prophylactic HPV vaccination.

SECTION 1: HUMAN PAPILLOMAVIRUS

Evidence for Causal Relationship

HPV was first proposed as a causative agent in the development of cervical cancer in the 1970s when Dr. Harald zur Hausen, a German physician and virologist, suggested that the same viral particles noted in genital warts may also be responsible for genital tract malignancies (3). This was a departure from the prevailing theory that a herpes simplex virus might be the causative agent. In 1983, he isolated HPV type 16 and implicated it in the development of cervical cancer (4). One year later, he had isolated HPV-18, thus discovering the two HPV types that cause approximately 70% of cervical cancers worldwide (5). For this body of important work, zur Hausen was awarded the Nobel Prize in Medicine in 2008.

In 1991, the International Agency for Research on Cancer (IARC) and the World Health Organization (WHO) concluded beyond a reasonable doubt that there is an association between HPV and cervical cancer (6). Though factors such as tobacco use, parity, contraceptive use, and sexual history may increase one's risk for development of the disease, persistent high-risk HPV infection is indisputably the most important risk factor.

Classification of HPV

Papillomaviruses are double-stranded DNA viruses that are members of the *Alpha* genus of the family Papovaviridae. Papillomaviruses are highly species-specific and infect a wide range of vertebrate hosts. All papillomaviruses have regulatory, early (E), and late (L) genomic regions. Within a given host species, many types of papillomaviruses exist and this phylogenetic subdivision is determined by the extent of DNA relatedness.

HPVs are epitheliotropic-infecting epithelial cells of the skin and mucous membranes and cause epithelial proliferation at the site of infection. HPV is currently divided into 120 distinct genotypes, and this list continues to expand (**Fig. 7.1**) (7). Over 40 types of HPV infect the anogenital tract (8). Traditionally, specific HPV types have been classified as high-risk types based on their potential to cause preinvasive and invasive disease. The most recent meeting of the IARC described 12 α-1 HPV types as high risk. These include HPV-16, -18, -31, -33, -35, -39, -45, -51, -52, -56, -58, and -59. Additionally, HPV-68, in the group α-2A, is categorized as probably carcinogenic (9).

Biology of HPV

HPV is a nonenveloped virus with a proteinaceous coat, which encases and protects the viral DNA. More specifically, the particle is composed of 72 capsomeres made of the viral proteins L1 and L2, also known as the major and minor capsid proteins, respectively. In addition to providing protection for the viral nucleic acid, the capsomeres also serve as the initial interaction site of the viral particle with the host cell.

The HPV genome is circular and double stranded and contains nearly 8,000 base pairs (**Fig. 7.2**). The overall organization of various HPV types is similar. The genome contains eight open reading frames, which are transcribed as a single polycistronic messenger RNA (mRNA), and through alternative splicing mechanisms and ribosomal scanning, this mRNA is translated into the eight proteins E1, E2, E4, E5, E6, E7, L1, and L2.

The HPV genome can be divided into three regions. The first region is the upstream regulatory region (URR), composed of nearly 1,000 base pairs. The URR does not code for proteins but contains binding sites for different cellular transcriptional activators and repressors, which then regulate the expression of the early viral genes (10). This region also contains binding sites for the viral proteins E1 and E2, which initiate viral replication and transcription (11). The URR is necessary for the regulation of gene expression, replication of the genome, and packaging of virus particles.

The URR primarily regulates the transcription of proteins in early infection including proteins E6, E7, E1, and E2. The late promoter is activated during the productive phase of the viral life cycle and results in transcription of the capsid proteins (L1 and L2) as well as E1, E2, E4, and E5.

HPV Life Cycle

Like other viruses, HPV must deliver its genome to the host cell and subsequently exploit the cellular machinery for its own purposes. HPV infects the host at sites of epithelial microtrauma, where the HPV particle can gain access to the actively proliferating basal cells of the epithelium (**Fig. 7.3**). The mechanisms of cell entry are complex and continue to be better elucidated (12). The HPV particle interacts with the cell surface via its major and minor capsid proteins (L1 and L2). α-6-Integrin had initially been suggested as a receptor; however, controversies exist regarding its interaction with HPV (13,14). Attachment receptors for HPV particles are likely heparan sulfate proteoglycans (HSPGs), specifically syndecan-1, which is found in the extracellular matrix of epithelial cells (13). Laminin-5 may be another specific extracellular matrix receptor

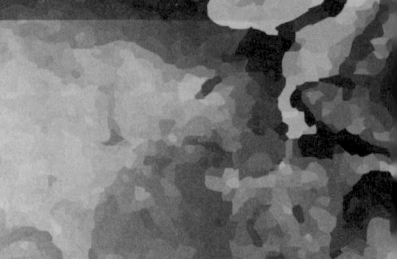

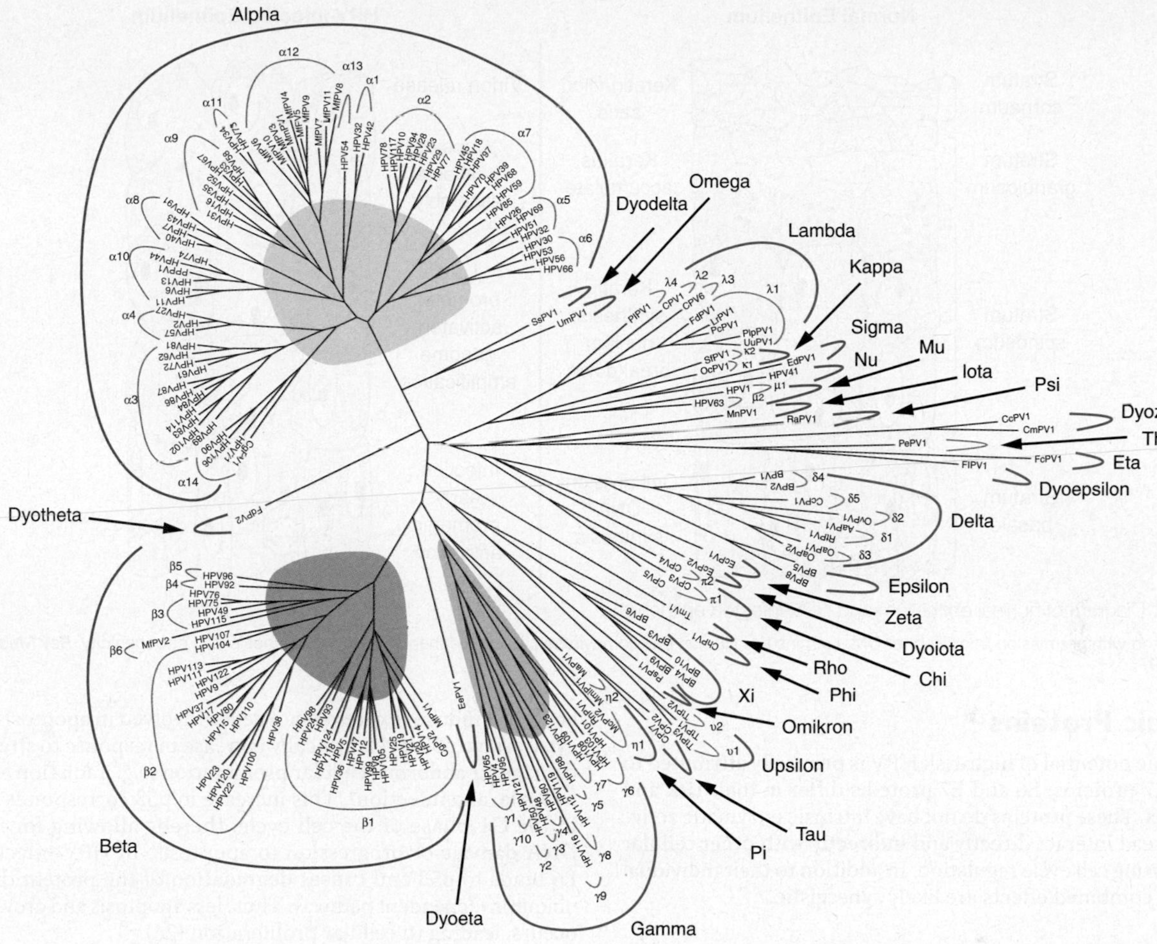

Figure 7.1. Papillomavirus phylogenic tree.

Source: Reprinted with permission from Bernard HU, Burk RD, Chen Z, et al. Classification of papillomaviruses (PVs) based on 189 PV types and proposal of taxonomic amendments. *Virology.* 2010;401:70–79.

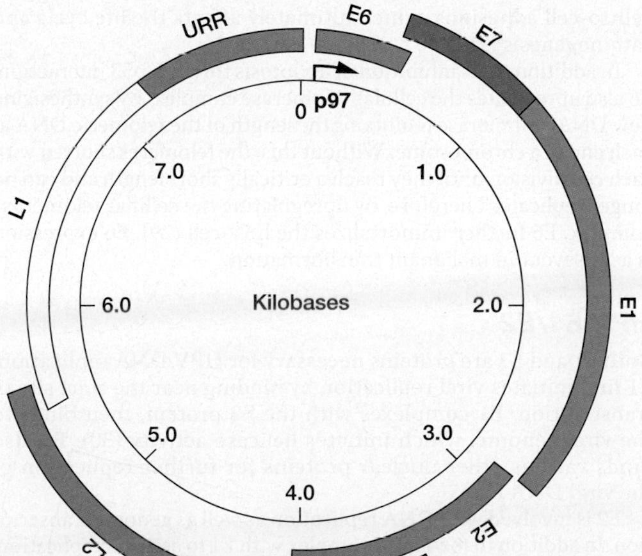

Figure 7.2. Schematic of genomic organization of HPV.

Source: Reprinted with permission from Wright TC, Ferenzy AF, Kurman RJ. Precancerous lesions of the cervix. In: Kurman RJ, ed. *Blaustein's Pathology of the Female Genital Tract.* 4th Ed. New York, NY: Springer-Verlag; 1994:229–241.

involved in binding and cell entry (15). Although the main target of HPV is the keratinocytes of the epithelium, HPV virus-like particles (VLPs) have also been shown to attach to cells important in immune function such as dendritic cells and Langerhans cells (16).

The binding of HPV to cell surface receptors in the basal cells over the basement membrane then initiates conformational changes in L2, which exposes additional binding sites (17,18). HPV then enters the cells via endocytosis. Most studies suggest clathrin- or caveolin-dependent endocytosis (19), although internalization independent of these proteins has also been described (20).

Once inside the basal epithelial cells, the viral genome begins to replicate. The life cycle of HPV is closely linked to the state of differentiation of the squamous epithelium of the host tissue. In normal squamous human epithelium, the basal layers (stratum basale) are the areas of active cell division. After division, the daughter cells migrate away from the basal cells (stratum spinosum) and no longer progress through the cell cycle. Instead, these terminally differentiated cells produce high-molecular-weight keratins until eventually the nuclear envelope breaks down and the cells become empty keratin-filled sacs (stratum corneum).

HPV-infected cells migrate away from the basal layer, and as the cells reach higher epithelial layers, the late promoter is activated and late gene transcription and translation occur. There is high-level amplification of the viral genome in these layers, and in the uppermost layer DNA is packaged into capsids and the infectious virions are assembled. Typical HPV-associated cytopathic changes such as koilocytosis, multinucleation, and nuclear enlargement are due to the assembly of the viral particles in the upper epithelial layers. The epithelium is then shed and HPV particles are released, which can then infect a new host.

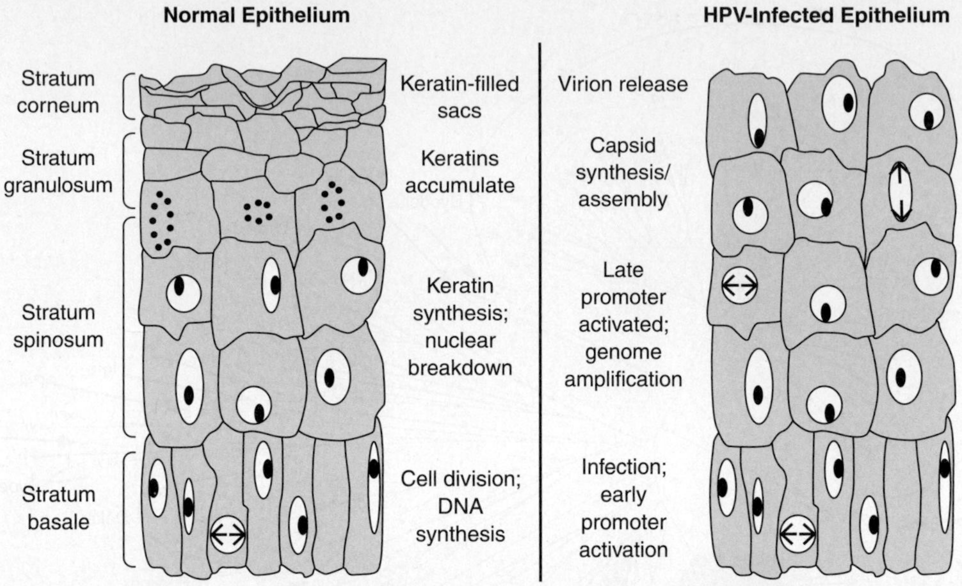

Figure 7.3. Diagram of normal epithelium and HPV-infected epithelium.

Source: Reprinted with permission from Hebner CM, Laimins LA. Human papillomaviruses: basic mechanisms of pathogenesis and oncogenicity. *Rev Med Virol.* 2006;16(2):83–97.

Oncogenic Proteins

The oncogenic potential of high-risk HPV is primarily attributed to the E6 and E7 proteins. E6 and E7 proteins differ in high-risk and low-risk types. These proteins do not have intrinsic enzymatic activities, but instead interact directly and indirectly with other cellular proteins affecting cell cycle regulation. In addition to their individual effects, their combined effects are likely synergistic.

HPV E7

The E7 protein is responsible for immortalizing cells infected with HPV, primarily by affecting the cell's transition from G1 into S-phase. E7 has a variety of targets, including the retinoblastoma (Rb) protein family, histone deacetylases (HDACs), cyclins, cyclin-dependent kinases (cdks), and cdk inhibitors (21).

Rb proteins regulate the cell cycle by controlling the transition at the G1/S-phase. Rb is hypophosphorylated and bound to E2F, a cellular transcription factor. In its bound state, Rb and E2F inhibit cellular proliferation. In normal proliferating cells, cyclin–kinase complexes phosphorylate Rb, E2F is then released, and transcription of S-phase genes occurs. E7 competes for Rb binding, thereby freeing E2F, which results in expression of S-phase genes and uncontrolled cell cycle proliferation (22,23).

The zinc finger region of E7 can interact with the class I HDACs. Through deacetylation of histones, HDACs induce chromatin remodeling (24). E7 binding to HDACs causes progression into S-phase, thereby lengthening the life of the cell.

Independent of these effects, continuous activity of the E7 protein leads to increasing genomic instability, which leads to more dysregulated cell growth and eventually cancer. It has been observed that cells expressing E7 show irregularities in numerous centrosomes leading to aberrant mitotic spindle poles, thereby affecting chromosome number during replication (25). E7 expression is a late event in malignant transformation.

HPV E6

Like E7, E6 is a small 151 amino acid protein that induces important changes in the host cell. It also lacks endogenous enzymatic activity and binds to cell cycle regulatory proteins, affecting life cycle and immortalization.

E6's most notable effect is its ability to bind to p53. p53 is a transcriptional activator and is an important tumor suppressor gene. p53 induces expression of genes involved in apoptosis and cell cycle arrest. p53 levels typically increase in response to stress, DNA damage, or abnormal cellular proliferation (e.g., radiation exposure, hypoxia, and infection). This increase in p53 corresponds to arrest in the G1-phase of the cell cycle, thereby allowing for repair of DNA damage or progression to apoptosis. In HPV-infected cells, E6 binds to p53 and causes degradation of the protein through a ubiquitin-dependent pathway. Thus, less apoptosis and growth arrest occurs, leading to cellular proliferation (26).

E6 has also been shown to interact with other proteins that are involved in a variety of cellular functions. E6 binds to transcriptional coactivators CREB-binding protein/p300, further downregulating p53-mediated transcription (27). E6 also interacts with the PDZ proteins, which are involved in cell signaling and cell-to-cell adhesions, which ultimately affects the life cycle and carcinogenesis (28).

In addition to its inhibition of apoptosis through p53 interaction, E6 also upregulates the cellular telomerase complex. By synthesizing new DNA, telomerase maintains the length of the telomeric DNA at each end of a chromosome. Without this, the telomeres shorten with each cell division until they reach a critically short length and can no longer replicate. Therefore, by upregulating the cellular telomerase complex, E6 further immortalizes the host cell (29). E6 expression is a late event in malignant transformation.

HPV E1/E2

Both E1 and E2 are proteins necessary for HPV DNA replication. E1 first initiates viral replication by binding near the start site of transcription. E1 complexes with the E2 protein, then binds to the viral genome, which initiates helicase activity (30). E1 also binds various other nuclear proteins for further replication of the viral DNA (31).

E2 is involved with DNA replication as well as genome transcription. In addition to forming a complex with E1 to assist in replication, E2 also works on the upper regulatory region to affect transcription of early genes (32). High concentrations of E2 repress transcription and low levels activate transcription. E2 therefore regulates E6 and E7 and loss of E2 expression can lead to carcinoma due to the unrestricted effects of E6 and E7. Like E1, other interactions have been noted between E2 and various proteins involved with transcription as well as mitosis and cell division. E1 and E2 expressions are early events in the natural history of cervical dysplasia.

Viral Integration and Transformation to Malignancy

HPV genomes infect the cell via circular extrachromosomal copies; however, over time, its viral genome can become inserted into host cell DNA, a process called integration. In low-grade cervical intraepithelial neoplasia (CIN), the HPV DNA is maintained in its closed, circular, episomal shape. However, in most high-grade CIN and cancers, the HPV DNA becomes integrated in the host chromosomal DNA (33,34). Many believe that this is a necessary event in cervical carcinogenesis. Integrated HPV has been found to be present in 83% of invasive cervical cancers, as compared with 8% of low-grade CIN, suggesting that integration is highly associated with the transition of low-grade to high-grade lesions (35,36).

SECTION 2: EPIDEMIOLOGY OF HPV INFECTIONS

Prevalence

HPV is the most common of all sexually transmitted infections; while age, race, geographic region, and other modifiable risk factors correlate with new infections, age and sexual behaviors are most clearly linked to new HPV infections. Early studies likely underestimated the prevalence of HPV infections. As newer molecular technologies have been developed, detection of viral infection improved, even at low levels. In addition to variability surrounding detection methods, HPV positivity may be episodic, corresponding to times of viral shedding.

Utilizing polymerase chain reactions on self-collected cervicovaginal specimens from over 4,000 US females, aged 14 to 49, the prevalence of HPV infection was estimated as part of the 2011 National Health and Nutrition Examination Survey (NHANES) (1) (**Fig. 7.4**). The overall prevalence of the 37 separate types was 42.5%. Prevalence was lower among females aged 14 to 19 (32.9%) and highest among females 20 to 24 years (53.8%), which is the peak age of new exposures. In that study, prevalence varied by race, with non-Hispanic Blacks having the highest prevalence (59.2%) followed by Mexican Americans (44.2%) and non-Hispanic Whites (39.2%). HPV positivity was significantly associated with poverty, sexual activity (including number of partners, age, and first encounter), and history of genital warts. In the United States, it is estimated that almost 85% to 90% of men and women will acquire HPV at some point in their lifetime (2).

HPV Prevalence Worldwide

Worldwide age-related trends are similar to US cohorts. Women less than 25 years of age have the highest prevalence of HPV infection. In most regions of the world, there is a decrease in prevalence with increasing age. In Africa, prevalence ranges from 12% to 55%, although

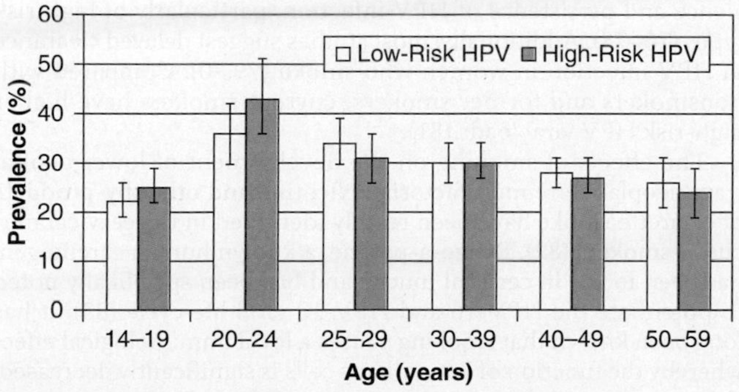

Figure 7.4. US prevalence of HPV infections in women.

Source: Reprinted with permission from Hariri S, Unger ER, Sternberg M, et al. Prevalence of genital human papillomavirus among females in the United States, the National Health and Nutrition Examination Survey, 2003–2006. *J Infect Dis.* 2011;204:566–573.

most studies consisted of cohorts of younger women. In Central and South America, prevalence has been reported to be as high as 64%, and interestingly, many studies showed an overall decrease in prevalence with age followed by an upward trend in women over age 50. Canadian prevalence was lower than that in the United States, with a peak incidence of 25%. Chinese trials showed a range of 6% to 53%, while Japanese trials generally reported prevalence of less than 15%. Studies of Indian women show ranges from 0% to 45%. European prevalence was almost consistently lower than in the United States, with a peak of approximately 20% in young women (37).

HPV Prevalence in Men

The trends in prevalence and clearance in men are inextricably linked to the epidemiology of HPV infections in women. HPV testing in men has limited yield when compared with HPV testing in women, because of the generally keratinized genital surfaces where HPV infection is present in men. A large population-based trial investigating HPV infection in American, Mexican, and Brazilian men demonstrated a 50% prevalence of any type of HPV infection. Specifically, high-risk HPV infections were found in 30%, with HPV 16 (7%) and HPV 51 (6%) being the most common (38,39). Additional data from the NHANES survey showed that men have a higher incidence of oral HPV infection of 10% versus 4% (40). In contrast to trends in women, prevalence of any HPV infection was not affected by age. Clearance of HPV infections seems to occur quicker in men, with an average clearance time of any HPV infection of approximately 6 months. In one study, nearly two-thirds of HPV infections in men were cleared within 1 year, and 90% within 2 years. Clearance was slowest in men aged 18 to 30 (38). Male circumcision significantly reduces genital HPV prevalence in men, which has led some to suggest circumcision as a method to reduce HPV-related disease burden in endemic communities where vaccination and screening is not yet feasible (41). In contrast to squamous cell carcinomas (SCC) of the female genital tract, HPV has only been detected in half of invasive penile SCC (42).

Natural History of HPV Infection (Rates of Abnormal Cytology, CIN, Cancer)

Despite its high prevalence, the majority of HPV infections are cleared by the body's immune system. Only a minority of persistent high-risk HPV infections result in CIN, and an even smaller subset progresses to invasive cancer.

Determining the exact rate of HPV clearance is complex. Some trials examine existing infections (prevalence trials), while others follow women who develop new infections (incident trials). Even within incidence-based trials, methods vary and any subject may have a combination of low-risk, high-risk, preexisting, or incident HPV infections. It is important to also note that though a negative HPV test likely represents clearance of infection, it may also represent a latent, subclinical infection. This concept is derived from a number of sources including data examining HIV positive women who became HPV positive in the absence of new sexual exposures, suggesting a reactivation of viral shedding during periods of immunodeficiency (43). Also, in long-term cohort studies, recurrent infections are often HPV types that the patient has previously had, suggesting reactivation (44,45). However, once cleared, very few HPV type-specific infections reappear and far fewer lead to clinically relevant disease such as high-grade CIN or cervical cancer (46).

The 1-year clearance rate of incident HPV infection ranges from 40% to 70%. Two- to 5-year clearance rates are as high as 70% to 100% in young women (47–50). This rate may be significantly lower in older women; one Chilean trial showed no clearance of high-risk HPV infections in women over the age of 70 (47). Young women are more likely to clear infections than older women, and low-risk HPV infections clear more quickly than high-risk HPV infections (49). The longest course of persistent infection is seen with HPV types 16, 31, 53, and 54 (49) (**Table 7.1**).

TABLE 7.1. HPV Persistence

Study	Year	Average Age	Type of Infection	HPV Persistence at 1 Year	HPV Persistence at 2 Years
Richardson et al.	2003	23	Incident, high risk	61%	x
Ho et al.	1998	20	Incident, high and low risk	30%	9%
Dalstein et al.	2003	32	Prevalent, high risk	60%	50%
Bae et al.	2009	48	Prevalent, high risk	X	41%

Sources: Richardson H, Kelsall G, Tellier P, et al. The natural history of type-specific human papillomavirus infections in female university students. *Cancer Epidemiol Biomarkers Prev*. 2003;12:485–490. Ho GY, Bierman R, Beardsley L, et al. Natural history of cervicovaginal papillomavirus infection in young women. *N Engl J Med*. 1998;338:423–428. Dalstein V, Riethmuller D, Pretet JL, et al. Persistence and load of high-risk HPV are predictors for development of high-grade cervical lesions: a longitudinal French cohort study. *Int J Cancer*. 2003;106:396–403. Bae J, Seo SS, Park YS, et al. Natural history of persistent high-risk human papillomavirus infections in Korean women. *Gynecol Oncol*. 2009;115:75–80.

The majority of women who acquire HPV infections do not develop CIN or invasive cancer. Of women who have persistent high-risk HPV infections, trials report variable rates of progression to CIN 2/3 from 8% to 28% (51–53).

Transmission

HPV infections are almost exclusively acquired during sexual exposure. Areas of microtrauma within the skin and mucosal surfaces are the likely sites of initial infection. Many natural history studies of HPV negative women at baseline who initiated intercourse confirm precedent sexual activity with new HPV infections (54). HPV has been detected in the oral mucosa and genital tract of young women who have not reported a history of vaginal intercourse. This may be the result of underreporting of sexual activity or noncoital sexual behaviors as a route for HPV transmission (55,56).

The rate of HPV acquisition correlates with increasing number of sexual partners (57). Transmission may occur more readily from women to men than from men to women, although data are conflicting (58,59). Data regarding concordance and HPV transmission efficacy among couples are also conflicting. In studies of young women and their male partners, HPV concordance ranged from 40% to 60%. Specific mechanisms that determine the efficiency of HPV transmission and concordance are poorly understood, although it appears that length of sexual activity may increase concordance (60–62). In addition to cervical, vaginal, and penile detection, HPV has been detected on areas of unprotected genital skin such as the vulva and scrotum, providing an explanation as to why condoms offer some but not complete protection against HPV infection (63).

SECTION 3: ADDITIONAL RISK FACTORS FOR DEVELOPMENT OF PREINVASIVE LESIONS OF THE LOWER GENITAL TRACT

Although HPV has been implicated as the most important and necessary risk factor for the development of preinvasive lesions of the lower genital tract, other risk factors have been identified that either increase the risk of HPV infection or potentiate the progression of HPV infection to malignant transformation.

Sexual History

Even before data convincingly linked HPV to the development of cervical cancer, it was well recognized that various aspects of a patient's sexual history put women at increased risk for developing preinvasive and subsequent invasive lesions of the cervix, vagina, and vulva.

Sexual history and behaviors strongly correlate with risk of acquiring HPV infection and developing preinvasive lesions (54). Overall, the number of recent and total lifetime male partners increases the rate of HPV infection, particularly high-risk HPV infection (64,65).

Early onset of sexual activity has also been shown as an independent risk factor for HPV infection in some studies (65). Some studies suggest that frequency of intercourse with one's partner may also play a role (54). Characteristics of the partner, including number of lifetime partners and multiple coincidental partners, have all been implicated in risk of HPV acquisition (54,64). The rate of having new partners and having known a new partner for shorter periods of time before having vaginal intercourse are also associated with increased risk of HPV infection (64).

Additionally, coinfection with other sexually transmitted diseases and vaginal infections has been associated with increased susceptibility to HPV infection. Both bacterial vaginosis and trichomoniasis are associated with HPV infection, although the correlation is not as strong with development of CIN (66,67). A history of herpes simplex virus infection and vulvar warts also increase the incidence of HPV infection (50). A history of previous chlamydial infection has long been implicated in the development of invasive SCC of the cervix (68,69). Hypotheses regarding pathogenesis include induction of squamous metaplasia at the transformation zone, increase in microabrasions, as well as interference with immune surveillance (68,70). More recent cohort studies have found that the role of chlamydia in carcinogenesis is likely related to both in promoting the acquisition and persistence of HPV infections (71,72).

Tobacco

In 2004, the IARC added cervical cancer to the list of cancers causally related to smoking based on analysis of numerous studies in the prior decade (73). As more epidemiologic and natural history studies were performed, conflicting data emerged on the association between cigarette smoking and HPV acquisition, persistence, and progression. Confounding variables have also been a factor; women who smoke are less likely to be compliant with screening guidelines (74) and more likely to have social stressors (75).

Most studies confirm that current smoking increases the prevalence and persistence of HPV infection, particularly of high-risk types (76–78). Additionally, most studies suggest delayed clearance of HPV infection in women who smoke (79,80). Compared with nonsmokers and former smokers, current smokers have higher high-risk HPV viral loads (81).

The effects of smoking on the development of lower genital tract neoplasia are multifactorial. Nicotine and other by-products of cigarette smoke have been readily identified in the cervical mucus of smokers (82). Benzo-a-pyrene, a known human carcinogen, has been found in cervical mucus and has been specifically noted to potentiate the HPV-16 and HPV-18 viral life cycle (83). It has long been known that smoking causes a local immunological effect whereby the function of Langerhans cells is significantly decreased, thus affecting the innate immune system (84). Studies of women with preinvasive and invasive disease have shown that compared with nonsmokers, smokers show aberrant methylation of p16, a tumor suppressor (85). Other recently identified tumor markers in smokers with CIN include overexpression of cyclooxygenase-2 and Ki-67 and underexpression of p53, interleukin-10, and fragile histidine triad (86).

Oral Contraceptive Pills

The association between oral contraceptive pills (OCPs) and preinvasive and invasive diseases of the lower genital tract has been conflicting and controversial. The largest population-based study, which pooled data from trials involving over 50,000 women worldwide, showed an increased risk of preinvasive and invasive disease in current users of OCPs, although this risk was eliminated when OCP use was discontinued (87). This study is criticized for heterogeneity between trials and the possible confounding effects of sexual behavior in women on OCPs—thus, many have questioned the conclusions. More recent large trials have shown that OCP use is not an independent risk factor for development of abnormal cytology, CIN, adenocarcinoma *in situ* (AIS), or invasive disease (88,89).

HIV and Immunosuppression

HIV infection is strongly associated with HPV infection and with more severe preinvasive and invasive disease (90). Additionally, HIV coinfection in one partner impacts the prevalence of HPV infection in the other partner (91). Higher incidence and prevalence as well as prolonged persistence of HPV are all more frequent in women who are HIV positive (92,93). CD4 count and HIV RNA levels correlate with high-risk HPV positivity (43). Although highly active antiretroviral therapy (HAART) has not been shown definitively to affect the incidence or persistence of HPV infections, it has been associated with better CIN outcomes and improves overall life expectancy of HIV positive women (94).

In a large prospective US-based study that followed more than 3,000 HIV-infected women and HIV-uninfected controls, high rates of HPV positivity were found in both HIV+ and HIV− women (92% vs. 66%, $p < 0.001$). CIN 3 or worse was found in 5% of HIV+ women compared with 2% of HIV− women ($p < 0.001$). Detection rate fell after 2 years of study, suggesting that although HIV+ women have higher rates of CIN 3+, it is still uncommon, especially after the initiation of regular cervical cancer screening and HAART (92,95).

In addition to its effect on prevalence of HPV infection, other mechanisms related to coinfection of HPV and HIV have been proposed. Primarily, it is noted that a functional immune system is required to keep HPV in a latent and subclinical state. Thus, HIV infection, in addition to other forms of immunosuppression, predisposes to progression and reactivation of HPV infection (43). Additionally, different molecular pathways have been proposed for HIV-related preinvasive lesions including a higher frequency of microsatellite instability as well as promotion of viral oncogenesis in HIV-associated CIN (96). Based on patterns of local pro-inflammatory immune markers, it appears that persistent HPV infection might make someone more susceptible to HIV infection as well.

Another group of women known to be at high risk for preinvasive HPV-associated lesions is transplant recipients and other patients on chronic immunosuppressive therapy such as those with systemic lupus erythematosus. Small, early studies noted a higher incidence of HPV infections and up to 16 times the rate of invasive cervical cancer in women with a history of renal transplant compared with controls (97). However, these data are limited by less effective methods of HPV testing and lack of control for covariates. In a recent prospective 10-year study of 48 Italian women with renal transplants, no increased risk of HPV infection, high-grade cytology, or preinvasive lesions was observed (98). A large Swedish cohort study found that the rate of vulvar malignancy in women who had undergone solid organ transplant was 26 times higher than the general population. Additionally, the rate of vaginal cancer was 16 times higher. Rates of cervical cancer were not statistically higher, and preinvasive lesions were only marginally increased (99). A US cohort of transplant recipients was analyzed, and only vulvar carcinoma demonstrated a statistically significant higher incidence in transplant recipients. In fact, the incidence of vulvar carcinoma following a solid organ transplant was higher than the incidence of cervical cancer (7.5 vs. 5.8 per 100,000 person years) (100). This may reflect improved cervical cancer surveillance in this population. However, it may also reflect the different pathology of vulvar lesions in immunocompromised women. Smaller studies suggest rates of 90% to 100% HPV positivity in preinvasive and invasive vulvar lesions in women with transplants (101,102).

Racial Disparities

For reasons not well understood, there are higher rates of cervical cancer as well as worse prognosis in both the primary and recurrent setting in African American women compared with non–African American women. Emerging data suggest there may be racial differences in the immunologic response to HPV infection. In one of the HPV vaccine trials, African American women were more likely to have non–HPV-16– or HPV-18–related infections (specifically, they were more likely to be infected with subtypes 35 and 58) (103). In another trial of HPV clearance in college-aged women, African American women were less likely to clear high-risk HPV infection compared with White women. Specifically, it took 601 days versus 316 days for 50% of women to clear their infection (104).

SECTION 4: PATHOLOGY OF PREINVASIVE LESIONS

Cervix

The nomenclature of preinvasive lesions has undergone many changes. Formerly known as cervical dysplasia and carcinoma *in situ* (CIS), preinvasive squamous cell lesions of the cervix were then categorized as various levels of CIN. More specifically, mild, moderate, and severe dysplasia/CIS were termed *CIN 1*, *CIN 2*, and *CIN 3*, respectively. In 2012, the College of American Pathologists and the American Society for Colposcopy and Cervical Pathology (ASCCP) convened and recommended a new standard nomenclature: the Lower Anogenital Squamous Terminology (LAST) (105). A single set of diagnostic terms is now recommended for all HPV-related preinvasive lesions of the lower genital tract. Lesions should be low-grade squamous intraepithelial lesions (LGSIL) or high-grade squamous intraepithelial lesions (HGSIL). When it cannot be determined based on routine stains if a lesion is high grade or low grade, biomarkers such as p16 should be used (105). Presence of p16 positivity on immunohistochemistry confirms that an indeterminate lesion is likely high grade (**Fig. 7.5**).

CIN Localization

The vast majority of CIN/SIL develop in the transformation zone of the cervix, located at the squamocolumnar junction between the columnar epithelium of the endocervix and the squamous epithelium of the ectocervix. This area has been "transformed" due to the process of metaplasia (**Fig. 7.6**). Prior to menarche, the transformation zone does not exist. The squamocolumnar junction occurs exactly at the level of the external cervical os. During menarche (as well as during pregnancy), the columnar epithelium of the endocervix appears on the ectocervix and is termed an "ectropion" or "cervical ectopy." This columnar epithelium gradually becomes replaced by stratified squamous epithelium due to a variety of factors including alterations in pH and other hormonal changes. This area of former columnar, now squamous, epithelium that lies between the original squamocolumnar junction and the new squamocolumnar junction is termed the *transformation zone*. The transformation zone is the primary site for inducing cell-mediated immunity in the lower genital tract, and its role in the acquisition of not only HPV infections, but also HIV infections, is still being elucidated (106,107).

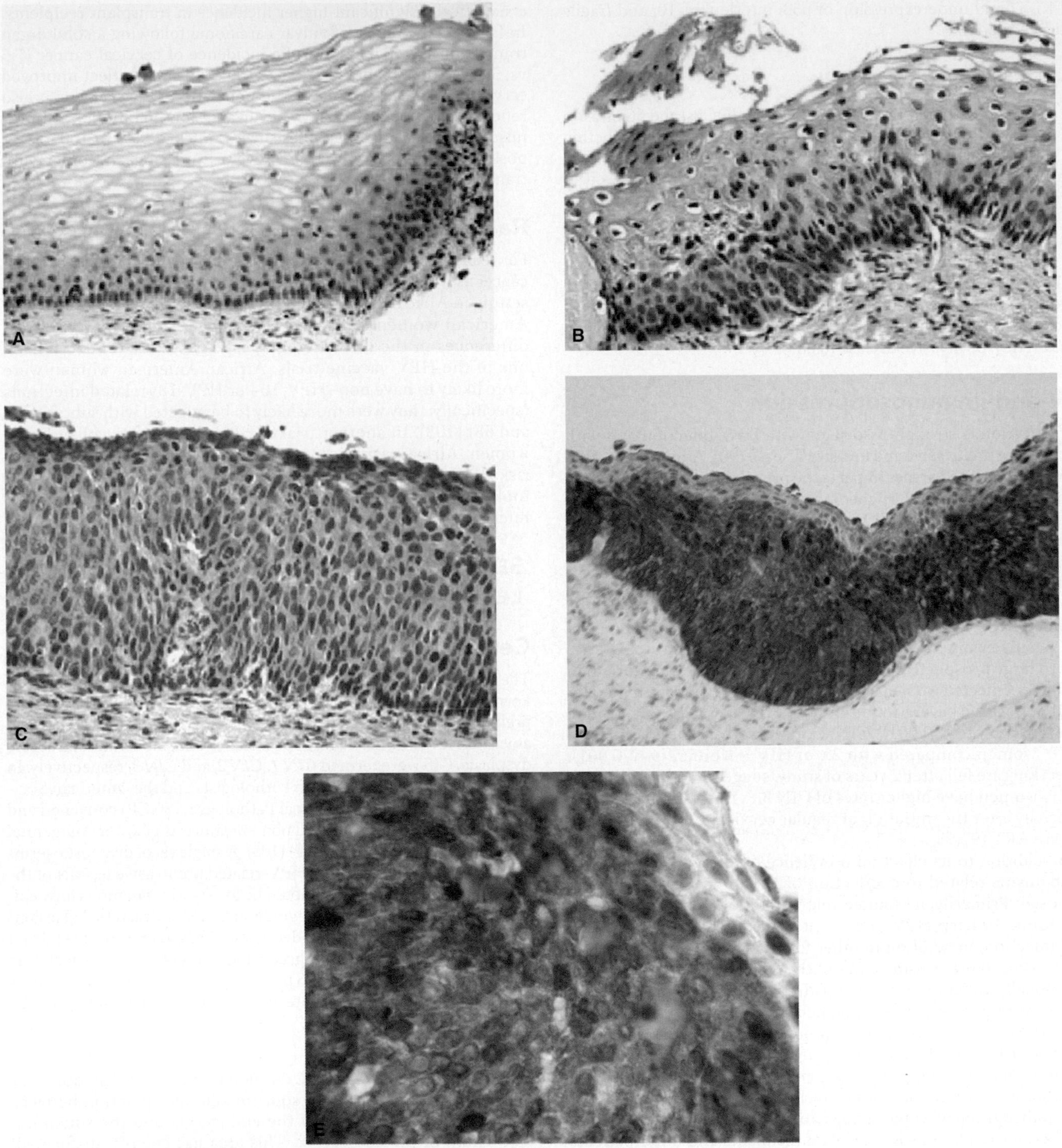

Figure 7.5. A: Normal squamous epithelium. **B:** CIN 1/LGSIL. **C:** CIN 3/HGSIL. **D:** Low-power view of p16 staining on cervical biopsy containing HGSIL. **E:** High-power view of p16 staining on cervical biopsy containing CIN 2/HGSIL.

Source: Images courtesy of University of Alabama at Birmingham.

Microscopic Appearance of CIN/SIL

Nuclear atypia is a prominent feature of CIN/SIL, which can occur at any level of dysplastic severity. It occurs as a result of enhanced proliferation, replication, and intracellular assembly of viral particles in HPV-infected cells. The nuclei are hyperchromatic and frequently multinucleated; additionally, the nuclear outline is often irregular rather than round. The swollen appearance of the cells is a result of viral particles present in the episomal area of the cell.

In addition to nuclear atypia, CIN 1 to 3 (low-grade to high-grade SIL) histology shows aberrant cytoplasmic differentiation. The basaloid cells, which are normally found as a single layer in contact with the basement membrane, replace the normal epithelium. These cells display nuclear crowding, loss of normal cell polarity, pleomorphism, and abnormal mitotic figures. The extent of these abnormal basaloid cells determines the grade of CIN/SIL.

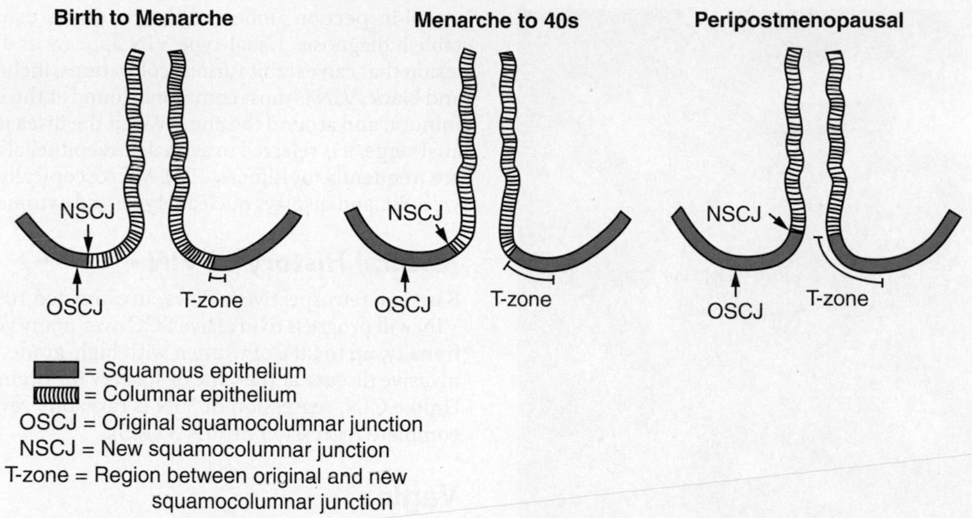

Figure 7.6. Impact of age on the location of the squamocolumnar junction. As females age, the location of the squamocolumnar junction on the cervix moves. The movement of the squamocolumnar junction defines the transformation zone.

This classification system was developed when all of CIN was thought to be a spectrum of disease. Now we understand that CIN 1/low-grade CIN 1/LGSIL usually represents a benign process that is merely a cytomorphologic representation of an active HPV infection, whereas high-grade SIL (formerly CIN 2 or 3) is truly premalignant. CIN 2 was traditionally a poorly reproducible category, with high levels of interobserver variability (108). In one trial, agreement between pathologists was as low as 13% in the category of CIN 2 compared with 81% agreement with CIN 3 lesions (109). Because of limitations surrounding reproducibility, it is now recommended that lesions be dichotomously classified as either low-grade or high-grade SIL, with the addition of molecular markers to improve clinically relevant disease ascertainment (105) (**Fig. 7.5**).

In CIN 1/LGSIL, the lower portion of the epithelium displays nuclear atypia of immature basaloid cells, while the remainder of the epithelium often shows additional cytopathic effects, termed *koilocytosis*, which are directly related to an active HPV infection. Koilocytes are cells with atypical nuclei and perinuclear clearing, also known as vacuolization. The large, perinuclear vacuole is often a result of activation of viral E5 and E6 proteins (110).

Natural History of CIN

CIN 1/LGSIL is the most common histologic diagnosis after colposcopic biopsy. Fortunately, very few of these lesions actually progress to a higher-grade lesion. Most will remain persistent or regress spontaneously as the HPV infection is cleared. In both prospective and retrospective trials, the incidence of CIN 2/3 18 to 24 months after diagnosis of CIN 1 ranges from 4% to 10% (111,112). A retrospective analysis of the ASCUS-LSIL Triage Study (ALTS) found that a diagnosis of CIN 1 on pathology (compared with a negative biopsy, or no biopsy taken) was not a risk factor for developing CIN 3 (113). Therefore, CIN 1/LGSIL is considered a non-neoplastic lesion and is not a disease that should require any extirpative treatment.

Without treatment, HGSIL has at least a 30% probability of becoming invasive cancer. This was shown in an unfortunate prospective study of a cohort of women with untreated CIN 3 followed over a 30-year period beginning in the 1960s in New Zealand. If adequately treated, however, very few women with HGSIL will recur or develop invasive cancer (114).

Glandular Dysplasia and AIS

Although the majority of preinvasive cervical lesions are of squamous cell histology, approximately 3% represent precursors to invasive adenocarcinoma (115). While HPV-16 is the most commonly identified subtype in glandular lesions, HPV-18 causes a greater proportion of glandular as compared with squamous lesions (116). Contrary to popular conceptions regarding preinvasive glandular lesions, the majority are solitary. Multifocal (or "skip lesions") do occur, but only in 10% to 15% of cases. Though glandular lesions can be found higher in the endocervical canal, the majority occur at the squamocolumnar junction (117).

Preinvasive glandular lesions can be divided into the categories of endocervical glandular dysplasia and AIS. These categories differ by degree of nuclear stratification, nuclear atypia, and numbers of mitosis and apoptosis. Additionally, immunohistochemistry, such as staining for a proliferative marker, Ki-67, may also be used to help differentiate between the two categories (118). An additional category, termed glandular atypia, encompasses nonpremalignant lesions with atypia associated with inflammation or previous radiotherapy. Rare variants of AIS have been described including endometrioid, intestinal, serous, and clear cell histologies.

Histologically, AIS is characterized by enlarged glandular cells with large, hyperchromatic nuclei (**Fig. 7.7**). Unlike the cytopathic effect of koilocytosis seen in HPV-infected squamous cells, endocervical cells show decreased cytoplasm and minimal intracellular mucin. Structurally, glandular cells are crowded with pseudostratification. Unlike squamous lesions, apoptosis is a common feature in glandular lesions and is seen in higher frequency in AIS compared with invasive adenocarcinoma (119).

Diagnosing early invasive endocervical adenocarcinoma is sometimes more challenging than diagnosing squamous lesions due to the complex growth patterns of endocervical glands. Atypical glands that extend greater than 5 mm from the uninvolved glands are usually termed invasive, whereas lesions within 5 mm are considered early invasive disease. Other features distinguish invasion from *in situ* lesions, including stromal reaction (desmoplasia, inflammation), confluence of glands, and solid components.

Vulva

Vulvar intraepithelial neoplasia (VIN) is increasing in incidence in the United States, with a 400% increase in preinvasive lesions and a 20% increase in invasive lesions between 1973 and 2000 (120). Classification of preinvasive vulvar disease has undergone many changes. In 2003, the WHO classified VIN in a three-grade system. Then, in 2004, the International Society for the Study of Vulvovaginal Disease (ISSVD) reclassified VIN into two categories: usual-type VIN, which is associated with HPV infection; and differentiated VIN, which is usually not associated with HPV infection (121). VIN 1 was abandoned in terminology primarily due to its high rate of misclassification into clinically relevant disease. Usual-type VIN includes

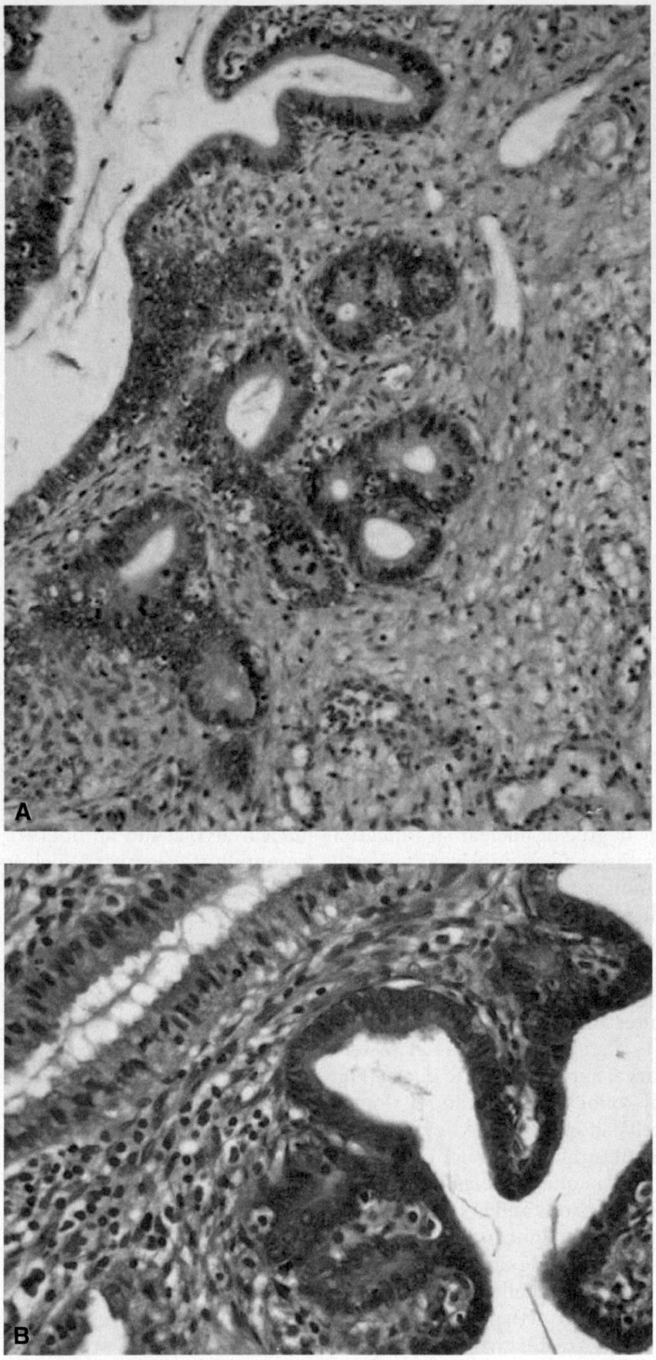

Figure 7.7. Adenocarcinoma *in situ* (AIS). **A:** High-power view. **B:** Low-power view. Normal endocervical glands in the upper left.
Source: Images courtesy of the University of Alabama at Birmingham.

only high-grade VIN and is composed of warty, basaloid, and mixed histologies. In addition to being an HPV-associated lesion, usual-type VIN shares the same risk factors as those for CIN including tobacco use and immunodeficiency. Differentiated VIN, sometimes referred to as "keratinizing type," occurs most commonly in older women and is often associated with lichen sclerosis. p53 mutations and microsatellite instability have been implicated in its pathogenesis. Five percent of women with lichen sclerosis develop invasive SCC with an average interval of 10 years (122). Differentiated VIN has a greater propensity to progress to invasive disease, and time to progression is shorter than that of usual-type VIN.

The differential diagnosis for vulvar lesions is broad and diverse. Distinguishing benign from preinvasive lesions can be difficult by visual inspection alone and thus biopsy is usually necessary to establish diagnosis. Usual-type VIN appears as a sharply demarcated lesion that can exhibit various colorations, including white, gray, red, and black. VIN is most commonly found at the introitus, on the labia minora, and around the anus. When the disease spreads beyond the anal verge, it is referred to as anal intraepithelial neoplasia and lesions are frequently multifocal (123). Microscopically, VIN resembles cervical SIL and displays nuclear atypia and cytoplasmic differentiation.

Natural History of VIN

Based on retrospective reviews, an estimated 10% to 15% of untreated VIN will progress to invasive SCC over many years (124,125). Additionally, up to 20% of women with high-grade VIN will have occult invasive disease at the time of surgery for preinvasive disease (126). Unlike CIN, regression of VIN is rare; one review noted only a 1% complete regression of VIN 3 (125).

Vagina

Vaginal intraepithelial neoplasia (VAIN) is another lesion that is part of the HPV spectrum in the lower genital tract. Its occurrence is less common and represents only 0.5% of all lower genital tract intraepithelial neoplasias. VAIN is most often found in the upper vagina and is most often multifocal. Many cases occur after hysterectomy, and occult vaginal malignancy is uncommon (127). Recurrence is more common with multifocal disease and ranges from 20% to 60% after treatment with laser or 5-fluorouracil (127). Recurrence is uncommon after partial vaginectomy (128). HPV infection is implicated in the pathogenesis of over half of VAIN (129). The histologic features of VAIN are similar to those of CIN and VIN. Because of its infrequency, there are no current recommendations for vaginal cancer screening in low-risk populations. Most screening recommendations do not recommend performing vaginal cuff cytology after a hysterectomy unless the hysterectomy was for CIN or cervical cancer (130).

SECTION 5: SCREENING

With the advent of successful screening for preinvasive disease of the lower genital tract, effective treatments of precancerous lesions have also emerged, subsequently affecting the overall disease burden of invasive lower genital tract malignancies.

Cervical cancer screening is hailed as one of the major public health advances in the 20th century. Initially seeking determinants of the ovulation cycle in guinea pigs, Dr. George Papanicolaou evaluated the vaginal smear as an indicator of hormone status. Eventually, he studied human subjects and incidentally found a malignancy on a vaginal smear. More than a decade later, Dr. Papanicolaou and his colleague Dr. Herbert Traut published *The Diagnostic Value of Vaginal Smears in Carcinoma of the Uterus*, which forever changed the landscape of cancer screening for women (131). The Papanicolaou, or Pap smear, is now used worldwide for cervical and vaginal cancer screening, and its utility and efficacy continue to be validated as newer molecular technologies emerge, particularly testing for HPV DNA.

It should be noted that the utility of the Pap smear as a screening test has not been based on randomized, controlled trials. Being the first such screening test in the modern era, the Pap smear never had to prove its clinical benefit through an evidence-based approach, as many modern screening tests are evaluated today.

Despite a lack of level I evidence, international epidemiologic data are quite convincing (132–135). In developed countries, the incidence of cervical cancer has declined dramatically since the acceptance and utilization of cervical cytology–based screening. In the United States, rates declined from 36.3 per 100,000 in the 1930s to 7.2 per 100,000 in the beginning of the 21st century—a reduction of over 80%. The greatest rate of decline occurred from the 1950s to the 1970s when rates dropped by over 3% per year (136). This correlates with the widespread adoption of routine cervical cancer cytology–based screening programs in the United States.

However, despite the widespread acceptance of cervical cancer screening tests, it is estimated that there are still over 12,000 new cases of cervical cancer diagnosed in the United States annually (137). Reports estimate that 20% to 30% of cases will be in women who have had proper screening (137,138). Thus, as effective as the Pap smear may be, it is evident that some cases of cervical cancer and premalignant lesions are not detected, suggesting that it can be further optimized.

There are elements inherent to cytology that may inhibit its success as a screening test. This includes poor cellularity due to collection or transfer. Also, Pap smears may be read as unsatisfactory due to inflammation, scant cellularity, or obscuring blood, thereby limiting diagnostic ability. The rate of unsatisfactory Pap smears ranges from 1% to 8% (139,140), and on reevaluation, a significant number of these show cytologic atypia, including high-grade lesions and carcinoma (139). This is usually overcome with liquid-based cytology, which is the more commonly used cervical cytology platform due to the ability to also perform molecular testing for pathogens like HPV from the same collection vial. One of the suggested approaches to overcoming human error in the analysis of Pap smears is HPV testing, which is highly sensitive and is not dependent on any subjective evaluation.

Despite rigorous international standards, the interpretation of cytology is subject to interobserver variability. Discrepancies between low- and high-grade lesions among various laboratories and personnel may be as high as 15% (141). Moreover, it is well established that the category of atypical squamous cells of undetermined significance (ASC-US) remains a poorly reproducible category. Attempts have been made to improve its low positive predictive value including HPV triage testing, but nonetheless, much variability exists regarding cytologic interpretation (108).

Even under the best circumstances when sampling is adequate, and interpretation is performed by experienced cytologists, the sensitivity and specificity of the Pap smear at baseline limit its functionality as a screening test. A pooled analysis of European and Canadian studies noted that though the specificity of the Pap smear in detecting high-grade dysplasia (CIN 2 or greater) was 96%, the sensitivity was only 53% (142). In another systematic review, the sensitivity of the Pap smear ranged from 30% to 87% and specificity ranged from 86% to 100% (143).

Currently, the American Cancer Society (ACS), the ASCCP, and the American Society of Clinical Pathology (ASCP) recommend that women should begin cytology screening starting at age 21, regardless of risk factors (**Table 7.2**). Cytology should be performed every 3 years until age 30 (130). Based on modeling studies in this age group, and taking into consideration the natural history of the disease (including high rates of regression and long periods required before invasion), there is no increased risk of death due to cervical cancer associated with screening every 3 years versus every 2 years. Moreover, there is a 40% increase in the rate of colposcopy when screening is performed every 2 years compared with every 3 years, with no increase in cancer detection with more testing (144).

At age 30, combined concurrent testing (or cotesting) with cytology and HPV testing is the preferred method of screening. If both tests are negative, screening can occur every 5 years (130). Cotesting improves sensitivity of detection of CIN 2/3 and lowers the false-negative rate of cytology alone (145,146). HPV testing also improves the detection of glandular lesions, which often go undetected with conventional cytology alone (147). If no HPV testing is performed, cytology alone every 3 years is acceptable. Women older than 65 and women with a previous hysterectomy for benign indications no longer need screening for cervical or vaginal cancer.

Cervical Cytology

Figure 7.8 shows the distribution of abnormal cervical cytology. ASC-US is the most common cytologic abnormality but the most poorly reproducible category. Other cytologic results include low-grade squamous epithelial lesion, high-grade squamous epithelial lesion, atypical squamous cells that cannot exclude high-grade SIL (ASC-H), and atypical glandular cells. Management algorithms will not be reviewed here, but can be referenced from society websites such as the ASCCP (http://www.asccp.org/guidelines).

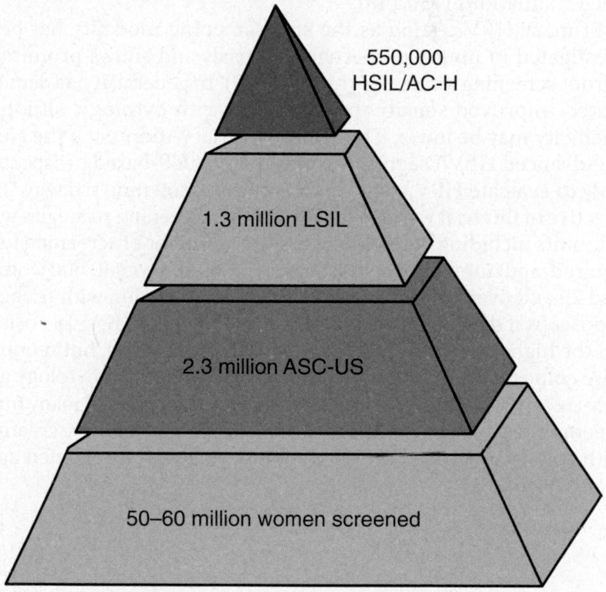

Figure 7.8. Distribution of abnormal cervical cytology.
Source: Adapted from Davey DD, et al. Bethesda 2001 implementation and reporting rates: 2003 practices of participants in the College of American Pathologists Interlaboratory Comparison Program in Cervicovaginal Cytology. *Arch Pathol Lab Med.* 2004;128(11):1224–1229, with permission.

TABLE 7.2. Cervical Cancer Screening Recommendations

Age	Screening Method	Comments
<21 years	No screening recommended	HPV testing is not recommended in this age group
21–29 years	Cytology alone every 3 years	HPV testing is not recommended in this age group
30–65 years	Preferred = "Cotesting" (HPV and cytology) *or* Acceptable = Cytology alone every 3 years	
>65 years	No screening following adequate negative prior screening	If history of CIN 2+, continue screening for 20 years
After hysterectomy	No screening	Applies only to women with no cervix and no history of CIN 2+
HPV vaccinated	Follow age-specific recommendations (same as unvaccinated women)	

Source: Adapted from Saslow D, Solomon D, Lawson HW, et al. American Cancer Society, American Society for Colposcopy and Cervical Pathology, and American Society for Clinical Pathology screening guidelines for the prevention and early detection of cervical cancer. *J Low Genit Tract Dis*. 2012;16(3):175–204, with permission.

Detection Methods

Molecular technologies for HPV detection have developed rapidly and been widely implemented clinically. The U.S. Food and Drug Administration (FDA) has approved five tests for detecting HPV. The first, Hybrid Capture II (HCII) assay (Qiagen, Germantown, MD), was approved in 2003; it detects 13 high-risk HPV types through nucleic acid hybridization assays using signal amplification and chemiluminescence. In 2009, the FDA approved two additional HPV DNA tests: Cervista HPV HR (Hologic, Bedford, MA), which detects 14 high-risk types, and Cervista HPV-16/18 (Hologic, Bedford, MA), which detects HPV types 16 and 18. In 2011, the Cobas HPV test (Roche Molecular Systems, Pleasanton, CA) was approved for the identification of HPV-16 and -18 while concurrently detecting 12 other high-risk HPV types. Most recently, the APTIMA HPV assay (GenProbe, San Diego, CA) was approved for cytology triage and cotesting. This assay detects the messenger RNA of the oncogenic E6 and E7 proteins of 14 high-risk HPV types (**Table 7.3**).

After over 60 years of cervical cancer screening with the Pap smear alone, guidelines have been modified to reflect an improved understanding of the role of high-risk HPV in the development of cervical cancer and the role of HPV testing in cervical cancer screening. The ASCCP recommends HPV testing in a variety of specific situations (130,148).

Primary HPV testing as the sole screening modality has been investigated in multiple international trials and shows promise in upfront screening strategies (146,149,150). In general, it has demonstrated improved sensitivity compared with cytology, although specificity may be lower. The ATHENA trial (Addressing the Need for Advanced HPV Diagnostics) was the first US-based prospective study to evaluate HPV testing as an upfront screening strategy. The objective of this trial was to evaluate various screening strategies with endpoints including detection of CIN2+, number of screening tests required, and number of colposcopies required. Over 40,000 women aged 25 and over were enrolled. Primary HPV testing with triage to colposcopy if the patient was specifically HPV-16 or HPV-18 positive had the highest sensitivity of CIN 2+ detection (80%), but required more colposcopic exams. Cotesting with both upfront cytology and high-risk HPV testing had similar sensitivity, but required many more screening tests (150). These data support primary HPV screening (with colposcopy based on HPV subtype analysis) for women aged 25 and over (151).

Additional Screening Strategies

In addition to cervical cytology and HPV testing from liquid-based cytologic specimens, other innovative techniques are being used in populations with limited access to standard screening approaches. In an attempt to make high-risk HPV testing more efficient, less invasive, and less costly, self-HPV testing has developed. Self-sampling demonstrates high concordance with physician collected samples (152). Prospective trials involving women who did not attend routine cervical screening programs in the Netherlands showed that, because of higher participation rates, the detection rate of CIN was higher than in the regularly screened population (153,154).

In developing nations where the cost of frequent follow-up exams and testing is prohibitive, visual inspection tests have emerged as an important method of screening and treatment. With a bright halogen lamp, visual inspection with acetic acid (VIA) or Lugol's iodine (VILI) is performed and positive lesions are referred to colposcopy with directed biopsy. Additionally, positive lesions can be treated immediately, bypassing the need for follow-up colposcopy. This is an efficient method of screening and treatment, and health care providers can be trained easily in visual inspection, further improving its feasibility (155). Although significant verification bias exists in a see-and-treat strategy, pooled analysis of trials utilizing visual inspection in developing nations revealed a sensitivity of 62% to 80% and specificity of 77% to 84% in detecting high-grade CIN (156).

VIA and VILI with see-and-treat strategies appear to be cost-effective. A study that modeled screening strategies in India, Kenya, Peru, South Africa, and Thailand showed that screening women once per lifetime with visual inspection effectively reduced cervical cancer mortality by over 25% at an acceptably low cost in relation to each nation's gross domestic product (157). Population-based studies on VIA have yielded mixed results. In a South Indian population, cervical cancer mortality was reduced by 25% with VIA compared to no screening (158). In the largest prospective trial enrolling over 130,000 women in rural India, one-time screening methods of HPV testing, cytology, and VIA were compared. Compared with a control group, only HPV testing reduced the rate of cervical cancer (159). Thus, once per lifetime HPV testing in women over 30 has been proposed as an effective method of cervical cancer reduction in low-resource settings.

TABLE 7.3. Cervical Cancer Screening

Name	Company	HPV Genotype Detection	Uses	FDA Approval Date
Digene Hybrid Capture 2 High-Risk HPV DNA Test	QIAGEN, Germantown, MD	16, 18, 31, 33, 35, 39, 45, 51, 52, 56, 58, 59, and 68	ASC-US triage Cotesting in women >30 years old	March 2003
Cervista HPV HR	Hologic, Bedford, MA	16, 18, 31, 33, 35, 39, 45, 51, 52, 56, 58, 59, 66, and 68	ASC-US triage Cotesting in women >30 years old	March 2009
Cervista HPV 16/18	Hologic, Bedford, MA	16, 18	Triage for follow-up of women >30 years old with negative cytology and positive high-risk HPV	March 2009
Cobas HPV Test	Roche Molecular Systems, Pleasanton, CA	Specifically identifies 16 and 18 while concurrently testing for 31, 33, 35, 39, 51, 52, 56, 58, 59, 66, and 68	ASC-US triage Cotesting in women >30 years old Triage for follow-up of women >30 years old with negative cytology and positive high-risk HPV testing	April 2011
APTIMA HPV assay	GenProbe, San Diego, CA	16, 18, 31, 33, 35, 39, 45, 51, 52, 56, 58, 59, 66, and 68	ASC-US triage Cotesting in women >30 years old	February 2012

Source: Adapted from Saslow D, Solomon D, Lawson HW, et al. American Cancer Society, American Society for Colposcopy and Cervical Pathology, and American Society for Clinical Pathology screening guidelines for the prevention and early detection of cervical cancer. *J Low Genit Tract Dis*. 2012;16(3):175–204, with permission.

SECTION 6: HPV VACCINATION

With an improved understanding of the role of HPV infection in the natural history of preinvasive and invasive lesions of the lower genital tract, prophylactic vaccination has emerged as an important element in cervical cancer prevention (**Table 7.4**).

The L1 capsid protein, which is one of two viral capsid proteins of the HPV virus, is the primary target for prophylactic vaccination. Vaccines consist of recombinant L1 proteins that form VLPs, which are combined with different adjuvants. Adjuvants stimulate the immune system and increase the response to vaccination and are aluminum based. VLPs primarily induce a humoral response with neutralizing antibodies, but they also induce cell-mediated immune responses. Neutralizing antibody responses are logs higher than that generated from a response to a new HPV infection.

Currently, three vaccines are approved in the United States for the prevention of cervical cancer. The quadrivalent vaccine (Merck & Co., Inc., Whitehouse Station, NJ, USA) contains VLPs to HPV types 6, 11, 16, and 18, and the bivalent vaccine (GlaxoSmithKline, Rixenstart, Belgium) contains VLPs to HPV types 16 and 18. In addition to the types covered in the quadrivalent vaccine, the newest 9-valent vaccine (Gardasil 9, Merck & Co., Inc., Whitehouse Station, NJ, USA) contains additional VLPs to the HPV types 31, 33, 45, 52, and 58, which combined account for about 20% of cervical cancers.

The FDA originally approved the quadrivalent vaccine in 2006 for girls and women aged between 15 and 25 years for the prevention of cervical cancer caused by HPV types 16 and 18; precancerous genital lesions caused by HPV types 6, 11, 16, and 18; and genital warts caused by HPV types 6 and 11. The federal Advisory Committee on Immunization Practices (ACIP) recommended routine vaccination of all 11- and 12-year-old girls. The three-shot vaccination series can begin as young as age 9 and can be given to women up to age 26. In 2008, the quadrivalent vaccine was also approved for the prevention of vaginal and vulvar cancer in this same population. The following year, its use was expanded to the prevention of genital warts due to HPV type 6 and 11 in boys and men aged between 15 and 25. In 2010, the FDA further expanded the indications to include the prevention of anal cancer and associated premalignant lesions caused by these same HPV types. In 2011, the ACIP recommended routine vaccination of all boys. The vaccine series can be given to boys as young as age 9 and up through age 22 for most men. The FDA approved the bivalent vaccine in 2009 for the prevention of cervical cancer and precancerous lesions caused by HPV-16 and -18 in women from 15 to 25 years of age. The ACIP recommendations for the bivalent vaccine mirror those for the quadrivalent vaccine, except that the bivalent vaccine is not approved for use in males. The 9-valent was approved in December 2014 for females aged 9 to 26 and males aged 9 to 15 for the prevention of cervical, vulvar, vaginal, and anal cancers and genital warts caused by the nine HPV types.

Multiple phase III trials have been conducted to evaluate the efficacy of these vaccines (160–162). These trials were blinded, placebo-controlled trials with endpoints that included development of CIN as well as external genital lesions for the quadrivalent vaccine. In an international trial that enrolled over 17,000 women aged between 16 and 26, the quadrivalent vaccine was 99% effective in preventing HPV-16 and -18 preinvasive or invasive lesions in a 3-year follow-up period in women who were HPV-naive at baseline. In an intent-to-treat analysis including women with preexisting infections, there was considerably less efficacy against incidence of CIN 2/3 or AIS due to any HPV type, thus proving that it works primarily as a prophylactic vaccine (161). This trial also showed that the quadrivalent vaccine was effective in preventing 96% of CIN 1, 100% of VIN 1, and 99% of condyloma in HPV-naive women (160).

The 4-year follow-up of a bivalent HPV vaccine trial, which enrolled over 18,000 young women, showed similar efficacy against development of CIN 3 and AIS. Specifically, efficacy against HPV-16– and HPV-18–mediated CIN 3 lesions was 100% in women who were HPV negative at the time of vaccination. The vaccine was also effective against other lesions caused by HPV types 31, 33, and 45, which are closely related to HPV-16 and -18 (163).

An international trial compared the efficacy of the quadrivalent vaccine with the 9-valent vaccine in women aged 16 to 26 years old (164). The rate of high-grade preinvasive genital tract disease was the same in both arms (14 per 1,000 person years), although there was a significant reduction in disease related to the five additional HPV types in the 9-valent arm. Antibody responses to HPV types 6, 11, 16, and 18 were noninferior in the 9-valent arm compared with the quadrivalent arm.

HPV vaccination has not been shown to be therapeutic against preexisting HPV infections. Therefore, HPV vaccine is most effective if it is administered prior to the onset of sexual activity. Additionally, the vaccine is not infectious, does not contain anything that would be teratogenic, and is considered teratogenicity category B. Routine pregnancy testing prior to administration is not necessary and lactating women can safely receive the vaccine (165). Based on the natural history of HPV infection and development of preinvasive and invasive disease, it may take at least 15 years before there is a significant impact on the incidence of high-grade SIL and perhaps 30 years before there is a change in cervical cancer incidence.

HPV vaccination programs are being instituted worldwide. HPV vaccination presents unique challenges in both high- and low-resource settings, including an older age of vaccination, a three-dose regimen

TABLE 7.4. HPV Vaccines

	Gardasil[a]	Cervarix[b]	Gardasil-9[a]
VLP types	HPV-6, -11, -16, -18	HPV-16, -18	HPV-6, -11, -16, -18, -31, -33, -45, -52, -58
Adjuvant	Aluminum salt	Aluminum salt plus monophosphoryl lipid A	Aluminum salt
Injection schedule	Three injections: 0, 2, 6 months	Three injections: 0, 1, 6 months	Three injections: 0, 2, 6 months
FDA approval	Females: prevention of vaginal, vulvar, and cervical cancer and their premalignant lesions (HPV-16, -18) Females and males: preventions of genital warts (HPV-6 and -11), anal cancer, and premalignant lesions (HPV-16, -18)	Females: prevention of cervical cancer and premalignant cervical lesions (HPV-16, -18)	Females: prevention of vaginal, vulvar, and cervical cancer and their premalignant lesions (HPV-16, -18, -31, -33, -45, -52, -58) Females and males: prevention of genital warts (HPV-6 and -11), anal cancer, and premalignant lesions
Additional benefits	Safe in lactation	Safe in lactation Efficacy against HPV-31, -33, -45	Safe in lactation

[a]Merck Sharp & Dohme Corp., Inc., Whitehouse Station, NJ, USA.
[b]GlaxoSmithKline, Rixenstart, Belgium.

at a high cost relative to other childhood vaccines, and potential sociocultural concerns about HPV being a sexually transmitted disease. Uptake of vaccination seems to be most affected by coverage of the vaccine at the state or national level. In the United States, it is estimated that almost 50% of adolescents received at least one dose and only 32% received all three. Vaccine uptake varies significantly by state, likely a reflection of variability of state funding (166). Worldwide, rates are slightly higher in other high-resource settings. In Manchester, United Kingdom, the uptake of two doses was reported at 55%; three-dose coverage in southern Australia was 69% and in Denmark, 62% (167–169). Despite many barriers to HPV vaccination, it is apparent that when communities make a focused effort to promote vaccination through financial coverage or public health awareness, high levels of vaccine uptake are noted.

Over 85% of cervical cancer cases occur in the developing world (170), yet patients in these nations are less likely to receive HPV vaccination. Despite its high cost relative to other childhood vaccines, in nations with high incidence, emerging models suggest that vaccination is cost-effective (171). Moreover, HPV vaccination has recently been made more affordable at a subsidized price of 5 US dollars per dose (166). This has prompted research into the most effective strategies for large-scale vaccination. In a large international trial of developing nations, HPV vaccination programs were integrated into preexisting health center-based and school-based vaccination programs in communities in India, Peru, Uganda, and Vietnam. Remarkably, complete vaccination (i.e., all three doses) was achieved in 68% to 96% of eligible girls (166). This study confirmed that a range of HPV vaccine delivery strategies were effective in achieving HPV immunization among eligible girls.

REFERENCES

1. Hariri S, Unger ER, Sternberg M, et al. Prevalence of genital human papillomavirus among females in the United States, the National Health And Nutrition Examination Survey, 2003-2006. *J Infect Dis.* 2011;204:566–573.
2. Chesson HW, Dunne EF, Hariri S, et al. The estimated lifetime probability of acquiring human papillomavirus in the United States. *Sex Transm Dis.* 2014;41:660–664.
3. Zur Hausen H. Condylomata acuminata and human genital cancer. *Cancer Res.* 1974;36:794.
4. Durst M, Gissmann L, Ikenberg H, et al. A papillomavirus DNA from a cervical carcinoma and its prevalence in cancer biopsy samples from different geographic regions. *Proc Natl Acad Sci U S A.* 1983;80:3812–3815.
5. Boshart M, Gissmann L, Ikenberg H, et al. A new type of papillomavirus DNA, its presence in genital cancer biopsies and in cell lines derived from cervical cancer. *EMBO J.* 1984;3:1151–1157.
6. Bosch FX, Munoz N, Shah KV, et al. Second International Workshop on the epidemiology of cervical cancer and human papillomaviruses. *Int J Cancer.* 1992;52:171–173.
7. Bernard HU, Burk RD, Chen Z, et al. Classification of papillomaviruses (PVs) based on 189 PV types and proposal of taxonomic amendments. *Virology.* 2010;401:70–79.
8. Munoz N, Castellsague X, de Gonzalez AB, et al. Chapter 1: HPV in the etiology of human cancer. *Vaccine.* 2006;24(Suppl 3):S3/1–10.
9. Bouvard V, Baan R, Straif K, et al. A review of human carcinogens—Part B: biological agents. *Lancet Oncol.* 2009;10:321–322.
10. Sen E, Alam S, Meyers C. Genetic and biochemical analysis of cis regulatory elements within the keratinocyte enhancer region of the human papillomavirus type 31 upstream regulatory region during different stages of the viral life cycle. *J Virol.* 2004;78:612–629.
11. Hubert WG, Kanaya T, Laimins LA. DNA replication of human papillomavirus type 31 is modulated by elements of the upstream regulatory region that lie 5' of the minimal origin. *J Virol.* 1999;73:1835–1845.
12. Horvath CA, Boulet GA, Renoux VM, et al. Mechanisms of cell entry by human papillomaviruses: an overview. *Virol J.* 2010;7:11.
13. Shafti-Keramat S, Handisurya A, Kriehuber E, et al. Different heparan sulfate proteoglycans serve as cellular receptors for human papillomaviruses. *J Virol.* 2003;77:13125–1335.
14. Evander M, Frazer IH, Payne E, et al. Identification of the alpha6 integrin as a candidate receptor for papillomaviruses. *J Virol.* 1997;71:2449–2456.
15. Culp TD, Budgeon LR, Marinkovich MP, et al. Keratinocyte-secreted laminin 5 can function as a transient receptor for human papillomaviruses by binding virions and transferring them to adjacent cells. *J Virol.* 2006;80:8940–8950.
16. Da Silva DM, Fausch SC, Verbeek JS, et al. Uptake of human papillomavirus virus-like particles by dendritic cells is mediated by Fcgamma receptors and contributes to acquisition of T cell immunity. *J Immunol.* 2007;178:7587–7597.
17. Day PM, Lowy DR, Schiller JT. Heparan sulfate-independent cell binding and infection with furin-precleaved papillomavirus capsids. *J Virol.* 2008;82:12565–12568.
18. Schelhaas M, Ewers H, Rajamaki ML, et al. Human papillomavirus type 16 entry: retrograde cell surface transport along actin-rich protrusions. *PLoS Pathog.* 2008;4:e1000148.
19. Day PM, Lowy DR, Schiller JT. Papillomaviruses infect cells via a clathrin-dependent pathway. *Virology.* 2003;307:1–11.
20. Spoden G, Freitag K, Husmann M, et al. Clathrin- and caveolin-independent entry of human papillomavirus type 16--involvement of tetraspanin-enriched microdomains (TEMs). *PLoS One.* 2008;3:e3313.
21. Wise-Draper TM, Wells SI. Papillomavirus E6 and E7 proteins and their cellular targets. *Front Biosci.* 2008;13:1003–1017.
22. Boyer SN, Wazer DE, Band V. E7 protein of human papilloma virus-16 induces degradation of retinoblastoma protein through the ubiquitin-proteasome pathway. *Cancer Res.* 1996;56:4620–4624.
23. Huang PS, Patrick DR, Edwards G, et al. Protein domains governing interactions between E2F, the retinoblastoma gene product, and human papillomavirus type 16 E7 protein. *Mol Cell Biol.* 1993;13:953–960.
24. Longworth MS, Laimins LA. The binding of histone deacetylases and the integrity of zinc finger-like motifs of the E7 protein are essential for the life cycle of human papillomavirus type 31. *J Virol.* 2004;78:3533–3541.
25. Duensing S, Lee LY, Duensing A, et al. The human papillomavirus type 16 E6 and E7 oncoproteins cooperate to induce mitotic defects and genomic instability by uncoupling centrosome duplication from the cell division cycle. *Proc Natl Acad Sci U S A.* 2000;97:10002–10007.
26. Thomas M, Pim D, Banks L. The role of the E6-p53 interaction in the molecular pathogenesis of HPV. *Oncogene.* 1999;18:7690–7700.
27. Thomas MC, Chiang CM. E6 oncoprotein represses p53-dependent gene activation via inhibition of protein acetylation independently of inducing p53 degradation. *Mol Cell.* 2005;17:251–264.
28. Massimi P, Gammoh N, Thomas M, et al. HPV E6 specifically targets different cellular pools of its PDZ domain-containing tumour suppressor substrates for proteasome-mediated degradation. *Oncogene.* 2004;23:8033–8039.
29. Veldman T, Horikawa I, Barrett JC, et al. Transcriptional activation of the telomerase hTERT gene by human papillomavirus type 16 E6 oncoprotein. *J Virol.* 2001;75:4467–4472.
30. Frattini MG, Laimins LA. The role of the E1 and E2 proteins in the replication of human papillomavirus type 31b. *Virology.* 1994;204:799–804.
31. Ma T, Zou N, Lin BY, et al. Interaction between cyclin-dependent kinases and human papillomavirus replication-initiation protein E1 is required for efficient viral replication. *Proc Natl Acad Sci U S A.* 1999;96:382–387.
32. Bouvard V, Storey A, Pim D, et al. Characterization of the human papillomavirus E2 protein: evidence of trans-activation and trans-repression in cervical keratinocytes. *EMBO J.* 1994;13:5451–5459.
33. Jeon S, Allen-Hoffmann BL, Lambert PF. Integration of human papillomavirus type 16 into the human genome correlates with a selective growth advantage of cells. *J Virol.* 1995;69:2989–2997.
34. Ho CM, Lee BH, Chang SF, et al. Integration of human papillomavirus correlates with high levels of viral oncogene transcripts in cervical carcinogenesis. *Virus Res.* 2011;161:124–130.
35. Tonon SA, Picconi MA, Bos PD, et al. Physical status of the E2 human papilloma virus 16 viral gene in cervical preneoplastic and neoplastic lesions. *J Clin Virol.* 2001;21:129–134.
36. Hopman AH, Smedts F, Dignef W, et al. Transition of high-grade cervical intraepithelial neoplasia to micro-invasive carcinoma is characterized by integration of HPV 16/18 and numerical chromosome abnormalities. *J Pathol.* 2004;202:23–33.
37. Smith JS, Melendy A, Rana RK, et al. Age-specific prevalence of infection with human papillomavirus in females: a global review. *J Adolesc Health.* 2008;43:S5–S25, S25 e1–e41.
38. Giuliano AR, Lee JH, Fulp W, et al. Incidence and clearance of genital human papillomavirus infection in men (HIM): a cohort study. *Lancet.* 2011;377:932–940.
39. Giuliano AR, Lazcano-Ponce E, Villa LL, et al. The human papillomavirus infection in men study: human papillomavirus prevalence and type distribution among men residing in Brazil, Mexico, and the United States. *Cancer Epidemiol Biomarkers Prev.* 2008;17:2036–2043.

40. Gillison ML, Broutian T, Pickard RK, et al. Prevalence of oral HPV infection in the United States, 2009–2010. *JAMA*. 2012;307:693–703.
41. Albero G, Castellsague X, Giuliano AR, et al. Male circumcision and genital human papillomavirus: a systematic review and meta-analysis. *Sex Transm Dis*. 2012;39:104–113.
42. Backes DM, Kurman RJ, Pimenta JM, et al. Systematic review of human papillomavirus prevalence in invasive penile cancer. *Cancer Causes Control*. 2009;20:449–457.
43. Strickler HD, Burk RD, Fazzari M, et al. Natural history and possible reactivation of human papillomavirus in human immunodeficiency virus-positive women. *J Natl Cancer Inst*. 2005;97:577–586.
44. Gonzalez P, Hildesheim A, Rodriguez AC, et al. Behavioral/lifestyle and immunologic factors associated with HPV infection among women older than 45 years. *Cancer Epidemiol Biomarkers Prev*. 2010;19:3044–3054.
45. Winer RL, Hughes JP, Feng Q, et al. Early natural history of incident, type-specific human papillomavirus infections in newly sexually active young women. *Cancer Epidemiol Biomarkers Prev*. 2011;20:699–707.
46. Rodriguez AC, Schiffman M, Herrero R, et al. Low risk of type-specific carcinogenic HPV re-appearance with subsequent cervical intraepithelial neoplasia grade 2/3. *Int J Cancer*. 2012;131(8):1874–1881.
47. Ferreccio C, Van De Wyngard V, Olcay F, et al. High-risk HPV infection after five years in a population-based cohort of Chilean women. *Infect Agent Cancer*. 2011;6:21.
48. Dalstein V, Riethmuller D, Pretet JL, et al. Persistence and load of high-risk HPV are predictors for development of high-grade cervical lesions: a longitudinal French cohort study. *Int J Cancer*. 2003;106:396–403.
49. Richardson H, Kelsall G, Tellier P, et al. The natural history of type-specific human papillomavirus infections in female university students. *Cancer Epidemiol Biomarkers Prev*. 2003;12:485–490.
50. Moscicki AB, Hills N, Shiboski S, et al. Risks for incident human papillomavirus infection and low-grade squamous intraepithelial lesion development in young females. *JAMA*. 2001;285:2995–3002.
51. Bae J, Seo SS, Park YS, et al. Natural history of persistent high-risk human papillomavirus infections in Korean women. *Gynecol Oncol*. 2009;115:75–80.
52. Koutsky LA, Holmes KK, Critchlow CW, et al. A cohort study of the risk of cervical intraepithelial neoplasia grade 2 or 3 in relation to papillomavirus infection. *N Engl J Med*. 1992;327:1272–1278.
53. Bory JP, Cucherousset J, Lorenzato M, et al. Recurrent human papillomavirus infection detected with the hybrid capture II assay selects women with normal cervical smears at risk for developing high grade cervical lesions: a longitudinal study of 3,091 women. *Int J Cancer*. 2002;102:519–525.
54. Ho GY, Bierman R, Beardsley L, et al. Natural history of cervicovaginal papillomavirus infection in young women. *N Engl J Med*. 1998;338:423–428.
55. Houlihan CF, de Sanjose S, Baisley K, et al. Prevalence of human papillomavirus in adolescent girls before reported sexual debut. *J Infect Dis*. 2014;210:837–845.
56. Shew ML, Weaver B, Tu W, et al. High frequency of human papillomavirus detection in the vagina before first vaginal intercourse among females enrolled in a longitudinal cohort study. *J Infect Dis*. 2013;207:1012–1015.
57. Kjaer SK, Chackerian B, van den Brule AJ, et al. High-risk human papillomavirus is sexually transmitted: evidence from a follow-up study of virgins starting sexual activity (intercourse). *Cancer Epidemiol Biomarkers Prev*. 2001;10:101–106.
58. Nyitray AG, Menezes L, Lu B, et al. Genital Human Papillomavirus (HPV) Concordance in Heterosexual Couples. *J Infect Dis*. 2012;206(2):202–211.
59. Burchell AN, Coutlee F, Tellier PP, et al. Genital transmission of human papillomavirus in recently formed heterosexual couples. *J Infect Dis*. 2011;204:1723–1729.
60. Bleeker MC, Hogewoning CJ, Berkhof J, et al. Concordance of specific human papillomavirus types in sex partners is more prevalent than would be expected by chance and is associated with increased viral loads. *Clin Infect Dis*. 2005;41:612–620.
61. Burchell AN, Tellier PP, Hanley J, et al. Human papillomavirus infections among couples in new sexual relationships. *Epidemiology*. 2010;21:31–37.
62. Benevolo M, Mottolese M, Marandino F, et al. HPV prevalence among healthy Italian male sexual partners of women with cervical HPV infection. *J Med Virol*. 2008;80:1275–1281.
63. Winer RL, Hughes JP, Feng Q, et al. Condom use and the risk of genital human papillomavirus infection in young women. *N Engl J Med*. 2006;354:2645–2654.
64. Winer RL, Lee SK, Hughes JP, et al. Genital human papillomavirus infection: incidence and risk factors in a cohort of female university students. *Am J Epidemiol*. 2003;157:218–226.
65. Franco EL, Villa LL, Ruiz A, et al. Transmission of cervical human papillomavirus infection by sexual activity: differences between low and high oncogenic risk types. *J Infect Dis*. 1995;172:756–763.
66. Watts DH, Fazzari M, Minkoff H, et al. Effects of bacterial vaginosis and other genital infections on the natural history of human papillomavirus infection in HIV-1-infected and high-risk HIV-1-uninfected women. *J Infect Dis*. 2005;191:1129–1139.
67. King CC, Jamieson DJ, Wiener J, et al. Bacterial vaginosis and the natural history of human papillomavirus. *Infect Dis Obstet Gynecol*. 2011;2011:319460.
68. Quint KD, de Koning MN, Geraets DT, et al. Comprehensive analysis of Human Papillomavirus and *Chlamydia trachomatis* in in-situ and invasive cervical adenocarcinoma. *Gynecol Oncol*. 2009;114:390–394.
69. Anttila T, Saikku P, Koskela P, et al. Serotypes of *Chlamydia trachomatis* and risk for development of cervical squamous cell carcinoma. *JAMA*. 2001;285:47–51.
70. Lehtinen M, Ault KA, Lyytikainen E, et al. *Chlamydia trachomatis* infection and risk of cervical intraepithelial neoplasia. *Sex Transm Infect*. 2011;87:372–376.
71. Samoff E, Koumans EH, Markowitz LE, et al. Association of *Chlamydia trachomatis* with persistence of high-risk types of human papillomavirus in a cohort of female adolescents. *Am J Epidemiol*. 2005;162:668–675.
72. Silins I, Ryd W, Strand A, et al. *Chlamydia trachomatis* infection and persistence of human papillomavirus. *Int J Cancer*. 2005;116:110–115.
73. IARC Working Group on the Evaluation of Carcinogenic Risks to Humans. Tobacco smoke and involuntary smoking. *IARC Monogr Eval Carcinog Risks Hum*. 2004;83:1–1438.
74. Byrne MM, Davila EP, Zhao W, et al. Cancer screening behaviors among smokers and non-smokers. *Cancer Epidemiol*. 2010;34:611–617.
75. Wilkerson JE, Bailey JM, Bieniasz ME, et al. Psychosocial factors in risk of cervical intraepithelial lesions. *J Womens Health (Larchmt)*. 2009;18:513–518.
76. Vaccarella S, Herrero R, Snijders PJ, et al. Smoking and human papillomavirus infection: pooled analysis of the International Agency for Research on Cancer HPV Prevalence Surveys. *Int J Epidemiol*. 2008;37:536–546.
77. Collins S, Rollason TP, Young LS, et al. Cigarette smoking is an independent risk factor for cervical intraepithelial neoplasia in young women: a longitudinal study. *Eur J Cancer*. 2010;46:405–411.
78. Ho GY, Kadish AS, Burk RD, et al. HPV 16 and cigarette smoking as risk factors for high-grade cervical intra-epithelial neoplasia. *Int J Cancer*. 1998;78:281–285.
79. Koshiol J, Schroeder J, Jamieson DJ, et al. Smoking and time to clearance of human papillomavirus infection in HIV-seropositive and HIV-seronegative women. *Am J Epidemiol*. 2006;164:176–183.
80. Giuliano AR, Sedjo RL, Roe DJ, et al. Clearance of oncogenic human papillomavirus (HPV) infection: effect of smoking (United States). *Cancer Causes Control*. 2002;13:839–846.
81. Xi LF, Koutsky LA, Castle PE, et al. Relationship between cigarette smoking and human papilloma virus types 16 and 18 DNA load. *Cancer Epidemiol Biomarkers Prev*. 2009;18:3490–3496.
82. Prokopczyk B, Cox JE, Hoffmann D, et al. Identification of tobacco-specific carcinogen in the cervical mucus of smokers and nonsmokers. *J Natl Cancer Inst*. 1997;89:868–873.
83. Alam S, Conway MJ, Chen HS, et al. The cigarette smoke carcinogen benzo[a]pyrene enhances human papillomavirus synthesis. *J Virol*. 2008;82:1053–1058.
84. Barton SE, Maddox PH, Jenkins D, et al. Effect of cigarette smoking on cervical epithelial immunity: a mechanism for neoplastic change? *Lancet*. 1988;2:652–654.
85. Lea JS, Coleman R, Kurien A, et al. Aberrant p16 methylation is a biomarker for tobacco exposure in cervical squamous cell carcinogenesis. *Am J Obstet Gynecol*. 2004;190:674–679.
86. Samir R, Asplund A, Tot T, et al. Tissue tumor marker expression in smokers, including serum cotinine concentrations, in women with cervical intraepithelial neoplasia or normal squamous cervical epithelium. *Am J Obstet Gynecol*. 2010;202:579 e1–e7.
87. Appleby P, Beral V, Berrington de Gonzalez A, et al. Cervical cancer and hormonal contraceptives: collaborative reanalysis of individual data for 16,573 women with cervical cancer and 35,509 women without cervical cancer from 24 epidemiological studies. *Lancet*. 2007;370:1609–1621.
88. Longatto-Filho A, Hammes LS, Sarian LO, et al. Hormonal contraceptives and the length of their use are not independent risk factors for high-risk HPV infections or high-grade CIN. *Gynecol Obstet Invest*. 2011;71:93–103.
89. International Collaboration of Epidemiological Studies of Cervical Cancer. Comparison of risk factors for invasive squamous cell carcinoma and adenocarcinoma of the cervix: collaborative reanalysis of individual data on 8,097 women with squamous cell carcinoma and 1,374 women with adenocarcinoma from 12 epidemiological studies. *Int J Cancer*. 2007;120:885–891.

90. Maiman M, Fruchter RG, Serur E, et al. Human immunodeficiency virus infection and cervical neoplasia. *Gynecol Oncol.* 1990;38:377–382.
91. Mbulawa ZZ, Coetzee D, Marais DJ, et al. Genital human papillomavirus prevalence and human papillomavirus concordance in heterosexual couples are positively associated with human immunodeficiency virus coinfection. *J Infect Dis.* 2009;199:1514–1524.
92. Massad LS, Xie X, Burk R, et al. Long-term cumulative detection of human papillomavirus among HIV seropositive women. *AIDS.* 2014;28:2601–2608.
93. De Vuyst H, Lillo F, Broutet N, et al. HIV, human papillomavirus, and cervical neoplasia and cancer in the era of highly active antiretroviral therapy. *Eur J Cancer Prev.* 2008;17:545–554.
94. Bratcher LF, Sahasrabuddhe VV. The impact of antiretroviral therapy on HPV and cervical intraepithelial neoplasia: current evidence and directions for future research. *Infect Agent Cancer.* 2010;5:8.
95. Massad LS, Xie X, D'Souza G, et al. Incidence of cervical precancers among HIV-seropositive women. *Am J Obstet Gynecol.* 2015;212:606. e1–e8.
96. Wistuba, II, Syed S, Behrens C, et al. Comparison of molecular changes in cervical intraepithelial neoplasia in HIV-positive and HIV-indeterminate subjects. *Gynecol Oncol.* 1999;74:519–526.
97. Halpert R, Fruchter RG, Sedlis A, et al. Human papillomavirus and lower genital neoplasia in renal transplant patients. *Obstet Gynecol.* 1986;68:251–258.
98. Origoni M, Stefani C, Dell'Antonio G, et al. Cervical Human Papillomavirus in transplanted Italian women: a long-term prospective follow-up study. *J Clin Virol.* 2011;51:250–254.
99. Adami J, Gabel H, Lindelof B, et al. Cancer risk following organ transplantation: a nationwide cohort study in Sweden. *Br J Cancer.* 2003;89:1221–1227.
100. Engels EA, Pfeiffer RM, Fraumeni JF Jr, et al. Spectrum of cancer risk among US solid organ transplant recipients. *JAMA.* 2011;306:1891–1901.
101. Meeuwis KA, Melchers WJ, Bouten H, et al. Anogenital malignancies in women after renal transplantation over 40 years in a single center. *Transplantation.* 2012;93(9):914–922.
102. Brown MR, Noffsinger A, First MR, et al. HPV subtype analysis in lower genital tract neoplasms of female renal transplant recipients. *Gynecol Oncol.* 2000;79:220–224.
103. Hariri S, Unger ER, Powell SE, et al. Human papillomavirus genotypes in high-grade cervical lesions in the United States. *J Infect Dis.* 2012;206:1878–1886.
104. Banister CE, Messersmith AR, Cai B, et al. Disparity in the persistence of high-risk human papillomavirus genotypes between African American and European American women of college age. *J Infect Dis.* 2015;211:100–108.
105. Darragh TM, Colgan TJ, Cox JT, et al. The Lower Anogenital Squamous Terminology Standardization Project for HPV-associated lesions: background and consensus recommendations from the College of American Pathologists and the American Society for Colposcopy and Cervical Pathology. *J Low Genit Tract Dis.* 2012;16:205–242.
106. Scott ME, Ma Y, Kuzmich L, et al. Diminished IFN-gamma and IL-10 and elevated Foxp3 mRNA expression in the cervix are associated with CIN 2 or 3. *Int J Cancer.* 2009;124:1379–1383.
107. Pudney J, Quayle AJ, Anderson DJ. Immunological microenvironments in the human vagina and cervix: mediators of cellular immunity are concentrated in the cervical transformation zone. *Biol Reprod.* 2005;73:1253–1263.
108. Stoler MH, Schiffman M. Interobserver reproducibility of cervical cytologic and histologic interpretations: realistic estimates from the ASCUS-LSIL Triage Study. *JAMA.* 2001;285:1500–1505.
109. Carreon JD, Sherman ME, Guillen D, et al. CIN2 is a much less reproducible and less valid diagnosis than CIN3: results from a histological review of population-based cervical samples. *Int J Gynecol Pathol.* 2007;26:441–446.
110. Krawczyk E, Suprynowicz FA, Liu X, et al. Koilocytosis: a cooperative interaction between the human papillomavirus E5 and E6 oncoproteins. *Am J Pathol.* 2008;173:682–688.
111. Castle PE, Gage JC, Wheeler CM, et al. The clinical meaning of a cervical intraepithelial neoplasia grade 1 biopsy. *Obstet Gynecol.* 2011;118:1222–1229.
112. Elit L, Levine MN, Julian JA, et al. Expectant management versus immediate treatment for low-grade cervical intraepithelial neoplasia: a randomized trial in Canada and Brazil. *Cancer.* 2011;117:1438–1445.
113. Cox JT, Schiffman M, Solomon D. Prospective follow-up suggests similar risk of subsequent cervical intraepithelial neoplasia grade 2 or 3 among women with cervical intraepithelial neoplasia grade 1 or negative colposcopy and directed biopsy. *Am J Obstet Gynecol.* 2003;188:1406–1412.
114. McCredie MR, Sharples KJ, Paul C, et al. Natural history of cervical neoplasia and risk of invasive cancer in women with cervical intraepithelial neoplasia 3: a retrospective cohort study. *Lancet Oncol.* 2008;9:425–434.
115. Wang SS, Sherman ME, Hildesheim A, et al. Cervical adenocarcinoma and squamous cell carcinoma incidence trends among white women and black women in the United States for 1976–2000. *Cancer.* 2004;100:1035–1044.
116. de Sanjose S, Quint WG, Alemany L, et al. Human papillomavirus genotype attribution in invasive cervical cancer: a retrospective cross-sectional worldwide study. *Lancet Oncol.* 2010;11:1048–1056.
117. Zaino RJ. Symposium part I: adenocarcinoma in situ, glandular dysplasia, and early invasive adenocarcinoma of the uterine cervix. *Int J Gynecol Pathol.* 2002;21:314–326.
118. Pavlakis K, Messini I, Athanassiadou S, et al. Endocervical glandular lesions: a diagnostic approach combining a semi-quantitative scoring method to the expression of CEA, MIB-1 and p16. *Gynecol Oncol.* 2006;103:971–976.
119. Moritani S, Ioffe OB, Sagae S, et al. Mitotic activity and apoptosis in endocervical glandular lesions. *Int J Gynecol Pathol.* 2002;21:125–133.
120. Judson PL, Habermann EB, Baxter NN, et al. Trends in the incidence of invasive and in situ vulvar carcinoma. *Obstet Gynecol.* 2006;107:1018–1022.
121. Sideri M, Jones RW, Wilkinson EJ, et al. Squamous vulvar intraepithelial neoplasia: 2004 modified terminology, ISSVD Vulvar Oncology Subcommittee. *J Reprod Med.* 2005;50:807–810.
122. Carlson JA, Ambros R, Malfetano J, et al. Vulvar lichen sclerosus and squamous cell carcinoma: a cohort, case control, and investigational study with historical perspective; implications for chronic inflammation and sclerosis in the development of neoplasia. *Hum Pathol.* 1998;29:932–948.
123. McNally OM, Mulvany NJ, Pagano R, et al. VIN 3: a clinicopathologic review. *Int J Gynecol Cancer.* 2002;12:490–495.
124. Jones RW, Rowan DM, Stewart AW. Vulvar intraepithelial neoplasia: aspects of the natural history and outcome in 405 women. *Obstet Gynecol.* 2005;106:1319–1326.
125. van Seters M, van Beurden M, de Craen AJ. Is the assumed natural history of vulvar intraepithelial neoplasia III based on enough evidence? A systematic review of 3322 published patients. *Gynecol Oncol.* 2005;97:645–651.
126. Husseinzadeh N, Recinto C. Frequency of invasive cancer in surgically excised vulvar lesions with intraepithelial neoplasia (VIN 3). *Gynecol Oncol.* 1999;73:119–120.
127. Diakomanolis E, Stefanidis K, Rodolakis A, et al. Vaginal intraepithelial neoplasia: report of 102 cases. *Eur J Gynaecol Oncol.* 2002;23:457–459.
128. Dodge JA, Eltabbakh GH, Mount SL, et al. Clinical features and risk of recurrence among patients with vaginal intraepithelial neoplasia. *Gynecol Oncol.* 2001;83:363–369.
129. Tsimplaki E, Argyri E, Michala L, et al. Human papillomavirus genotyping and e6/e7 mRNA expression in Greek women with intraepithelial neoplasia and squamous cell carcinoma of the vagina and vulva. *J Oncol.* 2012;2012:893275.
130. Saslow D, Solomon D, Lawson HW, et al. American Cancer Society, American Society for Colposcopy and Cervical Pathology, and American Society for Clinical Pathology screening guidelines for the prevention and early detection of cervical cancer. *J Low Genit Tract Dis.* 2012;16(3):175–204.
131. Papanicolaou GN, Traut HF. The diagnostic value of vaginal smears in carcinoma of the uterus. 1941. *Arch Pathol Lab Med.* 1997;121:211–224.
132. Sasieni P, Adams J. Effect of screening on cervical cancer mortality in England and Wales: analysis of trends with an age period cohort model. *BMJ.* 1999;318:1244–1245.
133. Quinn M, Babb P, Jones J, et al. Effect of screening on incidence of and mortality from cancer of cervix in England: evaluation based on routinely collected statistics. *BMJ.* 1999;318:904–908.
134. van der Aa MA, Pukkala E, Coebergh JW, et al. Mass screening programmes and trends in cervical cancer in Finland and the Netherlands. *Int J Cancer.* 2008;122:1854–1858.
135. Katki HA, Kinney WK, Fetterman B, et al. Cervical cancer risk for women undergoing concurrent testing for human papillomavirus and cervical cytology: a population-based study in routine clinical practice. *Lancet Oncol.* 2011;12:663–672.
136. Wingo PA, Cardinez CJ, Landis SH, et al. Long-term trends in cancer mortality in the United States, 1930–1998. *Cancer.* 2003;97:3133–3275.
137. Siegel RL, Miller KD, Jemal A. Cancer statistics, 2015. *CA Cancer J Clin.* 2015;65:5–29.
138. Subramaniam A, Fauci JM, Schneider KE, et al. Invasive cervical cancer and screening: what are the rates of unscreened and underscreened women in the modern era? *J Low Genit Tract Dis.* 2011;15:110–113.

139. Islam S, West AM, Saboorian MH, et al. Reprocessing unsatisfactory ThinPrep Papanicolaou test specimens increases sample adequacy and detection of significant cervicovaginal lesions. *Cancer.* 2004;102:67–73.
140. Bentz JS, Rowe LR, Gopez EV, et al. The unsatisfactory ThinPrep Pap Test: missed opportunity for disease detection? *Am J Clin Pathol.* 2002;117:457–463.
141. Woodhouse SL, Stastny JF, Styer PE, et al. Interobserver variability in subclassification of squamous intraepithelial lesions: results of the College of American Pathologists Interlaboratory Comparison Program in cervicovaginal cytology. *Arch Pathol Lab Med.* 1999;123:1079–1084.
142. Cuzick J, Clavel C, Petry KU, et al. Overview of the European and North American studies on HPV testing in primary cervical cancer screening. *Int J Cancer.* 2006;119:1095–1101.
143. Nanda K, McCrory DC, Myers ER, et al. Accuracy of the papanicolaou test in screening for and follow-up of cervical cytologic abnormalities: a systematic review. *Ann Intern Med.* 2000;132:810–819.
144. Stout NK, Goldhaber-Fiebert JD, Ortendahl JD, et al. Trade-offs in cervical cancer prevention: balancing benefits and risks. *Arch Intern Med.* 2008;168:1881–1889.
145. Bulkmans NW, Berkhof J, Rozendaal L, et al. Human papillomavirus DNA testing for the detection of cervical intraepithelial neoplasia grade 3 and cancer: 5-year follow-up of a randomised controlled implementation trial. *Lancet.* 2007;370:1764–1772.
146. Ronco G, Giorgi-Rossi P, Carozzi F, et al. Efficacy of human papillomavirus testing for the detection of invasive cervical cancers and cervical intraepithelial neoplasia: a randomised controlled trial. *Lancet Oncol.* 2010;11:249–257.
147. Anttila A, Kotaniemi-Talonen L, Leinonen M, et al. Rate of cervical cancer, severe intraepithelial neoplasia, and adenocarcinoma in situ in primary HPV DNA screening with cytology triage: randomised study within organised screening programme. *BMJ.* 2010;340:c1804.
148. Massad LS, Einstein MH, Huh WK, et al. 2012 updated consensus guidelines for the management of abnormal cervical cancer screening tests and cancer precursors. *Obstet Gynecol.* 2013;121:829–846.
149. Mayrand MH, Duarte-Franco E, Rodrigues I, et al. Human papillomavirus DNA versus Papanicolaou screening tests for cervical cancer. *N Engl J Med.* 2007;357:1579–1588.
150. Wright TC, Stoler MH, Behrens CM, et al. Primary cervical cancer screening with human papillomavirus: end of study results from the ATHENA study using HPV as the first-line screening test. *Gynecol Oncol.* 2015;136:189–197.
151. Huh WK, Ault KA, Chelmow D, et al. Use of primary high-risk human papillomavirus testing for cervical cancer screening: interim clinical guidance. *Gynecol Oncol.* 2015;136:178–182.
152. Petignat P, Faltin DL, Bruchim I, et al. Are self-collected samples comparable to physician-collected cervical specimens for human papillomavirus DNA testing? A systematic review and meta-analysis. *Gynecol Oncol.* 2007;105:530–535.
153. Gok M, Heideman DA, van Kemenade FJ, et al. HPV testing on self collected cervicovaginal lavage specimens as screening method for women who do not attend cervical screening: cohort study. *BMJ.* 2010;340:c1040.
154. Bais AG, van Kemenade FJ, Berkhof J, et al. Human papillomavirus testing on self-sampled cervicovaginal brushes: an effective alternative to protect nonresponders in cervical screening programs. *Int J Cancer.* 2007;120:1505–1510.
155. Blumenthal PD, Lauterbach M, Sellors JW, et al. Training for cervical cancer prevention programs in low-resource settings: focus on visual inspection with acetic acid and cryotherapy. *Int J Gynaecol Obstet.* 2005;89(Suppl 2):S30–S37.
156. Sankaranarayanan R, Gaffikin L, Jacob M, et al. A critical assessment of screening methods for cervical neoplasia. *Int J Gynaecol Obstet.* 2005;89(Suppl 2):S4–S12.
157. Goldie SJ, Gaffikin L, Goldhaber-Fiebert JD, et al. Cost-effectiveness of cervical-cancer screening in five developing countries. *N Engl J Med.* 2005;353:2158–2168.
158. Sankaranarayanan R, Esmy PO, Rajkumar R, et al. Effect of visual screening on cervical cancer incidence and mortality in Tamil Nadu, India: a cluster-randomised trial. *Lancet.* 2007;370:398–406.
159. Sankaranarayanan R, Nene BM, Shastri SS, et al. HPV screening for cervical cancer in rural India. *N Engl J Med.* 2009,360:1385–1394.
160. Dillner J, Kjaer SK, Wheeler CM, et al. Four year efficacy of prophylactic human papillomavirus quadrivalent vaccine against low grade cervical, vulvar, and vaginal intraepithelial neoplasia and anogenital warts: randomised controlled trial. *BMJ.* 2010;341:c3493.
161. Ault KA. Effect of prophylactic human papillomavirus L1 virus-like-particle vaccine on risk of cervical intraepithelial neoplasia grade 2, grade 3, and adenocarcinoma in situ: a combined analysis of four randomised clinical trials. *Lancet.* 2007;369:1861–1868.
162. Paavonen J, Jenkins D, Bosch FX, et al. Efficacy of a prophylactic adjuvanted bivalent L1 virus-like-particle vaccine against infection with human papillomavirus types 16 and 18 in young women: an interim analysis of a phase III double-blind, randomised controlled trial. *Lancet.* 2007;369:2161–2170.
163. Wheeler CM, Hunt WC, Joste NE, et al. Human papillomavirus genotype distributions: implications for vaccination and cancer screening in the United States. *J Natl Cancer Inst.* 2009;101:475–487.
164. Joura EA, Giuliano AR, Iversen OE, et al. A 9-valent HPV vaccine against infection and intraepithelial neoplasia in women. *N Engl J Med.* 2015;372:711–723.
165. Committee opinion no. 467: human papillomavirus vaccination. *Obstet Gynecol.* 2010;116:800–803.
166. LaMontagne DS, Barge S, Le NT, et al. Human papillomavirus vaccine delivery strategies that achieved high coverage in low- and middle-income countries. *Bull World Health Organ.* 2011;89:821–830.
167. Watson M, Shaw D, Molchanoff L, et al. Challenges, lessons learned and results following the implementation of a human papilloma virus school vaccination program in South Australia. *Aust N Z J Public Health.* 2009;33:365–370.
168. Brabin L, Roberts SA, Stretch R, et al. Uptake of first two doses of human papillomavirus vaccine by adolescent schoolgirls in Manchester: prospective cohort study. *BMJ.* 2008;336:1056–1058.
169. Widgren K, Simonsen J, Valentiner-Branth P, et al. Uptake of the human papillomavirus-vaccination within the free-of-charge childhood vaccination programme in Denmark. *Vaccine.* 2011;29:9663–9667.
170. Ferlay J, Shin HR, Bray F, et al. Estimates of worldwide burden of cancer in 2008: GLOBOCAN 2008. *Int J Cancer.* 2010;127:2893–2917.
171. Termrungruanglert W, Havanond P, Khemapech N, et al. Cost and effectiveness evaluation of prophylactic HPV vaccine in developing countries. *Value Health.* 2012;15:S29–S34.

CHAPTER 8

Perioperative and Critical Care

James J. Burke II, Scott C. Purinton, and Heather MacNew

INTRODUCTION

Surgery remains the mainstay of treatment for women with gynecologic malignancies regardless of whether an open or minimally invasive approach is utilized. Ultimately, outcomes of the surgical intervention rest with the gynecologic oncologist in concert with anesthesiologists, nursing staff, stomal therapists, physical therapists, pharmacists, social workers, and the social network/support of the patient, as well as others. Careful assessment of the patient prior to surgery can lead to improved outcomes and minimize surprises in the postoperative period. Should the need arise, prudent consultation with other medical specialists prior to or following surgery can further enhance patient care and result in better outcomes.

The chapter has been divided into two sections: preoperative care/risk recognition and postoperative care/critical care. Within each section, clinical information has been arranged by organ system, and recommendations are based on evidence (when available). As has become the norm with hospitals in the United States, most intensive care units (ICUs) have become "closed," meaning that when a patient is admitted to the ICU, the patient is cared for by a team led by a critical care specialist/intensivist. Thus, the critical care section provides basic yet practical information for the reader so that comanagement of the critically ill gynecologic oncology patient with an intensivist may be seamless.

PREOPERATIVE RISK ASSESSMENT

Initial Preoperative Evaluation

At the initial consultation for patients with known or suspected gynecologic malignancies, the gynecologic oncologist should take a thorough history, assessing for comorbid conditions, which may impact perioperative risk (1). Similarly, a thorough physical examination, looking for signs of diseases of which the patient is unaware, will aid in finding diseases that can impact surgical outcome. Review of accompanying medical records and radiographs is important. Ultimately, patients who will benefit from surgery are identified and will be deemed operable, operable but requiring further evaluation from specialists prior to surgery, or inoperable.

Subsequent discussions should focus on the course of treatment. If surgical, the planned operative procedure should be described to the patient in nonmedical terminology. Attendant risks of the procedure, as well as alternatives for therapy (if they exist), should be described to the patient. The length of time for the operation and length of anticipated hospital stay should be estimated for the patient and her family. Further time to recovery from the planned operative procedure should be estimated for the patient. Ideally, this information should be given in oral and written form for the patient. These elements of the treatment plan constitute *informed consent* and should be documented in the medical record by the physician at the initial consultation. Preferably, this "consenting" should be done before the patient is in the preoperative holding area on the day of her surgery. Should further evaluation be needed from a specialist (e.g., a cardiologist or a pulmonologist), a letter outlining the proposed surgical intervention should be sent to the consultant. However, the impact of these consultations, or "preoperative clearances," on perioperative outcomes is unclear (2–4).

If the patient's condition is such that a stoma(s) (ileostomy, colostomy, or urostomy) may be required, consultation with an enterostomal therapist for marking of the planned stoma(s) should be considered. During this visit, the therapist will take into account the location of the patient's waist, abdominal creases, how she wears her clothing, the types of clothing she wears, and the location of the future stoma when she stands or sits. In addition, the therapist can initiate education on the function and care of the stoma(s).

Should the proposed surgery result in a marked change of body image or possible sexual dysfunction (e.g., exenteration, radical vulvectomy, or vaginal reconstruction), consultation with prior patients who have successfully recovered from similar operations may be warranted. In addition, these patients may benefit from psychological counseling prior to their surgery. ***Best practice: Although quality evidence is lacking, most studies show that counseling provides beneficial effects with no evidence of harm. It is recommended that patients should routinely receive dedicated preoperative counseling.***

Ideally, preoperative laboratory testing will be dictated by findings from the history and physical examination. Unfortunately, unnecessary and inappropriate preoperative testing has been done in an effort to reduce poor perioperative outcomes, whereas evidence to support this practice is lacking and the cost to complete these unnecessary tests has been estimated to be over $3 billion (5). In order to standardize preoperative testing, evidence-based guidelines have been developed (6). The National Institute for Health and Care Excellence [formally known as the Institute for Health and Clinical Excellence] (NICE), an independent organization in the United Kingdom that produces evidence-based guidelines for the promotion of good health and treatment of disease, developed guidelines for preoperative testing. These guidelines take into account the patient's age, type of surgery, associated comorbidities, and the American Society of Anesthesiologists (ASA) grade for anesthesia risk (7) (**Table 8.1**). St. Clair et al. performed a retrospective study assessing adherence to the NICE guidelines for preoperative testing in patients having gynecologic surgery between 2005 and 2007. The authors found that among 1,402 patients evaluated, inappropriate preoperative testing resulted in costs over $418,000 (8).

CARDIAC RISK ASSESSMENT

Any gynecologic oncologist must be aware of the significance of cardiac disease in women when evaluating cardiac risk preoperatively. In 1999, the American Heart Association (AHA) published the first women-specific recommendations on the prevention of cardiovascular

TABLE 8.1. National Institute for Health and Clinical Excellence Recommendations for Preoperative Testing

Study	Age (years)	Recommendation
Chest X-ray	Any age	Cardiovascular surgery
	60 or older	Grade 4 surgery and ASA 3 or greater with cardiovascular disease
Electrocardiogram	16–39	ASA 2 or greater with cardiovascular disease or cardiovascular surgery
	40–59	As above, plus grade 4 surgery if ASA 2 or greater with renal disease, or ASA 3 with respiratory disease
	60–79	As above, plus grade 2 surgery if ASA 2 or greater with renal disease, or ASA 3+ with respiratory disease or grade 3 surgery or greater
	80 or older	Consider deferring if grade 1 surgery
Full blood count	16–59	ASA 3 with renal disease, or grade 3 or greater surgery
	60 or older	As above, plus grade 2 or greater surgery
Hemostasis	16 or older	Never recommend, may be considered
Renal function	15–59	ASA 2 or greater with renal disease, ASA 3 or greater with cardiovascular disease, ASA 2 or greater with cardiovascular disease, with grade 3 or greater surgery, ASA 3 or greater with respiratory disease, with grade 3 or greater surgery
	60 or older	As above, plus ASA 2 with cardiovascular disease, with grade 2 or greater surgery, or any grade 3 surgery
Urinalysis	16 or older	Never recommended, may be considered

ASA, American Society of Anesthesiologists.

ASA grade: ASA 1, normal/healthy; ASA 2, mild systemic disease; ASA 3, severe systemic disease.

Surgery grade: grade 1, minor surgery; grade 2, intermediate surgery; grade 3, major surgery; grade 4, extensive surgery.

Source: From St. Clair CM, Shah M, Diver EJ, et al. Adherence to evidence-based guidelines for preoperative testing in women undergoing gynecologic surgery. *Obstet Gynecol*. 2010;116(3):694–700, with permission.

disease (CVD) (9). These recommendations were updated in 2011 (10). Over the past 15 years, significant improvements have been made in the recognition and treatment of CVD in women; however, in recent years, the rate of death from coronary heart disease in women aged 35 to 54 years has been increasing. This increase is thought to be secondary to the alarming rise of obesity in the United States (11). Because of hormonal differences related to pregnancy and hormonal therapy, women are at higher risks for cerebrovascular events. The recently updated guidelines classify women in one of three groups: at high risk, at risk, or at ideal cardiovascular health. Preventative measures focus on normalization of cholesterol levels, treatment of hypertension, maintenance of a normal body mass index (BMI), smoking cessation, and consistent physical activity.

Cardiac risk factors are certainly one of the top concerns for surgeons when assessing perioperative risk. There are numerous reviews and systems that have been created for the purpose of evaluating cardiac risk among patients undergoing noncardiac surgery (12–16). The first large, prospective, multivariate analysis of patients undergoing noncardiac surgery was published by Goldman et al. in 1977 (17). They used definite endpoints of cardiac death, ventricular tachycardia, pulmonary edema, and myocardial infarction (MI). The assessment involves nine independent risk factors to create a point risk index and predict morbidity and mortality (**Tables 8.2** and **8.3**). One weakness of this index is that it underestimates risk in vascular surgery patients. To overcome this, newer cardiac risk assessment tools have been created. These include the Revised Cardiac Risk Index (RCRI) and the American College of Surgeons' National Surgical Quality Improvement Program (NSQIP) (18,19). The RCRI is a validated tool that assesses the risk of major cardiac complications in the perioperative period using six predictors of risk. The American College of Surgeons' NSQIP tool is different in that it adjusts risks depending on the type of surgery.

In response to a shift in the literature from calculation of risk with indices to clinical decision making, especially in regard to the need for preoperative evaluation, the American College of Cardiology/American Heart Association (ACC/AHA) guidelines for the prevention of CVD in women were developed (20). This document provides risk classification of CVD, based on clinical criteria and/or the Framingham 10-year global risk score (**Table 8.4**). This CVD risk stratification has not been assessed specifically for preoperative risk assessment, but provides classification of women who may need further (noninvasive or invasive) evaluation. The updated 2011 guidelines change the definition of a high-risk patient to include one who is at 10% or higher risk for a CVD event within 10 years (10).

TABLE 8.2. Multifactorial Index of Cardiac Risk

Risk Factor	Points
S3 gallop or increased jugular venous pressure	11
Myocardial infarction in previous 6 months	10
More than five premature ventricular ectopic beats per minute	7
Rhythm other than sinus or premature atrial contractions	7
Age >70 years	5
Emergency noncardiac operative procedure	4
Significant aortic stenosis	3
Poor general health status	3
Abdominal or thoracic surgery	3
Possible total	53

Source: Adapted from Goldman L, Caldera DL, Nussbaum SR, et al. Multifactorial index of cardiac risk in noncardiac surgical procedures. *N Engl J Med*. 1977;297:845–880, with permission.

TABLE 8.3. Multifactorial Index of Cardiac Risk, Cardiac Risk Class, Morbidity, and Mortality

Cardiac Risk	Total Points	Morbidity (%)	Mortality
Class I	0–5	0.7	0.2
Class II	6–12	5.0	1.6
Class III	12–25	11.5	2.3
Class IV	>26	22.2	55.6

Source: Adapted from Goldman L, Caldera DL, Nussbaum SR, et al. Multifactorial index of cardiac risk in noncardiac surgical procedures. *N Engl J Med*. 1977;297:845–850, with permission.

TABLE 8.4. Classification of CVD Risk in Women

Risk Status	Criteria
High risk	Established coronary heart disease Cerebrovascular disease Peripheral arterial disease Abdominal aortic aneurysm End-stage or chronic renal disease Diabetes mellitus 10-year Framingham global risk >20%[a]
At risk	≥1 major risk factors for CVD, including: Cigarette smoking Poor diet Physical inactivity Obesity, especially central adiposity Family history of premature CVD (CVD at <55 years of age in male relative and <65 years of age in female relative) Evidence of subclinical vascular disease (e.g., coronary calcification) Metabolic syndrome Poor exercise capacity on treadmill test and/or abnormal heart rate recovery after stopping exercise
Optimal risk	Framingham global risk <10% and a healthy lifestyle, with no risk factors

CVD, coronary vascular disease.

[a]OR at high risk on the basis of another population-adapted tool used to assess global risk.

Source: Adapted from Mosca L, Banka CL, Benjamin EJ, et al. Evidence-based guidelines for cardiovascular disease prevention in women: 2007 update. *Circulation*. 2007;115:1481–1501, with permission.

Clearly, the approach to the patient must include a careful history and physical examination. Some risk calculators determine that age alone is an independent risk factor for perioperative morbidity secondary to major adverse coronary events (19). Age greater than 62 years is an independent risk factor for perioperative stroke (21). Any prior history of cardiac disease such as angina, MI, arrhythmia, congestive heart failure (CHF), or valvular disease must be evaluated. Patients with unstable angina, recent MI, class III–IV heart failure, decompensated congestive failure, or aortic stenosis (AS) present the highest risk. These patients will likely require further invasive testing. Severe AS must be identified preoperatively because the risk of perioperative morbidity is as high as 30% (22).

In patients without overt cardiac risks, other factors, such as insulin-dependent diabetes mellitus, elevated preoperative serum creatinine, and history of cerebrovascular disease, need to be considered for uncovering subclinical disease. These risk factors are identified in the risk prediction models (18,19).

In 2014, the ACC/AHA published revised guidelines to direct invasive or interventional evaluations (16). The guidelines utilize functional capacity in terms of metabolic equivalents, with a level <4 being considered poor. An example would be a patient's ability to climb one flight of stairs or walk up a hill, which would classify the patient in the >4 group.

Testing available for further evaluation includes both invasive and noninvasive methods. The routine resting electrocardiogram (ECG) is a valuable screening tool for patients in whom history of coronary artery disease is unknown (23). It can potentially identify a prior MI, which may prompt further evaluation of coronary artery disease. Echocardiography can predict postoperative CHF in patients with ejection fractions (EFs) less than 35% (24). Although echocardiography cannot reliably predict ischemia, it may be quite useful in the evaluation of valvular diseases or for follow-up of patients with known left ventricular (LV) dysfunction. Additionally, elevated preoperative brain natriuretic peptide is an independent predictor of 30-day adverse cardiovascular outcomes after noncardiac surgery (25). Exercise or pharmacologic stress testing provides valuable information for perioperative ischemic risk. Nuclear scintigraphy with evaluation of perfusion defects has shown a positive predictive value of 12% to 16% and a negative predictive value of 99% (26). Dobutamine stress echocardiography has shown similar predictive values.

The ACC/AHA recommendations provide a mechanism to segregate patients whose surgery must be delayed for further cardiac evaluation because of a recent MI; those who should have their CHF optimized; or those who should have optimized control of dysrhythmias. In selected patients, coronary revascularization, angioplasty, stent placement, or valve replacement may be prudent before the planned noncardiac surgery (16).

The risk of reinfarction after a recent MI is directly related to the interval between the MI and an event which could precipitate an MI. However, these rates have been declining due to improved perioperative care. Reinfarction rates have dropped from 37% in patients undergoing noncardiac surgery within 3 months following MI to 5% to 10% more recently. Reinfarction rates continue to decline as the interval from the original MI increases, with rates of reinfarction being 2% to 3% and 1% to 2%, 4 to 6 months and greater than 6 months, respectively, following the acute event (27). Elective surgery should be postponed for 6 months following an acute MI; however, an urgent operation may be performed 4 to 6 weeks after infarction if stress testing is favorable and the patient receives cardiac monitoring in the perioperative period.

Perioperative β-Blockade

In 1996, a multicenter, randomized, placebo-controlled trial was published that evaluated the use of β-blockade with atenolol versus placebo in patients undergoing noncardiac surgery. Although no difference in perioperative mortality or MI was seen, the atenolol group had significantly fewer ischemic episodes (24% vs. 39%). Furthermore, at 6 and 24 months, the atenolol group had decreased mortality (9 vs. 21 deaths) and decreased number of cardiac events (16 vs. 32) (28). The Perioperative ISchemic Evaluation (POISE) trial showed that the use of β-blockers in the perioperative period reduces the risk of the composite outcome of cardiovascular death, nonfatal MI, and nonfatal cardiac arrest at 30 days. However, it also showed that bradycardic episodes and clinically significant hypotensive events resulted in an increased rate of strokes and death (29). The current recommendations from the ACC/AHA are that perioperative β-blockers should be continued on patients who are on β-blockers chronically. It may be reasonable to begin β-blockers on patients with intermediate- or high-risk myocardial ischemia; however, this must be guided by clinical circumstances (16).

PULMONARY RISK ASSESSMENT

Postoperative pulmonary complications (PPCs) represent a significant cause for morbidity and mortality in patients undergoing elective surgery. Additionally, they are one of the costliest of major postoperative complications (30). The incidence of pulmonary complications after nonthoracic surgery ranges from 2% to 19% (31). Laparotomy results in a 45% decrease in vital capacity and a 30% reduction in functional residual capacity (FRC) (32,33). When the patient is in the supine position, FRC is reduced below alveolar closing volume (i.e., the volume at which point alveoli start closing), which results in atelectasis (34).

When examining risk factors for postoperative pulmonary problems, a number of issues surface. General medical status (e.g., functional status, obesity, nutrition) is related to PPCs. A history of

CHF, renal failure, poor mental status, and immunosuppression is associated with a higher PPC rate (35). Surgical issues such as the type of procedure (open or minimally invasive), the type of incision (thoracic and upper abdominal being worse than midline or lower abdominal), duration of anesthetic (>2 hours), the use of a nasogastric tube (NGT; increased risk), and the use of parenteral (increased risk) versus epidural (decreased risk) analgesics are all correlated with PPC incidence (36,37). All patients undergoing noncardiothoracic surgery should be evaluated for the presence of the following risk factors for PPCs to receive pre- and postoperative interventions to reduce risk: chronic obstructive pulmonary disease (COPD), CHF, ASA class of II or greater, functional dependence, and age older than 60 years. In terms of direct pulmonary risk factors, the most common preexisting pulmonary disease is COPD (38). These patients retain carbon dioxide, have poor gas exchange, and have an increased residual volume. Smoking and history of dyspnea, pneumonia, and sleep apnea are other risk categories (36).

When interpreting the usual preoperative radiographic and laboratory values, several caveats must be kept in mind. A preoperative chest radiograph in normal adults has no predictive value other than providing essential baseline data for an at-risk patient. Arterial blood gas analysis has not been shown to be useful in providing risk stratification (39). A low serum albumin is a powerful marker of increased risk and should be considered in patients with one or more risk factors for PPCs (40). Preoperative pulmonary function tests (PFTs) are rarely useful for risk stratification and are not indicated prior to surgery. A consensus statement from the American College of Physicians in 2006 recommended that preoperative PFTs or chest radiography may be appropriate in patients with a previous diagnosis of COPD or asthma (38). Such testing may provide valuable baseline data and aid in risk stratification for patients with moderate to severe COPD who are undergoing major abdominal surgery.

Perioperative strategies for reducing the risk of PPCs include lung expansion techniques, smoking cessation, and optimization of gas exchange. Although preoperative and postoperative incentive spirometry has shown mixed results in reducing the rate of PPCs, it continues to be widely recommended (41), and it should be considered as a preventive strategy for any patient undergoing laparotomy. In order to maximize patient compliance, preoperative counseling and education are necessary. Clearly, COPD must be managed by controlling infection and optimizing medical regimens. Reactive airway disease should be prevented with the use of perioperative inhalation therapy such as β agonists. Steroid therapy is generally reserved for patients already utilizing these drugs as part of their medical regimen. These steroid-dependent patients will need stress-dose steroids to prevent insufficiency (see "Adrenal Suppression" section). Prophylactic antibiotics are not indicated in COPD patients to prevent pulmonary infections.

Smokers have significantly more postoperative complications, including pneumonia, surgical site infections, and death (42). Smoking-cessation programs have had an unclear effect on PPCs (43). Although data from poorly controlled trials have shown that short-term abstinence (<8 weeks from the time of surgery) may actually increase the complication rate, these results are controversial (44). However, abstinence for greater than 10 weeks demonstrated complication rates similar to those for nonsmokers (45). Unfortunately, the long-term success rate of smoking-cessation programs is low, and in the case of malignancy, the gynecologic oncologist rarely has the opportunity to delay the operation for 8 to 10 weeks.

Risk prediction tools for PPCs are available and can be useful in guiding the clinician's perioperative care (35,46–48).

Endocrinologic Risk Assessment

Diabetes

The prevalence of diabetes has reached epidemic proportions in the United States. In 2011, the Centers for Disease Control and Prevention reported that 25.8 million people or 8.3% of the population have diabetes (49). Diabetes accounts for the fourth leading comorbid condition among hospital discharges (50). One-fifth of surgical patients will have diabetes and people with known diabetes have a 50% risk of undergoing surgery at some point in their lifetime (51). Interestingly, one-third to one-half of patients hospitalized are unaware that they have diabetes and are currently receiving no treatment. It is only during preoperative evaluation for elective surgery or acute hospitalization that these patients will be diagnosed (52). Because of this prevalence, some authors have suggested that all surgical patients be regarded as dysglycemic until proven otherwise (53). Understanding the basic physiology of diabetes and how it impacts perioperative risk is crucial for the surgeon.

There are two types of diabetes. Type 1 diabetes occurs as a result of insulinopenia, with all type 1 diabetics being insulin dependent. In the absence of sufficient insulin, these patients develop ketoacidosis. Type 1 diabetics account for approximately 10% of all diabetics. Type 2 diabetes occurs as a result of insulin resistance and impaired insulin secretion. Type 2 diabetics may be treated with diet alone, oral hypoglycemic agents, noninsulin injectable medications, or insulin. These patients account for approximately 90% of all diabetics (54). However, approximately 30% of hospitalized patients will have a prediabetic condition consisting of impaired fasting glucose levels or impaired glucose tolerance (52). Thus, perioperative glycemic control will be dictated by known (or newly discovered) diabetic status.

When evaluating patients with known diabetes for surgery, attention should be directed toward the patient's diabetic status (i.e., type of glucose control; number of hypoglycemic events, etc.) and the long-term complications caused by diabetes, since this end organ damage can impact perioperative outcome. Most complications of diabetes are related to microvascular changes, such as diabetic retinopathy, neuropathy, nephropathy, and CVD (55). In addition to a thorough history and physical examination, preoperative studies should include an ECG to rule out a prior "silent" MI (especially in patients with diabetes for more than 10 years), serum creatinine, blood urea nitrogen, urinary analyses to assess renal function, and glycosylated hemoglobin (HbA_{1C}) to evaluate recent glycemic control. HbA_{1C} levels reflect the level of hyperglycemia that red blood cells (RBC) have been exposed to. Because the average lifespan of an RBC is 120 days, HbA_{1C} is an indicator of glycemic control over that period of time (54). As mentioned earlier, because of the prevalence of dysglycemia among hospitalized adults in the United States, measurement of HbA_{1C}, as a screening for diabetes, may identify patients with undiagnosed diabetes or impaired glucose metabolism (53). HbA_{1C} levels ≤6.5% are associated with good long-term glucose control and have been associated with decreased rates of infectious complications across a variety of surgical procedures (56,57). However, HbA_{1C} levels >6.5% are diagnostic for diabetes and evidence of poor glycemic control in known diabetics (58,59). Ultimately, the type of diabetes, preoperative glycemic control, the extent and magnitude of the intended surgery, the elective or emergent nature of said surgery, and other comorbid medical conditions will affect the metabolic changes these patients face intra- and postoperatively (53).

Another entity that has come to light in the last decade among hospitalized patients is that of stress-induced hyperglycemia (SIH). This disease is defined as an inpatient fasting glucose measurement ≥126 mg/dL or a random glucose measurement of more than 200 mg/dL, which returns to normal after discharge (51,60). A growing body of evidence suggests that SIH and diabetic hyperglycemia are different diseases (61), and SIH confers a higher risk of adverse outcomes, such as an increased risk of in-hospital mortality (59,62,63) and longer lengths of stay compared with nondiabetic or hyperglycemic diabetic patients (60).

The armamentarium available for treatment of diabetes has expanded over the last decade. Type 1 diabetics will most likely be using a combination of insulin therapies for glycemic control, whereas type 2 diabetics may be on oral therapy alone, insulin therapy alone, injectable noninsulin therapy alone, or some combination therapy of all the aforementioned agents. **Table 8.5** outlines some of these

■ **TABLE 8.5. Management of Diabetes Medications before Surgery in Patients Who Must Be NPO**

Medication Type	Night before Surgery	Morning of Surgery
Oral agents		
Sulfonyl-urea		Hold
Glyburide	Give with meal	
Glipizide		
Glimepiride		
Metformin (contraindicated in women with creatinine levels >1.4)	Hold	Hold; can induce lactic acidosis and should be held in procedures that require IV contrast
Thiazolidinediones	Hold	Hold; Can cause fluid retention in the postoperative period
Rosiglitazone		
Pioglitazone		
Meglitinides	Give with meal	Hold
Repaglinide		
Nateglinide		
α-Glucosidase inhibitors	Give with meal	Hold
Acarbose		
Miglitol		
Dipeptidal peptidase-IV inhibitor	Give with meal	Hold
Sitagliptin		
Noninsulin injectable		
Incretin mimetics	Give 30–60 minutes before meal	Hold
Exenatide		
Amylin analog	Give immediately before meal	Hold
Pramlintide		
Insulin		
Regular insulin	Give full dose	Give half dose
Humulin R		
Novolin R		
ReliOn R		
NPH insulin	Give full dose	Give half dose
Humulin N		
Novolin N		
ReliOn N		
Premixed insulins	Give full dose	Give half dose
Humulin 70/30		
Novolin 70/30		
Humalog 75/25		
Novolog 70/30		
Rapid-acting insulin	Give full dose with meals	Hold
Aspart		
Glulisine		
Lispro		
Inhaled insulin		
Basal insulin (long-acting)	If patient is on basal insulin and rapid-acting insulin, give full dose. If patient is on oral diabetes medication plus basal insulin or basal insulin only, give half dose	If patient is on basal insulin and rapid-acting insulin, give full dose. If patient is on oral diabetes medication plus basal insulin or basal insulin only, give half dose
Glargine		
Detemir		
Continuous subcutaneous insulin pump	Continue current settings	Switch to continuous insulin infusion and titrate

Source: From Meneghini LF. Perioperative management of diabetes: translating evident into practice. *Cleveland Clin J Med*. 2009;76(4):S53–S59 and Khan NA, Ghali WA, Spratt SE, et al. Perioperative management of diabetes mellitus. Physicians' Information and Education Resources. American College of Physicians, 31 Aug. 2009. 26 Apr. 2012. http://pier.acponline.org/physicians/public/periopr879/tables/periopr879-tl.html, with permission.

drugs and the timing for stopping these medications prior to surgical procedures because of their pharmacologic half-lives (64).

The physiologic changes that diabetic patients encounter during surgery result in a hyperglycemic state due to insulin resistance. The stress of surgery increases secretion of epinephrine, norepinephrine, cortisol, and growth hormone, all of which directly antagonize insulin action (53–55). In addition, gluconeogenesis and lipolysis are increased with mobilization of glucose precursors, and a net protein catabolism ensues. Glycemic control perioperatively will depend on the type of diabetes or impaired glucose tolerance the patient has, as well as the medications that have/have not been utilized to control such disease states. Recently, the Clinical Guidelines Subcommittee of The Endocrinology Society published treatment guidelines for noncritically ill patients hospitalized and subsequently found to be hyperglycemic (known diabetes vs. unknown). The authors would direct the reader to review these guidelines, and recommendations from this group, for perioperative care of patients with hyperglycemia undergoing surgical interventions, are listed in **Table 8.6** (65).

There are several case–control studies that demonstrate an increased risk for adverse outcomes in patients undergoing elective noncardiac surgery who have either preoperative or postoperative hyperglycemia (66–70). Postoperative glucose levels greater than 200 mg/dL are associated with prolonged hospital stays and increased risk of postoperative complications including wound infections and cardiac arrhythmias (67–69). Although diabetic patients with vascular disease are at risk of silent postoperative MI and acute renal failure (ARF), postoperative infections (respiratory, urinary, wound infections, etc.) account for about two-thirds of all postoperative complications and 20% of all postoperative deaths among diabetics undergoing surgery (56). Hyperglycemia has been shown to impair phagocytic function and chemotaxis of granulocytes when glucose levels are higher than 250 mg/dL (71).

Although glycemic control is important, the jury is still out on when control should be achieved (pre-, intra-, or postoperatively or throughout the entire perioperative period), what glucose levels should be achieved for maximum benefit, and which insulin regimen is most effective (53). The landmark publication by Van den Berghe et al. in 2001 showed, in a randomized, prospective fashion, that aggressive glycemic control through intensive insulin therapy (IIT) (maintaining glucose levels between 80 and 110 mg/dL) versus conventional insulin therapy (glucose levels between 180 and 200 mg/dL) in critically ill postoperative patients (more than 60% were cardiac surgery patients) reduced episodes of septicemia and in-hospital mortality by 46% and 34%, respectively (72). Despite the enthusiasm for tighter glucose control, subsequent studies over the last decade, with a heterogeneous population of acutely ill patients, have failed to confirm the results of Van den Berghe's work (53,60). In fact, the multinational, multidisciplinary **N**ormoglycemia in **I**ntensive **C**are **E**valuation and **S**urvival **U**sing **G**lucose **A**lgorithm **R**egulation (NICE-SUGAR) trial in 6,104 ICU patients reported increased mortality rates (27.5% [IIT] vs. 24.9% [control]) in patients who were kept at blood glucose levels of 81 to 108 mg/dL versus <180 mg/dL. The increased mortality was driven by increased rates of hypoglycemia (blood glucose <40 mg/dL) among patients with the tightest blood glucose control (6.8% [IIT] vs. 0.5% [control]) (73). Because of the NICE-SUGAR study, and others (60), recommendations for blood glucose targets have relaxed somewhat depending upon the condition of the patient.

TABLE 8.6. Perioperative Blood Glucose Control: An Endocrine Society Clinical Practice Guideline

Recommendation Number	
5.3.1	All patients with type 1 diabetes who undergo minor or major surgical procedures receive either continuous insulin infusion or subcutaneous basal insulin with bolus insulin as required to prevent hyperglycemia during the perioperative period
5.3.2	Patients with diabetes should discontinue oral and noninsulin injectable antidiabetic agents before surgery with initiation of insulin therapy in those patients that develop hyperglycemia during the perioperative period
5.3.3	When instituting subcutaneous insulin therapy in the postsurgical setting, basal (for patients who are NPO) or basal bolus (for patients who are eating) insulin therapy is the preferred approach. Sliding scale insulin (SSI) should not be used

Source: Umpierrez GE, Hellman R, Korytkoski MT, et al. Management of hyperglycemia in hospitalized patients in non-critical care setting: an Endocrine Society Clinical Practice Guideline. *J Clin Endocrinol Metab*. 2012;97:16–38.

Intravenous (IV) insulin therapy should be instituted in critically ill patients when blood glucose levels exceed 180 mg/dL, with the goal of maintaining glucose control between 140 and 180 mg/dL. For noncritically ill patients, the preprandial goal for glucose level is less than 140 mg/dL (74), with maintenance of blood glucose at these levels while minimizing hypoglycemia. Attaining these levels of glycemic control will depend upon the patient's type of diabetes, her medical condition, and her oral intake status.

Individual institutional policy will vary as to where patients may receive IV insulin therapy (ICU vs. step-down units vs. routine hospital floors). If the patient is receiving IV insulin, then transition to a subcutaneous route must be started before discontinuing the IV route. Most patients can be converted to long-acting basal insulin, with the dose usually being 50% to 80% of the prior day's IV insulin dose. An insulin regimen utilizing a subcutaneous basal/bolus approach outperforms traditional sliding scale regular insulin regimens. Umpierrez et al. expanded their previous work (75) by conducting a prospective randomized trial comparing subcutaneous basal/bolus insulin replacement to traditional subcutaneous sliding scale insulin (SSI) replacement for patients with type 2 diabetes undergoing general surgery, not expected to be admitted to the ICU, and whose glucose levels exceeded 140 mg/dL. In the group randomized to the basal/bolus insulin, the starting daily dose was 0.5 U/kg/day, with half of the dose being given as basal insulin (insulin glargine) once daily and half given as rapid-acting insulin analog (insulin glulisine) in fixed doses prior to meals. If the patient was nil per os (NPO), then the insulin glargine dose was given and the insulin glulisine was held until meals were resumed. For supplementation, the rapid-acting analog was used. Among the 211 patients studied, those in the basal/bolus group received higher daily doses of insulin, had lower daily mean blood glucose levels (27 mg/dL), had the same risk of hypoglycemic episodes (blood glucose levels <40 mg/dL), and more often achieved the glycemic goal of <140 mg/dL. In addition, the basal/bolus group had fewer wound infections, pneumonias, episodes of bacteremia, respiratory failure, and ARF as compared with the SSI group. There also was a nonsignificant trend toward fewer postsurgical ICU admissions and shorter ICU stays than in the SSI group (76). **Table 8.7** demonstrates the basal/bolus method to control hyperglycemia in type 2 diabetics postoperatively. Use of oral diabetic agents in hospitalized patients is not recommended (77). ***Best Practice: Perioperative maintenance of blood glucose levels (<180 to 200 mg/dL) results in improved perioperative outcomes. Glucose levels above this range should be treated with insulin infusions and regular blood glucose monitoring to avoid the risk of hypoglycemia.***

Thyroid Disorders

When patients give a history of hypothyroidism or hyperthyroidism during evaluation for surgery, thyroid-stimulating hormone (TSH) and thyroxine (T4) levels should be obtained. The primary objective is to determine whether the patient is euthyroid or not, prior to

TABLE 8.7. Basal/Bolus Insulin Treatment Protocol

<table>
<tr><th>Starting Insulin Doses (Insulin Glargine)</th><th colspan="4">Supplemental Insulin (Insulin Glulisine)</th><th>Insulin Adjustment</th></tr>
<tr><td>Discontinue all oral antidiabetic and noninsulin injectable medications</td><td colspan="4">Give supplemental insulin glulisine according to the sliding scale (below) for blood glucose >140 mg/dL</td><td>If the fasting and predinner BG is between 100 and 140 mg/dL and no hypoglycemia the previous day: no changes</td></tr>
<tr><td>Starting total daily dose (TDD): 0.5 units/kg actual body weight</td><td colspan="4">If patient is able and expected to eat, give supplemental glulisine before each meal and at bedtime following the "usual" column</td><td>If the fasting and predinner BG is between 140 and 180 mg/dL and no hypoglycemia the previous day: increase insulin TDD by 10% every day</td></tr>
<tr><td>Reduce TDD to 0.3 units/kg actual body weight in patients ≥70 years of age and/or serum creatinine ≥2.0 mg/dL</td><td colspan="4">If the patient is not able to eat, give supplemental glulisine every 6 hours (6–12 to 6–12) following the "sensitive" column</td><td>If the fasting and predinner BG is >180 mg/dL and no hypoglycemia the previous day: increase insulin TDD by 20% every day</td></tr>
<tr><td rowspan="8">Give half of the TDD as insulin glargine, at the same time once daily and half as insulin glulisine in three equally divided doses before each meal. Hold insulin glulisine if patient not able to eat</td><th>Blood Glucose (mg/dL)</th><th>Insulin Sensitive (units)</th><th>Usual (units)</th><th>Insulin Resistant (units)</th><td rowspan="4">If the fasting and predinner BG is between 70 and 99 mg/dL and no hypoglycemia: decrease insulin TDD by 10% every day</td></tr>
<tr><td>141–180</td><td>2</td><td>4</td><td>6</td></tr>
<tr><td>181–220</td><td>4</td><td>6</td><td>8</td></tr>
<tr><td>221–260</td><td>6</td><td>8</td><td>10</td></tr>
<tr><td>261–300</td><td>8</td><td>10</td><td>12</td><td rowspan="4">If the patient develops hypoglycemia BG <70 mg/dL: decrease insulin TDD by 20%</td></tr>
<tr><td>301–350</td><td>10</td><td>12</td><td>14</td></tr>
<tr><td>351–400</td><td>12</td><td>14</td><td>16</td></tr>
<tr><td>>400</td><td>14</td><td>16</td><td>18</td></tr>
</table>

TDD, total daily dose; BG, blood glucose

Source: Adapted from Umpierrez GE, Smiley D, Jacobs S, et al. Randomized study of basal-bolus insulin therapy in the inpatient management of patients with Type 2 diabetes undergoing general surgery (RABBIT 2 Surgery). *Diabetes Care*. 2011;34:256–261, with permission.

surgical intervention, so as to avoid the complications of myxedema or thyroid storm in the postoperative period.

Hypothyroidism is a common condition in the United States, affecting approximately 1% of all patients and 5% of the population over the age of 50, and it develops 10 times more often in women than in men (78). Decision to operate on patients with hypothyroidism will depend upon the level of hypothyroidism and the urgency of the surgery. Hypothyroidism can influence many physiologic functions, such as myocardial function, respiration, gastrointestinal (GI) motility, hemostasis, and free water balance (53,79). Although there have been no prospective, randomized studies looking at the surgical outcome of hypothyroid patients versus controls, several retrospective case-matched control studies have evaluated hypothyroid patients undergoing surgery. A study by Weinberg et al. demonstrated no differences between hypothyroid and euthyroid controls for perioperative complications. In addition, no differences in outcome were seen when hypothyroidism was stratified by T4 levels. The investigators concluded that patients with mild to moderate hypothyroidism should not be denied needed surgery in order to correct the metabolic problem. They further stated that insufficient numbers of patients with severe hypothyroidism precluded recommendations for perioperative care of these patients (80). In another retrospective study, Ladenson et al. reviewed perioperative complications among hypothyroid patients undergoing surgery, finding more intraoperative hypotension in noncardiac surgery, more heart failure in cardiac surgery, and more GI and neuropsychiatric complications. They also noted that patients were unable to mount fever in the face of infection, although infection rates were not different. Further more, no differences were found in the duration of hospitalization, perioperative arrhythmias, delayed anesthesia recovery, pulmonary complications, or mortality (81).

Patients with mild to moderate hypothyroidism requiring urgent surgery may have it without delay. These patients may have more minor complications of ileus, postoperative delirium, or infection without fever. Patients with severe hypothyroidism (myxedema coma, decreased mentation, pericardial effusions, heart failure, or very low levels of T4) who are to undergo urgent/emergent surgery will need IV levothyroxine (200 to 500 µg given during 30 minutes) followed by daily doses of 50 to 100 µg IV. These patients will likely need stress-dose glucocorticoids (see "Adrenal Suppression" section) started prior to, during, and continued after surgery due to coexisting adrenal insufficiency (AI; or due to the fact that IV replacement with levothyroxine may precipitate AI) (53,81,82).

Myxedema coma is a rare condition, with an incidence of 0.22 per million patients per year. Most of the cases (80%) occur among hospitalized, elderly (older than 60 years) women with long-standing hypothyroidism, but it can occur at any age (83). A majority of the cases will occur in the postoperative period due to inciting causes such as infections, cold exposure, sedatives, analgesics, and other medications. The mortality from this disease is high (80%), but has been decreasing in recent years due to increased awareness, testing, and improved perioperative care (84–86). Myxedema coma is characterized by severely depressed mental status, seizure, hypothermia, bradycardia, hyponatremia, heart failure, and hypopnea. Although maintenance of normothermia by warming is tempting, the resulting vasodilation may cause cardiovascular collapse in patients with intravascular volume depletion, cardiac insufficiency, and pericardial effusion/tamponade and should be performed carefully if at all (84). Myxedema coma is a medical emergency and necessitates urgent administration of levothyroxine. An initial IV bolus of 200 to 500 µg should be given, followed by 50 to 100 µg IV daily. Dehydration is frequently present and aggressive volume resuscitation with dextrose and normal saline should be instituted. IV glucocorticoids should be administered (50 mg hydrocortisone IV, four times daily) because of frequent AI. Resolution of symptoms, if properly treated, should begin within 24 hours.

Patients using thyroid replacement preparations can have their doses held during the immediate postoperative period until they are able to tolerate oral intake, as the half-life of these drugs is 5 to 9 days (79).

The causes of hyperthyroidism are many, but the most common cause is Graves disease. This autoimmune disorder, caused by an antibody directed to TSH receptors, results in increased thyroid hormone production. The clinical signs of hyperthyroidism include tachycardia, atrial fibrillation, fever, tremor, goiter, and ophthalmopathy (54). Most complications occurring in hyperthyroid patients undergoing surgery involve cardiac function, as T4 and T3 have direct inotropic and chronotropic effect on the heart and a vasodilatory effect on peripheral vasculature, resulting in the activation of the renin–angiotensin–aldosterone system. All of these events result in a high cardiac output state, which increases cardiac work and oxygen requirements and can result in MI (83). Arrhythmias are very common in the face of hyperthyroidism, with atrial fibrillation occurring in 10% to 20% of patients (87–90). Again, level of control prior to the operation will determine the perioperative outcome for the patient. Patients with controlled hyperthyroidism should be instructed to take their antithyroid medications in the morning of the day of surgery. Patients with mild hyperthyroidism may have surgery with preoperative β-blockers. However, patients with moderate or severe disease should have surgery canceled until a euthyroid state is attained (91).

The greatest perioperative risk for patients who have undiagnosed hyperthyroidism or who are inadequately treated is a rare, yet life-threatening condition known as thyroid storm. This “thyroid emergency” usually occurs intraoperatively or 48 hours postoperatively. The mortality of thyroid storm is 10% to 75% and requires treatment in a critical care environment (78). Symptoms are nonspecific and include hyperpyrexia, tachycardia, delirium, nausea and vomiting, and diarrhea (92). Treatment of thyroid storm is aimed at stopping production of thyroid hormone and treating the systemic effects of the decompensated patient. Antithyroid medications such as carbimazole, methimazole, and propylthiouracil (PTU) are used to inhibit the new synthesis of thyroid hormones. Unfortunately, there are no IV preparations for these compounds, so they must be administered enterally or per rectum as retention enemas or suppositories. Recent guidelines from the American Thyroid Association and the Association of Clinical Endocrinologists recommend that PTU be started with a loading dose of 500 to 1,000 mg followed by 250 mg every 4 hours, and methimazole should be administered at daily doses of 60 to 80 mg (93). Administering these drugs in this sequence will provide more rapid clinical improvement because PTU has the added advantage of inhibiting conversion of T4 to T3, which methimazole does not do. These drugs prevent synthesis of new thyroid hormone, but will not stop release of stored thyroid hormone. Either inorganic iodine or lithium carbonate (for patients who are allergic to iodine; 300 mg orally every 6 hours) must be given. Lugol’s solution or a saturated solution of potassium iodide (3 to 5 drops orally, every 6 hours) may be used, but must not be given sooner than 1 hour after the administration of the thionamide dosage; otherwise thyroid hormone synthesis will be enhanced by the iodine treatment. In severe cases of thyroid storm, plasmapheresis and therapeutic plasma exchange may be needed. β-Blockade is critical to ameliorate the manifestations of thyroid excess and does so by correcting the heart rate, reducing cardiac oxygen demand, and decreasing agitation, convulsions, psychotic behavior, and tremors. Propranolol is the most commonly used agent and dosages of 60 to 80 mg given orally every 4 hours or 0.5 to 1 mg IV followed by subsequent doses of 2 to 3 mg every several hours are recommended. Another theoretic benefit of β-blockade is the inhibition of conversion of T4 to T3. One other medication that has a high therapeutic benefit is the administration of corticosteroids, which not only inhibits the conversion of T4 to T3, but also treats AI, which may have occurred due to the rapid turnover of cortisol. Acetaminophen is preferred to salicylates, as the latter may exacerbate thyrotoxicosis by decreasing thyroid protein binding and increasing free T3 and T4. Finally, a thorough search for the precipitating cause of the thyroid storm should be undertaken immediately, with the most common cause in the perioperative period being infection (83).

Adrenal Suppression

How patients respond to stress is directly related to the hypothalamic-pituitary axis (HPA), and any defect in this cycle can have dramatic effects in the perioperative period. The most common cause of primary AI is autoimmune adrenalitis, where the adrenal cortex is destroyed and the patient’s endogenous production of glucocorticoid steroids is reduced or ceases. Secondary AI is characterized by atrophy of the adrenal cortex as a result of deficient adrenocorticotrophic hormone (ACTH) stimulation. The most common cause of secondary AI is administration of exogenous corticosteroids, which feeds back to cause a decrease in hypothalamic corticotropin-releasing hormone and subsequent decreased pituitary ACTH secretion. Although there is remarkable variability in individual response to a particular dose and length of treatment with steroids, in general, any patient who received the equivalent of 20 mg per day of prednisone for more than 5 days is at risk for HPA suppression. If the duration of steroid treatment is 1 month or longer, the patient will have HPA suppression, which can last for 6 to 12 months after stopping therapy, whereas an equivalent dose of prednisone 5 mg (or less) for any period of time will not usually suppress the HPA axis (94–96). Assessment of adrenal function (ACTH stimulation tests) in the perioperative period has not been shown to be sensitive or specific in identifying patients who are at risk for AI and who might respond to supplemental corticosteroids (97–100).

Recently, Marik and Varon performed a meta-analysis of the world literature concerning perioperative stress doses of corticosteroids for patients who take corticosteroids chronically. Their search revealed two randomized controlled trials (RCTs) and seven cohort studies, for a total of 315 patients. Although the number of patients is small, the two RCTs showed no differences in the hemodynamic profiles of patients receiving stress doses of corticosteroids, compared with patients receiving only their usual daily dose of corticosteroid. Similarly, in five of the seven cohort studies, patients who continued to receive their usual daily doses of corticosteroids without additional stress doses did not develop unexplained hypotension or adrenal crisis perioperatively. The remaining two cohort studies each had one patient who stopped his or her usual daily dose of corticosteroid preoperatively, and each developed unexplained postoperative hypotension, which responded to hydrocortisone and fluid therapy. The authors recommend that patients receiving therapeutic doses of corticosteroids, who undergo surgery, do not routinely need stress doses of corticosteroids as long as their usual daily dose is continued. In addition, adrenal function testing is not recommended for these patients because the test is overly sensitive and does not predict which patient will develop adrenal crisis. Further more, patients who have primary AI and who are taking physiologic replacement doses of corticosteroids will require supplemental stress doses of corticosteroids in the perioperative period (101).

Figure 8.1 outlines an algorithm that may be helpful in guiding clinicians in their decision-making about stress-dose steroids for patients who take them chronically. Giving stress-dose glucocorticoids needs to be weighed against the potential side effects of the drug (such as poor wound healing, fluid retention, and increased risk of infection) versus the benefits of supporting the HPA axis in a surgically stressed patient.

Renal Risk Assessment

Chronic kidney disease (CKD) affects over 13 million Americans (20 years and older; CKD stage 2 or worse) (102), with most having a glomerular filtration rate (GFR) of less than 60 mL/min/1.73 m^2 (103). The most common form of renal failure facing the surgeon is acute kidney injury (AKI) occurring during the postoperative period, which will be discussed in the section on postoperative/critical care. Since 2002, a uniform classification system for CKD was introduced, stratifying CKD into five stages based on estimation

Primary adrenal insufficiency (AI)

Hyponatremia

Hyperkalemia

Hypotension

Eosinophilia

OR

Secondary adrenal insufficiency (AI)

Patients taking 20 mg prednisone (or equivalent) for 5 days

Procedure	Emergent Surgery	Urgent or Elective Surgery
Minor Procedures performed under local anesthesia or less than 1 hour	25 mg IV Hydrocortisone (or equivalent)	1)No stress dose corticosteroids 2)Continue usual daily dose 3)If signs and symptoms of AI intraoperatively, 25 mg IV hydrocortisone (or equivalent)
Moderate Most vascular and orthopedic procedures	50 mg IV Hydrocortisone (or equivalent)	Preoperative short ACTH stim test[a] a)If appropriate response, no stress dose steroids. Continue usual daily dose b)If inappropriate response or suspected AI intraoperatively, 50 mg IV hydrocortisone (or equivalent)
Major Extensive procedures which last more than 2 hours and any procedure using cardiopulmonary bypass	100 mg IV Hydrocortisone (or equivalent)	Preoperative short ACTH stim test[a] a)If appropriate response, no stress dose steroids. Continue usual daily dose b)If inappropriate response or suspected AI intraoperatively, 100 mg IV hydrocortisone (or equivalent)

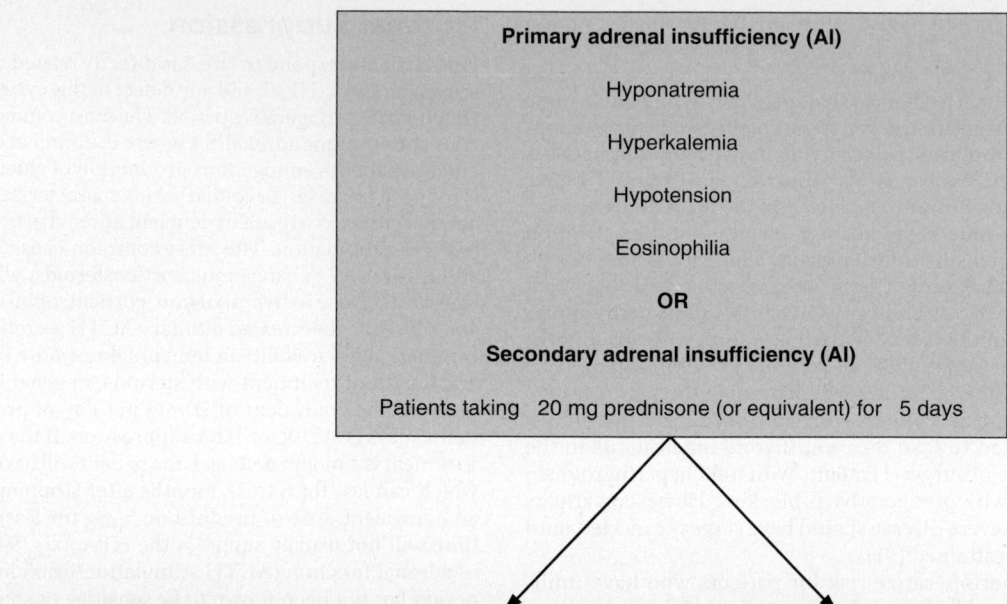

Figure 8.1. Algorithm for adrenal insufficiency. ACTH, adrenocorticotrophic hormone.

[a]The short ACTH stimulation involves IV administration of 250 μg synthetic ACTH (Cortrosyn, cosyntropin) followed by plasma cortisol collection 30 minutes later. Normal cortisol levels after stimulation greater than 18 μg/dL.

When given intraoperatively, steroid doses are continued every 8 hours for 48 hours.

Source: Adapted from Kohl BA, Schwartz S. How to manage perioperative endocrine insufficiency. *Anesthesiol Clin*. 2010;28:139–155, with permission.

of GFR and documentation of renal injury (103). Class 5 CKD, or end-stage renal disease (ESRD), includes patients who require renal replacement therapy (usually dialysis) for treatment (102). With the aging population, increasing prevalence of diabetes and hypertension, and advances in dialytic therapy, the number of patients living with CKD is increasing (102). Therefore, surgeons must be cognizant of the potential perioperative risks associated with these patients.

The predominant causes of CKD are diabetes and hypertension, accounting for 71% of all patients who are dialysis dependent (102). Patients with these underlying diseases tend to have other comorbid conditions such as coronary artery disease and peripheral vascular disease. Evaluation of CKD patients undergoing surgery should focus on four areas: cardiac evaluation, fluid and electrolyte management, anemia, and bleeding diatheses. Of course, glycemic control for diabetics and blood pressure control for hypertensive patients is obvious.

CVD has long been recognized as the leading cause of death among ESRD patients, which occurs in 50% of patients (102,104,105). However, patients with other stages of CKD, even minor derangements, have an increased risk of CVD. A recent study correlated the stage of CKD with odds ratios (ORs) for cardiovascular risk, demonstrating a graded increase in risk with increasing stage of CKD (OR 15 for stage I to OR 20 to 1,000 for stage V) (105). The disease factors which contribute to CVD among CKD patients include microalbuminuria/proteinuria, hypertension, diabetes, dsylipidemia, and smoking (106). In addition, many CKD patients will have coronary artery disease (23% to 40%) (107–109), and many ESRD patients (70% to 80%) will develop ventricular hypertrophy due to hypertension and severe anemia. This hypertrophy results in a decreased myocardial capillary density and diastolic and systolic dysfunction, all of which leads to disturbances in intraventricular conduction, electrical excitability, and ventricular arrhythmias (110). Therefore, these patients may benefit from a formal cardiac clearance from a cardiologist prior to surgical intervention.

The capacity of the failing kidney to maintain volume and electrolyte homeostasis is achieved through adaptive processes, which are limited in their ability to respond to physiologic stresses, placing well-compensated patients, in the premorbid state, at increased risk of fluid and electrolyte disturbances during the perioperative period (111). Intraoperative and perioperative fluid management in patients with CKD must therefore take into account the reduced capacity for both water excretion and conservation. Excessive free water administration must be avoided to prevent iatrogenic hypotonicity, while providing sufficient free water to prevent hypertonicity. Electrolyte status should be monitored frequently and water administration adjusted if hypo- or hypernatremia ensues (112). ESRD patients who are dependent upon dialysis will need to be euvolemic prior to surgery. Thus, communication with the patient's nephrologist is paramount. Details about the operation should be discussed, with planned preoperative dialysis (without heparin 24 hours prior to surgery) and postoperative dialysis on the day of surgery for large intraoperative fluid loads. Electrolytes should be monitored in the immediate postoperative period, with hyperkalemia being aggressively managed with dialysis, or medically if necessary. Acute hyperkalemia may be treated with glucose and insulin, which will drive the Na/K-ATPase pump resulting in an increase of intracellular potassium and lowering of extracellular potassium. Ten milliliters of calcium gluconate can afford cardioprotection and membrane stabilization in patients with abnormal ECGs (113). Decreasing total body potassium is the final step in the treatment of hyperkalemia. In nonoliguric patients, renal potassium excretion may be enhanced with loop-acting diuretics. Sodium polystyrene sulfonate (Kionex, Kayexalate) may be used as an exchange resin in the GI tract. Forty grams dissolved in 80 mL of sorbitol (or more to promote elimination) and given orally will bind one millimole of potassium for each gram given. Alternatively, 50 to 100 g of sodium polystyrene sulfonate may be dissolved in 200 mL of water and given rectally as a retention enema by inserting a Foley catheter into the rectum and filling the balloon (112). These administrations should be repeated every 2 to 4 hours until the potassium level is in a normal range (see section on potassium derangements). Caution with the use of this resin in postoperative patients is urged, as intestinal necrosis has been reported (114).

Most patients with CKD have or will develop anemia due to erythropoietin deficiency during the course of their disease and, prior to the introduction of erythropoietin stimulating agents (ESAs), were transfusion dependent. In recent years, the use of ESAs has come under scrutiny. Recent reviews have demonstrated that raising the hemoglobin levels above 11 g/dL in patients with CKD resulted in a 1.14-fold increase in OR deaths. These results highlight the need to carefully manage hemoglobin levels with ESAs within a recommended range of 9 to 11 g/dL (115,116). In urgent situations, transfusion of blood is necessary to maintain hemoglobin prior to and during surgery.

CKD patients have an increased risk of bleeding complications. Platelet dysfunction caused by renal failure is multifactorial, with retained uremic toxins, abnormal binding of von Willebrand factor, abnormal platelet arachidonic acid metabolism, and excess vascular prostacyclin and nitric oxide production all being implicated (117). The bleeding time provides the best correlation with risk of clinical bleeding in CKD patients. If a patient has demonstrated prior bleeding because of uremic platelet dysfunction, these patients must be treated with 1-deamino-8-D-arginine vasopressin IV, or intranasally, and with cryoprecipitate to prevent bleeding during surgery (118). In addition, patients may be treated with IV conjugated estrogens (0.6 mg/kg) if they are given 4 to 5 days prior to surgery (112,119).

Furthermore, with reduced or absent renal function, these patients metabolize drugs such as antibiotics, anesthetics, and analgesics poorly. Drug administration in ESRD must be done judiciously, with careful attention to the pharmacokinetics of particular drugs. Multiple guidelines exist that can direct drug dose reductions for patients with ESRD (120,121).

HEPATIC RISK ASSESSMENT

An increasing number of patients with chronic liver disease (CLD), advanced or end stage, will require nonliver transplant surgery (122). Reasons for this increase are an aging population, better long-term survival of patients with liver cirrhosis, and continuously improving outcomes after surgery and critical care medicine (123). Historically, liver dysfunction was related to chronic viral or alcoholic hepatitis. While the incidence of these conditions has not changed dramatically in recent years, the rising rate of obesity has led to nonalcoholic fatty liver disease, which is increasingly recognized as the most common cause of CLD in the United States (124).

As mentioned earlier, thorough preoperative evaluation of patients includes a comprehensive history and physical examination, with laboratory testing based upon historical and physical findings. Routine testing of liver function or coagulation in asymptomatic patients rarely yields abnormal results or changes in perioperative management (7). However, patients with a history of liver disease, jaundice, blood transfusions, the use of alcohol or other recreational drugs, hepatitis, or physical findings of icterus, hepatosplenomegaly, palmar erythema, or spider nevi should be tested to rule out occult or active liver diseases (123).

Patients with acute hepatitis (viral or alcohol induced) should have their surgery delayed until the acute phase of the disease process has passed and liver function tests have returned to normal. Mortality rates among these patients can range from 10% to 58% if surgery is pursued. Patients with acute liver failure/fulminant liver failure, defined as the development of jaundice, coagulopathy, and hepatic encephalopathy within 26 weeks in a patient with acute liver injury and without preexisting liver disease, are critically ill, and all surgery other than liver transplantation is contraindicated in these patients (125). Contrarily, patients with chronic infectious hepatitis, which is stable, tolerate surgery with minimal mortality (122,126,127). Of course the operator should practice universal precautions with all surgical interventions, regardless of the patient's known infectivity status.

Assessing the severity of the underlying liver disease is important to determine the perioperative outcome, which has been correlated with two classification systems: the Child-Turcotte-Pugh (CTP) classification and the model of end-stage liver disease (MELD) score. The CTP score was the first predictor of surgical risk/mortality for patients undergoing surgical intervention, specifically, patients having portacaval shunts. The system was modified by Pugh and colleagues to include prothrombin time in place of the subjective assessment of nutritional status, for use in patients undergoing esophageal transections for bleeding varices (128,129). Although widely known for classifying liver disease, this system has been criticized for utilizing subjective variables (ascites and encephalopathy) in developing a score. However, the CTP score correlates with mortality in patients undergoing differing types of surgery (123,130) (**Table 8.8**). The MELD score was originally devised as a prognostic measure of short-term mortality in patients with cirrhosis undergoing placement of a transjugular intrahepatic portosystemic shunt (131). The MELD score is derived from a complex formula which incorporates three biochemical variables (serum total bilirubin, serum creatinine, and the international normalized ratio [INR]) and assigns the patient a score of 8 to 40 (**Table 8.9**). The risk of morbidity and mortality in patients with liver disease depends upon the type of surgery and has been correlated to the aforementioned classification systems (**Tables 8.8 and 8.9**) (130). However, it is likely that over the last two

TABLE 8.8. Child-Turcotte-Pugh (CTP) Classification of Liver Disease and Operative Mortality

	Score		
Component	**1 Point**	**2 Points**	**3 Points**
Ascites	None	Controlled with medication	Treatment refractory
Encephalopathy	Absent	Grade I–II; controlled with medication	Grade III–IV; treatment refractory
Albumin, g/L	>3.5	2.8–3.5	<2.8
Bilirubin, mg/dL	<2	2–3	>3
INR	<1.7	1.7–2.3	>2.3
CTP Classification	Class A (5–6 points)	Class B (7–9 points)	Class C (10–15 points)
90-day mortality risk (abdominal surgery)	2%–10%	2%–30%	12%–76%

Source: Adapted from Hanje AJ, Patel T. Preoperative evaluation of patients with liver disease. *Nat Clin Pract Gastroenterol Hepatol*. 2007;4:266–276; Muir AJ. Surgical clearance for the patient with chronic liver disease. *Clin Liver Dis*. 2012;16:421–433; and Hoetzel A, Ryan H, Schmidt R. Anesthetic considerations for the patient with liver disease. *Curr Opin Anesthesiol*. 2012;25(3):340–347, with permission.

TABLE 8.9. Model for End-Stage Liver Disease (MELD) Score

MELD Score = (9.6 × $\log_e$[Creatinine]) + (3.8 × $\log_e$[Bilirubin]) + (11.2 × $\log_e$[INR]) + 6.4			
Creatinine levels above 4.0 mg/dL are assigned 4.0 mg/dL. Levels under 1.0 mg/dL are assigned 1.0 mg/dL. If the patient has had dialysis twice in the previous week, the value is assigned 4.0 mg/dL			
Bilirubin levels below 1.0 mg/dL are assigned 1.0 mg/dL			
INR levels below 1.0 are assigned 1.0			
The maximum score is 40. Scores calculated greater than 40 are assigned a value of 40			
MELD Score	Less than 10	10–15	Greater than 15
	Low Risk	Intermediate Risk	1. High Risk
30-Day Mortality (Abdominal/cardiac/orthopedic surgery)	5%–5.7%	10%	2. >50%

Source: Adapted from Hanje AJ, Patel T. Preoperative evaluation of patients with liver disease. *Nat Clin Pract Gastroenterol Hepatol*. 2007;4:266–276, Malik SM, Ahmad J. Preoperative risk assessment for patients with liver disease. *Med Clin North Am*. 2009;93:917–929, and Friedman LS. Surgery in the patient with liver disease. *Trans Am Clin Climatol Assoc*. 2010;121:192–204, with permission.

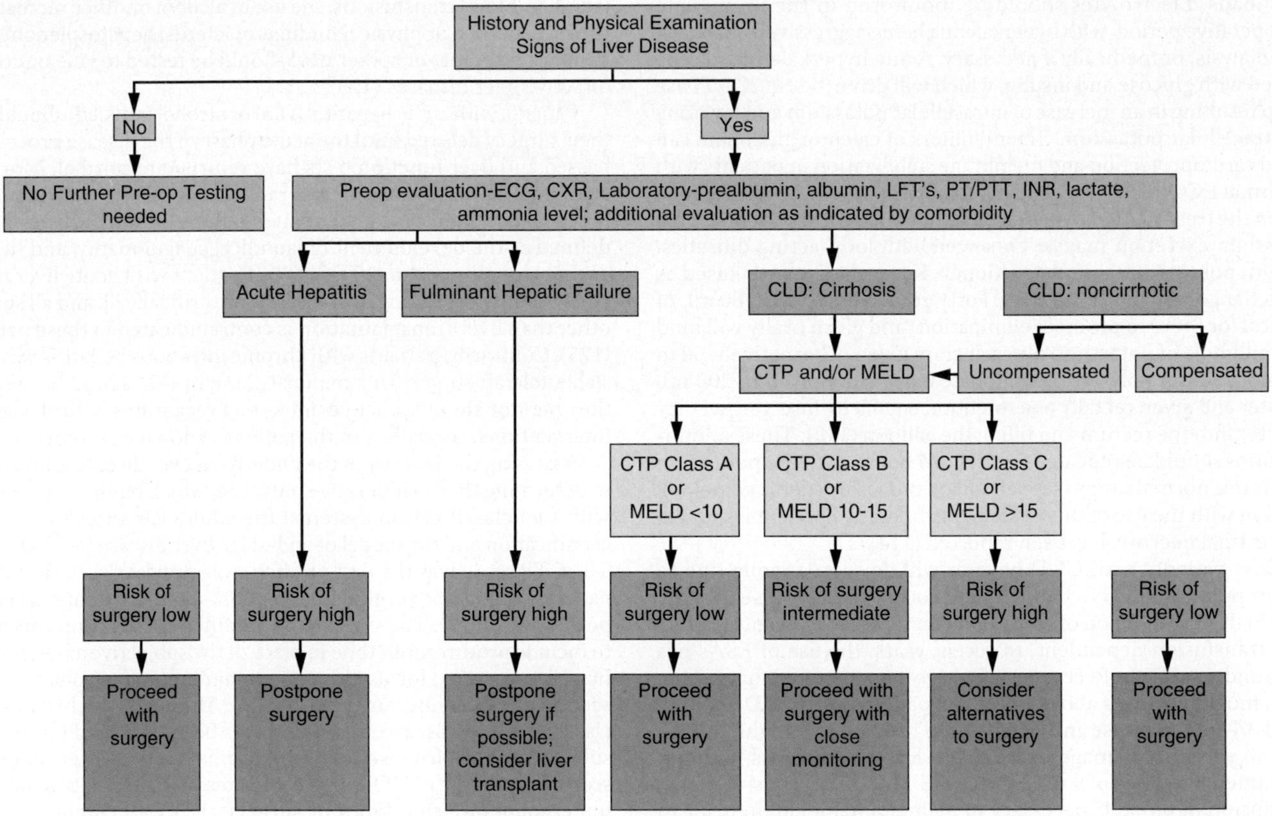

Figure 8.2. Preoperative evaluation and risk stratification in suspected liver disease. ECG, electrocardiogram; LFTs, liver function tests; ALT, alanine aminotransferase; AP, alkaline phosphatase; AST, aspartate aminotransferase; PT, prothrombin time; PTT, partial prothrombin time; INR, international normalization ratio; CLD, chronic liver disease; CTP, Childs–Turcotte–Pugh; MELD, model for end-stage liver disease.

Source: Adapted from Hanje AJ, Patel T. Preoperative evaluation of patients with liver disease. *Nat Clin Pract Gastroenterol Hepatol*. 2007;4:266–276 and Hoetzel A, Ryan H, Schmidt R. Anesthetic considerations for the patient with liver disease. *Curr Opin Anesthesiol*. 2012;25(3):340–347.

decades, mortality rates have decreased, despite the absence of large studies confirming this assumption (123).

Patients with cirrhosis of the liver also have coagulopathies, which need to be corrected prior to surgery. Vitamin K, fresh frozen plasma, or cryoprecipitate may be administered to correct the prothrombin time to within 3 seconds of normal. **Figure 8.2** presents an algorithm for patients with liver disease facing surgery.

Finally, selection of medications in patients with hepatic dysfunction needs to be done carefully, from types of perioperative antibiotics to anesthetic agents and analgesics. Patients with liver dysfunction are particularly susceptible to anesthetic effects such as changes in hepatic metabolism of medications and changes in hepatic blood flow. Alterations of the type and the dose of an agent are necessary to avoid postoperative hepatic dysfunction and hepatitis. Postoperative pain management with narcotic agents needs to be reduced by as much as 50% to account for the altered hepatic metabolism in these patients (132).

Preoperative Nutritional Assessment

There is a clear correlation between degree of malnutrition and increased risk of perioperative complications in cancer patients undergoing surgery (133). The broader consideration of nutrition in the gynecologic cancer patient is discussed in Chapter 32. The intent of this section is to present the concepts of preoperative nutritional evaluation and support of the gynecologic oncology patient undergoing surgery. Early refeeding and enteral and parenteral nutritional support in the postoperative patient will be discussed later.

The incidence of malnutrition among cancer patients has been estimated to be 20% to 80%, with the prevalence among gynecologic oncology patients being approximately 20%. For example, ovarian cancer patients are 19 times more likely to have moderate malnutrition when compared with patients with other gynecologic malignancies or benign conditions (134,135). Malnourished gynecologic oncology patients have been found to have an increased risk of postoperative complications, longer lengths of stay, hospital readmissions, reoperations, earlier cancer recurrences, and residual tumor after initial surgery (135–137). The methods for assessing malnutrition have varied among investigators and have included weight loss over a given time, various objective anthropometric parameters (e.g., weight loss, BMI, triceps skinfold thickness, and arm circumference), biochemical testing (e.g., serum albumin, prealbumin, total protein, transferrin, hemoglobin, and vitamins), and immunologic testing (skin sensitivity tests) (**Table 8.10**) (138).

Nutrition screening refers to the initial clinical evaluation that can quickly identify patients at high risk for malnutrition and who, later, may undergo a more formal and extensive nutritional assessment. Such instruments are the Malnutrition Screening Tool and the Malnutrition Universal Screening Tool, which have been used in oncology patients (**Table 8.11**). Logically, identifying patients at nutritional risk, by screening, will mark them for subsequent formal nutrition assessment and identify opportunities for medical nutrition therapy, which ultimately should improve patient outcomes. Unfortunately, this sequence of assumptions has never been subjected to prospective confirmation in clinical trials (139).

Many nutrition assessment tools have been developed, including subjective and objective data to assign risk, and some have been validated in cancer patients, including gynecologic cancer patients. Those instruments that have been used in cancer patients include the Subjective Global Assessment (SGA), the Patient-Generated Subjective Global Assessment (PG-SGA), Nutrition Risk Index (NRI), the Mini Nutritional Assessment (MNA), Prognostic Nutritional Index (PNI), and the Nutritional Risk Screening 2002 (NRS 2002) (**Table 8.11**). Although these are just examples of the many assessment tools available, none has emerged as the "gold standard" for nutritional screening and/or nutritional assessment among cancer patients, and their use depends upon which organization endorses a particular tool.

The SGA tool, originally described by Detsky in 1987, uses history and physical examination to assign a nutrition risk score. The PG-SGA was adapted from the SGA by Ottery, and later modified by McCallum and Polisena to give a numerical score of 0 to 47, specifically for the oncology population (140–143). It consists of two sections, one of which is done by the patient. This portion elicits information related to weight history, symptoms, food intake, and activity level. The other section, completed by a health care professional, includes an evaluation of metabolic demand, diagnosis, and comorbidities in relation to nutrition requirements and elements

TABLE 8.10. Measurement of Nutritional Depletion

	Depletion		
Parameters	**Mild**	**Moderate**	**Severe**
Triceps skin fold (TSF) % Standard	50–90	30–50	<30
Mid-arm muscle circumference (MAMC) % Standard	80–90	70–80	<70
Albumin, g/dL	3.0–3.4	2.1–3.0	<2.1
Total lymphocyte count (TLC), cmm	1,200–1,500	800–1,200	<800
Weight loss, % initial			
In 1 week	<1	1–2	>2
In 1 month	<2	2–5	>5
In 3 months	<5	5.0–7.5	>7.5
In 6 months	<7.5	7.5–10.0	>10.0

TABLE 8.11. Nutritional Screening and Assessment Tools

Tool	Components
Screening Instruments	
Malnutrition Screening Tool (MST)	3 items: weight, percentage weight loss, appetite
Malnutrition Universal Screening Tool (MUST)	3 items: BMI, percentage weight loss, acute disease effect
Nutritional Risk Screening 2002 (NRS 2002)	4 items: reduced BMI, percentage weight loss, decreased dietary intake, acute disease effect
Assessment Instruments	
Patient-Generated Subjective Global Assessment (PG-SGA)	Patient (4 questions): weight history, symptoms, food intake, activity level; Health care provider: metabolic demand, diagnosis and comorbidities, physical examination
Subjective Global Assessment (SGA)	History and physical examination to assign nutrition score
Prognostic Nutritional Index (PNI)	Equation: PNI Score (%) = 158 – 16.6 (albumin level in g/dL) – 0.78 (triceps skin fold in mm) – 0.2 (transferrin level in mg/dL) – 5.8 (Grade of delayed hypersensitivity)
Nutrition Risk Index (NRI)	Equation: NRI = 1.519 (serum albumin; g/dL) + 41.7 (current weight/usual weight) × 100
Mini Nutritional Assessment (MNA)	18 items: Screening portion (6 questions): food intake, weight loss, mobility stress, BMI; Assessment (12 questions): medical history, eating habits, anthropometric measurements

Source: Adapted from Huhmann MB, August DA. Review of American Society for Parenteral and Enteral Nutrition (ASPEN) clinical guidelines for nutrition support in cancer patients: nutrition screening and assessment. *Nutr Clin Pract.* 2008;23:182–188, with permission.

of physical examination. Every portion of the tool is given a numeric score, including the patient's portion, which is used to triage intervention. Laky and colleagues in 2007 showed, in a prospective fashion, that the PG-SGA could be easily administered to identify gynecologic cancer patients at risk for malnutrition. Their work established a prevalence of malnutrition among their patients in Brisbane, Australia. Among 145 patients with known or suspected gynecologic cancer, 116 patients were classified as well nourished (PG-SGA A), 29 patients were moderately malnourished (PG-SGA B), and none of the patients were severely malnourished (PG-SGA C). These investigators found that ovarian cancer patients were 19 times more likely to be malnourished, compared with patients with other gynecologic malignancies or benign conditions. In addition, they found that preoperative serum albumin levels correlated with the PG-SGA B score among ovarian cancer patients, similar to other previous reports (136,137,143), and may be a good indicator of malnutrition among gynecologic cancer patients in the absence of a full nutritional assessment (134). In 2008, Laky found that the scored PG-SGA, albumin level, triceps skinfold thickness, and total body potassium could predict the SGA better than chance. The authors concluded that the scored PG-SGA is the most appropriate tool for identifying malnutrition in gynecologic cancer patients.

The NRI was used to stratify nutrition risk in the Veterans Affairs Total Parenteral Nutrition Cooperative Study Group trial of perioperative parenteral nutrition. It is a simple equation that uses albumin and weight to classify individuals as either well nourished or malnourished. The equation:

$$\text{NRI} = 1.519\ (\text{serum albumin; g/dL}) + 41.7\ (\text{current weight/usual weight}) \times 100$$

A score less than 100 is considered malnourished (144). This particular tool has not been studied in gynecologic oncology patients.

The MNA is an 18-item tool that is divided into two sections: screening and assessment. The screening segment contains six questions related to food intake, weight loss, mobility, stress, and BMI. If this score is 11 or less, then a health care provider will complete the remaining 12-item assessment. A total score of <17 indicates malnutrition and a score between 17 and 23.5 indicates risk for malnutrition. This instrument has been validated in the elderly population, but its use among cancer patients is limited, and nonexistent among gynecologic cancer patients.

The PNI is an objective evaluation of nutritional status that includes anthropometric measurements and laboratory testing and an assessment of cell-mediated immunity by testing for mumps, tuberculin, and *Candida* (the grade of response is 0—nonreactive; 1—<5 mm induration; 2—≥5 mm induration) (145). The information gathered is put into the formula below:

$$\begin{aligned}\text{PNI Score (\%)} = {} & 158 - 16.6\ (\text{albumin level in g/dL}) - \\ & 0.78\ (\text{triceps skin fold in mm}) - \\ & 0.2\ (\text{transferrin level in mg/dL}) - \\ & 5.8\ (\text{Grade of delayed hypersensitivity})\end{aligned}$$

If the PNI is <40%, then the patient is determined to have normal nutritional status; PNI 40% to 49% indicates mild malnutrition; PNI >50% is severe malnutrition. Santoso et al. compared this objective, yet cumbersome and expensive, method with the SGA for gynecologic malignancies. They found that agreement between the two methods was only fair to moderate, with the SGA methodology trending toward underreporting when compared with the objective method (146).

The NRS 2002 was developed to include measures of current malnutrition and disease severity. This scoring system assesses current malnutrition by scoring the amount and duration of weight loss, reduced BMI, and recent decrease in dietary intake. In addition, the severity of illness is graded as a reflection of increased nutritional requirements. A score is calculated for each part of the assessment and added together for the final score. A score ≥3 indicates the need to start nutritional support. This NRS 2002 is recommended by the European Society for Clinical Nutrition and Metabolism (ESPEN) for the screening of hospitalized patients and has been widely accepted in Europe. It is important to note that this tool is useful in identifying patients who will benefit from nutrition intervention, but does not categorize the risk of malnutrition. This tool has not been evaluated among patients with gynecologic malignancies undergoing surgery (147).

Currently, the American Society of Parenteral and Enteral Nutrition (ASPEN) and the ESPEN do not recommend routine nutrition support therapy (NST-parenteral or enteral) in patients undergoing major cancer operations. The risks and costs of routine perioperative NST outweigh benefits in terms of surgical outcomes in cancer patients (133,147,148).

Several RCTs have been conducted to evaluate NST in cancer patients undergoing surgery. The largest trial, the Veterans Affairs Cooperative Study, randomized 395 surgical (abdominal or noncardiac thoracic surgeries) patients, mostly male, to receive at least 7 days of preoperative and 3 days of postoperative total parenteral nutrition (TPN) or to receive no perioperative nutritional supplementation. The TPN group had a greater number of infectious complications, mostly among patients classified as borderline or mildly malnourished compared with the unfed patients (14.1% vs. 6.4%). However, a subset of severely malnourished patients derived benefit from lower operative complication rates (5% vs. 43%, $p = 0.03$) without incurring an increase in infectious complications. The overall 30- and 90-day mortality rates were not different between the groups (144). Meijerink et al. completed a trial of preoperative nutrition among 151 patients undergoing surgery for gastric or colorectal cancer and randomized to preoperative TPN versus enteral nutrition (EN) versus standard oral diet (SOD). The authors found that there was no difference in mortality among the groups. However, patients who were severely malnourished and received either TPN or EN had fewer intra-abdominal abscesses than the SOD, but there was a difference in infectious morbidity between the TPN and EN groups (149). A similar study by Bozzetti et al. randomized severely malnourished patients undergoing resection of gastric or colonic malignancies to 10 days of preoperative and 9 days of postoperative TPN or SOD with hypocaloric TPN postoperatively only. The TPN only group showed lower noninfectious postoperative complication rates and mortality (150). And finally, Wu et al. randomized 468 patients to pre- and postoperative TPN/EN versus postoperative hypocaloric PN among moderately to severely malnourished patients undergoing surgery for GI cancers. The investigators found fewer complications, lower mortality, and shorter lengths of stay among the full nutrition support group (151). Because of the findings of these trials, ASPEN and ESPEN suggest that perioperative NST may be beneficial in moderately or severely malnourished patients if administered for 7 to 14 days preoperatively. The potential benefits of NST must be weighed against the potential risks of the NST itself and of delaying the operation. The authors direct the reader to reviews of these recommendations, which have been done by Huhman and August (for ASPEN) (133) and Braga et al. (for ESPEN) (148).

PREPARATION FOR SURGERY

Enhanced Recovery Pathway

In the last decade, enhanced recovery pathways (ERPs) or enhanced recovery after surgery (ERAS) protocols have been developed and implemented. These have improved surgical outcomes as well as realized significant cost savings in colorectal surgery, among other surgical specialties (152–155). These approaches were founded by European surgeons who challenged traditional surgical paradigms such as preoperative bowel preparation, the overnight fasting rule, and delayed postoperative feeding. The researchers found that most of these practices lacked scientific evidence and actually interfered with patients' preoperative preparation and recovery. Recent reviews of these protocols in colorectal surgery have demonstrated a reduction in length of stay of 2.5 days, a decrease in complications by as much as 50%, and a mean savings of $2,245 per patient (156–158). The basic principles of ERP are to attenuate the stress response to surgery by omitting bowel preparation, maintaining euvolemia, starting early postoperative feeding, and avoiding IV opioids (152, 159,160) (**Fig. 8.3**). These programs are protocols that must be followed to obtain the greatest benefit, without omitting any of the steps along the way. The barriers to implementation come from long-held biases, based on lack of evidence, and the fact that the patient will encounter multiple people from various specialties (preoperative nursing, anesthesia, residents, postoperative nursing, etc.) through her journey of surgery. Critical to the success of these programs is auditing of the process to identify areas where protocol deviations occur, and to identify areas for improvement.

Although literature about ERP in gynecologic oncology is sparse, and mostly retrospective, interest in implementing such programs is growing. One such study done at the Mayo Clinic in Rochester, MN, by Kalogera et al. demonstrated that the use of patient-controlled anesthesia decreased over 60%, with an 80% reduction of opioid use in the first 48 hours, without change of pain scores among enhanced recovery patients as compared with historic controls. In addition, the authors showed a 4-day reduction in length of hospital stay, with stable readmission rates and a 30-day cost saving of more than $7,600 per patient on the ERP. Further more, there were no differences in the rate of or complexity of postoperative complications among the enhanced recovery patients (160). With the adoption and success of such ERP programs in colorectal surgery, and with the likelihood that these programs would yield similar benefits in other surgical specialties, the ERAS Society was founded in 2010 in an effort to reach other surgical specialists and subspecialists and publish guidelines. As a result, the Society recently published a two-part series on ERAS in *Gynecologic Oncology*. The authors direct readers to these guidelines for further details (161,162). In this chapter, we will point out best practice for ERAS.

Medication Management

In preparation for surgery, patients may need to decrease or stop taking certain medications, especially those associated with higher incidence of anticoagulation risks. Appropriate notice and clear instructions should be given to patients in this case, as some medications require several days of cessation to produce the desired results. For patients with INR levels between 2.0 and 3.0, it will take approximately 4 days after warfarin therapy is discontinued for the INR to reach 1.5. Many patients on warfarin do not need to be covered with heparin therapy preoperatively. Administration of treatment-dose IV heparin or low-molecular-weight heparin (LMWH) while the INR is subtherapeutic is recommended for patients with a history of mechanical mitral valve, ball and cage valve, acute venous or arterial thromboembolism within 3 months of surgery, or atrial fibrillation with a history of thromboembolic stroke (163). A thorough discussion pertaining to usage of over-the-counter medications and herbal supplements is crucial in presurgery medication management. Patients should be counseled on the use of nonprescription medications, such as aspirin, nonsteroidal anti-inflammatories, ginkgo biloba, saw palmetto, garlic, ginseng, and vitamin E, as they have antiplatelet components and may enhance bleeding risk (164,165). If possible, anemia should be corrected preoperatively. The use of recombinant human erythropoietin with concurrent iron and folic acid supplementation 2 to 3 weeks preoperatively has been shown to reduce allogeneic blood transfusions in patients undergoing elective surgery (166). It has been estimated that 60% of all blood transfused in the United States is given to surgical patients.

Numerous studies have shown the benefit of starting medications, such as statins and β-blockers, in the preoperative setting to reduce cardiac risk (167). The perioperative use of β-blockers has been shown to reduce the incidence of postoperative myocardial ischemia, MI, and cardiac mortality by decreasing myocardial oxygen consumption and workload, although this has not been studied specifically in the morbidly obese population (167). Current ACC/AHA guidelines recommend that β-blockers should be continued in patients undergoing surgery who are receiving β-blockers to treat angina, symptomatic arrhythmias, hypertension, or other ACC/AHA class I guideline indications (168). For high-risk patients not receiving β-blockade, therapy should start before elective surgery, with the dose titrated to achieve a heart rate at rest of 50 to 60 beats/min (169). The perioperative use of β-blockers in high-risk patients undergoing major noncardiac surgery is supported by published data. However, studies have questioned the benefits of this approach in moderate-risk patients and report that the potential harm in low-risk groups might outweigh the benefit, highlighting the importance of patient selection (170).

Statins have also been shown to be effective cardioprotective drugs in the perioperative setting (167). Statins have been shown to act as plaque stabilizers and therefore possibly decrease the risk of thromboembolic events (167,171). With their low side effect profile and well documented benefits, statins should be strongly considered for all obese patients with elevated serum cholesterol or triglycerides (172).

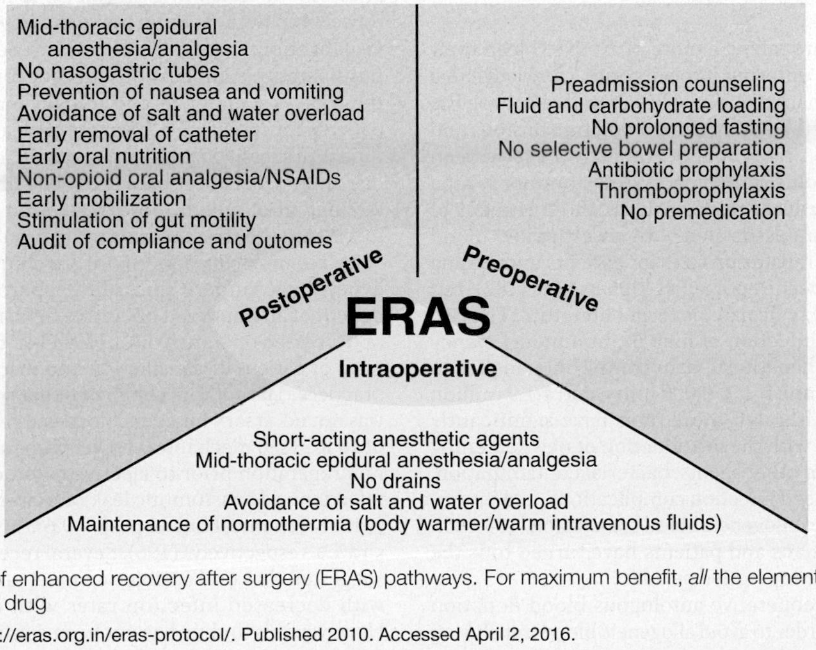

Figure 8.3. The elements of enhanced recovery after surgery (ERAS) pathways. For maximum benefit, *all* the elements must be followed. NSAID, nonsteroidal anti-inflammatory drug

Source: ERAS Protocol (EP). http://eras.org.in/eras-protocol/. Published 2010. Accessed April 2, 2016.

Close to 2 million patients undergo coronary angioplasty each year in Western countries, and >90% of these patients will have coronary stents placed as part of their intervention (173,174). Patients with bare metal stents are normally taking low-dose aspirin 81 mg. It is recommended that they stop taking aspirin 7 days before surgery (175,176).

Patients with drug-eluting stents take oral aspirin 81 mg, or even aspirin 325 mg, and, for the first 12 months after stent placement, daily oral clopidogrel 75 mg (176,177). Ideally, these patients should not undergo elective surgery, within the first 12 months after stenting. After the first 12 months, both medications are recommended to be stopped 7 days before surgery to reduce the risk of intra- and postoperative bleeding (175).

It is not uncommon for gynecologic oncology patients to undergo neoadjuvant chemotherapy. Most gynecologic oncologists would agree that the timing of surgery in relation to chemotherapy is crucial. In most cases, the surgical intervention should replace a cycle of chemotherapy. With regard to bevacizumab, special considerations should be taken into account since there is the added risk of bowel perforation and poor wound healing. The incidence, type, and timing of postsurgical bleeding events and wound healing complications were assessed in surgical patients in the AVastin And DOcetaxel (AVADO) and Avastin THErapy for advaNced breAst cancer (ATHENA) trials. Both study protocols followed recommendations to withhold bevacizumab for at least 6 weeks before elective surgery, and to wait 28 days (or until the wound was fully healed) after major surgery before recommencing bevacizumab therapy (178). Another study by Erinjeri et al. investigated how the timing of administration of bevacizumab affected the risk of wound healing in patients undergoing chest wall port placement. They concluded that the risk of a wound dehiscence requiring a chest wall port explant in patients treated with bevacizumab was inversely proportional to the interval between bevacizumab administration and port placement, with significantly higher risk seen when the interval is less than 14 days (179). Scappaticci et al. assessed postoperative wound healing complications in two randomized trials of 5 mg/kg bevacizumab in colorectal cancer treatment. Bevacizumab administered in combination with 5-fluorouracil/leucovorin-based chemotherapy 28 to 60 days after primary cancer surgery caused no increased risk of wound healing complications compared with chemotherapy alone. While wound healing complications were increased in patients who had major surgery during bevacizumab therapy, the majority of bevacizumab-treated patients experienced no complications (180).

Blood Banking

Patients and their families are taking a more proactive role in their health care and thereby are entering into surgeries knowledgeable of risks and expecting alternative options. Preoperative counseling should include discussion of the potential for blood transfusions and associated risks. Transfusion rates of approximately 5% have been reported for patients undergoing abdominal hysterectomy for benign disease (181). Radical procedures performed for the treatment of gynecologic malignancies are associated with an estimated blood loss of 1,000 mL or greater. Transfusion rates for patients undergoing radical hysterectomy have been reported as high as 80% (182), but rates of 10% to 20% are more typical in the recent literature. The risk of transfusion-transmitted infection of human immunodeficiency virus, hepatitis B virus, and hepatitis C virus from RBC transfusion is estimated at 1:2.1 million units, 1:250,000 units, and 1:1.9 million units, respectively (183). Although these rates have significantly decreased in the last decade with the introduction of new screening technologies, transmission of other agents, bacterial contamination, transfusion reactions, increased infection complications, and immunosuppression remain risks of allogeneic blood transfusion (184,185). One alternative both physicians and patients have turned to is the use of donor blood in the perioperative period.

Since the mid-1980s, preoperative autologous blood donation (PABD) has been utilized in order to avoid allogeneic blood transfusion in patients undergoing elective surgery where excessive blood loss is anticipated. Although this practice decreases homologous blood use, 15% of autologous donors will still receive allogeneic transfusions, and 50% of units collected are not used and must be discarded (186). Furthermore, PABD greatly increases the likelihood of any transfusion being necessary and is not without medical risks. Severe reactions during autologous donation occurred at a rate of 0.32% per unit collected and 0.75% per donor. Serious incidents during blood collection that required hospitalization were 12 times more likely in PABD compared with allogeneic donors (187). Transfusions to the wrong recipient, bacterial contamination, febrile nonhemolytic reactions, and allergic reactions have also been reported with autologous transfusion. The cost-effectiveness of PABD has been found to be extremely poor and has steadily deteriorated over the decade (186–189).

Acute normovolemic hemodilution (ANH) is an autologous blood-procurement strategy that is equivalent to PABD in reducing allogeneic transfusion needs. Its clinical utility has been extensively studied in patients undergoing radical prostatectomy, total joint replacement, and, more recently, major colorectal surgery. During ANH, blood is procured in the holding or operating room and replaced simultaneously with colloid and crystalloid until a target hematocrit level of 28% is reached or blood volume of 1,500 mL is removed (190). The patient's blood becomes diluted and the amount of actual red cell mass lost during surgery is reduced. ANH obviates the costs of blood testing, storage, or wastage because all blood collected during ANH is kept in the operating room and returned to the patient before the end of surgery. It is simple to perform and more convenient for the patient. Since the blood is collected at point-of-care, there is no possibility for clerical error or contamination. ANH has been shown to be a cost-effective yet underutilized strategy to reduce allogeneic blood transfusions (190–192). ANH in which the blood is kept in a continuous circuit with the patient is often a workable alternative for a Jehovah's Witness patient (190,193).

The utilization of erythropoietin in oncology patients should be on a case-by-case basis due to recent evidence of adverse effects in oncology patients (194).

Bowel Preparation and Preoperative Fasting

Older thinking had been that in anticipation of colorectal surgery, bowel preparation would decrease the risks of infection and anastomotic leaks. In gynecology, it was thought that mechanical bowel preparation would make the bowel easier to handle, improve visualization, especially with laparoscopic surgery, and decrease postoperative complications. Recent studies have demonstrated that these views are not true and actually may impede the preparation of patients for surgery. The process of cleansing the bowel with liters of fluid is distressing to patients, causing nausea and vomiting, physical discomfort, dehydration, electrolyte abnormalities, and prolonged fasting, all of which increase insulin resistance and catabolism, increasing the stress of the surgical process.

A recent meta-analysis of mechanical bowel preparation for gynecologic surgery (including laparoscopic surgery) showed no benefit of an improved operative field, better handling of the bowel, or decreased operative time. However, the analysis did show that the rates of patient dissatisfaction and discomfort were high with such practices. The authors concluded that mechanical bowel preparation was not necessary for gynecologic surgery (195). A systematic review of 18 RCTs of mechanical bowel preparation or rectal enemas versus no preparation prior to elective colorectal surgery showed that the infection and anastomotic leak rates were similar between the groups (with mechanical bowel prep—9.6% and 4.4%; without prep—8.5% and 4%, respectively) (196). Several recent retrospective studies have suggested that oral antibiotic bowel preparation may be associated with decreased infection rates with elective colorectal surgery. However, this finding has not been confirmed with randomized trials

(161,197). Finally, a recent RCT assessing the benefit of mechanical bowel preparation versus no prep for patients undergoing low anterior resections for rectal carcinoma demonstrated higher infectious morbidity for the no prep group, but no difference in anastomotic leaks (198). Clearly, further study of this topic will be needed. ***Best Practice: Routine oral mechanical bowel preparation should not be used in gynecologic/oncologic surgery, including patients with planned enteric resection.***

Fear of aspiration drove "dogma" within the specialties of anesthesiology and surgery to instruct patients to fast for 12 or more hours before surgery. The thinking was that a prolonged fast prior to surgery would reduce the amount of acid and gastric contents in the stomach, thus preventing aspiration at the time of induction (199). A Cochrane review of 22 randomized clinical trials has shown that shortened fasting periods did not increase the risk of aspiration, regurgitation, or related morbidity (200). Thus, the ASA recommends a fast of 6 hours preoperatively for solid foods and that clear liquids be consumed for up to 2 hours prior to surgery (201). A prolonged preoperative fast for up to 12 hours will cause the patient to deplete her glycogen stores, which leads to insulin resistance and hyperglycemia, which can increase postoperative complications and morbidity. Carbohydrate loading drinks given to patients 2 to 3 hours prior to surgery can prevent insulin resistance, decrease hyperglycemia, and attenuate the stress response to surgery. These complex carbohydrate solutions are emptied by the stomach within 30 to 90 minutes and have been shown to reduce patient anxiety, thirst, and hunger (199). An RCT of carbohydrate loading versus no loading in patients undergoing colorectal surgery showed a significant reduction in length of stay (202). ***Best Practice: Patients should be permitted to drink clear liquids until 2 hours before anesthesia and surgery. Patients should abstain from oral intake of solids 6 hours prior to induction of anesthesia. Oral carbohydrate loading reduces postoperative insulin resistance, improves preoperative well-being, and should be used routinely in nondiabetic patients.***

Infection Prophylaxis

The use of prophylactic antimicrobials plays a large role in reducing the rates of surgical site infections (SSIs) and should be used in clean or clean-contaminated operations, which include most procedures performed by gynecologic oncologists. Radical pelvic surgery introduces women to a higher risk of postoperative infection secondary to several potential factors: lengthened operating time, average age of patient requiring this specific surgery, increased blood loss, anemia, potential hypothermia, probable poor nutritional status, the presence of tumor, prior pelvic irradiation, diabetes, obesity, peripheral vascular disease, and a history of postsurgical infection (203,204). Prophylactic antibiotics should provide coverage consistent with the microbial milieu most likely to be encountered. In gynecologic oncology surgery, the most common infecting organisms are coliforms, enterococci, streptococci, clostridia, and bacteroides.

Several guidelines for antibiotic prophylaxis in surgery have been published (203,205–207). Most reports recommend cefazolin for gynecologic procedures. Although no longer available, cefotetan had been the preferred antibiotic for prophylaxis in longer radical gynecologic operations, as well as for prophylaxis prior to colorectal surgery, due to longer half-life and broad-spectrum coverage (208). An appropriate alternative for surgical procedures with a higher chance of bowel resection or injury is cefazolin plus metronidazole or ampicillin-sulbactam (207). Cefoxitin is another option, but availability has been limited. Most patients with a penicillin allergy can be treated with cefazolin; however, when allergy prohibits the administration of a cephalosporin, alternative regimens are clindamycin with gentamicin, a fluoroquinolone, or aztreonam (205). Itani et al. reported on a randomized, double-blinded trial in patients undergoing elective colorectal surgery that suggested ertapenem as an effective alternative to cefotetan (209). Ertapenem has received the Food and Drug Administration approval for prophylaxis for elective colon resection; however, the 2006 Medical Letter guidelines caution against the routine use of ertapenem for surgical prophylaxis due to cost and concerns that this practice may result in increased rates of antibiotic resistance (207).

When considering dosing orders to achieve and maintain effective tissue levels, parenteral antibiotics should be given within 1 hour (between 1 and 2 hours for fluoroquinolones and vancomycin) prior to skin incision as a loading dose (205). For patients weighing >70 kg, the dosage should be doubled (i.e., cefazolin 2 g IV) or weight-based dosing should be used. Repeat doses should be given intraoperatively for surgeries lasting longer than 3 to 4 hours or when blood loss exceeds 1,000 mL (207,208). Guidelines from the National Surgical Site Infection Project recommend that prophylactic antibiotic use for abdominal or vaginal procedures end within 24 hours of the operation (205). The majority of the published evidence supports the use of an appropriately timed administration of a single dose of antibiotic and indicates that repeat doses postoperatively are unnecessary and subject the patient to the potential emergence of resistant organisms (203,205–207).

The American College of Surgeons and the National Surgical Quality Improvement Plan employ a prospective, peer-reviewed database to quantify 30-day risk-adjusted surgical outcomes that encompass such variables as preoperative risk factors and postoperative mortality and morbidity, allowing comparison of outcomes among all hospitals in the program. Enrolled hospitals abstract case data into the database, the data are quantified, and the database generates comprehensive semiannual reports to the hospitals as well as real-time, continuously updated, online benchmarking reports (210).

SSIs account for nearly 40% of nosocomial infections in surgical patients and occur in up to 20% of patients undergoing abdominal surgery (203,205). They are a significant source of postoperative morbidity, resulting in longer hospital stays, increased rates of ICU admissions, hospital readmissions, and subsequently increased costs. Mortality rates increase two to three times for patients with an SSI as compared with patients who do not develop an SSI (211,212). In addition to the administration of preoperative antimicrobial prophylaxis, preoperative skin preparation is used to reduce the risk of SSI by decreasing the microbial count at the projected site of incision. A meta-analysis of six trials concluded that although whole-body scrubs or showers with antiseptic agents such as chlorhexidine or povidone-iodine prior to surgery reduce bacterial counts on the skin, this practice did not reduce wound infection rates (213). Surgical infection occurrences are noted to be influenced by both patient and operative environmental factors. Therefore, patients undergoing surgery should be instructed to bathe or shower normally the night or morning prior to surgery, removing any debris from the skin surface and decreasing environmental contaminants.

Inappropriate hair removal techniques can traumatize the skin and provide an opportunity for colonization of microorganisms. There is no evidence that hair removal prior to surgery will prevent or reduce SSI. To the contrary, meta-analysis evaluating hair removal techniques demonstrated a twofold increase in SSI when patients underwent hair removal by shaving versus clipping (214). Hair is generally sterile and therefore does not need to be removed unless the hair around the incision will interfere with the operation. When hair removal is necessary, the simplest and least irritating method of hair removal is an electric or battery-powered clipper with a disposable head (203,214). Some infection control experts advocate removing all razors from hospitals and operating rooms (215). ***Best Practice: IV antibiotics should be administered routinely within 60 minutes before skin incision. The dose should be repeated in the case of a prolonged operation or severe blood loss; the dose should be increased in obese patients. Hair clipping is preferred if hair removal is mandatory. Chlorhexidine-alcohol is preferred to aqueous povidone-iodine solution for skin cleansing.***

Special Considerations for Obese Patients

A heightened awareness of potential comorbidities should be extended when preparing morbidly obese patients for surgery. Coexisting disorders, such as coronary artery disease, hypertension, obesity-hypoventilation syndrome, obstructive sleep apnea, adult-onset diabetes mellitus, pulmonary hypertension, gastroesophageal reflux, impaired cardiac function, and hypercoagulability are common in morbidly obese patients and may be undiagnosed at the time of surgery. Certain symptoms of such comorbidities may not manifest themselves until the patient undergoes physiologic stress related to surgery thereby increasing perioperative morbidity and mortality. For example, baseline pulmonary function studies of markedly obese patients demonstrate mild hypoxemia; decreased vital capacity, tidal volume, and expiratory reserve volume; increased resistance; and ventilation-perfusion inequalities (216). During the postoperative period, severe hypoxemia may occur secondary to sedation, pain, immobility, atelectasis, and anemia, leading to cardiac arrhythmia or ischemia. A thorough preoperative medical history and physical examination should be performed to increase the findings of coexisting disease and minimize surgical risk. A comprehensive review of the pathophysiology associated with morbid obesity is beyond the scope of this chapter, and we direct the reader elsewhere for a thorough review (217).

Surgery in morbidly obese patients poses many challenges for teams on both sides of the surgical drape. The primary concern of the anesthesiologist is gaining adequate control of the airway. The combined problems of increased aspiration risk, rapid oxygen desaturation caused by decreased FRC, baseline hypoxemia, and increased oxygen demand, in addition to technical difficulties due to anatomic fat deposits, make intubation a high-risk procedure. An awake, fiberoptic-assisted intubation is often the technique of choice for obtaining an airway. Extubation should be delayed until the patient is fully awake and ideally sitting upright (218). There are technical operating room and instrumentation issues, which need to be addressed as well. Standard operating tables, stretchers, and hospital beds have weight limits, which have prompted specifically designed wider and sturdier models for the obese patient. Staff and patient safety during transfer of the patient from the operating table to the bed or gurney is also a concern in the extremely obese patient and must be taken into consideration. Proper retractors and extra-long instruments are essential and may not be available in all hospitals. Although these practical considerations are ostensibly mundane, failure to prepare may prevent a successful outcome, cause frustration to all involved, and possibly put the patient at risk.

Recent reports in the gynecologic oncology literature suggest performing panniculectomy to improve exposure of the peritoneal cavity and pelvic structures (219–221). Although this is a relatively straightforward procedure, it does require some experience and planning for optimal results. Hospital credentialing of surgical privileges may require the involvement of a plastic surgeon or proctoring until proficiency is demonstrated. In addition, since panniculectomy is considered a cosmetic procedure, many insurers may require prior authorization with documentation of medical necessity, or they may deny any reimbursement.

Critical Care and Postoperative Management

Cardiovascular Issues

Monitoring Issues

There are many tools at the hands of the modern-day clinician when it comes to monitoring the cardiovascular function of the patient. Clinical examination, heart rate, blood pressure measurement, and ECG are a few. In the critical care setting, the addition of the arterial catheter, central venous pressure (CVP), and pulmonary artery (PA) catheter increases sophistication. Most patients in the ICU can be managed with simple clinical parameters. Fluid status can be assessed by daily weights, pulse rate, blood pressure, and urine output. Continuous ECG monitoring is helpful for detecting arrhythmias and ischemia. CVP is often used for assessment of volume status and a crude estimation of cardiac function. If a patient has a central line, one of the ports can be continuously transduced for CVP. It is a common mistake among novices to evaluate a single reading of CVP rather than reviewing the trend. When the CVP is correlated with volume status, the resulting graph is a scatter graph (i.e., no correlation). There is correlation over time and in response to fluid challenges, blood transfusion, or medical therapy. One must remember that the CVP is a pressure measurement and not the desired measurement of volume (preload). Therefore, only crude estimations of fluid status can be made with results from this instrumentation. When the status of a patient's cardiac output or fluid state is unclear, a minimally invasive hemodynamic monitor or an invasive PA catheter (e.g., Swan-Ganz catheter) may be helpful. A minimally invasive hemodynamic monitor connects to an existing arterial catheter and performs continuous self-calibration. The sensor provides information on stroke volume, stroke volume variation, and cardiac output (222).

PA catheters are placed via a central vein (subclavian or jugular) as a central line. The catheter has a balloon-tipped transducer and is "floated" into the PA. Waveforms of the right ventricle, PA, and pulmonary capillary wedge pressure (PCWP) are directly visualized as the catheter progresses through the heart (**Fig. 8.4**), and confirmed placement is verified by chest radiograph (**Fig. 8.5**). Complications of placement include pneumothorax, arrhythmia, line sepsis, and rarely PA rupture. The PA catheter allows the measurement of cardiac output and oxygen delivery and estimation of preload by obtaining the pulmonary artery occlusive pressure (PAOP) or PCWP, the "wedge."

A number of formulas for calculation of hemodynamic parameters are crucial in utilizing the PA catheter for the care of the critically ill patient (**Table 8.12**). Assessment of preload is desirable for determining fluid administration or diuretic requirements for patients. The ideal measure of preload would be LV end-diastolic volume; however, this value is unobtainable with current technology and intensivists settle for "the wedge" as an estimation. By inflating the balloon placed in the PA, a direct column of standing fluid exists between the left atrium, through the pulmonary vasculature, and back to the balloon (transducer). The PAOP can be measured and is a crude reflection of left atrial pressure. If the PAOP is elevated, the preload is adequate (or excessive). If the measurement is low, the patient may be volume depleted. These measurements, as previously mentioned with CVP, are dynamic and trend is important. For example, if the PAOP is low and a fluid bolus is given, the PAOP should increase if the diagnosis of volume depletion was correct.

Thermodilution techniques are used to calculate cardiac output by injecting saline via a proximal port in the PA catheter and measuring the thermal changes at the distal tip of the PA catheter. By combining the preload assessment provided by the PAOP and the calculated cardiac output, differentiation between volume depletion and cardiogenic disease states can be made (see section on shock). Currently, there are PA catheters that can calculate right ventricular EF.

Taking a blood sample from the tip of the PA catheter, the most desaturated blood in the body is retrieved. In normal circulation, the blood from the superior and inferior vena cava mix and the blood from the coronary sinus is added to give a sample known as the mixed venous blood. By evaluating the oxygen saturation of this blood, oxygen delivery can be calculated (**Table 8.12**). This measurement is perhaps the most important function of the PA catheter. Current technology allows this function to be continuous via an infrared sensor at the tip of the PA catheter. For example, if oxygen delivery is determined to be low, there are only three situations that the clinician can influence: increase cardiac output (with fluid, chronotropes, or inotropes), increase the hemoglobin, or increase the oxygen saturation. In a patient with multiple medical comorbidities and following a major abdominal operation, the measurement of a normal oxygen delivery provides reassurance to the clinician that end organs are being perfused.

Calculation of the systemic vascular resistance (SVR) is also possible with a PA catheter. Because the SVR is a calculated value and not directly measured, inaccuracies are inherent and overinterpretation

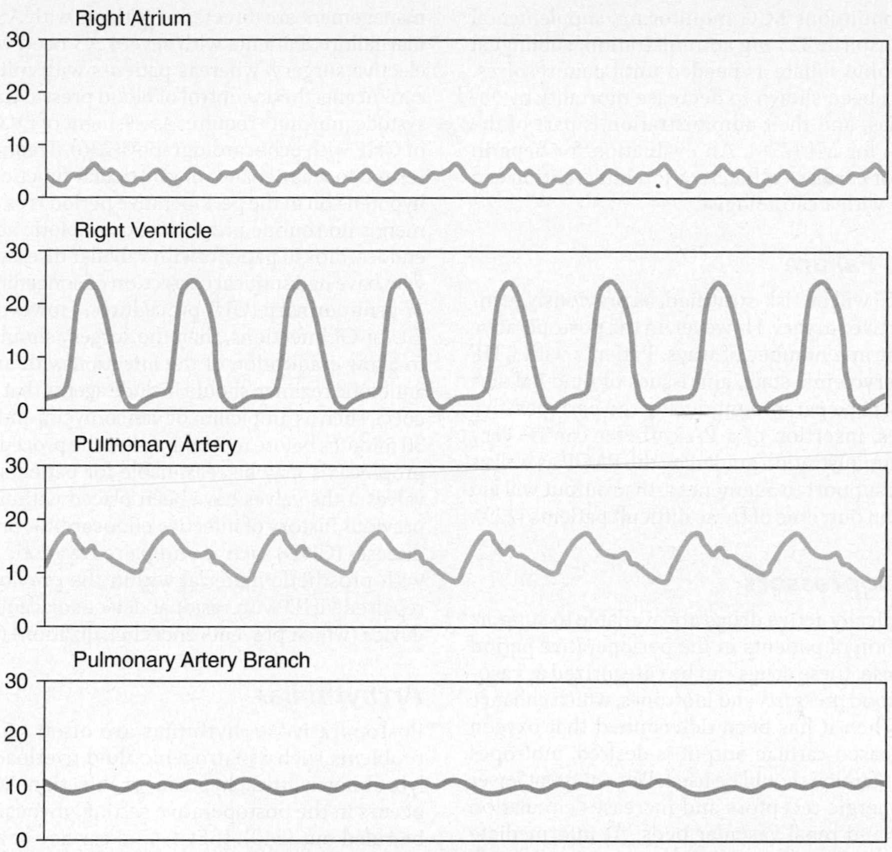

Figure 8.4. Pulmonary artery catheter waveform readings as the catheter passes through the heart into the pulmonary artery. *Y*-axis is reading in millimeters of mercury (mm Hg).

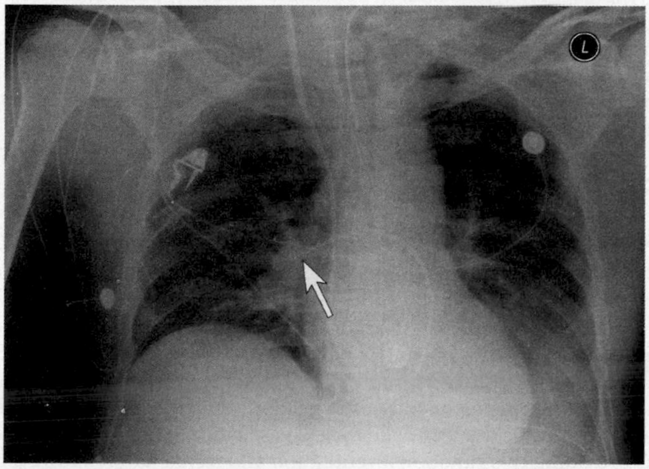

Figure 8.5. Chest radiograph showing proper placement of pulmonary artery catheter in the pulmonary artery (*arrow* shows tip of pulmonary catheter).

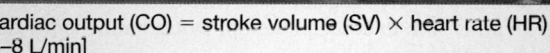

TABLE 8.12. Hemodynamic Formulas

Cardiac output (CO) = stroke volume (SV) × heart rate (HR) [4–8 L/min]
Cardiac index (CI) = CO/body surface area (BSA)
Systemic vascular resistance (SVR) = Mean arterial pressure (MAP) – Central venous pressure (CVP) × 80/CO [800–1,200 dynes - sec/cm^{-5}/m^2]
Arterial O_2 content (CaO_2) = (1.36) (hemoglobin) (oxygen saturation) + 0.003 (partial pressure of oxygen) [20 mL O_2/dL]
O_2 delivery (DO_2) = CO × CaO_2 × 10 [600–1,000 mL O_2/min]
O_2 availability (O_2AVI) = CI × CaO_2 × 10 [500–600 mL/min/m^2]
O_2 extraction ratio = (CaO_2 – CvO_2)/CaO_2 [25%]

Values in brackets are normal values.

of this value is cautioned. Rather than relying on the calculated SVR, the clinician should have a complete understanding of the measured blood pressure and cardiac output (SVR combines the two previously mentioned measured variables).

In one study of ovarian cancer patients undergoing cytoreductive surgery, 18% of patients had indications for PA catheter use (223). Because of the issues of volume status in these patients, PA catheter placement for postoperative fluid management may be especially helpful.

Recently, the use of PA catheters has become less common (224). Continuous dynamic measurements are possible with analysis of arterial and plethysmographic waveforms. Stroke volume variation can be used for goal-directed therapy (225). Other noninvasive or minimally invasive monitors have been developed, which include carbon dioxide rebreathing techniques to calculate cardiac output, esophageal Doppler among others (226).

Acute Postoperative MI

MI usually manifests with acute chest discomfort, elevated cardiac enzymes (troponin, creatinine phosphokinase, etc.), and ECG changes. Dyspnea, diaphoresis, nausea, and anxiety may also be associated. The MI definition is based on a rise of cardiac enzymes (troponin) in the setting of myocardial ischemia as evidenced by clinical symptoms, imaging findings, or ECG changes (227). Treatment includes

ICU monitoring with continuous ECG monitoring, supplemental oxygen, immediate oral aspirin 325 mg administration, sublingual nitroglycerin, and morphine sulfate as needed until pain resolves. Beta-blocker therapy has been shown to decrease mortality by decreasing fatal arrhythmias, and their administration is part of the early treatment regimen for MI (228). An evaluation for heparin therapy, thrombolytics, or cardiac catheterization intervention can be made in consultation with a cardiologist.

Congestive Heart Failure

Patients with known CHF will be risk-stratified, as previously mentioned, before major elective surgery. However, in the postoperative setting, CHF will present in a number of ways. Patients with CHF are in a continuous hypervolemic state, and issues of fluid balance (strict "ins" and "outs") will be paramount during the perioperative period. In difficult cases, insertion of a PA catheter can be very helpful. Judicious fluid administration guided by the PAOP as well as selective use of inotropic support to augment cardiac output will aid the clinician in a successful outcome of these difficult patients (229).

Inotropes and Vasopressors

A variety of hemodynamically active drugs are available to support the cardiovascular function of patients in the perioperative period (230). In the broadest sense, these drugs can be categorized as vasopressors, which elevate blood pressure, and inotropes, which enhance cardiac output (231). When it has been determined that oxygen delivery is low and increased cardiac output is desired, inotropes such as dopamine or dobutamine should be used. Dopamine, at lower doses, activates dopaminergic receptors and increases circulation in mesenteric, cerebral, and renal vascular beds. At intermediate doses, dopamine stimulates β-receptors in the heart and peripheral circulation. This activation causes tachycardia, increased stroke volume, and increased cardiac output. Increasing cardiac output in this fashion also increases demands for myocardial oxygen and could precipitate angina or MI (232). At high doses, dopamine acts as an α-agonist, causing vasoconstriction. Dobutamine is a β-1 agonist with much greater inotropic effect than dopamine and causes peripheral arterial vasodilation, decreasing afterload (this dilation can be abrupt and cause hypotension in some patients). Dobutamine is the drug of choice for severe heart failure.

Epinephrine is a potent sympathomimetic with β-mimetic effects at lower doses and α-mimetic effects at higher doses. This drug causes an acute increase in myocardial oxygen demand and is used in the setting of cardiac arrest or severe circulatory failure. Norepinephrine and phenylephrine are pure α-mimetic agents, utilized for vasoconstriction (neurogenic shock). In most situations of shock, fluid resuscitation is preferred to administration of α-agents. Although these agents will give a false sense of security that the blood pressure is normal, one must remember that the vasoconstriction underperfuses capillary beds and leads to renal hypoperfusion (acute renal injury), splanchnic hypoperfusion (resulting in translocation of gut flora), as well as a myriad of other problems (231,232).

Vasopressin is an option similar to epinephrine, with some important differences. This antidiuretic hormone (ADH) in high doses provides potent vasoconstriction and leads to improved cerebral and coronary blood flow in shock states. Unlike epinephrine, there is less myocardial oxygen demand and less propensity for inducing arrhythmias (233).

Amrinone (or inamrinone) and milrinone are phosphodiesterase inhibitors that provide a positive inotropic effect on cardiac musculature while causing systemic vasodilation. They are used in refractory cardiac failure (234).

Valvular Disease

AS is an independent risk factor for poor operative outcome from cardiac complications following noncardiac surgery. The risk depends on the severity of AS (235). Important considerations in perioperative management are directed at patients with AS and the level of ventricular failure. Patients with severe AS need valve replacement before elective surgery, whereas patients with mild to moderate AS need careful anesthetic control of blood pressure. The presence of ejection systolic murmurs requires assessment of LV function for the presence of CHF with echocardiography (236). Treatment and support will be related to maintenance of ventricular function. Avoidance of systemic hypotension in the perioperative period is essential. The AHA recommends no routine prophylactic antibiotic administration to prevent endocarditis in patients with valvular disease, with artificial valves, or who have had surgical correction of congenital defects undergoing GI or genitourinary (GU) procedures. However, if patients have active GU or GI infections, then the surgery should be delayed, if possible, to allow eradication of the infection with antibiotic treatment. Any antibiotic regimen should include agents that are active against enterococci, such as ampicillin or vancomycin, and should be administered 30 minutes before to 2 hours after the procedure (237,238). Antibiotic prophylaxis may be reasonable for patients with prosthetic cardiac valves if the valves have been placed within the previous 6 months; previous history of infective endocarditis; or certain congenital heart diseases (CHD) such as unrepaired cyanotic CHD, any repaired CHD with prosthetic material within the previous six months, and any repaired CHD with residual defect adjacent to a prosthetic patch or device (which prevents endothelialization) (239).

Arrhythmias

Postoperative arrhythmias are often secondary to noncardiac problems such as iatrogenic fluid overload, hypotension, electrolyte abnormalities, hypoxia, or infection. Whenever an arrhythmia occurs in the postoperative setting, myocardial ischemia must first be ruled out (240). If ECG and cardiac enzyme measurements are normal, the arrhythmia is not likely to be due to myocardial ischemia. Fortunately, most arrhythmias in the postoperative period are transient and self-resolving. Asymptomatic arrhythmias, except in the preoperative period, are generally of little clinical significance. Hypercapnia, hypoxemia, hypokalemia, acidosis, inadequate analgesia, and anemia can all promote cardiac arrhythmias. Supraventricular tachycardia is the most common rhythm disturbance seen in the postoperative period (241). Treatment with calcium channel blockers (such as diltiazem) or a β-blocker is usually the first-line recommended treatment for atrial fibrillation (242).

Pulmonary Issues

Ventilator Management

The ability to provide ventilatory support to the surgical patient has been a tremendous advance in postoperative care. Mechanical ventilators have enabled oncologic surgeons to perform major operations for aggressive control of lesions that were once considered to be unresectable. Although preemptive preoperative therapies attempt to avoid postoperative mechanical ventilation, some patients will require this therapy. Mechanical ventilation must be thought of as providing two functions: ventilation and oxygenation. However, these two functions must be separated and applied independently to each particular situation. A more difficult concept for residents and fellows to understand is that ventilation has nothing to do with oxygenation. Many patients decompensate on the ward despite supplemental oxygen and 100% oxygen saturation because tidal volumes were low and the patient was not ventilating.

When contemplating mechanical ventilation, one must ask two questions: is the patient able to oxygenate her tissues adequately, and can she ventilate adequately to maintain normal partial pressure of carbon dioxide (P_{CO_2}) and acid–base function? Adequate oxygenation can be determined by measurement of oxygen saturation and arterial partial pressure of oxygen (P_{O_2}). Targets are generally an O_2 saturation >92% or P_{O_2} greater than 65 mm Hg. Poor oxygenation may be caused by fluid overload, depressed mental status, underlying pulmonary disease, or shunt. Evaluation of the arterial blood gas will also give a pH and Pco_2 measurement. Patients may hypoventilate for a number of reasons. Postoperative pain may prohibit deep inspiration and the overuse of pain medication may depress the level of consciousness, leading to fewer and poorer respirations. Atelectasis, pneumonia, and poor pulmonary compliance all lead to difficulties in ventilation. Finally, a bronchial mucous plug or a pneumothorax will lead to life-threatening ventilatory compromise. A respiratory rate greater than 35 per minute or a Pco_2 greater than 55 mm Hg are accepted indications for intubation and mechanical ventilation.

When intubating patients, the size of the endotracheal tube must be considered, as this may impact removal and discontinuation of mechanical ventilation later. The larger the tube, the less resistance and the easier it will be for the patient to participate in "weaning" trials for discontinuing ventilatory support (243). Typical recommendations are a 7.5-mm tube for women and an 8.0-mm tube for men.

Traditionally, there are pressure-cycled ventilators and volume-cycled ventilators. Pressure-cycled ventilators are used routinely in neonatal ICU patients because overinflation can be dangerous to neonates. In the adult ICU, most ventilators are volume cycled, meaning that the clinician sets the tidal volume, and regardless of the pressures necessary to give the volume, the volume will be delivered. In patients in whom pulmonary compliance is reduced (i.e., due to a stiff lung or acute respiratory distress syndrome [ARDS]), efforts at controlling pressure are important. When setting the ventilator, a number of decisions must be made. The mode of delivery, tidal volume, and rate will determine ventilation, whereas the fraction of inspired oxygen (Fio_2) and positive end-expiratory pressure (PEEP) will determine oxygenation.

Mode

There are a number of ventilator modes. The first developed was controlled mechanical ventilation, where the tidal volume and rate are set and that is exactly what the patient receives—no more and no less. This mode is very good for patients under general anesthesia or who are paralyzed. However, this mode is very disturbing to the patient who wishes to participate, however slightly, in her own ventilation. This mode has evolved into the current assist/control (AC) mode, whereby the patient is guaranteed the fixed rate and tidal volume but can also trigger breaths in between with a similar tidal volume. In addition, the machine will synchronize the breath when the patient triggers such a breath. This mode provides complete rest for the patient by performing all the work of breathing and is generally used for patients in the immediate postoperative period or for patients who have critical illnesses such as organ failure or sepsis.

Intermittent mandatory ventilation (IMV) is a mode whereby the clinician sets a rate and a tidal volume, which the machine delivers. Any breath initiated by the patient is delivered in relation to the amount of effort the patient puts forth, meaning a strong effort gives the patient a large breath and a meager effort a smaller one. This is sometimes called a weaning mode. The patient is given full support with rate and tidal volume until she is stronger. The rate is slowly turned down, allowing the patient more frequent, spontaneous breaths until extubation. Synchronized IMV (SIMV) ensures that a machine-delivered breath does not stack onto a patient-initiated breath.

Pressure support ventilation (PSV) is a mode where patient-initiated breaths are given support from the ventilator only during the beginning of ventilation (inspiratory phase). The support is meant to help the patient overcome the large amount of resistance present in the valves of the machine, the ventilator circuit, and the endotracheal tube. By titrating PSV to the spontaneous tidal volume produced by the patient, one can fully or partially support patient breathing and overcome the work of breathing. This mode of ventilation is important during the "weaning" process.

Work of Breathing

When conceptualizing the job of the ventilator, the different types of work must be defined (243). In addition to the physiologic work of breathing that all humans do on a daily basis, huge workloads are imposed from the resistance of the ventilator equipment (e.g., breathing through a straw analogy). Finally, there is the pathologic work of breathing from pneumonia, the incision, etc. The intent of mechanical ventilation during disease states is to assume the last two types of "work" so that the patient may convalesce. As a patient improves and the pathologic work has been removed, the patient should be able to resume normal, physiologic work.

More Advanced Modes of Ventilation

With advanced circuitry and computer microprocessors, newer ventilator modes have been developed. Pressure-regulated volume control (PRVC) has largely replaced AC ventilation. PRVC provides the same function as AC while preventing overinflation. Recent data have shown that preventing overinflation (or stretch) of alveoli prevents trauma and decreases the incidence of ARDS (244). PRVC delivers the same tidal volume but changes the flow rate to prevent high pressures by measuring the pressure on a breath-to-breath basis. Volume control ventilation is a mode whereby a tidal volume target is set and the ventilator continually titrates the amount of PSV to provide this volume. This mode has been termed "autowean" or "weekend" mode because as the patient gets stronger, he or she will be able to meet the tidal volume setting. In situations where difficulties in ventilation are encountered, such as ARDS, hypercarbia, and acidosis, pressure control is used. This mode is similar to the neonatal pressure-cycled ventilator where the maximum pressure is set and the flow rate is decreased but the inspiratory time is lengthened to achieve proper ventilation. Airway pressure release ventilation, high-frequency jet ventilation, and inverse ratio ventilation are other advanced modes, the discussion of which is beyond the scope of this chapter.

Setting the Ventilator

Initial ventilator settings require a rate of 12 to 14 breaths per minute, with a tidal volume of 6 to 8 cc/kg. This is a departure from the traditional 12 cc/kg, which has been determined to result in greater alveolar trauma and increased risk for the development of ARDS (245). After initial setting of the ventilator, measurements of pH, Po_2, and Pco_2 from arterial blood gas are used to make further ventilator adjustments.

Oxygenation

Oxygenation is controlled by two settings: Fio_2 and PEEP. The inspired oxygen content can easily be controlled with the ventilator, to keep blood oxygen saturation greater than 92%. Inspired oxygen concentration greater than 60% is considered to be potentially toxic and may be the etiologic reason for pathologic changes similar to ARDS. In patients with normal lung function, studies have shown that higher concentrations of inspired oxygen can cause acute inflammation and fibroproliferative changes, resulting in toxic effects to lung tissue. Similar studies in patients with underlying lung disease are lacking (246,247). If it is necessary to have oxygen concentrations above 60%, the recommendation is to wean these levels as soon as possible. PEEP is another mechanism for improving oxygenation. In normal physiology, the glottis closes before full expiration, creating a PEEP of approximately 4 cm H_2O, and is termed physiologic PEEP. When ventilating patients, the addition of 5 cm H_2O PEEP is used as a baseline and is increased if added oxygen delivery is required. Increasing PEEP is the preferred method for improving oxygenation in postsurgical patients as opposed to increasing the Fio_2. Postsurgical patients have atelectasis and shunting secondary to operative pain and anesthesia. The addition of PEEP recruits collapsed alveoli, improving oxygenation and lung compliance. However, the use of PEEP must be balanced by potential adverse effects, which include decreased cardiac output and the risk for barotrauma.

Weaning from Ventilator

Multiple opinions exist on the techniques of weaning patients from mechanical ventilation. T-piece trials, spontaneous breathing trials, SIMV, and PSV are just a few. The best method of weaning is a pathway agreed upon by clinicians, nurses, and respiratory therapists. Before discontinuing mechanical ventilation, the disease process that required ventilation should have resolved and patients should have proper mental status and the ability to generate a cough. Copious secretions are often an initial reason not to consider weaning or extubation. Criteria for extubation, whether on T-piece or minimal PSV, have traditionally included a respiratory rate less than 35, a P_{CO_2} less than 50 mm Hg, and a negative inspiratory force greater than −20 cm H_2O. Rapid shallow breathing, defined as the respiratory frequency divided by the tidal volume in liters over a minute, is the most accurate predictor of failure in weaning patients from mechanical ventilation (248).

Acute Respiratory Distress Syndrome

ARDS is a condition that has been well recognized and extensively studied (249–251). This disease is a form of refractory hypoxemia that is caused by a variety of insults, which incites an inflammatory response consisting of increased production of cytokines, leukotrienes, endothelial adhesion molecules, and interleukins. These molecules, which are useful in the defense of the host organism, are particularly detrimental to pulmonary endothelium. ARDS is the result of some inciting cause and does not arise *de novo* as a primary problem. A study of patients who develop multiple organ dysfunction syndrome (MODS), a state where sequential organ failure leads to patient death, has shown that the lung may be the first organ system susceptible to these circulating inflammatory mediators (252). In addition to supportive treatment for ARDS, operative injuries or postoperative complications (e.g., intra-abdominal abscess, anastomotic leak) must be sought and ruled out.

In 1994, a consensus of American and European intensivists defined the criteria for ARDS and a lesser form of the disease described as acute lung injury (ALI) (250). Criteria include (a) acute onset after defined insult; (b) bilateral diffuse infiltrates on chest radiograph; (c) no evidence of left atrial hypertension, CHF, or a PAOP $\leq$ 18 mm Hg; and, most importantly, (d) impaired oxygenation. Impaired oxygenation was classified as ALI if the partial pressure of arterial oxygen (Pa_{O_2})/F_{IO_2} ratio was $\geq$300 mm Hg and ARDS if the Pa_{O_2}/F_{IO_2} ratio was $\geq$200 mm Hg. The Berlin definition of ARDS replaced the 1994 definition by removing the term ALI and removing the PAOP criteria (253). Postmortem examination of lungs with ARDS shows atelectasis, edema, inflammation, hyaline membrane deposition, and fibrosis. The mortality of ARDS is 30% to 40%. Treatment of these severely hypoxemic patients consists of mechanical ventilatory support with F_{IO_2} and PEEP. Because of alveolar damage, ventilation/perfusion mismatch occurs, resulting in a worsening shunt fraction and increasing dead space. As ALI/ARDS progresses, ventilation, due to decreased pulmonary compliance, becomes difficult and oxygenation progressively worsens. The end result is a hypercapnic state and respiratory acidosis.

The ARDS NET trial comparing high tidal volume, in order to maintain normocapnia, to low tidal volume, to prevent barotrauma, showed significantly improved survival among patients in the low tidal volume group (250). Current strategies employ tidal volumes of 6 cc/kg, while accepting elevated P_{CO_2} levels (permissive hypercapnia) (254).

Pneumonia

Pneumonia is a significant complication in postsurgical patients. Patients requiring mechanical ventilation are particularly susceptible to pneumonia (ventilator-acquired pneumonia [VAP]), with rates as high as 30% after 72 hours of ventilation. The mortality rate from VAP ranges from 25% to 50%. The pathogens are often gram-negative bacteria and are resistant to multiple antibiotics. High clinical suspicion and aggressive treatment of VAP are crucial. A review of this complicated topic by Chastre and Fagon is recommended for further reading (255).

Pulmonary Embolism and Deep Venous Thrombosis Prophylaxis

The prevention of venous thromboembolism is an important component of perioperative management of the gynecologic oncology patient. The American College of Chest Physicians consensus statement published in 2012 reviews the data extensively and provides recommendations (256). Patients undergoing major gynecologic surgery without venous thromboembolism prophylaxis have a risk of deep vein thrombosis (DVT) between 17% and 40% (257). Surgery for cancer, advanced age, previous VTE, prior pelvic radiation therapy, and abdominal resection (in contrast to vaginal resection) appears to increase the thromboembolic risk after gynecologic surgery (258). The incidence of pulmonary embolism (PE) is 1.6%, with the rate of fatal PE being 0.9%. In trials comparing low-dose unfractionated heparin (LDUH) with no therapy in general surgical patients, the DVT rate decreased from 25% to 8%. These studies also produced a 50% decrease in the rate of fatal PE (259). Comparisons of LMWH versus LDUH have shown equal efficacy. LMWH may have fewer complications (mostly wound hematomas) and greater ease of use with once-daily dosing.

Sequential pneumatic compression devices (PCDs) are attractive for patients at risk for bleeding complications. In trials comparing PCD with LDUH, both have shown efficacy. Elastic stockings T.E.D. hose and aspirin usage are not currently recommended for DVT prophylaxis. Studies have shown that the presence of D-dimer positivity in the face of DVT and/or PE, but the presence of any released blood or hematoma (i.e., in any postoperative patient) makes the D-dimer positivity nonspecific. In the surgical patient, a negative D-dimer makes DVT or PE highly unlikely; however, a positive test is essentially useless.

Patients at low risk (age less than 40 years, no risk factors, and minor surgery) need no prophylaxis, but early ambulation is encouraged. Moderate-risk patients (minor surgery in a patient with risk factors, major surgery with no risk factors) should receive PCD, LMWH, or LDUH, with equal results. High-risk patients require LWMH in addition to PCD.

Recently, the American College of Chest Physicians updated their recommendations for antithrombotic therapy for VTE disease (260). Diagnosis of DVT is performed by duplex ultrasonography, and treatment is with either heparinization to 1.5 times control prothrombin time or therapeutic doses of LMWH. Diagnosis of PE was traditionally made by pulmonary arteriogram. This practice has been abandoned because dynamic contrast-enhanced computerized tomography has better sensitivity. Once diagnosis is confirmed, the patient is anticoagulated with IV heparin or LMWH. Ultimately, since most of these patients have cancer, the updated recommendation is that these patients be treated with LMWH over warfarin (Coumadin) or any of the non–vitamin K oral anticoagulants (dabigatran, rivaroxaban, apixaban, or edoxaban) for at least 3 months in the case of DVT and PE (260). ***Best Practice: All gynecologic oncology patients with a major surgery >30 minutes should receive VTE prophylaxis with either LMWH or heparin, with prophylaxis being started preoperatively and continued intra- and postoperatively in combination PCD. Extended prophylaxis with LMWH heparin should be continued for 28 days after laparotomy in patients with abdominal or pelvic malignancies.***

Fluid and Electrolyte Issues

Understanding fluid and electrolyte physiology in gynecologic oncology is paramount because of the underlying disease processes that face the gynecologic oncologist and the ultimate, radical surgical interventions that are needed to treat them. These treatments result in great fluid shifts perioperatively, requiring careful attention to input of fluids (volume and content/type) as well as output from renal and GI sources, insensible sources, and drains. Since extensive discussions of these topics can be found elsewhere, this section presents a brief review of normal fluid and electrolyte physiology and discusses strategies for fluid resuscitation and correction of electrolyte deficiencies.

Total body water (TBW) can be calculated by a variety of methods and varies directly with the amount of adipose or lean tissue present in an individual patient. TBW estimates, therefore, must be adjusted based on the adiposity of the patients. In women, TBW accounts for approximately 60% of a patient's weight. TBW is distributed into extracellular fluid (ECF) and intracellular fluid (ICF), with the ECF being further divided into intravascular (one-quarter of the ECF) and interstitial (three quarters of the ECF) compartments. The ECF accounts for approximately one-third of the TBW, whereas ICF accounts for two-thirds (261,262). Direct measurement of the ECF and TBW is possible, with the resulting difference being an estimated ICF. **Table 8.13** describes the body fluid compartments and their contributions to body weight. Despite these arbitrary compartments (and electrolyte concentration differences between compartments, which are discussed in the paragraph below), water flows freely across all compartments. Thus, a derangement in one compartment will result in a compensatory change in another (263).

The electrolyte composition of the various compartments is different. Sodium is the predominant cation in the ECF and potassium is the predominant cation of the ICF. **Table 8.14** describes the various concentrations of electrolytes in the various fluid compartments. Because of the Donnan principle of equilibration, the content of cations and anions in the interstitial compartment is slightly higher than that in the intravascular compartment. This principle describes the unique relation between solutions of permeable and impermeable complex anions when these anions are unevenly distributed across a semipermeable membrane. Water, on the other hand, as mentioned earlier, freely equilibrates between the compartments (263).

Effective circulating volume (ECV) is a term used to describe the portion of the ECF that perfuses the organs of the body and affects baroreceptors (see next paragraph). In healthy patients, the ECV equates to the intravascular volume/compartment. But in disease states that increase "third spacing" such as sepsis (leaky capillaries), ascites due to intra-abdominal metastasis, or bowel obstruction with resulting edema and transudation, the interstitial compartment increases at the expense of the intravascular compartment, decreasing the ECV (261).

The osmotic activity of a fluid compartment is affected by the component ions and is described in milliosmoles (mOsm). Normal serum osmolality (in the ECF, of course) averages 290 mOsm/kg of H_2O. Osmoreceptors in the hypothalamus respond to small changes in serum osmolality, increasing or decreasing secretion of ADH and modifying the thirst response. These receptors are responsible for the day-to-day fine-tuning of fluid balance. Baroreceptors, on the other hand, in the intrathoracic vena cava, the atria, the aortic arch, the carotid arteries, and the renal parenchyma, sense volume changes by changes in pressure. These receptors begin a cascade of mediators such as aldosterone, atrial natriuretic peptide (ANP), prostaglandins, and the renin–angiotensin system, which ultimately result in changes of water and sodium balance mediated through the kidneys. These baroreceptors have little to do with the day-to-day fluid management and require intravascular losses of 10% to 20% to initiate activity (263).

The goal of fluid resuscitation is to maintain the ECV and keep or return the patient to euvolemia. Many gynecologic oncology procedures are lengthy and can result in large blood losses requiring immediate intraoperative replacement. In addition, following procedures where evacuation of large amounts of ascites has occurred and/or "peritoneal stripping" has left denuded surfaces, these patients may have large fluid shifts into the interstitial compartment, requiring large volumes of fluid to maintain the ECV. Finally, losses are not water alone and include electrolytes and clotting factors, which may need repletion. Selecting fluids to administer to a given patient is akin to selecting the correct IV medication to give; not *all* fluids are for *all* patients. The physician should understand the amount of daily maintenance fluid and electrolytes required by patients, calculate losses (fluid and electrolytes), determine ongoing fluid and electrolyte losses, and replace them with the appropriate fluid and electrolyte combinations and volumes. It is easy to fall into the trap of giving all patients an 8-hour rate (125 mL/hour) of maintenance fluid. However, an octogenarian, even with normal cardiac and renal function, weighing 50 kg, does not need that much maintenance fluid. "Formulas" for calculating appropriate maintenance fluid requirements exist (263).

With new enhanced recovery protocols in colorectal surgery, restricting fluids intraoperatively and postoperatively has been shown to reduce cardiopulmonary complications (7% vs. 24%; $p < 0.001$) and overall morbidity (OR 0.41; $p = 0.005$) (264,265). It is important to note that these improvements in morbidity were not seen if the fluid restrictions were instituted postoperatively. However, extreme restriction of fluids can lead to increased morbidity and mortality. So a fine line must be walked in an effort to keep the patient normovolemic during the surgical procedure. If, however, the surgical procedure planned will result in large blood loss or the patient has SIRS, advanced hemodynamic monitoring may be helpful in managing fluid resuscitation to maintain euvolemia (net zero

TABLE 8.13. Body Fluid Compartments

Total Body Water	Body Weight (%)	Total Body Water (%)
Total	60	100
Intracellular	40	67
Extracellular	20	33
Intravascular	5	8
Interstitial	15	25

Source: From Wait RB, Kahng KU, Dresner LS. Fluids and electrolytes and acid-base balance. In: Greenfield LJ, Mulholland M, Oldham KT, et al. eds. *Surgery: Scientific Principles and Practice*. 2nd ed. Philadelphia, PA: Lippincott–Raven Publishers; 1997;242–266, with permission.

TABLE 8.14. Electrolyte Concentrations in the Various Fluid Compartments

	Extracellular Fluid		
	Plasma	Interstitial Fluid	Intracellular Fluid
Cations			
Na^+	140	146	12
K^+	4	4	150
Ca^{2+}	5	3	10^{-7}
Mg^{2+}	2	1	7
Anions			
Cl^-	103	114	3
HCO_3^-	24	27	10
SO_4^{2-}	1	1	—
HPO_4^{3-}	2	2	116
Protein	16	5	40
Organic anions	5	5	—

Source: From Wait RB, Kahng KU, Dresner LS. Fluids and electrolytes and acid-base balance. In: Greenfield LJ, Mulholland M, Oldham KT, et al. eds. *Surgery: Scientific Principles and Practice*. 2nd ed. Philadelphia, PA: Lippincott–Raven Publishers; 1997;242–266, with permission.

sum: fluids out = fluids in). Extrapolation to gynecologic oncologic surgery would be expected to have these same results.

In general, the normal maintenance requirement of sodium is 1 to 2 mEq/kg/day and for potassium 0.5 to 1.0 mEq/kg/day. **Table 8.15** lists the various IV fluid preparations available for fluid resuscitation. Which fluid to be used is controversial and driven, in more instances, by "dogma," varying from physician to physician and institution to institution, rather than by evidence. Controversy over which fluid type to use in fluid resuscitation continues to this day. Several meta-analyses have shown no advantage of colloid over crystalloid for resuscitation in surgical patients (266–273). The use of colloid has been shown to be advantageous in conditions of hypoproteinemia, or in malnourished states where patients require plasma volume expansion and cannot tolerate large amounts of fluid (273).

Most of the time patients are given isotonic solutions, such as lactated Ringer's solution, to cover intraoperative losses. Again, the goal is to maintain euvolemia. If necessary, colloid can be used to maintain blood pressure over crystalloid. In general, the need for postoperative IV fluids beyond 12 to 24 hours following the procedure is rare in uncomplicated recovery. In the cases of continued IV fluid administration, a total hourly rate of 1.2 mL/kg (including drugs) should be given. Balanced crystalloid solutions are preferred over 0.9% saline solutions to reduce the risk of hyperchloremic acidosis. ***Best Practice: Very restrictive or liberal fluid regimens should be avoided in favor of euvolemia. In major open surgery and for high-risk patients where there is large blood loss (>7 mL/kg) or a SIRS response, the use of advanced hemodynamic monitoring to facilitate individualized fluid therapy and optimize oxygen delivery through the perioperative period is recommended. Oral intake of fluid should be started on the day of surgery. IV fluids should be terminated within 24 hours after surgery. Balanced crystalloid solutions (e.g., LR) are preferred to 0.9% normal saline.***

Sodium Derangements

Hyponatremia is the most common electrolyte abnormality seen in postoperative patients and is caused by excess free water rather than a depletion of sodium. Increases in free water absorption are mediated by a self-limited, physiologic increase in the secretion of ADH in response to the stress of surgery. Serum sodium levels rarely fall below 130 mEq/L, but may be further exacerbated by IV administration of large volumes of hypotonic solutions (i.e., 0.2%, 0.33%, and 0.45% sodium solutions). Other disease states can result in a hyperosmolar condition, resulting in a hyperosmolar ECF, causing fluid to shift from the ICF and lowering the sodium levels. These conditions include hyperglycemia; mannitol, ethylene glycol, or ethanol ingestion; and uremia. For each increase of 180 mg/dL of glucose above 100 mg/dL, there is a concomitant decrease in the serum sodium of 5 mEq/L (272). In addition, during situations where potassium is low, there is a compensatory exchange of sodium for potassium, resulting in hyponatremia. In either of these prior cases, total body sodium does not change. Finally, patients with hyperproteinemia or hyperlipidemia may have falsely low sodium values, which result from errors in the laboratory measurement of sodium. This *pseudohyponatremia* does not result in any symptoms of hyponatremia (263).

TABLE 8.15. Electrolyte Content of Commonly Used Intravenous Electrolyte Solutions

Solution	Electrolyte Concentration (mEq/L)					
	Na^+	K^+	Ca_2^+	Mg_2^+	Cl^-	HCO_3^-
Lactated Ringer's solution	130	4	4	—	109	28
0.2% NaCl	34	—	—	—	34	—
0.33% NaCl	56	—	—	—	56	—
0.45% NaCl	77	—	—	—	77	—
0.9% NaCl	154	—	—	—	154	—
3.0% NaCl	513	—	—	—	513	—
5.0% NaCl	855	—	—	—	855	—

Source: Adapted from Wait RB, Kahng KU, Dresner LS. Fluids and electrolytes and acid-base balance. In: Greenfield LJ, Mulholland M, Oldham KT, et al. eds. *Surgery: Scientific Principles and Practice.* 2nd ed. Philadelphia, PA: Lippincott-Raven Publishers; 1997;242–266, with permission.

The symptoms of hyponatremia are driven by cellular water intoxication and are related to the central nervous system (CNS) (e.g., lethargy, headaches, confusion, delirium, weakness, muscle cramps). The rate at which hyponatremia occurs also determines the symptoms. Chronic hyponatremia tends to be asymptomatic, whereas acute drops in serum sodium (levels 120 to 130) result in the symptoms listed above. Correction of hyponatremia must be done carefully to avoid central pontine myelinolysis, which results in the "locked-in syndrome."

Because most hyponatremia is related to dehydration (low ECV), simple correction of this state will increase the sodium plasma level. If the patient has a high ECV (such as the syndrome of inappropriate antidiuretic hormone secretion) or is in an edematous state, free water restriction should normalize the sodium level. However, if patients have symptoms of hyponatremia, aggressive replacement of sodium is prudent should the duration of the hyponatremia be determined to be no longer than 48 hours. Hyponatremic states lasting longer than 48 hours increase the risk of central pontine myelinolysis. Chronic cases need replacement at rates not exceeding 0.5 mEq/L/hour. Acute cases may be replaced at rates of 5 mEq/L/hour.

Hypernatremia is an uncommon finding and is related to large volumes of free water loss (through insensible routes such as breathing, sweating, and ventilation), diabetes insipidus, adrenal hyperfunction, or ingestion or administration of increased sodium solutions. Again, the symptoms are predominantly CNS oriented because of brain cell dehydration. Symptoms rarely occur until serum sodium levels exceed 160 mEq/L. In addition, the rapidity at which the derangement occurs determines the symptoms manifested. Treatment is carefully done with replacement of free water. Replacement too rapidly can cause cerebral edema and herniation. Patients with chronic hypernatremia need free water administration, which decreases the serum sodium no faster than 0.7 mEq/L.

Potassium Derangements

Whereas sodium is the major extracellular cation, potassium is the major intracellular cation by a ratio of 30:1. The intracellular potassium concentrations tend to be relatively constant, whereas the extracellular concentrations vary depending upon renal function/excretion. The majority of potassium secretion occurs in the distal tubule and the collecting duct of the nephron. Secretion is stimulated by increased urine flow, increased sodium delivery, high potassium levels, alkalosis, aldosterone, vasopressin, and β-adrenergic agonists. Insulin causes potassium to move into cells (as previously mentioned), reducing the extracellular concentration of potassium. Serum potassium levels are further affected by the acid–base status of patients. In alkalotic states, the potassium shifts into cells in exchange for hydrogen ions, whereas in acidotic states the exchange is opposite.

The predominant reason for hyperkalemia in a postoperative patient is renal dysfunction or failure. When these patients become critically ill, serum potassium concentrations can increase by 0.3 to 0.5 mEq/L/day in noncatabolic patients and 0.7 mEq/L/day in catabolic patients. It is important to rule out a spuriously elevated level secondary to hemolysis at the time of the blood draw either from too small a gauge of needle or simply from the application of the tourniquet and squeezing (263).

Hyperkalemia changes the membrane potential established by differences between the intracellular and extracellular milieu. This increased concentration has deleterious effects on cardiac muscle function, causing peaked T waves, flattened P waves, prolonged QRS complexes, and deep S waves on the ECG, and possibly resulting in ventricular fibrillation and cardiac arrest. Skeletal musculature is also affected with paresthesias and weakness, which can progress to a flaccid paralysis.

Treatment for hyperkalemia has been outlined in the section on renal risk factors. The mainstay is saline diuresis unless ECG changes are present, then infusion of calcium gluconate can be lifesaving. Utilization of 25 to 50 g of glucose and 10 to 20 units of regular insulin can drive potassium intracellularly and transiently lower plasma levels. Ultimately, definitive therapy relies upon increased excretion of potassium. For each gram of sodium polystyrene sulfonate (Kayexalate, given in the doses previously mentioned) used either orally or rectally, 0.5 mEq of potassium will be removed. Finally, in patients not responding to these therapies or patients with renal failure, hemodialysis may be indicated.

Hypokalemia is caused by decreased intake, increased GI losses (vomiting, diarrhea, fistulae), excessive renal losses (metabolic alkalosis, magnesium deficiency, hyperaldosteronism), a shift of potassium into the intracellular space (acute or uncompensated metabolic alkalosis, glucose and insulin administration, catecholamines), or any combination thereof. A reduction of serum potassium by 1 mEq/L represents a total body deficiency of about 100 to 200 mEq. (Remember that total exchangeable potassium is approximately 3,000 mEq, with the majority being intracellular and thus the majority of the loss [263].) Symptoms of hypokalemia cause ECG changes, with flattening of the T waves, depression of S-T segments, prominent U waves, and prolongation of the Q-T interval. Treatment is accomplished by replacement of potassium either orally or IV, depending upon the severity of symptoms and whether or not the patient is able to take oral preparations. IV replacement of potassium can be done at approximately 10 mEq/hour and should not be more concentrated than 40 mEq/L. If less fluid is desired, 20 mEq can be placed in 100 mL, but administration should not exceed 40 mEq/hour (263).

Magnesium Derangements

Most magnesium in the body is confined to the intracellular space and bone. Less than 1% of total body magnesium is in the serum. Of the magnesium in the serum, 60% is ionized, 25% is protein bound, and 15% is complexed with nonprotein anionic species (247). Magnesium is absorbed in the small intestine, directed by levels of vitamin D, and filtered by the kidney for excretion. Approximately 40% of renally excreted magnesium is reabsorbed in the ascending loop of Henle. Loop diuretics, hypermagnesemia, hypercalcemia, acidosis, and phosphate depletion result in increased excretion of magnesium.

Patients with renal failure and receiving magnesium-containing antacids or laxatives can become hypermagnesemic. In addition, patients with acidosis and dehydration may become hypermagnesemic. Patients present with CNS depression, loss of deep tendon reflexes, and ECG changes (prolonged P-R interval and QRS complex) in the face of elevated magnesium levels (greater than 8 mg/dL). As levels rise, patients will develop coma, respiratory failure, and/or cardiac arrest. Acute treatment of hypermagnesemia is slow IV infusion of 5 to 10 mEq of calcium. Because the etiology of this condition is usually renal failure, withholding magnesium-containing preparations may be all that is necessary. In severe instances, hemodialysis is required.

In gynecologic oncology patients, the overwhelming reason for hypomagnesemia is a history of cisplatin administration. However, other conditions such as hypoparathyroidism, malabsorptive states, chronic loop diuretic use, and the diuretic phase of ARF can cause hypomagnesemia. Symptoms are similar to hypocalcemia, with muscle weakness, fasciculations, tetany, hypokalemia, and ECG changes (Q-T prolongation, torsade de pointes). Treatment can be accomplished with oral preparations in less acute situations. However, large doses may produce diarrhea, worsening the situation. IV boluses of 2 to 3 g followed by infusions of 1 to 2 mEq/kg/day can be utilized for patients with severe symptoms.

Calcium Derangements

Almost all the calcium in the body is in bone, stored as hydroxyapatite crystals, and provides a supply that can be exchanged to the serum. Calcium homeostasis is controlled by parathyroid hormone (PTH), controlling intestinal absorption of calcium, renal excretion of calcium, and exchange of calcium from the bone. In the serum, calcium exists in three phases: 45% as an ionized form, which is responsible for most of the physiologic function of calcium; 40% in a protein-bound form, bound mostly to albumin; and 15% in a nonionized form, complexed with nonprotein anions that do not easily dissociate. A serum total calcium level is usually obtained when assessing calcium homeostasis, as measurement of ionized calcium is cumbersome. The total calcium levels change by 0.8 g/dL for each 1 g/dL change of albumin (up or down) (263).

In gynecologic oncology patients with hypercalcemia, the underlying malignancy is usually the etiologic agent. Hypercalcemia may be caused by direct bony involvement or, more commonly, secretion of PTH-like peptides and/or other humoral factors, which increase serum calcium levels. Other reasons for hypercalcemia include primary, secondary, or tertiary hyperparathyroidism, thiazide diuretic use, or lithium usage (263,274). Patients present with muscle fatigue, weakness, confusion, coma, ECG changes (shortening of the Q-T interval), nausea, and vomiting. The goal of treatment is to increase calcium excretion and stop bone turnover in order to decrease serum total calcium. Initial measures include vigorous hydration (200 mL/hour) with 0.9% or 0.45% saline solutions. Furosemide or other loop diuretics may be helpful in patients with borderline cardiac function or in patients with fluid overload. If the underlying malignancy is a breast carcinoma, patients may respond to high doses of steroids to reduce calcium levels. Other pharmacologic agents have been developed to stop bone resorption and reduce serum calcium levels. Calcitonin (4 IU/kg every 12 hours via subcutaneous or intramuscular injection) has a rapid onset of action and works by interfering with osteoclast maturation at several points (274). However, the duration of response is usually about 48 hours because of downregulation of calcitonin receptors by osteoclasts. Bisphosphonates have emerged as the drug of choice for treatment of hypercalcemia in malignancy. These agents work by inhibiting osteoclast activity and survival. The nitrogen-containing bisphosphonates are the most potent. Pamidronate (approved in 1991) and zoledronic acid (approved in 2001) are utilized in the United States. Another agent, ibandronate, is utilized in Europe but has not been approved for use in the United States. Zoledronic acid is the current drug of choice because of its proven superiority over pamidronate (275). The effective dose of zoledronic acid is 4 mg infused over 15 minutes and dosed every 3 to 4 weeks. Serum calcium levels return to normal in approximately 10 days and duration of response lasts approximately 40 days (276). Surgical resection is the treatment of choice for primary, secondary, or tertiary hyperparathyroidism (262,256).

Hypocalcemia is caused by hypoparathyroidism, hypomagnesemia, pancreatitis, and malnutrition. Patients present with tetany, hyperactive deep tendon reflexes, a positive Chvostek sign, positive Trousseau sign, and ECG changes (prolonged Q-T interval, prolonged S-T segment). Low levels of calcium may be present because of low albumin levels, but these levels do not affect the ionized portion of calcium and usually do not cause symptoms. Symptomatic hypocalcemia can be treated with IV infusion of either calcium gluconate or calcium chloride at a rate not exceeding 50 mg/min. Calcium chloride dissociates into the ionized form of calcium more readily and is the treatment of choice to raise serum ionized calcium level.

Acid–Base Disturbances

Optimum cellular function requires a very narrow range of pH for chemical reactions to occur normally. Several buffering systems exist within the body to maintain this optimum pH. The predominant buffering system is the carbonic acid–bicarbonate buffering system. Derangements in the concentration of bicarbonate (HCO_3^-) or in concentrations of carbon dioxide (CO_2) result in acid–base disorders.

Because the kidneys control excretion/generation of bicarbonate and the lungs exchange CO_2, these organs play a central role in the compensation of any acid–base disorder. Therefore, four situations arise in acid–base balance: metabolic acidosis and alkalosis, and respiratory acidosis and alkalosis. Compensatory mechanisms exist in each situation in order to blunt the effect on pH (**Table 8.16**).

Metabolic Acidosis

Most clinically significant metabolic acidosis occurs with a net loss of bicarbonate either due to direct loss or when consumption is greater than generation. Situations where extra renal losses of bicarbonate occur include diarrhea, GI fistulae, and urinary diversions (ureterosigmoidostomy or ureteroileostomy, which result in reabsorption of NH_4Cl from urine). Certain disease states result in the production of organic acids (ketoacidosis and lactic acidosis), which consume bicarbonate and outpace the renal compensatory mechanisms. Similarly, overdoses of certain drugs (e.g., aspirin) or ingestion of toxins (e.g., ethylene glycol, methanol) consume bicarbonate and outpace the renal compensatory mechanisms. Renal acidosis occurs when the intrinsic acid-excreting function of the kidney malfunctions, resulting in retention of acid and consumption of bicarbonate without concomitant regeneration of bicarbonate. These are classified as renal tubular acidosis (RTA I, distal tubule dysfunction; or RTA II, proximal tubule dysfunction). Cardiac effects are the major findings in metabolic acidosis (peripheral arteriolar dilation, decreased cardiac contractility, and central venous constriction). Other manifestations of metabolic acidosis include gastric distension, abdominal pain, nausea, and vomiting. In surgical patients, lactic acidosis is the primary cause of metabolic acidosis and results from tissue hypoperfusion. Therefore, treatment should be aimed at increasing tissue perfusion with fluid and blood administration. The use of bicarbonate is best reserved for patients with other, not easily reversible causes of metabolic acidosis. Older patients and patients with CVD may benefit from administration of bicarbonate. Administration should be instituted when the pH is 7.1 to 7.2. One or two ampules of bicarbonate (approximately 55 mEq/amp) can be administered IV, with further administrations being dictated by the pH obtained from an arterial blood gas measurement. In diabetic ketoacidosis, treatment with insulin and glucose infusion should not only reverse the acidosis but also treat the hyperglycemia.

Metabolic Alkalosis

Sustained metabolic alkalosis is an uncommon clinical entity and is related to renal dysfunction. Loss of HCl is the most common reason for an increase in extracellular bicarbonate. This situation occurs with prolonged nausea and vomiting or prolonged nasogastric suctioning of gastric contents. As acid is removed from the GI tract, a net gain of bicarbonate occurs. Other situations that can result in metabolic alkalosis include volume contraction, exogenous administration of bicarbonate or bicarbonate precursors (citrate, lactate, or calcium carbonate), hypokalemia, hypercalcemia, hypochloremia, excess mineralocorticoid usage, and high P_{CO_2}. Patients rarely present with symptoms, as metabolic alkalosis occurs gradually. However, in patients who develop this situation acutely, most symptoms are CNS oriented (e.g., confusion, stupor, coma, muscle fasiculations, tetany). Correction of the underlying disease state usually corrects the metabolic alkalosis. Repletion of electrolyte abnormalities and infusion of appropriate fluids (chloride-containing) restore volume and result in normal renal excretion of excess bicarbonate.

■ TABLE 8.16. Concentrations of HCO_3^- and P_{CO_2} in Primary Acid–Base Derangements and the Compensatory Response

	Primary		Compensatory Response		
Disorder	**pH**	**HCO_3^-**	**P_{CO_2}**	**HCO_3^-**	**P_{CO_2}**
Metabolic acidosis	↓	↓			↓
Metabolic alkalosis	→	→			→
Respiratory acidosis	↓		→	→	
Respiratory alkalosis	→		↓	↓	

Source: Adapted from Wait RB, Kahng KU, Dresner LS. Fluids and electrolytes and acid-base balance. In: Greenfield LJ, Mulholland M, Oldham KT, et al. eds. Surgery: Scientific Principles and Practice. 2nd ed. Philadelphia, PA: Lippincott–Raven Publishers; 1997;242–266, with permission.

Respiratory Acidosis

A depression of the pH occurs when there is hypoventilation. This occurs secondary to airway obstruction, COPD, depression of the respiratory center, impaired excursion of the thorax, or inappropriate ventilatory management in the mechanically ventilated patient. Development of symptoms depends upon the chronicity or acute nature of the event. If chronic, most patients have no symptoms. If it is an acute change, drowsiness, restlessness, headache, or development of a flapping tremor may occur. Treatment of this condition is aimed at the underlying cause of the hypoventilation. In chronic conditions, the hypoxemia, and subsequent hypercapnia, resulting from the hypoventilation, may be the sole drive for the patient's respirations. Correction of the hypoxemia may further worsen the respiratory acidosis and must be considered. In general, correction of the P_{CO_2} must be done slowly because reequilibration of cerebral bicarbonate concentration lags behind systemic changes (263).

Respiratory Alkalosis

Respiratory alkalosis occurs when the P_{CO_2} decreases with hyperventilation. Hyperventilation may occur because of hypoxia, drugs, decreased lung compliance, and mechanical ventilation. With drops in the arterial P_{O_2}, the peripheral chemoreceptors (in the carotid and aortic body) sense this change and result in hyperventilation to increase arterial P_{O_2}, with a resulting decrease in P_{CO_2}. Because of renal compensatory mechanisms, this condition is usually asymptomatic. However, in acute situations, patients may have a sensation of breathlessness, dizziness, nervousness with altered levels of consciousness, and tetany. Treatment of underlying hypoxia should address the hyperventilation. If acute symptoms are present, having the patient rebreathe expired air should temporarily relieve the symptoms.

Postoperative Nutritional Issues

As mentioned earlier, the full consideration of nutrition in the gynecologic oncology patient is presented in Chapter 31. In this section, we will discuss early refeeding in the postoperative gynecologic oncology patient, indications for EN, and TPN.

Although malnutrition has been shown to be prevalent among gynecologic oncology patients (134,135), many patients are adequately nourished, undergo surgery uneventfully, and have return of bowel function in 1 to 5 days while simultaneously resuming oral intake. Recently, several prospective randomized trials have been conducted that demonstrate the utility of early refeeding in the postoperative period. In these studies, patients in the early feeding group were fed on the first postoperative day, with 90% or more tolerating diets. The underlying malignancies, types of operations, and complications occurred at similar rates between the early refeeding and the "traditionally fed" patients in all the studies. The placement of NGTs for intolerance of diet was low among the studies (less than 10% incidence). Finally, length of hospital stay was shorter among the earlier fed patients (277–282). It is important to note that early feeding is associated with a higher rate of nausea, but not vomiting, abdominal distension or NGT use. ***Best Practice: A regular diet within the first 24 hours after gynecologic/oncologic surgery is recommended.***

The use of the enteral route is preferred in sustaining or repleting patients in the postoperative period after extensive procedures. EN utilizes normal physiologic absorptive mechanisms, maintains gut epithelial integrity, and reduces infectious morbidity (283,284). Studies on nutrition have found that the splanchnic circulation and support of the mucosal integrity of the small bowel may prevent progression to MODS. Specifically, the intestinal mucosa will atrophy secondary to lack of luminal nutrients and intermittent activation of the destructive cytokine pathways, and/or intermittent translocation of bacteria into the bloodstream will occur. These events result in "priming" neutrophils, which ultimately leads to a full-blown systemic inflammatory response, causing organ damage. A number of well-designed randomized trials have compared early enteral feeds to TPN in patients with pancreatitis, major elective surgery, and trauma (283,284). All of these studies have shown a clear benefit for early enteral feeding, with a decrease in infectious complications (284).

Although considered a nonessential amino acid in nourished, healthy patients, glutamine has emerged as an essential amino acid in patients who are stressed and critically ill. This amino acid has been shown to be an important component in maintaining enterocyte integrity and has now been added to most enteral preparations (283,284).

Enteral feeds may be given in a variety of fashions, and each is associated with its own type and number of complications. Intragastric feeds may be accomplished with NGTs, orogastric tubes, or percutaneous endoscopic gastrostomy tubes. Intragastric feeding has the advantage of utilizing the stomach as a reservoir for bolus feeding. In addition, stretching of the stomach stimulates the biliary-pancreatic axis, which may be trophic to the small bowel. Finally, the gastric secretions mix with the feeding material and decrease the osmolarity, thus reducing the incidence of diarrhea. The main disadvantage of this route of enteral feeding is the increased risk of gastric overdistension with high residual amounts of feeding material and the increased risk of aspiration pneumonia (283). Enteral feeds may also be accomplished through the placement of nasal tubes, which are positioned into the pylorus, duodenum, or jejunum (such as Dobhoff tubes). These tubes have the advantage of being placed (or migrating) more distal in the upper GI tract, greatly reducing the risk of aspiration. These types of tubes are preferred in patients who require long-term ventilation. Because of advances in endoscopic instrumentation, many of the tubes can be placed via this method. At the time of laparotomy, gastrostomy, or jejunostomy, tubes (such as a Stamm or Witzel tube) may be placed. These have the advantage of being placed at the time of major abdominal surgery under direct visualization/palpation. The techniques are described in other texts (283,285). Several enteral feeding preparations are available, but vary from hospital to hospital depending upon formulary makeup. The use of the enteral route is contraindicated in patients with mechanical intestinal obstructions, and for these patients nutritional support can be accomplished through the parenteral route.

TPN took the forefront in nutritional sustenance and replacement in the 1980s. The basic premise of TPN is to provide dietary precursors to maintain anabolic function. TPN can be broken into three components of replacement: glucose and lipid preparations for normal or increased energy expenditures, and amino acid preparations for protein synthesis. Because of the higher osmolar load presented by these preparations, central venous access is necessary for administration. Subclavian, internal jugular, or peripherally inserted central catheters will need to be placed, and they present the first of several potential complications associated with TPN administration. At the time of placement, pneumothorax, intubation of arterial structures, air embolism, or cardiac arrhythmias may occur. Later complications include the possibility of infection at the skin entrance site or line sepsis. Should these infectious complications occur, removal of the catheter and antibiotic administration will be necessary (284).

The Harris-Benedict equation is utilized to calculate basal energy expenditure (BEE) for patients and approximates the BEE of a sedentary, fasting, nonstressed individual (286):

$$\text{BEE} = 666 + (9.6 \times \text{weight [kg]}) + (1.7 \times \text{height [cm]}) - (4.7 \times \text{age [yr]})$$

Because stress of disease and surgical intervention need to be considered, "stress factors" have been developed and are multiplied by the BEE to arrive at kilocalories per day. Stress level multipliers are 1.2 for a resting individual, 1.3 for an ambulatory individual or moderate stress (e.g., systemic inflammatory response syndrome [SIRS], sepsis), and 1.5 for severe stress/burn patients.

After calculation of caloric requirements, the composition of the TPN solution to be administered should be determined. Because there are many different types of TPN preparations available, consultation with the nutrition team or pharmacists in an individual hospital is necessary to arrive at the desired solution.

In aerobic situations, glucose is the primary substrate for energy expenditure. It provides 3.4 kcal/g and is usually given in a concentrated form in order to provide 70% of the calculated calories. The remaining 30% of calories is provided by lipid preparations. Not only does this component have denser caloric content (it provides 9 kcal/g), but administration precludes the development of a fatty acid deficiency. Adjustment of the composition of TPN may be necessary depending upon the disease state (e.g., more contribution of kilocalories from fat vs. carbohydrate in a ventilated patient because of the respiratory quotient of fat vs. glucose).

Protein requirements are provided by amino acid solutions and are determined by the patient's age, sex, nutritional status, ongoing stress, and comorbid conditions. In general, 25% of protein requirements are obtained by normal oral intake. The remaining protein comes from breakdown of serum and organic proteins. Thus, periods of prolonged malnutrition, with decreased protein intake, and increased stress of disease will lead to breakdown of visceral protein. An estimate of maintenance protein requirements is 1 g nitrogen per kilogram of body weight. In situations of increased stress, the patient may need 1.2 to 1.5 g/kg in order to maintain and/or replace protein losses. **Table 8.17** shows serum protein measurements and their respective half-lives, which are useful for determining anabolic versus catabolic response to TPN

TABLE 8.17. Visceral Proteins Utilized as Indicators for Nutritional Status during Nutritional Repletion

Protein	Normal Range	Half-Life (days)	Levels Low In	Levels High In
Albumin	3.5–5.4 g/dL	18	Liver disease, pregnancy, overhydration, nephrotic syndrome	Dehydration
Transferrin	200–400 mg/dL	8	Chronic infection, chronic inflammation, liver disease, iron overload, nephrotic syndrome	Iron deficiency, pregnancy
Prealbumin	20–40 mg/dL	2	Liver disease, inflammation, surgery, nephrotic syndrome	
Retinol-binding protein (RBP)	3–6 mg/dL	0.5	Liver disease, hyperthyroidism, zinc deficiency, nephrotic syndrome	Renal insufficiency

treatment. Another method to assess nitrogen balance (positive or negative) is (283):

Nitrogen balance = protein intake / 6.25 – (urinary urea nitrogen + 4)

The amount of protein intake is divided by 6.25 to give the grams of nitrogen taken in. The urinary urea nitrogen is expressed in grams based upon a 24-hour collection. The correction factor of 4 is meant to adjust for the grams of nitrogen lost in the stool or nonurea nitrogen losses.

In addition to these three main components of TPN, daily requirements of vitamins, trace elements, and insulin are necessary to maintain/regain nourishment. Again, these preparations vary by hospital formulary and need consultation with resident pharmacists.

The rate of infusion of TPN needs to be titrated upward to take into account the large glucose load that the patient will be receiving. This lower rate allows the pancreas time to increase insulin secretion in order to meet the glucose load being presented. Similarly, the rate of infusion needs to be decreased when TPN is being stopped to prevent hypoglycemia. During TPN administration, blood glucose measurements by finger stick are required so that hyperglycemia is avoided. For the first several days, measurement of serum electrolytes, with adjustments being made daily, is necessary.

As previously mentioned, complications from venous access are some of the drawbacks of TPN administration. Other complications include metabolic derangements, which most often are mild but need correcting as soon as they are identified, abnormalities of liver function tests, the clinical significance of which is unclear (285), and cholelithiasis/cholecystitis secondary to gallbladder sludge.

Renal Issues

AKI is an abrupt decrease in kidney function that includes, but is not limited to, ARF. A number of etiologies for AKI have been described and include prerenal azotemia, acute tubular necrosis (ATN), acute postrenal obstructive nephropathy, and others (287). The incidence of AKI among hospitalized patients has been estimated to be 5% to 7.5%, with 30% to 40% of these cases occurring during the perioperative period (288). The prevalence of AKI among gynecologic surgeries is associated with the primary indication for the surgery, with malignant procedures being the highest (benign procedures 5% and malignant procedures 18%) (289). Epidemiologic evidence supports that even mild, reversible AKI has important clinical consequences, including increased risk of death (290,291). In their retrospective, observational study, Vaught et al. demonstrated that women with AKI after gynecologic surgery had a nine times higher adjusted OR of major adverse events compared with women without AKI (OR 8.95; 95% confidence interval 5.27 to 15.22). Further, they showed that the OR increased as the severity (Risk, Injury, Failure, Loss, and End-stage kidney disease [RIFLE] stage) of AKI increased (289).

There are three definitions of AKI that have evolved since 2004 and assess renal dysfunction by two parameters: changes in the serum creatinine level of estimated GFR (eGFR) from a baseline value and urine output per kilogram of body weight over a specific time period (292). In 2004, a consensus group, the Acute Dialysis Quality Initiative (ADQI), developed the RIFLE system (293). The next iteration at defining AKI was a modification of the RIFLE staging system by the Acute Kidney Injury Network (AKIN) in 2007. This modification added an absolute change in serum creatinine, eGFR criteria, and the inclusion of a time constraint of the rise in creatinine (294). Finally, in 2012, the Kidney Disease: Improving Global Outcomes (KDIGO) further revised the RIFLE and AKIN staging systems for a unified definition of AKI (**Table 8.18**) (295).

When AKI presents in the postoperative patient, causes can be divided into three parts: prerenal, renal, or postrenal (inflow, parenchymal, and outflow). The function of glomeruli to create the urinary filtrate depends upon adequate renal perfusion and represents the prerenal component. If the renal mean arterial pressure (MAP) falls below 80 mm Hg, perfusion of the glomeruli decreases (some disease states require the renal MAP to be higher for adequate perfusion). Many situations can decrease renal MAP and include anesthetics, atherosclerotic emboli, decreased vascular resistance, hypotension, intravascular volume contraction, mechanical ventilation, sepsis, and any form of shock. Autoregulation of the glomeruli can be disrupted by nonsteroidal anti-inflammatory drugs (NSAIDs), angiotensin-converting enzyme inhibitors, calcium channel blockers (diltiazem or verapamil), and endotoxins produced by gram-negative sepsis.

TABLE 8.18. Classification of Acute Kidney Injury according to KDIGO

Stage	Serum Creatinine	Urine Output
I	1.5–1.9 times baseline OR ≥0.3 mg/dL increase	<0.5 mL/kg/h for 6–12 hours
II	2.0–2.9 times baseline	<0.5 mL/kg/h for ≥12 hours
III	3.0 times baseline OR Increase in serum creatinine to ≥4.0 mg/dL OR Initiation of renal replacement therapy OR In patients < 18 years, decrease of eGFR to <35 mL/min per 1.73 m^2	<0.3 mL/kg/h for ≥24 hours OR Anuria for ≥12 hours

eGFR, estimated glomerular filtration rate

Source: Kellum JA and Lameire N. Diagnosis, evaluation and management of acute kidney injury: a KDIGO summary (part 1). *Crit Care.* 2013;17:204.

Renal parenchymal damage occurs most commonly in the postoperative patient because of prolonged hypotension or direct injury from inflammatory responses initiated by sepsis. In general, if the hypoperfusion is corrected quickly, reversible azotemia, creatinine elevation, and decreased urine output may be the only manifestations. However, prolonged hypoperfusion can cause ATN, which results in sloughing of renal tubular cells into the tubular lumen and obstruction. In addition, the production of Tamm-Horsfall proteins forms coarse granular casts, inciting an intense inflammatory response, further injuring the renal parenchyma (296,297). Other agents that can induce ATN include aminoglycoside antibiotics and iodinated contrast media. Approximately 15% of patients who receive aminoglycosides will have nephrotoxicity, and serum levels of these antibiotics need to be carefully monitored (298). Iodinated contrast media, used in multiple radiographic procedures, induces ATN by impairing nitric oxide production and increasing free radical formation (299,300). Diabetic patients with creatinine clearance rates less than 50 mL/min are at particularly high risk (301).

The final reason for ARF in the postoperative gynecologic oncology patient is outflow obstruction. Because of the radical pelvic procedures performed by gynecologic oncologists, ureteral injury is possible and needs to be excluded early in the evaluation of patients with AKI. Prompt reversal of the obstruction can further limit renal damage.

In general, expected postoperative urinary output should be maintained at 0.5 mL/kg of weight per hour. Most oliguria can be treated with careful intravascular expansion in the first 24 to 48 hours postsurgery. Hypoperfusion of the renal parenchyma must be avoided to prevent ATN from occurring. Once diagnosed, calculating the fractional excretion of sodium (FENa) or chloride can help to discern between prerenal causes or renal causes (hypoperfusions vs. ATN). The formula is presented below (302):

FENa = (urine Na level × serum Cr level) / (serum Na level × urine Cr level) × 100%

If the FENa is less than 1% and the urine specific gravity is greater than 1.025, the diagnosis is hypoperfusion. However, if ischemia has occurred, the FENa will be greater than 4% and the urine specific gravity will fall to 1.010 because of tubular damage and loss of renal concentrating mechanisms. One cannot calculate FENa in patients who have received diuretics or hyperosmotic agents (e.g., mannitol or contrast media). If prerenal and renal causes of low urine output have been excluded, ultrasonography may be useful in evaluating for outflow obstruction.

Once the underlying causes for AKI have been eliminated (e.g., hypoperfusion, obstruction, sepsis), only time can be offered as treatment. Therapies such as low-dose dopamine, furosemide, or mannitol administration, or ANP use have not demonstrated prevention of or improved recovery from AKI (303–308), and recent guidelines recommend avoidance of such treatments (287). Dialysis remains the only intervention that can support patients until return of renal function. Indications for dialysis include (a) hyperkalemia, metabolic acidosis, or volume expansion that cannot be controlled; (b) symptoms of uremia or encephalopathy; or (c) platelet dysfunction inducing a bleeding diathesis (302).

Shock

Definition

Shock is defined in its simplest terms as a decrease in tissue perfusion below the lowest metabolic needs of the tissue bed. This usually results in a depletion of stored energy and an increase in anaerobic metabolism with buildup of lactic acid and other toxic waste products. Hypotension is incorrectly thought of as a defining component of shock. Hypotension often leads to hypoperfusion, but the hypotensive patient is not in shock until evidence of hypoperfusion occurs. Various types of shock exist.

Hemorrhagic Shock

The first thought for a surgeon managing a postoperative patient who manifests signs and symptoms of shock is hemorrhage. Hypovolemic shock secondary to inadequate preload can be the result of excessive or ongoing blood loss or inadequate replacement or both. Certainly, after radical debulking procedures or major extirpative procedures, the potential for postoperative hemorrhage exists. Tachycardia, hypotension, and oliguria are typical clinical signs. In the face of these clinical signs, the surgeon should have high suspicion for active bleeding and be prepared to return the patient to the operating room for correction. Measurement of hemoglobin or hematocrit can be normal in the setting of acute blood loss since a decrease in red cells is accompanied by a decrease in mass. Once fluid is given for resuscitation, dilution will occur and the hemoglobin/hematocrit will fall. With invasive monitoring, the CVP will be low, as will cardiac output and the PAOP. As the stroke volume decreases to inadequate levels, the heart compensates by increasing the heart rate in order to maintain cardiac output. The treatment in these cases is aggressive volume resuscitation and control of ongoing blood loss. The controversy between resuscitation with colloid (albumin, plasma) and crystalloid (normal saline or lactated Ringer's solution) remains ongoing. The SAFE study is a large, randomized controlled double blind study that compared albumin with saline infusion in the ICU. It failed to demonstrate a beneficial effect (309).

Endpoints of resuscitation include normalization of serum lactic acid and base deficit. Measurement of the base deficit via an arterial blood gas analysis has become an effective means for following response to resuscitation. Following large operations where patients are admitted to the ICU and where large fluid shifts occur, the base deficit should be monitored serially until it has returned to normal. If a patient has a worsening base deficit (i.e., becomes more negative), then a search for other problems, such as ongoing hemorrhage, subacute anastomotic leak(s), or tissue ischemia, must be made and be addressed before the base deficit will normalize. The base deficit should normalize within the first 24 hours after surgery.

In the case of continued or rapid bleeding, the obvious course of treatment is reoperation. A number of options are now available intraoperatively in these situations. Obvious bleeding is controlled and ligated. Raw surfaces can be coagulated, treated with fibrin sealants or absorbable hemostatic powders. Damage control packing has been shown to increase survival in the direst situations. Massive transfusion, defined as greater than 1.5 blood volumes, presents a number of additional problems. These patients will have a dilutional coagulopathy, hypocalcemia, and hyperkalemia. After six to eight RBC transfusions have been given in rapid fashion for massive bleeding, some would advocate empiric fresh frozen plasma and platelets. Platelet transfusion is indicated for a platelet count <50,000 in the actively bleeding patient. The trauma literature supports the use of high product ratio during massive transfusion to improve mortality; however, this has yet to be demonstrated in the general surgical population (310). Attention to delivery of warm transfusions is critical as hypothermia and acidosis will promote coagulopathy and worsen bleeding. Once any of the "lethal triad" (hypothermia, acidosis, and coagulopathy) is manifested, then the operation needs to be quickly terminated even if this means damage control packing and transporting back to the ICU setting.

Cardiogenic Shock

A patient with adequate preload who shows signs of poor perfusion secondary to poor cardiac output is categorized as being in cardiogenic shock. The etiology may be a decrease in contractility (secondary to MI) or an increase in afterload (severe hypertension). Typically, "pump failure" results in decreased stroke volume and backup of fluid into the pulmonary circulation. This leads to pulmonary edema and decreased oxygen delivery. The most common provocation for pump failure is the overadministration of fluid in a patient with compromised ventricular function. Treatment consists of diuresis and optimization of cardiac output without increasing myocardial oxygen demand (a difficult task). In the case where significant failure has led to hypotension, dopamine and dobutamine are usually the drugs of choice. The usage of these drugs was discussed previously. Digoxin is commonly used for increasing contractility, but its effects are minor in the acute setting. In addition to inotropic support, correction of electrolyte disturbances (particularly potassium, calcium, and magnesium), maintenance of proper systemic oxygen saturation, and analgesia are important factors in decreasing myocardial stress.

Septic Shock

Septic shock has commonly been defined as hypotension related to infection, with eventual organ failure secondary to hypoperfusion despite adequate fluid resuscitation. This definition has changed with that of SIRS and is discussed in the section on "Sepsis and Systemic Inflammatory Response Syndrome." Sepsis is defined as a subset of patients with SIRS who have a documented infectious process. Resuscitation should be guided according to the recommendations in the Surviving Sepsis Campaign (311).

Infectious Disease Issues

Nosocomial Infections

Infections in the critically ill patient population are a significant cause of morbidity and mortality. Patients in the ICU are particularly vulnerable to infection because of decreased host defenses and the high incidence of resistant bacterial isolates found in ICU settings. In addition, the presence of indwelling catheters and IV lines lowers the inoculum needed to cause infection and provides portals of entry (312). Nosocomial infections are commonly associated with complications of medical or surgical therapy. Approximately 45% of ICU patients will have an infection and approximately half of those will have acquired the infection while in the ICU (312). Treatment includes identifying and eradicating the source of infection and promptly initiating empirical antibiotic therapy aimed at multidrug-resistant gram-negative and gram-positive organisms. If an intra-abdominal or pelvic source is suspected, empiric antibiotic therapy should include anaerobic coverage. Appropriate antibiotic classes include carbapenems, extended-spectrum penicillins, fluoroquinolone-metronidazole, aminoglycoside-metronidazole, or clindamycin combinations (313). In Chapter 28, the management of infections in the gynecologic cancer patient is discussed; therefore, information here is limited to infections pertaining to the critically ill patient.

Fungal Infections

Systemic fungal infections are of great concern for severely ill patients and are linked to an increased risk of morbidity and mortality. Diagnosis of a systemic candidal infection is not based on a unique presentation and therefore can be difficult to definitively pronounce at onset. Although a positive blood culture is the gold standard for diagnosis, blood culture techniques are relatively insensitive and clinicians frequently must rely on clinical judgment about the probability that candidemia is responsible for a patient's symptoms. Patients who have persistent fever, hypothermia, or unexplained hypotension, despite broad-spectrum antibiotic coverage, may have candidemia. Risk factors that have been associated with candidemia and invasive candidiasis include treatment with multiple antibiotics for extended periods, the presence of central venous catheters, the use of TPN, abdominal surgery, prolonged ICU stay, and compromised immune status (314). The initial choice of therapeutic agents depends on the epidemiologic characteristics of the particular ICU and host factors such as the severity of illness, infection site(s), neutropenia, and organ dysfunction. Fluconazole has excellent activity against *Candida albicans*, but infections caused by *Candida glabrata* or *Candida krusei* must be treated with amphotericin B or caspofungin. Amphotericin B should not be used in patients with renal failure, and azoles and echinocandins (caspofungin) should be used with caution in patients with hepatic dysfunction. Antifungal therapy should be continued for 14 days past the first negative blood culture for candidemia or until clinical microbiologic or radiographic resolution of the infection (315). In addition to antifungal therapy, it is generally recommended that all patients with candidemia have a dilated eye exam by an ophthalmologist and that all catheters be removed if possible (although tunneled catheters are at less risk) (314).

Abdominal Infections

The diagnosis of an intra-abdominal source of infection can be challenging in critically ill patients. Not all patients exhibit the same classic symptoms, as they may be masked by other disease processes or medical interventions. For example, abdominal pain and peritoneal signs may not be apparent in patients who are obtunded or sedated and ventilated. Fever and leukocytosis may be absent in 35% and 55% of patients with peritoneal infections (316). Ultrasonography is a useful diagnostic test that can be performed in the ICU and may assist with therapeutic intervention as well. It is extremely sensitive for evaluations of the pelvis and right upper quadrant, but evaluation of the entire abdomen can be limited by bowel gas, surgical dressings, and operator experience. For many of these reasons, a computed tomographic (CT) scan is the preferred study for the evaluation of patients with suspected intra-abdominal infection. To avoid misdiagnosing fluid-filled bowel as a possible abnormal fluid collection, it is essential that contrast agents be used when performing these studies. CT also has limitations, especially when used in the critically ill population. The presence of renal insufficiency precludes the use of IV contrast, and ileus or bowel obstruction may prevent complete opacification of the GI tract. Diagnostic laparoscopy can be performed in the ICU with minimal anesthesia and is a safe, accurate, and cost-effective alternative to laparotomy when managing suspected intra-abdominal processes (317).

Once identified, an intra-abdominal abscess must be fully evacuated and the source controlled. Radiologically assisted percutaneous drainage has become the preferred method for treating most abscesses located in the abdomen and pelvis. For well-delineated unilocular fluid collections, percutaneous drainage has a success rate better than 80% (318). Percutaneous drainage of complex abscesses or those with an enteric communication has a lower success rate, but remains a reasonable alternative treatment for the high-risk patient (319).

In some cases, surgery may be the only appropriate lifesaving intervention. Timely laparotomy in the critically ill patient with diffuse peritonitis allows for peritoneal toilet, debridement of infected and necrotic tissue, and control or repair of the source. Laparoscopic drainage of complex intra-abdominal abscess has also been reported with good success rates (320). Complex intra-abdominal infections that cannot be effectively controlled by a single laparotomy may be managed best with an open abdomen approach with temporary wound closure utilizing a composite, negative pressure (vacuum-pack) dressing (321). Potential advantages of the open abdomen approach include facilitation of repeated debridement, effective drainage, repeat exploration of the peritoneal cavity (at the ICU bedside if necessary), and reduction in intra-abdominal pressure (IAP). In general, the intervention that accomplishes the source control objective with the least physiologic upset should be employed (322).

Sepsis and SIRS

Inflammation is the body's initial response to tissue injury produced by chemical, mechanical, or microbial stimuli. Inflammation is an exceedingly complex cellular and humoral response involving interaction between the complement, kinin, coagulation, and fibrolytic cascades. The goal of inflammation is to enhance the movement of nutrients and phagocytic cells to the injury site in order to prevent invasion of microbes and limit the extension of injury. As a local response, this is beneficial, but appropriate regulation is necessary to prevent a pathologic, exaggerated systemic response, which is clinically identified as SIRS. Sepsis is the clinical syndrome of SIRS that is due to severe infection. The mediator response in SIRS can be divided into four phases based on the cytokine/cellular response: induction, triggering of cytokine synthesis, evolution of cytokine and coagulation cascade, and elaboration of secondary mediators leading to cellular injury. The three most important mediators operating in SIRS appear to be tumor necrosis factor-α, interleukin-1 (IL-1), and IL-6. The microcirculation endothelium is the key target for injury in the sepsis syndrome (323).

In 1992, the American College of Chest Physicians and the Society of Critical Care Medicine published definitions for SIRS and sepsis (**Table 8.19**), with the goal of standardizing terminology to aid clinicians in the diagnosis and treatment and to aid in the interpretation of research in this field (324). Many have criticized the 1992 consensus definitions as too nonspecific to be of use. In 2001, a group of experts reconvened and expanded the list of signs and symptoms of sepsis to reflect clinical bedside experience. In addition to the original criteria, altered mental status, oliguria, skin mottling, coagulopathy, hypoxemia, hyperglycemia in the absence of diabetes, thrombocytopenia, and altered liver function tests can also be used to establish the diagnosis of sepsis (324).

The host response, more than the pathogen, is the primary determinant of patient outcome. Failure to develop a fever, leukopenia, and hypothermia are associated with increased fatality rates in patients with sepsis and are thought to represent abnormalities in the host's inflammatory response. Other risk factors for mortality from sepsis include age greater than 40, underlying medical conditions, malnutrition, immune suppression, and cancer. The presence or absence of a positive blood culture does not influence outcomes; however, sepsis due to a nosocomial infection has a higher mortality than community-acquired infection (325).

Sepsis with acute organ dysfunction (severe sepsis) is a complex condition that represents a major challenge to the critical care team and carries a crude mortality rate of 28% to 50% (326). Gram-negative and gram-positive organisms as well as fungi cause systemic sepsis and septic shock. Early recognition is crucial to patient survival

■ **TABLE 8.19. Definitions for Systemic Inflammatory Response and Sepsis (SIRS)**

SIRS	Two or more of the following in the setting of a known cause of inflammation: Temperature >38°C or <36°C Pulse >90 Respirations >20/min or $PaCO_2$ <32 mm Hg WBC count >12,000 or <4,000 cells/mm^3 or >10% band forms
Sepsis	SIRS due to known infection
Severe sepsis	Sepsis with evidence of organ dysfunction, hypoperfusion, or hypotension
Septic shock	Sepsis with hypotension despite adequate fluid resuscitation

Source: Adapted from 1991 American College of Chest Physicians/Society of Critical Care Medicine Consensus Conference definitions, with permission.

because mortality rates are exceedingly high if the full clinical picture of shock and organ dysfunction develops. Septic shock is divided into an early hyperdynamic state and a late hypodynamic state.

Low SVR, splanchnic vasoconstriction, and increased cardiac output characterize the hyperdynamic phase of shock. Venous capacitance is increased and results in diminished effectiveness of the circulating blood volume. Aggressive volume resuscitation must be provided to restore cardiac preload and ventricular filling. These patients are best managed in an ICU with the placement of an arterial line, a PA catheter, and a bladder catheter. Appropriate cultures should be obtained and IV broad-spectrum antibiotics should be started within the first hour of recognition of severe sepsis. Laboratory tests of immediate concern include arterial blood gas determinations, creatinine, electrolytes, lactate, coagulation panel, and a complete blood count. Oxygenation and ventilation should be optimized with mechanical ventilation if indicated. If hypotension persists after optimization of the PCWP, the use of norepinephrine or dopamine may be necessary. Surgical debridement or manipulation of infected material should not be performed until the patient has been stabilized.

Early goal-directed therapy of the septic patient has been shown to improve survival. During the first 6 hours of resuscitation, the goals of therapy as outlined by the Surviving Sepsis Campaign guidelines include CVP of 8 to 12 mm Hg, MAP ≥65 mm Hg, urine output ≥0.5 mL/kg/hour, and central venous or mixed venous oxygen saturation ≥70%. If during the first 6 hours oxygen saturation goals are not achieved despite appropriate CVP, then transfusion of RBCs to achieve a hematocrit >30% and/or initiation of a dobutamine infusion is the next step (327).

In the hypodynamic phase of septic shock, hypotension results from cardiac output deterioration. The patient is often cool, mottled, oliguric, diaphoretic, and confused. The etiology of the hypodynamic cardiovascular response to sepsis may be inadequate volume resuscitation, underlying cardiac disease, or myocardial dysfunction associated with sepsis. This is a state of gross decompensation with global tissue hypoxia and is associated with greater mortality.

Numerous clinical trials have attempted to find specific agents that could modulate the underlying disease process in sepsis. Candidate therapies included agents that target mediators of inflammatory response, agents that boost the immune system, and prostaglandin inhibitors, but none was shown to be beneficial. One such agent, drotrecogin alfa (activated Xigris), is a recombinant form of human activated protein C, an endogenous protein with antithrombotic, profibrinolytic, and anti-inflammatory properties that is frequently deficient in sepsis. Although initial studies (The Recombinant Human Activated Protein C Worldwide Evaluation in Severe Sepsis—PROWESS) showed a clinically significant reduction in the 28-day all-cause mortality rate due to severe sepsis (328), results from a subsequent trial, the PROWESS-SHOCK trial, failed to demonstrate any significant benefit in 28-day all-cause mortality. The drug was subsequently withdrawn from the market in October 2011 (329).

In addition to early goal-directed therapy with hemodynamic interventions that balance systemic oxygen delivery with oxygen demand, other management strategies have shown in randomized, controlled trials to reduce mortality associated with severe sepsis. These include limiting the tidal volume to 6 to 7 mL/kg ideal body weight for patients requiring mechanical ventilation for ARDS, the use of moderate-dose corticosteroids (hydrocortisone 200 to 300 mg and fludrocortisone 50 μg daily) for 7 days in patients with refractory septic shock, and maintaining serum glucose levels <180 mg/dL (327). These therapies are not mutually exclusive, and optimal patient management may require a combination of approaches. Some of these strategies vary dramatically from traditional approaches and will require education and established protocols to safely incorporate them into practice.

Multiple Organ Dysfunction Syndrome

MODS is defined as the development of progressive physiologic dysfunction of two or more organ systems after an acute threat to systemic homeostasis (330). An acute threat can include SIRS, sepsis, massive trauma, burns, ischemia, or reperfusion injury. Patients usually present with pulmonary dysfunction, which typically develops early in the course of SIRS or sepsis. Renal dysfunction will present as a prerenal azotemia unless the initial insult stimulated a sudden oliguric ATN. Hyperbilirubinemia is the earliest indication of hepatic dysfunction. GI abnormalities include ileus, stress ulcers, diarrhea, and mucosal atrophy. The platelet count has been used as a surrogate marker of the hematologic system. Cardiac function is often measured by the severity of hypotension or the need for vasopressors. Deterioration of the nervous system is manifested by encephalopathy and peripheral neuropathies. The treatment of MODS is support of individual organ function and aggressive therapies aimed at correcting the underlying process. Mortality is related to the number of dysfunctional systems and is greater than 80% once four organ systems fail (331).

The Acute Physiology and Chronic Health Evaluation (APACHE) provided population-based estimates of mortality for the day of ICU admission (332). Several versions of the APACHE scoring system have been utilized, most recently APACHE IV. Organ failure scores, such as the Sequential Organ Failure Assessment (SOFA), can help assess organ dysfunction over time and are useful to evaluate morbidity. Independent of the initial value, an increase of the SOFA score during the first 48 hours of an ICU admission predicts a mortality rate of 50% or greater, and improvement of cardiovascular, renal, or respiratory SOFA score from baseline through day 1 of ICU admission is significantly related to greater survival (333). It is important to note that these and other outcome prediction models were designed as tools to be used in critical care research in order to stratify patients by severity of illness. They have not been validated for making decisions relating to individual patients.

Abdominal compartment syndrome (ACS) is an important but often unrecognized cause of acute deterioration of a patient after massive fluid resuscitation for septic or hypovolemic shock. Although ACS can impair the function of every organ system, it is generally manifested as hypotension, reduced urine output, and decreased pulmonary compliance. Most commonly associated with trauma patients, it has also been observed in patients with massive ascites, bowel obstruction or ileus, peritonitis, pancreatitis, and intraperitoneal blood. IAP is usually measured indirectly by a balloon-tipped catheter in the bladder. Intra-abdominal hypertension is defined as an IAP of 12 mm Hg or greater recorded by a minimum of three standard measurements conducted 4 to 6 hours apart (334). ACS is defined by an IAP of 20 mm Hg or greater and single or multiple organ failure that was not previously present. Operative decompression of the abdominal cavity with maintenance of an open abdomen via use of temporary closure techniques such as a vacuum pack is the only treatment that reverses the physiologic abnormalities resulting from ACS.

Neurologic Issues

Emotional and mental health of critically ill patients can affect their physical well-being, pain tolerance, and recovery. Stress and strain can be exacerbated by the unknown, pain, wounds, preexisting disease, infection, invasive medical interventions, and routine nursing care such as airway suctioning, repositioning, or dressing changes. The restlessness and distress often associated with critical illness must be quelled with analgesia, sedation, and neuromuscular blockade as a last resort. The Society of Critical Care Medicine and American Society of Health-System Pharmacists (ASHP) clinical practice guidelines for sedation, analgesia, and neuromuscular blockade of the critically ill adult were revised in 2002. This comprehensive document is available online at www.ashp.org (335,336).

Analgesia

Pain management for critically ill patients is a universal goal for all involved in their care. Patients who are not satisfied with the treatment they receive for pain may become more stressed and irritable, sleep less, and have a poor opinion of the care they are receiving on the whole. Pain may contribute to pulmonary dysfunction through localized guarding and generalized muscle rigidity that restricts movement of the chest wall and diaphragm. Unrelieved pain also evokes a stress response characterized by tachycardia, increased myocardial oxygen consumption, hypercoagulability, immunosuppression, and persistent catabolism (337). The combined use of effective analgesia and sedation may ameliorate the stress response and diminish pulmonary complications in postoperative critically ill patients. A comprehensive overview of pain management is covered in Chapter 30; therefore, only key aspects of pain management applicable to patients in the ICU will be addressed.

Pharmacologic therapies include opioids, NSAIDs, and acetaminophen. ASHP guidelines recommend fentanyl, hydromorphone, and morphine given as a continuous infusion or scheduled doses rather than "as needed." Fentanyl has the most rapid onset and shortest duration, but repeated dosing may cause accumulation and prolonged effects. Fentanyl may also be administered via a transdermal patch to hemodynamically stable patients with more chronic analgesic needs, but it is not recommended for the management of acute pain. Morphine has a quick onset but longer duration of action, so intermittent doses may be given. However, morphine causes histamine release, which contributes to hypotension, especially in a hemodynamically unstable patient. Hydromorphone's duration of action is similar to morphine but lacks an active metabolite or histamine release, making it an ideal drug for continuous infusion and for use in patients who cannot tolerate hypotension. Meperidine has an active metabolite that causes neuroexcitation including apprehension, tremors, delirium, and seizures, so its use is not recommended in critically ill patients who may need repeated doses. The characteristics of analgesics and sedatives commonly used in ICU patients are summarized in **Table 8.20**.

Sedation

To further combat anxiety and agitation associated with hospitalization and pain, sedatives are commonly added to routine medication administration. The physical environment of the ICU, limited ability to communicate, sleep deprivation, and medical circumstances precipitating the ICU admission are contributing factors creating anxiety in critically ill patients. Efforts to reduce anxiety, including frequent reorientation, provision of adequate analgesia, and optimization of the environment may be supplemented with sedatives. Agitation is also common in ICU patients; however, not all patients with anxiety will exhibit agitation. Sedatives reduce the stress response and improve tolerance to routine ICU procedures. For example, the use of sedation medication may be necessary to facilitate mechanical ventilation. Generally, sedatives should be administered intermittently to determine the dose needed to achieve the sedation goal, but they may be given as a continuous infusion if necessary. Daily interruption of sedative infusion is associated with shorter duration of mechanical ventilation, shorter ICU stays, and fewer instances of posttraumatic stress disorder (338,339). Benzodiazepines are sedatives and hypnotics that cause anterograde amnesia but lack analgesic properties. Midazolam has a rapid onset and short duration of effect with single doses, making it ideal for treating acutely agitated patients or for brief sedation with invasive procedures. Lorazepam has a slower onset but fewer potential drug interactions because of its metabolism via glucuronidation (**Table 8.20**).

Propofol is an IV general anesthetic that has sedative and hypnotic properties at lower doses. Like the benzodiazepines, propofol has no analgesic properties. Propofol has a rapid onset and short duration of sedation once discontinued. Propofol is a phospholipid emulsion that provides 1.1 kcal/mL from fat and should be counted as a caloric source. Long-term infusions may result in hypertriglyceridemia, and monitoring is recommended after 2 days of use (335). Physiologic dependence and potential withdrawal symptoms have been described in ICU patients who have been exposed to more than 1 week of sedative or narcotic therapy, including the use of propofol (340).

TABLE 8.20. Characteristics of Selected Analgesics and Sedatives Frequently Used in Critically Ill Patients

Agent	Indication	Active Metabolites (Effect)	Adverse Effects	Intermittent Dose (IV)[a]	Infusion Dose Range
Fentanyl	Pain	No metabolite, patient accumulates	Rigidity with high doses	0.35–1.5 μg/kg q 0.5–1 h	0.7–10 μg/kg/h
Hydromorphone	Pain	None	–	10–30 μg/kg q 1–2 h	7–15 μg/kg/h
Morphine	Pain	Yes (sedation)	Histamine release	0.01–0.15 mg/kg q 1–2 h	0.07–0.5 mg/kg/h
Ketorolac	Pain	None	GI bleeding, renal	15–30 mg q 6 h; decrease if >65 years; avoid >5 day use	–
Midazolam	Acute agitation	Yes (prolonged sedation)	–	0.02–0.08 mg/kg q 0.5–2 h	0.04–0.2 mg/kg/h
Lorazepam	Sedation	None	Solvent-related acidosis/renal failure in high doses	0.02–0.06 mg/kg q 2–6 h	0.01–0.1 mg/kg/h
Propofol	Sedation	None	Elevated triglycerides	–	5–80 μg/kg/min
Haloperidol	Delirium	Yes (EPS)	QT interval prolongation	0.03–0.15 mg/kg q 0.5–6 h	0.04–0.15 mg/kg/h

EPS, extrapyramidal symptoms; GI, gastrointestinal; IV, intravenous.

[a]More frequent doses may be needed for acute management in mechanically ventilated patients.

Neuromuscular Blockade

Neuromuscular blocking agents (NMBAs) can be used in conjunction with sedatives to facilitate mechanical ventilation, to manage intracranial pressure in head trauma, to ablate muscle spasms, and to decrease oxygen consumption only when all other means to accomplish these aims have failed (336). Pancuronium is a long-acting NMBA that is effective for up to 90 minutes after IV bolus dose of 0.06 to 0.1 mg/kg. It can be used as a continuous infusion by adjusting the dose to the degree of neuromuscular blockade that is desired. Since pancuronium is vagolytic, 90% of patients will have an increase in heart rate of greater than 10 beats per minute. For patients who cannot tolerate an increase in heart rate, vecuronium can be used. If neuromuscular blockade is necessary for patients with significant hepatic or renal failure, cisatracurium or atracurium should be used. Patients receiving any NMBA should be assessed using electronic twitch monitoring with a goal of adjusting the blockade to achieve one or two twitches. Before initiating neuromuscular blockade, patients should be adequately medicated with sedative and analgesic drugs, as it is difficult to assess pain and anxiety after NMBAs are given. Furthermore, neuromuscular paralysis without sedation is an extremely frightening and unpleasant experience.

Acute quadriplegic myopathy syndrome, also referred to as postparalytic quadriparesis, is a clinical triad of acute paresis, myonecrosis with increased creatine phosphokinase concentration, and abnormal electromyography that is related to prolonged exposure to NMBAs. This is a devastating complication of NMBA therapy and one of the reasons that indiscriminate use of these agents is discouraged. Increased risk of acute quadriplegic myopathy is associated with the concurrent use of corticosteroids; drug "holidays" may decrease the risk (341).

ICU Syndrome/Delirium

First reported in the 1960s, the term ICU syndrome, or psychosis, refers to a multitude of psychological disturbances exhibited by many critically ill patients (342). It has also been labeled postoperative delirium. The ICU syndrome has been defined as an altered emotional state occurring in a highly stressful environment that may manifest itself in a variety of psychological reactions including fear, memory disturbance, anxiety, confusion, withdrawal, despair, agitation, and disorientation. Factors such as sleep deprivation, noise, constant light exposure, restriction of movement, limited ability to communicate, as well as the patient's preadmission mental state and coping ability have all been reported as contributing causes of ICU syndrome. Current medical literature challenges this concept and argues that what is being called ICU syndrome or psychosis is diagnostic of delirium and not due to the ICU environment *per se*. Concerns have been raised that using the term *ICU syndrome* implies that confusion can be expected in the ICU setting and may reduce the vigilance necessary to recognize delirium and identify and treat the physiologic disturbances leading to it (343). Delirium is found in as many as 80% of critically ill patients and is associated with longer ICU admissions and increased mortality (344,345).

Delirium in the ICU setting is commonly caused by metabolic disturbances, hypoxia, electrolyte imbalances, alcohol or drug withdrawal, acute infection, and medications (**Table 8.21**) (343,345). Many drugs have anticholinergic properties that can exert an additive effect, causing neurotoxicity, especially in elderly patients. Anticholinergic-related delirium can be differentiated from other causes of delirium if the mental status clears after administration of the cholinesterase inhibitor physostigmine. Delirium presents in both a hypoactive and hyperactive form. Hypoactive delirium, which is associated with the worst prognosis, is characterized by psychomotor retardation, represents more global cerebral dysfunction, and is manifested by a calm appearance, inattention, and obtundation in extreme cases. Hyperactive delirium is more easily recognized by agitation and combative behaviors. Elderly patients may pose a particular diagnostic challenge when delirium is superimposed on baseline dementia.

TABLE 8.21. Commonly Used Intensive Care Unit Drugs Associated with Delirium[a]

Anesthetics	Anticonvulsants	Atropine[b]
Lidocaine	Carbamazepine	Cimetidine[b]
Propofol	Phenobarbital	Corticosteroids[b]
	Phenytoin	Digoxin[b]
Antibiotics		
Amphotericin B	Antihypertensives	Narcotic analgesics
Aztreonam	Diltiazem	Fentanyl
Cephalosporins	Enalapril	Meperidine[b]
Ciprofloxacin	Hydralazine	Morphine
Doxycycline	Methyldopa	
Imipenem	Propranolol	Nitroprusside
Metronidazole	Verapamil	Phenylephrine
Penicillins		Procainamide[b]
Tobramycin		Scopolamine[b]
		Tricyclic antidepressants[b]

[a]Listing is not intended to be all inclusive.
[b]Drugs known to have significant anticholinergic properties.

The medical management of delirium consists of finding and treating underlying medical conditions and then controlling any behavioral disturbances if necessary. Neuroleptic drugs are the first-line agents for the treatment of delirium. When causes are related to alcohol withdrawal syndrome, management is with benzodiazepines. Haloperidol is the neuroleptic of choice because it has minimal anticholinergic or hypotensive effects. A dose of 2 to 10 mg IV can be given every 20 to 30 minutes until agitation resolves. Once the delirium is controlled, scheduled doses every 4 to 6 hours consisting of 25% of necessary loading doses can be used and tapered off over several days. A continuous infusion can also be used (**Table 8.20**). Patients receiving repeat doses of haloperidol should be monitored for electrocardiographic changes. Extrapyramidal side effects such as rigidity, tremor, or facial tics can be managed with diphenhydramine hydrochloride (335).

End-of-Life Considerations

Despite valiant efforts and adherence to best practices of care, patients, families, and health care professionals are often faced with the difficult decision to withdraw life-sustaining treatment and care. The ethical aspect of foregoing treatment resides in the legal and ethical right of the patient to self-determination. Unfortunately, the majority of critically ill patients are unable to speak for themselves when decisions need to be made to withhold treatment. Living wills, power of attorney status, and advance directives must be acknowledged and honored regarding end-of-life considerations. If a medical power of attorney is not in place, some states stipulate who the surrogate will be by a legal hierarchy. The ethical basis for identification of an appropriate surrogate is primary if none of the preceding legal bases apply. In this situation, the physician and other health care providers have the responsibility to help identify the person or persons who have knowledge of the patient's values and preferences in order to assist with medical decisions on the patient's behalf. This process can become difficult in circumstances when family members or others close to the patient are in disagreement as to who should be the surrogate or what the patient would prefer. In these cases, health care providers should be knowledgeable of applicable legal directives and their ethical responsibility to act in their patient's best interest. Consultation with the institution's ethics committee may be helpful in trying to reach consensus (346). Although not responsible for the patient's death, those close to the patient often are left with feelings of guilt and anxiety in addition to their bereavement. It is important that the health care providers support the family both before and after the decision to withhold or withdraw life-sustaining treatment has been made, not imparting any personal bias.

End-of-life care of patients in the ICU requires a dramatic paradigm shift in attitude and interventions from intensive rescue-type care to intensive palliative care. When considering the array of interventions that may be discontinued or held, physicians and surrogates should focus on clearly articulating the goals of care. For example, a goal for survival until the patient's important loved ones can gather to say their good-byes may justify short-term continuation of ventilator support. If the only goal is patient comfort, then such treatment should be stopped. The withdrawal of life-sustaining treatment is a clinical procedure that deserves the same preparation and expectation of quality as other medical procedures. Honest, caring, and culturally sensitive communication with the patient's loved ones and the patient, if competent, should include explanations of how therapies will be withdrawn, what symptoms are expected, strategies to assess and ensure the patient's comfort, and information about the expected survival after interventions are withdrawn. Informed consent should be documented along with a formulated plan for withdrawing care (347). Adequate analgesia and sedation should be prescribed to relieve symptoms of pain, dyspnea, and anxiety during the dying process. IV opioids and shorter acting benzodiazepines are the drugs of choice. The clinician's primary goal should be to prevent suffering and ensure the patient's comfort even if doing so unintentionally hastens the patient's death. For this reason, palliative care teams might be useful (347).

REFERENCES

1. Dean MM, Finan MA, Kline RC. Predictors of complications and hospital stay in gynecologic cancer surgery. *Obstet Gynecol.* 2001;97:721–724.
2. Wijeysundera DN, Beattie WS, Austin PC, et al. Epidural anaesthesia and survival after intermediate-to-high risk non-cardiac surgery: a population-based cohort study. *Lancet.* 2008;372:562–569.
3. Auerbach AD, Rasic MA, Sehgal N, et al. Opportunity missed: medical consultation, resource use and quality of care of patients undergoing major surgery. *Arch Intern Med.* 2007;167:2338–2344.
4. Macpherson DS, Lofgren RP. Outpatient internal medicine preoperative evaluation: a randomized clinical trial. *Med Care.* 1994;32:498–507.
5. Fisher SP. Cost-effective preoperative evaluation and testing. *Chest.* 1999;115:96S–100S.
6. Card R, Sawyer M, Degnan B, et al. Institute for Clinical Systems Improvement (ICSI). Perioperative protocol. Updated March 2014.
7. National Institute for Clinical Excellence (NICE). *The Use of Routine Preoperative Tests for Elective Surgery. NICE Clinical Guidance No. 3.* London, England: National Institute for Clinical Excellence; 2003.
8. St Clair CM, Shah M, Diver EJ, et al. Adherence to evidence-based guidelines for preoperative testing in women undergoing gynecologic surgery. *Obstet Gynecol.* 2010;116:694–700.
9. Mosca L, Frundy SM, Judelson D, et al. Guide to preventive cardiology for women: AHA/ACC Scientific Statement Consensus panel statement. *Circulation.* 1999;99:2480–2484.
10. Mosca L, Benjamin EJ, Berra K, et al. Effectiveness-based guidelines for the prevention of cardiovascular disease in women 2011 update: a guideline from the American Heart Association. *Circulation.* 2011;123:1243–1262.
11. Ford ES, Ajani UA, Croft JB, et al. Explaining the decrease in U.S. deaths from coronary disease, 1980–*N Engl J Med.* 2007;356:2388–2398.
12. Pregler J, Freund KM, Kleinman M, et al. The heart truth professional education campaign on women and heart disease: needs assessment and evaluation results. *J Womens Health.* 2009;18(10):1541–1547.
13. Poon S, Goodman SG, Yan RT, et al. Bridging the gender gap: insights from a contemporary analysis of sex-related differences in the treatment and outcomes of patients with acute coronary syndromes. *Am Heart J.* 2012;163(1):66–73.
14. Hollenberg SM. Preoperative cardiac risk assessment. *Chest.* 1999;115(Suppl 5):51–57.
15. Freeman WK, Gibbons RJ. Perioperative assessment of cardiac patients undergoing noncardiac surgery. *Mayo Clin Proc.* 2009;84:79–90.
16. Fleisher LA, Beckman JA, Brown KA, et al. ACC/AHA 2007 Guidelines on perioperative cardiovascular evaluation and care for noncardiac surgery: executive summary: a report of the American College of Cardiology/American Heart Association Task Force on practice guidelines (Writing Committee to Revise the 2002 guidelines on perioperative cardiovascular evaluation for noncardiac surgery). *J Am Coll Cardiol.* 2007;50:1707–1732.
17. Goldman L, Caldera DL, Nussbaum SR, et al. Multifactorial index of cardiac risk in noncardiac surgical procedures. *N Engl J Med.* 1977;297:845–850.
18. Lee TH, Marcantonio ER, Mangione CM, et al. Derivation and prospective validation of a simple index for prediction of cardiac risk of major noncardiac surgery. *Circulation.* 1999;100:1043–1049.
19. Bilimoria KY, Liu Y, Paruch JL, et al. Development and evaluation of the universal ACS NSQIP surgical risk calculator: a decision aid and informed consent tool for patients and surgeons. *J Am Coll Surg.* 2013;217:833–842.e1–e3.
20. Mosca L, Banka CL, Benjamin EJ, et al. Evidence-based guidelines for cardiovascular disease prevention in women: 2007 update. *Circulation.* 2007;115:1481–1501.
21. Mashour GA, Shanks AM, Kheterpal S. Perioperative stroke and associated mortality after noncardiac, nonneurologic surgery. *Anesthesiology.* 2011;114:1289–1296.
22. Kertai MD, Bountioukos M, Boersma E, et al. Aortic stenosis: an underestimated risk factor for perioperative complications in patients undergoing noncardiac surgery. *Am J Med.* 2004;116:8–13.
23. Cohen ME, Ko CY, Bilimoria KY, et al. Optimizing ACS NSQIP modeling for evaluation of surgical quality and risk: patient risk adjustment, procedure mix adjustment, shrinkage adjustment, and surgical focus. *J Am Coll Surg.* 2013;217(2):336–346.e1.
24. Halm EA, Browner WS, Tubau JF, et al. Echocardiography for assessing cardiac risk in patients having noncardiac surgery. *Ann Intern Med.* 1996;125:433–441.
25. Karthikeyan G, Moncur RA, Levine O, et al. Is a pre-operative brain natriuretic peptide or N-terminal pro-B-type natriuretic peptide measurement an independent predictor of adverse cardiovascular outcomes within 30 days of noncardiac surgery? A systemic review and meta-analysis of observational studies. *J Am Coll Cardiol.* 2009;54(17):1599–1606.
26. Ferreira MJ. The role of nuclear cardiology for preoperative risk assessment prior to noncardiac surgery. *Rev Port Cardiol.* 2001;19(Suppl 1):163–169.
27. Ashton CM, Petersen NJ, Wray NP, et al. The incidence of perioperative myocardial infarction in men undergoing noncardiac surgery. *Ann Intern Med.* 1993;188:504–510.
28. Mangano DT, Layug EL, Wallace A, et al. Effect of atenolol on mortality and cardiovascular morbidity after noncardiac surgery. *N Engl J Med.* 1996;335:1713–1720.
29. POISE Study Group, Devereaux PJ, Yang H, et al. Effects of extended-release metoprolol succinate in patients undergoing non-cardiac surgery (POISE trial): a randomized controlled trial. *Lancet.* 2008;371(9627):1839–1847.
30. Dimick JB, Chen SL, Taheri PA, et al. Hospital costs associated with surgical complications: a report from the private-sector National Surgical Quality Improvement Program. *J Am Coll Surg.* 2004;199(4):531.
31. Fisher BW, Majumdar SR, McAlistar FA. Predicting pulmonary complications after nonthoracic surgery: a systematic review of blinded studies. *Am J Med.* 2002;112:219–225.
32. Meyers JR, Lembeck L, O'Kane H, et al. Changes in functional residual capacity of the lung after operation. *Arch Surg.* 1975;110:576.
33. Craig DB. Postoperative recovery of pulmonary function. *Anesth Analg.* 1981;60:46.
34. Ibañez J, Raurich JM. Normal values of functional residual capacity in the sitting and supine positions. *Intensive Care Med.* 1982;8(4):173–177.
35. Arozullah AM, Khuri SF, Henderson WG, et al. Development and validation of a multifactorial risk index for predicting postoperative pneumonia after major noncardiac surgery. *Ann Intern Med.* 2001;135:847–857.
36. Smetana FW, Lawrence VA, Cornell JE. Preoperative pulmonary risk stratification for noncardiothoracic surgery: systematic review for the American College of Physicians. *Ann Intern Med.* 2006;144:581–595.
37. Mitchell CK, Smoger SH, Pfeifer MP, et al. Multivariate analysis of factors associated with postoperative pulmonary complications following general elective surgery. *Arch Surg.* 1998;133:194–198.
38. Qaseem A, Snow V, Fitterman N, et al. Risk assessment for and strategies to reduce perioperative pulmonary complications for patients undergoing noncardiothoracic surgery: a guideline from the American College of Physicians. *Ann Intern Med.* 2006;144(8):575–578.
39. Latimer RG, Dickman M, Day WC, et al. Ventilatory patterns and pulmonary complications after upper abdominal surgery determined by preoperative and postoperative computerized spirometry and blood gas analysis. *Am J Surg.* 1971;122:622–632.

40. Gibbs J. Preoperative serum albumin level as a predictor of operative mortality and morbidity: results from the National VA Surgical Risk Study. *Acrh Surg*. 1999;134:36–42.
41. Restrepo RD, Wettstein R, Wittnebel L, et al. Incentive spirometry: 2011. *Respir Care*. 2011;56(10):1600–1604.
42. Hawn MT, Houston TK, Campagna EJ, et al. The attributable risk of smoking on surgical complications. *Ann Surg*. 2011;254(6):914–920.
43. Bluman LG, Mosca L, Newman N, et al. Preoperative smoking habits and postoperative pulmonary complications. *Chest*. 1998;113:883–889.
44. Shi U, Warner D. Brief preoperative smoking abstinence: is there a dilemma? *Anesth Analg*. 2011;113:1348–1351.
45. Nakagawa M, Tanaka H, Tsukuma H, et al. Relationship between the duration of the preoperative smoke-free period and the incidence of postoperative pulmonary complications after pulmonary surgery. *Chest*. 2001;120:705–710.
46. Mazo V, Sabaté S, Canet J, et al. Prospective external validation of a predictive score for postoperative pulmonary complications. *Anesthesiology*. 2014;121:219.
47. Gupta H, Gupta PK, Fang X, et al. Development and validation of a risk calculator predicting postoperative respiratory failure. *Chest*. 2011;140:1207.
48. Canet J, Gallart L, Gomar C, et al. Prediction of postoperative pulmonary complications in a population-based surgical cohort. *Anesthesiology*. 2010;113:1338.
49. Centers for Disease Control and Prevention. *National Diabetes Fact Sheet: National Estimates and General Information on Diabetes and Prediabetes in the United States*. Atlanta, GA: U.S. Department of Health and Human Services; 2011.
50. Elixhauser A, Yu K, Steiner C, et al. *Hospitalization in the United States, 1997. Healthcare Costs and Utilization. Project Fact Book No. 1. AHRQ Publication No. 00-0031*. Rockville, MD: Agency for Healthcare Research and Quality; 2000.
51. Clement S, Braithwaite SS, Magee MF, et al. Management of diabetes and hyperglycemia in hospitals. *Diabetes Care*. 2004;27:553–591.
52. Cowie CC, Rust KF, Ford ES, et al. Full accounting of diabetes and pre-diabetes in the U.S. population in 1988–1994 and 2005–2006. *Diabetes Care*. 2009;32:287–294.
53. Sheehy AM, Gabbay RA. An overview of preoperative glucose evaluation, management and perioperative impact. *J Diabetes Sci Technol*. 2009;3:1261–1269.
54. Kohl BA, Schwartz S. How to manage perioperative endocrine insufficiency. *Anesthesiol Clin*. 2010;28:139–155.
55. Meneghini LF. Perioperative management of diabetes: translating evident into practice. *Cleveland Clin J Med*. 2009;76:S53–S59.
56. Dronge AS, Perkal MF, Kancir S, et al. Long-term glycemic control and postoperative infectious complications. *Arch Surg*. 2006;141:375–380.
57. Raju TA, Torjman MC, Goldberg ME. Perioperative blood glucose monitoring in the general surgical population. *J Diabetes Sci Technol*. 2009;3:1282–1287.
58. The International Expert Committee report on the role of the A1C assay in the diagnosis of diabetes. *Diabetes Care*. 2009;32(7):1327–1334.
59. American Diabetes Association. Standards of medical care in diabetes-2009. *Diabetes Care*. 2009;32(Suppl 1):S13–S61.
60. Fahy BG, Sheehy AM, Coursin MD. Glucose control in the intensive care unit. *Crit Care Med*. 2009;37:1769–1776.
61. Egi M, Bellomo R, Stachowski E, et al. Blood glucose concentration and outcome of critical illness: the impact of diabetes. *Crit Care Med*. 2008;3:2249–2255.
62. Rady MY, Johnson DJ, Patel BM, et al. Influence of individual characteristics on outcome of glycemic control in intensive care unit patients with or without diabetes mellitus. *Mayo Clin Pro*. 2005;80:1558–1567.
63. Umpierrez GE, Smiley D, Jacobs S, et al. Randomized study of basal/bolus insulin therapy in the inpatient management of patients with type 2 diabetes undergoing general surgery (RABBIT 2 Surgery). *Diabetes Care*. 2011;34:256–261.
64. Khan NA, Ghali WA, Spratt SE, et al. *Perioperative Management of Diabetes Mellitus. Physicians' Information and Education Resources*. American College of Physicians, 2009. http://pier.acponline.org/physicians/public/periopr879/tables/periopr879-tl.html. Accessed April 26, 2012.
65. Umpierrez GE, Hellman R, Korytkowski MT, et al. Management of hyperglycemia in hospitalized patients in non-critical care setting: an Endocrine Society Clinical Practice Guideline. *J Clin Endocrinol Metab*. 2012;97:16–38.
66. Pompocelli JJ, Baxter JK, Babineau TJ, et al. Early postoperative glucose control predicts nosocomial infection rate in diabetic patients. *JPEN J Parenter Enteral Nutr*. 1998;22:77–81.
67. Frisch A, Chandra P, Smiley D, et al. Prevalence and clinical outcome of hyperglycemia in the perioperative period in non-cardiac surgery. *Diabetes Care*. 2010;33:1783–1788.
68. Noordzij PG, Boersma E, Schreiner F, et al. Increased preoperative glucose levels are associated with perioperative mortality in patients undergoing non-cardiac, non-vascular surgery. *Eur J Endocrinol*. 2007;156:137–142.
69. Ramos M, Khalpey Z, Lipsitz S, et al. Relationship of perioperative hyperglycemia and postoperative infections in patients who undergo general and vascular surgery. *Ann Surg*. 2008;248:585–591.
70. Sato H, Carvalho G, Sato T, et al. The association of preoperative glycemic control, intraoperative insulin sensitivity and outcomes after cardiac surgery. *J Clin Encocrinol Metab*. 2010;95:4338–4344.
71. Gallacher SJ, Thomason F, Fraser WD, et al. Neutrophil bactericidal function in diabetes mellitus: evidence for association with blood glucose control. *Diabet Med*. 1995;12:916–920.
72. Van Den Berghe G, Wouters P, Weekers F, et al. Intensive insulin therapy in critically ill patients. *N Engl J Med*. 2001;345:1359–1367.
73. Finfer S, Chittock DR, Su SY, et al. Intensive versus conventional glucose control in critically ill patients. *N Engl J Med*. 2009;360(13):1283–1297.
74. Moghissi ES, Korytowski MT, DiNardo M, et al. American Association of Clinical Endocrinologists and American Diabetes Association consensus statement on inpatient glycemic control. *Endocr Pract*. 2009;15:353–369.
75. Umpierrez GE, Smiley D, Zisman A, et al. Randomized study of basal-bolus insulin therapy in the inpatient management of patients with type 2 diabetes (RABBIT 2 trial). *Diabetes Care*. 2007;30:2181–2186.
76. Umpierrez GE, Smiley D, Jacobs S, et al. Randomized study of basal/bolus insulin therapy in the inpatient management of patients with type 2 diabetes undergoing general surgery (RABBIT 2 Surgery). *Diabetes Care*. 2011;34:256–261.
77. Miller JD, Richman DC. Preoperative evaluation of patients with diabetes mellitus. *Anesthesiology Clin*. 2016;34:155–169.
78. Ringle MD. Management of hypothyroidism and hyperthyroidism in the intensive care unit. *Crit Care Clin*. 2001;17:59–74.
79. Schiff RL, Welsh GA. Perioperative evaluation and management of the patient with endocrine dysfunction. *Med Clin N Am*. 2003;87:175–192.
80. Weinberg AD, Brennan MD, Gorman CA. Outcome of anesthesia and surgery in hypothyroid patients. *Arch Intern Med*. 1983;143:893–897.
81. Ladenson PW, Levin AA, Ridgway EC, et al. Complications of surgery in hypothyroid patients. *Am J Med*. 1984;77(2):261–266.
82. Bennett-Guerrero E, Kramer DC, Schwinn DA. Effect of chronic and acute thyroid reduction on perioperative outcome. *Anesth Analg*. 1997;85:30–36.
83. Klubo-Gwiezdzinska J, Wartofsky L. Thyroid emergencies. *Med Clin N Am*. 2012;96:385–403.
84. Conner LE, Coursin DB. Assessment and therapy of selected endocrine disorders. *Anesthesiol Clin N Am*. 2004;22:93–123.
85. Warofsky L. Myxedema coma. *Endocrinol Metab Clin North Am*. 2006;35:687–698, vii–viii.
86. Dutta P, Bhanasali A, Masoodi SR, et al. Predictors of outcome in myxedema coma: a study from a tertiary care centre. *Crit Care*. 2008;12(1):R1.
87. Forfar JC, Muir AL, Sawrers SA, et al. Abnormal left ventricular function in hyperthyroidism. *N Engl J Med*. 1982;307:1165–1170.
88. Klein I, Ojamaa K. Mechanisms of disease: thyroid hormone and the cardiovascular system. *N Engl J Med*. 2001;344:501–509.
89. Sawin CT, Geller A, Wolf PA. Low serum thyrotropin concentration as a risk factor for atrial fibrillation in older patients. *N Engl J Med*. 1994;331:1249–1252.
90. Woeber KA. Thyrotoxicosis and the heart. *N Engl J Med*. 1992;327:94–97.
91. Furlong D, Ahmed I, Jabbour S. Perioperative management of endocrine disorders. In: Merli GJ, Weitz HH, eds. *Medical Management of the Surgical Patient*, Chapter 12. 3rd Ed. Philadelphia, PA: Elsevier Saunders; 2007:411–452.
92. Nayak B, Burman K. Thyrotoxicosis and thyroid storm. *Endocrinol Metab Clinc North Am*. 2006;35(4):663–686, vii.
93. Bahn RS, Burch HB, Cooper DS, et al. Hyperthyroidism and other causes of thyrotoxicosis: management guidelines of the American Thyroid Association and American Association of Clinical Endocrinologists. *Thyroid*. 2011;21(6):593–646.
94. Nicholson G, Burrin JM, Hall GM. Perioperative steroid supplementation. *Anaesthesia*. 1998;53:1091–1104.
95. Henzen C, Suter A, Lerch E, et al. Suppression and recovery of adrenal response after short-term, high dose glucocorticoid treatment. *Lancet*. 2000;355:542–545.
96. Hopkins RL, Leinung MC. Exogenous Cushing's syndrome and glucocorticoid withdrawal. *Endocrinol Metab Clin North Am*. 2005;34:371–384.

97. Axelrod L. Perioperative management of patients treated with glucocorticoids. *Endocrinol Metab Clin North Am*. 2003;32:367–383.
98. Kehlet H, Binder C. Value of an ACTH test in assessing hypothalamic-pituitary-adrenocortical function in glucocorticoid-treated patients. *BMJ*. 1973;2:147–149.
99. Knudsen L, Christiansen LA, Lorentzen JE. Hypotension during and after operation in glucocorticoid-treated patients. *Br J Anaesth*. 1981;53:295–301.
100. Plumpton FS, Besser GM, Cole PV. Corticosteroid treatment and surgery. 1. An investigation of the indications for steroid cover. *Anaesthesia*. 1969;24:3–11.
101. Marik PE, Varon J. Requirment of perioperative stress doses of corticosteroids. *Arch Surg*. 2008;143(12):1222–1226.
102. U.S. Renal Data System. *USRDS 2011 Annual Data Report: Atlas of Chronic Kidney Disease and End-Stage Renal Disease in the United States*. Bethesda, MD: National Institutes of Health, National Institute of Diabetes and Digestive and Kidney Diseases; 2011.
103. Levey AS, Coresh J, Balk E, et al. National Kidney Foundation practice guidelines for chronic kidney disease: evaluation, classification, and stratification. *Ann Intern Med*. 2003;139(2):137–147.
104. Go AS, Chertow GM, Fan D, et al. Chronic kidney disease and the risks of death, cardiovascular events and hospitalization. *N Engl J Med*. 2004;351:1296–1305.
105. Schiffrin EL, Lipman ML, Mann JFE. Chronic kidney disease: effects on the cardiovascular system. *Circulation*. 2007;116:85–97.
106. Weir MR. Recognizing the link between chronic kidney disease and cardiovascular disease. *Am J Manag Care*. 2011;17:S396–S402.
107. Conlon PJ, Krucoff MW, Minda S, et al. Incidence and long-term significance of transient S-T segment deviation in hemodialysis patients. *Clin Nephrol*. 1998;49(4):236–239.
108. Pochmalicki G, Jan F, Fouchard I. Frequency of painless myocardial ischemia during hemodialysis in 50 patients with chronic kidney failure. *Arch Mal Coeur Vaiss*. 1990;83:1671–1675.
109. Pun PH, Smarz TR, Honeycutt EF, et al. Chronic kidney disease is associated with increased risk of sudden cardiac death among patients with coronary artery disease. *Kidney Int*. 2009;76:653–658.
110. De Bie MK, Maurits SB, Ton JR, et al. How to reduce sudden cardiac death in patients with renal failure. *Heart*. 2012;98:335–341.
111. Wallia R, Greenberg A, Piraino B, et al. Serum electrolyte patterns in end stage renal disease. *Am J Kidney Dis*. 1986;8:98–104.
112. Palevsky PM. Perioperative management of patients with chronic kidney disease or ESRD. *Best Pract Res Clin Anaesthesiol*. 2004;18(1):129–144.
113. Greenberg A. Hyperkalemia: treatment options. *Semin Nephrol*. 1998;18:46–57.
114. Joseph AJ, Cohn SL. Perioperative care of the patient with renal failure. *Med Clin North Am*. 2003;87:193–210.
115. Clement FM, Klarenbach S, Tonelli M, et al. An economic evaluation of erythropoiesis-stimulating agents in CKD. *Am J Kidney Dis*. 2010;56:1050–1061.
116. Esbach JW, Kelly MR, Haley NR, et al. Treatment of the anemia of progressive renal failure with recombinant human erythropoietin. *N Engl J Med*. 1989;321:158–163.
117. Rabelink TJ, Zwaginga JJ, Koomans HA, et al. Thrombosis and hemostasis in renal disease. *Kidney Int*. 1994;46:287–296.
118. Mannucci PM, Remuzzi G, Pusineri F, et al. Deamino-8-arginine vasopressin shortens the bleeding time in uremia. *N Engl J Med*. 1983;308:8–12.
119. Livio M, Mannucci PM, Vigano G, et al. Conjugated estrogens for the management of bleeding associated with renal failure. *N Engl J Med*. 1986;315:731–735.
120. Aronoff GR, Bennett WM, Berns JS, et al. *Drug Prescribing in Renal Failure: Dosing Guidelines for Adults and Children*. 5th Ed. Philadelphia, PA: American College of Physicians; 2007.
121. Matzke GR, Aronoff GR, Atkinson AJ, et al. Drug dosing consideration in patients with acute and chronic kidney disease-a clinical update from Kidney Disease: Improving Global Outcomes (KDIGO). *Kidney Int*. 2011;80:1122–1137.
122. Hanje AJ, Patel T. Preoperative evaluation of patients with liver disease. *Nat Clin Pract Gastroenterol Hepatol*. 2007;4:266–276.
123. Hoetzel A, Ryan H, Schmidt R. Anesthetic considerations for the patient with liver disease. *Curr Opin Anesthesiol*. 2012;25(3):340–347.
124. Muilenburg DJ, Singh A, Torzilli G, et al. Surgery in the patient with liver disease. *Med Clin North Am*. 2009;93:1065–1081.
125. Friedman LS. Surgery in the patient with liver disease. *Trans Am Clin Climatol Assoc*. 2010;121:192–204.
126. Runyon BA. Surgical procedures are well tolerated by patients with asymptomatic chronic hepatitis. *J Clin Gastroenterol*. 1986;8:542–544.
127. O'sullivan MJ, Envoy D, O'Donnell C, et al. Gallstones and laparoscopic cholecystectomy in hepatitis C patients. *Ir Med J*. 2001;94:114–117.
128. Child CG, Turcotte JG. Surgery and portal hypertension. *Major Probl Clin Surg*. 1964;1:1–85.
129. Pugh RN, Murray-Lyon IM, Dawson JL, et al. Transection of the oesophagus for bleeding oesophageal varices. *Br J Surg*. 1973;60(8): 646–649.
130. Muir AJ. Surgical clearance for the patient with chronic liver disease. *Clin Liver Dis*. 2012;16:421–433.
131. Malinchoc M, Kamath PS, Gordon FD, et al. A model to predict poor survival in patients undergoing transjugular intrahepatic portosystemic shunts. *Hepatology*. 2000;31(4):864–871.
132. Amarapurkar DM. Prescribing medications in patients with decompensated liver cirrhosis. *Int J Hepatol*. 2011;2011:519526. doi:10.4061/2011/519526.
133. Huhmann MB, August DA. Nutrition support in surgical oncology. *Nutr Clin Pract*. 2009;24:520–526.
134. Laky B, Janda M, Bauer J, et al. Malnutrition among gynecological cancer patients. *Eur J Clin Nutr*. 2007;61:642–646.
135. Gupta D, Vashi PG, Lammersfeld, et al. Role of nutritional status in predicting the length of stay in cancer: a systematic review of the epidemiological literature. *Ann Nutr Metab*. 2011;59:96–106.
136. Kathiresan AS, Brookfield KF, Schuman SI, et al. Malnutrition as a predictor of poor postoperative outcomes in gynecologic cancer patients. *Arch Gynecol Obstet*. 2011;284:445–451.
137. Obermair A, Hagenauer S, Tamandl D, et al. Safety and efficacy of low anterior en bloc resection as part of cytoreductive surgery for patients with ovarian cancer. *Gynecol Oncol*. 2001;83:115–120.
138. Laky B, Janda M, Cleghorn G, et al. Comparison of different nutritional assessments and body composition measurements in detecting malnutrition among gynecologic cancer patients. *Am J Clin Nutr*. 2008;87:1678–1685.
139. Huhmann MB, August DA. Review of American Society for Parenteral and Enteral Nutrition (ASPEN) clinical guidelines for nutrition support in cancer patients: nutrition screening and assessment. *Nutr Clin Pract*. 2008;23:182–188.
140. Detsky AS, McLaughlin JR, Baker JP, et al. What is subjective global assessment of nutritional status? *JPEN J Parenter Enteral Nutr*. 1987;11: 8–13.
141. Ottery FD. Definition of standardized nutritional assessment and interventional pathways in oncology. *Nutrition*. 1996;12:S15–S19.
142. MaCallum PD, Polisena CG. *The Clinical Guide to Oncology Nutrition*. Chicago, IL: The American Dietetic Association; 2000.
143. Donato D, Angelides A, Irani H, et al. Infectious complications after gastrointestinal surgery in patients with ovarian carcinoma and malignant ascites. *Gynecol Oncol*. 1992;44:40–47.
144. The VA Total Parenteral Nutrition Cooperative Study Group. Perioperative total parenteral nutrition in surgical patients. *N Engl J Med*. 1991;325:525–532.
145. Buzby GP, Mullen JL, Matthews DC, et al. Prognostic nutritional index in gastrointestinal surgery. *Am J Surg*. 1980;139:160–167.
146. Santoso JT, Cannada T, O'Farrel B, et al. Subjective versus objective nutritional assessment study in women with gynecological cancer: a prospective cohort trial. *Int J Gynecol Cancer*. 2004;14:220–223.
147. Anthony PS. Nutrition screening tools for hospitalized patients. *Nutr Clin Pract*. 2008;23:373–382.
148. Braga M, Ljungqvist O, Soeters P, et al. ESPEN guidelines on parenteral nutrition: surgery. *Clin Nutr*. 2009;28:378–386.
149. Meijerink WJ, von Meyenfeldt MF, Rouflart MM, et al. Efficacy of perioperative nutritional support. *Lancet*. 1992;340:187–188.
150. Bozzetti F, Gavazzi C, Miceli R, et al. Perioperative total parenteral nutrition in malnourished, gastrointestinal cancer patients: a randomized, clinical trial. *JPEN J Parenter Enteral Nutr*. 2000;24:7–14.
151. Wu GH, Liu ZH, Wu ZH, et al. Perioperative artificial nutrition in malnourished gastrointestinal cancer patients. *World J Gastroenterol*. 2006;12:2441–2444.
152. Nelson G, Kalogera E, Dowdy SC. Enhanced recovery pathways in gynecologic oncology. *Gynecol Oncol*. 2014;135:586–594.
153. Gustafsson UO, Scott MJ, Schwenk W, et al. Guidelines for perioperative care in elective colonic surgery: Enhanced Recovery After Surgery (ERAS®) Society recommendations. *World J Surg*. 2013;37:259–284.
154. Lassen K, Coolsen MM, Slim K, et al. Guidelines for perioperative care in pancreaticoduodenectomy: Enhanced Recovery After Surgery (ERAS®) Society recommendations. *World J Surg*. 2013;37:240–258.
155. Nygren J, Thacker J, Carli F, et al. Guidelines for perioperative care in elective rectal/pelvic surgery: Enhanced Recovery After Surgery (ERAS®) Society recommendations. *World J Surg*. 2013;37:285–305.

156. Chambers D, Paton F, Wilson P, et al. An overview and methodological assessment of systematic reviews and meta-anlysis of enhanced recovery programmes in colorectal surgery. *BMJ Open*. 2014;4:e005014.
157. Varadhan KK, Neal KR, Dejong CH, et al. The enhanced recovery after surgery (ERAS) pathway for patients undergoing major elective open colorectal surgery: a meta-analysis of randomized controlled trials. *Clin Nutr*. 2010;29:434–440.
158. Roulin D, Donadini A, Gander S, et al. Cost-effectiveness of the implementation of an enhanced recovery protocol for colorectal surgery. *Br J Surg*. 2013;100:1108–1114.
159. ERAS Protocol (EP). http://eras.org.in/eras-protocol/. Published 2010. Accessed April 2, 2016.
160. Kalogera E, Bakkum-Gamez JN, Jankowski CJ, et al. Enhanced recovery in gynecologic surgery. *Obstet Gynecol*. 2013;122:319–328.
161. Nelson, G, Altman AD, Nick A, et al. Guidelines for pre-and intra-operative care in gynecologic/oncology surgery: Enhanced Recovery After Surgery (ERAS®) Society recommendations-Part I. *Gynecol Oncol*. 2016;140:313–322.
162. Nelson G, Altman AD, Nick A, et al. Guidelines for postoperative care in gynecologic/oncology surgery: Enhanced Recovery After Surgery (ERAS®) Society recommendations-Part II. *Gynecol Oncol*. 2016;140:323–332.
163. Douketis JD. Perioperative management of patients who are receiving warfarin therapy: an evidence-based and practical approach. *Blood*. 2011;117:5044.
164. Destro MW, Speranzini MB, Cavalheiro Filho C, et al. Bilateral haematoma after rhytidoplasty and blepharoplasty following chronic use of Ginkgo biloba. *Br J Plast Surg*. 2005;58:100.
165. Cheema P, El-Mefty O, Jazieh AR. Intraoperative haemorrhage associated with the use of extract of Saw Palmetto herb: a case report and review of literature. *J Intern Med*. 2001;250:167.
166. Crosby E. Perioperative use of erythropoietin. *Am J Ther*. 2002;9:371–376.
167. Feringa HH, Bax JJ, Poldermans D. Perioperative medical management of ischemic heart disease in patients undergoing noncardiac surgery. *Curr Opin Anaesthesiol*. 2007;20:254–260.
168. Fleisher LA, Beckman JA, Brown KA, et al. ACC/AHA 2007 guidelines on perioperative cardiovascular evaluation and care for noncardiac surgery: a report of the American College of Cardiology/American Heart Association Task Force on Practice Guidelines (Writing Committee to Revise the 2002 guidelines on perioperative cardiovascular evaluation for noncardiac surgery) developed in collaboration with the American Society of Echocardiography, American Society of Nuclear Cardiology, Heart Rhythm Society, Society of Cardiovascular Anesthesiologists, Society for Cardiovascular Angiography and Interventions, Society for Vascular Medicine and Biology, and Society for Vascular Surgery. *J Am Coll Cardiol*. 2007;50:e159–e241.
169. Eagle KA, Berger PB, Calkins H, et al. ACC/AHA guideline update for perioperative cardiovascular evaluation for noncardiac surgery – executive summary a report of the American College of Cardiology/American Heart Association Task Force on practice guidelines (Committee to Update the 1996 guidelines on perioperative cardiovascular evaluation for noncardiac surgery). *Circulation*. 2002;105:1257–1267.
170. Lindenauer PK, Pekow P, Wang K, et al. Perioperative beta-blocker therapy and mortality after major noncardiac surgery. *N Engl J Med*. 2005;353:349–361.
171. Howard-Alpe GM, Sear JW, Foex P. Methods of detecting atherosclerosis in non-cardiac surgical patients: the role of biochemical markers. *Br J Anaesth*. 2006;97:758–769.
172. O'Neil-Callahan K, Katsimaglis G, Tepper MR, et al. Statins decrease perioperative cardiac complications in patients undergoing noncardiac vascular surgery: the statins for risk reduction in surgery (StaRRS) study. *J Am Coll Cardiol*. 2005;45:336–342.
173. Chassot PG, Delabays A, Spahn DR. Perioperative antiplatelet therapy: the case for continuing therapy in patients at risk of myocardial infarction. *Br J Anaesth*. 2007;99:316–328.
174. Steinhubl SR, Berger PB, Mann JT III, et al. Early and sustained dual oral antiplatelet therapy following percutaneous coronary intervention: a randomized controlled trial. *JAMA*. 2002;288:2411–2420.
175. Thachil J, Gatt A, Martlew V. Management of surgical patients receiving anticoagulation and antiplatelet agents. *Br J Surg*. 2008;95:1437–1448.
176. Korte W, Cattaneo M, Chassot PG, et al. Peri-operative management of antiplatelet therapy in patients with coronary artery disease: joint position paper by members of the working group on Perioperative Haemostasis of the Society on Thrombosis and Haemostasis Research (GTH), the working group on Perioperative Coagulation of the Austrian Society for Anesthesiology, Resuscitation and Intensive Care (OGARI) and the Working Group Thrombosis of the European Society for Cardiology (ESC). *Thromb Haemost*. 2011;105:743–749.
177. Patrono C, Baigent C, Hirsh J, et al. Antiplatelet drugs: American College of Chest Physicians evidence-based clinical practice guidelines (8th edition). *Chest*. 2008;133(Suppl 6):199–233.
178. Cortés J, Caralt M, Delaloge S, et al. Safety of bevacizumab in metastatic breast cancer patients undergoing surgery. *Eur J Cancer*. 2012;48(4):475–481.
179. Erinjeri JP, Fong AJ, Kemeny NE, et al. Timing of administration of bevacizumab chemotherapy affects wound healing after chest wall port placement. *Cancer*. 2011;117(6):1296–1301.
180. Scappaticci FA, Fehrenbacher L, Cartwright T, et al. Surgical wound healing complications in metastatic colorectal cancer patients treated with bevacizumab. *J Surg Oncol*. 2005;91(3):173–180.
181. Ng SP. Blood transfusion requirements for abdominal hysterectomy: 3-year experience in a district hospital (1993–1995). *Aust N Z J Obstet Gynaecol*. 1997;37:452–457.
182. Lentz SS, Shelton BJ, Toy NJ. Effects of perioperative blood transfusion on prognosis in early-stage cervical cancer. *Ann Surg Oncol*. 1998;5:216–219.
183. Dodd RY, Notari EP, Stramer SL. Current prevalence and incidence of infectious disease markers and estimated window-period risk in the American Red Cross blood donor population. *Transfusion*. 2002;42:975–979.
184. Dunne JR, Malone D, Tracy JK, et al. Perioperative anemia: an independent risk factor for infection, mortality, and resource utilization in surgery. *J Surg Res*. 2002;102:237–244.
185. Taylor RW, Manganaro L, O'Brien J, et al. Impact of allogenic packed red blood cell transfusion on nosocomial infection rates in the critically ill patient. *Crit Care Med*. 2002;30:2249–2254.
186. Vanderlinde ES, Heal JM, Blumberg N. Autologous transfusion. *BMJ*. 2002;324:772–775.
187. Popovsky MA, Whitaker B, Arnold NL. Severe outcomes of allogeneic and autologous blood donation: frequency and characterization. *Transfusion*. 1995;35:734–737.
188. Goldman M, Savard R, Long A, et al. Declining value of preoperative autologous donation. *Transfusion*. 2002;42:819–823.
189. Horowitz NS, Gibb RK, Menegakis NE, et al. Utility and cost effectiveness of preoperative autologous blood donation in gynecologic and gynecologic oncology patients. *Obstet Gynecol*. 2002;5:771–776.
190. Shander A, Rijhwani TS. Acute normovolemic hemodilution. *Transfusion*. 2004;44:26S–34S.
191. Monk TG, Goodnough LT, Brecher ME, et al. A prospective randomized comparison of three blood conservation strategies for radical prostatectomy. *Anesthesiology*. 1999;91:24–33.
192. Goodnough LT, Despotis GJ, Merkel K, et al. A randomized trial comparing acute normovolemic hemodilution and preoperative autologous blood donation in total hip arthroplasty. *Transfusion*. 2000;40:1054–1057.
193. Naunheim KS, Bridges CR, Sade RM. Should a Jehovah's Witness patient who faces imminent exsanguination be transfused? *Ann Thorac Surg*. 2011;92(5):1559–1564.
194. Aapro M, Jelkmann W, Constantinescu SN, et al. Effects of erythropoietin receptors and erythropoiesis-stimulating agents on disease progression in cancer. *Br J Cancer*. 2012;106(7):124.
195. Arnold A, Aitchison LP, Abbott J. Preoperative mechanical bowel preparation for abdominal, laparoscopic and vaginal surgery: a systematic review. *J Minim Invasive Gynecol*. 2015;22:737–752.
196. Guenaga KF, Matos D, Wille-Jorgensen P. Mechanical bowel preparation for elective colorectal surgery. *Cochrane Database Syst Rev*. 2011;(9):CD001544.
197. Toneva, FD, Deierhoi RJ, Morris M, et al. Oral antibiotic bowel preparation reduces length of stay and readmissions after colorectal surgery. *J Am Coll Surg*. 2013;216:756–762.
198. Bretagnol F, Panis Y, Rullier P, et al. Rectal cancer surgery with or without bowel preparation: the French FRECCAR III multicenter single-blinded randomized trial. *Ann Surg*. 2010;252:863e8.
199. Barber EL, van Le L. Enhanced recovery pathways in gynecology and gynecologic oncology. *Obstet Gynecol Survey*. 2015:70(12):780–792.
200. Brady M, Kinn S, Stuart P. Preoperative fasting for adults to prevent perioperative complication. *Cochrane Database Syst Rev*. 2003;(4):CD004423.
201. American Society of Anesthesiologists. Practice guidelines for preoperative fasting and the use of pharmacologic agents to reduce the risk of pulmonary aspiration: application to health patients undergoing elective procedures; a report by the American Society of Anesthesiologists Task Force on Preoperative Fasting. *Anesthesiology*. 1999:90:896–905.
202. Noblett SE, Watson DS, Huong H, et al. Pre-operative oral carbohydrate loading in colorectal surgery: a randomized controlled trial. *Colorectal Dis*. 2006;8:563–569.
203. Bratzler DW, Dellinger EP, Olsen KM, et al. Clinical practice guidelines for antimicrobial prophylaxis in surgery. *Surg Infect (Larchmt)*. 2013;14:73.

204. Malone DL, Genuit T, Tracy JK, et al. Surgical site infections: reanalysis of risk factors. *J Surg Res*. 2002;103:89–95.
205. Bratzler DW, Houck PM. Antimicrobial prophylaxis for surgery: an advisory statement from the National Surgical Infection Prevention Project. *Am J Surg*. 2005;189:395–404.
206. ACOG Practice Bulletin No.74: antibiotic prophylaxis for gynecologic procedures. *Obstet Gynecol*. 2006;108:225–234.
207. Antimicrobial prophylaxis for surgery. *Treat Guidel Med Lett*. 2006;4:83–88.
208. ASHP therapeutic guidelines on antimicrobial prophylaxis in surgery. *Am J Health Syst Pharm*. 1999;56:1839–1888.
209. Itani K, Wilson S, Awad S, et al. Ertapenem versus cefotetan prophylaxis in elective colorectal surgery. *N Engl J Med*. 2006;355:2640–2651.
210. Ingraham AM, Cohen ME, Bilimoria KY, et al. Association of surgical care improvement project infection-related process measure compliance with risk-adjusted outcomes: implications for quality measurement. *J Am Coll Surg*. 2010;211(6):705–714.
211. Kirkland KB, Briggs JP, Trivette L, et al. The impact of surgical-site infections in the 1990s: attributable mortality, excess length of hospitalization, and extra costs. *Infect Control Hosp Epidemiol*. 1999;20:725–730.
212. Perencevich EN, Sands KE, Cosgrove SE, et al. Health and economic impact of surgical site infections diagnosed after hospital discharge. *Emerg Infect Dis*. 2003;9:196–203.
213. Webster J, Osborne S. Preoperative bathing or showering with skin antiseptics to prevent surgical site infection. *Cochrane Database Syst Rev*. 2007;(2):CD004985. doi:10.1002/14651858. CD004985.pub3.
214. Tanner J, Woodings D, Moncaster K. Preoperative hair removal to reduce surgical site infection. *Cochrane Database Syst Rev*. 2006;(3):CD004122. doi:10.1002/14651858.CD004122.pub3.
215. Bratzler DW, Hunt DR. The surgical infection prevention and surgical care improvement projects: national initiatives to improve outcomes of patients having surgery. *Clin Infect Dis*. 2006;43:322–330.
216. Koenig SM. Pulmonary complications of obesity. *Am J Med Sci*. 2001;321:249–279.
217. Haslam DW, James WP. Obesity. *Lancet*. 2005;366:1197–1209.
218. Gaszynski T. Anesthetic complications of gross obesity. *Curr Opin Anaesthesiol*. 2004;17:271–276.
219. Hopkins MP, Shriner AM, Parker MG, et al. Panniculectomy at the time of gynecologic surgery in morbidly obese patients. *Am J Obstet Gynecol*. 2000;182:1502–1505.
220. Pearl ML, Valea FA, Disilvestro PA, et al. Panniculectomy in morbidly obese gynecologic oncology patients. *Int J Surg Invest*. 2000;2:59–64.
221. Tillmanns TD, Kamelle SA, Abudayyeh I, et al. Panniculectomy with simultaneous gynecologic oncology surgery. *Gynecol Oncol*. 2001;83:518–522.
222. Marik PE, Monnet X, Teboul JL. Hemodynamic parameters to guide fluid therapy. *Ann Intensive Care*. 2011;1(1):1.
223. Eisner RF, Montz FJ, Berek JS. Cytoreductive surgery for advanced ovarian cancer: cardiovascular evaluation with pulmonary artery catheter. *Gynecol Oncol*. 1990;37:11.
224. McGee WT, Mailloux P, Jodka P, et al. The pulmonary artery catheter in critical care. *Semin Dial*. 2006;19:480–491.
225. McGee WT. A simple physiologic algorithm for managing hemodynamics using stroke volume and stroke volume variation: physiologic optimization program. *J Intensive Care Med*. 2009;24:352–360.
226. Marik PE. Noninvasive cardiac output monitors: a state-of the- art review. *J Cardiothorac Vasc Anesth*. 2013;27:121–134.
227. Thygesen K, Alpert JS, White HD; for the Joint ESC/ACCF/AHA/WHF Task Force for the Redefinition of Myocardial Infarction. Universal definition of myocardial infarction. *J Am Coll Cardiol*. 2007;50:2173–2195.
228. Thygesen K, Alpert JS, White HD, for the Joint ESC/ACCF/AHA/WHF Task Force for the Redefinition of Myocardial Infarction. Universal definition of myocardial infarction. *J Am Coll Cardiol*. 2007;50:2173–2195.
229. Ho K, Pinsky JL, Kannel WB, et al. The epidemiology of heart failure: the Framingham Study. *J Am Coll Cardiol*. 1993;22:6A–13A.
230. Zaloga GP, Prielipp RC, Butterworth JF, et al. Pharmacologic cardiovascular support. *Crit Care Clin*. 1993;9:335–362.
231. Overgaard CB, Dzavik V. Inotropes and vasopressors. Review of physiology and clinical use in cardiovascular disease. *Circulation*. 2008;188:1047–1056.
232. Chiolero R, Flatt JP, Revelly JP, et al. Effects of catecholamines on oxygen consumption and oxygen delivery in critically ill patients. *Chest*. 1991;100:1676–1684.
233. Sharman A, Lowe J. Vasopressin and its role in critical care. *Contin Educ Anaesth Crit Care Pain*. 2008;8(4):134–137.
234. Yancy CW, Jessup M, Bozkurt B, et al. 2013 ACCF/AHA guideline for the management of heart failure: executive summary: a report of the American College of Cardiology Foundation/American Heart Association Task Force on practice guidelines. *Circulation*. 2013;128:1810.
235. Samarendra P, Mangione MP. Aortic stenosis and perioperative risk with noncardiac surgery. *J Am Coll Cardiol*. 2015;65(3):295–302.
236. Torsher LC, Shub C, Rettke SR, et al. Risk of patients with severe aortic stenosis undergoing noncardiac surgery. *Am J Cardiol*. 1998;81:448–452.
237. Wilson W, Taubert KA, Gewitz M, et al. Prevention of infective endocarditis: guidelines from the American Heart Association: a guideline from the American Heart Association Rheumatic Fever, Endocarditis, and Kawasaki Disease Committee, Council on Cardiovascular Disease in the Young, and the Council on Clinical Cardiology, Council on Cardiovascular Surgery and Anesthesia, and the Quality of Care and Outcomes Research Interdisciplinary Working Group. *Circulation*. 2007;116(15):1736–1754.
238. Nishimura RA, Clase A, Carabello DP, et al. ACC/AHA 2008 guideline update on valvular heart disease: focused update on infective endocarditis. *Circulation*. 2008;118:887–896.
239. Allen U. Infective endocarditis: updated guidelines. *Can J Infect Dis Med Microbiol*. 2010;21(2):74–77.
240. Christians KK, Wu B, Quebbeman EJ, et al. Postoperative atrial fibrillation in noncardiothoracic surgical patients. *Am J Surg*. 2001;182:713–715.
241. Balser JR, Martinez EA, Winters BD, et al. Beta-adrenergic blockade accelerates conversion of postoperative supraventricular tachyarrhythmias. *Anesthesiology*. 1998;89:1052–1059.
242. January CT, Wann L, Alpert JS, et al. 2014 AHA/ACC/HRS guideline for the management of patients with atrial fibrillation: Executive summary: A report of the American College of Cardiology/American Heart Association Task Force on practice guidelines and the Heart Rhythm Society. *J Am Coll Cardiol*. 2014;64(21):2246–2280.
243. Mehta S, Heffer MJ, Maham N, et al. Impact of endotracheal tube size on preextubation respiratory variables. *J Crit Care*. 2010;25(3):483–488.
244. Banner MJ, Jaeger MJ, Kirby RR. Components of the work of breathing and implications for monitoring ventilator-dependent patients. *Crit Care Med*. 1994;22:515–518.
245. Stewart T, Meade M, Cook D, et al. Evaluation of a ventilation strategy to prevent barotrauma in patients at high risk for acute respiratory distress syndrome. *N Engl J Med*. 1998;338:356–361.
246. Amoto M, Barbas C, Medeiros D, et al. Effect of a protective-ventilation strategy on mortality in the acute respiratory distress syndrome. *N Engl J Med*. 1998;338:347–354.
247. Lodat R. Oxygen toxicity. *Crit Care Clin*. 1990;6:749–765.
248. Yang KL, Tobin MJ. A prospective study of indexes predicting the outcome of trials of weaning from mechanical ventilation. *N Engl J Med*. 1991;324:1445–1450.
249. Rosenberg AL, Dechert RE, Park PK, et al. Review of a large clinical series: association of cumulative fluid balance on outcome in acute lung injury: a retrospective review of the ARDSnet tidal volume study cohort. *J Intensive Care Med*. 2009;24(1):35–46.
250. Bernard G, Artigas A, Brigham KL, et al. Report of the American-European Consensus Conference on acute respiratory distress syndrome: definitions, mechanisms, relevant outcomes, and clinical trial coordination. Consensus Committee. *J Crit Care*. 1994;9:72–81.
251. Luce J. Acute lung injury and the acute respiratory distress syndrome. *Crit Care Med*. 1998;26:369–376.
252. Marshall J, Cook D, Christou N, et al. Multiple organ dysfunction score: a reliable descriptor of a complex clinical outcome. *Crit Care Med*. 1995;23:1638–1652.
253. Artigas A, Bernard GR, Carlet J, et al. The American-European Consensus Conference on ARDS, part 2: Ventilatory, pharmacologic, supportive therapy, study design strategies, and issues related to recovery and remodeling. Acute respiratory distress syndrome. *Am J Respir Crit Care Med*. 1998;157(4 pt 1):1332–1347.
254. The Acute Respiratory Distress Syndrome Network. Ventilation with lower tidal volumes as compared with traditional tidal volumes for acute lung injury and the acute respiratory distress syndrome. *N Engl J Med*. 2000;342:1301–1308.
255. Chastre J, Fagon JY. Ventilator-associated pneumonia. *Am J Respir Crit Care Med*. 2002;165:867–903.
256. Guyatt GH, Akl EA, Crowther M, et al. Executive summary. Antithrombotic therapy and prevention of thrombosis, 9th Ed: American College of Chest Physicians evidence-based clinical practice guidelines. *Chest*. 2012;141(2):7s–47s.
257. Clarke-Pearson DL, Synan IS, et al. The natural history of postoperative venous thromboemboli in gynecologic oncology: a prospective study of 382 patients. *Am J Obstet Gynecol*. 1984;148:1051–1054.

258. Clarke-Pearson DL, Dodge RK, et al. Venous thromboembolism prophylaxis: patients at high risk to fail intermittent pneumatic compression. *Obstet Gynecol.* 2003;101:157–163.
259. Collins R, Scrimgeour A, Yusuf S, et al. Reduction in fatal pulmonary embolism and venous thrombosis by perioperative administration of subcutaneous heparin. Overview of results of randomized trials in general, orthopedic, and urologic surgery. *N Engl J Med.* 1988;318:1162.
260. Kearon C, Akl EA, Ornelas J, et al. Antithrombotic therapy for VTE disease: CHEST guideline and expert panel report. *Chest.* 2016;149(2):315–352.
261. Pestana C. *Fluids and Electrolytes in the Surgical Patient.* 4th Ed. Baltimore, MD: Lippincott Williams & Wilkins; 1989.
262. Vanatta JC, Fogelman MJ, eds. *Moyer's Fluid Balance: A Clinical Manual.* 2nd Ed. Chicago, IL: Year Book; 1976.
263. Wait RB, Kahng KU, Dresner LS. Fluids and electrolytes and acid-base balance. In: Greenfield LJ, Mulholland M, Oldham KT, et al. eds. *Surgery: Scientific Principles and Practice.* 2nd Ed. Philadelphia, PA: Lippincott–Raven Publishers; 1997:242–266.
264. Brandstrup B, Tonnesen H, Beier-Holgersen R, et al. Effects of intravenous fluid restriction on postoperative complications; comparison of two perioperative fluid regimens: a randomized assessor-blinded multicenter trial. *Ann Surg.* 2003;238:641–648.
265. Rahbari NN, Zimmermann JB, Schmidt T, et al. Meta-analysis of standard, restrictive and supplemental fluid administration in colorectal surgery. *Br J Surg.* 2009;96(4):331–341.
266. Lowe RJ, Moss GS, Jilek J, et al. Crystalloid versus colloid in the etiology of pulmonary failure after trauma. A randomized trial in man. *Surgery.* 1977;81:676–683.
267. Virgilio RW, Rice CL, Smith DE, et al. Crystalloid versus colloid resuscitation: is one better? A randomized clinical study. *Surgery.* 1979;85:129–139.
268. Weinstein PD, Doerfler ME. Systemic complications of fluid resuscitation. *Crit Care Clin.* 1992;8:439–448.
269. Metildi LA, Shackford SR, Virgilio RW, et al. Crystalloid versus colloid in fluid resuscitation of patients with severe pulmonary insufficiency. *Surg Gynecol Obstet.* 1984;158:207–212.
270. Rizoli SB. Crystalloids and colloids in trauma resuscitation: a brief overview of the current debate. *J Trauma.* 2003;54(Suppl 5):S82–S88.
271. Alderson P, Schierhout G, Roberts I, et al. Colloids versus crystalloids for fluid resuscitation in critically ill patients. *Cochrane Database Syst Rev.* 2000;(2):CD000567.
272. Choi PT, Yip G, Quinonez LG, et al. Crystalloids vs. colloids in fluid resuscitation: a systematic review. *Crit Care Med.* 1999;27:200–210.
273. Roberts JS, Bratton SL. Colloid volume expanders. Problems, pitfalls and possibilities. *Drugs.* 1998;55:621–630.
274. Berenson JR. Treatment of hypercalcemia of malignancy with bisphosphonates. *Semin Oncol.* 2002;29(Suppl 21):12–18.
275. Mundy GR. Hypercalcemia. In: Mundy GR, ed. *Bone Remodeling and Its Disorders.* 2nd Ed. London, England: Martin Dunitz; 1999:107–122.
276. Major P, Lortholary A, Hon J, et al. Zolendronic acid is superior to pamidronate in the treatment of hypercalcemia of malignancy: a pooled analysis of two randomized, controlled clinical trials. *J Clin Oncol.* 2001;19:558–567.
277. Pearl ML, Frandina M, Mahler L, et al. A randomized controlled trial of a regular diet as the first meal in gynecologic oncology patients undergoing intraabdominal surgery. *Obstet Gynecol.* 2002;100:230–234.
278. Pearl ML, Valea FA, Fischer M, et al. A randomized controlled trial of early postoperative feeding in gynecologic oncology patients undergoing intra-abdominal surgery. *Obstet Gynecol.* 1998;92:94–97.
279. Cutillo G, Maneschi F, Franchi M, et al. Early feeding compared with nasogastric decompression after major oncologic gynecologic surgery: a randomized study. *Obstet Gynecol.* 1999;93:41–45.
280. MacMillan SL, Kammerer-Doak D, Rogers RG, et al. Early feeding and the incidence of gastrointestinal symptoms after major gynecologic surgery. *Obstet Gynecol.* 2000;96:604–608.
281. Steed HL, Capstick V, Flood C, et al. A randomized controlled trial of early versus "traditional" postoperative oral intake after major abdominal gynecologic surgery. *Am J Obstet Gynecol.* 2002;186:861–865.
282. Schilder JM, Hurteau JA, Look KY, et al. A prospective controlled trial of early postoperative oral intake following major abdominal gynecologic surgery. *Gynecol Oncol.* 1997;67:235–240.
283. Souba WW, Austen WG Jr. Nutrition and metabolism. In: Greenfield LJ, Mulholland M, Oldham KT, et al. eds. *Surgery: Scientific Principles and Practice.* 2nd Ed. Philadelphia, PA: Lippincott–Raven Publishers; 1997:42–67.
284. Marik PE, Zaloga GP. Early enteral nutrition in acutely ill patients: a systematic review. *Crit Care Med.* 2001;29:2264–2270.
285. Morrow CP, Curtin JP. *Gynecologic Cancer Surgery.* New York, NY: Churchill Livingstone; 1996:194–205.
286. Blackburn GL, Bistrian BR, Moini BS, et al. Nutritional and metabolic assessment of the hospitalized patient. *JPEN J Parenter Enteral Nutr.* 1977;1:11–22.
287. Kellum JA, Lameire N. Diagnosis, evaluation and management of acute kidney injury: a KIDGO summary (part 1). *Critical Care.* 2013;17:204.
288. Thakkar C. Perioperative acute kidney injury. *Adv Chronic Kidney Dis.* 2013;20(1):67–75.
289. Vaught AJ, Ozrazgat-Baslant T, Javed A, et al. Acute kidney injury in major gynaecological surgery: an observational study. *BJOG.* 2015;122:1340–1348.
290. Hoste EA, Clermont G, Kersten A, et al. RIFLE criteria for acute kidney injury are associated with hospital mortality in critically ill patients: a cohort analysis. *Critical Care.* 2006;10:R73.
291. Uchino S, Bellomo R, Goldsmith D, et al. An assessment of the RIFLE criteria for acute renal failure in hospitalized patients. *Crit Care Med.* 2006;34:1913–1917.
292. Lameire N. The definitions and staging systems of acute kidney injury and their limitations in practice. *Arab J Nephrol Transplant.* 2013;6(3):145–152.
293. Bellomo R, Ronco C, Kellum J, et al. Acute Dialysis Quality Initiative workgroup. Acute renal failure: definitions, outcome measures, animal models, fluid therapy and information technology need: the Second International Consensus Conference of the Acute Dialysis Quality Initiative (ADQI) Group. *Crit Care.* 2004;8(4):R204–R212.
294. Mehta RL, Kellum JA, Shah SV, et al. Acute kidney injury network: report of an initiative to improve outcomes in acute kidney injury. *Crit Care.* 2007;11(2):R31.
295. Kidney Disease: Improving Global Outcomes (KDIGO) Acute Kidney Injury Work Group. KDIGO clinical practice guidelines for acute kidney injury. *Kidney Int.* 2012;2(Suppl 1):1–138.
296. Klausner JM, Paterson IS, Goldman G, et al. Postischemic renal injury is mediated by neutrophils and leukotrienes. *Am J Physiol.* 1989;256(5 pt 2):F794–F802.
297. Kribben A, Edelstein CL, Schrier RW. Pathophysiology of acute renal failure. *J Nephrol.* 1999;12(Suppl 2):S142–S151.
298. Prins JM, Buller HR, Kuijper EJ, et al. Once versus thrice daily gentamicin in patients with serious infections. *Lancet.* 1993;341(8841):335–339.
299. Murphy SW, Barrett BJ, Parfrey PS. Contrast nephropathy. *J Am Soc Nephrol.* 2000;11:177–182.
300. Rudnick MR, Berns JS, Cohen RM, et al. Contrast media-associated nephrotoxicity. *Semin Nephrol.* 1997;17:15–26.
301. McCullough PA, Wolyn R, Rocher LL, et al. Acute renal failure after coronary intervention: incidence, risk factors and relationship to mortality. *Am J Med.* 1997;103:368–375.
302. Edwards BF. Postoperative renal insufficiency. *Med Clin North Am.* 2001;85:1241–1254.
303. Baldwin L, Henderson A, Hickman P. Effect of postoperative low-dose dopamine on renal function after elective major vascular surgery. *Ann Intern Med.* 1994;120:744–747.
304. Dishart MK, Kellum JA. An evaluation of pharmacological strategies for the prevention and treatment of acute renal failure. *Drugs.* 2000;59:79–91.
305. Lassnigg A, Donner E, Grubhofer G, et al. Lack of renoprotective effects of dopamine and furosemide during cardiac surgery. *J Am Soc Nephrol.* 2000;11:97–104.
306. Marik PE, Iglesias J. Low-dose dopamine does not prevent acute renal failure in patients with septic shock and oliguria. NORASEPT II Study Investigators. *Am J Med.* 1999;107:387–390.
307. Sirivella S, Gielchinsky I, Parsonnet V. Mannitol, furosemide and dopamine infusion in postoperative renal failure complicating cardiac surgery. *Ann Thorac Surg.* 2000;69:501–506.
308. Allgren RL, Marbury TC, Rahman SM, et al. Anaritide in acute tubular necrosis. Auriculin Anaritide Acute Renal Failure Study Group. *N Engl J Med.* 1997;336:828–834.
309. The SAFE Study Investigators. A comparison of albumin and saline for fluid resuscitation in the intensive care unit. *N Engl J Med.* 2004;350:2247–2256.
310. Roswell SE, Barbosa RR, Diggs BS, et al. Effect of high product ratio massive transfusion on mortality in blunt and penetrating trauma patients. *J Trauma.* 2011;71(2 Suppl 3):S353–S357.
311. Dellinger RP, Levy MM, et al. Surviving sepsis Campaign: international guidelines for management of severe sepsis and septic shock: 2008. *Crit Care Med.* 2008;36:1394–1396.

312. National Nosocomial Infections Surveillance (NNIS). System report, data summary from January 1992 through June 2004, issued October 2004. *Am J Infect Control*. 2004;32:470–485.
313. Vincent JL, Rello J, Marshall J, et al. International study of the prevalence and outcomes of infection in intensive care units. *JAMA*. 2009;302(21):2323.
314. Ostrosky-Zeichner L, Pappas PG. Invasive candidiasis in the intensive care unit. *Crit Care Med*. 2006;34:857–863.
315. Pappas PG, Rex JH, Sobel JD, et al. Guidelines for treatment of candidiasis. *Clin Infect Dis*. 2004;38:161–189.
316. Crabtree TD, Pelletier SJ, Antevil JL, et al. Cohort study of fever and leukocytosis as diagnostic and prognostic indicators in infected surgical patients. *World J Surg*. 2001;25:739–744.
317. Jaramillo EJ, Trevino JM, Berghoff KR, et al. Bedside diagnostic laparoscopy in the intensive care unit: a 13-year experience. *JSLS*. 2006;10:155–159.
318. Cinat ME, Wilson SE, Din AM. Determinants of successful percutaneous image-guided drainage of intra-abdominal abscess. *Arch Surg*. 2002;137:845–849.
319. Garvais DA, Ho CH, O'Neill MJ, et al. Recurrent abdominal and pelvic abscesses: incidence, results of repeated percutaneous drainage, and underlying causes in 956 drainages. *Am J Roentgenol*. 2004;182:463–466.
320. Kok KY, Yapp SK. Laparoscopic drainage of postoperative complicated intra-abdominal abscess. *Surg Laparosc Endosc Percutan Tech*. 2000;10:311–313.
321. Schecter WP, Ivatury RR, Rotondo MF, et al. Open abdomen after trauma and abdominal sepsis: a strategy for management. *J Am Coll Surg*. 2006;203:390–396.
322. Marshall JC, Maier RV, Jimenez M, et al. Source control in the management of severe sepsis and septic shock: an evidence-based review. *Crit Care Med*. 2004;32(Suppl 11):S513–S526.
323. Aird WC. The role of endothelium in severe sepsis and multiple organ dysfunction syndrome. *Blood*. 2003;101:3765–3777.
324. Levy MM, Fink MP, Marshall JC, et al. 2001 SCCM/ESICM/ACCP/ATS/SIS International Sepsis Definitions Conference. *Crit Care Med*. 2003;31:1250–1256.
325. Shorr AF, Tabak YP, Killian AD, et al. Healthcare-associated bloodstream infection: a distinct entity? Insights from a large U.S. database. *Crit Care Med*. 2006;34:2588–2595.
326. Angus DC, Linde-Zwirble WT, Lidicker J, et al. Epidemiology of severe sepsis in the United States: analysis of incidence, outcome, and associated costs of care. *Crit Care Med*. 2001;29:1303–1310.
327. Martí-Carvajal AJ, Solà I, Lathyris D, et al. Human recombinant activated protein C for severe sepsis. *Cochrane Database Sys Rev*. 2012;(3):CD004388.
328. Bernard GR, Vincent JL, Laterre PF, et al. Efficacy and safety of recombinant human activated protein C for severe sepsis. *N Engl J Med*. 2001;344:699–709.
329. Xigris [drotrecogin alfa (activated)]: market withdrawal–failure to show survival benefit, 2011. http://www.fda.gov/Drugs/DrugSafety/ucm277114.htm. Accessed September 13, 2016.
330. American College of Chest Physicians/Society of Critical Care Medicine Consensus Conference. Definitions for sepsis and organ failure and guidelines for the use of innovative therapies in sepsis. *Crit Care Med*. 1992;20:864–874.
331. Vincent JL, de Mendonca A, Cantraine F, et al. Use of the SOFA score to assess the incidence of organ dysfunction/failure in intensive care units: results of a multicenter, prospective study. Working group on "sepsis-related problems" of the European Society of Intensive Care Medicine. *Crit Care Med*. 1998;26:1793–1800.
332. Zimmerman JE, Kramer AA, McNair DS, et al. Acute Physiology and Chronic Health Evaluation (APACHE) IV: Hospital mortality assessment for today's critically ill patients. *Crit Care Med*. 2006;34:1297–1310.
333. Levy MM, Macias WL, Vincent JL, et al. Early changes in organ function predict eventual survival in severe sepsis. *Crit Care Med*. 2005;33:2194–2201.
334. Vidal MG, Ruiz Weisser J, Gonzalez F, et al. Incidence and clinical effects of intra-abdominal hypertension in critically ill patients. *Crit Care Med*. 2008;36(6):1823.
335. Society of Critical Care Medicine and American Society of Health-System Pharmacists. Clinical practice guidelines for the sustained use of sedatives and analgesics in the critically ill adult. *Am J Health Syst Pharm*. 2002;59:150–178.
336. Society of Critical Care Medicine and American Society of Health-System Pharmacists. Clinical practice guidelines for sustained neuromuscular blockade in the adult critically ill patient. *Am J Health Syst Pharm*. 2002;59:179–195.
337. Epstein J, Breslow MJ. The stress response of critical illness. *Crit Care Clin*. 1999;15:17–33.
338. Kress JP, Gehlbach B, Lacy M, et al. The long-term psychological effects of daily sedative interruption on critically ill patients. *Am J Respir Crit Care Med*. 2003;168:1457–1461.
339. Kress JP, Pohlman AS, O'Connor MF, et al. Daily interruption of sedative infusions in critically ill patients undergoing mechanical ventilation. *N Engl J Med*. 2000;342:1471–1477.
340. Cammarano WB, Pittet JF, Weitz S, et al. Acute withdrawal syndrome related to the administration of analgesic and sedative medications in adult intensive care unit patients. *Crit Care Med*. 1998;26:676–684.
341. Bird SJ. Diagnosis and management of critical illness polyneuropathy and critical illness myopathy. *Curr Treat Options Neurol*. 2007;9:85–92.
342. McKegney FP. The intensive care syndrome. The definition, treatment and prevention of a new "disease of medical progress." *Conn Med*. 1966;30:633–636.
343. McGuire BE, Basten CJ, Ryan CJ, et al. Intensive care unit syndrome: a dangerous misnomer. *Arch Intern Med*. 2000;160:906–909.
344. Ely EW, Inouye SK, Bernard GR, et al. Delirium in mechanically ventilated patients: validity and reliability of the confusion assessment method for the intensive care unit (CAM-ICU). *JAMA*. 2001;286:2703–2710.
345. Thomason J, Shintani A, Peterson J, et al. Intensive care unit delirium is an independent predictor of longer hospital stay: a prospective study of 261 nonventilated patients. *Crit Care*. 2005;94:R375–R381.
346. Way J, Back AL, Curtis JR. Withdrawing life support and resolution of conflict with families. *BMJ*. 2002;325:1342–1345.
347. Nelson JE, Azoulay E, Curtis JR, et al. Palliative care in the ICU. *J Palliat Med*. 2012;15(2):168–174.

CHAPTER 9

Surgical Principles in Gynecologic Oncology

Yukio Sonoda, David Cibula, Denis Querleu, Eric Leblanc, and Oliver Zivanovic

Treatment of gynecologic malignancies involves multimodal therapy. Surgery may be the only mode of therapy required for some early gynecologic cancers; however, the majority of gynecologic malignancies require a combination of surgery with chemotherapy and/or irradiation.

This chapter will review the principles of surgery as a separate discipline and as an integral part of multimodal therapeutic planning. Specific operations and novel surgical techniques are discussed, but many procedures are addressed more completely in surgical texts and atlases (1–3). This textbook is also accompanied by narrated videos on a wide variety of surgical procedures. The role of surgical intervention in the treatment of gynecologic cancers is addressed herein with a more philosophic approach than would be taken in a surgical atlas. Key illustrations and tips are included that have enabled us to approach various radical procedures more confidently and safely. The focus of this chapter is to provide the reader with an appreciation and understanding of the surgical principles of the subspecialty of gynecologic oncology and the incorporation of minimally invasive surgery.

TECHNICAL ASPECTS OF SURGERY

Mastering the skills of surgery involves a thorough understanding of proper technique as well as knowledge of surgical anatomy. Maintaining sound technique requires consistent practice to keep surgical maneuvers well honed. This entails a sufficient case load to ensure adequate practice of the techniques while minimizing associated complications. The surgeon should also keep abreast of new technical developments and be able to modify his or her technique to incorporate these developments. A prime example has been the rapid growth of minimally invasive surgery and now robotics in gynecologic oncology.

Anatomy

Knowledge of anatomy is the basis for mastering surgery. Although gynecologic malignancies originate in the pelvis, the gynecologic oncologist must be completely familiar with the pelvis, abdomen, retroperitoneum, and the lymphatic drainage of the female genital tract because gynecologic cancers can affect all of these areas.

Lymphatic drainage from the cervix follows the uterine arteries and cardinal ligaments to the pelvic lymph nodes that include the external iliac, internal iliac (hypogastric), and obturator node groups (**Fig. 9.1**). From these pelvic lymph nodes, the drainage proceeds superiorly through the common iliac and presacral lymph nodes and then up to the para-aortic nodes.

The lymphatic drainage from both the uterine corpus and the ovaries follows one of three routes (**Fig. 9.1**): (a) along the uterine arteries in the broad ligaments to the pelvic nodes, (b) in channels following the round ligaments to the inguinal lymph nodes, or (c) along the ovarian lymphatics in the infundibulopelvic ligaments directly up to the para-aortic nodes.

The anatomy of the para-aortic lymph nodes has been well described by Fowler and Johnson (4). The para-aortic lymph nodes are part of the lumbar lymph node group. Usually, six subgroups of retroperitoneal nodes in the para-aortic region are recognized: paracaval, retrocaval, interaorto-caval, preaortic, para-aortic (left side), and retroaortic. The preaortic group drains the abdominal part of the gastrointestinal tract down to the mid rectum, whereas the retrocaval and retroaortic groups have no special area of drainage. The paracaval, interaorto-caval, and para-aortic (left side) receive lymphatic drainage from the iliac lymph nodes, ovaries, and other pelvic viscera (apart from the alimentary tract), and therefore it is these groups of nodes that are sampled in the surgical staging of gynecologic malignancies. However, systematic para-aortic lymphadenectomy should address all major regions, including paracaval, retrocaval, interaorto-caval, preaortic, para-aortic and retroaortic nodes.

There are typically 15 to 20 paracaval and para-aortic nodes per side. They are located adjacent to the inferior vena cava (IVC) and aorta, anterior to the lumbar spine, extending bilaterally to the medial margins of the psoas major muscles, and up to the diaphragmatic crura (4). The paracaval and para-aortic nodes usually dissected in gynecologic oncology span the region from the aortic bifurcation up to either the inferior mesenteric artery (IMA) or the renal veins.

The first major blood vessel encountered during a caudad-to-cephalad para-aortic node dissection is the IMA (**Fig. 9.1**). The IMA originates from the anterior surface of the aorta approximately 3 to 4 cm above the aortic bifurcation. Next, the right and left ovarian arteries arise from their respective sides of the aorta about 5 to 6 cm above the bifurcation (**Fig. 9.1**). The right ovarian vein inserts into the right side of the IVC approximately 1 cm below the right renal vein. The left ovarian vein does not insert directly into the IVC, but rather follows a path close to the left ureter inserting into the left renal vein lateral to the left border of the aorta. Three to four pairs of lumbar arteries and veins arise from the posterior surfaces of the aorta and IVC, respectively.

The gynecologic oncologist who operates on patients with advanced ovarian carcinoma often encounters disease spread involving upper abdominal structures such as the diaphragm, liver, pancreas, and spleen. Debulking of tumor from these areas has been demonstrated to improve the rate of optimal cytoreduction and subsequent survival (5,6). Anatomic considerations for diaphragm surgery include the relevant hepatic attachments and the underlying central vasculature (7,8) (**Fig. 9.2**). The anterior hepatic attachment is the falciform ligament, which contains the ligamentum teres in its infrahepatic portion, and attaches the liver to the anterior abdominal wall in its membranous hepatic portion. As the falciform ligament continues superiorly, its peritoneal surface divides laterally on each side to form the anterior right and left coronary ligaments. These coronary ligaments reflect off the liver capsule and delineate the posterior extent of peritoneum covering the superior diaphragm. The IVC lies to the right side of this falciform ligament division. The right and left hepatic veins drain into the anterior surface of the IVC at the level of this peritoneal reflection. The anterior coronary ligaments continue laterally and inferiorly along the posterior liver edge, where they join the posterior right and left coronary ligaments to form the right and left triangular ligaments, respectively. The right triangular ligament reflects from the liver to the diaphragm, right kidney, and right adrenal gland. The left triangular ligament reflects primarily to the diaphragm; the posterior left coronary ligament lies higher than the esophageal hiatus and the

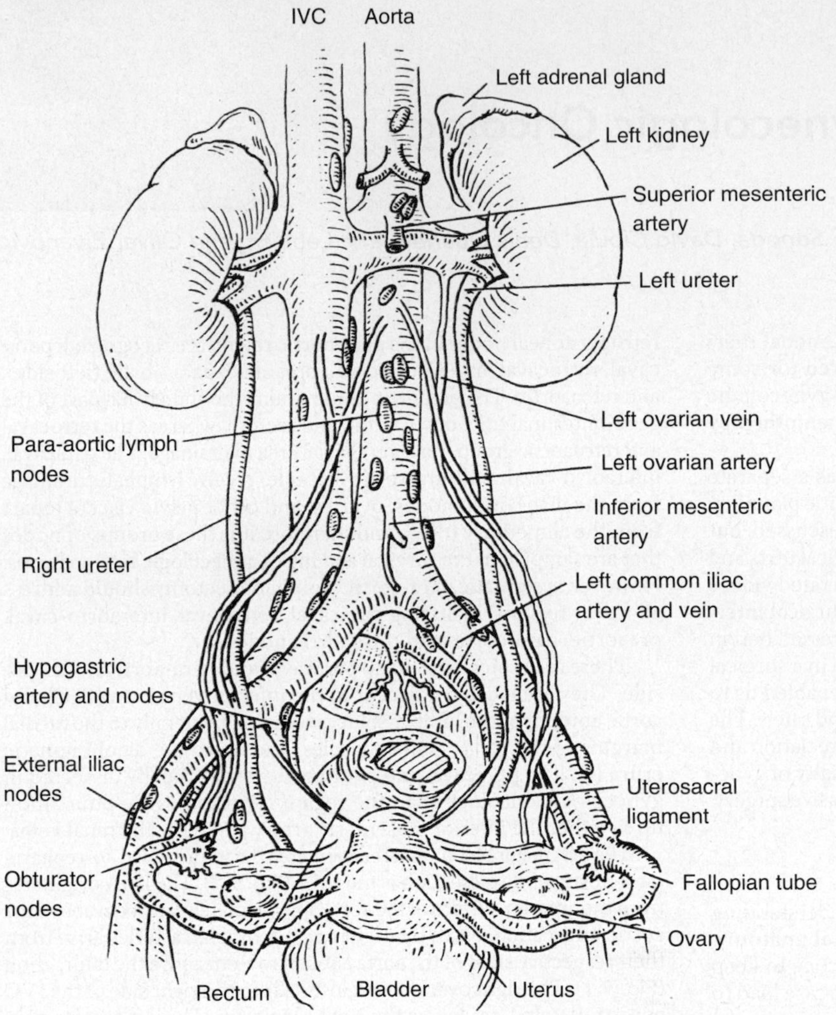

Figure 9.1. The pelvic and para-aortic lymph nodes and their relationship to the major retroperitoneal vessels.

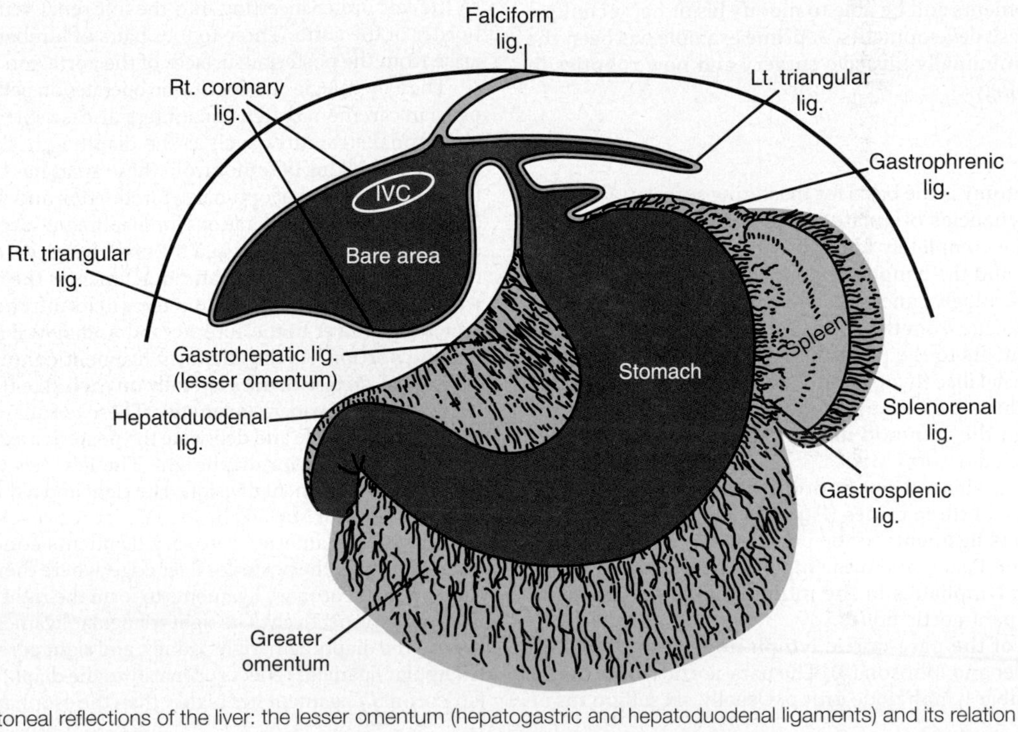

Figure 9.2. Peritoneal reflections of the liver: the lesser omentum (hepatogastric and hepatoduodenal ligaments) and its relation to the coronary ligament of the liver and diaphragm.

Source: Reprinted with permission from Skandalakis JE, Gray SW, Rowe JR, eds. *Anatomical Complications in General Surgery.* New York, NY: McGraw-Hill; 1983.

esophagus is generally not encountered. The coronary ligaments on each side delineate the larger "bare area" of the liver on the right and a smaller "bare area" on the left, which underlie the central tendon of the diaphragm. The right phrenic nerve penetrates this central tendon lateral to the vena caval foramen on the right and is usually not encountered until the "bare area" is exposed. The left phrenic nerve may penetrate the left diaphragm muscle above the central tendon and is a consideration during left-sided anterior diaphragm surgery.

In the left upper quadrant of the abdomen, the spleen lies under the 9th, 10th, and 11th ribs. It is situated adjacent and slightly deep to the stomach and colon, lateral to the pancreas, and sits on the superior aspect of the left kidney. The posterior aspect of the spleen is in contact with the adrenal gland as well as Gerota fascia of the kidney. The tail of the pancreas often approaches the splenic hilum and sometimes contacts the spleen. The spleen varies in size between individuals, but in general measures 12 cm in length, 7 cm in width, and 3 to 4 cm in width. The peritoneum creates folds that form the suspensory ligaments of the spleen. The four main "suspensory" ligaments are gastrosplenic, splenorenal, splenophrenic, and splenocolic ligaments. The splenophrenic and splenocolic ligaments are avascular. The gastrosplenic ligament contains the short gastric vessels. The splenorenal ligament has an anterior and posterior aspect and surrounds the splenic hilum. The splenic hilum contains the splenic artery, splenic vein, and sometimes the tail of the pancreas. The splenic vessels sometimes branch before entering the spleen. The splenic artery is tortuous and is one of the three branches of the celiac trunk. It runs along the superior aspect of the pancreas and gives rise to the short gastric arteries prior to entering the spleen, which course in the gastrosplenic ligament and supply the portion of the greater curvature of the stomach superior to the splenic artery (**Fig. 9.3**) (9). The splenic artery also gives rise to the left gastroepiploic artery, which supplies the remainder of the greater curvature of the stomach and the gastrocolic omentum. The splenic vein is slightly inferior and follows the course and branching of the artery.

Patient Positioning

The success of surgical procedure begins with patient positioning. This is often critical in improving exposure, particularly in obese patients. For most women undergoing radical hysterectomy, ovarian cancer cytoreduction, or pelvic exenterative procedures, we prefer the low lithotomy position using stirrups (**Fig. 9.4**) (1). The buttocks

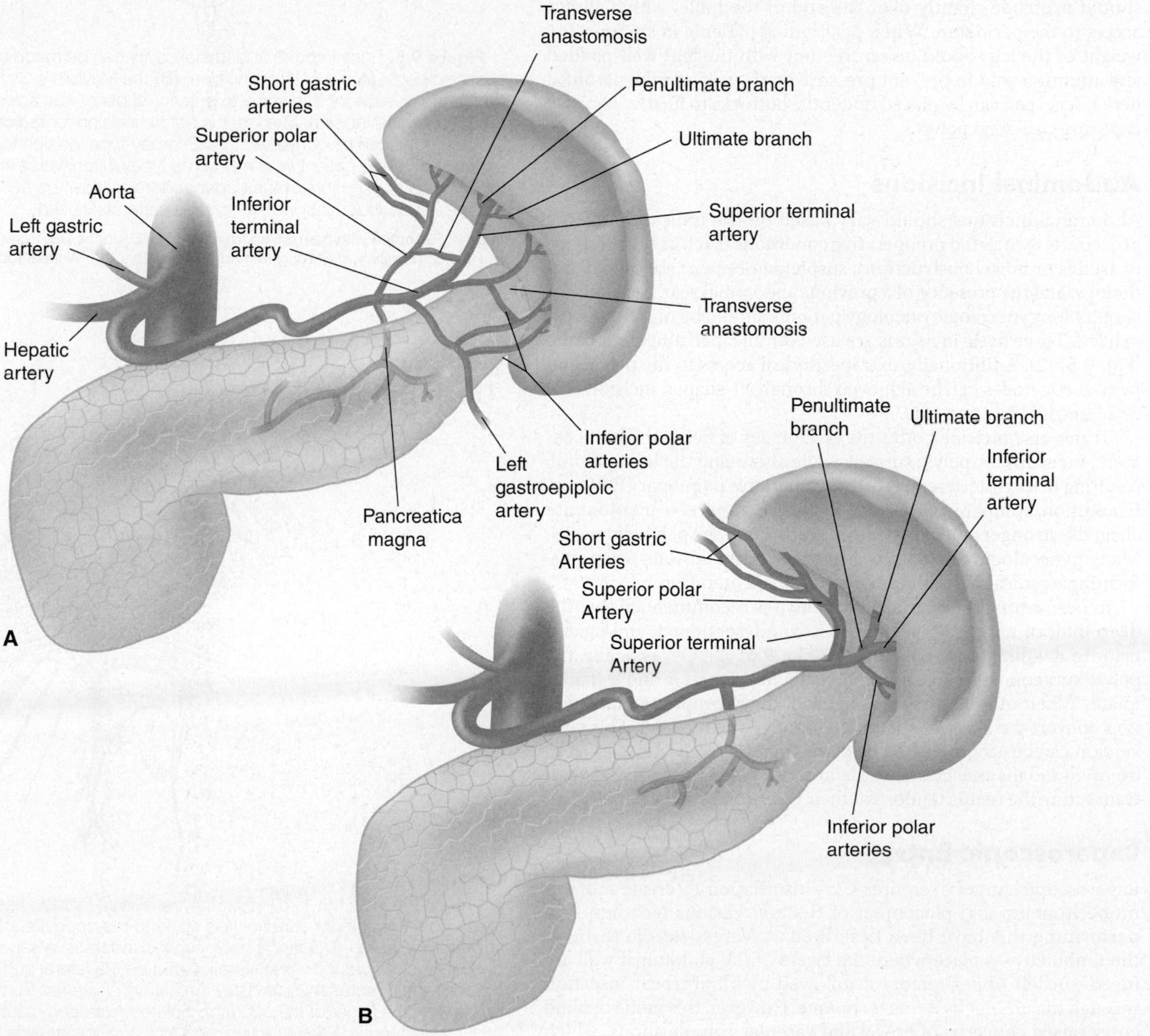

Figure 9.3. (A, B) Variations on splenic vascularization.

Source: Reprinted with permission from Poulin EC, Schlachta DM, Mazza J. Splenectomy. Gastroinestinal tract and abdomen. In: Souba WW, Fink MJ, Jurkovich GJ, et al., eds. *ACS Surgery*. New York, NY: WebMd; 2005.

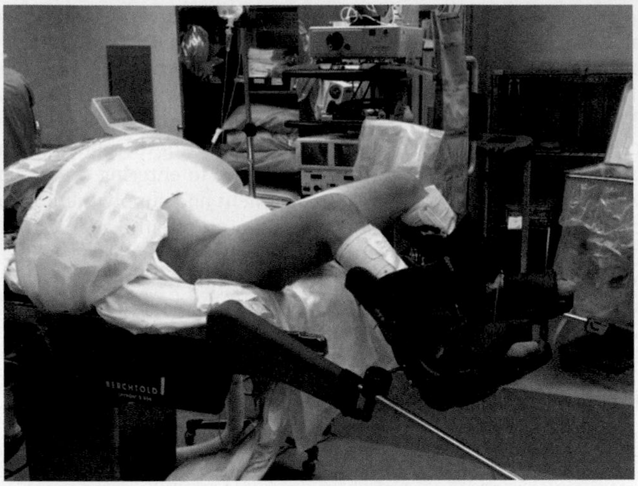

Figure 9.4. Low lithotomy position using Allen stirrups.

Source: Reprinted with permission from Morrow CP, Curtin JP, eds. *Gynecologic Cancer Surgery*. New York, NY: Churchill Livingstone; 1996.

should protrude slightly over the end of the table, which allows access to the perineum. When positioning patients in stirrups, the weight of the leg should be on the foot with the legs well-padded and attention paid to prevent pressure on the calf and the peroneal nerve. A gel pad can be placed under the buttocks to further improve exposure to a deep pelvis.

Abdominal Incisions

Abdominal incisions should vary based on the indication for the procedure, associated preoperative conditions (such as the presence of ascites or bowel obstruction), suspicion of upper abdominal pathology, and the presence of a previous abdominal scar. Incisions for surgery for gynecologic oncology patients should be highly individualized. Three basic incisions are used for intraperitoneal exposure (**Fig. 9.5**) (2). Additionally, extraperitoneal access to the pelvic and para-aortic nodes can be achieved through a J-shaped incision (10) or a "sunrise" incision (11).

Transverse incisions offer the advantages of being the best cosmetic incisions for pelvic surgery while also being the least painful, resulting in less interference with postoperative pulmonary function. In addition, compared to vertical incisions, transverse incisions are allegedly stronger and allow better exposure to the pelvic sidewalls. Many gynecologic oncologists use transverse incisions when performing a radical hysterectomy or pelvic exenteration.

In performing the Maylard incision, it is recommended that the deep inferior epigastric vessels be isolated, sectioned, and ligated prior to dividing the rectus muscle (**Fig. 9.6**) (2). Occasionally, the pelvic surgeon will make a Pfannenstiel incision and find it inadequate. When more exposure is needed, the appropriate maneuver is to convert the Pfannenstiel to a Cherney-type incision. This conversion can be accomplished by dissecting the rectus muscles from the pyramidalis muscles and the anterior rectus sheath and then transecting the rectus tendons at their insertion into the pubic bone.

Laparoscopic Entry

Laparoscopic surgery requires CO_2 insufflation to create a pneumoperitoneum and placement of trocars. Various techniques of performing this have been described. A Veress needle through the umbilicus—a place where the layers of the abdominal wall are fused—or left upper quadrant followed by blind trocar insertion through the umbilicus is one technique. However, this mode of blind entry raised concerns of bowel and vascular complications, which ultimately can be lethal. This is of particular concern because the majority of complications following laparoscopic surgery are related to trocar insertion.

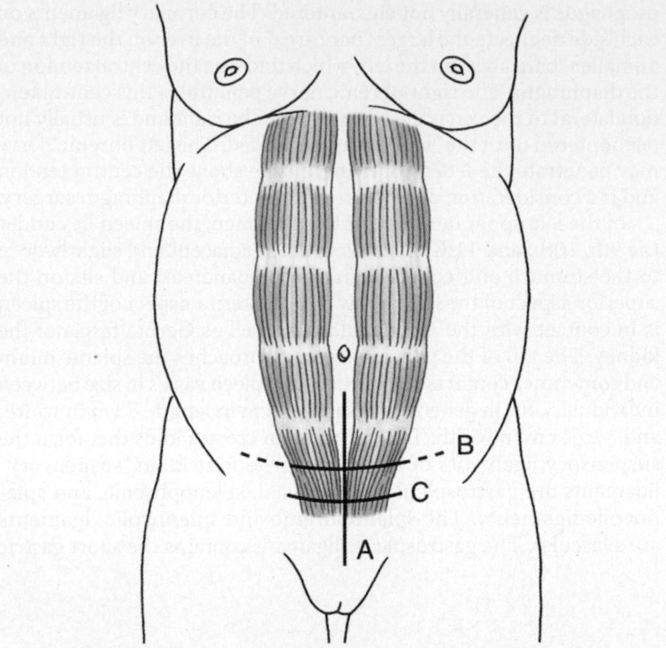

Figure 9.5. Entry into the abdominal cavity can be made by three basic incisions: **(A)** the midline incision; **(B)** the Maylard incision is made from anterior-superior iliac spine to anterior-superior iliac spine; and **(C)** the Pfannenstiel incision. The latter is not an incision for radical pelvic surgery, but it can be converted to a Cherney-type incision for improved exposure. For the patient who has some type of transverse incision, and for whom later exposure of the upper abdominal cavity is necessary, a midline upper abdominal incision can be separately used.

Source: Reprinted with permission from Fischer JE, Jones DB, Pomposelli FB, et al. *Fischer's Mastery of Surgery.* 6th ed. Philadelphia, PA: Wolters Kluwer; 2011.

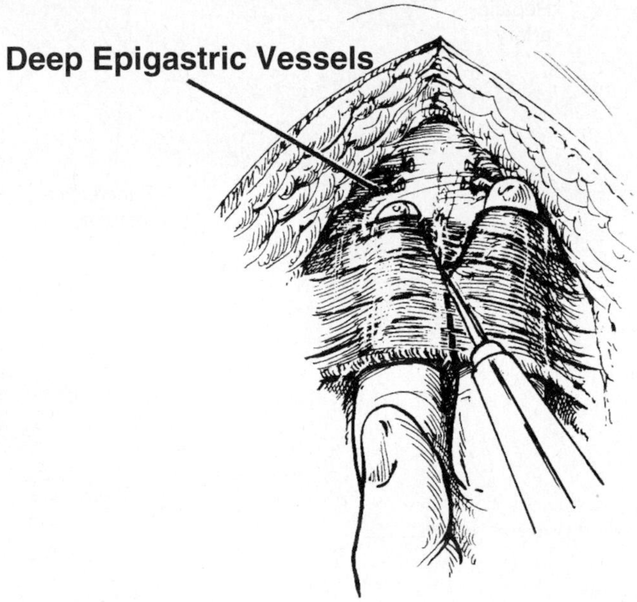

Figure 9.6. The Maylard incision. A transverse incision has been made from the anterior-superior iliac spine to the opposite anterior-superior iliac spine. The fascia has been incised transversely. The deep inferior epigastric vessels are located on the lateral and posterior borders of the rectus muscle. They are bluntly dissected from this position by the finger of the operator, isolated, clamped, sectioned, and tied. Only afterwards they are tied, should the rectus muscle be incised. This can be done with the Bovie.

Source: Reprinted with permission from Rock JA, Jones HW. *Te Linde's Operative Gynecology.* 10th ed. Philadelphia, PA: Wolters Kluwer; 2008.

To avoid a blind entry, the "open" technique in which the fascia and the peritoneum are surgically opened and the trocar inserted under direct visualization can be used, and is considered by many to be the safest access technique. A large literature review comparing data between 12,444 open laparoscopic and 489,335 closed laparoscopic cases revealed that rates of visceral and vascular injury were 0.083% and 0.075%, respectively, after closed laparoscopy, and 0.048% and 0.0%, respectively, after open laparoscopy ($p = 0.002$). Mortality rates were 0.003% for the closed and 0.0% for the open laparoscopy technique (12). However, a recent Cochran review of over 7,000 patients failed to reveal a difference in visceral or vascular injury between methods of entry. The open technique was associated with a reduction in failed entry rate when compared to the closed technique (13).

Once the pneumoperitoneum is established and the endoscope is placed, the ancillary trocars are placed under direct vision. Most gynecologic oncology procedures can be performed using a diamond trocar arrangement with one 10-mm suprapubic trocar, two 5-mm lateral trocars located just medial and superior to the iliac crest, and the umbilical trocar (14). Trocar positioning is of extreme importance because it must allow access to the entire abdomen, from the pelvis to the diaphragm. Traditional "straight stick" laparoscopy relies on the principle of triangulation. Selected trocar placement must provide an adequate angulation between instruments to perform the intended operation and positioning may be adapted to each specific situation.

Lymph Node Dissection

Dissection of the pelvic and para-aortic lymph nodes generally involves either a transperitoneal or extraperitoneal approach. The approach selected is dictated by the primary site of disease and the planned accompanying procedure. When a hysterectomy and/or surgical debulking is required, the approach is invariably transperitoneal. In certain situations such as the pretreatment surgical staging of patients with advanced-stage cervical cancer, the extraperitoneal approach is favored because the transperitoneal approach has been associated with significant radiation-induced intestinal morbidity due to postoperative adhesion formation (15).

Pelvic Lymph Node Dissection

Whether a transperitoneal or extraperitoneal approach is used, the pelvic lymphatic basin can be divided into five specific anatomical regions. Most surgeons initially remove pelvic nodes from the *external iliac region*. Lymphatic-fatty tissue is removed cranially, laterally, and medially from both external iliac vessels and between them. The medial border is formed by the paravesical space. The lateral border is the psoas muscle, the ventral is commonly indicated as the origin of the deep circumflex iliac vein, and the cranial border is the level of the common iliac artery bifurcation, where the lymphatic trunk continues as the superficial common iliac region (**Fig. 9.7**) (2). The genitofemoral nerve courses laterally to the external iliac artery and should be identified and preserved prior to excising the lymphatic tissue. It usually forms two branches, one running on the surface of the psoas muscle, while the second runs through the lymphatic tissue on the external iliac vessels, where it can be easily cut or injured.

Mobilization and retraction of the external iliac vessels allows access to the *obturator region*. The cranial border is formed by the common iliac vessels bifurcation, where the lymphatic trunk continues cranially as the deep common iliac region. The medial anatomical border is the paravesical space and the ventral border is formed by the pubic bone together with levator ani and obturator muscles, where the obturator nerve leaves the pelvis through the obturator canal. The lateral border is formed by the obturator internal muscle, and the caudal anatomical landmarks are the obturator vessels. The obturator nodes are most easily teased away from the nerve and vessels if one begins the dissection caudally (**Fig. 9.8**) (2). Usually the last dissected area is the *internal iliac region*, where the tissue is removed medially from the internal iliac vein.

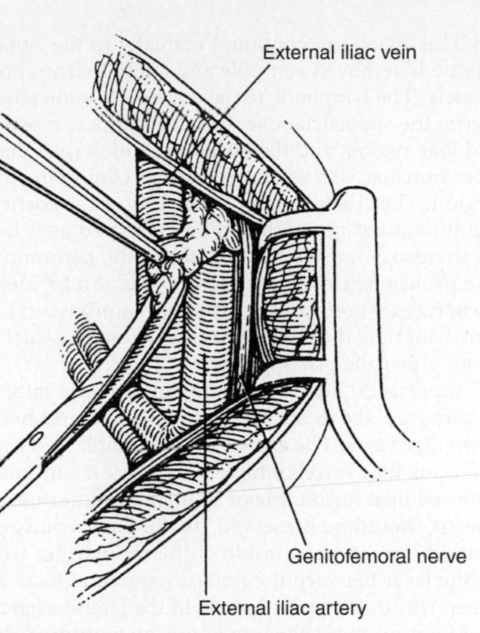

Figure 9.7. Starting at the bifurcation of the common iliac vessels, the loose areolar tissue over the vein is excised from cephalad to caudad. Clips should be used at the bifurcation of the common iliac to avoid troublesome bleeding.

Source: Reprinted with permission from Gallup DG, Talledo OE. *Surgical Atlas of Gynecologic Oncology.* Philadelphia, PA: WB Saunders Co.; 1994:57.

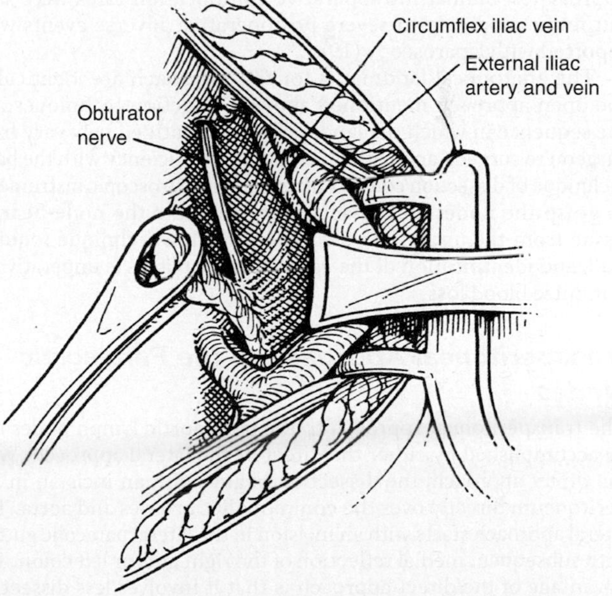

Figure 9.8. A vein retractor is used to retract the external iliac veins anterior and lateral to expose the obturator space. Lymphatic tissue is gently teased from the psoas muscle. The entire lymphatic bundle is clamped, sectioned at its caudal end, and ligated at the pelvic sidewall. With the use of the Singley forceps, the lymphatic bundle is bluntly dissected from the obturator nerve and mobilized superiorly. Often, the obturator vein and artery must be sacrificed to obtain access to tissue posterior and lateral to the nerve. Once the tissue is mobilized superiorly, all areolar tissue is cleaned off the hypogastric vessels to the level of the bifurcation of the common iliac artery. The large tissue bundle is clamped and removed en bloc. A tie or clips may be used at the level of the bifurcation.

Source: Reprinted with permission from Gallup DG, Talledo OE. *Surgical Atlas of Gynecologic Oncology.* Philadelphia, PA: WB Saunders Co.; 1994:58.

The dissection continues cranially to the *common iliac region.* Tissue is removed ventrally and laterally from both common iliac vessels. The lymphatic tissue can be anatomically divided into two parts: the superficial one, which continues mostly from the external iliac region; and the deep one, which runs deeply between the common iliac vein and psoas muscle, continuing from the obturator region. The cranial border is the level of the aortic bifurcation. The genitofemoral nerve should be preserved as it lies on the surface of the psoas muscle. Deeply below the common iliac vessels and the psoas muscle, on the sacral bone, can be identified two nerve structures—the cranial part of the lumbosacral trunk (L4 + L5) (medially) and the obturator nerve (laterally), which enters the region from under the psoas muscle.

If presacral nodes are to be removed the fatty-lymphatic tissue is removed above the sacral bone below and between both common iliac veins. The caudal border is indicated by the level of right common iliac vessels bifurcation, where it continues caudally as the internal iliac region. Major branches of inferior nerve hypogastric plexus should be preserved, as the plexus runs medially on both sides, below ureters, inside of the mesoureter which forms a thin tissue layer between the medial pararectal fossa and large vessels. Deep within the psoas muscle in the lateral aspect are branches of the femoral nerve, generally not encountered during traditional lymphadenectomy; however, in select cases of soft tissue involvement of the psoas muscle requiring a resection, care must be taken to avoid injury to the femoral nerve.

Laparoscopic transperitoneal lymphadenectomy remains the most popular approach employed by gynecologic oncologists. The early reports of this technique came from France in the late 1980s and early 1990s (16–18). The GOG LAP 2 study was a large prospective randomized trial comparing laparoscopic to open surgical staging in patients with uterine cancer. This study demonstrated that the lymph node yield was similar between the laparoscopic and open approaches. Similar intraoperative complication rates were seen but fewer moderate-to-severe postoperative adverse events were reported with laparoscopy (19).

The anatomical landmarks for this approach are identical to the open approach mentioned above. Dissection techniques and the sequence in which the landmarks are identified may vary from surgeon to surgeon and patient to patient. Proficiency with the basic technique of dissection consists of using the laparoscopic instruments to grasp the nodes and dissection to separate the node-bearing tissue from the underlying structures. Such a technique requires skill, and identification of the correct tissue planes is imperative to minimize blood loss.

Transperitoneal Approach to the Para-aortic Nodes

The transperitoneal approach to the para-aortic lymph nodes can be accomplished by either the direct or the lateral approach. With the direct approach, the dissection begins with an incision in the peritoneum directly over the common iliac arteries and aorta. The lateral approach starts with an incision in the lateral paracolic gutters with subsequent medial reflection of the right and/or left colon. The advantage of the direct approach is that it involves less dissection at the root of the small intestine mesentery and ureter; however, it is associated with a greater degree of difficulty in exposing the high left para-aortic nodes. Surgeons should be familiar with both approaches and may need to perform the approach best suited for the specific situation.

With the direct approach to the right para-aortic nodes, an incision is made in the peritoneum overlying the right common iliac artery (**Fig. 9.9**). The incision is carried up over the aorta to the level of the duodenum. If the nodal dissection is to be carried out only to the level of the IMA, it may not be necessary to mobilize the duodenum. Using blunt dissection, the ureter and ovarian vessels are identified and mobilized laterally. The lymphatic tissue lateral to the right common iliac artery is elevated and the dissection then proceeds in a caudad-to-cephalad direction. A plane is created between the IVC and the lymphatic pedicle. The majority of the right para-aortic nodes overlie the IVC and are generally easily dissected off the vessel. However, there is a fairly constant small vein within the lymphatics anterior to the IVC that inserts just above its bifurcation. If care is not taken to identify and ligate this so-called "fellow's" vein early in the dissection, it can easily be torn, with resultant, significant bleeding (1) requiring IVC repair. When the most cephalad extent of the dissection is reached, the pedicle is secured and divided (**Fig. 9.10**).

If the nodes above the IMA must be sampled, the third portion of the duodenum is mobilized by bilaterally incising the peritoneum around it and then sharply dissecting the areolar tissue underneath (4). The superior portion of the peritoneal incision can be carried up as high as the ligament of Treitz, which can also be divided if needed. Inferiorly, the peritoneal incision is extended over the right ureter around the cecum and up along the right paracolic gutter to mobilize the small bowel mesentery and part of the right colon (**Fig. 9.11**) (4). The small bowel can then be packed into the upper abdomen or

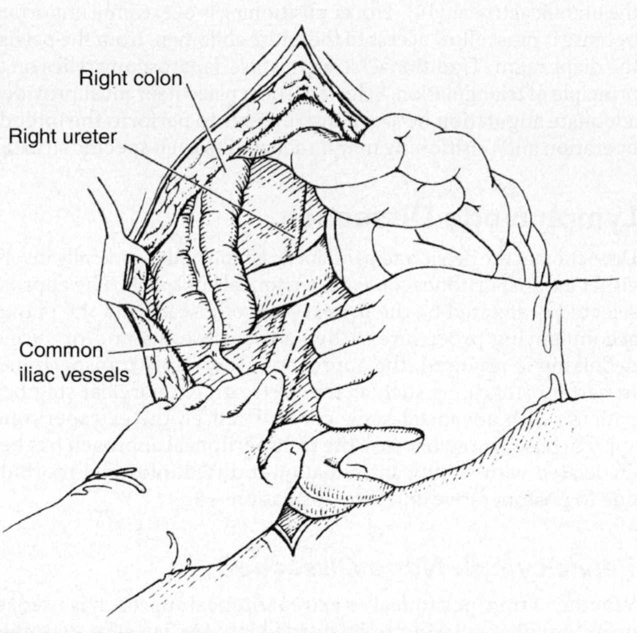

Figure 9.9. The small bowel is elevated out of the pelvis, placing the mesentery on gentle traction. The right ureter and common iliac artery are identified and the peritoneum overlying the artery is incised.

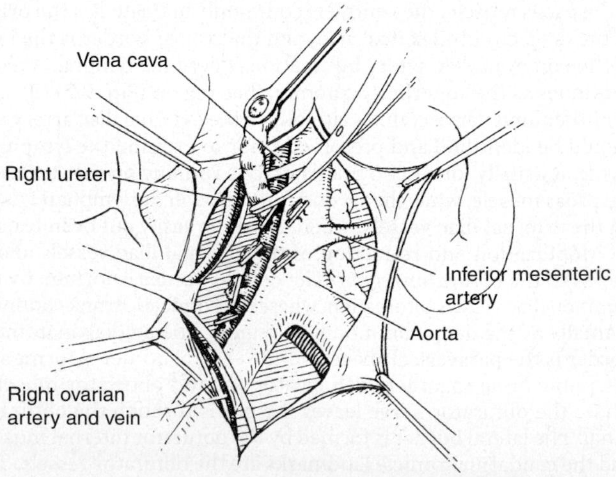

Figure 9.10. The specimen is dissected in a cephalad direction. Hemostatic clips are used on either side of the developing pedicle as it is mobilized and divided, and also at the most cephalad extent of the dissection before the specimen is removed.

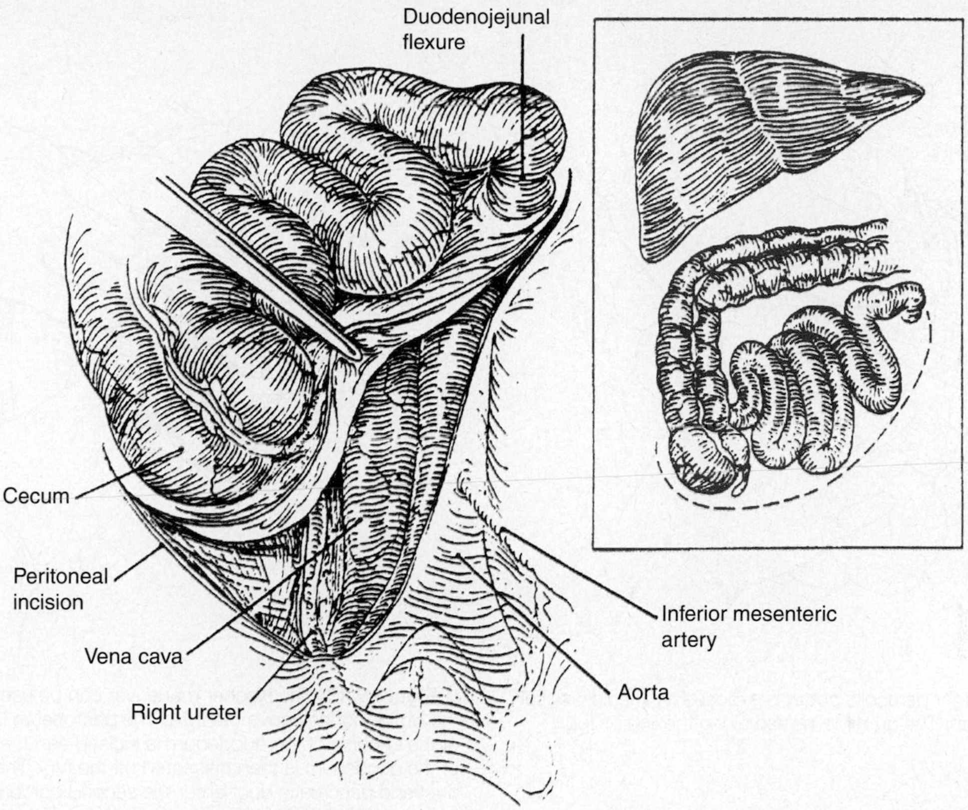

Figure 9.11. Extended peritoneal incision. The peritoneal incision is extended over the right ureter around the cecum and the cephalad along the right paracolic gutter. This allows for mobilization of the small bowel mesentery as well as the ascending colon.

Source: Reprinted with permission from Fowler JM, Johnson PR. Transperitoneal para-aortic lymphadenectomy. *Oper Tech Gynecol Surg.* 1996;1:9.

completely removed from the peritoneal cavity and stabilized outside of the abdominal cavity, or put into a bowel bag outside the abdomen. The duodenum is retracted superiorly, allowing identification and ligation of the right ovarian artery and vein. The lymphatic tissue can then be safely dissected off of the right side of the aorta and the anterior surface of the IVC up to the level of the renal veins.

The left para-aortic lymph nodes may be removed through the same peritoneal incision. The left common iliac artery, left side of the aorta, IMA, left ureter, and left psoas muscle are identified (**Fig. 9.12**). The ureter is mobilized laterally, and the lymphatic tissue lateral to the left common iliac artery and aorta is then removed in a caudad-to-cephalad direction. The left para-aortic lymph nodes lie lateral and partially behind the aorta. In dissecting these nodes, troublesome bleeding from the lumbar vessels can occasionally be encountered. Safe removal of the lymph nodes above the IMA frequently requires identification and division of the left ovarian artery and vein, and occasionally ligation of the IMA.

To remove right-sided para-aortic nodes via the lateral approach, the right paracolic gutter is incised along the line of Toldt (**Fig. 9.13**). The peritoneum is elevated off the psoas muscle and the incision is extended up to the hepatic flexure of the colon. The right colon is reflected medially. The ureter and ovarian vessels that remain are located on the undersurface of the reflected peritoneum. They may be left attached or mobilized laterally for better exposure. Mobilization of the colon medically exposes the IVC and aorta. After identifying the essential structures, the lymphatic tissue can then be dissected as previously described in a caudad-to-cephalad direction up to the third portion of the duodenum (**Fig. 9.14**).

To remove lymph nodes above the IMA, the Kocher maneuver is used to reflect the duodenum medially. The peritoneum lateral to the convexity of the C-curve of the duodenum is incised and the second portion of the duodenum is then dissected off the IVC. For further exposure, it may be necessary to extend the peritoneal

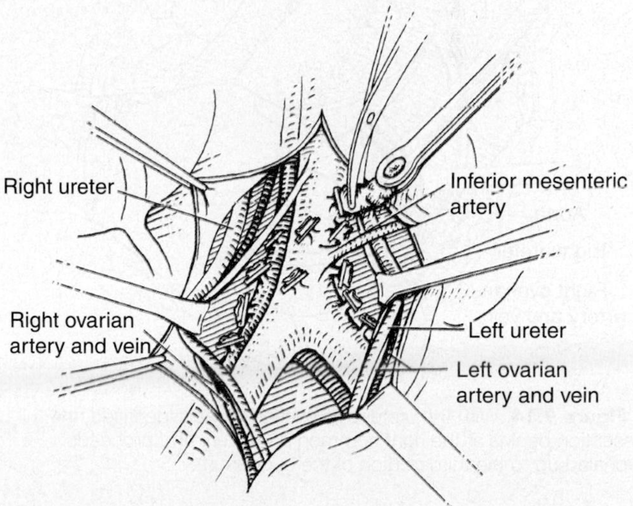

Figure 9.12. Removal of the left para-aortic nodes through the same peritoneal incision. The dissection also proceeds in a cephalad direction, again using hemostatic clips on the lateral and medial margins. Care should be taken to avoid injury to the inferior mesenteric artery that arises approximately 3 to 4 cm above the aortic bifurcation.

incision along the line of Toldt cephalad to mobilize completely the hepatic flexure of the colon (**Fig. 9.15**). The right ovarian artery and vein are identified and divided. The right-sided para-aortic lymph nodes can then be dissected off of the IVC and right aorta up to the level of the renal vessels.

The lateral approach to the left para-aortic lymph nodes is accomplished in a similar fashion by incising along the line of Toldt and mobilizing the left colon medially (**Fig. 9.16**). Again, the ureter

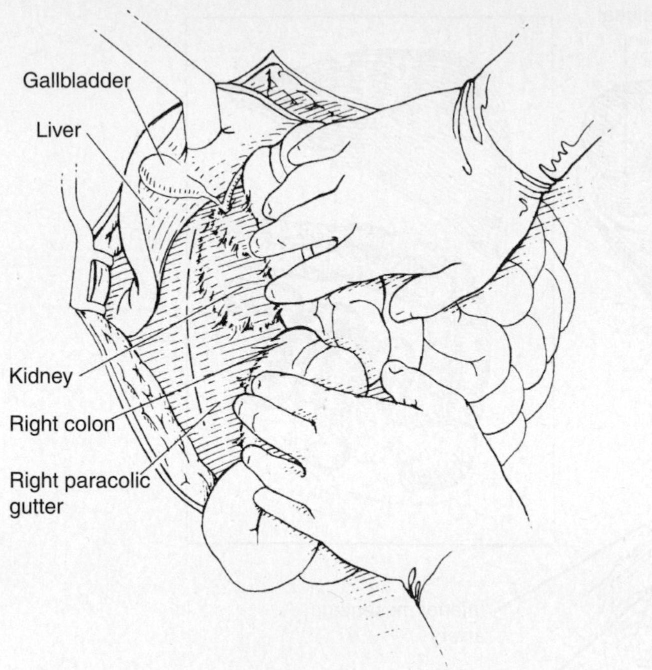

Figure 9.13. The right paracolic gutter is exposed by medial traction on the ascending colon. The gutter is incised along the line of Toldt.

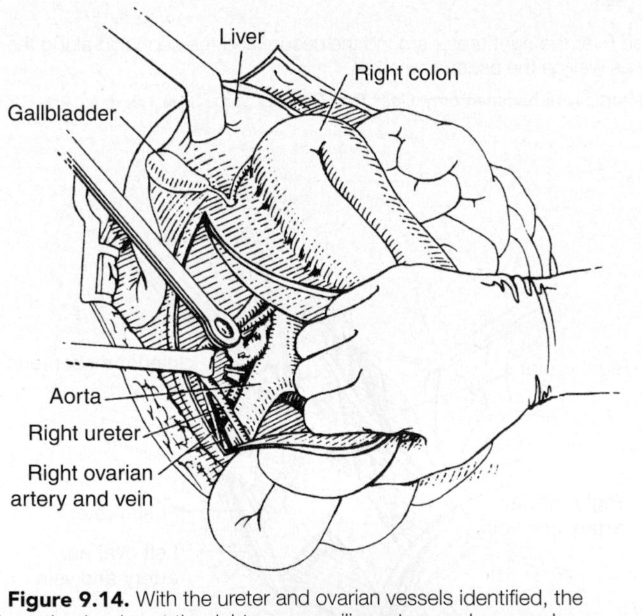

Figure 9.14. With the ureter and ovarian vessels identified, the dissection begins at the right common iliac artery and proceeds cephalad up to the third portion of the duodenum.

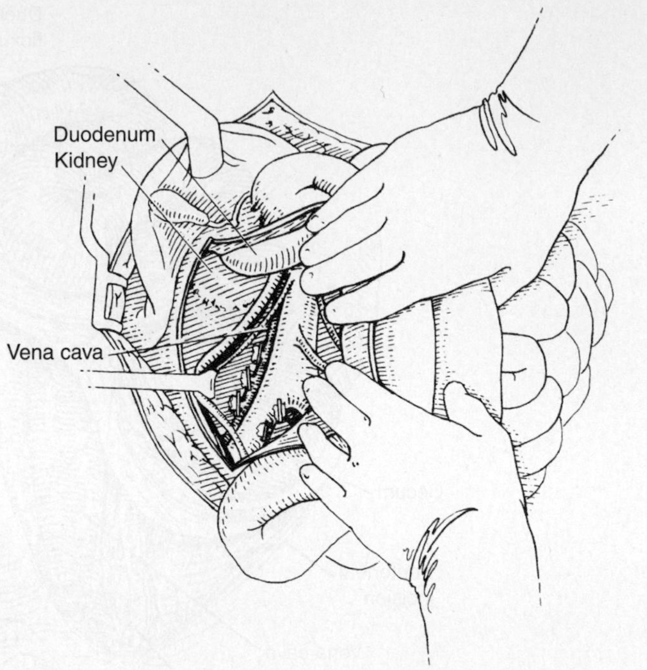

Figure 9.15. The Kocher maneuver can be used to gain access to the lymph nodes above the IMA. The peritoneum lateral to the convexity of the C-curve of the duodenum is incised and the second portion of the duodenum is then dissected off the IVC. The common bile duct and pancreatic duct enter the second portion of the duodenum posteromedially. For further exposure, the incision along the line of Toldt can be extended cephalad to completely mobilize the hepatic flexure of the colon.

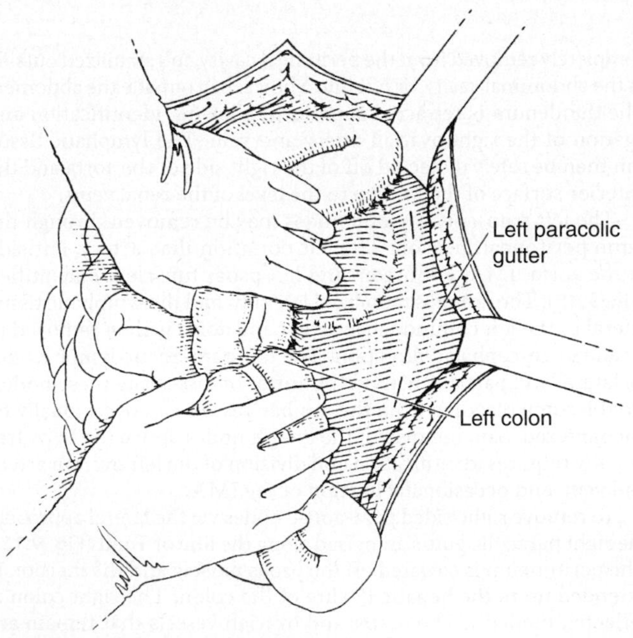

Figure 9.16. The lateral approach to the left para-aortic nodes is accomplished by retracting the descending colon medially and incising along the line of Toldt.

and ovarian vessels are identified on the undersurface of the reflected peritoneum, and may be left attached or mobilized laterally for better exposure (**Fig. 9.17**). After further mobilization of the left colon and identification of the aorta and the IMA, the left-sided nodes are removed in a caudad-to-cephalad direction (**Fig. 9.18**). Dissection of the nodes above the IMA requires mobilization of the splenic flexure of the colon, division of the left ovarian artery and vein, and occasionally ligation of the IMA.

The transperitoneal approach was the first described technique for laparoscopic removal of the aortic nodes (20,21). It mimics the open surgical approach. As for every upper abdominal procedure, the bowel loops are packed along with the omentum in the left upper quadrant. The dorsal peritoneum is opened alongside the axis of the right common iliac vessels and extended along the lower aorta. The upper peritoneal flap is elevated along with the third part of the duodenum. The anatomical landmarks for the dissection should be carefully identified. The aorta and IVC are the main landmarks. On the right side of the IVC, the right ureter is identified and then retracted laterally. The right ovarian vessels are identified to their

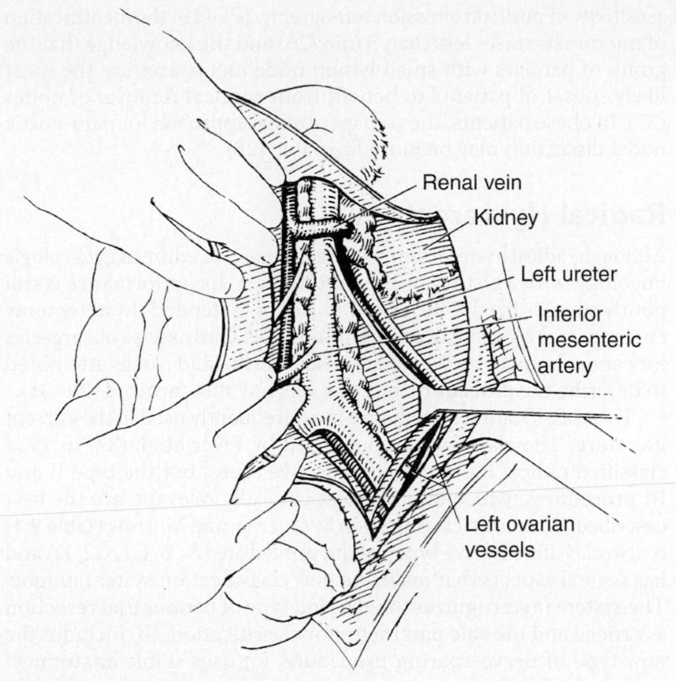

Figure 9.17. Using sharp and blunt dissection, the left colon can be mobilized medially, exposing the left ureter, ovarian vessels, and aorta.

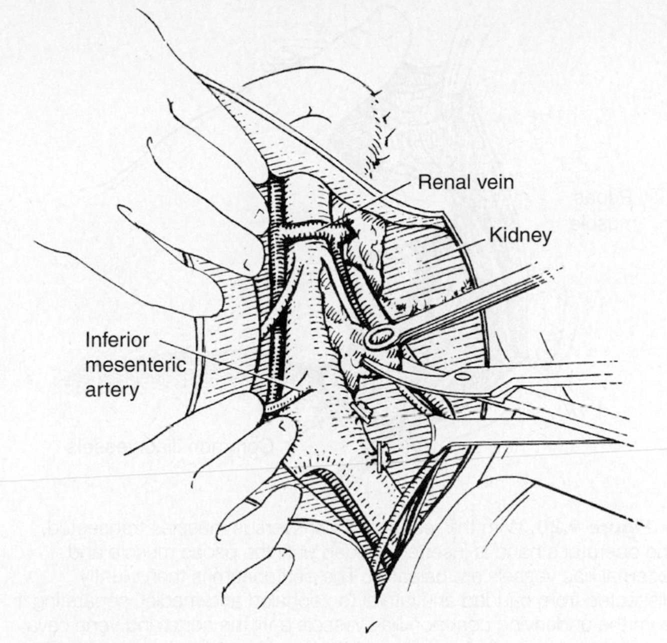

Figure 9.18. Dissection begins at the left common iliac artery and proceeds cephalad using hemostatic clips. Care should be taken to avoid injury to the inferior mesenteric artery that arises approximately 3 to 4 cm above the aortic bifurcation.

insertion into the IVC and aorta. The ventral aspect of the aorta is dissected, and the origin of the IMA is identified. The left renal vein is then identified, and this typically requires that the third part of the duodenum be elevated. Finally, the left ureter is identified and retracted laterally. The left ovarian vein is identified and traced to its insertion into the left renal vein.

High para-aortic nodes can be removed using the transperitoneal laparoscopic approach, with acceptable morbidity (22). When comparing the transperitoneal infrarenal lymphadenectomy to the inframesenteric lymphadenectomy, the extended para-aortic lymphadenectomy only took an additional 31 minutes on average and significantly increased the mean node counts from 9.0 to 19.6 (23).

Extraperitoneal Approach to the Para-aortic Nodes

The extraperitoneal approach to the para-aortic lymph nodes by means of a supraumbilical transverse sunrise incision was initially described by Gallup et al. (11). The skin incision is made 6 cm above the umbilicus in the midline and is carried laterally and caudad to the level of the iliac crests bilaterally (**Fig. 9.19**) (2).

The fascia is incised transversely. The rectus muscles are dissected off the anterior-lying fascia cephalad and caudad. The right rectus muscle is transected. The right transversus muscle is then identified and transected caudally and laterally. The hand of the operator is inserted deep into the incision until the right psoas muscle and external iliac vessels are palpated. The peritoneum is then bluntly dissected from caudad and lateral to cephalad and medial, separating it from the underlying common iliac vessels until the great vessels are exposed (**Fig. 9.20**) (2). If the peritoneum is inadvertently entered, it must be closed immediately.

After identification of the right ureter and ovarian vessels, the right para-aortic nodes can be removed. In thin patients, it may be possible to remove the left para-aortic nodes through a right abdominal approach. However, if exposure is difficult, the left rectus and transversus muscles can be transected and the peritoneum mobilized medially in a similar fashion to gain access to the left para-aortic nodes.

The laparoscopic extraperitoneal aortic approach was initially described in a porcine model (24). Subsequently, additional clinical

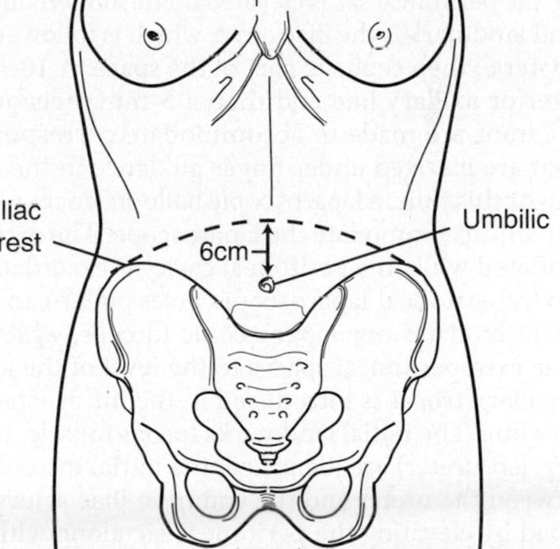

Figure 9.19. The "sunrise" incision. In the center, the incision is approximately 6 cm above the umbilicus. The incision is carried laterally in a downward fashion to the level of the iliac crests.

After Gallup DG, Talledo OE. *Surgical Atlas of Gynecologic Oncology.* Philadelphia, PA: WB Saunders Co.; 1994:118.

series using this approach have been described (25). The left lateral approach has several advantages over the right-sided approach during the dissection: (1) the upper part of the dissection, which is the left infrarenal area, is easier to reach; (2) the precaval and laterocaval nodes can be easily reached from the left side by compressing the IVC. The laparoscopic extraperitoneal approach to the aortic nodes is begun by using a 3-cm incision made in the left lower quadrant, medial to the iliac spine. The dissection is carried down to the

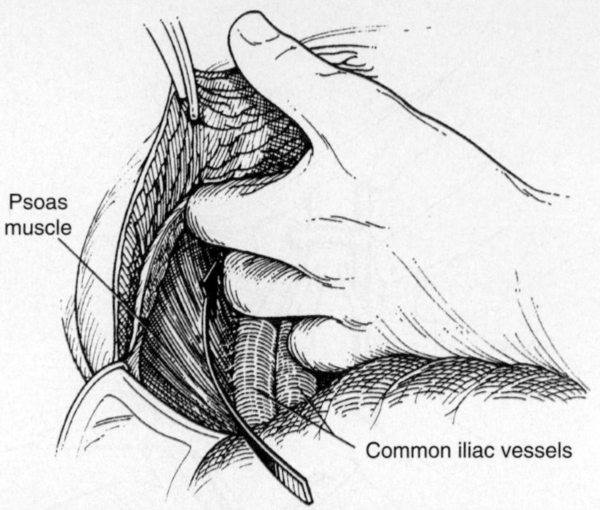

Figure 9.20. With the rectus and transversus muscles transected, the operator's hand is inserted caudad until the psoas muscle and external iliac vessels are palpated. The peritoneum is then bluntly dissected from caudad and lateral to cephalad and medial, separating it from the underlying common iliac vessels until the aorta and vena cava are exposed.

Source: Reprinted with permission from Gallup DG, Talledo OE. *Surgical Atlas of Gynecologic Oncology.* Philadelphia, PA: WB Saunders Co.; 1994:121.

preperitoneal space and, as in the open approach, care should be taken to leave the peritoneum intact. Transperitoneal laparoscopic guidance can be used to properly develop this space. Once the parietal fascia is opened, the surgeon's forefinger is introduced into the extraperitoneal space, and develops the retroperitoneal space along the psoas muscle and common iliac artery. With gentle blunt dissection, the peritoneal sac is elevated off the underlying structures. The second landmark is the iliac crest, which is followed laterally to open the lateral, then cephalic part of the space. A 10-mm incision of the anterior axillary line and then a 5-mm incision in the left upper quadrant are made to accommodate corresponding blunt trocars that are inserted under finger guidance in the extraperitoneal space. At this time, a laparoscopic balloon trocar is introduced. The trocar will accommodate the laparoscope. The extraperitoneal space is inflated while the peritoneal cavity is exsufflated, drained, and the extraperitoneal laparoscopic assessment can begin. This trocar accommodates one laparoscopic forceps, which is used to develop the extraperitoneal spaces to the level of the lower ribs. A second ancillary trocar is introduced in the infracostal area in the midaxillary line. The initial landmarks (psoas muscle, left common iliac artery, left ureter) are identified; the initial dissection plane is found between the ureter and the common iliac artery. The space is developed by elevating the peritoneal sac along with the ureter. Access is gained to the presacral area, then to the right common iliac area. Further development is obtained in the cephalic direction by clearing the connective tissue from the psoas muscle and the lateral aspect of the left common iliac artery, then of the aorta. The IMA and then the left renal vein, generally identified by following the left ovarian vein up to the point where it ends, are identified. The nodes are then separated from the vessels and from the sympathetic chain by a combination of sharp and blunt dissection with cauterization of small vessels. Multifunction instruments are best suited for this dissection, as they prevent changing instruments and overcome the fact that only two ancillary instruments can routinely be placed in the narrow retroperitoneal space.

The typical indication for extraperitoneal aortic dissection is in the patient with locally advanced cervical carcinoma. Knowledge of the status of the aortic nodes allows tailoring of the radiation therapy fields. In these cases, common iliac nodes are generally removed along with the para-aortic nodes. The potential benefit of surgical staging of locally advanced cervical cancer is based on the lack of sensitivity of positron emission tomography (PET) in the identification of micrometastases less than 5 mm (26) and the knowledge that the group of patients with small lymph node metastases are the most likely subset of patients to benefit from surgical removal of nodes (27). In obese patients, the transperitoneal approach for para-aortic nodal dissection may be more favorable (28).

Radical Hysterectomy

Although radical hysterectomy is a traditional procedure in gynecologic oncology, with a history of almost 100 years, its performance is still poorly standardized. The term "radical" or "extended" hysterectomy encompasses a variety of different surgeries. Early series of surgeries for cervical cancer by Wertheim, Okabayashi, and Meigs attempted to describe the procedure, but this was not standardized (29–31).

Two classification systems are most frequently used in the current literature. The classical one published by Piver et al. (32) in 1974 classified radical hysterectomy into five types, but the type II and III procedures, which are the most clinically relevant, are the best described. The recent classification by Querleu and Morrow (**Table 9.1**) is also classified by five types of the procedure (A, B, C1, C2, D) and has several aspects that make the new classification system unique. The system (a) recognizes the size and type of parametrial resection as crucial and the sole parameter for classification, (b) includes the new type of nerve-sparing procedure, (c) uses stable anatomical landmarks for the description of surgical resection margins, (d) identifies surgical landmarks in three planes—frontal, sagittal, and horizontal (**Fig. 9.21**) (33,34).

The type B radical hysterectomy corresponds mostly to the type II or modified radical hysterectomy. The aim of the procedure is to remove limited parts of the lateral and dorsal parametria (**Figs. 9.22–9.24**). The ureter must be identified in the parametrium, unroofed, dissected from the cervix, and displaced laterally. The resection margin is indicated by the ureteral bed. The ureteral artery, branching from the uterine artery at its crossing of the ureter, can serve as a helpful lateral landmark. Dorsally, type B aims at the resection of 1 to 2 cm of the dorsal parametria. Identification of autonomic nerves is not required, as they remains preserved in the parametria deeply below the resection margins.

A major intention of the nerve-sparing (C1) radical hysterectomy is to remove corresponding parts of ventral, lateral, and dorsal parametria but, at the same time, preserve major autonomic nerve supply to urinary bladder, upper vagina, and rectum (**Figs. 9.22–9.24**). Two types of vegetative nerves can be identified and spared: (a) the inferior hypogastric plexus, running in the lateral part of the dorsal parametrium, laterally to the cervix below the ureter at the level of the vaginal fornix and ventrally in the infraureteral part of the ventral parametrium toward the urinary bladder; (b) the splanchnic nerves localized at the bottom of the lateral pararectal space and in the caudal part of the lateral parametrium below the parametrial veins. Surgical margins for the nerve-sparing procedure must be kept above the course of the nerve structures in the ventral, lateral, and dorsal parametrium. Dorsally, the nerve-sparing procedure requires a dissection of two parts of the dorsal parametrium. The mesoureter (a fine structure stretched between the ureter and the sacral bone), containing major branches of hypogastric plexus, is separated laterally from the uterosacral ligament, which allows for an adequate resection of the latter. On the lateral parametrium, the caudal resection margin is indicated by the vaginal vein, the largest parametrial vein, which guarantees the preservation of splanchnic nerves in the caudal part of the lateral parametrium. Ventrally, the ureter is only partially dissected from the ventral parametrium, allowing for limited resection of the proximal supraureteral part of the ventral parametrium.

The radicality of the C2 procedure, which corresponds to the type III radical hysterectomy, is different from the nerve-sparing procedure, aiming at removal of the majority of all three parametrial parts (**Figs. 9.22–9.24**). The C2 procedure requires complete dissection of the ureter from the lateral and ventral parametria and

TABLE 9.1. Proposed Classification System and Corresponding Historical Types of Radical Hysterectomy

New Classification System	Corresponding Types
A	Extrafascial hysterectomy
B	Modified radical hysterectomy Type II radical hysterectomy
C1	Nerve-sparing radical hysterectomy
C2	Type III radical hysterectomy Classical/standard radical hysterectomy
D	Laterally extended parametrectomy

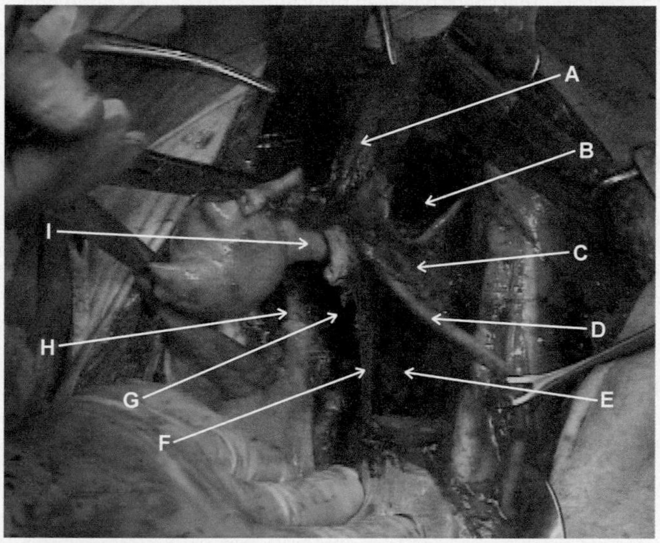

Figure 9.21. Three parts of the parametria. **A**—ventral parametrium; **B**—paravesical space; **C**—lateral parametrium; **D**—ureter; **E**—pararectal fossa; **F**—dorsal parametrium; **G**—sacrouterine space; **H**—rectum; **I**—cervix.

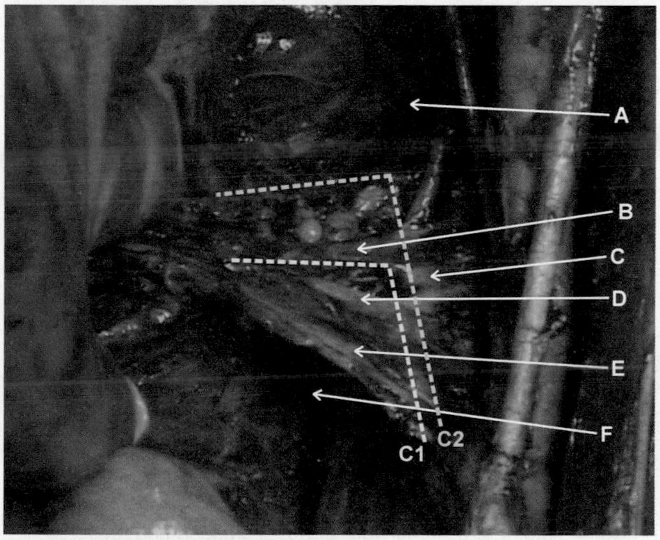

Figure 9.22. Resection lines for types B, C1, and C2 radical hysterectomy on the lateral parametrium. **A**—paravesical space; **B**—vaginal vein; **C**—internal iliac vein; **D**—uterine vein; **E**—uterine artery; **E**—pararectal fossa.

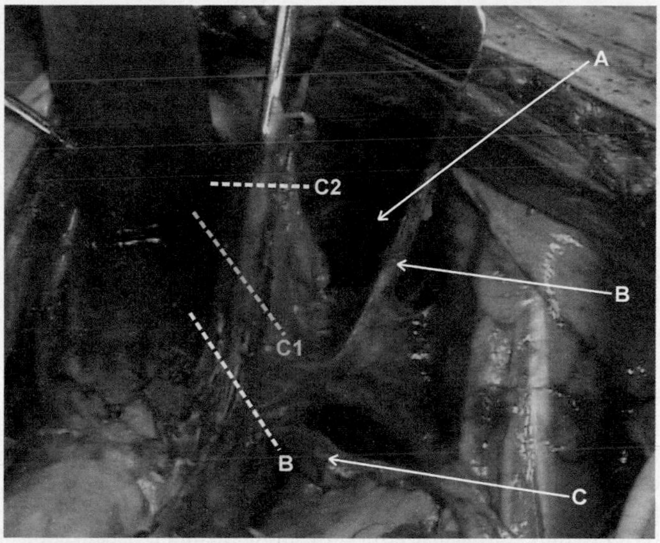

Figure 9.23. Resection lines for types B, C1, and C2 radical hysterectomy on the ventral parametrium. **A**—paravesical space; **B**—umbilical ligament; **C**—ureter.

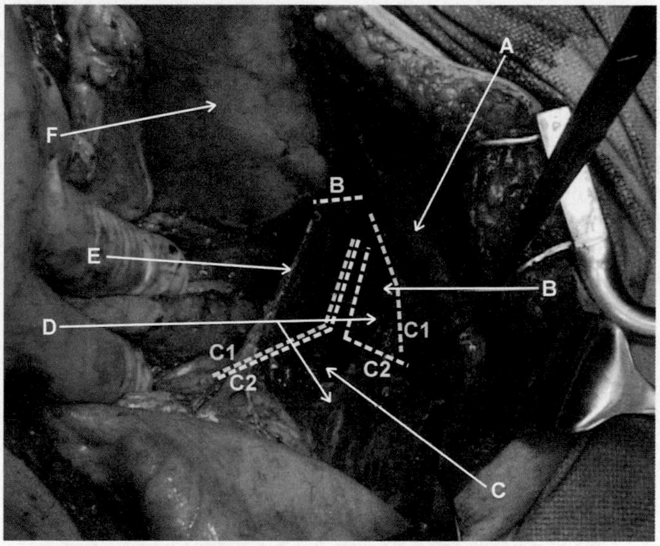

Figure 9.24. Resection lines for types B, C1, and C2 radical hysterectomy on the dorsal parametrium after dissection of the mesoureter from the sacrouterine ligament. **A**—ureter; **B**—mesoureter; **C**—space between the sacrouterine ligament and mesoureter; **D**—branches of the hypogastric plexus (white strips); **E**—sacrouterine ligament; **F**—cervix.

deeper dissection of the rectum from the dorsal parametria. The resection line on the dorsal parametria is deep below the former rectal attachment, causing unavoidable damage of the hypogastric plexus, so the dissection of the nerve from the uterosacral ligament is not required. The lateral parametrium is completely separated from the pelvic sidewall until the sacral bone is reached. On the ventral parametrium the ventral resection margin is formed by the urinary bladder. As a consequence, major branches of vegetative nerves are sacrificed during the C2-type procedure.

The technique of minimally invasive radical hysterectomy has evolved in the same way as simple hysterectomy. The vaginal approach (Schauta operation) was historically the first approach used. Laparotomy (Wertheim operation) soon took over, as radical vaginal surgery requires specific training and did not provide surgical access for lymph node dissection. Laparoscopic surgery provided a minimally invasive approach to lymph node dissection and led to a revival of the Schauta operation (35). Laparoscopic techniques were used to perform part of the radical dissection prior to completing the vaginal portion of the surgery (36–38). As technology and minimally invasive laparoscopic skills improved, reports of total laparoscopic hysterectomy appeared (39).

Ovarian Cancer Debulking

The goal of ovarian cancer debulking or cytoreduction is to remove all, or as close as possible to all, grossly visible and palpable tumor (40). The surgeon undertaking these complex surgeries should be familiar with the techniques used to remove tumor from the pelvis and the upper abdomen.

Removal of Pelvic Disease

Because ovarian malignancy often presents with large masses filling the pelvis and obliterating the cul-de-sac, a retroperitoneal approach can be used to identify important structures and secure vascular pedicles. An initial incision over the lateral pelvic sidewall just anterior to the external iliac artery will allow adequate visualization of the ureter and the ovarian vessels (**Fig. 9.25**). The paracolic gutters can be incised cephalad along the avascular line of Toldt for more adequate exposure of the retroperitoneal space. To avoid further troublesome hemorrhage the gonadal and uterine vessels can be identified, secured, and divided in the retroperitoneal space. If the anatomy is distorted by peritoneal implants, it may be prudent to identify the ureters, free them, lateralize them, and retract them laterally prior to removal of the uterus.

In cases where the pouch of Douglas is deeply infiltrated by disease or if there is involvement of the rectosigmoid colon, a reverse hysterectomy can facilitate complete removal of this disease. Entering the rectovaginal space allows for identification of the peritoneal reflection and often spares several cm of distal rectum in preparation for the transection and anastomosis. Here, gentle handling of the pararectal fatty tissue is of great importance. The rectal wall should not be skeletonized and devascularized. Rather than dissecting the perirectal fat, leaving a fat plane on the rectal surface allows for optimal distal perfusion. The term "modified posterior exenteration" is commonly used for the above procedure, as it entails an en bloc removal of the uterus, adnexa, infiltrated peritoneum, and the rectum. The procedure starts with the incision of the vesical peritoneal plica and dissection of the urinary bladder down to the level of the vaginal fornix. In cases of carcinomatosis on the peritoneal plica, a ventral peritonectomy—complete dissection of the infiltrated peritoneum from the urinary bladder—is part of the procedure. The retroperitoneum is opened laterally above the large vessels, both round ligaments are cut, the ureters are identified, and then the ovarian vessels are ligated and cut. The ureters are freed from the overlying peritoneum and the sigmoid colon is divided above the level of tumor infiltration. Occasionally, the complete removal of the tumor requires mobilization of the ureter in its parametrial part, and its dissection from the cervix and infiltrated parametria, similar to when performed during a radical hysterectomy. Once the uterine vessels are ligated bilaterally, the rectovaginal space between the vagina and the infiltrated pouch of Douglas is opened, the uterosacral ligaments are cut, and a reverse hysterectomy is completed by the incision of the vagina at the level of the vaginal fornix (**Fig. 9.26**). At this stage, the specimen is fixed in the pelvis only by the rectum and pararectal ligaments. The specimen is retracted cephalad, the infiltrated pouch of Douglas can be further dissected from the rectum, thus preserving a larger part of the rectum for anastomosis. After dividing the pararectal ligaments, the modified posterior exenteration is completed by division of the rectum below the level of tumor involvement. Low rectal anastomosis in this setting is generally performed and associated with a low rate of complications in well-trained hands (41,42).

Upper Abdominal Disease

Bristow et al. (43) demonstrated that expert centers with primary optimal cytoreduction rates of 75% or greater provided their patients with a 50% improvement in overall survival when compared to less

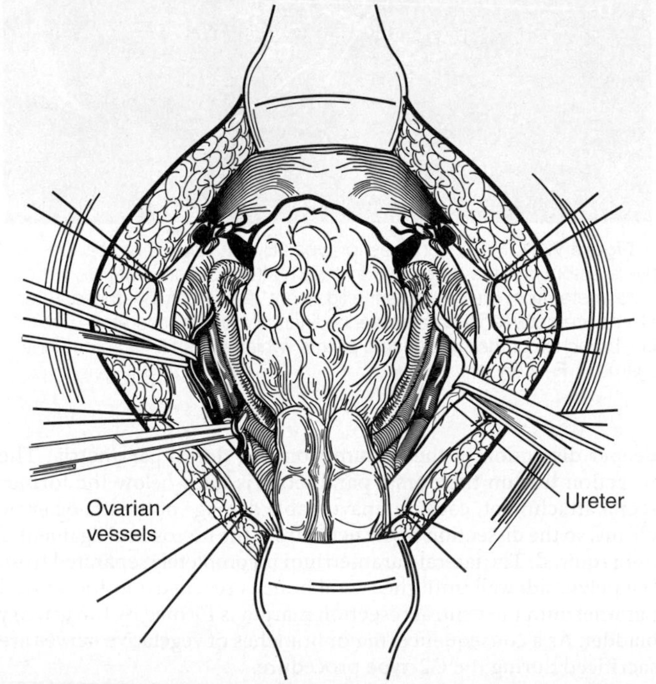

Figure 9.25. The ovarian vessels are skeletonized and divided at the pelvic brim. Early control of these vessels will help reduce blood loss during the later dissection. The ureter can be mobilized off the medial leaf of the broad ligament and retracted laterally on a Penrose drain or vessel loop.

After Gallup DG, Talledo OE. *Surgical Atlas of Gynecologic Oncology.* Philadelphia, PA: WB Saunders Co.; 1994:92.

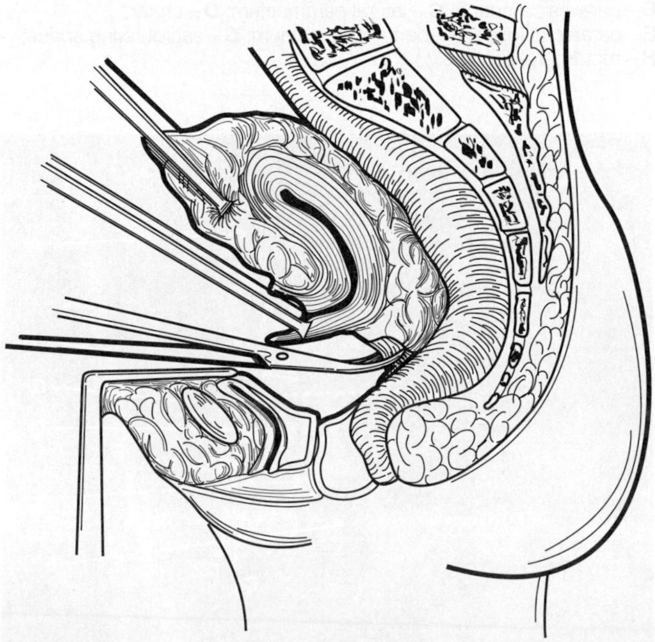

Figure 9.26. The posterior vaginal wall is grasped and retracted cephalad. The uterus can now be sharply dissected off of the rectosigmoid.

After Gallup DG, Talledo OE. *Surgical Atlas of Gynecologic Oncology.* Philadelphia, PA: WB Saunders Co.; 1994:103.

experienced centers with primary optimal cytoreduction rates of 25% or less. To achieve primary optimal cytoreduction rates of 75% or more in advanced-stage ovarian cancer patients, the surgeon should have the ability to remove disease involving upper abdominal structures such as the liver, diaphragm, spleen, and pancreas (5).

Adequate exposure is the most important factor in determining whether resection of diaphragm disease can be performed safely (7). In most cases, this can be done through a midline incision to the xiphoid, or in some cases the xiphoid can be removed.

Liver mobilization is almost universally essential when removing large volume disease on the right hemidiaphragm since a greater proportion of the right hemidiaphragm is obscured by the liver. A right-sided liver mobilization will be described primarily since tumor involvement on the left diaphragm is more easily resected without fully mobilizing the liver. In certain cases, metastatic deposits on the left diaphragm may be contiguous with the splenic capsule requiring splenectomy.

The infrahepatic edge of the falciform ligament containing the ligamentum teres is divided and ligated. The divided pedicle can be used to provide downward traction of the liver and remaining falciform ligament. The falciform ligament should be transected all the way to the coronary ligament. The coronary ligament is incised from the falciform to the right triangular ligament. Careful attention should be directed at the area of the hepatic notch that contains the right hepatic vein as it enters the IVC. It is found lateral to the union of the falciform and coronary ligaments. If further mobilization of the liver is necessary, the lateral attachments may be incised and the liver bluntly lifted off Gerota fascia of the right kidney and diaphragm.

The extent of diaphragm peritonectomy can be tailored according to the distribution of disease. When a full right diaphragm peritonectomy is performed, the peritoneum on the anterior edge of the diaphragm is incised along the costal margin. This edge is grasped and retracted inferiorly to visualize the line of attachment between the diaphragm and its overlying peritoneum. The plane between is developed with a combination of blunt and sharp dissection; however, this may not be possible if the tumor has extended through the peritoneum and diaphragm.

If tumor implants are securely fixed to the diaphragm muscle and/or are suspicious for full thickness diaphragm involvement, diaphragm resection can be performed. The technique for diaphragm resection depends largely on the size of the lesion to be resected. Small penetrating lesions can be resected using the Endo GIA stapler alone without entering the pleural cavity. The lesion is grasped with clamps, the diaphragm tented downward away from the lung, and the Endo GIA is used to staple and divide the tented diaphragm and invasive lesion while closing off the residual diaphragm. Larger lesions require entry into the pleural space. This is done carefully to avoid injury to the underlying lung. Once entered and the lung visualized/retracted, the lesion is resected en bloc with the peritoneal, muscular, and pleural layers. The defect can frequently be closed primarily with limited tension, using permanent sutures. Larger defects that are not amenable to primary closure should be closed with a permanent mesh secured to the peritoneal diaphragm surface (44). The majority of patients undergoing limited diaphragm resection can have their pleural cavity closed and the air from the thorax evacuated using a Red Rubber Robinson catheter. A purse-string suture is placed widely around the hole and a #14 French Red Rubber Robinson catheter is passed through the hole into the pleural cavity. The anesthesiologist is asked to give the patient a maximal inspiration, suction may be applied to the catheter, and the catheter is pulled as the purse-string suture is tied down. For patients undergoing more extensive resections or with other reasons to benefit from prolonged pleural drainage, such as pleurodesis, a chest tube can be placed in the operating room.

To remove tumor from the left upper quadrant, occasionally a splenectomy with or without distal pancreatectomy is required. The lesser sac can be entered to evaluate the posterior aspect of the stomach and pancreas. The gastrosplenic ligament and then the short gastrics are carefully divided. The spleen is mobilized medially and out of the left upper quadrant by dividing the splenophrenic and splenocolic ligaments and the other attachments to the adrenal gland and Gerota fascia of the left kidney. The spleen can now be elevated out of the splenic bed and into the incision. The splenic hilum is now grasped between the fingers to identify the splenic artery and vein as well as palpate the tail of the pancreas. These vessels should be ligated and divided. If needed, a linear stapler may be placed across the tail of the pancreas to remove tumor involving the distal pancreas and/or splenic hilum. Reinforcement of this staple line with 3-0 delayed absorbable suture, either continuously or interrupted, is optional. Use of staplers with a buttress may be associated with fewer pancreatic leaks (45).

Urinary Diversion

Over the past three decades, interest in performing continent urinary diversions for patients with gynecologic malignancies has emerged. Most gynecologic oncologists will use a modification of the Indiana (46) or Miami (47) pouch.

A modification of these pouches is shown in **Figures 9.27** to **9.29** (2). The colon is transected just proximal to the hepatic flexure (**Fig. 9.27**). The colon is then detubularized by a longitudinal incision along the tinea. The continent mechanism is created by two maneuvers. First, the terminal ileal segment is tapered down over a #14 French Foley catheter by using a gastrointestinal anastomosis (GIA) stapling device along the antimesenteric border of the ileum. The second maneuver is to plicate the ileocecal valve by placing concentric purse-string permanent sutures around it. The ureters are then implanted under direct vision (**Fig. 9.28**) (2). After closing the pouch, the ileal stoma can be brought out in several areas of the abdominal wall (**Fig. 9.29**) (2). Some use the umbilicus as the exit site. The ureteral stents can exit the abdomen via the ileal stoma or through separate incisions in the pouch and abdominal wall. The use of a Foley drain and a cecostomy tube for irrigation to remove mucus is generally employed.

Poor candidates for continent urinary diversion include those who are physically or psychologically unable to perform frequent self-catheterization and maintenance of the pouch. For these patients, an ileal conduit has been the preferred alternative. However, in patients who will also require a colostomy, performing a double barrel wet colostomy has been reported. This combined urinary and fecal diversion employs a loop colostomy with the proximal limb serving as an end colostomy and the distal limb as a sigmoid conduit. This double-barreled wet colostomy may be associated with fewer complications than performing separate urinary and fecal diversions (48).

SURGICAL MANAGEMENT OF GYNECOLOGIC CANCER

The gynecologic oncologist must be able to evaluate the woman with a genital tract malignancy, direct her management, perform the necessary surgical procedures, and supervise her postoperative care and surveillance. A patient who is managed by a surgeon not trained in gynecologic oncology may receive an inappropriate or inadequate operation. This was demonstrated in a series of 291 women with primary ovarian cancer who underwent intraoperative evaluation. Ninety-seven percent of the patients who underwent surgery by a gynecologic oncologist received complete staging operations, but in patients undergoing staging operations by an obstetrician-gynecologist or general surgeon, only 52% and 35%, respectively, had adequate operations (49).

Two more recent British studies retrospectively analyzed the outcomes of over 1,800 patients with ovarian cancer (50,51). Both studies found on multivariate analysis that patients' survival was adversely impacted when their initial operation was performed by a general surgeon as opposed to a gynecologic surgeon. These results are similar to those obtained by Nguyen et al. (52) in an American national survey of ovarian carcinoma. Eisenkop et al. (53) analyzed the outcomes of 263 patients with stages IIIC and IV ovarian

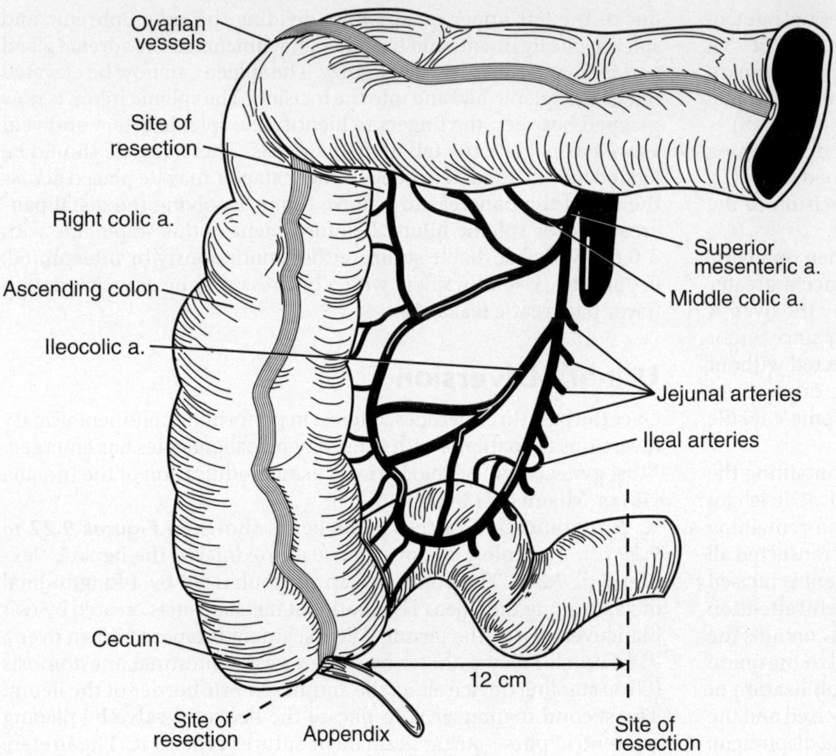

Figure 9.27. The anatomic location and vascularity of the right colon segment utilized for formation of the continent urinary pouch. Illustrated are the anatomic sites of division for creation of the continent pouch. The ascending colon is divided distal to the right colic artery. The terminal ileum is divided approximately 12 cm from the ileocecal valve. The resection can be accomplished with the use of surgical staplers or by intestinal clamps. If the appendix is present, it should be removed. The ileocecal segment has a rich blood supply derived from the right colic artery and the ileocolic artery. If one is performing the Miami pouch type of urinary diversion, the transverse colon would be divided distal to the middle colic artery.

After Gallup DG, Talledo OE. *Surgical Atlas of Gynecologic Oncology.* Philadelphia, PA: WB Saunders Co.; 1994:186.

carcinoma. When the primary surgery was performed by gynecologic oncologists, as compared to general obstetricians-gynecologists and general surgeons, the rate of optimal cytoreduction was significantly higher, the operative mortality substantially lower, and the median survival significantly longer.

Accordingly, other countries have attempted to centralize the care of patients with ovarian cancer so that they are primarily operated on by gynecologic oncologists (54,55). However, patterns of care studies in the United States have demonstrated that a significant percentage of women with ovarian cancer are not receiving their primary treatment from gynecologic oncologists (56,57). Consequently, in the United States, many women with ovarian cancer are still not receiving the recommended comprehensive primary surgery (58,59).

In the four decades since the establishment of gynecologic oncology as a subspecialty, cancer therapy has become increasingly sophisticated and complex, and it is difficult for any one physician to master all the skills necessary for treating gynecologic malignancies. More often, we must use multimodal therapy and participate in multidisciplinary care. There are many medical and radiation oncologists who have specialized in gynecologic cancer, and they are integral members of the multidisciplinary team. The Gynecologic Oncology Group, with its emphasis on multidisciplinary research, has demonstrated the effectiveness of such an approach.

Another important factor in providing optimal patient care is the environment in which gynecologic oncology is practiced. The facilities used by the gynecologic oncologist should offer state-of-the-art radiation therapy and chemotherapy. Patients should receive care tailored to the type and extent of their disease and their care not be determined by the limitations of the available facilities. Mortality rates for complex oncologic procedures, such as pelvic exenteration, have been demonstrated to be significantly lower in hospitals where a relatively high volume of procedures are performed, compared to hospitals in which the procedures are performed infrequently (60). The recent meta-analysis performed by Bristow et al. (43) evaluated 81 studies involving 6,885 patients with advanced ovarian cancer. This study demonstrated a 50% increase in median survival if patients' primary surgery was performed at an "expert" center compared to less experienced centers. In a recent review of the literature, Cowan et al. (61) concluded that patients with invasive epithelial ovarian cancer had improved optimal debulking rates, guideline adherence, and overall survival when cared for in high volume centers by high volume physicians.

Diagnosis and Staging

The diagnosis of any gynecologic cancer requires a surgical biopsy. The manner in which the histologic diagnosis is obtained varies with the disease and the clinical situation. A punch biopsy or an instrument biopsy may be sufficient for the diagnosis of an invasive cancer of the vulva, vagina, or cervix, but an excisional biopsy is necessary for the diagnosis of microinvasive or preinvasive cancer. A fine-needle aspiration biopsy for cytologic analysis may be adequate for establishing the extent of spread of a cancer, but may not be sufficient to provide histologic cell type and grade for the primary diagnosis. Core needle biopsy or surgical exploration may be required to provide this information for diagnosis.

The current International Federation of Gynecology and Obstetrics (FIGO) staging system of gynecologic cancers requires surgical staging for vulvar, endometrial, and ovarian cancer. Cervical cancer remains a clinically staged disease, although many centers use surgical staging (by laparotomy or laparoscopy) for treatment planning. **Table 9.2** lists the current methods of staging for the various gynecologic malignancies.

The initial surgical procedure in a patient with known or suspected gynecologic cancer should be performed by a trained gynecologic oncologist because the accuracy of diagnosis and staging significantly influences subsequent prognosis and therapy. Numerous studies have demonstrated that ovarian cancer staging operations performed by general obstetricians-gynecologists or general surgeons are inadequate much more frequently than if the

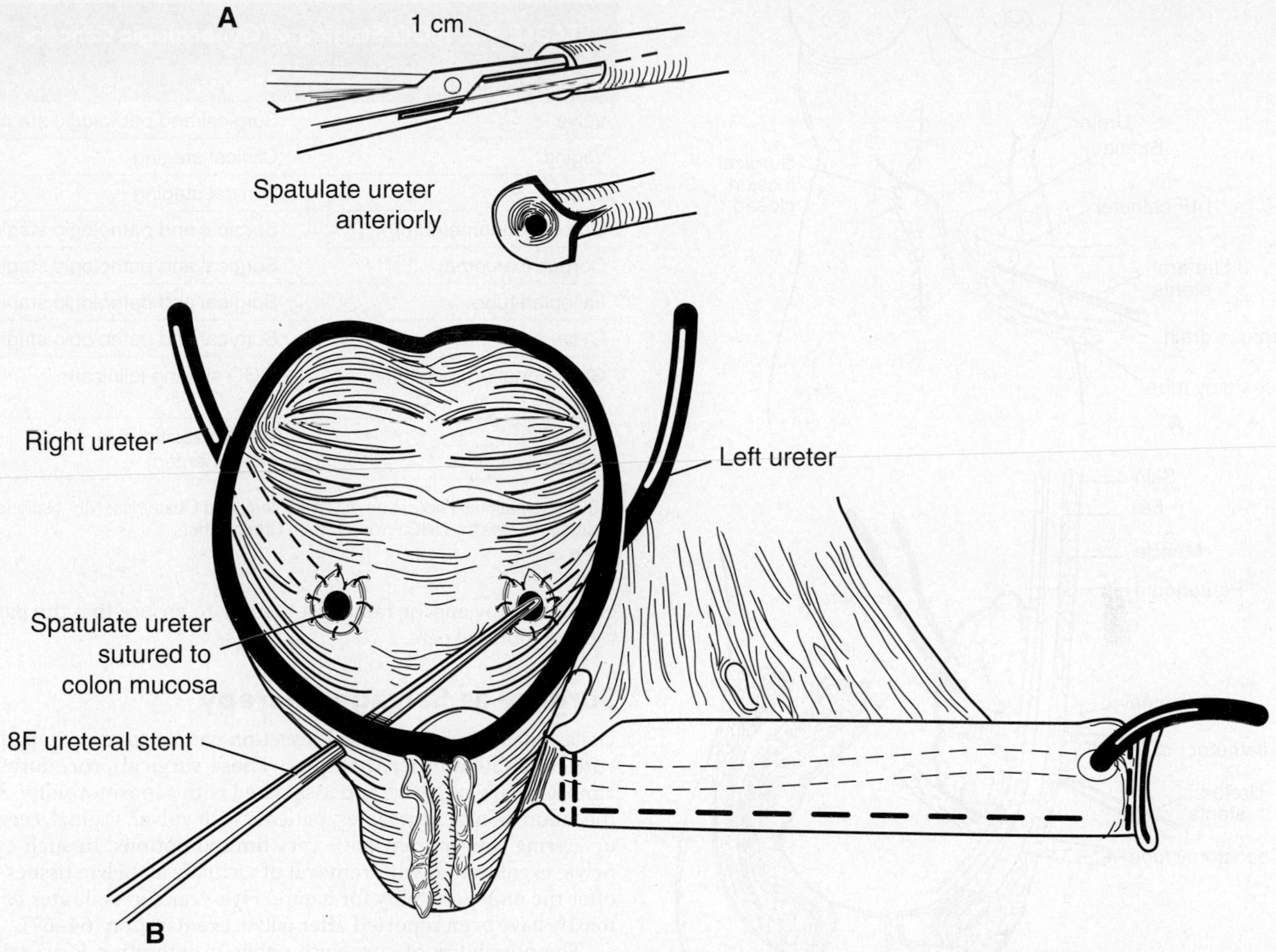

Figure 9.28. (A, B) Prior to beginning the continent diversion, the ureters have been transected (usually at the pelvic brim) and mobilized so that they can be brought to the area where the continent pouch will be located without tension. If necessary, the left ureter can be brought through or under the mesentery of the colon to facilitate its placement into the urinary pouch. An appropriate site is selected on what will be the posterior wall of the pouch, and a long thin clamp is used to perforate the colon and pull the ureter through. An approximately 1-cm segment of ureter is brought into the pouch. For ease of ureterointestinal anastomosis, the ureter should be secured posteriorly to the pouch by suturing the adventitial tissue of the ureter to the seromuscular layers of the pouch with three or four permanent 3-0 sutures. The ureter is spatulated to increase the lumen diameter. The ureter is sutured directly to the colon and is not tunneled. We use 4-0 polyglycolic suture. This is a full thickness approximation of the colon and ureter. Once both ureters have been sutured into the pouch, two #8 French ureterointestinal stents or long pediatric feeding tubes are placed retrograde into the renal pelvis. If a feeding tube is used, it should be sutured to the ureter with 4-0 chromic to ensure against displacement due to ureteral peristalsis. Note the three concentric sutures at the ileocecal valve.

After Gallup DG, Talledo OE. *Surgical Atlas of Gynecologic Oncology.* Philadelphia, PA: WB Saunders Co.; 1994:191.

operation is performed by a gynecologic oncologist. Young et al. (62) reported excellent survival in patients with early ovarian cancer, but stressed that these data were applicable only to patients with adequate surgical staging.

In addition to the anatomic site and stage of disease, the plan of therapy for most gynecologic malignancies is also influenced by the histologic cell type and histologic grade of the cancer. The collaboration of the surgeon, pathologist, and cytologist cannot be overemphasized in the diagnosis and staging of cancer. Communication about clinical history and desired information from the anatomic specimen is important in directing the clinical care of the patient.

Surgery as Primary Therapy

Surgery is usually the treatment method of choice for preinvasive diseases of the vulva, vagina, and cervix, for which local excision is both diagnostic and curative. Surgical margins should clear only gross and microscopic disease. In vulvar cancer, excision with a 1-cm normal tissue margin is appropriate (63).

Localized disease, such as stage I vulvar cancer, stage I posterior vaginal cancer, and stage IA2/IB1 cervical cancer, are usually managed by radical resection of the primary tumor and regional lymph node evaluation. Lymphadenectomy has traditionally been the standard method of evaluation; however, some centers have adopted sentinel lymph node evaluation instead. In these settings, the operations themselves are designed to be curative without adjunctive therapy unless high-risk conditions are identified. As described in the chapter on vulvar cancer, there is a trend toward more conservative therapy for vulvar malignancies. This allows preservation of normal tissues and prevents some of the disfigurement that can be associated with this surgery. Surgery may be curative without adjuvant therapy for other cancers as well, including early-stage endometrial cancer, stage IA ovarian cancer, and early sarcomas of the uterus.

Findings at surgery may identify patients who may benefit from additional treatment (adjuvant therapy). It is administered because of the potential for occult spread of disease based on a surgical finding (e.g., positive lymph nodes). The use of adjuvant therapy requires that information be available to allow the selection of patients with

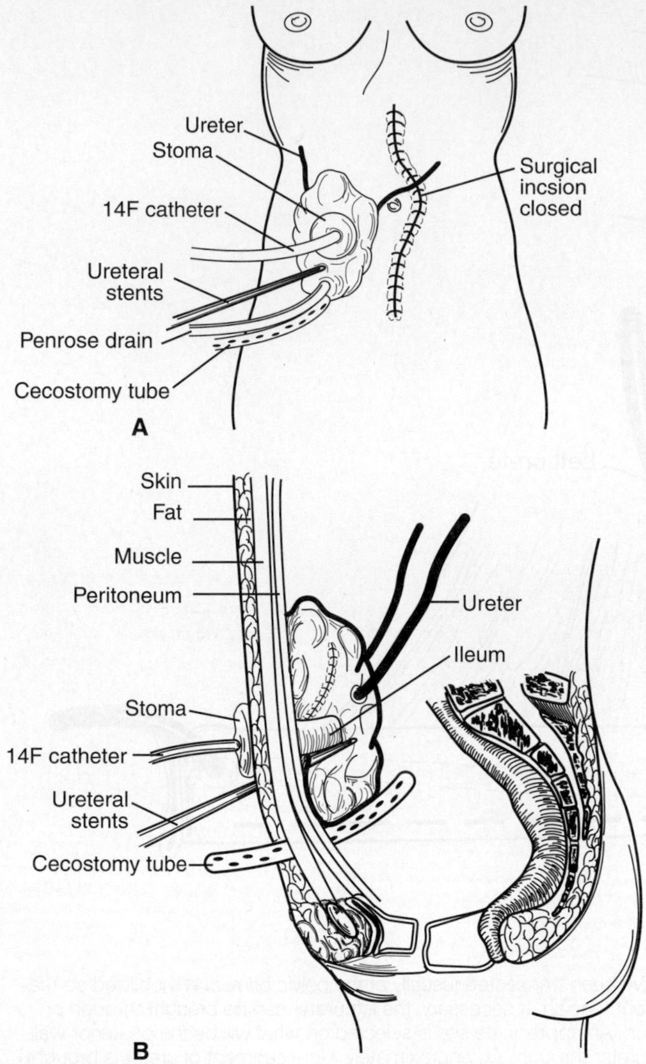

Figure 9.29. (A, B) The site for the ileal stoma is selected on the anterior abdominal wall and then incised through all abdominal tissue layers. The stoma is created for catheterization and the #14 French catheter should exit the pouch through this stoma. It is critical that the ileal segment be at a 90° angle with the abdominal wall so that catheterization is a "straight shot." The pouch may be sutured to the abdominal wall to accomplish this. All stents and drainage tubes are brought out through the anterior abdominal wall and secured. The pouch may also be anchored posteriorly (i.e., to the sacrum).

After Gallup DG, Talledo OE. *Surgical Atlas of Gynecologic Oncology.* Philadelphia, PA: WB Saunders Co.; 1994:193.

a high risk of recurrence. These risk groups are defined for each disease site in the appropriate chapters of this book.

Surgery Combined with Other Therapies

In some gynecologic cancers, surgery remains the cornerstone of treatment but may not be curative when used alone. Primary surgical cytoreduction of gross disease is vital in advanced ovarian cancer, but it is of little benefit without adjuvant chemotherapy. For patients with early-stage endometrial and cervical cancer, surgical removal of the uterus can be curative in many cases. However, depending on the histopathologic findings of the surgical specimens, additional regional radiotherapy and/or chemotherapy may be indicated. The gynecologic oncologist should be aware of which patients may benefit from adjuvant therapy, and be able to coordinate adjuvant chemotherapy and/or radiation therapy to ensure that the patient receives optimal care.

TABLE 9.2. FIGO Staging of Gynecologic Cancers

Site	Staging
Vulva	Surgical and pathologic staging
Vagina	Clinical staging
Cervix	Clinical staging
Corpus (endometrium)	Surgical and pathologic staging
Corpus (sarcoma)	Surgical and pathologic staging
Fallopian tube	Surgical and pathologic staging
Ovary	Surgical and pathologic staging
Gestational trophoblastic disease	FIGO staging (clinical)
	WHO classification (risk-oriented)

FIGO, International Federation of Gynecology and Obstetrics; NIH, National Institutes of Health; WHO, World Health Organization.

Surgery as Salvage Therapy

Occasionally, radical surgical resection can be curative in patients who have failed other therapies. These surgical procedures are almost always extensive and associated with some morbidity. After the failure of other therapies, patients with vulvar, vaginal, cervical, or uterine cancers may have very limited options. In such cases, pelvic exenteration with removal of virtually all pelvic tissues may offer the only possibility for a cure. Five-year survival rates of 23% to 61% have been reported after pelvic exenteration (64–67).

The possibility of cure with pelvic exenteration is associated with high morbidity and changes in bodily functions. The loss of the bladder and the rectum often requires permanent stomas, and sexual function is impaired or lost in many patients. For some patients, reconstructive techniques can prevent the need for stomas and may also restore sexual function. During the last three decades, improvements in initial surgery and radiation therapy along with refinements in selection criteria have made operations like pelvic exenteration infrequent (68). Today, most patients experience distant failure rather than regional failure, and they are therefore not candidates for attempts at curative pelvic exenteration.

Surgery as salvage therapy may also play an important role in the management of ovarian, fallopian tube, and some endometrial cancers. For patients who have failed initial therapy and chemotherapy, second attempts at cytoreduction may be beneficial, provided that reasonable salvage therapy is available (69–71).

Surgery for Metastatic Disease

In selected cases, distant metastases from gynecologic tumors may be curable by surgical resection, or the resection may produce a prolonged disease-free interval. Fuller et al. (72) reported on 15 patients who underwent pulmonary resection of distant metastases from a variety of gynecologic malignancies. They reported a 5-year survival rate of 36% and a 10-year survival rate of 26%. Patients with solitary metastases had a median survival of 64 months, with a median survival of 48 months for those with multiple metastases. Levenback et al. (73) reported their experience with 45 patients who underwent pulmonary resection of metastases from uterine sarcomas. From the date of the pulmonary resection, the 5-year survival rate was 41%, with a 10-year survival rate of 35%. They found a statistically improved chance of survival for patients who developed pulmonary metastases 1 year or longer from their original therapy, and for those with unilateral metastases. There was no statistical difference in survival based on the number of nodules (in one lung), the size of the lesion, the age of the patient, or the use of post-resection adjunctive therapy. However, the small numbers of patients in this study precluded adequate evaluation of these factors.

There is increasing evidence that salvage therapy in ovarian and fallopian tube cancers is likely to be more effective in patients with minimal residual disease. Secondary cytoreduction may play an important role in the treatment of select patients with recurrent disease (70). Recent reports have demonstrated promising results with surgical resection of isolated metastases to the parenchyma of the liver and spleen (74,75).

Surgery for Reconstruction

Reconstructive surgery may be performed at the time of resection of the cancer, as a delayed procedure, or as required therapy to correct a complication of treatment. Vulvar reconstruction is usually done at the time of initial resection and may involve the use of free skin grafts, rotational flaps of adjacent skin and fat tissue, or myocutaneous grafts from the thigh, buttocks, or anterior abdominal wall. Vaginal reconstruction may also be performed, usually as a planned, delayed phase of reconstruction. Vaginal reconstruction requires free skin grafts or myocutaneous flaps, depending on the size of the defect and whether or not there has been previous irradiation of the vaginal bed. The techniques of vulvar and vaginal reconstruction are explained in detail in other chapters of this book.

Reconstruction as therapy for complications of treatment may be required for the closure of defects from improper wound healing, radiation necrosis, or tissue loss after extravasation of chemotherapeutic agents. Although free skin grafts may be used to reconstruct surgical wound disruption or tissue loss due to chemotherapy extravasation, radiation necrosis usually requires the use of myocutaneous flaps because of a lack of adequate blood supply in the area of the injury.

Surgery for Palliation

Surgery for palliation may involve resection of tumor to relieve symptoms, or it may involve diversion or bypass of portions of the gastrointestinal or urinary tract to prolong life and provide comfort. Consideration of surgery for palliation must take into account the risks of the procedure and the degree of successful palliation. In many cases, these patients will have a limited life span; however, the gynecologic oncologist should not uniformly dismiss the concept of surgical palliation. A surgical procedure may provide quick relief of symptoms as compared to palliative administration of a chemotherapeutic agent for 6 to 12 months, which may or may not result in minor tumor shrinkage or stabilization of disease despite the side effects. The gynecologic oncologist must use astute surgical judgment and a realistic assessment of the patient's condition and wishes when deciding on palliative surgery.

Palliative surgery is more frequently used to relieve specific dysfunctions, such as obstruction of the urinary or intestinal tract. Relief of urinary tract obstruction may be accomplished by ureteroneocystostomy or by urinary conduit, depending on the location of the obstruction and the location or extent of disease. A urinary conduit can provide immediate and permanent relief to the patient who has a ureterovaginal, vesicovaginal, or urethrovaginal fistula. It may also provide relief of urinary obstruction, which will prolong life and allow for the administration of additional chemotherapy or irradiation. The judgment of the surgeon and the desires of the patient become essential factors in this decision-making process. For the patient suffering from constant urinary leakage or who may benefit from additional therapy, the decision to perform a urinary diversion is quite simple. If diversion is done to prolong life, however, the decision must be weighed carefully. For a patient who has a limited life expectancy or is in uncontrollable pain, performing a urinary diversion may do more harm than good.

In certain situations, one must also consider the relative benefits of nonsurgical urinary diversion, such as placement of a ureteral stent or a percutaneous nephrostomy. Nonoperative management options may be more attractive and may prove to be better choices than surgical intervention if they can resolve the urinary problem. This is particularly true if the aim is to employ adjunctive chemotherapy or irradiation, or if a surgical procedure is not feasible because of medical conditions or other considerations. Unfortunately, a percutaneous nephrostomy may not help the patient with a fistula because the nephrostomy may not totally divert the urine.

Placement of a ureteral stent, by cystoscopy or antegrade through a percutaneous nephrostomy, is usually better and safer than urinary diversion for the relief of obstruction. Current technology allows the placement of stents that can be left in place for months and can be changed easily over a guide wire by means of the cystoscope.

Intestinal obstruction is a common finding in patients with ovarian cancer. Deciding whether the operation is feasible can be more difficult in this setting, particularly since the radiologic studies may not reveal the true extent of disease. For the patient with localized disease, a diverting colostomy or an intestinal bypass is usually possible. For the patient with intra-abdominal carcinomatosis, the decision to operate should be weighed against the chance of success and the surgical risks.

Pothuri et al. (76) evaluated 68 palliative operations performed on 64 patients with recurrent ovarian cancer and intestinal obstruction. In 84% of cases, a corrective surgical procedure could performed, whereas no corrective surgical procedure was possible for the remaining 16%. Of the 57 cases where corrective surgery was possible, 71% were successfully palliated ("successful palliation" is defined as the ability to tolerate a regular or low-residue diet at least 60 days postoperatively). If surgery resulted in successful palliation, median survival was 11.6 months compared to 3.9 months for all other patients.

THE FUTURE OF GYNECOLOGIC ONCOLOGY

Gynecologic oncologists must continue to advance the efficacy of the surgical management of patients with gynecologic cancers. Recent trends in this field have focused on minimizing surgical-related morbidity without compromising oncologic outcomes.

Changes in Surgical Therapy

Technology will continue to expand surgical capabilities in the management of gynecologic cancers. Oncologic surgery in general has moved toward using minimally invasive techniques to perform surgical resection. There was a rapid increase in the use of laparoscopic surgery in the field of gynecologic oncology in the 1990s. Recent improvements in technology, in particular robotics, have further shifted the management of several gynecologic cancers away from open surgery to minimally invasive surgery.

Despite multiple reports that malignancies of the uterine corpus and cervix could be managed using a minimally invasive approach with traditional laparoscopy, the gynecologic oncology community was slow to adopt this technique. In a survey on the use of laparoscopy by members of the Society of Gynecologic Oncology in 2004, only 10% of respondents identified endometrial cancer surgery as the most commonly performed laparoscopic procedure (77). Advanced traditional laparoscopic procedures were not uniformly adopted by all gynecologic oncologists, and only a minority routinely performed advanced procedures. This was likely due to the need to acquire new surgical skills sets, the noncomplementary movements of the laparoscopic instruments compared to the surgeon's movements, and the limited range of motion of the currently available instruments. Laparoscopic technology only provided the surgeon with two-dimensional images, poor ergonomics for lengthy procedures, and difficulty in suturing. It may be technical and mentally challenging to complete many complex procedures in a minimally invasive fashion. The robotic surgical platform was initially developed for use by the military. In 2005, the U.S. Food and Drug Administration approved its use for gynecologic conditions. This led to a major shift in the surgical management of patients with gynecologic cancers, in particular, cancers of the uterine corpus and cervix. The advent of robotic technology has overcome many of the above-mentioned limitations associated with traditional laparoscopy. In an update of a previous survey of the members of the Society of Gynecologic Oncology, Conrad et al. reported that 70% of respondents in 2012 identified endometrial cancer surgery as the most commonly performed laparoscopic procedure. Much of this change may be related to the increase in use of robotic surgery for total hysterectomy and staging of endometrial cancer (78).

Sentinel lymph node evaluation is another example of the movement in the specialty to minimize surgical morbidity associated with cancer treatment. Lymphadenectomy has been an integral part of the surgical management of gynecologic malignancies. The identification of nodal metastases has profound effects on postoperative management and adjuvant therapy. However, this comes with a cost in that lymphadenectomy has been associated with long-term morbidity (79).

A more targeted approach to lymph node evaluation may eventually do away with the need to perform lymph node sampling to any degree. Sentinel lymph node mapping was first reported for penile cancer in 1977 (80). This method of assessing the lymph nodes has been widely used in the management of breast cancer and melanoma. Use of this technique in the management of vulvar and endometrial cancer was first reported in the 1990s (81,82). Sentinel node mapping has become a topic of debate, as it may provide diagnostic accuracy while minimizing the morbidity associated with complete lymphadenectomy (83,84). Although no large randomized study exists to support the use of sentinel node mapping for apparent early-stage cervical and endometrial cancers, there are large studies that do support this novel technique (85,86).

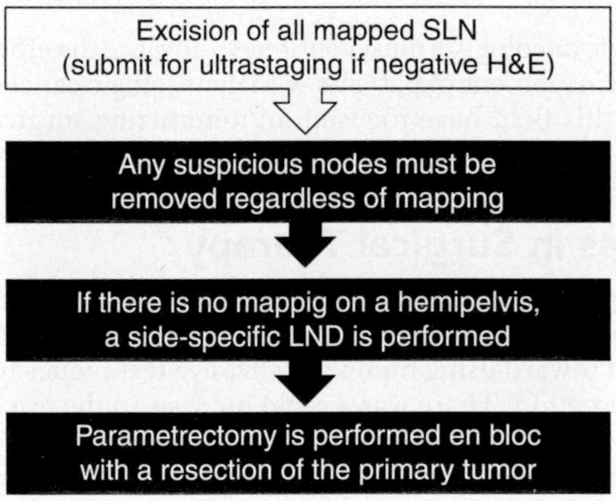

Figure 9.30. Sentinel lymph node algorithm for early-stage cervical cancer. H&E, hematoxylin and eosin (stain); SLN, sentinel lymph node; LND, lymph node dissection.

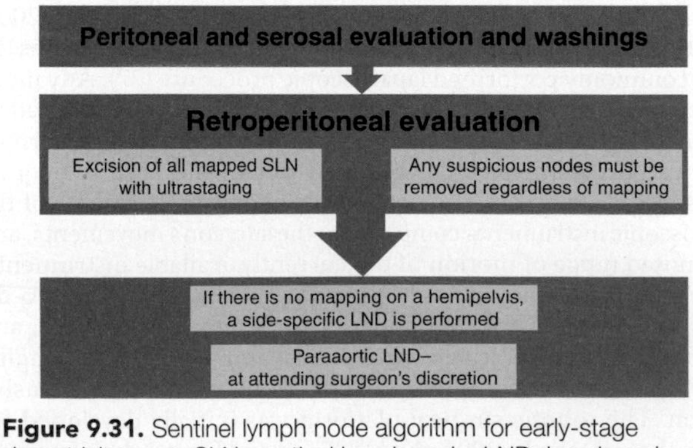

Figure 9.31. Sentinel lymph node algorithm for early-stage endometrial cancer. SLN, sentinel lymph node; LND, lymph node dissection.

Some have advocated using sentinel node mapping as part of a specific algorithm in the management of cervical and uterine cancers (**Figs. 9.30** and **9.31**) (87,88). In brief, these algorithms consist of retroperitoneal evaluation, including excision of all mapped sentinel nodes and suspicious nodes regardless of mapping; if there is no mapping on a hemipelvis, a side-specific lymph node dissection is performed. By employing such an algorithm, false-negative rates can be lowered, nodal counts minimized, and accuracy in the detection rate of lymph node metastases maintained (89).

Different techniques have been described for sentinel node mapping in endometrial cancer. Currently, there have been three injection sites described for this procedure. A cervical injection, a subserosal/myometrial, and a hysteroscopic endometrial injection have all been described. Cervical injection appears to be the easiest and most convenient technique; however, some have questioned its accuracy (90). The use of superior imaging technology such as fluorescence may also increase the detection rate of the sentinel nodes (91).

Innovative management pathways have been developed to hasten recovery and attenuate the stress response associated with surgery. Components of these pathways include preoperative patient education, reduction of preoperative fasting, omission of bowel preparation, perioperative normovolemia, limited use of nasogastric tubes and drains, early removal of urinary catheters, minimizing opiate use, early postoperative mobilization, enhanced gastrointestinal motility with prokinetics, and early enteral nutrition. Together, these components comprise an enhanced recovery pathway that has been adopted by many gynecologic oncologists and has resulted in decreased length of stay and cost (92,93).

Changes in the Indications for Surgery

Early diagnosis will change the indications for surgery and the types of procedures that should be done. It then follows that gynecologic oncologists will be able to treat more patients with less morbidity and with greater preservation of function. The use of minimally invasive surgery for patients with early-stage uterine cancer is a prime example of how patients can be effectively treated with less morbidity and improved quality of life.

Better adjunctive therapies will increase the importance of initial surgical therapy. More patients will benefit from surgical cytoreduction to minimize disease. The availability of effective irradiation, chemotherapeutic regimens, and biologic regimens will make adjuvant therapy feasible in more cases, and it will become more important for us to identify groups of high-risk patients who are likely to develop recurrent disease after surgery.

CONCLUSION

In 1969, the American Board of Obstetrics and Gynecology recommended the development of the subspecialty of gynecologic oncology, and in 1973, the American Board of Medical Specialties approved this unique specialty. The gynecologic oncologist should be viewed as a surgical oncologist who possesses sufficient familiarity with radiation oncology and medical oncology to ensure the proper integration of all modalities of treatment. In many cases, the gynecologic oncologist is able to apply surgical skills for primary therapy, secondary therapy, reconstruction, and palliation.

Many battles had to be won for gynecologic oncologists to perform the surgical procedures that are traditionally done by general surgeons and urologists. Although management of gynecologic cancers requires integration of surgery with the specialties of medical oncology and radiation oncology, advancement of the surgical management of patients with gynecologic malignancies remains solely within our specialty. We are primarily surgeons and must perform surgical procedures at the highest level. The advancement of the surgical management of patients with gynecologic malignancies remains solely within this specialty.

REFERENCES

1. Morrow CP, Curtin JP, eds. *Gynecologic Cancer Surgery*. New York, NY: Churchill Livingstone; 1996.
2. Gallup DG, Talledo OE, eds. *Surgical Atlas of Gynecologic Oncology*. Philadelphia, PA: WB Saunders; 1994.
3. Abu-Rustum NR, Barakat RR, Levine DA. *Atlas of Procedures in Gynecologic Oncology*, 3rd ed. London, UK: Informa Healthcare; 2013.
4. Fowler JM, Johnson PR. Transperitoneal para-aortic lymphadenectomy. *Oper Tech Gynecol Surg*. 1996;1:8–12.
5. Eisenhauer EL, Abu-Rustum NR, Sonoda Y, et al. The addition of extensive upper abdominal surgery to achieve optimal cytoreduction improves survival in patients with stage IIIC–IV epithelial ovarian cancer. *Gynecol Oncol*. 2006;103:1083–1090.
6. Chi DS, Eisenhauer EL, Zivanovic O, et al. Improved progression-free and overall survival in advanced ovarian cancer as a result of a change in surgical paradigm. *Gynecol Oncol*. 2009;114:26–31.
7. Eisenhauer EL, Chi DS. Liver mobilization and diaphragm peritonectomy/resection. *Gynecol Oncol*. 2007;104(2):S25–S28.
8. Skandalakis JE, Gray SW, Rowe JR, eds. *Anatomical Complications in General Surgery*. New York, NY: McGraw-Hill; 1983.
9. Poulin EC, Schlachta DM, Maazza J. Splenectomy. Gastroinestinal tract and abdomen. In: Souba WW, Fink MJ, Jurkovich GJ, et al., eds. *ACS Surgery: Principles and Practice*, 7th ed. Philadelphia, PA: BC Decker, Inc.; 2014.
10. Berman ML, Lagasse LD, Watring WG, et al. The operative evaluation of patients with cervical cancer by an extraperitoneal approach. *Obstet Gynecol*. 1977;50:658–664.
11. Gallup DG, King LA, Messing MJ, et al. Paraaortic lymph node sampling by means of an extraperitoneal approach with a supraumbilical transverse "sunrise" incision. *Am J Obstet Gynecol*. 1993;169:307–312.
12. Bonjer HJ, Hazebroek EJ, Kazemier G, et al. Open versus closed establishment of pneumoperitoneum in laparoscopic surgery. *Br J Surg*. 1997;84:599–602.
13. Ahmad G, Gent D, Henderson D, et al. Laparoscopic entry techniques. *Cochrane Database Syst Rev*. 2015;8:CD006583. doi:10.1002/14651858.CD006583.
14. Abu-Rustum NR, Sonoda Y. Transperitoneal laparoscopic staging with aortic and pelvic lymph node dissection for gynecologic malignancies. *Gynecol Oncol*. 2007;104(2 Suppl 1):5–8. Erratum in: *Gynecol Oncol*. 2007;107(3):598.
15. Weiser EB, Bundy BN, Hoskins WJ, et al. Extraperitoneal versus transperitoneal selective paraaortic lymphadenectomy in the pretreatment surgical staging of advanced cervical carcinoma: a Gynecologic Oncology Group study. *Gynecol Oncol*. 1989;33:283–289.
16. Dargent D, Salvat J. Envahissement ganglionnaire pelvien: place de la pelviscopie rétropéritonéale. In: Dargent D, Salvat J, eds. *L'Envahissement Ganglionnaire Pelvien*. Paris, France: Medsi McGraw-Hill; 1989.
17. Querleu D. Laparoscopic lymphadenectomy. Presented at the Second World Congress of Gynecologic Endoscopy, Clermont-Ferrand, France, June 5–8, 1989.
18. Querleu D, Leblanc E, Castelain B. Laparoscopic pelvic lymphadenectomy in the staging of early carcinoma of the cervix. *Am J Obstet Gynecol*. 1991;164:579–583.
19. Walker JL, Piedmonte MR, Spirtos NM, et al. Laparoscopy compared with laparotomy for comprehensive surgical staging of uterine cancer: Gynecologic Oncology Group Study LAP2. *J Clin Oncol*. 2009;27(32):5331–5336. doi:10.1200/JCO.2009.22.3248.
20. Childers JM, Surwit EA. Combined laparoscopic and vaginal surgery for the management of two cases of stage I endometrial cancer. *Gynecol Oncol*. 1992;45:46–48.
21. Querleu D, Leblanc E. Laparoscopic infrarenal paraaortic lymph node dissection for restaging of carcinoma of the ovary or fallopian tube. *Cancer*. 1994;73:1467–1471.
22. Querleu D, Leblanc E, Cartron G, et al. Audit of preoperative and early complications of laparoscopic lymph node dissection in 1000 gynecologic cancer patients. *Am J Obstet Gynecol*. 2006;195:1287–1292.
23. Kohler C, Klemm P, Schau A, et al. Introduction of transperitoneal lymphadenectomy in a gynecologic oncology center: analysis of 650 laparoscopic pelvic and/or paraaortic transperitoneal lymphadenectomies. *Gynecol Oncol*. 2004;95:52–61.
24. Vasilev SA, McGonigle KF. Extraperitoneal laparoscopic paraaortic lymph node dissection: development of a technique. *J Laparoendosc Surg*. 1995;5(2):85–90.
25. Querleu D, Dargent D, Ansquer Y, et al. Extraperitoneal endosurgical aortic and common iliac dissection in the staging of bulky or advanced cervical carcinomas. *Cancer*. 2000;88:883–891.
26. Leblanc E, Gauthier H, Querleu D, et al. Accuracy of 18-fluoro-2-deoxy-D-glucose positron emission tomography in the pretherapeutic detection of occult para-aortic node involvement in patients with a locally advanced cervical carcinoma [published online February 23, 2011]. *Ann Surg Oncol*. 2011.
27. Leblanc E, Narducci F, Frumovitz M, et al. Therapeutic value of pretherapeutic extraperitoneal laparoscopic staging of locally advanced cervical carcinoma. *Gynecol Oncol*. 2007;105:304–311.
28. Dowdy SC, Aletti G, Cliby WA, et al. Extra-peritoneal laparoscopic para-aortic lymphadenectomy—a prospective cohort study of 293 patients with endometrial cancer. *Gynecol Oncol*. 2008;111(3):418–424. doi:10.1016/j.ygyno.2008.08.021.
29. Wertheim E. The extended abdominal operation for carcinoma uteri (based on 500 operative cases). *Am J Obstet Dis Women Child*. 1912;66:169–232.
30. Okabayashi H. Radical abdominal hysterectomy for cancer of the cervix uteri. *Surg Gynecol Obstet*. 1921;33:335–341.
31. Meigs JV. Carcinoma of the cervix—the Wertheim operation. *Surg Gynecol Obstet*. 1944;78:195–198.
32. Piver MS, Rutledge F, Smith JP. Five classes of extended hysterectomy for women with cervical cancer. *Obstet Gynecol*. 1974;44(2):265–272.
33. Querleu D, Morrow CP. Classification of radical hysterectomy. *Lancet Oncol*. 2008;9(3):297–303.
34. Cibula D, Abu-Rustum NR, Benedetti-Panici P, et al. New classification system of radical hysterectomy: emphasis on a three-dimensional anatomic template for parametrial resection. *Gynecol Oncol*. 2011;122:264–268.
35. Dargent D. A new future for Schauta's operation through pre-surgical retroperitoneal pelviscopy. *Eur J Gynecol Oncol*. 1987;8:292–296.
36. Querleu D. Radical hysterectomies by the Schauta–Amreich and Schauta–Stoeckel techniques assisted by coelioscopy. *J Gynecol Obstet Biol Reprod (Paris)*. 1991;20:747–748.
37. Querleu D. Laparoscopically assisted radical vaginal hysterectomy. *Gynecol Oncol*. 1993;51:248–254.
38. Canis M, Mage G, Wattiez A, et al. Does endoscopic surgery have a role in radical surgery of cancer of the cervix uteri? *J Gynecol Obstet Biol Reprod (Paris)*. 1990;19:921.
39. Nezhat CR, Burrell MO, Nezhat FR, et al. Laparoscopic radical hysterectomy with paraaortic and pelvic node dissection. *Am J Obstet Gynecol*. 1992;166:864–866.
40. Chi DS, Eisenhauer EL, Lang J, et al. What is the optimal goal of primary cytoreductive surgery for bulky stage IIIC epithelial ovarian carcinoma? *Gynecol Oncol*. 2006;103:559–564.
41. Bristow RE, del Carmen MG, Kaufman JS, et al. Radical oophorectomy with primary stapled colorectal anastomosis for resection of locally advanced epithelial ovarian cancer. *J Am Coll Surg*. 2003;197(4):565–574.
42. Mourton SM, Temple LK, Abu-Rustum NR, et al. Morbidity of rectosigmoid resection and anastomosis in high risk patients undergoing primary cytoreductive surgery for advanced epithelial ovarian cancer. *Gynecol Oncol*. 2005;99:608–614.
43. Bristow RE, Tomacruz RS, Armstrong DK, et al. Survival effect of maximal cytoreductive surgery for advanced ovarian carcinoma during the platinum era: a meta-analysis. *J Clin Oncol*. 2002;20:1248–1259.
44. Juretzka M, Abu-Rustum NR, Sonoda Y, et al. Full thickness diaphragmatic resection for stage IV ovarian carcinoma using the EndoGIA stapling device with diaphragmatic reconstruction using a gortex graft: a case report and review of the literature. *Gynecol Oncol*. 2006;100:618–620.
45. Yamamoto M, Hayashi MS, Nguyen NT, et al. Use of Seamguard to prevent pancreatic leak following distal pancreatectomy. *Arch Surg*. 2009;144(10):894–899. doi:10.1001/archsurg.2009.39.
46. Rowland RG, Mitchell ME, Bihrle R, et al. Indiana continent urinary reservoir. *J Urol*. 1987;137:1136–1139.
47. Penalver MA, Benjany DE, Averette HE, et al. Continent urinary diversion in gynecologic oncology. *Gynecol Oncol*. 1989;34:274–288.
48. Backes FJ, Tierney BJ, Eisenhauer EL, et al. Complications after double-barreled wet colostomy compared to separate urinary and fecal diversion during pelvic exenteration: time to change back? *Gynecol Oncol*. 2013;128(1):60–64. doi:10.1016/j.ygyno.2012.08.004.
49. McGowan L, Lesher LP, Norris HJ, et al. Misstaging of ovarian cancer. *Obstet Gynecol*. 1985;65:568–572.
50. Kehoe S, Powell J, Wilson S, et al. The influence of the operating surgeon's specialization on patient survival in ovarian cancer. *Br J Cancer*. 1994;70:1014–1017.
51. Woodman C, Baghdady A, Collins S, et al. What changes in the organization of cancer services will improve the outcome for women with ovarian cancer? *Br J Obstet Gynecol*. 1997;104:135–139.
52. Nguyen HN, Averette HE, Hoskins W, et al. National survey of ovarian carcinoma. Part V: The impact of physician's specialty on patient's survival. *Cancer*. 1993;72:3663–3670.

53. Eisenkop SM, Spirtos NM, Montag TW, et al. The impact of subspecialty training on the management of advanced ovarian cancer. *Gynecol Oncol.* 1992;47:203–209.
54. Tingsulstad S, Skjeldestad FE, Hagen B. The effect of centralization of primary surgery on survival in ovarian cancer patients. *Obset Gynecol.* 2003;102:499–505.
55. Andersen ES, Knudsen A, Svarrer T, et al. The results of treatment of epithelial ovarian cancer after centralisation of primary surgery. Results from North Jutland, Denmark. *Gynecol Oncol.* 2005;99:552–556.
56. Harlan LC, Clegg LX, Trimble EL. Trends in surgery and chemotherapy for women diagnosed with ovarian cancer in the United States. *J Clin Oncol.* 2003;21:3488–3494.
57. Goff BA, Matthews BJ, Wynn M, et al. Ovarian cancer: patterns of surgical care across the United States. *Gynecol Oncol.* 2006;103:383–390.
58. Chan JK, Kapp DS, Shin JY, et al. Influence of the gynecologic oncologist on the survival of ovarian cancer patients. *Obstet Gynecol.* 2007;109:1342–1350.
59. Goff BA, Matthews BJ, Larson EH, et al. Predictors of comprehensive surgical treatment in patients with ovarian cancer. *Cancer.* 2007;109(10):2031–2042.
60. Begg CB, Cramer LD, Hoskins WJ, et al. Impact of hospital volume on operative mortality for major cancer surgery. *JAMA.* 1998;280:1747–1751.
61. Cowan RA, O'Cearbhaill RE, Gardner GJ, et al. Is it time to centralize ovarian cancer care in the United States? *Ann Surg Oncol.* 2016;23(3):989–993. doi:10.1245/s10434-015-4938-9.
62. Young RC, Walton LA, Ellenberg SS, et al. Adjuvant therapy in stage I and stage II epithelial ovarian cancer: results of two prospective randomized trials. *N Engl J Med.* 1990;332:1021–1027.
63. Heaps JM, Fu YS, Montz FJ, et al. Surgical-pathologic variables predictive of local recurrence in squamous cell carcinoma of the vulva. *Gynecol Oncol.* 1990;38(3):309–314.
64. Lawhead RA, Clark GC, Smith DH, et al. Pelvic exenteration for recurrent or persistent gynecologic malignancies: a 10-year review of the Memorial Sloan-Kettering Cancer Center Experience (1972–1981). *Gynecol Oncol.* 1989;33:279–282.
65. Morley GW, Hopkins MP, Lindenauer SM, et al. Pelvic exenteration, University of Michigan: 100 patients at 5 years. *Obstet Gynecol.* 1989;74:934–943.
66. Matthews CM, Morris M, Burke TW, et al. Pelvic exenteration in the elderly patient. *Obstet Gynecol.* 1992;79:773.
67. Khoury-Collado F, Einstein MH, Bochner BH, et al. Pelvic exenteration with curative intent for recurrent uterine malignancies. *Gynecol Oncol.* 2012;124(1):42–47. doi:10.1016/j.ygyno.2011.09.031.
68. Chi DS, Gemignani ML, Curtin JP, et al. Long-term experience in the surgical management of cancer of the uterine cervix. *Semin Surg Oncol.* 1999;17:161–167.
69. Eisenkop SM, Friedman RL, Spirtos NM. The role of secondary cytoreductive surgery in the treatment of patients with recurrent epithelial ovarian carcinoma. *Cancer.* 2000;88:144–153.
70. Chi DS, McCaughty K, Schwabenbauer S, et al. Guidelines and selection criteria for secondary cytoreductive surgery in patients with recurrent platinum sensitive epithelial ovarian carcinoma. *Cancer.* 2006;106(9):1933–1939.
71. Barlin JN, Puri I, Bristow RE. Cytoreductive surgery for advanced or recurrent endometrial cancer: a meta-analysis. *Gynecol Oncol.* 2010;118(1):14–18.
72. Fuller AF, Scannell JG, Wilkins W Jr. Pulmonary resection for metastases from gynecologic cancers: MGH experience, 1943–1982. *Gynecol Oncol.* 1985;22:174–180.
73. Levenback C, Rubin SC, McCormack PM, et al. Resection of pulmonary metastases from uterine sarcomas. *Gynecol Oncol.* 1992;45:202–205.
74. Yoon SS, Jarnagin WR, DeMatteo RP, et al. Resection of recurrent ovarian or fallopian tube carcinoma involving the liver. *Gynecol Oncol.* 2003;91(2):383–388.
75. Gemignani ML, Chi DS, Gurin CC, et al. Splenectomy in recurrent epithelial ovarian cancer. *Gynecol Oncol.* 1999;72:407–410.
76. Pothuri B, Vaidya A, Aghajanian C, et al. Palliative surgery for bowel obstruction in recurrent ovarian cancer: an updated series. *Gynecol Oncol.* 2003;89:306–313.
77. Frumovitz M, Ramirez PT, Greer M, et al. Laparoscopic training and practice in gynecologic oncology among Society of Gynecologic Oncologists members and fellows-in-training. *Gynecol Oncol.* 2004;94(3):746–753.
78. Conrad LB, Ramirez PT, Burke W, et al. Role of minimally invasive surgery in gynecologic oncology: an updated survey of members of the Society of Gynecologic Oncology. *Int J Gynecol Cancer.* 2015;25(6):1121–1127. doi:10.1097/IGC.0000000000000450.
79. Carlson JW, Kauderer J, Walker JL, et al. A randomized phase III trial of VH fibrin sealant to reduce lymphedema after inguinal lymph node dissection: a Gynecologic Oncology Group study. *Gynecol Oncol.* 2008;110(1):76–82. doi:10.1016/j.ygyno.2008.03.005.
80. Cabanas RM. An approach for the treatment of penile carcinoma. *Cancer.* 1977;39(2):456–466.
81. Levenback C, Burke TW, Gershenson DM, et al. Intraoperative lymphatic mapping for vulvar cancer. *Obstet Gynecol.* 1994;84(2):163–167.
82. Burke TW, Levenback C, Tornos C, et al. Intra-abdominal lymphatic mapping to direct selective pelvic and paraaortic lymphadenectomy in women with high-risk endometrial cancer: results of a pilot study. *Gynecol Oncol.* 1996;62(2):169–173.
83. Van der Zee AG, Oonk MH, de Hullu JA, et al. Sentinel node dissection is safe in the treatment of early-stage vulvar cancer. *J Clin Oncol.* 2008;26:884–889.
84. Levenback CF, Ali S, Coleman RL, et al. Lymphatic mapping and sentinel lymph node biopsy in women with squamous cell carcinoma of the vulva: a Gynecologic Oncology Group study. *J Clin Oncol.* 2012;30(31):3786–3791. doi:10.1200/JCO.2011.41.2528.
85. Ballester M, Dubernard G, Lécuru F, et al. Detection rate and diagnostic accuracy of sentinel-node biopsy in early stage endometrial cancer: a prospective multicentre study (SENTI-ENDO). *Lancet Oncol.* 2011;12(5):469–476. doi:10.1016/S1470-2045(11)70070-5.
86. Lécuru F, Mathevet P, Querleu D, et al. Bilateral negative sentinel nodes accurately predict absence of lymph node metastasis in early cervical cancer: results of the SENTICOL study. *J Clin Oncol.* 2011;29(13):1686–1691. doi:10.1200/JCO.2010.32.0432.
87. Barlin JN, Khoury-Collado F, Kim CH, et al. The importance of applying a sentinel lymph node mapping algorithm in endometrial cancer staging: beyond removal of blue nodes. *Gynecol Oncol.* 2012;125(3):531–535. doi:10.1016/j.ygyno.2012.02.021.
88. Cormier B, Diaz JP, Shih K, et al. Establishing a sentinel lymph node mapping algorithm for the treatment of early cervical cancer. *Gynecol Oncol.* 2011;122(2):275–280. doi:10.1016/j.ygyno.2011.04.023.
89. Leitao MM Jr, Khoury-Collado F, Gardner G, et al. Impact of incorporating an algorithm that utilizes sentinel lymph node mapping during minimally invasive procedures on the detection of stage IIIC endometrial cancer. *Gynecol Oncol.* 2013;129(1):38–41. doi:10.1016/j.ygyno.2013.01.002.
90. Khoury-Collado F, St Clair C, Abu-Rustum NR. Sentinel lymph node mapping in endometrial cancer: an update. *Oncologist.* 2016;21(4):461–466. doi:10.1634/theoncologist.2015-0473.
91. Jewell EL, Huang JJ, Abu-Rustum NR, et al. Detection of sentinel lymph nodes in minimally invasive surgery using indocyanine green and near-infrared fluorescence imaging for uterine and cervical malignancies. *Gynecol Oncol.* 2014;133(2):274–277. doi:10.1016/j.ygyno.2014.02.028.
92. Kalogera E, Bakkum-Gamez JN, Jankowski CJ, et al. Enhanced recovery in gynecologic surgery. *Obstet Gynecol.* 2013;122(2 pt 1):319–328. doi:10.1097/AOG.0b013e31829aa780.
93. Nelson G, Kalogera E, Dowdy SC. Enhanced recovery pathways in gynecologic oncology. *Gynecol Oncol.* 2014;135(3):586–594. doi:10.1016/j.ygyno.2014.10.006.

CHAPTER 10

Diagnostic Imaging

Shaunagh McDermott, Leslie K. Lee, and Susanna I. Lee

INTRODUCTION

The objectives of imaging in gynecologic oncology are detecting primary tumor, defining extent of tumor spread for treatment planning, monitoring treatment response, and detecting tumor recurrence. Comprehensive imaging of the gynecologic cancer patients can be achieved using a combination of pelvic ultrasound; chest, abdominal, and pelvic computed tomography; pelvic magnetic resonance imaging; and whole-body 2-[^{18}F]-fluoro-2-deoxy-D-glucose positron emission tomography integrated with CT (FDG-PET-CT). The choice of imaging exam depends on the clinical question (**Table 10.1**).

IMAGING MODALITIES

Ultrasound

Ultrasound (US) is a widely available imaging modality and can even be performed, if necessary, at the bedside. Another advantage is that no ionizing radiation is involved. Because it easily produces real-time imaging, US allows for rapid image-guided procedures when targets can be visualized. It provides the best combination of spatial and soft tissue resolution and contrast of all the various imaging modalities. However, because US does not penetrate through many tissues, its ability to image deep visceral organs and evaluate large lesions is limited. A reliable field of view for US is typically ≤5 cm. As a diagnostic test, its reported performance is widely variable, likely secondary to operator dependence. As exam performance does not require volumetric imaging, sample representative images are obtained during the exam in most practices. Hence, reader variability cannot be assessed nor is post hoc exam review feasible.

Transvaginal ultrasound (TVUS) brings the transducer closer to the uterus and can afford excellent evaluation of the endometrium in a nonenlarged uterus. Sonohysterogram, which utilizes TVUS while distending the endometrial cavity with fluid, can be used to evaluate for focal endocavitary lesions such as polyps, subserosal fibroids, and adhesions.

Computed Tomography

Computed tomography (CT) is also widely available in clinical practice. It can image most tissue types (bone, soft tissue, fat, and air) with high spatial resolution and reproducibility. Because image acquisition is rapid, CT is useful even in patients unable to cooperate with the exam (e.g., obtunded, pediatric). Images are acquired axially relative to the patient's long axis, but multidetector CT technology allows for high-quality image reformation into other planes. The most important drawback is ionizing radiation exposure, and this should be considered when imaging young patients and those without a cancer diagnosis. Although the effective doses associated with a diagnostic CT have not been directly shown to pose a health risk, an added lifetime fatal cancer risk of approximately 1:1,000 in an adult undergoing an abdominal CT has been extrapolated from higher doses (1). The risk is thought to be additive with each exam. Overall, though, the risk–benefit analysis for symptomatic patients favors scanning, especially in those with a diagnosis of malignancy. In patients undergoing body CT exams, the mortality risk posed by the underlying clinical condition has been shown to be more than an order of magnitude greater than risk from CT-induced cancer (2).

Intravenous iodinated contrast is used to improve soft tissue contrast, which is otherwise markedly limited with CT. Intravenous contrast is necessary to evaluate the gynecologic pelvis, solid upper abdominal organs (e.g., liver, kidneys), and vascular structures. For cancer indications, contrast administration is considered standard of care unless contraindicated. Iodinated intravenous contrast is associated with an overall 3% incidence of allergic reaction. The vast majority of these reactions are mild and self-limiting (e.g., urticaria pruritus); however, up to 0.04% are severe (e.g., bronchospasm, anaphylaxis), requiring hospitalization (3). Acute kidney injury, especially in patients with renal insufficiency, can be another potential complication of intravenous contrast. Renal function deterioration is usually temporary, with a serum creatinine peaking typically 24 to 48 hours after contrast administration. Common predisposing risk factors include age >70 years, diabetes, congestive heart failure, and nephrotoxic medications.

Magnetic Resonance Imaging

Magnetic resonance imaging (MRI) affords the best soft tissue contrast of any of the radiologic modalities. Thus, tumor conspicuity with solid organs is optimized. Images can be primarily acquired in multiple planes, with the more recent scanner models allowing for acquisition of volumetric image datasets and post hoc high-resolution multiplanar reconstruction. MRI involves no ionizing radiation and hence does not confer a cancer risk to pediatric and pregnant patients. The most important disadvantage of MRI is its long image acquisition time. Most examinations take 20 to 40 minutes, during which time the patient lies in an enclosed scanner. Inability of the patient to lie still or to follow instructions hinders successful image acquisition. A wider-bore or "open" scanner is an option if the patient is claustrophobic. But for abdominopelvic imaging, the resulting images are markedly lower in signal and, because of longer patient table times, are often degraded by motion. MRI uses an electromagnetic field and is therefore contraindicated in patients with pacemakers, cochlear implants, certain vascular clips, metallic objects in the eye, and neural stimulators. Patients are also screened for other indwelling foreign bodies such as orthopedic hardware, surgical clips, and intrauterine devices prior to the exam, and its compatibility with a high-field-strength magnet is ascertained prior to scanning. Even when deemed safe, most metallic foreign bodies included within the field of view result in distortion and degradation of the image quality.

A gadolinium-based contrast agent can be administered to better evaluate the solid viscera and improve the conspicuity of neoplasms. However, because MRI inherently affords better soft tissue contrast

TABLE 10.1. Imaging Modality Choice for Detection, Treatment Planning, and Follow-up of Gynecologic Cancers

Indication	CT[a]	MRI[a]	FDG-PET-CT[b]
Uterine cervical cancer: pretreatment			
Early detection	Poor	Poor	Poor
Differential diagnosis (benign vs. malignant)	Poor	Possible	Poor
Extent of tumor spread			
Tumor size	Poor	Best	Poor
Endocervical margin distance	Poor	Best	Poor
Parametrial involvement	Possible	Best	Possible
Lower third of vaginal involvement	Poor	Possible	Poor
Pelvic sidewall involvement	Possible	Possible	Possible
Hydronephrosis	Possible	Possible	Possible
Bladder mucosal involvement	Poor	Possible	Poor
Rectal mucosal involvement	Poor	Possible	Poor
Pelvic and para-aortic adenopathy	Possible	Possible	Best
Distant metastases (lymph node, bone)	Poor	Possible	Best
Distant metastases (liver)	Possible	Best	Possible
Distant metastases (lung)	Best	Poor	Possible
Uterine endometrial cancer: pretreatment			
Early detection	Poor	Poor	Poor
Differential diagnosis (benign vs. malignant)	Poor	Possible	Possible
Extent of tumor spread			
Greater than half thickness of myometrium extension	Poor	Best	Possible
Cervical stromal involvement	Poor	Best	Possible
Uterine serosal or adnexal involvement	Possible	Best	Possible
Vaginal or parametrial involvement	Possible	Best	Possible
Pelvic and para-aortic adenopathy	Possible	Possible	Best
Bladder mucosal involvement	Poor	Possible	Poor
Bowel mucosal involvement	Poor	Possible	Poor
Distant metastases (lymph node, bone)	Possible	Possible	Best
Distant metastases (liver)	Possible	Best	Possible
Distant metastases (lung)	Best	Poor	Possible
Uterine sarcoma: pretreatment			
Early detection	Poor	Poor	Poor
Differential diagnosis (benign vs. malignant)	Poor	Possible	Poor
Extent of tumor spread			
Tumor size	Poor	Best	Possible
Adnexal involvement	Possible	Best	Possible
Extrauterine pelvic tissue extension	Possible	Best	Possible
Abdominal tissue involvement	Possible	Possible	Possible
Pelvic and para-aortic adenopathy	Possible	Possible	Best
Bladder mucosal involvement	Poor	Possible	Poor
Bowel mucosal involvement	Poor	Possible	Poor
Distant metastases (lymph node, bone)	Possible	Possible	Best
Distant metastases (liver)	Possible	Best	Possible
Distant metastases (lung)	Best	Poor	Possible
Gestational trophoblastic disease: pretreatment			
Early detection	Poor	Poor	Poor
Differential diagnosis (benign vs. malignant)	Poor	Possible	Possible

TABLE10.1. Imaging Modality Choice for Detection, Treatment Planning, and Follow-up of Gynecologic Cancers (*continued*)

Indication	CT[a]	MRI[a]	FDG-PET-CT[b]
Extent of tumor spread			
Tumor size	Poor	Best	Possible
Extrauterine extension	Possible	Best	Possible
Distant metastases (lung)	Best	Poor	Possible
Distant metastases (other)	Possible	Poor	Best
Vulvar cancer: pretreatment			
Early detection	Poor	Poor	Poor
Differential diagnosis (benign vs. malignant)	Poor	Possible	Possible
Extent of tumor spread			
Tumor size	Possible	Best	Possible
Adjacent perineal organ involvement	Poor	Possible	Poor
Inguino-femoral adenopathy	Possible	Possible	Best
Upper urethra mucosal involvement	Poor	Possible	Poor
Upper vagina mucosal involvement	Poor	Possible	Poor
Bladder mucosal involvement	Poor	Possible	Poor
Bowel mucosal involvement	Poor	Possible	Poor
Fixation to pelvic bones	Possible	Best	Possible
Distant metastases (lymph node, bone)	Possible	Possible	Best
Distant metastases (liver)	Possible	Best	Possible
Distant metastases (lung)	Best	Poor	Possible
Ovarian cancer: pretreatment			
Early detection	Poor	Poor	Poor
Differential diagnosis (benign vs. malignant)	Possible	Best	Poor
Extent of tumor spread			
Ovary confined	Poor	Possible	Poor
Pelvis confined	Possible	Possible	Possible
Abdominal involvement	Possible	Possible	Possible
Retroperitoneal adenopathy	Possible	Possible	Best
Peritoneal or pleural effusion	Possible	Possible	Poor
Distant metastases (lymph node, bone)	Possible	Possible	Best
Distant metastases (liver)	Possible	Best	Possible
Distant metastases (lung)	Best	Poor	Possible
All cancers: post primary therapy			
Local or regional	Possible	Best	Poor
Lung	Best	Poor	Possible
Whole body	Possible	Poor	Best

[a]CT and MRI ratings assume that intravenous contrast is administered.

[b]PET-CT ratings assume that the PET exam is performed with a concurrent CT that is of sufficient beam strength to be of diagnostic quality (i.e., not a low-dose attenuation correction CT) either without or with intravenous contrast.

than CT, even a noncontrast exam, if that is the only possible option, yields diagnostic information. Intravenous gadolinium is associated with a much lower incidence of allergic reaction than iodinated contrast (0.07% vs. 3%) (4), with severe life-threatening reactions being extremely rare. However, in patients with renal failure, the administration of some gadolinium contrast agents has been associated with nephrogenic systemic fibrosis, a syndrome resulting in progressive fibrosis of the skin, joints, eyes, and organs, which is uniformly fatal.

Positron Emission Tomography

Positron emission tomography (PET) uses a physiologically active tracer and therefore provides functional information. The most commonly used tracer is 2-[^{18}F]-fluoro-2-deoxy-D-glucose (FDG), which is a glucose analog and therefore approximates tissue metabolism. The uptake of FDG at pathologic sites is dependent on tracer availability, and careful attention to patient preparation is required to ensure that tracer preferentially localizes to tumor rather than to normally hypermetabolic tissue (e.g., skeletal muscle, brown fat). The patient is instructed to avoid strenuous exercise and activity the day before the examination and to fast 4 to 6 hours prior to FDG administration to keep insulin levels low. Serum glucose is measured, as the exam is unlikely to yield accurate image data if values exceed 200 mg/dL. Immediately prior to and after FDG administration, patients are kept comfortably warm to minimize physiologic brown fat activation. Image acquisition typically requires 30 minutes, necessitating a degree of patient cooperation.

FDG-PET does not have the same spatial resolution or soft tissue contrast as the other imaging modalities, but this is mitigated by fusing PET images with concurrently acquired anatomic images (e.g., PET-CT). Accurate tracer localization to minimize false-positive and false-negative errors requires that the concurrent CT images be acquired with sufficient beam energy to be anatomically interpretable (5). Abdomen and pelvis represents a particularly common site for mislocalization errors, as this is the body part where tracer normally accumulates and is excreted through mobile peristaltic organs (e.g., urinary collecting system, bowel). However, as diagnostic-quality anatomic imaging is not mandated by practice standards (6), the CT image quality is a major source of variability in PET-CT practice (7).

Disadvantages of FDG-PET are false-positive results from inflammatory or infectious etiologies, reactive lymphadenopathy, chronic inflammatory disorders (e.g., sarcoid), and tissue response following surgery, radiotherapy, and chemotherapy. Posttreatment changes vary greatly in their degree and extent, but can be expected to contribute to PET appearances in the first 6 to 8 weeks and have been described as a source for interpretation error beyond 6 months. PET provides limited spatial resolution, which can result in false-negatives. Modern clinical PET scanners have a resolution limit of 4 mm (full width at half maximum [FWHM]); effectively, small structures up to 0.7 to 10 mm in diameter may not be reliably detected (8).

UTERINE CERVICAL CANCER

Detection

Imaging plays no role in the detection of cervical cancer, which is usually detected at Pap smear or by physical examination. On occasion, it will be detected on TVUS for abnormal vaginal bleeding in a patient who has not been undergoing screening.

Primary Treatment Planning

The Federation of Gynecology and Obstetrics (FIGO) staging of cervical cancer is based on clinical findings at physical exam (9). Imaging is not explicitly described, although its use is implied in assessment of pelvic sidewall involvement, hydronephrosis, and distant disease. Moreover, for advanced (beyond stage IB) disease, lymphadenopathy (while not included in FIGO staging) is a major factor in treatment planning. Therefore, in its 2009 revision, the FIGO staging committee has encouraged the incorporation of cross-sectional imaging techniques into the evaluation of patients with cervical cancer, where available (10). The National Comprehensive Cancer Network (NCCN) practice guidelines for cervical cancer work-up include chest radiography, CT or PET-CT, and MR imaging as indicated (11).

Two standard primary treatment options for invasive cervical cancer are radical hysterectomy and lymphadenectomy in early-stage disease (IA, IB1, and IIA1), and primary radical radiotherapy with concurrent administration of platinum-based chemotherapy for patients with bulky IB2/IIA2 disease (tumors greater than 4 cm) or those with locally advanced disease (stage IIB or greater). Imaging findings that usually triage a patient to chemoradiation are tumor size and parametrial extension, best assessed with MRI, and lymphadenopathy, best assessed with PET-CT (**Table 10.1**). The choice of optimal primary therapy that minimizes morbidity is achieved when both tests are included in the pretreatment evaluation (12).

MRI is the best imaging modality for visualizing the extent of primary tumor in the soft tissues of the central pelvis (**Fig. 10.1**). It can determine the tumor location and size, presence of invasion into the parametria, pelvic sidewall, or adjacent organs. An intergroup multicenter study in the United States showed that in patients with early-stage tumor intended for curative radical hysterectomy MRI had a sensitivity and specificity for detecting disease stage IIB or higher (i.e., parametrial tumor extension) of 53% and 75%, respectively, compared with clinical assessment, which demonstrated sensitivity and specificity of 29% and 99%, respectively (13). For measuring tumor size, MR imaging was shown to be superior to CT or clinical examination (14).

The presence of metastatic lymph nodes is the major factor driving treatment planning and is the best indicator of prognosis. For patients with clinically visible tumor, FDG-PET-CT is more sensitive than either CT or MRI in the evaluation of nodal involvement (**Fig. 10.2**

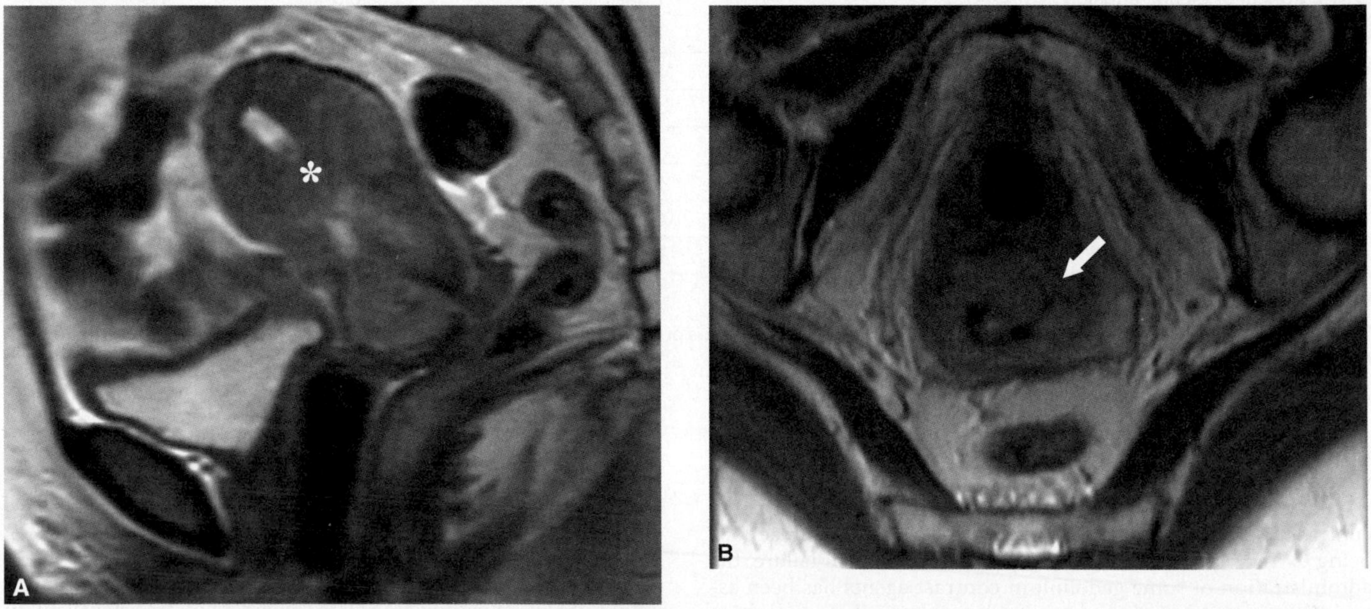

Figure 10.1. Cervical cancer pretreatment MRI. Sagittal **(A)** and axial **(B)** FSE T2-weighted images of the pelvis in a 55-year-old woman with squamous cell carcinoma of the cervix demonstrate a tumor measuring 5.5 cm extending into the uterine corpus (*asterisk*) and into the left parametria (*arrow*). Patient was classified as stage IIB and treated with chemoradiation. FSE, fast spin-echo.

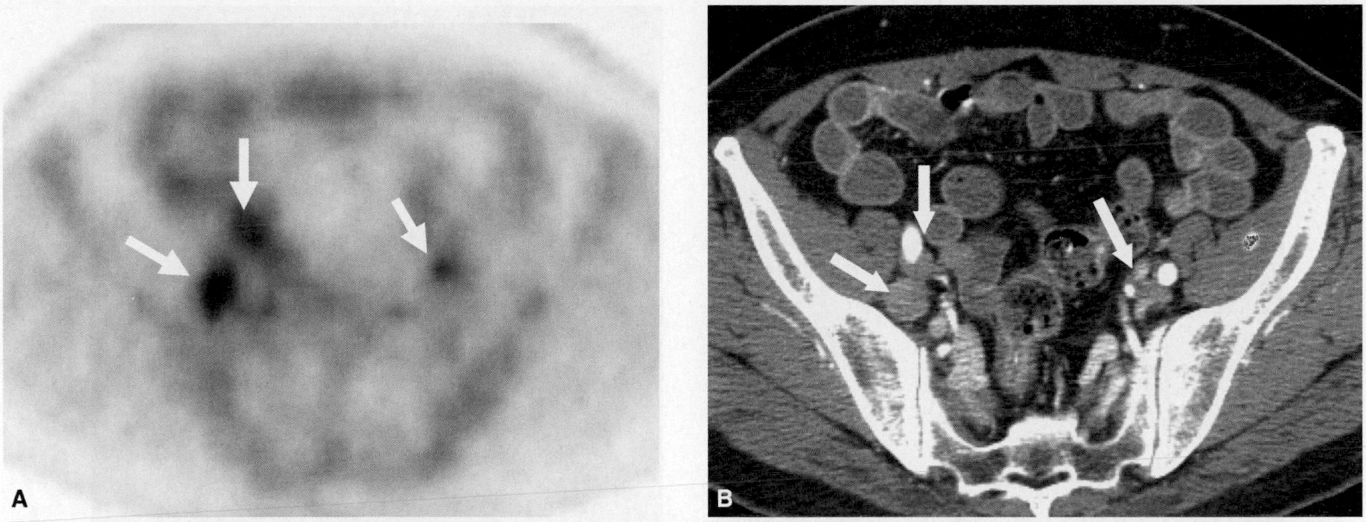

Figure 10.2. Cervical cancer lymphadenopathy detected on pretreatment PET-CT. Axial PET **(A)** of a 67-year-old woman with squamous cell carcinoma of the cervix demonstrates bilateral pelvic sidewall hypermetabolic foci (*arrows*) that localize on CT **(B)** to pelvic sidewall lymph nodes (*arrows*), most of which measure <1 cm in short axis. Biopsy confirmed lymph node metastases, and the patient was treated with chemoradiation.

and **Table 10.2**) (13,15–17,27). A recent meta-analysis comparing the diagnostic performance of PET or PET-CT, MRI, and CT in the detection of metastatic lymph nodes in patients with cervical cancer found that, in a patient-based data analysis, pooled sensitivity and specificity were highest at 82% and 95%, respectively, for PET or PET-CT, 50% and 92%, respectively, for CT, and 56% and 91%, respectively, for MRI. In region- or node-based data analysis, sensitivities of PET or PET-CT (54%) and CT (52%) were significantly higher than that of MRI (38%), while specificities of PET or PET-CT (97%) and MRI (97%) were higher than that of CT (92%) (28). Another meta-analysis also found that PET had a higher sensitivity (75%) and specificity (98%) than did MRI (56% and 93%, respectively) or CT (58% and 92%, respectively) (15).

Beyond the abdominopelvic nodes, FDG-PET also improves initial staging in advanced disease by revealing unexpected sites of distant disease such as supraclavicular lymph nodes. PET or PET-CT has been found to alter management in a significant number of patients with advanced disease (stage IIB–IVB) at presentation (29). In addition, the extent of lymph node involvement on PET and PET-CT has been shown to be a strong predictor of disease-specific survival. The risk of recurrent disease increases incrementally on the basis of the most distant level of PET lymph node involvement, with a hazard ratio of 2.40 (95% confidence interval [CI], 1.63 to 3.52) for pelvic, 5.88 (3.80 to 9.09) for para-aortic, and 30.27 (16.56 to 55.34) for supraclavicular involvement (30).

The ability to detect small-volume disease is especially important if fertility-preserving radical trachelectomy and lymphadenectomy is being contemplated (**Fig. 10.3**). Eligibility requirements include tumor smaller than 2 cm, distance from tumor margin to internal cervical os of more than 1 cm, and absence of lymph node metastases. MRI assesses the extent of local tumor with high accuracy and is routinely used for patient selection (31). PET-CT is also used in many institutions to evaluate for lymphadenopathy. But as the exam performs with low (32%) sensitivity in early-stage disease, its purpose is to identify ineligible candidates (32).

TABLE10 .2. Diagnostic Performance in Detection of Lymphadenopathy

Disease and Modality[a,b]	Sensitivity (%)	Specificity (%)
Uterine cervical cancer		
CT (13,15)	31–57	92–97
MRI (13,15)	37–55	93–94
PET-CT (16,17)	73–100	97–99
Uterine endometrial cancer		
CT (18)	45	88
MRI (19,20)	59–72	93–97
PET-CT (19,20)	67–74	93–99
Vulvar cancer		
CT (21)	60	90
MRI (22–24)	52–89	85–91
PET-CT (25,26)	50–92	91–100

[a]Intravenous contrast for CT and MRI is not necessary but may marginally improve performance.

[b]PET exam should be performed with a concurrent diagnostic-quality CT (i.e., not a low-dose attenuation correction only CT).

Post Primary Therapy

Recurrent cervical cancer usually occurs early in the course of disease, with 60% to 70% of cases occurring within 2 years of commencing treatment (33). No consensus recommendations advocate surveillance imaging. However, because ^{18}F-FDG-PET results have been shown to be prognostic of survival, the NCCN guidelines state that a single PET-CT examination can be performed 3 to 6 months after chemoradiation (**Fig. 10.4**). Patients with new, residual, or no disease on posttreatment FDG-PET imaging demonstrate a 3-year progression-free survival of 0%, 33%, and 78%, respectively (34), and a 5-year overall survival of 0%, 46%, and 92%, respectively (35).

Imaging is typically undertaken if clinical symptoms or signs suggest recurrence. Choice of exam is driven by the anatomic site(s) of suspected disease (**Table 10.1**). MRI is more accurate than PET-CT for detection of small-volume central pelvic recurrence that would be amenable to salvage resection (**Fig. 10.5**). However, particularly within the first 6 months after chemoradiation, MRI does not reliably differentiate posttreatment effects from recurrent tumor (36). Accuracy improves in patients with a remote history of radiation (>1 year), with one study reporting a sensitivity of 86% and a specificity of 94% for the detection of recurrent cervical cancer by MRI (37). Whole-body imaging with PET-CT is also routinely performed prior to pelvic exenteration to evaluate for occult distant metastases.

Following trachelectomy, surveillance with pelvic MRI at 6, 12, and 24 months has been suggested to evaluate for recurrent tumor

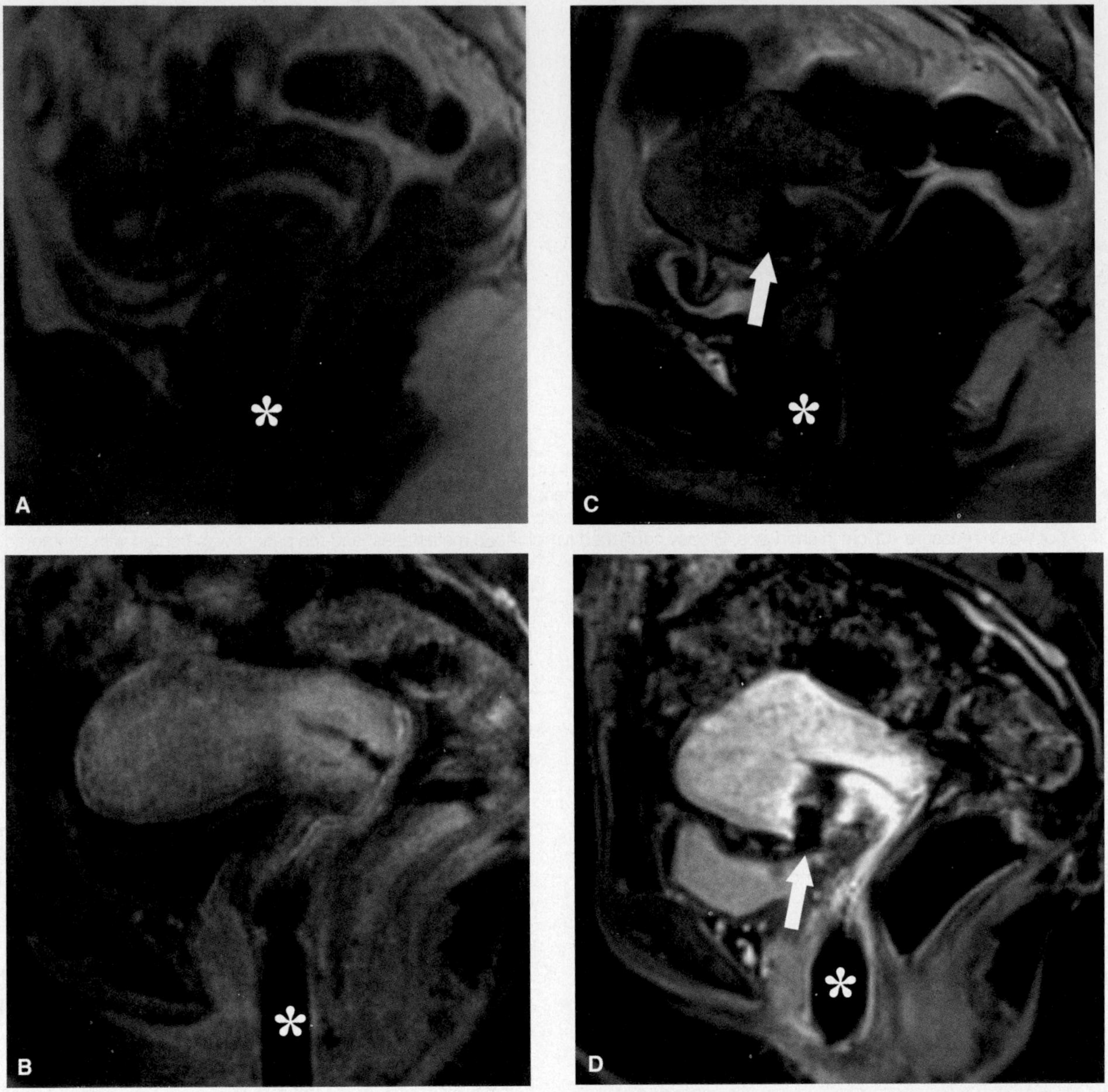

Figure 10.3. Pre- and posttrachelectomy pelvic MRI. Sagittal FSE T2-weighted **(A and C)** and postgadolinium T1-weighted with fat saturation **(B and D)** images with a tampon (*asterisk*) in the vagina in a 31-year-old woman show no visible tumor following a LEEP of a 1.2-cm cervical adenocarcinoma **(A and B)**. Following trachelectomy, the resection margin is indicated by the susceptibility artifact (*arrow*) from sutures. LEEP, loop electrosurgical excision procedure, FSE, fast spin-echo.

(38). Given that the uterus or the pelvic sidewall represent all the sites reported for posttrachelectomy recurrence (39,40), the choice of exam is logical. However, whether surveillance imaging is effective in early detection is yet to be demonstrated.

Uterine Endometrial Cancer

Detection

In postmenopausal women with abnormal vaginal bleeding, TVUS is used to identify those who need further evaluation with endometrial biopsy to assess for cancer (**Fig. 10.6**). Endometrial appearance is evaluated by both thickness and morphology. A large meta-analysis including 35 studies with 5,892 women demonstrated that ≥5 mm thickness defined as abnormal demonstrated sensitivity of 96% for endometrial cancer, whether or not the women were on hormone replacement therapy (41). Women with a 10% pretest probability of endometrial cancer and a negative TVUS had a posttest probability of endometrial cancer of only 1%. Thus, TVUS demonstrates very high sensitivity, and the likelihood ratio with a negative TVUS exam is much lower than that of more invasive techniques (42–44) (**Table 10.3**). It serves as an excellent screening test to obviate the need for endometrial biopsy in the majority of women with benign causes of postmenopausal bleeding.

As the role of TVUS is to screen women with postmenopausal bleeding for further work-up, the test has been optimized for high sensitivity but with moderate to low specificity. Thus, endometrial thickness cutoff ≥5 mm demonstrates low specificity, ranging from 59% to 63% (41,45), especially in women on hormone replacement therapy. Conversely, a normal endometrial thickness does not exclude endometrial cancer, as the test is predicted to miss 4 in 100 cancers. A study of women with postmenopausal bleeding who were not on tamoxifen found that half of the patients with endometrial cancer had an endometrial thickness between 3 and 4 mm (46). Therefore, even in patients with normal endometrial thickness, any persistent or recurrent bleeding, especially in women with clinical risk factors

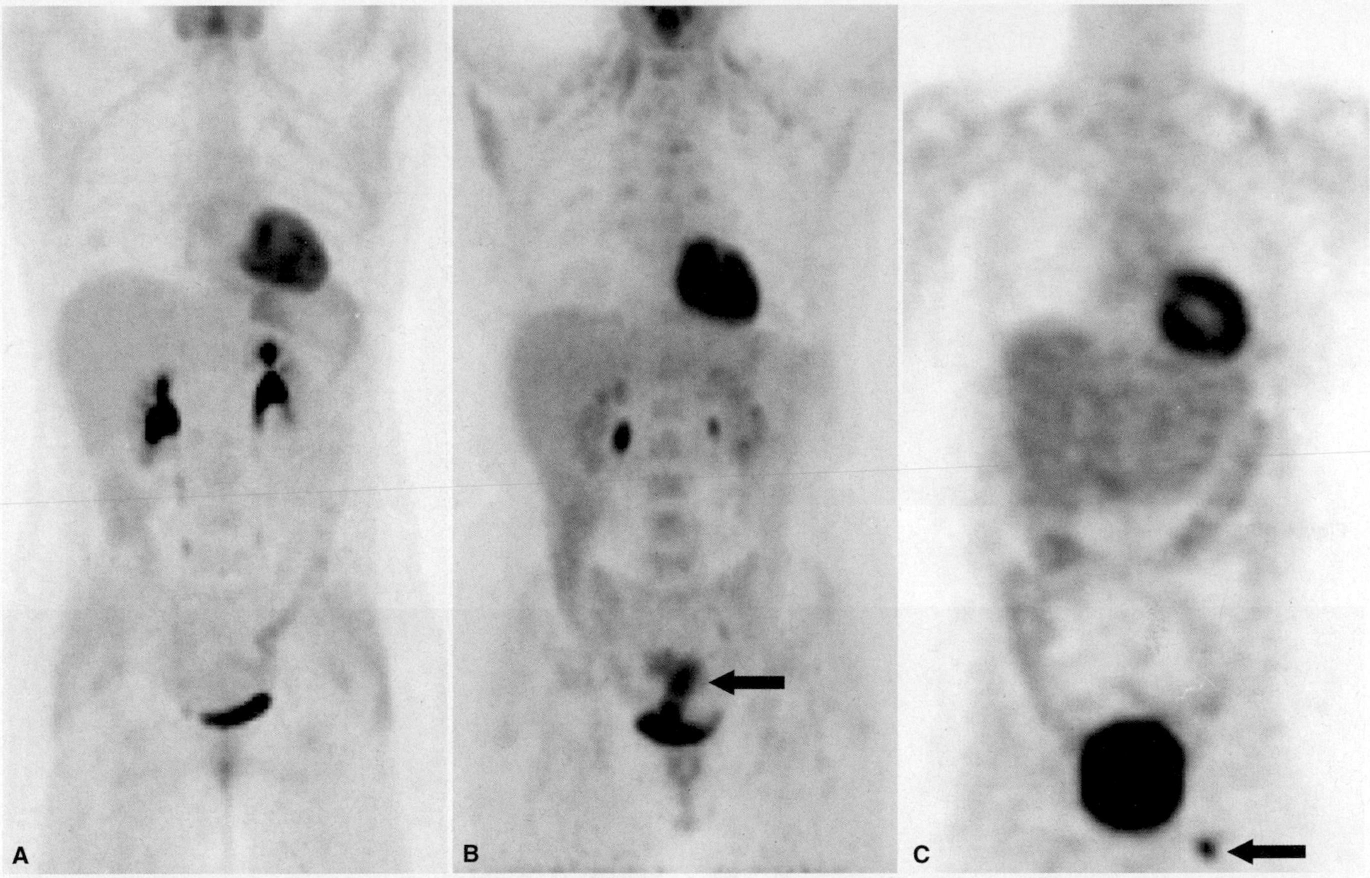

Figure 10.4. Posttherapy PET for cervical cancer prognosis. Coronal whole-body PET images in three different women obtained 3 to 4 months postchemoradiotherapy for advanced cervical cancer demonstrate no residual **(A)**, persistent **(B**, *arrow***)**, and new **(C**, *arrow)* disease. Corresponding predicted 3-year progression-free survival rates are 78%, 33%, and 0%, respectively.

Source: Schwarz JK, Siegel BA, Dehdashti F, et al. Association of posttherapy positron emission tomography with tumor response and survival in cervical carcinoma. *JAMA*. 2007;298(19):2289–2295.

for cancer, should be further evaluated to definitely identify the cause of the symptoms.

In premenopausal women with abnormal bleeding, endometrial thickness measurements with TVUS are less useful for cancer detection (47). MRI plays only a limited role in cancer detection and is reserved for women in whom TVUS or biopsy is precluded because of cervical or vaginal stenosis.

Primary Treatment Planning

Complete FIGO staging of endometrial cancer calls for a total abdominal hysterectomy (TAH), bilateral salpingo-oophorectomy (BSO), peritoneal washings, and retroperitoneal lymph node dissection (9). Because lymphadenectomy can incur perioperative complications and long-term morbidity such as lymphedema, some centers have

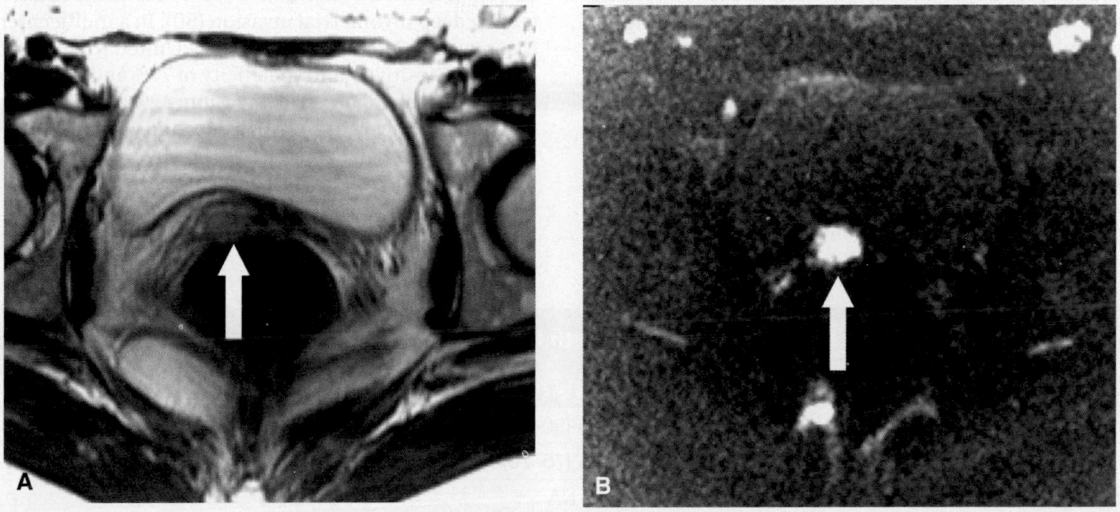

Figure 10.5. Local recurrence of cervical cancer detected on MRI vs. PET-CT. Axial FSE T2 **(A)** and diffusion **(B)** MR images demonstrate a 1.3 cm nodule above the vaginal vault (*arrow*) in a 34-year old woman with stage IB adenocarcinoma of the cervix treated 2 years ago. This nodule is much less apparent on the corresponding CT **(C)** image (*arrow*), which lacks tissue contrast and on the PET image **(D)** where the signal (*arrow*) is obscured by bladder tracer accumulation. Biopsy demonstrated recurrence.

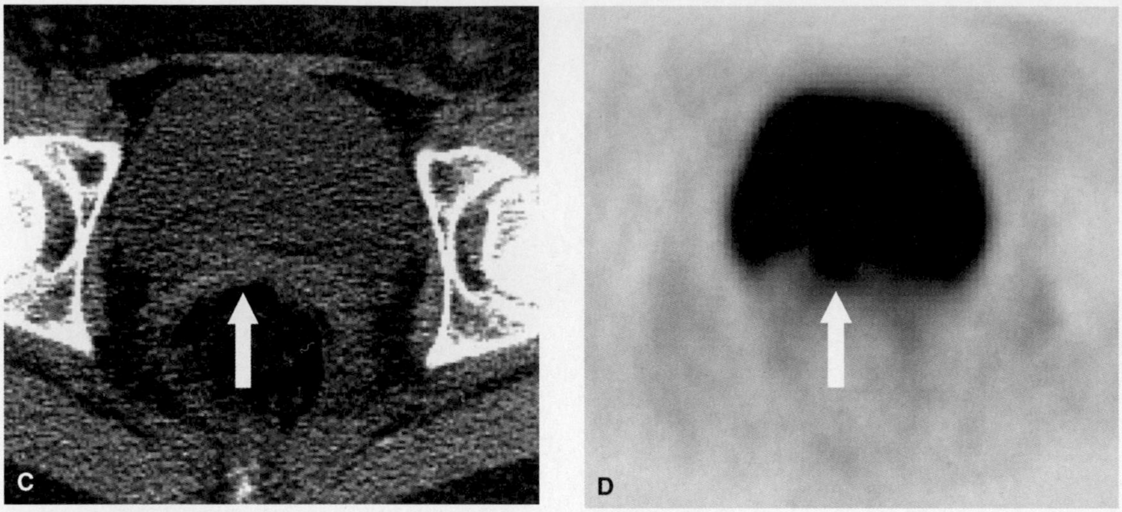

Figure 10.5. (*continued*)

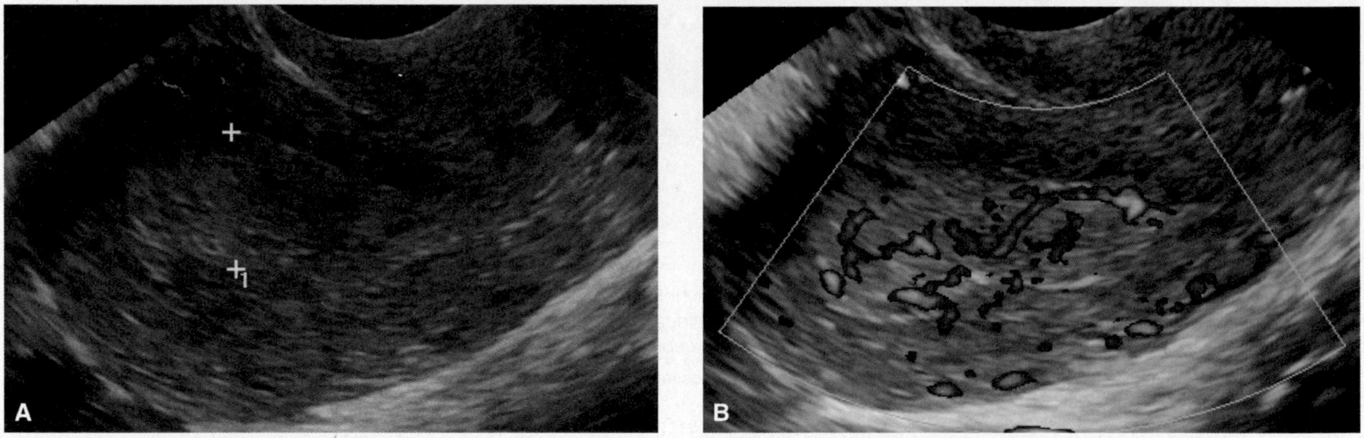

Figure 10.6. Endometrial cancer detected on transvaginal US. Sagittal gray-scale **(A)** and power Doppler **(B)** images of the uterus in a 65-year-old woman with postmenopausal bleeding demonstrate an abnormally thickened endometrium (calipers) measuring 10.9 mm and internal diffuse hypervascularity. Biopsy revealed endometrioid adenocarcinoma.

chosen to selectively perform the procedure only when the primary tumor demonstrates high-risk features (48). Imaging serves in surgical planning to evaluate for nodal and distant metastases. The NCCN guidelines for endometrial cancer work-up specify chest imaging and also consideration of MRI, CT, and FDG-PET in patients suspected to have extrauterine disease (49).

Because features of the primary tumor predict the likelihood of nodal metastases, sites with expertise in frozen section diagnosis often choose to forego imaging and make the decision to perform lymphadenectomy intraoperatively, based on the hysterectomy specimen (48). However, many institutions opt for preoperative MR imaging to evaluate the primary tumor size and intrauterine spread that predict whether lymphadenectomy will likely be required (**Fig. 10.7**). A meta-analysis found that contrast-enhanced MRI, CT, or US performed better than their noncontrast counterparts in detecting deep myometrial invasion (50). In a multicenter audit of 775 cases over a 12-month period in the United Kingdom, MRI demonstrated a sensitivity and specificity of 77% and 88%, respectively, for detecting deep myometrial invasion; 42% and 97%, respectively, for detecting cervical stromal invasion; and 64% and 96%, respectively, for diagnosing pelvic lymphadenopathy (51).

MRI is also used in the minority of endometrial cancer patients in whom hysterectomy is not intended as the primary therapy. It is used to screen patients with low-grade endometrial carcinoma

TABLE10.3. Endometrial Cancer Detection in Women with Postmenopausal Vaginal Bleeding

Modality	Sensitivity (95% CI)	Specificity (95% CI)	LR of Positive Test	LR of Negative Test
TVUS not on HRT(41)	96% (94–98)	92% (90–94)	11.9	0.05
TVUS on HRT (41)	96% (94–98)	77% (75–79)	4.0	0.12
Nonfocal biopsy (42)	NA	NA	66.5	0.14
Hysteroscopy (43)	86% (84–89)	99% (99–99)	60.9	0.15

HRT, hormone replacement therapy; NA, not available; LR, likelihood ratio.

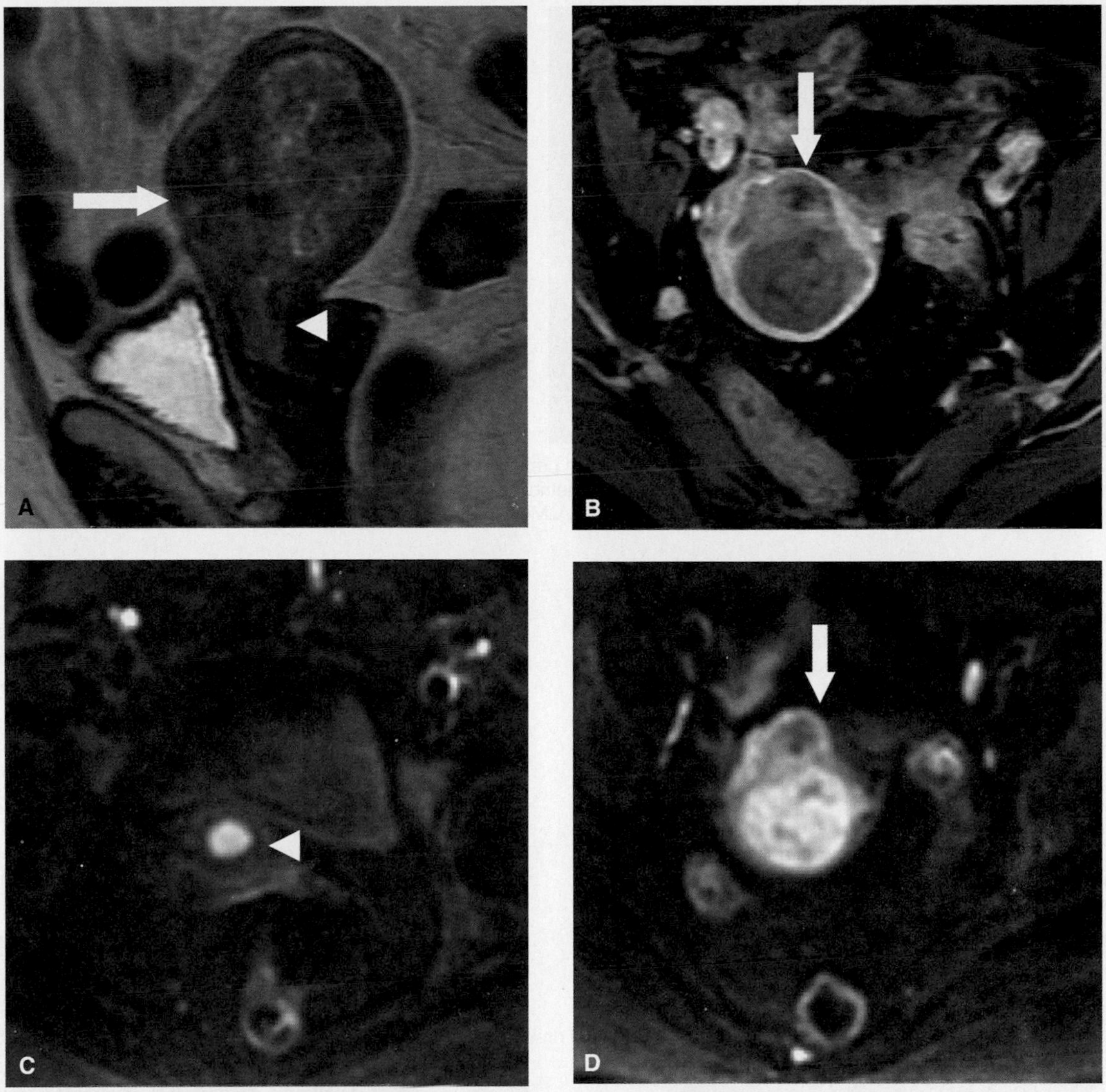

Figure 10.7. Endometrial cancer pretreatment MRI. Sagittal FSE T2-weighted **(A)**, axial postgadolinium T1-weighted **(B)**, and axial diffusion-weighted **(C and D)** images of a 71-year-old woman with endometrioid adenocarcinoma of the endometrium demonstrate an 8-cm tumor that extends >50% thickness into the anterior myometrium (*arrow*) and grows into the cervix (*arrowhead*). Note that intrauterine tumor extent is best seen only after contrast administration or with diffusion-weighted imaging. Imaging findings were confirmed on surgical pathology. FSE, fast spin-echo.

for fertility-sparing treatment (52). The purpose of imaging in such cases is to evaluate for evidence of myometrial invasion that would preclude treatment with high-dose progesterone. In patients with medical comorbidities that preclude surgery or in those with tumor invading the bladder or bowel (stage IVA), MRI delineates fields for radiotherapy, which represents the alternative initial therapy.

CT has no role in defining tumor spread in the central pelvic soft tissues. Contrast-enhanced CT can be useful in evaluating for nodal (stage IIIC) and distant metastases (stage IVB), when integrated FDG-PET-CT, a more accurate modality for this purpose, is not available. It more reliably detects distant parenchymal metastases, peritoneal implants, and malignant ascites (stage IVB) compared with MRI, the resolution of which is sometimes compromised by bowel or patient motion (53).

Most endometrial cancers are abnormally hypermetabolic on PET-CT; however, low-grade cancers can demonstrate little-to-no FDG avidity (54). Conversely, nonmalignant endometrial conditions, as in the proliferative phase of menstruation or menses, infection, and benign tumors (55), can demonstrate increased FDG avidity and should not be mistaken for cancer. For detection of lymphadenopathy, PET-CT is more sensitive than CT or MRI (**Fig. 10.8** and **Table 10.2**) (18–20) as it allows for detection of tumor involvement in lymph nodes that measure <1 cm in short axis, the size threshold for morphologic assessment of lymphadenopathy. Nevertheless, resolution is a limiting factor for PET-CT sensitivity: 17% for nodes ≤4 mm, 67% for nodes 5 to 9 mm, and 93% for nodes ≥10 mm (56). Consequently, although detection of FDG-avid nodes allows for surgical planning and resection for histologic confirmation, staging lymphadenectomy should still be performed in patients with primary tumors with high-risk features, without evidence of extrauterine disease, for detection of micrometastases.

Between 3% and 5% of patients with high-grade tumor histology harbor disease beyond the uterus and abdominopelvic nodes, such as intrathoracic or bony metastases (stage IVB) (57). The added value of FDG-PET-CT in this setting is to detect unsuspected distant metastatic deposits, for which it has been found to have a sensitivity of 100% and a specificity of 94% (**Fig. 10.9**) (58) Such findings would triage a patient away from the morbidity of an unnecessarily aggressive staging operation (59). PET-CT has been shown to be more sensitive than CT for detection of distant disease that alters the treatment plan to minimize morbidity (59).

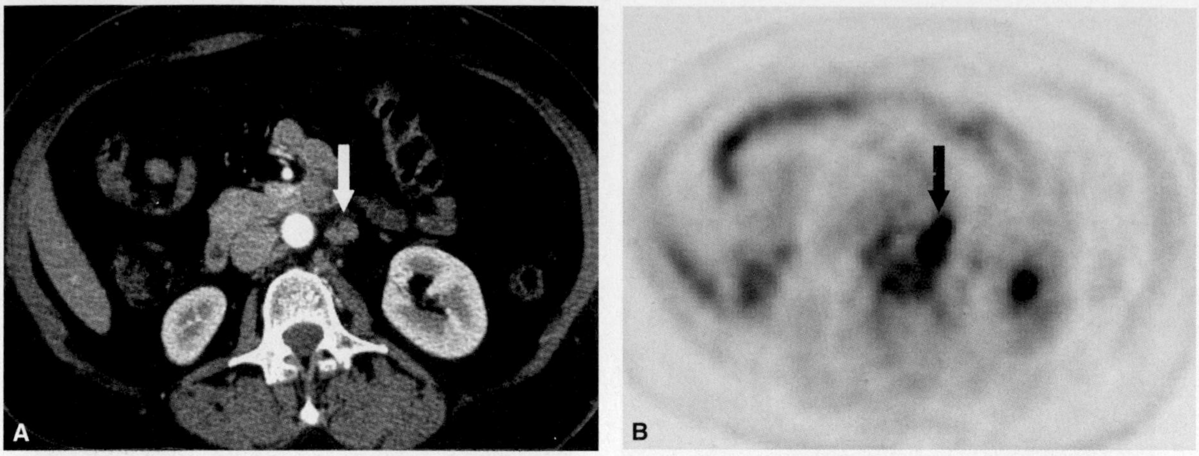

Figure 10.8. Endometrial cancer lymph node metastases detected on pretreatment PET-CT. Contrast-enhanced CT **(A)** and axial PET **(B)** images of a 60-year-old woman with adenocarcinoma (mixed serous and endometrioid cell types) of the endometrium demonstrate left para-aortic lymph nodes that measure < 1 cm short axis but appear hypermetabolic (*arrow*). Metastases were confirmed with surgical resection.

Post Primary Therapy

The use of imaging and its impact on the follow-up of endometrial cancer patients are not well defined. Endometrial cancer has a low rate of recurrence of 4% to 16% (60). Following primary surgery, 64% of recurrences occur within 2 years and 87% within 3 years. The most common sites of recurrence are lymph nodes (46%), best detected with PET-CT, and the vaginal vault (42%), best detected with pelvic exam (61). Less frequently, recurrent disease may manifest as peritoneal carcinomatosis (28%) or distant metastases in liver, lung, or bone (61). Although 20% present with clinically occult metastases (62), the role of surveillance imaging in patients at high risk for recurrence remains controversial.

Imaging is indicated in patients with clinically suspected recurrence. MRI is used to plan salvage surgery or radiotherapy for tumor in the central pelvis (**Fig. 10.10**). Whole-body PET or integrated PET-CT demonstrates 92% to 93% sensitivity and 93% to 100% specificity in detecting recurrent disease (63,64). A study measuring the added value of FDG-PET in addition to CT or MRI for posttherapy surveillance found that FDG-PET showed better diagnostic performance (accuracy 93%) compared with combined conventional imaging (accuracy 85%) and tumor markers (accuracy 83%) (64). Thus, if loco-regional therapy for recurrence is being contemplated, PET-CT is indicated to exclude occult distant metastases.

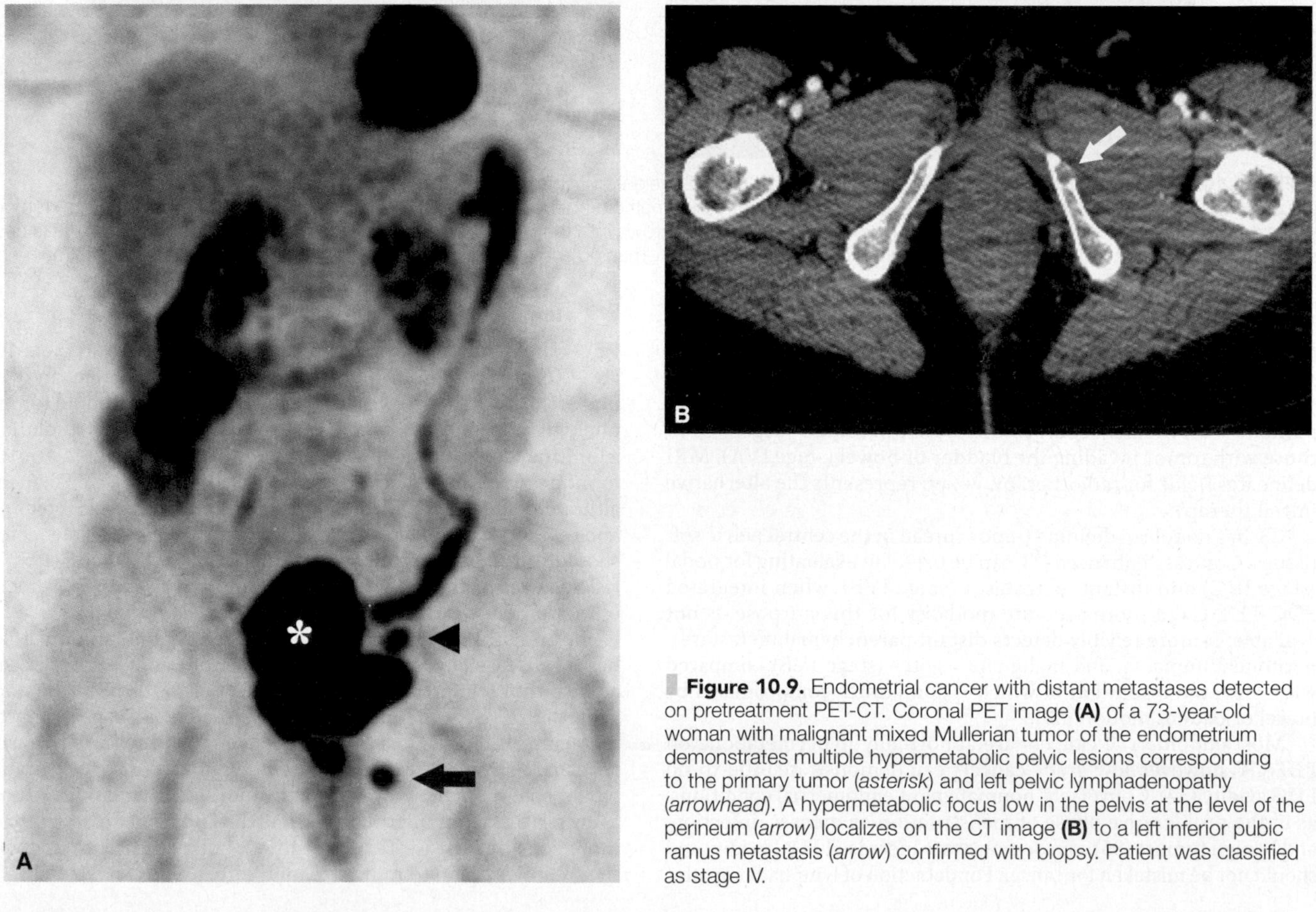

Figure 10.9. Endometrial cancer with distant metastases detected on pretreatment PET-CT. Coronal PET image **(A)** of a 73-year-old woman with malignant mixed Mullerian tumor of the endometrium demonstrates multiple hypermetabolic pelvic lesions corresponding to the primary tumor (*asterisk*) and left pelvic lymphadenopathy (*arrowhead*). A hypermetabolic focus low in the pelvis at the level of the perineum (*arrow*) localizes on the CT image **(B)** to a left inferior pubic ramus metastasis (*arrow*) confirmed with biopsy. Patient was classified as stage IV.

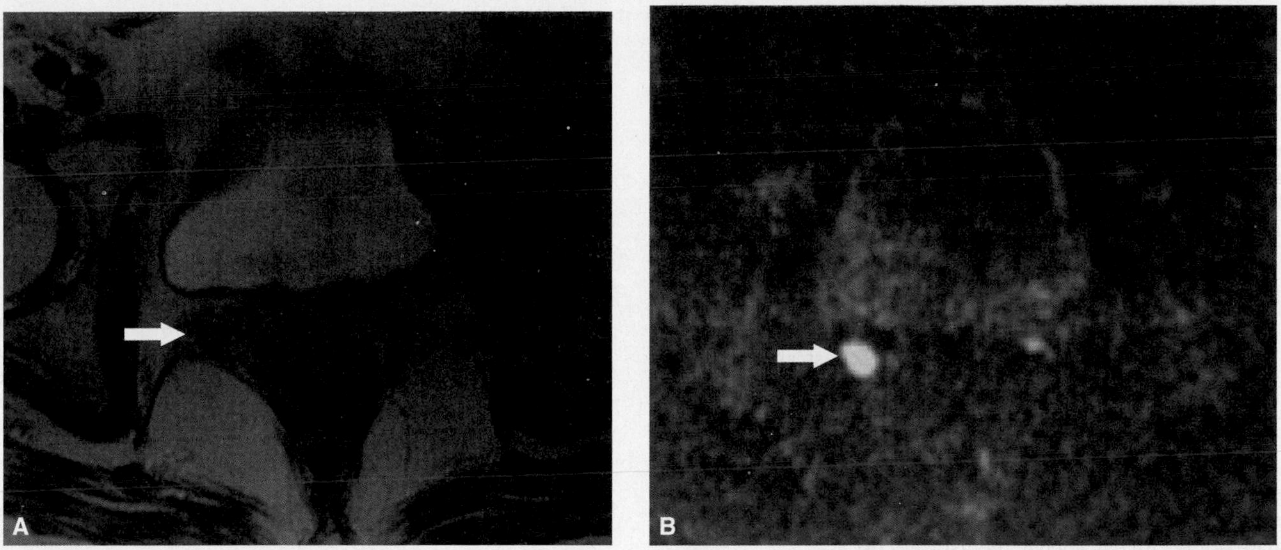

Figure 10.10. Local recurrence of endometrial cancer on MRI. Axial FSE T2-weighted **(A)** and diffusion-weighted **(B)** pelvic images of a 83-year-old woman treated for stage II endometrioid adenocarcinoma endometrial cancer 3 years ago reveal a 1-cm diffusion-restricted nodule (*arrow*) at the right vaginal vault. Biopsy confirmed recurrent tumor. FSE, fast spin-echo.

UTERINE SARCOMA

Detection

Pelvic sonography cannot distinguish a uterus enlarged from fibroids versus cancer. Consequently, recent reviews reveal a very low but not negligible risk of malignancy in women undergoing surgery for presumed benign fibroids. Most recently, the Food and Drug Administration (FDA) analyzed available data and found the prevalence of unsuspected sarcoma in women undergoing surgery for fibroids to be 1 in 352 (65). This statistic has been challenged as an overestimate, with an alternative analysis reporting an incidence of leiomyosarcoma (LMS) of 1 in 7,450 (66).

MRI is the modality recommended for treatment planning of an enlarged symptomatic uterus (67,68). It delineates tumor size, margins, and anatomic extent. The large field of view allows for detection of extrauterine growth such as lymphadenopathy, vascular invasion, peritoneal dissemination, and bone metastases. But although MRI can identify tumor growth outside the uterus, it is less accurate in differentiating a benign leiomyoma from a myometrium-confined LMS (**Fig. 10.11**). Sensitivity and specificity of MRI, measured in retrospective series enriched for LMS, have been reported as 56% to 100% and 93% to 94%, respectively (69,70). Extrapolating the best-case scenario of 100% sensitivity and 94% specificity to the real-world population yields a positive predictive value of <4%, indicating that the majority of uterine-confined LMS diagnosed by MRI will still

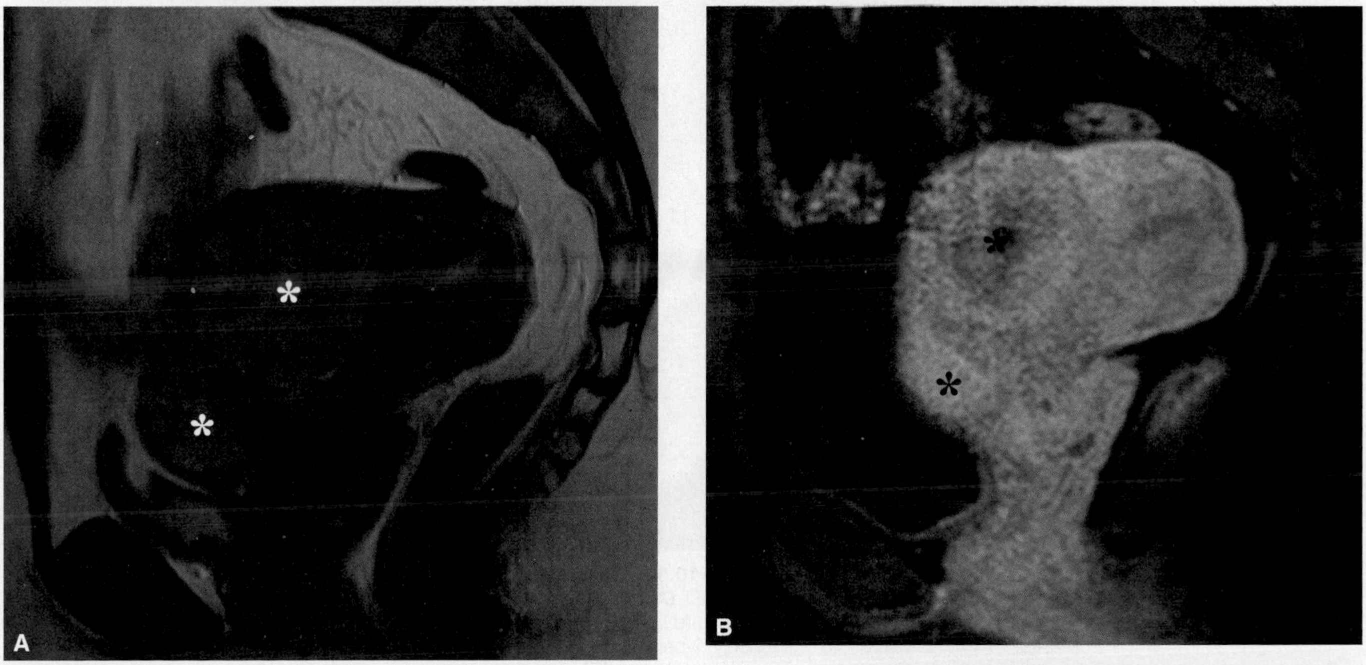

Figure 10.11. Leiomyosarcoma mimics leiomyoma. Sagittal FSE T2-weighted **(A)** and postgadolinium T1-weighted **(B)** images of the uterus in a 44-year-old woman with abnormal vaginal bleeding demonstrate a homogeneous, well-circumscribed, bilobed mass (*asterisk*) that enhances similarly to the myometrium. Mass is confined to the uterine myometrium, and no metastases are seen. Surgical pathology revealed a uterine-confined grade 2 leiomyosarcoma.

prove to be benign. However, when a uterine mass is diagnosed as LMS on MRI, the likelihood of underlying malignancy increases up to 15-fold, and this should be taken into account in treatment planning.

FDG-PET is not useful in differentiating benign from malignant uterine smooth muscle tumors. Tracer accumulation in fibroids is widely variable (71) and intense uptake that can mimic high-grade sarcoma has been reported in women older than 80 years (72). If all other imaging features are consistent with a fibroid, a markedly FDG-avid uterine myometrial mass is likely to represent a benign leiomyoma and not an LMS (**Fig. 10.12**).

Primary Treatment Planning

The NCCN guidelines recommend a CT of the chest, abdomen, and pelvis; an MRI; or PET-CT for the evaluation of uterine sarcoma regardless of how it is diagnosed (73). Chest imaging is necessary as soft tissue sarcomas, including LMS, demonstrate propensity for pulmonary metastases and, on occasion, will present as a primary lung mass in a woman with presumed fibroids (**Fig. 10.13**). For defining tumor extent, PET-CT is the most accurate modality to evaluate nodal and extrapelvic metastases (74).

Post Primary Therapy

The most common sites of metastatic disease from LMS are lung, followed by peritoneal cavity, bone, and liver (75–77). There is little evidence on which to base recommendations for imaging follow-up, although surveillance imaging with chest, abdomen, and pelvic CT is the usual practice (78). Anecdotal experience from small series suggests that FDG-PET identifies more sites of extrapelvic metastatic disease below the diaphragm, compared with CT (79).

GESTATIONAL TROPHOBLASTIC DISEASE

Detection

An elevated serum human chorionic gonadotropin (hCG), typically following a molar, ectopic, or failed pregnancy, is the usual presenting feature. TVUS is used to confirm suspected diagnosis and to exclude a normal pregnancy.

Primary Treatment Planning

Gestational trophoblastic disease (GTD) is staged anatomically using the FIGO classification (80). In addition, a World Health Organization Prognostic Scoring System, which requires assessment of tumor size, sites, and number of metastases, is allotted to each patient, as it best predicts clinical outcome (80). Lungs are the most common sites of metastases, and hence, chest imaging should be routinely performed either with a radiograph or CT (**Fig. 10.14A, B**). The latter is more accurate and can demonstrate hemorrhage, a common complication of this tumor (81). In cases of uterine enlargement, pelvic MRI can be used to assess tumor size and risk for perforation (**Fig. 10.14C, D**). Additional imaging may be indicated to confirm suspected metastases in the torso or central nervous system with CT or MRI, respectively.

Post Primary Therapy

Serial quantitative hCG is used to follow treatment response and to diagnose remission. Imaging is not routinely performed unless tumor markers suggest resistance to therapy or recurrence. Arteriovenous

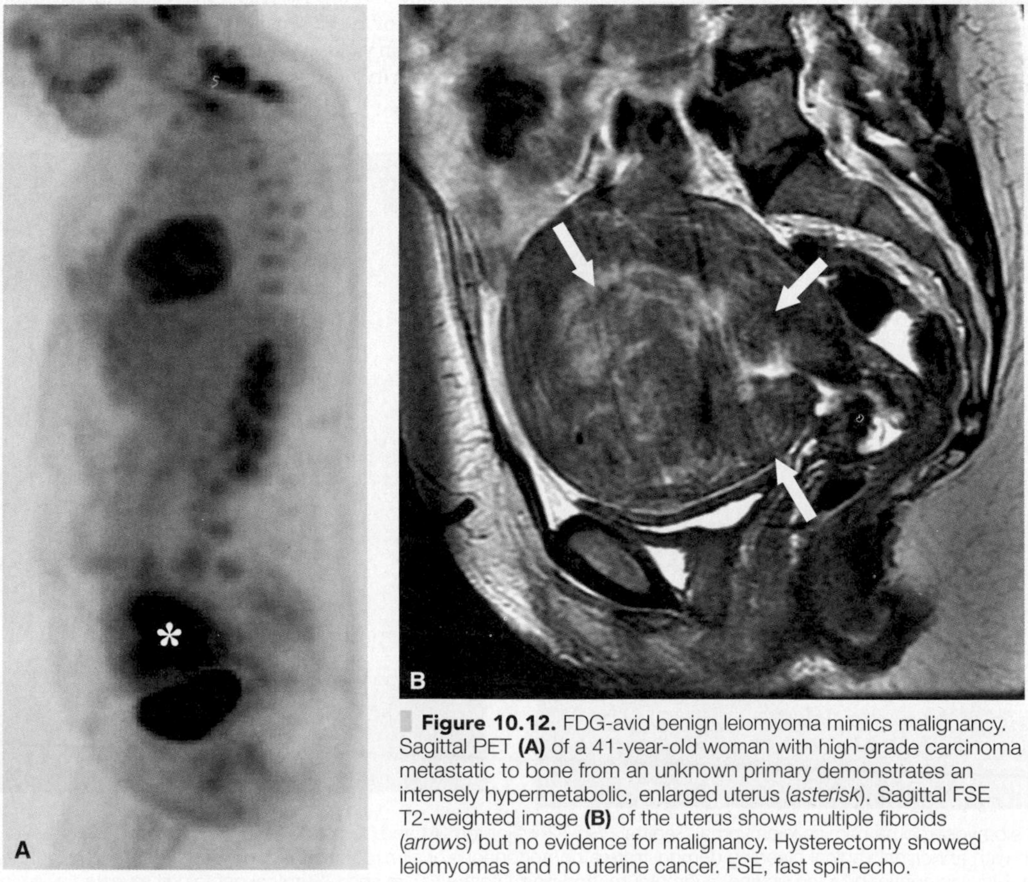

Figure 10.12. FDG-avid benign leiomyoma mimics malignancy. Sagittal PET **(A)** of a 41-year-old woman with high-grade carcinoma metastatic to bone from an unknown primary demonstrates an intensely hypermetabolic, enlarged uterus (*asterisk*). Sagittal FSE T2-weighted image **(B)** of the uterus shows multiple fibroids (*arrows*) but no evidence for malignancy. Hysterectomy showed leiomyomas and no uterine cancer. FSE, fast spin-echo.

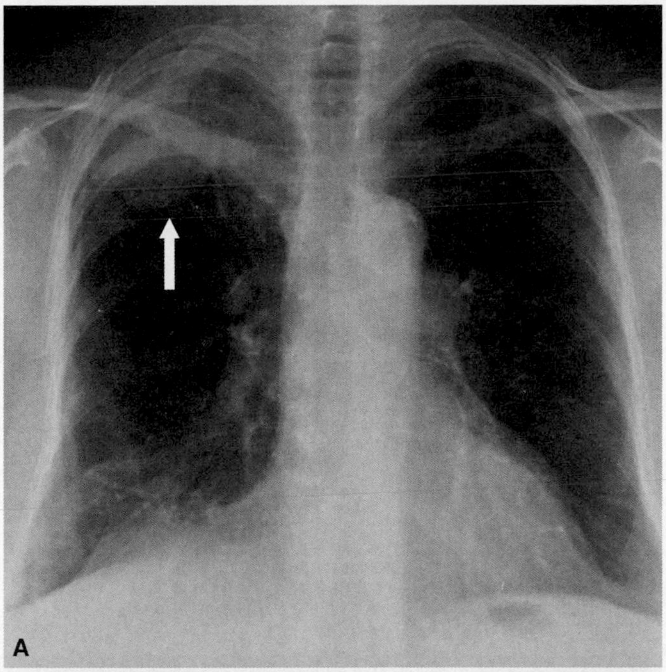

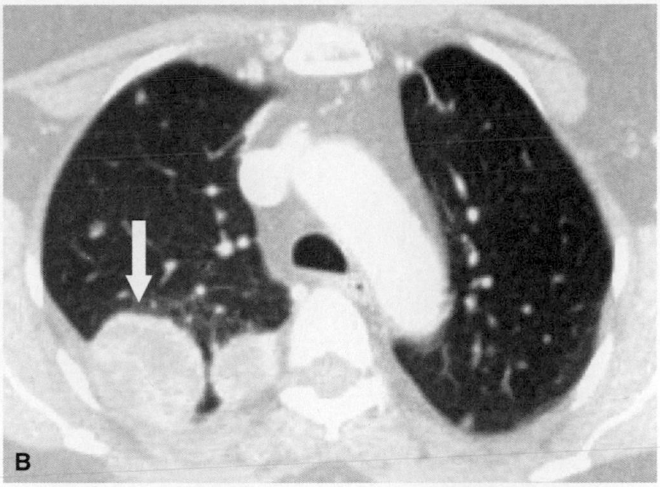

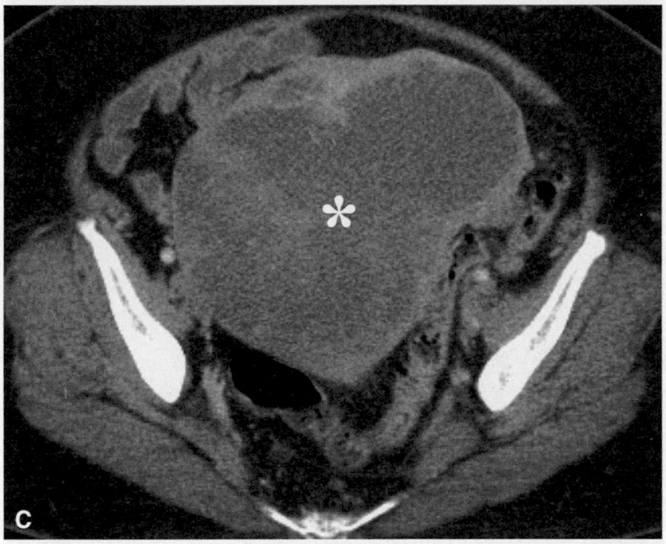

Figure 10.13. Leiomyosarcoma presents as lung mass. Posterior-anterior chest radiograph **(A)** obtained in a 62-year-old woman scheduled to undergo hysterectomy for symptomatic fibroids demonstrates a 3.5-cm right upper lobe mass (*arrow*). Chest CT **(B)** again demonstrates the mass (*arrow*) and other smaller bilateral pulmonary nodules. Abdominopelvic CT **(C)** shows an enlarged 17-cm uterus (*asterisk*) with heterogeneous areas of enhancement and necrosis but no evidence of extrauterine tumor. Lung mass biopsy revealed metastatic leiomyosarcoma.

malformation, a complication of tumors invasive into the myometrium, is best diagnosed with Doppler TVUS (**Fig. 10.15**) (82) and can be treated with angiographic embolization (83).

VULVAR CANCER

Detection

Imaging plays no role in diagnosis of vulvar cancer, which is detected on pelvic exam and confirmed with biopsy.

Primary Treatment Planning

The most recent revisions on the FIGO staging of vulvar cancer give better prognostic discrimination between stages (9). Features at presentation that predict patient outcome are the tumor size, depth of invasion, status of lymph node metastases, and distant metastases. Because of the morbidity associated with a radical surgery that includes inguinofemoral lymphadenopathy, noninvasive methods, such as imaging, to evaluate disease extent are becoming more popular. Performances of CT, MRI (**Fig. 10.16 A, B**), and PET-CT for nodal assessment have all been reported (**Table 10.2**) (21–26). In selected patients with early-stage squamous cell carcinoma (tumor <4 cm in diameter and clinically nonsuspicious groin nodes), sentinel lymph node excision is recommended (84,85). However, in patients with advanced loco-regional tumor, PET-CT is used to evaluate for stage IV disease (**Fig. 10.16 C, D**) (5).

Post Primary Therapy

Squamous cell carcinoma of the vulva is seen to recur in 30% to 50% of patients within 2 years. The majority of these are local; however, recurrences in the groin are associated with a poor prognosis (86,87). MRI can help in evaluating the extent of the local recurrence and guide salvage therapy. If loco-regional therapy is planned, PET-CT is used to evaluate for distant disease that would alter management.

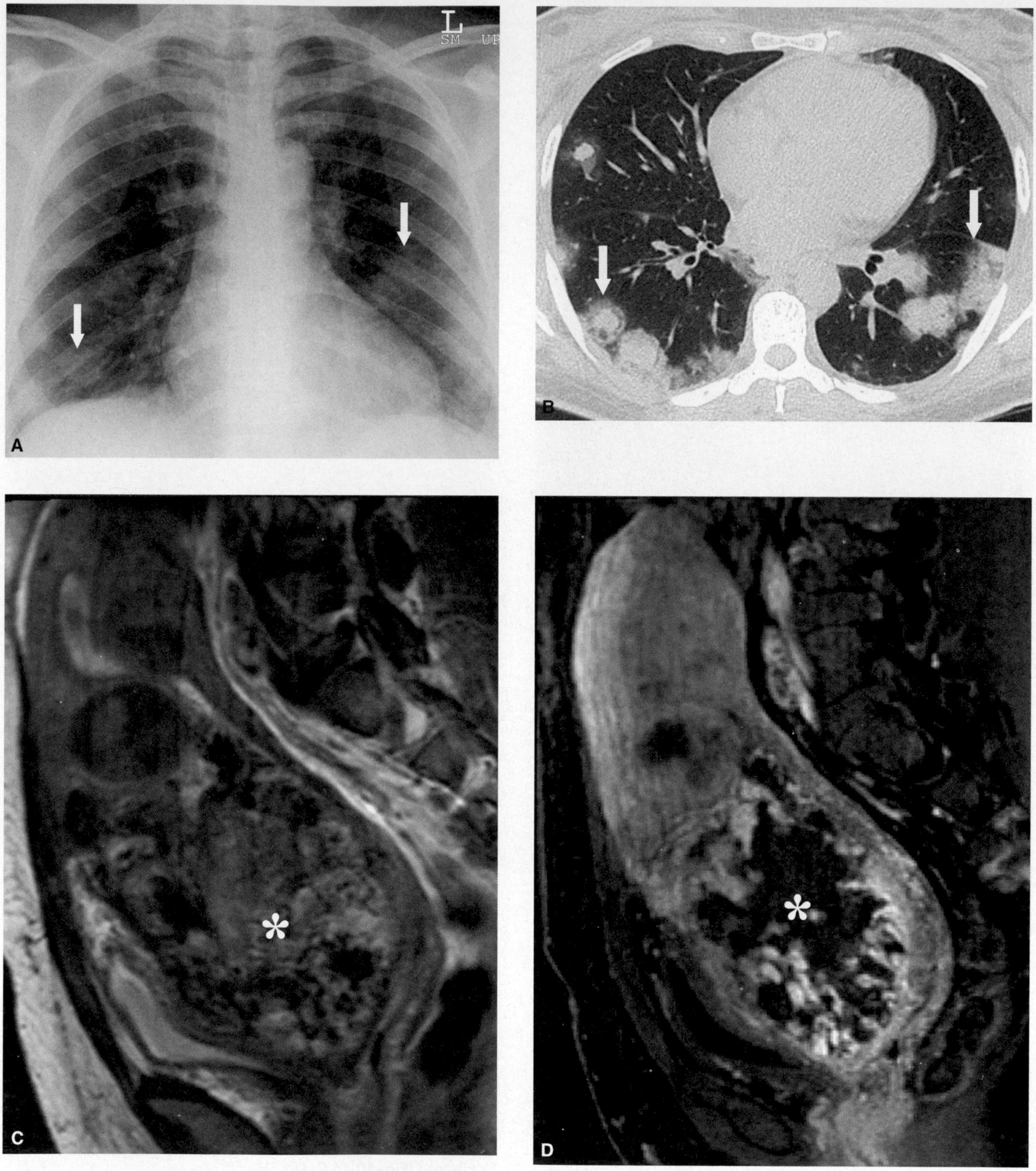

Figure 10.14. Choriocarcinoma presenting as pulmonary nodules. Posterior-anterior chest radiography **(A)** and CT **(B)** of a 49-year-old woman presenting with hemoptysis demonstrates bilateral nodules measuring up to 5 cm (*arrow*). Note the "ground glass halo" around the nodules on the chest CT indicating hemorrhage. Sagittal FSE T2-weighted **(C)** and postgadolinium T1-weighted **(D)** images reveal a 10-cm hypervascular mass (*asterisk*) with central necrosis that involves the lower endometrial cavity and the anterior myometrial wall. Biopsy revealed choriocarcinoma. FSE, fast spin-echo.

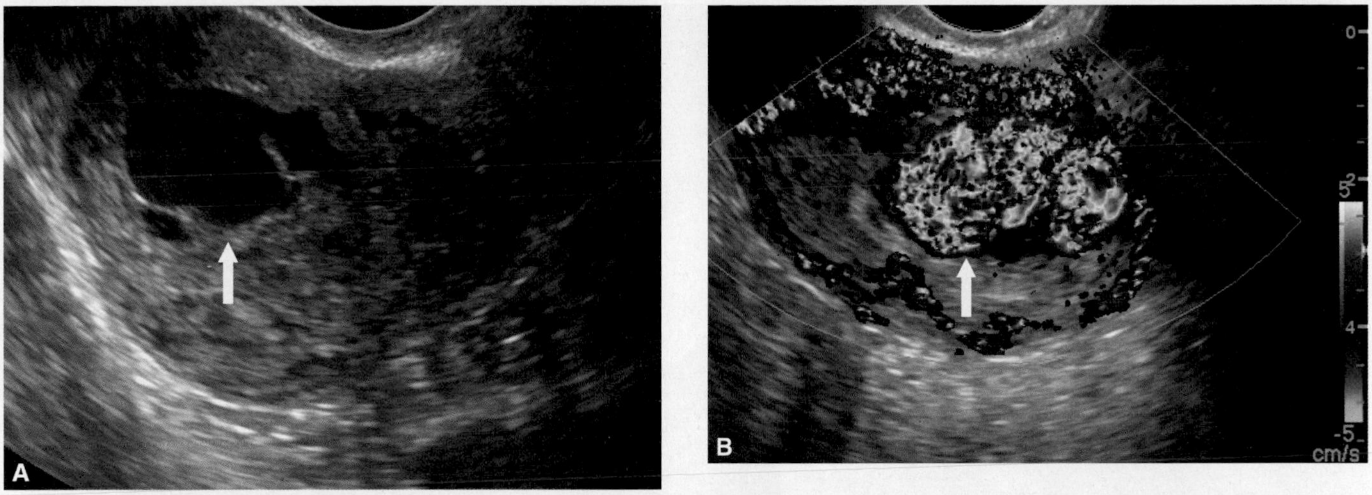

Figure 10.15. Uterine arteriovenous malformation on transvaginal US. Sagittal gray-scale **(A)** and transverse color Doppler **(B)** images of the uterus in a 33-year-old woman following therapy for high-risk GTD now presenting with abnormal bleeding show cystic spaces that demonstrate high-velocity turbulent flow (*arrows*). Diagnosis was confirmed and treated with angiography and embolization.

OVARIAN CANCER

Detection

Large randomized trials have shown that routine screening for ovarian cancer using a combination of physical examination, cancer antigen 125 (CA-125), and TVUS does not meaningfully decrease disease-specific mortality (88,89). These trials have shown that benign adnexal lesions are common, with a reported incidence of complex ovarian cysts of 3.2% in women over age 50 years (90,91), whereas ovarian cancer is rare, with 12.1 cases per 100,000 women (92). This high incidence of benign adnexal lesions coupled with the low incidence of ovarian cancer in the general population means that diagnostic testing algorithm with 100% sensitivity and 99% specificity is estimated to have a positive predictive value of <5% (93). In contrast, sensitivities and specificities of 85% to 100% and 52% to 100%, respectively, have been reported for detection of ovarian malignancies using US (94–96). Screening trials have also shown that the majority of ovarian cancers show rapid progression from early-stage sonographically detectable lesions to extraovarian spread with short lag times (**Fig. 10.17**). In one trial, all 10 of the ovarian cancers detected were at stage III or IV, having developed within the 6-month interval between screening exams (97). Consequently, the U.S. Preventative Services Task Force currently recommends against screening, given the scant evidence for any benefit and the morbidity incurred from unnecessary interventions (98).

A benign adnexal mass is diagnosed in 5% of CTs in postmenarchal women (99) and in 4% of CTs in women greater than 50 years (100).

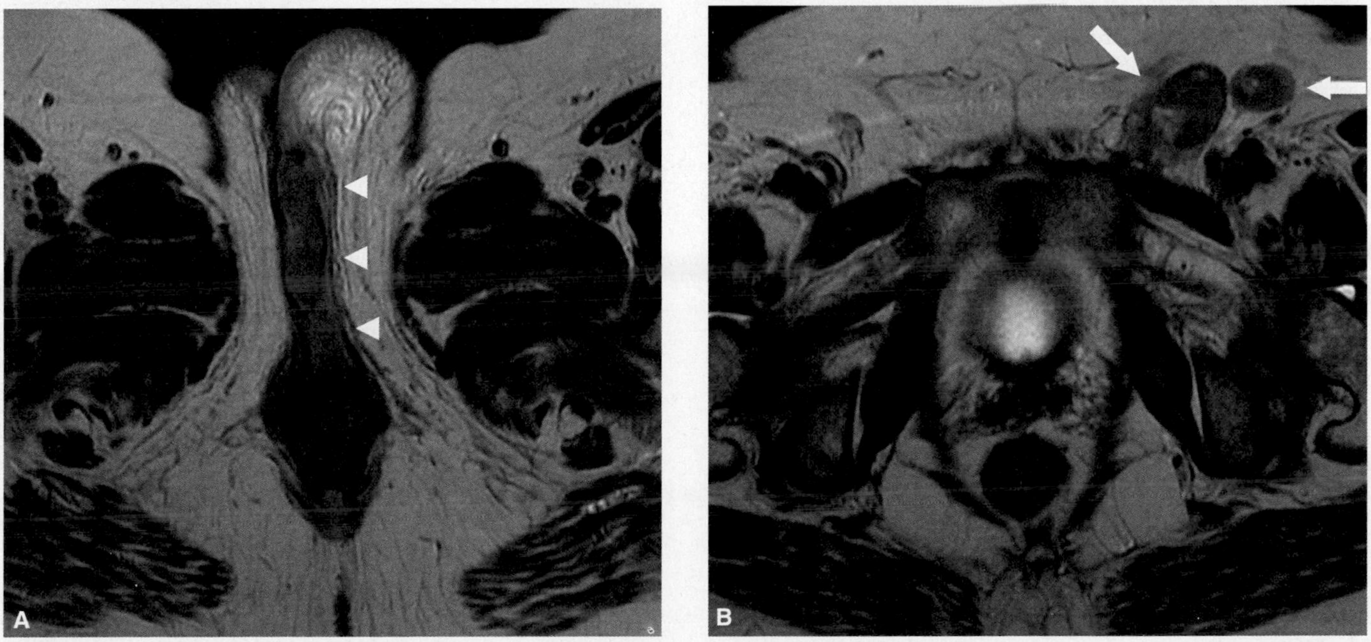

Figure 10.16. Vulvar cancer stage IV detected on PET-CT. Axial FSE T2-weighted images of the pelvic floor **(A and B)** of 66-year-old woman with squamous cell carcinoma of the vulva demonstrate a 7.8 × 1.5 cm left vulvar mass (*arrowheads*) and abnormally enlarged left inguinal nodes. Coronal PET **(C)** image again demonstrates hypermetabolic foci corresponding to the primary tumor (*asterisk*) and bilateral inguinal adenopathy. However, tracer accumulation higher in the left pelvis (*arrow*) localizes on concurrent CT **(D)** to metastases in the obturator nodes (*arrow*) confirmed with biopsy. FSE, fast spin-echo.

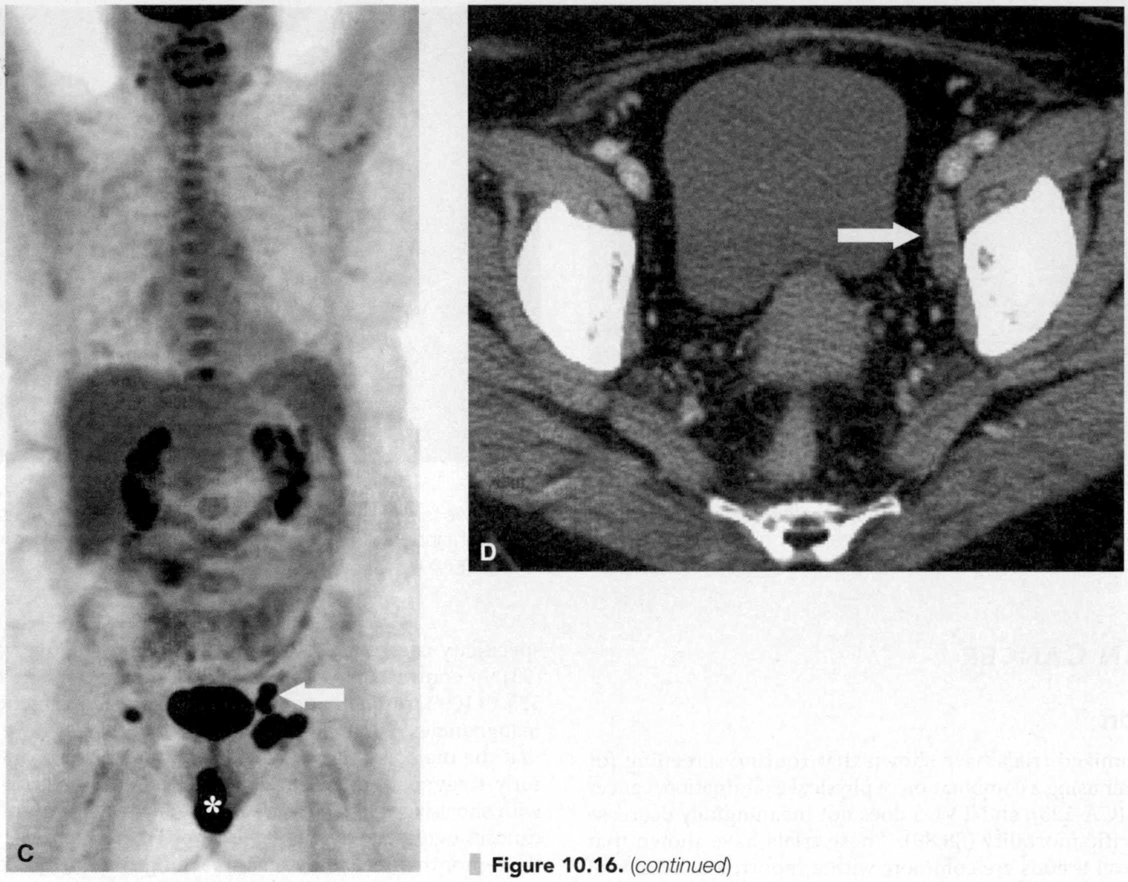

Figure 10.16. *(continued)*

A woman in the United States has a 5% to 10% lifetime chance of undergoing an oophorectomy for a benign adnexal mass (101), with resultant long-term morbidity of decreased fertility and premature menopause (102,103). Incidental adnexal masses represent a wide variety of pathologies, including functional cysts, mature teratoma, endometrioma, benign, borderline or malignant primary neoplasms, and extraovarian processes such as hydrosalpinx, peritoneal inclusion cyst, and fibroid (104). Given the high prevalence of incidental adnexal lesions, the role of imaging is to definitively characterize them as benign and minimize the number of unnecessary interventions.

MRI is the best modality to more definitively characterize incidental adnexal lesions likely to be benign. A meta-analysis evaluating the incremental value of a second test for adnexal mass deemed indeterminate on gray-scale US found that MRI changed the posttest probability of ovarian cancer in both pre- and postmenopausal women more than CT or combined gray-scale and Doppler US (105). The contribution of MRI in adnexal mass evaluation is its specificity, because it provides greater tissue characterization and localization of benign lesions. In a prospective study of women with suspected adnexal masses, both Doppler US and MRI were highly sensitive for identifying malignant lesions (US, 100%; MRI 96.6%), but the specificity of MRI was significantly greater (US, 39.5%; MRI 83.7%). Thus, women who clinically have a low risk of malignancy but have indeterminate lesions on US are the ones most likely to benefit from MRI (106).

Primary Treatment Planning

The FIGO staging system for ovarian cancer is based on surgery and pathology (107). Although it does not formally include imaging, it encourages the use of imaging to assess for important prognostic factors such as disease resectability and lymph node status. Thus, pretreatment imaging is used to define tumor extent, and to identify patients for whom primary surgery is unlikely to achieve optimal cytoreduction. NCCN guidelines include abdominopelvic CT or MRI in this context (108). The importance of imaging in helping to triage patients for appropriate management has increased because the use of neoadjuvant chemotherapy followed by interval cytoreductive surgery as a suitable alternative has been supported by multicenter randomized controlled trials (109,110).

CT is the primary imaging modality used to assess tumor spread and plan therapy for advanced ovarian cancer patients (**Fig. 10.18**). Imaging features that favor neoadjuvant chemotherapy include diffuse peritoneal thickening, peritoneal implants exceeding 2 cm in diameter, lesser sac and small-bowel mesentery involvement, pelvic sidewall involvement, large-volume ascites, and suprarenal retroperitoneal adenopathy (111–113). However, diagnostic accuracies have been reported over a wide range and are yet to be validated across multiple surgeons and institutions.

The ability to detect peritoneal implants depends on their size, with CT having a sensitivity of 14% to 27% for the detection of deposits less than 1 cm, especially in the absence of ascites (114,115). The sensitivity of CT for the detection of omental metastases is higher and reported to be 80% to 86% (114,115). The most commonly involved lymph nodes with ovarian cancer are at the para-aortic and aorto-caval locations at the level of the renal hilum. In general, a 1-cm short-axis diameter threshold is used to define an enlarged node. Hematogenous spread is the least common mode of spread in ovarian cancer but typically occurs in the solid abdominal organs such as the liver, spleen, kidneys, and adrenals; in the brain; and in the bones. CT has a sensitivity of 95% to 100% for the detection of liver disease and 50% to 60% for the detection of nodal disease (114,115).

Other modalities such as MRI or PET-CT can also be used with equal efficacy in planning cytoreductive surgery. A multicenter

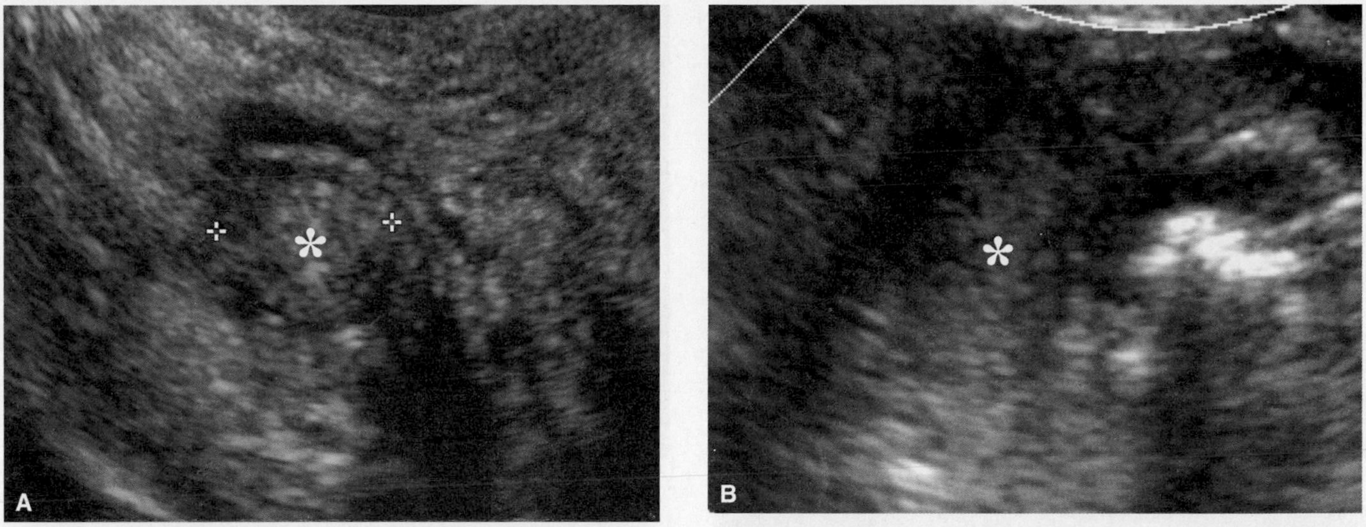

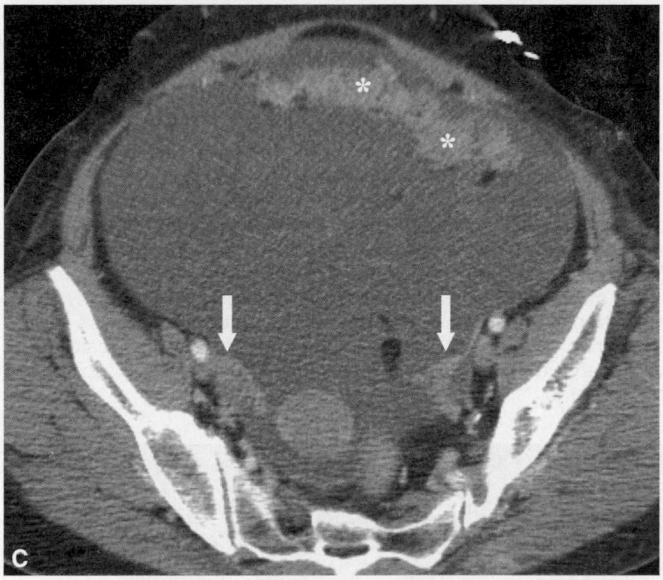

Figure 10.17. High-grade ovarian carcinoma at presentation. Endovaginal US images of the right **(A)** and left **(B)** ovaries (*asterisks*) of a 62-year-old woman with abdominal discomfort demonstrate normal ovaries and no ascites. Contrast-enhanced CT image **(C)** of the pelvis obtained 5 months later for worsening symptoms reveals interval development of enlarged ovaries (*arrows*), enhancing omental soft tissue (*asterisk*) and large amount of ascites. Stage III serous ovarian adenocarcinoma was confirmed with surgery and pathology.

trial of 280 patients with advanced ovarian cancer reported equal accuracy for CT and MR imaging (area under the curve [AUC], 0.96 for both) in diagnosing intraperitoneal tumor implants (116). FDG-PET-CT reportedly has sensitivities ranging from 62% to 100% and improves overall diagnostic accuracy by 5% to 22% compared with CT alone, mostly by identifying extra-abdominopelvic disease (**Fig. 10.19**) (117–119). But because CT is most widely available, is better tolerated, and yields higher-resolution anatomic information, it is the most commonly used modality across most institutions.

Post Primary Therapy

Although most patients will respond to primary therapy, 60% to 85% will eventually relapse (120), and almost all of them will die from the disease. The combination of clinical assessment and CA-125 measurement is routinely used to monitor patients treated for ovarian cancer in many institutions (121). However, CA-125, although useful, has limitations, since normal values do not exclude disease and elevated values do not define disease extent (122–124). In the 10% subgroup of biochemically "silent" patients, imaging is the primary means of assessing treatment response and of follow-up for recurrence.

Traditionally, CT and, less commonly, MRI are used to evaluate for suspected relapse, with a rise in CA-125 levels, which typically precedes imaging findings by several months. The sensitivity of CT ranges from 51% to 84%, and its specificity ranges from 81% to 93% (125–127). The sensitivity of CT for disease detection is proportional to lesion size. Many studies report limitations in the detection of small tumor nodules in the mesentery and along peritoneal surfaces (125,127). However, sagittal and coronal reformatted images available with multidetector scanning improve the detection of peritoneal implants (128).

More recently, because of its superior sensitivity, specificity, and reader agreement (129), PET-CT has become the preferred modality for detecting recurrent tumor and planning subsequent therapy (**Fig. 10.20** and **Table 10.4**). In two meta-analyses, PET-CT had the highest pooled sensitivity and specificity (91% and 86%, respectively) compared with PET and CT alone, MRI, and CA-125 (130,131). In prospective studies, PET-CT upstaged disease, compared with purely anatomic imaging, in 55% to 64% of patients by depicting additional sites of disease, and altered decisions on clinical management in 34% to 59% (132–135).

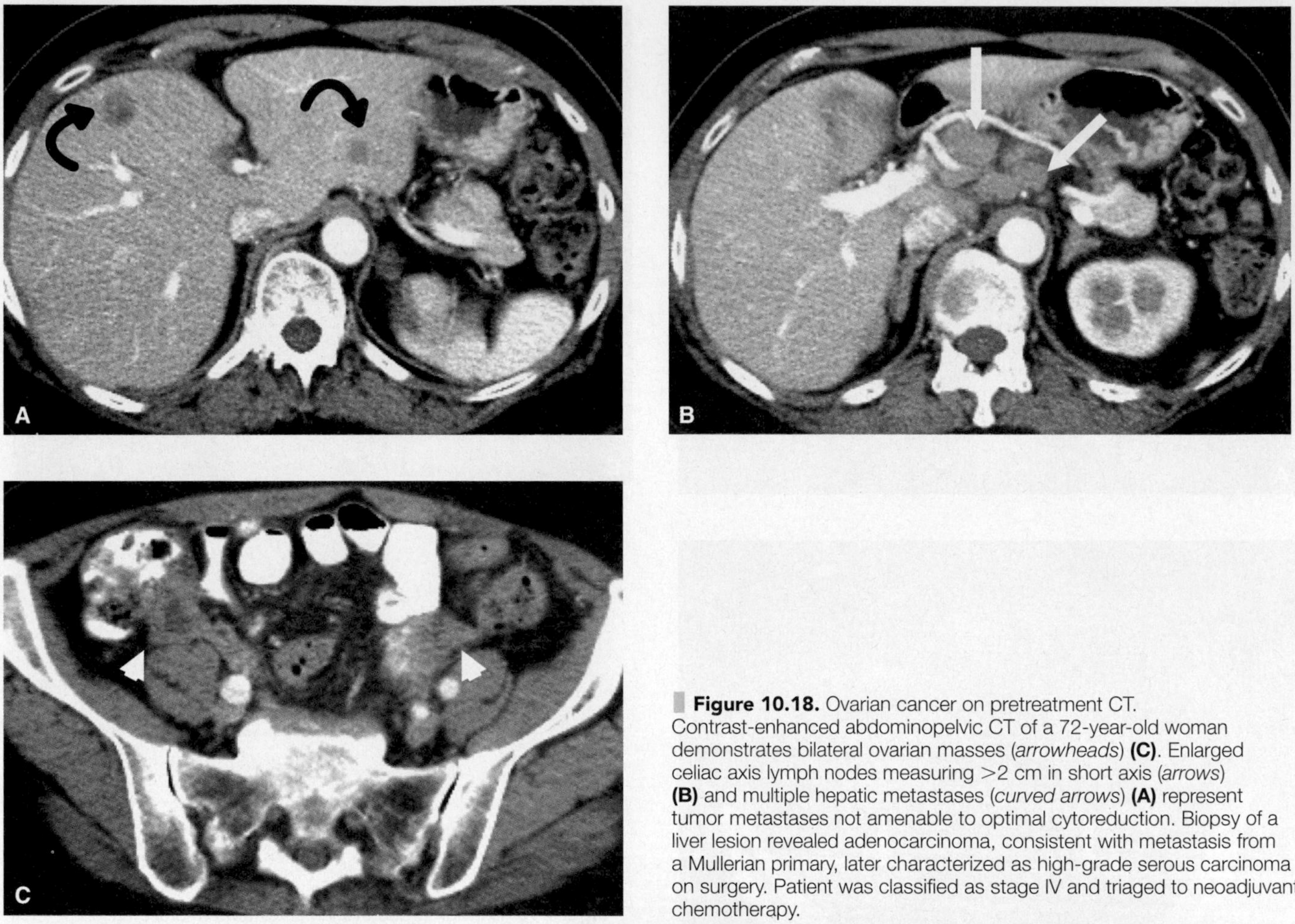

Figure 10.18. Ovarian cancer on pretreatment CT. Contrast-enhanced abdominopelvic CT of a 72-year-old woman demonstrates bilateral ovarian masses (*arrowheads*) **(C)**. Enlarged celiac axis lymph nodes measuring >2 cm in short axis (*arrows*) **(B)** and multiple hepatic metastases (*curved arrows*) **(A)** represent tumor metastases not amenable to optimal cytoreduction. Biopsy of a liver lesion revealed adenocarcinoma, consistent with metastasis from a Mullerian primary, later characterized as high-grade serous carcinoma on surgery. Patient was classified as stage IV and triaged to neoadjuvant chemotherapy.

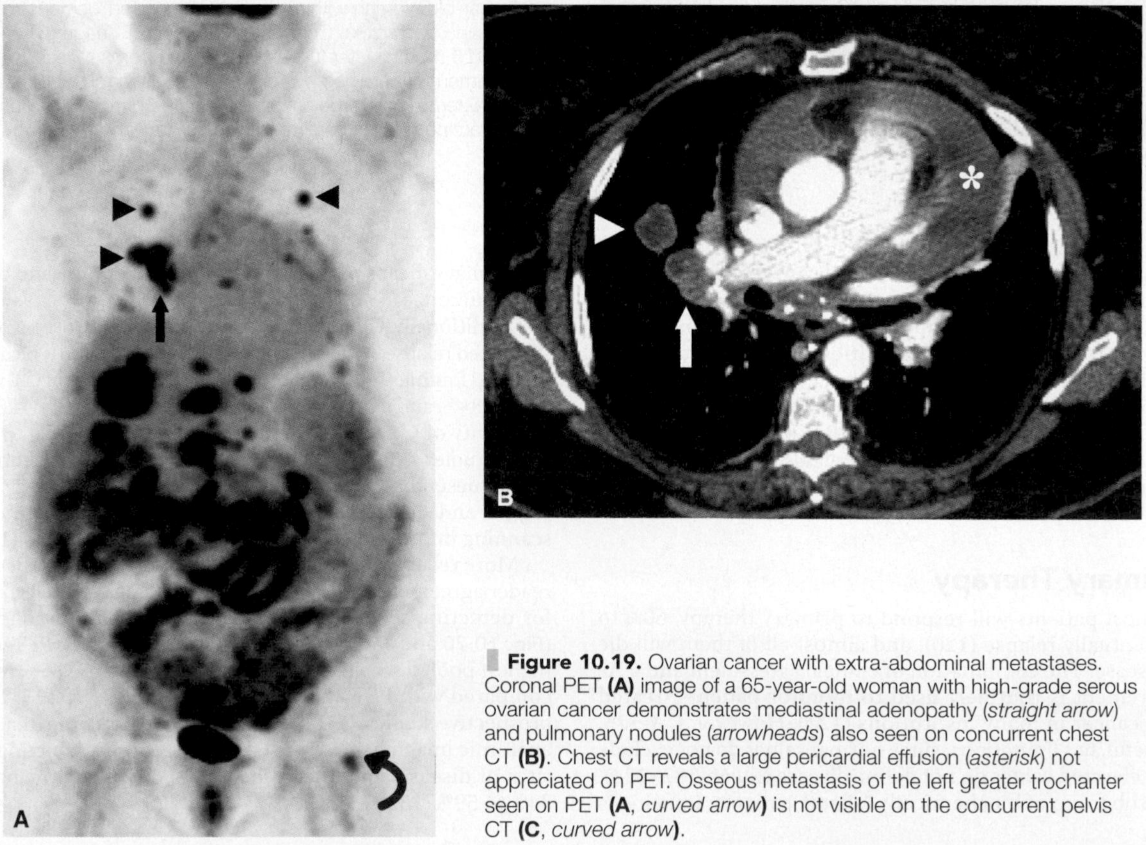

Figure 10.19. Ovarian cancer with extra-abdominal metastases. Coronal PET **(A)** image of a 65-year-old woman with high-grade serous ovarian cancer demonstrates mediastinal adenopathy (*straight arrow*) and pulmonary nodules (*arrowheads*) also seen on concurrent chest CT **(B)**. Chest CT reveals a large pericardial effusion (*asterisk*) not appreciated on PET. Osseous metastasis of the left greater trochanter seen on PET (**A**, *curved arrow*) is not visible on the concurrent pelvis CT (**C**, *curved arrow*).

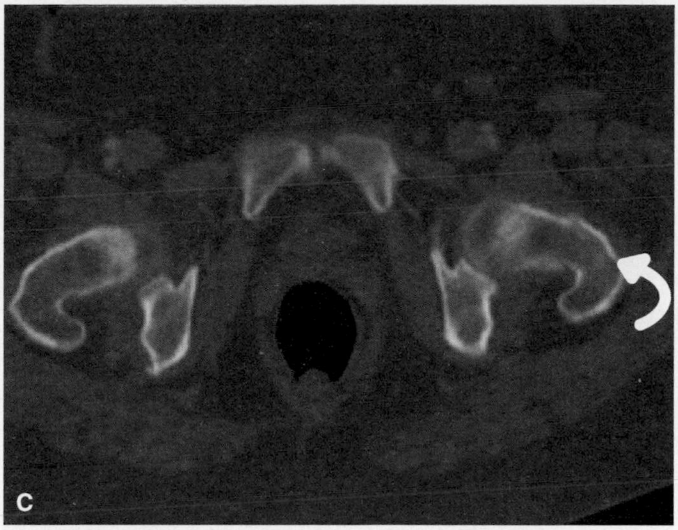

■ **Figure 10.19.** (*continued*)

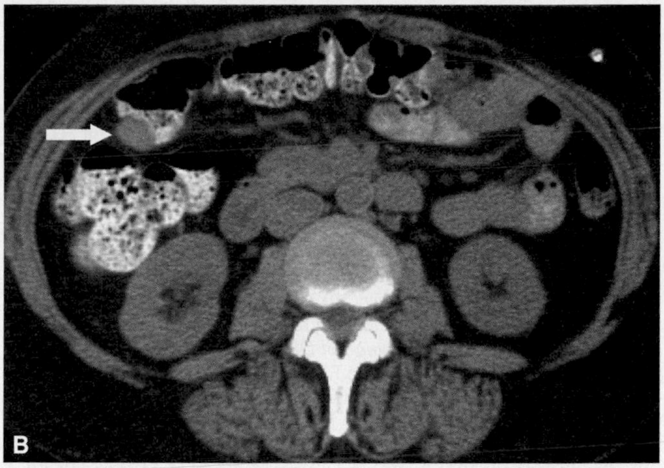

■ **Figure 10.20.** (*continued*)

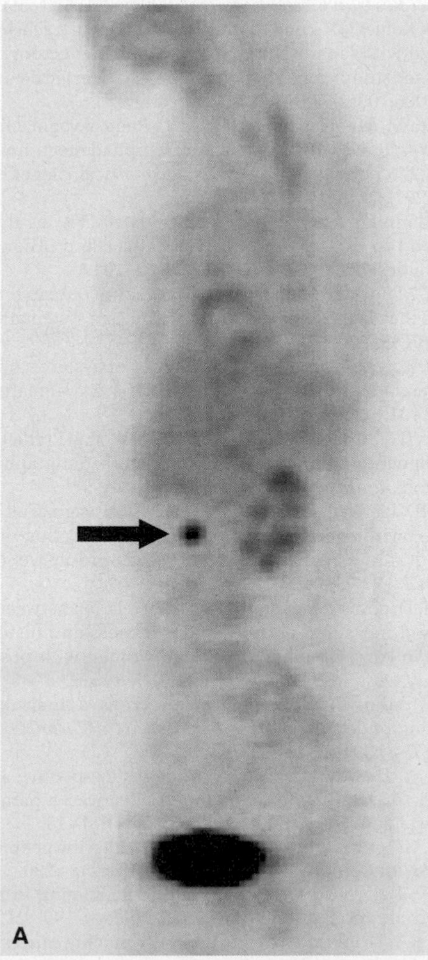

■ **Figure 10.20.** Recurrent ovarian cancer detected on PET-CT. Sagittal PET image **(A)** of a 62-year-old woman who initially presented 8 years ago with poorly differentiated (transitional and serous types) ovarian carcinoma and now with a rising CA-125 serum marker reveals a hypermetabolic focus in the mid abdomen. On concurrent CT **(B)**, the tracer localizes to a 1-cm peritoneal nodule (*arrow*), which was overlooked on a CT several days before.

TABLE 10.4. Diagnostic Performance in Detecting Ovarian Cancer Recurrence (130)

Modality	Sensitivity (95% CI)	Specificity (95% CI)	AUC
CT	79% (74–84)	84% (76–90)	0.885
MRI	75% (69–80)	78% (70–85)	0.796
PET-CT	91% (88–94)	88% (81–93)	0.956

From Gu P, Pan LL, Wu SQ, et al. CA 125, PET alone, PET-CT, CT and MRI in diagnosing recurrent ovarian carcinoma: a systematic review and meta-analysis. *Eur J Radiol*. 2009;71(1):164–174, with permission.

CONCLUSION

Imaging is central in many phases of gynecologic cancer care. In cancer detection, imaging (e.g., pelvic US with postmenopausal bleeding, pelvic MRI with indeterminate adnexal masses) serves as a screening tool to reassure those with benign disease and to triage others for further work-up. In primary treatment planning of all gynecologic cancers, body CT, pelvic MRI, or whole-body FDG-PET-CT defines tumor extent and aids in selection of a treatment strategy that optimizes patient outcome while minimizing morbidity. Following primary therapy, these imaging exams are used to assess therapy response, detect suspected recurrence, and select candidates for salvage therapy.

REFERENCES

1. National Research Council. *Health Risks from Exposure to Low Levels of Ionizing Radiation: BEIR VII Phase 2*. Washington, DC: The National Academies Press; 2006.
2. Zondervan RL, Hahn PF, Sadow CA, et al. Body CT scanning in young adults: examination indications, patient outcomes, and risk of radiation-induced cancer. *Radiology*. 2013;267(2):460–469.
3. Namasivayam S, Kalra MK, Torres WE, et al. Adverse reactions to intravenous iodinated contrast media: a primer for radiologists. *Emerg Radiol*. 2006;12(5):210–215.

4. Dillman JR, Ellis JH, Cohan RH, et al. Frequency and severity of acute allergic-like reactions to gadolinium-containing i.v. contrast media in children and adults. *AJR Am J Roentgenol.* 2007;189(6):1533–1538.
5. Prabhakar HB, Kraeft JJ, Schorge JO, et al. FDG PET-CT of gynecologic cancers: pearls and pitfalls. *Abdom Imaging.* 2015;40(7):2472–2485.
6. American College of Radiology. ACR–SPR Practice parameter for performing FDG-PET/CT in oncology 2007. Updated 2014. Available from: http://www.acr.org/~/media/71B746780F934F6D8A1BA5CCA5167EDB.pdf.
7. Graham MM, Badawi RD, Wahl RL. Variations in PET/CT methodology for oncologic imaging at U.S. academic medical centers: an imaging response assessment team survey. *J Nucl Med.* 2011;52(2):311–317.
8. Erdi YE. Limits of tumor detectability in nuclear medicine and PET. *Mol Imaging Radionucl Ther.* 2012;21(1):23–28.
9. Pecorelli S. Revised FIGO staging for carcinoma of the vulva, cervix, and endometrium. *Int J Gynaecol Obstet.* 2009;105(2):103–104.
10. Pecorelli S, Zigliani L, Odicino F. Revised FIGO staging for carcinoma of the cervix. *Int J Gynaecol Obstet.* 2009;105(2):107–108.
11. Koh WJ, Greer BE, Abu-Rustum NR, et al. Cervical cancer. *J Natl Compr Canc Netw.* 2013;11(3):320–343.
12. Pandharipande PV, Choy G, del Carmen MG, et al. MRI and PET/CT for triaging stage IB clinically operable cervical cancer to appropriate therapy: decision analysis to assess patient outcomes. *AJR Am J Roentgenol.* 2009;192(3):802–814.
13. Hricak H, Gatsonis C, Chi DS, et al. Role of imaging in pretreatment evaluation of early invasive cervical cancer: results of the intergroup study American College of Radiology Imaging Network 6651–Gynecologic Oncology Group 183. *J Clin Oncol.* 2005;23(36):9329–9337.
14. Mitchell DG, Snyder B, Coakley F, et al. Early invasive cervical cancer: tumor delineation by magnetic resonance imaging, computed tomography, and clinical examination, verified by pathologic results, in the ACRIN 6651/GOG 183 Intergroup Study. *J Clin Oncol.* 2006;24(36):5687–5694.
15. Selman TJ, Mann C, Zamora J, et al. Diagnostic accuracy of tests for lymph node status in primary cervical cancer: a systematic review and meta-analysis. *CMAJ.* 2008;178(7):855–862.
16. Sironi S, Buda A, Picchio M, et al. Lymph node metastasis in patients with clinical early-stage cervical cancer: detection with integrated FDG PET/CT. *Radiology.* 2006;238(1):272–279.
17. Loft A, Berthelsen AK, Roed H, et al. The diagnostic value of PET/CT scanning in patients with cervical cancer: a prospective study. *Gynecol Oncol.* 2007;106(1):29–34.
18. Selman TJ, Mann CH, Zamora J, et al. A systematic review of tests for lymph node status in primary endometrial cancer. *BMC Womens Health.* 2008;8:8.
19. Antonsen SL, Jensen LN, Loft A, et al. MRI, PET/CT and ultrasound in the preoperative staging of endometrial cancer—a multicenter prospective comparative study. *Gynecol Oncol.* 2013;128(2):300–308.
20. Signorelli M, Guerra L, Buda A, et al. Role of the integrated FDG PET/CT in the surgical management of patients with high risk clinical early stage endometrial cancer: detection of pelvic nodal metastases. *Gynecol Oncol.* 2009;115(2):231–235.
21. Andersen K, Zobbe V, Thranov IR, et al. Relevance of computerized tomography in the preoperative evaluation of patients with vulvar cancer: a prospective study. *Cancer Imaging.* 2015;15:8.
22. Hawnaur JM, Reynolds K, Wilson G, et al. Identification of inguinal lymph node metastases from vulval carcinoma by magnetic resonance imaging: an initial report. *Clin Radiol.* 2002;57(11):995–1000.
23. Bipat S, Fransen GA, Spijkerboer AM, et al. Is there a role for magnetic resonance imaging in the evaluation of inguinal lymph node metastases in patients with vulva carcinoma? *Gynecol Oncol.* 2006;103(3):1001–1006.
24. Kataoka MY, Sala E, Baldwin P, et al. The accuracy of magnetic resonance imaging in staging of vulvar cancer: a retrospective multi-center study. *Gynecol Oncol.* 2010;117(1):82–87.
25. Kamran MW, O'Toole F, Meghen K, et al. Whole-body [18F]fluoro-2-deoxyglucose positron emission tomography scan as combined PET-CT staging prior to planned radical vulvectomy and inguinofemoral lymphadenectomy for squamous vulvar cancer: a correlation with groin node metastasis. *Eur J Gynaecol Oncol.* 2014;35(3):230–235.
26. Lin G, Chen CY, Liu FY, et al. Computed tomography, magnetic resonance imaging and FDG positron emission tomography in the management of vulvar malignancies. *Eur Radiol.* 2015;25(5):1267–1278.
27. Atri M, Zhang Z, Dehdashti F, et al. Utility of PET-CT vs CT alone to evaluate retroperitoneal lymph node metastasis in advanced cervical cancer. *J Clin Oncol.* 2015;33(Suppl):5585.
28. Choi HJ, Ju W, Myung SK, et al. Diagnostic performance of computer tomography, magnetic resonance imaging, and positron emission tomography or positron emission tomography/computer tomography for detection of metastatic lymph nodes in patients with cervical cancer: meta-analysis. *Cancer Sci.* 2010;101(6):1471–1479.
29. Chao A, Ho KC, Wang CC, et al. Positron emission tomography in evaluating the feasibility of curative intent in cervical cancer patients with limited distant lymph node metastases. *Gynecol Oncol.* 2008;110(2):172–178.
30. Kidd EA, Siegel BA, Dehdashti F, et al. Lymph node staging by positron emission tomography in cervical cancer: relationship to prognosis. *J Clin Oncol.* 2010;28(12):2108–2113.
31. Lakhman Y, Akin O, Park KJ, et al. Stage IB1 cervical cancer: role of preoperative MR imaging in selection of patients for fertility-sparing radical trachelectomy. *Radiology.* 2013;269(1):149–158.
32. Signorelli M, Guerra L, Montanelli L, et al. Preoperative staging of cervical cancer: Is 18-FDG-PET/CT really effective in patients with early stage disease? *Gynecol Oncol.* 2011;123(2):236–240.
33. Babar S, Rockall A, Goode A, et al. Magnetic resonance imaging appearances of recurrent cervical carcinoma. *Int J Gynecol Cancer.* 2007;17(3):637–645.
34. Schwarz JK, Siegel BA, Dehdashti F, et al. Association of posttherapy positron emission tomography with tumor response and survival in cervical carcinoma. *JAMA.* 2007;298(19):2289–2295.
35. Grigsby PW, Siegel BA, Dehdashti F, et al. Posttherapy [18F] fluorodeoxyglucose positron emission tomography in carcinoma of the cervix: response and outcome. *J Clin Oncol.* 2004;22(11):2167–2171.
36. Vincens E, Balleyguier C, Rey A, et al. Accuracy of magnetic resonance imaging in predicting residual disease in patients treated for stage IB2/II cervical carcinoma with chemoradiation therapy: correlation of radiologic findings with surgicopathologic results. *Cancer.* 2008;113(8):2158–2165.
37. Weber TM, Sostman HD, Spritzer CE, et al. Cervical carcinoma: determination of recurrent tumor extent versus radiation changes with MR imaging. *Radiology.* 1995;194(1):135–139.
38. Shepherd JH. Uterus-conserving surgery for invasive cervical cancer. *Best Pract Res Clin Obstet Gynaecol.* 2005;19(4):577–590.
39. Hertel H, Kohler C, Grund D, et al. Radical vaginal trachelectomy (RVT) combined with laparoscopic pelvic lymphadenectomy: prospective multicenter study of 100 patients with early cervical cancer. *Gynecol Oncol.* 2006;103(2):506–511.
40. Lanowska M, Mangler M, Spek A, et al. Radical vaginal trachelectomy (RVT) combined with laparoscopic lymphadenectomy: prospective study of 225 patients with early-stage cervical cancer. *Int J Gynecol Cancer.* 2011;21(8):1458–1464.
41. Smith-Bindman R, Kerlikowske K, Feldstein VA, et al. Endovaginal ultrasound to exclude endometrial cancer and other endometrial abnormalities. *JAMA.* 1998;280(17):1510–1517.
42. Clark TJ, Mann CH, Shah N, et al. Accuracy of outpatient endometrial biopsy in the diagnosis of endometrial cancer: a systematic quantitative review. *BJOG.* 2002;109(3):313–321.
43. Clark TJ, Voit D, Gupta JK, et al. Accuracy of hysteroscopy in the diagnosis of endometrial cancer and hyperplasia: a systematic quantitative review. *JAMA.* 2002;288(13):1610–1621.
44. Dubinsky TJ, Stroehlein K, Abu-Ghazzeh Y, et al. Prediction of benign and malignant endometrial disease: hysterosonographic-pathologic correlation. *Radiology.* 1999;210(2):393–397.
45. Langer RD, Pierce JJ, O'Hanlan KA, et al. Transvaginal ultrasonography compared with endometrial biopsy for the detection of endometrial disease. Postmenopausal Estrogen/Progestin Interventions Trial. *N Engl J Med.* 1997;337(25):1792–1798.
46. Phillip H, Dacosta V, Fletcher H, et al. Correlation between transvaginal ultrasound measured endometrial thickness and histopathological findings in Afro-Caribbean Jamaican women with postmenopausal bleeding. *J Obstet Gynaecol.* 2004;24(5):568–572.
47. Smith P, Bakos O, Heimer G, et al. Transvaginal ultrasound for identifying endometrial abnormality. *Acta Obstet Gynecol Scand.* 1991;70(7–8):591–594.
48. Mariani A, Dowdy SC, Cliby WA, et al. Prospective assessment of lymphatic dissemination in endometrial cancer: a paradigm shift in surgical staging. *Gynecol Oncol.* 2008;109(1):11–18.
49. Koh WJ, Greer BE, Abu-Rustum NR, et al. Uterine neoplasms, version 1.2014. *J Natl Compr Canc Netw.* 2014;12(2):248–280.
50. Kinkel K, Kaji Y, Yu KK, et al. Radiologic staging in patients with endometrial cancer: a meta-analysis. *Radiology.* 1999;212(3):711–718.
51. Duncan KA, Drinkwater KJ, Frost C, et al. Staging cancer of the uterus: a national audit of MRI accuracy. *Clin Radiol.* 2012;67(6):523–530.
52. Ushijima K, Yahata H, Yoshikawa H, et al. Multicenter phase II study of fertility-sparing treatment with medroxyprogesterone acetate for endometrial carcinoma and atypical hyperplasia in young women. *J Clin Oncol.* 2007;25(19):2798–2803.
53. Russell AH, Anderson M, Walter J, et al. The integration of computed tomography and magnetic resonance imaging in treatment planning for gynecologic cancer. *Clin Obstet Gynecol.* 1992;35(1):55–72.

54. Nakamura K, Kodama J, Okumura Y, et al. The SUVmax of 18F-FDG PET correlates with histological grade in endometrial cancer. *Int J Gynecol Cancer*. 2010;20(1):110–115.
55. Liu Y. Benign ovarian and endometrial uptake on FDG PET-CT: patterns and pitfalls. *Ann Nucl Med*. 2009;23(2):107–112.
56. Kitajima K, Murakami K, Yamasaki E, et al. Accuracy of 18F-FDG PET/CT in detecting pelvic and paraaortic lymph node metastasis in patients with endometrial cancer. *AJR Am J Roentgenol*. 2008;190(6):1652–1658.
57. Keys HM, Roberts JA, Brunetto VL, et al. A phase III trial of surgery with or without adjunctive external pelvic radiation therapy in intermediate risk endometrial adenocarcinoma: a Gynecologic Oncology Group study. *Gynecol Oncol*. 2004;92(3):744–751.
58. Park JY, Kim EN, Kim DY, et al. Comparison of the validity of magnetic resonance imaging and positron emission tomography/computed tomography in the preoperative evaluation of patients with uterine corpus cancer. *Gynecol Oncol*. 2008;108(3):486–492.
59. Picchio M, Mangili G, Samanes Gajate AM, et al. High-grade endometrial cancer: value of [(18)F]FDG PET/CT in preoperative staging. *Nucl Med Commun*. 2010;31(6):506–512.
60. Todo Y, Kato H, Kaneuchi M, et al. Survival effect of para-aortic lymphadenectomy in endometrial cancer (SEPAL study): a retrospective cohort analysis. *Lancet*. 2010;375(9721):1165–1172.
61. Sohaib SA, Houghton SL, Meroni R, et al. Recurrent endometrial cancer: patterns of recurrent disease and assessment of prognosis. *Clin Radiol*. 2007;62(1):28–34; discussion 5–6.
62. Berchuck A, Anspach C, Evans AC, et al. Postsurgical surveillance of patients with FIGO stage I/II endometrial adenocarcinoma. *Gynecol Oncol*. 1995;59(1):20–24.
63. Kitajima K, Murakami K, Yamasaki E, et al. Performance of FDG-PET/CT in the diagnosis of recurrent endometrial cancer. *Ann Nucl Med*. 2008;22(2):103–109.
64. Sironi S, Picchio M, Landoni C, et al. Post-therapy surveillance of patients with uterine cancers: value of integrated FDG PET/CT in the detection of recurrence. *Eur J Nucl Med Mol Imaging*. 2007;34(4):472–479.
65. Food and Drug Administration. Quantitative assessment of the prevalence of unsuspected uterine sarcoma in women undergoing treatment of uterine fibroids: summary and key findings, 2014. Available from: http://www.fda.gov/downloads/MedicalDevices/Safety/AlertsandNotices/UCM393589.pdf
66. Society of Interventional Radiology. FDA-2014-N-0736: Comments on laparoscopic power morcellation devices, 2014. Available from: http://www.sirweb.org/misc/SIR LetterFDA-2014-N-0736.pdf
67. Kido A, Togashi K, Koyama T, et al. Diffusely enlarged uterus: evaluation with MR imaging. *Radiographics*. 2003;23(6):1423–1439.
68. Khan AT, Shehmar M, Gupta JK. Uterine fibroids: current perspectives. *Int J Womens Health*. 2014;6:95–114.
69. Cornfeld D, Israel G, Martel M, et al. MRI appearance of mesenchymal tumors of the uterus. *Eur J Radiol*. 2010;74(1):241–249.
70. Goto A, Takeuchi S, Sugimura K, et al. Usefulness of Gd-DTPA contrast-enhanced dynamic MRI and serum determination of LDH and its isozymes in the differential diagnosis of leiomyosarcoma from degenerated leiomyoma of the uterus. *Int J Gynecol Cancer*. 2002;12(4):354–361.
71. Chura JC, Truskinovsky AM, Judson PL, et al. Positron emission tomography and leiomyomas: clinicopathologic analysis of 3 cases of PET scan-positive leiomyomas and literature review. *Gynecol Oncol*. 2007;104(1):247–252.
72. Kitajima K, Murakami K, Yamasaki E, et al. Standardized uptake values of uterine leiomyoma with 18F-FDG PET/CT: variation with age, size, degeneration, and contrast enhancement on MRI. *Ann Nucl Med*. 2008;22(6):505–512.
73. Koh WJ, Greer BE, Abu-Rustum NR, et al. Uterine sarcoma, Version 1.2016. *J Natl Compr Canc Netw*. 2015;13(11):1321–1331.
74. Ho KC, Lai CH, Wu TI, et al. 18F-fluorodeoxyglucose positron emission tomography in uterine carcinosarcoma. *Eur J Nucl Med Mol Imaging*. 2008;35(3):484–492.
75. Tirumani SH, Deaver P, Shinagare AB, et al. Metastatic pattern of uterine leiomyosarcoma: retrospective analysis of the predictors and outcome in 113 patients. *J Gynecol Oncol*. 2014;25(4):306–312.
76. Gadducci A, Landoni F, Sartori E, et al. Uterine leiomyosarcoma: analysis of treatment failures and survival. *Gynecol Oncol*. 1996;62(1):25–32.
77. Mayerhofer K, Obermair A, Windbichler G, et al. Leiomyosarcoma of the uterus: a clinicopathologic multicenter study of 71 cases. *Gynecol Oncol*. 1999;74(2):196–201.
78. National Comprehensive Cancer Network. NCCN Clinical practice guidelines in oncology: uterine neoplasms, 2016. Available from: http://www.nccn.org/professionals/physician_gls/pdf/uterine.pdf
79. Sung PL, Chen YJ, Liu RS, et al. Whole-body positron emission tomography with 18F-fluorodeoxyglucose is an effective method to detect extra-pelvic recurrence in uterine sarcomas. *Eur J Gynaecol Oncol*. 2008;29(3):246–251.
80. FIGO Committee on Gynecologic Oncology. Current FIGO staging for cancer of the vagina, fallopian tube, ovary, and gestational trophoblastic neoplasia. *Int J Gynaecol Obstet*. 2009;105(1):3–4.
81. Miyasaka Y, Hachiya J, Furuya Y, et al. CT evaluation of invasive trophoblastic disease. *J Comput Assist Tomogr*. 1985;9(3):459–462.
82. O'Brien P, Neyastani A, Buckley AR, et al. Uterine arteriovenous malformations: from diagnosis to treatment. *J Ultrasound Med*. 2006;25(11):1387–1392; quiz 94–95.
83. Lim AK, Agarwal R, Seckl MJ, et al. Embolization of bleeding residual uterine vascular malformations in patients with treated gestational trophoblastic tumors. *Radiology*. 2002;222(3):640–644.
84. Van der Zee AG, Oonk MH, De Hullu JA, et al. Sentinel node dissection is safe in the treatment of early-stage vulvar cancer. *J Clin Oncol*. 2008;26(6):884–889.
85. Levenback C, Coleman RL, Burke TW, et al. Intraoperative lymphatic mapping and sentinel node identification with blue dye in patients with vulvar cancer. *Gynecol Oncol*. 2001;83(2):276–281.
86. Cormio G, Loizzi V, Carriero C, et al. Groin recurrence in carcinoma of the vulva: management and outcome. *Eur J Cancer Care (Engl)*. 2010;19(3):302–307.
87. Fonseca-Moutinho JA. Recurrent vulvar cancer. *Clin Obstet Gynecol*. 2005;48(4):879–883.
88. Buys SS, Partridge E, Black A, et al. Effect of screening on ovarian cancer mortality: the Prostate, Lung, Colorectal and Ovarian (PLCO) Cancer Screening Randomized Controlled Trial. *JAMA*. 2011;305(22):2295–2303.
89. Jacobs IJ, Menon U, Ryan A, et al. Ovarian cancer screening and mortality in the UK Collaborative Trial of Ovarian Cancer Screening (UKCTOCS): a randomized controlled trial. *Lancet*. 2016;387(10022):945–956.
90. Bailey CL, Ueland FR, Land GL, et al. The malignant potential of small cystic ovarian tumors in women over 50 years of age. *Gynecol Oncol*. 1998;69(1):3–7.
91. van Nagell JR Jr, DePriest PD, Reedy MB, et al. The efficacy of transvaginal sonographic screening in asymptomatic women at risk for ovarian cancer. *Gynecol Oncol*. 2000;77(3):350–356.
92. National Cancer Institute. SEER Stat Fact Sheets: Ovary Cancer. Available from: http://seer.cancer.gov/statfacts/html/ovary.html
93. American College of Obstetricians and Gynecologists. ACOG Committee Opinion: number 280, December 2002. The role of the generalist obstetrician–gynecologist in the early detection of ovarian cancer. *Obstet Gynecol*. 2002;100(6):1413–1416.
94. Brown DL, Doubilet PM, Miller FH, et al. Benign and malignant ovarian masses: selection of the most discriminating gray-scale and Doppler sonographic features. *Radiology*. 1998;208(1):103–110.
95. Alcazar JL, Jurado M. Using a logistic model to predict malignancy of adnexal masses based on menopausal status, ultrasound morphology, and color Doppler findings. *Gynecol Oncol*. 1998;69(2):146–150.
96. Rehn M, Lohmann K, Rempen A. Transvaginal ultrasonography of pelvic masses: evaluation of B-mode technique and Doppler ultrasonography. *Am J Obstet Gynecol*. 1996;175(1):97–104.
97. Fishman DA, Cohen L, Blank SV, et al. The role of ultrasound evaluation in the detection of early-stage epithelial ovarian cancer. *Am J Obstet Gynecol*. 2005;192(4):1214–1221; discussion: 21–2.
98. Moyer VA, U.S. Preventive Services Task Force. Screening for ovarian cancer: U.S. Preventive Services Task Force reaffirmation recommendation statement. *Ann Intern Med*. 2012;157(12):900–904.
99. Slanetz PJ, Hahn PF, Hall DA, et al. The frequency and significance of adnexal lesions incidentally revealed by CT. *AJR Am J Roentgenol*. 1997;168(3):647–650.
100. Pickhardt PJ, Hanson ME. Incidental adnexal masses detected at low-dose unenhanced CT in asymptomatic women age 50 and older: implications for clinical management and ovarian cancer screening. *Radiology*. 2010;257(1):144–150.
101. National Institutes of Health Consensus Development Conference Statement. Ovarian cancer: screening, treatment, and follow-up. *Gynecol Oncol*. 1994;55(3, pt 2):S4–S14.
102. Lass A. The fertility potential of women with a single ovary. *Hum Reprod Update*. 1999;5(5):546–550.
103. Shuster LT, Gostout BS, Grossardt BR, et al. Prophylactic oophorectomy in premenopausal women and long-term health. *Menopause Int*. 2008;14(3):111–116.
104. Iyer VR, Lee SI. MRI, CT, and PET/CT for ovarian cancer detection and adnexal lesion characterization. *AJR Am J Roentgenol*. 2010;194(2):311–321.
105. Kinkel K, Lu Y, Mehdizade A, et al. Indeterminate ovarian mass at US: incremental value of second imaging test for characterization—meta-analysis and Bayesian analysis. *Radiology*. 2005;236(1):85–94.

106. Sohaib SA, Mills TD, Sahdev A, et al. The role of magnetic resonance imaging and ultrasound in patients with adnexal masses. *Clin Radiol.* 2005;60(3):340–348.
107. Mutch DG, Prat J. 2014 FIGO staging for ovarian, fallopian tube and peritoneal cancer. *Gynecol Oncol.* 2014;133(3):401–404.
108. Morgan RJ Jr, Alvarez RD, Armstrong DK, et al. Ovarian cancer, version 3.2012. *J Natl Compr Canc Netw.* 2012;10(11):1339–1349.
109. van der Burg ME, van Lent M, Buyse M, et al. The effect of debulking surgery after induction chemotherapy on the prognosis in advanced epithelial ovarian cancer: Gynecological Cancer Cooperative Group of the European Organization for Research and Treatment of Cancer. *N Engl J Med.* 1995;332(10):629–634.
110. Vergote I, Trope CG, Amant F, et al. Neoadjuvant chemotherapy or primary surgery in stage IIIC or IV ovarian cancer. *N Engl J Med.* 2010;363(10):943–953.
111. Suidan RS, Ramirez PT, Sarasohn DM, et al. A multicenter prospective trial evaluating the ability of preoperative computed tomography scan and serum CA-125 to predict suboptimal cytoreduction at primary debulking surgery for advanced ovarian, fallopian tube, and peritoneal cancer. *Gynecol Oncol.* 2014;134(3):455–461.
112. Bristow RE, Duska LR, Lambrou NC, et al. A model for predicting surgical outcome in patients with advanced ovarian carcinoma using computed tomography. *Cancer.* 2000;89(7):1532–1540.
113. Dowdy SC, Mullany SA, Brandt KR, et al. The utility of computed tomography scans in predicting suboptimal cytoreductive surgery in women with advanced ovarian carcinoma. *Cancer.* 2004;101(2):346–352.
114. Meyer JI, Kennedy AW, Friedman R, et al. Ovarian carcinoma: value of CT in predicting success of debulking surgery. *AJR Am J Roentgenol.* 1995;165(4):875–878.
115. Forstner R, Hricak H, Occhipinti KA, et al. Ovarian cancer: staging with CT and MR imaging. *Radiology.* 1995;197(3):619–626.
116. Tempany CM, Zou KH, Silverman SG, et al. Staging of advanced ovarian cancer: comparison of imaging modalities—report from the Radiological Diagnostic Oncology Group. *Radiology.* 2000;215(3):761–767.
117. Dirisamer A, Schima W, Heinisch M, et al. Detection of histologically proven peritoneal carcinomatosis with fused 18F-FDG-PET/MDCT. *Eur J Radiol.* 2009;69(3):536–541.
118. Kitajima K, Murakami K, Yamasaki E, et al. Diagnostic accuracy of integrated FDG-PET/contrast-enhanced CT in staging ovarian cancer: comparison with enhanced CT. *Eur J Nucl Med Mol Imaging.* 2008;35(10):1912–1920.
119. Yoshida Y, Kurokawa T, Kawahara K, et al. Incremental benefits of FDG positron emission tomography over CT alone for the preoperative staging of ovarian cancer. *AJR Am J Roentgenol.* 2004;182(1):227–233.
120. Berek JS, Trope C, Vergote I. Surgery during chemotherapy and at relapse of ovarian cancer. *Ann Oncol.* 1999;10(Suppl 1):3–7.
121. Gadducci A, Cosio S. Surveillance of patients after initial treatment of ovarian cancer. *Crit Rev Oncol Hematol.* 2009;71(1):43–52.
122. Folk JJ, Botsford M, Musa AG. Monitoring cancer antigen 125 levels in induction chemotherapy for epithelial ovarian carcinoma and predicting outcome of second-look procedure. *Gynecol Oncol.* 1995;57(2):178–182.
123. Patsner B, Orr JW Jr, Mann WJ Jr, et al. Does serum CA-125 level prior to second-look laparotomy for invasive ovarian adenocarcinoma predict size of residual disease? *Gynecol Oncol.* 1990;38(3):373–376.
124. Rubin SC, Hoskins WJ, Hakes TB, et al. Serum CA 125 levels and surgical findings in patients undergoing secondary operations for epithelial ovarian cancer. *Am J Obstet Gynecol.* 1989;160(3):667–671.
125. Funt SA, Hricak H, Abu-Rustum N, et al. Role of CT in the management of recurrent ovarian cancer. *AJR Am J Roentgenol.* 2004;182(2):393–398.
126. Prayer L, Kainz C, Kramer J, et al. CT and MR accuracy in the detection of tumor recurrence in patients treated for ovarian cancer. *J Comput Assist Tomogr.* 1993;17(4):626–632.
127. Sala E, Kataoka M, Pandit-Taskar N, et al. Recurrent ovarian cancer: use of contrast-enhanced CT and PET/CT to accurately localize tumor recurrence and to predict patients' survival. *Radiology.* 2010;257(1):125–134.
128. Pannu HK, Bristow RE, Montz FJ, et al. Multidetector CT of peritoneal carcinomatosis from ovarian cancer. *Radiographics.* 2003;23(3):687–701.
129. Sebastian S, Lee SI, Horowitz NS, et al. PET-CT vs. CT alone in ovarian cancer recurrence. *Abdom Imaging.* 2008;33(1):112–118.
130. Gu P, Pan LL, Wu SQ, et al. CA 125, PET alone, PET-CT, CT and MRI in diagnosing recurrent ovarian carcinoma: a systematic review and meta-analysis. *Eur J Radiol.* 2009;71(1):164–174.
131. Havrilesky LJ, Kulasingam SL, Matchar DB, et al. FDG-PET for management of cervical and ovarian cancer. *Gynecol Oncol.* 2005;97(1):183–191.
132. Fulham MJ, Carter J, Baldey A, et al. The impact of PET-CT in suspected recurrent ovarian cancer: a prospective multi-center study as part of the Australian PET Data Collection Project. *Gynecol Oncol.* 2009;112(3):462–468.
133. Mangili G, Picchio M, Sironi S, et al. Integrated PET/CT as a first-line re-staging modality in patients with suspected recurrence of ovarian cancer. *Eur J Nucl Med Mol Imaging.* 2007;34(5):658–666.
134. Simcock B, Neesham D, Quinn M, et al. The impact of PET/CT in the management of recurrent ovarian cancer. *Gynecol Oncol.* 2006;103(1):271–276.
135. Soussan M, Wartski M, Cherel P, et al. Impact of FDG PET-CT imaging on the decision making in the biologic suspicion of ovarian carcinoma recurrence. *Gynecol Oncol.* 2008;108(1):160–165.

CHAPTER 11

Biologic and Physical Principles of Radiation Oncology

Beth A. Erickson, Meena Bedi, Firas Mourtada, and Sunil J. Advani

RADIATION ONCOLOGY AS A SPECIALTY

Radiation oncology is a specialty focused primarily on the treatment of malignancies, although there are a number of benign diseases for which radiation can be used. Training in radiation oncology begins with internship, followed by 4 years of residency. Board certification follows, requiring successful completion of both written and oral exams. Residency training includes an in-depth understanding of the natural history and treatment of all malignancies, including the roles of surgery and systemic therapy in this era of multimodality therapies. An in-depth understanding of surgical procedures, pathology, and radiologic anatomy, as well as the efficacies and toxicities of systemic therapy, is required. Formal instruction in physics and radiobiology is also part of the residency training. Subspecialization with a specific practice focus on gynecologic or other cancers may follow. Only a few centers sponsor fellowships, which are usually focused on brachytherapy or other special procedures. Brachytherapy skills are especially important in the curative treatment of patients with gynecologic cancer. In addition, contemporary treatment of gynecologic malignances requires mastery of rapidly evolving technology for delivering external beam irradiation with techniques such as intensity-modulated radiation therapy (IMRT) and image-guided radiation therapy (IGRT). Radiation oncologists are important contributors to the management of individual patients and participate on multidisciplinary tumor boards. Having a knowledgeable and subspecialized radiation oncologist and gynecologic oncologist paired is a great benefit to all. In addition to radiation oncologists, other allied health professionals are integral to the radiation oncology department and treatment delivery. Radiation therapists are the individuals who actually operate the radiation equipment and deliver radiation treatments. Some of them will obtain a Bachelor of Science degree followed by a 13-month training program in radiation therapy. Alternatively, a 2-year associate degree in diagnostic radiology can be obtained followed by 1 to 2 years in radiation therapy training. Dosimetrists are primarily responsible for planning the radiation therapy or dosimetry prior to treatment delivery. Most of these individuals are former radiation therapists. An additional 1 to 2 years of training under a physicist and board-certified dosimetrist and additional years of practice are required to be eligible for board certification. Radiation physicists supervise and review the work of dosimetrists. Physicists are also integral to the introduction and maintenance of the rapidly evolving technology in radiation oncology departments. They are very involved with quality assurance and radiation safety. They can be Master's-level or PhD-level physicists and should be board certified.

INTRODUCTION TO RADIOBIOLOGY

Radiobiology is the study of how ionizing radiation (IR) interacts with biologic processes (1). The physics of IR delivery allows for dose deposition to be sculpted to targeted tumor tissues (2). However, for IR to reach tumors deep in the body, it passes through a number of normal tissues. Therefore, it is important for radiation oncologists to deliver the optimal dose of IR in order to eradicate the tumor while minimizing the risk of injury to surrounding normal structures (such as bladder and bowel) that are within the radiation field. As with most medical treatments, the clinical utility of IR is based on a therapeutic ratio, that is, IR's ability to destroy targeted tumor tissue is greater than its toxicity to normal tissues. The effect of the dose–response relationship of IR on cancerous and normal tissues can be depicted as a pair of sigmoidal curves (**Fig. 11.1**). At low doses of IR, there is little effect on tumor control but also a low risk for complications. With very high doses of IR, the likelihood for tumor control is high but there is also an unacceptably high rate of normal tissue complications. In between these two extremes, as the dose of IR increases, effects on both cancerous and normal tissues increase rapidly. A key feature in this part of the dose–response curve is that the tumor kill curve is shifted to the left of the normal tissue complication curve. Thus, for a given dose of IR, the probability of tumor kill is greater than the probability of normal tissue damage. It is in this dose range that the therapeutic ratio of IR can be exploited to cure cancer with an acceptable toxicity profile.

An understanding of radiobiology allows us to appreciate the rationale for how radiotherapy is used in gynecologic cancers and in the development of novel therapies. For example, radiosensitizing drugs increase tissue sensitivity to IR, which is graphically represented by shifting of the tissue response curves to the left (**Fig. 11.1**) (2,3). The implication of this is that a lower dose of IR is required in the presence of the radiosensitizer to achieve a similar degree of tissue response when compared to IR alone. Of clinical importance is that certain chemotherapies can preferentially radiosensitize tumors,

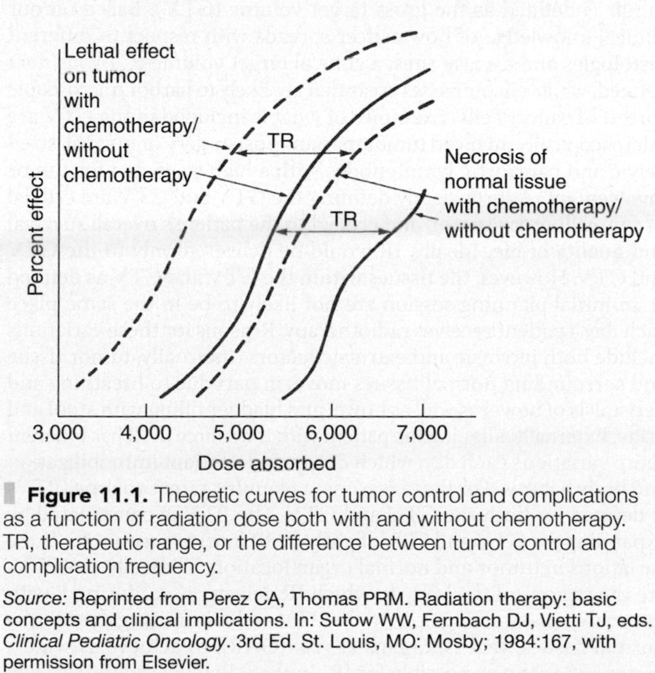

Figure 11.1. Theoretic curves for tumor control and complications as a function of radiation dose both with and without chemotherapy. TR, therapeutic range, or the difference between tumor control and complication frequency.

Source: Reprinted from Perez CA, Thomas PRM. Radiation therapy: basic concepts and clinical implications. In: Sutow WW, Fernbach DJ, Vietti TJ, eds. *Clinical Pediatric Oncology*. 3rd Ed. St. Louis, MO: Mosby; 1984:167, with permission from Elsevier.

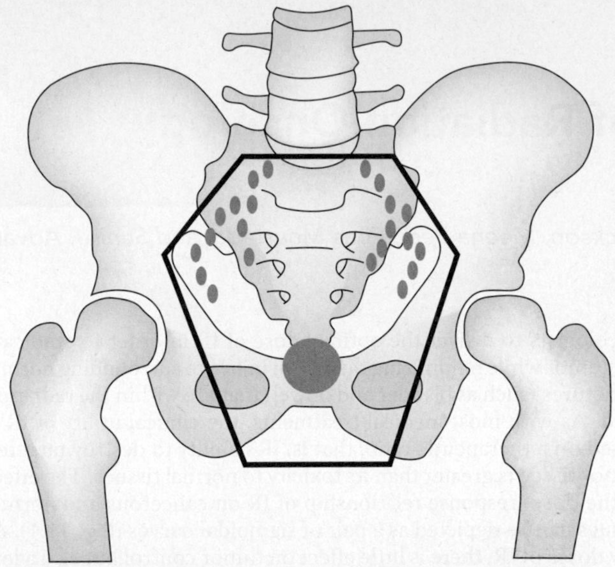

Figure 11.2. Target definition in radiation treatment planning for cervical cancer. The solid circle represents the GTV, which is the cervical primary defined both clinically and radiographically. The CTV is the pelvic lymph nodes, which have a high probability of at least microscopic involvement. The PTV is shown as the outer solid line and represents the margin added to the CTV to account for organ motion and daily setup error.

and therefore shift the tumor kill control curve farther to the left than the normal tissue complication curve (4). This widens the therapeutic ratio of IR, with improved tumor control and decreased normal tissue toxicity.

While defining tumor control and normal tissue response lies at the center of radiotherapy, in clinical practice radiotherapy is delivered to defined targeted volumes (**Fig. 11.2**) (5). These volumes are contoured (drawn) by a radiation oncologist based on both physical exam and radiographic imaging (computed tomography [CT], ultrasound, magnetic resonance imaging [MRI], and positron emission tomography [PET]). The area of clinical/radiographic evident tumor is defined as the gross target volume (GTV). Based on our clinical knowledge of how cancer spreads with respect to different histologies and disease sites, a clinical target volume (CTV) is next defined, which encompasses areas that are likely to harbor microscopic spread of cancer cells. Examples of what is included in the CTV are microscopically involved tumor margins postsurgery or normal-sized pelvic and paraaortic lymph nodes with a high suspicion for tumor involvement. Appropriately defining the GTV and CTV are crucial to controlling the tumor, and crucial to the patient's overall survival and quality of life. Ideally, IR would be delivered only to the GTV and CTV. However, the tissues within the GTV and CTV as defined at an initial planning session are not likely to be in the same place each day a patient receives radiotherapy. Reasons for these variations include both intrinsic and extrinsic factors. Internally, tumor tissue and surrounding normal tissues move, in part due to breathing and peristalsis of bowel as well as bowel and bladder filling with stool and urine. Externally, aligning the patient with the source of IR has inherent setup variations each day, which can include patient immobilization and body habitus. For these reasons, a planning target volume (PTV) is defined for both the GTV and CTV. The PTV is constructed by expanding the GTV and CTV slightly (≤10 mm) to account for these variations in tumor and normal organ location. Clinically, the PTVs are the regions of the body to which IR delivery is conformed, with the goal of maximizing dose to the PTV and minimizing dose to the normal tissues, that is, organs at risk (OAR), to achieve as wide a therapeutic ratio as possible for IR. In the following section, we will go over the radiobiologic principles that underlie the biologic basis of radiotherapy. An understanding of basic radiobiologic principles and of preclinical research allows for continued advancement and refinement of the use of radiotherapy in gynecologic cancers.

Interaction of IR with Tissue and DNA Damage

Radiotherapy utilizes IR, which is part of the electromagnetic spectrum of radiation (**Fig. 11.3**) (1). This spectrum is composed of a broad range of waves ranging from radio waves to visible light and IR. In the electromagnetic spectrum, the energy, wavelength, and frequency of waves are related by the following equations:

$$\text{Energy in electron volts (eV)} = h \times \nu$$
$$c = \lambda \times \nu$$

h = Planck's constant, 4.14×10^{-15} eV seconds
c = speed of light, 3×10^{8} m/sec
λ = wavelength (m)
ν = frequency of wave (1/sec)

Thus, the high-energy waves located in the IR part of the electromagnetic spectrum are of high frequencies and short wavelengths. This radiation is called ionizing, because it deposits a sufficient amount of energy into the tissue to eject electrons from atoms and generate ions. At the high energies of IR used in radiation oncology, IR interacts with atoms through the Compton process (**Fig. 11.4**). In the Compton process, IR ejects electrons from the outer shells of atoms. These liberated electrons mediate tissue responses to IR. The electrons can directly hit targets within the cell, resulting in damage, that is, direct effect. However, it is the indirect effect of the electrons that predominates. In the indirect effect, the ejected electrons first interact with intracellular water generating hydroxyl radicals. These hydroxyl radicals are highly reactive and damage many components of irradiated tissue through oxidative stress and DNA damage. It should be noted that the timescale of these interactions of IR with tissue is less than seconds, as ionizations and electrons are unstable and are quick to chemically react. However, the downstream effects of IR persist and result in both tumor cell death and normal tissue toxicity. Initial biochemical cellular responses occur within minutes to days following exposure to IR; tumor regression occurs in the ensuing weeks to months; and finally radiation-induced cancers manifest years following the initial exposure to IR.

IR-induced free radicals can cause all types of damage to cells. However, for conventional fractionated IR doses (<10 Gy/day), DNA is the major target of IR-generated free radicals. The evidence for DNA as one of the targets for radiation is substantial: (a) incorporation of

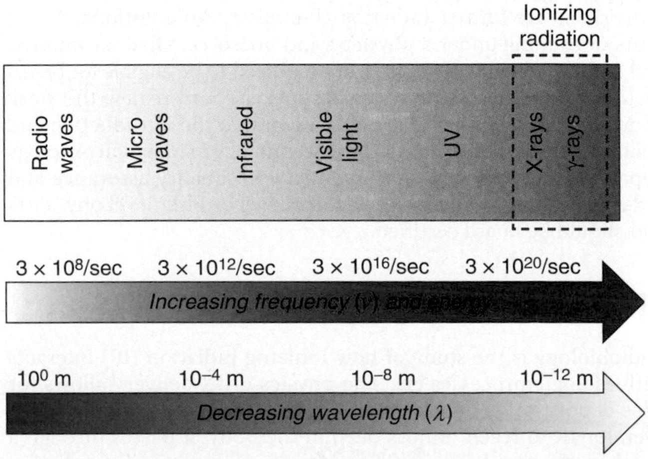

Figure 11.3. Electromagnetic spectrum. X-ray and γ-ray ionizing radiation are located in the short-wavelength, high-frequency, and high-energy part of the spectrum.

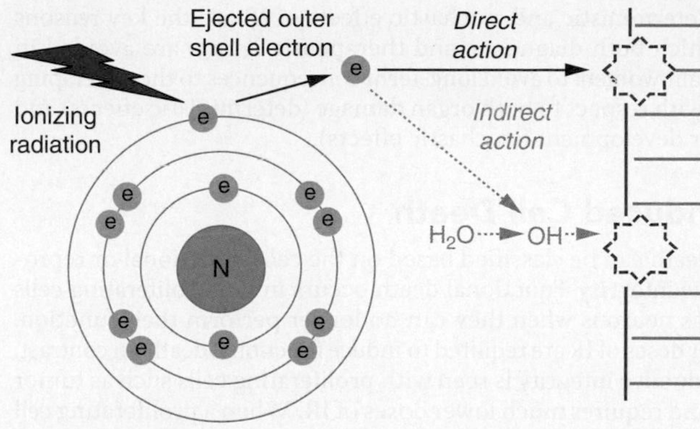

Figure 11.4. Interaction of ionizing radiation with matter. High-energy photons used in radiotherapy result in ejection of outer shell electrons through the Compton process. These ejected electrons then mediate tissue response to radiotherapy by causing oxidative and DNA damage. They can interact directly with DNA (Direct Action) or more likely through interaction with water to and generation of hydroxyl radicals (Indirect Action).

radioactive tritium into DNA causes cell death at greater rates than cytoplasmic tritium; (b) halogenated pyrimidines, when present in DNA, increase the cell's inherent radiosensitivity in an amount proportionate to the degree of incorporation; (c) a correlation between radiation, DNA double-stranded break repair, and clonogenic survival has also been observed; (d) the concentration of DNA in the nucleus correlates positively with radiosensitivity; (e) microirradiation techniques have shown the nucleus to be the most radiosensitive organelle (6–8). Free radical damage to DNA results in cross-links, base damage, single-strand breaks, and double-strand breaks (**Fig. 11.5**). These DNA double-strand breaks constitute the "lethal hit" of IR that is responsible for killing cells. IR-induced DNA double-strand breaks can be directly visualized using a single-cell gel electrophoresis assay, also known as neutral comet assay, in which DNA double-strand breaks appear as smaller fragments of DNA that move across the electrical field and form a "tail" to the "comet head" of the larger undamaged DNA strands (**Fig. 11.6**) (9). While highly valuable in laboratory studies on IR, neutral comet assays are limited to use in cell culture radiobiology basic science research. To assess IR DNA damage in tissue, DNA damage response signaling can be interrogated. IR-induced DNA double-strand breaks result in activation of signaling cascades to deal with the damage. One such response is phosphorylation of histone 2A on serine 139, termed γH2AX. Within the nucleus of irradiated cells, γH2AX foci formation can be quantitated (**Fig. 11.7**).

Once DNA double-strand breaks are created, cells attempt to fix the damage. Resolution of DNA double-strand breaks can result in chromosomal aberrations that are classified as lethal or nonlethal (**Fig. 11.8**) (10). These aberrations are readily apparent in chromosomes of people exposed to IR, by either direct visualization of metaphase chromosome spreads or more advanced techniques of fluorescence in situ hybridization (FISH), in which each chromosome is "painted" a different color. Nonlethal chromosomal aberrations include translocations and deletions. While genetic information is lost in these two cases, cells are still potentially capable of surviving and proliferating. Lethal resolutions of DNA double-strand breaks include dicentric and ring chromosome formation. The commonality of lethal resolutions is that an acentric DNA fragment is created such that during cell division at mitosis, one daughter cell loses an entire chromosome, resulting in cell death. Mechanistically, cells have evolved two major processes for repairing DNA double-strand breaks, nonhomologous end joining (NHEJ) and homologous recombination (HR) (11). NHEJ is the simplest type of repair mechanism. In NHEJ, two ends of broken DNA are processed and then ligated together. It does not utilize or require an undamaged DNA template. Therefore, NHEJ is error-prone and can result in mutations introduced in the genome through insertions or deletions of genetic material. In contrast to NHEJ, HR is an error-free DNA double-strand break repair

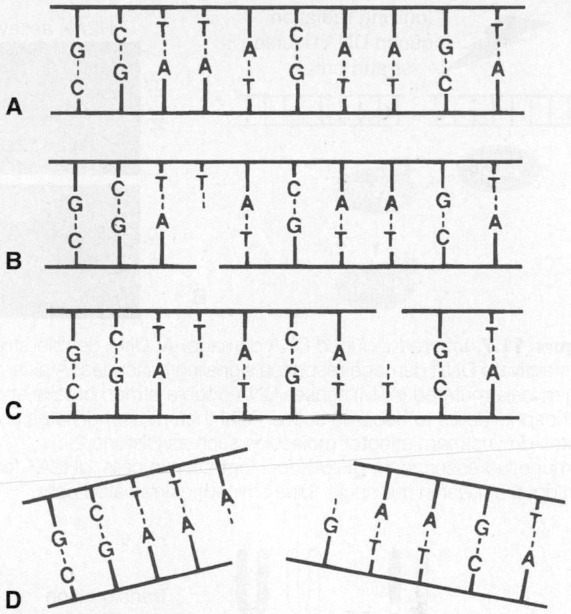

Figure 11.5. Diagrams of single- and double-strand DNA breaks caused by radiation. **A:** Two-dimensional representation of the normal DNA double helix. The base pairs carrying the genetic code are complementary (i.e., adenine pairs with thymine, guanine pairs with cytosine). **B:** A break in one strand is of little significance because it is readily repaired, using the opposite strand as a template. **C:** Breaks in both strands, if well separated, are repaired as independent breaks. **D:** If breaks occur in both strands and are directly opposite or separated by only a few base pairs, this may lead to a double-strand break, when the chromatin snaps into two pieces.

Source: Courtesy of Dr. John Ward. From Hall EJ. *Radiobiology for the Radiologist*. 4th Ed. Philadelphia, PA: JB Lippincott; 1994, with permission.

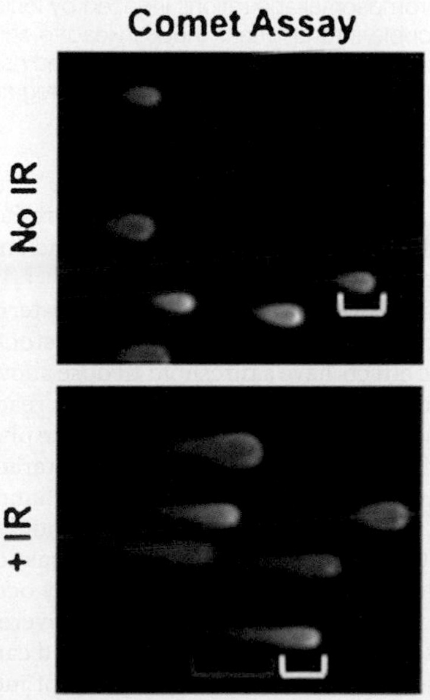

Figure 11.6. Measurement of infrared-induced DNA double-strand breaks. Cells were irradiated and analyzed by neutral comet assay. In nonirradiated cells, intact DNA appears as a nucleoid (comet head), yellow bracketed area. Following IR, DNA double-strand migrate in the electrical field and form a comet tail, red bracketed area.

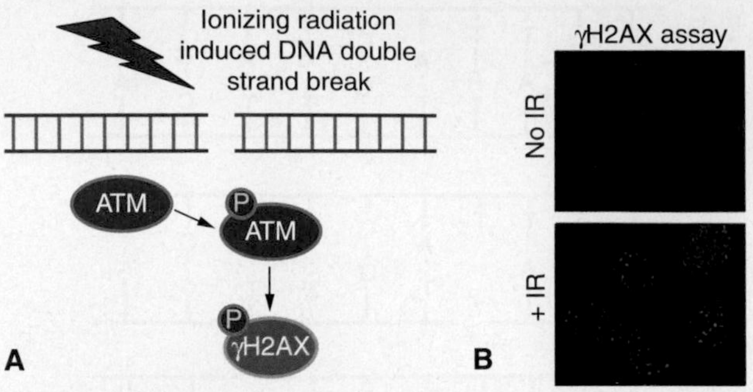

Figure 11.7. Infrared-induced DNA damage. **A:** DNA double-strand breaks activate DNA damage response signaling cascades. Ataxia telangiectasia mutated (ATM) senses DNA double-strand breaks and autophosphorylates to become active. ATM then phosphorylates and activates downstream effector molecules such as Histone 2.
B: Immunofluorescence for gH2AX foci formation in cells. gH2AX foci (green dots) appear in the nuclei (blue stained) of irradiated cells.

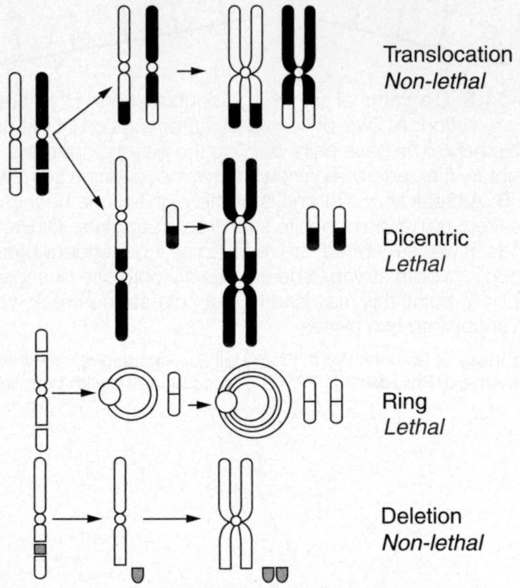

Figure 11.8. Chromosomal aberrations induced by ionizing radiation. IR results in DNA double-strand breaks that can lead to chromosomal aberrations. Chromosomal aberrations can be classified as lethal or nonlethal based on the ability of chromosomes to segregate to daughter cells in mitosis.

process. HR requires a DNA template, and therefore can only occur when cells are in the S/G_2 phase of the cell cycle and an undamaged template DNA strand exists.

Following repair of IR-induced damage, the long-term impacts on surviving tissue are classified as deterministic and stochastic effects (12). Deterministic effects have a threshold IR dose above which they are typically observed. Once the threshold dose is reached, further increases in IR dose result in increased severity of the phenotype. The classic example of an IR deterministic effect is cataract formation. At very low doses of IR to the lens of the eye, the chance of cataract formation is next to zero. However, once a threshold dose of IR is delivered, cataracts can develop. In contrast, stochastic effects have no threshold IR dose at which they can potentially occur and their severity does not increase as more IR dose is delivered. The most troubling stochastic effect of IR is radiation-induced carcinogenesis. In principle, any dose of IR is randomly capable of inducing DNA damage with resulting genetic mutations that lead to cancer development. Like deterministic effects, stochastic effects are more likely to occur as IR dose increases due to the probabilistic manner in which IR interacts with tissue. With these concerning late effects of IR, every effort is made to judiciously apply IR to a patient's situation.

The deterministic and stochastic effects of IR are the key reasons for which both diagnostic and therapeutic X-rays are avoided in pregnant women: to avoid long-term consequences to the developing fetus with respect to both organ damage (deterministic effects) and cancer development (stochastic effects).

IR-Induced Cell Death

Cell death can be classified based on the cells' functional or reproductive integrity. Functional death occurs in nonproliferating cells such as neurons when they can no longer perform their function. Higher doses of IR are required to induce functional death. In contrast, reproductive integrity is seen with proliferating cells such as tumor cells and requires much lower doses of IR. When a proliferating cell is irradiated, there are three possible outcomes: survival, senescence, or death. Survival requires repair of damaged DNA such as through NHEJ or HR described earlier. However, even after recovering from the initial irradiation, surviving cells may have mutations and damage resulting in deterministic or stochastic effects. While survival of irradiated cells in normal tissue is paramount, the ultimate goal of radiotherapy is the death of tumor cells, or, more precisely, preventing tumor cells from replicating. Replicative senescence can occur after DNA damage when cells permanently exit the cell cycle and do not replicate. Senescence is a mechanism of self-preservation for damaged cells, since cellular division would result in death. It should be noted that senescence is different than quiescence. Quiescence is a temporary exit from the cell cycle at G_1 into the G_0 phase. Cells in G_0 are not preparing to divide but can still perform their function. Under appropriate stimuli, cells in quiescence reenter the cell cycle and divide. While not a mechanism of cell death, if tumor cells undergo senescence, the patient is in essence cured of her tumor. For cell death, mechanisms following irradiation include apoptosis, autophagy, and mitotic catastrophe.

Apoptosis, or programmed cell death, follows an orderly cascade (13). It is an energy-dependent process that requires intact molecular biologic pathways. Apoptosis can be initiated by two distinct mechanisms: (a) extrinsic pathway, where the apoptotic stimulus occurs extracellularly, or (b) intrinsic pathway, where the cascade of events is mediated by intracellular events (**Fig. 11.9**). Mechanistically, apoptosis is mediated by caspases that are expressed as inactive precursors (procaspases). Upon apoptotic stimuli, proteolytic cleavage of procaspases results in active caspases, which then cleave downstream effector proteins. The extrinsic pathway begins by binding of a specific ligand such as Fas-L or tumor necrosis factor (TNF) to a membrane death receptor. The intrinsic pathway, on the other hand, requires disruption of the mitochondrial membrane and release of cytochrome c from the mitochondria to the cytoplasm. While the upstream activation of apoptosis through extrinsic or intrinsic pathways differs, both pathways converge on cleaving and activating procaspase 3. A number of methods have been developed to measure apoptosis including caspase cleavage, DNA fragmentation, and cellular membrane changes. If apoptosis occurs, it is evident within hours of IR by activation of caspases and loss of cell membrane polarity. However, while conventional fractionated radiotherapy does not induce significant apoptosis in solid tumors, recent preclinical evidence suggests that larger single fractions of radiotherapy ($>$10 Gy) can induce apoptosis in irradiated endothelial cells (14,15). Given the location of gynecologic cancers, such large fractions of IR have not typically been employed. However, with advances in brachytherapy planning and delivery, such higher doses may provide a way to target the tumor vasculature. Autophagy occurs during nutrient deprivation and metabolic stress (16). The goal of autophagy is catabolism of cellular structures to provide a source of nutrients to cells and help them survive periods of stress. Its role in IR-induced death is under investigation.

Mitotic catastrophe is the predominant mechanism of cell death induced by IR (17). In mitotic catastrophe, cells die as a result of trying to replicate. As mentioned above, IR-induced DNA double-strand breaks results in chromosome and chromatid aberrations. If not

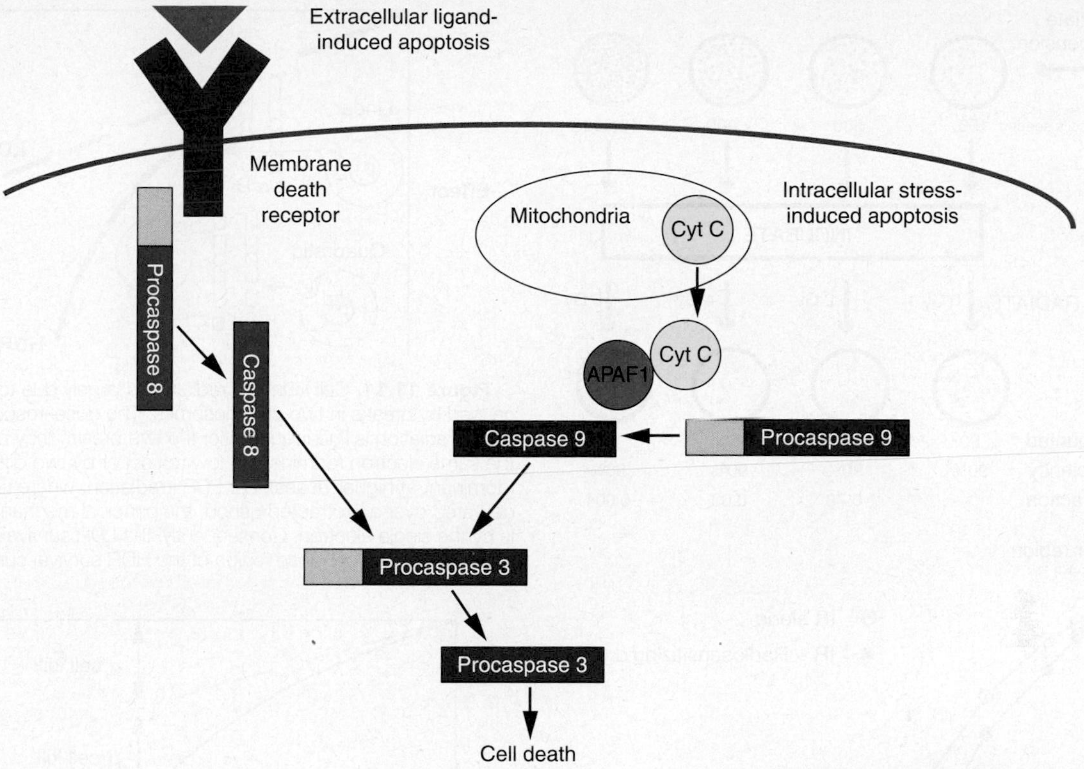

Figure 11.9. Apoptotic pathways of cell death. In the extrinsic pathway, death receptor binding of ligand activates initiator caspase 8. In the intrinsic pathways, intracellular stress results in mitochondrial release of cytochrome C (cyt C), which binds to apoptotic protease activating factor 1 (APAF1) to activate initiator caspase 9. Both pathways converge on activating effector caspases, i.e., caspase 3, which result in apoptotic cell death.

dividing, the full complement of genetic material remains within the cell. However, when cells pass through mitosis and divide into two daughter cells, certain chromosome and chromatid aberrations (e.g., ring and dicentric chromosomes) do not result in equal segregation of the genetic material to the two daughter cells. In addition, DNA double-strand breaks result in increasing genomic instability of dividing cells. Therefore, cells may replicate a few times, after which the loss of increasing genetic material results in cell death. In contrast to the orderly process of apoptosis, mitotic catastrophe is energy-independent and results in necrosis and inflammation. Since it requires cells to divide, mitotic catastrophe is not evident as quickly as apoptosis.

Cell Survival Curves and Tumor Control Probability

The gold standard technique used to measure IR-induced cell kill is the clonogenic assay (**Fig. 11.10**) (18). The clonogenic assay is particularly useful for measuring cell death through mitotic catastrophe. In principle, it measures the reproductive ability of individual cells following different doses of IR. Cells are seeded at low density and allowed to replicate for 10 to 14 days, over which time each cell forms a colony of >50 daughter cells. As cells undergo mitotic catastrophe they stop dividing and do not form a colony of >50 daughter cells. Since it is such a crucial technique for measuring sensitivity of cells to IR, we will review the technique in some detail. It first involves creating a suspension containing the target population of cells at a known concentration. An aliquot with a known number of cells is plated on growth media and allowed to incubate. As one would expect, not all the cells successfully form a colony, and so plating efficiency must be calculated by dividing the number of formed colonies by the starting number of cells. The experiment is repeated, but after plating and before incubation, the Petri dish is irradiated. The number of colonies formed is divided by the starting number of cells, which is then divided by plating efficiency to yield the ratio of surviving cells. This experiment is repeated over a range of doses of radiation and under various conditions to yield a cell survival curve. An important feature of the cell survival curve is that it uses a logarithmic scale on the *y*-axis. This correlates with mathematical modeling of cell survival as a function of radiation dose.

The simplest model one can envision for the sterilization of cancer cells by radiation in a given volume is the log cell kill model. A typical course of radiation therapy is given in 10 to 40 fractions administered over 2 to 8 weeks. Each fraction kills a fixed percentage of cells. One term that can be used for this is D_{10}, the dose that kills 90% of the cells. If there are 100 cells and a D_{10} dose is administered, 10 viable cells remain. Consider a tumor 1 g in size, which has 10^9 cells. If the D_{10} for this tumor is 3 Gy, how many fractions are required for a 90% chance of sterilization? The log cell kill model gets slightly more complicated when dealing in fractions, as 1/10 of a viable cell does not exist. Instead, 0.1 cells represent a 10% chance that a viable cell will exist at the end of therapy. Therefore, a tumor with 10^9 cells requires 10 decades of cell kill for a 90% chance of tumor control. Three Gy $\times$ 10 fractions = 30 Gy total dose. This model makes a number of invalid assumptions such as D_{10} remaining constant throughout the course of radiation, but highlights the logarithmic nature of fractionated radiation kill. Instead of D_{10}, D_0 is the more commonly used term in radiobiology and is based on natural logarithm, where base e = 2.72. D_0 is the dose of radiation where 1/e (37%) cells survive or 63% (1 − 1/e) of cells are killed. D_0 is related to D_{10} by the following formula: $D_{10} = 2.3 \times D_0$. For most tumors, the D_0 is estimated to be 1 to 2 Gy, and in fractionated external beam radiation we typically deliver 1.8 or 2 Gy with each fraction.

Two theoretical experimental cell survival curves are shown in **Figure 11.11** under either LDR (low-dose-rate) or HDR (high-dose-rate) radiation conditions. The curve for LDR is best fit by a straight line, while the HDR curve is shown to have two components, an earlier linear component mirroring the LDR curve followed by a quadratic component. At higher doses of radiation, the HDR curve always has a higher proportion of cell kill than the LDR curve for any given dose.

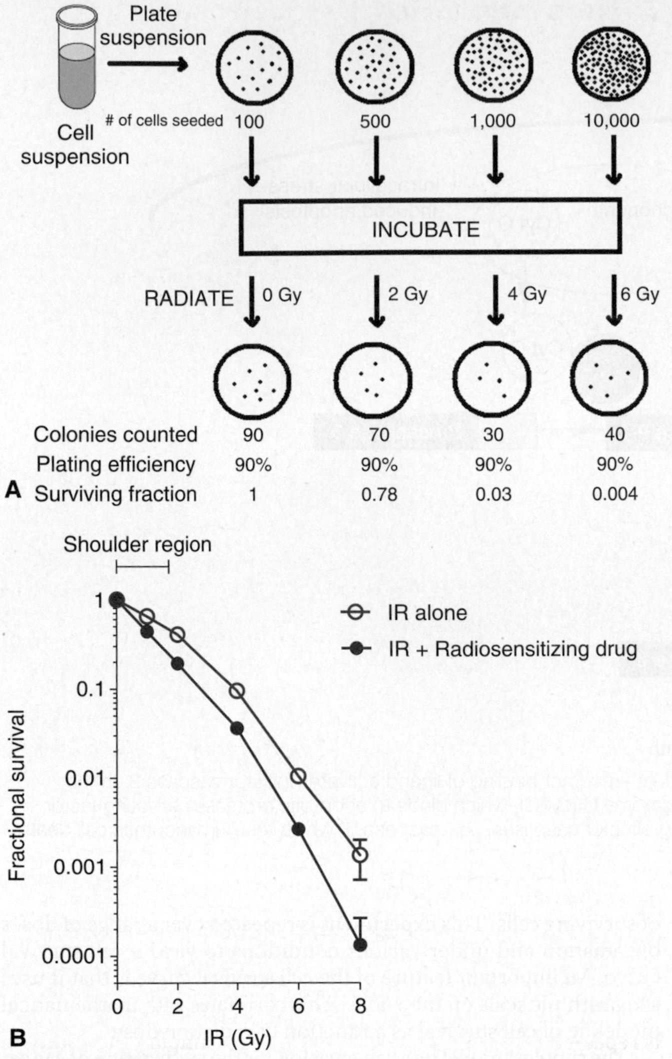

Figure 11.10. Clonogenic survival curves. Surviving fraction of irradiated cells. **A:** Cell culture technique used for clonogenic assays. A cell suspension of a known concentration of cells is used to seed differing number of cells in cell culture dishes. The cells are allowed to settle and are then irradiated. Viable cells will replicate and form colonies visible to the naked eye. The plating efficiency is calculated in the nonirradiated condition and used to normalize the surviving fraction of irradiated cells. **B:** The surviving fraction is then plotted logarithmically on the *y*-axis and an IR dose is plotted linearly on the *x*-axis (*blue line*). Red line shows decreased survival of cells that were treated with a radiosensitizer prior to irradiation.

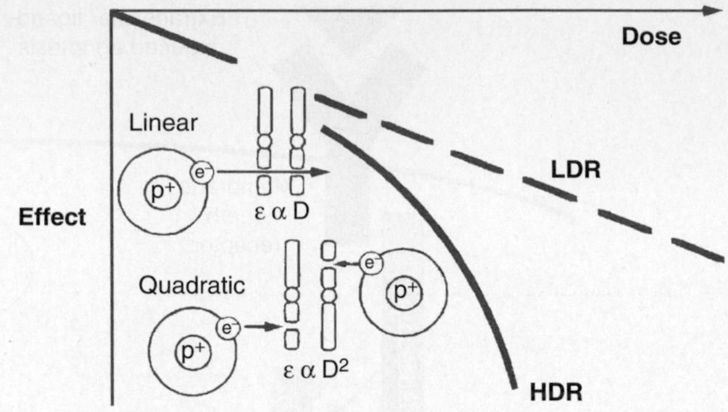

Figure 11.11. Cell killing by radiation is largely due to aberrations caused by breaks in two chromosomes. The dose–response curve for HDR irradiation is linear quadratic: the two breaks may be caused by the same electron (dominant at low doses) or by two different electrons (dominant at higher doses). For LDR irradiation, where radiation is delivered over a protracted period, the principal mechanism of cell killing is by the single electron. Consequently, the LDR survival curve is an extension of the low-dose region of the HDR survival curve.

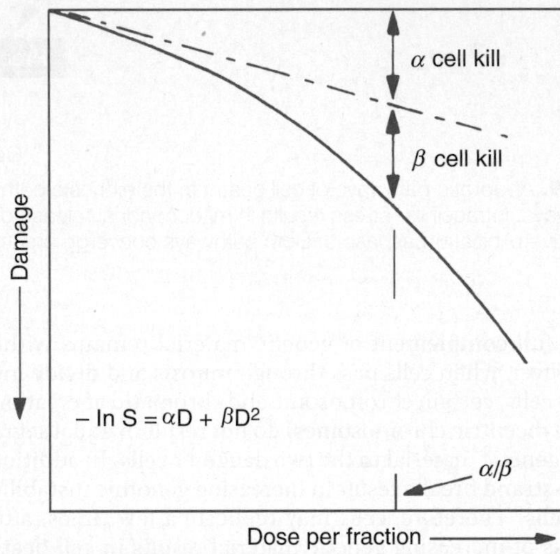

Figure 11.12. At a dose equal to the α/β ratio, the log cell kill due to the α process (nonreparable) is equal to that due to the β process (reparable injury): α/β is thus a measure of how soon the survival curve begins to bend over significantly.

Source: Reprinted from Fowler JR. Fractionation and therapeutic gain. In: Steel GG, Adams GE, Peckham MJ, eds. *Biologic Basis of Radiotherapy*. Amsterdam, The Netherlands: Elsevier Science; 1983:181–194, with permission from Elsevier.

The rate at which radiation is delivered causes dramatic differences in the shape of the cell survival curve. This is best described by considering the linear quadratic model with DNA as the lethal target. In the linear quadratic model:

$$\text{Surviving fraction} = e^{-\alpha D - \beta D2}$$

α: constant for proportion of cell survival due to linear component

β: constant for proportion of cell survival due to quadratic component

D: dose of IR

The linear component is due to a single ejected electron causing both DSBs. The important point is that the degree of the linear component of cell kill, also known as α kill, is proportional to D since only one photon/electron is involved. The linear quadratic model also shows two chromosomal breaks, the result of two separate ejected Compton electrons by radiation. Cell kill accounted for by the quadratic portion, or β kill, is proportional to D^2 because two photons/electrons are involved. Looking at the HDR curve at low doses of radiation, there is very little β kill; however, at higher doses, the β component increases exponentially because of D^2. Under LDR conditions, the β component is absent, leaving only α kill. This is best explained by the idea that β kill involves damage to one chromosome and so is more easily repaired, provided that the radiation dose rate and rate of DSB formation are not significantly greater than the cell's repair capacity. The linear quadratic formula was used to generate **Figure 11.12**. The dashed line represents the α component and is generated by extrapolating the initial slope of the curve to higher doses of radiation. The point at which the α and β kill are equal is shown, and the dose at which this occurs is called the α/β ratio. It is worth noting that the α/β ratio is a bit of a misnomer, as ratios typically are unitless values. However, α/β has the units of Gy. The α/β ratio for early side effects and tumor tissue is thought to be higher, approximately 10 Gy, than for late side effects, which is estimated to be 3 Gy.

Of clinical relevance is the α/β ratio, which helps to calculate biologically effective doses (BED). It is clear from **Figure 11.4** that both the total dose of radiation and the speed at which it is delivered can produce very different outcomes. The same holds true for fractionated courses of radiation. For example, 16 Gy delivered in a single treatment, as is the case for radiosurgery, can sterilize a small cancerous tumor of cancer cells. However, the same treatment delivered over 8 days would be clinically insignificant. **Figure 11.9** shows theoretical cell survival curves for early and late reactions under two separate experimental conditions, single fraction and multifraction regimens. A formula that normalizes a biologic endpoint under various dose-fractionation schemes is necessary (5). The α/β ratio from the linear quadratic equation has enabled the prediction of various biologic endpoints with different fractionation schemes, and is given by the following equation:

$$BED = nd(1 + d/(\alpha/\beta))$$

BED = biologically effective dose
n = number of fractions
d = dose per fraction
α/β = dose where the α component of cell kill equals the β component

BED calculations allow for comparison of two different dose-fractionation schemes in terms of tumor control/acute toxicity if α/β is 3, or late tissue complications when α/β is set to 10. An extension of this BED calculation is the ability to calculate the total dose delivered in 2 Gy fractions. This is particularly useful in gynecologic oncology patients where the radiation dose is delivered as both external beam radiotherapy and brachytherapy. A measure of the total dose delivered, if delivered as 2 Gy fractions, can be calculated using the EQD2 formula:

$$EQD2 = (BED_{EBRT} + BED_{BT})/(1 + 2/\alpha/\beta)$$

BED_{EBRT}: External beam contribution to BED
BED_{BT}: Brachytherapy contribution BED

EQD2 calculations are a tool to allow for meaningful comparisons of different IR fractionation schemes. In principle, if the EQD2 is the same for two different IR regimens, they should yield similar patient outcomes.

While these mathematical models of radiation cell kill all have their limitations, they do provide a foundation for how radiation oncologists approach the total dose delivered and the fraction size used. Moreover, the basic concepts of radiation log kill are reflected in the administered treatments. Consider, for example, curative therapy for cervical cancer. While the CTV has a high likelihood of harboring malignancy, it does not have clinically evident disease. For cervical cancer, this could be normal-sized pelvic and possibly paraaortic lymph nodes or an area of positive margin. The CTV typically requires a lower dose of radiation for control, ranging from 45 to 54 Gy, as there are potentially fewer cancer cells that to eradicate. In contrast, the GTV with its known bulky disease requires a higher dose of radiation, such as 80 to 90 Gy, to sterilize the larger number of tumor cells. Attaining such doses of radiation while respecting normal tissue tolerance is not feasible with EBRT alone and therefore brachytherapy is required. In contrast, if a patient undergoes a hysterectomy in which bulk tumor is removed, then there is no GTV, and brachytherapy is often not needed because dose to the CTV can be safely administered by external beam radiation therapy or lower doses of brachytherapy alone.

Factors Influencing Tissue Sensitivity to Radiation Therapy

The above discussion provides the general biologic basis of how IR interacts with cells. However, the clinical utility of radiation therapy is dependent on tumor and normal tissue characteristics that play a pivotal role in how radiotherapy is delivered, and its efficacy. There are four classic factors that have been termed the "4 R's" of radiobiology: (1) Repair, (2) Repopulation, (3) Reassortment, and (4) Reoxygenation. These "4 R's" provide a rationale and framework for the fundamental basis of using fractionated radiotherapy.

Repair

With DNA being the critical target, radiation therapy needs to selectively damage the DNA of tumor cells yet spare the surrounding normal tissues. The simplest solution would be to deposit IR dose to tumor cells and not to normal tissues. Current technology using IMRT and brachytherapy techniques makes it possible for IR doses to better conform to tumors and spare the critical normal tissues in close proximity. Radiobiologically, tumor and normal tissue often have a differential capacity for DNA damage repair that can be exploited to widen the therapeutic ratio of IR. In survival curves of irradiated cells, a "shoulder" region is apparent at lower doses. Following IR, cells attempt to repair the DNA damage. At high doses, the repair processes are overwhelmed and cell death occurs in an exponential manner. However, at lower doses, cells are able to repair the DNA damage if sufficient time is given prior to the delivery of another dose of IR. Therefore, this "shoulder" region of the survival curve represents sublethal damage repair (19). The dose range of IR within the shoulder region is often within the clinically relevant doses of D_0. A consequence of genomic instability within cancer cells is decreased DNA damage repair capacity compared to normal tissue. Graphically, the "shoulder" region of irradiation survival curves is wider in noncancerous cells compared to cancer cells (**Fig. 11.13**). Therefore, instead of delivering one large dose of IR, the total IR dose is split into smaller doses that are delivered over weeks. Note that by breaking up the radiotherapy in fractions, the shoulder of the cell survival curve is repeated and by doing this, we are able to amplify the ability of normal tissue to repair and tolerate IR damage while tumor cells are preferentially killed. Also of importance is that sublethal DNA damage repair takes hours to occur and provides a rationale for delivering fractionated external beam radiotherapy once daily, to allow time for normal tissues to recover from radiation-induced DNA damage.

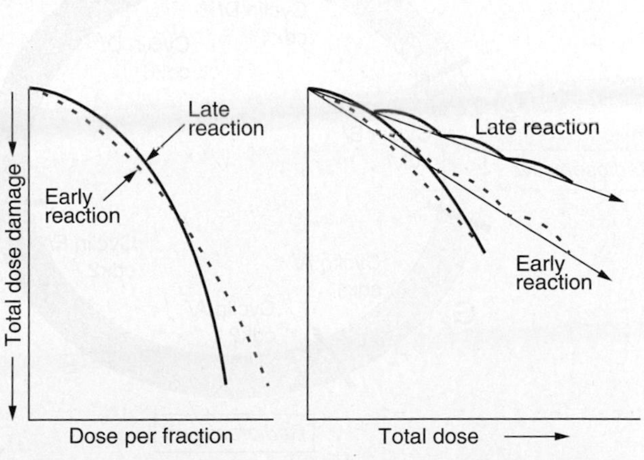

Figure 11.13. Difference in cell survival curves for acute and late radiation effects with single or multifractionated doses of irradiation.

Source: Reprinted from Fowler JF. Fractionation and therapeutic gain. In: Steel GG, Adams GE, Peckham MT, eds. *Biologic Basis of Radiotherapy*. Amsterdam, The Netherlands: Elsevier Science; 1983:181, with permission from Elsevier.

Repopulation

While fractionating IR allows for sublethal damage repair in normal tissue, it needs to be balanced against the concept of tumor repopulation. Following tumor irradiation, a phenomenon of accelerated repopulation has been demonstrated to occur (20,21). In accelerated repopulation, stress responses and death of a proportion of the tumor result in surviving tumor cells proliferating more rapidly. To combat this, the overall time in which the total radiotherapy package (external beam and brachytherapy) is delivered to patients should be minimized. Avoidance of treatment breaks due to acute radiotherapy/chemotherapy side effects to the normal tissues (bowel, bladder, bone marrow) is paramount, as treatment breaks may compromise patient outcomes by allowing cancerous cells to proliferate, negating the goals of therapy. Clinical data support such a concept in patients with cervical cancer, where an increase in overall radiotherapy treatment time has been shown to negatively affect outcomes.

Reassortment

Interestingly, intrinsic sensitivity to IR varies with the cell cycle. The cell cycle is an orderly progression resulting in DNA replication and division into two daughter cells (**Fig. 11.14**) (22,23). S phase stands for "synthesis" and is where DNA replication occurs. M phase stands for "mitosis" and is when cellular division occurs to create two daughter cells. In between are the G_1 and G_2 phases, standing for "gap 1" and "gap 2." Late S phase tends to be the most radioresistant phase of the cell cycle because the DNA repair machinery for replication can also repair radiation damage. In contrast, the M phase is also the most radiosensitive phase of the cell cycle because once the cell enters into M phase, it will attempt to divide without arresting. Therefore, any DNA damage caused in M phase is likely to be passed along to the daughter cells and may be fatal. This is another important reason why rapidly dividing cells such as cancer cells are radiosensitive as opposed to slower proliferating normal tissue. While M phase is the most radiosensitive it is also unfortunately the portion of the cell cycle in which cells spend the least amount of time. Approximately 15% of cycling tumor cells are in G_2/M at a given moment. Therefore, the majority of tumor cells are in a relatively radioresistant phase of the cell cycle on any given day radiation is delivered. Fractionating and delivering IR over multiple days takes advantage of the fact that different populations of the tumor will be in G_2/M during each day's treatment and will have increased sensitivity to IR. In addition, IR-induced DNA damage results in cell cycle checkpoints, and in particular the G_2/M checkpoint. Checkpoints take cells temporarily out of the cell cycle so they can assess and respond to their damage. IR can synchronize tumor cells so that the following day a greater fraction will be in the radiosensitive G_2/M phase of the cell cycle.

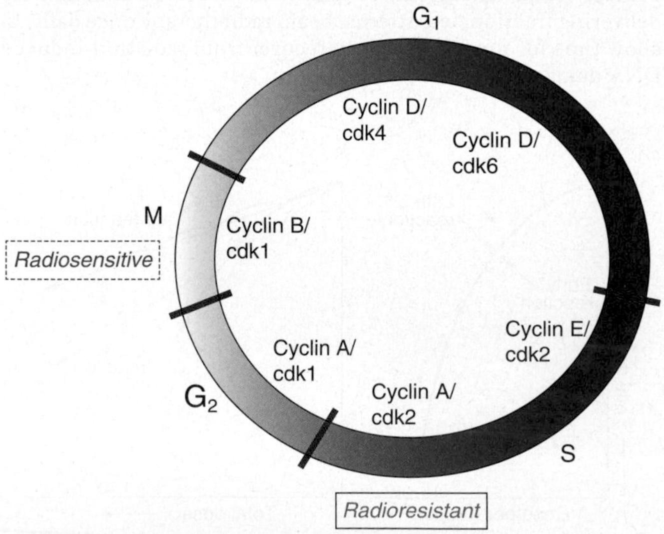

Figure 11.14. Cell cycle and variation in radiosensitivity. As cells replicate they pass through phases of the cell cycle where a unique cyclin and cyclin-dependent kinase (cdk) heterodimer is formed. Each cyclin/cdk heterodimer phosphorylates and activates a unique set of proteins required for completion of that phase. DNA synthesis occurs in S phase, which is the most radioresistant phase. Cell division occurs in M phase, which is the most radiosensitive phase of the cell cycle.

Reoxygenation

Oxygen within tumor cells alters sensitivity to radiation (24,25). Under hypoxic conditions, cells are relatively resistant to radiation compared to oxygenated tumors. The oxygen enhancement ratio (OER) for radiation is approximately 3, which implies the dose of radiation required under hypoxic conditions is three times that needed under aerated conditions to create a similar level of cell kill. Oxygen is known to chemically modify radiation-induced DNA damage by creating a DNA–peroxide bond, thereby making it very difficult to repair by the cell. This is known as the oxygen fixation hypothesis (26). Therefore, under hypoxic conditions, one would expect DNA damage repair to be more effective, and higher dose would therefore be required to kill cells.

Tumor hypoxia can be categorized as either acute or chronic. Acute hypoxia is perfusion limited and occurs due to temporary closures of vasculature secondary to temporary vasospasms and malformed tumor blood vessels. As with tumor reassortment, areas of acute hypoxia within the tumor will vary from day to day, as do the cells in G_2/M. Areas of the tumor that were acutely hypoxic on a given day may have increased blood flow and oxygen delivery on subsequent days of radiation. In contrast to the perfusion limits of acute hypoxia, chronic hypoxia is defined as diffusion limited and occurs as tumor growth outstrips its vasculature. In tissue, oxygen can diffuse a distance of 70 to 100 µm from blood vessels. Therefore, tumor cells that are located further from the vasculature have decreased oxygen delivery and are relatively resistant to IR.

Combining Radiotherapy with Systemic Therapies

For locally advanced cancers, patient outcomes are improved when radiotherapy is combined with chemotherapy (2–4). Rationales for delivery of chemotherapy concurrently with radiotherapy are: (1) it allows delivery of the entire treatment package in a more compact time frame; (2) radiotherapy and chemotherapy kill cancer cells by different mechanisms, making it more difficult for resistant tumor clones to survive; (3) certain chemotherapy drugs sensitize tumor cells to IR-mediated DNA damage and cell death. Cytotoxic chemotherapies such as cisplatin, 5-fluorouracil (5-FU), and paclitaxel function as radiosensitizers and have been used in patients with locally advanced cervical cancer to improve tumor control. As the molecular events that drive cancers are elucidated, more targeted approaches to radiosensitization are being evaluated (27–29). An example of this is the epidermal growth factor receptor (EGFR). EGFR is a member of the ErbB family of cell surface receptors. Certain tumors overexpress EGFR. Binding of EGFR to its ligand results in intracellular signaling promoting tumor growth and resistance to radiotherapy. EGFR has been pharmacologically targeted with antibodies (cetuximab) and small molecule inhibitors (erlotinib, gefitinib). Preclinical research has shown that EGFR inhibition radiosensitizes tumor cells.

Another radiosensitization strategy moves away from targeting tumor cells and instead targets the tumor vasculature (30,31). Tumor angiogenesis is crucial to the continued growth of tumors as they grow larger than 70 to 100 µm. Tumor vessel growth relies on vascular endothelial growth factors (VEGFs). Bevacizumab is a monoclonal antibody that binds VEGF-A, which then prevents VEGF-A from binding to VEGF receptors located on endothelial cells. Preclinical data suggest that treating tumors with bevacizumab can also radiosensitize them. Bevacizumab can potentially interact with IR in two distinct fashions. First, via the decrease in VEGF receptor signaling endothelial cells are more likely to be killed by IR (32). Second, treating tumors with bevacizumab results in "renormalization" of the tumor vasculature (30). Tumor vasculature is more chaotically organized than blood vessels in normal tissue due to an imbalance of pro- and antiangiogenesis factors. This results in increased permeability and interstitial pressure within tumors and has the untoward consequence of decreasing both chemotherapy and oxygen delivery to tumor cells. Bevacizumab helps to restore the balance of pro- and antiangiogenesis factors. By increasing cytotoxic chemotherapy and oxygen delivery to tumors, bevacizumab can also increase the sensitivity of tumor cells to IR-mediated cell death.

Finally, immunotherapy is emerging as a paradigm-shifting approach to cancer therapy that can be combined with radiotherapy (31,33,34). While the concept is not new, elucidation of mechanisms involved in immune tolerance of tumor growth has resulted in the discovery of new pharmacologic targets. As cancers evolve they develop strategies to hide from the immune system through immune checkpoints that downregulate immune responses. Two checkpoint inhibitors have begun to show clinical efficacy. Ipilimumab is an antibody against cytotoxic T-lymphocyte antigen 4 (CTLA-4). Nivolumab and pembrolizumab are antibodies against programmed cell death protein-1 (PD-1). While antibodies to CTLA-4 and PD-1 reverse tumor immune suppression, they do so by distinct nonoverlapping mechanisms. Interestingly, IR has also been shown to evoke a tumor immune response that results in an abscopal effect. In preclinical animal models that harbor multiple tumors, localized treatment of a single tumor with IR can result in tumor shrinkage in the other nonirradiated tumors (i.e., abscopal effect). More recently, trials in cancer patients with metastatic disease suggest that radiotherapy to a single tumor site, in combination with activation of the immune system by either interleukin (IL)-2 or checkpoint inhibitors, can result in abscopal responses (35,36). The abscopal effect is a phenomenon observed in metastatic cancer patients, where treating only a single metastasis with focal radiotherapy also results in distant nontreated tumors shrinking. While these data are early, they do suggest a novel and important role for radiotherapy in modulating tumor immune responses in patients that are distinct from IR's conventional role of being a local therapy that kills cancer cells by inducing DNA damage. As these and other targeted approaches are translated from the laboratory to clinical testing, the development of more personalized approaches to using radiotherapy in cancer patients will improve tumor control and decrease toxicity to normal tissue.

INTRODUCTION TO RADIATION PHYSICS

Radiation physics is the study of the interaction of radiation with matter. In the treatment of patients with radiation, this matter is either tumor tissue or normal tissues such as the skin, the internal organs, or the supporting tissues and structures.

Units Used in Radiation and Radiation Therapy

Radiation is a term that refers to "energy in transit." In a general sense, it can be categorized as ionizing or nonionizing (such as the visible light). IR is used in radiation therapy, a process where neutral atoms acquire a positive or a negative charge. This process can take numerous forms. The most common forms of IR used in radiation therapy are X-rays, γ-rays, neutrons (electromagnetic radiation), electrons, and protons (particulate radiation). X-rays and γ-rays are also known as photons or packets of energy and are used to treat most body sites where radiation is deemed efficacious. Other particles or forms of radiation, such as protons, neutrons, and heavier α particles, are less commonly used in radiation therapy except in select clinical situations. Protons, other heavy charged particles, and neutrons have a higher linear energy transfer coefficient when compared to high-energy photons and therefore are more efficient at transferring or depositing their energy in tissue. Protons are used increasingly in the treatment of prostate cancers, choroidal melanomas, skull base and paraspinal tumors, and pediatric tumors. Neutrons have been used for salivary gland tumors, sarcomas, and prostate cancers. Protons are positively charged particles that can be accelerated in an electric field to high energies. The primary characteristic of a proton beam is its Bragg peak. The Bragg peak describes the depth at which the majority of a proton's energy is deposited. Prior to the depth of the Bragg peak, only a very small amount of the proton energy is deposited. The Bragg peak depth is determined by the energy of the incident protons, and covers only very small width of tissue at that depth. In order to cover more tissue, the energy of the incoming proton beam is varied. The net dose deposition results in a low entrance dose and a finely controlled width of treatment dose at depth. This makes proton treatments an excellent choice for the treatment of tumors adjacent to critical structures. Neutrons are relatively massive uncharged particles that can be generated by cyclotrons. Poor treatment geometry and dose distributions have limited the enthusiasm for neutron beam therapy (37).

X-rays and γ-rays are forms of electromagnetic radiation, similar to visible light, but with a much smaller wavelength, that is, greater energy. The only difference between X-rays and γ-rays is their respective origins. X-rays are derived from interactions in the atom that are outside the nucleus, typically by bombardment of the atom or target with high-speed electrons. This is the source of radiation produced by most modern radiotherapy treatment machines known as linear accelerators or LINACS. Their name derives from acceleration of these electrons. γ-Rays arise from a process within the nucleus of the atom called radioactive decay, which occurs in brachytherapy sources and cobalt (^{60}Co) teletherapy treatment machines. This type of electromagnetic radiation can penetrate several millimeters to centimeters of normal tissue in close proximity to tumors or tissues at risk. There is increased penetration as the energy of the gamma rays is increased. The X-rays produced by LINACs are much more penetrating (due to their high energy) than ^{60}Co gamma rays and are used to treat tumors or tissues at a distance from the LINAC, such as deep within the pelvis or abdomen.

Electrons are forms of particulate radiation and considered to be small (compared to the nucleus), negatively charged particles. Because of their inherent charge, these particles interact more strongly with the atoms found in tissue. Electrons will usually only penetrate a few millimeters to centimeters in tissue. Similar to photons, the higher the energy of the electron, the farther it will penetrate into the tissue. Electrons are used to treat tumors or tissues close to the skin surface such as superficial inguinal nodes and tumors of the skin, including vulvar cancers.

Regarding photon interactions with tissue, the dominant process at energies used in radiation therapy is termed the Compton effect (**Fig. 11.15**). The probability that a photon will interact with a target atom is inversely proportional to the energy of the incident

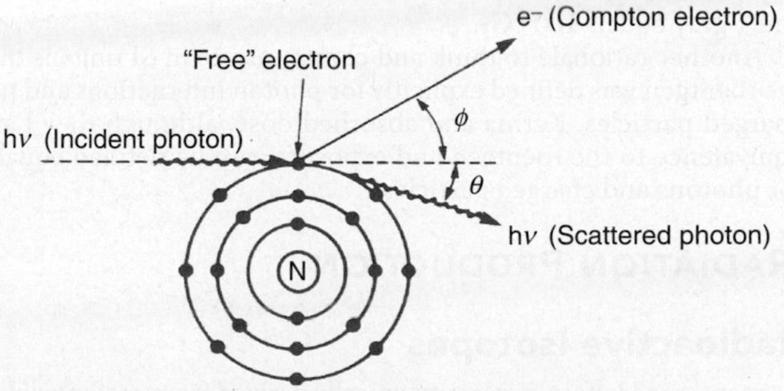

Figure 11.15. Schematic drawing illustrating the process of the Compton effect. The incident photon interacts with one of the atom's outer electrons, and the energy is shared between the ejected electron and a scattered photon.

Source: From Purdy JA. Principles of radiologic physics, dosimetry, and treatment planning. In: Perez CA, Brady LW, eds. *Principles and Practice of Radiation Oncology*. 3rd Ed. Philadelphia, PA: Lippincott-Raven Publishers; 1998, with permission.

TABLE 11.1. SI Units for Radiation Therapy

Quantity	SI Unit (Special Name)	Non-SI Unit	Conversion Factor
Exposure	C kg^{-1}	roentgen (R)	1 C kg^{-1} ≈ 3,876 R
Absorbed dose, kerma	J kg^{-1} (gray [Gy])	rad	1 Gy = 100 rad
Dose equivalent	J kg^{-1} (sievert [Sv])	rem	1 Sv = 100 rem
Activity	s^{-1} (becquerel [Bq])	curie	1 Bq = 2.7 × 10^{-11} Ci

photon and nearly independent of the atomic number of the target material. As a result, at the energies used in radiation therapy, termed megavoltage (MV), the absorbed dose in normal tissues is comparable to that in nearby bone. At much lower energies, termed kilovoltage (kV), the absorbed dose would scale with the atomic number of the target with higher absorbed dose in bone compared to normal soft tissues.

At the second International Congress of Radiology in 1928, the basic unit of radiation exposure, the roentgen (R), was defined (37). Although the original definition evolved over time, the fundamental idea remained the same. The roentgen is the amount of photon radiation that causes 0.001293 g of air to produce one electrostatic unit of positive or negative charge (esu). The value of 0.001293 g is the mass of 1 cc of air at a temperature of 0°C and a pressure of 760 mm Hg. The definition of the roentgen can also be expressed in other equivalent terms:

$$1 \text{ R} = 2.58 \times 10^{-4} \text{ C/kg air}$$

or, conversely, expressed in SI units, the unit of exposure is defined by

$$1 \text{ C/kg} = 3{,}876 \text{ R}$$

Table 11.1 lists some basic units of radiation and radiation therapy, both in historic context and in terms of modern SI units. Kerma (kinetic energy release per unit mass) defines the transfer of energy from photons to directly ionized particles. These directly ionized particles, in turn, transfer some of their energy to the medium (usually tissue). This transfer of energy is defined as the absorbed dose to the medium from the radiation beam. The SI unit for kerma is joule per kilogram (J/kg) or gray (Gy). In a slightly confusing definition, the SI unit for absorbed dose is also joule per kilogram or gray. The term gray has replaced the previously used term "rad." Oftentimes, the term centigray (cGy) is used. The cGy is equivalent to the rad and 1 gray equals 100 cGy.

Another rationale to think and communicate in SI units is that the roentgen was defined explicitly for photon interactions and not charged particles. Kerma and absorbed dose, although they have equivalence to the roentgen and exposure, can be defined equally for photons and charged particles.

RADIATION PRODUCTION

Radioactive Isotopes

As mentioned before, γ-rays are typically derived from radionuclides, such as ^{60}Co. Electrons or beta particles also come from radionuclides. In fact, most radioactive material produces a combination of photons (gamma rays) and electrons during the decay process. Radioactivity is the result of an atom changing its "energy" state, usually to a lower "energy" state, by the emission/absorption/internal conversion of photons or electrons in the atom. These processes result in disintegrations or radioactive decay, whereby the atom releases photons or electrons or both during the change in "energy" states. The release of these particles is a form of radiation (or energy) that can be used to irradiate tissues. The absorbed dose resulting from this radiation depends on the energy and particle type as mentioned above, as well as the tissue in which it interacts.

Radioactivity, or activity, is denoted by the symbol *A* and is defined as the number of disintegrations per unit of time. The following relationship defines activity, the decay constant, and ultimately the half-life for a radioactive material:

$$A = N/t = \gamma N$$

This equation is solved using an exponential solution:

$$A = A_o e{-}\lambda^t$$

where *A* is the initial activity, λ is the decay constant, and *t* is some unit of time later. Other important concepts for radioactivity and radioactive decay are the half-life, $T_{1/2}$, and the average life, T_a. The half-life is the amount of time needed to reduce the original amount of material by half. This is also equivalent to reducing the original activity by half. $T_{1/2}$ is related to the decay constant by $T_{1/2} = 0.693/\lambda$. The average life represents the period of time that a hypothetical source would need, if it retained its original activity for a fixed period of time (T_a) before suddenly decaying to zero activity, to produce the same number of disintegrations over an infinite amount of time by the same source if it decayed exponentially. T_a is related to the decay constant and the half-life by $T_a = 1/\lambda = 1.44\ T_{1/2}$.

Radionuclides can occur naturally or be created artificially. Artificially created radionuclides are usually created by neutron bombardment of otherwise stable isotopes. The resulting interactions produce atoms that are inherently unstable and will decay to a more stable form with a predictable half-life, releasing energy or radiation through this decay. Naturally occurring radionuclides originally come from one of three standard series—the uranium series, the actinium series, and the thorium series—so named because of a dominant radionuclide in each series. In general, the higher the atomic number, the more likely an isotope will be radioactive. **Table 11.2** lists many of the common radionuclides used in brachytherapy, along with their physical properties. For gynecologic cancers, use of radium 226 (^{226}Ra) sources is now historic. Though cost-effective because of its long half-life (1,622 years), radium releases a by-product, radon gas, if the mechanical integrity of the source capsule is compromised. This could require closure of hospital wards due to radon gas contamination. Cesium 137 (^{137}Cs) has replaced radium as a safer yet effective radionuclide. Less shielding is required for cesium than radium, and there is no risk of radon gas leakage. With a half-life of 30 years, it is also cost-effective due to the infrequent need for replacement. Cesium can be used clinically for years without replacement, but the treatment duration must be adjusted to allow for radioactive decay (38). It is typically used for LDR gynecologic brachytherapy in tandem and ovoid and cylinder applicators. Iridium 192 (^{192}Ir) is produced in various source strengths and can be used for interstitial and intracavitary gynecologic implants. ^{192}Ir half-life of 74.2 days requires frequent replacement and, typically, this is custom ordered individually for each implant rather than stored in the radiation oncology department like ^{137}Cs sources. High-activity ^{192}Ir (10Ci) sources are used for HDR brachytherapy and are replaced every 3 months, and lower activity ^{192}Ir sources are used for LDR brachytherapy.

Linear Accelerators

LINACS are another method of producing radiation for treatment of malignancies. LINACS can produce both photon and electron beams of different energies, depending on their construction. The principles behind a LINAC involve accelerating an initial beam of electrons across a variable electric field. The greater the strength of the electric field, the more energetic the electron beam. This electron

TABLE 11.2. Physical Properties and Uses of Brachytherapy Radionuclides

Element	Isotope	Energy (MeV)	Half-Life	HVL-Lead (mm)	Source Form	Clinical Application
Obsolete Sealed Sources of Historic Significance						
Radium	^{226}Ra	0.83 (avg)	1,626 years	16	Radium salt encapsulated in tubes and needles	LDR intracavitary and interstitial
Radon	^{222}Rn	0.83 (avg)	3.83 days	16	Radon	Permanent interstitial; temporary molds
Currently Used Sealed Sources						
Cesium	^{137}Cs	0.662	30 years	6.5	Cesium salt encapsulated in tubes and needles	LDR intracavitary and interstitial
Iridium	^{192}Ir	0.397 (avg)	74 days	6	Seeds in nylon ribbon; encapsulated source on steel cable	LDR temporary interstitial; HDR interstitial and intracavitary
Cobalt	^{60}Co	1.25	5.26 years	11	Encapsulated spheres	HDR intracavitary
Iodine	^{125}I	0.028	59.6 days	0.025	Seeds	Permanent interstitial
Palladium	^{103}Pd	0.020	17 days	0.013	Seeds	Permanent interstitial
Gold	^{198}Au	0.412	2.7 days	6	Seeds	Permanent interstitial
Strontium	$^{90}Sr–^{90}Y$	2.24 MeV β_{max}	28.9 years	—	Plaque	Superficial ocular lesions
Cesium-131	131Cs	0.030 MeV	9.7 days	0.042	Seeds	Permanent interstitial
Developmental Sealed Sources						
Americium	^{241}Am	0.060	432 years	0.12	Tubes	LDR intracavitary
Ytterbium	^{169}Yb	0.093	32 days	0.48	Seeds	LDR temporary interstitial
Californium	^{252}Cf	2.4 (avg) neutrons	2.65 years	—	—	—
Samarium	^{145}Sm	0.043	340 days	0.060	Seeds	LDR temporary interstitial
Unsealed Radioisotopes Used for Radiopharmaceutical Therapy						
Strontium	^{89}Sr	1.4 MeV β_{max}	51 days	—	$SrCl_2$ IV solution	Diffuse bone metastases
Iodine	^{131}I	0.61 MeV β_{max} 0.364 MeV g	8.06 days	—	Capsule NaI oral solution	Thyroid cancer
Phosphorus	^{32}P	1.71 MeV β_{max}	14.3 days	—	Chromic phosphate colloid instillation; Na_2PO_3 solution	Ovarian cancer seeding: peritoneal surface; polycythemia vera, chronic leukemia

HDR, high dose rate; LDR, low dose rate.

beam can be adjusted to control its shape and intensity before delivery to the patient. Alternatively, the electron beam can be directed to a tungsten target. The electron–target interaction creates a forward scattered photon beam or X-ray. The resulting photon beam can then be modified by the machine using filters and collimators to produce the desired radiation field shape.

Photon beams of different energies have a different absorbed dose pattern within tissues. This pattern is normally characterized as a percent depth dose or variation of dose as a function of depth within tissue, as shown in **Figures 11.16** and **11.17**, and by dose profiles, or variation of dose as a function of lateral distance at a given depth (**Fig. 11.18**). The key feature in all of the figures is that higher-energy photons deposit dose at greater depths. Because of the way dose is deposited and absorbed in tissue, the higher the photon energy, the lesser the dose deposited at shallow depths toward the surface of the patient. This is called "skin sparing" and is a characteristic of high-energy photons. In fact, the higher the photon energy, the deeper the point at which the maximum absorbed dose is deposited. After this D_{max}, the absorbed dose decreases because the photon beam is attenuated by the tissues through which it passes.

Figure 11.19 shows a simplified drawing of a LINAC. The gantry (or part of the LINAC where radiation exits the machine) can rotate 360° around the patient on the treatment table. The table can also be rotated about the vertical axis of the radiation beam. This

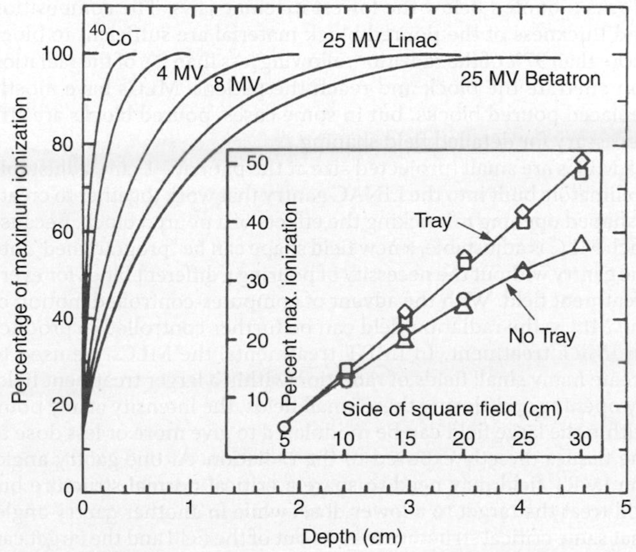

Figure 11.16. ^{60}Co to 25-MV X-rays.

Source: From Velkley DE, Manson DJ, Purdy JA, et al. Build-up region of megavoltage photon radiation sources. *Med Phys*. 1975;2:14–19, with permission.

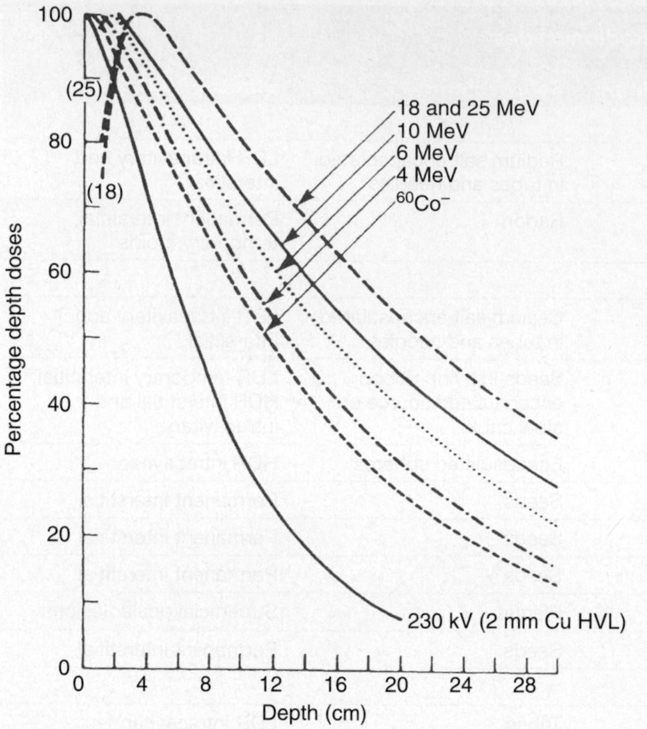

Figure 11.17. Typical X-ray or photon beam central axis percentage depth–dose curves for a 10 × 10 cm beam for 230 kV (2 mm Cu HVL) at 50 cm SSD; ^{60}Co and 4 MV at 80 cm SSD; and 6, 10, 18, and 25 MV at 100 cm SSD. The last two beams coincide at most depths but do not coincide in the first few millimeters of the built-up region. The 4, 6, 18, and 25-MV data are for the Varian Clinic 4, 6, 20, and 35 units, respectively, at the Department of Radiation Oncology, Washington University in St. Louis.

Source: From Cohen M, Jones DEA, Greene D. Central axis depth dose data for use in radiotherapy. *Br J Radiol*. 1972;11:21, with permission.

combination of angles allows the radiation to be directed to almost any part of a patient's body.

Modern LINACS are equipped with multileaf collimators (MLCs) and asymmetric jaws to control the shape of the radiation beam directed before it reaches the patient (**Fig. 11.20**). Prior to asymmetric jaws and MLCs, photon beam shaping was achieved using poured blocks mounted below the lowest machine jaws. The composition and thickness of the poured block material are sufficient to block more than 97% of the radiation, allowing less than 3% of the radiation to penetrate the block and reach the patient. MLCs have mostly replaced poured blocks, but in some cases, poured blocks are still necessary for detailed field shaping.

MLCs are small (projected size at the patient ~1 cm), adjustable collimators built into the LINAC gantry that work together to create a shaped opening mimicking the effects of a poured block. Because each MLC is adjustable, a new field shape can be "programmed" into the gantry without the necessity of pouring a different block for every treatment field. With the advent of computer-controlled motion of the MLCs, the radiation field can be further controlled to produce an IMRT treatment. In IMRT treatments, the MLCs are used to create many small fields of radiation within a larger treatment field. By opening and closing these small fields, the intensity at any point within the large field can be modulated to give more or less dose to the tissues directly exposed to the radiation. At one gantry angle, the IMRT field may need to spare a critical normal structure but still treat the target to a lower dose, while in another gantry angle, that same critical structure may be out of the field and the target can receive a higher intensity to compensate for the lowered intensity in the first field. This adaptability allows the radiation treatment planner to create and deliver very complex treatment fields that improve target coverage, while attempting to spare normal tissues.

In practical terms, IMRT treatment plans are an improvement of the more conventional three-dimensional (3-D) conformal treatment plans. 3-D conformal treatment plans use fewer fields to achieve nominal coverage of the treatment target. At each gantry angle, the radiation is either hitting the target/normal tissue or not with a simple shaped treatment field. Normal tissues may be impossible to spare, relative to adjacent targets. IMRT treatment plans may use similar gantry angle setups, but with the additional intensity modulation, the IMRT fields can create a complicated dose distribution within the patient. In some cases, where the normal tissues are relatively far from the target tissues, there may be no benefit or rationale for the more complex IMRT treatment plan compared to 3-D conformal treatment plans. In cases where the proximity of normal tissues and target varies across a field and between gantry angles, IMRT may prove the more efficient treatment plan to protect normal tissues while focusing dose onto the target (**Figs. 11.21** and **11.22**). National guidelines have been created for the safe and appropriate use of IMRT (39,40). IMRT may be appropriate and ideal for the treatment of gynecologic cancers (41).

A pivotal treatment technique for the success of IMRT is IGRT (42–44). Historically, treatment setups were verified by orthogonal radiographs and treatment fields by port films or X-rays of the treatment fields superimposed on the patient. Modern LINACS have added onboard imaging (OBI) that facilitates electronic recording of the treatment fields at every treatment setup using an electronic portal imaging device (EPID). By comparing computer-generated radiographs (DRRs or digitally reconstructed radiographs) with the actual patient images, discrepancies in field shape and patient setup can be corrected before the delivered treatment. This type of corrective behavior before treatment is the foundation of IGRT. Over the last decade, the addition of CT imaging within the LINAC was implemented to verify the correct 3-D alignment of the patient on the treatment table prior to each fraction delivery within minutes. Partial CT scans (not full 360° rotation) are obtained prior to each treatment. In some LINACS, the CT scans are obtained and constructed based on the therapeutic photon beams (MV). In other approaches, an X-ray source (kV) is used to acquire the CT scans. Because megavoltage CT (MV-cone beam computed tomography [CBCT]) uses the therapeutic high-energy photon beam (6 MV), the image quality suffers because of poor soft tissue contrast. On the other hand, kV-CBCT has a lower energy photon source (<140 keV) which is used to acquire and reconstruct the patient image. kV-CBCT has better soft tissue contrast than MV-CBCT, but is prone to distorting artifacts from high-density objects within the patient, such as hip prostheses. For either image modality, the CT image at the time of treatment and its corresponding isocenter location are compared to the treatment planning CT and isocenter for agreement. Adjustments for rotation, lateral, vertical, and longitudinal discrepancies are made prior to treatment. The intent of these IGRT methods is to improve the accuracy of the treatment setup on a daily basis relative to the original treatment plan. This enables decreasing the size of the radiation fields, as there is not as much need for a large margin on the target, which can decrease normal tissue irradiation and even allow for dose escalation to the target. Guidelines for use of IGRT have been published by the American Society for Radiation Oncology (ASTRO) and the American College of Radiology (ACR) (45). Online MR imaging has recently been added to the LINAC (Elekta) or a Cobalt-60-based LINAC (ViewRay) to allow for real-time IGRT with superior soft tissue resolution as compared to kV-CBCT of intact cancers such as cervical or vaginal cancers to guide treatment accuracy.

Volumetric-modulated arc therapy (VMAT) has been used to deliver IMRT. TomoTherapy is one form of arc therapy. TomoTherapy (AccuRay, Madison, WI) (**Fig. 11.23**) is a special type of LINAC/helical CT combination (44). TomoTherapy units were the first commercially available treatment machines that directly combined CT (MVCT in this case) with highly complex MLCs to deliver IMRT using IGRT. Each day, the patient receives an MVCT, a comparison using 3-D fusion to the original treatment plan is made, adjustments

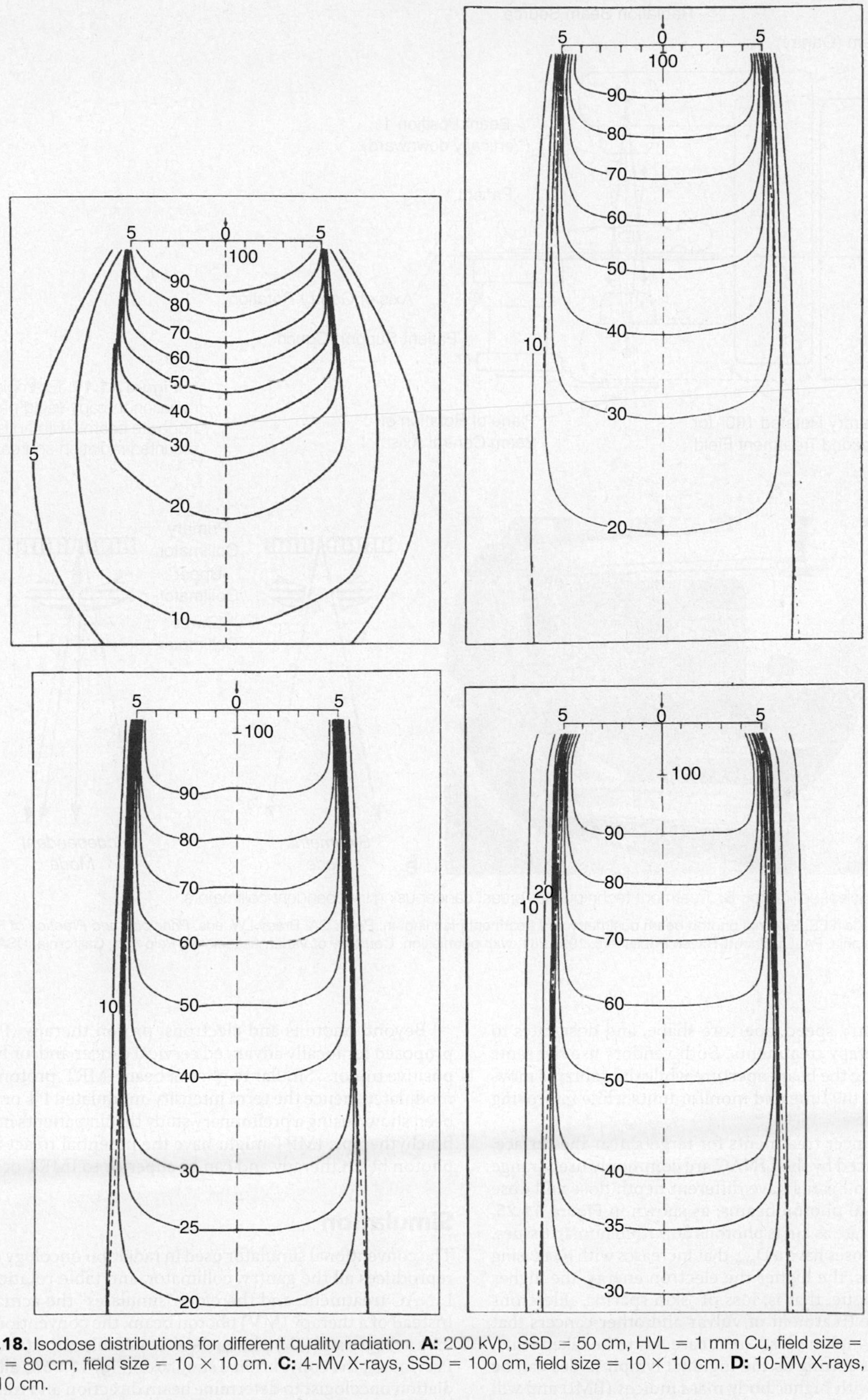

Figure 11.18. Isodose distributions for different quality radiation. **A:** 200 kVp, SSD = 50 cm, HVL = 1 mm Cu, field size = 10 × 10 cm. **B:** ^{60}Co, SSD = 80 cm, field size = 10 × 10 cm. **C:** 4-MV X-rays, SSD = 100 cm, field size = 10 × 10 cm. **D:** 10-MV X-rays, SSD = 100 cm, field size = 10 × 10 cm.

Source: From Khan FM. *The Physics of Radiation Therapy*. 2nd Ed. Baltimore, MD: Williams & Wilkins; 1994, with permission.

to the patient position are made, and IMRT treatment is delivered without the patient needing to change machines. Corrections to the delivered dose can even be modeled based on the patient's current anatomy as visualized by the MVCT built into the TomoTherapy machine. This enables treatment of complex presentations such as paraaortic adenopathy with the closely positioned kidneys and bowel (**Fig. 11.24**). Excellent clinical outcomes have been published with rotational therapy for these types of presentations (46). Currently, all modern LINACS can deliver sophisticated and dynamic radiation arcs; examples are the Varian (RapidArc) and Elekta (VMAT). The

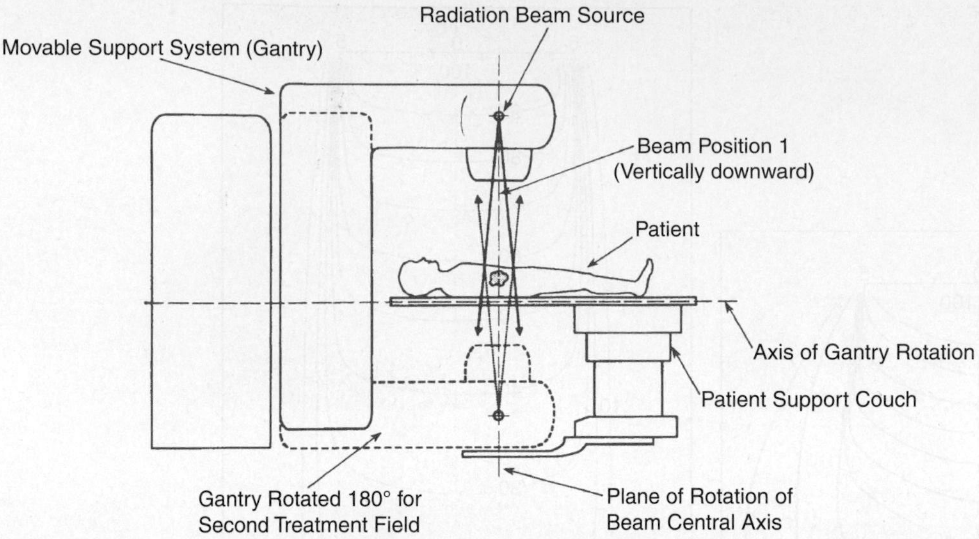

Figure 11.19. Example of multifield radiation therapy using parallel opposite beams with an isocentrically mounted radiation source.

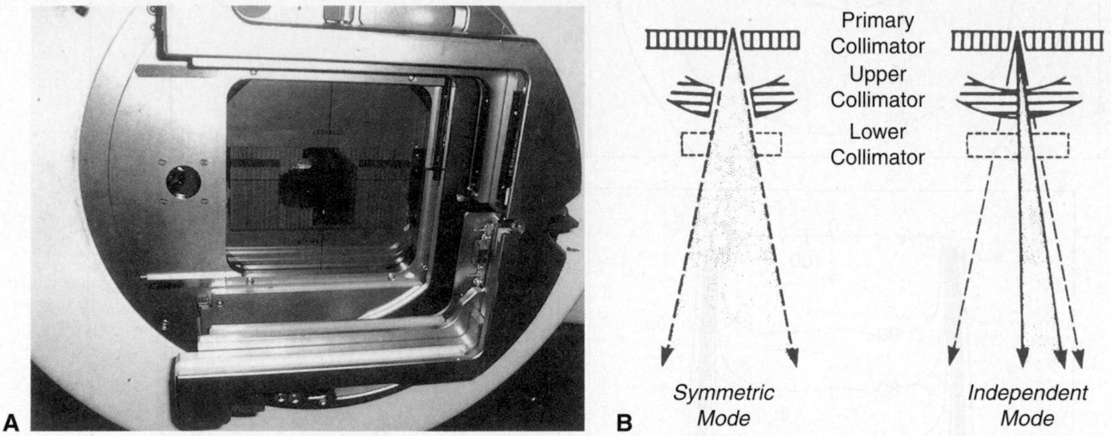

Figure 11.20. A: Multileaf collimator. **B:** Treatment technique for breast cancer using independent collimators.

Source: From Purday JA, Klein EE. External photon beam dosimetry and treatment planning. In: Perez CA, Brady LW, eds. *Principles and Practice of Radiation Oncology*. 3rd Ed. Philadelphia, PA: Lippincott-Raven Publishers; 1998:281, with permission. Courtesy of Varian Associates, Palo Alto, California, USA.

LINACS controls gantry speed, aperture shape, and dose rates to generate their arc therapy treatments. Both vendors use the same principle of modulating the beam aperture while the gantry is moving in arc to minimize the time and monitor units while improving dose conformality.

For gynecologic cancer treatments for targets near the surface, electron beams produced by the LINAC are commonly used (range 4 to 21 MeV). Electron beams have different depth dose and dose profiles as compared to photon beams, as shown in **Figure 11.25**, electrons do not penetrate as far as photons do within human tissues. While electron depth doses have a D_{max} that increases with increasing energy, unlike photons, the higher the electron energy, the higher the surface dose to tissue, that is, loss of "skin sparing." Electrons have been used in the treatment of vulvar and other cancers that involve the inguinal lymph nodes. Great care has to be taken when using electrons in this setting as the inguinal lymph nodes can be very deep in women with higher body mass indices (BMI) and will under dose nodes at a depth >3 cm. This resulted in an increased risk of inguinal failures in the Gynecologic Oncology Group (GOG) 88 study (47). Electrons can be used to treat the vulva in patients with close or positive vulvar margins or in combination with higher-energy beams to treat the inguinal nodes in patients with lower BMI. Proper delineation of the inguinal lymph nodes is essential in determining the most appropriate technique to treat them (48).

Beyond photons and electrons, proton therapy (PT) has been proposed for locally advanced cervical cancer and/or lymph node–positive tumors. Similar to photon beam IMRT, protons can also be modulated, hence the term intensity-modulated PT or IMPT. It has been shown using a preliminary study that in patients not eligible for brachytherapy, IMPT might have the potential to act as a boost to photon beam therapy and can be superior to IMRT or VMAT (49).

Simulation

The conventional simulator used in radiation oncology departments reproduces all the gantry, collimator, and table rotations used in a LINAC treatment, and therefore "simulates" the actual treatment. Instead of a therapy (MV) photon beam, the conventional simulator uses a diagnostic (kV) photon beam to simulate the treatment beam. Previously, the conventional simulator (**Fig. 11.26A**) allowed the radiation oncologist to determine beam direction and treatment fields that would be needed for a radiotherapy treatment based on X-ray fluoroscopy. The radiographic visualization of internal structures allowed special shielding (poured blocks) to be constructed. All the geometric parameters of the conventional simulator are nearly identical to the actual treatment LINACS. The intersections of the gantry rotation axis, collimator rotation axis (the machine isocenter), and patient location are identified and marked on the patient's skin

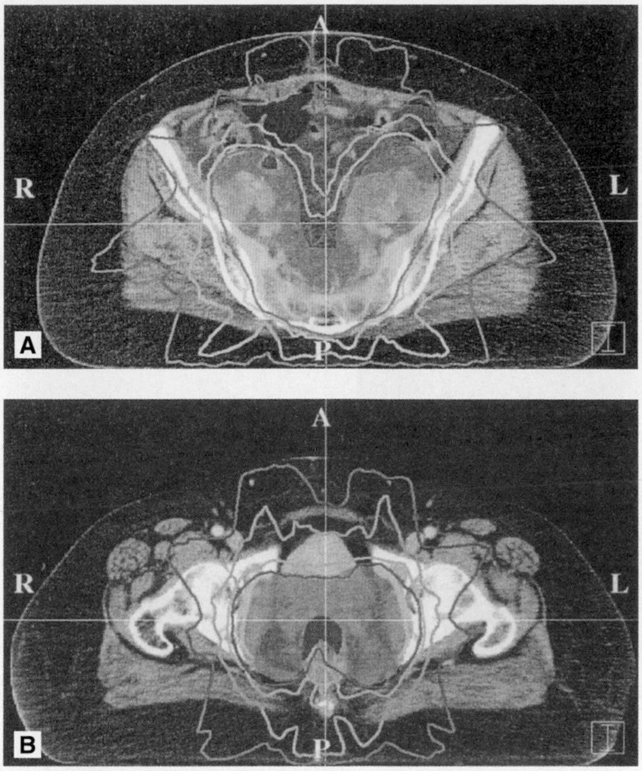

Figure 11.21. A: Isodose curves from a whole-pelvic intensity-modulated radiation therapy plan superimposed on an axial CT slide through the upper pelvis. Highlighted are the 100%, 90%, 70%, and 50% isodose curves. **B:** Isodose curves from a whole-pelvic intensity-modulated radiation therapy plan superimposed on an axial CT slide through the lower pelvis. Highlighted are the 100%, 90%, 70%, and 50% isodose curves.

Source: Reprinted from Mundt AJ, Lujan AE, Rotmensch J, et al. Intensity-modulated whole pelvic radiotherapy in women with gynecologic malignancies. *Int J Radiat Oncol Biol Phys*. 2002;52:1330, with permission from Elsevier.

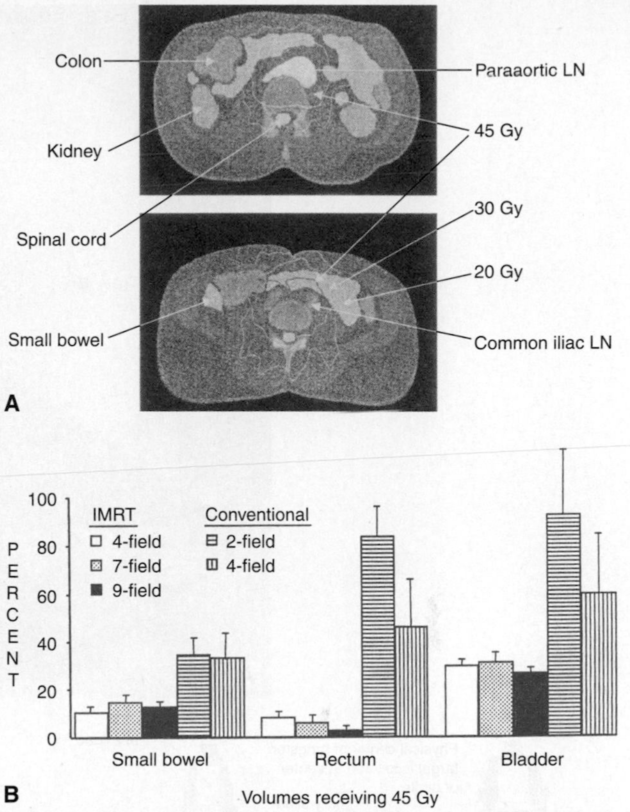

Figure 11.22. A: Axial views of intensity-modulated radiation therapy dose distribution. **B:** The functional volume of the small bowel, rectum, and bladder receiving ≥45 Gy with intensity-modulated radiation therapy and conventional techniques when 100% of the target volume (uterus) receives ≥95% of the prescription dose (45 Gy).

Source: Reprinted from Portelance L, Chao KSCC, Grigsby PW, et al. Intensity-modulated radiation therapy (IMRT) reduces small bowel and bladder doses in patients with cervical cancer receiving pelvic and paraaortic irradiation. *Int J Radiat Oncol Biol Phys*. 2001;51:261–266, with permission from Elsevier.

with removable ink or a permanent series of tattoos. These marks facilitate the reproduction of the same clinical setup for the patient each day of treatment. Hard-copy radiographs can also be used to document the expected treatment fields for comparison with port films obtained on the treatment LINAC.

CT-based simulators ("CTSims") have largely replaced conventional simulators in most radiation oncology departments. CTSims (**Fig. 11.26B**) combine a diagnostic CT scanner with a software package that allows for the simulation of the patient setup in the virtual world of the computer. All of the necessary gantry angles and table angles are modeled in the computer. Computer-controlled room lasers tied into the CTSim software allow the simulator therapist to identify the treatment isocenter in a fashion similar to the conventional simulator (Virtual Sims). DRRs are created for later comparison to actual treatment images. The treatment isocenter and the full CT images can then be transferred to the computer planning system for further treatment planning. Some departments are also equipped with MR or PET scanners for treatment planning. Fusion of CT images with PET or MR images enables CT-based treatment planning with the benefit of improved tumor definition with PET or MR to reduce margin size or increase dose (50,51).

Computerized Dosimetry

In a modern radiotherapy department, computers are necessary to accurately calculate the absorbed doses to tissues. These absorbed doses within tissues are termed isodoses, or lines of the same dose. To initiate this process, CT images of the area of interest at a pretreatment planning session or simulation are acquired. These scans are typically obtained on the CT simulator. Treatment targets such as pelvic/paraaortic lymph nodes, the uterus, or vagina are identified through contouring on these images by the radiation oncologist, as are normal tissues such as the rectosigmoid, bladder, large and small bowel, kidneys, stomach, and spinal cord. Dose goals and constraints are identified for the targets and normal tissues, respectively. A dosimetrist uses this information to design the radiation treatment plan. Treatment beams are planned and the resulting dosimetry is reviewed by the treating physician and a qualified medical physicist (QMP). The radiation plan is optimized as needed to best address the tumor and avoid the normal organs and tissues. In order for a computer treatment planning system to do all this, the depth dose and dose profiles for all of the treatment beams (photons and electrons) must be accurately entered into the planning system. This process is referred to as treatment planning commission, a task which is carefully performed by the QMP.

There are varying complexities of treatment plans that might be used. For simple targets, such as metastatic cancer to the spine, a simple single field or parallel opposed, two-dimensional (2-D) plan might be all that is required. Complexities of internal anatomy and external surface contours can be ignored while still successfully delivering a palliative treatment plan to the patient. More complicated target definitions might require specific and accurate knowledge of adjacent internal anatomy and the details of the patient's surface in order to accurately deliver a successful treatment plan. In these cases, a 3-D conformal treatment plan is developed. In still more complicated target/normal tissue regions, IMRT/VMAT/IMPT treatment planning might be required in order to give sufficient

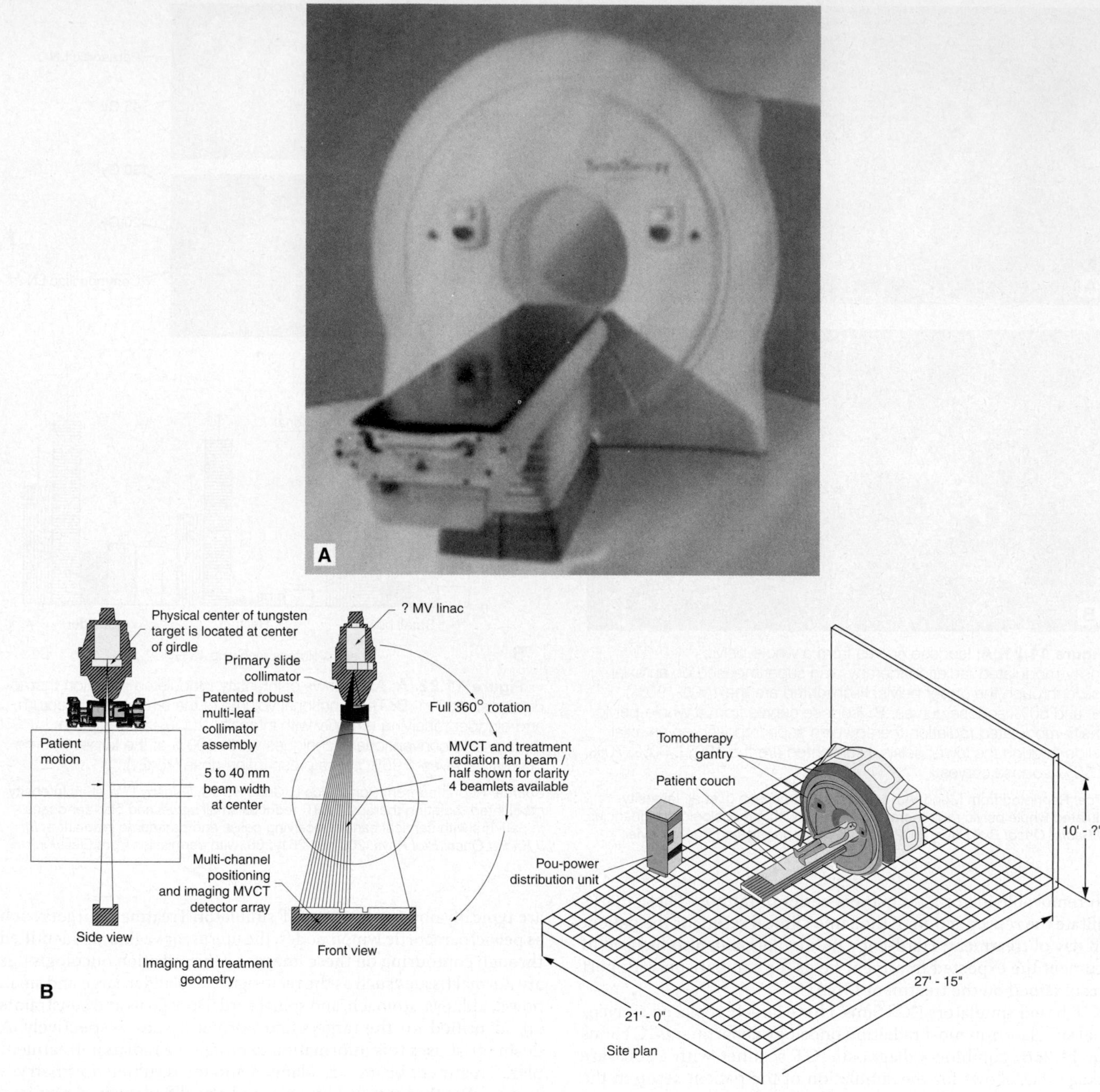

Figure 11.23. A: Helical TomoTherapy device commercially available for IMRT. **B:** Diagrammatic representation of the device.
Source: Courtesy of TomoTherapy Inc., Madison, Wisconsin, USA.

dose to the target while minimizing the dose to an adjacent normal tissue. The goal for most treatment plans is to treat the target to a specified dose while minimizing dose to adjacent normal tissues.

In all of these examples, the word "target" is used. The goal is to encompass the target with the desired dose. Targets are more formally defined in ICRU 50 (52). **Figure 11.27** illustrates the GTV, the CTV, the PTV, and the treated volume. Each of the target or tumor volumes is larger than the previous target volume by some margin. The CTV includes all of the GTV plus possible microscopic extensions. The PTV includes all of the CTV plus a margin to account for possible geometric uncertainties of the patient or treatment margin. The irradiated volume includes all of the PTV plus any margins that might be included in the treatment plan to provide minimum dose coverage to the PTV.

Brachytherapy Principles

Brachytherapy is a term with Greek roots where "brachy" means "short distance." With brachytherapy, a highly concentrated dose of radiation is delivered to immediately surrounding tissues within millimeters to several centimeters of the applicators that carry the radioactive sources (53). This allows for delivery of a high dose of radiation to closely approximated tumor while relatively sparing surrounding normal tissues such as the rectosigmoid, bladder, and small bowel. This is in comparison to teletherapy, where "tele" means "far distance" and refers to external beam irradiation discussed above (photons/electron/protons), where the radiation source is at a greater distance from the patient (100 cm) than with brachytherapy, where sources are near the target. With external beam irradiation, the tumor

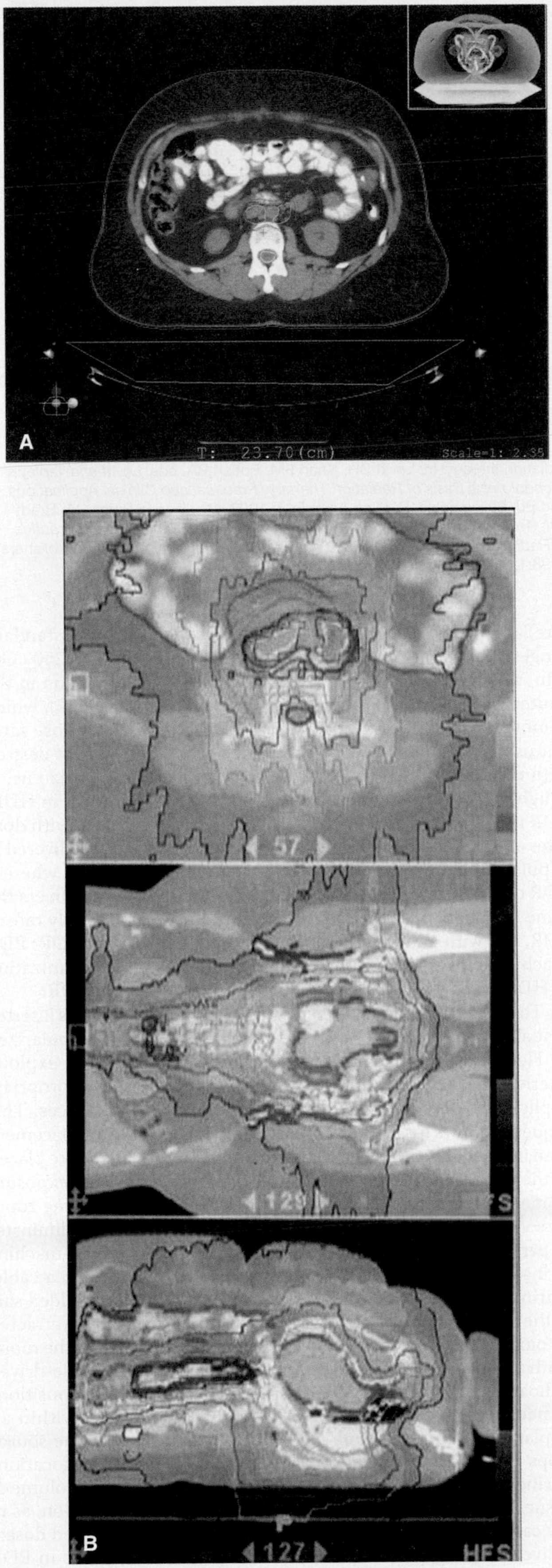

Figure 11.24. A: Contours of enlarged paraaortic nodes with margin are shown in close proximity to the small bowel. **B:** IMRT plan for extended-field irradiation in axial, coronal, and sagittal projections.

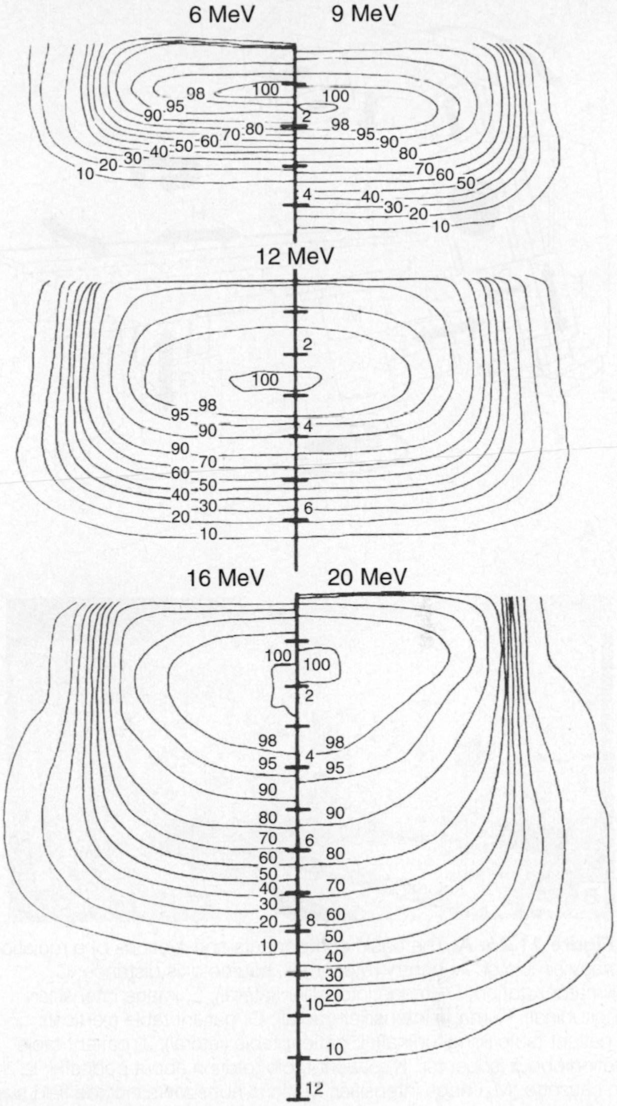

Figure 11.25. Electron beam central axis isodose curves for a 10 × 10 cm field at 100 cm SSD. These data are for the Varian Clinac 20 at the Department of Radiation Oncology, Washington University in St. Louis, MO.

Source: From Glasgow GP, Purdy JA. External beam dosimetry and treatment planning. In: Perez CA, Brady LW, eds. *Principles and Practice of Radiation Oncology*. 2nd Ed. Philadelphia, PA: JB Lippincott; 1992:208–245, with permission.

and/or tumor bed are typically irradiated along with adjacent tissues at risk, such as lymph nodes. External beam irradiation typically is much more penetrating than brachytherapy unless electron beam external irradiation is used. With electron beam therapy, superficial structures such as the skin and/or superficial lymph nodes are optimally treated, unlike the deep abdominopelvic tissues, which are best irradiated with the penetrating photons produced by a LINAC.

There are different types of brachytherapy or radioactive implants (53,54). Temporary implants are used most frequently and are categorized as interstitial or intracavitary. With interstitial brachytherapy, the radioactive sources are transiently inserted into tumor-bearing tissues directly through placement in hollow needles or tubes. With intracavitary brachytherapy, radioactive sources are placed into naturally occurring body cavities or orifices, such as the vagina or uterus, using commercially available hollow applicators such as a vaginal cylinder or tandem and ovoids. Temporary surface applications or plesiotherapy for ophthalmic or skin tumors and intraluminal applications in the esophagus, bronchus, and bile duct are other possible approaches. Permanent interstitial implants entail

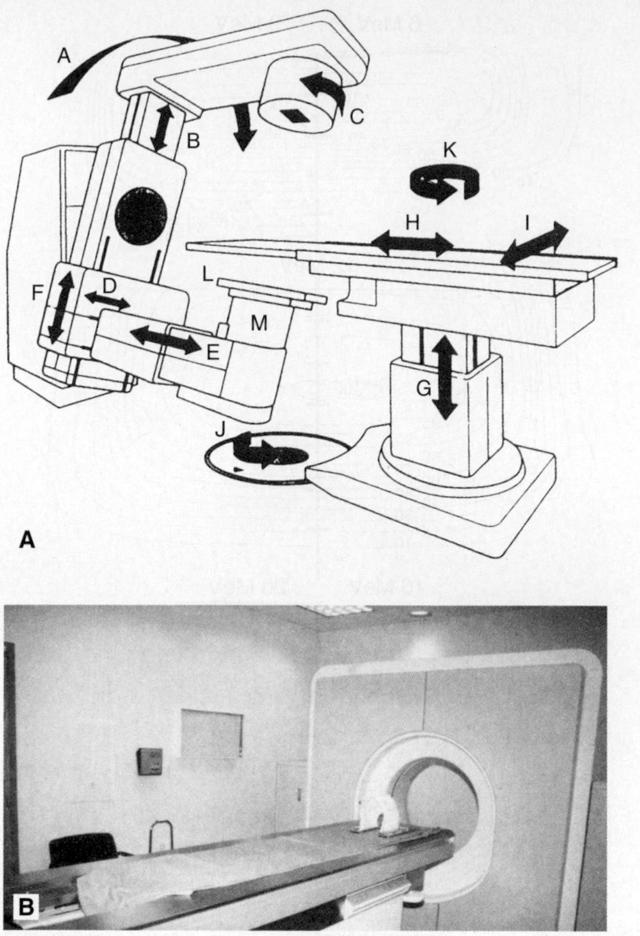

Figure 11.26. A: The basic components and motions of a radiation therapy simulator. A, gantry rotation; B, source-axis distance; C, collimator rotation; D, image intensifier (lateral); E, image intensifier (longitudinal); F, image intensifier (radial); G, patient table (vertical); H, patient table (longitudinal); I, patient table (lateral); J, patient table rotation about isocenter; K, patient table rotation about pedestal; L, film cassette; M, image intensifier. Motions not shown include field size delineation, radiation beam diaphragms, and source-tray distance. **B:** Three-dimensional simulator that is basically a modified CT scanner with a flat couch suite for treatment planning.

Source: From Van Dyk J, Mah K. Simulators and CT scanners. In: Williams JR, Thwaites DI, eds. *Radiotherapy Physics*. New York, NY: Oxford Medical Publications; 1993:118 (**Fig. 7.3**). Reprinted by permission of Oxford University Press.

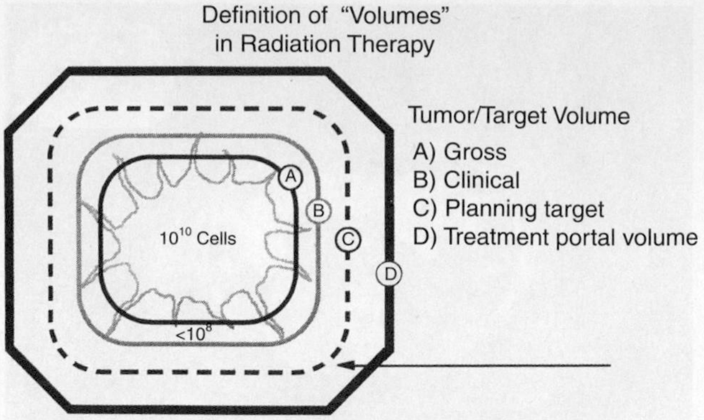

Figure 11.27. Schematic representation of "volumes" in radiation therapy. The treatment portal volume includes the GTV, potential areas of local and regional microscopic disease around the tumor (clinical), and a margin of surrounding normal tissue (planning).

Source: From Perez CA, Purdy JA. Rationale for treatment planning in radiation therapy. In: Levitt SH, Khan FM, Potish RA, eds. *Levitt and Tapley's Technological Basis of Radiation Therapy: Practical and Clinical Applications*. 2nd Ed. Philadelphia, PA: Lea & Febiger; 1992. Modified in Perez CA, Brady LW, Roti JL. Overview. In: Perez CA, Brady LW, eds. *Principles and Practice of Radiation Oncology*. 3rd Ed. Philadelphia, PA: Lippincott-Raven Publishers; 1998:1, with permission.

insertion of radioactive seeds (iodine 125 [^{125}I]; gold 198 [^{198}Au]; palladium 103 [^{103}Pd]) directly into tumor-bearing tissues to emit radiation continuously as they decay to a nonradioactive form (53). Radioactive sources are also described as sealed or unsealed, referring to whether they are solid (^{137}Cs; ^{192}Ir) or liquid radioisotopes (phosphorus 32 [^{32}P]). The most common sealed radioactive sources used for gynecologic brachytherapy are ^{192}Ir and ^{137}Cs. Historically, unsealed radioactive sources such as ^{32}P have been used to treat the entire peritoneal cavity in ovarian cancer. The limitation of this source was that the beta rays emitted penetrated only a distance of 3 mm, making it useful only for patients with microscopic or very thin residual tumor deposits following debulking.

Dose rate is also an important variable in brachytherapy. Traditional LDR irradiation has been used for decades in gynecologic cancers using ^{226}Ra and ^{137}Cs sources for intracavitary insertions and low-activity ^{192}Ir sources for interstitial insertions. HDR brachytherapy has gradually been introduced over the last several decades and entails the use of a highly radioactive (10-Ci) ^{192}Ir source. There are several definitions for the dose rates used in brachytherapy. The ICRU 38 classifies LDR as 0.4 to 2 Gy/hr, MDR (medium dose rate) as 2 to 12 Gy/hr, and HDR as >12 Gy/hr (55). More standard ranges for LDR are 40 to 100 cGy/hr, and for HDR 20 to 250 cGy/min, which is 1,200 to 15,000 cGy/hr. MDR is not common in the United States. Another approach is pulsed dose rate (PDR), which is mostly popular in Europe (56,57). PDR mimics ^{137}Cs dose rates but uses ^{192}Ir sources and afterloading technology. PDR is desired with the scarcity of available new ^{137}Cs sources. Rather than using a high-activity 10-Ci ^{192}Ir source with short dwell times as in HDR, PDR uses a medium-strength ^{192}Ir source of 0.5 to 1.0 Ci with dose rates of up to 3 Gy/hr. The radiation with PDR is typically delivered in a "pulsed" method over only 10 to 30 minutes of each hour, whereas LDR delivers 30 to 100 cGy/hr continuously (57). PDR delivers the same total dose over the same total time at the same hourly rate as LDR, but with an instantaneous dose rate higher than LDR. PDR brachytherapy was developed to combine the isodose optimization of HDR brachytherapy with the biologic advantages of LDR.

The term "afterloading," whereby an unloaded applicator is inserted first and the radioactive sources introduced later, was popularized by Henschke (53). Nearly every modern brachytherapy exploits afterloading. An ideal implant is established with the appropriate applicator before being loaded with the radioactive sources. This sequence allows for more careful and accurate applicator placement than inherent to earlier "hot loaded" applicators, which were placed in the operating room preloaded with radium. Radiation exposure to medical personnel is reduced and exposure of operating room personnel is totally eliminated. Remote afterloading, which eliminates all personnel exposure, entails the use of a computer-driven machine to insert and retract the source(s), which are attached to a cable. During treatment, the source is transported from its shielded safe to the patient's applicators via a transfer tube. Sources are retracted automatically whenever visitors or hospital personnel enter the room. With modern remote afterloading techniques, a single cable-driven radioactive source is propelled through an array of dwell positions in needles, plastic tubes, or intracavitary applicators within an implanted volume. Through computerized dosimetry, the source stops for a specified duration at a preselected number of locations during its transit, delivering a specified dose to a defined volume of tissue. This dose may be delivered rapidly in a large fraction, as in the case of HDR brachytherapy, or a series of small "pulsed doses" delivered at a given frequency over a period of days, as in PDR brachytherapy (56,57). Typically, these treatment units are housed in shielded rooms in the hospital (LDR or PDR) or the radiation oncology department (HDR) (53).

Radiation Protection

The amount of radiation that a person other than patients under treatment can receive is governed by state and federal regulations. The actual values depend on whether the person is considered part of the general public or an occupationally exposed worker. These values can change with different regulations. The National Council on Radiation Protection and Measurements (58) set the following recommendations for limits on exposure to IR:

Public exposures <1 mSv or 0.1 rem annually
Occupational exposures <50 mSv or 5 rem annually

Additionally, NCRP Report #91 (58) placed limits on embryo-fetus exposures:

Total dose limit <5 mSv or 0.5 rem
Dose equivalent limit in 1 month <0.5 mSv or 0.05 rem

These recommended limits were adopted by the Nuclear Regulatory Commission (U.S. Nuclear Regulatory Commission, 10 CFR 20, Standards for Protection against Radiation).

LINACS produce radiation using electrical power. Once the LINAC is turned "off," there is little, if any, radiation exposure risk to staff. Radioactive isotopes, used most often for brachytherapy, however, do not have an "off" switch. They are always undergoing radioactive decay with the resultant radiation production of X-rays, γ-rays, electrons, and other particles.

Radiation safety is an important focus for patients and health care workers. All hospitals that house radioactive sources or LINACs will have a special department termed radiation safety. Radiation personnel are responsible for monitoring radiation exposure in hospitals and clinics. All health care workers exposed to radiation must wear badges that track radiation exposure. There are three words that encompass all of the important aspects of radiation safety and protection: time, distance, and shielding. All three can be used to reduce radiation exposure. The dose delivered to a target from a radioactive source is directly proportional to the amount of time the target is exposed to the radioactive source (59). The dose delivered to a target is inversely proportional to the square of the distance from the radioactive source, double the distance, and the dose is reduced by a factor of four:

$$\text{Dose} \sim \text{time}$$

$$\text{Dose} \sim 1/r^2$$

This is the inverse square rule. The relationship between shielding and absorbed dose is more complicated. The simplest explanation is that the absorbed dose is reduced in an exponential relationship to the physical amount of shielding. The exact relationship (μ) depends on the energy of radiation and the specific material, such as concrete or lead, used to provide the protection. More material (x) means more protection. Less energy means more protection for the same thickness (x) of material:

$$\text{Dose} \sim e^{-}\mu^{x}$$

Minimizing time, maximizing distance, and maximizing shielding will reduce one's absorbed radiation dose. Fortunately, there is relatively little exposure to radiation for most health care providers. The LINACs in radiation oncology are strategically located and shielded to minimize radiation to anyone other than the treated patient. Many brachytherapy insertions are typically performed with remote afterloading to minimize exposure, and often outpatient brachytherapy can be realized because of HDR techniques. This takes the patient off the hospital ward and thereby avoids exposure to the health professional caring for inpatients. The shielded rooms in the radiation oncology department protect the attendant staff from exposure as well.

Occupational Exposure Management of Female Radiation Workers

Pregnancy declaration is optional, but once declared, the employee is required to formally inform her employer. Furthermore, the radiation safety officer should interview her, her employment should be evaluated for exposure history, and steps should be taken to minimize exposure for the current work duties. The National Council on Radiological Protection (58) recommends that the embryo/fetus has limited exposure to less than 0.5 Sv/month.

CLINICAL APPLICATIONS

Historical Background

The use of radiation in the treatment of gynecologic cancers has a rich history. Roentgen rays were used externally as early as 1902 to treat cervical carcinoma and "radium rays" in 1906. In Europe, the use of intracavitary radium was reported in 1903 for the treatment of inoperable uterine cancers (60). In those early years, there was little knowledge of the biologic effects of radiation on the normal and tumor tissues. Typically, a uterine tandem was used alone without vaginal colpostats. There was also little understanding of the dose distribution in the tumor and surrounding normal tissues, and implant duration, and thereby dose, was entirely empirical. As such, complications and failures were common. Since these early years, there has been a tremendous accumulation of knowledge relative to both external beam irradiation and brachytherapy, which will be reviewed.

EXTERNAL BEAM IRRADIATION FOR GYNECOLOGIC CANCERS

Cervical and Vaginal Cancers

In cervical and vaginal cancers, the role of external beam irradiation is to shrink bulky tumor prior to implantation to bring it within range of the high-dose portion of the intracavitary dose distribution, improve tumor geometry by shrinking tumor that may distort anatomy and prevent optimal brachytherapy, and sterilize paracentral and nodal disease that lies beyond reach of the intracavitary system (61). Some institutions maximize the brachytherapy component of the treatment regimen and perform the first intracavitary insertion after 10 to 20 Gy with subsequent external beam delivered with a central block (62). Other institutions treat the whole pelvis to 40 to 50 Gy and perform brachytherapy once the external beam is completed (61). The total dose at point A or the HR CTV, however, should remain the same, stage for stage. Implementing brachytherapy early with subsequent reliance on only the implant to treat the central disease may be considered an advantage as a greater portion of the central dose is delivered with the implant, with relative sparing of the bladder and rectum, perhaps permitting delivery of a higher central dose over a shorter period of time (62). More reliance, however, is placed on the extremely complex match between the intracavitary system and the edge of the midline block, if used, making good implant geometry imperative when brachytherapy constitutes a large portion of the central dose. Those who prefer to deliver an initial 40 to 45 Gy of external beam first believe that the ability to deliver a homogeneous distribution to the entire region at risk for microscopic disease, and the ability to have more shrinkage of central disease prior to intracavitary irradiation, outweigh other considerations. The brachytherapy dose is accordingly decreased to respect normal tissue tolerance. In addition to causing regression of central disease, the external beam fields are also directed at the regional lymph nodes at risk. In cervical and vaginal cancer, the risk of pelvic lymph node involvement is related to the stage of disease, tumor size, and lymphatic vascular space invasion. Other histomorphologic factors influencing lymph node involvement in cervical cancer include pathologic tumor diameter, depth of stromal invasion, uterine body involvement, parametrial spread, and the number of cervical quadrants involved by tumor (62). Early necropsy studies reported the lymphatic pathways for patients with cervical cancer (63). The primary lymphatic pathway is to the parametrial and paracervical nodes, and the obturator and internal and external iliac nodes. Secondary spread can occur to the sacral and common iliac nodes, with subsequent spread to the paraaortic nodes. Unlike in endometrial cancer, paraaortic lymph node involvement in the absence of pelvic lymph node involvement is rare. Inguinal lymph node involvement occurs with distal vaginal spread of disease or via the round ligament if there is extensive involvement of the corpus. The cervical lymphatics are located in three plexuses in the mucosa, muscularis, and serosa of the cervix, and anastomose extensively with the lymphatics of the uterine isthmus. This interconnected lymphatic supply is one of the reasons why the entire uterus should be within the external beam fields when treating cervical cancer. Additionally, there may also be lower uterine segment and endometrial extension of tumor. There are lymph vessels running posteriorly in the uterosacral ligaments to lymph nodes located in the sacrum between the rectum and the internal iliac vessels. These posterior nodes may terminate in the common iliac, subaortic, or paraaortic lymph nodes (64). For all gynecologic cancers, these patterns of lymphatic spread influence the external beam field borders. Traditionally, design of "standard" pelvic fields, as shown in many radiation oncology textbooks, has been based primarily on skeletal landmarks and considered quite simple and straightforward. The skeletal landmarks are not sufficient for field design (65). Traditionally, many institutions have used the "four-field box" technique to treat the pelvis with typical anterior-posterior (AP)–posterior-anterior (PA) field sizes of 15 × 15 cm and lateral field widths of 8 to 9 cm (**Fig. 11.28**) (61). The intent of the four fields is to use rather narrow lateral beams to avoid some of the small bowel anteriorly and a portion of the rectum posteriorly. Surgical and imaging series using CT (66), MRI, (67,68), and lymphangiograms (LAG) (65) have revealed that fields of these sizes can easily miss the primary tumor and its extensions and the regional lymphatics at risk, and design of the pelvic fields needs to be done with care and use of confirmatory imaging (67). Plain films do not visualize the important soft tissues such as the cervical tumor and its extensions, the uterus, or the lymph nodes at risk. Additionally, bladder and rectal contrast and a vaginal obturator or cervical markers have been used to guide field design, but are not sufficient. As with the brachytherapy component of treatment, the adequacy of the external beam fields and margins has a direct relationship with local and regional control. What may be considered a mysterious failure following definitive irradiation, perhaps caused by "radiation resistance," may actually be the result of a marginal miss due to external beam field design. Placement of radiation fields must take into account the alteration of the spatial relationship between the tumor and normal anatomy due to individual anatomic, tumor-induced, or treatment-related positional variations of the uterus and cervix, as well as knowledge of the location of the regional lymphatics (67). Radiation oncologists must be aware of these patterns of disease spread and must have an in-depth understanding of CT anatomy when designing radiation fields following CT simulation. Identification and contouring of enlarged nodes in nodal regions at risk and identification of the iliac vessels, which serve as surrogates for the location of unenlarged lymph nodes, are important in subsequently defining radiation field borders (**Fig. 11.29**) (69). Additionally, contouring of the entire uterus and portions of the vagina will also ensure that these tissues are included in the radiation fields (**Fig. 11.29**). Reliance on bony anatomy alone for radiation field design rather than on CT-defined targets is discouraged. Generally, the superior border of the pelvic fields is at the S1–L5 interspace for early-stage disease (i.e., nonbulky IB or IIA) or at the L4–5 interspace for more advanced disease. The latter is used if one wants to cover the common iliac lymph nodes. Interestingly, Greer et al. evaluated "standard" pelvic fields (AP–PA, 15 × 15 cm; lateral, 8 to 9 cm wide) for the treatment of cervical cancer in relationship to intraoperative findings.

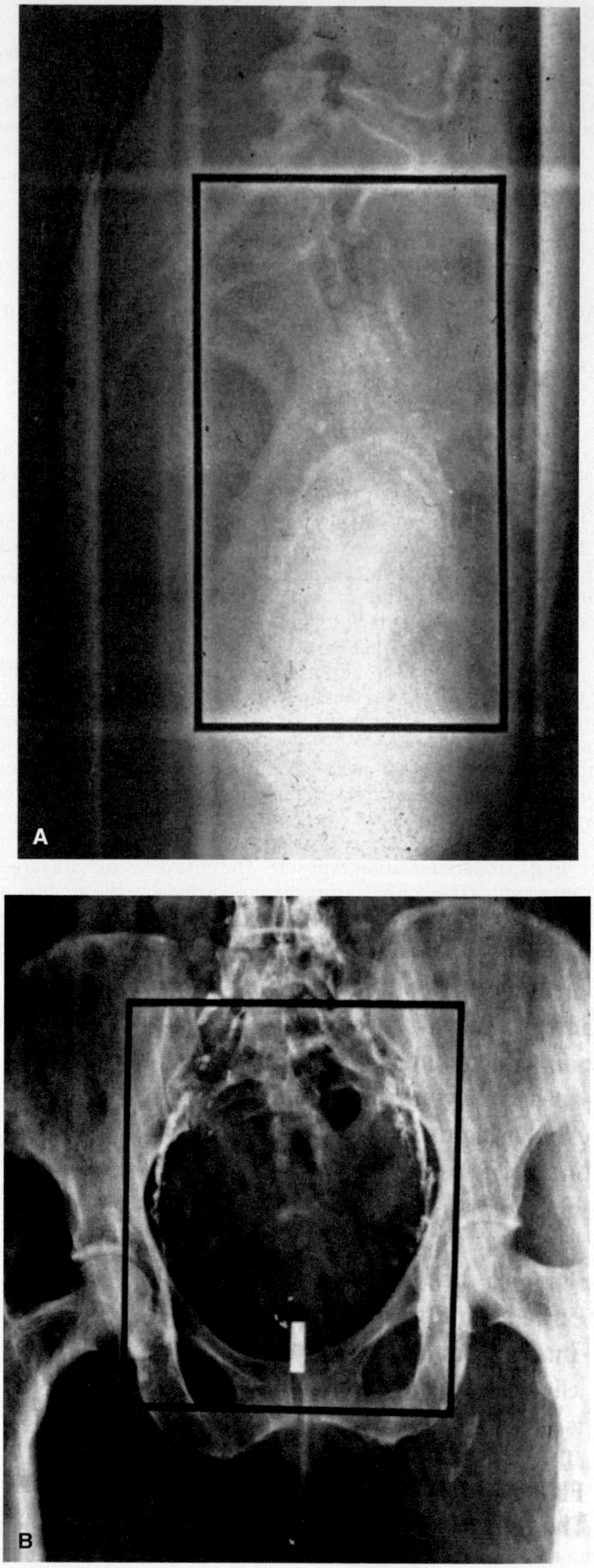

Figure 11.28. Traditional four-field pelvic box technique with short and narrow fields, with the potential to miss the uterine fundus and the pelvic lymph nodes.

Source: Reprinted with permission from Fletcher GH, ed. *Textbook of Radiotherapy*. 3rd Ed. Philadelphia, PA: Lea & Febiger; 1980:761–762.

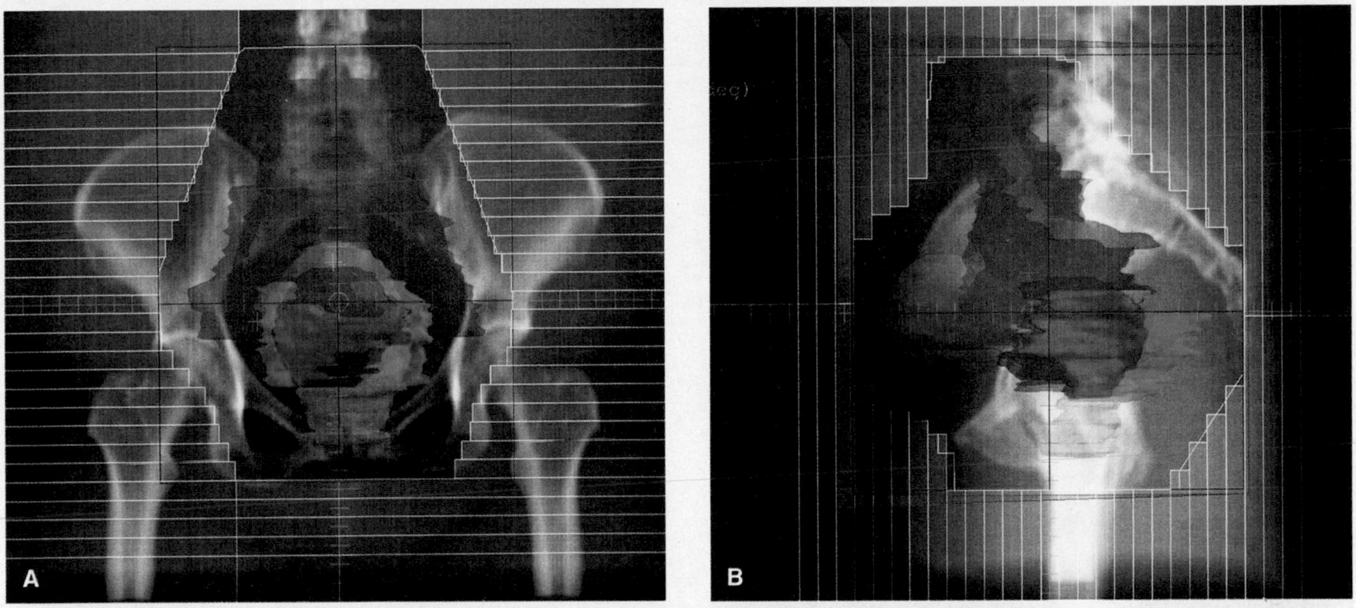

Figure 11.29. Digitally reconstructed AP (**A**) and lateral (**B**) radiographs with associated contoured targets including the pelvic lymph nodes and uterus/cervix/parametria and vagina. Note the multileaf collimator leaves defining the field shape in accordance with coverage of the targets of interest.

Based on intraoperative measurements of the location of the aortic bifurcation and the bifurcation of the common iliac arteries relative to the lumbosacral prominence (the anterior caudal border of L5), Greer et al. concluded that anterior and posterior treatment fields with a superior border at the L4–5 interspace are required to cover the internal iliac, external iliac, and obturator nodes, as the bifurcations of the common iliac arteries were above the lumbosacral prominence in 87% of the patients studied. Coverage of the common iliacs could require extending the upper field border to the L3–4 interspace or even the L2–3 interspace in some patients (70). Obviously, with CT-based dosimetry, it is imperative to outline the vessels and/or nodes in these areas to determine the appropriate field borders because unnecessary irradiation of bowel could occur if all patients were treated to the L2–3 interspace, based on this assumption (**Fig. 11.29**). CT is an excellent tool for identifying pathologically enlarged nodes, multiple small lymph nodes that by increased number rather than size are suspicious, or in the absence of nodes, the aortic and iliac bifurcations and the iliac vessels (66). The inferior border of the pelvic field is usually at the bottom of the ischial tuberosities or 3 to 4 cm below the most distal vaginal component of disease. Inguinal nodes are included if there is distal vaginal spread, in which case treatment of the vaginal introitus with margin would also be required. MRI is especially helpful in imaging vaginal tumor extension (71). The lateral borders of the AP–PA fields must be designed carefully as the normally recommended 1.5 to 2.0-cm margin from the pelvic brim may be too narrow. Using lymphangiography, Bonin et al. (65) found that a margin of at least 2.6 cm on each pelvic brim was needed in order to cover all pelvic lymph nodes if bony landmarks were used. The lateral fields are even more prone to marginal misses than the AP–PA fields, as demonstrated in multiple series that have compared the standard textbook lateral fields (8 to 12 cm wide) to fields designed based on CT and MRI images (**Fig. 11.30**) (67). For the lateral fields, a commonly employed guideline is to place the posterior border in a horizontal line, parallel to the treatment couch that divides the mid-rectum and intersects the sacrum between the second and third sacral segments (S2–3 interspace), and the anterior border by a horizontal line, parallel to the treatment couch from the anteroinferior lip of L5 to the anterior aspect of the pubic symphysis. These "standard" lateral fields are too narrow. For the lateral fields, careful consideration needs to be given to the anterior border to include the external iliac nodes. Based on lymphangiography, Bonin et al. (65) found that, in order to cover the external iliac nodes, the anterior border of the lateral field was sometimes as much as 2 cm anterior to the pubic symphysis. Taylor et al. (69) showed that a modified 7-mm margin typically covers 99% of the pelvic lymph nodes. Additionally, the anterior border must also be drawn to include the entire uterus, given the interconnecting lymphatics of the uterus and cervix and the possibility of lower uterine segment/endometrial extension (**Fig. 11.30**) (67). Enlargement of the uterine fundus by the presence of hematometra or massive fundal extension of cancer can displace the fundus anteriorly and cephalad, as can an anteverted or retroverted uterus (68). The prone position may accentuate this displacement (67). The anterior field border should be based on CT or MRI delineation of the tumor and/or normal anatomical variants to avoid underdosing of these structures (68). The posterior border of the lateral fields must be designed carefully. Based on intraoperative findings, Greer et al. showed that the cardinal and uterosacral ligaments extend posterior to the rectum and sigmoid in their attachments to the sacrum. As part of the parametria, these tissues often contain nodes, even in early disease (IB and II, 22.5%) or are involved by direct extension and need to be covered in most patients by including the entire sacrum in the lateral fields (70). If there is uterosacral ligament involvement, it is especially important to include the entire sacrum in the lateral fields, although some institutions will use this as a criterion for AP–PA fields alone (64). The internal iliac lymph nodes may lie very close to the rectum, and splitting of the rectum can result in a marginal miss of these nodes (**Fig. 11.31**) (66). In the setting of posterior cervical lesions, there may also be direct extension to the superior rectal nodes or sacral lymph nodes. Tumor can also extend directly around the rectum. Kim et al. found that the most common site of an inadequate margin was near the portion of the lateral field blocking the rectum. On CT, it was found that tumor often fell along the lateral aspect of the rectum. The second most common site of inadequate margin was the posterior border at the S2–3 interspace. Zunino et al. (68) also found inadequate posterior border margins when the uterus was both retroverted and anteverted (**Fig. 11.30**). The reason for narrow lateral fields is typically concern over the rectum and the small bowel. Greer et al. (70) reported no increase in late rectal complications when including the entire sacrum in the field. It may also be a mistake to avoid the chance of a marginal miss by treating just with anterior and posterior fields, as in most cases some of the small bowel can be omitted from

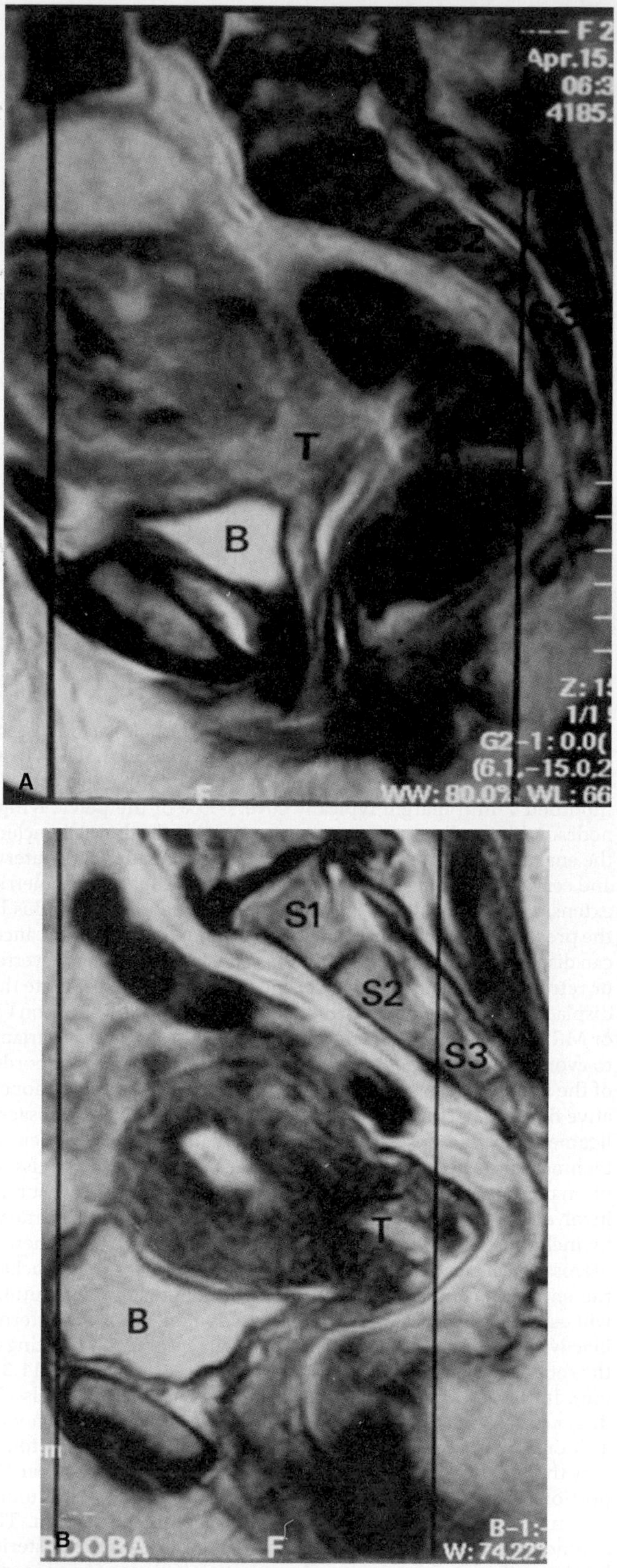

■ **Figure 11.30.** (**A, B**): Traditional lateral fields are superimposed on sagittal MRI scans to evaluate target coverage with traditional fields. Note that (**A**) the traditional lateral fields would not completely cover the uterine fundus. and (**B**) the traditional lateral field would cut through cervical tumor within the anteverted uterus.

Source: Reprinted with permission from Zunino S, Rosato O, Lucino S, et al. Anatomic study of the pelvis and carcinoma of the uterine cervix as related to the box technique. *Int J Radiat Oncol Biol Phys*. 1999;44(1):56–57.

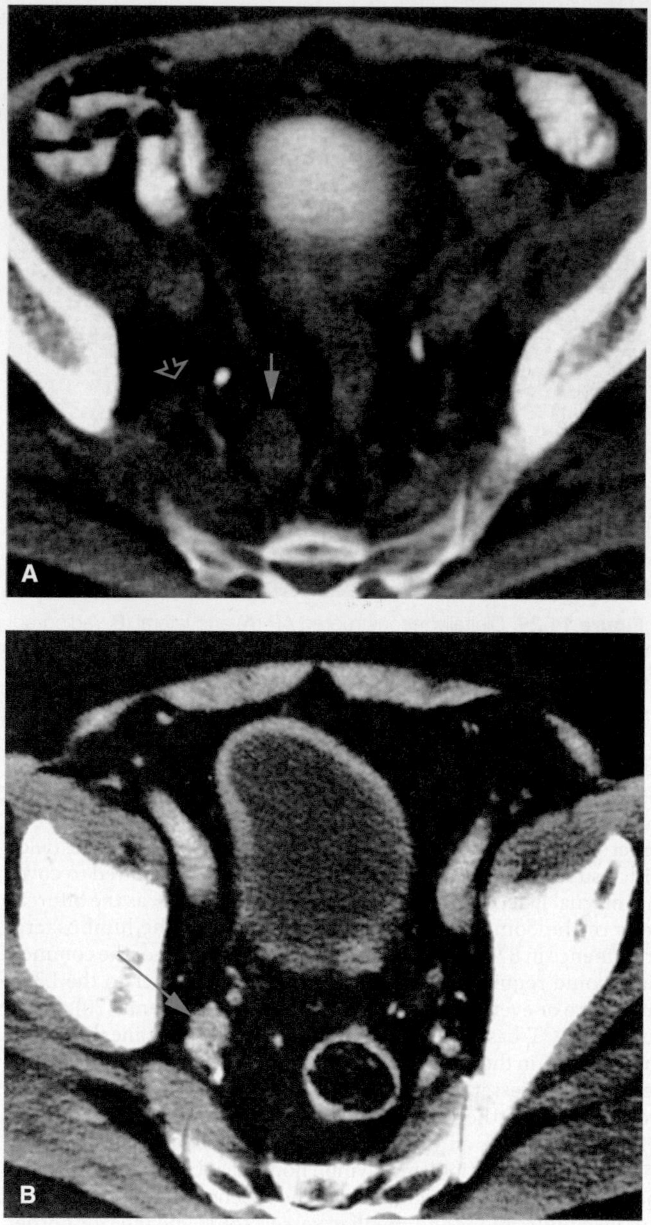

■ **Figure 11.31. A:** The location of the presacral lymph nodes mandates including the entire sacrum to cover disease in the uterosacral and cardinal ligaments and superior rectal (presacral) nodes. The right lateral sacral node *(solid arrow)* is medial to the hypogastric vessels *(open arrow)*. **B:** Note the proximity of the internal iliac lymph node *(solid arrow)* to the rectum. This spatial relationship would exclude partial blocking of the rectum on the lateral fields.

Source: Reprinted with permission from Park J, Charnsangavej C, Yoshimitsu K, et al. Pathways of nodal metastases from pelvic tumors: CT demonstration. *Radiographics*. 1994;14(6):1311.

the lateral fields when using imaged-based planning. MRI has been found to be an invaluable tool for delineating normal anatomy and the extent of cervical tumor involvement because of its superior soft tissue contrast compared to CT. MRI also allows direct imaging in sagittal, coronal, and transverse plains (68). Sagittal MRI images are exceedingly helpful in designing radiation fields (**Fig. 11.30**). Design of the anterior and posterior borders of the lateral fields can be especially influenced by these images. Thomas et al. (67) performed MRI rather than CT in the treatment position and found better delineation of the tumor volume due to the superior contrast resolution. PET/CT scans have largely replaced LAGs at most institutions with Medicare approval and can detect involved pelvic and paraaortic lymph nodes better than CT alone (72,73). Unlike CT, PET does not rely on lymph node size alone, but rather on metabolic alterations for detection of disease. PET has better accuracy than can be achieved with CT or MRI, with a sensitivity of 85% to 90%, a specificity of 95% to 100%, and overall accuracy of 90% to 95%. Nodes as small as 6 mm can be imaged with PET, providing information to guide therapy and predict outcome.

Midline Blocks

Midline blocks have been used historically at various points in time at many institutions (**Fig. 11.32**). It is important to understand when the midline block is placed, as this will influence the HDR fraction size. Higher whole pelvis doses can be utilized without a midline block, but the HDR doses have to be appropriately reduced. HDR and external beam fractions should not be given on the same day. Use of midline blocks is controversial, as there can be an increased risk of rectosigmoid, bladder, and small bowel complications if careful attention is not given to tracking and limiting the total dose in these OAR (74–76).

A midline block may be used during external beam to avoid regions of excessive dose adjacent to the brachytherapy implant and to deliver an adequate dose to potential tumor-bearing regions outside of the implant. When using a midline block early in the treatment course, more reliance is placed on the extremely complex match between the intracavitary system and the edge of the midline block. There are some important safety issues to consider when using midline blocks (74–76). The midline block position should be based on films with similar isocenters. If patients receive external beam irradiation in the prone position, it may be wise to simulate them in the supine position for their parametrial boosts so that they are in the same position as they are for their implants. Midline blocks can be positioned to account for applicator deviation. Alignment along the midplane of the patient can be problematic if the tandem is deviated. Midline blocks that are too narrow may not adequately shield the bladder and rectosigmoid, given their ability to move in and out of the blocked field. Filling and emptying of these organs may also alter their position relative to the block. Eifel et al. point out that the distance between the distal ureters is usually 4 to 5 cm. A narrow block may fail to shield a portion of the ureters during external beam (77). Reviewing the M.D. Anderson experience, Eifel et al. detected an increase in complications in patients with midline blocks (4 cm) used throughout the course of external beam. Since the ureters are typically 2 to 3 cm from the midline, the explanation for the ureteral stenosis could have been an overlap between the external beam fields and the high-dose region of the intracavitary implants (77). A margin of 0.5 cm lateral to the lateral ovoid surface is recommended in designing the width of the midline block for each patient to protect the implanted volume. If the intracavitary system is broad, a wide midline block may potentially shield the external iliac lymph nodes. If tissues immediately adjacent to the colpostats and tandem tip are not shielded, portions of the ileocecal junction and rectosigmoid may be overdosed (78). Huang et al. (78) recommended avoiding a combination of parametrial boost doses of ≥54 Gy and a cumulative rectal biologically effective dose (CRBED) ≥100 Gy_3 to decrease the risk of radiation-induced bowel complications. When a midline block is inserted prior to 40 Gy, it should not extend to the top of the field since it will shield the common iliac and presacral lymph nodes, which will be underdosed. When there is suspicion of uterosacral ligament involvement, it is safer to avoid early placement of the midline block, which will shield disease lying posterior to the implant (64). Due to concern over rectal tolerance, the rectum is shielded after a certain amount of external beam radiation therapy, which can block tumor in the perirectal area and uterosacral space. The geometric configuration of the intracavitary implant emphasizes lateral rather than posterior coverage and does not effectively treat the perirectal and uterosacral space effectively. This can lead to underdosing of tissues in this area and an increased risk of central recurrence. Higher whole pelvis external beam doses, interstitial implantation, or addition of a supplemental posterior oblique external beam boost may offer ways to compensate dose in this area (64). Given the potential for risk, some would advocate abandoning the midline block in favor of other options (74–76). Fenkell et al. (76) showed that 66.7% of patients had a greater than 50% increase in doses to the rectum, bladder (D2cc) of the sigmoid with the use of a midline block. Use of IMRT with low central doses near the bladder and rectosigmoid and higher doses covering the pelvic nodes has been described as a replacement for the more antiquated midline block (50).

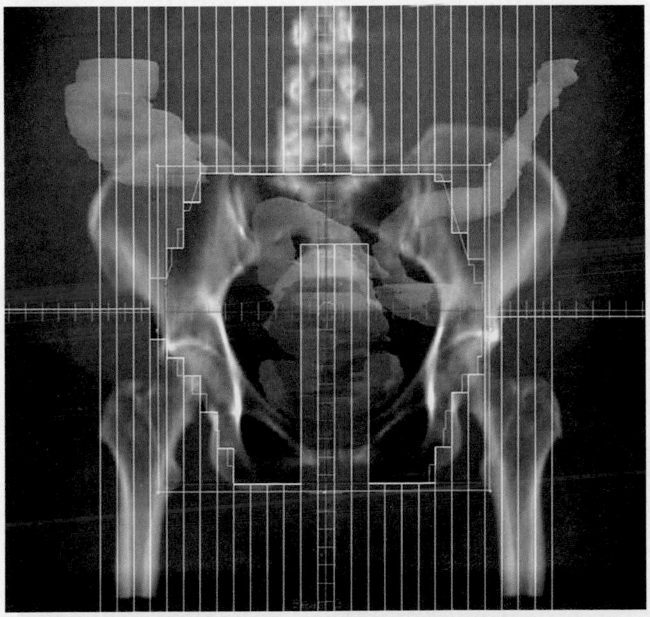

Figure 11.32. Midline blocks: A midline block defined by the leaves of the multileaf collimator used to shield the central pelvic structures. Note the unblocked bladder and sigmoid that may receive some of the brachytherapy dose and all of the external beam dose.

Parametrial/Nodal Boosting in Cervical Cancer

Parametrial boosting is often recommended for patients with bulky parametrial or sidewall disease, after completion of the whole pelvis field and midline block fields, as the parametria are a common site of failure. The need for boosting is usually based on the status of disease regression following whole pelvis irradiation. MRI may be helpful in making this assessment both before and during radiation. Logsdson and Eifel (79) suggest boosting residual lateral pelvic wall disease after 40 to 45 Gy whole pelvis to 60 to 62 Gy to small volumes. Perez et al. (80,81) found a trend toward increased pelvic control with point B doses (defined as 6 cm lateral to the central axis) >45 Gy. Perez et al. found that the incidence of pelvic recurrence was correlated with tumor size and dose of irradiation delivered to the lateral parametrium. There was an increase in the incidence of pelvic recurrence in patients receiving less than 50 Gy, but no correlation with increasing doses of irradiation (82). Doses needed to eradicate parametrial disease in the literature are typically around 60 Gy, combining the external beam doses with the implant doses. The proximity of small bowel can make this a risky proposition. Perez et al. (83) noted that with doses below 50 Gy to the lateral pelvic wall, the risk of small bowel complications was about 1% and somewhat higher with larger doses. In a later series, grade 3 small bowel sequelae were 1% with doses of 50 Gy and 2% to 4% with doses over 60 Gy ($p = 0.04$) (84). Perez et al. recommend limiting the small bowel doses to less than 60 Gy. When there is uterosacral space involvement, thought should be given to the use of a supplemental posterior oblique external beam boost (64). Grigsby et al. used PET/

CT scans to evaluate lymph node size, irradiation dose, and patterns of failure. The parametrial and lymph node boost doses used were in the range of 9.0 to 14.4 Gy following large field doses of 50.4 Gy. Radiation dose and lymph node size were not significant predicators of lymph node failure. The risk of an isolated lymph node failure was <2% (85). A reoperation series following definitive irradiation and chemotherapy was reported by Houvenaegel et al. After 45 Gy and whole pelvis and selective parametrial or nodal boosting to 55 to 60 Gy, 15.9% of patients had biopsy-proven residual disease in the pelvic nodes and 11.7% of paraaortic nodes (86). Use of IMRT may be a method to increase dose to bulky nodes or residual parametrial disease while sparing adjacent normal structures (50,87).

Endometrial Cancer

The need for postoperative external beam radiation therapy in endometrial cancer is well described in the ASTRO consensus guidelines (88). Patients with grade 3 and ≥50% myometrial invasion or grade 1 to 2, ≥50% myometrial invasion, and other risk factors such as age >60 with or without lymphovascular space invasion may benefit from pelvic external beam radiation. External beam radiation is recommended in patients with stage III–IV disease because it improves survival. Chemotherapy should also be considered in patients with locally advanced disease and delivered concurrently, sequentially, or in an interdigitated manner (88). For endometrial cancer, many of the same nodes are at risk as in cervical cancer, but the spread of disease is not as predictable with the paraaortic nodes independently at risk. The presacral nodes are also not at risk unless there is cervical involvement. Both the pelvic and paraaortic nodes are at risk in all sites of uterine involvement, and grade, myometrial invasion, and lymphatic vascular space invasion are more predictive of risk than is location (89,90). Cervical and lower uterine segment involvement increases the likelihood of pelvic and paraaortic lymph node metastases compared to fundal location, as do increasing histologic grade and myometrial invasion. In the surgical staging series of Boronow et al. (90), 18 of 222 patients had lower uterine segment involvement and 6 (33%) had pelvic lymph node metastases. In the final GOG surgical staging series report, by location, patients with fundal lesions had a 4% risk of paraaortic and 8% risk of pelvic lymph node involvement, whereas patients with lower uterine segment involvement had a 16% risk of pelvic and 14% risk of paraaortic lymph node involvement.

In endometrial cancer, external beam irradiation is generally recommended for patients thought to be at significant risk for lymph node metastases and/or a vaginal cuff recurrence. Traditionally, this has been recommended in the absence of a lymph node dissection or a limited lymph node sampling. External beam irradiation is still delivered at many institutions in the setting of a negative lymph node dissection when high-risk features such as deep myometrial invasion, high grade, lymphatic vascular space invasion, lower uterine segment involvement, or cervical invasion are present (88).

External beam irradiation typically covers the upper one-half to two-thirds of the vagina, the pelvic lymph node regions, and the surgical bed (**Fig. 11.33**). External beam field design must necessarily include the pelvic lymphatics with exclusion of as much small bowel as possible. Treatment of the patient in the prone position with a full bladder will help to exclude at least some small bowel in most patients unless these loops are fixed in the pelvis (**Fig. 11.34**). It is important, however, for the lateral fields to cover the course of the external iliac nodes, which are quite anterior in the pelvis and require inclusion of some small bowel in the lateral fields to be adequately covered. Doses of 45 to 50.4 Gy are typical, with some institutions treating to 40 Gy and as high as 60 Gy to reduced fields in the setting of nodal disease. Whole-pelvic fields are generally reduced or a midline block is added after variable doses.

Prone techniques have been used in the treatment of many other pelvic malignancies in an attempt to exclude small bowel from the field. Use of a belly board device to further enhance small bowel displacement has become standard practice in the treatment of many pelvic malignancies. Use of prone position with or without a belly board for the treatment of patients with cervical cancer has been reported in a few series, in the postoperative (91) and definitive settings (92). Prone positioning with the belly board has been used extensively for patients with rectal cancers when using a PA and two lateral fields. Concern over this technique for patients with gynecologic malignancies when adding a fourth field (AP) to cover the external iliac nodes has been raised by Ghosh et al., due to the uncertainty in source to skin distance (SSD) and variation in tissue thickness from the anterior field. In patients who underwent postoperative irradiation for cervical cancer, they observed that the small bowel was best excluded from the AP–PA fields when the patient was positioned prone without the belly board, thereby compressing the small bowel laterally out of the AP–PA fields. They recommended an alternating routine (93). Bladder distention can also help to optimally displace bowel when using the belly board (94). Concern over use of the belly board in patients treated with definitive versus postoperative irradiation for cervical cancer is also raised due to the potential change in position of the uterus when prone, the impact and variability of bladder filling, and the potential daily variation in the setup (93). CT-based dosimetry has documented that the prone position, particularly with bladder filling, can alter the position of the uterus within the radiation field (67). Hence, if patients are

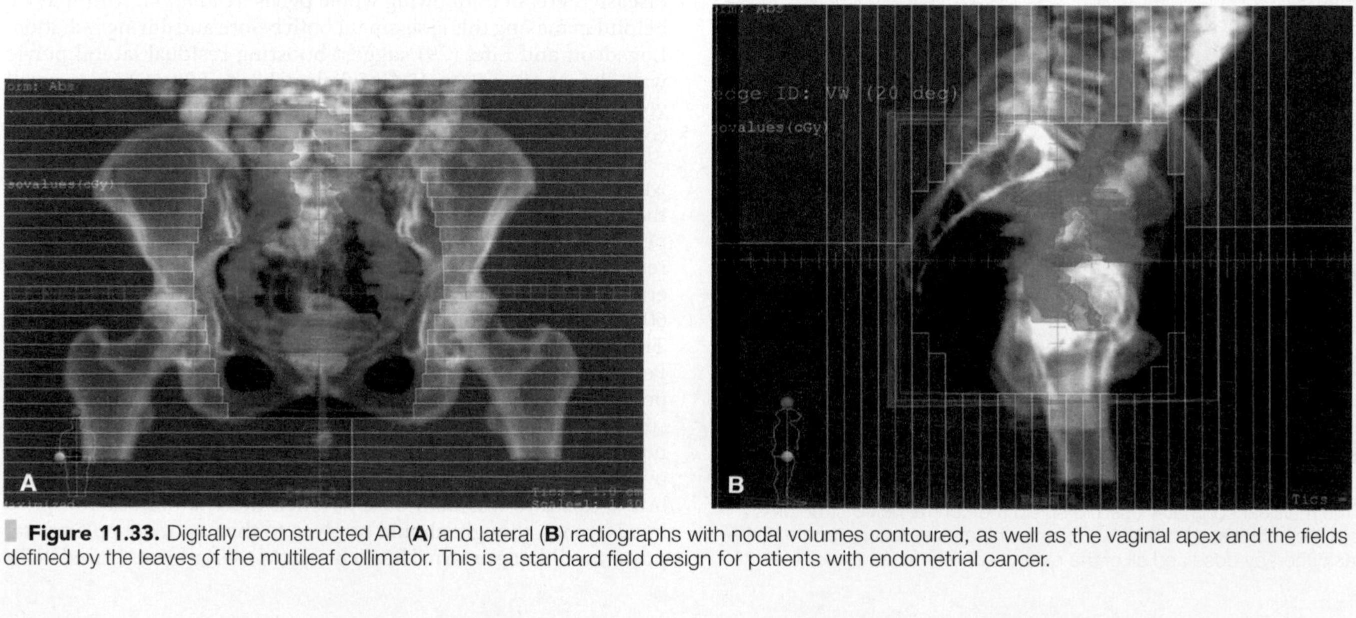

Figure 11.33. Digitally reconstructed AP (**A**) and lateral (**B**) radiographs with nodal volumes contoured, as well as the vaginal apex and the fields defined by the leaves of the multileaf collimator. This is a standard field design for patients with endometrial cancer.

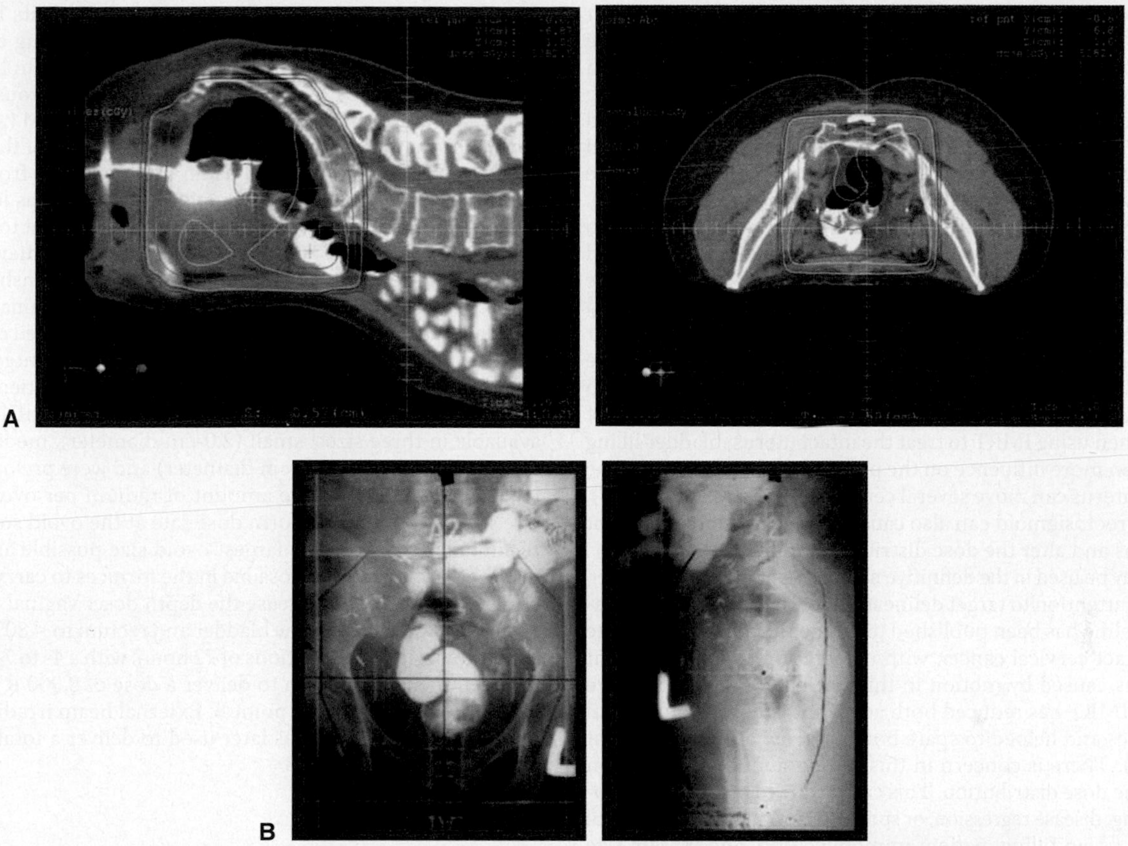

Figure 11.34. A: Utility of the prone technique for small bowel displacement as shown on a sagittal and axial CT scan of a patient with endometrial cancer planned in the prone position. B: Radiographs of the pelvis showing significant amount of small bowel in the radiation fields.

simulated prone, it is even more imperative to use CT- or MRI-based dosimetry in the prone position to make sure that the entire uterus is in the pelvic fields, and it is also imperative to consistently fill or empty the bladder (95). IGRT may also be helpful in ensuring that the daily setup is reproducible and reliable.

Extended-Field Irradiation

Extended-field irradiation refers to inclusion of both the pelvic and paraaortic nodes in the radiation fields. Common indications for extended-field irradiation in gynecologic cancers include patients with positive paraaortic nodes or those with positive pelvic nodes or bulky primary lesions feared to be at risk for microscopic paraaortic disease (**Fig. 11.35**). Extended fields include more normal organs than pelvic fields alone. Limitation of dose to the small bowel, kidneys, liver, stomach, and spinal cord are essential. Three-dimensional conformal techniques are helpful in achieving an acceptable therapeutic ratio. Use of IMRT has recently been piloted in this setting, with further attempts to decrease acute and late toxicity (**Fig. 11.20**). Selective boosting of gross nodal disease may allow for safer dose escalation (87).

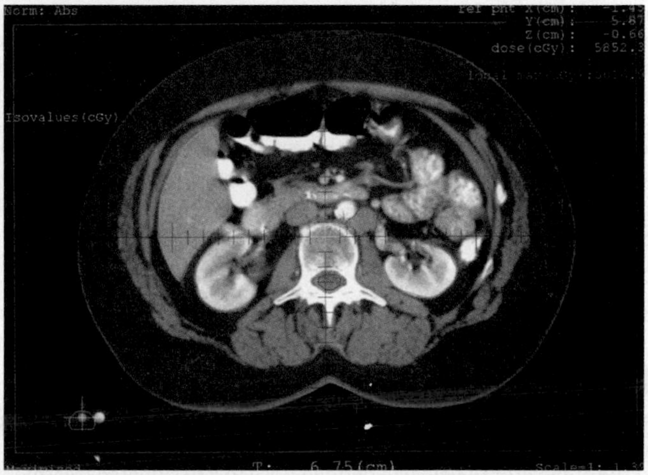

Figure 11.35. Axial CT scan demonstrating an enlarged periaortic lymph node near the left renal hilum.

Pelvic and Inguinal Irradiation

External beam fields will necessarily include the inguinal lymph nodes in patients with vulvar cancer or distal vaginal cancers, or when cancer of the cervix or endometrium involves the distal vagina. Risk of femoral head necrosis or femoral neck fractures is increased in this setting. Recent use of IMRT to treat vulvar and vaginal cancers has been published with success (96,97).

Intensity-Modulated Radiation Therapy

IMRT is an excellent treatment method for gynecologic cancers. The setting where IMRT may be the most helpful and the most widely accepted is postoperatively for select endometrial and cervical cancer presentations (98). Results of the Radiation Therapy Oncology Group (RTOG) 0418 study "A Phase II Study of Intensity-Modulated Radiation Therapy (IMRT) to the Pelvis with or without Chemotherapy for Postoperative Patients with either Endometrial or Cervical Carcinoma" showed a decrease in both acute and late toxicity in the postoperative setting in patients with either cervical or endometrial cancers (99). Other prospective and single institutional studies have confirmed this (46,100). In the postoperative setting, there is often a significant amount of small bowel in the pelvis , which can be avoided to a greater degree with IMRT than with 3-D conformal radiation techniques (**Fig. 11.22**). Bone marrow sparing can also be improved over a 3-D conformal approach (101,102). Bladder and rectosigmoid doses can be reduced. Margin sizes around the target and bladder and rectal filling are important considerations, as are immobilization techniques when using IMRT. Target delineation and normal organ delineation are extremely important when using IMRT. What is not defined is either not adequately treated, or spared (51). RTOG 0418 defined parameters for contouring of targets and normal organs, margin size, and dose volume constraints in the postoperative setting in early cervical or endometrial cancers (103). An online atlas available on the RTOG website was developed to improve consistency between multiple contouring physicians, and continues to be used to guide in target delineation even though the protocol has been completed (104). This same atlas has been used in GOG/NRG studies, which include IMRT techniques with minor modifications over time. A normal tissue-contouring atlas is available on the RTOG/NRG website (105). Other atlases are also available to guide radiation oncologists in defining these structures of interest (69,106). When using IMRT to treat the intact uterus, bladder filling can have even more influence on the position of the uterus, and the vagina and uterus can move several centimeters as a result (51,107). Stool in the rectosigmoid can also cause movement of the adjacent pelvic organs and alter the dose distribution in the rectosigmoid.

IMRT may be used in the definitive management of cervical cancer, with careful attention to target delineation as well as motion. A consensus guideline has been published to define the most appropriate CTV for intact cervical cancer, with recognition of the significant uncertainties caused by motion in this setting (108). Studies have shown that IMRT has reduced both acute and late gastrointestinal (GI) toxicities and helped to spare bone marrow during treatment (50,102,109). There is concern in this setting about organ motion relative to the dose distribution. This can be due to bladder or rectosigmoid filling, disease regression, or sporadic motion (43,110). Careful attention to organ filling, patient immobilization, and margin size can help to minimize such motion, which could compromise target and normal organ doses (42). Daily CT imaging prior to treatment can also help to assess for this motion and adapt the treatment plan as needed. Use of IMRT for extended-field irradiation to treat the pelvic and paraaortic region is successfully implemented to decrease dose to the small bowel, kidneys, liver, spinal cord, and bone marrow (**Fig. 11.20**). Selective boosting of gross nodal disease may allow for safer dose escalation (87,111). IMRT techniques have also been used for vulvar cancers to help spare the upper femur as well as the small bowel and bone marrow (47,96,97).

Brachytherapy Systems for the Treatment of Cervical Cancer

Brachytherapy is essential in the treatment of many gynecologic cancers. Intracavitary brachytherapy for cervical carcinoma was profoundly impacted by the development of various "systems" that attempted to combine empiricism with a more scientific and systematic approach. A dosimetric system refers to a set of rules concerning a specific applicator type, radioactive isotope, and distribution of the sources in the applicator to deliver a defined dose to a designated treatment region (55). Within any system, specification of treatment in terms of dose, timing, and administration is necessary to implement the prescription in a consistent manner. Three systems were developed in Europe, including the Paris, Stockholm, and Manchester system (112–114). The Manchester system principles are an integral part of modern brachytherapy (114).

The Manchester System

The Manchester system was developed in 1932 by Tod and Meredith (114) and was later modified in 1953 (115) at the Holt Radium Institute. It standardized treatment with predetermined doses and dose rates directed at fixed points in the pelvis. The fixed points A and B were selected on the theory that the dose in the paracervical triangle impacted normal tissue tolerance rather than the actual doses to the bladder, rectum, and vagina. The paracervical triangle was described as a pyramidal-shaped area with its base resting on the lateral vaginal fornices and its apex curving around with the anteverted uterus. "Point A" was defined as 2 cm lateral to the central canal of the uterus and 2 cm from the mucous membrane of the lateral fornix in the axis of the uterus (**Fig. 11.36**). It often correlates anatomically with the point of crossage of the ureter and uterine artery and was taken as an average point from which to assess dose in the paracervical region. "Point B" was located 5 cm from midline at the level of point A, and was thought to correspond to the location of the obturator lymph nodes. To achieve consistent dose rates, a set of strict rules dictating the relationship, position, and activity of radium sources in the uterine and vaginal applicators was devised. The amount of radium would vary based on ovoid size and uterine length such that the same dose in roentgen would be delivered to point A regardless of the size of the patient or the size and shape of the tumor, uterus, and vagina. The vaginal ovoids were available in three sizes: small (2.0-cm diameter), medium (2.5-cm diameter), and large (3.0-cm diameter) and were preloaded or "hot loaded" with radium. The amount of radium per ovoid varied by size so as to obtain a uniform dose rate at the ovoid surface. It was recommended to use the largest ovoid size possible and place the ovoids as far laterally as possible in the fornices to carry the radium closer to point B and increase the depth dose. Vaginal packing was used to limit the dose to the bladder and rectum to <80% of point A. Two intracavitary applications of 72 hours with a 4- to 7-day interval between them were given to deliver a dose of 8,000 R at 55.5 R/hr to point A and 3,000 R to point B. External beam irradiation with a midline block in place was later used to deliver a total cumulative dose of 6,000 R to point B.

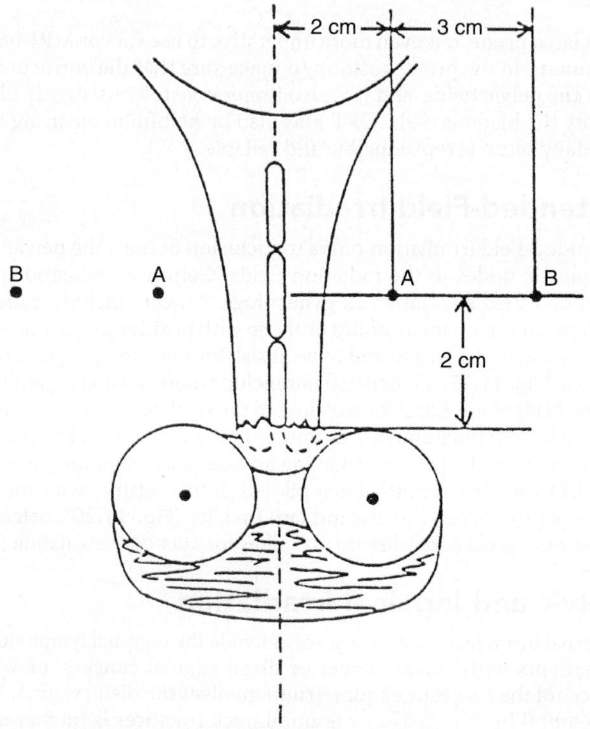

Figure 11.36. The Manchester system. Definitions of points A and B in the classical Manchester system are found in the text. In a typical application, the loading of intrauterine applicators varied: between 20 and 35 mg of radium and between 15 and 25 mg of radium for each vaginal ovoid. The resultant treatment time to deliver 8,000 R at point A was 140 hours.

Source: From Meredith WJ. *Radium Dosage: The Manchester System.* Edinburgh, UK: Livingstone; 1967, with permission.

The Manchester system is the basis for contemporary intracavitary techniques and dose specification. With current LDR applications using cesium rather than radium, it is considered standard to have a point A dose rate of 50 to 60 cGy/hr and to deliver a total dose of 85 Gy to point A and 60 Gy to point B when combined with external beam therapy while limiting the normal tissues to <80% of the point A dose.

The Fletcher (M.D. Anderson) System

The Fletcher system was established at M.D. Anderson Hospital in the 1940s (116). The Fletcher applicator was subsequently developed and remains an integral part of gynecologic brachytherapy (**Fig. 11.37**) (117). The initial dosimetric work at M.D. Anderson was done prior to the development of computerized dosimetry in the 1960s as in the Paris system; milligram-hours (mg-hr) was used for dose prescription with the premise that with any geometric arrangement of specified sources, dose at any point is proportional to the amount of radioactivity and the implant duration. Though previous systems (Paris and Stockholm) had used mg-hr, clinical experience alone determined the amount of radium tolerable to the tissues. Fletcher et al. (118) predicted that better results and less morbidity could be obtained if knowledge of the energy absorbed at various points in the pelvis ("measured data") such as the bladder and rectum and pelvic lymph nodes could be determined. According to Fletcher, a dosimetric approach should meet the following requirements: (a) ensure that the primary disease in the cervix and fornices and immediate extensions into the paracervical triangle are adequately treated; (b) guide treatments in such a way that the bladder and rectum are not overdosed (respect mucosal tolerance); and (c) determine the dose received by the various lymph node groups. Individualization to fit the anatomical situation was an essential aspect of this system.

The primary prescription parameter in the Fletcher system was tumor volume, and prescription rules were based on maximum mg-hrs and maximum time, taking into account the total external beam dose and the calculated sigmoid dose. An application was left in place until either of these two maximums was reached. Large mg-hr implants were halted by the mg-hr prescription while smaller mg-hr implants were terminated by time. A set of maxima of mg-hrs was established for combinations with external irradiation, which were published in tables (119,120). Standardized source arrangements and limits on the vaginal surface dose and mg-hrs were all used to help specify treatment.

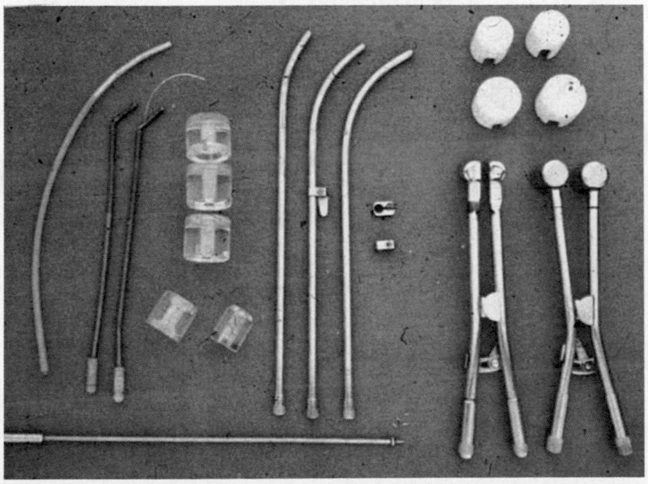

Figure 11.37. Fletcher-Suit-Delclos LDR applicators. **Left to right:** Afterloading colpostats, mini-ovoids, tandems, cylinders, and source inserters.

Source: Reprinted with permission from Fletcher GH, ed. *Textbook of Radiotherapy*. 3rd Ed. Philadelphia, PA: Lea & Febiger; 1980:741.

Despite a more elaborate dosimetry system, the Fletcher system combined many elements of the Paris and Manchester systems, including using the largest size ovoid possible, positioned as far laterally and cephalad as possible, to deliver the highest tumor dose at depth for a given mucosal dose. By using a larger ovoid, the radium–mucous membrane distance was increased, allowing a greater increase in the total number of mg-hrs and a greater volume of adequate irradiation (116). The Fletcher colpostats were actually a further evolution of the Manchester ovoids and were made with the same diameters of 2, 2.5, and 3 cm but were more cylindrical than Manchester "ovoids" and were attached to handles, with shielding in the direction of the bladder and rectum. Initially these were preloaded with radium, but later an afterloading model was developed and loaded instead with ^{137}Cs (121). Recommended loadings were 15, 20, and 25 mg of radium for the 2-, 2.5-, and 3-cm colpostats, respectively, and 5 to 10 mg for the mini-ovoids (122). As in earlier systems, it was also recommended that the longest tandem available be used and loaded so that sources reached the uterine fundus in order to provide an adequate distribution in the lower uterine segment and paracervical areas, and to increase the dose to the obturator lymph nodes. Additionally, a high position of the applicator in the pelvis and a wide separation of the ovoids were thought to increase the dose to the pelvic wall. Tight packing was also recommended to displace the system upward and centrally and to decrease the dose to the bladder and rectum (116). Recommended tandem loadings were usually 15, 10, and 10 mg of radium, with the amount of radium in the tandem usually greater than that in the ovoids. The distal source in the tandem was to be positioned to produce an even pear-shaped dose distribution with no drop in dose rate between the tandem and ovoids, without excessive overlap that would result in a hot spot on the adjacent bladder or rectal mucosa. With the ovoids well positioned, this was usually accomplished by placing the physical end of the distal source at or a few millimeters beyond the external os of the cervix. A 10-mg protruding source was recommended if the vaginal ovoids were separated by more than 5 cm or displaced caudally, with each ovoid then decreased by 5 mg.

A careful review of implant films was outlined (**Fig. 11.38**). It was recommended to keep the tandem in the axis of the pelvis, equidistant from the sacral promontory and pubis and the lateral pelvic walls, to avoid overdosage to the bladder, sigmoid, or one ureter. The tandem was recommended to bisect the ovoids on the AP films and bisect their height on the lateral films. The flange of the tandem was to be flush against the cervix and the ovoids surrounding it, verified by confirming the proximity of the applicators to radiopaque cervical seeds. Radiopaque vaginal packing was used to hold the system in place and displace the bladder and rectum. Scrutiny of implant films prior to treatment remains an important tenet of brachytherapy. Two or more intracavitary insertions were thought to make more efficient use of the inverse square law such that the second and third implants would deliver intense radiation to the tumor periphery because of interval tumor regression. A recent retrospective review of implant geometry has confirmed the consistency of the M.D. Anderson approach and the good outcomes achieved when attention is paid to applicator position in the pelvis (123).

The M.D. Anderson approach to treatment specification reflects a policy of treating advanced cervical carcinoma to normal tissue tolerance (124). This includes integrating standard loadings and mg-hrs with calculated doses to the bladder, rectum, sigmoid, and vaginal surface. The activity in the ovoids is limited by the vaginal surface dose, which is kept below 140 Gy. Calculated bladder and rectal doses are noted and are sometimes used to limit the duration of the intracavitary system, with the combined external beam and implant doses for the bladder kept at <75 to 80 Gy and for the rectum at <70 to 75 Gy. Mg-Ra-eq-hrs are usually limited to 6,000 to 6,500 after 40 to 45 Gy external beam. Though mg-hrs have usually been used to guide and report doses at M.D. Anderson, recent retrospective reviews have also reported point doses, though these have not been used to plan or prescribe treatment. With the implant loadings and durations outlined by Fletcher, typical dose rates at point A are approximately 57 cGy/hour and vaginal surface dose rates are

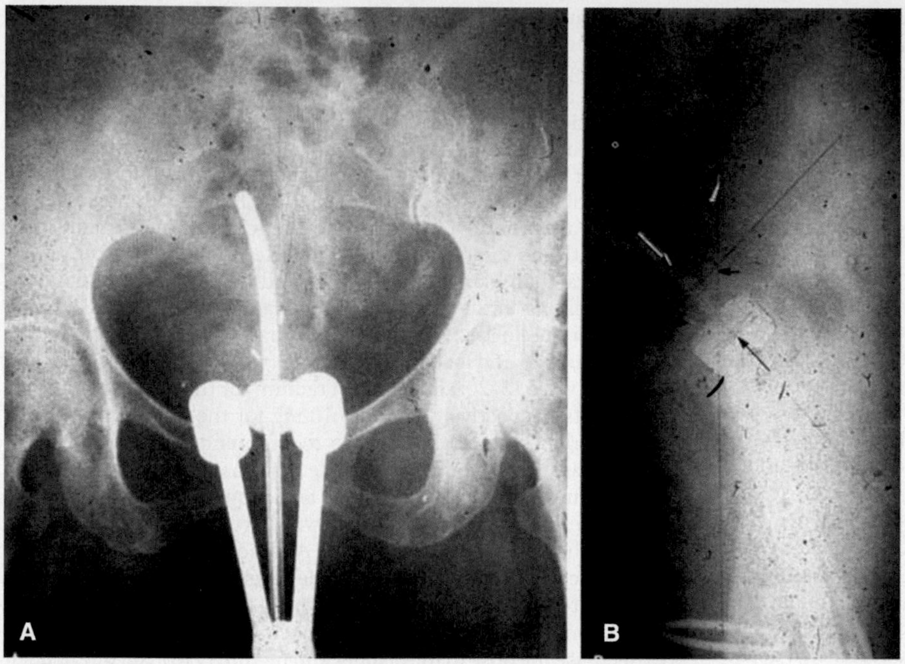

Figure 11.38. Ideal position of tandem and ovoid applicator on an AP radiograph (**A**) and on a lateral radiograph (**B**). Note the metallic seeds inserted into the cervix.

Source: Reprinted with permission from Fletcher GH, ed. *Textbook of Radiotherapy*. 3rd Ed. Philadelphia, PA: Lea & Febiger; 1980:745.

100 cGy/hour (79,123). The median doses to point B and to the International Commission on Radiation Units and Measurements (ICRU) rectal and bladder reference points averaged 28%, 59%, and 60% of the point A doses, respectively. The median total dose to point A from external beam and intracavitary irradiation was 87 Gy, and the median doses to the bladder and rectum were 68 and 70 Gy. The total dose delivered to the vaginal surface was limited to 120 to 140 Gy or 1.4 to 2.0 times the point A dose. These total doses to point A and the vagina, bladder, and rectum are used as contemporary guidelines for determining implant duration and, therefore, dose.

Point A Redefined

The failure of localization radiographs to show the surfaces of the ovoids made implementation of the initial definition of point A difficult. The definition of point A was modified in 1953 to be "2 cm up from the lower end of the intrauterine source and 2 cm laterally in the plane of the uterus, as the external os was assumed to be at the level of the vaginal fornices" (**Fig. 11.39**) (115). This definition of point A is currently used at many institutions (125,126). A seed or marker ball placed near the exocervix and coincident with the tandem flange is used to identify the exocervix on the localization films. This definition, however, becomes problematic when the cervix protrudes between the ovoids (**Fig. 11.40**). This causes a resultant increase in dose rate at point A because point A lies in the higher dose "bulge" around the ovoids (127). The variation of point A often occurs in a high-gradient region of the isodose distribution. A consistent location for dose specification should fall sufficiently superior to the ovoids where the dose distribution runs parallel to the tandem (**Fig. 11.41**). In patients with deep vaginal fornices, reverting to use of the ovoid surface rather than the exocervix can help to solve this problem (127).

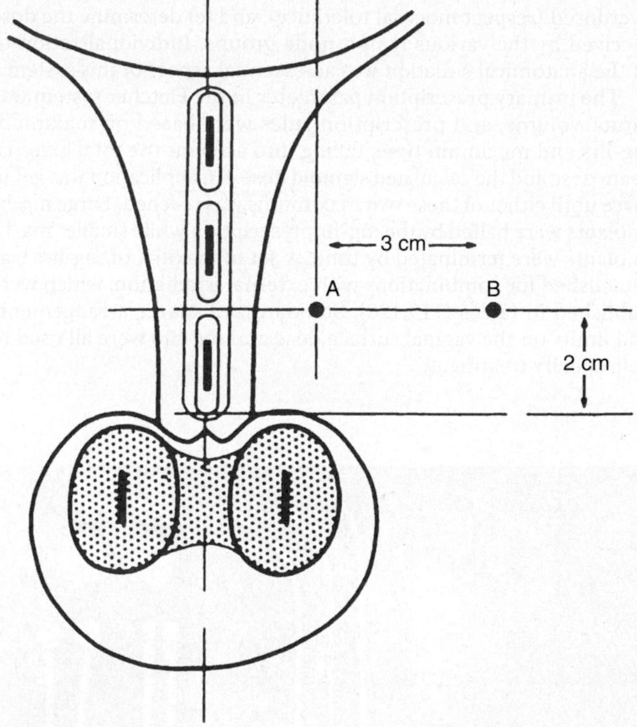

Figure 11.39. Revised Manchester system definition of point A.

Source: From Morita K. Cancer of the cervix. In: Vahrson HW, ed. *Radiation Oncology of Gynecologic Cancers*. 1st Ed. Berlin, Heidelberg: Springer-Verlag; 1997:185, with permission.

Limitations of Brachytherapy Systems: Point A

It has become clear over time that points A and B are not anatomic sites. The actual specification is related to the position of the intracavitary sources rather than to an anatomical structure. Lewis et al. also demonstrated that point A does not maintain a constant relationship to any specific structure and its position varies with the type of applicator, individual tumor anatomy, and age of the patient. No correlation was found between point B and the pelvic wall (128,129). Potish also questions the validity of point A, as its position bears no fixed relationship to tumor or normal tissue anatomy, and is in a steep dose gradient and sensitive to displacement (130). Point A can be identical for implants that differ in fundamental ways and deliver different overall 3-D dose distributions.

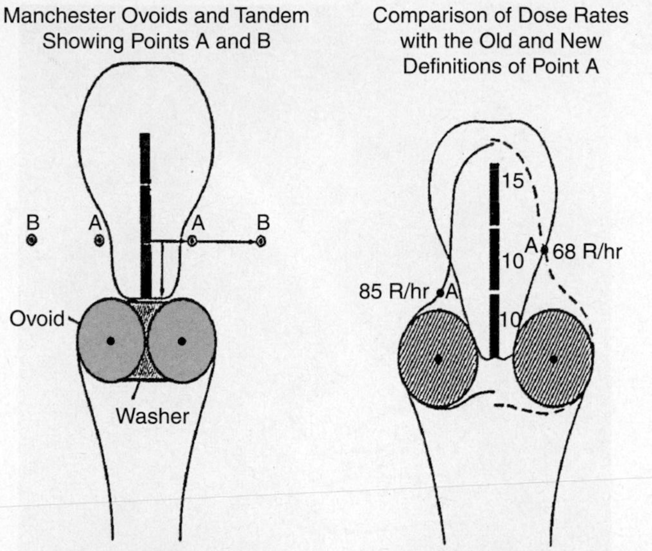

Figure 11.40. The definition of point A using the revised Manchester definition becomes problematic when the cervix protrudes between the ovoids, causing an increase in dose rate at point A. Use of the classical Manchester definition of point A (point A defined from the level of the upper vaginal fornices rather than the location of the exocervix) may be helpful.

Source: Reprinted with permission from Batley F, Constable WC. The use of the Manchester system for treatment of cancer of the uterine cervix with modern afterloading radium applicators. *Am J Roentgenol Rad Ther*. 1967;18:397.

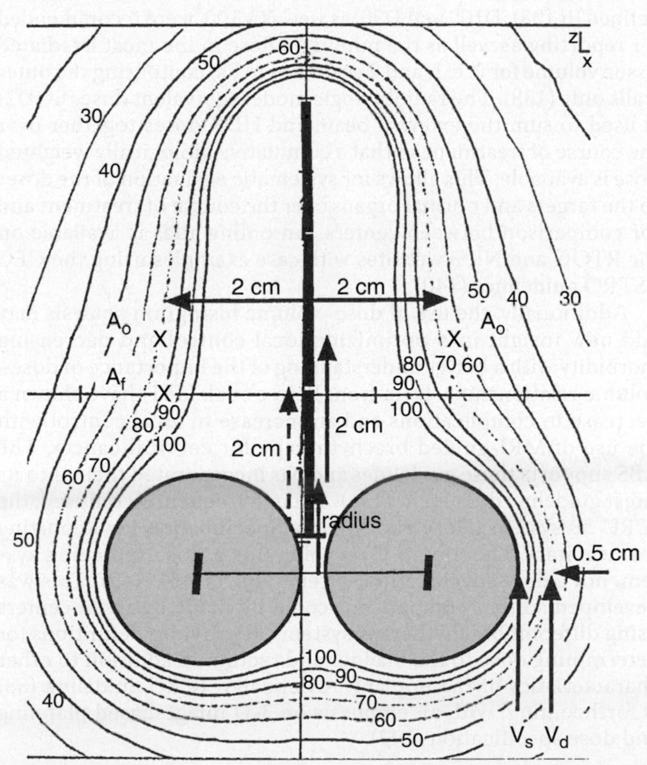

Figure 11.41. Variations of point A based on definition. A consistent location for dose specification should fall superior to the ovoids, where the dose distribution runs parallel to the tandem and not close to bulge of the pear.

Source: Reprinted with permission from Nag S, Chao C, Erickson B, et al. American Brachytherapy Society recommendations for low-dose rate brachytherapy for carcinoma of the cervix. *Int J Radiat Oncol Biol Phys*. 2002;52(1):38.

Limitations of Brachytherapy Systems: mg-hr Systems

The use of mg-hr systems at many institutions also continues to guide the choice of source strength and duration of the implant, estimate the risk of complications, compare treatment between patients and institutions, and estimate efficacy (131). In the past, little attempt was made to obtain dose information to anatomical structures, and mg-hr prescriptions were not necessarily accompanied by isodose distributions, so that the dose prescription was not related to patient anatomy.

Contemporary Dose Specification for Cervical Cancer

With LDR brachytherapy, the basic principle of 2-D film-based intracavitary prescription is to leave a specific loading of sources in for a definite time, determined by empirical experience, prescription rules, and computerized dosimetry which provides the dose at several anatomic points and isodose distributions (**Fig. 11.42**). The intracavitary dose is based on the extent of disease and is altered if computer calculations indicated high doses to surrounding critical structures. The rectum and bladder are viewed as tolerance points, compared to point A, which is a treatment dose specification point (57). A combination of both mg-hrs and point doses is used at some institutions to guide implant duration (127). Though these definitions vary from institution to institution, most will attempt to quantify doses in the paracervical region (point A), and at either point B or the pelvic wall (C or E), and the rectum and bladder (57,125,126). Although intracavitary point dose calculations are not recorded as often for the sigmoid, vaginal mucosa, or cervix, dose evaluation at these points is also helpful. Maruyama et al. (132) defined a point T (tumor dose) located 1 cm above the cervical marker and 1 cm lateral to the tandem, which is usually two to three times the dose at point A. Vaginal surface dose rates, defined at the lateral ovoid surface, will vary based on applicator diameter and available source strengths and should be in the range of 1.4 to 2.0 (the point A dose) (123,133).

It has become clear that 2-D orthogonal film-based dose distribution analysis, in which single or multiple reference points are chosen on films at the interface of the organs closest to the applicators and at select dose specification points, is inadequate for gynecologic brachytherapy. Single tumor reference points such as point A, chosen from localization films, do not give sufficient information about the dose distribution throughout the tumor volume. Nor do the reference points for the bladder and rectosigmoid accurately reflect the dose distribution within these organs. Additionally, there is no recognition of the volume of tumor and normal tissues receiving these doses (51). With the advent of MRI- and CT-compatible applicators and the presence of CT simulators and MR scanners in radiation oncology departments, as well as DICOM image transfer from scanners to treatment planning systems, 3-D image–guided brachytherapy is becoming the standard. Image-based brachytherapy entails defining both the disease and the OAR and then shaping the dose distribution to optimally cover disease and exclude the normal tissues (**Fig. 11.43**) (51,134,135). Directly relating the intracavitary system to the anatomy through use of CT and MRI is the next step in the lineage of dosimetric systems. The American Brachytherapy Society (ABS) has been pivotal in developing guidelines for the treatment of gynecologic cancers, with a special emphasis on image-based techniques (57,136).

CT is excellent for delineating the normal pelvic organs, but poor in defining tumor in the cervix or vagina. With CT-based computerized dosimetry, rectosigmoid and bladder doses can more accurately be determined than with localization films. Even when using CT-compatible applicators, however, the boundaries between structures of interest are poorly defined (134). The value of MR in the imaging of gynecologic cancers lies in its multiplanar capability and superior soft tissue resolution, compared to CT, enabling

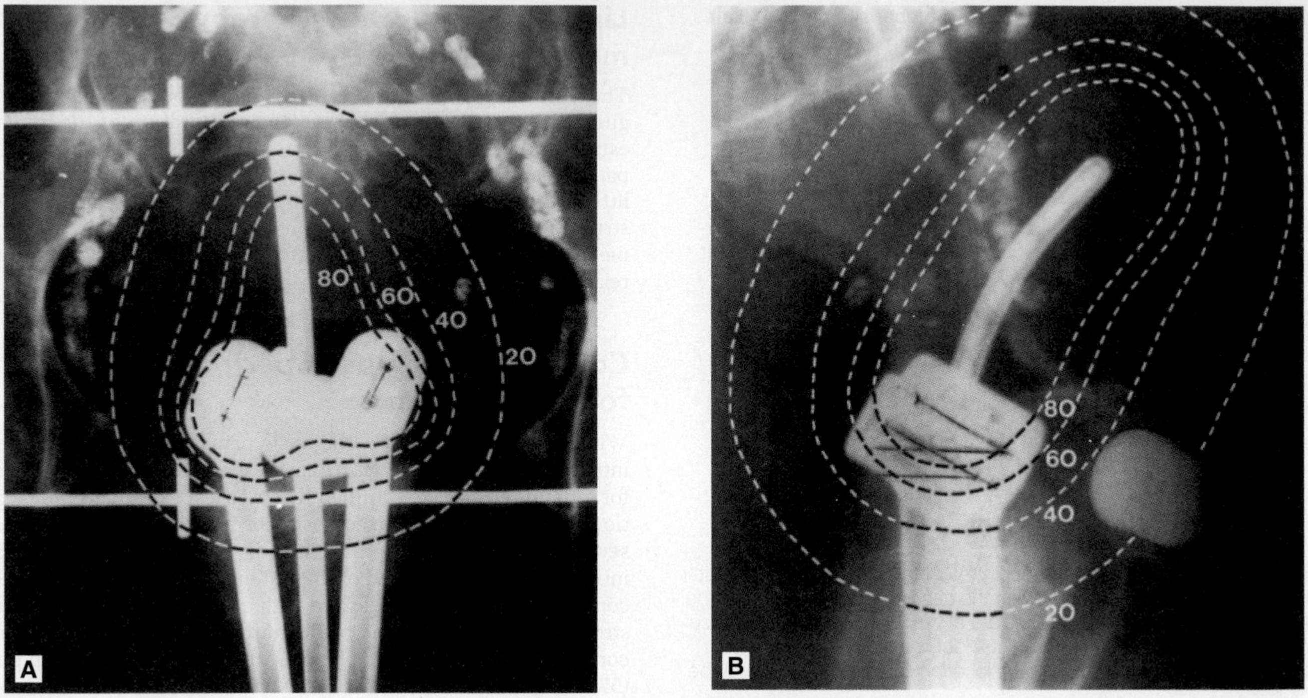

Figure 11.42. A: AP view of intracavitary insertion for carcinoma of the uterine cervix. **B:** Lateral view of same implant. Isodose curves (cGy/hr) are superimposed.

Source: From Perez CA, Grigsby PW, Williamson JF. Clinical applications of brachytherapy. I: Low dose-rate. In: Perez CA, Brady LW, eds. *Principles and Practice of Radiation Oncology*. 3rd Ed. Philadelphia, PA: Lippincott-Raven Publishers; 1998:487, with permission.

delineation of tumor within the cervix, uterus, and vagina as well as within the parametrial and vaginal tissues (134,137). Tumors of the cervix display moderately increased signal on T2-weighted images relative to normal cervical stroma, permitting definition of tumor volume. This is an advantage during brachytherapy, as one can assess the proximity of the tumor to the applicator and the subsequent dose distribution throughout the tumor volume. The excellent soft tissue resolution of MRI allows visualization of residual tumor in relation to the isodose distribution around the MRI-compatible brachytherapy applicators (**Fig. 11.44**) (134,137,138). The dose distribution can then be optimally conformed to the defined target volume while accurately defining and limiting the dose to the adjacent normal OAR. The Gyn GEC ESTRO working group began to develop guidelines for recording and reporting 3-D image-based treatment planning for cervical cancer brachytherapy in 2000. The guidelines were published in 2005, and described a methodology using MRI at the time of brachytherapy to define the GTV and CTV (5,139). The gross tumor volume (GTV) at the time of brachytherapy was defined as residual tumor following external beam on clinical examination, as well as the high-signal regions on T2 fast spin echo (FSE) images in the cervix and paracervical tissues. The high-risk clinical target volume (HRCTV) included the GTV as well as the entire cervix and the extracervical tumor spread at the time of brachytherapy. The "high-risk" volume refers to tissues with a major risk of local recurrence because of residual macroscopic disease, which require a high dose of radiation, similar to that delivered traditionally to point A. The intermediate-risk CTV (IRCTV) was defined as encompassing the HRCTV with a margin of 5 to 15 mm, and refers to tissues carrying a significant microscopic tumor load. Doses of approximately 60 Gy are intended for this volume. With these different regions of risk defined according to physical examination and MR at the time of brachytherapy, dose volume parameters were defined for the GTV, HRCTV, IRCTV, and the OAR. For the rectum, contouring included the outer wall from the anorectal junction to the rectosigmoid flexure, and the sigmoid contour continued alone until the sigmoid was approximately 2 cm from the uterus. The small bowel was contoured only if within 2 cm of the uterus. The outer contours of the bladder were also defined (5,138). D100 and D90, as well as V100, were recommended for reporting as well as the minimum dose in the most irradiated tissue volume for 0.1, 1, and 2 cc of the OARs, contouring the outer walls only (138). The radiobiologic model equivalent dose (EQD2) is used to sum the external beam and HDR doses together over the course of treatment so that a cumulative biologically weighted dose is available. This allows for systematic evaluation of the doses to the targets and normal organs over the course of treatment and for comparison between centers. An online atlas is available on the RTOG and NRG websites with case examples using the GEC ESTRO guidelines (140).

Additionally, the use of dose–volume histogram analysis may add new insight into optimizing local control and decreasing morbidity with a better understanding of the importance of dose–volume relationships. Data from Potter et al. (141) have shown a decrease in complications and an increase in local control with the use of MRI-guided brachytherapy for cervical cancer. The ABS supports these guidelines and has incorporated them into its latest guideline document (136). Though frequently confused, the ICRU 38 system (Dose and Volume Specification for Reporting Intracavitary Therapy in Gynecology) is a dose reporting system, not a dose specification system (**Fig. 11.45**) (142). This was developed so that comparisons could be made between centers using different brachytherapy systems. It provides definitions for determining dose to the bladder and rectum in addition to other characteristics of the implant. An updated ICRU guideline (88) is forthcoming, with an emphasis on 3-D image-based planning and dose specification (142).

Importance of Brachytherapy in Cervical Cancer

When curative treatment is planned, the standard of care for patients with cervical carcinoma treated with definitive irradiation is a combination of external beam irradiation and brachytherapy (143–145). As revealed in the Quality Research in

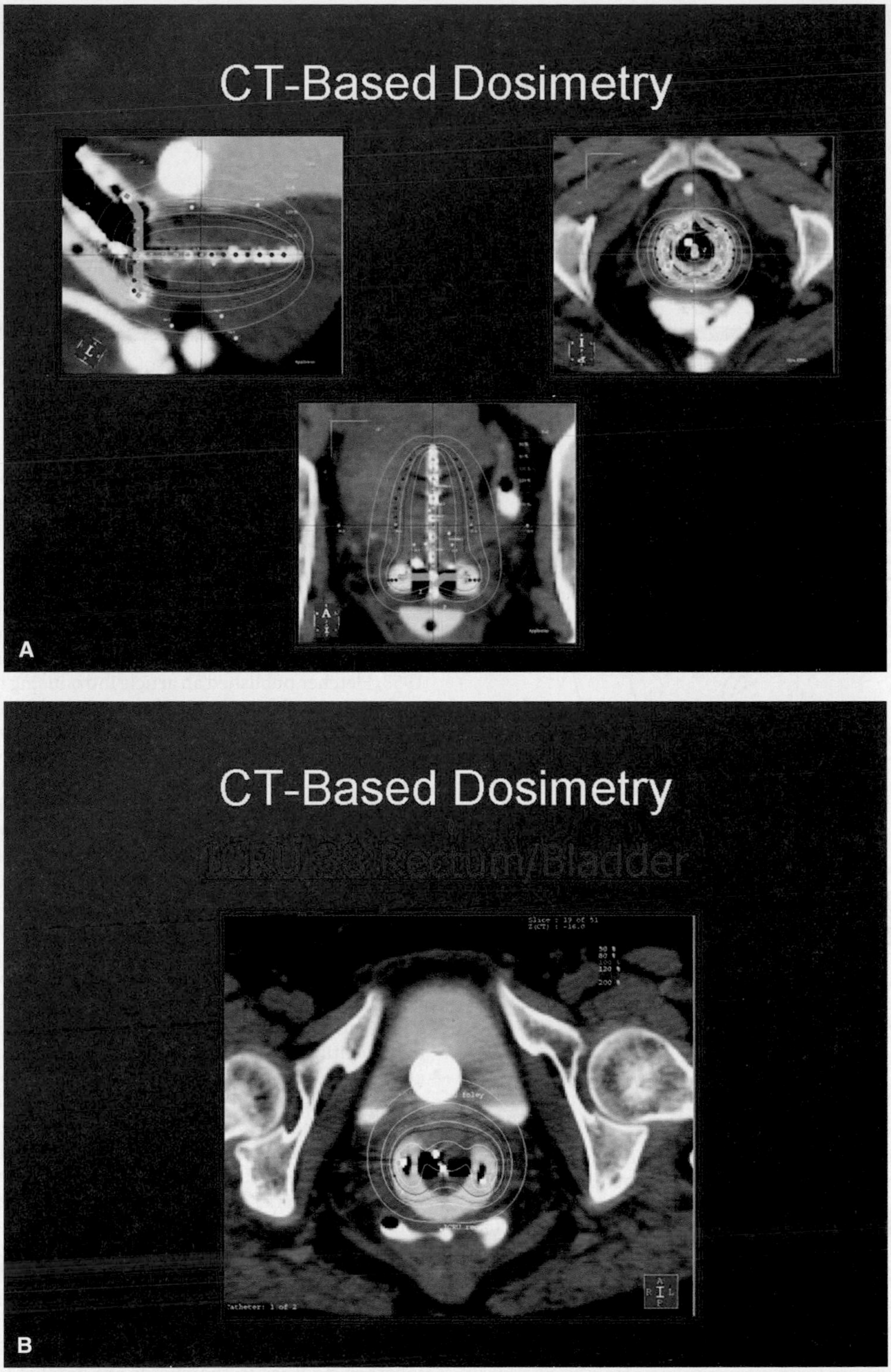

Figure 11.43. A: Sagittal, coronal, and axial CT images with MRI/CT-compatible applicator in place showing the isodose distribution around the applicator and within the surrounding tissues. **B:** Axial CT at the level of the Foley catheter bulb near the traditional ICRU 38 bladder and rectal points. Contrast is present within the bladder and rectum as well as the bladder catheter bulb.

Radiation Oncology (former Patterns of Care Studies [PCS]) and retrospective series, recurrences and complications are decreased when brachytherapy is used in addition to external beam (79,80, 143–145). Retrospective series with external beam alone have demonstrated marginal outcomes with this approach (146,147). Common reasons for avoidance of brachytherapy include inability to negotiate the endocervical canal or poor performance status. Inability to negotiate the endocervical canal should be rare with the use of intraoperative ultrasound, and when this occurs, interstitial implantation is a much better option. Even with IMRT and the ability to customize and escalate the dose to specific volumes, brachytherapy cannot be replaced (134,147). The efficacy of brachytherapy is attributable to the ability of radioactive implants to deliver a higher concentrated radiation dose more precisely to tissues than external beam alone, by treating from the "inside out" due to the close proximity of the radioactive source(s) to the

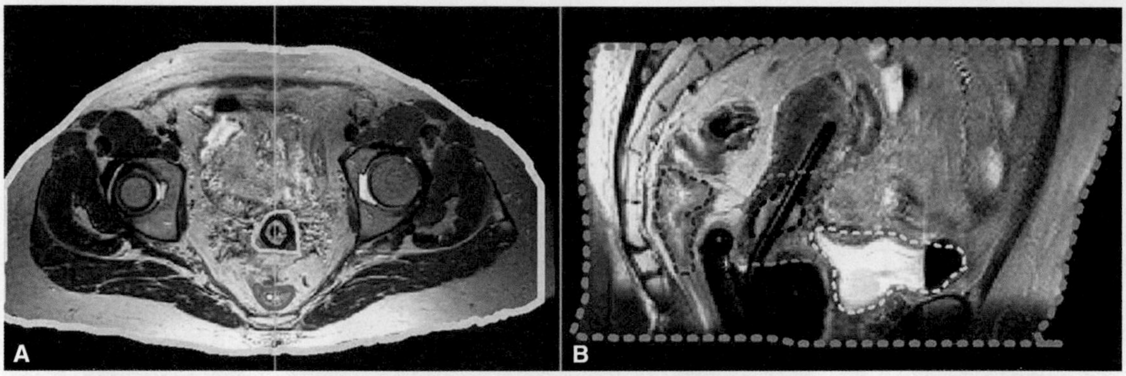

Figure 11.44. Axial (**A**) and sagittal (**B**) MRI images with MRI-compatible applicator in place with contours of the GTV and HRCTV as well as the rectum, sigmoid, and bladder.

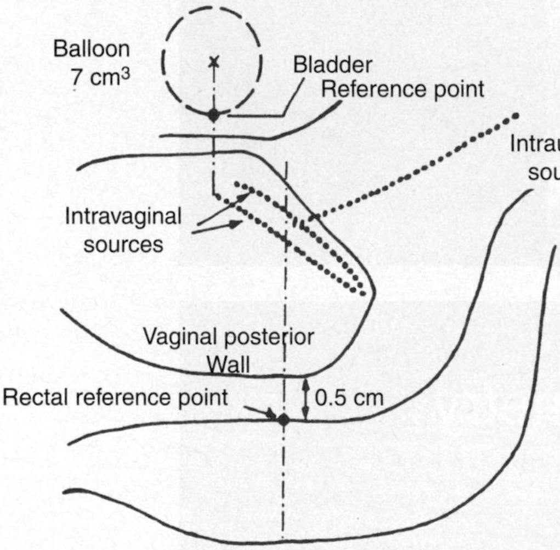

Figure 11.45. Reference points for bladder and rectal brachytherapy doses proposed by the ICRU.

Source: From Commission on Radiation Units and Measurements. Report 38: Dose and Volume Specification for Reporting Intracavitary Therapy in Gynecology. Bethesda, MD: International Commission on Radiation Units; 1985:11, Reprinted with permission of the International Commission on Radiation Units and Measurements, http://ICRU.org.

tumor, which contributes to improved local control and survival. At the same time, surrounding healthy tissues such as the bladder and rectosigmoid are relatively spared due to the rapid fall-off of dose around the applicators with distance. With IMRT, dose will necessarily be distributed in the surrounding normal tissues as it makes its way to the cervix, as the dose is delivered from the "outside in." The external beam component of treatment is, however, very important because it addresses tissues at a distance from the brachytherapy applicator, such as the pelvic lymph nodes. The external beam also brings about tumor regression in intact cervical and vaginal cancers such that the residual tissue is brought within the range of the pear-shaped or cylindrical-shaped radiation dose distribution around standard applicators (53,54).

Brachytherapy Applicators

Given the significance of brachytherapy, it is important to select the appropriate applicator to accommodate patient anatomy and the disease, and shape the associated isodose distribution to encompass the disease entirely. Tumor volume and patient anatomy are key in this decision. Tumor size and shape are variable, and there is a multitude of applicators available to address these diverse presentations.

Intracavitary Applicators: Cervical Cancer

Low Dose Rate

There are various LDR applicators available for intracavitary brachytherapy (54). The best known are the Fletcher-Suit and Henschke tandem and ovoid (colpostat) applicators (**Fig. 11.37**). In 1953, Fletcher published an article introducing his preloaded radium applicator, which was designed to produce the largest possible volume of adequate radiation in each of the common directions of spread of disease—the uterine body, parametria, and paravaginal tissues—with relative sparing of the bladder trigone and anterior rectum due to the addition of shielding (116,117). The applicator was modified in the 1960s for afterloading (Fletcher-Suit applicator) (121) and in the 1970s to accommodate ^{137}Cs sources (121). In the 1970s, the Delclos mini-ovoid was developed for use in narrow vaginal vaults (**Fig. 11.37**) (122). The mini-colpostats have a diameter of 1.6 cm and a flat inner surface. The mini-ovoids do not have additional shielding inside the colpostat, and this together with their smaller diameter produces a higher surface dose than regular ovoids, with resultant higher doses to the rectum and bladder. Appropriate source strength and treatment duration adjustment are important considerations in preventing complications. Fletcher tandems are available in four curvatures, with the greatest curvature used for cavities measuring >6 cm and lesser curvatures used for smaller cavities (**Fig. 11.37**). A flange with keel is added to the tandem once the uterine canal is sounded, which approximates the exocervix and defines the length of source train needed. The keel prevents rotation of the tandem after packing. The distal end of the tandem near the cap is marked so that rotation of the tandem after insertion can be assessed. PDR-adapted applicators are also available but are much more like HDR applicators than their LDR equivalents (61).

The Henschke tandem and ovoid applicator was initially unshielded (128) but later modified with rectal and bladder shielding (148). It consists of hemispheroidal ovoids with the ovoids and tandem fixed together. Sources in the ovoids are parallel to the sources in the uterine tandem. The Henschke applicator may be easier to insert into shallow vaginal fornices compared to Fletcher ovoids.

The Fletcher-Suit-Delclos tandem and cylinder applicator was designed to accommodate narrow vaginas where ovoids may be contraindicated and to treat varying lengths of the vagina when mandated by vaginal spread of disease (122). The cylinders vary in size from 2 to 5 cm to accommodate varying vaginal sizes (**Fig. 11.37**). A narrow vagina poses a therapeutic challenge (149). Use of vaginal cylinders may lead to a higher rate of local failure as the dose to the lateral cervix and pelvic sidewall is reduced in the absence of ovoids, which produce the optimum pear-shaped distribution. These patients also tend to receive lower total doses due to the proximity of the rectum and bladder (**Fig. 11.46**) (124).

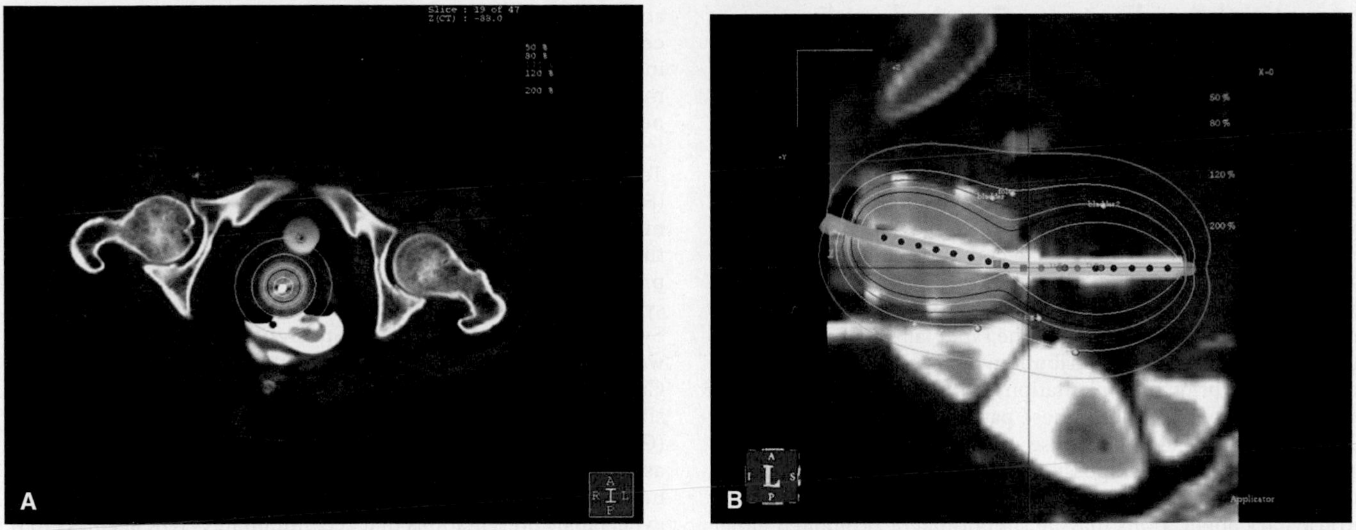

Figure 11.46. MRI/CT-compatible tandem and cylinder applicator with associated isodose distribution in axial (**A**) and sagittal (**B**) views demonstrating the close proximity to the rectum due to the absence of packing or rectal retraction.

There is less of a dose gradient between the vaginal mucosa and the bladder and rectum than in a patient with a wider vagina (149). Additionally, packing cannot be used with cylinders to decrease the rectal and bladder doses (150,151). Vaginal cylinders increase the length of vagina and rectum treated, with an associated increase in complications. Vaginal fistulas, rectal ulcers, and strictures are reported with increased frequency when vaginal cylinders are used (152). Pourquier et al. (153) indicated that doses should be reduced with the use of vaginal cylinders and mini-ovoids to reduce complications, as these applicators have no shielding. Interstitial implantation should also be a consideration for patients with a narrow vagina or with distal vaginal disease.

The Importance of Optimal Applicator Placement

Geometrically optimal intracavitary implants improve outcome over suboptimal implants. Corn et al. reported an analysis of the 1978 and 1983 PCS, which attempted to analyze the outcomes of cervical cancer patients based on the technical quality of the implant. A technically good implant correlated significantly with improved local control, with a trend toward improved survival (154). In a review of the RTOG 0116 and 0128 trials, the quality of applicator placement was statistically related to the risk of local recurrence and disease-free survival (155). Perez et al. (80) observed that "inadequate" insertions increased the incidence of pelvic failures and that the quality of the intracavitary insertion had a measurable impact on the incidence of complications (83). Attention to the details of implant geometry has been linked to improved outcome in the series of Katz and Eifel at M.D. Anderson (123). Prior to afterloading, it was much more difficult to obtain adequate applicator placement, due to the need to complete the insertion quickly to avoid excessive exposure to the sources in the preloaded applicators. In the era of afterloading, applicator placement can be more methodical. Orthogonal films or other imaging (CT, MRI) should always be obtained following applicator placement to assess applicator geometry and the need for adjustment to ensure optimum placement (119). Optimum applicator placement is pivotal in maximizing local control. Placement of the brachytherapy applicators in direct proximity to the cervix is necessary to avoid underdosage. There will be a cold spot if the ovoids or other vaginal applicators are displaced away from the cervix (**Fig. 11.47**). Proper applicator selection is important in avoiding malpositioning. It is extremely important to place metallic markers on the cervix so that the flange of the tandem and the ovoids/cylinder dome are positioned in close proximity to these markers as confirmed on orthogonal check films (57,123).

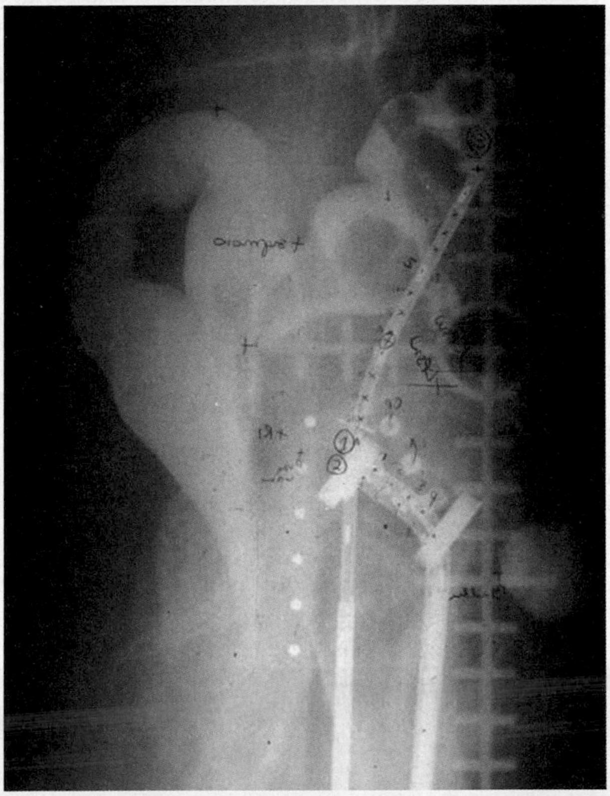

Figure 11.47. Lateral radiograph of a poorly positioned HDR tandem and ovoid applicator. Note that the tandem does not bisect the ovoids and that the ovoid appears to be displaced inferiorly from the cervical marker balls.

Likewise, suboptimal applicator placement can increase the risk of complications. Applicators that are too close to the bladder and rectum can increase rectal and bladder complications. Sources in the tandem can give very high doses of radiation to the small bowel (ileum), sigmoid, and upper bladder, often not revealed by orthogonal X-rays. Tandems that have perforated through the uterus can cause severe hot spots in the nearby normal organs.

Interstitial Applicators: Cervical and Vaginal Cancers—LDR and HDR

The size of the reference pear-shaped isodose achieved with tandem and ovoids is not variable except by increasing the duration (dose) of the implant. The shape of the reference pear-shaped isodose can be altered to some degree by varying the source strengths and applicator type, but it may not be able to encompass a bulky tumor, particularly when there is bulky parametrial or vaginal disease. In these settings, the disease may be better accommodated by an interstitial application (**Fig. 11.48**) (156). Patients with large, bulky lesions will have a higher rate of local failure because of a decrease in dose to the periphery of the tumor due to the rapid fall-off of dose beyond the relevant pear-shaped distribution. The use of higher doses of external beam prior to implantation and interstitial techniques is an important consideration. These patients should not be treated with external beam alone, because achieving the curative radiation doses required may be impossible due to the limited tolerance of the interposed small bowel, rectum, and bladder (146,147). Standard intracavitary applications may be suboptimal or prohibited either by tumor bulk or by distorted normal anatomy, and these patients should not be treated with geometrically unfavorable intracavitary implants (154,155).

The limitations of intracavitary techniques contrast with the strengths of interstitial techniques in certain settings. It is important to determine which approach is best on a patient-by-patient basis. Interstitial implantation is appropriate in select patients with bulky tumors, anatomical distortion such as an obliterated endocervical canal or narrow vagina, or recurrent disease (54,156). Interstitial implantation is used in <10% of patients with gynecologic cancers (157). Attention to patient comfort during and after the procedure, integration of appropriate imaging for ideal needle insertion relative to the tumor and dose specification/fractionation, and minimization of both acute and late morbidity are key in achieving a successful outcome. Typically, these are performed in higher volume centers through the combined efforts of Radiation Oncology and Gynecologic Oncology (158). The ABS has recently published consensus guidelines for LDR and HDR interstitial brachytherapy for cervical and vaginal cancers summarizing the most current recommendations (57,159).

The development of prefabricated perineal templates, through which stainless steel needles were inserted and afterloaded with ^{192}Ir or ^{125}I, was pivotal in advancing interstitial techniques for the treatment of cervical and vaginal cancers. With these interstitial techniques, rather than doing a freehand implant, the template concept allows for a predictable distribution of needles inserted across the entire perineum through a perforated template according to an optimum pattern. Commercially available and institution-specific templates are used in these patients to accommodate varying disease presentations. Stainless steel and plastic needles are used, which are afterloaded with low- or high-activity ^{192}Ir sources. The MUPIT (Martinez Universal Perineal Interstitial Template, Beaumont Hospital, Royal Oak, Michigan, USA) template (**Fig. 11.49**) accommodates implantation of multiple pelvic-perineal malignancies (prostate, anorectal, gynecologic) (53,160,161). In this system, one template accommodates many different disease presentations. Recent modifications of this template and needle system enabling HDR implants have become available (162). The Syed-Neblett (Best Industries, Springfield, Virginia) is the other well-known commercially available template system (53,163,164). Currently, there are three LDR Syed-Neblett templates of varying size and shape for use in implantation of gynecologic malignances (GYN 1 to 36 needles, GYN 2 to 44 needles, GYN 3 to 53 needles), as well as templates for implantation of the anus, prostate, and urethra (53) (**Fig. 11.50**). There is also a disposable template for gynecologic presentations that accommodates HDR needles (165).

The Syed-Neblett and MUPIT templates are particularly suited for treatment of vaginal disease, as the vaginal obturator needles can be strategically loaded to encompass disease from the fornices to the introitus. Additionally, the obturator needles can be advanced directly into the cervix, along with a uterine tandem, and may be essential to deliver tumoricidal radiation doses to the cervix by preventing a central "cold spot," especially if an intrauterine tandem is not used (158,159). Use of an intrauterine tandem along with interstitial needles has been statistically associated with an improvement in overall survival in stage IIIB cervical cancer (166). The more peripheral needles are used for implantation of the parametria, which is often underdosed in intracavitary approaches. Modifications of these standard templates have evolved and other innovative templates have been developed for vulvar, vaginal, and cervical carcinomas (53). Attention to the depth of needle insertion as well as to the number and location of needles is key in achieving an optimum implant (53,158). Additionally, modification of the ring and ovoid applicators to accommodate a limited number of needles to improve tumor coverage has been reported recently, with improved local control in patients with bulky IIB and IIIB disease (141,167,168). In these applications, only 10% to 20% of the dwell time is contributed from source positions in the needles, and the remainder by the intracavitary component of the applicator (136). Individualized computer-generated dosimetry is an integral part of interstitial dose delivery. CT imaging following needle implantation has proven very helpful in identifying tumor volume and critical normal structures, confirming the adequacy of needle placement in relation to these structures or needed adjustments, analyzing and manipulating the dose distribution related to these structures, and assisting with dose specification and the integration of external beam irradiation (53,169). Postprocedure epidural anesthesia provides optimal pain control and allows the needles and tandem to be manipulated outside the operating room if necessary. Modification of the planned source placement based upon the location of specific needles and critical structures can therefore be made before or after source loading (158).

With LDR techniques, traditional LDRs are the goal, achieved through differential loading (core sources ≤1/2 activity of peripheral sources) of low-activity sources. "Reference" dose rates of 60 to 80 cGy/hr are optimal (57). The implant dose rates as well as the dose homogeneity and distribution can be manipulated by selectively changing the activity associated with a particular needle or needles or by selectively unloading, either immediately or during the implant, strategic needles in the pattern. With HDR techniques, optimization of the dose distribution with predetermined parameters for the reference dose, normal organ doses, and dose homogeneity can produce even more ideal implant dosimetry (**Fig. 11.51**). Typically, total LDR doses to the tumor volume or reference isodose from the implant range from 23 to 40 Gy over 2 to 4 days, for a total dose of

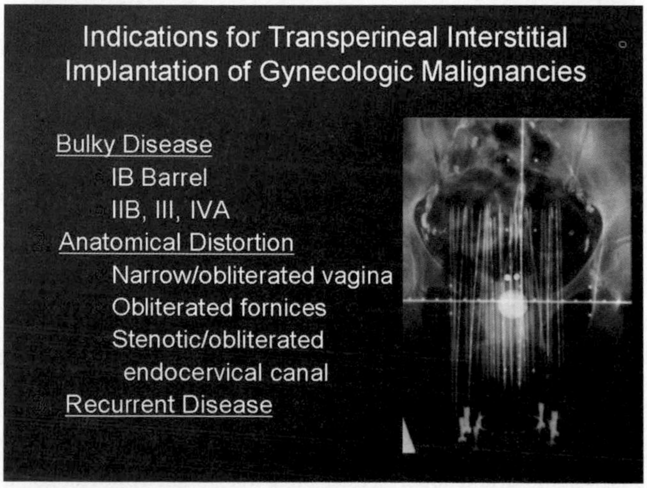

Figure 11.48. Indications for interstitial implantation and associated AP radiograph of the implanted needles.

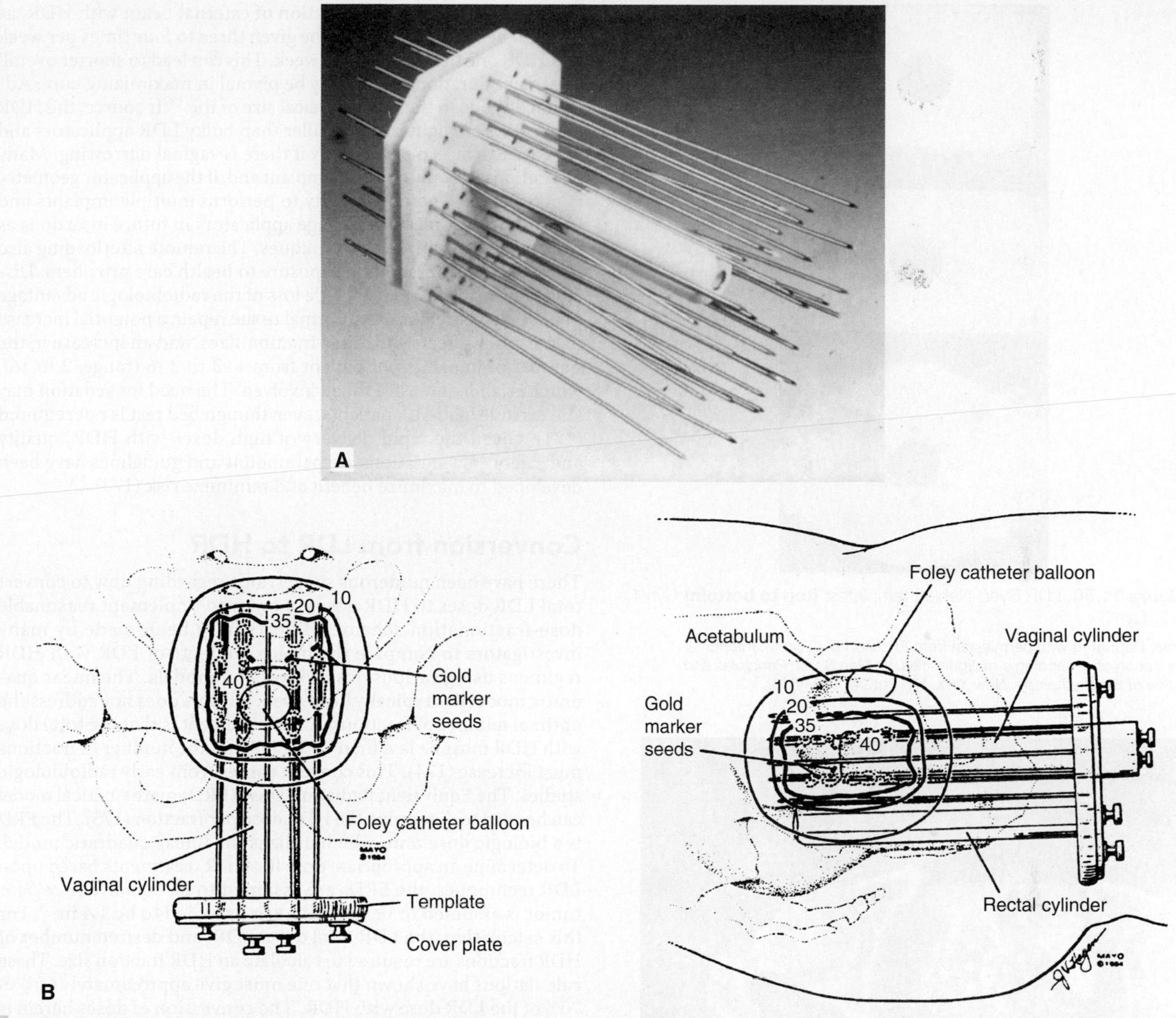

Figure 11.49. A: Martinez Universal Perineal Interstitial Template (MUPIT). **B:** Diagrammatic representation in coronal and sagittal planes of the same template.

Source: **A:** Courtesy of Dr. Alvaro Martinez, William Beaumont Hospital, Detroit, Michigan, USA. **B:** Reprinted from Martinez A, Edmundson GK, Cox RS, et al. Combination of external beam irradiation and multiple-site perineal applicator (MUPIT) for treatment of locally advanced or recurrent prostatic, anorectal, and gynecologic malignancies. *Int J Radiat Oncol Biol Phys.* 1985;11:391–398, with permission from Elsevier.

70 to 80 Gy (53,57,169). The total HDR dose will be approximately 60% of the total LDR dose and will be given in divided fractions. There is not a consistent data relative to EQD2 doses when using 3-D image-based HDR interstitial brachytherapy techniques. These seems to be a consensus that the doses are lower than with combined intracavitay HDR and external beam, perhaps on the order of an EQD2 of 75 to 80 Gy (136,159). With either approach, careful attention to significant hot spots within the implant and doses to the bladder, rectosigmoid, and vaginal surface are requisite to obtaining the best outcome (158,159,165).

External whole-pelvic irradiation (39.6 to 45.0 Gy) generally precedes implantation. For either LDR or HDR, one or two template implants can be done 1 to 2 weeks following external beam. With HDR, one to two fractions can be delivered per day over a period of 2 to 5 days, whereas with LDR, continuous hourly radiation is delivered. After the implant, selective external irradiation boosting can be done as needed. The total LDR dose to the reference volume from the combined implant and external beam approximates 70 to 85 Gy over 8 weeks (158).

HDR Brachytherapy for Cervical Cancer

Though LDR techniques have been the traditional standard for decades for gynecologic brachytherapy, there appear to be some inherent advantages to HDR techniques (170–172). Because the treatment time is very short, treatment is performed on an outpatient basis without the need for several days of bed rest, and with greater patient acceptance and comfort. This allows treatment of some patients with medical comorbidities, that would prohibit use of LDR techniques because of the prolonged bed rest they would subsequently require. With the shorter treatment time, the implant reproducibility is superior to traditional LDR approaches because more stable positioning of applicators is possible. The shortened treatment time provides a greater degree of certainty that the sources will remain in the 3-D positions documented in the isodose distributions, and that applicator displacement as a function of time will be decreased. The use of applicator fixation devices allows more constant and reproducible geometry of source positioning. The newer systems, which allow a single source to "dwell" at a site

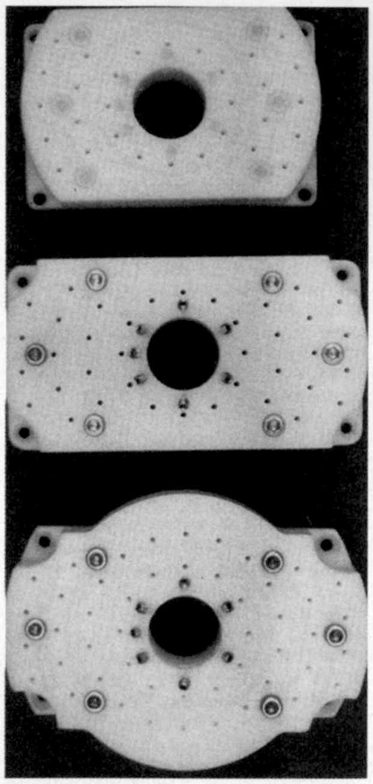

Figure 11.50. LDR Syed-Neblett templates: **(top to bottom)** Gyn 1, Gyn 2, Gyn 3.

Source: Reprinted with permission from Erickson B, Gillin M. Interstitial implantation of gynecologic malignancies. In: Nag S, ed. *Principles and Practice of Brachytherapy*. New York, NY: Futura; 1997:518.

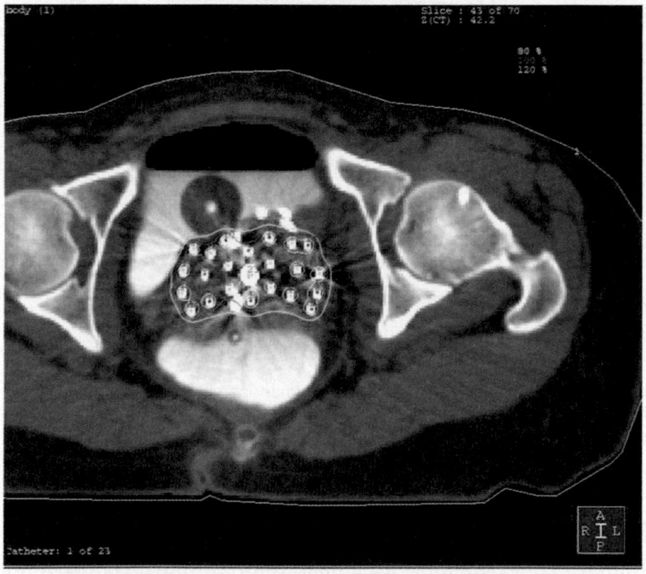

Figure 11.51. Axial CT scan with needles inserted into the cervical and paracervical tissues between the bladder and rectum. Isodose curves shown are 80%, 100%, and 120% of the prescription dose.

for a calculated period of time, combined with dose optimization software programs, provide a significant improvement in the ability to shape the dose distribution. The small source size allows for finer increments in source location and relative weighting for each source location than with the fixed source sizes and activities inherent to the LDR ^{137}Cs sources. This allows for greater precision coupled with greater flexibility and, perhaps, a reduction in normal tissues doses. Additionally, the rectal retraction devices available with the HDR applicators maximize displacement of the rectum for short periods of time and may give superior and more predictable displacement than traditional vaginal gauze packing. These factors lead to improved dose delivery to the tumor relative to surrounding normal tissues.

There is also increased integration of external beam with HDR, as external beam irradiation can be given three to four times per week and HDR one to two times per week. This can lead to shorter overall treatment duration, which may be pivotal in maximizing cure. Additionally, due to the small physical size of the ^{192}Ir source, the HDR applicators are lighter and smaller than bulky LDR applicators and are easier to insert, particularly if there is vaginal narrowing. Many institutions use only one LDR implant and, if the applicator geometry is poor, there is no opportunity to perform multiple implants and improve the geometry or change applicators in future insertions as can be realized with HDR techniques. The remote afterloading also provides a lack of radiation exposure to health care providers. Disadvantages of HDR may include loss of the radiobiologic advantage of LDR, decreased time for normal tissue repair, a potential increase in late tissue effects with large fraction sizes, and an increase in the number of implants per patient from 1–3 to 3–6 (range, 2 to 16), which is labor-intensive for all involved. The need for sedation may still exclude high-risk patients, even though bed rest is not required (171). Given the rapid delivery of high doses with HDR, quality and safety considerations are paramount and guidelines have been developed to maximize benefit and minimize risk (173).

Conversion from LDR to HDR

There have been numerous suggestions regarding how to convert total LDR doses to HDR doses in order to implement reasonable dose-fractionation schemes. Efforts have been made by many investigators to compare the biologic effects of LDR with HDR regimens using various dose conversion models. The linear quadratic model has typically been used, but this does not address the optimal number of fractions. A basic concept is that the total dose with HDR must be less than with LDR and the number of fractions must increase (174). This concept comes from early radiobiologic studies. The Equivalent Radiation Dose (ERD) mathematical model can be used to determine the HDR dose per fraction (175). The ERD is a biologic dose unit, which utilizes the linear quadratic model. To determine an appropriate dose for HDR treatments based upon LDR techniques, the ERDs are assumed to be equal. The α/β for tumor is assumed to be 10, while μ is assumed to be 1.4 hr^{-1}. For this calculation, the LDR total dose, LDR, and desired number of HDR fractions are required to calculate an HDR fraction size. These calculations have shown that one must give approximately 60% to 70% of the LDR dose with HDR. The conversion of doses herein is strictly for the brachytherapy component of the treatment course. More recently, there has been interest in calculating the equivalent dose (EQD2) at 2 Gy/fraction for both the radiation targets (point

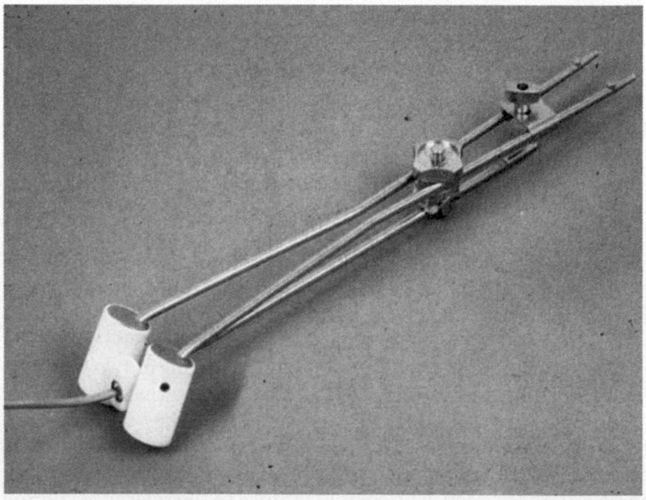

Figure 11.52. HDR tandem and ovoids.

Source: Courtesy of Nucletron.

A, HRCTV) and the OAR when adding together both the external beam and the brachytherapy components of treatment. This can be done for LDR, PDR, and HDR. This interactive worksheet is available through the American Brachytherapy website (136).

HDR Applicators

The tandems and ovoids used with HDR are variations of the traditional Fletcher and Henschke LDR applicators but are lighter, narrower, and smaller (**Fig. 11.52**) (54,136). The ovoids are 2.0, 2.5, and 3.0 cm in diameter with and without shielding. The relationship of the colpostat to the handle is different between HDR and LDR colpostats, so that the cable-driven HDR source can negotiate the angle between the handle and the colpostat. The Selectron colpostats are angled at 60° to the applicator handles. Standard Fletcher-Suit LDR colpostats are angled most often at 15° and sometimes at 30° with respect to the colpostat handles (**Fig. 11.53**). This can lead to a different relationship between the tandem and the colpostats and between the colpostats and the cervix, best seen on the lateral orthogonal X-rays taken for dosimetry after applicator insertion. As previously mentioned, these applicators have also been adapted for needle insertion for bulkier tumors (167).

The ring applicator, which is an adaptation of the Stockholm technique, has become a popular applicator (176) (**Fig. 11.54**). The plastic caps that come with the ring applicator place the vaginal mucosa 0.6 cm from the source path, compared to the caps for the ovoids, which place the vaginal mucosa from the source path at a distance of 1 to 1.5 cm. The short distance from the ring to vaginal mucosa can result in very high surface doses if fixed weighting, nonoptimized techniques are used (172,176). The bladder and rectum may also receive higher doses with fixed weighting nonoptimized dosimetry. It is important not to activate all the positions in the ring, as this will increase the dose to the rectum, bladder, and vaginal mucosa. Typically, four dwells are activated on each side of the smallest ring (36 mm), five on each side of the medium ring (40 mm), and six on each side of the large ring (44 mm). The tandems are available in lengths of 2 to 8 cm. Four ring-tandem angles are available, including 30°, 45°, 60°, and 90°. The shape of the isodose curves comparing the ring with tandem and ovoids will also have a different shape and the volume of tissue irradiated will also differ (176). The ring applicator is ideal for patients without lateral vaginal fornices. Its ease of insertion and predictable geometry make it a popular alternative to tandem and ovoids. As previously mentioned, the ring applicator has also been adapted to accommodate needles for patients with bulky tumors (141,168).

Tandem and cylinder applicators are used in the setting of a narrow vagina or vaginal extension of disease, and are available in diameters of 2.0 to 4.0 cm (**Fig. 11.55**) (54). In most cases, rectal and bladder displacement are not possible with this applicator, although some of the cylinders have built-in shielding. A posterior speculum blade to displace the rectum can be used if there is no posterior vaginal disease. As with LDR tandem and cylinder applicators, the bladder and rectal doses may increase with this applicator, and the dose distribution will be more cylindrical than pear-shaped, which can underdose bulky tumors (**Fig. 11.46**). Careful attention to normal tissue doses and target coverage is necessary in this setting (136).

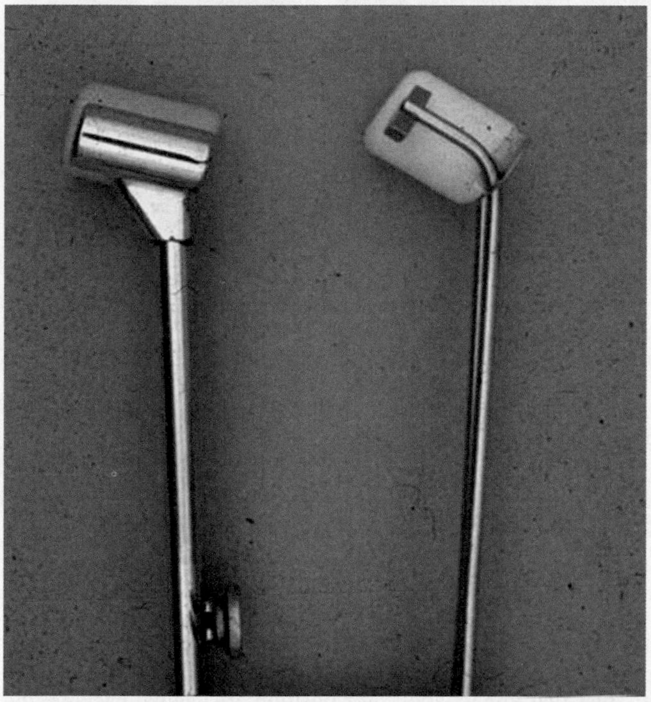

Figure 11.53. LDR versus HDR ovoid angles. The LDR ovoids are positioned at 15° or 30° to the vaginal axis versus 60° in the HDR ovoids

Source: Courtesy of Nucletron.

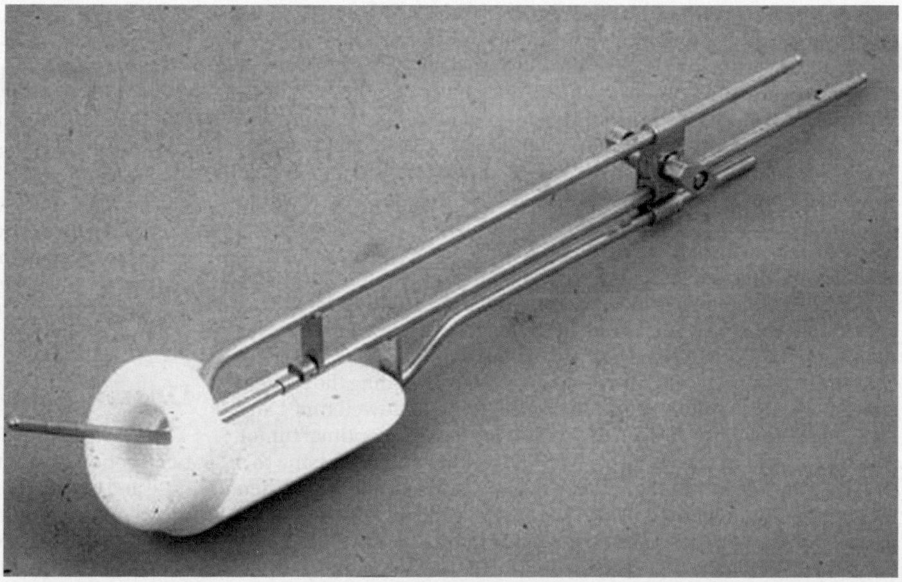

Figure 11.54. Tandem and ring applicator with associated rectal retractor.

Source: Courtesy of Nucletron.

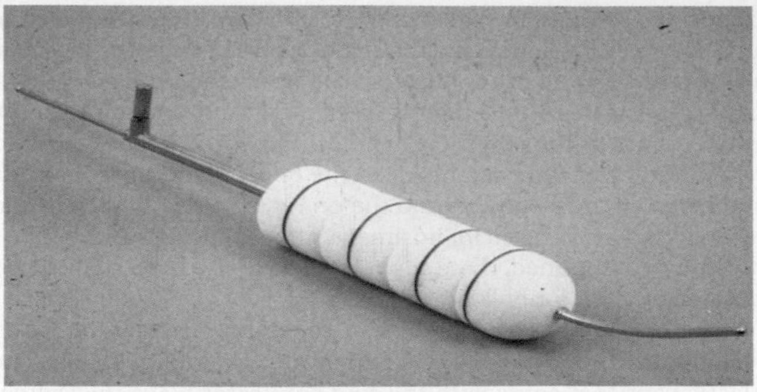

Figure 11.55. Tandem and cylinder applicator.
Source: Courtesy of Nucletron.

HDR Treatment Planning

The dose distribution with HDR tandem and ovoids and tandem and ring applicators models the LDR pear-shaped isodose distribution. HDR regimens use a paracervical dose specification point (A), rather than mg-hrs, or a volume-based dose specification such as the HRCTV (136). Rectal, bladder, sigmoid, and vaginal surface doses should always be specified or documented, and some assessment of dose to the pelvic lymph nodes and lateral parametria should be documented.

The HDR system utilizes special vocabulary to describe certain functions and applications. A "dwell position" is a position at which the source is driven to stop or dwell. Dwell positions can be 2.5 and 5 mm apart. An active length will be converted into a number of dwell positions. "Patient points" are points of interest at which the dose is calculated; they are defined on the orthogonal implant films. Examples include bladder, rectum, and sigmoid. "Applicator points" are points of interest at which the dose is calculated; they are defined by manually inputting the coordinates. Typically, applicator points include point A and points on the lateral surface of a ring, ovoid, or cylinder. "Dose points" are points at which the dose is optimized. In general, doses are specified using dose points. The optimization program then attempts to give the prescription dose at each of these points. With the tandem and ring, a similar system is used. The entire ring should never be activated, as this will cause high rectal, bladder, and vaginal doses. For the tandem and cylinder, again, a similar system is used, with the exception that at the cylinder interface, dose points are entered laterally from the dwell positions at the distances representing the cylinder surface. Due to the close proximity of the bladder and rectum in women requiring vaginal cylinders because of a narrow vagina, dose specification needs to be done with great care so as not to give excessive doses to the bladder and rectum. Dose specification at point A alone can result in underdosing of target tissue and overdosing of dose-limiting tissues (177,178). If using 2-D planning, in addition to point A, specifying dose at the vaginal applicator surface is important. If using a volume-based approach, dose specification to the HRCTV while negotiating the doses to 2 cc of the bladder and rectosigmoid is key. With either approach, optimization of the dose distribution follows and enables design of a more ideal dose distribution (**Fig. 11.56**). The term "optimization" refers to the process of achieving certain dose values at points or volumes within the implant. It is not the simple generation of a standard dose distribution by using fixed dose points around the applicator (136). The goal is to match the dose distribution to point A or the HR CTV while simultaneously avoiding the OAR. Inherent to optimization is starting with a standard plan of loading the tandem and the vaginal applicator and then modifying the dwell times and dwell weights to reduce dose to the OAR and ensure optimal tumor coverage (136). Excessive optimization can alter the pear shape to a less desirable configuration with the same point A dose (178). When altering the standard dwell times and weights, it is important to also monitor changes in the dose, dose/volume parameters, and the spatial dose distribution that result from the modified loading pattern.

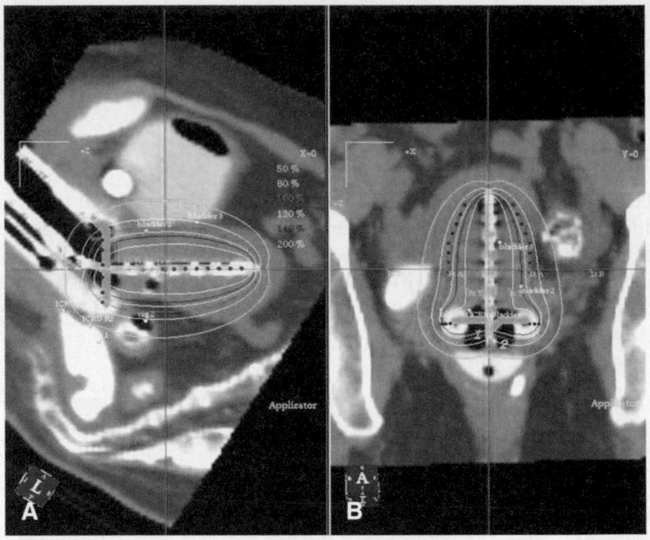

Figure 11.56. Dose distribution around a tandem and ring applicator in sagittal (**A**) and coronal (**B**) projections with dose specified at the ring surface and at the level of point A.

Reliance on dose volume histograms alone can be dangerous if if one does not also evaluate the spatial dose distribution (136). The entire length of the tandem does not always need to be treated and should be guided by the definition of remaining tumor at the time of brachytherapy, as seen on MR or CT. This can reduce dose to the OARs (179). Likewise, activation of dwell positions in the vaginal applicator should also be considered carefully, in light of the closely approximated bladder and rectum and vaginal target.

HDR Dosimetry Generation

It is important to perform dosimetry for each fraction of an HDR tandem and vaginal applicator regimen even if the same applicator is used, as there may be quite a bit of variation in applicator position with each fraction (136,180). There is also applicator deformation of the adjacent structures, which varies with applicator position (181). Variables that impact applicator position are vaginal packing, the presence and effectiveness of sedation/anesthesia, and use of the dorsal lithotomic versus legs down position. The bladder and rectosigmoid may also change configuration due to changes in filling and position, and doses to these organs will vary from fraction to fraction. Uterine and sigmoid mobility may also impact the dose distribution in these organs. Additionally, disease regression and vaginal narrowing will vary from fraction to fraction and can result in changes in dose distribution. A change in applicator can also result in changes in dose distribution, as can changing the ovoid or ring size, ovoid separation, and tandem curvature. The ovoids may also change in separation, and their relative position to the tandem over time if there is no fixed relationship between the tandem and ovoids. Jones et al. (180) found that when treatment planning was not performed for each fraction and only the initial dosimetry was used, there was increased dose to at-risk normal organs. This is also true when using a tandem and ring, even though it has a fixed geometry. The applicator position relative to the pelvic organs is the important factor rather than the relationship of the tandem to the ring (**Fig. 11.57**).

Dose-Fractionation Schemes

There is no consensus as to the optimal number of fractions and dose per fraction except that the choice will depend on the external beam dose and on whether central shielding is used as well as normal tissue doses, medical comorbidities, and the stage of disease. The linear quadratic model was suggested as a guide to formulate the regimens chosen at each institution (182). Currently, the GOG protocols define

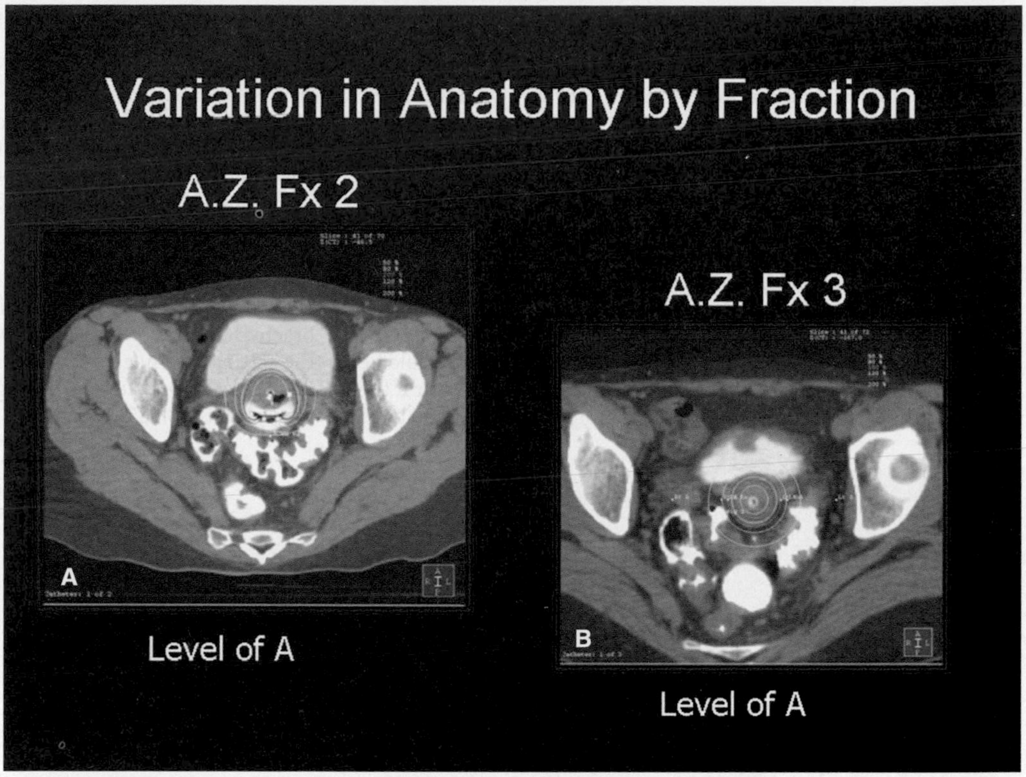

Figure 11.57. Variation in anatomy between fraction 2 (**A**) and fraction 3 (**B**) of a five-fraction HDR course. Note the difference in the position of normal organs at the level of point A between fractions 2 and 3.

a dose/fractionation scheme of 5.6 to 6.3 Gy × 5 to point A with whole pelvis doses of 41.4 to 45 Gy. RTOG protocols allow fraction sizes of 5.3 to 7.4 Gy when using four to seven fractions, depending on the external beam dose. Tables for combining various external beam doses with varying HDR fractions using the linear quadratic formula and normal-tissue-modifying factor have been provided with these protocols (182). There has been increasing concern that 6 Gy times 5 to point A may result in excessive toxicity to the rectum and sigmoid when combined with whole pelvis doses of 45 G, and a dose of 5.5 Gy times 5 to point A may be more reasonable (136). In the United States, the most common HDR intracavitary regimen prescribes two fractions per week for a total of five fractions, with 5 to 6 Gy/fraction (136,183). Internationally the most common dose per fraction was between 5 and 7 Gy, with the higher dose per fraction associated with a decrease in fraction number (three to five fractions) (157). When using volumetric image-guided brachytherapy, the dose at point A can still be tracked but the goal is to deliver 80-90 Gy to the HRCTV, depending on the volume of disease, while limiting dose to the OAR to an acceptable level. The EQD2 limit to the D2cc (the minimum dose in the most irradiated 2 cm^3 normal tissue volume for the rectum and sigmoid) is 70 to 75 Gy, and for the bladder 80 to 90 Gy (136).

Sequencing of External Beam Radiation with Brachytherapy

In nonbulky disease presentations, HDR insertions are often integrated early in the treatment course after approximately 20 Gy of external beam radiation therapy. Alternatively, some institutions choose to take the whole pelvis to 40 to 45 Gy initially, preceding the five HDR insertions, unless the patient has very early disease or evidence of early vaginal stenosis. This allows for maximum disease regression prior to brachytherapy. When delivering 40 to 45 Gy to the whole pelvis before initiation of HDR, it is important to avoid treatment prolongation by giving two HDR fractions per week to complete the radiation within 50 to 56 days (136). Compressing the duration of treatment to <60 days may be desirable (183).

Brachytherapy for Endometrial Cancer

Hysterectomy is the cornerstone of treatment for endometrial carcinoma. Selective use of vaginal brachytherapy, external beam irradiation, or both in the postoperative setting is based on the histopathologic risk factors identified in the tissues removed at the time of surgical staging (184,185). Vaginal brachytherapy is typically performed using Fletcher colpostats, or a variety of vaginal cylinders (Delclos, Burnett). Both LDR and HDR techniques are used (186,187) (**Fig. 11.58**). The choice of ovoids versus cylinders is individual and both have relative advantages and disadvantages (51). Vaginal ovoids are available in diameters of 2 to 3 cm with associated caps and shielding. Vaginal cylinders are available in diameters of 2 to 5 cm, with or without shielding. Vaginal ovoids generally require sedation for insertion, whereas cylinders do not. The length of the vagina treated with vaginal ovoids is approximately the upper third, whereas vaginal cylinders can treat a portion of or the entire vagina. Though rare, when present, distal vaginal metastases tend to be located in the periurethral area (188). Poorly differentiated tumors may recur earlier and present in the distal vagina or distant disease sites, whereas well-differentiated lesions tend to recur later and are often in the upper vagina (189). Distal vaginal recurrences or metastases, however, are rare after radiation and have been noted to occur in 0.5% to 1% of patients when the upper vagina was treated. It is therefore not suggested to treat more than the upper half of the vagina routinely. Typically, the length of vagina treated with vaginal cylinders is between 4 and 5 cm, perhaps favoring a longer length when using brachytherapy alone (186,187). Packing is typically used to displace the rectum and bladder with ovoids and not with cylinders. Due to the longer length of vagina treated and the lack of packing, a larger volume of rectum and bladder will be treated with cylinders. Vaginal ovoids may be prohibited in a narrow vagina, whereas vaginal cylinders may not be in close approximation with all of the vaginal mucosa in the setting of a wide vaginal apex or if the cuff has been closed with “dog ears” rather than in a cylindrical shape.

Most vaginal brachytherapy for endometrial cancer is performed with vaginal cylinders using HDR techniques (**Fig. 11.58**) (186,187). The dose distribution should ideally conform to the shape of the cylinder (187,190). Dose is typically specified either at the vaginal applicator surface (mucosal surface) or at a depth of 0.5 cm from the applicator or vaginal mucosal surface (186,187). Dose prescription at 0.5 cm can lead to excessively high mucosal doses, and surface doses should also be tracked (187,191). Additionally, careful assessment of dose to the rectum and bladder through use of computerized dosimetry should be performed for the first fraction of radiation delivered (**Fig. 11.58**). CT-based planning allows for an excellent assessment of the doses to the bladder and rectum as well as evaluation of air gaps at the interface of the applicator surface and vaginal mucosa, but is only needed for the first fraction (187,192). Choo et al. (193) have revealed that 95% of the vaginal lymphatic channels are located within 3 mm of the vaginal surface and that dose prescription to a depth of less than 5 mm may be adequate. For LDR insertions, dose rates at the surface of the applicator should be in the range of 80 to 100 cGy/hr, and perhaps 50 to 70 cGy/hr if the prescription is at 0.5 cm (190). Total vaginal surface doses of 50 to 80 Gy are reported most frequently in the literature. When used with external beam, cumulative doses of 60 to 100 Gy at the vaginal surface are reported in the literature. Doses in excess of 80 Gy to the vaginal mucosa are not necessary in the setting of adjuvant therapy, and can be associated with increased morbidity. For a vaginal recurrence of endometrial cancer, doses of 80 Gy and higher may be needed when combining external beam and brachytherapy (194).

Vaginal brachytherapy alone is generally considered an option for patients treated with hysterectomy, with either no or selective lymph node sampling, who are thought to be at low risk for lymph node metastases. These patients typically have grade 1 or 2 disease without significant myometrial invasion (<1/3) (88,185). Vaginal brachytherapy alone is considered an option at some institutions in the setting of a negative pelvic lymph node dissection, even when high-risk factors such as high-grade or deep myometrial invasion are present (88,185).

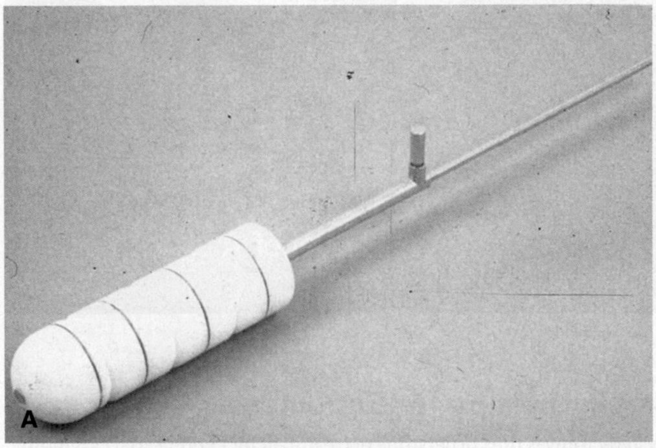

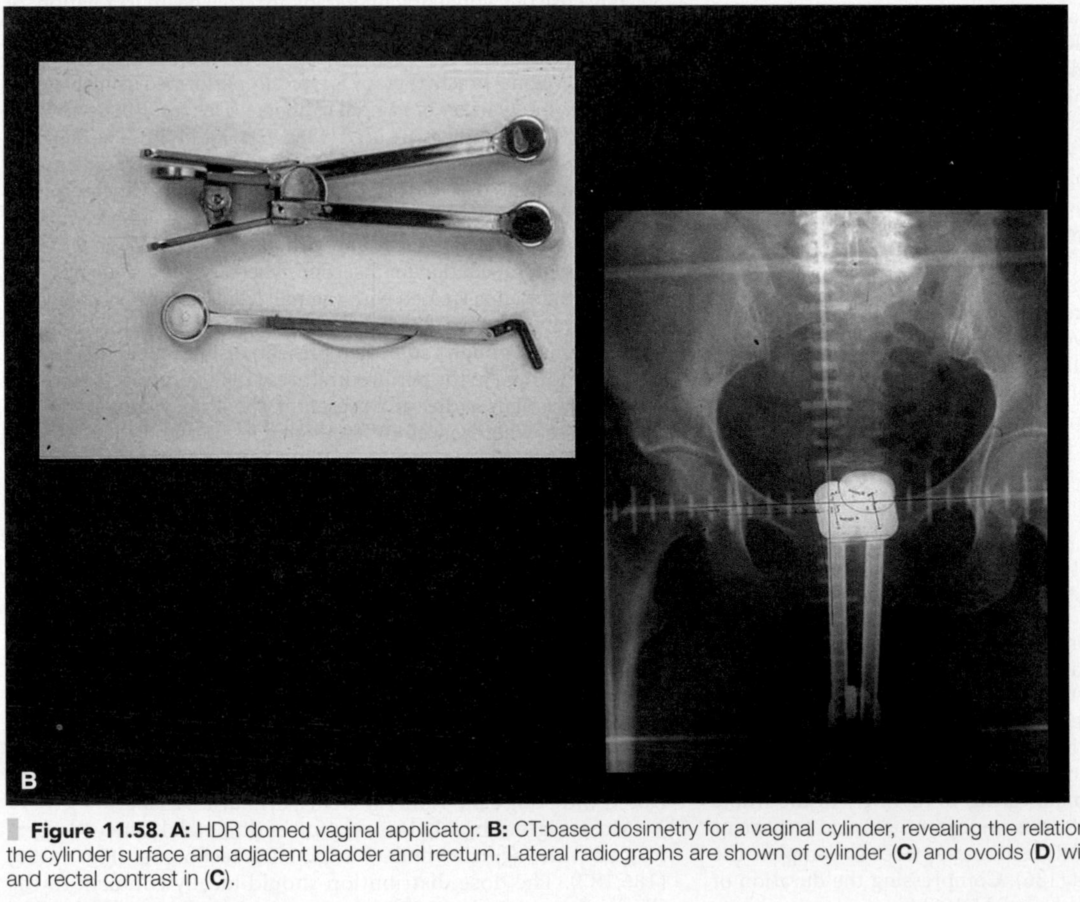

Figure 11.58. A: HDR domed vaginal applicator. **B:** CT-based dosimetry for a vaginal cylinder, revealing the relationship of the dose distribution to the cylinder surface and adjacent bladder and rectum. Lateral radiographs are shown of cylinder (**C**) and ovoids (**D**) with bladder bulb contrast in both and rectal contrast in (**C**).

Source: Courtesy of Nucletron.

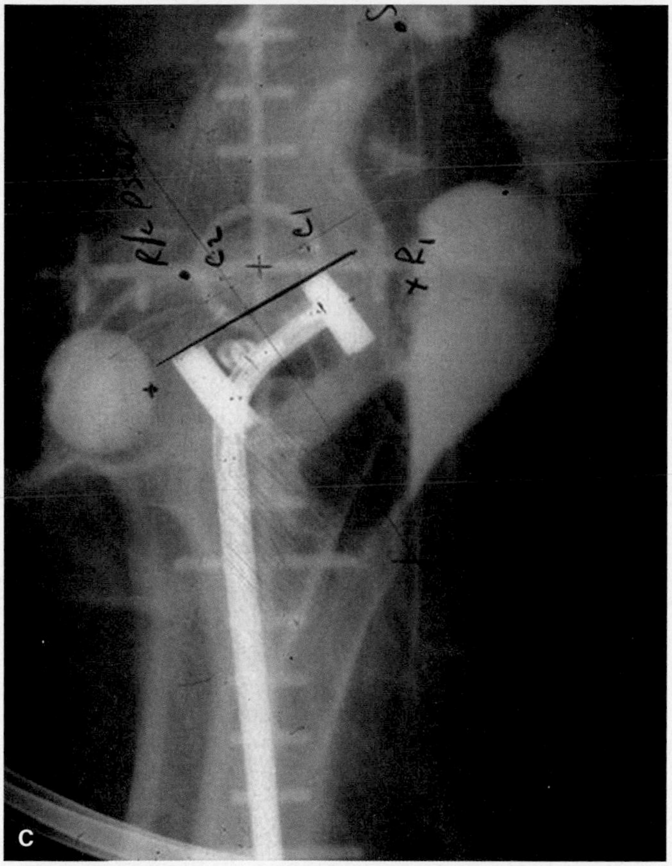

Figure 11.58. *(continued)*

There is great debate about whether a vaginal cuff boost is routinely necessary in addition to external beam irradiation for early-stage endometrial cancer; there is little data to support it (88,184). Practice patterns are based more on institutional tradition and individual preference rather than prospective randomized trials. The rationale for use of a vaginal boost is the supposition that there may be a critical dose needed at the vaginal apex to optimally decrease the likelihood of a vaginal apex recurrence. Doses in excess of the 45 to 50 Gy typically delivered with external beam may be necessary if there are microscopic tumor cells embedded in the hypoxic vaginal cuff.

In some clinical situations more complex brachytherapy procedures are required to treat endometrial cancer. Patients with bulky stage II endometrial cancers may benefit from preoperative radiation with external beam alone, brachytherapy alone, or a combination of the two. Tandem and ovoids or tandem and ring or cylinder applicators are used in this setting. Medically inoperable endometrial cancer is a rare phenomenon in the current era of aggressive surgical staging. When encountered, it may require the use of sophisticated radiation techniques (195). The ABS released guidelines specific to patients who have inoperable endometrial cancer (196). The ABS recommends MRI if available, or CT, to determine the uterine wall thickness and for volume-based brachytherapy. The ABS recommends brachytherapy alone in patients with stage I, grade 1 to 2 endometrial cancer with minimal myometrial invasion on MRI. If MRI is not available, then external beam radiation in conjunction with brachytherapy should be used. In patients with stage I disease and deep myometrial invasion based on MRI, or stage II or stage III disease, external beam radiation to a total dose of 45 to 50 Gy is recommended, followed by brachytherapy (195,196).

Tandem and ovoids or a tandem and ring or cylinder may be appropriate if the uterine cavity is small. If the uterus is large or if there is more extensive disease, special uterine applicators such as dual and triple tandems or Heyman-Simons capsules may be helpful (**Fig. 11.59**) (195). There is better coverage of the entire endometrial cavity with these applicators, and dose can be delivered through the uterine wall to the serosa of the uterus. HDR and LDR techniques can be used.

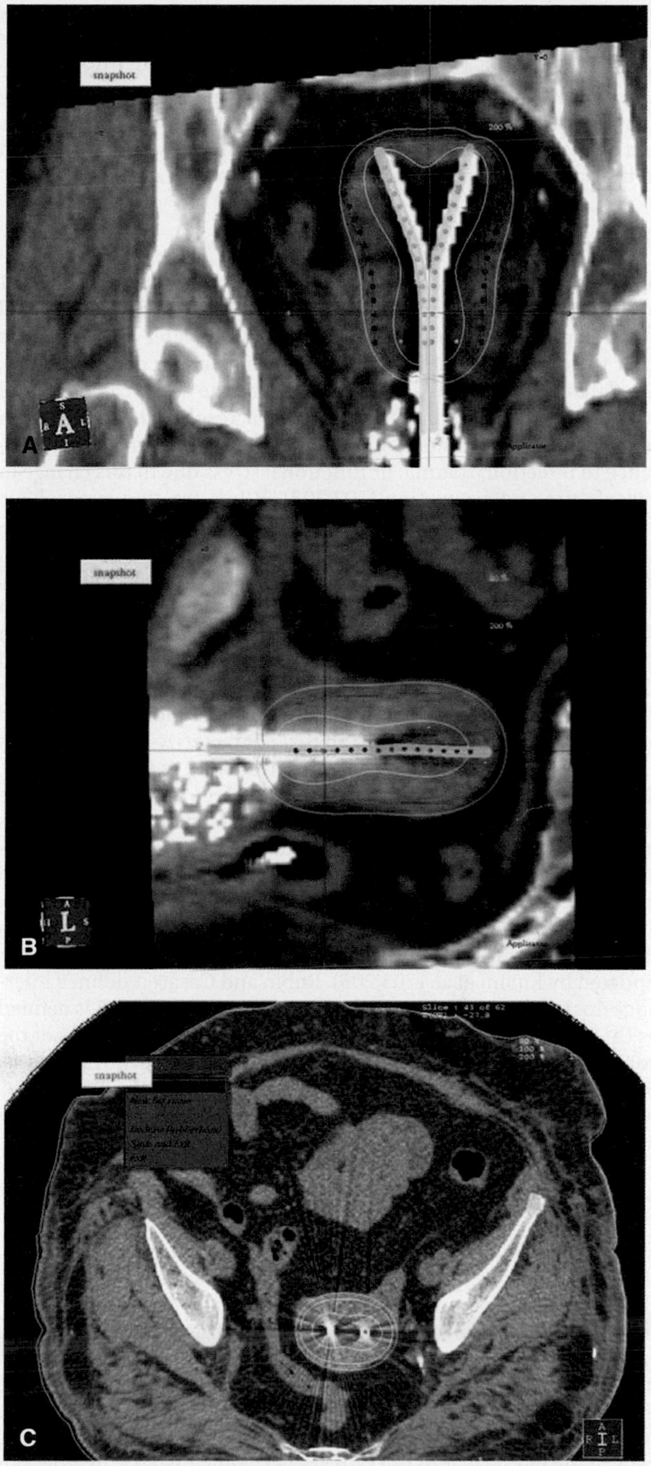

Figure 11.59. Brachytherapy plan for a patient with medically inoperable endometrial cancer in coronal (**A**), sagittal (**B**), and axial (**C**) dimensions. Note dual tandems on the coronal image (**A**).

Patients with recurrent endometrial cancer usually benefit from both external beam and brachytherapy. Doses in excess of 80 Gy may lead to better local control in these patients (194). In patients with residual vaginal disease less than 0.5 cm in maximum thickness, vaginal cylinders or ovoids can be used, whereas in patients with thicker lesions following external beam, interstitial techniques are needed.

For apical lesions, laparotomy or laparoscopy or imaged-guided brachytherapy may be required for optimum needle placement, and to avoid small bowel tethered to the pelvic floor (53,197,198). Similar brachytherapy techniques can be used for patients with primary cancer of the vagina (51,159,199). Multichannel vaginal cylinders can be very helpful in this setting to direct dose to where it is needed in the vagina and spare uninvolved walls the high dose (200,201).

Radiation-Induced Tissue Effects

Side effects that develop during the course of radiation and persist for 3 months or less following completion of radiation are termed acute side effects. Those toxicities that develop later than 3 months after the completion of radiation are termed late or chronic effects. The late effects of radiation are due to damage at the capillary level where there is endothelial cell proliferation, resulting in less diffusion of oxygen into the tissues with resulting fibrosis. There is less resistance to infection, trauma, or functional stress due to this change in vasculature and circulation (202,203). When treating gynecologic cancers, the normal tissues in the pelvis that are most often irradiated incidentally are the rectosigmoid, small bowel, bladder, vagina, pelvic bones and bone marrow. In the upper abdomen the kidneys, liver, stomach, small bowel, large bowel, and spinal cord may be in the radiation field. The response of a tissue or organ to radiation depends on two factors: (a) the inherent sensitivity of the individual cells, and (b) the kinetics of the population as a whole, of which the cells are a part. These factors combine to account for the substantial variations in response to radiation that characterize different tissues (1). Additionally, the volume of tissue irradiated as well as the dose, dose rate, and fractionation scheme will affect both acute and late toxicities. The addition of chemotherapy or other systemic agents may impact toxicity, as may other medical comorbidities such as diabetes, hypertension, collagen vascular diseases, Crohn's disease, and ulcerative colitis, as well as social risk factors such as smoking (204). The most comprehensive data describing the effects of radiation on the normal tissues were published by Rubin and Casarett and later updated by Emani et al. (203,205). Rubin and Casarett defined tolerance doses (TDs) for almost all of the tissues. The TD 5/5 is defined as the probability of a 5% risk of complications within 5 years of the completion of radiation, and TD 5/50 as the probability of a 50% risk of complications within 5 years (203). More recently, the QUANTEC (Quantitative Analyses of Normal Tissue Effects in the Clinic) guidelines have been published with updated recommendations (206,207).

Skin

When undergoing radiation treatment for abdominopelvic tumors, the patient often experiences minimal skin reactions; this is due to the skin-sparing quality of the high-energy radiation beams used to treat these sites deep within the body. In contrast, when undergoing radiation treatment of the vulvar and inguinal regions, for which electrons or lower energy X-rays are more often used, there may be marked skin reactions. Skin reactions are also more likely to develop in skin folds such as the inguinal creases or intergluteal fold. The cells in the basal layer of the skin are very sensitive to radiation, but because of the time required for these differentiating cells to move from the basal layer to the keratinized layer of skin, there is a 2- to 3-week delay between the start of radiation and the appearance of skin reactions. Erythema is the first visible skin reaction, and is due to dilation of the small capillaries ; it is usually seen about the third week of radiation. Other skin reactions include dry desquamation and moist desquamation, occurring after the fourth week of radiation. Moist desquamation occurs with transient loss of the epidermis and exposure of the dermis. Serous fluid often oozes from the exposed and inflamed dermis (203,208). These effects may be enhanced by the combination of irradiation and some chemotherapeutic agents, particularly actinomycin D and doxorubicin (Adriamycin) (209). It is also well known that chemotherapy agents such as Adriamycin or gemcitabine can "recall" radiation reactions after the original reaction has subsided (210). Radiation-induced skin reactions are treated with various topical ointments and creams as well as with sitz baths and special emphasis on cleansing all stool and urine gently from the perineum. Additionally, if the distal vagina or vulva is in the radiation field, patients may also complain of dysuria or painful defecation, which is due to the caustic effects of the urine and stool on the denuded epithelium of the distal vagina, perianal area, and vulva. Diarrhea control and use of barrier creams to protect the irritated skin from stool and urine will help to minimize discomfort and hasten skin healing. Sulfa-based creams and Domeboro soaks can be used to expedite healing. Return of the epidermis can take 10 to 14 days. Residual surviving basal cells form islands of regeneration, which proliferate to reepithelialize the area. Islands of skin forming in the desquamated skin herald skin renewal. The new skin is thin and pink, with gradual return to normal in 2 to 3 weeks (203). Late manifestations of radiation on the skin include depigmentation, subcutaneous fibrosis, dryness and thinning with loss of apocrine and sebaceous glands, thinning or loss of hair, and telangiectasias. Necrosis of the skin is rare and generally occurs only with very high doses of radiation in excess of 60 Gy (203,209).

Bone Marrow/Pelvic Bones

The lymphocytes are the most radiosensitive cells in the bone marrow. The rate of fall of the various components of the marrow is a function of the half-lives of the mature cells. These half-lives are as follows: erythrocytes, 120 days; granulocytes, 6.6 hours; and platelets, 8 to 10 days (203). Pelvic irradiation may cause transient lymphopenia. This is even more of an issue when whole-abdominal or extended-field irradiation is used, due to the increased bone marrow in the radiation fields. This decrease in lymphocytes is thought to be the result of irradiation of the lymphocytes circulating through the vascular bed, and may not be indicative of bone marrow reserve depletion. Prior or concurrent chemotherapy will also lead to increased bone marrow toxicity. Frequent monitoring of the complete blood count is considered standard of care with pelvic or abdominal irradiation. Permanent chronic changes are noted even when small segments of the bone marrow are irradiated to doses over 30 Gy, and recovery may take up to 18 months or longer in a proportion of patients with good reparative capacity.

Insufficiency fractures can also develop in irradiated pelvic bones (211,212). These most commonly involve the sacrum and ileum, followed by the pubic bones, and rarely the acetabulum. Patients may complain of sudden onset of back or groin pain, which worsens with weight bearing and changes in position. MRI is the best imaging modality to detect them and also rule out recurrent disease. Sometimes edema will be reported in the absence of actual fractures, and in other cases, actual fractures will be seen. It is important not to confuse these changes with metastatic disease, as further palliative irradiation would worsen the integrity of the bone. Symptoms from these changes in the pelvic bones will often improve over time, but patients may also suffer future symptoms from exacerbation of these fractures or development of new fractures over time. Percutaneous cementing of the injured bone can be used if patients remain symptomatic. Narcotics and changes in activity are often required. Femoral neck complications can include avascular necrosis as well as fracture. This is a rare complication following irradiation of the inguinal nodes. Hip replacement surgery is required to resolve this problem (213). The skeletal health of at-risk patients undergoing radiation should be considered pretreatment with baseline bone densities and referral for medical intervention.

Liver

During whole-abdominal irradiation or paraaortic irradiation, the liver is in the radiation field and dose must be limited to this critical organ. Clinical and pathologic studies have shown that the liver is not a radioresistant organ (214). Veno-occlusive disease is the pathologic entity caused by radiation. Necrosis and atrophy of the hepatic cells result from this change in blood supply (203). CT scanning following radiation can show changes in perfusion of the liver corresponding to the radiation fields. These changes are not always associated with toxicity. The clinical course and liver changes depend on the dose-fractionation scheme and volume of irradiation as well as the presence of chemotherapy and preexisting liver disease. During radiation, the liver enzymes may be elevated. This can continue following completion of radiation. Signs of radiation hepatitis can include a marked elevation of alkaline phosphatase (3 to 10 times normal), with much less elevation of the transaminases (normal to two times normal) (203,214). Liver enlargement and varying amount of ascites can also evolve. If the doses and volumes are high enough, liver failure can occur. The TD 5/5 for whole liver is 30 Gy in 2 Gy fractions (203,205). Small portions of the liver can receive up to 70 to 90 Gy. Mean liver doses of <28 to 32 Gy at 2 Gy/fraction are recommended (215).

Kidney

The kidneys are very sensitive to small doses of radiation, and a common goal is to avoid greater than 18 to 20 Gy whole kidney dose. When delivering whole-abdominal irradiation, the kidneys are at risk and must be blocked at acceptable doses to prevent renal failure. When delivering paraaortic irradiation, the kidneys are also at risk, and treatment planning CT scans can help to define which beam angles would best irradiate the nodal regions while avoiding the kidneys. When planning radiation fields, sometimes one kidney will need to be irradiated more than the other and the equivalent of one kidney must be spared. Chemotherapy can lower kidney tolerance to radiation as can increasing age. Irradiation of only one kidney does not necessarily reduce the risk of renal complications (216). Functional renal studies prior to radiation are important in documenting unexpected perfusion or excretion abnormalities and in determining how much each kidney contributes to total renal function. Functional changes have been described after exposure of the kidney to more than 20 Gy, and signs and symptoms of renal dysfunction can follow, including hypertension, leg edema, and urinalysis showing albuminuria and low specific gravity (216). A normocytic, normochromic anemia may also appear. Renal function studies will ultimately show decreased blood flow and filtration rates. CT scans may reveal a small kidney if one kidney has been preferentially irradiated to protect the other (203). Current dose–volume recommendations are found in the QUANTEC data (216).

Ovaries

In premenopausal patients treated with definitive irradiation, the ovaries will be irradiated incidentally and ovarian failure will occur. Hot flashes and other menopausal symptoms can develop during radiation. Hormone replacement therapy is an important consideration in women younger than 50. Alternatively, midline oophoropexy has been used in young women requiring irradiation for Hodgkin's disease, in an effort to spare the ovaries. The ovaries can also be elevated out of the radiation field and placed above the true pelvis to attempt to protect them when treating cervical cancer. The radiosensitivity of the ovarian cells varies considerably with age. The dose necessary to castrate a woman depends on her age. A larger dose is required during the period of more active follicular proliferation. A single dose of 4.0 to 8.0 Gy or fractionated doses of 12 to 20 Gy (depending on age) are known to produce permanent castration and sterility in most patients (202,203,209).

Vagina

There are few noticeable acute reactions when treating the upper two-thirds of the vagina with radiation. Some patients may notice a white-yellow vaginal discharge, which is due to mucositis of the vaginal mucosa. This may be evident during and can continue for several months after radiation (203). The lower third of the vagina, however, will become quite irritated when irradiated, in part due to irradiation of the vulva and urethra as described above. The distal vagina is less tolerant of radiation than the proximal, and the TDs are in the range of 80 to 90 Gy versus 120 to 150 Gy, respectively (217). There are, however, no studies that have successfully correlated dose-volume histogram (DVH) parameters with morbidity (218). Vaginal narrowing and shortening is a late sequela of radiation, which can alter and impede sexual function. Combined brachytherapy and external beam irradiation will cause more late effects than either modality alone. Use of a vaginal dilator or intercourse two to three times per week can help to keep the vagina open. Use of lubrication with intercourse as well as estrogen creams to build up the vaginal mucosa can also make intercourse more comfortable (209,219). Rarely, with excessive doses of radiation, patients can develop vaginal necrosis. This is due to a change in blood supply to the vaginal tissues and is much more common at the introitus than at the vaginal apex, perhaps due to the vascular supply of the vagina. The posterior vaginal wall is most frequently involved (217). Interstitial implants are more likely to cause necrosis than intracavitary implants. Hydrogen peroxide douches, antibiotics, and hyperbaric oxygen therapy can help the vaginal tissues to heal (220). Narcotics are often necessary to control the associated pain until healing has occurred. Trental (pentoxifylline) can also help soft tissue necrosis to heal (221). The uterus is very resistant to high doses of radiation, as is evident in patients treated with external beam and brachytherapy for cervical cancer. Rare cervical necrosis can occur, and will respond readily to hyperbaric oxygen treatments and pentoxifylline (220,209). There may be an increased risk of this in patients using cocaine. Necrosis can also be caused by recurrent tumor; distinguishing recurrent disease from necrosis can be very difficult and sometimes requires surgical intervention (203).

Stomach, Small and Large Intestines

The stomach is lined with a mucous membrane comprising columnar epithelium which is sensitive to radiation. Like the small and large bowel reactions, the stomach lining develops erosions and thinning, and subsequent edema and ulceration. Symptoms may include nausea, vomiting, reflux, and pain. Use of prophylactic antiemetics and proton pump inhibitors can decrease the acute effects of radiation. Acid production can be decreased during radiation and for up to 1 to 2 years after. Late effects can include gastritis and ulceration with associated bleeding. Progressive fibrosis can lead to gastric outlet obstruction and rarely, perforation, all of which are dose and volume dependent (203). The entire stomach can tolerate doses of 45 to 50 Gy, but data on maximum tolerated doses are inadequate (222).

The acute effects of radiation on the small intestine are due to the inherent radiation sensitivity of the rapidly dividing undifferentiated crypt of Lieberkühn cells. The normal lining of the GI tract is a self-renewing tissue. These undifferentiated stem cells normally migrate and differentiate upward from the lower half of the crypts to the tips of the intestinal villi as they mature, providing a continuous supply of surface cells as they divide. Their function is to primarily form absorptive cells but also mucous-secreting goblet cells and endocrine cells (202,203,208). The mature cells at the surface of the villi are repeatedly sloughed and replaced by the cells that originate in the crypts. These undifferentiated crypt cells are the most sensitive to radiation and are preferentially depleted, leading to loss of mature replacement cells at the surface of the villi. When these mature mucosal cells cannot be replaced, the villi shorten and the loss of absorptive function of the small intestine occurs. This loss of function results in fluid and nutrient wasting, diarrhea, and dehydration. This constellation of symptoms is termed acute radiation enteritis. Fortunately, reepithelialization occurs within several days due to recovery of the rapidly dividing crypt cells (208). Mucosal healing will occur within 10 to 14 days if radiation is terminated, and symptoms will accordingly improve and resolve in most patients. It is common to observe watery diarrhea with intermittent abdominal cramping starting in the second or third week of abdominal or pelvic irradiation. Increased peristalsis, disturbance of the absorption mechanisms, and decreased transit time may also occur. Patients will report increased flatulence and noisy bowel sounds. Rarely, patients will report nausea. Implementation of a low-residue diet, hydration, and use of antimotility agents can be very helpful. Some patients may be lactose and fat intolerant as well. Judicious use of narcotics to calm the bowel can also be helpful. Concurrent 5-FU or gemcitabine can worsen small bowel toxicity; diarrhea from 5-FU often appears before the radiation enteritis has had time to evolve. The late effects of radiation on the small bowel may be a continuation of the acute effects (222). Some patients will experience chronic diarrhea, requiring a permanent change in diet. Certain foods may trigger diarrhea, such as those high in fiber or fat. Spicy foods and monosodium glutamate may also trigger diarrhea. Areas of narrowing corresponding to regions of high dose or adhesions can occur in the small bowel loops and lead to partial obstruction of the small bowel. Patients may report abdominal pain and distention followed by diarrhea and relief of these symptoms. A complete bowel obstruction would also be characterized by abdominal pain and distention in addition to vomiting and lack of bowel movements. Small bowel obstructions occur in approximately 5% of irradiated patients, and surgical intervention is required in some to relieve these obstructions. Prior surgeries or a history of perforated appendix, pelvic abscess, or inflammatory bowel disease may increase the risk of small bowel toxicity, as can the use of chemotherapy. Hypertension and diabetes can also be risk factors, as can thin body habitus. Radiation to large volumes of bowel or high doses to even small volumes of bowel can lead to bowel obstructions. The ileum is the most common loop of bowel involved (203). Malabsorption of fats, carbohydrates, protein, B_{12}, and lactose may occur in some patients. Excessive bile salts can reach the colon and act as a cathartic, and medications such as cholestyramine may be helpful in controlling the resultant loose stools.

Small bowel doses should be limited to 45 to 50 Gy with 60 Gy maximum (84). Current recommendations for small bowel dose/volume constraints are as follows: The absolute volume of small bowel receiving >15 Gy should be <120 cc when delineating individual loops of bowel. If the entire peritoneal space is defined, the volume of small bowel receiving >45 Gy should be <195 cc (222).

The rectosigmoid mucosa is a rapid renewal system similar to the small bowel. When the rectum is included in the irradiated volume, there is rectal discomfort with tenesmus and production of mucous, sometimes mixed with blood in the stools (203). Patients may report frequent and sometimes painful evacuations of only small amounts of stool mixed with mucus. Hemorrhoids may worsen during radiation. This constellation of symptoms is termed "proctitis." Medications to decrease the number of stools as well as antispasmodic agents can be helpful. Suppositories or foams with steroids can be helpful, as can topical perianal skin ointments and lotions. Uncontrolled radiation enteritis can worsen radiation proctitis due to frequent stooling through the irritated rectum. With respect to late effects, if the dose of radiation is large enough, it may cause temporary or permanent ulceration and bleeding due to telangiectasias (**Fig. 11.60**) (223). Cortisone-containing rectal suppositories and foams or sulfasalazine instillations can also help to heal the bleeding and ulcerated rectal mucosa, as can argon laser ablation of the telangiectasias.

Hyperbaric oxygen therapy can be helpful in controlling severe bleeding (224,225). Fibrosis, stenosis, perforation, and fistula formation are rarer (**Fig. 11.61**). In general, doses in excess of 60 Gy are necessary to produce this more advanced radiation damage to the small bowel and rectosigmoid (223). Fecal diversion may be necessary in the setting of stenosis, necrosis, or fistula formation. Retrospective analyses have shown that limited surfaces of the rectum can tolerate point doses of about 75 Gy (external beam and brachytherapy) with acceptable morbidity (77,84). Volumetric data on dose tolerances for the rectum and sigmoid are currently being validated in image-guided series.

Bladder/Ureters/Urethra

The bladder and ureters have a rapidly renewing transitional epithelium. The effect of radiation is early denudation similar to the skin due to injury to the rapidly dividing basal cells. Epithelial desquamation leads to focal ulcerations, hyperemia, and edema of the bladder wall, which is visible at cystoscopy (203,208,226). Acute and transient radiation cystitis may be observed with moderate doses of irradiation (>30 Gy), and usually requires no specific treatment. Patients will report urinary frequency and urgency and mild dysuria, as well as decreased bladder capacity. However, with higher radiation doses, more severe symptoms of cystitis develop, such as severe dysuria and hematuria, which may require treatment. Agents such as Pyridium may help lessen these symptoms. Significant spasms of the bladder musculature, which can be improved with administration of smooth muscle relaxants, may also occur. It is important to rule out the presence of a concomitant bacterial infection, which may exacerbate the symptoms. Infections are seen at an increased rate in irradiated patients, perhaps in part due to radiation-induced diarrhea and contamination of the perineum. Urinalysis and urine cultures obtained under sterile conditions, when indicated, should be obtained before institution of antibiotic therapy. Radiation cystitis is characterized by the presence of white cells and red cells without bacteria on urinalysis.

With doses above 60 Gy, chronic cystitis and hematuria may be observed due to telangiectasias, which can develop in the bladder lining (227). With higher doses, more severe chronic cystitis, fibrosis, and decreased bladder capacity may occur. Rarely, bladder neck contractures as well as fistulas may occur, which can necessitate surgical intervention. Fistulas are more likely to occur if there is invasion of the bladder wall by tumor, or in the setting of interstitial implants. Surgery may be required to deal with some of these complications (203). Hyperbaric oxygen therapy can be very helpful with hemorrhagic cystitis, as can the drug pentosan polysulfate (Elmiron), which has been used for interstitial cystitis (220,228). The ureters are quite resistant to radiation and, although rare ureteral stenosis is reported in some series (226,229). This may require stenting or, rarely, diversion. Interstitial implants, or early placement of a narrow midline block, are more likely than intracavitary implants to cause this (77). Urethral stenosis is also rare and is also more likely to occur with interstitial than intracavitary approaches. Careful dilation can be helpful in sustaining bladder outflow (226).

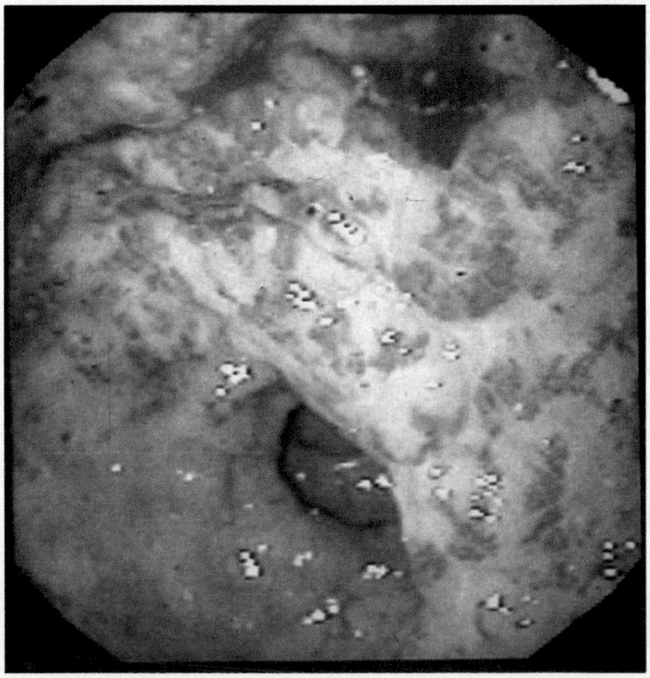

Figure 11.60. Radiation-induced telangiectasias of the rectum consistent with radiation proctitis.

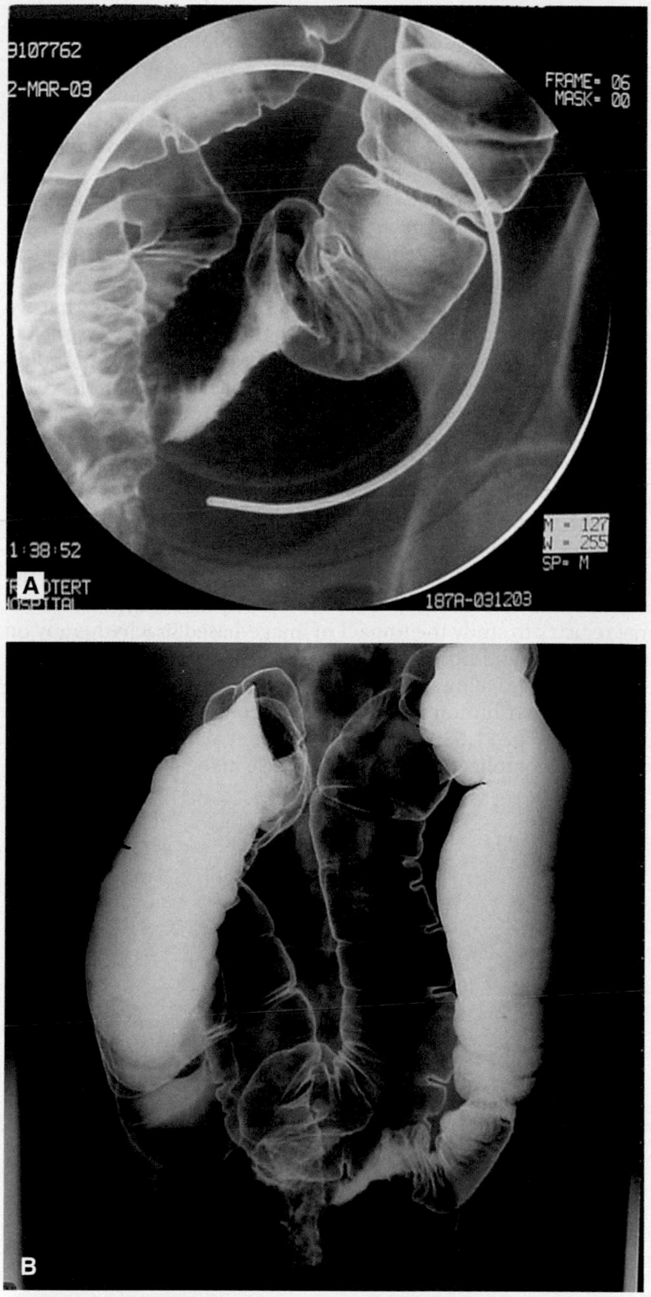

Figure 11.61. Radiation-induced sigmoid stricture noted on a contrast study: **A:** full view, **B:** magnified view, following definitive chemoradiation.

Bladder and Rectosigmoid—LDR

The bladder and rectosigmoid are the organs of concern in the setting of combined external beam irradiation and brachytherapy for gynecologic cancers. Dose and volume are considered two important variables related to complications. Dose has been thought to be an important determinant of normal tissue complications. Attempts have been made to determine the maximum tolerable normal tissue dose with an acceptable risk of complications. There is no consensus as to what these values should be. Point doses may or may not coincide with complication risk, as they do not account for the volume of organ irradiated. They are also not defined consistently. Maximum bladder point doses of 75 to 80 Gy and rectal doses of 70 to 75 Gy are guidelines (84,227,223). The ratio of dose to the rectal point and bladder point and dose to point A is also important, with a low incidence of rectal (0.3% vs. 5%) and bladder (2% vs. 2% to 5%) complications when this ratio is less than 80% (84). Other factors such as external beam dose and intracavitary dose rate are also important in the etiology of complications. The volume of rectum and bladder irradiated is an important variable in the development of complications in addition to the cumulative dose (230). Both external beam and use of tandem and cylinder applicators can increase the volume of bladder and rectum treated. Stage, patient age, and medical comorbidities such as hypertension, diabetes, diverticulitis, or inflammatory bowel disease may also increase the risk of complications, as can the administration of chemotherapy. Individual radiosensitivity may also impact complication risk.

Bladder and Rectosigmoid—HDR

Acceptable normal tissue doses are even more debatable in HDR than LDR. Using HDR techniques, the therapeutic range is narrower and the risk of complications seems to rise faster than the rate of improved tumor control. Available clinical data also suggest that in addition to total HDR dose, the most important factor in late complication development is the dose per fraction and the number of fractions (231). The organ most at risk for complications is the rectosigmoid, whereas the bladder complication risk is comparatively low. Rectal and sigmoid complications occur earlier than bladder complications (77). Rectal bleeding is the most frequent rectal morbidity occurring in approximately 30% of patients (77). To avoid excessive morbidity, better physical dose distributions must be achieved with HDR to reduce doses to critical normal structures. This implies the use of rectal and bladder displacement. Rectal retractors have become an integral component of insertion techniques and perhaps improve the effectiveness and reproducibility of rectal displacement over gauze vaginal packing (172). Various disparate recommendations concerning normal tissue fraction size and total dose exist in the literature. Sakata et al. (232) found that the probability of rectal complications increased dramatically above a maximal rectal dose (Deq) of 60 Gy. Cheng et al. (233) found that patients with >62 Gy of summed external beam and intracavitary doses to the proximal rectum and >110 Gy maximal proximal rectal BED had significant increase in complications. Various recommendations for rectal and bladder TDs are in the literature using point doses and time–dose-fractionation and biologically effective dose (BED) values (204). Use of film-based point doses is becoming less common than use of image-based methods using CT or MR. If using film-based dosimetry, it is very important to choose points related to critical structures very carefully on the orthogonal films. Rectum above the level of the vaginal applicators and rectal retractor should be identified and sigmoid in addition to rectal points should be evaluated, as should bladder and vaginal points. When possible, the doses to the normal critical structures should be less than the dose at point A, perhaps in the range of 50% to 80%. The portions of the rectum and sigmoid that are above the range of the rectal retractor are most often the hot spots, and every effort must be made to decrease the dose to the rectosigmoid relative to the point A dose. Consideration to decreasing the dwell times or turning off dwell positions in the tandem should be given. Tandem lengths of 6 to 8 cm are typical. If there is endometrial extension, a longer tandem may be needed. Additionally, use of a tapered tandem will decrease sigmoid, bladder, and small bowel doses (133). Contrast in the sigmoid is helpful in making these decisions. CT scanning after applicator placement is exceedingly helpful and much more reliable in assessing the proximity of the sigmoid to the tandem and in manipulating the dose distribution (**Fig. 11.62**). Sigmoid doses can often be higher than the rectal ICRU doses (233). Dose volume data appear to be more helpful than point dose data in predicting for complications. Using CT- or MR-based volume planning, the EQD2 limit to the D2cc (the minimum dose in the most irradiated 2 cm^3 normal tissue volume for the rectum and sigmoid) is 70 to 75 Gy and for the bladder is 80 to 90 Gy (5,139,141,157). Georg et al. found that for the rectum, a significant dose effect was found for all DVH parameters for any grade of complication as well as for G2 to G4 side effects with the exception of the D0.1cc. For G2 to G4 rectal toxicity, a threshold of 60 Gy (EQD2)

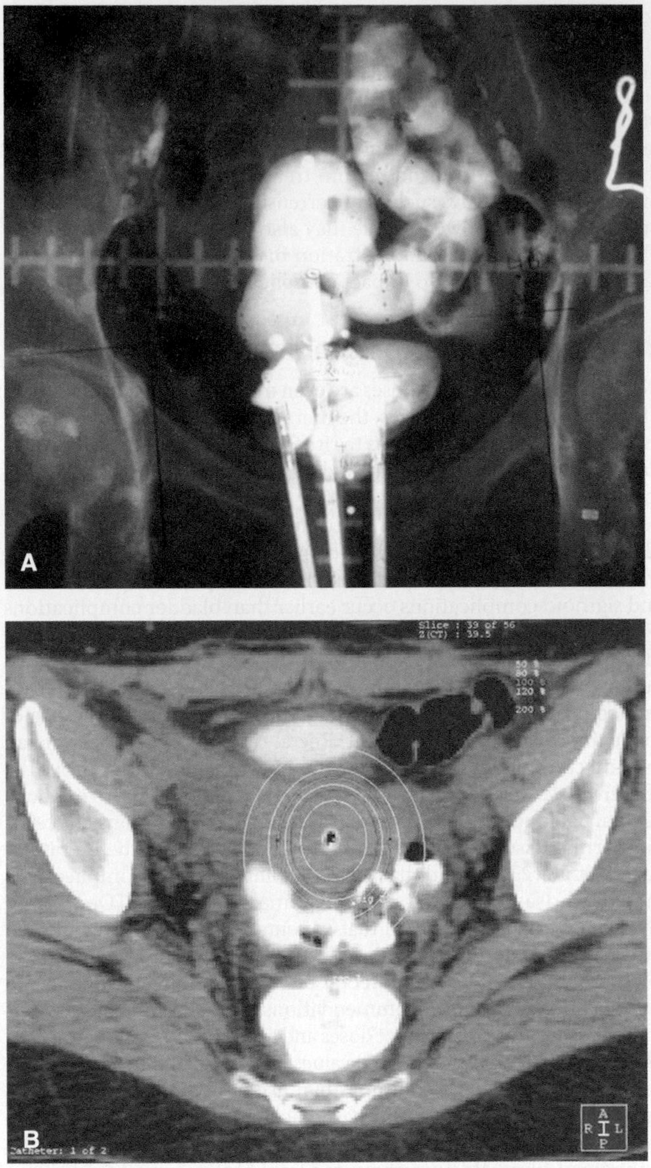

Figure 11.62. Radiograph of the pelvis with a tandem and ovoid applicator in place demonstrates the circuitous course of the sigmoid (**A**). The axial CT scan (**B**) demonstrates a more accurate relationship of the sigmoid to the uterine tandem, and the need to limit dose to this loop of sigmoid positioned very close to the high-dose region of the implant.

was observed, with a 10% incidence at 78 Gy and a 20% incidence at 90 Gy. For bladder, no significant dose–response was observed for G1 to G4 side effects, but for complications of >G2, dose effect curves could be generated for all DVH parameters that were statistically significant. For bladder, there was a 5% risk of G2 to G4 morbidity with a D2cc of 70 Gy, a 10% risk of G2 to G4 morbidity with a D2cc of 101 Gy, and a 20% risk of G2 to G4 morbidity with a D2cc of 134 Gy (234,235). Late bladder sequelae have been infrequent in patients with such doses but longer follow-up is needed to be certain as the late effects in the bladder can be quite delayed in their appearance (141). Georg et al. and Kook et al. also found a correlation between rectal dose volume parameters and endoscopically defined mucosal changes as well as clinical side effects (236,237).

FUTURE FOCUS

Reduction of morbidity and improvement in local control and cure is a common goal in the treatment of patients with gynecologic cancers. Use of 3-D and functional imaging will be increasingly important to define tumor and normal tissues. This can perhaps allow escalation of dose to the tumor and reduction of dose to the critical normal tissues. There has been, however, a reluctance to vary from traditional dose specification as good outcomes have been published at institutions skilled in the care of gynecologic patients. It is potentially dangerous to optimize therapy to such an extent that the dose distribution looks dramatically different from the traditional "pear shape," which effectively encompasses the primary tumor and parametria in cervical cancer presentations. Making this pear too narrow to avoid critical structures may lead to a higher rate of local recurrence. Yet it is important to treat the disease and not just strive for an ideal dose distribution. Studies using CT indicate that we underestimate normal tissue doses with the present 2-D dosimetric analysis used at most institutions. Whether this information should change the way we prescribe doses remains debatable. Directly relating the intracavitary system to the anatomy through use of CT and MRI seems to be the next step in the lineage of dosimetric systems (**Fig. 11.63**). The GEC ESTRO GYN Working Group guidelines for defining and contouring tumor volumes and normal tissues on MRI scans with the brachytherapy applicators in place, as well as specifying and tracking dose to volumes rather than points, are being used worldwide (5,139). These guidelines are now incorporated into the EMBRACE I and II studies, which are actively accruing patients in a large registry to study the impact of image-based brachytherapy on tumor control and normal tissue toxicity. The excellent soft tissue resolution of MRI allows visualization of residual tumor in relation to the isodose distribution around the MRI-compatible brachytherapy applicators (**Fig. 11.63**). Data from Potter et al. (141) have shown a decrease in complications and an increase in local control with the

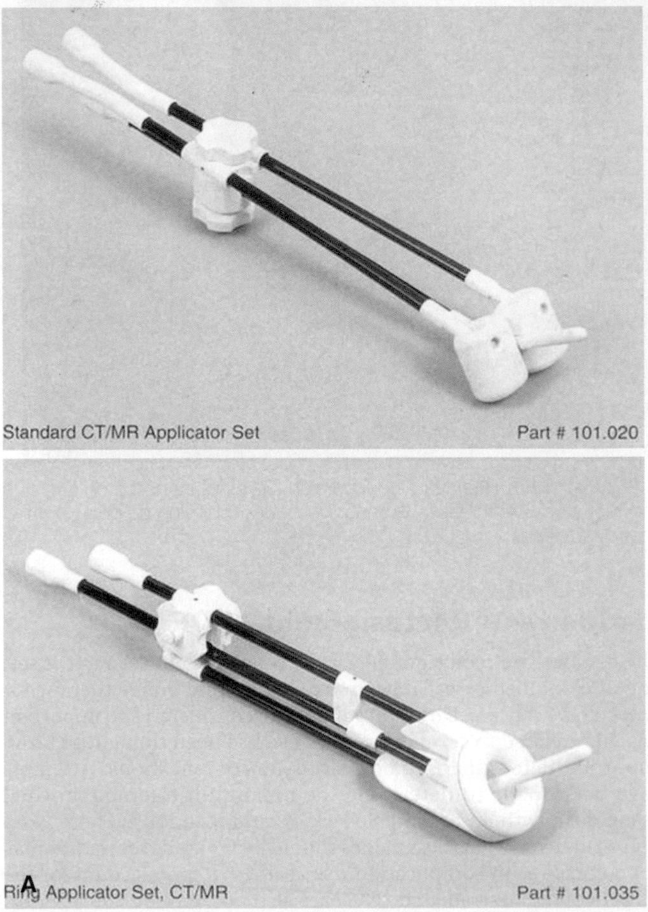

Figure 11.63. A: MRI-compatible applicators. **B, C:** MRI of the pelvis with an MRI/CT-compatible applicator ring (**B**) and ovoids (**C**) in place. Note the associated dose distribution relative to visible tumor within the cervix and the bladder, rectum, and sigmoid.

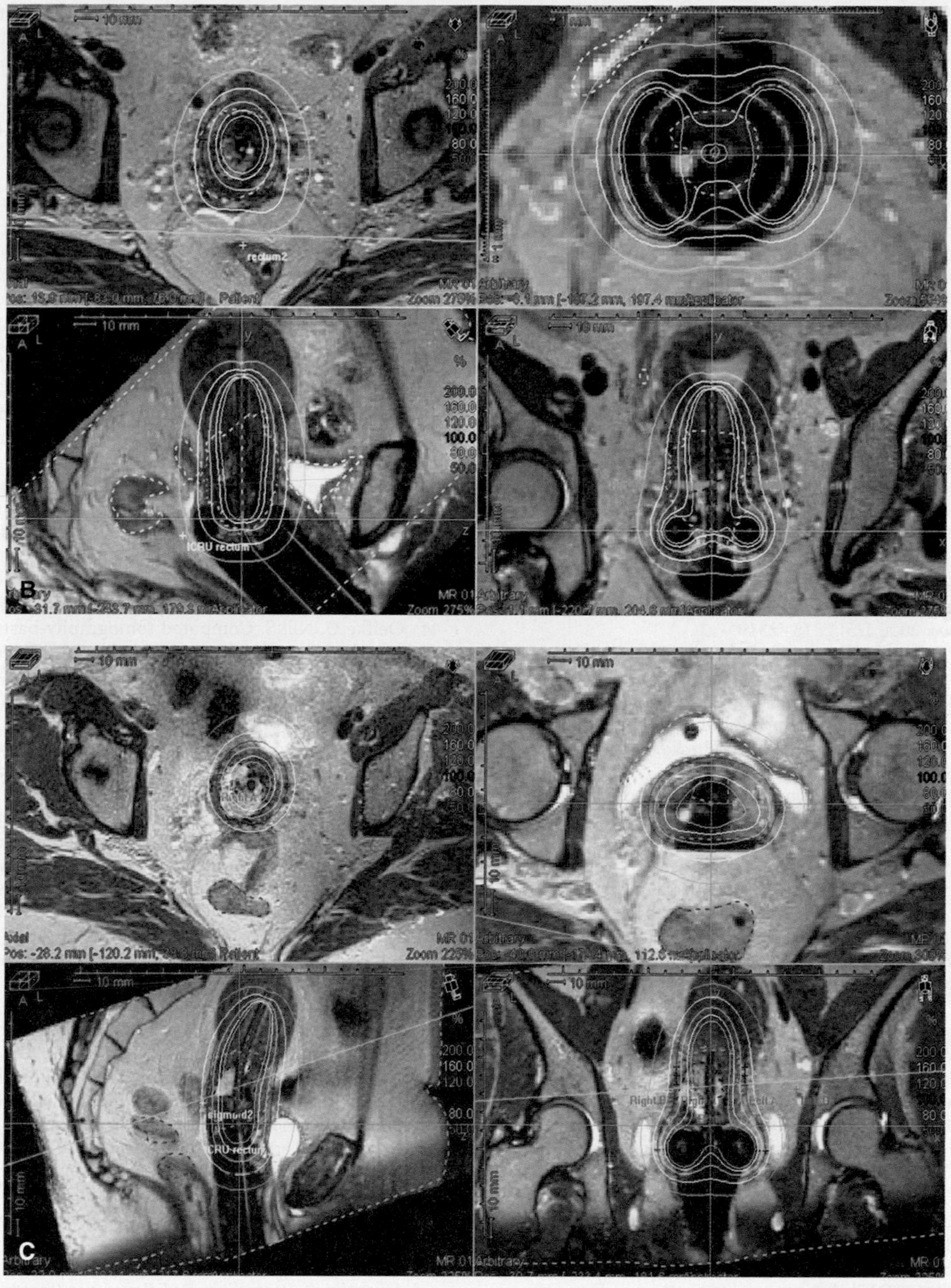

Figure 11.63. *(continued)*

use of MRI-guided brachytherapy for cervical cancer. Additionally, the use of dose–volume histogram analysis may add new insight into optimizing local control and decreasing morbidity with a better understanding of the importance of dose–volume relationships. This may be a powerful tool to help improve the therapeutic ratio in patients with gynecologic cancer and will best be achieved through collaboration of radiation oncologists, gynecologic oncologists, and diagnostic radiologists.

REFERENCES

1. Hall EJ, Giaccia AJ. *Radiobiology for the Radiologist*. 7th Ed. Philadelphia, PA: Wolters Kluwer Health/Lippincott Williams & Wilkins; 2012.
2. Liauw SL, Connell PP, Weichselbaum RR. New paradigms and future challenges in radiation oncology: an update of biological targets and technology. *Sci Transl Med*. 2013;5(173):173sr2. doi:10.1126/scitranslmed.3005148.
3. Moding EJ, Kastan MB, Kirsch DG. Strategies for optimizing the response of cancer and normal tissues to radiation. *Nat Rev Drug Discov*. 2013;12(7):526–542. doi:10.1038/nrd4003.
4. Klopp AH, Eifel PJ. Chemoradiotherapy for cervical cancer in 2010. *Curr Oncol Rep*. 2011;13(1):77–85. doi:10.1007/s11912-010-0134-z.
5. Pötter R, Haie-Meder C, Van Limbergen E, et al. Recommendations from gynaecological (GYN) GEC ESTRO working group (II): concepts and terms in 3D image-based treatment planning in cervix cancer brachytherapy-3D dose volume parameters and aspects of 3D image-based anatomy, radiation physics, and radiobiology. *Radiother Oncol*. 2006;78(1):67–77.
6. Warters RL, Hofer KG, Harris CR, Smith JM. Radionuclide toxicity in cultured mammalian cells: elucidation of the primary site of radiation damage. *Curr Top Radiat Res Q*. 1978;12(1–4):389–407.
7. Hawkins RB. The influence of concentration of DNA on the radiosensitivity of mammalian cells. *Int J Radiat Oncol Biol Phys*. 2005;63(2):529–535.
8. Cremer C, Cremer T, Zorn C, et al. Induction of chromosome shattering by ultraviolet irradiation and caffeine: comparison of whole-cell and partial-cell irradiation. *Mutat Res*. 1981;84(2):331–348.

9. Sak A, Stuschke M. Use of γH2AX and other biomarkers of double-strand breaks during radiotherapy. *Semin Radiat Oncol.* 2010;20(4):223–231. doi:10.1016/j.semradonc.2010.05.004.
10. Lloyd DC, Dolphin GW. Radiation-induced chromosome damage in human lymphocytes. *Br J Ind Med.* 1977;34(4):261–273.
11. Shrivastav M, De Haro LP, Nickoloff JA. Regulation of DNA double-strand break repair pathway choice. *Cell Res.* 2008;18(1):134–147.
12. Hamada N, Fujimichi Y. Classification of radiation effects for dose limitation purposes: history, current situation and future prospects. *J Radiat Res.* 2014;55(4):629–640. doi:10.1093/jrr/rru019.
13. Khan KH, Blanco-Codesido M, Molife LR. Cancer therapeutics: targeting the apoptotic pathway. *Crit Rev Oncol Hematol.* 2014;90(3):200–219. doi:10.1016/j.critrevonc.2013.12.012.
14. Brown JM, Carlson DJ, Brenner DJ. The tumor radiobiology of SRS and SBRT: are more than the 5 Rs involved? *Int J Radiat Oncol Biol Phys.* 2014;88(2):254–262. doi:10.1016/j.ijrobp.2013.07.022.
15. Rao SS, Thompson C, Cheng J, et al. Axitinib sensitization of high Single Dose Radiotherapy. *Radiother Oncol.* 2014;111(1):88–93. doi:10.1016/j.radonc.2014.02.010.
16. Hönscheid P, Datta K, Muders MH. Autophagy: detection, regulation and its role in cancer and therapy response. *Int J Radiat Biol.* 2014;90(8):628–635. doi:10.3109/09553002.2014.907932.
17. Vakifahmetoglu H, Olsson M, Zhivotovsky B. Death through a tragedy: mitotic catastrophe. *Cell Death Differ.* 2008;15(7):1153–1162. doi:10.1038/cdd.2008.47.
18. Franken NA, Rodermond HM, Stap J, et al. Clonogenic assay of cells in vitro. *Nat Protoc.* 2006;1(5):2315–2319.
19. van der Schueren E, Landuyt W, Scalliet P. Repair of 'sublethal damage': key factor in normal tissue tolerance to fractionated and low dose rate irradiation. *Front Radiat Ther Oncol.* 1989;23:60–74.
20. Durand RE. Tumor repopulation during radiotherapy: quantitation in two xenografted human tumors. *Int J Radiat Oncol Biol Phys.* 1997;39(4):803–808.
21. Huang Z, Mayr NA, Gao M, et al. Onset time of tumor repopulation for cervical cancer: first evidence from clinical data. *Int J Radiat Oncol Biol Phys.* 2012;84(2):478–484. doi:10.1016/j.ijrobp.2011.12.037.
22. Terasima T, Tolmach LJ. Changes in x-ray sensitivity of HeLa cells during the division cycle. *Nature.* 1961;190:1210–1211.
23. Dillon MT, Good JS, Harrington KJ. Selective targeting of the G2/M cell cycle checkpoint to improve the therapeutic index of radiotherapy. *Clin Oncol (R Coll Radiol).* 2014;26(5):257–265. doi:10.1016/j.clon.2014.01.009.
24. Coleman CN. Hypoxia in tumors: a paradigm for the approach to biochemical and physiologic heterogeneity. *J Natl Cancer Inst.* 1988; 80(5):310–317.
25. Kim CK, Park SY, Park BK, et al. Blood oxygenation level-dependent MR imaging as a predictor of therapeutic response to concurrent chemoradiotherapy in cervical cancer: a preliminary experience. *Eur Radiol.* 2014;24(7):1514–1520. doi:10.1007/s00330-014-3167.
26. Ewing D. The oxygen fixation hypothesis: a reevaluation. *Am J Clin Oncol.* 1998;21(4):355–361.
27. Lin SH, George TJ, Ben-Josef E, et al. Opportunities and challenges in the era of molecularly targeted agents and radiation therapy. *J Natl Cancer Inst.* 2013;105(10):686–693. doi:10.1093/jnci/djt055.
28. Raleigh DR, Haas-Kogan DA. Molecular targets and mechanisms of radiosensitization using DNA damage response pathways. *Future Oncol.* 2013;9(2):219–233. doi:10.2217/fon.12.185.
29. Tomao F, Di Tucci C, Imperiale L, et al. Cervical cancer: are there potential new targets? An update on preclinical and clinical results. *Curr Drug Targets.* 2014;15(12):1107–1120.
30. Jain RK. Normalizing tumor microenvironment to treat cancer: bench to bedside to biomarkers. *J Clin Oncol.* 2013;31(17):2205–2218. doi:10.1200/JCO.2012.46.3653.
31. Tewari KS, Monk BJ. New strategies in advanced cervical cancer: from angiogenesis blockade to immunotherapy. *Clin Cancer Res.* 2014;20(21):5349–5358. doi:10.1158/1078-0432.CCR-14-1099.
32. Gao H, Xue J, Zhou L, et al. Bevacizumab radiosensitizes non-small cell lung cancer xenografts by inhibiting DNA double-strand break repair in endothelial cells. *Cancer Lett.* 2015;365(1):79–88. doi:10.1016/j.canlet.2015.05.011.
33. Burnette B, Weichselbaum RR. Radiation as an immune modulator. *Semin Radiat Oncol.* 2013;23(4):273–280. doi:10.1016/j.semradonc.2013.05.009.
34. Sharabi AB, Lim M, DeWeese TL, et al. Radiation and checkpoint blockade immunotherapy: radiosensitisation and potential mechanisms of synergy. *Lancet Oncol.* 2015;16(13):e498–e509. doi:10.1016/S1470-2045(15)00007-8.
35. Seung SK, Curti BD, Crittenden M, et al. Phase 1 study of stereotactic body radiotherapy and interleukin-2—tumor and immunological responses. *Sci Transl Med.* 2012;4(137):137ra74. doi:10.1126/scitranslmed.3003649.
36. Twyman-Saint Victor C, Rech AJ, Maity A, et al. Radiation and dual checkpoint blockade activate non-redundant immune mechanisms in cancer. *Nature.* 2015;520(7547):373–377. doi:10.1038/nature14292.
37. Johns HE, Cunningham JR. *The Physics of Radiology.* 4th Ed. Springfield, IL: Charles C. Thomas; 1983.
38. Khan FM. *The Physics of Radiation Therapy.* 4th Ed. Philadelphia, PA: Lippincott Williams and Wilkins; 2009.
39. Holmes T, Das R, Low D, et al. American Society of Radiation Oncology recommendations for documenting intensity-modulated radiation therapy treatments. *Int J Radiat Oncol Biol Phys.* 2009;74(5):1311–1318.
40. Hartford A, Palisca M, Eichler T, et al. American Society for Therapeutic Radiology and Oncology (ASTRO) and American College of Radiology (ACR) practice guidelines for intensity-modulated radiation therapy (IMRT). *Int J Radiat Oncol Biol Phys.* 2009;73(1):9–14.
41. Wagner A, Jhingran A, Gaffney D. Intensity modulated radiotherapy in gynecologic cancers: hope, hype or hyperbole? *Gynecol Oncol.* 2013;130(1):229–223.
42. Tyagi N, Lewis JH, Yashar CM, et al. Daily online cone beam computed tomography to assess interfractional motion in patients with intact cervical cancer. *Int J Radiat Oncol Biol Phys.* 2011;80(1):273–280.
43. Haripotepornkul NH, Nath SK, Scanderbeg D, et al. Evaluation of intra- and inter-fraction movement of the cervix during intensity modulated radiation therapy. *Radiother Oncol.* 2011;98:347–351.
44. Oelfke U, Nill S. Computed tomography-based image-guided radiation therapy technology. In: Hendee R, Li X, eds. *Imaging in Medical Diagnosis and Therapy: Adaptive Radiation Therapy.* Boca Raton, FL: Taylor Francis Group; 2011:141–156.
45. Potters L, Gaspar L, Kavanagh B, et al. American Society for Therapeutic Radiology and Oncology (ASTRO) and American College of Radiology (ACR) practice guidelines for image-guided radiation therapy (IGRT). *Int J Radiat Oncol Biol Phys.* 2010;76(2):319–325.
46. Schwarz JK, Wahab S, Grigsby PW. Prospective phase I-II trial of helical tomotherapy with or without chemotherapy for postoperative cervical cancer patients. *Int J Radiat Oncol Biol Phys.* 2011;81(5):1258–1263.
47. Eifel PJ. Regional treatment of vulvar cancer; lessons from the past and lessons for the future. *Pract Radiat Oncol.* 2012;2:279–281.
48. Kim CH, Olson AC, Kim Y, et al. Contouring inguinal and femoral nodes; how much margin is needed around the vessels? *Pract Radiat Oncol.* 2012;2(4):274–278.
49. Clivio A, Kluge A, Cozzi L, et al. Intensity modulated proton beam radiation for brachytherapy in patients with cervical carcinoma. *Int J Radiat Oncol Biol Phys.* 2013;87(5):897–903.
50. Kidd EA, Siegel BA, Dehdashiti F, et al. Clinical outcomes of definitive intensity-modulated radiation therapy with fluorodeoxyglucose-positron emission tomography simulation in patients with locally advanced cervical cancer. *Int J Radiat Oncol Biol Phys.* 2010;77(4):1085–1091.
51. Erickson B, Lim K, Steward J, et al. Adaptive radiation therapy for gynecologic cancers. In: Hendee R, Li X, eds. *Imaging in Medical Diagnosis and Therapy: Adaptive Radiation Therapy.* Boca Raton, FL: Taylor & Francis Group; 2011:351–368.
52. *International Commission on Radiation Units and Measurements, Prescribing, Recording, and Reporting Photon Beam Therapy.* ICRU Report 50. Bethesda, MD: International Commission on Radiation Units and Measurements; 1993.
53. Erickson B, Wilson JF. Clinical indications for brachytherapy. *J Surg Oncol.* 1997;65:218–227.
54. Erickson B, Kudrimoti M, Haiemeder C. Brachytherapy for gynecologic cancers. In: Venselaar J, Meigooni A, Baltas D, Hoskin PJ, eds. *Comprehensive Brachytherapy. Physical and Clinical Aspects,* Chapter 21. Boca Raton, FL:Taylor & Francis; 2013:295–318.
55. International Commission on Radiation Units and Measurements. Dose and Volume Specification for Reporting Intracavitary Therapy in Gynecology. ICRU Report 38. Bethesda, MD: International Commission on Radiation Units and Measurements; 1985.
56. Castelnau-Marchand P, Chargari C, Maroun P, et al. Clinical outcomes of definitive chemoradiation followed by intracavitary pulsed-dose rate image-guided adaptive brachytherapy in locally advanced cervical cancer. *Gynecol Oncol.* 2015;139(2):288–294.
57. Lee L, Das I, Higgins S, et al. American Brachytherapy Society consensus guidelines for locally advanced carcinoma of the cervix. Part III: low-dose-rate and pulsed-dose-rate brachytherapy. *Brachytherapy.* 2012;11:53–57.

58. *Recommendation on Limits for Exposure to Ionizing Radiation.* Report No. 91. Bethesda, MD: National Council on Radiation Protection and Measurements; 1987.
59. Nath R, Anderson L, Luxton G, et al. Dosimetry of interstitial brachytherapy sources: recommendations of AAPM Radiation Therapy Committee Task Group No. 43. *Med Phys.* 1995;22:209–234.
60. Vahrson H, Glaser FH. History of HDR afterloading in brachytherapy. *Strahlenther Onkol.* 1988;82(Suppl):2–6.
61. Fletcher GH, Rutledge FN, Chau PM. Policies of treatment in cancer of the cervix uteri. Am *J Roentgenol.* 1962;87:6–21.
62. Perez CA, Camel HM, Kuske RR, et al. Radiation therapy alone in the treatment of carcinoma of the uterine cervix: a 20-year experience. *Gynecol Oncol.* 1986;23:127–140.
63. Hendriksen E. The lymphatic spread of carcinoma of the cervix and of the body of the uterus. A study of 420 necropsies. *Am J Obstet Gynecol.* 1949;58(5):924–942.
64. Chao C, Williamson J, Grigsby P, et al. Uterosacral space involvement in locally advanced carcinoma of the uterine cervix. *Int J Radiat Oncol Biol Phys.* 1998;40(2):397–403.
65. Bonin S, Lanciano R, Corn B, et al. Bony landmarks are not an adequate substitute for lymphangiography in defining pelvic lymph node location for the treatment of cervical cancer with radiotherapy. *Int J Radiat Oncol Biol Phys.* 1996;34(1):167–172.
66. Park J, Charnsangavej C, Yoshimitsu K, et al. Pathways of nodal metastasis from pelvic tumors: CT demonstration. *RadioGraphics.* 1994;14(6):1309–1321.
67. Thomas L, Chacon B, Kind M, et al. Magnetic resonance imaging in the treatment planning of radiation therapy in carcinoma of the cervix treated with the four-field pelvic technique. *Int J Radiat Oncol Biol Phys.* 1997;37(4):827–832.
68. Zunino S, Rosato O, Lucino S, et al. Anatomic study of the pelvis in carcinoma of the uterine cervix as related to the box technique. *Int J Radiat Oncol Biol Phys.* 1999;44(1):53–59.
69. Taylor A, Rockall A, Reznek R, et al. Mapping pelvic lymph nodes: guidelines for delineation in intensity-modulated radiotherapy. *Int J Radiat Oncol Biol Phys.* 2005;63(5):1604–1612.
70. Greer B, Koh W, Stelzer K, et al. Expanded pelvic radiotherapy fields for treatment of local-regionally advanced carcinoma of the cervix: outcome and complications. *Am J Obstet Gynecol.* 1996;174(4):1141–1150.
71. Balleyguier C, Sala E, Da Cunha T, et al. Staging of uterine cervical cancer with MRI: guidelines of the European Society of Urogenital Radiology. *Eur Radiol.* 2011;21(5):1102–1110.
72. Kidd EA, Siegel BA, Dehdashti F, et al. Lymph node staging by positron emission tomography in cervical cancer: relationship to prognosis. *J Clin Oncol.* 2010;28(12):2108–2113.
73. Fontanilla HP, Klopp AH, Lindberg ME, et al. Anatomic distribution of [(18)F]fluorodeoxyglucose-avid lymph nodes in patients with cervical cancer. *Pract Radiat Oncol.* 2013;3(1):45–53.
74. Lindegaard J, Tanderup K. Counterpoint: time to retire the parametrial boost. *Brachytherapy.* 2012;11:80–83.
75. Good J, Lalondrelle S, Blake P. Point: parametrial irradiation in locally advanced cervix cancer can be achieved effectively with a variety of external beam techniques. *Brachytherapy.* 2012;11:77–79.
76. Fenkell L, Assenholt M, Nielsen S, et al. Parametrial boost using midline shielding results in an unpredictable dose to tumor and organs at risk in combined external beam radiotherapy and brachytherapy for locally advanced cervical cancer. *Int J Radiat Oncol Biol Phys.* 2011;79(5):1572–1579.
77. Eifel PJ, Levenback C, Wharton JT, et al. Time course and incidence of late complications in patients treated with radiation therapy for FIGO stage IB carcinoma of the uterine cervix. *Int J Radiat Oncol Biol Phys.* 1995;32:1289–1300.
78. Huang EY, Wang CJ, Hsu HC, et al. Dosimetric factors predicting severe radiation-induced bowel complications in patients with cervical cancer: combined effect of external parametrial dose and cumulative rectal dose. *Gynecol Oncol.* 2004;95:101–108.
79. Logsdson M, Eifel P. FIGO IIIB squamous cell carcinoma of the cervix: an analysis of prognostic factors emphasizing the balance between external beam and intracavitary radiation therapy. *Int J Radiat Oncol Biol Phys.* 1999;43(4):763–775.
80. Perez CA, Breaux S, Madoc-Jones H, et al. Radiation therapy alone in the treatment of carcinoma of the uterine cervix I. Analysis of tumor recurrence. *Cancer.* 1983;51:1393–1402.
81. Perez CA, Fox S, Lockett MA, et al. Impact of dose in outcome of irradiation alone in carcinoma of the uterine cervix: analysis of two different methods. *Int J Radiat Oncol Biol Phys.* 1991;21:885–898.
82. Perez C, Grigsby P, Chao C, et al. Tumor size, irradiation dose, and long-term outcome of carcinoma of uterine cervix. *Int J Radiat Oncol Biol Phys.* 1998;41(2):307–317.
83. Perez CA, Breaux S, Bedwinek JM, et al. Radiation therapy alone in the treatment of carcinoma of the uterine cervix. II. Analysis of complications. *Cancer.* 1984;54:235–246.
84. Perez C, Grigsby P, Lockett M, et al. Radiation therapy morbidity in carcinoma of the uterine cervix: dosimetric and clinical correlation. *Int J Radiat Oncol Biol Phys.* 1999;44(4):855–866.
85. Grigsby P, Singh A, Siegel B, et al. Lymph node control in cervical cancer. *Int J Radiat Oncol Biol Phys.* 2004;59(3):706–712.
86. Houvenaegel G, Lelievre L, Rigouard A, et al. Residual pelvic lymph node involvement after concomitant chemoradiation for locally advanced cervical cancer. *Gynecol Oncol.* 2006;102:74–79.
87. Vargo JA, Kim H, Choi S, et al. Extended field intensity modulated radiation therapy with concomitant boost for lymph node-positive cervical cancer: analysis of regional control and recurrence patterns in the positron emission tomography/computed tomography ear. *Int J Radiat Oncol Biol Phys.* 2014;90(5):1091–1098.
88. Klopp A, Smith BD, Alektiar K, et al. The role of postoperative radiation therapy for endometrial cancer: executive summary of an American Society for Radiation Oncology evidence-based guideline. *Pract Radiat Oncol.* 2014;4(3);137–144.
89. Creasman WT, Boronow RC, Morrow CP, et al. Adenocarcinoma of the endometrium: its metastatic lymph node potential. *Gynecol Oncol.* 1976;4:239–243.
90. Boronow RC, Morrow CP, Creasman WT, et al. Surgical staging in endometrial cancer: clinical–pathologic findings of a prospective study. *Obstet Gynecol.* 1984;63(6):825–832.
91. Olofsen-van Acht M, van den Berg H, Quint S, et al. Reduction of irradiated small bowel volume and accurate patient positioning by use of a belly board device in pelvic radiotherapy of gynecologic cancer patients. *Radiother Oncol.* 2001;59:87–93.
92. Ahmad R, Hoogeman MS, Quint S, et al. Residual setup errors caused by rotation and non-rigid motion in prone-treated cervical cancer patients after online CBCT image-guidance. *Radiother Oncol.* 2012;103:322–326.
93. Ghosh K, Padilla L, Murray K, et al. Using a belly board device to reduce the small bowel volume within pelvic radiation fields in women with post-operatively treated cervical carcinoma. *Gynecol Oncol.* 2001;83:271–275.
94. Bondar L, Hoggeman M, Mens JW, et al. Toward an individualized target motion management for IMRT of cervical cancer based on model-predicted cervix-uterus shape and position. *Radiother Oncol.* 2011;99(2):240–245.
95. Buchali A, Koswig S, Dinges S, et al. Impact of the filling status of the bladder and rectum on their integral dose distribution and movement of the uterus in the treatment planning of gynaecological cancer. *Radiother Oncol.* 1999;52:29–34.
96. Hacker NF, Eifel PJ, van der Velden J. FIGO Cancer Report 2015. Cancer of the vulva. *Int J Gynaecol Obstet.* 2015;131:S76–S83.
97. Beriwal S, Shukla G, Shinde A, et al. Preoperative intensity modulated radiation therapy and chemotherapy for locally advanced vulvar carcinoma: analysis of pattern of relapse. *Int J Radiat Oncol Biol Phys.* 2013;85(5):1269–1274.
98. Hasselle MD, Rose BS, Kochanski JD, et al. Clinical outcomes of intensity-modulated pelvic radiation therapy for carcinoma of the cervix. *Int J Radiat Oncol Biol Phys.* 2011;80(5):1436–1445.
99. Jhingran A, Winter K, Portelance L, et al. A phase II study of intensity modulated radiation therapy to the pelvis for postoperative patients with endometrial carcinoma: Radiation Therapy Oncology Group Trial 0418. *Int J Radiat Oncol Biol Phys.* 2012;84(1)e23–e28.
100. Barillot I, Tavernier E, Peignaux K, et al. Impact of post-operative intensity modulated radiotherapy on acute gastro-intestinal toxicity for patients with endometrial cancer: results of the phase II RTCMIENDOMETRE French multicentre trial. *Radiother Oncol.* 2014;111(1):138–143.
101. Klopp AH, Moughan J, Portelance L, et al. Hematologic toxicity in RTOG 0418: a phase 2 study of postoperative IMRT for gynecologic cancer. *Int J Radiat Oncol Biol Phys.* 2013;86(1):83–90.
102. Albuquerque K, Giangreco D, Morrison C, et al. Radiation-related predictors of hematologic toxicity after concurrent chemoradiation for cervical cancer and implications for bone marrow-sparing pelvic IMRT. *Int J Radiat Oncol Biol Phys.* 2011;79(4):1043–1047.
103. Small Jr W, Mell L, Anderson P, et al. Consensus guidelines for the delineation of the clinical target volume for intensity modulated pelvic radiotherapy in the postoperative treatment of endometrial and cervical cancer. *Int J Radiat Oncol Biol Phys.* 2008;71(2):428–434.

104. Small W, Mundt A. *Gynecologic Pelvis Atlas*. RTOG Radiation Therapy Oncology Group; 2007. http://www.rtog.org/gynatlas/main.html. Accessed January 9, 2009.
105. Gay H, Barthold H, O'Meara E, et al. Pelvic normal tissue contouring guidelines for radiation therapy: a Radiation Therapy Oncology Group Consensus Panel Atlas. *Int J Radiat Oncol Biol Phys*. 2012;83(3):e353–e362.
106. Martinez-Monge R, Fernandes P, Gupta N, et al. Cross-sectional nodal atlas: a tool for the definition of clinical target volumes in three-dimensional radiation therapy planning. *Radiology*. 1999;211:815–828.
107. Jhingran A, Salehpour M, Sam M, et al. Vaginal motion and bladder and rectal volumes during pelvic intensity-modulated radiation therapy after hysterectomy. *Int J Radiat Oncol Biol Phys*. 2012;82(1):256–262.
108. Lim K, Small W Jr, Portelance L, et al. Consensus guidelines for delineation of clinical target volume for intensity-modulated pelvic radiotherapy for the definitive treatment of cervix cancer. *Int J Radiat Oncol Biol Phys*. 2011;79(2):348–355.
109. Gandhi AK, Sharma DN, Rath GK, et al. Early clinical outcomes and toxicity of intensity modulated versus conventional pelvic radiation therapy for locally advanced cervix carcinoma: a prospective randomized study. *Int J Radiat Oncol Biol Phys*. 2013;87(3):542–548.
110. Langerak T, Mens JW, Quint S, et al. Cervix motion in 50 cervical cancer patients assessed by daily cone beam computed tomographic imaging of a new type of marker. *Int J Radiat Oncol Biol Phys*. 2015;93(3):532–539.
111. Cihoric N, Tapia C, Kruger K, et al. IMRT with ^{18}FDG-PET\CT based simultaneous integrated boost for treatment of nodal positive cervical cancer. *Radiat Oncol*. 2014;9:83.
112. Heyman J. The so-called Stockholm method and the results of treatment of uterine cancer at the Radiumhemmet. *Acta Radiol*. 1935;16:129–147.
113. Lenz M. Radiotherapy of cancer of the cervix at the Radium Institute, Paris, France. *Am J Roentgenol Radium Ther Nucl Med*. 1927;17:335–342.
114. Tod MC, Meredith WJ. A dosage system for use in the treatment of cancer of the uterine cervix. *Br J Radiol*. 1938;11:809–824.
115. Tod M, Meredith WJ. Treatment of cancer of the cervix uteri—a revised "Manchester method." *Br J Radiol*. 1953;26:252–257.
116. Fletcher GH, Shalek RJ, Wall JA, et al. A physical approach to the design of applicators in radium therapy of cancer of the cervix uteri. *Am J Roentgenol*. 1952;68:935–949.
117. Fletcher GH. Cervical radium applicators with screening the direction of bladder and rectum. *Radiology*. 1953;60:77–84.
118. Fletcher GH, Brown TC, Rutledge FN. Clinical significance of rectal and bladder dose measurements in radium therapy of cancer of the uterine cervix. *Am J Roentgenol Radium Ther Nucl Med*. 1958;79:421–450.
119. Fletcher GH, Rutledge FN, Chau PM. Policies of treatment in cancer of the cervix uteri. *Am J Roentgenol*. 1962;87:6–21.
120. Fletcher GH. Cancer of the uterine cervix: Janeway lecture, 1970. *Am J Roentgenol Radium Ther Nucl Med*. 1971;3:225–242.
121. Haas JS, Dean RD, Mansfield CM. Dosimetric comparison of the Fletcher family of gynecologic colpostats 1950–1980. *Int J Radiat Oncol Biol Phys*. 1985;11:1317–1321.
122. Delclos L, Fletcher GH, Moore EB, et al. Minicolpostats, dome cylinders, other additions and improvements of the Fletcher-Suit afterloadable system: indications and limitations of their use. *Int J Radiat Oncol Biol Phys*. 1980;6:1195–1206.
123. Katz A, Eifel P. Quantification of intracavitary brachytherapy parameters and correlation with outcome in patients with carcinoma of the cervix. *Int J Radiat Oncol Biol Phys*. 2000;48(5):1417–1425.
124. Eifel PJ, Morris M, Wharton JT, et al. The influence of tumor size and morphology on the outcome of patients with FIGO stage IB squamous cell carcinoma of the uterine cervix. *Int J Radiat Oncol Biol Phys*. 1994;29:9–16.
125. Potish RA, Gerbi BJ. Cervical cancer: intracavitary dose specification and prescription. *Radiology*. 1987;165:555–560.
126. Potish RA. The effect of applicator geometry on dose specification in cervical cancer. *Int J Radiat Oncol Biol Phys*. 1990;18:1513–1520.
127. Batley F, Constable WC. The use of the Manchester system for treatment of cancer of the uterine cervix with modern after-loading radium applicators. *Am J Roentgenol Radium Ther Nucl Med*. 1967;18:396–400.
128. Lewis GC, Raaventos A, Half J. Space dose relationships for points A and B in the radium therapy of cancer of the uterine cervix. *Am J Roentgenol Radium Ther Nucl Med*. 1960;83:432–446.
129. Gebara W, Weeks K, Jones E, et al. Carcinoma of the uterine cervix: a 3D-CT analysis of dose to the internal, external and common iliac nodes in tandem and ovoid applications. *Radiother Oncol*. 2000;56:43–48.
130. Potish RA, Gerbi BJ. Role of point A in the era of computerized dosimetry. *Radiology*. 1986;158:827–831.
131. Cunningham DE, Stryker JA, Velkley DE, et al. Intracavitary dosimetry: a comparison of mg-hr prescription to doses at points A and B in cervical cancer. *Int J Radiat Oncol Biol Phys*. 1981;7:121–123.
132. Maruyama Y, Van Nagell Jr, Wrede DE, et al. Approaches to optimization of dose in radiation therapy of cervix carcinoma. *Radiology*. 1976;120:389–398.
133. Decker W, Erickson B, Albano K, et al. Comparison of traditional low dose rate to optimized and nonoptimized high dose rate tandem and ovoid dosimetry. *Int J Radiat Oncol Biol Phys*. 2001;50(2):561–567.
134. Viswanathan AN, Erickson BA. Seeing is saving: the benefit of 3D imaging in gynecologic brachytherapy. *Gynecol Oncol*. 2015;138:207–215.
135. Harkenrider MM, Alite F, Silva SR, et al. Image-based brachytherapy for the treatment of cervical cancer. *Int J Radiat Oncol Biol Phys*. 2015;92(4):921–934.
136. Viswanathan A, Beriwal S, DeLosSantos J, et al. American Brachytherapy Society consensus guidelines for locally advanced carcinoma of the cervix. Part II: High-dose-rate brachytherapy. *Brachytherapy*. 2012;11:47–52.
137. Dimopoulos JCA, Petrow P, Tanderup K, et al. Recommendations from Gynaecological (GYN) GEC-ESTRO Working Group (IV): basic principles and parameters for MR imaging within the frame of image based adaptive cervix cancer brachytherapy. *Radiother Oncol*. 2012;103(1):113–122.
138. Kirisits C, Potter R, Lang S, et al. Dose and volume parameters for MRI-based treatment planning in intracavitary brachytherapy for cervical cancer. *Int J Radiat Oncol Biol Phys*. 2005;62(3):901–911.
139. Haie-Meder C, Potter R, Van Limbergen E, et al. Recommendations for Gynecological (GYN) GEC-ESTRO Working Group (I): concepts and terms in 3D image-based 3D treatment planning in cervix cancer brachytherapy with emphasis on MRI assessment of GTV and CTV. *Radiother Oncol*. 2005;74:235–245.
140. Viswanathan AN, Erickson B, Gaffney DK, et al. Comparison and consensus guidelines for delineation of clinical target volume for CT- and MR-based brachytherapy in locally advanced cervical cancer. *Int J Radiat Oncol Biol Phys*. 2014;90:320–328.
141. Potter R, Georg P, Dimopoulos JCA, et al. Clinical outcome of protocol based image (MRI) guided adaptive brachytherapy combined with 3D conformal radiotherapy with or without chemotherapy in patients with locally advanced cervical cancer. *Radiother Oncol*. 2011;100(1):116–123.
142. International Commission on Radiation Units and Measurements. Prescribing, recording and reporting brachytherapy for cancer of the cervix (ICRU Report 89). *J ICRU*. 2013;13(1-2).
143. Eifel P, Moughan J, Erickson B, et al. Patterns of radiotherapy practice for patients with carcinoma of the uterine cervix. A Patterns of Care Study. *Int J Radiat Oncol Biol Phys*. 2004;60(4):1144–1153.
144. Eifel PJ, Ho A, Khalid N, et al. Patterns of radiation therapy practice for patients treated for intact cervical cancer in 2005 to 2007: a quality research in radiation oncology study. *Int J Radiat Oncol Biol Phys*. 2014;89(2):249–256.
145. Smith GL, Jiang J, Giordano SH, et al. Trends in the quality of treatment for patients with intact cervical cancer in the United States, 1999 through 2011. *Int J Radiat Oncol Biol Phys*. 2015;92(2):260–267.
146. Barraclough L, Swindell R, Livsey J, et al. External beam boost for cancer of the cervix uteri when intracavitary therapy cannot be performed. *Int J Radiat Oncol Biol Phys*. 2008;71(3):772–778.
147. Chen CC, Lin JC, Jan JS, et al. Definitive intensity-modulated radiation therapy with concurrent chemotherapy for patients with locally advanced cervical cancer. *Gyn Oncol*. 2011;122:9–13.
148. Hilaris BS, Nori D, Anderson LL. Brachytherapy in cancer of the cervix. In: Hilaris BS, Nori D, Anderson LL, eds. *Atlas of Brachytherapy*. New York, NY: Macmillan Publishing; 1988;244–256.
149. Kagan AR, DiSaia PJ, Wollin M, et al. The narrow vagina, the antecedent for irradiation injury. *Gynecol Oncol*. 1976;4:291–298.
150. Crook JM, Esche BA, Chaplain G, et al. Dose-volume analysis and the prevention of radiation sequelae in cervical cancer. *Radiother Oncol*. 1987;8:321–332.
151. Cunningham DE, Stryker JA, Velkley DE, et al. Routine clinical estimation of rectal, rectosigmoidal, and bladder doses from intracavitary brachytherapy in the treatment of carcinoma of the cervix. *Int J Radiat Oncol Biol Phys*. 1981;7:653–660.
152. Hamberger AD, Unal A, Gershenson DM, et al. Analysis of the severe complications of irradiation of carcinoma of the cervix: whole pelvis irradiation and intracavitary radium. *Int J Radiat Oncol Biol Phys*. 1983;9:367–371.
153. Pourquier H, Dubois JB, Delard R. Exclusive use of radiotherapy in cancer of the cervix prevention of late pelvic complications. *Cervix*. 1990;8:61–74.
154. Corn BW, Hanlon AL, Pajak TF, et al. Technically accurate intracavitary insertions improve pelvic control and survival among patients with locally advanced carcinoma of the uterine cervix. *Gynecol Oncol*. 1994;53:294–300.

155. Viswanathan AN, Moughan J, Small Jr W, et al. The quality of cervical cancer brachytherapy implantation and the impact on local recurrence and disease-free survival in Radiation Therapy Oncology Group Prospective Trials 0116 and 0128. *Int J Gyn Cancer*. 2012;22(1):123–131.
156. Erickson B, Gillin M. Interstitial implantation of gynecologic malignancies. *J Surg Oncol*. 1997;66:285–295.
157. Viswanathan A, Creutzberg C, Craighead P, et al. International brachytherapy practice patterns: a survey of the Gynecologic Cancer Intergroup (GCIG). *Int J Radiat Oncol Biol Phys*. 2012;82(1):250–255.
158. Viswanathan AN, Erickson BE, Rownd J. Image-based approaches to interstitial brachytherapy. In: Viswanathan AN, Kirisits C, Erickson BE, et al., eds. *Gynecologic Radiation Therapy. Novel Approaches to Image-Guidance and Management*. New York, NY: Springer; 2011:247–259.
159. Beriwal S, Demanes DJ, Erickson B, et al. American Brachytherapy Society consensus guidelines for interstitial brachytherapy for vaginal cancer. *Brachytherapy*. 2012;11:68–75.
160. Gupta A, Vicini F, Frazier A, et al. Iridium-192 transperineal interstitial brachytherapy for locally advanced or recurrent gynecologic malignancies. *Int J Radiat Oncol Biol Phys*. 1999;43(5):1055–1060.
161. Martinez A, Cox RS, Edmundson GK. A multiple site perineal applicator (MUPIT) for treatment of prostatic, anorectal, and gynecologic malignancies. *Int J Radiat Oncol Biol Phys*. 1984;10:297–305.
162. Inoue T, Inoue T, Tanaka E, et al. High dose rate fractionated interstitial brachytherapy as the sole treatment for recurrent carcinoma of the uterus. *J Brachyther Int*. 1999;15:161–167.
163. Syed AMN, Puthawala AA, Neblett D, et al. Transperineal interstitial-intracavitary "Syed-Neblett" applicator in the treatment of carcinoma of the uterine cervix. *Endocuriether Hypertherm Oncol*. 1986;2:1–13.
164. Syed A, Puthawala A, Abdelaziz N, et al. Long-term results of low-dose-rate interstitial-intracavitary brachytherapy in the treatment of carcinoma of the cervix. *Int J Radiat Oncol Biol Phys*. 2002;54(1):67–78.
165. Beriwal S, Rwigema JC, Higgins E, et al. Three-dimensional image-based high-dose-rate interstitial brachytherapy for vaginal cancer. *Brachytherapy*. 2012;11:176–180.
166. Viswanathan AN, Cormack R, Rawal B, et al. Increasing brachytherapy dose predicts survival for interstitial and tandem-based radiation for stage IIIB cervical cancer. *Int J Gyn Cancer*. 2009;19(8):1402–1406.
167. Nomden C, deLeeuw A, Moerland M, et al. Clinical use of the Utrecht applicator for combined intracavitary/interstitial brachytherapy treatment in locally advanced cervical cancer. *Int J Radiat Oncol Biol Phys*. 2012;84(4):1424–1430.
168. Dimopoulos J, Kirisits C, Petric P, et al. The Vienna applicator for combined intracavitary and interstitial brachytherapy of cervical cancer: clinical feasibility and preliminary results. *Int J Radiat Oncol Biol Phys*. 2006;66:83–90.
169. Erickson B, Albano K, Gillin M. CT-guided interstitial implantation of gynecologic malignancies. *Int J Radiat Oncol Biol Phys*. 1996;36(3):699–709.
170. Orton C. High and low dose rate brachytherapy for cervical carcinoma. *Acta Oncol*. 1998;37(2):117–125.
171. Stewart A, Viswanathan A. Current controversies in high-dose-rate versus low-dose-rate brachytherapy for cervical cancer. *Cancer*. 2006;107(5):908–915.
172. Sarkaria JN, Petereit DG, Stitt JA, et al. A comparison of the efficacy and complication rates of low dose-rate versus high dose-rate brachytherapy in the treatment of uterine cervical carcinoma. *Int J Radiat Oncol Biol Phys*. 1994;30:75–82.
173. Erickson BA, Demanes DJ, Ibbott GS, et al. American Society for Radiation Oncology (ASTRO) and American College of Radiology (ACR) practice guideline for the performance of high-dose-rate brachytherapy. *Int J Radiat Oncol Biol Phys*. 2011;79(3):641–649.
174. Brenner DJ, Huang Y, Hall EJ. Fractionated high dose-rate versus low dose-rate regimens for intracavitary brachytherapy of the cervix: equivalent regimens for combined brachytherapy and external irradiation. *Int J Radiat Oncol Biol Phys*. 1991;21:1415–1423.
175. Orton CG. Biologic treatment planning. In: Martinez AA, Orton CG, Mould RF, eds. *Brachytherapy HDR and LDR*. Columbia, MD: Nucletron; 1990:205–215.
176. Erickson B, Jones R, Rownd J, et al. Is the tandem and ring applicator a suitable alternative to the high dose rate Selectron tandem and ovoid applicator? *J Brachyther Int*. 2000;16:31–144.
177. Mai J, Erickson B, Rownd J, et al. Comparison of four different dose specification methods for high dose rate intracavitary radiation for treatment of cervical cancer. *Int J Radiat Oncol Biol Phys*. 2001;51(4):1131–1141.
178. Cetingoz R, Ataman O, Tuncel N, et al. Optimization in high dose rate brachytherapy for utero-vaginal applications. *Radiother Oncol*. 2001;58:31–36.
179. Anker C, Cachoeira C, Boucher K, et al. Does the entire uterus need to be treated in cancer of the cervix? Role of adaptive brachytherapy. *Int J Radiat Oncol Biol Phys*. 2010;76(3):704–712.
180. Jones N, Rankin J, Gaffney D. Is simulation necessary for each high-dose-rate tandem and ovoid insertion in carcinoma of the cervix? *Brachytherapy*. 2004;3:120–124.
181. Christensen G, Carlson B, Chao C, et al. Imaged-based dose planning of intracavitary brachytherapy: registration of serial-imaging studies using deformable anatomic templates. *Int J Radiat Oncol Biol Phys*. 2001;51(1):227–243.
182. Nag S, Gupta N. A simple method of obtaining equivalent doses for use in HDR brachytherapy. *Int J Radiat Oncol Biol Phys*. 2000;46(2):507–513.
183. Erickson B, Eifel P, Moughan J, et al. Patterns of brachytherapy practice for patients with carcinoma of the cervix (1996–1999): a Patterns of Care study. *Int J Radiat Oncol Biol Phys*. 2005;63(4):1083–1092.
184. Mitra D, Klopp AH, Viswanathan AN. Pros and cons of vaginal brachytherapy after external beam radiation therapy in endometrial cancer. *Gynecol Oncol*. 2016;140(1):167–75.
185. Harkenrider MM, Block AM, Siddiqui ZA, et al. The role of vaginal cuff brachytherapy in endometrial cancer. *Gynecol Oncol*. 2015;136(2):365–72.
186. Small W, Erickson B, Kwakwa F. American Brachytherapy Society survey regarding practice patterns of post-operative irradiation for endometrial cancer: current status of vaginal brachytherapy. *Int J Radiat Oncol Biol Phys*. 2005;63(5):1502–1507.
187. Small Jr W, Beriwal S, Demanes D, et al. American Brachytherapy Society consensus guidelines for adjuvant vaginal cuff brachytherapy after hysterectomy. *Brachytherapy*. 2012;11:58–67.
188. Dobbie BMW. Vaginal recurrences in carcinoma of the body of the uterus and their prevention. *J Obstet Gynaecol Br Emp*. 1953;60:702–705.
189. Price JJ, Hahn GA, Rominger CJ. Vaginal involvement in endometrial carcinoma. *Am J Obstet Gynecol*. 1965;91(8):1060–1065.
190. Gore E, Gillin M, Albano K, et al. Comparison of high dose rate and low dose rate dose distributions for vaginal cancers. *Int J Radiat Oncol Biol Phys*. 1995;31(1):165–170.
191. Li S, Aref I, Walker E, et al. Effects of prescription depth, cylinder size, treatment length, tip space, and curved end on doses in high-dose-rate vaginal brachytherapy. *Int J Radiat Oncol Biol Phys*. 2007;67(4):1268–1277.
192. Russo J, Armeson K, Richardson S. Comparison of 2D and 3D imaging and treatment planning for postoperative vaginal apex high-dose rate brachytherapy for endometrial cancer. *Int J Radiat Oncol Biol Phys*. 2012;83(1):e75–e80.
193. Choo J, Scudiere J, Bitterman P, et al. Vaginal lymphatic channel location and its implication for intracavitary brachytherapy radiation treatment. *Brachytherapy*. 2005;4:236–240.
194. Jhingran A, Burke T, Eifel, P. Definitive radiotherapy for patients with isolated vaginal recurrence of endometrial carcinoma after hysterectomy. *Int J Radiat Oncol Biol Phys*. 2003;56(5):1366–1372.
195. Gill BS, Chapman BV, Hansen KJ, et al. Primary radiotherapy for non-surgically managed Stage I endometrial cancer: utilization and impact of brachytherapy. *Brachytherapy*. 2015;14(3):373–379.
196. Schwarz JK, Beriwal S, Esthappan J, et al. Consensus statement for brachytherapy for the treatment of medically inoperable endometrial cancer. *Brachytherapy*. 2015;14(5):587–599.
197. Viswanathan A, Cormack R, Holloway C, et al. Magnetic resonance-guided interstitial therapy for vaginal recurrence of endometrial cancer. *Int J Radiat Oncol Biol Phys*. 2006;66(1):91–99.
198. Vargo JA, Kim H, Houser CJ, et al. Definitive salvage for vaginal recurrence of endometrial cancer: the impact of modern intensity-modulated-radiotherapy with image-based HDR brachytherapy and the interplay of the PORTEC 1 risk stratification. *Radiother Oncol*. 2014;113(1):126–131.
199. Glaser S, Beriwal S. Brachytherapy for malignancies of the vagina in the 3D ear. *J Contemp Brachytherapy*. 2015;7(4):312–318.
200. Vargo JA, Kim H, Houser CJ, et al. Image-based multichannel vaginal cylinder brachytherapy for vaginal cancer. *Brachytherapy*. 2015;14(1):9–15.
201. Glaser SM, Kim H, Beriwal S. Multichannel vaginal cylinder brachytherapy—impact of tumor thickness and location on dose to organs at risk. *Brachytherapy*. 2015;14(6)913–918.
202. Rotman M, Aziz H, Choi K. Radiation damage of normal tissues in the treatment of gynecologic cancers. *Front Radiat Ther Oncol*. 1989;23:349–366.
203. Rubin P, Casarett G. *Clinical Radiation Pathology*. Vol. 1–2. Philadelphia, PA: WB Saunders; 1968.
204. Viswanathan AN, Lee LJ, Eswara JR, et al. Complications of pelvic radiation in patients treated for gynecologic malignancies. *Cancer*. 2014;120:3870–3883.
205. Emani B, Lyman J, Brown A, et al. Tolerance to therapeutic irradiation. *Int J Radiat Oncol Biol Phys*. 1991;21:109–122.

206. Bentzen S, Constine L, Deasy J, et al. Quantitative analyses of normal tissue effects in the clinic (QUANTEC): an introduction to the scientific issues. *Int J Radiat Oncol Biol Phys.* 2010;76(3):S3–S9.
207. Marks L, Yorke E, Jackson A, et al. Use of normal tissue complication probability models in the clinic. *Int J Radiat Oncol Biol Phys.* 2010;76(3):S10–S19.
208. Cox J, Ang K, eds. *Radiation Oncology: Rationale, Technique, Results.* 8th Ed. St. Louis, MO: Mosby; 2003.
209. Grigsby P, Russell A, Bruner D, et al. Late injury of cancer therapy on the female reproductive tract. *Int J Radiat Oncol Biol Phys.* 1995;31(5):1289–1299.
210. Camidge R, Price A. Characterizing the phenomenon of radiation recall dermatitis. *Radiother Oncol.* 2001;59:237–245.
211. Tai P, Hammond A, Van Dyk J, et al. Pelvic fractures following irradiation of endometrial and vaginal cancer—a case series and review of lecture. *Radiother Oncol.* 2000;56:23–28.
212. Huh S, Kim B, Kang M, et al. Pelvic insufficiency fracture after pelvic irradiation in uterine cervix cancer. *Gynecol Oncol.* 2002;86:264–268.
213. Grigsby P, Roberts H, Perez C. Femoral head fracture following groin irradiation. *Int J Radiat Oncol Biol Phys.* 1995;32(1):63–67.
214. Lawrence T, Robertson J, Anscher M, et al. Hepatic toxicity resulting from cancer treatment. *Int J Radiat Oncol Biol Phys.* 1995;31(5):1237–1248.
215. Pan C, Kavanagh B, Dawson L, et al. Radiation-associated liver injury. *Int J Radiat Oncol Biol Phys.* 2010;76(3):S94–S100.
216. Dawson L, Kavanagh B, Paulino A, et al. Radiation-associated kidney injury. *Int J Radiat Oncol Biol Phys.* 2010;76(3):S108–S115.
217. Hintz BL, Kagan AR, Chan P, et al. Radiation tolerance of the vaginal mucosa. *Int J Radiat Oncol Biol Phys.* 1980;6:711–716.
218. Fidarova E, Berger D, Schussler S, et al. Dose volume parameter D_{2cc} does not correlate with vaginal side effects in individual patients with cervical cancer treated within a defined treatment protocol with very high brachytherapy doses. *Radiother Oncol.* 2010;97:76–79.
219. Au S, Grigsby P. The irradiation tolerance dose of the proximal vagina. *Radiother Oncol.* 2003;67:77–85.
220. Pasquier D, Hoelscher T, Schmutz J, et al. Hyperbaric oxygen therapy in the treatment of radio-induced lesions in normal tissues: a literature review. *Radiother Oncol.* 2004;72:1–13.
221. Okunieff P, Augustine E, Hicks J, et al. Pentoxifylline in the treatment of radiation-induced fibrosis. *J Clin Oncol.* 2004;22(11):2207–2213.
222. Kavanagh B, Pan C, Dawson L, et al. Radiation dose-volume effects in the stomach and small bowel. *Int J Radiat Oncol Biol Phys.* 2010;76(3):S101–S107.
223. Michalski J, Gay H, Jackson A, et al. Radiation dose-volume effects in radiation-induced rectal injury. *Int J Radiat Oncol Biol Phys.* 2010;76(3):S123–S129.
224. Mayer R, Klemen H, Quehenberger F, et al. Hyperbaric oxygen—an effective tool to treat radiation morbidity in prostate cancer. *Radiother Oncol.* 2001;61:151–156.
225. Woo TCS, Joseph D, Oxer H, et al. Hyperbaric oxygen treatment for radiation proctitis. *Int J Radiat Oncol Biol Phys.* 1997;38(3):619–622.
226. Marks L, Carroll P, Dugan T, et al. The response of the urinary bladder, urethra, and ureter to radiation and chemotherapy. *Int J Radiat Oncol Biol Phys.* 1995;31(5):1257–1280.
227. Viswanathan A, Yorke E, Marks L, et al. Radiation dose-volume effects of the urinary bladder. *Int J Radiat Oncol Biol Phys.* 2010;76(3):S116–S122.
228. Bevers RFM, Bakker D, Kurth KH. Hyperbaric oxygen treatment for haemorrhagic radiation cystitis. *Lancet.* 1995;346:803–804.
229. McIntyre J, Eifel P, Levenback C, et al. Ureteral stricture as a late complication of radiotherapy for stage IB carcinoma of the uterine cervix. *Cancer.* 1995;75(3):836–843.
230. Roeske J, Mundt A, Halpern H, et al. Late rectal sequelae following definitive radiation therapy for carcinoma of the uterine cervix: a dosimetric analysis. *Int J Radiat Oncol Biol Phys.* 1997;37(2):351–358.
231. Wang C, Leung S, Chen H, et al. High-dose rate intracavitary brachytherapy (HDR-IC) in treatment of cervical carcinoma: 5-year results and implication of increased low-grade rectal complication on initiation of an HDR-IC fractionation scheme. *Int J Radiat Oncol Biol Phys.* 1997;38(2):391–398.
232. Sakata KI, Nagakura H, Oouchi A, et al. High-dose-rate intracavitary brachytherapy: results of analyses of late rectal complications. *Int J Radiat Oncol Biol Phys.* 2002;54(5):1369–1376.
233. Cheng JCH, Peng LC, Chen YH, et al. Unique role of proximal rectal dose in late rectal complications for patients with cervical cancer undergoing high-dose-rate intracavitary brachytherapy. *Int J Radiat Oncol Biol Phys.* 2003;57(4):1010–1018.
234. Georg P, Potter R, Georg D, et al. Dose effect relationship for late side effects of the rectum and urinary bladder in magnetic resonance image-guided adaptive cervix cancer brachytherapy. *Int J Radiat Oncol Biol Phys.* 2012;82(2):653–657.
235. Georg P, Lang S, Dimopoulos J, et al. Dose-volume histogram parameters and late side effects in magnetic resonance image-guided adaptive cervical cancer brachytherapy. *Int J Radiat Oncol Biol Phys.* 2011;79(2):356–362.
236. Koom W, Sohn D, Kim JY, et al. Computed tomography-based high-dose-rate intracavitary brachytherapy for uterine cervical cancer: preliminary demonstration of correlation between dose-volume parameters and rectal mucosal changes observed by flexible sigmoidoscopy. *Int J Radiat Oncol Biol Phys.* 2007;68(5):1446–1454.
237. Georg P, Kirisits C, Goldner G, et al. Correlation of dose-volume parameters, endoscopic and clinical rectal side effects in cervix cancer patients treated with definitive radiotherapy including MRI-based brachytherapy. *Radiother Oncol.* 2009;91:173–180.

CHAPTER 12

Targeted Therapies in Gynecologic Cancers

Stephanie Lheureux and Amit M. Oza

INTRODUCTION

Biologic Foundations of Cancer

Normal cellular function and growth requires a complex interplay of intracellular and microenvironmental processes, which are precisely regulated by processes that have developed through evolution with internal controls and redundancies. Aberrations in cellular regulatory processes may result in major effects on the macromolecular or cellular environment. There are inbuilt corrective mechanisms, such as cell death, to maintain homeostasis and balance however, cancers develop when these homeostatic mechanisms fail or cells evade normal controls. Development of cancer is the product of biologic insults exerted individually and collectively on the genome, the proteome, *via* modulation of the microenvironment, or evasion of the immune system. For example, insults to master regulatory genes responsible for safeguarding cellular integrity (such as *p53, BRCA1/2, myc, ras,* or *src*) result in well-characterized downstream aberrations to cell signaling. Evidence of this can be seen through:

i. deregulated cell death that enables an unyielding rate of growth and metastatic spread of cancerous cells;
ii. rewiring of cell signaling that allows for redirection or diversion of cancer-specific nutrients;
iii. evasion of the immune system that permits undetected and uncontrolled growth.

Cancer that escapes these internal self-regulatory mechanisms can develop increasing clonal and genomic diversity, with resulting cellular heterogeneity in space and over time. This cancer cell evolution and the difficulty in defining this real time, contributes to difficulty for therapeutic targeting. Understanding the contribution of each of these elements to the development and progression of cancer is essential for developing targeted or precision therapies. Elucidating the precise magnitude that each element contributes to clinical behavior, sensitivity, and resistance is essential to understanding biology and improving precision of targeted therapy in cancer. The focus of this chapter will be on the involvement of these elements in gynecologic malignancies and the development and adoption of targeted therapies in ovarian, endometrial, and cervical cancers. This is a dynamic area with new developments and discoveries that are being incorporated into therapeutic targeting. The goal of precision medicine is to improve the accuracy of our understanding of cancer biology and use this knowledge to intelligently develop tools and techniques that not only predict therapeutic effect, but also match with treatment in an attempt to increase efficacy and reduce toxicity.

WHAT IS A TARGET AND WHAT DEFINES A TARGET?

Hanahan and Weinberg (1,2) described the six basic hallmarks of cancer that not only define its behavior—including distinctive and complementary capabilities that enable tumor growth and metastatic dissemination—but provide a roadmap for targeted drug development against key regulatory/survival processes in cancer cells (**Fig. 12.1**).

Targets can further be classified as prognostic or predictive in nature. Prognostic factors are clinical or biologic characteristics that are objectively measurable and provide information on the likely outcome of disease in an untreated individual; in contrast, a predictive marker is a clinical or biologic characteristic that provides information on the likely benefit from treatment (either in terms of tumor shrinkage or survival) (3). Excellent guidelines on identifying and validating biomarkers and accuracy of prediction have been published by the National Cancer Institute (NCI) and the US Food and Drug Administration (FDA), and serve to improve accuracy and reliability in clinical decision making (4, http://www.fda.gov/MedicalDevices/DeviceRegulationandGuidance/Overview/default.htm).

Biology of Gynecologic Cancers

Gynecologic cancers show genomic and clonal diversity and heterogeneity in space and time, and can lead to considerable differences in clinical behavior. There is also considerable variation in pathology, even within ostensibly similar diagnoses. For example, epithelial ovarian cancer (EOC) consists of five distinct histologic types that include high-grade serous ovarian cancers (HGSOC) and low-grade serous ovarian cancers (LGSOC), mucinous, clear cell, and endometrioid subtypes; while sex cord stromal and others such as germ cell comprise the non-epithelial group (5). Endometrial cancer (EC) has been segregated into Type I estrogen-dependent cancer such as endometrioid and Type 2, which consists of estrogen-independent non-EC carcinomas such as serous, clear cell carcinoma, carcinosarcoma, mucinous adenocarcinoma, squamous cell carcinoma, and mixed adenocarcinoma. These histologic subtypes reflect independent mechanisms of carcinogenesis and distinct disease biology. As such, histologic confirmation of disease subtype by an expert gynecologic pathologist is essential for accurate diagnosis, and ultimately, to inform decisions about therapy. The increasing assessment of subtype-specific mutations or molecular aberrations, particularly by The Cancer Genome Atlas (TCGA), has shed light on the genomic foundation of ovarian (2011) and endometrial (2013)

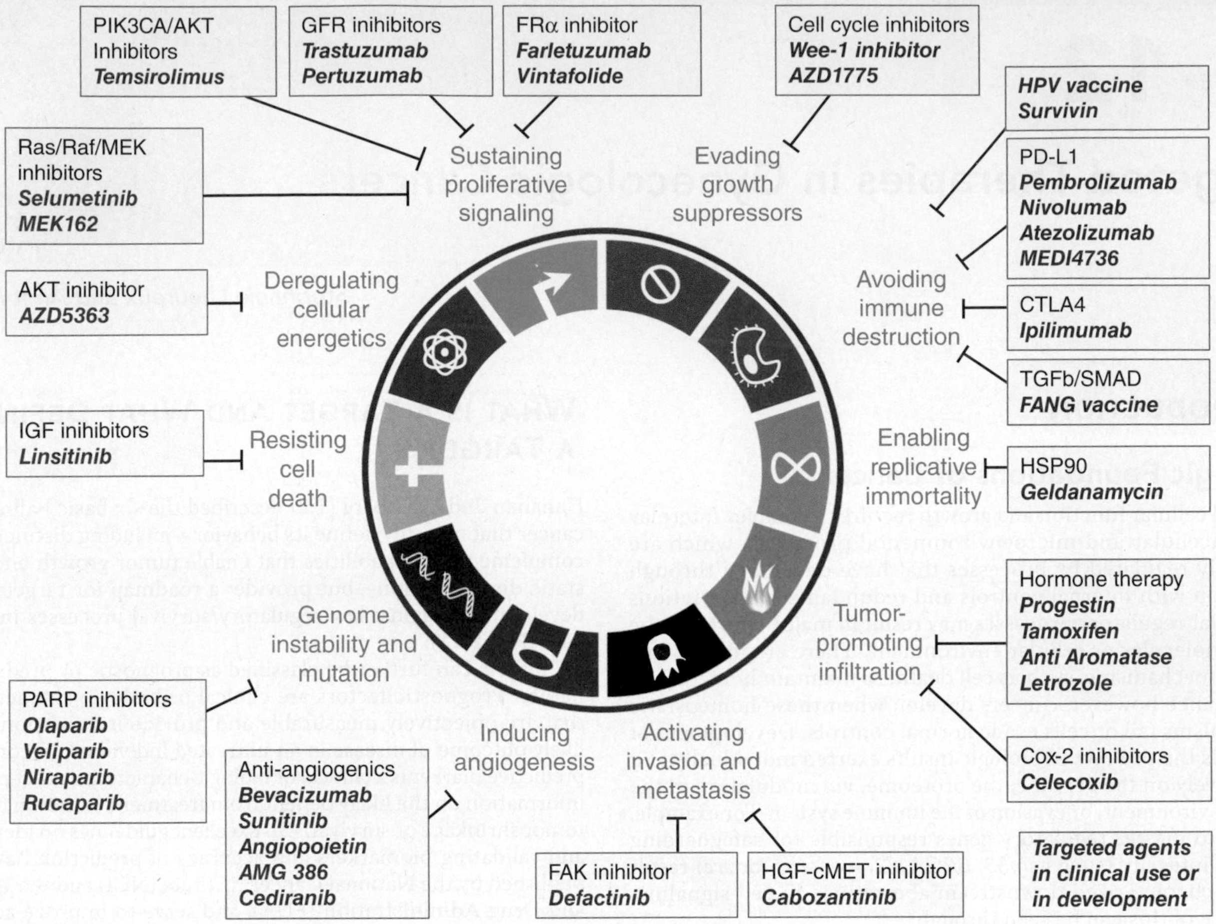

Figure 12.1. Hallmarks of cancer and therapeutic targets in gynecologic cancers. Adapted from Hanahan D, Weinberg RA. Hallmarks of cancer: the next generation. *Cell*. 2011;144(5):646–674.

cancers (6,7), alongside similar profiling efforts in cervical cancer (2014) (8). The availability of reliable data identifying contributions from point mutations in heritable and nonheritable genes and, in some cases, significant aberrations in oncogenic pathways contributing to disease, has led to the concerted development of research studies with targeted therapies in gynecologic cancers. The key findings from TCGA analyses in gynecologic cancers are summarized in **Table 12.1**.

Target Identification, Validation, and Measurement

It is important to note that identification of potential targets, their validation, and subsequent incorporation into predictive biomarkers for clinical trials or standard therapy must be conducted in a methodologically rigorous manner to warrant confidence in the results. One of the major challenges is to identify the role of the target in carcinogenesis and cancer growth, determine its functionality, and distinguish its role between driver or passenger abnormalities. Biomarkers which may guide therapy must be measured in regulated conditions (CLIA, CAP) and are subject to regulatory oversight. Precision of biomarker development and incorporation are beyond the scope of this chapter, but excellent references which guide development, validation, incorporation into clinical trials, and standard therapy are included (4).

Targeting the Targets

Improved understanding of disease biology has led to the development of numerous potential targets and biomarkers to improve precision of therapy. Target engagement can be through several different modalities that modulate or interact with cell surface receptors (monoclonal antibodies), intracellular cascade pathways and signaling (small molecule tyrosine kinase inhibitors), or microenvironment effects related to tumor vasculature or hypoxia. There have also been some interesting results using antibody–drug conjugates that are being leveraged for treatment in gynecologic malignancies. Modulating the immune environment with dynamic changes in cancer cell interaction with T cells or NK cells is a very active area of study, including cellular therapy using *ex-vivo* propagation of immune cells, vaccines, and checkpoint inhibitors. Finally, improved delivery of targeted agents to cancer cells using nanoparticles such as porphysomes presents tremendous opportunity for precision bombing of cancer cells and reducing bystander or collateral toxicity (9).

Genetic Factors Contributing to Gynecologic Malignancies

TP53

TP53 is one of the most important tumor suppressor genes and is frequently mutated in human cancers. Generally, p53 functions as a transcription factor that is stabilized and activated by various genotoxic and cellular stress signals, such as DNA damage, hypoxia, oncogene activation, and nutrient deprivation, consequently leading to cell cycle arrest, apoptosis, senescence, and metabolic adaptation (10). *TP53* somatic mutations are a defining early event in HGSOC (6,11) as well as in serous endometrial cancer (12). p53 seems an attractive target in gynecologic cancers; contemporary strategies targeting p53 have been developed, including gene therapy to restore

TABLE 12.1. Integrated Genomic Analyses of Ovarian and Endometrial Cancers Conducted by TCGA Network

TCGA Target Population	Major Study Findings
HGSOC (6)	• Characterized by *TP53* mutations in almost all tumors (96%); • Low prevalence but statistically recurrent somatic mutations in nine further genes including: *NF1*, *BRCA1*, *BRCA2*, *RB1*, and *CDK12*; • 113 significant focal DNA copy number aberrations; • Promoter methylation events involving 168 genes; • Four ovarian cancer transcriptional subtypes, three microRNA subtypes, four promoter methylation subtypes, and a transcriptional signature associated with survival duration; • Impact of tumors with *BRCA1/2* (*BRCA1* or *BRCA2*) and *CCNE1* aberrations on survival; • Homologous recombination is defective in about half of the tumors analyzed; and • NOTCH and FOXM1 signaling involved in serous ovarian cancer pathophysiology.
Endometrial carcinoma (7)	• Uterine serous tumors and ~25% of high-grade endometrioid tumors had extensive copy number alterations, few DNA methylation changes, low ER/PR levels, and frequent *TP53* mutations; • Most endometrioid tumors had few copy number alterations or *TP53* mutations, but frequent mutations in *PTEN*, *CTNNB1*, *PIK3CA*, *ARID1A*, and *KRAS* and novel mutations in the SWI/SNF chromatin remodeling complex gene *ARID5B*; • A subset of endometrioid tumors had a markedly increased transversion mutation frequency and newly identified hotspot mutations in DNA polymerase epsilon (POLE); • Novel Classification System: o POLE ultramutation, o Microsatellite instability hypermutation, o Copy number low, and o Copy number high. • Uterine serous carcinomas share genomic features with ovarian serous and basal-like breast carcinomas.

Cervical cancer data are yet to be published.

p53 function, inhibition of p53–MDM2 interaction, restoration of mutant p53 to wild-type p53 or targeting p53 family proteins. However, p53-targeted therapy remains challenging (10). Different types of *TP53* mutations have been described but the functionality of this mutation is complex (13). Most *TP53* mutations are missense mutations that result in single amino acid substitutions in p53 and expression of high levels of dysfunctional p53 protein (14). Some types of *TP*53 mutations are termed gain-of-function or loss-of-function mutations. The impact on patient outcome and response to treatment is not well established, and investigations remain ongoing.

Cell Cycle

The cell cycle is a complex process involving numerous regulatory proteins from which the cyclin-dependent kinases (CDK) are central (**Fig. 12.2**). These proteins regulate the cell's progression through

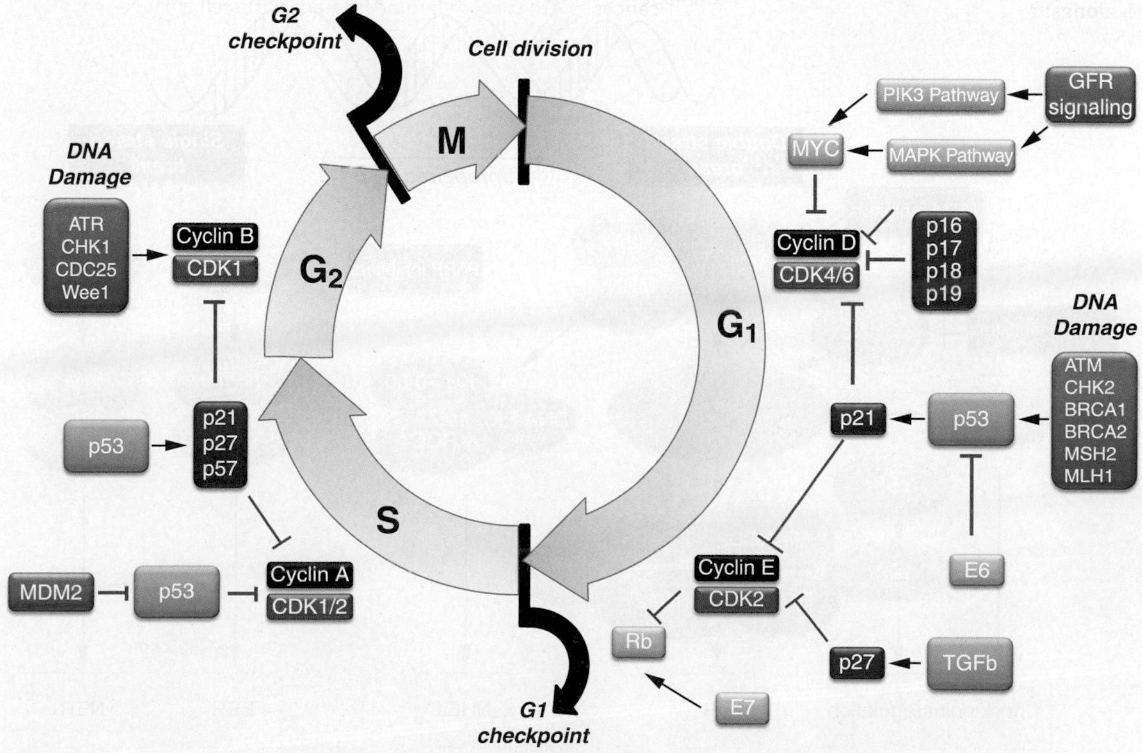

Figure 12.2. Cell cycle regulation. Cyclins and CDKs promote cell cycle progression and are mediated by inhibitory molecules.

the stages of the cell cycle and in turn, are regulated by numerous proteins, including p53, p21, p16, and cdc25. Downstream targets of cyclin–CDK complexes include pRb and E2F (15). The cell cycle is particularly altered in gynecologic cancers due to alterations either in oncogenes that indirectly affect the cell cycle or in tumor suppressor genes or oncogenes that directly impact cell cycle regulation, such as p53, p16, or viral infection including papillomavirus (HPV)-associated cervical and vulvar carcinomas (the manifold effects of the viral oncogenes E6 and E7 on cell cycle control). Tumor-associated cell cycle defects are often mediated by alterations in CDK activity. Misregulated CDKs induce unscheduled proliferation as well as genomic and chromosomal instabilities. Emerging evidence suggests that tumor cells may also require specific interphase CDKs for proliferation. Selective CDK inhibition may provide therapeutic benefit against certain human neoplasias (16). Therefore, the cell cycle has become an intense subject of research in recent years. Any drug or toxin with DNA-damaging ability would be expected to alter cell cycle progression.

DNA Repair and Homologous Recombination Pathway

In the DNA repair pathway, important targets in ovarian cancer, particularly in HGSOC, are the *breast cancer gene 1* (*BRCA1*) or 2 (*BRCA2*) genes (17) (**Fig. 12.3**). Mutations in these genes predispose germline carriers to breast and ovarian cancer as well as many other malignancies—the lifetime risk of developing ovarian cancer is 40% to 60% and 11% to 27% for *BRCA1* and *BRCA2* pathogenic mutation carriers, respectively (18). These particular mutations are implicated in 10% to 15% of all ovarian cancer cases and almost 20% of HGSOC histology (19), including women without a family history of breast or ovarian cancer. The diagnosis of HGOSC should lead to germline testing for all patients.

An increasing body of evidence indicates the benefit of targeting pathways involved in maintaining DNA integrity, including *BRCA1* and *BRCA2* signaling (20). Harboring a germline *BRCA1/2* mutation is described as predictive of platinum sensitivity (21) and confers predictable sensitivity to poly ADP-ribose polymerase (PARP) inhibitors, as impairment in DNA repair conferred by pathogenic *BRCA1/2* mutations can be leveraged into therapeutic effect by blocking poly ADP-ribose polymerase, another major enzyme in DNA repair. This simultaneous promotion of DNA double-strand breaks (DSBs) and hindrance of DSB repair by inhibition of PARP protein expression (22,23) has led to accelerated development of inhibitors of PARP protein. This effect, dubbed "synthetic lethality," was demonstrated preclinically and confirmed clinically, and has led to the initial approval of olaparib in the treatment of *BRCA1/2*-mutated HGSOC. Germline and somatic testing for *BRCA1/2* provides important information about predisposition as well as predictive biomarker for therapy using PARP inhibitors in women with ovarian cancer, and has led to clinical implementation and approval.

The ability to leverage deficiencies in homologous recombination has been shown to extend beyond *BRCA1/2* mutation with phenotypic features of those tumors exhibiting *BRCA*-like behavior. Studies conducted by Walsh et al. (24,25) using targeted, massively parallel next-generation sequencing—the BROCA panel sequenced 21 tumor suppressor genes, including *BRCA1/2* and other genes known to cause inherited breast or ovarian cancers—screened 360 patients with ovarian, peritoneal, or fallopian tube carcinomas for germline mutations, and showed that 18% of patients have germline mutations in *BRCA1/2* and another 6% have a non-*BRCA1/2* germline mutation. They identified mutations in every evaluable Fanconi Anemia pathway gene including *NBN, MRE11, RAD50, RAD51C, PALB2, BARD1*, and *BRIP1* (25). There are also a unique subset of tumors that harbor mutations in the homologous recombination (HR) pathway other than *BRCA1/2*, exhibiting a *BRCA*-like

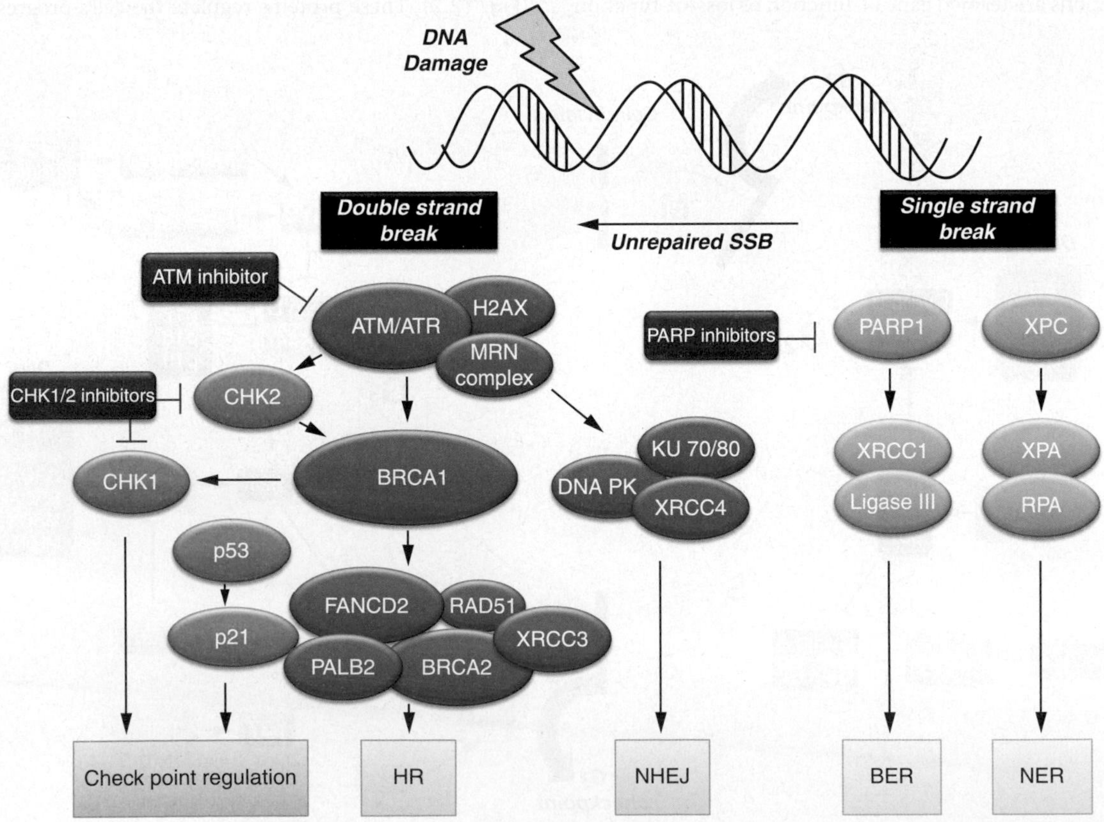

Figure 12.3. DNA repair pathway and therapeutic targets in cancer.

profile—specific phenotype with features and behavior similar to *BRCA*-related ovarian cancers, including sensitivity to platinum (DNA-damaging agents), improved progression-free survival (PFS) and survival rates, and HGSOC histology (26). Similar to the above, genes involved in the *BRCA*-like profile include *RAD51*, *PALB2*, *CHEK2*, *Mre11* complex, and *BARD1* (26). A study investigating rucaparib (another PARP inhibitor) monotherapy in patients with recurrent platinum-sensitive HGSOC has confirmed *BRCA1/2* mutation as a biomarker of response as well as genomic loss of heterozygosity (LOH), a potential predictive surrogate marker for HR deficiency (27). It was hypothesized that the inability of the cell to perform HR leads to genomic scarring and LOH, thus enabling the use of high LOH as a signature of HR deficiency.

Defects in DNA repair are also found in Lynch syndrome—an autosomal dominant, inherited cancer-susceptibility syndrome in women with endometrial cancer involving several genes including: *MLH1*, mutS homologue 2 (*MSH2*), *MSH6*, *PMS1* homologue 2; (*PMS2*) (mutations of DNA mismatch repair [MMR] system component), and others (28). Similar to *BRCA1/2*, family history is inadequate to identify affected individuals; and as such, the clinical and research communities are increasing screening strategies to identify germline carriers who are at increased risk of disease. These approaches include screening immunohistochemistry (IHC) for the presence of MMR proteins in all colorectal and endometrial cancers and for those patients with loss of MMR detected, they can then subsequently be referred for germline testing (28). Similar to other gynecologic cancers, testing for somatic or epigenetic changes may provide predictive or prognostic information; however, additional studies to validate this approach are warranted. As is expected, most centers favor MMR IHC for practicality—family testing, interpretation, cost, normal tissue not required—with an increasing number of centers growing their IHC testing platform to include MMR IHC using two to four antibodies on all endometrial cancers (28–30).

PI3K/AKT/mTOR

The phosphatidylinositol 3-kinase (PI3K)/AKT/mammalian target of rapamycin (mTOR) pathway plays a critical role in the malignant transformation of human tumors and their subsequent growth, proliferation, and metastasis (31). The PI3K/AKT/mTOR signaling pathway regulates central aspects of cancer biology such as metabolism, cellular growth, and survival (32). Upon stimulation of receptor tyrosine kinases, PI3K phosphorylates phosphatidylinositol-4,5-bis-phosphate 2 (PIP2) into PIP3, resulting in the activation of AKT. Among its targets, AKT controls the activation of the downstream pathway effector, the mammalian target of rapamycin (mTOR), which activates two key substrates 4EBP1 and p70S6K. This results in increased translation of target genes involved in angiogenesis (VEGF) and cell cycle progression (cyclin D1, c-Myc). The primary negative regulator of the PI3K pathway is the tumor suppressor phosphatase and tensin homologue (PTEN). PTEN can dephosphorylate PIP3, reversing AKT activation and inhibiting further downstream signaling; however, in the absence of PTEN inhibition, AKT phosphorylates, leading to mTOR activation. This is one of the most commonly altered pathways in EC; it is described in 92% and 60% of type I and II tumors, respectively. EC has more frequent mutations in the PI3K/AKT pathway than any other tumor type studied by TCGA (7). Activation of the PI3K/AKT pathway occurs frequently in type I EC through a variety of mechanisms such as the loss of PTEN that occurs in up to 70% of cases and/or PI3K mutations occurring in upward of 36% of cases. *PTEN* mutation is also frequently observed (27.3%) in clear cell EOC (33). More recently, frequent alteration of *ARID1A* and *PIK3CA* have been reported in this rare histology subtype. The AKT/mTOR pathway is thought to be the most important passage for tumor growth in clear cell ovarian cancer (34). Mutations in the beta-catenin and *PTEN* genes as well as the tumor suppressor genes *PID3CA* and *ARID1A* have been identified in EC. Recently, it has been reported that *KRAS* and *PIK3CA* gene mutations may be important players in the oncogenesis of these tumors, and their role in treatment in this subgroup should be explored (35).

Mitogen-Activated Protein Kinase

The mitogen-activated protein kinase (MAPK) pathway is activated and appears to play a prominent role in the pathogenesis of LGSOC (36). Approximately 20% to 40% of low-grade serous carcinomas have a *KRAS* mutation, whereas *BRAF* mutations are rare (approximately 5%). *KRAS* is a frequent mutation detected in advanced LGSOC, and the *BRAF* V600E mutation is associated with serous borderline tumors and early-stage LGSOC (37). As a result, the V600E mutation is associated with a better clinical outcome. The MAPK cascade is triggered by the binding of a ligand that ultimately leads to phosphorylation of ERK. Thus, MEK is a good candidate for targeted therapy, and a number of MEK inhibitors (MEKi) have been developed (34).

Others

The driver mutation in *FOXL2* and dysregulation of the PI3K/AKT pathway have been implicated in granulosa cell tumor development. In preclinical data, mTOR inhibitor may be a useful pharmacologic target for the treatment of this disease (38).

ROLE OF THE IMMUNE SYSTEM IN GYNECOLOGIC MALIGNANCIES

Immune Evasion

The presence of tumor-infiltrating lymphocytes (TILs) was associated with favorable outcome in gynecologic cancers. POLE ultramutation and microsatellite instability (MSI) are associated with high neo-antigen loads and number of TILs, which is counterbalanced by overexpression of PD-1 and PD-L1. MSI is more frequent in endometrioid than in non-endometrioid tumors, and occurs in roughly 30% of sporadic cases of EC.

Early phase clinical trials using checkpoint inhibitors to modulate immune cells in gynecologic cancer are yielding interesting results in ovarian and endometrial cancers, with initial evidence of objective responses and prolonged disease control. There are several agents in active development as single agents, or in combination with chemotherapy, targeted agents, monoclonal antibodies, and vaccines (**Fig. 12.4**).

Viral Contributions to Disease—The Human Papillomavirus Connection

Viral infections have been shown to contribute to the development of gynecologic cancers (39). Human Papillomavirus (HPV) has been implicated in the majority of cervical cancers, up to 70% of squamous cell carcinomas of the vulva, 60% of squamous cell carcinomas of the vagina (40), and appears to have a high prevalence in ovarian cancer patients, based on a meta-analysis of 24 primary studies of 889 patients across 11 countries on 3 continents (41).

Historically, cervical cancer has been the most actively studied gynecologic cancer because HPV16 and 18 are responsible for the majority of HPV-related cancers. As with viral infections, HPV infects epithelial cells and initiates production of proteins E6 and E7 (high risk) that are considered oncoproteins, interfering with cell death and promoting continued cell proliferation (42).

Based on evidence that host-dependent immunologic status and HPV-induced immune evasion are responsible for persistent HPV infection, the causal factor of cervical cancer, immunotherapy is an attractive strategy. HPV integration into the host's cellular genome allows permanent expression of viral oncoproteins, promoting cell transformation into cancerous cells, inactivation of tumor suppressor genes, and finally, cell growth and tumor proliferation. HPV

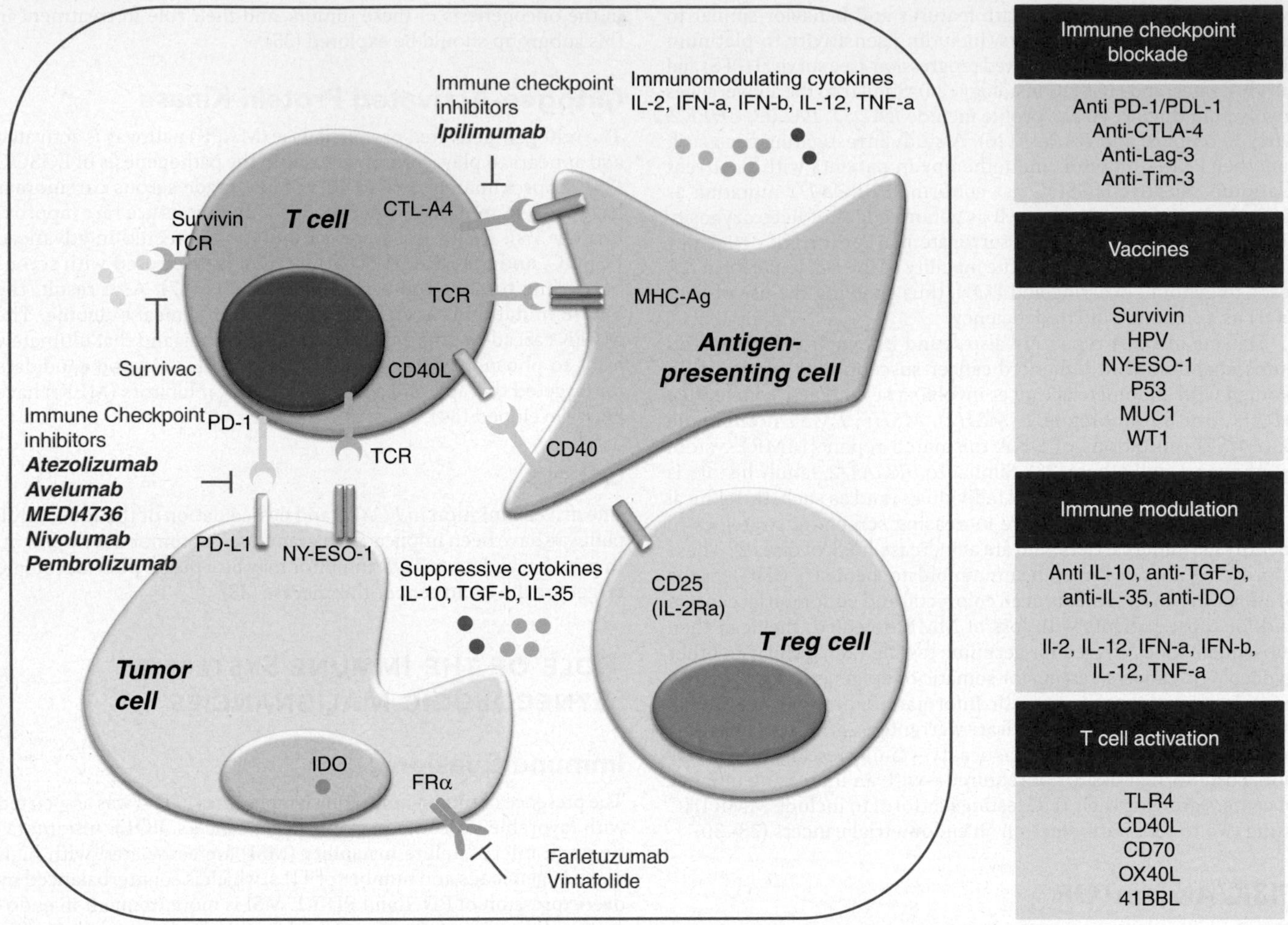

Figure 12.4. Immune response and targets of immunotherapy in gynecologic cancers.

infection also invokes a cellular immune response with regulatory T cells involved in the immune-suppressive status of HPV-associated malignancies (43). The role of immunotherapy for the treatment of cervical cancer is evolving. Several strategies are being evaluated; most are in early phase clinical trials.

MICROENVIRONMENT IN GYNECOLOGIC MALIGNANCIES

It has been increasingly recognized that the tumor microenvironment plays a complex role in tumor growth, development, and metastasis. Growth of malignant tumors requires a functional blood supply to provide nutrients, and this is facilitated and regulated by selection of proangiogenic peptides and growth factors in a complex interplay with regulatory antiangiogenic factors (44). Tumor vasculature is a field of intense study, pioneered by Judah Folkman, Bob Kerbel, and Rakesh Jain. Vascular endothelial growth factor (VEGF) is a key driver of angiogenesis and has been recognized as an important mechanism of tumor growth, survival, and metastasis in gynecologic cancers. VEGF overexpression has been consistently demonstrated in EC, EOC, and cervical cancers, and overexpression of VEGF is likely responsible for some of the pathognomic features of advanced ovarian cancer like ascites, secondary to capillary leakiness caused by excessive VEGF (45). It is also apparent that tumors and metastases often have disorganized internal vasculature, and unchecked cellular growth often leads to intratumoral hypoxia, which is a strong prognostic indicator of resistance to chemotherapy and radiation.

The microenvironment features of cancer growth have been incorporated into therapeutic strategies that impact on growth of tumors through modulation. The most successful strategies have been through incorporation of bevacizumab, a VEGF inhibitor in conjunction with chemotherapy in ovarian and cervical cancer. Beyond VEGF, different targets are under investigation such as platelet-derived growth factor, fibroblast growth factor, angiopoietin, and Ephrin type-A receptor 2 (46). Several other VEGF-targeting strategies have also led to positive results in randomized clinical trials, but as yet have not resulted in major changes in clinical practice.

PROTEOMIC ALTERATIONS AND TARGETING DISEASE

Hormonal Therapy

Hormonal therapy is an attractive strategy in treating gynecologic cancers. In endometrial cancer, a significant proportion of type 1 tumors express estrogen receptor (ER) or progesterone receptor (PR), and have been described as predictors of favorable survival (47,48). To date, the agents that have been investigated in this setting include: progestogens, selective ER modulators (SERM), aromatase inhibitors (AI), and GnRH inhibitors. The most common hormonal treatment has been progestational agents, which demonstrates anti-tumor responses in as many as 15% to 30% of patients (47,49). These responses are associated with clinical benefits (50) and (51), particularly in patients with well-differentiated tumors, and positive PR status has a higher response rate (RR) (52). In fact, progestogens have demonstrated

■ TABLE 12.2. Summary of GOG218 and ICON7 Landmark Studies with Bevacizumab in the Front-Line Setting

Trial	GOG-0218	ICON7
Setting/design	Double-blinded, placebo-controlled Three arms Bevacizumab for 15 months Bevacizumab 15 mg/kg q3w	Open-label Two arms Bevacizumab for 12 months Bevacizumab 7.5 mg/kg q3w
Patient population	Stage III (optimal, visual/palpable) Stage III (suboptimal) Stage IV	Stage I or IIA (grade 3 or clear cell histology) Stages IIB–IV (all)
End point analyses	Progression: RECIST and CA-125 OS analysis (formal testing at time of PFS) Independent Radiologic Confirmation (IRC)	Progression: RECIST Defined final OS analysis (end 2012) No IRC
Time of PFS analysis	Total no. of PFS events in control arm	Total no. of PFS events in both arms and 1 year after last patient randomized
Patients on therapy at time of PFS analysis	14% arm I, 17% arm II, 24% arm III	Two patients in bevacizumab arm
No. of events/no. of patients	783/1,248 (arm I and III)	759/1,528
Analysis methods	One-sided log-rank test Non-proportional hazards not yet presented	Two-sided log-rank test Non-proportional hazards explored

OS, overall survival; PFS, progression-free survival; RECIST, Response Evaluation Criteria in Solid Tumors.

favorable tolerability and efficacy with RRs of 22% overall (53,54) and it has been shown that positive receptor status (in particular PR) is correlated with response (55). Low-grade histology is also predictive of response (50); however, a small number of receptor-negative patients may still benefit, providing the rationale for exploring the mechanisms involved in treatment response (56).

AIs and tamoxifen (SERMs) have demonstrated overall RRs of ~10% (57–59). Following subgroup analysis, tamoxifen showed higher RRs of 23% and 14% in grade I and II patients, respectively (57). A phase II trial of mifepristone—a selective PR modulator agent—was evaluated in PR-positive advanced or recurrent endometrial cancer and was shown to achieve only stable disease as a single agent (60). The combination of tamoxifen and megestrol has been proposed to be more efficacious due to upregulation of the PR by tamoxifen but in practice no clear benefit has been seen to date (61,62). The overall RR was 27%, with a median PFS of 2.7 months and an overall survival (OS) of 14 months (62).

In the setting of advanced disease, there have been no improvements in survival in women with EC treated with hormonal therapy, as reported in the *Cochrane Review* (63). The publication has postulated that this finding may be due to the fact that many of the studies were conducted years ago, and advancements in technology and hormone receptor measurements have occurred since then, as well as response assessment criteria that make it difficult to compare against recent trial findings. As such, efforts continue to refine the role of hormonal therapy in endometrial cancer in the upfront and advanced settings (47).

PRECISION THERAPY IN CLINICAL PRACTICE

Antiangiogenics—Bevacizumab

Targeting the tumor microenvironment through inhibition of tumor-associated angiogenesis has been an effective strategy in gynecologic malignancies. Bevacizumab is a humanized monoclonal antibody against VEGF, was the first clinically available antiangiogenic in North America, and the first to show striking activity as a single agent, as well as in combinations, in ovarian cancer. Early phase clinical trials showed important clinical activity in women with platinum-resistant ovarian cancer, both as a single agent and in combination with metronomic chemotherapy with oral cyclophosphamide. The agent also allowed opportunities for palliation/control of ascites, which responded quickly (as it is related to VEGF); however, there were important side effects that initially led to concerns about the viability of bevacizumab in ovarian cancer. In one of the initial trials in women with advanced bulky recurrent disease, bowel perforation was seen in 11% with bevacizumab therapy, and more likely to be seen in relation to number of prior lines of therapy, disease bulk, or bowel involvement. Subsequent studies have been more selective with women who have bulky disease or bowel involvement, and perforation rates have come down considerably. A detailed assessment by Burger et al. (64) based on GOG218 showed the overall risk of bowel perforation to be 3.2% in a first-line setting, risk factors being a history of inflammatory bowel disease and bowel surgery.

The first randomized trials in a front-line setting were conducted by the Gynecologic Oncology Group (GOG, now NSABP, RTOG, and GOG—NRG) and by the MRC Clinical Trials Group from the United Kingdom. The complementary studies evaluated concurrent and maintenance bevacizumab in women with optimally and suboptimally debulked ovarian cancer, at two different doses and for different duration (**Table 12.2**).

Both of these pivotal trials were positive for their primary end points of PFS with concurrent and maintenance bevacizumab, a very acceptable toxicity profile. The magnitude of benefit seemed to be related to the duration of therapy more than dose. Continuation of bevacizumab alone in the adjuvant setting for 12 or 15 months following chemotherapy first-line treatment in combination with bevacizumab showed a modest but significant PFS benefit in two phase III studies (GOG218 (64) and ICON7 (65)) (**Figs. 12.5** and **12.6**). The benefit seen with bevacizumab in ICON7 was associated with increasing burden of disease, as patients with suboptimal and stage IV disease derived the maximum benefit. ICON7 was also powered and conducted to evaluate OS. There was no difference in OS with the addition of bevacizumab to the entire group of patients, but in a preplanned survival analysis, patients at high risk (suboptimally debulked stage III/IV, non-operated patients) had improved median OS by 9.4 months. This has led to further refinement of approval in Canada and many European countries for the incorporation of bevacizumab in women with high risk, suboptimally debulked or metastatic disease at presentation (**Fig. 12.7**).

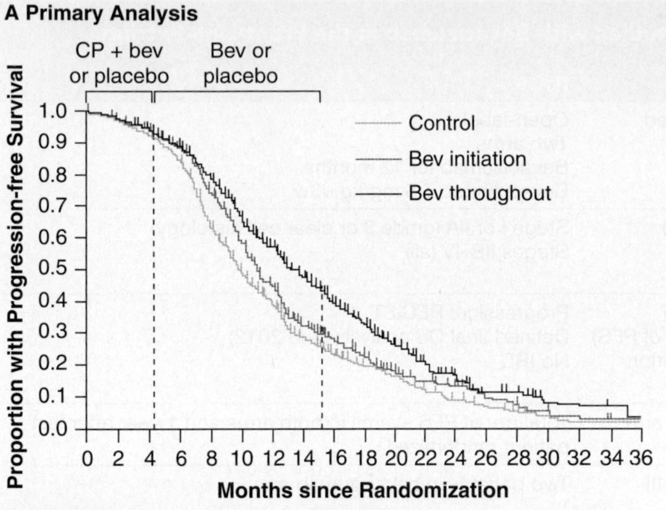

No. at Risk				
Control	625	199	33	8
Bev initiation	625	219	29	6
Bev through-out	625	254	38	8

Figure 12.5. GOG PFS showing the results of primary analysis of PFS for all 1,873 patients randomly assigned to receive chemotherapy with carboplatin and paclitaxel (CP) plus placebo, followed by placebo alone (the control group), CP plus bevacizumab (bev) followed by placebo (the bevacizumab-initiation group), or CP plus bevacizumab followed by bevacizumab (the bevacizumab-throughout group). There was a significant, time-dependent decrease in the hazard of progression in the bevacizumab-throughout group as compared with the control group (hazard ratio [HR], 0.717; 95% confidence interval [CI], 0.625 to 0.824; $p < 0.001$).

From Burger RA, Brady MF, Bookman MA, et al; Gynecologic Oncology Group. Incorporation of bevacizumab in the primary treatment of ovarian cancer. *N Engl J Med*. 2011;365:2473–2483.

The improvement in PFS has led to approval of bevacizumab in a front-line setting in more than 50 countries internationally, except the United States. Many candidate biomarkers have been evaluated to predict which patients could be identified pre-therapy; yet at this stage, the clinical predictive algorithm for high risk remains the best defined predictor of benefit in a first-line setting. Additional trials in a first-line setting will define the optimal duration of maintenance therapy to confirm whether or not prolonged duration of administration further improves PFS. Studies have also shown safety in combining bevacizumab with IP therapy or administering bevacizumab following neo-adjuvant chemotherapy.

In platinum-sensitive recurrent ovarian cancer, Aghajanian et al., (66) demonstrated very striking improvement in PFS when bevacizumab was added at 15 mg/kg to carboplatin (AUC 4) and gemcitabine (1,000 mg/m^2), and continued to progression, with a hazard ratio of 0.48 (66). In platinum-resistant disease, the Aurelia trial also showed striking improvement with the addition of bevacizumab 15 mg/kg to a choice of chemotherapy regimens—weekly paclitaxel, topotecan, or liposomal doxorubicin. The most durable benefit was seen in women who received weekly paclitaxel, with indications of improved in OS in this group (67).

Randomized trials incorporating bevacizumab concurrently with chemotherapy and continuing with bevacizumab beyond chemotherapy in first-line and platinum-sensitive recurrence have all shown significant improvement in progression as well as subgroups that show improvement extending to OS. As a consequence, bevacizumab has become an approved standard in ovarian cancer treatment, though there are some regulatory differences in approval in different countries. National Comprehensive Cancer Network (NCCN) guidelines in epithelial ovarian, fallopian tube, primary peritoneal cancers, and less common histopathologies (carcinosarcoma, clear cell, mucinous,

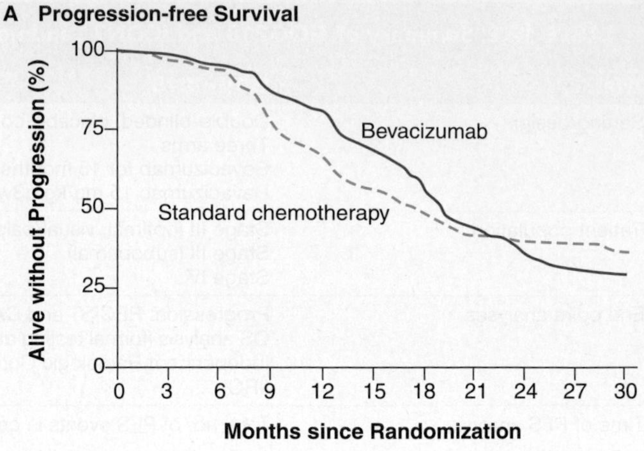

No. at Risk						
Standard chemotherapy	764	693	464	216	91	25
Bevacizumab	764	715	585	263	73	19

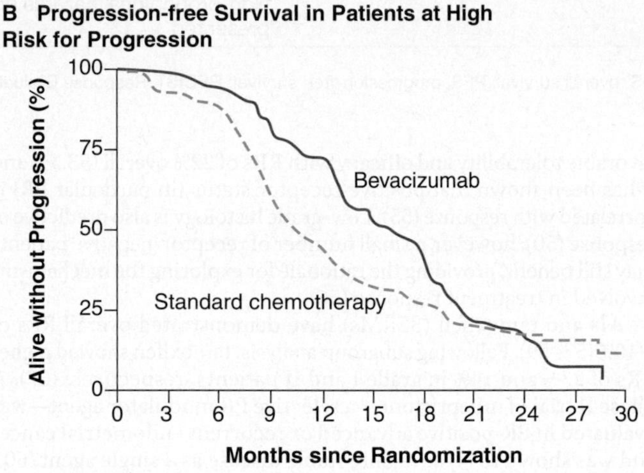

No. at Risk						
Standard chemotherapy	234	205	98	36	14	2
Bevacizumab	231	213	159	56	10	1

Figure 12.6. ICON7 PFS and OS curves. **A:** Differences in PFS according to treatment group in the total study population. **B:** PFS in patients at risk of disease progression. PFS, progression-free survival; OS, overall survival.

From Perren TJ, Swart AM, Pfisterer J, et al; for the ICON7 Investigators. A phase 3 trial of bevacizumab in ovarian cancer. *N Engl J Med*. 2011;365:2484–2496.

borderline epithelial, grade 1 low-grade serous, endometrioid) stage II–IV according to ICON-7 and GOG218 schedules. In cervical cancer, recently updated NCCN guidelines suggest cisplatin/paclitaxel/bevacizumab first-line combination therapy in the setting of recurrent or metastatic disease, as well as bevacizumab single agent during second-line therapy (68).

In a phase III trial, targeting this angiogenesis pathway with bevacizumab in combination with standard chemotherapy in advanced recurrent cervical cancer has showed an increased objective RR from 36% to 48% ($p = 0.008$) and an OS benefit compared to standard regimen (OS increased from 13.3 to 17 months). Bevacizumab was associated with a reasonable toxicity profile. The side effects were consistent with those previously associated with bevacizumab, including hypertension, neutropenia, and thromboembolism, or formation of blood clots. Specifically, treatment with bevacizumab was associated with more grade 3 to 4 bleeding, thrombosis/embolism,

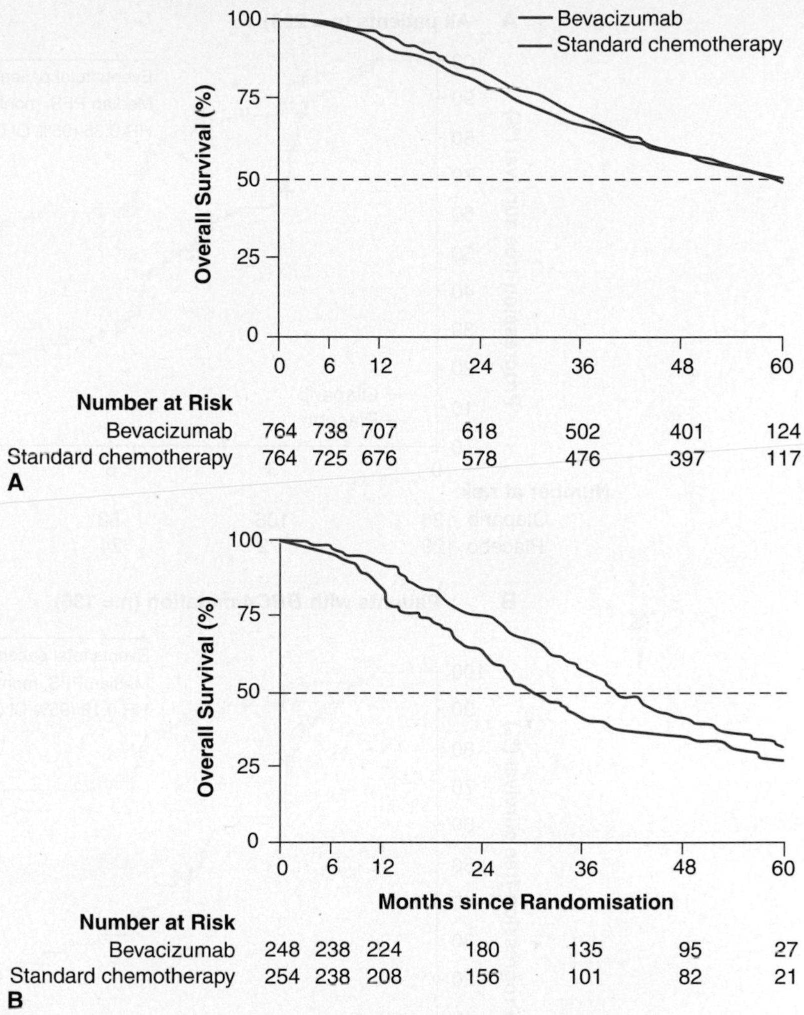

Figure 12.7. Overall survival (OS). **A:** Overall survival in all patients. **B:** Overall survival in high-risk patients.

From Oza AM, Cook AD, Pfisterer J, et al. Standard chemotherapy with or without bevacizumab for women with newly diagnosed ovarian cancer (ICON7): overall survival results of a phase 3 randomized trial. *Lancet Oncol*. 2015;16(8):928–936.

and gastrointestinal fistula. This OS improvement has led to the first U.S. FDA-approved anti-VEGF agent, bevacizumab, for the treatment of advanced stage, persistent, or recurrent cervical cancer. This advancement with bevacizumab did not lead to identify biomarkers of response, and the median OS survival remains low at 17 months, highlighting the need for innovative treatment strategies (69).

PARP Inhibitors

Approximately 50% of women with grade serous ovarian cancer have evidence of homologous recombination deficiency, and 15% to 20% have *BRCA1/2* mutations. This genomic profile and susceptibility to impaired DNA repair has been leveraged for therapy using PARP inhibitors, with evidence of clinical activity as a single agent (70, Clovis Ariel 2 from JCO presentation). A pivotal international, multicenter, randomized, phase II study that evaluated olaparib (a PARP inhibitor) as maintenance treatment in women with HGSOC who had responded to platinum-based chemotherapy (71) showed important clinical activity in improving PFS. Preplanned retrospective analysis of outcomes by *BRCA1/2* status in this study demonstrated that *BRCA*-mutated patients had better PFS with olaparib maintenance compared to those receiving placebo (11.2 vs 4.3 months; HR 0.18; $p < 0.0001$) (72) (**Fig. 12.8**). The PFS benefit was still observed when somatic *BRCA*-mutated patients were included in the analysis. Additional evidence supporting the role of olaparib as maintenance therapy was reported in an international, multicenter, randomized, open-label study of women with platinum-sensitive relapsed HGSOC (73). In this phase II trial, olaparib was given with carboplatin/paclitaxel chemotherapy and continued as maintenance monotherapy. Overall, study findings show a significant PFS improvement when compared to chemotherapy alone (12.2 and 9.6 median PFS, respectively; HR 0.51; 95% CI 0.34 to 0.77; $p = 0.0012$). A greater benefit was detected in patients with a *BRCA1/2* mutation (PFS HR 0.21; 95% CI 0.08 to 0.55; $p = 0.015$) than in those without a *BRCA1/2* mutation. Further, study analysis revealed strong evidence that olaparib maintenance is most likely a key contributor to the improvement in PFS in this patient population (73). There are numerous ongoing PARP inhibitor studies investigating women with *BRCA1/2* mutations as well as mutations in other homologous recombination-deficient (HRD) genes, as data has shown HRD genes to exhibit *BRCA*-like behavior (6). To date, the use of olaparib maintenance has been approved in Europe after response to platinum-based chemotherapy in women with platinum-sensitive HGSOC who harbor a germline or somatic *BRCA1/2* mutation (72) and in the United States, as single-agent therapy after three lines of chemotherapy in patients with germline *BRCA1/2* mutation HGSOC (74).

TARGETED THERAPY SIDE EFFECTS AND MANAGEMENT STRATEGIES

Bevacizumab

The most common toxicities observed are hypertension, proteinuria, and epistaxis, which are known side effects of bevacizumab treatment. There is an increased risk of thromboembolism events and rare case of gastrointestinal perforation; however, it is important to note that patient-related outcome is favorable (75). Within clinical practice, a review analyzing data from 156 patients with recurrent ovarian cancer

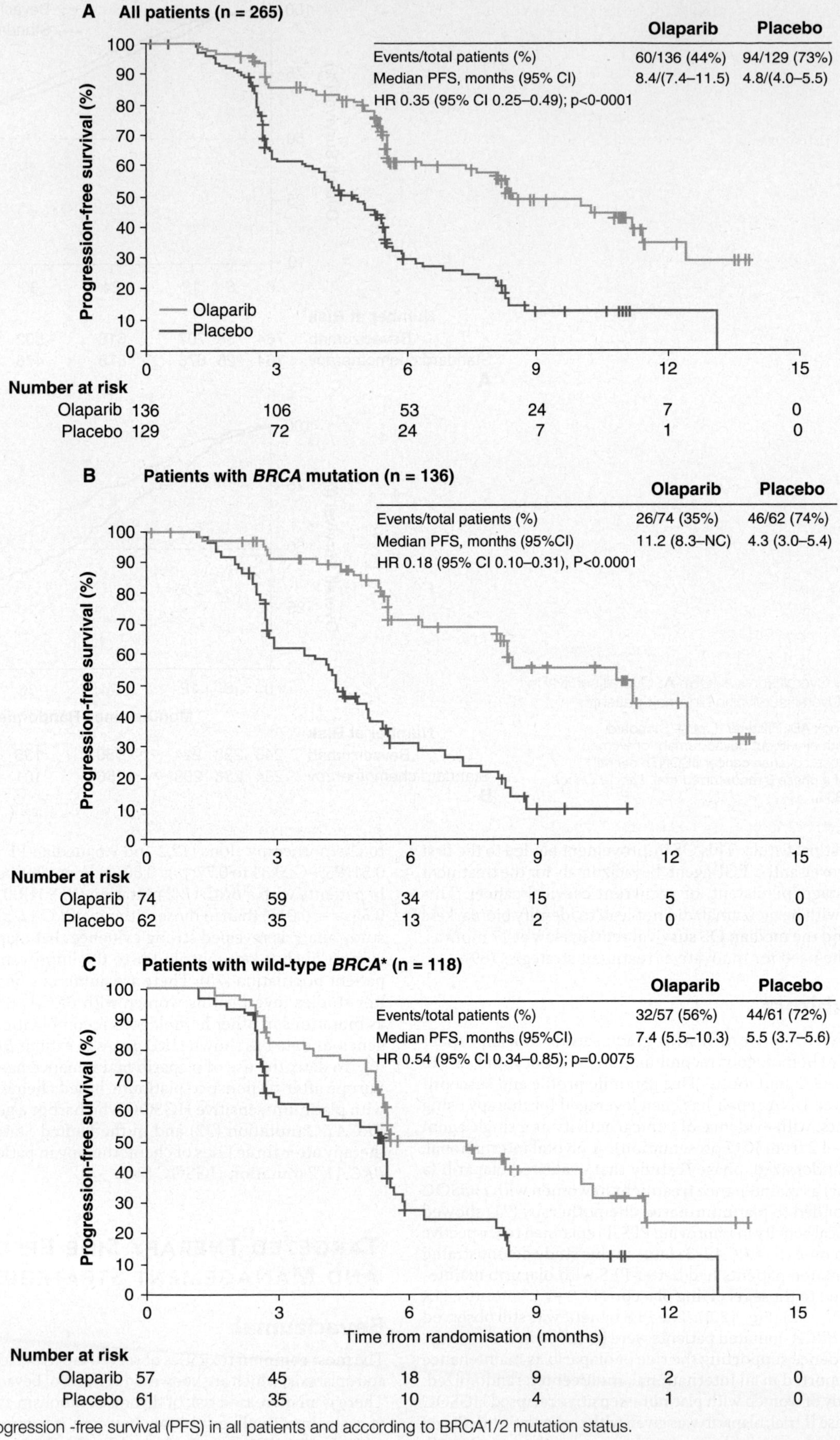

Figure 12.8. Progression -free survival (PFS) in all patients and according to BRCA1/2 mutation status.

From Ledermann J, Harter P, Gourley C, et al; Olaparib maintenance therapy in patients with platinum-sensitive relapsed serous ovarian cancer: a preplanned retrospective analysis of outcomes by BRCA status in a randomized phase 2 trial. *Lancet Oncol*. 2014;15(8):852-861.

who had received bevacizumab between January 2006 and June 2009 were retrospectively identified from institutional records of five French centers and examined toxicity data (76). Findings reported by Selle et al. (76) confirm the effect of heavy pretreatment on the occurrence of serious and fatal adverse events in clinical practice as reported in clinical trials and other retrospective studies, and that medical history of hypertension is an independent predictive risk factor for the development of high-grade hypertension during bevacizumab treatment (76). As such, treating physicians should exercise caution and consider all risk factors for managing bevacizumab toxicity prior to introduction including time to bevacizumab introduction, history of hypertension, and low incidence of preexisting obstructive disease (76).

Olaparib

The most common toxicities seen with olaparib—and similar amongst other PARP inhibitors in development—include nausea, vomiting, fatigue, and myelosuppression [PMID: 26051946]. In practice, these toxicities are manageable and require patient education. Additional information regarding the potential increased risk of myelodysplasia syndrome and acute myeloid leukemia are being collected.

Targeted Agents in the Maintenance Setting

Given the high rate of recurrence in gynecologic cancers, attempting to maintain disease control post standard chemotherapy is a new area of investigation to lower tumor burden. A meta-analysis of 13 randomized controlled trials published between 2006 and 2014 indicated that while both PFS and OS were statistically and significantly improved in the targeted maintenance therapy group as compared to the control group (PFS: HR 0.84, 95% CI 0.75 to 0.95, $p = 0.001$; OS: HR 0.91, 95% CI 0.84 to 0.98, $p = 0.02$), targeted agents were also significantly correlated with increased risk of fatigue, diarrhea, nausea, vomiting, and hypertension (77). Importantly, the meta-analysis also provided evidence illustrating that no significant differences were found in incidence rates of abdominal pain, constipation, or joint pain (77). As such, this novel treatment approach necessitates the education of patients in regard to drug management as chronic disease.

In October 2016, promising results were published using the PARP inhibitor, Niraparib as maintenance treatment for women with platinum-sensitive, recurrent ovarian cancer (78). In this trial, two independent cohorts were categorized based on the presence or absence of a germline *BRCA* (*gBRCA*) mutation; women without a *gBRCA* were further subgrouped based on whether they were positive for homologous recombination deficiency (HRD) using a commercially available genomic assay. All patients had platinum-sensitive recurrent ovarian cancer and were enrolled no later than 8 weeks after completing their last dose of platinum-based chemotherapy. Using a 2:1 randomization design, patients were assigned treatment with niraparib (300 mg) or placebo, orally administered on a daily basis for 28-day cycles.

With a median duration of follow-up of 17 months, compared to placebo, the median duration of progression-free survival (PFS) was significantly prolonged with niraparib in women with a *gBRCA* (21 versus 5.5 months; HR 0.27, 95%CI 0.17-0.41), without a *gBRCA* but HRD-positive (13 versus 4 months, HR 0.38, 95%CI 0.24-0.59), and those without a *gBRCA* mutation and HRD-negative (9 versus 4 months, 95%CI 0.34-0.61). Overall survival results were not mature at the time of publication. Of note, the rate of treatment discontinuation was higher in women taking niraparib versus placebo (15.5 versus 2%) but no on-study deaths were reported. Major toxicities associated with niraparib included thrombocytopenia, and anemia, neutropenia, with a 1.4% incidence of myelodysplastic syndrome reported. Patient reported outcomes were similar in both groups. These results suggest that maintenance niraparib may benefit all women with platinum-sensitive ovarian cancer, regardless of whether or not they harbor a *gBRCA*, though those women with a *gBRCA* and/or HRD on genomic assessment of their tumor stand to benefit the most.

REFERENCES

1. Hanahan D, Weinberg RA. The hallmarks of cancer. *Cell.* 2000;100(1):57–70.
2. Hanahan D, Weinberg RA. Hallmarks of cancer: the next generation. *Cell.* 2011;144(5):646–674.
3. Italiano A. Prognostic or predictive? It is time to get back to definitions! *J Clin Oncol.* 2011;29(35):4718; author reply 4718–4719.
4. Dancey JE, Dobbin KK, Groshen S, et al; Biomarkers Task Force of the NCI Investigational Drug Steering Committee. Guidelines for the development and incorporation of biomarker studies in early clinical trials of novel agents. *Clin Cancer Res.* 2010;16(6):1745–1755.
5. Banerjee S, Kaye SB. New strategies in the treatment of ovarian cancer: current clinical perspectives and future potential. *Clin Cancer Res.* 2013;19(5):961–968.
6. Cancer Genome Atlas Research Network. Integrated genomic analyses of ovarian carcinoma. *Nature.* 2011;474(7353):609–615.
7. Cancer Genome Atlas Research Network, Kandoth C, Schultz N, et al. Integrated genomic characterization of endometrial carcinoma. *Nature.* 2013;497(7447):67–73.
8. Ojesina AI, Lichtenstein L, Freeman SS, et al. Landscape of genomic alterations in cervical carcinomas. *Nature.* 2014;506(7488):371–375.
9. Raghavan R, Brady ML, Sampson JH. Delivering therapy to target: improving the odds for successful drug development. *Ther Deliv.* 2016;7(7):457–481.
10. Hong B, van den Heuvel AP, Prabhu VV, et al. Targeting tumor suppressor p53 for cancer therapy: strategies, challenges and opportunities. *Curr Drug Targets.* 2014;15(1):80–89.
11. Vang R, Levine DA, Soslow RA, et al. Molecular alterations of TP53 are a defining feature of ovarian high-grade serous carcinoma: a rereview of cases lacking TP53 mutations in The Cancer Genome Atlas Ovarian Study. *Int J Gynecol Pathol.* 2016;35(1):48–55.
12. Schultheis AM, Martelotto LG, De Filippo MR, et al. TP53 mutational spectrum in endometrioid and serous endometrial cancers. *Int J Gynecol Pathol.* 2016;35(4):289–300.
13. Seagle BL, Yang CP, Eng KH, et al. TP53 hot spot mutations in ovarian cancer: selective resistance to microtubule stabilizers in vitro and differential survival outcomes from The Cancer Genome Atlas. *Gynecol Oncol.* 2015;138(1):159–164.
14. Bykov VJ, Wiman KG. Mutant p53 reactivation by small molecules makes its way to the clinic. *FEBS Lett.* 2014;588(16):2622–2627.
15. Santo L, Siu KT, Raje N. Targeting cyclin-dependent kinases and cell cycle progression in human cancers. *Semin Oncol.* 2015;42(6):788–800.
16. Malumbres M, Barbacid M. Cell cycle, CDKs and cancer: a changing paradigm. *Nat Rev Cancer.* 2009;9(3):153–166.
17. Karakasis K, Burnier JV, Bowering V, et al. Ovarian cancer and BRCA1/2 testing: opportunities to improve clinical care and disease prevention. *Front Oncol.* 2016;6:119. doi:10.3389/fonc.2016.00119. eCollection 2016.
18. Chen S, Parmigiani G. Meta-analysis of BRCA1 and BRCA2 penetrance. *J Clin Oncol.* 2007;25(11):1329–1333.
19. Alsop K, Fereday S, Meldrum C, et al. BRCA mutation frequency and patterns of treatment response in BRCA mutation-positive women with ovarian cancer: a report from the Australian Ovarian Cancer Study Group. *J Clin Oncol.* 2012;30(21):2654–2663.
20. McCabe N, Turner NC, Lord CJ, et al. Deficiency in the repair of DNA damage by homologous recombination and sensitivity to poly(ADP-ribose) polymerase inhibition. *Cancer Res.* 2006;66(16):8109–8115.
21. Pennington KP, Walsh T, Harrell MI, et al. Germline and somatic mutations in homologous recombination genes predict platinum response and survival in ovarian, fallopian tube, and peritoneal carcinomas. *Clin Cancer Res.* 2014;20(3):764–775.
22. Ashworth A. A synthetic lethal therapeutic approach: poly(ADP) ribose polymerase inhibitors for the treatment of cancers deficient in DNA double-strand break repair. *J Clin Oncol.* 2008;26(22):3785–3790.
23. Farmer H, McCabe N, Lord CJ, et al. Targeting the DNA repair defect in BRCA mutant cells as a therapeutic strategy. *Nature.* 2005;434(7035):917–921.
24. Walsh T, Lee MK, Casadei S, et al. Detection of inherited mutations for breast and ovarian cancer using genomic capture and massively parallel sequencing. *Proc Natl Acad Sci U S A.* 2010;107(28):12629–12633.
25. Walsh T, Casadei S, Lee MK, et al. Mutations in 12 genes for inherited ovarian, fallopian tube, and peritoneal carcinoma identified by massively parallel sequencing. *Proc Natl Acad Sci U S A.* 2011;108(44):18032–18037.
26. Toss A, Tomasello C, Razzaboni E, et al. Hereditary ovarian cancer: not only BRCA 1 and 2 genes. *Biomed Res Int.* 2015;2015:341723.
27. McNeish IA, Oza AM, Coleman RL, et al; ASCO. Results of ARIEL2: a Phase 2 trial to prospectively identify ovarian cancer patients likely to respond to rucaparib using tumor genetic analysis. 2015 ASCO Annual Meeting (oral presentation); 2015.

28. McAlpine JN, Temkin SM, Mackay HJ. Endometrial cancer: not your grandmother's cancer. *Cancer*. 2016;122(18):2787–2798.
29. Rabban JT, Calkins SM, Karnezis AN, et al. Association of tumor morphology with mismatch-repair protein status in older endometrial cancer patients: implications for universal versus selective screening strategies for Lynch syndrome. *Am J Surg Pathol*. 2014;38(6):793–800.
30. Goodfellow PJ, Billingsley CC, Lankes HA, et al. Combined microsatellite instability, MLH1 methylation analysis, and immunohistochemistry for Lynch syndrome screening in endometrial cancers from GOG210: an NRG Oncology and Gynecologic Oncology Group Study. *J Clin Oncol*. 2015;33(36):4301–4308.
31. Mabuchi S, Kuroda H, Takahashi R, et al. The PI3K/AKT/mTOR pathway as a therapeutic target in ovarian cancer. *Gynecol Oncol*. 2015;137(1):173–179.
32. Engelman JA, Luo J, Cantley LC. The evolution of phosphatidylinositol 3-kinases as regulators of growth and metabolism. *Nat Rev Genet*. 2006;7(8):606–619.
33. Sato N, Tsunoda H, Nishida M, et al. Loss of heterozygosity on 10q23.3 and mutation of the tumor suppressor gene PTEN in benign endometrial cyst of the ovary: possible sequence progression from benign endometrial cyst to endometrioid carcinoma and clear cell carcinoma of the ovary. *Cancer Res*. 2000;60(24):7052–7056.
34. Fujiwara K, McAlpine JN, Lheureux S, et al. Paradigm shift in the management strategy for epithelial ovarian cancer. *Am Soc Clin Oncol Educ Book*. 2016;35:e247–e257.
35. Wright AA, Howitt BE, Myers AP, et al. Oncogenic mutations in cervical cancer: genomic differences between adenocarcinomas and squamous cell carcinomas of the cervix. *Cancer*. 2013;119(21):3776–3783.
36. Romero I, Sun CC, Wong KK, et al. Low-grade serous carcinoma: new concepts and emerging therapies. *Gynecol Oncol*. 2013;130(3):660–666.
37. Grisham RN, Iyer G, Garg K, et al. BRAF mutation is associated with early stage disease and improved outcome in patients with low-grade serous ovarian cancer. *Cancer*. 2013;119(3):548–554.
38. Goulvent T, Ray-Coquard I, Borel S, et al. DICER1 and FOXL2 mutations in ovarian sex cord-stromal tumors: a GINECO Group study. *Histopathology*. 2016;68(2):279–285.
39. Butkus ME, Prundeanu LB, Oliver DB. Translocon "pulling" of nascent SecM controls the duration of its translational pause and secretion-responsive secA regulation. *J Bacteriol*. 2003;185(22):6719–6722.
40. Growdon WB, Del Carmen M. Human papillomavirus-related gynecologic neoplasms: screening and prevention. *Rev Obstet Gynecol*. 2008;1(4):154–161.
41. Rosa MI, Silva GD, de Azedo Simões PW, et al. The prevalence of human papillomavirus in ovarian cancer: a systematic review. *Int J Gynecol Cancer*. 2013;23(3):437–441.
42. Bhat P, Mattarollo SR, Gosmann C, et al. Regulation of immune responses to HPV infection and during HPV-directed immunotherapy. *Immunol Rev*. 2011;239(1):85–98.
43. Song D, Li H, Li H, et al. Effect of human papillomavirus infection on the immune system and its role in the course of cervical cancer. *Oncol Lett*. 2015;10(2):600–606.
44. Niu G, Chen X. Vascular endothelial growth factor as an anti-angiogenic target for cancer therapy. *Curr Drug Targets*. 2010;11(8):1000–1017.
45. Gavalas NG, Liontos M, Trachana SP, et al. Angiogenesis-related pathways in the pathogenesis of ovarian cancer. *Int J Mol Sci*. 2013;14(8):15885–15909.
46. Tomao F, Papa A, Rossi L, et al. Beyond bevacizumab: investigating new angiogenesis inhibitors in ovarian cancer. *Expert Opin Investig Drugs*. 2014;23(1):37–53.
47. Lheureux S, Oza AM. Endometrial cancer-targeted therapies myth or reality? Review of current targeted treatments. *Eur J Cancer*. 2016;59:99–108.
48. Zhang Y, Zhao D, Gong C, et al. Prognostic role of hormone receptors in endometrial cancer: a systematic review and meta-analysis. *World J Surg Oncol*. 2015;13:208.
49. Podratz KC, O'Brien PC, Malkasian GD Jr, et al. Effects of progestational agents in treatment of endometrial carcinoma. *Obstet Gynecol*. 1985;66(1):106–110.
50. Thigpen JT, Brady MF, Alvarez RD, et al. Oral medroxyprogesterone acetate in the treatment of advanced or recurrent endometrial carcinoma: a dose-response study by the Gynecologic Oncology Group. *J Clin Oncol*. 1999;17(6):1736–1744.
51. Temkin SM, Fleming G. Current treatment of metastatic endometrial cancer. *Cancer Control*. 2009;16(1):38–45.
52. Carlson MJ, Thiel KW, Leslie KK. Past, present, and future of hormonal therapy in recurrent endometrial cancer. *Int J Womens Health*. 2014;6:429–435. doi:10.2147/IJWH.S40942. eCollection 2014.
53. Wright JD, Barrena Medel NI, Sehouli J, et al. Contemporary management of endometrial cancer. *Lancet*. 2012;379(9823):1352–1360.
54. Tsoref D, Oza AM. Recent advances in systemic therapy for advanced endometrial cancer. *Curr Opin Oncol*. 2011;23(5):494–500.
55. Decruze SB, Green JA. Hormone therapy in advanced and recurrent endometrial cancer: a systematic review. *Int J Gynecol Cancer*. 2007;17(5):964–978.
56. Zaino RJ, Brady WE, Todd W, et al. Histologic effects of medroxyprogesterone acetate on endometrioid endometrial adenocarcinoma: a Gynecologic Oncology Group study. *Int J Gynecol Pathol*. 2014;33(6):543–553.
57. Thigpen T, Brady MF, Homesley HD, et al. Tamoxifen in the treatment of advanced or recurrent endometrial carcinoma: a Gynecologic Oncology Group study. *J Clin Oncol*. 2001;19(2):364–367.
58. Ma BB, Oza A, Eisenhauer E, et al. The activity of letrozole in patients with advanced or recurrent endometrial cancer and correlation with biological markers—a study of the National Cancer Institute of Canada Clinical Trials Group. *Int J Gynecol Cancer*. 2004;14(4):650–658.
59. Rose PG, Brunetto VL, VanLe L, et al. A phase II trial of anastrozole in advanced recurrent or persistent endometrial carcinoma: a Gynecologic Oncology Group study. *Gynecol Oncol*. 2000;78(2):212–216.
60. Ramondetta LM, Johnson AJ, Sun CC, et al. Phase 2 trial of mifepristone (RU-486) in advanced or recurrent endometrioid adenocarcinoma or low-grade endometrial stromal sarcoma. *Cancer*. 2009;115(9):1867–1874.
61. Whitney CW, Brunetto VL, Zaino RJ, et al; Gynecologic Oncology Group study. Phase II study of medroxyprogesterone acetate plus tamoxifen in advanced endometrial carcinoma: a Gynecologic Oncology Group study. *Gynecol Oncol*. 2004;92(1):4–9.
62. Fiorica JV, Brunetto VL, Hanjani P, et al; Gynecologic Oncology Group study. Phase II trial of alternating courses of megestrol acetate and tamoxifen in advanced endometrial carcinoma: a Gynecologic Oncology Group study. *Gynecol Oncol*. 2004;92(1):10–14.
63. Kokka F, Brockbank E, Oram D, et al. Hormonal therapy in advanced or recurrent endometrial cancer. *Cochrane Database Syst Rev*. 2010;(12):CD007926. doi:10.1002/14651858.CD007926.pub2.
64. Burger RA, Brady MF, Bookman MA, et al; Gynecologic Oncology Group. Incorporation of bevacizumab in the primary treatment of ovarian cancer. *N Engl J Med*. 2011;365(26):2473–2483.
65. Perren TJ, Swart AM, Pfisterer J, et al; ICON7 Investigators. A phase 3 trial of bevacizumab in ovarian cancer. *N Engl J Med*. 2011;365(26):2484–2496.
66. Aghajanian C, Blank SV, Goff BA, et al. OCEANS: a randomized, double-blind, placebo-controlled phase III trial of chemotherapy with or without bevacizumab in patients with platinum-sensitive recurrent epithelial ovarian, primary peritoneal, or fallopian tube cancer. *J Clin Oncol*. 2012;30(17):2039–2045.
67. Pujade-Lauraine E, Hilpert F, Weber B, et al. Bevacizumab combined with chemotherapy for platinum-resistant recurrent ovarian cancer: The AURELIA open-label randomized phase III trial. *J Clin Oncol*. 2014;32(13):1302–1308.
68. Koh WJ, Greer BE, Abu-Rustum NR, et al. Cervical cancer, version 2.2015. *J Natl Compr Canc Netw*. 2015;13(4):395–404; quiz 404.
69. Tewari KS, Sill MW, Long HJ 3rd, et al. Improved survival with bevacizumab in advanced cervical cancer. *N Engl J Med*. 2014;370(8):734–743.
70. Gelmon KA, Tischkowitz M, Mackay H, et al. Olaparib in patients with recurrent high-grade serous or poorly differentiated ovarian carcinoma or triple-negative breast cancer: a phase 2, multicentre, open-label, non-randomized study. *Lancet Oncol*. 2011;12(9):852–861.
71. Ledermann J, Harter P, Gourley C, et al. Olaparib maintenance therapy in platinum-sensitive relapsed ovarian cancer. *N Engl J Med*. 2012;366(15):1382–1392.
72. Ledermann J, Harter P, Gourley C, et al. Olaparib maintenance therapy in patients with platinum-sensitive relapsed serous ovarian cancer: a preplanned retrospective analysis of outcomes by BRCA status in a randomized phase 2 trial. *Lancet Oncol*. 2014;15(8):852–861.
73. Oza AM, Cibula D, Benzaquen AO, et al. Olaparib combined with chemotherapy for recurrent platinum-sensitive ovarian cancer: a randomized phase 2 trial. *Lancet Oncol*. 2015;16(1):87–97.
74. Kaufman B, Shapira-Frommer R, Schmutzler RK, et al. Olaparib monotherapy in patients with advanced cancer and a germline BRCA1/2 mutation. *J Clin Oncol*. 2015;33(3):244–250.
75. Stockler MR, Hilpert F, Friedlander M, et al. Patient-reported outcome results from the open-label phase III AURELIA trial evaluating bevacizumab-containing therapy for platinum-resistant ovarian cancer. *J Clin Oncol*. 2014;32(13):1309–1316.
76. Selle F, Emile G, Pautier P, et al. Safety of bevacizumab in clinical practice for recurrent ovarian cancer: a retrospective cohort study. *Oncol Lett*. 2016;11(3):1859–1865.
77. Qian X, Qin J, Pan S, et al. Maintenance therapy in ovarian cancer with targeted agents improves PFS and OS: a systematic review and meta-analysis. *PLoS One*. 2015;10(9):e0139026.
78. Mirza MR, Monk BJ, Herrstedt J, et al. Niraparib maintenance therapy in platinum-sensitive, recurrent ovarian cancer. *N Engl J Med*. 2016; doi:10.1056/NEJMoa1611310.

CHAPTER 13

Principles of Chemotherapy in Gynecologic Cancer

Stéphanie L. Gaillard and Michael A. Bookman

HISTORICAL OVERVIEW OF CANCER CHEMOTHERAPY

We are in the midst of an important transition from conventional cytotoxic agents to new strategies that incorporate mechanism-based molecular-targeted therapeutics. Even with these changes in our treatment paradigm, several conventional cytotoxic agents maintain a central role in the care of women with gynecologic cancers. In that context, a brief review of drug development provides a framework for understanding the evolving balance between toxicity, efficacy, and design of treatment regimens.

First reports of a drug-mediated tumor response were noted 150 years ago using Fowler solution (arsenic trioxide in potassium bicarbonate) in patients with Hodgkin disease and leukemia (1). Arsenic compounds had been used for various medicinal purposes for over 2,000 years, and cyclic hematologic toxicity was observed following arsenic administration in normal individuals and patients with leukemia (2), establishing a close association between tumor response and host toxicity that still exists today. Cumulative dose-limiting toxicity (arsenic poisoning) was also described following expanded utilization of arsenic in chronic myelogenous leukemia (3).

The term *chemotherapy* has been attributed to Paul Ehrlich, a Nobel laureate physician and bacteriologist, who developed *in vivo* rodent models of infection and introduced Salvarsan, an organic arsenical originally used to cure syphilis in 1910. His early *in vivo* modeling also encouraged the development of inbred transplantable rodent tumors, thereby establishing a paradigm that has been widely adopted for screening new antitumor agents.

Although the topical vesicant properties of sulfur mustard received much attention during World War I, multiple systemic effects, including leukopenia, bone marrow aplasia, and mucosal ulceration, also emerged. Cancer chemotherapy, in the traditional sense, began with the demonstration that nitrogen mustard had reproducible activity against transplanted lymphoma in mice, prompting clinical trials as early as 1942 (4). However, owing to World War II, much of the research remained classified until 1946. Following the demonstration by Farber and Diamond (5) in 1948 that aminopterin, an antifolate, could induce temporary remission in childhood leukemia, antimetabolites became the next major category of agents to be developed, and were ultimately associated with cures in women with choriocarcinoma (6). Research during the 1940s also included the Nobel Prize–winning observations of Huggins and Hodges (7) regarding the antitumor effect of estrogens in prostate cancer.

Conventional Cytotoxic Agents

Cytotoxic agents commonly used in the treatment of gynecologic malignancies are listed in **Table 13.1**, spanning a period of development beginning in 1945, including analogs with more favorable toxicity profiles. Attention has also been directed at alternative formulations of standard agents, including liposomal or polymer-based encapsulation, protein conjugation, nanoparticles, or lipid solubilization, to modify drug disposition, tumor targeting, and the potential for host toxicity. A timeline of key US and EU regulatory approvals in ovarian cancer is summarized in **Figure 13.1**.

With the availability of multiple agents, each with a different molecular target, mechanism of action, pattern of resistance, and spectrum of host toxicity, we have also seen frequent utilization of multidrug combinations, particularly as primary therapy for advanced disease. The use of adjuvant therapy, including concurrent chemoradiation for early-stage disease, has been greatly expanded in selected clinical situations, with the result that a larger proportion of patients are exposed to chemotherapy at an earlier point in

TABLE 13.1. Common Cytotoxic Agents Used in the Treatment of Gynecologic Malignancies

Agent	Classification	Primary Mechanism of Action	Notable Side Effects (% Frequency)	Management Considerations
Altretamine	Alkylating agent	Requires hepatic microsomal activation to form DNA cross-links	Delayed nadir Neurotoxicity: somnolence, mood changes, lethargy, depression, agitation, hallucinations (25%)	Oral
Bleomycin	Antitumor Antibiotic	Generates oxygen free radical species leading to DNA breaks	Pulmonary toxicity (10%): increased risk with cumulative dose >400 units, smoking history, underlying lung disease, and oxygen exposure; Skin toxicity Hypersensitivity reactions (25%) Rare vascular events (MI, stroke, Raynaud)	Obtain CXR and PFTs with DLCO/vital capacity at start of therapy, and then as clinically indicated; discontinue if PFT parameters decrease ≥15% or pulmonary infiltrates develop; avoid exposure to high FiO_2, which can enhance pulmonary damage; avoid smoking

(continued)

■ **TABLE 13.1. Common Cytotoxic Agents Used in the Treatment of Gynecologic Malignancies (*continued*)**

Agent	Classification	Primary Mechanism of Action	Notable Side Effects (% Frequency)	Management Considerations
Capecitabine	Antimetabolite	Prodrug of 5-fluorourocil involving liver and tumor enzymatic reactions, inhibits thymidylate synthase	GI: diarrhea (dose-limiting in 55%), mucositis, N/V (≤50%), elevated LFTs (≤40%) Derm: PPE (severe in 15%–20%) Vascular: rare cardiac vasospasm, risk higher with prior MI	Oral administration Interacts with warfarin
Carboplatin	Organoplatinum analog	Activated by aquation and forms DNA adducts	Myelosuppression: particularly thrombocytopenia (nadir day 21) Hypersensitivity (allergic) reactions (maximal risk during subsequent courses of therapy) Sterility/ovarian failure	Predominant renal clearance, dosed by target AUC using Calvert formula based on estimated GFR, should be administered after paclitaxel if used in combination
Cisplatin	Platinum analog	Rapid activation by aquation, Forms DNA adducts	Nephrotoxicity: 10–20 days post dose (35%–40%), but cleared predominantly by non-renal mechanisms Electrolyte loss: magnesium, calcium, potassium GI: acute and delayed emesis Myelosuppression Neurotoxicity: peripheral sensory neuropathy (common, cumulative); ototoxicity; encephalopathy/ seizures/motor dysfunction (rare) Vascular (rare): MI, arteritis, stroke, Raynaud Sterility/ovarian failure	Often used as a radiosensitizing agent
Cyclophosphamide	Alkylating agent	Hepatic microsomal activation, forms DNA cross-links	Myelosuppression Hemorrhagic cystitis/dysuria (5%–10%) Sterility/ovarian failure Increased risk of secondary malignancies	Commonly given on daily low-dose (metronomic) schedule for ovarian cancer
Dacarbazine	Alkylating agent	Inhibits DNA, RNA, and protein synthesis	Flu-like syndrome CNS toxicity (paresthesias, ataxia, lethargy, seizures) Photosensitivity	Vesicant
Dactinomycin	Antitumor Antibiotic	Generates activated oxygen free radical species leading to DNA breaks	GI: severe N/V, mucositis/diarrhea Skin hyperpigmentation Radiation recall reaction	Vesicant
Docetaxel	Antimicrotubule agent	Enhances tubulin polymerization, inhibits mitosis and cell division	Hypersensitivity reactions Fluid retention syndrome with edema, pleural effusion, ascites (50%), GI: mucositis/diarrhea (40%) Compared to paclitaxel: peripheral neuropathy less common, but increased myelosuppression	Hypersensitivity and fluid retention syndrome can be reduced with steroid pretreatment Vesicant
Doxorubicin	Antitumor Antibiotic	Intercalates into DNA inhibiting synthesis and function, inhibits topoisomerase-II, formation of free radicals and DNA breaks	Cardiotoxicity: acute arrhythmias or conduction abnormalities, chronic congestive heart failure Radiation recall Photosensitivity Red–orange discoloration of urine	Monitor LVEF at baseline and periodically, cumulative doses ≥450 mg/m^2 associated with higher risk Strong vesicant
Epirubicin	Antitumor Antibiotic	Derivative of doxorubicin (see previous row)	Cardiotoxicity: acute arrhythmias or conduction abnormalities, chronic congestive heart failure Radiation recall Photosensitivity Red–orange discoloration of urine	Monitor LVEF at baseline and periodically, cumulative doses ≥900 mg/m^2 associated with higher risk Strong vesicant

■ **TABLE 13.1. Common Cytotoxic Agents Used in the Treatment of Gynecologic Malignancies (*continued*)**

Agent	Classification	Primary Mechanism of Action	Notable Side Effects (% Frequency)	Management Considerations
Etoposide	Topoisomerase-II inhibitor	Inhibits topoisomerase-II preventing DNA unwinding	GI: emesis (30%–40%), more common with oral administration Increased risk of secondary malignancies (5–8 years posttreatment)	Oral administration common for ovarian cancer
5-Fluorouricil	Antimetabolite	Requires tissue activation, inhibits thymidylate synthase with impact on DNA synthesis and function	GI: mucositis/diarrhea, can be severe Derm: Palmar-plantar erythrodysesthesia Neurologic: confusion, seizures, somnolence, ataxia, encephalopathy (rare) Cardiac: chest pain, EKG changes, enzyme elevation (attributed to coronary vasospasm)	Patients with underlying deficiency in dihydropyrimidine dehydrogenase may experience severe myelosuppression, GI toxicity, and/or neurologic toxicity
Gemcitabine	Antimetabolite	Metabolized into triphosphate nucleotide with incorporation into DNA, inhibiting synthesis and function	Myelosuppression: often dose-limiting GI: diarrhea, stomatitis, mucositis (15%–20%) Fever or flu-like syndrome (20%–40%) Pneumonitis Maculopapular rash	Potent radiosensitizer
Ifosfamide	Alkylating agent	Microsomal hepatic activation, forms DNA cross-links	Myelosuppression: often dose-limiting Hemorrhagic cystitis Neurotoxicity: lethargy/confusion, seizure, cerebellar ataxia, weakness, hallucinations, cranial nerve dysfunction Infertility	Prevent hemorrhagic cystitis with Mesna and hydration Higher risk of neurotoxicity with high-dose therapy and impaired renal function, older age, and low albumin
Irinotecan	Topoisomerase-I inhibitor	Equilibrium conversion to active metabolite SN-38 which binds to topoisomerase-I, preventing DNA synthesis	GI: diarrhea both acute (during or within 24 hours of infusion) and late, can be severe	Acute diarrhea secondary to cholinergic effect (can be managed with atropine); late diarrhea must be managed aggressively to prevent dehydration and electrolyte loss; UGT1A1 7/7 genotype increases risk for GI toxicity and myelosuppression
PEGylated liposomal doxorubicin	Antitumor Antibiotic	Polyethyline glycosylated liposomal formulation of doxorubicin (see above)	Much lower risk of cardiotoxicity compared to parent doxorubicin, higher risk of palmar plantar erythrodysesthesia	May not be substituted for doxorubicin
Melphalan	Alkylating agent	DNA cross-linking	Myelosuppression: nadir 4–6 weeks post-therapy GI: nausea/emesis, mucositis, diarrhea Increased risk of secondary malignancies	
Mitomycin	Antitumor Antibiotic	DNA cross-linking	Myelosuppression: nadir 4–6 weeks post-therapy Mucositis Hemolytic-uremic syndrome (<2%, however can be fatal) Interstitial pneumonitis Hepatic veno-occlusive disease	Vesicant
Oxaliplatin	Platinum analog	DNA cross-linking	Neurotoxicity: frequently dose-limiting, can manifest as sensory neuropathy, gait abnormalities, cognitive dysfunction, or difficulty breathing Intolerance to cold (including ingestion of cold liquids) Hypersensitivity reactions GI: N/V, diarrhea	Careful monitoring of neurologic function necessary Neurotoxicity more frequently reversible than with cisplatin (3–4 months)

(continued)

■ **TABLE 13.1. Common Cytotoxic Agents Used in the Treatment of Gynecologic Malignancies (*continued*)**

Agent	Classification	Primary Mechanism of Action	Notable Side Effects (% Frequency)	Management Considerations
Paclitaxel	Taxane, anti-microtubule agent	Enhances tubulin polymerization, inhibits mitosis and cell division	Myelosuppression Hypersensitivity reactions: (most common with first or second dose) Sensory neuropathy Transient asymptomatic sinus bradycardia GI: mucositis/diarrhea (when administered by prolonged infusion), transient LFT elevations Onycholysis (more common with weekly dosing)	May be dosed weekly or every 3 weeks
Pemetrexed	Antimetabolite	Multitargeted anti-folate: Inhibition of the folate-dependent enzymes. thymidylate synthase, and DNA synthesis	Myelosuppression: often dose-limiting Derm: rash, frequently PPE GI: N/V, mucositis, diarrhea, transient LFT elevations	Insufficient folate intake increases toxicity risk, prevent with vitamin B12 and folate supplementation; steroids may be used prophylactically to prevent skin rash NSAIDs and aspirin inhibit renal clearance of pemetrexed, discontinue use in days leading up to and following pemetrexed administration
Temozolomide	Alkylating agent	Structurally and functionally similar to dacarbazine	Myelosuppression: dose-limiting Photosensitivity GI: N/V	Monitor for development of lymphopenia, increased risk of PCP (consider prophylaxis)
Topotecan	Topoisomerase-I inhibitor	Inhibits topoisomerase-I leading to dsDNA breaks	Myelosuppression: dose-limiting GI: N/V (80%) Microscopic hematuria (10%)	Administered either weekly, or day 1–5 every 3 weeks
Vinblastine	Antimicrotubule agent	Inhibits tubulin polymerization disrupting microtubule assembly during mitosis	Myelosuppression: neutrophil nadir days 4–6 GI: mucositis/stomatitis, constipation Neurologic: peripheral sensory neuropathy, autonomic dysfunction (including hypertension), seizures/coma (rare) Vascular events (stroke, MI, Raynaud, acute pulmonary edema) Pulm: bronchospasm, respiratory distress (rare)	Vesicant (not for intrathecal administration) Attentive to early management of constipation
Vincristine	Antimicrotubule agent	Inhibits tubulin polymerization disrupting microtubule assembly during mitosis	Neurotoxicity (most common DLT): peripheral neuropathy, autonomic dysfunction, cranial nerve palsies, cortical blindness, seizures/coma GI: constipation, paralytic ileus, abdominal pain Myelosuppression: generally mild	Vesicant (not for intrathecal administration) Attentive to early management of constipation
Vinorelbine	Antimicrotubule agent	Inhibits tubulin polymerization disrupting microtubule assembly during mitosis	Myelosuppression: nadir day 7 GI: N/V, constipation, diarrhea, stomatitis, anorexia, transient LFT elevation Neurotoxicity: usually mild Hypersensitivity reactions Fatigue	Vesicant (not for intrathecal administration)

the natural history of their disease. On the basis of a combination of intrinsic and acquired factors, the majority of advanced tumors eventually demonstrate broad resistance to conventional cytotoxic chemotherapy, and there has been renewed interest in novel biologic and immunologic approaches with non–cross-resistant mechanisms. In addition, with improved understanding of the mechanisms associated with drug resistance, newer agents have been developed that may partially reverse resistant phenotypes through blockade of specific pathways, inhibition of DNA repair, or promotion of cellular apoptosis.

Exploration of the biologic mechanisms associated with tumor growth, maintenance, metastasis, and resistance to chemotherapy has led to the development of molecular-targeted therapeutics. In general, novel targeted agents exhibit toxicities that are distinct from conventional cytotoxic chemotherapy, often sparing proliferative compartments, such as bone marrow and mucosal epithelium. However, there is still the potential for serious toxicity, including drug interactions, alterations in hepatic or renal function, bleeding, thrombosis, pneumonitis, leukoencephalitis, and autoimmunity. Thus far, the addition of novel targeted agents to conventional

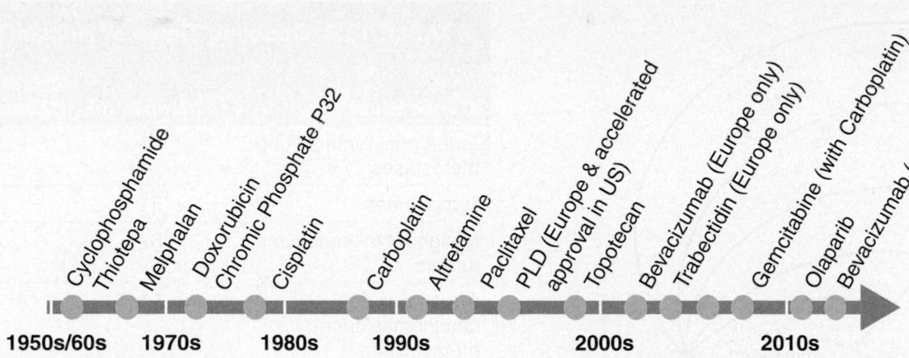

Figure 13.1. Approval timeline of chemotherapeutic agents commonly used in the treatment of ovarian cancer.

chemotherapy for gynecologic malignancies has resulted in only modest improvements in long-term clinical outcomes.

TUMOR BIOLOGY IN RELATION TO CHEMOTHERAPY

Tumor Growth and Cellular Kinetics

Many of the principles of modern chemotherapy are derived from knowledge of the growth characteristics of normal and tumor tissues. Exploitation of the differences between normal and tumor tissues has provided the historical basis for utilization of radiation and chemotherapy. The cellular kinetics of normal tissues also explains many of the toxicities associated with chemotherapy. All normal tissues, particularly during fetal development and variably during adult life, possess the capacity for cellular division and growth.

The *static* population includes well-differentiated cells that arise from pluripotent fetal stem cells and rarely undergo cell division during adult life (**Table 13.2**). Oocytes represent a specialized static population. Damage to these cells can have long-term consequences and has prompted interest in stem cell biology. The *expanding* population of normal tissues retains the capacity to grow, but in their adult state, they are normally quiescent. Under stress, especially after injury, a proliferative burst is followed by return to quiescence. The *renewing* cell population is in a continuous proliferative state, with ongoing cell division balanced by cell loss and terminal differentiation.

The patterns of normal cell growth partially explain some of the toxic effects of cytotoxic therapy and why some tissues are commonly spared (8,9). Renewing cell populations with constant turnover are most sensitive to acute injury from conventional chemotherapy or irradiation. This is reflected by the frequent occurrence of dose-limiting bone marrow suppression, mucositis, and azoospermia during cytotoxic drug treatment, with relative sparing of nonproliferative compartments, such as brain, muscle, kidney, bone, and oocytes. However, even nondividing tissues can experience late chronic effects related to DNA damage.

Dysregulated growth of cancer cells occurs because of altered growth factor signaling and/or disruption of normal checkpoint mechanisms. Despite a capacity for continuous growth, the actual process of cancer cell division is not more rapid than division in normal cells.

Programmed cell death, or apoptosis, has emerged as a major mechanism for regulating growth and development of tissues. Furthermore, certain oncogenes, like *MYC* and *BCL2,* and tumor suppressor genes (anti-oncogenes), including *RB* and *TP53,* are central to the regulation of apoptosis. Expression of these genes can alter the sensitivity of cancer cells to treatment with chemotherapy and radiation. For instance, overexpression of functional bcl-2 and nonfunctional p53 genes can render tumor cells resistant to a number of chemotherapeutic agents (10), suggesting that efforts to restore apoptotic signaling may improve chemosensitivity.

TABLE 13.2. Growth Patterns of Normal Cell Populations

Static	Expanding	Renewing
Striated muscle	Hepatocytes	Bone marrow
Neurons	Bile duct epithelium	Epidermis
Nephrons	Vascular endothelium	Gastrointestinal epithelium
Oocytes		Spermatocytes

Emerging data have also described stem-like behavior in subpopulations of ovarian cancer cells, including dormant cells with a low mitotic index that exclude cytotoxic drugs from their cytoplasm and demonstrate increased resistance to chemotherapy (11,12). These stem-like cells are generally enriched during the repopulation that occurs following primary chemotherapy, and targeting of these distinct cell populations has become an important area of research.

Cell Cycle Kinetics

An understanding of the kinetic behavior of individual tumor cells is also important in understanding tumor growth. **Figure 13.2** is a schematic view of the cell cycle. Cells can remain in a non-cycling postmitotic compartment (G_0) for extended periods of time, but retain the ability to reenter active cycling when triggered by growth factors or other local signals. The point of entry, or first gap phase (G_1), can be of variable length and associated with diverse cellular activities, including protein and RNA synthesis, DNA repair, and cell growth. After passing the first checkpoint in G_1, the cell enters the DNA synthetic phase (S), during which a complete copy of the cellular DNA is created through replication. The second gap phase (G_2) provides another opportunity for checkpoint control before entering active mitosis (M), during which the nuclear membrane disappears and the chromosomes condense (prophase) and align (metaphase) in conjunction with the appearance of the mitotic apparatus, consisting of microtubules, centrioles, and the kinetochore. Mitotic alignment is associated with one final checkpoint prior to actual separation (anaphase), followed by dissolution of the mitotic apparatus (telophase) and creation of daughter cells through cytokinesis. The postmitotic period (G_1) is variable, and cells can further differentiate, enter a non-cycling state (G_0), or initiate another cycle.

Cell cycle events have important implications, as most chemotherapeutic agents disrupt DNA, RNA, or protein synthesis. Rapidly proliferating cells (i.e., short G_1) are most sensitive to chemotherapy, whereas cells that slowly proliferate (i.e., G_0 or long G_1) are generally less sensitive. Nondividing cells, such as the differentiated elements

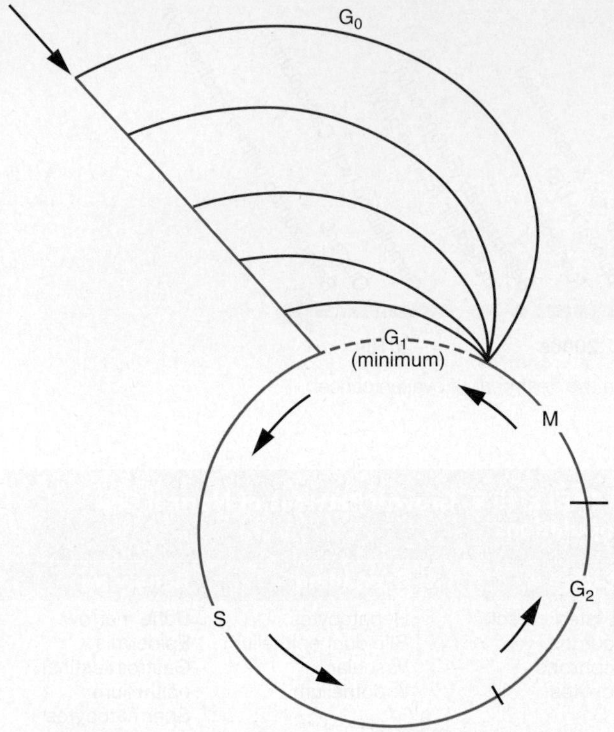

Figure 13.2. Phases of the cell cycle, beginning with M (mitosis) and proceeding through G_1 (postmitotic phase), S (DNA synthetic phase), and G_2 (premitotic phase). As G_1 becomes progressively longer, it is known as G_0.

of a mature teratoma, may occupy space and contribute to tumor bulk and symptoms, but are relatively insensitive to chemotherapy.

Cell cycle times may be estimated by performing labeled mitotic curves *in vivo* or *in vitro,* and appear to be relatively similar for many solid tumors, with cycle times ranging from 10 to 31 hours (13). When contrasted with the wide variation in observed human tumor doubling times (**Table 13.3**), it suggests that variations in clinical tumor growth cannot be simply ascribed to variations in the cell cycle.

Growth fraction and programmed cell death also influence the overall tumor growth rate and response to therapy. The growth fraction is the proportion of tumor cells that are actively cycling. Often, these proliferating cells are located proximal to small blood vessels. Growth fractions in human tumors are quite variable, ranging from 25% to 95%. Although it may seem paradoxical, the rate of cell loss is usually very high in human tumors, ranging from 70% to more than 95%, and small changes in cell loss could produce major changes in apparent tumor growth (14).

Host–Tumor Interactions

Ultimately, dysregulated growth exceeds local resources, and the tumor becomes dependent on the manipulation of host angiogenic pathways for delivery of oxygen, access to nutrients, and removal of waste products. Tumors generally grow without structured lymphatic drainage and are characterized by increased interstitial pressures as a consequence of disordered capillary proliferation with leaky vessels and accumulation of extracellular fluid. Together, these factors result in regional hypoxia, acidosis, and necrosis that can limit the effective delivery of chemotherapy, and may protect viable tumor cells that are more distant from functional capillaries. One of the potential benefits observed with anti-angiogenic therapy has been normalization of tumor vessels with reduced interstitial pressures and improved drug delivery (15).

Log Cell Kill

In principle, the rational use of chemotherapy relies on basic concepts of cellular kinetics, but the translation from preclinical models to solid tumors has been challenging. In animals, the curability of transplanted tumors is inversely proportional to the tumor cell number and size, and timing of treatment initiation. In part, this is the result of important tumor–host interactions, such as the time required to establish a blood supply. However, this is also an illustration of first-order cell kill kinetics, whereby a constant fraction of exposed cells is killed, rather than a constant number. Using first-order kinetics, a single treatment for a tumor weighing 1 g (approximately 10^9 cells) might yield 90% cell kill and would decrease the tumor population by only one log, leaving 10^8 viable cells. Without further treatment, the tumor would grow back at a constant rate, with only a modest delay in lethality. Only when the log cell kill is very large (>99%), and repetitive, can chemotherapy be curative or capable of reducing residual disease to less than 10^4 cells. Certain cancers, such as choriocarcinoma, can be cured with a single application of a single drug. However, the majority of cancers are intrinsically less sensitive and require multiagent chemotherapy over multiple cycles to achieve clinical benefit. Distribution of treatment over multiple cycles allows for host recovery while still achieving the cumulative cell kill required for tumor regression and cure.

An important modification to the log-kill theory is that the fraction of cells killed is not independent of tumor size, but inversely proportional to it (16). Termed the Norton–Simon hypothesis, it proposes that a dose effective at killing a high proportion of cells in a faster growing, small tumor, may be ineffective on the identical tumor cells when present in a larger, slower growing tumor. This hypothesis is at the basis of the development of "dose-dense" regimens, in which chemotherapy doses are administered at shorter intervals to prevent recovery of the cancer cells between doses (see section on Dose Intensity, Density, and Regimen Complexity).

TABLE 13.3. Doubling Times of Human Tumors

Tumor Histology	Patients (n)	Doubling Time (Mean ± 2 SD, Days)
Embryonal tumors (lung metastases)	76	27 ± 5
Lymphomas	51	29 ± 6
Malignant mesenchymal tumors	87	41 ± 7
Squamous cell carcinomas (lung metastases)	51	58 ± 9
Squamous cell carcinomas (primary tumors)	97	82 ± 14
Adenocarcinomas (lung metastases)	4	83 ± 12
Adenocarcinomas (primary tumors)	34	166 ± 48

Cell Cycle Specificity

Chemotherapeutic agents have complex mechanisms of action with an impact on multiple intracellular pathways. Nevertheless, certain anticancer drugs are known to be proliferation-dependent and cell cycle–specific. Other drugs are cycle nonspecific, and are capable of killing in all phases of the cell cycle, generally without dependence on the proliferative rate. Examples of cycle nonspecific drugs include alkylating agents, particularly nitrogen mustard, which are effective against a variety of solid tumors, including those with low growth fractions. Cell cycle–specific agents depend on the proliferative fraction of the tumor and phase of the cell cycle. A typical example is hydroxyurea, which inhibits ribonucleotide reductase. Not surprisingly, cell cycle–specific drugs tend to be more effective against tumors with a high proliferative rate and growth fractions.

The interaction of specific cytotoxic agents with the cell cycle is summarized in **Table 13.4**.

Modeling Tumor Growth Kinetics

Multiple tumor growth patterns have been described and mathematically modeled, primarily based on *in vitro* and animal data (17). A classic model is based on Gompertz law. This model proposes that during initial cell divisions, tumor growth follows an exponential pattern; however, as the tumor grows larger, the rate of growth also slows exponentially and the time required to double the tumor volume also increases (**Fig. 13.3**). Other conclusions of clinical relevance can also be derived from this model. First, metastatic spread may occur well before obvious evidence of the primary lesion (18). Second, at later stages of tumor growth, a small number of doublings can produce a marked change in tumor size, with an increased potential for adverse clinical consequences. For instance, a 1-cm mass (at least 30 prior doublings) becomes a 4-cm mass after just two more doublings. Third, since chemotherapy preferentially targets rapidly proliferating cells, the model implies that chemotherapy would be more effective during the exponential phase of tumor growth.

There is limited information regarding the actual doubling times of human tumors *in vivo* (19,20), as summarized in **Table 13.3**. For this historical analysis, untreated tumors were relatively circumscribed and serially measured by radiographic imaging, often as pulmonary metastases. It is clear that embryonal tumors, lymphomas, and mesenchymal tumors have shorter doubling times than adenocarcinomas or squamous cell carcinomas. In addition, metastases generally have faster doubling times than their corresponding primary lesions.

Other models have sought to recapitulate the multiple complex factors leading to carcinogenesis by incorporating the multistep acquisition of growth-enhancing genetic mutations, the balance between replication and cell death, nutrient availability, immune evasion, and the capacity to induce angiogenesis (17). However, cancer behavior is diverse, and a single tumor may exhibit different growth kinetics during various phases of its development. Nevertheless, understanding tumor growth kinetics may elucidate critical processes necessary for tumor progression, metastases, and drug resistance while identifying new opportunities for therapeutic intervention.

GENERAL PRINCIPLES OF CHEMOTHERAPY

Treatment Objectives

Although certain general principles guide the clinician in choosing the appropriate classes of drugs or combinations, the decision to

TABLE 13.4. Relationship of Chemotherapy Agents to Intracellular Targets and Cell Cycle Progression

Classification	Cell Cycle Specificity	Cellular Targets and Mechanisms	Examples
Inhibition of DNA synthesis and repair	G_1, S	Inhibition of nucleotide synthesis and metabolism. Inhibition of thymidylate synthase, thymidylate phosphorylase, dihydrofolate reductase, ribonucleotide reductase	Antifolates (methotrexate, pemetrexed), nucleoside analogs (6-mercaptopurine, 5-fluorouracil, cytarabine, fludarabine, gemcitabine), hydroxyurea
	S	Stabilization of DNA-topoisomerase-II cleavable complex, DNA intercalation, +/− free radical formation	Anthracyclines (doxorubicin, daunomycin, idarubicin, epirubicin), anthracenediones (mitoxantrone), epipodophyllotoxins (etoposide), actinomycin D
	S	Stabilization of DNA-topoisomerase-I cleavable complex	Camptothecins (topotecan, irinotecan)
Alkylating agents and related compounds	G_1, G_2, S	Direct DNA damage, DNA adduct formation, free radical production, strand breakage	Radiation, platinum compounds (cisplatin, carboplatin, oxaliplatin), bleomycin, mitomycin C, nitrogen mustard, nitrosoureas, ecteinascidin
Antimicrotubule reagents	M	Inhibition of tubulin polymerization	Vinca alkaloids (vincristine, vinblastine, vinorelbine), colchicine
		Promotion of tubulin polymerization	Taxanes (paclitaxel, docetaxel), epothilones
		Kinesin spindle proteins	Investigational agents
Cell cycle agents	G_1, S, G_2, M	Mitotic checkpoint control, cyclin-dependent kinases (CDK), aurora kinases	Flavopiridol, palbociclib
Signal transduction modulators	G_0, G_1, S, G_2	Growth factor sequestration, receptor blockade	Trastuzumab, cetuximab, pertuzumab, aflibercept, bevacizumab
		Inhibition of tyrosine kinase–mediated signal transduction	Erlotinib, gefitinib, dasatinib, imatinib, sorafenib, sunitinib, lapatinib
		Modulation of protein kinase C	Bryostatin, enzastaurin
		Inhibition of hormonal pathways	Tamoxifen, raloxifene, anastrazole, letrozole, fulvestrant, megestrol, mifepristone, flutamide, leuprolide
Gene regulation	NA	Gene regulation by inhibition of promoter methylation, DNA methyltransferase, or histone deacetylase	Azacytidine, suberoylanilide hydroxamic acid (vorinostat, belinostat)
Protein modifications	NA	Posttranslational protein modifications, inhibition of farnesylation	Tipifarnib, bisphosphonates
		Inhibition of the proteasome complex and clearance of ubiquinated proteins	Bortezomib

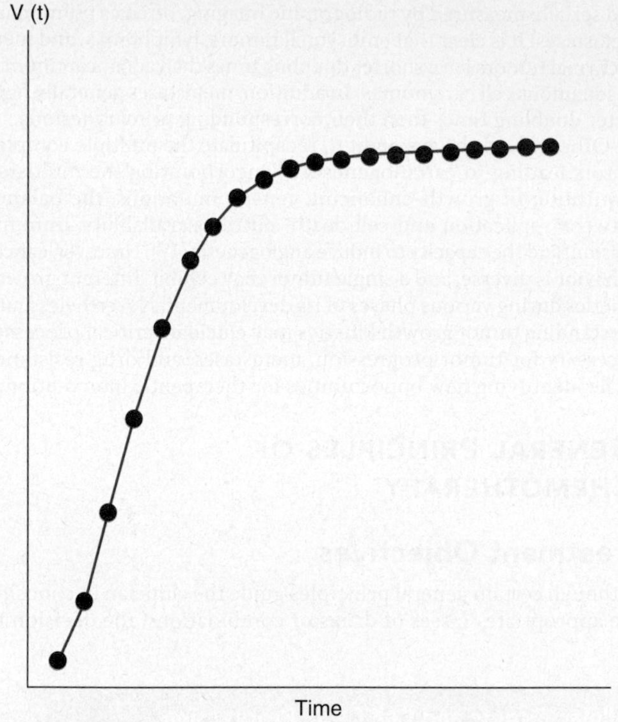

Figure 13.3. Hypothetical Gompertzian tumor growth curve. Exponential tumor growth with exponential growth retardation. The vertical axis is tumor volume and the horizontal axis is time.

TABLE 13.5. Important Considerations before Using Antineoplastic Drugs

Natural history of the malignancy
Biopsy proof of malignancy
Identification of primary site
Rate of progression or grade
Stage of disease, patterns of spread
Patient characteristics
Physiologic age, nutritional status, performance status
Vital organ function; bone marrow reserve
Comorbid conditions
Extent of previous treatment
Supportive care
Adequate facilities to evaluate, monitor, and treat potential drug toxicities
Emotional, social, and financial status; support from family
Collaboration with referring physician
Treatment goals
Parameters to monitor objective response to treatment
Potential benefits
Curative intent
Improved or sustained quality of life
Control of disease
Palliation of symptoms

use these agents *at all* must be considered carefully. The critical factors involved in formulating a recommendation are reviewed in **Table 13.5**.

Natural History

Antineoplastic agents should be used only in patients whose malignancy has been established via pathologic examination, and with thoughtful consideration of the expected natural history, based on the primary tumor site, extent of disease, and rate of progression. Individual factors that could have an impact on tolerance for therapy must be evaluated in the context of treatment goals, including physiologic age (as reflected by vital organ function), general health, performance status, nutritional status, desire for treatment, and the presence of underlying illness. Prior history, including any previous cancer treatment and residual functional impairment, as well as patterns of recurrence, should also be considered. Finally, the emotional, social, and financial concerns of the patient and family must be respected (**Table 13.5**). Recommendations and goals should be presented to the patient and family in conjunction with a realistic analysis of potential risks and benefits, which contributes to the process of informed consent and which should be followed by sharing of written information for future reference.

Clinical Assessment

In view of the potential for serious toxicity, it is desirable to have some objective means of measuring tumor response by physical examination, radiographic imaging, and/or analysis of serum tumor markers. However, it is not uncommon to administer multiple cycles of adjuvant or postoperative chemotherapy without any direct means of documenting tumor response. In these circumstances, the physician should be alert for any clinical evidence of tumor recurrence or progression during treatment. In patients with evaluable disease, continued administration of chemotherapy requires verification of ongoing benefit.

Expectations

The likelihood of achieving clinical benefit influences the choice of treatment and the acceptance of potential toxicity. Primary tumors (and recurrence after surgical resection or radiation without prior chemotherapy) can generally be grouped according to the likelihood of achieving a durable response. While the use of chemotherapy is supported by data from phase 3 clinical trials, it is also apparent that research findings are often extended to populations with lower risk, and more patients are being exposed to platinum-based therapy at earlier points in the natural history of their disease, with an increased risk of treatment-resistant disease at the time of recurrence.

Most importantly, there is a group of tumors for which primary chemotherapy has been curative in the majority of patients, including choriocarcinoma and ovarian germ cell tumors. These patients should be treated aggressively with curative intent. Toxicity in this setting is acceptable, assuming that it is reversible, as the probability of long-term survival is high.

A second group, including advanced epithelial ovarian carcinoma, has high response rates to primary therapy (exceeding 75%), with prolongation of disease-free and median overall survival, but with only a modest improvement in overall mortality. Patients with these tumors usually benefit from therapy in terms of extended survival or quality-adjusted survival, and they should receive primary treatment at full doses unless contraindicated.

A third group of cancers, including advanced (or recurrent) endometrial cancer, cervical cancer, low-grade serous carcinoma, and uterine carcinosarcoma (mixed Müllerian tumors), have intermediate or lower response rates to primary chemotherapy, with shorter duration of remission and limited improvement in overall survival. Treatment with an initial course of therapy is reasonable, with careful monitoring of toxicity and response.

Other tumors, including uterine leiomyosarcoma, are more resistant to primary therapy, achieving a low frequency of objective response without prolongation of survival. In this setting, the use of chemotherapy should be carefully considered and particular emphasis placed on including these patients in well-structured clinical trials to evaluate innovative treatments.

In patients with recurrent or progressive disease (PD) after prior chemotherapy, the expectations of response are reduced due to the emergence of drug resistance and the impact of prior therapy and/or disease on performance status and vital organ function. As such, treatment goals are usually aimed at control or palliation, with attention to quality of life and control of symptoms. In this population, the frequency of stable disease usually exceeds the objective response rate. With appropriate chemotherapy regimens that avoid cumulative toxicity, patients without further disease progression may remain on therapy for prolonged periods of time with an acceptable quality of life.

Choice of Specific Chemotherapeutic Regimens

Once the decision to use chemotherapy has been made, the appropriate regimen must be selected. The physician is aided in this task by the results of randomized trials and evolving standards of care, including published practice guidelines. However, not every patient can receive "standard" therapy because of idiosyncratic reactions, vital organ dysfunction, prior treatment, geographic location, or other factors. Practical individualized decisions are facilitated by the logical grouping of chemotherapeutic agents in several classes with similar pharmacologic properties, mechanisms of action, and spectrum of toxicity. The most important classes are the platinum-based alkylating agents, non-platinum alkylating agents, antimetabolites, antitumor antibiotics, antimicrotubule agents, nucleoside analogs, hormones, and newer molecular-targeted therapies (**Table 13.1**).

A number of combination regimens have been evaluated in the management of gynecologic cancer, and some have been widely adopted as "standard of care" for primary management of advanced-stage or recurrent disease. Phase 3 trials have demonstrated the superiority of specific regimens, such as paclitaxel with either cisplatin (21) or carboplatin (22) in ovarian cancer; a combination of carboplatin and paclitaxel in endometrial cancer (23); cisplatin and bevacizumab with either paclitaxel or topotecan in cervical cancer (24); and ifosfamide with paclitaxel in uterine carcinosarcoma (25).

However, none of the standard combinations for advanced ovarian, endometrial, or cervical cancer has been directly compared to sequential therapy with the best active single agents, and the superiority of combination therapy, while widely endorsed, has not been fully established. For example, in the setting of ovarian cancer, phase 3 trials have suggested that sequential therapy with platinum followed by paclitaxel may offer similar long-term outcomes to a combination of platinum and paclitaxel (26). Although the initial frequency of tumor response is often increased with combination therapy, long-term outcomes such as overall survival and symptom-adjusted quality of life can be similar for patients who receive optimal sequential therapy with single agents. This is primarily related to the advanced stage of disease at the time of initial treatment with systemic chemotherapy and the lack of curative therapy for the majority of patients. As such, if individual patient circumstances contraindicate the use of a standard combination regimen, it remains a reasonable option to begin therapy with one of the active single agents. Combinations can also be employed as adjuvant therapy for patients with early-stage disease who are at increased risk for recurrence, and for patients with late recurrence after good response to initial therapy.

Adjuvant chemotherapy refers to the initial use of systemic chemotherapy after surgery and/or radiation therapy has been performed with curative intent, and there is no evidence of residual disease. Adjuvant chemotherapy is considered if the subsequent risk for recurrence after initial definitive therapy is relatively high (generally greater than 20%), but it is not routinely recommended when the risk of recurrence is less than 10%. In the adjuvant therapy of epithelial ovarian cancer, long-term results from randomized trials have documented a reduction in the risk of recurrence after platinum-based chemotherapy (27,28). However, in carefully staged patients (to exclude occult advanced-stage disease), it has been difficult to establish an advantage in overall survival. Phase 3 studies in endometrial cancer (29) and uterine carcinosarcoma (30) have documented improved survival with the use of adjuvant combination chemotherapy compared to whole abdomen radiation in selected patients with high-risk disease, increasing the overall proportion of patients who receive adjuvant therapy.

Concurrent chemotherapy with radiation (chemoradiation) refers to the use of chemotherapy to sensitize the tumor to the effects of radiation delivered with curative intent. This has been most extensively studied in the primary management of locally advanced cervical cancer, where platinum-based chemoradiation has been proven superior to radiation alone (31). In general, the duration of chemotherapy coincides with the duration of external beam radiation. Although the preferred weekly dose of cisplatin might appear to be low, these regimens generally exceed the overall dose intensity of cisplatin when used to treat advanced disease, and patients require monitoring to avoid cumulative toxicity and treatment interruptions.

Neoadjuvant chemotherapy generally refers to the use of chemotherapy in the management of locally advanced disease, in situations where it would be difficult or impractical to perform immediate surgery or radiation. Following a response to initial chemotherapy, there is an expectation that morbidity associated with the overall treatment program can be minimized in conjunction with a reduction in radiation treatment volume or extent of surgery. With support from two phase 3 randomized trials, the use of neoadjuvant chemotherapy in advanced ovarian cancer has emerged as an acceptable option, particularly in patients with extensive disease not amenable to optimal cytoreduction, or in the presence of comorbidities that might increase surgical risk (32,33).

Monitoring of Tumor Response

Generally accepted criteria for evaluation of responses are necessary to facilitate treatment decisions and comparisons among different regimens. Several standards have been used, including those developed by the World Health Organization (WHO). However, in 2000, an international working group including the European Organization for Research and Treatment of Cancer, the National Cancer Institute of Canada, and the National Cancer Institute (NCI) of the United States developed, validated, and published new Response Evaluation Criteria in Solid Tumors (RECIST 1.0), which were widely adopted within clinical trials and updated as RECIST 1.1 in 2009 (34).

Positron emission tomography (PET) data are not included in RECIST, but the computed tomography (CT) component of a PET-CT study can be used for RECIST if the CT is of sufficient diagnostic quality. PET Response Criteria in Solid Tumors (PERCIST) have been developed, but have not been widely adopted (35). An overview of RECIST determinations is provided in **Table 13.6**.

Where available, tumor markers are not sufficient to declare response but, if initially elevated, must normalize to designate a complete response. International criteria to declare disease progression on the basis of a serial elevation in CA-125 have been widely adopted, but there is incomplete agreement on criteria to define a partial response during treatment (36). Changes in CA-125 alone, without other evidence of disease, are not recognized within the RECIST paradigm and are not validated for seeking regulatory approval of new treatments. Overall, RECIST is more detailed and specific than previous response criteria, and is also more demanding of the clinical team and radiologist.

Complete regressions of cancer are generally associated with a prolongation of survival. Partial remissions are generally accompanied by improved well-being for a period of time but are not expected to improve overall survival. While a variety of terms have been used to designate lesser responses (e.g., minor response, objective regression), these are rarely associated with any significant clinical benefit. Disease stabilization is an acceptable goal in the setting of palliative therapy for recurrent disease provided that symptoms have not progressed and the patient can tolerate continued therapy.

Changes in the volume of ascites or pleural fluid are not usually considered in the measurement of response, as a number of factors unrelated to cancer can influence third-space fluid accumulation, such as nutritional status, renal function, and treatment-related toxicity. However, appearance of a new fluid collection with cytologic verification would represent PD. Similarly, the appearance of new symptoms, such as a partial small bowel obstruction, does not

TABLE 13.6. Evaluation of Overall Disease Response (RECIST 1.1)

Complete Response (CR)[a]	Disappearance of all *target*[b] and *non-target* lesions, absence of new lesions, and normalization of tumor marker levels (if appropriate). Pathologic lymph nodes must have a reduction in short axis to <10 mm.
Partial Response (PR)	Disappearance of all *target* lesions, without progression of *non-target* lesions, without appearance of new lesions, and with persistence of abnormal tumor marker levels. Or At least a 30% decrease in the sum LD of *target* lesions (taking as reference the baseline sum LD) without progression of *non-target* lesions or appearance of new lesions.
PD	At least a 20% increase in the sum LD of *target* lesions, taking as reference the smallest sum LD recorded since the start of treatment, or the appearance of one or more new lesions, or progression of any *non-target* lesion. The sum LD must demonstrate an increase ≥5 mm.
SD[c]	Neither sufficient shrinkage of *target* lesions to qualify for PR nor sufficient increase to qualify for PD, taking as reference the smallest sum LD since the start of treatment. No appearance of new lesions (*target* or *non-target*).

Note: Measurable lesions can be accurately measured in at least one dimension with longest diameter (LD) ≥20 mm using conventional radiography, or ≥10 mm with spiral CT scan, or ≥10 mm with calipers on physical examination. Lymph nodes must be ≥15 mm along the short axis to be considered pathologic or measureable.

Non-measurable lesions consist of all other lesions, including small lesions (longest diameter <20 mm with conventional imaging techniques or <10 mm with spiral CT scan), bone lesions, leptomeningeal disease, ascites, pleural/pericardial effusion, inflammatory breast disease, lymphangitis, cystic lesions, and abdominal masses that are not confirmed or followed by imaging techniques.

[a]To be assigned PR or CR, changes in tumor measurements must be confirmed by repeat assessments no less than 4 weeks after the criteria for response are first met. The duration of overall response is measured from the time that criteria are met for CR or PR (whichever status is recorded first) until the first date that recurrence or PD is objectively documented, taking as reference for PD the smallest measurements recorded since the treatment started.

[b]Target lesions include measurable lesions up to a maximum of two lesions per organ and five lesions in total, representing all involved organs, selected on the basis of size (lesions with the longest diameter) and suitability for accurate repeated measurements. Non-target lesions include all other lesions (or sites of disease) to be identified and recorded at baseline. Serial measurements of these lesions are not required, but the presence or absence of each should be noted throughout follow-up.

[c]In the case of SD, follow-up measurements must have met the SD criteria at least once after study entry at a minimum interval (in general, not less than 6 to 8 weeks) that is defined in the study protocol. SD is measured from the start of the treatment until the criteria for disease progression are met, taking as reference the smallest measurements recorded since the treatment started.

always indicate progression of disease but could be related to prior surgery, irradiation, chemotherapy, or infection. Overall monitoring of small-volume intraperitoneal, diaphragmatic, or intrapleural disease is not adequately addressed within RECIST.

PHARMACOLOGIC PRINCIPLES OF CHEMOTHERAPY

Many factors may influence the effectiveness and/or toxicity of chemotherapy, including dose, frequency of administration, absorption, distribution, metabolism, and excretion, as well as clinical complications, such as renal impairment, malnutrition, or drug–drug interactions.

Dose Intensity, Density, and Regimen Complexity

The dose and frequency of drug administration can contribute to the overall effectiveness of a treatment regimen, as well as the spectrum and severity of toxicity. Dose intensity is a standardized measure of the amount of drug administered over time, most commonly expressed as mg/m²/week.

Preclinical studies demonstrate a sigmoidal relationship between dose and tumor response (**Fig. 13.4**). This is characterized by a *lag phase* and a lower limit *threshold* for observing benefit; a *linear phase,* where increases in dose are matched by improved efficacy; and a *plateau,* where toxicity continues to increase but there is no incremental improvement in response. In highly responsive tumors (e.g., choriocarcinoma, dysgerminoma), the entire dose–response curve is shifted to the left, with the result that standard chemotherapy doses are already situated near the upper plateau, and further dose increases are unlikely to achieve any improvement in clinical outcomes. In resistant tumors (e.g., previously treated cervical cancer), the curve is shifted to the right, and is also flattened, reducing the maximal potential benefit and increasing the risk of toxicity.

The dose intensity hypothesis has been extensively evaluated in the setting of advanced ovarian cancer, beginning with a series of

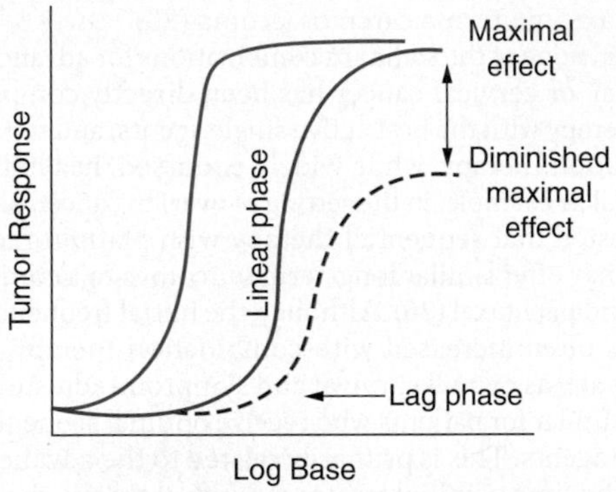

Figure 13.4. Theoretical dose–response curve. The vertical axis is the tumor response and the horizontal axis is the log of the dose. A hypothetical dose-response curve is illustrated by the green line. The blue line represents a highly responsive tumor (e.g., choriocarcinoma), in which the dose–response curve is shifted to the left. The red line represents a resistant tumor (e.g., previously treated cervical cancer) in which treatment response is diminished.

retrospective reports (37). However, within practical dose ranges that can be achieved in the clinical setting, prospective randomized trials have not demonstrated significant improvements in either disease-free or overall survival (38). While frontline studies focused on platinum dose intensity, the question of paclitaxel dose intensity was also addressed in the setting of recurrent disease, again without evidence of improved outcomes.

Dose intensity is limited by acute (single cycle) and cumulative (multi cycle) nonhematologic and hematologic toxicities. Although multiple cycles of high-dose carboplatin and paclitaxel (with or without topotecan or gemcitabine) can be safely administered with hematopoietic progenitor and growth factor support, it is more difficult to overcome serious non-hematologic toxicities. Thus far, there is no evidence that a two- to threefold increase in carboplatin dose intensity and cumulative dose delivery is associated with a substantial improvement in clinical outcomes (39), and it is unlikely that this approach will be further evaluated. In contrast, there is renewed interest in "dose-dense" therapy, in which a series of two or three individual single agents are sequentially administered at maximal tolerated doses using short cycle intervals. This approach has been favorably evaluated in the adjuvant therapy of breast cancer (40) and ovarian cancer (41), though at a cost of increased hematologic toxicity. Short cycle intervals may offer a safer approach for intensification by reinforcing normal biologic rhythms that can accelerate repair and minimize host toxicity. Further data on adjuvant treatment in ovarian cancer is discussed elsewhere.

In theory, another approach to improve outcomes would be to incorporate a third cytotoxic drug. This concept has been extensively evaluated in the primary therapy of advanced-stage ovarian cancer, with a series of definitive phase 3 trials. For example, GOG0182-ICON5 was a five-arm phase 3 international cooperative group trial exploring triplet and sequential doublet combinations that included gemcitabine, topotecan, or PEG-liposomal doxorubicin (42). There was no benefit in progression-free or overall survival from the addition of a third cytotoxic drug compared to a conventional combination of carboplatin and paclitaxel. Similarly, in advanced or metastatic endometrial cancer, the triplet regimen of cisplatin, paclitaxel, and doxorubicin was not superior to conventional carboplatin and paclitaxel (23).

Absorption, Distribution, and Transport

Drugs may be given by many different routes, depending on solubility, biologic barriers, requirements for drug activation, local tissue tolerance, feasibility for an individual patient, and optimal tumor drug exposure, which is estimated as the area under the concentration time curve (AUC) for the drug and active metabolites. The ultimate effectiveness of any chemotherapeutic agent depends on optimizing the AUC at critical tumor sites. However, there are no established techniques for noninvasive measurement of active drug concentration at these critical sites, and we are forced to extrapolate tumor drug exposure from preclinical models and plasma or fluid concentrations over time. Techniques such as magnetic resonance spectroscopy, microcapillary sampling, and PET can potentially provide information on drug distribution and tumor metabolism, but they require a substantial investment in technology and specialized reagents.

The increasing utilization of oral chemotherapy and development of oral molecular-targeted agents has renewed interest in bioavailability in the setting of meals and other factors that can modulate local intestinal transport. In most cases, initial dose and schedule guidelines from Food and Drug Administration (FDA)–approved labeling reflect data from large phase 3 trials, rather than smaller studies that might examine dietary or drug interactions. For example, the bioavailability of one tyrosine kinase inhibitor could be increased over threefold in the setting of a high-fat meal (43), but the label recommends taking the drug on an empty stomach. With the high cost of chronic medication, it is apparent that there could also be substantial economic implications to these pharmacokinetic observations (44).

Some natural compounds, such as those found in grapefruit juice, can inhibit the cytochrome P450 isozyme CYP3A4 within the intestinal mucosa (45), as well as the drug efflux pump p-glycoprotein. Drugs that are substrates for either of these compounds, including cyclosporine, erythromycin, calcium channel blockers, and benzodiazepines, can be more efficiently absorbed after ingestion of grapefruit juice, due to reduced local metabolism, leading to increased serum levels that may have clinical consequences.

The extent of drug binding to serum proteins, as well as physical properties, such as lipid solubility, diffusion, or molecular weight, may have an impact on tumor drug exposure. In addition, some areas of the body, particularly the brain, are actively protected from drug exposure and can serve as pharmacologic tumor sanctuaries, where small numbers of sequestered cancer cells may survive otherwise curative systemic therapy. Larger solid tumors eventually disrupt the blood–brain barrier, restoring access to conventional chemotherapy. In this manner, even drugs that are normally excluded from the central nervous system, such as carboplatin, can achieve dramatic reductions in metastatic disease (46).

In addition to achieving local delivery, most drugs must be internalized within tumor cells to achieve cytotoxicity. Internalization can be accomplished by passive diffusion, active transport, pinocytosis, or receptor-mediated endocytosis. Molecular targeting has also been utilized to enhance the delivery of conventional cytotoxic agents to tumors, based on expression of tumor-associated antigens, or the presence of specific receptors. For example, ado-trastuzumab emtansine is a HER2-targeted antibody drug conjugate linked to a cytotoxic agent that is inactive until internalized and released within the HER2-expressing cancer cell. These strategies have resulted in improved efficacy with decreased toxicity compared to conventional therapy (47).

Many chemotherapeutic agents are lipophilic and highly protein bound in plasma, particularly to albumin. Commonly used agents with greater than 95% protein binding include cisplatin, paclitaxel, docetaxel, etoposide, and the active metabolite of irinotecan (SN-38). Agents with less protein binding include doxorubicin (75%), topotecan (35%), gemcitabine (10%), carboplatin (<5%), and ifosfamide (<5%). It is generally the unbound "free" drug that mediates toxicity, and any condition associated with variability in protein binding can have an impact on cumulative drug exposure. For example, the toxicity of chemotherapy is frequently accentuated in patients with poor nutritional status, which is associated with reduced protein levels and other metabolic changes (48). Docetaxel offers an interesting example for potential interactions, due to extensive binding to albumin, lipoproteins, and α-acidic glycoprotein, which has been correlated with changes in drug clearance, prompting further evaluation of optimized dosing (49).

Intraperitoneal Chemotherapy

Although most chemotherapy is administered by the systemic route, there are unique situations in which the regional use of chemotherapy has been studied, with intraperitoneal administration being a specific example. If primary tumors or their metastases are anatomically confined to specific organs or particular regions of the body, or if unique pharmacokinetic circumstances exist that favor regional clearance, there is a theoretical rationale for regional chemotherapy. For example, intra-arterial drug administration has been studied in cervical cancer, localized recurrence of rectal carcinoma, melanoma, and head and neck cancer. Local complications are potentially serious, including arterial thrombosis, wound slough, lymphedema, and osteonecrosis caused by the shared arterial blood supply between the tumor and neighboring normal tissues. While high response rates can be achieved in selected patients, larger randomized trials are needed to evaluate overall risks and long-term outcomes.

Intracavitary chemotherapy has been used for tumors confined to the peritoneum, pleura, or pericardium. The rationale for this approach is based on the fact that clearance from a body cavity is delayed compared to the systemic circulation, achieving more prolonged exposure to higher regional concentrations of active agents. This technique has been most extensively studied in ovarian cancer, with evaluation of many agents, including 5-fluorouracil, doxorubicin, cisplatin, carboplatin, cytarabine, melphalan, etoposide, and paclitaxel (50). Phase 1–2 studies have uniformly demonstrated a pharmacologic advantage favoring the intraperitoneal compartment but have not documented enhanced drug delivery to actual sites of disease. Of key importance, penetration of peritoneal tumor nodules by passive diffusion is limited by fibrotic adhesions, tumor encapsulation, and high interstitial pressures as a consequence of intratumoral capillary leak without functional lymphatic drainage. In addition, both cisplatin and carboplatin are rapidly cleared from the peritoneal compartment and recirculated through the blood, limiting the window for direct tumor penetration, exposing the host to systemic toxicity, and raising questions about the clinical importance of the local pharmacokinetic advantage. On the basis of these observations, it has been postulated that the major role for intracavitary therapy would be in patients with minimal residual disease.

Cisplatin has received the greatest attention for intraperitoneal delivery in ovarian cancer, particularly for the primary treatment of small-volume residual disease following initial cytoreductive surgery (51). In view of the risk of systemic non-hematologic toxicity from intraperitoneal cisplatin, there has been renewed interest in the substitution of intraperitoneal carboplatin, which differs in terms of reduced protein binding and increased overall time required for *in situ* activation (via aquation), with the possibility that clinical outcomes could be different between the two agents. This question is currently under investigation in two phase 3 randomized trials (GOG0252 and JGOG iPOCC).

In contrast to cisplatin, paclitaxel is poorly absorbed from the peritoneal compartment, suggesting that patients might benefit from combined intravenous and intraperitoneal administration to optimize tumor drug exposure. As a single-agent, intraperitoneal paclitaxel demonstrated a 61% pathology-confirmed complete response rate among 28 assessable patients with initial microscopic disease (52). However, only 1 of 31 patients (3%) with greater than microscopic disease achieved a complete response, emphasizing the limitations of drug access and penetration by diffusion from the peritoneal space.

Intraperitoneal therapy could also have an impact on the tumor–host relationship through alterations in local cytokine production, angiogenic response, or immunoregulation. Hopefully, future studies will evaluate some of these biologic parameters to assist with optimization of therapy. In this regard, it is also possible that intraperitoneal therapy could have clinical benefit regardless of the extent of disease, and current randomized trials have enrolled a subset of patients with suboptimal residual disease following primary cytoreductive surgery.

Biotransformation

Some agents, such as cyclophosphamide, ifosfamide, and capecitabine, are administered as true prodrugs and must undergo irreversible metabolism to the active form, most commonly in the liver, but also in tumor or other host tissues. For many of these agents, intraperitoneal or intra-arterial administration would be ineffective, as it would achieve high local concentrations of the native compound, but without an opportunity for bioconversion. Other agents are in reversible equilibrium with reactive intermediates, such as irinotecan and SN-38 (7-ethyl-10-hydroxycamptothecin), with dependencies on local pH and presence of specific enzymes, such as carboxyesterase. Cisplatin and carboplatin both require activation through irreversible aquation to a reactive intermediary before they can initiate DNA adduct formation. Although the final reactive compounds are identical, the rate of aquation and adduct formation is much slower with carboplatin (53), but can be accelerated in the presence of activating nucleophiles, such as glutathione (54), even though the same nucleophiles can partially block cisplatin-DNA adduct formation at higher concentrations.

Renal Excretion and Physiologic Age

Drug inactivation, elimination, or excretion can dramatically influence cumulative exposure, which significantly affects antitumor activity and host toxicity. Inactivation and excretion of chemotherapeutic agents occurs primarily through the liver, kidneys, and body tissues, with lesser elimination through the stool. While any impairment of normal liver or kidney function can disturb drug metabolism and excretion, the most common problem encountered in the setting of gynecologic cancer is acute or chronic renal insufficiency due to tumor-mediated obstruction, drug-induced toxicity, advanced age, or preexisting comorbidities.

The use of combination chemotherapy in the elderly patient can pose a number of challenges related to bone marrow reserve and vital organ function (55). Although the risk of hematologic toxicity is generally increased, overall benefits from active chemotherapy regimens can still be demonstrated, as illustrated by the analysis of data from several breast cancer trials (56). Studies in ovarian cancer have indicated that age is an adverse prognostic factor, but there are insufficient data to determine how the benefits of treatment change with age. In part, this is related to the underutilization of chemotherapy in elderly patients and reduced enrollment of elderly patients on clinical trials (57). From that perspective, it is important to define tolerable and effective treatment regimens that can be safely administered in elderly patients, incorporating supportive care, geriatric assessment, and adjustments for age-related changes in vital organ function (58).

In surveying the general nondiabetic female population, the incidence of moderate renal insufficiency dramatically increases with age, which is of particular relevance to the care of women with gynecologic cancer (59). For example, in the 60- to 69-year age group, over one-third of women have an estimated glomerular filtration rate (GFR) of less than 60 mL/min/1.73 m^2 (**Fig. 13.5**). In addition, serum creatinine levels can be inappropriately low in women with gynecologic

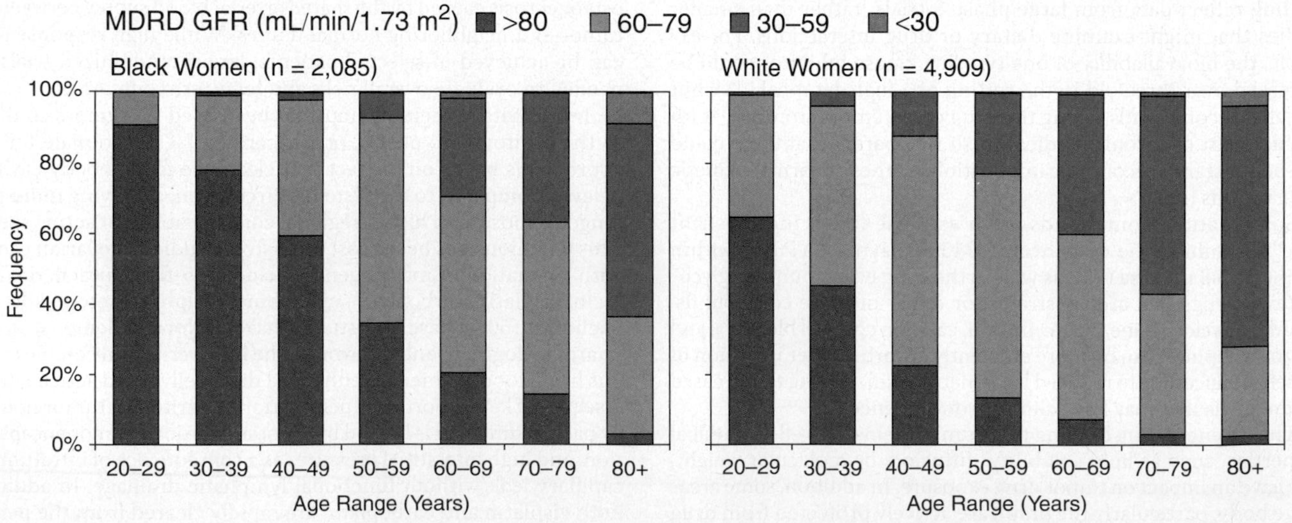

Figure 13.5. Distribution of renal function in nondiabetic adults. Weighted distribution of predicted GFR (mL/min/1.73 m^2) based on the MDRD formula from the Third National Health and Nutrition Examination Survey (NHANES III).

Source: From Clase CM, Garg AX, Kiberd BA. Prevalence of low glomerular filtration rate in nondiabetic Americans: Third National Health and Nutrition Examination Survey (NHANES III). *J Am Soc Nephrol.* 2002;13:1338–1349, with permission.

cancer, as a consequence of reduced muscle mass, malnutrition, postoperative recovery, or third-space fluid accumulation. In those settings, any of the standard formulae will overestimate GFR, with potential clinical consequences. Clearly, universal caution in dosing drugs with high renal clearance, especially carboplatin, is required.

Several methods are available to estimate GFR and classify the extent of renal injury based on age, sex, serum creatinine, and other factors (60–62). In general, serum creatinine is the dominant factor, and it remains unclear whether minor differences between formulae might have meaningful and/or consistent clinical consequences with regard to drug dosing. In most cases, it is sufficient to estimate GFR rather than obtain a precise measurement. However, all of these formulae are based on stable normalized biologic parameters and are less useful in the setting of dynamic changes following acute renal injury, or other non-renal fluctuations in serum creatinine.

While urine collection for estimation of creatinine clearance (based on measured creatinine in the urine over a period of time) might appear to provide a better estimate of GFR, it is also subject to clinical variability, due to different rates of creatinine tubular secretion. Utilization of direct techniques to measure actual GFR, such as clearance of ^{51}Cr-ethylenediaminetetraacetic acid or inulin, remains the standard for comparison with indirect estimates, but these assays are rarely used in clinical practice due to cost and complexity.

Staging of chronic renal disease has been used to reflect overall severity and guide management decisions, including dose modifications. The most commonly used staging system is from the National Kidney Foundation (63). The formula derived from the Modification of Diet in Renal Disease (MDRD) study has been incorporated in standardized laboratory reports (60). However, the MDRD has not generally been validated for actual drug dosing. As a result, the Cockcroft–Gault (61) and Jelliffe (62) formulae are more commonly used for drug dose calculation (**Table 13.7**).

The situation has become further complicated by an international effort to recalibrate creatinine standards based on isotope dilution mass spectrometry (IDMS). These new standards have now been adopted by all major vendors and commercial laboratories. The relationship between old (pre-IDMS) and new (IDMS) creatinine values within the same patient is variable, depending on the specific vendor and equipment. In general, IDMS standards will lower the serum creatinine value by approximately 12%. Using the IDMS creatinine value will therefore increase the estimated GFR, and could lead to higher doses of chemotherapy, particularly carboplatin, with an impact on hematologic toxicity (64). These changes prompted a review by the FDA, the NCI, and the national cooperative groups, followed by distribution of safe initial dose recommendations in 2010 for patients enrolled in clinical trials, as detailed in **Table 13.8**, incorporating recommendations from the legacy GOG (65).

Specific guidelines exist for modifying drug doses for patients with renal impairment (66), with special attention to a growing list of agents with renal-dominant clearance (**Table 13.9**). Dosing parameters for patients on dialysis receiving individual drugs, such as cisplatin (67) and carboplatin (68), are also available. However, owing to the rapid introduction of new agents, clinicians are urged to consult updated prescribing information and online database resources.

TABLE 13.7. Commonly Utilized Formulae to Estimate Creatinine Clearance

Formula Name	Estimation of Creatinine Clearance (CrCl)
Cockcroft–Gault formula (39)	CrCl (mL/min) = (140 – age) × weight (kg) × (0.85 if female)/serum Cr (mg/dL) × 72
Jelliffe formula (40)	CrCl (mL/min) = {98 – [0.8 × (age – 20)]} × (0.9 if female)/serum Cr (mg/dL)
MDRD formula (38)	GFR (mL/min/1.73 m^2) = 170 × [serum Cr (mg/dL)]$^{-0.999}$ × (age)$^{-0.176}$ × (0.762 if female) × (1.180 if African American) × [SUN (mg/dL)]$^{-0.170}$ × [Alb (g/dL)]$^{+0.318}$

Alb, serum albumin concentration; Cr, creatinine; GFR, glomerular filtration rate; MDRD formula, the Modification of Diet in Renal Disease study equation; SUN, serum urea nitrogen concentration.

Metabolism and Pharmacogenomics

Drugs can be metabolized in the liver, in other normal host tissues, or within tumors. Aside from those agents with extensive renal clearance, hepatic metabolism usually predominates. A large number of microsomal and cytoplasmic enzymes contribute to this process, with associated genetic polymorphisms that can account for individual variability in clearance, efficacy, resistance, and the risk of hepatic or non-hepatic toxicity. Techniques for screening and identification of pharmacogenomic elements are expanding, with potential implications for individualized drug selection, dosing, prediction of efficacy, and risk of toxicity.

With awareness of polymorphisms in key enzymes, it has been possible to identify individuals with a dramatically increased risk of toxicity (**Table 13.10**). Preemptive screening is controversial and not

TABLE 13.8. Initial Carboplatin Dose Recommendations based on IDMS Creatinine Values[a]

Calculate using Calvert formula[b]	Carboplatin Total Dose (mg) = Target AUC (mg × min/mL) × [GFR + 25] (mL/min)
Estimate GFR using Cockcroft–Gault equation[c]	Creatinine Clearance (mL/min) = $\frac{[140 - \text{Age years})] \times \text{Weight (kg)} \times 0.85 \text{ (for women)}]}{72 \times \text{Serum Creatinine (mg / dL)}}$
Body Weight: For body mass index (BMI) <25, use actual body weight For BMI >25[d], use adjusted body weight	Adjusted Weight (kg) = (Actual Weight – Ideal Weight) × 0.40) + Ideal Weight) Ideal Weight (kg) = ([Height in cm/2.54] – 60) × 2.3) + 45.5
For abnormally low serum creatinine values, GFR should be capped at a maximum value of 125 mL/min or estimated GFR can be calculated using the lower limit of normal for the serum creatinine test utilized.	Maximum Carboplatin Dose: AUC 6 = 900 mg AUC 5 = 750 AUC 4 = 600

[a]Subsequent modifications are based on hematologic toxicity or recalculation in the event of a change in renal function or body weight.

[b]Although developed with measured GFR, estimated GFR is routinely employed in clinical practice.

[c]Of note, although the Cockcroft–Gault equation was developed and validated for drug dosing using pre-IDMS creatinine values, it is the preferred formula for estimating GFR.

[d]The BMI cutoff for using adjusted body weight is under review; revised guidelines with a higher cutoff are expected.

TABLE 13.9. Modifications in the Setting of Renal and Hepatic Dysfunction

Agents that Should Be Considered for Modification in the Presence of Moderate Renal Dysfunction	Agents that Generally do not Require Modification in the Presence of Moderate Renal Dysfunction	Agents that Should be Considered for Modification in the Presence of Hepatic Dysfunction
Actinomycin D	Anastrozole	Docetaxel
Bleomycin	Bevacizumab	Doxorubicin
Capecitabine	Cabazitaxel	Epirubicin
Carboplatin	Cetuximab	Mitoxantrone
Cisplatin[a]	Docetaxel	NAB-paclitaxel
Cyclophosphamide	Doxorubicin	Paclitaxel
Etoposide	Epirubicin	PEG-liposomal doxorubicin
Hydroxyurea	Erlotinib	Vinblastine
Ifosfamide	Fluorouracil	Vincristine
Melphalan	Gefitinib	Vinorelbine
Methotrexate	Gemcitabine	
Pemetrexed	Irinotecan	
Topotecan	Letrozole	
	Leucovorin	
	Leuprorelin	
	Megestrol	
	Mitomycin	
	NAB-paclitaxel	
	Oxaliplatin	
	Paclitaxel	
	PEG-liposomal doxorubicin	
	Tamoxifen	
	Temozolomide	
	Trastuzumab	
	Vinblastine	
	Vincristine	
	Vinorelbine	

[a]Can be administered at full doses in anephric patients receiving hemodialysis.

widely performed. The potential reduction in risk must be balanced against the costs of a widespread screening program (69).

Dose modifications should be considered for patients with liver disease (70), particularly for drugs that are primarily metabolized in the liver and/or excreted in the bile, such as paclitaxel, docetaxel, nanoparticle albumin-bound paclitaxel (71), doxorubicin, and the Vinca alkaloids (vincristine, vinblastine, and vinorelbine) (**Table 13.9**). Excessive toxicity may occur with doses that would ordinarily be acceptable, and guidelines for treating patients with impaired liver function should be consulted. However, variability in non-hepatic clearance, compensatory host adaptations, and interactions with other drugs, make these recommendations less reliable than those provided for patients with renal dysfunction. For example, dose reduction of etoposide in the setting of biliary obstruction remains controversial and may not be required (72).

Drug Interactions

During routine care, patients may receive a variety of drugs, including antiemetics, antihistamines (H_1 and H_2), steroids, nonsteroidal anti-inflammatory agents, anticoagulants, narcotics, and anti-infective agents. In addition, older patients frequently receive medication to manage underlying comorbidities, such as diabetes, hypertension, and elevated cholesterol. In view of the number and diversity of medications in common use, it is somewhat surprising that most interactions with cytotoxic chemotherapy appear to be of little consequence. However, prospective studies of chemotherapy administration in non-cancer volunteers are impractical, and many potential interactions have not been fully explored. In fact, patients are likely to be excluded from enrollment on clinical trials on the basis of concomitant medications, due to the lack of prospective collection of valuable data to document safety or the need for treatment modifications. In clinical practice, the occurrence of excessive hematologic and/or non-hematologic toxicity in an individual patient is usually attributed directly to the chemotherapy and managed with treatment modifications, rather than ascribed to a potential drug interaction.

When they occur, drug interactions can be critical, and some of the more important interactions are listed in **Table 13.11**. Particular attention should be paid to drugs that could alter renal function, such as aminoglycoside antibiotics, nonsteroidal anti-inflammatory agents, and diuretics, in patients with reduced fluid intake. Typical interactions relevant in gynecologic cancer chemotherapy are the displacement of methotrexate from its transport protein by aspirin or sulfonamides, suppression of pseudocholinesterase by alkylating agents with increased apnea duration during succinylcholine-assisted general anesthesia, impairment of doxorubicin clearance by pre-administration of paclitaxel, and impairment of paclitaxel clearance by pre-administration of cisplatin.

Increased attention has been focused on drug metabolism and potential interactions with CYP isozymes, particularly CYP3A4, which

TABLE 13.10. Pharmacogenomic Variants Affecting Cytotoxic Chemotherapy Metabolism

Enzyme	Drug	Most Common Allelic Variant	Clinical Implication
DPD	5-FU, capecitabine	>100 exist resulting in enzyme deficiency	Severe deficiency can prolong half-life by >100-fold resulting in severe mucositis, diarrhea, and pancytopenia
TS	5-FU, capecitabine	*TYMS* 2R/2R	Higher expression may lead to inadequate response
		TYMS 3R/3R	Low expression can increase toxicity
CYP3A5	Vincristine	*CYP3A5**3	Allelic variants reduce expression and increase risk of neurotoxicity
UGT1A	Irinotecan	*UGT1A1**28	Increased risk of life-threatening diarrhea and pancytopenia, includes patients with Gilbert syndrome
TPMT	6-MP	*TPMT**2, *3A, or *3C	Increases risk for pancytopenia

5-FU, fluorouracil; CYP3A5, cytochrome P450 3A5; DPD, dihydropyrimidine dehydrogenase; TPMT, thiopurine-*S*-methyltransferase; TS, thymidylate synthase; TYMS, thymidylate synthase; UGT1A1, uridinediphosphate glucuronosyl transferase 1A1.

■ **TABLE 13.11. Physiologic and Pharmacologic Interactions in Cancer Chemotherapy**

Physiologic Condition	Causation	Impact and Examples
Renal insufficiency	Obstruction, chronic kidney disease, hypovolemia, hypotension, non-steroidals, nephrotoxins (aminoglycosides, cisplatin)	Decreased clearance of methotrexate, carboplatin, and other agents
Hepatobiliary dysfunction	Biliary obstruction, hepatitis, cirrhosis	Decreased clearance of doxorubicin, mitoxantrone, vincristine, vinblastine, etoposide, paclitaxel, docetaxel
	Gilbert syndrome, impaired glucuronidation and polymorphisms (UGTA1A)	Increased exposure to SN-38 (from irinotecan)
	Decreased microsomal activity	Impaired activation of cyclophosphamide and ifosfamide
Reduced protein binding	Carrier displacement (sulfonamide, salicylates, phenytoin)	Increased toxicity, higher free drug levels (methotrexate)
	Reduced carrier proteins (malnutrition)	Increased toxicity, higher free drug levels (cisplatin, paclitaxel, docetaxel, etoposide, SN-38)
Altered intestinal absorption	Oral antibiotics (neomycin)	Decreased absorption of methotrexate
	High-fat meal	Increased bioavailability of lapatinib
		Decreased bioavailability of capecitabine
	Grapefruit juice (intestinal CYP3A4 inhibition)	Increased bioavailability (cyclosporine, erythromycin, benzodiazepines)
Decreased metabolism	Caused by allopurinol	Delayed clearance of 6-mercaptopurine
	Dihydropyrimidine dehydrogenase (DPD) deficiency	Lethal toxicity from 5-fluorouracil
Cholinesterase inhibition	Caused by cyclophosphamide	Decreased clearance of succinylcholine
Monoamine oxidase inhibition	Caused by procarbazine	Neurotoxicity and seizures (tricyclic antidepressants and phenothiazines)
MDR-1 competition	Associated with natural products and other substrates, including verapamil, cyclosporine, tamoxifen	Decreased efflux and increased toxicity from natural products (doxorubicin, vincristine, paclitaxel, docetaxel)
CYP2C9 Inhibition	Caused by capecitabine	Increased AUC of warfarin
CYP3A4 Induction	Caused by glucocorticoids, barbiturates, rifampin	Increased activation of cyclophosphamide
Inhibition	Caused by ketoconazole, itraconazole, fluconazole, erythromycin	Decreased metabolism of substrates (potentially significant)
Substrate competition	Caused by cyclophosphamide, ifosfamide, paclitaxel, docetaxel, etoposide, vincristine, vinblastine, tamoxifen, gefitinib	Decreased metabolism of other substrates (usually not clinically significant)

has been linked to the metabolism of nearly half of all pharmaceutical agents (73). These interactions are guided by several common principles. Drugs that are *substrates* for the same isozyme may competitively inhibit metabolism, but these interactions are usually not of clinical consequence. Drugs that *directly inhibit* CYP isozymes without being a substrate for that isozyme are more likely to have clinical consequences. In this regard, itraconazole, ketoconazole, and fluconazole can inhibit CYP3A4 at low concentrations, and erythromycin can inhibit CYP3A4 via covalent binding and inactivation. Other drugs act as *inducers* of CYP isozymes by increasing gene expression or protein levels, such as glucocorticoids, barbiturates, and rifampin, which can increase the net activity of CYP3A4, resulting in decreased concentrations of susceptible compounds. In addition, many drugs that interact with CYP3A4 are natural products and may also interact with ABC family drug efflux pumps, including MDR-1. Among the anticancer agents that are substrates for CYP3A4 are cyclophosphamide, ifosfamide, docetaxel, etoposide, paclitaxel (also CYP2C8), docetaxel, vincristine, vinblastine, and tamoxifen (74). Many tyrosine kinase inhibitors inhibit CYP enzymes. Cyclosporine and verapamil can increase concentrations of doxorubicin and etoposide, probably through blockade of the P170 drug efflux pump.

Owing to the diversity and rapid adoption of new compounds, information regarding drug interactions is best obtained from online databases, the package insert, or directly from the manufacturer.

Prolongation of the cardiac QT interval has emerged as another important area of drug interactions and potential life-threatening toxicity. Congenital syndromes with prolonged QT interval are generally associated with mutations in protein channels involved with ion transport, most commonly inward potassium flux through the hERG (human ether-a-go-go) channel (75). Risks of polymorphic ventricular tachycardia, including Torsades de Pointes, can be accentuated by exposure to cytotoxic and/or supportive care medications that interact with these pathways. However, the effects are unpredictable, and drugs that prolong QT may have a low risk of inducing ventricular tachycardia, while other drugs, such as terfenadine, with minimal impact on the QT interval, can trigger life-threatening arrhythmias. Of particular relevance in gynecologic oncology, women tend to have a greater risk than men, with longer baseline QT intervals following puberty. In addition to direct drug-mediated effects on QT interval, it is also important to be attentive to the indirect impact of CYP isoenzymes (as discussed above), which can result in a pharmacokinetic interaction with clinical consequences.

Again, knowledge of specific drugs associated with QT prolongation is evolving, and information is best obtained from organizations that have maintained a tabulated list, such as Credible Meds (https://www.crediblemeds.org/pdftemp/pdf/CompositeList.pdf). Avoidance of concomitant high-risk medications is often a component of early-phase studies, until adequate safety data is available, and this has prevented some patients from enrolling on clinical trials.

DRUG RESISTANCE AND TUMOR CELL HETEROGENEITY

The curative potential of chemotherapy is limited by the emergence of drug resistance, which can be either intrinsic or acquired, and may involve one drug or multiple agents (pleiotropic resistance). Of interest, tumors with intrinsic or primary drug resistance to natural products often arise from duct cells or cells lining excretory organs (76). These cells, which normally detoxify, transport, and excrete a wide variety of toxic compounds, may retain these normal functions after transformation, manifesting as chemoresistance.

Intrinsic drug resistance is inferred based on clonal survival of tumor populations after initial chemotherapy exposure. Solid tumors are thought to consist of a mixture of clonal variants with different preexisting mutations and patterns of resistance. Following repetitive cycles of chemotherapy, a process of clonal selection can occur, enriching for resistant populations, even while there could be a reduction in clinical tumor volume secondary to elimination of more sensitive tumor elements.

Acquired resistance develops from cumulative somatic mutations, regulation of gene expression (including epigenetic processes), or other phenotypic alterations, over a period of time. From a clinical perspective, the end result of this process is indistinguishable from intrinsic resistance. However, acquired resistance is more likely to have a reversible component that could influence the timing and selection of subsequent chemotherapy. The best specific example is amplification of the dihydrofolate reductase (*DHFR*) gene, which is associated with acquired resistance to methotrexate (77). *DHFR* gene amplification is not generally observed prior to methotrexate exposure and can be reversed in the absence of drug exposure.

For each chemotherapeutic agent, resistance can develop via multiple mechanisms. Common mechanisms of resistance are listed in **Table 13.12** and include (1) decreased uptake or increased efflux of the compound, preventing accumulation in the neoplastic cells, (2) impaired activation of the compound to its active metabolite or increased metabolism of drug to inactive metabolites, (3) alterations to the target (via changes in expression or mutation), and (4) adaptations to the therapeutic effect (improved DNA repair or tolerance of damage).

Multidrug Resistance

Broad-based multidrug, or pleiotropic, drug resistance has been associated with overexpression of MDR1 (P 170 glycoprotein) and/or other ABC family membrane-associated transport proteins (78). After exposure to a potential MDR or transport protein substrate, tumor cells will develop cross-resistance to a variety of structurally and functionally unrelated agents. This multidrug resistance phenotype has maximal impact on natural products and their analogs, including the anthracyclines, Vinca alkaloids, and taxanes, and is associated with increased drug efflux and a net lowering of intracellular drug concentration. Although relatively uncommon in newly diagnosed ovarian cancer (79,80), with increased utilization of natural products, including taxanes, etoposide, and liposomal doxorubicin, this pattern of resistance generally emerges over time. A number of efflux inhibitors have been evaluated in combination with chemotherapy. However, none of these have been FDA approved for clinical use because of a tendency to accentuate host toxicity, which then requires a compensatory dose reduction. Recently, small molecule tyrosine kinase inhibitors (e.g., erlotinib, sunitinib), phosphodiesterase-5 inhibitors (e.g., sildenafil), and other naturally occurring compounds have been identified as MDR-ABC transporter antagonists and warrant further investigation, particularly if their effects can be tumor-targeted to avoid increased hematologic and mucosal toxicity (78).

TABLE 13.12. Specific Mechanisms of Tumor Drug Resistance

Resistance Mechanism	Examples	Specific Cellular Target or Effects
Impaired activation	5-Fluorouracil	Reduced levels of thymidylate synthase, thymidylate phosphorylase, or dihydropyrimidine dehydrogenase
	Methotrexate	Reduced intracellular polyglutamation
	Doxorubicin	Low P450 enzymes
	Cyclophosphamide, ifosfamide	Decreased microsomal transformation
	Gemcitabine	Decreased deoxycytidine kinase
Increased drug efflux	Natural products	Increased *MDR1* (P 170)
	Topotecan, mitoxantrone	Increased *BCRP* (ABCG2)
Increased drug inactivation	Alkylating agents, platinum	Elevated glutathione and other cellular thiols
Accelerated DNA repair	Alkylating agents, platinum, radiation	Induction of DNA repair enzymes
Increased damage tolerance	Alkylating agents, platinum, radiation	Loss of DNA mismatch repair
Transport defects	Melphalan	Reduced carrier-mediated uptake
	Gemcitabine	Decreased nucleoside transporter
	Platinum	Decreased copper transporter-1
Target alterations	Methotrexate	*DHFR* gene amplification
	Paclitaxel, docetaxel	Increased tubulin-β3 isoforms or mutations
	Hydroxyurea, gemcitabine	Decreased ribonucleotide reductase
	Glucocorticoids	Decreased receptor binding
	Camptothecins	Decreased topoisomerase-I
	Anthracyclines, etoposide	Decreased topoisomerase-II

Platinum Resistance and DNA Repair

Although a number of DNA alkylating agents and radiation are used in the treatment of gynecologic cancer, platinum derivatives remain the most important compounds in clinical practice. However, the dramatic success of platinum-based therapy is nearly overshadowed by the emergence of platinum resistance, and this observation has stimulated a substantial body of research over the last 35 years.

Platinum compounds are administered as inactive prodrugs that undergo aquation to form a reactive intermediate, a process that occurs more rapidly with cisplatin, compared to carboplatin, which has larger organic leaving groups. The primary cytotoxic effect involves formation of platinum-DNA adducts followed by activation of the DNA damage response and induction of apoptosis. Platinum can also form adducts with cellular proteins, but this is much less likely to result in tumor cytotoxicity. Resistance mechanisms have been identified at each point, and include decreases in intracellular accumulation, inactivation by sequestration by glutathione and other nucleophilic scavengers, increased repair of DNA adducts and/or double-strand breaks, increased tolerance of unrepaired adducts, and defects in apoptotic signaling (81). The major transporter involved in copper homeostasis, copper transporter-1 (CTR1), has a substantial role in cellular platinum uptake. Downregulation of CTR1 expression, which can be triggered by platinum in a feedback loop, leads to reduced intracellular accumulation and efficacy. Similarly, increased expression of multidrug resistance proteins can lead to resistance by increasing platinum export. Platinum analogs that do not require CTR1 for internalization and methods to increase platinum accumulation are being investigated.

Another mechanism of resistance revolves around the inactivation of aquated platinum agents by glutathione (GSH) and other cysteine-rich nucleophilic proteins. Increases in enzymes involved in GSH synthesis (gamma-glutamylcysteine synthetase) and conjugation of GSH to cisplatin (glutathione S-transferase) have also been implicated as resistance mechanisms. The exact mechanism by which GSH and other thiol compounds modulate cytotoxicity is unknown, although they can interfere with the formation of DNA-platinum adducts (82).

As noted, enhanced capacity for DNA damage tolerance and accelerated repair can play a role in resistance. Nucleotide excision repair (NER) is the major DNA repair pathway associated with removal of platinum-induced DNA adducts. Expression of ERCC1, a critical NER component, has been associated with reduced antitumor efficacy of platinum agents (83). In lung cancer, immunohistochemical evaluation of *ERCC1* levels was also predictive for survival following cisplatin-based adjuvant therapy, with improved survival in patients with *ERCC1*-negative tumors (84). However, *ERCC1* may also have prognostic significance independent of chemotherapy, as patients assigned to observation with *ERCC1*-positive tumors had better survival compared to those with *ERCC1*-negative tumors (85). Randomized trials to prospectively assign chemotherapy for lung cancer based on *ERCC1* status have suggested that higher response rates can be achieved, but without a difference in progression-free or overall survival (86). The role of *ERCC1* as a prognostic or selective factor in women with ovarian cancer seems less clear (87). Similarly, resistance can develop because of increased damage tolerance, often due to defects in adduct detection or intracellular signaling, such as loss of mismatch repair proteins (e.g., MLH1 and MSH2) (88).

Interestingly, tumors associated with germline or somatic BRCA1/2 mutations have defects in homologous recombination high-fidelity DNA repair, and tend to remain highly sensitive to platinum agents over multiple courses of treatment (89). These tumors are also more sensitive to PARP inhibition, but may develop a secondary mutation that partially restores BRCA function, generating an unusual mechanism of resistance to platinum and PARP inhibitors.

Finally, alterations in the apoptotic machinery (loss of pro-apoptotic factors or overexpression of anti-apoptotic factors) can lead to decreased triggering of apoptosis in response to platinum agents, leading to the development of resistance. Clearly, the multifactorial development of platinum resistance mechanisms remains a major challenge in the treatment of gynecologic cancers, particularly high-grade serous ovarian cancer.

Taxane Resistance

Similar to platinum resistance, multiple mechanisms are associated with taxane resistance. Overexpression of the drug efflux protein MDR-1 has been consistently associated with resistance to paclitaxel in cell lines and in retrospective analysis of clinical outcomes (90). Alterations in microtubule dynamics through mutations in tubulin subunits, changes in subunit proportions, or shifts in expression level or phosphorylation status of microtubule-associated proteins (MAPs) are also associated with paclitaxel resistance (91). Many of these mechanisms lead to resistance to the broader class of microtubule-stabilizing agents, in addition to taxanes. Importantly, however, this is not universally true. For example, alteration of the proportion of tubulin-β3 isoforms has been implicated in resistance to paclitaxel, while retaining sensitivity to non-taxane anti-tubulin agents, such as the epothilones (92). Unfortunately, prospective randomized trials using an inhibitor of MDR-1 with paclitaxel, or with a combination of paclitaxel and carboplatin, failed to improve clinical outcomes, and required a reduction in paclitaxel dosing, due to increased hematologic toxicity (93,94). Recent preclinical studies suggest that tyrosine kinase inhibitors may be beneficial in combination with paclitaxel through their effect on MAP phosphorylation or inhibition of MDR proteins (95,96).

Neither induction of MDR proteins nor alterations in microtubule dynamics adequately explains the clinical behavior associated with weekly scheduling of paclitaxel therapy in women with ovarian cancer. For example, patients can still respond to weekly paclitaxel after progressing within 6 months of receiving three-weekly paclitaxel as a component of primary therapy (97). Preclinical studies are examining a number of diverse pathways, including angiogenesis, cytokine networks, autophagy, the apoptotic machinery, and microRNAs.

Other Mechanisms of Agent-Specific Resistance

A number of specific alterations have been identified in the setting of individual drugs (**Table 13.12**). For example, *DHFR* gene amplification was demonstrated in a patient with methotrexate-resistant ovarian cancer who had localized *DHFR* gene copies on an abnormally staining region of chromosome 4q (98). Methotrexate resistance has also been associated with defects in polyglutamation, limiting intracellular methotrexate accumulation (99). The action of nucleoside analogs, such as gemcitabine (2,2-difluorodideoxycytidine), is dependent on active membrane transport for uptake, which is followed by double phosphorylation and potential incorporation in DNA. This complex process offers several opportunities for development of resistance, such as decreased activity of specific nucleoside transport proteins or reduced phosphorylation by depletion of deoxycytidine kinase (100). In addition, the main enzymatic target of phosphorylated gemcitabine, the M2 subunit of ribonucleotide reductase, can undergo gene amplification in resistant cell lines (101) similar to the primary mechanism of resistance to hydroxyurea, an inhibitor of ribonucleotide reductase. Of interest, sensitivity to gemcitabine can actually be increased severalfold by prior exposure to flavopiridol, an inhibitor of cyclin-dependent kinase activity, which has been shown to accelerate catabolism of the M2 subunit protein through the proteasome complex (102). Increased levels of target gene expression or protein, including thymidylate synthase, thymidylate phosphorylase, and dihydropyrimidine dehydrogenase, have also been associated with resistance to 5-fluorouracil in colon cancer, and have been correlated with clinical outcomes following 5-fluorouracil treatment (103,104). Even a superficial analysis of these specific examples would suggest potential strategies for screening of tumor tissue to guide the selection of optimal chemotherapy regimens, providing a basis for the application of tissue, gene, and protein arrays.

Tumor Profiling

Solid tumors have traditionally been considered a homogeneous collection of clonally derived cells with similar features, but it is now clear that tumors are composed of subpopulations with diverse biologic characteristics. Through genetic instability and epigenetic processes, such as gene promoter methylation and histone modifications, these subpopulations may exhibit different properties, with an impact on chemotherapy response. In addition, there can be variability in the potential for metastatic spread among cells that appear to be similar at a morphologic and genetic level (105). Recognition of tumor heterogeneity has altered our understanding of tumor behavior, with broad implications for multiagent and multimodality treatment programs.

Following the development of model systems for screening new anticancer compounds, it is not surprising that attention was focused on the process of screening actual human tumor cells for sensitivity and resistance to chemotherapy agents (106). A variety of methods were developed utilizing clonogenic survival, ^{3}H-thymidine incorporation, vital dye exclusion, treatment of transplanted tumor xenografts, and colorimetric analysis of adenosine triphosphate levels. Although there is relatively good correlation between high-level resistance to individual agents demonstrated *in vitro* and lack of a clinical response *in vivo*, it is more difficult to predict sensitivity to specific agents, or to guide the utilization of drug combinations (107), reflecting tumor cell heterogeneity, assay complexity, and inability to evaluate the tumor–host relationship, including the impact of angiogenesis, cytokines, and immune response. A nonrandomized trial in recurrent ovarian cancer suggested good correlation between *ex vivo* assay sensitivity and clinical response (108), but this may be no better than selecting reasonable agents based on routine clinical factors, especially in the setting of recurrent disease. Importantly, there is a lack of prospective randomized data to validate these approaches, as well as concerns regarding cost-effectiveness and the logistical challenges associated with obtaining and shipping fresh tumor tissue.

With the rapid development of gene expression and proteomic arrays, mutational analysis, RNA sequencing, whole genome scanning, and whole genome sequencing, these questions have been carried to a new level of sophistication, as illustrated by The Cancer Genome Atlas project (109). In addition, as drug development has shifted toward molecular-targeted agents, there has been a request from the FDA to incorporate predictive or selective biomarkers in regulatory filing, even though the cellular pathways and regulatory networks are not always well understood. Finally, large population-based molecular data repositories are under development, with the potential to rapidly identify targets, select patients, and evaluate new drugs without randomized trials. This raises a number of interesting questions.

MANAGEMENT OF CHEMOTOXICITIES

Dose Selection, Toxicity Assessment, and Supportive Care

Chemotherapeutic regimens are universally toxic, with a narrow therapeutic index, and it is generally necessary to adjust individual doses in accordance with patient tolerance. Initial dosing is derived from body surface area (BSA), weight, renal function, and hepatic function. However, a number of other factors could further influence tolerance, including nutritional status, performance status, extent of disease, exposure to prior therapy, third-space fluid accumulations, metabolic polymorphisms, and uncharacterized drug interactions. Current dose algorithms generally fail to address these factors, although emerging pharmacodynamic and pharmacogenomic research has improved individualized dosing in selected cases.

Optimal dosing in obese patients has also been questioned, as the distribution and metabolism of drugs within adipose tissue could vary from other compartments. Obesity is a risk factor for cancer development and is common in the setting of endometrial cancer. In addition, obesity is associated with a number of other comorbidities or metabolic conditions that could alter drug kinetics or the risk of toxicity. For these reasons, and in view of toxicity observed within previously radiated endometrial cancer patients, GOG had previously capped the BSA used for initial drug dosing to a value of 2 m^2. However, actual data to reinforce this decision are limited (110,111), and a more recent ASCO guidelines panel has recommended that obese patients should receive full weight-based dosing without arbitrary reductions or caps (112).

Consistent and standardized monitoring of host toxicity will help to prevent life-threatening events and assist in the implementation of dose adjustments. The Cancer Therapy Evaluation Program (CTEP) of the NCI has developed a detailed and comprehensive set of guidelines for the description and grading of acute and chronic organ-specific toxicity in collaboration with the FDA, international cooperative groups, and the pharmaceutical industry. Most clinical research protocols have incorporated these criteria, which are also applicable to the grading of toxicity for standard chemotherapy regimens outside of a clinical trial. The current version of the Common Terminology Criteria for Adverse Events (CTCAE) is available in electronic format from CTEP (http://ctep.cancer.gov/protocolDevelopment/adverse_effects.htm). Basic hematologic parameters from CTCAE version 4 have been summarized in **Table 13.13**.

An unintended consequence of our current regulatory environment is that most new medications receive single-agent FDA approval at a dose and schedule that is close to the maximally tolerated dose (MTD), increasing the likelihood of host toxicity, particularly when administered over multiple cycles. The association between dose and toxicity is usually dramatic at levels close to the MTD. As such, a modest reduction in dose or an adjustment in schedule can have a substantial impact on acute and cumulative toxicities. The impact of these minor modifications on efficacy is generally unknown, but is unlikely to be as dramatic as the impact on toxicity, and many clinicians frequently make modifications to the starting dose and/or schedule of single agents or combinations, essentially in variance from FDA-approved indications. As these modifications become integrated with clinical practice, limited supporting data emerge, usually from nonrandomized trials, but it is important to recognize that the primary FDA-approved dose and schedule is rarely changed. Many agents in common use today, including polyethylene glycol

TABLE 13.13. CTCAE Grading of Myelosuppression

Adverse Event Terminology	Grade 1	2	3	4
White Blood Cell Decreased (per mm^3)	LLN to 3,000	<3,000 to 2,000	<2,000 to 1,000	<1,000
Neutrophil Count Decreased (per mm^3)	LLN to 1,500	<1,500 to 1,000	<1,000 to 500	<500
Anemia (Hemoglobin) (g/dL)	LLN to 10.0	<10.0 to 8.0	<8.0; transfusion indicated	Life-threatening consequences, urgent intervention indicated
Platelet Count Decreased (per mm^3)	LLN to 75,000	<75,000 to 50,000	<50,000 to 25,000	<25,000

LLN, lower limit normal (institutional).

Source: CTCAE, Common Terminology Criteria for Adverse Events, version 4.03, Cancer Therapy Evaluation Program, National Cancer Institute. http://ctep.cancer.gov/protocolDevelopment/. Published June 14, 2010.

(PEG)-liposomal doxorubicin, topotecan, paclitaxel, docetaxel, and gemcitabine, are frequently modified in accordance with emerging clinical experience, but without changes in the FDA-approved regimen. It is thus important for the clinician to be aware of these emerging clinical profiles, as well as data from pivotal trials that were used to support original FDA registration.

In view of the narrow safety margin for chemotherapy, it is important that all orders be reviewed by a nurse and pharmacist with oncology experience. Height, weight, calculation of BSA, ideal weight adjustments (if appropriate), pertinent laboratory values, and methods of dose calculation should be clearly indicated and verifiable. Templated orders encourage systematic review and can reduce the risk of error. In addition, it is preferable to have defined dose levels to account for expected treatment modifications rather than relying on percentage-based modifications. For example, it is not always obvious if a percentage refers to the degree of dose reduction or the amount of drug to be administered, which becomes compounded over multiple cycles, with the potential for more than one modification. One convenient method of structured dose modification is illustrated in **Table 13.14**. With this approach, modifications for the subsequent course of therapy are implemented according to the degree (grade), duration, and timing of toxicity experienced during the preceding course. Although treatment can be delayed on a week-by-week basis to allow for recovery, delays of greater than 2 weeks should be avoided through dose modification and utilization of hematopoietic growth factors. With expanded utilization of combination regimens, it is also helpful to know the patterns of toxicity associated with individual drugs, as it might be appropriate to modify one component rather than an entire regimen.

Bone Marrow Toxicity

Bone marrow toxicity is the most common dose-limiting side effect associated with cytotoxic drugs, and neutropenia is the most common manifestation of bone marrow toxicity, occurring 7 to 14 days after initial drug treatment and persisting for 3 to 10 days. Notable exceptions to this timeline include chlorambucil, mitomycin C, and melphalan; which can have prolonged and cumulative myelosuppression with nadirs typically 4 to 6 weeks after therapy. CTCAE grading criteria are summarized in **Table 13.13**. For purposes of dose modification, the absolute neutrophil count (ANC) is preferred over total white blood count, as this more accurately reflects dose tolerance and risk of infection, which is correlated with the duration of grade 4 neutropenia (ANC $\leq 500/mm^3$). Dose-limiting thrombocytopenia is less common than neutropenia, but has become more frequent with wider utilization of carboplatin and carboplatin-based combinations. A systematic approach to management of hematologic toxicity can help to reduce the risk of error and facilitate overall compliance with a treatment regimen (**Table 13.14**).

Radiation, alkylating agents (e.g., melphalan, carboplatin), and other DNA-damaging agents (e.g., nitrosoureas, mitomycin C), can have cumulative long-term effects on bone marrow reserve. Most other agents, including the taxanes and topotecan, show no evidence of cumulative toxicity and can be administered for multiple cycles without dose modification, once a tolerable dose is established.

In view of the frequent occurrence of neutropenia and the risk of infectious complications, utilization of G-CSF, including filgrastim or the longer-acting PEG-filgrastim, has increased. Although these agents promote more rapid granulocyte recovery, thus avoiding potential complications and facilitating the maintenance of dose intensity, their use has not been shown to improve long-term survival for patients with gynecologic cancer, compared to conservative management with modest dose reductions and cycle delay. The American Society of Clinical Oncology and European Society for Medical Oncology have published guidelines on the use of hematopoietic growth factors (113,114); key recommendations are listed in **Table 13.15**.

It is important to remember that G-CSF is not effective in the management of thrombocytopenia and may actually increase the degree of thrombocytopenia by diversion of immature marrow elements, a particular problem after multiple cycles of carboplatin. Recombinant megakaryocyte growth factor was evaluated as an option to maintain platelet counts in patients with protracted chemotherapy-induced thrombocytopenia (115). However, current treatment programs for gynecologic malignancies are not generally associated with a high frequency of complicated grade 4 thrombocytopenia, and the value of aggressive support appears to be limited.

TABLE 13.14. Representative Drug Dose Modifications for Hematologic Toxicity

Category (Timing)	Parameters	CTCAE Grade	Dose or Schedule Modifications
Granulocytes (day of therapy)	$>1,500/mm^3$	0, 1	Full doses of all drugs.
	$<1,500/mm^3$	2, 3, 4	Delay until recovered. If delay >7 days, reduce doses by one level or add G-CSF. If delay >14 days, reduce doses by one level and add G-CSF.
Platelets (day of therapy)	WNL	0	Full doses of all drugs.
	<LLN to $75,000/mm^3$	1	Delay until recovered.
	$<75,000/mm^3$	2, 3, 4	Delay until recovered. If delay >7 days, reduce doses by one level.
Granulocytes (cycle nadir)	$>1,000/mm^3$	0, 1, 2	Full doses of all drugs.
	$<500/mm^3$ for ≥7 days	4	Reduce doses by one level. If already reduced, add G-CSF for future cycles.
	$<1,000/mm^3$ with fever	3, 4	Add G-CSF for current episode, reduce doses by one level for future cycles. If already reduced, add G-CSF for future cycles.
Platelets (cycle nadir)	$\geq 50,000/mm^3$	3	Full doses of all drugs.
	$<50,000/mm^3$ with bleed	3, 4	Reduce doses by one level.
	$<25,000/mm^3$	4	Reduce doses by one level.

CTCAE, Common Terminology Criteria for Adverse Events; G-CSF, granulocyte colony-stimulating factor; LLN, lower limit normal; WNL, within normal limits.

Dose reductions for individual drugs within a combination regimen should be based on the likelihood that a particular drug contributes to the observed hematologic toxicity.

TABLE 13.15. General Guidelines for Hematopoietic Growth Factor Use

Primary prophylaxis	When risk of febrile neutropenia is ≥20% or with certain dose-dense or high-dose intensity regimens
Secondary prophylaxis	Neutropenic complication from prior cycle in which reduced dose or treatment delay may compromise outcome
Neutropenia	Should not be routinely used in patients who are afebrile
Febrile neutropenia	Should not be routinely used; consider in patients at high risk for infection-related complications or poor prognostic factors

Moderate degrees of anemia, which may contribute to chronic fatigue, are quite common in cancer patients receiving chemotherapy. With increased recognition of blood–borne viral pathogens and limited supplies of banked blood, frequent transfusions are not practical or recommended, and many patients will adapt to chronic anemia with minimal symptoms. While recombinant erythropoiesis-stimulating agents are available, the potential risks including cardiovascular events, thrombosis, and reduced tumor-related survival in placebo-controlled, randomized trials (116), have led to guidelines limiting use and prompted the FDA to implement specific Risk Evaluation and Mitigation Strategies that require physician training, registration, and auditing (117,118). Patients with anemia should undergo evaluation of iron stores, with appropriate use of iron replacement, as early as possible, particularly in the setting of endometrial and cervical cancers, which can be associated with vaginal bleeding.

Gastrointestinal Toxicity

Most anticancer agents are associated with some degree of nausea, vomiting, and anorexia. There are three major categories of nausea and vomiting: *anticipatory*, occurring prior to actual administration of chemotherapy; *acute onset*, beginning within 1 hour of chemotherapy administration and persisting for less than 24 hours; and *delayed*, beginning more than 1 day after chemotherapy administration and persisting for several days. Prophylactic management of these adverse effects improves patient acceptance and facilitates completion of therapy with full doses on schedule.

The antiemetic regimen is tailored to the emetogenic potential of the treatment, which reflects the incorporation of specific drugs, as well as the dose and schedule of drug administration. Mild nausea and vomiting can often be managed effectively with H_1 antihistamines (diphenhydramine), phenothiazines (prochlorperazine or thiethylperazine), butyrophenones (haloperidol), steroids (dexamethasone or methylprednisolone), benzamides (metoclopramide), or benzodiazepines (lorazepam). These are likely to be sufficient with drugs such as bleomycin, docetaxel, paclitaxel, Vinca alkaloids, 5-fluorouracil, methotrexate, mitomycin C, gemcitabine, PEG-liposomal doxorubicin, and topotecan.

For drugs with more severe emetogenic potential, including cisplatin, carboplatin, cyclophosphamide, or dactinomycin, a more aggressive prophylactic regimen is required. In general, these patients should receive a 5-hydroxytryptamine (5-HT3) receptor antagonist, such as ondansetron, prior to chemotherapy and repeated at 8- to 12-hour intervals for 3 days. Both compounds are also available in an oral formulation, which has been helpful in the management of delayed and/or chronic nausea after chemotherapy or nausea associated with multiday oral chemotherapy regimens. Longer-acting 5-HT3 antagonists, which require only a single intravenous or oral dose prior to chemotherapy have also become available. As a group, the 5-HT3 antagonists have been quite effective in controlling severe emesis, with few side effects, but are more expensive than prochlorperazine (119). Chronic nausea and vomiting can be a particular problem after several cycles of cisplatin and occasionally carboplatin (120). The mechanism is poorly understood, and symptoms can be difficult to control with currently available medications, prompting the use of extended steroid administration, cannabinoids, repeated dosing with 5-HT3 receptor antagonists, or utilization of substance P antagonists that block the neurokinin-1 (NK1) receptor, such as aprepitant and rolapitant.

Anticipatory nausea and vomiting can become a significant problem during repeated cycles of chemotherapy, as patients associate environmental cues (such as odor, carpeting, or paint colors) with nausea. In addition to behavioral modification, it can sometimes be modulated by pretreatment with antiemetics and amnesic drugs, such as benzodiazepines, administered orally at home prior to arriving at the treatment center. Lorazepam (0.05 mg/kg) can also be given by slow intravenous push 1 hour before therapy, with doses being continued as needed every 4 hours for up to 6 doses (121). Unfortunately, this particular schedule produces significant sedation and can be used only in hospitalized patients or outpatients with independent transportation.

Diarrhea, oral stomatitis, esophagitis, and gastroenteritis are also potential problems. Patients with significant oral or esophagogastric symptoms may have their symptoms managed with oral viscous lidocaine (2%), other topical anesthetics, or parenteral narcotics in severe cases. In general, dose-limiting mucosal injury is uncommon with platinum-based combinations, taxanes, and other single agents used in the treatment of gynecologic cancer. In refractory cases of mucositis, patients should be screened for secondary infectious complications, such as candidiasis and herpes simplex. Following treatment with irinotecan, noninfectious secretory diarrhea is a well-recognized dose-limiting toxicity associated with local exposure to the active metabolite SN-38 and is generally managed with prophylactic antimotility agents and intravenous hydration, with utilization of octreotide in severe cases. Diarrhea can also result from diffuse mucosal injury following administration of doxorubicin (including PEG-liposomal doxorubicin), 5-fluorouracil, methotrexate, and other agents. In the setting of recent surgery and chemotherapy, patients are also at increased risk for infectious diarrhea, and screening for *Clostridium difficile* is appropriate.

Alopecia

Scalp alopecia is one of the most emotionally taxing side effects of chemotherapy. Aside from long-lasting alopecia that follows cranial irradiation, it is almost always reversible, but it can be a major deterrent to successful chemotherapy. Total scalp alopecia is particularly common with drugs like doxorubicin and paclitaxel, and there is generally some degree of partial alopecia with cisplatin, carboplatin, cyclophosphamide, docetaxel, Vinca alkaloids, and 5-fluorouracil. In a minority of cases, patients treated with paclitaxel will also experience loss of eyelashes, eyebrows, and other body hair, which can be particularly distressing. A variety of physical techniques have been devised to minimize alopecia, including scalp tourniquets and ice caps designed to decrease scalp blood flow. Although partially effective, they are rarely successful with extended chemotherapy.

Skin Toxicity

Skin toxicities that occur during chemotherapy include allergic or hypersensitivity reactions (HSR), skin hyperpigmentation, photosensitivity, radiation recall reactions, nail abnormalities, folliculitis, palmar-plantar erythrodysesthesia (PPE, hand–foot syndrome), and local extravasation necrosis. Many of these are drug specific and self-limited, but occasionally they may be dose limiting.

PPE is a reversible but painful erythema, scaling, swelling, or ulceration involving the hands and feet. This occurs more often with chronic oral or intravenous medications, weekly treatment regimens, and formulations that increase drug circulation time, such as prolonged oral etoposide, weekly and continuous-infusion 5-fluorouracil, capecitabine, and PEG-liposomal doxorubicin, where it has emerged as a major dose-limiting toxicity (122).

Extravasation necrosis is a serious complication seen after tissue infiltration of vesicant drugs such as doxorubicin, dactinomycin, mitomycin C, and vincristine (123). These drugs should always be administered through a freely flowing intravenous line with careful monitoring. Caution is also required during utilization of central venous ports, as malfunctions in the needle, hub, or tubing can be associated with gradual extravasation that will not be apparent for several hours (124). Small series have reported a limited experience with local infiltration or topical application of steroids, *n*-acetylcysteine, dimethyl sulfoxide, and hyaluronidase, with variable results, and recommendations are imprecise. However, single or multiple intravenous doses of dexrazoxane, a topoisomerase-II catalytic inhibitor, appear to offer specific protection against injury from anthracyclines, including doxorubicin and daunorubicin (125,126). Severe skin necrosis from some extravasations may require surgical debridement and skin grafting.

Neurotoxicity

Peripheral neuropathy is the most common neurotoxicity encountered in gynecologic oncology and is a particular risk with administration of cisplatin, paclitaxel, docetaxel, nanoparticle albumin-bound (NAB) paclitaxel, epothilones, Vinca alkaloids, and hexamethylmelamine (127,128). Although neuropathy is less common with carboplatin than cisplatin, it can still occur, particularly in combination with paclitaxel. Peripheral neuropathy generally begins with symptoms of paresthesia accompanied by loss of vibratory and position sense in longer nerves associated with the feet and hands. It then progresses to functional impairment, with gait unsteadiness and loss of fine motor coordination, such as trouble buttoning clothes and writing. This is closely followed by loss of deep tendon reflexes and eventual development of motor weakness. With paclitaxel and other non-platinum agents, this is almost always reversible but may require several months posttherapy for substantial improvement. In more severe cases, accompanied by neuronal injury or demyelination, recovery may require active neuronal regeneration over an extended period of time, and symptoms may persist for the patient's lifetime.

In current clinical practice, neurotoxicity from widely utilized microtubule-stabilizing agents is predominant (129,130). The frequency of moderate-to-severe toxicity is more common with paclitaxel, compared to docetaxel or epothilones. Risk appears related to peak levels associated with individual doses, as well as cumulative doses over multiple cycles, which is further complicated by alternative schedules and newer drug formulations. For example, although the risk associated with NAB-paclitaxel on the FDA-approved 3-week schedule is at least as high as paclitaxel (131), the risk is reduced with NAB-paclitaxel administered on a weekly schedule, even with higher cumulative doses. In addition, as the primary means of assessment is clinical, reported frequencies vary widely in clinical trials, reflecting variability in documenting history, and subjective and objective findings.

If related to cisplatin, neuropathy can continue to progress after therapy has been discontinued owing to ongoing axonal demyelination and loss, with long-term persistence of symptoms. Cisplatin has also been associated with permanent ototoxicity and, at higher doses, with loss of color vision (132) and autonomic neuropathy. Oxaliplatin can produce a long-term peripheral neuropathy similar to cisplatin (133), but it is also associated with transient acute reactions, including paresthesia and cold-sensitive laryngeal dysesthesia (134), which may reflect blockade of membrane ion channels (135). While the mechanism of oxaliplatin-induced neuropathy is thought to be related to chelation of calcium, ASCO recommends against infusions of calcium and magnesium as a preventative measure (136).

Although some patients report transient distal paresthesia after a single dose of paclitaxel, the onset of persistent neuropathy is generally more gradual. Neuropathy can become clinically apparent after two to three courses of therapy, with mild symptoms that resolve between cycles. Careful questioning and examination may reveal subtle findings at an earlier stage, and functional assessments have been developed that demonstrate good concordance with actual neuropathy (137). Patients with underlying neurologic problems, such as those secondary to diabetes, alcoholism, or carpal tunnel syndrome, are particularly susceptible, and substitution of docetaxel for paclitaxel can be a useful strategy in some situations. All patients who receive potentially neurotoxic therapy, especially cisplatin and paclitaxel, should be routinely queried regarding proprioception and fine motor tasks and examined for loss of vibratory sense, high-frequency hearing, and deep tendon reflexes.

In view of the frequency of neurotoxicity and the impact on daily life, there has been interest in agents that might prevent nerve damage, encourage recovery, or ameliorate symptoms; however, little high-quality data is available to recommend use of preventative agents (136). Among the agents used to ameliorate symptoms, duloxetine appears to be the most beneficial, although amitriptyline, gabapentin, and pregabalin are also commonly used.

Other neurotoxicities include acute and chronic encephalopathies, usually associated with intrathecal chemotherapy, acute cerebellar syndromes, autonomic dysfunction, inappropriate secretion of antidiuretic hormone, and cranial nerve paresis. Of particular relevance to the gynecologic cancer population, an acute reversible metabolic encephalopathy has been well-described in association with ifosfamide and attributed to the toxic metabolite chloroacetaldehyde. Risk factors for development of ifosfamide-induced encephalopathy include renal dysfunction, low serum albumin, older age, and concomitant use of aprepitant. Symptoms may improve with benzodiazepines or methylene blue (138), which may act through inhibition of monoamine oxidase activity reducing chloroacetaldehyde formation in the liver.

Genitourinary Toxicity

Renal toxicity is a well-recognized side effect of cisplatin, with implication of specific local metabolites, even though only a small fraction of cisplatin is cleared by renal excretion. In contrast, carboplatin undergoes extensive renal clearance with little risk of toxicity. Indeed, with increased substitution of carboplatin for cisplatin, and with a reduction in overall cisplatin dose intensity, there has been a decline in clinical familiarity with cisplatin-mediated nephrotoxicity. However, the expanded utilization of concurrent cisplatin and pelvic radiation for management of early-stage cervical cancer has renewed awareness of this potential problem, particularly as commonly utilized weekly dosing can exceed 100 mg/m^2 over a 3-week period. Careful attention to hydration status and saline-driven urinary output before, during, and immediately after therapy is required to reduce the risk associated with this serious complication (139).

Another troublesome side effect is hemorrhagic cystitis, which can be seen with cyclophosphamide or ifosfamide, attributed to the metabolite acrolein. With moderate-dose cyclophosphamide, this complication can be prevented by maintaining high urinary output, which reduces overall urothelial exposure to the toxic metabolites. However, patients receiving combination regimens often have reduced oral intake post-chemotherapy, and selected patients receiving cyclophosphamide might benefit from supplemental intravenous hydration. The risk of cystitis is essentially 100% with ifosfamide, even with aggressive hydration, but this can be prevented with simultaneous administration of mesna, which binds and neutralizes acrolein in the urine (140).

Hypersensitivity Reactions

Increased utilization of paclitaxel, a natural product with poor solubility, has focused attention on the risk of HSR. For intravenous administration, paclitaxel is formulated in Cremophor-EL, a mixture of polyoxyethylated castor oil and dehydrated alcohol, which has been associated with mast cell degranulation and clinical HSR. Over 80% of reactions occur within minutes during either the first or second cycle of drug administration, and can usually be managed with prophylactic medication (corticosteroids, histamine H_1/H_2 blockade) followed by rechallenge beginning at a lower rate of infusion (141,142). Similar reactions have been reported with docetaxel and PEG-liposomal doxorubicin, but with lower frequency in the absence of Cremophor-EL. Emerging data with NAB-paclitaxel indicate a marked reduction in the risk of HSR, further emphasizing the role of formulation, vehicle, and carriers.

With improved survival and an increased utilization of second-line therapy, patients may also experience more traditional allergic reactions to selected chemotherapy agents. Carboplatin, an organoplatinum compound, has emerged as a major source of late allergic reactions. These occur most often during the second cycle of a second course of therapy, suggesting a process of antigen recall and priming of the immune response (143). Patients receiving a second course of carboplatin-based therapy should be closely monitored for early signs of hypersensitivity, to avoid more serious reactions. Unlike the situation with paclitaxel, carboplatin reactions are not readily prevented or circumvented with prophylactic medication, although inpatient

(144) and outpatient strategies (145) for desensitization have been successfully utilized. It is important to note that the desensitization routine does not eliminate the allergic process, and must generally be repeated with each cycle of treatment. Of interest, the combination of carboplatin with PEG-liposomal doxorubicin has a much lower incidence of carboplatin allergy, compared to a combination of carboplatin and paclitaxel or single-agent carboplatin, and might be preferred in the management of recurrent disease (146).

Other Significant Toxicities

A comprehensive discussion of all potential toxicities associated with currently available chemotherapeutic agents is beyond the scope of this chapter. Nevertheless, a variety of other important toxicities are occasionally encountered in regimens commonly used in gynecologic oncology. These include cardiac toxicity from cumulative doxorubicin exposure, radiation recall vasculitis from doxorubicin, pulmonary fibrosis from bleomycin, gonadal dysfunction in premenopausal women from alkylating agents, and secondary acute leukemia from the chronic administration of alkylating agents, particularly melphalan, in ovarian cancer.

DEVELOPMENTAL CHEMOTHERAPY

Background

The identification, evaluation, and regulatory approval of effective drugs for cancer treatment is a long, complicated, and expensive process. Promising candidates are identified and prioritized through preclinical screening, utilizing derivatives of previously defined active agents or established drug classes or new compounds engineered to interact with a specific target. In addition, there continues to be broad screening of natural products isolated from terrestrial and marine sources. Some evidence of antitumor activity during screening must be demonstrated before clinical trials are undertaken. Thus far, all useful antitumor agents have demonstrated antitumor activity using *in vitro* or *in vivo* screening systems.

These traditional approaches are being increasingly challenged because of the large number of new genes and potential targets identified through molecular biology, genomics, and proteomics. Principles of genomic libraries, solid-phase organic synthesis, and combinatorial chemical library generation have been adopted by the pharmaceutical industry to promote high-throughput screening. As new targets are identified, a large number of related compounds can be created, beginning with lead natural products or known reagents, and then screened for improved target binding and/or inhibition of target function. Substantial bioinformatics resources are required to manage and analyze the large amount of data generated from these processes, but the accumulation of gene expression and proteomic data can facilitate "pre-discovery" modeling of potential targets and reagents prior to decision-making about actual development. To some extent, these processes have evolved in parallel, as it is clear that agents generated from a library or a database will still require some form of biologic validation prior to entering complex and expensive clinical studies.

After antitumor activity has been identified, the new agent must be formulated for human use and produced in sufficient quantities to support clinical trials. This is never a trivial achievement, as was evident from the natural supply limitations and formulation problems encountered in early trials with paclitaxel and the camptothecins. Clinical-grade material is then subjected to detailed preclinical toxicology tests in animals. These toxicology trials are done in several animal species and may explore different schedules of drug administration to provide a basis for clinical development. As such, they are time-consuming, complex, and expensive.

After all of the steps of preclinical testing are completed, new agents can enter clinical evaluation. As such, clinical trials are the primary means utilized to evaluate new agents in a systematic manner. All physicians and patients are urged to consider participation in clinical trials, which are available for almost all diagnoses and treatment circumstances. Sponsors of clinical trials include the NCI in collaboration with individual institutions and national groups, such as NRG Oncology, as well as the pharmaceutical industry and individual institutions.

Clinical Trials

Detailed rationale and methodology for clinical trials design has been covered in other sections. This section highlights key concepts related to the evolving paradigm of investigational drug development. In the traditional development of an investigational agent, phase 1 trials are designed to identify the dose, schedule, and safety profile of the agent; phase 2 trials test the safety and efficacy of a fixed dose of the drug in a larger population with a single cancer type, and determine whether the drug warrants further development; and phase 3 trials are used to validate drugs that have shown promise in phase 2 trials. However, the focus in the modern era on identification of biomarkers of treatment efficacy and development of targeted therapies has led to adaptations to the conventional clinical trial designs (**Table 13.16**).

Adaptations to Traditional Clinical Trial Design in the Modern Era

Recognizing that many agents, such as human monoclonal antibodies, may not demonstrate traditional dose-limiting toxicities (DLT) to define the MTD, some phase 1 trials have adapted their end points to include defining dose based on target engagement or biologic effect. Others have included an expanded cohort to confirm safety and targeting, or an embedded phase 2 component to estimate clinical activity. Still others are selecting patients based on molecular markers to increase likelihood of biologic effect or target engagement. Phase 1 studies can also serve to evaluate new combinations that build on standardized chemotherapy regimens, to establish feasibility and tolerability of the proposed regimen before embarking on larger trials. In certain situations, such as epithelial ovarian cancer, phase 1 trials may enroll newly diagnosed patients without prior therapy, as the experimental combinations generally incorporate other known active agents.

Traditional phase 2 studies test a single agent in patients with a specific cancer diagnosis, usually in the setting of measurable disease after one (or two) prior chemotherapy regimens. Surrogate end points thought to reflect potential clinical benefit, such as response rate, disease stabilization rate, biochemical (tumor

TABLE 13.16. Adaptations to Traditional Clinical Trial Designs

	Traditional	Adaptations
Phase 1	Identification of MTD, DLTs, PKs	Defining dose based on target engagement or biologic effect Expansion cohorts (may be disease specific) to confirm safety and targeting or embedded phase 2 to evaluate efficacy Patient selection based on molecular markers
Phase 2	Evaluate efficacy and safety profile of a fixed-dose regimen in a single tumor type utilizing a single arm without randomization	Randomized phase 2 Enrichment strategies Basket trials Umbrella trials Phase 2/3
Phase 3	Randomized, double blinded trial with standard of care comparator arm	Adaptive designs Group sequential designs

marker) response rate, or the proportion of patients alive and progression-free at a specific time interval, are typically used to evaluate efficacy and are compared to historic comparators. Due to changes in clinical care over time (i.e., improvements in supportive care, earlier detection of recurrence, or changes in treatment standard of care), historical data may no longer reflect current expected clinical outcomes, particularly in terms of time to event (progression-free interval or overall survival) end points. In these cases, randomized phase 2 designs incorporating a control arm may be more appropriate (147).

Randomized phase 2 designs can also be used to allocate patients among two or more treatment arms to minimize potential differences in prognostic factors or other variables. Each arm is then independently tested against the same historical threshold value. Using this approach, one or both arms can be selected for further clinical development. Such randomized trials are generally underpowered for direct comparison of response rate and survival between each arm, owing to the limited number of patients.

Adaptive enrichment strategies allow for the modification of enrollment criteria, based on interim assessments of benefit in subpopulations as determined by a molecular screening approach (148). For example, at the start of the study, a companion molecular test may be performed but not used to define eligibility. If interim analyses support the hypothesis that using the molecular test predicts response to the trial agent, the eligibility criteria may be adapted to exclude patients who would not be expected to benefit.

Umbrella trials provide a centralized infrastructure to test different targeted therapies in a single tumor type in multiple sub-trials. Assignment to a sub-trial is guided by the detection of molecularly defined subsets using a centralized screening platform. In contrast, basket trials typically test a single targeted agent and enroll patients based on specific tumor molecular abnormalities regardless of tissue of origin or histology. Both of these approaches require substantial validation of the companion diagnostic test and confirmation of its link to efficacy of the study agent. However, these can be powerful approaches to studying rare molecular subtypes or rare disease types for which it would normally not be possible to conduct a randomized clinical trial. These, and other integrated strategies are intended to conserve patient resources while accelerating the overall development process, allowing for the discontinuation of arms based on interim assessments of futility (148).

Clearly, the advent of molecular diagnostics has changed the face of clinical trial designs. Though it has been suggested that the traditional sequential phase 1→2→3 trial paradigm is no longer necessary (149), at this point validation of a regimen in a rigorous, randomized phase 3 clinical trial is still required for FDA approval. In a phase 3 randomized trial, a study regimen is directly compared with an existing standard regimen in a particular clinical setting, as defined by the type of cancer, stage of disease, and prior therapy. The size and duration of the trial depends on the primary end point (progression-free survival, overall survival, or quality-adjusted survival), anticipated effect size, and the power and precision of the statistical design. Generally, this is also a collaborative process, which combines scientific, clinical, and regulatory objectives.

Recently, adaptive designs, particularly those that allow for adaptation of study sample size or statistical objective, to maintain study power have been used to enhance the chances that the study will answer the posed question. With the push toward targeted therapy and individualized treatments, there has also been increased pressure from regulatory agencies to include companion diagnostics in phase 3 trials, to predict the likelihood of response and to select appropriate patients. However, not all presumptive biomarkers will be validated, and it is sometimes more useful to include a wider variety of patients with tumor specimens that can be studied for multiple markers and pathways. In addition, if the patient population is too narrowly defined, it may be more difficult to randomize patients to a treatment arm that does not include access to a particular drug.

FDA Approval and Post-marketing Studies

Following a successful phase 3 trial or, preferably, a group of related trials, a sponsor can apply to the FDA for marketing approval for a specific disease indication. This triggers a detailed review of data by the Oncology Drug Advisory Committee (ODAC), which then issues a recommendation to the FDA, followed by formal review and a decision by the FDA, which may grant approval or request additional data. In the United States, all commercial marketing requires FDA approval for at least one specific indication. The average time from initial drug discovery to application for an FDA-approved indication is 10 to 12 years, involving considerable expense and effort, as noted above. Supplemental phase 4 or post-marketing studies can be required by the FDA as part of the approval process, or may be performed by the sponsor to evaluate alternative drug formulations or resolve questions regarding dose, schedule, or toxicity. In addition, phase 4 studies may involve substitution of the new agent in combination with chemotherapeutic regimens already established for the disease. These studies are not commonly employed in the development of new chemotherapeutic regimens, but may provide confirmatory evidence of safety and efficacy.

Drug Interactions, Scheduling, and Sequence

Drugs should be used in their optimal dose and schedule. However, new combinations have the potential to alter the pharmacokinetics, bioavailability, toxicity, and efficacy of individual components based on substrate-dependent effects, such as a reduction in nucleotide pools or altered metabolism. Therefore, the optimal dose and schedule for individual agents within a combination might differ from their use as single agents.

As an illustration, the impact of sequence variations using cisplatin or carboplatin with either paclitaxel or topotecan has been explored in preclinical models and phase 1 clinical trials. Preclinical models showed enhanced cytotoxicity when paclitaxel was administered prior to cisplatin and antagonism by the reverse (150,151). In a phase 1 trial, administration of cisplatin prior to a 24-hour infusion of paclitaxel delayed subsequent clearance of paclitaxel, leading to more profound neutropenia compared to the reverse sequence (150). The mechanism for this effect is unknown, but it is not attributable to platinum-associated renal dysfunction. Instead, it may be related to cisplatin-mediated inhibition of cytochrome P450 mixed-function oxidases that participate in paclitaxel metabolism. Thus, the schedule ultimately adopted in clinical practice (paclitaxel followed by cisplatin) is less toxic, potentially more efficacious, and was predicted by preclinical modeling. Although carboplatin does not inhibit the cytochrome P450 mixed-function oxidases, the sequence was empirically extended to carboplatin-based combinations. In part, this sequence was based on practical considerations related to the risk of acute paclitaxel HSR, which can require interruption of treatment, and it was more acceptable to administer the carboplatin after it was clear that the patient had already tolerated the paclitaxel.

A different pattern was observed with sequences of platinum and topotecan. Preclinical models have consistently favored the sequence of cisplatin followed by topotecan, which has been postulated to interfere with repair of platinum-mediated DNA damage. However, in a phase 1 clinical trial, treatment with cisplatin on day 1, prior to a 5-day course of topotecan, was associated with increased toxicity, compared with administration of cisplatin on day 5 after completing the 5-day course of topotecan (152). In this instance, the sequence recommended by preclinical modeling was more toxic, and the question of antitumor efficacy remains to be resolved. A similar sequence-dependent relationship was identified with carboplatin (153). However, toxicity is reduced when docetaxel is administered prior to topotecan (154), emphasizing that each new combination may require independent evaluation.

Even with a single drug, the schedule of administration can have a significant impact on host toxicity and potential efficacy. Early

TABLE 13.17A. Impact of Paclitaxel Infusion Duration and Schedule on Toxicity and Efficacy

Paclitaxel Dose and Schedule			*Dose-Limiting Toxicities*				
Infusion Duration (Hours)	**Dose Interval (Weeks)**	**Single-Agent Unit Dose (mg/m²/day)**	**Neutropenia**	**Mucositis**	**Alopecia**	**Neuropathy**	**Antitumor Efficacy**
96	3–4	80–120	+++	++	+++	+	+++
24	3	135	++	0	+++	++	+++
3	3	175	+	0	+++	+++	+++
1	1	60–80	0	0	+	+	+++

TABLE 13.17B. Impact of Topotecan Infusion Duration and Schedule on Toxicity and Efficacy

Topotecan Dose and Schedule			*Dose-Limiting Toxicities*				
Infusion Duration (Days)	**Dose Interval (Weeks)**	**Single-Agent Unit Dose (mg/m²/day)**	**Neutropenia**	**Mucositis**	**Alopecia**	**Neuropathy**	**Antitumor Efficacy**
21	4	0.40	+++	0	0	0	+++
5	3–4	1.25	+++	0	0	0	+++
3	3	2.00	+++	0	0	0	++
1	3	8.50	+++	0	0	0	+
1	1	1.75	++	0	0	0	–
1	1	4.00	+	0	0	0	+

studies with paclitaxel utilized an arbitrary 24-hour infusion, which was selected to reduce the risk of HSR (**Table 13.17**). Subsequent preclinical data suggested that prolonged exposure (96 hours) might have greater efficacy. Owing to increased bone marrow and mucosal toxicity, the MTD was lowered, and the frequency of serious neuropathy was reduced. However, the 96-hour regimen did not demonstrate significant activity in patients with recurrent ovarian cancer (155). In addition, the efficacy of a 3-hour infusion was comparable to a 24-hour infusion in a phase 3 trial (156), reinforcing a clinical shift toward the convenient 3-hour schedule, which achieved a higher MTD, primarily due to a marked decrease in bone marrow toxicity, but with an increased incidence of neuropathy. This was followed by a phase 1 evaluation of a weekly low-dose 1-hour infusion, which was almost devoid of serious toxicity, including a decreased incidence of alopecia, with maintenance of clinical efficacy (157). Thus, the optimal preclinical regimen (96-hour exposure) was superseded in the clinical setting by an unexpected series of observations from empiric phase 1 trials, yielding decreased toxicity, improved convenience, and the potential for increased efficacy.

With topotecan, a different relationship was defined (**Table 13.17B**). Initial studies utilized an inconvenient daily infusion for 5 consecutive days, which was based on preclinical data suggesting that prolonged exposure would be more efficacious. This 5-day regimen achieved a 33% response rate in a GOG phase 2 trial in recurrent platinum-sensitive ovarian cancer with expected dose-limiting neutropenia and thrombocytopenia (158). This was followed by the evaluation of a single 24-hour infusion once every 3 weeks, achieving only a 7% response rate in a similar population (159). An attempt to define an intermediate 3-day regimen achieved only a 14% response rate (160). Topotecan was also evaluated as a prolonged intravenous infusion for 21 days to maximize the duration of exposure (161). Although the study was conducted in a different patient population, the overall response rate (35%) was similar to the 5-day regimen, and once again there was equivalent hematologic toxicity without dose-limiting non-hematologic toxicity. When evaluated as a weekly treatment program, tolerability and acceptance were improved, but the overall efficacy was reduced (162,163). In this situation, changes in drug schedule, over a wide range, were associated with substantial differences in efficacy, but without any change in the spectrum or severity of host toxicity, with the exception of reduced hematologic toxicity on the weekly schedule. Thus, each new agent must be independently evaluated in the appropriate clinical setting to select the optimal dose and schedule for cancer treatment.

Development of Combination Regimens

With some notable exceptions, single agents are not sufficient to achieve prolonged survival or cure. Combinations of conventional cytotoxics can approach maximal cell kill by including drugs with minimal overlap of toxicities, such that antitumor effects can be summed but the toxicities dispersed. Combinations are also more likely to demonstrate activity against heterogeneous tumor populations, and effective combinations could prevent the emergence of drug resistance. However, in practice it may also encourage greater resistance among surviving cell fractions.

No direct evidence currently exists to indicate whether optimal combinations should utilize sequential single agents, doublets, or triplets. Several combinations including triplet cytotoxic therapy and sequential doublet chemotherapy were evaluated in epithelial ovarian cancer in an effort to improve on the results obtained with a standard combination of carboplatin and paclitaxel. However, based on completed phase 3 trials in approximately 12,000 women, none of the combinations achieved an improvement in clinical outcomes, providing additional support for a shift in developmental priorities toward molecular-targeted agents and other novel approaches (164).

Development of combination regimens has been guided by several principles (**Table 13.18**) and recommendations for phase 1 development of combination regimens have been made by the Clinical Trial Design Task Force of the NCI Investigational Drug Steering Committee (165).

TABLE 13.18. Principles of Combination Chemotherapy

Each component should have Activity against the target tumor as a single agent A different mechanism of action and cellular target A biochemical basis for additive or synergistic effects in combination with at least one of the other agents No evidence of antagonistic interactions Distinct patterns of resistance to discourage the emergence of drug-resistant phenotypes
Optimal dose, schedule, and sequence of drug administration should be determined from preclinical data and early clinical trials to maximize tumor response and minimize host toxicity.
Minimal overlap of non-hematologic toxicity is desirable to safely maintain full therapeutic doses of each component over multiple cycles.

A Contemporary Challenge: Drug Shortages

Trends in drug development within the academic community and pharmaceutical industry have dramatically changed over the last 2 decades, and we are now seeing an abundance of new molecular-targeted agents, with only a limited investment in conventional cytotoxics. Many of our most widely utilized standard chemotherapeutic agents have exceeded the period of patent protection and are now produced and distributed as generic compounds. With reductions in insurance reimbursement rates and the rising expense associated with manufacturing and quality control, the profitability of generic medications and the number of generic manufacturing facilities have declined. This has contributed to intermittent and chronic shortages of a number of compounds, including cisplatin, paclitaxel, 5-fluorouracil, leucovorin, bleomycin, polyethylene-glycosylated liposomal doxorubicin, antiemetics, and steroids. Consequences include greater costs to obtain drugs through alternate sources, omission of specific drugs from standard treatment regimens, and closure or delay of important clinical trials. Solutions to this international problem are complex, and it is likely that important shortages will manifest for a number of years to come. Information on current drug shortages can be obtained from the U.S. FDA and the American Society of Health-System Pharmacists:

http://www.fda.gov/Drugs/DrugSafety/DrugShortages/default.htm
http://www.ashp.org/DrugShortages/Current

Conclusion

Although there have been significant advances in understanding the molecular biology of gynecologic malignancies, chemotherapy remains the mainstay of treatment for these cancers. Understanding the pharmacologic principles underpinning their efficacy, mechanisms of resistance, and toxicity, optimal dosing sequencing, and timing of therapy, will allow for the strategic development of combination regimens (including molecularly targeted agents) to improve outcomes for women with gynecologic malignancies.

References

1. Lissauer H. Zwei Falle von Leucaemie. *Berl Klin Wochenschr*. 1865;2:403–404.
2. Cutler EG, Bradford EH. Action of iron, cod-liver oil, and arsenic on the globular richness of the blood. *Am J Med Sci*. 1878;75:74–84.
3. Kandel EV, LeRoy GV. Chronic arsenical poisoning during the treatment of chronic myeloid leukemia. *Arch Intern Med*. 1937;60(5):846–866.
4. Gilman A. The initial clinical trial of nitrogen mustard. *Am J Surg*. 1963;105:574–578.
5. Farber S, Diamond LK. Temporary remissions in acute leukemia in children produced by folic acid antagonist, 4-aminopteroyl-glutamic acid. *N Engl J Med*. 1948;238(23):787–793.
6. Hertz R, Ross GT, Lipsett MB. Primary chemotherapy of nonmetastatic trophoblastic disease in women. *Am J Obstet Gynecol*. 1963;86:808–814.
7. Huggins C, Hodges CV. Studies on prostatic cancer. I. The effect of castration, of estrogen and androgen injection on serum phosphatases in metastatic carcinoma of the prostate. *CA Cancer J Clin*. 1972;22(4):232–240.
8. Tannock I, Frei E III. Possible role of cell kinetics in prediction of the response to cancer therapy. *Natl Cancer Inst Monogr*. 1971;34:19–24.
9. Lampkin BC, Nagao T, Mauer AM. Synchronization and recruitment in acute leukemia. *J Clin Invest*. 1971;50(10):2204–2214.
10. Lotem J, Sachs L. Regulation by bcl-2, c-myc, and p53 of susceptibility to induction of apoptosis by heat shock and cancer chemotherapy compounds in differentiation-competent and -defective myeloid leukemic cells. *Cell Growth Differ*. 1993;4(1):41–47.
11. Szotek PP, Pieretti-Vanmarcke R, Masiakos PT, et al. Ovarian cancer side population defines cells with stem cell-like characteristics and Mullerian Inhibiting Substance responsiveness. *Proc Natl Acad Sci U S A*. 2006;103(30):11154–11159.
12. Glinsky GV. "Stemness" genomics law governs clinical behavior of human cancer: implications for decision making in disease management. *J Clin Oncol*. 2008;26(17):2846–2853.
13. Tannock I. Cell kinetics and chemotherapy: a critical review. *Cancer Treat Rep*. 1978;62(8):1117–1133.
14. Steel GG. Cell loss as a factor in the growth rate of human tumours. *Eur J Cancer*. 1967;3(4):381–387.
15. Jain RK. Normalization of tumor vasculature: an emerging concept in antiangiogenic therapy. *Science*. 2005;307(5706):58–62.
16. Norton L. Cancer log-kill revisited. *Am Soc Clin Oncol Educ Book*. 2014:3–7.
17. Rodriguez-Brenes IA, Komarova NL, Wodarz D. Tumor growth dynamics: insights into evolutionary processes. *Trends Ecol Evol*. 2013;28(10):597–604.
18. Hanin L, Bunimovich-Mendrazitsky S. Reconstruction of the natural history of metastatic cancer and assessment of the effects of surgery: Gompertzian growth of the primary tumor. *Math Biosci*. 2014;247:47–58.
19. Charbit A, Malaise EP, Tubiana M. Relation between the pathological nature and the growth rate of human tumors. *Eur J Cancer*. 1971;7(4):307–315.
20. Baserga R. The relationship of the cell cycle to tumor growth and control of cell division: a review. *Cancer Res*. 1965;25:581–595.
21. McGuire WP, Hoskins WJ, Brady MF, et al. Cyclophosphamide and cisplatin compared with paclitaxel and cisplatin in patients with stage III and stage IV ovarian cancer. *N Engl J Med*. 1996;334(1):1–6.
22. Bookman MA, Greer BE, Ozols RF. Optimal therapy of advanced ovarian cancer: carboplatin and paclitaxel vs. cisplatin and paclitaxel (GOG 158) and an update on GOG0 182-ICON5. *Int J Gynecol Cancer*. 2003;13(6):735–740.
23. Miller D, Filiaci V, Fleming G, et al. Randomized phase III noninferiority trial of first line chemotherapy for metastatic or recurrent endometrial carcinoma: A Gynecologic Oncology Group study. *Gynecol Oncol*. 2012;125(3):771.
24. Tewari KS, Sill MW, Long HJ III, et al. Improved survival with bevacizumab in advanced cervical cancer. *N Engl J Med*. 2014;370(8):734–743.
25. Homesley HD, Filiaci V, Markman M, et al. Phase III trial of ifosfamide with or without paclitaxel in advanced uterine carcinosarcoma: a Gynecologic Oncology Group study. *J Clin Oncol*. 2007;25(5):526–531.
26. Muggia FM, Braly PS, Brady MF, et al. Phase III randomized study of cisplatin versus paclitaxel versus cisplatin and paclitaxel in patients with suboptimal stage III or IV ovarian cancer: a Gynecologic Oncology Group study. *J Clin Oncol*. 2000;18(1):106–115.
27. Young RC, Brady MF, Nieberg RK, et al. Adjuvant treatment for early ovarian cancer: a randomized phase III trial of intraperitoneal 32P or intravenous cyclophosphamide and cisplatin—a Gynecologic Oncology Group Study. *J Clin Oncol*. 2003;21(23):4350–4355.
28. Trimbos JB, Vergote I, Bolis G, et al. Impact of adjuvant chemotherapy and surgical staging in early-stage ovarian carcinoma: European Organisation for Research and Treatment of Cancer-Adjuvant ChemoTherapy in Ovarian Neoplasm trial. *J Natl Cancer Inst*. 2003;95(2):113–125.
29. Randall ME, Filiaci VL, Muss H, et al. Randomized phase III trial of whole-abdominal irradiation versus doxorubicin and cisplatin chemotherapy in advanced endometrial carcinoma: a Gynecologic Oncology Group study. *J Clin Oncol*. 2006;24(1):36–44.
30. Wolfson AH, Brady MF, Rocereto T, et al. A gynecologic oncology group randomized phase III trial of whole abdominal irradiation (WAI) vs. cisplatin-ifosfamide and mesna (CIM) as post-surgical therapy in stage I–IV carcinosarcoma (CS) of the uterus. *Gynecol Oncol*. 2007;107(2):177–185.

31. Rose PG, Ali S, Watkins E, et al. Long-term follow-up of a randomized trial comparing concurrent single agent cisplatin, cisplatin-based combination chemotherapy, or hydroxyurea during pelvic irradiation for locally advanced cervical cancer: a Gynecologic Oncology Group study. *J Clin Oncol*. 2007;25(19):2804–2810.
32. Vergote I, Trope CG, Amant F, et al. Neoadjuvant chemotherapy or primary surgery in stage IIIC or IV ovarian cancer. *N Engl J Med*. 2010;363(10):943–953.
33. Kehoe S, Hook J, Nankivell M, et al. Primary chemotherapy versus primary surgery for newly diagnosed advanced ovarian cancer (CHORUS): an open-label, randomised, controlled, non-inferiority trial. *Lancet*. 2015;386(9990):249–257.
34. Eisenhauer EA, Therasse P, Bogaerts J, et al. New response evaluation criteria in solid tumours: revised RECIST guideline (version 1.1). *Eur J Cancer*. 2009;45(2):228–247.
35. Wahl RL, Jacene H, Kasamon Y, et al. From RECIST to PERCIST: evolving considerations for PET response criteria in solid tumors. *J Nucl Med*. 2009;50(Suppl 1):122S–150S.
36. Rustin GJ, Vergote I, Eisenhauer E, et al. Definitions for response and progression in ovarian cancer clinical trials incorporating RECIST 1.1 and CA 125 agreed by the Gynecological Cancer Intergroup (GCIG). *Int J Gynecol Cancer*. 2011;21(2):419–423.
37. Levin L, Hryniuk WM. Dose intensity analysis of chemotherapy regimens in ovarian carcinoma. *J Clin Oncol*. 1987;5(5):756–767.
38. McGuire WP, Hoskins WJ, Brady MF, et al. Assessment of dose-intensive therapy in suboptimally debulked ovarian cancer: a Gynecologic Oncology Group study. *J Clin Oncol*. 1995;13(7):1589–1599.
39. Havrilesky LJ, Reiner M, Morrow PK, et al. A review of relative dose intensity and survival in patients with metastatic solid tumors. *Crit Rev Oncol Hematol*. 2015;93(3):203–210.
40. Kummel S, Krocker J, Kohls A, et al. Randomised trial: survival benefit and safety of adjuvant dose-dense chemotherapy for node-positive breast cancer. *Br J Cancer*. 2006;94(9):1237–1244.
41. Katsumata N, Yasuda M, Isonishi S, et al. Long-term results of dose-dense paclitaxel and carboplatin versus conventional paclitaxel and carboplatin for treatment of advanced epithelial ovarian, fallopian tube, or primary peritoneal cancer (JGOG 3016): a randomised, controlled, open-label trial. *Lancet Oncol*. 2013;14(10):1020–1106.
42. Bookman MA, Brady MF, McGuire WP, et al. Evaluation of new platinum-based treatment regimens in advanced-stage ovarian cancer: a Phase III Trial of the Gynecologic Cancer Intergroup. *J Clin Oncol*. 2009;27(9):1419–1425.
43. Koch KM, Reddy NJ, Cohen RB, et al. Effects of food on the relative bioavailability of lapatinib in cancer patients. *J Clin Oncol*. 2009;27(8):1191–1196.
44. Ratain MJ, Cohen EE. The value meal: how to save $1,700 per month or more on lapatinib. *J Clin Oncol*. 2007;25(23):3397–3398.
45. Lown KS, Bailey DG, Fontana RJ, et al. Grapefruit juice increases felodipine oral availability in humans by decreasing intestinal CYP3A protein expression. *J Clin Invest*. 1997;99(10):2545–2553.
46. Cormio G, Gabriele A, Maneo A, et al. Complete remission of brain metastases from ovarian carcinoma with carboplatin. *Eur J Obstet Gynecol Reprod Biol*. 1998;78(1):91–93.
47. Wong DJ, Hurvitz SA. Recent advances in the development of anti-HER2 antibodies and antibody-drug conjugates. *Ann Transl Med*. 2014; 2(12):122.
48. Vandebroek AJ. Nutritional status in relation to treatment modalities. *EJC Suppl*. 2013;11(2):296–298.
49. Engels FK, Sparreboom A, Mathot RA, et al. Potential for improvement of docetaxel-based chemotherapy: a pharmacological review. *Br J Cancer*. 2005;93(2):173–177.
50. Markman M. Intraperitoneal antineoplastic drug delivery: rationale and results. *Lancet Oncol*. 2003;4(5):277–283.
51. Jaaback K, Johnson N, Lawrie TA. Intraperitoneal chemotherapy for the initial management of primary epithelial ovarian cancer. *Cochrane Database Syst Rev*. 2011;11:CD005340.
52. Markman M, Brady MF, Spirtos NM, et al. Phase II trial of intraperitoneal paclitaxel in carcinoma of the ovary, tube, and peritoneum: a Gynecologic Oncology Group study. *J Clin Oncol*. 1998;16(8):2620–2624.
53. Knox RJ, Friedlos F, Lydall DA, et al. Mechanism of cytotoxicity of anticancer platinum drugs: evidence that cis-diamminedichloroplatinum(II) and cis-diammine-(1,1-cyclobutanedicarboxylato)platinum(II) differ only in the kinetics of their interaction with DNA. *Cancer Res*. 1986;46(4 pt 2):1972–1979.
54. Natarajan G, Malathi R, Holler E. Increased DNA-binding activity of cis-1,1-cyclobutanedicarboxylatodiammineplatinum(II) (carboplatin) in the presence of nucleophiles and human breast cancer MCF-7 cell cytoplasmic extracts: activation theory revisited. *Biochem Pharmacol*. 1999;58(10):1625–1629.
55. Hurria A, Lichtman SM. Pharmacokinetics of chemotherapy in the older patient. *Cancer Control*. 2007;14(1):32–43.
56. Muss HB, Biganzoli L, Sargent DJ, et al. Adjuvant therapy in the elderly: making the right decision. *J Clin Oncol*. 2007;25(14):1870–1875.
57. Tew WP, Fleming GF. Treatment of ovarian cancer in the older woman. *Gynecol Oncol*. 2015;136(1):136–142.
58. Freyer G, Tinker AV. Clinical trials and treatment of the elderly diagnosed with ovarian cancer. *Int J Gynecol Cancer*. 2011;21(4):776–781.
59. Clase CM, Garg AX, Kiberd BA. Prevalence of low glomerular filtration rate in nondiabetic Americans: Third National Health and Nutrition Examination Survey (NHANES III). *J Am Soc Nephrol*. 2002;13(5):1338–1349.
60. Levey AS, Bosch JP, Lewis JB, et al. A more accurate method to estimate glomerular filtration rate from serum creatinine: a new prediction equation. Modification of Diet in Renal Disease Study Group. *Ann Intern Med*. 1999;130(6):461–470.
61. Cockcroft DW, Gault MH. Prediction of creatinine clearance from serum creatinine. *Nephron*. 1976;16(1):31–41.
62. Jelliffe RW. Letter: creatinine clearance: bedside estimate. *Ann Intern Med*. 1973;79(4):604–605.
63. National Kidney Foundation. K/DOQI clinical practice guidelines for chronic kidney disease: evaluation, classification, and stratification. *Am J Kidney Dis*. 2002;39(2 Suppl 1):S1–S266.
64. Murray B, Bates J, Buie L. Impact of a new assay for measuring serum creatinine levels on carboplatin dosing. *Am J Health Syst Pharm*. 2012;69(13):1136–1141.
65. Ivy SP, Zwiebel J, Mooney M. Follow-up for information letter regarding AUC-based dosing of carboplatin. Investigational Drug Branch, Cancer Therapy Evaluation Program, Division of Cancer Treatment and Diagnosis, National Cancer Institute. http://ctep.cancer.gov/content/docs/Carboplatin_Information_Letter.pdf. Accessed December 10, 2015.
66. Li YF, Fu S, Hu W, et al. Systemic anticancer therapy in gynecological cancer patients with renal dysfunction. *Int J Gynecol Cancer*. 2007;17(4):739–763.
67. Gouyette A, Lemoine R, Adhemar JP, et al. Kinetics of cisplatin in an anuric patient undergoing hemofiltration dialysis. *Cancer Treat Rep*. 1981;65(7–8):665–668.
68. Motzer RJ, Niedzwiecki D, Isaacs M, et al. Carboplatin-based chemotherapy with pharmacokinetic analysis for patients with hemodialysis-dependent renal insufficiency. *Cancer Chemother Pharmacol*. 1990;27(3):234–238.
69. Boisdron-Celle M, Remaud G, Traore S, et al. 5-Fluorouracil-related severe toxicity: a comparison of different methods for the pretherapeutic detection of dihydropyrimidine dehydrogenase deficiency. *Cancer Lett*. 2007;249(2):271–282.
70. Powis G. Effect of human renal and hepatic disease on the pharmacokinetics of anticancer drugs. *Cancer Treat Rev*. 1982;9(2):85–124.
71. Villano JL, Mehta D, Radhakrishnan L. Abraxane induced life-threatening toxicities with metastatic breast cancer and hepatic insufficiency. *Invest New Drugs*. 2006;24(5):455–456.
72. Hande KR, Wolff SN, Greco FA, et al. Etoposide kinetics in patients with obstructive jaundice. *J Clin Oncol*. 1990;8(6):1101–1107.
73. Tanaka E. Clinically important pharmacokinetic drug–drug interactions: role of cytochrome P450 enzymes. *J Clin Pharm Ther*. 1998;23(6):403–416.
74. Kivisto KT, Kroemer HK, Eichelbaum M. The role of human cytochrome P450 enzymes in the metabolism of anticancer agents: implications for drug interactions. *Br J Clin Pharmacol*. 1995;40(6):523–530.
75. Nachimuthu S, Assar MD, Schussler JM. Drug-induced QT interval prolongation: mechanisms and clinical management. *Ther Adv Drug Saf*. 2012;3(5):241–253.
76. Fojo AT, Ueda K, Slamon DJ, et al. Expression of a multidrug-resistance gene in human tumors and tissues. *Proc Natl Acad Sci U S A*. 1987;84(1):265–269.
77. Nunberg JH, Kaufman RJ, Schimke RT, et al. Amplified dihydrofolate reductase genes are localized to a homogeneously staining region of a single chromosome in a methotrexate-resistant Chinese hamster ovary cell line. *Proc Natl Acad Sci U S A*. 1978;75(11):5553–5556.
78. Kathawala RJ, Gupta P, Ashby CR Jr, et al. The modulation of ABC transporter-mediated multidrug resistance in cancer: a review of the past decade. *Drug Resist Updat*. 2015;18:1–17.
79. Schondorf T, Scharl A, Kurbacher CM, et al. Amplification of the mdr1-gene is uncommon in recurrent ovarian carcinomas. *Cancer Lett*. 1999;146(2):195–199.
80. Rubin SC, Finstad CL, Hoskins WJ, et al. Expression of P-glycoprotein in epithelial ovarian cancer: evaluation as a marker of multidrug resistance. *Am J Obstet Gynecol*. 1990;163(1 pt 1):69–73.

81. Galluzzi L, Senovilla L, Vitale I, et al. Molecular mechanisms of cisplatin resistance. *Oncogene*. 2012;31(15):1869–1883.
82. Sadowitz PD, Hubbard BA, Dabrowiak JC, et al. Kinetics of cisplatin binding to cellular DNA and modulations by thiol-blocking agents and thiol drugs. *Drug Metab Dispos*. 2002;30(2):183–190.
83. Dabholkar M, Bostick-Bruton F, Weber C, et al. ERCC1 and ERCC2 expression in malignant tissues from ovarian cancer patients. *J Natl Cancer Inst*. 1992;84(19):1512–1517.
84. Olaussen KA, Dunant A, Fouret P, et al. DNA repair by ERCC1 in non-small-cell lung cancer and cisplatin-based adjuvant chemotherapy. *N Engl J Med*. 2006;355(10):983–991.
85. Zheng Z, Chen T, Li X, et al. DNA synthesis and repair genes RRM1 and ERCC1 in lung cancer. *N Engl J Med*. 2007;356(8):800–808.
86. Cobo M, Isla D, Massuti B, et al. Customizing cisplatin based on quantitative excision repair cross-complementing 1 mRNA expression: a phase III trial in non-small-cell lung cancer. *J Clin Oncol*. 2007;25(19):2747–2754.
87. Rubatt JM, Darcy KM, Tian C, et al. Pre-treatment tumor expression of ERCC1 in women with advanced stage epithelial ovarian cancer is not predictive of clinical outcomes: a Gynecologic Oncology Group study. *Gynecol Oncol*. 2012;125(2):421–426.
88. Aebi S, Kurdi-Haidar B, Gordon R, et al. Loss of DNA mismatch repair in acquired resistance to cisplatin. *Cancer Res*. 1996;56(13):3087–3090.
89. Bolton KL, Chenevix-Trench G, Goh C, et al. Association between BRCA1 and BRCA2 mutations and survival in women with invasive epithelial ovarian cancer. *JAMA*. 2012;307(4):382–390.
90. Penson RT, Oliva E, Skates SJ, et al. Expression of multidrug resistance-1 protein inversely correlates with paclitaxel response and survival in ovarian cancer patients: a study in serial samples. *Gynecol Oncol*. 2004;93(1):98–106.
91. Barbuti AM, Chen ZS. Paclitaxel through the ages of anticancer therapy: exploring its role in chemoresistance and radiation therapy. *Cancers (Basel)*. 2015;7(4):2360–2371.
92. Carrara L, Guzzo F, Roque DM, et al. Differential in vitro sensitivity to patupilone versus paclitaxel in uterine and ovarian carcinosarcoma cell lines is linked to tubulin-beta-III expression. *Gynecol Oncol*. 2012;125(1):231–236.
93. Fracasso PM, Brady MF, Moore DH, et al. Phase II study of paclitaxel and valspodar (PSC 833) in refractory ovarian carcinoma: a gynecologic oncology group study. *J Clin Oncol*. 2001;19(12):2975–2982.
94. Lhomme C, Joly F, Walker JL, et al. Phase III study of valspodar (PSC 833) combined with paclitaxel and carboplatin compared with paclitaxel and carboplatin alone in patients with stage IV or suboptimally debulked stage III epithelial ovarian cancer or primary peritoneal cancer. *J Clin Oncol*. 2008;26(16):2674–2682.
95. Sun YL, Kumar P, Sodani K, et al. Ponatinib enhances anticancer drug sensitivity in MRP7-overexpressing cells. *Oncol Rep*. 2014;31(4):1605–1612.
96. Yu Y, Gaillard S, Phillip JM, et al. Inhibition of spleen tyrosine kinase potentiates paclitaxel-induced cytotoxicity in ovarian cancer cells by stabilizing microtubules. *Cancer Cell*. 2015;28(1):82–96.
97. Markman M, Blessing J, Rubin SC, et al. Phase II trial of weekly paclitaxel (80 mg/m^2) in platinum and paclitaxel-resistant ovarian and primary peritoneal cancers: a Gynecologic Oncology Group study. *Gynecol Oncol*. 2006;101(3):436–440.
98. Trent JM, Buick RN, Olson S, et al. Cytologic evidence for gene amplification in methotrexate-resistant cells obtained from a patient with ovarian adenocarcinoma. *J Clin Oncol*. 1984;2(1):8–15.
99. Cowan KH, Jolivet J. A methotrexate-resistant human breast cancer cell line with multiple defects, including diminished formation of methotrexate polyglutamates. *J Biol Chem*. 1984;259(17):10793–10800.
100. Obata T, Endo Y, Murata D, et al. The molecular targets of antitumor 2′-deoxycytidine analogues. *Curr Drug Targets*. 2003;4(4):305–313.
101. Zhou B, Mo X, Liu X, et al. Human ribonucleotide reductase M2 subunit gene amplification and transcriptional regulation in a homogeneous staining chromosome region responsible for the mechanism of drug resistance. *Cytogenet Cell Genet*. 2001;95(1–2):34–42.
102. Jung CP, Motwani MV, Schwartz GK. Flavopiridol increases sensitization to gemcitabine in human gastrointestinal cancer cell lines and correlates with down-regulation of ribonucleotide reductase M2 subunit. *Clin Cancer Res*. 2001;7(8):2527–2536.
103. Johnston PG, Lenz HJ, Leichman CG, et al. Thymidylate synthase gene and protein expression correlate and are associated with response to 5-fluorouracil in human colorectal and gastric tumors. *Cancer Res*. 1995;55(7):1407–1412.
104. Salonga D, Danenberg KD, Johnson M, et al. Colorectal tumors responding to 5-fluorouracil have low gene expression levels of dihydropyrimidine dehydrogenase, thymidylate synthase, and thymidine phosphorylase. *Clin Cancer Res*. 2000;6(4):1322–1327.
105. Fidler IJ, Kripke ML. Metastasis results from preexisting variant cells within a malignant tumor. *Science*. 1977;197(4306):893–895.
106. Kern DH, Weisenthal LM. Highly specific prediction of antineoplastic drug resistance with an in vitro assay using suprapharmacologic drug exposures. *J Natl Cancer Inst*. 1990;82(7):582–588.
107. Cortazar P, Johnson BE. Review of the efficacy of individualized chemotherapy selected by in vitro drug sensitivity testing for patients with cancer. *J Clin Oncol*. 1999;17(5):1625–1631.
108. Nagourney RA, Brewer CA, Radecki S, et al. Phase II trial of gemcitabine plus cisplatin repeating doublet therapy in previously treated, relapsed ovarian cancer patients. *Gynecol Oncol*. 2003;88(1):35–39.
109. The Cancer Genome Atlas Research Network. Integrated genomic analyses of ovarian carcinoma. *Nature*. 2011;474(7353):609–615.
110. Hunter RJ, Navo MA, Thaker PH, et al. Dosing chemotherapy in obese patients: actual versus assigned body surface area (BSA). *Cancer Treat Rev*. 2009;35(1):69–78.
111. Bandera EV, Lee VS, Rodriguez-Rodriguez L, et al. Impact of chemotherapy dosing on ovarian cancer survival according to body mass index. *JAMA Oncol*. 2015;1(6):737–745.
112. Griggs JJ, Mangu PB, Temin S, et al. Appropriate chemotherapy dosing for obese adult patients with cancer: American Society of Clinical Oncology Clinical Practice Guideline. *J Oncol Pract*. 2012;8(4):e59–e61.
113. Crawford J, Caserta C, Roila F, et al. Hematopoietic growth factors: ESMO Clinical Practice Guidelines for the applications. *Ann Oncol*. 2010;(21 Suppl 5):v248–v251.
114. Smith TJ, Bohlke K, Lyman GH, et al. Recommendations for the use of WBC growth factors: American Society of Clinical Oncology Clinical Practice Guideline Update. *J Clin Oncol*. 2015;33(28):3199–3212.
115. Parameswaran R, Lunning M, Mantha S, et al. Romiplostim for management of chemotherapy-induced thrombocytopenia. *Support Care Cancer*. 2014;22(5):1217–1222.
116. Tonia T, Mettler A, Robert N, et al. Erythropoietin or darbepoetin for patients with cancer. *Cochrane Database Syst Rev*. 2012;12:CD003407.
117. Rizzo JD, Brouwers M, Hurley P, et al. American Society of Clinical Oncology/American Society of Hematology clinical practice guideline update on the use of epoetin and darbepoetin in adult patients with cancer. *J Clin Oncol*. 2010;28(33):4996–5010.
118. Schrijvers D, De Samblanx H, Roila F, et al. Erythropoiesis-stimulating agents in the treatment of anaemia in cancer patients: ESMO Clinical Practice Guidelines for use. *Ann Oncol*. 2010;(21 Suppl 5):v244–v247.
119. Bonneterre J, Chevallier B, Metz R, et al. A randomized double-blind comparison of ondansetron and metoclopramide in the prophylaxis of emesis induced by cyclophosphamide, fluorouracil, and doxorubicin or epirubicin chemotherapy. *J Clin Oncol*. 1990;8(6):1063–1069.
120. du Bois A, Vach W, Kiechle M, et al. Pathophysiology, severity, pattern, and risk factors for carboplatin-induced emesis. *Oncology*. 1996;(53 Suppl 1):46–50.
121. Friedlander ML, Sims K, Kearsley JH. Impairment of recall improves tolerance of cytotoxic chemotherapy. *Lancet*. 1983;2(8351):686.
122. Muggia FM, Hainsworth JD, Jeffers S, et al. Phase II study of liposomal doxorubicin in refractory ovarian cancer: antitumor activity and toxicity modification by liposomal encapsulation. *J Clin Oncol*. 1997;15(3):987–993.
123. Kassner E. Evaluation and treatment of chemotherapy extravasation injuries. *J Pediatr Oncol Nurs*. 2000;17(3):135–148.
124. Schulmeister L, Camp-Sorrell D. Chemotherapy extravasation from implanted ports. *Oncol Nurs Forum*. 2000;27(3):531–538; quiz 539–540.
125. Langer SW, Sehested M, Jensen PB. Treatment of anthracycline extravasation with dexrazoxane. *Clin Cancer Res*. 2000;6(9):3680–3686.
126. Mouridsen HT, Langer SW, Buter J, et al. Treatment of anthracycline extravasation with Savene (dexrazoxane): results from two prospective clinical multicentre studies. *Ann Oncol*. 2007;18(3):546–550.
127. Verstappen CC, Heimans JJ, Hoekman K, et al. Neurotoxic complications of chemotherapy in patients with cancer: clinical signs and optimal management. *Drugs*. 2003;63(15):1549–1563.
128. Quasthoff S, Hartung HP. Chemotherapy-induced peripheral neuropathy. *J Neurol*. 2002;249(1):9–17.
129. Lee JJ, Swain SM. Peripheral neuropathy induced by microtubule-stabilizing agents. *J Clin Oncol*. 2006;24(10):1633–1642.
130. Hausheer FH, Schilsky RL, Bain S, et al. Diagnosis, management, and evaluation of chemotherapy-induced peripheral neuropathy. *Semin Oncol*. 2006;33(1):15–49.
131. Gradishar WJ, Tjulandin S, Davidson N, et al. Phase III trial of nanoparticle albumin-bound paclitaxel compared with polyethylated castor oil-based paclitaxel in women with breast cancer. *J Clin Oncol*. 2005;23(31):7794–7803.
132. Wilding G, Caruso R, Lawrence TS, et al. Retinal toxicity after high-dose cisplatin therapy. *J Clin Oncol*. 1985;3(12):1683–1689.

133. Land SR, Kopec JA, Cecchini RS, et al. Neurotoxicity from oxaliplatin combined with weekly bolus fluorouracil and leucovorin as surgical adjuvant chemotherapy for stage II and III colon cancer: NSABP C-07. *J Clin Oncol.* 2007;25(16):2205–2211.
134. Pasetto LM, D'Andrea MR, Rossi E, et al. Oxaliplatin-related neurotoxicity: how and why? *Crit Rev Oncol Hematol.* 2006;59(2):159–168.
135. Krishnan AV, Goldstein D, Friedlander M, et al. Oxaliplatin and axonal Na^+ channel function in vivo. *Clin Cancer Res.* 2006;12(15):4481–4484.
136. Hershman DL, Lacchetti C, Dworkin RH, et al. Prevention and management of chemotherapy-induced peripheral neuropathy in survivors of adult cancers: American Society of Clinical Oncology clinical practice guideline. *J Clin Oncol.* 2014;32(18):1941–1967.
137. Calhoun EA, Welshman EE, Chang CH, et al. Psychometric evaluation of the Functional Assessment of Cancer Therapy/Gynecologic Oncology Group-Neurotoxicity (Fact/GOG-Ntx) questionnaire for patients receiving systemic chemotherapy. *Int J Gynecol Cancer.* 2003;13(6):741–748.
138. Soffietti R, Trevisan E, Ruda R. Neurologic complications of chemotherapy and other newer and experimental approaches. *Handb Clin Neurol.* 2014;121:1199–1218.
139. Santoso JT, Lucci JA III, Coleman RL, et al. Saline, mannitol, and furosemide hydration in acute cisplatin nephrotoxicity: a randomized trial. *Cancer Chemother Pharmacol.* 2003;52(1):13–18.
140. Andriole GL, Sandlund JT, Miser JS, et al. The efficacy of mesna (2-mercaptoethane sodium sulfonate) as a uroprotectant in patients with hemorrhagic cystitis receiving further oxazaphosphorine chemotherapy. *J Clin Oncol.* 1987;5(5):799–803.
141. Bookman MA, Kloth DD, Kover PE, et al. Short-course intravenous prophylaxis for paclitaxel-related hypersensitivity reactions. *Ann Oncol.* 1997;8(6):611–614.
142. Weiss RB, Donehower RC, Wiernik PH, et al. Hypersensitivity reactions from taxol. *J Clin Oncol.* 1990;8(7):1263–1268.
143. Markman M, Kennedy A, Webster K, et al. Clinical features of hypersensitivity reactions to carboplatin. *J Clin Oncol.* 1999;17(4):1141.
144. Rose PG, Fusco N, Smrekar M, et al. Successful administration of carboplatin in patients with clinically documented carboplatin hypersensitivity. *Gynecol Oncol.* 2003;89(3):429–433.
145. Lee CW, Matulonis UA, Castells MC. Rapid inpatient/outpatient desensitization for chemotherapy hypersensitivity: standard protocol effective in 57 patients for 255 courses. *Gynecol Oncol.* 2005;99(2):393–399.
146. Joly F, Ray-Coquard I, Fabbro M, et al. Decreased hypersensitivity reactions with carboplatin-pegylated liposomal doxorubicin compared to carboplatin-paclitaxel combination: analysis from the GCIG CALYPSO relapsing ovarian cancer trial. *Gynecol Oncol.* 2011;122(2):226–232.
147. Rubinstein L, Crowley J, Ivy P, et al. Randomized phase II designs. *Clin Cancer Res.* 2009;15(6):1883–1890.
148. Mandrekar SJ, Dahlberg SE, Simon R. Improving clinical trial efficiency: thinking outside the box. *Am Soc Clin Oncol Educ Book.* 2015:e141–e147.
149. Verweij J. Clinical trials in drug development: a minimalistic approach. *Curr Opin Oncol.* 2012;24(3):332–337.
150. Rowinsky EK, Gilbert MR, McGuire WP, et al. Sequences of taxol and cisplatin: a phase I and pharmacologic study. *J Clin Oncol.* 1991;9(9):1692–1703.
151. Jekunen AP, Christen RD, Shalinsky DR, et al. Synergistic interaction between cisplatin and taxol in human ovarian carcinoma cells in vitro. *Br J Cancer.* 1994;69(2):299–306.
152. Rowinsky EK, Kaufmann SH, Baker SD, et al. Sequences of topotecan and cisplatin: phase I, pharmacologic, and in vitro studies to examine sequence dependence. *J Clin Oncol.* 1996;14(12):3074–3084.
153. Bookman MA, McMeekin DS, Fracasso PM. Sequence dependence of hematologic toxicity using carboplatin and topotecan for primary therapy of advanced epithelial ovarian cancer: a phase I study of the Gynecologic Oncology Group. *Gynecol Oncol.* 2006;103(2):473–478.
154. Zamboni WC, Egorin MJ, Van Echo DA, et al. Pharmacokinetic and pharmacodynamic study of the combination of docetaxel and topotecan in patients with solid tumors. *J Clin Oncol.* 2000;18(18):3288–3294.
155. Markman M, Rose PG, Jones E, et al. Ninety-six-hour infusional paclitaxel as salvage therapy of ovarian cancer patients previously failing treatment with 3-hour or 24-hour paclitaxel infusion regimens. *J Clin Oncol.* 1998;16(5):1849–1851.
156. Eisenhauer EA, ten Bokkel Huinink WW, Swenerton KD, et al. European-Canadian randomized trial of paclitaxel in relapsed ovarian cancer: high-dose versus low-dose and long versus short infusion. *J Clin Oncol.* 1994;12(12):2654–2666.
157. Fennelly D, Aghajanian C, Shapiro F, et al. Phase I and pharmacologic study of paclitaxel administered weekly in patients with relapsed ovarian cancer. *J Clin Oncol.* 1997;15(1):187–192.
158. McGuire WP, Blessing JA, Bookman MA, et al. Topotecan has substantial antitumor activity as first-line salvage therapy in platinum-sensitive epithelial ovarian carcinoma: a Gynecologic Oncology Group study. *J Clin Oncol.* 2000;18(5):1062–1067.
159. Markman M, Blessing JA, Alvarez RD, et al. Phase II evaluation of 24-h continuous infusion topotecan in recurrent, potentially platinum-sensitive ovarian cancer: a Gynecologic Oncology Group study. *Gynecol Oncol.* 2000;77(1):112–115.
160. Miller DS, Blessing JA, Lentz SS, et al. Phase II evaluation of three-day topotecan in recurrent platinum-sensitive ovarian carcinoma: a Gynecologic Oncology Group study. *Cancer.* 2003;98(8):1664–1669.
161. Hochster H, Wadler S, Runowicz C, et al. Activity and pharmacodynamics of 21-day topotecan infusion in patients with ovarian cancer previously treated with platinum-based chemotherapy. New York Gynecologic Oncology Group. *J Clin Oncol.* 1999;17(8):2553–2561.
162. Herzog TJ, Sill MW, Walker JL, et al. A phase II study of two topotecan regimens evaluated in recurrent platinum-sensitive ovarian, fallopian tube or primary peritoneal cancer: a Gynecologic Oncology Group study (GOG 146Q). *Gynecol Oncol.* 2011;120(3):454–458.
163. Sehouli J, Stengel D, Harter P, et al. Topotecan weekly versus conventional 5-day schedule in patients with platinum-resistant ovarian cancer: a randomized multicenter phase II trial of the North-Eastern German Society of Gynecological Oncology Ovarian Cancer Study Group. *J Clin Oncol.* 2011;29(2):242–248.
164. Bookman MA. First-line chemotherapy in epithelial ovarian cancer. *Clin Obstet Gynecol.* 2012;55(1):96–113.
165. Paller CJ, Bradbury PA, Ivy SP, et al. Design of phase I combination trials: recommendations of the Clinical Trial Design Task Force of the NCI Investigational Drug Steering Committee. *Clin Cancer Res.* 2014;20(16):4210–4217.

CHAPTER 14

Pharmacology and Therapeutics in Gynecologic Cancer

David S. Alberts, Hilary Calvert, Maria Lluria-Prevatt, Paul H. Sugarbaker, and Bradley J. Monk

The determinants of effective cancer drug therapies include drug disposition, tumor kinetics, and drug resistance. These factors profoundly influence the cytotoxicity of each anticancer drug and must be considered in designing therapeutic regimens. These principles are discussed in Chapter 15. In this chapter, we elaborate the basic and clinical pharmacology of cancer chemotherapeutic and biologic agents and provide a limited discussion of cytotoxic, molecularly targeted, antiangiogenetic, and modulating/supportive care drugs useful in the treatment of patients with gynecologic cancer.

Determinants of Effective Drug Therapies

Drug Disposition Factors

The term *pharmacokinetics* describes the time course of drug disposition in body fluids and tissues through the use of mathematical models. These models use an equation or set of equations to describe the concentration versus time profile of a specific drug after administration into the body. The models are often illustrated by box diagrams, with each box or compartment corresponding to a region of the body, although the compartments may not represent real anatomic regions. A drug is considered to be uniformly distributed within a compartment if its concentration within tissues has reached homogeneity.

Pharmacokinetic models may be useful in predicting the plasma or tissue concentrations of drugs in the body after any one of several routes or methods of drug administration. The simplest model has one compartment into which the drug is assumed to be instantaneously introduced, and elimination occurs by one linear route. The disappearance of the drug from this compartment can be described by a straight line if plotted on semilogarithmic graph paper. As discussed by Tozer (1), no one-compartment pharmacokinetic model can be used to describe the disposition of commonly used anticancer drugs; nevertheless, the one-compartment pharmacokinetic model lends itself to an understanding of the concept of plasma half-life (i.e., $t_{1/2}$), which represents the time required for the concentration of a drug at any point on the plasma concentration time elimination curve to achieve half its value. This constant may be applied repeatedly, so that, for instance, only 25% of the drug remains in two half-lives. The equation for plasma half-life that can be applied to any linear plasma concentration–time elimination curve is as follows: $t_{1/2}z = 0.693/$ slope of the linear elimination curve (i.e., λ_z or rate constant for that part of the curve). Unfortunately, the determination of the terminal half-life of a drug is often poorly reproducible because it is highly dependent on measuring multiple plasma levels, often at the limit of drug assay sensitivity.

Pharmacokinetic Models

The pharmacokinetics of virtually all anticancer drugs require two- or three-compartment models for their mathematic description. These models are commonly referred to as biphasic or triphasic models (i.e., two or three phases observed on semilogarithmic plots). Conceptually, the one-compartment model relates to a drug that remains confined to the intravascular space after intravenous (IV) injection, and the two- or three-compartment model allows the pharmacokinetic description of anticancer drugs whose ultimate targets are beyond the intravascular space in tumor tissues.

Drug Clearance and Area Under the Curve (AUC)

Wisdom dictates using the simplest mathematical model that can provide the "best" fit of the actual plasma concentration time data using nonlinear least squares regression. After the mathematical model is selected, it is possible to generate the important pharmacokinetic parameters that describe the disposition of a specific anticancer drug within the body. Besides the determination of the terminal-phase plasma half-life (i.e., half-life related to the second or third phase of biphasic or triphasic plasma concentration time data), the area under the plasma disappearance curve ($AUC_0\infty$) and total body plasma clearance (Cl_T) are the most significant and clinically useful pharmacokinetic parameters. The relationship between AUC and clearance is simplified to: dose = clearance × area.

Although the height of an anticancer drug's peak plasma level (C_{max}) generally correlates with peak dose and the degree of toxicity, the drug's plasma AUC tends to correlate better with its ultimate antitumor activity and normal tissue side effects. For example, when identical doses of melphalan are administered first orally and then intravenously at a 1-month interval, because of its poor oral availability, the melphalan plasma AUC after the oral dose would be only one-third of that after the IV dose (**Fig. 14.1**). As would be anticipated, the equivalent IV dose of melphalan was associated with a twofold to threefold deeper nadir in granulocytes and a greater than twofold increase in objective response rates in various cancer types (e.g., myeloma).

The plasma AUC (in mg/mL · h) can be estimated through the use of a pharmacokinetic model or measured directly by plotting the drug's plasma concentrations against time on semilogarithmic graph paper. Then, it is possible to calculate the areas of successive trapezoids under the concentration × time curve wherein the upper surface of the trapezoid is a line that connects two successive plasma concentration data points. By convention, when the plasma AUC is measured in this way, the terminal part of the AUC is calculated using a triangular area, rather than a trapezoid.

After the plasma AUC has been determined, it is possible to derive the anticancer drug's total body clearance rate based on the following formula: $Cl_T = \text{dose (mg)}/\text{AUC (mg/mL} \cdot \text{h)}$. The resulting Cl_T is measured in units of milliliters or liters per minutes or hours, sometimes with normalization to the body surface area. The total body clearance of an anticancer drug depends on the drug's dose and plasma AUC and represents the rate at which the drug is eliminated from the entire body. The drug's total body clearance is made up of the combination of renal clearance (Cl_R) plus nonrenal clearance (Cl_{NR}). The renal clearance of a drug can be calculated by the following equation: $Cl_R = Ae_c/AUC$, where Ae_c is the total amount of the unchanged drug that is excreted in the urine. For many drugs

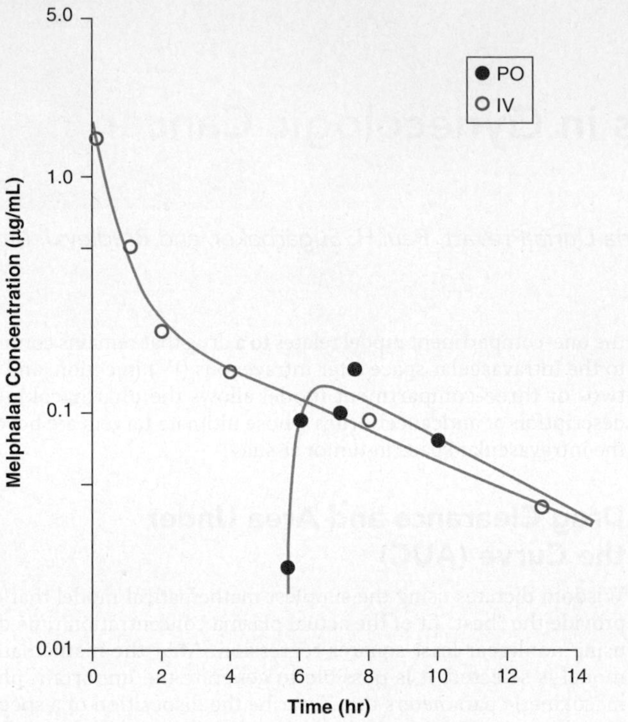

Figure 14.1. Plasma disappearance curves for IV and oral (tablets) melphalan (0.6 mg/kg) in a patient with ovarian cancer. The melphalan plasma AUC associated with the bolus oral dose was only one-third of that associated with the IV dose.

Source: Reprinted with permission from Alberts DS, Chang SY, Chen HS, et al. Oral melphalan kinetics. *Clin Pharmacol Ther*. 1979;26:737–745.

that are glomerularly filtered but not reabsorbed, renal clearance is proportional to creatinine clearance (CrCl). In a patient with severe renal impairment, if nonrenal clearance is unaltered, the total body clearance of the drug is diminished significantly. This phenomenon is observed in patients with relatively severe renal impairment who receive drugs like methotrexate and carboplatin, both of which are eliminated mainly through renal excretion.

Volume of Distribution

The volume of distribution (Vd) of an anticancer drug is another important pharmacokinetic parameter that relates the drug plasma concentration (measured at the time of administration through extrapolation of the terminal phase of the concentration–time curve to 0 time) to the total amount of drug in the body. Thus, Vd_{area} represents the volume of distribution of a drug in the terminal phase of its elimination from the body and in its simplest form, Vd = amount of drug in the body ÷ plasma concentration. Since drug levels are typically measured only in the plasma compartment and not in tissues, most reported Vd values represent the "apparent" Vd of the drug in the plasma. Thus, these Vd values represent a theoretic plasma volume that would account for the drug's plasma levels after administration. The Vd in the terminal phase can be derived using the following equation: Vd_{area} = dose/AUC slope (λ_z), where λ_z is the rate constant in the terminal phase of a biphasic or triphasic elimination curve.

Linear and Nonlinear Kinetics

Most drugs exhibit linear pharmacokinetics, which in its simplest configuration means that the C_{max} and AUC are proportionate to the dose, and the $T_{½}$ Vd and clearance are constant, that is, they do not change with the dose. Linearity helps make predictions about the effects of changes in doses since the AUC (and the biologic effects) of the drug should change in proportion to the dose. Drugs with nonlinear pharmacokinetics such as aspirin, ethanol, and phenytoin have saturable elimination patterns. This means that small dose changes can disproportionately increase the AUC and the drug's biologic effects. Drugs with nonlinear pharmacokinetic patterns may therefore have longer $T_{½}$s and much lower clearance values when the dose is increased.

As discussed by Collins and Dedrick (2), there are at least two explanations for nonlinear kinetics. First, nonlinearity may be caused by changes in drug excretion at high doses. For example, at extremely high doses of methotrexate (i.e., 7 to 8 g/m^2), the drug load outstrips renal tubular secretion capacity. Second, nonlinearity may be observed for drugs that depend almost completely on elimination through a specific degradative enzyme system (e.g., antimetabolites). Drugs like cytarabine and 5-fluorouracil administered in high doses may overcome the capacity of their respective degradative enzymes with a resultant decrease in their total body clearance rates and an increase in plasma levels that are more than proportionate to their doses.

Intraperitoneal Drug Pharmacokinetics

The administration of chemotherapy directly into the abdominal cavity (i.e., intraperitoneal [IP]) is a standard option, particularly for women with optimally cytoreduced ovarian cancer. Anticancer drugs with known activity against ovarian cancer that undergo slow clearance from the IP space into the systemic circulation without causing significant chemical peritonitis are the favored IP compounds. The most commonly administered agent is cisplatin, though both paclitaxel and carboplatin have also been effectively administered via the IP route. The IP administration of cisplatin likely results in approximately 20-fold greater concentrations of cisplatin into the IP space than are achievable with IV administration. Additionally, the IP administration of paclitaxel results in 1,000-fold greater concentration time products in the IP space than is achievable with IV administration (3). Caution must be taken when considering other agents for research-based IP administration, as some cytotoxic agents have not demonstrated efficacy and have been associated with excessive toxicity when given IP (e.g., mitoxantrone, doxorubicin) (4–7).

As with IV administration of anticancer drugs, the drug clearance rate from the IP space is the most useful pharmacokinetic parameter for comparing drugs that are administered by the IP route in the treatment of ovarian cancer. The peritoneal clearance rate can be calculated by dividing the drug dose by its IP concentration · time product, which must be measured with repeated IP fluid content sampling. Intraperitoneal drugs with slow clearance rates are favored because they result in prolonged exposure of the IP tumor bed to high concentrations of anticancer drug. It is also possible to assess the pharmacokinetic characteristics of drug doses by comparing their peak IP concentration with peak plasma concentration after IP dosing or comparing their IP concentration · time product (AUC_{IP}), with their plasma concentration · time products (AUC_{IV}) after IP dosing. Virtually all commonly used drugs administered IP in patients with ovarian cancer have peak or concentration · time product ratios of more than 20. In some cases, the peritoneal exposures can be much greater. For example, paclitaxel IP exposure with IP therapy is 300 to nearly 3,000 times greater than with IV treatment (8).

Except for drugs whose cytotoxicity depends on continuous exposure, such as cytarabine and methotrexate, drugs used by the IP route should be administered relatively rapidly in at least 2 L of peritoneal dialysate and should remain within the peritoneal space without removal. For schedule-independent drugs, it is important to maintain high concentrations as long as possible within the IP space to improve efficacy. It is of considerable interest that as the IP dialysate volume decreases, a drug's IP clearance rate increases rapidly. Thus, large volumes of IP fluid increase the chances for uniform drug distribution throughout the IP space and optimize clearance rates. Generally, it is suggested to administer the IP drug dose in the first liter of peritoneal dialysate, followed by a second liter of dialysate to the point of mild abdominal discomfort.

Ultimately, the effectiveness of IP therapy depends on the inherent cytotoxic potency of the individual agent and its ability to penetrate from the outer surface to the inner core of IP tumors. The degree of tumor penetration depends on the molecular weight, charge, and chemical structure of the compound. There is an inverse relationship between molecular weight and tumor penetration. The higher the molecular weight of the anticancer drug, the lower the degree of tumor penetration.

Hyperthermic Intraoperative Peritoneal Chemotherapy (HIPEC)

For women with advanced ovarian cancer, the ultimate goal of treatment is to manage and prevent peritoneal metastases. However, the same is true for other gynecologic cancers, including endometrial cancer and uterine sarcoma. Cytoreductive surgery with perioperative chemotherapy is a treatment option for these patients. For women undergoing surgical cytoreduction, hyperthermic intraperitoneal chemotherapy (HIPEC) has been used in the operating room as part of the surgical procedure. An alternative procedure is for normothermic early postoperative intraperitoneal chemotherapy (EPIC), which, in contrast, is administered in the first few postoperative days. As surgeons have ascended the learning curve for this combination of extensive surgery combined with perioperative chemotherapy, the mortality has been reduced to 1% or less. Also, the grade III and grade IV adverse events have been reduced to 20% (9). Most recent publications associate the morbidity and mortality with the extensive cytoreductive surgery, and estimate the adverse outcomes from the perioperative chemotherapy to be unusual. Of course, knowledgeable management of both aspects of the combined treatment is an absolute requirement for success.

For HIPEC, agents whose maximal cytotoxic effect is completed with a 60- to 120-minute treatment in the operating room are the ones most often chosen. These chemotherapy agents should be augmented by moderate heat of approximately 42°C, which is maintained in the whole abdomen through the use of a hyperthermia pump (10). The chemotherapy agents used through an IP route or through an IV route in a multiagent HIPEC regimen are listed in **Table 14.1** (11–19).

An important consideration for HIPEC and EPIC concerns the selection of cancer chemotherapy agents that may show drug synergy. The bidirectional treatment with HIPEC and the continuing treatment postoperatively with EPIC present an opportunity to eradicate the peritoneal surface component of gastrointestinal malignancy from the natural history of the disease. As surgeons learn to modify their surgical procedures to ensure a safe cytoreductive procedure, more effective combinations of both IV and IP chemotherapy used in HIPEC become the foci of promising clinical investigations.

TABLE 14.1. Agents Used in HIPEC Therapy AUC Ratio Will Vary With Total Volume of Chemotherapy Solution and Type of Carrier Solution (Colloid vs. Crystalloid)

Agent	Dose (mg/m²)	AUC Ratio (Approximate) (Peritoneal:Plasma)
Mitomycin C	15–30	25
Cisplatin	75–250	8
Doxorubicin	15	150
Melphalan	60	33
Gemcitabine	1,000	500
Oxaliplatin	200–460	16
Ifosfamide (IV)	1,300	–5
5-Fluorouracil (IV)	600	2.3
Paclitaxel	175	1,000
Docetaxel	60	550

Clinical Pharmacology of Active Drugs Against Gynecologic Cancers

We discuss below in alphabetical order the clinical pharmacology of cytotoxic, and modulating/supportive care drugs with demonstrated activity against gynecologic cancers. We also include several Food and Drug Administration (FDA)–approved drugs for other indications that may prove active against gynecologic cancers. Targeted therapies are discussed separately in Chapter 12.

Cytotoxic Agents

Albumin-bound Paclitaxel

Albumin-bound paclitaxel is FDA approved for the treatment of breast cancer after failure of treatment for metastatic disease or recurrence within 6 months of adjuvant chemotherapy. Phase III trials have demonstrated superior efficacy to castor oil–based paclitaxel and a more favorable toxicity profile (20).

Chemistry. Albumin-bound paclitaxel (Abraxane, ABI-007) is a protein-bound form of paclitaxel that measures approximately 130 nanometers. Each vial of albumin-bound paclitaxel contains 100 mg of paclitaxel and 900 mg of human albumin. The chemical name of paclitaxel is 5β,20-Epoxy-1,2α,4,7β,10β,13α-hexahydroxytax-11-en-9-one 4,10-diacetate 2-benzoate 13-ester with (2*R*,3*S*)- *N*-benzoyl-3-phenylisoserine, and the empirical formula and molecular weight are $C_{47}H_{51}NO_{14}$ and 853.91, respectively.

Administration and Dosage. The recommended dosage of albumin-bound paclitaxel is 260 mg/m² IV over 30 minutes every 3 weeks. No premedication to prevent hypersensitivity reactions is needed. Each mL of the reconstituted formulation contains 5 mg/mL paclitaxel. The exact total dosing volume of 5 mg/mL for the patient should be calculated using the following formula: total dose (mg) ÷ 5 (mg/mL). Reconstituted agent should be used immediately, but can be refrigerated for up to 8 hours. If precipitates are observed, the solution should be discarded.

Side Effects and Toxicities. Neutropenia and sensory neuropathy are dose-dependent. In drug-approval studies, grade 4 neutropenia occurred among approximately 9% of patients, as compared with 22% of patients receiving 175 mg/m² paclitaxel. Infection (generally oral candidiasis and respiratory system events) occurred in approximately 23% of patients receiving albumin-bound paclitaxel. Anemia occurred among 33% of patients (severe anemia in 1%). Severe cardiotoxicity occurred in approximately 3% of patients. Dyspnea (12%) and cough (6%) were also reported among patients receiving albumin-bound paclitaxel. Patients with neutrophil counts of less than 1,500 cells/mm³ should not receive albumin-bound paclitaxel, as it may lead to bone marrow suppression, which can result in infection.

Altretamine

Altretamine (hexamethylmelamine, Hexalen), a synthetic cytotoxic antineoplastic s-triazine derivative, has FDA approval for treatment of persistent or recurrent ovarian cancer after first-line chemotherapy with cisplatin or other alkylating agents. The drug also exhibits antitumor activity against breast cancer, lymphomas, small cell carcinoma of the lung, and endometrial and cervical cancer.

Chemistry. The empiric formula of altretamine is $C_9H_{18}N_6$ (molecular weight = 210.28).

Mechanism of Action. The mechanism of action of altretamine is not completely elucidated. Although it bears structural similarity to and cross-reactivity with triethylenemelamine, a classic alkylating agent, evidence demonstrating altretamine to be an alkylating agent is inconclusive. Altretamine does not consistently demonstrate cross-resistance with classic alkylating agents used in rodent tumors or in human cancer treatment, but its clinical antitumor spectrum resembles that of an alkylating agent.

Rutty and Connors (21,22) presented definitive evidence that metabolic activation of altretamine is necessary for its cytotoxic activity. It is extensively demethylated *in vivo* in the presence of liver enzymes, and these *N*-methylolmelamine derivatives are more cytotoxic than the parent compound (22). Additional studies have shown that the reactive methyl intermediates, formed during altretamine *N*-demethylations, covalently bind to tissue macromolecules, including DNA, and that the cytotoxicity against certain human solid tumor cells *in vitro* is dependent on the metabolic formation of the reactive intermediates or their direct addition to cell culture incubate(23).

Drug Disposition. Altretamine is practically insoluble in water and, therefore, it has only been administered orally, precluding absolute bioavailability studies. After administration of altretamine to laboratory animals by any route, urinary recovery of parent drug was very low (<1%), and urinary recovery of total dose or total radioactivity after administration of ^{14}C-labeled drug was as high as 90%. Ames (23) determined that the bioavailability of the parent compound in rabbits after oral administration was 25% of that obtained after IV administration. Moreover, after giving the rabbits labeled altretamine by stomach tube, 85% of labeled drug equivalents was recovered in the urine. The high rate of recovery suggests efficient gastrointestinal absorption.

The urinary recovery and bioavailability data demonstrate that altretamine is well absorbed after oral administration and that the drug is extensively metabolized regardless of route of administration. The low bioavailability of intact altretamine is due to first-pass metabolism rather than to poor absorption.

After oral administration in doses of 120 to 300 mg/m^2, peak plasma levels, measured by gas chromatographic assay, from 0.2 to 20.8 mg/L are reached between 0.5 and 3 hours. The terminal phase plasma half-life ranges from 4.7 to 10.2 hours (24). The interpatient variability of AUCs, ranging from 1.2 to 60.1 mg/L · h, is most likely due to the differences in the rate at which the drug is metabolized.

Administration and Dosage. The recommended dose for altretamine as a single agent for use in ovarian cancer is 260 mg/m^2/d, orally, for 14 to 21 consecutive days in a 28-day cycle (25). The total daily doses should be given as four divided oral doses after meals and at bedtime. In combination regimens, altretamine is typically used at a dose of 150 mg/m^2/d for 7 to 14 days of monthly cycles (26,27).

Side Effects and Toxicities. With high, continuous daily dosing, nausea and vomiting were the dose-limiting toxic effects, and a form of reversible peripheral neurotoxicity occurred occasionally. Myelosuppression was mild to moderate. Leukocyte and platelet counts usually recovered within 1 week of therapy discontinuation.

In a study of 395 patients with advanced ovarian cancer treated with altretamine-containing combination regimens with or without cisplatin, no additional effect of altretamine on the incidence or severity of neurotoxicity could be demonstrated (28). Peripheral neuropathy and central nervous system (CNS) symptoms are more likely to occur in patients receiving continuous, high-dose daily altretamine administered on an intermittent schedule than in those receiving moderate doses. Neurologic toxicity reverses after the drug is discontinued. Pyridoxine should not be used concomitantly with altretamine to reduce neurotoxicity because clinical trials data suggest it may inhibit cytotoxic activity. Concurrent administration of altretamine and antidepressants of the monoamine oxidase inhibitor class may cause severe orthostatic hypotension. Cimetidine, an inhibitor of microsomal drug metabolism, increased altretamine's half-life and toxicity in a rat model.

In two phase II studies of single-agent altretamine, at a dose of 260 mg/m^2 for 14 to 21 days of each monthly cycle, the most common toxicity was grade 2 to 3 nausea (23%) (29,30). In a consolidation therapy phase II trial, only three patients (4%) experienced any grade 4 toxicity: granulocytopenia (two patients) and anxiety/depression (one patient). The most common grade 3 toxicities were malaise, fatigue, or lethargy in seven patients (7%) and nausea in six patients (6%). Aside from these, there were no other grade 3 or 4 toxicities that occurred in more than 5% of patients (30).

With continuous high-dose daily drug administration, nausea and vomiting of gradual onset occur frequently. Although in most instances these symptoms are controllable with antiemetics, the severity sometimes requires altretamine dose reduction or, rarely, discontinuation.

Altretamine should be temporarily discontinued for 14 days or longer and subsequently restarted with a 20% to 25% dose reduction for any of the following side effects: gastrointestinal intolerance unresponsive to symptomatic measures, leukocyte count less than 2,000/mm^3 or granulocyte count less than 1,000/mm^3, platelet count less than 75,000/mm^3, or progressive neurotoxicity. If neurologic symptoms fail to stabilize on the reduced-dose schedule, altretamine should be discontinued.

Bleomycin

Bleomycin is used as palliative treatment in patients with advanced cervical (31) and vulvar cancers. Other clinical indications include squamous cell carcinomas of the head and neck, gestational trophoblast neoplasia, lymphomas, germ cell and sex cord stromal tumors.

Chemistry. Bleomycin (Blenoxane), an antineoplastic, is a mixture of complex glycopeptides originally isolated from a strain of the fungus *Streptomyces verticillis*. The primary components are bleomycins A_2 and B_2. The family of bleomycin glycopeptides have a relatively high molecular weight and are quantitated in units of cytotoxic activity (i.e., roughly 1 U/1 mg of polypeptide protein). The molecular formula of bleomycin A_2 is $C_{55}H_{84}N_{17}O_{21}S_3$ (molecular weight = 1,414), and the molecular formula of bleomycin B_2 is $C_{55}H_{84}N_{20}O_{21}S_2$ (molecular weight = 1,425).

Mechanism of Action. Although the exact mechanism of action is unknown, a key to its activity is the isolation of native compounds from *S. verticillis* as coordinated Cu(II) complexes, which are inactive as antitumor agents. When complexed with ferrous iron, bleomycin becomes a potent oxidase, producing DNA strand breaks by oxygen free radicals. Its unique mechanism of action is schedule dependent and cell cycle dependent for the G_2 phase.

The oxygen radicals produced by the bleomycin–iron complex bound to DNA primarily cause single-strand breaks and a lesser degree of double-strand breaks. There is a subsequent release of base propenals of all four DNA bases: guanine, thymine, adenine, and cytosine. These modified free bases result from cleavage of the deoxyribose sugar at the 3′-4′ bond. There is an apparent specificity for the release of thymine and for DNA binding at guanine-rich sequences in actively transcribed genes (32). The linker regions of DNA between nucleosomes comprise an important site for specific strand cleavage by bleomycin (33). Several mechanisms have been theorized to explain the development of resistance to bleomycin. Less important mechanisms appear to include DNA repair, membrane alterations, and decreased drug accumulation. The primary mechanism probably involves metabolic inactivation of bleomycin by a cytosolic hydrolase, which is in the cysteine proteinase family. The enzyme inactivates bleomycin by replacing a terminal amine with a hydroxyl group. The distribution of bleomycin hydrolase appears to explain some of the relative resistance and sensitivity to bleomycin in normal tissues. Normal tissues with high intrinsic hydrolase activities, such as the liver, spleen, intestine, and bone marrow, are not targets for bleomycin's toxic effects. In contrast, lung tissues and skin have low levels of hydrolase activity and are particularly susceptible to bleomycin-induced toxicity. However, there appears to be no direct correlation between hydroxylase levels in tumor cells and bleomycin-induced cytotoxicity (33). The development of other methods of bleomycin metabolism by tumor cells may be responsible for the emergence of drug resistance (34).

Drug Disposition. Bleomycin is eliminated predominantly by urinary excretion. This accounts for 45% to 62% of a dose after 24 hours. In the blood, the drug is rapidly cleared, and two phases of elimination are apparent. As a practical point, this means that over 95% of a dose has been completely eliminated by 24 hours (about six half-lives) (35). If administered by an intracavitary route, a large percentage of a bleomycin dose is absorbed, and the fractional systemic bioavailability is about 45% for intrapleural or IP injections. The drug appears to efflux more slowly from the peritoneal cavity. This suggests that there is significantly greater local drug retention in the IP space. This may explain some of the drug's unique efficacy by intracavitary administration (36,37). An increased exposure to drug in these local compartments is also reflected by the tenfold higher drug levels achieved with IP or intrapleural therapy than with equivalent IV dosing.

Renal insufficiency markedly alters bleomycin elimination (38,39). This effect becomes most pronounced in patients with CrCl values less than 25 to 35 mL/min (38). In these patients, the Vd is unaltered at about 20 L, but the half-life varies as the inverse exponent of CrCl. Thus, significant bleomycin dose reductions are required in all patients with reduced renal function.

Dosage. Bleomycin (in combination with cisplatin and etoposide or vinblastine) is used most commonly by bolus IV administration at dosages of as high as 30 mg/wk for up to 12 weeks in the treatment of patients with germ cell tumors of the ovary. These 30-mg doses often are associated with delayed febrile episodes that can be inhibited successfully with a morning dose of dexamethasone or prednisone.

Bleomycin continues to be used commonly by continuous IV infusion at dosages of 10 mg/m^2/d for 4 consecutive days, with courses repeated every 4 weeks. This schedule has proven successful in the treatment of women with metastatic cervical cancer. Total bleomycin doses should usually not exceed 400 mg to avoid serious pulmonary toxicity.

Bleomycin can also be administered by the intramuscular (IM) route in doses of 15 to 30 mg. Absorption appears to be complete, and because of its lack of vesicant activity, the IM route has proven to be extremely safe (40).

Side Effects and Toxicities. Bleomycin's dose-limiting side effect is pulmonary toxicity, which occurs in approximately 10% of treated patients and in rare instances can result in death. The likelihood of lung damage increases with advanced age, chest irradiation (41), hyperoxia during surgical anesthesia (42,43), renal insufficiency, and cumulative doses greater than 400 U. However, pulmonary toxicity is variable and may occur in younger patients following low cumulative doses. Bleomycin-induced lung damage presents as pneumonitis with dry cough, dyspnea, and rales and may progress within weeks to pulmonary fibrosis. Bleomycin should be discontinued at the first clinical signs of lung toxicity. Acute pneumonitis is often responsive to corticosteroid therapy; however, there is no effective therapy for the chronic pulmonary fibrosis that may result for bleomycin therapy (44). As a result, pulmonary function tests should be obtained before the initiation of treatment, and on day one of each subsequent cycle.

Bleomycin is nonmyelosuppressive (a factor that facilitates its use in combination chemotherapeutic regimens). Mucocutaneous toxicities, including mucositis, are the primary acute side effects of bleomycin. Manifestations of cutaneous reactions include hyperpigmentation, erythema, rash, striae, pruritus, thickening of the nail beds, and, in rare instances, scleroderma (45). Fever, chills, and alopecia are common. Mild nausea, vomiting, and anorexia may also occur, but are typically self-limiting. Infrequent side effects include headache, pain at tumor site, and anaphylactoid reactions. An idiosyncratic reaction consisting primarily of mucositis and skin rash has also been reported (46).

Because up to 70% of a bleomycin dose is eliminated by renal excretion, bleomycin dose should be reduced for individuals with severe renal insufficiency. Unfortunately, there are no prospectively evaluated dosing nomograms for bleomycin dose adjustment. An empirical dose-adjustment formula has been described (38). The percentage dose reductions that are indicated by applying this formula to a "normal" CrCl of 120 mL/min and a fractional urinary drug excretion of 0.45 are: CrCl >35 mL/min, no dose reduction required; CrCl = 20 mL/min, 50% dose reduction; CrCl = 15 mL/min, 52% dose reduction; CrCl = 10 mL/min, 55% dose reduction; and CrCl = 5 mL/min, 60% dose reduction. This is only a general guide, and it has not been clinically validated in a prospective study or retrospective analysis. Patients over 65 years of age may be at increased risk of developing orthostatic hypotension, especially when the recommended rate of IV infusion is exceeded.

Drug Interactions. Nephrotoxic drugs may significantly reduce the rate of bleomycin clearance and thus increase toxicity. Yee and coworkers (47) observed markedly reduced bleomycin clearance in children who had received six courses of a regimen including cisplatin (cumulative dose 300 mg/m^2). In another case report, fatal bleomycin pulmonary toxicity occurred in a patient with cisplatin-induced acute renal failure (48). Similar toxic interactions should be anticipated for combinations of bleomycin with other nephrotoxic drugs, such as aminoglycosides, amphotericin, or cyclosporine.

Capecitabine

Capecitabine (Xeloda) is an orally administered antineoplastic agent. In patients with metastatic breast cancer, capecitabine in combination with docetaxel is indicated after failure of prior anthracycline-containing chemotherapy, and monotherapy is indicated for those who are resistant to paclitaxel and are resistant to anthyracycline-containing chemotherapy (or further anthyracycline-containing chemotherapy is not indicated).

Chemistry. Capecitabine is a fluoropyrimidine carbamate prodrug form of 5′-deoxy-5-fluorouridine (5′-DFUR) that is enzymatically converted to 5-flurouracil (5-FU) *in vivo*. Its chemical name is 5′-deoxy-5-fluoro-*N*-[(pentyloxy) carbonyl]-cytidine, and its molecular weight is 359.35.

Mechanism of Action. Capecitabine itself is inactive, but after absorption in the gastrointestinal tract is metabolized to 5-FU by three enzymes: carboxylesterase, which converts capecitabine to 5′-deoxy-5-fluorocytidine in the liver; is converted to 5′-deoxy-5-fluorouridine by cytidine deaminase in the liver and tumor tissue; and thymidine phosphorylase, which in many cases is highly expressed in tumors, completes the final step of conversion to 5-FU. Theoretically, capecitabine therapy is likely to be most effective in patients with tumors that express high concentrations of thymidine phosphorylase (resulting in greater 5-FU being generated in the tumor) and low concentrations of dihydropyrimidine dehydrogenase (which rapidly breaks down 5-FU) (49). 5-FU acts as a false pyrimidine or antimetabolite ultimately to inhibit the formation of the DNA-specific nucleoside base thymidine. The metabolites of 5-FU, 5-fluoro-21-deoxyuridine-5′-monophosphate (FdUMP) and 5-fluorouridine triphosphate (FUTP), inhibit thymidylate synthase (TS) and are incorporated into cellular RNA. DNA synthesis and function are inhibited by the incorporation of FdUNP into cellular DNA (50). A pharmacogenetic study of capecitabine in 105 consecutive patients has shown an increase in toxicity in patients homozygous for the TS 3RG allele, also showing that a patient with a DPD IVS14 + 1G>A mutation died from toxicity, emphasizing the importance of polymorphisms in the metabolizing enzymes of this drug (51).

Drug Disposition. After oral administration, capecitabine reaches peak blood levels in about 1.5 hours, and peak 5-FU levels are reached at about 2 hours. Food reduces the rate and extent of absorption for both capecitabine and 5-FU. Plasma protein binding is not dose dependent and is less than 60% for capecitabine and its metabolites. Capecitabine (95.5% of administered dose) and its metabolites are excreted in urine. Capecitabine has no effect on the pharmacokinetics of docetaxel or vice versa. The precise pharmacokinetics of capecitabine have been difficult to establish, which is thought to be due to the large interindividual and intraindividual variation in expression of the enzyme dihydropyrimidine dehydrogenase (49).

Administration and Dosage. Capecitabine is available as 150- and 500-mg tablets for oral use. The recommended dose is 2,500 mg/m^2 daily to be administered as two doses: 1,250 mg/m^2 in the morning and 1,250 mg/m^2 in the evening for 2 weeks, followed by a 1-week rest (21-day cycle). Because of the high rate of grade 2 or greater capecitabine-induced palmar–plantar erythrodysesthesia (PPE), recommendations have been made to reduce the starting dose to 2,000 mg/m^2 daily. It should be taken with water within 30 minutes after a meal. The same dosage of capecitabine should be used when combined with docetaxel, which should be administered at 75 mg/m^2 as a 1-hour infusion on day 1 of the 21-day cycle. Premedication (per docetaxel labeling) should be started prior to docetaxel administration for patients receiving the combination therapy.

Side Effects and Toxicities. The only side effect that occurs more frequently with capecitabine than with IV 5-FU is PPE (15% to 20% of patients). The other more common side effects of capecitabine include diarrhea (40%) and nausea and vomiting (30% to 40%). Grade 3 hyperbilirubinemia occurred in 15.2% and grade 4 in 3.9% of patients in the clinical safety database of Xeloda. Of those patients experiencing grades 3 and 4 hyperbilirubinemia, many (64% and 71%, respectively) had liver metastases at baseline, and 57.5% and 35.5% had elevations in alkaline phosphatase or transaminases, respectively. Other less common side effects include myelosuppression (less frequent than with IV 5-FU), leukopenia, and cardiotoxicity. In general, capecitabine is relatively well tolerated.

Carboplatin

Carboplatin (Paraplatin) is a platinum-based agent that is approved by the FDA for the treatment of patients with advanced ovarian cancer of epithelial origin. It is also active against metastatic endometrial and cervical cancer.

Chemistry. Carboplatin has a molecular formula of $C_6H_{12}N_2O_4Pt$ and a molecular weight of 371.25. Its chemical name is cis-diammine-(1,1-cyclobutanedicarboxylato) platinum(II). The water solubility of carboplatin (14 mg/mL) is approximately 10 times that of cisplatin.

Mechanism of Action. Carboplatin, like cisplatin, produces an equal number of predominantly interstrand DNA cross-links rather than DNA-protein cross-links, causing equivalent lesions and biologic effects. The differences in potencies appear to be related to the aquation rate, which is significantly higher for cisplatin as compared with carboplatin (52). It covalently binds to DNA with preferential binding to the N-7 position of guanine and adenine (50). Like cisplatin, carboplatin must first undergo sequential losses of the nonamine carboxylato ligands. Although this process proceeds readily with the loss of the chlorides in cisplatin, the rate of leaving or "opening" of the carboxylato moieties in carboplatin is much slower (53). The molar potency of carboplatin in creating DNA lesions and cytotoxicity was observed to be roughly 2% of cisplatin *in vitro* and 25% to 33% of cisplatin *in vivo* (54,55). A more striking difference is the markedly delayed onset of peak cross-linking for carboplatin compared with cisplatin. With carboplatin, maximal DNA cross-linking occurs 18 hours after exposure compared with 6 to 12 hours for cisplatin (55). In addition, carboplatin-induced DNA cross-links appear to have a slower rate of resolution than cisplatin-induced cross-links. This slower onset and offset of carboplatin cross-linking is believed to be a direct result of a slow rate of monofunctional adduct formation or a slower rate of conversion of monoadducts to cross-links.

Although the final DNA adducts formed by cisplatin and carboplatin are the same, there are large differences in the kinetics of their formation and the rate of conversion of mono- to di- adducts (56) that could impact on the ability of various DNA repair enzymes to cause resistance. Further, cell membrane transport proteins are thought to be critical determinants of platinum drug sensitivity and resistance. It is known that cisplatin and carboplatin differ in their transport characteristics (57). Leblanc et al. (58) showed that substantial hepatic P450 induction occurred in rats following cisplatin treatment, but not following carboplatin. Waxman et al. (59) showed that cisplatin induced glutathione S-transferase (GST) Yc expression in the liver of rats, but carboplatin did not. These data may be significant because GSTs are thought to contribute to platinum resistance. Natarajan et al. (60) extended the latter observation by showing that S-containing nucleophiles (thiourea, glutathione, and human breast cancer MCF-7 cell cytoplasmic extracts) significantly decreased the formation of DNA platinum adducts from cisplatin, but significantly increased them from carboplatin. Despite the pharmacokinetic and mechanistic differences between carboplatin and cisplatin, phase III studies and meta-analyses of clinical studies reveal equivalent activity between carboplatin and cisplatin in all prognostic subgroups of ovarian cancer patients (61,62). However, meta-analysis is performed on pooled data. It is entirely plausible that subsets of ovarian cancers with differing genetic phenotypes will respond differentially to cisplatin and carboplatin.

Harrap (63) described nuclear protein phosphorylation after treatment with both cisplatin and carboplatin. These events appear to correlate with cell killing (64). Carboplatin reacts with two sites on DNA to produce cross-links, as has been observed with cisplatin (65). The formation of DNA adducts results in the inhibition of DNA synthesis and function and inhibits transcription (50). These lesions involve a bifunctional platinum adduct to a single-strand DNA. This may produce transcriptional miscoding and an inhibition of DNA synthesis. It is possible that the cytotoxic effects of carboplatin are the result of binding to nuclear and cytoplasmic proteins. Carboplatin-induced cytotoxicity is not cell cycle phase specific, but it can be maximized by exposing cells in S phase to the drug.

Drug Disposition. The pharmacokinetics of carboplatin differ significantly from those of cisplatin. **Table 14.2** shows that the plasma clearance of carboplatin is biphasic and slower than that of cisplatin, with a much higher percentage of drug being excreted in the urine. Unlike cisplatin, carboplatin binds to plasma proteins relatively slowly so that in the first 24 hours after administration, there is a considerable concentration of the free drug circulating. The major route of elimination of carboplatin is glomerular filtration and tubular secretion. There is little or no true metabolism of the drug. The carboxylato bonds in carboplatin are slowly hydrolyzed to yield transient aquated intermediates. These activated platinum species are believed to lead directly to irreversible adducts to DNA or protein. Overall, the rate of hydrolysis of carboplatin is significantly slower than that of cisplatin, leading to much slower reactivity with DNA (66). Because at least 65% of a carboplatin dose is excreted in the urine, significant dose adjustments are recommended for patients with CrCl values less than 60 mL/min. However, since the widespread use of formula-based dosing (see Administration and

TABLE 14.2. Carboplatin Pharmacokinetics

Cumulative 24-hour Urinary Excretion	65% (if Creatinine Clearance >60 mL/min)
In vitro half-life (H_2O)	~24 hours
Plasma half-life β phase (free drug)	180 minutes
Protein-bound drug	>5 days
Volume of distribution	16–20 L
Protein binding	30% (slow equilibration)

Dosage section, below), these reductions are implicit in the use of the formula and need not be separately calculated.

Carboplatin is widely distributed in body fluids and achieves good penetration into pleural effusions and ascites fluid (67,68). Pharmacokinetic studies in patients receiving continuous carboplatin infusions show that, although total platinum levels increase over the course of the infusion, free or active platinum levels can decrease from 78% on day 1 to 38% on day 4 of a 4-day infusion.

Administration and Dosage. Carboplatin is usually administered as a brief infusion in a solution of 0.9% sodium chloride or 5% dextrose in water. The drug is typically diluted in 500 mL of fluid and infused IV over 15 to 30 minutes to 1 hour without further hydration (69,70). Carboplatin has also been administered as a continuous 24-hour IV infusion for 1, 4, or 5 days or as a continuous IV infusion for 21 days.

The Calvert equation is the most frequently used formula for carboplatin dosing, inasmuch as it requires minimal calculations, results in predictable levels of myelosuppression, and prevents underdosing or overdosing in patients with excellent or poor renal function, respectively (71). The Calvert formula appears below along with general guidelines for selecting the specific carboplatin AUC.

Carboplatin total dose (mg) = AUC (mg/mL · min) × [GFR (mL/min) + 25] AUC = 7 when carboplatin is used as a single agent in patients with good bone marrow reserve; 6 when carboplatin is used in combination regimens in patients with good bone marrow reserve or when used as a single agent in patients who have had prior moderate chemotherapy; and 4 when carboplatin is used as a single agent in patients with prior heavy chemotherapy exposure.

Glomerular filtration rate (GFR) can be determined by measuring CrCl (i.e., [^{51}Cr]-ethylenediamine-tetraacetic acid) for all patients or estimated CrCl for patients who have had no prior cisplatin exposure or have not had cisplatin for at least 2 months before carboplatin dose determination.

As an example, if the desired carboplatin AUC is 6 for a patient with an estimated CrClof 75 mL/min, the total carboplatin dose would equal 6 × (75 + 25), or 600 mg.

As already noted,, the Calvert formula uses the following estimate of carboplatin clearance: Cl = GFR + 25. Although the method may be optimal (72), isotopic determination of the GFR as measured by [^{51}Cr]-ethylenediamine-tetraacetic acid (^{51}Cr-EDTA) is not available in many countries, and the estimated CrCl is often substituted for the GFR. A commonly used method for estimating CrCl is the Cockroft–Gault (CG) equation (73):

$$CrCl = \frac{(140 - Age) \times Wt \times (1 - 0.15 \times Sex)}{(72 \times SCr \times 0.0113)}$$

CrCl = Creatinine clearance; Age = Age in years; Sex = 1 if female, 0 if male; SCr = Serum
Creatinine in mmol/L; Wt = Weight in kg.

Both the CG calculation of CrCl and the CrCl based on a 24-hour urine collection result in a systematic underestimation of the carboplatin AUC by approximately 10% (74–76). This level of bias may be deemed acceptable in view of the clinical utility of substituting CrCl for GFR. Significantly, the accuracy of the CG calculation depends on the method used for measuring creatinine. When the CG formula was derived, a colorimetric reaction was used that significantly overestimates the plasma level of creatinine. A more accurate measurement uses an enzymatic method (77). The use of a more accurate method combined with the CG formula leads to an unexpectedly high dose of carboplatin. Recently, creatinine measurements in the USA have been standardized using isotope dilution mass spectrometry, leading to potential overdosage in some trial protocols and a recommendation for a dose cap (78). The issue of using a creatinine-based estimate of the GFR has been approached by Wright et al. (77) where alternatives to the CG formula are proposed for use with differing creatinine assays.

The Calvert formula was prospectively evaluated by Sorenson et al. (79) in 24 previously untreated ovarian cancer patients and was found to predict more accurately carboplatin exposure than calculation of dose based on body surface area. The AUC of carboplatin as calculated by the Calvert formula accurately predicted the level of myelosuppression as determined by the relative decrease in the platelet count (79).

Side Effects and Toxicities. Although the activity is comparable to cisplatin, carboplatin is better tolerated, as measured by toxicity (e.g., low incidence of alopecia [80]) and quality-of-life analysis (62). The usual dose-limiting toxicity of carboplatin is bone marrow suppression, particularly thrombocytopenia (81). Leukopenia and anemia also occur but are less severe.

The platelet nadir is achieved 2 to 3 weeks after an IV bolus injection, and recovery is generally complete 4 to 5 weeks after dosing. However, patients with poor bone marrow reserve from previous chemotherapy or radiation therapy can have more profound thrombocytopenia and leukopenia with carboplatin treatment. Cell depletion may persist for several weeks after dosing.

Nausea and vomiting induced by carboplatin is much less severe than with cisplatin and rarely lasts beyond 24 hours. In a study of 943 ovarian cancer patients randomized to carboplatin, only 9% experienced greater than grade 2 nausea and/or vomiting (80). Emesis can usually be blocked entirely with aggressive therapy using antiemetic drug combinations (82). Diarrhea has been reported in only 6% of patients, and constipation in 3% of carboplatin-treated patients (83).

Nephrotoxicity has been reported with carboplatin, but it is much less common and less severe than with cisplatin. In a large review, transient elevations in serum creatinine and blood urea nitrogen were described in 7% and 16% of patients, respectively (83). Measured CrCl s dropped in 25% of patients, and a slight increase in uric acid was described in the same percentage of patients. However, there can be a significant loss of serum electrolytes, including potassium (16% of patients) and magnesium (37%). Serum calcium is only rarely decreased after carboplatin (83).

A few cases of carboplatin-induced hematuria have been described. Hepatic enzyme elevations occasionally occur with carboplatin (83). Alkaline phosphatase was transiently increased in 36% of patients, and serum glutamic oxaloacetic transaminase (SGOT) or serum glutamic pyruvic transaminase (SGPT) in about 15% of patients. Serum bilirubin levels are rarely elevated (4%) (83).

Neurotoxicity is uncommon after carboplatin and was described in only 25 of 428 (6%) patients treated on a variety of schedules for different tumor types (83). Mild paresthesias have been reported in a few patients receiving cumulative carboplatin doses of more than 1.6 g/m^2 (81). Unlike cisplatin, these peripheral nerve toxicities rarely produce any disabling symptoms. In most cases, no neurotoxicity was attributed to the drug.

Ototoxicity does not appear to be problematic with carboplatin, and only 8 of 710 (1.1%) patients have described clinical hearing deficits, mainly tinnitus (83). However, if pretreatment and serial audiometric tests are performed, as many as 15% of the patients may have some decrease in audio acuity. Fortunately, ototoxicity from carboplatin sometimes improves after therapy is halted. Like cisplatin, greater ototoxicity from carboplatin can be expected in patients with preexisting hearing loss or in those concurrently being given other ototoxic drugs, such as aminoglycosides.

Other rare carboplatin toxicities include alopecia (2% of patients), mucositis (2%), skin rash (1.7%), injection site irritation without extravasation necrosis (0.4%), and a flu-like syndrome (1.3%) (83). The same study described alterations in taste sensation. Skin disorders from carboplatin treatment may appear as an erythematous rash in exposed areas, and do not occur in all patients who had developed similar rashes on cisplatin (81).

Although carboplatin-associated hypersensitivity reactions rarely occur when the drug is administered as part of an initial chemotherapeutic regimen, subsequent administration of carboplatin in the setting of second-line or salvage therapy is associated with an increased risk of hypersensitivity. It has been estimated that over 25% of patients who receive more than six courses of platinum-based (i.e., cisplatin or carboplatin) chemotherapy develop sensitivity to carboplatin (84). The onset of symptoms may occur during the carboplatin infusion or up to 3 days after drug administration. Mild reactions consist of localized itching and erythema, primarily of the palms and soles, and/or facial flushing, whereas severe reactions can cause diffuse erythema, tachycardia, wheezing, facial edema, chills, rigors, throat and chest tightness, dyspnea, vomiting, alterations in blood pressure (both hypotension and hypertension), and, in extreme cases, respiratory arrest. Mild cases may respond to IV diphenhydramine (50 mg) or oral diphenhydramine (25 to 50 mg every 4 to 6 hours), and additional courses of carboplatin can be administered. Severe hypersensitivity reactions typically necessitate the discontinuance of carboplatin; however, some patients are able to receive additional courses of carboplatin preceded by the administration of corticosteroids for several days prior to carboplatin administration. Hypersensitivity reactions may also occur when carboplatin is administered by the IP route (85).

Platinum-based chemotherapy (either cisplatin or carboplatin) has been shown to increase the risk of leukemia in ovarian cancer patients (86) Following carboplatin-based chemotherapy, the estimated relative risk of leukemia is 6.5 (95% CI, 1.1 to 9.4). The relative risk increases as a function of both cumulative dose and duration of treatment. Patients who receive 4,000 mg or greater of carboplatin have a relative risk of 7.6 of developing leukemia, whereas patients who receive more than 12 months of carboplatin-based chemotherapy have a relative risk of 7. Although radiation therapy alone does not increase the risk of leukemia, radiation therapy administered in combination with platinum-based chemotherapy is associated with a significantly higher risk of leukemia than platinum-based chemotherapy without radiation ($p = 0.006$). The average time to onset of secondary leukemia is 4 years after the diagnosis of ovarian cancer. Although the potential benefits of platinum-based chemotherapy for ovarian cancer far outweigh the risk of secondary leukemia, the dose-dependent leukemogenic potential of platinum-based chemotherapy should be considered during its administration to patients with early-stage disease.

Drug Interactions. Although the pharmacokinetics of carboplatin are not altered by coadministration of paclitaxel, patients who receive combination chemotherapy with carboplatin plus paclitaxel experience less thrombocytopenia than would be predicted if carboplatin was administered as a single agent (74,87). The relationship between free platinum exposure and thrombocytopenia following carboplatin/paclitaxel chemotherapy can be described by a sigmoid maximum effect model (74). In that the degree of neutropenia appears to be unaffected by coadministration of paclitaxel and carboplatin, this pharmacodynamic interaction is believed to occur at the megakaryocyte level (87).

The cytoprotective agent amifostine reduces carboplatin-induced thrombocytopenia (88) but also extends the plasma half-life of carboplatin (89). In a randomized trial of carboplatin with or without amifostine, the median platelet nadir of patients treated with carboplatin 500 mg/m^2 was 88,000/μL, whereas the nadir in patients who received amifostine 910 mg/m^2 was 127,000/μL ($p = 0.023$) (88). Pharmacokinetic studies have shown that amifostine administered just before the carboplatin infusion and 2 to 4 hours thereafter is associated with a significant increase in the terminal half-life of the ultrafiltrable platinum species (e.g., in patients with a CrCl less than 80 mL/min, the platinum half-life increased from 4.2 to 5.6 hours with the addition of amifostine). In patients with good renal function, the impact of the increase in terminal half-life was associated with a minimal effect on the AUC. However, patients with impaired renal function experienced significant increases in the AUC of the ultrafiltrable platinum species (89).

Special Applications. Patients with advanced ovarian cancer have been treated with IP carboplatin in doses ranging from 200 to 650 mg/m^2 (90). Pharmacologic studies have demonstrated that serum concentrations are equivalent between IV and IP carboplatin regimens, but IP administration results in more than 10 times the concentration in the peritoneal cavity as compared with IV administration (91). However, cisplatin may be a better choice for IP delivery in that it appears to have significantly better penetration into tumor masses than carboplatin (92). Several early-phase trials show potentially promising results (93,94); however, there is a need for phase 3 research to determine the possible efficacy of IP carboplatin, and trials to determine the optimal dosing schedule.

Cisplatin

Cisplatin (Platinol, *cis*-diamminedichloroplatinum II) is a primary drug in the treatment of advanced cancer of the ovary, cervix, and endometrium.

Chemistry. Cisplatin has the molecular formula $PtCl_2H_6N_2$ (molecular weight = 300.1). It is a planar inorganic heavy metal complex containing a central atom of platinum surrounded by two chloride atoms and two ammonia molecules in the *cis* position. It is soluble in water at a concentration of 1 mg/mL. Only the *cis*-isomer is therapeutically active.

Mechanism of Action. Cisplatin's interaction with DNA is probably its primary mode of action. The antitumor effect of cisplatin has been correlated with binding to DNA and the production of intrastrand cross-links and formation of DNA adducts, similar to carboplatin (65,95). Intrastrand cisplatin adducts can cause changes in DNA conformation that may affect DNA replication (96). Platinum DNA adduct levels have been measured in patients' leukocytes and correlated with clinical response (95).

Mechanisms of cisplatin drug resistance are the foci of concentrated research. Methods by which tumor cells may develop resistance to platinum agents include decreased drug accumulation, increased glutathione levels, enhanced DNA repair, and increased capacity to tolerate DNA damage (97,98).

The ERCC1 repair protein is part of the nucleotide excision repair system, which takes part in single-strand break repair. It is thought that this system may be responsible for the removal of intrastrand DNA platinum adducts from DNA. High expression of ERCC1 has been associated with platinum resistance and poorer survival in ovarian cancer patients treated with platinum-based regimens (99) [H10]. ERCC-1 has also been identified as playing a critical role in the synergy of gemcitabine and cisplatin. Phase 2 data suggest that gemcitabine may reverse cisplatin resistance, as gemcitabine–cisplatin combination therapy was active in platinum-resistant ovarian cancer patients (100).

Resistance to platinum drugs has also been associated with the activity of the double-strand break repair system, homologous recombination (HR) repair. Tumors arising in patients with germline *BRCA1* and *BRCA2* mutations respond better to platinum-based therapy and survive longer on treatment than their BRCA wild-type counterparts (101–103). Both *BRCA1* and *BRCA2* are involved in HR, and patients whose tumors contain somatic *BRCA*1/2 mutations or who show impaired HR ("BRCA-ness") also respond better and survive longer on platinum-based therapy than case controls (104,105). The idea that platinum resistance may be mediated by HR is supported by the observation of secondary mutations that reactivate either the *BRCA1* (106) or the *BRCA2* (107,108) proteins when these patients eventually become resistant to platinum drugs.

In vitro studies have shown that the copper transporter, CTR1, plays a regulatory role with respect to the uptake of platinum drugs (109). In a study of 40 patients with ovarian carcinoma, Yoo-Young Lee et al. (110) showed that high CTR1 expression was specifically associated with sensitivity to platinum-based therapy and prolonged progression-free survival while low CTR1 expression and high STR2 expression were associated with resistance to platinum-based therapy and shorter survival.

Mechanisms of resistance also include the increased inactivation of thiol-containing proteins such as glutathione and glutathione-related enzymes, a deficiency in mismatch repair enzymes (e.g., hMHL1, hMSH2), and decreased drug accumulation due to alterations in cellular transport (50).

A study of hMLH1 methylation in the plasma DNA of ovarian cancer patients at presentation and relapse showed no correlation with outcome at presentation, but high methylation was associated with poorer outcome following relapse (111). Whether this was due to resistance to platinum drugs is not clear because the report does not document the treatments given following relapse. Further, a follow-on randomized Phase 2 study using decitabine to induce demethylation of the HMLH1 promoter showed an inferior outcome in the decitabine arm (112). The clinical relevance of mismatch repair defects in the response to platinum agents remains uncertain.

Recent evidence also suggests that resistance to platinum and other agents may be mediated by factors in the tumor environment rather than in the tumor cell itself. Roodhart et al. (113) have identified two distinct platinum-induced polyunsaturated fatty acids, 12-oxo-5,8,10-heptadecatrienoic acid (KHT), and hexadeca-4,7,10,13-tetraenoic acid (16:4(n-3)), that in minute quantities induce resistance to a broad spectrum of chemotherapeutic agents, including platinum agents.

Drug Disposition. Cisplatin demonstrates a triphasic disappearance curve with a $t_{1/2\alpha}$ of 20 minutes, a $t_{1/2\beta}$ of 48 to 70 minutes, and a terminal-phase half-life of 24 hours (114). The first two phases of disappearance represent clearance of free drug from the plasma, and the third phase is probably removal of drug from the plasma proteins. The ratio of cisplatin to total free platinum in plasma has a great deal of interpatient variability: from 0.5 to 1.1 after a dose of 100 mg/m^2. Three hours after a bolus injection and 2 hours after a 3-hour infusion, 90% of the plasma protein is bound to the platinum in cisplatin, not the cisplatin itself. The complexes between albumin and platinum are slowly eliminated with a minimum half-life of 5 days or more (115). Ninety percent of the drug that is excreted is removed by renal mechanisms (i.e., glomerular filtration and tubular secretion), and less than 10% is removed by biliary excretion. Fecal excretion appears to be insignificant. The total proportion of a given dose that is excreted is variable and has been reported to be between 31 and 85% after 51 days (116). The remainder remains bound to tissues for very long periods. Schierl et al. (117) reported two long-term biologic half-lives of platinum of 16 and 720 days and showed that, of an administered dose of 800-mg cisplatin, 1 mg remained in a long-term pool after 3,000 days. There is a potential for accumulation of ultrafilterable platinum plasma concentrations whenever cisplatin is administered on a daily basis but not when dosed on an intermittent schedule.

Administration and Dosage. Cisplatin may be administered intravenously or intraperitoneally. Cisplatin should be mixed only in solutions containing 0.9% or more sodium chloride, because drug stability is directly related to the concentration of the salt. When admixed with dextrose-containing solutions, by chromatographic analysis, the drug appears to be relatively unstable, with decomposition evident by 2 hours (118). Platinum also can form significant, colored complexes if directly admixed with mannitol and stored for 2 to 3 days (119). Short-term (<24 hour) admixtures, however, have been successfully used. Needles or IV sets containing aluminum should not be used in the preparation or administration of cisplatin, because this drug rapidly reacts with aluminum, resulting in a loss of drug potency and the formation of a black precipitate (120).

To protect against nephrotoxicity, it is critical that a high urinary output be maintained during cisplatin therapy. Several methods of accomplishing this have been recommended; however, the most widely practiced method involves prehydration and mannitol diuresis (121). If cisplatin is administered in a hospital setting, patients should receive hydration with 1 to 2 L of fluid prior to cisplatin. Mannitol diuresis is accomplished by diluting the cisplatin in 2 L of normal saline containing 37.5 g of mannitol. The solution is then infused over 6 to 8 hours. Adequate hydration and urinary output should be maintained during the next 24 hours. A safe outpatient procedure using concurrent mannitol that appears to prevent serious nephrotoxicity has also been reported (122). The desired dose of cisplatin plus 50 g mannitol is diluted to 1 L with 5% dextrose plus 0.45% sodium chloride, USP. This solution may then be infused at a rate of no greater than 1 mg/min. For patients with known cardiac disease, the dose may be placed in 200 mL of a 10% mannitol solution and infused at a rate of no greater than 1 mg/min. This is followed by 200 mL of additional 10% mannitol. An alternative is to add the drug to 400 mL of 10% mannitol that is then brought up to a 1-L volume with normal saline containing 3 g of magnesium sulfate and administered intravenously over 1 hour (123).

Intraperitoneal cisplatin administration requires that an implantable device (IV port, such as single-lumen venous-access catheter: 9.6F, Port-A-Cath or Bardport) be surgically placed in the IP space. It is important to note that peritoneal or fenestrated catheters can lead to fibrous sheath formation, small bowel obstruction and perforation, and should be avoided (124). Day 2 IP administration requires that cisplatin be mixed in 1 L of normal saline and then warmed to body temperature. The 1-L cisplatin solution is instilled as rapidly as possible into the IP space via the catheter, and should be followed by up to 1 additional liter of saline to the point of mild abdominal discomfort. The cisplatin solution is allowed to remain in the IP cavity (i.e., the fluid is not drained). Concurrently, at least 1 L normal saline must be administered IV along with 40-g mannitol to assure a brisk diuresis to eliminate the cisplatin. Since cisplatin has the potential to be highly emetogenic, it is important to consider an aggressive antiemetic regimen (125,126).

Retrospective analysis by Levin and Hryniuk (127) strongly suggests that the cisplatin efficacy against ovarian cancer is directly correlated with cisplatin dose intensity (i.e., mg/m^2/wk). Typical high-dose regimens include 20 mg/m^2 daily for 5 days repeated every 3 weeks, 100 to 120 mg/m^2 IV every 3 to 4 weeks, or 100 mg/m^2 on day 1 and day 8 repeated every 20 days (128,129). Holleran and DeGregorio (130) prepared an excellent review of high-dose (200 mg/m^2/course) cisplatin. Dose-limiting toxicities with the higher dose regimens include severe, relatively irreversible neurotoxicity and myelosuppression. Responses have been seen in conventional-dose cisplatin-refractory patients, but they generally are of relatively short duration.

Side Effects and Toxicities. Dose-related nephrotoxicity is the major dose-limiting toxicity of cisplatin. It is manifested by renal tubular damage resulting in an elevation of the BUN or serum creatinine. The peak detrimental effect on renal function usually occurs between the 10th and 20th days after treatment. The renal damage is usually reversible. Patients concomitantly receiving gentamicin and cephalothin have been shown to be at greater risk of developing acute renal failure (131).

Madias and Harrington (132) have characterized the renal damage of cisplatin as being similar to mercury nephrotoxicity. Pathologically, renal tubular necrosis, degeneration, and interstitial edema without glomerular changes are observed. Although clinically overt renal toxicity may be common, it is usually reversible. However, some degree of long-term damage is likely. The renal-protective effect of hydration and mannitol is well established in animals and humans, and renal impairment can be prevented (122).

Ototoxicity, manifested by high-frequency hearing loss (above the frequency of normal speech), may be seen in as many as 30% of patients treated with cisplatin (133). Hearing impairment may be dose related and can be unilateral or bilateral. Occasional tinnitus (but not vestibular dysfunction) has been reported. The ototoxicity may be partially reduced by adequate hydration and the use of mannitol diuresis. Patients with lower than average threshold before chemotherapy with cisplatin were more likely to experience greater threshold shifts (133).

Neurotoxicity can be a dose-limiting side effect of cisplatin, particularly with high-dose regimens (134). The range of cisplatin-induced neurologic deficits includes peripheral sensory neuropathy, ototoxicity, autonomic neuropathy manifested by orthostatic hypotension and gastric paresis, Lhermitte syndrome, and rarely focal encephalopathy, often accompanied by cortical blindness. Peripheral neuropathy is by far the most common cisplatin-induced neurotoxicity. Neurotoxicity is dose dependent, with symptoms typically developing after cumulative doses of 300 mg/m^2 or greater. A review of published literature (135) found that neurotoxicity occurred in 85% of patients at cumulative doses of 300 mg/m^2 or greater, but occurred in only 15% of patients who had received a cumulative dose below this level. Initial symptoms are usually numbness and tingling in the distal fingers and toes. If cisplatin is continued, proximal extension of the peripheral neuropathy occurs, and the sense of joint position becomes impaired, resulting in more severe neurologic symptoms, including ataxia, gait disturbances, loss of manual dexterity, and wheelchair dependency. Symptoms may begin and progress up to four or more months after discontinuation of cisplatin. In 30% to 50% of patients, cisplatin neuropathy is irreversible.

Symptomatic hypomagnesemia frequently occurs with cisplatin. In a study to determine the effects of magnesium supplementation on cisplatin-induced hypomagnesemia, the administration of magnesium (oral and IV) with cisplatin to one group of patients produced less renal tubular damage and no compromise in efficacy than that seen in a group not supplemented with magnesium (136).

Without adequate antiemetic therapy, most patients who receive cisplatin experience nausea and vomiting. This reaction may be severe and usually starts within the first hour after treatment, and may persist for 24 to 48 hours. Delayed nausea and vomiting, lasting from 3 to 5 days, may also occur. The combination of a 5-HT3 inhibitor (e.g., ondansetron or granisetron) with dexamethasone (10 to 40 mg IV) has reduced the incidence of severe nausea and vomiting by as much as 75% (137). Delayed nausea and vomiting can be eradicated by continuation of oral low-dose dexamethasone (with or without a 5-HT3 inhibitor) for the first 5 days after platinum treatment (138). Other less effective antiemetic regimens to prevent cisplatin-induced nausea and vomiting include prochlorperazine, dexamethasone, and lorazepam; metoclopramide and dexamethasone; metoclopramide and methylprednisolone; or metoclopramide and lorazepam (82,139).

Anaphylactic hypersensitivity reactions consisting of tachycardia, wheezing, hypotension, and facial edema occurring within a few minutes of IV administration have occurred occasionally after a dose of cisplatin given to previously treated patients (140,141). These hypersensitivity reactions have been controlled with corticosteroids, epinephrine, or antihistamines. Wiesenfeld and colleagues (142) reported successful retreatment with cisplatin after apparent allergic reactions in two patients. *In vivo* and *in vitro* tests in one patient could not demonstrate an immunologic basis for the initial reaction. Both patients were successfully rechallenged with cisplatin after only diphenhydramine pretreatment. This suggests a nonallergic cause of the acute hypersensitivity reactions occasionally seen with platinum.

Myelosuppression occurs in 25% to 30% of patients receiving the recommended dose, and is more pronounced at higher doses. Coombs-positive hemolytic anemia also occurs as a result of cisplatin treatment. Cisplatin-induced anemia has been shown to respond to recombinant erythropoietin (143).

Drug Interactions. When cisplatin is given in combination with other agents, the order of drug sequence can affect the severity of drug-induced myelosuppression. Rowinsky and Donehower (144) conducted a phase 1 study of sequential escalating doses of paclitaxel and cisplatin therapy and determined that myelosuppression was more severe when cisplatin administration preceded paclitaxel than when given after paclitaxel. Another phase 1 study was conducted to evaluate the effects of drug sequence of treatment with cisplatin in combination with topotecan (145). This study also found a significantly higher incidence of myelosuppression when cisplatin was administered first.

Cisplatin-induced nephrotoxicity should be considered whenever this agent is given prior to or in combination with other cytotoxic drugs that are cleared by renal elimination (e.g., bleomycin, ifosfamide, etoposide, methotrexate). Cisplatin reduces the renal clearance of these agents, resulting in an increased accumulation of these drugs. Yee and coworkers (47) observed markedly reduced bleomycin clearance in children who had received six courses of a regimen including cisplatin (cumulative dose 300 mg/m^2). In another case report, fatal bleomycin pulmonary toxicity occurred in a patient with cisplatin-induced acute renal failure (48).

Cisplatin is directly inactivated by mesna and amifostine (50). The FDA has approved amifostine to reduce the cumulative renal toxicity associated with repeated administration of cisplatin in patients with advanced ovarian cancer. In a phase 3 randomized study of ovarian cancer patients, amifostine treatment, prior to IV cisplatin plus cyclophospham, did not appear to reduce cisplatin's anticancer activity (146). However, there are only limited data in other chemotherapeutic settings, and the FDA recommends that amifostine should not be administered to patients in settings where chemotherapy could produce a significant survival advantage or cure except in a clinical trial (147).

Cyclophosphamide

Cyclophosphamide (Cytoxan, Neosar, CTX, CPM, and Endoxan) is an alkylating agent that, before the advent of paclitaxel, was used in the primary chemotherapy of advanced, epithelial-type ovarian and endometrial cancer. At this time, it is uncommonly used in the treatment of gynecologic cancers because of the more effective agents currently available (e.g., paclitaxel). It is occasionally used in the third-line treatment of ovarian cancer and as a second-line agent in the treatment of choriocarcinoma.

Chemistry. Cyclophosphamide is a cyclic phosphamide ester of nitrogen mustard and is referred to chemically as 2-[bis-(2-chloroethyl) amino]tetrahydro-2H-1,3,2,-oxazaphosphorine 2-oxide monohydrate. Its molecular weight is 279.1. The monohydrate is un-ionized and lipid soluble; in normal saline or water, it is soluble to a maximum of 4% at room temperature.

Mechanism of Action. Cyclophosphamide, a bifunctional substituted nitrogen mustard, was synthesized in 1958 in an attempt to achieve greater selective toxicity for tumor tissue. The *N*-methyl moiety of nitrogen mustard is replaced with a cyclic phosphamide group, resulting in a stable, inactive compound. The bis-(2-chloroethyl) group cannot ionize until the cyclic phosphamide is opened at the phosphorus-nitrogen linkage.

Activation of cyclophosphamide is a multistep process. The liver microsomal P450 mixed-function oxidase system converts the parent drug to 4-hydroxycyclophosphamide. This metabolite exists in equilibrium with the acyclic tautomer, aldophosphamide. These compounds may be further oxidized by hepatic aldehyde oxidase to the inactive metabolites of carboxyphosphamide and 4-ketocyclophosphamide. Nonenzymatic conversion to the cytotoxic compounds of phosphoramide mustard and acrolein occurs in susceptible peripheral tissues.

Most of the alkylating agents, like cyclophosphamide, are bifunctional, which facilitates their reaction with two cellular molecules. Accordingly, they can cross-link the two opposite strands of DNA to give an interstrand cross-link, react with two sites on the same strand (intrastrand cross-link), or cross-link DNA to protein. The latter type of lesion is generally considered to be innocuous, but the relative significance of the other cross-links is still in contention. DNA intrastrand cross-links are more frequent than interstrand cross-links and are more often considered to be the critical lesions.

These two classes can be differentiated by the structure of the cross-links in DNA. Generally, the entire mustard is involved in the cross-link, with the two mustard "arms" linked usually to the N7 position of guanine. Because these guanines can be separated by several bases in DNA, the linkages represent particularly bulky lesions.

Drug Disposition. After IV administration, approximately 15% of the drug is excreted unchanged in the urine, and the remainder as metabolites. The plasma half-life of the parent compound after doses of 6 to 80 mg/kg appears to range from 4 to 6.5 hours (148,149). Approximately 50% of the alkylating metabolites (but not parent drug) is bound to plasma proteins.

Although cyclophosphamide is exclusively excreted by the kidneys, because of the un-ionized nature of the intact drug molecule, tubular reabsorption is avid. Hepatic inactivation appears to be the major mechanism of active drug elimination. The mean renal clearance of intact drug is approximately 11 mL/min, or 15% of CrCl, but renal elimination remains the major route of disposition of the more polar, less lipid-soluble metabolites (150). There can be significantly prolonged retention of active (alkylating) metabolites in patients with severe renal failure, and doses should be adjusted accordingly.

Dosage. Cyclophosphamide is active in many different types of malignancies. The dosing schemes are numerous and depend on the particular disease. Two general categories of treatment schedules exist. In the method generally used to treat ovarian and endometrial cancers, an intermediate dose (600 to 1,000 mg/m^2) is given all at once over a short period. This treatment approach usually involves other drugs, such as cisplatin, carboplatin, or doxorubicin, whose additive toxic effects must be considered in selecting the dose and frequency of cyclophosphamide administration. Adequate hydration for 72 hours before and following high-dose treatment with cyclophosphamide is recommended to reduce cyclophosphamide-induced hemorrhagic cystitis (151).

An alternative continuous low-dose regimen for cyclophosphamide has been developed. Doses of 25 to 50 mg/d are given on a continuous basis. Used in this way, it was originally thought that cyclophosphamide acted as an "accidental" antiangiogenic agent (152). It is usually well tolerated with few side effects. Colleoni and colleagues published a trial of continuous low-dose cyclophosphamide with methotrexate in breast cancer and showed antitumor activity that correlated with vascular endothelial growth factor (VEGF) levels (153). Further, Miscoria and colleagues found an association between progression-free survival and thymidine phosphorylase levels (154). A suggestion has been made that the acrolein metabolite of cyclophosphamide acts as an antiangiogenic agent (155). The use of cyclophosphamide in this way has come to be known as "metronomic" dosing. In addition to the antiangiogenic effect, metronomic cyclophosphamide may also have an immune regulatory function (156). Ge et al. (157) showed that metronomic cyclophosphamide induced an increase in the number of breast cancer reactive t-cells and that this correlated with disease stabilization in breast cancer.

There have been a large number of trials of the metronomic approach in a range of tumor types, including ovarian cancer. These have been reviewed (158). Activity is frequently reported, but the heterogeneous nature of the trials, the frequent combination with established antiangiogenic agents, and the lack of randomized trials makes the overall role of this approach currently undefined.

Side Effects and Toxicities. Myelosuppression consisting primarily of leukopenia is the usual dose-limiting toxic effect of cyclophosphamide. Both the nadir and time of bone marrow recovery are rapid at 8 to 14 and 18 to 21 days, respectively. Although this drug has long been considered to be "platelet sparing," significant thrombocytopenia can also occur at very high doses (>1.5 g/m^2).

Acute, sterile hemorrhagic cystitis, believed to be due to the acrolein metabolite, is an infrequent toxic manifestation, but is occasionally dose limiting. It is understandably more common in poorly hydrated or renally compromised patients. The onset of this complication may be delayed from 24 hours to several weeks. It is detected by gross hematuria or a microscopic hematuria of greater than 20 erythrocytes per high-power field. The bleeding may persist but is usually transient. Prophylactic hydration with intake of at least 3 L/d appears to offer the best protection. With continued therapy, patients characteristically develop a fibrotic "small bladder," and urinary frequency may become a permanent problem. There is a definite increase in the risk of bladder cancer in these patients. The availability of the sulfhydryl mesna as a prophylactic treatment of patients at high risk for developing cyclophosphamide-induced cystitis has almost completely eliminated this side effect.

A syndrome of inappropriate antidiuretic hormone (SIADH), or "water intoxication," has been reported after cyclophosphamide treatment. This is more common with IV doses greater than 50 mg/kg and is both a limitation to and consequence of fluid loading (159). Alopecia occurs to some degree in all patients receiving cyclophosphamide and is significant in at least half of all patients treated. Regrowth of hair may occur even with continuing treatment. Gastrointestinal problems are more common with high doses given orally. Anorexia, nausea, and vomiting are all common reactions, but they are usually controlled with IV antiemetic regimens. A rare pulmonary toxic effect has been reported with a pneumonitis picture similar to "busulfan lung." The typical clinical presentation is that of an interstitial pneumonitis, usually occurring after long-term and continuous low-dose therapy (160). The onset of symptoms is insidious. Pathologically, there can be alveolitis with eventual fibrosis and atypical type II pneumocytes. Steroids may be beneficial. Other toxic effects include testicular atrophy, sometimes with reversible oligospermia and azoospermia. Amenorrhea also has been reported. As with all alkylating agents, drug-induced congenital abnormalities are possible. With high-dose therapy used for bone marrow transplant (120 to 180 mg/kg), cyclophosphamide-associated cardiac toxicity has been reported (161).

Special Precautions. It is important to keep the patient well hydrated during cyclophosphamide therapy to reduce the potential for hemorrhagic cystitis. It is advisable to administer at least 1 L of additional IV fluids (usually normal saline) to ensure an adequate urine volume to excrete the cyclophosphamide metabolite acrolein, which can otherwise alkylate bladder mucosa and cause hemorrhagic cystitis. The patient should be instructed to drink at least eight glasses of fluid daily during the 2 days after cyclophosphamide administration. In patients prone to developing cystitis, consider administering prophylactic IV mesna, a sulfhydryl-containing compound that can neutralize acrolein.

Drug Interactions. Cyclophosphamide must be metabolized to be active. Although some cyclophosphamide may be activated by phosphatases and phosphamidases peripherally, most of the drug is metabolized by microsomal enzymes in the liver (162,163). These enzymes may be activated by drugs such as phenobarbital or inhibited by drugs such as proadifen (SKF 525A). Because active and toxic metabolites are generated by the reactions of these enzymes and cyclophosphamide, many potential drug interactions may exist.

Barbiturates and other inducers of hepatic microsomal enzymes, such as phenytoin and chloral hydrate, may increase the rate of hepatic conversion of cyclophosphamide to its toxic metabolites. Similarly, cyclophosphamide may block the metabolism of barbiturates, increasing sedative effects. Although the clinical significance of these reactions is not clear, cyclophosphamide toxicity may be increased by the H_2-histamine blocker cimetidine (164). Cimetidine, but not ranitidine, may increase cyclophosphamide's myelotoxicity through an increase in the concentration time product of its active metabolites (e.g., 4-hydroxycyclophosphamide and phosphoramide mustard) (165). Thus, H_2-blockers like ranitidine may be safer to use than cimetidine when high doses of cyclophosphamide are administered.

Dactinomycin

Dactinomycin (actinomycin D, ACT-D, Cosmegen) has been shown to be active in the treatment of patients with germ cell tumors of the ovary and endometrium, and in gestational trophoblastic disease (166–168).

Chemistry. Dactinomycin has a molecular weight of 1,255 and an empiric formula of $C_{62}H_{86}N_{12}O_{16}$. The drug is an antitumor antibiotic isolated from *Streptomyces parvulus*. The molecular structure includes two peptide loops linked to a three-ring chromophoric phenoxazone ring system (actinocin). The drug is highly soluble in water, forming an amber- to gold-colored solution.

Mechanism of Action. Dactinomycin becomes anchored into or around a purine-pyrimidine base pair in DNA by intercalation. DNA-dependent ribosomal RNA synthesis and new messenger RNA synthesis is inhibited. The peptide loops appear to allow tight drug binding to DNA because the actinocin (phenoxazone) moiety alone is inactive. This can occur adjacent to any G-C pair in DNA.

Bound dactinomycin molecules dissociate very slowly from DNA owing to electrostatic interactions of the cyclic peptide rings with each strand of the DNA double helix. This process, which stabilizes the intercalative interaction, appears to be crucial for cytotoxicity.

Dactinomycin on a molar basis is one of the most potent antineoplastic agents available. The drug possesses some hypocalcemic activity, similar to mithramycin. Although maximal cell killing is observed in the G_1 phase, the cytotoxic action is thought to be primarily cell cycle-nonspecific. Actively proliferating cells are more sensitive than quiescent cells to the lethal effects of the drug (169).

In that dactinomycin is a natural product, it is not surprising that the primary mode of tumor cell resistance to dactinomycin is mediated through overexpression of P-glycoprotein (170).

Drug Disposition. Tattersall and colleagues (171) studied the pharmacokinetics of radiolabeled [^3H] dactinomycin in patients. They reported that the drug appeared to be only minimally metabolized, and was concentrated in nucleated cells. There was a greater drug uptake into bone marrow than in plasma. Drug penetration into the CNS was not observed. Urinary and fecal recovery totaled only 30% each after 9 days, and there was significant drug retention in lymphocytes and granulocytes. This may explain the prolonged terminal plasma half-life of 36 hours observed after single dactinomycin doses. There appears to be little metabolism because approximately 90% of excreted drug is collected as the intact molecule. Some monolactone forms of dactinomycin are recovered in the urine.

Using a more specific radioimmunoassay, a much shorter dactinomycin half-life is described ($t_{1/2\alpha} = 0.78$ minutes, $t_{1/2\beta} = 3.5$ hours) (172). The discrepancies between these and Tattersall's findings reflect the differences in the assays used.

Administration and Dosage. Dactinomycin is administered intravenously by slow IV push or, preferably, into the tubing of a freely running IV solution. A 5- to 10-mL flush of 5% dextrose in water (D_5W) or normal saline is recommended before and after IV push administration to assure vein patency and to flush any remaining drug from the tubing.

Dactinomycin is commonly given intravenously in short "pulse" doses of 500 μg/m^2 daily for as long as 5 days in adults. The dose for each 2-week cycle should not exceed 15 μg/kg/d or 400 to 600 μg/m^2/d for 5 days.

A wide variety of dosing regimens have been employed. Several clinical studies have documented equal efficacy and toxicity for single-dose dactinomycin regimens (173,174). In nonmetastatic gestational trophoblastic cancer, a single IV dose of 1.25 mg/m^2 every 14 days produced a 99% remission rate after four courses of therapy (174). Compared with five divided doses of 500 μg/m^2/d, the single-dose method produced slightly greater mild-to-moderate toxic effects.

Side Effects and Toxicities. Bone marrow depression is the usual dose-limiting toxic effect of dactinomycin. It is usually manifested 7 to 10 days after dosing. All blood elements are affected, but primarily the platelets and leukocytes are depressed. Combined with gastrointestinal reactions, myelosuppression appears to be dose-limiting as well as dose-dependent (175). Immunosuppression is another well-known effect of dactinomycin. Patients should not receive this drug during viral infection because of the risk of developing disseminated disease.

Severe gastrointestinal consequences, such as vomiting, may occasionally represent the acute dose-limiting toxic effects of dactinomycin. Vomiting can persist for 4 to 20 hours, but it can be controlled by combination antiemetic regimens (176). Mucositis may also be severe. It is characterized by severe oral ulcerations and diarrhea in 30% of patients. Reversible alopecia may occur with dactinomycin. A variety of other skin manifestations have been reported, including acneiform changes, erythema, and hyperpigmentation.

Dactinomycin is toxicologically similar to the anthracyclines and characteristically interacts with radiation therapy, producing delayed "radiation recall" skin damage. Previously irradiated or even irritated skin may become reddened and inflamed after drug administration. Frank necrosis is sometimes reported. Oral ulcers may also develop after radiation therapy. These reactions may occur months after radiation therapy. Experimentally, radiation therapy given after dactinomycin does not produce this effect.

Dactinomycin potentiates pulmonary radiation and decreases radiation tolerance by at least 20%. Reintroduction of dactinomycin following pulmonary radiation has resulted in fatal pulmonary fibrosis (177). As noted in the "Special Precautions" section below, dactinomycin is highly ulcerogenic if extravasated.

Special Precautions. Dactinomycin is extremely damaging to soft tissue, and every effort should be made to assure vein patency during administration. Extravasations characteristically result in immediate pain and swelling followed by indolent, poorly healing necrotic ulcers (176).

Dactinomycin is highly potent and is typically dosed in micrograms per kilogram. Doses must be calculated and prepared carefully to prevent inadvertent overdosage of this drug. No specific antidote to overdosage is known, although granulocyte colony–stimulating factors may be useful.

Dactinomycin is a potent immunosuppressant and can inhibit the effectiveness of vaccinations given after drug administration. The drug also produces radiation recall skin and soft tissue damage if given after ionizing radiation.

Docetaxel

Docetaxel (Taxotere) is a semisynthetic analog of paclitaxel and has an FDA-approved indication for locally advanced or metastatic breast cancer after failure of prior chemotherapy. It is also FDA approved for locally advanced or metastatic non–small cell lung cancer after failure of prior platinum-based chemotherapy. It has shown marked antitumor activity against a variety of solid tumors, including both platinum-sensitive and platinum-refractory epithelial ovarian cancer (178,179).

Chemistry. The natural component of docetaxel is 10-deacetyl baccatin III, which is extracted from the needles of the European yew tree (*Taxus baccata* L.) (179). Docetaxel has a molecular weight of 861.9 and the empirical formula $C_{43}H_{53}NO_{14} \cdot 3H_2O$. Unlike paclitaxel, which uses a polyoxyl compound (Cremophor) as a diluent, docetaxel is formulated in Tween 80 and alcohol.

Mechanism of Action. In a manner similar to paclitaxel, docetaxel promotes microtubule assembly and inhibits the depolymerization of tubulin. However, compared with paclitaxel, the microtubules formed by docetaxel are more slowly reversible, and there are differential effects on tau binding sites and on microtubule-associated proteins. Docetaxel-induced stabilization of microtubules halts cellular division in M phase, thereby preventing cell replication.

Drug Disposition. The pharmacokinetics of docetaxel when administered as an IV infusion lasting from 1 to 24 hours have been investigated in a number of studies (180). When administered as a typical 1-hour infusion at doses of 70 to 100 mg/m^2, pharmacokinetics reveals triphasic elimination with a plasma AUC of 3.13 to 4.83 mg/mL/h, a peak plasma concentration of 2.57 to 3.67 μg/mL, and a terminal-phase plasma half-life of 13.6 hours. There is very limited renal excretion of docetaxel; the 24-hour urinary excretion was 1.4% of the dose administered. Plasma drug clearance was determined to be 21.3 L/h/m^2 (181).

Administration and Dosage. All patients receiving docetaxel should be premedicated with oral corticosteroids such as dexamethasone 16 mg/d (e.g., 8 mg b.i.d) for 3 days, beginning 1 day prior to docetaxel administration, to reduce fluid retention and the risk of hypersensitivity reactions.

Docetaxel is commercially available in single-dose 20- and 80-mg vials with accompanying diluent vials. Both the docetaxel vials and the diluent vials should stand at room temperature for approximately 5 minutes before mixing. The entire contents of the diluent vial should be aseptically transferred to the docetaxel vial, and the resulting contents should be gently rotated for 15 seconds to promote complete mixture. The resulting concentration of docetaxel is 10 mg/mL. Foam may be present owing to the Tween 80; however, it should largely dissipate within a few minutes. The infusion solution is prepared by aseptically withdrawing the proper amount of docetaxel with a calibrated syringe and adding it to a 250-mL infusion bag or bottle containing either 0.9% sodium chloride or 5% dextrose solution to produce a final concentration of 0.3 to 0.9 mg/mL. The infusion solution should be mixed by manual rotation and inspected for particulate formation and/or discoloration. Solutions that are cloudy or that contain particulate matter should be discarded.

The recommended dose of docetaxel for chemotherapy in women with metastatic breast cancer ranges from 60 to 100 mg/m^2 IV as a continuous 1-hour infusion every 3 weeks. For non–small cell lung cancer, the recommended dose is 75 mg/m^2 IV as a continuous 1-hour infusion every 3 weeks.

The optimal dosing schedule for docetaxel in gynecologic cancers is presently undefined. A 100-mg/m^2 dose administered as a 1-hour infusion every 3 weeks has been used in phase 2 trials. Other tolerable docetaxel dose schedules that have been identified in phase 1 studies are: 50 mg/m^2/d on days 1 and 8 every 3 weeks; 70 to 90 mg/m^2 by 24-hour continuous IV infusion every 3 weeks; 80 to 100 mg/m^2 by 6-hour infusion every 3 weeks; 14 mg/m^2/d for 5 days by 1-hour infusion every 21 days (182); and 30 to 35 mg/m^2 weekly (183,184). Docetaxel has been administered in combination with cisplatin using the following schedule: docetaxel 85 to 100 mg/m^2 as a 1-hour IV infusion followed (3 hours after completion) by cisplatin 75 mg/m^2 as a 3-hour IV infusion, with cycles repeated every 3 weeks (185).

Side Effects and Toxicities. The major dose-limiting toxicity of docetaxel is neutropenia, which is noncumulative and generally resolves within 7 to 8 days. The combined results of early phase 2 studies of docetaxel (without steroid premedication) in ovarian cancer revealed that at a dose level of 100 mg/m^2 every 3 weeks, over 90% of patients developed grades 3 to 4 neutropenia, with febrile neutropenia occurring in 8% to 44% of patients (186). The incidence of other grade 3 to 4 toxicities were stomatitis (0% to 5%), diarrhea (6% to 20%), dermatitis (4% to 8%), acute hypersensitivity reactions (7% to 12%), and fluid retention (8% to 12%). Other docetaxel-induced side effects include alopecia, anemia, neurosensory effects (paresthesia, dysesthesia, pain), and asthenia (182).

In early phase 2 studies, slow-onset (i.e., after three to five courses), cumulative fluid retention leading to peripheral or generalized edema with possible development of pleural effusion and/or ascites was a common dose-limiting toxicity. However, a 5-day premedication regimen with corticosteroids, starting the day before docetaxel administration, significantly reduces this side effect. In a retrospective analysis, severe fluid retention occurred in 20% of patients who received no premedication compared with 5% of patients who received steroid prophylaxis. Additionally, the percentage of patients who discontinued treatment secondary to fluid retention was reduced from 32% to 2% ($p < 0.00001$) with the use of a 5-day corticosteroid regimen (182). Steroid prophylaxis also reduces the incidence and severity of dermatologic side effects and hypersensitivity reactions.

The spectrum of docetaxel-induced hypersensitivity reactions is less severe than that associated with paclitaxel. In the absence of prophylactic medication, mild hypersensitivity reaction as characterized by flushing, rash, and pruritus occurs in approximately 5% of docetaxel administrations. Moderate reactions with dyspnea and/or slight hypertension occur in 8% of treatments, and severe reactions (with bronchospasm, angioedema, and/or severe hypertension) occur in less than 2% of docetaxel administrations (187). Initial symptoms of hypersensitivity to docetaxel therapy generally occur within minutes of the start of the first or second course of docetaxel, and resolve rapidly with interruption of the infusion. Patients can be successfully rechallenged with docetaxel therapy following medication with corticosteroids, antihistamines, and H_2-agonists.

Dermatologic toxicities typically appear as maculopapular eruptions and desquamation generally localized to the extremities. Nail changes, including onycholysis, may also occur. Skin changes are largely self-limiting and may be alleviated with glycerin/chlorhexidine ointment or oral pyridoxine. This side effect can often be prevented with prophylactic oral steroids and H_1- and H_2-agonists (188). Recurrent skin toxicity refractory to oral prophylactic medication and pyridoxine therapy may respond to local hypothermia during docetaxel administration (189).

Special Precautions. Patients with impaired liver function have a significant reduction in docetaxel clearance and an increased risk of life-threatening side effects. Analysis of the overall safety database revealed that patients with moderately impaired liver function (defined as transaminase levels more than 1.5 times the upper limit of normal and alkaline phosphatase more than 2.5 times the upper limit of normal) have a 27% reduction in docetaxel clearance and a 38% increase in the area under the concentration–time curve (182). When compared with patients with normal liver function, patients with at least moderately impaired liver function had a significantly greater incidence of febrile neutropenia (40% vs. 16%) and toxic death (20% vs. 1.4%). Grades 3 to 4 nausea/vomiting, stomatitis, and thrombocytopenia were also increased in patients with impaired liver function (182).

The recommended docetaxel dose level for a patient with moderate hepatic impairment (defined as transaminases between 1.5 and 3.5 times the upper limit of normal and an alkaline phosphatase between 2.5 and 6.0 times the upper limit of normal) is 75 mg/m^2 over 1 hour. No safe docetaxel dose can be recommended for patients with greater than moderate liver impairment (190).

Doxorubicin

Doxorubicin (Adriamycin) is FDA approved for the treatment of many cancers, including sarcoma and breast cancer. In addition, it is a commonly employed agent in the treatment of metastatic endometrial cancer and advanced ovarian cancer.

Chemistry. Doxorubicin is an anthracycline antibiotic obtained from *Streptomyces peucetius* var. *caesius*. It has a molecular weight of 580. The doxorubicin structure includes a water-soluble basic reducing amino sugar, daunosamine, linked by a glycosidic bond to carbon atom number 7 on the D-ring of the water-insoluble chromophore aglycone, adrimycinone.

Structural changes in the side groups of doxorubicin alter antitumor potency and pharmacokinetic properties. The aglycone is inactive, and modifications in the amino sugar substituents can also alter antitumor or toxic potency (191).

In DNA, the amino sugar projects into the minor groove and can interact electrostatically with negatively charged phosphate groups in the DNA strand to stabilize the aglycone moiety. Doxorubicin can also form complexes with iron or copper by means of the hydroquinone moieties (192). Metal-iron doxorubicin complexes may contribute to cardiotoxicity by enhancing redox cycling of the quinone moiety to produce membrane-damaging oxygen free radicals (193).

Doxorubicin hydrochloride is freely soluble in water, slightly soluble in normal saline, and very slightly soluble in alcohol.

Doxorubicin is also commercially available in a polyethylene glycol (PEG)–coated (pegylated, Stealth) liposomal form (see Liposomal Encapsulated Doxorubicin section below).

Mechanisms of Action. DNA Binding. The anthracyclines, including doxorubicin, probably have several modes of action. The anthracycline portion of the molecule appears to intercalate between stacked nucleotide pairs in the DNA helix by means of P-P–type bonds (194). The drug may also bind ionically around certain base pairs of DNA (adlineation). The overall effect of this is interference with nucleic acid synthesis, specifically an inhibition of DNA synthesis (195). However, preribosomal RNA synthesis is also affected by the drug binding to DNA, preventing DNA-directed RNA and DNA transcription (196).

Mechanisms other than intercalation may also contribute to the antitumor effect of the doxorubicin molecule. The contribution of alkylation to antitumor effects has not been established.

Free Radical Formation. Oxygen free radical intermediates containing an unpaired electron can be formed by doxorubicin. This can react rapidly with oxygen to form superperoxide, and with hydrogen peroxide, highly reactive hydroxyl radicals can form. These radicals damage membrane lipids by peroxidation, break DNA strands by attacking ribose-phosphate bonds, and directly oxidize purine or pyrimidine bases, thiols, and amines (193,197). Free-radical mechanisms have most often been associated with cardiotoxicity.

Doxorubicin appears to be active in all phases of the cell cycle, and although maximally cytotoxic in S phase, it is not phase-specific (198). Cells exposed to lethal doxorubicin concentrations in G_1 can proceed through S phase but are then blocked and die in G_2. Higher concentrations can also produce an S-phase blockade (199).

Inhibition of DNA Topoisomerase II. Topoisomerases are enzymes capable of covalent binding to DNA, forming transient breaks in one strand (TOPO-I) or two strands (TOPO-II). This activity is highly phase-dependent for G_2, and in the case of TOPO-II, normally mediates strand passage to facilitate DNA condensation or decondensation (200). Doxorubicin and other DNA intercalators inhibit the strand-passing activity of TOPO-II by increasing and stabilizing the initial enzyme-DNA (cleavable) complexes. This leads to protein-linked DNA double-strand breaks that are roughly proportional to the cytotoxic potency of the drug *in vitro* (201).

Drug Disposition. Doxorubicin pharmacokinetics is usually described using a two-compartment or three-compartment open model. The drug is rapidly distributed in body tissues, and about 75% of the drug is bound to plasma proteins, principally albumin (202). In the blood, the free doxorubicin fraction depends on the hematocrit, with more free drug being available in patients with a reduced hematocrit (203). The avid binding to DNA is believed to explain the prolonged terminal elimination half-life of 30 to 40 hours, the large apparent Vd of up to 28 L/kg, and the incomplete (50%) total recovery of drug in urine, bile, and feces (204). Human tissues with high drug concentrations (in descending order) include liver, lymph nodes, muscle, bone marrow, fat, and skin (205). The drug does not distribute into the CNS.

There is a significant distribution of doxorubicin into human breast milk (206). Doxorubicin levels of 0.24 μM and 0.2 μM of doxorubicinol have been measured in human milk. They produce cumulative AUCs in breast milk of 9.9 and 16.5 μM · h, respectively. Both of these values are greater than concurrent plasma AUC values. However, doxorubicin does not appear to pass the placenta consistently. Except for one study reporting low drug levels in placental blood of 0.78 to 1.19 nmol/g and no drug in cord blood plasma, several other trials detected no drug in amniotic fluid after doxorubicin administration to pregnant patients (207–209).

Doxorubicin is extensively metabolized and eliminated primarily as glucuronide conjugates of the parent aglycone or its hydroxylated congener doxorubicinol (204,210). The conjugated metabolites are exclusively excreted in the bile and feces. Overall, biliary excretion accounts for about 40% of an administered dose (211). Approximately 42% of the biliary drug is parent doxorubicin, 22% is doxorubicinol, and 36% comprises other metabolites (211). Only 5% to 10% of the administered drug is excreted in the urine as doxorubicin (40%), doxorubicinol (29%), and other metabolites (31%).

In liver disease, patients with cholestasis have delayed doxorubicin clearance and experience exaggerated toxic reactions from standard doses (212). However, hepatoma patients with cirrhosis or simple hepatocellular enzyme elevation appear to have normal doxorubicin clearance and toxic effects from standard doses (213). Although obesity reduces clearance of doxorubicin in adult cancer patients (214), there were no differences in doxorubicin toxicity between normal, mildly obese, and obese patients.

There is some evidence that repeated doxorubicin dosing alters pharmacokinetics (215,216). In these reports, doxorubicin levels were lower after repeated dosing, which suggests increased drug clearance. However, because neither toxicity nor response rates were altered, the clinical significance of these observations has not been established. Age may also be a factor. In one trial, the highest clearances of doxorubicin were observed in the younger patients (217). These observations suggest that higher peak doxorubicin levels may be achieved in older patients.

The hepatic extraction ratio for doxorubicin in humans is 0.45 to 0.5, and systemic drug levels are about 25% lower with intra-arterial administration compared with IV dosing (218). Several studies have shown that the pharmacokinetics of intra-arterial drug are similar to those seen after IV doses (205,219). The relatively low hepatic extraction rate and similar overall disposition patterns provide little pharmacokinetic rationale for intra-arterial administration as a means of localizing doxorubicin effects to the liver (220).

Administration and Dosage. Short IV push infusions and IV bolus injections have been used with doxorubicin. A slow IV push over several minutes with constant monitoring of the patient and blood return can help minimize the chance of serious tissue damage due to extravasation. A 5- to 10-mL flush of normal saline or D_5W before and after administration is strongly recommended to test vein patency and flush any remaining drug from the tubing. Alternatively, injection into the side port of a running IV infusion has also been recommended. The patient should be asked to report immediately any change in sensation during the administration. Old venipuncture sites or infusion sites previously used for administering blood, antibiotics, or other medications should not be used to administer doxorubicin. Heparin locks (unless recently inserted) are not recommended because the drug is chemically incompatible with sodium heparin.

Prolonged infusions increase the incidence and severity of stomatitis and dermatologic reactions. Administration through tunneled central venous catheters or indwelling vascular access ports is mandatory for all prolonged infusions. Careful patient and site monitoring are required, because of the risk of doxorubicin extravasation from central vascular access devices.

Numerous dosing schedules have been reported. The individual doxorubicin dose depends on clinical variables, including the cumulative dose administered to date and the potential for interaction with other drugs or radiation (**Table 14.3**). As a single agent, doses of 60 to 75 mg/m^2 as a single IV injection have been used and repeated no more often than every 3 weeks. An alternative scheme uses 20 to 30 mg/m^2 given daily for 3 consecutive days, repeated in 3 weeks (221). When used in combination therapy, the most commonly used dosage is 40 to 60 mg/m^2 given as a single IV injection every 21 to 28 days.

Both the dose and rate of dosing (dose intensity) can have therapeutic impacts for different agents and tumors (222). Clinical studies with doxorubicin show that greater dose intensity is associated with

■ **TABLE 14.3. Intravenous Dosing Guidelines for Doxorubicin**

Dose (mg/m²)[a]	Intravenous Method	Schedule	Average Cumulative Tolerable Dose[c] (mg/m²)
60–75[b]	Bolus	Every 3 weeks	550
30	Bolus	3 successive days, every 3 weeks	550
20	Bolus	Weekly	750
60	96-hour infusion	Every 3–4 weeks	1,000

[a]Lower doses should be administered to patients with hepatobiliary dysfunction and for poor bone marrow reserve or performance status.

[b]Allows for greater dose intensity in breast cancer.

[c]Represents average total **cumulative dose tolerated without clinical evidence of** doxorubicin cardiotoxicity.

enhanced response rates in breast cancer (223). The doses compared in this trial were 70 mg/m^2 every 21 days for 8 cycles versus 35 mg/m^2 every 21 days for 16 cycles.

Dose adjustments are required in a number of clinical settings (**Table 14.4**), specifically in the case of hyperbilirubinemia. A 50% dose reduction is indicated if plasma bilirubin concentration is 1.2 to 3.0 mg/dL, and the dose must be reduced by 75% if plasma bilirubin concentration reaches 3.1 to 5.0 mg/dL.

Side Effects and Toxicities. The single acute dose-limiting toxicity for doxorubicin is bone marrow suppression. The most common seen dose-limiting toxicity is leukopenia, with a nadir at 10 to 14 days. Other hematologic toxicities, such as anemia and thrombocytopenia, have been reported, but they are rare and generally less severe. Recovery from myelosuppression is usually prompt, and often resolves within about 1 week after the nadir.

Doxorubicin is known to produce local skin and deep-tissue damage at the site of inadvertent extravasations (226,227). Ulcers may result after 33% of extravasations. The lesions undergo a slow, indolent expansion and occasionally involve tendons and other deep structures. They characteristically do not heal and are associated with prolonged local drug retention (228). Reilly and colleagues (226) recommend early surgical debridement, with skin grafting and tendon repair for serious infiltrations. Numerous pharmacologic antidotes have been evaluated, but few have demonstrated unequivocal clinical efficacy. The application of cold, topical dimethyl sulfoxide (DMSO) is recommended (229).

■ **TABLE 14.4. Modifications of Doxorubicin Doses**

Condition	Recommended Dose Modification
Prior doxorubicin	Limit total cumulative lifetime dose (by IV bolus) to 550 mg/m² (224)
Prior chest radiation therapy	Reduce total dose limit to 300–350 mg/m²
Obesity	Base dose on ideal body weight (214)
Hepatobiliary dysfunction	Reduce dose for elevated serum bilirubin (give 50% of dose for serum bilirubin of 1.2–1.9 mg/dL, and give 25% of dose for serum bilirubin ≥ 3.0 mg/dL (225)
	Use Indocyanine green disappearance rate as an indicator of doxorubicin clearance
Infusion method	Greater cumulative (total) dose may be afforded by weekly bolus doses or continuous (96-hour) infusions[a] (Legha, 1982)

Note: Average safe cumulative doxorubicin dose is 750 mg/m² using standard infusion schedules.

[a]Average safe cumulative doxorubicin dose is 1,000 mg/m² when administered with a 96-hour infusion schedule.

Cardiac consequences from the drug have included acute effects, such as a rare pericarditis–myocarditis syndrome or electrophysiologic aberrations, and a total dose–related cardiomyopathy (230,231). Nonspecific electrocardiographic changes during infusion or immediately afterward may be seen. These include T-wave flattening, ST depression, supraventricular tachyarrhythmias, and extra systolic contractions (232). These conduction abnormalities are generally transient, not associated with severe morbidity, and do not require dose modification.

Cardiomyopathy from doxorubicin is dose related. It presents initially as a clinical syndrome identical to classic congestive heart failure. It is usually irreversible, but symptoms can be managed with standard medical therapy involving digitalis, glycosides, and diuretics. Potential risk factors for doxorubicin cardiotoxicity include cumulative doses greater than 550 mg/m^2, prior mediastinal irradiation (≥20 Gy), age greater than 70 years, and preexisting cardiovascular diseases, such as prior myocardial infarction or long-standing hypertension (225). Anthracycline-induced cardiomyopathy can also occur 4 to 20 years after the drug is stopped at standard dose limits (233). The administration of anthracyclines incorporated into liposomes is one method that may significantly reduce the risk of cardiac toxicity (see Liposomal Encapsulated Doxorubicin section below) (234).

At total doses under 500 mg/m^2, the incidence of cardiomyopathy is less than 1%; between 501 and 600 mg/m^2, 11% are affected; and the incidence is 30% for doses above 600 mg/m^2. In a retrospective cardiotoxicity study of 4,018 patient records, Von Hoff and associates (224) described an overall incidence of 2.2% for doxorubicin-induced congestive heart failure. In this analysis, performance status, sex, race, and tumor type did not influence the incidence of cardiomyopathy. However, elderly patients were at greater risk, even after adjustment for the normally decreased cardiac function in this group. The major determinants were the dose, the schedule of administration, and the age of the patient. A weekly doxorubicin dosing schedule was associated with significantly less congestive heart failure than an every-3-weeks dosing schedule. Continuous IV infusions over 96 hours can also significantly lessen doxorubicin cardiotoxicity (235).

Dexrazoxane (Zinecard) is a chemoprotective agent with an FDA-approved indication for reducing doxorubicin-associated cardiomyopathy in women with metastatic breast cancer who have received a cumulative doxorubicin dose of ≥300 mg/m^2 and who, in their physician's opinion, would benefit from further doxorubicin therapy.

There is evidence that doxorubicin is a radiosensitizing or radiomimetic agent and can cause reactivation of tissue reactions in areas previously irradiated (236,237). Radiation recall reactions have also been reported in areas of previous drug infiltration. A particularly sensitive area for serious recall toxicity is the esophagus (238).

Other toxic effects are observed in rapidly proliferating normal tissues. These include marked alopecia in all hairy body areas. Stomatitis may occur at high doses and is more pronounced when the drug is given on consecutive days. It generally begins in the sublingual and lateral tongue regions as a burning sensation with noticeable erythema. The initial inflammation typically progresses to ulceration after a few days. Anal fissures or proctitis have been rarely reported. Nausea and vomiting are common but of moderate intensity. Diarrhea is rare with consecutive daily dosing, and the emetic effects are generally limited to the first day of treatment. Hyperpigmentation of the skin, especially the nail beds, may occur. Extravasations of doxorubicin are known to cause severe ulceration and soft tissue necrosis (226,227). Vein patency should be assured before injection and constantly monitored during administration.

Drug Interactions. Doxorubicin is believed to interact with numerous other drugs. Most of these effects have been described only in experimental systems, and their clinical significance is, therefore, unknown. However, several potentially significant interactions have been described in cancer patients. Altered doxorubicin disposition is postulated with α-interferon, and substantial doxorubicin dose reductions are required (239). The combination of doxorubicin with H_2-antihistamines, such as ranitidine or cimetidine, may also increase toxicities significantly and necessitate drug dose reduction.

Eribulin

Eribulin is licensed for the third-line treatment of metastatic breast cancer and was also approved for the treatment of unresectable liposarcoma.

Chemistry. Eribulin is a synthetic derivative of the natural product, Halichondrin B, a product originally isolated from a marine sponge. It acts as a microtubule dynamics inhibitor. The chemical name for eribulin mesylate (the injectable form) is 11,15:18,21:24,28-Triepoxy-7,9-ethano-12,15-methano-9H,15H-furo[3,2-i]furo[2',3':5,6]pyrano[4,3-b][1,4]dioxacyclopentacosin-5(4H)-one, 2-[(2S)-3-amino-2-hydroxypropyl]hexacosahydro-3-methoxy-26-methyl-20,27-bis(methylene)-,(2R,3R,3aS,7R,8aS,9S,10aR,11S,12R,13aR,13bS,15S,18S,21S,24S,26R,28R,29aS)-,methanesulfonate (salt). It has a molecular weight of 826.0 (729.9 for free base). The empirical formula is C40H59NO11•CH4O3S.

Mechanism of Action. Eribulin binds to tubulin and sequesters it into nonproductive aggregates, thereby inhibiting mitosis and causing a G2/M cell cycle block.

Drug Disposition. Eribulin is administered intravenously. The majority of the dose is excreted unchanged in the feces, with only about 9% in the urine. There is little metabolism, with about 90% of the drug being excreted unchanged. The Vd is approximately 40 L, and the half-life about 40 hours.

Dosage. The recommended dose of eribulin for patients with normal hepatic function is 1.4 mg/m^2, administered intravenously over 2 to 5 minutes on Days 1 and 8 of a 21-day cycle. Dose reductions to 0.7 mg/m^2 are recommended for patients with mild hepatic impairment, and to 1.1 mg/m^2 for patients with moderate renal impairment.

Further dose reductions are recommended according to the level of myelosuppression encountered during treatment.

Side Effects and Toxicities. The dose-limiting toxicity of eribulin is myelosuppression. Peripheral neuropathy also occurs. QT prolongation has also been reported. Other adverse events that have been reported in >10% of patients are asthenia, constipation, diarrhea, nausea, and vomiting.

Drug Interactions. As already noted, there is little CYP-mediated metabolism of eribulin, and no significant drug interactions are expected [H71].

Etoposide

Intravenous etoposide (VP-16) is commonly used in combination chemotherapy regimens for the treatment of patients with germ cell tumors of the ovary (168). Oral etoposide has activity for refractory or recurrent ovarian cancer (240).

Chemistry. Etoposide is a semisynthetic epipodophyllotoxin derived from the root of *Podophyllum* (the May apple plant, or mandrake). The chemical name is demethylepipodophyllotoxin 9-[4,6-O-(R)-ethylidene-β-D-glucopyranoside]. Etoposide has the molecular formula of $C_{29}H_{32}O_{13}$ and a molecular weight of 588.58. It is highly soluble in methanol and chloroform, slightly soluble in ethanol, and sparingly soluble in water. Because of poor water solubility, the commercial drug is dissolved in an ethanol-based cosolvent system.

Etoposide was originally synthesized from *P. embodi* (241). Structure-activity studies show that the hydroxyl group at the C-4′ position is required for activity, and that alterations at this site can dramatically affect activity.

Mechanism of Action. There is marked schedule dependence for etoposide cell killing, and cytotoxic effects are maximal in G_2 phase (242). There is also some activity against cells in late S phase, and the drug can halt cell cycle traverse at the S-G_2 interphase (243).

Etoposide produces protein-linked DNA strand breaks by inhibiting DNA TOPO-II enzymes (244). This normal mammalian enzyme mediates double-strand–passing activities in G_2 phase to condense or decondense supercoiled DNA (245). Drug-induced inhibition of TOPO-II is an energy-dependent process that is influenced by dose and duration of exposure.

Etoposide does not bind directly to DNA, but rather stabilizes a transition form of the DNA–TOPO-II complex (244). The number of single and double DNA strand breaks reflects the cytotoxic dose-response curve (246). Etoposide and intercalative drugs such as doxorubicin "poison" TOPO-II enzymes by stabilizing an otherwise transient form of TOPO-II covalently linked with DNA (201). Normal TOPO-II strand-passing activity is thereby blocked, and cell progression out of G_2 phase is halted (200,247). The production of cytotoxicity by etoposide may ultimately involve chromosomal breaks characterized as sister chromatid exchanges (248).

Another postulated etoposide mechanism involves microsomal activation to reactive intermediates capable of generating oxygen-free radicals (246). Nucleoside transport is also inhibited at high drug concentrations, but whether this makes a major contribution to the antitumor effect is unknown (249).

Drug Disposition. A two-compartment open pharmacokinetic model appears to adequately describe etoposide disposition in cancer patients (250). The terminal half-life of the drug appears to be about 7 hours and is independent of the dose, route, or method of administration (251). Renal excretion appears to account for about 30% of overall drug elimination. Forty-two percent to 66% of radiolabeled drug is recovered in the urine, of which less than half is parent etoposide.

With standard doses of etoposide, no drug is detectable in the cerebrospinal fluid (CSF), and even after doses of 400 to 800 mg/m^2, CSF levels are less than 2% of concurrent plasma levels (252). Despite the low distribution of drug into the CSF, mean levels of 1.4 μg/g (range undetectable to 5.9 μg/g) have been measured in brain tumor tissue (253). The drug also distributes into myometrial carcinoma and normal myometrium, achieving relatively high levels in these tissues (254).

Biliary secretion of parent drug accounts for 2% or less of the dose, although fecal recovery of drug and metabolites is variable, ranging from 1.5% to 16.3% (255). However, patients with obstructive jaundice excrete a larger fraction of the dose in urine (46%) than do unaffected patients (35%), which suggests that there is a slight decrease in hepatic drug metabolism with a commensurate increase in renal clearance (252).

The plasma protein binding of etoposide is normally high, averaging 95% in typical patients (256). The free (unbound) fraction of etoposide can vary from 6% to 37%. Patients with increased bilirubin or decreased albumin may have an increase in the free fraction, even though systemic clearance is unaltered (256). Myelosuppression may also be increased commensurately in these patients. Other conditions that may decrease etoposide clearance include prior cisplatin therapy, obesity, and elevated alkaline phosphatase levels (257).

The absolute oral bioavailability of etoposide gelatin capsules ranges from 25% to 74%, with a mean of 48% (258). Some patients experience a 30% change in overall bioavailability (both increased and decreased) with repeat dosing. Neither food nor other chemotherapeutic agents appear to alter etoposide absorption (259).

Wide variations in peak levels and AUC values were also described in this trial.

Administration and Dosage. Etoposide must be diluted before use with either 0.5% dextrose or 0.9% sodium chloride to give a final concentration of 0.2 to 0.4 mg/mL. Etoposide should be given by IV infusion over a 30- to 60-minute period. Severe hypotension may occur if the drug is given too rapidly. Although not a vesicant, extravasation of the drug should be avoided (260). Examine all solutions for fine precipitates; mix before use. Precipitation may occur if the solution is prepared 0.4 mg/mL. Continuous infusions of etoposide have been used as a means of enhancing efficacy because of its phase-specific mode of antitumor action. Most infusions have used 5-day courses, although 72-hour infusions have also been employed (261,262). Oral administration of etoposide capsules may be useful if patient compliance is high and low-emetogenic drug regimens are used. The capsules may be taken all at once to achieve the desired dose. Neither food nor other chemotherapeutic drugs appear to alter oral absorption of the drug (259).

The variety of doses and schedules that have been used with etoposide are presented in **Table 14.5**. General principles of dosing include more frequent administration to take advantage of cell cycle–dependent cytotoxicity, an approximate doubling of oral doses due to 50% bioavailability for the gelatin capsules, and significant dose reductions for combinations of etoposide with other myelosuppressive drugs, or for patients with poor bone marrow reserve or poor performance status. In general, etoposide doses can be repeated every 3 to 4 weeks, depending on the leukocyte count. A pharmacokinetic study in patients with obstructive jaundice showed that no significant dose reductions are needed if renal function is normal (263).

Side Effects and Toxicities. Side effects and toxicities for oral and IV administration of etoposide as a single agent are similar. The principal toxicity of etoposide is dose-related and dose-limiting bone marrow suppression. Leukopenia and thrombocytopenia occur, but leukopenia consistently predominates, with a nadir at approximately 16 days and with recovery usually beginning by days 20 to 22.

Gastrointestinal complaints of nausea, vomiting, or anorexia are usually minor and are more frequent with the oral preparations (264). Other adverse effects include alopecia in 20% to 90% of patients, headache, fever, and hypotension (265). Severe hypotension can occur if the drug is infused too rapidly (<30 minutes) (255). Stomatitis has been reported infrequently. There have been rare instances of generalized allergic reactions and anaphylaxis (266). A few episodes of cardiotoxicity, including myocardial infarction and congestive heart failure, have been described (267). Immune suppression appears to be minimal with this drug (265). Bronchospasm with severe wheezing has been observed rarely, and has usually been responsive to antihistamines and glucocorticosteroids. Chemical phlebitis has also been associated with etoposide, although this reaction is most likely related to solubilizers in the diluent. Diluted solutions of etoposide are not vesicants. For inadvertent extravasations of highly concentrated etoposide solution, hyaluronidase may be effective (268).

Neurotoxicity has rarely been reported with etoposide. This has consisted of somnolence and fatigue in 3% of patients and peripheral neuropathy in less than 1% of patients. However, the drug may exacerbate preexisting neuropathy caused by vincristine (269). Predisposing factors include advanced age, impaired nutritional status, and poor performance status. Degradation of myelin lamellae has been observed in affected nerves.

5-Fluorouracil and Floxuridine

5-Fluorouracil (5-FU) is a fluorinated pyrimidine differing from the normal DNA substrate, uracil, by a fluorinated number 5 carbon (chemically, 5-fluoro-2,4(1H,3H)-pyrimidinedione). 5-FU has activity as a second-line agent in advanced ovarian and cervical cancers and, in combination with cisplatin, is used as an adjunct to radiation therapy in women with locally advanced cervical cancer.

Chemistry. Floxuridine (FUDR) is highly similar to its prodrug, 5-FU. The discussion of FUDR in this chapter will be limited to its special application as an intraperitoneally administered agent in salvage therapy for ovarian cancer. 5-FU is light-sensitive and precipitates at low temperatures or, occasionally, with prolonged standing at room temperature. It has the molecular formula of $C_4H_3FN_2O_2$ and a molecular weight of 130.08.

Mechanism of Action. 5-FU acts as a false pyrimidine or antimetabolite to inhibit the formation of the DNA-specific nucleoside base thymidine. There are at least three mechanisms of action: inhibition of TS by 5-fluoro21-deoxyuridine-5′-monophosphate (FdUMP), the active metabolite of 5-FU; incorporation of FUTP into cellular RNA; and incorporation of FUTP into cellular DNA (270). 5-FU is a cell cycle phase–specific agent with cytotoxic effects seen maximally in S phase.

Drug Disposition. There is disagreement over whether 5-FU is eliminated by a two-compartment or three-compartment model

TABLE 14.5. Intravenous and Oral Dosing Schedules for Etoposide

Administration Method	Dose mg/m²/d	Dose Days	Repeat Dosing Interval (weeks)	Clinical Application
Short single-dose IV infusion	200–250	1	7	Single agent, small cell lung cancer
Short multiple-dose IV infusion	100	1–5	3–4	Testicular cancer
	100	1, 3, 5	3–4	With other drugs
	45	1–7	3	Phase I
Continuous IV infusion	125	1–5	4	Phase I, single agent
	30	1–5	4	With cisplatin in advanced cancer
	80	1–5	4	Phase I, good-risk patients
	50	1–5	4	Poor-risk patients
	125	1–3	4	Adult patients with advanced cancer (240)
	500	1 (24-hour)	3	Small cell lung cancer
Oral	160	1–5	3–4	Small cell lung cancer
	50	1–21	4	Ovarian cancer (243)

(2,271,272). Fraile and associates (273) demonstrated that plasma levels of 5-FU after oral administration are quite erratic. Schaaf and colleagues (274) documented that the pharmacokinetic characteristics of 5-FU are nonlinear. Doubling of the dose was accompanied by a decrease in nonrenal clearance. The half-life from the high dose was twice as long as that for the low dose of 5-FU. Their data were compatible with a product-inhibition model. Yoshida and coworkers (275) found positive correlations between the dose and serum steady-state levels (C_{SS}) and areas under the concentration–time curves (AUC). Patients who developed toxic reactions had greater C_{SS}s and AUCs. However, there were no correlations between serum levels and patient response to therapy.

5-FU and FUDR are extensively metabolized in the liver (hepatic metabolism can detoxify up to 80% of the total dose). However, there is no absolute documentation that patients with impaired liver function require dose reductions of 5-FU (276); however, patients should be monitored as they may be at increased risk of toxicity. As much as 15% of a dose may be found intact in the urine by 6 hours, with 90% excreted in the first hour. Depressed renal function does not generally require dosage adjustment for 5-FU.

5-FU distributes to all areas of body water by simple diffusion. Significant quantities of the drug may enter the CNS, and after 15 mg/kg given through IV, CSF levels of 6 to 8×10^{-6} M are obtained after 30 minutes. These levels persist for several hours and slowly subside. Although distribution to brain tissue is less rapid, abnormal areas, such as those with neoplasms, may more readily take up drug.

5-FU achieves high and persistent levels in effusions after IV administration. Hepatic administration through the portal vein or artery also achieves high concentrations in the liver parenchyma and produces relatively low systemic levels.

Santini and colleagues (277) showed that therapeutic monitoring of 5-FU levels in patients with head and neck cancer can be used to improve the therapeutic index of the drug (i.e., less toxicity with maximal efficacy).

Administration and Dosage. Doses of 5-FU to be given by the IV push route do not require further dilution from the commercial solution. Vein patency should be assured before administering a dose, with a 5- to 10-mL flush of normal saline or D_5W and another flush after the dose to rinse the remaining drug from the tubing. For short infusion (less than 24 hours), the rate of administration is not critical, and the dose should be given at a rate compatible with the particular vein selected. The patient should be continuously monitored to guard against extravasation. Most doses can be conveniently given over 1 to 2 minutes in this fashion.

Continuous infusions (over 4 to 5 days) may maximize the efficacy of this cycle-specific drug and lessen hematologic toxicity (278–280). Infusions of the drug may be added to a convenient volume of D_5W or normal saline, and each reconstituted daily dose can be administered over 24 hours. Commonly, the daily dose is added to 1 L, although volume is not critical.

Regimens reported for the use of 5-FU include the use of a loading dose, weekly IV bolus, continuous infusions over 4 to 5 days or over 6 weeks, and oral dosing. 5-FU may be administered intravenously as a bolus, rapid injection on a monthly (425 to 450 mg/m^2 IV on days 1 to 5 every 28 days) or a weekly schedule (500 to 600 mg/m^2 every week for 6 weeks every 8 weeks), or continuous IV infusion (24-hour infusion 2,400 to 2,600 mg/m^2 every week; 96-hour infusion 800 to 1,000 mg/m^2/d; or 120-hour infusion 1,000 mg/m^2/d on days 1 to 5 every 21 to 28 days) (50).

The loading dose scheme calls for one course of 400 to 500 mg/m^2 (12 mg/kg; maximum of 800 mg) daily for 5 days every 28 days, given as a single daily bolus injection or as a 4-day continuous infusion. This is followed by a weekly maintenance regimen. Horton and coresearchers (281) and Jacobs and coworkers (282), however, strongly associated the use of the loading dose with significant morbidity and occasional fatalities, and suggested that it offers no greater antitumor efficacy over a weekly bolus injection of 15 mg/kg given via IV.

Maintenance 5-FU dosing regimens include the following: 200 to 250 mg/m^2 (6 mg/kg) every other day for 4 days, repeated in 4 weeks (if toxicity has resolved); or 500 to 600 mg/m^2 (15 mg/kg), given by IV weekly as a continuous infusion or bolus injection (with and without the loading dose).

By continuous infusion, higher daily doses have been successfully used, and many investigators have reported lessened hematologic toxicity and enhanced efficacy. Most of a dose is eliminated by the liver, and the remainder by the kidney. Therefore, marked dysfunction in either system probably requires a dose reduction.

There are two commonly used dosing regimens for 5-FU combined with leucovorin: 370 mg/m^2/d of 5-FU for 5 days plus leucovorin given as a continuous infusion of 500 mg/m^2/d, beginning 24 hours before the first dose of 5-FU and continuing for 12 hours after completion of therapy; or 5-FU given at doses of 500 to 1,000 mg/m^2 every 2 weeks, preceded by calcium leucovorin at a dose of 20 mg/m^2 given as a 10-minute infusion (283,284).

Side Effects and Toxicities. The most pronounced and dose-limiting toxic effects of 5-FU are on the normal, rapidly proliferating tissues of the bone marrow and the lining of the gastrointestinal tract. Some nausea and vomiting can be expected. These adverse effects may respond relatively well to antiemetic treatment. Stomatitis, however, is usually an early sign of impending severe toxicity that may become evident after 5 to 8 days of therapy. Symptoms include soreness, erythema, or ulceration of the oral cavity or dysphagia. Other reported gastrointestinal symptoms are diarrhea, proctitis, and esophagitis.

Leukopenia, primarily granulocytopenia and thrombocytopenia, occur with a nadir at 9 to 14 days for the granulocytes and 7 to 14 days for platelets. Patients who are poor candidates for 5-FU therapy are those with a total leukocyte count of 2,000/mm^3 or less or a platelet count of 100,000/mm^3 or less, or those with poor nutritional status at the outset of therapy.

Some degree of alopecia is expected, although hair regrowth has occurred even when successive doses are given. Partial loss of nails and hyperpigmentation of the nail beds and other body areas (e.g., face, hands) have been reported. These may resemble the hyperpigmentation seen in Addison disease. A maculopapular rash may occur on the extremities and sometimes the trunk. The rash is usually reversible. Sunlight may heighten or initiate many dermatologic reactions to 5-FU.

Various series have reported PPEs in association with very long continuous infusion 5-FU (over several weeks). in 42% to 82% of patients. The syndrome is progressive and disrupts treatment (285). This has encouraged the development of prodrugs of 5-FU, such as 5′-deoxy-5-fluorouridine, capecitabine, BOF-A2, ftorafur, UFT, and S-1 (286,287). Although there is no indicated treatment for PPE, the incidence has been reduced to a few percentage points by limiting 5-FU continuous infusion durations to 21 days with at least one additional week off drug. Possible therapies that have yet to be evaluated in clinical trials include DMSO, systemic corticosteroids, and pyridoxine (vitamin B_6) (286,288).

Hyperpigmentation over the veins used for 5-FU administration has been observed (289). In one the veins remained patent, but there was marked darkening of the skin immediately over the vein.

5-FU may also cause an acute cerebellar syndrome that can persist beyond the period of actual treatment (290,291). Neurotoxicity may be evidenced by headache, minor visual disturbances, cerebellar ataxia, or all three. This is a rare complication. The neurotoxic metabolite is probably fluorocitrate.

Cardiotoxicity is a rare but potentially serious toxicity attributable to 5-FU. The incidence of cardiotoxicity may vary from 1.2% to 18% of patients (292) and includes cases of myocardial infarction, angina, dysrhythmias, cardiogenic shock, sudden death, and electrocardiographic changes. The mechanism producing 5-FU–induced cardiotoxicity is unknown.

Special Precautions. 5-FU should never be given to pregnant women. 5-FU may increase the cortisone requirement in patients who have had an adrenalectomy (e.g., for breast cancer), and consideration should be given to increased doses of cortisone for patients receiving 5-FU.

Because dihydropyrimidine dehydrogenase is the rate-limiting enzyme in the metabolism of 5-FU, patients with a familial deficiency of dihydropyrimidine dehydrogenase (familial pyrimidinemia) should not receive 5-FU. The administration of 5-FU to patients with this enzyme deficiency has led to severe toxicity and even death (293,294).

Accidental splashing of 5-FU on the skin or eyes of personnel should be treated with immediate irrigation with saline solution or water. There have been no long-term sequelae of these accidents (295).

Because of the alkaline nature of the drug, admixture with any acidic agents (amino acids, penicillin, multivitamins, insulin, tetracycline) represents a theoretic incompatibility.

Gemcitabine

Gemcitabine (Gemzar) was approved by the FDA in 1995 for treatment of patients with advanced pancreatic cancer, based on an increase in survival and clinical benefit (improvement in pain and performance status). The combination of gemcitabine plus cisplatin is also is FDA-approved and is considered standard therapy for patients with advanced non–small cell lung cancer. Gemcitabine has demonstrated significant activity in advanced ovarian cancer patients and is active against refractory ovarian cancer and cervical cancer, as well as other solid tumors (296–300).

Chemistry. Gemcitabine is a synthetic nucleoside analog with a structure that is highly similar to deoxycitidine and cytosine arabinoside (ara-C). Gemcitabine HCl is 2′-deoxy-2′,2′-difluorocytidine monohydrochloride (β isomer). The empirical formula for gemcitabine is $C_9H_{11}F_2N_3O_4{\cdot}HCl$, and the agent has a molecular weight of 299.66.

Mechanism of Action. Gemcitabine is a prodrug and undergoes multiple phosphorylations by deoxycytidine kinase at the intracellular level to form the active diphosphate and triphosphate metabolites. The triphosphate is incorporated into DNA as a fraudulent base pair. Following the insertion of gemcitabine, one additional deoxynucleotide is added to the end of the DNA chain before replication is terminated. This process is known as "masked chain termination" and prevents exonucleases from excising off the fraudulent base pair (301,302). The diphosphate inhibits ribonucleotide reductase and thereby depletes the deoxynucleotide pools that are necessary for DNA synthesis and repair (303). Inactivation of gemcitabine occurs when the drug is metabolized by cytidine deaminase (both intracellulary and extracellulary) to form difluorodeoxyuridine (304).

Drug Disposition. Following administration of gemcitabine 1,000 mg/m^2 by 30-minute IV infusion, the parent compound undergoes rapid clearance in a diphasic manner. The plasma half-life and clearance are dose, age, and gender dependent. Gemcitabine pharmacokinetics were evaluated in 353 patients with varied solid tumors, using short infusions (<70 minutes) and long infusions (70 to 285 minutes) at various total doses (500 to 3,600 mg/m^2) (305). There is a three- to fourfold interpatient variability in pharmacokinetics. As already noted, gemcitabine is metabolized intracellularly by deoxycytidine kinase to form the active diphosphate and triphosphate metabolites. The drug is inactivated both intracellularly and extracellularly by cytidine deaminase to form difluorodeoxyuridine (dFdU). Of the administered gemcitabine dose, 99% is excreted in the urine either as the parent compound (<10%) or as dFdU (306,307).

Dutch researchers have performed a pharmacokinetic schedule-finding study of gemcitabine plus cisplatin. Gemcitabine 800 mg/m^2 was administered as a 30-minute infusion 4 hours before, 24 hours before, 4 hours after, or 24 hours after administration of cisplatin 50 mg/m^2 by 1-hour IV infusion. Neither of the dosing schedules that used a 4-hour interval between drug administrations resulted in significant pharmacokinetic or pharmacologic differences. However, when gemcitabine was administered 24 hours before cisplatin, there was a twofold decrease in the plasma AUC of platinum. Furthermore, when the order of the drugs was reversed (i.e., cisplatin was administered 24 hours before gemcitabine), there was a 1.5-fold increase in the concentration–time product of the active triphosphate metabolite of gemcitabine within white blood cells. On the basis of these results, the investigators are conducting a phase 2 study of the cisplatin/gemcitabine combination, wherein cisplatin is administered 24 hours prior to gemcitabine (308).

Administration and Dosage. Gemcitabine should be diluted in 0.9% sodium chloride to a concentration of no greater than 40 mg/mL (higher drug concentrations may result in incomplete dissolution). Gemcitabine is generally administered as a 30-minute IV infusion at a dose of 1,000 mg/m^2; infusion durations of greater than 60 minutes are associated with dose-limiting flu-like symptoms (309).

The standard dosing schedule used for treatment of pancreatic cancer is 1,000 mg/m^2 by 30-minute IV infusion once weekly for 7 weeks for cycle 1, followed by a 1-week rest, then 1,000 mg/m^2 once weekly for 3 weeks, followed by a 1-week rest for subsequent cycles (310).

In vitro studies have shown synergism between gemcitabine and cisplatin in a variety of human cancer cell lines (311,312). It is believed that this synergism is primarily the result of increased platinum–DNA adduct formation (312). An increase in DNA–platinum adducts has also been demonstrated for the combination in the clinical arena (313) [H64]. As noted (see Drug Disposition section), the interval between cisplatin and gemcitabine administration can affect both pharmacokinetic and pharmacologic parameters (308). This combination appears to be especially promising for patients with advanced ovarian cancer.

Side Effects and Toxicities. Gemcitabine-induced toxicity is highly schedule-dependent; small daily doses are associated with greater toxicity than large doses administered on a weekly basis (314). The dose, schedule, and duration of infusion of gemcitabine directly affects the toxicity profile (314). Infusion durations of greater than 60 minutes are associated with increased myelosuppression and hepatic toxicity, whereas the administration of small daily doses results in dose-limiting flu-like symptoms (304,309). When gemcitabine is administered using the standard weekly dosing schedule, therapy is generally well tolerated, and bone marrow suppression is the major dose-limiting toxicity.

Analysis of safety data from 22 completed clinical trials, in which gemcitabine was administered on a weekly basis to 979 patients, revealed that neutropenia was the most significant hematologic side effect. Six percent of patients experienced grade 4 neutropenia, and an additional 20% experienced grade 3 neutropenia. Grade 4 leukopenia was experienced by less than 1% of patients. Decreases in white blood cell counts were noncumulative, short-lived, and rarely resulted in complications. Only 6 of the 979 patients (1.1%) developed severe infections, and no patient developed a life-threatening infection. Grades 3 and 4 anemia were experienced by 6.8% and 1.3% of patients, respectively, and only 2 of the 979 patients discontinued gemcitabine secondary to anemia. Grades 3 and 4 thrombocytopenia occurred in 4.1% and 1.1% of patients, respectively. Less than 1% of patients received platelet transfusions, and only 4 patients (0.4%) discontinued therapy because of thrombocytopenia (314).

Gemcitabine is associated with a low incidence of hepatic toxicity. Grade 3 elevations in alkaline phosphatase, alanine aminotransferase (ALT), or aspartate aminotransferase (AST) occurred in less than 8% of patients. Grade 4 elevations in these liver enzymes occurred in 2% or less of patients. Grade 3 or 4 increases in bilirubin occurred in 1.8% and 0.8% of patients, respectively. It is noteworthy that one-third of patients in this study population had documented liver metastases (314).

Clinically significant renal toxicity rarely occurs with gemcitabine therapy. However, rare cases of hemolytic uremic syndrome have been reported with gemcitabine therapy. The incidence is believed to be approximately 0.6% (314,315).

Other nonhematologic toxicities that were reported in more than 5% of patients were nausea/vomiting (64.3% overall, 17.1% grade 3, 1.2% grade 4), fever (37.3% overall, 0.7% severe), edema (greater than 20% of patients), flu-like symptoms (18.9%, 0.9% severe), cutaneous reactions (24.8%, 0.2% severe), alopecia (14.1%, 0.4% severe), diarrhea (12.1%, 0.7% severe), somnolence (9.1%, 0.9% severe), infection (8.7%, 1.1% severe), mucositis (8.4%, 0.2% severe), constipation (7.8%, 0.7% severe), and dyspnea (7.7%, 1.2% severe). Nausea and vomiting were rarely dose-limiting, and only 2 (0.2%) patients discontinued gemcitabine therapy because of nausea. Fever was a fairly frequent toxicity and sometimes occurred in the absence of flu-like symptoms or infection. Subcutaneous edema, including peripheral edema and facial edema, occurred in a significant number of patients. Edema was generally mild to moderate in nature; few patients (0.6%) discontinued gemcitabine because of this side effect, and the edema resolved after drug discontinuation. Flu-like symptoms consisted of headache, back pain, chills, myalgia, asthenia, and anorexia, and were generally short-lived. Paracetamol reportedly provided relief to some patients. Cutaneous reactions consisted of erythema in mild cases (15.5%) and dry desquamation, vesiculation, and/or pruritus in moderate cases (9.1%). Only 1 patient developed severe cutaneous toxicity that was characterized as moist desquamation and ulceration. Dyspnea (with or without bronchospasm) occurs in less than 10% of patients following gemcitabine administration. This toxicity generally occurs within a few hours of treatment and resolves within 6 hours (314).

Fatal pulmonary toxicity (acute respiratory distress syndrome) has been reported as a rare side effect of gemcitabine therapy (316). Symptoms include progressive dyspnea, tachypnea, marked hypoxemia, and bilateral interstitial infiltrates consistent with pulmonary edema. Some patients have responded to the termination of gemcitabine therapy and treatment with corticosteroids and diuretics. Prior radiation therapy to the mediastinum may be a risk factor for gemcitabine-induced pulmonary edema (316,317).

Ifosfamide

In combination with cisplatin, ifosfamide (IFEX, Holoxan) has been administered to patients with advanced cancer of the cervix, and in combination chemotherapy, it is a second-line treatment for patients with advanced cancer of the ovary (318,319). It also has activity in advanced or recurrent endometrial cancer (320).

Chemistry. Chemically, ifosfamide is 3-(2-chloroethyl)-2-[(2-chloroethyl)amino]-tetrahydro- 2H-1,3,2-oxazaphosphorine-2-oxide, and is chemically related to the nitrogen mustards and a structural analog of cyclophosphamide. It differs only in the position of one of the two chloroethyl groups, which is transposed to the endocyclic (ring) nitrogen in ifosfamide. The molecular formula is $C_7H_{15}Cl_2N_2O_2P$, and the compound has a molecular weight of 261.1.

Mechanism of Action. Ifosfamide is a metabolically activated alkylating agent. Like cyclophosphamide, it must first undergo hydroxylation by microsomal (mixed-function oxidase) enzyme systems (321). The activation of ifosfamide occurs more slowly than that of cyclophosphamide, and there is quantitatively greater oxidation of the chloroethyl side chains with ifosfamide. This leads to a greater production of chloracetaldehyde, a possible neurotoxin.

The activation process generates highly reactive metabolites, particularly 4-hydroxyifosfamide, which are capable of cellular uptake and, ultimately, covalent binding to protein and to DNA (322). Metabolites can spontaneously break down to yield the bladder irritant acrolein and the active alkylating moiety, ifosforamide mustard. Cross-linking of DNA strands proceeds from ifosforamide mustard, but acrolein binds nonspecifically and covalently to bladder epithelium. The DNA–cross-link distance is greater for ifosfamide (seven atoms) compared with cyclophosphamide (five atoms). Furthermore, the aziridine forms more slowly and is less reactive because it lacks a positive charge (323). Chain scission of DNA and inhibition of thymidine uptake also occur with ifosfamide. The primary mechanism of alkylation is not cell cycle-specific.

Drug Disposition. The pharmacokinetics of ifosfamide appears to be qualitatively similar to those of cyclophosphamide. Creaven and coworkers (324) found a plasma half-life of radiolabeled ifosfamide (5,000 mg/m^2) of 13.8 hours, with 82% urinary (radioactivity) recovery.

The plasma decay pattern appears to be biexponential (two-compartment model) for large bolus doses and monoexponential (one-compartment model) with fractionated doses. In contrast to single-dose pharmacokinetics studies, Allen and associates (325) found that with sequential daily administration of 2,400 mg/m^2/d for 3 days, there is monoexponential plasma decay with a half-life of 6.9 hours and a metabolized urinary recovery fraction of 72.8%, in contrast to the biexponential decay (plasma half-life 15.2 hours) of a single-bolus dose of ifosfamide (5,000 mg/m^2). This finding suggests that the metabolic disposition of the drug may be dose-dependent. These half-lives are approximately twice those reported for cyclophosphamide. Of note, a longer ifosfamide half-life may be seen in obese patients who are more than 20% over ideal body weight. The renal clearance rate of ifosfamide is about twice that for cyclophosphamide: 21.3 versus 10.7 mL/min in bolus dosing and 18.7 versus 10.7 mL/min with fractionated doses. Only about half of an ifosfamide dose is metabolized. Compared with about 90% for cyclophosphamide. This reflects a substantial difference in the metabolic clearance capacity for the two analogs. Although more intact (inactive) ifosfamide than cyclophosphamide is renally excreted, urinary alkylating activity persists longer with ifosfamide.

Creaven and coworkers (324) demonstrated that, because unchanged ifosfamide, but not metabolites, penetrates the blood–brain barrier, alkylating activity in the CSF may occur but is probably negligible.

Administration and Dosage. Ifosfamide is reconstituted by the addition of sterile water to the vial, which should be shaken to dissolve. Ifosfamide may be further diluted to a concentration of 0.6 to 29 mg/mL in 5% dextrose or 0.9% sodium chloride. It is administered intravenously, usually by a short infusion. Ifosfamide may also be administered by slow IV push in a 75-mL minimal volume of sterile saline solution, but not water, and infused over at least 30 minutes or by continuous infusion over 5 days. Large single doses of ifosfamide produce much more toxicity than fractionated schedules, which are therefore preferred in solid-tumor treatment regimens. Adequate hydration of the patient before and for 72 hours after ifosfamide therapy is recommended to reduce the incidence of drug-induced hemorrhagic cystitis. The use of a concurrent prophylactic agent for hemorrhagic cystitis, such as mesna (Mesnex), is required to prevent severe hematuria from high-dose ifosfamide. At least 2 L of fluid each day is recommended to produce a copious urine output.

Continuous infusions of ifosfamide over 24 hours have also been given every 3 weeks (326). Mesna can be given concurrently in the same infusion container or as a 4-hour intermittent IV bolus (327). However, renal toxicities may be increased with the single, large infusions. Extravasation of the drug should not cause tissue necrosis, but one case report has been described (328).

The FDA-approved dose for testicular cancer is 1,200 mg/m^2/d for 5 consecutive days every 21 days. Other dosage schedules include 2,000 mg/m^2 IV continuous infusion on days 1 to 3 every 21 days as part of the MAID regimen (mesna, Adriamycin, ifosfamide, dacarbazine) for soft tissue sarcoma; 1,000 mg/m^2 on days 1 and 2 every 28 days as part of the ICE regimen (ifosfamide, carboplatin, etoposide) for non-Hodgkin lymphoma; and 1,000 mg/m^2 on days 1 to 3 every 21 to 28 days as part of the TIC regimen (paclitaxel, ifosfamide, carboplatin) for head and neck cancer (50).

Side Effects and Toxicities. Creaven and associates (324) reviewed the clinical toxicity of ifosfamide administered as a large bolus injection (200 to 10,000 mg/m^2) and in a fractionated 3-day (2,400 mg/m^2/d) schedule. Urinary tract toxicity is the dose-limiting factor with both schedules. The clinical hallmark is hemorrhagic cystitis, which is caused by excretion of active alkylating metabolites into the urinary bladder. Vigorous hydration with oral and IV fluids and concomitant mesna are needed to prevent serious ifosfamide-induced bladder damage. Hydration may also overcome the antidiuretic effects of this drug. Nelson and colleagues (327) used IV furosemide (20 to 40 mg) to maintain adequate urine flow in a phase 1 study of ifosfamide. Diuretic responses usually occurred within 1 hour.

Symptoms of dysuria and urinary frequency appear to parallel those of hematuria. The onset of symptoms is 1 to 2 days after injection, with an average duration of 9 days (range 1 to 41 days) (329). Dose-related ifosfamide-induced nephrotoxicity was detected by elevation of the BUN, producing a subsequent dose-related uremia in 66% of patients receiving 150 mg/kg. Other lesions seen at autopsy (4 of 7 patients) included evidence of acute tubular necrosis and pyelonephritis. At low daily doses, granular cylindruria was seen in all patients, denoting marked tubular damage. The cylindruria cleared within 10 days of drug discontinuance (329). DeFronzo and coresearchers (330) also described glomerular dysfunction and a Fanconi-type picture in a patient treated with ifosfamide. Prior cisplatin therapy may also increase ifosfamide-induced nephrotoxicity (331,332).

Nausea and vomiting are common and are more severe after a rapid injection of large ifosfamide doses. Emesis typically begins within a few hours of administration and persists an average of 3 days (range 1 to 28 days) (329).

Hematologic toxicity from ifosfamide usually involves only a mild-to-moderate degree of leukopenia in most patients. In a review by Creaven and coworkers (324), significant thrombocytopenia was not encountered for any of the dose schedules used.

Lethargy and confusion are seen with high doses of ifosfamide and may be caused by the chloracetaldehyde metabolite. Nelson and associates (327) observed that this lasted from 1 to 8 hours, was spontaneously reversible, and was related to the passage of intact drug into the CNS. Seizures, ataxia, stupor, and weakness have been reported after ifosfamide. These effects may be increased by concomitant neurotoxic drugs, such as certain antiemetics, tranquilizers, narcotics, and antihistamines. There is a single case report of nonconvulsive status epilepticus associated with ifosfamide therapy. The patient responded to discontinuation of the ifosfamide and phenytoin therapy (333). Although alkylating metabolites appear to penetrate the blood–brain barrier, the levels achieved are too low to be useful in the treatment of CNS tumors (324).

Alopecia is usually seen with ifosfamide, especially when large bolus doses are used. In a study by Van Dyk et al. (329), the average onset of maximal hair loss was 19 days (range 11 to 32 days) after the start of treatment.

Hepatic enzyme elevations have been described in some patients. The elevations in alkaline phosphatase and serum transaminase are transient and typically resolve rapidly without sequelae.

Special Precautions. The patient must be kept well-hydrated during ifosfamide therapy to reduce the potential for hemorrhagic cystitis. The use of mesna given intravenously or orally is required to prevent hemorrhagic cystitis. **Table 14.6** outlines the recommended mesna schedule for ifosfamide uroprotection.

Patients who have received previous or concurrent therapy with radiation or cytotoxic drugs may require significant ifosfamide dosage reductions. Dose reductions should also be considered for patients with impaired renal function and/or serum albumin concentrations below 3.5 g/dL.

Drug Interactions. Several drug interactions are possible with ifosfamide. Because the compound undergoes hepatic activation by microsomal enzymes, induction is potentially possible by pretreatment with various enzyme-inducing drugs, such as phenobarbital, phenytoin, and chloral hydrate.

Nephrotoxic drugs like cisplatin may significantly increase ifosfamide renal damage (331). Other drug interactions reported for cyclophosphamide that may also occur with ifosfamide include reactions with metabolic alteration of H_2-antihistamines, such as cimetidine.

TABLE 14.6. Dosing Schedules for Mesna Combined with Ifosfamide

Route of Mesna Administration	Dose (mg/kg) as a Percentage of Ifosfamide Dose at Times before and after Ifosfamide		
	15 minutes before	***4 hours after***	***8 hours after***
Intravenous	20%	20%	20%
Oral[a]	Not recommended; use IV route	0%	0%

[a]For highly reliable patients with total emetic control, mesna solution can be diluted 1:1 to 1:10 in carbonated cola drinks or in chilled fruit juices (e.g., apple, grape, tomato, and orange juice) and administered orally.

Ixabepilone

Ixabepilone is FDA-approved for use as monotherapy in the treatment of metastatic or locally advanced breast cancer after the failure of an anthracycline, a taxane, and capecitabine, or in combination with capecitabine after the failure of an anthracycline and a taxane.

Chemistry. Ixabepilone is a semisynthetic epothilone microtubule inhibitor. Epothilone is a natural product isolated from a myxobacterium, *Sorangium cellulosum*. Ixabepilone is modified by replacing the naturally occurring lactone in the macrocycle by a lactam, intended to reduce the rate of metabolism of the ring. The chemical name for ixabepilone is (1S,3S,7S,10R,11S,12S,16R)-7,11-dihydroxy-8,8,10,12,16-pentamethyl-3-[(1E)-1-methyl-2-(2-methyl-4-thiazolyl) ethenyl]-17-oxa-4-azabicyclo[14.1.0] heptadecane-5,9-dione, and it has a molecular weight of 506.7.

Mechanism of Action. Ixabepilone stabilizes αβ-II and αβ-III microtubules leading to the death of proliferating cells via a block in the mitotic phase of the cell cycle. Ixabepilone has a low affinity for the efflux pump proteins MRP1 and P-glycoprotein, which are a known cause of resistance to taxanes. It is also active in human tumor xenografts that overexpress βIII tubulin isoforms or have tubulin mutations conferring resistance to taxanes. Furthermore, it is active in human tumor xenograft models that are resistant to other commonly used anticancer drugs such as anthracyclines and vinca alkaloids.

Drug Disposition. Following IV injection of ixabepilone, the mean Vd is reported in excess of 1,000 L, indicating a very high tissue distribution. The clearance has been reported as 475 ± 247 mL/min/m^2, the half-life at 14 hours. Plasma protein binding was in the region of 67% to 77%. Ixabepilone is eliminated primarily as the metabolized drug in the feces. Approximately 86% of an administered dose was eliminated in 7 days, with 65% of the dose in the feces and 21% of the dose in the urine. Unchanged ixabepilone was 1.6% of the dose in the feces and 5.6% of the dose in the urine of the recovered dose, respectively. Ixabepilone is extensively metabolized in the liver, and studies with human liver microsomes suggest that CYP3A4 is the primary route.

Dosage. The recommended dosage of ixabepilone is 40 mg/m^2 administered intravenously over 3 hours every 3 weeks. Dose adjustments are recommended for hematologic and neurologic toxicities. One of the license indications for ixabepilone is for use in combination with capecitabine. Ixabepilone with capecitabine is contraindicated in patients with AST or ALT >2.5 × ULN or bilirubin >1 × ULN because of increased risk of toxicity and neutropenia-related death.

To minimize the chance of hypersensitivity reactions, it is recommended that all patients receive premedication with an H1 and H2 inhibitor. Patients who experience a hypersensitivity reaction should receive treatment with corticosteriods.

Side Effects and Toxicities. Dose-dependent myelosuppression is seen with grade 4 neutropenia, reported in 36% of patients. Myelosuppression is more severe in patients with hepatic impairment. Peripheral neuropathy is common and has been reported in approximately 65% of patients, with 14% to 21% grade 3/4.

Drug Interactions. Drug interactions are to be expected with other drugs that are metabolized by (e.g., ketoconazole) or induce (e.g., rifampin) CYP3A4. These two drugs have been shown to increase and decrease the exposure to ixabepilone by +79% and −43%, respectively. It is recommended that strong inhibitors or inducers of CYP3A4 be avoided where possible and dose modifications considered when any strong or weak inducer of inhibitor is used.

Liposomal Encapsulated Doxorubicin

Liposomal doxorubicin (Doxil, Caelyx) is FDA-approved for the treatment of patients with metastatic, refractory ovarian cancer, and AIDS-related Kaposi sarcoma.

Chemistry. Doxorubicin HCl, which is the established name for (8*S*,10*S*)-10-[(3-amino-2,3,6- trideoxy-α-L-*lyxo*-hexopyranosyl) oxy]-8-glycolyl-7,8,9,10-tetrahydro-6,8,11-trihydroxy-1- methoxy-5,12-naphthacenedione hydrochloride, has a molecular weight of 579.99 and the molecular formula $C_{27}H_{29}NO_{11} \cdot HCl$. The liposomal carriers are composed of *N*-(carbonyl-methoxypolyethylene glycol 2000)-1,2distearoyl- *sn*-glycero-3-phosphoethanolamine sodium salt (MPEG-DSPE), 3.19 mg/mL; fully hydrogenated soy phosphatidylcholine, 9.58 mg/mL; and cholesterol, 3.19 mg/mL. Greater than 90% of the drug is encapsulated in the liposomes. The liposomal encapsulation of doxorubicin dramatically alters the pharmacokinetic and toxicity profiles of the drug.

Mechanism of Action. The mechanism of action of doxorubicin mirrors that of doxorubicin. Liposomes are microscopic vesicles composed of a phospholipid bilayer that are capable of encapsulating active drugs. The liposomes of the encapsulated form of doxorubicin are formulated with surface-bound MPEG, a process often referred to as pegylation, to protect liposomes from detection by the mononuclear phagocyte system and to increase blood circulation time (334).

Drug Disposition. Liposomal doxorubicin is associated with a much longer plasma half-life, slower plasma clearance, and reduced Vd than free doxorubicin. In a pharmacokinetics study performed in 6 patients with solid tumors, the area under the plasma disappearance curve was 1.0 mg/L hour versus 609 mg/L hour when 25 mg/m^2 of doxorubicin was administered as free drug or as a pegylated liposomal form, respectively. The initial half-life was 0.07 versus 3.2 hours, and the terminal half-life was 8.7 versus 45.2 hours for the free and liposomal forms of doxorubicin, respectively. Additionally, the steady-state Vd was 254 L versus 4.1 L for the free and liposomal forms, respectively (335). Liposomal encapsulation of doxorubicin has also been shown to result in fourfold to 16-fold increases in tumor-tissue drug concentrations relative to that achieved following administration of the free form.

Administration and Dosage. Liposomal doxorubicin must be diluted in 250 mL of 5% dextrose before administration. Because liposomal doxorubicin contains no preservative or bacteriostatic agent, aseptic technique must be strictly observed. Liposomal doxorubicin may be administered as an IV infusion over 30 to 60 minutes. In that liposomal doxorubicin is not a vesicant, extravasation of the drug is not a critical concern. For ovarian cancer patients, liposomal doxorubicin should be administered at a dose of 50 mg/m^2 (every 4 weeks) at an initial rate of 1 mg/min to reduce the risk of infusion reactions. The rate may be increased to a 60-minute infusion if no adverse events are noted; however, in clinical practice, a dose of 40 mg/m^2 is more commonly employed.

Side Effects and Toxicities. Unlike the parent drug, liposomal doxorubicin is not a vesicant and is associated with minimal cardiotoxicity, alopecia, and nausea/vomiting. However, the liposomal encapsulation results in acute infusion reactions, and an increased rate of PPE and stomatitis (336). PPE is a dose-limiting toxicity that can occur in 26% of patients who receive 50 mg/m^2 every 4 weeks (337). Stomatitis is a second dose-limiting toxicity associated with liposomal doxorubicin. Current methods to prevent PPE and stomatitis include dose reduction and discontinuation (grade 1—redose. If the patient has experienced previous grade 3 or 4 toxicity, delay the treatment by 2 weeks until resolution to grades 0 to 1, and reduce dose by 25% before returning to original dose level; grades 2 to 4—delay up to 2 weeks until resolved, if no resolution to grades 0 to 1, discontinue; grades 3 to 4—after delay and resolution to grades 0 to 1, decrease dose by 25%, if no resolution, discontinue). To help relieve pain from PPE, topical wound care, elevation, and cold compresses may be used as supportive care (288). Topical DMSO has been used to treat skin extravations (99% DMSO four times daily up to 14 days), but has yet to be evaluated in a randomized trial (286). Other possible therapies that have yet to be evaluated in clinical trials include systemic corticosteroids and pyridoxine (vitamin B_6) (288).

Infusion-related reactions occur in less than 10% of patients treated with liposomal doxorubicin and are most common during the first course of treatment. Symptoms may include flushing, shortness of breath, facial swelling, headache, chills, back pain, tightness in the chest and throat, and hypotension. Alopecia has been observed in only 15% of ovarian cancer patients treated with liposomal doxorubicin.

Methotrexate

Methotrexate is an active drug in the first-line treatment of gestational choriocarcinoma, chorioadenoma destruens, and hydatidiform mole. It is used in the prophylaxis and treatment of meningeal leukemia, and in combination with other agents for the treatment of breast cancer, epidermoid cancers of the head and neck, advanced mycosis fungoides, advanced non-Hodgkin lymphoma, lung cancer, and metastatic squamous cell cancer of the cervix.

Chemistry. Methotrexate is a cell cycle–specific antifolate analog, which differs from folic acid in two substitutions: an amino group for a hydroxyl in the pteridine portion of the molecule and a methyl group on the amino nitrogen between the pteridine nucleus and the benzoyl group of 4-amino-10-methyl folic acid. Chemically, methotrexate is *N*-[4-[[(2,4-diamino-6-pteridinyl)methyl]benzoyl]-L-glutamic acid. It is a weak acid with a molecular weight of 454.45 and a molecular formula of $C_{20}H_{22}N_8O_5$. It is only slightly soluble in water and alcohol. Sodium methotrexate is water soluble and is used in injectable preparations.

Mechanism of Action. Free intracellular methotrexate tightly binds to dihydrofolate reductase (DHFR), blocking the reduction of dihydrofolate to tetrahydrofolic acid, the active form of folic acid. As a result, thymidylate synthetase and various steps in de novo purine synthesis that require 1-carbon transfer reactions are halted. This in turn arrests DNA, RNA, and protein synthesis.

Amino acid syntheses blocked by methotrexate include those requiring 1-carbon transfer, such as the conversion of glycine to serine and homocysteine to methionine. Experimental studies have shown that thymidylate synthetase is inhibited at methotrexate concentrations of 10^{-8} M or less, but inhibition of purine synthesis requires concentrations of 10^{-7} M or greater (338).

Methotrexate undergoes a variable degree of polyglutamation intracellularly. The polyglutamated forms of the drug are positively charged and do not readily pass through cell membranes. Methotrexate polyglutamates form an intracellular pool of active drug that is retained for long periods, sometimes months, after a single dose (339). The ability of tumor cells to add t-glutamyl residues to methotrexate may be a key determinant of antitumor activity.

The effects of methotrexate are rapidly reversible as free methotrexate leaves the cells. The normal intracellular levels of dihydrofolate are very low (10^{-8} M) but increase greatly after methotrexate administration.

Resistance to methotrexate may develop as a result of elevated DHFR activity or defective transport of methotrexate into malignant cells. Increased DHFR enzyme levels may also result from amplification of the DHFR gene, a process associated with homogeneously staining regions of chromosomes and an unstable inheritance mediated by double minutes or extra chromosomal DNA fragments (340). Certain quinazolines have been shown to be effective inhibitors of thymidylate synthetase and may be useful clinically in overcoming this type of resistance (341). *In vitro* studies and clinical experimentation with high-dose therapy indicate that a major mechanism of resistance is probably secondary to decreased cellular uptake.

Methotrexate is classified as a cell cycle phase–specific antimetabolite with activity mostly in S phase. Experimentally, methotrexate synchronizes tumor cells in S phase about 36 to 72 hours after administration (342).

The enhanced toxic effect on tumors compared with normal tissue from high-dose methotrexate with leucovorin rescue may be a result of bypassing normal carrier-mediated cell membrane transport of methotrexate. Leucovorin and its metabolite, 5-methyltetrahydrofolate, share a common influx transport site with methotrexate. There appear to be at least two active transport carrier systems involved in the influx and efflux of methotrexate and folates (343). If normal cells are rescued with calcium leucovorin, methotrexate can then exert a relatively greater toxic effect on the tumor cells. Selective rescue of normal cells may be mediated by a slower rate of DNA synthesis relative to the tumor cell or to tissue-specific differences in transmembrane transport.

Drug Disposition. Orally administered methotrexate is rapidly but incompletely absorbed from the gastrointestinal tract. It reaches peak blood levels in approximately 1 hour. Approximately 50% to 60% of the drug in the blood is bound to plasma proteins. Methotrexate is widely distributed to body tissues. In conventional doses, methotrexate is excreted unchanged in the urine. In high doses, it is partially metabolized to 7-hydromethotrexate, which is only slightly soluble in acidic solutions. About 1% to 11% of a dose is excreted as the 7-hydroxy metabolite, and this may comprise as much as 35% of the drug level in the terminal elimination phase. Only about one-third of an oral dose is absorbed, but IM absorption is almost 100% (344).

The hepatic extraction coefficient for methotrexate appears to be very low, and intra-arterial hepatic doses show metabolism and pharmacokinetics similar to IV doses (345). Methotrexate is both filtered at the glomerulus and actively secreted by the renal tubule. Drugs that interfere with renal excretion of weak acids, such as probenecid, sulfinpyrazone, and salicylates, may be expected to reduce the rate of methotrexate excretion. Probenecid has been used successfully in one study to produce a prolonged elevation of plasma methotrexate levels from otherwise low doses of methotrexate (346).

Plasma decay of methotrexate levels have reportedly been biphasic and possibly triphasic. Huffman and associates (347) reported half-lives after a 30 mg/m^2 dose to be triphasic: 0.750 ± 0.11, 3.49 ± 0.55, and 26.99 ± 4.44 hours, respectively. Stoller and colleagues (348) reported a biphasic plasma decay for high-dose therapy of 2.06 ± 0.16 and 10.4 ± 1.8 hours. Wang and coresearchers (349) reported age-dependent biphasic elimination of high-dose methotrexate.

Patients with pleural effusions may accumulate methotrexate that slowly distributes from this compartment back into the plasma to increase systemic exposure and the risk of toxicity (350). Effusions should be drained before administration of methotrexate.

Administration and Dosage. Methotrexate may be given by the oral, IM, IV (IV infusion or push), intra-arterial, or intrathecal routes. For treatment of neoplastic disease, oral administration of low-dose methotrexate is preferred because of rapid absorption of the tablet form of the agent. Methotrexate has been administered by numerous dosing schedules. The usual starting doses are adjusted based on clinical response and hematologic monitoring. In general, methotrexate is administered orally or intramuscularly in doses of 15 to 30 mg daily for a 5-day course. Courses are usually repeated three to five times as required, with rest periods of 1 or more weeks between courses until toxicities subside (351). Leucovorin is indicated following treatment with higher doses of methotrexate, to diminish toxicity.

If the IV formulation is administered, the dose should be reduced by 50% for patients with renal insufficiency (BUN ≥30 mg/L). Similar dose reductions should be made for the oral form, although no specific guidelines are available. Methotrexate administration is contraindicated in patients with a CrCl less than 40 mL/min and/or a serum creatinine greater than 2 mg/dL.

Side Effects and Toxicities. Hematologic effects of methotrexate include leukopenia, thrombocytopenia, and anemia. They occur rapidly and depend on the dose and schedule used. The nadir of hemoglobin depression occurs after 6 to 13 days and of reticulocyte at 2 to 7 days, with rebound between 9 and 19 days. Leukocyte nadir occurs within 4 to 7 days, followed by partial recovery and then, in rare instances, a second decrease in the leukocyte counts occurs during days 12 to 21. The platelet nadir is reached in 5 to 12 days. Hypogammaglobulinemia may also occur after methotrexate administration.

Nausea, vomiting, and anorexia are usually the earliest gastrointestinal symptoms. Gingivitis, glossitis, pharyngitis, stomatitis, and ulcerations with bleeding of the mucosal membranes of the mouth or other portions of the gastrointestinal tract may occur. If ulcerative stomatitis or diarrhea occurs, methotrexate therapy must be interrupted to prevent severe hemorrhagic enteritis or intestinal perforation.

Hepatotoxicity is more common in patients receiving high-dose therapy and in those receiving frequent small doses. Hepatocellular injury is indicated in liver function tests by a rise in SGOT and SGPT, usually within the first 12 hours. Prothrombin times may rise with a decrease in plasma factor VII activity, and indirect hyperbilirubinemia may develop. All of these usually return to normal within 1 week. Hepatocytes appear to be protected by fractionated high-dose methotrexate treatments with leucovorin rescue if treatments are administered at intervals of less than 1 week. This may be due to leucovorin activity remaining from prior doses. Various pathologic hepatic changes can occur, including atrophy, necrosis, fatty changes, fibrosis, and cirrhosis. Liver biopsy is the only reliable means of assessing the degree of methotrexate hepatotoxicity.

Dermatologic side effects include erythematous rashes, pruritus, urticaria, folliculitis, vasculitis, photosensitivity, depigmentation, or hyperpigmentation. Alopecia may occur, with several months being required for regrowth. CNS effects include dizziness, malaise, and blurred vision. Encephalopathy also has been reported. Intrathecal administration has been followed by increased CSF pressure, convulsions, paresis, and a syndrome resembling the Guillain–Barré syndrome (352). Deaths have been reported after intrathecal therapy. Renal failure may occur in patients receiving methotrexate, especially in high doses. This risk may be decreased by alkalinization of the urine to increase methotrexate solubility and by giving large quantities of fluid. Other reactions rarely reported include chills and fever, osteoporosis, and pulmonary reactions, mainly fibrosis (353).

Drug Interactions. Potential drug interactions have been postulated to occur with other protein-bound drugs, such as salicylates, sulfonamides, phenytoin, and *p*-aminobenzoic acid. These drugs displace methotrexate from its protein-binding site in the blood, causing an increase in the levels of the free drug. However, the overall degree of binding is probably not high enough for major displacement interactions.

Antibiotics used in gut sterilization may also alter methotrexate pharmacokinetics in humans, eliminating the slow phase of excretion (354). Salicylates and probenecid may also compete with methotrexate for renal tubular secretion and increase its serum half-life.

Ethyl alcohol may increase the possibility of methotrexate-induced hepatotoxicity. Oral anticoagulants, such as warfarin, may be greatly potentiated by methotrexate. Methotrexate may alter the liver metabolism of these drugs.

There are several drug interactions described for methotrexate with other chemotherapeutic agents. For example, a clinically significant interaction between methotrexate and L-asparaginase involves the administration of methotrexate 3 to 24 hours before L-asparaginase. The methotrexate treatment is believed to block protein synthesis and reduce asparaginase toxicities, allowing larger doses to be given. Some sequential methotrexate combinations may produce enhanced therapeutic activity. For example, methotrexate given 4 to 9 hours before 5-FU may produce enhanced antitumor activity in breast cancer, but with a commensurate increase in toxic effects (163,355). The mechanism of this interaction involves a significant increase in 5-FU for at least 3 hours (355). The reverse sequence decreases therapeutic activity (356).

Methotrexate activity is enhanced, and thus toxicity increased, when it is used with aspirin, penicillins, nonsteroidal anti-inflammatory agents, cephalosporins, or phenytoin. These agents inhibit the renal excretion of methotrexate (50).

Mitomycin

Mitomycin (Mutamycin, mitomycin C) is a purple antibiotic isolated from *Streptomyces caespitosus* that is indicated for disseminated adenocarcinoma of the stomach or pancreas in combination with other agents and as palliative treatment. It has also proved useful in combination chemotherapy as a third-line agent in the treatment of advanced cervical cancer.

Chemistry. The chemical name for mitomycin is [1*aR*]6-amino-8-[[(aminocarbonyl)oxy]methyl]- 1,1*a*,2,8,8*a*,8*b*-hexahydro-8*a*-methoxy-5-methylazirino[2′,3′:3,4]-pyrrolo[1,2-*a*]indole-4,7-dione, and it has a molecular weight of 334. Mitomycin is heat stable, is soluble in water and other organic solvents, and has a unique absorption peak at 365 nM (357). In solution, it is slowly inactivated by visible but not ultraviolet light. It is very unstable in acidic and highly basic conditions. The aziridine and carbamate groups on mitomycin are necessary for alkylating activity but not for antibacterial activity. The compound is activated by reduction of the quinone moiety, which releases a methanol residue from the molecule. This allows the aziridine ring to open, exposing an electrophilic carbon at C_1 (alkylating site). The second (cross-linking) site for alkylation is exposed at C_{10} after an enzymatic or chemically mediated loss of the carbamate side chain.

Mechanism of Action. Mitomycin is activated *in vivo* to an alkylating agent that cross-links complementary DNA strands, halting DNA synthesis. DNA is the major site of mitomycin activity, although at extremely high concentrations, RNA synthesis may also be affected. The active metabolites of mitomycin resulting from reduction of the quinone moiety yield an opened aziridine ring exposing the primary alkylating site at C_1. A second alkylating site at C_{10} is exposed with the enzymatic loss of the carbamate side chain (358). The molecular site of DNA binding has been identified at the N_2 and O_6 positions of adjacent guanines in the minor groove of DNA (359).

Activation of the drug can be mediated by chemical reducing agents, by microsomal enzymes, or even by brief exposure to an acidic pH. The extent of DNA binding appears to be related to the guanine and cytosine content of the particular DNA. Cytotoxicity probably results directly from DNA synthesis inhibition secondary to alkylation.

Oxygen free radicals may also contribute to the cytotoxicity of mitomycin by producing DNA strand breaks (360). Oxygen free radicals are produced by cyclic redox reactions of the quinone moiety. Mitomycin's cytotoxic action is not cell cycle phase–specific, but cytotoxic effects are maximized if cells are treated in late G_1 and early S phase. In addition to the direct cytotoxic effects of the drug, mitomycin also causes chromosomal aberrations (mutagenic activity), and in experimental systems, it is a potent carcinogen and teratogen.

Kennedy and coworkers (361) described selective activation of mitomycin by hypoxic cells, suggesting some drug selectivity for hypoxic tumors. Resistance to mitomycin involves an increase in specific cytosolic proteins (possibly a glutathione transferase) and collateral resistance with anthracyclines and dactinomycin (362,363). The latter type of multidrug resistance is mediated by P-glycoprotein expression, with resultant enhanced drug efflux, as observed in mitomycin C–resistant L-1210 cells (364).

Drug Disposition. Mitomycin is cleared rapidly from the vascular compartment. Peak serum concentrations of about 1 μg/mL are typically achieved after IV bolus doses of 10 mg/m^2 (365). Less than 10% of the dose is excreted into the urine, and this is complete within a few hours after administration. Mitomycin has also been detected in the bile and feces, although animal studies demonstrate that the highest drug levels occur in the kidneys. Detectable levels were also found in muscle, lung, intestine, stomach, and eye, but not in the brain, spleen, or liver (357).

The primary means of mitomycin elimination is by liver metabolism, but the specific enzymes responsible are unknown. However, the enzymes responsible for metabolism do not appear to involve the P450 mixed-function oxide family. *In vitro* studies demonstrate drug inactivation on contact with tissue preparations from the spleen, liver, kidney, brain, and heart. This inactivation is further augmented by anaerobic conditions (357).

There is no detectable change in mitomycin pharmacokinetics in patients with altered hepatic function nor when other drugs, including furosemide, are given concurrently (365,366). Schilcher and colleagues (367) showed that the pharmacokinetics of mitomycin do not change after the administration of high doses.

Mitomycin distribution into bile and ascites fluids has been quantitated in patients receiving standard IV doses. The maximum biliary level of 0.5 μg/mL was achieved after 2 hours and was five- to eightfold higher than simultaneous plasma levels during the elimination phase (368). Mitomycin also rapidly penetrates into ascites fluid and reaches maximal concentrations of 0.05 μg/mL 1 hour after administration. This distribution represents about 40% of the total plasma exposure. The drug also appears to concentrate slightly in cervical tissues after IV administration (369).

With intra-arterial administration, the hepatic extraction of mitomycin averages only 23% (370). The calculated relative advantage for hepatic arterial infusions is only 2.5- to 3.6-fold greater than for other methods.

Administration and Dosage. Sterile water (10 mL) should be added to each 5-mg vial of mitomycin and shaken gently to dissolve. Mitomycin should be administered intravenously to avoid extravasation of the drug. If extravasation occurs, severe local tissue necrosis may occur (371). The drug is usually given by a slow IV push, with continuous patient monitoring to lessen the chance of extravasation. Short infusions in 100 to 150 mL of D_5W or normal saline have also been used. Vein patency should be checked before the administration of any dose, using 5 to 10 mL of fluid that does not contain the drug. The same procedure should follow the dose. This flushes any remaining drug from the tubing and the venipuncture site.

The recommended dose of mitomycin used as a single agent is 20 mg/m^2 given IV every 6 to 8 weeks. In combination with other myelosuppressive drugs, mitomycin doses are typically limited to 10 mg/m^2 every 6 to 8 weeks. Bolus doses greater than 20 mg/m^2 produce severe toxicity without greatly enhancing efficacy.

Repeat dosing of mitomycin should be based on adequate marrow recovery, including leukocytes, platelets, and erythrocytes. Leukocyte count should return to 4,000/mm^3, and platelet count to 100,000/mm^3.

An ambulatory continuous infusion of mitomycin has been administered at 0.75 $mg/m^2/d$ for consecutive 50-day dosing (372). A dosing regimen of 3 $mg/m^2/d$ for 5 days every 4 to 6 weeks has also been used (372). These regimens are believed to deliver greater dose intensity by reducing myelosuppression. Intra-arterial perfusion doses of 20 mg/m^2 have been given every 6 to 8 weeks (373).

Side Effects and Toxicities. Bone marrow suppression involving platelets, leukocytes, and erythrocytes is the most serious toxicity, and it can continue for 3 to 8 weeks after drug administration is halted (357). Myelosuppression, particularly anemia, can be cumulative. This has been minimized by keeping total lifetime doses under 50 to 60 mg/m^2.

Gastrointestinal disturbances in the form of nausea, vomiting, and anorexia occasionally develop. These reactions are usually not severe and have an onset within 1 to 2 hours after administration. They may persist for several hours. Stomatitis may also occur, but it is generally not severe.

Renal toxicity detected by increasing serum BUN and creatinine levels with glomerular dysfunction is occasionally seen. This does not appear to be dose- or treatment-duration related, and it is usually not severe. However, mitomycin can also induce a microangiopathic hemolytic anemia with progressive renal failure (hemolytic-uremic syndrome) and cardiopulmonary decompensation. This disease is fatal within 3 to 4 weeks of diagnosis, although the onset is typically delayed for months after mitomycin administration (374). The incidence of this toxic effect may approach 10% among patients given large cumulative doses (374). In one series, renal complications from mitomycin developed in 1.6% of 63 patients receiving a total dose of 50 mg/m^2 or less, 11% of 37 patients receiving 50 to 69 mg/m^2, and 28% of 18 patients receiving total doses greater than 70 mg/m^2 (375). This suggests that a threshold for inducing microangiopathic hemolytic anemia may be a cumulative dose of about 50 mg/m^2 of mitomycin. Signs of the disease include thrombocytopenia, circulating schistocytes, and acute renal failure. Histopathologic examinations of the kidneys reveal fibrin thrombi in arterioles, tubular atrophy, and widespread glomerular necrosis.

Veno-occlusive disease of the liver has been reported after high-dose mitomycin therapy and autologous bone marrow transplantation (376). Signs include progressive hepatic dysfunction, abdominal pain, and ascites. Although this has rarely been observed with low-dose therapy, it appears to be much more frequent after high-dose regimens.

Alopecia may occur after mitomycin therapy, but it is usually not severe. Rarely, purple bands in the nail beds correspond to sequential doses of the drug. Lethargy or weakness may occur and can last from several days to 3 weeks. Fatigue and some drowsiness or confusion have also been observed. Dose-related skin reactions and fever with drug administration are occasionally seen.

Severe soft tissue ulcers may also be expected if the drug escapes the vein during administration. Mitomycin extravasation injuries can result in chronic ulcers that can expand over months (377). Particularly distressing aspects of some mitomycin extravasations include the delayed (3 to 4 months) and sometimes distal occurrence of soft tissue ulceration after uneventful injections in a peripheral vein (377,378). In animals, the only effective antidote to mitomycin skin reactions was topical DMSO (99% DMSO). Mitomycin extravasations may be empirically treated with topical application of 1.5 mL of DMSO every 6 hours for 14 days (379).

Interstitial pneumonia thought to be secondary to mitomycin has been reported in a small number of patients. These patients showed rapid improvement after treatment with corticosteroids (380).

Special Precautions. Myelosuppression may be cumulative with successive doses of mitomycin and may necessitate dose reductions. Careful monitoring of blood counts is critical. Serious local ulceration may occur if the drug is delivered outside the vein. Extravasation of mitomycin must be avoided.

Clinically significant antitumor drug synergy in humans has yet to be described for mitomycin, although it is probably at least additive in several drug combinations, including the FAM regimen (5-FU, doxorubicin, mitomycin) used in gastrointestinal cancer, the MOB regimen [mitomycin, vincristine (Oncovin), bleomycin] used in carcinoma of the uterine cervix, and megestrol acetate in patients with advanced breast cancer.

Paclitaxel

Paclitaxel (Taxol) is one of the most commonly used drugs in oncology, with FDA approval for primary and subsequent treatment of epithelial ovarian cancer, as salvage therapy for metastatic breast cancer, in second-line treatment of AIDS-related Kaposi sarcoma, and in the treatment of non–small cell lung cancer. It is also active against a variety of other solid tumors, including cervical and endometrial cancer (381–384).

Chemistry. It is a diterpene plant product derived from the bark of the Pacific yew, *Taxus baccata*. It has a molecular weight of 853.9, is insoluble in water, and has an empirical formula of $C_{47}H_{51}NO_{14}$. Its chemical name is 5β,20-epoxy-1,2α,4,7β,10β,13α-hexahydroxytax- 11-en-9-one4,10-diacetate 2-benzoate 13-ester with (2*R*,3*S*)-*N*-benzoyl-3-phenylisoserine.

Mechanism of Action. Paclitaxel acts as a mitotic spindle poison. In a manner contrary to known mitotic spindle inhibitors, such as colchicine and podophyllotoxin, paclitaxel promotes assembly of microtubules and stabilizes them, preventing depolymerization. This inability to depolymerize microtubules prevents cellular replication (144).

Drug Disposition. Early pharmacokinetic studies using standard doses and a 24-hour infusion suggested that paclitaxel pharmacokinetics were linear; however, with short infusions and/or high dose levels, paclitaxel's nonlinear pharmacokinetics become readily apparent (190). The nonlinearity is due to saturable distribution, metabolism, and elimination. Terminal elimination half-life is largely dependent on the dose and administration schedule. At a dose level of 175 mg/m^2 with a 3-hour infusion, mean pharmacokinetic parameters of paclitaxel include the following: plasma $t_{1/2\alpha}$, 16 minutes; plasma $t_{1/2\beta}$, 140 minutes; plasma $t_{1/2\gamma}$, 18.75 hours; plasma clearance, 12.69 $L/h/m^2$; plasma AUC, 16.81 μmol/L · h; 48-hour urinary excretion, <10% of dose; and 48-hour fecal excretion, 70% of dose (190).

Clearance is rapid and not due to urinary excretion; the major route of paclitaxel elimination is believed to be via hepatic metabolism and subsequent biliary excretion (382). About 70% to 80% of the drug is eliminated by fecal excretion.

Administration and Dosage. All patients undergoing paclitaxel therapy should receive premedication to prevent severe hypersensitivity reactions. A recommended regimen is dexamethasone (either 20 mg orally the night before treatment and the morning of treatment or 20 mg IV 30 minutes before paclitaxel delivery) plus diphenhydramine (50 mg) and famotidine (20 mg) IV 30 minutes before chemotherapy (386). For the majority of patients, administration of dexamethasone 20 mg IV 30 to 60 minutes before paclitaxel is sufficient and has been proved effective in preventing hypersensitivity reactions.

Paclitaxel is commercially available as an injection concentrate in 30-mg (5 mL), 100-mg (16.7 mL), and 300-mg (50 mL) multidose vials. Before infusion, paclitaxel must be diluted with 0.9% sodium chloride, 5% dextrose, 5% dextrose and 0.9% sodium chloride injection, or 5% dextrose in Ringer's injection to a final concentration of 0.3 to 1.2 mg/mL. The solution is stable for up to 27 hours at room temperature. Paclitaxel should be administered through an in-line filter with a microporous membrane not greater than 0.22 μ to remove particulates that are present in paclitaxel solutions. Although particulate formation does not indicate loss of drug potency, solutions exhibiting excess particulate matter formation should be discarded. Because of the possibility of leaching of phthalate plasticizers with paclitaxel solutions, only nonpolyvinylchloride (such as polyethylene or polyolefin) IV administration sets should be used.

As a result of an unacceptable level of severe hypersensitivity reactions in early phase I studies (most likely related to the Cremaphor EL vehicle), a 24-hour infusion schedule and a premedication regimen with corticosteroids and histamine H_1- and H_2-antagonists were used in all phase 2 and 3 clinical trials conducted in the United States from 1987 to 1992. Later clinical studies established that a 3-hour paclitaxel infusion schedule can be administered safely without a significant increase in major hypersensitivity reactions and that the shortened infusion schedule is associated with significantly less grade 4 neutropenia than the 24-hour infusion (i.e., 71% vs. 18% for the 24- and 3-hour infusions, respectively) (352). Follow-up studies have determined that a 1-hour infusion schedule is also feasible; however, infusion durations of less than 1 hour are associated with a prohibitively high rate of hypersensitivity reactions (387).

The FDA-approved recommended therapeutic regimen for patients with platinum-refractory ovarian cancer is paclitaxel 135 or 175 mg/m^2 administered IV over 3 hours every 3 weeks, but the optimal regimen has not been clearly established. Paclitaxel has been administered by various other schedules during investigational studies in patients with solid tumors, including 135 to 250 mg/m^2 as a 24-hour continuous infusion every 3 weeks; 212 to 225 mg/m^2 as a 6-hour infusion every 3 weeks; 30 mg/m^2 as a 1-hour infusion daily for 5 days every 3 weeks; 30 mg/m^2 as a 6-hour infusion daily for 5 days every 3 weeks; 120 to 140 mg/m^2 as a 96-hour infusion every 3 weeks; and 150 mg/m^2 as a 120-hour infusion every 3 weeks (144).

Weekly schedules of paclitaxel have been explored extensively, particularly in combination with carboplatin, and this has emerged as a reasonable option for the treatment of ovarian cancer. They are generally better tolerated than the higher dose used with every 3-week dosing (388,389).

Special Precautions. Before the institution of standard prophylactic medications, the incidence of major hypersensitivity reactions associated with paclitaxel therapy approached 25% to 30%. With premedication, the incidence of severe hypersensitivity reactions has decreased to less than 2%. The majority of paclitaxel-induced hypersensitivity reactions can be categorized as grade 1, with symptoms of dyspnea with bronchospasm, urticaria, and hypotension. Major sensitivity reactions usually occur within the first 10 minutes after the first or second dose of paclitaxel (144). Minor symptoms of flushing and rashes are not predictive of the future development of severe manifestations (144,352). According to National Cancer Institute guidelines for paclitaxel administration, emergency equipment must be available, and medical personnel should be in attendance during paclitaxel infusion, especially during the first 15 minutes of the first and second courses. Vital signs should be periodically monitored during the first several hours of drug infusion. The paclitaxel infusion should be discontinued immediately if symptoms of a major hypersensitivity reaction occur (including respiratory distress, hypotension, generalized urticaria, and angioedema). Severe hypersensitivity reactions may be treated with IV epinephrine, IV diphenhydramine, IV fluids, and nebulized beta-agonists. Steroid therapy may be helpful in the resolution of recurrent symptoms (390). There is strong evidence that patients who develop major hypersensitivity reactions may be successfully retreated with slow, low-dose infusions of paclitaxel after premedication with multiple high doses of corticosteroids and antihistamines (391).

Drug Interactions. Paclitaxel therapy appears to modify the hematologic toxicity associated with platinum agents. Rowinsky et al. (392) conducted a phase 1 study of sequential escalating doses of paclitaxel and cisplatin therapy, and determined that myelosuppression was more severe when paclitaxel was administered immediately after cisplatin therapy than when given before cisplatin.

Concomitant medications that contain substrates or inhibitors of hepatic enzymes, principally cytochrome P450 isoenzymes CYP_2C_8 and CYP_3A_4, may increase paclitaxel clearance, and caution should be exercised when administering paclitaxel. In a study by Chang et al. (393), the pharmacokinetics of paclitaxel were significantly altered by the concomitant use of anticonvulsants (i.e., phenytoin, carbamazapine, and phenobarbital), and the maximum tolerated doses of paclitaxel in malignant glioma patients were 360 mg/m^2 for those on anticonvulsant therapy versus 240 mg/m^2 for those not receiving anticonvulsants. There was also a significant difference in paclitaxel metabolite and toxicity profiles between the two groups. Central neurotoxicity, rather than neutropenia, was the dose-limiting toxicity in patients on anticonvulsant therapy who received paclitaxel at a dose greater than 350 mg/m^2.

Pemetrexed

Pemetrexed is FDA-approved for combination therapy with cisplatin for malignant pleural mesothelioma, and for single-agent therapy for non–small cell lung cancer. However, it has shown promise as a treatment for ovarian and cervical cancers.

Chemistry. Pemetrexed (Alimta) is an antifolate antineoplastic agent with the chemical name of L-Glutamic acid, N-[4-[2-(2-amino-4,7-dihydro-4-oxo-1*H*-pyrrolo[2,3-*d*]pyrimidin-5-yl)ethyl]benzoyl]-, disodium salt, heptahydrate. It has a molecular weight of 597.49 and the molecular formula $C_{20}H_{19}N_5Na_2O_6 \cdot 7H_2O$.

Mechanism of Action. Pemetrexed inhibits the folate-dependent enzymes TS, DHFR, and glycinamide ribonucleotide formyltransferase (GARFT). The inhibition of GARFT, for example, is directly associated with a decrease in the rate of tumor cells (394). Although methotrexate was an early but potent inhibitor of DHFR, the antifolate activity of pemetrexed is quite different. The K_m for pemetrexed is 100th that of methotrexate for folylpolyglutamate synthetase, making it possible to rapidly and completely block TS activity, whereas methotrexate acts in a more gradual and cumulative process, only impacting cellular proliferation at the point where more than 95% of the enzyme is inhibited (394). Additional details regarding the unique mechanism of action of pemetrexed, including features of membrane transport, its maintained activity in loss of transport activity, and its comparison with other antifolates (e.g., 5-FU, methotrexate, raltitrexed) are discussed in more detail elsewhere (394).

Drug Disposition. Pemetrexed is primarily excreted in the urine and is only minimally metabolized. The elimination half-life is approximately 3.5 hours among patients with normal renal function. Pemetrexed exposure increases with decreasing renal function. Pemetrexed is 81% bound to plasma proteins, and binding is not affected by renal function.

Administration and Dosage. Pemetrexed is administered IV at 500 mg/m^2 over 10 minutes on day 1 of every 21-day cycle. When used in combination therapy, cisplatin (75 mg/m^2 over 2 hours) should begin 30 minutes after the pemetrexed administration. The premedication regimen with pemetrexed includes corticosteroids (dexamethasone) to reduce skin rash reactions, and folate-containing vitamin supplementation (daily for at least 7 days before pemetrexed administration) to reduce some toxicities.

Side Effects and Toxicities. The most commonly occurring side effects associated with pemetrexed treatment include hematologic toxicity, fever and infection, stomatitis, pharyngitis, and rash. Although many toxicities appeared to be significantly less frequent among patients receiving folate supplementation (e.g., neutropenia, nausea, vomiting, fever, infection), rates of hypertension (11% vs. 3%), chest pain (8% vs. 6%), and thrombosis/embolism (6% vs. 3%) were higher among those receiving supplementation. Rare cases of colitis have been reported in postmarketing studies.

Topotecan

Topotecan (Hycamtin, topotecan hydrochloride) was approved by the FDA in 1996 for the treatment of ovarian cancer patients after failure of primary chemotherapy. It is also indicated in the treatment of small cell lung cancer after the failure of first-line chemotherapy.

Chemistry. Topotecan is a semisynthetic analog of camptothecin. The parent compound is derived from the bark of an ornamental tree native to Asia, *Camptotheca acuminata.* Sodium camptothecin was studied in clinical trials in the late 1960s through the early 1970s. However, clinical development of this agent was halted despite evidence of a variety of tumor responses because of severe and unpredictable toxicities (e.g., myelosuppression and hemorrhagic cystitis) (395). Topotecan and other camptothecin analogs (e.g., irinotecan) have been formulated in an effort to overcome unacceptable toxicities and to increase cytotoxicity and water solubility. Topotecan incorporates a stable basic side chain at the 9-position of the A-ring of 10-hydroxycamptothecin, which increases aqueous solubility. The molecular weight is 457.9 (the HCl salt), and the formula is $C_{23}H_{23}N_3O_5 \cdot HCl$ (the free base has a molecular weight of 421.5). The chemical name of topotecan is (*S*)-10-[(dimethylamino)methyl]-4-ethyl-4,9-dihydroxy-1*H*-pyrano[3′,4′:6,7] indolizino [1,2-*b*]quinoline-3,14-(4*H*,12*H*)-dione monohydrochloride.

Mechanism of Action. In a manner similar to camptothecin, topotecan's cytotoxicity results from the inhibition of TOPO-I, an enzyme that induces reversible single-strand breaks during DNA replication. Camptothecin analogs bind with and stabilize the transient TOPO-I–DNA complex, preventing religation of the single-strand breakage. The interaction of the ternary topotecan–TOPO-I–DNA complex with replication enzymes results in double-strand DNA breaks and cellular death. Topotecan exists in a pH-dependent equilibrium as both a closed lactone ring and a hydroxy acid; the hydroxy acid is formed by hydrolysis of the lactone ring. The active lactone form predominates at a pH below 7, and at a pH of 6, over 80% of topotecan exists in the lactone form. Slow reaction kinetics studies have shown that the hydroxy acid is inactive and that only the closed lactone bonds with the TOPO-I–DNA complex (396).

Drug Disposition. After IV administration, plasma pharmacokinetics show that the lactone form, which is active as an inhibitor of TOPO-I, is rapidly converted to the hydroxy acid form. At the end of a brief infusion, approximately half of the dose administered exits as hydroxy acid (397). One hour after administration, less than 30% of the dose remains in the lactone form. Topotecan does not inhibit TOPO-II.

Both forms of topotecan are subject to rapid biphasic elimination. In a summary of pharmacokinetics studies, the mean half-life of topotecan lactone was only 3 hours (range 1.2 to 4.9 hours) (396). Binding to plasma proteins is approximately 35%. Renal excretion appears to account for 40% to 70% of drug clearance (50,151).

When topotecan was administered as a weekly 24-hour IV infusion of 1 to 2 mg/m², the plasma steady-state concentration and the AUC increased linearly with dose. The lactone-to–total drug concentration ratio was constant, which suggests that the total drug concentration may be used as a measure of active lactone exposure with weekly, long infusions (398). In addition, comparison of day 1 pharmacokinetics values with blood counts showed that both the topotecan AUC and the lactone AUC were predictive of the level of neutrophil reduction on days 15, 22, and 29 using the sigmoid E_{max} model (398). This led the investigators to suggest that topotecan-induced myelosuppression is noncumulative, and that elimination probably remains unchanged with repeat dosing in individual patients. Other studies have also found a correlation between the topotecan AUC and the level of neutropenia (397,399).

Limited sampling models for topotecan pharmacokinetics have been proposed that may facilitate tailoring of topotecan drug doses in individual patients and large pharmacodynamic studies of topotecan (400,401). Plasma concentrations of the lactone and hydroxy acid forms of topotecan at 2 hours, after a 30-minute infusion, reliably predicted the lactone form AUC, the hydroxy acid AUC, the total topotecan AUC, and the clearance rate.

Administration and Dosage. Each 4-mg vial of topotecan should be reconstituted with 4 mL of sterile water. The resulting solution can be further diluted with either 0.9% sodium chloride or 5% dextrose. Because the active lactone form of topotecan is subject to a pH-dependent hydrolysis to the inactive hydroxy acid, consideration should be given to maintenance of an acidic pH during drug infusion. When the topotecan lactone is dissolved in 5% dextrose, only approximately 10% is converted to the hydroxy acid (397). Because the product does not contain an antibacterial preservative, it should be used immediately once constituted.

Parenteral topotecan has been administered by IV infusions varying in length from 30 minutes to 21 days (396). The standard FDA-approved dosing regimen is 1.5 mg/m²/d × 5 days by 30-minute IV infusion every 21 days, for a minimum of four courses owing to delayed tumor response, as tolerated (in the absence of tumor progression). However, this dosing schedule is associated with a more than 80% incidence of grade IV neutropenia. Many oncologists, therefore, use a dose of 1.25 mg/m²/d for 5 days and/or administer prophylactic G-CSF. Today, a weekly dosing schedule is more often utilized because of equivalent efficacy, less toxicity, and better acceptability by patients (402,403).

Side Effects and Toxicities. Toxicity data are available from a phase III, randomized study of topotecan 1.5 mg/m²/d for 5 days every 21 days versus paclitaxel 175 mg/m² IV over 3 hours every 21 days in ovarian cancer patients with progressive or recurrent disease following primary platinum-based chemotherapy (404). Neutropenia was the predominant toxicity in this study: 79% of patients experienced grade 4 neutropenia, 25% of patients experienced febrile neutropenia, and 5% of patients developed sepsis [two patients (2%) died of sepsis]. The onset of grade 4 neutropenia was on days 9 through 15 of a chemotherapy cycle, and it did respond to G-CSF therapy. Thrombocytopenia also occurred frequently: 50% of patients experienced grades 3 to 4 thrombocytopenia (25% experienced grade 4). Grade 4 anemia occurred in 3.6% of patients.

The most common nonhematologic toxicities were cumulative, dose-related alopecia (76%) and nausea/vomiting (10% grades 3 to 4), which was amenable to antiemetic therapy. Other frequent toxicities were fatigue (41%), constipation (43%), diarrhea (40%), abdominal pain (27%), fever in the absence of neutropenia (29%), stomatitis (24%), dyspnea (24%), and asthenia (22%) (404).

Special Precautions. Because topotecan has a high rate of renal excretion and a modest hepatic clearance, a clinical study was conducted to evaluate the impact of renal and hepatic dysfunction on toxicity in patients undergoing treatment with topotecan on a daily × 5 dosing schedule (405,406). Pharmacokinetic analyses showed clear correlations between CrCl and plasma clearance of both topotecan and topotecan lactone ($r^2 = 0.65$, $p < 0.0001$). Although the standard dose for patients with good renal function is 1.5 mg/m²/d × 5 days, this study determined that the recommended starting dose for patients with moderate hepatic dysfunction (CrCl of 20 to 39 mL/min) was 0.75 mg/m². The investigators urged extreme caution with topotecan administration in patients with more profound renal insufficiency and recommended further dose reductions for heavily pretreated patients (405). Hepatic insufficiency did not appear to exacerbate hematologic toxicity (405). Nonhematologic toxicity appeared to be unaffected by either renal or hepatic insufficiency.

Vinorelbine

Vinorelbine (Navelbine) is a third-generation semisynthetic vinca alkaloid that has been commercially available in the United States since 1994 for treatment of non–small cell lung cancer. Vinorelbine also appears to have significant activity in breast cancer patients (407,408) and moderate activity in patients with cervical or ovarian cancer (409,410), as well as other tumor types (411).

Chemistry. It has a molecular formula of $C_{45}H_{54}N_4O_8 \cdot 2C_4H_6O_6$ and a molecular weight of 1079.12. Vinorelbine's structure differs from that of the parent compounds, vincristine and vinblastine, in that it contains a nine-member (rather than eight-member) catharanthine ring (412). Its chemical name is 3′,4′-didehydro-4′-deoxy-*C*′-norvincaleukoblastine[*R*-(*R**,*R**)-2,3-dihydroxybutanedioate-(1:2)(salt)].

Mechanism of Action. Like other vinca alkaloids, vinorelbine is classified as a "spindle poison" because it interacts with tubulin with resulting inhibition of microtubule assembly and cellular division during mitosis (413). Vinelorbine blocks cell cycle progression specifically in G_2 and M phases (151).

Drug Disposition. The pharmacokinetics of vinorelbine show large interpatient variability and are best described by a triphasic model. Following IV administration of a 30-mg/m^2 dose, a peak plasma level of 1,000 ng/mL is achieved, but the plasma level declines to 100 ng/mL within 2 hours. Vinorelbine rapidly binds to platelets (78% of total dose) and plasma proteins (13.5%), and only 1.7% is available as free drug (413). The drug readily diffuses into other tissues, and has a large Vd (75.61 L/kg). The terminal half-life is approximately 45 hours (414).

The primary means of vinorelbine clearance appears to be hepatic metabolism. Approximately 18% and 46% is recovered in the urine and feces, respectively; however, recovery was incomplete in pharmacokinetic studies (415,416).

Administration and Dosage. Vinorelbine is a vesicant and requires careful administration. The drug should be diluted in a syringe or IV bag to a concentration of 1.5 to 3.0 mg/mL (syringe) or 0.5 to 2 mg/mL (IV bag). When using a syringe or IV bag, vinorelbine should be diluted with dextrose (5%) or sodium chloride (0.9%). When using an IV bag, it may also be diluted with sodium chloride (0.45%), Ringer injection, or lactated Ringer injection. Diluted vinorelbine should be administered over 6 to 10 minutes into a side port of a free-flowing IV line closest to the IV bag. Following vinorelbine administration, the vein should be flushed with at least 75 to 125 mL of IV solution. Longer IV infusions (e.g., 20 minutes) are associated with a higher incidence of phlebitis (417).

Vinorelbine solution is incompatible with fluorouracil, mitomycin, and thiotepa. It is also incompatible with several antibiotics (including a number of cephalosporins, amphotericin B, ampicillin, piperacillin, and trimethoprim-sulfamethoxazole), acyclovir, furosemide, ganciclovir, methylprednisolone, and sodium bicarbonate (418).

Vinorelbine is generally administered at a dose of 30 mg/m^2 every week. This dosing schedule has been used in combination chemotherapeutic regimens; however, the recommended dosing schedule in combination with cisplatin (100 mg/m^2 every 4 weeks) is weekly administration of vinorelbine at a dose of 25 mg/m^2. Attempts to increase vinorelbine dose intensity using a daily × 3 every 21 days dosing schedule with or without G-CSF have not been successful (419,420). However, Weiss et al. (421) have reported that continuous infusion of vinorelbine at doses of 8 to 10 mg/m^2/d with concurrent administration of G-CSF results in a twofold increase in vinorelbine dose intensity without increasing toxicity.

Side Effects and Toxicities. The primary dose-limiting toxicity of vinorelbine is myelosuppression, chiefly granulocytopenia (36% of patients, <500 cells/mm^3). A safety summary of data from North American clinical trials reported that when vinorelbine was administered at a dose of 30 mg/m^2/week to patients with breast cancer and non–small cell lung cancer, 64% of patients experienced grades 3 to 4 granulocytopenia, 50% experienced grades 3 to 4 leukopenia, and 9% developed grades 3 to 4 anemia. Despite the high incidence of granulocytopenia, most events were uncomplicated, and only 7% of patients required hospitalization for fever and/or infection. The death rate due to sepsis was 1% to 2%. Myelosuppression was noncumulative, and the incidence of grades 3 and 4 granulocytopenia declined during later cycles of vinorelbine therapy. The granulocyte nadir typically occurred on day 14 of treatment, with recovery of the granulocyte count within 7 days (422).

Vinorelbine therapy is frequently associated with transient increases in liver enzymes, especially alkaline phosphatase. Virtually all patients experience a rise in alkaline phosphatase, with approximately 25% developing grade 3 toxicity and an additional 2% experiencing grade 4 elevations. Increases in AST and ALT also occur in more than half of all patients. However, most patients with liver enzyme increases remain asymptomatic and do not require dose modification of vinorelbine. Total bilirubin can also be elevated: 10% of patients experience some degree of increased bilirubin, with 2% experiencing grade 4 elevation. Because of the high incidence of liver and bone metastases in the study population (breast cancer and non–small cell lung cancer patients), the proportion of these toxicities that is directly attributable to vinorelbine therapy is unknown (422).

Other common toxicities associated with vinorelbine when administered as a single agent at a dose of 30 mg/m^2/wk by a 20-minute IV infusion include nausea (38% overall, 2% severe), vomiting (17% overall, 2% severe), constipation (31%, 3% severe), asthenia (29%, 5% severe), injection site reactions (26%, 2% severe), anorexia (15%, 1% severe), diarrhea (15%, 1% severe), stomatitis (14%, 0% severe), pain (13%, 2% severe), paresthesia (13%, <1% severe), fever (11%, 1% severe), and alopecia (10%, <1% severe) (422). Vinorelbine-induced nausea and vomiting are generally mild and are readily controlled with standard antiemetic medication (422). Injection site reactions include erythema, warmth, pain, and phlebitis. Repeated administration of vinorelbine can result in discoloration of the vein. As discussed above, shortening the injection duration to 6 to 10 minutes significantly reduces the incidence of injection site reactions (417).

Injection site pain and pain of unspecified etiology has been reported with administration of vinorelbine as a single agent (422). In addition, acute tumor pain has been reported in several cancer patients who received treatment with vinorelbine plus a platinum-containing agent (either carboplatin or cisplatin) (423,424).

Pulmonary toxicity is an infrequent side effect of vinorelbine. Approximately 5% of patients experience dyspnea. Some cases of dyspnea are characterized by rapid onset during administration and resolve with bronchodilator therapy. Other cases occur usually within 1 hour of vinorelbine infusion and are characterized by life-threatening progressive dyspnea and the development of interstitial infiltrates (422,425). The coadministration of mitomycin may increase the pulmonary toxicity of vinorelbine (425).

Rare side effects of vinorelbine include pancreatitis, PPE (with prolonged infusions), paralytic ileus, and syndrome of inappropriate ADH secretion (381,426–428).

Special Precautions. Vinorelbine extravasation can result in severe local irritation, tissue necrosis, and phlebitis. If extravasation occurs, the injection should be halted immediately, and any remaining portion of the dose should be injected into a different vein. Specific antidotes for vinorelbine extravasation have not been studied; however, vinblastine extravasation reactions may be ameliorated with the use of corticosteroid injections followed by cold compresses (382).

Drug Interactions. In that vinca alkaloids are metabolized by the cytochrome P450 3A system, coadministration of strong P450 inhibitors, such as erythromycin and ketoconazole, could potentially reduce vinorelbine clearance and increase toxicity (429,430). Doxorubicin and etoposide are also metabolized by the P450 system, and coadministration of these drugs with vinorelbine could potentially affect vinorelbine metabolism (429).

Mitomycin is known to exacerbate vinca alkaloid–induced pulmonary toxicity (431), and the combination of high-dose vinorelbine (50 mg/m^2 on days 1 and 21) plus mitomycin (15 mg/m^2 on day 1) has been associated with life-threatening acute pulmonary toxicity characterized by rapid onset of severe, progressive dyspnea and the development of bilateral interstitial infiltrates (425).

The combination of paclitaxel and vinorelbine has been associated with severe neurotoxicity including grade 4 motor neuropathy, irreversible ototoxicity, and vocal cord paresis (432,433). In one report of clinical experience in five patients with preexisting, mild-to-moderate, paclitaxel-induced sensory neuropathy, the combination of vinorelbine 25 to 30 mg/m^2 followed by paclitaxel 150 mg/m^2 by 3-hour infusion every 2 weeks resulted in severe, slowly reversing motor neuropathy in all five patients. Four of the five patients required the use of a wheelchair (432).

ENDOCRINE AGENTS

Aromatase Inhibitors

Anastrozole

Anastrozole (Arimidex) is FDA approved in three settings to treat postmenopausal breast cancer: 1) for the adjuvant treatment of postmenopausal patients with estrogen receptor–positive (ER+) early breast cancers; 2) for the first-line treatment of postmenopausal women with ER+ or hormone receptor unknown locally advanced or metastatic breast cancer; and 3) for second-line treatment following tamoxifen therapy. It is one of many available aromatase inhibitors (AI) but is unique in that it is a nonsteroidal AI. Anastrozole is rarely associated with response in ER-negative disease. Anastrozole has been shown to have fewer side effects and a significant survival advantage as compared with megestrol acetate in the treatment of postmenopausal patients with breast cancer (434).

Chemistry. Chemically, it is 1,3-benzenediacetonitrile, α,α,α′,α′-tetramethyl-5-(1H-1,2,4-triazol-1-ylmethyl). It has a molecular formula of $C_{17}H_{19}N_5$ and a molecular weight of 293.4.

Mechanism of Action. Anastrozole is a nonsteroidal AI that prevents the peripheral conversion of androgens (androstenedione and testosterone) to estrogens (estrone, estrone sulfate, and estradiol) (50). Anastrozole has a significant effect on serum estradiol; as low as 1 mg/d has caused estradiol levels to be undetectable (435). In patients receiving 5 mg and 10 mg of anastrozole, there was no effect on adrenal corticosteroids or aldosterone.

Drug Disposition. Following oral administration, anastrozole is well absorbed into the systemic circulation and not affected by food ingestion. Pharmacokinetics are linear and not affected by repeated dosing. Steady-state concentration levels are achieved after approximately 7 days of treatment.

Administration and Dosage. Anastrozole is administered orally at a dose of 1 mg/d. For advanced disease, treatment should continue until disease progression.

Side Effects and Toxicities. When compared in a controlled clinical study with megestrol acetate, the principal side effect of anastrozole was diarrhea (occurred in 8.4% vs. 2.8% of patients treated with megestrol acetate). In general, it is very well tolerated, with the most frequent side effects (any grade) being asthenia (18%), nausea (18%), headache (14%), hot flushes (13.2%), and pain (10%).

Special Precautions. Anastrozole is contraindicated in pregnancy and premenopausal women as well as those who have shown a hypersensitivity to the drug or its excipients. In women with preexisting ischemic heart disease, an increased incidence of ischemic cardiovascular events has been seen. It can also cause a decrease in bone mineral density and an elevation in serum cholesterol.

Drug Interactions. Coadministration of anastrozole and tamoxifen in breast cancer patients reduced anastrozole plasma concentrations by 27%. Estrogen-containing regimens should not be coadministered because they may diminish its pharmacologic action. The drug does not appear to alter the effect of warfarin or inhibit cytochrome P450.

Special Applications. According to the National Comprehensive Cancer Network Clinical Practice Guidelines in Oncology for Uterine Neoplasms (436), anastrozole (as well as other AIs) is listed as a possible "substitute" for progestational agents or tamoxifen in treating "asymptomatic or low-grade metastases." It is hypothesized that anastrozole may play a role on a molecular level in the endometrium. Most endometrial carcinomas are associated with endometrial hyperplasia and are estrogen receptor (ER) and progesterone receptor (PR) positive. In addition to ER/PR status, there is a progressive increase in the expression of the protein pS2 from normal to hyperplastic to well-differentiated carcinoma (437). Aromatase inhibition may be able to alter the course of disease by preventing the endometrium from being exposed to estrogen. This may in turn alter the expression of the pS2 protein because there is a strong association between ER/PR expression and expression of pS2 protein (437). Aromatase activity has been demonstrated in both ER/PR–positive and ER/PR– negative endometrial carcinomas (438). Although much research has yet to be done, phase I and II trials have demonstrated safety and minimal activity in an unselected population of recurrent endometrial carcinoma patients (439,440). There is some evidence that it may have benefit in the treatment of endometrial hyperplasia as well as endometrial stromal sarcomas (441).

Finally, the National Comprehensive Cancer Network (NCCN) Clinical Practice Guidelines in Oncology for Ovarian Cancer (442) mentions anastrozole as well as other "hormonal therapies" (443) as "potentially active." Case reports have also noted responses in recurrent and metastatic ovarian sex cord stromal cancers such as granulosa cell tumors (444).

Letrozole

Letrozole (Femara) is a nonsteroidal AI that is FDA approved for the adjuvant treatment of postmenopausal women with hormone receptor–positive early breast cancer as well as the first- and second-line treatment of advanced or metastatic breast cancer (hormone receptor positive or hormone receptor unknown). Letrozole is also used for the treatment of advanced breast cancer in postmenopausal women whose disease has progressed following antiestrogen therapy.

Chemistry. The chemical name of letrozole is 4,4′-(1H- 9,1,2,4-Triazol-1-ylmethylene) dibenzonitrile, and the empirical formula is C17H11N5.

Drug Disposition. Letrozole is not affected by food intake, and is rapidly and completely absorbed through the gastrointestinal tract. The terminal elimination half-life is two days. The major excretion route is via the kidneys. Steady-state plasma concentration is reached in 2 to 6 weeks of daily 2.5 mg dosing. These concentrations are up to two times higher than after a single dose. Steady-state levels can be maintained for long periods of time without continuous accumulation of letrozole.

Administration and Dosage. Letrozole is administered orally, at 2.5 mg per day. Letrozole can be taken at any time during the day regardless of food intake. Treatment is indicated until disease progression.

Side Effects and Toxicities. Letrozole has a more favorable toxicity profile as compared with tamoxifen, with greater or equivalent efficacy in breast cancer patients (445). The most common side effects (>20%) include hot flashes and arthralgia. Bone pain, flushing, sweating, asthenia, edema, back pain, nausea, hypercholesterolemia, and dyspnea each occur in no more than 20% of patients.

Special Precautions. Letrozole may cause a decrease in bone mineral density to a much greater degree than tamoxifen. Increases in serum cholesterol have also been observed with letrozole as well as hepatic impairment. Since it causes fatigue, dizziness, and somnolence, caution should be advised when driving or using machinery. Letrozole is contraindicated in pregnancy.

Special Applications. Like anastrozole, the NCCN Clinical Practice Guidelines in Oncology for Ovarian Cancer (442) mention letrozole along with other "hormonal therapies" (443) as "potentially active." (446,447). Finally, the NCCN Clinical Practice Guidelines in Oncology for Uterine Neoplasms (436) lists letrozole (as well as other AIs) as a possible "substitute" for progestational agents or tamoxifen in treating "asymptomatic or low-grade metastases" from endometrioid endometrial cancers.

PROGESTATIONAL AGENTS

Medroxyprogesterone

Medroxyprogesterone acetate (MPA) therapy is indicated for the treatment of secondary amenorrhea and abnormal uterine bleeding due to hormonal imbalance in the absence of organic pathology, such as fibroids or uterine cancer. In addition, MPA is indicated along with estrogen therapy for therapeutic use in women to reduce the incidence of endometrial hyperplasia. MPA is not approved as a therapeutic approach to any solid tumor.

Chemistry

The chemical name of the progestational agent, MPA (Provera), is Pregn-4-ene-3,20-dione,17-(acetyloxy)-6-methyl-,(6α)-. Its empirical formula is $C_{24}H_{34}O_4$, with a molecular weight of 386.53.

Drug Disposition

MPA is absorbed through the gastrointestinal tract, and is primarily metabolized by the liver. Maximum concentrations are reached within 2 to 4 hours after oral administration. Food intake enhances the bioavailability of MPA (C_{max} by up to 70% and AUC up to 33% increase), but does not affect its half-life (12 to 16 hours).

Administration and Dosage

MPA is administered at 5 or 10 mg/d for endometrial hyperplasia for 12 to 14 consecutive days every month. For abnormal uterine bleeding or amenorrhea, MPA is generally administered for a shorter duration (e.g., 5 to 10 consecutive days). Patients experience withdrawal bleeding for 3 to 5 days following the treatment cycle. Medroxyprogesterone acetate is recommended to be used with 0.625 mg conjugated estrogens in women with a uterus to avoid the risk of endometrial cancer. Women without a uterus may receive estrogen without a progestin. In addition to the tablet form for oral intake, there is an IM depot formulation that may permit alternative treatment regimens. The IM formulation of MPA was compared with oral megestrol acetate for the treatment of menopausal symptoms in breast cancer patients. In this short-term study, the IM formulation provided superior benefit to patients and may be an alternative to long-term oral progestin therapy (448).

Side Effects and Toxicities

Medroxyprogesterone acetate, similar to other progestins (e.g., megestrol acetate), may cause abnormal uterine bleeding, breast tenderness, or nausea. The Women's Health Initiative study found that estrogen plus progesterone was associated with an increased risk of myocardial infarction, stroke, invasive breast cancer, pulmonary emboli, and deep vein thrombosis in postmenopausal women (449). A memory study embedded within the Women's Health Initiative found that this combination may also be associated with an increased risk of developing dementia in women over the age of 65 (450). A black box warning now included on the MPA package insert recommends that estrogen/progesterone be used at the lowest possible dose for the shortest duration possible for the specific treatment goals of the patient.

Special Precautions

MPA is almost exclusively metabolized in the liver, with the glucuronide conjugate metabolites being excreted in the urine. Thus, MPA should be used with extreme caution in renal insufficiency or hepatic impairment. MPA is contraindicated in women with undiagnosed genital bleeding, breast cancer, suspected estrogen- or progesterone-dependent neoplasia, active venous or arterial thrombosis, missed abortion, pregnancy, or known hypersensitivity to MPA.

Drug Interactions

No formal pharmacokinetic drug interaction studies of MPA have been performed.

Special Applications

There is some evidence that MPA may be used for endometrial hyperplasia or stage I endometrial cancer as an alternative to surgery to preserve fertility (451,452). Medroxyprogesterone acetate has also demonstrated activity when used with other agents in advanced or recurrent endometrial cancer (453,454). Along with AIs and tamoxifen, MPA and other progestational agents are listed as an option in treating recurrent or advanced endometrial cancer by the NCCN (436). The NCCN does not list MPA as an active agent in epithelial ovarian cancer.

Megestrol Acetate

Megestrol acetate is an FDA-approved progestin that is used for the palliative treatment of advanced carcinoma of the breast or endometrium (i.e., recurrent, inoperable, or metastatic disease).

Chemistry

The chemical name of megestrol acetate (Megace) is 17 •-acetyloxy-6-methylpregna-4,6-diene-3,20-dione. Similar to MPA, it has the empirical formula $C_{24}H_{34}O_4$, and has a molecular weight of 384.51. The precise mechanism by which megestrol acetate produces its antineoplastic effects against endometrial carcinoma is unknown. However, there is evidence to suggest a local effect as a result of the marked changes brought about by the direct instillation of progestational agents into the endometrial cavity. The antineoplastic action of megestrol acetate on carcinoma of the breast is better understood.

Progestational agents like megestrol acetate modify the action of other steroid hormones and exert a direct cytotoxic effect on tumor cells. Pharmacologic doses of megestrol acetate not only decrease the number of hormone-dependent human breast cancer cells but are also capable of modifying and abolishing the stimulatory effects of estrogen on these cells. It has been suggested that progestins may inhibit cell growth in one of two ways: by interfering with the stability, availability, or turnover of the ER complex in its interaction with genes or in conjunction with the progestin receptor complex, by interacting directly with the genome to turn off specific estrogen-responsive genes.

Drug Disposition

Megestrol acetate is primarily excreted in the urine, and oral absorption rates are variable. Time to peak concentration ranges from 1 to 3 hours, and the plasma elimination half-life ranges from 13 to 104.9 hours. Steady-state plasma concentrations have not yet been established.

Administration and Dosage

Megestrol acetate is supplied in 20 mg and 40 mg tablets for oral intake. Although the recommended dosage for breast cancer is 160 mg/d (40 mg q.i.d.), and for endometrial carcinoma it is 40 to 320 mg/d in divided doses, there are a wide variety of dose and schedules implemented therapeutically for precancerous conditions (e.g., AEH).

Side Effects and Toxicities

The side-effect profiles of the progestational agents such as megestrol acetate or medroxyprogesterone acetate are similar. However, weight gain is a common side effect with megestrol acetate. Thrombophlebitis and pulmonary embolism have been reported with megestrol acetate. Other toxicities include heart failure, nausea and vomiting, edema, breakthrough menstrual bleeding, dyspnea, tumor flare (with or without hypercalcemia), hyperglycemia, glucose intolerance, alopecia, hypertension, carpal tunnel syndrome, mood changes, hot flashes, malaise, asthenia, lethargy, sweating, and rash. In general, there are only rare severe toxicities reported with progestational agents.

Special Precautions

Megestrol acetate should be used with caution in patients with a history of thromboembolic disease. Exacerbation of preexisting diabetes with increased insulin requirements has also been reported in association with the use of megestrol acetate.

SELECTIVE ER MODULATORS

Tamoxifen Citrate

Tamoxifen citrate (Nolvadex) is a nonsteroidal agent with antiestrogenic properties. It is indicated for the treatment of metastatic breast cancer in men and women. In premenopausal women, it is an alternative to oophorectomy or ovarian irradiation. ER+ tumors are more likely to respond. Tamoxifen is also indicated as adjuvant treatment in node-positive and node-negative breast cancer in. It is indicated in women with ductal carcinoma *in situ* (DCIS) to reduce the risk of invasive carcinoma. Finally, it is approved to reduce the incidence of breast cancer among high-risk women. Tamoxifen competes with estrogen for binding sites, which explains its increased effectiveness in ER+ tumors.

Chemistry

The chemical formula of tamoxifen is (Z)2-[4-(1,2-diphenyl-1-butenyl) phenoxy]-*N*,*N*-dimethylethanamine 2-hydroxy-1,2,3-propanetricarboxylate (1:1), and has a molecular weight of 563.62.

Mechanism of Action

Tamoxifen, like raloxifene and toremifene, is a nonsteroidal selective ER modulator (SERM). All three agents are competitive inhibitors of estrogen binding to ER, and all have mixed agonist and antagonist activity, depending on the target tissue. These mixed activities have led to the redesignation of this class of compounds from "antiestrogens" to SERMs.

SERMs provide some protection against menopausal bone loss, presumably because of their partial agonist activity. However, the increase in bone density is substantially less than that seen with estrogen. SERMs lower serum total and low-density lipoprotein-cholesterol concentrations (by 12% and 19%, respectively, in one report), although they do not increase serum HDL-cholesterol. Tamoxifen's antagonist effect is particularly prominent with respect to breast cancer. Finally, tamoxifen is an estrogen agonist in the endometrium.

Most receptors of the steroid family, with the exception of the ER, are classically viewed as "translocating receptors," that is, they move from a principally cytoplasmic distribution in the absence of hormone to a predominantly nuclear localization in hormone-stimulated cells. However, the ER appears to be predominantly nuclear both in the presence and in the absence of hormone. The ER operates as a ligand-dependent transcription factor; attachment of estrogen hormone to the ER's ligand-binding domain results in either direct binding of the ER to estrogen response elements in the promoter of target genes or to a protein–protein interaction with coactivators at their respective promoter sites (455). Subsequently, the hormone–receptor complex is able to bind to estrogen-specific response elements that activate or repress expression of genes whose protein products are responsible for the physiologic actions of the hormone. Estrogen exerts its effect through two receptors, ERα and ERβ. The exact function of ERα and ERβ is under study, but they appear to have different biologic functions, as indicated by their distinct expression patterns.

Drug Disposition

Peak plasma concentrations (average 40 ng/mL) take place approximately 5 hours after dosing. The decline in plasma concentrations is biphasic with a terminal elimination half-life of about 6 days. Steady-state concentrations for tamoxifen are achieved in about 4 weeks after initiation of therapy. Tamoxifen is extensively metabolized, with *N*-desmethyl tamoxifen being the major metabolite. Approximately 65% of the administered dose is eliminated in the feces within 2 weeks (456).

Administration and Dosage

Tamoxifen is available in 10- and 20-mg tablets for oral administration. The recommended dosage is 20 to 40 mg/d; when the higher daily dose is prescribed, it should be divided into two doses of 20 mg (morning and evening).

Side Effects and Toxicities

Tamoxifen causes estrogenic changes of the vaginal and cervical squamous epithelium and increases the incidence of cervical and endometrial polyps (457). It is associated with an increased risk of uterine malignancies (endometrial adenocarcinoma and uterine sarcoma). Other serious adverse events associated with tamoxifen treatment include stroke, deep vein thrombosis, and pulmonary embolism. A discussion weighing the benefits versus the risks should take place before treatment with tamoxifen; however, the benefits have been determined to outweigh the risks in women who take tamoxifen to reduce the risk of breast cancer recurrence.

Serious and life-threatening events associated with tamoxifen include uterine malignancies, stroke, and pulmonary embolism. Tamoxifen is contraindicated in patients with known hypersensitivity to the drug or any of its ingredients. In the treatment of DCIS, tamoxifen is contraindicated in women who require concomitant anticoagulant therapy or in women with a history of deep vein thrombosis or pulmonary embolus. As with other additive hormonal therapies (estrogens and androgens), hypercalcemia has been reported in some breast cancer patients with bone metastases within a few weeks of starting treatment with tamoxifen. Tamoxifen has been associated with changes in liver enzyme levels, and on rare occasions, a spectrum of more severe liver abnormalities including fatty liver, cholestasis, hepatitis, and hepatic necrosis. Ocular disturbances, including corneal changes, decrement in color vision perception, retinal vein thrombosis, and retinopathy have been reported in patients receiving tamoxifen. An increased incidence of cataracts and the need for cataract surgery have been reported in patients receiving tamoxifen.

GONADOTROPIN-RELEASING HORMONE ANALOGS

Leuprolide Acetate

Leuprolide acetate (Lupron) is a synthetic nonapeptide analog of naturally occurring gonadotropin-releasing hormone (GnRH), also known as luteinizing-hormone-releasing hormone. The analog possesses greater potency than the natural hormone. It is indicated in the palliative treatment of advanced prostate cancer and is used in the treatment of early hormone receptor–positive breast cancer occurring in premenopausal women.

Chemistry

The chemical name is 5-oxo-L-prolyl-L-histidyl-L-tryptophyl-L-seryl-L-tyrosyl-D-leucyl-L-leucyl-L-arginyl-*N*-ethyl-L-prolinamideacetate. GnRH agonists are synthetically modeled after the natural GnRH decapeptide with specific amino acid substitutions typically in positions 6 and 10. Other than leuprolide acetate, other agonists include: 1. buserelin (Suprefact, Suprecor); 2. nafarelin (Synarel) (only a single substitution at position 6); 3. histrelin (Supprelin LA, Vantas); 4. goserelin (Zoladex); 5. deslorelin (Suprelorin, Ovuplant). These medications can be administered intranasally, by injection, or by implant. Injectables have been formulated for daily, monthly, and quarterly use; and implants can last from 1 to 12 months.

Mechanism of Action

GnRH agonists do not quickly dissociate from the GnRH receptor. As a result, initially there is an increase in FSH and LH secretion (so-called "flare effect"). However, after about 10 days, a profound hypogonadal effect (i.e., decrease in FSH and LH) is achieved through receptor downregulation by internalization of receptors. Generally, this induced and reversible hypogonadism is the therapeutic goal.

Drug Disposition

Following a single injection of 7.5 mg of leuprolide acetate (depot Lupron), the mean plasma leuprolide concentration is almost 20 ng/mL at 4 hours and 0.36 ng/mL at 4 weeks. The mean steady-state

Vd of leuprolide following IV bolus administration to healthy male volunteers was 27 L. *In vitro* binding to human plasma proteins ranged from 43% to 49%. In healthy male volunteers, a 1 mg bolus of leuprolide administered intravenously revealed that the mean systemic clearance was 7.6 L/h, with a terminal elimination half-life of approximately 3 hours based on a two-compartment model. Following administration of depot Lupron 3.75 mg to three patients, less than 5% of the dose was recovered as parent or one of its major metabolites in the urine.

Administration and Dosage

The recommended dose of depot Lupron has traditionally been 7.5 mg monthly. Other recently approved doses and schedules include 22.5 mg every 3 months, 30 mg every 4 months, or 45 mg every 6 months.

Side Effects and Toxicity

Side effects of GnRH agonists are signs and symptoms of hypoestrogenism, including hot flashes, headaches, and osteoporosis.

Special Precautions

Leuprolide acetate is contraindicated in individuals with known hypersensitivity to GnRH agonists or any of the excipients in Lupron. Reports of anaphylactic reactions to GnRH agonist analogs have been reported in the medical literature. Leuprolide acetate and other GnRH analogs may cause fetal harm when administered to a pregnant woman. GnRH analogs is contraindicated in women who are or may become pregnant. Hyperglycemia and an increased risk of developing diabetes have been reported in men receiving GnRH agonists. Increased risk of developing myocardial infarction, sudden cardiac death, and stroke has been reported in association with use of GnRH agonists in men.

Drug Interactions

No pharmacokinetic-based drug–drug interaction studies have been conducted with GnRH agonists. However, because leuprolide acetate is a peptide that is primarily degraded by peptidase and not by cytochrome P-450 enzymes as noted in specific studies, and the drug is only about 46% bound to plasma proteins, drug interactions would not be expected to occur.

Special Applications

In gynecologic cancers, leuprolide acetate is listed as an active agent in endometrial cancer by the NCCN (436) although the results of clinical trials have been mixed (458,459). Approximately 80% of human ovarian and endometrial cancers and 50% of breast cancers express GnRH and its receptor as part of an autocrine regulatory system (460). The classic GnRH receptor signal-transduction mechanisms, known to operate in the pituitary, are not involved in the mediation of antiproliferative effects of GnRH analogs in these cancer cells. The GnRH receptor rather interacts with the mitogenic signal transduction of growth factor receptors and related oncogene products associated with tyrosine kinase activity via activation of a phosphotyrosine phosphatase resulting in downregulation of cancer cell proliferation. In addition, GnRH activates nucleus factor kappaB (NFkappaB) and protects the cancer cells from apoptosis. Furthermore, GnRH induces activation of the c-Jun N-terminal kinase/activator protein-1 (JNK/AP-1) pathway independent of the known AP-1 activators, protein kinase C (PKC) or mitogen-activated protein kinase (MAPK/ERK) (461).

MODULATING AGENTS/SUPPORTIVE CARE DRUGS USED IN THE TREATMENT OF GYNECOLOGIC CANCERS

Defining approaches to improve the therapeutic index of cancer chemotherapy, such that tumor cell kill is enhanced while toxicity to normal cells is minimized remains a fundamental goal of cancer treatment. A major limiting factor in successful cancer therapy is the ability of the tumor to develop resistance to the drugs used for treatment. A second fundamental problem faced by the oncologist treating patients with chemotherapy is the acute and chronic toxic effects of the drugs to the normal tissues. One approach that holds promise for the improvement of the therapeutic index is the concept of modulation, or the use of drugs with little or no cytotoxic activity to modulate the efficacy of standard anticancer drugs. Modulating agents can be divided into three main classes based on their ability to: (a) protect host tissue from the toxic effects of the cancer drugs; (b) potentiate anticancer drugs; and (c) reverse acquired drug resistance. In this section, we discuss agents with chemoprotective abilities used with chemotherapy in the treatment of gynecologic cancers.

Chemoprotective Agents

Leucovorin

Chemistry. Leucovorin, a chemically reduced derivative of folic acid, also known as citrovorum factor or folinic acid, was the original chemoprotective agent employed to overcome high-dose methotrexate-induced bone marrow toxicity (462,463). Leucovorin calcium tablets contain either 5-mg or 25-mg leucovorin as the calcium salt of N-[4-[[(2-amino-5-formyl-1, 4, 5, 6, 7, 8-hexahydro-4-oxo-6-pteridinyl)methyl] amino]benzoyl]-L-glutamic acid.

Mechanism of Action. Leucovorin can serve as a substitute for the endogenous reduced-folate cofactor (N^5,N^{10}-methylene tetrahydrofolate) that is diminished by methotrexate. Thus, leucovorin can "rescue" cells by replenishing intracellular reduced-folate pools and preventing methotrexate toxicity via blockade of thymidine synthesis. Leucovorin acts in a dose- and time-dependent fashion and must be given within 48 hours of methotrexate to elicit its rescue effects.

Leucovorin is also a successful modulatory agent used clinically to potentiate the antitumor activity of 5-FU (464). Leucovorin can enhance the DNA toxicity induced by 5-FU through the formation of a stable tertiary complex of 5,10-methylene tetrahydrofolate, TS, and fluorodeoxyuridine monophosphate. Compared with 5-FU alone, this combination has been shown to produce higher response rates and, in some cases, longer survival for patients with metastatic gastrointestinal malignancies (465). The combination of 5-FU and leucovorin currently is being tested extensively in other malignancies, including metastatic breast cancer (466). A complete review of leucovorin as a modulating agent is beyond the scope of this chapter, and the reader is referred to a number of excellent reviews on this topic (464,467).

Drug Disposition. Both IV and IM leucovorin produce rapid increases in serum concentrations of biologically active folates; these rises are sustained over time and are still detectable at 24 hours after drug administration. The bioavailability of IV and IM doses are comparable based on area under the serum concentration–time curve, although for IM administration, the peak concentration was lower and the time to peak concentration is longer. The initial rise in serum folate associated with IV and IM dosing is represented as 5-formyltetrahydrofolate; this falls concomitantly with the appearance of 5-methyltetrahydrofolate. Oral leucovorin is 92% bioavailable compared with IV administration and produces a predictably different pattern of circulating folates, 5-methyltetrahydrofolate being the predominant form. Terminal elimination half-life, apparent Vd, and clearance of total folate were not significantly different among the three treatments.

Administration and Dosage. Leucovorin calcium rescue is indicated after high-dose methotrexate therapy in treatment of some gynecologic cancers. Leucovorin calcium is also indicated to diminish the toxicity and counteract the effects of impaired methotrexate elimination and of inadvertent overdosages of folic acid antagonists.

Leucovorin calcium is indicated in the treatment of megaloblastic anemias due to folic acid deficiency when oral therapy is not feasible.

Leucovorin is also indicated for use in combination with 5-fluorouracil to prolong survival in the palliative treatment of patients with advanced colorectal cancer. In advanced colorectal cancer, either of the following two regimens is recommended:

1. Leucovorin is administered at 200 mg/m^2 by slow IV injection over a minimum of 3 minutes, followed by 5-fluorouracil at 370 mg/m^2 by IV injection.
2. Leucovorin is administered at 20 mg/m^2 by IV injection followed by 5-fluorouracil at 425 mg/m^2 by IV injection. 5-Fluorouracil and leucovorin should be administered separately to avoid the formation of a precipitate. Treatment is repeated daily for 5 days. This 5-day treatment course may be repeated at 4-week (28-day) intervals for two courses and then repeated at 4- to 5-week (28–35 day) intervals provided that the patient has completely recovered from the toxic effects of the prior treatment course. In subsequent treatment courses, the dosage of 5-fluorouracil should be adjusted based on patient tolerance of the prior treatment course. The daily dosage of 5-fluorouracil should be reduced by 20% for patients who experienced moderate hematologic or gastrointestinal toxicity in the prior treatment course, and by 30% for patients who experienced severe toxicity.

Leucovorin calcium tablets are indicated to diminish the toxicity and counteract the effects of impaired methotrexate elimination and of inadvertent overdosages of folic acid antagonists. Because absorption is saturable, oral administration of daily doses greater than 25 mg is not recommended.

Side Effects and Toxicity. Allergic sensitization, including anaphylactoid reactions and urticaria, has been reported following administration of both oral and parenteral leucovorin. No other adverse reactions have been attributed to the use of leucovorin *per se.*

Special Precautions. Parenteral administration is preferable to oral dosing if there is a possibility that the patient may vomit or not absorb the leucovorin. Leucovorin has no effect on other established toxicities of methotrexate such as the nephrotoxicity resulting from drug and/or metabolite precipitation in the kidney.

Drug Interactions. Folic acid in large amounts may counteract the antiepileptic effect of phenobarbital, phenytoin, and primidone, and increase the frequency of seizures in susceptible children.

Preliminary animal and human studies have shown that small quantities of systemically administered leucovorin enter CSF primarily as 5-methyltetrahydrofolate and, in humans, remain 1 to 3 orders of magnitude lower than usual methotrexate concentrations following intrathecal administration. However, high doses of leucovorin may reduce the efficacy of intrathecally administered methotrexate. Leucovorin may enhance the toxicity of fluorouracil.

Special Applications. In gynecologic cancer, leucovorin is primarily used with high-dose methotrexate for gestational trophoblastic disease (468–470).

Mesna

Mesna (Mesnex) is used clinically as a specific chemoprotective agent against bladder toxicity resulting from oxazophosphorine-based alkylating agents, such as cyclophosphamide and ifosfamide. It is sodium-2-mercaptoethane sulfonate, with the molecular formula $C_2H_5NaO_3S_2$ and a molecular weight of 164.18.

Mechanism of Action. Mesna inactivates the protein-reactive aldehyde, acrolein metabolite of ifosfamide and cyclophosphamide, which accumulates in the urinary bladder and results in dose-limiting urotoxicity (268). Plasma conversion of mesna to its inactive disulfide metabolite, dimesna, allows for the pretreatment and simultaneous administration of mesna as a urinary protector for ifosfamide and cyclophosphamide (high dose). Following renal filtration and secretion, dimesna is converted back to the active parent compound by glutathione reductase, which is subsequently delivered to the bladder. The mesna free sulfhydryl groups in the urinary bladder can directly complex to and thus neutralize acrolein, in addition to potentially blocking acrolein formation in the urinary tract (471). The metabolic characteristic of mesna should preclude any potential protection to tumors. Indeed, there is no clinical evidence that mesna coadministration with ifosfamide results in decreased antitumor activity. However, mesna has been shown to prevent the cytotoxicity of platinum agents when given simultaneously with them in *in vitro* models. As such, careful scheduling of mesna is warranted for clinical trials using ifosfamide in combination with platinum compounds. In addition, mesna should not be given simultaneously with cisplatin.

Drug Disposition. Proper scheduling of mesna has been based on pharmacokinetic analysis, which showed that mesna and dimesna have relatively short half-lives of approximately 1 hour and that peak urinary thiol accumulation following IV or oral mesna occurs at 1 and 3 hours, respectively (472). Because the half-life of mesna is much shorter than that of acrolein, it must be administered beyond the completion of ifosfamide.

Administration and Dosage. Mesna is available for IV bolus injection (100 mg/mL) or for oral use, available as 400-mg tablets. For IV administration, it should be diluted to obtain a final concentration of 20 mg/mL. The diluted solution is stable for 24 hours at room temperature. The approved schedule for IV administration of mesna is as a bolus dose (20% of the ifosfamide dose) before ifosfamide, and two additional doses 4 and 8 hours after ifosfamide treatment (319). A combination of IV and oral mesna has been used to simplify outpatient ifosfamide therapy. The oral dose of mesna is given equal to 40% of the ifosfamide dosage in two doses at 2 and 6 hours after ifosfamide administration, based on a 50% urinary bioavailability of oral mesna. Oral doses of 3 g/m^2 have been well tolerated in patients; however, nausea was observed in healthy volunteers receiving oral doses greater than 2 g/m^2. Goren (473) reviewed the dosing schedules and incidence of hematuria in 47 clinical studies in which oral mesna was administered to 1,986 patients who received greater than 6,475 courses of ifosfamide. Compilation of the data showed that a variety of doses and schedules of oral and IV mesna were effective at preventing hemorrhagic cystitis in patients treated with a number of different ifosfamide regimens. Although an optimal dose and schedule of mesna have not been established, adequate protection against ifosfamide-induced cystitis can be achieved using an initial IV dose of mesna that is equal to 20% of the ifosfamide dose, followed by two oral doses of mesna, each equal to 40% of the ifosfamide dose.

Side Effects and Toxicities. The most common side effects of mesna include headache, injection site reactions, flushing, dizziness, nausea, vomiting, flu-like symptoms, and coughing. Patients may develop hematuria (up to 6%) when administered ifosfamine plus mesna; a urine sample should be evaluated for hematuria each day prior to ifosfamide therapy.

Special Precautions. Health care providers should advise patients taking mesna to drink at least a quart of liquid a day. Patients should be informed to report if their urine has turned a pink or red color, if they vomit within 2 hours of taking oral mesna, or if they miss a dose of oral mesna.

Drug Interactions. No clinical drug studies have been conducted.

Special Applications. The superiority of mesna as a chemoprotectant against ifosfamide- and cyclophosphamide-induced bladder toxicity has been demonstrated in a number of clinical trials (319). In a comparative study of patients treated with ifosfamide at a dose of 2 g/m^2/d for 5 days, only 20% of the patients treated with mesna (400 mg/m^2) exhibited hematuria compared with 60% of those treated with *N*-acetylcysteine (NAC, 1.5 g/m^2) (473). In a phase II trial of ifosfamide and mesna in patients with platinum/paclitaxel–refractory ovarian cancer, there were no documented episodes of hemorrhagic cystitis, but one patient experienced treatment-related microscopic hematuria (318).

Subcutaneous administration of mesna is also being explored as an alternative to IV and oral dosing (474). Patients with gynecologic cancers receiving ifosfamide were treated with an initial IV dose of mesna at 20% of the ifosfamide dose. A subcutaneous infusion of mesna was given approximately 30 minutes after the completion of the ifosfamide infusion. A total dose of mesna equal to 40% of the ifosfamide dose was infused at a rate of 4 mL/h over 8 hours. The subcutaneous infusion of mesna was well tolerated, and no episodes of gross hematuria were observed.

REFERENCES

1. Tozer N. Pharmacokinetics concepts basic to cancer chemotherapy. In: Ames MM, Powis G, Covach JS, eds. *Pharmacokinetics of Anti-Cancer Agents in Humans*. New York, NY: Elsevier; 1983.
2. Collins JM, Dedrick RL. Pharmacokinetics of anticancer drugs. In: Chabner BE, ed. Pharmacologic principles of cancer treatment. Philadelphia, PA: WB Saunders; 1982:73.
3. Markman M. Intraperitoneal therapy of ovarian cancer. *Semin Oncol.* 1998;25(3):356–360.
4. Markman M, Hakes T, Reichman B, et al. Phase II trial of weekly or biweekly intraperitoneal mitoxantrone in epithelial ovarian cancer. *J Clin Oncol.* 1991;9(6):978–982.
5. Deppe G, Malviya VK, Boike G, et al. Intraperitoneal doxorubicin in combination with systemic cisplatinum and cyclophosphamide in the treatment of stage III ovarian cancer. *Eur J Gynaecol Oncol.* 1991;12(2):93–97.
6. Frasci G, Tortoriello A, Facchini G, et al. Intraperitoneal (ip) cisplatin-mitoxantrone-interferon-alpha 2b in ovarian cancer patients with minimal residual disease. *Gynecol Oncol.* 1993;50(1):60–67.
7. Muggia FM. New and emerging intraperitoneal (IP) drugs for ovarian cancer treatment. *Semin Oncol.* 2006;33(6 suppl 12):S18–S24.
8. Markman M, Rowinsky E, Hakes T, et al. Phase I trial of intraperitoneal taxol: a Gynecoloic Oncology Group study. *J Clin Oncol.* 1992;10(9):1485–1491.
9. Sugarbaker P, Van der Speeten K, Stuart O, et al. Patient-and treatment-related variables, adverse events and their statistical relationship for treatment of pertoneal metastases. In: Sugarbaker P, ed. *Cytoreductive Surgery and Perioperative Chemotherapy for Peritoneal Surface Malignancy: Textbook and Video Atlas.* Woodbury, CT: Ciné-Med Inc.; 2012.
10. Esquivel J. Technology of hyperthermic intraperitoneal chemotherapy in the United States, Europe, China, Japan, and Korea. *Cancer J.* 2009;15(3):249–254.
11. Alexander HR, Hanna N, Pingpank JF. Clinical results of cytoreduction and HIPEC for malignant peritoneal mesothelioma. *Cancer Treat Res.* 2007;134:343–355.
12. Elias DM, Sideris L. Pharmacokinetics of heated intraoperative intraperitoneal oxaliplatin after complete resection of peritoneal carcinomatosis. *Surg Oncol Clin N Am.* 2003;12(3):755–769.
13. Howell SB, Pfeifle CE, Olshen RA. Intraperitoneal chemotherapy with melphalan. *Ann Intern Med.* 1984;101(1):14–18.
14. Mohamed F, Sugarbaker PH. Intraperitoneal taxanes. *Surg Oncol Clin N Am.* 2003;12(3):825–833.
15. Richards WG, Zellos L, Bueno R, et al. Phase I to II study of pleurectomy/decortication and intraoperative intracavitary hyperthermic cisplatin lavage for mesothelioma. *J Clin Oncol.* 2006;24(10):1561–1567.
16. Sugarbaker PH, Stuart OA, Bijelic L. Intraperitoneal gemcitabine chemotherapy treament for patients with resected pancreatic cancer, rationale and report of early data. *Int J Surg Oncol.* 2011;2011:161862.
17. Van der Speetin K, Stuart OA, Chang D, et al. Changes induced by surgical and clinical factors in the pharmacology of intraperitoneal mitomycin C in 145 patients with peritoneal carcinomatosis. *Cancer.* 2010;68(1):147–156.
18. Van der Speetin K, Stuart OA, Mahteme H, et al. Pharmacokinetic study of perioperative intravenous Ifosfamide. *Int J Surg Oncol.* 2011;2011:185092.
19. Zylberberg B, Dormont D, Madelenat P, et al. First-line intraperitoneal cisplatin-paclitaxel and intravenous ifosfamide in Stage IIIc ovarian epithelial cancer. *Eur J Gynaecol Oncol.* 2004;25(3):327–332.
20. Gradishar WJ, Tjulandin S, Davidson N, et al. Phase III trial of nanoparticle albumin-bound paclitaxel compared with polyethylated castor oil-based paclitaxel in women with breast cancer. *J Clin Oncol.* 2005;23(31):7794–7803.
21. Rutty CJ, Connors TA. In vitro studies with hexamethylmelamine. *Biochem Pharmacol.* 1977;26(24):2385–2391.
22. Rutty CJ, Connors TA, Nguyen Hoang N, et al. In vivo studies with hexamethylmelamine. *Eur J Cancer.* 1978;14(6):713–720.
23. Ames MM, Powis G, Kovach JS, et al. Disposition and metabolism of pentamethylmelamine and hexamethylmelamine in rabbits and humans. *Cancer Res.* 1979;39(12):5016–5021.
24. D'Incalci M, Bolis G, Mangioni C, et al. Variable oral absorption of hexamethylmelamine in man. *Cancer Treat Rep.* 1978;62(12):2117–2119.
25. Markman M, Blessing JA, Moore D, et al. Altretamine (hexamethylmelamine) in platinum-resistant and platinum-refractory ovarian cancer: a Gynecologic Oncology Group phase II trial. *Gynecologic Oncol.* 1998;69(3):226–229.
26. Frasci G, Comella G, Comella P, et al. Carboplatin (CBDCA)-hexamethylmelamine (HMM)-oral etoposide (VP-16) first-line treatment of ovarian cancer patients with bulky disease: a phase II study. *Gynecol Oncol.* 1995;58(1):68–73.
27. Kristensen GB, Baekelandt M, Vergote IB, et al. A phase II study of carboplatin and hexamethylmelamine as induction chemotherapy in advanced epithelial ovarian carcinoma. *Eur J Cancer.* 1995;31A(11):1778–1780.
28. van der Hoop RG, van der Burg ME, ten Bokkel Huinink WW, et al. Incidence of neuropathy in 395 patients with ovarian cancer treated with or without cisplatin. *Cancer.* 1990;66(8):1697–1702.
29. Keldsen N, Havsteen H, Vergote I, et al. Altretamine (hexamethylmelamine) in the treatment of platinum-resistant ovarian cancer: a phase II study. *Gynecol Oncol.* 2003;88(2):118–122.
30. Rothenberg ML, Liu PY, Wilczynski S, et al. Phase II trial of oral altretamine for consolidation of clinical complete remission in women with stage III epithelial ovarian cancer: a Southwest Oncology Group trial (SWOG-9326). *Gynecol Oncol.* 2001;82(2):317–322.
31. Baker LH, Opipari MI, Wilson H, et al. Mitomycin C, vincristine, and bleomycin therapy for advanced cervical cancer. *Obstet Gynecol.* 1978;52(2):146–150.
32. Mirabelli CK, Huang CH, Crooke ST. Role of deoxyribonucleic acid topology in altering the site/sequence specificity of cleavage of deoxyribonucleic acid by bleomycin and talisomycin. *Biochemistry.* 1983;22(2):300–306.
33. Dorr RT. Bleomycin pharmacology: mechanism of action and resistance, and clinical pharmacokinetics. *Semin Oncol.* 1992;19(2 suppl 5):3–8.
34. Sebti SM, Jani JP, Mistry JS, et al. Metabolic inactivation: a mechanism of human tumor resistance to bleomycin. *Cancer Res.* 1991;51(1):227–232.
35. Alberts DS, Chen HS, Liu R, et al. Bleomycin pharmacokinetics in man. I. Intravenous administration. *Cancer Chemother Pharmacol.* 1978;1(3):177–181.
36. Ostrowski MJ. Intracavitary therapy with bleomycin for the treatment of malignant pleural effusions. *J Surg Oncol Suppl.* 1989;1:7–13.
37. Ruckdeschel JC, Moores D, Lee JY, et al. Intrapleural therapy for malignant pleural effusions. A randomized comparison of bleomycin and tetracycline. *Chest.* 1991;100(6):1528–1535.
38. Crooke ST, Comis RL, Einhorn LH, et al. Effects of variations in renal function on the clinical pharmacology of bleomycin administered as an iv bolus. *Cancer Treat Rep.* 1977;61(9):1631–1636.
39. Crooke ST, Luft F, Broughton A, et al. Bleomycin serum pharmacokinetics as determined by a radioimmunoassay and a microbiologic assay in a patient with compromised renal function. *Cancer.* 1977;39(4):1430–1434.
40. Oken MM, Crooke ST, Elson MK, et al. Pharmacokinetics of bleomycin after im administration in man. *Cancer Treat Rep.* 1981;65(5–6):485–489.
41. Samuels ML, Johnson DE, Holoye PY, et al. Large-dose bleomycin therapy and pulmonary toxicity. A possible role of prior radiotherapy. *JAMA.* 1976;235(11):1117–1120.
42. Ingrassia TS III, Ryu JH, Trastek VF, et al. Oxygen-exacerbated bleomycin pulmonary toxicity. *Mayo Clin Proc.* 1991;66(2):173–178.
43. Katz EJ, Andrews PA, Howell SB. The effect of DNA polymerase inhibitors on the cytotoxicity of cisplatin in human ovarian carcinoma cells. *Cancer Commun.* 1990;2(4):159–164.
44. Maher J, Daly PA. Severe bleomycin lung toxicity: reversal with high dose corticosteroids. *Thorax.* 1993;48(1):92–94.
45. Kerr LD, Spiera H. Scleroderma in association with the use of bleomycin: a report of 3 cases. *J Rheumatol.* 1992;19(2):294–296.
46. Haerslev T, Avnstorp C, Joergensen M. Sudden onset of adverse effects due to low-dosage bleomycin indicates an idiosyncratic reaction. *Cutis.* 1993;52(1):45–46.
47. Yee GC, Crom WR, Champion JE, et al. Cisplatin-induced changes in bleomycin elimination. *Cancer Treat Rep.* 1983;67(6):587–589.
48. Bennett WM, Pastore L, Houghton DC. Fatal pulmonary bleomycin toxicity in cisplatin-induced acute renal failure. *Cancer Treat Rep.* 1980;64(8–9):921–924.
49. Gerbrecht BM. Current Canadian experience with capecitabine: partnering with patients to optimize therapy. *Cancer Nurs.* 2003;26(2):161–167.

50. Chu E, DeVita VT. *Physicians' Cancer Chemotherapy Drug Manual 2003*. Sudbury, Canada: Jones and Bartlett Publishers; 2003.
51. Largillier R, Etienne-Grimaldi MC, Formento JL, et al. Pharmacogenetics of capecitabine in advanced breast cancer patients. *Clin Cancer Res*. 2006;12:5496–5502.
52. Knox R, Friedlos F, Lydall D, et al. Mechanism of cytotoxicity of anticancer platinum drugs: evidence that cis-diamminedichloroplatinum(II) and cis-diammine-(1,1-cyclobutanedicarboxylato)platinum(II) differ only in the kinetics of their interaction with DNA. *Cancer Res*. 1986;46(4 pt 2):1972–1979.
53. Horacek P, Drobnik J. Interaction of cis-dichlorodiammineplatinum (II) with DNA. *Biochim Biophys Acta*. 1971;254(2):341–347.
54. DeNeve W, Valeriote F, Tapazoglou E, et al. Discrepancy between cytotoxicity and DNA interstrand crosslinking of carboplatin and cisplatin in vivo. *Invest New Drugs*. 1990;8(1):17–24.
55. Micetich KC, Barnes D, Erickson LC. A comparative study of the cytotoxicity and DNA-damaging effects of cis-(diammino)(1,1-cyclobutanedicarboxylato)-platinum(II) and cis-diamminedichloroplatinum(II) on L1210 cells. *Cancer Res*. 1985;45(9):4043–4047.
56. Fichtingerschepman A, Vandijkknijnenburg H, Vanderveldevisser S, et al. Cisplatin-DNA-adducts and Carboplatin-DNA-adducts - is PT-AG the cytotoxic lesion? *Carcinogenesis*. 1995;16(10):2447–2453.
57. Burger H, Zoumaro-Djayoon A, Boersma A, et al. Differential transport of platinum compounds by the human organic cation transporter hOCT2 (hSLC22A2). *Br J Pharmacol*. 2010;159(4):898–908.
58. LeBlanc GA, Sundseth SS, Weber GF, et al. Platinum anticancer drugs modulate P-450 messenger RNA levels and differntially alter hepatic drugs and steroid-hormone metabolism in male and female rats. *Cancer Res*. 1992;52(3):540–547.
59. Waxma D, Sundseth S, Srivastava P, et al. Gene specific oligonuleotide probes for alpha, Mu, Pi and microsomal rat glutathione s-transferases-analysis of liver transferase expression and its modulation by hepatic enzyme inducers and platinum anticancer drugs. *Cancer Res*. 1992;52(20):5797–5802.
60. Natarajan G, Malathi R, Holler E. Increased DNA binding activity of cis-1,1-cyclobutanedicarboxylatodiammineplatinum(II) (Carboplatin) in the presence of nucleophiles and human breast cancer MCF-7 cell cytoplasmic extracts: activation theory revisited. *Biochem Pharmacol*. 1999;58(20):5797–5802.
61. Aabo K, Adams M, Adnitt P, et al. Chemotherapy in advanced ovarian cancer: four systematic meta-analyses of individual patient data from 37 randomized trials. Advanced Ovarian Cancer Trialists' Group. *Br J Cancer*. 1998;78(11):1479–1487.
62. du Bois A, Luck HJ, Meier W, et al. Carboplatin/paclitaxel versus cisplatin/paclitaxel as first-line chemotherapy in advanced ovarian cancer: an interim analysis of a randomized phase III trial of the Arbeitsgemeinschaft Gynakologische Onkologie Ovarian Cancer Study Group. *Semin Oncol*. 1997;24(5 suppl 15):S15-44–S15-52.
63. Harrap KR. Preclinical studies identifying carboplatin as a viable cisplatin alternative. *Cancer Treat Rev*. 1985;12 suppl A:21–33.
64. Wilkinson R, Cox PJ, Jones M, et al. Selection of potential second generation platinum compounds. *Biochem J*. 1978;60:851.
65. Zwelling LA, Kohn KW. Mechanism of action of cis-dichlorodiammineplatinum(II). *Cancer Treat Rep*. 1979;63(9–10):1439–1444.
66. Gaver RC, George AM, Deeb G. In vitro stability, plasma protein binding and blood cell partitioning of 14C-carboplatin. *Cancer Chemother Pharmacol*. 1987;20(4):271–276.
67. Shea TC, Flaherty M, Elias A, et al. A phase I clinical and pharmacokinetic study of carboplatin and autologous bone marrow support. *J Clin Oncol*. 1989;7(5):651–661.
68. Van Echo DA, Egorin MJ, Whitacre MY, et al. Phase I clinical and pharmacologic trial of carboplatin daily for 5 days. *Cancer Treat Rep*. 1984;68(9):1103–1114.
69. Horwich A, Dearnaley DP, Duchesne GM, et al. Simple nontoxic treatment of advanced metastatic seminoma with carboplatin. *J Clin Oncol*. 1989;7(8):1150–1156.
70. Misset B, Escudier B, Leclercq B, et al. Acute myocardiotoxicity during 5-fluorouracil therapy. *Intensive Care Med*. 1990;16(3):210–211.
71. Calvert AH, Newell DR, Gumbrell LA, et al. Carboplatin dosage: prospective evaluation of a simple formula based on renal function. *J Clin Oncol*. 1989;7(11):1748–1756.
72. Martino G, Frusciante V, Varraso A, et al. Efficacy of 51Cr-EDTA clearance to tailor a carboplatin therapeutic regimen in ovarian cancer patients. *Anticancer Res*. 1999;19(6C):5587–5591.
73. Cockroft DW, Gault MH. Prediction of creatinine clearance for serum creatinine. *Nephron*. 1976;16(1):31–41.
74. Belani CP, Kearns CM, Zuhowski EG, et al. Phase I trial, including pharmacokinetic and pharmacodynamic correlations, of combination paclitaxel and carboplatin in patients with metastatic non-small-cell lung cancer. *J Clin Oncol*. 1999;17(2):676–684.
75. Calvert AH, Boddy A, Bailey NP, et al. Carboplatin in combination with paclitaxel in advanced ovarian cancer: dose determination and pharmacokinetic and pharmacodynamic interactions. *Semin Oncol*. 1995;22(5 suppl 12):91–98; discussion 9–100.
76. Okamoto H, Nagatomo A, Kunitoh H, et al. Prediction of carboplatin clearance calculated by patient characteristics or 24-hour creatinine clearance: a comparison of the performance of three formulae. *Cancer Chemother Pharmacol*. 1998;42(4):307–312.
77. Wright J, Boddy A, Highley M, et al. Estimation of glomerular filtration rate in cancer patients. *Br J Cancer*. 2001;84(4):452–459.
78. Goldberg P, ed. *New Creatinine Test Raises Questions about Accuracy of Carboplatin Dosing*. 2010.
79. Sorensen BT, Stromgren A, Jakobsen P, et al. Dose-toxicity relationship of carboplatin in combination with cyclophosphamide in ovarian cancer patients. *Cancer Chemother Pharmacol*. 1991;28(5):397–401.
80. The International Collaborative Ovarian Neoplasm Group. Paclitaxel plus carboplatin versus standard chemotherapy with either single-agent carboplatin or cyclophosphamide, doxorubicin, and cisplatin in women with ovarian cancer: the ICON3 randomised trial.[comment]. *Lancet*. 2002;360(9332):505–515.
81. Calvert AH, Harland SJ, Newell DR, et al. Early clinical studies with cis-diammine-1,1-cyclobutane dicarboxylate platinum II. *Cancer Chemother Pharmacol*. 1982;9(3):140–147.
82. Plezia PM, Alberts DS, Kessler J, et al. Immediate termination of intractable vomiting induced by cisplatin combination chemotherapy using an intensive five-drug antiemetic regimen. *Cancer Treat Rep*. 1984;68(12):1493–1495.
83. Canetta R, Rozencweig M, Carter SK. Carboplatin: the clinical spectrum to date. *Cancer Treat Rev*. 1985;12 suppl A:125–136.
84. Markman M, Kennedy A, Webster K, et al. Clinical features of hypersensitivity reactions to carboplatin. *J Clin Oncol*. 1999;17(4):1141.
85. Shukunami K, Kurokawa T, Kawakami Y, et al. Hypersensitivity reactions to intraperitoneal administration of carboplatin in ovarian cancer: the first report of a case. *Gynecol Oncol*. 1999;72(3):431–432.
86. Travis LB, Holowaty EJ, Bergfeldt K, et al. Risk of leukemia after platinum-based chemotherapy for ovarian cancer. *N Engl J Med*. 1999;340(5):351–357.
87. Calvert AH. A review of the pharmacokinetics and pharmacodynamics of combination carboplatin/paclitaxel. *Semin Oncol*. 1997;24(1 suppl 2):S2-85–S2-90.
88. Budd GT, Ganapathi R, Adelstein DJ, et al. Randomized trial of carboplatin plus amifostine versus carboplatin alone in patients with advanced solid tumors. *Cancer*. 1997;80(6):1134–1140.
89. Korst AE, van der Sterre ML, Eeltink CM, et al. Pharmacokinetics of carboplatin with and without amifostine in patients with solid tumors. *Clin Cancer Res*. 1997;3(5):697–703.
90. Markman M, Reichman B, Hakes T, et al. Evidence supporting the superiority of intraperitoneal cisplatin compared to intraperitoneal carboplatin for salvage therapy of small-volume residual ovarian cancer. *Gynecol Oncol*. 1993;50(1):100–104.
91. Miyagi Y, Fujiwara K, Kigawa J, et al. Intraperitoneal carboplatin infusion may be a pharmacologically more reasonable route than intravenous administration as a systemic chemotherapy. A comparative pharmacokinetic analysis of platinum using a new mathematical model after intraperitoneal vs. intravenous infusion of carboplatin—a Sankai Gynecology Study Group (SGSG) study. *Gynecol Oncol*. 2005;99(3):591–596.
92. Los G, Verdegaal EM, Mutsaers PH, et al. Penetration of carboplatin and cisplatin into rat peritoneal tumor nodules after intraperitoneal chemotherapy. *Cancer Chemother Pharmacol*. 1991;28(3):159–165.
93. Muggia FM, Groshen S, Russell C, et al. Intraperitoneal carboplatin and etoposide for persistent epithelial ovarian cancer: analysis of results by prior sensitivity to platinum-based regimens. *Gynecol Oncol*. 1993;50(2):232–238.
94. Fujiwara K, Suzuki S, Ishikawa H, et al. Preliminary toxicity analysis of intraperitoneal carboplatin in combination with intravenous paclitaxel chemotherapy for patients with carcinoma of the ovary, peritoneum, or fallopian tube. *Int J Gynecol Cancer*. 2005;15(3):426–431.
95. Reed E, Ozols RF, Tarone R, et al. Platinum-DNA adducts in leukocyte DNA correlate with disease response in ovarian cancer patients receiving platinum-based chemotherapy. *Proc Natl Acad Sci U S A*. 1987;84(14):5024–5028.
96. Rice JA, Crothers DM, Pinto AL, et al. The major adduct of the antitumor drug cis-diamminedichloroplatinum(II) with DNA bends the duplex by approximately equal to 40 degrees toward the major groove. *Proc Natl Acad Sci U S A*. 1988;85(12):4158–4161.

97. Perez RP. Cellular and molecular determinants of cisplatin resistance. *Eur J Cancer.* 1998;34(10):1535–1542.
98. Reed E. Platinum-DNA adduct, nucleotide excision repair and platinum based anti-cancer chemotherapy. *Cancer Treat Rev.* 1998;24(5):331–344.
99. Steffensen KD, Waldstrom M, Jakobsen A. The relationship of platinum resistance and ERCC1 protein expression in epithelial ovarian cancer. *Int J Gynecol Cancer.* 2009;19(5):820–825.
100. Rose PG, Mossbruger K, Fusco N, et al. Gemcitabine reverses cisplatin resistance: demonstration of activity in platinum- and multidrug-resistant ovarian and peritoneal carcinoma. *Gynecol Oncol.* 2003;88(1):17–21.
101. Cannistra SA. Cancer of the ovary. *N Engl J Med.* 2004;351(24):2519–2529.
102. Cass I, Baldwin RL, Varkey T, et al. Improved survival in women with BRCA-associated ovarian carcinoma. *Cancer.* 2003;97(9):2187–2195.
103. Tan DS, Rothermundt C, Thomas K, et al. "BRCAness" syndrome in ovarian cancer: a case-control study describing the clinical features and outcome of patients with epithelial ovarian cancer associated with BRCA1 and BRCA2 mutations. *J Clin Oncol.* 2008;26(34):5530–5536.
104. Hennessy BT, Timms KM, Carey MS, et al. Somatic mutations in BRCA1 and BRCA2 could expand the number of patients that benefit from poly (ADP ribose) polymerase inhibitors in ovarian cancer. *J Clin Oncol.* 2010;28(22):3570–3576.
105. Konstantinopoulos PA, Spentzos D, Karlan BY, et al. Gene expression profile of BRCAness that correlates with responsiveness to chemotherapy and with outcome in patients with epithelial ovarian cancer. *J Clin Oncol.* 2010;28(22):3555–3561.
106. Swisher EM, Sakai W, Karlan BY, et al. Secondary BRCA1 mutations in BRCA1-mutated ovarian carcinomas with platinum resistance. *Cancer Res.* 2008;68(8):2581–2586.
107. Edwards SL, Brough R, Lord CJ, et al. Resistance to therapy caused by intragenic deletion in BRCA2. *Nature.* 2008;451(7182):1111–1115.
108. Sakai W, Swisher EM, Karlan BY, et al. Secondary mutations as a mechanism of cisplatin resistance in BRCA2-mutated cancers. *Nature.* 2008;451(7182):1116–1120.
109. Safaei R. Role of copper transporters in the uptake and efflux of platinum containing drugs. *Cancer Lett.* 2006;234:34–39.
110. Lee YY, Choi CH, Do IG, et al. Prognostic value of the copper transporters, CTR1 and CTR2, in patients with ovarian carcinoma receiving platinum-based chemotherapy. *Gynecol Oncol.* 2011;122(2):361–365.
111. Gifford G, Paul J, Vasey PA, et al. The acquisition of hMLH1 methylation in plasma DNA after chemotherapy predicts poor survival for ovarian cancer patients. *Clin Cancer Res.* 2004;10(13):4420–4426.
112. Glasspool RM, Gore M, Rustin G, et al. Randomized phase II study of decitabine in combination with carboplatin compared with carboplatin alone in patients with recurrent advanced ovarian cancer. *J Clin Oncol.* 2009;27(15s):5562.
113. Roodhart JM, Daenen LG, Stigter EC, et al. Mesenchymal stem cells induce resistance to chemotherapy through the release of platinum-induced fatty acids. *Cancer Cell.* 1016;20(3):370–383.
114. DeConti RC, Toftness BR, Lange RC, et al. Clinical and pharmacological studies with cis-diamminedichloroplatinum (II). *Cancer Res.* 1973;33(6):1310–1315.
115. Cisplatin [package insert]. Irvine, CA: Gensia Sicor Pharmaceuticals; 2000.
116. Ehninger G, Haag C, Wilms K. Die Pharmakokinetik von cis-Diaminodichloroplatin. *Tumor Diagn Ther.* 1984;5:147.
117. Schierl R, Rohrer B, Hohnloser J. Long-term platinum excretion in patients treated with cisplatin. *Cancer Chemother Pharmacol.* 1995;36:75–78.
118. Earhart RH. Instability of cis-dichlorodiammineplatinum in dextrose solution. *Cancer Treat Rev.* 1979;6(62):1105.
119. Eshaque M, McKay MJ, Theophande T, et al. p-Mannitol platinum complexes. *Wadley Med Bull.* 1976;7:338.
120. Prestayko AW, Cadiz M, Crooke ST. Incompatibility of aluminum-containing iv administration equipment with cis-dichlorodiammineplatinum(II) administration. *Cancer Treat Rep.* 1979;63(11–12):2118–2119.
121. Hayes DM, Cvitkovic E, Golbey RB, et al. High dose cis-platinum diammine dichloride: amelioration of renal toxicity by mannitol diuresis. *Cancer.* 1977;39(4):1372–1381.
122. Rainey JM, Alberts DS. Safe, rapid administration schedule for cis-platinum-mannitol. *Med Pediatr Oncol.* 1978;4(4):371–375.
123. Brock J, Alberts DS. Safe, rapid administration of cisplatin in the outpatient clinic. *Cancer Treat Rep.* 1986;70(12):1409–1414.
124. Walker JL, Armstrong DK, Huang HQ, et al. Intraperitoneal catheter outcomes in a phase III trial of intravenous versus intraperitoneal chemotherapy in optimal stage III ovarian and primary peritoneal cancer: a Gynecologic Oncology Group Study. *Gynecol Oncol.* 2006;100(1):27–32.
125. Alberts DS, Delforge A. Maximizing the delivery of intraperitoneal therapy while minimizing drug toxicity and maintaining quality of life. *Semin Oncol.* 2006;33(6 suppl 12):S8–S17.
126. NCCN. NCCN Antiemesis Guidelines version 2.2006 2006 [3/11/2006]. Available from. http://www.nccn.org/professionals/physican_gls/PDF/antiemesis.pdf.
127. Levin L, Hryniuk WM. Dose intensity analysis of chemotherapy regimens in ovarian carcinoma. *J Clin Oncol.* 1987;5(5):756–767.
128. Bonomi P, Blessing JA, Stehman FB, et al. Randomized trial of three cisplatin dose schedules in squamous-cell carcinoma of the cervix: a Gynecologic Oncology Group study. *J Clin Oncol.* 1985;3(8):1079–1085.
129. Gandara DR, Wold H, Perez EA, et al. Cisplatin dose intensity in non-small cell lung cancer: phase II results of a day 1 and day 8 high-dose regimen. *J Natl Cancer Inst.* 1989;81(10):790–794.
130. Holleran WM, DeGregorio MW. Evolution of high-dose cisplatin. *Invest New Drugs.* 1988;6(2):135–142.
131. Gonzalez-Vitale JC, Hayes DM, Cvitkovic E, et al. Acute renal failure after cis-dichlorodiammineplatinum(II) and gentamicin-cephalothin therapies. *Cancer Treat Rep.* 1978;62(5):693–698.
132. Madias NE, Harrington JT. Platinum nephrotoxicity. *Am J Med.* 1978;65(2):307–314.
133. Fleming S, Peppard S, Ratanatharathorn V, et al. Ototoxicity from cis-platinum in patients with stages III and IV previously untreated squamous cell cancer of the head and neck. *Am J Clin Oncol.* 1985;8(4):302–306.
134. Alberts DS, Noel JK. Cisplatin-associated neurotoxicity: can it be prevented? *Anticancer Drugs.* 1995;6(3):369–383.
135. Cersosimo RJ. Cisplatin neurotoxicity. *Cancer Treat Rev.* 1989;16(4):195–211.
136. Willox JC, McAllister EJ, Sangster G, et al. Effects of magnesium supplementation in testicular cancer patients receiving cis-platin: a randomised trial. *Br J Cancer.* 1986;54(1):19–23.
137. Morrow GR, Hickok JT, Rosenthal SN. Progress in reducing nausea and emesis. Comparisons of ondansetron (Zofran), granisetron (Kytril), and tropisetron (Navoban). *Cancer.* 1995;76(3):343–357.
138. Latreille J, Pater J, Johnston D, et al. Use of dexamethasone and granisetron in the control of delayed emesis for patients who receive highly emetogenic chemotherapy. National Cancer Institute of Canada Clinical Trials Group. *J Clin Oncol.* 1998;16(3):1174–1178.
139. Kris MG, Gralla RJ, Tyson LB, et al. Controlling delayed vomiting: double-blind, randomized trial comparing placebo, dexamethasone alone, and metoclopramide plus dexamethasone in patients receiving cisplatin. *J Clin Oncol.* 1989;7(1):108–1014.
140. Khan A, Hill JM, Grater W, et al. Atopic hypersensitivity to cis-dichlorodiammineplatinum(II) and other platinum complexes. *Cancer Res.* 1975;35(10):2766–2770.
141. Von Hoff DD, Slavik M, Muggia FM. Letter: allergic reactions to cis platinum. *Lancet.* 1976;1(7950):90.
142. Wiesenfeld M, Reinders E, Corder M, et al. Successful re-treatment with cis-dichlorodiammineplatinum(II) after apparent allergic reactions. *Cancer Treat Rep.* 1979;63(2):219–221.
143. Abels RI. Use of recombinant human erythropoietin in the treatment of anemia in patients who have cancer. *Semin Oncol.* 1992;19(3 suppl 8):29–35.
144. Rowinsky EK, Donehower RC. Paclitaxel (taxol). *N Engl J Med.* 1995;332(15):1004–1014.
145. de Jonge MJ, Loos WJ, Gelderblom H, et al. Phase I pharmacologic study of oral topotecan and intravenous cisplatin: sequence-dependent hematologic side effects. *J Clin Oncol.* 2000;18(10):2104–2115.
146. Kemp G, Rose P, Lurain J, et al. Amifostine pretreatment for protection against cyclophosphamide-induced and cisplatin-induced toxicities: results of a randomized control trial in patients with advanced ovarian cancer. *J Clin Oncol.* 1996;14(7):2101–2112.
147. Schuchter LM, Hensley ML, Meropol NJ, et al. 2002 update of recommendations for the use of chemotherapy and radiotherapy protectants: clinical practice guidelines of the American Society of Clinical Oncology. *J Clin Oncol.* 2002;20(12):2895–2903.
148. Bagley CM Jr, Bostick FW, DeVita VT Jr. Clinical pharmacology of cyclophosphamide. *Cancer Res.* 1973;33(2):226–233.
149. Struck RF, Alberts DS, Horne K, et al. Plasma pharmacokinetics of cyclophosphamide and its cytotoxic metabolites after intravenous versus oral administration in a randomized, crossover trial. *Cancer Res.* 1987;47(10):2723–2726.
150. Cohen JL, Jao JY, Jusko WJ. Pharmacokinetics of cyclophosphamide in man. *Br J Pharmacol.* 1971;43(3):677–680.
151. Dorr RT, Von Hoff DD. *Cancer Chemotherapy Handbook*, 2 ed. Norwalk, CT: Appleton & Lange; 1994.

152. Kerbel RS, Viloria-Petit A, Klement G, et al. 'Accidental' anti-angiogenic drugs. Anti-oncogene directed signal transduction inhibitors and conventional chemotherapeutic agents as examples. *Eur J Cancer.* 2000;36(10):1248–1257.
153. Colleoni M, Rocca A, Sandri MT, et al. Low-dose oral methotrexate and cyclophosphamide in metastatic breast cancer: antitumor activity and correlation with vascular endothelial growth factor levels. *Ann Oncol.* 2002;13(1):73–80.
154. Miscoria M, Tonetto F, Deroma L, et al. Exploratory predictive and prognostic factors in advanced breast cancer treated with metronomic chemotherapy. *Anticancer Drugs.* 2012;23:326–334.
155. Gunther M, Wagner E, Ogris M. Acrolein: unwanted side product or contribution to antiangiogenic properties of metronomic cyclophosphamide therapy? *J Cell Mol Med.* 2008;12(6B):2704–2716.
156. Ghiringhelli F, Menard C, Puig PE, et al. Metronomic cyclophosphamide regimen selectively depletes CD4+CD25+ regulatory T cells and restores T and NK effector functions in end stage cancer patients. *Cancer Immunol Immunother.* 2007;56(5):641–648.
157. Ge Y, Domschke C, Stoiber N, et al. Metronomic cyclophosphamide treatment in metastasized breast cancer patients: immunological effects and clinical outcome. *Cancer.* 2012;61(3):353–362.
158. Penel N, Adenis A, Bocci G. Cyclophosphamide-based metronomic chemotherapy: after 10 years of experience, where do we stand and where are we going? *Crit Rev Oncol Hematol.* 2012;82(1):40–50.
159. DeFronzo RA, Braine H, Colvin M, et al. Water intoxication in man after cyclophosphamide therapy. Time course and relation to drug activation. *Ann Intern Med.* 1973;78(6):861–869.
160. Topilow AA, Rothenberg SP, Cottrell TS. Interstitial pneumonia after prolonged treatment with cyclophosphamide. *Am Rev Respir Dis.* 1973;108(1):114–117.
161. Braverman AC, Antin JH, Plappert MT, et al. Cyclophosphamide cardiotoxicity in bone marrow transplantation: a prospective evaluation of new dosing regimens. *J Clin Oncol.* 1991;9(7):1215–1223.
162. Connors TA, Cox PJ, Farmer PB, et al. Some studies of the active intermediates formed in the microsomal metabolism of cyclophosphamide and isophosphamide. *Biochem Pharmacol.* 1974;23(1):115–129.
163. Wiemann MC, Cummings FJ, Kaplan HG, et al. Clinical and pharmacological studies of methotrexate-minimal leucovorin rescue plus fluorouracil. *Cancer Res.* 1982;42(9):3896–3900.
164. Dorr RT, Soble MJ, Alberts DS. Interaction of cimetidine but not ranitidine with cyclophosphamide in mice. *Cancer Res.* 1986;46(4 pt 1):1795–1799.
165. Struck RF, Alberts DS, Plezia PM, et al. Effect of the antiulcer drug ranitidine on the pharmacokinetics and hematologic toxicity of cyclophosphamide and its cytotoxic metabolites in patients. [Abstract]. *Proc AACR.* 1988;29:187.
166. Harris NL, Brenner DE, Anthony LB, et al. The influence of ranitidine on the pharmacokinetics and toxicity of doxorubicin in rabbits. *Cancer Chemother Pharmacol.* 1988;21(4):323–328.
167. Homesley HD. Single-agent therapy for nonmetastatic and low-risk gestational trophoblastic disease. *J Reprod Med.* 1998;43(1):69–74.
168. Williams SD. Ovarian germ cell tumors: an update. *Semin Oncol.* 1998;25(3):407–413.
169. Schwartz HS. Some determinants of the therapeutic efficacy of actinomycin D (NSC-3053), adriamycin (NSC-123127), and daunorubicin (NSC-83142). *Cancer Chemother Rep.* 1974;58(1):55–62.
170. Knutsen T, Mickley LA, Ried T, et al. Cytogenetic and molecular characterization of random chromosomal rearrangements activating the drug resistance gene, MDR1/P-glycoprotein, in drug-selected cell lines and patients with drug refractory ALL. *Genes Chromosomes Cancer.* 1998;23(1):44–54.
171. Tattersall MH, Sodergren JE, Dengupta SK, et al. Pharmacokinetics of actinoymcin D in patients with malignant melanoma. *Clin Pharmacol Ther.* 1975;17(6):701–708.
172. Brothman AR, Davis TP, Duffy JJ, et al. Development of an antibody to actinomycin D and its application for the detection of serum levels by radioimmunoassay. *Cancer Res.* 1982;42(3):1184–1187.
173. Blatt J, Trigg ME, Pizzo PA, et al. Tolerance to single-dose dactinomycin in combination chemotherapy for solid tumors. *Cancer Treat Rep.* 1981;65(1–2):145–147.
174. Petrilli ES, Twiggs LB, Blessing JA, et al. Single-dose actinomycin-D treatment for nonmetastatic gestational trophoblastic disease. A prospective phase II trial of the Gynecologic Oncology Group. *Cancer.* 1987;60(9):2173–2176.
175. Philips RS, Schwartz HS, Sternberg SS, et al. The toxicity of actinomycin D. *Ann N Y Acad Sci.* 1970;89:348.
176. Frei E III. The clinical use of actinomycin. *Cancer Chemother Rep.* 1974;58(1):49–54.
177. Cohen IJ, Loven D, Schoenfeld T, et al. Dactinomycin potentiation of radiation pneumonitis: a forgotten interaction. *Pediatr Hematol Oncol.* 1991;8(2):187–192.
178. Francis P, Schneider J, Hann L, et al. Phase II trial of docetaxel in patients with platinum-refractory advanced ovarian cancer. *J Clin Oncol.* 1994;12(11):2301–2308.
179. Gelmon K. The taxoids: paclitaxel and docetaxel. *Lancet.* 1994;344(8932):1267–1272.
180. Bruno R, Sanderink GJ. Pharmacokinetics and metabolism of Taxotere (docetaxel). *Cancer Surv.* 1993;17:305–313.
181. Aapro MS. Phase I and pharmacokinetic study of RP 56976 in a new ethanol-free formulation of Taxotere. *Ann Oncol.* 1992;3:208.
182. Von Hoff DD. The taxoids: same roots, different drugs. *Semin Oncol.* 1997;24(4 suppl 13):S13-3–S13-10.
183. Maisano R, Mare M, Zavettieri M, et al. Is weekly docetaxel an active and gentle chemotherapy in the treatment of metastatic breast cancer? *Anticancer Res.* 2003;23(2C):1923–1926.
184. Stemmler HJ, Gutschow K, Sommer H, et al. Weekly docetaxel (Taxotere) in patients with metastatic breast cancer. *Ann Oncol.* 2001;12(10):1393–1398.
185. Pronk LC, Schellens JH, Planting AS, et al. Phase I and pharmacologic study of docetaxel and cisplatin in patients with advanced solid tumors. *J Clin Oncol.* 1997;15(3):1071–1079.
186. Kaye SB, Piccart M, Aapro M, et al. Phase II trials of docetaxel (Taxotere) in advanced ovarian cancer-an updated overview. *Eur J Cancer.* 1997;33(13):2167–2170.
187. Wanders J, Schrijvers D, Bruntsch U, et al. The EORTC-ECTG experience with acute hypersensitivity reactions (HSR) in Taxotere studies. [Abstract]. *Proc ASCO.* 1993;12:73.
188. Galindo E, Kavanagh J, Fossella F, et al. Docetaxel (Taxotere) toxicities: analysis of a single institution experience with 168 patients (623 courses). *Proc Am Soc Clin Oncol.* 1994;13:164.
189. Zimmerman GC, Keeling JH, Lowry M, et al. Prevention of docetaxel-induced erythrodysesthesia with local hypothermia. *J Natl Cancer Inst.* 1994;86(7):557–558.
190. Eisenhauer EA, Vermorken JB. The taxoids. Comparative clinical pharmacology and therapeutic potential. *Drugs.* 1998;55(1):5–30.
191. Henry DW. Structure-activity relationships among daunorubicin and adriamycin analogs. *Cancer Treat Rep.* 1979;63(5):845–854.
192. Hasinoff BB, Davey JP. Adriamycin and its iron(III) and copper(II) complexes. Glutathione-induced dissociation; cytochrome c oxidase inactivation and protection; binding to cardiolipin. *Biochem Pharmacol.* 1988;37(19):3663–3669.
193. Myers CE, Gianni L, Simone CB, et al. Oxidative destruction of erythrocyte ghost membranes catalyzed by the doxorubicin-iron complex. *Biochemistry.* 1982;21(8):1707–1712.
194. Di Marco A, Zunino F, Silverstrini R, et al. Interaction of some daunomycin derivatives with deoxyribonucleic acid and their biological activity. *Biochem Pharmacol.* 1971;20(6):1323–1328.
195. Painter RB. Inhibition of DNA replicon initiation by 4-nitroquinoline 1-oxide, adriamycin, and ethyleneimine. *Cancer Res.* 1978;38(12):4445–4449.
196. Driscoll JS, Hazard GF, Jr, Wood HB, Jr, Goldin A. Structure-antitumor activity relationships among quinone derivatives. *Cancer Chemother Rep.* 1974;4(2):1–362.
197. Goodman J, Hochstein P. Generation of free radicals and lipid peroxidation by redox cycling of adriamycin and daunomycin. *Biochem Biophys Res Commun.* 1977;77(2):797–803.
198. Kim SH, Kim JH. Lethal effect of adriamycin on the division cycle of HeLa cells. *Cancer Res.* 1972;32(2):323–325.
199. Ritch PS, Occhipinti SJ, Cunningham RE, et al. Schedule-dependent synergism of combinations of hydroxyurea with adriamycin and 1-beta-D-arabinofuranosylcytosine with adriamycin. *Cancer Res.* 1981;41(10):3881–3884.
200. Glisson BS, Ross WE. DNA topoisomerase II: a primer on the enzyme and its unique role as a multidrug target in cancer chemotherapy. *Pharmacol Ther.* 1987;32(2):89–106.
201. Tewey KM, Chen GL, Nelson EM, et al. Intercalative antitumor drugs interfere with the breakage-reunion reaction of mammalian DNA topoisomerase II. *J Biol Chem.* 1984;259(14):9182–9187.
202. Eksborg S, Ehrsson H, Ekqvist B. Protein binding of anthraquinone glycosides, with special reference to adriamycin. *Cancer Chemother Pharmacol.* 1982;10(1):7–10.
203. Piazza E, Broggini M, Trabattoni A, et al. Adriamycin distribution in plasma and blood cells of cancer patients with altered hematocrit. *Eur J Cancer Clin Oncol.* 1981;17(10):1089–1096.

204. Benjamin RS, Riggs CE, Jr, Bachur NR. Plasma pharmacokinetics of adriamycin and its metabolites in humans with normal hepatic and renal function. *Cancer Res.* 1977;37(5):1416–1420.
205. Lee YT, Chan KK, Harris PA, et al. Distribution of adriamycin in cancer patients: tissue uptakes, plasma concentration after IV and hepatic IA administration. *Cancer.* 1980;45(9):2231–2239.
206. Egan PC, Costanza ME, Dodion P, et al. Doxorubicin and cisplatin excretion into human milk. *Cancer Treat Rep.* 1985;69(12):1387–1389.
207. D'Incalci M, Broggini M, Buscaglia M, et al. Transplacental passage of doxorubicin. *Lancet.* 1983;1(8314–8315):75.
208. Karp GI, von Oeyen P, Valone F, et al. Doxorubicin in pregnancy: possible transplacental passage. *Cancer Treat Rep.* 1983;67(9):773–777.
209. Roboz J, Gleicher N, Wu K, et al. Does doxorubicin cross the placenta? Lancet. 1979;2(8156–8157):1382–1383.
210. Bachur NR. Adriamycin (NSC-123127) pharmacology. *Cancer Chemother Rep.* 1975;6:153.
211. Riggs CE, Jr, Benjamin RS, Serpick AA, et al. Bilary disposition of adriamycin. *Clin Pharmacol Ther.* 1977;22(2):234–241.
212. Benjamin RS. A practical approach to Adriamycin (NSC-123127). *Cancer Chemother Rep.* 1975;6:191.
213. Chan KK, Chlebowski RT, Tong M, et al. Clinical pharmacokinetics of adriamycin in hepatoma patients with cirrhosis. *Cancer Res.* 1980;40(4):1263–1268.
214. Rodvold KA, Rushing DA, Tewksbury DA. Doxorubicin clearance in the obese. *J Clin Oncol.* 1988;6(8):1321–1327.
215. Gessner T, Robert J, Bolanowska W, et al. Effects of prior therapy on plasma levels of adriamycin during subsequent therapy. *J Med.* 1981;12(2–3):183–193.
216. Morris RG, Reece PA, Dale BM, et al. Alteration in doxorubicin and doxorubicinol plasma concentrations with repeated courses to patients. *Ther Drug Monit.* 1989;11(4):380–383.
217. Robert J, Hoerni B. Age dependence of the early-phase pharmacokinetics of doxorubicin. *Cancer Res.* 1983;43(9):4467–4469.
218. Garnick MB, Ensminger WD, Israel M. A clinical-pharmacological evaluation of hepatic arterial infusion of adriamycin. *Cancer Res.* 1979;39(10):4105–4110.
219. Bern MM, McDermott W, Jr, Cady B, et al. Intraaterial hepatic infusion and intravenous adriamycin for treatment of hepatocellular carcinoma: a clinical and pharmacology report. *Cancer.* 1978;42(2):399–405.
220. Chen HS, Gross JF. Intra-arterial infusion of anticancer drugs: theoretic aspects of drug delivery and review of responses. *Cancer Treat Rep.* 1980;64(1):31–40.
221. Creasey WA, McIntosh LS, Brescia T, et al. Clinical effects and pharmacokinetics of different dosage schedules of adriamycin. *Cancer Res.* 1976;36(1):216–221.
222. Hryniuk W, Levine MN. Analysis of dose intensity for adjuvant chemotherapy trials in stage II breast cancer. *J Clin Oncol.* 1986;4(8):1162–1170.
223. Carmo-Pereira J, Costa FO, Henriques E, et al. A comparison of two doses of adriamycin in the primary chemotherapy of disseminated breast carcinoma. *Br J Cancer.* 1987;56(4):471–473.
224. Von Hoff DD, Layard MW, Basa P, et al. Risk factors for doxorubicin-induced congestive heart failure. *Ann Intern Med.* 1979;91(5):710–717.
225. Minow RA, Benjamin RS, Gottlieb JA. Adriamycin (NSC-123127) cardiomyopathy—an overview with determinants of risk factors. *Cancer Chemother Rep.* 1975(6):195.
226. Reilly JJ, Neifeld JP, Rosenberg SA. Clinical course and management of accidental adriamycin extravasation. *Cancer.* 1977;40(5):2053–2056.
227. Rudolph R, Stein RS, Pattillo RA. Skin ulcers due to adriamycin. *Cancer.* 1976;38(3):1087–1094.
228. Dorr RT, Dordal MS, Koenig LM, et al. High levels of doxorubicin in the tissues of a patient experiencing extravasation during a 4-day infusion. *Cancer.* 1989;64(12):2462–2464.
229. Dorr RT. Antidotes to vesicant chemotherapy extravasations. *Blood Rev.* 1990;4(1):41–60.
230. Lefrak EA, Pitha J, Rosenheim S, et al. Adriamycin (NSC-123127) cardiomyopathy. *Cancer Chemother Rep.* 1975;6:203.
231. Lenaz L, Page JA. Cardiotoxicity of adriamycin and related anthracyclines. *Cancer Treat Rev.* 1976;3(3):111–120.
232. Rinehart JJ, Lewis RP, Balcerzak SP. Adriamycin cardiotoxicity in man. *Ann Intern Med.* 1974;81(4):475–478.
233. Steinherz LJ, Steinherz PG, Tan CT, et al. Cardiac toxicity 4 to 20 years after completing anthracycline therapy. *JAMA.* 1991;266(12):1672–1677.
234. Speyer J, Wasserheit C. Strategies for reduction of anthracycline cardiac toxicity. *Semin Oncol.* 1998;25(5):525–537.
235. Bielack SS, Erttmann R, Winkler K, et al. Doxorubicin: effect of different schedules on toxicity and anti-tumor efficacy. *Eur J Cancer Clin Oncol.* 1989;25(5):873–882.
236. Donaldson SS, Glick JM, Wilbur JR. Letter: adriamycin activating a recall phenomenon after radiation therapy. *Ann Intern Med.* 1974;81(3):407–408.
237. Greco FA, Brereton HD, Kent H, et al. Adriamycin and enhanced radiation reaction in normal esophagus and skin. *Ann Intern Med.* 1976;85(3):294–298.
238. Newburger PE, Cassady JR, Jaffe N. Esophagitis due to adriamycin and radiation therapy for childhood malignancy. *Cancer.* 1978;42(2):417–423.
239. Sarosy GA, Brown TD, Von Hoff DD, et al. Phase I study of alpha 2-interferon plus doxorubicin in patients with solid tumors. *Cancer Res.* 1986;46(10):5368–5371.
240. Rose PG, Blessing JA, Buller RE, et al. Prolonged oral etoposide in recurrent or advanced non-squamous cell carcinoma of the cervix: a Gynecologic Oncology Group study. *Gynecol Oncol.* 2003;89(2):267–270.
241. Keller-Juslen C, Kuhn M, Stahelin H, von Wartburg A. Synthesis and antimitotic activity of glycosidic lignan derivatives related to podophyllotoxin. *J Med Chem.* 1971;14(10):936–940.
242. Misra NC, Roberts DW. Inhibition by 4'-demethyl-epipodophyllotoxin 9-(4,6-O-2-thenylidene-beta-D-glucopyranoside) of human lymphoblast cultures in G2 phase of the cell cycle. *Cancer Res.* 1975;35(1):99–105.
243. Krishan A, Paika K, Frei E, III. Cytofluorometric studies on the action of podophyllotoxin and epipodophyllotoxins (VM-26, VP-16-213) on the cell cycle traverse of human lymphoblasts. *J Cell Biol.* 1975;66(3):521–530.
244. Ross W, Rowe T, Glisson B, et al. Role of topoisomerase II in mediating epipodophyllotoxin-induced DNA cleavage. *Cancer Res.* 1984;44(12 pt 1):5857–5860.
245. Chen AY, Liu LF. DNA topoisomerases: essential enzymes and lethal targets. *Annu Rev Pharmacol Toxicol.* 1994;34:191–218.
246. 24Wozniak AJ, Ross WE. DNA damage as a basis for 4'-demethylepipodophyllotoxin-9-(4,6-O-ethylidene-beta-D-glucopyranoside) (etoposide) cytotoxicity. *Cancer Res.* 1983;43(1):120–124.
247. Smith PJ, Anderson CO, Watson JV. Predominant role for DNA damage in etoposide-induced cytotoxicity and cell cycle perturbation in human SV40-transformed fibroblasts. *Cancer Res.* 1986;46(11):5641–5645.
248. Chatterjee S, Trivedi D, Petzold SJ, et al. Mechanism of epipodophyllotoxin-induced cell death in poly(adenosine diphosphate-ribose) synthesis-deficient V79 Chinese hamster cell lines. *Cancer Res.* 1990;50(9):2713–2718.
249. Wozniak AJ, Glisson BS, Hande KR, et al. Inhibition of etoposide-induced DNA damage and cytotoxicity in L1210 cells by dehydrogenase inhibitors and other agents. *Cancer Res.* 1984;44(2):626–632.
250. Allen LM, Creaven PJ. Comparison of the human pharmacokinetics of VM-26 and VP-16, two antineoplastic epipodophyllotixin glucopyranoside derivatives. *Eur J Cancer.* 1975;11(10):697–707.
251. D'Incalci M, Farina P, Sessa C, et al. Pharmacokinetics of VP16-213 given by different administration methods. *Cancer Chemother Pharmacol.* 1982;7(2–3):141–145.
252. Hande KR, Wedlund PJ, Noone RM, et al. Pharmacokinetics of high-dose etoposide (VP-16-213) administered to cancer patients. *Cancer Res.* 1984;44(1):379–382.
253. Stewart DJ, Richard MT, Hugenholtz H, et al. Penetration of VP-16 (etoposide) into human intracerebral and extracerebral tumors. *J Neurooncol.* 1984;2(2):133–139.
254. D'Incalci M, Sessa C, Rossi C, et al. Pharmacokinetics of etoposide in gestochoriocarcinoma. *Cancer Treat Rep.* 1985;69(1):69–72.
255. Creaven PJ, Newman SJ, Selawry OS, et al. Phase I clinical trial of weekly administration of 4'-demethylepipodophyllotoxin 9-(4,6-O-ethylidene-beta-D-glucopyranoside) (NSC-141540; VP-16-213). *Cancer Chemother Rep.* 1974;58(6):901–907.
256. Stewart CF, Arbuck SG, Fleming RA, et al. Changes in the clearance of total and unbound etoposide in patients with liver dysfunction. *J Clin Oncol.* 1990;8(11):1874–1879.
257. Pfluger KH, Schmidt L, Merkel M, et al. Drug monitoring of etoposide (VP16-213). Correlation of pharmacokinetic parameters to clinical and biochemical data from patients receiving etoposide. *Cancer Chemother Pharmacol.* 1987;20(1):59–66.
258. Smyth RD, Pfeffer M, Scalzo A, et al. Bioavailability and pharmacokinetics of etoposide (VP-16). *Semin Oncol.* 1985;12(1 suppl 2):48–51.
259. Harvey VJ, Slevin ML, Joel SP, et al. The effect of food and concurrent chemotherapy on the bioavailability of oral etoposide. *Br J Cancer.* 1985;52(3):363–367.
260. Dorr RT, Alberts DS. Skin ulceration potential without therapeutic anticancer activity for epipodophyllotoxin commercial diluents. *Invest New Drugs.* 1983;1(2):151–159.
261. Ozols RF. Oral etoposide for the treatment of recurrent ovarian cancer. Drugs. 1999;58(suppl 3):43–49.

262. Steward WP, Thatcher N, Edmundson JM, et al. Etoposide infusions for treatment of metastatic lung cancer. *Cancer Treat Rep.* 1984;68(6):897–899.
263. Hande KR, Wolff SN, Greco FA, et al. Etoposide kinetics in patients with obstructive jaundice. *J Clin Oncol.* 1990;8(6):1101–1107.
264. Rozencweig M, Von Hoff DD, Henney JE, et al. VM 26 and VP 16-213: a comparative analysis. *Cancer.* 1977;40(1):334–342.
265. Epipodophyllotoxin VP 16213 in treatment of acute leukaemias, haematosarcomas, and solid tumours. *Br Med J.* 1973;3(5873):199–202.
266. Dombernowsky P, Nissen NI, Larsen V. Clinical investigation of a new podophyllum derivative, epipodophyllotoxin, 4′-demethyl-9-(4,6-O-2-thenylidene- -D-glucopyranoside) (NSC-122819), in patients with malignant lymphomas and solid tumors. *Cancer Chemother Rep.* 1972;56(1):71–82.
267. Aisner J, Whitacre M, VanEcho DA, et al. Doxorubicin, Cyclophosphamide and VP16-213 (ACE) in the treatment of small cell lung cancer. *Cancer Chemother Pharmacol.* 1982;7(2–3):187–193.
268. Dorr RT. Chemoprotectants for cancer chemotherapy. Semin Oncol. 1991;18(1 suppl 2):48–58.
269. Thant M, Hawley RJ, Smith MT, et al. Possible enhancement of vincristine neuropathy by VP 16. *Cancer.* 1982;49(5):859–864.
270. Rustum YM. Biochemical rationale for the 5-fluorouracil leucovorin combination and update of clinical experience. *J Chemother.* 1990;2 suppl 1:5–11.
271. Collins JM, Dedrick RL, King FG, et al. Nonlinear pharmacokinetic models for 5-fluorouracil in man: intravenous and intraperitoneal routes. *Clin Pharmacol Ther.* 1980;28(2):235–246.
272. McDermott BJ, van den Berg HW, Murphy RF. Nonlinear pharmacokinetics for the elimination of 5-fluorouracil after intravenous administration in cancer patients. *Cancer Chemother Pharmacol.* 1982;9(3):173–178.
273. Fraile RJ, Baker LH, Buroker TR, et al. Pharmacokinetics of 5-fluorouracil administered orally, by rapid intravenous and by slow infusion. *Cancer Res.* 1980;40(7):2223–2228.
274. Schaaf LJ, Dobbs BR, Edwards IR, et al. Nonlinear pharmacokinetic characteristics of 5-fluorouracil (5-FU) in colorectal cancer patients. *Eur J Clin Pharmacol.* 1987;32(4):411–418.
275. Yoshida T, Araki E, Iigo M, et al. Clinical significance of monitoring serum levels of 5-fluorouracil by continuous infusion in patients with advanced colonic cancer. *Cancer Chemother Pharmacol.* 1990;26(5):352–354.
276. Floyd RA, Hornbeck CL, Byfield JE, et al. Clearance of continuously infused 5-fluorouracil in adults having lung or gastrointestinal carcinoma with or without hepatic metastases. *Drug Intell Clin Pharm.* 1982;16(9):665–667.
277. Santini J, Milano G, Thyss A, et al. 5-FU therapeutic monitoring with dose adjustment leads to an improved therapeutic index in head and neck cancer. *Br J Cancer.* 1989;59(2):287–290.
278. Lokich JJ, Ahlgren JD, Gullo JJ, et al. A prospective randomized comparison of continuous infusion fluorouracil with a conventional bolus schedule in metastatic colorectal carcinoma: a Mid-Atlantic Oncology Program Study. *J Clin Oncol.* 1989;7(4):425–432.
279. Moertel CG. Chemotherapy of gastrointestinal cancer. *N Engl J Med.* 1978;299(19):1049–1052.
280. Moertel CG, Schutt AJ, Reitemeier RJ, et al. A comparison of 5-fluorouracil administered by slow infusion and rapid injection. *Cancer Res.* 1972;32(12):2717–2719.
281. Horton J, Olson KB, Sullivan J, et al. 5-FU in cancer: an improved regimen. *Ann Intern Med.* 1970;73:897.
282. Jacobs EM, Reeves WJ, Jr, Wood DA, et al. Treatment of cancer with weekly intravenous 5-fluorouracil. Study by the Western Cooperative Cancer Chemotherapy Group (WCCCG). *Cancer.* 1971;27(6):1302–1305.
283. Bruckner HW, Glass LL, Chesser MR. Dose-dependent leucovorin efficacy with an intermittent high-dose 5-fluorouracil schedule. *Cancer Invest.* 1990;8(3–4):321–326.
284. Doroshow JH, Multhauf P, Leong L, et al. Prospective randomized comparison of fluorouracil versus fluorouracil and high-dose continuous infusion leucovorin calcium for the treatment of advanced measurable colorectal cancer in patients previously unexposed to chemotherapy. *J Clin Oncol.* 1990;8(3):491–501.
285. Curran CF, Luce JK. Fluorouracil and palmar-plantar erythrodysesthesia. *Ann Intern Med.* 1989;111(10):858.
286. Lopez AM, Wallace L, Dorr RT, et al. Topical DMSO treatment for pegylated liposomal doxorubicin-induced palmar-plantar erythrodysesthesia. *Cancer Chemother Pharmacol.* 1999;44(4):303–306.
287. Malet-Martino M, Martino R. Clinical studies of three oral prodrugs of 5-fluorouracil (capecitabine, UFT, S-1): a review. *Oncologist.* 2002;7(4):288–323.
288. Nagore E, Insa A, Sanmartin O. Antineoplastic therapy-induced palmar-plantar erythrodysesthesia ('hand-foot') syndrome. Incidence, recognition and management. *Am J Clin Dermatol.* 2000;1(4):225–234.
289. Hrushesky WJ. Serpentine supravenous 5-fluorouracil (NSC-19893) hyperpigmentation. *Cancer Treat Rep.* 1976;60(5):639.
290. Boileau G, Piro AJ, Lahiri SR, et al. Cerebellar ataxia during 5-fluorouracil (NSC-19893) therapy. *Cancer Chemother Rep.* 1971;55(5):595–598.
291. Gottlieb JA, Luce JK. Cerebellar ataxia with weekly 5-fluorouracil administration. *Lancet.* 1971;1(7690):138–139.
292. Cianci G, Morelli MF, Cannita K, et al. Prophylactic options in patients with 5-fluorouracil-associated cardiotoxicity. *Br J Cancer.* 2003;88(10):1507–1509.
293. Diasio RB, Beavers TL, Carpenter JT. Familial deficiency of dihydropyrimidine dehydrogenase. Biochemical basis for familial pyrimidinemia and severe 5-fluorouracil-induced toxicity. *J Clin Invest.* 1988;81(1):47–51.
294. Lu Z, Zhang R, Diasio RB. Population characteristics of hepatic dihydropyrimidine dehydrogenase activity, a key metabolic enzyme in 5-fluorouracil chemotherapy. *Clin Pharmacol Ther.* 1995;58(5):512–522.
295. Curran CF, Luce JK. Accidental acute exposure to fluorouracil. *Oncol Nurs Forum.* 1989;16(4):468.
296. Belpomme D, Krakowski I, Beauduin M, et al. Gemcitabine combined with cisplatin as first-line treatment in patients with epithelial ovarian cancer: a phase II study. *Gynecol Oncol.* 2003;91(1):32–38.
297. Fowler WC, Jr, Van Le L. Gemcitabine as a single-agent treatment for ovarian cancer. *Gynecol Oncol.* 2003;90(2 pt 2):S21–S23.
298. Hansen SW, Tuxen MK, Sessa C. Gemcitabine in the treatment of ovarian cancer. *Ann Oncol.* 1999;10 suppl 1:51–53.
299. Markman M, Webster K, Zanotti K, et al. Phase 2 trial of single-agent gemcitabine in platinum-paclitaxel refractory ovarian cancer. *Gynecol Oncol.* 2003;90(3):593–596.
300. Zarba JJ, Jaremtchuk AV, Gonzalez Jazey P, et al. A phase I-II study of weekly cisplatin and gemcitabine with concurrent radiotherapy in locally advanced cervical carcinoma. *Ann Oncol.* 2003;14(8):1285–1290.
301. Huang P, Chubb S, Hertel LW, et al. Action of 2′,2′-difluorodeoxycytidine on DNA synthesis. *Cancer Res.* 1991;51(22):6110–6117.
302. Plunkett W, Huang P, Gandhi V. Preclinical characteristics of gemcitabine. *Anticancer Drugs.* 1995;6 suppl 6:7–13.
303. Heinemann V, Xu YZ, Chubb S, et al. Inhibition of ribonucleotide reduction in CCRF-CEM cells by 2′,2′-difluorodeoxycytidine. *Mol Pharmacol.* 1990;38(4):567–572.
304. Abbruzzese JL, Grunewald R, Weeks EA, et al. A phase I clinical, plasma, and cellular pharmacology study of gemcitabine. *J Clin Oncol.* 1991;9(3):491–498.
305. Eli Lilly and Company. Gemzar (Gemcitabine HCI) for Injection 2003 [11/5/03]. Available from: http://pi.lilly.com/us/gemzar.pdf.
306. Allerheiligen S, Johnson R, Hatcher B, et al. Gemcitabine pharmacokinetics are influenced by gender, body surface area, amd duration of infusion. [Abstract]. *Proc ASCO.* 1994;13:136.
307. Storniolo AM, Allerheiligen SR, Pearce HL. Preclinical, pharmacologic, and phase I studies of gemcitabine. *Semin Oncol.* 1997;24(2 suppl 7):S7-2–S7-7.
308. van Moorsel CJ, Kroep JR, Pinedo HM, et al. Pharmacokinetic schedule finding study of the combination of gemcitabine and cisplatin in patients with solid tumors. *Ann Oncol.* 1999;10(4):441–448.
309. O'Rourke TJ, Brown TD, Havlin K, et al. Phase I clinical trial of gemcitabine given as an intravenous bolus on 5 consecutive days. *Eur J Cancer.* 1994;30A(3):417–418.
310. Hui YF, Reitz J. Gemcitabine: a cytidine analogue active against solid tumors. *Am J Health Syst Pharm.* 1997;54(2):162–170; quiz 97–98.
311. Bergmann AM, Ruiz van Haperen VM, Veerman G, et al. Synergistic interaction between cisplatin and gemcitabine in vitro. *Clin Cancer Res.* 1996;2:521.
312. van Moorsel CJ, Pinedo HM, Veerman G, et al. Mechanisms of synergism between cisplatin and gemcitabine in ovarian and non-small cell lung cancer cell lines. *Br J Cancer.* 1999;80:981.
313. Ledermann JA, Gabra H, Jayson GC, et al. Inhibition of carboplatin-induced DNA interstrand cross-link repair by gemcitabine in patients receiving these drugs for platinum-resistant ovarian cancer. *Clin Cancer Res.* 2010;16(19):4899–4905.
314. Aapro MS, Martin C, Hatty S. Gemcitabine-a safety review. *Anticancer Drugs.* 1998;9(3):191–201.
315. Serke S, Riess H, Oettle H, et al. Elevated reticulocyte count—a clue to the diagnosis of haemolytic-uraemic syndrome (HUS) associated with gemcitabine therapy for metastatic duodenal papillary carcinoma: a case report. *Br J Cancer.* 1999;79(9–10):1519–1521.

316. Pavlakis N, Bell DR, Millward MJ, et al. Fatal pulmonary toxicity resulting from treatment with gemcitabine. *Cancer.* 1997;80(2):286–291.
317. Sauer-Heilborn A, Kath R, Schneider CP, et al. Severe non-haematological toxicity after treatment with gemcitabine. *J Cancer Res Clin Oncol.* 1999;125(11):637–640.
318. Markman M, Kennedy A, Sutton G, et al. Phase 2 trial of single agent ifosfamide/mesna in patients with platinum/paclitaxel refractory ovarian cancer who have not previously been treated with an alkylating agent. *Gynecol Oncol.* 1998;70(2):272–274.
319. Sutton G. Ifosfamide and mesna in epithelial ovarian carcinoma. *Gynecol Oncol.* 1993;51(1):104–108.
320. Sutton GP, Blessing JA, DeMars LR, et al. A phase II Gynecologic Oncology Group trial of ifosfamide and mesna in advanced or recurrent adenocarcinoma of the endometrium. *Gynecol Oncol.* 1996;63(1):25–27.
321. Allen LM, Creaven PJ. Activation of the antineoplastic drug isophosphamide by rat liver microsomes. *J Pharm Pharmacol.* 1972;24(7):585–586.
322. Allen LM, Creaven PJ. Interaction of mechlorethamine and isophosphamide with bovine serum albumin and rat liver microsomes. *J Pharm Sci.* 1973;62(5):854–856.
323. Boal JH, Williamson M, Boyd VL, et al. 31P NMR studies of the kinetics of bisalkylation by isophosphoramide mustard: comparisons with phosphoramide mustard. *J Med Chem.* 1989;32(8):1768–1773.
324. Creaven PJ, Allen LM, Cohen MH, et al. Studies on the clinical pharmacology and toxicology of isophosphamide (NSC-109724). *Cancer Treat Rep.* 1976;60(4):445–449.
325. Allen LM, Creaven PJ, Nelson RL. Studies on the human pharmacokinetics of isophosphamide (NSC-109724). *Cancer Treat Rep.* 1976;60(4):451–458.
326. Stuart-Harris RC, Harper PG, Parsons CA, et al. High-dose alkylation therapy using ifosfamide infusion with mesna in the treatment of adult advanced soft-tissue sarcoma. *Cancer Chemother Pharmacol.* 1983;11(2):69–72.
327. Nelson RL, Creaven PJ, Cohen MH, et al. Phase I clinical trial of a 3-day divided dose schedule of ifosfamide (NSC 109724). *Eur J Cancer.* 1976;12(3):195–198.
328. Mateu J, Alzamora M, Franco M, et al. Ifosfamide extravasation. *Ann Pharmacother.* 1994;28(11):1243–1244.
329. Van Dyk JJ, Falkson HC, Van der Merwe AM, et al. Unexpected toxicity in patients treated with iphosphamide. *Cancer Res.* 1972;32(5):921–924.
330. DeFronzo RA, Abeloff M, Braine H, et al. Renal dysfunction after treatment with isophosphamide (NSC-109724). *Cancer Chemother Rep.* 1974;58(3):375–382.
331. Goren MP, Wright RK, Pratt CB, et al. Potentiation of ifosfamide neurotoxicity, hematotoxicity, and tubular nephrotoxicity by prior cis-diamminedichloroplatinum(II) therapy. *Cancer Res.* 1987;47(5):1457–1460.
332. Hacke M, Schmoll HJ, Alt JM, et al. Nephrotoxicity of cis-diamminedichloroplatinum with or without ifosfamide in cancer treatment. *Clin Physiol Biochem.* 1983;1(1):17–26.
333. Bhardwaj A, Badesha PS. Ifosfamide-induced nonconvulsive status epilepticus. *Ann Pharmacother.* 1995;29(12):1237–1239.
334. DOXIL (doxorubicin HCl liposome injection) [package insert]. Mountain View, CA: Alza Corporation; 2001.
335. Gabizon A, Catane R, Uziely B, et al. Prolonged circulation time and enhanced accumulation in malignant exudates of doxorubicin encapsulated in polyethylene glycol–coated liposomes. *Cancer Res.* 1994;54(4):987–992.
336. Alberts DS, Garcia DJ. Safety aspects of pegylated liposomal doxorubicin in patients with cancer. *Drugs.* 1997;54 suppl 4:30–35.
337. Gordon AN, Fleagle JT, Guthrie D, et al. Recurrent epithelial ovarian carcinoma: a randomized phase III study of pegylated liposomal doxorubicin versus topotecan. *J Clin Oncol.* 2001;19(14):3312–3322.
338. Zaharko DS, Fung WP, Yang KH. Relative biochemical aspects of low and high doses of methotrexate in mice. *Cancer Res.* 1977;37(6):1602–1607.
339. Jolivet J, Schilsky RL, Bailey BD, et al. Synthesis, retention, and biological activity of methotrexate polyglutamates in cultured human breast cancer cells. *J Clin Invest.* 1982;70(2):351–360.
340. Alt FW, Kellems RE, Bertino JR, et al. Selective multiplication of dihydrofolate reductase genes in methotrexate-resistant variants of cultured murine cells. 1978. *Biotechnology.* 1992;24:397–410.
341. Calvert AH, Jones TR, Jackman AL, et al. 2-Amino-4-hydroxyquinazolines with dual metabolic loci in methotrexate resistant cells. [Abstract]. *Proc AACR.* 1979;20:24.
342. Weinstein G, Newburger A, Troner M. Cell kinetic synchronization of human malignant melanoma (MM) with low-dose methotrexate (MTX) in vivo. [Abstract]. *Proc AACR.* 1979;20:403.
343. Chello PL, Sirotnak FM, Dorick DM. Alterations in the kinetics of methotrexate transport during growth of L1210 murine leukemia cells in culture. *Mol Pharmacol.* 1980;18(2):274–280.
344. Campbell MA, Perrier DG, Dorr RT, et al. Methotrexate: bioavailability and pharmacokinetics. *Cancer Treat Rep.* 1985;69(7–8):833–838.
345. Ignoffo RJ, Oie S, Friedman MA. Pharmacokinetics of methotrexate administered via the hepatic artery. *Cancer Chemother Pharmacol.* 1981;5(4):217–220.
346. Aherne GW, Piall E, Marks V, et al. Prolongation and enhancement of serum methotrexate concentrations by probenecid. *Br Med J.* 1978;1(6120):1097–1099.
347. Huffman DH, Wan SH, Azarnoff DL, et al. Pharmacokinetics of methotrexate. *Clin Pharmacol Ther.* 1973;14(4):572–579.
348. Stoller RG, Jacobs SA, Drake JC, et al. Pharmacokinetics of high-dose methotrexate (NSC-740). *Cancer Chemother Rep.* 1975;6:91.
349. Wang YM, Sutow WW, Romsdahl MM, et al. Age-related pharmacokinetics of high-dose methotrexate in patients with osteosarcoma. *Cancer Treat Rep.* 1979;63(3):405–410.
350. Evans WE, Pratt CB. Effect of pleural effusion on high-dose methotrexate kinetics. *Clin Pharmacol Ther.* 1978;23(1):68–72.
351. Methotrexate Injection, USP [package insert]. Bedford, OH: Ben Venue Laboratories; 2000.
352. Eisenhauer EA, ten Bokkel Huinink WW, Swenerton KD, et al. European-Canadian randomized trial of paclitaxel in relapsed ovarian cancer: high-dose versus low-dose and long versus short infusion. *J Clin Oncol.* 1994;12(12):2654–2666.
353. Everts CS, Westcott JL, Bragg DG. Methotrexate therapy and pulmonary disease. *Radiology.* 1973;107(3):539–543.
354. Creaven GB, Morgan RG. Alteration of methotrexate (MTX) pharamacokinetics by gut sterilization in man. [Abstract]. *Proc AACR.* 1975;16:134.
355. Cadman E, Heimer R, Davis L. Enhanced 5-fluorouracil nucleotide formation after methotrexate administration: explanation for drug synergism. *Science.* 1979;205(4411):1135–1137.
356. Bowen D, White JC, Goldman ID. A basis for fluoropyrimidine-induced antagonism to methotrexate in Ehrlich ascites tumor cells in vitro. *Cancer Res.* 1978;38(1):219–222.
357. Crooke ST, Bradner WT. Mitomycin C: a review. *Cancer Treat Rev.* 1976;3(3):121–139.
358. Lown JW, Weir G. Studies related to antitumor antibiotics. Part XIV. Reactions of mitomycin B with DNA. *Can J Biochem.* 1978;56(5):269–304.
359. Tomasz M, Chowdary D, Lipman R, et al. Reaction of DNA with chemically or enzymatically activated mitomycin C: isolation and structure of the major covalent adduct. [Abstract]. *Proc Natl Acad Sci U S A.* 1986;83:6702.
360. Dusre L, Covey JM, Collins C, et al. DNA damage, cytotoxicity and free radical formation by mitomycin C in human cells. *Chem Biol Interact.* 1989;71(1):63–78.
361. Kennedy KA, Rockwell S, Sartorelli AC. Preferential activation of mitomycin C to cytotoxic metabolites by hypoxic tumor cells. *Cancer Res.* 1980;40(7):2356–2360.
362. Matsumoto S, Shigeoka T, Takakura Y, et al. Cellular interaction and in vitro antitumor effect of various mitomycin C prodrugs in mitomycin C-resistant L1210 leukemia cell lines. *Chem Pharm Bull (Tokyo).* 1987;35(9):3792–3799.
363. Taylor CW, Brattain MG, Yeoman LC. Occurrence of cytosolic protein and phosphoprotein changes in human colon tumor cells with the development of resistance to mitomycin C. *Cancer Res.* 1985;45(9):4422–4427.
364. Dorr RT, Liddil JD, Trent JM, et al. Mitomycin C resistant L1210 leukemia cells: association with pleiotropic drug resistance. *Biochem Pharmacol.* 1987;36(19):3115–3120.
365. van Hazel GA, Scott M, Rubin J, et al. Pharmacokinetics of mitomycin C in patients receiving the drug alone or in combination. *Cancer Treat Rep.* 1983;67(9):805–810.
366. Verweij J, den Hartigh J, Stuurman M, et al. Relationship between clinical parameters and pharmacokinetics of mitomycin C. *J Cancer Res Clin Oncol.* 1987;113(1):91–94.
367. Schilcher RB, Young JD, Ratanatharathorn V, et al. Clinical pharmacokinetics of high-dose mitomycin C. *Cancer Chemother Pharmacol.* 1984;13(3):186–190.
368. den Hartigh J, McVie JG, van Oort WJ, et al. Pharmacokinetics of mitomycin C in humans. *Cancer Res.* 1983;43(10):5017–5021.
369. Malviya VK, Young JD, Boike G, et al. Pharmacokinetics of mitomycin-C in plasma and tumor tissue of cervical cancer patients and in selected tissues of female rats. *Gynecol Oncol.* 1986;25(2):160–170.
370. Hu E, Howell SB. Pharmacokinetics of intra-arterial mitomycin C in humans. *Cancer Res.* 1983;43(9):4474–4477.

371. Argenta LC, Manders EK. Mitomycin C extravasation injuries. *Cancer.* 1983;51(6):1080–1082.
372. Lokich J, Perri J, Fine N, et al. Mitomycin C: phase I study of a constant infusion ambulatory treatment schedule. *Am J Clin Oncol.* 1982;5(4):443–447.
373. Tseng MH, Luch J, Mittelman A. Regional intra-arterial mitomycin C infusion in previously treated patients with metastatic colorectal cancer and concomitant measurement of serum drug level. *Cancer Treat Rep.* 1984;68(11):1319–1324.
374. Hanna WT, Krauss S, Regester RF, et al. Renal disease after mitomycin C therapy. *Cancer.* 1981;48(12):2583–2588.
375. Valavaara R, Nordman E. Renal complications of mitomycin C therapy with special reference to the total dose. *Cancer.* 1985;55(1):47–50.
376. Lazarus HM, Gottfried MR, Herzig RH, et al. Veno-occlusive disease of the liver after high-dose mitomycin C therapy and autologous bone marrow transplantation. *Cancer.* 1982;49(9):1789–1795.
377. Johnston-Early A, Cohen MH. Mitomycin C-induced skin ulceration remote from infusion site. *Cancer Treat Rep.* 1981;65(5–6):529.
378. Wood HA, Ellerhorst-Ryan JM. Delayed adverse skin reactions associated with mitomycin-C administration. *Oncol Nurs Forum.* 1984;11(4):14–18.
379. Olver IN, Aisner J, Hament A, et al. A prospective study of topical dimethyl sulfoxide for treating anthracycline extravasation. *J Clin Oncol.* 1988;6(11):1732–1735.
380. Chang AY, Kuebler JP, Pandya KJ, et al. Pulmonary toxicity induced by mitomycin C is highly responsive to glucocorticoids. *Cancer.* 1986;57(12):2285–2290.
381. Raderer M, Kornek G, Scheithauer W. Re: Vinorelbine-induced pancreatitis: a case report. *J Natl Cancer Inst.* 1998;90(4):329.
382. Dorr RT, Alberts DS. Vinca alkaloid skin toxicity: antidote and drug disposition studies in the mouse. *J Natl Cancer Inst.* 1985;74(1):113–120.
383. Chang SY, Evans TL, Alberts DS. The stability of melphalan in the presence of chloride ion. *J Pharm Pharmacol.* 1979;31(12):853–854.
384. Goodman GE, Chang SE, Alberts DS, eds. The antitumor activity of melphalan and its hydrolysis products. *Proc AACR.* 1980;21(1207):301.
385. Dorr RT. Pharmacology of the taxanes. *Pharmacotherapy.* 1997;17(5 pt 2):96S–104S.
386. Markman M, Kennedy A, Webster K, et al. Paclitaxel-associated hypersensitivity reactions: experience of the gynecologic oncology program of the Cleveland Clinic Cancer Center. *J Clin Oncol.* 2000;18(1):102–105.
387. Tsavaris NB, Kosmas C. Risk of severe acute hypersensitivity reactions after rapid paclitaxel infusion of less than 1-h duration. *Cancer Chemother Pharmacol.* 1998;42(6):509–511.
388. Boruta DM, II, Fowler WC, Jr, Gehrig PA, et al. Weekly paclitaxel infusion as salvage therapy in ovarian cancer. *Cancer Invest.* 2003;21(5):675–681.
389. Sharma R, Graham J, Blagden S, et al. Sustained platelet-sparing effect of weekly low dose paclitaxel allows effective, tolerable delivery of extended dose dense weekly carboplatin in platinum resistant/refractory epithelial ovarian cancer. *BMC.* 2011;11:289.
390. Rowinsky EK, Eisenhauer EA, Chaudhry V, et al. Clinical toxicities encountered with paclitaxel (Taxol). *Semin Oncol.* 1993;20(4 suppl 3):1–15.
391. Peereboom DM, Donehower RC, Eisenhauer EA, et al. Successful re-treatment with taxol after major hypersensitivity reactions. *J Clin Oncol.* 1993;11(5):885–890.
392. Rowinsky EK, Kaufmann SH, Baker SD, et al. Sequences of topotecan and cisplatin: phase I, pharmacologic, and in vitro studies to examine sequence dependence. *J Clin Oncol.* 1996;14(12):3074–3084.
393. Chang SM, Kuhn JG, Rizzo J, et al. Phase I study of paclitaxel in patients with recurrent malignant glioma: a North American Brain Tumor Consortium report. *J Clin Oncol.* 1998;16(6):2188–2194.
394. Chattopadhyay S, Moran RG, Goldman ID. Pemetrexed: biochemical and cellular pharmacology, mechanisms, and clinical applications. *Mol Cancer Ther.* 2007;6(2):404–417.
395. Slichenmyer WJ, Rowinsky EK, Donehower RC, et al. The current status of camptothecin analogues as antitumor agents. *J Natl Cancer Inst.* 1993;85(4):271–291.
396. Creemers GJ, Lund B, Verweij J. Topoisomerase I inhibitors: topotecan and irenotecan. *Cancer Treat Rev.* 1994;20(1):73–96.
397. Rowinsky EK, Grochow LB, Ettinger DS, et al. Phase I and pharmacological study of the novel topoisomerase I inhibitor 7-ethyl-10-[4-(1-piperidino)-1-piperidino]carbonyloxycamptothecin (CPT-11) administered as a ninety-minute infusion every 3 weeks. *Cancer Res.* 1994;54(2):427–436.
398. O'Dwyer PJ, LaCreta FP, Haas NB, et al. Clinical, pharmacokinetic and biological studies of topotecan. *Cancer Chemother Pharmacol.* 1994;34 suppl:S46–S52.
399. Stewart CF, Baker SD, Heideman RL, et al. Clinical pharmacodynamics of continuous infusion topotecan in children: systemic exposure predicts hematologic toxicity. *J Clin Oncol.* 1994;12(9):1946–1954.
400. Minami H, Beijnen JH, Verweij J, et al. Limited sampling model for area under the concentration time curve of total topotecan. *Clin Cancer Res.* 1996;2(1):43–46.
401. van Warmerdam LJ, Verweij J, Rosing H, et al. Limited sampling models for topotecan pharmacokinetics. *Ann Oncol.* 1994;5(3):259–264.
402. Morris RT. Weekly topotecan in the management of ovarian cancer. *Gynecol Oncol.* 2003;90(3 pt 2):S34–S38.
403. Rowinsky EK. Weekly topotecan: an alternative to topotecan's standard daily x 5 schedule? *Oncologist.* 2002;7(4):324–330.
404. ten Bokkel Huinink W, Gore M, Carmichael J, et al. Topotecan versus paclitaxel for the treatment of recurrent epithelial ovarian cancer. *J Clin Oncol.* 1997;15(6):2183–2193.
405. O'Reilly S, Rowinsky EK, Slichenmyer W, et al. Phase I and pharmacologic study of topotecan in patients with impaired renal function. *J Clin Oncol.* 1996;14(12):3062–3073.
406. O'Reilly S, Rowinsky E, Slichenmyer W, et al. Phase I and pharmacologic studies of topotecan in patients with impaired hepatic function. *J Natl Cancer Inst.* 1996;88(12):817–824.
407. Blajman C, Balbiani L, Block J, et al. A prospective, randomized Phase III trial comparing combination chemotherapy with cyclophosphamide, doxorubicin, and 5-fluorouracil with vinorelbine plus doxorubicin in the treatment of advanced breast carcinoma. *Cancer.* 1999;85(5):1091–1097.
408. Llombart-Cussac A, Pivot X, Rhor-Alvarado A, et al. First-line vinorelbine-mitoxantrone combination in metastatic breast cancer patients relapsing after an adjuvant anthracycline regimen: results of a phase II study. *Oncology.* 1998;55(5):384–390.
409. Burger RA, DiSaia PJ, Roberts JA, et al. Phase II trial of vinorelbine in recurrent and progressive epithelial ovarian cancer. *Gynecol Oncol.* 1999;72(2):148–153.
410. Morris M, Brader KR, Levenback C, et al. Phase II study of vinorelbine in advanced and recurrent squamous cell carcinoma of the cervix. *J Clin Oncol.* 1998;16(3):1094–1098.
411. Peacock NW, Burris HA, Dieras V, et al. A phase I trial of vinorelbine in combination with mitoxantrone in patients with refractory solid tumors. *Invest New Drugs.* 1998;16(1):37–43.
412. Mangeney P, Andriamialisoa RZ, Lallemand JY, et al. 5'Nor-anhydrovinblastine, prototype of a new class of vinblastine derivatives. *Tetrahedron.* 1979;35:2175.
413. Johnson SA, Harper P, Hortobagyi GN, et al. Vinorelbine: an overview. *Cancer Treat Rev.* 1996;22(2):127–142.
414. Marquet P, Lachatre G, Debord J, et al. Pharmacokinetics of vinorelbine in man. *Eur J Clin Pharmacol.* 1992;42(5):545–547.
415. Wargin WA, Lucas VS. The clinical pharmacokinetics of vinorelbine (Navelbine). *Semin Oncol.* 1994;21(5 suppl 10):21–27.
416. Leveque D, Jehl F. Clinical pharmacokinetics of vinorelbine. *Clin Pharmacokinet.* 1996;31(3):184–197.
417. Lozano M, Muro H, Triguboff E, et al. A randomized trial for effective prevention of Navelbine (NVB) related phlebitis. [Abstract]. *Proc ASCO.* 1995;14:535.
418. Trissel LA, Martinez JF. Visual, turbidimetric, and particle-content assessment of compatibility of vinorelbine tartrate with selected drugs during simulated Y-site injection. *Am J Hosp Pharm.* 1994;51(4):495–499.
419. Gershenson DM, Burke TW, Morris M, et al. A phase I study of a daily x3 schedule of intravenous vinorelbine for refractory epithelial ovarian cancer. *Gynecol Oncol.* 1998;70(3):404–409.
420. Havlin KA, Ramirez MJ, Legler CM, et al. Inability to escalate vinorelbine dose intensity using a daily x3 schedule with and without filgrastim in patients with metastatic breast cancer. *Cancer Chemother Pharmacol.* 1999;43(1):68–72.
421. Weiss AJ, Sabol J, Lackman RD. Concurrent administration of vinorelbine with recombinant human granulocyte colony–stimulating factor: an effective method of increasing dose intensity. *Am J Clin Oncol.* 1999;22(1):38–41.
422. Hohneker JA. A summary of vinorelbine (Navelbine) safety data from North American clinical trials. *Semin Oncol.* 1994;21(5 suppl 10):42–46; discussion 6–7.
423. Gebbia V, Testa A, Valenza R, et al. Acute pain syndrome at tumour site in neoplastic patients treated with vinorelbine: report of unusual toxicity. *Eur J Cancer.* 1994;30A(6):889.
424. Kornek GV, Kornfehl H, Hejna M, et al. Acute tumor pain in patients with head and neck cancer treated with vinorelbine. *J Natl Cancer Inst.* 1996;88(21):1593.

425. Raderer M, Kornek G, Hejna M, et al. Acute pulmonary toxicity associated with high-dose vinorelbine and mitomycin C. *Ann Oncol.* 1996;7(9):973–975.
426. Garrett CA, Simpson TA Jr. Syndrome of inappropriate antidiuretic hormone associated with vinorelbine therapy. *Ann Pharmacother.* 1998;32(12):1306–1309.
427. Hoff PM, Valero V, Ibrahim N, et al. Hand-foot syndrome following prolonged infusion of high doses of vinorelbine. *Cancer.* 1998;82(5):965–969.
428. Liebmann J, Friedman K. Adynamic ileus in a patient with non-small-cell lung cancer after treatment with vinorelbine. *Am J Med.* 1996;101(6):658–659.
429. Budman DR. Vinorelbine (Navelbine): a third-generation vinca alkaloid. *Cancer Invest.* 1997;15(5):475–490.
430. Zhou-Pan XR, Seree E, Zhou XJ, et al. Involvement of human liver cytochrome P450 3A in vinblastine metabolism: drug interactions. *Cancer Res.* 1993;53(21):5121–5126.
431. Ozols RF, Hogan WM, Ostchega Y, et al. MVP (mitomycin, vinblastine, and progesterone): a second-line regimen in ovarian cancer with a high incidence of pulmonary toxicity. *Cancer Treat Rep.* 1983;67(7–8):721–722.
432. Parimoo D, Jeffers S, Muggia FM. Severe neurotoxicity from vinorelbine-paclitaxel combinations. *J Natl Cancer Inst.* 1996;88(15):1079–1080.
433. Tibaldi C, Pazzagli I, Berrettini S, et al. A case of ototoxicity in a patient with metastatic carcinoma of the breast treated with paclitaxel and vinorelbine. *Eur J Cancer.* 1998;34(7):1133–1134.
434. Buzdar AU, Jonat W, Howell A, et al. Anastrozole versus megestrol acetate in the treatment of postmenopausal women with advanced breast carcinoma: results of a survival update based on a combined analysis of data from two mature phase III trials. Arimidex Study Group. *Cancer.* 1998;83(6):1142–1152.
435. Plourde PV, Dyroff M, Dukes M. Arimidex: a potent and selective fourth-generation aromatase inhibitor. *Breast Cancer Res Treat.* 1994;30(1):103–111.
436. NCCN Clinical Practice Guidelines in Oncology: Uterine Neoplasms. 2012 Contract No.: http://www.nccn.org/professionals/physician_gls/f_guidelines.asp#uterine.
437. Koshiyama M, Yoshida M, Konishi M, et al. Expression of pS2 protein in endometrial carcinomas: correlation with clinicopathologic features and sex steroid receptor status. *Int J Cancer.* 1997;74(3):237–244.
438. Watanabe K, Sasano H, Harada N, et al. Aromatase in human endometrial carcinoma and hyperplasia. Immunohistochemical, in situ hybridization, and biochemical studies. *Am J Pathol.* 1995;146(2):491–500.
439. Rose PG, Brunetto VL, VanLe L, et al. A phase II trial of anastrozole in advanced recurrent or persistent endometrial carcinoma: a Gynecologic Oncology Group study. *Gynecol Oncol.* 2000;78(2):212–216.
440. Tredway DR, Buraglio M, Hemsey G, et al. A phase I study of the pharmacokinetics, pharmacodynamics, and safety of single- and multiple-dose anastrozole in healthy, premenopausal female volunteers. *Fertil Steril.* 2004;82(6):1587–1593.
441. Agorastos T, Vaitsi V, Pantazis K, et al. Aromatase inhibitor anastrozole for treating endometrial hyperplasia in obese postmenopausal women. *Eur J Obstet Gynecol Reprod Biol.* 2005;118(2):239–240.
442. NCCN Clinical Practice Guidelines in Oncology: Ovarian Cancer Including Fallopian Tube Cancer and Primary Peritoneal Cancer. 2012 Contract No.: http://www.nccn.org/professionals/physician_gls/f_guidelines.asp#ovarian.
443. Rao GG, Miller DS. Clinical applications of hormonal therapy in ovarian cancer. *Curr Treat Options Oncol.* 2005;6(2):97–102.
444. Freeman SA, Modesitt SC. Anastrozole therapy in recurrent ovarian adult granulosa cell tumors: a report of 2 cases. *Gynecol Oncol.* 2006;103(2):755–758.
445. Li YF, Fu S, Hu W, et al. Systemic anticancer therapy in gynecological cancer patients with renal dysfunction. *Int J Gynecol Cancer.* 2007.
446. Smyth JF, Gourley C, Walker G, et al. Antiestrogen therapy is active in selected ovarian cancer cases: the use of letrozole in estrogen receptor-positive patients. *Clin Cancer Res.* 2007;13(12):3617–3622.
447. Rao GG, Miller DS. Hormonal therapy in epithelial ovarian cancer. *Expert Rev Anticancer Ther.* 2006;6(1):43–47.
448. Bertelli G, Venturini M, Del Mastro L, et al. Intramuscular depot medroxyprogesterone versus oral megestrol for the control of postmenopausal hot flashes in breast cancer patients: a randomized study. *Ann Oncol.* 2002;13(6):883–888.
449. Rossouw JE, Anderson GL, Prentice RL, et al. Risks and benefits of estrogen plus progestin in healthy postmenopausal women: principal results From the Women's Health Initiative randomized controlled trial. *JAMA.* 2002;288(3):321–333.
450. Shumaker SA, Legault C, Rapp SR, et al. Estrogen plus progestin and the incidence of dementia and mild cognitive impairment in postmenopausal women: the Women's Health Initiative Memory Study: a randomized controlled trial. *JAMA.* 2003;289(20):2651–2662.
451. Imai M, Jobo T, Sato R, et al. Medroxyprogesterone acetate therapy for patients with adenocarcinoma of the endometrium who wish to preserve the uterus-usefulness and limitations. *Eur J Gynaecol Oncol.* 2001;22(3):217–220.
452. Kobiashvili H, Charkviani L, Charkviani T. Organ preserving method in the management of atypical endometrial hyperplasia. *Eur J Gynaecol Oncol.* 2001;22(4):297–299.
453. Bafaloukos D, Aravantinos G, Samonis G, et al. Carboplatin, methotrexate and 5-fluorouracil in combination with medroxyprogesterone acetate (JMF-M) in the treatment of advanced or recurrent endometrial carcinoma: A Hellenic cooperative oncology group study. *Oncology.* 1999;56(3):198–201.
454. Thigpen JT, Brady MF, Alvarez RD, et al. Oral medroxyprogesterone acetate in the treatment of advanced or recurrent endometrial carcinoma: a dose-response study by the Gynecologic Oncology Group. *J Clin Oncol.* 1999;17(6):1736–1744.
455. Katzenellenbogen BS, Choi I, Delage-Mourroux R, et al. Molecular mechanisms of estrogen action: selective ligands and receptor pharmacology. *J Steroid Biochem Mol Biol.* 2000;74(5):279–285.
456. Thomas Medical Economics, Vol 6.0.0a. PDR Electronic Library; 2003.
457. Varras M, Polyzos D, Akrivis C. Effects of tamoxifen on the human female genital tract: review of the literature. *Eur J Gynaecol Oncol.* 2003;24(3–4):258–268.
458. Covens A, Thomas G, Shaw P, et al. A phase II study of leuprolide in advanced/recurrent endometrial cancer. *Gynecol Oncol.* 1997;64(1):126–129.
459. Lhomme C, Vennin P, Callet N, et al. A multicenter phase II study with triptorelin (sustained-release LHRH agonist) in advanced or recurrent endometrial carcinoma: a French anticancer federation study. *Gynecol Oncol.* 1999;75(2):187–193.
460. Marelli MM, Moretti RM, Januszkiewicz-Caulier J, et al. Gonadotropin-releasing hormone (GnRH) receptors in tumors: a new rationale for the therapeutical application of GnRH analogs in cancer patients? *Curr Cancer Drug Targets.* 2006;6(3):257–269.
461. Grundker C, Emons G. Role of gonadotropin-releasing hormone (GnRH) in ovarian cancer. *Reprod Biol Endocrinol.* 2003;1:65.
462. Bertino JR. "Rescue" techniques in cancer chemotherapy: use of leucovorin and other rescue agents after methotrexate treatment. *Semin Oncol.* 1977;4(2):203–216.
463. Kamen BA, Winick NJ. High dose methotrexate therapy: insecure rationale? *Biochem Pharmacol.* 1988;37(14):2713–2715.
464. Tew KD, Houghton PJ, Houghton JA. Preclincial and clinical modulation of anticancer drugs. Boca Raton, Fl: CRC Press; 1993.
465. Erlichman C. Fluorouracil and leucovorin for metastatic colorectal cancer. *J Chemother.* 1990;2 suppl 1:38–40.
466. Zaniboni A, Arcangeli G, Meriggi F, et al. Low-dose 6-S leucovorin and5-fluorouracil as salvage treatment in metastatic breast cancer. [Abstract]. *Proc ASCO.* 1994;13:91.
467. Kobayashi K, Schilsky RL. Update on biochemical modulation of chemotherapeutic agents. *Oncology (Huntingt).* 1993;7(5):99–106, 9; discussion 10–14, 17.
468. Barnhart K, Coutifaris C, Esposito M. The pharmacology of methotrexate. *Expert Opin Pharmacother.* 2001;2(3):409–417.
469. Elit L, Covens A, Osborne R, et al. High-dose methotrexate for gestational trophoblastic disease. *Gynecol Oncol.* 1994;54(3):282–287.
470. Sekharan PK, Sreedevi NS, Radhadevi VP, et al. Management of postmolar gestational trophoblastic disease with methotrexate and folinic acid: 15 years of experience. *J Reprod Med.* 2006;51(10):835–840.
471. Brock N, Pohl J, Stekar J, et al. Studies on the urotoxicity of oxazaphosphorine cytostatics and its prevention—III. Profile of action of sodium 2-mercaptoethane sulfonate (mesna). *Eur J Cancer Clin Oncol.* 1982;18(12):1377–1387.
472. Burkert H. Clinical overview of mesna. *Cancer Treat Rev.* 1983;10 suppl A:175–181.
473. Goren MP, McKenna LM, Goodman TL. Combined intravenous and oral mesna in outpatients treated with ifosfamide. *Cancer Chemother Pharmacol.* 1997;40(5):371–375.
474. Markman M, Kennedy A, Webster K, et al. Continuous subcutaneous administration of mesna to prevent ifosfamide-induced hemorrhagic cystitis. *Semin Oncol.* 1996;23(3 suppl 6):97–98.

CHAPTER 15

Immunotherapy of Gynecologic Malignancies

Paul J. Sabbatini, Kunle Odunsi, Jacobus Pfisterer, and Dmitriy Zamarin

Patients with ovarian cancer are particularly well-suited for participation in studies evaluating immune-based treatment strategies, due, in part, to the natural history of this disease. The historical data indicates that 70% of patients with advanced disease are in complete clinical remission following initial cytoreductive surgery and platinum- and taxane-based primary chemotherapy (1). However, only 30% of optimally debulked stage III patients will remain disease-free, and there is a median progression-free interval of approximately 24 months (2). Despite the high relapse rate, many patients return to a complete or partial clinical remission following additional chemotherapy, but ever-shortening intervals of response are seen (3). Despite this chronic course of relapse and response, in a study evaluating intraperitoneal (IP) therapy as part of primary treatment, the median survival of optimally debulked patients exceed 60 months (4). Neither higher doses, nor protracted schedules, nor non–cross-resistant consolidation chemotherapy has provided additional benefits. Ovarian cancer patients with minimal disease burdens are therefore appropriate candidates for clinical trials evaluating immune-based therapy.

With regard to other gynecologic malignancies, a significant proportion of immune strategies being evaluated in patients with cervical cancer target human papillomavirus, and this subject is covered separately in Chapter 20 (5). The evaluation of immune-based approaches for the treatment of endometrial cancer has been limited, but interest is growing (6). Targets such as human trophoblast cell surface marker (TROP-2), Wilms Tumor Gene (WT-1), and a variety of cancer testis (CT) antigens have been shown to be expressed in endometrial cancers, which has prompted early stage trials with dendritic cell (DC) vaccines and adoptive cellular therapy as two examples (7,8). In addition, contemporary data show enhanced efficacy with PD-1 blockade in patients having tumors with mismatch repair deficiency, which includes patients with endometrioid uterine carcinoma (9).

Cancer Immunology: Overview

The immune system evolved to fight foreign invaders such as bacteria, viruses, and parasites. However, strong evidence suggests that it also plays a crucial role in controlling or rejecting incipient cancers. William B. Coley (10) first observed regression in patients with sarcoma contracting "accidental erysipelas" as early as 1893. Because patients with competent immune systems still develop cancers, and spontaneous remission of tumors is rare, enthusiasm for the effectiveness of immune system control has waxed and waned over the decades. The fact that animal models with a variety of deficiencies in immunologic components consistently develop carcinoma has allowed the concept of immunosurveillance to be sustained and developed (11,12). Observations in patients with ovarian cancer strongly support a role for immune system involvement in patient outcome. For example, 5-year overall survival (OS) in epithelial ovarian cancer has been correlated with the presence or absence of tumor-infiltrating lymphocytes (TIL) (38% vs. 4.5%, $p < 0.001$) (13). A second study also showed improved survival in patients with increased frequencies of intraepithelial $CD8^+$ TIL (55 vs. 26 months; HR = 0.33; 95% CI, 0.18 to 0.60; $p = 0.0003$) (14). Finally, data show that cancer cells and TILs in ovarian high-grade serous carcinoma suggest that expression of programmed cell death (PD-1) and PD-ligand 1 (PDL-1) may have prognostic impact, particularly when this feature is expressed at higher levels (15). In contrast, patients with increased numbers of immune suppressive $CD4^+CD25HI$ regulatory T cells (Tregs) have reduced survival (15). The process is made more complex when we recognize that not only can the immune system protect the host against tumor development, but it is also thought to select cancer cells of lower immunogenicity that can escape early immunity because of changes in gene expression. This actually leads to an outgrowth of tumors with the capacity to escape recognition, and this process has been termed immunoediting (16). The immunoediting or "immune sculpting" process, therefore, is responsible for shaping the immunogenicity of the tumors that will eventually form. Considering the effectors of the immune system in the context of both of these processes is important in order to develop immune-directed therapies with the greatest chance of success (17,18).

The mechanism by which tumors escape from immune surveillance is complex (19). An alteration in nearly all known effectors required for immune activation has been proposed as being responsible for immune evasion. In some cases, antigen presentation is downregulated, or gene deletions or rearrangements may cause reduced expression of the major histocompatibility (MHC I) complex, thus preventing T-lymphocyte activation (20,21). Tumors can also secrete proteins that inhibit T-cell effector action or that promote the development of regulatory T cells that suppress immune function (22). It has been shown that certain melanomas can actually remodel their stromal microenvironment so as to resemble lymphoid tissue, recruiting regulatory cells to promote tolerance and allow tumor progression (23). Other mechanisms include the downregulation of intracellular adhesion molecules (24), changes in molecules responsible for apoptosis signaling (25), or the development of peripheral tolerance (26). Due to the increasing number of interacting mechanisms with putative activity enabling immune escape, approaches directed against multiple mechanisms will likely be needed to eradicate immune-tolerant tumor cells (27).

Innate Immunity

The immune system is broadly divided into two arms: innate and active immunity, but there are multiple examples of cross-communication between them. Recent data, for example, show that neutrophil survival is influenced by T-cell responses (28). *Innate immunity* is present at birth and does not require adaptation to react against microorganisms or tumors. It includes physical barriers (mucous membranes, skin), chemical components (complement, hydrolytic enzymes), and multiple other cellular components. Natural killer cells are lymphocytes programmed to recognize and destroy tissues that have been altered or placed under stress; for example, by viruses or by malignant transformation (29). They do not have antigen-specific receptors, but instead have inhibiting receptors that can recognize MHC class I molecules on normal cells, which prevents their activation (30). MHC

I expression is aberrant or absent on many virus- and tumor-infected cells (31). Another component includes macrophages, which play many roles in immunity and inflammation, including production of a multitude of soluble secreted proinflammatory proteins; these proteins act as growth factors for other cells of the immune system, for neovasculature, and for cancer cells. The growth factors include *cytokines* and *chemokines*, and they support the growth, movement, and survival of immune and inflammatory cells. Macrophages play important roles in tissue remodeling during wound healing, mediating inflammatory responses, sampling molecules from the environment through internalization, and presenting antigens to stimulate T cells. Macrophages can also play a counterproductive role through production of molecules that promote tumor growth and angiogenesis (e.g., vascular endothelial growth factor [VEGF] and basic fibroblast growth factor) (32). Macrophages can also inhibit immune responses through production of cytokines and other molecules that downregulate immunity, such as prostaglandins E2, arginase I, and transforming growth factor-β. Thus, the role of macrophages in tumors is complex, and provides an additional means of communication between traditionally defined innate and acquired immunity effectors (33). DCs have some properties that are similar to macrophages, including production of cytokines and sampling of molecules from the environment. Most importantly, DCs are one of the key links between the innate immune system and the adaptive or acquired immune system through presentation of antigens (professional antigen-presenting cells [APC]) to initiate T-cell activation.

Adaptive Immunity

Adaptive immunity is characterized by adaptation to antigens; for example, antigens of infectious pathogens (or potentially cancer). This arm of the immune system is not mature or activated at birth, but rather adapts through maturation in response to antigens of pathogens. It is characterized by receptors encoded by the immunoglobulin (Ig) gene family. These receptors have the capacity to rearrange, creating enormous diversity ($>10^{11-12}$ different receptors). This provides a system that generates enormous specificity, recognizing and responding to a wide range of antigens that have not previously been encountered.

The two major cell types of acquired immunity are *T lymphocytes* (T cells) and *B lymphocytes* (B cells). T cells have the capacity to recognize antigens sequestered in different compartments within cells; for example, antigens generated in the cytoplasm or nucleus by viral infections (34). T cells recognize antigens as short peptides, 8 to 16 amino acids in length. These peptides must be complexed with and presented by specialized antigen-presenting molecules, the MHC molecules, to T-cell receptors (TCRs). In humans, MHC molecules are the human leukocyte antigens (HLAs) expressed on virtually every cell in the body. On the other hand, B cells produce secreted *antibodies* that can recognize soluble and cell surface molecules. Both T cells and B cells initially develop with a limited range of receptors for immune recognition. However, in response to antigen (e.g., from a virus or cancer cell) presented by a professional APC, T cells or B cells that have receptors with the best "fit" to the antigen itself (for B cells) or antigen/MHC complex (for T cells) are stimulated to proliferate, and this subpopulation is quickly expanded (35).

Humoral Immunity

B cells usually recognize antigens in their natural configuration (34). An individual host has a repertoire of B cells that are capable of generating antibodies against the full range of pathogens encountered in the environment. To do this, the total population of B lymphocytes expresses a diverse repertoire of immunoglobulins. Each B cell expresses immunoglobulin against a single antigenic determinant; the immunoglobulin is expressed at the cell surface of the B cell, where it acts as a specific receptor to transduce signals in response to that antigen (36). Once activated, the B cell creates an individual monoclonal antibody (mAb). The diversity of specificities in different B cells is generated by rearrangements of the immunoglobulin genes, and new antibody specificities continue to be generated in response to new antigens (37). During development, B cells with high-avidity immunoglobulins against ubiquitous self-antigens are eliminated. This elimination of B cells reactive with autoantigens is not absolute, however, as a broad array of antibodies against autoantigens is found in the blood of humans. Peripheral blood B cells consist of naïve and relatively short-lived B cells, long-lived memory B cells resulting from maturation in response to antigenic stimulation, and a small population of B cells expressing germline immunoglobulins that have not undergone rearrangement (these are found in the $CD5^+$ B-cell population) (14).

B cells are mobile, and after developing in the bone marrow, they migrate through the peripheral blood to B-cell-rich areas in lymphoid organs; for example, the follicles of lymph nodes, spleen, and gastrointestinal tract. Many B cells continue recirculating in the blood. If cognate antigen is encountered in lymphoid organs, the B lymphocyte migrates to the T-cell-rich areas, where appropriate T-cell help can be provided to promote increased antibody diversity and increased affinity through immunoglobulin gene rearrangements (38). This T-cell help does not have to be induced by the same antigen. Chemical conjugation of the antibody-recognized antigen to highly immunogenic bacterial or xenogeneic proteins, or, alternatively, expression of the antigen in bacterial or viral vectors, is a widely used approach to ensure adequate T-cell help in vaccines. The result of T-cell help is generation of plasma cells, the most mature form of B cell with the highest capacity for antibody production. In addition, T-cell help promotes formation of germinal centers in lymphoid organs where hypermutation in immunoglobulin genes and class and subclass switching occur to generate antibodies with higher affinities for antigen. Class switching refers to changes in antibody class during an immune response, with the IgM class of antibodies appearing first, generally followed by antibodies of the IgG class (different subclasses of IgG antibodies have different blood half-lives and different capacities for effector functions, such as fixation of complement or binding to Fc receptors). The consequence is plasma cells secreting increasingly higher affinity IgG antibodies as the immune response matures over time (39). In addition, some B cells that generally recognize nonprotein antigens. For example, carbohydrate or glycolipid antigens can be stimulated to proliferate in the absence of T-cell help. The immunoglobulin variable region (called the Fv region) determines antibody specificity and is located in the Fab domain of immunoglobulins. This region mediates effective binding to antigens. However, the constant region (Fc), where antibody class and subclass are determined, is equally critical. Binding of antibody to antigen results in a conformational change in the Fc portion, leading to activation of several effector mechanisms, including complement activation (discussed below). IgM antibodies are synthesized early in the response. If T-cell help is available, antibody responses mature through immunoglobulin gene rearrangements into the higher affinity IgG classes. These are capable of improved binding to antigen as well as receptors on the bone marrow–derived cells for the Fc domain, expanding potential effector functions. The responses to most nonprotein antigens are IgM class and generally do not mature to IgG responses. The IgM pentamer structure is specialized to increase avidity of binding to multimeric antigens and to efficiently activate effector functions such as complement (40). Activation of complement, which includes blood components with different enzymatic properties, results in opsonization (coating of pathogens by complement components), recognition by complement receptors on macrophages, monocytes, neutrophils, and DCs, with subsequent activation of these cells leading to phagocytosis and/or killing. In addition, complement can form a membrane attack complex, which creates holes in membranes of target pathogens and cancer cells, producing complement-dependent cytotoxicity (CDC) (41,42). IgG antibodies are synthesized following immunoglobulin gene rearrangements, with switches in Fc domains, as the B cell matures in response to T-cell help. IgG antibodies usually have higher affinity, and can be found in the extracellular space as well as in the blood. IgG1 and IgG3 antibodies in humans are especially effective at activating complement and also at sensitizing pathogens for killing by NK cells, macrophages, and other cells with complement receptors and immunoglobulin Fc receptors (43).

Opsonization for ingestion and destruction by phagocytes can occur through complement activation, but also occurs directly as a consequence of engagement of Fc receptors on phagocytic cells. Antibodies complexed to antigen bind to Fc receptors, which can lead to activation signals through activating Fc receptors (e.g., FcRIII), but activation can be countered by IgG binding to the inhibitory Fc receptor, FcRIIB. Fc receptors, which are bound effectively by IgG1 and IgG3 subclasses of human antibodies, are expressed on monocytes, macrophages, NK cells, neutrophils, mast cells, and other cells. Cross-linking of Fc receptors leads to activation of the cells, in some cases leading to antibody-dependent cell-mediated cytotoxicity (ADCC) of tumor cells through production of cytotoxic molecules; for example, perforin and granzyme by NK cells and reactive molecular species by macrophages (44–46). Monoclonal antibodies are commonly used for cancer therapy. Antitumor effects can be mediated in part by antibody binding to critical molecules on the surface of tumor cells; for example, by inhibiting tumor cell attachment or growth receptors. Generally, however, interactions of antibodies with cell antigens are not very effective unless Fc receptor–mediated effector mechanisms are also activated.

Cellular Immunity

T lymphocytes recognize processed (digested) molecules that complex with MHC molecules within APCs. The antigen/MHC molecules are then trafficked to the cell surface for recognition by TCRs, which are encoded by genes of the immunoglobulin family. Similar to generation of antibodies, great diversity of TCRs is generated by rearrangements of these immunoglobulin family genes. Each monoclonal TCR must bind to its cognate antigen/MHC complex (CD4 cells bind to MHC class II molecules, and CD8 cells bind to MHC class I molecules) presented on the surface of APCs (47,48). Signaling from the TCR following engagement of antigen/MHC complex is insufficient to activate the T cell. Additional signals are required (costimulatory signals or "signal 2"). The most important costimulatory signal in T cells comes from the T-cell surface molecule CD28, which engages B7 molecules (CD80 and CD86) on APCs (49–51). Engagement of TCR by antigen/MHC in conjunction with CD28 engagement of B7 is sufficient to activate naïve T cells. Within several days following T-cell activation, a second molecule, CTLA-4, appears on the T-cell surface to provide a brake to the T-cell response. CTLA-4 also binds B7 molecules, but with much higher affinity, therefore displacing CD28 activation signals. CTLA-4 signaling leads to downregulation of the T-cell response. The manipulation of CTLA-4 activity has been shown to have therapeutic efficacy, with initial data showing tumor responses in patients with melanoma (52,53). Other studies have shown responses in a variety of tumor types, including gynecologic cancers (54). PD-1, a co-inhibitory immune signal receptor, has also shown promising activity in patients with platinum-resistant ovarian cancer (55). A variety of other costimulatory molecules are upregulated on the surface of activated T cells, including OX40 and 4-1BB (CD137), which promote survival of T cells and help generate long-lived T-cell memory responses (56,57). Once T cells are activated by professional APCs (primarily DCs), they gain a variety of effector functions, including the production of cytokines and cytotoxic molecules, which lead to the death of target cells.

Antigen-Presenting Cells

Dendritic cells are the prototype of professional APCs and are the critical link between innate immunity and acquired immunity. These are phagocytic cells that sit on epidermal surfaces, including skin and mucosal membranes, constantly sampling their environment to search for infectious organisms. Although DCs continuously ingest molecules from their environment, uptake of antigen is insufficient to activate DCs. Rather, DCs have a set of receptors, most notably the toll-like receptors (TLRs), which can recognize lipid-containing molecules and CpG-rich DNA and poly-U RNA sequences produced specifically by microbial organisms. Engagement of TLR signals for activation of the DC, with increased expression of MHC and B7 molecules, and movement of cells with captured antigen to draining lymph nodes. It is in draining lymph nodes that DCs activate appropriate T cells that recognize the specific antigens presented by MHC molecules. Subsequently, activated T cells can travel from the draining lymph node to distant sites of infection or tumor to carry out the effector functions. One of the central problems for cancer immunology is that DCs may ingest and process cancer antigens, but without activation through TLRs or other receptors, the DCs remain incapable of activating T cells (because of insufficient expression of costimulatory molecules, such as B7) and do not move to draining lymph nodes. In fact, insufficiently activated DCs presenting antigens can induce anergy, a form of immune tolerance in which T cells become paralyzed and incapable of responding to cognate antigens. This is one of the mechanisms used to maintain immune tolerance to self, to prevent autoimmunity, but it also presents a major hurdle for cancer immunity. Cancer cells do not have any readily apparent mechanism to activate DCs, although several self-molecules, including heat shock protein, hyaluronate, and uric acid crystals, have been suggested to cause activation.

Helper and Regulatory T Cells

Several types of T cells are activated by DCs, and the type is influenced by whether antigens are presented by MHC class I or MHC class II molecules on APCs. MHC class I molecules complexed with antigen stimulate $CD8^+$ T cells that are cytotoxic and kill target cells (infected cells or tumor cells). Antigens presented by class II MHC molecules stimulate $CD4^+$ helper T cells. Helper T cells produce chemokines and cytokines to help recruit and orchestrate other components of the immune system. Helper T cells come in several types, and different cytokines in the milieu determine what type of T cell is generated. Each type of helper T cell mediates different types of immune responses with different characteristics. Th1 T cells produce interferon (IFN)-γ to activate cytotoxic T cells and macrophages for *cellular immune responses.* On the other hand, Th2 helper T cells produce interleukin (IL)-4 and other cytokines that favor antibody responses, or *humoral immunity*. The newly discovered Th17 $CD4^+$ T cell produces IL-17 to mediate inflammatory autoimmune diseases, such as arthritis, colitis, and encephalitis, and may play a role in cancer pathogenesis, either by promoting cancer progression or by destroying tumors. Another type of $CD4^+$ T cell restricted by MHC II presentation negatively regulates immune responses. These are regulatory T cells or Tregs. Tregs recognize self-antigens, are dependent on IL-2, and produce inhibitory molecules such as IL-10 and transforming growth factor-β. Th1 cellular immunity may be particularly effective at attacking tumors in tissues, whereas humoral immunity may have an advantage in controlling circulating metastatic tumor cells. Infiltration of ovarian cancers and other cancers by Treg cells is associated with a poorer prognosis (52,58).

CANCER IMMUNITY AND IMMUNOTHERAPY

Studies over the past 3 decades have shown that the immune system can recognize and destroy cancers, but this typically involves interactions between multiple arms of the immune system. For instance, simple recognition by T cells, antibodies, or NK cells is usually not sufficient to reject cancers. Cytotoxic T cells and NK cells produce soluble and cell surface molecules that induce death of target tumor cells. Helper T cells can produce cytokines and chemokines that recruit not only cytotoxic T cells or B cells to make antibodies, but also inflammatory cells that mediate tissue destruction. Checkpoints are responsible for the maintenance of the effector response. Antibodies can activate NK cells, macrophages, or other cells that have receptors for the antibodies' Fc domain, leading to activation of the recruited cells, a mechanism implicated in the antitumor effects of monoclonal antibody therapies. Antibodies can also activate complement proteins in the blood that can directly kill tumor cells and activate inflammatory cells at the tumor site.

There is evolving and expansive data confirming that the immune system can recognize antigens on tumor cells and that immunity may be sufficient to destroy tumors, and this provides the impetus to develop new strategies for *immunotherapy*. These approaches can be broadly divided into three groups. First, *immune modulation* uses more broad approaches to treat cancer. Traditional examples include cytokines such as IL-2, IL-12, or IFNs, and more recently, more targeted approaches such as those interfering with CTLA-4 or PD-1 (53). Secondly, *passive therapy* refers to the transfer of specific components from the acquired immune system to the host with cancer. The best examples are monoclonal antibodies directed against antigens expressed on the surface of cancer cells such as rituximab against the CD20 antigen, or trastuzumab (Herceptin) directed toward the HER 2 receptor in breast cancer. It should be noted that although the antitumor effects of trastuzumab probably involve, in part, inhibition of signaling by the HER2 tyrosine kinase oncogene, evidence strongly supports a major role for immune activation of Fc receptor–positive cells by both rituximab and trastuzumab (59). Another example of passive immunotherapy is adoptive cellular therapy, in which cells from the blood or bone marrow donor are purified, cultured, and/or manipulated outside the body and reinfused into the same patient (autologous) or a different patient (allogeneic). Cellular therapy has particularly focused on T cells and, more recently, on NK cells. Finally, *active immunization* refers to vaccines that trigger an immune response in the patient. Both passive and active immunotherapy must be directed against specific antigens on cancer cells, and the notion of an integrated immune response with effectors that include antibodies and T cells, as well as some component of immunomodulation, is increasingly becoming the goal of immunotherapeutic strategies (60).

With regard to potential targets, ongoing advances utilizing newer technologies including serologic analysis of recombinant cDNA expression libraries (SEREX) (61,62), robust applications of bioinformatics (63), and seromic profiling techniques (64) have allowed further characterization of tumor-associated antigens in multiple tumor types. There are over 2,000 candidate tumor-associated antigens and they are generally classified as follows (65): (1) differentiation antigens (66), (2) mutational antigens (67) (which are altered forms of proteins), (3) amplification antigens (68), (4) splice variant antigens (69), (5) glycolipid antigens (70), (6) viral antigens (71), and (7) CT antigens (72). Representative examples of each group are seen in **Table 15.1**.

In addition to selecting the appropriate targets, it is necessary to select the strategy to be used for immunotherapy. Multiple approaches have been considered from giving the effector cells directly to including antigens of a variety of types given alone or with adjuvants, administering modified or unmodified tumor cell lysates (autologous or allogeneic), priming DCs with a variety of agents, making tumor hybrids with APCs, or administering DNA alone or in a recombinant fashion. A sample of cancer vaccine strategies are listed in **Table 15.2**.

A critical component of any immune approach is a consideration of immune escape. Tumors escape destruction by the immune system *via* a variety of active, regulatory mechanisms. These include downregulation of MHC and tumor antigen loss (81), stimulation of the inhibitory receptors on T cells such as CTLA-4 (82), PD-1, and LAG-3 (83), tumor overproduction of indoleamine 2,3-dioxygenase (IDO) (84), induction of increased tumor infiltration by regulatory $CD4^+$ $CD25^+$ $CD25^+$ T cells (T_{regs}) (85), and also certain types of natural killer T (NKT) cells that inhibit tumor immune destruction (86). Overcoming these mechanisms is the goal of immunomodulation.

TABLE 15.1. Antigens for Immunotherapy

Antigen Category	Representative Examples
Differentiation antigens	Tyrosinase (66), Melan-Mart-1 (73), gp-100 (74)
Mutational antigens	CD4 (67), β-catenin (75), caspase (76)
Amplification antigens	Her2/neu (68), P53 (77)
Slice variant antigens	NY-CO-37/PDZ 45 (69), ING1 (78)
Glycolipid antigens	MUC1 (70)
Viral antigens	HPV (71)
CT antigens	MAGE (72), NY-ESO-1 (79), LAGE-1 (80)

CT, cancer testis.

TABLE 15.2. Examples of Vaccine Approaches

I. Antigens alone, with, or without adjuvants Peptides Protein Gangliosides Immunoglobulin idiotypes
II. Dendritic cells Peptides, immunoglobulin idiotype Tumor lysates DNA or RNA Protein
III. Tumor cells unmodified or modified Autologous Allogeneic Mixed autologous–allogeneic
IV. Tumor–APCs hybrid
V. DNA alone (naked DNA)
VI. Recombinant viruses (adenovirus, vaccinia, others)
VII. Bacteria (e.g., Listeria)

IMMUNOMODULATION

Multiple potential difficulties remain in developing new immunotherapy approaches, including insufficient activation of DCs by cancer cells, inhibition of responses by Treg cells, and both intrinsic and extrinsic mechanisms that downregulate T-cell responses; for example, signaling through CTLA-4. These checkpoints all participate in dampening immune responses against cancer. Modulating immune checkpoints by activation of effector cells, depletion of Tregs, or activation of professional APCs could substantially improve the therapeutic efficacy of vaccines or adoptively transferred T cells. The development of functional antibodies is now enabling effective immunomodulation as shown in **Figure 15.1**. Passive therapy with monoclonal antibodies or with adoptive cellular treatments may also prove capable of bypassing some of these checkpoints.

Dendritic Cell Activation

The main mechanism of immune stimulation by CD 40 ligands is activation of DCs resulting in increased survival, upregulation of costimulatory molecules, and secretion of critical cytokines to T-cell priming such as IL-12. This promotes antigen presentation, priming, and cross-priming of $CD4^+$ and $CD8^+$ effector T cells (87). However, agonistic anti-CD40 antibody is best used in combination with vaccines or toll-like receptor agonists (87,88), because alone it can accelerate the deletion of tumor-specific cytotoxic lymphocytes (89). Additional value of CD40 ligation is provided by the fact

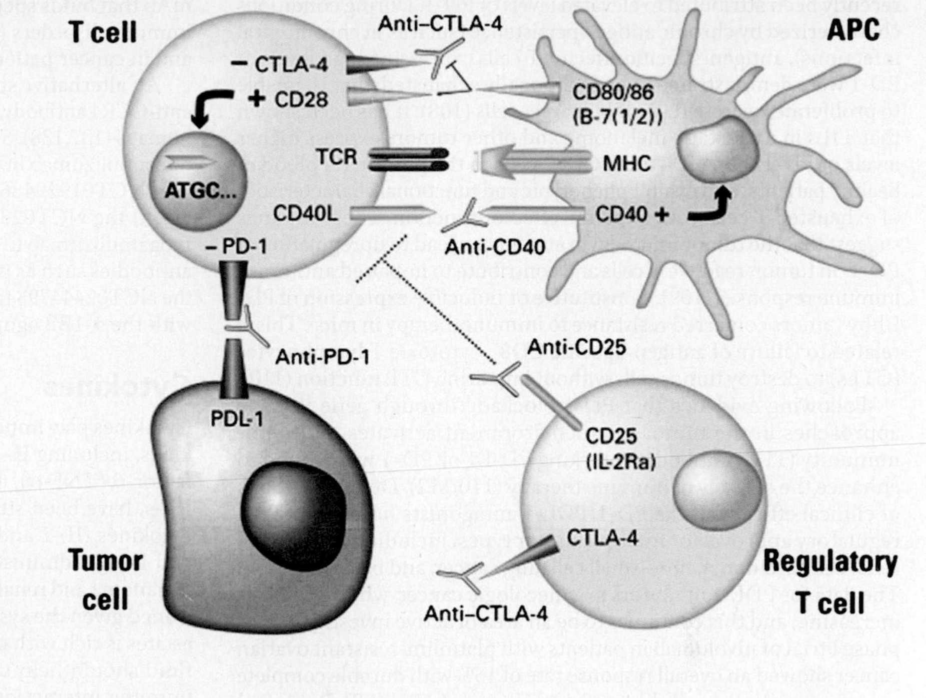

Figure 15.1. The modulation of immune checkpoints.

Source: From Kandalaft LE, Powell DJ Jr, Singh N, et al. Immunotherapy for ovarian cancer: what's next? *J Clin Oncol*. 2011;29:925–933, with permission.

that ovarian cancers, like many tumors, express the CD40 receptor (90–93) and respond to CD40 agonists with apoptosis and growth inhibition *in vitro* and *in vivo* (94).

Effector T-cell Activation

T-cell activation is triggered through the TCR by recognition of the cognate antigen complexed with MHC. This activation is regulated by complex signals downstream of CD28 family immune receptors, which include costimulatory (CD28 and ICOS) and inhibitory receptors (CTLA-4, PD-1, and BTLA). PD-1 and CTLA-4 are induced on T cells following a TCR signal, and result in cell cycle arrest and termination of T-cell activation. The use of blocking CTLA-4 or PD-1 mAbs can sustain the activation and proliferation of tumor-specific T cells, preventing anergy or exhaustion, thereby permitting the development of an effective tumor-specific immune response.

CTLA-4 Blockade

CTLA-4 is the best characterized of the inhibitory B7 receptors. As with CD28, CTLA-4 also binds CD80 and 86 expressed by APCs, but provides inhibitory signals to the T cell, serving as a negative feedback loop. CTLA-4 knockout mice develop uncontrolled lymphoproliferation with early lethality. Furthermore, administration of CTLA-4 blockade significantly enhanced antitumor immunity in a variety of mouse models and with various therapeutic combinations including vaccine, TLR agonists, chemotherapy and radiation therapy. Although Treg constitutively express CTLA-4, CTLA-4 blockade had no effect on the number or function of Treg in cancer patients. CTLA-4 blockade activates CD4 and CD8$^+$ T effector cells by removing an inhibitory checkpoint on proliferation and function (95,96). The combination of direct enhancement of Teff cell function and inhibition of Treg activity is important for mediating the full therapeutic effects of anti-CTLA-4 antibodies during cancer immunotherapy (97).

On the basis of these data, multiple clinical studies have been undertaken to assess the efficacy of a CTLA-4 antagonist antibody in the setting of human cancer. The initial clinical data emerged from studies in patients with melanoma (98). Randomized phase III trials showed an OS advantage for ipilimumab over conventional chemotherapy in patients with melanoma, and regulatory approval was obtained in 2011 (53,99). In patients with melanoma, the most common grade 3 to 4 adverse events were colitis/enterocolitis (increased frequency of diarrhea/stools), dermatitis, and hypophysitis. Significant progress has been made in standardizing treatment approaches to the unique adverse events common to checkpoint blockade (9,100).

Ipilimumab has been evaluated in patients with gynecologic cancers, although the experience remains limited. For example, 11 patients with ovarian carcinoma, previously vaccinated with GM-CSF modified, irradiated autologous tumor cells (GVAX), received ipilimumab (1 month to 3 years following GVAX). Significant antitumor effects were observed in a minority of the patients. One patient achieved a dramatic fall in CA-125 levels several months after an initial dose of ipilimumab. Nine additional infusions of the anti-CTLA-4 antibody spaced at 3- to 5-month intervals over nearly 4 years maintained disease control, with grade 1 rash as the only adverse event (101). In contrast to the melanoma cohort, a single dose of 3 mg/kg ipilimumab triggered two cases of grade 3 gastrointestinal inflammation among the nine ovarian carcinoma patients, associated with significant diarrhea. Endoscopic biopsies revealed mucosal damage associated with abundant granulocytes, macrophages, CD4$^+$ and CD8$^+$ T cells, and FoxP3$^+$ Treg. The remaining seven patients showed only minor inflammatory toxicities including papular rash or urticarial-like reactions at sites of prior vaccination (101). Tumor regression in these patients correlated with the CD8$^+$/Treg ratio, suggesting that other forms of therapy targeting Treg depletion may provide an effective treatment when combined with the tumor vaccine and CTLA-4 antibody approaches (101). A phase II clinical trial of ipilimumab in relapsed platinum-sensitive ovarian cancer with measurable disease is ongoing (NCT01611558).

PD-1 Blockade

Programmed death receptor-1 is a negative regulator of cell activation, primarily expressed on both B and T lymphocytes, which binds PD-L1 and PD-L2 ligands. PD-L2 is restricted to professional APCs, whereas PD-L1 is expressed on many tissues, and plays a pivotal role in maintaining peripheral tolerance (102). A variety of epithelial cancers express PD-L1 (103–105) including ovarian carcinoma cells as well as tumor-infiltrating tolerogenic DCs and myeloid-derived suppressor cells (MDSCs) (106,107). Furthermore, expression levels correlate with disease course. Although PD-1 signaling can occur at very low levels of receptor expression, functional significance has recently been attributed to elevated levels of PD-1. During conditions characterized by chronic antigen persistence (such as in chronic viral infections), antigen-specific effector T cells expressing high levels of PD-1 were demonstrated to be functionally exhausted; that is, unable to proliferate, secrete IL-2, or kill target cells (108). It has been shown that TILs in metastatic melanoma and other tumors express higher levels of PD-1 than $CD4^+$ and $CD8^+$ cells in the peripheral blood of healthy patients, and exhibit phenotypic and functional characteristics of exhausted T cells with impaired effector function. These findings suggest that the tumor microenvironment can lead to upregulation of PD-1 on tumor-reactive T cells and contribute to impaired antitumor immune responses (109). Constitutive or inducible expression of PD-L1 by tumors conferred resistance to immunotherapy in mice. This is related to failure of antigen-specific $CD8^+$ cytotoxic T lymphocytes (CTLs) to destroy tumor cells without impairing CTL function (110).

Following evidence that PD-1 blockade through gene therapy approaches in the tumor microenvironment activates antitumor immunity (111), antibodies blocking PD-L1 or PD-1 were found to enhance the efficacy of immune therapy (110,112). Demonstrations of clinical efficacy of the PD-1/PDL-1 antagonists have resulted in regulatory approval for multiple tumor types, including melanoma, renal cell carcinoma, non–small cell lung cancer, and bladder cancer. The data for PDL-1 inhibitors in gynecologic cancer, while limited, is increasing, and this continues to be an area of active investigation. A phase I trial of nivolumab in patients with platinum-resistant ovarian cancer showed an overall response rate of 15% with durable complete responses with overall disease control rate of 45% (55). A second phase Ib study evaluating pembrolizumab in 26 previously treated PDL-1 + ovarian cancer patients showed 1 patient with complete response (CR) and 2 with partial response (PR) (113). Finally, a study of the PDL-1 antagonist avelumab showed an overall response rate of 10.7% and a disease control rate of 54.7% (114).

Despite their similarities, the regulatory roles of CTLA-4 and PD-1 differ. For example, CTLA-4 ligation does not inhibit PI3-kinase signaling, whereas PD-1 engagement blocks the induction of PI3K activity. PD-1-mediated signaling blocks T-cell activation more effectively than CTLA-4–mediated signaling. In addition, PD-1 signaling may be related to T-cell apoptosis. Whereas the ligands for CTLA-4, CD80, and CD86 are primarily expressed by mature APCs, PD-L1 (on tumor cells or myeloid cells) and PD-1 (on effector T cells) are significantly upregulated in the tumor microenvironment. The effects of PD-1 blockade are therefore more pronounced in the tumor than in periphery. Thus, given the differing but potentially synergistic mechanisms, combination therapy of PD-1 and CTLA4 blockade has been evaluated and was recently shown to be beneficial in patients with melanoma (115). A clinical trial for patients with ovarian cancer (NCT01772004) is ongoing (116).

T Regulatory Cell Depletion

$CD4^+$ $CD25^+$ $Foxp3^+$ T regulatory cells are responsible for maintaining peripheral tolerance by inhibiting T-cell activity. A number of Treg-depleting strategies have been investigated (117–121). An example is the use of low-dose oral or intravenous cyclophosphamide (122,123). Other strategies for Treg depletion are through targeting the IL-2 receptor alpha chain, also known as CD25. In mouse models, the use of anti-CD25 monoclonal antibody before vaccination led to complete tumor rejection and establishment of long-lasting tumor immunity, with no autoimmune complications (124,125). Administration of anti-CD25 antibody linked to a potent proinflammatory toxin showed significant but transient reduction in $CD4^+$ $CD25^+$ Treg cells in patients with metastatic melanoma (126). Another clinical approach of targeting CD25 is through Denileukin diftitox, a fusion protein of IL-2 and diphtheria toxin that targets CD25-expressing cells used in patients with melanoma, ovarian cancer, and renal cell carcinoma (127–130). Although effective in short-term infusions, these conjugates are quite immunogenic and induce neutralizing antibodies, which hamper their long-term application. Another agent is Daclizumab, which is an FDA-approved humanized IgG1-kappa mAb that binds specifically to CD25 (131). It has been used in autoimmune disorders (132,133), acute graft-versus-host disease (134), and in cancer patients with $CD25^+$ T-cell malignancies (135,136).

An alternative strategy has been suggested through the use of an anti-CCR4 antibody, which selectively depletes regulatory T cells from humans (137,138). Several phase 1 studies on the anti-CCR4 antibody mogamulizumab in patients with solid tumors are currently ongoing. The NCT01929486 trial is evaluating mogamulizumab as a single agent; the NCT02301130 and NCT02705105 trials are examining mogamulizumab in combination with immune checkpoint blocking antibodies such as tremelimumab, durvalumab, and nivolumab; and the NCT02444793 trial is evaluating mogamulizumab in combination with the 4-1BB agonist PF-05082566.

Cytokines

Cytokines play important roles in immune modulation. Many cytokines, including IL-2, IL-3, IL-4, IL-6, IL-10, IL-12, tumor necrosis factor-α (TNF-α), macrophage colony-stimulating final factor, and IFNs, have been studied for their roles in tumor treatment. Some cytokines (IL-2 and IFN-α) have been approved by the U.S. Food and Drug Administration (FDA) specifically for the treatment of melanoma and renal cell carcinoma, although enthusiasm for use has waned given the systemic toxicity profile (139,140). Ovarian cancer ascites is rich with cytokine expression, and the study of this ascitic fluid should help us gain a better understanding of the complex immune interactions between tumor and host. A recent analysis showed ascites to be high in proinflammatory cytokines IL-6, IL-8, and the immune suppressive cytokines IL-10, CCL22, and TGF-B in most samples. Interestingly, high IL-6 expression predicted residual disease after debulking and was highest at recurrence (141).

Interferons

Although the full extent of action of IFN in patients with ovarian cancer is unknown, several mechanisms have been proposed: (a) stimulation of NK cells and macrophages, both of which are known to have antitumor properties (21); (b) antiangiogenic effects; and (c) inhibition of expression of dysregulated oncogenes (such as *HER2/neu*), thereby improving the responsiveness of cisplatin-resistant cells (142). A Gynecologic Oncology Group Study evaluated administration of systemic IFN-α to patients with advanced ovarian cancer in which patients with measurable disease showed a low response rate of approximately 10% (143). The role of intravenous IFN-α as a maintenance treatment after initial surgical resection and chemotherapy was also evaluated in a randomized phase 3 study and showed no benefit (144). Systemic IFN-α was also associated with frequent dose-limiting toxicity. Because of the poor response rate and frequent toxicity of systemic administration, further studies were focused on IP administration of IFN-α. Multiple clinical trials with IP IFN therapy were carried out, leading to a randomized trial (by the Southwest Oncology Group) of adjuvant IP IFN-α in stage III ovarian cancer patients who showed no evidence of disease after primary surgery and chemotherapy (145). The trial was closed early, but there was no difference between the study arms with regard to progression-free survival ($p = 0.56$). In cervical cancer, monotherapy with IFN-α had minimal activity (146). Studies evaluating intralesional IFN in human papillomavirus (HPV)–associated diseases (cervix and vulvar cancer) have waned as directly targeted immunologic approaches against the virus have emerged. Nonetheless, a study utilizing intralesional IFN = alpha 2b in high-grade cervical intraepithelial neoplasia showed a 60% response rate. Treated patients also expressed more Th1 (IFN-γ, TNF-α, IL-2) cytokines, with a significant reduction in the viral load of high-risk HPV ($p = 0.0313$) (147).

Interleukin-2

IL-2 is a T-cell growth factor that plays a central role in the immune system, with data showing IL-2-induced $CD4^+$ T-cell expansion in patients with HIV infection (144) as well as clinical responses in renal cell cancer and malignant melanoma, resulting in FDA approval of IL-2 in treatment for these tumors (148,149). It has been shown to activate tumor-associated macrophages and upregulate IFN-stimulated genes (150). Because of the toxicity of intravenous IL-2 administration, studies in ovarian cancer focused on IP administration. A phase 2-3 study (151) of IP IL-2 in patients with laparotomy-confirmed persistent or recurrent ovarian cancer after ≥6 courses of prior platinum-based chemotherapy reported an overall response rate of 25.7%, with an overall 5-year survival probability of 13.9%. A more recent study shows that IP IL-2 administration in patients with ovarian cancer increases $CD4^{+}CD25$ high T cells that highly express FOXP3 and suppress Treg cells. This suggests that IL-2 has a critical role in maintaining the Treg pool as well as enforcing Treg cell tumor trafficking in humans, and may lend itself to combination studies of other agents targeting different immune checkpoints (152,153). A disadvantage of frequent administration of intravenous high-dose IL-2 is the occurrence of dose-limiting side effects. Therefore, delivery of IL-2 from an expression plasmid has been evaluated for the treatment of ovarian cancer. IP treatment of ovarian tumors with an IL-2–expressing plasmid resulted in an increase in local IL-2 levels, a change in the cytokine profile of the tumor ascites, and a significant antitumor effect in a mouse model (154). An *in vitro* study on colorectal cancer showed the ability of plasmids expressing murine IL-2 to enhance the antitumor activity of viral vector immunization against a cancer mucosa antigen, showing the tolerability and possibility of combining plasmid-derived IL-2 production with other immunotherapeutic strategies as well (155).

Interleukin-12

IL-12 is a cytokine produced mainly by activated monocytes, tissue macrophages, and B cells. It can induce IFN-γ and together with IL-2 becomes a potent activator of CTLs and NK cells (156,157). Whereas IL-4 and IL-10 mediate the development of Th2-type immunity, IL-12 initiates the differentiation to the Th1 phenotype. In addition, IL-12 production can be negatively or positively regulated by cytokines. For example, IL-10 and IL-4 have been shown to inhibit the production of IL-12 (158), whereas IL-2 and IFN-α enhance its production. In addition, IL-12 has potent antimetastatic and antitumor effects in several murine tumor models, as well as in human tumor cells *in vitro* and *in vivo* (159). Ascitic IL-12 had been shown to be an independent prognostic factor for adverse outcome in ovarian cancer (160), although later there was uncertainty over this finding as a result of a possible statistical flaw (161). A phase 2 GOG clinical trial (162) evaluated intravenously administered recombinant human IL-12 in patients with recurrent or refractory ovarian cancer. Myelotoxicity and capillary leak syndrome were the major adverse events. Partial response rate was 3.8%, with no complete responders. Recent focus has shifted to evaluating the administration of IL-12 expressing DNA. Two studies have evaluated this strategy in patients with malignant melanoma, showing response of greater than 30% in 5 of 12 patients receiving intratumoral injections; or CR in 2 of 19 and PR or stable disease (SD) in 8 of 19 patients using electroporation of plasmid coding IL-12 (163,164).

ANTIBODY-MEDIATED THERAPY OF CANCER

Antibodies are the primary mechanism for eliminating infectious pathogens from the bloodstream. The effect of most commonly used vaccines against infectious agents is thought to be primarily a consequence of antibody induction with subsequent complement-mediated inflammation and cytotoxicity (156). In addition, tumor antigen-specific autoantibodies are found in the sera of patients with solid tumors, and generally increase with tumor burden (165,166). As one example, the presence of p53 autoantibodies was detected in 41.7% of patients with serous cancer, and detectable p53 antibodies were associated with improved OS ($p = 0.04$; HR, 0.57; 95% CI, 0.33 to 0.97) (167). It is unknown whether this finding represents a biomarker for prognosis, or whether the antibodies exert immunologic control of tumor. Another example is found in the presence of natural antibodies (i.e., prior to vaccination or administration) in paraneoplastic syndromes. In a series of 100 patients with small cell lung cancer, patients with autoantibodies causing the Lambert–Eaton myasthenic syndrome had improved survival (19.6 months) versus those who were antibody negative (8.9) (168). In platinum-resistant ovarian cancer patients, another study showed that anti-MUC1 IgM antibodies correlated with OS at both early ($p = 0.052$) and late ($p = 0.009$) time points (169). These results provide the possibility that functionally effective antibodies may confer a survival advantage. The possibility that these represent a biomarker for better outcome instead cannot be excluded from this data. The ability of antibodies to mediate protection from tumor recurrence has also been suggested in experimental animal models (170). The administration of monoclonal antibody 3F8 against GD2 or induction of GD2 antibodies by vaccination after challenge with EL4 lymphoma (which expresses GD2) showed prolonged survival in mice receiving antibody ($p < 0.004$) or vaccination ($p < 0.008$) (170). Trials in gynecologic cancers have included the administration of murine or humanized antibodies directly targeting tumor-associated antigens, indirect approaches utilizing anti-idiotypic antibodies, or antibodies conjugated to radionuclides, cytokines, or other immunotoxins. The greatest success in the antibody-mediated treatment of cancer to date has come from a series of monoclonal antibodies against antigens expressed at the cell surface of cancer cells, with clinical efficacy in both the advanced disease and the adjuvant settings. Monoclonal antibodies are produced by hybridoma cells. They have evolved from simple murine-derived antibodies with recombinant engineering techniques that now permit monoclonal antibodies of various sizes, configurations, valences, and target effector functions (171). Examples of agents of their efficacy continue to grow and include an ever-increasing list such as rituximab, ibritumomab, and tositumomab for B-cell lymphomas; gemtuzumab for acute myelocytic leukemias; alemtuzumab for chronic lymphocytic leukemias; cetuximab for colorectal and head and neck squamous cell carcinomas; and trastuzumab for breast cancer (171,172). Several mechanisms of action have been postulated: (1) monoclonal antibodies can mediate effector cells by having an activating or suppressive function in pathways such as with CTLA-4 (53), (2) they may target tumor supportive molecules such as VEGF with bevacizumab (173), or (3) they may recognize tumor-specific receptors and by binding may activate or repress signaling pathways. Preclinical studies suggest that antibodies may have the most efficacy in the adjuvant setting. Because many gynecologic cancer patients are initially rendered free of detectable disease by surgery and/or chemotherapy after initial diagnosis, the administration of effective mAbs or vaccines with antibodies as part of the effector repertoire would have broad applicability. There are a variety of potential antigen targets for antibodies on gynecologic cancers. Screening for this purpose was traditionally limited to surface antigens because antibodies recognize antigens primarily at the cell surface. A previous study screened a series of 40 mAbs against 25 common antigens that are potential targets for antibody-mediated immunotherapy, as listed in **Table 15.3** (70,174,175). The antigens expressed by ovarian and endometrial cancers are similar, and quite different from those expressed by melanomas, and similar to, although not the same as, those expressed by prostatic cancers. The 18 excluded antigens (including CEA and *HER2/neu*) were expressed in one or zero of five specimens. The expression of these antigens on normal tissues is essentially restricted to apical epithelial cells at luminal borders, a site that appears not to be accessible to the immune system. In addition to these overexpressed tumor-associated antigens, other targets have included overexpressed growth factor receptors (e.g., *HER2/neu* [erbB2], epidermal growth factor receptor [EGFR], VEGF); and mutated tumor suppressor genes (e.g., *p53* and *BRCA-1*). Binding of mAb to these antigens may have antitumor effect generated through a variety of possible mechanisms including: (a) antibody-mediated recruitment of human effector mechanisms *in situ*, ADCC against the tumor cells; (b) development of tumor-specific CTLs; (c) activation of the complement system; (d) stimulation of

■ TABLE 15.3. Potential Antigens for Antibody-Directed Therapy

	Antigen (mAb)[a]									
Tumor	sTn (CC49)	sTn (B72.3)	TF (49H.8)	Le^y (3S193)	Le^y (BR96)	GM2 (696)	Globo-H (Mbr1)	MUC-1 (HMFG2)	KSA (GA7333)	MUC-16/ (CA-125)
Ovarian	4/5	3/5	5/5	4/5	99/133[b]	5/5	18/19	5/5	5/5	53/62[c]
Endometrial	4/5	2/5	4/5	3/5	2/5	5/5	4/5	3/5	5/5	—
Melanoma	0/5	0/5	0/5	0/5	0/5	10/10	0/10	0/5	0/5	0/4
Small cell Lung	0/5	0/5	0/5	2/5	1/5	6/6	4/6	2/5	4/5	0/2
Prostate	4/5	3/5	1/5	3/5	3/5	5/5	2/5	1/5	5/5	0/5

[a]All the tumor tissues were stained by avidin–biotin complex immunoperoxidase methods (173). Figures are the number of tumor specimens with >50% positive tumor cells by immunohistochemistry.

[b]From Federici MF, Kudryashov V, Saigo PE, et al. Selection of carbohydrate antigens in human epithelial ovarian cancers as targets for immunotherapy: serous and mucinous tumors exhibit distinctive patterns of expression. *Int J Cancer*. 1999;81(2):193–198.

[c]From Kabawat SE, Bast RC, Welch WR, et al. Immunopathologic characterization of a monoclonal antibody that recognizes common surface antigens of human ovarian tumors of serous, endometrioid, and clear cell types. *Am J Clin Pathol*. 1983;79(1):98–104.

granulocytes cytotoxic to the cancer cells; and (e) induction of an anti-idiotypic antibody that can elicit active immunity.

The extensive expression of CA-125 in over 80% of serous and endometrioid ovarian cancers has been well documented since the early 1980s (176). Following the successful cloning of CA-125 and identification of it as a complex mucin, it has been termed MUC-16 (177,178). Multiple efforts focusing on MUC 16 as a logical target for immunotherapy are underway.

Antibody Conjugates

In an attempt to add to the efficacy of unconjugated antibodies, efforts have been made to optimize the antitumor activity by conjugating with radionuclides, toxins, cytotoxic drugs, or second antibodies. The choice of conjugates and specific antibodies is influenced by features such as antigen internalization, lysosomal degradation, shedding, and heterogeneity of expression. The mechanism can be complex in that for some, internalization is a prerequisite for cellular toxicity, whereas in others, it may result in reduced efficacy and increased host toxicity due to intracellular catabolism (179).

Radionuclides

A variety of radionuclides have been conjugated with antibodies for imaging and treatment. The optimal radionuclide for cancer therapy is dependent on many factors (180). Radioconjugates with β (i.e., ^{131}I and ^{90}Y) and α (i.e., ^{211}At and ^{212}Bi) emitters have been proposed for regional therapy of peritoneal implants (181). Estimates of dosimetry suggest that adequate therapy (i.e., 20 Gy) could be delivered to tumors with a depth <300 μg using ^{211}At, <0.1 cm using ^{131}I, and <1 cm using ^{90}Y when conjugated to antibodies. The relatively low radiation dose makes the IP delivery route attractive in the setting of ovarian cancer, placing the source close to the tumor implants in the case of ovarian cancer. Delivery of effective radiation dose is greatly influenced by the extent of tumor binding, depth of tumor penetration, catabolism, and relative distribution between tumor and normal tissues. Antibody-radionuclide conjugates have been successfully developed for non-Hodgkin lymphoma, resulting in drug approvals with CD20 targeted agents (182). Randomized clinical data in ovarian cancer are sparse, with two larger studies having been reported. A randomized trial of 251 patients with stage Ia or Ib grade 3, or Ic, or grade 2 ovarian cancer with no macroscopic residual disease were randomized to IP radioactive chromic phosphate (32P) versus cisplatin and cyclophosphamide chemotherapy. The cumulative incidence of recurrence at 10 years was 35% (95% CI, 27% to 45%) versus 28% (95% CI, 21% to 38%), favoring chemotherapy (p = ns). The toxicity profile of 32P was worse (183).

The SMART study was a large randomized trial that evaluated IP yttrium-90-labeled HMFG1 murine monoclonal antibody in patients with ovarian cancer after a surgically defined complete remission. The MUC 1 antigen targeted by ^{90}Y-muHMFG1 is well established as an immunotherapy target, and is overexpressed on 90% of adenocarcinomas, including ovarian cancer. The phase 2 data supporting the use of ^{90}Y-muHMFG1 administered intraperitoneally in patients in first remission was promising, with a Cox model estimate of 10-year survival at 70% compared to 32% of case-matched controls ($p = 0.003$) (184). Patients were stratified using a second surgical assessment, as disease status at second look remains a powerful predictor of ultimate progression-free and OS (185). Despite the strong preclinical and clinical data supporting this approach, at a median follow-up of 3.5 years, relapses occurred in 98 versus 104 patients (p = ns). Although there is no randomized evidence supporting the efficacy of radioconjugates in gynecologic malignancies to date, the number of candidate agents for investigation continues to increase.

Immunotoxins, Drugs, and Cytokines

Drugs, toxins, and cytokines conjugated to mAbs have been evaluated in numerous cancers. Immunotoxins incorporate an antibody-binding domain and a toxin joined by a chemical cross-linker, peptide, or disulfide bond. The specific targeting afforded by mAbs and the relative potency of the toxin moiety present potential therapeutic advantages. Early conjugates, which have generally not been successful, linked antibodies to standard anticancer drugs such as doxorubicin or vinblastine. It is generally not possible to deliver comparable levels of cytotoxic agents as intravenous administration using this approach. This field is advancing by replacing murine antibodies with humanized versions and conjugating agents that are both specific and functional at lower doses (57,186). Multiple agents are being evaluated, although none have proven effective in gynecologic tumors to date.

Other Selected Clinical Trials with Monoclonal Antibodies

Monoclonal Antibodies for Patients with Ovarian Cancer

CA-125, a tumor-specific antigen that is found in 97% of patients with late-stage ovarian cancer, was first described by Bast et al. (176) as an antigen that is elevated in the serum of patients with epithelial ovarian cancer. CA-125 has been cloned and identified as the mucin MUC-16 (187), as shown in **Figure 15.2**. Studies have shown that MUC-16 has a variety of functions and contributes to ovarian cancer

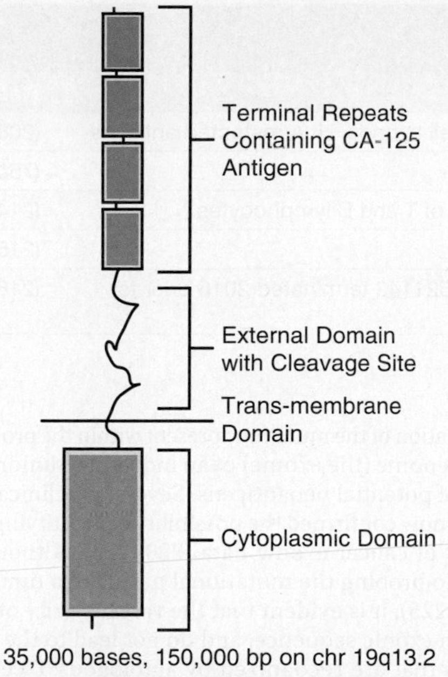

Figure 15.2. Proposed MUC-16 structure.

TABLE 15.4. Monoclonal Antibodies for Patients with Ovarian Cancer

Antibody	Target	Results	References
Oregovomab	CA125	No benefit. PFS 1st line 13.3 vs. 10.3 months, $p = 0.71$	(190)
Abagovomab	CA125	No benefit. HR for PFS 1.099 (95% CI, 0.919–1.315; $p = 0.301$); OS 1.150 (95% CI, 0.872–1.518; $p = 0.322$).	(191)
Matuzumab	EGF	No benefit. Phase 2 trial (n = 75) with no activity.	(192)
Trastuzumab	Her 2/neu	No benefit. 45 Her 2 + patients had RR 7.3% with PFS 2 months.	(193)

cell growth, survival, and invasiveness (188). Recent data suggest that expression is extended to digestive tract adenocarcinomas, and moderate expression likewise correlates with poor survival ($p < 0.001$) (189). The sheer size of the MUC-16 complex has made selecting appropriate sequences for incorporation into vaccines difficult, and initial studies focused on antibodies that could be raised against CA-125. In addition to antibodies targeting CA-125 for patients with ovarian cancer, others have been directed toward EGF, Her2/neu, and VEGF (see **Table 15.4**). (The role of antivascular agents is discussed in Chapters 23, 20, and 21 for the treatment of ovarian, cervical, and endometrial cancers.)

Monoclonal Antibodies for Patients with Cervical and Endometrial Cancers

There are no approved antibody strategies targeting antigens in cervical or endometrial cancers to date. VEGF-targeted approaches are ongoing in patients with cervical carcinoma and endometrial cancer, and these are discussed in the appropriate chapters. EGF-targeted approaches have also been evaluated in patients with cervical cancer. EGFR is overexpressed in 85% of patients with invasive cervical cancer (194). Cetuximab is a chimeric IgG1 mAb that antagonizes normal ligand receptor interactions. A phase 2 trial by the Gynecology Oncology Group evaluated single agent cetuximab in 38 patients. No clinical responses were detected (195). Cetuximab was also evaluated in 76 patients in combination with cisplatin chemotherapy in treated and chemotherapy-naïve patients. Response rates of 9% and 16%, respectively, were seen, with no evidence that there is any advantage to cetuximab over cisplatin alone (196).

CANCER VACCINES

Vaccines continue to be evaluated as an approach to immunotherapy (197–201). Similar to experiences in other immunogenic tumors (202), vaccines have shown limited efficacy as monotherapy in patients with advanced recurrent disease. Current efforts to improve vaccines are directed broadly toward: (a) optimizing the choice of antigens; (b) improving vaccine delivery systems to maximize the magnitude and quality (phenotype and polarization) of antibody and T-cell responses; and (c) developing combinatorial approaches with adoptive T-cell or immunomodulation therapy to maximize activation and function of vaccine-primed effector cells *in vivo*.

Vaccines Designed Primarily to Generate Antibody Responses

Most current vaccines seek to generate cellular responses (often with an accompanying humoral or integrated response). However, based on the cell surface target antigen selection process appropriate for antibody recognition described earlier, and advances in the chemical and enzymatic synthesis of carbohydrate and glycopeptide antigens and optimization of adjuvant use, the exploration of a variety of synthetic antigen vaccines with antibody production as one end point has been performed. In one example, a pilot trial of a heptavalent vaccine-KLH conjugate (GM2, GLOBO-H, LeY, TN-MUC1, Tn(c), sTn and TF) plus QS-21 in patients with epithelial ovarian, fallopian tube, or peritoneal cancer in a second or subsequent remission was evaluated (200). Fluorescence-activated cell sorting (FACS) and CDC analysis showed increased reactivity against MCF7 cells in 7 of 9 patients, with some increase seen in all patients. This led to Gynecology Oncology Group Trial 255 (NCT00693342), which was a randomized trial in ovarian cancer patients with second or third complete clinical remission receiving either the adjuvant alone (OPT-821) or the multivalent antigen construct + OPT-821. The end point was the proportion of patients who were disease-free at 12 months (35% vs. 50%). 171 patients were enrolled and randomized. The estimated hazard ratio for PFS of the vaccine conjugate + opt-821 to the opt-821 reference arm was 0.98 (95% CI, 0.71 to 1.36). At a current follow-up of 34 months, the median OS for the opt-821 arm was 47 months and had not yet been reached for the vaccine conjugate + opt-821. Therefore, the study did not meet its primary PFS endpoint, and the secondary OS endpoint requires further follow-up (203).

On the basis of this lack of activity, additional to the development of vaccine now seek to produce cellular or integrated responses.

Vaccines Primarily Designed to Produce Cellular or Integrated Responses

There are a wide range of options for augmenting the immunogenicity of the antigenic targets for T-cell immunity, and this remains the primary goal for tumor immunotherapy (204,205). This now includes the possibility of genetically modifying T cells themselves to express both tumor-associated antigens and DC-activating molecules (205). For the antigens, the options include (a) the full proteins or MHC-restricted peptides modified by amino acid substitutions to increase immunogenicity; (b) genes or mini-genes for these proteins or peptides used as DNA vaccines; or (c) genes expressed in viral or bacterial vectors. Costimulatory molecules, cytokines, or molecules

TABLE 15.5. Select Vaccines for Patients with Ovarian Cancer

Vaccine	Target	References
DC	Tumor derived, DC tumor cell hybrids, HLA restricted antigens	(208–210)
NY-ESO-1 (proteins, peptides, epigenetic potentiation)	CT antigen	(75,211–213)
GM-CSF secreting vaccines	Inducing T cells, expansion of T and B lymphocytes	(214)
Farletuzumab	Folate Receptor Targeting	(215)
MUC-1 targeted	MUC-1 (recent Trial NCT01521143 terminated 2015 prior to completion)	(216)

CT, cancer testis; DC, dendritic cell; HLA, human leukocyte antigen.

targeting antigens to particular processing compartments can be incorporated into these vaccines. DNA vaccines are appealing in this regard because of ease of production, versatility, and adaptability to such combinations (190). Most of these approaches can also be applied to expressing these antigens in APCs, such as DCs, that are then used to vaccinate the patient. Furthermore, because many tumor-rejection antigens detected by T cells in experimental animals are individually unique (mutated), a variety of individualized vaccines are being tested. Whole-cell vaccines can be prepared from a specific patient (if accessible tumor is available), and immunogenicity may be increased by the use of an immunologic adjuvant and transduction with genes for cytokines or costimulatory molecules, or treatment with haptens such as dinitrophenyl (DNP) (206). Other approaches attempting to increase the immunogenicity of unique and shared antigens include the use of heat shock proteins that may carry the full range of cancer peptides, and DNA or messenger RNA vaccines that may be obtained from smaller biopsy specimens (207). See **Table 15.5** for further information.

WHOLE TUMOR VACCINES

Several groups have used viruses to increase tumor cell immunogenicity for whole tumor cell vaccination. An alternative approach to deliver effectively whole tumor antigen is by using DCs. Although whole tumor vaccines offer distinct advantages, some drawbacks warrant consideration. First, surgical procurement of large numbers of autologous tumor cells may not be possible in many patients. Alternatives to this limitation exist, including use of allogeneic cell lines or the use of tumor mRNA. RNA electroporation of DCs is a convenient approach to generate a potent tumor vaccine (206). An additional concern with whole tumor vaccination relates to the inclusion of a large number of "self" antigens, which could potentially drive tolerogenic responses, that is, expand Treg rather than cytotoxic lymphocyte responses. Other work has demonstrated that DCs can be polarized *ex vivo* with the use of IFNs, TLR agonists, or p38 mitogen-activated protein kinase inhibitors to drive cytotoxic lymphocytes and Th17 effector cells at the expense of Treg activity (217). On the other hand, if immunization is successful, there may be increased concern for breaking tolerance to "self" antigens, leading to immunopathology. To date, pilot studies with whole tumor vaccines have reported no autoimmunity in patients with ovarian cancer.

NEOANTIGEN VACCINES

Advances in next-generation sequencing and epitope prediction now permit the rapid identification of mutant tumor neoantigens. This has led to efforts in utilizing these mutant tumor neoantigens for personalizing cancer immunotherapies. Indirect support for this approach comes from studies demonstrating that (i) infusion of autologous *ex vivo* expanded TILs can induce objective clinical responses in metastatic melanoma (218) and (ii) the relationship between pretherapy $CD8^+$ T-cell infiltrates and response to checkpoint blockade in melanoma (219). Deep-sequencing technologies permit easy identification of the mutations present within the protein-encoding part of the genome (the exome) of an individual tumor, allowing for prediction of potential neoantigens. Several preclinical and clinical studies have now confirmed the possibility of identifying neoantigens on the basis of cancer exome data (220–223). Although there are limitations to probing the mutational profile of a tumor in a single biopsy (224,225), it is evident that the vast majority of neoantigens occur within exonic sequence, and do not lead to the formation of neoantigens that are recognized by autologous T cells (225,226). Consequently, a robust pipeline for filtering the cancer exome data is essential. Epitope presentation of neoantigens by MHC class I molecules may be predicted using previously established algorithms that analyze critical features such as the likelihood of proteasomal processing, transport into the endoplasmic reticulum, and affinity for the relevant MHC class I alleles. To predict epitope abundance, gene and/or protein expression levels can also be integrated into the analysis. It therefore appears useful to stimulate neoantigen-specific T-cell responses in cancer patients using two possible approaches. The first is to synthesize long peptide vaccines that encode a set of predicted neoantigens. The second approach is to identify and expand preexisting neoantigen-specific T-cell populations to create either bulk neoantigen-specific T-cell products or TCR-engineered T cells for adoptive therapy.

ADOPTIVE CELLULAR THERAPY

Effective cancer immunotherapy is dependent on the presence of large numbers of antitumor lymphocytes with appropriate homing and effector functions that enable them to seek out and destroy cancer cells *in vivo*. The adoptive transfer of *ex vivo* expanded tumor-reactive T cells holds the potential of achieving this condition in a short period of time, as shown in **Figure 15.3**. Clinical trials testing spontaneous or induced polyclonal or oligoclonal T cells conducted in the past have provided crucial lessons that can guide further optimization. The use of *ex vivo* expanded TILs has yielded the best clinical immunotherapy results to date. The advantages of TIL-based adoptive therapy include the presence of spontaneously occurring T cells with natural avidity against tumors that have escaped thymic deletion; the use of a polyclonal population of T cells that can limit immunologic escape of tumors; and the natural selection of patients whose tumor microenvironment is already conducive to T-cell homing. Initial studies using TILs in the treatment of metastatic melanoma during the late 1980s and early 1990s demonstrated objective antitumor responses, but these were short-lived. Based on animal studies showing that host lymphodepletion before T-cell transfer enhances persistence of T cells and antitumor response, a scheme of incremental lymphodepletion through high-dose nonmyeloablative chemotherapy and whole body radiation was tested. Infused cells were both long-lived and highly penetrating, showing regression of voluminous metastatic tumors, with recent reports showing up to 16% complete response and 72% overall objective response rates with maximal lymphodepletion and radiation. T-cell persistence correlated with long-lasting responses (120,202). Although these are phase 1 studies accruing a highly selected cohort of patients with

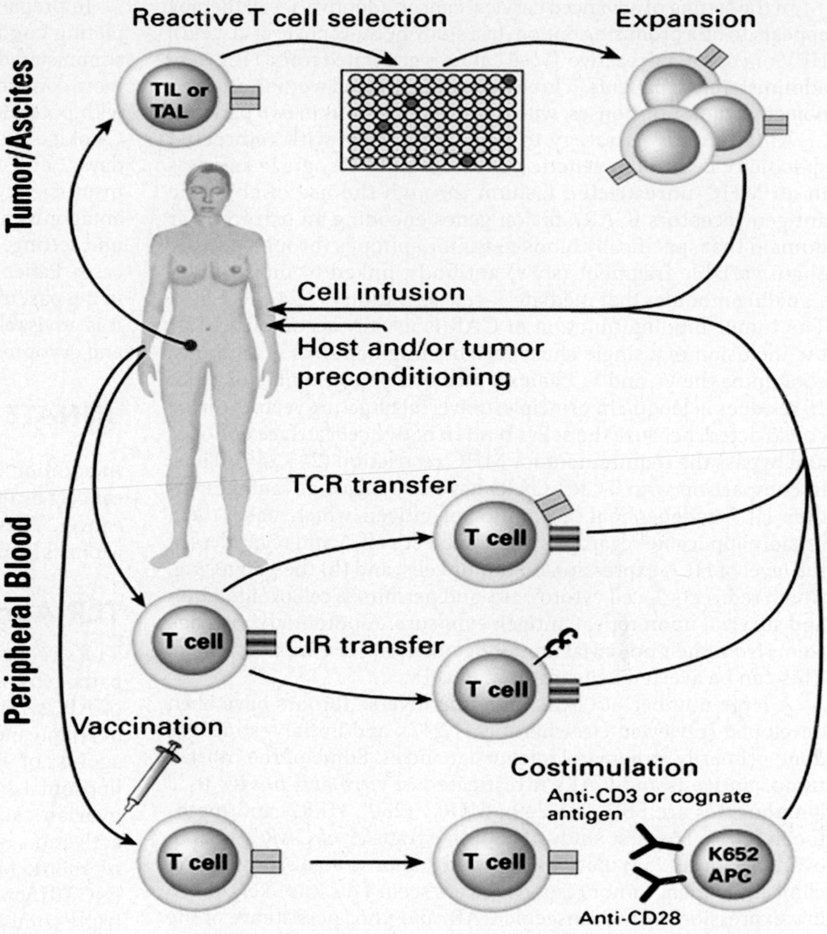

Figure 15.3. Cellular therapy.

Source: From Kandalaft LE, Powell DJ Jr, Singh N, et al. Immunotherapy for ovarian cancer: what's next? *J Clin Oncol*. 2011;29:925–933, with permission.

metastatic melanoma, with preexisting antitumor immunity, whose tumors yield tumor-reactive TILs, the results clearly demonstrate the power of adoptive immunotherapy and dispel the assumption that immunotherapy can control only small tumors (227). Interestingly, adoptive transfer of $CD8^+$ clones expanded *ex vivo* to large numbers, and transferred following lymphodepletion, did not result in objective tumor response in melanoma, indicating that polyclonal T cells, a mixture of memory and effector cells, and $CD4^+$ cells are necessary for tumor rejection (228).

Although TIL-based adoptive therapy has been tested mainly in melanoma or in hematologic malignancies, there is evidence that it also presents an important opportunity in ovarian cancer. In the early 1990s, ovarian cancers were found to yield reactive TILs after IL-2 culturing *in vitro* that might be amenable to adoptive transfer (229,230). Moreover, pilot clinical trials of adjuvant therapy with adoptive transfer of tumor-derived lymphocytes expanded *ex vivo* with IL-2, following surgical debulking and frontline chemotherapy, showed a marked survival advantage (231,232). Stage III EOC patients treated with consolidation adoptive transfer of expanded TILs after completion of cisplatin-based frontline chemotherapy ($n = 13$) had a 3-year OS rate of 100%, whereas 3-year OS in a control group of patients ($n = 10$) receiving only chemotherapy was 67.5% ($p < 0.01$). The 3-year disease-free survival of the patients in the TIL group and in the control group was 82.1% and 54.5%, respectively. Although these results can be limited by the lack of randomization, they nevertheless support the feasibility of adoptive therapy for ovarian cancer (231).

Optimization of adoptive TIL therapy is a matter of intense investigation, currently directed at: (a) optimizing methods to select tumor-reactive TIL and expand them under optimal costimulation conditions that allow preferential expansion of specific T-cell phenotypes; and (b) optimizing host and/or tumor conditioning. As shown in the melanoma trials, although infused cells had an effector phenotype ($CD27^-$ $CD28^-$ $CD45RA^-$ $CD62L^-$ $CCR7^-$), TILs that persist at 2 months in association with tumor regression were characterized by a less differentiated phenotype ($CD27^+$ $CD28^+$ $CD45RA^+$ but $CD62L^-$ $CCR7^-$) and longer telomeres (233–237). These results argue that use of memory rather than effector cells may be more convenient for adoptive transfer (238), which has been confirmed by mouse models (239). Because TILs comprise a large number of tumor-reactive effector cells, identification of culture conditions that preferentially expand memory phenotypes is a priority. Recent technological advances with the development of artificial APCs (aAPCs) expressing a variable repertoire of costimulatory molecules and cytokines have generated new opportunities to provide the desired costimulatory molecules and cytokines to re-educate TILs, improving their potency and function *in vivo*. More recent work has described the development of a next-generation K562-based aAPC platform capable of expressing multiple gene inserts, including HLA-A2, CD64 (the high-affinity Fc receptor), CD80, CD83, CD86, CD137L (4-1BBL), and CD252 (Ox40L), and a variety of T-cell supporting cytokines (240). Cell-based aAPCs have proven to be more efficient at activating and expanding $CD8^+$ $CD28^-$ T cells, and antigen-specific T cells, than the magnetic bead-based aAPC (240).

One strategy to overcome the daunting task of raising large numbers of tumor-reactive T cells is by engineering T cells to redirect their specificity. This can be accomplished by transducing lymphocytes to express a cloned TCR with a high affinity for tumor-associated epitopes. In this case, the cloned heterodimeric TCR is transduced to mixed peripheral blood T cells isolated from the patient, creating a large amount of bispecific T cells, which are polyclonal with respect to their original TCR, but potentially monoclonal for the cloned TCR (if recombination with endogenous TCR is minimized) (241). Alternatively, T cells can be transduced with a chimeric immunoreceptor.

In the setting of advanced cervical cancer, adoptive T-cell therapy appears to be a promising option. In a study by Stevanović et al. (242), HPV oncoprotein-reactive T-cell cultures generated from TILs were administered to patients. Three out of nine treated women attained objective tumor responses, with durable remissions in two patients.

An alternative strategy to engineer T cells with redirected specificity is through genetic modification to recognize antigens in an MHC-unrestricted fashion through the use of chimeric antigen receptors (CAR), fusion genes encoding an extracellular domain that specifically binds to tumor epitopes through a single chain variable fragment (scFv) antibody, linked to intracellular signaling modules that mediate T-cell activation (57,241,243,244). The tumor binding function of CAR is usually accomplished by the inclusion of a single chain variable fragment (scFv) antibody, containing the V_H and V_L chains joined by a peptide linker of about 15 residues in length. In principle, universal targeting vectors can be constructed, because the scFvs bind to native cell surface epitopes and bypass the requirement for MHC restriction (245,246). Thus, in comparison with TCRs, CARs have two major advantages: (a) their HLA-independent recognition of antigen, which makes them broadly applicable regardless of the subject's HLA and regardless of the level of HLA expression on tumor cells, and (b) their signaling, which redirects T-cell cytotoxicity and permits T-cell proliferation and survival upon repeat antigen exposure. A potential drawback stems from their potential immunogenicity, if scFv are nonhuman. This can be averted by using human scFv.

A large number of CARs targeting diverse tumors have been developed (reviewed elsewhere) (241,247), and initial testing was done primarily in hematologic malignancies. Some of the ovarian tumor antigens and CARs investigated *in vitro* and *in vivo* in T lymphocytes are FBP (248,249), MUC1 (250), HER2, and mesothelin (251). The first study of adoptive transfer of CAR T cells in ovarian cancer (252) that was reported demonstrated safety, but no clinically evident tumor responses were seen. This was likely due to low expression of the transgenic CAR, and poor persistence of the transferred T cells (252). Persistence can be dramatically improved by using human scFv and by adding costimulatory signaling capabilities to the intracytoplasmic domain of CARs (253). One issue that must be addressed with CARs is that signaling through the cytosolic domain of the usual scFv-TCRz single chain construct does not fully replicate the multichain TCR signaling complex. This is solved by incorporating additional signaling modules in the cytoplasmic domain of the chimeric receptor. Efficient lentiviral and tissue culture technology also now enables highly efficient transduction of primary T cells (254). Other preclinical studies in which the T cells were engineered to express an MUC-16–specific CAR were associated with complete eradication of orthotopic ovarian xenografts (253). Additional studies evaluating T cells targeting other ovarian cancer–associated targets such as folate receptor, mesothelin, and NY-ESO-1 are ongoing.

Reports also indicate that T cells that are expanded *ex vivo* to maintain more stem-like T-cell populations, known as T stem cell memory (Tscm) cells, are capable of a more sustained response by replenishing effectors (255). A clear benefit of transferring less mature, more stem-like cells is likely due to the increased persistence and replenishing capability of these cells *in vivo*. Next-generation autologous car-T cell (ACT) protocols are focused on (i) using less mature cells up to and including hematopoietic stem cells to provide a long-lasting, potentially life-long supply of effector T cells engineered against tumor antigens by TCR genes; (ii) incorporation of suicide genes in the gene-modification that could add an extra level of safety; (iii) incorporation of switch receptors that allow recognition of multiple antigenic targets; (iv) conversion of inhibitory signaling (e.g., *via* the PD-1 receptor) into an agonist signal by modifying the costimulatory domain of CAR T cells against the ligand; and (v) genetic labeling with bioluminescence imaging and positron emission tomography reporter genes to allow real-time visualization of transgenic T cell traffic into the tumor and its correlation with antitumor responses (256).

In preparation for the ACT, patients usually receive lymphodepleting conditioning chemotherapy, and low- or high-dose IL2 is administered after the transfer for T-cell expansion. As ACT becomes more common, it becomes very important that all centers are familiar with potential adverse events that may occur and its management. Cytokine release syndrome, typically occurring between postinfusion days 2 and 10, manifested as fever, hypotension, and respiratory insufficiency, can be managed with tocilizumab, an IL6-receptor antagonist and general supportive treatment in an intensive care unit setting. High-dose steroids are administered to life-threatening cases. Patients who have undergone multiple cycles of chemotherapy in the past may end up with persistent pancytopenia, and therefore, it is advisable to decrease the dose of conditioning chemotherapy and cryopreserve stem cell reserve for backup.

INNATE IMMUNE AGONISTS

In addition to vaccines, several strategies targeting recognition of cancers by the innate immune system have been explored in ovarian cancer. These strategies include type I IFN discussed earlier, TLR agonists, and microbial agents such as oncolytic viruses and bacteria.

TLR Agonists

TLRs recognize signature molecules broadly shared by various pathogens, which leads to production of type I IFNs and maturation of APCs. TLR ligands are being explored as anticancer agents in ovarian cancer (257). VTX-2337 (motolimod) is a small molecule agonist of TLR8, which has been evaluated in combination with liposomal doxorubicin in a phase 1 study in patients with advanced ovarian cancer. The study had evidence of safety and immune activation with clinical benefit (258). A phase 2 study evaluating motolimod in combination with liposomal doxorubicin is ongoing (NCT01666444), and an additional study is currently evaluating a triple combination of motolimod, liposomal doxorubicin, and the PD-L1 targeting antibody durvalumab (NCT02431559).

Oncolytic Viruses

Oncolytic viruses are viruses that have an inherent preferential predilection for replication in cancer cells as opposed to normal tissues. In addition to having tumor-debulking properties, the viruses serve as strong activators of innate immunity through provision of TLR agonists, release of tumor antigens and danger signals, and production of type I IFN. Several trials using oncolytic viruses administered intraperitoneally have been conducted in patients with advanced ovarian cancer, with most of the studies demonstrating good tolerability and durable disease stabilization in some patients (259–265). These studies suggest that IP oncolytic viruses present a viable therapeutic strategy in ovarian cancer, although for optimal efficacy, their evaluation in combination with other modalities (e.g., chemotherapy, other immunotherapies) is likely warranted.

Listeria

Live-attenuated *Listeria monocytogenes* (Lm)–based vaccines use a genetically modified form of the bacteria. Several studies have explored Lm-based vaccine encoding HPV-16 E7 protein in the setting of advanced cervical cancer. A prospective phase 2 study conducted in India was designed to evaluate the safety and efficacy of this vector (ADXS11-001) with and without cisplatin chemotherapy in patients with advanced cervical cancer. The results, presented at the ASCO 2014 meeting, demonstrated a 36% 12-month survival and an 11% response rate, suggesting that ADXS11-001 is an active agent in recurrent cervical cancer (266). A GOG phase II trial (protocol 265) evaluating the use of ADXS11-001 in the treatment of persistent or recurrent squamous or nonsquamous cell carcinoma of the cervix is ongoing (267).

CONCLUSIONS

Many patients with cervical, endometrial, or ovarian cancer who eventually develop treatment-resistant disease can initially be rendered free of clinically detectable disease by surgery, radiation therapy, and/or chemotherapy for varying periods of time. This setting, where the targets are circulating tumor cells or micrometastasis rather than bulk disease, is ideal for treatment with immune-based interventions. Significant advances have been made in the field of cancer immunotherapy over the last decade. It has been equally important to identify tumor antigens with immunogenic potential, as well as the application of a variety of approaches to augment the antitumor response in particular, using immunomodulatory strategies such as checkpoint blockade. Although there is clear evidence of long-lasting benefit in isolated groups of patients, there are numerous steps to take to continue to improve the outcomes for patients: (1) biomarkers for response must be developed, such as characterization of predictive genomic signatures, (2) broadening early success with checkpoint blockade by targeting Ox 40, ICOS, and others; (3) consideration of combinations with other modalities such as radiation, chemotherapy, or cryotherapy , to enhance antigen presentation, (4) consideration of the use of oncolytic viruses, (5) combinations with a variety of targeted agents exploiting the immune-modulating effect of the targeted drugs, and (6) evaluation of agents targeting other immune inhibitory mechanisms such as regulatory T cells, IDO, and MDSCs.

We must move ahead with discovery-oriented translational research in the form of clinical trials that quickly assess alternative vaccine strategies, immunomodulation approaches, combination strategies, immunologic monitoring methods, and tumor escape mechanisms. The key to success will depend on the continued development of organized multidisciplinary groups with the adoption of standardized patient populations (e.g., second or third remission), as well as standardized monitoring to enable the comparison of single variables such as the constitution of an antigen (protein, peptide, viral vectors, or DNA); the method, frequency, and intensity of antigen delivery; the effect of different adjuvants; and the characteristics of the effectors. In concert, a combination of strategies with the aim of achieving an integrated response (antibody and T-cell effectors) along with immunomodulatory approaches seems most likely to provide a meaningful clinical benefit in the future.

REFERENCES

1. McGuire WP, Hoskins WJ, Brady MF, et al. Cyclophosphamide and cisplatin compared with paclitaxel and cisplatin in patients with stage III and stage IV ovarian cancer. *N Engl J Med*. 1996;334:1–6.
2. Muggia FM, Braly PS, Brady MF, et al. Phase III randomized study of cisplatin versus paclitaxel versus cisplatin and paclitaxel in patients with suboptimal stage III or IV ovarian cancer: a Gynecologic Oncology Group study. *J Clin Oncol*. 2000;18(1):106–115.
3. Markman M, Markman J, Webster K, et al. Duration of response to second-line, platinum-based chemotherapy for ovarian cancer: implications for patient management and clinical trial design. *J Clin Oncol*. 2004;22(15):3120–3125.
4. Armstrong DK, Bundy B, Wenzel L, et al. Intraperitoneal cisplatin and paclitaxel in ovarian cancer. *N Engl J Med*. 2006;354(1):34–43.
5. Koutsky LA, Ault KA, Wheeler CM, et al. A controlled trial of a human papillomavirus type 16 vaccine. *N Engl J Med*. 2002;347(21):1645–1651.
6. Brooks N, Pouniotis DS. Immunomodulation in endometrial cancer. *Int J Gynecol Cancer*. 2009;19(4):734–740.
7. Coosemans, A, Wölfl M, Berneman ZN, et al. Immunological response after therapeutic vaccination with WT1 mRNA-loaded dendritic cells in end-stage endometrial carcinoma. *Anticancer Res*. 2010:30(9):3709–3714.
8. Bignotti E, Ravaggi A, Romani C, et al. Trop-2 overexpression in poorly differentiated endometrial endometrioid carcinoma: implications for immunotherapy with hRS7, a humanized anti-trop-2 monoclonal antibody. *Int J Gynecol Cancer*. 2011;21(9):1613–1621.
9. Champiat S, Lambotte O, Barreau E, et al. Management of immune checkpoint blockade dysimmune toxicities: a collaborative position paper. *Ann Oncol*. 2016;27(4):559–574.
10. Coley WB. V. Sarcoma of the clavicle: end-results following total excision. *Ann Surg*. 1910;52(6):776–796.
11. Dunn GP, Bruce AT, Ikeda H, et al. Cancer immunoediting: from immunosurveillance to tumor escape. *Nat Immunol*. 2002;3(11):991–998.
12. Bui JD, Schreiber RD. Cancer immunosurveillance, immunoediting and inflammation: independent or interdependent processes? *Curr Opin Immunol*. 2007;19(2):203–208.
13. Zhang L, Conejo-Garcia JR, Katsaros D, et al. Intratumoral T cells, recurrence, and survival in epithelial ovarian cancer. *N Engl J Med*. 2003;348(3):203–213.
14. Curiel TJ, Coukos G, Zou L, et al. Specific recruitment of regulatory T cells in ovarian carcinoma fosters immune privilege and predicts reduced survival. *Nat Med*. 2004;10(9):942–949.
15. Dietl J, Engel JB, Wischhusen J. The role of regulatory T cells in ovarian cancer. *Int J Gynecol Cancer*. 2007;17(4):764–770.
16. Shankaran V, Ikeda H, Bruce AT, et al. IFNgamma and lymphocytes prevent primary tumour development and shape tumour immunogenicity. *Nature*. 2001;410(6832):1107–1111.
17. Smyth MJ, Dunn GP, Schreiber RD. Cancer immunosurveillance and immunoediting: the roles of immunity in suppressing tumor development and shaping tumor immunogenicity. *Adv Immunol*. 2006;90:1–50.
18. Koebel CM, Vermi W, Swann JB, et al. Adaptive immunity maintains occult cancer in an equilibrium state. *Nature*. 2007;450(7171):903–907.
19. Muenst S, Läubli H, Soysal SD, et al. The immune system and cancer evasion strategies: therapeutic concepts. *J Intern Med*. 2016;279(6):541–562.
20. Meissner M, Reichert TE, Kunkel M, et al. Defects in the human leukocyte antigen class I antigen processing machinery in head and neck squamous cell carcinoma: association with clinical outcome. *Clin Cancer Res*. 2005;11(7):2552–2560.
21. Hicklin DJ, Marincola FM, Ferrone S. HLA class I antigen downregulation in human cancers: T-cell immunotherapy revives an old story. *Mol Med Today*. 1999;5(4):178–186.
22. Shevach EM. Fatal attraction: tumors beckon regulatory T cells. *Nat Med*. 2004;10(9):900–901.
23. Shields JD, Kourtis IC, Tomei AA, et al. Induction of lymphoidlike stroma and immune escape by tumors that express the chemokine CCL21. *Science*. 2010;328(5979):749–752.
24. Liu Z, Guo B, Lopez RD. Expression of intercellular adhesion molecule (ICAM)-1 or ICAM-2 is critical in determining sensitivity of pancreatic cancer cells to cytolysis by human gammadelta-T cells: implications in the design of gammadelta-T-cell-based immunotherapies for pancreatic cancer. *J Gastroenterol Hepatol*. 2009;24(5):900–911.
25. Igney FH, Krammer PH. Immune escape of tumors: apoptosis resistance and tumor counterattack. *J Leukoc Biol*. 2002;71(6):907–920.
26. Staveley-O'Carroll K, Sotomayor E, Montgomery J, et al. Induction of antigen-specific T cell anergy: an early event in the course of tumor progression. *Proc Natl Acad Sci U S A*. 1998;95(3):1178–1183.
27. Yigit R, Massuger LF, Figdor CG, et al. Ovarian cancer creates a suppressive microenvironment to escape immune elimination. *Gynecol Oncol*. 2010;117(2):366–372.
28. Pelletier M, Micheletti A, Cassatella MA. Modulation of human neutrophil survival and antigen expression by activated CD4+ and CD8+ T cells. *J Leukoc Biol*. 2010;117(2):366–372.
29. Cooley S, Weisdorf DS. Natural killer cells and tumor control. *Curr Opin Hematol*. 2010;17(6):514–521.
30. Joncker NT, Shifrin N, Delebecque F, et al. Mature natural killer cells reset their responsiveness when exposed to an altered MHC environment. *J Exp Med*. 2010;207(10):2065–2072.
31. Garrido C, Algarra I, Maleno I, et al. Alterations of HLA class I expression in human melanoma xenografts in immunodeficient mice occur frequently and are associated with higher tumorigenicity. *Cancer Immunol Immunother*. 2010;59(1):13–26.
32. Veillat V, Carli C, Metz CN, et al. Macrophage migration inhibitory factor elicits an angiogenic phenotype in human ectopic endometrial cells and triggers the production of major angiogenic factors via CD44, CD74, and MAPK signaling pathways. *J Clin Endocrinol Metab*. 2010;95(12):E403–E412.
33. Qualls JE, Murray PJ. A double agent in cancer: stopping macrophages wounds tumors. *Nat Med*. 2010;16(8):863–864.
34. Davies DR, Cohen GH. Interactions of protein antigens with antibodies. *Proc Natl Acad Sci U S A*. 1996;93(1):7–12.
35. Mauro C, Fu H, Marelli-Berg F. T cell trafficking and metabolism: novel mechanisms and targets for immunomodulation. *Curr Opin Pharmacol*. 2012;12(4):452–457.
36. Chan TD, Gardam S, Gatto D, et al. In vivo control of B-cell survival and antigen-specific B-cell responses. *Immunol Rev*. 2010;237(1):90–103.

37. Boyd SD, Gaëta BA, Jackson KJ, et al. Individual variation in the germline Ig gene repertoire inferred from variable region gene rearrangements. *J Immunol.* 2010;184(12):6986–6992.
38. Vinuesa CG, Sze DM, Cook MC, et al. Recirculating and germinal center B cells differentiate into cells responsive to polysaccharide antigens. *Eur J Immunol.* 2003;33(2):297–305.
39. Pone EJ, Zhang J, Mai T, et al. BCR-signalling synergizes with TLR-signalling for induction of AID and immunoglobulin class-switching through the non-canonical NF-kappaB pathway. *Nat Commun.* 2012;3:767.
40. Wang SY, Weiner G. Complement and cellular cytotoxicity in antibody therapy of cancer. *Expert Opin Biol Ther.* 2008;8(6):759–768.
41. Walport MJ. Complement. First of two parts. *N Engl J Med.* 2001;344(14):1058–1066.
42. Walport MJ. Complement. Second of two parts. *N Engl J Med.* 2001;344(15):1140–1144.
43. Azeredo da Silveira S, Kikuchi S, Fossati-Jimack L, et al. Complement activation selectively potentiates the pathogenicity of the IgG2b and IgG3 isotypes of a high affinity anti-erythrocyte autoantibody. *J Exp Med.* 2002;195(6):665–672.
44. Chan AC, Carter PJ. Therapeutic antibodies for autoimmunity and inflammation. *Nat Rev Immunol.* 2010;10(5):301–316.
45. Lv M, Lin Z, Qiao C, et al. Novel anti-CD20 antibody TGLA with enhanced antibody-dependent cell-mediated cytotoxicity mediates potent anti-lymphoma activity. *Cancer Lett.* 2010;294(1):66–73.
46. Natsume A, Niwa R, Satoh M. Improving effector functions of antibodies for cancer treatment: enhancing ADCC and CDC. *Drug Des Devel Ther.* 2009;3:7–16.
47. Coico R, Sunshine G. *Immunology: A Short Course.* Hoboken, NJ: John Wiley and Sons.; 2009:391.
48. Bjorkman PJ, Saper MA, Samraoui B, et al. Structure of the human class I histocompatibility antigen, HLA-A2. *J Immunol.* 2005;174(1):6–19.
49. Trombetta ES, Mellman I. Cell biology of antigen processing in vitro and in vivo. *Annu Rev Immunol.* 2005;23:975–1028.
50. Cohn M. Does the signal for the activation of T cells originate from the antigen-presenting cell or the effector T-helper? *Cell Immunol.* 2006;241(1):1–6.
51. Smith-Garvin JE, Koretzky GA, Jordan MS. T cell activation. *Annu Rev Immunol.* 2009;27:591–619.
52. Hong H, Gu Y, Zhang H, et al. Depletion of CD4+CD25+ regulatory T cells enhances natural killer T cell-mediated anti-tumour immunity in a murine mammary breast cancer model. *Clin Exp Immunol.* 2010;159(1):93–99.
53. Hodi FS, O'Day SJ, McDermott DF, et al. Improved survival with ipilimumab in patients with metastatic melanoma. *N Engl J Med.* 2010;363(8):711–723.
54. Bourla AB, Zamarin D. Immunotherapy: new strategies for the treatment of gynecologic malignancies. *Oncology (Williston Park).* 2016;30(1):59–66, 69.
55. Hamanishi J, Mandai M, Ikeda T, et al. Safety and antitumor activity of Anti-PD-1 antibody, nivolumab, in patients with platinum-resistant ovarian cancer. *J Clin Oncol.* 2015;33(34):4015–4022.
56. Sharma RK, Schabowsky RH, Srivastava AK, et al. 4-1BB ligand as an effective multifunctional immunomodulator and antigen delivery vehicle for the development of therapeutic cancer vaccines. *Cancer Res.* 2010;70(10):3945–3954.
57. Moran AE, Kovacsovics-Bankowski M, Weinberg AD. The TNFRs OX40, 4-1BB, and CD40 as targets for cancer immunotherapy. *Curr Opin Immunol.* 2013;25(2):230–237.
58. Li Y, Liu S, Margolin K, et al. Summary of the primer on tumor immunology and the biological therapy of cancer. *J Transl Med.* 2009;7:11.
59. Clynes RA, Towers TL, Presta LG, et al. Inhibitory Fc receptors modulate in vivo cytotoxicity against tumor targets. *Nat Med.* 2000;6(4):443–446.
60. Topalian SL, Weiner GJ, Pardoll DM. Cancer immunotherapy comes of age. *J Clin Oncol.* 2011;29(36):4828–4836.
61. Kohler ME, Johnson BD, Palen K, et al. Tumor antigen analysis in neuroblastoma by serological interrogation of bioinformatic data. *Cancer Sci.* 2010;101(11):2316–2324.
62. Sahin U, Türeci O, Schmitt H, et al. Human neoplasms elicit multiple specific immune responses in the autologous host. *Proc Natl Acad Sci U S A.* 1995;92(25):11810–11813.
63. Chatterjee M, Wojciechowski J, Tainsky MA. Discovery of antibody biomarkers using protein microarrays of tumor antigens cloned in high throughput. *Methods Mol Biol.* 2009;520:21–38.
64. Gnjatic S, Ritter E, Büchler MW, et al. Seromic profiling of ovarian and pancreatic cancer. *Proc Natl Acad Sci U S A.* 2010;107(11):5088–5093.
65. Piura B, Piura E. Autoantibodies to tumor-associated antigens in epithelial ovarian carcinoma. *J Oncol.* 2009;2009:581939.
66. Brichard V, Van Pel A, Wölfel T, et al. The tyrosinase gene codes for an antigen recognized by autologous cytolytic T lymphocytes on HLA-A2 melanomas. *J Exp Med.* 1993;178(2):489–495.
67. Wolfel T, Hauer M, Schneider J, et al. A p16INK4a-insensitive CDK4 mutant targeted by cytolytic T lymphocytes in a human melanoma. *Science.* 1995;269(5228):1281–1284.
68. Cheever MA, Disis ML, Bernhard H, et al. Immunity to oncogenic proteins. *Immunol Rev.* 1995;145:33–59.
69. Scanlan MJ, Chen YT, Williamson B, et al. Characterization of human colon cancer antigens recognized by autologous antibodies. *Int J Cancer.* 1998;76(5):652–658.
70. Zhang S, Cordon-Cardo C, Zhang HS, et al. Selection of carbohydrate tumor antigens as targets for immune attack using immunotherapy. I. Focus on gangliosides. *Int J Cancer.* 1997;73:42–49.
71. Tindle RW. Human papillomavirus vaccines for cervical cancer. *Curr Opin Immunol.* 1996;8(5):643–650.
72. Boon T, van der Bruggen P. Human tumor antigens recognized by T lymphocytes. *J Exp Med.* 1996;183(3):725–729.
73. Coulie PG, Brichard V, Van Pel A, et al. A new gene coding for a differentiation antigen recognized by autologous cytolytic T lymphocytes on HLA-A2 melanomas. *J Exp Med.* 1994;180(1):35–42.
74. Salgaller ML, Afshar A, Marincola FM, et al. Recognition of multiple epitopes in the human melanoma antigen gp100 by peripheral blood lymphocytes stimulated in vitro with synthetic peptides. *Cancer Res.* 1995;55(21):4972–4979.
75. Robbins PF, El-Gamil M, Li YF, et al. A mutated beta-catenin gene encodes a melanoma-specific antigen recognized by tumor infiltrating lymphocytes. *J Exp Med.* 1996;183(3):1185–1192.
76. Mandruzzato S, Brasseur F, Andry G, et al. A CASP-8 mutation recognized by cytolytic T lymphocytes on a human head and neck carcinoma. *J Exp Med.* 1997;186(5):785–793.
77. Gnjatic S, Cai Z, Viguier M, et al. Accumulation of the p53 protein allows recognition by human CTL of a wild-type p53 epitope presented by breast carcinomas and melanomas. *J Immunol.* 1998;160(1):328–333.
78. Jager E, Jager D, Knuth A. CTL-defined cancer vaccines: perspectives for active immunotherapeutic interventions in minimal residual disease. *Cancer Metastasis Rev.* 1999;18(1):143–150.
79. Chen YT, Scanlan MJ, Sahin U, et al. A testicular antigen aberrantly expressed in human cancers detected by autologous antibody screening. *Proc Natl Acad Sci U S A.* 1997;94(5):1914–1918.
80. Lethe B, Lucas S, Michaux L, et al. LAGE-1, a new gene with tumor specificity. *Int J Cancer.* 1998;76(6):903–908.
81. Dudley ME, Wunderlich JR, Yang JC, et al. A phase I study of nonmyeloablative chemotherapy and adoptive transfer of autologous tumor antigen-specific T lymphocytes in patients with metastatic melanoma. *J Immunother.* 2002;25(3):243–251.
82. Hurwitz AA, Yu TF, Leach DR, et al. CTLA-4 blockade synergizes with tumor-derived granulocyte-macrophage colony-stimulating factor for treatment of an experimental mammary carcinoma. *Proc Natl Acad Sci U S A.* 1998;95(17):10067–10071.
83. Matsuzaki J, Gnjatic S, Mhawech-Fauceglia P, et al. Tumor-infiltrating NY-ESO-1-specific CD8+ T cells are negatively regulated by LAG-3 and PD-1 in human ovarian cancer. *Proc Natl Acad Sci U S A.* 2010;107(17):7875–7880.
84. Uyttenhove C, Pilotte L, Théate I, et al. Evidence for a tumoral immune resistance mechanism based on tryptophan degradation by indoleamine 2,3-dioxygenase. *Nat Med.* 2003;9(10):1269–1274.
85. Fujii S, Fujimoto K, Shimizu K, et al. Presentation of tumor antigens by phagocytic dendritic cell clusters generated from human CD34+ hematopoietic progenitor cells: induction of autologous cytotoxic T lymphocytes against leukemic cells in acute myelogenous leukemia patients. *Cancer Res.* 1999;59(9):2150–2158.
86. Terabe M, Matsui S, Noben-Trauth N, et al. NKT cell-mediated repression of tumor immunosurveillance by IL-13 and the IL-4R-STAT6 pathway. *Nat Immunol.* 2000;1(6):515–520.
87. Elgueta R, Benson MJ, de Vries VC, et al. Molecular mechanism and function of CD40/CD40L engagement in the immune system. *Immunol Rev.* 2009;229(1):152–172.
88. Scarlett UK, Cubillos-Ruiz JR, Nesbeth YC, et al. In situ stimulation of CD40 and toll-like receptor 3 transforms ovarian cancer-infiltrating dendritic cells from immunosuppressive to immunostimulatory cells. *Cancer Res.* 2009;69(18):7329–7337.
89. Kedl RM, Jordan M, Potter T, et al. CD40 stimulation accelerates deletion of tumor-specific CD8(+) T cells in the absence of tumor-antigen vaccination. *Proc Natl Acad Sci U S A.* 2001;98(19):10811–10816.
90. Melichar B, Patenia R, Gallardo S, et al. Expression of CD40 and growth-inhibitory activity of CD40 ligand in ovarian cancer cell lines. *Gynecol Oncol.* 2007;104(3):707–713.

91. Hakkarainen T, Hemminki A, Pereboev AV, et al. CD40 is expressed on ovarian cancer cells and can be utilized for targeting adenoviruses. *Clin Cancer Res.* 2003;9(2):619–624.
92. Gallagher NJ, Eliopoulos AG, Agathangelo A, et al. CD40 activation in epithelial ovarian carcinoma cells modulates growth, apoptosis, and cytokine secretion. *Mol Pathol.* 2002;55(2):110–120.
93. Ciaravino G, Bhat M, Manbeian CA, et al. Differential expression of CD40 and CD95 in ovarian carcinoma. *Eur J Gynaecol Oncol.* 2004;25(1):27–32.
94. Toutirais O, Gervais A, Cabillic F, et al. Effects of CD40 binding on ovarian carcinoma cell growth and cytokine production in vitro. *Clin Exp Immunol.* 2007;149(2):372–377.
95. Qureshi OS, Zheng Y, Nakamura K, et al. Trans-endocytosis of CD80 and CD86: a molecular basis for the cell-extrinsic function of CTLA-4. *Science.* 2011;332(6029):600–603.
96. Korman AJ, Peggs KS, Allison JP. Checkpoint blockade in cancer immunotherapy. *Adv Immunol.* 2006;90:297–339.
97. Peggs KS, Quezada SA, Chambers CA, et al. Blockade of CTLA-4 on both effector and regulatory T cell compartments contributes to the antitumor activity of anti-CTLA-4 antibodies. *J Exp Med.* 2009;206(8):1717–1725.
98. Fong L, Small EJ. Anti-cytotoxic T-lymphocyte antigen-4 antibody: the first in an emerging class of immunomodulatory antibodies for cancer treatment. *J Clin Oncol.* 2008;26(32):5275–5283.
99. Robert C, Thomas L, Bondarenko I, et al. Ipilimumab plus dacarbazine for previously untreated metastatic melanoma. *N Engl J Med.* 2011;364(26):2517–2526.
100. Michot JM, Bigenwald C, Champiat S, et al. Immune-related adverse events with immune checkpoint blockade: a comprehensive review. *Eur J Cancer.* 2016;54:139–148.
101. Hodi FS, et al. Immunologic and clinical effects of antibody blockade of cytotoxic T lymphocyte-associated antigen 4 in previously vaccinated cancer patients. *Proc Natl Acad Sci U S A.* 2008;105(8):3005–3010.
102. Iwai Y, Ishida M, Tanaka Y, et al. Involvement of PD-L1 on tumor cells in the escape from host immune system and tumor immunotherapy by PD-L1 blockade. *Proc Natl Acad Sci U S A.* 2002;99(19):12293–12297.
103. Nakanishi J, Wada Y, Matsumoto K, et al. Overexpression of B7-H1 (PD-L1) significantly associates with tumor grade and postoperative prognosis in human urothelial cancers. *Cancer Immunol Immunother.* 2007;56(8):1173–1182.
104. Thompson RH, Dong H, Lohse CM, et al. PD-1 is expressed by tumor-infiltrating immune cells and is associated with poor outcome for patients with renal cell carcinoma. *Clin Cancer Res.* 2007;13(6):1757–1761.
105. Gao Q, Wang XY, Qiu SJ, et al. Overexpression of PD-L1 significantly associates with tumor aggressiveness and postoperative recurrence in human hepatocellular carcinoma. *Clin Cancer Res.* 2009;15(3):971–979.
106. Curiel TJ, Wei S, Dong H, et al. Blockade of B7-H1 improves myeloid dendritic cell-mediated antitumor immunity. *Nat Med.* 2003;9(5):562–567.
107. Javeed A, Zhang B, Qu Y, et al. The significantly enhanced frequency of functional CD4+CD25+Foxp3+ T regulatory cells in therapeutic dose aspirin-treated mice. *Transpl Immunol.* 2009;20(4):253–260.
108. Kaufmann DE, Walker BD. PD-1 and CTLA-4 inhibitory cosignaling pathways in HIV infection and the potential for therapeutic intervention. *J Immunol.* 2009;182(10):5891–5897.
109. Blank C, Mackensen A. Contribution of the PD-L1/PD-1 pathway to T-cell exhaustion: an update on implications for chronic infections and tumor evasion. *Cancer Immunol Immunother.* 2007;56(5):739–745.
110. Hirano F, Kaneko K, Tamura H, et al. Blockade of B7-H1 and PD-1 by monoclonal antibodies potentiates cancer therapeutic immunity. *Cancer Res.* 2005;65(3):1089–1096.
111. He YF, Zhang GM, Wang XH, et al. Blocking programmed death-1 ligand-PD-1 interactions by local gene therapy results in enhancement of antitumor effect of secondary lymphoid tissue chemokine. *J Immunol.* 2004;173(8):4919–4928.
112. Blank C, Kuball J, Voelkl S, et al. Blockade of PD-L1 (B7-H1) augments human tumor-specific T cell responses in vitro. *Int J Cancer.* 2006;119(2):317–327.
113. Varga A, Piha-Paul SA, Ott PA, et al. Antitumor activity and safety of pembrolizumab in patients with PDL-1 positive advanced ovarian cancer: intermim results of a phase Ib study. *J Clin Oncol.* 2015;33(15):5510.
114. Disis ML, Patel MR, Pant S. Avelumab, an anti PDL-1 antibody in patients with previously treated, recurrent or refractory ovarian cnacer, a phase Ib open label expansion trial. *J Clin Oncol.* 2015;33(15):5509.
115. Larkin J, Hodi FS, Wolchok JD. Combined nivolumab and ipilimumab or monotherapy in untreated melanoma. *N Engl J Med.* 2015;373(13):1270–1271.
116. Berger R, Rotem-Yehudar R, Slama G, et al. Phase I safety and pharmacokinetic study of CT-011, a humanized antibody interacting with PD-1, in patients with advanced hematologic malignancies. *Clin Cancer Res.* 2008;14(10):3044–3051.
117. Berd D, Sato T, Maguire HC Jr, et al. Immunopharmacologic analysis of an autologous, hapten-modified human melanoma vaccine. *J Clin Oncol.* 2004;22(3):403–415.
118. Dudley ME, Wunderlich JR, Robbins PF, et al. Cancer regression and autoimmunity in patients after clonal repopulation with antitumor lymphocytes. *Science.* 2002;298(5594):850–854.
119. Machiels JP, Reilly RT, Emens LA, et al. Cyclophosphamide, doxorubicin, and paclitaxel enhance the antitumor immune response of granulocyte/macrophage-colony stimulating factor-secreting whole-cell vaccines in HER-2/neu tolerized mice. *Cancer Res.* 2001;61(9):3689–3697.
120. Dudley ME, Wunderlich JR, Yang JC, et al. Adoptive cell transfer therapy following non-myeloablative but lymphodepleting chemotherapy for the treatment of patients with refractory metastatic melanoma. *J Clin Oncol.* 2005;23(10):2346–2357.
121. Klebanoff CA, Wunderlich JR, Yang JC, et al. Sinks, suppressors and antigen presenters: how lymphodepletion enhances T cell-mediated tumor immunotherapy. *Trends Immunol.* 2005;26(2):111–117.
122. Berd D, Maguire HC Jr, Mastrangelo MJ. Induction of cell-mediated immunity to autologous melanoma cells and regression of metastases after treatment with a melanoma cell vaccine preceded by cyclophosphamide. *Cancer Res.* 1986;46(5):2572–2577.
123. MacLean GD, Reddish MA, Koganty RR, et al. Antibodies against mucin-associated sialyl-Tn epitopes correlate with survival of metastatic adenocarcinoma patients undergoing active specific immunotherapy with synthetic STn vaccine. *J Immunother Emphasis Tumor Immunol.* 1996;19(1):59–68.
124. Benencia F, Coukos G, Regulatory Cell T. Depletion can boost DC-based vaccines. *Cancer Biol Ther.* 2005;4(6):628–630.
125. Prasad SJ, Farrand KJ, Matthews SA, et al. Dendritic cells loaded with stressed tumor cells elicit long-lasting protective tumor immunity in mice depleted of CD4+CD25+ regulatory T cells. *J Immunol.* 2005;174(1):90–98.
126. Powell DJ Jr, Attia P, Ghetie V, et al. Partial reduction of human FOXP3+ CD4 T cells in vivo after CD25-directed recombinant immunotoxin administration. *J Immunother.* 2008;31(2):189–198.
127. Dannull J, Su Z, Rizzieri D, et al. Enhancement of vaccine-mediated antitumor immunity in cancer patients after depletion of regulatory T cells. *J Clin Invest.* 2005;115(12):3623–3633.
128. Barnett B, Kryczek I, Cheng P, et al. Regulatory T cells in ovarian cancer: biology and therapeutic potential. *Am J Reprod Immunol.* 2005;54(6):369–377.
129. Mahnke K, Schönfeld K, Fondel S, et al. Depletion of CD4+CD25+ human regulatory T cells in vivo: kinetics of Treg depletion and alterations in immune functions in vivo and in vitro. *Int J Cancer.* 2007;120(12):2723–2733.
130. Rasku MA, Clem AL, Telang S, et al. Transient T cell depletion causes regression of melanoma metastases. *J Transl Med.* 2008;6:12.
131. Waldmann TA. Daclizumab (anti-Tac, Zenapax) in the treatment of leukemia/lymphoma. *Oncogene.* 2007;26(25):3699–3703.
132. Kreijveld E, Koenen HJ, Klasen IS, et al. Following anti-CD25 treatment, a functional CD4+CD25+ regulatory T-cell pool is present in renal transplant recipients. *Am J Transplant.* 2007;7(1):249–255.
133. Nussenblatt RB, Fortin E, Schiffman R, et al. Treatment of noninfectious intermediate and posterior uveitis with the humanized anti-Tac mAb: a phase I/II clinical trial. *Proc Natl Acad Sci U S A.* 1999;96(13):7462–7466.
134. Przepiorka D, Kernan NA, Ippoliti C, et al. Daclizumab, a humanized anti-interleukin-2 receptor alpha chain antibody, for treatment of acute graft-versus-host disease. *Blood.* 2000;95(1):83–89.
135. Lehky TJ, Levin MC, Kubota R, et al. Reduction in HTLV-I proviral load and spontaneous lymphoproliferation in HTLV-I-associated myelopathy/tropical spastic paraparesis patients treated with humanized anti-Tac. *Ann Neurol.* 1998;44(6):942–947.
136. Vincenti F, Nashan B, Light S. Daclizumab: outcome of phase III trials and mechanism of action. Double Therapy and the Triple Therapy Study Groups. *Transplant Proc.* 1998;30(5):2155–21558.
137. Sugiyama D, Nishikawa H, Maeda Y, et al. Anti-CCR4 mAb selectively depletes effector-type FoxP3+CD4+ regulatory T cells, evoking antitumor immune responses in humans. *Proc Natl Acad Sci U S A.* 2013;110(44):17945–17950.
138. Ogura MI, Ishida T, Hatake K, et al. Multicenter phase II study of mogamulizumab (KW-0761), a defucosylated anti-cc chemokine receptor 4 antibody, in patients with relapsed peripheral T-cell lymphoma and cutaneous T-cell lymphoma. *J Clin Oncol.* 2014;32(11):1157–1163.
139. Fyfe GA, Fisher RI, Rosenberg SA, et al. Long-term response data for 255 patients with metastatic renal cell carcinoma treated with high-dose recombinant interleukin-2 therapy. *J Clin Oncol.* 1996;14(8):2410–2411.

140. Chang E, Rosenberg SA. Patients with melanoma metastases at cutaneous and subcutaneous sites are highly susceptible to interleukin-2-based therapy. *J Immunother.* 2001;24(1):88–90.
141. Yigit R, Figdor CG, Zusterzeel PL, et al. Cytokine analysis as a tool to understand tumour–host interaction in ovarian cancer. *Eur J Cancer.* 2011;47(12):1883–1889.
142. Marth C, Windbichler GH, Hausmaninger H, et al. Interferon-gamma in combination with carboplatin and paclitaxel as a safe and effective first-line treatment option for advanced ovarian cancer: results of a phase I/II study. *Int J Gynecol Cancer.* 2006;16(4):1522–1528.
143. Abdulhay G, DiSaia PJ, Blessing JA, et al. Human lymphoblastoid interferon in the treatment of advanced epithelial ovarian malignancies: a Gynecologic Oncology Group study. *Am J Obstet Gynecol.* 1985;152(4):418–423.
144. Sereti I, Anthony KB, Martinez-Wilson H, et al. IL-2-induced CD4+ T-cell expansion in HIV-infected patients is associated with long-term decreases in T-cell proliferation. *Blood.* 2004;104(3):775–780.
145. Alberts DS, Hannigan EV, Liu PY, et al. Randomized trial of adjuvant intraperitoneal alpha-interferon in stage III ovarian cancer patients who have no evidence of disease after primary surgery and chemotherapy: an intergroup study. *Gynecol Oncol.* 2006;100(1):133–138.
146. Wadler S, Burk RD, Neuberg D, et al. Lack of efficacy of interferon-alpha therapy in recurrent, advanced cervical cancer. *J Interferon Cytokine Res.* 1995;15(12):1011–1016.
147. Ramos MC, Mardegan MC, Peghini BC, et al. Expression of cytokines in cervical stroma in patients with high-grade cervical intraepithelial neoplasia after treatment with intralesional interferon alpha-2b. *Eur J Gynaecol Oncol.* 2010;31(5):522–529.
148. Fisher RI, Rosenberg SA, Fyfe G. Long-term survival update for high-dose recombinant interleukin-2 in patients with renal cell carcinoma. *Cancer J Sci Am.* 2000;6(Suppl 1):S55–S57.
149. Chang X, Zheng P, Liu Y. Selective elimination of autoreactive T cells in vivo by the regulatory T cells. *Clin Immunol.* 2009;130(1):61–73.
150. Weiss GR, Grosh WW, Chianese-Bullock KA, et al. Molecular insights on the peripheral and intratumoral effects of systemic high-dose rIL-2 (aldesleukin) administration for the treatment of metastatic melanoma. *Clin Cancer Res.* 2011;17(23):7440–7450.
151. Edwards RP, Gooding W, Lembersky BC, et al. Comparison of toxicity and survival following intraperitoneal recombinant interleukin-2 for persistent ovarian cancer after platinum: twenty-four-hour versus 7-day infusion. *J Clin Oncol.* 1997;15(11):3399–3407.
152. Wei S, Kryczek I, Edwards RP, et al. Interleukin-2 administration alters the CD4+FOXP3+ T-cell pool and tumor trafficking in patients with ovarian carcinoma. *Cancer Res.* 2007;67(15):7487–7494.
153. Peng DJ, Liu R, Zou W. Regulatory T cells in human ovarian cancer. *J Oncol.* 2012;2012:345164.
154. Horton HM, Dorigo O, Hernandez P, et al. IL-2 plasmid therapy of murine ovarian carcinoma inhibits the growth of tumor ascites and alters its cytokine profile. *J Immunol.* 1999;163(12):6378–6385.
155. Snook AE, Huang L, Schulz S, et al. Cytokine adjuvanation of therapeutic anti-tumor immunity targeted to cancer mucosa antigens. *Clin Transl Sci.* 2008;1(3):263–264.
156. Raff HV, Bradley C, Brady W, et al. Comparison of functional activities between IgG1 and IgM class-switched human monoclonal antibodies reactive with group B streptococci or *Escherichia coli* K1. *J Infect Dis.* 1991;163(2):346–354.
157. Trinchieri G. Interleukin-12: a cytokine produced by antigen-presenting cells with immunoregulatory functions in the generation of T-helper cells type 1 and cytotoxic lymphocytes. *Blood.* 1994;84(12):4008–4027.
158. Nash MA, Lenzi R, Edwards CL, et al. Differential expression of cytokine transcripts in human epithelial ovarian carcinoma by solid tumour specimens, peritoneal exudate cells containing tumour, tumour-infiltrating lymphocyte (TIL)-derived T cell lines and established tumour cell lines. *Clin Exp Immunol.* 1998;112(2):172–180.
159. Whitworth JM, Alvarez RD. Evaluating the role of IL-12 based therapies in ovarian cancer: a review of the literature. *Expert Opin Biol Ther.* 2011;11(6):751–762.
160. Zeimet AG, Widschwendter M, Knabbe C, et al. Ascitic interleukin-12 is an independent prognostic factor in ovarian cancer. *J Clin Oncol.* 1998;16(5):1861–1868.
161. Kudelka AP, Lenzi R, Atkinson EN, et al. Is ascitic fluid interleukin-12 an independent prognostic factor in ovarian cancer? The necessity of correction milligram P values for multiple comparisons. *J Clin Oncol.* 1998;16(9):3208–3209.
162. Hurteau JA, Blessing JA, DeCesare SL, et al. Evaluation of recombinant human interleukin-12 in patients with recurrent or refractory ovarian cancer: a Gynecologic Oncology Group study. *Gynecol Oncol.* 2001;82(1):7–10.
163. Mahvi DM, Henry MB, Albertini MR, et al. Intratumoral injection of IL-12 plasmid DNA-results of a phase I/IB clinical trial. *Cancer Gene Ther.* 2007;14(8):717–723.
164. Daud AI, DeConti RC, Andrews S, et al. Phase I trial of interleukin-12 plasmid electroporation in patients with metastatic melanoma. *J Clin Oncol.* 2008;26(36):5896–5903.
165. Chapman C, Murray A, Chakrabarti J, et al. Autoantibodies in breast cancer: their use as an aid to early diagnosis. *Ann Oncol.* 2007;18(5):868–873.
166. Chatterjee M, Mohapatra S, Ionan A, et al. Diagnostic markers of ovarian cancer by high-throughput antigen cloning and detection on arrays. *Cancer Res.* 2006;66(2):1181–1190.
167. Anderson KS, Wong J, Vitonis A, et al. p53 autoantibodies as potential detection and prognostic biomarkers in serous ovarian cancer. *Cancer Epidemiol Biomarkers Prev.* 2010;19(3):859–868.
168. Maddison P, Lang B. Paraneoplastic neurological autoimmunity and survival in small-cell lung cancer. *J Neuroimmunol.* 2008;201–202:159–162.
169. Budiu RA, Mantia-Smaldone G, Elishaev E, et al. Soluble MUC1 and serum MUC1-specific antibodies are potential prognostic biomarkers for platinum-resistant ovarian cancer. *Cancer Immunol Immunother.* 2011;60(7):975–984.
170. Zhang H, Zhang S, Cheung NK, et al. Antibodies can eradicate cancer micrometastasis. *Cancer Res.* 1998;58:2844–2899.
171. Bellati F, Napoletano C, Gasparri ML, et al. Monoclonal antibodies in gynecological cancer: a critical point of view. *Clin Dev Immunol.* 2011;2011:890758.
172. Reichert JM, Dhimolea E. The future of antibodies as cancer drugs. *Drug Discov Today.* 2012;17(17–18):954–963.
173. Burger RA, Brady MF, Bookman MA, et al. Phase III trial of bevacizumab in the primary treatment of advanced epithelial ovarian cancer, primary peritoneal cancer, or fallopian tube cancer: a Gynecology Oncology Group study. *J Clin Oncol.* 2010;28(18s):946s.
174. Zhang S, Zhang HS, Cordon-Cardo C, et al. Selection of tumor antigens as targets for immune attack using immunohistochemistry: protein antigens. *Clin Cancer Res.* 1998;4:2669–2676.
175. Zhang S, Zhang HS, Cordon-Cardo C, et al. Selection of tumor antigens as targets for immune attack using immunohistochemistry: II. Blood group related antigens. *Int J Cancer.* 1997;73:50–56.
176. Bast RC Jr, Feeney M, Lazarus H, et al. Reactivity of a monoclonal antibody with human ovarian carcinoma. *J Clin Invest.* 1981;68(5):1331–1337.
177. Yin BW, Dnistrian A, Lloyd KO. Ovarian cancer antigen CA125 is encoded by the MUC16 mucin gene. *Int J Cancer.* 2002;98(5):737–740.
178. O'Brien TJ, Beard JB, Underwood LJ, et al. The CA 125 gene: an extracellular superstructure dominated by repeat sequences. *Tumour Biol.* 2001;22(6):348–366.
179. Teicher BA. Antibody-drug conjugate targets. *Curr Cancer Drug Targets.* 2009;9(8):982–1004.
180. Teicher BA, Chari RV. Antibody conjugate therapeutics: challenges and potential. *Clin Cancer Res.* 2011;17(20):6389–6397.
181. Meredith RF, Buchsbaum DJ, Alvarez RD, et al. Brief overview of preclinical and clinical studies in the development of intraperitoneal radioimmunotherapy for ovarian cancer. *Clin Cancer Res.* 2007;13(18 pt 2):5643s–5645s.
182. Maloney D, Morschhauser F, Linden O, et al. Diversity in antibody-based approaches to non-Hodgkin lymphoma. *Leuk Lymphoma.* 2010;51(Suppl 1):20–27.
183. Young RC, Brady MF, Nieberg RK, et al. Adjuvant treatment for early ovarian cancer: a randomized phase III trial of intraperitoneal 32P or intravenous cyclophosphamide and cisplatin—a Gynecologic Oncology Group study. *J Clin Oncol.* 2003;21(23):4350–4355.
184. Nicholson S, Gooden CS, Hird V, et al. Radioimmunotherapy after chemotherapy compared to chemotherapy alone in the treatment of advanced ovarian cancer: a matched analysis. *Oncol Rep.* 1998;5(1):223–226.
185. Barakat RR, Sabbatini P, Bhaskaran D, et al. Intraperitoneal chemotherapy for ovarian carcinoma: results of long-term follow-up. *J Clin Oncol.* 2002;20(3):694–698.
186. Chari RV. Targeted delivery of chemotherapeutics: tumor-activated prodrug therapy. *Adv Drug Deliv Rev.* 1998;31(1–2):89–104.
187. Yin BW, Lloyd KO. Molecular cloning of the ca125 ovarian cancer antigen: identification as a new mucin, muc 16. *J Biol Chem.* 2001;276(29):27371–27375.
188. Bafna S, Kaur S, Batra SK. Membrane-bound mucins: the mechanistic basis for alterations in the growth and survival of cancer cells. *Oncogene.* 2010;29(20):2893–2904.

189. Streppel MM, Vincent A, Mukherjee R, et al. Mucin 16 (cancer antigen 125) expression in human tissues and cell lines and correlation with clinical outcome in adenocarcinomas of the pancreas, esophagus, stomach, and colon. *Hum Pathol*. 2012;43(10):1755–1763.
190. Berek J, Taylor P, McGuire W, et al. Oregovomab maintenance monoimmunotherapy does not improve outcomes in advanced ovarian cancer. *J Clin Oncol*. 2009;27(3):418–425.
191. Sabbatini P, Berek JS, Casado A, et al. Abagovomab maintenance therapy in patients with epithelial ovarian cancer after complete response post first line chemotherapy: preliminary results of the randomized double blind, placebo controlled multi-center MIMOSA trial. *J Clin Oncol*. 2010;28(15 Suppl):5036.
192. Zeineldin R, Muller CY, Stack MS, et al. Targeting the EGF receptor for ovarian cancer therapy. *J Oncol*. 2010;2010:414676.
193. Bookman MA, Darcy KM, Clarke-Pearson D, et al. Evaluation of monoclonal humanized anti-HER2 antibody, trastuzumab, in patients with recurrent or refractory ovarian or primary peritoneal carcinoma with overexpression of HER2: a phase II trial of the Gynecologic Oncology Group. *J Clin Oncol*. 2003;21(2):283–290.
194. Kim GE, Kim YB, Cho NH, et al. Synchronous coexpression of epidermal growth factor receptor and cyclooxygenase-2 in carcinomas of the uterine cervix: a potential predictor of poor survival. *Clin Cancer Res*. 2004;10(4):1366–1374.
195. Santin AD, Sill MW, McMeekin DS, et al. Phase II trial of cetuximab in the treatment of persistent or recurrent squamous or non-squamous cell carcinoma of the cervix: a Gynecologic Oncology Group study. *Gynecol Oncol*. 2011;122(3):495–500.
196. Farley J, Sill MW, Birrer M, et al. Phase II study of cisplatin plus cetuximab in advanced, recurrent, and previously treated cancers of the cervix and evaluation of epidermal growth factor receptor immunohistochemical expression: a Gynecologic Oncology Group study. *Gynecol Oncol*. 2011;121(2):303–308.
197. Leffers N, Daemen T, Helfrich W, et al. Antigen-specific active immunotherapy for ovarian cancer. *Cochrane Database Syst Rev*. 2014;(9):CD007287. doi:10.1002/14651858.CD007287.pub3.
198. Chu CS, Kim SH, June CH, et al. Immunotherapy opportunities in ovarian cancer. *Expert Rev Anticancer Ther*. 2008;8(2):243–257.
199. Odunsi K, Sabbatini P. Harnessing the immune system for ovarian cancer therapy. *Am J Reprod Immunol*. 2008;59(1):62–74.
200. Sabbatini P, Odunsi K. Immunologic approaches to ovarian cancer treatment. *J Clin Oncol*. 2007;25(20):2884–2893.
201. Hung CF, Wu TC, Monie A, et al. Antigen-specific immunotherapy of cervical and ovarian cancer. *Immunol Rev*. 2008;222:43–69.
202. Rosenberg SA, Yang JC, Restifo NP. Cancer immunotherapy: moving beyond current vaccines. *Nat Med*. 2004;10(9):909–915.
203. Sabbatini P, Chen L, Lucci JA, et al. A phase II randomized, double-blind trial of a polyvalent vaccine-KLH conjugate (NSC 748933 IND# 14384) + OPT-821 versus OPT-821 in patients with epithelial ovarian (EOC), fallopian tube, or peritoneal cancer who are in second or third complete remission. *J Clin Oncol*. 2016;34(15 Suppl):5517.
204. Trumpfheller C, Longhi MP, Caskey M, et al. Dendritic cell-targeted protein vaccines: a novel approach to induce T-cell immunity. *J Intern Med*. 2012;271(2):183–192.
205. Bear AS, Cruz CR, Foster AE. T cells as vehicles for cancer vaccination. *J Biomed Biotechnol*. 2011;2011:417403.
206. Benencia F, Courreges MC, Coukos G. Whole tumor antigen vaccination using dendritic cells: comparison of RNA electroporation and pulsing with UV-irradiated tumor cells. *J Transl Med*. 2008;6:21.
207. Murshid A, Gong J, Stevenson MA, et al. Heat shock proteins and cancer vaccines: developments in the past decade and chaperoning in the decade to come. *Expert Rev Vaccines*. 2011;10(11):1553–1568.
208. Zom GG, Khan S, Filippov DV, et al. TLR ligand-peptide conjugate vaccines: toward clinical application. *Adv Immunol*. 2012;114:177–201.
209. Markowicz S, Nowecki ZI, Rutkowski P, et al. Adjuvant vaccination with melanoma antigen-pulsed dendritic cells in stage III melanoma patients. *Med Oncol*. 2012;29(4):2966–2977.
210. Fujii S, Takayama T, Asakura M, et al. Dendritic cell-based cancer immunotherapies. *Arch Immunol Ther Exp (Warsz)*. 2009;57(3):189–198.
211. Sabbatini P, Tsuji T, Ferran L, et al. Phase I trial of overlapping long peptides from a tumor self-antigen and poly-ICLC shows rapid induction of integrated immune response in ovarian cancer patients. *Clin Cancer Res*. 2012;18(23):6497–6508.
212. Odunsi K, Matsuzaki J, James SR, et al. Epigenetic potentiation of NY-ESO-1 vaccine therapy in human ovarian cancer. *Cancer Immunol Res*. 2014;2(1):37–49.
213. Odunsi K, Matsuzaki J, Karbach J, et al. Efficacy of vaccination with recombinant vaccinia and fowlpox vectors expressing NY-ESO-1 antigen in ovarian cancer and melanoma patients. *Proc Natl Acad Sci U S A*. 2012;109(15):5797–5802.
214. Higano CS, Corman JM, Smith DC, et al. Phase 1/2 dose-escalation study of a GM-CSF-secreting, allogeneic, cellular immunotherapy for metastatic hormone-refractory prostate cancer. *Cancer*. 2008;113(5):975–984.
215. Vergote I, Armstrong D, Scambia G, et al. A randomized, double-blind, placebo-controlled, phase III study to assess efficacy and safety of weekly farletuzumab in combination with carboplatin and taxane in patients with ovarian cancer in first platinum-sensitive relapse. *J Clin Oncol*. 2016;34(19):2271–2278.
216. Loveland BE, Zhao A, White S, et al. Mannan-MUC1-pulsed dendritic cell immunotherapy: a phase I trial in patients with adenocarcinoma. *Clin Cancer Res*. 2006;12(3 pt 1):869–877.
217. Cannon MJ, O'Brien TJ. Cellular immunotherapy for ovarian cancer. *Expert Opin Biol Ther*. 2009;9(6):677–688.
218. Dudley ME, Gross CA, Somerville RP, et al. Randomized selection design trial evaluating CD8+-enriched versus unselected tumor-infiltrating lymphocytes for adoptive cell therapy for patients with melanoma. *J Clin Oncol*. 2013;31(17):2152–2159.
219. Tumeh PC, Harview CL, Yearley JH, et al. PD-1 blockade induces responses by inhibiting adaptive immune resistance. *Nature*. 2014;515(7528):568–571.
220. Castle JC, Kreiter S, Diekmann J, et al. Exploiting the mutanome for tumor vaccination. *Cancer Res*. 2012;72(5):1081–1091.
221. Gubin MM, Zhang X, Schuster H, et al. Checkpoint blockade cancer immunotherapy targets tumour-specific mutant antigens. *Nature*. 2014;515(7528):577–581.
222. Wick DA, Webb JR, Nielsen JS, et al. Surveillance of the tumor mutanome by T cells during progression from primary to recurrent ovarian cancer. *Clin Cancer Res*. 2014;20(5):1125–1134.
223. Rizvi NA, Hellmann MD, Snyder A, et al. Cancer immunology. Mutational landscape determines sensitivity to PD-1 blockade in non-small cell lung cancer. *Science*. 2015;348(6230):124–128.
224. Gerlinger M, Rowan AJ, Horswell S, et al. Intratumor heterogeneity and branched evolution revealed by multiregion sequencing. *N Engl J Med*. 2012;366(10):883–892. doi:10.1056/NEJMoa1113205.
225. Linnemann C, van Buuren MM, Bies L, et al. High-throughput epitope discovery reveals frequent recognition of neo-antigens by CD4+ T cells in human melanoma. *Nat Med*. 2015;21(1):81–85.
226. Lu YC, Yao X, Crystal JS, et al. Efficient identification of mutated cancer antigens recognized by T cells associated with durable tumor regressions. *Clin Cancer Res*. 2014;20(13):3401–3410.
227. Rosenberg SA, Dudley ME. Adoptive cell therapy for the treatment of patients with metastatic melanoma. *Curr Opin Immunol*. 2009;21(2):233–240.
228. Yee C, Thompson JA, Byrd D, et al. Adoptive T cell therapy using antigen-specific CD8+ T cell clones for the treatment of patients with metastatic melanoma: in vivo persistence, migration, and antitumor effect of transferred T cells. *Proc Natl Acad Sci U S A*. 2002;99(25):16168–16173.
229. Freedman RS, Edwards CL, Kavanagh JJ, et al. Intraperitoneal adoptive immunotherapy of ovarian carcinoma with tumor-infiltrating lymphocytes and low-dose recombinant interleukin-2: a pilot trial. *J Immunother Emphasis Tumor Immunol*. 1994;16(3):198–210.
230. Ioannides CG, Den Otter W. Concepts in immunotherapy of cancer: introduction. *In Vivo*. 1991;5(6):551–552.
231. Fujita K, Ikarashi H, Takakuwa K, et al. Prolonged disease-free period in patients with advanced epithelial ovarian cancer after adoptive transfer of tumor-infiltrating lymphocytes. *Clin Cancer Res*. 1995;1(5):501–507.
232. Aoki Y, Takakuwa K, Kodama S, et al. Use of adoptive transfer of tumor-infiltrating lymphocytes alone or in combination with cisplatin-containing chemotherapy in patients with epithelial ovarian cancer. *Cancer Res*. 1991;51(7):1934–1939.
233. Gattinoni L, Finkelstein SE, Klebanoff CA, et al. Removal of homeostatic cytokine sinks by lymphodepletion enhances the efficacy of adoptively transferred tumor-specific CD8+ T cells. *J Exp Med*. 2005;202(7):907–912.
234. Huang J, Kerstann KW, Ahmadzadeh M, et al. Modulation by IL-2 of CD70 and CD27 expression on CD8+ T cells: importance for the therapeutic effectiveness of cell transfer immunotherapy. *J Immunol*. 2006;176(12):7726–7735.
235. Powell DJ Jr, Dudley ME, Robbins PF, et al. Transition of late-stage effector T cells to CD27+ CD28+ tumor-reactive effector memory T cells in humans after adoptive cell transfer therapy. *Blood*. 2005;105(1):241–250.
236. Shen X, Zhou J, Hathcock KS, et al. Persistence of tumor infiltrating lymphocytes in adoptive immunotherapy correlates with telomere length. *J Immunother*. 2007;30(1):123–129.

237. Zhou J, Shen X, Huang J, et al. Telomere length of transferred lymphocytes correlates with in vivo persistence and tumor regression in melanoma patients receiving cell transfer therapy. *J Immunol.* 2005;175(10):7046–7052.
238. Perret R, Ronchese F. Memory T cells in cancer immunotherapy: which CD8 T-cell population provides the best protection against tumours? *Tissue Antigens.* 2008;72(3):187–194.
239. Hinrichs CS, Borman ZA, Cassard L, et al. Adoptively transferred effector cells derived from naive rather than central memory CD8+ T cells mediate superior antitumor immunity. *Proc Natl Acad Sci U S A.* 2009;106(41):17469–17474.
240. Suhoski MM, Golovina TN, Aqui NA, et al. Engineering artificial antigen-presenting cells to express a diverse array of co-stimulatory molecules. *Mol Ther.* 2007;15(5):981–988.
241. Sadelain M, Riviere I, Brentjens R. Targeting tumours with genetically enhanced T lymphocytes. *Nat Rev Cancer.* 2003;3(1):35–45.
242. Stevanović S, Draper LM, Langhan MM, et al. Complete regression of metastatic cervical cancer after treatment with human papillomavirus-targeted tumor-infiltrating T cells. *J Clin Oncol.* 2015;33(14):1543–1550.
243. Walker RE, Bechtel CM, Natarajan V, et al. Long-term in vivo survival of receptor-modified syngeneic T cells in patients with human immunodeficiency virus infection. *Blood.* 2000;96(2):467–474.
244. Brocker T, Karjalainen K. Adoptive tumor immunity mediated by lymphocytes bearing modified antigen-specific receptors. *Adv Immunol.* 1998;68:257–269.
245. Gross G, Waks T, Eshhar Z. Expression of immunoglobulin-T-cell receptor chimeric molecules as functional receptors with antibody-type specificity. *Proc Natl Acad Sci U S A.* 1989;86(24):10024–10028.
246. Pinthus JH, Waks T, Kaufman-Francis K, et al. Immuno-gene therapy of established prostate tumors using chimeric receptor-redirected human lymphocytes. *Cancer Res.* 2003;63(10):2470–2476.
247. Sadelain M, Brentjens R, Riviere I. The promise and potential pitfalls of chimeric antigen receptors. *Curr Opin Immunol.* 2009;21(2):215–223.
248. Wang G, Chopra RK, Royal RE, et al. A T cell-independent antitumor response in mice with bone marrow cells retrovirally transduced with an antibody/Fc-gamma chain chimeric receptor gene recognizing a human ovarian cancer antigen. *Nat Med.* 1998;4(2):168–172.
249. Parker LL, Do MT, Westwood JA, et al. Expansion and characterization of T cells transduced with a chimeric receptor against ovarian cancer. *Hum Gene Ther.* 2000;11(17):2377–2387.
250. Wilkie S, Picco G, Foster J, et al. Retargeting of human T cells to tumor-associated MUC1: the evolution of a chimeric antigen receptor. *J Immunol.* 2008;180(7):4901–4909.
251. Carpenito C, Milone MC, Hassan R, et al. Control of large, established tumor xenografts with genetically retargeted human T cells containing CD28 and CD137 domains. *Proc Natl Acad Sci U S A.* 2009;106(9):3360–3365.
252. Kershaw MH, Westwood JA, Parker LL, et al. A phase I study on adoptive immunotherapy using gene-modified T cells for ovarian cancer. *Clin Cancer Res.* 2006;12(20 pt 1):6106–6115.
253. Koneru M, O'Cearbhaill R, Pendharkar S, et al. A phase I clinical trial of adoptive T cell therapy using IL-12 secreting MUC-16(ecto) directed chimeric antigen receptors for recurrent ovarian cancer. *J Transl Med.* 2015;13:102.
254. June CH, Blazar BR, Riley JL. Engineering lymphocyte subsets: tools, trials and tribulations. *Nat Rev Immunol.* 2009;9(10):704–716.
255. Gattinoni L, Lugli E, Ji Y, et al. A human memory T cell subset with stem cell-like properties. *Nat Med.* 2011;17(10):1290–1297.
256. Kimura T, Koya RC, Anselmi L, et al. Lentiviral vectors with CMV or MHCII promoters administered in vivo: immune reactivity versus persistence of expression. *Mol Ther.* 2007;15(7):1390–1399.
257. Muccioli M, Benencia F. Toll-like receptors in ovarian cancer as targets for immunotherapies. *Front Immunol.* 2014;5:341. doi:10.3389/fimmu.2014.00341.
258. Monk BJ, Brady WE, Lankes HA, et al. VTX-2337, a TLR8 agonist, plus chemotherapy in recurrent ovarian cancer: preclinical and phase I data by the Gynecologic Oncology Group. 2013 ASCO Annual Meeting. *J Clin Oncol.* 2013;31:3077.
259. Kim KH, Dmitriev IP, Saddekni S, et al. A phase I clinical trial of Ad5/3-Δ24, a novel serotype-chimeric, infectivity-enhanced, conditionally-replicative adenovirus (CRAd), in patients with recurrent ovarian cancer. *Gynecol Oncol.* 2013;130(3):518–524. doi:10.1016/j.ygyno.2013.06.003.
260. Kim KH, Dmitriev I, O'Malley JP, et al. A phase I clinical trial of Ad5.SSTR/TK.RGD, a novel infectivity-enhanced bicistronic adenovirus, in patients with recurrent gynecologic cancer. *Clin Cancer Res.* 2012;18(12):3440–3451.
261. Kimball KJ, Preuss MA, Barnes MN, et al. A phase I study of a tropism-modified conditionally replicative adenovirus for recurrent malignant gynecologic diseases. *Clin Cancer Res.* 2010;16(21):5277–5287.
262. Galanis E, Hartmann LC, Cliby WA, et al. Phase I trial of intraperitoneal administration of an oncolytic measles virus strain engineered to express carcinoembryonic antigen for recurrent ovarian cancer. *Cancer Res.* 2010;70(3):875–882.
263. Vasey PA, Shulman LN, Campos S, et al. Phase I trial of intraperitoneal injection of the E1B-55-kd-gene-deleted adenovirus ONYX-015 (dl1520) given on days 1 through 5 every 3 weeks in patients with recurrent/refractory epithelial ovarian cancer. *J Clin Oncol.* 2002;20(6):1562–1569.
264. Hasenburg A, Fischer DC, Tong XW, et al. Adenovirus-mediated thymidine kinase gene therapy for recurrent ovarian cancer: expression of coxsackie-adenovirus receptor and integrins alphavbeta3 and alphavbeta5. *J Soc Gynecol Invest.* 2002;9(3):174–180.
265. Hasenburg A, Tong XW, Fischer DC, et al. Adenovirus-mediated thymidine kinase gene therapy in combination with topotecan for patients with recurrent ovarian cancer: 2.5-year follow-up. *Gynecol Oncol.* 2001;83(3):549–554.
266. Basu P, Mehta AO, Jain MM, et al. ADXS11-001 immunotherapy targeting HPV-E7: final results from a phase 2 study in Indian women with recurrent cervical cancer. 2014 ASCO Annual Meeting. *J Clin Oncol.* 2014; 32(5, Suppl):5610.
267. Huh WK, Dizon DS, Powell MA, et al. ADXS11-001 immunotherapy in squamous or non-squamous persistent/recurrent metastatic cervical cancer: results from stage I of the phase II GOG/NRG0265 study. 2016 ASCO Annual Meeting. *J Clin Oncol.* 2016;34:5516.

CHAPTER 16

Clinical Trials Methodology and Biostatistics

Mark F. Brady, Jeffrey C. Miecznikowski, and Virginia L. Filiaci

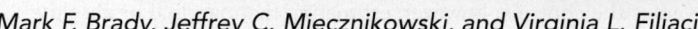

Clinicians make treatment recommendations daily. These recommendations arise from culling information from standardized clinical guidelines, published reports, expert opinion, or personal experiences. The synthesis of information from these sources into a particular recommendation for an individual patient is based on a clinician's personal judgment. But what constitutes reliable and valid information worthy of consideration? It has long been recognized that properly planned and conducted clinical trials are important sources of empirical evidence for shaping clinical judgment. This chapter begins by describing a general system for classifying clinical study designs. The components of a clinical trial and essential considerations for developing new trials are then presented. Because translational research (TR) objectives are incorporated into many modern cancer trials, some issues related to design and analyses of these components are also presented.

CLASSIFICATION OF STUDY DESIGNS

In general, a clinical study is any experiment involving human subjects that evaluates an intervention that attempts to reduce the impact of a specific disease in a particular population. The term clinical trial is usually limited to prospective studies where individuals receive an intervention and then followed to assess their health status. When an intervention is applied to prevent the onset of a particular disease, the trial is classified as a primary prevention trial. For example, a primary prevention trial may evaluate healthy lifestyles or a vitamin supplement in a population of individuals who are considered to be at risk of a particular disease. Secondary prevention trials evaluate interventions that are applied to individuals with early stages of a disease to reduce their risk of progressing to more advanced stages. Tertiary intervention trials are aimed at evaluating interventions that reduce the risk of morbidity or mortality due to a particular disease.

Clinical trials that evaluate methods for detecting disease in a preclinical state are called **screening trials**. Early detection may mean diagnosing a malignancy in an early stage (e.g., the use of mammography in the detection of breast cancer) or in a premalignant state (e.g., the use of Papanicolaou smear in the detection of cervical intraepithelial neoplasia). There are typically two types of interventions in a screening trial. The first intervention is the screening program (e.g., annual mammograms) that involves individuals who appear to be free of the disease. However, once the disease is detected in an individual, a secondary intervention (e.g., surgery) is performed in hopes of stopping the disease from progressing to more advanced stages. Consequently, screening trials require *both* interventions to be effective. An effective screening procedure is useless if the secondary intervention does not alter the course of the disease. On the other hand, an ineffective screening procedure would cause the secondary intervention to be applied indiscriminately or too late for the treatment to be effective.

Nonexperimental studies (or **observational studies**) can be classified into three broad design categories: cohort (or **prospective**), case–control (or **retrospective**), and **cross-sectional**. In cohort studies, individuals are initially grouped according to their exposure status, which can be based on environmental, genetic, lifestyle, or therapeutic treatment factors. These individuals are then followed to determine who develops the disease of interest. The aim of these studies is to assess whether the exposure is associated with the incidence of the disease under study. This design is in contrast to the case–control study that retrospectively identifies individuals on the basis of whether they have the disease and then measures and compares their exposure histories. General discussions of case–control studies tend to use the term exposure, but this term can encompass the status of a particular protein or genetic biomarker. Measuring exposure may be as simple as questioning the individuals about their personal or employment history, or it may involve a more sophisticated assessment such as analyzing the individual's biologic specimens for biomarkers. Though the case–control study has drawbacks, it has the advantage of often being less expensive, easier, and quicker to perform than a cohort study, especially when the disease is rare. The power of the case–control design is clearly demonstrated in the study reported by Herbst et al. (1) that demonstrated that mothers taking diethylstilbestrol during pregnancy increases the risk of vaginal cancers occurring in their daughters exposed *in utero*.

There is a special type of case–control study that is nested within a cohort of exposed and unexposed individuals. For instance, suppose a large prospective clinical trial is conducted within a specific population and blood or tissue samples are banked for each of the individuals who were enrolled into the study cohort. After the study has been completed, the investigators may be interested in determining whether a biomarker is associated with the subjects' outcome. Instead of assessing the biomarker for all the individuals in the cohort study, when the outcome is uncommon it is usually more efficient to assess the new biomarker in those individuals who experienced the outcome of interest (cases), and only a subset of those who did not experience the outcome (controls). In this type of study, the case–control study is said to be **nested** within a cohort study.

There are several approaches to selecting the controls from the cohort, and each approach offers advantages and disadvantages. First, controls can simply be a randomly selected subset of all of the control subjects. This is the traditional case–control procedure. Alternatively, one or more controls could be randomly selected from the subset of controls that have risk factors matching each case (individual matching). This is the matched case–control design. The variables that are selected for matching should be associated with the disease and the exposure of interest. These variables are considered potential confounders. Matching on variables that are only associated with the exposure will undermine the efficiency of the study design. The goal of matching is to increase the study's efficiency by forcing cases and controls to have similar distributions of the confounders. Because time at risk of developing a disease (e.g., age) is frequently associated with both risk of disease and exposure, nested case–control studies frequently match on the time that an individual is at risk. In this case, each case is matched to a control that has been at risk of developing the disease for at least as long as the time until the matched case developed the disease. While the most often stated reason for matching is to reduce confounding, it actually tends to provide an important increase in efficiency. It is important to recognize, however, that following the matching process the selected controls are no longer representative of the controls in the target population. In particular, the distribution of the confounding variables and the exposure (e.g., the new biomarker of interest) in the control sample will be shifted toward that of the cases (2). Matched case–control studies can provide valid estimates of the conditional relative odds of the new biomarker for diseased cases versus the controls; however, estimating the marginal or absolute effects of the biomarker in the target population requires complex weighting procedures (3).

The **case–cohort design** provides another approach to selecting individuals from an established cohort (4). All of the individuals in the cohort who develop the disease outcome are selected and designated as cases. Then a subcohort of individuals is randomly selected from the entire cohort, which provides the controls. One of the primary advantages of the case–cohort approach is that the same subcohort can be used for the analyses of multiple disease outcomes. In contrast, a matched case–control study would need to identify matches for each of the cases that is selected for each type of outcome studied.

It should be noted that the goal of the cross-sectional study is to describe the prevalence of a disease and an exposure in a population during a specific period of time. These studies can often be conducted more quickly and less expensively than both the cohort or case–control studies, but they are seldom used when the time between exposure and disease onset is long, as it is for cancer.

COMPONENTS OF A CLINICAL TRIAL

Objectives

In clinical oncology research, the ultimate purpose is to accomplish a defined objective, whether it be to develop a treatment plan that puts the patients into a disease-free state, reduce the risk of cancer recurrence, or allow patients to return to their normal lifestyle within a reasonable period of time. When it comes to a particular clinical trial, however, objectives need to be more precisely defined. In general, they typically incorporate three elements: the interventions to be evaluated, the "yardstick" to be used to measure treatment benefit (see End Points), and a brief description of the target population (see Eligibility Criteria). These three elements (i.e., "what," "how," and "who") should be stated in the most precise, clear, and concise terms possible. An open dialogue among expert investigators remains the most effective approach for establishing the objectives of any clinical trial.

End Points

The end points of a trial typically consist of a measurable and reproducible entity in the patient's disease process that can be used to assess the efficacy of an intervention. A study may assess more than one end point, but in these instances the end point of primary interest should be clearly specified or else the study design should carefully reflect the complexity of interpreting multiple outcomes. End points can also be a composite measure of multiple outcomes. For instance, some studies assessing health-related quality of life aggregate patient-reported scores from several related items or domains that are all considered components of a larger concept called quality of life.

End points should be a valid (unbiased) measure of the treatment effect on the disease process. They should not be susceptible to a systematic error that favors one treatment, which would lead to biased estimates of the treatment's effect. For instance, trials assessing time to disease progression, in which the schedule for CT scans is different for each treatment group, are susceptible to assessment bias. Second, the measurement of an end point should be reliable and not susceptible to subjective interpretation. Third, end points that are directly relevant to the patient are preferable, although valid surrogate end points are considered indirectly relevant to the patient. Finally, end points which are not too expensive or inconvenient for the patient are preferred. It is not always possible for a single end point to exhibit all of these characteristics simultaneously. For example, avoiding death is very relevant to a patient with a lethal disease like advanced gynecologic cancer. Also, survival can usually be measured very reliably. However, most cancer patients will not only receive the treatments prescribed by the study, but after exhibiting signs of disease progression, they also receive other anticancer therapies. In this case, the validity of overall survival (OS) comparisons is suspected because they not only reflect the effects of the study treatment, but also the effects of other therapies that are external to the study.

End points may be classified as: categorical (e.g., clinical response), continuous (e.g., serum CA-125 values), or time-to-event (e.g., survival time). A time-to-event end point includes both time (a continuous measure) and censoring status (categorical measure). The data type influences the methods of analysis.

Measurement Errors

The susceptibility of an outcome to measurement errors is an important consideration when choosing an end point. These can be characterized as random or systematic errors. Random error refers to variation that occurs among measurements that is not predictable, and appears to be due to chance alone. For example, a serum sample could be divided into 10 aliquots and submitted to the laboratory for CA-125 determinations. If the laboratory returns nearly the same value for each aliquot, then the associated random error is low, and the measurement may be deemed reproducible. On the other hand, if the CA-125 values vary considerably among aliquots, perhaps because of inconsistent laboratory procedures, then individual values may be considered unreliable. In this case, taking the average CA-125 measurement across all 10 aliquots is expected to be a better estimate of the patient's true CA-125 value than any single measurement.

Deviations from the true value that occur in a regular fashion are termed systematic errors, or bias. For example, suppose an investigator initiates a randomized trial comparing two treatments with time to disease progression being the primary end point. The protocol indicates that the patient should be assessed after each cycle of therapy. However, suppose that a treatment cycle duration is 2 weeks for one treatment group and 4 weeks for the second treatment group. Using a more intense assessment schedule for the group being treated on 2-week cycles would tend to detect progressions earlier than in the group being treated every 4 weeks. Therefore, the time to failure comparison between treatments would systematically favor the treatment group with a longer interval between assessments.

When there are recognized sources of error, it is important that the study design implements procedures to avoid or minimize their effects. For example, random error in many cases can be accommodated by either increasing the number of individuals in the study (the sample size), or in some cases by increasing the number of assessments performed on each individual. Systematic measurement error cannot be addressed by increasing the sample size. In fact, increasing the sample size may exacerbate the problem because small systematic errors in large comparative trials contribute to the chances of erroneously concluding that the treatment effect is statistically significant. The approaches to controlling sources of systematic error tend to be procedural. For example, treatment randomization is used to control selection bias, placebos are used to control observer bias, standardized assessment procedures and schedules are used to control measurement bias, and stratified analyses are used to control biases due to confounding. For an extensive description of biases that can occur in analytic research, see Sackett, 1979 (5).

Surrogate End Points

Surrogate end points do not necessarily have direct clinical relevance to the patient. Instead, surrogate end points are often intermediate events in the etiologic pathway to other events that are directly relevant to the patient (6). The degree to which a treatment's effect on a surrogate end point predicts the treatment's effect on a clinically relevant end point is a measure of the surrogate's validity. The ideal surrogate end point is an observable event that is a necessary and sufficient precursor in the causal pathway to a clinically relevant event. Additionally, the treatment's ability to alter the surrogate end point must be directly related to its impact on the true end point. It is important that the validity and reliability of a surrogate end point be established and not simply presupposed (7,8). Surrogate end points are sometimes justified on the basis of an analysis that demonstrates a statistical correlation between the surrogate event and a true end point. However, while such a correlation is a necessary condition, it is not a sufficient condition to justify using a particular surrogate as an end point in a clinical trial. For example, CA-125 levels following three cycles of treatment of ovarian cancer have been shown to be associated with OS (9). However, it has not (yet) been demonstrated that the degree to which any particular treatment reduces CA-125 levels reliably predicts its effects on clinically relevant end points, like overall survival.

Primary End Points in Gynecologic Oncology Treatment Trials

The United States Food and Drug Administration organized a conference to consider end points for trials involving women diagnosed with advanced ovarian cancer (10). Meta-analyses were presented that indicated that progression-free survival (PFS) can be considered a valid end point for trials involving women with advanced ovarian cancer. However, while the general validity of PFS for predicting OS has been established, PFS comparisons in a particular study can be biased because of differences in disease assessment schedules among treatment groups, either intentionally or unintentionally. In contrast, overall survival time is generally not susceptible to this source of bias.

The progression-free interval (PFI) may be a reasonable end point in trials involving patients with early or locally advanced cancer. The difference between PFI and PFS resides in how patients, who die without any evidence of disease progression, are handled in an analysis. Patients who die without evidence of progression are censored at the time of their death in a PFI analysis, but are considered an uncensored event in a PFS analysis. If deaths due to non-cancer–related causes are common, then selecting PFI as the study end point will generally increase the study's sensitivity for detecting active treatments. In this case, however, the analysis needs to consider procedures that will account for treatment-related deaths, as well as deaths from competing causes, which may occur prior to disease recurrence. Simply censoring the time to recurrence in these cases can make a very toxic treatment appear more effective than it actually is.

A number of studies have provided evidence that a new treatment increases the duration of PFS, but not OS. For example, OVAR 2.2, a second-line treatment trial involving patients with platinum-sensitive ovarian cancer, indicated that carboplatin and gemcitabine significantly decreased the hazard of first progression or death by 28% (hazard ratio $= 0.72$, $p = 0.003$) when compared to carboplatin alone (11). However, there was no appreciable difference between the treatment groups with regard to the duration of OS (hazard ratio $= 0.96$, $p = 0.735$). Also, three trials evaluating maintenance bevacizumab for first- or second-line treatment of ovarian cancer reported significant prolongation in the duration of PFS (12–14), but no difference in overall survival. PFS may be a good surrogate for OS, but it appears to be susceptible to a small but not insignificant chance of false-positive prediction. Despite this, it is very rare for the results of an oncology trial to indicate that a new treatment prolongs OS but does not delay the onset of recurrence or progression.

It seems reasonable to expect that an anticancer treatment that prolongs survival should exert its influence by delaying the onset of new or progressive disease. This has prompted some investigators to recommend using both PFS and OS as trial end points (15–17). Specifically, trials involving patients with advanced stage cancer are designed to assess OS in the final analysis, but PFS is monitored at scheduled interim analyses. If the trial's evolving evidence indicates that there is insufficient PFS benefit, then the trial may be stopped early with the conclusion that the treatment has insufficient activity to warrant further investigation in the target population. This procedure tends to halt trials of inactive treatments early, but continues trials of active agents to completion.

To date, PFS has not been formally validated for use in trials involving patients with metastatic cervical, endometrial, or vulvar cancers. In the absence of a formally validated surrogate end point, OS or symptom relief remain reasonable end points. Because relief from symptoms is susceptible to assessment bias, trials utilizing these end points should use validated instruments (see Measurement Errors) and consider blinding the study treatments whenever possible.

Response (disease status) assessed via reassessment laparotomy following treatment has been proposed for use as a study end point in ovarian cancer trials (18). The justification is that those patients with no pathologic evidence of disease are more likely to experience longer survival than those with evidence of disease. The principal drawback to this end point is that reassessment laparotomy is a very onerous procedure for the patient; many patients refuse reassessment surgery, or the surgery may become medically contraindicated. Even among patients of surgeons who are strong proponents of reassessment surgery, the percentage of patients not reassessed is typically greater than 15%. These missing evaluations can significantly undermine the interpretability of the study.

In summary, the ideal primary end point provides valid and reliable evidence about the intervention's impact on the disease. It is, itself, either clinically relevant to the patient, or a validated surrogate of a clinically relevant outcome. It should be convenient and cost-effective to measure. Unfortunately, in some trials, these features are not always available simultaneously. If a surrogate end point is used, then its validity should be established, not presumed.

Eligibility Criteria

The eligibility criteria serve two purposes in a clinical trial. The immediate purpose is to define those patients with a particular disease, clinical history, and personal and medical characteristics who may be considered for enrollment. The subsequent purpose of eligibility criteria is typically evident after the clinical trial is completed and the results are available. At this time physicians need to carefully consider to whom the results apply. Therefore, during study development, investigators should be cognizant of the generalizability of any results that are ultimately reported. A potentially useful approach for determining the necessity of a particular eligibility criterion is to clearly identify its function. In addition to defining the target population, there are four distinct functions that an eligibility criterion may serve: benefit-morbidity equipoise (safety), homogeneity of benefit (scientific), logistics and regulatory compliance (19).

Ideally, each patient who meets the eligibility criteria of a clinical trial would be asked to participate. However, this is seldom possible for multiple reasons. **Figure 16.1** displays common restrictions that can limit the entry of patients to a clinical trial. In particular, restricted access to the study may contribute to distorted sampling from the target population, which is called selection bias. For example, participating investigators at university hospitals might tend to enroll disproportionately more patients with cancer who have undergone more aggressive initial cytoreductive surgeries than their counterparts at community hospitals.

Eligibility criteria applied for safety are in place to eliminate patients for whom the risk of adverse effects from treatment is not commensurate with the potential for benefit. An example of this may be to restrict eligibility to patients with normal organ function based on concern that a trial therapeutic may be too toxic in such

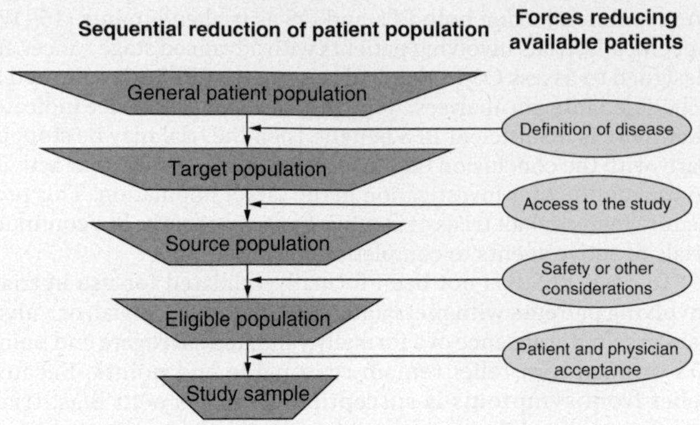

Figure 16.1. Sequential reduction of patient population.

patients. Eligibility criteria may also be warranted when there is a scientific or biologic rationale for a variation in treatment benefit across patient subgroups, particularly if the effect of a new therapy may be expected to be dramatically inconsistent across the entire spectrum of the target population, so much so that statistical power can be compromised (19). One example of this type of exclusion criterion is found in GOG Protocol 152 (A Phase 3 Randomized Study of Cisplatin [NSC#119875] and Taxol [Paclitaxel][NSC#125973] with Interval Secondary Cytoreduction versus Cisplatin and Paclitaxel in Patients with Suboptimal Stage III & IV Epithelial Ovarian Carcinoma). This study was designed to assess the value of secondary cytoreductive surgery in patients with Stage III ovarian cancer. All patients entered into this study were to receive three courses of cisplatin and paclitaxel. After completing this therapy they were then randomized to either three additional courses of chemotherapy or interval secondary cytoreductive surgery followed by three additional courses of chemotherapy. The eligibility criteria excluded patients who had only microscopic residual disease following their primary cytoreductive surgery, because there is no scientific reason to expect that interval cytoreduction would be of any value to patients with no gross residual disease. In addition, the desire to accrue a study population with homogeneous prognosis is a common reason for eligibility criteria. In fact, eligibility criteria should be as broad as possible to enhance generalizability.

Eligibility criteria based on regulatory considerations include those institutional and governmental regulations that require a signed and witnessed informed consent and study approval by the local Institutional Review Board. These restrictions are required in most research settings and are not subject to the investigator's discretion. Finally, they can be justified by logistic considerations. For example, a study that requires frequent clinic visits for proper evaluation or toxicity monitoring may restrict patients who are unable to arrange reliable transportation. The potential problem with such a restriction is how it is structured. A criterion requiring that the patient have a car at her disposal is probably too restrictive, because some patients from resource-poor areas may not have access to private transportation. Such a restriction tends to erode the generalizability of the trial by oversampling from resource-rich communities.

Many biostatisticians believe that eligibility criteria in oncology trials tend to be too restrictive and complicated (19,20). Overly restrictive or complex eligibility criteria hamper accrual, prolong the study's duration, and delay the reporting of results, and therefore should be avoided. The Medical Research Council has demonstrated that it is possible to conduct trials with simple and few eligibility criteria (21). As an example, the International Collaborative Ovarian Neoplasms (ICON 3) trial compared standard carboplatin or cisplatin–adriamycin–cyclophosphamide regimen to paclitaxel plus carboplatin in women with newly diagnosed ovarian cancer. This trial employed only six eligibility criteria, three of which were for safety (fit to receive chemotherapy, absence of sepsis, and bilirubin less than twice the normal level). This was in sharp contrast to GOG Protocol 162 (A Phase 3 Randomized Trial of Cisplatin (NSC #119875) with Paclitaxel (NSC #125973) Administered by Either 24-Hour Infusion or 96-Hour Infusion in Patients with Selected Stage III and Stage IV Epithelial Ovarian Cancer), which had 34 eligibility criteria.

PHASES OF THERAPEUTIC INTERVENTION TRIALS

The traditional approach to identifying and evaluating new drugs has relied on sequential evidence from phase 1, 2, and 3 clinical trials. Each of these study designs stem from very distinct study objectives. Phase 2 trials build on the evidence gathered from phase 1 trial results, and similarly phase 3 trials build on phase 2 and phase 1 trial results. The investigation of a given treatment may be halted at any phase, due to safety and/or efficacy issues. Depending upon the underlying investigation, the time from the initiation of a phase 1 trial for a given treatment to the completion of a phase 3 trial often spans several years. Trials can also include multiple phases. Although this may cut down on the overall duration as compared to developing and running individual trials, additional upfront development time is increased, with no guarantee that the additional phases will ever complete.

Phase 1 Trials

The purpose of a phase 1 trial is to determine an acceptable dose or schedule for a new therapy as determined by toxicity and/or pharmacokinetics. Because of the limited number of patients involved in phase 1 trials, outcome measures such as response and survival are not the primary interests in these studies. In general, the phase 1 trial marks the first use of a new experimental agent in humans. Most escalate dose or schedule of the new agent either after a prespecified number of consecutive patients have been successfully treated or within an individual as each dose is determined to be tolerable.

The usual phase 1 trial of a cytotoxic agent attempts to balance the delivery of the greatest dose intensity against an acceptable risk of dose-limiting toxicity (DLT). The conventional approach is to increase the dose of the new agent after demonstrating that a small cohort of consecutive patients (three to six) was able to tolerate the regimen. However, once an unacceptable level of toxicity occurs (e.g., two or three patients experiencing DLT), the previously acceptable dose level is used to treat additional patients to provide further evidence that the current dose has an acceptable risk of DLT. If this dose is regarded as acceptable, it is called the recommended dose level (RDL) for further development. The RDL should not be confused with the maximum tolerated dose (MTD). The MTD is a theoretical concept used to design phase 1 trials, whereas the RDL is an *estimate* of the MTD, and may or may not be accurate.

Alternative strategies for estimating the MTD have been proposed. The primary motivation for these newer strategies is to reduce the number of patients treated at therapeutically inferior doses and to reduce the overall size of the study. One of these alternatives implements a Bayesian approach and is referred to as the continual reassessment method (CRM) (22). It has the attractive feature of determining the dose level for the next patient based on statistical modeling of the toxicity experience of previously treated patients. While the traditional approach has been criticized for treating too many patients at subtherapeutic doses and providing unreliable estimates of the MTD, CRM has been criticized for tending to treat too many patients at doses higher than the MTD (23). Refinements to CRM have been proposed (24) and found to have good properties compared to alternative dose-seeking strategies (25).

Another family of designs termed the accelerated titration design (ATD) allows doses to be escalated within each patient and incorporates toxicity or pharmacologic information from each course of therapy into the decision regarding whether or not to pursue further escalation (26). Both the modified-CRM and ATD designs can provide significant advantages over the conventional phase 1 design. Finally, phase I studies to identify doses for combinations of agents may require the consideration of potential pharmacokinetic or pharmacodynamic interactions (27).

Other phase I study designs are often utilized for trials involving precision therapies. These studies often incorporate a biomarker end point that signals either the activation or deactivation of a targeted pathway. As the dose is increased for small cohorts of individuals, the biomarker is measured and toxicity monitored simultaneously. Then, statistical models are used to determine a safe dose where the targeted pathway is consistently activated or inhibited (28).

Even though the majority of phase 1 trials in cancer research follow what has been described above, alternative phase 1 trials may arise in other settings such as medical device trials, prevention trials, education intervention trials, behavior modification trials, in which the first phase of investigation may actually utilize healthy subjects, such as studies designed to determine the utility of a new educational intervention on smoking cessation. The phase 1 trial may simply be utilized as an approach toward gaining some experience with the intervention prior to moving forward to the next phase of investigation.

Phase 2 Trials

Once a dose and schedule for a new regimen have been determined, the reasonable next step is to seek evidence that the new regimen is worthy of further evaluation in a prespecified patient population. The principle goal of a phase 2 trial is to prospectively quantify the potential efficacy of the new therapy. Because a phase 2 trial treats more patients at the RDL than in a phase 1 trial, it also provides an opportunity to more reliably assess toxicities. A phase 2 trial is often referred to as a screening trial because it attempts to judiciously identify active treatments worthy of further study in much the same way a clinician screens patients for possibly a more extensive disease evaluation. The study should have adequate sensitivity to detect active treatments and adequate specificity for rejecting inactive treatments. A phase 2 trial may evaluate a single new treatment or incorporate randomization to evaluate several new therapies or treatment schedules simultaneously.

Traditionally, phase 2 trials have been designed as a single-arm trial, but the randomized phase 2 trial has been utilized with increasing frequency. However, investigators should consider several factors when designing the phase 2 trial as a single-arm or a multi-arm randomized trial. While the required sample size is smaller for the single-arm trial, strong and sometimes unwarranted assumptions are required in the design (29). Single-arm trials assume that the probability of response to standard treatment in the target population is known with certainty, which is often suspect, because of unanticipated or unknown differences between the study sample and historical sample(s). For instance, there may be differences in the patients' prognoses unintentionally introduced by the study's eligibility criteria or changes in patient referral patterns. Differences in the response assessment schedule, the modalities for evaluation, or the definition of response may change over time and therefore distort comparisons with historical results. Therefore, whenever possible, we prefer the randomized controlled phase 2 design of a novel agent against an accepted standard treatment. However, when the probability of response to standard treatment is widely accepted to be very low (e.g., $<5\%$), a single-arm trial makes sense.

Phase 2 trials can have a single-stage or a multistage design. In a single-stage design, a fixed number of patients are treated with the new therapy. The goal of the single-stage design is to achieve a predetermined level of precision in estimating the end point. Although precision is one important goal in cancer trials, investigators and trial experts aim to reduce the number of patients exposed to inferior (or inactive) therapies. For this reason, many phase 2 cancer trials use multistage designs. Multistage designs implement planned interim analyses of the data and apply predetermined rules to assess whether there is sufficient evidence to warrant continuing the trial. These rules are in place to stop accrual in trials with regimens having less than the desired activity while allowing regimens having at least a minimally acceptable level of activity to proceed to completion. Two-stage designs that minimize the expected sample size when the new treatment has a clinically uninteresting level of activity have been proposed for single-arm studies (30) and multi-arm studies (31). In the cooperative group setting there is often a need for flexibility in specifying exactly when the interim analysis will occur. This is because of the significant administrative and logistic overhead of coordinating the study in several clinics. Therefore, designs that do not require the interim analyses to occur after a precise number of patients are entered are useful particularly in the multi-institutional setting (32).

Regardless of the measure of treatment efficacy, toxicity is a secondary end point in phase 2 trials. This approach is not likely to be appropriate in phase 2 trials of very aggressive treatments in which stopping rules may explicitly consider both response and the cumulative incidence of certain toxicities (33–35). Bayesian designs that permit continuous monitoring of both toxicity and response have also been proposed (36). Other designs account for simultaneous assessment of two outcomes (e.g., response rate and survival), also referred to as a bivariate outcome (37).

The approach to clinical trials utilizing biomarker-driven selection and molecularly targeted therapies is discussed below.

Phase 3 Trials

The goal of a phase 3 trial is to prospectively and definitively determine the effects of a new therapy relative to a standard therapy in a well-defined patient population. Phase 3 trials are also used to determine an acceptable standard therapy when there is no prior consensus on the appropriate standard therapy. It is useful to distinguish phase 3 objectives as having an efficacy, equivalency, or non-inferiority design consideration. An **efficacy** design is characterized by the search for an intervention strategy that provides a therapeutic advantage over the current standard of care. An **equivalency** trial seeks to demonstrate that two interventions can be considered sufficiently similar on the basis of outcome such that one can be reasonably substituted for the other. **Non-inferiority** trials seek to identify new treatments that reduce toxicity, patient inconvenience, or treatment costs without significantly compromising efficacy.

Efficacy Trials

From the outset of efficacy trials, it is recognized that the benefit of a novel treatment (which is being evaluated) may be accompanied by an increased risk of toxicity, inconvenience, or financial cost, when compared to the standard of care. However, it is hoped that the benefits will be sufficiently large to offset these drawbacks. This is illustrated in **Figure 16.2**. Suppose treatment A is the standard of care for a particular target disease population. The quantitative *difference in efficacy* between treatments with respect to a particular outcome (B-A) can be described on a horizontal axis as in **Figure 16.2**. If we are reasonably certain that the difference between treatments is less than zero (left of 0), then we would consider treatment A to be better. On the other hand, if the treatment difference is greater than zero (right of 0), then we would conclude that the new treatment, B, is better. Furthermore, we can use dotted lines on this graph to demarcate a region in which the difference between A and B is small enough to warrant no clinical preference for A or B. Consider the results from a trial expressed as the estimated *difference between treatments* and the corresponding 95% or 99% confidence interval (CI) superimposed on this graph. The CI depicts those values of the treatment difference that can be reasonably considered consistent with the data from the trial. When the CIs are sufficiently broad that the data cannot distinguish between the treatments being tested, the trial is determined to be inconclusive (**Fig. 16.2**). This is a typical consequence of a small trial. On the other hand, if the CI entirely excludes the region where treatment A is better than treatment B, then we can conclude that treatment B is significantly better than treatment A (**Fig. 16.2**). Note that in this case the lower bound of

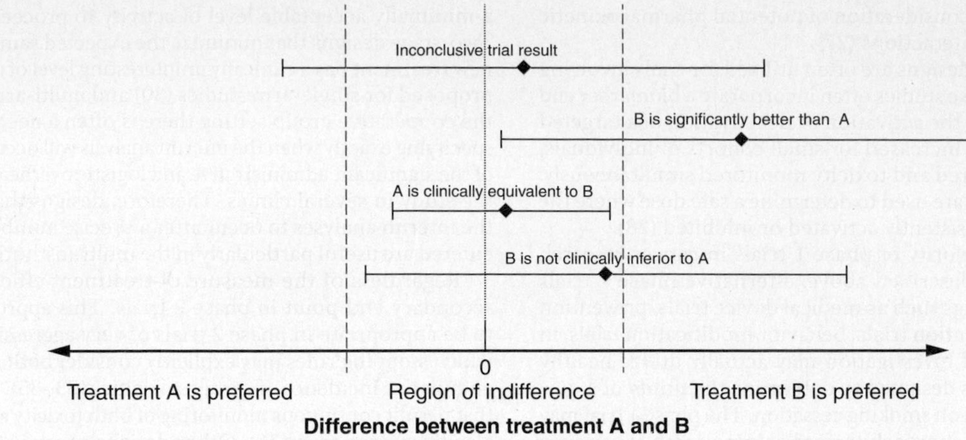

Figure 16.2. Graphical representation of the point estimates and confidence intervals describing the *difference* in efficacy between the standard treatment **(A)** and a new experimental regimen **(B)** from five hypothetical trials.

the CI may extend into the region of clinical indifference, but the CI must exclude the region below (left of) 0 difference.

When an efficacy trial fails to demonstrate that a new experimental regimen is statistically superior to the control regimen, this should not be interpreted as demonstrating that these regimens are equally effective. Even though the estimated difference between two treatments may be near zero, the CI may not rule out treatment differences that are clinically relevant. Therefore, we advocate cautious interpretation from efficacy studies that conclude "therapeutic equivalency" when only a small difference between treatments with regard to the outcome is observed. Careful inspection of the CIs, such as those in **Figure 16.2**, is appropriate, as well as where one personally considers where the region of clinical indifference is located.

Equivalency Trials

The equivalency study design is perhaps a misnomer, because it is impractical to generate enough data from any trial to definitively claim that the two treatments are equivalent. Instead, an investigator typically defines the limits for treatment differences that can be interpreted as clinically irrelevant. If it is a matter of opinion for what differences in effect sizes can be considered clinically irrelevant, this issue can become a major source of controversy in the final interpretation of the trial results. Bioequivalency designs are occasionally conducted to demonstrate that two treatments exert similar influence on the expression of a biomarker. In this case, an investigator should have some notion about the acceptable range of biomarker expression that can be considered clinically equivalent. These studies are designed so that, within tolerable limits, the treatments can be considered as having similar biologic effects.

Non-inferiority Trials

A non-inferiority study design may be considered when the currently accepted standard treatment is associated with significant toxicity and a new and less toxic treatment becomes available. The goal of this type of study is to demonstrate that substituting the new treatment for the current standard treatment does not compromise efficacy appreciably (38–41). Referring to **Figure 16.2**, the trial seeks to provide sufficient evidence to be reasonably certain that the difference between A and B lies above the lower boundary of the indifference region. This lower boundary is often called the "non-inferiority margin." If the CI for the difference in efficacy fails to exclude the region where the standard regimen, A, is preferred, then there is insufficient evidence to conclude that the new regimen is not inferior to standard treatment.

The justification for the non-inferiority margin selected in a particular study is often controversial. If this margin is set too low, then the study has an unacceptably high probability of recommending an inferior treatment. If it is too high, then the trial utilizes too many clinical and financial resources. To select an appropriate margin of non-inferiority it is important to recognize that even though a non-inferiority trial may explicitly compare only two treatments, implicitly there is a third treatment to be considered. For example, suppose that several historical studies indicate that treatment A is better than a placebo for treating a specific disease. In this case, the goal of a non-inferiority study is to demonstrate that a new experimental treatment, B, does not significantly compromise efficacy when compared to the currently accepted active standard treatment, A. However, it should also demonstrate that B would have been better than a placebo, if a placebo had been included in the current trial. In other words, the current trial will directly estimate the effectiveness of B relative to A, but it must also indirectly consider the effectiveness of B relative to the previous control treatment (placebo in this case). This indirect comparison relies on obtaining a reliable and unbiased estimate of the effectiveness of the current active control to the previous control from previous trials.

Sometimes the margin of non-inferiority is expressed as a proportion of the effectiveness of A relative to the previous standard treatment. For example, a non-inferiority study could be designed to have a high probability of concluding that a new treatment retains at least 50% of the activity of the standard regimen, A. Note that an investigator may wish to be highly confident that none of the efficacious benefits of the current standard treatment be sacrificed. In this case, the margin of non-inferiority is set at 0 (**Fig. 16.2**) and the design is the same as the efficacy trial. Indeed, an efficacy trial can be considered a study in which the investigator is willing to accept the new treatment B, only if the trial results indicate that B is statistically superior to A.

Obtaining reliable estimates for the activity of the currently accepted active standard treatment can be a very troublesome aspect of non-inferiority oncology trials. For example, cisplatin 75 mg/m^2 and paclitaxel 135 mg/m^2 infused over 24 hours was the first platinum–taxane combination to demonstrate activity in the treatment of advanced ovarian cancer (42). Subsequently, several trials were conducted to assesses whether carboplatin could be safely substituted for cisplatin (43–45) or whether Taxotere could be substituted for paclitaxel (46). However, there has been some controversy about the amount of benefit provided by paclitaxel (47). An investigator can reasonably ask: "what is the effect size of paclitaxel and how much of this effect can I be reasonably certain is preserved by Taxotere?"

Randomized Trials

There are several design features to consider when developing a phase 3 trial concept. One important feature to consider is treatment randomization. The randomized clinical trial (RCT) has several scientific advantages. First, both the known and unknown prognostic factors tend to be distributed similarly across the treatment groups when a trial implements randomized treatments. Second, a potential source of differential selection bias is eliminated. This bias could occur when there is an association between treatment choice and prognosis—it need not be intentional. When a physician's interest in a trial or a patient's decision to participate in the trial depends on the assigned treatment, a nonrandom association between treatment and prognosis can be introduced. Finally, randomization provides the theoretical underpinning for the significance test (48). In other words, the probability of a false-positive trial as stated in the study design is justified with randomization. It is important to recognize that the advantages provided by randomizing the study treatments are forfeited when all of the randomized patients are not included in the final analyses.

It is sometimes argued that because many factors influencing prognosis are known, perhaps other approaches to allocating treatments can be considered, and statistical models used to adjust for any imbalances in prognosis. However, the conclusions from this type of trial must be based on the completeness of knowledge about the disease and acceptability of the modeling assumptions. If the disease is moderately unpredictable with regard to the outcome, or the statistical model is inappropriate, then the conclusions are suspect.

Kunz and Oxman (49) have compared the results from overviews of randomized and nonrandomized clinical trials that evaluated the same intervention, and reported that nonrandomized studies tended to overestimate the treatment effect compared to randomized trials by 76% to 160%. Schulz et al. (50) compared 33 randomized controlled trials that had inadequate concealment of the random treatment assignments, to those studies that had adequate concealment. They found that even those with inadequate concealment tended to overestimate the treatment effect (relative odds) by 40%. Some investigators do not appreciate the importance of concealment and will go to considerable lengths to subvert it (51). When the randomization technique requires pre-generated random treatment assignments, one must guarantee that the investigators, who are enrolling patients, do not have access to the assignment lists.

It should be acknowledged that the patient–physician relationship can occasionally be challenged by introducing the concept of treatment randomization (52). Patients may prefer a sense of confidence from their physician regarding the "best" therapy for them. However, physicians involved in an RCT must honestly acknowledge that the best therapy is unknown and that an RCT is preferable to continued ignorance. One survey of 600 women seen in a breast clinic suggests that 90% of women prefer their doctor to admit uncertainty about the best treatment option, rather than give them false hope (53).

Randomization Techniques. The simplest approach to randomization is to assign treatments based on a coin flip, sequential digits from random number tables, or computerized pseudorandom number generators. On average, each individual has a defined probability of being allocated to a particular study treatment, when they enter the study. While this approach is simple, the statistical efficiency of the analyses can be enhanced by constraining the randomization so that each treatment is allocated an equal number of times. Permuted block randomization is sometimes used to promote equal treatment group sizes. A block can be created by shuffling a fixed number of cards for each treatment and then assigning the patients according to the random order of the deck. After completing each block there are an equal number of patients assigned to the treatment groups. For example, consider a trial comparing treatments A and B. There are six possible ways the block can be ordered when the block size is four: AABB, ABBA, BBAA, BABA, ABAB, and BAAB. A sufficient number of assignments for an RCT can be created by randomly selecting a series of blocks from the six distinct possibilities.

There are three features of blocked randomization to be considered. First, the probability of a particular treatment being allocated is not the same throughout the study, as in simple randomization. Taking the example above, every fourth treatment is predetermined by the previous three allocations. Second, the use of small blocks in a single-clinic study may undermine concealment and allow an investigator to deduce the next treatment. This potential problem can be corrected by continually changing the block size throughout the assignment list. Third, large block sizes can undermine the benefits of blocking. As block sizes increase, the procedure resembles simple randomization.

The statistical efficiency of the study can be further enhanced by stratifying patients into groups with similar prognoses and using separate lists of blocked treatments for each stratum. This procedure is called stratified permuted block randomization. It is worth noting that using simple randomization within stratum would defeat the purpose of stratification, because this is equivalent to using simple randomization for all patients. Likewise, trials that stratify on too many prognostic factors are likely to have many uncompleted treatment blocks at the end of the study, which also defeats the intent of blocking (54).

When it is desirable to balance more than a few prognostic factors, an alternative is dynamic treatment allocation; one particular type being minimization. Whereas stratified block randomization will balance treatment assignments within each combination of the various factor levels, minimization tends to balance treatments within each level of the factor, separately. Each time a new patient is entered into the study, the number of individuals who share any of the prognostic characteristics of the new patient is tabulated. A metric, which measures the imbalance of these factors among the study treatments, is computed as if the new patients were allocated to each of the study treatments in turn. The patient is then allocated to the treatment that would favor the greatest degree of balance (55). In the event that the procedure indicates equal preference for two or more possible treatment allocations, simple randomization can be used to determine the individual's treatment assignment. Regardless of the degree of imbalance, however, this randomization process should not be deterministic. Instead, the treatments that restore the greatest degree of balance are more likely to be allocated.

Concealment during the randomization process refers to the procedure in which the assigned study treatment is not revealed to the patient or the investigator until after the subject has successfully enrolled onto the study. The purpose of concealment is to eliminate a bias that can arise from an individual's decision to participate in the study depending on the treatment assignment (56). Concealment is an essential component of RCTs.

Blinding is a procedure that prevents the patient or physician from knowing which treatment is being used. In a single-blinded study, the patient is unaware of which study treatments she is receiving. A double-blinded study results in a situation in which neither the patient nor the health care provider is aware of that information. One purpose of blinding is to avoid measurement bias, particularly differential measurement bias (see End Points section). This type of bias occurs when the value of a measurement is influenced by the knowledge of the treatment being received. It can occur when the measurement of an end point is in part or totally subjective. Most methods for assessing pain are subjective, and require treatment blinding to promote the study's validity.

Oncology trials frequently do not implement blinding for several reasons. It is rather difficult to blind treatments when various treatment modalities are used (e.g., surgery versus radiation therapy, or intravenous versus oral administrations), when good medical practice is jeopardized (e.g., special tests are required to monitor toxicity due to particular treatments), or when it is logistically difficult (e.g., the evaluating physician must be kept isolated from the treatment of patient). In the absence of blinding, care should be taken that the method of measuring the end point is precisely stated in the protocol and consistently applied to each patient uniformly. Trials that assess quality of life or relief from symptoms should give serious consideration to treatment blinding. Schulz et al. (57) have reviewed 110 RCTs published between 1990 and 1991 from four journals dedicated to obstetrics and gynecology. Thirty-one of these trials reported being double-blinded. Schultz et al. conclude that blinding should have been used more often, despite frequent impediments. Moreover, blinding seemed to have been compromised in at least three of the trials where it was implemented.

Placebos blind the patient, and usually the physician as well, as to whether they are receiving an experimental or inert treatment. Placebos are frequently used in trials where there is no accepted standard treatment and the end point is susceptible to measurement bias. The use of a placebo is also important when the end point can be affected by the patient's psychological response to the knowledge of receiving therapy, combined with a belief that the therapy is effective. This phenomenon is aptly named the "placebo effect." In such circumstances, the use of a placebo provides a treatment-to-control comparison that measures only the therapeutic effect. Note that the "placebo effect" is a distinctly different type of measurement bias from those that have been previously discussed. Careful ethical considerations must precede the use of a placebo or sham procedure in any clinical trial (58).

Trials with Historical Controls

The strict definition of a phase 3 trial does not necessarily require concurrent controls (i.e., prospectively enrolled patients assigned the standard treatment) or randomization (i.e., random treatment allocation). However, these two features are almost synonymous with phase 3 trials today.

The principal drawback from inferring treatment differences from a historically controlled trial is that the treatment groups may differ in a variety of characteristics that are not apparent. Differences in outcome, which are in fact due to differences in characteristics between the groups, may be erroneously attributed to the treatment. Although statistical models are often used to adjust for some potential biases, adjustments are possible only for factors that have been recorded accurately and consistently from both samples. Shifts in medical practice over time, differences in the definition of the disease, eligibility criteria, follow-up procedures, or recording methods can all contribute to a differential bias. Unlike random error, this type of error cannot be reduced by increasing the sample size. Moreover, the undesirable consequences of moderate biases may be exacerbated with larger sample sizes. When a trial includes *concurrent* controls, the definition of disease and the eligibility criteria can be applied consistently to both treatment groups. Also, the standard procedures for measuring the end point can be uniformly applied to all patients.

Factorial Designs

Factorial designs are used when several interventions are to be studied simultaneously. The term *factorial* arises from historical terminology in which the treatments were referred to as factors. Each factor has corresponding levels; for example, an investigator may wish to compare a study agent administered at three dose levels: high dose, medium dose, and none. The total number of factor combinations being studied is the product of the number of levels for each factor or treatment. For example, a trial that evaluates treatment A at three levels and treatment B at two levels is called a 3-by-2 (denoted 3×2) factorial design. If the relative effects due to the various levels of treatment A are independent of the levels of B, the two treatments (A and B) can be evaluated simultaneously. The factorial design provides a significant reduction in the required sample size when compared to trials that study A and B separately. The key assumption necessary for a factorial design is that all treatments can be given simultaneously, without interaction or interference.

The most commonly utilized factorial design is the 2×2 factorial design that includes two distinct treatment regimens at each of two factor levels. For example, suppose individuals entering a cancer prevention trial are randomly assigned to receive vitamin E (placebo-A or 50 mg/day) and beta carotene (placebo-B or 20mg/day) in a study designed as a 2×2 factorial. In this case, the factors are vitamin E and beta carotene, whereas the respective factor levels are placebo-A or 50 mg/day for vitamin E, and placebo-B or 20 mg/day for beta carotene. There are four treatment combinations. In a standard 2×2 design, the main effect of vitamin E can be ascertained by utilizing information from each of the four treatment groups. In some studies, however, the main effects may be of secondary importance compared to the "interaction" between each factor. An interaction exists when the effect due to one of the factors (i.e., treatment A) depends on the level of the other factor (treatment B). In drug discovery, a "positive" interaction may imply a synergistic effect of two drugs in combination; that is, the effect of the combination therapy is greater than the sum of the individual additive effects. Reliable tests of an interaction require a relatively large number of patients in each of the four treatment groups. If potential treatment interaction cannot reasonably be ruled out or there is interest in possible interactions, then attention to the statistical power of such tests is an important part of designing and interpreting the study results (59).

HYPOTHESIS TEST

A hypothesis is a conjecture based on prior experiences that leads to refutable predictions (60). A hypothesis is frequently framed in the context of either a null or an alternative hypothesis. In a therapeutic efficacy trial, a null hypothesis may postulate that a treatment does not influence patients' outcome. The alternative hypothesis is that a particular, well-defined treatment approach will influence the patients' outcome to a prespecified degree. These hypotheses cast the purpose of the trial into a clear framework. During the study design, the investigators select a test statistic from an appropriate statistical procedure (e.g., an F-statistic from an analysis of variance, or a chi-square statistic from a logistic model) that evaluates the degree to which the study data support the null hypothesis. A type I error is committed when the null hypothesis is in fact true, but the test statistic leads the investigator to incorrectly conclude it is false. Committing the type I error would be disastrous if it means discontinuing the use of an active control treatment that is well tolerated and substituting an experimental therapy that is more toxic, but in reality, no better. A type II error is committed when the null hypothesis is not true, but the test statistic lead the investigator to erroneously conclude that it is true. Type II errors commonly occur in studies that involve too few subjects to reliably estimate clinically important treatment effects. Prospectively specifying the null hypothesis, the appropriate statistical method for the analysis, the test statistic, and quantifying the acceptable probabilities of type I error (i.e., α-level) and type II error are essential elements for determining the appropriate design and sample size for a particular trial.

p-Value

At times statisticians play the role of the conservative physician, cautiously prescribing a significance test only when it is appropriate. There is a general concern that the *p*-value is overused, even abused, and overemphasized. A common misconception is that the *p*-value is the probability that the null hypothesis is true. The null hypothesis is either true or false, and so it is therefore not subject to a probability statement. It is the inference that an investigator makes, based on his data, that is susceptible to error. The *p*-value is simply the probability that the test statistic would be as extreme or even more extreme, if the null hypothesis was in fact true (see Hypothesis Test section).

Misconceptions about the *p*-value may arise in part from a poor distinction between the *p*-value and the α-level of a study (61). The α-level is the probability of the test statistic rejecting the null hypothesis when it is true. It is specified during the design phase of the study, and is unaltered by the results obtained. The *p*-value results from a statistical test performed on the observed data.

TRANSLATIONAL RESEARCH

Many modern clinical trials involve the systematic collection and banking of biologic materials from the participants. These materials may include serum, plasma, urine, buccal cells, or tumor tissue, which are collected and stored in a biorepository. The biologic materials together with the clinical data can then be used to understand how a biologic effect translates into the treatment effect on the patient population. This translation gives rise to the concept of translational research (TR). In TR, discoveries in laboratory science are translated into practical applications. The flow of information from TR studies is a two-way street: (1) more complete understanding of tumor biology and (2) more effective treatments for patients.

The goal in this section is to provide clinical and laboratory scientists with some fundamental information needed to design, implement, and analyze the data from TR studies. The following sections develop the concepts for: (1) biomarker discovery and verification, and (2) biomarker validation. Insights are provided into the goals and expectations a researcher can have when performing a biomarker study. With this knowledge at hand, the reader can avoid some of the mistakes, errors, and biases that have plagued TR and have led to false, misreported, or misleading reports.

It is important to understand that biomarkers can be used to diagnose a disease, to assess prognosis, to select appropriate treatments (predictive), or to assess treatment outcomes (surrogate end point). Thus, biomarkers can be incorporated into many aspects of clinical practice and research once validated. There are two types of biomarker validation to consider: analytic and clinical validation. Analytic validation refers to obtaining evidence that the biomarker assay result is reproducible under a variety of conditions and that the assay is shown to accurately measure the intended analyte. This is essential before a biomarker can be clinically validated. Clinical validation involves demonstrating that the biomarker is "fit for purpose." That is, it functions properly for its intended use as a diagnostic, prognostic, treatment selective, or surrogate marker. The rigor needed to evaluate the clinical utility of a biomarker has recently been emphasized in light of several failed attempts at validating complex biomarkers (62–64).

Biospecimen Collection

The biologic specimens used in a study are typically gathered either prospectively or retrospectively. In the prospective approach, patients are identified and followed forward in time. There are several advantages with the prospective approach. First, patient enrollment can focus on enrolling individuals only from the intended target population. Second, the procedures for collecting and preparing specimens can be tailored to the intended laboratory procedures. Third, the quality control procedures for collecting the clinical data can target those data items that are required for the specific study objectives. Fourth, the patient's treatment and follow-up assessments can be standardized and optimized in accordance with the goals of the study. When samples are retrospectively collected, the laboratory analysis is performed using previously archived specimens that may have been originally collected for another intended purpose. The investigator using a retrospective approach is a prisoner to the procedures that were set down before the current study goals were contemplated; therefore, they may not be optimal for his or her intended objectives. For instance, the samples may have come from patients who are not representative of the target population. This reduces the validity of the study results. The specimens may have been obtained, prepared, or stored using outdated or less-than-optimal procedures for laboratory tests. This could introduce biases in the measurements or reduce the power of the study.

Biomarker Development Process

A widely used definition of a biomarker is: "A characteristic that is objectively measured and evaluated as an indicator of normal biological processes, pathogenic processes, or pharmacologic responses to an intervention" (65). Biomarkers can be measurements of macromolecules (DNA, RNA, proteins, lipids), cells, or processes that describe a normal or abnormal biologic state in a patient. From the paradigm of TR described above, biomarkers can inform investigators about a patient's disease diagnosis, prognosis, prediction of response to therapy (i.e., effect modifier), or prediction of a clinical outcome (i.e., surrogate end point).

Generally speaking, biomarkers can be diagnostic, prognostic, or predictive. A diagnostic biomarker is designed to identify the presence of a disease or other condition, while a prognostic biomarker is an indicator that helps researchers in predicting the course of a patient's disease. Prognostic biomarkers are used to estimate the risk of a future clinical outcome; examples include: state of the disease, histology of the tumor, or patient's performance status. A biomarker may also be deemed predictive, and as such, it can be used to modify the estimated risk of a future outcome only when a particular type of treatment is taken. In breast cancer patients, examples of predictive biomarkers are: estrogen receptor status when the treatment is tamoxifen, or HER2/neu status when the treatment is trastuzumab. The phrase "treatment selection marker" may be preferable terminology for a predictive biomarker, to avoid confusion with other uses of the word predictive. For immediate purposes here, predictive markers are viewed as a special class of prognostic markers and we primarily focus on prognostic biomarker studies in general. Only in the section describing studies involving targeted therapies will the distinction be made.

In the following sections, a common biomarker development strategy is discussed that includes: (1) Biomarker discovery, and (2) Biomarker validation. In short, these steps are presented in **Table 16.1** (Discovery and Test Validation Stage) (66).

Discovery Phase

Regardless of whether the samples were retrospectively or prospectively collected, many studies are designed to discover biomarkers with clinical utility, from among many potentially useful biomarkers.

Since the invention of microarray technology and related high-throughput (HT) technologies, researchers have been able to compile large amounts of information and an enormous pool of potential biomarkers. These so-called HT platforms have become commonly used experimental platforms in the biologic realm (67). A HT platform is designed to measure large numbers (thousands or millions) of signatures in a biologic organism at a given time point. These platforms are a function of the postgenomic era and are often used to determine how genomic expression is regulated or involved in biologic processes. The technologies in **Table 16.2** use hybridization and sequence-based platforms such as gene expression microarrays and RNA-Seq to obtain data matrices.

TABLE 16.1. Biomarker Development for HT Technologies

Classifier Development Phase
- **Probe Discovery:** Identify a subset of genes/proteins associated with the clinical outcome of interest.
- **Probe Verification:** Confirm measurements on selected genes/proteins using alternate laboratory techniques, like IHC or Rt-PCR.
- **Classifier Development:** Use the confirmed genes/proteins to develop a model (classifier) that appears to predict clinical outcome.

Classifier Verification Phase
- **Model Verification:** Confirm the model's properties using a small independent sample of individuals or cross-classification techniques.
- **Document Classifier:** Document the computational procedures and criteria for interpreting the lockdown model.

Classifier Validation
- **Validation:** Evaluate the model's predictive accuracy in a sample of individuals representative of the target population. Any changes to the procedures or the lockdown model to improve the classifier will require further validation.

For additional information, see National Research Council. *Evolution of Translational Omics: Lessons Learned and the Path Forward.* Washington, DC: The National Academies Press, 2012.

■ TABLE 16.2. A Summary of Discovery Platforms, the Material Analyzed in the Platform, and the Recent Cancer Biomarker Discovery Studies using the Given Platform

Platform	Material	Cancer studies
aCGH microarray	DNA	Albertson et al. (68), Hodgson et al. (69), Pollack et al. (70), Albertson (71), Albertson et al. (72), Hackett et al. (73), Garnis et al. (74), Veltman et al. (75), Pinkel and Albertson (76), Rossi et al. (77), Idbaih et al. (78)
Gene expression microarray	mRNA	Ramaswamy et al. (79), Gordon et al. (80), Tibshirani et al. (81), Statnikov et al. (82), Glas et al. (83), Van't Veer et al. (84), Sotiriou et al. (85), Michiels et al. (86), Barrier et al. (87), Miecznikowski et al. (88)
RNA – Seq	Transcriptomics	Levin et al. (89), Pflueger et al. (90)
DNA methylation	DNA	Portela and Esteller (91)
Mass spectrometry	Peptide/proteomics	Paweletz et al. (92), Koopmann et al. (93), Kolch et al. (94), Lan et al. (95), Diamandis (96,97)

Several of the common HT assay platforms used in experiments designed for cancer diagnosis are listed in **Table 16.2**. These platforms were chosen to illustrate the diversity of platforms available for interrogating DNA, RNA, or proteins.

Preprocessing HT Platforms

In short, preprocessing algorithms are required in nearly all of the HT technologies listed in **Table 16.2**. This is due to the fact that HT platforms measure both biologic signal and technical signal. Therefore, the goal of preprocessing algorithms is removal of the technical signal. This technical signal can be considered in terms of background correction and normalization to adjust across experiments. The background corrections and normalization account for technical artifacts that can occur due to either the array construction or laboratory procedures that introduce systematic errors in the signal on individual arrays or across arrays. Often these preprocessing techniques are specific to the platform employed (e.g., Miecznikowski et al. [98]), and therefore it is impractical to review all of the available preprocessing methods here.

Type I Error and Multiple Testing

The experiments performed in the HT discovery phase often have a goal of simply narrowing down the genome or proteome to a subset of potentially relevant biomarkers. In this sense, the scientists are performing a data reduction where the goal is to choose a subset of markers from the HT scope that are related to or associated with clinical outcome. The association with outcome is assessed using a null hypothesis for each biomarker and summarizing "significance" with a *p*-value. In this case, the interpretation of each *p*-value differs slightly from a study with a single null hypothesis (See Hypothesis Test and *p*-value sections).

When the type I error is limited to 5% for a single hypothesis, there is only a 1-in-20 chance of rejecting that null hypothesis, if it is in fact true. When 10,000 null hypotheses are tested, as may be typical in some HT studies even if all of the null hypotheses were true, one would expect 500 null hypotheses to be rejected at the 5% significance level. The large number of false rejections would make the downstream analysis of confirmation and verification frustrating and impractical.

Therefore, during the discovery phase of an HT experiment, the goal is to limit the Type I error rate. That is, HT studies are designed to limit the number of false-positives, denoted by V in **Table 16.3A**. **Table 16.3B** lists some alternative approaches to controlling the Type I error rate during the discovery phase of the experiment. Statistically significant or interesting markers are determined from hypothesis testing in light of controlling one of the Type I error rates listed in **Table 16.3B**.

■ TABLE 16.3A. A Summary of Results from Analyzing Multiple Hypothesis Tests

	H_0 Retained	H_0 Rejected	Total
H_0 True	U	V	M_0
H_0 False	T	Q	M_1
	M – R	R	M

M_0 and M_1 are considered as fixed (unknown) parameters representing the number of true nulls and the number of true alternatives, respectively. The random variables U and Q represent the number of the correct decisions, whereas the random variables T and V represent the number of incorrect decisions. V is the number of false-positives.

■ TABLE 16.3B. Summaries of Type I Errors Using Random Variables Defined in Table 16-3A

Abbreviation	Name	Quantity
FWER	Family wise error rate	$Pr(V \geq 1)$
k-FWER	Generalized family wise error rate	$Pr(V \geq k)$
FDR	False discovery rate	E[V/R]
k-FDR	Generalized false discovery rate	$E[VI(V \geq k)/(MAX(R,1))]$
PCER	Per comparison error rate	E[V]/M
TPPFP	Tail probabilities for the proportion of false-positives	$Pr(V/R) > q$

Pr( ), probability of; E[ ], expectation of.

Confirmation and Verification

To have reasonable power in light of multiple testing, the Type I errors in **Table 16.3B** tend to be more liberal (more likely to reject null hypotheses) than standard scientific significance testing procedures. Thus, any markers from the discovery phase should be confirmed or verified using other methods, such as immunohistochemical (IHC) assays or reverse transcription polymerase chain reaction (RT-PCR). These verification platforms could use either the same samples from the discovery phase or a new independent set of samples. The goal for this step is to confirm that the biomarker signal from the discovery platform is accurately measuring the expression of the desired gene, protein, or RNA.

Including a confirmation step ensures researchers that their discovery markers can be confirmed using other platforms. This provides some reassurance in the ability of the markers to be confirmed on independent samples from possibly different institutions with, possibly, differing methods of assessment. Methods that describe how to correlate RT-PCR and IHC signals with their microarray counterparts can be found in Press et al. (99), van den Broek and van de Vijver (100), McShane et al. (101), Esteban et al. (102).

In certain IHC assays, the results should be performed by at least two different observers who are blinded to the clinical data. This may alleviate the subjectivity in these experiments, because IHC assays require selection of best regions to score, and subjective measurements of staining intensity and percentage of stained cells.

Validation Phase

Various statistical models can be fit using the data in the discovery phase. At the end of the discovery phase, there should be a complete specification of the marker assay method and model, and thorough documentation of the (final) lockdown model. The fully specified precise lockdown model will be evaluated using a validation dataset. Note, for example, that this must include specifying all coefficients in the classification model and any of the rules for deciding the level of a biomarker.

Validation in biomarker experiments should always involve an independent dataset, that is, data from patients who were not included in any of the discovery dataset(s). Note that internal validation procedures such as cross-validation, bootstrapping, or other data resampling methods are useful to give insights into issues such as bias and variance of regression parameter estimates and stability of the model derived. In these internal validation procedures, some portion of the data is held out (test set), while a model is built on the remaining portion (training set). A limitation of these internal procedures is that there may be biases that affect the training and test sets equally. For example, if the set of specimens for confirmation are collected in the same laboratory, processed by the same technician, and run on the same equipment, then peculiarities of the data (equipment, lab, and technician) will be shared between the samples used to develop the model and the samples used to evaluate the model.

Even with the requirement of an independent dataset, there may still be levels of validation evidence. For example, a lower level of validation evidence may be independent sets of specimens and clinical data collected at a single institution using carefully controlled protocols, with samples from the same patient population. Meanwhile, a higher level of validation evidence would be independent sets of specimens and clinical data collected at multiple institutions.

Additionally, it should be stressed that the independent validation dataset must be relevant to the intended use of the candidate biomarker test. Patients in the independent dataset should have the same type of disease, the same stage, and should be in the same clinical setting in which the candidate test should be used in the future. Ideally, the specimens for independent confirmation will have been collected at different points in time, at different institutions, from different patient populations, with samples processed in a different laboratory to demonstrate that the test has broad applicability and is not over-fit to any particular situation.

Publicly Available Data

Publicly available datasets can help with the development process; furthermore, they can fill in gaps regarding knowledge of systems biology; for example, providing the proteomics story when an individual investigation generates only genomic data. They can be used in an integrative analysis and a meta-analysis. These meta-analyses can strengthen the conclusions drawn from an individual researcher's study. They may also offer insights from other study populations. As DNA microarray technology has been widely applied to detect gene activity changes in many areas of biomedical research, development and curation of online microarray data repositories are at the forefront of research endeavors to use and reuse this mounting deluge of data. Several representative repositories of microarray datasets are available (**Table 16.4**). A somewhat recent comparison of the available microarray databases was provided in Gardiner-Garden and Littlejohn (106). Computer programs like Anduril (107) provide procedures for organizing, storing, and analyzing massive genomic data. Statistical packages in R have also been created that allow users to easily import data from database like ArrayExpress into Bioconductor packages (108).

TABLE 16.4. Repositories of Microarray Datasets

ArrayExpress (103)	http://www.ebi.ac.uk/arrayexpress/
Gene Expression Omnibus (GEO)(104)	http://www.ncbi.nlm.nih.gov/geo/
Center for Information Biology Gene Expression Database (CIBEX)(105)	http://cibex.nig.ac.jp/data/index.html
TCGA	http://tcga-data.nci.nih.gov/tcga/tcgaHome2.jsp or https://gdc-portal.nci.nih.gov/

Concordant with the development of online data repositories, researchers have developed specific data standards required for microarray analysis. The data standard concept describes the minimum information about a microarray experiment (MIAME) that is needed to enable the interpretation of the results of the experiment and to potentially reproduce the experiment (109). MIAME compliance will ensure that biologic properties of the samples and the phenotypes that were assayed were correctly recorded, thus ensuring that the data can be quickly assessed for its suitability in studying new questions. The public repositories including ArrayExpress (103), GEO (110), and CIBEX (105) are all designed to hold MIAME compliant microarray data.

Especially exciting for oncologists, multiple platforms of microarray data from The Cancer Genome Atlas (TCGA) are now available. The TCGA project is further described in Stratton et al. (111), but, in short, represents one of the first large-scale attempts to study the multiple types of genetic mutations involved in multiple cancer types from different cohorts of patients. Initially, the pilot projects studied glioblastoma multiforme and ovarian serous cystadenocarcinoma, but have now expanded to cover roughly 25 different cancer types. For each cancer type, the patient cohorts (collected from different sites) include several hundred individuals, and the platform techniques include gene expression profiling, copy number variation profiling, single nucleotide polymorphism (SNP) genotyping, methylation profiling, and microRNA profiling. These data have been made publicly available, making TCGA dataset a great resource for research using meta-analysis and integrative analysis techniques that were not previously available.

DEVELOPING TR STUDIES AND REPORTING RESULTS

Guidelines have been developed to promote accurate and complete reporting of results from biomarker studies. Throughout this section, the importance of having well-defined questions for the proposed data is stressed. In other words, serious thought, planning, and discussions among a team of scientists are necessary in order to successfully perform biomarker analysis including discovery, verification, and validation.

In the discovery phase it is important that the proposed technology has been validated; for example, technical replication studies in Strand et al. (112), Callesen et al. (113), Leyland-Jones et al. (114), De Cecco et al. (115), Hicks et al. (116), Benton et al. (117), Freidin et al. (118), Lawrie et al. (119). During the discovery phase, it is also important to consider differences in material preparation; for example, frozen tissue samples versus paraffin-embedded tissues as discussed in Nowak et al. (120), Mittempergher et al. (121). During the verification phase these issues may also play a role; however, other concerns may arise, such as the level of concordance in signal necessary between the discovery platform and the verification platform. Ultimately, after discovery and verification, a lockdown model is carried forth to validation. This so-called lockdown model can be interpreted in a decision theoretic setting; each future sample must be classified or the outcome predicted based only on the model and a given sample signal from the intended technology.

In the validation phase, it is important to note that there is a major difference between answering *a priori* defined hypotheses and providing conclusions from exploratory analyses. Conclusions drawn from exploratory data analysis are descriptive results and typically need to be confirmed in a validation dataset, while an *a priori* hypothesis leads to stronger conclusions and does not necessarily need an external validation. Care should be given in reporting unanticipated significant effects, as these are most likely due to chance and thus unlikely to be validated in other studies. Most importantly, researchers should keep in mind that, in the long term, the success of biomarker studies should be measured by clinical improvement in patient outcomes.

A prodigious number of prodigious number of biomarker studies reported in the literature; however, a surprising number of these results are irreproducible. The reasons for these discrepancies may lie in differences in methodological procedures, inadequate control of false-positive findings, improper validation procedures, variability in the patient sampling, or any number of other differences in study design, conduct, or analytical procedures. Many published studies lack adequate information that would allow an evaluation of quality or comparability. To promote clear and complete reporting of biomarker studies, the REMARK guidelines have been developed (122). These guidelines make specific recommendations for preparing TR presentations, reports, and publications with regard to describing patient and sample characteristics, assay methodology, study design, methods of data analysis, and results. While these recommendations

TABLE 16.5. REporting Recommendations for Tumor MARKer Prognostic Studies (REMARK)

Introduction
1. State the marker examined, the study objectives, and any prespecified hypotheses
Materials and methods
Patients
1. Describe the characteristics (e.g., disease stage or comorbidities) of the study patients, including their source and inclusion and exclusion criteria.
2. Describe treatments received and how they were chosen (e.g., randomized or rule-based).
Specimen characteristics
1. Describe type of biologic material used (including control samples) and methods of preservation and storage.
Assay methods
1. Specify the assay method used and provide (or reference) a detailed protocol, including specific reagents or kits used, quality control procedures, reproducibility assessments, quantitation methods, and scoring and reporting protocols. Specify whether and how assays were performed blinded to the study end point.
Study design
1. State the method of case selection, including whether prospective or retrospective and whether stratification or matching (e.g., by stage of disease or age) was used. Specify the time period from which cases were taken, the end of the follow-up period, and the median follow-up time.
2. Precisely define all clinical end points examined.
3. List all candidate variables initially examined.
4. Give rationale for sample size; if the study was designed to detect a specific effect size, give the target power and effect size.
Statistical analysis methods
1. Specify all statistical methods, including details of any variable selection procedures and other model-building issues, how model assumptions were verified, and how missing data were handled.
2. Clarify how marker values were handled in the analyses; if relevant, describe methods used for cut-point determination.
Results
Data
1. Describe the flow of patients through the study, including the number of patients included in each stage of the analysis (a diagram may be helpful) and reasons for dropout. Specifically, for both overall and for each subgroup extensively examined, report the number of patients and the number of events.
2. Report distribution of basic demographic characteristics (at least age and sex), standard (disease-specific) prognostic variables, and tumor marker, including numbers of missing values.
Analysis and presentation
1. Show the relation of the marker to standard prognostic variables.
2. Present univariate analyses showing the relation between the marker and outcome, with the estimated effect (e.g., hazard ratio and survival probability). Preferably provide similar analyses for all other variables being analyzed. For the effect of a tumor marker on a time-to-event outcome, a Kaplan–Meier plot is recommended.
3. For key multivariate analyses, report estimated effects (e.g., hazard ratio) with confidence intervals for the marker and, at least for the final model, all other variables in the model.
4. Among reported results, provide estimated effects with confidence intervals from an analysis in which the marker and standard prognostic variables are included, regardless of their statistical significance.
5. If done, report results of further investigations, such as checking assumptions, sensitivity analyses, and internal validation.
Discussion
1. Interpret the results in the context of the prespecified hypotheses and other relevant study; include a discussion of limitations of the study.
2. Discuss implications for future research and clinical value.

Source: Reprinted from REMARK criteria: REporting recommendations for tumor MARKer prognostic studies (REMARK) for the Statistics Subcommittee of the NCI Working Group on Cancer Diagnostics. McShane LM, Altman DG, Sauerbrei W, et al. REporting recommendations for tumor MARKer prognostic studies (REMARK). *Nat Clin Pract Oncol*. 2005;2(8):416–422.

have been distilled into bullets in **Table 16.5**, useful additional information can be found in the REMARK document (122).

Clinical Trials Involving Targeted Therapies

A clinically useful biomarker can identify patients with diseases that are either resistant or sensitive to a specific targeted therapy. As such, they can be used to improve the efficiency of a study and provide more precise treatment for specific subgroups of patients. This concept is illustrated in **Table 16.6**. Suppose the probability of response to standard treatment is 20% in the general patient population. Furthermore, suppose that 20% of the individuals in the general patient population are very responsive to a new targeted treatment, such that, when the targeted agent is added to the standard treatment, the probability of response is 60% among this sensitive subgroup, but unchanged in the nonsensitive subgroup. If the new treatment is combined with standard treatment in the general population, regardless of their sensitivity status, then the expected probability of response would only be 28% (i.e., 20% of population has 60% response rate, and 80% has 20% response rate $= 0.20 \times 0.60 + 0.80 \times 0.20 = 0.28$). If a randomized trial was now designed to compare standard treatment versus standard treatment with the new agent, then over 1,000 patients would need to be enrolled to reliably detect this size of a treatment effect (**Table 16.6**). On the other hand, if the study used a perfectly accurate biomarker (sensitivity = 100% and specificity = 100%) to restrict enrollment to treatment-sensitive patients, then only 60 patients would be needed for the study (**Table 16.6**) and the expected number of patients needed for screening would be about 300. In the real world, biomarkers are seldom perfect. A biomarker with 80% sensitivity and 80% specificity could still be used to increase the prevalence of treatment-sensitive patients (e.g., **Fig. 16.3**). In this case, the probability of response to the standard regimen with the new targeted agent in the enriched study population would be 40% ($0.50 \times 0.60 + 0.50 \times 0.20 = 0.40$). The two-arm trial designed with this imperfect biomarker to select sensitive patients would require 220 enrolled patients in order to reliably detect the difference in response rates (**Table 16.6**), and the expected number of patients needed for screening would be about 688.

In any study design where a biomarker is used to enrich the study sample with individuals considered most likely to respond, it may not be possible to differentiate between an ineffective treatment and a clinically invalid biomarker. Misspecification of the treatment target and misclassification of the tumor state are fundamental reasons for study failure. There can be a mismatch between the agent and the patient selection process in an enrichment design because of inadequate understanding of a potentially complex biologic pathway, or the true target of the agent under study, or use of an invalid surrogate end point biomarker (**Fig. 16.4**). A successful study depends on the degree to which the biomarker accurately measures the true state of the treatment's target(s). Ideally, measuring the agent's effect through the biomarker should measure the agent's effect through the targeted pathway (highlighted in indigo in **Figure 16.4**). If the

TABLE 16.6. Required Sample Size for a Randomized Trials with a Target Prevalence = 20%

	Probability of Response				Assumptions	
Patient Population	Standard Therapy (P_0)	Standard + Targeted Therapy (P_1)	Sample Size	Screen Size	Sensitivity	Specificity
Ideal Target Population	0.2	0.6	60	300	100	100
General Population	0.2	0.28	1022	1022	—	—
Enriched Population	0.2	0.4	220	688	80	80

Design parameters: H_0: $P_0 \geq P_1$, $\alpha = 0.05$, $\beta = 0.1$

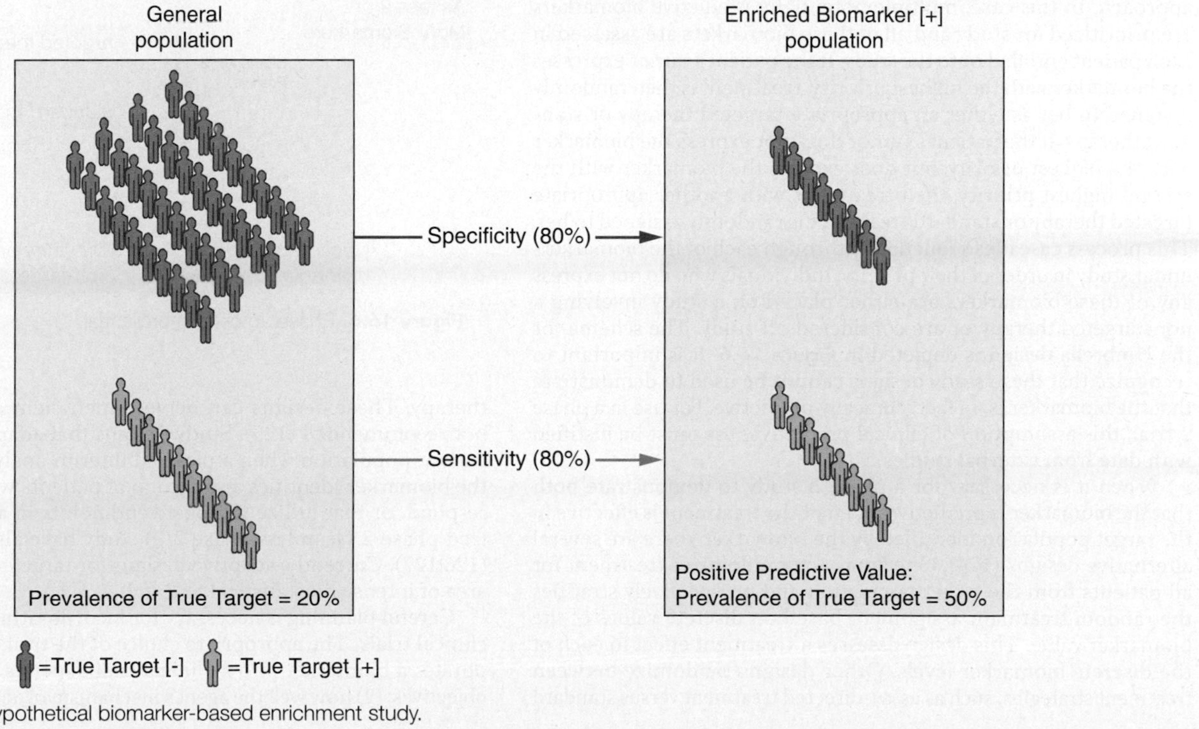

Figure 16.3. Hypothetical biomarker-based enrichment study.

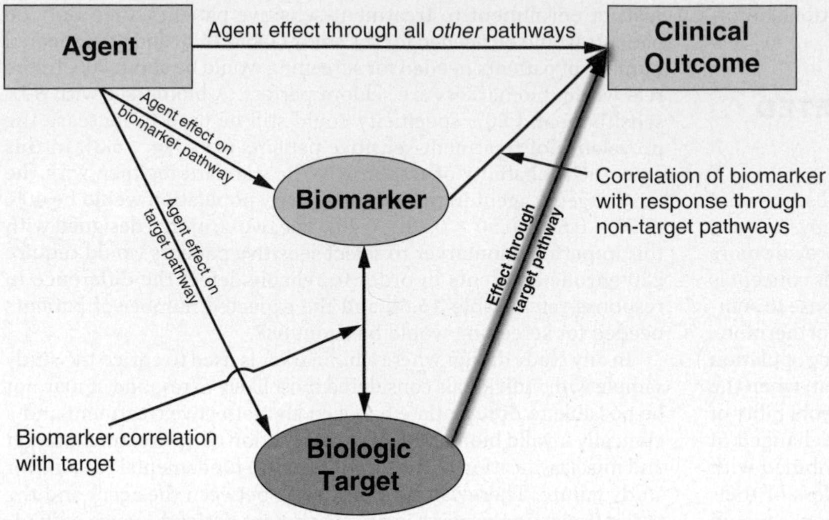

Figure 16.4. Schematic of the causal relationships and correlations between treatment, biomarker, biologic target, and clinical outcome.

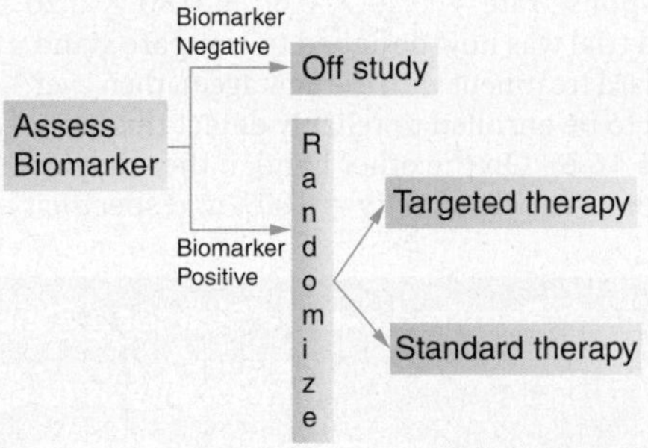

Figure 16.5. Phase 2b or 3 biomarker-enriched randomized treatment trial.

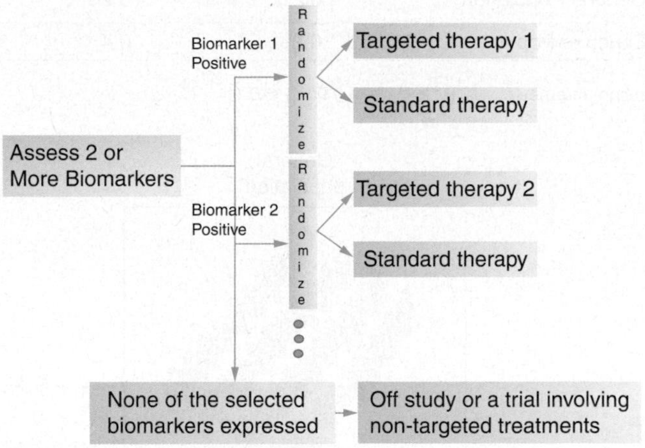

Figure 16.6. Phase 2b or 3 umbrella trial.

treatment can influence the disease through pathways that are not captured by the biomarker, then the activity of the agent will be underestimated and potentially missed. For example, in ovarian cancer, mutations in the *BRCA1* and *BRCA2* genes identify tumors likely to respond to a class of agents referred to as Poly-ADP ribose polymerase inhibitors (PARPi). However, responses to PARPi have been observed among patients with no *BRCA* mutations (123). This suggests that markers of other biologic pathways will be needed to identify PARPi-sensitive tumors, such as markers for methylation of the *BRCA* genes or other types of dysfunction in the homologous recombination mechanism. Therefore, if the biomarkers that are used to define PARPi sensitivity included only *BRCA* mutation status, then sensitivity is sacrificed. On the other hand, if the markers for determining PARPi sensitivity include inconsequential mutations in the *BRCA* genes, specificity is diminished. In enrichment studies, loss of sensitivity and specificity decreases the predictive value of the marker, which in turn decreases the chances that a study will identify active targeted agents (**Table 16.6** and **Fig. 16.3**). The schema for a biomarker-enriched randomized phase 2b or 3 trial is presented in **Figure 16.5**. The "Umbrella design" generalizes this enrichment approach. In this case, multiple potentially predictive biomarkers are prioritized for study and all of these biomarkers are assessed in each patient enrolled onto the study. If the patient's tumor expresses the biomarker with the highest priority, treatment is then randomly assigned to her as either an appropriate targeted therapy or standard therapy. If the patient's tumor does not express the biomarker with the highest priority, but does express the biomarker with the second highest priority, then treatment with another appropriate targeted therapy or standard treatment is randomly assigned to her. This process cascades sequentially through each of the biomarkers under study in order of their priority. Individuals who do not express any of these biomarkers are either placed on a study involving a non-targeted therapy or are considered off study. The schema for the Umbrella design is depicted in **Figure 16.6**. It is important to recognize that these study designs cannot be used to demonstrate that the biomarker is, in fact, clinically predictive. For use in a phase 3 trial, this assumption of clinical predictiveness must be justified with data from external studies.

When it is necessary for a phase 3 study to demonstrate both that the biomarker is predictive and that the treatment is effective in the target population identified by the biomarker, there are several alternative designs (124). One approach randomizes treatment for all patients from the target population and prospectively stratifies the random treatment assignment based on discrete values of the biomarker value. This design assesses a treatment effect in each of the discrete biomarker levels. Other designs randomize between treatment strategies, such as assay-directed treatment versus standard therapy. These designs can be very inefficient and are generally not recommended (125). Study designs that adaptively modify the patient population when a planned interim analysis indicates that the biomarker identifies a subgroup of patients who are unlikely to respond, or that utilize surrogate end points in a lead-in randomized phase 2 (seamless phase 2/3) study have also been proposed (126,127). Currently, adaptive designs for targeted therapies are an area of intense biostatistical research.

Careful planning is necessary for incorporating biomarkers into clinical trials. The appropriate choice of the trial design that incorporates a biomarker into a clinical trial depends on (1) the study's objectives, (2) how well the agent's mechanism of action is understood,

(3) how well the role of the target is understood, and (4) how well the selected biomarker captures the state of the drug's true target(s).

CONCLUSION

The complexity of clinical trial design, conduct, analysis, and reporting has increased considerably over the past 60 years, since randomized treatment trials and public screening trials first began. It is difficult for a single clinician to consider initiating a large-scale clinical study because it often requires extensive collaboration with other physicians, as well as professionals from disciplines such as biology, statistics, ethics, psychology, and economics.

REFERENCES

1. Herbst AL, Ulfelder H, Poskanzer DC. Adenocarcinoma of the vagina. Association of maternal stilbestrol therapy with tumor appearance in young women. *N Engl J Med.* 1971;284(15):878–881.
2. Rothman K, Greenland S. *Modern Epidemiology*. Philadelphia, PA: Lippincott-Raven Publishers; 1998.
3. Rose S, Laan MJ. Why match? Investigating matched case-control study designs with causal effect estimation. *Int J Biostat.* 2009;5(1):Article 1.
4. Wacholder S. Practical considerations in choosing between the case-cohort and nested case-control designs. *Epidemiology.* 1991;2(2):155–158.
5. Sackett DL. Bias in analytic research. *J Chronic Dis.* 1979;32(1–2):51–63.
6. Fleming TR, DeMets DL. Surrogate end points in clinical trials: are we being misled? *Ann Intern Med.* 1996;125(7):605–613.
7. Buyse M, Molenberghs G, Burzykowski T, et al. The validation of surrogate endpoints in meta-analyses of randomized experiments. *Biostatistics.* 2000;1(1):49–67.
8. Lesko LJ, Atkinson AJ Jr. Use of biomarkers and surrogate endpoints in drug development and regulatory decision making: criteria, validation, strategies. *Annu Rev Pharmacol Toxicol.* 2001;41:347–366.
9. Skaznik-Wikiel ME, Sukumvanich P, Beriwal S, et al. Possible use of CA-125 level normalization after the third chemotherapy cycle in deciding on chemotherapy regimen in patients with epithelial ovarian cancer: brief report. *Int J Gynecol Cancer.* 2011;21(6):1013–1017.
10. FDA and the American Society of Clinical Oncology (ASCO), with co-sponsorship by the American Association for Cancer Research (AACR) Public Workshop on Endpoints for Ovarian Cancer. http://www.fda.gov/Drugs/DevelopmentApprovalProcess/DevelopmentResources/CancerDrugs/ucm094586.htm. Accessed 2006.
11. Pfisterer JM, Plante M, Vergote I, et al. Gemcitabine plus carboplatin compared with carboplatin in patients with platinum-sensitive recurrent ovarian cancer: an intergroup trial of the AGO-OVAR, the NCIC CTG, and the EORTC GCG. *J Clin Oncol.* 2006;24(29):4699–4707.
12. Burger RA, Brady MF, Bookman MA, et al. Incorporation of bevacizumab in the primary treatment of ovarian cancer. *N Engl J Med.* 2011;365(26):2473–2483.
13. Perren TJ, Swart AM, Pfisterer J, et al. A phase 3 trial of bevacizumab in ovarian cancer. *N Engl J Med.* 2011;365(26):2484–2496.
14. Aghajanian C, Blank SV, Goff BA, et al. OCEANS: a randomized, double-blind, placebo-controlled phase iii trial of chemotherapy with or without bevacizumab in patients with platinum-sensitive recurrent epithelial ovarian, primary peritoneal, or fallopian tube cancer. *J Clin Oncol.* 2012;30(17):2039–2045.
15. Royston P, Parmar MK, Qian W. Novel designs for multi-arm clinical trials with survival outcomes with an application in ovarian cancer. *Stat Med.* 2003;22(14):2239–2256.
16. Parmar MK, Barthel FM, Sydes M, et al. Speeding up the evaluation of new agents in cancer. *J Natl Cancer Inst.* 2008;100(17):1204–1214.
17. Oza AM, Castonguay V, Tsoref D, et al. Progression-free survival in advanced ovarian cancer: a Canadian review and expert panel perspective. *Curr Oncol.* 2011;18 (Suppl 2):S20–S27.
18. Creasman WT. Second-look laparotomy in ovarian cancer. *Gynecol Oncol.* 1994;55(3, pt 2):S122–S127.
19. George SL. Reducing patient eligibility criteria in cancer clinical trials. *J Clin Oncol.* 1996;14(4):1364–1370.
20. Begg CB, Engstrom PF. Eligibility and extrapolation in cancer clinical trials. *J Clin Oncol.* 1987;5(6):962–968.
21. International Collaborative Ovarian Neoplasm Group. Paclitaxel plus carboplatin versus standard chemotherapy with either single-agent carboplatin or cyclophosphamide, doxorubicin, and cisplatin in women with ovarian cancer: the ICON3 randomised trial. *Lancet.* 2002;360(9332):505–515.
22. O'Quigley J, Pepe M, Fisher L. Continual reassessment method: a practical design for phase I clinical trials in cancer. *Biometrics.* 1990;46:33–48.
23. Korn EL, Midthune D, Chen TT, et al. A comparison of two phase I trial designs. *Stat Med.* 1994;13(18):1799–1806.
24. Goodman SN, Zahurak ML, Piantadosi S. Some practical improvements in the continual reassessment method for phase I studies. *Stat Med.* 1995;14(11):1149–1161.
25. Ahn C. An evaluation of phase I cancer clinical trial designs. *Stat Med.* 1998;17:1537–1549.
26. Simon R, Freidlin B, Rubinstein L, et al. Accelerated titration designs for phase I clinical trials in oncology. *J Natl Cancer Inst.* 1997;89:1138–1147.
27. Paller CJ, Bradbury PA, Ivy SP, et al. Design of phase I combination trials: recommendations of the clinical trial design task force of the NCI investigational drug steering committee. *Clin Cancer Res.* 2014;20(16):4210–4217.
28. Mandrekar SJ, Qin R, Sargent DJ. Model-based phase I designs incorporating toxicity and efficacy for single and dual agent drug combinations: methods and challenges. *Stat Med.* 2010;29(10):1077–1083.
29. Mandrekar SJ, Sargent DJ. Randomized phase II trials: time for a new era in clinical trial design. *J Thorac Oncol.* 2010;5(7):932–934.
30. Simon R. Optimal two-stage designs for phase II clinical trials. *Contr Clin Trials.* 1989;10:1–10.
31. Wieand S, Therneau T. A two-stage design for randomized trials with binary outcomes. *Control Clin Trials.* 1987;8:20–28.
32. Chen TT, Ng TH. Optimal flexible designs in phase II clinical trials. *Stat Med.* 1998;17:2301–2312.
33. Jennison C, Turnbull BW. Group sequential tests for bivariate response: interim analyses of clinical trials with both efficacy and safety endpoints. *Biometrics.* 1993;49:741–752.
34. Bryant J, Day R. Incorporating toxicity considerations into the design of two-stage phase II clinical trials. *Biometrics.* 1995;51:1372–1383.
35. Conaway MR, Petroni GR. Designs for the phase II trials allowing for a trade off between response and toxicity. *Biometrics.* 1996;52:1375–1386.
36. Thall P, Simon RM, Estey EH. New statistical strategy for monitoring safety and efficacy in single-arm clinical trials. *J Clin Oncol.* 1996;14(1):296–303.
37. Sill MW, Yothers G. A method for utilizing bivariate efficacy outcome measures to screen agents for activity in 2-stage phase II clinical trials. Technical Report. State University of New York at Buffalo, Buffalo; 2006:1–9.
38. Durrleman S, Simon R. Planning and monitoring of equivalence studies. *Biometrics.* 1990;46:329–336.
39. Senn S. Inherent difficulties with active control equivalence studies. *Stat Med.* 1993;12:2367–2375.
40. Wiens B. Choosing an equivalence limit for noninferiority or equivalence studies. *Contr Clin Trials.* 2002;23:2–14.
41. Rothmann M, Li N, Chen G, et al. Design and analysis of non-inferiority mortality trials in oncology. *Stat Med.* 2003;22(2):239–264.
42. McGuire WP, Hoskins WJ, Brady MF, et al. A phase III trial comparing cisplatin/cytoxan and cisplatin/paclitaxel in advanced ovarian cancer. *Proc Am Soc Clin Oncol.* 1993;12:abstract 808.
43. Neijt JP, Engelholm SA, Tuxen MK, et al. Exploratory phase III study of paclitaxel and cisplatin versus paclitaxel and carboplatin in advanced ovarian cancer. *J Clin Oncol.* 2000;18(17):3084–3092.
44. du Bois A, Lück HJ, Meier W, et al. A randomized clinical trial of cisplatin/paclitaxel versus carboplatin/paclitaxel as first-line treatment of ovarian cancer. *J Natl Cancer Inst.* 2003;95(17):1320–1329.
45. Ozols RF, Bundy BN, Greer BE, et al. Phase III trial of carboplatin and paclitaxel compared with cisplatin and paclitaxel in patients with optimally resected stage III ovarian cancer: a Gynecologic Oncology Group study. *J Clin Oncol.* 2003;21(17):3194–3200.
46. Vasey PA. Role of docetaxel in the treatment of newly diagnosed advanced ovarian cancer. *J Clin Oncol.* 2003;21(10 Suppl):136–144.
47. Sandercock J, Parmar MK, Torri V, et al. First-line treatment for advanced ovarian cancer: paclitaxel, platinum and the evidence. *Br J Cancer.* 2002;87(8):815–824.
48. Byar DP, Simon RM, Friedewald WT, et al. Randomized clinical trials. Perspectives on some recent ideas. *N Engl J Med.* 1976;295:74–80.
49. Kunz R, Oxman A. The unpredictability paradox: review of empirical comparisons of randomised and non-randomised clinical trials. *Br Med J.* 1998;317:1185–1190.
50. Schulz KF, Chalmers I, Hayes RJ, et al. Empirical evidence of bias. Dimensions of methodological quality associated with estimates of treatment effects in controlled trials. *JAMA.* 1995;273(5):408–412.
51. Schulz KF. Subverting randomization in controlled trials. *JAMA.* 1995;274(18):1456–1458.
52. Emanuel EJ, Patterson WB. Ethics of randomized clinical trials. *J Clin Oncol.* 1998;16(1):365–371.

53. Ellis PM, Coates AS. Ethics of randomized clinical trials. *J Clin Oncol.* 1998;16(7):2570.
54. Therneau TM. How many stratification factors are "too many" to use in a randomization plan? *Contr Clin Trials.* 1993;14(2):98–108.
55. Pocock SJ, Simon R. Sequential treatment assignment with balancing for prognostic factors in the controlled clinical trial. *Biometrics.* 1975;31(1):103–115.
56. Schulz KF, Altman DG, Moher D. Allocation concealment in clinical trials. *JAMA.* 2002;288(19):2406–2407; author reply 2408–2409.
57. Schulz KF, Grimes DA, Altman DG, et al. Blinding and exclusions after allocation in randomized controlled trials: survey of published parallel group trials in obstetrics and gynaecology. *Br Med J.* 1996;312:742–744.
58. Rothman KJ, Michels KB. The continuing unethical use of placebo controls. *N Engl J Med.* 1994;331(6):394–398.
59. Green S, Liu PY, O'Sullivan J. Factorial design considerations. *J Clin Oncol.* 2002;20(16):3424–3430.
60. Last, Ed. *A Dictionary of Epidemiology.* New York, NY, Oxford University Press; 1995.
61. Goodman SN. p Values, hypothesis tests, and likelihood: Implications for epidemiology of a neglected historical debate. *Am J Epidemiol.* 1993;137(5):485–499.
62. Ransohoff DF. Lessons from controversy: ovarian cancer screening and serum proteomics. *J Natl Cancer Inst.* 2005;97(4):315–319.
63. IOM. Evaluation of biomarkers and surrogate endpoints in chronic disease. http://www.iom.edu/Reports/2010/Evaluation-of-Biomarkers-and-Surrogate-Endpoints-in-Chronic-Disease.aspx. Accessed 2010.
64. Goozner M. Duke scandal highlights need for genomics research criteria. *J Natl Cancer Inst.* 2011;103(12):916–917.
65. Biomarkers Definitions Working Group. Biomarkers and surrogate endpoints: preferred definitions and conceptual framework. *Clin Pharmacol Ther.* 2001;69(3):89–95.
66. National Research Council. *Evolution of Translational Omics: Lessons Learned and the Path Forward.* Washington, DC: The National Academies Press; 2012.
67. Rajan S, Djambazian H, Dang HC, et al. The living microarray: a high-throughput platform for measuring transcription dynamics in single cells. *BMC Genomics.* 2011;12:115.
68. Albertson DG, Ylstra B, Segraves R, et al. Quantitative mapping of amplicon structure by array CGH identifies CYP24 as a candidate oncogene. *Nat Genet.* 2000;25(2):144–146.
69. Hodgson G, Hager JH, Volik S, et al. Genome scanning with array CGH delineates regional alterations in mouse islet carcinomas. *Nat Genet.* 2001;29(4):459–464.
70. Pollack JR, Sorlie T, Perou CM, et al. Microarray analysis reveals a major direct role of DNA copy number alteration in the transcriptional program of human breast tumors. *Proc Natl Acad Sci U S A.* 2002;99(20):12963–12968.
71. Albertson DG. Profiling breast cancer by array CGH. *Breast Cancer Res Treat.* 2003;78(3):289–298.
72. Albertson DG, Collins C, McCormick F, et al. Chromosome aberrations in solid tumors. *Nat Genet.* 2003;34(4):369–376.
73. Hackett CS, Hodgson JG, Law ME, et al. Genome-wide array CGH analysis of murine neuroblastoma reveals distinct genomic aberrations which parallel those in human tumors. *Cancer Res.* 2003;63(17):5266–5273.
74. Garnis C, Coe BP, Zhang L, et al. Overexpression of LRP12, a gene contained within an 8q22 amplicon identified by high-resolution array CGH analysis of oral squamous cell carcinomas. *Oncogene.* 2004;23(14):2582–2586.
75. Veltman JA, Fridlyand J, Pejavar S, et al. Array-based comparative genomic hybridization for genome-wide screening of DNA copy number in bladder tumors. *Cancer Res.* 2003;63(11):2872–2880.
76. Pinkel D, Albertson DG. Array comparative genomic hybridization and its applications in cancer. *Nat Genet.* 2005;37(Suppl):S11–S17.
77. Rossi MR, Conroy J, McQuaid D, et al. Array CGH analysis of pediatric medulloblastomas. *Genes Chromosomes Cancer.* 2006;45(3):290–303.
78. Idbaih A, Marie Y, Lucchesi C, et al. BAC array CGH distinguishes mutually exclusive alterations that define clinicogenetic subtypes of gliomas. *Int J Cancer.* 2008;122(8):1778–1786.
79. Ramaswamy S, Tamayo P, Rifkin R, et al. Multiclass cancer diagnosis using tumor gene expression signatures. *Proc Natl Acad Sci U S A.* 2001;98(26):15149–15154.
80. Gordon GJ, Jensen RV, Hsiao LL, et al. Translation of microarray data into clinically relevant cancer diagnostic tests using gene expression ratios in lung cancer and mesothelioma. *Cancer Res.* 2002;62(17):4963–4967.
81. Tibshirani R, Hastie T, Narasimhan B, et al. Diagnosis of multiple cancer types by shrunken centroids of gene expression. *Proc Natl Acad Sci U S A.* 2002;99(10):6567–6572.
82. Statnikov A, Aliferis CF, Tsamardinos I, et al. A comprehensive evaluation of multicategory classification methods for microarray gene expression cancer diagnosis. *Bioinformatics.* 2005;21(5):631–643.
83. Glas AM, Floore A, Delahaye LJ, et al. Converting a breast cancer microarray signature into a high-throughput diagnostic test. *BMC Genomics.* 2006;7:278.
84. van 't Veer LJ, Dai H, van de Vijver MJ, et al. Gene expression profiling predicts clinical outcome of breast cancer. *Nature.* 2002;415(6871):530–536.
85. Sotiriou C, Neo SY, McShane LM, et al. Breast cancer classification and prognosis based on gene expression profiles from a population-based study. *Proc Natl Acad Sci U S A.* 2003;100(18):10393–10398.
86. Michiels S, Koscielny S, Hill C. Prediction of cancer outcome with microarrays: a multiple random validation strategy. *Lancet.* 2005;365(9458):488–492.
87. Barrier A, Boelle PY, Roser F, et al. Stage II colon cancer prognosis prediction by tumor gene expression profiling. *J Clin Oncol.* 2006;24(29):4685–4691.
88. Miecznikowski JC, Wang D, Liu S, et al. Comparative survival analysis of breast cancer microarray studies identifies important prognostic genetic pathways. *BMC Cancer.* 2010;10:573.
89. Levin JZ, Berger MF, Adiconis X, et al. (2009). Targeted next-generation sequencing of a cancer transcriptome enhances detection of sequence variants and novel fusion transcripts. *Genome Biol.* 2009;10(10):R115.
90. Pflueger D, Rickman DS, Sboner A, et al. N-myc downstream regulated gene 1 (NDRG1) is fused to ERG in prostate cancer. *Neoplasia.* 2009;11(8):804–811.
91. Portela A, Esteller M. Epigenetic modifications and human disease. *Nat Biotechnol.* 2010;28(10):1057–1068.
92. Paweletz CP, Trock B, Pennanen M, et al. Proteomic patterns of nipple aspirate fluids obtained by SELDI-TOF: potential for new biomarkers to aid in the diagnosis of breast cancer. *Dis Markers.* 2001;17(4):301–307.
93. Koopmann J, Zhang Z, White N, et al. Serum diagnosis of pancreatic adenocarcinoma using surface-enhanced laser desorption and ionization mass spectrometry. *Clin Cancer Res.* 2004;10(3):860–868.
94. Kolch W, Neususs C, Pelzing M, et al. Capillary electrophoresis-mass spectrometry as a powerful tool in clinical diagnosis and biomarker discovery. *Mass Spectrom Rev.* 2005;24(6):959–977.
95. Lan KK, Rosenberger WF, Lachin JM. Sequential monitoring of survival data with the Wilcoxon statistic. *Biometrics.* 1995;51(3):1175–1183.
96. Diamandis EP. Analysis of serum proteomic patterns for early cancer diagnosis: drawing attention to potential problems. *J Natl Cancer Inst.* 2004;96(5):353–356.
97. Diamandis EP. Mass spectrometry as a diagnostic and a cancer biomarker discovery tool: opportunities and potential limitations. *Mol Cell Proteomics.* 2004;3(4):367–378.
98. Miecznikowski JC, Gaile DP, Liu S, et al. A new normalizing algorithm for BAC CGH arrays with quality control metrics. *J Biomed Biotechnol.* 2011;2011:860732.
99. Press MF, Hung G, Godolphin W, et al. Sensitivity of HER-2/neu antibodies in archival tissue samples: potential source of error in immunohistochemical studies of oncogene expression. *Cancer Res.* 1994;54(10):2771–2777.
100. van den Broek LJ, van de Vijver MJ. Assessment of problems in diagnostic and research immunohistochemistry associated with epitope instability in stored paraffin sections. *Appl Immunohistochem Mol Morphol.* 2000;8(4):316–321.
101. McShane LM, Aamodt R, Cordon-Cardo C, et al. Reproducibility of p53 immunohistochemistry in bladder tumors. National Cancer Institute, Bladder Tumor Marker Network. *Clin Cancer Res.* 2000;6(5):1854–1864.
102. Esteban J, Baker J, Cronin M, et al. Tumor gene expression and prognosis in breast cancer: multi-gene RT-PCR assay of paraffin-embedded tissue. *Proc Am Soc Clin Oncol.* 2003;22:A3416.
103. European Bioinformatics Institute. ArrayExpress. http://www.ebi.ac.uk/arrayexpress/. Accessed 2012.
104. Edgar R, Domrachev M, Lash AE. Gene expression omnibus: NCBI gene expression and hybridization array data repository. *Nucleic Acids Res.* 2002;30(1):207–210.
105. Ikeo K, Ishi-i J, Tamura T, et al. CIBEX: Center for Information Biology Gene Expression Database. *C R Biol.* 2003;326(10–11):1079–1082.
106. Gardiner-Garden M, Littlejohn TG. A comparison of microarray databases. *Brief Bioinform.* 2001;2(2):143–158.

107. Ovaska K, Laakso M, Haapa-Paananen S, et al. Large-scale data integration framework provides a comprehensive view on glioblastoma multiforme. *Genome Med.* 2010;2(9):65.
108. Huber W, Carey VJ, Gentleman R, et al. Orchestrating high-throughput genomic analysis with bioconductor. *Nat Methods.* 2015;12(2):115–121.
109. Brazma A, Hingamp P, Quackenbush J, et al. Minimum information about a microarray experiment (MIAME)-toward standards for microarray data. *Nat Genet.* 2001;29(4):365–371.
110. National Center for Biotechnology Information. GEO: Gene Expression Omnibus. http://www.ncbi.nlm.nih.gov/geo/. 2012.
111. Stratton MR, Campbell PJ, Futreal PA. The cancer genome. *Nature.* 2009;458(7239):719–724.
112. Strand C, Enell J, Hedenfalk I, et al. RNA quality in frozen breast cancer samples and the influence on gene expression analysis-a comparison of three evaluation methods using microcapillary electrophoresis traces. *BMC Mol Biol.* 2007;8:38.
113. Callesen AK, Vach W, Jørgensen PE, et al. Reproducibility of mass spectrometry based protein profiles for diagnosis of breast cancer across clinical studies: a systematic review. *J Proteome Res.* 2008;7(4):1395–1402.
114. Leyland-Jones BR, Ambrosone CB, Bartlett J, et al. Recommendations for collection and handling of specimens from group breast cancer clinical trials. *J Clin Oncol.* 2008;26(34):5638–5644.
115. De Cecco L, Musella V, Veneroni S, et al. Impact of biospecimens handling on biomarker research in breast cancer. *BMC Cancer.* 2009;9:409.
116. Hicks DG, Kushner L, McCarthy K. Breast cancer predictive factor testing: the challenges and importance of standardizing tissue handling. *J Natl Cancer Inst Monogr.* 2011;2011(42):43–45.
117. Benton HP, Want E, Keun HC, et al. Intra-and inter-laboratory reproducibility of ultra performance liquid chromatography-time-of-flight mass spectrometry for urinary metabolic profiling. *Anal Chem.* 2012;29(4):2424–2432.
118. Freidin MB, Bhudia N, Lim E, et al. Impact of collection and storage of lung tumor tissue on whole genome expression profiling. *J Mol Diagn.* 2012;14(2):140–148.
119. Lawrie CH, Ballabio E, Soilleux E, et al. Inter- and intra-observational variability in immunohistochemistry: a multicentre analysis of diffuse large B-cell lymphoma staining. *Histopathology.* 2012;61(1):18–25.
120. Nowak NJ, Miecznikowski J, Moore SR, et al. Challenges in array comparative genomic hybridization for the analysis of cancer samples. *Genet Med.* 2007;9(9):585–595.
121. Mittempergher L, de Ronde JJ, Nieuwland M, et al. Gene expression profiles from formalin fixed paraffin embedded breast cancer tissue are largely comparable to fresh frozen matched tissue. *PLoS One.* 2011;6(2):e17163.
122. McShane LM, Altman DG, Sauerbrei W, et al. REporting recommendations for tumor MARKer prognostic studies (REMARK). *Nat Clin Pract Oncol.* 2005;2(8):416–422.
123. Sessa C. Update on PARP1 inhibitors in ovarian cancer. *Ann Oncol.* 2011;22(Suppl 8):viii72–viii76.
124. Simon R. Clinical trial designs for evaluating the medical utility of prognostic and predictive biomarkers in oncology. *Per Med.* 2010;7(1):33–47.
125. Freidlin B, McShane LM, Korn EL. Randomized clinical trials with biomarkers: design issues. *J Natl Cancer Inst.* 2010;102(3):152–160.
126. Wang SJ, O'Neill RT, Hung HM. Approaches to evaluation of treatment effect in randomized clinical trials with genomic subset. *Pharm Stat.* 2007;6(3):227–244.
127. Jenkins M, Stone A, Jennison C. An adaptive seamless phase II/III design for oncology trials with subpopulation selection using correlated survival endpoints. *Pharm Stat.* 2011;10(4):347–356.

CHAPTER 17

Cost-Effective and Value-Based Gynecologic Cancer Care

Laura J. Havrilesky, Shalini L. Kulasingam, Elizabeth L. Jewell, and David E. Cohn

OVERVIEW OF COST, QUALITY, AND VALUE IN HEALTH CARE

The cost of health care in the United States continues to rise and is expected to encompass 20% of the gross domestic product by 2020. Despite rising costs, there has not been a commensurate increase in the quality of care delivered in the United States. For this reason, there has been increasing pressure on health systems and providers to demonstrate "value," defined by high-quality and cost-effective care. In this chapter, we will review the historical backdrop that has led to the current level of scrutiny being applied to health care providers to deliver value-based (high-quality and cost-conscious) care. We will define value in health care and describe current and proposed methods to measure value. We will review the methodology of cost-effectiveness analyses (CEAs) and the current evidence regarding the cost-effectiveness of specific interventions in gynecologic cancers.

Cost and Comparative Effectiveness

Given that the ideal infrastructure for measuring value does not yet exist, how can we conduct outcomes-based research with the goal of improving health care quality? Comparative effectiveness research (CER) is defined by the National Academy of Medicine (NAM, previously named the Institute of Medicine) as "the generation and synthesis of evidence that compares the benefits and harms of alternative methods to prevent, diagnose, treat and monitor a clinical condition, or to improve the delivery of care." With this broad definition, the NAM provides a framework for CER to exist, for example, in the development of a model to better understand the potential impact of an intervention (generation of evidence) or in the form of the comparison of two existing treatments of a condition (synthesis of evidence). Congress, in the American Recovery and Reinvestment Act (ARRA) of 2009, appropriated $1.1 billion to jump-start the nation's efforts to accelerate CER. Furthermore, ARRA created the Patient-Centered Outcomes Research Institute (PCORI), a public–private organization charged with setting national priorities for CER.

As the field of CER has become integrated into health care policy and coverage decisions, there has concurrently been increasing concern that CER will lead to denial of certain health care interventions. As a result of concerns raised about resource rationing and the devaluation of life in health states with a high burden of disability, the Affordable Care Act (ACA) of 2010 stated that "The Patient-Centered Outcomes Research Institute (PCORI) . . . shall not develop or employ a dollars per quality-adjusted life year (or similar measure that discounts the value of a life because of an individual's disability) as a threshold to establish what type of health care is cost-effective or recommended." (1) This means that PCORI, the institute that was created in response to concerns about the high cost of health care in the United States, is prohibited from sponsoring studies that include considerations of cost-effectiveness. Despite this, experts have argued that the funding of CER still provides quality evidence for employment in standard CEAs and will therefore ultimately inform the question of value in health care (2).

Summary

With increasing pressure to control the costs and improve the quality of health care, measurement of value will be an important means by which different treatments can be critically evaluated.

DEFINING AND MEASURING VALUE IN ONCOLOGY

Value can be defined broadly as the desirable health outcomes achieved per monetary unit spent (3). The United States is currently transitioning to a value-based reimbursement system to replace the current system of payment for services provided. In March 2013, the National Commission on Physician Payment Reform published recommendations to transition to a blended payment system (4). These recommendations include elimination of stand-alone fee-for-service payment to medical practices and a transition to an approach based on quality and value. By 2019, physicians will enter an alternative payment model (APM) track or a Merit-Based Incentive Payment System (MIPS) track based on eligibility (5). These impending changes in the reimbursement of medical care make it imperative that physicians understand the principals of defining quality and value in health care.

Status Quo Measurement of Value in Health Care

Health care quality measures have come into the spotlight on a national level as directed by the Patient Protection and ACA, with the goal of understanding and optimizing the correlation between health care spending and quality care. To this end, mandatory reporting of quality measures was included in section 2701 of the ACA (1). However, the implementation of an effective and clinically relevant reporting system is limited by the complex process by which these quality measures are identified, vetted, and applied.

On April 16, 2015, the US Senate passed legislation to repeal the Sustainable Growth Rate formula, which governed provider payment under Medicare's Physician Fee Schedule (6). In its place, the enactment of the Medicare Access and Children's Health Insurance Program Reauthorization Act of 2015 has accelerated the movement toward value-based rather than volume-based payments by 2019 through the introduction of two tracks: the MIPS and APM. Under MIPS, four weighted categories (quality, resource use, clinical practice improvement activities, and meaningful use of electronic health record technology) are used to calculate an overall MIPS score, which is linked to provider payment adjustment based on performance. Providers can also opt out of MIPS by choosing to participate in an APM, which utilizes bundled payment arrangements for episodes of care and accountable care organizations to financially incentivize controlling cost growth while maintaining quality care over time. The Department of Health and Human Services (DHHS) announced goals for 30% of Medicare payments to be value based by the end of 2016 and 50% by the end of 2018 (7). However, many of the quality measures used in these value-based payment models have yet to be fully defined.

Other potential opportunities to achieve value in health care may be related to the elimination of the use of therapies that are not cost-effective (e.g., those that are more expensive, less effective, or both, than alternative treatments). While there is no established agency in the United States that evaluates the cost-effectiveness of health care interventions, such models do exist in the United Kingdom, Canada, Australia, France, and Germany through "value determination" reviews (8). An additional focus on value through the reduction in readmission rates has gained increasing attention; readmissions are a major contributor to health care costs and are estimated to account for approximately $17 billion annually (9); it is estimated that up to 75% of all readmissions are preventable (10). As such, the US government has made reducing readmissions a priority to improve patient care, reduce health care spending, and therefore increase value. To address this goal, the Hospital Readmissions Reduction Program was established to limit reimbursements to hospitals with excess readmission ratios. Additionally, the Bundled Payments for Care Improvement initiative was established to determine payments based upon episodes of care (rather than for individual services) when patients are readmitted within 30 days of their index hospitalization (11–14).

Proposed Methods of Value Measurement in Oncology Care

In this section, we will describe two innovative methods that have been proposed for assessment of value in oncology health care.

ASCO Value Framework

A high proportion of all health care spending occurs in oncology. While in the past, patients with insurance may have been shielded from the increasing costs of cancer treatments beyond their responsibility for out-of-pocket copayments, changes in the structure of insurance policies with shared payment plans have led to an increasing experience of "financial toxicity," resulting in lower quality of life and an increasing rate of bankruptcy due to health care expenditures. Evidence indicates that cancer patients want information about the comparative effectiveness of available treatments as well as information on their relative costs. ASCO's Value in Cancer Care task force, first convened in 2007, has identified lists of common practices in oncology that were considered "low value" due to their expense and a lack of high-level evidence supporting their use (15,16). These lists, developed as part of the American Board of Internal Medicine Foundation's "Choosing Wisely" campaign, included avoidance of unnecessary imaging following an early-stage cancer diagnosis, avoidance of the provision of prophylactic antiemetic and bone marrow support regimens in low-risk settings, and avoidance of routine screening studies in patients with a low life expectancy. Of note, in 2013 the Society of Gynecologic Oncology published its own "top five" list of low-value interventions to avoid: (1) the screening of asymptomatic, low-risk women for ovarian cancer, (2) the use of Pap smear as a surveillance strategy for endometrial cancer, (3) the performance of colposcopy for low-grade squamous intraepithelial lesion Pap smear results in patients with a history of cervical cancer, (4) the use of routine surveillance imaging in patients with a history of gynecologic cancers, and (5) the delay of palliative care for women with advanced or relapsed cancer (17).

In 2015, the task force presented a framework for comparing the relative clinical benefit, toxicity, and cost of novel treatments in the medical oncology setting. The purpose of the framework is "to provide a standardized approach to assist physicians and patients in assessing the value of a new drug treatment for cancer as compared with one or several prevailing standards of care" and to provide oncologists with "information and physician-guided tools necessary to assess the relative value of cancer therapies as an element of shared decision making with their patients." The ASCO "value framework" was designed to define the value of medical interventions for the treatment of malignancy for which there exists phase III randomized controlled trial (RCT) data to inform outcomes. The framework provides the tools to calculate the net health benefits (NHBs) of a novel therapy (compared with standard of care therapy) for advanced or metastatic cancer using four criteria: (1) clinical benefit based on improvement in overall survival (OS), progression-free survival (PFS), or response rate; (2) toxicity differences; (3) symptom palliation; and (4) treatment-free interval. The clinical benefit calculation employs ASCO-assigned importance weights for OS (using a multiplier of 16), PFS (multiplier 11), or response rate (multiplier 8). In its current form, the framework assigns importance weights based on the opinions of task force members. The maximum possible NHB score for each therapy is 130 points. NHBs are intended to be presented alongside the drug-acquisition cost and, if available, the patient's out-of-pocket cost for each therapy. Value snapshots are calculated differently for treatments with curative intent as compared with those for metastatic disease. **Figure 17.1** depicts an example of a value snapshot constructed using the ASCO format for the comparison of standard chemotherapy with chemotherapy plus bevacizumab for recurrent, platinum-resistant ovarian cancer, using the AURELIA clinical trial results (18).

ASCO presents the framework as a starting point for conversations about value between oncologist and patient and points out that the presentation of such data is a responsibility of all practitioners of oncology. An open comment period regarding the value framework was solicited, and it is anticipated that future iterations may include a more transparent, evidence-based foundation of the weighting methods used to calculate NHB.

The Porter Value Framework

Harvard Business School economist Michael E. Porter argues that the definition and demonstration of value are integral to reining in costs and to overall health care reform. He states, "the absence of comprehensive and rigorous outcome and cost measurement is arguably the biggest weakness standing in the way of health care improvement" (3). He argues that surrogate measures of quality, such as the measurement of compliance to guidelines or even of patient satisfaction, do not necessarily indicate quality of care. In order to truly assess quality, the outcomes important to each disease must be defined and measured.

In an effort to begin to define high-quality outcomes, Porter has developed an idealized outcomes measures hierarchy, in which specific health outcomes are multitiered and defined for each disease. In oncology, the highest priority is assigned to survival, followed by functional status achieved, recovery times following treatment, effects of the treatment process on function and quality of life, and sustainability of the cancer-free state. In the Porter value framework, costs are defined as they apply to a full optimal "cycle of care" for a given medical condition, usually representing periods of a year or more. Responsibility for outcomes and reimbursements is shared by all participating providers for a given heath condition.

Ultimately, Porter argues, "Improving value requires either improving one or more outcomes without raising costs or lowering costs without compromising outcomes, or both." (19). Porter's strategic agenda for a high-value health care delivery system includes six components: (1) organization of care in disease-related integrated practice units; (2) measurement of outcomes and costs for every patient; (3) bundled payments for care cycles; (4) integration of care delivery across facilities; (5) expansion of services across geography; and (6) building an enabling information technology platform.

Conclusions—Value in Health Care

Significant progress has been made in the understanding of "value" in health care. Additionally, recent developments in the measurement and quantification of value have led to an expanded effort to tie quality, outcomes, and value-based cancer care to payment models for health systems and providers. Continued understanding of the factors that

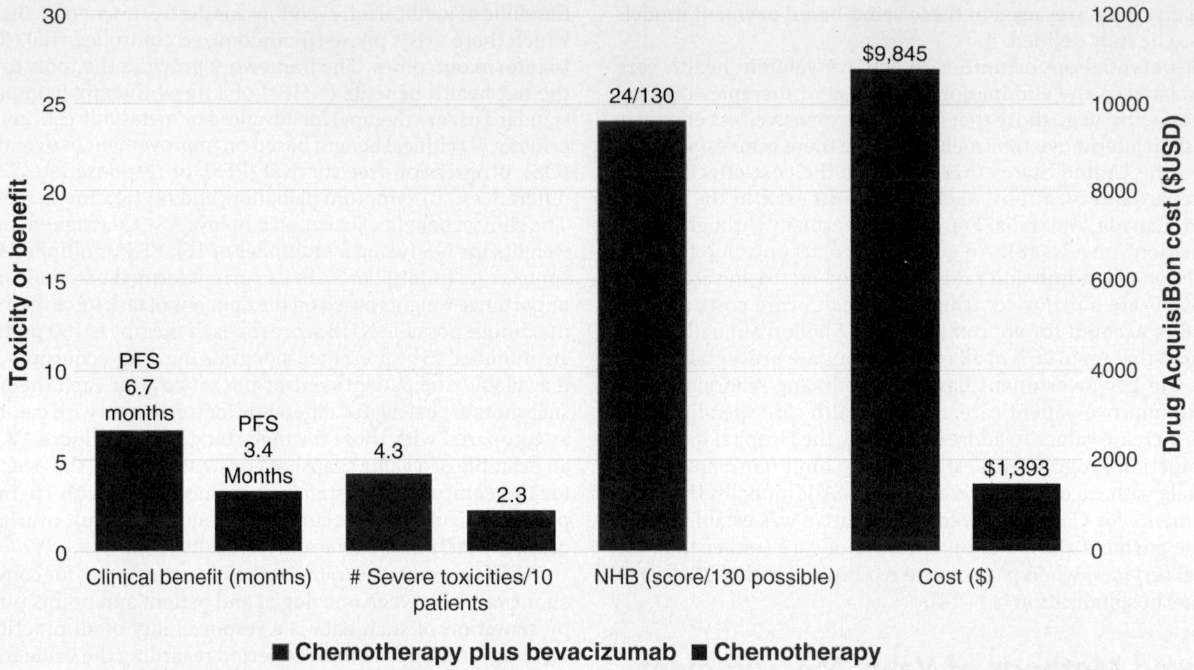

Figure 17.1. Value snapshot representing the benefits and costs of standard chemotherapy using weekly paclitaxel compared with standard chemotherapy plus bevacizumab for the treatment of platinum-resistant recurrent ovarian cancer.

drive value will be critical to cancer care, including that related to gynecologic cancers. In 2015, the Society for Gynecologic Oncology (SGO) had begun to develop strategies for the development of an APM for endometrial cancer, and subsequently ovarian cancer. This SGO effort is critical in that the DHHS's MIPS and APM programs will be implemented on or after January 1, 2019. Development of a cancer-specific strategy by experts in treating these diseases is critical to the ultimate relevance and success of any APM.

PRINCIPALS OF HEALTH ECONOMIC ANALYSES

This section will introduce basic types of health economic studies. The term "cost-effectiveness analysis" is commonly used as a catchall term for any health economic analysis. In fact, there are several distinct forms of health economic evaluation, including CEA, cost-utility analysis (CUA), and cost-minimization analysis (CMA). CEA and CUA are the most frequently used health economic analyses. CEAs compare alternative interventions using a cost per unit of effectiveness such as a year of life gained (20). CUAs examine cost, effectiveness, and preferences for health outcomes. CMAs compare only cost (20).

Cost-Effectiveness Analyses

CEA is defined by the UK's National Institute for Health and Clinical Excellence (NICE) as an economic study design in which the consequences of different interventions are measured using a single outcome (e.g., years of life gained, deaths avoided) (21). A CEA is used to help prioritize the allocation of resources and to decide between two or more treatments or interventions. It compares a standard of care strategy with its more costly alternatives in terms of the additional cost per unit of effectiveness. Units of effectiveness in oncology CEA are most commonly expressed as additional survival time but may also be expressed in other terms; for example, the number of adverse events or additional procedures avoided or the number of cases of cancer prevented. This type of study is commonly used when a decision or health policy maker is operating within a given budget and is considering a limited range of options (20). When an intervention costs more and is also more effective than its alternative, the cost-effectiveness comparison is expressed as an incremental cost-effectiveness ratio (ICER), or the ratio of the difference in costs to the difference in effectiveness between two strategies.

Cost-Minimization Analyses

In some cases, alternative medical decisions have approximately equivalent effectiveness but potentially different costs. In such cases, the effectiveness component of a CEA may not be needed. CMAs assume comparable effectiveness between strategies and choose a preferred strategy based on the mean cost of each (22). For example, a decision analysis comparing the costs of three different surgical approaches to endometrial cancer staging assumed equal survival outcomes between strategies and therefore did not incorporate effectiveness (23).

Cost-Utility Analyses

CUA is a form of CEA in which effectiveness is adjusted based on the quality of life that is associated with each strategy. In CUAs, *utilities* are the measurement used for quality of life and represent the preferences of an individual or a society for a particular health outcome. A utility is a number between 0 and 1, with 1 representing perfect health and 0 representing death. The most common metric used for comparison of strategies in a CUA is a quality-adjusted life year (QALY). The QALY quantifies both differences in survival and in quality of life between strategies. In an oncology CUA, the QALY is usually derived as the product of the length of survival in a specific health state and the utility representing the quality of life in that state. For example, 1 year of additional survival in a health state of utility 0.8 is equivalent to 0.8 QALYs. CUAs are preferred when both morbidity and mortality are affected by the proposed medical intervention or when quality of life related to the intervention being examined is a major concern. QALYs are the recommended outcome for health economic analyses if utility scores are available (24).

Methods for Development of a Health Economic Decision Model

This section will address specific methods used in the development of a health economic decision model, with an emphasis on the two most common types of models, CEA and CUA.

Define the Model's Perspective

The perspective of a health economic model is the first important consideration as costs are calculated differently based on the perspective taken. Most CEAs are performed from a third-party payer or a societal perspective. In a third-party-payer perspective model, costs assumed by an insurance company or by Medicare are incorporated. These may include professional fees for encounters and procedures, reimbursements to the hospital or ambulatory surgical center for postoperative care, or reimbursements for home health or rehabilitation care. A societal perspective is usually most appropriate as it accounts not only for all costs included from a third-party-payer perspective, but also for costs related to a patient's lost productivity and the caregiver's expense. For example, if one surgical approach results in a faster return to work, this will be associated with less cost that is due to lost productivity. Use of the societal perspective has led to the recognition that minimally invasive surgery results in cost savings to society (23,25). Other perspectives of health economic models include the *patient* and *hospital* perspectives. A hospital perspective model might be used to inform the decision to purchase expensive equipment such as robotic surgery platforms or an intraoperative radiotherapy facility.

Define the Question

Once the model's perspective has been determined, the clinical problem, standard approach, and any alternatives must be defined (26). The alternatives to the intervention of interest should always include a standard of care approach or even a "do nothing" approach. Next, a conceptual model for the analysis is developed, which outlines the possible consequences of each intervention. Decision models are often used as the conceptual framework for CEAs and have become an integral part of CEA studies.

Develop a Decision Tree

A simple decision tree begins with a *decision node* representing the primary clinical decision being examined. Two or more strategies may be examined using one decision tree. The subsequent nodes in the tree are termed *chance nodes* and define the probability of each possible clinical event that follows from the initial decision. For example, if the decision node concerns the clinical question of whether to accept a blood transfusion, the first chance node may define the probability that the patient will be infected with a blood borne infection such as HIV if she accepts. Another chance node may define the risk of death if transfusion is refused (**Fig. 17.2**). Probabilities defined at chance nodes are usually derived from the literature or from clinical trial data. At the end of each branch of a decision tree is the *terminal node*, at which a payoff representing the effectiveness of that strategy occurs. In the blood transfusion example, the terminal nodes define three states: life, death, or life with a blood borne infection such as HIV. The payoff for life is 1, for death is 0, and for infection is a utility representing a lifetime spent with the infection. The expected value of each strategy, or its effectiveness, is calculated as the weighted average of the probabilities and payoffs associated with each terminal branch of the tree. The strategy resulting in the highest expected value is said to be the most effective. The payoff in an oncology model is usually expressed as a survival time. In a CUA, the effectiveness might be the product of survival time and the quality of life–based preference score, or utility.

Once all possible clinical events and their probabilities and payoffs have been defined by chance nodes, the costs of tests, treatments, and adverse events may be incorporated at each node. The cost associated with each strategy is calculated as a weighted average of the costs and probabilities associated with each branch of the tree.

Analysis of Model

After cost and effectiveness information have been collected and incorporated into the model, the analyses are performed. Results of cost-effectiveness models are expressed in terms of a comparison of two or more strategies. When one strategy is both more costly and less effective than an alternative strategy, it is said to be *dominated* and should not be considered. Likewise, a strategy that is both more effective and less costly is considered to be *dominant* and should be the treatment of choice. In these two cases, a numeric cost-effectiveness quantification is not needed. When one strategy is both more costly and more effective than an alternative, an ICER is calculated. This is expressed as the difference in the mean cost divided by the difference in the mean effectiveness between strategies.

The ICER for comparison of intervention A with intervention B is defined as

$$\text{ICER} = \frac{\text{Cost}_A - \text{Cost}_B}{\text{Effect}_A - \text{Effect}_B}$$

It is important to note that the ICER is *not* estimated by dividing the cost of one intervention by the measure of its own effectiveness. This average cost-effectiveness ratio is not comparable to the ICER and is not a useful metric in CEAs (27).

In the United States, an intervention has traditionally been considered cost-effective relative to an alternative strategy if the ICER is less than $50,000 per year of life saved (YLS)/QALY (22). Although ICER thresholds of $50,000 per YLS are theoretically used in decision making, they are not strictly applied. Social norms may raise this value such that interventions costing up to $100,000 or even greater per QALY have sometimes been considered cost-effective (28). The term "cost-effective" does not mean that a strategy saves money but

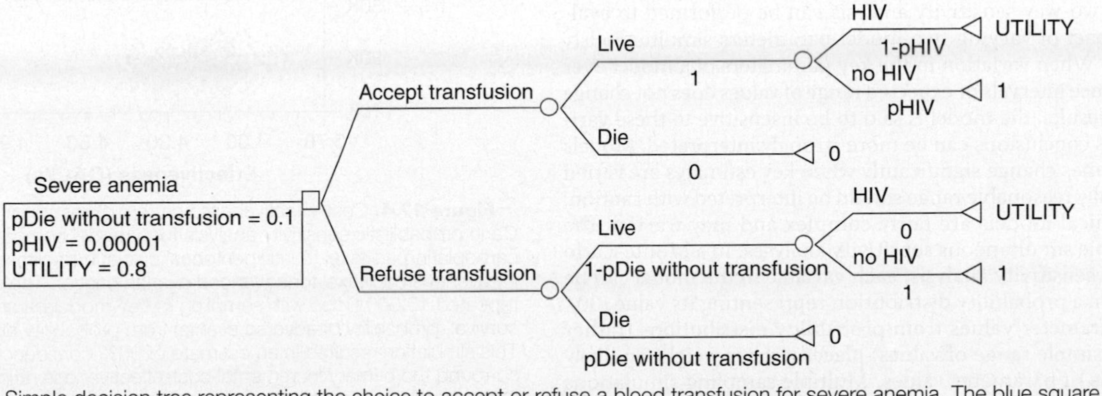

Figure 17.2. Simple decision tree representing the choice to accept or refuse a blood transfusion for severe anemia. The blue square is the decision node, green circles are chance nodes, and the red triangles are terminal nodes. Probabilities of events are depicted beneath each branch. Payoffs are listed to the right of terminal nodes. Three parameters are modeled as variables and have been given numeric values defined beneath the decision node: pHIV is the probability of being infected with HIV should the patient accept a transfusion. pDie Without Transfusion is the probability of death from severe anemia without a transfusion. UTILITY is the quality of life–related value of living with HIV, where 0 represents death and 1, perfect health.

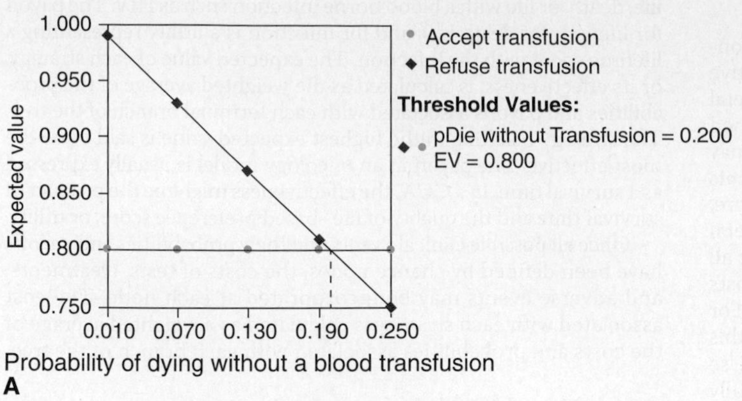

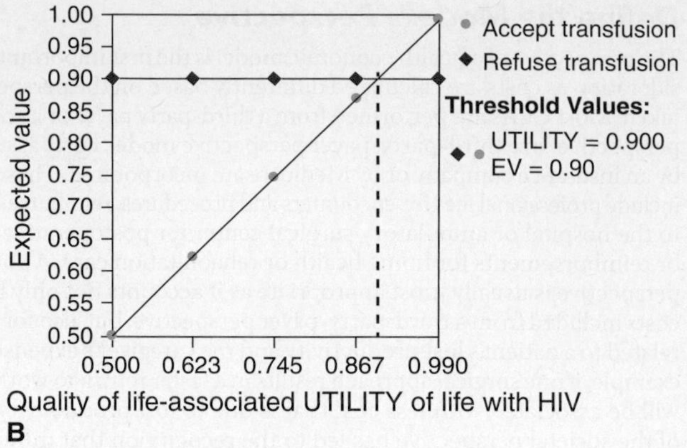

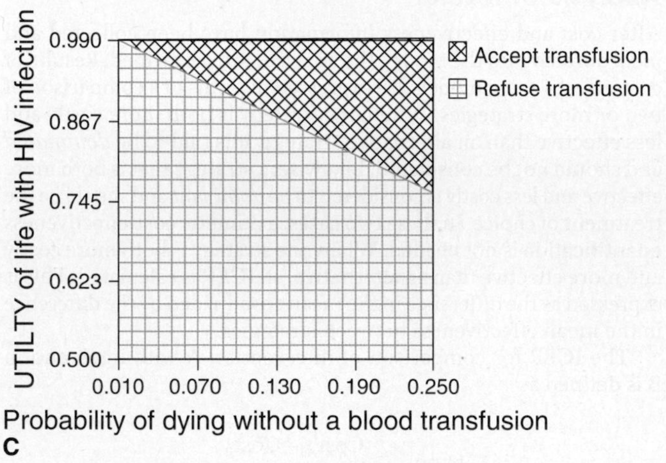

Figure 17.3. A: One-way sensitivity analysis on the probability of death from anemia without a blood transfusion. When the probability of death from anemia exceeds the threshold value of 0.2, the expected value of accepting the transfusion exceeds that of refusing transfusion, and the correct choice is to accept the transfusion. **B:** One-way sensitivity analysis on the quality of life–related utility of living with HIV. When the utility exceeds the threshold value of 0.9, the expected value of accepting the transfusion exceeds that of refusing transfusion, and the correct choice is to accept the transfusion. **C:** Two-way sensitivity analysis in which the utility associated with HIV infection and the probability of death without transfusion are varied simultaneously. The blue shaded area represents values for which acceptance of a transfusion results in the highest expected value (payoff) and is the preferred choice. Green shaded area represents combinations for which refusal of transfusion is the preferred choice.

rather that the additional cost of the intervention is worthwhile, usually from the perspective of society.

Sensitivity Analyses

Uncertainty in health economic analyses may exist about such input parameters as cost, survival, or clinical probabilities. To assess the impact of such uncertainty on the findings of a decision model, a sensitivity analysis can be performed. The simplest form of sensitivity analysis is a one-way analysis. Estimates are varied one parameter at a time to evaluate the impact changes make on the outcome or conclusions of the model (29). For example, in the simple model describing the decision to accept or refuse a blood transfusion, varying the probability of death due to anemia or the utility related to quality of life with HIV has an impact on the expected value of each decision (**Fig. 17.3A,B**). Likewise, a two-way sensitivity analysis can be performed to evaluate the impact of varying two model parameters simultaneously (**Fig. 17.3C**). When variation in the key parameters of a model over their confidence intervals or expected range of values does not change the model's results, the model is said to be insensitive to these variations and its conclusions can be more strongly interpreted. Models whose outcomes change significantly when key estimates are varied over a clinically reasonable range should be interpreted with caution.

Most clinical models are fairly complex and may warrant the use of multiple simultaneous sensitivity analyses. In a Monte Carlo probabilistic sensitivity analysis, each variable in the model can be sampled from a probability distribution representing its value (30). Sampling parameter values from probability distributions (rather than from a simple range of values) places greater weight on likely combinations of parameter values. Multiple sampling simulations of the model may then be run, each of which results in an individual cost-effectiveness comparison or estimate. Multiple simulations allow for construction of a cost-effectiveness scatterplot and the ability to express confidence intervals around the ICER estimate (**Fig. 17.4**), which effectively allows quantification of the total impact

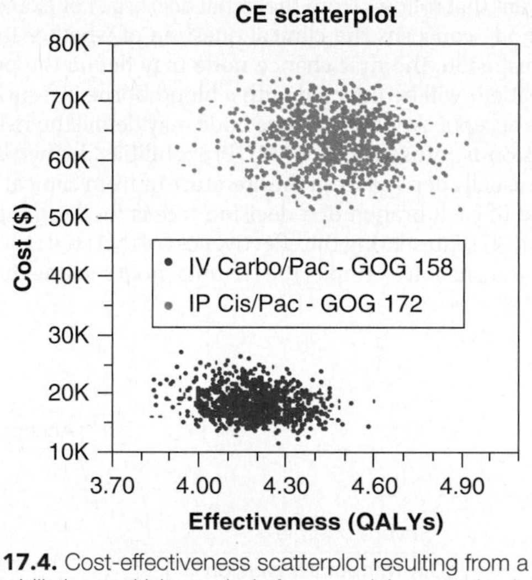

Figure 17.4. Cost-effectiveness scatterplot resulting from a Monte Carlo probabilistic sensitivity analysis for a model comparing intravenous carboplatin/paclitaxel to intraperitoneal cisplatin/paclitaxel and intravenous paclitaxel for advanced ovarian cancer. The simulation was repeated 10,000 times with sampling of key model parameters (cost, survival, probability of adverse events) from probability distributions. This simulation resulted in an estimate of 95% confidence intervals to surround the primary incremental cost-effectiveness ratio estimate. QALY, quality-adjusted life year.

Source: Reprinted with permission. © 2008 American Society of Clinical Oncology. All rights reserved. Havrilesky LJ, Alvarez-Secord A, Darcy KM, et al. Cost effectiveness of intraperitoneal compared with intravenous chemotherapy for women with optimally resected stage III cancer: A Gynecologic Oncology Group study. *J Clin Oncol.* 2008;26(25):4144–4150.

of uncertainty on the model and the confidence that can be placed in the analysis results.

INPUT DEVELOPMENT FOR HEALTH ECONOMIC MODELS

The following section details methods for the development of input data for health economic models.

Estimation of Costs

Cost Definitions

The costs incorporated into a CEA depend on the study's perspective. The standard CEA or CUA is performed from a societal perspective (22). However, alternative perspectives include those of the patient, hospital, or a third-party payer. In a societal perspective analysis, the costs included are all of those borne by society and should therefore include both direct and indirect costs. Direct costs include direct medical costs (e.g., professional and hospital costs, diagnostic tests and procedures) and direct nonmedical costs (such as travel to receive care). Indirect costs account for lost productivity due to time off work for illness, both for the patient and any caregivers. When a health economic model is performed from a nonsocietal perspective, the scope of the costs included may be narrower. For example, in an analysis performed from a third-party-payer perspective, lost productivity would not be included.

Costs versus Charges

When performing a health economic analysis, it is important to distinguish costs from charges. Charges represent what the provider or hospital asks an individual to pay for a service, and not the reimbursement provided by either a private third-party payer or Medicare. Because reimbursements by the Centers for Medicare and Medicaid Services (CMS) are generally considered to approximate the cost of providing a service, it is standard to use national Medicare reimbursements to approximate the costs of medical tests, procedures, or services in a health economic analysis (31). If a Medicare reimbursement is not available for a particular aspect of medical costs, charges may be used to calculate costs using a cost-charge ratio. Cost-charge ratios allow a calculation of the proportion of hospital charges that represent cost to the hospital. Cost-charge ratios are specific to individual hospital departments and may be available from CMS (http://www.cms.gov).

Surgical Costs

Health economic analyses in gynecologic oncology may include an estimate of the costs of surgical procedures. CMS reimbursements may be used to approximate these costs from a societal perspective. Direct surgical costs include professional fees (surgeon, anesthesiologist, pathologist), the cost of hospital recovery, and the costs of any tests or procedures performed in the postoperative period. Postoperative outpatient care is usually part of a global fee that includes the first 90 days of postoperative care and is therefore not included separately. Likewise, the reimbursement for recovery in the hospital or ambulatory surgery center is usually determined by a CMS code, and this reimbursement covers tests and inpatient care. However, additional procedures performed postoperatively are associated with additional professional fees.

Costs of Hospitalization

The cost of a hospitalization may be estimated for health economic models using the Diagnosis Related Group, a CMS code that takes into account the primary diagnosis and the patient's comorbidities and is used to determine the reimbursement Medicare provides to the hospital. An alternative method for estimating the cost of an inpatient hospital stay is to use the Agency for Healthcare Research and Quality's Healthcare Cost and Utilization Project Nationwide Inpatient Sample (http://www.hcup-us.ahrq.gov/). This large all-payer public database provides inpatient data from a national sample of over 1,000 hospitals in 44 states and is released annually. Mean and median charges and costs of all hospitalizations for a specific primary or secondary diagnosis can be obtained by entering the International Classification of Diseases, Ninth Revision (ICD-9) codes. Results can be stratified by demographic information.

Outpatient Treatment Costs

Outpatient treatments in gynecologic oncology often refer to chemotherapy. Cost tabulation should include the CMS reimbursements for the individual chemotherapy drugs and any other medications infused based on the designated J code for each drug. Tests performed routinely over the course of a cycle of treatment should also be included. Finally, the costs of infusion at an outpatient facility should be included using appropriate current procedural terminology codes.

Adverse Events

When two or more strategies are compared using a health economic model, it is critical that the adverse events associated with each strategy be accounted for. Specifically, when severe adverse events result in additional medical or nonmedical costs, these costs should be incorporated as well. For example, if one chemotherapy strategy results in a higher rate of febrile neutropenia, the cost of a hospitalization for this diagnosis should be incorporated into the cost of each strategy in proportion to the probability of the event in each treatment group. Adverse events whose frequencies are not significantly different between strategies or that do not generate additional cost (e.g., grade 1 anemia) may reasonably be omitted from a CEA. However, models should adjust for quality of life differences resulting from adverse events.

Cost Collection as a Component of Phase III Trials

While many cost-effectiveness studies are performed following completion of the clinical trials from which the data are derived, such analyses are ideally planned and executed in conjunction with prospective phase III trials. The International Society for Pharmacoeconomics and Outcomes Research Task Force on Good Research Practices recommends that collection of health economic data should be fully integrated into phase III studies (31). In a phase III trial, prospective economic data are usually collected by accounting for differences in health resource utilization between treatment groups. Ideally, this might include an accounting of all health-related encounters in each treatment group. However, logistical considerations during trial planning often require prioritization as to which data elements will be collected. Therefore, it is often appropriate to choose to focus on "big ticket" items as well as resources that are expected to differ between treatment arms. Resource utilization collection is accomplished by means of subject diaries in which outpatient and inpatient encounters as well as travel and caregiver time may be recorded. Once resource utilization collection is accomplished, national fee schedules and reimbursements are generally used to assign costs to each element.

Modeling Effectiveness

Effectiveness in CEA should be reported in units of relevant clinical outcomes. For example, in oncology studies, effectiveness might be expressed as the number of cases of cancer prevented, the number of unnecessary surgical procedures avoided, or the number of cancer recurrences prevented. However, it is most common in oncology CEA to quantify effectiveness using survival. Thus, in CEAs, the comparison of alternative strategies might be described in terms of the cost per additional year of life, or QALY, saved. While OS is a standard outcome in both CEA and clinical trials, PFS may also be reported.

Modeling Survival

Survival outcomes may be modeled in several ways. One simple method is to assign a survival time (e.g., mean survival in years) to each relevant branch of a simple decision tree. While this method accomplishes the assignment of a survival "value" to each branch of the model, it does not account for additional costs or changes in quality of life that may need to be applied only to subjects who are still alive at a later time. For example, it may be useful to apply the cost of additional cycles of treatment or adverse events to only those individuals remaining alive or progression free at a specific time point. An alternative, and more common, method is to use a modified Markov state transition model to represent survival (see Construction of a Markov Natural History Model section). When a modified Markov approach is used, costs of events that are applied only if a subject is alive or has relapsed may be applied at each relevant time point. Likewise, changes in quality of life during or after treatment may also be quantified. In the context of comparing effectiveness results of a prospective clinical trial, raw survival data can be used to model Kaplan–Meier survival curves directly (**Fig. 17.5**).

Modeling Quality of Life

Medical interventions in oncology may improve quality of life without extending life or may extend life but worsen quality during treatment. Economic analyses that are based only on cost and efficacy do not fully account for the value of many treatments and interventions. CUAs account for the morbidity, physical well-being, and emotional well-being associated with medical treatments. CUAs may be used when the interventions being considered affect both quality of life and survival or when there is no expected difference in survival but a difference in quality of life is anticipated (20).

In CUAs, quality of life is represented by a utility. A utility is a measure of the desirability or preference that individuals or societies place on a given health outcome (32,33). Utility scores are usually linked to judgments about the value of a particular health state. The anchor health states are 0 for death and 1 for perfect health. Applying utility scores to a cost-effectiveness model allows the outcome of the economic analysis, now the CUA, to be reported in QALYs.

Eliciting Preferences for Calculation of Utility Scores

Use of utility scores in a cost-utility model requires a defined health state for each distinct outcome of the intervention and its alternative (34). For example, health states of interest in an ovarian cancer CUA may include (1) newly diagnosed ovarian cancer starting primary chemotherapy; (2) completed primary therapy, no evidence of disease; (3) progressive disease on treatment; or (4) end-stage ovarian cancer. Descriptions of health states are needed to derive utilities. The description of each health state includes information about levels of physical health, emotional health, activities of daily living, and overall well-being (35). A rater provides preferences for each health state and a utility score is created. Raters are selected according to the perspective of the study. For example, if a societal perspective is taken, then representatives of the general population should be used to score the preference (22). The preferences of individuals with conditions of interest (such as patients) or of physicians are important ancillary information that might be incorporated into studies performed from alternative perspectives, but these cannot be substituted for societal preferences when the model's perspective is societal (26). Several rigorous formal approaches to the direct measurement of preferences and calculation of utility scores for health states have been developed, of which the most commonly used are the standard gamble (SG) and the time trade-off (TTO) methods.

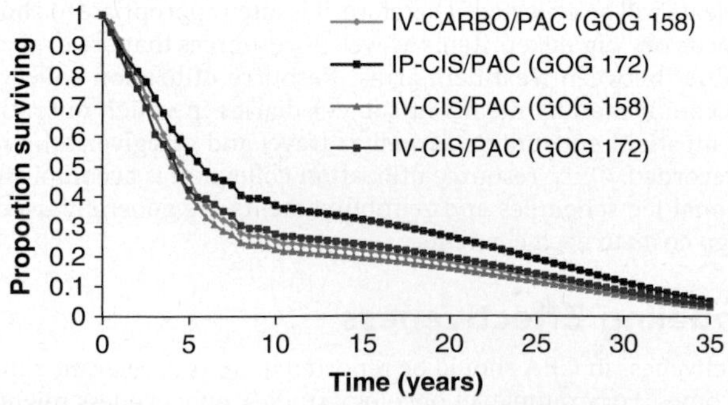

Figure 17.5. Survival curve output from a modified Markov state transition model designed to compare the cost-effectiveness of chemotherapy regimens studied in two randomized phase III trials.

Source: Reprinted with permission. Havrilesky LJ, Alvarez-Secord A, Darcy KM, et al. Cost effectiveness of intraperitoneal compared with intravenous chemotherapy for women with optimally resected stage III cancer: A Gynecologic Oncology Group study. *J Clin Oncol.* 2008;26(25):4144–4150.

The TTO method presents the rater with a choice between two health states, both of which have a certain outcome (36). Raters choose between a set number of years of life in a certain health state (i.e., with disease) and a shorter number of years of life in perfect health. The shortest period of time in perfect health that a rater would accept in exchange for a lifetime in the diseased state determines the utility score. For example, if the rater would accept living the next 20 years (but no less) in perfect health instead of living the next 30 years in the diseased health state, the utility score for the health state would be 20/30 or 0.67. The TTO method is relatively easy for raters to comprehend.

In the SG, raters are asked to choose between two alternatives: one with a guaranteed outcome and an alternative containing uncertainty or a "gamble." The guaranteed outcome is the less-than-perfect health state that is being rated. The alternative consists of a treatment that has two possible results: perfect health, with a probability of p, or a worst state (such as death) with a probability $1-p$. The value of p is then varied until the rater is indifferent between the choices of the alternative outcome. While there is some debate concerning consistency of results between the SG and TTO, they are both considered standard methods for eliciting utilities (33,34,37).

Use of Quality of Life Instruments and Health Status Classification Systems to Derive Utilities for CER

Measuring preferences for health outcomes using the direct SG and TTO methods is not a simple exercise and is beyond the scope of most clinical trials for which a CUA might be desirable. There exist a number of prescored health status classification systems to allow indirect assignment of utilities based on questionnaires, and calibrated using prior studies of societal preferences. For example, EuroQoL-5D (EQ-5D) is a simple questionnaire in which raters report no problem, some problem, or a major problem in five dimensions: mobility, self-care, usual activities, pain/discomfort, anxiety/depression (38). The ratings are scores from 0 (dead) to 1 (perfect health) and have been measured against the TTO technique on a random sample of 3,000 members of the adult population in the United Kingdom (39). The score obtained from the EQ-5D may be directly applied to health economic models and is the method preferred by the UK NICE.

The Functional Assessment of Cancer Therapy (FACT) is a 33-item scale developed to measure quality of life in patients undergoing cancer treatment (40). It is commonly used in RCTs of gynecologic cancers. The FACT consists of a core instrument (FACT-G) that can be supplemented by various subscales based on the malignancy of interest. While conversion of FACT scores to utilities has been studied, these methods have not been fully validated (41).

To date, the TTO and SG methods are the most accepted methods to develop utility scores. Although the use of quality of life instruments eases the labor intensiveness of collecting preferences using the TTO and SG methods, many question the validity of the use of indirect methods such as quality of life instruments to construct CUAs. At present, there is no clearly superior method for determining utility scores, either direct or indirect methods. Moreover, some believe that utilities should best be derived from patients as patients really know their disease condition best (42). Others feel that the preferences of the general public are most relevant because society as a whole must delegate distribution of its health care resources (43). As economic analyses evolve, the limitations of preference ratings should be examined and a consistent method of developing utility scores should be determined to allow for better comparisons to be made across cost-utility studies.

MODELING APPROACHES TO SCREENING FOR GYNECOLOGIC CANCERS

In the following section, methods for the development of natural history models of cancer and their use in screening decision analyses will be described. The current state of evidence for cervical and ovarian cancer screening as informed by the current literature as well as simulation modeling will then be reviewed.

Modeling the Natural History of Cancer

In order to evaluate the effectiveness of a proposed cancer screening test for which no phase III clinical trials have been completed, a model can be created that simulates the natural history of the disease with and without screening. The simplest model is a decision tree. Although decision trees are useful for modeling outcomes that occur over a short period of time, such as a year, they can become unwieldy when trying to model a disease that occurs over a longer period or that involves recurrent events such as multiple episodes of screening or multiple cycles of treatment. Markov models are used for events that recur or occur in a predictable manner over time (44). They are particularly well suited to depicting the events associated with cancer, especially cancers that have a screening component.

Construction of a Markov Natural History Model

For creation of a Markov model, the natural history of a cancer is broken up into a defined, mutually exclusive, and exhaustive set of states. For cervical cancer, these states could include Well, Human Papillomavirus (HPV) Infection, Preinvasive Disease, Undetected Invasive Cancer (Stages I though IV), Detected Invasive Cancer (Stages I though IV), Cancer Death, and Death from Other Causes. For epithelial ovarian cancer, which does not have a universal preinvasive state, natural history states might include Well, Undetected and Detected Invasive Cancer (Stages I through IV), Cancer Death, and Death from Other Causes (**Fig. 17.6**). Once the states have been defined, movement (usually referred to as "transition") between the states is defined based on knowledge of the cancer's natural history. The probabilities of moving from one state to another over a fixed period of time are then used to populate the model. These are usually obtained from the epidemiologic literature, an analysis of an epidemiologic study, or expert opinion. Together, the states, allowed transitions and probabilities constitute the model. Once programmed, the model can be used to calculate different outcomes such as the lifetime risk of developing or dying from cancer. The outcomes are usually calculated for a cohort (or cohorts) of women who are assumed to enter the model at a given age and are then followed until death or a later age (i.e., 100 years).

Calibration

An important step in developing a model is obtaining probabilities or estimates for key variables (referred to as parameters) from the literature. However, often there are few available estimates, estimates of varying degrees of quality, or even no existing estimates for a given model parameter. The selection of a given clinical estimate is important since this affects the credibility of the model's aggregate result. Calibration is a process that involves comparing the model-predicted results with observed data to ensure a reasonably good fit of one to the other. Model calibration involves several steps: (1) identification

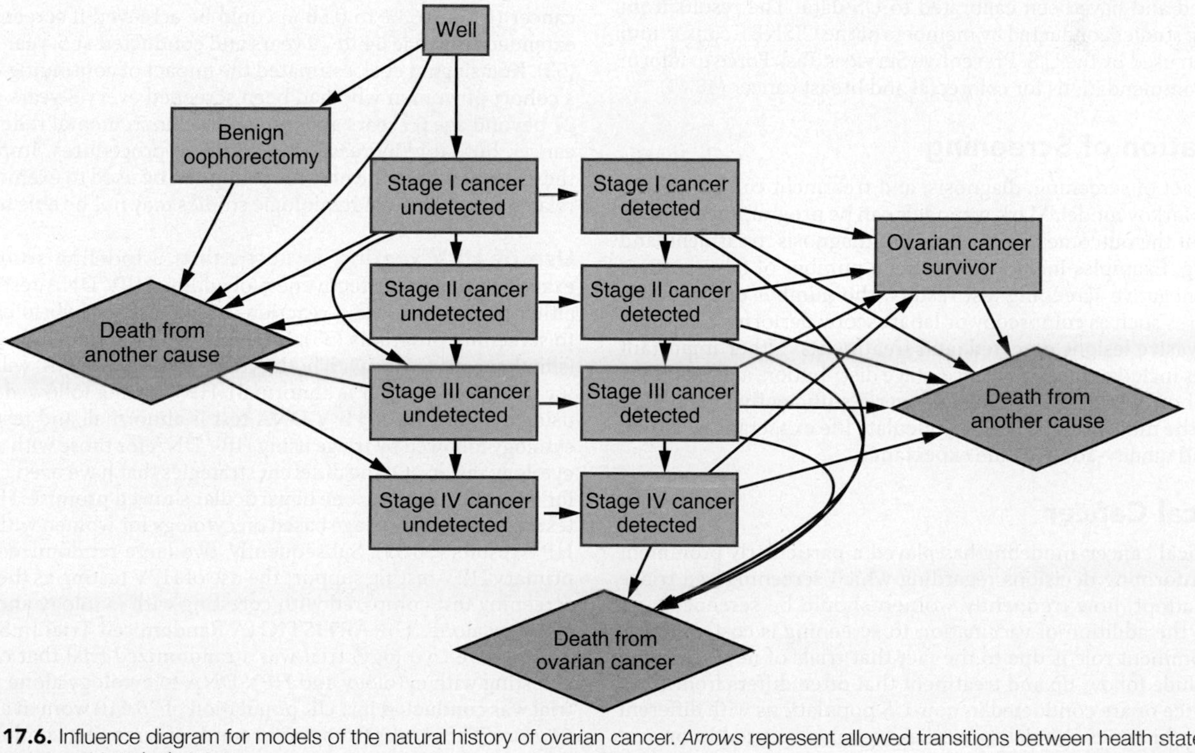

Figure 17.6. Influence diagram for models of the natural history of ovarian cancer. *Arrows* represent allowed transitions between health states. Diamonds represent terminal states.

Source: Reprinted with permission from Havrilesky LJ, Sanders GD, Lulasingam S, et al. Development of an ovarian cancer screening decision model that incorporates disease heterogeneity: implications for potential mortality reduction. *Cancer.* 2011;117(3):545–553.

of calibration endpoints (for cancer this usually means age-specific cancer incidence, but can also include stage distribution and age-specific mortality curve); (2) establishment of criteria for determining how well the model-predicted data fit the observed data (this may be visual inspection or using a statistical goodness of fit test); (3) adjustment of the set of model input parameters (i.e., probabilities); and (4) comparison of model-predicted outcomes to observed outcomes using the prespecified criteria and repeating steps 3 and 4 until a satisfactory calibration is achieved (45,46).

Validation

Model validation (confirmation that the calibrated model predicts results that are consistent with observed results from screening trials) can be achieved in a number of ways. The most robust method is to compare model-predicted outcomes with actual outcomes. For example, Havrilesky et al. constructed a natural history model accounting for the observed heterogeneity of epithelial ovarian cancers. Validation was performed by simulating the prevalence screen phase of the UK Collaborative Trial of Ovarian Cancer Screening (UKCTOCS) ovarian cancer screening trial. The model predicted the stage distribution of cancers detected by screening and the positive predictive value of the multimodality prevalence screen within their reported 95% confidence intervals (47). To the degree that simulated results do not reproduce those observed in a clinical trial, the question arises whether there are key input parameters or model structural differences that affect the conclusions. A model can then be revised to determine whether the prediction is improved in an iterative process. Usually, the initial decision to conduct a modeling study is based on the fact that there is no observed data that exist to answer a given question. In this case, model validation is achieved by comparing the results from models built by different, independent groups, to evaluate for similarity. This approach has been adopted by the Cancer Intervention and Surveillance Modeling Network (CISNET). CISNET is a consortium of National Cancer Institute–sponsored investigators who use statistical modeling to study cancer control interventions in prevention, screening, and treatment and their effects on population trends in incidence and mortality. The models in this consortium were independently developed and have been calibrated to US data. The results from modeling studies conducted by members of the CISNET consortium have been used by the U.S. Preventive Services Task Force to inform their recommendations for colorectal and breast cancer (48,49).

Simulation of Screening

The impact of screening, diagnosis, and treatment can be tracked using a Markov model. Markov models can be programmed to keep a count of the outcomes associated with diagnosis, treatment, and screening. Examples include the average number of false-positive or false-negative screening test results, the number of diagnostic procedures such as colposcopy or laparoscopy performed, number of preinvasive lesions detected, and treatments. Other important outcomes include cancer incidence, stage distribution, and mortality. If the cohort of women is modeled over a sufficiently long period of time, the model can be used to calculate life expectancy, lifetime costs, and quality-adjusted life expectancy.

Cervical Cancer

For cervical cancer, modeling has played a particularly prominent role in informing decisions regarding which screening and triage tests to adopt, how frequently women should be screened, and whether the addition of vaccination to screening is cost-effective. This prominent role is due to the fact that trials of new screening tests include follow-up and treatment that often differs from clinical practice or are conducted in non-US populations with different screening histories. Modeling studies can also be used to project both short- and long-term results from trials. For example, trials for the HPV vaccines used cervical intraepithelial neoplasia (CIN) grade 2 or higher as primary outcomes. However, cancer incidence and death are more important outcomes for policy makers. Modeling has been used to estimate the potential cost-effectiveness of adding vaccination to screening. More recently, modeling has been used to justify the expanded coverage of HPV vaccines to include boys. The following sections describe how models of HPV and cervical cancer have been used to enhance clinical data and inform policies regarding screening and vaccination for cervical cancer prevention.

Questions Addressed by Cervical Cancer Models

Appropriate age to begin/end and screening interval with cytology. A mathematical model of cervical cancer, developed in the 1980s by David Eddy, was used to examine the relationship between Pap smear screening interval and cancer incidence (50). This modeling study showed that screening every 2 or 3 years would result in 95% to 99% of the cancer reduction benefit of screening every year, but with lower costs and fewer procedures. In terms of the ages to begin and end screening, these have for the most part been based on epidemiologic data showing that cancer incidence peaks in the late 30s to mid-40s but that the incidence of CIN peaks in the 20s (51,52). More recently, modeling has been used to help inform changes to recommendations regarding the age to begin or end screening but also to quantify the trade-offs in terms of burdens and benefits of screening at different ages. An example is from Canfell et al. who modeled the impact of changing the UK screening guidelines to begin at age 25 years instead of age 21 years (53). They found that if the age to begin screening was delayed until 25 years, the lifetime risk of cancer would be minimally affected (cumulative lifetime incidence decreasing from 0.63% to 0.61%) due to the low incidence of cancer in young women (53). More recently, Kulasingam et al. modeled the impact of varying the age to begin screening in 1-year increments from age 15 to 25 years on cancer incidence and mortality (54). They showed that screening in the teens was associated with a high number of additional diagnostic procedures, but very small reductions in lifetime risk of cancer, when compared with beginning screening in the 20s. In terms of the age to end screening, Canfell et al. showed that further reductions in lifetime incidence of cancer (from 0.63% to 0.56%) could be achieved if screening were extended from age 64 to 79 years and conducted at 5-year intervals (53). Kulasingam et al. estimated the impact of continuing to screen a cohort of women who had been screened every 3 years since age 21 beyond age 65 years and also showed incremental reductions in cancer, but large increases in additional procedures. Importantly, these studies illustrate how modeling can be used to examine issues related to age that epidemiologic studies may not be able to answer.

Use of HPV testing in screening. Modeling studies have examined the cost-effectiveness of adding HPV DNA testing (with either polymerase chain reaction–based tests or hybrid capture 2) to screening programs (55). Strategies examined include cotesting (simultaneous testing with both cytology and HPV DNA, with referral for treatment if either is abnormal), HPV testing followed by triage using cytology if the HPV DNA test is abnormal, and testing with cytology followed by triage using HPV DNA for those with abnormal cytology results. Of the different strategies that have been compared for cost-effectiveness, one in particular showed promise: HPV DNA testing followed by triage based on cytology for women with positive HPV results (56,57). Subsequently, two large randomized trials of primary HPV testing support the use of HPV testing as the primary screening test compared with cotesting with cytology and HPV or cytology alone. The ARTISTIC (A Randomised Trial In Screening To Improve Cytology) trial was a randomized trial that compared cotesting with cytology and HPV DNA to cytology alone (58). The trial was conducted in a UK population of 25,410 women aged 20 to 64 years. The results from three rounds of screening conducted over 6 years were used in combination with a decision model to compare the following screening strategies: (1) screening with cytology alone; (2) screening with HPV followed by triage of HPV-positive women with cytology; (3) screening with HPV followed by triage with genotyping for HPV-16/18 or cytology for other high-risk HPV-positive women; and (4) cotesting with cytology and HPV. The model predicted that primary screening with HPV DNA (strategies 2 or 3) is more effective and potentially cost-saving compared with screening with cytology alone (59).

In the United States, the Addressing the Need for Advanced HPV Diagnostics (ATHENA) study is a prospective 3-year cervical cancer screening trial of 47,208 women aged 21 years and older that compared the performance of the cobas HPV test (Roche Molecular Diagnostics, Pleasanton, CA), which detects 12 HPV types and also provides separate results for HPV-16 and -18, alone and in combination with cervical cytology (60). An analysis restricted to women aged 25 years and older showed that primary screening with HPV, and use of genotyping and cytology for triage of HPV-positive women, was more sensitive with a similar positive predictive value than cytology using an ASCUS cut-point for referral to colposcopy. Based, in part, on these results, the Food and Drug Administration (FDA) in 2014 approved the use of the cobas HPV test as a stand-alone screening test for cervical cancer screening in women aged 25 years and older. Interim guidelines on the use of this test recommend immediate colposcopy for women who are HPV-16 and/or -18 positive or the use of cytology for triage of women who are positive for the other 12 HPV types (61). To date, modeling studies of this new strategy have not been conducted; however, such studies will be needed to quantify the potential impact on cancer and cancer deaths that this new screening option will have compared to currently recommended strategies, namely, screening every 3 years with cytology beginning at age 21 years and ending at age 65 years or switching to cotesting every 5 years beginning at age 30 years.

Quantifying the impact of HPV vaccination. Two types of models have been used to explore HPV vaccine effectiveness: Markov state transition cohort models (described above) and dynamic transmission models, with a third category—hybrid models—that uses a combination of the two (62). Dynamic models track population changes over time by taking into account births as well as deaths. Importantly, dynamic transmission models also account for how infection with HPV depends on patterns of sexual behavior and the distribution of infection in the population (63). As such, a strength of dynamic models is that they can be used to determine herd immunity, explore the relative value of vaccinating boys in addition to girls, and explore how sexual mixing patterns (how men and women form partnerships and how these affect transmission) affect the age at which vaccination should begin and age(s) for catch-up programs (i.e., vaccination offered to girls and/or women who are not part of the optimal age group but who may still derive a benefit). A recent modeling study conducted using multiple, independently developed HPV and cervical cancer hybrid, Markov and fully dynamic models concluded that vaccination of girls prior to the age of sexual debut has the potential to considerably reduce the burden of CIN and cervical cancer (64). This is especially true if a long duration of vaccine efficacy and high vaccine coverage are modeled. Vaccine price has also consistently been shown to impact the cost-effectiveness of adding vaccination to screening or adding HPV vaccines to existing vaccine programs. Indeed, if HPV vaccines are priced below certain thresholds for different countries, HPV vaccination could potentially be cost-saving compared with not screening (65). Of note, across a range of analyses, vaccination of girls only prior to onset of sexual activity, as opposed to vaccination of boys and girls plus catch-up vaccination, has been shown to have the most attractive cost-effectiveness profile. However, under conditions of low coverage, as has occurred in the United States, extending vaccination to boys is potentially cost-effective (66). Based on these results, and survey data showing low uptake of the HPV vaccines in the United States, the Centers for Disease Control and Prevention Advisory Committee on Immunization Practices (ACIP) decided to extend HPV vaccine recommendations to include boys in addition to girls in 2009 (67). In 2015, the FDA approved a nonavalent HPV vaccine targeted against seven high-risk and two low-risk HPV types associated with approximately 80% of cervical cancers. Modeling by Brisson et al. was conducted to determine the impact of recommending this vaccine in a US population and was included in the recommendation for use of this vaccine by the ACIP (68). Their modeling study predicts that use of the 9vHPV in both males and females will be cost-saving when compared with 4vHPV if the cost of the new vaccine is at most $13 greater than the cost of the 4vHPV vaccine. The 9vHPV was cost-saving in a number of scenarios, and the cost per QALY gained did not exceed $25,000 in any scenario across a range of assumptions about HPV natural history, cervical cancer screening, vaccine coverage, vaccine duration of protection, and health care costs. However, the cost-effectiveness of the 9vHPV was sensitive to assumptions about cost of the vaccine.

Screening in the era of HPV vaccines. The issue of whether and how screening should change in the era of HPV vaccines is complex and will depend on a number of factors that are still unknown. These include, but are not limited to, the performance of cytology and HPV tests in vaccinated women, whether predicted reductions in CIN and cancer are achieved, and whether vaccination will affect screening behavior, in particular screening participation. Under the assumption that vaccines will markedly reduce cancer incidence and mortality, potentially cost-effective approaches to screening vaccinated cohorts of women include strategies that use a less frequent screening interval, delayed age of first screening, and/or use of a strategy based on HPV DNA testing followed by cytology (56,69). Of note, preliminary modeling to examine the impact of cross protection and broad spectrum vaccines suggests that far fewer screens than currently recommended will be needed to continue to achieve significant reductions in cervical cancer (70). However, with low vaccine coverage continuing to be an issue in the United States, changes to screening for vaccinated cohorts have yet to be instituted and may well be decades off (71).

Modeling has been used extensively in cervical cancer to inform how we should approach screening and add HPV vaccination programs to screening programs. Given the development of new tests for cervical cancer and new vaccines that cover more HPV types than the first generation of HPV vaccines, modeling will continue to play a key role in determining the most effective and cost-effective strategies for prevention of cervical cancer.

Ovarian Cancer

Because the majority of ovarian cancers are diagnosed at an advanced stage, there has been considerable interest in designing screening strategies to diagnose and treat women earlier in the hopes of improving survival outcomes. Several key parameters may impact the success of any cancer screening program: (1) Availability of effective treatment for screen positive individuals; (2) Sufficiently high disease prevalence; (3) Existence of an effective screening test; and (4) Acceptable cost or cost-effectiveness of the screening program. Each of these parameters is addressed below in the context of development of a screening test for epithelial ovarian cancer.

Effectiveness of Treatment

Pathologic and genetic data now suggest that epithelial ovarian cancer is a heterogeneous disease, with a number of different precursor lesions. Many high-grade serous ovarian cancers likely originate in the fallopian tubes, whereas some clear cell and endometrioid lesions may originate in the endometrium. Because there is no universal, clearly defined precursor lesion for all epithelial ovarian cancer, the target lesion for the screening tests that are currently in phase III trials is stage I disease. Targeting early-stage disease may be appropriate because survival from epithelial ovarian cancer diagnosed at stage I is encouraging. Women with stage I disease with low-risk features may be cured without the need for adjuvant treatment, while those with higher risk stage I disease may still achieve excellent outcomes following three to six cycles of platinum- and taxane-based chemotherapy (72).

Disease Prevalence

Perhaps the biggest challenge to development of a successful ovarian cancer screening program is the low prevalence of this disease. The lifetime incidence of ovarian cancer in the United States is approximately 1.4%. In postmenopausal women, the most likely target population for a screening program, its prevalence is approximately 40 per 100,000 women. Disease prevalence has a direct impact on the achievable positive predictive value of a screening test, which defines the number of diagnostic procedures or surgeries that would be required to diagnose one case of ovarian cancer. Expert opinion suggests that the minimal acceptable positive predictive value for an ovarian cancer screening test should be 10%. To achieve this value in the postmenopausal population, a screening test needs to have a specificity exceeding 99.6%.

Effectiveness of Screening Test

To date, no screening test for ovarian cancer has been proven effective in reducing mortality from this disease. Two large randomized trials have recently been performed to evaluate screening strategies utilizing the CA125 serum test and transvaginal ultrasound. The Prostate, Lung, Colorectal and Ovarian (PLCO) screening trial randomized 78,216 women to either usual care or a combination of annual CA125 for six consecutive years and annual transvaginal ultrasound for four consecutive years (73). After a median follow-up of 12.4 years, there was no difference in ovarian cancer mortality between the screened and unscreened groups. However, there was evidence of possible harm due to the screening intervention, in the form of a 15% rate of serious adverse events among women with false-positive screening tests who underwent surgical procedures. The authors concluded that simultaneous screening with CA125 and ultrasound does not reduce ovarian cancer mortality and may introduce harms (74).

A second large screening trial, the UKCTOCS study, randomized 202,638 postmenopausal women to no intervention, annual transvaginal ultrasound, or a multimodality algorithm incorporating annual CA125 and second-line transvaginal ultrasound. Mortality was 15% lower, but not statistically significantly so, in the multimodality screening group. However, a planned analysis excluding all cancers diagnosed during the prevalence screen of the trial demonstrated significant ovarian cancer mortality reduction. The authors concluded that further clinical follow-up was needed to make judgment about both the clinical efficacy and cost-effectiveness of the screening algorithm (75).

Comparative Effectiveness of Screening

Several groups have used mathematical modeling to determine the likely success and cost-effectiveness of screening strategies. Skates and Singer designed the first reported stochastic simulation model of the natural history of ovarian cancer. This model suggested that screening using CA125 could potentially save 3.4 years of life per case of cancer detected (76). Urban et al. subsequently modified the Skates and Singer model and performed a cost-effectiveness assessment of several screening strategies. The authors reported that multimodality screening with CA125 followed by transvaginal ultrasound only if CA125 was positive or doubling was potentially cost-effective compared with single test strategies and no screening (77).

More recent screening models have incorporated new data about the pathophysiology and progression of ovarian cancer. Havrilesky et al. constructed a natural history model that, based on the physical proximity of the ovaries to upper abdominal organs such as small bowel and omentum, allowed progression of stage I cancers either to stage II or directly to stage III (78). Disease incidence, mortality, and stage distribution were calibrated to reflect Surveillance, Epidemiology, and End Results (SEER) data. A modified version of this model was designed to account for the heterogeneity of ovarian cancer by modeling aggressive and indolent phenotypes with different rates of progression (47). These models highlighted factors that are important to the success of a screening program. For example, increasing the frequency of screening had a more favorable impact on reducing cancer mortality than increasing the sensitivity of the individual screening test. However, due to the increased cost of screening more frequently, increasing the frequency actually reduced cost-effectiveness. Both models reinforced the important link between specificity and positive predictive value. An annual screening test with a sensitivity of 85% and specificity of less than 99% would have a positive predictive value not exceeding 4%. However, at a specificity of 99.9%, the positive predictive value for annual screening was excellent at 22%. Annual screening of a population of women aged 50 to 85 years at average risk of ovarian cancer with a test at 85% sensitivity and 95% specificity was predicted to improve life expectancy 2.92 days on average, with an ICER of $73,469 per YLS compared with no screening. However, simulated screening of a "high risk" population of women aged 50 to 85 years with a relative risk of developing ovarian cancer of 2 resulted in an improvement in the predicted ICER to $36,025/YLS when compared with no screening. In sensitivity analysis, key factors in achieving a cost-effective screening test (defined as an ICER of less than $50,000 per YLS) were an inexpensive test, a very high test specificity, and infrequent (annual or less) testing. Screening appeared to be potentially most cost-effective when the test specificity was well above 99% and the testing interval was annually or less frequently (78).

These prior models confirm that very high test specificity is required to achieve acceptable positive predictive values, while mortality reduction is sensitive to screening frequency. Annual screening for ovarian cancer appears to be potentially cost-effective in high-risk populations and at very high screening test specificities. For women at average risk, both long-term mortality data and final analysis of the costs of the multimodality screening algorithm in the UKCTOCS trial are critical to any assessment of the costs, benefits, and potential cost-effectiveness of currently available screening strategies. Moreover, because none of the health economic models of screening performed to date have taken quality of life into account, any health economic assessments of ovarian cancer screening would be premature.

COST-EFFECTIVENESS OF THERAPEUTICS IN GYNECOLOGIC CANCERS

In the next section, the value and cost-effectiveness literature regarding therapeutic interventions for gynecologic malignancies are reviewed.

Ovarian Cancer

Chemotherapy for Newly Diagnosed Ovarian Cancer

The standard treatment for ovarian cancer is primary surgical staging with maximum possible cytoreduction followed by chemotherapy.

Introduction of taxanes. The first cost-effectiveness studies in ovarian cancer chemotherapy were performed in response to the introduction of taxanes into the front-line chemotherapy regimen for this disease. Two independent RCTs, conducted by the Gynecological Oncology Group (GOG 111) and the European-Canadian Intergroup (OV-10), demonstrated that cisplatin plus paclitaxel as primary chemotherapy is superior to previous therapy of cisplatin plus cyclophosphamide in clinical response rate, PFS, and OS (79–81). When first introduced, paclitaxel–cisplatin was a more expensive therapy than the old standard of cyclophosphamide–cisplatin. A number of cost-effectiveness investigations were performed using data from GOG 111. From the perspective of a US oncology practice, the total drug costs for cisplatin plus paclitaxel were four times higher than those for cisplatin plus cyclophosphamide ($9,918 vs. $2,527; year of costing not specified) (82). Compared with cisplatin plus cyclophosphamide, the incremental costs per year of life gained for cisplatin plus paclitaxel therapy were $19,820 for inpatient treatment and $21,222 for outpatient treatment. These incremental costs fall well within the generally accepted cost-effective range for new therapies.

Carboplatin and paclitaxel are now both marketed as generics; older studies are therefore less applicable than when originally published. Given the current low cost of paclitaxel, any clinically superior regimen using this drug is also likely to be found cost-effective. Chan et al. have recently performed an economic analysis based on results of a phase III Japanese GOG trial (83) demonstrating that weekly dose-dense paclitaxel is cost-effective compared with an every 3-week regimen in the setting of primary treatment (84).

Intraperitoneal chemotherapy. The NCCN guidelines for ovarian cancer recommend intraperitoneal (IP) chemotherapy as primary/adjuvant therapy for optimally debulked (<1 cm) stage II or greater ovarian cancer treatment (85). Several phase III clinical trials have identified advantages of the use of IP chemotherapy for adjuvant treatment of stage III ovarian cancer; the most recent of these studies demonstrated an OS advantage of 16 months in the IP arm at the expense of increased risk of adverse events and a significant reduction in quality of life (86). Long-term follow-up of GOG trials shows that the survival advantage associated with IP chemotherapy persists past 10 years (87).

Two analyses have evaluated the cost-effectiveness of IP chemotherapy for the primary treatment of stage III ovarian cancer. When comparing IP with intravenous (IV) chemotherapy, Bristow et al. reported that IP chemotherapy was potentially cost-effective compared with IV, with an ICER of US$37,454 per QALY (88). Havrilesky et al. reported an estimate of US$180,022 per QALY when using a 7-year time horizon, which was consistent with the current duration of survival results from GOG 172 (89). However, when the time horizon was extended to a lifetime under the assumption that any survival advantage realized with IP chemo would persist over that period, the ICER of IP chemotherapy dropped to US$32,053 per QALY. While both studies informally incorporated quality of life based on the FACT surveys administered to patients enrolled on GOG trials of chemotherapy, neither performed a validated utility assessment. Conclusions that may be drawn from these studies are that IP chemotherapy is potentially cost-effective for women with stage III disease, but that more formal incorporation of quality of life and investigation of less costly outpatient IP regimens, as were incorporated into the more recently accrued GOG 252 trial, would strengthen this conclusion (88,89).

Bevacizumab. Bevacizumab is an anti–vascular endothelial growth factor inhibitor of angiogenesis and is FDA approved for treatment of a number of different cancers, including platinum-resistant ovarian cancer. With regard to the primary treatment of ovarian cancer, the ICON7 and GOG 218 phase III clinical trials of newly diagnosed ovarian cancer independently and simultaneously reported a small 2- to 6-month OS advantage to the addition of bevacizumab to primary combination of carboplatin/paclitaxel, followed by 14 to 22 additional cycles of consolidation bevacizumab in the absence of progression (90,91). Even prior to the initial presentation of the data in ovarian cancer, questions were raised about the cost of universal bevacizumab. Cohn et al. performed CEAs examining the likely clinical benefit of bevacizumab and the cost of the drug as well as its associated adverse events. These analyses demonstrated that there was no reasonable scenario under which bevacizumab could be considered cost-effective by existing measures (92,93). A subset analysis of the ICON7 data revealed that the main benefit of bevacizumab appears to be confined to women with high-risk disease such as those suboptimally cytoreduced and those with stage IV disease (90). While ideally treatment of a smaller subset of women with ovarian cancer who are most likely to benefit would make this drug more cost-effective, initial attempts at modeling this scenario did not demonstrate this to be a cost-effective alternative (94).

Consolidation therapy. Consolidation regimens that have been studied for ovarian cancer include paclitaxel and bevacizumab; both have a proven PFS benefit but neither has demonstrated an OS benefit. Lesnock et al. performed a CEA of consolidation therapy following carboplatin/paclitaxel, comparing 12 months additional paclitaxel to 17 cycles of additional bevacizumab. Clinical data were derived from the PFS results of GOG 178 and GOG 218. Consolidation therapy with paclitaxel was found to be cost-effective; bevacizumab consolidation was dominated (less effective and more costly) by paclitaxel consolidation (95).

Treatment of Recurrent Ovarian Cancer

Most women with ovarian cancer will achieve clinical remission following primary treatment but will eventually experience recurrence.

Platinum-sensitive recurrence. Patients who experience recurrence more than 6 months after completing a first-line chemotherapy regimen are considered to have "platinum-sensitive" ovarian cancer and have an excellent response rate when re-treated with platinum agents (96,97). Two large RCTs have compared the use of single-agent therapy with combination regimens for platinum-sensitive ovarian cancer. These studies identified a PFS advantage for the combination regimens of gemcitabine plus carboplatin and paclitaxel plus platinum chemotherapy regimens (as well as an OS advantage for paclitaxel plus platinum) compared with platinum alone, and the authors suggested that the combination regimens should be considered standard of care (98,99).

Based on these two studies, Havrilesky et al. designed a Markov state transition model that evaluated the optimal treatment strategy for patients with recurrent platinum-sensitive ovarian cancer. Paclitaxel plus carboplatin had an ICER of $15,564 per additional progression-free year compared with single-agent carboplatin, while gemcitabine plus carboplatin has a less attractive ICER of $278,388 per additional progression-free year compared with paclitaxel plus carboplatin (100). Given that both carboplatin and paclitaxel are now available as generic drugs in the United States, their cost advantage is not surprising. Neurological and hematological toxicities of the regimens were incorporated into a sensitivity analysis that varied the severity and costs associated with treatment. Over a reasonable range of utility scores, paclitaxel plus carboplatin was still cost-effective compared with carboplatin alone, and gemcitabine plus carboplatin remained non-cost-effective (100). These results must be interpreted on an individual basis with an individual's prior adverse event profile in mind; for example, it is unlikely that a patient with severe neurotoxicity due to prior taxane treatment would be re-treated with the same drug.

Platinum-resistant recurrence. Recurrent ovarian cancer that occurs within 6 months of completing a first-line chemotherapy regimen has a poor prognosis, with cure being very unlikely. Rocconi et al. performed a CEA of treatment options for recurrent platinum-resistant ovarian cancer and concluded that only best supportive care (no chemotherapy) was clearly cost-effective, while second-line monotherapy was possibly marginally cost-effective (ICER $64,104 per YLS) as well (101). Even without incorporation of toxicity rates and costs, the authors found that combination chemotherapy regimens were never cost-effective for platinum-resistant disease due to unfavorable ICERs.

Finally, bevacizumab is now FDA approved for platinum-resistant recurrent ovarian cancer based on the results of the AURELIA trial which demonstrated superior PFS when bevacizumab was added to standard of care single-agent chemotherapy (18). Cost-effectiveness evaluations are forthcoming but as yet unpublished in this clinical setting.

Targeted therapies. In the era of personalized medicine, the use of molecular and/or genomic tumor testing to individually tailor cancer treatments has become popular. However, very few targeted treatments have been demonstrated to perform better than nontargeted treatments. The exception in ovarian cancer is the use of polyADP ribose polymerase inhibitors. Women with germline BRCA mutations have been shown to have significantly improved PFS when treated with maintenance olaparib following standard chemotherapy for platinum-sensitive recurrence. In a study by Secord et al., BRCA testing performed specifically to direct the use of maintenance olaparib for platinum-sensitive disease did not appear to be cost-effective when compared with no testing (102). However, consideration of genetic testing is now recommended for all women with ovarian cancer. As germline and/or somatic tumor testing become more prevalent and the costs of targeted agents drop, targeted therapies should become increasingly attractive from an economic standpoint.

Cervical Cancer

Primary Treatment

The standard treatment of cervical cancer has been established for very early-stage and locally advanced-stage disease. However, there is continued debate over the appropriate treatment of stage IB2 disease (103). Current options include primary surgery with radical hysterectomy and lymphadenectomy followed by tailored chemoradiation, primary chemoradiation, and primary chemoradiation followed by simple hysterectomy. The choice of therapy depends on many factors including available resources, costs, patient characteristics, and physician and patient preferences.

Two groups have developed health economic models to inform the treatment of stage IB2 cervical cancer. Rocconi et al. developed a decision model with a third-party-payer perspective to compare three strategies: (1) radical hysterectomy followed by tailored therapy; (2) primary chemoradiation; and (3) neoadjuvant chemotherapy followed by simple hysterectomy. Radical hysterectomy was the least costly strategy per survivor at $41,212; chemoradiation and neoadjuvant chemotherapy followed by simple hysterectomy cost $43,197 and $72,613 per survivor, respectively (104). The authors concluded that radical hysterectomy is the most cost-effective treatment for stage IB2 cervical cancer.

In a second analysis, Jewell et al. used a modified Markov state transition decision model from a third-party-payer perspective to compare primary chemoradiation with primary radical hysterectomy with tailored adjuvant therapy (RH+TA) for the treatment of stage IB2 cervical cancer. Patients undergoing completed radical hysterectomy were divided into three risk groups to determine adjuvant treatment based on surgical pathologic risk features. Adverse events and their costs were included. The model predicted 5-year OS of 79.6% in the RH+TA arm and 78.9% in the chemoradiation arm. The mean cost of RH+TA was $27,840 compared with $21,403 for chemoradiation. The ICER comparing RH+TA with chemoradiation was $63,689 per additional YLS (105). While Rocconi et al. found RH+TA therapy to be the least expensive option, Jewell et al. found that RH+TA was the costlier treatment option in the base case. The difference in the outcomes of the two decision models may be related to differences in assumptions about the frequency of adjuvant radiotherapy and in cost estimates for radiotherapy. These studies demonstrate how the assumptions, inputs, and design of a model are critical to its results.

Use of Radiation Therapy in Cervical Cancer

Intracavitary radiation treatment is recognized to play a significant and important role in the standard radiotherapy treatment of cervical carcinoma. The majority of centers worldwide use either low dose rate (LDR) or high dose rate (HDR) methods. Randomized trials have confirmed the apparent equivalence of HDR and LDR in terms of the incidence of adverse effects, tumor control, and survival (106). HDR is becoming more prevalent, possibly based on its outpatient nature, the ability to treat a greater number of patients, the ability to treat tumors at different sites, and the perceived cost savings to the health care system due mainly to the outpatient nature of the treatment. However, HDR treatment costs per insertion are frequently greater than those for LDR, and increasing attention is now being paid to thorough health economic analysis by health care professionals in an attempt to reduce escalating health care costs.

Jones et al. undertook a formal analysis of LDR versus HDR brachytherapy from a Canadian hospital perspective (107). Fixed and direct costs arising from equipment purchases, equipment maintenance fees, patient care, and operating costs including the staff, hospitalization, and operating room costs of LDR and HDR insertions were incorporated into a cost model. This study demonstrated that the LDR technique is less expensive when treating up to 80 patients per year. However, the ability to treat a significantly greater number of patients and the potential to treat other sites made use of an HDR unit a more reasonable choice for high-volume centers where over 80 cervical cancer patients are treated annually.

Recurrence and Metastasis

Following the publication of the phase 3 GOG 240 trial, which demonstrated a significant, 3.7-month OS advantage to incorporation of bevacizumab into the chemotherapy treatment of advanced and recurrent cervical cancer, several authors have assessed the economic impact of bevacizumab in cervical cancer treatment. Minion et al. developed a Markov-based decision model and estimated the ICER of therapy with bevacizumab to be $295,164/QALY (108). Phippen et al. performed a similar analysis in their model, identifying an ICER of $155,000/QALY (109). Both groups identified the cost of bevacizumab as the main constraint on the cost-effectiveness of the new regimen.

Preferences for Treatment and Its Effects

Jewell et al. elicited preferences for calculation of utility scores from cervical cancer survivors and from women without cancer. The authors created descriptions of health states that included detailed information about available treatments for early-stage cervical cancer. Surgical scenarios ranged from minimally invasive radical hysterectomy with low-risk pathology requiring no additional treatment to aborted radical hysterectomy due to locally advanced disease followed by primary chemoradiation and brachytherapy. Primary chemoradiation (including teletherapy and brachytherapy) was also evaluated. Physical and emotional aspects of each treatment were outlined and, where appropriate, details about initial postoperative recovery, outpatient whole pelvic radiation, outpatient chemotherapy, and inpatient brachytherapy were described in each health state scenario. Common side effects were incorporated into each description. The TTO method was used. Health states describing primary chemoradiation were less preferred than those describing primary surgery, regardless of whether postoperative adjuvant chemoradiation was described (**Table 17.1**). Even in health scenarios with similar 5-year survival, subjects ranked surgery followed by tailored adjuvant treatment as equivalent or slightly preferred over primary chemoradiation. Subjects ranked a minimally invasive approach as most preferred, suggesting that an overnight hospitalization, smaller incision sites, and faster return to activities of daily living are preferred (110). Preferences were also elicited for adverse events related to treatment; subjects ranked severe radiation-related events such as radiation proctitis and gastrointestinal fistula as the least preferred outcomes (111).

Endometrial Cancer

Endometrial cancer is a disease in which outcomes research can be challenging; despite the high incidence of disease, the event rate (recurrence or death) is low. As such, randomized clinical trials for low- or intermediate-risk disease require a large number of subjects and long-term follow-up to demonstrate significance. CER approaches, therefore, may be quite relevant in endometrial cancer. CER in endometrial cancer spans aspects of surgical management, the use of adjuvant radiation and chemotherapy, surveillance for disease recurrence, and the evaluation and management of individuals at risk for or diagnosed with Lynch syndrome–associated cancers.

Preoperative Testing

The use of preoperative imaging in patients with clinical stage I endometrial cancer has, in certain circumstances, been demonstrated to identify disease that might not be amenable to resection. While certain authors supported the strategy of preoperative computed

■ **TABLE 17.1. Utility Scores Elicited from Members of the Public and Cervical Cancer Survivors for Health States Related to the Treatment of Newly Diagnosed Cervical Cancer**

Rank	Treatment	Mean	95% Confidence Intervals
1	Minimally invasive radical hysterectomy No adjuvant treatment	0.94	0.89–0.99
2	Radical hysterectomy Low-risk features No adjuvant treatment	0.89	0.82–0.97
3	Radical hysterectomy Intermediate-risk features No adjuvant treatment	0.89	0.82–0.96
4	Radical hysterectomy Intermediate-risk features Adjuvant chemoradiation	0.80	0.72–0.89
5	Radical hysterectomy High-risk features Adjuvant chemoradiation High dose rate brachytherapy	0.78	0.69–0.87
6	Primary chemoradiation	0.76	0.66–0.85
7	Aborted radical hysterectomy due to extent of disease Primary chemoradiation	0.68	0.57–0.79

Source: Reprinted from Jewell EL, Smrtka M, Broadwater G, et al. Utility scores and treatment preferences for clinical early-stage cervical cancer. *Value Health.* 2011;13(4):582–586, with permission from Elsevier.

tomography (CT) in patients planned to undergo surgery for endometrial cancer, others questioned the effectiveness and cost of this intervention. Bansal et al. performed a study evaluating patients with endometrial cancer who underwent a preoperative CT of the abdomen and pelvis (112). In 7/250 (3%) of patients, the CT results led to an alteration of the surgical plan. In patients with high-risk histology (serous, clear cell, and sarcoma), the plan was changed in up to 13% of cases. When the cost of imaging was incorporated into their model, the authors estimated that more than $17,000 was expended to alter the management of one patient. As such, the authors argued that routine preoperative CT in patients with clinical stage I endometrial cancer was not cost-effective.

Laparotomy versus Minimally Invasive Surgery

Over the last few decades, minimally invasive surgery has been incorporated into the management of many malignancies, including endometrial cancer. Randomized trials of laparotomy versus laparoscopy were reported from the Netherlands (113), Australia (114), and the United States (115), all demonstrating similar oncologic outcomes between groups. These trials demonstrated that laparoscopy was associated with a modest improvement in quality of life compared with laparotomy (116,117). Investigators from the Netherlands evaluated the cost of treatment relative to survival and quality of life of subjects undergoing laparotomy or laparoscopic staging of their endometrial cancer (118). Despite a slightly increased cost for minimally invasive surgery (higher operative costs but lower hospital stay costs), total laparoscopic hysterectomy remained cost-effective because of the low rate of complications seen in the minimally invasive arm compared with laparotomy. This group also performed a meta-analysis of 12 trials of laparoscopic endometrial cancer surgery and reached the conclusion that laparoscopy was cost-effective compared with laparotomy (25).

Laparoscopy versus Robot-Assisted Laparoscopy

In 2006, the FDA cleared the first computer-aided (robotic) surgical system for hysterectomy. There has subsequently been a rapid incorporation of robotic surgery into gynecologic cancer practices, mainly for the treatment of endometrial cancer. Initial reports of this surgical approach demonstrated feasibility and acceptable toxicity. However, the initial purchase price of the robot (greater than $1 million), yearly maintenance contract (greater than $100,000 annually), and limited use of disposable instruments add a fixed cost to this procedure over laparoscopy or laparotomy. Given the expense of robotic surgery, analyses of the cost of robotic surgery have been published, often with differing conclusions. Initially, Bell et al. described a series of patients who underwent abdominal, laparoscopic, or robotic staging for endometrial cancer, with the robotic approach being found less costly compared with laparotomy, but not significantly more expensive than laparoscopy (119). Subsequent to this report, other approaches have been utilized to assess the cost-effectiveness and comparative effectiveness of robotic surgery compared with other surgical approaches. Barnett et al. utilized decision modeling from the perspectives of both society and the hospital (with and without the cost of the purchase of the robot incorporated) to assess the impact of surgical approach (laparotomy, laparoscopy, and robotic) for staging of endometrial cancer (23). These authors concluded that while laparoscopy is the least expensive approach, the decreased societal cost associated with an early return to normal function makes robotic surgery less expensive than laparotomy. In sensitivity analysis, when the costs of disposable instruments and equipment are minimized to less than one half their current cost, robotic surgery becomes the least costly approach. The modeling approach with sensitivity analyses is critically important in helping to understand which factors drive cost in endometrial cancer surgery and to acknowledge that the perspective from which the analysis is taken significantly impacts the conclusions that can be drawn. Additionally, a population-based CER analysis was undertaken by Wright et al. describing more than 2,400 women who underwent minimally invasive surgery for endometrial cancer, 58% robotically and 42% laparoscopically (120). These authors found similar rates of complications but an increased cost with robotic surgery and concluded that longer-term outcome data regarding robotic surgery are necessary before this approach should be considered standard for the management of endometrial cancer. Collectively, the data regarding robotic endometrial cancer surgery suggest an increased cost, decreased morbidity compared with laparotomy, and cost-effectiveness that varies based on the perspective from which the data are interpreted.

Lymphadenectomy for Surgical Staging

Following two randomized trials suggesting that lymphadenectomy for unselected endometrial cancer does not improve survival outcomes (121,122), the role of this procedure in the routine management of endometrial cancer has undergone increased scrutiny. Various strategies have been proposed to identify patients who are at highest risk for metastasis to the lymph nodes, generally incorporating tumor grade, depth of myometrial invasion, histology, and tumor size. Kwon et al. found that as tumor grade increases, lymphadenectomy is more cost-effective than its omission, mainly due to the reduced rate of radiation in node-negative patients (123). Modeling of grade 3 endometrial cancer by Havrilesky et al. demonstrated that lymph node dissection had an ICER of $40,183/QALY compared with no lymph node dissection (124). Cohn et al. modeled grade 1 cancers and found that even in this group of patients at low risk for lymph node metastasis, routine lymphadenectomy was cost-effective compared with a strategy of selective lymphadenectomy, based on the assumption of a lower rate of adjuvant radiation in the surgically staged patients (125). Conversely, Lee et al. demonstrated that when preoperative prediction models classified patients as low risk, selective lymphadenectomy was less costly and more effective than routine lymphadenectomy (126). Havrilesky et al. modeled a hypothetical test that could reliably predict lymph node metastasis, finding that such a test could be cost-effective as long as it was fairly inexpensive (127). Collectively, the cost-effectiveness data suggest that strategies to select a high-risk group for lymphadenectomy are more likely to be cost-effective. Sentinel lymph node mapping is a technique recently incorporated into endometrial cancer staging that reduces the number of lymph nodes removed while retaining sensitivity to identify metastatic disease (128). The cost-effectiveness of sentinel lymph node mapping compared with full lymph node dissection for endometrial cancer has not yet been formally reported.

Surveillance for Endometrial Cancer Recurrence

Given that the OS of women with endometrial cancer is approximately 85%, investigators have challenged the notion that routine intermittent surveillance for pelvic examination and vaginal cytology (with or without chest imaging) is cost-effective or even necessary for most women with endometrial cancer. In support of the trend toward decreased intensity of surveillance, it has been estimated that the cost of routine vaginal cytology to identify a single asymptomatic recurrence is more than $44,000 (129). Whether the identification of these asymptomatic individuals leads to improved outcomes is even less certain (130).

Lynch Syndrome

It is estimated that 2.3% of patients with endometrial cancer have Lynch syndrome as the cause of their disease (131). Given the relatively low prevalence of the disease, the ability to distinguish these patients from all those with sporadic disease would be enormously beneficial, as the probands and their families could be introduced to prevention and screening interventions that might decrease the risk of dying from Lynch-related malignancies. However, the clinical Amsterdam criteria are relatively insensitive and nonspecific in identifying Lynch syndrome. Thus, many institutions have begun utilizing immunohistochemistry (IHC) for the DNA mismatch repair genes as an initial screen for Lynch syndrome. Health economic studies of this strategy have demonstrated that utilizing IHC in patients with a first-degree relative with a Lynch-associated cancer is cost-effective (132). Other investigators have shown that the routine use of IHC with genetic testing for patients, with a triage to genetic testing based on a proband's age <60 years, is more cost-effective than other screening strategies (133). Additionally, the cost-effectiveness of strategies to prevent the disease in probands with known Lynch syndrome has been evaluated. Kwon et al. demonstrated that in this population, annual surveillance with endometrial biopsy, pelvic ultrasound, and CA125 at 30 years plus risk-reducing hysterectomy and oophorectomy at 40 years is the most effective strategy, though substantially more expensive than preventative surgery alone or screening alone, with an additional $194,000 spent per increase in year of survival compared with the next best strategy (134). The cost-effectiveness of risk-reducing surgery has also been confirmed by Yang et al., who demonstrated that this intervention is more cost-effective than either yearly examination or yearly invasive screening for malignancy (135).

CHAPTER SUMMARY

Gynecologic oncology provides a rich opportunity to investigate the cost-effectiveness and value of various diagnostic, therapeutic, screening, and preventative strategies. While the field is still relatively young, substantial knowledge about these strategies has been gained through CER techniques and modeling. Continued investigation with refinement of tools for the investigation of value-based gynecologic cancer care is needed to advance the state of knowledge.

KEY POINTS

1. There is increasing pressure on health systems and providers in the United States to demonstrate "value," as defined by high-quality and cost-effective care.
2. CER provides the framework for studies that compare the potential harms and benefits of strategies to prevent, diagnose, or treat gynecologic malignancy.
3. Health economic studies, including CEA and CUA, compare medical interventions on the basis of their relative costs as well as their potential harms and benefits.
4. A key factor in the development of a cost-utility model is the incorporation of quality of life, which requires a preference-based utility. The utility may be derived using a variety of quality of life–related instruments. Use of the utility allows the results of a model to be expressed in QALYs, which are a standard effectiveness outcome.
5. The results of health economic decision models are highly dependent on their perspective and the assumptions made in their construction.
6. Uncertainty in health economic models is best described using multiple sensitivity analyses.
7. There is a growing body of evidence to guide clinical and resource allocation decisions in gynecologic oncology.

REFERENCES

1. Congress USt. Patient Protection and Affordable Care Act. 2009.
2. Chandra A, Jena AB, Skinner JS. The pragmatist's guide to comparative effectiveness research. *J Econ Perspect.* 2011;25(2):27–46.
3. Porter ME. What is value in health care? *N Engl J Med.* 2010;363(26):2477–2481.
4. Report of the National Commission on Physician Payment Reform. 2013; http://physicianpaymentcommission.org/wp-content/uploads/2013/03/physician_payment_report.pdf. Accessed November 22, 2015.
5. Medicare Physician Payment Reform. http://www.ama-assn.org/ama/pub/advocacy/topics/medicare-physician-payment-reform.page. Accessed November 22, 2015.
6. Congress USt. Medicare Access and CHIP Reauthorization Act of 2015. 2015.
7. Services DoHaH. Request for Information Regarding Implementation of the Merit-Based Incentive Payment System, Promotion of Alternative Payment Models, and Incentive Payments for Participation in Eligible Alternative Payment Models. 2015.
8. Schnipper LE, Davidson NE, Wollins DS, et al. American Society of Clinical Oncology statement: a conceptual framework to assess the value of cancer treatment options. *J Clin Oncol.* 2015;33(23):2563–2577.
9. Jencks SF, Williams MV, Coleman EA. Rehospitalizations among patients in the Medicare fee-for-service program. *N Engl J Med.* 2009;360(14):1418–1428.
10. van Walraven C, Bennett C, Jennings A, et al. Proportion of hospital readmissions deemed avoidable: a systematic review. *CMAJ.* 2011;183(7):E391–E402.
11. Services CfMaM. Readmission reduction program. 2013.
12. Services CfMaM. Centers for Medicare & Medicaid Services (US). Bundled Payments for Care Improvement (BPCI) initiative: general information. 2013.
13. Epstein AM. Revisiting readmissions–changing the incentives for shared accountability. *N Engl J Med.* 2009;360(14):1457–1459.

14. Hackbarth G, Reischauer R, Mutti A. Collective accountability for medical care–toward bundled Medicare payments. *N Engl J Med.* 2008;359(1):3–5.
15. Schnipper LE, Smith TJ, Raghavan D, et al. American Society of Clinical Oncology identifies five key opportunities to improve care and reduce costs: the top five list for oncology. *J Clin Oncol.* 2012;30(14):1715–1724.
16. Schnipper LE, Lyman GH, Blayney DW, et al. American Society of Clinical Oncology 2013 top five list in oncology. *J Clin Oncol.* 2013;31(34):4362–4370.
17. Five things physicians and patients should question. *Choosing Wisely.* http://www.choosingwisely.org/societies/society-of-gynecologic-oncology/. Accessed January 6, 2015.
18. Pujade-Lauraine E, Hilpert F, Weber B, et al. Bevacizumab combined with chemotherapy for platinum-resistant recurrent ovarian cancer: The AURELIA open-label randomized phase III trial. *J Clin Oncol.* 2014;32(13):1302–1308.
19. Porter ME, Lee, TH. The strategy that will fix health care. *Harv Bus Rev.* 2013;19(10):50–70.
20. Drummond MF, Sculpher MJ, Torrance GW, et al. *Methods for the Economic Evaluation of Health Care Programmes.* 3rd Ed. Oxford, UK: Oxford University Press; 2005.
21. Excellence NIfHaC. Guide to the methods of technology appraisal. 2008. http://www.nice.org.uk/media/B52/A7/TAMethodsGuideUpdatedJune2008.pdf.
22. Gold M SJ, Russell L, Weinstein M. *Cost-Effectiveness in Health and Medicine.* New York, NY: Oxford University Press; 1996.
23. Barnett JC, Judd JP, Wu JM, et al. Cost comparison among robotic, laparoscopic, and open hysterectomy for endometrial cancer. *Obstet Gynecol.* 2010;116(3):685–693.
24. Williams A. Priority setting in public and private health care. A guide through the ideological jungle. *J Health Econ.* 1988;7(2):173–183.
25. Bijen CB, Vermeulen KM, Mourits MJ, et al. Costs and effects of abdominal versus laparoscopic hysterectomy: systematic review of controlled trials. *PLoS One.* 2009;4(10):e7340.
26. Petitti DB. *Meta-Analysis, Decision Analysis, and Cost-Effectiveness Analysis: Methods for Quantitative Synthesis in Medicine.* 2nd Ed. New York, NY: Oxford University Press; 2000.
27. Detsky AS, Naglie IG. A clinician's guide to cost-effectiveness analysis. *Ann Intern Med.* 1990;113(2):147–154.
28. Yabroff KR, Lamont EB, Mariotto A, et al. Cost of care for elderly cancer patients in the United States. *J Natl Cancer Inst.* 2008;100(9):630–641.
29. Drummond MF, O'Brien B, Stoddart GL, et al. *Methods for the Economic Evaluation of Health Care Programmes.* 2nd Ed. New York, NY: Oxford University Press; 1997.
30. Doubilet P, Begg CB, Weinstein MC, et al. Probabilistic sensitivity analysis using Monte Carlo simulation. A practical approach. *Med Decis Making.* 1985;5(2):157–177.
31. Ramsey S, Willke R, Briggs A, et al. Good research practices for cost-effectiveness analysis alongside clinical trials: the ISPOR RCT-CEA Task Force report. *Value Health.* 2005;8(5):521–533.
32. Torrance GW. Utility approach to measuring health-related quality of life. *J Chronic Dis.* 1987;40(6):593–603.
33. Froberg DG, Kane RL. Methodology for measuring health-state preferences–II: scaling methods. *J Clin Epidemiol.* 1989;42(5):459–471.
34. Torrance GW. Measurement of health state utilities for economic appraisal. *J Health Econ.* 1986;5(1):1–30.
35. Ware JE Jr. Standards for validating health measures: definition and content. *J Chronic Dis.* 1987;40(6):473–480.
36. Torrance GW, Thomas WH, Sackett DL. A utility maximization model for evaluation of health care programs. *Health Serv Res.* 1972;7(2):118–133.
37. Llewellyn-Thomas H, Sutherland HJ, Tibshirani R, et al. The measurement of patients' values in medicine. *Med Decis Making.* 1982;2(4):449–462.
38. Brooks R. EuroQol: the current state of play. *Health Policy.* 1996;37(1):53–72.
39. Dolan P, Gudex C, Kind P, et al. The time trade-off method: results from a general population study. *Health Econ.* 1996;5(2):141–154.
40. Cella DF, Tulsky DS, Gray G, et al. The functional assessment of cancer therapy scale: development and validation of the general measure. *J Clin Oncol.* 1993;11(3):570–579.
41. Hess LM, Brady WE, Havrilesky LJ, et al. Comparison of methods to estimate health state utilities for ovarian cancer using quality of life data: a Gynecologic Oncology Group study. *Gynecol Oncol.* 2013;128(2):175–180.
42. Ubel PA, Loewenstein G, Jepson C. Whose quality of life? A commentary exploring discrepancies between health state evaluations of patients and the general public. *Qual Life Res.* 2003;12(6):599–607.
43. Arnold D, Girling A, Stevens A, et al. Comparison of direct and indirect methods of estimating health state utilities for resource allocation: review and empirical analysis. *BMJ.* 2009;339:b2688.
44. Sonnenberg FA, Beck JR. Markov models in medical decision making: a practical guide. *Med Decis Making.* 1993;13(4):322–338.
45. Taylor DC, Pawar V, Kruzikas D, et al. Methods of model calibration: observations from a mathematical model of cervical cancer. *Pharmacoeconomics.* 2010;28(11):995–1000.
46. Choi YH, Jit M, Gay N, et al. Transmission dynamic modelling of the impact of human papillomavirus vaccination in the United Kingdom. *Vaccine.* 2010;28(24):4091–4102.
47. Havrilesky LJ, Sanders GD, Kulasingam S, et al. Development of an ovarian cancer screening decision model that incorporates disease heterogeneity. *Cancer.* 2011;117(3):545–553.
48. Zauber AG, Lansdorp-Vogelaar I, Knudsen AB, et al. Evaluating test strategies for colorectal cancer screening: a decision analysis for the U.S. Preventive Services Task Force. *Ann Intern Med.* 2008;149(9):659–669.
49. Mandelblatt JS, Cronin KA, Bailey S, et al. Effects of mammography screening under different screening schedules: model estimates of potential benefits and harms. *Ann Intern Med.* 2009;151(10):738–747.
50. Eddy DM. The frequency of cervical cancer screening. Comparison of a mathematical model with empirical data. *Cancer.* 1987;60(5):1117–1122.
51. ACOG Committee on Practice Bulletins–Gynecology. ACOG Practice Bulletin no. 109: Cervical cytology screening. *Obstet Gynecol.* 2009;114(6):1409–1420.
52. Smith RA, Cokkinides V, Brooks D, et al. Cancer screening in the United States, 2010: a review of current American Cancer Society guidelines and issues in cancer screening. *CA Cancer J Clin.* 2010;60(2):99–119.
53. Canfell K, Barnabas R, Patnick J, et al. The predicted effect of changes in cervical screening practice in the UK: results from a modelling study. *Br J Cancer.* 2004;91(3):530–536.
54. Kulasingam SL, Havrilesky L, Ghebre R, et al. *Cervical Cancer: A Decision Analysis for the U.S. Preventive Services Task Force.* Rockville, MD: Agency for Healthcare Research and Quality; 2011.
55. Muhlberger N, Sroczynski G, Esteban E, et al. Cost-effectiveness of primarily human papillomavirus-based cervical cancer screening in settings with currently established Pap screening: a systematic review commissioned by the German Federal Ministry of Health. *Int J Technol Assess Health Care.* 2008;24(2):184–192.
56. Goldhaber-Fiebert JD, Stout NK, Salomon JA, et al. Cost-effectiveness of cervical cancer screening with human papillomavirus DNA testing and HPV-16,18 vaccination. *J Natl Cancer Inst.* 2008;100(5):308–320.
57. Berkhof J, Coupe VM, Bogaards JA, et al. The health and economic effects of HPV DNA screening in The Netherlands. *Int J Cancer.* 2010;127(9):2147–2158.
58. Kitchener HC, Almonte M, Thomson C, et al. HPV testing in combination with liquid-based cytology in primary cervical screening (ARTISTIC): a randomised controlled trial. *Lancet Oncol.* 2009;10(7):672–682.
59. Kitchener H, Canfell K, Gilham C, et al. The clinical effectiveness and cost-effectiveness of primary human papillomavirus cervical screening in England: extended follow-up of the ARTISTIC randomised trial cohort through three screening rounds. *Health Technol Assess.* 2014;18(23):1–196.
60. Ogilvie GS, van Niekerk DJ, Krajden M, et al. A randomized controlled trial of Human Papillomavirus (HPV) testing for cervical cancer screening: trial design and preliminary results (HPV FOCAL Trial). *BMC Cancer.* 2010;10:111.
61. Huh WK, Ault KA, Chelmow D, et al. Use of primary high-risk human papillomavirus testing for cervical cancer screening: interim clinical guidance. *Obstet Gynecol.* 2015;125(2):330–337.
62. Dasbach EJ, Elbasha EH, Insinga RP. Mathematical models for predicting the epidemiologic and economic impact of vaccination against human papillomavirus infection and disease. *Epidemiol Rev.* 2006;28:88–100.
63. Garnett GP, Kim JJ, French K, et al. Chapter 21: Modelling the impact of HPV vaccines on cervical cancer and screening programmes. *Vaccine.* 2006;24(Suppl 3):S3/178–S3/186.
64. Jit M, Demarteau N, Elbasha E, et al. Human papillomavirus vaccine introduction in low-income and middle-income countries: guidance on the use of cost-effectiveness models. *BMC Med.* 2011;9:54.
65. Goldie SJ, O'Shea M, Campos NG, et al. Health and economic outcomes of HPV 16,18 vaccination in 72 GAVI-eligible countries. *Vaccine.* 2008;26(32):4080–4093.
66. Kim JJ, Goldie SJ. Cost effectiveness analysis of including boys in a human papillomavirus vaccination programme in the United States. *BMJ.* 2009;339:b3884.
67. Centers for Disease Control and Prevention (CDC). FDA Licensure of Quadrivalent Human Papillomavirus Vaccine (HPV4, Gardasil) for use in males and guidance from the Advisory Committee on Immunization Practices (ACIP). *MMWR Morb Mortal Wkly Rep.* 2010;59(20):630–632.

68. Brisson M. Cost-effectiveness of 9-valent HPV vaccination. Presentation before the Advisory Committee on Immunization Practices (ACIP), October 30, 2014. Atlanta, GA: US Department of Health and Human Services, CDC; 2014.
69. Tully SP, Anonychuk AM, Sanchez DM, et al. Time for change? An economic evaluation of integrated cervical screening and HPV immunization programs in Canada. *Vaccine.* 2012;30(2):425–435.
70. Coupe VM, Bogaards JA, Meijer CJ, et al. Impact of vaccine protection against multiple HPV types on the cost-effectiveness of cervical screening. *Vaccine.* 2012;30(10):1813–1822.
71. Ng J, Ye F, Roth L, et al. Human Papillomavirus Vaccination coverage among female adolescents in managed care plans - United States, 2013. *MMWR Morb Mortal Wkly Rep.* 2015;64(42):1185–1189.
72. Bell J, Brady MF, Young RC, et al. Randomized phase III trial of three versus six cycles of adjuvant carboplatin and paclitaxel in early stage epithelial ovarian carcinoma: a Gynecologic Oncology Group study. *Gynecol Oncol.* 2006;102(3):432–439.
73. Buys SS, Partridge E, Greene MH, et al. Ovarian cancer screening in the Prostate, Lung, Colorectal and Ovarian (PLCO) cancer screening trial: findings from the initial screen of a randomized trial. *Am J Obstet Gynecol.* 2005;193(5):1630–1639.
74. Buys SS, Partridge E, Black A, et al. Effect of screening on ovarian cancer mortality: the Prostate, Lung, Colorectal and Ovarian (PLCO) Cancer Screening Randomized Controlled Trial. *JAMA.* 2011;305(22):2295–2303.
75. Jacobs IJ, Menon U, Ryan A, et al. Ovarian cancer screening and mortality in the UK Collaborative Trial of Ovarian Cancer Screening (UKCTOCS): a randomised controlled trial. *Lancet.* 2015;387(10022):945–956.
76. Skates SJ, Singer DE. Quantifying the potential benefit of CA 125 screening for ovarian cancer. *J Clin Epidemiol.* 1991;44(4–5):365–380.
77. Urban N, Drescher C, Etzioni R, et al. Use of a stochastic simulation model to identify an efficient protocol for ovarian cancer screening. *Control Clin Trials.* 1997;18(3):251–270.
78. Havrilesky LJ, Sanders GD, Kulasingam S, et al. Reducing ovarian cancer mortality through screening: Is it possible, and can we afford it? *Gynecol Oncol.* 2008;111(2):179–187.
79. McGuire WP, Hoskins WJ, Brady MF, et al. Cyclophosphamide and cisplatin compared with paclitaxel and cisplatin in patients with stage III and stage IV ovarian cancer. *N Engl J Med.* 1996;334(1):1–6.
80. Piccart MJ, Bertelsen K, James K, et al. Randomized intergroup trial of cisplatin-paclitaxel versus cisplatin-cyclophosphamide in women with advanced epithelial ovarian cancer: three-year results. *J Natl Cancer Inst.* 2000;92(9):699–708.
81. Piccart MJ, Bertelsen K, Stuart G, et al. Long-term follow-up confirms a survival advantage of the paclitaxel-cisplatin regimen over the cyclophosphamide-cisplatin combination in advanced ovarian cancer. *Int J Gynecol Cancer.* 2003;13(Suppl 2):144–148.
82. McGuire W, Neugut AI, Arikian S, et al. Analysis of the cost-effectiveness of paclitaxel as alternative combination therapy for advanced ovarian cancer. *J Clin Oncol.* 1997;15(2):640–645.
83. Katsumata N, Yasuda M, Takahashi F, et al. Dose-dense paclitaxel once a week in combination with carboplatin every 3 weeks for advanced ovarian cancer: a phase 3, open-label, randomised controlled trial. *Lancet.* 2009;374(9698):1331–1338.
84. Dalton HJ, Yu X, Hu L, et al. An economic analysis of dose dense weekly paclitaxel plus carboplatin versus every-3-week paclitaxel plus carboplatin in the treatment of advanced ovarian cancer. *Gynecol Oncol.* 2012;124(2):199–204.
85. Morgan RJ Jr, Alvarez RD, Armstrong DK, et al. NCCN Clinical Practice Guidelines in Oncology: epithelial ovarian cancer. *J Natl Compr Canc Netw.* 2011;9(1):82–113.
86. Armstrong DK, Bundy B, Wenzel L, et al. Intraperitoneal cisplatin and paclitaxel in ovarian cancer. *N Engl J Med.* 2006;354(1):34–43.
87. Tewari D, Java JJ, Salani R, et al. Long-term survival advantage and prognostic factors associated with intraperitoneal chemotherapy treatment in advanced ovarian cancer: a gynecologic oncology group study. *J Clin Oncol.* 2015;33(13):1460–1466.
88. Bristow RE, Santillan A, Salani R, et al. Intraperitoneal cisplatin and paclitaxel versus intravenous carboplatin and paclitaxel chemotherapy for Stage III ovarian cancer: a cost-effectiveness analysis. *Gynecol Oncol.* 2007;106(3):476–481.
89. Havrilesky LJ, Alvarez Secord A, Darcy KM, et al. Cost effectiveness of intraperitoneal compared with intravenous chemotherapy for women with optimally resected stage III ovarian cancer: a Gynecologic Oncology Group Study. *J Clin Oncol.* 2008;26(25):4144–4150.
90. Perren TJ, Swart AM, Pfisterer J, et al. A phase 3 trial of bevacizumab in ovarian cancer. *N Engl J Med.* 2011;365(26):2484–2496.
91. Burger RA, Brady MF, Bookman MA, et al. Incorporation of bevacizumab in the primary treatment of ovarian cancer. *N Engl J Med.* 2011;365(26):2473–2483.
92. Cohn DE, Kim KH, Resnick KE, et al. At what cost does a potential survival advantage of bevacizumab make sense for the primary treatment of ovarian cancer? A cost-effectiveness analysis. *J Clin Oncol.* 2011;29(10):1247–1251.
93. Cohn DE, Barnett JC, Wenzel L, et al. A cost-utility analysis of NRG Oncology/Gynecologic Oncology Group Protocol 218: incorporating prospectively collected quality-of-life scores in an economic model of treatment of ovarian cancer. *Gynecol Oncol.* 2015;136(2):293–299.
94. Barnett JC, Alvarez-Secord A, Cohn D, et al. Cost-effectiveness of a predictive biomarker for bevacizumab responsiveness in the primary treatment of ovarian cancer. *Gynecol Oncol.* 2012;125(Suppl 1):S66.
95. Lesnock JL, Farris C, Krivak TC, et al. Consolidation paclitaxel is more cost-effective than bevacizumab following upfront treatment of advanced epithelial ovarian cancer. *Gynecol Oncol.* 2011;122(3):473–478.
96. Rose PG, Fusco N, Fluellen L, et al. Second-line therapy with paclitaxel and carboplatin for recurrent disease following first-line therapy with paclitaxel and platinum in ovarian or peritoneal carcinoma. *J Clin Oncol.* 1998;16(4):1494–1497.
97. Dizon DS, Hensley ML, Poynor EA, et al. Retrospective analysis of carboplatin and paclitaxel as initial second-line therapy for recurrent epithelial ovarian carcinoma: application toward a dynamic disease state model of ovarian cancer. *J Clin Oncol.* 2002;20(5):1238–1247.
98. Parmar MK, Ledermann JA, Colombo N, et al. Paclitaxel plus platinum-based chemotherapy versus conventional platinum-based chemotherapy in women with relapsed ovarian cancer: the ICON4/AGO-OVAR-2.2 trial. *Lancet.* 2003;361(9375):2099–2106.
99. Pfisterer J, Plante M, Vergote I, et al. Gemcitabine plus carboplatin compared with carboplatin in patients with platinum-sensitive recurrent ovarian cancer: an intergroup trial of the AGO-OVAR, the NCIC CTG, and the EORTC GCG. *J Clin Oncol.* 2006;24(29):4699–4707.
100. Havrilesky LJ, Secord AA, Kulasingam S, et al. Management of platinum-sensitive recurrent ovarian cancer: a cost-effectiveness analysis. *Gynecol Oncol.* 2007;107(2):211–218.
101. Rocconi RP, Case AS, Straughn JM Jr, et al. Role of chemotherapy for patients with recurrent platinum-resistant advanced epithelial ovarian cancer: a cost-effectiveness analysis. *Cancer.* 2006;107(3):536–543.
102. Secord AA, Barnett JC, Ledermann JA, et al. Cost-Effectiveness of BRCA1 and BRCA2 mutation testing to target PARP inhibitor use in platinum-sensitive recurrent ovarian cancer. *Int J Gynecol Cancer.* 2013;23(5):846–852.
103. Grigsby PW. Primary radiotherapy for stage IB or IIA cervical cancer. *J Natl Cancer Inst Monogr.* 1996;21:61–64.
104. Rocconi RP, Estes JM, Leath CA III, et al. Management strategies for stage IB2 cervical cancer: a cost-effectiveness analysis. *Gynecol Oncol.* 2005;97(2):387–394.
105. Jewell EL, Kulasingam S, Myers ER, et al. Primary surgery versus chemoradiation in the treatment of IB2 cervical carcinoma: a cost effectiveness analysis. *Gynecol Oncol.* 2007;107(3):532–540.
106. Shigematsu Y, Nishiyama K, Masaki N, et al. Treatment of carcinoma of the uterine cervix by remotely controlled afterloading intracavitary radiotherapy with high-dose rate: a comparative study with a low-dose rate system. *Int J Radiat Oncol Biol Phys.* 1983;9(3):351–356.
107. Jones G, Lukka H, O'Brien B. High dose rate versus low dose rate brachytherapy for squamous cell carcinoma of the cervix: an economic analysis. *Br J Radiol.* 1994;67(803):1113–1120.
108. Minion LE, Bai J, Monk BJ, et al. A Markov model to evaluate cost-effectiveness of antiangiogenesis therapy using bevacizumab in advanced cervical cancer. *Gynecol Oncol.* 2015;137(3):490–496.
109. Phippen NT, Leath CA III, Havrilesky LJ, et al. Bevacizumab in recurrent, persistent, or advanced stage carcinoma of the cervix: is it cost-effective? *Gynecol Oncol.* 2015;136(1):43–47.
110. Jewell EL, Smrtka M, Broadwater G, et al. Utility scores and treatment preferences for clinical early-stage cervical cancer. *Value Health.* 2011;14(4):582–586.
111. Jewell EL, Smrtka M, Broadwater G, et al. Preference-based utility scores for adverse events associated with the treatment of gynecologic cancers. *Int J Gynecol Cancer.* 2013;23(6):1158–1166.
112. Bansal N, Herzog TJ, Brunner-Brown A, et al. The utility and cost effectiveness of preoperative computed tomography for patients with uterine malignancies. *Gynecol Oncol.* 2008;111(2):208–212.
113. Mourits MJ, Bijen CB, Arts HJ, et al. Safety of laparoscopy versus laparotomy in early-stage endometrial cancer: a randomised trial. *Lancet Oncol.* 2010;11(8):763–771.

114. Kondalsamy-Chennakesavan S, Janda M, Gebski V, et al. Risk factors to predict the incidence of surgical adverse events following open or laparoscopic surgery for apparent early stage endometrial cancer: results from a randomised controlled trial. *Eur J Cancer.* 2012;48(14):2155–2162.
115. Walker JL, Piedmonte MR, Spirtos NM, et al. Recurrence and survival after random assignment to laparoscopy versus laparotomy for comprehensive surgical staging of uterine cancer: Gynecologic Oncology Group LAP2 Study. *J Clin Oncol.* 2012;30(7):695–700.
116. Janda M, Gebski V, Brand A, et al. Quality of life after total laparoscopic hysterectomy versus total abdominal hysterectomy for stage I endometrial cancer (LACE): a randomised trial. *Lancet Oncol.* 2010;11(8):772–780.
117. Kornblith AB, Huang HQ, Walker JL, et al. Quality of life of patients with endometrial cancer undergoing laparoscopic international federation of gynecology and obstetrics staging compared with laparotomy: a Gynecologic Oncology Group Study. *J Clin Oncol.* 2009;27(32):5337–5342.
118. Bijen CB, Vermeulen KM, Mourits MJ, et al. Cost effectiveness of laparoscopy versus laparotomy in early stage endometrial cancer: a randomised trial. *Gynecol Oncol.* 2011;121(1):76–82.
119. Bell MC, Torgerson J, Seshadri-Kreaden U, et al. Comparison of outcomes and cost for endometrial cancer staging via traditional laparotomy, standard laparoscopy and robotic techniques. *Gynecol Oncol.* 2008;111(3):407–411.
120. Wright JD, Burke WM, Wilde ET, et al. Comparative effectiveness of robotic versus laparoscopic hysterectomy for endometrial cancer. *J Clin Oncol.* 2012;30(8):783–791.
121. Panici PB, Maggioni A, Hacker N, et al. Systematic aortic and pelvic lymphadenectomy versus resection of bulky nodes only in optimally debulked advanced ovarian cancer: a randomized clinical trial. *J Natl Cancer Inst.* 2005;97(8):560–566.
122. Kitchener H, Swart AM, Qian Q, et al. Efficacy of systematic pelvic lymphadenectomy in endometrial cancer (MRC ASTEC trial): a randomised study. *Lancet.* 2009;373(9658):125–136.
123. Kwon JS, Carey MS, Goldie SJ, et al. Cost-effectiveness analysis of treatment strategies for Stage I and II endometrial cancer. *J Obstet Gynaecol Can.* 2007;29(2):131–139.
124. Havrilesky LJ, Chino J, Myers ER. How much is another randomized trial of lymph node dissection in endometrial cancer worth? A value of information analysis. *Gynecol Oncol.* 2013;131(1):140–146.
125. Cohn DE, Huh WK, Fowler JM, et al. Cost-effectiveness analysis of strategies for the surgical management of grade 1 endometrial adenocarcinoma. *Obstet Gynecol.* 2007;109(6):1388–1395.
126. Lee JY, Cohn DE, Kim Y, et al. The cost-effectiveness of selective lymphadenectomy based on a preoperative prediction model in patients with endometrial cancer: insights from the US and Korean healthcare systems. *Gynecol Oncol.* 2014;135(3):518–524.
127. Havrilesky LJ, Maxwell GL, Chan JK, et al. Cost effectiveness of a test to detect metastases for endometrial cancer. *Gynecol Oncol.* 2009;112(3):526–530.
128. Leitao MM Jr, Khoury-Collado F, Gardner G, et al. Impact of incorporating an algorithm that utilizes sentinel lymph node mapping during minimally invasive procedures on the detection of stage IIIC endometrial cancer. *Gynecol Oncol.* 2013;129(1):38–41.
129. Bristow RE, Purinton SC, Santillan A, et al. Cost-effectiveness of routine vaginal cytology for endometrial cancer surveillance. *Gynecol Oncol.* 2006;103(2):709–713.
130. Salani R, Backes FJ, Fung MF, et al. Posttreatment surveillance and diagnosis of recurrence in women with gynecologic malignancies: Society of Gynecologic Oncologists recommendations. *Am J Obstet Gynecol.* 2011;204(6):466–478.
131. Hampel H, Panescu J, Lockman J, et al. Comment on: Screening for Lynch syndrome (hereditary nonpolyposis colorectal cancer) among endometrial cancer patients. *Cancer Res.* 2007;67(19):9603.
132. Kwon JS, Scott JL, Gilks CB, et al. Testing women with endometrial cancer to detect Lynch syndrome. *J Clin Oncol.* 2011;29(16):2247–2252.
133. Resnick K, Straughn JM Jr, Backes F, et al. Lynch syndrome screening strategies among newly diagnosed endometrial cancer patients. *Obstet Gynecol.* 2009;114(3):530–536.
134. Kwon JS, Sun CC, Peterson SK, et al. Cost-effectiveness analysis of prevention strategies for gynecologic cancers in Lynch syndrome. *Cancer.* 2008;113(2):326–335.
135. Yang KY, Caughey AB, Little SE, et al. A cost-effectiveness analysis of prophylactic surgery versus gynecologic surveillance for women from hereditary non-polyposis colorectal cancer (HNPCC) Families. *Familial Cancer.* 2011;10(3):535–543.

CHAPTER 18

Vulva

Emily Penick, Sushil Beriwal, Edward J. Wilkinson, and John W. Moroney*

INTRODUCTION

Malignant tumors of the vulva are rare and account for less than 5% of all cancers of the female genital tract. In 2015, there were an estimated 5,150 new cases of and 1,080 deaths from invasive vulvar carcinoma in the United States (1). Because of its low incidence, most primary care providers will never encounter a patient with vulvar cancer. Although a rare patient with vulvar cancer will present without symptoms, most women with vulvar cancer initially present with complaints such as vulvar irritation, pruritus, pain, or a mass that does not resolve. The interval between the onset of symptoms and the diagnosis of cancer can be protracted if a woman who is embarrassed by new vulvar symptoms delays seeking care, or if a physician prescribes empiric topical therapies without a proper physical examination or tissue biopsy confirmation. Jones and Joura (2) evaluated the clinical events preceding the diagnosis of squamous cell carcinoma of the vulva and found that 88% of patients had experienced symptoms for more than 6 months, 31% of women had three or more medical consultations before the diagnosis of vulvar carcinoma, and 27% had applied topical estrogen or corticosteroids to the vulva.

The vulva is covered by keratinized squamous epithelium; accordingly, most malignant vulvar tumors are squamous cell carcinomas (SCCs). Consequently, our current understanding of the epidemiology, spread patterns, prognostic factors, and survival data for vulvar cancer is largely derived from experience with SCCs. Malignant melanoma is the second most common cancer of the vulva. Although there is some consensus regarding the behavior and treatment of vulvar melanoma, its rarity has thus far precluded robust, prospective clinical trials. A number of other malignant tumors, both epithelial and stromal in origin, arise from normal vulvar tissue and are discussed in detail later in this chapter. Finally, the vulva may be secondarily involved with malignant disease originating in the cervix, bladder, anorectum, colon, breast, or other organs.

The traditional therapeutic approach to vulvar cancer has been radical surgical excision of the primary tumor and inguinofemoral lymphadenectomy. Experience has shown that survival is improved with the administration of postoperative radiation therapy (RT) to selected patients deemed to be at high risk for locoregional failure. More recently, the use of neoadjuvant radiotherapy (RT) with concomitant radiosensitizing chemotherapy (CT) has proven to be effective in treating vulvar cancer patients for whom radical surgery would be either too morbid or technically not feasible. New surgical techniques, including sentinel lymph node (SLN) biopsy, hold the promise of better outcomes for patients with early disease. An individualized approach to vulvar cancer management, often employing multiple modalities in an effort to achieve disease control with better cosmetic results and sexual function, is now the norm. This chapter deals with these and other topics pertinent to the principles of management of women with vulvar cancer.

ANATOMY

The vulva consists of the external genital organs—including the mons pubis, labia minora and majora, clitoris, vaginal vestibule, and perineal body—and their supporting subcutaneous tissues. The vulva is bordered superiorly by the anterior abdominal wall, laterally by the labiocrural fold at the medial thigh, and inferiorly by the anus. The vagina and urethra open onto the vulva. The mons pubis is a prominent mound of hair-bearing skin and subcutaneous adipose and connective tissue that is located anterior to the pubic symphysis. The labia majora are two elongated skin folds that course posterior from the mons pubis and blend into the perineal body. The labia minora are a smaller pair of skin folds medial and parallel to the labia majora that extend inferiorly to form the margin of the vaginal vestibule. Superiorly, the labia minora separate into two components that course above and below the clitoris, fusing with those of the opposite side to form the prepuce and frenulum, respectively. The skin of the labia minora contains sebaceous glands near its junction with the labia majora, but it is not hair-bearing and it has little or no underlying adipose tissue. The clitoris is supported externally by the fusion of the labia minora (prepuce and frenulum) and is approximately 2 to 3 cm anterior to the urethral meatus. It is composed of erectile tissue organized into the glans, body, and two crura. Two loosely fused corpora cavernosa form the body of the clitoris and extend superiorly from the glans, ultimately dividing into the two crura. The crura course laterally beneath the ischiocavernosus muscles and attach to the ischial rami.

The vaginal vestibule is situated in the center of the vulva and is homologous to the male distal urethra. It has squamous mucosal epithelium that is demarcated bilaterally and posteriorly by the junction with the keratinized epithelium at Hart's line, located on the medial labia minora and inferiorly on the perineal body. The vagina, urethra, periurethral glands, minor vestibular glands, and the Bartholin's glands open onto the vestibule. Anteriorly, the minor small vestibular glands are located beneath the vestibular mucosa and open onto its surface, predominantly on the more anterior vestibule. The vestibular bulbs, a loose collection of bilateral erectile tissue covered superficially by the bulbocavernosus muscle, are located laterally. The Bartholin glands, two small, mucus-secreting glands situated within the subcutaneous tissue of the posterior labia majora, have ducts opening onto the posterolateral portion of the vestibule. The perineal body is a 3 to 4 cm band of skin and subcutaneous tissue located between the posterior extensions of the labia majora. It separates the vaginal vestibule from the anus and forms the posterior margin of the vulva.

* Charles F. Levenback, David H. Moore, Wui-Jin Koh, and William P. McGuire contributed to prior editions of this chapter.

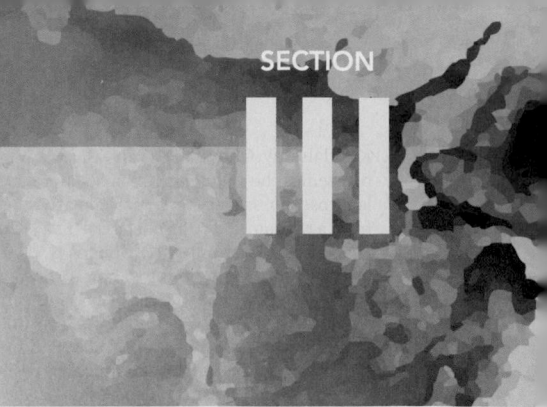

Vascular Anatomy and Neurologic Innervation

The vulva has a rich blood supply derived primarily from the internal pudendal artery, which arises from the anterior division of the internal iliac (hypogastric) artery, and the superficial and deep external pudendal arteries, which arise from the femoral artery. The internal pudendal artery exits the pelvis and passes behind the ischial spine to reach the posterolateral vulva, where it divides into several small branches to the ischiocavernosus and bulbocavernosus muscles, the perineal artery, artery of the bulb, urethral artery, and dorsal and deep arteries of the clitoris. Both external pudendal arteries travel medially to supply the labia majora and their deep structures. These vessels anastomose freely with branches from the internal pudendal artery. Innervation of the vulva is derived from multiple sources and spinal cord levels. The mons pubis and upper labia majora are innervated by the ilioinguinal nerve (L1) and the genital branch of the genitofemoral nerve (L1–2). Either of these nerves may be easily injured during pelvic lymph node dissection, with resulting paresthesias. The pudendal nerve (S2–4) enters the vulva parallel to the internal pudendal artery and gives rise to several branches that innervate the lower vagina, labia, clitoris, perineal body, and their supporting structures.

Groin Anatomy and Lymphatic Drainage

Vulvar lymphatics run anteriorly through the labia majora, turn laterally at the mons pubis, and drain primarily into the superficial inguinal LNs. Dye studies by Parry-Jones demonstrated that vulvar lymphatic channels do not extend laterally to the labiocrural folds and do not cross the midline, unless the site of dye injection is at the clitoris or perineal body (3).

The vulvar lymphatics drain to the superficial inguinal LNs located within the femoral triangle formed by the inguinal ligament superiorly, the border of the sartorius muscle laterally, and the border of the adductor longus muscle medially. There are 8 to 10 inguinal LNs lying along the saphenous vein and its branches between Camper's fascia and fascia overlying the femoral vessels (**Fig. 18.1A–C**) (3). The first draining LN is the SLN and can be identified using various lymphatic mapping techniques. The SLN is frequently found medial to the femoral vein just above the adductor muscle. Second echelon LNs may be in the groin or pelvis. The Cloquet's node, or the most superior inguinal LN, is located under the inguinal ligament. Lymphatic drainage from the SLN is sequential to the external iliac, common iliac, and aortic LNs (**Fig. 18.1A–C**).

The fossa ovalis is a crescent-shaped terminus of the fascia lata and the site where vascular and lymphatic structures meet with the femoral vessels. The cribriform fascia is a term widely used in the literature describing the anatomy of the groin and is said to cover the fossa ovalis. The cribriform fascia is hard to identify and is more of a "lamina" than an actual fascia. SLN biopsy with lymphatic mapping deemphasizes the need to identify the cribriform structure and focuses the surgeon's attention on functional *in vivo* surgical anatomy rather than textbook descriptions of LN locations (3).

EPIDEMIOLOGY

An estimated 5,150 women were diagnosed with vulvar cancer in the United States in 2015, and approximately 1,050 died of the disease. Vulvar SCC accounts for approximately 3% to 5% of all gynecologic malignancies and 1% of all carcinomas in women, with an incidence rate of 1 to 2 per 100,000 women (1). Most vulvar cancers occur in postmenopausal women in the seventh decade, although more recent reports have identified a trend toward younger age at diagnosis (4,5). Earlier observational studies suggested associations between hypertension, diabetes mellitus, and obesity and vulvar carcinoma; however, subsequent analyses have not confirmed the prognostic significance of these diagnoses (5).

NATURAL HISTORY (PATTERNS OF SPREAD)

Several infectious agents have been proposed as possible etiologic agents in vulvar carcinoma, including granulomatous infections, herpes simplex virus, and, most notably, human papillomavirus (HPV). HPV infection is present in virtually 100% of women with cervical cancer. The relationship between HPV infection and vulvar cancer is much less straightforward. This is likely due to the different etiologic pathways that are believed to be responsible for vulvar cancer. These different etiologic pathways are discussed in detail in the chapter on preinvasive disease; however, because of subject matter overlap, some of the data related to HPV and invasive squamous cell carcinoma of the vulva are discussed here.

Vulvar condyloma acuminata have a well-described relationship with HPV as the causal agent, most commonly HPV-6 or -11, and strong associations between vulvar condylomas and the later development of vulvar cancer have been identified (6). The role of HPV in the development of premalignant and malignant lesions of the vulva has become clearer as molecular techniques for HPV detection and mutational analyses have improved. Earlier studies identified HPV DNA in both invasive and carcinoma *in situ* lesions via immunohistochemistry. More recent studies have used DNA detection methods such as polymerase chain reaction and *in situ* hybridization to detect high-risk serotypes (7). Among HPV serotypes, HPV- 16 is the most common; however, many other serotypes, including -18, -33, and -52, have been reported. HPV DNA can be identified in approximately 85% to 97% of intraepithelial lesions (HSIL/VIN 2–3), but is seen in 10% to 69% of invasive lesions (8). Such a wide range of associated HPV is seen in association with HSIL/vulvar intraepithelial neoplasia (VIN) and invasive vulvar carcinoma primarily because of differences in detection methods, with newer molecular methods having greater sensitivity and specificity. There are also differences between studies regarding the distribution of HSIL/VIN subtypes (usual or differentiated) and histologic types of carcinomas. This work continues in clinical investigations. In a recent clinical trial of 12,021 women using a 9-valent HPV vaccine, the number of HPV-related external genital biopsies was reduced by 92.3% for follow-up to 54 months (9).

Although HPV DNA is associated with most intraepithelial lesions (85% to 97%), it is much less commonly seen in association with invasive lesions (~27% to 50%) (8,10). Marked differences between HPV positivity in VIN and vulvar cancers are also seen with respect to age. Basta et al. (11) conducted a retrospective case control study examining the coexistence of HPV and the incidence of both VIN and stage I vulvar cancer. HPV infection was present in 61.5% of cases of VIN and vulvar cancer in women aged 45 years or less, and in 17.5% of women older than 45 years.

In 2004, the International Society for the Study of Vulvovaginal Disease (ISSVD) proposed a modified terminology for VIN as two distinct processes: the "usual type (uVIN) encompasses high-grade lesions (VIN 2 and 3) and are caused by HPV (12). The differentiated type of VIN (dVIN) is not caused by HPV. VIN1 lesions are considered to be condyloma and should be managed accordingly as discussed by the 2011 American College of Obstetrician Gynecologists (ACOG)–American Society for Colposcopy and Cervical Pathology (ASCCP) (13). The most common VIN type occurs more frequently in younger women, tends to be multifocal, and has association with HPV serotypes 16, 33, and 18. In contrast, dVIN is less common (2% to 10% of all VIN), generally not related to HPV, and is shown to be unifocal and associated with other vulvar dermatoses such as lichen sclerosus and lichen planus (10,14).

The incidence of HPV-associated VIN has been increasing over the past 20 years, particularly in women of reproductive age, with the highest frequency reported in women aged 20 to 35 (15). The development of condyloma acuminatum/genital warts is attributed to infection with HPV-6 or -11, with the median time between infection and development of lesions at 5 to 6 months. In patients

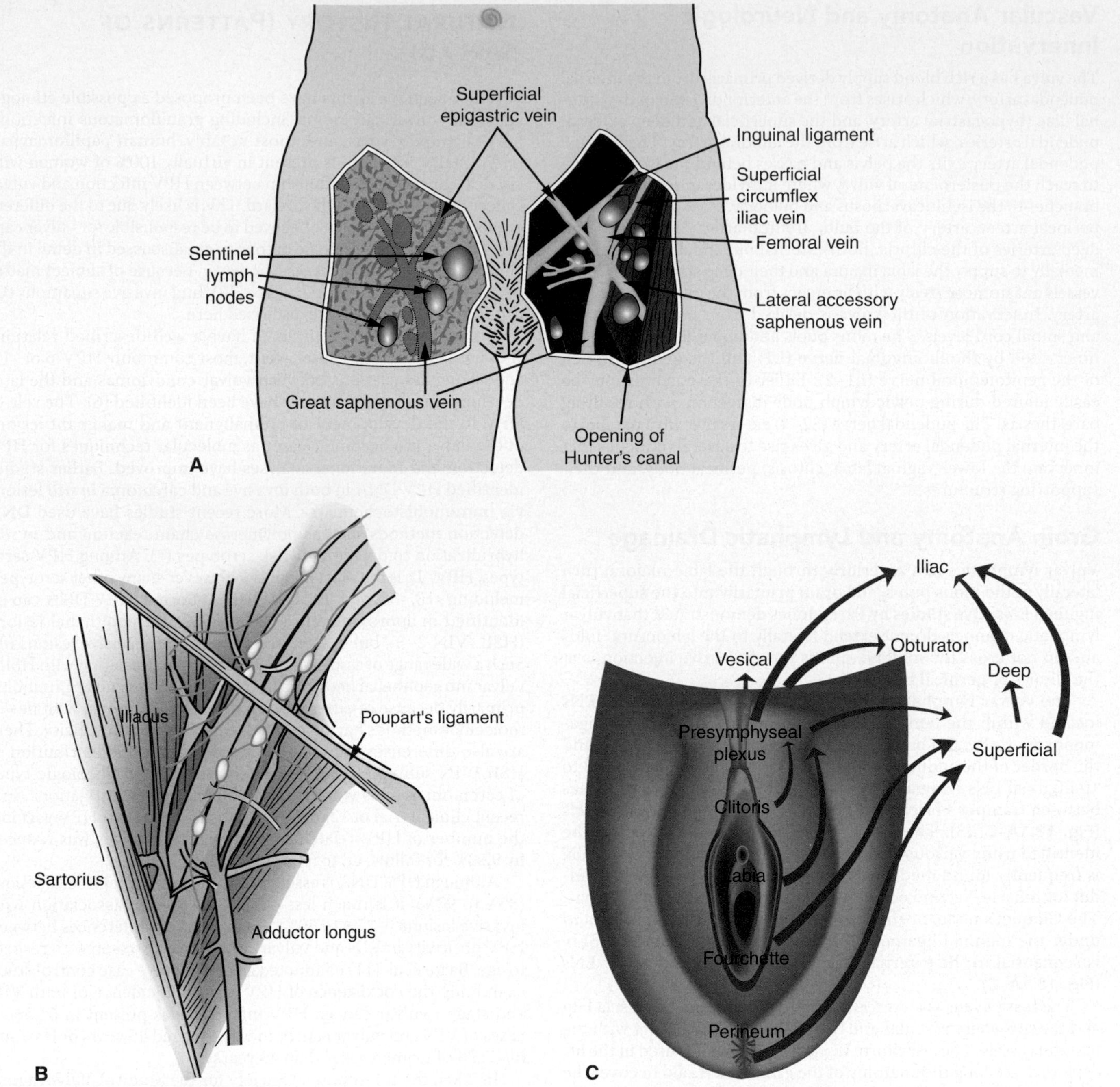

Figure 18.1. These historic figures illustrate some of the problems depicting the lymphatic anatomy of the groin accurately. **A, B:** Vessels, muscles, and nerves. **A:** Sentinel nodes; however, this is based on location rather than a mapping procedure, which is misleading. **B:** Nodes between the femoral artery and the vein. Lymph nodes between the vessels are common in the pelvis but not in the groin. **C:** Direct drainage from the clitoral area of the vulva to pelvic lymph nodes. This drainage pattern is not observed with preoperative or intraoperative lymphatic mapping studies.

with a history of cervical or vaginal cancer, the vulva should be examined as part of a surveillance exam. In those patients with a history of VIN or lichen sclerosus, self-examination with a mirror should be taught (16).

Chronic immunosuppression and tobacco smoking have also been linked as cofactors for the development of invasive vulvar cancer. Vulvar cancer incidence is increased in female renal transplant patients, as well as women with HIV and AIDS (17,18). Smoking is an independent risk factor for the development of SCC of the vulva, although the reason for this is unclear. One hypothesis is that genetic variations in T-cell-mediated IL-2 responses among smokers may explain differential susceptibility to the development of squamous vulvar carcinomas (19).

Chronic vulvar inflammatory lesions, such as vulvar dermatoses, including lichen sclerosus (LS), lichen planus, lichen simplex chronicus (including squamous cell hyperplasia), and vulvar intraepithelial neoplasia (HSIL/VIN 2–3 (usual as well as differentiated types), particularly dVIN, have been suggested as precursors of invasive squamous cancers (15). Carli et al. (16) suggested a possible role of LS as a precursor to vulvar cancer, based on their observation that 32% of vulvar cancer cases not related to HPV were associated with LS. More recently, in a pathologic reevaluation of patients with a diagnosis of LS who were followed clinically for a minimum of 10 years, van de Nieuwenhof and colleagues identified concordant diagnoses of LS in 58/61 patients who did not progress to cancer, and concordant diagnoses of LS in only 29/60 patients who were identified with a subsequent diagnosis of vulvar cancer. Most patients reclassified as having something other than LS were considered to have dVIN (25/31 patients). This study highlights dVIN as a uniquely at-risk histology that deserves prompt treatment and close follow-up. Differentiated VIN is often found in lesions, previously diagnosed as LS, that have progressed to vulvar SCC (15). In a more recent long-term follow-up study of women with LS, those identified with LS had a progressively increased frequency of vulvar SCC with increasing duration of the disease. In this study, most squamous carcinomas were superficially invasive. At 24 months of follow-up, 1.2% had carcinoma, whereas at 300 months, 36.8% had carcinoma (20). Despite this association, however, LS is not considered a true premalignant condition like HSIL/VIN 2–3. Standard clinical management of LS, including chronic, as-needed topical steroid use, periodic surveillance examinations, and selective biopsies of discrete lesions, has been reported to reduce the risk of vulvar carcinoma (21).

Vulvar lichen planus (LP), like LS, is also recognized as being associated with an increased risk of a subsequent diagnosis of vulvar SCC. In a long-term Finnish study (follow-up >43 years) evaluating more than 12,144 women with LS and 9,030 women with LP, both diagnoses were associated with an increased risk of vulvar carcinoma. Among women with LS, many of those who subsequently presented with vulvar carcinoma presented within 5 years of the beginning of the study, with 993 (8%) women subsequently having carcinoma. Among women with LP, 919 (10%) subsequently developed carcinoma (22).

In a study of 405 patients noted to have VIN 2–3, Jones et al. (23) found that 3.8% of patients had developed invasive cancer despite therapy, and 10 untreated patients developed invasive cancer between 1.1 and 7.3 years (mean, 3.9 years) from the time of initial observation. In a recent retrospective study of 240 women with vulvar squamous lesions, 213 with HSIL/VIN 2–3 were treated with surgical excision. Among these patients, 21 (9.8%) were found to have an associated invasive squamous carcinoma within the surgical specimen. Most tumors were superficial, varying in size from 0.1 to 2 cm. On follow-up, 25% of the patients with positive margins had local recurrence of HSIL, whereas 16.6% of those with negative surgical margins were identified with a recurrence (22). Although some intraepithelial lesions regress spontaneously, it appears that a significant number persist or progress to invasive cancer.

Differentiated VIN is recognized as a precursor of vulvar SCC and is associated with LS in many cases. In a retrospective study involving 240 patients with vulvar squamous lesions, 27 were found to be dVIN, and 19 of these cases (70.4%) had associated SCC (22). In a retrospective study of 18 dVIN cases, 14 were found to have associated SCC, and of these, 12 had associated vulvar LS (24). Trimble et al. (25) postulated that SCC of the vulva may represent a final common endpoint of heterogeneous etiologic pathways. According to their studies, two histologic subtypes, those with basaloid or warty features, are associated with HPV, whereas keratinizing squamous carcinomas are not. Furthermore, basaloid or warty carcinomas are associated with classic risk factors for cervical carcinoma, including age at first intercourse, lifetime number of sexual partners, prior abnormal Pap smears, smoking, and lower socioeconomic status. Keratinizing squamous carcinomas are weakly linked to these factors, and in some cases not at all.

Mitchell et al. evaluated 169 women with invasive vulvar cancers and noted that second genital squamous neoplasms occurred in 13% of cases. The risk of a second primary tumor was significantly increased in cancer cases with HPV DNA, intraepithelioid growth pattern, or adjacent dysplasia (26). These observations support the concept that some squamous lesions may be initiated by neoplastic etiologies that produce change within the entire field of the lower genital tract (field effect). The obvious clinical implication of this observation is that a patient with an established squamous lesion of the vulva, vagina, or cervix needs to be evaluated and monitored for new or coexistent lesions at other genital sites.

Vulvar cancers metastasize in three ways: (a) local growth and extension into adjacent organs, (b) lymphatic embolization to regional lymph nodes in the groin, and (c) hematogenous dissemination to distant sites. Inguinal node metastasis can be predicted by the presence of multiple risk factors, including tumor diameter, higher histologic grade, depth of stromal invasion, and lymph-vascular space invasion (27). Clinically important observations regarding nodal metastases include the following: (a) Inguinal nodes are the most frequent site of lymphatic metastasis; (b) In-transit metastases within vulvar epithelium and deep tissues are exceedingly rare, suggesting that most initial lymphatic metastases represent embolic phenomena; (c) Metastasis to the contralateral groin or deep pelvic nodes are unusual in the absence of ipsilateral groin metastases; (d) Nodal involvement generally proceeds in a stepwise fashion from the superficial inguinal to the deep inguinal and then to the pelvic nodes (27).

Spread beyond the inguinal lymph nodes is considered distant metastasis (stage IVB). The occurrence of such metastases are due to either sequential lymphatic spread to secondary and tertiary nodal groups or as a result of hematogenous dissemination to more distant sites, such as bone, lung, or liver. Distant metastases are uncommon at initial presentation and are usually seen in the setting of recurrent disease.

Clinical Presentation

Most women with vulvar cancer present with pruritus or vulvar discomfort and a recognizable, exophytic or endophytic ulcerated lesion. Selecting the most appropriate site for biopsy in women with condyloma, chronic vulvar LS, multifocal high-grade squamous intraepithelial lesions (VIN 3), or Paget's disease can be difficult, and multiple biopsies may be required. Optimal management for any patient presenting with a suspicious lesion is to proceed directly to biopsy under local analgesia. Tissue biopsies should include the cutaneous lesion in question and representative contiguous underlying stroma, so that the presence and depth of invasion (DOI) can be accurately assessed. Because DOI is a central issue in the management of vulvar cancer, punch biopsies are encouraged and shave biopsies are generally discouraged in the diagnosis of vulvar lesions. If invasion is suspected and a punch biopsy fails to confirm the clinical suspicion, then an incisional or excisional biopsy should be performed. Primary care physicians should be encouraged not to excise an entire lesion if avoidable, in order to facilitate a subsequent sentinel node procedure by a gynecologic oncologist. **Figure 18.2** illustrates an early-stage vulvar cancer.

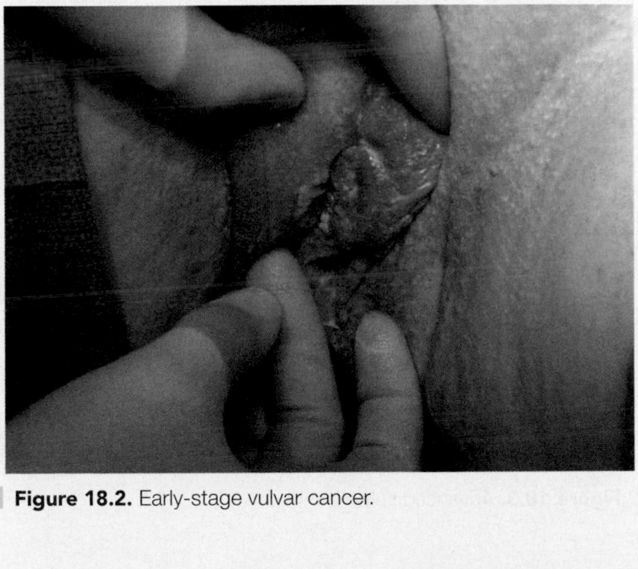

Figure 18.2. Early-stage vulvar cancer.

DIAGNOSTIC EVALUATION

The evaluation of a patient with vulvar cancer must consider the clinical extent of disease and the presence of coexisting medical illnesses. Initial evaluation should include a detailed physical examination with measurements of the primary tumor, assessment for extension to adjacent mucosal or bony structures, and clinical evaluation of the inguinal LNs. It is helpful to record the distance from vital structures such as the clitoris, urethral meatus, and anus, since these structures limit the ability to obtain adequate surgical margins. Diagnostic imaging is not required in women with small primary lesions and normal body habitus. In obese women, the inguinal nodes are difficult to palpate, and imaging may help identify the presence of lymphadenopathy. Patients with large or fixed tumors, and those who are difficult to examine in the clinic, may benefit from an exam under anesthesia with cystourethroscopy and proctosigmoidoscopy. **Figure 18.3** illustrates an advanced tumor, for which such an approach can help determine resectability.

Radiographic studies that have been described as beneficial are computed tomography (CT), magnetic resonance imaging (MRI), positron emission tomography (PET), ultrasound, and single photon emission CT. While newer imaging modalities can benefit treatment planning, it is also important to note that published series are small, and no individual modality has been shown to be superior to others in terms of detecting metastatic or recurrent disease (28–31). The best modality might differ depending on the practice situation and skills of the diagnostic imaging consultants. Suspicious lymph nodes should be biopsied if the findings would alter the surgical plan. Because neoplasia of the female genital tract is often multifocal, evaluation of the vagina and cervix, including cervical cytologic screening, should always be performed in women with vulvar neoplasms (32). Lymphoscintigraphy (LSG) is discussed later in this chapter.

STAGING

The International Federation of Gynecology and Obstetrics (FIGO) adopted a modified surgical staging system for vulvar cancer in 1989, which was revised in 1995 and more recently in 2009 (**Table 18.1**). The 2009 revision was performed to address issues such as the lack of a useful prognostic spread among stages, and significant prognostic heterogeneity among stage III patients. After the 1995 revision, much has been learned about the significance of the number of involved nodes, the size of inguinal metastases, and nodal morphology (33,34).

The technique recommended by the ISSVD, the International Society of Gynecologic Pathologists (ISGYP), the College of American Pathologists (CAP), and the World Health Organization (WHO) to assess depth of stromal invasion is to measure from the base of the epithelium (epithelial–stromal junction) at the nearest superficial dermal papillae to the deepest point of tumor penetration. These definitions and methods of measurement are supported by the recent CAP-ASCCP Lower Anogenital Squamous Terminology (LAST) project (**Fig. 18.4**) (35).

Among SCCs limited to the vulva, those with a DOI ≤ 1 mm are associated with a <1% risk for lymph node metastasis. Tumors with a DOI of 1.1 to 3 mm are associated with lymph node metastases in 6% to 12% of patients, and approximately 15% to 20% of tumors with a DOI of 3.1 to 5 mm are associated with positive lymph nodes (36).

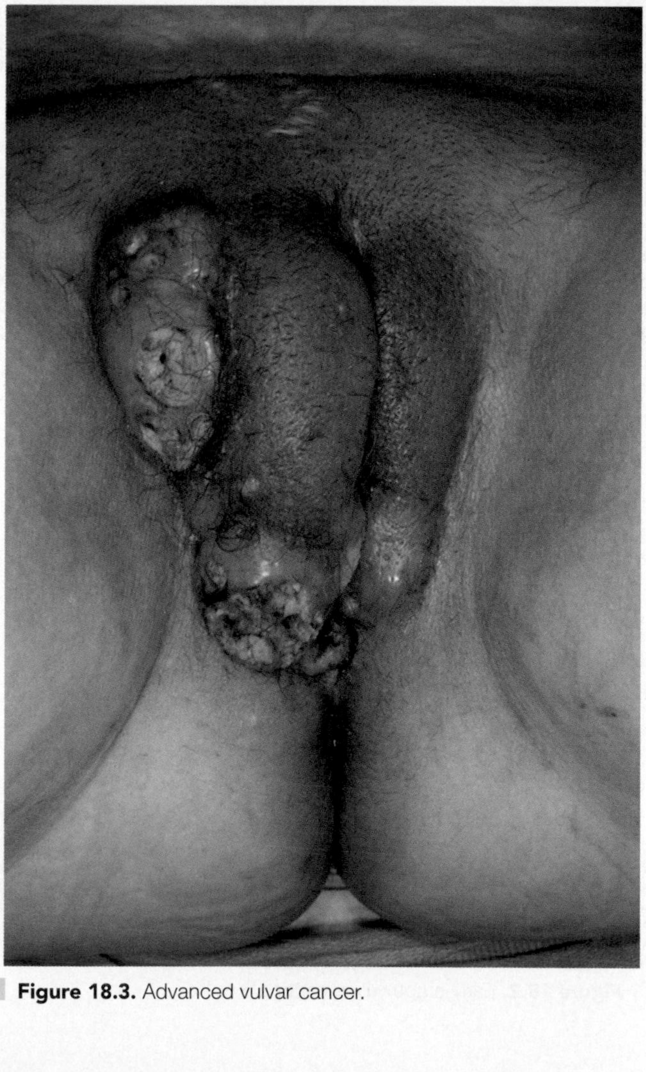

Figure 18.3. Advanced vulvar cancer.

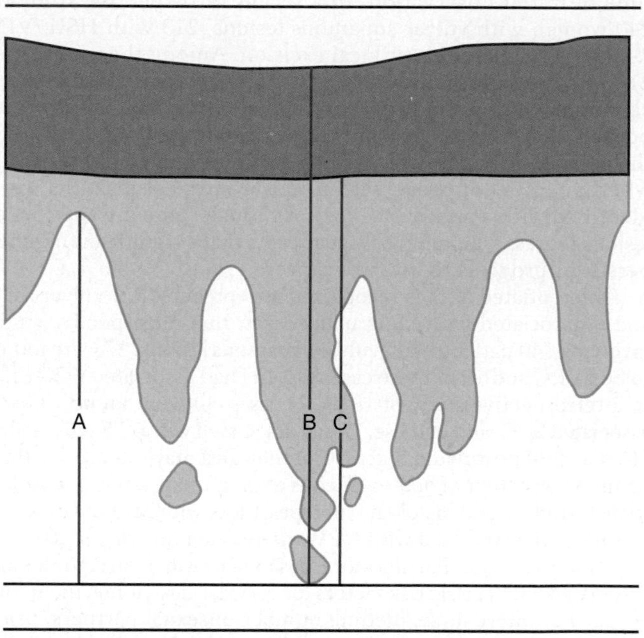

Figure 18.4. Methods for measurement of vulvar superficially invasive carcinomas. Depth of invasion. **A**: The measurement from the epithelial stromal junction of the most superficial dermal papillae to the deepest point of invasion. This measurement is defined as the depth of invasion and is used to define stage IA vulvar carcinoma. **B**: The measurement is the thickness of the tumor from the surface of the lesion to the deepest point of invasion. **C**: Measurement is from the bottom of the granular layer to the deepest point of invasion. This is also defined as thickness of the tumor in cases where there is a keratinized surface. The International Society of Gynecological Pathologists and the World Health Organization recommend that both the depth of invasion and the thickness of tumor, as well as the method of measurement, be defined in the pathology reports.

Source: Reprinted with permission from Wilkinson EJ. Superficial invasive carcinoma of the vulva. *Clin Obstet Gynecol*. 1985;28:188–192.

In the 2009 revision, all stage I and stage II patients by definition have uninvolved LNs. With respect to inguinal lymphadenectomy, there is no clear definition of how many LNs constitute an adequate evaluation. SLN biopsy is not mentioned as a requirement; however, the emphasis on the size of micrometastases in stage III implies that an SLN biopsy is performed either alone or as part of a lymphadenectomy.

The 2009 staging system added three pathologic groupings within stage III (a, b, and c), each of which contains prognostic significance. These three groups are the number of positive nodes, the size of the largest inguinal node metastasis, and the presence or absence of extracapsular extension. These pathologic features have been shown in multiple studies to be the strongest predictors of mortality related to vulvar cancer (34,37). The other notable difference in the 2009 schema is the absence of stage difference based on unilaterality versus bilaterality of groin involvement; any groin metastasis is considered to be stage III disease. The 2009 FIGO staging guidelines for vulvar cancer were devised with correlation for the American Joint Committee on Cancer (AJCC) tumor node metastasis (TNM) classification scheme (**Table 18.1**) (34). Tumor assessment is based on physical examination, with endoscopy in cases of bulky disease. Nodal status is determined by the surgical evaluation of the groin. The presence or absence of distant metastases should be determined on the basis of an individualized diagnostic workup based on the patient's clinical presentation (33).

Because of the infrequent incidence of vulvar melanoma, there has historically been a paucity of data to guide staging algorithms for patients with this disease. Recent data, however, support an assertion that AJCC staging guidelines (updated in 2010) for cutaneous melanoma should be applied to vulvar melanoma. Moxley et al. examined 77 cases of vulvar melanoma from five academic medical centers, applying the 2002 modifications of the AJCC staging system for cutaneous melanoma, Breslow thickness, and Clark level to all patients. Breslow's thickness was associated with recurrence ($p = 0.002$) but not survival; however, the AJCC-2002 staging system was predictive of overall survival (OS) ($p = 0.006$) in patients with vulvar melanoma (38). It is important that primary tumor thickness (using Breslow's method) and nodal status are the primary determinants of survival in this disease. Also important, however, are the presence or absence of ulceration and mitotic rate; these descriptors also factor prominently in the staging of cutaneous melanoma (**Tables 18.2A** and **18.2B**).

TABLE 18.1. Integrated 2009 FIGO and AJCC Staging System for Squamous Cell Carcinoma of the Vulva

FIGO		AJCC		
		T	N	M
		Tis: No invasion past basement membrane (not in FIGO system)		
I: Tumor confined to the vulva				
1A	Lesions ≤2 cm in size, confined to vulva or perineum and with stromal invasion ≤1 mm, no nodal metastasis	T1a	N0	M0
1B	Lesions >2 cm in size or with stromal invasion >1 mm, confined to the vulva or perineum, with negative nodes	T1b	N0	M0
II	Tumor of any size with extension to adjacent perineal structures (1/3 lower urethra, 1/3 lower vagina, anus), with negative nodes	T2	N0	M0
III	Tumor of any size with or without extension to adjacent perineal structures (1/3 lower urethra, 1/3 lower vagina, anus), with positive inguinofemoral lymph nodes	T1 or T2	N1–N3	M0
IIIA	(i) 1–2 lymph node metastasis(es) (<5 mm), or (ii) 1 lymph node metastasis (≥5 mm)	T1 or T2	N1a = (i) N1b = (ii)	M0
IIIB	(i) 3 or more lymph node metastases (<5 mm) or (ii) 2 or more lymph node metastases (≥5 mm)	T1 or T2	N2a = (i) N2b = (ii)	M0
IIIC	Positive nodes with extracapsular spread	T1 or T2	N2c N3 = inguinal skin ulceration or fixed nodes	M0
IV	Tumor invades other regional (2/3 upper urethra, 2/3 upper vagina), or distant structures	T3 = any size, involves upper urethra, bladder, rectum, bone		
IVA	Tumor invades (i) upper urethral and/or vaginal mucosa, bladder mucosa, rectal mucosa, or fixed to pelvic bone, or (ii) fixed or ulcerated inguinofemoral lymph nodes	T3		M0
IVB	Distant metastasis: includes pelvic nodes	T1, T2, or T3		M1

AJCC stage groupings

Stage	T, N, M combination
0	Tis, N0, M0
IA	T1a, N0, M0
IB	T1b, N0, M0
II	T2, N0, M0
IIIA	T1 or T2, N1a or N1b, M0
IIIB	T1 or T2, N2a or N2b, M0
IIIC	T1 or T2, N2c, M0
IVA	Either T1 or T2, N3, M0 or T2, any N, M0
IVB	any T, any N, M1

TABLE 18.2A. TNM Staging Categories for Cutaneous Melanoma

Classification	Thickness (mm)	Ulceration Status/Mitoses
Tis	NA	NA
T1	≤1	a: Without ulceration and mitosis < 1/mm^2 b: With ulceration or mitoses ≥ 1/mm^2
T2	1.01–2	a: Without ulceration b: With ulceration
T3	2.01–4	a: Without ulceration b: With ulceration
T4	>4	a: Without ulceration b: With ulceration
N	**No. of metastatic nodes**	**Nodal metastatic burden**
N0	0	NA
N1	1	a: Micrometastasis[a] b: Macrometastasis[b]
N2	2–3	a: Micrometastasis[a] b: Macrometastasis[b] c: In-transit metastases/satellites without metastatic nodes
N3	4+ metastatic nodes, or matted nodes, or in-transit metastases/satellites with metastatic nodes	
M	**Site**	**Serum LDH**
M0	No distant metastases	NA
M1a	Distant skin, subcutaneous, or nodal metastases	Normal
M1b	Lung metastases	Normal
M1c	All other visceral metastases	Normal
	Any distant metastasis	Elevated

LDH, lactate dehydrogenase; NA, not applicable.

[a]Micrometastases are diagnosed after sentinel lymph node biopsy.

[b]Micrometastases are defined as clinically detectable nodal metastases confirmed pathologically.

TABLE 18.2B. TNM Stage Grouping for Cutaneous Melanoma

Clinical Staging				Pathologic Staging			
	T	N	M		T	N	M
0	Tis	N0	M0	0	Tis	N0	M0
IA	T1a	N0	M0	IA	T1a	N0	M0
IB	T1b	N0	M0	IB	T1b	N0	M0
	T2a	N0	M0		T2a	N0	M0
IIA	T2b	N0	M0	IIA	T2b	N0	M0
	T3a	N0	M0		T3a	N0	M0
IIB	T3b	N0	M0	IIB	T3b	N0	M0
	T4a	N0	M0		T4a	N0	M0
IIC	T4b	N0	M0	IIC	T4b	N0	M0
III	Any T	>N0	M0	IIIA	T1-4a	N1a	M0
					T1-4a	N2a	M0
				IIIB	T1-4b	N1a	M0
					T1-4b	N2a	M0
					T1-4a	N1b	M0
					T1-4a	N2b	M0
					T1-4a	N2c	M0

■ **TABLE 18.2B. TNM Stage Grouping for Cutaneous Melanoma (*continued*)**

Clinical Staging				Pathologic Staging			
				IIIC	T1-4b	N1b	M0
					T1-4b	N2b	M0
					T1-4b	N2c	M0
					Any T	N3	M0
IV	Any T	Any N	M1	IV	Any T	Any N	M1

Clinical staging includes microstaging of the primary melanoma and clinical/radiologic evaluation for metastases. By convention, it should be used after complete excision of the primary melanoma with clinical assessment for regional and distant metastases.

Source: Reprinted with permission from Edge SB, Byrd DR, Compton CC, et al. *AJCC Cancer Staging Manual.* New York, NY: Springer; 2009.

PATHOLOGY

Most vulvar malignancies arise within squamous epithelium. Although the vulva does not have an identifiable transformation zone, as the cervix does, squamous neoplasms arise most commonly on the labia minora, clitoris, posterior fourchette, perineal body, or medial aspects of the labia majora. Within the vulvar vestibule and fourchette, squamous neoplasia may arise where keratinized stratified squamous epithelium transitions to the nonkeratinized squamous mucosa of the vestibule, also known as Hart's line (39).

Most vulvar squamous carcinomas arise within areas of epithelium associated with a recognizable epithelial cell abnormality. Approximately 60% of cases have adjacent HSIL (VIN 3). In cases of superficially invasive squamous carcinoma of the vulva, the frequency of adjacent HSIL (VIN 3) approaches 85% (14). Lichen sclerosus, usually with associated hyperplastic features, dVIN, or HSIL (VIN 3) can be found adjacent to vulvar SCC in 15% to 40% of the cases (40,41). Granulomatous disease is also associated with vulvar SCC; however, this is not a commonly associated finding in the United States. Thus, vulvar SCC precursors can be considered in distinct groups: those associated with HPV, "usual" VIN, and those that are not (e.g., those associated with LS, chronic granulomatous disease) (see Epidemiology section).

EPITHELIAL CARCINOMAS

Squamous Cell Carcinomas

Stage I squamous carcinomas of the vulva with a DOI of 3 mm have a LN metastasis rate averaging 12%. Tumors with a DOI of 5 mm or more have a LN metastasis rate of at least 15%. Tumors with a DOI $\leq$ 1 mm carry little risk of LN metastasis (42). DOI and tumor thickness are separately defined and measured because considerable variations can exist among measurements from various superficial points in tumors of approximately 1 mm (41). When evaluating an ulcerated tumor thought to be superficially invasive, measurement from the surface of the ulcer, rather than from the adjacent dermal papillae as recommended for the DOI measurement, may result in serious underestimation, and understaging, of the tumor. When there is epithelial acanthosis, thickening, or hyperkeratosis, measurement of invasion from the overlying surface epithelium of the tumor, that is, measuring the thickness of the tumor rather than DOI, can result in overstaging. With large tumors, and some tumors with invasion deeper than 1 mm, thickness may be the only reliable measurement because of the lack of identifiable adjacent dermal papillae (41).

In addition to tumor stage and depth or thickness, other pathologic features include vascular space invasion, growth pattern of the tumor, grade of the tumor, and tumor type. Vascular space involvement can be defined as tumor within an endothelial lined vascular space. Strict pathologic criteria require that the tumor be attached to the wall of the vessel, but this is not observed in all cases. Vascular space involvement by SCC of the vulva is associated with a higher frequency of LN metastasis and a lower overall 5-year survival rate. No reliable methods unambiguously predict LN metastasis by quantitation of vascular space involvement by tumor.

Tumor growth pattern influences the rate of LN metastasis and survival in tumors >1 mm in DOI. In stage IA vulvar carcinomas, tumor growth pattern does not influence the risk of node involvement. Three factors describe tumor growth patterns: confluent; compact (pushing pattern); and fingerlike (or spray or diffuse), a pattern also described as poorly differentiated (36). Confluent growth is defined as a tumor mass composed of interconnected tumor >1 mm in dimension (**Fig. 18.5**). Confluent growth is characteristic of deeply invasive SCCs that are associated with stromal desmoplasia, resulting in fibrovascular stromal changes adjacent to the interconnected cords of tumor.

Compact (pushing; well differentiated) growth is squamous tumor growth that maintains continuity with the overlying epithelium and infiltrates as a well-defined and well-circumscribed tumor mass, without islands of infiltrating tumor remote from the tumor mass. Tumors with compact growth typically have a thickness $\leq$5 mm and rarely invade vascular space. They are characteristically well differentiated, with the tumor cells resembling the squamous cells of the adjacent and overlying epithelium. There is usually minimal stromal desmoplasia, although there may be a lymphocytic inflammatory cell infiltrate (39).

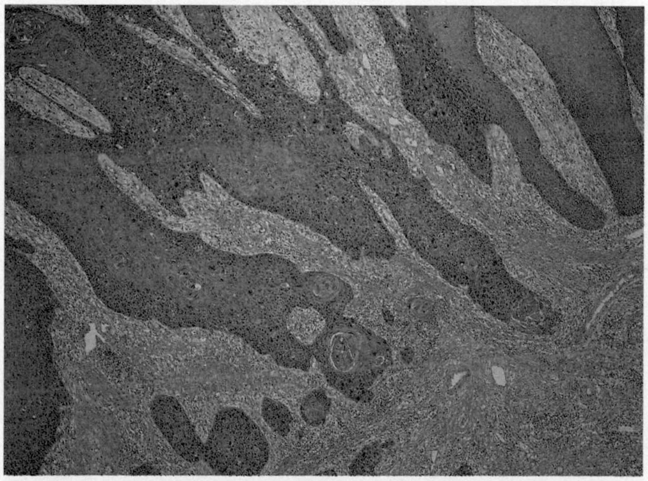

Figure 18.5. Confluent pattern of invasion. The tumor has a compact, pushing growth pattern with a well-defined tumor–dermal interface. The tumor diameter exceeds 1 cm, and has fingerlike growth pattern, with small, variable-sized tumor nests within the adjacent dermis. The adjacent dermis has a desmoplastic, fibrotic appearance.

Fingerlike (spray or diffuse; poorly differentiated) growth is characterized by a trabecular appearance, with small islands of poorly differentiated tumor cells found within the dermis or submucosa deeper than the bulk of the tumor mass. Tumors with this growth pattern are typically associated with a desmoplastic stromal response (**Fig. 18.6**) and a lymphocytic inflammatory cell infiltrate. In tumors with a DOI <5 mm, the fingerlike pattern of growth is associated with a higher frequency of inguinal lymph node metastasis (39).

In some cases, a single tumor may have both compact and fingerlike growth patterns. Mixed patterns, in our experience, are more commonly encountered in frankly invasive vulvar carcinomas and are rarely seen in superficially invasive tumors. The Gynecologic Oncology Group (GOG) has referred to tumors with a compact pattern of growth as well differentiated, and to tumors with the fingerlike pattern of growth as poorly differentiated. Using this terminology, the GOG proposed the following grading system for vulvar SCC:

- Grade 1 tumors are composed of well differentiated tumor and contain no poorly differentiated element.
- Grade 2 tumors contain both patterns, with the poorly differentiated portions making up one-third or less of the tumor.
- Grade 3 tumors also contain both components, with the poorly differentiated portion composing more than one-third but less than one-half of the tumor.
- Grade 4 tumors have one-half or more of the tumor composed of the poorly differentiated elements.

The ISGYP Committee of Terminology for Non-neoplastic Epithelial Disorders and Tumors recommended that the following information be included in the pathology report of all excised vulvar SCCs, information also supported by the CAP, and often used by tumor registries (43):

1. Depth of tumor invasion in millimeters
2. Thickness of the tumor in millimeters
3. Method of measurement of the DOI and thickness
4. Presence or absence of vascular space (lymphatic) involvement by tumor
5. Diameter of the tumor, measured from the specimen in the fresh or fixed state
6. Clinical measurement of the tumor diameter, if available

Several histopathologic types of vulvar SCC are recognized. The usual types include SCC, keratinizing type; SCC, nonkeratinizing type; basaloid carcinoma; and warty (condylomatous) carcinoma (42). Less common types include acantholytic SCC, SCC with tumor giant cells and spindle cell squamous carcinoma, SCC with sarcoma-like stroma, sebaceous carcinoma, verrucous carcinoma, and other rarer types (41,42).

Adenoid squamous carcinoma (pseudoangiosarcomatous carcinoma, acantholytic SCC, pseudoglandular SCC) refers to SCCs with pseudoglandular features. These tumors are characterized by small gland-like spaces within a tumor that otherwise appears to be a poorly differentiated SCC. It is considered a highly aggressive variant of vulvar SCC (44). This tumor should be differentiated from adenosquamous carcinomas that contain an obvious adenocarcinoma component (40). Adenoid squamous carcinoma does not contain sialomucin, but adenosquamous carcinoma typically does contain mucin within the adenocarcinoma component.

SCC with tumor giant cells has multinucleated tumor giant cells intermixed within the squamous carcinoma. This tumor may resemble amelanotic melanoma. SCC with tumor giant cells, unlike melanoma, does not express S100 antigen, HMB45, or Melan-A on immunoperoxidase studies. This tumor does express low molecular weight keratin, similar to other squamous carcinomas (45).

Sebaceous Carcinoma of the Vulva

These tumors, which arise from the sebaceous glands of the vulvar skin, may be associated with VIN. This rare tumor is aggressive. The tumor cells are relatively large, with large nuclei, and prominent nucleoli with prominent cytoplasm. The cytoplasm, related to its lipid content, has a finely vacuolated appearance. The tumor may have the appearance of a SCC intermixed with sebaceous elements. Deep invasion and lymph node or other metastases may be present on initial presentation (46,47).

Spindle Cell Squamous Cell Carcinomas

These tumors consist of poorly differentiated neoplastic epithelial cells that have an elongated spindle shape and may mimic a spindle cell melanoma or a sarcoma (**Fig. 18.7**) (48). SCC with spindle cell stroma is associated with a sarcoma-like stromal/dermal response that may mimic a primary sarcoma. Spindle cell SCCs can be differentiated from sarcomas by immunoperoxidase techniques. Like other SCCs, the spindle cell variant contains keratin and lacks the antigens distinctive to sarcomas of various origins. S100 antigen, HMB45, and Melan-A are usually immune-reactive in a spindle cell melanoma and lacking in a spindle cell squamous carcinoma.

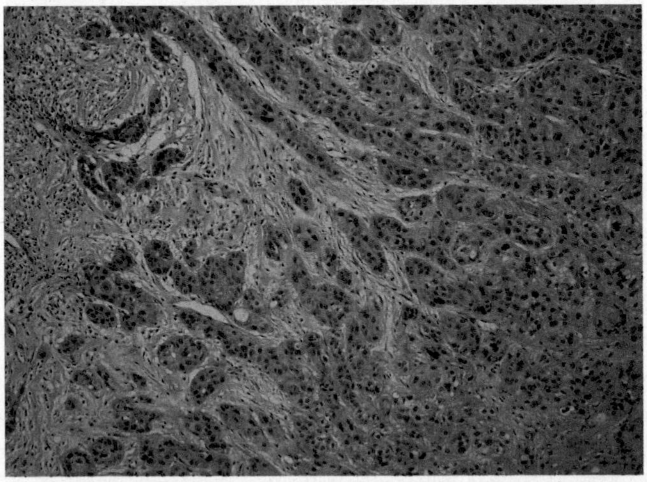

Figure 18.6. Fingerlike growth. The tumor forms small nests surrounded by a desmoplastic stroma.

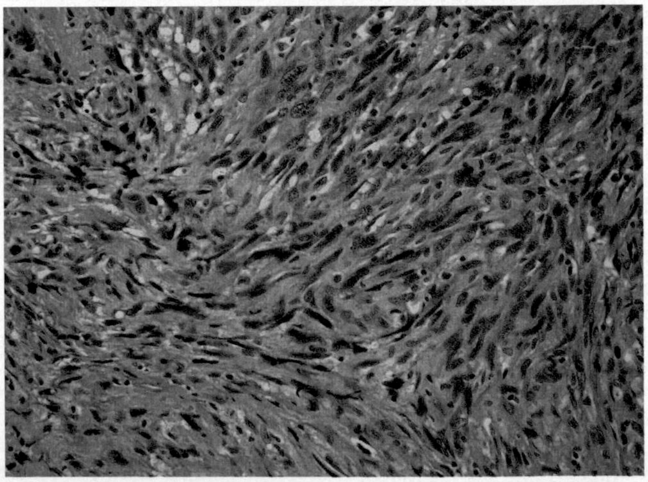

Figure 18.7. Spindle cell squamous carcinoma. The tumor cells have a spindle shape and poorly defined cell junctions.

Verrucous Carcinoma

Verrucous carcinoma of the vulva typically presents as an exophytic appearing growth that can be locally destructive. Clinically, it may resemble condyloma acuminatum. The so-called Buschke-Lowenstein giant condyloma is classified as a variant of verrucous carcinoma by WHO (42). Microscopically, verrucous carcinoma is characterized by well differentiated epithelial cells. The tumor growth pattern is characterized by a "pushing" tumor–dermal interface with minimal stroma between the acanthotic epithelium (**Fig. 18.8**). The surface is often hyperkeratotic, and there may be parakeratosis. Observed mitoses are characteristically normal. Within the dermis, a mild lymphocytic inflammatory cell response is usually seen. Vascular space involvement by tumor is characteristically lacking. Because of its excellent prognosis, strict histologic criteria should be used in the diagnosis of verrucous carcinoma. Squamous carcinomas with focal verrucous features should not be described or diagnosed as verrucous carcinoma.

Verrucous carcinomas are characteristically diploid, unlike typical SCCs of the vulva, which are usually aneuploid by DNA analysis. The major differential diagnosis of verrucous carcinoma includes keratoacanthomas, pseudocarcinomatous hyperplasia, epithelioid sarcoma, and malignant rhabdoid tumor.

Basal Cell Carcinoma

Basal cell carcinoma (BCC) is a relatively rare tumor in the vulva, accounting for 2% to 4% of infiltrative neoplasms (49). These tumors are most commonly found in elderly women with a median age of 75 years, as compared with 67 years of age for SCCs, as noted in a recent study (50). The tumor may be a plaque or papule. Vulvar BCC most commonly arises on the labia majora and is typically relatively small, ranging from 0.2 to 2.5 cm, with a median size ≤0.85 cm in a recent study of 35 cases (50). The surface of the tumor appears granular and is well circumscribed.

The epithelial cells composing BCC are typically small and vary in form, with small hyperchromatic nuclei that may exhibit some nuclear pleomorphism. These tumors may have a variety of growth patterns (e.g., trabecular, insular), although peripheral nuclear palisading is a relatively consistent finding. BCCs often have an intraepithelial component that is contiguous with the infiltrative component, if present.

Metatypical Basal Cell Carcinoma

This is a variant of BCC that usually occurs at mucocutaneous junctions. The term *basosquamous carcinoma* is applied to these tumors because of their microscopic features, which include BCC intermixed with a SCC component. Nuclear pleomorphism is usually seen in metatypical BCC and in the basal cell and squamous cell components of the tumor. The deeper tumor cells, close to the underlying stroma, have the greatest degree of nuclear pleomorphism and the more prominent squamous features. These tumors have a more aggressive clinical behavior than typical BCC (39).

The differential diagnosis of metatypical BCC includes basaloid SCC, Merkel cell tumor of the skin, and metastatic small cell carcinoma. Basaloid SCC can be distinguished by its lack of characteristic basal cell growth pattern, and the presence of intracellular bridges. Nuclear pleomorphism is typically much greater in basaloid SCC than in BCC. BCCs express BerEP4 on histochemical study, an antigen not expressed by basaloid SCCs (41). Basaloid SCCs are typically associated with HPV-16, which is not typically associated with BCC. Merkel cell tumors and other neuroendocrine tumors of the vulva are typically subcutaneous or dermal nodules, and not intraepithelial lesions (see section on neuroendocrine tumors).

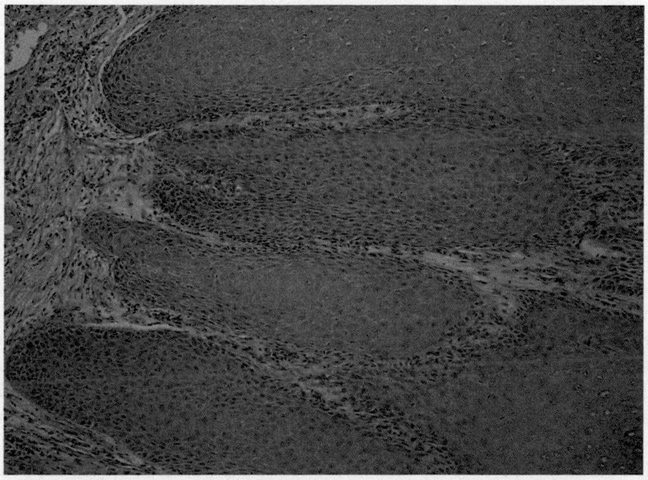

■ **Figure 18.8.** Verrucous carcinoma. The epithelial cells are well differentiated, and the tumor has a "pushing border" with a delicate vascular core between the epithelial elements.

Neuroendocrine and Neuroectodermal Tumors: Merkel Cell Tumors and Peripheral Neuroectodermal Tumor/Extraosseous Ewing Sarcoma

High-Grade Neuroendocrine Carcinoma/ Merkel Cell Tumor

The WHO classifies high-grade neuroendocrine carcinoma tumors into three categories: small cell neuroendocrine carcinoma (small cell carcinoma/SCNEC); large cell neuroendocrine carcinoma; and Merkel cell tumor (51). Although SCNEC tumors are well recognized in the lung, vagina, and cervix, they are extremely rare in the vulva. The WHO recommends that the term "small cell carcinoma" be used only for high-grade neuroendocrine tumors of small cell type, which would be a very rare finding in the vulva. Most of the high-grade neuroendocrine carcinomas reported in the vulva are Merkel cell tumors of the skin that typically occur within the dermis. They are rare, and may have a deceptive appearance as single or multiple cutaneous nodules. Ulceration may occur. The tumors may occur concurrently with vulvar SCC and/or VIN (51). These tumors can be divided into two major types: those composed predominantly of small, relatively uniform cells with little cytoplasm and a hyperchromatic, punctate nuclear chromatin pattern. The second type has cellular features resembling low-grade neuroendocrine tumors, with round to polygonal cells, little cytoplasm, and pale finely granular nuclear chromatin. Both types usually have a high mitotic count. Merkel cell tumors can also be subclassified as carcinoid-like (trabecular), intermediate type, and small cell (oat cell) type. By immunohistochemistry (IHC), these tumors typically express neuron-specific enolase (NSE), NCAM/CD56, cytokeratin CAM 5.2, cytokeratin 20, and AE1/AE3 (51). They may also express synaptophysin and chromogranin. Cytokeratin study, such as with cytokeratin 20, demonstrates a distinct perinuclear cytoplasmic dot. Dense core neurosecretory granules are seen by electron microscopy. These features differentiate it from BCC or SCC (41). Merkel cell tumors frequently have both regional LN and distant metastases, and are associated with a poor prognosis.

Peripheral Neuroectodermal Tumor/ Extraosseous Ewing Sarcoma

Peripheral neuroectodermal tumor (PNET) is a rare neuroendocrine vulvar neoplasm that has been reported in children, and women of reproductive age. The tumor may present as a subcutaneous or polypoid mass in the labia minora or majora, and clinically may resemble a Bartholin's cyst, or be ulcerated. On microscopic examination, the tumor is circumscribed multi-lobulated, and contain small cells with hyperchromatic nuclei and scant cytoplasm. Some cells have small nucleoli, and mitotic figures are usually common, with mitotic counts from 3 to exceeding 10 per 10 high power fields (HPFs). Numerous patterns of growth may be seen with highly cellular undifferentiated areas, areas with cyst formation containing eosinophilic proteinaceous material, Homer-Wright rosettes, and follicle-like structures. The cells of PNET have periodic acid-Schiff (PAS) staining cytoplasm that digests with diastase, and typically express CD99 and vimentin. Although, as in Merkel cell tumors, focal reactivity for synaptophysin and NSE may be present, cytokeratin reactivity is absent but may be focally immuno-reactive in some cases; dense core neurosecretory granules, as seen in Merkel cell tumor by electron microscopy, are not present (52–54).

Urothelial/Transitional Cell Carcinoma

Urothelial carcinoma may be a primary tumor of the vulva, usually arising within the Bartholin's glands. More commonly, urothelial carcinoma is metastatic to the vulva, having arisen within the bladder or urethra. In rare instances, the tumor presents as a Paget-like lesion of the vulva (see section on Paget's disease) (55). Microscopically, urothelial carcinomas are composed of relatively uniform cells; nuclear pleomorphisms may be marked in high-grade urothelial neoplasms. The cytoplasm is eosinophilic without apparent inclusions or keratin formations, although focal keratin formation may be seen. The tumors may exhibit papillary-like growth.

Adenocarcinoma and carcinoma of Bartholin's glands: Most primary adenocarcinomas of the vulva arise within Bartholin's glands. Adenocarcinoma may also arise from other glands or skin appendages of the vulva, including sweat glands and Skene's glands (42). Invasive vulvar Paget's disease has also given rise to adenocarcinoma (**Fig. 18.9**). Primary malignant tumors arising within Bartholin's glands include SCC (88%) and adenocarcinoma (12%) (56).

Carcinomas of Bartholin's glands generally occur in older women and are rare in women younger than 50. Therefore, it is generally advisable to excise an enlarged Bartholin's gland in women 50 years of age or older, especially if there is no known history of prior Bartholin's cyst. If a cyst is drained and a palpable mass persists, excision of the gland is indicated.

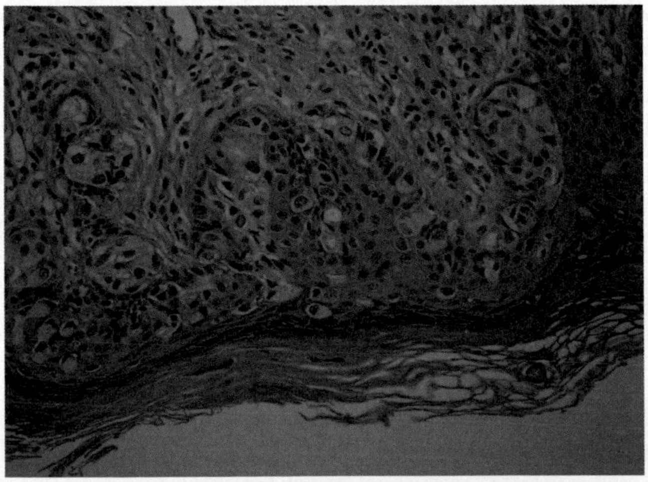

Figure 18.9. Paget's disease. The large cells with prominent cytoplasm and large nuclei represent the intraepithelial Paget's cells. A few small gland-like intraepithelial structures are formed by the Paget's cells.

Primary carcinomas within Bartholin's glands are usually solid tumors and are often deeply infiltrative. A variety of histologic types of adenocarcinoma have been described within Bartholin's glands, such as mucinous, papillary, and mucoepidermoid carcinoma tumor types, in addition to adenosquamous, squamous, and transitional cell carcinoma. Adenocarcinoma of Bartholin's glands is typically immuno-reactive for carcinoembryonic antigen (CEA). Histopathologic features that identify a carcinoma arising in Bartholin's glands include a recognizable transition from a Bartholin's gland to tumor. The histopathologic tumor type must be consistent with origin from a Bartholin's gland, and the tumor must not appear to be metastatic to gland. These malignancies are characteristically deep and difficult to detect in their early growth. Approximately 20% of women with primary carcinoma of Bartholin's glands have metastatic tumor to the inguinal lymph nodes at the time of primary tumor diagnosis (56).

Vulvar Paget's Disease and Paget-like Lesions. Vulvar Paget's disease typically presents as an eczematoid, red, weeping area on the vulva, often localized to the labia majora, perineal body, clitoral area, or other sites. This disease typically occurs in older, postmenopausal Caucasian women, although it has been described in a premenopausal woman (56a,b). Because of its eczematoid, erythematous and/or ulcerated appearance, it is not unusual for vulvar Paget's disease to be misdiagnosed as eczema or contact dermatitis. Approximately 15% of women with vulvar Paget's disease have underlying primary adenocarcinoma, usually arising within apocrine glands or the underlying Bartholin's glands. The Wilkinson and Brown etiologic classification of vulvar Paget's disease divides Paget's disease into two main groups: those of cutaneous origin and those of noncutaneous origin (55). The two most common types of noncutaneous Paget's disease are those associated with colorectal adenocarcinoma and those associated with bladder urothelial carcinoma. Women with Paget's disease of the colorectal type usually present with a lesion that involves the perianal skin, and this lesion is a manifestation of underlying colon or rectal adenocarcinoma. Women with Paget-like disease (pagetoid urothelial intraepithelial neoplasia [PUIN]) typically present with a lesion involving the periurethral area and vulvar vestibule (55,57). In these cases, there is associated bladder and/or urethral urothelial carcinoma, with extension of the neoplastic urothelial cells to the epithelium of the vulva. In cases of PUIN, wide local excision is an acceptable surgical treatment because there is no associated underlying cutaneous adenocarcinoma. The tumor cells are from the bladder and/or urethra, representing an intraepithelial transitional cell neoplasm extending from the bladder and/or urethra (55).

Cutaneous Paget's disease is most commonly a primary intraepithelial neoplasm, and in such cases, the intraepithelial Paget's disease may have an associated invasive Paget's disease. In rare cases, cutaneous Paget's disease may be a manifestation of an underlying cutaneous adenocarcinoma (55). Cutaneous Paget's disease is characterized by the presence of Paget's cells found within the involved epithelium. A Paget's cell is relatively large, with a prominent nucleus that typically has coarse chromatin and a prominent nucleolus. On hematoxylin and eosin (H & E) staining, the cytoplasm is distinctly pale compared with the surrounding keratinocytes. The cytoplasm may be vacuolated or appear foamy, and typically is somewhat basophilic (**Fig. 18.9**).

Paget's cells of cutaneous origin are rich in CEA, which can be identified with immunoperoxidase techniques. Paget's cells also express cytokeratin 7 (CK-7) and gross cystic disease fluid protein 15 (GCDFP-15) (55). Paget's cells infrequently express CA-125, and estrogen receptor is generally negative. Immunohistochemical staining for CK-7 is useful in many cases to identify the Paget's cells that are strongly CK-7 positive, whereas the adjacent epithelial cells are negative. Invasive Paget's disease ≤1 mm in DOI has reportedly little risk for recurrence (58).

The differential diagnosis of Paget's disease of cutaneous origin includes PUIN/Paget's disease of urothelial origin, Paget's disease of colorectal origin/or other related adenocarcinoma, superficial spreading malignant melanoma, pagetoid reticulosis, and the pagetoid variant of VIN, which are keratinocytic cells resembling Paget's cells. These can all be differentiated by immunoperoxidase techniques because melanomas do not express cytokeratin, but usually express S100 protein, HMB45, and Melan-A, which are absent in Paget's cells (55). The Paget-like cells in PUIN express uroplakin-2 and uroplakin-3, whereas uroplakins are not expressed in Paget's disease of cutaneous origin. The PUIN lesions do not express GCDFP-15. In a study of 15 cutaneous Paget's disease and 3 PUIN cases, GATA-3 was found to be reactive in both lesions and did not distinguish between them (59). Adenocarcinoma cells of colonic, anal, or rectal origin express CEA, as well as caudal homeobox (CDX), whereas Paget's disease of cutaneous origin does not express CDX. HSIL (VIN 3) of pagetoid type may microscopically resemble Paget's disease or melanoma, but the cells of LSIL or HSIL (VIN 1, VIN 2–3) do not express CEA, S100, or melanoma antigen (55,57).

Vulvar Malignant Melanoma. Malignant melanoma of the vulva accounts for approximately 9% of all primary malignant neoplasms on the vulva, and vulvar melanoma accounts for approximately 3% of all melanomas in women. This tumor occurs predominantly in Caucasian women, with approximately one-third of the cases occurring in women younger than 50; the mean age at diagnosis is 55 years (60). Peak frequency occurs between the sixth and seventh decades, and the highest incidence is in women 75 years of age or older, where the age-specific incidence is reported to be 1.28/100,000 (61). The most common presenting symptom is bleeding; however, symptoms may include pruritus, pain, dysuria, and a palpable mass (62,63). The tumor may arise from a preexisting pigmented lesion or from normal-appearing skin. The primary site on the vulva may be the clitoris, labia minora, and labia majora, where melanomas occur with approximately equal frequency (64). The tumor may be elevated, nodular, or ulcerated. Although tumors are usually pigmented, approximately one-fourth are amelanotic (**Fig 18.10**). In the clinical setting, the differential diagnosis includes pigmented condyloma acuminatum, pigmented HSIL VIN, atypical genital nevus, melanosis of the vulva, or other malignant tumors, including malignant soft tissue tumors.

Historically, vulvar malignant melanomas have been subclassified histopathologically into three categories: superficial spreading malignant melanoma, nodular melanoma, and mucosal lentiginous melanoma, which is also referred to as mucosal/acral lentiginous melanoma (65). Mucosal lentiginous melanomas are the type most commonly reported on the vulva, accounting for over one-half of the cases in larger series (61,65). Nodular melanomas are second in frequency, accounting for approximately one-fifth of the cases, and have the overall worst prognosis of the melanoma types, usually related to the greater thickness and deeper invasion at the time of presentation. Although it can be useful to be aware of these histopathologic categories because of persistent use in some centers, their clinical utility is limited, replaced by more objective and reproducible pathologic tumor characteristics such as DOI, ulceration, and mitotic rate (66).

Tumor thickness is the most important measurement in evaluating malignant melanoma. Historically, Clark's levels and Breslow's thickness definitions, which describe the extent of dermal and subcutaneous involvement by invasive melanoma lesions, were used to triage patients with T1 lesions into different prognostic groups for treatment (64). More recently, however, the 2009 AJCC Melanoma Staging and Classification update (seventh edition) recommended discontinuation of the use of these methods for characterization of T1 invasive melanoma lesions (66).

Melanomas arising in the vulva may metastasize to other sites within the lower female genital tract, including the cervix, vagina, urethra, and rectum. Distant metastasis is common with disseminated disease. Survival after recurrence is poor, approximately 5%.

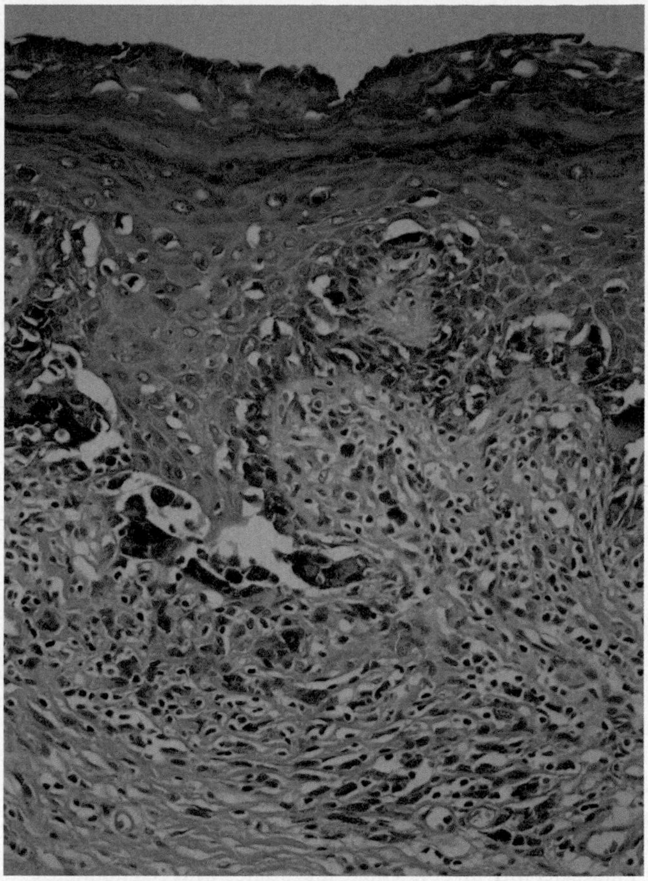

Figure 18.10. Malignant melanoma. The tumor is within the dermis and contains dark melanin pigment. Junctional growth is seen within the overlying epithelial dermal junction.

Vulvar Sarcomas

Leiomyosarcoma

Leiomyosarcoma (LMS) is the most frequent primary vulvar sarcoma, although sarcomas of the vulva are relatively rare. It occurs in women in the fourth or fifth decade of life and most commonly arises in the labia majora or Bartholin's gland area. The tumors are generally larger than 5 cm in diameter when first diagnosed, presenting as an enlarging mass. It may be deep within the subcutaneous tissue and painful in some circumstances.

On microscopic examination, these tumors are composed of interlacing spindle-shaped cells, sometimes with an epithelioid appearance. Histopathologic criteria for malignancy require at least three of the following features: size >5 cm, evidence of infiltrative growth into adjacent tissue, cytologic atypia of a moderate to severe degree, and mitotic count > 5 mitoses per 10 high power fields (HPFs). In cases with minimal pleomorphism, but with most of the other criteria, it is generally accepted that the diagnosis of LMS can be made with a mitotic count of 10 or more per 10 high power fields (HPFs). Tumors that have an infiltrating border or nuclear atypia with pleomorphism and mitotic count of 5 or more per 10 HPFs are classified as LMS (67).

Malignant Fibrous Histiocytoma

Malignant fibrous histiocytoma (MFH) arises from histiocytes with fibroblastic differentiation. It is considered the second most common sarcoma of the vulva and has its peak frequency in women of middle age. MFH typically presents as a solitary mass that may appear somewhat brownish or pigmented, secondary to areas of focal hemorrhage within the tumor.

On microscopic examination, the tumor is characterized by a complex interlacing cellular growth pattern with marked nuclear pleomorphism, including multinucleated cells and large bizarre cells. Abnormal mitotic figures may be apparent. On immunoperoxidase study, these tumors contain α_1 antitrypsin and α_1 antichymotrypsin. MFH is typically infiltrative, and may involve the underlying fascia. Involvement of the fascia is associated with a higher risk of local spread and distant metastasis (68).

Epithelioid Sarcoma

Epithelioid sarcoma may arise within the labia majora, subclitoral area, and clitoris. Its microscopic features may resemble squamous carcinoma, malignant melanoma, malignant rhabdoid tumor, or lymphoma. Epithelioid sarcoma is usually relatively superficial, arising in and involving the reticular dermis, but it may occur in deeper structures (69).

On microscopic examination, the tumor is nodular and may have areas of necrosis. The tumor cells have an epithelioid appearance with eosinophilic cytoplasm, but there may be metaplastic components, including cartilage and bone. On immunohistochemistry, this tumor contains cytokeratin, which does not distinguish it from epithelial tumors, but is of value in differentiating it from malignant melanoma or other types of soft tissue tumors. Epithelioid sarcoma rarely metastasizes, although local recurrence is a risk. Immunoperoxidase studies are of value in differentiation, but not in differentiating epithelioid sarcoma from malignant rhabdoid tumor. The distinction of these two tumors is based primarily on microscopic features (69).

Malignant Rhabdoid Tumor

Malignant rhabdoid tumor has been described in the vulva, and, like epithelioid sarcoma, may be relatively superficial and contain tumor cells with an epithelioid appearance with eosinophilic cytoplasm. Unlike epithelioid sarcoma, malignant rhabdoid tumors have relatively pleomorphic nuclei. Metaplastic elements are usually not present. Malignant rhabdoid tumor also has eosinophilic cytoplasmic inclusions, which are not present in epithelioid sarcoma. These inclusions give some of the cells the appearance of signet ring cells. Malignant rhabdoid tumor has a lobulated architecture but lacks necrosis or granulomatous features, which are often found in epithelioid sarcoma (70,71).

Aggressive Angiomyxoma

Aggressive angiomyxoma is a primary soft tissue tumor of the vulva and pelvis that occurs predominantly in women of reproductive age. It is locally aggressive but rarely metastatic (72). It typically presents as a deep soft tissue mass or pelvic mass, sometimes mimicking a Bartholin's cyst or inguinal hernia. In the pelvis, it may displace other pelvic organs and may be best appreciated on radiologic studies.

This tumor is typically poorly circumscribed and difficult to discriminate from adjacent soft tissue. On microscopic examination, the tumor has many blood vessels. It consists predominantly of spindle- to stellate-shaped cells, with relatively small uniform nuclei representing predominantly fibroblasts and myofibroblasts. Mitotic figures are very rare. The tumor stroma varies from myxoid to densely collagenous. Nerves, small glandular structures with mucin-secreting columnar cells, and other epithelial elements may be found trapped within the tumor. The differential diagnosis is as for angiomyofibroblastoma (AMF), summarized next.

AMF

AMF is a rare, benign tumor of soft tissue origin that occurs predominantly in the female genital tract. When involving the vulva, it usually presents as a soft subcutaneous mass, but may occasionally be pedunculated (73).

On microscopic examination, the tumor usually has well-demarcated borders. Variable cellularity is present, with an edematous appearance. The cells are spindle shaped, plasmacytoid or epithelioid in appearance, and mitotic figures are rare. Cells are present in most cases and may be clustered about blood vessels. The tumor is vascular, with small- to medium-sized vessels. Some inflammatory cells, commonly lymphocytes or mast cells, may be seen around the vessels.

Tumors Metastatic to the Vulva

Most metastatic tumors to the vulva involve the labia majora or Bartholin's glands. In the vulva, they most often present as multiple intradermal or subcutaneous nodules but may present as a Bartholin's gland mass (74–76). Metastatic tumors account for approximately 8% of all vulvar tumors, and in approximately one-half of the cases the primary tumor is in the lower genital tract, including the cervix, vagina, endometrium, and ovary. Cervical carcinoma is the most common origin of contiguous metastasis. Local metastasis secondary to contiguous involvement of the vulva from urothelial carcinoma of the bladder or urethra, or anorectal carcinoma, may involve the vulva and present as a Paget-like lesion (see Paget's disease and Paget-like lesions in this section) or a vulvar or groin node mass. Remote metastases have been observed from tumors arising in breast, kidney, stomach, lung, and other sites (76).

PROGNOSTIC FACTORS (INFLUENCING CHOICE OF TREATMENT)

Prognostic information collected during the diagnostic workup of SCCs of the vulva serves as a basis for both patient counseling and treatment decisions. Fundamental decisions regarding goals of therapy (cure vs. palliation) and sequencing of primary treatment (primary surgery vs. chemoradiation (CRT)) should be based on four factors: (a) historical and demographic risk factors; (b) characteristics of the primary tumor, including location, laterality, size (cm), DOI, lymph-vascular space invasion and margin width; (c) clinical ± radiographic assessment of the inguinal LNs; and (d) probability of distant metastatic disease.

After resection of the primary tumor and surgical evaluation of the inguinal LNs, additional information obtained from intraoperative observations and the final pathologic specimens serve to guide decisions regarding adjuvant therapy. The most important prognostic factors for the adjuvant management of SCC of the vulva have been incorporated into the FIGO and AJCC staging systems (**Table 18.1**). Among the many factors that affect recurrence risk and disease-specific mortality, nodal status, particularly the number of positive nodes, size of the largest metastasis, and the presence or absence of extracapsular extension, are the most important (77). It is impossible to accurately detect LN involvement on physical exam; therefore, the FIGO staging of vulvar cancer changed from a clinical to a surgical and histopathologic approach, with evaluation of extranodal extension (ENE) also taken into account. Each of the above risk factors is discussed in relation to its temporal presentation (presurgical vs. postsurgical resection). Prognostic factors associated with the resection specimen and inguinal lymph node evaluation following surgery are also discussed.

Presurgery

DOI, tumor size, and lymph-vascular space invasion are the primary determinants of a patient's risk for nodal metastases, and the presence of nodal involvement is the single most important determinant of disease-specific mortality. Multiple studies have demonstrated a direct correlation between lymph-vascular space invasion, increasing stromal invasion, and the presence of involved inguinal LNs (78–80).

Postsurgery

Following surgery, intraoperative findings and final pathologic analysis are used to estimate recurrence risk and subsequently guide decisions regarding adjuvant therapy. Among the many pathologic findings (in addition to tumor size, lymph-vascular space invasion, and DOI) that have been shown to affect recurrence risk, surgical nodal status is the most important (78–80).

Risk of local recurrence (LR), although associated with tumor size and extent, is also related to the adequacy of the surgical resection margins. Heaps et al. (81), in their analysis of formalin-fixed tissue specimens, were able to demonstrate a sharp rise in the incidence of LR for tumors with microscopic margins <8 mm. They suggested that this would correspond to a minimum margin of 1 cm in fresh, unfixed tissue. These observations were confirmed in a retrospective multivariate analysis of clinical data by Chan et al. (80), who showed that pathologic margin distance ≤8 mm is an important predictor of LR; de Hullu et al. (82) reported nine LRs among 40 patients with tumor-free margins ≤8 mm compared with no LRs among 39 patients with margins >8 mm. To aid the surgeon in planning surgical margins of resection, Hoffman et al. (83) measured the radial occult microscopic spread of tumor in patients with invasive SCC of the vulva. They found that the gross and microscopic peripheries of most cancers were approximately the same; however, ulcerative tumors with an infiltrative pattern of invasion were more likely to extend beyond what is grossly apparent. The prognostic impact of ENE has also been evaluated. ENE is the dissemination of LN metastasis through the lymph node capsule and into the surrounding soft tissue. A study performed by Luchini et al. (84) evaluated the presence of ENE, with those individuals with ENE having significantly higher rates of all-cause mortality.

The single most important prognostic factor for recurrence and OS in women with vulvar cancer is metastasis to the inguinal LNs; most recurrences happen within 2 years of primary treatment (77,79). A number of imaging modalities have been studied for the preoperative evaluation of inguinal LN metastasis, including MRI, CT, PET, SPECT, and ultrasound. Currently, there is no imaging modality with a sufficiently high negative predictive value to allow for exclusion of surgical groin LN evaluation (85,86).

GENERAL MANAGEMENT

Historical Background

Development of the en bloc technique of radical vulvectomy with bilateral inguinofemoral lymphadenectomy during the 1940s and 1950s was a dramatic improvement over prior surgical options, and greatly enhanced survival, particularly for women with smaller tumors and negative LNs (87). In this era before effective RT that could provide local and regional disease control, the ability to successfully resect vulvar tumors reduced the occurrence of terminal progression dominated by intractable pain, immobility, malodorous drainage, and bleeding. Long-term survival of 85% to 90% can now be routinely obtained with radical surgery. Unfortunately, en bloc radical vulvectomy with inguinofemoral lymphadenectomy is associated with very morbid postoperative complications such as wound breakdown, lymphedema, disfigurement, and loss of sexual function. Appropriate indications for this procedure in the primary treatment of vulvar cancer are very rare.

Presently, smaller vulvar tumors can be acceptably managed by less radical, double or triple incision surgical approaches, and many authors have proposed more limited resections for certain subsets considered to represent early or low-risk disease (88). The advantages of such approaches include retention of a significant portion of the uninvolved vulva, preservation of body image and sexual function, less operative morbidity, and fewer complications later. Multimodality programs that incorporate radiation, surgery, and chemotherapy have now been validated in women with high-risk tumors, based on success with similar approaches in women with squamous cancers of the cervix and anus (88,89).

Sentinel Inguinal Lymph Node Biopsy

The SLN is defined as the first draining LN of a tumor, and can be identified using a lymphatic mapping technique. This is based on the observation that peritumoral injection of a liquid-based material results in superficial cutaneous lymphatic channel absorption of this material followed quickly by transport to the SLN. Either a vital blue dye, or radiocolloid, or both, can be used to facilitate SLN identification by direct visualization and/or detection of low levels of radioactivity by a handheld radiation detection device or imaging study (**Figs. 18.11** and **18.12**). The modern SLN concept was first described by Morton and colleagues in patients with cutaneous melanoma; shortly thereafter, it was described in patients with vulvar cancer (90,91). Preliminary experience with both intraoperative lymphatic dye and radioisotope injections confirmed that the SLN of the vulva is always in the inguinal LN basin and can be identified in most patients (92,93). This early experience supported the concept that the successful assessment of lymphatic metastases may ultimately be accomplished with resection/biopsy of one or two SLNs.

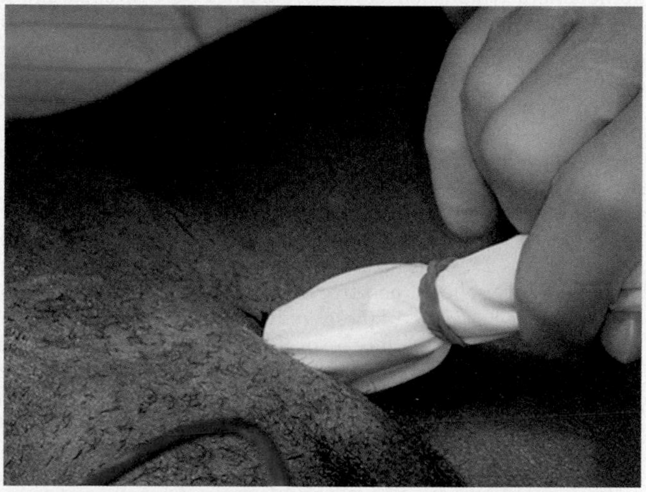

Figure 18.11. Transdermal localization of a sentinel node using a handheld gamma counter. The probe has a collimator and is pointed away from the primary tumor. Radioactivity will fall off rapidly until the sentinel node is encountered. Mark the site of an increase in activity.

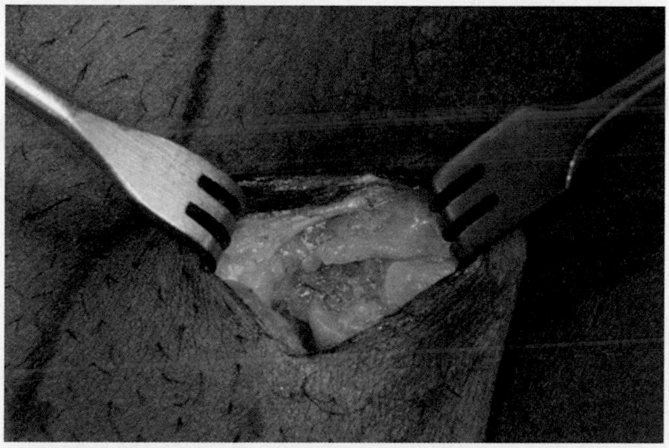

Figure 18.12. A hot, blue sentinel node identified through a small incision. Frozen section is requested only if the sentinel node is grossly suspicious. Immunohistochemical staining is performed if the routine hematoxylin and eosin staining does not reveal metastatic disease. After a sentinel node is removed, the wound is explored with the gamma counter to assure that there is no other sentinel node in the field.

Based on these pilot study results, two large multi-institutional trials were initiated to determine the utility of SLN biopsy (SLNB) in women with vulvar cancer. The Groningen International Study on Sentinel Nodes in Vulvar Cancer (GROINSS-V) trial used a prospective, observational design, enrolling 403 evaluable women with tumors ≤4 cm who underwent SLNB alone. Of these, 276 women had a negative SLNB and were closely observed for recurrence during a 2-year follow-up period. Eight patients (2.9%) suffered a groin relapse. When patients with multifocal primary tumors were removed from the analysis, the relapse rate was only 2.3% (94). Long-term results in 377 patients with unifocal disease from this same study were recently reported, detailing 36.4% and 46.4% ($p = 0.03$) 10-year local recurrence rate for sentinel node-negative and sentinel node-positive patients, respectively. In addition, they found that isolated groin recurrence rate was 2.5% for sentinel node-negative patients and 8% for sentinel node-positive patients at 5 years. The authors concluded that although survival is favorable for sentinel node-negative patients, the high rate of LR in these patients is of concern (95).

The second study, GOG 173, employed a validation design. All women underwent SLNB followed by unilateral or bilateral inguinofemoral lymphadenectomy: 515 women were enrolled, and 418 were evaluable. If the primary tumor was more than 2 cm from the midline, a unilateral SLNB and inguinofemoral lymphadenectomy were performed. If the tumor was within 2 cm of the midline, or involved the midline, bilateral inguinal lymphadenectomies were performed. The false-negative rate was 8.3%, and the false-negative predictive value (FNPV) was 3.7% for the entire cohort. The FNPV is a prediction of the chance of a positive non-SLN when the SLN is free of tumor and a lymphadenectomy has not been performed. In GOG 173, the FNPV by groin was 2.7%; for patients with tumors <4 cm, it was 2%. This means that a patient with a tumor <4 cm, no palpable LNs, and a negative SLNB has a 2% chance of a groin relapse (96). The results of these studies indicate that, for appropriately selected women in the care of a surgeon experienced with this technique, the risk of groin relapse following a negative SLNB is 2% to 3% (**Table 18.3**). This compares favorably with superficial inguinal lymphadenectomy, as reported by Stehman et al. (97) for the GOG. As with all surgical innovations, individual practitioners must use care when implementing new procedures. Gynecologic oncologists can learn the procedure from peers or from surgical oncologists treating melanoma or breast cancer patients. Prior to adopting this as his or her standard, each gynecologic oncologist should determine his or her own false-negative rate by performing SLNB followed by inguinofemoral lymphadenectomy in approximately 10 cases. Some practices see very few vulvar cancer patients, in which case referral is appropriate. Considered together, the GROINS V and GOG 173 trials strongly support an assertion that, under the appropriate circumstances, SLNB should be offered to eligible women with vulvar cancer.

It is important to note that the largest SLN evaluations to date have all involved pathologic ultrastaging with serial sectioning and immunohistochemical (IHC) staining if routine H & E staining does not reveal metastatic disease. In most studies, including GOG 173 and GROINS V, approximately half of the LN metastases were detected by immunohistochemical staining. SLNB has the promise of reducing the number of unnecessary lymphadenectomies performed in node-negative women, while at the same time identifying additional women who may benefit from adjuvant therapy.

The combination of local vulvar resection and SLNB holds the promise of improved outcomes for many women with vulvar cancer. Preservation of sexual function and body image, a reduction in the risk of lymphedema, and more focused use of adjuvant therapy are all possible.

Patients with Clinical Stage I/II Tumors at Presentation

Tumors demonstrating a DOI ≤1 mm have minimal risk for lymphatic dissemination. Excisional procedures that incorporate a 1 cm normal tissue margin are likely to provide curative results (88,98). Patients in this category represent the only subset for whom surgical evaluation of the inguinal LNs can be omitted. These superficially invasive carcinomas tend to arise in younger patients with HSIL/VIN lesions that are commonly associated with oncogenic HPV infections. Occult invasion in lesions thought to be intraepithelial is common (99,100). Consequently, the entire lower genital tract and vulva should be carefully evaluated before surgical resection of these lesions is attempted. The risk of vulvar recurrence or development of a new lesion at another vulvar site is significant. After primary therapy, these patients should undergo frequent follow-up examinations.

Management of clinical stage I and II vulvar cancer includes wide radical excision of the primary tumor with unilateral or bilateral SLNB, with or without inguinofemoral lymphadenectomy. The operation removes the primary tumor with a wide radial margin of normal skin (2 cm), along with a deep margin to the deep perineal

TABLE 18.3. Sentinel Lymph Node Biopsy Sensitivity Analysis

Analysis	SLNB Result	Present	Absent	Total	Sensitivity	90% CI	NPV (%)	90% CI	FNPV (%)	90% CI
By patients	Positive	121	0	121						
	Negative	11	286	297						
	Total	132	286	418	91.7	86.7–95.3	96.3	93.9–97.9	3.7	2.1–6.1
By groin	Positive	140	0	140						
	Negative	12	441	453						
	Total	152	441	593	92.1	87.5–95.4	97.4	95.7–98.5	2.7	1.5–4.3
In tumors <4 cm	Positive	67	0	67						
	Negative	4	198	202						
	Total	71	198	269					2.0	0.7–4.5
In tumors >4 cm	Positive	54	0	54						
	Negative	7	88	95						
	Total	61	88	149					7.4	3.5–13.4

CI, confidence interval; FNPV, false-negative predictive value; NPV, negative predictive value; SLNB, sentinel lymph node biopsy.

Source: Reprinted with permission from Levenback CF, Ali S, Coleman RL, et al. Lymphatic mapping and sentinel lymph node biopsy in women with squamous cell carcinoma of the vulva: a Gynecologic Oncology Group study. *J Clin Oncol*. 2012;30(31):3786–3791.

fascia; thus, the vulvar specimen will contain tumor, skin, subcutaneous fat, vascular perforators, and dermal lymphatics. This approach provides excellent long-term survival and local control in approximately 88% of patients (101). Every attempt should be made to preserve structures such as the clitoris and urethral meatus. Deep margins are rarely a problem except on the perineum, where there is little or no subcutaneous fat. In this case, removal of the capsule of the anus or some of the sphincter muscle itself can be performed without loss of anal function.

Vulvar defects for small primary tumors can usually be closed with simple mobilization of the skin and fat surrounding the vulva. In cases where primary closure is not possible, any one of a number of plastic closures is useful (discussed later). Consultation with a plastic surgeon in such cases can be invaluable.

A subanalysis of GOG 173 data also provided guidance regarding when unilateral groin evaluation is safe. GOG 173 required bilateral LN evaluation except when the tumor was more than 2 cm from a midline structure. There were 234 women enrolled on GOG 173 who had a preoperative LSG, and at least one SLN was identified during surgery. There were 105 women with midline primary tumors; 32 of these women had unilateral drainage on preoperative LSG. Four of these patients had LN metastases on the side that did not have LSG drainage. There were 65 women with tumors located within 2 cm of the midline but not directly involving a midline structure; 27 women (42%) had unilateral drainage on LSG and bilateral surgical groin evaluation. None of these patients had metastases to the side without LSG drainage. These data support the time-honored oncologic surgical experience that midline tumors can have bilateral drainage and a unilateral LSG should not result in omission of one side (102). Conversely, if the tumor is lateralized (>2 cm from midline) and unilateral drainage is confirmed by LSG, unilateral SLNB is appropriate. The authors routinely obtain preoperative LSG, preferably by SPECT/CT (see **Fig. 18.16**), regardless of the location of the primary, because it helps confirm the location of the SLN in three dimensions as well as the lymphatic drainage pattern.

Overall survival for women following an adequate resection of a primary squamous carcinoma limited to the vulva and with uninvolved inguinal LNs is >90%. Stage II patients who have negative margins and uninvolved nodes but involvement of the lower vagina or urethra should obtain similar results.

Clinical Stage III and IV Cancers at Presentation

Some women have LN metastases detected by preoperative physical examination or diagnostic imaging, or at the time of their primary surgery. If a node is grossly involved at this point, most gynecologic oncologists will proceed with inguinofemoral lymphadenectomy on the assumption that there is a high likelihood of additional positive LNs.

Clinical stage II/III tumors that extend to adjacent mucosal structures often involve inguinal LNs. Many are bulky; however, some are of modest size but are considered high risk because of proximity to critical midline structures. Some primary tumors can be curatively excised by radical vulvectomy or by some variation of PE and vulvectomy. Surgical resection of 1 to 1.5 cm of the distal urethra to achieve a negative surgical margin does not appear to compromise bladder continence (103). Although radical surgery is an option for patients with locally advanced tumors, contemporary therapeutic strategies have centered on sequenced RT or CRT followed by radical surgery as a means to preserve either urinary or fecal continence or both. Vulvar cancers are sufficiently sensitive to therapeutic radiation such that function-sparing operations are feasible in selected patients with advanced disease who receive combined modality treatment (89). For patients with stage IVA tumors, similar experiences have been reported; ultraradical (exenterative) resections may also be considered for selected patients. Although occasional cures have been described with innovative combinations of surgery, radiation, and chemoradiation, treatment of patients with stage IVB vulvar cancer should be considered palliative.

Node-Positive Cancers

An optimal management strategy for clinically apparent node-positive patients is yet to be defined. Two factors impact management of regional disease: radiation can have a significant impact on sterilizing or eradicating small-volume nodal disease; surgical resection of bulky nodal disease improves regional control, and probably enhances the curative potential of RT. In multivariate analysis, Hyde et al. (104) found that, for patients with clinically positive groin nodes who underwent surgery followed by RT, the method of surgical groin node dissection (nodal "debulking" vs. full groin dissection) had no prognostic significance.

Patients who undergo bilateral inguinofemoral lymphadenectomy as initial therapy and are found to have positive nodes—clearly those with more than one positive node—benefit from postoperative irradiation to the groin and lower pelvis. RT is superior to surgery in the management of patients with positive pelvic nodes. The morbidity of combining inguinofemoral lymphadenectomy with radiation may be substantial. The highest incidences of chronic groin and extremity complications, primarily lymphedema, are seen in such cases (105).

The optimal management of patients found with a single involved lymph node has been a matter of controversy since the publication of GOG-37. In the interim, multiple retrospective studies have tried to establish whether or not such patients benefit from adjuvant RT (106,107). Recently, Mahner et al. published a retrospective analysis of 1,618 patients with vulvar cancer, among which 495 patients were noted to have (+) inguinal nodes; 447 of these patients received surgical groin staging; 244 and 169 did and did not receive adjuvant therapy, respectively; 172 patients were found to have a single (+) LN, and 77 of these received adjuvant therapy. Multivariate regression was unable to identify a significant survival advantage in this population of patients who received adjuvant RT. The authors postulated that this could be attributable to the small number of patients in this subgroup; however, lack of benefit could not be excluded (108). Similarly, several management options are available for patients found to have positive nodes during the course of an inguinal lymphadenectomy when performed as a staging procedure: (a) no further surgical therapy may be performed; (b) the lymphadenectomy can be extended to include the ipsilateral deep nodes, the contralateral groin nodes, or both; or (c) postoperative irradiation can be added to any of these surgical options. Given the heterogeneity of vulvar cancer presentations, treatment individualization is necessary. If postoperative RT to the inguinal nodes is ultimately deemed necessary, it would be reasonable to limit resection to grossly positive nodes. Here the intent would be to minimize the likelihood of lymphedema following combined radical surgery and radiation. Excellent local control and minimal morbidity have been achieved when selective inguinal lymphadenectomy and tailored postoperative adjuvant therapy were administered to carefully selected patients (101).

The ideal management for a patient with a microscopically positive SLN who did not have a full lymphadenectomy at primary surgery is unknown and is being investigated in the GROINS VII/GOG 270 trial. In this trial, women with a negative SLN are observed, women with a metastasis ≤2 mm receive postoperative RT, and women with larger metastases are managed with inguinofemoral lymphadenectomy and RT. Concurrent radiosensitizing cisplatin is optional. Until these results are reported, uncertainty will remain about the management of SLNB-positive patients.

Management of Recurrent Squamous Vulvar Cancers

Vulvar cancer recurrences can be categorized into three clinical groups: local (vulva), groin, and distant. Published experience with a localized vulvar recurrence is surprisingly good. Recurrence-free survival (RFS) can be obtained in up to 75% of cases when the recurrence is limited to the vulva and can be excised with a gross clinical margin (109). The observation that many of these recurrences arise at sites remote from the initial primary tumor or that they occur years after apparently successful primary treatment suggests that some recurrences probably represent new primary tumors rather than the development of new disease. Recurrences in the groin, however, are almost universally fatal. A few patients may be saved by resection of bulky disease and local radiation, perhaps even using intensity-modulated RT (IMRT) in patients who have had prior pelvic radiation. Patients who develop distant metastases are candidates for palliative systemic cytotoxic or targeted CT or transition to comfort care.

Management of Nonsquamous Vulvar Cancers

Malignant Melanoma

Malignant melanoma is the second most common vulvar malignancy, and it is most commonly seen in postmenopausal Caucasian women. Typical presentations include either an asymptomatic pigmented lesion identified during a routine exam or pruritic or painful vulvar mass (**Fig. 18.13**) (110). A definitive diagnosis is established with a biopsy. IHC staining for melanoma-specific antigen and S100 may be helpful in uncertain cases. Melanomas may arise from existing pigmented vulvar lesions or as new isolated primary tumors. Consequently, any pigmented vulvar lesion should be considered for biopsy. Cutaneous melanoma has evolved significantly over the past 45 years. Because of the rarity of vulvar melanoma, it has not been clear whether extrapolation of prognostic and treatment data from cutaneous nonvulvar disease is appropriate for vulvar melanoma patients. Thus, until recently, multiple authors have described their experience with vulvar melanoma using one or more different staging systems (e.g., Breslow's depth, Clark's levels, AJCC staging), making standardization of prognostic groups and treatment strategies difficult. Moxley et al. reported a multi-institutional retrospective examination of 77 patients with vulvar melanoma. Patient stages were determined using the AJCC Staging Guidelines (6th edition) (2002), Breslow's thickness, and Clark's levels, and treatments were correlated with outcomes, specifically recurrence and overall survival. Among the three staging methods, only AJCC staging was significantly correlated with OS, although Breslow's thickness was significantly associated with likelihood of recurrence (38). For this reason, the 2009 AJCC Melanoma Staging and Classification revision

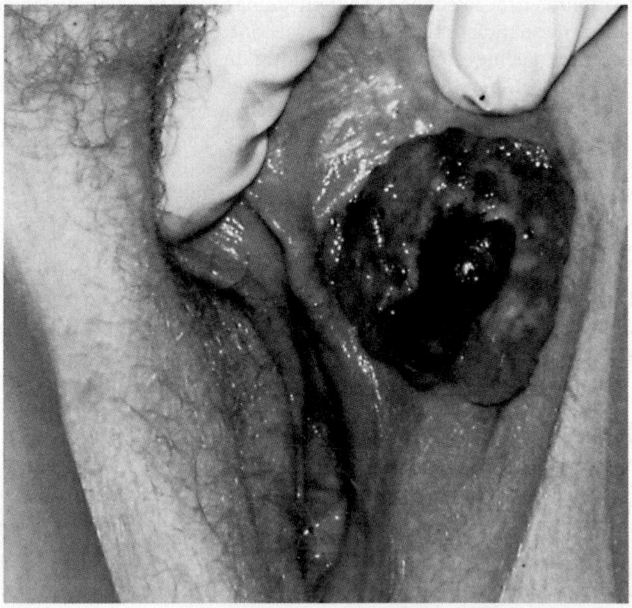

Figure 18.13. Nodular, darkly pigmented malignant melanoma of the left labium majus.

recommended against continued use of Clark's level and Breslow's thickness for management of T1 invasive melanoma lesions (66).

The primary treatment modality for vulvar melanoma is surgical excision. Radical vulvectomy with bilateral inguinofemoral lymphadenectomy has been the historical treatment of choice (111). Because most failures are distant, radical local resection does not appear to enhance survival. Furthermore, many patients with vulvar melanoma are elderly, with coexisting medical problems, making less radical and morbid surgery compelling. More recent reviews recommend some form of hemi-vulvectomy or wide local excision along with inguinal lymphadenectomy or SLN mapping (38,63). DOI, mitotic activity, and the presence of ulceration are prognostically significant and should be considered in treatment planning. Based on information derived from large series of patients with cutaneous melanomas at nongenital sites, regional lymphadenectomy should probably be considered a prognostic rather than a therapeutic procedure. In a multivariate analysis of 644 patients with vulvar melanoma, Sugiyama et al. (110) reported 5-year disease-specific survival rates of 68%, 29%, and 19% for patients with zero, one, and two or more positive LNs, respectively. Lymphadenectomy can be avoided in patients with superficial melanomas (<1 mm), for whom the risk of metastatic disease is negligible. SLN identification and biopsy have been increasingly applied to the surgical management of cutaneous malignant melanomas, and multiple authors assert that for those surgeons who are competent with the technique, SLN mapping and biopsy should be considered a standard practice, with false-negative rates extrapolated from squamous carcinoma of the vulva comparable to other disease sites as are typical in breast cancer and cutaneous, nonvulvar melanoma (38,63).

High-Risk Vulva-Localized and Metastatic Melanoma

Until more recently, systemic therapy for high-risk localized or metastatic melanoma was considered strictly palliative; durable responses were rare, and adverse effects were considerable. Interferon α-2b, dacarbazine, temozolomide, and platinum-based cytotoxic therapies have shown activity in patients with small-volume tumor burden; however, toxicities are considerable, with limited improvements in survival (63). More recently, with improved molecular characterization of cutaneous (nonvulvar) melanomas and the development of multiple targeted inhibitors that have dramatically improved survival for this disease, systemic therapies for high-risk localized as well as metastatic and recurrent melanoma follow the evolving treatment paradigms of nonvulvar malignant melanoma. Examples of such targets with associated inhibitors are B-Raf (vemurafenib), c-Kit (imatinib), and CTLA-4 (ipilimumab) (112). A more involved discussion of systemic therapy for melanoma is beyond the scope of this chapter. For those gynecologic oncologists without considerable experience in the treatment of melanoma patients, we recommend early referral for high-risk localized vulvar or metastatic melanoma patients to a medical oncologist or gynecologic oncology center that specializes in the systemic care of malignant melanoma patients.

Patients with superficial lesions have an excellent chance for cure after surgical resection; however, patients with deeper lesions, or metastases at the time of diagnosis, have a worse prognosis. These patients are good candidates for investigational trials.

Basal Cell Carcinoma

BCCs should be removed by excisional biopsy using a minimum surgical margin of 1 cm. Lymphatic or distant spread is exceedingly rare (113). Local recurrence may happen, particularly in tumors removed with suboptimal resection margins.

Adenocarcinoma

Patients presenting with vulvar adenocarcinoma should first undergo a clinical evaluation to determine whether the lesion in question is a vulvar cancer or a metastasis. Despite the paucity of data regarding the evaluation and treatment of vulvar adenocarcinoma, resection of localized disease with a radical margin is recommended by radical wide excision, and hemi-vulvectomy or radical vulvectomy seem appropriate (88). Some form of inguinal lymphadenectomy should be included with primary surgical resection. RT may have a role in enhancing local control for women with large primary tumors or inguinal metastases.

Paget's Disease

Paget's disease is associated with a concurrent underlying invasive adenocarcinoma component in approximately 15% of cases (114). As many as 20% to 30% of these patients will have or will later develop an adenocarcinoma at another nonvulvar location (115,116), although more recent series suggest a lower incidence of secondary malignancies (117). Observed sites of nonvulvar malignancies developing in patients with extramammary Paget's disease include breast, lung, colorectum, gastric area, pancreas, and upper female genital tract. Screening and surveillance for tumors at these sites should be considered in patients with Paget's disease.

Paget's disease should be resected with at least a 1 cm margin. If underlying invasion is suspected, the deep margins should be extended to the perineal fascia. Black et al. (118) showed that patients with microscopically positive margins had a significantly higher rate of recurrence; however, with extended follow-up, all patients eventually recurred. Others have shown that despite surgical efforts to the contrary, microscopically positive margins are frequent, and disease recurrence is common regardless of margin status. Repeat local excision of recurrent disease is usually effective in the absence of invasion (116).

NONSURGICAL THERAPY

Imiquimod is an immune modulator that is believed to affect the function of the Toll-like receptor (Tlr) as a costimulatory molecule for T cell-mediated immune response to malignant cells. It has well-documented activity for treatment of genital warts as well as vulvar dysplasia. Reportedly, it also has activity in extramammary Paget's disease. In several small case series, complete response (CR) rates of as much as 92% have been reported (119,120).

Tumors Metastatic to the Vulva

Treatment of tumors metastatic to the vulva have a uniformly poor prognosis, and treatment should focus on local control. As with bulky, primary site vulvar cancers, a multimodal approach seems to provide some opportunity for long-term survival, as well as enhanced local tumor control and organ preservation.

Cutaneous vulvar lymphatic metastases may occur as in-transit tumor emboli from anorectal tumors, or as retrograde flow metastases when bulky tumors of the cervix or uterus obstruct the normal lymphatic drainage patterns (**Fig. 18.14**). These metastases are multiple and are often bilateral. Their histology reflects that of the primary tumor. Because this metastatic pattern is associated with advanced tumors, the primary tumor is usually readily detectable by examination.

SURGICAL TECHNIQUES

In planning a surgical approach, it is important to take into account the patient's age, medical comorbidities, desire for sexual function preservation, tumor size, and disease stage. In the case of a locoregional vulvar cancer, surgery will remain the first choice of therapy (121).

Wide Radical Excision

Several names have been applied to the procedures used to resect small vulvar cancers: partial deep excision, radical wide excision, radical local excision, wide local excision, modified radical vulvectomy, and hemi-vulvectomy. Regardless of the preferred nomenclature, the surgical procedure should be adequately defined and described. Surgical incisions are devised to allow for at least a 1 to 2 cm resection margin encompassing the primary lesion (**Fig. 18.15**). Dissection is carried to the deep perineal fascia. Tumors located close to the anus or anal sphincter can be managed by radical wide excision with sphincter or flap repair, or they can be treated with combined modality therapy, as outlined in the RT section. Most wide radical excision sites can be closed primarily. In some patients, fasciocutaneous pedicle flaps can be used to facilitate coverage of the vulvar defect. Some form of inguinal lymphadenectomy, performed through a separate incision, is generally combined with radical wide excision.

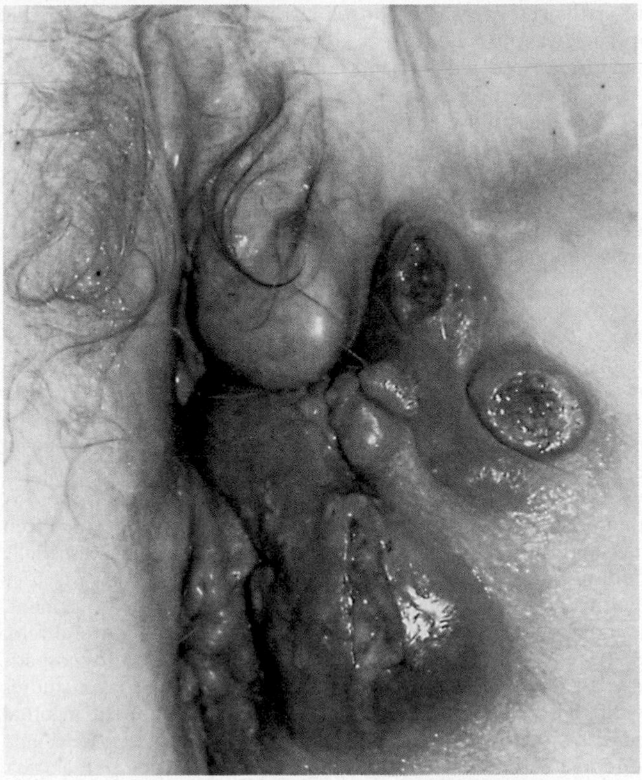

Figure 18.14. Multiple in-transit lymphatic metastases from a cloacogenic carcinoma of the rectum. A large constricting lesion was evident on rectal examination.

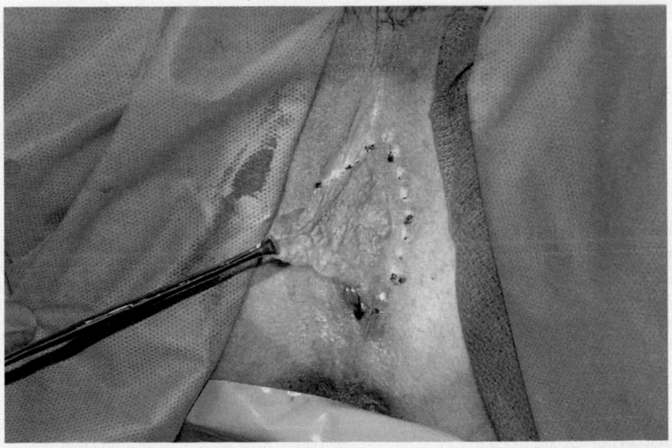

Figure 18.15. An early vulvar cancer identified in a background of VIN III. A planned 2-cm margin is outlined.

Ambulation is begun, if possible, on the day of surgery. Perineal irrigation and air (natural or forced) drying is started within 24 hours of the surgery. The average hospital stay for patients undergoing radical wide excision is usually one to two days. Wound breakdown, usually of minor degree, is reported in at least 15% of cases (122). The incidence and severity of groin complications is proportional to the extent of the lymphadenectomy.

Inguinofemoral Lymphadenectomy

Appropriate surgical management of the groin nodes has been evolving for many years. Original descriptions of radical vulvectomy included en bloc resection of the vulva with inguinal and pelvic lymph nodes. The extent of lymphadenectomy was steadily reduced, first eliminating the pelvic node dissection and then reducing the extent of the groin dissection. The concept of superficial inguinal lymphadenectomy was proposed in the late 1970s; however, this approach was ultimately rejected by gynecologic oncologists owing to an unexpectedly high relapse rate (**Table 18.4**) (123).

The most common current approach starts with an incision parallel to and just above or below the inguinal ligament. The incision is carried through Camper's fascia, and small flaps are elevated to expose the lymph node-bearing fat and preserve blood supply to the skin. There is no need to skeletonize the femoral artery; however, identification of the medial wall of the femoral vein helps ensure removal of the medial fat pad, where the SLN is frequently found. The dissection can usually be performed solely with electrocautery or a small vessel-sealing device. The saphenous vein is encountered at the lower medial margin of the dissection, and whenever possible, should be preserved to reduce the risk for postoperative lymphedema. The dissected specimen is removed for pathologic assessment. The skin incision can be closed with either staples or absorbable sutures. A closed-suction drain is placed and removed when output is <25 mL/day.

Unfortunately, historic nomenclature for performance of inguinofemoral lymphadenectomy has been inconsistent and often confusing. The authors find the terms "deep" and "superficial" especially troubling and, in the SLN era, largely meaningless. A satisfactory groin dissection has been performed when the inguinal ligament, adductor longus, saphenous vein, medial wall of the femoral vein, and the fossa ovalis have been identified, and the LNs and most adipose tissue within these boundaries are removed. Cadaver studies identify 8 to 10 LNs in the femoral triangle defined by the inguinal ligament, sartorius muscle, and adductor longus. Surgical node counts are dependent on the thoroughness of the surgeon and pathologist.

Sentinel Lymph Node Biopsy Technique

As discussed previously, SLNB should be offered as an alternative to inguinofemoral lymphadenectomy as part of primary management in women with tumors ≤4 cm, with no suspicious LNs on physical examination or imaging and no prior groin surgery or radiation that might interfere with lymphatic drainage pathways. There is insufficient evidence to make a recommendation regarding SLNBs in women who have tumors >4 cm, or multifocal disease (128,129).

TABLE 18.4. Unanticipated Groin Failure in Patients with Negative Superficial Lymphadenectomy

Investigators	No.	%
Burke et al. (124)	4/76	5.2
Berman et al. (125)	0/50	0
Stehman et al. (126)	6/121	5.0
Gordinier et al. (127)	9/104	8.6
Total	19/351	5.4

The authors obtain an LSG in most patients. If possible, the surgeon should perform the injection for vulvar cancer or ensure that the nuclear medicine specialist is comfortable with injecting the vulva. The injection is painful; EMLA cream can be helpful in decreasing the associated discomfort. SLNs can be identified using a dye such as isosulfan blue, blue violet, or methylene blue, or a radioactive tracer called technetium-99m (99mTc) with LSG; the blue dye and radiotracer can be used alone or in combination. If using technetium-99m, 0.1 to 0.5 mCi radiolabeled filtered Tc-99m is generally injected one day prior to surgery, followed by the performance of a preoperative scintigraphy (usually on the morning of surgery) (130).

Various techniques have been described for SLN. de Hullu et al. described their technique involving a combination of technetium-99m as well as blue dye. In their protocol, 0.2 to 0.6 mL of 60 MBq technetium-99m-labeled nanocolloid is injected circumferentially around the tumor and LSG is performed, and skin sites correlating with the findings of the lymphoscintigram SLN location are marked with a pencil. On the morning of surgery, following induction of anesthesia, 2.0 mL of patent blue dye (2.5% in aqueous solution containing 0.6% sodium chloride and 0.05% disodium hydrogen phosphate) is injected in the same locations. SLNs are then identified using a handheld gamma probe. For SLN dissections employing only blue dye, 4 mL of isosulfan blue can be injected adjacent to the primary tumor. Following injection, the tissues can be massaged to aid with dye dispersal. After approximately 5 minutes, a groin incision can be made and LN dissection carried out. In those patients with midline tumors, bilateral injections should be performed (130).

The half-life of the radiocolloid is approximately 6 hours, so a patient can be injected in the morning and operated on the same day. Frequently, this is not possible, and a second injection is necessary. If blue dye is utilized, it is visible in the SLN for only 45 minutes. The authors typically inject the radiocolloid prior to sterile prepping and draping, and inject the blue dye only when the team is prepared to make an incision. All injections are intradermal, 0.5 to 1.0 cm from the tumor itself. Intratumoral or subcutaneous injections will most likely result in a failure to identify the SLN. Transdermal localization of the SLN using a handheld gamma counter is possible in most patients. The SLN is identified using a tenfold higher measured radiation than the basal count at the primary injection site (130).

There are pros and cons to the various methods and injection materials used in SLN dissection. If using blue dye, the color becomes visible in the nodes and lymphatic channels, quickly allowing for rapid SLN dissection (101). There is a low rate of hypersensitivity reactions to blue dye, and the dye is also inexpensive (131,132). The disadvantage of using blue dye is that it rapidly passes through the lymphatics, and so it is possible to miss the SLN (131). The advantages of LSG include the ability to determine the number and location of the SLNs preoperatively and to detect a SLN outside the nodal basin; however, the cost of equipment associated with the use of a radiotracer, as well as the involvement of nuclear medicine, requires more coordination between the operating room and radiology departments (131).

SPECT/CT is also valuable for locating the SLN in relation to the femoral vessels (**Fig. 18.16**). A small incision is made over the location of the SLN. Although data are limited, clinical experience indicates that the SLN is commonly medial to the femoral vein and just above the adductor longus muscle. Once the SLN is removed, the wound is scanned for any residual radioactivity. It is imperative that all SLNs in the groin are removed. The gamma counter may detect second echelon nodes in the pelvis just above the inguinal ligament. If blue lymphatic channels lead to a node that is not hot or blue, it is still considered an SLN.

Studies in vulvar cancer in which SLN dissection was performed, followed by a completion inguinofemoral lymphadenectomy, suggest that the SLN is accurate in identifying LN metastasis with a NPV approaching 100% (132). A meta-analysis undertaken by Mead et al. evaluated SLN detection rates between blue dye, radiotracer, and combination injection. Within this meta-analysis, combined blue

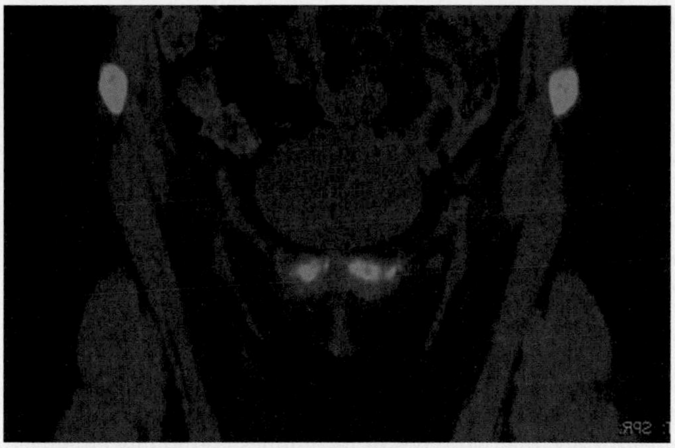

Figure 18.16. SPECT/CT demonstrating left sentinel lymph node just medial to the femoral vein. SPECT/CT provides superior localization of sentinel lymph nodes compared with 2-dimensional lymphoscintigraphy. The number of sentinel nodes identified should correspond to the number removed at surgery.

dye and 99mTc testing had the highest rate of SLN detection; pooled rates are 94.0% for 99mTc (95% confidence interval [CI], 90.5 to 96.4), 68.7% for blue dye alone (95% CI, 63.1 to 74.0) and 97.7 (95% CI, 96.6 to 98.5) for 99mTc and blue dye combined (133).

Within the pathology laboratory, the evaluation of SLNs requires detailed and systematic evaluation of the submitted specimen. The LN sample submitted requires proper identification of patient name, source, name of the surgeon submitting, node location, date, and number of nodes identified.

In sectioning SLNs, it is recognized that, to achieve close to 100% identification of all metastases, the section spacing must be one-half the diameter of the tumor to be detected (133). The LN or nodes are sliced in 1 to 2 mm slices, cutting the LN at right angles to the long axis of the node. All of the LN tissue (slices) should be submitted for study.

Once the nodal tissue is embedded in the paraffin block, the node slices can be cut at closer intervals to improve tumor detection. Although there are some variations on this sectioning method, our approach is to cut three sections from each block. After facing the block to get a full face of the sectioned nodal tissue, the first 5-μm section is cut. This section is stained with H&E. We then cut 100 microns into the block and cut another 5-μm section. This second slide is held for additional H&E staining, or IHC, if the first and last H&E sections have equivocal findings. We then cut an additional 100 microns into the block and take the third section. This slide is stained with H&E. The pathologist reviews the two H&E slides, and if the findings are equivocal, the held second slide is then studied.

Limited information is available regarding ideal surveillance following SLNB. Our preferred technique is ultrasound, since it is noninvasive and the internal architecture of the LNs can be imaged (**Fig. 18.17A,B**). Early detection of a groin failure may help improve outcomes with multimodality treatment.

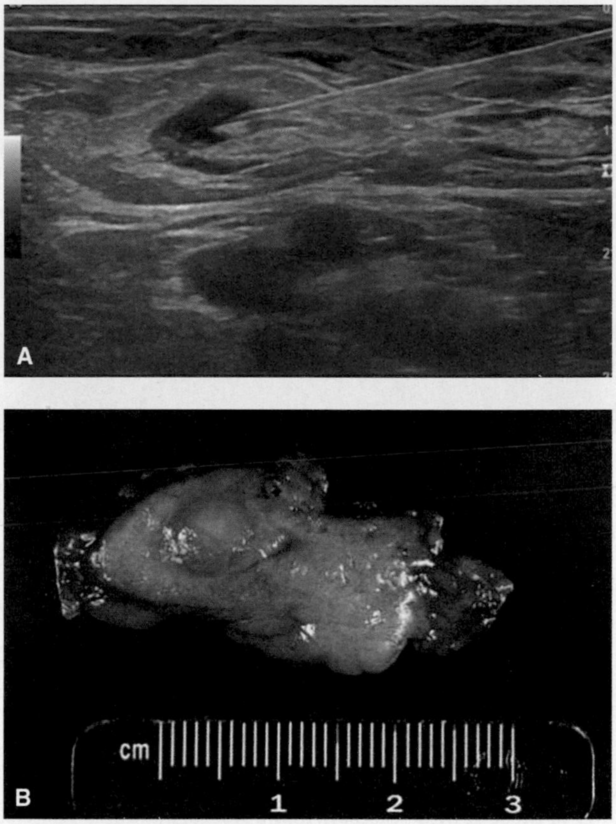

Figure 18.17. Close surveillance following sentinel lymph node biopsy is recommended because groin relapse is difficult to treat. Physical examination is very unreliable. **A:** Ultrasound can be very effective, as illustrated here. Six months after negative sentinel lymph node biopsy, ultrasound detected a 5-mm metastasis. Fine needle aspiration confirmed metastatic disease. **B:** The patient underwent inguinal femoral lymphadenectomy and radiation therapy. She remains disease free at 2 years.

Surgical Resection for Recurrent Disease

The site and volume of recurrent vulvar lesions dictate both resectability and potential for cure. Recurrences can be categorized as local (vulvar), inguinal, or distant (pelvis, lower extremity, or beyond). Surgical therapy plays a curative or palliative role in selected subsets of patients with recurrent disease.

Wide Radical Excision

As many as 75% of patients with recurrent disease limited to the vulva can be salvaged by radical wide excision (partial deep vulvectomy) or reexcision of the tumor (109,134). Surgical principles of recurrent vulvar tumors are identical to those for primary tumors: wide excision with a measured normal tissue margin of at least 1 to 2 cm. Particular attention is also focused on obtaining a clear deep margin. Because most patients have had prior operative therapy, primary closure of the vulvar defect is frequently more difficult. More complex reconstructive efforts may be needed to restore tissue integrity.

Radical Vulvectomy

Rarely, radical vulvectomy may be indicated for recurrent vulvar cancer. The classic description of en bloc radical vulvectomy and bilateral lymphadenectomy can be based on either a "butterfly" or "longhorn" approach. The butterfly incisions use convex "wings" over the groin and around the anus to facilitate closure of the defect (**Fig. 18.18**). The longhorn incisions were developed to limit skin resection over the groin in an attempt to reduce wound breakdown (135). The arcing superior incision is placed from the lateral margins of the groin dissection across the mons pubis. The lateral vulvar incisions are placed at the labiocrural folds, because these topographical landmarks represent the most lateral location of the superficial vulvar lymphatics. The perianal incision is placed to allow resection of the perineal body. These incisions are taken to the level of the deep inguinal and perineal fascia and permit en bloc removal of both superficial and deep groin nodes, the entire vulva, and an intervening skin bridge.

After removal of the specimen, the skin and mucosal edges are undermined to permit mobilization and primary closure with delayed absorbable suture. Some degree of tension at the suture lines

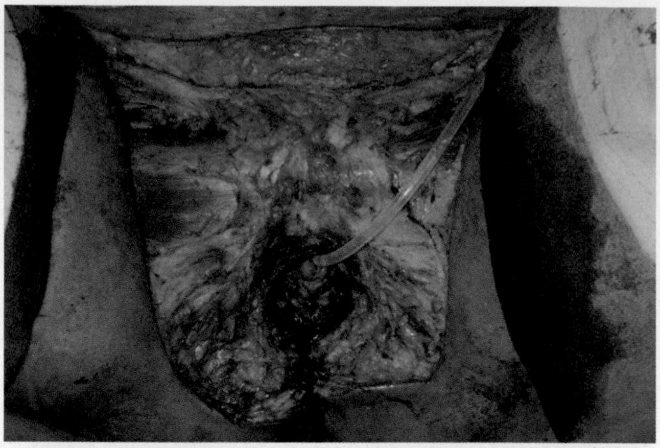

Figure 18.18. Butterfly incision described for a traditional radical vulvectomy with bilateral inguinal lymphadenectomy. Modern indications for radical vulvectomy are exceedingly rare. The patient shown in **Figure 18.5** was treated with concurrent chemoradiation and still had bilateral gross tumor. This figure demonstrates the field following resection.

is unavoidable, particularly in the perineal body and periurethral areas. Closed-suction drains are usually placed in the groin sites to remove excess lymphatic and serous fluid accumulations, and are usually removed when drain output is minimal (5 to 14 days).

A small degree of wound breakdown is seen in approximately 50% of patients. Local wound care results in satisfactory secondary healing in most of these cases. Lymphocyst formation is relatively common and frequently presents as a tense but nontender groin mass. Percutaneous needle drainage is usually sufficient, but occasionally replacement of a groin drain may be required. Inguinal cellulitis, lower extremity lymphangitis, and lymphedema are uncommon late sequelae. The incidence of these complications is related to the extent of groin therapy, and is highest in patients treated with superficial and deep lymphadenectomy followed by inguinal RT. The 3-incision concept preserves the radicality of the vulvar resection while retaining skin over the groin. Consequently, the incidence of major wound breakdown is significantly reduced to approximately 15% to 20% of cases (136). As with other techniques, the incidence and severity of groin complications such as infection, wound breakdown, or lymphocyst formation remain high (122).

Pelvic Exenteration

Curative resection may still be possible when vulvar recurrence extends to the vagina, proximal urethra, or anus. Selected patients have achieved long-term survival after PE for such recurrences (137,138). The surgical approach in these cases should be individualized to the size and location of the recurrent tumor, prior therapies, and the age and overall health of the patient. Patients considered for PE should have a thorough preoperative evaluation to exclude the presence of regional and/or distant metastases. Frequently, anterior or posterior exenteration with an extended vulvar phase will provide excellent resection margins, while allowing preservation of either urinary or fecal continence. The techniques used to perform the exenteration are identical to those routinely used for the treatment of women with recurrent cervical carcinoma. Multiple vulvar and perineal reconstructive techniques have been described for coverage of large surgical defects (139–141).

Resection of Groin Recurrence

Patients who develop isolated groin recurrence should be treated with multimodality treatment if radiotherapy is still an option. Surgical resection should be viewed with caution in the previously irradiated patient. A resection with negative margins usually requires the resection of vessels or bone with plastic reconstruction. Ultraradical surgery attempted in young patients with outstanding performance status and a small relapse in an irradiated groin that appears resectable on preoperative imaging is associated with high morbidity. Extended survival is possible for the few patients who achieve control of recurrent disease in the groin and do not later manifest distant metastasis (142). Isolated groin recurrence is a rare event, so the data to support the efficacy of this treatment are anecdotal.

Vulvar Reconstruction

With careful planning and adequate tissue mobilization, most vulvar defects can be closed primarily. When large portions of the vulva have been resected, when tissue mobility is poor, or when RT has been administered previously, primary closure may not be feasible. Alternate tissue sources must be considered for these difficult cases. Categorically, the two types of techniques commonly employed for extensive vulvar reconstruction are fasciocutaneous flaps and myocutaneous flaps. Local advancement flaps can be used for smaller defects, and pedicled flaps harvested from the inner thigh, gluteal fold, and the abdomen are used for larger defects. The techniques referenced in the next section should be employed only by surgeons who are regularly practiced in their use.

Fasciocutaneous Advancement Flaps. A variety of fasciocutaneous advancement flaps are described for vulvar reconstruction. These flaps include skin, underlying subcutaneous tissue, and underlying fascia. Nearly all of them are based on the rich, redundant blood supply from the internal pudendal artery and subsequent superficial perineal artery perforators that approach the vulva and perineum, primarily from the posterior and lateral directions. This is significant because most vulvar fasciocutaneous flaps are designed to preserve fasciocutaneous perforators from these directions. Studies performed by John et al. have evaluated approaches to perineal reconstruction following resection of large portions of the vulva and perineum. Following a wide local excision, the most common reconstructive method is the local flap. If larger amounts of tissue are removed, the next choice for reconstruction is the V-Y advancement flap, with or without incorporation of the gracilis muscle (143).

Among gynecologic oncologists, the most widely utilized pedicle flap has been the rhomboid flap; however, lotus pedicle flaps are also commonly used by plastic surgeons for closure of large vulvar defects. The lotus petal fasciocutaneous flap, irrespective of the specific design, is supplied primarily by perforating branches of the internal pudendal artery, and also through nonperforating branches of the inferior gluteal artery. The lotus petal flap best respects a natural anatomic fold at the donor site leading to the most cosmetic donor site closure (144). Although a detailed discussion of the techniques employed for these flaps is outside the scope of this chapter, references for multiple fasciocutaneous flaps that have been employed by these authors are referenced here (140,145,146).

Myocutaneous Flaps. Myocutaneous flaps, in comparison with fasciocutaneous advancement flaps, include a segment of muscle, and usually receive their blood supply and innervation through an identifiable, named neurovascular pedicle. These are usually large, thick tissue sources that are best suited for the reconstruction of substantial defects. Each of the following listed flaps has notable advantages and disadvantages. Several types of myocutaneous flaps, namely the gracilis, gluteus maximus, tensor fascia lata, vastus lateralis, and vertical rectus abdominus flaps, have been used to repair and reconstruct large vulvar and groin defects (141). Historically, the gracilis flap was used to fill large vulvar and urogenital defects; however, in recent decades, the myocutaneous flap most commonly described for extensive vulvar reconstruction is the transverse rectus abdominis muscle (TRAM) flap based on the robust inferior epigastric pedicle. TRAM flaps are useful for repairing defects in the anterior vulvar regions (147). As with fasciocutaneous flaps, a detailed description of each flap is beyond the scope of this chapter; however, a number of techniques are referenced here (145,148).

Vulvar reconstruction with myocutaneous flaps has numerous disadvantages when compared with fasciocutaneous flaps, namely, increased intraoperative complexity, requirement for meticulous wound care postoperatively, and requirement for larger incisions. Myocutaneous flaps require the sacrifice of functional muscles. Fasciocutaneous flaps, in contrast, do not sacrifice muscle and can be performed with a more modest-sized flap thickness, resulting in less morbidity (147). Regardless of method or type of flap performed, it is important to monitor patients in the postoperative period for wound dehiscence and flap necrosis (143).

RADIATION THERAPY

Early accounts of poor survival rates after primary RT of vulvar carcinomas led some investigators to surmise that radiotherapy had a narrow therapeutic role in the curative management of patients with vulvar cancer (149). The use of high doses of radiation alone, delivered with low-energy ^{60}cobalt photons and en face electron boosts, in patients who were mostly poor surgical candidates, resulted in a suboptimal therapeutic benefit between tumor control probability and normal tissue complications (150). More modern-day practices, such as incorporating consecutive daily fractionation, attention to dosimetric planning detail, and appreciation of vulvar and low pelvic radiation tissue tolerance limits, have undoubtedly shown that relatively high doses of radiation can be delivered safely. RT is now accepted as an important element in the multidisciplinary management of patients with vulvar cancer.

Adjuvant Radiotherapy to the Vulva

Following initial resection of a vulvar primary tumor, various surgico-pathologic features are associated with a higher risk of local recurrence, including tumor margins <8 mm after tissue fixation (deep or at the skin surface), lymph-vascular space invasion, and deep tumor penetration (80,81,151).

Avoidance of local recurrence is critical given poor salvage rates, particularly among those with nodal relapse. Although no prospective trials of postoperative vulvar site RT have been completed, adjuvant radiation of the primary tumor bed in selected patients with close/positive margins or multiple other high-risk features (LVSI, depth >1 cm, or size >4 cm with high-grade histology) does improve vulvar tumor control (152,153). For example, in a retrospective series by Faul et al., (152) patients with positive surgical margins had a significant reduction (33% vs. 69%) in the risk of locoregional recurrence, if receiving adjuvant RT. A similar benefit was seen for patients with close surgical margins (5% vs. 31%). Recent data also highlighted a dose–response relationship for patients with close (≤5 mm) or positive margins, where patients receiving ≥56 Gy had lower rates of vulvar recurrence compared with ≤50.4 Gy (21% vs. 34%, $p = 0.046$) (153). In combination, the data suggest that patients with close/positive margins benefit from adjuvant RT to the vulva to reduce risk of relapse. Nonetheless, after RT, the rates of locoregional relapse remain elevated (16% to 35.7%), suggesting that reexcision, when feasible, may be appropriate (152,153).

Adjuvant Regional Radiotherapy

The requirement for surgical evaluation of the LNs depends largely on the risk of involvement, which is driven predominantly by DOI and clinical tumor size (88). In general, well-lateralized T1a lesions (<2 cm in size with ≤1 mm stromal invasion) have a low probability of nodal involvement. The application of sentinel node biopsy for T1b lesions (≥2 cm in size or >1 mm stromal invasion) enables avoidance of the morbidity of inguinal dissection, although the role of completion dissection versus adjuvant RT alone in sentinel node-positive disease is the question being addressed in GROINSS-VII.

GROINSS-VII was initially designed to have women with negative SLNs observed, whereas patients with positive SLN(s) were to receive adjuvant RT with or without CT. Interim analysis demonstrated a high rate of recurrences based on the size of LN metastases (2.1% for LN ≤ 2 mm vs. 20% for LN > 2 mm) (94). Based on these findings, the trial protocol was modified to mandate completion dissection and then possible adjuvant RT for patients with macrometastases defined as >2 mm. Although these interim results suggest suboptimal efficacy of RT for macrometastases, some concerns have been raised regarding contouring and target volume delineation described in the protocol, prompting modification of RT contouring details (154). Additional controversy exists regarding the definition of macrometastases, with GROINSS-VII identifying this entity as metastases >2 mm. With most patient accrual completed, the final results of this trial, including detailed analysis of dose and volume, will help guide the treatment of sentinel node-positive patients. With the interim findings, patients with macrometastases in sentinel nodes should be considered for inguinal node dissection followed by assessment for adjuvant RT.

GOG 88 attempted to define the optimal approach to clinically negative inguinal nodes in a trial that randomized patients between inguinal node irradiation and radical lymphadenectomy (followed by inguinopelvic radiation in patients with positive nodes) after resection of the primary tumor (155). This study was closed after the entry of only 58 patients when there appeared to be a higher rate of groin recurrence in the RT arm (0% vs. 18.5%). However, a number of criticisms arose from the treatment protocol because of lack of CT-based planning, underdosing of the inguinal nodes due to technique, and lack of radiographic staging. Review of treatment delivery revealed that all five patients who failed had inadequate tumor doses (<47 Gy), reflecting the unaccounted for depth of inguinal nodes (mean 6.1 vs. 3 cm prescribed depth) (156,157). Appropriate volume-based contouring guidelines have now been established on the basis of patterns of recurrences (158).

Despite GOG 88 findings, a number of retrospective studies have suggested that regional prophylactic RT is an effective method of preventing groin recurrences with minimal morbidity when appropriately delivered (158–161). In a large single-institution retrospective analysis, Katz et al. (158) reported no differences in the inguinal relapse rates for patients treated with prophylactic groin irradiation compared with those undergoing lymph node dissection. Combined across retrospective series, the incidence of groin recurrence following treatment of the undissected nodal region appears to be 0% to 12%, the lowest occurring in a series using three-dimensional treatment planning and intensity-modulated RT. Improved and greater application of pretreatment radiographic staging may further contribute to lower inguinal recurrence rates.

Although the role of prophylactic RT in the undissected but high-risk groin remains controversial, there is strong evidence that adjuvant RT after surgical assessment improves regional tumor control and survival in patients who have documented nodal metastases following inguinal node dissection. Retrospective studies suggested that patients with metastases to multiple nodes or extranodal tumor extension had an increased risk of groin recurrence after radical surgery, and therefore may benefit from RT (162). However, the critical role of RT was not appreciated until 1986, when Homesley et al. (163) published prospective GOG trial results.

In GOG 37, 114 patients with involved inguinal nodes underwent radical vulvectomy and inguinal lymphadenectomy. Patients who had positive inguinal nodes were randomized intraoperatively to receive either pelvic node dissection or postoperative irradiation to the pelvic and inguinal nodes. This trial was closed before the projected accrual goal, based on interim analysis identifying a significant survival benefit with RT (68% vs. 54%, $p = 0.03$). The differences between the 2-year survival rates of patients treated with RT or pelvic dissection were most marked for patients presenting with clinically positive nodes (59% vs. 31%, respectively) and for those with two or more positive groin nodes (63% vs. 37%, respectively). Extended follow-up showed a nonsignificant 6-year overall survival benefit to the radiation arm (51% vs. 41%). Yet the cancer-related death rate was significantly higher for pelvic node resection than for radiation (HR, 0.49 [95% CI, 0.28 to 0.87]; 51% vs. 29%) (105). Coupled with higher rates of inguinal failure for patients treated with surgery alone (24% vs. 5%), these results emphasized the poor salvage rate seen in patients developing groin recurrences. Interestingly, 8% of patients in both treatment arms had recurrences at the primary site, even though the vulva was not included in the radiotherapy field, raising the question of whether selective radiation to the vulva may have further increased the benefit of radiation.

The largest challenge at present is whether RT should be applied to patients with a single node with an adequate dissection and without ulceration or extracapsular extension. On unplanned subset analysis in GOG 37, the survival benefit seen with radiation was maintained for those with N2/3 disease, $\geq$2 positive lymph nodes, or inadequate nodal dissection (defined as node positivity $\geq$20% of dissected nodes). On the other hand, no significant difference in survival was seen for patients with one microscopically positive node; the authors later commented that the number of patients in this subset was insufficient for reliable analysis. Retrospective data suggest that patients with even a single positive inguinal nodal metastasis benefit from adjuvant radiation, particularly if the groin dissection was less extensive in scope or if a nodal positive ratio is >20% (105,106,108,164). More recent analyses from SEER and a retrospective multicenter cohort study from Germany suggest a benefit to adjuvant RT even in patients with a single positive node (108,164). Another indication that radiation may be useful in the single positive inguinal lymph node patient is derived from data in the GROINSS-V study (165). Patients with a single sentinel node metastasis larger than 2 mm had a lower DSS (69.5%) than patients with a single sentinel node metastasis $\leq$2 mm (94.4%, $p = 0.001$). Overall, these findings suggest that patients with N2/3 disease, $\geq$2 positive LNs, or inadequate nodal dissection should receive adjuvant radiation. In addition, patients with a single positive LN should be strongly considered to receive radiation based on suboptimal outcomes and supportive retrospective data.

Despite nodal dissection and adjuvant radiation, outcomes are poor in node-positive patients, even in the modern era. In GOG 37, the 6-year overall survival was only 51%, while retrospective data show similarly suboptimal survival (105,106,108,164). Other prospective GOG trials have proven high rates of distant relapse among node-positive patients, particularly in those with multiple node involvement (89,105). With this appreciation and the growing application of concurrent CT in the preoperative setting, the role of CT postoperatively has yet to be clearly addressed. Recent registry-based data using the National Cancer Database (NCDB) illustrated a benefit with predominantly concurrent CT (HR, 0.62, $p < 0.001$), providing further suggestion of the potential role of CT.

Preoperative Radiotherapy

In patients who present with more advanced primary tumors, RT may be delivered preoperatively. Advocates of this approach have listed several theoretical advantages for patients with locally advanced vulvar carcinomas:

1. Less radical resection of the vulva may be adequate to achieve local tumor control after preoperative treatment of the vulva with radiation;
2. Tumor regression during radiation may allow the surgeon to obtain adequate tumor-free surgical margins without sacrificing important pelvic structures such as the urethra, anus, and the clitoris;
3. RT alone may be sufficient to sterilize microscopic regional disease when the inguinal nodes are not radiographically determined to be involved and may mobilize fixed and matted nodes, facilitating subsequent surgical excision.

Although the published experiences with preoperative single-modality RT are small, several investigators have reported excellent responses and high local control rates after treatment of advanced tumors with relatively modest doses of radiation followed by local resection (162,166). These early reports provided evidence that radiation could significantly debulk advanced local disease and allow for more conservative, viscera-sparing surgery, while preserving good local control.

Data has since emerged that support the therapeutic benefit of concurrent CT with radiation, typically followed by limited surgical resection, in managing locally advanced disease (89,167,168). Typical regimens have included combinations of radiation coadministered with 5-fluorouracil (5-FU), and cisplatin or mitomycin C. Most investigators have observed remarkable regressions of bulky lesions with concurrent CT with RT, suggesting that therapeutic responses may be better than would be expected with RT alone. Randomized trials of the role of concurrent CT have not been done and are unlikely to be feasible within this disease, given the small number of patients and heterogeneity of clinical presentation. However, recent single experimental arm trials have demonstrated improved local control and survival when concurrent cisplatin CT was added to radiation in locally advanced vulvar cancers (89,167).

The most compelling data in support of concurrent CRT in the management of locally advanced disease come from two large prospective phase 2 trials performed by the GOG. In the first study (GOG protocol 101), 71 evaluable patients with locally advanced T3 or T4 disease who were deemed not resectable by standard radical vulvectomy underwent preoperative CRT (167). CT consisted of two cycles of 5-FU and cisplatin. Radiation was delivered to a dose of 47.6 Gy, using a planned split-course regimen, with part of the radiation given twice daily during the 5-FU infusion. Patients underwent planned resection of the residual vulvar tumor, or incisional biopsy of the original tumor site in the case of complete clinical response (cCR), 4 to 8 weeks after CRT. A cCR was noted in 33 of 71 patients (47%). Following vulvar excision or biopsy, 22 patients (31%) were found to have no residual tumor in the pathologic specimen. In all, only 2 of 71 patients (3%) had unresectable disease after CRT, and in only 3 patients was it impossible to preserve urinary and/or gastrointestinal continuity following complete resection of the primary tumor. With a median follow-up interval of 50 months, 11 patients (16%) have developed locally recurrent disease in the vulva (167). These results are all the more notable considering the relatively low dose of radiation used in these typically bulky, advanced tumors.

Building on this experience, investigators sought to study weekly cisplatin (40 mg/m^2) coadministered with radiation (GOG protocol 205). Additionally, this study eliminated the break in RT and increased RT dose to 57.6 Gy. On this trial, 58 evaluable patients with untreated locally advanced T3 or T4 disease not amenable to standard radical vulvectomy underwent preoperative radiation with concurrent CT (89). Following preoperative therapy, 64% had a clinical CR and 50% had a pathologic complete response (pCR), a notable improvement compared with the regimen used in GOG 101. In an attempt to further improve on the pCR rate, GOG 279 has been designed with use of concurrent gemcitabine with cisplatin, integration of IMRT, and dose escalation to 64 Gy. This trial is currently accruing patients.

Following preoperative chemoradiation for locally advanced disease, it remains unclear whether surgery is necessary in those who achieve cCR. In GOG 101, approximately 70% of patients who achieved cCR were found to have no pathologic residual in the surgical specimen (167). In GOG 205, 34 of 37 patients (92%) underwent surgical biopsy only to assess treatment response (169). Of these 34 women, 29 (78%) had biopsies showing a CR. Based on this 22% to 30% risk of discordant findings between CR and PR, at minimum, an excisional biopsy of the primary site should be completed to confirm a CR to treatment.

The role of preoperative CRT has been assessed in patients who present with bulky, unresectable inguinal adenopathy. In GOG 101 (study of preoperative CRT for local regionally advanced vulvar cancer), there was a cohort of 42 evaluable patients with N2 or N3 nodal disease who were deemed initially unresectable. Patients received 47.6 Gy of RT in split-course fashion, with two concurrent cycles of 5-FU and cisplatin, as described above. Planned inguinofemoral LN dissection was performed 3 to 8 weeks later. In only 2 patients (5%) did nodal disease remain unresectable. The surgical specimen showed histologic clearance of nodal disease in 15 patients (36%). At a median follow-up of 78 months, only 1 of 37 patients (3%) who completed the fully prescribed regimen of preoperative therapy and bilateral inguinofemoral node dissection relapsed in the groin. This study, while nonrandomized, provides further evidence of the efficacy of combined CRT in the management of local regionally advanced vulvar cancer and of patients with significant regional adenopathy.

Definitive Radiotherapy

Historical data evaluating the use of RT alone for vulvar cancer was generally disappointing, with a significant number of recurrences and considerable toxicity. With integration of more modern, advanced techniques and favorable results from preoperative radiotherapy, some have reexplored the role of definitive radiotherapy using higher cumulative doses. Two of these series have shown that doses exceeding 55 to 56 Gy independently predict for improved local control (170,171). Based on these findings, radiotherapy alone may be an option for patients not suitable for surgery, assuming intent to reach relatively high doses.

In an effort to reach these doses when treating definitively, few studies have assessed the role of interstitial brachytherapy, either alone or after external beam radiotherapy (EBRT) (172,173). When delivering a high dose via EBRT (mean dose, 50.4 Gy) and an interstitial brachytherapy boost (mean dose, 28.7 Gy), Tewari et al. (173) illustrated no local failures among patients with primary advanced vulvar SCC. Hoffman et al. (172) similarly evaluated patients treated with interstitial brachytherapy with or without EBRT, demonstrating disease control in 7 of 10 patients receiving 70 to 90 Gy, albeit with high rates of necrosis. The considerable hot spot at the skin achieved with brachytherapy may account for this high rate of soft tissue necrosis. Brachytherapy boost should therefore be used cautiously and possibly selectively for patients with significant vaginal extension.

Radiation Therapy Technique

Conventional (Two- and Three-dimensional) Radiotherapy

Radiation techniques used for treatment of vulvar carcinoma reflect a need to cover the vulva plus lower pelvic and inguinal nodes, while simultaneously minimizing radiation dose to the femoral heads. Conventional approaches utilized an anterior field that encompasses the inguinal regions, lower pelvic nodes, and vulva, and a narrower posterior field that encompasses the lower pelvic nodes and vulva but excludes most of the femoral heads. The intent here is to cover one nodal echelon proximal to the nodal echelon with metastatic vulvar cancer disease. The inferior-most borders of the fields should extend 2 to 3 cm caudal to the saphenous and femoral vein junction. If the fields are evenly weighted to the midplane of the pelvis using 6 MV photons, the contribution of the anterior field to the groin nodes at a depth of 3 to 5 cm will generally be 60% to 70% of the dose to the mid pelvis. Some choose to use 6 MV from the anterior field and 15 MV from the posterior field to save posterior organs at risk. The difference may be made up by supplementing the dose to the lateral groins with anterior electron fields of appropriate energy.

Currently, CT scans obtained in the process of radiation dose planning are used to detect enlarged nodes that may not be appreciated on clinical exam and to determine the appropriate electron energy. Based on patterns of relapse, institutional contouring guidelines have been established to ensure adequate coverage (174) (**Fig 18.19**). Gross disease in the groin or vulva may be boosted with en face electron fields or conformal photon RT. If radiation is directed to the regional nodes only, with intentional sparing of the vulva, care must be taken to avoid a large "midline" block, which may lead to higher medial groin and vulvar failures.

Intensity-Modulated Radiotherapy

The complex anatomy of the vulva and its regional lymphatics have led some investigators to propose the use of IMRT in the management of vulvar cancer (**Fig. 18.20**) (175,176). To whom IMRT should be offered remains debated, although this modality is now being incorporated in clinical trials (i.e., GOG 279). In modern practice, IMRT may replace conventional external beam approaches used in the treatment of vulvar cancer; however, outcome data remain limited. Most data come from experience extrapolated from the treatment of anal carcinoma in multi-institutional clinical trials or limited single-institution series (169,176,177). IMRT is gradually being used more for radiotherapeutic management of gynecologic

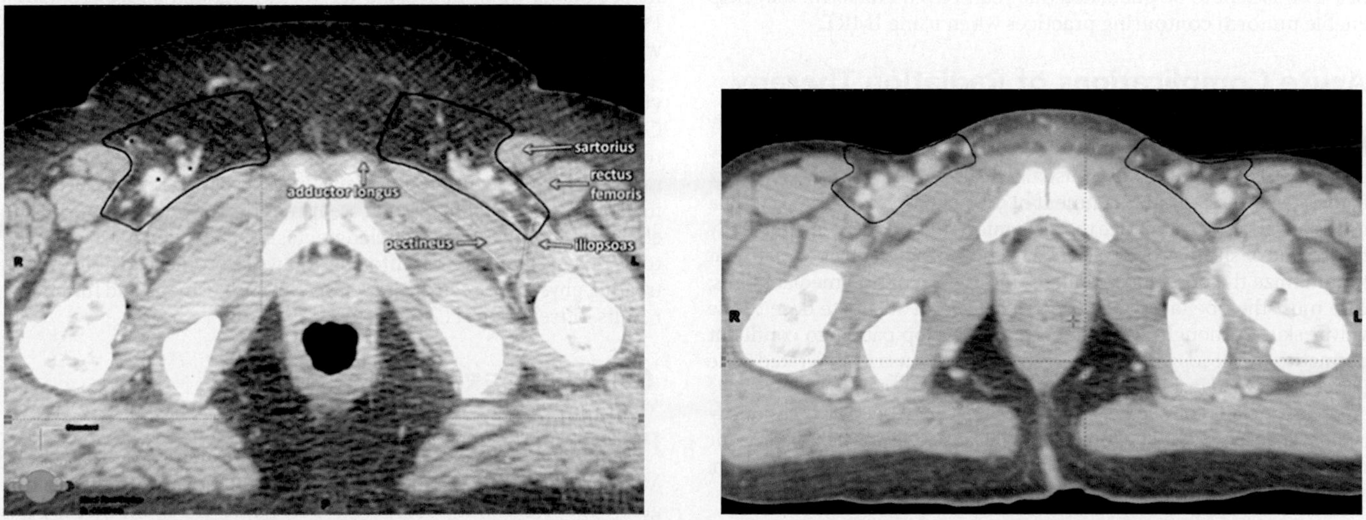

Figure 18.19. Location of nodal involvement within the inguinal region (**left**) and respective contouring guidelines for inguinal clinical target volume to encompass potential subclinical disease (**right**).

Source: Reprinted with permission from Kim CH, Olson AC, Kim H, et al. Contouring inguinal and femoral nodes; how much margin is needed around the vessels? *Pract Radiat Oncol.* 2012;2:274–278.

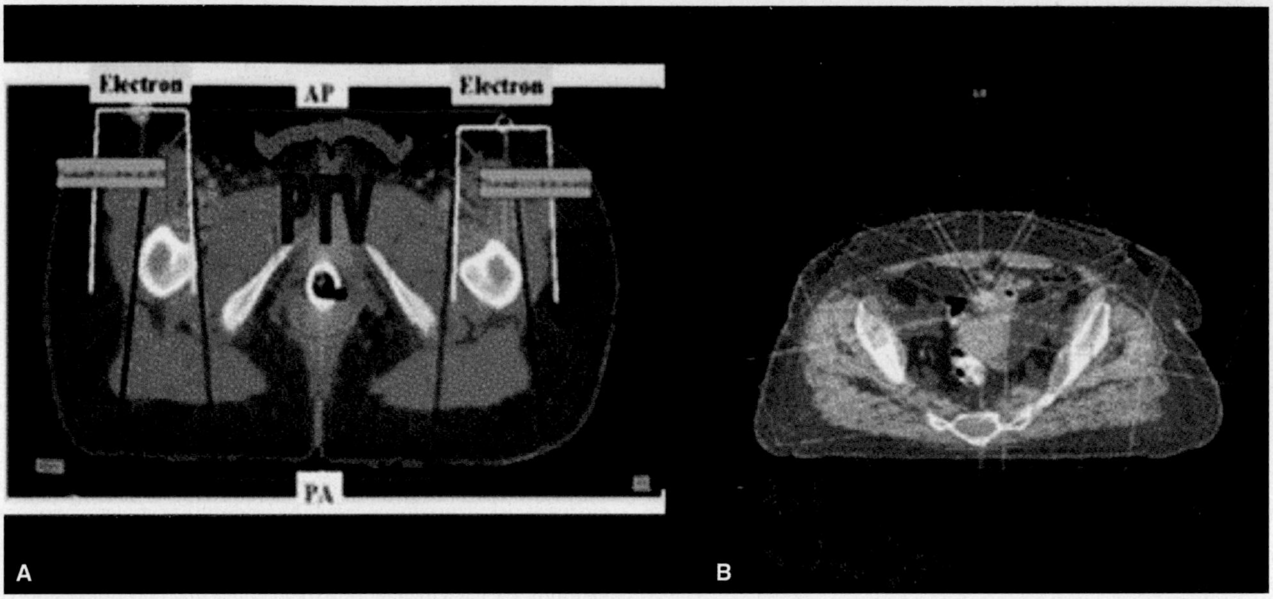

Figure 18.20. A: Conventional radiotherapy. **B**: Intensity-modulated radiation therapy in the management of vulvar cancer.

Source: Reprinted with permission from Beriwal S, Heron D, Kim H, et al. Intensity-modulated radiotherapy for the treatment of vulvar carcinoma: a comparative dosimetric study with early clinical outcome. *Int J Radiat Oncol Biol phys*. 2006;64:1395–1400.

malignancies, including vulvar cancer. It is an attractive approach to RT in the pelvis because of its ability to escalate radiation dose while decreasing radiation dose to nearby healthy normal tissue, improving the therapeutic window for radiation.

Although radiobiologically effective, IMRT has some practical limitations. Uncertainties in patient setup and target volume definition when using IMRT techniques have been raised. Vulvar and groin target motion resulting from quiet breathing during treatment is expected to be minimal, as are shifting bladder and rectal volumes unlikely to substantially modify primary disease position during beam-on time. Again borrowing from overall RT experience, it is not unreasonable to conclude that daily repositioning of women prior to radiation delivery, using such devices as on-board cone beam CT, will adjust for setup inconsistencies. Single-institution data evaluating patterns of inguinal relapse have better clarified challenges with target delineation (174). Presently, consensus group contouring guidelines for volume and dose have been presented in a national meeting in anticipation of a manuscript to be published this year. This manuscript may help enable uniform contouring practices when using IMRT.

Acute Complications of Radiation Therapy

Acute radiation reactions are brisk, and doses of 35 to 45 Gy routinely induce patchy or confluent moist desquamation. However, with adequate local care, this acute reaction usually heals within 3 to 4 weeks. Sitz baths, steroid cream, and treatment of possible superimposed Candida infection all help to minimize the discomfort. If the patient is sufficiently flexible, he or she may be placed in a frog-leg position during treatment to minimize the dose and ensuing skin reaction on the medial thighs; care must then be taken, however, to deliver an adequate dose to the vulvar skin. Although most patients will develop patchy to confluent dermatitis by the fourth week of treatment, this is usually tolerated if the patient is warned in advance and assured that the discomfort will resolve after treatment is completed. Although a treatment break is occasionally required, delays should be minimized, because they may allow time for repopulation of tumor cells. IMRT helps reduce dose to uninvolved skin, especially in groin regions, which also helps reduce dermatitis (176).

Late Complications of Radiation Therapy

Many factors add to the late morbidity of RT in patients with vulvar carcinoma. Patients with advanced vulvar carcinomas are often treated with RT following radical surgery, which may include extensive dissection of the inguinal and possibly pelvic nodes. Large ulcerative cutaneous lesions frequently have superimposed infection. Patients are often elderly and may have complicating medical conditions, such as diabetes, multiple prior surgeries, and osteoporosis. The contribution of concurrent CT to local morbidity is not yet clearly defined, but may contribute to bowel and bone complications (178). Conversely, the addition of complex treatment planning such as IMRT may further reduce the risk of skin, small bowel, bone and bone marrow toxicities, with a single-institution series showing no severe (grade $\geq$ 3) late complications for vulvar cancer patients (177,179).

The incidence of lower extremity edema after inguinal irradiation alone appears to be small (155). RT is likely to contribute to the cumulative incidence of peripheral leg edema following radical node dissection, but there was no difference evident in the GOG randomized study of radiation (16%) versus pelvic node dissection (22%) (163). Other complications include the risk of pelvic and femoral head fracture, most notably when delivering RT to the inguinal nodes (180,181). Previous techniques provided substantial dose to the femoral heads, which can be decreased by techniques such as IMRT (175,177).

The effect of RT on the long-term cosmesis and function of the vulva is poorly understood. Although treatment with radiation or CRT and wide excision is becoming a more accepted alternative to extensive surgery for selected patients, and major complication rates appear to be acceptable, very little has been reported regarding subtler late effects of such treatment in the vulva. Possible late effects include atrophy and telangiectasias. Late effects are expected to be dose-related. Better information will become available only as treating physicians record and report the late cosmetic and functional results of treatment (178).

Chemotherapy

Primary Treatment of Advanced Disease

Most patients diagnosed with vulvar cancer can be cured with surgery with or without postoperative RT; thus, CT monotherapy has traditionally been used solely for salvage. Patients with advanced vulvar cancers tend to be older, with significant medical comorbidities, making them poor candidates for cytotoxic therapy because of concomitant diseases that increase the likelihood of significant adverse effects. Furthermore, recurrent vulvar cancer often occurs in the setting of extensive prior surgery and/or RT, making tolerance to cytotoxic therapy poor.

Cytotoxic Chemotherapy

Neoadjuvant Chemotherapy

Squamous carcinoma is the only histologic type of vulvar cancer for which there are significant data assessing the utility of cytotoxic CT in recurrent or advanced primary vulvar cancer not initially amenable to surgery or RT. In order to reduce morbidity of subsequent curative intent surgical therapy, a number of smaller studies have been performed to assess the feasibility of this approach. Geisler et al. subjected 13 patients to neoadjuvant CT with cisplatin (50 mg/m^2) and 5-FU (1,000 mg/m^2/24 hours) q3w (n = 10 cisplatin and 5-FU, n = 3 cisplatin only). The combination achieved CRs in 100% of patients (10% CR); 9/10 patients then underwent radical vulvar resection and inguinofemoral lymphadenectomy. In all patients, preservation of anal and urethral sphincter function was achieved; 9/9 patients who completed both neoadjuvant CT and surgery remained alive and free of disease at 49 months (182).

In a more recent prospective study of 10 patients with advanced primary vulvar cancer whose only curative option was PE combined with neoadjuvant CT, patients were offered either paclitaxel (175 mg/m^2, d1 + ifosfamide (5 mg/m^2, d2) + cisplatin (70 mg/m^2, d1) [TIP], or paclitaxel (175 mg/m^2, d1) + cisplatin (70 mg/m^2, d1) [TP] at the discretion of the treating physician (TIP n = 4, TP n = 5). Overall response rate (ORR) was 80% with one CR, two persistent carcinoma *in situ* and 6 patients with PR >50% tumor regression; 9/9 patients underwent radical surgery with inguinofemoral lymphadenectomy, and all were disease-free at completion of primary combined therapy. Ultimately, 6/9 patients recurred with a PFS = 14 months from surgery (multiple different salvage therapies were utilized). After a median follow-up of 40 months, 56% of patients were alive and without evidence of disease (NED) (178).

A prospective multicenter trial compared four cisplatin-based regimens and one bleomycin-based regimen in 35 patients with advanced vulvar cancer; 33 of 35 patients completed CT, with PRs noted in 30 patients and stable disease noted in 3 patients; 27 patients subsequently underwent radical surgery (25 with inguinofemoral lymphadenectomy). Of 16 patients with clinically apparent nodes before treatment, 11 were found with residual nodal disease, and they then underwent CRT. At a median of 49 months of follow-up, 24 of 27 patients remained NED. Because of the overall number of patients treated, as well as the multiple different cytotoxic regimens used, the authors could not establish a clear standard for recommendation; however, the results suggest a possible role for neoadjuvant CT for advanced vulvar cancers initially not amenable to surgery (179).

Before neoadjuvant therapy is considered a standard approach in advanced patients, further study involving larger numbers of patients and more controlled therapy regimens is recommended.

Systemic Treatment of Metastatic and Recurrent Vulvar Cancer

Despite the success of curative intent therapies in advanced vulvar cancer patients, a significant minority of patients will recur (40% to 50%), and 5-year overall survival (OS) in this group of patients is <10% (167,185). Unfortunately, in view of the rarity of this disease and difficulty with a prospective study of an even more infrequently encountered group of patients, there is no clear standard for treatment of patients with metastatic or recurrent disease who are not amenable to surgery or RT. As a result, most patients are treated with regimens extrapolated from study of CT in metastatic SCC of the cervix. Accordingly, most patients are treated with cisplatin-based combination regimens, and there is interest in the use of bevacizumab in vulvar cancer.

Early studies in vulvar cancer with single-agent cytotoxic chemotherapies such as piperazinedione, cisplatin (50 mg/m^2, q21d), and mitoxantrone were disappointing, with no responses noted (186,187).

A prospective phase 2 study evaluated the use of cisplatin (80 mg/m^2, q21d) + vinorelbine (25 mg/m^2, d1, d8) in 16 chemotherapy-naïve patients; 15 patients were evaluable for response, and ORR was 40%, with 4 CRs, 2 PRs, and 5 patients with stable disease. Median PFS was 10 months, with a median OS of 19 months. Toxicity was considered manageable, with nausea/vomiting and leukopenia the primary grade 3 and 4 toxicities (188).

Single-agent therapy with paclitaxel (175 mg/m^2 q21d) was evaluated in 31 heavily pretreated patients with advanced, recurrent, or metastatic vulvar cancer who were not amenable to surgery or RT. In 29 evaluable patients, ORR was 14% (189). Based on this, further study of single-agent paclitaxel in this population has not been attempted.

Receptor Targeted Therapies

Epidermal Growth Factor Receptor (EGFR) Inhibitors

Recognition of the fact that EGFR expression via IHC staining is elevated in malignant vulvar tumors has led to the use of EGFR tyrosine kinase inhibitors (TKIs) as monotherapy and in combination with cytotoxic CT in palliation of advanced and recurrent vulvar cancer patients. Olawaiye et al. (190,191) reported two dramatic PRs to single-agent erlotinib in women with advanced, treatment-refractory disease; Bacha subsequently reported a PR in a woman with advanced disease. A phase 2 prospective GOG trial using erlotinib in 41 patients with advanced or recurrent vulvar cancer described PRs in 28% and SD in 40% of patients. Unfortunately, responses were not durable, and grade 3 and 4 toxicities (diarrhea, dehydration, and renal failure) were notable (191).

Vascular Endothelial Growth Factor Receptor (VEGF) Targeting

Recent advances in the treatment of cervical cancer with antiangiogenic therapies, most notably bevacizumab, have led to significant interest in application of similar antiangiogenic therapies in the treatment of vulvar cancer (192). As approximately 40% of vulvar cancers are believed to be a result of HPV infection, there is hope that similar efficacy for this classically chemo-refractory disease will be possible. To date, though, there are no published reports of activity for antiangiogenic therapies in vulvar cancer.

Results of Therapy

The overall results of therapy for women with squamous cancers of the vulva are excellent, largely because approximately two-thirds of patients present with early-stage tumors. Five-year survival rates for vulvar cancer have improved over the past two decades. Landrum et al. used GOG data to perform an historical comparison between patients treated between 1977 and 1984 (n = 577) and patients treated between 1990 and 2005 (n = 175). Stratification into "minimal, low, intermediate, and high-risk" groups was performed to enable comparisons. Patients treated in the era of less radical surgery and modern CRT fared better than historical comparisons, with 5-year survival by risk group (minimal → high) of 100% versus 97.9%, 97% versus 87.4%, 82% versus 74.8%, and 100% versus 29.0% (193).

Several strategies to enhance survival for women with vulvar cancer are evident. High-risk patients can be educated and screened more consistently for the development of early cancer. Women with HPV infections, *in situ* vulvar disease, long smoking history, and other genital neoplasms are at risk for developing vulvar cancer (194). Careful screening targeted at women with these high-risk factors may lead to improvements in early diagnosis (195).

The survival rate for women with nodal spread is one-half that for women without nodal disease who have similarly sized primary tumors. Improvements in the use of molecular markers for metastatic disease and biologic aggressiveness would be helpful for triaging higher-risk patients into more effective adjuvant therapies. And, of course, there is a dire need for better treatment options for node-positive patients.

SEQUELAE OF TREATMENT

Immediate complications such as wound infection and lymphocysts were common in the radical vulvectomy era. These occur much less frequently now because of the use of multimodal primary therapies, less radical surgery, and innovations such as prophylactic antibiotics and closed-suction drains. Breakdown of the vulvar incision is increased in patients who are smokers, as well as those with vasculopathy.

Lymphedema starts to appear within weeks of surgery. The severity is related to the extent of groin surgery, wound complications, postoperative RT, and preexisting conditions of the lower extremities. Lymphedema is not always limited to the lower leg and thigh. It may also include the mons, groins, and hips. The use of SLNB reduces but does not eliminate wound complications and lymphedema. Pressure stockings, sequential compression devices, lymphedema massage, and microvascular surgery have been used to manage lower extremity lymphedema, with limited results. *Prevention* of lymphedema with the use of SLNB is the best strategy for limiting its adverse effects (132).

All gynecologic surgery, especially surgery for vulvar cancer, can have an adverse effect on body image and sexual function. Informed consent obtained for vulvar cancer surgery should include a discussion regarding these risks. No assumptions regarding a woman's sexual activity should be made on the basis of age or marital status. We have found that preoperative consultation with a sexual health expert can be invaluable for many women.

FUTURE DIRECTIONS (RESEARCH, POTENTIAL MANAGEMENT CHANGES)

The incorporation of SLNB into the care of women with vulvar cancer raises many new questions regarding treatment of lymph node-positive patients. Should a woman with a microscopically positive SLN undergo full regional lymphadenectomy? How does the size of a groin metastasis impact survival, and how should it affect decisions regarding adjuvant treatment? Are isolated tumor cells clinically relevant (129,196)?

The GROINSVII/GOG 270 protocol, which is being conducted in Europe and North America, seeks to answer some of these questions. The original study design called for SLN-positive patients to be treated with 50-Gy RT to the groin. Early stopping rules were met because there were an unexpected number of patients with groin relapse following SLNB and RT. On further analysis, there were no groin relapses among patients with metastases <2 mm. The study has been amended to require inguinofemoral lymphadenectomy for women with metastases over 2 mm and postoperative RT of 56 Gy. The role of adjuvant CT is unclear. GROINSVII/GOG 270 allows the use of concurrent cisplatin during RT, albeit at the discretion of the treating physician.

Another area of significant interest will be targeted therapy. Large phase II/III trials in vulvar cancer are unlikely because of population size; however, lessons learned from squamous carcinomas of the anus, head and neck, cervix, and cutaneous melanoma will likely provide significant insights into novel therapies for vulvar cancer patients.

SUMMARY

Most patients with vulvar cancer are potentially curable at the time of presentation for care. The major challenge for providers is how to balance providing curative therapy with preserving quality of life, including organ function, sexual function, and body image.

The preferred therapy for patients with early disease is surgery alone. The morbidity of surgery can be reduced with the use of SLNB as an alternative to regional lymphadenectomy. This approach has proved very successful in the treatment of patients with breast cancer and cutaneous melanoma. There is now enough clinical evidence to support routine use in patients with vulvar cancer. Further investigation is needed to determine the ideal management of patients with a positive SLN.

Women with advanced disease usually benefit from multimodality therapy. The exact combination and order of treatment rely on consultation with a team including a gynecologic oncologist, radiation oncologist, pathologist, and diagnostic imager. Vulvar cancer is sufficiently infrequent for even busy clinicians to consider referral to a high-volume center when considering the care of women with this disease.

INTERNATIONAL PERSPECTIVES

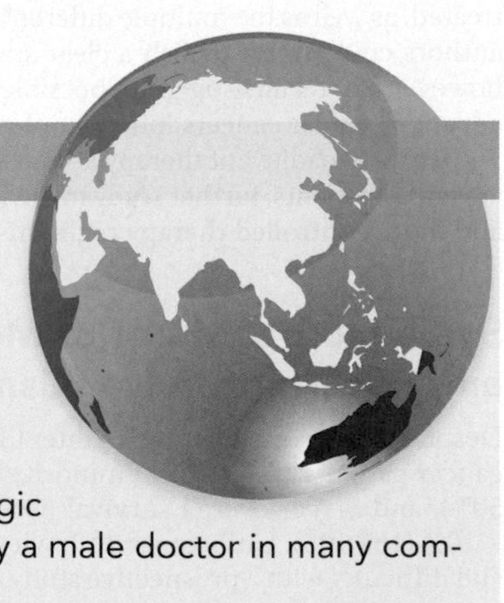

Vulvar Cancer in the Developing World

Adriana Bermudez, MD

The incidence of vulvar cancer in the developing world is unknown, because most of these countries have no reliable tumor registries.

Screening programs for gynecologic cancers are not readily available in low-resource settings. Furthermore, cultural and religious reasons make gynecologic cancer diagnoses more difficult, because patients feel ashamed to be attended by a male doctor in many communities. This is especially true for older patients with vulvar lesions.

Because most female cancer patients are managed by general gynecologists, once vulvar cancer is diagnosed, treatment is often not on hand. Radical surgery cannot be performed for want of infrastructure and necessary skill sets, and RT machines are usually saved for younger patients.

Opioids and morphine are also not available in many countries in the developing world. As a result, many women with vulvar cancer in these countries die without treatment or palliative care.

INTERNATIONAL PERSPECTIVES

Vulvar Cancer in Chile

Jorge Brañes Yunusic, MD

The incidence of vulvar cancer in Chile, as in other regions of the world, is relatively low, accounting for 3% to 5% of all genital tract malignancies. Mortality rates are also similar, and have been unchanged for the last two decades at approximately 0.5/100,000 women (1).

According to local data, compared with that of international publications, patient characteristics are almost identical in many respects (e.g., mean age at diagnosis, histology, body mass index, etc.), except for stage at diagnosis, because our patients usually present with more advanced disease. In one series of patients, the average size of the primary tumor was 4 cm (personal communication). Along the same lines, 68% of patients from another cohort presented with stage III disease at diagnosis (2). These two issues, along with the disease's relatively low frequency, influence the way we treat our patients.

In most centers, sentinel lymph node (SLN) detection is not routinely performed. The main reasons for this are the following: (a) low number of cases per center, which minimizes a surgeon's chances of getting accustomed to and mastering the technique, and (b) as mentioned above, the high number of patients presenting with advanced disease at diagnosis—a group of patients in whom the method has not been entirely validated.

Besides complete blood tests, the preoperative workup should include a CT scan of the abdomen and pelvis. When involvement of the midline structure is suspected, MRI can help guide treatment between surgery and RT for the primary tumor.

Clinical management of stage IA disease is wide local excision without evaluation of the inguinofemoral LNs. Stage I/II disease, other than IA, is managed with wide local excision or radical vulvectomy for the primary tumor and unilateral or bilateral inguinofemoral lymphadenectomy.

In case of involvement of midline structures, where urinary or fecal continence cannot be assured, CRT followed by resection of residual disease is preferred. Postoperative RT to the pelvis and inguinal nodes is indicated in the case of two or more positive inguinal nodes.

In conclusion, the 5-year overall survival rate reported in a Chilean retrospective cohort study of 86 patients with vulvar cancer was 57%. Among the studied variables, stage was the independent factor in the analysis (2).

(1) Donoso E. Cambio del perfil epidemiológico y demográfico determina un mayor riesgo de cáncer ginecológico en la mujer chilena. *Rev Chil Obstet Ginecol.* 2012;77(4):247–248.

(2) Carcamo M, Orellana JJ, Gayan P, Valenzuela MT. Survival of patients with vulvar cancer. *Rev Med Chile.* 2010;138:723–728.

INTERNATIONAL PERSPECTIVES

Vulvar Cancer in Latin America

Gustavo Ferraris, MD, PhD

Vulvar cancer is rare in Latin America, representing 3% to 5% of all gynecologic tumors. Characteristic of postmenopausal women, the percentage of patients younger than 50 years is progressively increasing in the region, showing a strong association with HPV infection.

The workup is similar to what is mentioned elsewhere the chapter, with the exception of the use of cystoscopy and sigmoidoscopy, which is reserved for advanced cases. In Latin America, most of the patients present with advanced disease at the time of diagnosis, and the standard treatment is CRT, most commonly a modification of the Nigro protocol for anal cancer (5-FU CI days 1 to 4, and mytomicin C, day 1, two cycles 21 days) plus radiation (50 Gy beginning first cycle; boost 20 to 25 Gy in residual disease). The same treatment scheme is also used for recurrent tumors larger than 5 cm, or tumors in any location where surgical resection

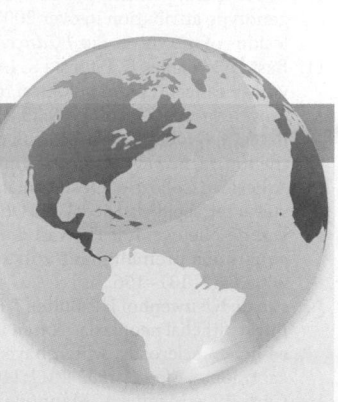

(*continued*)

INTERNATIONAL PERSPECTIVES (*continued*)

may not allow for appropriate margins. For operable disease, a sentinel node biopsy technique is used in cases of squamous histology, tumors smaller than 4 cm, unifocal tumors, and nonpalpable or cytology-negative inguinal nodes.

Single-institution reports (1) of combined modality therapy in advanced disease show an actuarial 5-year survival rate of 60.5%. Analyzing the impact of nodal status on survival, 5-year survival in patients with negative nodes was 80%, and 74.5% for patients with a single node-positive, dropping to less than 7% in the setting of multiple metastatic nodes.

(1) Pautas en Oncología, Diagnóstico, Tratamiento y Seguimiento del Cáncer. Instituto Oncológico Angel Roffo, Universidad de Buenos Aires, Capítulo Cáncer de vulva, page 241- 249- ISBN 987-97055-9-9, 2015.

REFERENCES

1. Siegel RL, Miller KD, Jemal A. Cancer statistics, 2015. *CA Cancer J Clin.* 2015;65(1):5–29.
2. Jones RW, Joura EA. Analyzing prior clinical events at presentation in 102 women with vulvar carcinoma: evidence of diagnostic delays. *J Reprod Med.* 1999;44(9):766–768.
3. Plentl AA, Friedman EA. Lymphatic system of the female genitalia: the morphologic basis of oncologic diagnosis and therapy. *Major Probl Obstet Gynecol.* 1971;2:1–223.
4. Joura EA, Losch A, Haider-Angeler MG, et al. Trends in vulvar neoplasia: increasing incidence of vulvar intraepithelial neoplasia and squamous cell carcinoma of the vulva in young women. *J Reprod Med.* 2000;45(8):613–615.
5. Lanneau GS, Argenta PA, Lanneau MS, et al. Vulvar cancer in young women: demographic features and outcome evaluation. *Am J Obstet Gynecol.* 2009;200(6):645. e641–e645.
6. Blomberg M, Friis S, Munk C, et al. Genital warts and risk of cancer: a Danish study of nearly 50 000 patients with genital warts. *J Infect Dis.* 2012;205(10):1544–1553.
7. van de Nieuwenhof HP, van Kempen LC, de Hullu JA, et al. The etiologic role of HPV in vulvar squamous cell carcinoma fine tuned. *Cancer Epidemiol Biomarkers Prev.* 2009;18(7):2061–2067.
8. Gargano JW, Wilkinson EJ, Unger ER, et al. Prevalence of human papillomavirus (HPV) types in vulvar cancer and VIN 3 in the United States before vaccine introduction. *J Low Genit Tract Dis.* 2012;16(4):471–479.
9. Joura EA, Garland S, Giuliano A, et al. End of study efficacy for vulvovaginal disease of a novel 9-valent HPV L1 virus-like particle vaccine in 26 year old women. *J Low Genit Tract Dis.* 2015;19(3 Suppl 1):S10.
10. de Sanjose S, Alemany L, Ordi J, et al. Worldwide human papillomavirus genotype attribution in over 2000 cases of intraepithelial and invasive lesions of the vulva. *Eur J Cancer.* 2013;49(16):3450–3461.
11. Basta A, Adamek K, Pitynski K. Intraepithelial neoplasia and early stage vulvar cancer. Epidemiological, clinical and virological observations. *Eur J Gynaecol Oncol.* 1999;20(2):111–114.
12. Preti M, Igidbashian S, Costa S, et al. VIN usual type-from the past to the future. *Ecancermedicalscience.* 2015;9:531.
13. American College of Obstetricians and Gynecologists. Management of vulvar intraepithelial neoplasia. *Obstet Gynecol.* 2014;118(509):1192–1194.
14. van de Nieuwenhof HP, van der Avoort IA, de Hullu JA. Review of squamous premalignant vulvar lesions. *Crit Rev Oncol Hematol.* 2008;68(2):131–156.
15. van de Nieuwenhof HP, Bulten J, Hollema H, et al. Differentiated vulvar intraepithelial neoplasia is often found in lesions, previously diagnosed as lichen sclerosus, which have progressed to vulvar squamous cell carcinoma. *Mod Pathol.* 2011;24(2):297–305.
16. Carli P, De Magnis A, Mannone F, et al. Vulvar carcinoma associated with lichen sclerosus: experience at the Florence, Italy, Vulvar Clinic. *J Reprod Med.* 2003;48(5):313–318.
17. Brown JE, Sunborg MJ, Kost E, et al. Vulvar cancer in human immunodeficiency virus-seropositive premenopausal women: a case series and review of the literature. *J Low Genit Tract Dis.* 2005;9(1):7–10.
18. Chaturvedi AK, Madeleine MM, Biggar RJ, et al. Risk of human papillomavirus-associated cancers among persons with AIDS. *J Natl Cancer Inst.* 2009;101(16):1120–1130.
19. Hussain SK, Madeleine MM, Johnson LG, et al. Cervical and vulvar cancer risk in relation to the joint effects of cigarette smoking and genetic variation in interleukin 2. *Cancer Epidemiol Biomarkers Prev.* 2008;17(7):1790–1799.
20. Micheletti L, Preti M, Radici G, et al. Vulvar lichen sclerosus and malignant transformation: a retrospective study of 976 cases. *J Low Genit Tract Dis.* 2016;20(3 Suppl 1):S8.
21. Lee A, Brandford J, Fisher G. Long-term management of adult vulvar lichen sclerosus. *J Low Genit Tract Dis.* 2015;19(3 Suppl 1):S23.
22. Preti M, Micheletti L, Ghiringhello B, et al. Squamous intraepithelial lesions of the vulva: 30 years of experience of a single center. *J Low Genit Tract Dis.* 2015;19(3 Suppl 1):S10.
23. Jones RW, Rowan DM, Stewart AW. Vulvar intraepithelial neoplasia: aspects of the natural history and outcome in 405 women. *Obstet Gynecol.* 2005;106(6):1319–1326.
24. Loch JR, Rush DS, Wilkinson EJ. Differentiated (simplex) vulvar intraepithelial neoplasia: a study of 18 cases with analysis of phosphohistone-H3 (PHH3), P53 and P16ink4a studies. *J Low Genit Tract Dis.* 2015;19 (3 Suppl 1):S5.
25. Trimble CL, Hildesheim A, Brinton LA, et al. Heterogeneous etiology of squamous carcinoma of the vulva. *Obstet Gynecol.* 1996;87(1):59–64.
26. Mitchell MF, Prasad CJ, Silva EG, et al. Second genital primary squamous neoplasms in vulvar carcinoma: viral and histopathologic correlates. *Obstet Gynecol.* 1993;81(1):13–18.
27. Gonzalez Bosquet J, Magrina JF, Magtibay PM, et al. Patterns of inguinal groin metastases in squamous cell carcinoma of the vulva. *Gynecol Oncol.* 2007;105(3):742–746.
28. Cohn DE, Dehdashti F, Gibb RK, et al. Prospective evaluation of positron emission tomography for the detection of groin node metastases from vulvar cancer. *Gynecol Oncol.* 2002;85(1):179–184.
29. Beneder C, Fuechsel FG, Krause T, et al. The role of 3D fusion imaging in sentinel lymphadenectomy for vulvar cancer. *Gynecol Oncol.* 2008;109(1):76–80.
30. Kobayashi K, Ramirez PT, Kim EE, et al. Sentinel node mapping in vulvovaginal melanoma using SPECT/CT lymphoscintigraphy. *Clin Nucl Med.* 2009;34(12):859–861.
31. Kataoka MY, Sala E, Baldwin P, et al. The accuracy of magnetic resonance imaging in staging of vulvar cancer: a retrospective multi-centre study. *Gynecol Oncol.* 2010;117(1):82–87.
32. de Bie RP, van de Nieuwenhof HP, Bekkers RL, et al. Patients with usual vulvar intraepithelial neoplasia-related vulvar cancer have an increased risk of cervical abnormalities. *Br J Cancer.* 2009;101(1):27–31.
33. Pecorelli S. Revised FIGO staging for carcinoma of the vulva, cervix, and endometrium. *Int J Gynecol Obstet.* 2009;105(2):103–104.
34. Hacker NF. Revised FIGO staging for carcinoma of the vulva. *Int J Gynaecol Obstet.* 2009;105(2):105–106.
35. Darragh TM, Colgan TJ, Cox JT, et al. The lower anogenital squamous terminology standardization project for HPV-associated lesions: background and consensus recommendations from the College of American Pathologists and the American Society for Colposcopy and Cervical Pathology. *J Low Genit Tract Dis.* 2012;16(3):205–242.
36. Yoder BJ, Rufforny I, Massoll NA, et al. Stage IA vulvar squamous cell carcinoma—an analysis of tumor invasive characteristics and risk. *Am J Surg Pathol.* 2008;32(5):765–772.
37. Edge S, Byrd DR, Compton CC, et al. *AJCC Cancer Staging Manual.* New York, NY: Springer; 2009.

38. Moxley KM, Fader AN, Rose PG, et al. Malignant melanoma of the vulva: an extension of cutaneous melanoma? *Gynecol Oncol.* 2011;122(3):612–617.
39. Wilkinson EJ, Stone IK. *Atlas of Vulvar Disease.* 3rd ed. New York, NY: Wolters Kluwer/Lippincott Williams & Wilkins Philadelphia; 2012.
40. Jones RW, Sadler L, Grant S, et al. Clinically identifying women with vulvar lichen sclerosus at increased risk of squamous cell carcinoma: a case-control study. *J Reprod Med.* 2004;49(10):808–811.
41. Kurman RJ, Ronnett J, Sherman ME, et al. *Tumors of the Cervix, Vagina, and Vulva.* Washington, DC: Armed Forces Institute of Pathology; 2010.
42. Crum CP, Hereington CS, McCluggage WG, et al. *Epithelial Tumors.* 4th ed. Lyon, France: IRAC; 2014.
43. Wilkinson EJ. Protocol for the examination of specimens from patients with carcinomas and malignant melanomas of the vulva: a basis for checklists. Cancer Committee of the American College of Pathologists. *Arch Pathol Lab Med.* 2000;124(1):51–56.
44. Horn LC, Liebert UG, Edelmann J, et al. Adenoid squamous carcinoma (pseudoangiosarcomatous carcinoma) of the vulva: a rare but highly aggressive variant of squamous cell carcinoma-report of a case and review of the literature. *Int J Gynecol Pathol.* 2008;27(2):288–291.
45. Wilkinson EJ, Croker BP, Friedrich EG, Jr, et al. Two distinct pathologic types of giant cell tumor of the vulva: a report of two cases. *J Reprod Med.* 1988;33(6):519–522.
46. Carlson JW, McGlennen RC, Gomez R, et al. Sebaceous carcinoma of the vulva: a case report and review of the literature. *Gynecol Oncol.* 1996;60(3):489–491.
47. Escalonilla P, Grilli R, Canamero M, et al. Sebaceous carcinoma of the vulva. *Am J Dermatopathol.* 1999;21(5):468–472.
48. Copas P, Dyer M, Comas FV, et al. Spindle cell carcinoma of the vulva. *Diagn Gynecol Obstet.* 1982;4(3):235–241.
49. de Giorgi V, Salvini C, Massi D, et al. Vulvar basal cell carcinoma: retrospective study and review of literature. *Gynecol Oncol.* 2005;97(1):192–194.
50. Sinn HP, Mayer C, Kommoss F. Clinical presentation and pathologic features of vulvar basal cell carcinomas. *J Low Genit Tract Dis.* 2015;19 (3 Suppl 1):S22.
51. Crum CP, Herrington CS, McGluggage WG, et al. *Neuroendocrine Tumors.* 4th ed. Lyon, France: IRAC; 2014.
52. Vang R, Taubenberger JK, Mannion CM, et al. Primary vulvar and vaginal extraosseous Ewing's sarcoma/peripheral neuroectodermal tumor: diagnostic confirmation with CD99 immunostaining and reverse transcriptase-polymerase chain reaction. *Int J Gynecol Pathol.* 2000;19(2):103–109.
53. Takeshima N, Tabata T, Nishida H, et al. Peripheral primitive neuroectodermal tumor of the vulva: report of a case with imprint cytology. *Acta Cytol.* 2001;45(6):1049–1052.
54. Wilkinson EJ, Crum CP, Herrington CS, et al. *Neuroectodermal Tumors.* 4th ed. Lyon, France: IRAC; 2014.
55. Wilkinson EJ, Brown HM. Vulvar Paget disease of urothelial origin: a report of three cases and a proposed classification of vulvar Paget disease. *Hum Pathol.* 2002;33(5):549–554.
56. Bhalwal AB, Nick AM, Dos Reis R, et al. Carcinoma of the bartholin gland: a review of 33 cases. *Int J Gynecol Cancer.* 2016;26(4):785–789.
56a. Delport ES. Extramammary Paget's disease of the vulva: an annotated review of the current literature. *Australas J Dermatol.* 2013;54(1):9–21.
56b. Jones IS, Crandon A, Sanday K. Paget's disease of the vulva: diagnosis and follow-up key to management; a retrospective study of 50 cases from Queensland. 2011;122(1):42–44.
57. Malik SN, Wilkinson EJ. Pseudo-Paget's disease of the vulva: a case report. *J Low Genit Tract Dis.* 1999;3(1):55.
58. Crawford D, Nimmo M, Clement PB, et al. Prognostic factors in Paget's disease of the vulva: a study of 21 cases. *Int J Gynecol Pathol.* 1999;18(4):351–359.
59. Newsom K, Alizadeh L, Al-Quran SZ, et al. Use of GATA-3 and uroplakin-II in differentiating primary cutaneous vulvar paget disease from pagetoid urothelial intraepithelial neoplasia. *J Low Genit Tract Dis.* 2015;19(3 Suppl 1):S6.
60. Panizzon RG. Vulvar melanoma. *Semin Dermatol.* 1996;15(1):67–70.
61. Ragnarsson-Olding BK, Nilsson BR, Kanter-Lewensohn LR, et al. Malignant melanoma of the vulva in a nationwide, 25-year study of 219 Swedish females: predictors of survival. *Cancer.* 1999;86(7):1285–1293.
62. Raspagliesi F, Ditto A, Paladini D, et al. Prognostic indicators in melanoma of the vulva. *Ann Surg Oncol.* 2000;7(10):738–742.
63. Wechter ME, Reynolds RK, Haefner HK, et al. Vulvar melanoma: review of diagnosis, staging, and therapy. *J Low Genit Tract Dis.* 2004;8(1):58–69.
64. Piura B, Rabinovich A, Dgani R. Malignant melanoma of the vulva: report of six cases and review of the literature. *Eur J Gynaecol Oncol.* 1999;20(3):182–186.
65. Benda JA, Platz CE, Anderson B. Malignant melanoma of the vulva: a clinical-pathologic review of 16 cases. *Int J Gynecol Pathol.* 1986;5(3):202–216.
66. Balch CM, Gershenwald JE, Soong SJ, et al. Final version of 2009 AJCC melanoma staging and classification. *J Clin Oncol.* 2009;27(36):6199–6206.
67. Nucci MR, Ganesan R, McGluggage WG, et al. *Soft Tissue Tumors.* 4th ed. Lyon, France: IRAC; 2014.
68. Vural B, Ozkan S, Yildiz K, et al. Malignant fibrous histiocytoma of the vulva: a case report. *Arch Gynecol Obstet.* 2005;273(2):122–125.
69. Han CH, Li X, Khanna N. Epithelioid sarcoma of the vulva and its clinical implication: a case report and review of the literature. *Gynecol Oncol Rep.* 2016;15:31–33.
70. Nucci MR, Fletcher CD. Vulvovaginal soft tissue tumours: update and review. *Histopathology.* 2000;36(2):97–108.
71. Chokoeva AA, Tchernev G, Cardoso JC, et al. Vulvar sarcomas—short guideline for histopathological recognition and clinical management. Part 1. *Int J Immunopathol Pharmacol.* 2015;28(2):178–186.
72. Nielsen GP, Young RH. Mesenchymal tumors and tumor-like lesions of the female genital tract: a selective review with emphasis on recently described entities. *Int J Gynecol Pathol.* 2001;20(2):105–127.
73. Sims SM, Stinson K, McLean FW, et al. Angiomyofibroblastoma of the vulva: a case report of a pedunculated variant and review of the literature. *J Low Genit Tract Dis.* 2012;16(2):149–154.
74. Lerner LB, Andrews SJ, Gonzalez JL, et al. Vulvar metastases secondary to transitional cell carcinoma of the bladder: a case report. *J Reprod Med.* 1999;44(8):729–732.
75. Vang R, Medeiros LJ, Malpica A, et al. Non-Hodgkin's lymphoma involving the vulva. *Int J Gynecol Pathol.* 2000;19(3):236–242.
76. Neto AG, Deavers MT, Silva EG, et al. Metastatic tumors of the vulva: a clinicopathologic study of 66 cases. *Am J Surg Pathol.* 2003;27(6): 799–804.
77. Raspagliesi F, Hanozet F, Ditto A, et al. Clinical and pathological prognostic factors in squamous cell carcinoma of the vulva. *Gynecol Oncol.* 2006;102(2):333–337.
78. Maggino T, Landoni F, Sartori E, et al. Patterns of recurrence in patints with squamous cell carcinoma of the vulva: a multicenter CTF Study. *Cancer.* 2000;89(1):116–122.
79. Gonzalez Bosquet J, Magrina JF, Gaffey TA, et al. Long-term survival and disease recurrence in patients with primary squamous cell carcinoma of the vulva. *Gynecol Oncol.* 2005;97(3):828–833.
80. Chan JK, Sugiyama V, Pham H, et al. Margin distance and other clinico-pathologic prognostic factors in vulvar carcinoma: a multivariate analysis. *Gynecol Oncol.* 2007;104(3):636–641.
81. Heaps JM, Fu YS, Montz FJ, et al. Surgical-pathologic variables predictive of local recurrence in squamous cell carcinoma of the vulva. *Gynecol Oncol.* 1990;38(3):309–314.
82. De Hullu JA, Hollema H, Lolkema S, et al. Vulvar carcinoma: the price of less radical surgery. *Cancer.* 2002;95(11):2331–2338.
83. Hoffman MS, Gunesakaran S, Arango H, et al. Lateral microscopic extension of squamous cell carcinoma of the vulva. *Gynecol Oncol.* 1999;73(1):72–75.
84. Luchini C, Nottegar A, Solmi M, et al. Prognostic implications of extranodal extension in node-positive squamous cell carcinoma of the vulva: a systematic review and meta-analysis. *Surg Oncol.* 2016;25(1):60–65.
85. Oonk MH, Hollema H, de Hullu JA, et al. Prediction of lymph node metastases in vulvar cancer: a review. *Int J Gynecol Cancer.* 2006;16(3):963–971.
86. Bipat S, Fransen GA, Spijkerboer AM, et al. Is there a role for magnetic resonance imaging in the evaluation of inguinal lymph node metastases in patients with vulva carcinoma? *Gynecol Oncol.* 2006;103(3):1001–1006.
87. Taussig LR, Torrey FA. Malignant melanoma: a statistical and pathological review of thirty-five cases. *Cal West Med.* 1940;52(1):15–18.
88. Fuh KC, Berek JS. Current management of vulvar cancer. *Hematol Oncol Clin North Am.* 2012;26(1):45–62.
89. Moore DH, Ali S, Koh WJ, et al. A phase II trial of radiation therapy and weekly cisplatin chemotherapy for the treatment of locally-advanced squamous cell carcinoma of the vulva: a gynecologic oncology group study. *Gynecol Oncol.* 2012;124(3):529–533.
90. Morton DL, Wen DR, Foshag LJ, et al. Intraoperative lymphatic mapping and selective cervical lymphadenectomy for early-stage melanomas of the head and neck. *J Clin Oncol.* 1993;11(9):1751–1756.
91. Levenback C, Burke TW, Gershenson DM, et al. Intraoperative lymphatic mapping for vulvar cancer. *Obstet Gynecol.* 1994;84(2):163–167.
92. Levenback C, Burke TW, Morris M, et al. Potential applications of intraoperative lymphatic mapping in vulvar cancer. *Gynecol Oncol.* 1995;59(2):216–220.

93. Decesare SL, Fiorica JV, Roberts WS, et al. A pilot study utilizing intraoperative lymphoscintigraphy for identification of the sentinel lymph nodes in vulvar cancer. *Gynecol Oncol.* 1997;66(3):425–428.
94. Van der Zee AG, Oonk MH, De Hullu JA, et al. Sentinel node dissection is safe in the treatment of early-stage vulvar cancer. *J Clin Oncol.* 2008;26(6):884–889.
95. te Grootenhuis NC, van der Zee AG, van Doorn HC, et al. Sentinel nodes in vulvar cancer: long-term follow-up of the GROningen INternational Study on Sentinel nodes in Vulvar cancer (GROINSS-V) I. *Gynecol Oncol.* 2016;140(1):8–14.
96. Levenback CF, Ali S, Coleman RL, et al. Lymphatic mapping and sentinel lymph node biopsy in women with squamous cell carcinoma of the vulva: a gynecologic oncology group study. *J Clin Oncol.* 2012;30(31):3786–3791.
97. Stehman FB, Ali S, DiSaia PJ. Node count and groin recurrence in early vulvar cancer: a gynecologic oncology group study. *Gynecol Oncol.* 2009;113(1):52–56.
98. Barton DP, Berman C, Cavanagh D, et al. Lymphoscintigraphy in vulvar cancer: a pilot study. *Gynecol Oncol.* 1992;46(3):341–344.
99. Chafe W, Richards A, Morgan L, et al. Unrecognized invasive carcinoma in vulvar intraepithelial neoplasia (VIN). *Gynecol Oncol.* 1988;31(1):154–165.
100. Modesitt SC, Waters AB, Walton L, et al. Vulvar intraepithelial neoplasia III: occult cancer and the impact of margin status on recurrence. *Obstet Gynecol.* 1998;92(6):962–966.
101. Burke TW, Levenback CF, Coleman RC. Surgical therapy of T1 and T2 vulvar carcinoma—further experience with radical wide excision and selective inguinal lymphadenectomy. *Gynecol Oncol.* 1995;57:215–219.
102. Coleman RL, Ali S, Levenback CF, et al. Is bilateral lymphadenectomy for midline squamous carcinoma of the vulva always necessary? An analysis from Gynecologic Oncology Group (GOG) 173. *Gynecol Oncol.* 2013;128(2):155–159.
103. de Mooij Y, Burger MP, Schilthuis MS, et al. Partial urethral resection in the surgical treatment of vulvar cancer does not have a significant impact on urinary continence. A confirmation of an authority-based opinion. *Int J Gynecol Cancer.* 2007;17(1):294–297.
104. Hyde SE, Valmadre S, Hacker NF, et al. Squamous cell carcinoma of the vulva with bulky positive groin nodes-nodal debulking versus full groin dissection prior to radiation therapy. *Int J Gynecol Cancer.* 2007;17(1):154–158.
105. Kunos C, Simpkins F, Gibbons H, et al. Radiation therapy compared with pelvic node resection for node-positive vulvar cancer—a randomized controlled trial. *Obstet Gynecol.* 2009;114(3):537–546.
106. Parthasarathy A, Cheung MK, Osann K, et al. The benefit of adjuvant radiation therapy in single-node-positive squamous cell vulvar carcinoma. *Gynecol Oncol.* 2006;103(3):1095–1099.
107. Shylasree T, Bryant A, Howells R. Chemoradiation for advanced primary vulval cancer [review]. *Cochrane Database Syst Rev.* 2011;(4):CD003752.
108. Mahner S, Jueckstock J, Hilpert F, et al. Adjuvant therapy in lymph node-positive vulvar cancer: the AGO-CaRE-1 study. *J Natl Cancer Inst.* 2015;107(3).
109. Piura B, Masotina A, Murdoch J, et al. Recurrent squamous cell carcinoma of the vulva: a study of 73 cases. *Gynecol Oncol.* 1993;48(2):189–195.
110. Sugiyama VE, Chan JK, Shin JY, et al. Vulvar melanoma: a multivariable analysis of 644 patients. *Obstet Gynecol.* 2007;110(2 pt 1):296–301.
111. Phillips GL, Bundy BN, Okagaki T, et al. Malignant melanoma of the vulva treated by radical hemivulvectomy. A prospective study of the Gynecologic Oncology Group. *Cancer.* 1994;73(10):2626–2632.
112. Janco JM, Markovic SN, Weaver AL, et al. Vulvar and vaginal melanoma: case series and review of current management options including neoadjuvant chemotherapy. *Gynecol Oncol.* 2013;129(3):533–537.
113. Lui PC, Fan YS, Lau PP, et al. Vulvar basal cell carcinoma in China: a 13-year review. *Am J Obstet Gynecol.* 2009;200(5):514. e511–e515.
114. Creasman WT, Gallager HS, Rutledge F. Paget's disease of the vulva. *Gynecol Oncol.* 1975;3(2):133–148.
115. Fanning J, Lambert HC, Hale TM, et al. Paget's disease of the vulva: prevalence of associated vulvar adenocarcinoma, invasive Paget's disease, and recurrence after surgical excision. *Am J Obstet Gynecol.* 1999;180(1 pt 1):24–27.
116. Ciavattini A, Sopracordevole F, Di Giuseppe J. Surgical treatment of Paget disease of the vulva- prognostic significance of stromal invasion and surgical margin status. *J Low Genit Tract Dis.* 2016;20(2):1–5.
117. Niikura H, Yoshida H, Ito K, et al. Paget's disease of the vulva: clinicopathologic study of type 1 cases treated at a single institution. *Int J Gynecol Cancer.* 2006;16(3):1212–1215.
118. Black D, Tornos C, Soslow RA, et al. The outcomes of patients with positive margins after excision for intraepithelial Paget's disease of the vulva. *Gynecol Oncol.* 2007;104(3):547–550.
119. Ho SA, Aw DC. Extramammary Paget's disease treated with topical imiquimod 5% cream. *Dermatol Ther.* 2010;23(4):423–427.
120. Feldmeyer L, Kerl K, Kamarashev J, et al. Treatment of vulvar Paget disease with topical imiquimod: a case report and review of the literature. *J Dermatol Case Rep.* 2011;5(3):42–46.
121. Zweizig S, Korets S, Cain JM. Key concepts in management of vulvar cancer. *Best Pract Res Clin Obstet Gynaecol.* 2014;28(7):959–966.
122. Gaarenstroom KN, Kenter GG, Trimbos JB, et al. Postoperative complications after vulvectomy and inguinofemoral lymphadenectomy using separate groin incisions. *Int J Gynecol Cancer.* 2003;13(4):522–527.
123. Burke TW, Stringer CA, Gershenson DM, et al. Radical wide excision and selective inguinal node dissection for squamous cell carcinoma of the vulva. *Gynecol Oncol.* 1990;38(3):328–332.
124. Burke TW, Levenback C, Coleman RL, et al. Surgical therapy of T1 and T2 vulvar carcinoma: further experience with radical wide excision and selective inguinal lymphadenectomy. *Gynecol Oncol.* 1995;57(2):215–220.
125. Berman ML, Soper JT, Creasman WT, et al. Conservative surgical management of superficially invasive stage I vulvar carcinoma. *Gynecol Oncol.* 1989;35(3):352–357
126. Stehman FB, Bundy BN, Dvoretsky PM, et al. Early stage I carcinoma of the vulva treated with ipsilateral superficial inguinal lymphadenectomy and modified radical hemivulvectomy: a prospective study of the Gynecologic Oncology Group. *Obstet Gynecol.* 1992;79(4):490–497.
127. Gordinier ME, Malpica A, Burke TW, et al. Groin recurrence in patients with vulvar cancer with negative nodes on superficial inguinal lymphadenectomy. *Gynecol Oncol.* 2003;90(3):625–628.
128. Slomovitz BM, Coleman RL, Oonk MH, et al. Update on sentinel lymph node biopsy for early-stage vulvar cancer. *Gynecol Oncol.* 2015;138(2):472–477.
129. Covens A, Vella ET, Kennedy EB, et al. Sentinel lymph node biopsy in vulvar cancer: Systematic review, meta-analysis and guideline recommendations. *Gynecol Oncol.* 2015;137(2):351–361.
130. de Hullu JA, Hollema H, Piers DA, et al. Sentinel lymph node procedure is highly accurate in squamous cell carcinoma of the vulva. *J Clin Oncol.* 2000;18(15):2811–2816.
131. Levenback C, Coleman RL, Burke TW, et al. Intraoperative lymphatic mapping and sentinel node identification with blue dye in patients with vulvar cancer. *Gynecol Oncol.* 2001;83(2):276–281.
132. Zivanovic O, Khoury-Collado F, Abu-Rustum NR, et al. Sentinel lymph node biopsy in the management of vulvar carcinoma, cervical cancer, and endometrial cancer. *Oncologist.* 2009;14(7):695–705.
133. Meads C, Sutton AJ, Rosenthal AN, et al. Sentinel lymph node biopsy in vulval cancer: systematic review and meta-analysis. *Br J Cancer.* 2014;110(12):2837–2846.
134. Hopkins MP, Reid GC, Morley GW. The surgical management of recurrent squamous cell carcinoma of the vulva. *Obstet Gynecol.* 1990;75(6):1001–1005.
135. Abitbol MM. Carcinoma of the vulva: improvements in the surgical approach. *Am J Obstet Gynecol.* 1973;117(4):483–489.
136. Hacker NF, Eifel PJ, van der Velden J. Cancer of the vulva. *Int J Gynaecol Obstet.* 2012;119(suppl 2):S90–S96.
137. Miller B, Morris M, Levenback C, et al. Pelvic exenteration for primary and recurrent vulvar cancer. *Gynecol Oncol.* 1995;58(2):202–205.
138. Forner DM, Lampe B. Exenteration in the treatment of stage III/IV vulvar cancer. *Gynecol Oncol.* 2012;124(1):87–91.
139. Yii NW, Niranjan NS. Lotus petal flaps in vulvo-vaginal reconstruction. *Br J Plast Surg.* 1996;49(8):547–554.
140. Sawada M, Kimata Y, Kasamatsu T, et al. Versatile lotus petal flap for vulvoperineal reconstruction after gynecological ablative surgery. *Gynecol Oncol.* 2004;95(2):330–335.
141. McMenamin DM, Clements D, Edwards TJ, et al. Rectus abdominis myocutaneous flaps for perineal reconstruction: modifications to the technique based on a large single-centre experience. *Ann R Coll Surg Engl.* 2011;93(5):375–381.
142. Cormio G, Loizzi V, Carriero C, et al. Groin recurrence in carcinoma of the vulva: management and outcome. *Eur J Cancer Care (Engl).* 2010;19(3):302–307.
143. John HE, Jessop ZM, Di Candia M, et al. An algorithmic approach to perineal reconstruction after cancer resection—experience from two international centers. *Ann Plast Surg.* 2013;71(1):96–102.
144. Argenta PA, Lindsay R, Aldridge RB, et al. Vulvar reconstruction using the "lotus petal" fascio-cutaneous flap. *Gynecol Oncol.* 2013;131(3):726–729.
145. Franchelli S, Leone MS, Bruzzone M, et al. The gluteal fold fascio-cutaneous flap for reconstruction after radical excision of primary vulvar cancers. *Gynecol Oncol.* 2009;113(2):245–248.
146. Buda A, Confalonieri PL, Rovati LC, et al. Tunneled modified lotus petal flap for surgical reconstruction of severe introital stenosis after radical vulvectomy. *Int J Surg Case Rep.* 2012;3(7):299–301.

147. Vitale SG, Valenti G, Biondi A, et al. Recent trends in surgical and reconstructive management of vulvar cancer: review of literature. *Updates Surg.* 2015;67(4):367–371.
148. Petrie N, Branagan G, McGuiness C, et al. Reconstruction of the perineum following anorectal cancer excision. *Int J Colorectal Dis.* 2009;24(1):97–104.
149. Helgason NM, Hass AC, Latourette HB. Radiation therapy in carcinoma of the vulva: a review of 53 patients. *Cancer.* 1972;30(4):997–1000.
150. Busch M, Wagener B, Duhmke E. Long-term results of radiotherapy alone for carcinoma of the vulva. *Adv Ther.* 1999;16(2):89–100.
151. Binder SW, Huang I, Fu YS, et al. Risk factors for the development of lymph node metastasis in vulvar squamous cell carcinoma. *Gynecol Oncol.* 1990;37(1):9–16.
152. Faul CM, Mirmow D, Huang Q, et al. Adjuvant radiation for vulvar carcinoma: improved local control. *Int J Radiat Oncol Biol Phys.* 1997;38(2):381–389.
153. Viswanathan AN, Pinto AP, Schultz D, et al. Relationship of margin status and radiation dose to recurrence in post-operative vulvar carcinoma. *Gynecol Oncol.* 2013;130(3):545–549.
154. Glaser S, Olawaiye A, Huang M, et al. Inguinal nodal region radiotherapy for vulvar cancer: are we missing the target again? *Gynecol Oncol.* 2014;135(3):583–585.
155. Stehman FB, Bundy BN, Thomas G, et al. Groin dissection versus groin radiation in carcinoma of the vulva: a Gynecologic Oncology Group study. *Int J Radiat Oncol Biol Phys.* 1992;24(2):389–396.
156. Koh WJ, Chiu M, Stelzer KJ, et al. Femoral vessel depth and the implications for groin node radiation. *Int J Radiat Oncol Biol Phys.* 1993;27(4):969–974.
157. Eifel PJ. Vulvar carcinoma: radiotherapy or surgery for the lymphatics? *Front Radiat Ther Oncol.* 1994;28:218–225.
158. Katz A, Eifel PJ, Jhingran A, et al. The role of radiation therapy in preventing regional recurrences of invasive squamous cell carcinoma of the vulva. *Int J Radiat Oncol Biol Phys.* 2003;57(2):409–418.
159. Leiserowitz GS, Russell AH, Kinney WK, et al. Prophylactic chemoradiation of inguinofemoral lymph nodes in patients with locally extensive vulvar cancer. *Gynecol Oncol.* 1997;66(3):509–514.
160. Manavi M, Berger A, Kucera E, Vavra N, Kucera H. Does T1, N0-1 vulvar cancer treated by vulvectomy but not lymphadenectomy need inguinofemoral radiation? *Int J Radiat Oncol Biol Phys.* 1997;38(4):749–753.
161. Beriwal S, Shukla G, Shinde A, et al. Preoperative intensity modulated radiation therapy and chemotherapy for locally advanced vulvar carcinoma: analysis of pattern of relapse. *Int J Radiat Oncol Biol Phys.* 2013;85(5):1269–1274.
162. Hacker NF, Berek JS, Juillard GJ, et al. Preoperative radiation therapy for locally advanced vulvar cancer. *Cancer.* 1984;54(10):2056–2061.
163. Homesley HD, Bundy BN, Sedlis A, et al. Radiation therapy versus pelvic node resection for carcinoma of the vulva with positive groin nodes. *Obstet Gynecol.* 1986;68(6):733–740.
164. Xanthopoulos E, Mitra N, Grover S, et al. Adjuvant radiation therapy in node-positive vulvar cancer. *Int J Radiat Oncol Biol Phys.* 2013;87(2):S128–S129.
165. Oonk MH, van Hemel BM, Hollema H, et al. Size of sentinel-node metastasis and chances of non-sentinel-node involvement and survival in early stage vulvar cancer: results from GROINSS-V, a multicentre observational study. *Lancet Oncol.* 2010;11(7):646–652.
166. Jafari K, Magalotti F, Magalotti M. Radiation therapy in carcinoma of the vulva. *Cancer.* 1981;47(4):686–691.
167. Moore DH, Thomas GM, Montana GS, et al. Preoperative chemoradiation for advanced vulvar cancer—a phase II study of the gynecologic oncology group. *Int J Radiat Oncol Biol Phys.* 1998;42(1):79–85.
168. Mak RH, Halasz LM, Tanaka CK, et al. Outcomes after radiation therapy with concurrent weekly platinum-based chemotherapy or every-3-4-week 5-fluorouracil-containing regimens for squamous cell carcinoma of the vulva. *Gynecol Oncol.* 2011;120(1):101–107.
169. DeFoe SG, Beriwal S, Jones H, et al. Concurrent chemotherapy and intensity-modulated radiation therapy for anal carcinoma-clinical outcomes in a large National Cancer Institute-designated integrated cancer centre network. *Clin Oncol (R Coll Radiol).* 2012;24(6):424–431.
170. Prempree T, Amornmarn R. Radiation treatment of recurrent carcinoma of the vulva. *Cancer.* 1984;54(9):1943–1949.
171. Koay EJ, Jhingran A, Klopp AH, et al. Definitive radiation therapy of locally advanced squamous cell carcinoma of the vulva: factors associated with vulvar disease control. *Int J Radiat Oncol Biol Phys.* 2012;84(3):S460.
172. Hoffman M, Greenberg S, Greenberg H, et al. Interstitial radiotherapy for the treatment of advanced or recurrent vulvar and distal vaginal malignancy. *Am J Obstet Gynecol.* 1990;162(5):1278–1282.
173. Tewari K, Cappuccini F, Syed AM, et al. Interstitial brachytherapy in the treatment of advanced and recurrent vulvar cancer. *Am J Obstet Gynecol.* 1999;181(1):91–98.
174. Kim CH, Olson AC, Kim H, et al. Contouring inguinal and femoral nodes; how much margin is needed around the vessels? *Pract Radiat Oncol.* 2012;2(4):274–278.
175. Beriwal S, Heron DE, Kim H, et al. Intensity-modulated radiotherapy for the treatment of vulvar carcinoma: a comparative dosimetric study with early clinical outcome. *Int J Radiat Oncol Biol Phys.* 2006;64(5):1395–1400.
176. Beriwal S, Coon D, Heron DE, et al. Preoperative intensity-modulated radiotherapy and chemotherapy for locally advanced vulvar carcinoma. *Gynecol Oncol.* 2008;109(2):291–295.
177. Kachnic LA, Winter K, Myerson RJ, et al. RTOG 0529: a phase 2 evaluation of dose-painted intensity modulated radiation therapy in combination with 5-fluorouracil and mitomycin-C for the reduction of acute morbidity in carcinoma of the anal canal. *Int J Radiat Oncol Biol Phys.* 2013;86(1):27–33.
178. Barton DP. The prevention and management of treatment related morbidity in vulval cancer. *Best Pract Res Clin Obstet Gynaecol.* 2003;17(4):683–701.
179. Klopp AH, Moughan J, Portelance L, et al. Hematologic toxicity in RTOG 0418: a phase 2 study of postoperative IMRT for gynecologic cancer. *Int J Radiat Oncol Biol Phys.* 2013;86(1):83–90.
180. Baxter NN, Habermann EB, Tepper JE, et al. Risk of pelvic fractures in older women following pelvic irradiation. *JAMA.* 2005;294(20):2587–2593.
181. Ikushima H, Osaki K, Furutani S, et al. Pelvic bone complications following radiation therapy of gynecologic malignancies: clinical evaluation of radiation-induced pelvic insufficiency fractures. *Gynecol Oncol.* 2006;103(3):1100–1104.
182. Geisler JP, Manahan KJ, Buller RE. Neoadjuvant chemotherapy in vulvar cancer: avoiding primary exenteration. *Gynecol Oncol.* 2006;100(1):53–57.
183. Raspagliesi F, Zanaboni F, Martinelli F, et al. Role of paclitaxel and cisplatin as the neoadjuvant treatment for locally advanced squamous cell carcinoma of the vulva. *J Gynecol Oncol.* 2014;25(1):22–29.
184. Aragona AM, Cuneo N, Soderini AH, et al. Tailoring the treatment of locally advanced squamous cell carcinoma of the vulva: neoadjuvant chemotherapy followed by radical surgery: results from a multicenter study. *Int J Gynecol Cancer.* 2012;22(7):1258–1263.
185. Witteveen PO, van der Velden J, Vergote I, et al. Phase II study on paclitaxel in patients with recurrent, metastatic or locally advanced vulvar cancer not amenable to surgery or radiotherapy: a study of the EORTC-GCG (European Organisation for Research and Treatment of Cancer--Gynaecological Cancer Group). *Ann Oncol.* 2009;20(9):1511–1516.
186. Thigpen JT, Blessing JA, Homesley HD, et al. Phase II trials of cisplatin and piperazinedione in advanced or recurrent squamous cell carcinoma of the vulva: a Gynecologic Oncology Group Study. *Gynecol Oncol.* 1986;23(3):358–363.
187. Muss HB, Bundy BN, Christopherson WA. Mitoxantrone in the treatment of advanced vulvar and vaginal carcinoma: a gynecologic oncology group study. *Am J Clin Oncol.* 1989;12(2):142–144.
188. Cormio G, Loizzi V, Gissi F, et al. Cisplatin and vinorelbine chemotherapy in recurrent vulvar carcinoma. *Oncology.* 2009;77(5):281–284.
189. Akl A, Akl M, Boike G, et al. Preliminary results of chemoradiation as a primary treatment for vulvar carcinoma. *Int J Radiat Oncol Biol Phys.* 2000;48(2):415–420.
190. Olawaiye A, Lee LM, Krasner C, et al. Treatment of squamous cell vulvar cancer with the anti-EGFR tyrosine kinase inhibitor Tarceva. *Gynecol Oncol.* 2007;106(3):628–630.
191. Bacha OM, Levesque E, Renaud MC, et al. A case of recurrent vulvar carcinoma treated with erlotinib, an EGFR inhibitor. *Eur J Gynaecol Oncol.* 2011;32(4):423–424.
192. Tewari KS, Sill MW, Long HJ, III, et al. Improved survival with bevacizumab in advanced cervical cancer. *N Engl J Med.* 2014;370(8):734–743.
193. Landrum LM, Lanneau GS, Skaggs VJ, et al. Gynecologic Oncology Group risk groups for vulvar carcinoma: improvement in survival in the modern era. *Gynecol Oncol.* 2007;106(3):521–525.
194. Clifford GM, Polesel J, Rickenbach M, et al. Cancer risk in the Swiss HIV Cohort Study: associations with immunodeficiency, smoking, and highly active antiretroviral therapy. *J Natl Cancer Inst.* 2005;97(6):425–432.
195. Santoso JT, Crigger M, English E, et al. Smoking cessation counseling in women with genital intraepithelial neoplasia. *Gynecol Oncol.* 2012;125(3):716–719.
196. Graebe K, Garcia-Soto A, Aziz M, et al. Incidental power morcellation of malignancy: a retrospective cohort study. *Gynecol Oncol.* 2015;136(2):274–277.

CHAPTER 19

Vaginal Cancer

Josephine Kang, Amanda N. Fader, and Akila Viswanathan

ANATOMY

The vagina is a fibromuscular tube that extends from the cervix down to the vestibule, or cleft, between the labia minora. The average length of the vagina is 3 to 4 inches. Superiorly, it joins the uterine cervix at an angle and, as a result, the posterior vaginal wall is longer than the anterior wall. The upper aspect of the posterior vaginal wall is separated from the rectum by a peritoneal reflection known as the pouch of Douglas. Invaginations between the vaginal mucosa and cervix form the anterior, posterior, and lateral fornices. Laterally, the vagina is adjacent to the pelvic fascia and levator ani muscles. Inferiorly, the vagina extends through the urogenital diaphragm to lie dorsal to the urethra and ventral to the rectum. The fibromuscular perineal body separates the vagina from the anal canal. At the introitus, the vagina has a perforated fold of thin connective tissue and mucous membrane known as the hymen (**Fig. 19.1**).

The vaginal wall comprises the mucosa, muscularis, and adventitia. The innermost lining of the vagina is formed by a nonkeratinizing, stratified squamous epithelium overlying a basement membrane. Underneath the mucosa is connective tissue composed of elastin, and a thick muscularis layer composed of two layers of smooth muscle. The inner layer is arranged circularly, whereas the outer layer is arranged longitudinally. This muscular layer is covered by the third layer, a thin adventitia that merges with neighboring organs. This epithelial mucosa lacks glandular structures, and instead receives lubrication from mucous secretions originating in the cervix.

The vagina has a complex, extensive network of lymphatic drainage, with vessels that course through the submucosal and muscularis layer.

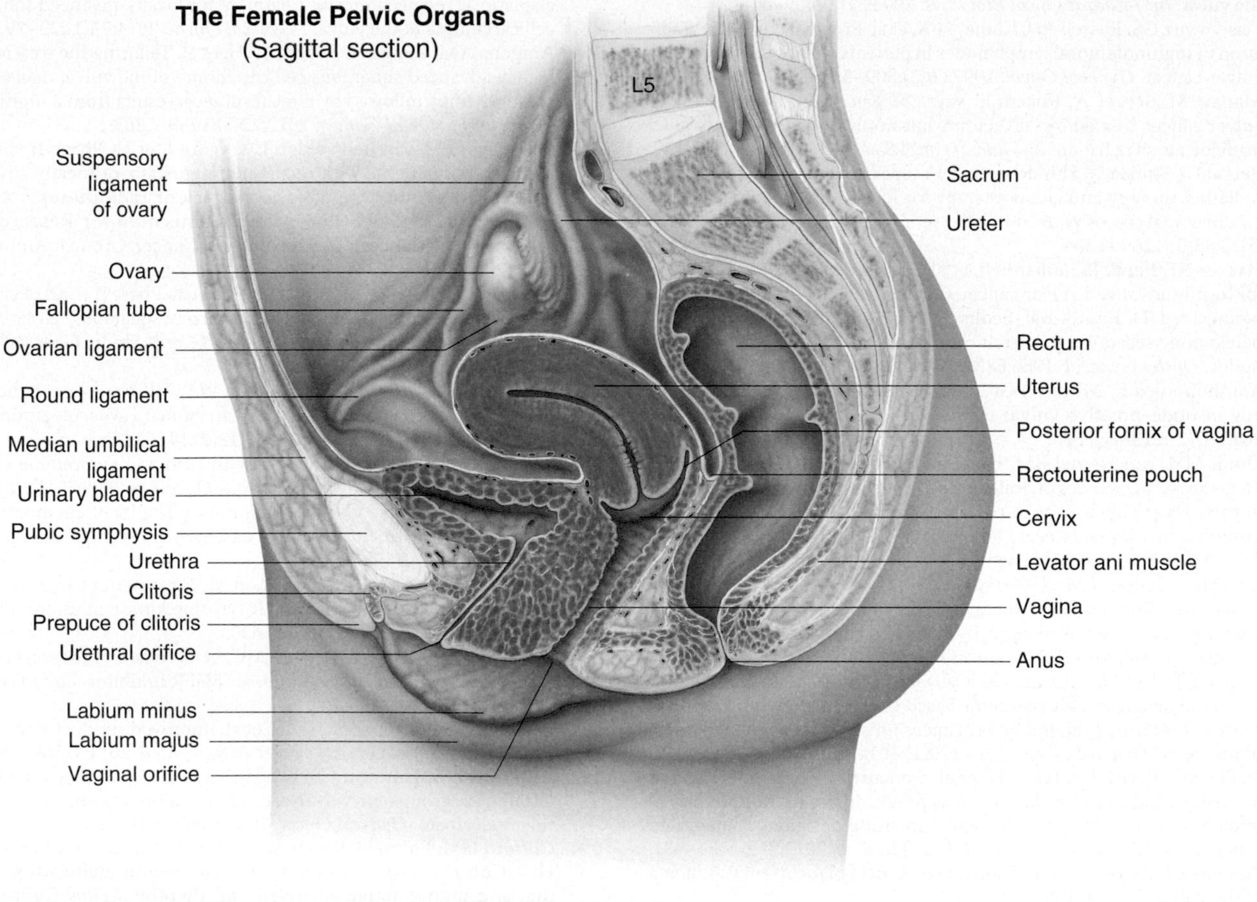

Figure 19.1. The lower female pelvis in sagittal view. The vagina is a fibromuscular tube situated posterior to the bladder and urethra and anterior to the rectum. The anterior and posterior fornices are formed by protrusion of the cervix into the vaginal canal.

Source: Reproduced from Anatomical Chart Company, Female Reproductive System Anatomical Chart, Philadelphia, PA: Wolters Kluwer Health, 2001.

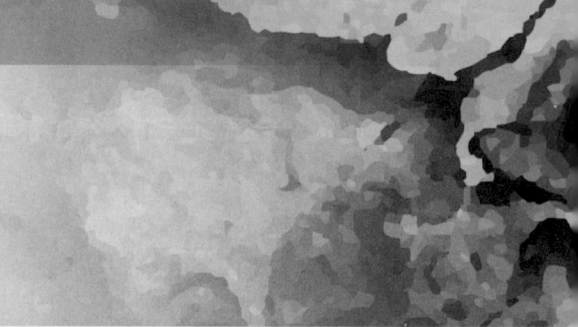

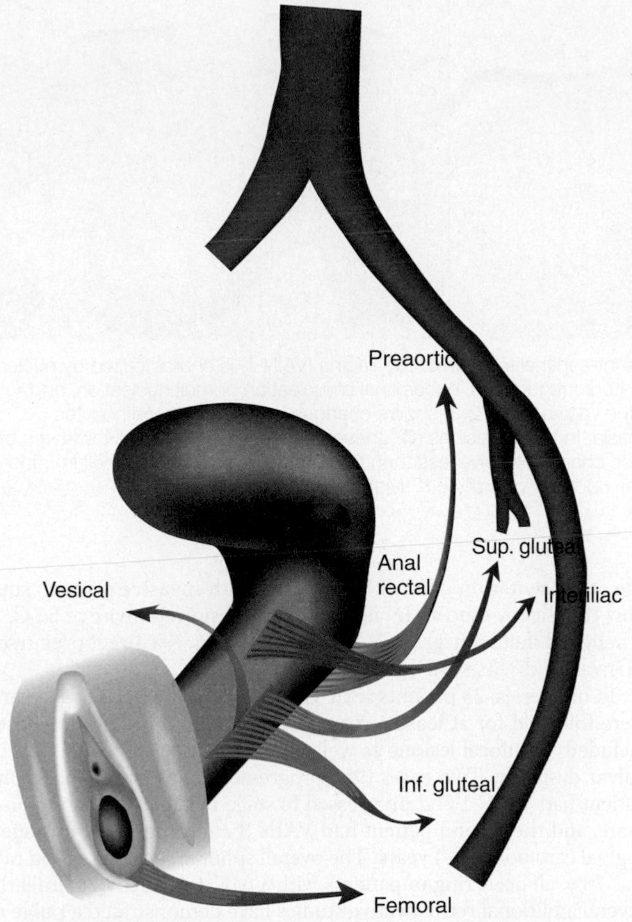

Figure 19.2. Lymphatic drainage of the vagina.

Source: Reproduced from Plentl AA, Friedman EA. Lymphatic system of the female genitalia. In: Plentl AA, Friedman EA, eds. *The Morphologic Basis of Oncologic Diagnosis and Therapy*. Philadelphia, PA: WB Saunders; 1971:55, Figure 5-2. Used with permission.

The uppermost portion drains primarily via cervical lymphatics. The superior anterior vagina drains along cervical channels to the interiliac and parametrial nodes, and the posterior upper vagina drains into the inferior gluteal, presacral, and anorectal nodes (**Fig. 19.2**). The inferior aspect of the vagina drains into the inguinal and femoral nodes, and ultimately to the pelvic nodes, following the drainage patterns of the vulva. Lesions in the midvagina have been shown to drain either way (1). Lesions infiltrating the rectovaginal septum may spread to the pararectal and presacral nodes. Because there are multiple interconnections between lymphatic channels, the pattern of drainage cannot be reliably predicted based on location of the primary tumor.

Proximally, the vagina is supplied by the vaginal artery, which arises from the cervical branch of the uterine artery and runs lateral to the vagina until it anastomoses with the inferior vesical and middle rectal arteries. The venous plexus runs parallel to the arteries, draining into the internal iliac vein. The vaginal vault is innervated by the lumbar plexus and pudendal nerve, with branches from sacral roots 2 to 4 (2). Embryologically, the vagina is believed to be of dual origin, with the upper third derived from the uterine canal, while the lower two-thirds are derived from the urogenital sinus (3).

Epidemiology, Presentation, and Management

According to the American Cancer Society estimates for 2016 (4), there will be approximately 4,600 new cases and 950 deaths from primary vaginal cancer. Primary vaginal cancer is a rare malignancy, constituting 1% to 2% of all gynecologic malignancies (5). According to compiled data from US population–based cancer registries spanning 1998 to 2003, the incidence of all vaginal cancers was 0.18 per 100,000 females for in situ cases and 0.69 per 100,000 females for invasive cases (6).

Most primary vaginal malignancies are squamous cell carcinomas (SCC). According to a National Cancer Data Base (NCDB) report (7), which evaluated 4,885 patients with primary vaginal cancer registered from 1985 to 1994, approximately 92% of patients were diagnosed with in situ or invasive SCC or adenocarcinomas, 4% with melanomas, 3% with sarcomas, and 1% with other/unspecified types of cancer. Sixty-six percent of all vaginal cancers were invasive, with SCC representing 79% of all invasive cases.

The peak incidence of primary vaginal cancer is in the sixth and seventh decades of life. According to data from the Surveillance, Epidemiology and End Results (SEER) Program (8), 2,149 women in the United States were diagnosed with primary vaginal cancer from 1990 to 2004. The mean age at diagnosis was 65 +/− 14 years, and incidence rates increased with age. There has been an overall decrease in the incidence of primary vaginal tumors, possibly secondary to earlier detection and to implementation of strict exclusion criteria in the International Federation of Obstetrics and Gynecology (FIGO) staging system.

At the same time, there has been a steady increase in the diagnosis of vaginal intraepithelial neoplasia (VAIN) over the past several decades, perhaps as a result of expanded cytologic screening and increased awareness (5). It is hypothesized that VAIN is a precursor lesion to SCC of the vagina (9).

Most malignant lesions in the vagina are attributable to direct spread or metastases from other gynecologic malignancies, and are classified accordingly. According to the FIGO staging system, any tumor involving both the vagina and the cervix should be classified as a cervical carcinoma. Similarly, any tumor involving both the vagina and the vulva is to be classified as a vulvar carcinoma (10). A malignant vaginal lesion in a patient with a prior history of invasive cervical carcinoma within the past 5 years also excludes diagnosis as a primary vaginal cancer (11). As a result, only a minority of vaginal carcinomas meet the criteria of a primary vaginal cancer. According to one study of 141 vaginal carcinoma cases, only 26% could be classified as such (12).

Owing to infrequent presentation, treatment recommendations are based on results from relatively small retrospective series comprising heterogeneous patient populations and treatments. Given the low incidence of vaginal cancer, it is unlikely that randomized clinical trials will be undertaken.

Vaginal Intraepithelial Neoplasia

Epidemiology

Hummer and colleagues first reported VAIN in 1933 and defined it as atypical squamous cells without evidence of stromal invasion (9). The incidence of VAIN is estimated to be 0.2 to 0.3 cases per 100,000, with peak incidence found in women who are 40 and 60 years of age (5,9,13,14). VAIN is further characterized according to depth of epithelial involvement from one third, two thirds and greater than two thirds thickness as VAIN 1, 2, and 3, respectively. Several series report that the median age at diagnosis for patients with VAIN 1 or 2 is lower than that for VAIN 3 (15–17), but this has not been corroborated by other series (9,18).

Involvement of the full thickness of the epithelium is known as in situ vaginal cancer and is included as VAIN 3 (**Fig. 19.3**). The incidence of in situ vaginal cancer is estimated to be 0.1 per 100,000 women, with peak incidence between ages 70 and 79, according to data from the U.S. Centers for Disease Control and Prevention's National Program of Cancer Registries, and the National Cancer Institute's SEER Program (19). These numbers are similar to data from US population–based cancer registries encompassing the years from 1998 to 2003, which report incidence of in situ vaginal cancer to be 0.18 per 100,000 females (6). The peak age of in situ vaginal cancer is slightly higher than that for primary vaginal cancer.

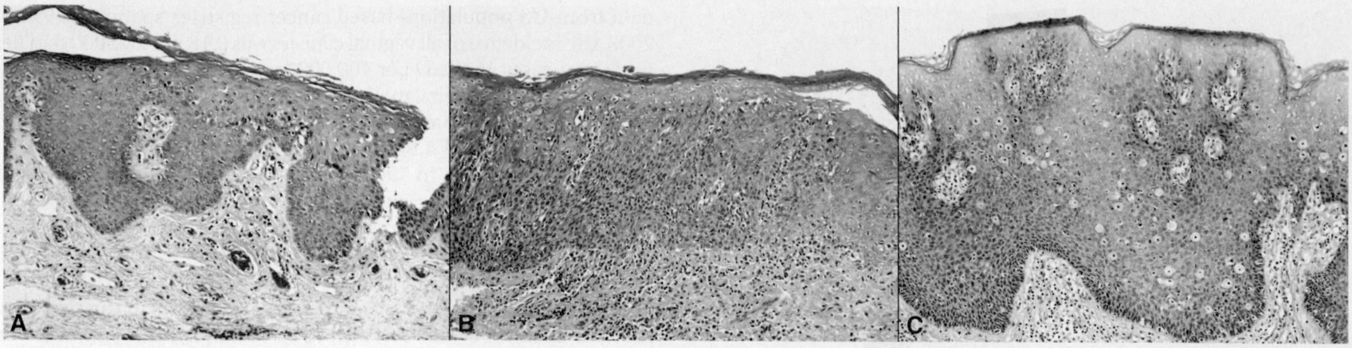

Figure 19.3. Vaginal intraepithelial neoplasia (VAIN) **A:** Low-grade squamous intraepithelial lesion of the vagina (VAIN 1) is characterized by nuclear enlargement in the upper one-third of the squamous epithelium with nuclear contour irregularities, occasional binucleation or multinucleation, and distinct cytoplasmic halos. **B, C:** High-grade squamous intraepithelial lesion of the vagina (VAIN 2-3) shows changes in the basal keratinocytes including nuclear pleomorphism with high N:C ratio, crowding, and hyperchromasia. In VAIN 3 lesions (**C**), these changes involve the full thickness of the epithelium, and frequent mitoses are usually seen. In VAIN 2 lesions (**B**), these changes involve less than the full thickness of the epithelium, and mitoses, when present, are confined to the lower levels of the epithelium. Images courtesy of Emily E.K. Meserve.

Source: Images courtesy of Emily E.K. Meserve.

There are multiple risk factors for VAIN; the most common are low socioeconomic level, history of genital warts, hysterectomy at an early age, history of cervical intraepithelial neoplasia (CIN), immunosuppression, prior pelvic radiation, smoking, exposure to diethylsilbestrol (DES), and history of sexually transmissible diseases (STD) and/or human papillomavirus (HPV) infection (15,20–22). HPV is implicated in the development of VAIN, and the relationship between HPV and development of intraepithelial neoplasia has also been best demonstrated for cervical lesions. HPV 16 and 18 are the most prevalent subtypes associated with VAIN (23). A review of 232 published VAIN cases documented a high prevalence of HPV using identified on PCR or hybrid capture assays for detection, with 98.5% and 92.6% of VAIN 1 and VAIN 2/3 cases positive for HPV (24). A series by Sugase et al. (25) examining 71 biopsy specimens of VAIN found HPV in 100% of samples. Fifteen different known subtypes were identified (HPV 16, 18, 30, 31, 35, 40, 42, 43, 51, 52, 53, 54, 56, 58, 66). It is estimated that HPV 16/18 is identified in 40% of VAIN 1 and 60% of high-grade VAIN 2/3 cases (24).

The diagnosis of VAIN is associated with prior or concurrent neoplasia elsewhere in the lower genital tract. Multiple series suggest approximately 50% to 90% of patients with VAIN have concurrent or prior history of intraepithelial neoplasia or carcinoma of the cervix or vulva (13,15,26). Immunosuppression from human immunodeficiency virus (HIV) is also a risk factor for both VAIN and HPV, though a higher incidence of invasive vaginal cancer in infected women has not been demonstrated (27–29). The role of pelvic radiation in the development of secondary vaginal neoplasia is unclear, with conflicting data suggesting that a history of ionizing radiation may predispose to VAIN or vaginal cancer after a latency period of many years (30–32). In utero exposure to DES may double the risk of VAIN, thought to be due to transformation zone enlargement, increasing the risk of HPV infection (33). With widespread implementation of HPV vaccination, it is anticipated that the incidence of VAIN will start to decline. It is predicted that HPV vaccination will ultimately prevent up to 70% of VAIN cases (34,35).

Although the pathogenesis of both VAIN and CIN is attributable to HPV infection, the incidence of VAIN is notably lower. One study reported a 100-fold difference in incidence (15). It is speculated that the mature, squamous epithelium of the vagina is less vulnerable to persistent dysplasia than the metaplastic transformation zone of the cervix (9,15).

Natural History

Although the likelihood of VAIN progressing to invasive disease is difficult to predict in individual cases, multiple clinical series have demonstrated a significant overall increase in risk of invasive vaginal cancer after a diagnosis of VAIN (26,32,36,37). Similar risk factors for VAIN and invasive vaginal cancer, as well as the younger average age at presentation of VAIN compared with invasive disease, support the theory that VAIN is a precursor lesion to invasive SCC. It is believed that high-grade VAIN, in particular, is a direct precursor to invasive disease (9).

In one series, 23 patients with VAIN, with a mean age of 41 years, were followed for at least 3 years without treatment (26); the cases included multifocal lesions as well as lesions associated with CIN or vulvar dysplasia. Two cases (9%) progressed to invasive cancer; one patient had VAIN 1 and progressed to stage I vaginal carcinoma in 5 years, and the second patient had VAIN 3 and progressed to stage I vaginal carcinoma in 4 years. The overall spontaneous regression rate was 78%, all occurring in patients with VAIN 1 or VAIN 2. Similarly, several additional retrospective studies have demonstrated a range of 2% to 20% of patients with VAIN progressing to invasive vaginal cancer (26,32,36,38–40). The rate of occult invasive disease in patients with VAIN 3 is reportedly as high as 28% (41). The risk of malignant transformation in VAIN 1 and 2 is less clearly elucidated (18,20).

Histopathology

VAIN is defined as the presence of squamous cell atypia without evidence of invasion. Histopathologically, most lesions are epidermoid and exhibit full-thickness alterations with atypical mitoses and hyperchromatism (42). Punctation and mosaic patterns are often noted in high-grade VAIN (18). Most lesions are multifocal and can involve all surfaces of the vagina, although the superior one-third of the vagina is most common (26,32).

VAIN is further classified into low-grade (VAIN 1) and high-grade (VAIN 2-3). VAIN 1 is characterized by cytomorphologic changes limited to the upper one-third of the epithelium. Such changes include nuclear enlargement, nuclear hyperchromasia, cytoplasmic halos, and occasional binucleation. VAIN 2-3 is characterized by cytomorphologic changes in the basal keratinocytes, including nuclear pleomorphism, nuclear hyperchromasia and crowding, and mitotic figures (including atypical forms). VAIN 2 and 3 are distinguished by depth of cytologic change. Cytologic changes confined to the lower two-thirds of the epithelium are designated VAIN 2, whereas changes involving the full thickness of the epithelium are VAIN 3. Carcinoma in situ encompasses the full epithelial thickness and is included under VAIN 3.

Excluded from the diagnosis of VAIN is the presence of glandular intraepithelial dysplasia, or atypical vaginal adenosis; these entities are associated with in utero DES exposure and are deemed to be precursors of DES-associated clear cell adenocarcinoma (43).

Clinical Presentation

VAIN is usually asymptomatic (32) and most commonly detected after cytologic evaluation as part of surveillance in patients with a history of CIN or invasive cervical carcinoma. Vaginal colposcopy with iodine stain is important when patients present with an abnormal pap smear but no gross abnormality. Any colposcopically abnormal area warrants a directed biopsy. Around the vaginal vault, where occult carcinoma may be found, excisional biopsies are recommended (44). According to the 2002 American Cancer Society guidelines, surveillance cytology for VAIN in posthysterectomy patients is recommended if there is a history of cervical pathology, although it is low yield (45). The optimal incorporation of HPV testing into screening is not yet known (46). At present, evidence does not support routine surveillance in patients without a history of CIN or invasive cervical cancer.

Prognostic Factors

A significant association between higher viral load of HPV and likelihood of persistent disease after treatment was demonstrated by So et al. (47). There is also a significant association between risk of relapse in patients positive for high-risk HPV versus those who are negative (48). Of such patients, a retrospective review of 33 patients with VAIN treated at the University of Pennsylvania (38) found patients with a history of radiation therapy (RT) to be more refractory to treatment, with a significantly higher likelihood of recurrence after surgical and ablative therapy. Patients with a history of RT had an odds ratio of 3.6 for recurrent disease (95% CI, 1.5 to 9.0) compared to patients without a history of RT.

Treatment Options

There is currently no consensus on optimal treatment modality, as reported data are generally retrospective and based on decades of experience with various treatments and patient characteristics; thus, it is difficult to compare different therapeutic modalities (**Table 19.1**). Treatment approaches include local excision, partial or total vaginectomy, laser vaporization, electrocoagulation, topical 5% fluorouracil (5-FU) administration, topical 5% imiquimod, and

TABLE 19.1. Local Control of Vaginal Intraepithelial Neoplasia by Treatment Modality

Series	Year	# Patients	% Recurrence	Follow-up	Treatment Notes
Surgery					
Benedet (49)	1984	136	25%	>5 years	WLE, PV, TV
Lenehan (32)	1986	19	16%	5–112 months	PV, TV
Ireland (50)	1988	25	4%	3 months–11 years	PV, TV
Hoffman (41)	1992	32	17%	6–73 months	PV; 28% invasive cancer
Fanning (51)	1999	15	0%	22 months	PV; 6.6% invasive cancer
Cheng (13)	1999	35	34%	1–124 months	WLE
Dodge (20)	2001	13	0%	>7 months	PV
Indermaur (52)	2005	105	12%	2–9 months	PV, 12% invasive cancer
Terzakis (53)	2010	23	25%	24 months	
Gunderson (9)	2013	44	27%	1–194 months	PV, LE
Laser therapy					
Jobson (54)	1983	24	17%	6–27 months	
Audet-LaPoint (55)	1990	32	28%	7–85 months	3.8% invasive cancer at excision 3 of 11 w/invasive cancer at recurrence
Hoffman (56)	1991	26	42%	2.2 years (mean)	
Diakomanolis (57)	1996	25	32%	35–82 months	
Campagnutta (58)	1999	39	23%	13–90 months	
Dodge (20)	2001	42	38%	>7 months	
Perotta (59)	2013	21	14%	12–78 months	
Gunderson (9)	2013	34	47%	1–194 months	
Topical 5-FU					
Woodruff (60)	1975	9	11%	3–7 years	1%–2% 5-FU q month
Petrilli (61)	1980	15	20%	2–60 months	BID × 5 d
Kirwan (62)	1985	14	7%	4–42 months	q week × 10 weeks
Krebs (63)	1989	37	19%	12–84 months	q week × 10 weeks
Audet-Lapointe (55)	1990	12	17%	9–42 months	q d × 5 days
Dodge (20)	2001	22	59%	>7 months	
Topical imiquimod					
Diakomonolis (64)	2002	3	See note		3 × weekly × 8weeks 3 pts with high-grade disease, therapy revealed regression to VAIN1 (*n* = 2) or cure (*n* = 1)
Buck (65)	2003	56	14%		0.25 g q week × 3 weeks

■ **TABLE 19.1. Local Control of Vaginal Intraepithelial Neoplasia by Treatment Modality (*continued*)**

Series	Year	# Patients	% Recurrence	Follow-up	Treatment Notes
Radiation					
Prempree (66)	1977	7	0%		ICB 70–80 Gy
Chyle (67)	1996	37	17%		ICB or orthovoltage radiation
MacLeod (68)	1997	14	14%	46 months (mean)	HDR-ICB, 34–45 Gy to vaginal surface, 4–10 fx
Ogino (69)	1998	6	0%	13–153 months	HDR-ICB, mean dose 23.3 Gy
Perez (70)	1999	20	6%		ICB 60–70 Gy
Graham (71)	2007	22	14%	77 months	MDR-ICB, 48 Gy to point Z
Blanchard (72)	2011	28	7%	79 months	LDR, 60 Gy to 5 mm below mucosa
Song (73)	2014	34	6%	48 months	HDR-ICB, 40 Gy in 8 fx
Zolciak-Siwinska (74)	2015	20	10%	39 months	HDR-ICB, 6–7.5 Gy x 3–5 fx

Fx, fractions; HDR, high dose rate; ICB, intracavitary brachytherapy; LDR, low dose rate; MDR, medium dose rate; PV, partial vaginectomy; TV, total vaginectomy; WLE, wide local excision.

radiation (15–18,20,52,61,71,75–77). Reported success rates for different approaches range from 48% to 100% for laser vaporization (56,78,79), 52% to 100% for colpectomy (41,52,57), 75% to 100% for topical 5-FU (60–63,80–83), 57% to 86% for topical 5% imiquimod (77), and 83% to 100% for radiation (68,69,72,76,84). Given the breadth of available therapies, an individualized approach to patient management is advised, with consideration given to the patient's overall health, desire to preserve sexual function, candidacy for surgery, disease multifocality, and prior treatment failures.

Most patients with VAIN 1 are offered close surveillance. Lesions often regress spontaneously; in one study by Aho et al. (26), 78% of patients with VAIN 1 or VAIN 2 had spontaneous regression of disease without treatment. However, over time, VAIN 1 can recur or progress. In one study by Gunderson et al. (9) on 37 patients with VAIN 1, 54% of patients who were observed developed recurrent, persistent, or progressive disease, versus 73% of patients who were treated with excision or ablation. Overall, disease recurrence/progression occurred at a median time of 17 months. Appropriate treatment for VAIN 2 should be determined on an individual basis, based on disease extent and associated patient factors. Therapy for VAIN 3 should be more aggressive, as there is a higher likelihood of progression to invasive disease, including occult invasive disease (41,52).

Surgical and Ablative Therapies. Surgical excision for VAIN is an option in select cases, particularly for vaginal vault lesions. Approaches include local excision, partial vaginectomy, and, in rare cases, total vaginectomy for highly extensive disease, which provides the advantage of obtaining a complete pathologic diagnosis. Most resections can be performed through a transvaginal approach. Location of VAIN in the vaginal vault or posthysterectomy suture recesses may require partial vaginectomy for complete resection, because redundancy of the vaginal mucosa makes it difficult to rule out occult disease with biopsy alone.

Excision of smaller lesions can be achieved through a cold-knife approach, electrosurgical loop excision, laser, or ultrasonic surgical aspiration (85–87). The CO_2 laser has been used for ablation of local tissue, with multiple treatments required in approximately one-third of patients (55,56,58,63,79,88,89). Complications include postoperative pain, scarring, and bleeding; however, the treatment is fairly well tolerated overall, with minimum impact on sexual function (90). Diakomanolis et al. (57) reported that of 52 patients who underwent laser treatment or partial vaginectomy, the results favored laser ablation for multifocal disease and partial vaginectomy for unifocal disease. Ultrasonic surgical aspiration is another technique with the same efficacy as that of laser ablation; in one series of 110 patients, 1-year recurrence-free survival rates were 24% and 26%, respectively (52).

Series on surgical treatment of VAIN report recurrence rates in the range of 0% to 50%, with follow-up ranging from 3 months to 18 years (13,15,32,41,49). Overall, series that specifically examine upper vaginectomy report control rates of 68% to 88% (17,36,41,52,57). For example, Hoffman et al. (41) reported that 83% of patients with VAIN 3 remained free of disease at a mean follow-up time of 38 months. Of note, 28% of all patients were found to have occult invasive disease upon upper vaginectomy. A subsequent study by Indermaur et al. (52), which retrospectively reviewed 36 patients treated with upper vaginectomy for VAIN, reported 88% to be free of recurrence at a mean follow-up time of 25 months. Thirteen patients (12%) were found to have invasive cancer: 8 had frank invasive disease, and 5 had microinvasive carcinoma. Complication rates of upper vaginectomy have been variably reported; in the series by Indermaur, there was a 9% complication rate. Potential complications from surgery depend on the extent and method of surgical resection, and range from vaginal shortening and stenosis to standard postoperative morbidity associated with abdominal procedures. It should be noted that patients with a history of RT are at higher risk of postoperative complications, with a higher rate of fistula formation reported in one study (13).

Topical Treatments. Topical therapies have been utilized in patients with early-stage lesions, multifocal disease, or multiple comorbidities that render them non-ideal surgical candidates. Topical creams are favored in the management of young, HPV-positive women presenting with multifocal lesions (91). Topical applications have also been utilized before surgery to reduce lesion size and improve stripping of neoplastic epithelial cells from underlying stroma (15). Treatments include topical 5-FU and 5% imiquimod cream, with response rates of up to 86% for imiquimod and 41% to 88% for 5-FU (60,62–65,76,81,82,92,93). Imiquimod increases levels of interferon-alpha, interleukin 12, and tumor necrosis factor (64), resulting in immunomodulation of the vaginal mucosa. Side effects of topical treatments include local irritation, with burning and ulceration being the most commonly reported adverse events (60,81).

Radiation Therapy. In general, RT is reserved for patients who relapse after more conservative treatments. RT is an alternate treatment with a long history of efficacy, with several small series over the past 20 to 30 years reporting control rates ranging from 80% to 100% (16,32,55,69,71,72,76,84,94,95). High dose rate (HDR), medium dose rate (MDR), and low dose rate (LDR) techniques have reportedly yielded acceptable results, although it is difficult to compare regimens because of small patient numbers, generally short follow-up times, and overall lack of uniformity among series. Drawbacks to RT include potential undertreatment of occult invasive disease, the risk of secondary malignancy, and long-term morbidity, although there are no prospective data available regarding the impact of treatment on sexual function and quality of life.

Overall, excellent local control and low toxicity have been reported for LDR brachytherapy. LDR treatment is delivered with an intracavitary vaginal cylinder using cesium 137. Typically, a dose of 60 Gy is delivered to the vaginal mucosa, but a wide range of doses, depending on depth of dose prescription, as well as a variety of techniques, have been reported (70,72,76,84,95). Chyle et al. (67) prescribed 70 to 80 Gy to the vaginal surface, and reported a 17% recurrence rate at 10 years in their series of 37 patients. Perez et al. (70) treated patients with a dose of 60 to 70 Gy to the vaginal surface, and reported one recurrence out of 20 patients. The recurrence occurred in the distal vagina and was noted to be marginal. Blanchard et al. (72) published a series on 28 patients with VAIN 3 treated at Institut Gustave Roussy from 1985 to 2008. Patients were treated with LDR brachytherapy, using a vaginal mold technique, to a dose of 60 Gy prescribed 5 mm below the vaginal surface; 18 patients received treatment to the upper half of the vagina, 6 were treated to the upper two-thirds, and 4 were treated to the whole vaginal length. With a median follow-up time of 41 months, the authors report only one in-field recurrence, and a 10-year local control rate of 93%. Treatment with LDR brachytherapy is well tolerated overall; in the Blanchard et al. series, there were no grade 3 or 4 late toxicities, and only one grade 2 gastrointestinal toxicity noted. This is consistent with the Perez series, in which there was only one grade 3 urinary complication among 40 patients with VAIN 3 or stage 1 vaginal cancer treated with LDR (70).

There are limited data on the use of MDR brachytherapy treatment for VAIN. Graham et al. (71) reviewed their experience using MDR intracavitary brachytherapy for VAIN 3 at the Beatson Oncology Center in Glasgow, UK. Using a MDR Selectron, 48 Gy was prescribed 0.5 cm lateral to the ovoid surface (point Z) over two insertions, spaced 1 week apart. Ovoids were chosen over vaginal cylinder placement in order to adequately cover epithelium sutured into the superolateral vagina at hysterectomy. With a median follow-up of 77 months, recurrent/residual VAIN 3 was documented in three patients, two of whom subsequently developed invasive or microinvasive vaginal carcinoma. One other patient developed late progression 14 years after treatment. There were minimal acute effects during treatment; however, with longer follow-up, all patients were noted to have grade 1–2 mucosal atrophy, dryness, and telangiectasia. Four patients developed grade 3 toxicity with severe vaginal stenosis, and one patient developed a grade 4 vaginal ulcer that presented 2 years after treatment. One other patient developed grade 3 urinary toxicity with urethral stricture, requiring intermittent self-catheterization.

Several series have reported promising results for HDR brachytherapy, with disease-free survival (DFS) rates of 90% or greater. HDR brachytherapy is generally reserved for patients with VAIN 3, particularly if there is an in situ disease component. Ogino et al. (69) reported their experience treating six patients with VAIN 3 at Kanagawa Cancer Center from 1983 to 1993, with a mean dose of 23.3 Gy (range 15–30 Gy); most treatments were delivered in five fractions using two ovoids, with dose calculated to a point 1 cm superior to the vaginal apex. Lesions distal to the vaginal vault had doses calculated 1 cm beyond the plane of the vaginal cylinder in order to deliver adequate dose to the entire vagina. Median follow-up was 90.5 months, and there was no evidence of disease recurrence in the treated patients. Two patients developed moderate to severe vaginal stenosis, and three patients developed rectal bleeding, that resolved. MacLeod et al. (68) reviewed their experience treating 14 patients with VAIN 3 from 1985 to 1995. The total dose was 34 to 45 Gy to the vaginal surface, in 8.5-Gy fractions delivered twice a week, or 4.5-Gy fractions delivered four times a week. One patient developed invasive cancer, and one patient had persistent VAIN 3. There were no major acute toxicities, and two patients developed late grade 3 vaginal atrophy and stenosis. According to one study that evaluated toxicity after use of HDR brachytherapy for VAIN in 20 patients, utilizing the CTCAE scale, a biologically equivalent dose of 70 Gy or greater results in significantly greater toxicity. The most common toxicities were decreased libido, vaginal discharge, dryness, mucositis, stenosis, and vaginitis (74).

Malignant Tumors of the Vagina: Squamous Cell Carcinoma

Epidemiology

The NCDB review by Creasman et al., for the period 1985 to 1994, revealed 3,244 cases of invasive primary vaginal carcinoma, with 24% of patients presenting with American Joint Committee on Cancer (AJCC) stage I disease, 20% AJCC stage II, 24% AJCC stages III–IV, and 32% unknown. Most tumors were moderately (28%) or poorly (28%) differentiated at presentation. Consistent with this data, a review of five series, including a total of 1,375 cases of vaginal cancer, reported the FIGO stage distribution as follows: 26% stage I, 37% stage II, 24% stage III, and 13% stage IV (96).

According to the SEER study by Shah and colleagues (8), most women diagnosed with primary vaginal cancer are non-Hispanic Whites (66%), followed by African Americans (14%), Hispanic Whites (12%), Asian/Pacific Islanders (7%), and others (1%). Incidence rates were highest for African American women (1.24/100,000 person-years) and lowest for Asian/Pacific Islanders (0.64/100,000 person-years). The greatest proportion of women (36%) presented with stage I disease, and 65% had squamous histology, consistent with other reports.

Risk Factors

Risk factors for primary vaginal SCC are similar to those for VAIN and cervical neoplasia. Commonly cited factors include HPV infection and/or history of cervical or vulvar intraepithelial neoplasia, immunosuppression, multiple sexual partners, and early age at first intercourse. It is believed that most cases of vaginal cancer can be attributed to HPV infection. According to a meta-analyses comprising 14 studies, the overall HPV prevalence was 70% for vaginal carcinomas, with the most common subtypes as follows: HPV 16 (53.7%), HPV 18 (7.6%), and HPV 31 (5.6%). Multiple subtypes of HPV were identified in 3.4% of cases (97).

In a population-based case–control study of 156 women with VAIN or invasive cancer, significant risk factors included early age at intercourse, increased number of lifetime sexual partners, and current smoking. HPV DNA was detectable in 80% of patients with in situ disease and in 60% of those with invasive disease; 30% of patients reported a history of treatment for invasive malignancy, most commonly cervix, or in situ anogenital neoplasia (37). A case–control study of 41 women with in situ disease or invasive carcinoma identified low socioeconomic status, history of genital warts, vaginal discharge or irritation, history of abnormal cytology, prior hysterectomy, and vaginal trauma as potential risk factors (98). A larger case–control study of 36,856 women found an increased risk of vaginal cancer in alcoholics, likely associated with a higher incidence of other lifestyle factors, such as promiscuity and smoking, which are also associated with a higher incidence of HPV infection. Early hysterectomy appears to be a risk factor in some studies, if performed for malignant or premalignant disease (37,99).

Patients with a history of cervical cancer have a significantly higher risk of developing in situ as well as invasive carcinoma of the vagina. Studies suggest that 10% to 50% of patients with a history of VAIN or invasive carcinoma of the vagina have undergone treatment for in situ or invasive cervical carcinoma (32,67,100–106), with the interval from treatment of cervical disease to development of vaginal carcinoma averaging approximately 14 years (102,107). HIV-infected women are also at higher risk of developing vaginal carcinoma, which tends to behave more aggressively in HIV-positive than in HIV-negative patients (108).

The role of ionizing radiation to the pelvis in the development of vaginal carcinoma is unclear, with conflicting reports. According to one study that analyzed 1,200 patients treated over a 20-year period for carcinoma of the cervix, prior RT was not shown to result in increased secondary pelvic neoplasms (31). A second study by Boice et al. (30), however, reported a 14-fold increased risk of vaginal cancer in women with a history of pelvic irradiation before the age of 45, with a significant dose–response relationship.

Another potential risk factor is chronic irritation of the vaginal mucosa, resulting in chronic inflammation, hyperkeratosis, thickening, and acanthosis (108), with subsequent metaplastic and dysplastic changes; however, this is not proven. Although older studies showed that more vaginal cancers arise from the posterior vaginal wall, other studies report approximately equal distribution of invasive carcinomas on the anterior and posterior walls (36,102,109–111); this poses an argument against the theory that pooling of irritating substances in the posterior fornix contributes to the development of vaginal cancers, particularly on the posterior wall. Chronic irritation from the use of vaginal pessaries has also been implicated as a factor in vaginal cancer development (112,113).

Clinical Presentation

Up to 65% of patients with vaginal cancer present with irregular vaginal bleeding as their primary symptom (102,114,115). Vaginal discharge is the second most common symptom, occurring in 10% to 15% of patients. Less frequent symptoms, associated with locally advanced disease, include the presence of a mass; pain; urinary symptoms including frequency, dysuria, or hematuria; or gastrointestinal complaints such as tenesmus, constipation, or melena. Because of the proximity of anterior wall lesions to the urethra and bladder, urinary symptoms can be seen more commonly in vaginal cancer than in cervical cancer. Up to 20% of women are asymptomatic at the time of diagnosis (102,116), with lesions detected via cytologic screening or by speculum examination.

Vaginal cancer most frequently involves the superior one-third of the vaginal canal, with series reporting 50% to 83% of cases occurring in this region (36,110,111,117–120). A high proportion of patients have a history of prior hysterectomy. There is approximately equal involvement of the middle and inferior thirds (36), although some studies suggest that involvement of the lower third is more common than involvement of the middle third (102,111). The lateral walls are less frequently involved. Tumors may exhibit an exophytic or ulcerative, infiltrating growth pattern.

Vaginal tumors can spread along the vaginal walls to involve the cervix or vulva, but involvement of the cervix or vulva at the time of diagnosis excludes classification as a primary vaginal cancer. Lesions can extend radially, either into the lumen to form exophytic masses or through the vaginal wall to invade surrounding musculature and organs. Anterior wall lesions can infiltrate the vesicovaginal septum and/or urethra. Posterior wall lesions can infiltrate the rectovaginal septum and involve the rectal mucosa. Advanced disease can extend laterally toward the parametrium and paracolpal tissues, or into the urogenital diaphragm, levator ani muscles, or pelvic fascia, and eventually to the pelvic sidewall.

Distant metastases can occur with advanced disease at presentation, or on recurrence after primary therapy. The most frequent site of hematogenous metastasis is the lung, whereas less commonly noted sites are the liver and bone (67). In a series by Perez et al. (105), the incidence of distant metastasis was 16% for stage I, 31% for stage II, 46% for stage IIB, 62% for stage III, and 50% for stage IV. Some histologies may have a higher likelihood of distant metastases than others. Chyle et al. (67) noted a higher incidence of distant metastases in patients with adenocarcinoma (48%) than in those with SCC (10%), with correspondingly lower 10-year survival rates (20% vs. 50%).

Histopathology

Grossly, SCC of the vagina can present as nodular, ulcerated, indurated, exophytic or endophytic lesions, and it is difficult to histologically distinguish a primary vaginal SCC from recurrent cervical or vulvar carcinoma. Histologically, tumors are graded as well, moderately, or poorly differentiated, and have been described as keratinizing, nonkeratinizing, basaloid, warty, or verrucous. Most of these lesions are nonkeratinizing and moderately differentiated (121) (**Fig. 19.4**).

Verrucous carcinoma is a distinct histologic variant of vaginal SCC (122). It commonly presents as a well-circumscribed, soft, cauliflower-like mass that is microscopically well differentiated, with a papillary growth pattern and acanthotic epithelium (**Fig. 19.5**). There is surface maturation with parakeratosis or hyperkeratosis without koilocytosis. This variant of SCC exhibits less aggressive behavior, and rarely metastasizes (122–125). Therefore it should be considered an entity distinct from other vaginal SCC.

Sarcomatoid SCC is a rare subset of vaginal SCC, comprising 2% of all cases (**Fig. 19.6**). It is characterized by spindle-shaped neoplastic cells that may initially be mistaken for sarcoma. However, positive

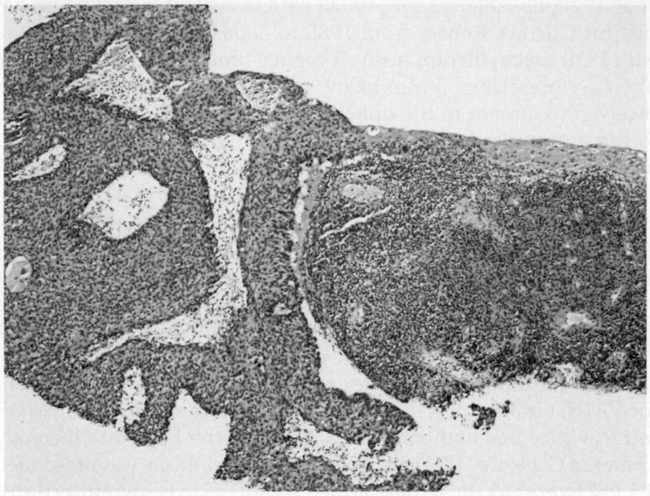

Figure 19.4. Moderately differentiated squamous cell carcinoma of the vagina. Invasive squamous cell carcinoma may appear as nests of atypical keratinocytes, or, alternatively, may appear as complex, redundant strips of neoplastic epithelium. In moderately differentiated squamous cell carcinoma, the keratinocytes show nuclear atypia, nuclear hyperchromasia, and high N:C ratio, often with easily identifiable mitoses, and limited evidence of squamous maturation, as expected in well-differentiated examples. Images courtesy of Emily E.K. Meserve.

Source: Images courtesy of Emily E.K. Meserve.

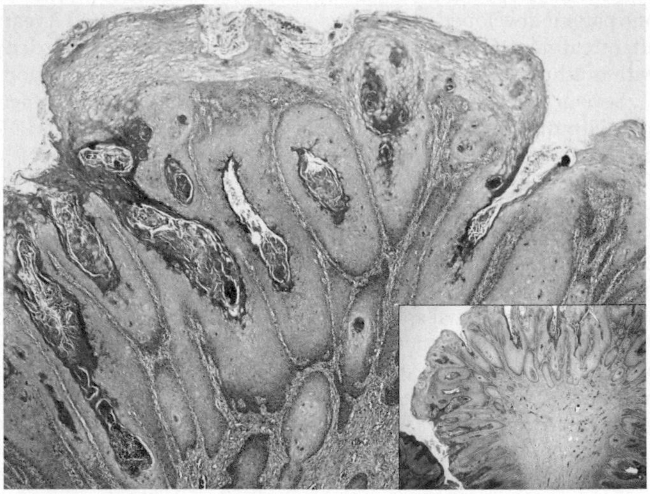

Figure 19.5. Verrucous squamous cell carcinoma. Verrucous squamous cell carcinoma is a rare subtype of extremely well-differentiated squamous cell carcinoma. Tumors are often exophytic (inset) with very bland and uniform cytologic features and often a "pushing" pattern of invasion, rather than invasion by irregular nests or single cells as seen more frequently in conventional SCC. Images courtesy of Emily E.K. Meserve.

Source: Images courtesy of Emily E.K. Meserve.

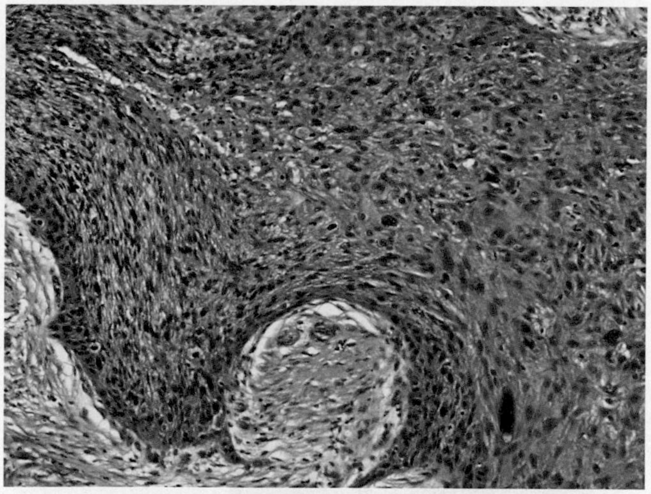

Figure 19.6. Sarcomatoid squamous cell carcinoma. Sarcomatoid squamous cell carcinoma is a type of poorly differentiated squamous cell carcinoma wherein neoplastic squamous epithelial cells exhibit a spindle cell morphology. Keratin expression is less consistent in areas of spindle cell morphology, but continuity with areas of more conventional poorly differentiated SCC, with prominent nuclear pleomorphism and necrosis, helps confirm the diagnosis of carcinoma. Images courtesy of Emily E.K. Meserve.

Source: Images courtesy of Emily E.K. Meserve.

stains for cytokeratin help distinguish sarcomatoid SCC as a poorly differentiated variant of vaginal SCC (126).

Patterns of Lymphatic Drainage

The vagina has a complex pattern of lymphatic drainage, with multiple interconnections. The upper vagina drains to the obturator and hypogastric nodes, similar to the cervix. The lower vagina drains to the inguinal, femoral, and external iliac nodes, and posteriorly situated lesions can drain to the inferior gluteal, presacral, or perirectal nodes. Lymphatic channels in the mucosa run parallel to networks of channels in the submucosa and muscular layer, ultimately converging to form trunks at the vaginal wall periphery, which subsequently drain to major pelvic nodal groups.

In view of considerable crossover drainage, the location of the primary tumor is not a reliable indicator of drainage site. Frumovitz et al. (127) utilized lymphoscintigraphy to determine patterns of lymphatic drainage in 14 women diagnosed with primary vaginal cancers, and found a substantial degree of anomalous drainage, resulting in a change in RT for 33% of patients. For example, among four women with lesions located in the upper third of the vagina, which is predicted to drain along the cervical lymphatic chains to the pelvis, two (50%) were found to have a sentinel node in the inguinal region. Among five women with lesions located at the vaginal introitus, a location predicted to drain along the vulvar lymphatic chains to the inguinal triangle, three (60%) were found to have a sentinel node in the pelvis.

The risk of nodal metastasis appears to increase significantly with stage. Sparse data on nodal metastases are derived from series in which exploratory laparotomies and lymphadenectomies were performed (107). However, the true incidence of positive lymph nodes is difficult to determine because most patients receive treatment with RT and do not undergo surgical lymphadenectomy. The incidence of lymph node involvement has been reported as 0% to 14% in stage I and 21% to 32% in stage II disease (107,128,129). The incidence of nodal involvement in stages III and IV is reportedly as high as 78% and 83%, respectively (111). At diagnosis, up to 20% of patients have clinically positive inguinal nodes, with reported ranges of 5.3% to 20% (70,105). The risk of nodal failure increases significantly with local recurrence. Chyle et al. (67) reported 10-year inguinal and pelvic failure rates of 16% and 28%, respectively, in patients with local recurrence, in contrast to 2% and 4%, respectively, in patients without local recurrence.

Diagnostic Workup

The diagnostic workup should start with a thorough history and physical examination, giving careful attention to the pelvis. Complete assessment of tumor extent and assessment of vaginal walls is facilitated by examination under anesthesia. During speculum examination, the speculum blades can obscure the anterior and posterior walls, so it is essential to rotate the speculum for visualization of all four walls from the introitus to the apex. Bimanual examination, with careful digital palpation, should be performed, assessing for parametrial and pelvic sidewall involvement and invasion of tumor to the rectal mucosa.

Inguinal nodes should be palpated for disease involvement, particularly if the primary lesion is situated in the lower portion of the vagina, because 5% to 20% of patients reportedly have involved inguinal nodes at presentation (70,105). Suspicious nodes warrant a biopsy. Laboratory tests include a complete blood count with differential and assessment of renal and hepatic function.

A definitive diagnosis is achieved with biopsy of suspected lesions, which can present as an exophytic mass, plaque, or ulcer. If a lesion is not visible in the setting of abnormal cytology, colposcopy with acetic acid, followed by Lugol's iodine stain, is conducted. Biopsies of white epithelium or atypical vascularity should be obtained after application of acetic acid. Iodine will identify Schiller-positive regions, which are nonstaining, and should correspond to areas identified following application of acetic acid. Adequate biopsies should include the cervix, if present, to rule out a cervical primary. Patients can present with multiple regions of abnormality. The differential diagnosis of a vaginal mass includes endometriosis, vaginal polyp, vaginal adenosis, or Gardner's duct cyst.

FIGO staging of vaginal cancer is clinical, and may include chest x-ray, intravenous pyelography (IVP), barium enema, cystoscopy, and proctosigmoidoscopy. Cystoscopy or proctosigmoidoscopy may be necessary in patients with symptoms suggestive of bladder or rectal infiltration. Computed tomographic (CT) imaging and magnetic resonance imaging (MRI) do not affect FIGO stage assignment, but are commonly used. CT of the pelvis is obtained in place of IVP to assess the renal parenchyma, and also to obtain information on the extent of local disease and lymph node status. MRI can provide salient treatment planning information by characterizing extent of invasion and differentiating malignant tumor, which is isointense to muscle on T1 and hyperintense on T2, from normal structures and/or fibrosis (130). Advantages of MRI over other imaging modalities include superior soft tissue contrast resolution, allowing accurate assessment of tumor volume, extent of local invasion, and accurate assessment of pelvic nodal involvement. In general, MRI is regarded as superior to CT for staging of gynecologic malignancies, and should be obtained when available.

Positron emission tomography (PET) has shown efficacy in detecting the extent of primary tumor and abnormal lymph nodes in vaginal cancer with higher sensitivity than CT (**Fig. 19.7**), as is the case in cervical carcinoma (131). Primary vaginal carcinoma and metastatic lesions demonstrate avid uptake of 2[fluorine 18]-fluoro-2-deoxy-D-glucose (FDG). In one study, 23 patients with primary vaginal carcinoma received both PET and CT during staging. CT identified the primary tumor in only 43% of patients, whereas PET identified the tumor in 100%. PET identified suspicious uptake in groin and pelvic nodes in 8 of 23 patients, compared to 4 of 23 with CT. Treatment planning was modified in 14% of patients because of findings from PET, and the authors concluded that PET detects primary tumor and abnormal lymph nodes more often than CT (131). It is important that the patient have an empty bladder before imaging, as physiologic FDG activity in a filled bladder can potentially interfere with accurate estimation of vaginal involvement. In practice, most patients undergoing planning for RT are assessed with CT as well as MRI and/or PET, based on extrapolation from studies of other gynecologic malignances as well.

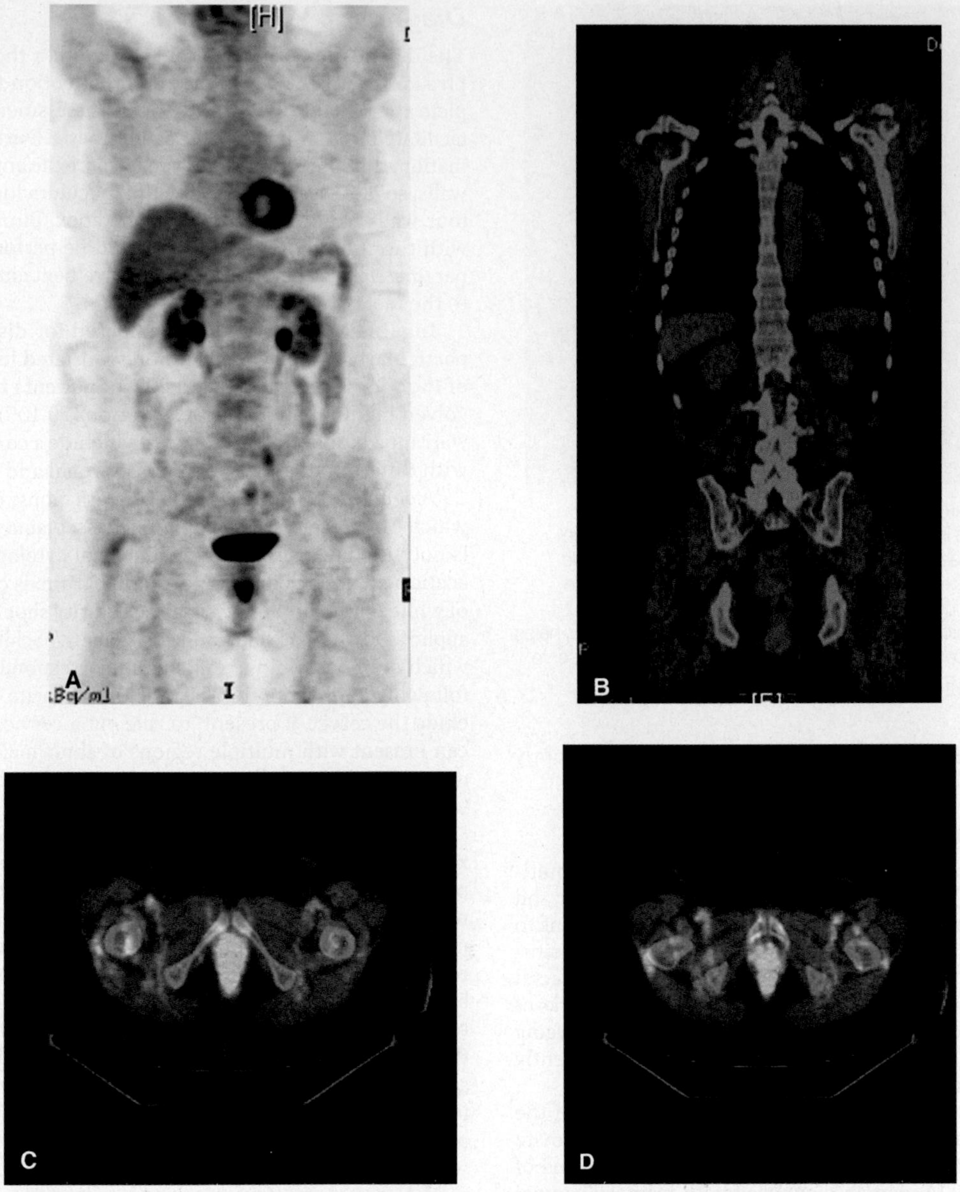

Figure 19.7. CT/PET fusion images of vaginal carcinoma. **A, B:** Coronal **C, D**: Axial images of a localized invasive vaginal carcinoma, extending into the central and lower one-third portion of the vagina above the introitus (*see arrows*).

Staging

The AJCC (132) and FIGO (10) systems are used to stage vaginal cancer (**Tables 19.2 and 19.3**). Primary vaginal melanomas and lymphomas are staged according to the AJCC staging systems for melanomas and lymphomas, respectively (132).

For patients with a prior gynecologic malignancy, a 5-year disease-free period is generally considered adequate to allow for distinction between recurrent disease and a new primary vaginal cancer. FIGO no longer recognizes carcinoma in situ as stage 0.

Stage I disease is defined as limited to the vaginal wall, and stage II disease involves subvaginal tissue without extension to the pelvic wall. Discriminating between stages I and II can be subjective; thin tumors <0.5 cm are generally classified as stage I, whereas thicker infiltrating tumors or those with paravaginal nodularity are classified as stage II. Perez et al. proposed a modification to the FIGO system in 1973, distinguishing tumors with paravaginal submucosal extension only (stage IIA) from tumors with parametrial infiltration (stage IIB) (70). The study reported a 20% 5-year survival difference (55% vs. 35%) between stages IIA and IIB. This modification has not been adopted into FIGO staging; however, some investigators consider the distinction to be prognostically relevant (66,105).

Prognostic Factors

Stage at time of presentation is the most significant prognostic factor, according to numerous studies (8,70,103,133–136). According to the NCDB study, the largest population-based series on vaginal cancer thus far, 5-year survival rates are as follows: 96% for stage 0, 73% for stage I, 58% for stage II, and 36% for stages III/IV disease (7). The series by Shah et al. (8), based on SEER data for women diagnosed between 1990 and 2004, also reveals the correlation between stage and outcome, with 5-year disease-specific survival (DSS) rates of 84% for stage I, 75% for stage II, and 57% for stages III/IV; the adjusted hazard ratio for mortality, on multivariate analysis, was 4.67. In the Perez et al. (105) series, 165 patients with primary vaginal cancer were treated with definitive RT, and had 10-year actuarial DFS rates of 94% for stage 0, 75% for stage I, 55% for stage IIA, 43% for stage IIB, 32% for stage III, and 0% for stage IV (137).

TABLE 19.2. International Federation of Gynecology and Obstetrics Staging System for Carcinoma of the Vagina

Stage	Description
Stage I	Carcinoma is limited to vaginal wall
Stage II	Carcinoma has involved the subvaginal tissue but has not extended to the pelvic wall[a]
Stage III	Carcinoma has extended to the pelvic wall
Stage IV	Carcinoma has extended beyond the true pelvis or has involved the mucosa of the bladder or rectum; bullous edema as such does not permit a case to be allotted to Stage IV
Stage IVA	Tumor invades bladder and/or rectal mucosa and/or direct extension beyond the true pelvis

Source: From FIGO Committee on Gynecologic Oncology. Current FIGO staging for cancer of the vagina, fallopian tube, ovary, and gestational trophoblastic neoplasia. *Int J Gynaecol Obstet.* 2009;105:1.

[a]Pelvic wall is defined as muscle, fascia, neurovascular structures, or skeletal portions of the bony pelvis.

TABLE 19.3. American Joint Commission on Cancer Staging of Vaginal Cancer

Primary tumor (T)	
Tx	Primary tumor cannot be assessed
T0	No evidence of primary tumor
Tis/0	Carcinoma in situ
T1/I	Tumor confined to the vagina
T2/II	Tumor invades paravaginal tissues but not the pelvic wall
T3/III	Tumor extends to the pelvic wall*
T4/IVA	Tumor invades mucosa of the bladder or rectum and/ or extends beyond the pelvis (bullous edema is not sufficient to classify a tumor as T4)
Regional lymph nodes (N)	
Nx	Regional lymph nodes cannot be assessed
N0	No regional lymph nodes
N1/IVB	Pelvic or inguinal lymph node metastasis
Distant metastasis (M)	
Mx	Distant metastasis cannot be assessed
M0	No distant metastasis
M1/IVB	Distant metastasis
Stage groupings	
Stage 0	Tis N0 M0
Stage I	T1 N0 M0
Stage II	T2 N0 M0
Stage III	T1-3 N1 M0, T3 N0 M0
Stage IVA	T4, any N, M0
Stage IVB	Any T, any N, M1

Used with the permission of the American Joint Committee on Cancer (AJCC), Chicago, Illinois. The original source for this material is the AJCC Cancer Staging Manual, Seventh Edition (2010) published by Springer-Verlag New York, www.springer.com.

Size of the initial lesion is a prognostic factor that has shown significance in several series. The SEER database study (8), which included 2,149 women with primary vaginal cancer, noted a significantly lower 5-year survival rate in women with tumors ≥4 cm than in those with tumors <4 cm (65% vs. 84%); however, size information was missing for 52% of women. After multivariate analysis, patients with the larger tumors had an adjusted hazard ratio of 1.71 for mortality. Chyle et al. (67), in their review of 301 patients treated at M.D. Anderson Cancer Center (MDACC) from 1953 to 1991, found that women with lesions larger than 5 cm in maximum diameter had a significantly higher 10-year local recurrence rate than those with smaller lesions (40% vs. 20%). The series by Hellman et al. (135), with 314 patients treated at the Karolinska University Hospital from 1956 to 1996, found that only three factors independently predicted poor survival on multivariate analysis: advanced age, tumor size ≥4 cm, and advanced stage. Tumors comprising two-thirds or more of the vagina and tumors growing circumferentially were associated with an extremely poor prognosis. The series by Tran et al. (138), which reviewed records of 78 patients with SCC treated at Stanford University Medical Center from 1959 to 2005, also found size to be a prognostic factor for DFS on multivariate analysis, along with stage, prior hysterectomy, and pretreatment hemoglobin level. Smaller series by Tjalma et al. (139) and Kirkbride et al. (103) also describe adverse outcomes with larger tumor size. Other series have failed to show significance, but are likely hindered by small numbers, difficulties in accurate assessment of size, and treatment heterogeneity.

Extent of vaginal canal involvement has also been identified as significant, perhaps because it is a surrogate for tumor size. In a series by Stock et al. (110) that examined 100 cases of primary vaginal carcinoma treated at Magee-Women's Hospital from 1962 to 1992, patients with involvement of one-third of the vaginal canal or less had a significantly higher 5-year disease-free survival rate (61%) than patients with more extensive involvement (25%).

Several studies suggest HPV status is an indicator of favorable prognosis. Fuste and colleagues found a trend toward longer survival in women with HPV-positive tumors in their series of 32 patients, with median survival times of 113.9 months versus 19.7 months for women with HPV-positive and HPV-negative tumors, respectively ($p = 0.15$) (140). Alonso et al. (141) evaluated a total of 57 patients, of whom 70.2% had evidence of high-risk HPV. On multivariate analysis (MVA), HPV-positive status was a favorable prognostic variable for overall survival (OS) (HR 0.35, $p = 0.038$). Brunner et al. (142) evaluated 35 patients with primary invasive SCC of the vagina. Using in situ hybridization, HPV was detected in 51.4% of cases. There was no significant influence on clinical stage, grade, or tumor size, nor did prognosis differ between HPV-positive and HPV-negative tumors. However, in a subset of patients with FIGO stage III or higher disease, HPV positivity was found to correlate with improved DFS and overall survival (OS), with p values of 0.004 and 0.023, respectively.

There is conflicting evidence concerning the impact of lesion location on prognosis; it has been noted in some (67,117,143–145) but not all (105,120,146) reports. In an analysis of 110 patients by Kucera (147), 5-year survival rates were 60% for lesions of the upper third of the vagina, 37.5% for lesions of the middle third, and 37% for the lower third. Chyle et al. (67) noted a 17% rate of pelvic relapse in patients with tumors in the upper third of the vagina, 36% for patients with tumors in the middle or lower third, and 42% for patients with whole vaginal involvement. Lesions in the posterior wall were also associated with a worse prognosis than lesions involving the anterior vaginal wall (67), with 10-year recurrence rates of 32% versus 19% on univariate analysis ($p < 0.007$). The Hellman series (135), however, found no difference in prognosis between anterior and posterior tumors. Similarly, histologic grade has been an independent significant predictor of survival in several series (103,117,145), but not others (135). Hellman et al. evaluated the impact of tumor grade and other histopathologic variables (mitotic activity, koilocytosis, growth in vessels, lymphocytic reactions) and found no correlation with survival.

Several series suggest a correlation between older age and decreased survival (9,135,145). For example, age was also noted to be a significant prognostic factor in the Urbanski et al. (145) series, with 5-year survival rates of 83% for patients younger than 60 compared with 25% for those 60 years of age or older ($p < 0.0001$). Age >60 years was negatively associated with survival in the series by Gunderson et al., (9) which examined a total of 110 patients (HR 2.16; $p = 0.0339$). Other series have failed to demonstrate the statistical significance of age (70,148).

Other possible prognostic factors include hemoglobin levels, prior hysterectomy, and smoking status. Tran et al. reviewed records of 78 patients with primary SCC of the vagina treated at Stanford University Hospital, and found a hemoglobin level <12.5 g/dL prior to definitive treatment to be prognostic for worse pelvic control and DSS (128); 5-year DSS rates were 55% for women with Hg levels <12.5 g/dL and 76% for those with levels ≥12.5 g/dL. This remained significant after multivariate analysis, along with prior hysterectomy, stage, and tumor size. The study by Tran et al. (138) is the first to identify prior hysterectomy as a favorable prognostic factor on multivariate analysis. This may reflect more rigorous surveillance in posthysterectomy patients, resulting in tumors discovered at an earlier stage, or may be a reflection of less overall vaginal tissue as a substrate for tumorigenesis. Two subsequent studies have identified hysterectomy as a significant prognostic factor, but only on univariate analysis (67,135).

For patients treated with radiation, treatment time may be a significant factor impacting tumor control (149,150). Lee et al. (150) found overall treatment time of ≤9 weeks to be associated with a pelvic tumor control rate of 97%, compared with 57% for treatment time >9 weeks ($p < 0.01$). Pingley et al. (149) also noted a correlation between treatment time and outcome; patients receiving brachytherapy within 4 weeks of external beam RT (EBRT) had a 5-year DFS rate of 60%, compared with 30% in patients who had an interval greater than 4 weeks.

Treatment: Surgery

For most patients with invasive vaginal cancer, surgery has a limited role, and radiation is the treatment of choice. Owing to the rarity of these lesions, and the required individualization of treatment, it is recommended that patients be referred to a tertiary center with experienced practitioners. In general, surgery is considered useful in the following specific scenarios.

For example, patients with early-stage lesions may have acceptable outcomes if a potentially curative resection can be achieved without extensive functional morbidity. Typically, amenable lesions are small, superficially invasive, and well demarcated, and localized to the upper vagina. A wide local excision can be performed for in situ lesions. For more invasive lesions, a radical upper vaginectomy and pelvic lymphadenectomy can be considered. If the uterus is still present, a radical hysterectomy is also recommended; the goal is to achieve at least 1 cm margins (11).

Surgery can be considered for previously irradiated patients who cannot receive further radiation. Typically, such cases require pelvic exenteration.

Surgery is also a consideration for select patients with stage IVA disease. Extensive lesions in the proximal aspect of the vaginal canal require radical hysterectomy, upper vaginectomy, and bilateral pelvic lymphadenectomy. Older surgical series often required pelvic exenteration in 40% to 50% of cases to obtain negative margins (107,111). Anterior exenteration removes the vagina, urethra, and bladder, and is often necessary to achieve negative margins for invasive anterior wall lesions. Posterior exenteration requires resection of the vagina and rectum. Deeply invasive, circumferential lesions may require a total exenteration in order to achieve clear margins. With positive margins, adjuvant radiation should be offered. Lesions that extend to the inferior vagina require a total vaginectomy with radical hysterectomy, pelvic lymphadenectomy, and possibly vulvovaginectomy and inguinofemoral lymphadenectomy (101,102,110,111). It is not uncommon for relatively small lesions to invade the rectum or urethra early in the disease course, given the close proximity of the vagina to these structures. Given the potentially devastating functional results associated with radical surgery, definitive radiation is the treatment of choice for most patients with invasive vaginal cancer, and has largely replaced surgery as the primary therapeutic modality.

Reported 5-year OS rates for stage I vaginal cancer treated with surgery range from 75% to 100% (**Table 19.4**) (7,101,107,110,139,151). The distinction between stage I and II disease is made clinically, based on physical examination, and it can vary. The NCDB review for cancers of the vagina noted superior survival rates in patients treated with surgery (7), though this likely reflects selection of healthier patients with good performance status for radical surgery. A more recent analysis utilizing the SEER database (8) found women with stage I disease treated with surgery only to have a lower risk of mortality than those treated with radiation only, combined modalities, or no treatment; however, this difference did not reach statistical significance. For stage II vaginal cancer patients, there was a similar trend toward increased mortality in women who did not have surgery alone as their primary treatment modality, but values once again did not reach statistical significance in their multivariate adjusted model.

Ling et al., (152) in a small series consisting of four patients with stage I disease, report their experience using laparoscopic radical hysterectomy with vaginectomy and reconstruction of the vagina. With follow-up times ranging from 40 to 54 months, they report that all patients were free of disease, with satisfactory sexual function. The authors suggest that laparoscopic surgery may be an option for select patients with early-stage disease, with good outcomes.

TABLE 19.4. Early-Stage Vaginal Cancer Treated with Primary Surgery

Series	Stage	# of Pts	Outcomes	Column1	Notes
Creasman (1985–1994) (7)	I	76	5y OS 90%		
	II	34	5y OS 70%		
Tjalma (1974–1999) (139)	I	26	5y OS 91%		4 pts received adjuvant RT 5 LE, 19 htx, 2 ext
Rubin (1957–1980) (111)	I/II	9	5y OS 75%		
Davis (1960–1987) (107)	I/II	52	5y OS 85%		21 ext
Otton (1982–1998) (151)	I	8	5y OS 100%		6 PV; 2 htx + removal of vaginal cuff
Stock (1962–1992) (110)	I	17	5y DFS 56%		6 LE, 7 PV, 4 RV
	II	33	5y DFS 68%		6 ext, 17 RV, 8 PV, 2 LE
Ball (1947–1978) (101)	I	19	5y OS 84%		4 ext
	II	8	5y OS 63%		1 ext

Ext, exenteration; htx, hysterectomy; LE, local excision; pts, patients; PV, partial vaginectomy; RV, radical vaginectomy.

Other series also report excellent results with primary surgical therapy, though authors acknowledge bias resulting from selection of healthier patients with less extensive disease for primary surgery over radiation. In a review of 100 cases by Stock et al. (110), with 85 SCC cases, surgical treatment was noted to be a significantly favorable prognostic factor for DFS, compared with RT alone. For stage I patients, DFS rates were 56% and 80% for patients treated with surgery versus RT, respectively. For stage II patients, survival rates were 68% and 31% after surgery and RT, respectively, though this likely reflects selection bias, with patients with more extensive involvement offered RT. Overall 5-year survival was 47%. Stock et al. concluded that surgery consisting of radical hysterectomy, pelvic lymphadenectomy, and upper vaginectomy could be reasonable for stage I lesions and select stage II lesions, with RT being the preferred primary modality for patients with stage IIB disease. It should be noted, however, that 23 of 33 stage II patients (70%) treated with surgery required a total vaginectomy or exenterative procedure, which carries significant morbidity and functional impairment.

Smaller series also support use of surgery in select patients with early-stage disease. Tjalma et al. (139) reported on 55 cases of primary vaginal SCC. Of 27 patients with stage I disease, 26 received surgery, with 4 subsequently receiving some form of adjuvant RT. With a median follow-up time of 45 months, 5-year survival was reported to be 91%. Otton et al. (151), in their retrospective review of 70 patients with stage I–II vaginal carcinoma treated at Queensland Center for Gynaecological Cancer between 1982 and 1998, report that patients treated with surgery alone, or a combination of surgery and RT, had significantly longer survival times than patients treated with radiation alone. The authors suggest that surgery may be effective in a select subset of patients with small, localized tumors that permit clear surgical margins. Peters et al. (120) reviewed records of 86 patients with vaginal carcinoma, including 68 SCC cases, treated at the University of Michigan Medical Center. Twelve selected patients had surgery as primary therapy, with a 75% survival rate. Similarly, Rubin et al. (111) reported on eight patients with stage I or II disease who received surgery as primary treatment; 5-year survival was 75%, and the overall local control rate for the stage I patients was 80%, suggesting that highly selected patients can achieve excellent outcomes with surgery. Davis et al. (107) reported on 89 patients with vaginal carcinoma, treated primarily at the Mayo Clinic from 1960 to 1987. A total of 52 patients were treated with surgery as primary therapy, with 5-year survival of 85%, compared with 65% for patients who received RT alone. In the stage II patients, the 5-year survival rates were 49%, 50%, and 69% for surgery, radiation, and combined treatment with surgery and RT, respectively. However, treatment modalities cannot be effectively compared using retrospective series, given selection biases.

Several series report their experience using surgery for advanced-stage III or IV patients, with most cases requiring radical excision, typically pelvic exenteration (101,102,110,111). Control rates, at best, are around 50%, even with highly selected patients. In practice, given the overall poor prognosis and morbidity associated with surgery, advanced-stage patients should receive definitive RT, typically in combination with chemotherapy (CT).

Another approach that has been proposed involves neoadjuvant CT followed by radical surgery (153,154). Benedetti et al. (153) reported 11 patients with stage II SCC of the vagina treated by using three cycles of neoadjuvant paclitaxel and cisplatin followed by surgical resection. Ninety-one percent of patients obtained a partial or complete response to neoadjuvant CT; 27% achieved a complete response. All patients had disease-free resection margins after surgery, and only one patient had positive lymph nodes. At a median follow-up time of 75 months, 10 of 11 patients (91%) were alive, and of those, eight (73%) were free of disease. Postoperative complications were mild.

A case report documented the use of neoadjuvant CT consisting of bleomycin and cisplatin, followed by radical surgery, for one patient with stage II SCC of the vagina. The patient was free of disease, with satisfactory sexual function, at 30 months (153). However, it is necessary to evaluate the feasibility of this treatment in larger series of patients, with longer follow-up.

Treatment: Radiation

For most patients, RT is the treatment of choice given the desire for organ preservation and the significant morbidity that may be incurred by exenterative surgery. It is important to individualize RT techniques based on size, depth, and location of the lesion. The outcomes of retrospective series on use of RT for vaginal cancer are summarized in **Table 19.5**, and are addressed in detail in the next section.

Stage I. Brachytherapy alone is an option for select patients presenting with small, superficial tumors (see treatment algorithm in **Fig. 19.8**). Reported local control rates range from 62% to 100% (104,105,109,115,117,145,162–164). Perez et al. (70) reported pelvic tumor control of 88% in patients with stage I disease who received brachytherapy alone, using a dose of 60 to 70 Gy prescribed 5 mm beyond the plane of the implant or vaginal mucosa, with a vaginal surface dose of 80 to 120 Gy. Notably, tumor control in stage I vaginal carcinoma was similar to that of brachytherapy alone, versus brachytherapy plus EBRT. This observation is consistent with reports from some groups (70,147,165), but not others (115,164). Other series suggest high locoregional failure rates with brachytherapy alone. Kanayama et al. report that three of eight (38%) patients with stage I vaginal cancer, treated with brachytherapy alone, developed lymph node recurrence. Frank et al. (115) reported on 21 patients with stage I disease who were treated with local radiation only, without regional node coverage. Nine received brachytherapy alone, 11 received EBRT with or without brachytherapy, and one received local EBRT using a transvaginal orthovoltage cone. Three of nine patients treated with brachytherapy alone developed recurrent disease in the pelvis, resulting in a 10-year pelvic disease control rate of 67%. Patients who received EBRT with or without brachytherapy did not have pelvic recurrences. A pelvic relapse rate of 18% at 10 years was noted by Frank and colleagues (115), with all pelvic failures occurring in patients treated with brachytherapy alone. Overall, these results suggest a need for caution when brachytherapy alone is used without prophylactic lymph node irradiation, given the fairly high rates of lymph node recurrence. Appropriate patient selection is critical, particularly because the distinction between stages I and II is based on clinical exam, and can vary between providers.

Poorly differentiated or extensively infiltrating stage I lesions should be treated with a combination of EBRT and brachytherapy. Given possible underestimation of submucosal disease and/or nodal disease, resulting in a potentially high likelihood of recurrence with brachytherapy alone, some groups recommend incorporating EBRT into treatment of all stage I patients, except for those with very small, superficial lesions (115,164). In their series of patients with vaginal cancer treated at MDCC between 1970 and 2000, Frank et al. (115), noted a trend toward increasing use of EBRT for stage I vaginal SCC over time.

Actuarial 5-year survival rates for stage I disease range from 60% to 85% (8,105,115,138). DSS rates for stage I disease, treated with definitive radiation, range from 75% to 95% (67,70,106). The 10-year pelvic relapse rate, comprising local, pelvic nodal, and inguinal nodal failures, was reportedly 16% (115) for stage I patients. Most failures are locoregional. Distant metastases are uncommon and occur in about 5% of patients (70,107,162).

With LDR, treatment can be delivered in two applications, the first designed to treat the entire vaginal wall, and the second to cover the tumor volume. When HDR brachytherapy is the primary treatment, the entire length of the vagina is typically treated to a mucosal dose of 60 to 65 Gy, with an additional mucosal dose of 20 to 30 Gy delivered to the area of tumor involvement (166). Treatment can be delivered with a shielded vaginal cylinder or with a multichannel HDR cylinder to treat the tumor with a 2-cm margin and

■ TABLE 19.5. Outcomes for Vaginal Cancer Treated with Primary Radiation

Series	Outcome	Stage I	Stage II	Stage III	Stage IV	Treatment
Dixit (1985–1989) (147)	2y DSS	100%	70%	19%	0%	EBRT and/or BT
Fine (1963–1991) (155)	5y OS	42%	68%	58%	0%	EBRT and/or BT
Kucera (1975–1984) (146)	5y OS	81%	44%	35%	32%,0%[a]	EBRT and/or BT
Perez (1953–1991) (70)	PC	85%	66%,56%[b]	65%	27%	EBRT and/or BT
	10y DFS	80%	55%,35%[b]	38%	0%	
de Crevoisier (1970–2001) (156)	5y PC	79%		62%		EBRT and/or BT
Lee (1964–1990) (149)	5y PC	87%	88%,68%[b]	80%	67%	EBRT and/or BT
	5y CSS	94%	80%,39%[b]	79%	62%	
Frank (1970–2000) (115)	5y PC	86%	84%	71%		EBRT + BT (n = 119), EBRT (n = 63)
	5y DSS	85%	78%	58%		
Chyle (1953–1991) (67)	10y PC	84%	75%	60%	40%	EBRT + BT (n = 121), EBRT (n = 95), BT (n = 26),
	10y OS	55%	51%	37%	40%	transvaginal cone (n = 2)
Stryker (1976–1994) (157)	5y DSS	78%	63%	33%	50%	EBRT + BT (n = 25), EBRT (n = 7), BT (n = 2)
Lian (1986–2006) (158)	5y DSS	90%	87%	32%	26%	EBRT + BT (n = 28), EBRT (n = 17), BT (n = 4), S+RT (n = 6)
Tran (1959–2005) (137)	5y PC	83%	76%	62%	30%	EBRT + BT (n = 43), EBRT (n = 22), BT (n = 10)
	5y DSS	92%	68%	44%	13%	
Mock (1986–1999) (94)	5y DSS	92%	57%	59%	0%	EBRT + BT (n = 55), EBRT (n = 5), BT (n = 26)
Urbanski (1965–1988) (144)	5y DFS	73%	54%	23%	0%	EBRT + BT (n = 77), BT (n = 11), EBRT (n = 15)
Beriwal (2000–2006) (159)	2y crude LC		100%	100%	100%	EBRT + HDR BT
Creasman (1985–1994) (7)	5y OS	73%	58%	36%		RT and/or S
Kirkbride (1974–1989) (103)	5y DSS	72%	70%	53%	42%	RT and/or S
Rubin (1958–1980) (111)	5y OS	75%	48%	54%	0%	RT and/or S
Stock (1962–1992) (110)	5y LC	72%	62%	0%	21%	RT and/or S
	5y DFS	67%	53%	0%	15%	
Shah (1990–2004) (8)	5y DSS	84%	75%	57%		RT and/or S
Hellman (1956–1996) (160)	5y DSS	75%	36%	36%	20%,0%[a]	RT and/or S
Miyamoto (1972–2009) (161)	3y OS	56% (Combined I-IV)				RT ± S

[a]Outcomes for stage IVA, IVB respectively.

[b]Outcomes for stage IIA, IIB respectively.

5-FU, 5-fluorouracil; AWD, alive with disease; BT, brachytherapy; cis, cisplatin; CSS, cause-specific survival; DFS, disease-free survival; DID, died of intercurrent disease; DOD, died of disease; DSS, disease-specific survival; EBRT, external beam radiation; HDR, high dose rate; LC, local control; MMC, mitomycin C; NED, no evidence of disease; OS, overall survival; PC, pelvic control; RT, radiotherapy (any form); S, surgery.

block uninvolved mucosal surfaces (167). HDR can also be used to treat superficial lesions.

Use of a multichannel HDR cylinder is an alternative technique with favorable local control and low toxicity. The standard multichannel HDR cylinder consists of a central channel with 6 to 12 peripheral channels, allowing preferential dosing to the target but decreasing dose to normal structures. Vargo et al. (168) reported outcomes for 41 patients with vaginal cancer treated with this technique to a median equivalent dose in 2 Gy fractions (EQD2) of 77.1 Gy. Definitive treatment consisted of EBRT followed by brachytherapy. Most (71%) patients had FIGO 1 disease. At 2 years, there was 93% local control, and 4% overall late grade 3 or higher toxicity, demonstrating comparable results to historical treatments. A tumor thickness cutoff of 5 mm for the apex and posterior vagina, and 7 mm for other locations, was utilized.

Guidelines from the American Brachytherapy Society recommend a cumulative D90 (dose to 90% of volume) EQD2 of 70 to 85 Gy to the vaginal tumor (169). Various regimens can be used to achieve this dose, with commonly utilized schedules of 45 Gy in 25 fractions EBRT followed by HDR brachytherapy in five fractions of 4.5 to 5.5 Gy (EQD2 = 71.4 to 79.8 Gy), or 9 to 10 fractions of 3 Gy (EQD2 = 73.5 to 76.8 Gy).

Stage II. Stage II vaginal carcinoma involves the subvaginal tissue, but does not extend to the pelvic sidewall. The primary treatment for stage II disease is radiation, most commonly as a combination of EBRT followed by vaginal brachytherapy; CT can also be considered. Outcomes with brachytherapy alone have been poor, and thus this approach is not recommended. With brachytherapy alone, Perez et al. (70) noted a 36% pelvic tumor control rate in stage II patients,

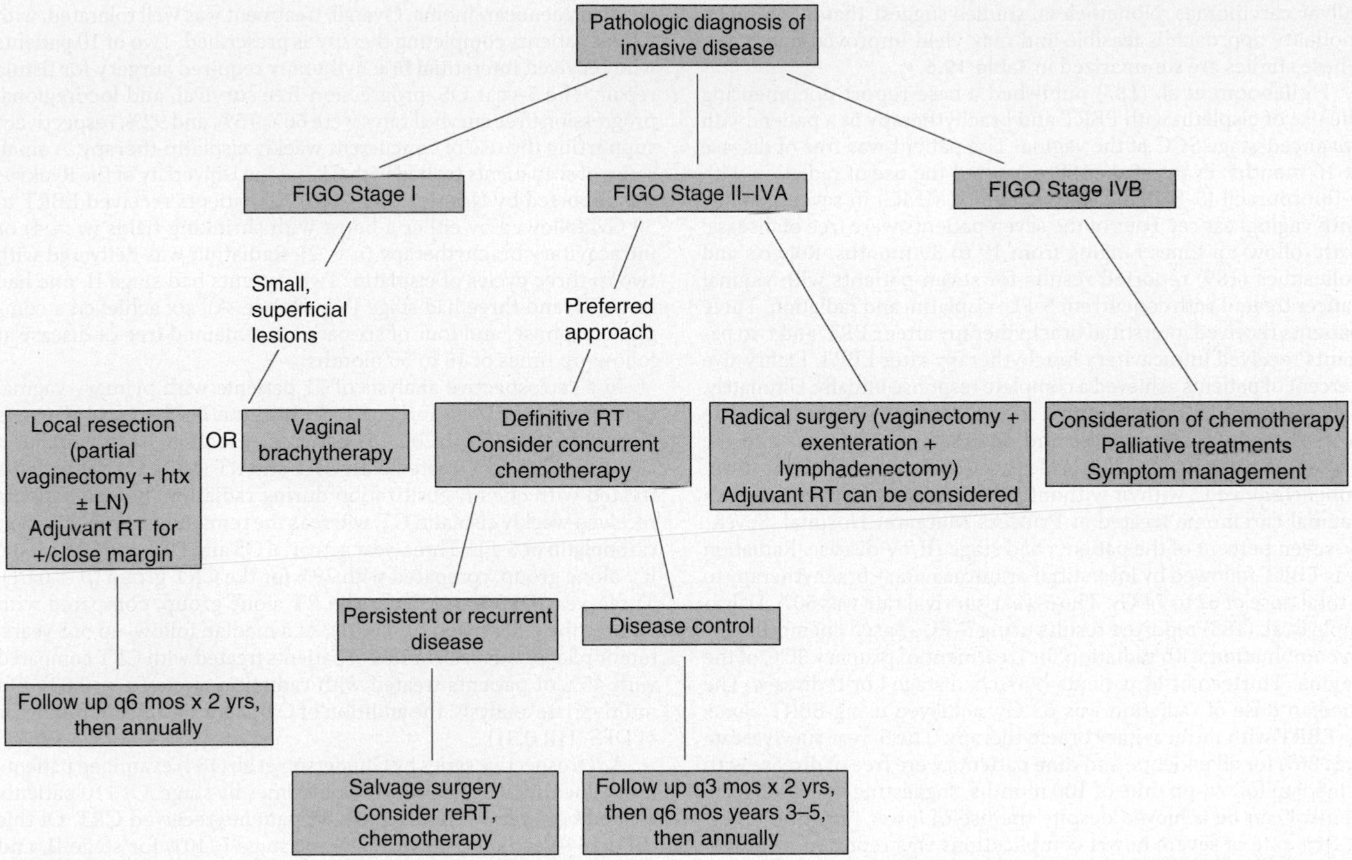

Figure 19.8. Proposed treatment algorithm for invasive squamous cell cancer of the vagina. htx, hysterectomy; LN, lymphadenectomy; RT, radiation treatment.

compared with 67% in patients treated with a combination of EBRT and brachytherapy. The benefit of combining EBRT and brachytherapy, as opposed to using either alone, has been shown in other series as well (67,110).

During EBRT, the pelvis generally receives 45 to 50.4 Gy in 1.8 Gy fractions, with consideration of a parametrial boost if there is extensive primary infiltration or high suspicion of nodal disease. Inguinal lymph nodes are included in a modified whole pelvic field for lesions involving the distal one-third of the vaginal canal.

Brachytherapy should be carefully delivered to ensure adequate coverage of tumor volume. An interstitial technique, ideally with three dimensional (3D) imaging for treatment planning, is required for tumors >5 mm in depth (104,170). Extensive tumors, or deeply infiltrating tumors with nondistinct margins, may be poor candidates for brachytherapy. In such cases, boosting tumors with conformal techniques or intensity-modulated RT (IMRT) may be preferred, and may yield better outcomes than suboptimal brachytherapy (115). The tumor volume should receive a minimum of 75 to 80 Gy using combined EBRT and brachytherapy. Fleming et al. (171) and Puthawala and colleagues (172) both report improved outcomes with higher doses of 80 to 100 Gy.

The 5-year survival rate for patients with stage II disease treated with RT alone ranges from 35% to 70% for stage IIA, and 35% to 60% for stage IIB (29,151,173). Pelvic relapse at 10 years has been reported at 25% by Frank et al., which is consistent with recent series reporting 5-year pelvic control rates ranging from 76% to 84% (115,138). The likelihood of distant metastasis is higher for stage IIB lesions compared with stage IIA (105,165), with overall reported rates ranging from 22% to 46% (105,107).

Stages III and IVA. Locally advanced vaginal cancer is treated with a combined modality approach of RT and consideration of CT, extrapolating from favorable outcomes with use of chemoradiation therapy (CRT) in cervical cancer patients (174,175). Radiation is delivered as pelvic EBRT, followed by additional parametrial boost when warranted. If adequate tumor coverage can be achieved without undue toxicity, interstitial brachytherapy is employed to deliver a minimum tumor dose of 75 to 80 Gy. If brachytherapy is not feasible because of extensive tumor infiltration of the rectovaginal septum or bladder, a shrinking-field technique or IMRT have been used to deliver additional dose to the primary lesion (176,177). The overall cure rate for patients with stage III disease ranges from 30% to 50%. Stage IVA carries a worse prognosis. In highly selected patients with small-volume stage IV disease, pelvic exenteration can yield good long-term control; however, in practice, EBRT remains the primary treatment (7,8,70,110,111,115,145, 178,179). Five-year actuarial survival rates for women with stage III disease range from 25% to 58% (7,8,180), with local failure rates of 30% to 75% (105,115,138). Outcomes for stage IV disease are worse, with survival rates of 0% to 40% (67,110,155). Despite treatment with EBRT and brachytherapy, only 20% to 30% of patients with stages III-IV disease achieve local control. Pelvic recurrences are more frequent than distant recurrences (115). A combination approach utilizing CT with concurrent RT has shown favorable outcomes. A single-institution retrospective review of patients treated with RT alone, versus CRT, showed that use of concurrent CT to improve DFS on multivariate analysis (HR 0.31; $p = 0.04$) (178).

Role of Chemotherapy and Radiation

CT has been incorporated with radiation for treatment of vaginal cancer, extrapolating from studies in cervical cancer showing improved PFS and OS when cisplatin is added to RT (70,161,174,175,181,182). Given the rarity of vaginal cancer, there are no randomized trials comparing RT alone with RT plus CT. Retrospective series are limited by small numbers or inclusion of other cancers, such as cervical and vulvar carcinomas. Nonetheless, studies suggest that a combined modality approach is feasible and may yield improved outcomes. These studies are summarized in **Table 19.6.**

Holleboom et al. (187) published a case report documenting the use of cisplatin with EBRT and brachytherapy in a patient with advanced-stage SCC of the vagina. The patient was free of disease at 16 months. Evans et al. (188) reported the use of radiation with 5-fluorouracil (5-FU) and mitomycin C (MMC) in seven patients with vaginal cancer. Four of the seven patients were free of disease, with follow-up times ranging from 19 to 39 months. Roberts and colleagues (189) reported results for seven patients with vaginal cancer treated with concurrent 5-FU, cisplatin, and radiation. Three patients received interstitial brachytherapy after EBRT, and two patients received intracavitary brachytherapy after EBRT. Eighty-five percent of patients achieved a complete response initially. Ultimately, 61% recurred, at a median time to recurrence of 6 months. There were three local recurrences and one distant metastasis and the 5-year OS rate was 22%. Kirkbride et al. (103) reported on the use of concurrent 5-FU, with or without MMC, in 26 of 153 patients with vaginal carcinoma treated at Princess Margaret Hospital. Seventy-seven percent of the patients had stage III/IV disease. Radiation was EBRT followed by interstitial or intracavitary brachytherapy to a total dose of 62 to 74 Gy. The 5-year survival rate was 50%. Dalrymple et al. (183) reported results using 5-FU–based chemotherapy in combination with radiation for treatment of primary SCC of the vagina. Thirteen of 14 patients (93%) had stage I or II disease. The median dose of radiation was 63 Gy, achieved using EBRT alone, or EBRT with intracavitary brachytherapy. The 5-year survival rate was 86% for all patients, and nine patients were free of disease with a median follow-up time of 100 months, suggesting that good local control can be achieved despite the use of lower radiation doses. A 31% rate of severe bowel complications was reported, with two deaths as a result of bowel obstruction.

A retrospective series from MDACC by Frank and colleagues (115) included nine patients with stage II–IVA SCC of the vagina treated with RT and concurrent cisplatin-based CRT. With a mean follow-up time of 129 months, improved local control with the use of chemotherapy was noted, with 44% of patients treated with concurrent CRT remaining free of disease. Samant et al. (185) published a review of 12 vaginal cancer patients, stage II–IVA, treated with concurrent weekly cisplatin at a dose of 40 mg/m^2 for 5 weeks. Patients received concurrent EBRT to a median dose of 45 Gy, with LDR interstitial or HDR intracavitary brachytherapy boost of median dose 30 Gy. Six patients had stage II disease, four had stage III disease, and two had stage IVA disease. Ten of 12 patients (83%) had SCC; the other two had adenocarcinoma. Overall, treatment was well tolerated, with 92% of patients completing therapy as prescribed. Two of 10 patients who received interstitial brachytherapy required surgery for fistula repair. The 5-year OS, progression-free survival, and locoregional progression-free survival rates were 66%, 75%, and 92%, respectively, supporting the use of concurrent weekly cisplatin therapy. A small series of six patients treated with CRT at the University of the Ryukyus was reported by Nashiro et al. (186) All patients received EBRT to 50 Gy, followed by either a boost with shrinking fields (n = 4) or intracavitary brachytherapy (n = 2). Radiation was delivered with two to three cycles of cisplatin. Two patients had stage II, one had stage III, and three had stage IVA disease. All six achieved a complete response, and four of six patients remained free of disease at follow-up times of 18 to 55 months.

In a retrospective analysis of 71 patients with primary vaginal cancer treated at Dana-Farber Cancer Institute/Brigham and Women's Hospital from 1972 to 2009, 51 patients were treated with radiation alone, and 20 were treated with CRT and RT (182). Of the patients treated with chemosensitization during radiation, 85% of patients received weekly cisplatin CT, whereas the remainder received either carboplatin or 5-FU. Three-year actuarial OS and DFS was 56% for the RT-alone group, compared with 79% for the CRT group (p = 0.01). Three-year DFS was 43% for the RT alone group, compared with 73% for the CRT group (p = 0.01). At a median follow-up of 3 years, tumor relapse was seen in 15% of patients treated with CRT compared with 45% of patients treated with radiation alone (p = 0.03). On multivariate analysis, the addition of CT was a significant predictor of DFS (HR 0.31).

A retrospective series by Gunderson et al. (184) examined patients treated with CRT and reported outcomes by stage. Of 110 patients treated between 1990 and 2004, 41 patients received CRT. Of this cohort, 4-year survival was 64% for stage I, 40% for stage II, and 12% for stage III/IV.

Ghia et al. (190) published a retrospective patterns-of-care analysis using the SEER database, analyzing data on women with primary vaginal cancer treated with EBRT and/or brachytherapy between 1991 and 2005. Of the 326 women in the study cohort, 80.4% had SCC. It was noted that CRT was used in 7.5% of patients treated before 1999 compared with 36.1% of those treated afterward ($p < 0.001$). Cisplatin was the most frequently utilized agent, accounting for 59% of CRT treatments. CT was significantly less likely to be used in conjunction with RT for women older than 80 years of age; otherwise, there was no difference for race, stage, grade, histologic diagnosis, comorbidities, or brachytherapy use. On multivariate analysis, CRT was not found to correlate with improved cause-specific or OS.

TABLE 19.6. Select Series with Outcomes for Combined Chemotherapy and Radiation for Vaginal Cancer

Series	Outcomes	Stage	Notes
Miyamoto (1972–2009) (161)	3y OS 79%	St I, n = 18; St II, n = 19, St III, n = 8, St IVA, n = 6	RT+cis, 5FU or carboplatin
Dalrymple (1986–1996) (183)	NED n = 9 (FU 74–168 months); DOD n = 1 (12 months); DID n = 4 (46–109 months)	St I, n = 1; St II, n = 10, St III, n = 1	RT+5-FU, cis/5FU or MMC
Gunderson (1990–2004) (184)	4y OS 64% (Stage I), 40% (Stage II), 12% (Stage III/IV)	St I, n = 31; St II, n = 30; St III/IV, n = 69	CRT, n = 87; S + CRT, n = 43
Samant (1999–2004) (185)	5y OS 66%	St II, n = 6; St III, n = 4; St IVA, n = 2	RT+cis
Nashiro (2002–2005) (186)	DOD n = 1 (25 months); NED n = 4 (FU 19–54 months); AWD n = 1 (FU 19 months)	St II, n = 2; St III, n = 1; St IVA, n = 3	RT+cis or cis/5FU

AC, adenocarinoma; B, brachytherapy; CRT, chemoradiation; EBRT, external beam radiation; FU, fluorouracil; LR PFS, locoregional progression-free survival; NED, no evidence of disease; OS, overall survival; SCC, squamous cell carcinoma.

Outcomes

According to SEER-based data, outcomes for vaginal cancer may be improving. A recent study by Shah et al. (8) analyzed records from the SEER database of 2,149 women diagnosed with primary vaginal cancer between 1990 and 2004. The risk of mortality was noted to decrease over time, with a 17% decrease in the risk of death for women diagnosed after 2000 relative to those diagnosed between 1990 and 1994. The authors reported 5-year DSS rates of 84% for stage I, 75% for stage II, and 57% for stages III–IV. An older study by Creasman et al. (7) focused on 4,885 women diagnosed with vaginal cancer between 1985 and 1994, and reported 5-year survival rates of 96% for stage 0, 73% for stage I, 58% for stage II, and 36% for stages III–IV, with 85% of invasive cases being SCC.

In general, the rate of locoregional recurrence ranges from 10% to 20% for stage I and 30% to 40% for stage II. Patients with advanced disease often have persistent disease despite treatment. In a series by Dixit et al. (148), 68% of failures in stage III patients were due to persistent disease. Most treatment failures occur within 5 years, with a median time to recurrence of 6 to 12 months (115,191), and local recurrence is the most common pattern of treatment failure in most published series. Extravaginal recurrences in the pelvic lymph nodes are less common. The reported rates of distant metastasis vary, ranging from 7% to 33% and usually occur later in the course of disease, with approximately half of all distant metastases presenting at the time of local recurrence (104,105,118,148).

Clear Cell Adenocarcinoma

Epidemiology

Clear cell adenocarcinoma of the vagina was first reported in 1971 by Herbst and Scully (192), who documented six cases of primary vaginal clear cell carcinoma in patients 15 to 22 years of age: five of the six had been exposed to the synthetic estrogen DES in utero during the first trimester. This was the first report suggesting that in utero exposure to DES, prescribed during the mid-1940s to 1960s for high-risk pregnancies, could result in an increased risk of clear cell adenocarcinoma. DES-related clear cell adenocarcinoma presents at a young age, with studies documenting median age at presentation to be within the second or third decade of life (192,193). Studies suggest that there is a bimodal distribution for clear cell adenocarcinoma of the vagina, the first peak comprising young women with a mean age of 26, most of whom were exposed to DES in utero, and a second peak comprising women with a mean age of 71 years, not exposed to DES (192,194). Most patients present with stages I–II disease (192,195).

Risk Factors

In 45% to 95% of cases, clear cell adenocarcinoma of the vagina is associated with vaginal adenosis, defined as the abnormal presence of glandular epithelium in the vagina (196,197). Vaginal adenosis has three patterns: endocervical, tuboendometrial, and embryonic (44,197,198). Grossly, vaginal adenosis appears as red, velvety, grapelike clusters in the vagina. Glandular columnar epithelium of Mullerin type either appears beneath the squamous epithelium or replaces it, undergoing progressive squamous metaplasia (199).

Vaginal adenosis is believed to be a precursor lesion to clear cell adenocarcinoma of the vagina. It is a common histologic abnormality in women who have been exposed to DES in utero, presenting in up to 95% of such women (196,197). However, it is not strictly confined to this population (200).

The risk of developing clear cell adenocarcinoma in DES-exposed women is estimated to be 1 in 1,000 (195), suggesting that there are multiple factors contributing to pathogenesis. Additional factors associated with increased risk include DES exposure before the 12th week of pregnancy, a maternal history of prior miscarriage, birth in autumn, and prematurity (170).

Histopathology

Clear cell adenocarcinoma of the vagina is most often located in the upper third of the anterior vagina and may vary greatly in size. These cancers can also arise in the cervix. Grossly, they exhibit exophytic growth and are superficially invasive (201). Microscopically, they are composed of vacuolated, glycogen-rich cells; hence the term clear cell carcinoma (**Fig. 19.9**). The most common histologic pattern is tubulocystic, although solid, papillary, and mixed cell patterns have also been described (129,202). Cells are cuboidal or columnar in shape, with large, atypical protruding nuclei, rimmed by a small amount of vacuolated cytoplasm.

Clinical Presentation

Patients with clear cell adenocarcinoma most often present with abnormal vaginal bleeding (192), which is found in 50% to 75% of cases. Cytology is not reliable, revealing abnormality in only 33% of cases; therefore, careful assessment of the entire vaginal vault to assess for submucosal irregularity is recommended, in addition to four-quadrant cytologic assessment (203). Abnormal discharge, urinary symptoms, and lower gastrointestinal complaints can also be noted, particularly in advanced cases. The differential diagnosis of vaginal adenocarcinoma is often challenging, because it must be distinguished from metastases from distant sites.

Prognostic Factors

For clear cell adenocarcinoma, prognostic variables associated with worse survival include advanced-stage, nontubulocystic pattern of histology, size >3 cm, and depth of invasion >3 mm (201). A study of 21 women with clear cell carcinoma of the vagina and cervix reported that overexpression of wild-type p53 was associated with a more favorable prognosis (204). Primary adenocarcinoma of the vagina not associated with DES exposure is extremely rare. In a review of 26 such cases by Frank et al., (205) 5-year OS was 34%, significantly worse than in patients with SCC. A recent series described five cases of clear cell adenocarcinoma in patients without prior DES exposure, treated between 1990 and 2013 (206). The patients were all older than 40 years of age. There was high incidence of distant spread, especially to the lungs; OS at 5 years was 55%.

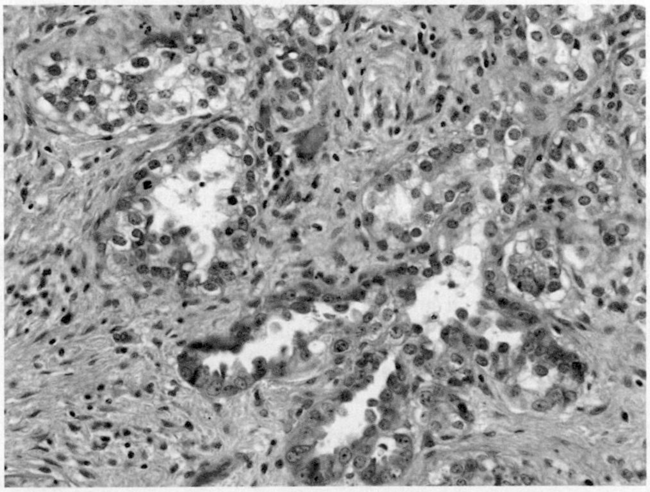

Figure 19.9. Clear cell carcinoma. Clear cell carcinoma (CCC) of the vagina appears as nests and irregular glands lined by cells with characteristic clear to pale eosinophilic cytoplasm. CCC may show a mixture of architectural patterns including papillary, tubulopapillary, and tubulocytic patterns, and cytologic features may be variable from round to oval nuclei with prominent nucleoli (as seen in this example) to more significant nuclear pleomorphism and conspicuous mitoses.

Source: Images courtesy of Emily E.K. Meserve.

Treatment Options

The optimal management of clear cell adenocarcinoma is unclear. There are several published series on DES-related clear cell adenocarcinomas (129,201,207–209) using conventional treatments similar to those used for SCC of the vagina for stage I and II disease, including surgery with radical hysterectomy, vaginectomy and lymphadenectomy with construction of a neovagina, or definitive RT and consideration of radiosensitizing concurrent CT (210,211). In these series, there has been an emphasis on preservation of ovarian and vaginal function, owing to the earlier age at diagnosis in DES-exposed patients. According to data from the United States Registry for Research on Hormonal Transplacental Carcinogenesis, approximately one half of all vaginal clear cell adenocarcinoma cases were treated with radical surgery alone (212).

Wharton et al. (213) report the use of intracavitary or transvaginal irradiation for early-stage disease, with excellent tumor control and preservation of ovarian function. Herbst et al. (214) reported on 142 cases of stage I clear cell adenocarcinoma. For the 117 patients treated with radical surgery, there was an 8% risk of recurrence and 87% OS. For patients treated with radiation, there was a 36% risk of recurrence. The authors acknowledge that it is difficult to compare surgery with radiation, as radiation was most likely used in patients with larger lesions less amenable to resection.

A series by Senekjian et al. (208) reported on 219 cases of stage I clear cell vaginal adenocarcinoma. Forty-three patients received local therapy alone, consisting of vaginectomy, local excision or local irradiation with or without excision, and the remaining patients had conventional radical surgery. At 10 years, the actuarial survival rates were equivalent (88% vs. 90%). However, the actuarial recurrence rate was significantly higher (40% vs. 13%) with local excision alone. Patients who received local irradiation, with or without local excision, had decreased local recurrence compared to those treated with excision alone ($p < 0.03$).

A subsequent series by Senekjian et al. (129) reviewed 76 cases of stage II clear cell adenocarcinoma. The 10-year OS rate was 65%. The 5-year survival rates were 80% for patients treated with surgery, 87% for patients treated with radiation, and 85% for patients treated with both. The authors advocate treatment with combination EBRT and brachytherapy for stage II disease, with surgery reserved for smaller, more easily resectable lesions in the upper vagina. The use of pelvic exenteration for primary and recurrent lesions has been reported by Senekjian and colleagues (209). Survival outcomes were comparable to those of patients treated with other modalities. Thus, to minimize morbidity and preserve quality of life, exenterative approaches are advocated only for patients with disease recurrence after RT. Herbst et al. reported a 5-year survival rate after pelvic relapse was reportedly 40% (207).

Most recurrences occur within 3 years of therapy, although recurrences 10 to 20 years after treatment have been reported (215). Most recurrences are local or locoregional, with approximately one-third detected at distant sites, most commonly in the lungs or extrapelvic lymph nodes, although there have been rare cases of central nervous system (CNS) metastases manifesting years after treatment (216). The 10-year actuarial survival rate for clear cell adenocarcinoma of the vagina is 79%. For stage I and II disease, survival rates are 90% and 80%, respectively.

Other Adenocarcinomas

Most adenocarcinomas that present in the vagina are attributed to metastatic spread from other sites. Vaginal metastases from adenocarcinoma of the breast, kidneys, or other gynecologic primary sites have been described (217–219). Primary non-CCA of the vagina is extremely rare, and occurs predominantly in postmenopausal women. Histologic variants include endometrioid, mucinous, mesonephric, and papillary serous adenocarcinoma (**Fig. 19.10**). Vaginal endometrioid adenocarcinoma is the most common non-clear cell subtype, and presents most often in women with a history of endometriosis.

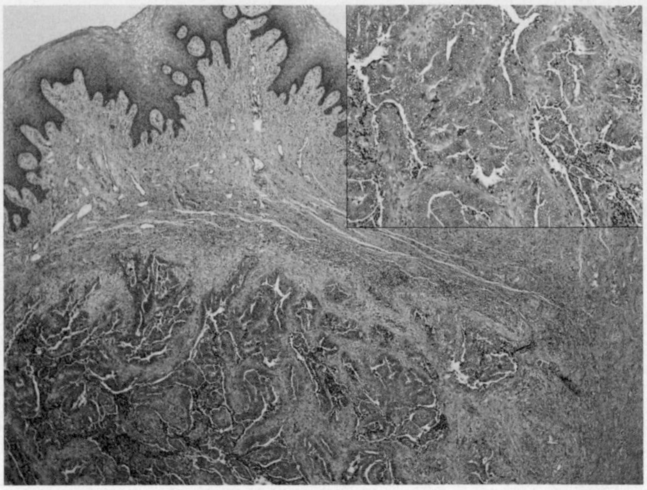

Figure 19.10. Vaginal adenocarcinoma. Vaginal adenocarcinoma appears as irregular glands infiltrating beneath unremarkable squamous mucosa often associated with endometriosis. Cytologically (inset), the cells are oriented around the glandular lumen and show nuclear pleomorphism, coarse to vesicular chromatin, and often frequent mitoses. Images courtesy of Emily E.K. Meserve.

Source: Images courtesy of Emily E.K. Meserve.

Only a handful of case reports or series have been published in detail about endometrioid adenocarcinoma of the vagina (220–230). In one series of 18 cases of primary vaginal endometrioid adenocarcinoma (220), 10 cases arose from the apex; 14 of 18 cases had vaginal endometriosis, which is important in indicating a primary vaginal tumor rather than secondary spread from the endothelium. Median age at presentation was 57, with a range from 45 to 81 years. There have been case reports of mucinous adenocarcinoma of the vagina (221–233), with at least one arising from a focus of endocervicosis (234).

On gross exam, endometrioid adenocarcinomas can be polypoid, papillary, rough, granular, fungating, exophytic, or flat, and most arise from the superior aspect of the vagina. Microscopically, tumors display a predominant component of typical endometrioid carcinoma, with tubular glands lined by columnar cells with moderate amounts of eosinophilic cytoplasm, and large elongated nuclei. Only a handful of cases of mucinous adenocarcinoma have been described (218,231–233), including rare cases arising in neovaginas (235) or arising from endocervicosis (234). Mesonephric adenocarcinoma arises from mesonephric duct remnants situated in the lateral vaginal wall (236,237). Primary papillary serous adenocarcinoma of the vagina has rarely been reported (238).

Melanoma

According to the NCDB report by Creasman et al. (7), vaginal melanomas comprise 4% of all primary vaginal cancers. Melanomas arising from the vaginal mucosa are rare, accounting for 2.8% to 5% of all vaginal neoplasms (239–241), with just over 100 new cases reported each year in the United States. Melanomas arising from the vaginal mucosa are thought to originate from mucosal melanocytes in regions of melanosis or from atypical melanocytic hyperplasia.

The incidence of vaginal melanoma has remained stable and is reportedly 0.26 per million (242). Most reported cases are in Caucasian women; one study of 37 women with primary melanoma of the vagina reported that 84% of patients were Caucasian and only 3% African American (239). According to a report by Hu et al. (243) analyzing SEER data from 1992 to 2005 on 125 cases of vaginal melanoma with known race/ethnicity, there is no significant difference in incidence of vaginal melanoma between Caucasian and African American women, with a White/Black ratio of 1.02 after age adjustment. In the report by Creasman and colleagues, most patients were of advanced age at presentation, with only 23% of patients diagnosed before the age of 60; 28% were diagnosed between the ages of 60 and 69, 28% were diagnosed between the ages of 70 and 79, and 22% were diagnosed at age 80 or older (7).

Grossly, melanoma of the vagina tends to be pigmented, and may present as a dark mass, plaque, or ulceration; multifocal presentation is also common. The most common appearance is polypoid nodular (244). The most common location at presentation is the anterior vaginal wall and lower one-third of the vagina (239,240,245).

In a case series of 37 women with primary vaginal melanoma reported by Frumovitz et al. (239), median tumor size at presentation was 3 cm (range 0.4 to 5 cm), with median depth of invasion of 7 mm (range 1 to 21 mm). Twenty-one percent of patients presented with multifocal disease. Twenty-four patients (65%) presented with lesions in the distal third of the vagina or introitus.

Microscopically, tumors may be composed of epithelioid, spindle or nevus-like cells, and stain frequently positive for S-100 protein, HMB-45, and Melan A (**Fig. 19.11**). When S-100 is negative or only focally positive, tyrosinase and MART-1 are useful markers. Poorly differentiated tumors may be difficult to distinguish from carcinomas or sarcomas. Tumor thickness correlates with prognosis and may be measured by Breslow's methods (246).

Vaginal melanoma is a highly malignant disease with a propensity for early hematogenous spread. The most common presenting symptoms are slight vaginal bleeding and usually blood-tinged, foul-smelling, or purulent vaginal discharge (247). Reid et al. (248) reviewed 115 patients with primary melanoma of the vagina, and found depth of invasion and lesion size >3 cm to be negative prognostic factors. Stage was not found to be prognostic for outcome, but only 42 of the 115 patients had this information available. Compared to women with SCC, patients with vaginal melanoma have a significant 1.5-fold increased risk of mortality (8).

Treatment Options

Primary vaginal melanoma is uncommon; as a result, treatment outcomes for only a small number of patients have been reported (239,247,248–253), and it is difficult to make definitive treatment recommendations. Treatments used in published series include wide local excision, radical surgery, RT, and CT, or a combination of modalities.

Regardless of primary treatment, outcomes have been disappointing. Overall prognosis is poor, with historic 5-year survival rates ranging from 5% to 30% regardless of treatment modality or extent of surgical resection (248,249,252). There is a high rate of distant metastases, ranging from 66% to 100% (249,254,255).

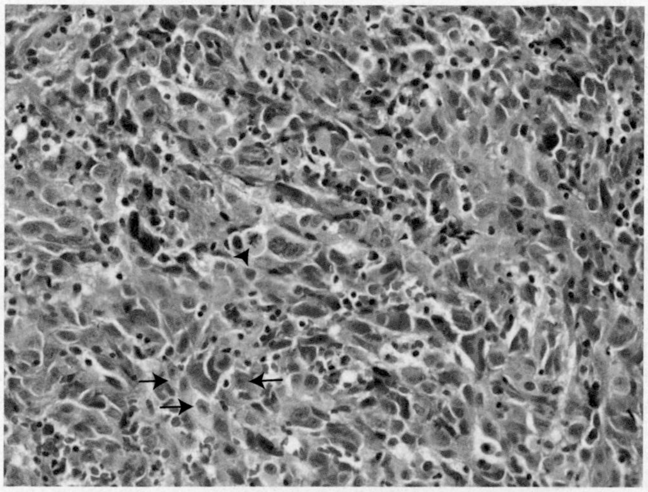

Figure 19.11. Vaginal melanoma. Malignant melanoma exhibits variable morphology. This example shows a vaguely nested to discohesive epithelioid neoplasm with characteristic eosinophilic nucleoli (*arrows*), significant nuclear pleomorphism, and mitoses (*arrowhead*). The presence of melanin pigment and immunohistochemistry can be helpful to confirm the diagnosis. Images courtesy of Emily E.K. Meserve.
Source: Images courtesy of Emily E.K. Meserve.

Some authors advocate incorporation of radical surgical resection into the treatment paradigm, when feasible (256–258). Surgery is favored over RT because melanoma tends to be radioresistant. Geisler et al. (256) recommend primary pelvic exenteration for vaginal melanomas with invasion >3 mm, reporting a 5-year survival rate of 50% if pelvic nodes are free of disease. Morrow and DiSaia (258), in their review of gynecologic melanoma, recommend radical surgery based on a review of the literature that revealed 3 out of 19 long-term survivors after exenteration with wide local excision. Chung and colleagues (249) reviewed 19 cases of primary vaginal melanoma treated between 1934 and 1976. All patients who received wide local excision developed recurrence. Five-year survival was only 21%. Miner and colleagues (259) reported on 35 patients treated at Memorial Sloan Kettering Cancer Center from 1977 to 2001: 69% underwent surgery, which was either en bloc removal of the involved pelvic organs, wide excision, or total vaginectomy, with elective pelvic lymph node dissection in 74% of cases. Thirty-one percent of patients received definitive RT. Primary surgical therapy was significantly associated with a longer OS (25 vs. 13 months). Recurrence-free survival was not found to correlate with surgical extent. A study by Huang et al. (300) found 5-year OS to be 32%, but as high as 47% in patients who underwent surgical treatment.

Several series comparing radical surgery and local excision find equivalent outcomes (247,250,261,262). In general, treatment modality does not appear to significantly affect survival. Bonner et al. (263) reported on nine cases of vaginal melanoma. Three patients were treated with wide local excision, and six underwent radical surgery. All nine patients developed locoregional recurrence. Therefore, the authors suggest adding pelvic RT to improve local control. The use of wide local excision followed by postoperative EBRT and brachytherapy has been proposed. A more recent review by Frumovitz and colleagues (239) reported that RT after wide local excision can reduce local recurrences. However, most patients develop distant metastases, most commonly in the lungs and liver.

Retrospective data suggest that RT may improve local control for vaginal melanoma (247,264). Among the few long-term survivors reported in the literature are a handful of patients who were treated with radiation. Harwood and Cummings (265) described a complete response in four patients with vaginal melanoma treated with radiation, although two subsequently relapsed. Rogo et al. (266), in their series of 22 cases of vulvovaginal melanoma, reported comparable results for surgery and RT, with eight patients (36%) alive 5 years after treatment. Petru et al. (264), in their series documenting 14 patients treated for primary malignant melanoma of the vagina, noted that three of nine patients treated with radiation, either as primary treatment ($n = 2$) or in the postoperative setting ($n = 1$), survived longer than 5 years. Median OS for all patients was 10 months, with a 5-year DFS rate of 14% and an OS rate of 21%.

Given the high rates of distant metastases, CT has been used, either alone or in conjunction with RT (239,267). The use of systemic CT and/or immunotherapy has not consistently been shown to improve patient outcomes thus far (267). Frumovitz et al., in their review of 37 women with stage I melanoma of the vagina treated at MDACC between 1980 and 2009, report very poor prognosis even in this group of patients with localized disease, with a 5-year OS rate of 20%. In that study, 10% of patients received nonsurgical treatment with RT, CT, or both. Patients treated surgically had significantly longer survival times compared with those treated nonsurgically. RT delivered after wide local excision reduced local recurrence and demonstrated a trend toward longer survival times, from 16.1 months to 29.4 months. A study by Xia et al. (253) evaluated 44 women, diagnosed and treated for vaginal melanoma between 2002 and 2011. There was no difference in OS between local excision and radical surgery. However, the authors noted increased PFS with the addition of adjuvant CT and RT (8.6 vs. 16.0 months, $p = 0.038$). Other reports have described the use of immunotherapy after surgery, and reveal that the best outcomes are achieved with this approach (260).

Based on limited but promising data suggesting an improvement in local control with the addition of adjuvant RT, treatment can be considered. However, there is no general recommendation for the treatment of primary vaginal melanoma. When RT is administered, vaginal melanoma is treated similarly to vaginal carcinoma, with volumes and doses ranging from 50 Gy for subclinical disease to 75 Gy for gross tumor.

Sarcoma

Sarcomas represent 3% of all primary vaginal cancers (7). In a report based on data from the NCDB between 1985 and 1994 (7), there were 135 cases of primary vaginal sarcoma, of heterogeneous histologies and varying age. Twenty-two percent of patients were under 14 years of age, with a median age at presentation of approximately 50 years. Consistent with this, a recent analysis of the SEER database identified 221 patients with primary vaginal sarcoma, diagnosed between 1988 and 2010, with a mean age of 54.9 (268). Compared with other vaginal cancers, sarcomas tend to be larger, with decreased likelihood of lymph node involvement, and are more commonly treated with primary surgery without RT. It was estimated that, after adjusting for other variables, patients vaginal sarcomas had a 69% greater risk of cancer-related mortality when compared with SCC.

Vaginal sarcoma most frequently presents as an asymptomatic vaginal mass (269). In one series, this was the most common system, and was, found in 35% of patients, followed by vaginal, rectal, or bladder pain (26%), bleeding or serosanguinous discharge from the vagina or rectum (18%), leucorrhea (9%), dyspareunia (7%), or difficulty in micturition (7%).

Leiomyosarcoma (LMS) is the most common histology in adults, representing up to 65% of all vaginal sarcoma cases; however, overall numbers are very small, with fewer than 150 published reports in the literature (269). Vaginal leiomyosarcomas originate from the smooth muscle of the vaginal wall, but may also develop from smooth muscle cells in tissues adjacent to the vagina. Grossly, patients present with a palpable submucosal nodule, although advanced tumors may demonstrate palpable necrosis or exophytic polypoid tissue (270). Criteria to distinguish between benign leiomyoma and leiomyosarcoma include greater than five mitoses per 10 high-power fields (HPF), moderate or marked cytologic atypia, and infiltrating margins (271) (**Fig. 19.12**). In view of considerable variation in smooth muscle tumors from area to area, adequate sampling is recommended to achieve an accurate diagnosis. Microscopically, leiomyosarcomas demonstrate interlacing bundles of spindle-shaped cells, with blunt-ended nuclei and fibrillar cytoplasm (247,271). Leiomyosarcomas have a predilection for the posterior vaginal wall, with published reports suggesting approximately 43% to 45% in the posterior vagina, 17% to 21% anteriorly, and 34% to 39% laterally (269,272). Leiomyosarcomas are also aggressive; they undergo early hematogenous dissemination, frequently recur locally (7,269), and often demonstrate pulmonary metastases (273).

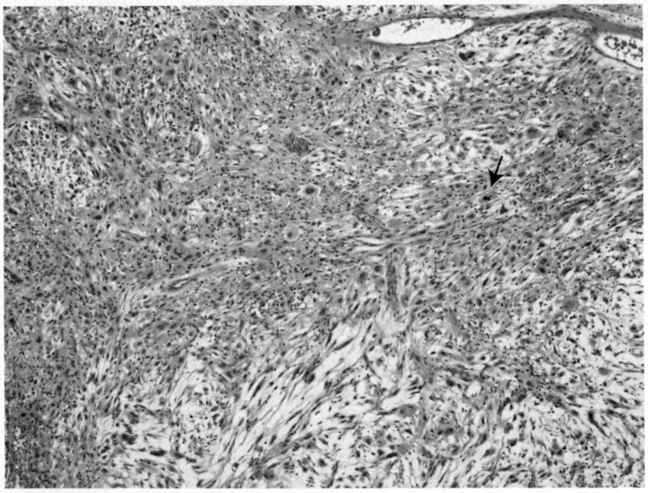

Figure 19.12. Leiomyosarcoma. Leiomyosarcoma of the vagina appears similar to malignant smooth muscle tumors in other anatomic sites and shows spindled to epithelioid (when morphologically higher grade) cells in a fascicular architecture. There is significant nuclear atypia with nuclear hyperchromasia and numerous mitotic figures, including atypical forms (*arrow*). Images courtesy of Emily E.K. Meserve.

Source: Images courtesy of Emily E.K. Meserve.

Other less common histologies include malignant mixed Mullerian tumor (MMT), endometrial stromal sarcoma, and angiosarcoma (274,275). MMTs, also called carcinosarcomas, are highly aggressive, biphasic neoplasms composed of an epithelial component as well as a sarcomatous component. The epithelial component in vaginal MMT is most often SCC (274). The sarcomatous component may be composed of fibroblasts and smooth muscle, or include cartilage, striated muscle, bone, and other heterologous tissues. The metaplastic carcinoma theory suggests that there is a common cell of origin for MMT, with carcinoma giving rise to the sarcomatous component via metaplasia (276). The most common differential diagnosis is sarcomatoid carcinoma. The spindle and carcinomatous components are positive for cytokeratin in sarcomatous carcinoma, whereas MMT demonstrates a sarcomatous component that is positive for vimentin, with the carcinomatous component positive for cytokeratin (274).

The first case of vaginal MMT was described in 1975 by Davis et al. (277), after which only 11 cases have been reported in the literature, with patients' age ranging from 57 to 74 years (274,278–282). At least one case report of MMT of the vagina detected high-risk HPV in both the carcinomatous and sarcomatous components, suggesting that some vaginal MMTs may be related to HPV (278). Fewer than 10 cases of angiosarcoma of the vagina have been reported in the literature (283,284). A history of pelvic RT is a risk factor for pelvic sarcomas, particularly angiosarcoma (275).

In the pediatric population, embryonal rhabdomyosarcoma/sarcoma botryoides is the most common histology (285), with 90% of cases occurring in children younger than 5 years of age (286).

Prognostic Factors

Review of the literature indicates that vaginal sarcomas undergo early hematogenous dissemination as well as frequent local recurrence. Pulmonary metastases are common (269,272). Adverse prognostic factors for vaginal sarcoma include high histologic grade, stage, size >3 cm, infiltrative borders, and cytologic atypia (273).

Treatment Options

Despite surgery and the use of adjuvant RT in select cases, sarcoma patients sustain poor outcomes due to a high incidence of local recurrence and distant metastasis. Locoregional control is especially important for vaginal leiomyosarcoma. A series by Peters et al. (287) reported on 17 cases, comprising 10 patients with leiomyosarcoma, 4 with MMT, and three with other types of sarcomas. There were only three patients alive and free of disease with follow-up times of 84 to 161 months. All three patients had undergone pelvic exenteration. Patients who received other forms of primary therapy all died of recurrence, with the pelvis as the first site of recurrence in all cases. In 50% of cases, the pelvis was the only site of failure, stressing the importance of local treatment. OS of 8 and 10 years following wide local excision have been reported (272).

Postoperative RT has been used to manage soft tissue sarcomas in other sites to reduce locoregional recurrence rates (288). Results from adjuvant radiation for high-grade sarcoma in other regions of the body have been extrapolated to vaginal cancer. In patients with involved margins, high doses above 62.5 Gy are generally required to achieve local control (289). Systemic treatment with doxorubicin is standard for leiomyosarcoma (290).

Outcomes

In the SEER analysis, 5-year survival was 89% for stage I, and under 50% for stage II vaginal sarcomas of all types (268). Other series describe similarly poor outcomes. Five-year survival was 36% for patients with leiomyosarcoma in the Peters et al. (287) series. The survival rate for patients with MMT was even lower, at 17%. There are only a few case reports and small series detailing treatment of primary vaginal MMT. Neesham and colleagues (280) published a case report of a 74-year-old patient treated with wide local excision and radiation for a 5.5-cm stage I MMT. She developed distant metastases within 6 months of local therapy. Analysis of patterns of failure suggests that local therapy does not have a significant impact on survival owing to early distant spread. Therefore, CT is typically administered after surgery for MMT in other sites, and should be considered for primary vaginal lesions, along with adjuvant RT as warranted. Platinum-based CT has been used for MMT occurring elsewhere in the pelvis. It has not yet been determined whether platinum agents are best administered alone or in combination with other agents. Combination regimens include a platinum agent and/or paclitaxel and/or ifosfamide (291–294).

Lymphoma

Lymphomas of the female genital tract are rare, accounting for only 1% of all primary extranodal lymphomas (295). Lymphomas of the vagina are exceedingly uncommon, with fewer than 30 cases reported in the literature thus far (296–315). In one review from the Armed Forces Institute of Pathology, only 4 of 9,500 cases of lymphoma were determined to originate from the vagina (316). Diffuse large B cell lymphoma is the most common histology, though there have also been reports of lymphoplasmacytic, Burkitt's, and mucosa-associated lymphoid tissue (MALT) lymphomas (303).

On exam, the tumor is typically palpable, with infiltrative thickening and/or ulceration of the vaginal wall (311). Immunohistochemical analyses are valuable techniques for confirming diagnosis, with tumors typically expressing CD20 (304,314). The most common symptom at presentation is vaginal bleeding. Leukemic infiltrates may be difficult to distinguish from lymphoma; therefore, chloroacetate esterase or myeloperoxidase staining may be useful. Although there is no established treatment protocol for primary lymphoma of the vagina, it seems reasonable to extrapolate from results for extranodal lymphomas elsewhere in the body and to use similar chemotherapeutic and response-based RT regimens. For patients wishing to retain fertility, CT alone may be an option in select cases.

If diagnosed at an early stage, the prognosis for vaginal lymphoma is excellent, with 5-year survival rates of up to 90%. Of 10 cases reported in the literature between 1994 and 2007, all patients except one were cured of disease after treatment with CT or a combination of RT and CT (302,304,308,310,317–320). Follow-up periods for these 10 cases ranged from 6 to 120 months, and one patient died from other causes. Eight patients had Ann Arbor stage IEA disease, one had IIEA, and one did not have stage reported. The most common CT regimen was cyclophosphamide, doxorubicin, vincristine, and prednisone (CHOP). Complete remission was also achieved using methotrexate, doxorubicin, cyclophosphamide, vincristine, prednisone, and bleomycin (MACOP-B) in one patient. Half of the patients did not receive RT because of an excellent response to CT alone.

Small Cell Carcinoma of the Vagina and Other Rare Histologies

Primary small cell carcinoma of the vagina is a rare entity, with fewer than 25 cases reported in the literature (321). Mean age at diagnosis is 59 years, with poor outcome due to early widespread dissemination. Eighty-five percent of patients die within 1 year of diagnosis (322,323). Neuroendocrine differentiation is often manifested by secretory granules, argyrophilia, and expression of neuroendocrine markers (324,325), staining positive for cytokeratin, neuron-specific enolase, chromogranin A, and serotonin (**Fig. 19.13**). Thyroid transcription factor 1 can also be positive, and should not be used to differentiate primary from metastatic disease (326). Microscopically, it is indistinguishable from that of the lung. These tumors can occur in pure form or be associated with squamous or glandular elements (322,324). Ectopic Cushing's syndrome has been documented in primary small cell carcinoma of the vagina (325). Treatment typically follows general principles for small cell carcinomas of the cervix, with aggressive therapy, including combination cisplatin-based CT, RT, brachytherapy, and surgery if feasible.

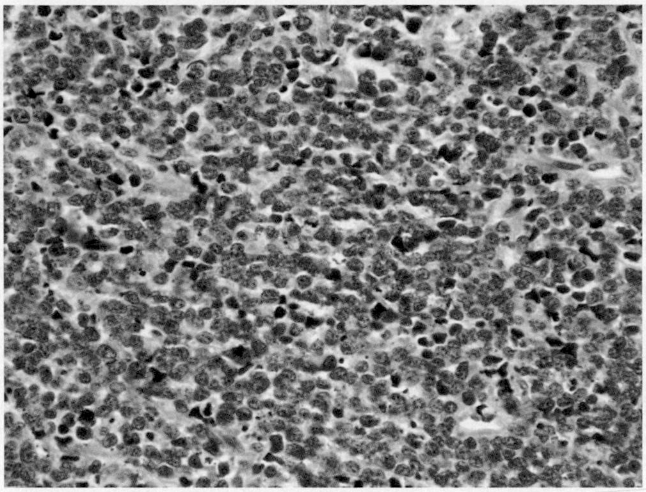

Figure 19.13. Neuroendocrine carcinoma of the vagina. Small cell carcinoma of the vagina is a poorly differentiated neuroendocrine carcinoma showing small blue cells with round to irregularly shaped nuclei with coarse ("salt and pepper") chromatin, very scant cytoplasm, and numerous mitotic and apoptotic figures. Importantly, designation as a primary small cell carcinoma of the vagina is possible only after exclusion of metastasis from other anatomic sites (i.e., lung). Immunohistochemical markers are generally not helpful in establishing site of origin in neuroendocrine carcinomas. Images courtesy of Emily E.K. Meserve.

Source: Images courtesy of Emily E.K. Meserve.

Vaginal paraganglioma is a rare neuroendocrine tumor, with fewer than 10 cases reported in the literature in younger women, with median age at presentation of 31 years (327–329). It is thought to be an indolent tumor, managed surgically. The tumor can manifest with catecholamine secretion, similarly to paragangliomas elsewhere in the body (327).

Adenosquamous carcinoma of the vagina is also uncommon. Microscopically, tumor cells are composed of glandular and squamous elements. One case report described adenosquamous carcinoma associated with small cell carcinoma of the endometrium in a 64-year-old female (330). Treatment approaches similar to those used for SCC of the vagina, including consideration of combination CRT for patients with gross disease.

RADIOTHERAPY TECHNIQUES

Definitive treatment of primary vaginal cancer with RT typically involves a combination of EBRT and brachytherapy. Owing to advances in conformal RT, tumor dose can be escalated while the dose to surrounding normal structures, such as small bowel, rectum, bladder, urethra, and the femoral heads, can be minimized. The use of 3D imaging to guide brachytherapy treatment planning is evolving, and recent results for vaginal cancer show excellent outcomes (331,332). Brachytherapy can be delivered via intracavitary or interstitial approaches, using LDR or HDR techniques.

External Beam Radiotherapy

The treatment technique, dose prescription, and selection of the appropriate energy level must be individualized for each patient. In general, when radiation is delivered as primary therapy, EBRT is prescribed prior to or, in some cases, without brachytherapy for a subset of patients with stage I, and all patients with stages II–IVA disease.

At the time of simulation, it may be helpful to identify the distal tumor margin with a radio-opaque marker. Unless contraindicated, the use of oral and intravenous contrast can be helpful, allowing delineation of vascular structures and facilitating the contouring of bladder, small bowel, and rectum. CT simulation allows contouring of vessels as a surrogate for lymph node localization, allowing more precise and individualized field delineation relative to pelvic bony anatomy (333,334). When available, fusion of diagnostic pelvic MRI or PET–CT to the treatment plan can assist in defining the tumor (**Fig. 19.7**). If inguinal nodes are to be treated, a "frog leg" position can be considered.

Two-Dimensional Treatment Planning

Before the widespread availability of 3D treatment planning, EBRT was delivered with two-dimensional (2D) techniques. Opposed anterior and posterior fields (AP/PA) were a common beam arrangement, though four-field plans incorporating lateral fields with small bowel blocks can be advantageous for avoiding bowel. If lateral fields are used, avoid shielding any potential regions of nodal involvement, including the presacral, perirectal, and anterior external iliac nodes. Selection of higher photon energy is preferred for superior dose distribution.

The target volume for EBRT is influenced by diagnostic imaging results and stage of disease. Treatment fields are designed to ensure coverage of the vagina and common iliac, external iliac, hypogastric, and obturator lymph nodes. A standard field has the L5-S1 interspace as the superior border, which ensures coverage of retroperitoneal nodes that lie caudal to the common iliac bifurcation (335,336). However, because many initial failures occur predominantly in the vagina, paracolpos, and parametria, some authors suggest setting the superior border 1 to 2 cm superior to the inferior margin of the sacroiliac joints in patients with negative imaging of regional nodes, in order to minimize treatment toxicity (337). If there are positive pelvic lymph nodes, the superior border should be raised to the L4-L5 interspace or higher to cover the common iliac nodes. The inferior border lies at the introitus to ensure coverage of the entire vagina, or 4 cm distal to the most caudal aspect of the vaginal tumor. Lateral borders are 1.5 to 2.0 cm lateral to the pelvic brim. Lateral fields, when utilized, should extend anteriorly to the pubic symphysis and posteriorly to the junction of the S2-S3 interspace. The border should be extended accordingly to include the inguinal nodes, if warranted. The dose to the inguinal nodes should be calculated during treatment planning to ensure appropriate coverage. When designing treatment fields, the interconnectivity of vaginal lymph node drainage should be kept in mind. Unexpected nodal drainage is possible, and should be considered. In a study of 14 women with vaginal cancer who received pretreatment lymphatic mapping with sentinel lymph node identification, two out of four women with a lesion in the upper one-third of the vagina were found to have a sentinel lymph node in the inguinal region (127).

Several techniques can be considered when treating the inguinal region to minimize dose to the femoral heads. An electron boost can be used to raise the inguinal dose to appropriate levels. Alternately, unequally weighted beams (2:1, AP:PA) or a combination of low- and high-energy photons (4 to 6 MV AP; 15 to 18 MV PA) can be used. Another method uses a wide AP and a narrow PA field, with a daily photon boost to the inguinal nodes delivered with asymmetric collimator jaws (338).

Three-D Conformal Treatment

The use of 3D imaging in simulation and treatment planning has increased dramatically over the past two decades and is currently used at almost all centers. This allows treatment fields to be tailored to a patient's specific anatomy. The gross tumor volume (GTV) is defined as the extent of gross disease found on clinical examination, as well as palpable lymph nodes and suspicious lymph nodes and regions seen on CT, MRI, and/or PET. The GTV is expanded by 1 to 2 cm to form the clinical target volume (CTV), which also includes the entire length of the vagina, paravaginal tissue up to the pelvic sidewall, and bilateral pelvic lymph nodes. Visualization of vessels allows approximation of lymph node locations. The pelvic nodal CTV can be defined as a 1- to 2-cm margin around blood vessels, and should include the common iliac, external iliac, internal iliac, obturator, perirectal, and presacral lymph node regions. For distal vaginal involvement, inguinal lymph nodes are commonly included, with the inferior border set at the lowest aspect of the ischial tuberosity or lesser trochanter. The CTV is expanded by 1 cm to form the planning target volume (PTV). The small bowel, bladder, and rectum are contoured, and doses to normal structures calculated.

Standard dose to the pelvis is 45 to 50.4 Gy in 1.8-Gy fractions, followed in select cases by a parametrial boost ranging from 50 to 65 Gy. Elective nodal irradiation of the inguinal nodes may be delivered up to 45 to 50 Gy. Gross nodal disease should receive 60 to 65 Gy, if feasible, using conformal therapy. For clinically palpable inguinal nodes, this can be achieved with reduced portals, using low-energy photons or electrons.

The location of the tumor, its size, extent of disease, and treatment response should be considered when individualizing treatment for each patient. After EBRT to the pelvis, tumors of the vaginal apex >0.5 cm in depth should be considered for interstitial brachytherapy or external beam boost; tumors <0.5 cm should be treated with intracavitary brachytherapy. Depending on location, tumors of the mid-vagina can be treated with external beam boost or considered for freehand interstitial brachytherapy, particularly if they are located anteriorly or laterally. Tumors of the distal vagina are also amenable to treatment with interstitial brachytherapy, especially if the tumor is relatively confined. In general, brachytherapy is delivered upon completion of EBRT, and allows dose escalation to the vaginal tumor up to 70 to 80 Gy.

Intensity-Modulated Radiation Therapy

Intensity-modulated RT (IMRT) may allow dose escalation to gross disease in areas such as inguinal or pelvic lymph nodes, diffusely infiltrative disease, or sidewall tumors inaccessible to brachytherapy. Shrinking-field techniques, or IMRT, can be used for dose escalation if brachytherapy is not feasible (339,340). In such circumstances, a total dose of 70 to 75 Gy minimum should be delivered to gross disease. Higher doses are difficult to achieve without substantially increasing the risk of toxicity to adjacent normal tissues such as urethra, bladder, and rectum. Typical IMRT input parameters based on those used for postoperative endometrial cancer in the Radiation Therapy Oncology Group (RTOG) trial 0921 include the following: ≤30% of small bowel to receive ≤40 Gy, with a dose to 2 cc of the small bowel (D2cc) maximum of 55 Gy; ≤35% of bladder to receive ≤40 Gy with a D2cc maximum of 90 Gy; ≤60% of the rectum and sigmoid to receive ≤40 Gy with a D2cc maximum of 70 to 75 Gy; and the femoral heads 15% to receive ≤35 Gy. IMRT plans are optimized to minimize the volume of PTV that receives more than 110% of the prescribed dose (341).

When utilizing the IMRT technique, it is important to consider the possibility of significant shifts in tumor position due to constant normal tissue changes and rapid tumor regression. Therefore, we recommend contouring an integrated vaginal volume (IVV) that reflects the CTV volume, paying close attention to rectal and bladder filling, and contouring the position of the vagina with both bladder full and bladder empty (**Fig. 19.14**) (342). A PTV margin of 1 to 1.5 cm is recommended, given the degree of motion and uncertainties in target definition.

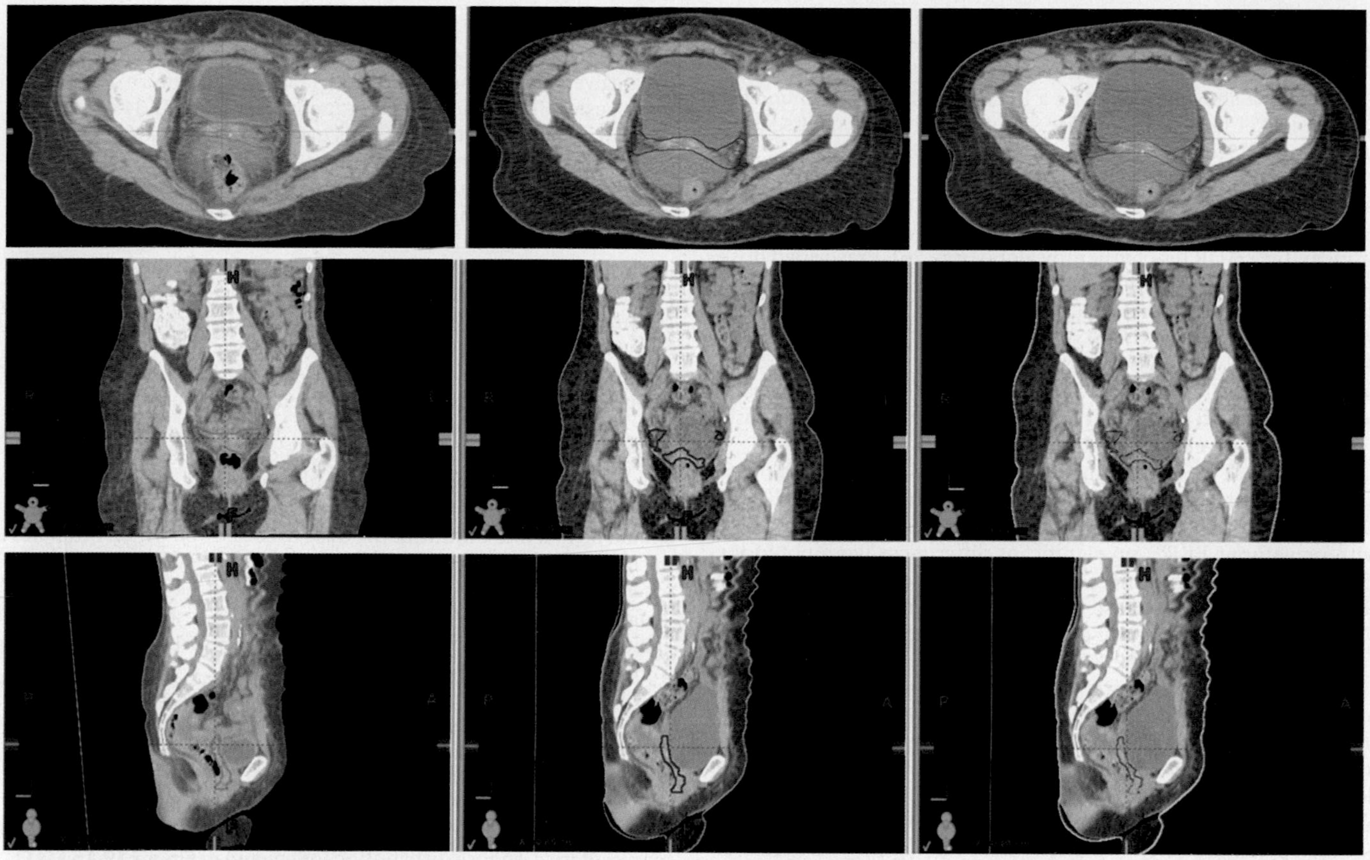

Figure 19.14. Displacement of the vagina with bladder filling. Axial, coronal, and sagittal images are shown for the same patient. The left panel shows a relatively empty bladder, with the vaginal cuff contoured in yellow. The middle panel shows a full bladder, with the vaginal cuff contoured in blue. The right panel shows a full bladder with the two vaginal contours superimposed, demonstrating the posterior deviation of the vaginal cuff that occurs with bladder filling.

Brachytherapy

Suitability for intracavitary or interstitial brachytherapy is assessed on the basis of tumor response to EBRT. In general, patients with superficial disease ≤5 mm in thickness can receive intracavitary treatment, whereas thicker lesions require interstitial brachytherapy in order to achieve adequate dose coverage. Intracavitary brachytherapy as monotherapy can be considered for patients with VAIN, and highly selected patients with minimally invasive stage I disease. In most cases, brachytherapy is offered after EBRT to boost the cumulative dose to 70 to 80 Gy.

Low Dose Rate Intracavitary Brachytherapy

Low dose rate intracavitary brachytherapy (LDR-ICB) is commonly performed using a vaginal cylinder loaded with cesium-137 radioactive sources. A variety of vaginal applicators are available, such as Burnett, Bloedorn, Delclos (343), or MIRALVA (344,345). Some cylinders have lead shielding to protect regions of the vagina, bladder, and rectum. Most applicators come in different diameters, and the largest diameter cylinder that can be comfortably accommodated by the patient should be used, to improve the ratio of mucosa to tumor dose. Usually, two to three cesium sources are placed along the central tandem of the cylinder. For LDR-ICB, the labia are typically sutured closed to secure the implant. It is important to avoid placing a source over the vulva, as this may increase skin toxicity. Use of LDR remote control afterloading can also minimize exposure of hospital personnel to radiation.

With appropriate selection of dose specification points, a uniform dose distribution can be achieved over the entire length of the vagina. In cases where disease is localized to the upper vagina or vaginal fornices, an intrauterine tandem can be used to anchor the vaginal cylinder, or used with vaginal colpostats. Vaginal colpostats can also be used alone to treat the upper vagina. Some institutions report good results utilizing custom vaginal molds (346).

A retrospective series by Pingley et al. (149) reported their experience treating 134 women with primary vaginal cancer. Only the 75 patients who completed treatment were analyzed. Most patients received EBRT to 50 Gy, and 59 patients received subsequent brachytherapy (30 with LDR-ICB, 29 interstitial). The 5-year DFS rate in patients treated with LDR-ICB was 53% and 30% for patients who did not receive brachytherapy. Patients who received brachytherapy within 4 weeks of EBRT had a DFS rate of 60%, compared with 30% in those who did not, suggesting that a shorter interval between EBRT and brachytherapy is preferable.

High Dose Rate Intracavitary Brachytherapy

High dose rate intracavitary brachytherapy (HDR-ICB) is typically performed using iridium 192, with applicators similar to those described for LDR. HDR-ICB delivers treatment over a span of several minutes, and has the potential advantages of limiting exposure to caregivers, as well as the ability to optimize dose distribution through varying dwell times (347,348). A variety of treatment regimens have been published, ranging from one to six insertions, with doses of 3 to 8 Gy per fraction (109,331,349). When HDR-ICB is administered, 3D treatment planning based on CT and/or MRI should be utilized to reduce dose to normal tissues.

Compared with LDR radiation, there is theoretically less potential sublethal damage repair and thus an increased likelihood of normal tissue toxicity. However, this has not been demonstrated in vaginal cancer, or in cervical cancer, where multiple prospective and retrospective studies have failed to note any significant difference in local control, survival, or toxicity outcomes between HDR and LDR brachytherapy (350).

Multiple single-institution studies with small numbers of patients have shown HDR to be a feasible and safe technique for vaginal cancer (159,351), and are summarized in the next section and in **Table 19.6**.

The largest series of HDR brachytherapy for vaginal cancer is from Vienna by Mock et al. (94) and reported on 86 patients. Patients with stage 0 to stage II disease received treatment with intracavitary HDR brachytherapy alone ($n = 26$). Prescribed dose per fraction ranged from 5 to 8 Gy, with a mean dose of 7 Gy, and the number of insertions ranged from two to six, with a median of five. In that series, the 5-year recurrence-free survival rates were 100%, 77%, and 50% for stages 0, I, and II, respectively. The authors noted similar local failure rates for HDR brachytherapy administered with or without EBRT for both stage I and II disease. Treatment was well tolerated.

Kucera et al. (352) described their experience with 80 patients who received treatment with HDR-ICB, with or without EBRT. Compared with a historical group of patients treated with LDR-ICB, with or without EBRT, no significant differences were noted for local and distant recurrences or rate of complications. Three-year actuarial overall and disease-specific survival rates were 51% and 61%, respectively. Three-year disease-specific survival rates for stage I and stage II patients were 83% and 66%, respectively.

Stock et al. (109) reported results for 49 patients treated with primary carcinoma of the vagina. Of this group, 15 patients were treated with EBRT and HDR brachytherapy for vaginal carcinoma, with dose per treatment ranging from 3 to 8 Gy. The total median dose delivered via HDR was 21 Gy, and the total median tumor dose overall was 63 Gy. No significant difference in outcome was noted between patients treated with LDR versus HDR. Five-year actuarial survival was reported to be 50% in the HDR brachytherapy group. In comparison, the 5-year survival rate for patients who received EBRT alone ($n = 11$) was 9% ($p < 0.001$), with a higher rate of stage IV disease in the EBRT-alone group (36%) compared with the brachytherapy group (5%).

Nanavati et al. (349) published their experience treating 13 patients with primary vaginal cancer with EBRT to 45 Gy followed by HDR-ICB of 20 to 28 Gy, delivered in three to four fractions and calculated 0.5 cm from the surface of the applicator. All 13 patients achieved a complete response; with a median follow-up time of 2.6 years, the local control rate was 92%. No grade 3 or 4 acute or chronic intestinal or bladder toxicity was noted during this short follow-up period, but 46% of patients developed moderate to severe vaginal stenosis. All patients had stage I or stage II disease, and the authors concluded that EBRT plus HDR-ICB is an acceptable treatment with a high response rate, good local control and survival, and minimal toxicity.

Beriwal and colleagues (351) described their experience using intracavitary HDR brachytherapy in five patients with either primary or recurrent vaginal cancer treated between 2000 and 2006. The median dose for intracavitary brachytherapy was 20 Gy in three to five fractions, prescribed 0.5 cm from the surface of the applicator. One patient received intracavitary brachytherapy only, because of prior RT with EBRT and HDR brachytherapy. Interpretation is limited because of short follow-up, and the results are combined with interstitial brachytherapy patients, but suggest that EBRT followed by HDR brachytherapy is efficacious and safe.

Interstitial Brachytherapy

Any paravaginal extension at the time of diagnosis, regardless of treatment response, merits consideration of interstitial brachytherapy, as a vaginal cylinder is unable to deliver sufficient coverage to this region. Other candidates for interstitial brachytherapy include patients with lesions thicker than 5 mm, distal vaginal extension, or those with a vagina that is unable to accommodate standard intracavitary applicators.

High Dose Rate Interstitial Brachytherapy

HDR interstitial brachytherapy has the advantage of limiting exposure to caregivers and visitors, and offers the ability to optimize dose distribution using 3D image-based treatment planning (331,348,353). Use of permanent radioactive implants using gold 198 or iodine 125 has also been reported for smaller volume disease (354), and can provide long-lasting control in elderly or previously irradiated patients. In general, temporary implants are preferred over permanent implants because of their relative safety/simplicity, cost effectiveness, easy applicability, readily controlled distribution of sources, and easier modification of dose distribution. Given the close proximity of the rectum and bladder, it is important to minimize treatment toxicity by avoiding overdosing of critical normal structures. However, underdosing the target volume is also a serious risk; thus, it is critical to optimize target localization and needle placement (355).

Dosing. Vaginal cancer with gross residual disease at the time of brachytherapy is prescribed a cumulative EQD2 dose of 70 to 90 Gy, with 60 Gy prescribed to the entire vaginal surface. Special care should be taken to minimize the dose to the bowel, which often lies in close proximity to gross disease. Image-based planning software, when available, allows the dose to conform to the target areas yet avoid organs at risk. As a result, optimal dose distribution can be achieved. Image-guided technique should be utilized when possible to reduce toxicity and improve local control.

Given the difficulty of insertion, physicians may insert the applicator once and treat patients over a several-day inpatient hospitalization. Twice-a-day regimens range from 9 to 10 fractions of 200 to 300 cGy per fraction, BID, or three to six fractions, ranging from 450 to 650 cGy, BID, with at least 6 hours between fractions. It is also feasible to perform two separate insertions with two hospitalizations. A representative isodose distribution is depicted in **Figure 19.15** (341).

Proposed dose schedules for HDR interstitial brachytherapy, depending on dose of initial EBRT, have been released by the American Brachytherapy Society (169). The number of fractions range from 3 to 10 (**Table 19.7**), with the goal of delivering total EQD2 of over 70 Gy to the CTV.

For CT- or MRI-based 3D treatment planning, the D90, D100, V100, V150, and V200 are parameters used to describe tumor volumes and the doses to those volumes. D90 and D100 are defined as the minimum dose delivered to 90% and 100% of the volume, respectively. V100, V150, and V200 are defined as the volumes receiving 100%, 150%, and 200% of the prescribed physical dose, respectively (356).

When MRI-guided adaptive brachytherapy is utilized, the high-risk CTV (HRCTV) is defined as clinically palpable disease, plus any residual disease seen on MRI, and the entire circumference of the adjacent vagina at the level of the residual tumor. The intermediate-risk CTV (IRCTV) includes the region of initial tumor extension and the remaining vagina in order to encompass potential submucosal tumor spread. The low-risk CTV (LRCTV) is the remaining vagina.

The use of MRI-guided adaptive brachytherapy in locally advanced vaginal cancer was reported by Dimopoulos et al. (357) with excellent outcomes, supporting the use of the following parameters for image-guided adaptive brachytherapy: for HRCTV, D90 of ≥85 Gy; for IRCTV, D90 ~60 Gy; and for LRCTV, D90 of ~50 Gy. Thirteen patients with stages II–IV disease were treated. Mean D2cc doses to the bladder, urethra, rectum, and sigmoid colon were 80, 76, 70, and 60 Gy, respectively. Toxicity was acceptable, with two fistulas reported and one case of periurethral necrosis. The 3-year local control and OS rates were 92% and 85%, respectively, with a mean D90 to the HRCTV of 86 (±13) Gy.

The bladder, rectum, sigmoid, urethra, and, when necessary, small bowel are contoured as volumes at risk, and the D2cc and D0.1cc calculated (358). The recommended maximum equivalent dose in 2-Gy fractions (EQD2) D2cc to the rectum and sigmoid is 70 to 75 Gy, and should be less than 70 Gy when feasible (169). Maximum EQD2 D2cc for the bladder should be 90 Gy.

There are no DVH parameters specific to the female urethra, but in general, the D2cc should be comparable to parameters for

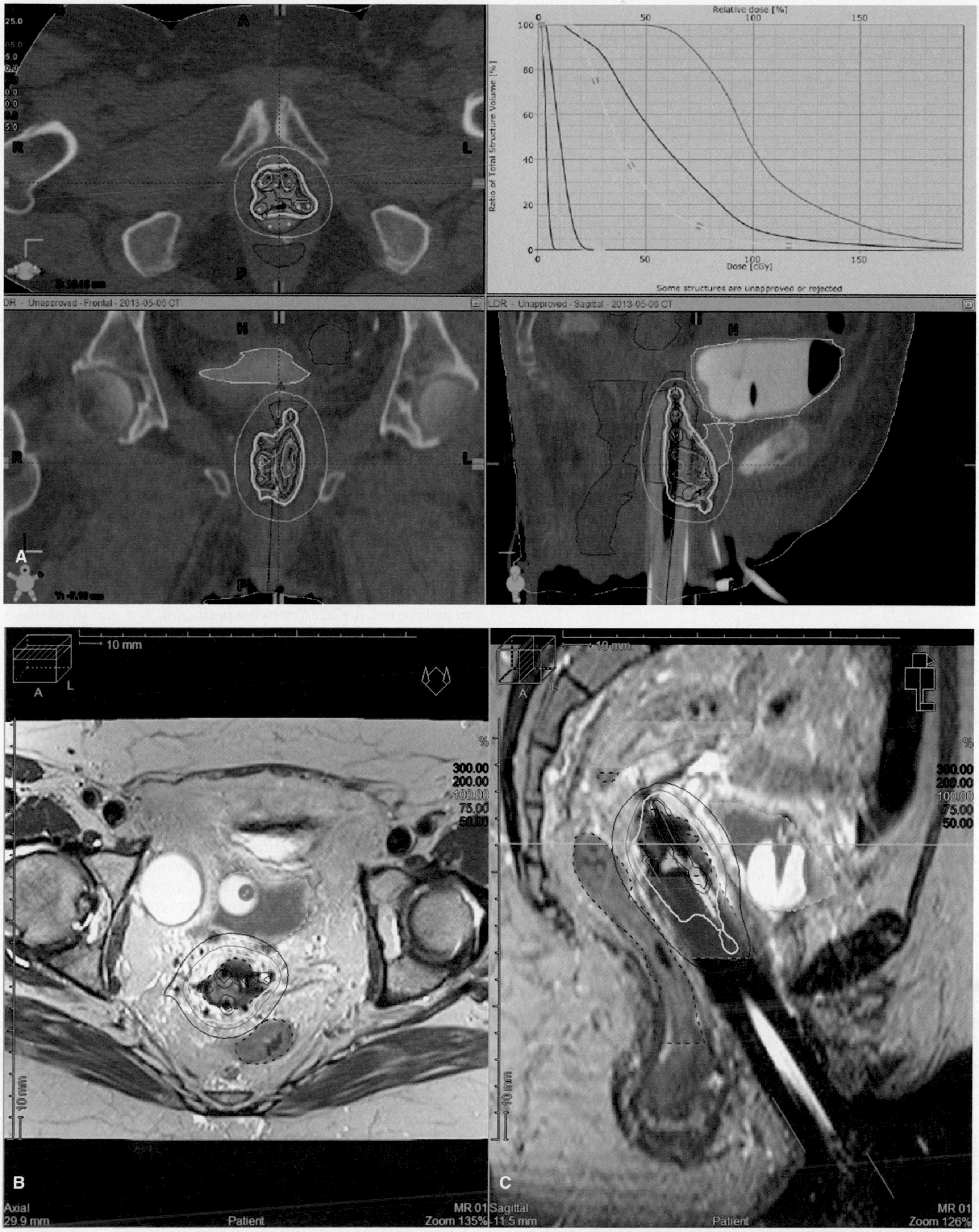

Figure 19.15. Interstitial implantation of a vaginal tumor extending above the vaginal obdurator at the inguinal apex. The vaginal length is treated with the prescription dose in this case. **A, B, C**: Axial, sagittal, and coronal isodose distributions are depicted with a dose-volume histogram.

TABLE 19.7. Dose Schedules for HDR Interstitial Brachytherapy in Combination with EBRT, Modified by Beriwal et al, American Brachytherapy Society (165)

EBRT		HDR		EQD2
Total Dose	# Fx	Dose per Fx	# Fx	CTV
36 Gy[a]	18	5.0 Gy	6	72.9
		5.5 Gy	6	87
39.6 Gy[a]	22	5.0 Gy	6	76.4
		5.5 Gy	6	81.5
45 Gy	25	3.0 Gy	9	73.6
		3.0 Gy	10	76.8
		4.5 Gy	5	71.5
		5.0 Gy	5	75.5
		5.5 Gy	5	79.8
		7.0 Gy	3	74.1
50.4 Gy	28	4.0 Gy	5	72.9
		4.5 Gy	5	76.8
		5.0 Gy	5	80.9
		7.0 Gy	3	79.4

[a]Assumes midline block after 36–39.6 Gy, with total pelvic dose to 50.4 Gy.

EBRT, external beam radiation; EQD2, equivalent dose in 2 Gy fractions; Fx, fractions; HDR, high dose rate.

bladder and rectum. A study from Brigham and Women's Hospital reported the incidence of grade 3 or higher complication rates in 51 women undergoing HDR 3D-planned interstitial brachytherapy (359). Median D2cc for bladder, rectum, and sigmoid were 64.6, 61.0, and 51.9 Gy, respectively. The actuarial rates of grade 3 to 4 complications at 2 years were 20% gastrointestinal, 9% vaginal, 6% skin, 3% musculoskeletal, and 2% lymphatic. The D2cc for the rectum was significantly higher in patients with grade 2 or more gastrointestinal toxicity. On univariate analysis, D2cc and D0.1cc for rectum and sigmoid, tumor size and tumor volume at the time of brachytherapy were associated with gastrointestinal complications. This analysis validated the recommended D0.1cc and D2cc for the rectum and sigmoid.

Preoperative Assessment

Clinical examination provides an imprecise estimate of tumor thickness. T1- with gadolinium and T2-weighted MRI may be obtained if possible after EBRT to assess residual disease. MRI is superior to other imaging modalities for determining tumor thickness. Use of a radio-opaque marker in the vagina placed at the time of diagnosis and after external beam will facilitate assessment of the lesion on CT imaging. Contrast, such as ultrasound gel placed to distend the vagina, may also aid in visualization of the tumor.

The patient should be assessed for general, epidural, or spinal anesthesia. Patients with a history of laminectomy, significant degenerative disease, or labile blood pressure are suboptimal candidates for epidural anesthesia. Epidural anesthesia allows the patient to control the degree of pelvic anesthesia, yet avoid the systemic effects, somnolence, and potential mental status changes that may occur with a peripheral patient-controlled anesthesia device. When feasible, a combination of general anesthesia during the insertion followed by an epidural patient-controlled anesthesia approach that continues during the entire inpatient hospitalization maximizes pain relief.

Patients on anticoagulation with medications such as warfarin should switch to low molecular weight (LMR) heparin approximately 1 week before the procedure; LMR heparin may be discontinued 24 hours before insertion time and withheld for the duration of the implant, although subcutaneous heparin for thrombosis prophylaxis may be initiated after the procedure is completed. Patients may have a gentle bowel preparation orally or an enema before the procedure.

Applicator Selection

Template systems are available to secure the position of the needles in the target volumes, and include the Syed-Neblett template, the modified Syed-Neblett, and the Martinez Universal Perineal Interstitial Template (MUPIT) (360). These systems consist of a perineal template, a vaginal cylindrical obturator, and hollow guides for loading radionuclide sources. The perineal template requires suturing to perineal skin. The vaginal obturator allows for placement of a tandem, making it possible to combine interstitial with intracavitary treatment if desired. A freehand technique is best reserved for lower vaginal tumors, where the mass can be readily palpated and visualized.

Procedure

The insertion procedure is performed with the patient in a dorsal lithotomy position. The physician should be mindful that slight needle displacement can occur when legs are lowered back to the supine position. A digital and speculum examination allows assessment of vaginal width, tumor size and location, amount and thickness of residual parametrial or paravaginal disease, and presence of any fistulas. A sterile setup is used at the time of insertion. A Foley catheter is placed for bladder drainage. For patients with an intact uterus, a central tandem may be inserted to anchor the applicator. A vaginal central plastic cylinder is placed over the tandem and secured. The template, which contains multiple openings through which needles can be inserted, is placed onto the perineum. The tumor volume is implanted by inserting the needles through the holes of the template, with the goal of covering the GTV with a 1- to 2-cm margin, utilizing 3D imaging afterward to confirm proper needle location and uniform dose distribution around the tumor volume.

When possible, utilizing image guidance to perform implants is ideal to improve target localization and guide needle placement. Available modalities include laparoscopic guidance, ultrasound, CT, and MRI. Results associated with these various techniques are summarized.

Real-time transrectal ultrasound is one method of visualization, reported by Stock and colleagues (361). The ultrasound probe can be brought close to the vagina, parametria, and cervix, and the longitudinal mode of the ultrasound probe is useful in determining the optimum depth of needle insertion. Transverse imaging is also utilized during the procedure to ensure coverage of the target area and to avoid entry into the bladder, rectum, or small bowel. Through the use of this technique, invasive laparotomy or laparoscopy can often be avoided.

Several investigators have used laparoscopic guidance or laparotomy (360–365) to improve the accuracy and safety of interstitial implant placement. With open laparotomy, the bladder and urethra can be visualized during needle placement. The bladder and rectum can be protected either by using slings or tissue expanders or by lysis of adhesions. Disaia and Creasman (366) described the creation of an "omental carpet," where a section of omentum is placed along the descending colon into the pelvis to separate the bladder and rectum from the implant and prevent small bowel adhesions. If laparotomy is performed in a two-application course of treatment, it is typically done for the first application only. As expected, there is higher associated morbidity with the use of laparotomy compared with other techniques, as a result of increased operative time, longer postoperative recovery, risk of bleeding, and ileus.

Laparoscopic visualization may sometimes be an alternative to open laparotomy. Although laparoscopy is less invasive, both laparoscopic approaches and open laparotomy are limited by an inability to visualize extraperitoneal structures, such as parts of the bladder, uterus, and cervix, as well as the vagina and paravaginal tissues.

However, these techniques can be considered when CT or MRI are not available during brachytherapy, to avoid needle insertion through the small bowel and sigmoid.

The use of 3D imaging during brachytherapy has increased with the rise of CT and MR availability, and is a favored approach when available owing to lower morbidity and invasiveness compared with historic approaches (367). Only a few institutions have access to real-time image guidance during brachytherapy (368); most scan patients after insertion is complete, with readjustment of inappropriately placed needles after CT and MRI.

The integration of 3D imaging during brachytherapy allows determination of depth and location of insertion, and enables repositioning if perforation into the bladder or rectum is detected. Treatment planning based on 3D imaging allows high dose to be delivered to the tumor volume, yet spares critical adjacent organs. The use of 3D image-based HDR brachytherapy has been shown to improve local control and decrease treatment-related toxicities (369,370). There are fewer published reports on 3D HDR brachytherapy for primary vaginal cancer, but results suggest similar outcomes (332).

It is not feasible at many institutions to obtain an MRI at the time of brachytherapy. A diagnostic MRI obtained after EBRT before brachytherapy can be used instead to assist with treatment planning. MRI provides superior tumor delineation, whereas CT images may result in overestimation of tumor extension (371). The use of MRI at the time of implant can be limited by lack of access, as well as the requirement for specific applicators and increased scanning time.

Precautions for Interstitial Patients

Appropriate measures should be taken to reduce the likelihood of needle displacement during hospitalization. Patients should be instructed to remain in bed, with the head of the bed raised no more than 15 degrees. To ensure there has been no needle displacement between fractions, the needle length protruding the template can be measured and validated before every treatment.

Skin care is also important. Given the risk of decubitus ulcer, it is advisable to utilize an air mattress, when available. To minimize skin abrasion, gauze or duoderm can be placed between the template and perineal skin.

To prevent the development of a deep vein thrombosis, patients should receive subcutaneous heparin and pneumoboots.

Patients should be seen in follow-up 2 to 4 weeks after implant removal for a skin check, then at 3-month intervals up to a year, then every 6 months. Dilute hydrogen peroxide douching is advised for patients with tissue necrosis development. Antibiotics with anaerobic coverage are recommended if a malodorous discharge accompanies the necrosis. Hyperbaric oxygen should be considered for those proven on biopsy not to have recurrent disease.

Outcomes with Interstitial Technique

There are only a handful of series describing outcomes for vaginal cancer treated with interstitial brachytherapy. They are summarized here.

Kushner et al. (372) reported outcomes of HDR brachytherapy in 19 patients with primary vaginal cancer. 2D treatment planning was performed, with interstitial brachytherapy delivered to 8 patients at a median dose of 23 Gy in four fractions. The 2-year OS rate for all patients was 66.1%. Three patients (15.8%) had serious late effects, including ureteral stenosis, vaginal necrosis, and small bowel obstruction; two of these patients were treated with interstitial brachytherapy.

A series by Tewari et al. (373) reviewed the long-term results of interstitial brachytherapy, with or without EBRT, in 71 patients with primary vaginal cancer. A Syed-Neblett template was used with an interstitial iridium 192 afterloading technique. Patients received a minimum of 20 Gy via implant, with a total tumor dose of approximately 80 Gy. With a median follow-up time of 66 months, 5-year DFS rates were reported to be 100%, 60%, 61%, 30%, and 0% for stage I, IIA, IIB, III, and IV patients, respectively. Significant complications were noted in 13% of patients, and included necrosis, fistula, and small bowel obstruction. Overall, 75% of patients achieved local control.

Beriwal and colleagues described results using 3D image-based HDR interstitial brachytherapy (331) at the University of Pittsburgh Cancer Institute. A total of 30 patients with primary vaginal cancer ($n = 17$) or recurrent gynecologic cancer to the vagina ($n = 13$) were treated using the Syed-Neblett template, with CT scan done after placement of needles for confirmation and treatment planning. Of the subset of 17 patients with primary vaginal cancer, the numbers of patients with stage I, II, III, and IVA disease were 2, 9, 5, and 1, respectively. Fifty-three percent of patients received concurrent chemotherapy with weekly cisplatin at 40 mg/m^2, and apical lesions had laparoscopic guidance during needle placement. The CTV and organs at risk were contoured on CT scan for treatment planning after placement of needles. Most patients (93.3%) received EBRT to a median dose of 45 Gy, followed by HDR interstitial brachytherapy at 3.75 to 5 Gy per fraction in five fractions to a median dose of 21.3 Gy. Overall median D90 to the high-risk CTV was 74.3 Gy, and median D2cc to the bladder, rectum, and sigmoid were 58.5, 57.2, and 50 Gy, respectively, showing excellent sparing of critical organs. At a median follow-up of 16.7 months, the 2-year locoregional control and OS rates were 78.8% and 70.2%, respectively, suggesting good local control. Overall, the treatment was fairly well tolerated. There were no grade 3 or higher gastrointestinal complications. One patient developed late grade 3 vaginal ulceration and another had grade 4 vaginal necrosis.

A study by Manuel et al. reviewed outcomes for 75 patients with vaginal cancer. Patients were treated with the image-guided ($n = 50$) or non–image-guided ($n = 25$) technique from 1973 to 2014 (332). With the use of the image-guided technique, there was a trend toward improved DFS (2 year DFS 77% vs. 42%, respectively; $p = 0.072$), improved OS (84% vs. 47%; $p = 0.26$), and decreased gastrointestinal and genitourinary toxicity, supporting incorporation of CT and/or MRI as image guidance when available.

Brachytherapy versus External Beam Boost

In select circumstances when patients are not appropriate candidates for brachytherapy, IMRT can be considered as an alternative for boost to residual gross disease. A retrospective dosimetric analysis from Princess Margaret Hospital (374) reported data comparing IMRT boost treatment plans with conventional and 4-field radiation boost plans for 12 patients with cervical ($n = 8$), endometrial ($n = 2$), or vaginal ($n = 2$) cancer. IMRT conferred a significant improvement in dose conformity, with overall improvement in rectal and bladder dose-volume distributions, relative to conformal radiation, though inferior to brachytherapy. However, when comparing an ideal photon or proton external beam boost to brachytherapy, brachytherapy provided the best coverage and normal tissue sparing (375).

Barraclough and colleagues (376) used an EBRT boost in 21 patients with cervical cancer who were unable to undergo intracavitary brachytherapy. A 3D conformal boost was used to deliver a total dose of 54 to 70 Gy. With a median follow-up of 2.3 years, 48% of patients had recurrent disease, with central recurrence in 16 of 21 patients, significantly higher than the 3% to 4% local recurrence rates reported with MR-planned brachytherapy. These results are dramatically inferior to those reported with brachytherapy, suggesting that external beam boosts should be considered as an alternative only when brachytherapy is not feasible.

Stereotactic body radiotherapy (SBRT) is a relatively newer treatment modality with very little data to support its use. A review by Higginson et al. (377) reported on two vaginal cancer patients treated with a SBRT boost instead of brachytherapy. Fiducial markers were placed into the paravaginal, parametrial, or cervical tissues during outpatient clinical examination. The two patients with vaginal cancer received 40 to 45 Gy EBRT followed by 25 Gy in five fractions of SBRT; one patient had a local recurrence at 5 months, and another developed distant disease 17 months posttreatment. Toxicity included one acute grade 2 cystitis and one late grade 3 rectal bleeding.

Treatment Toxicity and Management

Pathologic changes in the vaginal mucosa after RT include marked mucosal atrophy, with epithelial thinning and loss of the overlying stratified squamous layer. There can be hyalinization and collagenization of submucosal connective tissues, with fibrosis of the muscular layer and vasculature. Such changes result in compromised oxygenation of injured tissues, promoting ulceration and fistula formation. Cytologic abnormalities within the first 6 months after RT are common, and it is important to distinguish postradiation atypia from new or recurrent malignancy during posttreatment follow-up (378). Clinically, vaginal stenosis and shortening can manifest several months after RT, although presentation as late as 15 years posttreatment has been documented (379).

Acute injury to the vaginal mucosa should be managed symptomatically through hygiene, recognition and treatment of infection, and pain control. There should be a low threshold for starting antifungal medications, as Candida can exacerbate vaginitis. Sitz baths and topical ointments may be useful for radiation dermatitis, and both topical and oral analgesics can be prescribed for mucositis and general discomfort during RT.

The bladder and rectum are located close to the vagina, and patients commonly develop acute toxicity during treatment (380). Increased urinary frequency, urgency, and dysuria can be managed with phenazopyridine, a urinary tract analgesic, as well as oral anticholinergic and antispasmodic medications. Antidiarrheal medications such as loperamide and, in more severe cases, tincture of opium, should be prescribed for symptom management early in the development of symptoms. Irritation of the anal mucosa can cause exacerbation of hemorrhoids and occasional hemorrhagic spotting and discomfort with defecation; topical hemorrhoidal ointments or suppositories can be used.

Regular use of a vaginal dilator to decrease stenosis and shortening should be recommended shortly after completion of RT, because it is difficult to reverse stenosis and shortening once fibrosis has ensued. Topical estrogen, applied three times a week for 6 to 9 months after radiation, was shown in a randomized controlled trial, published in 1975, to reduce the incidence of stenosis, dyspareunia, and cytologic changes in vaginal epithelium (381). However, because of a small potential for systemic absorption with untoward effects on endometrial proliferation, the use of topical estrogens is not favored for all patients.

Radiation necrosis can be conservatively managed with local debridement, peroxide douches, antimicrobials, and estrogen. There is some evidence that hyperbaric oxygen can facilitate healing, with a greater than 50% reduction in vaginal ulceration noted in one series (382). Fistulas present more of a treatment challenge. Despite the use of interventions such as urinary or fecal diversions, additional surgical correction is often required for effective management, particularly in the setting of rectovaginal fistulas (383).

PATTERNS OF FAILURE

Most treatment failures occur within 5 years, with a median time to recurrence of 6 to 12 months (115,191), and local recurrence is the most common pattern of treatment failure in most published series. Extravaginal recurrences in the pelvic lymph nodes are less common.

Overall rates of locoregional recurrence, by stage, are shown in **Table 19.5**. In general, the rate of locoregional recurrence ranges from 10% to 20% for stage I and 30% to 40% for stage II disease. Patients with advanced disease often have persistent disease despite treatment, up to 68% according to one series (148).

The reported rates of distant metastasis vary, ranging from 7% to 33%, and usually occur later in the course of disease, with approximately half of all distant metastases presenting at the time of local recurrence (104,106,118,148).

GENERAL MANAGEMENT, TREATMENT OPTIONS, AND OUTCOME—SPECIAL SCENARIOS

The Posthysterectomy Patient

Approximately 60% of patients with primary vaginal cancer have had prior hysterectomy. This likely reflects the high proportion of patients with a history of cervical neoplasia and carcinoma requiring surgical management, as well as overall increased rates of hysterectomy in the general female population (384,385). Finding methods to improve target positioning during EBRT becomes especially important as treatment delivery becomes increasingly more conformal.

After hysterectomy, the small bowel tends to fall lower into the pelvis, increasing the likelihood of it being irradiated during treatment. There is also daily variation in vaginal vault position. A study by Jhingran et al. (342) evaluated the variations in vaginal vault position and bladder and rectal volumes in posthysterectomy patients undergoing IMRT, and found significant variations in the position of the vaginal vault depending on bladder and rectal filling. Patients were instructed to have a full bladder before radiation treatment; however, the study showed a median difference of 247 cc despite this. It is likely that bladder movement affects vaginal position. For patients with fiducial markers placed in the vagina, the median movement during treatment was 0.59 cm in the right–left direction, 1.46 cm in the anterior–posterior direction, and 1.2 cm in the superior–inferior direction. Thus, it is important to be mindful of target movement when delineating the treatment volume.

To minimize uncertainly, the treating physician can fuse planning CT scans taken with full and empty bladder in order to estimate the potential range of target volume positions during treatment. Another approach, though less practical, is to fill the bladder with a fixed volume of saline using a Foley catheter immediately before treatment, or to utilize fiducial markers for daily localization.

History of Prior Pelvic Radiation

As many as 10% to 50% of patients with VAIN or invasive carcinoma of the vagina have a previous diagnosis of cervical carcinoma (32,67,100–106), with an average interval of 14 years between diagnosis of cervical disease to development of vaginal carcinoma (102,107). As a result, a proportion of patients with vaginal cancer have a history of prior pelvic radiation. Reirradiation can be considered in this setting, but there is an increased risk of toxicity, particularly radionecrosis and fistula formation. Xiang et al. (386) published a series on 73 patients with a history of RT for cervical carcinoma who received a second diagnosis of vaginal malignancy 5 to 30 years later. All patients received EBRT and brachytherapy for treatment of their initial cancer. Reirradiation for the vaginal malignancy was planned according to site and volume of the vaginal tumor and location and dose of the prior radiation. Patients received brachytherapy, using either radium delivered to the tumor base (30 to 40 Gy in three to five fractions) or HDR with cobalt 60 to the tumor base (20 to 35 Gy in three to five fractions), followed by a dose to 0.5 cm below the vaginal mucosa at 20 to 30 Gy in four to six fractions delivered using a vaginal mold. For involvement of the vulva or groin, patients additionally received EBRT to a dose of 30 to 40 Gy. Most patients received RT alone; 11 also received CT, most typically cisplatin-based. The 5-year survival rate was 40.3%, and three patients survived more than 15 years.

There were significant side effects with reirradiation: 18 of 73 patients developed radionecrosis. Other side effects included one (1.4%) vesicovaginal fistula and eight (11%) rectovaginal fistulas, hematuria (12.3%), and moderate to severe rectal sequelae (13.6%).

Beriwal et al. (351) reported on the use of HDR interstitial and intracavitary brachytherapy for five patients with recurrent vaginal cancer and a history of prior pelvic RT. Significant grade 3 or higher toxicities were noted in patients who received total EQD2 dose above 140 Gy. Median time from prior RT to recurrence was 4 years (range 6 months to 18 years). The recurrence was within 2 cm of the prior field in two patients and within the previous field for four patients. All patients received EBRT to a median dose of 45 Gy, followed by brachytherapy. For the four patients with prior overlapping fields, the cumulative EQD2 to the vaginal mucosa ranged from 120.7 to 154.54 Gy. Of these patients, one developed a rectovaginal fistula 2 years after treatment, and another developed chronic vaginal ulceration with vaginal shortening to 2 cm; the EQD2values were 142.98 and 154 Gy, respectively.

Carcinoma of the Neovagina

The neovagina is a surgically constructed vaginal canal, typically described in patients with congenitally deformed or absent genitalia, or patients desiring reconstruction of a functional vagina after surgery for gynecologic malignancy. Various methods have been utilized for neovaginal construction, including split-skin grafts, myocutaneous flaps, and formation of an artificial canal between the rectum and the vagina (387). Given its overall rarity, there are very few reports of in situ or invasive carcinoma arising in the neovagina.

A review of published literature reveals six published reports of carcinoma in situ (388–393). The period of development of carcinoma in situ ranged from 6 months to 20 years after constructive surgery. Invasive carcinoma of the neovagina tends to be poorly differentiated, and most reported cases have been SCC. All reported patients have presented with large tumor masses and evidence of rapid progression, with poor overall outcomes (394,235,395–397).

Treatment options include radiation, with or without an attempt at radical resection, and, in select cases, lymph node dissection. Of 16 reported cases from a review by Steiner et al. (387), 9 received primary radiation alone, 1 received radiation followed by exenteration and intraoperative radiation, and 4 underwent exenteration. Recurrence status was not documented for all patients. Three were found to have rapid disease recurrence within several months. Two patients were free of disease at 10 and 18 months, respectively. One patient had a recurrence-free interval of 3 years, but died a year later from disease.

Although there is no optimal treatment, resection followed by consideration of adjuvant radiation is preferable to definitive radiation alone, as surgery can offer full pathologic diagnosis. The extent of disease, patient characteristics, and treatment goals should guide the choice of treatment.

Salvage Therapy for Recurrent or Persistent Disease

For patients with recurrent or persistent disease, it is important to determine whether there is a reasonable chance of cure with salvage treatment or whether the primary goal is palliation. Thus, multiple factors, including extent of disease, site, extent of recurrence, disease-free interval, status of systemic disease, patient age, comorbidities, and overall performance status, must be considered.

Early-stage lesions that recur after RT can be surgically salvaged. A retrospective review of pelvic exenteration for recurrent gynecologic malignancies at University of California Los Angeles Medical Center from 1956 to 2001 reported survival rates for patients with recurrent cervical and vaginal cancer to be 73% at 1 year and 54% at 5 years (398).

Patients with tumor persistence or recurrence after limited surgical procedures can be considered for more extensive surgery. If not, systemic chemotherapy and/or radiation can be administered.

Recurrent disease in advanced-stage patients is more challenging to treat. Most patients have received prior EBRT and thus have options limited to radical surgery or, in patients with localized disease, reirradiation. For patients with small pelvic recurrences, reirradiation with intracavitary or interstitial brachytherapy has been reported, with control rates between 50% and 75%, and grade 3 or higher complication rates between 7% and15% (342,386,399–402). Beriwal et al. evaluated HDR brachytherapy for primary and recurrent vaginal malignancy. In the subset of patients with a previous malignancy, crude local control rates were 100% for patients without prior RT and 67% for patients with a history of RT.

Palliative Therapy

Local treatment can provide symptomatic benefit for patients with advanced disease who have no curative options. Advanced disease can result in vaginal bleeding, pelvic pain, lymphedema, and visceral obstruction. Vaginal bleeding is a common symptom, which can become brisk if tumor erodes into a larger vessel. Large fractions of radiation delivered initially during the treatment course may be useful in achieving hemostasis for such cases. Other options include embolization, infusion of vasopressin, and balloon catheterization for severe hemodynamic losses.

FOLLOW-UP

Recommendations for posttreatment surveillance are based on Society of Gynecologic Oncology (SGO) guidelines for gynecologic malignancies (403). Patients with early-stage lesions, treated with surgery alone, can be followed every 6 months for 2 years, then annually thereafter. Patients with more advanced lesions are at higher risk of recurrence, and are recommended follow-up every 3 months for the first 2 years, then every 6 months for the next 3 years, and annually thereafter.

There is insufficient evidence to support the use of regular cervical or vaginal cytology to detect cancer recurrence. However, the SGO recommends annual cytology as surveillance to detect other gynecologic abnormalities. The routine use of CT or PET as surveillance is not recommended.

SUMMARY

Vaginal cancer is a rare disease, accounting for 1% to 2% of all gynecologic malignancies. Patients presenting with stage I disease should be considered for surgical excision if tumor is small and surgically accessible without undue morbidity. Patients with more advanced disease are managed primarily with RT, often in conjunction with CT. Surgical resection is typically reserved for treatment failures, given the extensive morbidity of pelvic exenteration.

INTERNATIONAL PERSPECTIVES

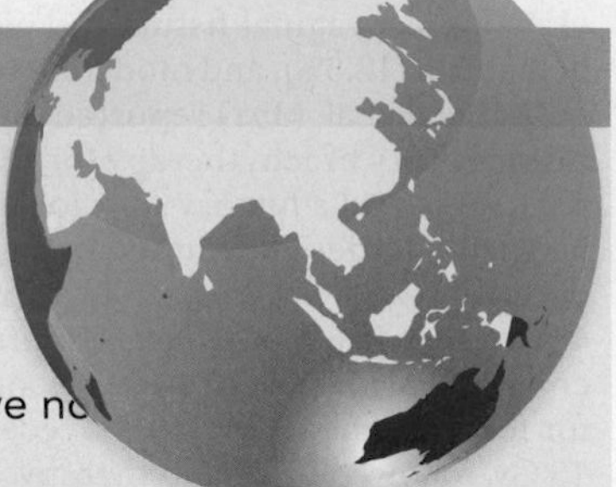

Vaginal Cancer in the Developing World

Adriana Bermudez, MD

Vaginal cancer is a rare malignancy even in developed countries. The incidence of this neoplasia in the developing world is unknown, because most of them have no reliable tumor registries.

Screening programs for gynecologic cancers are not readily available in low-resource settings. Furthermore, cultural and religious reasons make gynecologic cancer diagnoses more difficult, as patients feel uncomfortable if attended by a male doctor in many communities. This is especially true for older patients, and vaginal cancer occurs more often in women over 60 years of age.

Because most women cancer patients are managed by general gynecologists, once vaginal cancer is diagnosed, treatment is often not on hand. Radical surgery cannot be performed for want of infrastructure and necessary skill sets.

Opioids and morphine are also not available in many countries in the developing world. As a result, many women with vaginal cancer in these countries will die with no treatment and no palliative care.

INTERNATIONAL PERSPECTIVES

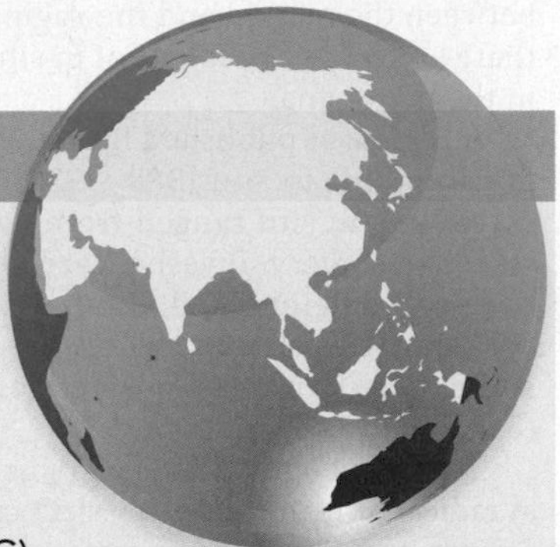

Vaginal Cancer in India

Umesh Mahantshetty, MBBS, DMRT, MD, DNB

The chapter on vaginal cancer is comprehensively written. I acknowledge the efforts of Josephine Kang and colleagues for this chapter. My views regarding different perspectives and/or unique variations in presentation, diagnosis, and management of vaginal cancer from the perspective of a low-/middle-income (LMIC) setting are as follows:

Vaginal cancer is a rare malignancy, accounting for <2% of gynecological malignancies in LMICs also. Primary vaginal cancers are also diagnosed at advanced stages, and because cervical cancer burden is high, vaginal cancer diagnosis is usually overlooked and hence may be underreported in LMICs. Although there are some guidelines for definition of primary vaginal cancer in routine clinical practice, except for older age group at presentation, the primary diagnosis poses a major challenge.

Management: The management guidelines for primary vaginal cancers are essentially based on the robust evidence from management of cervical cancers. Most radiation-naive patients undergo radical RT with/without concomitant cisplatin CT. The success of radical RT including brachytherapy depends on the clinical mapping and documentation of disease at diagnosis and brachytherapy. With a strong institutional background in brachytherapy, we have reported clinical outcomes in our patients treated with LDR brachytherapy (endovaginal and interstitial), which has been incorporated in chapter **(1).** Our protocol includes EBRT to a dose of 50 Gy/25# over 5 to 6 weeks with/without radiosensitizing cisplatin-based CT followed by HDR brachytherapy boost. In patients with complete or near-complete response HDR brachytherapy boost is delivered with single/multichannel vaginal cylinders to a dose of 12 Gy @ 6 Gy per fraction once weekly. In patients with significant residual disease, especially paracolpos/paravaginal tissues, interstitial template base (MUPIT/customized indigenous templates) to a dose of 3.5 to 4 Gy per fraction four to six times over 3 to 4 days in one application is offered, which results in optimal treatment outcome in our group of patients **(2).**

Patients with postradiation vaginal cancers are usually diagnosed at advanced stages, and radical surgery is seldom possible. In highly selective patients, salvage reirradiation with HDR brachytherapy is offered for posttreatment cervical and vaginal recurrences with promising results **(3).** The reirradiation dose depends on

INTERNATIONAL PERSPECTIVES (*continued*)

the initial RT interval, prior radiation doses, and the reirradiation protocol. In general, radiation doses more than 40 Gy EQD2 result in better outcome.

Posttreatment follow-up is similar to follow-up for cervical cancers, but poses a greater challenge because most women come from rural settings and low socioeconomic backgrounds.

(1) Pingley S, Shrivastava SK, Sarin R, et al. Primary carcinoma of the vagina: Tata Memorial Hospital experience. *Int J Radiat Oncol Biol Phys*. 2000;46(1):101–108.

(2) Mahantshetty U, Shrivastava S, Kalyani N, et al. Template-based high-dose-rate interstitial brachytherapy in gynecologic cancers: a single institutional experience. *Brachytherapy*. 2014;13(4):337–342.

(3) Mahantshetty U, Kalyani N, Engineer R, et al. Reirradiation using high-dose-rate brachytherapy in recurrent carcinoma of uterine cervix. *Brachytherapy*. 2014;13(6):548–553.

INTERNATIONAL PERSPECTIVES

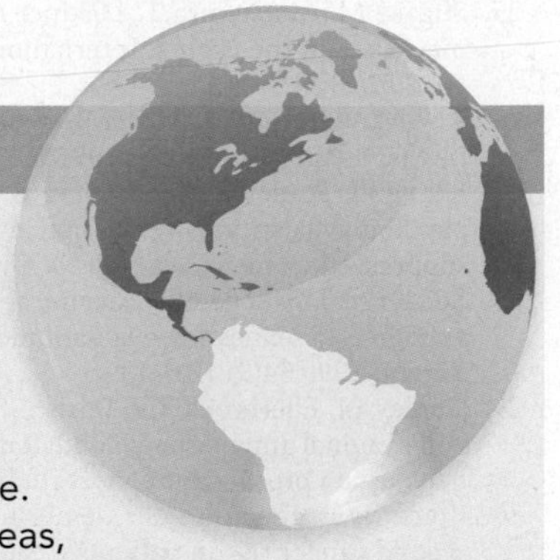

Vaginal Cancer in Latin America

Gustavo Ferraris, MD, PhD

Vaginal cancer is rare in Latin America, representing only 1% of all gynecologic tumors. As with cervical and vulvar cancers, vaginal intraepithelial neoplasia (VAIN) is associated with HPV infection, after which it progresses to invasive disease.

In Latin America, oncology services are generally concentrated in large urban areas, leaving rural areas mostly underserved. Furthermore, PAP screening and vaccination health policies are limited and not readily enforced. Risk factors in this area include the following: chronic vaginal irritation, lack of PAP smears, multiple lifetime sex partners, early age at first intercourse, and partners with penile HPV.

The workup is similar to that reported in other parts of the world, with the exception of the use of cystoscopy and sigmoidoscopy for stage II disease or symptoms, and PET is not routinely used.

In Latin America, as most patients present with advanced disease at the time of diagnosis, the standard treatment is RT without cisplatin-based CT. In general, the recommended treatment is EBRT 3DCRT or IMRT to whole pelvis +/− inguinal lymph node to 45 to 50 Gy plus intracavitary +/− interstitial brachytherapy boost to the tumor with 2 cm radial margin to 75 to 85 Gy. Midline blocks are used in case of 3DCRT. Smaller tumors (<0.5 cm thick, <2 cm) situated in the upper third of the vagina or in the introitus can be treated with surgery, as cervical and vulvar tumors are.

REFERENCES

1. Benson RC. Cancer of the female genital tract. *CA Cancer J Clin*. 1968;18(1):2–13.
2. Sedlis A, Robboy SJ. *Diseases of the Vagina, in Blaustein's Pathology of the Female Genital Tract*. Kurman RJ, Ed. New York, NY: Sringer-Verlag; 1987:98–140.
3. Cunha GR. The dual origin of vaginal epithelium. *Am J Anat*. 1975;143(3):387–392.
4. Siegel RL, Miller KD, Jemal A. Cancer statistics, 2016. *CA Cancer J Clin*. 2016;66(1):7–30.
5. Henson D, Tarone V. An epidemiologic study of cancer of the cervix, vagina, and vulva based on the Third National Cancer Survey in the United States. *Am J Obstet Gynecol*. 1977;129(5):525–532.
6. Wu X, Matanoski G, Chen VW, et al. Descriptive epidemiology of vaginal cancer incidence and survival by race, ethnicity, and age in the United States. *Cancer*. 2008;113(10 suppl):2873–2882.
7. Creasman WT, Phillips JL, Menck HR. The National Cancer Data Base report on cancer of the vagina. *Cancer*. 1998;83(5):1033–1040.
8. Shah CA, Goff BA, Lowe K, et al. Factors affecting risk of mortality in women with vaginal cancer. *Obstet Gynecol*. 2009;113(5):1038–1045.
9. Gunderson CC, Nugent EK, Elfrink SH, et al. A contemporary analysis of epidemiology and management of vaginal intraepithelial neoplasia. *Am J Obstet Gynecol*. 2013;208(5):410. e1–e6.
10. FIGO Committee on Gynecologic Oncology. Current FIGO staging for cancer of the vagina, fallopian tube, ovary, and gestational trophoblastic neoplasia. *Int J Gynaecol Obstet*. 2009;105(1):3–4.
11. Hacker NF, Eifel PJ, van der Velden J. Cancer of the vagina. *Int J Gynaecol Obstet*. 2012;119(suppl 2):S97–S99.
12. Murad TM, Durant JR, Maddox WA, et al. The pathologic behavior of primary vaginal carcinoma and its relationship to cervical cancer. *Cancer*. 1975;35(3):787–794.
13. Cheng D, Ng TY, Ngan HY, et al. Wide local excision (WLE) for vaginal intraepithelial neoplasia (VAIN). *Acta Obstet Gynecol Scand*. 1999;78(7):648–652.
14. Hampl M, Huppertz E, Schulz-Holstege O, et al. Economic burden of vulvar and vaginal intraepithelial neoplasia: retrospective cost study at a German dysplasia centre. *BMC Infect Dis*. 2011;11:73.
15. Sillman FH, Fruchter RG, Chen YS, et al. Vaginal intraepithelial neoplasia: risk factors for persistence, recurrence, and invasion and its management. *Am J Obstet Gynecol*. 1997;176(1 pt 1):93–99.
16. Rome RM, England PG. Management of vaginal intraepithelial neoplasia: A series of 132 cases with long-term follow-up. *Int J Gynecol Cancer*. 2000;10(5):382–390.
17. Diakomanolis E, Stefanidis K, Rodolakis A, et al. Vaginal intraepithelial neoplasia: report of 102 cases. *Eur J Gynaecol Oncol*. 2002;23(5):457–459.
18. Boonlikit S, Noinual N. Vaginal intraepithelial neoplasia: a retrospective analysis of clinical features and colpohistology. *J Obstet Gynaecol Res*. 2010;36(1):94–100.

19. Watson M, Saraiya M, Wu X. Update of HPV-associated female genital cancers in the United States, 1999-2004. *J Womens Health.* 2009;18(11):1731–1738.
20. Dodge JA, Eltabbakh GH, Mount SL, et al. Clinical features and risk of recurrence among patients with vaginal intraepithelial neoplasia. *Gynecol Oncol.* 2001;83(2):363–369.
21. Gonzalez Bosquet E, Torres A, Busquets M, et al. Prognostic factors for the development of vaginal intraepithelial neoplasia. *Eur J Gynaecol Oncol.* 2008;29(1):43–45.
22. Jamieson DJ, Paramsothy P, Cu-Uvin S, et al. Vulvar, vaginal, and perianal intraepithelial neoplasia in women with or at risk for human immunodeficiency virus. *Obstet Gynecol.* 2006;107(5):1023–1028.
23. Insinga RP, Liaw KL, Johnson LG, et al. A systematic review of the prevalence and attribution of human papillomavirus types among cervical, vaginal, and vulvar precancers and cancers in the United States. *Cancer Epidemiol Biomark Prev.* 2008;17(7):1611–1622.
24. Smith JS, Backes DM, Hoots BE, et al. Human papillomavirus type-distribution in vulvar and vaginal cancers and their associated precursors. *Obstet Gynecol.* 2009;113(4):917–924.
25. Sugase M, Matsukura T. Distinct manifestations of human papillomaviruses in the vagina. International journal of cancer. *J Int Cancer.* 1997;72(3):412–415.
26. Aho M, Vesterinen E, Meyer B, et al. Natural history of vaginal intraepithelial neoplasia. *Cancer.* 1991;68(1):195–197.
27. Sillman F, Stanek A, Sedlis A, et al. The relationship between human papillomavirus and lower genital intraepithelial neoplasia in immunosuppressed women. *Am J Obstet Gynecol.* 1984;150(3):300–308.
28. Spitzer M. Lower genital tract intraepithelial neoplasia in HIV-infected women: guidelines for evaluation and management. *Obstet Gynecol Survey.* 1999;54(2):131–137.
29. Conley LJ, Ellerbrock TV, Bush TJ, et al. HIV-1 infection and risk of vulvovaginal and perianal condylomata acuminata and intraepithelial neoplasia: a prospective cohort study. *Lancet.* 2002;359(9301):108–113.
30. Boice JD Jr, Engholm G, Kleinerman RA, et al. Radiation dose and second cancer risk in patients treated for cancer of the cervix. *Radiat Res.* 1988;116(1):3–55.
31. Lee JY, Perez CA, Ettinger N, et al. The risk of second primaries subsequent to irradiation for cervix cancer. *Int J Radiat Oncol Biol Phys.* 1982;8(2):207–211.
32. Lenehan PM, Meffe F, Lickrish GM. Vaginal intraepithelial neoplasia: biologic aspects and management. *Obstet Gynecol.* 1986;68(3):333–337.
33. Bornstein J, Adam E, Adler-Storthz K, et al. Development of cervical and vaginal squamous cell neoplasia as a late consequence of in utero exposure to diethylstilbestrol. *Obst Gynecol Survey.* 1988;43(1):15–21.
34. Dillner J, Dillner J, Kjaer SK, et al. Four year efficacy of prophylactic human papillomavirus quadrivalent vaccine against low grade cervical, vulvar, and vaginal intraepithelial neoplasia and anogenital warts: randomised controlled trial. *BMJ.* 2010;341:c3493.
35. Joura EA, Leodolter S, Hernandez-Avila M, et al. Efficacy of a quadrivalent prophylactic human papillomavirus (types 6, 11, 16, and 18) L1 virus-like-particle vaccine against high-grade vulval and vaginal lesions: a combined analysis of three randomised clinical trials. *Lancet.* 2007;369(9574):1693–1702.
36. Benedet JL, Murphy KJ, Fairey RN, et al. Primary invasive carcinoma of the vagina. *Obstet Gynecol.* 1983;62(6):715–719.
37. Daling JR, Madeleine MM, Schwartz SM, et al. A population-based study of squamous cell vaginal cancer: HPV and cofactors. *Gynecol Oncol.* 2002;84(2):263–270.
38. Liao JB, Jean S, Wilkinson-Ryan I, et al. Vaginal intraepithelial neoplasia (VAIN) after radiation therapy for gynecologic malignancies: a clinically recalcitrant entity. *Gynecol Oncol.* 2011;120(1):108–112.
39. Geelhoed GW, Henson DE, Taylor PT, et al. Carcinoma in situ of the vagina following treatment for carcinoma of the cervix: a distinctive clinical entity. *Am J Obstet Gynecol.* 1976;124(5):510–516.
40. Choo YC, Anderson DG. Neoplasms of the vagina following cervical carcinoma. *Gynecol Oncol.* 1982;14(1):125–132.
41. Hoffman MS, DeCesare SL, Roberts WS, et al. Upper vaginectomy for in situ and occult, superficially invasive carcinoma of the vagina. *Am J Obstet Gynecol.* 1992;166(1 pt 1):30–33.
42. Woodruff JD. Carcinoma in situ of the vagina. *Clin Obstet Gynecol.* 1981;24(2):485–501.
43. Robboy SJ, Young RH, Welch WR, et al. Atypical vaginal adenosis and cervical ectropion. Association with clear cell adenocarcinoma in diethylstilbestrol-exposed offspring. *Cancer.* 1984;54(5):869–875.
44. Hacker NF, Eifel PJ, van der Velden J. Cancer of the vagina. *Int J Gynaecol Obstet.* 2015;131(suppl 2):S84–S87.
45. Saslow D, Runowicz CD, Solomon D, et al. American Cancer Society Guideline for the Early Detection of Cervical Neoplasia and Cancer. *J Low Genit Tract Dis.* 2003;7(2):67–86.
46. Orr JM, Barnett JC, Leath CA III. Incidence of subsequent abnormal cytology in cervical cancer patients completing five-years of post treatment surveillance without evidence of recurrence. *Gynecol Oncol.* 2011;122(3):501–504.
47. So KA, Hong JH, Hwang JH, et al. The utility of the human papillomavirus DNA load for the diagnosis and prediction of persistent vaginal intraepithelial neoplasia. *J Gynecol Oncol.* 2009;20(4):232–237.
48. Jentschke M, Hoffmeister V, Soergel P, et al. Clinical presentation, treatment and outcome of vaginal intraepithelial neoplasia. *Arch Gynecol Obstet.* 2016;293(2):415–419.
49. Benedet JL, Sanders BH. Carcinoma in situ of the vagina. *Am J Obstet Gynecol.* 1984;148(5):695–700.
50. Ireland D, Monaghan JM. The management of the patient with abnormal vaginal cytology following hysterectomy. *Br J Obstet Gynaecol.* 1988;95(10):973–975.
51. Fanning J, Manahan KJ, McLean SA. Loop electrosurgical excision procedure for partial upper vaginectomy. *Am J Obstet Gynecol.* 1999;181(6):1382–1385.
52. Indermaur MD, Martino MA, Fiorica JV, et al. Upper vaginectomy for the treatment of vaginal intraepithelial neoplasia. *Am J Obstet Gynecol.* 2005;193(2):577–580; discussion 580–581.
53. Terzakis E, Androutsopoulos G, Zygouris D, et al. Loop electrosurgical excision procedure in Greek patients with vaginal intraepithelial neoplasia. *Eur J Gynaecol Oncol.* 2010;31(4):392–394.
54. Jobson VW, Homesley HD. Treatment of vaginal intraepithelial neoplasia with the carbon dioxide laser. *Obstet Gynecol.* 1983;62(1):90–93.
55. Audet-Lapointe P, Body G, Vauclair R, et al. Vaginal intraepithelial neoplasia. *Gynecol Oncol.* 1990;36(2):232–239.
56. Hoffman MS, Roberts WS, LaPolla JP, et al. Laser vaporization of grade 3 vaginal intraepithelial neoplasia. *Am J Obstet Gynecol.* 1991;165(5 pt 1):1342–1344.
57. Diakomanolis E, Rodolakis A, Boulgaris Z, et al. Treatment of vaginal intraepithelial neoplasia with laser ablation and upper vaginectomy. *Gynecol Obstet Invest.* 2002;54(1):17–20.
58. Campagnutta E, Parin A, De Piero G, et al. Treatment of vaginal intraepithelial neoplasia (VAIN) with the carbon dioxide laser. *Clin Exper Obstet Gynecol.* 1999;26(2):127–130.
59. Perotta M, Marchitelli CE, Velazco AF, et al. Use of CO2 laser vaporization for the treatment of high-grade vaginal intraethelial neoplasia. *J Low Genit Tract Dis.* 2013;17(1):23–27.
60. Woodruff JD, Parmley TH, Julian CG. Topical 5-fluorouracil in the treatment of vaginal carcinoma-in-situ. *Gynecol Oncol.* 1975;3(2):124–132.
61. Petrilli ES, Townsend DE, Morrow CP, et al. Vaginal intraepithelial neoplasia: Biologic aspects and treatment with topical 5-fluorouracil and the carbon dioxide laser. *Am J Obstet Gynecol.* 1980;138(3):321–328.
62. Kirwan P, Naftalin NJ. Topical 5-fluorouracil in the treatment of vaginal intraepithelial neoplasia. *Br J Obstet Gynaecol.* 1985;92(3):287–291.
63. Krebs HB. Treatment of vaginal intraepithelial neoplasia with laser and topical 5-fluorouracil. *Obstet Gynecol.* 1989;73(4):657–660.
64. Diakomanolis E, Haidopoulos D, Stefanidis K. Treatment of high-grade vaginal intraepithelial neoplasia with imiquimod cream. *N Engl J Med.* 2002;347(5):374.
65. Buck HW, Guth KJ. Treatment of vaginal intraepithelial neoplasia (primarily low grade) with imiquimod 5% cream. *J Low Genit Tract Dis.* 2003;7(4):290–293.
66. Prempree T, Viravathana T, Slawson RG, et al. Radiation management of primary carcinoma of the vagina. *Cancer.* 1977;40(1):109–118.
67. Chyle V, Zagars GK, Wheeler JA, et al. Definitive radiotherapy for carcinoma of the vagina: outcome and prognostic factors. *Int J Radiat Oncol Biol Phys.* 1996;35(5):891–905.
68. MacLeod C, Fowler A, Dalrymple C, et al. High-dose-rate brachytherapy in the management of high-grade intraepithelial neoplasia of the vagina. *Gynecol Oncol.* 1997;65(1):74–77.
69. Ogino I, Kitamura T, Okajima H, et al. High-dose-rate intracavitary brachytherapy in the management of cervical and vaginal intraepithelial neoplasia. *Int J Radiat Oncol Biol Phys.* 1998;40(4):881–887.
70. Perez CA, Grigsby PW, Garipagaoglu M, et al. Factors affecting long-term outcome of irradiation in carcinoma of the vagina. *Int J Radiat Oncol Biol Phys.* 1999;44(1):37–45.
71. Graham K, Wright K, Cadwallader B, et al. 20-year retrospective review of medium dose rate intracavitary brachytherapy in VAIN3. *Gynecol Oncol.* 2007;106(1):105–111.
72. Blanchard P, Monnier L, Dumas I, et al. Low-dose-rate definitive brachytherapy for high-grade vaginal intraepithelial neoplasia. *Oncologist.* 2011;16(2):182–188.
73. Song JH, Lee JH, Lee JH, et al. High-dose-rate brachytherapy for the treatment of vaginal intraepithelial neoplasia. *Cancer Res Treat.* 2014;46(1):74–780.

74. Zolciak-Siwinska A, Gruszczynska E, Jonska-Gmyrek J, et al. Brachytherapy for vaginal intraepithelial neoplasia. *Eur J Obstet Gynecol Reprod Biology*. 2015;194:73–77.
75. Cardosi RJ, Bomalaski JJ, Hoffman MS. Diagnosis and management of vulvar and vaginal intraepithelial neoplasia. *Obstet Gynecol Clin North Am*. 2001;28(4):685–702.
76. Murta EF, Neves Junior MA, Sempionato LR, et al. Vaginal intraepithelial neoplasia: clinical-therapeutic analysis of 33 cases. *Arch Gynecol Obstet*. 2005;272(4):261–264.
77. de Witte CJ, van de Sande AJ, van Beekhuizen HJ, et al. Imiquimod in cervical, vaginal and vulvar intraepithelial neoplasia: A review. *Gynecol Oncol*. 2015;139(2):377–384.
78. Stafl A, Wilkinson EJ, Mattingly RF. Laser treatment of cervical and vaginal neoplasia. *Am J Obstet Gynecol*. 1977;128(2):128–136.
79. Townsend DE, Levine RU, Crum CP, et al. Treatment of vaginal carcinoma in situ with the carbon dioxide laser. *Am J Obstet Gynecol*. 1982;143(5):565–568.
80. Piver MS, Barlow JJ, Tsukada Y, et al. Postirradiation squamous cell carcinoma in situ of the vagina: treatment by topical 20 percent 5-fluorouracil cream. *Am J Obstet Gynecol*. 1979;135(3):377–380.
81. Caglar H, Hertzog RW, Hreshchyshyn MM. Topical 5-fluorouracil treatment of vaginal intraepithelial neoplasia. *Obstet Gynecol*. 1981;58(5):580–583.
82. Daly JW, Ellis GF. Treatment of vaginal dysplasia and carcinoma in situ with topical 5-fluorouracil. *Obstet Gynecol*. 1980;55(3):350–352.
83. Hull MG, Bowen-Simpkins P, Paintin DB. Topical treatment of vaginal intraepithelial neoplasia. *Obstet Gynecol*. 1977;49(3):382.
84. WoodmanCB, Mould JJ, Jordan JA. Radiotherapy in the management of vaginal intraepithelial neoplasia after hysterectomy. *Br J Obstet Gynaecol*. 1988;95(10):976–979.
85. Patsner B. Treatment of vaginal dysplasia with loop excision: report of five cases. *Am J Obstet Gynecol*. 1993;169(1):179–180.
86. von Gruenigen VE, Gibbons HE, Gibbins K, et al. Surgical treatments for vulvar and vaginal dysplasia: a randomized controlled trial. *Obstet Gynecol*. 2007;109(4):942–947.
87. Robinson JB, Sun CC, Bodurka-Bevers D, et al. Cavitational ultrasonic surgical aspiration for the treatment of vaginal intraepithelial neoplasia. *Gynecol Oncol*. 2000;78(2):235–241.
88. Woodman CB, Jordan JA, Wade-Evans T. The management of vaginal intraepithelial neoplasia after hysterectomy. *Br J Obstet Gynaecol*. 1984;91(7):707–711.
89. Stuart GC, Flagler EA, Nation JG, et al. Laser vaporization of vaginal intraepithelial neoplasia. *Am J Obstet Gynecol*. 1988;158(2):240–243.
90. Sherman AI. Laser therapy for intraepithelial cancer of the vagina. *Am J Obstet Gynecol*. 1992;167(1):293–294.
91. Haidopoulos D, Diakomanolis E, Rodolakis A, et al. Can local application of imiquimod cream be an alternative mode of therapy for patients with high-grade intraepithelial lesions of the vagina? *Int J Gynecol Cancer*. 2005;15(5):898–902.
92. Iavazzo C, Pitsouni E, Athanasiou S, et al. Imiquimod for treatment of vulvar and vaginal intraepithelial neoplasia. *Int J Gynaecol Obstet*. 2008;101(1):3–10.
93. Stokes IM, Sworn MJ, Hawthorne JH. A new regimen for the treatment of vaginal carcinoma in situ using 5-fluorouracil. Case report. *Br J Obstet Gynaecol*. 1980;87(10):920–921.
94. Mock U, Kucera H, Fellner C, et al. High-dose-rate (HDR) brachytherapy with or without external beam radiotherapy in the treatment of primary vaginal carcinoma: long-term results and side effects. *Int J Radiat Oncol Biol Physics*. 2003;56(4):950–957.
95. Punnonen R, Grönroos M, Meurman L, et al. Diagnosis and treatment of primary vaginal carcinoma in situ and dysplasia. *Acta Obstet Gynecol Scand*. 1981;60(5):513–514.
96. Berek JS, Hacker NH. *Berek & Hacker's Gynecologic Oncology, 5th Edition*. Philadelphia, PA: Lippincott Williams & Wilkins; 2009.
97. De Vuyst H, Clifford GM, Nascimento MC, et al. Prevalence and type distribution of human papillomavirus in carcinoma and intraepithelial neoplasia of the vulva, vagina and anus: a meta-analysis. International journal of cancer. *J Int Cancer*. 2009;124(7):1626–1636.
98. Schiffman M, Kjaer SK. Chapter 2: Natural history of anogenital human papillomavirus infection and neoplasia. *J Natl Cancer Inst Monogr*. 2003(31):14–19.
99. Herman JM, Homesley HD, Dignan MB. Is hysterectomy a risk factor for vaginal cancer? *JAMA*. 1986;256(5):601–603.
100. Andersen ES. Primary carcinoma of the vagina: a study of 29 cases. *Gynecol Oncol*. 1989;33(3):317–320.
101. Ball HG, Berman ML. Management of primary vaginal carcinoma. *Gynecol Oncol*. 1982;14(2):154–163.
102. Gallup DG, Talledo OE, Shah KJ, et al. Invasive squamous cell carcinoma of the vagina: a 14-year study. *Obstet Gynecol*. 1987;69(5):782–785.
103. Kirkbride P, Fyles A, Rawlings GA, et al. Carcinoma of the vagina—experience at the Princess Margaret Hospital (1974-1989). *Gynecologic Oncology*. 1995;56(3):435–443.
104. Leung S, Sexton M. Radical radiation therapy for carcinoma of the vagina-impact of treatment modalities on outcome: Peter MacCallum Cancer Institute experience 1970-1990. *Int J Radiat Oncol Biol Phys*. 1993;25(3):413–418.
105. Perez CA, Camel HM, Galakatos AE, et al. Definitive irradiation in carcinoma of the vagina: long-term evaluation of results. *Int J Radiat Oncol Biol Phys*. 1988;15(6):1283–1290.
106. Spirtos NM, Doshi BP, Kapp DS, et al. Radiation therapy for primary squamous cell carcinoma of the vagina: Stanford University experience. *Gynecol Oncol*. 1989;35(1):20–26.
107. Davis KP, Stanhope CR, Garton GR, et al. Invasive vaginal carcinoma: analysis of early-stage disease. *Gynecol Oncol*. 1991;42(2):131–136.
108. Merino MJ. Vaginal cancer: the role of infectious and environmental factors. *Am J Obstet Gynecol*. 1991;165(4 pt 2):1255–1262.
109. Stock RG, Mychalczak B, Armstrong JG, et al. The importance of brachytherapy technique in the management of primary carcinoma of the vagina. *Int J Radiat Oncol Biol Phys*. 1992;24(4):747–753.
110. Stock RG, Chen AS, Seski J. A 30-year experience in the management of primary carcinoma of the vagina: analysis of prognostic factors and treatment modalities. *Gynecol Oncol*. 1995;56(1):45–52.
111. Rubin SC, Young J, Mikuta JJ. Squamous carcinoma of the vagina: treatment, complications, and long-term follow-up. *Gynecol Oncol*. 1985;20(3):346–353.
112. Jain A, Majoko F, Freites O. How innocent is the vaginal pessary? Two cases of vaginal cancer associated with pessary use. *J Obstet Gynaecol*. 2006;26(8):829–830.
113. Schraub S, Sun XS, Maingon P, et al. Cervical and vaginal cancer associated with pessary use. *Cancer*. 1992;69(10):2505–2509.
114. Eddy GL, Marks RD Jr, Miller MC III, et al. Primary invasive vaginal carcinoma. *Am J Obstet Gynecol*. 1991;165(2):292–296; discussion 296–298.
115. Frank SJ, Jhingran A, Levenback C, et al. Definitive radiation therapy for squamous cell carcinoma of the vagina. *Int J Radiat Oncol Biol Phys*. 2005;62(1):138–147.
116. Underwood PB Jr, Smith RT. Carcinoma of the vagina. *JAMA*. 1971;217(1):46–52.
117. Kucera H, Vavra N. Radiation management of primary carcinoma of the vagina: clinical and histopathological variables associated with survival. *Gynecol Oncol*. 1991;40(1):12–16.
118. Houghton CR, Iversen T. Squamous cell carcinoma of the vagina: a clinical study of the location of the tumor. *Gynecol Oncol*. 1982;13(3):365–372.
119. Eddy GL, Singh KP, Gansler TS. Superficially invasive carcinoma of the vagina following treatment for cervical cancer: a report of six cases. *Gynecol Oncol*. 1990;36(3):376–379.
120. Peters WA III, Kumar NB, Morley GW. Carcinoma of the vagina. Factors influencing treatment outcome. *Cancer*. 1985;55(4):892–897.
121. Perez CA, Arneson AN, Dehner LP, et al. Radiation therapy in carcinoma of the vagina. *Obstet Gynecol*. 1974;44(6):862–872.
122. Vayrynen M, Romppanen T, Koskela E, et al. Verrucous squamous cell carcinoma of the female genital tract. Report of three cases and survey of the literature. *Int J Gynaecol Obstet*. 1981;19(5):351–356.
123. Crowther ME, Lowe DG, Shepherd JH. Verrucous carcinoma of the female genital tract: a review. *Obstet Gynecol Survey*. 1988;43(5):263–280.
124. Robertson DI, Maung R, Duggan MA. Verrucous carcinoma of the genital tract: is it a distinct entity? Canadian journal of surgery. *Journal Canadien De Chirurgie*. 1993;36(2):147–151.
125. Andersen ES, Sorensen IM. Verrucous carcinoma of the female genital tract: report of a case and review of the literature. *Gynecol Oncol*. 1988;30(3):427–434.
126. Raptis S, Haber G, Ferenczy A. Vaginal squamous cell carcinoma with sarcomatoid spindle cell features. *Gynecol Oncol*. 1993;49(1):100–106.
127. Frumovitz M, Gayed IW, Jhingran A, et al. Lymphatic mapping and sentinel lymph node detection in women with vaginal cancer. *Gynecol Oncol*. 2008;108(3):478–481.
128. Al-Kurdi M, Monaghan JM. Thirty-two years experience in management of primary tumours of the vagina. *Br J Obstet Gynaecol*. 1981;88(11):1145–1150.
129. Senekjian EK, Frey KW, Stone C, et al. An evaluation of stage II vaginal clear cell adenocarcinoma according to substages. *Gynecol Oncol*. 1988;31(1):56–64.
130. Taylor MB, Dugar N, Davidson SE, et al. Magnetic resonance imaging of primary vaginal carcinoma. *Clin Radiol*. 2007;62(6):549–555.

131. Lamoreaux WT, Grigsby PW, Dehdashti F, et al. FDG-PET evaluation of vaginal carcinoma. *Int J Radiat Oncol Biol Physics*. 2005;62(3):733–737.
132. Edge SB, Byrd DR, Compton CC, et al. *AJCC Cancer Staging Manual. 6 ed*. New York, NY: Springer; 2010.
133. Tewari KS, Cappuccini F, Puthawala AA, et al. Primary invasive carcinoma of the vagina: treatment with interstitial brachytherapy. *Cancer*. 2001;91(4):758–770.
134. Nori D, Hilaris BS, Stanimir G, et al. Radiation therapy of primary vaginal carcinoma. *Int J Radiat Oncol Biol Phys*. 1983;9(10):1471–1475.
135. Hellman K, Lundell M, Silfversward C, et al. Clinical and histopathologic factors related to prognosis in primary squamous cell carcinoma of the vagina. *Int J Gynecol Cancer*. 2006;16(3):1201–1211.
136. Beller U, Sideri M, Maisonneuve P, et al. Carcinoma of the vagina. *J Epidemiol Biostat*. 2001;6(1):141–152.
137. Herbst AL, Green TH Jr, Ulfelder H. Primary carcinoma of the vagina. An analysis of 68 cases. *Am J Obstet Gynecol*. 1970;106(2):210–218.
138. Tran PT, Su Z, Lee P, et al. Prognostic factors for outcomes and complications for primary squamous cell carcinoma of the vagina treated with radiation. *Gynecol Oncol*. 2007;105(3):641–649.
139. Tjalma WA, Monaghan JM, de Barros Lopes A, et al. The role of surgery in invasive squamous carcinoma of the vagina. *Gynecol Oncol*. 2001;81(3):360–365.
140. Fuste V, Del Pino M, Perez A, et al. Primary squamous cell carcinoma of the vagina: human papillomavirus detection, p16(INK4A) overexpression and clinicopathological correlations. *Histopathology*. 2010;57(6):907–916.
141. Alonso I, Felix A, Torné A, et al. Human papillomavirus as a favorable prognostic biomarker in squamous cell carcinomas of the vagina. *Gynecol Oncol*. 2012;125(1):194–199.
142. Brunner AH, Grimm C, Polterauer S, et al. The prognostic role of human papillomavirus in patients with vaginal cancer. *Int J Gynecol Cancer*. 2011;21(5):923–929.
143. Ali MM, Huang DT, Goplerud DR, et al. Radiation alone for carcinoma of the vagina: variation in response related to the location of the primary tumor. *Cancer*. 1996;77(9):1934–1939.
144. Tarraza MH Jr, Muntz H, Decain M, et al. Patterns of recurrence of primary carcinoma of the vagina. *Eur J Gynaecol Oncol*. 1991;12(2):89–92.
145. Urbanski K, Kojs Z, Reinfuss M, et al. Primary invasive vaginal carcinoma treated with radiotherapy: analysis of prognostic factors. *Gynecol Oncol*. 1996;60(1):16–21.
146. Whelton J, Kottmeier HL. Primary carcinoma of the vagina: a study of a Radiumhemmet series of 145 cases. *Acta Obstet Gynecol Scand*. 1962;41:22–40.
147. Kucera H, Langer M, Smekal G, et al. Radiotherapy of primary carcinoma of the vagina: management and results of different therapy schemes. *Gynecol Oncol*. 1985;21(1):87–93.
148. Dixit S, Singhal S, Baboo HA. Squamous cell carcinoma of the vagina: a review of 70 cases. *Gynecol Oncol*. 1993;48(1):80–87.
149. Pingley S, Shrivastava SK, Sarin R, et al. Primary carcinoma of the vagina: Tata Memorial Hospital experience. *Int J Radiat Oncol Biol Phys*. 2000;46(1):101–108.
150. Lee WR, Marcus RB Jr, Sombeck MD, et al. Radiotherapy alone for carcinoma of the vagina: the importance of overall treatment time. *Int J Radiat Oncol Biol Phys*. 1994;29(5):983–988.
151. Otton GR, Nicklin JL, Dickie GJ, et al. Early-stage vaginal carcinoma—an analysis of 70 patients. *Int J Gynecol Cancer*. 2004;14(2):304–310.
152. Ling B, Gao Z, Sun M, et al. Laparoscopic radical hysterectomy with vaginectomy and reconstruction of vagina in patients with stage I of primary vaginal carcinoma. *Gynecol Oncol*. 2008;109(1):92–96.
153. Lv L, Sun Y, Liu H, et al. Neoadjuvant chemotherapy followed by radical surgery and reconstruction of the vagina in a patient with stage II primary vaginal squamous carcinoma. *J Obstet Gynaecol Res*. 2010;36(6):1245–1248.
154. Benedetti Panici P, Bellati F, Plotti F, et al. Neoadjuvant chemotherapy followed by radical surgery in patients affected by vaginal carcinoma. *Gynecol Oncol*. 2008;111(2):307–311.
155. Schäfer U, Micke O, Prott FJ, et al. The results of primary radiotherapy in vaginal carcinoma [in German]. *Strahlenther Onkol*. 1997;173(5):272–280.
156. de Crevoisier R, Sanfilippo N, Gerbaulet A, et al. Exclusive radiotherapy for primary squamous cell carcinoma of the vagina. *Radiother Oncol*. 2007;85(3):362–370.
157. Stryker JA. Radiotherapy for vaginal carcinoma: a 23-year review. *Br J Radiol*. 2000;73(875):1200–1205.
158. Lian J, Dundas G, Carlone M, et al. Twenty-year review of radiotherapy for vaginal cancer: an institutional experience. *Gynecol Oncol*. 2008;111(2):298–306.
159. Beriwal S, Bhatnagar A, Heron DE, et al. High-dose-rate interstitial brachytherapy for gynecologic malignancies. *Brachytherapy*. 2006;5(4):218–222.
160. Hellman K, Lundell M, Silfversward C, et al. Clinical and histopathologic factors related to prognosis in primary squamous cell carcinoma of the vagina. *Int J Gynecol Cancer*. 2006;16(3):1201–1211.
161. Miyamoto DT. Viswanathan, Concurrent chemoradiation for vaginal cancer. *Plos One*. 2013;8(6):e65048.
162. Dancuart F, Delclos L, Wharton JT, et al. Primary squamous cell carcinoma of the vagina treated by radiotherapy: a failures analysis—the M. D. Anderson Hospital experience 1955-1982. *Int J Radiat Oncol Biol Phys*. 1988;14(4):745–749.
163. Reddy S, Saxena VS, Reddy S, et al. Results of radiotherapeutic management of primary carcinoma of the vagina. *Int J Radiat Oncol Biol Phys*. 1991;21(4):1041–1044.
164. Kanayama N, Isohashi F, Yoshioka Y, et al. Definitive radiotherapy for primary vaginal cancer: correlation between treatment patterns and recurrence rate. *J Radiat Res*. 2015;56(2):346–353.
165. Prempree T, Amornmarn R. Radiation treatment of primary carcinoma of the vagina. Patterns of failures after definitive therapy. *Acta Radiol Oncol*. 1985;24(1):51–56.
166. Perez CA, Korba A, Sharma S. Dosimetric considerations in irradiation of carcinoma of the vagina. *Int J Radiat Oncol Biol Phys*. 1977;2(7–8):639–649.
167. Glaser SM, Beriwal S. Brachytherapy for malignancies of the vagina in the 3D era. *J Contemp Brachyther*. 2015;7(4):312–318.
168. Vargo JA, Kim H, Houser CJ, et al. Image-based multichannel vaginal cylinder brachytherapy for vaginal cancer. *Brachytherapy*. 2015;14(1):9–15.
169. Beriwal S, Demanes DJ, Erickson B, et al. American Brachytherapy Society consensus guidelines for interstitial brachytherapy for vaginal cancer. *Brachytherapy*. 2012;11(1):68–75.
170. Manetta A, Gutrecht EL, Berman ML, et al. Primary invasive carcinoma of the vagina. *Obstet Gynecol*. 1990;76(4):639–642.
171. Fleming P, Nisar Syed AM, Neblett D, et al. Description of an afterloading 192Ir interstitial-intracavitary technique in the treatment of carcinoma of the vagina. *Obstet Gynecol*. 1980;55(4):525–530.
172. Puthawala A, Syed AM, Nalick R, et al. Integrated external and interstitial radiation therapy for primary carcinoma of the vagina. *Obstet Gynecol*. 1983;62(3):367–372.
173. Herbst AL, Anderson S, Hubby MM, et al. Risk factors for the development of diethylstilbestrol-associated clear cell adenocarcinoma: a case-control study. *Am J Obstet Gynecol*. 1986;154(4):814–822.
174. Morris M, Eifel PJ, Lu J, et al. Pelvic radiation with concurrent chemotherapy compared with pelvic and para-aortic radiation for high-risk cervical cancer. *N Engl J Med*. 1999;340(15):1137–1143.
175. Rose PG, Bundy BN, Watkins EB, et al. Concurrent cisplatin-based radiotherapy and chemotherapy for locally advanced cervical cancer. *N Engl J Med*. 1999;340(15):1144–1153.
176. Mundt AJ, Mell LK, Roeske JC. Preliminary analysis of chronic gastrointestinal toxicity in gynecology patients treated with intensity-modulated whole pelvic radiation therapy. *Int J Radiat Oncol Biol Phys*. 2003;56(5):1354–1360.
177. Mundt AJ, Lujan AE, Rotmensch J, et al. Intensity-modulated whole pelvic radiotherapy in women with gynecologic malignancies. *Int J Radiat Oncol Biol Phys*. 2002;52(5):1330–1337.
178. Sinha B, Stehman F, Schilder J, et al. Indiana University experience in the management of vaginal cancer. *Int J Gynecol Cancer*. 2009;19(4):686–693.
179. Hegemann S, Schäfer U, Lellé R, et al. Long-term results of radiotherapy in primary carcinoma of the vagina. *Strahlenther Onkol*. 2009;185(3):184–189.
180. Fine BA, Piver MS, McAuley M, et al. The curative potential of radiation therapy in the treatment of primary vaginal carcinoma. *Am J Clin Oncol*. 1996;19(1):39–44.
181. National Cancer Institute. *NCI Clinical Announcement On Cervical Cancer: Chemotherapy Plus Radiation Improves Survival*. Bethesda, MD: United States Department of Health and Human Services, Public Health Service; 1999.
182. Keys HM, Bundy BN, Stehman FB, et al. Cisplatin, radiation, and adjuvant hysterectomy compared with radiation and adjuvant hysterectomy for bulky stage IB cervical carcinoma. *N Engl J Med*. 1999;340(15):1154–1161.
183. Dalrymple JL, Russell AH, Lee SW, et al. Chemoradiation for primary invasive squamous carcinoma of the vagina. *Int J Gynecol Cancer*. 2004;14(1):110–117.
184. Gunderson CC, Nugent EK, Yunker AC, et al. Vaginal cancer: the experience from 2 large academic centers during a 15-year period. *J Low Genit Tract Dis*. 2013;17(4):409–413.

185. Samant R, Lau B, E C, et al. Primary vaginal cancer treated with concurrent chemoradiation using Cis-platinum. *Int J Radiat Oncol Biol Phys.* 2007;69(3):746–750.
186. Nashiro T, Yagi C, Hirakawa M, et al. Concurrent chemoradiation for locally advanced squamous cell carcinoma of the vagina: case series and literature review. *Int J Clin Oncol.* 2008;13(4):335–339.
187. Holleboom CA, Kock HC, Nijs AM, et al. cis-Diaminechloroplatinum in the treatment of advanced primary squamous cell carcinoma of the vaginal wall: a case report. *Gynecol Oncol.* 1987;27(1):110–115.
188. Evans LS, Kersh CR, Constable WC, et al. Concomitant 5-fluorouracil, mitomycin-C, and radiotherapy for advanced gynecologic malignancies. *Int J Radiat Oncol Biol Phys.* 1988;15(4):901–906.
189. Roberts WS, Hoffman MS, Kavanagh JJ, et al. Further experience with radiation therapy and concomitant intravenous chemotherapy in advanced carcinoma of the lower female genital tract. *Gynecol Oncol.* 1991;43(3):233–236.
190. Ghia AJ, Gonzalez VJ, Tward JD, et al. Primary vaginal cancer and chemoradiotherapy: a patterns-of-care analysis. *Int J Gynecol Cancer.* 2011;21(2):378–384.
191. Tabata T, Takeshima N, Nishida H, et al. Treatment failure in vaginal cancer. *Gynecol Oncol.* 2002;84(2):309–314.
192. Herbst AL, Ulfelder H, Poskanzer DC. Adenocarcinoma of the vagina. Association of maternal stilbestrol therapy with tumor appearance in young women. *N Engl J Med.* 1971;284(15):878–881.
193. Herbst AL, Anderson D. Clear cell adenocarcinoma of the vagina and cervix secondary to intrauterine exposure to diethylstilbestrol. *Semin Surg Oncol.* 1990;6(6):343–346.
194. Herbst AL. Diethylstilbestrol and adenocarcinoma of the vagina. *Am J Obstet Gynecol.* 1999;181(6):1576–1578; discussion 1579.
195. Melnick S, Cole P, Anderson D, et al. Rates and risks of diethylstilbestrol-related clear-cell adenocarcinoma of the vagina and cervix. An update. *N Engl J Med.* 1987;316(9):514–516.
196. Robboy SJ, Scully RE, Herbst AL. Pathology of vaginal and cervical abnormalities associated with prenatal exposure to diethylstilbestrol (des). *J Reprod Med.* 1975;15(1):13–18.
197. Robboy SJ, Welch WR, Young RH, et al. Topographic relation of cervical ectropion and vaginal adenosis to clear cell adenocarcinoma. *Obstet Gynecol.* 1982;60(5):546–551.
198. Verloop J, Rookus MA, van Leeuwen FE. Prevalence of gynecologic cancer in women exposed to diethylstilbestrol in utero. *N Engl J Med.* 2000;342(24):1838–1839.
199. Robboy SJ, Welch WR, Young RH, et al. Dysplasia and cytologic findings in 4,589 young women enrolled in diethylstilbestrol-adenosis (DESAD) project. *Am J Obstet Gynecol.* 1981;140(5):579–586.
200. Robboy SJ, Hill EC, Sandberg EC, et al. Vaginal adenosis in women born prior to the diethylstilbestrol era. *Hum Pathol.* 1986;17(5):488–492.
201. Herbst AL, Robboy SJ, Scully RE, et al. Clear-cell adenocarcinoma of the vagina and cervix in girls: analysis of 170 registry cases. *Am J Obstet Gynecol.* 1974;119(5):713–724.
202. Jones WB, Koulos JP, Saigo PE, et al. Clear-cell adenocarcinoma of the lower genital tract: Memorial Hospital 1974-1984. *Obstet Gynecol.* 1987;70(4):573–577.
203. Hanselaar AG, Van Leusen ND, De Wilde PC, et al. Clear cell adenocarcinoma of the vagina and cervix. A report of the Central Netherlands Registry with emphasis on early detection and prognosis. *Cancer.* 1991;67(7):1971–1978.
204. Waggoner SE, Anderson SM, Luce MC, et al. p53 protein expression and gene analysis in clear cell adenocarcinoma of the vagina and cervix. *Gynecol Oncol.* 1996;60(3):339–344.
205. Frank SJ, Deavers MT, Jhingran A, et al. Primary adenocarcinoma of the vagina not associated with diethylstilbestrol (DES) exposure. *Gynecol Oncol.* 2007;105(2):470–474.
206. Nomura H, Maki M, Sanshiro O, et al. Clinical characteristics of non-squamous cell carcinoma of the vagina. *Int J Gynecol Cancer.* 2015;25(2):320–324.
207. Herbst AL, Norusis MJ, Rosenow PJ, et al. An analysis of 346 cases of clear cell adenocarcinoma of the vagina and cervix with emphasis on recurrence and survival. *Gynecol Oncol.* 1979;7(2):111–122.
208. Senekjian EK, Frey KW, Anderson D, et al. Local therapy in stage I clear cell adenocarcinoma of the vagina. *Cancer.* 1987;60(6):1319–1324.
209. Senekjian EK, Frey K, Herbst AL. Pelvic exenteration in clear cell adenocarcinoma of the vagina and cervix. *Gynecol Oncol.* 1989;34(3):413–416.
210. Guiou M, Hall WH, Konia T, et al. Primary clear cell adenocarcinoma of the rectovaginal septum treated with concurrent chemoradiation therapy: a case report. *Int J Gynecol Cancer.* 2008;18(5):1118–1121.
211. Miyamoto DT, Tanaka CK, Viswanathan AN. Concurrent chemoradiation improves survival in patients with vaginal cancer. 52nd American Society for Therapeutic Radiology and Oncology Annual Meeting. San Diego, CA; 2010.
212. Waggoner SE, Mittendorf R, Biney N, et al. Influence of in utero diethylstilbestrol exposure on the prognosis and biologic behavior of vaginal clear-cell adenocarcinoma. *Gynecol Oncol.* 1994;55(2):238–244.
213. Wharton JT, Tortolero-Luna G, Linares AC, et al. Vaginal intraepithelial neoplasia and vaginal cancer. *Obstet Gynecol Clin North Am.* 1996;23(2):325–345.
214. Herbst AL, Cole P, Norusis MJ, et al. Epidemiologic aspects and factors related to survival in 384 Registry cases of clear cell adenocarcinoma of the vagina and cervix. *Am J Obstet Gynecol.* 1979;135(7):876–886.
215. Fishman DA, Williams S, Small W Jr, et al. Late recurrences of vaginal clear cell adenocarcinoma. *Gynecol Oncol.* 1996;62(1):128–132.
216. Lin LM, Sciubba DM, Gallia GL, et al. Diethylstilbestrol (DES)-induced clear cell adenocarcinoma of the vagina metastasizing to the brain. *Gynecol Oncol.* 2007;105(1):273–276.
217. Tarraza HM Jr, Meltzer SE, DeCain M, et al. Vaginal metastases from renal cell carcinoma: report of four cases and review of the literature. *Eur J Gynaecol Oncol.* 1998;19(1):14–18.
218. Saitoh M, Hayasaka T, Ohmichi M, et al. Primary mucinous adenocarcinoma of the vagina: possibility of differentiating from metastatic adenocarcinomas. *Pathol Int.* 2005;55(6):372–375.
219. Nag S, Martínez-Monge R, Copeland LJ, et al. Perineal template interstitial brachytherapy salvage for recurrent endometrial adenocarcinoma metastatic to the vagina. *Gynecol Oncol.* 1997;66(1):16–19.
220. Staats PN, Clement PB, Young RH. Primary endometrioid adenocarcinoma of the vagina: a clinicopathologic study of 18 cases. *Am J Surg Pathol.* 2007;31(10):1490–1501.
221. Nomoto K, Hori T, Kiya C, et al. Endometrioid adenocarcinoma of the vagina with a microglandular pattern arising from endometriosis after hysterectomy. *Pathol Int.* 2010;60(9):636–641.
222. Haskel S, Chen SS, Spiegel G. Vaginal endometrioid adenocarcinoma arising in vaginal endometriosis: a case report and literature review. *Gynecol Oncol.* 1989;34(2):232–236.
223. Adjetey V, Ganesan R, Downey GP. Primary vaginal endometrioid carcinoma following unopposed estrogen administration. *J Obstet Gynaecol.* 2003;23(3):316–317.
224. Bamford DS. Primary adenocarcinoma of the vagina. *Proc R Soc Med.* 1967;60(10):999–1000.
225. Eckert R. Adenocarcinoma arising in endometriosis. *Am Fam Physician.* 2000;62(4):734, 736.
226. Granai CO, Walters MD, Safaii H, et al. Malignant transformation of vaginal endometriosis. *Obstet Gynecol.* 1984;64(4):592–595.
227. Hyman MP. Extraovarian endometrioid carcinoma. Review of the literature and report of two cases with unusual features. *Am J Clin Pathol.* 1977;68(4):522–527.
228. Orr JW Jr, Holimon JL, Sisson PF. Vaginal adenocarcinoma developing in residual pelvic endometriosis: a clinical dilemma. *Gynecol Oncol.* 1989;33(1):96–98.
229. Wirtheimer C. [2 Cases of Endometrial Adenocarcinoma of Different Origin]. *Bull Soc R Belge Gynecol Obstet.* 1964;34:117–129.
230. Tewari DS, McHale MT, Kuo JV,et al. Primary invasive vaginal cancer in the setting of the Mayer-Rokitansky-Kuster-Hauser syndrome. *Gynecol Oncol.* 2002;85(2):384–387.
231. Ebrahim S, Daponte A, Smith TH, et al. Primary mucinous adenocarcinoma of the vagina. *Gynecol Oncol.* 2001;80(1):89–92.
232. Nasu K, Kai K, Matsumoto H, et al. Primary mucinous adenocarcinoma of the vagina. *Eur J Gynaecol Oncol.* 2010;31(6):679–681.
233. Werner D, Wilkinson EJ, Ripley D, et al. Primary adenocarcinoma of the vagina with mucinous-enteric differentiation: a report of two cases with associated vaginal adenosis without history of diethylstilbestrol exposure. *J Low Genit Tract Dis.* 2004;8(1):38–42.
234. McCluggage WG, Price JH, Dobbs SP. Primary adenocarcinoma of the vagina arising in endocervicosis. *Int J Gynecol Pathol.* 2001;20(4):399–402.
235. Hiroi H, Yasugi T, Matsumoto K, et al. Mucinous adenocarcinoma arising in a neovagina using the sigmoid colon thirty years after operation: a case report. *J Surg Oncol.* 2001;77(1):61–64.
236. Droegemueller W, Makowski EL, Taylor ES. Vaginal mesonephric adenocarcinoma in two prepubertal children. *Am J Dis Child.* 1970;119(2):168–170.
237. Shaaban MM. Primary adenocarcinoma of the vagina of mesonephric pattern. Report of a case and review of literatur. *Aust N Z J Obstet Gynaecol.* 1970;10(1):55–58.
238. Riva C, Fabbri A, Facco C, et al. Primary serous papillary adenocarcinoma of the vagina: a case report. *Int J Gynecol Pathol.* 1997;16(3):286–290.
239. Frumovitz M, Etchepareborda M, Sun CC, et al. Primary malignant melanoma of the vagina. *Obstet Gynecol.* 2010;116(6):1358–1365.

240. Greggi S, Losito S, Pisano C, et al. Malignant melanoma of the vagina: report of two cases and review of the literature. *Int Surg.* 2010;95(2):120–125.
241. Ghosh A, Pradhan S, Swami R, et al. Primary malignant melanoma of vagina—a case report with review of literature. *JNMA J Nepal Med Assoc.* 2007;46(168):203–205.
242. Weinstock MA. Malignant melanoma of the vulva and vagina in the United States: patterns of incidence and population-based estimates of survival. *Am J Obstet Gynecol.* 1994;171(5):1225–1230.
243. Hu DN, Yu GP, McCormick SA. Population-based incidence of vulvar and vaginal melanoma in various races and ethnic groups with comparisons to other site-specific melanomas. *Melanoma Res.* 2010;20(2):153–158.
244. Gupta JC, Arora MM, Jungalwala BN, et al. Primary Melanoma of the Vagina. *J Obstet Gynaecol Br Commonwealth.* 1964;71:801–803.
245. Gokaslan H, Şişmanoğlu A, Pekin T, et al. Primary malignant melanoma of the vagina: a case report and review of the current treatment options. *Eur J Obstet Gynecol Reprod Biol.* 2005;121(2):243–248.
246. Breslow A. Tumor thickness, level of invasion and node dissection in stage I cutaneous melanoma. *Ann Surg.* 1975;182(5):572–575.
247. Irvin WP Jr, Bliss SA, Rice LW, et al. Malignant melanoma of the vagina and locoregional control: radical surgery revisited. *Gynecol Oncol.* 1998;71(3):476–480.
248. Reid GC, Schmidt RW, Roberts JA, et al. Primary melanoma of the vagina: a clinicopathologic analysis. *Obstet Gynecol.* 1989;74(2):190–199.
249. Chung AF, Casey MJ, Flannery JT, et al. Malignant melanoma of the vagina—report of 19 cases. *Obstet Gynecol.* 1980;55(6):720–727.
250. Buchanan DJ, Schlaerth J, Kurosaki T. Primary vaginal melanoma: thirteen-year disease-free survival after wide local excision and review of recent literature. *Am J Obstet Gynecol.* 1998;178(6):1177–1184.
251. Levitan Z, Gordon AN, Kaplan AL, et al. Primary malignant melanoma of the vagina: report of four cases and review of the literature. *Gynecol Oncol.* 1989;33(1):85–90.
252. Van Nostrand KM, Lucci JA III, Schell M, et al. Primary vaginal melanoma: improved survival with radical pelvic surgery. *Gynecol Oncol.* 1994;55(2):234–237.
253. Xia L, Han D, Yang W, et al. Primary malignant melanoma of the vagina: a retrospective clinicopathologic study of 44 cases. *Int J Gynecol Cancer.* 2014;24(1):149–155.
254. Jentys W, Sikorowa L, Mokrzanowski A. Primary melanoma of the vagina. Clinicopathologic study of 7 cases. *Oncology.* 1975;31(2):83–91.
255. Norris HJ, Taylor HB. Melanomas of the vagina. *Am J Clin Pathol.* 1966;46(4):420–426.
256. Geisler JP, Look KY, Moore DA, et al. Pelvic exenteration for malignant melanomas of the vagina or urethra with over 3 mm of invasion. *Gynecol Oncol.* 1995;59(3):338–341.
257. Stellato G, Iodice F, Casella G, et al. Primary malignant melanoma of the vagina: case report. *Eur J Gynaecol Oncol.* 1998;19(2):186–188.
258. Morrow CP, DiSaia PJ. Malignant melanoma of the female genitalia: a clinical analysis. *Obstet Gynecol Survey.* 1976;31(4):233–271.
259. Miner TJ, Delgado R, Zeisler J, et al. Primary vaginal melanoma: a critical analysis of therapy. *Ann Surg Oncol.* 2004;11(1):34–39.
260. Huang Q, Huang H, Wan T, et al. Clinical outcome of 31 patients with primary malignant melanoma of the vagina. *J Gynecol Oncol.* 2013;24(4):330–335.
261. DeMatos P, Tyler D, Seigler HF. Mucosal melanoma of the female genitalia: a clinicopathologic study of forty-three cases at Duke University Medical Center. *Surgery.* 1998;124(1):38–48.
262. Cobellis L, Calabrese E, Stefanon B, et al. Malignant melanoma of the vagina. A report of 15 cases. *Eur J Gynaecol Oncol.* 2000;21(3):295–297.
263. Bonner JA, Perez-Tamayo C, Reid GC, et al. The management of vaginal melanoma. *Cancer.* 1988;62(9):2066–2072.
264. Petru E, Nagele F, Czerwenka K, et al. Primary malignant melanoma of the vagina: long-term remission following radiation therapy. *Gynecol Oncol.* 1998;70(1):23–26.
265. Harwood AR, Cummings BJ. Radiotherapy for mucosal melanomas. *Int J Radiat Oncol Biol Phys.* 1982;8(7):1121–1126.
266. Rogo KO, Andersson R, Edbom G, et al. Conservative surgery for vulvovaginal melanoma. *Eur J Gynaecol Oncol.* 1991;12(2):113–119.
267. Brand E, Fu YS, Lagasse LD, et al. Vulvovaginal melanoma: report of seven cases and literature review. *Gynecol Oncol.* 1989;33(1):54–60.
268. Ghezelayagh T, Rauh-Hain JA, Growdon WB. Comparing mortality of vaginal sarcoma, squamous cell carcinoma, and adenocarcinoma in the surveillance, epidemiology, and end results database. *Obstet Gynecol.* 2015;125(6):1353–1361.
269. Ahram J, Lemus R, Schiavello HJ. Leiomyosarcoma of the vagina: case report and literature review. *Int J Gynecol Cancer.* 2006;16(2): 884–891.
270. Suh MJ, Park DC. Leiomyosarcoma of the vagina: a case report and review from the literature. *J Gynecol Oncol.* 2008;19(4):261–264.
271. Tavassoli FA, Norris HJ. Smooth muscle tumors of the vagina. *Obstet Gynecol.* 1979;53(6):689–693.
272. Ciaravino G, Kapp DS, Vela AM, et al. Primary leiomyosarcoma of the vagina. A case report and literature review. *Int J Gynecol Cancer.* 2000;10(4):340–347.
273. Curtin JP, Saigo P, Slucher B, et al. Soft-tissue sarcoma of the vagina and vulva: a clinicopathologic study. *Obstet Gynecol.* 1995;86(2): 269–272.
274. Ahuja A, Safaya R, Prakash G, et al. Primary mixed mullerian tumor of the vagina—a case report with review of the literature. *Pathol Res Pract.* 2011;207(4):253–255.
275. Prempree T, Tang CK, Hatef A, et al. Angiosarcoma of the vagina: a clinicopathologic report. A reappraisal of the radiation treatment of angiosarcomas of the female genital tract. *Cancer.* 1983;51(4):618–622.
276. Kounelis S, Jones MW, Papadaki H, et al. Carcinosarcomas (malignant mixed mullerian tumors) of the female genital tract: comparative molecular analysis of epithelial and mesenchymal components. *Hum Pathol.* 1998;29(1):82–87.
277. Davis PC, Franklin EW III. Cancer of the vagina. *South Med J.* 1975;68(10):1239–1242.
278. Sebenik M, Yan Z, Khalbuss WE, et al. Malignant mixed mullerian tumor of the vagina: case report with review of the literature, immunohistochemical study, and evaluation for human papilloma virus. *Hum Pathol.* 2007;38(8):1282–1288.
279. Sotiropoulou M, Haidopoulos D, Vlachos G, et al. Primary malignant mixed mullerian tumor of the vagina immunohistochemically confirmed. *Arch Gynecol Obstet.* 2005;271(3):264–266.
280. Neesham D, Kerdemelidis P, Scurry J. Primary malignant mixed Mullerian tumor of the vagina. *Gynecol Oncol.* 1998;70(2):303–307.
281. Shibata R, et al. Primary carcinosarcoma of the vagina. *Pathol Int.* 2003;53(2):106–110.
282. Garcia Coronel R, Diaz Palacios V, Amador Montelongo C. [Vaginal carcinosarcoma (report of a case)]. *Ginecologia y obstetricia de Mexico.* 1974;35(209):285–289.
283. McAdam JA, Stewart F, Reid R. Vaginal epithelioid angiosarcoma. *J Clin Pathol.* 1998;51(12):928–930.
284. Tohya T, Katabuchi H, Fukuma K, et al. Angiosarcoma of the vagina. A light and electronmicroscopy study. *Acta Obstet Gynecol Scand.* 1991;70(2):169–172.
285. Hays DM, Shimada H, Raney RB Jr, et al. Sarcomas of the vagina and uterus: the Intergroup Rhabdomyosarcoma Study. *J Pediatr Surg.* 1985;20(6):718–724.
286. Magne N, Oberlin O, Martelli H, et al. Vulval and vaginal rhabdomyosarcoma in children: update and reappraisal of Institut Gustave Roussy brachytherapy experience. *Int J Radiat Oncol Biol Phys.* 2008;72(3):878–883.
287. Peters WA III, Kumar NB, Andersen WA, et al. Primary sarcoma of the adult vagina: a clinicopathologic study. *Obstet Gynecol.* 1985;65(5): 699–704.
288. Suit HD, Mankin HJ, Wood WC, et al. Treatment of the patient with stage M0 soft tissue sarcoma. *J Clin Oncol.* 1988;6(5):854–862.
289. Fein DA, Lee WR, Lanciano RM, et al. Management of extremity soft tissue sarcomas with limb-sparing surgery and postoperative irradiation: do total dose, overall treatment time, and the surgery-radiotherapy interval impact on local control? *Int J Radiat Oncol Biol Phys.* 1995;32(4):969–976.
290. Nielsen OS, Dombernowsky P, Mouridsen H, et al. High-dose epirubicin is not an alternative to standard-dose doxorubicin in the treatment of advanced soft tissue sarcomas. A study of the EORTC soft tissue and bone sarcoma group. *Br J Cancer.* 1998;78(12):1634–1639.
291. Leiser AL, Chi DS, Ishill NM, et al. Carcinosarcoma of the ovary treated with platinum and taxane: the memorial Sloan-Kettering Cancer Center experience. *Gynecol Oncol.* 2007;105(3):657–661.
292. Mok JE, Kim YM, Jung MH, et al. Malignant mixed mullerian tumors of the ovary: experience with cytoreductive surgery and platinum-based combination chemotherapy. *Int J Gynecol Cancer.* 2006;16(1):101–105.
293. Muntz HG, Jones MA, Goff BA, et al. Malignant mixed mullerian tumors of the ovary: experience with surgical cytoreduction and combination chemotherapy. *Cancer.* 1995;76(7):1209–1213.
294. Rutledge TL, Gold MA, McMeekin DS, et al. Carcinosarcoma of the ovary-a case series. *Gynecol Oncol.* 2006;100(1):128–132.
295. Ferry JA, Young RH. Malignant lymphoma, pseudolymphoma, and hematopoietic disorders of the female genital tract. *Pathol Annu.* 1991;26(pt 1):227–263.

296. Liang R, Chiu E, Loke SL. Non-Hodgkin's lymphomas involving the female genital tract. *Hematol Oncol.* 1990;8(5):295–299.
297. Perren T, Farrant M, McCarthy K, et al. Lymphomas of the cervix and upper vagina: a report of five cases and a review of the literature. *Gynecol Oncol.* 1992;44(1):87–95.
298. Mahendran SM. Primary non-Hodgkin's lymphoma of the vagina masquerading as a uterine fibroid in pregnancy. *J Obstetr Gynaecol.* 2008;28(4):456–458.
299. Hussein IY, Said MR, Macheta A, et al. Primary non-Hodgkin's lymphoma of the vagina. *J Obstet Gynaecol.* 2007;27(7):752.
300. Cohn DE, Resnick KE, Eaton LA, et al. Non–Hodgkin's lymphoma mimicking gynecological malignancies of the vagina and cervix: a report of four cases. *Int J Gynecol Cancer.* 2007;17(1):274–279.
301. Zafar M, Mehmood A, Abassi MH, et al. Primary non-Hodgkin's lymphoma of vagina associated with pregnancy. *J Coll Physicians Surg Pak.* 2006;16(6):424–425.
302. Garavaglia E, Taccagni G, Montoli S, et al. Primary stage I-IIE non-Hodgkin's lymphoma of uterine cervix and upper vagina: evidence for a conservative approach in a study on three patients. *Gynecol Oncol.* 2005;97(1):214–218.
303. Yoshinaga K, Akahira J, Niikura H, et al. A case of primary mucosa-associated lymphoid tissue lymphoma of the vagina. *Hum Pathol.* 2004;35(9):1164–1166.
304. Engin H, Türker A, Abali H, et al. Successful treatment of primary non-Hodgkin's lymphoma of the vagina with chemotherapy. *Arch Gynecol Obstet.* 2004;269(3):208–210.
305. Raspagliesi F, Ditto A, Fontanelli R, et al. Primary non-Hodgkin's lymphoma of the vagina. *Haematologica.* 2000;85(6):666–667.
306. Vang R, Medeiros LJ, Silva EG, et al. Non-Hodgkin's lymphoma involving the vagina: a clinicopathologic analysis of 14 patients. *Am J Surg Pathol.* 2000;24(5):719–725.
307. Guarini A, Pavone V, Valentino T, et al. Primary non Hodgkin's lymphoma of the vagina. *Leuk Lymphoma.* 1999;35(5–6):619–622.
308. Skinnider BF, Clement PB, MacPherson N, et al. Primary non-Hodgkin's lymphoma and malakoplakia of the vagina: a case report. *Hum Pathol.* 1999;30(7):871–874.
309. Papadopoulos AJ, Pambakian H, Devaja O, et al. High grade non-Hodgkins stage IEB primary malignant lymphoma of the cervix and upper vagina. A case report. *Eur J Gynaecol Oncol.* 1996;17(6):484–486.
310. Hoffkes HG, Schumann A, Uppenkamp M, et al. Primary non-Hodgkin's lymphoma of the vagina. Case report and review of the literature. *Ann Hematol.* 1995;70(5):273–276.
311. Lonardi F, Ferrari V, Pavanato G, et al. Primary lymphoma of the vagina. A case report. *Haematologica.* 1994;79(2):182–183.
312. Prevot S, Hugol D, Audouin J, et al. Primary non Hodgkin's malignant lymphoma of the vagina. Report of 3 cases with review of the literature. *Pathol Res Pract.* 1992;188(1–2):78–85.
313. Bagella MP, Fadda G, Cherchi PL. Primary non-Hodgkin lymphoma of the vagina: case report. *Clin Exper Obstet Gynecol.* 1989;16(4):100–102.
314. Harris NL, Scully RE. Malignant lymphoma and granulocytic sarcoma of the uterus and vagina. A clinicopathologic analysis of 27 cases. *Cancer.* 1984;53(11):2530–2545.
315. Buchler DA, Kline JC. Primary lymphoma of the vagina. *Obstet Gynecol.* 1972;40(2):235–237.
316. Chorlton I, Karnei RF Jr, King FM, et al. Primary malignant reticuloendothelial disease involving the vagina, cervix, and corpus uteri. *Obstet Gynecol.* 1974;44(5):735–748.
317. McNicholas MM, Fennelly JJ, MacErlaine DP. Imaging of primary vaginal lymphoma. *Clin Radiol.* 1994;49(2):130–132.
318. Domingo S, Perales A, Torres V, et al. Epstein-Barr virus positivity in primary vaginal lymphoma. *Gynecol Oncol.* 2004;95(3):719–721.
319. Pham DC, Guthrie TH, Ndubisi B. HIV-associated primary cervical non-Hodgkin's lymphoma and two other cases of primary pelvic non-Hodgkin's lymphoma. *Gynecol Oncol.* 2003;90(1):204–206.
320. Signorelli M, Maneo A, Cammarota S, et al. Conservative management in primary genital lymphomas: the role of chemotherapy. *Gynecol Oncol.* 2007;104(2):416–421.
321. Gardner GJ, Reidy-Lagunes D, Gehrig PA. Neuroendocrine tumors of the gynecologic tract: A Society of Gynecologic Oncology (SGO) clinical document. *Gynecol Oncol.* 2011;122(1):190–198.
322. Kaminski JM, Anderson PR, Han AC, et al. Primary small cell carcinoma of the vagina. *Gynecol Oncol.* 2003;88(3):451–455.
323. Elsaleh H, Bydder S, Cassidy B, et al. Small cell carcinoma of the vagina. *Aust Radiol.* 2000;44(3):336–337.
324. Ulich TR, Liao SY, Layfield L, et al. Endocrine and tumor differentiation markers in poorly differentiated small-cell carcinoids of the cervix and vagina. *Arch Pathol Lab Med.* 1986;110(11):1054–1057.
325. Crowder S, Tuller E. Small cell carcinoma of the female genital tract. *Semin Oncol.* 2007;34(1):57–63.
326. Bing Z, Levine L, Lucci JA, et al. Primary small cell neuroendocrine carcinoma of the vagina: a clinicopathologic study. *Arch Pathol Lab Med.* 2004;128(8):857–862.
327. Cai T, Li Y, Jiang Q, et al. Paraganglioma of the vagina: a case report and review of the literature. *Oncol Targets Ther.* 2014;7:965–968.
328. Hassan A, Bennet A, Bhalla S, et al. Paraganglioma of the vagina: report of a case, including immunohistochemical and ultrastructural findings. *Int J Gynecol Pathol.* 2003;22(4):404–406.
329. Shen JG, Chen YX, Xu DY, et al. Vaginal paraganglioma presenting as a gynecologic mass: case report. *Eur J Gynaecol Oncol.* 2008;29(2):184–185.
330. Tohya T, Miyazaki K, Katabuchi H, et al. Small cell carcinoma of the endometrium associated with adenosquamous carcinoma: a light and electron microscopic study. *Gynecol Oncol.* 1986;25(3):363–371.
331. Beriwal S, Rwigema JM, Higgins E, et al. 3D image-based HDR interstitial brachytherapy for vaginal cancer. *Brachytherapy.* 2011.
332. Manuel M, Cho LP, Damato AL, et al. Are clinical outcomes improved with image guided interstitial brachytherapy for vaginal cancer? *Int J Radiat Oncol Biol Phys.* 2015;93(3):E285–E286.
333. Taylor A, Rockall AG, Reznek RH, et al. Mapping pelvic lymph nodes: guidelines for delineation in intensity-modulated radiotherapy. *Int J Radiat Oncol Biol Phys.* 2005;63(5):1604–1612.
334. Finlay MH, Ackerman I, Tirona RG, et al. Use of CT simulation for treatment of cervical cancer to assess the adequacy of lymph node coverage of conventional pelvic fields based on bony landmarks. *Int J Radiat Oncol Biol Phys.* 2006;64(1):205–209.
335. Greer BE, Koh WJ, Figge DC, et al. Gynecologic radiotherapy fields defined by intraoperative measurements. *Gynecol Oncol.* 1990;38(3):421–424.
336. McAlpine J, Schlaerth JB, Lim P,et al. Radiation fields in gynecologic oncology: correlation of soft tissue (surgical) to radiologic landmarks. *Gynecol Oncol.* 2004;92(1):25–30.
337. Yeh AM, Marcus RB Jr, Amdur RJ, et al. Patterns of failure in squamous cell carcinoma of the vagina treated with definitive radiotherapy alone: what is the appropriate treatment volume? International journal of cancer. *J Int Cancer.* 2001;96 suppl:109–116.
338. Dittmer PH, Randall ME. A technique for inguinal node boost using photon fields defined by asymmetric collimator jaws. *Radiother Oncol.* 2001;59(1):61–64.
339. Mundt AJ, Roeske JC, Lujan AE. Intensity-modulated radiation therapy in gynecologic malignancies. *Med Dosim.* 2002;27(2):131–136.
340. Roeske JC, Lujan A, Rotmensch J, et al. Intensity-modulated whole pelvic radiation therapy in patients with gynecologic malignancies. *Int J Radiat Oncol Biol Phys.* 2000;48(5):1613–1621.
341. Viswanathan AN, Kirisits C, Erickson BE, et al. *Gynecologic Radiation Therapy: Novel Approaches to Image-Guidance and Management. 1 ed.* Heidelberg, Germany: Springer-Verlag; 2011.
342. Jhingran A, Salehpour M, Sam M, et al. Vaginal motion and bladder and rectal volumes during pelvic intensity-modulated radiation therapy after hysterectomy. *Int J Radiat Oncol Biol Phys.* 2012:82(1):256–262.
343. Delclos L, Fletcher GH, Moore EB, et al. Minicolpostats, dome cylinders, other additions and improvements of the Fletcher-suit afterloadable system: indications and limitations of their use. *Int J Radiat Oncol Biol Phys.* 1980;6(9):1195–1206.
344. Perez CA, Slessinger E, Grigsby PW. Design of an afterloading vaginal applicator (MIRALVA). *Int J Radiat Oncol Biol Phys.* 1990;18(6):1503–1508.
345. Slessinger ED, Perez CA, Grigsby PW, et al. Dosimetry and dose specification for a new gynecological brachytherapy applicator. *Int J Radiat Oncol Biol Phys.* 1992;22(5):1117–1124.
346. Bertoni F, Bertoni G, Bignardi M. Vaginal molds for intracavitary curietherapy: a new method of preparation. *Int J Radiat Oncol Biol Phys.* 1983;9(10):1579–1582.
347. Nag S, Erickson B, Thomadsen B, et al. The American Brachytherapy Society recommendations for high-dose-rate brachytherapy for carcinoma of the cervix. *Int J Radiat Oncol Biol Phys.* 2000;48(1):201–211.
348. Orton CG. High-dose-rate brachytherapy may be radiobiologically superior to low-dose rate due to slow repair of late-responding normal tissue cells. *Int J Radiat Oncol Biol Phys.* 2001;49(1):183–189.
349. Nanavati PJ, Fanning J, Hilgers RD, et al. High-dose-rate brachytherapy in primary stage I and II vaginal cancer. *Gynecol Oncol.* 1993;51(1):67–71.
350. Stewart AJ, Viswanathan AC. Current controversies in high-dose-rate versus low-dose-rate brachytherapy for cervical cancer. *Cancer.* 2006;107:908–915.
351. Beriwal S, Heron DE, Mogus R, et al. High-dose rate brachytherapy (HDRB) for primary or recurrent cancer in the vagina. *Radiat Oncol.* 2008;3:7.
352. Kucera H, Mock U, Knocke TH, et al. Radiotherapy alone for invasive vaginal cancer: outcome with intracavitary high dose rate brachytherapy

versus conventional low dose rate brachytherapy. *Acta obstetricia et gynecologica Scandinavica.* 2001;80(4):355–360.

353. Nag S, Martínez-Monge R, Selman AE, et al. Interstitial brachytherapy in the management of primary carcinoma of the cervix and vagina. *Gynecol Oncol.* 1998;70(1):27–32.
354. Randall ME, Evans L, Greven KM, et al. Interstitial reirradiation for recurrent gynecologic malignancies: results and analysis of prognostic factors. *Gynecol Oncol.* 1993;48(1):23–31.
355. Subak LL, Hricak H, Powell CB, et al. Cervical carcinoma: computed tomography and magnetic resonance imaging for preoperative staging. *Obstet Gynecol.* 1995;86(1):43–50.
356. Potter R, Haie-Meder C, Van Limbergen E, et al. Recommendations from gynaecological (GYN) GEC ESTRO working group (II): concepts and terms in 3D image-based treatment planning in cervix cancer brachytherapy-3D dose volume parameters and aspects of 3D image-based anatomy, radiation physics, radiobiology. *Radiother Oncol.* 2006;78(1):67–77.
357. Dimopoulos JC, Schmid MP, Fidarova E, et al. Treatment of locally advanced vaginal cancer with radiochemotherapy and magnetic resonance image-guided adaptive brachytherapy: dose-volume parameters and first clinical results. *Int J Radiat Oncol Biol Physics.* 2012;82(5):1880–1888.
358. Kirisits C, Pötter R, Lang S, et al. Dose and volume parameters for MRI-based treatment planning in intracavitary brachytherapy for cervical cancer. *Int J Radiat Oncol Biol Phys.* 2005;62(3):901–911.
359. Lee LJ, Viswanathan AN. Predictors of toxicity after Image-guided high-dose-rate interstitial brachytherapy for gynecologic cancer. *Int J Radiat Oncol Biol Phys.* 2012;84(5):1192–1197.
360. Martinez A, Cox RS, Edmundson GK. A multiple-site perineal applicator (MUPIT) for treatment of prostatic, anorectal, and gynecologic malignancies. *Int J Radiat Oncol Biol Phys.* 1984;10(2):297–305.
361. Stock RG, Chan K, Terk M, et al. A new technique for performing Syed-Neblett template interstitial implants for gynecologic malignancies using transrectal-ultrasound guidance. *Int J Radiat Oncol Biol Phys.* 1997;37(4):819–825.
362. Corn BW, Lanciano RM, Rosenblum N, et al. Improved treatment planning for the Syed-Neblett template using endorectal-coil magnetic resonance and intraoperative (laparotomy/laparoscopy) guidance: a new integrated technique for hysterectomized women with vaginal tumors. *Gynecol Oncol.* 1995;56(2):255–261.
363. Childers JM, Surwit EA. Current status of operative laparoscopy in gynecologic oncology. *Oncology.* 1993;7(11):47–51; discussion 53–54, 57.
364. Orr JW Jr, Dosoretz DD, Mahoney D, et al. Surgically (laparotomy/laparoscopy) guided placement of high dose rate interstitial irradiation catheters (LG-HDRT): technique and outcome. *Gynecol Oncol.* 2006;100(1):145–148.
365. Paley PJ, Koh WJ, Stelzer KJ, et al. A new technique for performing Syed template interstitial implants for anterior vaginal tumors using an open retropubic approach. *Gynecol Oncol.* 1999;73(1):121–125.
366. Disaia PJ, Creasman WT. *Clinical Gynecologic Oncology. 4th ed.* St. Louis, MO: Mosby; 1993.
367. Viswanathan AN, Erickson BA. Three-dimensional imaging in gynecologic brachytherapy: a survey of the American Brachytherapy Society. *Int J Radiat Oncol Biol Phys.* 2010;76(1):104–109.
368. Viswanathan AN, Cormack R, Holloway CL, et al. Magnetic resonance-guided interstitial therapy for vaginal recurrence of endometrial cancer. *Int J Radiat Oncol Biol Phys.* 2006;66(1):91–99.
369. Potter R, Dimopoulos J, Bachtiary B, et al. 3D conformal HDR-brachy- and external beam therapy plus simultaneous cisplatin for high-risk cervical cancer: clinical experience with 3 year follow-up. *Radiother Oncol.* 2006;79(1):80–86.
370. Holloway CL, Racine ML, Cormack RA, et al. Sigmoid dose using 3D imaging in cervical-cancer brachytherapy. *Radiother Oncol.* 2009;93(2):307–310.
371. Viswanathan AN, Dimopoulos J, Kirisits C, et al. Computed tomography versus magnetic resonance imaging-based contouring in cervical cancer brachytherapy: results of a prospective trial and preliminary guidelines for standardized contours. *Int J Radiat Oncol Biol Phys.* 2007;68(2):491–498.
372. Kushner DM, Fleming PA, Kennedy AW, et al. High dose rate (192) Ir afterloading brachytherapy for cancer of the vagina. *Br J Radiol.* 2003;76(910):719–725.
373. Tewari K, Cappuccini F, Brewster WR, et al. Interstitial brachytherapy for vaginal recurrences of endometrial carcinoma. *Gynecol Oncol.* 1999;74(3):416–422.
374. Chan P, Yeo I, Perkins G, et al. Dosimetric comparison of intensity-modulated, conformal, and four-field pelvic radiotherapy boost plans for gynecologic cancer: a retrospective planning study. *Radiat Oncol.* 2006;1:13.
375. Georg D, Kirisits C, Hillbrand M, et al. Image-guided radiotherapy for cervix cancer: high-tech external beam therapy versus high-tech brachytherapy. *Int J Radiat Oncol Biol Phys.* 2008;71(4):1272–1278.
376. Barraclough LH, Swindell R, Livsey JE, et al. External beam boost for cancer of the cervix uteri when intracavitary therapy cannot be performed. *Int J Radiat Oncol Biol Phys.* 2008;71(3):772–778.
377. Higginson DS, Morris DE, Jones EL, et al. Stereotactic body radiotherapy (SBRT): Technological innovation and application in gynecologic oncology. *Gynecol Oncol.* 2011;120(3):404–412.
378. Gupta S, Gupta YN, Sanyal B. Radiation changes in vaginal and cervical cytology in carcinoma of the cervix uteri. *J Surg Oncol.* 1982;19(2):71–73.
379. Eifel PJ, Levenback C, Wharton JT, et al. Time course and incidence of late complications in patients treated with radiation therapy for FIGO stage IB carcinoma of the uterine cervix. *Int J Radiat Oncol Biol Phys.* 1995;32(5):1289–1300.
380. Shrieve DC, Loeffler JS. *Human Radiation Injury. 1st ed.* Philadelphia, PA: Lippincott Williams & Wilkins; 2011.
381. Pitkin RM, Buchsbaum HJ, Lenz H. Estrogen and the irradiated vagina. *Obstet Gynecol.* 1975;46(2):243–245.
382. Fink D, Chetty N, Lehm JP, et al. Hyperbaric oxygen therapy for delayed radiation injuries in gynecological cancers. *Int J Gynecol Cancer.* 2006;16(2):638–6342.
383. Piekarski JH, Jereczek-Fossa BA, Nejc D, et al. Does fecal diversion offer any chance for spontaneous closure of the radiation-induced rectovaginal fistula? *Int J Gynecol Cancer.* 2008;18(1):66–70.
384. Manetta A, Pinto JL, Larson JE, et al. Primary invasive carcinoma of the vagina. *Obstet Gynecol.* 1988;72(1):77–81.
385. Mawson AR. The place of hysterectomy in the management of benign uterine disease. *HMO Pract.* 1996;10(2):69–74.
386. Xiang EW, Shu-mo C, Ya-qin D, et al. Treatment of late recurrent vaginal malignancy after initial radiotherapy for carcinoma of the cervix: an analysis of 73 cases. *Gynecol Oncol.* 1998;69(2):125–129.
387. Steiner E, Woernle F, Kuhn W, et al. Carcinoma of the neovagina: case report and review of the literature. *Gynecol Oncol.* 2002;84(1):171–175.
388. Lathrop JC, Ree HJ, McDuff HC Jr. Intraepithelial neoplasia of the neovagina. *Obstet Gynecol.* 1985;65(3 suppl):91S–94S.
389. Gallup DG, Castle CA, Stock RJ. Recurrent carcinoma in situ of the vagina following split-thickness skin graft vaginoplasty. *Gynecol Oncol.* 1987;26(1):98–102.
390. Imrie JE, Kennedy JH, Holmes JD, et al. Intraepithelial neoplasia arising in an artificial vagina. Case report. *Br J Obstet Gynaecol.* 1986;93(8):886–888.
391. Wheelock JB, Schneider V, Goplerud DR. Malignancy arising in the transplanted vagina. *South Med J.* 1986;79(12):1585–1587.
392. Lowe MP, Ault KA, Sood AK. Recurrent carcinoma in situ of a neovagina. *Gynecol Oncol.* 2001;80(3):403–404.
393. Guven S, Guvendag Guven ES, Ayhan A, et al. Recurrence of high-grade squamous intraepithelial neoplasia in neovagina: case report and review of the literature. *Int J Gynecol Cancer.* 2005;15(6):1179–1182.
394. Munkarah A, Malone JM Jr, Budev HD, et al. Mucinous adenocarcinoma arising in a neovagina. *Gynecol Oncol.* 1994;52(2):272–275.
395. Jackson GW. Primary carcinoma of an artificial vagina. Report of a case. *Obstet Gynecol.* 1959;14:534–536.
396. Duckler L. Squamous cell carcinoma developing in an artificial vagina. *Obstet Gynecol.* 1972;40(1):35–38.
397. Rotmensch J, Rosenshein N, Dillon M, et al. Carcinoma arising in the neovagina: case report and review of the literature. *Obstet Gynecol.* 1983;61(4):534–536.
398. Berek JS, Howe C, Lagasse LD, et al. Pelvic exenteration for recurrent gynecologic malignancy: survival and morbidity analysis of the 45-year experience at UCLA. *Gynecol Oncol.* 2005;99(1):153–159.
399. Russell AH, Koh WJ, Markette K, et al. Radical reirradiation for recurrent or second primary carcinoma of the female reproductive tract. *Gynecol Oncol.* 1987;27(2):226–232.
400. Randall ME, Barrett RJ. Interstitial irradiation in the management of recurrent carcinoma of the cervix after previous radiation therapy. *North Carolina Med J.* 1988;49(6):306–308.
401. Gupta AK, Vicini FA, Frazier AJ, et al. Iridium-192 transperineal interstitial brachytherapy for locally advanced or recurrent gynecological malignancies. *Int J Radiat Oncol Biol Phys.* 1999;43(5):1055–1060.
402. Charra C, Roy P, Coquard R, et al. Outcome of treatment of upper third vaginal recurrences of cervical and endometrial carcinomas with interstitial brachytherapy. *Int J Radiat Oncol Biol Phys.* 1998;40(2):421–426.
403. Salani R, Backes FJ, Fung MF, et al. Posttreatment surveillance and diagnosis of recurrence in women with gynecologic malignancies: Society of Gynecologic Oncologists recommendations. *Am J Obstet Gynecol.* 2011;204(6):466–478.

CHAPTER 20

Cervix Uteri

Charles A. Kunos, Fadi W. Abdul-Karim, Don S. Dizon, and Robert Debernardo

EPIDEMIOLOGY

According to the World Health Organization, uterine cervix cancers were the fourth most common malignancy in women, and the seventh most common overall, with 528,000 new incident cases reported in 2012 (1). An estimated 266,000 women died around the world from uterine cervix cancer in 2012, accounting for almost 8% of all female cancer deaths (1). Nearly 9 out of every 10 women with uterine cervix cancer died in underdeveloped regions of the world (1). In the United States, the American Cancer Society (ACS) projected that 12,900 new cases of uterine cervix cancer would arise in American women in 2015, and an estimated 4,100 (32%) of those women would die (2). Based on these statistics, 1 (0.6%) in 154 American women would develop invasive uterine cervix cancer between birth and death (2). It has been claimed that these statistics likely underestimate a true worldwide uterine cervix cancer disease burden, mostly because inadequate medical resources in rural and economically depressed regions infrequently capture new incident cases of uterine cervix cancer. Indeed, uterine cervix cancer is only one of two cancers (the other, colorectal cancer) that can be effectively screened for as a precancerous lesion. Early detection of uterine cervix cancer is a paramount health care issue, as around 40% of newly diagnosed uterine cervix cancers in American women occur in women with no prior screening, and another 10% of new incident cases occur in women who have not had screening in the preceding 5 years (3).

Two specific American populations deserve mention, Hispanics and African-Americans. The United States Census Bureau recognized nearly 51 million Americans in 2010 as self-identified Hispanics or Latinos, accounting for 16% of the total US population (4). Hispanics are the largest, fastest-growing, and youngest minority group in the United States, with one of every two residents dwelling in the states of California, Florida, or Texas. The ACS estimated in 2012 that 2,100 (4%) new uterine cervix cancers befell Hispanic Americans, for a probability of developing uterine cervix cancer between birth and death of 1 (1.1%) in 95 Hispanic females (4). For the same year, 500 (24% of the 2,100 new cases) Hispanic Americans were anticipated to die from uterine cervix cancer (4). The 2012 incidence rate of uterine cervix cancer among Hispanic American women was 64% higher than among non-Hispanic Whites (4). The highest incidence rates were found among Hispanic women residing in the American Midwest, reportedly due to new immigrant populations (5). Efforts to improve early detection have been successful—the prevalence of Papanicolaou (Pap) testing rose from 64% among 18-year and older Hispanic women in 1987 to 75% in 2010 (4). Across Hispanic subpopulations, up to 80% of Cuban and Puerto Rican women undergo uterine cervix cancer screening (4). However, most US cancer data are reported for Hispanic Americans as an aggregate group, which hides critical differences that exist between subpopulations according to their country of origin.

African-Americans have the highest mortality and shortest cancer-specific survival for most cancers of any racial or ethnic group in the United States. In 2013, 42 million self-identified African-Americans resided in the United States (13% of the total US population), with one of every four residents living in the states of Florida, New York, or Texas (6). The ACS estimated that in 2013, 2,060 (3%) new uterine cervix cancer cases occurred in African-American women (6). In 2013, African-American females had a lifetime uterine cervix cancer diagnosis probability of 1 (0.85%) in 119 (6). Also in 2013, 720 (35% of the 2,060 new cases) uterine cervix cancer deaths were expected among African-Americans (6). This translates into a new uterine cervix cancer incident rate in 2013 that was 34% higher than among white women (6). Racial disparity in this disease has narrowed considerably, as new case rates have fallen precipitously in African-Americans due to more effective programmatic screening efforts (7). Between 2008 and 2010, the prevalence of Pap testing within the previous 3 years was similar among African-American and white American women (78%) (6).

ETIOLOGY AND RISK FACTORS

The etiology of uterine cervix cancer has been connected to sexual activity, although the exact molecular events implicated in its pathogenesis have not been fully known. Risk factors such as young age of coitarche (8), multiple sexual partners or male partners with multiple partners (9), and a history of sexually transmitted disease (10) correlate with a risk for uterine cervix cancer pathogenesis. Uterine cervix cancer is exceedingly uncommon among females not sexually active (11,12). Low income (13), low educational status (14), and a history of human papillomavirus (HPV) infection (15) are surrogate risk factors for uterine cervix cancer. Smoking (current smoker or former smoker or never smoker) has been associated with a risk for a malignant uterine cervix cell phenotype (16).

Molecular and clinical evidence have implicated HPV infection as at least one causative agent for uterine cervix cancer neoplasia. HPV subtypes 16, 18, 31, 33, 35, 45, 52, and 58 (**Table 20.1**) are the most virulent forms associated with cervical intraepithelial neoplasia (CIN) (now coined high-grade squamous intraepithelial lesion on biopsy) or cancer (15). HPV infections (single or multiple infections) account for as much as 86% of worldwide incidence of invasive uterine cervix cancer (15). Certainly, immune competence has a role in HPV-related carcinogenesis (17,18)—in as much as a uterine cervix cancer diagnosis might define an AIDS illness event (19). HPV subtyping screens have become sufficiently discriminating, with sensitivity and specificity of around 95% each (20,21), but HPV subtyping screens are not yet a primary stand-alone diagnostic tool in all women (22). For contrast, exfoliative cytology has a modest 53% sensitivity but high 97% specificity (23). The ATHENA trial of 47,208 women found that 10% of women testing positive for HPV 16 or HPV

TABLE 20.1. Human Papillomavirus (HPV) Genotypes

Low-Risk Oncogenic HPV	High-Risk Oncogenic HPV
6, 11, 42, 43, 44	16, 18, 31, 33, 35, 39, 45, 51, 52, 56, 58, 59, 68

18 had grade 3 CIN or worse undetected by cytology alone (24–26). According to 2015 consensus guidelines of the American Society for Colposcopy and Cervical Pathology, women 30 to 65 years should be cotested with exfoliative cytology and HPV testing every 5 years (22). If found to have negative cytology but a positive for high-risk HPV (16, 18, or 16/18), cotesting should be repeated in 12 months or HPV genotyping should be done. If the HPV genotyping assay is positive, women should submit to timely colposcopy (22). As such, HPV pathophysiology provides a context for the clinical management of uterine cervix cancer, and so attention is turned next to the known core molecular processes governing the disease process.

HPVs are nonenveloped viruses utilizing double-stranded closed circular DNA to replicate in the cutaneous and mucosal epithelia of the female and male anogenital tracts (27). HPV DNA encodes six early proteins (E1, E2, E4–E7) and two late proteins (L1, L2) that hijack host cell molecular pathways first to synthesize DNA and then to package it (27). HPV-E6 binds p53, causes its degradation, and thereby removes a G1/S-phase cell cycle restriction checkpoint (28–30). HPV-E6 also disrupts DNA building block output from the usual rate-limiter ribonucleotide reductase, in that the virus promotes more 2'-deoxyribonucleoside diphosphates (dNDPs) to be supplied freely when demanded (31–33). HPV-E7 degrades hypophosphorylated retinoblastoma protein through a proteosome-dependent pathway (34) that also promotes unchecked activation of a synthesis cell cycle transcription factor (E2F) (35). E2F turns on S-phase proteins critical to DNA replication, like ribonucleotide reductase M2 protein (36). Through an activated telomerase (37), HPV extends host cell life and thus increases HPV-infected cell numbers. Far-reaching outcomes of HPV overriding cell cycle checkpoints include instability of the host cell genome and susceptibility to neoplasia or to an oncogenic phenotype (27). Such observations suggest that throughout its evolution HPV has targeted at least transcriptional and protein–protein checkpoints in uterine cervix cells to unleash dNDP production by ribonucleotide reductase.

Uterine Cervix Anatomy

The *cervix uteri* (Latin: neck of the uterus) is centered in the pelvis, representing the lower narrowed segment of the uterus. The cervix assumes a conical shape, truncated at its distal apex, and has its long axis directed backward and downward. It projects posteriorly into the vagina, connecting the vaginal vault to the uterine body hollow (*corpus uteri*) by its endocervical canal (*canalis cervicis uteri*). The supravaginal portion of the cervix (*portio supravaginalis*) extends to the lower uterine segment (isthmus) and associates intimately with the bladder peritoneum forming the vesicouterine pouch, an anterior *cul-de-sac* that must be dissected and separated for surgical exposure. The peritoneum covers the supravaginal cervix posteriorly and is reflected upon the rectum, forming the posterior rectouterine cul-de-sac (pouch of Douglas). The vaginal portion of the cervix (*portio vaginalis*) protrudes into the vagina as a round extremity with a circular external aperture between the anterior and posterior vaginal fornices. The vaginal portion of the cervix has two lips, a short anterior and a long posterior. In length, the cervix ranges 2 to 5 cm.

The uterine cervix is fibrous, covered by membranes (*tunica mucosa*) of squamous cells when in contact with the vagina (ectocervix) and by columnar cells when communicating with the uterus (endocervix). A transition from stratified squamous to ciliated columnar cells, coined the transformation zone, occurs in the lower one third of the canal. The length of the transition zone changes throughout life, receding in old age. The preponderance of preneoplastic and neoplastic lesions of the uterine cervix arises from the transformation zone. The ciliated columnar cells secrete viscid alkaline mucus.

The uterine cervix has four cardinal ligaments: one anterior, one posterior, and two transverse (Mackenrodt). The anterior ligament involves the vesicouterine fold of peritoneum, anchoring the supravaginal cervix to the anterior pelvis via the anterior cul-de-sac. The posterior ligament consists of the rectouterine fold of peritoneum, connecting the supravaginal cervix by the rectum to fibrous tissue and nonstriped muscle constituting the uterosacral ligaments. The two transverse ligaments (*ligamentum transversali coli*) span either side of the uterine cervix, and continuously extend into the tissues of the pelvic sidewall surrounding the pelvis iliac blood vessels. The cardinal ligaments anatomically define two surgical spaces, the paravesical space anteriorly and the pararectal space posteriorly. Portions of the cardinal ligament overlie the pelvic ureter (below the uterine artery, above the uterine vein) about 2 cm superior and 2 cm lateral to the external os of the cervix, an anatomic triangle referred to in brachytherapy as prescription point A. For completeness, superior to the supravaginal cervix arise the two lateral or broad ligaments (*ligamentum latum uteri*) enveloping the uterine tubes, round ligament of the uterus, the ovary and its ligaments, the epoophoron and paroophoron. The innervation of the uterine cervix derives from sacral (S2–S4) nerve roots.

Blood supply to the uterine cervix and its return occurs through the uterine artery and vein, tributaries of the anterior branch of the hypogastric blood vessels. Collateral arterial anastomoses arise from the ovarian artery (descending aorta), internal pudendal artery (hypogastric artery tributary), and obturator artery (hypogastric artery tributary). A web of venous blood vessels returns blood to the bilateral gonadal and bilateral iliac veins.

The uterine cervix is considered an immunocompetent organ, capable of mounting an immune response to an external pathogen antigen (38–40). In some respects, the bulk of large uterine cervix cancers might represent normal cells, cancer cells, and tumor-infiltrating lymphocytes. In an orderly fashion, lymph vessel drainage from the uterine cervix flows to paracervical and obturator nodes, internal iliac nodes, external iliac nodes, common iliac nodes, and then paraaortic nodes. First nodal sites of disease include the paracervical and the iliac nodes (41). Left supraclavicular lymph nodes are next echelon extrapelvic distant sites of lymphatic spread. Uterine cervix immunocompetence (42) impacts anticancer proimmune drugs (43), and radiation-induced immune-mediated tumor abscopal response (44).

Uterine Cervix Disease Natural History

Preinvasive Disease

Uterine cervix cells acquire an oncogenic phenotype through what appears to be a methodical neoplastic process reflected in epithelial cell histology. For uterine cervix squamous cell disease, the histologic terms for preinvasive disease have been consolidated. Terminology describes (a) low-grade squamous intraepithelial lesions (LSIL) indicating microscopic acute HPV infection; (b) high-grade squamous intraepithelial lesions (HSIL) indicating precancerous lesions; and (c) cancer. Histologically, HSIL correlates with CIN grade 3 (CIN 3) and most cases of CIN grade 2 (CIN 2) (45).

Most LSIL cases and half of HSIL cases regress to normal cytology within 2 years of first diagnosis by cytology. Thus, a recommendation for active surveillance has been supported for women with CIN 1 or CIN 2 (22). There is prognostic value in labeling CIN 2 distinct from CIN 3 by histopathologists, and so, follow-up cytology evaluations must undergo greater scrutiny (22).

Invasive Disease

The oncogenic potential of uterine cervix cancers follows a more erratic evolution—disease benchmarks are not well chronicled. Uterine cervix cancers follow an International Federation of Gynecology and Obstetrics (FIGO) clinical staging system (**Table 20.2**) (46). Surgical findings or radiographic-guided biopsies of lymph nodes or lung metastasis must not be used to change or to modify clinical FIGO staging. All uterine cervix cancer histologies are included. If staging disagreements arise, earlier stage is given.

■ TABLE 20.2. Uterine Cervix Clinical Staging

TNM[a]	FIGO[a]	
Primary tumor (T)		
TX		Primary tumor cannot be assessed.
T0		No evidence of primary tumor
Tis	0	Carcinoma *in situ* (preinvasive carcinoma)
T1	I	Cervical carcinoma confined to uterus (extension to corpus should be disregarded)
T1a	IA	Invasive carcinoma diagnosed only by microscopy. Stromal invasion with a maximum depth of 5 mm measured from the base of the epithelium and a horizontal spread of ≤7 mm. Vascular space involvement, venous or lymphatic, does not affect classification.
T1a1	IA1	Measured stromal invasion ≤3 mm in depth and ≤7 mm in horizontal spread
T1a2	IA2	Measured stromal invasion >3 mm and ≤5 mm with a horizontal spread ≤7 mm
T1b	IB	Clinically visible lesion confined to the cervix or microscopic lesion >T1a/IA2
T1b1	IB1	Clinically visible lesion ≤4 cm in greatest dimension
T1b2	IB2	Clinically visible lesion >4 cm in greatest dimension
T2	II	Cervical carcinoma invades beyond uterus but not pelvic wall or lower third of vagina
T2a	IIA	Tumor without parametrial invasion
T2a1	IIA1	Clinically visible lesion ≤4 cm in greatest dimension
T2a2	IIA2	Clinically visible lesion >4 cm in greatest dimension
T2b	IIB	Tumor with parametrial invasion
T3	III	Tumor extends to pelvic wall and/or involves lower third of vagina, and/or causes hydronephrosis or nonfunctioning kidney.
T3a	IIIA	Tumor involves lower third of vagina, no extension to pelvic wall.
T3b	IIIB	Tumor extends to pelvic wall and/or causes hydronephrosis or nonfunctioning kidney.
T4	IVA	Tumor invades mucosa of bladder or rectum, and/or extends beyond true pelvis (bullous edema is not sufficient to classify a tumor as T4).
Regional lymph nodes (N)		
NX		Regional lymph nodes cannot be assessed.
N0		No regional lymph node metastasis
N1	IIIB	Regional lymph node metastasis
Distant metastasis (M)		
M0		No distant metastasis
M1	IVB	Distant metastasis (including peritoneal spread, involvement of supraclavicular, mediastinal, or paraaortic lymph nodes, lung, liver, or bone)

[a]The American Joint Committee on Cancer definitions of the T categories correspond to clinical stages accepted by the International Federation of Gynecology and Obstetrics (FIGO). Both systems are listed.

TNM, tumor-node-metastasis.

Source: AJCC. Cervix uteri. In: Edge SB, Byrd DR, Compton CC, et al, eds. *AJCC Cancer Staging Manual*. 7th ed. New York, NY: Springer; 2010:395–402.

Metastatic Disease

Patterns of spread of uterine cervix cancers are considered predictable and orderly, as pelvic lymph node metastases are low in the absence of deep stromal invasion of the uterine cervix (47–49) and paraaortic lymph node metastases are low when pelvic lymph nodes are uninvolved (50,51).

For instance, depth of stromal invasion elevates the risk for regional lymph node metastasis. Fifty-one women (1981 to 1984) who had conization of the cervix for cancer with 3 to 5 mm of invasion (width limited to 7 mm) followed by completion radical hysterectomy plus lymphadenectomy were found to have no lymph node metastases, no recurrences, and no cancer-related deaths over a 5-year observation period (47). Inner third, middle third, and outer third depth of invasion were associated with a frequency of pelvic lymph node metastases of 5% (9 of 199), 13% (28 of 210), and 26% (60 of 227) in a surgicopathologic study (1981 to 1984) of uterine cervix cancer patients (48). Invasion into adjoining parametria is associated with a frequency of pelvic lymph node metastases of 43% (19 of 44) (48). Also in this study, histologic grade 2 or grade 3 disease conferred 14% (52 of 373) and 22% (39 of 179) frequencies of pelvic lymph node metastases (48). Lymphovascular invasion was associated with a 25% (70 of 276) chance of pelvic lymph node metastases (48).

Indeed, lymph node metastases are an important clinical consideration even though nodal status is not considered in International FIGO staging of uterine cervical cancer. Take for an example an Italian Group study (1986 to 1991) that investigated 172 patients who had undergone radical abdominal hysterectomy for uterine cervix cancer stage IB or IIA patients (50). The study found a 25% (28 of 114) rate of pelvic node metastases when the cervical diameter measured ≤4 cm, whereas the rate was 31% (17 of 55) when the cervical diameter measured >4 cm. An American Gynecologic Oncology Group study (1973 to 1981) found paraaortic lymph node metastases associated with initial clinical stage, with rates of 5%, 16%, and 25% for stage IB, II, and III, respectively (51). For 98 patients who had paraaortic lymph node metastases found at staging laparotomy or at definitive operative management, a 15-month median survival and a 25% probability of 3-year survival was reported (51).

Metastasis to scalene lymph node occurs infrequently, unless uterine cervix cancer involves paraaortic lymph nodes (11% prevalence rate, [52]). Distant spread of uterine cervix cancers includes dissemination to the lungs or liver, and less commonly to the brain and axial or appendicular bones. After intervention, there are uterine cervix recurrences within 24 months, with a median of 20 months (50).

CLINICAL PRESENTATION AND DIAGNOSTIC EVALUATION

Preclinical Invasive Disease

Screening Cytology

Screening cytology is of high clinical benefit because of its ease of sample acquisition, test sensitivity, and ability to detect multiple phases of uterine cervix dysplasia. But, a single test may have limited sensitivity for uterine cervix cancer detection (45). Two primary sampling methods are used, the conventional Pap smear or liquid-based cytology.

Following its 2013 final recommendations, the United States Preventive Services Task Force (USPSTF) recommends uterine cervix dysplasia screening in women aged 21 to 65 years with Pap cytology every 3 years, or for women aged 30 to 65 years who desire a longer screening interval, screening by Pap cytology and HPV cotesting done every 5 years (53).

The ACS has addressed age-appropriate screening strategies in its view, including appropriateness of Pap cytology with or without HPV cotesting, follow-up of women after screening, the age at which to exit screening, and screening strategies for women vaccinated against HPV 16 or 18 infections (54). For women aged less than 21 years, no screening is recommended. Women aged 21 to 29 years should consider Pap cytology alone every 3 years. Women aged 30 to 65 years should preferably undergo Pap cytology and HPV cotesting every 5 years. In this category, women with cytology negative and HPV-positive testing undergo 12-month follow-up with cotesting, or if subsequently found positive for HPV 16 or 18 undergo colposcopy. Women aged 65 years or older exit screening if prior screening was negative. Hysterectomy prompts exit from further Pap cytology or HPV cotesting, that is, when the uterine cervix is surgically absent or a personal health history of CIN 2 or more (<20 years) and uterine cervix cancer (ever) are absent. HPV-vaccinated women follow their age-specific recommendations (same as unvaccinated women). The American College of Obstetricians and Gynecologists (ACOG) does not support changing screening intervals (55).

An updated standard terminology, the Bethesda system 2014, describes specimen adequacy and dysplastic cytologic abnormalities. For squamous cell epithelial cell abnormalities, it describes the following: (a) atypical squamous cells of undetermined significance (ASCUS) or atypical squamous cells—cannot rule out high-grade squamous intraepithelial lesion (ASCH); (b) LSIL; (c) HSIL (encompassing CIN 2 or CIN 3 or carcinoma *in situ*), and squamous cell carcinoma (56). For glandular epithelial cell abnormalities, it describes the following abnormalities: (a) atypical glandular cells (AGS, specifying endocervix, endometrial, or not otherwise specified origins); (b) AGS favoring neoplastic; (c) endocervical adenocarcinoma *in situ* (AIS); (d) adenocarcinoma (56).

A large multicenter trial (ASCUS/LSIL Triage Study [ALTS]) of 3,488 women begun in 1997 randomized immediate colposcopy versus triage to colposcopy according to Pap cytology and HPV cotesting (57). Pap cytology reported 86% of cases with an overall CIN 3 or worse diagnosis. HPV cotesting identified 92% (10 pg/mL cutoff) or 96% (1 pg/mL cutoff) of cases with an overall CIN 3 or worse diagnosis. The ALTS study established high-risk HPV testing as the most cost-effective triage test for ASCUS. After this study, the American Society of Colposcopy and Cervical Pathology (ASCCP) and American Society for Clinical Pathology (ASCP) have endorsed HPV cotesting as the preferred method of triage for ASCUS smears detected by liquid-based cytology for women 30 years or older (54).

HPV Testing

For women ≥30 years undergoing screening in the United States, a recommendation for HPV cotesting as an adjunct to cytology has been made to triage women with ASCUS (24,25). In European nations, HPV tests serve to triage women with ASCUS, to monitor them after CIN treatment, and even to be a stand-alone primary screening test without cytology (58). Australia (59) and the Netherlands (60) have accepted self-sampling HPV tests as primary screens for their national uterine cervix dysplasia and cancer screening programs. Detection of HPV DNA involves either hybrid capture 2 or polymerase chain reaction technologies. HPV cotesting has become more widespread as a diagnostic aid (26,57,61,62). **Table 20.3** catalogs the triage of cytology categories negative for intraepithelial lesion of malignancy (NILM) or ASCUS to CIN 3 or worse by HPV testing.

The effect of HPV cotesting as an adjunct to liquid-based cytology was evaluated by a large cohort study (ATHENA, 2008 to 2009) involving 47,208 American women (25). In that study, the combination of cytology and HPV cotesting was superior to cytology alone for the detection of CIN 3 or worse over a 3-year observation period. HPV testing alone identified 64% more CIN 3 or worse lesions (294, 95% confidence interval [CI]: 260 to 325) than cytology (179, 95% CI, 152 to 206) and 23% more than cotesting (240, 95% CI, 209 to 270). ATHENA is the first screening study in American women to support HPV primary screening with triage of HPV-positive women using HPV 16 or 18 genotyping and reflex cytology at age 25 years (25).

Reduced uterine cervix squamous intraepithelial lesion prevalence has arisen out of prophylactic HPV vaccination of adolescent women. A randomized trial reporting 42-month follow-up on 17,622 HPV-naive adolescent women (aged 16 to 26 years) has shown that a prophylactic quadrivalent HPV vaccine (types 6, 11, 16, 18) administered day 1, month 2, and month 6 sustains immunocompetence against HPV 16 and HPV 18 CIN in those receiving vaccine versus those receiving placebo (63). Long-term high efficacy, immunogenicity, and acceptable safety in adolescent women have been confirmed in a Nordic region extension of the original studies (64). Moreover, Australia instituted in 2007 a nationally funded vaccination program with the quadrivalent HPV vaccine. The initial program launched vaccination as a continuing component of a 12 to 13-year-old schoolgirl health program, and funded two catch-up programs targeting 13 to 17-year-old school adolescents and 18 to 26-year-old women in general practice and community well-woman evaluations (65). A 0.38% (95% CI, 0.16 to 0.61) decrease in a population-wide prevalence of CIN 2 or worse was noticed in the vaccinated cohort between 2007 and 2009, compared to incidence found in the Victorian Cervical Cytology registry (Australia, 2003 to 2009). In the United Sates, adolescent female vaccination rates are low, with only about 40% of adolescents reporting receiving the vaccine (66,67). HPV vaccination efforts remain aggressive (68,69).

Colposcopy

Colposcopy examines the lower genital tract by a colposcope with binocular magnification (5× to 30×) for visual diagnosis and biopsy of suspicious precancerous or cancerous lesions. Colposcopy is an important diagnostic tool in uterine cervix cancer prevention in women with an abnormal screening test (70). Acetic acid or Lugol solution highlights dysplastic change such as acetowhite plaques or vacuolar abnormalities (including punctations, mosaicism, and abnormal vessel branching) that may signify high-grade lesions. Indications for colposcopy include an abnormal-appearing cervix, persistent postcoital bleeding or discharge, persistent CIN 1, 2, or

■ TABLE 20.3. Cytologic Testing or Cotesting and Intervention According to Test Results

Cytology or Cotesting Result	Proportion (%) of Screening Result	Risk (%) of HSIL or Cancer	Suggested Intervention
Squamous cell carcinoma	<0.01	84	Immediate colposcopy
HPV+/HSIL	0.20	71	Immediate colposcopy
HSIL	0.21	69	Immediate colposcopy
HPV−/HSIL	0.01	49	Immediate colposcopy
HPV+/LSIL	0.81	19	Immediate colposcopy
LSIL	0.97	16	Immediate colposcopy
HPV−/LSIL	0.19	5	Repeat testing in 6–12 months
HPV+/AGC	0.05	45	Immediate colposcopy
AGC	0.21	13	Immediate colposcopy
HPV−/AGC	0.16	2	Immediate colposcopy
HPV+/ASC-H	0.12	45	Immediate colposcopy
ASC-H	0.17	35	Immediate colposcopy
HPV−/ASC-H	0.05	12	Immediate colposcopy
HPV+/ASCUS	1.10	18	Immediate colposcopy
ASCUS	2.80	7	Repeat testing in 6–12 months
HPV−/ASCUS	1.80	1	Repeat testing in 3 years
HPV+/Pap−	3.60	10	Repeat testing in 6–12 months
Pap−	96	0.68	Repeat testing in 3 years
HPV−/Pap−	92	0.27	Repeat testing in 5 years

AGC, atypical glandular cells; ASC-H, atypical squamous cells (cannot rule out high-grade lesion); ASCUS, atypical squamous cells of undetermined significance; HPV, human papillomavirus; HSIL, high-grade squamous intraepithelial lesion; LSIL, low-grade squamous intraepithelial lesion; Pap, Papanicolaou.

3 cytology, *in utero* exposure to diethylstilbestrol (DES, a synthetic estrogen), and ASCUS cytology with positive high-risk HPV 16, 18, or 45. Adequate colposcopy examinations involve full visualization of the uterine cervix and its transformation zone. Endocervical curettage (ECC) might be helpful, and yet, its routine practice remains debatable (71). Multiquadrant biopsy improves accuracy of colposcopy, especially when a lesion is not readily visualized (71,72).

Conization

Conization of the uterine cervix means surgical extirpation of the squamocolumnar junction (transformation zone). The procedure involves either cold knife conization in the operating room suite, or thermal cautery with loop excision in the outpatient office or in the operating room suite. Indications for conization include inadequate colposcopy, positive ECC, persistent CIN 1 (typically >1 year), CIN 2 or 3, carcinoma *in situ*, and discrepancy among cytology, colposcopy, and pathologic findings. After examination of 447 histopathologic slices from 97 patient conization procedures, small cone height was significantly associated with positive disease margin status: a 20-mm cone height was recommended (73).

Loop Diathermy

Outpatient thermal cautery with loop electrosurgical excision procedure (LEEP or loop diathermy) is an alternative to cold knife conization (74). Studies have demonstrated loop diathermy to be as effective as cold knife conization (75) and laser vaporization (76), with some gynecologists favoring loop diathermy in terms of cost, anesthesia, and ease of use. Thermal artifact obscures margin status. Return patient visits after loop diathermy might be due to incomplete excision complicated by thermal artifact, secondary hemorrhage, and findings of invasive cancer (74).

Clinical Invasive Disease

Symptoms and Complaints

Uterine cervix cancer presents most often with abnormal vaginal discharge, postcoital bleeding, or nonmenstrual vaginal bleeding. Well-woman visits might also discover asymptomatic lesions upon pelvic examination or cytologic evaluation. As a lesion grows in size, it might elicit local pelvic pain or disrupted urination or defecation. If disease were to spread to regional pelvic or paraaortic lymph nodes, back pain or unilateral leg swelling (or even bullous edema) might become evident.

Physical Findings

Abnormal contour of the uterine cervix on physical examination might be the first clue to disease, with necrotic or friable lesions being particularly suspicious. Palpable extension of disease onto the walls of the vagina must be described, if present. Parametrial, sidewall, and uterosacral ligament extension are best felt and described by rectovaginal examination. Nodal disease in the groin, femoral, and scalene lymph node regions should be assessed to guide intervention.

Diagnostic Biopsy

Biopsies should secure sufficient nonnecrotic tissue at depth for diagnosis of uterine cervix cancers. Marginal biopsy rather than central necrotic tissue biopsy yields superior results.

Staging

Clinical Staging Procedures

Pelvic examination with rectovaginal palpation provides the basis for clinical cancer staging. An examination under anesthesia, when needed, provides superior visual and manual examination when patients relay discomfort and pain with routine pelvic examination. Examination under anesthesia affords cystoscopy, proctoscopy, and special instrument biopsy when indicated.

Clinical Laboratory Studies

A complete peripheral blood count is indicated to assess anemia (<10 g/dL [77]), which might need packed red blood cell correction. Thrombocytopenia might be found in up to 30% of patients, which might need replacement prior to therapeutic intervention. Serum blood urea nitrogen and creatinine obtained as part of the chemistry panel assess renal insufficiency and dehydration, which might need stabilization and rehydration prior to cisplatin-based radiochemotherapy. Liver function panels are obtained generally prior to chemotherapy when indicated. A baseline urinalysis including pregnancy test are indicated to assess for pregnancy in potential childbearing patients.

Clinical Serum Tumor Markers

Table 20.4 lists actively investigated serum tumor markers for uterine cervix cancer (78–88). Uterine cervix cancers—represented mostly by HPV-competent squamous cell carcinoma or adenocarcinoma—express unique phenotypic fingerprints, which are possibly indicative of higher rates of nodal or visceral metastases and poorer disease-specific survival. Prospective trials randomizing go or no-go therapeutic decisions based on serum tumor markers remain elusive.

Clinical Radiographic Studies

The FIGO system for cancer staging relies only on clinical examination (46). Noninvasive chest radiography, intravenous pyelography (IVP), cystoscopy, sigmoidoscopy, and barium enema radiography may aid in clinical evaluation, but are not mandatory (46). Computed tomography (CT), 2-[^{18}F]fluoro-2-deoxy-D-glucose (FDG), positron emission tomography (PET), dual PET/CT, magnetic resonance imaging (MRI), and dual PET/MRI studies (89) are not yet integrated into formal staging criteria. In the United States and other countries, these studies are considered important in the care of women with uterine cervix cancer as they improve diagnostic accuracy.

When compared to operative staging, FIGO clinical stage for uterine cervix cancer understages 30% of stage IB, 25% of stage IIB, and 40% of stage IIIB patients (90). Abdominopelvic CT or MRI images help sort out cross-sectional anatomy and assist in evaluating prognostic features such as tumor size and lymph node metastasis. A 25-center intergroup trial conducted by the American College of Radiology Imaging Network and by the Gynecologic Oncology Group (ACRIN 6651/GOG 183]) begun in 2000 prospectively evaluated MRI, CT, clinical exam, and histopathologic analysis for their ability to predict lymph node involvement as verified by lymphadenectomy in 208 women with uterine cervix cancer (91–93). MRI correctly identified 20 (37%) of 54 of cases with surgicopathologic-confirmed lymph node metastases; CT correctly labeled 17 (31%) of 55 cases (93). The investigators concluded both modalities had an underperforming, low sensitivity for detecting lymph node metastases. However, MRI outperformed CT in the ability to measure uterine cervix cancer diameter (92), an important prognostic variable. MRI has therefore been associated with a positive predictive value of 61 (95% CI, 48%–73%) among women surgically confirmed for positive pelvic and paraaortic lymph node metastases, a negative predictive value of 66% (95% CI, 55%–75%) among women surgically confirmed for positive pelvic lymph nodes and negative paraaortic lymph nodes, and a negative predictive value of 86% (95% CI, 76%–92%) in women with surgically confirmed negative pelvic and paraaortic lymph nodes (94). In cases of parametrial extension, MRI provides superior detail of tumor-related anatomic invasion and affords best contour definition in brachytherapy radiation planning (95).

PET studies have shown that the radiotracer FDG associates with all measures of disease burden, including the prevalence of lymph node metastases, rates of objective (complete or partial) treatment

TABLE 20.4. Biologic Markers Predicting Lymph Node Metastasis in Uterine Cervix Cancer

Test	Cutoff (ng/mL)	Sensitivity (%)	Specificity (%)	% Node Metastasis	Test Used in Decision for	Reference
Squamous cell carcinoma antigen (SCC-Ag)	>3.5	81	65	35 (34 of 96)	BR	(78)
	>3.5	71	67	71 (15 of 21)	PR	(79)
	>2.0	64	69	64 (23 of 36)	PR	(80)
	>1.9	66	NR	66 (53 of 80)	AR	(81)
	>1.5	75	40	75 (215 of 286)	BR	(82)
Squamous cell carcinoma antigen (SCC-Ag)	>3.5	81	65	35 (34 of 96)	BR	(78)
	>3.5	71	67	71 (15 of 21)	PR	(79)
	>2.0	64	69	64 (23 of 36)	PR	(80)
	>1.9	66	NR	66 (53 of 80)	AR	(81)
	>1.5	75	40	75 (215 of 286)	BR	(82)
	>1.5	NR	NR	30 (35 of 116)	BR	(83)
Cytokeratin fragment 19 (CYFRA 21.1)	>3.30	36	90	36 (13 of 36)	PR	(80)
Cancer antigen 125 (CA 125)	≥30 U/mL	67	84	67 (6 of 9)	PR	(85)
Human cartilage glycoprotein 39 (YKL-40)	>92.2	21	71	21 (10 of 47)	ID	(86)
High mobility group box protein 1 (HMGB1)	>28.1	63	40	63 (45 of 71)	PR	(87)
Uterine cervix circulating tumor cells (CTCs)	E6/E7+	0	78	25 (3 of 12)	CTC	(88)

AR, adjuvant radiation; BR, biochemical response; CTC, E6+ or E7+ circulating tumor cells; ID, initial detection; NR, not reported; PR, predicting response.

response, and progression-free survival, in patients with uterine cervix cancer (96–99). FDG proves useful due to its "look-alike" sugar form, being "trapped" by intracellular hexokinase, and being concentrated in overactive cancer cells. A 32-patient surgicopathologic study (1994 to 1998) of presurgical abdominopelvic PET followed by open surgical lymphadenectomy showed a 75% sensitivity and 92% specificity for uterine cervix cancer metastases in paraaortic lymph nodes (96). A 101-patient radiographic study (1998 to 2000) of whole-body PET found that PET-avid paraaortic lymph nodes predicted progression-free survival (97). A 482 patient retrospective study (1997 to 2008) investigated imaging-only confirmed sites of lymph node metastases (98). It found 205 patients (43%) with no FDG-avid lymph nodes; 186 patients (39%) with FDG-avid pelvic lymph nodes only; 65 patients (13%) with FDG-avid pelvic and paraaortic lymph nodes; and 26 patients (5%) with FDG-avid pelvic, paraaortic, and supraclavicular lymph nodes. Among 51 uterine cervix cancer patients (2004 to 2009) in whom presurgical PET scans were obtained, a ≤0.33 posttherapy: pretherapy standard uptake value maximum ratio of primary cancer metabolic signal was associated in 88% of patients with an at least partial radiochemotherapy treatment response (99). A phase I trial (2006 to 2008) explored PET-assessed metabolic response to novel radiochemotherapy in uterine cervix cancer patients (100). Afterward, a prospective phase II clinical trial (2009 to 2011) in 25 women with advanced-stage uterine cervix or vaginal cancers used a 3-month posttherapy PET-assessed metabolic response as the primary efficacy endpoint (101,102).

Pretreatment Paraaortic Node Operative Staging

Paraaortic lymph node metastases indicate negative prognosis and short survival (96). It is debatable whether there is a therapeutic advantage to operative removal of paraaortic disease. An extraperitoneal approach or transperitoneal approach to paraaortic lymphadenectomy was of similar sensitivity and morbidity in a 288-patient (1977 to 1981) uterine cervix cancer surgical staging study (103). Knowledge of paraaortic lymph node disease has been shown to direct care away from surgery toward extended-field radiation therapy in up to 20% of patients (104). As part of a prospective, multicenter clinical trial (1999 to 2002), patients with histologically confirmed stage IB2, stage IIA ≥4 cm or stage IIB to IVA uterine cervix cancers underwent MRI prior to pelvic and abdominal lymphadenectomy (94). Lymph nodes <1 cm were bisected whereas those >1 cm were serially sectioned into 5-mm sections for microscopy. Thirty three patients had 94 metastasis-positive and 659 metastasis-negative lymph nodes removed. Mean size of the long axis of the 60 largest positive and the 209 negative lymph nodes removed did not differ (19 ± 9 mm vs. 19 ± 12 mm; $p = 0.47$). The authors suggested that the negative predictive value of MRI for paraaortic lymph nodes among patients reported to have negative pelvic and paraaortic lymph nodes on MRI is high enough that surgical evaluation and extended-field radiation therapy are not necessary. For all others, the positive and negative predictive values of MRI are too low to determine the need for extended-field radiation therapy without first performing surgical evaluation. A phase III international trial evaluating lymphadenectomy in locally advanced uterine cervix cancer study (LiLACS) is underway (105).

Sentinel Lymph Node Mapping in Early Uterine Cervix Cancer

The feasibility of sentinel lymph node mapping has been explored in 39 patients with invasive uterine cervix cancer undergoing radical hysterectomy and pelvic lymphadenectomy (106). All patients underwent presurgical lymphoscintigraphy and intraoperative mapping with both a blue dye and a handheld gamma probe. Lymphoscintigraphy revealed at least one sentinel lymph node in 33 (85%) patients, including 21 (55%) patients with bilateral sentinel lymph nodes. All 39 patients had at least one sentinel lymph node identified during surgery. The majority (80%) of sentinel lymph nodes were in iliac, obturator, and parametrial nodal basins (in descending order of frequency). The remainder was in either the common iliac or the paraaortic nodal basins. A total of 132 nodes were identified clinically as sentinel lymph nodes; 65 (49%) were both blue and hot, 35 (27%) were blue only, and 32 (24%) were hot only. The sensitivity of the sentinel node was 88% and the negative predictive value was 97%. The German AGO Study Group (1998 to 2006) identified a 93% sentinel lymph node detection rate, 77% sensitivity, and 94% negative predictive value in 590 women of all uterine cervix cancer stage who underwent lymph node detection after labeling with technetium, patent blue, or both (107). Obstacles to widespread adoption include sensitivity of frozen section preparation to detect lymph node metastasis, pathologic expertise, uniformity of surgicopathologic technique, and a determination of whether the clinical impact of presurgical tumor size affects the rate of sentinel lymph node event (41).

PATHOLOGY

Squamous Cell Carcinoma

Squamous cell carcinoma of the uterine cervix includes microinvasive and more deeply invasive squamous cancer cell variants that may differ in biologic behavior, such as verrucous, papillary squamous, transitional, warty, or lymphoepithelioma-like carcinoma.

Preinvasive Disease

High-grade squamous intraepithelial lesion describes full-thickness epithelial neoplasia of the cervix. The normal maturation steps of a squamous epithelium are absent. Cells often have enlarged oval nuclei, increased nuclear: cytoplasm ratios, and mitotic figures (**Fig. 20.1**). Persistent squamous cell carcinoma *in situ* became invasive cancer in 22% of New Zealand women over a five-year period (108).

Microinvasive Disease

Microinvasive squamous cell carcinoma typically arises from squamous intraepithelial neoplasia, originating from surface epithelium or from endocervical glands. Microinvasive carcinoma describes irregular, haphazardly arranged small nests of squamous cells that have penetrated the basement membrane of the surface or glandular epithelium. Cells are larger, have abundant eosinophilic cytoplasm, and are associated with a desmoplastic stromal reaction (**Fig. 20.2**).

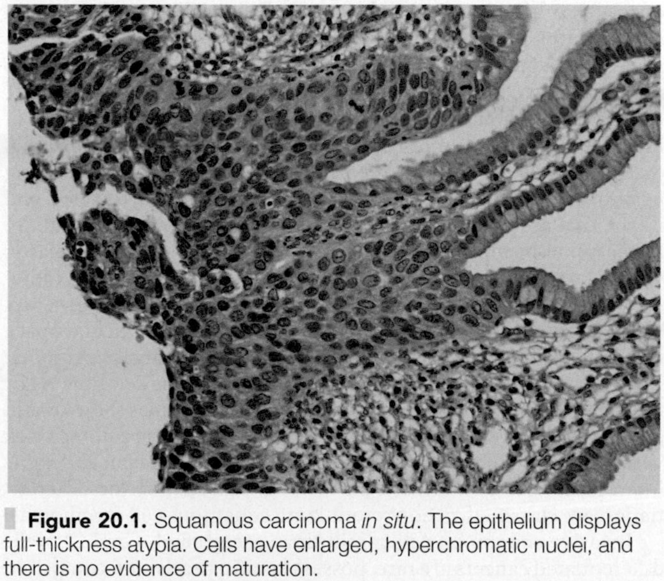

Figure 20.1. Squamous carcinoma *in situ*. The epithelium displays full-thickness atypia. Cells have enlarged, hyperchromatic nuclei, and there is no evidence of maturation.

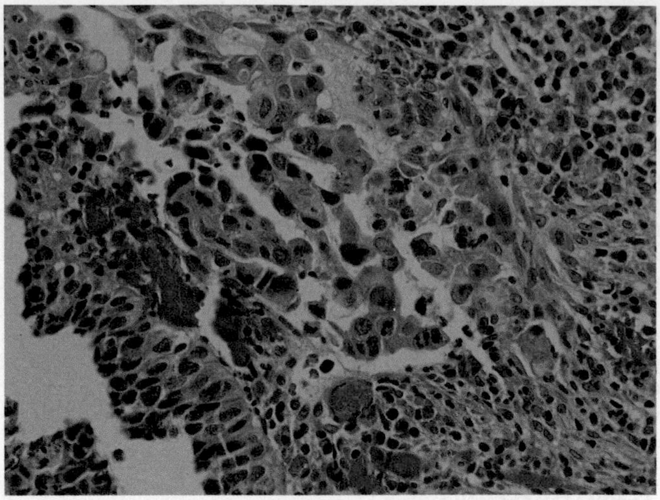

Figure 20.2. Microinvasive squamous carcinoma. There is an area of squamous carcinoma *in situ (lower left)*. A nest of invasive carcinoma cells *(center)* has broken through the basement membrane. The invasive cells are larger, with more abundant cytoplasm and larger, more pleomorphic nuclei. A desmoplastic stroma response is present *(right)*.

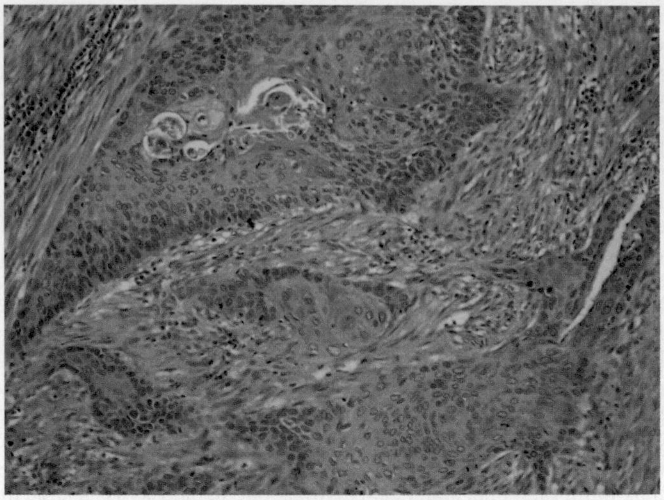

Figure 20.3. Invasive squamous carcinoma. Small, irregular nests of cells with markedly atypical nuclei are present. They are surrounded by desmoplastic stroma containing inflammatory cells.

Microinvasive squamous cell depth of invasion should be measured from the originating basement membrane. For instance, if carcinoma arises from the surface epithelium, depth is the distance from the basement membrane of the surface epithelium to the deepest nest of invasive cells. If carcinoma arises from an endocervical gland, depth is measured from the basement membrane of the gland. If the originating site is unclear, depth is measured from the basement membrane of the surface epithelium. Nests of superficially invasive squamous cells observed in small biopsies should be reported along with the dimensions of any invasive tumor. A diagnosis of microinvasive squamous cell carcinoma of the cervix requires a loop diathermy or conization biopsy that encircles the entire lesion with negative margin. In a 133-patient surgicopathologic microinvasive cancer of the uterine cervix study (1965 to 1976), tumor penetration was <1 mm in 38%, 1 to 2 mm in 30%, 2 to 3 mm in 17%, 3 to 4 mm in 12%, and ≥4 mm in 4% (109). No lymph node metastases were detected at the time of radical hysterectomy in 74 patients. Only two (1.5%) patients developed relapse (109).

Invasive Disease

Invasive squamous cell carcinoma of the uterine cervix arises most often from high-grade dysplasia, which initially may have been detected up to 10 years beforehand. It has been shown that CIN 2 progressed eight times more often and CIN 3 progressed 22 times more often to carcinoma *in situ* or invasive cancer than did CIN 1 (110). HPV is associated with invasive disease in more than 86% of incident cases (15). Tumors may be firm indurated masses, polypoid, or ulcerated. Under the microscope, irregular, haphazardly infiltrating nests of cells are apparent. Cells have an eosinophilic cytoplasm, and nuclei that are enlarged, atypical, and hyperchromatic (**Fig. 20.3**). Mitoses may be numerous and atypical. A pronounced desmoplastic stromal reaction occurs around invasive cell nests, perhaps indicative of host immune cell response to virally altered uterine cervix cells and manifesting as bulky tumor (111). Lymphovascular space invasion may be present, especially in more deeply invasive tumors.

Invasive squamous cell carcinomas are labeled as keratinizing or nonkeratinizing. Keratinizing squamous cell carcinomas show keratin pearl architecture. Nonkeratinizing squamous cell carcinomas lack keratin pearls, display abundant eosinophilic cytoplasm, and show intercellular bridges. Small cells lacking neuroendocrine differentiation are classified as nonkeratinizing squamous cell carcinomas.

Invasive squamous cell carcinomas are graded. Grade 1 well-differentiated cancers are rare, possess keratin pearls, and comprised of keratinized cells predominantly. Grade 1 cell nuclei show modest atypia and mitoses are uncommon. Grade 2 moderately differentiated cancers represent the majority, are typically nonkeratinizing squamous cell carcinomas, display nuclear pleomorphism and more numerous mitoses, and have an infiltrative pattern. Grade 3 poorly differentiated cancers either have smaller cells without neuroendocrine differentiation, or are pleomorphic with anaplastic nuclei. Grade 3 cancers have a propensity for spindle-shaped cells that must be distinguished from sarcoma by positive cytokeratin stains.

Squamous Cell Carcinoma Variants

Papillary Squamous and Transitional Cell Carcinoma

A papillary superficial architecture with substantial nuclear atypia occurs as one variant of uterine cervix cancer. The most common presenting symptoms are vaginal bleeding and abnormal Pap smears. Papillary, polypoid, or granular lesions are often evident on examination of the cervix.

Papillary squamous and transitional cell carcinomas have thin or thick papillae that contain connective tissue cores covered by highly atypical epithelium displaying keratinization. Occasionally, the epithelium consists of multiple layered cells with oval hyperchromatic nuclei without keratinization and resemble urothelial transitional cell epithelium. Nuclear grooves may be present. Immunohistochemical studies have shown that most of these tumors are cytokeratin 7 positive and cytokeratin 20 negative; these results are consistent with a squamous cell differentiation. HPV-16 DNA has been detected and these tumors have a shared uroplakin III negative, p63 positive, and $p16^{INK4A}$ positive immunophenotype regardless of light microscopic features (112).

Papillary squamous cell and transitional cell carcinomas of the uterine cervix are associated commonly with an underlying invasive squamous cell carcinoma. Other cases of invasive cancers have been described. Therefore, superficial biopsies displaying only a papillary portion of the neoplasm may be inconclusive. Loop diathermy or conization should be done to exclude an underlying invasive cancer.

Local relapse and systemic metastasis occur with these cancer types. Papillary squamous cell and transitional cell carcinomas must be separated from verrucous carcinomas, which display little cell atypia and have a much more indolent clinical course.

Verrucous Carcinoma

Verrucous carcinoma arises in a papillary excrescence of the cervix resembling condyloma acuminatum (perhaps the "giant condyloma of Buschke and Lowenstein"). Microscopic examination displays pointed "church spire" papillary fronds of squamous epithelium lacking connective tissue cores. Connective tissue beneath these fronds displays bulbous nests of squamous epithelium that invade the stroma with a pushing margin but minor cytologic atypia. Significant nuclear atypia identifies another form of uterine cervix carcinoma. The histopathologic distinction between verrucous carcinoma and squamous cell carcinoma is critical because verrucous carcinoma invades local tissues but does not metastasize elsewhere. A verrucous carcinoma diagnosis necessitates visual inspection of the invasive portion of the tumor; superficial biopsies are inconclusive.

Warty Carcinoma

Warty carcinomas are rare papillary neoplasms marked by condylomatous changes but possess histopathologic features of invasive squamous cell carcinoma at their deep margin (113). HPV-related cellular changes ("koilocytotic atypia") are shown in **Figure 20.4**.

Lymphoepithelioma-Like Carcinoma

Lymphoepithelioma-like carcinoma, most commonly seen in the nasopharynx, represents another variant of uterine cervix cancer. The clinical presentation ranges from a cervical tumor producing modest abnormal vaginal bleeding to nonvisible cervical tumors detected only by cervical cytology smears. Lymphoepithelioma-like carcinoma of the cervix presents most often in Asian women and is associated with Epstein–Barr virus infection in those patients (114). The latter observation remains controversial. Microscopic examination reveals nests of cells with pale eosinophilic cytoplasm and large vesicular nuclei with prominent eosinophilic nucleoli. Cell margins are indistinct, lending to a syncytial phenotype. A prominent inflammatory infiltrate comprising of lymphocytes, plasma cells, and eosinophils occurs. This carcinoma distinguishes itself from glassy cell carcinoma (also accompanied by prominent inflammation) by its indistinct cell margins and granular eosinophilic cytoplasm. The lymphocytic infiltrate contains predominantly CD8+ suppressor/cytotoxic T cells (115).

Adenosquamous Carcinoma

Adenosquamous carcinoma includes an admixture of malignant glandular cell and squamous cell elements. This term is not a basket classification for poorly differentiated squamous carcinomas, in which mucicarmine stains show only scattered mucin vacuoles. Likewise, this term is not descriptive of a true collision tumor, where an adenocarcinoma abuts a squamous cell carcinoma. An adenosquamous carcinoma has high tumor cell grade, presence of vascular invasion, and aggressive malignant potential.

Adenocarcinoma

Adenocarcinoma of the uterine cervix is on the rise, accounting for 25% of incident cancer cases (116). Two are described, endocervical AIS or adenocarcinoma (56). HPV types 18, 33, 35, 45, 51, 58, or 59 confer risk for adenocarcinoma, although HPV 16 occurs as well (117).

Adenocarcinoma In Situ

Under the microscope, AIS preserves overall endocervical gland architecture with varying degrees of cytologic atypia, including nuclear enlargement and stratification, nuclear hyperchromasia, and mitotic figures (**Fig. 20.5**). Most AISs occur near the transformation zone.

Adenocarcinoma

Adenocarcinoma of the uterine cervix shows altered endocervical gland architecture in the form of solid or cribriform nests of cells, architecturally irregular or incomplete glands lined by malignant cells, or small buds of highly atypical cells arising from glands involved by AIS. A desmoplastic stroma accompanies tumors. The FIGO definition of microinvasive carcinoma generally applies to all types of cancers, but the term has not been generally accepted for adenocarcinoma of the uterine cervix because an increased incidence of metastatic disease corresponds to incremental increases in depth of invasive disease.

Mucinous Adenocarcinoma

Mucinous adenocarcinoma of the uterine cervix includes endocervical, intestinal, signet ring cell, minimal deviation, and villoglandular variants. HPV DNA has been detected in 91% of mucinous adenocarcinomas of the cervix (118).

Mucinous Adenocarcinoma, Endocervical Variant

An endocervical variant of mucinous adenocarcinoma occurs most often. Irregular, haphazardly arranged tubuloracemose glands are lined by cells resembling those seen in normal endocervical glands,

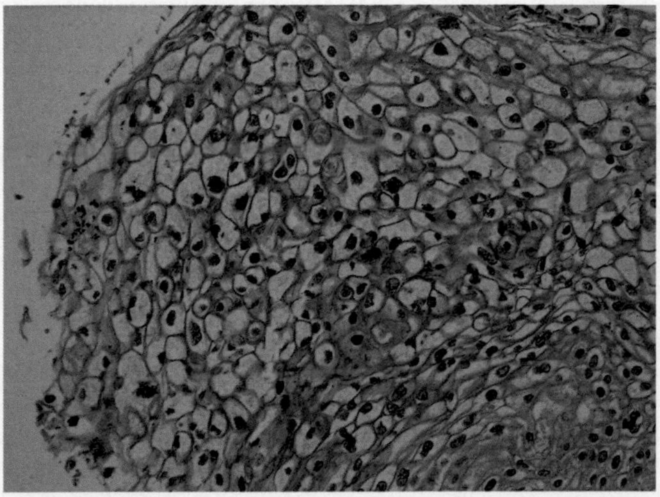

Figure 20.4. Human papillomavirus changes. This squamous epithelium displays cells with large halos surrounding atypical nuclei ("koilocytotic atypia").

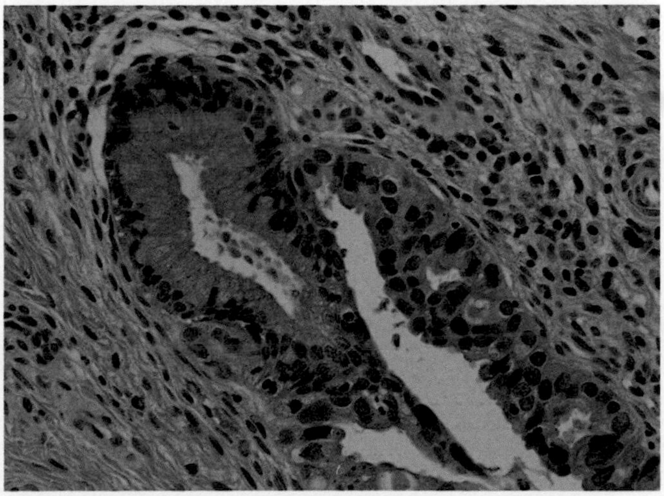

Figure 20.5. Adenocarcinoma *in situ*. Part of this endocervical gland is normal *(upper left corner)*. Stratified cells with atypical, large nuclei and mitotic figures have replaced the remainder of the gland.

but with limited amounts of cytoplasmic mucin. Nuclei are basally located, stratified, and atypical (**Fig. 20.6**). Mitoses are found. Grade 1 well-differentiated cancers have uniform nuclei with minimal stratification and few mitotic figures. Grade 2 moderately differentiated adenocarcinomas have more prominent cytologic atypia with more frequent mitoses. Grade 3 poorly differentiated adenocarcinomas contain prominent solid regions, pleomorphic nuclei, and many mitoses. A desmoplastic stromal response is variable.

Mucinous Adenocarcinoma, Intestinal Type, Signet Ring, and Colloid Variants

A rare form of uterine cervix adenocarcinoma has goblet cells in endocervical glands; these tumors possess intestinal differentiation. Malignant signet ring cells and colloid cells are rare in the uterine cervix; these adenocarcinoma variants must be distinguished from metastatic gastrointestinal tract cancers.

Mucinous Adenocarcinoma, Minimal Deviation Variant

The minimal deviation variant of mucinous adenocarcinoma represents only about 1% of uterine cervix adenocarcinomas (119) and is not associated with HPV infection (120). Firm, tan–yellow tumors are found in hysterectomy samples. Microscopic inspection finds disorganized glands infiltrating the cervical stroma, with budding contours or angular peaked outlines. The glands look deceptively benign on low-power magnification. A lack of cytologic atypia must be seen for this diagnosis. On high-power magnification, cells may have some nuclear enlargement, stratification, and rare mitotic figures. The infiltrating glands are devoid of substantial desmoplastic reaction.

Mucinous Adenocarcinoma, Well-Differentiated Villoglandular Variant

Well-differentiated villoglandular adenocarcinomas occur as polypoid or papillary endocervical masses. Microscopy reveals villous, papillary structures assuming long and slender forms or short and broad forms. A connective tissue core with inflammatory cells may be present. The overlying epithelium consists of a single stratified layer of cells with endocervical, endometrial, or intestinal differentiation. Nuclei are mildly atypical and mitotic figures are infrequent (**Fig. 20.7**). Invasive adenocarcinoma may be seen beneath papillary areas, characterized by branching glands lined by atypical cells and surrounded by desmoplastic stroma. This does not display marked nuclear atypia and epithelial tufting seen in the much more aggressive papillary serous carcinoma of the uterine cervix. This variant may be associated with typical AIS of the uterine cervix. Usually, a villoglandular uterine cervix cancer should not be suggested when only small biopsy specimens are available for review; a definitive diagnosis should be made only when viewing conization or hysterectomy surgical specimens. Villoglandular cancers having a high-grade cytologic component or an underlying obvious invasive adenocarcinoma may be linked to lymphovascular invasion, lymph node metastases, and higher probability of relapse (121).

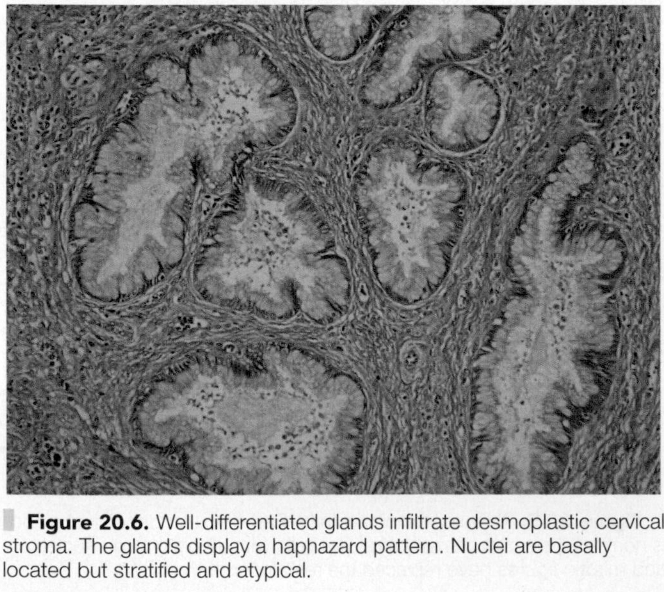

Figure 20.6. Well-differentiated glands infiltrate desmoplastic cervical stroma. The glands display a haphazard pattern. Nuclei are basally located but stratified and atypical.

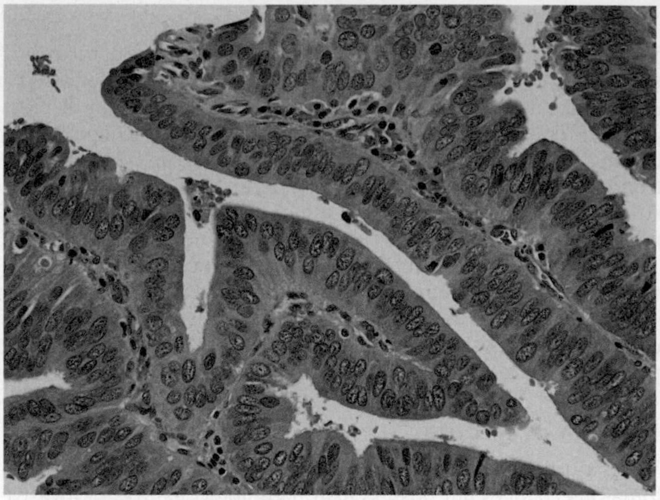

Figure 20.7. Well-differentiated villoglandular adenocarcinoma. Long, slender villous processes are covered with epithelium, displaying mild atypia. Nuclei are crowded, but they retain an oval shape and are uniform in size.

Adenocarcinoma, Endometrioid Variant

Endometrioid carcinomas of the uterine cervix are rare and overdiagnosed, accounting for 7% of all adenocarcinomas of the uterine cervix. These are "look-alike" malignancies sharing histopathologic features with endometrioid cancers of the uterine corpus. Thus, a primary endometrial adenocarcinoma with endocervical extension or drop metastasis masquerading as a uterine cervix cancer must be excluded. Immunohistochemical signature of carcinoembryonic antigen (CEA) positivity, estrogen receptor (ER) negativity, and vimentin negativity marks uterine endocervix primary cancers, while the opposite signature characterizes uterine corpus primary cancers. HPV markers (e.g., p16) also support a uterine endocervix primary cancer.

Adenocarcinoma, Clear Cell Variant

Clear cell cancers of the uterine cervix are linked to intrauterine DES exposure; however, clear cell cancers also occur in the absence of DES exposure. Histopathologic examination identifies solid sheets of cells containing abundant glycogen-rich clear cytoplasm, atypical nuclei, and numerous mitoses. A tubulocystic pattern involves alternating tubule and cystic spaces lined by oxyphilic, hobnail, or clear cells. A papillary pattern is uncommon and often mixed solid and tubulocystic areas are seen. Clear cell carcinomas of the cervix are not associated with HPV infection (120).

Adenocarcinoma, Papillary Serous Variant

Papillary serous uterine cervix cancers are not associated with HPV infection (120). There is a bimodal age distribution, occurring in patients younger than 40 years and patients older than 65 years. Gross pathologic examination reveals a nodular mass, an indurated cervix, or no visible abnormality. Under the microscope, these cancers appear identical to serous tumors of the ovary, endometrium, and primary peritoneal serous carcinomas. Exclusion of metastasis or extension of disease from another primary site, especially the endometrium, is paramount. Histopathologic examination identifies fibrous papillae lined by atypical epithelial cells; secondary papillae or tufts of malignant-appearing epithelial surface cells are often present (**Fig. 20.8**). Glandular structures have misshapen luminal borders because of cancer cell tufts. Nuclei show high-grade atypia and an abundant number of mitoses are observed. These aggressive cancers often metastasize to pelvic, paraaortic, and groin lymph nodes, and portend a worse prognosis.

Adenocarcinoma, Mesonephric Variant

Mesonephric duct remnants in the lateral aspects of the uterine cervix may be identified as lobules of small, round, glandular structures lined by flattened cuboidal epithelium with intraluminal periodic acid-Schiff stain (PAS)-positive material. These cells do not contain intracytoplasmic mucin, unlike cells lining endocervical glands. Mesonephric-variant adenocarcinomas arise from the lateral mesonephric duct remnants, with few cases reported. These cancers display ductal, tubular, retiform, solid, and sex cord–like patterns and cells that lack intracytoplasmic mucin.

Adenocarcinoma, Microcystic Endocervical Variant

Microcystic endocervical-variant adenocarcinoma is rare, as only eight cases are described (122). The hallmark pattern involves many low-power microscopic cystic and dilated glands. Magnification reveals abundant cytologic atypia and mitoses. Pockets of mucinous or intestinal endocervical adenocarcinoma are found; cells are deeply invasive. Postsurgical local relapses have been recorded.

Glassy Cell Carcinoma

Glassy cell carcinoma represents an uncommon variant of adenosquamous carcinoma, showing cells with eosinophilic cytoplasm, well-defined margins, and prominent nucleoli. A plasma cell infiltrate is often seen. Relapses of adenocarcinomas or adenosquamous carcinomas may assume a glassy cell carcinoma appearance when the original cells have been irradiated (116).

Adenoid Cystic Carcinoma

Adenoid cystic carcinoma of the uterine cervix is both rare and aggressive, presenting most often in elderly patients. Microscopy reveals a cribriform gland pattern, with glands enclosing hyaline or mucinous material. Nuclei are large and pleomorphic, both to a greater extent as compared to adenoid basal epithelioma. Mitoses are present. Necrosis might be seen. Cells stain with cytokeratin; in contrast to the salivary gland variant, this cancer does not exhibit myoepithelial cells, either by immunohistochemistry for S100 protein or by electron microscopy. Relapses and metastases occur.

Adenoid Basal Epithelioma (Carcinoma)

Adenoid basal epitheliomas are rare neoplasms of the uterine cervix. An indolent behavior led to the term "adenoid basal epithelioma." HPV 16 DNA integration has been observed (120). These lesions may be precursors for a variety of uterine cervix carcinomas. A subclassification as adenoid basal epitheliomas versus carcinomas should be used. Microscopically, adenoid basal epithelioma shows cell nests with a basaloid appearance and peripheral palisading. Gland lumina are found within nests, but the number of glands formed is variable. Squamous metaplasia and mitoses are seen infrequently. Adenoid basal epithelioma, in the absence of a coexisting invasive carcinoma, is benign. The disease must be distinguished from adenoid cystic carcinoma, given the profound difference in oncologic phenotype. Adenoid basal epitheliomas with carcinomatous components should be reported as cancers.

Neuroendocrine Cancers

Consistent labeling for neuroendocrine tumors of the uterine cervix facilitates epidemiology and natural history chronologies of these cancers (123). Immunohistochemical chromogranin or synaptophysin stains provide necessary evidence of neuroendocrine differentiation except in small cell carcinoma of the uterine cervix. Typical carcinoids of the uterine cervix are rare, identified with caution because most uterine cervix neuroendocrine tumors are aggressive, and too few cases describe the histopathology and natural history of this cancer variant. Atypical carcinoids of the uterine cervix are rare, display organoid cell nests, nuclear atypia, and have a mitotic rate of 5 to 10 foci per high powered microscope field of view. Necrosis may be present. Large cell neuroendocrine carcinomas of the uterine cervix (**Fig. 20.9**) possess organoid cell nests with peripheral palisading of nuclei, prominent nucleoli, variable levels of necrosis, eosinophilic cytoplasmic granules, and numerous mitotic figures (>10 foci per high powered microscope

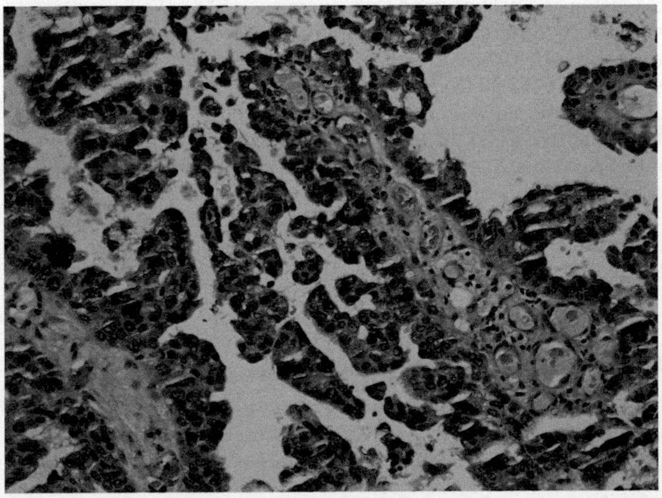

Figure 20.8. Serous adenocarcinoma. The papillary structures have a connective tissue core. There is marked tufting and stratification, and the nuclei are markedly atypical.

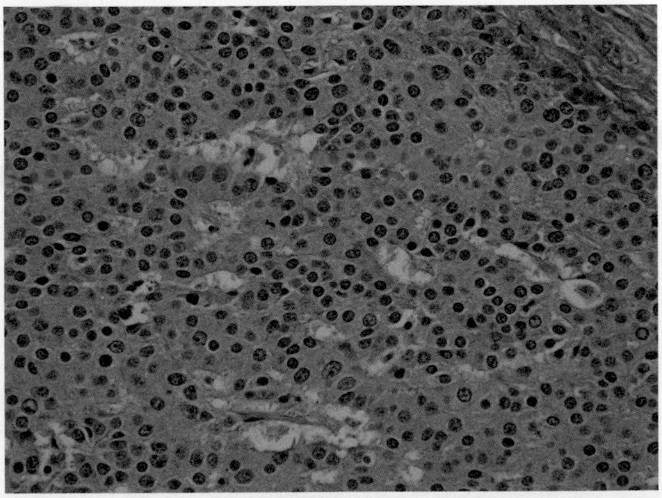

Figure 20.9. Large cell neuroendocrine carcinoma. This tumor displays organoid architecture. The tumor cells are much larger than those seen in small cell carcinoma. They have abundant eosinophilic cytoplasm, and there are numerous mitotic figures. Areas of necrosis were present elsewhere in the tumor.

field of view). Lymphovascular space involvement may be seen. Coexisting AIS or adenocarcinoma of the cervix is often found, marking these cancers as highly aggressive neoplasms. Evidence of neuroendocrine differentiation is required; chromogranin or synaptophysin immunoreactivity is used for diagnosis.

Small Cell Carcinoma

Most neuroendocrine cancers observed arising from the uterine cervix are small cell carcinomas. Small cell carcinomas have cells with scant cytoplasm, inconspicuous nuclei with finely stippled chromatin, nuclear molding, extensive necrosis, crush artifact, and numerous mitotic figures (**Fig. 20.10**). Single-cell infiltration of the stroma has been observed commonly. Lymphovascular space invasion is seen often. Small cell carcinomas can be difficult to treat and recurrences are common.

Mixed Epithelial and Mesenchymal Tumors

Mullerian adenosarcomas may arise from the uterine cervix (124). Polypoid or papillary masses often give rise to nonmenstrual bleeding. Cells form benign-appearing glands in a sarcomatous stroma. A periglandular cuff of condensed stroma may be present. The sarcomatous element shows a variable number of mitotic figures, and some instances display heterologous elements such as striated muscle or cartilage. Mullerian adenosarcomas confer a favorable prognosis; deep invasion and sarcomatous overgrowth are adverse prognostic factors. Malignant mixed mullerian tumors may involve the cervix, but only five cases have been reported (125).

Other Malignant Tumors

Sarcomas arising from the uterine cervix are observed but uncommon. A histopathologic review of 1,583 malignancies of the uterine cervix found only 8 (0.5%) sarcomas (126). Five were carcinosarcomas and three were unclassified, leiomyosarcomas, or endometrial stromal sarcomas. Extranodal lymphomas of the uterine cervix are typically of diffuse B-cell origin (127). Primitive neuroectodermal tumors (128) and desmoplastic small round cell tumors (129) also have been described.

Secondary tumors of the uterine cervix might represent neoplasms invading from contiguous organs (such as the uterine corpus, urinary bladder, or rectum) or metastases from other organ sites (such as the ovary, uterus, or other visceral organs).

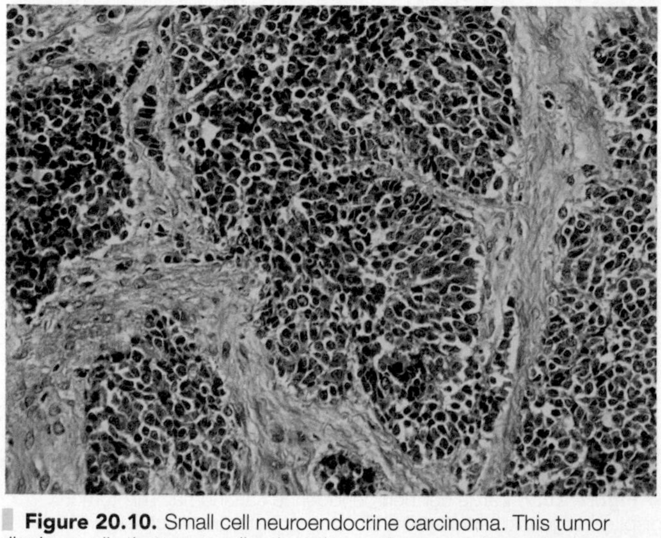

Figure 20.10. Small cell neuroendocrine carcinoma. This tumor displays cells that are smaller than those of squamous carcinoma. Nuclei are large and atypical with molding of adjacent nuclei. There is a very high mitotic rate.

UTERINE CERVIX CANCER PROGNOSTIC FACTORS

Surgicopathologic Factors

A prospective 732-patient surgicopathologic study (1981 to 1984) of untreated stage I squamous cell uterine cervix cancer evaluated prognostic factors and cancer outcome (48,49). The protocol stipulated radical hysterectomy, pelvic and paraaortic transperitoneal lymphadenectomy, and peritoneal cytology. Gross primary tumors were associated more often (85 [21%] of 477) with pelvic lymph node metastases than occult primary tumors (15 [9%] of 168, $p = 0.009$). Three-year disease-free survival estimates were 95% for occult tumors, 88% for tumors ≤3 cm, and 68% for tumors >3 cm.

In the same study, a risk of pelvic lymph node metastases was associated with the depth of invasion in fractional thirds more so than absolute tumor size in millimeters—5% for inner third (9 of 199), 13% for middle third (28 of 210), and 26% (60 of 227) for outer third ($p = 0.0001$). Three-year disease-free survival estimates were 94% for inner third, 85% for middle third, and 74% for outer third invasion. Lymphovascular space invasion is associated with risk of pelvic lymph node metastasis, as 25% (70 of 276) of positive invasion cases had nodal metastases versus 8% (30 of 366) when invasion was absent. Three-year disease-free survival was 77% in positive lymphovascular space invasion cases and 89% in negative cases. Invasion of the parametria by uterine cervix cancer was associated with risk for pelvic lymph node metastases. When present, 43% (194 of 44) of cases had pelvic lymph nodes with metastases. When absent, 14% (81 of 599) of cases had pelvic lymph nodes with metastases.

Age at diagnosis is the least dramatic significant factor contributing to risk of lymph node metastases (48), and loses more significance when 50 years is used as an arbitrary breakpoint (49). Following an example of a moderately differentiated uterine cervix cancer with middle third invasion and no lymphovascular space or parametrial invasion, the expected probabilities of lymph node metastases in women aged 35, 45, 55, or 65 years are 9%, 8%, 5%, and 3%, respectively (48).

Lymph Node Factors

Lymph node metastasis from uterine cervix cancer has long been identified as a major prognostic factor, with surgical and radiotherapeutic management decisions partially based on the risk for nodal disease. Six (3%) of 177 patients with ≤5 mm invasion had pelvic lymph node metastases, the lowest risk of nodal disease in a surgicopathologic study (48). Sixteen (22%) of 74 patients with uterine extension had pelvic lymph node metastases (48). Well, moderately, and poorly differentiated tumors had risk for pelvic lymph node metastases of 10% (9 of 93), 14% (52 of 373), and 22% (39 of 179), respectively (48); 545 patients with no pelvic node metastases had a 3-year disease-free interval estimate of 86%, while 100 patients with positive pelvic node metastases had a 3-year disease-free interval estimate of 74% (49). A larger number of removed pelvic node metastases did not correlate with a poorer prognosis, as the 3-year disease-free intervals were 72%, 86%, and 65% for one, two, and three or more positive pelvic nodes, respectively (49). Despite the significant impact of nodal status on prognosis, nodal metastasis is not included in the FIGO staging system.

Clinical Stage Factors

Clinical stage has been found to be a weak risk factor in an era where radiographic and pathologic information are more powerful prognostic factors. A multivariate analysis of prognostic variable among 626 women included in therapeutic clinical trials did find correlated clinical stage and progression-free interval (130). This retrospective study involved 150 patients who received radiation therapy alone, 136 patients who received radiation therapy and

Corynebacterium parvum, 156 patients who received radiation therapy plus misonidazole, and 184 patients who received radiation therapy and hydroxyurea. Paraaortic lymph node metastases were associated with sixfold risk for death and 11-fold risk for short progression-free interval (130). The investigators stated that with increased risk of node positivity, the distinction made by clinical stage falls. The investigators concluded that a combination of the most powerful risk factor (node status) with the most commonly used risk factor (clinical stage) presents a clear separation of patients in regard to uterine cervix cancer survival (130).

Histopathology Factors

In a study from the United States Military Health Care System, 185 women with adenocarcinoma and 88 women with adenosquamous carcinoma were studied for clinical outcomes. Adenosquamous histopathology was associated with a significantly decreased 5-year survival (65% vs. 83%; $p < 0.002$). In a 243-patient randomized clinical trial of radiation alone versus radiochemotherapy, histopathology lost its prognostic significance when chemotherapy was added (131). Among 182 women with adenocarcinoma or adenosquamous cancer treated by cisplatin radiochemotherapy, survival was not lower than the survival seen for 842 women with squamous cell cancer (132).

Hypoxia and Anemia Factors

Among 494 women treated on two consecutive prospective radiation therapy trials, 278 (56%) had stage II and 216 (44%) had stage III or IV disease. After adjusting patient age, race, performance status, cancer stage, tumor size, cell type, and duration of radiation, mean hemoglobin values during treatment were found to predict disease progression ($p < 0.0001$). Pretreatment values were not predictive of disease progression. When a 6-week treatment course was divided into 2-week periods (early, middle, and late), hemoglobin values during the late period were the most predictive of disease progression ($p = 0.0289$). Review of translational science confirms the same (133).

Anemia affects patterns of relapse and survival in women with uterine cervix cancer (134), and packed red blood cell infusions are recommended. Recombinant human erythropoietin has been used to stimulate red blood cell production and maintain hemoglobin levels above 12 g/dL. In a trial (135), women with stage IIB–IVA uterine cervix cancer and an initial hemoglobin less than 14 g/dL were randomly assigned to radiochemotherapy without or with recombinant human erythropoietin (40,000 units s.c. weekly). Erythropoietin was stopped if hemoglobin was greater than 14 g/dL. The study closed prematurely, with less than 25% of the planned accrual, due to thromboembolic events attributed to erythropoietin. Median follow-up was 37 months. Three-year progression-free and overall survivals were estimated at 65% and 75% after radiochemotherapy and at 58% and 61% after radiochemotherapy plus erythropoietin, respectively. Thromboembolic events occurred in 4 (8%) receiving radiochemotherapy and 11 (19%) receiving radiochemotherapy plus erythropoietin. All thromboembolic events were not treatment related. No deaths occurred from thromboembolic events. A second line of evidence deterring use of erythropoietin is from an 18-patient (1999 to 2002) surgicopathologic study. Erythropoietin receptor expression was found in 16 (89%) of 18 uterine cervix cancers (136), suggesting the possibility that erythropoietin agents might stimulate growth of uterine cervix cancer cells. As such, packed red blood cell infusions, not erythropoietin, are recommended to correct anemia in uterine cervix cancer patients.

Smoking may lead to tissue hypoxia. In a trial that randomized 328 women to cisplatin–radiation or to 5-FU–radiation, 133 (42%) were reported smokers of any kind and 111 (40%) were smokers of nicotine-based products (137). In a multivariate analysis, a significant increase in the risk of death (but not disease progression) was seen for reported smokers (hazard ratio [HR], 1.51; 95% CI, 1.01 to 2.27, $p = 0.04$) and for tobacco-derived smokers (HR, 1.57; 95% CI, 1.03 to 2.38, $p = 0.04$). The biologic mechanism of this phenomenon is still under investigation.

Uterine Cervix Cancer Biomarkers and Imaging Correlates

Uterine cervix cancer biomarkers are under investigation (**Table 20.4**), including ribonucleotide reductase subunit expression (138).

PET scans have been studied as imaging correlates in uterine cervix cancer trials. PET has 75% sensitivity and 92% specificity (96). Posttherapy FDG-avid uptake (persistent or new) is negatively associated with metabolic treatment response, developing metastatic disease, and death from uterine cervix cancer (139–141). Consensus recommendations for use of PET as an indicator of therapeutic response have been put forward (142)—a >25% increase in FDG standard uptake value indicates progressive metabolic disease, a ≤25% increase or a <15% decrease in FDG standard uptake value indicates stable metabolic response, a >15% reduction in FDG standard uptake value indicates partial metabolic response, and complete absence of FDG standard uptake value indicates complete metabolic response (143). In the modern era of radiotherapy, FDG responses >15% are seen in nearly all cases, and thus, makes use of FDG PET imaging to assess uterine cervix cancer response after radiotherapy challenging (99). A 51-patient radiochemotherapy study evaluated more rigorously a "true" metabolic response if a patient's posttherapy: pretherapy uptake ratio was ≤0.33 and found that this cutoff was more meaningful in assessing treatment response (99). A prospective phase II radiochemotherapy trial found that a posttherapy: pretherapy uptake ratio of ≤0.33 occurred in 96% (23 of 24 [95% CI, 80% to 90%]) of treated radiochemotherapy patients (101) and none has had local relapse.

Dynamic contrast-enhanced MRI (DCE-MRI), diffusion-weighted MRI (DWI-MRI), or MRI may be a useful biomarker for response to therapy, recurrence, and overall survival. Serial MRI scans before, during, and after radiation therapy were obtained in 115 women (144). Residual MRI volumes of 20% or more detected at 4,000 to 5,000 cGy were independently associated with inferior 5-year local control (53% vs. 97%, $p < 0.001$) and disease-specific survival rates (50% vs. 72%, $p = 0.009$). After all radiation delivery, patients having residual MRI volumes of 10% or more had no local control and a 17% disease-specific survival, compared with 91% local control and 72% disease-specific survival when less than 10% of tumor volume remained ($p < 0.001$).

General Management and Results of Treatment

Severe Dysplasia and Carcinoma *In Situ*

Women with CIN 2 or 3 or carcinoma *in situ* have no risk of lymph node metastases, and thus, are often treated by conization, loop diathermy, cryotherapy, simple hysterectomy, or rarely intracavitary brachytherapy. These techniques have similar efficacy.

In a 1,121-patient case series of carcinoma *in situ* (1951 to 1975), therapeutic conization was completed in 795 women, with only 19 (2%) recurrent carcinoma *in situ* cases and only 7 (1%) invasive cancer cases observed in follow-up (145). In this same study, therapeutic hysterectomy was performed in 238 women with only 3 (1%) recurrent carcinoma *in situ* and only 5 (2%) invasive cancers observed during follow-up. Therapeutic outpatient fine loop diathermy under local anesthesia (1988 to 1989) was done in 557 women, with 506 (91%) having normal cytology and 19 (3%) having persistent CIN at 6 months posttherapy (87). For seven low-morbidity surgical techniques used in 23 trials, there has been no obviously superior surgical technique for treating CIN (146). Conization is preferred to ablative procedures when endocervical curettage reveals malignant-appearing cells (147), when adenocarcinoma *in situ* is present (148), or when colposcopy is unsatisfactory. Uterus-sparing low-morbidity procedures might have adverse effects such as cervical stenosis, predisposition to preterm labor in subsequent pregnancies, persistent vaginal discharge, and possible infertility.

Cryotherapy

Cryosurgery involves use of a liquid nitrogen-containing probe fitting in the endocervical canal to cool abnormal cells to below −20°C and destroy abnormal tissues by forming an "ice-ball." In a retrospective study of 37,142 women treated for CIN 1, 2, or 3 (1986 to 2004) from the British Columbia Cancer Agency cytology database (149), cryotherapy was associated with the highest rate of posttherapy persistent or recurrent disease as compared to all other low-morbidity procedures (adjusted odds ratio for invasive cancer = 2.9, 95% CI = 2.1 to 4.6). For more conservative management of CIN, cryotherapy might be considered reserved for low medical resource practices.

Intracavitary Brachytherapy for the Poor Surgical Candidate

Women with CIN have almost no risk for metastases to pelvic lymph nodes, thus intracavitary brachytherapy is a treatment option when the patient is a poor surgical candidate. In a limited 21-patient case series (1959 to 1986), a disease control rate of 100% was reported with no significant adverse events (150). The average radiation dose to point A was 4,612 cGy and to the surface of the cervix 9,541 cGy.

Clinical Stage IA

Stage IA1 (or microinvasive) uterine cervix cancer has a 5% or lower risk of lymph node metastases or relapse and has been managed by surgical techniques ranging from cold knife conization to radical hysterectomy with a near 100% rate of disease control (109). Postsurgical confirmation of lymphovascular space invasion in a conization specimen may prompt definitive hysterectomy and lymphadenectomy (109). Technetium-99 and blue dye labeling for lymph node mapping was associated with high rates of sentinel lymph node detection, 92% sensitivity, and 98% negative predictive value for metastasis detection (151).

Stage IA2 uterine cervix cancer has a 5% to 13% chance association with pelvic lymph node metastases. Low-morbidity surgeries are not used often, deferring to modified radical hysterectomy and selective pelvic lymphadenectomy as standard. Sentinel node dissection is under investigation (151). Parametrial invasion remains a surgical planning concern in stage IA2 patients (152), as even limited parametrial invasion confers a high 43% risk for nodal metastases (48). Radical vaginal trachelectomy and extrafascial hysterectomy are being explored in those desiring fertility preservation.

Radical Vaginal Trachelectomy

A radical vaginal trachelectomy surgically removes the cervix, the upper part of the vagina, and pelvic lymph nodes. It is a two-step surgery. A pelvic lymphadenectomy is done first to exclude nodal metastases. If no nodal metastases are found, a trachelectomy is done. After completion of the trachelectomy, the uterus and vagina are reunited and a cerclage placed. The radical vaginal trachelectomy may be an option for younger women with small (≤2 cm in size) uterine cervix cancers who want to become pregnant (153,154). In a 137-patient case series (1994 to 2007), uterine cervix cancers had a median depth of invasion of 3 mm, lymphovascular space invasion present in 68%, and most (60%) were well differentiated (grade 1). After a median follow-up of 51 months, 5 (4%) developed a relapse for a 5-year recurrence-free survival estimate of 95% (153).

Intracavitary Brachytherapy for the Stage IA Poor Surgical Candidate

Women with stage IA have a 5% or less risk for metastases to pelvic lymph nodes, and so intracavitary brachytherapy is a treatment option when the patient is a poor surgical candidate. In a limited 34-patient case series (1959 to 1986), a 97% disease control rate was reported with a 6% rate of manageable adverse events (150). The average radiation dose to point A was 5,571 cGy and to the surface of the cervix was 10,430 cGy.

Nonbulky Clinical Stage IB–IIA

Clinical stage IB describes lesions confined to the uterine cervix, and is dichotomized into nonbulky IB1 (≤4 cm) or bulky IB2 (>4 cm) cancers. Nonbulky clinical stage IB1 and IIA uterine cervix cancers can be cured by radical surgery or by radiation therapy with similar effectiveness. Radical surgery offers an opportunity to study histopathologic factors for optimal risk group assignment. The 5-year survivals after surgery range from 83% to 92% (50,155). Radiation therapy is reasonable and effective in nearly all clinical stage IB to IIA patients, as 5-year survival after radiation therapy ranges from 83% to 91% (50,155). Patient health, tumor features, and clinical patterns of care influence treatment of choice.

Radical hysterectomy has been performed by abdominal, vaginal, laparoscopy and robot-assisted approaches. Since salpingo-oophorectomy is not part of a routine radical hysterectomy, surgical removal of the ovaries is based on a woman's age and other clinical factors such as menopausal status and medical illness—the rate of ovarian metastasis from uterine cervix cancer is less than 0.5% (156). A radical trachelectomy may be an option for young women with ≤2 cm uterine cervix cancers who desire future pregnancy (154).

Both radiation therapy and surgery are active against nonbulky uterine cervix cancer, and have been compared in a randomized trial among women with clinical stages IB to IIA cancer (50). In that study (1986 to 1991), radiation therapy involved two-field or more external pelvic radiation to deliver a median total dose of 4,700 cGy (range 4,000 to 5,300 cGy). After 2 weeks, one ^{137}cesium low dose rate (LDR) insertion was done to raise the point A dose to a median 7,600 cGy (range 7,000 to 9,000 cGy). Positive lymph node metastases had boosts of 500 to 1,000 cGy. In the same study, radical surgery involved a class III radical abdominal hysterectomy and lymphadenectomy. Adjuvant radiation therapy was given to surgical patients who had at least one risk factor—that is, surgical stage > pT2a, <3 mm of uninvolved cervical stroma, cut-through positive surgical margins, and presence of lymph node metastases. Adjuvant radiation involved the same multiportal field design and a total dose of 5,040 cGy to the pelvic-only fields. Extended-field paraaortic fields received 4,500 cGy when lymph node metastases were detected at surgery. Sixty-four percent (108 of 169) of the randomized radical hysterectomy group underwent adjuvant radiation; 5-year estimates for overall and disease-free survival were 83% and 74%, respectively, and did not differ significantly between the radiation therapy and radical hysterectomy groups (50). For patients whose tumors were ≤4 cm, the 5-year disease-free survival rate was 82% after radiation and 80% after surgery. For patients whose tumors were >4 cm, the 5-year disease-free survival rate was 57% after radiation and 63% after surgery. Between-group differences by tumor size were not significant. Among all patients, 86 (26%) patients developed relapse: 42 (25%) after surgery and 44 (26%) after radiation. Of the 86 patients with relapse, 50 (58%) patients had local or pelvic relapse—22 (52%) after surgery and 28 (64%) after radiation therapy ($p = 0.42$). Severe grade 2 or 3 morbidity was significantly higher in the surgery group (28%) as compared to the radiation therapy group (12%, $p = 0.0004$). The investigators concluded that there was no superior treatment of choice for nonbulky uterine cervix cancer (50).

Postoperative Node-Negative Patients with Intermediate-Risk Factors for Relapse

Postoperative pelvic radiation has been assessed in a randomized trial (1988 to 1995) of 277 women with clinical stage IB uterine cervix cancer with negative lymph nodes but also must have had two or more features including more than one third stromal invasion, lymphovascular space invasion, and tumor diameter ≥4 cm (**Table 20.5**) (157). Radical hysterectomy was required in all patients. For those randomized to radiation, a pelvis-only four-field box delivered 4,600

TABLE 20.5. Gynecologic Oncology Group Protocol 092 Eligibility Criteria

Lymphovascular Space Involvement	Cervix Stromal Invasion	Tumor Size
Positive	Deep 1/3	Any
Positive	Middle 1/3	≥2 cm
Positive	Superficial 1/3	≥5 cm
Negative	Deep or middle 1/3	≥4 cm

cGy to 5,040 cGy. No brachytherapy was done. Local and distant relapse rates were 21% and 9% after surgery and 14% and 3% after adjuvant radiation, respectively. A significant 46% reduction in the hazard for relapse (0.54, 95% CI, 0.35 to 0.81, $p = 0.007$) and 42% reduction in the hazard for progression-free survival (0.58, 95% CI, 0.40 to 0.85, $p = 0.009$) were observed; 3-year progression-free and overall survival estimates were 85% and 88% after radiation and 70% and 82% after observation, respectively. A 7% rate of grade 3 or above gastrointestinal complications was reported. The investigators concluded that radiation therapy is an option for women with node-negative stage IB uterine cervix cancer with two or more pathologic risk factors. There is currently an open randomized phase III trial by the Gynecologic Oncology Group trial (GOG 0263) evaluating the role of chemoradiation versus radiation alone in intermediate-risk, stage I/IIA cervical carcinoma with high-risk features as above.

Postoperative Patients with High-Risk Factors for Relapse

Indications for adding chemotherapy to adjuvant radiation include positive lymph nodes, parametrial invasion, or positive surgical margins (158). In a 243-patient trial (1991 to 1996), women who had IA2, IB, or IIA uterine cervix cancer initially treated with radical hysterectomy and lymphadenectomy and had positive pelvic lymph nodes or positive margins or parametrial invasion randomized to adjuvant radiation or adjuvant radiation plus chemotherapy. Radiation involved a pelvis-only four-field box delivered 4,930 cGy in 29 daily fractions; brachytherapy was not permitted. A paraaortic extended field was allowed for 4,500 cGy if high common iliac nodes were positive for metastases. Four cycles of chemotherapy were given, starting on day 1 of radiation therapy. One cycle included cisplatin (70 mg m^{-2}) by 2-hour infusion on day 1 and 5-fluorouracil (5-FU) (1,000 mg m^{-2}) as a 96-hour infusion over days 1 to 4. The third and fourth cycles began after radiation therapy, on days 43 and 64. Local and distant relapse rates were 9% and 10% after radiochemotherapy versus 22% and 16% after radiation alone, respectively ($p = 0.20$). A significant reduction in the hazard for progression or death (0.50) was observed, favoring radiochemotherapy ($p = 0.003$). A 16% rate of grade 3 or above gastrointestinal complications was reported. It was concluded that radiochemotherapy improved survival among women with early-stage uterine cervix cancer and postsurgical findings of positive pelvic lymph nodes, positive margins, or parametrial invasion. Later analyses suggested that clinical benefit arose most from adding chemotherapy among women with tumors >2 cm in diameter (+19%) or when two or more lymph nodes harbored metastases (+20%) (131).

Bulky Clinical Stage IB

Barrel-shaped bulky uterine cervix cancers were considered best addressed by hysterectomy rather than by intracavitary radiation because of awkward anatomic geometry and inhomogeneous tumor hypoxia from expanded cell bulk (159,160). The increased central pelvis relapse rate in women with bulky tumors was reportedly greatly lowered by hysterectomy, but data for improved survival was lacking. A 256-patient clinical trial (1984 to 1991) in women with bulky, >4 cm, stage IB uterine cervix cancers underwent pelvis-only radiation and were randomized to a radiation-only arm or to a radiation–surgery involving extrafascial hysterectomy (161). Two- or four-field external beam radiation therapy delivered 4,000 cGy in the radiation-only arm and 4,500 cGy in the radiation–surgery arm. Intracavitary brachytherapy prescribed to point A delivered 4,000 cGy in the radiation-only arm and 3,000 cGy in the radiation–surgery arm. Two to six weeks after radiation, extrafascial hysterectomy with removal of the fallopian tubes and ovaries and not contiguous parametrial tissue was done. Local and distant relapse rates were 35% and 15% in the radiation-only arm as compared to 17% and 19% in the radiation–surgery arm. No survival benefit was observed. Grade 3 or above gastrointestinal adverse events occurred in 6% of radiation-only patients and in 7% of radiation–surgery patients. The investigators concluded that extrafascial hysterectomy was of limited clinical benefit to women with bulky, >4 cm, stage IB uterine cervix cancers.

A second trial (1992 to 1997) studied 369 women with bulky ≥4 cm stage IB uterine cervix cancers randomly partitioned into radiochemotherapy plus hysterectomy versus radiation-only plus hysterectomy treatment arms (162). All patients underwent extrafascial hysterectomy 3 to 6 weeks after completion of radiation. A pelvis-only four-field box delivered 4,500 cGy; LDR brachytherapy delivered 3,000 cGy to point A. Cisplatin was infused once weekly at a 40 mg m^{-2} dose, for a maximum of six doses. Grade 3 or 4 gastrointestinal adverse events were 5% in the radiation–surgery arm and were 14% in the radiochemotherapy–surgery arm (162). Local and distant relapse proportions were 24% and 18% in the radiation–surgery arm and were 11% and 13% in the radiochemotherapy–surgery arm (163). At surgery, there were more radiochemotherapy patients (52%) with no microscopic residual cancer than radiation-only patients (42%). This finding likely confounded the observation of improved 5-year progression-free (76% vs. 60%) and overall (80% vs. 66%) survival estimates favoring radiochemotherapy. There was no significant difference in survival (HR, 0.89). Hysterectomy substituting for additional brachytherapy seemed to obscure results and the investigators suggested that a clinical benefit of adjuvant hysterectomy was doubtful (162,163).

A 288-patient trial randomly allocated women with bulky, ≥4 cm, stage IB uterine cervix cancers to neoadjuvant cisplatin–vincristine chemotherapy followed by radical hysterectomy or to radical hysterectomy alone (164). About half of all patients received postoperative radiation therapy for adverse risk factors persistent at the time of surgery. From this study, there was no evidence that this form of neoadjuvant chemotherapy provided clinical benefit in the bulky, ≥4 cm, stage IB uterine cervix cancer population.

Clinical Stages IIB, IIIB, and IVA

Radiochemotherapy is standard for women who have clinical stage IIB, IIIB, and IVA disease (**Table 20.6**). This is in due part to the observation that radiation therapy alone provides 5-year survival rates of 60%, 45%, and 30% for clinical stage IIB, IIIB, and IVA disease, respectively (165). The role of chemotherapy in the treatment of advanced-stage disease has been established in landmark clinical trials, with clear gains in survival benefit (up to +15% or more) seen over the past 25 years (166 to 176). Regardless of biologic mechanism, radiochemotherapy has been under intense clinical study. Cisplatin protracts repair of radiation-induced DNA damage (177), enhancing radiation-induced cell kill (32). Hydroxyurea, 5-FU, and gemcitabine interfere with DNA precursor supply by ribonucleotide reductase (178), and these drugs successfully have added to cisplatin–radiation effects (168,170,171,175). Tirapazamine undergoes one-electron reduction in hypoxic cells and elicits single-strand and double-strand DNA breaks (179), but was not found to be clinically useful (176).

Coadministration of weekly cisplatin during radiation therapy lowers the relative risk of relapse and death from disease by nearly 40%

TABLE 20.6. Randomized Radiochemotherapy Trials for Advanced-Stage Uterine Cervix Cancer

Trial	Clinical Stage	No.	RT Ctrl Agent	RT Exp Agent	Relapse HR[a]	p	3-Year OS	Reference
GOG-004 (1970–1976)	IIIB-IVA	190	Placebo	Hydroxyurea 80 mg kg^{-1} q3d	NR	<0.05	24% vs. 30%	(166)
Roswell Park (1977–1986)	IIIB	45	Placebo	Hydroxyurea 80 mg kg^{-1} q3d	NR	0.06	50% vs. 58%	(167)
RTOG 90-01 (1990–1997)	IIB, III, IVA or IB/IIA >5 cm LN+	388	Extended-field radiation	Cisplatin 75 mg m^{-2} q3wk 5-fluorouracil 4 g m^{-2} q3wk	0.48 (0.35–0.66)	<0.001	64% vs. 75%	(168)
GOG-85 (1986–1990)	IIB, III, IVA	368	Hydroxyurea 80 mg kg^{-1} q3d	Cisplatin 50 mg m^{-2} q3wk 5-fluorouracil 4 g m^{-2} q3wk	0.79 (0.62–0.99)	0.03	58% vs. 68%	(170)
GOG-120 (1992–1997)	IIB, III, IVA	526	Hydroxyurea 3 g m^{-2} q3d	Cisplatin 40 mg m^{-2} qwk	0.57 (0.42–0.78)	<0.001	48 v. 68%	(171)
			Hydroxyurea 3 g m^{-2} q3d	Cisplatin 50 mg m^{-2} q3wk 5-fluorouracil 4 g m^{-2} q3wk Hydroxyurea 2 g m^{-2} q3d	0.55 (0.40–0.75)	<0.001	48% vs. 68%	(171)
NCIC (1991–1996)	IIB, III, IVA or IB2/IIA >5 cm or LN+	253	pelvis-only, radiation, brachytherapy	Cisplatin 40 mg m^{-2} qwk	0.91 (0.62–1.35)	0.43	66% vs. 68%	(173)
GOG-165 (1997–2000)	IIB, III, IVA, paraaortic LN−	316	Cisplatin 40 mg m^{-2} qwk	5-fluorouracil 1125 mg m^{-2} qwk	1.25 (0.90–1.74)	>0.05	68% vs. 62%	(174)
Eli-Lilly (2002–2004)	IIB, III, IVA, paraaortic LN−	515	Cisplatin 40 mg m^{-2} qwk Gemcitabine 125 mg m^{-2} qwk	Cisplatin 40 mg m^{-2} qwk Gemcitabine 125 mg m^{-2} qwk+ Cisplatin 50 mg m^{-2} q3wk Gemcitabine 1 gm^{-2} d1,8 q3wk ×2 adjuvant cycles	0.68 (0.49–0.95)	0.02	70% vs. 78%	(175)
GOG-219 (2006–2009)	IIB, IIIB, IVA or IB2/IIA >4cm, paraaortic LN−	379	Cisplatin 40 mg m^{-2} qwk	Cisplatin 75 mg m^{-2} q3wk Tirapazamine 220 mg m^{-2} qwk	1.05 (0.75–1.47)	0.79	71% vs. 71%	(176)
GOG-123 (1992–1997)	IB2 (>4 cm)	369	Pelvis-only, radiation, extrafascial, hysterectomy	Cisplatin 40 mg m^{-2} qwk + same	0.51 (0.34–0.75)	0.001	76% vs. 84%	(162)
GOG-109 (1991–1996)	IA2, IB, IIA, LN+ margin+ para+	243	Radical hysterectomy, pelvis-only, radiation	same + Cisplatin 70 mg m^{-2} q3wk 5-fluorouracil 4 g m^{-2} q3wk+ ×2 adjuvant cycles	0.50 (0.29–0.84)	0.01	78% vs. 88%	(158)

[a]Hazard ratio with 95% confidence interval.

Ctrl, control; Exp, experimental; GOG, G Oncology Group; HR, hazard ratio; LN, lymph node; No., number; NCIC, National Cancer Institute of Canada; NR, not reported; OS, overall survival; Para, Parametria; RT, radiation therapy; RTOG, Radiation Therapy Oncology Group.

in women with advanced-stage uterine cervix cancer, compared with radiation therapy alone. Most disease progression and cancer-related death events are observed within the first 2 years after therapy, and the hazard falls to near zero after that interval making 3-year endpoints most relevant. Durable evidence from four randomized clinical trials confirms an advantage of cisplatin-based radiochemotherapy (131,163,169,170). All of the trials listed in **Table 20.6** share problems in logistics and in cross comparison. When taken in sum, trials indicate weekly cisplatin is standard for women with uterine cervix cancer who require radiation therapy.

One of two molecular changes relating to ribonucleotide reductase are found in uterine cervix cancers—cells have become addicted to HPV-related dNDP overproduction or mutated *p53* allows work-arounds to cell cycle restriction checkpoints (43). All four trials showing reduction in relapse and death are rooted in mitigating ribonucleotide reductase DNA precursor payout (178). Building on this notion, a promising series of triapine radiochemotherapy trials has been reported (100–102). Triapine blocks the M2/M2b subunit of ribonucleotide reductase, protracts cisplatin–radiation DNA damage, and increases uterine cervix cancer cell kill (31,32).

For 24 women with clinical stage II or III or with node-positive stage IB2 uterine cervix cancer (2006 to 2009), three times weekly triapine (25 mg m^{-2}) added to once weekly cisplatin (40 mg m^{-2}) and standard daily radiation resulted in a 3-year 96% pelvic disease control rate and 82% overall survival (102). Two (8%) cancer-related deaths occurred among these 24 women. No serious adverse events were encountered. A randomized phase II trial of triapine radiochemotherapy has begun (NCT01835171).

An alternative antiangiogenesis strategy has been studied to improve survival (180). Three-cycle bevacizumab (10 mg kg^{-1}) was added to once weekly cisplatin (25 mg m^{-2}) and standard daily radiation for treatment of 49 women with bulky stage IB or stage II–IIIB uterine cervix cancer. This phase II clinical trial (2006 to 2009) reported no serious adverse events. Three-year overall and disease-free survival estimates were 81% (95% CI, 67%–90%) and 69% (95% CI, 54%–80%), respectively. A 23% local relapse rate was noted, with six patients noted to have persistent disease at 12 months posttherapy. Bevacizumab radiochemotherapy warrants further primary therapy investigation.

Clinical Stage IIIA

Cervical carcinomas extending to the lower third of the vagina without pelvic sidewall extension or hydronephrosis are uncommon, representing only 3% of patients with uterine cervix cancer (181). A 5-year local control rate of 72% but survival rate of 37% was noted (181). Cisplatin-based radiochemotherapy is standard. Inguinal lymph nodes might harbor metastases, and should be irradiated prophylactically (4,500 to 5,040 cGy). Radiation dose can be escalated (>6,500 cGy) if inguinal lymph nodes are confirmed positive. Custom-designed radiation portals and intracavitary or interstitial brachytherapy are common (**Fig. 20.11**).

Clinical Stage IVB

Women with metastatic clinical stage IVB uterine cervix cancer, or even persistent or recurrent disease, have unmet therapeutic needs and quality of life assessments during chemotherapy. In a 284-patient randomized clinical trial with built-in quality of life study (182), 56% of enrollees died before or during the 9-month observation period. Cisplatin 50 mg m^{-2} is considered the most active drug with an up to 50% response rate (183). Bevacizumab 15 mg kg^{-1} has improved survival (184).

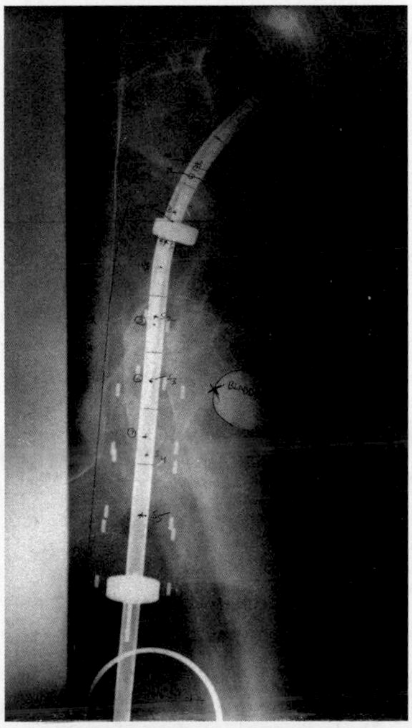

Figure 20.11. Lateral view of an intracavitary implant for a stage IIIA cervical carcinoma with extension to the lower third of the vagina. The tandem extends from the uterine fundus through the vagina. Delclos rings are placed over the tandem throughout its course in the vagina. This controls the distance from the radioactive sources (^{137}cesium in this case) and allows the vaginal radiation doses to be measured and controlled.

Cisplatin (cis-diamminedichloroplatinum II) as a single agent was evaluated in a 22-patient phase II clinical trial among women with advanced-stage or recurrent uterine cervix cancer (183). Cisplatin was administered as 50 mg m^{-2} over a 1 mg min^{-1} infusion every 3 weeks until adverse events precluded further treatment or disease progressed. Eleven (50%) of 22 women with no prior chemotherapy exposure had an objective response. Two (17%) of 12 women with prior chemotherapy treatment had an objective response. Median duration of response was 6 months. Adverse events included clinically significant leukopenia (3%), thrombocytopenia (3%), nausea or emesis (18%), and nephrotoxicity (10%). Three cisplatin dose schedules were tested in a 497-patient randomized trial (1978 to 1982): regimen 1 gave cisplatin 50 mg m^{-2} every 21 days, regimen 2 gave 100 mg m^{-2} every 21 days, and regimen 3 gave cisplatin 20 mg m^{-2} for five consecutive days repeated every 21 days (185). The regimens were tolerated, but with regimen 2 especially a 44% leukopenia rate and 14% nephrotoxicity rate was noted. Response rates were 21%, 31%, and 25% for regimens 1, 2, and 3 respectively; the response rate for regimen 2 versus regimen 1 was statistically significant ($p = 0.015$) but less than the magnitude initially considered clinically significant. The median duration of response was 5, 4, and 5 months for regimens 1, 2, and 3, respectively.

A cisplatin-paclitaxel combination has been evaluated in a 264-patient randomized clinical trial (1997 to 1999) of women with clinical stage IVB or persistent or recurrent uterine cervix cancer (186). Cisplatin (50 mg m^{-2}) was given as a 1 mg min^{-1} infusion every 21 days. Paclitaxel (135 mg m^{-2}) as a 24-hour infusion preceded cisplatin (50 mg m^{-2}) on day 1 of an every 21-day cycle. This was done to take advantage of possible G_1/S (cisplatin) and M-phase (paclitaxel) cell cycle–disrupting synergy among the agents. The 19% rate of response in the cisplatin-alone group was similar to the rate described in previous studies of cisplatin for metastatic uterine cervix cancer (range, 17%–31%). The addition of paclitaxel significantly increased the rate of response to 36% ($p = 0.002$), suggesting that paclitaxel introduces additional cytotoxicity in uterine cervix cancer. Grade 3 or 4 anemia (28% vs. 13%), thrombocytopenia (4% vs. 2%), and leukopenia (55% vs. 3%) were more common in the cisplatin–paclitaxel arm. The observation that nearly all patients eventually had disease progression and died within 2 years of treatment suggests an acquired resistance to a cisplatin-paclitaxel combination.

A cisplatin-topotecan combination has been tested in a 293-patient randomized clinical trial (1999 to 2002) of women with clinical stage IVB or persistent or recurrent uterine cervix cancer (187). Cisplatin (50 mg m^{-2}) was given as a 1 mg min^{-1} infusion every 21 days. Topotecan (0.75 mg m^{-2}) was given as a 30-minute infusion on days 1, 2, and 3 followed by cisplatin (50 mg m^{-2}) on day 1, repeated every 21 days. It was hypothesized that disruption of DNA replication forks by topotecan would slow DNA adduct repair and exacerbate cytotoxicity. The 13% response rate in the cisplatin-alone arm was lower than expected. Adding topotecan elevated the response rate significantly to 27% ($p = 0.004$), indicating synergy. Grade 3 or 4 thrombocytopenia (31% vs. 3%) and leukopenia (63% vs. 0.5%) were more common in the cisplatin-topotecan arm. Grade 3 or 4 anemia was similar (31% vs. 38%). All patients had disease progression and died within 3 years of study entry.

A trial of four cisplatin-containing doublets (2003 to 2007) randomized 513 women with clinical stage IVB or persistent or recurrent uterine cervix cancer to cisplatin-paclitaxel, cisplatin-vinorelbine, cisplatin-gemcitabine, or cisplatin-topotecan (188). Paclitaxel (135 mg m^{-2}) over 24 hours on day 1 preceded cisplatin (50 mg m^{-2}) on day 2 of an every 21-day cycle. Vinorelbine (30 mg m^{-2}) was given on days 1 and 8 plus cisplatin (50 mg m^{-2}) on day 1 every 3 weeks. Gemcitabine (1,000 mg m^{-2}) was infused on days 1 and 8 plus cisplatin

(50 mg m^{-2}) on day 1 every 3 weeks. Topotecan (0.75 mg m^{-2}) was administered on days 1, 2, and 3 plus cisplatin (50 mg m^{-2}) on day 1 every 3 weeks. The rates of response were 29% for cisplatin-paclitaxel, 26% for cisplatin-vinorelbine, 22% for cisplatin-gemcitabine, and 23% for cisplatin-topotecan. Grade 3 or 4 leukopenia was 63%, 68%, 43%, and 71% and grade 3 or 4 thrombocytopenia was 7%, 8%, 28%, and 35% for the cisplatin-paclitaxel, cisplatin-vinorelbine, cisplatin-gemcitabine, or cisplatin-topotecan regimens, respectively. None of the regimens was superior to cisplatin-paclitaxel, and trends for response, progression-free survival, and overall survival favored cisplatin-paclitaxel (188).

A two-by-two factorial design randomized clinical trial (2009 to 2012) of bevacizumab 15 mg kg^{-1} added to chemotherapy was completed in a 452-patient study (184). Chemotherapy consisted of cisplatin (50 mg m^{-2}) plus paclitaxel (135 mg m^{-2}), or cisplatin (50 mg m^{-2}) plus paclitaxel (135 mg m^{-2}) plus topotecan (0.75 mg m^{-2}). The rate of response was significantly higher for women who received bevacizumab (48%) than among those who did not receive bevacizumab (36%, $p = 0.008$). An added median survival of 3.7 months was observed (17.0 vs. 13.3 months, hazard ratio for death 0.71, 98% CI, 0.54 to 0.95). Gastrointestinal events (52% vs. 44%), fistula (6% vs. <1%), and neutropenia (35% vs. 26%) were observed. The observation that a cytostatic vascular endothelial growth factor-neutralizing antibody had an impact on overall survival in women with metastatic, persistent, or recurrent uterine cervix cancer was the most remarkable finding for this clinical trial.

Persistent or Recurrent Uterine Cervix Cancer

General Considerations

Uterine cervix cancer-related death occurs most often because of uncontrolled disease in the pelvis. Persistent disease after primary treatment or short-interval relapse of disease in the pelvis is often amenable to salvage surgery or radiation therapy; however, patient desire for treatment and selection of therapeutic intervention are often predicated on disease extent, disease-free interval, impact of prior therapy on pelvic anatomy, patient performance status, and patient comorbidities.

If curative salvage treatment is intended, a biopsy of the relapse and restaging radiographic imaging should be acquired. Sciatic pain, leg edema, and hydronephrosis are pathognomonic for pelvic sidewall involvement. PET may be the most accurate restaging test (189).

Radical Surgery for Pelvic Disease after Prior Radiation Therapy

Radical hysterectomy, not planned as part of initial care, has been used as a means of surgical salvage for small (<2 cm) persistent or recurrent uterine cervix cancers (190). But most often total pelvic exenteration has been performed for central pelvic relapses without evidence of extrapelvic disease, with up to one third of the procedures aborted at some point during the procedure. Exenteration operative time ranges up to 8 hours, average blood loss is 3L, and postprocedure hospital stay can be up to 23 days (191). Perioperative mortality rates are as high as 14% (192). Complications arise in up to 45% of patients (193), with bowel obstruction (22%), intestinal fistula (15%), and urogenital fistula (8%) as significant adverse events (191). In a 55-patient retrospective study (1998 to 2004), tumor-free exenteration surgical margin is associated with a 55% survival estimate, as compared to a 10% survival estimate when margins are positive for tumor (194). Overweight and obese women with recurrent disease undergoing exenteration experience longer operative times and higher wound separation rates than otherwise, but overall postsurgical survival appears equal to normal-weight women (195).

Pelvic anatomy reconstruction typically involves urostomy, colostomy, and muscle-flap neovagina. Diversion of urine flow by implanting the ureters into an isolated piece of ileum for a separate urostomy with bag reservoir is preferred over a wet colostomy involving implantation of the ureters into a colostomy diverting fecal flow (196). An ileal urostomy is incontinent. Continent internal reservoirs using bowel wall allow for self-catheterization, but are associated with a 50% to 65% rate of complication from pyelonephritis, ureteral stricture, leak or fistula, renal stone formation, and even rarely, renal failure (197–199). Muscle-flap reconstructions of a neovagina for sexual activity, pelvic tissue fill, and prevention of fistulas have been described (200–203).

Radical Radiation or Radiochemotherapy for Pelvic Disease after Prior Surgery

Small (<2 cm) persistent or recurrent disease, or vagina-only relapses are amenable to radiation therapy, with durable control exceeding 70% (204–206); 10-year survival estimates in radiotherapy-naive patients are as high as 35% (206). Interstitial brachytherapy (3,000 to 5,500 cGy) (207,208) and stereotactic body radiation therapy (2,400 cGy) (209) have been described for disease involving deep pelvic tissues. Use of carboplatin-gemcitabine chemotherapy and stereotactic body radiation therapy has been explored in a phase I trial (210).

For pelvic or paraaortic lymph node relapses after first-line surgery or radiochemotherapy, conventional radiochemotherapy (>4,500 cGy) (211) or stereotactic body radiation therapy (800 cGy × 3 doses) (209) have been used. Low toxicity and durable disease control rates exceeding 95% have been documented with either of these two techniques.

Intraoperative electron radiation therapy has been used during radical salvage surgery for persistent or recurrent uterine cervix cancer. The technique is attractive due to its direct exposure of at-risk tumor-harboring tissue to limited penetration electrons and because of its low radiation dose scatter to normal tissues retracted away or shielded during dose delivery. A single fraction of 1,500 cGy (range 625 to 2,500 cGy) was used most often in a case series of 86 patients (1983 to 2010) (212). Adverse events include peripheral neuropathy (19%), ureteral stenosis (5%), and bowel fistula or perforation (5%). Eleven (69%) of 16 women experiencing neuropathy after intraoperative radiation required long-term pain medication.

Chemotherapy and Biologic Targeted Agents for Persistent or Recurrent Uterine Cervix Cancer

Currently, chemotherapy and biologic targeted agents for persistent or recurrent uterine cervix cancer falls into a palliative role. These therapies may prolong 6-month progression-free survival in up to 24% of patients (213). However, there are no randomized trials that compare best supportive care against chemotherapy or biologic targeted agents to show that these therapies improve overall survival. Women with relatively good performance status are often presented with chemotherapy or biologic targeted agent treatments. Regimens used are discussed in the chemotherapy section of this chapter.

UNUSUAL CLINICAL SITUATIONS

Node-Positive Early-Stage (Operable) Cervical Carcinoma

Should the Hysterectomy Be Completed?

When lymph node metastases are detected and positive by clinical imaging or by surgical staging, should a completion hysterectomy be done? A surgicopathologic study evaluated 1,127 women with clinical stage IB uterine cervix cancers (214). At the time of surgery, 98 (9%) women were found to have extrauterine disease and the operation aborted at the discretion of the operating surgeon. Cited reasons for stopping the planned operation included extrapelvic disease (30) or pelvic extension (26), grossly positive pelvic lymph nodes (12), other pelvic tissue implants (8), and gross serosal extension (2).

Radiation therapy including brachytherapy was mostly done. The disease-free interval and overall survival was short at 10 months and 17 months, respectively, for abandoned-operation patients. Among the abandoned-operation patients, those with extrapelvic disease had the shortest progression-free interval and survival, and those with direct pelvic extension the longest progression-free interval and survival.

Evidence to conclude that completing a radical hysterectomy improves the outcome is otherwise limited and possibly detrimental (215) and may increase the risk of adverse side effects. Disadvantages of a completion radical hysterectomy include delay in starting radiochemotherapy, increasing morbidity, and duplication of local treatment when a single modern radiochemotherapy regimen would suffice. Leaving a uterus intact provides an appropriate conduit for intracavitary brachytherapy and probably lessens radiation-related bowel complications by preventing the bowel from resting in the low pelvis. It may be that the compromise, having the surgeon resect or debulk grossly positive pelvic lymph nodes and surgically stage paraaortic lymph nodes but abort the radical hysterectomy to preserve the brachytherapy conduit, is a treatment choice optimizing overall patient care. Postoperative radiochemotherapy would start soon after convalescence.

Should Bulky Pelvic Lymph Nodes Be Debulked?

Should a surgeon resect or debulk grossly positive pelvic lymph nodes? Case series reports indicate that a local pelvic control benefit has been observed when lymph nodes are removed (216,217), but since node positivity increases the hazard for occult distant organ metastases, a survival benefit seems unlikely. As mentioned above, debulking and staging nodal surgery with minimally invasive procedures that also preserve the uterus for brachytherapy may be an optimal compromise for overall care of a patient with bulky pelvic lymph nodes.

Should Invasive Uterine Cervix Cancer Be Treated by Simple Hysterectomy?

A simple hysterectomy may have been done for benign, CIN, carcinoma *in situ*, or even occult microinvasive disease of the uterine cervix. Whether to do additional second-look surgery or completion surgery to complete a classic radical hysterectomy remains debated. It is common practice that if only microinvasive carcinoma is found and there is no evidence of lymphovascular space invasion, no additional surgery is needed. However, in clinical situations where indicators for greater than microinvasive disease are present, the simple extrafascial abdominal hysterectomy is not satisfactory because parametrial soft tissue, vaginal cuff, and pelvic lymph nodes are not removed. Radical parametrectomy has been done in an attempt to complete radical surgery; rates of pelvic relapse are 7% or less after radical parametrectomy (218). Adjuvant radiation therapy for inadvertent invasive cancer discovered after simple hysterectomy, rather than additional surgery, has been done. In that clinical situation, a reported disease-free survival of 83% at 5 years posttherapy has been reported (219). Standard postoperative radiation doses (4,500 cGy–5,040 cGy) are recommended.

Guidelines suggest that inadvertently discovered clinical stage 1A1 uterine cervix cancer patients with no lymphovascular space invasion undergo surveillance whereas those with lymphovascular space invasion undergo radiation therapy (220). Inadvertently discovered clinical stage 1A2 or higher uterine cervix cancer patients should undergo completion surgery inclusive of parametrectomy, upper vaginectomy, and pelvic lymphadenectomy with paraaortic node sampling (220). Additional clinical decisions for radiation or radiochemotherapy are made based on surgicopathologic findings.

Small Cell Carcinoma of the Uterine Cervix

Small cell carcinomas of the uterine cervix are rare and share an oncologic phenotype with their counterparts in the lung. In one case series (221), 10 patients had IB1 disease (although two had radiographic nodal metastases) and 11 patients had stage IB2 to IIIB disease. Six patients underwent radical hysterectomy (five were stage IB1) and 15 patients had curative intent radiation therapy. Cisplatin-based chemotherapy was administered to 62% of patients, either neoadjuvantly or adjuvantly with or after radiation therapy. No patient whose initial clinical stage was higher than IB1 survived. Relapses in the radiation portals were uncommon, but elsewhere relapses were common. Many practitioners approach small cell carcinoma of the cervix like the lung variant, providing cisplatin-etoposide radiochemotherapy to pelvic disease followed by prophylactic cranial irradiation for complete responders (222). The 3-year survival rate after cisplatin-etoposide radiochemotherapy was 28%.

Extranodal Lymphoma of the Uterine Cervix

Extranodal lymphomas of the uterine cervix are rare and not typically detected by Pap cytology. B-cell lymphomas are most common. As with other lymphomas, involved-field radiochemotherapy offers best clinical outcomes (223). Standard chemotherapy regimens include cyclophosphamide, doxorubicin, vincristine, prednisone at doses, and schedules typical of non-Hodgkin lymphoma therapy. Rituximab has been added to this regimen to treat uterine cervix lymphoma (224), but use of rituximab is not yet considered mainstream. A role for radical or debulking surgery remains to be clarified (223), but in general is not indicated.

Sarcoma of the Uterine Cervix

Primary sarcomas arising in the uterine cervix are exceedingly rare. Radical hysterectomy or radiochemotherapy has been effective in patients with localized pelvic disease (126).

Uterine Cervix Stump Cancer

A prior supracervical hysterectomy has been performed in up to 7% of uterine cervix cancer patients (225). In one radiation therapy case series (226), the average time between supracervical hysterectomy and stump cancer diagnosis was 27 years. External beam radiation plus intracavitary brachytherapy prescribed to a typical point A dose resulted in 10-year progression-free survival rates of 100%, 100%, 79%, 100%, 66%, and 39% in clinical stages 0, IA, IB, IIA, IIB, and IIIB, respectively. Intracavitary brachytherapy can be tricky (**Fig. 20.12**). Tandem and ovoid brachytherapy applicators have reduced tandem lengths with the uterine fundus removed, limiting applied radiation dose to typical point A dose prescription points. Customized external beam radiation therapy and brachytherapy are commonplace in order to obtain relatively accepted radiotherapeutic goals.

Radiation Therapy Alone When Chemotherapy Cannot Be Administered

In a clinical situation where radiation therapy alone is planned, a single randomized clinical trial offers guidance for field design and radiation dose. Between 1979 and 1986, 337 women with clinical stage IB or IIA disease and a tumor diameter >4 cm or clinical stage IIB uterine cervix cancers were randomized to pelvic field–only irradiation or to pelvic field plus extended-field paraaortic lymph node irradiation (227). The midplane pelvic radiation dose was 4,000 cGy to 5,000 cGy. Paraaortic radiation dose was 4,400 cGy to 4,500 cGy. Intracavitary brachytherapy delivered 3,000 cGy to 4,000 cGy to point A; 10-year survival rates favored the extended-field arm (55%) as compared to the pelvic-only arm (44%). The site of first failure occurring outside of the pelvis was lower in the extended-field arm (16%) as compared to the pelvic-only arm (23%). More patients experienced grade 4 (10 vs. 5) and fatal grade 5 (4 vs. 1)

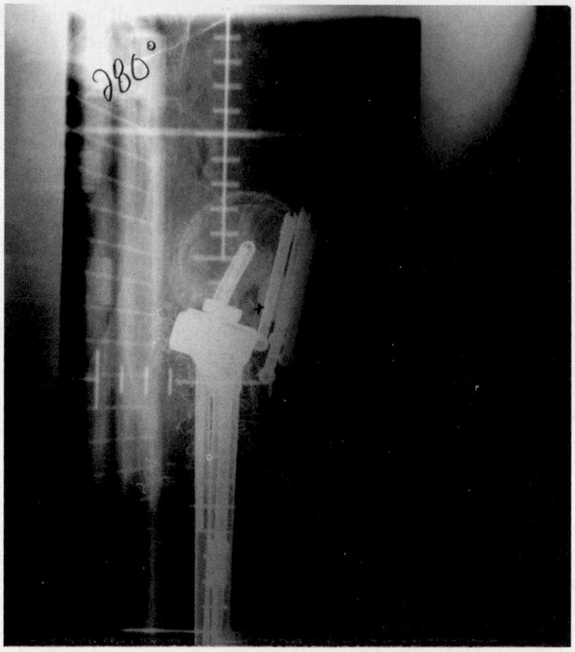

Figure 20.12. Approximately lateral view of intracavitary implant for a cervical stump carcinoma. The intrauterine length is only 2.5 cm, limiting the number of sources or source positions that can be placed into the uterus. The vaginal mucosa, anterior rectal wall, and bladder base will get relatively higher doses for an equivalent point A dose in most cases like this.

adverse events in the extended-field arm than in the pelvic-only arm. Abdominal surgery for any reason affected toxicity rates. In surgical patients undergoing extended-field radiation, the cumulative incidences of grade 4 or 5 toxicity were 9%, 11%, and 11% at 2, 5, and 10 years, respectively. In surgical patients undergoing pelvic-only radiation, the cumulative incidences were 2%, 2%, and 2% at 2, 5, and 10 years, respectively. The investigators concluded that the overall survival benefit of extended-field irradiation was explained by a lower incidence of distant relapse and better salvage in complete responders who later relapsed locally (227). Extended-field radiochemotherapy has not been compared to pelvis-only radiochemotherapy.

MANAGEMENT OF UTERINE CERVIX CANCER DURING PREGNANCY

Clinical Disease during Pregnancy

Of all women diagnosed with CIN or worse, less than 1% (0.1%) developed invasive cancer during pregnancy (228). Abnormal Pap cytology or abnormal vaginal bleeding had been observed in 9% of pregnant women (228). Use of an endocervical brush is safe. Curettage is not recommended, as risk for premature rupture of membranes is high. A 7,253-patient cohort study in Finland among women treated for CIN by cold knife or laser conization, cryotherapy, or loop diathermy between 1974 and 2001 found that treatment raised the risk for premature delivery—median duration of pregnancy was shorter in treated women than a reference population in Finland (229).

Clinical Diagnosis during Pregnancy

Any abnormal lesion of the uterine cervix during pregnancy necessitates a biopsy of the lesion. Colposcopy can be performed safely through the 20th week of pregnancy (230). Among 612 pregnant women, a colposcopy-directed biopsy was performed safely without complication in 449 women (73%), whereas 91 (15%) women did not have biopsies because of normal colposcopy and 72 patients (12%) had either CIN 1 or 2. Inability to visually inspect the entire squamocolumnar junction is not an indication to proceed to conization during pregnancy, as most repeat colposcopy procedures will be satisfactory because of squamocolumnar junction eversion as pregnancy progresses.

Management of Dysplasia during Pregnancy

Of dysplasia cases identified during pregnancy, up to 70% regress and resolve completely in the postpartum observation period (231). Persistence of CIN into the postpartum period is as high as 47% (231). Progression of CIN to high-grade lesions occurs in up to 30% (231) and to invasive cancer in up to 11% (232). Overall, a conservative management approach is safe, involves colposcopy every 8 weeks, and results in definitive management in the postpartum period (232).

Conization during Pregnancy

Cold knife conization during pregnancy was associated with a 24% rate of first trimester fetal loss and 10% rate of second trimester fetal loss among 180 studied pregnant women (233). Conization followed by vasopressin injection, lateral hemostatic sutures, and cerclage was found to be safe and without complication in a case study of 17 pregnant women (234). In 14 of those cases, the endocervical and ectocervical margins were negative. Two pregnant women with CIN and one pregnant woman with multifocal invasive cancer had positive conization margins. There were no second trimester fetal losses. Arguments against cerclage use include that the cerclage may be a nidus for infection and that the majority of postconization fetal deaths are delayed presumably due to chorioamnionitis and not necessarily due to a function of cervical incompetence.

Loop diathermy has been studied in 20 pregnant women with gestational ages ranging from 8 to 34 weeks (235). Fourteen (70%) of those 20 pregnant women had dysplasia encompassed by the loop diathermy specimen. Eight (57%) of those 14 pregnant women had involved margins. Nine (47%) of 20 had persistent dysplasia 3 months postpartum (including three women whose initial specimens were negative). Three preterm births, two postprocedure blood transfusions following loop diathermy, and one unexplained fetal loss occurring 4 weeks postprocedure were documented. The gestational age range of those women with procedure-related morbidity was 27 to 34 weeks. The investigators concluded that loop diathermy during pregnancy did not yield consistent diagnostic specimens and was associated with a high procedural complication rate. As such, if conization is indicated for treatment of cancer during pregnancy, a second trimester cold knife conization technique may be the preferred method.

Adenocarcinoma *In Situ* and Microinvasive Disease during Pregnancy

During pregnancy, the uterine cervix might show an Arias-Stella reaction, a benign change in the endometrium associated with the presence of chorionic tissue. With a colposcope and in smear or liquid cytology, the reactive cells appear malignant and, used to be labeled cancer. AIS and microinvasive disease of the uterine cervix are difficult to assess and treat adequately during pregnancy. Management guidelines are the same as for nonpregnant women. Vaginal delivery should be safe in women with microscopic disease, and definitive management may be delayed safely until the postpartum period.

Invasive Cancer during Pregnancy

Surgery and Route of Delivery

More than 75% of uterine cervix cancers that develop in pregnancy present as stage I disease (236). Cancer stage, tumor size, lymph node status, gestational age, and a woman's desire to maintain a pregnancy are important factors contributing to therapeutic decisions and interventions. Surgical therapeutic options can be dichotomized by gestational age of <20 weeks or >20 weeks.

Invasive uterine cervix cancers found <20 weeks gestation in a pregnant woman most often are managed immediately, resulting in fetal loss. Delays in surgical intervention have ranged between 3 and 12 weeks for a woman suspected of having stage I disease (231). Patients choosing to delay definitive surgical treatment of stage I disease until after delivery may safely undergo appropriate surgical treatment, including radical hysterectomy. Blood loss and postsurgical febrile illness may be more common after radical hysterectomy in pregnant versus nonpregnant women (237).

For stage I disease, radical hysterectomy can be safely performed at a gestational age >20 weeks when fetal lung maturity is documented and a third-trimester cesarean section is planned (238). Vaginal trachelectomy with cerclage and lymphadenectomy has been performed in pregnant women with stage IB uterine cervix cancers <2 cm expressing a desire to preserve pregnancy and fertility (239). After 72 procedures in this patient population, 50 subsequent pregnancies were observed in 31 women. A total of 36 (72%) of those 50 pregnancies reached the third trimester. Among the 36 third-trimester pregnancies, 3 (8%) ended prematurely at <32 weeks gestation, 5 (14%) delivered between 32 and 36 weeks, and 28 (78%) delivered at term (>37 weeks).

In a matched case-control study, 56 women had uterine cervix cancer diagnosed during pregnancy and another 27 women had cancer diagnosed within 6 months postpartum (240). One (14%) of seven patients who underwent cesarean section developed a local and a distant disease relapse. In contrast, 10 (59%) of 17 who underwent vaginal delivery developed relapses ($p = 0.04$). In multivariate analysis, vaginal delivery was the most significant predictor of relapse (odds ratio [OR], 6.91; 95% CI, 1.45 to 32.8), followed by high stage (OR, 4.66; 95% CI, 1.05 to 20.8). The investigators cautiously concluded that cesarean section was a preferred route of delivery in pregnant women with uterine cervix cancer.

Radiation Therapy during Pregnancy

Therapeutic radiation exposure of 2,000 cGy or more alters uterine organ function and may impair the uterine corpus's ability to support gestation (241). Spontaneous miscarriage has been reported at 4,000 cGy (242), a radiation dose much lower than that needed to control uterine cervix cancers. When pregnant women desire to keep the pregnancy, radiation therapy should be delayed until the postpartum period. For women desiring therapeutic intervention, surgery or chemotherapy is preferred.

Neoadjuvant Chemotherapy during Pregnancy

Neoadjuvant chemotherapy in a pregnant woman with uterine cervix cancer has been considered depending on gestational age, desire to maintain the pregnancy, cancer stage, lymph node status, and cancer histology. Cancer histology affects therapeutic decisions greatly. For instance, small cell carcinoma is associated with a very poor prognosis and termination of pregnancy in deference to treatment is considered most strongly (243). Conventional histopathologies including squamous cell, adenocarcinoma, and adenosquamous may be managed without pregnancy termination (243).

The European Society of Gynecological Oncology task force "Cancer in Pregnancy" has published recommendations for the successful management of invasive cancer during pregnancy (244). Multidisciplinary teams should avoid iatrogenic prematurity and aim for term delivery. Most standard regimens of chemotherapy can be administered from 14 weeks gestational age onward. Neoadjuvant platinum-based chemotherapy in pregnant women with uterine cervix cancer appears feasible and safe for both the mother and infant in limited case series (245–247).

Human Immunodeficiency Virus and Uterine Cervix Neoplasia

The United States Centers for Disease Control and Prevention (CDC) designated invasive cancers of the uterine cervix as an AIDS-defining illness in 1993 (248). HIV infection has a significant impact on HPV infection and the course of HPV-related disease. The CDC reports that HIV has infected 1,218,400 persons older than 13 years, taking account of 156,300 (13%) persons unaware of their HIV infection (249). Women accounted for 20% of new incident cases of HIV infection in 2010, became infected by heterosexual contact (84%) or by injection drug use (16%), and comprise 23% of those living with HIV infection in 2011 (249). HIV-infected women have an increased HPV prevalence (36%) and an increased risk of multiple concurrent HPV genotype infections (250).

Preinvasive Disease Prevalence and Risk of Progression

Compared to their HIV-uninfected counterparts, HIV-infected women have increased overall prevalence and persistence of high-risk HPV, multiple genotype infections, higher relative prevalence of nonvaccine oncogenic HPV genotypes, increased risk for progression of cervical neoplasia caused by HPV, and an increased risk of invasive cancer of the uterine cervix (250,251).

The Women's Interagency HIV Study (WIHS) begun in 1994 follows 2,056 HIV-positive and 569 HIV-negative women at six sites in the United States (251). In the WIHS cohort, women with the highest prevalence of HPV coinfection were those with a CD4 count of $<200\ mm^{-3}$ regardless of HIV viral load. When CD4 counts were $>200\ mm^{-3}$, a higher prevalence of HPV coinfection was found among women with an HIV viral load >20,000 copies/mL versus those with HIV viral load of <20,000 copies/mL. The lowest HPV coinfection rate was found in those women with a CD4 count $>500\ mm^{-3}$ and HIV viral load <4,000 copies/mL. High-risk HPV genotypes (18, 31, 33, 45, 51, 52, 56, 58, 59 >16) were observed at a threefold or higher rate in HIV-infected women as compared to non–HIV-infected women. HIV-infected women had a 36% rate of having two or more HPV coinfections.

A second prospective cohort study (1994 to 1999) tracked 1,639 HIV-seropositive and 452 seronegative women (252). Regardless of HIV-related immunosuppression, the likelihood of spontaneous regression of uterine cervix dysplasia was reduced among HIV-infected women. In marked contrast to other HIV-related neoplasms (i.e., Kaposi sarcoma and non-Hodgkin lymphoma), extreme immunosuppression is not necessary to see increases in invasive uterine cervix cancer in HIV-infected women. Indeed, most invasive cancers arise in women with CD4 counts $>200\ mm^{-3}$ (253).

Uterine Cervix Dysplasia Screening in HIV-Infected Women

Pap smears and liquid cytology are important tools in uterine cervix dysplasia screens despite controversies in overall test reliability. Women in the prospective HIV Epidemiology Research Study (HERS, 1993 to 1995) were monitored for uterine cervix dysplasia as one of the study endpoints (254). Among 189 HIV-infected women examined during 478 visits, 143 biopsies (30%) showed CIN. Of these, 8 (6%) were CIN II or CIN III disease. Among 95 HIV-uninfected women examined during 141 visits, 18 (13%) biopsies revealed CIN, and 2 (11%) were CIN II or CIN III disease. The investigators concluded that there was no difference in the accuracy of the Pap test by HIV infection status (254). According to USPSTF recommendations, women with HIV infection should undergo semiannual screening in the first 12 months after diagnosis, and then annually if the results are normal (53). If any abnormality is detected, then closer follow-up and colposcopy examination are warranted.

HPV Subtype Cotesting in HIV-Infected Women

Given the high prevalence of HPV in HIV-infected women, clinical triage of HPV cotesting was shown to be successful, but of unclear predictive or prognostic value (255). Obtaining HPV cotests during the first two Pap screens after a woman's initial HIV infection diagnosis may be cost-effective and informative. But, there is no consensus regarding HPV cotesting in HIV-infected women, and the best recommendation is to individualize cotesting need according to identified risk factors.

Vaginal Pap Cytology after Hysterectomy in HIV-Infected Women

HIV-infected women in the aforementioned HERS study had a 63% incidence of squamous intraepithelial lesions (SIL) after hysterectomy when evaluated by postsurgical vaginal Pap cytology (256). When CD4 counts were <200 mm^{-3} and HIV viral loads were $>10{,}000$ copies/mL, SIL vaginal cytology was seen most commonly. Of 102 HIV-infected women studied, 16 (16%) had biopsy-proven vaginal intraepithelial neoplasia. The high rate of SIL and vaginal intraepithelial neoplasia prompted the investigators to recommend vigilant surveillance of the lower genital tract by vaginal Pap cytology.

Effects of Highly Active Antiretroviral Therapy on Cancer Risk in HIV-Infected Women

Partial immune reconstitution afforded by highly active antiretroviral therapy (HAART) has reduced mortality and morbidity in HIV-infected women and has lowered rates of AIDS-associated cancers (Kaposi sarcoma and non-Hodgkin lymphoma). The impact of HAART on uterine cervix dysplasia and cancer has been equivocal. Registry data (1980 to 2004) on 499,230 HIV-infected AIDS patients spanning the pre-HAART and HAART eras were linked to 15 US cancer registries (253). The investigators observed among women with AIDS a standardized incidence ratio of 8.9 (95% CI = 8.0 to 9.9) for uterine cervix *in situ* and invasive cancer. In these women with AIDS, a relative risk per decline of 100 CD4 T cells per cubic millimeter was 1.32 (95% CI = 0.96 to 1.80; $p = 0.077$), indicating an increased risk for *in situ* and invasive cancer. Findings were similar in a Swiss HIV cohort study (257).

Human Papilloma Virus Vaccination and Its Effect on HIV-Infected Women

The AIDS Clinical Trials Group protocol A5240 (2008 to 2011) tested the immunogenicity and safety of the quadrivalent HPV vaccine (types 6, 11, 16, and 18) in 319 HIV-infected women in the United States, Brazil, and South Africa, where cohorts were based on screening CD4 counts: >350 mm^{-3} (stratum A), 201 to 350 mm^{-3} (stratum B), and ≤ 200 mm^{-3} (stratum C) (258). In the study, the median CD4 count was 310 mm^{-3} and 40% had undetectable HIV viral loads. No safety issues were observed. Seroconversion proportions among women at week 28 after administration for HPV types 6, 11,16, and 18 respectively were 96, 98, 99, and 91% for stratum A; 100%, 98%, 98%, and 85% for stratum B; and 84%, 92%, 93%, and 75% for stratum C. The investigators suggested that the quadrivalent HPV vaccine was safe and immunogenic in HIV-infected women aged 13 to 45 years. But, it was noted that women with viral loads $>10{,}000$ copies/mL or CD4 counts <200 mm^{-3} had lower seroconversion rates.

Treatment of Uterine Cervix Dysplasia in HIV-Infected Women

In HIV-infected women, CIN regressed to normal in 30% of cases (259). Immune-mediated regression may be observed with CD4 counts >500 mm^{-3} and HAART therapy may also contribute (259). For high-grade CIN, conization by cautery or by cold knife, or ablative cryotherapy or laser vaporization are adequate therapy when invasive disease has been excluded and satisfactory colposcopy has been documented.

Relapse is high in HIV-infected women. Loop diathermy was associated with relapse in 56% HIV-infected women versus 10% in HIV-uninfected women (260). The wide difference is an issue as 100% of HIV-infected women had positive loop diathermy margins as compared to only 32% of HIV-uninfected women.

Medical Therapy in HIV-Infected Women

A phase III unmasked clinical trial randomized 101 HIV-infected women either to receive 6 months of biweekly treatment with vaginal 5-FU cream (2 g) or underwent 6 months of observation after standard excisional or ablative uterine cervix treatment for CIN (261). In the trial, 38% of women developed recurrence—14 (28%) of 50 women in the 5-FU therapy group and 24 (47%) of 51 women in the observation group. 5-FU therapy was significantly associated with a lengthened time to positive CIN result. Observation patients were more likely to have high-grade recurrences, with 31% developing CIN II or III compared with 8% in the 5-FU treatment arm ($p = 0.014$). Disease recurred more quickly in observation patients. Baseline CD4 count related significantly to time to relapse, with 46% of patients with CD4 counts <200 mm^{-3} developing recurrence, versus 33% of patients with CD4 counts at least 200 mm^{-3}. Uterine cervix disease recurred more slowly in HIV-infected patients who had received antiretroviral therapy than in antiretroviral therapy–naive patients. There were no instances of grade 3 or 4 adverse events. 5-FU therapy compliance was satisfactory to the investigators.

Treatment of Invasive Cancer in HIV-Infected Women

The treatment of invasive uterine cervix cancer in HIV-infected women differs little from that for HIV-negative women. In a study from South Africa, 47 HIV-infected women (80%) and 291 HIV-uninfected women (90%) completed 6,800 cGy or more external beam radiation therapy and high dose rate (HDR) brachytherapy. Of the 333 women who underwent radiochemotherapy, 26 HIV-infected women (53%) and 212 HIV-uninfected women (75%) completed the anticipated four or more planned weekly cycles of platinum-based chemotherapy. More research studying treatment compliance and outcomes is needed.

SURGERY FOR UTERINE CERVIX CANCER

Surgical Hysterectomy Classification

Radical hysterectomy involves assessment of two important anatomic landmarks–the paravesical space and pararectal space. The relatively avascular paravesical space lies lateral to the bladder and is opened by surgical dissection underneath the insertion of the uterine round ligaments into the pelvic sidewall. The superior pubic ramus forms the anterior wall, the bladder and vagina bound the medial wall, the external iliac blood vessels and obturator fossa form the lateral wall, and the cardinal ligament encloses the posterior wall to distinguish this space from the pararectal space. The paravesical space can be continuous with the Retzius space found between the bladder and the pubic bone. The pararectal space lies between the ureter in the lateral aspect and the origin of the hypogastric artery in the medial aspect. The pararectal space follows the arc of the sacrum. The cardinal ligament bounds this space anteriorly, the hypogastric vessels laterally, the ureter medially, and the sacrum and levator muscles posteriorly. Descriptions for surgical hysterectomy classification are given in **Table 20.7**.

Class I: Extrafascial Hysterectomy

A class I extrafascial hysterectomy is the most common surgery for gynecologic illness. The procedure involves removal of the uterus

■ TABLE 20.7. Surgical Classifications for Hysterectomy

	Intrafascial	Extrafascial (I)	Modified Radical (II)	Radical (III)	Extended (IV)
Uterus	Removed	→	→	→	→
Uterine cervix	Partially removed	Completely removed	→	→	→
Uterine cervix fascia	Partially removed	Completely removed	→	→	→
Upper vagina	None	Small rim removed	Proximal 2 cm removed	Upper 1/3 to 1/2 removed	→
Bladder	Partially mobilized	→	→	Fully mobilized	Partially removed
Rectum	Not mobilized	Rectovaginal septum partially mobilized	→	Rectovaginal septum fully mobilized	→
Ureters	Not mobilized	→	Unroofed in ureteral tunnel	Completely dissected to bladder entry	Partially removed
Cardinal ligaments	Resected medial to ureters	→	Resected at level of ureter	Resected at pelvic sidewall	→
Uterosacral ligaments	Resected at cervix	→	Partially resected	Resected at sacral origin	→

by dissecting it from adnexal structures and round ligaments, separating it from the bladder at the vesicouterine fold and past the level of the cervix. Ligation of the uterine vessels at their insertion close to the cervicouterine junction is needed. Repeated application of surgical clamps along the uterine and cervical walls is needed as the parametria are separated. Removal is achieved with dissection of the uterine cervix off from the upper vagina, sparing as much of the vagina length as possible. The pubovesicocervical fascia is removed with the specimen. The open vagina is sewn closed with simple running or interrupted sutures. A class I hysterectomy is satisfactory treatment for high-grade CIN, carcinoma *in situ,* and clinical stage IA1 invasive cancers. Abdominal, vaginal, laparoscopic, or robot-assisted techniques are described.

Class II: Modified Radical Hysterectomy

A class II modified radical hysterectomy has gained popularity. The procedure involves opening and exploring the paravesical and pararectal spaces to determine ease of resection of the uterine cervix tumor with adequate negative surgical margins. This may be determined by index finger palpation of the paravesical space and by middle finger palpation of the pararectal space. Pelvic tissues bearing lymph nodes are felt for gross involvement. If determined to be amenable to surgical resection, the procedure moves forward to dissection of the uterine artery at its junction with the ureter. The bilateral ureters are partially dissected off the parametria and both tunneled to their bladder insertions. The bladder is peeled off the lower uterine segment past the uterine cervix. Parametrial tissue is extirpated medial to the two ureters. The ureterosacral ligaments are isolated and the proximal portions medial to the ureter are removed. A 2-cm margin of vagina is removed along with the uterine cervix. Pelvic lymphadenectomy accompanies the modified radical hysterectomy. A class II modified radical hysterectomy is carried out for small uterine cervix tumors (<2 cm), depending on surgical experience and preference. Abdominal, laparoscopic, or robot-assisted techniques are described.

Class III: Radical Hysterectomy

The class III abdominal radical hysterectomy distinguishes itself from the class II modified radical hysterectomy in its extent of parametrial resection. Paravesical space and pararectal space explorations are done as in the modified radical hysterectomy. Here, the uterine artery is ligated at its origin from the internal iliac (or hypogastric) artery. The ureters are tunneled fully to their insertion into the bladder trigone. The ureterosacral ligaments are isolated and tissue removed. The bladder is peeled off the anterior uterine cervix. The cardinal ligaments are resected to the pelvic sidewall and rectum mobilized to remove elements nearest the sacrum. The upper one third of vagina is removed, although this portion of the procedure may be tailored according to tumor size and the patient's pelvic anatomy. Pelvic lymphadenectomy and paraaortic node palpation and sampling are carried out. Abdominal, laparoscopic, or robot-assisted techniques have been routinely preformed; however, there are no cancer-related outcome data reported comparing these approaches.

Class IV: Extended Radical Hysterectomy

Indications for a class IV extended radical hysterectomy are few given availability of modern radiochemotherapy for advanced-stage uterine cervix cancers. The procedure involves all of the steps taken in a class III radical hysterectomy and adds complete dissection of the ureter off the vesicouterine ligament, ligation and removal of the superior vesicle artery, and removal of the upper three quarters of the vagina. Risks for bladder dysfunction and for fistula are much higher with this surgery than class I, II, or III hysterectomy. An open abdominal or robot-assisted operation is performed.

Class V: Extended Radical Hysterectomy or Pelvic Exenteration

A class V extended radical hysterectomy or pelvic exenteration follows all the steps of the class IV extended radical hysterectomy, but with removal of the distal ureter or bladder with reimplantation of proximal ureter into external or bowel conduits as needed. An open abdominal or robot-assisted operation is done. Only the bladder is removed in an anterior exenteration, and the rectum and anus are removed in a posterior exenteration.

New Classifications of Radical Hysterectomy

In 2008, new classifications for radical hysterectomy were put forward utilizing terminology based on lateral extent of surgical extirpation (262). There are four types listed, A through D.

Type A follows the class I extrafascial hysterectomy. In this surgery, the tissues around the uterine cervix are transected medial to each ureter and the uterine vessels are ligated at their cervicouterine union. A minimal vaginal margin is removed.

Type B follows the class II modified radical hysterectomy and involves surgical cuts through the parametria at the level of the ureter. Subtype B1 does not remove lateral paracervical lymph nodes. Subtype B2 includes lateral paracervical lymph nodes removal. The ureter is tunneled under the uterine artery and rolled to the lateral aspect. The parametria is then resected to the level of the rolled ureter. A 2-cm vaginal margin is taken.

Type C distinguishes itself from the class III radical hysterectomy. In the type C procedure, the parametria are removed at a more lateral margin next to the hypogastric vessels. Subtype C1 preserves nearby nerve bundles, while subtype C2 does not. Uterosacral ligaments are removed to the level of the rectum. The ureter is fully mobilized. Uterine vessels are ligated at their origin. The bladder branches of the hypogastric plexus near the bladder pillars are preserved.

Type D mimics the class IV extended radical hysterectomy and includes removal of the entire parametrial tissue. Subtype D1 involves parametrial resection with harvest of hypogastric vessels. Subtype D2 includes the steps in subtype D1, but adds greater removal of fascia and muscular structures. These are rare operations.

Alternative Operations for Uterine Cervix Cancer

Radical Vaginal Hysterectomy

A pelvic and paraaortic lymphadenectomy cannot be performed through the vagina, negating a radical vaginal hysterectomy for most cancer patients. With the introduction of minimally invasive laparoscopic or robot-assisted lymphadenectomy (263), radical vaginal hysterectomy has gained popularity as an oncologic surgical procedure, wherein the abdominal incision is omitted, thus quickening recovery.

A radical vaginal hysterectomy begins with a laparoscopic or robot-assisted lymphadenectomy. Both the paravesical space and pararectal space can be opened by laparoscopy or by robot-assisted procedures for exploration of the spaces and determination of surgical ease of uterine cervix tumor removal. A vaginal approach starts with outlining a 2-cm vaginal margin and its ringlike separation of the uterine cervix from the vagina. Vaginal mucosa folds over the uterine cervix and facilitates traction during downward removal of the specimen. The vesicouterine space is opened, bladder pillars are identified, and then ligated. The paravesical space is explored by digital dissection and the ureters are palpated. Uterine vessels are ligated at their origin from the hypogastric vessels. The pararectal space is opened and uterosacral ligaments are transected midway along their posterior expanse. Then, the ureters are moved laterally for parametrial tissue resection. The specimen is retracted downward and removed. The upper vagina is sewn closed in a typical fashion with delayed absorbable sutures.

Radical Trachelectomy

Abdominal, vaginal, and robot-assisted procedures have been described for radical trachelectomy (263). A radical trachelectomy begins with a laparoscopic or robot-assisted lymphadenectomy. The vaginal portion follows the radical vaginal hysterectomy except that the uterine fundus is retained. Amputating the uterine cervix at the level of the cervicouterine junction achieves the desired procedure—about 1 cm of cervix is left behind attached to the uterine fundus although some gynecologic oncologists prefer that all uterine cervix tissue is removed at surgery. Frozen section confirms margin-free status. A cerclage is fashioned at the cervicouterine junction and a probe opens any remaining endocervical canal. The pararectal space is closed and the upper vagina sewn to the uterine stump by interrupted sutures. Since cervix tissue might remain depending on the tailored surgical procedure done, Pap cytology and pelvic examinations are done per routine screening protocols.

Nerve-Sparing Radical Hysterectomy

A radical hysterectomy procedure can injure the hypogastric nerve plexus, disrupting bladder control and continence at a rate of 5%. Rectal incontinence also has been reported due to nerve injury. Nerve-sparing procedures have been described (264 to 266). A nerve-sparing procedure comprises avoiding the hypogastric nerve underneath the ureter lateral to the ureterosacral ligament and sidestepping the inferior hypogastric plexus during removal of the cardinal and the vesicouterine ligaments.

Total Pelvic Exenteration

Total pelvic exenteration has been completed in select clinical stage IVA uterine cervix cancer patients, but its main use is for management of central pelvic relapses without evidence of extrapelvic disease. Surgery includes *en bloc* removal of the uterine cervix, uterine corpus, bladder, rectum, and vagina. An anterior pelvic exenteration only removes the uterine cervix, uterine corpus, bladder, and vagina. A posterior pelvic exenteration only removes the uterine cervix, uterine corpus, rectum, and vagina. The procedure, tailored or not, is morbid—poor patient health, pelvic sidewall extension, hydronephrosis, and presence of extrapelvic metastases are contraindications to the procedure. Perioperative mortality occurs in up to 14% of surgical patients (192). Thorough radiographic imaging such as by PET is recommended to determine disease extent prior to surgery (267,268). Long-term sexual dysfunction and associated psychosocial impact must be considered by the patient and the surgeon before undertaking this procedure (269).

RADIATION THERAPY FOR UTERINE CERVIX CANCER

External Beam Radiation Therapy

Whole Pelvis Radiation

For a long time, the radiation dose target has been primary uterine cervix cancer and pelvic lymph nodes, whether involved or not by metastases (166,167). Radiation treatment fields or portals for the treatment of uterine cervix cancer were drawn arbitrarily using bony landmarks of vertebral spine interspaces or pelvic brim dimensions and possibly radiopaque markers for the uterine cervix, vagina, rectum, and bladder. Anteroposterior two-field or anteroposterior and lateral four-field treatment portals irradiate primary disease targets and node-bearing tissue. Intraoperative mapping done in 100 women undergoing radical surgery (270) found common iliac blood vessel bifurcation cephalad to the lumbosacral prominence in 87% of patients. As such, the superior border of anteroposterior portals is placed at the L4–L5 interspace to enclose external iliac and internal iliac (hypogastric) lymph nodes or is placed at the L2–L3 interspace to include common iliac lymph nodes. In the same study (270), pelvic width was 12 cm at the obturator fossae and 14 cm at the inguinal ring femoral arteries. Thus, the lateral border of anteroposterior portals is placed 2 cm lateral to the widest pelvic brim to ensure pelvic lymph node inclusion. The inferior border of anteroposterior portals is placed at the lowest extent of the obturator foramen, and at least 4 cm below the lowermost extent of uterine cervix disease. Lateral portals use the same superior and inferior border positions as in anteroposterior fields. The posterior border of lateral portals is placed behind the posterior aspect of the sacrum to ensure that the uterosacral and cardinal ligaments are entirely encompassed (270). The anterior border of lateral portals lies in front of the pubic symphysis inferiorly, and cuts in superiorly to limit bowel dose but maintains a 3-cm margin on the vertebral bodies so that iliac nodes are dosed appropriately. CT-based radiation therapy planning is standard nowadays (**Fig. 20.13**).

Groin Inguinal Lymph Node Radiation

For clinical stage IIIA uterine cervix cancer that involves the distal one third of the vagina, the radiation treatment portal must be widened in the low pelvis to enclose inguinal lymph nodes because of the increased likelihood of metastases. CT cross-sectional anatomy lends itself to measurement of nodal depth and adequate radiation dosing. Two-field radiation portals are commonly used to avoid

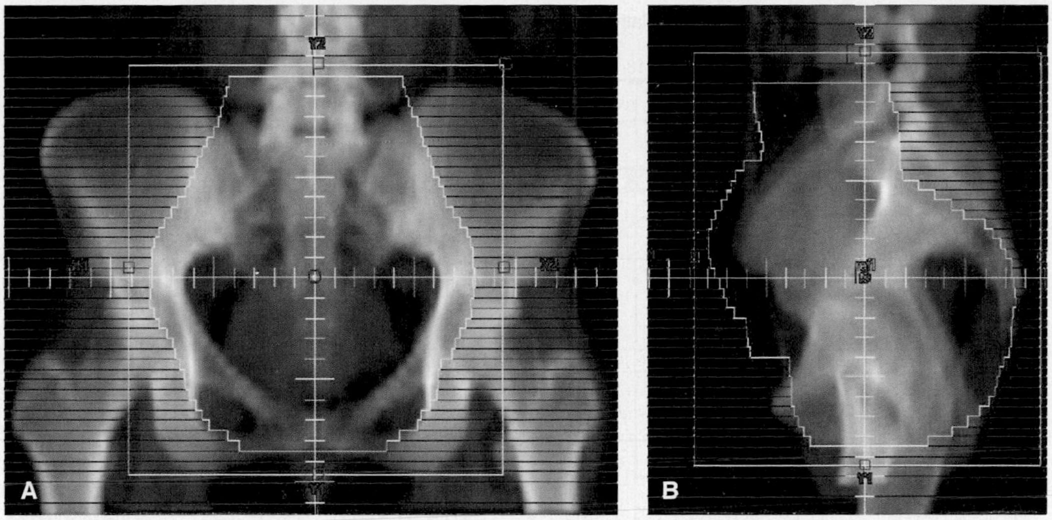

Figure 20.13. Standard fields for external beam whole pelvis radiation therapy. **A:** Anteroposterior port. **B:** Lateral port.

problems with underdosing and field junctions (271). Intensity modulated radiation therapy techniques have been described (272).

Midline Shield Use Prior to Brachytherapy

There is no consensus on the use of a 4 cm wide midline shield to protect the bladder and the rectum from excessive dose prior to brachytherapy (273). A midline shield has been used to block normal central pelvic tissues during a parametrial boost after a 4,500 cGy dose—a technique using standard two-field anteroposterior fields to boost radiation dose to pelvic sidewall lymph nodes (brachytherapy point B) while blocking midline anatomy. A midline shield places brachytherapy prescription point A on the shield edge. Practices introducing a midline shield at 3,000 to 4,000 cGy attempt to protect the bladder and the rectum from excessive delivered radiation dose prior to brachytherapy, realizing that disease is shielded. Proponents of an early shield argue that intracavitary brachytherapy dose provides sufficient make-up dose to sterilize central pelvic disease. Objectors of an early shield argue that central pelvic disease, once shielded, repairs, redistributes, reoxygenates, and repopulates uterine cervix cancer cells, essentially undoing therapeutic effects of already applied radiation dose.

Small Field Radiation

Radiation portals for occult postoperative disease or for intact disease have not varied much in 30 years because of high concern for central pelvic relapse of uterine cervix cancer. But, it has been suggested that in surgically staged node-negative patients, smaller than standard radiation portals might be useful and meaningful to lower radiation-related morbidity (274,275). Rather than small field radiation therapy portals, intensity modulated radiation therapy has become more commonplace.

Intensity Modulated Radiation Therapy for Uterine Cervix Cancer

Intensity modulated radiation therapy uses a multifield radiation beam arrangement with variable beam fluency to generate radiation dose clouds closely conforming to radiation targets. Radiation planning is CT-based. Magnetic resonance and PET image overlays are often used to ensure that targets are not missed due to precipitous radiation dose fall-off with the technique. Treatment machines might utilize "step-and-shoot" or "sliding-window" or helical tomotherapy or "volumetric-modulated arc therapy" to deliver the desired radiation dose. Anatomic atlases and contour guidelines are being defined, tested in clinical trials, and revised (272). An example of the intensity modulated radiation dose cloud is depicted in **Figure 20.14**. Dose–volume histograms plot the proportion of target volume or of an organ-at-risk volume planned to receive delivered dose over the course of the radiation prescription. Treating radiation oncologists use this information to balance sufficient delivery of radiation dose and hazard for organ injury. Intensity modulated radiation therapy often results in high target coverage by the prescription dose and low organ-at-risk exposure (**Fig. 20.15**).

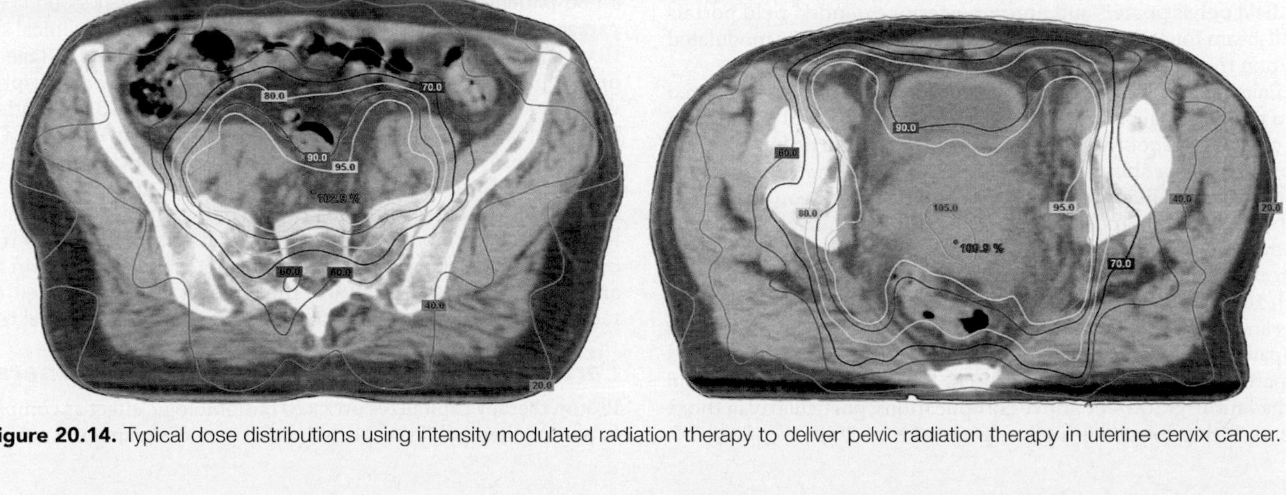

Figure 20.14. Typical dose distributions using intensity modulated radiation therapy to deliver pelvic radiation therapy in uterine cervix cancer.

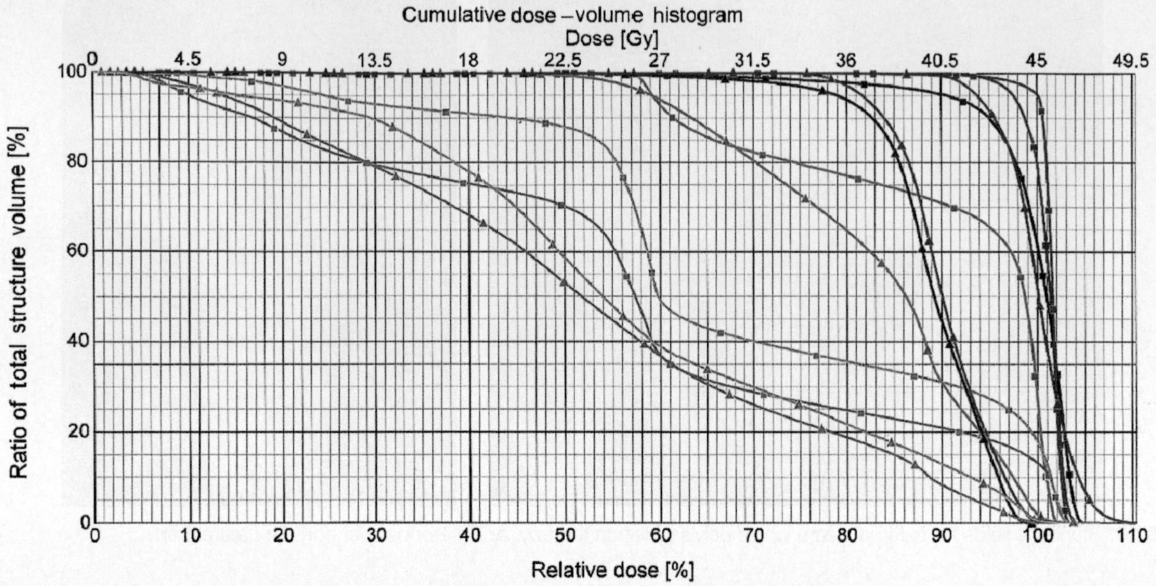

Figure 20.15. This dose–volume histogram (DVH) compares a four-field "box" arrangement *(squares)* with an intensity modulated radiation therapy plan *(triangles)*. The DVH plots doses to the planning target volume (PTV) and the organs at risk (OARs).

There are pitfalls that treating radiation oncologists must be aware of when using intensity modulated radiation therapy. Target and organ-at-risk motions due to respiration, bladder fill, and rectal fill have been documented (276). With applied radiation dose, central pelvic disease might regress such that intrapelvic target position rests outside the intensity modulated radiation therapy dose clouds (277). Clinical trials closely studying the use of intensity modulated radiation therapy in patients with intact uterine cervix cancers are needed. Consensus guidelines are emerging (272) and clinical experience grows (278,279). Early clinical experience suggests that gastrointestinal and marrow toxicities may be lower with intensity modulated radiation therapy (278,279).

Extended-Field Radiation Therapy for Uterine Cervix Cancer

Extended-field radiation therapy produces clinical benefit (227). Reluctance to use extended-field radiation portals centers on a perception of excessive radiation dose delivered to spinal cord, kidneys, and small intestine. Extended-field portals extend the superior border of pelvic radiation portals to include the 12th thoracic vertebral body. Anteroposterior two-field approaches are often done with differential weighting (70:30), but four-field variants are also used (**Fig. 20.16**). Modern techniques use half-beam matched pairs of four-field pelvis portals and anteroposterior extended-field portals or half-beam four-field pelvis portals matched to intensity modulated radiation therapy abdominal extended field.

Clinical stage IB, II, III, or IVA uterine cervix cancers are associated with a risk of paraaortic lymph node metastases in 5%, 21%, 31%, and 13% of cases, respectively (51). Hazard for paraaortic lymph node relapses has been shown to rise after pelvic field–only radiochemotherapy (169). Given orderly lymphatic dissemination of uterine cervix cancer, adjuvant extended-field radiation therapy is a logical treatment strategy that might avoid risks and delays associated with surgical staging of paraaortic lymph nodes. In a randomized trial (227), 10-year relapse rates in the pelvis were 35% for pelvic-only fields and 31% for extended fields. First sites of failure were distant (nonparaaortic metastases) more often in the pelvic-only arm as compared to the extended-field arm ($p = 0.05$). The extended-field arm had more grade 4 or above complications, particularly in those patients with prior abdominal surgery (11% vs. 2%).

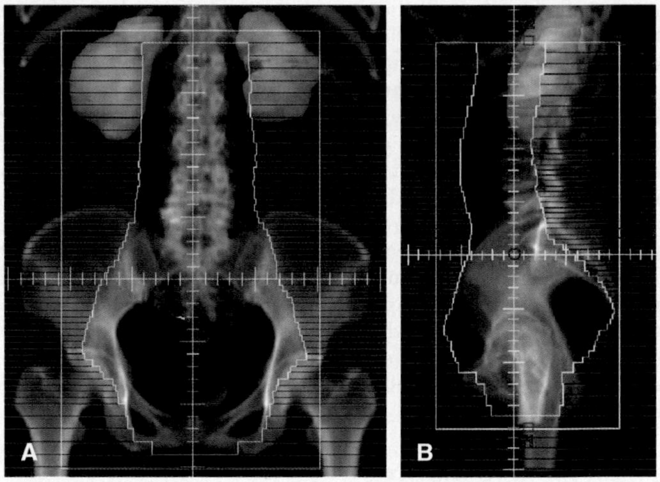

Figure 20.16. Portals of extended-field radiation therapy. **A:** Anteroposterior portal. **B:** Lateral portal. Yellow shadows indicate kidneys.

Extended-field radiochemotherapy has been delivered safely in an 86-patient clinical trial (280). Radiation involved 4,500 cGy to paraaortic lymph nodes in all, 3,960 cGy to the pelvis in clinical stage IB or IIB patients, and 4,860 cGy to the pelvis in clinical stage IIIB or IVA patients. Point A intracavitary brachytherapy prescriptions were 4,000 cGy in IB/IIB patients and 3,000 cGy in IIIB/IVA patients. Point B doses were raised to 6,000 cGy by parametrial boost. Chemotherapy involved cisplatin (50 mg m^{-2}) and 5-FU (4,000 mg m^{-2}) administered weeks one and five of radiation therapy. Grade 3 or above acute toxicities were mostly gastrointestinal (19%) or hematologic (15%). Late morbidity risk was 14% at 4 years for mostly rectal complications. Relapses were pelvis only in 21%, distant only in 21%, and pelvis plus distant in 11% of the patients. Other extended-field radiochemotherapy combinations are being tested in clinical trials.

Particle Beam External Beam Radiation Therapy

Proton therapy capitalizes on a x20 radiobiologic effect as compared to photon therapy. The reported use of particle beam external beam radiation therapy is extremely limited, with 25 patients treated in a single case series (281). Proton radiation therapy has been associated with a 10-year overall survival estimate and local control rate of 89% and 100%, respectively, for clinical stage IIB patients; 10-year overall survival estimate and local control rate of 40% and 61%, respectively, were seen for clinical stage IIIB or IVA patients; 4% of proton-treated patients had grade 4 or above late intestine or bladder complications at 5 years.

Uterine Cervix Brachytherapy

Brachytherapy refers to "short distance" radiation therapy. Uterine corpus and uterine cervix conduit anatomies lend themselves well to the placement of intracavitary applicators for high radiation dose delivery. ^{137}Cesium and ^{192}iridium are the most popular radioactive elements for LDR and HDR brachytherapy, respectively. Hollow afterloading intrauterine tandem and vaginal colpostats, rings, or cylinders are used in most brachytherapy practices. Interstitial implants possibly involve ^{137}cesium in intracavitary tandems and ^{192}iridium seed strings in peripheral needles, although ^{198}gold and ^{131}cesium have use. The American Brachytherapy Society provides guidelines for the practice of brachytherapy for advanced-stage uterine cervix cancer (282–284).

Intracavitary Brachytherapy Implants

Intracavitary brachytherapy implants usually accompany external beam radiation therapy treatments so that uterine cervix disease receives 8,000 cGy or more radiation dose. In early-stage disease, intracavitary brachytherapy implants may be used alone. LDR implants deliver radiation dose in rates measured by hours, whereas HDR implants are measured in minutes. LDR brachytherapy has been applied in uterine cervix cancer treatment from 1913 (285).

The Paris, Stockholm, and Manchester systems were developed around the same time to establish a set of standardized rules accounting for radioactive source strength and its geometry, application method, and duration of exposure. The three systems described an intrauterine component (tandem) and a vaginal applicator. Prescriptions were quantified in terms of milligram-hours, that is, the product of the total mass of ^{226}radium or radium equivalent (e.g., ^{137}cesium) contained in the sources, and the duration of the application in hours.

The Manchester system first used units of radiation exposure (Roentgens) rather than milligram-hours in radiation dose prescriptions. The dose in Roentgens was prescribed to specific points, termed point A and point B. Point A was defined as a point 2 cm lateral to the center of the uterine canal and 2 cm from the lateral vaginal fornix mucous membrane in the plane of the uterus. Point A served as a surrogate for average radiation dose delivered to the "paracervical triangle." Point B was defined as 5 cm lateral from the patient's midline at the same level as point A. Point B represented a surrogate for average radiation dose delivered to obturator lymph nodes. A variety of tandem and ovoid applicator loadings aimed for a relatively constant point A dose rate of 50 to 55 cGy/hour. The widely used Fletcher-Suit applicator system, loadings, and reference points A and B in US brachytherapy practices are all derived from the Manchester system.

Computer-assisted isodose curve determinations provide optimal means of point A, point B, bladder, and rectum radiation dose (**Fig. 20.17**). The International Commission on Radiation Units and Measurements (ICRU) Report No. 38 (ICRU-38) (286) defines radiation dose and volume specifications for the reporting of gynecologic intracavitary brachytherapy. ICRU-38 recommends that reference points such as point A not be used, because "such points are located in a region where the dose gradient is high and any inaccuracy in the determination of the distance results in large uncertainties in the absorbed doses evaluated at those points." Instead, ICRU-38 brought forth the concept of a 6,000 cGy reference volume (including the contribution of dose delivered by external beam treatment). A pear-shaped reference volume should be described in terms of its three dimensions according ICRU-38: height (maximum dimension along the intrauterine sources), width (maximum dimension perpendicular to the intrauterine sources), and thickness (maximum dimension perpendicular to the intrauterine sources in the oblique sagittal plane). Opponents of ICRU-38 reporting cite lack of rationale for a 6,000 cGy reference volume, leading to poor acceptance by brachytherapy practitioners (287). ICRU-38 bladder and rectal reference points are used.

Determination of the ICRU-38 bladder reference point involves the use of a Foley catheter placed in the bladder and the Foley balloon filled with 7 cm^3 of radiopaque fluid. On a lateral radiograph, the reference point is the posterior balloon surface. Overfill of the Foley balloon will lead to an underestimation of the bladder average dose and an overestimation of the bladder maximum dose. Underfill of the Foley balloon will lead to an overestimation of the bladder average dose and underestimation of the bladder maximum dose.

Determination of the ICRU-38 rectal reference point involves the use of a rectal marker or intravaginal radiopaque mold. On a lateral radiograph, the reference point is the anterior most point along the rectal marker closest to the uterine tandem or lies 5 mm posterior to the posterior aspect of an intravaginal mold or vaginal packing.

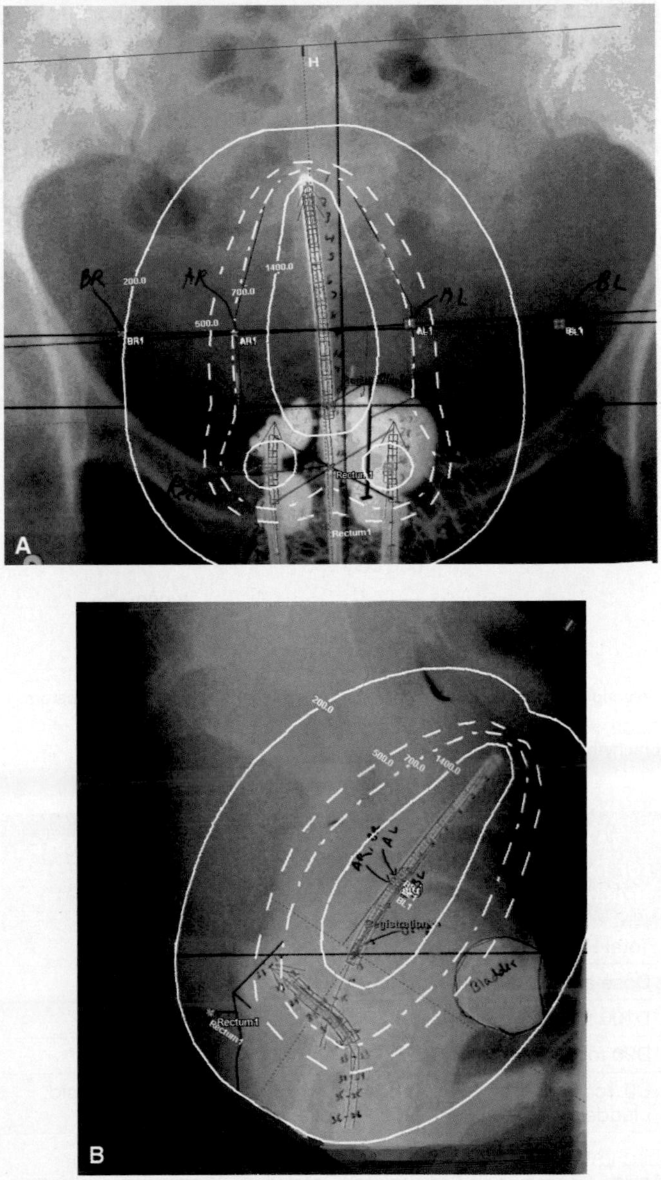

Figure 20.17. Axial **(A)** and **(B)** sagittal views of tandem and ovoids showing dose distribution superimposed on reconstructed CT images.

The first insertion of a LDR intracavitary implant occurs after 4,000 to 4,500 cGy of external beam radiation therapy. A prescription dose of 2,000 cGy is common, but might be raised for optimal geometry or might be lowered for suboptimal geometry. This is done to decrease lesion size and to improve applicator relationships of the uterine cervix and vagina. Midline shields are employed in some practices, as discussed earlier. A second insertion is performed 1 or 2 weeks later, with a prescription dose of 2,000 cGy or a dose needed to bring the total brachytherapy dose to 4,000 to 4,500 cGy most often. HDR implants are associated with a variety of radiation prescriptions (**Table 20.8**). A common practice involves five weekly insertions and a prescription of 600 cGy per fraction delivered to point A. HDR implants are scheduled in the fourth week of daily pelvic radiation. After completion of pelvic radiation, HDR implants might be given twice per week (3 days separating implants) so that all radiation is delivered within a total of 8 weeks.

Image-Guided Brachytherapy

Although an empiric point A prescription point has proven useful, better understanding of brachytherapy dose distribution using modern imaging techniques enables better radiation dose cloud coverage of tumor and delivery of less radiation does to normal organs. Guidelines (95,288) for image-based brachytherapy and its reporting have been written (**Table 20.9**). Investigators recommend T2-weighted MRI scans as the preferred method for scanning implant geometry. In an image-guided brachytherapy application, gross tumor volume (GTV), clinical tumor volume (CTV), and organs at risk (OAR) are contoured, allowing quantitative analysis of implant geometry through dose–volume histograms. In a 10-patient case series, MRI was similar to CT when contouring OARs, but CT overestimated uterine cervix tumor widths compared to MRI (289). Tumor width overestimates associated were adequate for contouring OARs. The investigators suggested that MRI was the preferred imaging modality for image-based brachytherapy since prescription doses were likely to be more accurate anatomically. Limited availability of MRI-compatible applicators and expense has slowed adoption of image-based brachytherapy. Recent studies and a consensus guideline have suggested that primarily CT-based planning can be sufficient for image-guided brachytherapy, although the addition of at least one MRI, with or without instrumentation, is informative in most patients (95,290).

TABLE 20.8. Suggested Schedules of HDR-ICBT in the United States

External Beam Radiation Therapy	HDR-ICBT (Point A)	EQD2 (Point A)
4,500 cGy in 25 fractions	700 cGy × 4	8,390 cGy
	600 cGy × 5	8,430 cGy
	550 cGy × 6	7,980 cGy
	500 cGy × 6	8180 cGy

Prescriptions intended for tandem and ovoid, or tandem and ring applicators.

EQD2, normalized dose; HDR-ICBT, high dose rate intracavitary brachytherapy.

TABLE 20.9. GEC-ESTRO Recommended Parameters for Recording and Reporting MRI Image-Guided Brachytherapy

Total Reference Air Kerma (TRAK)
Dose at point A (right, left, mean)
D100 for GTV, HR-CTV, and IR-CTV
D90 for GTV, HR-CTV, and IR-CTV
D0.1cc, D1cc, and D2cc for OAR (for example, rectum, sigmoid, bladder)

GEC-ESTRO, The Groupe Européen de Curiethérapie and the European Society for Therapeutic Radiology and Oncology; GTV, gross tumor volume; HR-CTV, high-risk clinical target volume; IR-CTV, intermediate-risk clinical target volume; MRI, magnetic resonance imaging; OAR, organ at risk.

Brachytherapy Dose Rate Considerations

Radiation dose rate impacts radiobiologic effectiveness (291). Conventional external beam radiation delivered by teletherapy machines deliver radiation dose at a rate ranging from 100 to 300 cGy/minute. Teletherapy radiation doses are fractionated. In contrast, brachytherapy doses can be delivered continuously or in fractions and over a much broader range of dose rates.

ICRU defines LDR brachytherapy as an exposure between 40 and 200 cGy/hour, medium dose rate brachytherapy as between 200 and 1,200 cGy/hour, and HDR brachytherapy as >1,200 cGy/hour. When dose rates are lowered, radiobiologic effects decrease due to enhanced sublethal DNA damage repair and cancer cell repopulation. Late-responding (slowly proliferating) tissues show enhanced sublethal DNA damage repair, while acute-responding (rapidly proliferating) tissues or cancers do not (33). During continuous LDR exposure, late-responding tissues show greater tolerance to radiation exposure. During HDR exposure, late-responding tissues show low tolerance to radiation exposure. Due to this phenomenon, HDR brachytherapy has a narrower therapeutic window than LDR brachytherapy. Because distance from a HDR source should be maximized to minimize effect on normal tissue, rectal retractors, vaginal speculums, and gauze packing are used in this technique. To allow easier access to the uterine cavity, cervical sleeves may be placed. Pulse dose rate brachytherapy provides a workaround of this radiobiologic phenomenon—hourly brief (5 minutes or so) exposures to HDR sources kill cancer cells but preserve late-responding tissues (292). Guidelines for pulse dose rate brachytherapy have been written (284). Isoeffective pulse dose rate brachytherapy has been reported (293,294). Local disease control rates and technique-related toxicity among LDR, pulse dose rate, and HDR brachytherapy techniques appear similar.

Interstitial Implants

Interstitial perineal implants are a treatment option when uterine intracavitary implants are not possible anatomically. Implants are planned and completed using a perineal template, such as the Syed-Neblett Interstitial Template (**Fig. 20.18**). Fluoroscopy or ultrasound aids in "straight" needle positioning during the procedure. Laparoscopy can be used to lower bowel perforation by deeply positioned needles. Interstitial brachytherapy may involve CT and magnetic resonance image fusion preplanning, operative placement of perineal needles using predetermined template maps, postprocedure CT-based planning, and afterloading therapy using ^{137}cesium and ^{192}iridium continuous LDR sources or ^{192}iridium HDR sources. Only experienced radiation oncologists should perform the procedure in centers familiar with the procedure.

Brachytherapy Radiation Doses for Uterine Cervix Cancer

American women with uterine cervix cancer often receive 4,500 cGy pelvic radiation for therapeutic intent prior to brachytherapy. LDR brachytherapy adds 4,000 cGy to point A over a single or two intracavitary insertions. A range in LDR brachytherapy dose has been accepted, with small <1 cm tumors receiving 3,000 cGy prescription doses while larger tumors receive 4,500 to 5,000 cGy prescription doses when normal anatomy permits.

An isoeffective HDR prescription dose may be 25% less than the typical LDR dose. A dose of 3,000 cGy in five equally divided 600

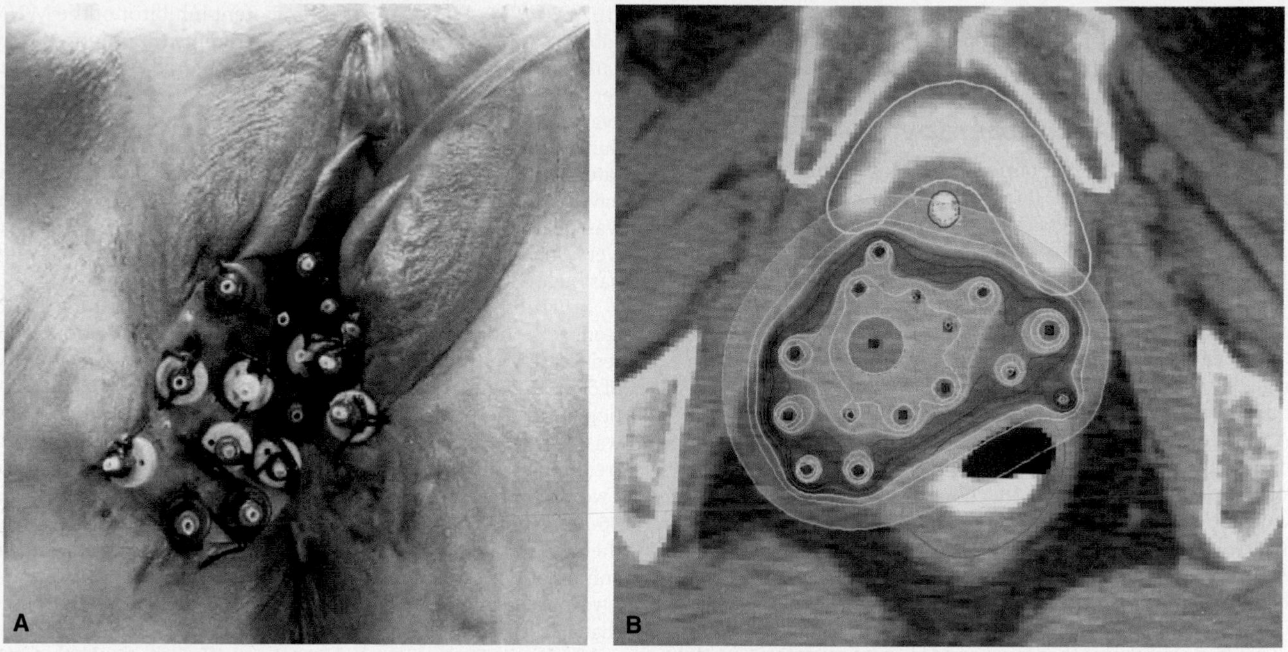

Figure 20.18. High dose rate interstitial brachytherapy for vaginal stump recurrence. **A:** External view of the application. Vinyl template applicators are used in this case. **B:** Dose distribution curves superimposed on a relevant CT image. Red line: 100% prescribed isodose line. Orange line: CTV. CTV, clinical tumor volume; CT, Computed tomography. (Special courtesy of Dr. K. Yoshida, Department of Radiology, Osaka National Hospital).

Source: Special courtesy of Dr. K. Yoshida, Department of Radiology, Osaka National Hospital.

cGy fractions is a common prescription (**Table 20.8**). For a median biologic equivalent dose at point A of 101 Gy10 (EQD2 [normalized dose] = 8,400 cGy), a 3-year local control rate as high as 97% has been reported (295). For the same dose, actuarial 3-year grade 3 or above adverse events occurred at a rate of 17%. Another case series found that an EQD2 of 8,500 cGy provided an at least 86% rate of local control and 2-year hazard for grade 3 or above adverse events of 14% (296).

Radiochemotherapy plus image-guided (MRI) adaptive intracavitary brachytherapy (700 cGy × 4 doses) for an EQD2 dose of at least 8,700 cGy as studied in a single-institution 156-patient trial (2001 to 2008) produced 3-year pelvic disease control rates of 95% in nonbulky stage IB/IIB and 85% in bulky stage IIB/III/IV uterine cervix cancer patients (297). Late morbidity totaled 188 grade 1 or 2 and 11 grade 3 or 4 late adverse events were documented in 143 assessable patients. Spatial distribution of radiation dose (298), MRI/CT planning techniques (299), and interfraction anatomic variation (300) impact results from radiochemotherapy plus image-guide adaptive intracavitary brachytherapy. An international study on MRI-guided brachytherapy in advanced uterine cervix cancer (EMBRACE, NCT00920920) was closed and EBRACE II is about to begin (301).

Altered Radiation Fractionation

Conventional external beam pelvic radiation therapy schedules use a 180 to 200 cGy fraction size delivered once per day, 5 days per week. Pelvic radiation therapy plus brachytherapy finishes at 56 ± 3 days. Nonstandard altered fractionation may employ hypofractionation (larger doses per fraction, lower total dose), hyperfractionation (smaller doses per fraction given more frequently, e.g., 2 or 3 small 120 cGy fractions per day), accelerated fractionation (standard fraction sizes given twice or more daily), or concomitant boosts (larger volume irradiation plus additional small fraction irradiation to a reduced volume on the same day). In an accelerated hyperfraction trial (1999 to 2002), 3,000 cGy pelvic radiation (150 cGy/fraction twice daily) plus 2,000 cGy pelvic radiation with a midline shield (200 cGy/fraction daily) was delivered (302). Two to four brachytherapy implants were done. Median treatment time was 35 days. Both a 5-year local control rate of 84% and 5% grade 3 or above adverse rate was reported.

Stereotactic body radiation therapy (SBRT) utilizes hypofractioned radiation therapy (800 cGy × 3 doses given on consecutive days) to treat persistent or recurrent uterine cervix cancer (209).

Total Radiation Therapy Treatment Time

Conventional pelvic external beam radiation therapy plus brachytherapy finishes in 56 ± 3 days. A loss of pelvic disease control of 1% per day is seen when complete radiation therapy exceeds this limit (303). In a 335-patient retrospective review of two prospective randomized clinical trials (304), prolonged radiation (delayed for any cause) was associated with poorer progression-free survival (HR, 1.98; 95% CI, 1.16 to 3.38, $p = 0.012$) and with overall survival (HR, 1.88; 95% CI, 1.08 to 3.26; $p = 0.024$).

Urgent Palliative Radiation for Uterine Cervix Cancer

Urgent palliation of pelvic pain, obstruction, or bleeding may be needed for the patient with uterine cervix cancer. For significant vaginal bleeding, vaginal packing and urgent start of 300 to 400 cGy fraction per day radiation therapy may be done. Three or four fractions of radiation allow for conventional CT-based radiation planning. Conventional dose and schedule of external beam radiation plus brachytherapy typically follows. Use of palliative radiochemotherapy has been explored (305).

Patients with stage IVB or incurable recurrent carcinoma often require palliation of pelvic pain or bleeding, and their general condition may not warrant a prolonged course of external irradiation. A 290-patient clinical trial (1985 to 1989) used a radiation dose of 4,440 cGy in 12 fractions (370 cGy BID) with a rest after 1,480 cGy and 2,960 cGy (306). The rest interval was randomly allocated between 2 and 4 weeks to determine effects on tumor control. No difference in tumor control was identified ($p = 0.59$). A 7% complication rate was noted at 18 months in survivors. This finding represents a significant lower rate of late complications as compared to a 49% rate seen with higher dose per fraction (1,000 cGy in one fraction repeated at 4-week intervals × 3 doses) in a prior trial (307).

Chemotherapy for Uterine Cervix Cancer

Single-Agent Chemotherapy

A unifying radiochemotherapeutic strategy for women with uterine cervix cancer remains elusive. It is now very well accepted that uterine cervix cancer cells overexpress DNA replication and repair machinery to meet 2'-deoxyribonucleoside triphosphate (dNTP) demand and supply economics (178). Although proliferating uterine cervix cancer cells demand large numbers of dNTPs for genome duplication, cancer cells sustaining DNA damage may need dNTPs more urgently. The number of dNTPs demanded is a function of the type of DNA damage. After radiation, many thousands of dNTPs are needed to repair the several thousand base damages in RNA, mitochondrial DNA, and genomic DNA, whereas DNA damage brought about by chemotherapy may demand only few hundred dNTPs for repair. In a neoplasm like uterine cervix cancer, where cells are overexpressing ribonucleotide reductase facilitating dNTP supply for DNA repair (308), the demand for dNTPs to repair chemotherapy-induced DNA damage is met quickly. This may be why single-agent cytotoxic DNA-damaging agents like cisplatin, carboplatin, nedaplatin, doxorubicin, and epirubicin have 10% to 18% single-agent activity. Targeted biologic chemotherapies appear to be cytostatic, as they alone do not overcome the uterine cancer cell dNTP supply machinery. Single-agent activity ranges between zero and 18%. Targeted biologic chemotherapies do significantly enhance the cytotoxic activity, as radiation–biologic agent activity ranges between 75% and 96% and chemotherapy–biologic agent activity ranges between 22% and 31%.

Combined Modality Chemotherapy

Evidence of Enhanced Chemotherapy Cytotoxicity after Radiochemotherapy

In one clinical trial (162) where women with clinical stage IB uterine cervix cancer were randomized to radiochemotherapy or to radiation prior to radical hysterectomy, more hysterectomy specimens without detectable cancer occurred in the radiochemotherapy group than in the radiation-alone group (52% vs. 41%, $p = 0.04$).

Evidence of Enhanced Radiochemotherapy Cytotoxicity in Uterine Cervix Cancer

Weekly infusions of cisplatin during daily radiation therapy have been assessed in phase II trials (309–312) and phase III randomized trials (171,174). The results of these trials have shown weekly cisplatin treatment to be well tolerated and easy to administer on an outpatient schedule. Cisplatin-containing radiochemotherapy improves survival and disease-free survival. Improvements appear to be a function of a lower rate of relapse in the pelvis. Radiochemotherapy is associated with higher adverse event rates that are dominated by hematologic and gastrointestinal complications, with no evidence of serious late adverse effects.

Other than cisplatin chemotherapy, agents that disrupt ribonucleotide reductase have been tested in women with uterine cervix cancer. Hydroxyurea reduces the tyrosyl radical of ribonucleotide reductase, rendering the enzyme inactive (313). One randomized trial tested twice weekly hydroxyurea (80 mg kg^{-1}) versus placebo during conventional pelvic radiation therapy. Because of hydroxyurea's disruption of ribonucleotide reductase, radiosensitization was expected, and indeed, the trial found a 68% pelvic disease control rate at 3 years after hydroxyurea radiation versus 49% after radiation alone (166). Three-year progression-free survival was 30% after hydroxyurea radiation as compared to 20% after radiation alone. A 26% rate of grade 3 or above neutropenia limited repeated hydroxyurea dosing. In addition to this trial, three other randomized trials have also found combining hydroxyurea and radiation therapy beneficial (167,170,171). A 1,000 times more potent inhibitor of the M2/M2b subunit of ribonucleotide reductase, triapine (3-aminopyridine-2-carboxaldehyde thiosemicarbazone) has entered early phase uterine cervix cancer clinical trial testing. A phase II trial (2009 to 2011) evaluated triapine 25 mg m^{-2} infused three times weekly (M W F) during cisplatin radiochemotherapy and found a 96% local control rate (101). In this trial, triapine was infused shortly after radiation to have optimal inhibitory effect on dNTP supply when dNTP demand was peak. Three-year disease-free and overall survival estimates were 80% and 82%, respectively (102). A randomized phase II trial has begun (NCT01835171).

5-FU obstructs thymidylate synthase, ultimately upsetting the dNTP feedback loop that guides the dNTP selectivity site of ribonucleotide reductase. One randomized trial evaluated protracted venous infusion of 5-FU (225 mg m^{-2} day^{-1} for five consecutive days) during conventional radiation therapy (174). Three-year progression-free survival was 60% for the 5-FU radiation arm. A 35% higher 5-FU radiation treatment failure rate than cisplatin–radiation suggested inferiority. Two randomized clinical trials evaluated protracted 5-FU (4 g over 96-hour infusion) plus cisplatin during conventional pelvic radiation therapy (168,170). The first trial found that a 5-FU–cisplatin–radiation combination resulted in a 75% rate of pelvic disease control and 60% 3-year progression-free survival benefit (170). The second trial observed that a 5-FU–cisplatin–radiation combination conferred a 3-year 81% pelvic disease control rate and 70% disease-free survival benefit (169).

Evidence of Enhanced Cytotoxicity after Neoadjuvant Chemotherapy before Surgery

In one clinical trial (314), women with clinical stage IB2, IIA2, or IIB squamous cell uterine cervix cancer were randomized to neoadjuvant chemotherapy, then radical surgery, or to radical surgery alone. Neoadjuvant chemotherapy involved 21-day bleomycin, vincristine, mitomycin, and cisplatin repeated for 2 to 4 cycles. The 134-patient trial was stopped early because survival was inferior with neoadjuvant chemotherapy. Five-year survival estimates were 70% after neoadjuvant chemotherapy, then surgery versus 74% after surgery alone. A 40% rate of response to neoadjuvant chemotherapy was seen in surgical specimens.

A 288-patient clinical trial of neoadjuvant vincristine-cisplatin chemotherapy was completed among women with clinical stage IB uterine cervix cancer having a tumor diameter ≥4 cm (164). Chemotherapy involved vincristine 1 mg m^{-2} and cisplatin 50 mg m^{-2} repeated every 10 days for 3 cycles. At the time of reporting, median follow-up was 62 months. The vincristine–cisplatin–surgery and surgery-alone groups had similar relapse rates (HR 0.998) and death rates (HR 1.008). There were 78% who had planned surgery in the vincristine–cisplatin–surgery group compared to 79% in the surgery-only group. In this trial, adjuvant radiation therapy was permitted for protocol-specific surgicopathologic risk factors; 45% needed adjuvant radiation in the vincristine–cisplatin–surgery group versus 52% in the surgery-only group ($p > 0.05$).

Two ongoing clinical trials are evaluating neoadjuvant platinum-based chemotherapy prior to surgery versus cisplatin-based radiochemotherapy (NCT00039338, NCT00193739). At this time, neoadjuvant chemotherapy is not recommended in the presurgical care of women with uterine cervix cancer outside of a clinical trial. See **Table 20.6**.

Evidence of Enhanced Cytotoxicity after Neoadjuvant Chemotherapy before Radiochemotherapy

Two clinical studies of dose-dense paclitaxel-carboplatin neoadjuvant chemotherapy before standard radiochemotherapy have shown promise. In one pilot study, a 92% response rate (23 complete responses in 24 patients) was observed (315). In another phase II trial, an 85% response rate (39 complete or partial responses in 46 patients) was reported (316). A prospective randomized clinical trial (INTERLACE, NCT01566240) tests improved survival after dose-dense paclitaxel-carboplatin neoadjuvant chemotherapy prior to radiochemotherapy versus radiochemotherapy alone. Currently, neoadjuvant chemotherapy before radiochemotherapy is not used in the management of women with uterine cervix cancer outside the context of a clinical trial.

Evidence of Uterine Cervix Cancer Cytotoxicity for Second-Line Chemotherapy

Cetuximab, an antibody that inhibits epidermal growth factor receptor activity, has been tested alone or in combination with cisplatin in clinical trials. Cetuximab has been given as a 400 mg m^{-2} loading dose followed by 250 mg m^{-2} on days 1, 8, and 15 of a 21-day cycle. As a single agent, cetuximab was given in a phase II trial (2007 to 2009) to women with pretreated persistent or recurrent uterine cervix cancer (317). No responses were observed and 14% survived free of progression for 6 months. In another phase II trial (2004 to 2008) for women with pretreated persistent or recurrent uterine cervix cancer, a cetuximab-cisplatin combination elicited a 9% rate of response in chemotherapy-exposed patients or 16% rate of response in chemotherapy-naive patients (318). Another inhibitor of epidermal growth factor receptor activity, erlotinib, resulted in no objective responders in a phase II trial among women with recurrent squamous cell carcinoma of the uterine cervix (319).

Paclitaxel, acting as an inhibitor of mitotic-spindle disassembly, has been given alone or in combination with cisplatin for treatment of uterine cervix cancer. In a phase II trial (1991 to 1993), chemotherapy-naive patients with advanced-stage uterine cervix cancer underwent 21-day paclitaxel (170 mg m^{-2} [135 mg m^{-2} in cases of prior pelvic radiation]) infusions over 24 hours (320). Paclitaxel resulted in two complete responders and seven partial responders, for a 17% overall response rate. Docetaxel and nab-paclitaxel have 9% and 29% activity, respectively (321,322). To test additive effects, a phase II trial (1996 to 1997) studied paclitaxel (135 mg m^{-2}) plus cisplatin (75 mg m^{-2}) given every 21 days in chemotherapy-naive patients with advanced-stage squamous cell uterine cervix cancer (323). Grade 3 or above neutropenia occurred in 77% of treated patients. Five complete responders and 14 partial responders made up the paclitaxel-cisplatin response group, giving a 46% overall response rate.

Pemetrexed acts as a folate antimetabolite, inhibiting thymidylate synthase, dihydrofolate reductase, and glycinamide ribonucleotide formyltransferase during purine and pyrimidine synthesis. Given as a single agent every 21 days, pemetrexed at a dose of 900 mg m^{-2} resulted in a 15% overall response rate in a phase II trial (2004 to 2006) for women with pretreated advanced-stage or recurrent uterine cervix cancer that had progressed on at least one prior chemotherapy treatment (324). Response was 25% in nonirradiated patients and 7% in previously irradiated patients. In another phase II trial (2008 to 2011), chemotherapy-naive patients with advanced-stage uterine cervix cancer underwent pemetrexed (500 mg m^{-2}) plus cisplatin (50 mg m^{-2}) treatment every 21 days (325). Grade 2 or above neutropenia occurred in 35% of treated patients. The overall response rate was 31%, with one complete and 16 partial responders observed.

Pharmacologic inhibition of stalled or collapsed DNA replication forks has been explored as a mechanism to accentuate topotecan-related cytotoxicity (326). It has been found that use of the poly adenosine diphosphate-ribose polymerase inhibitor veliparib, conceptually a DNA-strand break repair blocking agent, enhances topotecan-induced damage (326). Bringing this concept forward to the clinic, patients in a phase II clinical trial (2011 to 2013) of 27 heavily pretreated uterine cervix cancer patients underwent topotecan (0.6 mg m^{-2}) infusion and twice-daily 10 mg oral veliparib dose days 1 to 5 of each cycle, repeated every 21 days (327). Anemia (59%), leukopenia (22%), and thrombocytopenia (44%) were common grade 3 or 4 adverse events. Two partial responses (7%) and 10 stable disease responses (37%) were noted, suggesting a need for cisplatin coadministration with topotecan-veliparib to kill uterine cervix cancer cells.

Adjuvant Chemotherapy

Adjuvant chemotherapy seeks to treat occult spread of uterine cervix cancer. A meta-analysis using a random-effects model studied adjuvant cisplatin-based chemotherapy in 368 women with clinical stage IA2 to IIA uterine cervix cancer (328), with inclusion of an aforementioned cisplatin–radiation randomized trial (158). The meta-analysis study claims, built principally on the randomized clinical trial data, that the addition of chemotherapy to radiation therapy significantly improves cancer-related survival outcomes. What remains a question is whether adjuvant cycles of chemotherapy administered after radiochemotherapy provide clinical benefit.

A randomized clinical trial conducted in women with clinical stage IA2, IB, and IIA uterine cervix cancer who had positive pelvic nodes, positive margins, or parametrial invasion at the time of radical hysterectomy included four consecutive 21-day cycles of cisplatin 70 mg m^{-2} and 5-FU 4,000 mg m^{-2}, with cycles three and four given after radiochemotherapy (158). Estimated 5-year survival in the adjuvant chemotherapy cycles arm was 80% (131). Another randomized trial conducted in women with clinical stage IIB, III, or IVA uterine cervix cancer underwent radiochemotherapy and added two consecutive 21-day cycles of cisplatin 50 mg m^{-2} and gemcitabine 1,000 mg m^{-2} (175). Estimated five-year survival in the adjuvant chemotherapy cycles arm was 76%. Whether adding two adjuvant cycles contributed to clinical benefits could not be commented upon in either clinical trial.

Ongoing clinical trials test the hypothesis that adjuvant chemotherapy cycles meaningfully add clinical benefit in women with uterine cervix cancer. A United States-led international cooperative group prospective randomized trial (NCT00980954) evaluates adjuvant cycles of paclitaxel and carboplatin after radiochemotherapy in women with clinical stage IA2, IB, or IIA uterine cervix cancer. A Sun Yat-sen University-led multicenter prospective randomized trial (NCT00806117) studies adjuvant cycles of paclitaxel and cisplatin after sequential radiochemotherapy in women with clinical stage IB or IIA uterine cervix cancer. An Australian-led international cooperative group prospective randomized trial (NCT0141608) examines "outback" adjuvant cycles of paclitaxel and carboplatin after radiochemotherapy in women with paraaortic lymph node–negative clinical stage IB to IVA uterine cervix cancer. A United States-led phase I clinical trial (NCT01295502) tested tolerability of "outback" adjuvant cycles of paclitaxel and carboplatin after radiochemotherapy in women with paraaortic lymph node–positive clinical stage IB to IVA uterine cervix cancer, and is closed to accrual. Results are anticipated.

Given that uterine cervix cancer and HPV infection are linked, immunomodulatory treatment is attractive (43). A Japanese Gynecologic Oncology Group clinical trial randomized 249 women with clinical stage IIB to IVA squamous cell carcinoma of the uterine cervix to twice weekly 0.2 micrograms of Z-100, an immunomodulator extracted from human type tubercle bacilli, or placebo during radiation alone or radiochemotherapy (329). Z-100 was continued until disease progression or termination of the trial. The observed 5-year overall survival rate was 76% (95% CI, 66%–83%) for the Z-100 arm versus 66% (95% CI, 56%–74%) for the placebo arm ($p = 0.07$). No differences in adverse events were noted in the two arms. Similarly, an American cooperative group is investigating adjuvant cycles of CLTA-4 antibody ipilimumab after radiochemotherapy in a dose finding phase I trial (NCT01711515), and is already closed to accrual. Results are anticipated.

UTERINE CERVIX TREATMENT SEQUELAE

Surgery-Related Adverse Events

Pelvic surgery for uterine cervix cancer in any form has a risk for bleeding, infection, and inadvertent injury to nearby organs and tissues. For procedures less than a hysterectomy, incompetence of the uterine cervix and a predisposition to preterm labor exist. Grade

2 or above urogynecologic complications occur in up to 31% of patients undergoing radical hysterectomy for uterine cervix cancer (50). In one randomized trial, grade 2 or above toxicity was 31% in women undergoing radical hysterectomy for uterine cervix cancers measuring ≤4 cm and 33% in women having the same surgery for cancers >4 cm (50). In the same trial, surgical mortality was 0.6%, with one death attributed to spontaneous ileal perforation (11 months after surgery–radiation) and one death due to pulmonary embolism (17 days posttherapy). A 2% perioperative complication rate was reported—one vascular lesion during lymphadenectomy, one ureterovaginal fistula, and one fatal pulmonary embolism. Long-term neurogenic bladder symptoms persisted in 13% of surgical patients. Late-occurring severe actinic cystitis, stress incontinence, and other bladder complications were reported in 3%. Severe edema, pelvic lymphocyst, and abdominal hernia occurred in 0%, 8%, and 11% of patients long-term, respectively. Rectal dysfunction (e.g., incontinence or constipation) after surgery alone is infrequent (157). Age (330), obesity (331), and use of surgical drains (332) have not impacted complication rates after surgery.

Radiation-Related Adverse Events

Patients undergoing radiation therapy alone are counseled on risk for fatigue, skin erythema, dysuria from bladder irritation, and diarrhea from bowel irritation. Short-term muscle, bone, and nerve injury are uncommon. In a case series (333), a 20% frequency of grade 2 or above toxicity has been noted among patients receiving 6,000 cGy or more radiation dose. In a clinical trial, the frequency of patients experiencing grade 3 or above gastrointestinal or genitourinary complication was 2% after 7,000 cGy or more pelvic-only radiation dose (173). Long-term sexual dysfunction, lymphedema, lumbosacral plexopathy, and pelvic insufficiency fractures are likely to be underreported, but occur at a grade 4 or above rate in 4% of patients (227). In a 1,784-patient retrospective study (334), women having clinical stage IB uterine cervix cancer treated had an overall actuarial risk for any long-term complication of 14% at 20 years posttherapy. Significant urinary tract complications occurred in 0.7% per year up to 3 years posttherapy, then tapered to 0.25% per year for the next 22 years. Significant colorectal complications happened at a 1% rate per year in the first 2 years posttherapy, and then declined to 0.06% per year for the next 23 years.

Radiation-related adverse events are expected to be more common among women undergoing external beam radiation therapy plus intracavitary brachytherapy. Prolonged bed rest for intracavitary brachytherapy implants was associated with only a 0.3% risk of life-threatening thromboembolism (11 of 4,043 patients undergoing 7,662 implants) (335). Radiation therapy technique, more than prescribed radiation dose, is associated with radiation-related adverse events.

Sexual dysfunction is a concern after radiation therapy. In one study where sexual health surveys were obtained in 606 women treated between 1991 and 1992 (336), a total of 167 (68%) of 247 women with a history of uterine cervix cancer and 236 (72%) of 330 controls indicated that they engaged in regular vaginal intercourse. Insufficient lubrication (26% of cancer patients vs. 11% control patients), foreshortened vagina (26% vs. 3%), and an insufficiently elastic vagina (23% vs. 4%) were cited reasons for not engaging in regular vaginal intercourse; 26% of the cancer group reported moderate or much distress due to vaginal changes, as compared to 8% of the control group.

Insufficiency fracture of the sacroiliac joint occurs at a low rate in most patients. Patients aged 55 years or older, who weigh >55 kg, or received a radiation dose of 5,040 cGy or more with curative intent are more likely to sustain a pelvic insufficiency fracture (337). A 5-year cumulative incidence of pelvic insufficiency fracture was 20%, with 13% requiring narcotic analgesic or hospital admission for management of pain.

Pentoxifylline and vitamin E are medical therapies used to manage soft tissue late adverse events of pelvic radiation therapy (338,339). For medically refractory radiation-related ulceration and necrosis of soft tissues, hyperbaric oxygen therapy has been used (340,341).

Improved uterine cervix cancer survival has made long-term hazards from treatment more important, including the risk of developing a second cancer after radiation therapy. In the United States Surveillance, Epidemiology and End Results (SEER) cancer registries, 8% of all radiotherapy patients surviving longer than 1 year developed a second solid cancer that could be related to prior radiation therapy (342).

Combined Modality-Related Adverse Events

Radiation Followed by Surgery-Related Adverse Events

Radiation therapy predisposes to tissue hardening and fibrosis, especially because the tumor is sterilized and body healing thickens connective tissues. In one clinical trial (161), women randomly allocated to radiation followed by radical hysterectomy have the same incidence of grade 3 or above complications (10%) as compared to women treated by radiation alone (10%). The proportion of women experiencing any toxicity was higher in the radiation, then surgery arm (63%) as compared to the radiation-only arm (56%). In another study (162), women randomized to radiochemotherapy followed by radical hysterectomy had a 35% rate of grade 3 or above toxicity as compared to 13% in women randomized to radiation followed by radical hysterectomy. Gastrointestinal grade 3 or above short-term adverse events were unbalanced between the radiochemotherapy, then surgery arm (14%) versus radiation, then surgery arm (5%). Long-term effects on the skin, gastrointestinal tract, and genitourinary tract were more common after radiochemotherapy–surgery (4%, 5 fistulas, 1 colonic perforation, 1 intestinal perforation) than after radiation–surgery (2%, 5 fistulas [3 in 1 patient], and 1 intestinal obstruction) (163).

Surgery Followed by Radiation-Related Adverse Events

Operations involving radical hysterectomy result in pelvic intestinal adhesions along denuded organ surfaces, elevating the risk for adjuvant treatment complications. Postsurgical radiation therapy after paraaortic nodal staging exacerbates grade 2 or above complications, especially when a transperitoneal approach was taken as compared to when an extraperitoneal approach was used (103). An extraperitoneal approach was favorable compared to a transperitoneal approach in regard to bowel obstruction (4% vs. 12%), regional enteric injury (4% vs. 12%), and retroperitoneal fibrosis (2% vs. 3%). Regional fistula formation (1% vs. 0%) was similar. The overall incidence of any grade adverse event was 35% after an extraperitoneal approach versus 45% after a transperitoneal approach. For those women requiring interstitial brachytherapy, the incidence of any grade adverse event favored an extraperitoneal approach (30% vs. 45%).

In one clinical trial, women randomly allocated to radical hysterectomy also received adjuvant radiation therapy for adverse pathologic factors found at the time of surgery (50). The incidence of short-term grade 2 or above complications in the surgery, then radiation group (20%) was similar to the surgery-only group (16%) and exceeded that of the radiation-only (7%) group. For long-term complications, the proportions were 29%, 24%, and 16%, respectively, for the surgery, then radiation, surgery-only, and radiation-only groups. In another clinical trial, women randomized to postsurgical radiochemotherapy had a 17% hazard for grade 4 or above toxicity as compared to 4% after postsurgical radiation alone (158).

Radiochemotherapy-Related Adverse Events

Radiochemotherapy for women with advanced-stage uterine cervix cancer results in short- and long-term complications. Meta-analyses of radiochemotherapy versus radiotherapy alone in 24 randomized trials enrolling 4,921 women treated in the 1980s and 1990s show an increased hazard for adverse event after radiochemotherapy treatment (343).

Short-term hematologic (neutropenia) and gastrointestinal (nausea, emesis, and diarrhea) adverse events were significantly more common in radiochemotherapy treatment groups. Long-term complications and risks for second solid cancers attributable to radiochemotherapy were not well reported. Radiochemotherapy treatment-related deaths were rare—six deaths occurred from short-term complications (e.g., neutropenic sepsis) and four deaths happened from long-term complications (e.g., bowel perforation or fistula). Another 1,243-patient retrospective review (2001 to 2002) found grade 3 or above long-term gastrointestinal or genitourinary complications in 10% of patients receiving radiochemotherapy versus 8% of patients receiving radiation therapy alone (344). Most radiochemotherapy adverse events occur within the first 3 years posttherapy. Use of intensity modulated radiation therapy might lower radiochemotherapy-related gastrointestinal and marrow toxicities, a concept being tested in the international INTERTECC randomized trial (NCT01554397).

Thromboembolic Adverse Events

Venous thromboembolic adverse events among women with uterine cervix cancer occur at a rate ranging between 0% and 34% (345–347). Patient risk factors include age, weight, mobility, preexistent hypercoagulable conditions (e.g., factor V Leiden or prothrombin gene mutation), and personal history of prior thromboembolic event, venous stasis, or endothelial cell injury. Postsurgical reduced mobility, bed rest during LDR brachytherapy, and radiochemotherapy treatment itself may exacerbate venous stasis and led to thromboembolic events in 17% of patients (345). Tumor-related factors include pathophysiology, secretion of prothrombotic molecules, and clinical stage (345). Clinical stage is associated with thromboembolic events because direct pelvic sidewall invasion or metastasis resulting in bulky lymph nodes elicits lower extremity venous stasis and thrombus formation. In a clinical trial randomly allocating women with uterine cervix cancer to an erythropoietin-stimulating agent or to no agent, patients in the erythropoietin-stimulating agent arm had a 19% hazard for thromboembolism, whereas those in the no-agent arm had an 8% hazard (135). In the erythropoietin-stimulating agent arm, not all thromboembolic adverse events were linked to the agent (135). Still, erythropoietin-stimulating agents are not recommended for women with uterine cervix cancers. Most thromboembolic adverse events occur within the first 2 years posttherapy.

INTERNATIONAL PERSPECTIVES

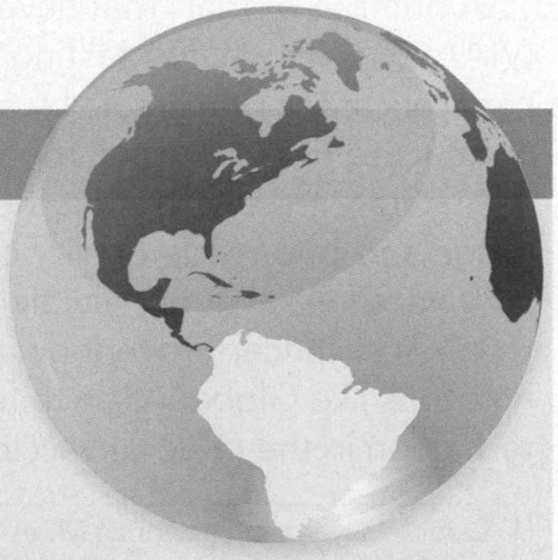

Cervical Cancer in Latin America

Fernando Cotait Maluf, MD (Brazil)

More than 500,000 women are diagnosed with cervical cancer each year and more than 275,000 succumb to disease globally, 88% of which occurs in low-income and middle-income countries (LMICs) (1,2). In Latin America, cervical cancer is the second most common cause of cancer-related deaths among women, with an annual reported incidence of 21.2 per 100,000 women (74,488 cases in 2015) and a mortality rate approaching 8.7 deaths per 100,000 women (31,303 CC deaths in 2015) (1). Mortality continues to rise in Latin America, with current projections estimating an increase of 45% by 2030 (3). Despite this, combating cervical cancer is not a United Nations' 2015 Millennium Development Goal (4). Most women in Latin America do not receive screening despite efforts within the past two decades to develop cytology-based screening programs (5). Many women continue to be diagnosed with advanced cervical cancer, often at ages <45 years (6). Among 37,638 cases diagnosed in Brazil between 2000 and 2009, 71% were stage IIB or higher (FIGO staging) (7).

Because deaths from cervical cancer are preventable by vaccination and screening, there is an urgent need for a cost-effective strategy to reduce cervical cancer mortality in Latin America. Currently, countries in Latin America appear eager to introduce the HPV vaccine, which is highly worthy but insufficient by itself. Latin American countries need to invest in both educational and adequate screening initiatives including timely follow-up and treatment of curable lesions, because only such a comprehensive plan against cervical cancer lead to reductions in mortality.

(1) Ferlay J, Shin HR, Bray F, et al. *GLOBOCAN 2010v2.0, Cancer Incidence and Mortality World- wide: IARC Cancer Base No. 10*. Lyon, France: IARC; 2014.

(2) Jemal A, Bray F, Center MM, et al. Global cancer statistics. *CA Cancer J Clin*. 2011;61(2):69–90.

(3) Pan American Health Organization. *Cervical Cancer*. http://www.paho.org/hq/index.php?option=com_topics&view=article&id=348&Itemid=40936&lang=en. Accessed July 21, 2014.

(4) United Nations. *Millennium Development Goals Report 2015*. http://www.un.org/millenniumgoals/2015_MDG_Report/pdf/MDG%20 2015%20rev%20(July%201).pdf. Accessed August 5, 2015.

(5) Stormo AR, Espey D, Glenn J, et al. Findings and lessons learned from a multi-partner collaboration to increase cervical cancer prevention efforts in Bolivia. *Rural Remote Health*. 2013;13(4):2595.

(6) Carmo CC, Luis RR. Survival of a cohort of women with cervical cancer diagnosed in a Brazilian cancer center. *Rev Saude Publica*. 2011;45(4):661–667.

(7) Thuler LC, de Aguiar SS, Bergmann A. Determinants of late stage diagnosis of cervical cancer in Brazil [in Portuguese]. *Rev Bras Ginecol Obstet*. 2014;36(6):237–243.

INTERNATIONAL PERSPECTIVES

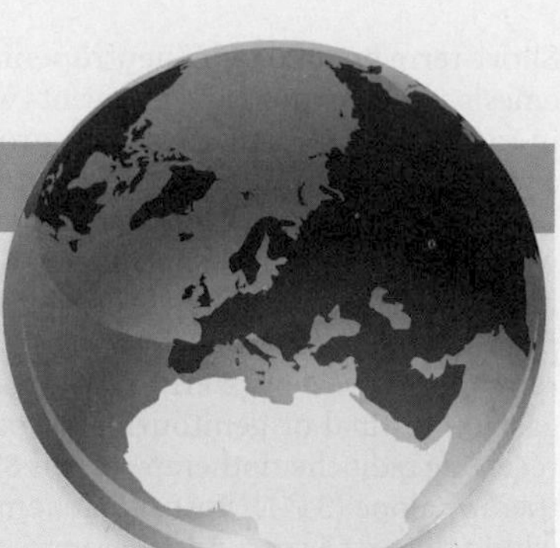

Cervical Cancer in South Africa

Lynette Denny, MD

As well illustrated in this chapter, cervical cancer is a potentially completely preventable disease, yet it remains the most or second most common cancer in many low- and middle-income countries (LMICs). Major contributors to the high incidence of cervical cancer and its mortality in these countries include the lack of preventative services, focus on communicable diseases, and maternal and neonatal mortality, among many others.

The requirements of cytology-based cervical cancer screening programs are far too complex for LMICs, which are characterized by competing health needs, poor health care infrastructure, limited financial and human resources, war, civil strife, environmental instability, and widespread poverty. As a consequence of these interconnected issues, researchers began focusing on alternative protocols and tests for screening women in LMICs, particularly in order to move into what was called "screen and treat" (1).

A number of trials that have randomly assigned women to screening with visual inspection with acetic acid (VIAA) or to HPV DNA testing and cytology have shown that HPV DNA testing coupled with treatment can reduce cervical cancer precursors by at least 75% and cervical cancer deaths by approximately 30%. One randomized trial, conducted over 12 years, reported that VIAA was associated with a reduction in deaths due to cervical cancer (2).

It is now imperative that these secondary prevention methods be implemented and upscaled to reach high coverage and to provide quality care to women over 30 years. The introduction of two, and soon a third, commercial HPV vaccines, all prophylactic and targeting the most important HPV types, is likely to provide an excellent solution to cervical cancer prevention in LMICs. There are still many challenges, but with the support of international organizations like Global Alliance for Vaccines and Immunization (GAVI) and buy-in from Ministries of Health, and the reduction in the price of vaccines, high coverage of young girls should make a dramatic difference in the future.

(1) Denny L, Kuhn L, De Souza M, et al. Screen-and-treat approaches for cervical cancer prevention in low-resource settings: a randomized controlled trial. *JAMA*. 2005;294(17):2173–2181.

(2) Sankaranarayanan R, Nene BM, Shastri SS, et al. HPV screening for cervical cancer in rural India. *NEJM*. 2009;360(14):1385–1394.

INTERNATIONAL PERSPECTIVES

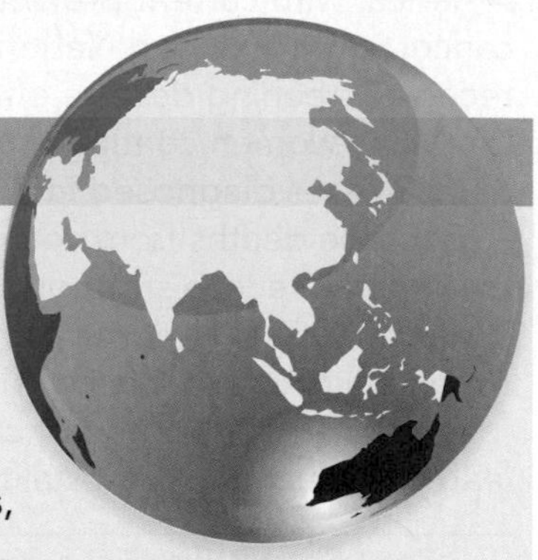

Cervical Cancer in India

Umesh Mahantshetty, MBBS, DMRT, MD, DNB

I acknowledge the efforts put in by Charles Kunos and colleagues for this comprehensively written chapter on cervical cancer. Following are my views regarding different perspectives and/or unique variations in presentation, diagnosis, and management of cervical cancer in low- and middle-income countries (LMIC).

Epidemiology, Presentation, and Diagnosis

Cervical cancer, a global disease, remains a major problem in LMICs including India. An estimated 470,000 (15%–51% of female cancer patients) new cases of cervical cancer are diagnosed each year worldwide and 80% of these occur in developing countries (1). Although, the incidence is on a decline, it is still estimated that about 100,000 new cases will be diagnosed in India in 2020 and more than two thirds are diagnosed at an advanced stage (2). There are no formal cervical cancer screening programs in most LMICs including India. Several research groups including IARC, Tata Memorial Hospital, and other Regional Cancer Centers in India have been involved in rural and urban scenarios in community research studies to explore cost-effective screening methods like visual inspection with acetic acid (VIA) or Lugol iodine (VILI) and HPV testing instead of the gold standard, cytology. VIA showed reduction in cervical cancer mortality in low-resource settings and now is being explored as a screening strategy nationwide (3). Tata Memorial Hospital being a tertiary cancer center, 1,200 to 1,300 new cervical cancer cases are registered, 500 to 600 patients are treated with radical intent with the remaining referred to their home town, other centers, or palliation.

INTERNATIONAL PERSPECTIVES

Management

Many of the international guidelines that exist for management of cervical cancer have been developed in the context of evidence and clinical practice pertinent to the developed world, with hardly any representation from the developing countries on the expert panels who formulate these guidelines. Clinical practice guidelines in developing countries continue to be largely guided by these guidelines since they are based on high-quality evidence and adopted to the local environment. However, many of these guidelines may not be applicable because of unique issues, resource constraints and/or lack of expertise. Consensus statements and expert appraisal of unique issues at various forums are formalized and adopted as guidelines (4,5). Regional Cancer Centers like Tata Memorial Hospital are involved in developing strategies, refining treatment protocols, generating evidence, and evaluating cost effectiveness. An example of evolution of treatment protocols and clinical outcome from the 1980s to 1990s for cervical cancers has been published elsewhere (6).

Various issues and lacunae in the existing evidence, for example, use of concomitant cisplatin-based chemoradiation, optimal utilization of brachytherapy, pelvic and/or paraaortic nodal disease at presentation, parametrial or nodal boost, follow-up strategies, etc., were part of a consensus discussion (7).

Concomitant Cisplatin Chemoradiotherapy

Although chemoradiation is regarded as the standard of care for women with cervical cancer, it is worth remembering that these results were obtained in a trial setting in women from affluent countries. However, concerns regarding the poor general condition, more prevalence of malnutrition, anemia, and compromised socioeconomic conditions in Indian women may lead to decreased tolerance to chemoradiation. Also in most of the international trials regarding chemoradiation, acute toxicity was seen to rise threefold. Hence, judicious use of adding chemotherapy to radiation is recommended with primary aim being to give adequate doses of radiation without unprecedented gaps and compromising the overall treatment time. Also, evidence for use of concomitant chemoradiation and exact benefit in IIIB is lacking in the literature: final analyses of 850-patient randomized trial from India are awaited *(CRACx study: NC00193791)*.

Brachytherapy

Brachytherapy forms an integral part of treatment for radical treatment of cervical cancer. Although we have around 300 HDR units, we have many challenges, such as, uneven distribution of units with fewer units in rural regions, lack of expertise and training, and high economic burden of running the brachytherapy units.

There have been recent developments and suggestion to move from conventional radiography-based brachytherapy to image-guided adaptive brachytherapy. However, the use of MR imaging for fractionated brachytherapy planning is not routinely practiced owing to the availability of MRI in radiotherapy setups, economic viability, etc. The use of alternate imaging modalities such as CT scan, ultrasonography (transabdominal and transrectal) is being evaluated currently with promising results. For low-income and resource-limited countries where cervical cancer is a major health problem, use of a simple, cost-effective imaging modality like ultrasonography would result in wider applicability to optimize cervical brachytherapy (8).

Posttreatment surveillance is a major challenge, given the fact that most women come from rural and low socioeconomic backgrounds. So, posttreatment optimal surveillance strategies in LMIC settings need further research.

(1) Stewart BS, Kleihues P. Cancers of female reproductive tract. In: Stewart BW, Kleihues P, eds., *World Cancer Report*. Lyon, France: World Health Organization, International Agency for Research in Cancer IARC Press; 2003;215–222.

(2) Dinshaw KA, Rao DN, Ganesh B. *Tata Memorial Hospital Cancer Registry Annual Report*. Mumbai, India: Department of Biostatistics and Epidemiology, Tata Memorial Hospital; 1999:52.

(3) Shastri SS. *ASCO 2013: Cervical Cancer using Visual Inspection with Vinegar reduces Mortality by 31% in India* (abstract no. 2); 2013.

(4) Shrivastava SK, Mahantshetty U, Narayan K. FIGO cancer report 2015: principles of radiation therapy in low-resource and well-developed settings, with particular reference to cervical cancer. *Int J Gynecol Obstet*. 2015;131(suppl 2):S153–S158.

(5) Mahantshetty U, Dinshaw KA, Shrivastava S, et al. Cervical cancer: clinical features, investigations, staging and prognosis. In: Ajitkumar T, Barrett A, Hatcher H, Cook N, eds., *Oxford Desk Reference*. Oxford: Oxford University Press; 2011:316 -327.

(6) Shrivastava SK, Mahantshetty U, Engineer R, et al. Treatment and outcome in cancer cervix patients treated between 1979 and 1994: a single institutional experience. *J Cancer Res Ther*. 2013;9(4):672–679.

(7) Mahantshetty U, Krishnatry R, Kumar S, et al. Consensus meeting and update on existing guidelines for management of cervical cancer with special emphasis on the practice in developing countries, including India: the expert panel at the 8th annual women's cancer initiative Tata Memorial Hospital Conference 2010-11. *Indian J Med Paediatr Oncol*. 2012;33(4):16–20.

(8) Mahantshetty U, Khanna N, Swamidas J, et al. Trans-abdominal ultrasound (US) and Magnetic Resonance Imaging (MRI) correlation for conformal intracavitary brachytherapy in carcinoma of the uterine cervix. *Radiother Oncol*. 2012;102(1):130–134.

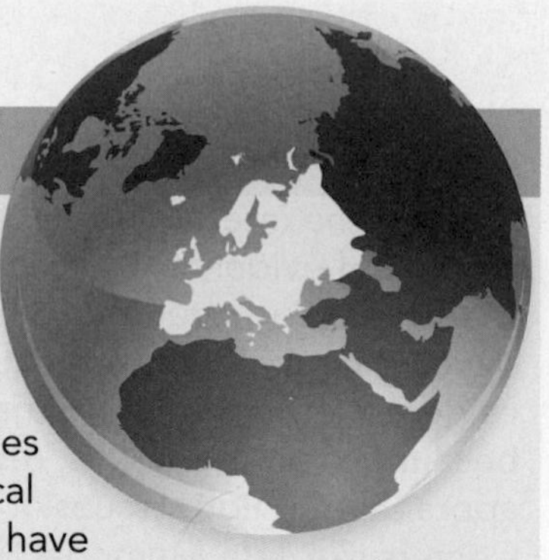

INTERNATIONAL PERSPECTIVES

Cervical Cancer in France

Denis Querleu, MD

Cervical cancer is one of the most common cancers found in women living in low- and middle-income countries (LMICs). Most diagnoses occur in developing countries where cases are detected in later stages with poorer prognoses. Mortality from cervical cancer has decreased only in countries where successful national screening programs have been established. Considered from an international perspective, cervical cancer is probably the most diverse of gynecologic malignancies in terms of geographical disparities. Access to care, access and adherence to screening, methods and standards of care are amazingly different across continents. Even within high-income countries, socioeconomic disparities create an obvious and ethically shocking contrast between populations who benefit from the access to vaccination, screening, specialized physicians, and advanced techniques, and those who do not.

The generalization of primary prevention using vaccination depends on cost, cultural, and religious issues. Attendance to screening is consistently poor in undereducated or disadvantaged populations due to lack of awareness, lack of health-seeking behaviors, mismatch between tradition, religion, and modernity, including denial of extramarital relationships and cultural taboos. Interestingly, simplified screening techniques like visual inspection with acetic acid, which are not standard in developed countries, seem to be effective in other countries. On the other hand, in Belgium, where the number of cytologic examinations is theoretically sufficient to cover more than the whole target population, the screening coverage does not exceed 61%. This reflects the fact that part of the population is uselessly overscreened whereas a significant proportion of women do not benefit from screening (1). It is worrying to observe that, in England, efforts to reduce screening inequalities have resulted in a significant improvement in equitable delivery of breast screening, although not of cervical screening (2).

The situation regarding management of the disease in LMICs is dismal. For example, there is only one radiation therapy machine for 10 million people in Northwest Africa.

Even in the United States, and possibly more in the United States than in other developed countries, where health insurance is generalized, disparities in the management and outcome of cervical cancer according to health insurance status are seen. Medicaid and uninsured patients experience increased overall mortality (3). Inequalities in access to care among ethnic and racial groups are well documented. The mortality rate for black women remains twice that for white women (4). Morbid obesity is an independent predictor of mortality in women with cervical cancer (5). However, the causes of such inequalities are complex and solutions are not straightforward.

Regression can also be observed in high-income countries. Significant disparities seem to have emerged for cervical cancer from 2004 in New South Wales (Australia) (6). In this area, approximately 13.4% of deaths from cancer could have been postponed had socioeconomic disparity been eliminated. Despite its established efficacy, brachytherapy is underused in the management of cervical cancers. Brachytherapy, a critical but technically challenging component of the management of advanced cervical cancer, is decreasingly used, resulting in insufficient training of radiation oncology residents. Along the same lines, surgical quality care is insufficiently fostered, and the decrease of incidence of invasive cervical cancer in some countries results in poor exposure of physicians and trainees.

Early diagnosis, access to specialist gynecologic oncologists, and treatment at a high-volume facility with advanced resources are still influenced by geographic barriers among countries worldwide, and within countries. Equity in cervical cancer care is a compelling objective for the future worldwide.

(1) Arbyn M, Fabri V, Temmerman M, et al. Attendance at cervical cancer screening and use of diagnostic and therapeutic procedures on the uterine cervix assessed from individual health insurance data (Belgium, 2002–2006). *PLoS One*. 2014;9(4):e92615.

(2) Douglas E, Waller J, Duffy SW, et al. Socioeconomic inequalities in breast and cervical screening coverage in England: are we closing the gap? *J Med Screen*. 2016;23(2):98–103.

(3) Churilla T, Egleston B, Dong Y, et al. Disparities in the management and outcome of cervical cancer in the United States according to health insurance status. *Gynecol Oncol*. 2016;141(3):516–523.

(4) Chatterjee S, Gupta D, Caputo TA, et al. Disparities in Gynecological Malignancies. *Front Oncol*. 2016;6:36. doi:10.3389/fonc.2016.00036.

(5) Frumovitz M, Jhingran A, Soliman PT, et al. Morbid obesity as an independent risk factor for disease-specific mortality in women with cervical cancer. *Obstet Gynecol*. 2014;124(6):1098–1104.

(6) Stanbury J, Baade P, Yu Y, et al. Cancer survival in New South Wales, Australia: socioeconomic disparities remain despite overall improvements. *BMC Cancer*. 2016;16(1):48.

REFERENCES

1. Ferlay J, Soerjomataram I, Ervik M, et al. *GLOBOCAN 2012 v1.0, Cancer Incidence and Mortality Worldwide*. Lyon, France: International Agency for Research on Cancer; 2013.
2. American Cancer Society. *Cancer Facts & Figures 2015*. Atlanta, GA: American Cancer Society; 2015.
3. Parham GP, Shaver M, Brown P, et al. Significance of a first-time atypical Papanicolaou smear in a young, high-risk African-American and Latino-American population. *J Natl Med Assoc*. 1994;86(4):273–277.
4. American Cancer Society. *Cancer Facts & Figures for Latinos: 2012-2014*. Atlanta, GA: American Cancer Society; 2012.
5. Watson M, Saraiya M, Benard V, et al. Burden of cervical cancer in the United States, 1998-2003. *Cancer*. 2008;113(suppl 10):2855–2864.
6. American Cancer Society. *Cancer Facts & Figures for African Americans: 2013-2014*. Atlanta, GA: American Cancer Society; 2013.
7. Jemal A, Simard EP, Dorell C, et al. Annual report to the nation on the status of cancer, 1975-2009, featuring the burden and trends in human papillomavirus(HPV)-associated cancers and HPV vaccination coverage levels. *J Natl Cancer Inst*. 2013;105(3):175–201.
8. Plummer M, Peto J, Franceschi S. Time since first sexual intercourse and the risk of cervical cancer. *Int J Cancer*. 2012;130(11):2638–2644.
9. Lu B, Viscidi RP, Lee JH, et al. Human papillomavirus (HPV) 6, 11, 16, and 18 seroprevalence is associated with sexual practice and age: results from the multinational HPV Infection in Men Study (HIM Study). *Cancer Epidemiol Biomarkers Prev*. 2011;20(5):990–1002.
10. Kjaer SK, Chackerian B, van den Brule AJ, et al. High-risk human papillomavirus is sexually transmitted: evidence from a follow-up study of virgins starting sexual activity (intercourse). *Cancer Epidemiol Biomarkers Prev*. 2001;10(2):101–106.
11. Taylor RS, Carroll BE, Lloyd JW. Mortality among women in 3 Catholic religious orders with special reference to cancer. *Cancer*. 1959;12:1207–1225.
12. Fraumeni JF Jr, Lloyd JW, Smith EM, et al. Cancer mortality among nuns: role of marital status in etiology of neoplastic disease in women. *J Natl Cancer Inst*. 1969;42(3):455–468.
13. McKinnon B, Harper S, Moore S. Decomposing income-related inequality in cervical screening in 67 countries. *Int J Public Health*. 2011;56(2):139–152.
14. Mazor KM, Williams AE, Roblin DW, et al. Health literacy and pap testing in insured women. *J Cancer Educ*. 2014;29(4):698–701.
15. Alemany L, de Sanjose S, Tous S, et al. Time trends of human papillomavirus types in invasive cervical cancer, from 1940 to 2007. *Int J Cancer*. 2014;135(1):88–95.
16. Waggoner SE, Darcy KM, Tian C, et al. Smoking behavior in women with locally advanced cervical carcinoma: a Gynecologic Oncology Group study. *Am J Obstet Gynecol*. 2010;202(3):283.e1–e7.
17. Wang SS, Bratti MC, Rodriguez AC, et al. Common variants in immune and DNA repair genes and risk for human papillomavirus persistence and progression to cervical cancer. *J Infect Dis*. 2009;199(1):20–30.
18. Wang SS, Gonzalez P, Yu K, et al. Common genetic variants and risk for HPV persistence and progression to cervical cancer. *PLoS One*. 2010;5(1):e8667.
19. Maiman M, Fruchter RG, Clark M, et al. Cervical cancer as an AIDS-defining illness. *Obstet Gynecol*. 1997;89(1):76–80.
20. Reid JL, Wright TC Jr, Stoler MH, et al. Human papillomavirus oncogenic mRNA testing for cervical cancer screening: baseline and longitudinal results from the CLEAR Study. *Am J Clin Pathol*. 2015;144(3):473–483.
21. Castle PE, Cuzick J, Stoler MH, et al. Detection of human papillomavirus 16, 18, and 45 in women with ASC-US cytology and the risk of cervical precancer: results from the CLEAR HPV study. *Am J Clin Pathol*. 2015;143(2):160–167.
22. Schlichte MJ, Guidry J. Current cervical carcinoma screening guidelines. *J Clin Med*. 2015;4(5):918–932.
23. Dillner J, Rebolj M, Birembaut P, et al. Long term predictive values of cytology and human papillomavirus testing in cervical cancer screening: joint European cohort study. *BMJ*. 2008;337:a1754.
24. Monsonego J, Cox JT, Behrens C, et al. Prevalence of high-risk human papilloma virus genotypes and associated risk of cervical precancerous lesions in a large U.S. screening population: data from the ATHENA trial. *Gynecol Oncol*. 2015;137(1):47–54.
25. Wright TC, Stoler MH, Behrens CM, et al. Primary cervical cancer screening with human papillomavirus: end of study results from the ATHENA study using HPV as the first-line screening test. *Gynecol Oncol*. 2015;136(2):189–197.
26. Wright TC Jr, Stoler MH, Sharma A, et al. Evaluation of HPV-16 and HPV-18 genotyping for the triage of women with high-risk HPV+ cytology-negative results. *Am J Clin Pathol*. 2011;136(4):578–586.
27. Hebner C, Laimins L. Human papillomaviruses: basic mechanisms and pathogenesis and oncogenicity. *Rev Med Virol*. 2006;16(2):83–97.
28. Cole S, Danos O. Nucleotide sequence and comparative analysis of the human papillomavirus type 18 genome: phylogeny of papillomaviruses and repeated structure of the E6 and E7 gene products. *J Mol Biol*. 1987;193(4):599–608.
29. Barbosa M, Lowy D, Schiller J. Papillomavirus polypeptides E6 and E7 are zinc-binding proteins. *J Virol*. 1989;63(3):1404–1407.
30. Werness B, Levine A, Howley P. Association of human papillomavirus type 16 and 18 E6 proteins with p53. *Science*. 1990;248:76–79.
31. Kunos C, Chiu S, Pink J, et al. Modulating radiation resistance by inhibiting ribonucleotide reductase in cancers with virally or mutationally silenced p53 protein. *Radiation Res*. 2009;172(6):666–676.
32. Kunos C, Radivoyevitch T, Pink J, et al. Ribonucleotide reductase inhibition enhances chemoradiosensitivity of human cervical cancers. *Radiation Res*. 2010;174(5):574–581.
33. Kunos C, Colussi V, Pink J, et al. Radiosensitization of human cervical cancer cells by inhibiting ribonucleotide reductase: enhanced radiation response at low dose rates. *Int J Radiat Oncol Biol Phys*. 2011;80(4):1198–1204.
34. Gonzalez S, Stremlau M, He X, et al. Degradation of the retinoblastoma tumor suppressor by the human papillomavirus type 16 E7 oncoprotein is important for functional inactivation and is separable from proteosomal degradation of E7. *J Virol*. 2001;75(16):7583–7591.
35. Huang P, Patrick D, Edwards G, et al. Protein domains governing interactions between E2F, the retinoblastoma gene product, and human papillomavirus type 16 E7 protein. *Mol Cell Biol*. 1993;13(2):953–960.
36. Chabes AL, Bjorklund S, Thelander L. S Phase-specific transcription of the mouse ribonucleotide reductase R2 gene requires both a proximal repressive E2F-binding site and an upstream promoter activating region. *J Biol Chem*. 2004;279(11):10796–10807.
37. Klingelhutz A, Foster S, McDougall J. Telomerase activation by the E6 gene product of human papillomavirus type 16. *Nature*. 1996;380(6569):79–82.
38. Hasan UA, Zannetti C, Parroche P, et al. The human papillomavirus type 16 E7 oncoprotein induces a transcriptional repressor complex on the Toll-like receptor 9 promoter. *J Exp Med*. 2013;210(7):1369–1387.
39. Vandermark ER, Deluca KA, Gardner CR, et al. Human papillomavirus type 16 E6 and E 7 proteins alter NF-kB in cultured cervical epithelial cells and inhibition of NF-kB promotes cell growth and immortalization. *Virology*. 2012;425(1):53–60.
40. de Vos van Steenwijk PJ, Heusinkveld M, Ramwadhdoebe TH, et al. An unexpectedly large polyclonal repertoire of HPV-specific T cells is poised for action in patients with cervical cancer. *Cancer Res*. 2010;70(7):2707–2717.
41. Holman LL, Levenback CF, Frumovitz M. Sentinel lymph node evaluation in women with cervical cancer. *J Minim Invasive Gynecol*. 2014;21(4):540–545.
42. Kobayashi A, Greenblatt RM, Anastos K, et al. Functional attributes of mucosal immunity in cervical intraepithelial neoplasia and effects of HIV infection. *Cancer Res*. 2004;64(18):6766–6774.
43. Kunos C. Novel biological radiochemotherapy approaches in locally advanced-stage cervical cancer management. *Discov Med*. 2014;17(94):179–186.
44. Golden EB, Chhabra A, Chachoua A, et al. Local radiotherapy and granulocyte-macrophage colony-stimulating factor to generate abscopal responses in patients with metastatic solid tumors: a proof-of-principle trial. *Lancet Oncol*. 2015;16(7):795–803.
45. Schiffman M, Solomon D. Clinical practice. Cervical-cancer screening with human papillomavirus and cytologic cotesting. *N Engl J Med*. 2013;369(24):2324–2331.
46. Pecorelli S, Zigliani L, Odicino F. Revised FIGO staging for carcinoma of the cervix. *Int J Gynecol Obstet*. 2009;105(2):107–108.
47. Creasman WT, Zaino RJ, Major FJ, et al. Early invasive carcinoma of the cervix (3 to 5 mm invasion): risk factors and prognosis. A Gynecologic Oncology Group study. *Am J Obstet Gynecol*. 1998;178(1 pt 1):62–65.
48. Delgado G, Bundy B, Fowler WJ, et al. A prospective surgical pathological study of stage I squamous carcinoma of the cervix: a Gynecologic Oncology Group Study. *Gynecol Oncol*. 1989;35(3):314–320.
49. Delgado G, Bundy B, Zaino R, et al. Prospective surgical-pathological study of disease-free interval in patients with stage IB squamous cell carcinoma of the cervix: a Gynecologic Oncology Group study. *Gynecol Oncol*. 1990;38(3):352–357.
50. Landoni F, Maneo A, Colombo A, et al. Randomized study of radical surgery versus radiotherapy for stage Ib-IIa cervical cancer. *Lancet*. 1997;350(9077):535–540.
51. Berman ML, Keys H, Creasman W, et al. Survival and patterns of recurrence in cervical cancer metastatic to periaortic lymph nodes (a Gynecologic Oncology Group study). *Gynecol Oncol*. 1984;19(1):8–16.

52. Burke TW, Heller PB, Hoskins WJ, et al. Evaluation of the scalene lymph nodes in primary and recurrent cervical carcinoma. *Gynecol Oncol.* 1987;28(3):312–317.
53. Moyer V, LeFevre M, Siu A, et al. Final recommendation statement: cervical cancer: screening. Rockville, MD: United States Preventive Services Task Force; 2013.
54. Saslow D, Solomon D, Lawson HW, et al. American Cancer Society, American Society for Colposcopy and Cervical Pathology, and American Society for Clinical Pathology screening guidelines for the prevention and early detection of cervical cancer. *CA Cancer J Clin.* 2012;62(3):147–172.
55. Committee on Practice Bulletins—Gynecology. ACOG practice bulletin number 131: screening for cervical cancer. *Obstet Gynecol.* 2012;120(5):1222–1238.
56. Nayar R, Wilbur DC. The Pap Test and Bethesda 2014. "The reports of my demise have been greatly exaggerated." (after a quotation from Mark Twain). *Acta Cytol.* 2015;59(2):121–132.
57. Sherman ME, Schiffman M, Cox JT. Effects of age and human papilloma viral load on colposcopy triage: data from the randomized atypical squamous cells of undetermined significance/low-grade squamous intraepithelial lesion triage study (ALTS). *J Natl Cancer Inst.* 2002;94(2):102–107.
58. Arbyn M, Anttila A, Jordan J, et al. European guidelines for quality assurance in cervical cancer screening. Second edition—summary document. *Ann Oncol.* 2010;21(3):448–458.
59. Sultana F, English DR, Simpson JA, et al. Rationale and design of the iPap trial: a randomized controlled trial of home-based HPV self-sampling for improving participation in cervical screening by never- and under-screened women in Australia. *BMC Cancer.* 2014;14:207.
60. Arbyn M, Castle PE. Offering self-sampling kits for HPV testing to reach women who do not attend in the regular cervical cancer screening program. *Cancer Epidemiol Biomarkers Prev.* 2015;24(5):769–772.
61. Sherman ME, Castle PE, Solomon D. Cervical cytology of atypical squamous cells-cannot exclude high-grade squamous intraepithelial lesion (ASC-H): characteristics and histologic outcomes. *Cancer.* 2006;108(5):298–305.
62. Lorenzato M, Clavel C, Masure M, et al. DNA image cytometry and human papillomavirus (HPV) detection help to select smears at high risk of high-grade cervical lesions. *J Pathol.* 2001;194(2):171–176.
63. Dillner J, Kjaer SK, Wheeler CM, et al. Four year efficacy of prophylactic human papillomavirus quadrivalent vaccine against low grade cervical, vulvar, and vaginal intraepithelial neoplasia and anogenital warts: randomised controlled trial. *BMJ.* 2010;341:c3493.
64. Nygard M, Saah A, Munk C, et al. Evaluation of the long-term anti-human papillomavirus 6 (HPV6), 11, 16, and 18 immune responses generated by the quadrivalent HPV vaccine. *Clin Vaccine Immunol.* 2015;22(8):943–948.
65. Brotherton JM, Fridman M, May CL, et al. Early effect of the HPV vaccination programme on cervical abnormalities in Victoria, Australia: an ecological study. *Lancet.* 2011;377(9783):2085–2092.
66. Daley EM, Vamos CA, Buhi ER, et al. Influences on human papillomavirus vaccination status among female college students. *J Women's Health.* 2010;19(10):1885–1891.
67. Liddon NC, Hood JE, Leichliter JS. Intent to receive HPV vaccine and reasons for not vaccinating among unvaccinated adolescent and young women: findings from the 2006-2008 National Survey of Family Growth. *Vaccine.* 2012;30(16):2676–2682.
68. Leval A, Herweijer E, Ploner A, et al. Quadrivalent human papillomavirus vaccine effectiveness: a Swedish national cohort study. *J Natl Cancer Inst.* 2013;105(7):469–474.
69. Castellsague X, Munoz N, Pitisuttithum P, et al. End-of-study safety, immunogenicity, and efficacy of quadrivalent HPV (types 6, 11, 16, 18) recombinant vaccine in adult women 24-45 years of age. *Br J Cancer.* 2011;105(1):28–37.
70. World Health Organization. *WHO Guidelines for Screening and Treatment of Precancerous Lesions for Cervical Cancer Prevention* (WHO Guidelines Approved by the Guidelines Review Committee). Geneva, Switzerland: World Health Organization; 2013.
71. Apgar BS, Kaufman AJ, Bettcher C, et al. Gynecologic procedures: colposcopy, treatments for cervical intraepithelial neoplasia and endometrial assessment. *Am Fam Physician.* 2013;87(12):836–843.
72. Davies KR, Cantor SB, Cox DD, et al. An alternative approach for estimating the accuracy of colposcopy in detecting cervical precancer. *PLoS One.* 2015;10(5):e0126573.
73. Kliemann LM, Silva M, Reinheimer M, et al. Minimal cold knife conization height for high-grade cervical squamous intraepithelial lesion treatment. *Eur J Obstet Gynecol Reprod Biol.* 2012;165(2):342–346.
74. Bigrigg MA, Codling BW, Pearson P, et al. Colposcopic diagnosis and treatment of cervical dysplasia at a single clinic visit. Experience of low-voltage diathermy loop in 1000 patients. *Lancet.* 1990;336(8709):229–231.
75. Luesley DM, Cullimore J, Redman CW, et al. Loop diathermy excision of the cervical transformation zone in patients with abnormal cervical smears. *BMJ.* 1990;300(6741):1690–1693.
76. Dey P, Gibbs A, Arnold DF, et al. Loop diathermy excision compared with cervical laser vaporisation for the treatment of intraepithelial neoplasia: a randomised controlled trial. *BJOG.* 2002;109(4):381–385.
77. Winter WE, Maxwell G, Tian C, et al. Association of hemoglobin level with survival in cervical carcinoma patients treated with concurrent cisplatin and radiotherapy: a Gynecologic Oncology Group Study. *Gynecol Oncol.* 2004;94(2):495–501.
78. Li X, Zhou J, Huang K, et al. The predictive value of serum squamous cell carcinoma antigen in patients with cervical cancer who receive neoadjuvant chemotherapy followed by radical surgery: a single-institute study. *PLoS One.* 2015;10(4):e0122361.
79. Duk JM, de Bruijn HW, Groenier KH, et al. Cancer of the uterine cervix: sensitivity and specificity of serum squamous cell carcinoma antigen determinations. *Gynecol Oncol.* 1990;39(2):186–194.
80. Molina R, Filella X, Auge JM, et al. CYFRA 21.1 in patients with cervical cancer: comparison with SCC and CEA. *Anticancer Res.* 2005;25(3a):1765–1771.
81. Reesink-Peters N, van der Velden J, Ten Hoor KA, et al. Preoperative serum squamous cell carcinoma antigen levels in clinical decision making for patients with early-stage cervical cancer. *J Clin Oncol.* 2005;23(7):1455–1462.
82. Jeong BK, Choi DH, Huh SJ, et al. The role of squamous cell carcinoma antigen as a prognostic and predictive factor in carcinoma of uterine cervix. *Radiat Oncol J.* 2011;29(3):191–198.
83. Kawaguchi R, Furukawa N, Kobayashi H, et al. Posttreatment cut-off levels of squamous cell carcinoma antigen as a prognostic factor in patients with locally advanced cervical cancer treated with radiotherapy. *J Gynecol Oncol.* 2013;24(4):313–320.
84. Gaarenstroom KN, Bonfrer JM, Kenter GG, et al. Clinical value of pretreatment serum Cyfra 21-1, tissue polypeptide antigen, and squamous cell carcinoma antigen levels in patients with cervical cancer. *Cancer.* 1995;76(5):807–813.
85. Bender DP, Sorosky JI, Buller RE, et al. Serum CA 125 is an independent prognostic factor in cervical adenocarcinoma. *Am J Obstet Gynecol.* 2003;189(1):113–117.
86. Mitsuhashi A, Matsui H, Usui H, et al. Serum YKL-40 as a marker for cervical adenocarcinoma. *Ann Oncol.* 2009;20(1):71–77.
87. Sheng X, Du X, Zhang X, et al. Clinical value of serum HMGB1 levels in early detection of recurrent squamous cell carcinoma of uterine cervix: comparison with serum SCCA, CYFRA21-1, and CEA levels. *Croat Med J.* 2009;50(5):455–464.
88. Weismann P, Weismanova E, Masak L, et al. The detection of circulating tumor cells expressing E6/E7 HR-HPV oncogenes in peripheral blood in cervical cancer patients after radical hysterectomy. *Neoplasma.* 2009;56(3):230–238.
89. Tian J, Fu L, Yin D, et al. Does the novel integrated PET/MRI offer the same diagnostic performance as PET/CT for oncological indications? *PLoS One.* 2014;9(6):e90844.
90. Lagasse LD, Creasman WT, Shingleton HM, et al. Results and complications of operative staging in cervical cancer: experience of the Gynecologic Oncology Group. *Gynecol Oncol.* 1980;9(1):90–98.
91. Mitchell DG, Snyder B, Coakley F, et al. Early invasive cervical cancer: MRI and CT predictors of lymphatic metastases in the ACRIN 6651/GOG 183 intergroup study. *Gynecol Oncol.* 2009;112(1):95–103.
92. Mitchell DG, Snyder B, Coakley F, et al. Early invasive cervical cancer: tumor delineation by magnetic resonance imaging, computed tomography, and clinical examination, verified by pathologic results, in the ACRIN 6651/GOG 183 Intergroup Study. *J Clin Oncol.* 2006;24(36):5687–5694.
93. Hricak H, Gatsonis C, Chi DS, et al. Role of imaging in pretreatment evaluation of early invasive cervical cancer: results of the intergroup study American College of Radiology Imaging Network 6651-Gynecologic Oncology Group 183. *J Clin Oncol.* 2005;23(36):9329–9337.
94. Gold M, Zhang Z, Marques H, et al. MRI prior to systematic lymphadenectomy in patients with locally advanced cervical cancer. *J Clin Oncol.* 2011;29(suppl 15):5042.
95. Viswanathan AN, Erickson B, Gaffney DK, et al. Comparison and consensus guidelines for delineation of clinical target volume for CT- and MR-based brachytherapy in locally advanced cervical cancer. *Int J Radiat Oncol Biol Phys.* 2014;90(2):320–328.
96. Rose PG, Adler LP, Rodriguez M, et al. Positron emission tomography for evaluating para-aortic nodal metastasis in locally advanced cervical cancer before surgical staging: a surgicopathologic study. *J Clin Oncol.* 1999;17(1):41–45.

97. Grigsby PW, Siegel BA, Dehdashti F. Lymph node staging by positron emission tomography in patients with carcinoma of the cervix. *J Clin Oncol.* 2001;19(17):3745–3749.
98. Kidd E, Siegel B, Dehdashti F, et al. The standardized uptake value for F-18 fluorodeoxyglucose is a sensitive predictive biomarker for cervical cancer treatment response and survival. *Cancer.* 2007;110(8):1738–1744.
99. Kunos C, Radivoyevitch T, Abdul-Karim F, et al. 18F-fluoro-2-deoxy-d-glucose positron emission tomography standard uptake value as an indicator of cervical cancer chemoradiation therapeutic response. *Int J Gynecol Cancer.* 2011;21(6):1117–1123.
100. Kunos C, Waggoner S, Von Gruenigen V, et al. Phase I trial of intravenous 3-aminopyridine-2-carboxaldehyde thiosemicarbazone (3-AP, NSC #663249) in combination with pelvic radiation therapy and weekly cisplatin chemotherapy for locally advanced cervical cancer. *Clin Cancer Res.* 2010;16(4):1298–1306.
101. Kunos C, Radivoyevitch T, Waggoner S, et al. Radiochemotherapy plus 3-aminopyridine-2-carboxaldehyde thiosemicarbazone (3-AP, NSC #663249) in advanced-stage cervical and vaginal cancers. *Gynecol Oncol.* 2013;130(1):75–80.
102. Kunos CA, Sherertz TM. Long-term disease control with triapine-based radiochemotherapy for patients with stage IB2-IIIB cervical cancer. *Front Oncol.* 2014;4:184.
103. Weiser E, Bundy B, Hoskins W, et al. Extraperitoneal versus transperitoneal selective paraaortic lymphadenectomy in the pretreatment surgical staging of advanced cervical carcinoma (A Gynecologic Oncology Group Study). *Gynecol Oncol.* 1989;33(3):283–289.
104. Leblanc E, Narducci F, Frumovitz M, et al. Therapeutic value of pretherapeutic extraperitoneal laparoscopic staging of locally advanced cervical carcinoma. *Gynecol Oncol.* 2007;105(2):304–311.
105. Frumovitz M, Querleu D, Gil-Moreno A, et al. Lymphadenectomy in locally advanced cervical cancer study (LiLACS): phase III clinical trial comparing surgical with radiologic staging in patients with stages IB2-IVA cervical cancer. *J Minim Invasive Gynecol.* 2014;21(1):3–8.
106. Levenback C, Coleman RL, Burke TW, et al. Lymphatic mapping and sentinel node identification in patients with cervix cancer undergoing radical hysterectomy and pelvic lymphadenectomy. *J Clin Oncol.* 2002;20(3):688–693.
107. Altgassen C, Hertel H, Brandstadt A, et al. Multicenter validation study of the sentinel lymph node concept in cervical cancer: AGO Study Group. *J Clin Oncol.* 2008;26(18):2943–2951.
108. McIndoe WA, McLean MR, Jones RW, et al. The invasive potential of carcinoma in situ of the cervix. *Obstet Gynecol.* 1984;64(4):451–458.
109. Sedlis A, Sall S, Tsukada Y, et al. Microinvasive carcinoma of the uterine cervix: a clinical-pathologic study. *Am J Obstet Gynecol.* 1979;133(1):64–74.
110. Holowaty P, Miller AB, Rohan T, et al. Natural history of dysplasia of the uterine cervix. *J Natl Cancer Inst.* 1999;91(3):252–258.
111. Sheu BC, Hsu SM, Ho HN, et al. Reversed CD4/CD8 ratios of tumor-infiltrating lymphocytes are correlated with the progression of human cervical carcinoma. *Cancer.* 1999;86(8):1537–1543.
112. Drew PA, Hong B, Massoll NA, et al. Characterization of papillary squamotransitional cell carcinoma of the cervix. *J Low Genit Tract Dis.* 2005;9(3):149–153.
113. Winkler B, Crum CP, Fujii T, et al. Koilocytotic lesions of the cervix. The relationship of mitotic abnormalities to the presence of papillomavirus antigens and nuclear DNA content. *Cancer.* 1984;53(5):1081–1087.
114. Tseng CJ, Pao CC, Tseng LH, et al. Lymphoepithelioma-like carcinoma of the uterine cervix: association with Epstein-Barr virus and human papillomavirus. *Cancer.* 1997;80(1):91–97.
115. Martorell MA, Julian JM, Calabuig C, et al. Lymphoepithelioma-like carcinoma of the uterine cervix. *Arch Pathol Lab Med.* 2002;126(12):1501–1505.
116. Young RH, Clement PB. Endocervical adenocarcinoma and its variants: their morphology and differential diagnosis. *Histopathology.* 2002;41(3):185–207.
117. Castellsague X, Diaz M, de Sanjose S, et al. Worldwide human papillomavirus etiology of cervical adenocarcinoma and its cofactors: implications for screening and prevention. *J Natl Cancer Inst.* 2006;98(5):303–315.
118. Pirog EC, Kleter B, Olgac S, et al. Prevalence of human papillomavirus DNA in different histological subtypes of cervical adenocarcinoma. *Am J Pathol.* 2000;157(4):1055–1062.
119. Hart WR. Symposium part II: special types of adenocarcinoma of the uterine cervix. *Int J Gynecol Pathol.* 2002;21(4):327–346.
120. An HJ, Kim KR, Kim IS, et al. Prevalence of human papillomavirus DNA in various histological subtypes of cervical adenocarcinoma: a population-based study. *Mod Pathol.* 2005;18(4):528–534.
121. Kim HJ, Sung JH, Lee E, et al. Prognostic factors influencing decisions about surgical treatment of villoglandular adenocarcinoma of the uterine cervix. *Int J Gynecol Cancer.* 2014;24(7):1299–305.
122. Tambouret R, Bell DA, Young RH. Microcystic endocervical adenocarcinomas: a report of eight cases. *Am J Surg Pathol.* 2000;24(3):369–374.
123. Albores-Saavedra J, Gersell D, Gilks CB, et al. Terminology of endocrine tumors of the uterine cervix: results of a workshop sponsored by the College of American Pathologists and the National Cancer Institute. *Arch Pathol Lab Med.* 1997;121(1):34–39.
124. McCluggage WG. Mullerian adenosarcoma of the female genital tract. *Adv Anat Pathol.* 2010;17(2):122–129.
125. Sharma NK, Sorosky JI, Bender D, et al. Malignant mixed mullerian tumor (MMMT) of the cervix. *Gynecol Oncol.* 2005;97(2):442–445.
126. Wright JD, Rosenblum K, Huettner PC, et al. Cervical sarcomas: an analysis of incidence and outcome. *Gynecol Oncol.* 2005;99(2):348–351.
127. Muntz HG, Ferry JA, Flynn D, et al. Stage IE primary malignant lymphomas of the uterine cervix. *Cancer.* 1991;68(9):2023–2032.
128. Malpica A, Moran CA. Primitive neuroectodermal tumor of the cervix: a clinicopathologic and immunohistochemical study of two cases. *Ann Diagn Pathol.* 2002;6(5):281–287.
129. Khalbuss WE, Bui M, Loya A. A 19-year-old woman with a cervicovaginal mass and elevated serum CA 125. Desmoplastic small round cell tumor. *Arch Pathol Lab Med.* 2006;130(4):e59–e61.
130. Stehman FB, Bundy BN, DiSaia PJ, et al. Carcinoma of the cervix treated with radiation therapy. I. A multi-variate analysis of prognostic variables in the Gynecologic Oncology Group. *Cancer.* 1991;67(11):2776–2785.
131. Monk BJ, Wang J, Im S, et al. Rethinking the use of radiation and chemotherapy after radical hysterectomy: a clinical-pathologic analysis of a Gynecologic Oncology Group/Southwest Oncology Group/Radiation Therapy Oncology Group trial. *Gynecol Oncol.* 2005;96(3):721–728.
132. Rose PG, Java JJ, Whitney CW, et al. Locally advanced adenocarcinoma and adenosquamous carcinomas of the cervix compared to squamous cell carcinomas of the cervix in gynecologic oncology group trials of cisplatin-based chemoradiation. *Gynecol Oncol.* 2014;135(2):208–212.
133. Fyles AW, Milosevic M, Pintilie M, et al. Anemia, hypoxia and transfusion in patients with cervix cancer: a review. *Radiother Oncol.* 2000;57(1):13–19.
134. Dunst J, Kuhnt T, Strauss HG, et al. Anemia in cervical cancers: impact on survival, patterns of relapse, and association with hypoxia and angiogenesis. *Int J Radiat Oncol Biol Phys.* 2003;56(3):778–787.
135. Thomas G, Ali S, Hoebers FJ, et al. Phase III trial to evaluate the efficacy of maintaining hemoglobin levels above 12.0 g/dL with erythropoietin vs above 10.0 g/dL without erythropoietin in anemic patients receiving concurrent radiation and cisplatin for cervical cancer. *Gynecol Oncol.* 2008;108(2):317–325.
136. Shenouda G, Mehio A, Souhami L, et al. Erythropoietin receptor expression in biopsy specimens from patients with uterine cervix squamous cell carcinoma. *Int J Gynecol Cancer.* 2006;16(2):752–756.
137. Waggoner S, Darcy K, Fuhrman B, et al. Association between cigarette smoking and prognosis in locally advanced cervical carcinoma treated with chemoradiation: a Gynecologic Oncology Group study. *Gynecol Oncol.* 2006;103(3):853–858.
138. Kunos C, Winter K, Dicker A, et al. Ribonucleotide reductase expression in cervical cancer: a radiation therapy oncology group translational science analysis. *Int J Gynecol Cancer.* 2013;23(4):615–621.
139. Grigsby PW, Siegel BA, Dehdashti F, et al. Posttherapy [18F] fluorodeoxyglucose positron emission tomography in carcinoma of the cervix: response and outcome. *J Clin Oncol.* 2004;22(11):2167–2171.
140. Schwartz J, Siegel B, Dehdashti F, et al. Association of post-therapy positron emission tomography with tumor response and survival in cervical carcinoma. *JAMA.* 2007;298(19):2289–2295.
141. Schwartz J, Grigsby P, Dehdashti F, et al. The role of ^{18}F-FDG PET in assessing therapy response in cancer of the cervix and ovaries. *J Nucl Med.* 2009;50(suppl 5):64S–73S.
142. Shankar L, Hoffman J, Bacharach S, et al. Consensus recommendations for the use of 18F-FDG PET as an indicator of therapeutic response in patients in National Cancer Institute Trials. *J Nucl Med.* 2006;47(6):1059–1066.
143. Young H, Baum R, Cremerius U, et al. Measurement of clinical and subclinical tumor response using 18F-fluorodeoxyglucose and positron emission tomography: review and 1999 EORTC recommendations. *Eur J Cancer.* 1999;35(13):1771–1782.
144. Mayr NA, Wang JZ, Lo SS, et al. Translating response during therapy into ultimate treatment outcome: a personalized 4-dimensional MRI tumor volumetric regression approach in cervical cancer. *Int J Radiat Oncol Biol Phys.* 2010;76(3):719–727.
145. Kolstad P, Klem V. Long-term followup of 1121 cases of carcinoma in situ. *Obstet Gynecol.* 1976;48(2):125–129.
146. Martin-Hirsch PL, Paraskevaidis E, Kitchener H. Surgery for cervical intraepithelial neoplasia. *Cochrane Database Syst Rev.* 2000;(2):CD001318. doi:10.1002/14651858.CD001318.

147. Temkin SM, Hellmann M, Lee YC, et al. Dysplastic endocervical curettings: a predictor of cervical squamous cell carcinoma. *Am J Obstet Gynecol.* 2007;196(5):469.e1–e4.
148. Costales AB, Milbourne AM, Rhodes HE, et al. Risk of residual disease and invasive carcinoma in women treated for adenocarcinoma in situ of the cervix. *Gynecol Oncol.* 2013;129(3):513–516.
149. Melnikow J, McGahan C, Sawaya GF, et al. Cervical intraepithelial neoplasia outcomes after treatment: long-term follow-up from the British Columbia Cohort Study. *J Natl Cancer Inst.* 2009;101(10):721–728.
150. Grigsby PW, Perez CA. Radiotherapy alone for medically inoperable carcinoma of the cervix: stage IA and carcinoma in situ. *Int J Radiat Oncol Biol Phys.* 1991;21(2):375–378.
151. Lecuru F, Mathevet P, Querleu D, et al. Bilateral negative sentinel nodes accurately predict absence of lymph node metastasis in early cervical cancer: results of the SENTICOL study. *J Clin Oncol.* 2011;29(13):1686–1691.
152. Covens A, Rosen B, Murphy J, et al. How important is removal of the parametrium at surgery for carcinoma of the cervix? *Gynecol Oncol.* 2002;84(1):145–149.
153. Beiner ME, Hauspy J, Rosen B, et al. Radical vaginal trachelectomy vs. radical hysterectomy for small early stage cervical cancer: a matched case-control study. *Gynecol Oncol.* 2008;110(2):168–171.
154. Dargent D. Radical trachelectomy: an operation that preserves the fertility of young women with invasive cervical cancer. *Bulletin de l'Academie nationale de medecine.* 2001;185(7):1295–1304; discussion 305–306.
155. Piver MS, Marchetti DL, Patton T, et al. Radical hysterectomy and pelvic lymphadenectomy versus radiation therapy for small (less than or equal to 3 cm) stage IB cervical carcinoma. *Am J Clin Oncol.* 1988;11(1):21–24.
156. Shimada M, Kigawa J, Nishimura R, et al. Ovarian metastasis in carcinoma of the uterine cervix. *Gynecol Oncol.* 2006;101(2):234–237.
157. Rotman M, Sedlis A, Piedmonte M, et al. A phase III randomized trial of postoperative pelvic irradiation in stage IB cervical carcinoma with poor prognostic features: follow-up of a Gynecologic Oncology Group study. *Int J Radiat Oncol Biol Phys.* 2006;65(1):169–176.
158. Peters WI, Liu P, Barrett R, et al. Concurrent chemotherapy and pelvic radiation therapy compared with pelvic radiation therapy alone as adjuvant therapy after radical surgery in high-risk early-stage cancer of the cervix. *J Clin Oncol.* 2000;18(8):1606–1613.
159. Durrance FY, Fletcher GH, Rutledge FN. Analysis of central recurrent disease in stages I and II squamous cell carcinomas of the cervix on intact uterus. *Am J Roentgenol Radium Ther Nucl Med.* 1969;106(4):831–838.
160. Nelson AJ 3rd, Feltcher GH, Wharton JT. Indications for adjunctive conservative extrafascial hysterectomy in selected cases of carcinoma of the uterine cervix. *Am J Roentgenol Radium Ther Nucl Med.* 1975;123(1):91–99.
161. Keys HM, Bundy BN, Stehman FB, et al. Radiation therapy with and without extrafascial hysterectomy for bulky stage IB cervical carcinoma: a randomized trial of the Gynecologic Oncology Group. *Gynecol Oncol.* 2003;89(3):343–353.
162. Keys HM, Bundy BN, Stehman FB, et al. Cisplatin, radiation, and adjuvant hysterectomy compared with radiation and adjuvant hysterectomy for bulky stage IB cervical carcinoma. *N Engl J Med.* 1999;340(15):1154–1161.
163. Stehman F, Ali S, Keys H, et al. Radiation therapy with or without weekly cisplatin for bulky stage 1B cervical carcinoma: follow-up of a Gynecologic Oncology Group trial. *Am J Obstet Gynecol.* 2007;197:503.e1–e6.
164. Eddy GL, Bundy BN, Creasman WT, et al. Treatment of ("bulky") stage IB cervical cancer with or without neoadjuvant vincristine and cisplatin prior to radical hysterectomy and pelvic/para-aortic lymphadenectomy: a phase III trial of the gynecologic oncology group. *Gynecol Oncol.* 2007;106(2):362–369.
165. Perez CA, Grigsby PW, Chao KS, et al. Tumor size, irradiation dose, and long-term outcome of carcinoma of uterine cervix. *Int J Radiat Oncol Biol Phys.* 1998;41(2):307–317.
166. Hreshchyshyn MM, Aron BS, Boronow RC, et al. Hydroxyurea or placebo combined with radiation to treat stages IIIB and IV cervical cancer confined to the pelvis. *Int J Radiat Oncol Biol Phys.* 1979;5(3):317–322.
167. Piver MS, Vongtama V, Emrich LJ. Hydroxyurea plus pelvic radiation versus placebo plus pelvic radiation in surgically staged stage IIIB cervical cancer. *J Surg Oncol.* 1987;35(2):129–134.
168. Morris M, Eifel P, Lu J, et al. Pelvic radiation with concurrent chemotherapy compared with pelvic and para-aortic radiation for high-risk cervical cancer. *N Engl J Med.* 1999;340(15):1137–1143.
169. Eifel PJ, Winter K, Morris M, et al. Pelvic irradiation with concurrent chemotherapy versus pelvic and para-aortic irradiation for high-risk cervical cancer: an update of radiation therapy oncology group trial (RTOG) 90-01. *J Clin Oncol.* 2004;22(5):872–880.
170. Whitney CW, Sause W, Bundy BN, et al. Randomized comparison of fluorouracil plus cisplatin versus hydroxyurea as an adjunct to radiation therapy in stage IIB-IVA carcinoma of the cervix with negative para-aortic lymph nodes: a Gynecologic Oncology Group and Southwest Oncology Group study. *J Clin Oncol.* 1999;17(5):1339–1348.
171. Rose PG, Bundy BN, Watkins EB, et al. Concurrent cisplatin-based radiotherapy and chemotherapy for locally advanced cervical cancer. *N Engl J Med.* 1999;340(15):1144–1153.
172. Rose P, Ali S, Watkins E, et al. Long-term follow-up of a randomized trial comparing concurrent single agent cisplatin, cisplatin-based combination chemotherapy, or hydroxyurea during pelvic irradiation for locally advanced cervical cancer: A Gynecologic Oncology Group Study. *J Clin Oncol.* 2007;25(19):2804–2810.
173. Pearcy R, Brundage M, Drouin P, et al. Phase III trial comparing radical radiotherapy with and without cisplatin chemotherapy in patients with advanced squamous cell cancer of the cervix. *J Clin Oncol.* 2002;20(4):966–972.
174. Lanciano R, Calkins A, Bundy BN, et al. Randomized comparison of weekly cisplatin or protracted venous infusion of fluorouracil in combination with pelvic radiation in advanced cervix cancer: a gynecologic oncology group study. *J Clin Oncol.* 2005;23(33):8289–8295.
175. Duenas-Gonzalez A, Zarba J, Patel F, et al. A phase III, open-label, randomized study comparing concurrent gemcitabine plus cisplatin and radiation followed by adjuvant gemcitabine and cisplatin versus concurrent cisplatin and radiation in patients with stage IIB to IVA carcinoma of the cervix. *J Clin Oncol.* 2011;29(13):1678–1685.
176. DiSilvestro PA, Ali S, Craighead PS, et al. Phase III randomized trial of weekly cisplatin and irradiation versus cisplatin and tirapazamine and irradiation in stages IB2, IIA, IIB, IIIB, and IVA cervical carcinoma limited to the pelvis: a Gynecologic Oncology Group study. *J Clin Oncol.* 2014;32(5):458–464.
177. Olive P, Banath J. Kinetics of H2AX phosphorylation after exposure to cisplatin. *Cytometry B.* 2009;76B(2):79–90.
178. Kunos C, Radivoyevitch T. Molecular strategies of deoxynucleotide triphosphate supply inhibition used in the treatment of gynecologic malignancies. *Gynecol Obstetric.* 2011;S4:001 doi:10.4172/2161-0932.S4-001.
179. Brown JM, Lemmon MJ. Potentiation by the hypoxic cytotoxin SR 4233 of cell killing produced by fractionated irradiation of mouse tumors. *Cancer Res.* 1990;50(24):7745–7749.
180. Schefter T, Winter K, Kwon J, et al. RTOG 0417: efficacy of bevacizumab in combination with definitive radiation therapy and cisplatin chemotherapy in untreated patients with locally advanced cervical carcinoma. *Int J Radiat Oncol Biol Phys.* 2014;88(1):101–105.
181. Kavadi VS, Eifel PJ. FIGO stage IIIA carcinoma of the uterine cervix. *Int J Radiat Oncol Biol Phys.* 1992;24(2):211–215.
182. Monk BJ, Huang HQ, Cella D, et al. Quality of life outcomes from a randomized phase III trial of cisplatin with or without topotecan in advanced carcinoma of the cervix: a Gynecologic Oncology Group Study. *J Clin Oncol.* 2005;23(21):4617–4625.
183. Thigpen J, Shingleton H, Homesley H, et al. Cis-platinum in treatment of advanced or recurrent squamous cell carcinoma of the cervix: a phase II study of the Gynecologic Oncology Group. *Cancer.* 1981;48(4):899–903.
184. Tewari K, Sill M, Long HJ 3rd, et al. Improved survival with bevacizumab in advanced cervical cancer. *N Engl J Med.* 2014;370(8):734–743.
185. Bonomi P, Blessing JA, Stehman FB, et al. Randomized trial of three cisplatin dose schedules in squamous-cell carcinoma of the cervix: a Gynecologic Oncology Group study. *J Clin Oncol.* 1985;3(8):1079–1085.
186. Moore DH, Blessing JA, McQuellon RP, et al. Phase III study of cisplatin with or without paclitaxel in stage IVB, recurrent, or persistent squamous cell carcinoma of the cervix: a gynecologic oncology group study. *J Clin Oncol.* 2004;22(15):3113–3119.
187. Long HJ 3rd, Bundy BN, Grendys EC Jr, et al. Randomized phase III trial of cisplatin with or without topotecan in carcinoma of the uterine cervix: a Gynecologic Oncology Group study. J Clin Oncol. 2005;23(21):4626–4633.
188. Monk B, Sill M, McMeekin D, et al. Phase III trial of four cisplatin-containing doublet combinations in stage IVB, recurrent, or persistent cervical carcinoma: a Gynecologic Oncology Group study. *J Clin Oncol.* 2009;27(28):4649–4655.
189. Chong A, Ha JM, Jeong SY, et al. Clinical usefulness of (18)F-FDG PET/CT in the detection of early recurrence in treated cervical cancer patients with unexplained elevation of serum tumor markers. *Chonnam Med J.* 2013;49(1):20–26.

190. Coleman RL, Keeney ED, Freedman RS, et al. Radical hysterectomy for recurrent carcinoma of the uterine cervix after radiotherapy. *Gynecol Oncol.* 1994;55(1):29–35.
191. Berek JS, Howe C, Lagasse LD, et al. Pelvic exenteration for recurrent gynecologic malignancy: survival and morbidity analysis of the 45-year experience at UCLA. *Gynecol Oncol.* 2005;99(1):153–159.
192. Petruzziello A, Kondo W, Hatschback SB, et al. Surgical results of pelvic exenteration in the treatment of gynecologic cancer. *World J Surg Oncol.* 2014;12:279.
193. Westin SN, Rallapalli V, Fellman B, et al. Overall survival after pelvic exenteration for gynecologic malignancy. *Gynecol Oncol.* 2014;134(3):546–551.
194. Marnitz S, Kohler C, Muller M, et al. Indications for primary and secondary exenterations in patients with cervical cancer. *Gynecol Oncol.* 2006;103(3):1023–1030.
195. Iglesias DA, Westin SN, Rallapalli V, et al. The effect of body mass index on surgical outcomes and survival following pelvic exenteration. *Gynecol Oncol.* 2012;125(2):336–42.
196. Bricker EM. Bladder substitution after pelvic evisceration. *Surg Clin North Am.* 1950;30(5):1511–1521.
197. Penalver MA, Angioli R, Mirhashemi R, et al. Management of early and late complications of ileocolonic continent urinary reservoir (Miami pouch). *Gynecol Oncol.* 1998;69(3):185–191.
198. Ramirez PT, Modesitt SC, Morris M, et al. Functional outcomes and complications of continent urinary diversions in patients with gynecologic malignancies. *Gynecol Oncol.* 2002;85(2):285–291.
199. Ungar L, Palfalvi L. Pelvic exenteration without external urinary or fecal diversion in gynecological cancer patients. *Int J Gynecol Cancer.* 2006;16(1):364–368.
200. McCraw JB, Massey FM, Shanklin KD, et al. Vaginal reconstruction with gracilis myocutaneous flaps. *Plast Reconstr Surg.* 1976;58(2):176–183.
201. O'Connell C, Mirhashemi R, Kassira N, et al. Formation of functional neovagina with vertical rectus abdominis musculocutaneous (VRAM) flap after total pelvic exenteration. *Ann Plast Surg.* 2005;55(5):470–473.
202. Soper JT, Havrilesky LJ, Secord AA, et al. Rectus abdominis myocutaneous flaps for neovaginal reconstruction after radical pelvic surgery. *Int J Gynecol Cancer.* 2005;15(3):542–548.
203. Sood AK, Cooper BC, Sorosky JI, et al. Novel modification of the vertical rectus abdominis myocutaneous flap for neovagina creation. *Obstet Gynecol.* 2005;105(3):514–518.
204. Ito H, Shigematsu N, Kawada T, et al. Radiotherapy for centrally recurrent cervical cancer of the vaginal stump following hysterectomy. *Gynecol Oncol.* 1997;67(2):154–161.
205. Ijaz T, Eifel PJ, Burke T, et al. Radiation therapy of pelvic recurrence after radical hysterectomy for cervical carcinoma. *Gynecol Oncol.* 1998;70(2):241–246.
206. Grigsby PW. Prospective phase I/II study of irradiation and concurrent chemotherapy for recurrent cervical cancer after radical hysterectomy. *Int J Gynecol Cancer.* 2004;14(5):860–864.
207. Randall ME, Evans L, Greven KM, et al. Interstitial reirradiation for recurrent gynecologic malignancies: results and analysis of prognostic factors. *Gynecol Oncol.* 1993;48(1):23–31.
208. Brabham JG, Cardenes HR. Permanent interstitial reirradiation with 198Au as salvage therapy for low volume recurrent gynecologic malignancies: a single institution experience. *Am J Clin Oncol.* 2009;32(4):417–422.
209. Kunos C, Brindle J, Waggoner S, et al. Phase II clinical trial of robotic stereotactic body radiosurgery for metastatic gynecologic malignancies. *Front Oncol.* 2012;2:181.
210. Kunos CA, Sherertz TM, Mislmani M, et al. Phase I Trial of carboplatin and gemcitabine chemotherapy and stereotactic ablative radiosurgery for the palliative treatment of persistent or recurrent gynecologic cancer. *Front Oncol.* 2015;5:126.
211. Grigsby PW, Vest ML, Perez CA. Recurrent carcinoma of the cervix exclusively in the paraaortic nodes following radiation therapy. *Int J Radiat Oncol Biol Phys.* 1994;28(2):451–455.
212. Barney BM, Petersen IA, Dowdy SC, et al. Intraoperative electron beam radiotherapy (IOERT) in the management of locally advanced or recurrent cervical cancer. *Radiat Oncol.* 2013;8:80.
213. Monk B, Sill M, Burger R, et al. Phase II trial of bevacizumab in the treatment of persistent or recurrent squamous cell carcinoma of the cervix: a gynecologic oncology group study. *J Clin Oncol.* 2009;27(7):1069–1074.
214. Whitney CW, Stehman FB. The abandoned radical hysterectomy: a Gynecologic Oncology Group Study. *Gynecol Oncol.* 2000;79(3):350–356.
215. Morice P, Rouanet P, Rey A, et al. Results of the GYNECO 02 study, an FNCLCC phase III trial comparing hysterectomy with no hysterectomy in patients with a (clinical and radiological) complete response after chemoradiation therapy for stage IB2 or II cervical cancer. *Oncologist.* 2012;17(1):64–71.
216. Cheung TH, Lo KW, Yim SF, et al. Debulking metastatic pelvic nodes before radiotherapy in cervical cancer patients: a long-term follow-up result. *Int J Clin Oncol.* 2011;16(5):546–552.
217. Tozzi R, Lavra F, Cassese T, et al. Laparoscopic debulking of bulky lymph nodes in women with cervical cancer: indication and surgical outcomes. *BJOG.* 2009;116(5):688–692.
218. Park JY, Kim DY, Kim JH, et al. Management of occult invasive cervical cancer found after simple hysterectomy. *Ann Oncol.* 2010;21(5):994–1000.
219. Chen SW, Liang JA, Yang SN, et al. Postoperative radiotherapy for patients with invasive cervical cancer following treatment with simple hysterectomy. *Jpn J Clin Oncol.* 2003;33(9):477–481.
220. National Comprehensive Cancer Network. *Cervical Cancer*; 2015. http://www.nccn.org 2015.
221. Viswanathan AN, Deavers MT, Jhingran A, et al. Small cell neuroendocrine carcinoma of the cervix: outcome and patterns of recurrence. *Gynecol Oncol.* 2004;93(1):27–33.
222. Hoskins PJ, Wong F, Swenerton KD, et al. Small cell carcinoma of the cervix treated with concurrent radiotherapy, cisplatin, and etoposide. *Gynecol Oncol.* 1995;56(2):218–225.
223. Stroh EL, Besa PC, Cox JD, et al. Treatment of patients with lymphomas of the uterus or cervix with combination chemotherapy and radiation therapy. *Cancer.* 1995;75(9):2392–2399.
224. Hashimoto A, Fujimi A, Kanisawa Y, et al. Primary diffuse large B-cell lymphoma of the uterine cervix successfully treated with rituximab plus cyclophosphamide, doxorubicin, vincristine, and prednisone chemotherapy-a case report. *Gan to kagaku ryoho.* 2013;40(13):2589–2592.
225. Hannoun-Levi JM, Peiffert D, Hoffstetter S, et al. Carcinoma of the cervical stump: retrospective analysis of 77 cases. *Radiother Oncol.* 1997;43(2):147–153.
226. Kovalic JJ, Grigsby PW, Perez CA, et al. Cervical stump carcinoma. *Int J Radiat Oncol Biol Phys.* 1991;20(5):933–938.
227. Rotman M, Pajak TF, Choi K, et al. Prophylactic extended-field irradiation of para-aortic lymph nodes in stages IIB and bulky IB and IIA cervical carcinomas. Ten-year treatment results of RTOG 79-20. *JAMA.* 1995;274(5):387–393.
228. Fauci JM, Schneider KE, Whitworth JM, et al. Referral patterns and incidence of cervical intraepithelial neoplasia in adolescent and pregnant patients: the impact of the 2006 guidelines. *J Low Genit Tract Dis.* 2011;15(2):124–127.
229. Kalliala I, Anttila A, Dyba T, et al. Pregnancy incidence and outcome among patients with cervical intraepithelial neoplasia: a retrospective cohort study. *BJOG.* 2012;119(2):227–235.
230. Economos K, Perez Veridiano N, Delke I, et al. Abnormal cervical cytology in pregnancy: a 17-year experience. *Obstet Gynecol.* 1993;81(6):915–918.
231. Frega A, Scirpa P, Corosu R, et al. Clinical management and follow-up of squamous intraepithelial cervical lesions during pregnancy and postpartum. *Anticancer Res.* 2007;27(4c):2743–2746.
232. Kaplan KJ, Dainty LA, Dolinsky B, et al. Prognosis and recurrence risk for patients with cervical squamous intraepithelial lesions diagnosed during pregnancy. *Cancer.* 2004;102(4):228–232.
233. Averette HE, Nasser N, Yankow SL, et al. Cervical conization in pregnancy. Analysis of 180 operations. *Am J Obstet Gynecol.* 1970;106(4):543–549.
234. Goldberg GL, Altaras MM, Block B. Cone cerclage in pregnancy. *Obstet Gynecol.* 1991;77(2):315–317.
235. Robinson WR, Webb S, Tirpack J, et al. Management of cervical intraepithelial neoplasia during pregnancy with LOOP excision. *Gynecol Oncol.* 1997;64(1):153–155.
236. Pettersson BF, Andersson S, Hellman K, et al. Invasive carcinoma of the uterine cervix associated with pregnancy: 90 years of experience. *Cancer.* 2010;116(10):2343–2349.
237. Leath CA 3rd, Bevis KS, Numnum TM, et al. Comparison of operative risks associated with radical hysterectomy in pregnant and nonpregnant women. *J Reprod Med.* 2013;58(7–8):279–284.
238. Karrberg C, Radberg T, Holmberg E, et al. Support for down-staging of pregnancy-associated cervical cancer. *Acta obstetricia et gynecologica Scandinavica.* 2015;94(6):654–659.
239. Plante M, Renaud MC, Hoskins IA, et al. Vaginal radical trachelectomy: a valuable fertility-preserving option in the management of early-stage cervical cancer. A series of 50 pregnancies and review of the literature. *Gynecol Oncol.* 2005;98(1):3–10.
240. Sood AK, Sorosky JI, Mayr N, et al. Cervical cancer diagnosed shortly after pregnancy: prognostic variables and delivery routes. *Obstet Gynecol.* 2000;95(6 pt 1):832–838.

241. Ghadjar P, Budach V, Kohler C, et al. Modern radiation therapy and potential fertility preservation strategies in patients with cervical cancer undergoing chemoradiation. *Radiat Oncol.* 2015;10:50.
242. Benhaim Y, Haie-Meder C, Lhomme C, et al. Chemoradiation therapy in pregnant patients treated for advanced-stage cervical carcinoma during the first trimester of pregnancy: report of two cases. *Int J Gynecol Cancer.* 2007;17(1):270–274.
243. Morice P, Uzan C, Gouy S, et al. Gynaecological cancers in pregnancy. *Lancet.* 2012;379(9815):558–569.
244. Amant F, Halaska MJ, Fumagalli M, et al. Gynecologic cancers in pregnancy: guidelines of a second international consensus meeting. *Int J Gynecol Cancer.* 2014;24(3):394–403.
245. Kong TW, Lee EJ, Lee Y, et al. Neoadjuvant and postoperative chemotherapy with paclitaxel plus cisplatin for the treatment of FIGO stage IB cervical cancer in pregnancy. *Obstet Gynecol Sci.* 2014;57(6):539–543.
246. Li J, Wang LJ, Zhang BZ, et al. Neoadjuvant chemotherapy with paclitaxel plus platinum for invasive cervical cancer in pregnancy: two case report and literature review. *Arch Gynecol Obstet.* 2011;284(3):779–783.
247. Tewari K, Cappuccini F, Gambino A, et al. Neoadjuvant chemotherapy in the treatment of locally advanced cervical carcinoma in pregnancy: a report of two cases and review of issues specific to the management of cervical carcinoma in pregnancy including planned delay of therapy. *Cancer.* 1998;82(8):1529–1534.
248. From the Centers for Disease Control and Prevention. 1993 revised classification system for HIV infection and expanded surveillance case definition for AIDS among adolescents and adults. *JAMA.* 1993;269(6):729–730.
249. HIV in the United States: At a Glance. Division of HIV/AIDS Prevention, National Center for HIV/AIDS, U.S. Department of Health & Human Services; 2015.
250. Clifford GM, Goncalves MA, Franceschi S. Human papillomavirus types among women infected with HIV: a meta-analysis. *AIDS.* 2006;20(18):2337–2344.
251. Palefsky JM, Minkoff H, Kalish LA, et al. Cervicovaginal human papillomavirus infection in human immunodeficiency virus-1 (HIV)-positive and high-risk HIV-negative women. *J Natl Cancer Inst.* 1999;91(3):226–236.
252. Massad LS, Ahdieh L, Benning L, et al. Evolution of cervical abnormalities among women with HIV-1: evidence from surveillance cytology in the women's interagency HIV study. *J Acquir Immune Defic Syndr.* 2001;27(5):432–442.
253. Chaturvedi AK, Madeleine MM, Biggar RJ, et al. Risk of human papillomavirus-associated cancers among persons with AIDS. *J Natl Cancer Inst.* 2009;101(16):1120–1130.
254. Anderson JR, Paramsothy P, Heilig C, et al. Accuracy of Papanicolaou test among HIV-infected women. *Clin Infect Dis.* 2006;42(4):562–568.
255. D'Souza G, Burk RD, Palefsky JM, et al. Cervical human papillomavirus testing to triage borderline abnormal pap tests in HIV-coinfected women. *AIDS.* 2014;28(11):1696–1698.
256. Paramsothy P, Duerr A, Heilig CM, et al. Abnormal vaginal cytology in HIV-infected and at-risk women after hysterectomy. *J Acquir Immune Defic Syndr.* 2004;35(5):484–491.
257. Clifford GM, Polesel J, Rickenbach M, et al. Cancer risk in the Swiss HIV Cohort Study: associations with immunodeficiency, smoking, and highly active antiretroviral therapy. *J Natl Cancer Inst.* 2005;97(6):425–432.
258. Kojic EM, Kang M, Cespedes MS, et al. Immunogenicity and safety of the quadrivalent human papillomavirus vaccine in HIV-1-infected women. *Clin Infect Dis.* 2014;59(1):127–135.
259. Delmas MC, Larsen C, van Benthem B, et al. Cervical squamous intraepithelial lesions in HIV-infected women: prevalence, incidence and regression. European Study Group on Natural History of HIV Infection in Women. *AIDS.* 2000;14(12):1775–1784.
260. Wright TC Jr, Koulos J, Schnoll F, et al. Cervical intraepithelial neoplasia in women infected with the human immunodeficiency virus: outcome after loop electrosurgical excision. *Gynecol Oncol.* 1994;55(2):253–258.
261. Maiman M, Watts DH, Andersen J, et al. Vaginal 5-fluorouracil for high-grade cervical dysplasia in human immunodeficiency virus infection: a randomized trial. *Obstet Gynecol.* 1999;94(6):954–961.
262. Querleu D, Morrow CP. Classification of radical hysterectomy. *Lancet Oncol.* 2008;9(3):297–303.
263. Debernardo R, Starks D, Barker N, et al. Robotic surgery in gynecologic oncology. *Obstet Gynecol Int.* 2011;2011:139867.
264. Ditto A, Martinelli F, Mattana F, et al. Class III nerve-sparing radical hysterectomy versus standard class III radical hysterectomy: an observational study. *Ann Surg Oncol.* 2011;18(12):3469–3478.
265. Charoenkwan K, Srisomboon J, Suprasert P, et al. Nerve-sparing class III radical hysterectomy: a modified technique to spare the pelvic autonomic nerves without compromising radicality. *Int J Gynecol Cancer.* 2006;16(4):1705–1712.
266. Raspagliesi F, Ditto A, Fontanelli R, et al. Type II versus Type III nerve-sparing radical hysterectomy: comparison of lower urinary tract dysfunctions. *Gynecol Oncol.* 2006;102(2):256–262.
267. Lakhman Y, Nougaret S, Micco M, et al. Role of MR Imaging and FDG PET/CT in selection and follow-up of patients treated with pelvic exenteration for gynecologic malignancies. *Radiographics.* 2015;35(4):1295–1313.
268. Burger IA, Vargas HA, Donati OF, et al. The value of 18F-FDG PET/CT in recurrent gynecologic malignancies prior to pelvic exenteration. *Gynecol Oncol.* 2013;129(3):586–592.
269. Rezk YA, Hurley KE, Carter J, et al. A prospective study of quality of life in patients undergoing pelvic exenteration: interim results. *Gynecol Oncol.* 2013;128(2):191–197.
270. Greer BE, Koh WJ, Figge DC, et al. Gynecologic radiotherapy fields defined by intraoperative measurements. *Gynecol Oncol.* 1990;38(3):421–424.
271. Dittmer PH, Randall ME. A technique for inguinal node boost using photon fields defined by asymmetric collimator jaws. *Radiother Oncol.* 2001;59(1):61–64.
272. Lim K, Small W Jr, Portelance L, et al. Consensus guidelines for delineation of clinical target volume for intensity-modulated pelvic radiotherapy for the definitive treatment of cervix cancer. *Int J Radiat Oncol Biol Phys.* 2011;79(2):348–355.
273. Fenkell L, Assenholt M, Nielsen SK, et al. Parametrial boost using midline shielding results in an unpredictable dose to tumor and organs at risk in combined external beam radiotherapy and brachytherapy for locally advanced cervical cancer. *Int J Radiat Oncol Biol Phys.* 2011;79(5):1572–1579.
274. Kridelka FJ, Berg DO, Neuman M, et al. Adjuvant small field pelvic radiation for patients with high risk, stage IB lymph node negative cervix carcinoma after radical hysterectomy and pelvic lymph node dissection. A pilot study. *Cancer.* 1999;86(10):2059–2065.
275. Ohara K, Tsunoda H, Nishida M, et al. Use of small pelvic field instead of whole pelvic field in postoperative radiotherapy for node-negative, high-risk stages I and II cervical squamous cell carcinoma. *Int J Gynecol Cancer.* 2003;13(2):170–176.
276. Randall ME, Ibbott GS. Intensity-modulated radiation therapy for gynecologic cancers: pitfalls, hazards, and cautions to be considered. *Semin Radiat Oncol.* 2006;16(3):138–143.
277. Beadle BM, Jhingran A, Salehpour M, et al. Cervix regression and motion during the course of external beam chemoradiation for cervical cancer. *Int J Radiat Oncol Biol Phys.* 2009;73(1):235–241.
278. Hasselle MD, Rose BS, Kochanski JD, et al. Clinical outcomes of intensity-modulated pelvic radiation therapy for carcinoma of the cervix. *Int J Radiat Oncol Biol Phys.* 2011;80(5):1436–1445.
279. Chen CC, Lin JC, Jan JS, et al. Definitive intensity-modulated radiation therapy with concurrent chemotherapy for patients with locally advanced cervical cancer. *Gynecol Oncol.* 2011;122(1):9–13.
280. Varia MA, Bundy BN, Deppe G, et al. Cervical carcinoma metastatic to para-aortic nodes: extended field radiation therapy with concomitant 5-fluorouracil and cisplatin chemotherapy: a Gynecologic Oncology Group study. *Int J Radiat Oncol Biol Phys.* 1998;42(5):1015–1023.
281. Kagei K, Tokuuye K, Okumura T, et al. Long-term results of proton beam therapy for carcinoma of the uterine cervix. *Int J Radiat Oncol Biol Phys.* 2003;55(5):1265–1271.
282. Viswanathan AN, Thomadsen B. American Brachytherapy Society consensus guidelines for locally advanced carcinoma of the cervix. Part I: general principles. *Brachytherapy.* 2012;11(1):33–46.
283. Viswanathan AN, Beriwal S, De Los Santos JF, et al. American Brachytherapy Society consensus guidelines for locally advanced carcinoma of the cervix. Part II: high-dose-rate brachytherapy. *Brachytherapy.* 2012;11(1):47–52.
284. Lee LJ, Das IJ, Higgins SA, et al. American Brachytherapy Society consensus guidelines for locally advanced carcinoma of the cervix. Part III: low-dose-rate and pulsed-dose-rate brachytherapy. *Brachytherapy.* 2012;11(1):53–57.
285. Heyman J. The combined radium and Rontgen treatment of cancer of the cervix uteri. *Ann Surg.* 1931;93(1):443–450.
286. International Commision on Radiation Units and Measurements. *ICRU Report 38: Dose and Volume Specification for Reporting Intracavitary Therapy in Gynecology*. Bethesda, MD: International Commission on Radiation Units and Measurements; 1985.
287. Potter R, Van Limbergen E, Gerstner N, et al. Survey of the use of the ICRU 38 in recording and reporting cervical cancer brachytherapy. *Radiother Oncol.* 2001;58(1):11–8.

288. Haie-Meder C, Potter R, Van Limbergen E, et al. Recommendations from Gynaecological (GYN) GEC-ESTRO Working Group (I): concepts and terms in 3D image based 3D treatment planning in cervix cancer brachytherapy with emphasis on MRI assessment of GTV and CTV. *Radiother Oncol*. 2005;74(3):235–245.
289. Viswanathan AN, Dimopoulos J, Kirisits C, et al. Computed tomography versus magnetic resonance imaging-based contouring in cervical cancer brachytherapy: results of a prospective trial and preliminary guidelines for standardized contours. *Int J Radiat Oncol Biol Phys*. 2007;68(2):491–498.
290. Eskander RN, Scanderbeg D, Saenz CC, et al. Comparison of computed tomography and magnetic resonance imaging in cervical cancer brachytherapy target and normal tissue contouring. *Int J Gynecol Cancer*. 2010;20(1):47–53.
291. Hall EJ. *Radiobiology for the Radiologist*. 5th ed. Philadelphia, PA: Lippincott Williams & Wilkins; 2000:588.
292. Fowler J, van Limbergen E. Biological effect of pulsed dose rate brachytherapy with stepping sources if short half-times of repair are present in tissues. *Int J Radiat Oncol Biol Phys*. 1997;37(4):877–883.
293. Swift P, Purser P, Roberts L, et al. Pulsed low dose rate brachytherapy for pelvic malignancies. *Int J Radiat Oncol Biol Phys*. 1997;37(4):811–817.
294. Rogers C, Freel J, Speiser B. Pulsed low dose rate brachytherapy for uterine cervix carcinoma. *Int J Radiat Oncol Biol Phys*. 1999;43(1):95–100.
295. Anker CJ, Cachoeira CV, Boucher KM, et al. Does the entire uterus need to be treated in cancer of the cervix? Role of adaptive brachytherapy. *Int J Radiat Oncol Biol Phys*. 2010;76(3):704–712.
296. Forrest JL, Ackerman I, Barbera L, et al. Patient outcome study of concurrent chemoradiation, external beam radiotherapy, and high-dose rate brachytherapy in locally advanced carcinoma of the cervix. *Int J Gynecol Cancer*. 2010;20(6):1074–1078.
297. Potter R, Georg P, Dimopoulos JC, et al. Clinical outcome of protocol based image (MRI) guided adaptive brachytherapy combined with 3D conformal radiotherapy with or without chemotherapy in patients with locally advanced cervical cancer. *Radiother Oncol*. 2011;100(1):116–123.
298. Schmid MP, Kirisits C, Nesvacil N, et al. Local recurrences in cervical cancer patients in the setting of image-guided brachytherapy: a comparison of spatial dose distribution within a matched-pair analysis. *Radiother Oncol*. 2011;100(3):468–472.
299. Nesvacil N, Potter R, Sturdza A, et al. Adaptive image guided brachytherapy for cervical cancer: a combined MRI-/CT-planning technique with MRI only at first fraction. *Radiother Oncol*. 2013;107(1):75–81.
300. Nesvacil N, Tanderup K, Hellebust TP, et al. A multicentre comparison of the dosimetric impact of inter- and intra-fractional anatomical variations in fractionated cervix cancer brachytherapy. *Radiother Oncol*. 2013;107(1):20–25.
301. Yoshida K, Jastaniyah N, Sturdza A, et al. Assessment of parametrial response by growth pattern in patients with international federation of gynecology and obstetrics stage IIB and IIIB cervical cancer: analysis of patients from a prospective, multicenter trial (EMBRACE). *Int J Radiat Oncol Biol Phys*. 2015;93(4):788–796.
302. Ohno T, Nakano T, Kato S, et al. Accelerated hyperfractionated radiotherapy for cervical cancer: multi-institutional prospective study of forum for nuclear cooperation in Asia among eight Asian countries. *Int J Radiat Oncol Biol Phys*. 2008;70(5):1522–1529.
303. Petereit D, Sakaria J, Chappell R, et al. The adverse effect of treatment prolongation in cervical carcinoma. *Int J Radiation Oncology Biol Phys*. 1995;32(5):1301–1307.
304. Monk BJ, Tian C, Rose PG, et al. Which clinical/pathologic factors matter in the era of chemoradiation as treatment for locally advanced cervical carcinoma? Analysis of two Gynecologic Oncology Group (GOG) trials. *Gynecol Oncol*. 2007;105(2):427–433.
305. Carrascosa LA, Yashar CM, Paris KJ, et al. Palliation of pelvic and head and neck cancer with paclitaxel and a novel radiotherapy regimen. *J Palliat Med*. 2007;10(4):877–881.
306. Spanos WJ Jr, Clery M, Perez CA, et al. Late effect of multiple daily fraction palliation schedule for advanced pelvic malignancies (RTOG 8502). *Int J Radiat Oncol Biol Phys*. 1994;29(5):961–967.
307. Spanos WJ Jr, Wasserman T, Meoz R, et al. Palliation of advanced pelvic malignant disease with large fraction pelvic radiation and misonidazole: final report of RTOG phase I/II study. *Int J Radiat Oncol Biol Phys*. 1987;13(10):1479–1482.
308. Kunos C, Radivoyevitch T, Kresak A, et al. Elevated ribonucleotide reductase levels associate with suppressed radiochemotherapy response in human cervical cancers. *Int J Gynecol Cancer*. 2012;22(9):1463–1469.
309. Runowicz CD, Wadler S, Rodriguez-Rodriguez L, et al. Concomitant cisplatin and radiotherapy in locally advanced cervical carcinoma. *Gynecol Oncol*. 1989;34(3):395–401.
310. Malfetano JH, Keys H. Aggressive multimodality treatment for cervical cancer with paraaortic lymph node metastases. *Gynecol Oncol*. 1991;42(1):44–47.
311. Malfetano J, Keys H, Kredentser D, et al. Weekly cisplatin and radical radiation therapy for advanced, recurrent, and poor prognosis cervical carcinoma. *Cancer*. 1993;71(11):3703–3706.
312. Malfetano JH, Keys H, Cunningham MJ, et al. Extended field radiation and cisplatin for stage IIB and IIIB cervical carcinoma. *Gynecol Oncol*. 1997;67(2):203–27.
313. Nyholm S, Thelander L, Graslund A. Reduction and loss of the iron center in the reaction of the small subunit of mouse ribonucleotide reductase with hydroxyurea. *Biochemistry*. 1993;32(43):11569–11574.
314. Katsumata N, Yoshikawa H, Kobayashi H, et al. Phase III randomised controlled trial of neoadjuvant chemotherapy plus radical surgery vs radical surgery alone for stages IB2, IIA2, and IIB cervical cancer: a Japan Clinical Oncology Group trial (JCOG 0102). *Br J Cancer*. 2013;108(10):1957–1963.
315. Singh RB, Chander S, Mohanti BK, et al. Neoadjuvant chemotherapy with weekly paclitaxel and carboplatin followed by chemoradiation in locally advanced cervical carcinoma: a pilot study. *Gynecol Oncol*. 2013;129(1):124–128.
316. McCormack M, Kadalayil L, Hackshaw A, et al. A phase II study of weekly neoadjuvant chemotherapy followed by radical chemoradiation for locally advanced cervical cancer. *Br J Cancer*. 2013;108(12):2464–2469.
317. Santin AD, Sill MW, McMeekin DS, et al. Phase II trial of cetuximab in the treatment of persistent or recurrent squamous or non-squamous cell carcinoma of the cervix: a Gynecologic Oncology Group study. *Gynecol Oncol*. 2011;122(3):495–500.
318. Farley J, Sill MW, Birrer M, et al. Phase II study of cisplatin plus cetuximab in advanced, recurrent, and previously treated cancers of the cervix and evaluation of epidermal growth factor receptor immunohistochemical expression: a Gynecologic Oncology Group study. *Gynecol Oncol*. 2011;121(2):303–308.
319. Schilder RJ, Sill MW, Lee YC, et al. A phase II trial of erlotinib in recurrent squamous cell carcinoma of the cervix: a Gynecologic Oncology Group Study. *Int J Gynecol Cancer*. 2009;19(5):929–933.
320. McGuire WP, Blessing JA, Moore D, et al. Paclitaxel has moderate activity in squamous cervix cancer. A Gynecologic Oncology Group study. *J Clin Oncol*. 1996;14(3):792–795.
321. Garcia AA, Blessing JA, Vaccarello L, et al. Phase II clinical trial of docetaxel in refractory squamous cell carcinoma of the cervix: a Gynecologic Oncology Group Study. *Am J Clin Oncol*. 2007;30(4):428–431.
322. Alberts DS, Blessing JA, Landrum LM, et al. Phase II trial of nab-paclitaxel in the treatment of recurrent or persistent advanced cervix cancer: a gynecologic oncology group study. *Gynecol Oncol*. 2012;127(3):451–455.
323. Rose PG, Blessing JA, Gershenson DM, et al. Paclitaxel and cisplatin as first-line therapy in recurrent or advanced squamous cell carcinoma of the cervix: a gynecologic oncology group study. *J Clin Oncol*. 1999;17(9):2676–2680.
324. Miller DS, Blessing JA, Bodurka DC, et al. Evaluation of pemetrexed (Alimta, LY231514) as second line chemotherapy in persistent or recurrent carcinoma of the cervix: a phase II study of the Gynecologic Oncology Group. *Gynecol Oncol*. 2008;110(1):65–70.
325. Miller DS, Blessing JA, Ramondetta LM, et al. Pemetrexed and cisplatin for the treatment of advanced, persistent, or recurrent carcinoma of the cervix: a limited access phase II trial of the gynecologic oncology group. *J Clin Oncol*. 2014;32(25):2744–2749.
326. Shunkwiler L, Ferris G, Kunos C. Inhibition of poly(ADP-Ribose) polymerase enhances radiochemosensitivity in cancers proficient in DNA double-strand break repair. *Int J Mol Sci*. 2013;14(2):3773–3785.
327. Kunos C, Deng W, Dawson D, et al. A phase I-II evaluation of veliparib (NSC #737664), topotecan, and filgrastim or pegfilgrastim in the treatment of persistent or recurrent carcinoma of the uterine cervix: an NRG Oncology/Gynecologic Oncology Group Study. *Int J Gynecol Cancer*. 2015;25(3):484–492.
328. Rosa DD, Medeiros LR, Edelweiss MI, et al. Adjuvant platinum-based chemotherapy for early stage cervical cancer. *Cochrane Database Syst Rev*. 2012;(6):CD005342. doi:10.1002/14651858.CD005342.pub3.
329. Sugiyama T, Fujiwara K, Ohashi Y, et al. Phase III placebo-controlled double-blind randomized trial of radiotherapy for stage IIB-IVA cervical cancer with or without immunomodulator Z-100: a JGOG study. *Ann Oncol*. 2014;25(5):1011–1017.
330. Levrant SG, Fruchter RG, Maiman M. Radical hysterectomy for cervical cancer: morbidity and survival in relation to weight and age. *Gynecol Oncol*. 1992;45(3):317–322.

331. Cohn DE, Swisher EM, Herzog TJ, et al. Radical hysterectomy for cervical cancer in obese women. *Obstet Gynecol.* 2000;96(5 pt 1):727–731.
332. Franchi M, Trimbos JB, Zanaboni F, et al. Randomised trial of drains versus no drains following radical hysterectomy and pelvic lymph node dissection: a European Organisation for Research and Treatment of Cancer-Gynaecological Cancer Group (EORTC-GCG) study in 234 patients. *Eur J Cancer.* 2007;43(8):1265–1268.
333. Perez CA, Grigsby PW, Lockett MA, et al. Radiation therapy morbidity in carcinoma of the uterine cervix: dosimetric and clinical correlation. *Int J Radiat Oncol Biol Phys.* 1999;44(4):855–866.
334. Eifel PJ, Levenback C, Wharton JT, et al. Time course and incidence of late complications in patients treated with radiation therapy for FIGO stage IB carcinoma of the uterine cervix. *Int J Radiat Oncol Biol Phys.* 1995;32(5):1289–1300.
335. Jhingran A, Eifel PJ. Perioperative and postoperative complications of intracavitary radiation for FIGO stage I-III carcinoma of the cervix. *Int J Radiat Oncol Biol Phys.* 2000;46(5):1177–1183.
336. Bergmark K, Avall-Lundqvist E, Dickman PW, et al. Vaginal changes and sexuality in women with a history of cervical cancer. *N Engl J Med.* 1999;340(18):1383–1389.
337. Oh D, Huh SJ, Nam H, et al. Pelvic insufficiency fracture after pelvic radiotherapy for cervical cancer: analysis of risk factors. *Int J Radiat Oncol Biol Phys.* 2008;70(4):1183–1188.
338. Gothard L, Cornes P, Brooker S, et al. Phase II study of vitamin E and pentoxifylline in patients with late side effects of pelvic radiotherapy. *Radiother Oncol.* 2005;75(3):334–341.
339. Chiao TB, Lee AJ. Role of pentoxifylline and vitamin E in attenuation of radiation-induced fibrosis. *Ann Pharmacother.* 2005;39(3):516–522.
340. Feldmeier J. Hyperbaric oxygen therapy for delayed radiation injuries. In: Neuman T, Thom S, eds. *Physiology and Medicine of Hyperbaric Oxygen Therapy.* Philadelphia, PA: Saunders Elsevier; 2008:231–256.
341. Fink D, Chetty N, Lehm JP, et al. Hyperbaric oxygen therapy for delayed radiation injuries in gynecological cancers. *Int J Gynecol Cancer.* 2006;16(2):638–642.
342. Berrington de Gonzalez A, Curtis RE, Kry SF, et al. Proportion of second cancers attributable to radiotherapy treatment in adults: a cohort study in the US SEER cancer registries. *Lancet Oncol.* 2011;12(4):353–360.
343. Green J, Kirwan J, Tierney J, et al. Concomitant chemotherapy and radiation therapy for cancer of the uterine cervix. *Cochrane Database Syst Rev.* 2005;20(3):CD002225.
344. Vale CL, Tierney JF, Davidson SE, et al. Substantial improvement in UK cervical cancer survival with chemoradiotherapy: results of a Royal College of Radiologists' audit. *Clin Oncol (R Coll Radiol).* 2010;22(7):590–601.
345. Barbera L, Thomas G. Venous thromboembolism in cervical cancer. *Lancet Oncol.* 2008;9(1):54–60.
346. Barbera L, Thomas G. Erythropoiesis stimulating agents, thrombosis and cancer. *Radiother Oncol.* 2010;95(3):269–276.
347. Jacobson G, Lammli J, Zamba G, et al. Thromboembolic events in patients with cervical carcinoma: Incidence and effect on survival. *Gynecol Oncol.* 2009;113(2):240–244.
348. Fairman J, Wijerathna S, Ahmad M, et al. Structural basis for allosteric regulation of human ribonucleotide reductase by nucleotide-induced oligomerization. *Nat Struct Mol Biol.* 2011;18(3):316–322.
349. Kolberg M, Strand KR, Graff P, et al. Structure, function, and mechanism of ribonucleotide reductases. *Biochim Biophys Acta.* 2004;1699(1–2):1–34.
350. Reece S, Hodgkiss J, Stubbe J, et al. Proton-coupled electron transfer: the mechanistic underpinning for radical transport and catalysis in biology. *Phil Trans R Soc B.* 2006;361:1351–1364.
351. Kunos C, Ferris G, Pyatka N, et al. Deoxynucleoside salvage facilitates DNA repair during ribonucleotide reductase blockade in human cervical cancers. *Radiat Res.* 2011;176(4):425–433.
352. Weinberg G, Ullman D, Martin D Jr. Mutator phenotypes in mammalian cell mutants with distinct biochemical defects and abnormal deoxyribonucleoside triphosphate pools. *Proc Natl Acad Sci U S A.* 1981;78(4):2447–2451.
353. Radivoyevitch T. Automated mass action model space generation and analysis methods for two-reactant combinatorially complex equilibriums: An analysis of ATP-induced ribonucleotide reductase R1 hexamerization data. *Biol Direct.* 2009;4(1):50.
354. Eriksson S, Graslund A, Skog S, et al. Cell cycle-dependent regulation of mammalian ribonucleotide reductase. The S phase-correlated increase in subunit M2 is regulated by de novo protein synthesis. *J Biol Chem.* 1984;259:11695–11700.
355. Chabes A, Thelander L. Controlled protein degradation regulates ribonucleotide reductase activity in proliferating mammalian cells during the normal cell cycle and in response to DNA damage and replication blocks. *J Biol Chem.* 2000;275(23):17747–17753.
356. Tanaka H, Arakawa H, Yamaguchi T, et al. A ribonucleotide reductase gene involved in a p53-dependent cell-cycle checkpoint for DNA damage. *Nature.* 2000;404(6773):42–49.
357. Xue L, Zhou B, Liu X, et al. Wild-type p53 regulates human ribonucleotide reductase by protein-protein interaction with p53R2 as well as hRRM2 subunits. *Cancer Res.* 2003;63(5):980–986.
358. Zhou B, Liu X, Mo X, et al. The human ribonucleotide reductase subunit hRRM2 complements p53R2 in response to UV-induced DNA repair in cells with mutant p53. *Cancer Res.* 2003;63(20):6583–6594.

CHAPTER 21

Corpus: Epithelial Tumors

Susana M. Campos, Larissa J. Lee, Marcela G. Del Carmen, and D. Scott McMeekin

Endometrial cancer accounts for nearly 50% of all new gynecologic cancers diagnosed in the United States. It is the fourth most common malignancy in women, and the eighth most common cause of cancer death. The American Cancer Society (ACS) estimated that there were 60,050 new cases of endometrial carcinoma and 10,470 deaths from advanced or recurrent disease in 2015 (including both endometrial cancers [EC] and uterine sarcomas) (1). Worldwide, EC is only second to cervical cancer in frequency. The ACS reported that the incidence of EC rose 13% from 1987 to 2012; however, the numbers of deaths rose ~250% in the same time period. Endometrial carcinoma occurs most often in the sixth and seventh decades of life, with an average age at onset of 60 years. It is estimated that 75% to 85% of the cases occur in women aged 50 years and older, and 95% occur in patients over 40 years of age (2,3). The disease, although reported in patients as young as age 16 years, is rare in women younger than 30 years of age.

Endometrial cancer is commonly confined to the uterus at diagnosis. Data from the National Cancer Institute's Surveillance, Epidemiology, and End Results (SEER) program demonstrated that stage I disease was found in 73% of patients, and 10% had stage II disease (4). The 26th Annual Report of the International Federation of Gynecology and Obstetrics (FIGO) on 9,386 EC patients demonstrated that 83% of patients were stage I–II (5). With the favorable disease distribution at presentation, it is not surprising that most patients have a favorable prognosis. Results from FIGO show that 85% to 91% of stage I patients are alive at 5 years, and patients in the SEER database with localized disease have 96% 5-year survival (4,5). As a result, EC has been considered a "good cancer"; that is, most patients present with early-stage, highly curable disease. Despite the favorable characteristics for most patients, those with high-risk factors, including increased age, higher tumor grade, aggressive histology, and advanced-stage face real challenges.

The management of EC continues to evolve. In the past, most patients received some form of pre- or postoperative radiation in combination with a simple hysterectomy. With a better understanding of the relationship between uterine factor and risk of nodal disease and recurrence, selective use of surgical staging was integrated. This was followed by an era during which, increasingly, surgical therapy expanded to include routine use of pelvic and para-aortic lymphadenectomy. Minimally invasive techniques were studied, and have been routinely adopted into the surgical management of women with EC. Today, greater emphasis is being placed on the selection of particular patients for whom lymphadenectomy may offer better outcomes, and whose avoidance may result in less morbidity. Understanding tumor biology as it relates to predicting recurrence and survival, and how genetic changes can be exploited to direct postoperative therapies, represent our current challenges. Over 10 years ago, the National Cancer Institute convened an expert panel to develop a national 5-year plan for research priorities in gynecologic cancers. The resulting report, Priorities of the Gynecologic Cancer Progress Review Group (PRG), specified that an understanding of tumor biology was the central key in controlling gynecologic cancers. For EC, one of the top research priorities defined by the PRG was to identify prognostic and predictive markers for treatment efficacy and toxicity. In a 2006 State of the Science Meeting in Manchester, UK, a series of research questions on prevention, adjuvant treatment, and treatment of advanced or recurrent disease were proposed for setting the stage for a clinical trials agenda over the next 5 years (6). In 2011, the Society of Gynecologic Oncologists convened a panel of experts that produced a report, "Pathway to Progress in Women's Cancers." That report detailed areas of research, by disease site, on which the women's cancer community should focus for the next decade. For EC, the recommended road map for the future would include research related to obesity, predicting risk of metastatic disease, targeting therapy based on risk factors and molecular characteristics of disease, and cost-effective care (7).

Current clinical controversies center on identifying which patient populations might benefit most from lymphadenectomy, developing alternatives to performing lymphadenectomy, and creating risk models to assist in selection of patients who may benefit most from adjuvant therapies. While we suspect that an increased use of surgical staging has translated to a better understanding of risk, data also suggest that despite negative nodes, uterine factors play a significant role in risk of recurrence. Current trends also suggest a less frequent use of pelvic radiation therapy (RT) or no use of any radiation (8). There have been important developments in chemotherapy (CT) for EC. Combination CT is increasingly used in the primary management of advanced and recurrent disease, and may hold promise in an adjuvant setting. How to best integrate RT, and which specific techniques to consider, are being studied in ongoing clinical trials. Hormonal therapy remains an important option, and our understanding of steroid receptors at a molecular level may help to determine which patients may benefit most (9). Enhanced understanding of biologically relevant targets has fostered the development of new classes of agents that target susceptible pathways in tumor cells, and targeted agents are being integrated into large clinical trials (10,11).

ANATOMY

The uterus is a fibromuscular pelvic organ situated between the bladder and the rectum and enveloped by peritoneal reflections. It is divided into the fundus, isthmus, and cervix. The uterine wall is composed of the outer smooth muscle myometrium and inner cavity lined by glandular endometrial epithelium with supporting stroma (endometrium). Five paired ligaments cover or support the uterus: broad, round, uterosacral, cardinal, and vesicouterine. The uterosacral and cardinal ligaments provide the greatest support within the pelvis and, contrary to cervical cancer, are infrequently involved with tumor spread. Blood is supplied to the uterus by the uterine artery, a branch of the hypogastric artery, which enters the wall of the uterus at the isthmus after it crosses over the ureter. It anastomoses with the ovarian artery in the ovarian ligament.

Malignant transformation of the endometrium is manifest in many fashions, based on the anatomic relationships. Tumor growth may be confined to the endometrium, invade the underlying myometrium, penetrate to the uterine serosal surface or adjacent bladder or rectum, or extend into the cervical canal and invade cervical glands or stroma. Peritoneal disease spread may occur via transmigration from the fallopian tubes or through serosal penetration. Hematogenous spread is not uncommon in EC.

The lymphatics of the myometrium drain into the subserosal network of lymphatics, which coalesce into larger channels before leaving the uterus. Lymph flows from the fundus toward the adnexa and infundibulopelvic ligaments. The lymph flow from the lower and middle thirds of the uterus tends to spread in the base of the broad ligaments toward the lateral pelvic sidewall (12). There are four drainage channels from the uterus: from the fundus, in the folds of the broad ligament, along the mesosalpinx and fallopian tubes, and along the round ligaments. The drainage sites are principally reflected in metastatic potential to pelvic and para-aortic lymph nodes (LN), and occasionally involve inguinal nodes.

Epidemiology and Risk Factors

The most important risk factor for the development of EC is age. Endometrial cancer is primarily a disease of postmenopausal woman, with median age at cancer diagnosis of 60 years (5). Approximately 85% of cases occur after the age of 50; the peak age-specific incidence is from 75 to 79 years (109 per 100,000), and only 5% of cases are reported in women younger than 40 years of age (2,3,13). The ACS has reported that the probability of developing a uterine cancer to be 1 in 142 from age 40 to 59, 1 in 124 from age 60 to 69, and 1 in 78 from age 70 and older (1). Not unexpectedly, with an aging U.S. population, the total number of cases of EC has increased yearly, whereas the annual age-adjusted incidence rate peaked in the mid-1970s (33.8 per 100,000) and has remained stable at 23 to 25 cases per 100,000 women over the last 10 years (1).

Race also appears to play a role in the development of EC. The rates of EC are highest in North America and northern Europe, lower in Eastern Europe and Latin America, and lowest in Asia and Africa (14). Factors accounting for these findings include differences in rates of obesity, use of hormone replacement therapy (HRT), and reproductive factors. In the U.S., non-Hispanic White women have the highest age-adjusted incidence of EC at 25.4 (per 100,000 women), compared to women of African American (19.5), Asian (15.8), or Hispanic (17) heritage (15). African American women, however, have a much higher mortality rate (7.1 vs. 3.9 per 100,000) and lower 5-year survival (61% vs. 84%) compared to non-Hispanic White women. Relative survival in White women exceeds that for African Americans by at least 7% at every stage of diagnosis (1). In the 2012 ACS report, incidence rates of uterine cancers in White women were noted to have stabilized; however, since 2004, incidence rates have increased by nearly 2% per year for African American women (1). Multiple explanations have been suggested to explain the differences in outcomes between racial groups, including differences in frequency of high-risk tumor types, differences in access to care (reduced use of surgery and radiation), and differences in medical comorbidities among races. Data from SEER demonstrated that African American women were more frequently diagnosed with higher stage, grade, and high-risk histologies than non-Hispanic White women, but there was no difference in the frequency of recommended therapy between races (4). In two analyses of nearly 1,200 patients with advanced or recurrent EC who participated in phase 3 chemotherapy trials conducted by the Gynecologic Oncology Group (GOG), African American race was independently associated with a lower likelihood of response to CT (relative odds of response 0.62) and decreased overall survival (OS; hazard ratio [HR], 1.26) compared to White women (16,17). These results suggest that racial disparity in outcomes exist even though patients were treated in similar fashion. Interestingly, one small study comparing microarray-based expression profiling between stage-, grade-, and histology-matched African American and Caucasian patients found no clear differences in global gene expression profiles, suggesting that environmental or social issues played a greater role in explaining disparity (18).

Most cases of endometrial carcinoma are thought to be sporadic; however, some cases clearly have a hereditary basis. Lynch syndrome (hereditary nonpolyposis colorectal cancer [HNPCC]) is an autosomal-dominant cancer susceptibility syndrome associated with early-onset colon, rectal, ovary, small bowel, ureter/renal pelvis cancers, and EC. Lynch syndrome–related ECs account for 2% to 5% of all ECs, and occur in nearly 10% of women diagnosed with EC at less than 50 years of age (19). The lifetime risk of EC in women with Lynch syndrome is 40% to 60%, a risk similar to that of developing colon cancer. The risk of ovarian cancer is 10% to 12%. In about 50% of cases where patients have both colonic and gynecologic cancers (endometrial or ovarian), the gynecologic cancer precedes the diagnosis of colon cancer (20). The syndrome is most commonly due to germ-line mutations of one of the DNA mismatch repair genes *MSH2, MLH1, or MSH6*. In one study, 23% of EC patients diagnosed at $<$50 years of age, with one relative having a Lynch-type cancer, had a mismatch repair gene mutation (21). Prophylactic hysterectomy and bilateral salpingo-oophorectomy has been shown to be an effective strategy for preventing ovarian and ECs in these high-risk patients (22).

Controversy exists regarding the relationship between *BRCA1* and *BRCA2* mutations and the risk of EC. Germ-line mutations of *BRCA1* and *BRCA2* account for a large proportion of hereditary breast and ovarian/primary peritoneal cancers. In 1999, Hornreich et al. (23) presented a case report of sisters with the same *BRCA1* mutation who were diagnosed with serous carcinomas of the uterus, and suggested a possible association. Several larger studies have attempted to address this hypothesis. In one study of 199 Ashkenazi Jewish patients with EC from a single institution, Levine et al. genotyped all patients for founder *BRCA1* and *BRCA2* mutations that existed in that patient population. The frequency of germ-line mutations (3 per 199, 1.5%) in EC patients was comparable to the baseline rate of 2% in the Ashkenazi population, suggesting no increased risk (24). In a large prospective study by Beiner et al., (25) 857 known *BRCA1* and *BRCA2* carriers aged 45 to 70 years were followed over time for the development of EC. With an average length of follow-up of 3.3 years, six women developed EC. Four of the six patients had used tamoxifen. Compared to the expected rate of EC in a general population, *BRCA* carriers who did not receive tamoxifen did not have a significant increase in risk of developing EC, whereas those patients who had received tamoxifen had an 11.6 incidence ratio ($p = 0.0004$). Barak evaluated 289 Jewish women with EC (80% type I, 20% type II tumors) for predominant mutations in Jewish populations (*BRCA1, BRCA2, MSH2, MSH6* selected mutations). Five women were found with *BRCA1/2* mutations, reflecting a rate similar to that seen in the general Ashkenazi Jewish population, and the authors indicated that the data did not support screening based on an EC diagnosis (26).

The clinical picture in endometrial carcinoma is varied, as are the associated risk factors for its development. One of the paradigms for bridging the gaps between epidemiologic, clinical pathologic, and molecular factors seen in EC types is the relatively simple, yet attractive classification system of ECs suggested by Bokhman in 1983 (27). Endometrial cancers are thought to broadly arise from one of two different pathways: estrogen dependent or estrogen independent (**Table 21.1**). On the basis of the clinical and histologic features, ECs have been divided into type I and type II tumors. Type I tumors are more common (85%), tend to be found in younger women, and develop via a precursor lesion of atypical hyperplasia. These tumors are associated with a predisposing history of hyperestrogenism. They tend to be well differentiated and have minimal myometrial invasion, and as a result typically have a favorable outcome. Type II tumors account for a small percentage of ECs, occur in an older population, and frequently develop in the setting of an atrophic endometrium. About half of all relapses occur in this group. Serous, clear cell, and perhaps grade 3 tumors fit into the type II category. Despite the broad generalizations of the two categories, translational science data lends support for distinguishing these groups at a molecular level. For example, mutations of *TP53* are common in uterine papillary serous carcinoma (UPSC), and rare in type I tumors (28). In type I tumors, tumor suppressor genes encoding the phosphatase

■ **TABLE 21.1. Comparison between Type I and Type II Endometrial Cancers**

	Type I	Type II
Clinical features		
Risk factors	Unopposed estrogen	Age
Race	White > Black	White = Black
Differentiation	Well differentiated	Poorly differentiated
Histology	Endometrioid	Non-endometrioid
Stage	I/II	III/IV
Prognosis	Favorable	Not favorable
Molecular features		
Ploidy	Diploid	Aneuploid
K-ras overexpression	Yes	Yes
HER2/neu overexpression	No	Yes
P53 overexpression	No	Yes
PTEN mutations	Yes	No
MSI	Yes	No

MSI, microsatellite instability.

and tensin homologue (*PTEN)* mutations are common, but are rare with UPSC tumors. Global gene expression profiles have also been shown to be different between type I and II tumors (29).

Endogenous or exogenous exposure to estrogen is believed to be an important risk factor for the development of endometrial hyperplasia and type I cancers (30). Estrogens not opposed by progestins lead to increased mitotic activity of endometrial cells, resulting in more frequent errors in DNA replication and somatic mutations (31,32). These genetic changes are manifest clinically in endometrial hyperplasia and cancer. Estrogen excess as an etiology for cancers is supported by epidemiologic features of the disease. Patients with chronic anovulation, nulliparity, early age of menarche, and late menopause have classically been identified with EC. Occasionally, endometrial hyperplasia or cancer develops in the setting of an estrogen-producing ovarian tumor (granulosa cell tumor) (33). The use of unopposed estrogens as part of hormone replacement strategies was first defined as an important risk factor in 1975, when the age-adjusted rate for EC peaked at nearly 33.8 per 100,000 (34,35). A meta-analysis of 30 studies showed that the relative risk of ever-users of estrogen therapy was 2.3 compared to non-users, and it increased to 9.5 in users of 10 or more years (36).

Obesity is an increasingly common problem in the U.S., and is estimated to account for 17% to 46% of EC in postmenopausal women (36). Studies have shown that plasma concentrations of androstenedione and estrogens are correlated with body weight in postmenopausal women (37,38). Aromatization of androstenedione to estrone in adipose cells is believed to be the principle mechanism of excess estrogen production (39). While much of the data suggests that the relationship is strongest between estrogen exposures and type I cancers, Weiss et al. demonstrated in a case–control study that the risk of more aggressive tumors (higher grade or higher stage) was also seen with unopposed estrogen therapy, obesity, low parity, and history of diabetes. The authors suggested that the risk of EC was influenced by similar risk factors regardless of tumor aggressiveness (40). Diabetes has also been associated classically with type I ECs (41,42). Only noninsulin-dependent diabetes (type 2 diabetes mellitus [DM]), characterized by insulin resistance and elevated insulin levels, appears to be associated with EC (43). Hyperinsulinemia and higher levels of insulin-like growth factor 1 are thought to have neoplastic potential and, coupled with increased estrogen, are responsible for cancer development (44–46).

Tamoxifen and Endometrial Cancer

Tamoxifen is a selective estrogen receptor modulator (SERM) with antiestrogenic properties in the breast and estrogenic effects in tissues such as bone, the cardiovascular system, and the uterus. It has been used in prevention and treatment for all stages of breast cancer. An association with tamoxifen and EC was first reported by Killackey et al. (47) in 1985. The strongest data initially implicating tamoxifen use and the subsequent development of EC were published in 1989 by Fornander et al. (48). The investigators reviewed the frequency of new primary cancers as recorded in the Swedish Cancer Registry for a group of 1,846 postmenopausal women with early breast cancer who were included in a randomized trial of adjuvant tamoxifen. They noted a 6.4-fold increase in the relative risk of EC in 931 tamoxifen-treated patients compared to 915 patients in the control group. The dose of tamoxifen in this study was 40 mg/d, and the greatest cumulative risk of developing EC was after 5 years of tamoxifen use.

Fisher et al. (49) published data regarding the association between tamoxifen use and the development of EC when they reported the findings of the National Surgical Adjuvant Breast and Bowel Project (NSABP) B-14 trial. Data regarding the rates of endometrial and other cancers were analyzed in 2,843 patients with node-negative, estrogen receptor (ER)-positive, invasive breast cancer randomly assigned to placebo or tamoxifen (20 mg/d), and on 1,220 tamoxifen-treated patients registered in NSABP B-14, subsequent to randomization. The average annual hazard rate for EC in the placebo group was 0.2 out of 1,000 and 1.6 out of 1,000 for the randomized tamoxifen-treated group. The relative risk of an EC occurring in the randomized, tamoxifen-treated group was 7.5. Similar results were seen in the 1,220 registered patients who received tamoxifen. The mean duration of tamoxifen therapy was 35 months, with 36% of the ECs developing within 2 years of therapy and six occurring less than 9 months after treatment was initiated, suggesting that some of the cancers may have been present prior to starting tamoxifen therapy.

Any conclusions drawn regarding the risks of tamoxifen treatment in inducing EC must weigh the benefits of tamoxifen in reducing breast cancer recurrence and new contralateral breast cancers. In the B-14 trial, the cumulative rate per 1,000 women with breast cancer relapse was reduced from 227.8 in the placebo group to 123.5 in the randomized tamoxifen-treated group. In addition, the cumulative rate of contralateral breast cancer was reduced from 40.5 to 23.5, respectively, in the two groups. Taking into account the increased cumulative rate of EC, there was a 38% reduction in the 5-year cumulative hazard rate in the tamoxifen-treated group. Thus, the benefit of tamoxifen therapy for breast cancer outweighs the potential increase in EC.

The suspected mechanism for EC development following tamoxifen exposure is thought to be related to its estrogenic effects on the endometrium. As such, type I, low-grade/early-stage cancers would be expected. A report from the Yale Tumor Registry by Magriples et al. (50) suggested that uterine cancers occurring in breast cancer patients on tamoxifen may behave more aggressively, and carry a worse prognosis. Other studies, however, have not been able to confirm these findings (**Table 21.2**) (49,51–53). It would appear from the available literature that there is no difference in the stage, grade, or prognosis of ECs associated with tamoxifen use.

More commonly, breast cancer patients are being managed with different strategies, which may reduce the impact of tamoxifen on EC risk. Next-generation SERM agents, such as raloxifene, are effective in preventing breast cancer and reducing osteoporosis. In a large case–control study of women with (547 cases) and without (1,410 controls) EC, raloxifene users had a 50% reduction in risk of EC compared to non-users, and tamoxifen users had three times the risk of developing EC compared to those who had used raloxifene

TABLE 21.2. Clinicopathologic Data from Series Reporting on Tamoxifen-Associated Uterine Cancer

	Magriples	Barakat	Fisher	van Leeuwen	van Leeuwen	Total (%)
No. patients	15	23	25	17	23	103
FIGO stage						
I	7	15	21	14	17	74 (71.8)
II	0	2	1	2	3	8 (7.8)
III	2	5	1	0	0	8 (7.8)
IV	0	1	1	1	0	3 (2.9)
Unstaged	6	0	1	0	3	10 (9.7)
Histology						
Endometrioid	9	17	18	16	17	77 (74.8)
High-risk[a]	6	6	7	1	6	26 (25.2)
Grade (adenocarcinoma)						
Low (grade 1,2)	5	13	18	15	Not given	51 (72.9)[b]
High (grade 3)	10	4	5	0	Not given	19 (27.1)[b]
Deaths from uterine cancer	5 (33%)	5 (22%)	4 (16%)	3 (10%)	0 (0%)	17 (16.5)

[a]Includes papillary serous, clear cell, sarcoma.

[b]Grade only known for 70 patients.

Source: Reprinted with permission from Barakat RR. The effect of tamoxifen on the endometrium. *Oncology.* 1995;9:129–134.

(54). Compared to SERMs, aromatase inhibitors prevent estrogen synthesis by inhibiting the conversion of androgens to estrogens. Third-generation aromatase inhibitors (anastrozole, letrozole, exemestane) are replacing tamoxifen for many breast cancer patients, with ~50% of postmenopausal ER-positive patients receiving aromatase inhibitors (53). In clinical trials, compared to tamoxifen, aromatase inhibitors are associated with lower incidences of vaginal bleeding or EC (54,55). In premenopausal patients, aromatase inhibitors have little activity, and tamoxifen will continue to play a role.

Protective Factors

Factors that reduce circulating estrogen levels (weight loss/exercise, cigarette smoking) appear to be protective against EC. Similarly, progestins antagonize the effects of estrogen on the endometrium and prevent the development of hyperplasia and cancer, when added to estrogens (endogenous or exogenous) (56). Combined estrogen–progestin HRT has been associated with reductions in the risk of EC in most, but not all, studies. Prior use of oral contraceptives also appears to be protective against the development of EC (57,58).

Natural History of Disease

A better understanding of the natural history of EC has developed through evaluation of the patterns of spread. In a landmark study, the GOG performed a surgical pathologic study (GOG 33) in 621 patients with clinical stage I–occult stage II EC who underwent a standardized surgical procedure including exploration of the abdomen with biopsy of suspicious findings, collection of peritoneal fluid for cytologic evaluation, abdominal hysterectomy and BSO, and pelvic and para-aortic nodal dissection (59). The results of this study demonstrated important relationships regarding uterine tumor characteristics and spread of disease, and should be ingrained into the memory of those caring for patients with ECs.

Overall, 22% of patients with seemingly uterine-confined disease were found to have extrauterine spread. Pelvic and/or para-aortic metastases were found in 11% of patients, 12% had positive peritoneal cytology, 5% had adnexal involvement, and 6% had gross intraperitoneal spread. Nodal metastases were related to tumor grade and depth of myometrial invasion, and patients with positive cytology, or adnexal or intraperitoneal spread also had increased frequency of nodal disease.

Patterns of failure in patients with recurrent EC demonstrate, alone or in combination, hematogenous, lymphatic, intraperitoneal, or local/contiguous spread. As attention has increasingly focused on therapies (surgical, radiation, CT) to reduce particular sites of recurrences, several have argued for defining relationships between initial disease spread and subsequent risk of recurrence (60). In GOG 33, treatment was not specified by protocol, but results showed that outcomes could be predicted by extent of disease found at surgery, thus demonstrating the important relationship between what is learned at surgical staging and recurrence risk (61).

Diagnostic Evaluation

Screening

Many ECs develop by way of a precursor lesion. Estrogen-related cancers frequently develop secondary to atypical endometrial hyperplasia (AEH) or demonstrate AEH in the uterus at the time of hysterectomy. Serous tumors may also develop through a precursor lesion, endometrial intraepithelial carcinoma (EIC) (62,63). Prompt recognition of precursor lesions, with institution of proper treatment, will prevent cancers and their sequelae. The relatively low prevalence of EC in the population (5 per 1,000 women >45 years) makes standardized screening inefficient. There are a few uncontrolled studies lending some support to the efficacy of screening programs (64,65). No randomized trials have been published. No health economic data have been presented in relation to the published reports. The American College of Obstetrics and Gynecology and the Society of Gynecologic Oncology do not recommend routine screening of patients for uterine cancer (66,67). The ACS does recommend annual endometrial biopsies starting at age 35 for women known to have or to be at risk for HNPCC.

In lieu of routine screening, prompt assessment of symptomatic patients and those at high risk should be considered. Because 95% of ECs occur in women aged 40 years and older, and because endometrial hyperplasia tends to occur in premenopausal and perimenopausal women, it is appropriate to evaluate individuals past their fourth decade of life if they experience abnormal bleeding. Similarly, a higher degree of suspicion should be held for younger patients with high-risk characteristics including significant obesity, polycystic ovarian syndrome/chronic anovulation, or tamoxifen exposure.

Prevention

Due to the increased risk of EC associated with unopposed estrogens, women with an intact uterus should rarely, if ever, be prescribed estrogen-only replacement therapy. The addition of progestins to the regimens of patients treated with exogenous estrogen may prevent endometrial hyperplasia and protect against the development of carcinoma (56,57). Continuous or sequential progestin regimens may be used, but the most important factor is administration of a progestin for at least 10 to 14 days each month. In patients with chronic endogenous estrogen exposure, such as obese women with polycystic ovarian syndrome or chronic anovulation, and perimenopausal women with menometrorrhagia, periodic treatment with a progestin to create scheduled withdrawal bleeding and prevent hyperplasia may be considered (68,69).

In most cases, patients with hyperplasia with atypia should be treated by vaginal or abdominal hysterectomy to prevent the development of EC (70). Surgery is the definitive therapy as it stops bleeding, prevents cancer, and alleviates the potential for medical failure. Patients with AEH remain at high risk for recurrence of AEH or cancer during their lifetime, even after successful medical therapy (71). Most importantly, despite a preoperative diagnosis of AEH, many patients will be found to have a cancer at the time of hysterectomy (71,72). Older data suggested that if the endometrial sample is obtained by a biopsy or curettage, 15% to 25% of patients with the diagnosis of atypical hyperplasia may have a uterine carcinoma (73,74). Prospective data from a large surgical–pathologic trial conducted by the GOG demonstrated that, of 289 patients with a community diagnosis of AEH, 40% had an EC (72). Neither the type of preoperative endometrial biopsy (office endometrial biopsy [EMB] or dilatation and curettage [D&C]), nor the use of an expert pathology panel, was associated with a better ability to predict who had cancer or not. Patients with significant medical comorbidities, advanced age, or those desiring future fertility may be managed with progestational therapy (75). It has been suggested that a D&C should be performed in patients who will be medically managed with progestins for therapeutic effect (surgical curettage of tissue) and to better define the risk of an unrecognized cancer, while the data to support these practices are limited. When progestins are used to manage AEH, the specific agents, doses, and schedules may mirror those used to manage dysfunctional uterine bleeding or advanced or recurrent cancer. To assess the success of medical therapy, endometrial biopsies should be performed at 3- to 4-month intervals, provided cancer is not identified (76,77).

Screening and prevention strategies for women on tamoxifen are more challenging. Women with intact uteri who are taking tamoxifen for either treatment or prevention of breast cancer should be informed of the increased relative risk of developing EC with the use of tamoxifen. This risk is balanced by the reductions in recurrence or development of a contralateral breast cancer. Women on tamoxifen should be encouraged to report abnormal bleeding or vaginal discharge. Screening of asymptomatic women on tamoxifen therapy with ultrasound or endometrial biopsies is not recommended (78,79).

Clinical Presentation

The classic symptom of endometrial carcinoma is abnormal uterine bleeding. A variety of conditions give rise to abnormal bleeding, but particular suspicion should be held for postmenopausal women, and women aged 40 years and over with high-risk factors. Approximately 10% of symptomatic postmenopausal patients are found to have a cancer on biopsy (80). In one series, using age >70 years, diabetes, or nulliparity as risk factors, patients with all three factors had an 87% chance of an AEH/carcinoma diagnosis, whereas only 3% had significant pathology in the absence of all risk factors (81). Additionally, patients with EC may present with vaginal discharge, or have a thickened endometrium that is incidentally noted on ultrasound performed for another reason. Pap smear screening is not designed to identify EC, but occasionally patients will have abnormal cervical cytology (atypical glandular cells of undetermined significance, adenocarcinoma *in situ*). Patients with intraperitoneal disease may present with similar complaints to patients with ovarian cancer, such as abdominal distention, pelvic pressure, and pain.

Historically, when EC was a clinically staged disease (FIGO 1971), fractional D&C was the procedure of choice to evaluate abnormal bleeding. Fractional D&C permitted assessment of uterine size and allowed for endocervical curettage, important steps in the staging process. The standard procedure starts with curettage of the endocervix prior to cervical dilatation. Careful sounding of the uterus is performed followed by dilatation of the cervix, followed by systematic curetting of the entire endometrial cavity. Cervical and endometrial specimens should be kept separate and forwarded for pathologic interpretation.

Pathologic evaluation of the endometrium provides histologic diagnosis and can identify other etiologies of bleeding such as chronic endometritis, atrophy, polyps, cervical cancer, or unusual histologic variants (carcinosarcoma, serous carcinoma, placental nodule), which may alter management. Tissue evaluation by office EMB or D&C offer similar information when adequately performed. Today EMB has largely replaced D&C as the diagnostic procedure of choice. In the GOG hyperplasia study, 63% of the specimens were from EMB (Vabra, Novak, Pipelle) and 37% were from D&C (72). Results of endometrial biopsies correlate well with endometrial curetting, and the accuracy in detecting cancer is 91% to 99% (82,83). The accuracy of identifying cancers with EMB is higher in postmenopausal patients than in premenopausal, and a positive study showing cancer is more accurate for identifying disease than it is in excluding it. If office biopsy cannot be obtained (cervical stenosis, patient intolerance of procedure) or results are nondiagnostic, it should be followed by D&C. In cases of abnormal bleeding that persists despite negative biopsy, additional investigation is warranted.

Hysteroscopy has been advocated as an adjuvant to D&C to improve detection of pathology in the evaluation of postmenopausal bleeding. Whether it improves the sensitivity to detect hyperplasia and cancers is controversial (84–86). Hysteroscopy is more accurate in postmenopausal patients, and is more accurate in detecting cancer versus other pathology than it is in identifying cancer or hyperplasia versus other pathology. One concern is that hysteroscopy may promote transtubal migration of tumor cells, which can be detected as malignant pelvic washings on cytology. In one retrospective study, an odds ratio (OR) of 3.88 for positive cytology was seen in hysteroscopic D&Cs compared to D&C alone, and the authors cautioned against hysteroscopy for evaluating EC (87). Similarly, a review of literature suggested that water-based hysteroscopy was associated with increased frequency of positive cytology at time of hysterectomy (88). Positive peritoneal cytology as the sole extrauterine factor is now longer recognized as a stage-defining characteristic under the FIGO 2009 system, however (89). No prospective studies have been performed to date, and it remains uncertain what effect positive washing produced by hysteroscopy has, if any, on prognosis.

Ultrasound is commonly used as a less invasive tool to evaluate abnormal bleeding. The measurement of endometrial thickness (ET) has been shown to best predict the absence of carcinoma, with a false-negative rate of 4%, using a threshold value of <5 mm (90,91). The specific ET used for a cutoff value depends on the menopausal status of the patient population evaluated and on the use of HRT. For example, postmenopausal patients on HRT have a median ET 2 to 3 mm more than those not on HRT (92,93). In a meta-analysis of 85 studies, Smith-Bindman et al. (91) reported that a cutoff level of >5 mm would detect 96% of cancers, and would have a 39% false-positive rate. Transvaginal ultrasound measuring the lining thickness of the endometrium has excellent negative predictive value for ruling out ECs or hyperplasia when the thickness is <5 mm, but provides less information when >5 mm. Given a pretest probability of having EC in a postmenopausal patient with vaginal bleeding of 10%, a normal endometrial stripe is associated with a 1% chance of a cancer. A consensus panel, composed of radiologists, pathologists, and gynecologic oncologists, suggested that when ET is <5 mm, the test can be considered negative for EC (94). For patients with ET >5 mm, EMB, D&C with hysteroscopy, or saline infusion sonohysteroscopy should be performed. Saline infusion sonohysteroscopy has been suggested as a more effective way to define findings in the endometrial cavity noted on ultrasound, and provide clearer distinction of polyps, fibroids, and cancers (95). It is more likely to be successful in pre- than postmenopausal patients. The role of vaginal ultrasound in the evaluation of bleeding remains somewhat controversial, due to the importance of histology in defining treatment (for benign and malignant conditions) and the concern about failing to identify cancers. Good clinical judgment would suggest that patients with ET <5 mm who have persistent bleeding undergo tissue biopsy.

DIAGNOSTIC WORKUP

Preoperative Assessment

Following a diagnosis of EC, the surgeon must assess the surgical risks of the patient, evaluate the patient for possible metastatic spread, and determine the most appropriate surgical procedure. EC patients are frequently elderly and suffer from obesity, hypertension, diabetes, or cardiac disease. In a series of 595 consecutive patients, Marziale et al. (96) found an operability rate of 87%. Preoperative assessment must be performed, occasionally requiring consultation with additional specialists. At a minimum, patients require a thorough examination to evaluate for evidence of cardiac or pulmonary disease, and to determine the surgical approach. A chest x-ray and electrocardiogram (EKG), complete blood count, and assessment of electrolytes and renal function are standard in this population. Preoperative counseling includes obtaining permission to remove the uterus, tubes, and ovaries, and permission for thorough intra-abdominal exploration with biopsy and tumor resection as indicated, including removal of the pelvic and para-aortic LN.

Evaluation of Metastatic Spread

A thorough physical examination may discover suspicious supraclavicular, inguinal, and/or occasional pelvic LN as well as suggest the presence of pleural effusions, ascites, or omental caking. The pelvic examination can suggest cervical, vaginal, or adnexal spread. An assessment of uterine size and mobility is important, particularly in patients being considered for vaginal approaches (laparoscopic-assisted vaginal hysterectomy [LAVH], total vaginal hysterectomy [TVH]). A chest radiograph is done to search for metastatic tumor as well as to evaluate the cardiopulmonary status of the patient. For patients without obvious extrauterine disease, surgery is the next step. In cases where intra-abdominal, gross cervical, or distant disease spread is suspected, additional studies such as computed tomography (CT) scans, magnetic resonance imaging (MRI), or cystoscopy and proctoscopy may be needed to assist with surgical planning.

In general, there is very limited need for imaging studies prior to surgery; findings typically do not result in management changes because most patients present with stage I–II disease, and the surgery is essentially the same for stage I–III patients. Imaging studies have significant limitations in detecting nodal disease, which tends to be microscopic in 90% of cases (97,98). In a small series of higher risk patients who underwent preoperative FDG PET/CT, Signrelli and colleagues showed a 78% sensitivity and 93% negative predictive value (99). The GOG is conducting an ongoing prospective assessment of PET/CT in patients with endometrial and cervical cancer (GOG 233). In a prospective blinded comparison of the accuracy of preoperative transvaginal ultrasound versus frozen section assessment of myometrial invasion, intraoperative frozen section outperformed ultrasound. The sensitivity and specificity of predicting invasion (none, <50%, >50%) of the ultrasound was 75% and 89%, respectively (100). Patient review of systems and clinical examination frequently lead to suspicion of gross extrauterine disease. Imaging studies may be of better use in certain situations. Serous and clear cell tumors have a greater frequency of extrauterine disease spread, and imaging studies may offer additional information in some cases. In some settings, imaging studies may help to determine whether to refer the patient to a gynecologic oncologist, or perform surgical staging when it would not otherwise be considered. In addition, imaging studies may be most useful in helping to counsel young patients who are considering fertility preservation options. It has been suggested that MRI has more value than CT scans in assessing myometrial invasion, cervical invasion, and nodal disease, with several reports indicating a 75% to 90% accuracy in determining muscle involvement (101–104). However, limitations do exist, making routine use more difficult to recommend (105,106). At the present time, the only way to accurately diagnose the extent and depth of intrauterine invasion is by histologic examination of the hysterectomy specimen.

Biomarkers that predict the presence of extrauterine disease spread might be useful in triaging patients to referral centers for consideration of surgical staging, or to define risk. A variety of biomarkers have been proposed as possible candidates, with CA-125 being the most studied (107–109). Attempts have been made to correlate CA-125 levels with extent of extrauterine disease, as serum levels are frequently elevated in patients with advanced or metastatic EC. This observation was first reported by Niloff et al. (110) in 1984. Values exceeding 35 U/mL were found in 14 (78%) of 18 patients with stage IV or recurrent disease, although none of 11 patients with stage I disease had elevated CA-125. Hsieh et al. (111) reviewed preoperative serum CA-125 levels, operative records, and pathologic reports in 141 patients diagnosed with EC to find out if the preoperative level of CA-125 can provide additional information for determining the extent of lymphadenectomy required in the surgical staging, and which cutoff is optimal in this respect. Of 141 patients, 124 were staged surgically and 24 (19%) were found to have LN metastasis. In the node-positive group, median preoperative serum levels were 94 U/mL (range, 17 to 363 U/mL). Multivariate analysis showed LN metastasis had the most significant effect on the elevation of CA-125 levels (>40 U/mL). The sensitivity and specificity for screening LN metastasis were 78% and 84%, respectively. The data of Hsieh et al. give evidence that preoperative CA-125 levels greater than 40 U/mL can be considered an indication for full pelvic and para-aortic lymphadenectomy in the surgical staging of EC. Rose et al. (112) found serial CA-125 measurements to be most useful in patients with high-risk disease whose initial stage was II, III, or IV, or whose tumor was grade 3 or of clear cell or serous histology. Fifteen (94%) of 16 patients with recurrent disease had an elevated CA-125 level. Serial measurements of CA-125 are also used to monitor for recurrence, and to assess response to tumor therapy in patients whose levels were initially elevated at diagnosis. In the LACE trial, which compared laparotomy to laparoscopy in the management of early-staged EC, 657 patients had preoperative CA-125 levels which were correlated with extrauterine disease spread. Using a cutoff of 30 U/mL, 15% were noted to have elevated CA-125 levels, and of these 37% had extrauterine disease (113). Ideally, serum biomarkers or tests which can be performed on diagnostic samples (EMB, D&C specimens) would be most useful.

Determining the Surgical Procedure

Of all the female pelvic malignancies, there are more advocates for different treatment plans for EC than any other. The standard treatment for this disease has been and remains total hysterectomy and concomitant removal of both ovaries and fallopian tubes. However, through the years, preoperative and postoperative irradiation has had an important role in the management of this disease. The first significant report of employing irradiation in the management of patients with EC was the publication of the "Stockholm technique" by Heyman in 1935 (114). The use of intracavitary implants using the Heyman method became increasingly popular in the ensuing years. Subsequently, reports comparing results in patients treated with a single intrauterine tandem versus those treated with multiple intrauterine capsules revealed a lower incidence of residual disease and an improved 5-year survival rate, in the patients treated with capsules (115–117). In cooperative studies in the late 1960s, Lewis et al. (118) showed that 25% of patients had deep myometrial invasion if treated initially by surgery, and only 8% had deep invasion if treated by preoperative irradiation. Patients frequently were managed with preoperative radiation (whole pelvic radiation [WPR], low-dose-rate [LDR] implant with or without WPR) followed within 4 to 6 weeks by a complete hysterectomy. While surgical evaluation of LN in EC was reported in the 1960s, it was not widely embraced (119–122). The GOG undertook the large surgical–pathologic study, GOG 33, of clinical stage I EC to better define patterns of spread, with the hope that defining pathologic relationships would lead to a tailored (rather than a universal) approach to radiation (59,61). The results of this study subsequently led to the incorporation of a surgical staging system (FIGO 1988). In 2009, FIGO updated staging for EC (**Tables 21.3** and **21.4**) (89)

Contemporary management of most patients with EC remains surgical and includes, at minimum, an initial surgical exploration with collection of peritoneal fluid for cytologic evaluation (intraperitoneal cell washings), through inspection of the abdominal and pelvic cavities, with biopsy or excision of any extrauterine lesions suspicious for tumor, and total extrafascial hysterectomy with BSO. In 2009, FIGO removed the status of cytology as a stage-defining criteria (IIIA, by FIGO 1988); however, there was no intent to discontinue the practice of cytologic evaluation. Whereas the traditional approach has been to perform this surgery abdominally (typically through a vertical midline incision), minimally invasive techniques have increasingly been integrated into the forefront. The uterus should be particularly observed for tumor breakthrough of the serosal surface. The distal ends of the fallopian tubes are clipped or ligated to prevent possible tumor spill during uterine manipulation. To complete the surgical staging of EC, the removal of bilateral pelvic and para-aortic LN is also required.

When surgical staging is indicated, a bilateral pelvic and para-aortic nodal lymphadenectomy is performed. The anatomic boundaries of the pelvic nodal dissection are comparable to what is used for a pelvic nodal dissection with cervical cancer, and is outlined by the margins of the circumflex iliac vein distally, the bifurcation of the iliac vessels proximally; the lateral margin is the genitofemoral nerve, and the medial margin is the superior vesical artery. The floor of the dissection is the obturator nerve. Nodal/fatty tissue is skeletonized from these structures. In cases of bulky nodal disease, complete resection/debulking, rather than biopsy to solely demonstrate metastatic disease, is favored where possible. The common iliac nodes can be removed as a separate specimen or divided at a midpoint along the vessels, submitting the inferior half with the pelvic nodes, and the superior half with the para-aortic nodes. Particularly on the left side, the common iliac nodes will be quite lateral in location, and sufficient mobilization will be required in order to visualize these nodes. Removal of para-aortic nodes can be performed through a midline peritoneal incision over the common iliac arteries and aorta, or by mobilizing the right and left colon medially (123,124). In each case, LN are resected along the upper common iliac vessels on either

TABLE 21.3. Corpus Cancer Surgical Staging, FIGO 1988

Stages/Grades	Characteristics
IA G123	Tumor limited to endometrium
IB G123	Invasion to less than half of the myometrium
IC G123	Invasion to less than half of the myometrium
IIA G123	Endocervical glandular involvement only
IIB G123	Cervical stromal invasion
IIIA G123	Tumor invades serosa or adnexa or positive peritoneal cytology
IIIB G123	Vaginal metastases
IIIC G123	Metastases to pelvic or para-aortic lymph nodes
IVA G123	Tumor invades bladder and/or bowel mucosa
IVB	Distant metastases including intra-abdominal and/or inguinal LN

LN, lymph node.

TABLE 21.4. Corpus Cancer Surgical Staging, FIGO 2009

Stages/Grades	Characteristics
IA G123	No or less than half myometrial invasion
IB G123	Invasion equal to or more than half of the myometrium
II G123	Tumor invades the cervical stroma but does not extend beyond the uterus
IIIA G123	Tumor invades serosa of the corpus uteri and/or adnexa
IIIB G123	Vaginal and/or parametrial involvement
IIIC1 G123 IIIC2 G123	Metastases to pelvic LN Metastases to para-aortic LN, with or without positive pelvic nodes
IVA G123	Tumor invades bladder and/or bowel mucosa
IVB	Distant metastases including intra-abdominal and/or inguinal LN
Histopathology, degree of differentiation	
Cases should be grouped by the degree of differentiation of the adenocarcinoma:	
G1	5% or less of a nonsquamous or nonmorular solid growth pattern
G2	6% to 50% of a nonsquamous or nonmorular solid growth pattern
G3	More than 50% of a nonsquamous or nonmorular solid growth pattern
Notes on pathologic grading	
Notable nuclear atypia, inappropriate for the architectural grade, raises the grade of a grade 1 or grade 2 tumor by 1.	
In serous adenocarcinomas, clear cell adenocarcinomas, and squamous cell carcinomas, nuclear grading takes precedence.	
Adenocarcinomas with squamous differentiation are graded according to the nuclear grade of the glandular component.	
Rules related to staging	
Because corpus cancer is now surgically staged, procedures previously used for determination of stages are no longer applicable, such as the finding of fractional D&C to differentiate between stages I and II.	
It is appreciated that there may be a small number of patients with corpus cancer who will be treated primarily with radiation therapy. If that is the case, the clinical staging adopted by FIGO in 1971 would still apply, but designation of that staging system would be noted.	
Ideally, width of the myometrium should be measured, along with the width of tumor invasion.	

D&C, dilatation and curettage; FIGO, International Federation of Gynecology and Obstetrics; LN, lymph node.

side and from the lower portion of the aorta and vena cava. At the present time, the inferior mesenteric artery is used to demark the superior extent of the para-aortic nodal dissection, although some prefer to routinely extend the dissection to the level of the renal vessels (125). If suspicious nodes extending to the renal vessels are identified, they should be removed if possible.

In cases with gross omental or intraperitoneal disease spread, cytoreductive surgery with total omentectomy, radical peritoneal stripping, and occasionally bowel resection are required. The goal of reducing the residual disease to no or small volumes, akin to what is performed for ovarian cancer, is increasingly considered. In cases complicated by medical comorbidity, advanced age, or obesity, or when nodal dissection cannot or will not be performed, TVH with or without laparoscopic/robotic assistance may also be utilized. Following surgical assessment, patients may be classified based on pathologic features as to their risk of recurrence, and those deemed to be at sufficient risk may be offered adjuvant therapies.

Nonsurgical Management

The principle management of most patients with EC is surgical. The decision to use surgery is a function of patient and disease status. Patients with significant medical comorbidities who are not acceptable candidates for surgery (markedly advanced age, diminished performance status, severe cardiac/pulmonary disease, massive obesity) may be managed by alternative means. Primary RT without surgery has been used, and is discussed later in this chapter. Progestational therapy may be used for those who are inoperable or in younger patients who elect for fertility preservation (75,126). Patients not undergoing surgery should be clinically staged according to the clinical staging system proposed by FIGO in 1971 (**Table 21.5**) (127). Those who do undergo initial hysterectomy are staged by the 2009 FIGO (revised 1988) system (**Table 21.4**) (89). Patients who are obese, but otherwise surgical candidates may undergo an abdominal panniculectomy to enhance surgical exposure to facilitate hysterectomy and nodal dissection (128,129). For patients presenting with disseminated or nonresectable disease, nonsurgical options including radiation, CT, or hormonal therapy have also been used. Surgery may be required to control vaginal bleeding in some of these cases.

Approximately 5% of women with EC are diagnosed under the age of 40 (4). For some younger women, the standard treatment of hysterectomy is unacceptable due to desires to maintain fertility. EC in younger women is usually associated with early-stage, low-grade disease and carries a favorable prognosis, making medical management an attractive option to some (76,77,126,130,131). Patients without myometrial invasion are thought to be the best candidates, and may undergo pelvic MRI to assess for myometrial involvement. Progestational therapy, most commonly with medroxyprogesterone acetate (MPA) or megestrol acetate, has been successful in reversing malignant changes in up to 76% of cases (126,130). Increasingly, there has been a consideration for progestin-based intrauterine devices, although the data is limited. In a 2012 systematic review of the literature, 74% of AEH and 72% of grade 1 EC patients achieved a pathologic complete response (CR) for 6 months or longer with oral progestins (132). The range of CRs for AEH was 50% to 95%, and for grade 1 cancer was 50% to 100%. The mean time required to achieve the CR was 6 months. Of 22 patients reported with grade 1 cancer treated with IUD, 68% achieved a CR. Because response may be temporary or incomplete, periodic sampling of the endometrium is advised. Penner and colleagues suggested that lack of response to progestin therapy is more common when the first response assessment shows lack of response, despite adjacent stromal decidualization (133).

TABLE 21.5. Corpus Cancer Clinical Staging, FIGO 1971

Stage	Characteristics
I	Carcinoma is confined to the corpus
IA	Length of the uterine cavity is 8 cm or less
IB	Length of the uterine cavity is more than 8 cm
Histologic subtypes of adenocarcinoma	
G1	Highly differentiated adenomatous carcinoma
G2	Differentiated adenomatous carcinoma with partly solid areas
G3	Predominantly solid or entirely undifferentiated carcinoma
II	Carcinoma involves the corpus and cervix
III	Carcinoma extends outside the uterus but not outside the true pelvis
IV	Carcinoma extends outside the true pelvis or involves the bladder or rectum

Vaginal Hysterectomy

Vaginal hysterectomy with or without postoperative radiation may be another option for managing complicated patients. Vaginal hysterectomy has often been cited as the simplest and least morbid approach to hysterectomy, and has produced similar treatment outcomes in patients with clinical stage I EC (134–136). It is often used as an alternative to an abdominal approach in obese and poor-surgical-risk patients (137,138). Limitations include the lack of exploration of the intraperitoneal cavity, inability to procure cytologic washings, greater difficulty in performing a salpingo-oophorectomy, and inability to assess LN status. Given that LN metastasis is related to such high-risk features as poor differentiation, unfavorable histologic subtypes, and deep myometrial invasion, the option of TVH for management of this cancer centers on preoperative uterine pathology and the need for comprehensive surgical staging (59). TVH is not appropriate for the management of EC in patients with concomitant adnexal pathology.

Nodal Dissection

The value of staging any malignancy relates to the ability to describe the extent of disease at diagnosis, and to define comparable patient populations for whom prognosis and therapy are similar. Given the inability to accurately detect disease spread for many gynecologic malignancies, solely based on clinical examination and imaging studies, surgical staging systems that require pathologic evaluation of sampled sites have been largely incorporated into practice. The value of surgical staging as it relates to ECs has been the subject of increased scrutiny and debate over the last several years. For ECs, the ability of surgical staging to accurately identify spread to draining LN basins and how this information (or lack of it) changes prognosis and alters the use of postoperative therapies are a source of controversy. Proponents of routine surgical staging suggest that the ability to identify otherwise unrecognized disease spread to the nodes changes the postoperative therapies that are given, and is the most accurate way to assess risk. Most controversial is the assertion that surgical staging has a therapeutic benefit independent of the node status (positive or negative for metastatic disease).

Fundamentally, surgeons must determine for themselves whether or not they believe that surgical staging has sufficient value to offer it for all patients or only selectively based on risk factors identified pre- and intraoperatively. If a patient will not be offered surgical staging/nodal dissection, then minimizing surgical morbidity with only total hysterectomy and bilateral salpingo-oophorectomy may be warranted. In this case, lower risk/quicker recovery comes at the cost of less information. In cases where nodal dissection is deemed necessary or potentially will be performed, patients must be adequately counseled regarding the risks and benefits. The principle risks attributable to nodal dissections include increased operative time, potential for blood loss associated with vascular injury, ileus,

■ **TABLE 21.6. Risks Associated with Nodal Dissection: Surgical Complication Rates Associated with Abdominal Hysterectomy + Pelvic and Para-Aortic Lymph Node Dissection**

Study	N	Hemorrhage (%)	GU Injury (%)	DVT/PE (%)	Lymphocyst (%)	Other
Morrow 1991(61)	895	2.2	0.4	2	1.2	—
Homesley 1992(140)	196	6% transfused	—	4	—	"Serious" 6%
Orr 1997(139)	396	4.2% transfused	0.6	1.5	1.2	—
Mariani 2006(142)	96 node (+) patients	—	1	1	3.1	—

DVT/PE, deep vein thrombosis/pulmonary embolism; GU, genitourinary.

and genitofemoral nerve injury with resulting numbness and paresthesias over medial thighs, lymphocyst formation, and lymphedema (**Table 21.6**) (61,139–141). In general, the risks associated with nodal dissections are low and acceptable. Patients who have nodal dissections and receive pelvic RT may be at a greater risk of bowel morbidity and chronic lymphedema than those without dissections (143,144). Nodal dissections also require the involvement of someone trained and skilled to perform the procedure. The principle advantage of comprehensive staging is that the physician and patient are provided with the greatest amount of information which may be critical in making recommendations with regards to the need for adjuvant therapy and prognosis. In the contemporary management of EC, this information results in less use of radiation, and substitution of vaginal cuff brachytherapy (VCB) for pelvic radiation (122,145,146).

The importance, extent, and technique of nodal dissection are hotly debated. Questions relate to which patients should be offered and could benefit from surgical staging (all, some, none), and what is the optimal surgical procedure to be performed (biopsy of enlarged/visible nodes, lymphadenectomy). Controversy also exists between those surgeons who perform only pelvic dissections and those who advocate pelvic and para-aortic nodal dissection. If para-aortic nodes are removed, are bilateral nodes required, and to what superior extent (inferior mesenteric artery, renal vessels) should the dissection proceed?

Nodal Dissection—None

In the United States, comprehensive surgical staging of EC is infrequently performed. Only 30% to 40% of patients undergo nodal assessment, indicating that the majority of U.S. patients are not staged (146,147). Many gynecologists are neither trained in the techniques of lymphadenectomy nor are familiar with the concept of full surgical staging. Full staging is more commonly performed by specialized surgeons, such as gynecologic oncologists (148,149). Philosophically, those opposed to nodal dissections suggest that most patients are at low risk for nodal disease, treatment decisions can be based on final pathologic information, and despite node dissection the majority of patients who are node-negative do not get benefit (150). Most patients with EC do present with low-risk features. In the entire GOG 33 study population of 621 patients, 75% had grade 1 to 2 tumors, 59% had inner one-third or less myometrial invasion, and only 9% of patients had positive LN (59). The Postoperative Radiation Therapy in Endometrial Cancer (PORTEC) trial evaluated patients with stage IC, grade 1; stage IB-C, grade 2; or stage IB, grade 3 who underwent hysterectomy without LN dissection and compared observation to postoperative pelvic radiation (151). Of note, on the basis of grade and depth of invasion, approximately 60% of patients enrolled in GOG 33 would have had disease characteristics required for eligibility in the PORTEC trial. This patient population managed without nodal dissection had favorable outcomes with or without RT (5-year survival rates of 85% observation, 81% with pelvic radiation) in the PORTEC study (151). In a follow-up study including 427 patients with higher risk disease (age >60 years plus either grade 1 to 2 and outer 50% invasion, or grade 3 with inner 50% invasion, or stage IIA (1988 FIGO) disease, the PORTEC 2 study compared pelvic RT to VCB. None of the patients underwent nodal assessment, and 5-year progression-free survival (PFS) (78% to 83%) and survival (80% to 85%) suggested that even intermediate-risk patients may be managed without lymphadenectomy, albeit at the cost of requiring adjuvant therapy, with resulting favorable outcomes (152). Trimble et al. (153) reported on data from stage I EC patients collected by SEER from 1988 to 1993 and showed that 5-year relative survival for patients without nodal dissection was 98% compared to 96% in those undergoing nodal dissection and suggested that nodal dissection did not convey a benefit for the overall population. Unfortunately, data on adjuvant therapy use was not available. It is suspected that increased use of radiation in unstaged patients may produce similar outcomes to patients who are staged and who avoid RT.

In a nonrandomized trial comparing hysterectomy with or without pelvic lymphadenectomy, followed by RT, 14% of patients (n = 207) with negative nodes treated with VCB recurred compared to 16% who did not have a lymphadenectomy (n = 660) (154). While the authors noted similar cancer-free survival between the groups, all patients who did not have nodal dissections received both pelvic radiation and VCB to attain these results.

Two randomized trials comparing hysterectomy with or without lymphadenectomy have been reported. A Study in the Treatment of Endometrial Cancer (ASTEC) randomized patients with 1,369 EC to hysterectomy with (LND group) or without (no-LND group) pelvic lymphadenectomy (155). Following surgery, patients with stage I-IIA disease were then randomized again to observation or pelvic RT if they had grade 3, serous, or clear cell histology; >50% myometrial invasion; or endocervical glandular invasion (stage IIA). Nodal status did not alter the use of RT such that node-positive patients could be assigned to observation. Treatment centers were also permitted to use VCB regardless of pelvic radiation assignment based on institutional preference. As a result, a patient with unknown nodal status could receive VCB and not be considered to have received RT. Of the LND group, 54 patients were found to positive nodes (9%) compared with 9 (1.3%) patients in the no-LND group. The quality of the nodal dissection has been criticized in this study as 8% of patients within the LND group did not get a nodal dissection, 12% had <5 nodes removed (median = 12 nodes), and para-aortic nodal dissection was not performed. There was no difference in PFS (HR, 1.0) or survival (HR, 1.25; $p = 0.14$) between the LND groups. Pelvic lymphadenectomy was associated with a longer operative time, and increased frequency of ileus (3% vs. 1%), deep venous thrombosis (1% vs. 0.1%), lymphocysts (1% vs. 0.3%), and wound complications (1% vs. 0.3%) compared to the no-LND group. The frequency of transfusions and length of hospitalization were comparable between groups. The authors concluded that the results suggest no evidence of benefit for PFS/OS for pelvic lymphadenectomy and that it "could not be recommended as a routine procedure for *therapeutic* purposes" (155).

A similar study was performed by Italian investigators (CONSORT trial). In this trial, 514 patients were assigned to hysterectomy with or without pelvic lymphadenectomy (156). Patients were required to have myometrial invasion, and patients with grade 1 tumors and <50% invasion were excluded. In the no-LND group, 22% of patients had nodal dissections due to clinical suspicion with 14% of these cases, or 3% of the entire no-LND arm, having node-positive disease. In the LND group, the median number of nodes removed was 26. Para-aortic dissection could be performed at the surgeon's discretion and was done 26% of cases. In the LND group, 13% were found to have positive nodes. Lymphocysts and lymphedema were more common in the LND group but other early and late complications were similar. Postoperative therapy was not protocol prescribed, but the use of RT was more common in the no-LND group (25% vs. 17%). The 5-year disease-free survival (DFS) was 81% in both groups, and 5-year survival was 90% in the no-LND group versus 86% in the LND group (HR 1.2, $p = 0.5$). The authors concluded that pelvic lymphadenectomy could not be recommended as a routine procedure for therapeutic purposes (156).

Both the ASTEC (A) and Italian (I) studies have been heavily criticized (157–159). Weaknesses of the studies relate to the absence of treatment in patients identified with positive nodes (A), lack of prescribed adjuvant therapy (I), limited power to show improvements in outcome if one truly existed (A, I), poor quality of the LND (A), absence of para-aortic nodal dissection (A, I), lack of quality-of-life assessment evaluating effect of both surgery and downstream use of adjuvant therapy (A, I), and the over representation of low-risk patients (A, I). Despite these limitations, these datasets provide the only level 1 evidence on the role of lymphadenectomy. The studies also suggest that the marginal benefit that lymphadenectomy may provide is likely to be modest for most patients. In addition, the data provide a strong argument that removing negative nodes is unlikely to significantly improve outcomes.

Without nodal information, physicians must rely on uterine factors to estimate the probability for nodal disease and pelvic failure to determine the need for postoperative radiation. Risk assessments may be based on nodal positivity estimates from GOG 33 or based on uterine factor–derived risk groups treated with or without RT (PORTEC, GOG 99; 962,146,153,162). Nodal positivity is not infrequent in patients with higher risk uterine factors based on GOG 99 or PORTEC models. Nugent and colleagues classified a series of 352 clinical stage 1, endometrioid adenocarcinoma patients into risk groups based on PORTEC and GOG 99 models. Nodal positivity rates were 20% with PORTEC and 35% with GOG 99 HIR criteria (151). Without specific nodal information, treatments must be based on estimates of risk/probability; this estimation can result in an increase in the use of radiation, particularly if the primary benefit of postoperative radiation is in node-positive patients. Complicating the issue of nodal dissection is that nodal status is only one of several important prognostic factors (160,161). Kwon and colleagues performed a population-based cohort study of 316 EC patients who underwent lymphadenectomy and reported that pelvic node status was not an independent determinant of survival, whereas prognosis was determined more by uterine factors (161).

The absence of nodal dissection may also lead to poorer outcomes. For example, a subset of 99 patients with stage IC, grade 3 EC, who did not have LN dissection, were not eligible, but were treated with pelvic radiation and followed prospectively within the PORTEC trial (162). Five-year survival for this group of patients was 58%, and 12% had vaginal or pelvic failures despite WPR. It is interesting to note that the outcome of this group is poorer than what has been reported in patients with stage IIIC EC managed by lymphadenectomy followed by radiation (163–165). If patients are not to have nodal dissection, then it would seem reasonable to consider minimally invasive or vaginal approaches to reduce morbidity.

Nodal Dissection—Selective

Surgical staging is the most accurate way to determine the extent of disease spread. Palpation of pelvic LN is not sufficiently accurate, with a sensitivity of 72% in a recent prospective study (166,167). The baseline rate of nodal disease in an "all comer" population of EC patients is roughly 9% (**Table 21.7**). Increasingly, the challenge has been how to identify the smaller portion of patients at high risk from the larger low-risk population. Clearly, subgroups of patients at very high risk (non-endometrioid histology, carcinosarcoma, gross cervical involvement, gross extrauterine disease spread) exist, but these represent a minority of the 400,000 cases of uterine cancer per year in the U.S. Many gynecologic oncologists consider nodal assessment to be a fundamental step in the evaluation and management of most women with EC, and nodal assessment has been incorporated into the surgical staging of EC since 1988.

Increasingly, there has been a discussion in the literature to attempt to describe which populations should be offered lymphadenectomy, and the optimal strategy for defining those at risk (tumor biomarkers, frozen section criteria, sentinel nodal evaluation). Many believe that nodal dissections should be reserved for those with sufficient risk of nodal disease (59,61,169,170). What risk of nodal disease (3%, 5%, 10%, etc.) warrants the procedure is debated—that is, at what level would one be comfortable missing unrecognized nodal spread. Equally important in the discussion is the understanding of whether uterine risk factors, independent of nodal status, should drive risk assessment and use of adjuvant therapy and whether adjuvant therapies given to those with node-positive or node status unknown perform similarly.

Historically, data from GOG 33 demonstrated important relationships between tumor grade and depth of invasion and frequency of nodal disease that can be used to decide whether to perform nodal assessments (**Tables 21.8** and **21.9**) (59). For example, the risk of pelvic nodal disease was 3% for all patients with grade 1 tumors, but was 11% with deeply invasive (outer one-third myometrial invasion) tumors. Patients with grade 3 tumors had a risk of pelvic nodal metastases of 18%, and 34% with deep invasion. With cervical invasion, the rate of pelvic nodal disease was 16%. Patients with serous or clear cell histology also warrant nodal dissection as ~30% to 50% will have nodal disease, and even in the absence of myometrial invasion,

TABLE 21.7. Frequency of Nodal Disease

Study	N	Frequency of Nodal Disease (%)
GOG 33 (59)		
ASTEC	621	9
(+LND)	686	9
(–) LND (155)	685	1
CONSORT		
(+ LND)	264	13
(–) LND (156)	250	3
LAP II (168)	2510	9
PORTEC HIR Criteria (160)	66	20
GOG 99 HIR Criteria (160)	188	35

TABLE 21.8. Histologic Grade and Depth of Invasion

	Grade, No. of Patients			
Depth	Grade 1 (%)	Grade 2 (%)	Grade 3 (%)	Total (% of Total)
Endometrium only	44 (24)	31 (11)	11 (7)	86 (14)
Superficial	96 (53)	131 (45)	54 (35)	281 (45)
Middle	22 (12)	69 (24)	24 (16)	115 (19)
Deep	18 (10)	57 (20)	64 (42)	139 (22)
Total	180 (100)	288 (100)	153 (100)	621 (100)

Source: Reprinted from Creasman WT, Morrow CP, Bundy BN, et al. Surgical pathologic spread patterns of endometrial cancer: a Gynecologic Oncology Group study. *Cancer.* 1987;60:2035–2041.

TABLE 21.9. Frequency of Nodal Metastasis among Risk Factors

Risk Factor	No. of Patients	Pelvic No. (%)	Aortic No. (%)
Histology			
Endometrioid adenocarcinoma	599	56 (9)	30 (5)
Others	22	2 (9)	4 (18)
Grade			
1 Well	180	5 (3)	3 (2)
2 Moderate	288	25 (9)	14 (5)
3 Poor	153	28 (18)	17 (11)
Myometrial invasion			
Endometrial	87	1 (1)	1 (1)
Superficial	279	15 (5)	8 (3)
Middle	116	7 (6)	1 (1)
Deep	139	35 (25)	24 (17)
Site of tumor location			
Fundus	524	42 (8)	20 (4)
Isthmus-cervix	97	16 (16)	14 (14)
CLS involvement			
Negative	528	37 (7)	19 (9)
Positive	93	21 (27)	15 (19)
Other extrauterine metastasis			
Negative	586	40 (7)	26 (4)
Positive	35	18 (51)	8 (23)
Peritoneal cytology[a]			
Negative	537	38 (7)	20 (4)
Positive	75	19 (25)	14 (19)

[a]Nine patients did not have cytology reported.

CLS, capillary-like space.

Source: Modified with permission from Creasman WT, Morrow CP, Bundy BN, et al. Surgical pathologic spread patterns of endometrial cancer: a Gynecologic Oncology Group study. *Cancer* 1987;60:2035.

nodal metastases have been reported in up to 36% of patients (171). Some advocate that LN need not be sampled for tumor limited to the endometrium, regardless of grade, because less than 1% of these patients have disease spread to pelvic or para-aortic LN (59,172). A gray zone in deciding about LN sampling is represented by patients whose only risk factor is inner one-half myometrial invasion, particularly if the grade is 2 or 3. This group has 5% or less chance of node positivity (59). In the most recent survey of Society for Gynecologic Oncology (SGO) members, 35% of respondents reported doing lymphadenectomy for grade 1 tumors; however, the use increased to 60% for grade 2 and 90% for grade 3 (125).

Increasingly, the debate has focused on appropriate selection of patients at such low risk for nodal metastasis that lymphadenectomy may be safely avoided. While flawed, the ASTEC and Italian studies have suggested that routine nodal dissection may have limited value. If the primary value of lymphadenectomy is to identify patients with positive nodes (as a "diagnostic test") which define patients who need additional/different postoperative therapy, there is value in defining populations at sufficiently low risk for whom no lymphadenectomy is required. In 2000, the Mayo group described a model which could classify a group with a low risk of nodal disease spread and high DFS based on frozen section evaluation of the uterus that showed grade 1 to 2 endometrioid tumor, inner 50% invasion, and tumor size < 2 cm (173). Mariani subsequently reported on a prospective experience of 422 patients and reported that 33% of patients with endometrioid-type tumors would qualify as low risk in this model. The authors also showed that 22% patients with risk factors outside of their low-risk model had positive nodal spread at time of lymphadenectomy (174). Several other investigators have attempted to validate these findings. Convery and colleagues tried to replicate the conditions of Mayo criteria (which are assessed intraoperatively by frozen section) by retrospectively evaluating 602 patients with grade 1 to 2 endometrioid EC and who had intraoperative assessment of tumor (for depth of invasion +/− tumor size) (175). The authors showed that 2/110 (1.8%) patients meeting the Mayo criteria who underwent a lymphadenectomy removing at least eight nodes were found to have metastatic spread to LN. Milam attempted to validate the Mayo criteria using a 971-patient surgical dataset from patients participating in the GOG Lap 2 trial (randomized trial of laparoscopy vs. open hysterectomy with pelvic and para-aortic lymphadenectomy [176]). Of 971 patients with endometrioid adenocarcinoma and complete data, 65 (7%) were identified with positive LN. Patients were classified into a "low risk" category based on three Mayo criteria; grade 1 to 2 tumor, <50% myometrial invasion, and tumor size < 2 cm. These risk characteristics were assigned based on final pathology report and not frozen section, however, as was used in the Mayo studies. Approximately 40% of patients met the low-risk criteria and of these 3/389 (0.8%) had positive LN.

Kang reporting for the Korean GOG retrospectively evaluated 540 patients with endometrioid-type cancers who had undergone preoperative EMB, CA-125 level, and MRI followed by hysterectomy and pelvic lymphadenectomy to create a risk model for predicting nodal disease (177). The model was developed on a 360-patient training set and validated against a 180-patient cohort. Interestingly, the logistic regression model included only data from the MRI and CA-125 level, grade was not an independently significant variable. The authors suggested that based on preoperative information, they could classify 53% of patients as low-risk (<50%) myometrial invasion and absence of enlarged nodes or extrauterine disease by MRI and CA-125 (<35 IU/mL). Of the low-risk group, only one patient had positive nodal disease (1.7% false-negative rate) suggesting that these patients may avoid an unnecessary lymphadenectomy.

Low-grade tumors appear to represent the most appropriate group for developing criteria to limit lymphadenectomy. Bernardini performed a retrospective comparison between two academic institutions preferences for management of preoperative grade 1 endometrioid EC (178). Of 483 cases with a preoperative grade 1 cancer, final pathology was grade 1 in 357/483 (74%) cases, and 20% were upgraded (grade 2, 18%; grade 3, 2%). In one institution, surgical staging was performed in 50% of cases, and four (3%) patients were identified with nodal disease. At the second institution, LN dissection was performed in only 12% of patients, and three (1.4%) were found to have positive nodal disease. At the second institution, postoperative use of RT was more common (21% vs. 7%), although older patient age, capillary space invasion, and cervical involvement were more common at the second site. Despite the differences in surgical practice, the 3-year survival was 96% at both centers. These data indicate that there is little margin to improve outcomes through strategies directed at all patients in this patient population.

Selective use of nodal dissection highlights the balance between the likelihood of identifying otherwise unrecognized disease against cost, morbidity, and use of adjuvant therapy (with downstream cost, morbidity). The overall surgical complication of lymphadenectomy is approximately 20%. The serious complication rate is ≤6%, and is likely to be lower with surgeons who more frequently perform the procedure (61,139–141). Downstream utilization of adjuvant therapy, which may occur more frequently in the absence of lymphadenectomy, must also be considered into this balance. While the proposed models predicting low-risk disease status appear to be accurate, it is important to understand that the pretest probability of having positive nodes in a large patient population with grade

1 to 2 endometrioid tumors is ~3% to 7%, illustrating the narrow margin in improved outcome (e.g., identify 100% of patients with positive nodes and then use adjuvant therapy which cures 100% of these) that lymphadenectomy may be able to offer in this population of patients. Lymphadenectomy perhaps allows for fine tuning the management of low-risk patients, but does not appear to be the driver of outcomes.

Intraoperative assessment of the uterus in patients with low-grade endometrioid adenocarcinoma of the endometrium has been used to guide the surgeon as to when to perform a nodal dissection. Gross inspection of the uterus immediately following its removal can be used to estimate the degree of myometrial invasion. If the uterus is opened by the operating surgeon, care should be employed to avoid distortion of the anatomy. Optimally, the unfixed uterus should be opened by the surgical pathologist, who can grossly estimate the depth of invasion, assess involvement of the cervix, and later sample the tumor for histologic assessment. There is no typical gross appearance of an EC. Most are polypoid or ulcerative. Carcinoma usually differs in texture and color from the surrounding normal endometrium. The normal endometrium is irregular and tan, but a carcinoma is usually shaggy, white to gray–white, and focally hemorrhagic. Areas of myometrial invasion may be visible as gray–white to white, with yellow areas disclosing necrosis (**Figs. 21.1** and **21.2**). The texture may be soft, friable, or firm depending on the degree of necrosis.

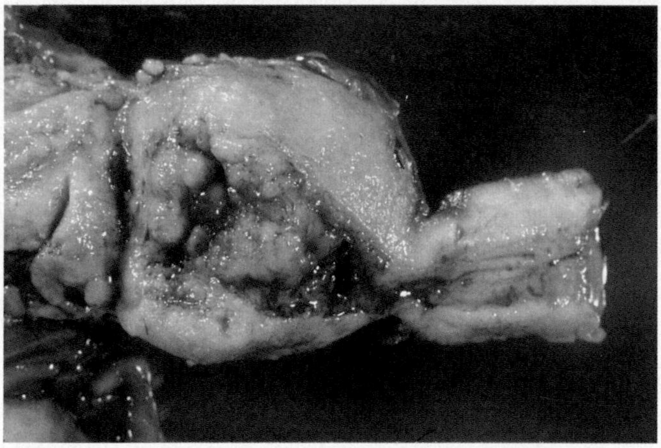

Figure 21.1. Endometrioid adenocarcinoma. A polypoid adenocarcinoma of the endometrium that fills much of the lumen and superficially invades the myometrium.

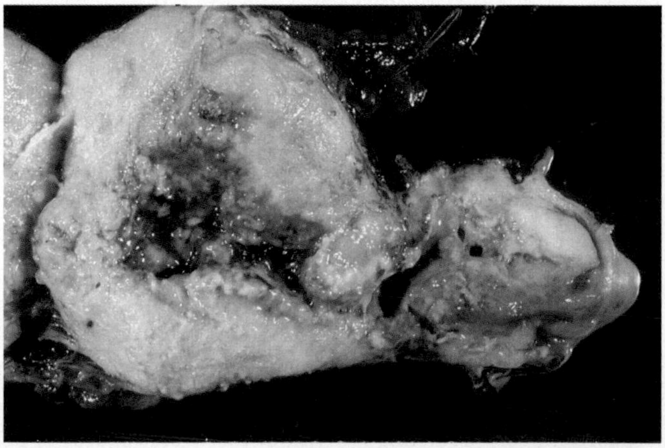

Figure 21.2. Endometrial adenocarcinoma. An ulcerating and deeply invasive adenocarcinoma that extends into the uterine cervix.

Doering et al. (179) reported a 91% accuracy rate for 148 patients for determining the depth of myometrial invasion by gross visual examination of the cut uterine surface. A prospective study indicated that visual inspection of < or >50% correlated with microscopic assessment in 85% cases (167). However, the sensitivity of determining >50% was lower at 72%. Invasion of the myometrium may be more extensive microscopically than is evident visibly because of the characteristic infiltrative growth pattern of the tumor. In a retrospective study by Goff and Riche, the gross estimation by pathologists of myometrial invasion in grades 2 and 3 tumors was poor (180). With invasion, the uterine cavity usually enlarges and the myometrium thickens, but a small uterus may have myometrial penetration to the serosa.

Nodal Dissection—Routine

Data from 1990–2000 provided support for performing uniform comprehensive surgical staging for nearly all patients with EC. The rationale for uniform staging includes the lack of a patient population for whom nodal disease is so low that nodes should be omitted, the inaccuracy of preoperative or intraoperative assessments predicting the risk for nodal disease, the potential for therapeutic benefit in node-positive and node-negative patients, and the lack of significant morbidity associated with the procedure. Postoperative adjuvant decisions are best made with the most complete information. If nodal assessment is the predominant factor by which to categorize patients into risk groups, routine nodal dissection is the best method by which to determine which few patients will require adjuvant therapy.

What constitutes an acceptable rate of nodal disease in EC to warrant the procedure is surgeon dependent. In cervical cancer, routine pelvic lymphadenectomy is advocated for all stage IA2 tumors where nodal positivity rates are 3% to 5% (181). For clinical stage I ovarian cancer, para-aortic dissection is recommended for all, given the 6% risk of para-aortic disease (182). In EC, major complication rates associated with nodal dissection are 2% to 6%, suggesting that this might be an appropriate level of risk to balance against the risk of nodal metastases. Data from GOG 33 show that only patients with tumor limited to the endometrium had a risk of pelvic nodal disease ≤3%, and this group accounted for only 14% of the entire study population.

Frozen section assessment has been the traditional tool to facilitate decisions on selective nodal dissections. Several studies have demonstrated inaccuracies with frozen sections in the interpretation of grade and depth of myometrial invasion compared to final pathology (183–185). In one prospective evaluation, frozen section determination of depth of invasion correlated with final pathology in 67% of cases but resulted in upstaging in 28% of cases (183). Patients with grade 1 EC or AEH were upstaged in 61% of cases. The clinical significance of these errors has been debated (150), but many believe that such unexpected upstaging justifies routine staging even in seemingly low-risk patients (183,184). Data also suggest that the strategy of routine nodal dissection is more cost-effective than either no staging or selective staging based on frozen section results (186,187).

The technique of nodal dissection has undergone evolution. In an era where everyone was to receive RT, there was little value for a complete evaluation of LN. Removal of palpably enlarged nodes, "plucking" of visibly noted nodes, and "sampling" have given way to a more thorough assessment. Only 10% of patients with metastases to LN will have grossly enlarged nodes, and frequently, even in these cases, direct palpation through the overlying peritoneum will fail to identify them (59). Today, adjuvant therapies are based on the extent of disease, and are often only reserved for node-positive patients. Nodal assessments should sufficiently examine sites at risk including external iliac, hypogastric, and obturator nodes in the pelvis, common iliac nodes, and para-aortic nodes. Moving from a sampling technique to a more thorough lymphadenectomy is not associated with increased complication rates (188). Nodal dissection should be bilateral given the frequency of both left and right para-aortic involvement (189,190). It is interesting to note that GOG 33 only specified right-sided para-aortic removal in the surgical protocol. Likewise, the nodal dissection is more apt to be representative when a larger number of nodes are removed.

An assessment of pelvic and para-aortic LN is required to assign stage according to FIGO 2009. The 2009 staging system now separates stage subcategories based on extent of nodal disease (IIIC1, pelvic positive, IIIC2, any para-aortic positive) (89). Two principal nodal basins drain the uterus; the lower and middle portion of the uterus drains laterally to the pelvic LN, the upper corpus and fundus drain to the para-aortic nodes. When LN are positive, para-aortic nodes are involved in ~50% of the time. Isolated para-aortic nodes with negative pelvic nodes are uncommon, particularly with grade 1 to 2 tumors, and are involved in only ~2% of cases (59,191,192). Para-aortic nodal dissection is more difficult to perform than pelvic dissection, by laparotomy or by laparoscopy, and is associated with greater risk. As such, some advocate for pelvic nodal dissections with only performing para-aortic nodal dissections selectively. In GOG 33, 46% of the positive para-aortic LN were enlarged, and 98% of the cases with aortic node metastases came from patients with positive pelvic nodes, adnexal or intra-abdominal metastases, or outer one-third myometrial invasion (59). These risk factors affected only 25% of the patients, yet they yielded most of the positive para-aortic node patients.

The importance of para-aortic nodal spread in node-positive EC cannot be ignored (**Table 21.10**). Data from GOG 33 showing that of all patients, isolated para-aortic nodal metastases occurred in 2% is often taken out of context (59). If the goal of nodal dissection is to identify the node-positive patient population and to remove involved nodes, para-aortic disease is seen in 40% to 66% of patients with node-positive/stage IIIC1/2 EC, including isolated positive para-aortic nodes in up to 7% to 21% of cases in certain groups. If only pelvic nodes are removed, when they are positive, para-aortic nodes will be positive in addition in nearly 30% to 40% of cases. It makes less sense to remove only pelvic or only para-aortic nodes given this data. Data would also suggest that when positive, outcomes are improved in patients who have complete surgical resection of para-aortic nodes. Chuang et al. (193) reported on their experience with selective pelvic and or para-aortic dissections and found that failure to systematically remove pelvic and para-aortic nodes resulted in an increased frequency of recurrence in undissected retroperitoneal sites. Similarly, Mariani et al. (188) showed that patients at high risk for para-aortic nodal disease (based on invasion >50%, palpable positive pelvic nodes, positive adnexa) who did not have para-aortic dissection or who had biopsy only and who were managed as though para-aortic nodes were positive had 5-year survival of 71% compared to 85% for those patients with positive para-aortic nodes who did undergo complete resection. Lymph node recurrences were detected in 37% of those not having para-aortic dissection compared to none in patients with positive but resected para-aortic nodes, suggesting a possible therapeutic effect of removing involved para-aortic nodes.

A provocative study from Japan (SEPAL study) was published in early 2010 that retrospectively compared the practices of two centers with regard to use of pelvic with or without para-aortic lymphadenectomy (194). At one center, systematic pelvic lymphadenectomy was performed in 325 patients. With a median of 34 pelvic nodes removed, the incidence of stage IIIC disease was 12%. At the second institution, 346 patients underwent pelvic and para-aortic lymphadenectomy. With a median of 59 pelvic and 23 para-aortic nodes resected, stage IIIC disease was identified in 16%. The centers were well matched for stage and tumor grade, but the center where para-aortic lymphadenectomy was performed used adjuvant CT more commonly (47% vs. 27%). Patients were classified into low-versus intermediate- to high-risk groups and outcomes were compared based on lymphadenectomy type. In the intermediate–high risk group (but not low risk), recurrence-free, DSS, and OS were significantly better in those women receiving para-aortic dissections. In a multivariate analysis, age, tumor type, nodal spread, and type of lymphadenectomy were independently associated with improved survival. The authors suggested that if future lymphadenectomy trials were to be conducted, both pelvic and para-aortic lymphadenectomy should be performed (194).

At the present time, the superior extent of para-aortic dissection should be at least to the level of the inferior mesenteric artery. Some suggest that dissections should proceed to the level of the renal vessels given the venous and lymphatic drainage following the infundibulopelvic ligament. In one series, 7 out of 11 patients had positive para-aortic nodes identified above the inferior mesenteric artery (195). The Mayo group noted that when para-aortic nodes were positive, 77% of cases had involvement above the IMA (174). This extended para-aortic dissection is feasible laparoscopically as well (196,197). Prospective data describing the frequency of high para-aortic/pararenal nodes are awaited.

The retrospective data suggesting a therapeutic benefit supports, but does not prove, the hypothesis that lymphadenectomy is therapeutic. These studies are largely from single institutions, have short follow-up, suffer from selection biases, and do not clearly account for stage migration. Despite these limitations, the therapeutic value of lymphadenectomy is supported by several reports. Kilgore et al. (198) were among the first to report a therapeutic effect of nodal dissections in a series of 649 clinical stage I–occult II patients who were classified based on the extent of nodal dissection. Patients who underwent multiple site pelvic nodal dissection (defined by nodal dissection of at least four pelvic nodal sites) and had a mean of 11 nodes removed had improved survival over those patients who did not have nodes sampled. The survival advantage for multiple site dissection persisted even when patients were stratified into low-risk (uterine-confined disease) and high-risk (extrauterine disease) groups who received radiation. An explanation for this may be the removal of unrecognized micrometastasis, which goes undetected by standard pathologic processing techniques. Girardi et al. (199) performed pelvic lymphadenectomy in 76 patients with EC (mean

TABLE 21.10. Relationship between Pelvic and Para-Aortic Nodal Involvement in Patients with Node-Positive Endometrial Cancer

Study	N	Surgical Technique	Pelvic (+) Only (%)	Pelvic and Para-aortic (+) (%)	Para-aortic Only (%)	Any Involvement of Para-aortic Nodes (%)
Creasman 1987	70	Routine: sampling	51	31	17	48
Schorge 1996	35	Selective: lymphadenectomy	74	17	9	26
Hirahatake 1997	42	Routine: systematic lymphadenectomy	57	38	5	42
Onda 1997	30	Routine: systematic lymphadenectomy	33	60	6.6	66
McMeekin 2001	47	Routine: lymphadenectomy	38	41	21	62
Otsuka 2002	23	Selective: systematic lymphadenectomy	66	33	10	43
Havrilesky 2005	96	Selective: lymphadenectomy	52	30	18	48

37 nodes removed) and reported a 36% nodal positivity rate. Nodal tissue was processed as step serial sections and 37% of positive nodes were <2 mm in diameter, suggesting that nodal metastases may be missed in a proportion of node-positive patients processed in a less extensive manner. Others have shown improvement in outcomes following a more complete nodal dissection in node-negative populations. Cragan et al. (200) evaluated 509 stage I–IIA patients who underwent selective pelvic+/− para-aortic lymphadenectomy and found a survival advantage for patients with grade 3 tumors who had >11 pelvic nodes removed, compared to those with ≤11 nodes removed (HR 0.25). For patients with high-risk features (grade 3, >50% myometrial invasion, serous/clear cell tumors) 5-year survival was 82% when >11 nodes were removed versus 64% when ≤11 nodes were removed. Chan et al. (201) reported on the effect of a more complete nodal dissection in over 12,000 women with EC tracked in the SEER data system. In patients with high-risk disease (IB/grade 3, IC, II–IV), 5-year survival was proportional to the number of nodes removed, increasing from 75% to 87% when 1 versus >20 nodes were removed. In a multivariate analysis, a more extensive nodal assessment was an independent predictor of survival. Prospective data from the ASTEC and Italian studies suggest that there is no therapeutic benefit to resecting negative LN (155,156). The use of postoperative adjuvant therapy in patients without nodal dissection may obscure potential benefit of lymphadenectomy, making benefit difficult to measure. Likewise, patients with low-risk uterine factors may be identified with nodal disease.

In patients with positive pelvic and/or para-aortic nodes, complete resection followed by adjuvant therapy results in superior outcomes. Havrilesky reported on 91 patients with Stage IIIc disease including 39 with microscopic involvement of the LN and 52 with grossly enlarged nodes. Five-year survival was 58% for patients with microscopic LN, 48% for those with grossly positive LN completely resected, and only 22% in cases where the nodes were not resected. The authors felt that this data suggested a therapeutic benefit for lymphadenectomy (202). Bristow evaluated 41 patients with bulky adenopathy who underwent complete resection of involved nodes. Compared with patients who had gross residual disease in LN remaining after surgery, those with resected disease had longer PFS (38 months vs. 9 months) (203). Mariani et al. (142) showed that pelvic sidewall failure at 5 years was 57% for patients who had inadequate nodal dissection and/or no adjuvant radiation compared to 10% when patients had adequate (removal >10 nodes) lymphadenectomy and received radiation. The best outcomes reported for node-positive patients follow complete nodal dissection. For example, in one series, of 30 stage IIIC patients managed with systematic pelvic and para-aortic lymphadenectomy (average number nodes removed, 66) followed by RT and CT, 5-year survival was 100% for patients with positive pelvic nodes and 75% for positive para-aortic nodes (163).

The most cogent argument for routine staging is that following thorough nodal assessment, most patients with node-negative disease can accurately be classified as low risk, and may avoid pelvic radiation or receive VCB in lieu of pelvic RT. Three randomized trials comparing radiation to observation have failed to demonstrate a survival advantage for adjuvant pelvic RT in patients with stage I–II disease, suggesting that in the absence of nodal disease no therapy is a reasonable option (144,151,204). Indeed, patients with negative nodes and low-risk uterine factors (which account for two-thirds of stage I–II EC patients) have incredibly low risk of recurrence and death (2% cancer specific death at 48 months, with or without pelvic radiation) (144). Retrospective studies have shown how the incorporation of a strategy using lymphadenectomy changes the use of postoperative radiation (122,139,145,205,206). In a SEER review of 26,043 women with EC, patients with intermediate-risk disease who underwent nodal assessment were less likely to receive external beam pelvic RT and more likely to receive vaginal brachytherapy compared to women who did not undergo nodal assessment (146). In the absence of nodal disease, recurrence risk is low and OS is high, with no radiation or with the substitution of VCB.

Alternatives to Lymphadenectomy

Given the debate as to the value of lymphadenectomy, a variety of alternative strategies have been evaluated. The concept of lymphatic mapping by sentinel LN dissection has been accepted into practice in patients with breast cancer and melanoma, and is increasingly being used in vulvar cancers. The technique uses a preoperative local injection of radioactive colloid 6 to 12 hours preoperatively followed by a lymphoscintigram, with or without an immediately preoperative injection of a colorimetric dye (isosulfan blue). The theory suggests that regional nodal spread first moves to a "sentinel" node(s) for which markers (lymphoscintigram, gamma counter, gross blue appearance of node) make apparent. By selectively resecting the sentinel node, the "at-risk node" is evaluated, but other nodes are retained *in situ*, thus reducing morbidity, length of surgery, blood loss. For sentinel mapping to be effective, reproducible techniques must be developed and validated, standard nodal processing (serial sectioning, immunohistochemical (IHC) evaluations) must be developed, and the false-negative rate must be low. Given that the pretest probability for nodal disease is low (~9%) in an all-comer population, large studies will be required to adequately evaluate sentinel node mapping.

The appropriate site of injection for colloid/blue dye is evident in vulvar cancers and cutaneous melanomas; however, there is debate on where to inject the uterus to delineate nodal drainage of the tumor. Possible sites of injection include the uterine fundus, cervix, or hysteroscopic injection of the tumor (207). As lymphatic drainage of the uterus is complex, it is unclear whether injections of the cervix mirror drainage of the uterus in general or specifically of the tumor. For example, there is discussion in the literature as to whether cervical injections may identify para-aortic sentinel nodal disease. In addition to the surgical technique, controversy exists as to the best way to process sentinel node specimens. Immunohistochemical processing to detect cytokeratin is important in that it increases the identification of micrometastatic implants, although the clinical significance of this type of disease is uncertain (208,209).

Investigators at Memorial Sloan Kettering have performed a series of sentinel node mapping surgeries on 266 patients, followed by pelvic +/− para-aortic lymphadenectomy. Using a cervical injection technique, they reported sentinel detection was possible in 84% of cases, 12% of cases had positive nodal disease, and metastatic cells were three times more likely in sentinel nodes than in non-sentinel nodes (210). In a meta-analysis of 26 series on sentinel node dissection, Kang estimated that the detection rate for sentinel nodes was 78% and the sensitivity was 93%. In a disease where baseline rates of nodal involvement are roughly 10%, this translates to a ~1% false-negative rate (211). As most of the series in the meta-analysis included small numbers of patients, the authors cautioned against routine substitution of sentinel nodal mapping for lymphadenectomy based on the current data.

Minimally Invasive Surgery for EC

After several years of debate and discussion, minimally invasive techniques have been integrated into the management of EC as a standard of care. Techniques utilized in the initial treatment of EC include LAVH, total laparoscopic hysterectomy (TLH), and robotic hysterectomy with concomitant salpingo-oophorectomy and pelvic and para-aortic nodal dissection to stage patients. Minimally invasive staging techniques include transperitoneal and extraperitoneal assessment of nodes and may be done at the time of hysterectomy or at a later time to restage patients following incomplete surgical staging. The decade of the 1990s advanced the use of minimally invasive surgery and introduced the laparoscopic techniques and tools required for comprehensive surgical staging of EC. As the initial debate on LAVH focused on whether laparoscopic techniques could be substituted for abdominal ones, in EC, debate has focused on whether laparoscopic surgical staging could be substituted for open procedures. Initial case reports and small single institutional series describing technique and demonstrating feasibility were replaced by large series, small randomized trials, and subsequently, multi-institutional randomized controlled trials (168,212–220).

Improvements in laparoscopic equipment facilitated the development of LAVH. Building on that experience, and coupled with the introduction of better optics for visualization, laparoscopic resection of LN became possible. Querleu et al. (221) were the first to report pelvic lymphadenectomy for cervical cancer in 1991, followed by Nezhat et al. (222) who reported in 1992 on the use of laparoscopic pelvic and para-aortic lymphadenectomy with radical hysterectomy in cervical cancer. When first utilized in EC, laparoscopic para-aortic node dissection only evaluated right-sided nodes (212). Techniques have subsequently been developed allowing for dissection to include the left para-aortic nodes, and facilitate extraperitoneal approaches. (196,197,223–225).

Childers et al. (212,213) described the initial experience of LAVH in 59 patients with clinical stage I endometrial carcinoma. Laparoscopic pelvic and right-sided aortic LN samplings were performed in patients with grade 2 or 3 lesions, or with grade 1 lesions, and greater than 50% myometrial invasion on frozen section. For the group, the mean weight was 153 pounds, and in two patients, laparoscopic lymphadenectomy was precluded by obesity. Six patients underwent conversion to an open procedure because of intraperitoneal disease, and two patients required laparotomy to manage complications, including a transected ureter and a cystotomy. The mean hospital stay was 2.9 days. Since that time many retrospective series have appeared in the literature describing techniques and presumed advantages (226–229). In general, mean operating times were longer for laparoscopy, but the overall complication rates, length of stay, and hospital charges were lower. With short follow-ups, there was no significant difference in disease recurrence between the two groups.

Prospective data has also emerged. A small prospective, randomized trial comparing laparoscopic-assisted vaginal versus abdominal surgery in patients with EC was reported by Malur et al. (217). They randomized 70 patients with EC FIGO stage I–III to laparoscopy-assisted simple or radical vaginal hysterectomy or simple or radical abdominal hysterectomy with or without LN resection. Blood loss and transfusion rates were significantly lower in the laparoscopic group. The number of pelvic and para-aortic LN, duration of surgery, and incidence of postoperative complications were similar for both groups. No significant differences in disease recurrence rate and long-term survival were found between the laparoscopic and laparotomy groups (97.3% vs. 93.3% and 83.9% vs. 90.9% for stages I, II, and III, respectively). Malzoni and colleagues reported on a 159-patient trial comparing TLH to TAH with lymphadenectomy. The authors reported less blood loss, shorter hospitalization, and less common ileus with TLH. Operative time was longer (136 minutes vs. 123 minutes) with TLH, but there was no difference in number of nodes removed, frequency of stage IIIC disease, ability to do para-aortic dissection, or in recurrence. The LACE trial compared TLH (n = 190) to TAH (n = 142) in 332 patients with stage I EC (with or without lymphadenectomy) (168).The preliminary report designed to specifically assess quality-of-life end points showed that 2.4% of laparoscopic cases required conversion to an open approach, operating time for TLH on average was 30 minutes longer, grade 3 to 4 adverse events were more frequent (23% vs. 12%) in the TAH groups, and quality-of-life assessments favored TLH for up to 6 months post surgery. Concurrent LN assessment was more common with TAH versus TLH (68% vs. 41%), and ~20% of patients participating in the study received some form of adjuvant therapy (CT, RT, or both).

The largest and most comprehensive dataset to date comes from the large prospective, randomized trial conducted by the GOG (Lap II trial) (220). The study was designed to compare laparoscopic hysterectomy with comprehensive surgical staging to the traditional laparotomy technique (using a 2:1 randomization favoring the laparoscopic arm) to determine the complete staging rates, safety, short-term surgical outcomes, and long-term cancer recurrence and survival. The study enrolled 920 patients to the open arm and 1,696 patients to laparoscopy. The rate of conversion from laparoscopy to open procedure was 26%, and was most frequently related to poor visibility (15%), extrauterine cancer spread (4%), and bleeding (3%). The conversion rate increased with increasing patient obesity, with the laparoscopic success rate being 90% with a body mass index (BMI) <20, 65% with BMI = 35, and 34% with BMI = 50. Median number of removed nodes was similar between each technique as were the frequencies of patients found to have positive LN. Complication rates (combined rates of vascular, urinary, bowel, nerve, or other complications) for those who had an open procedure were 7.6%, compared to 9.5% of patients randomized to laparoscopy. Of the 1,242 patients randomized to laparoscopy who had the procedure successfully completed laparoscopically, the complication rate was 4.9%. Comparing patients who underwent open surgery versus successful completion of laparoscopy, operative time was longer (median 70 minutes), but hospital time was shorter (2 days vs. 4 days) with laparoscopy. Postoperative arrhythmia, pneumonia, ileus, antibiotic use, and any complications > grade 2 were lower in the laparoscopic group. The authors concluded that laparoscopic surgical staging is an acceptable and possibly a better option, particularly when the surgery can be successfully completed laparoscopically.

Results of long-term survival in laparoscopically treated compared to laparotomy-treated EC patients suggest comparable outcomes. Tozzi reporting on the first prospective trial (n = 122 patients) reported DFS of 91% with LAVH and 94% with laparotomy, with survival of 86% versus 90%, respectively (230). In a subsequent evaluation of recurrence and survival data from the GOG LAP 2 trial published in 2012, 3-year recurrence rates were 11.4% with laparoscopy versus 10.2% with open surgery, and 5-year survival was 90% in each arm (231).

Age and obesity have been suggested as relative contraindications to laparoscopic surgery. In the GOG Lap II trial, the median age was 63 years. Scribner et al. (232) evaluated the surgical experience of uterine cancer patients with age ≥65 years who underwent LAVH with pelvic and para-aortic lymphadenectomy (n = 67) or abdominal hysterectomy with pelvic and para-aortic lymphadenectomy (n = 45). Laparoscopic staging could be completed in 78% of patients. In the laparoscopic group, the BMI was 29.5 kg/m^2 (range, 15.9 to 54.7), and 33% had a history of prior laparotomy. For the 22% of patients who required a conversion to laparotomy, obesity (10%), bleeding (6%), and intraperitoneal disease (5%) were the most frequent reasons. Similar nodal counts (29 laparoscopic, 29 open) were noted, the operative time was longer (236 minutes vs. 148 minutes), and hospital stay was shorter (median 3 days vs. 5.6 days) with laparoscopy. The authors concluded that with the anticipated growth of an aging patient population, laparoscopic management is a viable option.

It has been suggested that obese patients are poor laparoscopic candidates because of difficulties in establishing pneumoperitoneum, poorer visualization, inability to tolerate the steep Trendelenburg positioning needed to facilitate the surgery, and difficulties with ventilation. In the report by Childers et al., (212,213) mean patient weight was only 153 pounds. It is important to recognize that regardless of surgical approach, complete surgical staging is more difficult in an obese patient. Scribner et al. (233) compared 55 obese patients (median weight 96.6 kg, median BMI 40) who underwent LAVH with pelvic and para-aortic lymphadenectomy to 45 patients (median weight 101 kg, median BMI 39) who had abdominal hysterectomy with pelvic and para-aortic lymphadenectomy. Successful completion of laparoscopy was possible in 64%, with patients with a BMI <35 kg/m^2 having an 82% success rate compared to 44% when the BMI was >35 kg/m^2. Eltabbakh et al. (234) evaluated 40 women with BMI between 28 and 60 years who were treated with LAVH and compared them to 40 similar women treated by abdominal approach. Laparoscopic conversion was only required in 8% of patients. Laparoscopic surgery was associated with a longer operative time (195 minutes vs. 138 minutes), but more pelvic nodes (mean 11 vs. 5), less pain medicine requirement, and shorter hospital stay (2.5 days vs. 5.6 days) were recorded. TLH has also demonstrated feasibility in heavier patients (235). In the prospective GOG series, there was ≥80% success rate with patients with a BMI of 27 or less, but even at a BMI of 35, 65% were able have successful laparoscopic surgery (220).

Robotic surgery may represent the next step forward in minimally invasive surgery. Since FDA approval for hysterectomy and myomectomy procedures in 2005, there has been an increasing utilization of robotic surgery within gynecologic oncology. To date, greater than 15 series ranging in size from 4 to 405 patients have described robotic experience or compared outcomes to laparoscopy and/or open procedures (**Table 21.11**) (236–242). The proposed advantages of robotic surgery include improved visualization with 3-D optics, "wrist-like" motion of instruments allowing greater dexterity, reduction in tremor, easier learning curve for adoption compared to straight-stick laparoscopy and more comfortable ergonomics. Published data suggest comparable outcomes with respect to blood loss, nodal counts, and operative time compared to laparoscopy. Mean nodal counts and operative complications are comparable to laparoscopy, with several series suggesting lower postoperative complications compared to open surgery. As with new surgical techniques, there is a learning curve through which additional experience leads to quicker operative times and higher nodal retrieval rates. The Ohio State group has suggested that 20 procedures are required for proficiency (243).

Robotic surgery may offer unique opportunities for obese patients (244,245). Several series suggest that robotics may overcome some of the challenges of laparoscopy and may reduce the morbidity associated with open cases. Seamon and colleagues reported that in a series of 109 obese patients (mean BMI 40) treated by robotic hysterectomy and staging, the conversion rate was 16%. (244) The 92 patients successfully treated by robotic platform were compared to a matched cohort of 162 laparotomy patients. Total nodal counts (~24 nodes each group) and frequency of adequate lymphadenectomy (defined as at least 10 nodes removed) were similar in both groups, but blood transfusion rate, hospital stay, complications, and wound problems were reduced with robotic surgery.

Arguments have been advanced for and against each of the surgical approaches to EC. Vaginal hysterectomy was once a favored operation, but it did not allow for routine removal of the ovaries in some patients. It also did not permit for surgical resection of LN, inspection of the peritoneal cavity or the retroperitoneum for metastatic disease, or collection of peritoneal fluid for cytology (246). Laparoscopic-assisted or total laparoscopic approaches overcome these limitations, however. Compared to open procedures, LAVH/TLH are thought to lead to reduced incisional complications, wound infections, ileus, hospital stay, cost, and improved rate of recovery and quality of life (220,221,247). Data from prospective studies also showed that short-term (6 weeks to 6 months) patient-assessed quality-of-life assessments favor minimally invasive surgery (247). In patients requiring postoperative radiation, laparoscopic surgical staging followed by RT is suggested to result in fewer bowel adhesions and radiation-induced bowel injuries (226). Criticisms of LAVH/TLH with laparoscopic nodal dissection relate to the learning curve required to master new or unfamiliar procedures, the increased length of operative times, and concerns about the adequacy of the nodal dissection. Studies do suggest that with increased experience, operative times decrease and nodal counts increase (223,227). Laparoscopy also introduced different procedure-related complications (228,229). Rarely, the technique has been associated with port-site recurrences or intraperitoneal dissemination of disease by laparoscopic gas and/or uterine manipulation.

Whether a minimally invasive procedure is comparable to an open approach must be judged by the ability to accurately dissect appropriate nodal basins, to remove an adequate/representative number of LN, to identify metastatic disease, and by the rates of recurrence. The technique used to remove the uterus/ovaries is not the source of controversy, although TLH and robotic hysterectomy may facilitate removal of larger uteri or assist in cases with poor descensus compared to LAVH. Comprehensive surgical staging allows for appropriate risk stratification to make appropriate treatment recommendations. Multiple reports demonstrated similar node counts for open, laparoscopic, and robotic techniques in the surgical staging of EC (229,236). In the GOG Lap II trial, median numbers of nodes from pelvic and para-aortic basins, and frequencies of positive nodes were comparable in the surgical arms (220). If laparoscopic nodal dissection cannot be performed, conversion to laparotomy is advised to yield inadequate information for treatment planning.

Minimally invasive surgery must be performed with an acceptable complication rate in order to be considered a viable option. In one series reporting on complication rates with an institution's first 100 pelvic and para-aortic nodal dissections, conversion to manage complications was required in 5 to control bleeding, and 1 to repair a ureteral injury (248). In another group's experience with 150 patients, seven major vascular injuries were reported, but only 4 patients required laparotomy (249). Querleu et al. (250) reported on intraoperative and postoperative complications of laparoscopic node dissection from 1,192 pelvic and para-aortic nodal dissections. Only 13 open procedures were required to complete the nodal dissections, and a laparotomy was required in 7 cases to manage complications. Eleven intraoperative vascular injuries were noted, but none required management by laparotomy. In the GOG Lap 2 study, intraoperative complications were comparable (7.6% open, 9.5% randomized to laparoscopy, 4.9% successful completion of laparoscopy) (220). Postoperative complications and short-term quality-of-life improvements favored laparoscopy. A meta-analysis of robotic studies for gynecologic conditions noted that for endometrial series, robotic surgery was associated with less blood loss and less frequent conversions to open procedure compared to laparoscopy.

TABLE 21.11. Selected Robotic Surgery Series in EC

Study	N (Robot Cases)	Type of Study	Procedure	OR Time (min) (Mean/Median)	# Nodes (Mean/Median)
Boggess- 2008	103	Compare to LSC + Open	Hyst + PPALND	191	33
DeNardis-2008	87	Compare to LSC	Hyst + PPALND	177	19
Veljovich-2008	25	Compare to LSC + Open	Hyst +/– LND	283	18
Holloway- 2009	100	Case series	Hyst + PPALND	171	19
Seaman- 2009	105	Compare to LSC	Hyst + PPALND	242	31
Lowe- 2009	405	Case series	Hyst +/– LND	172	14
Lim-2011	122	Compare to LSC	Hyst + PPALND	147	25

EC, Endometrial Cancer; hyst, hysterectomy; LND, lymph node dissection unspecified; LSC, Laparoscopic; open, laparotomy; PPALND, Pelvic, para-aortic lymph node dissection.

Restaging

One of the more useful roles of minimally invasive surgery is in restaging patients who underwent hysterectomy only. Patients who undergo hysterectomy without nodal dissection and who have pathologic risk factors for potential nodal spread face a difficult dilemma. Patients may elect to receive radiation or chemotherapy (presuming nodes are positive), elect observation (presuming nodes are negative), or undergo a second operation. A second laparotomy can be difficult to accept. Laparoscopic staging offers a less invasive option for collecting information. Childers et al. (251) reported the initial experience with restaging in 13 patients, finding disease in 3 patients.

Recommendations for Minimally Invasive Surgery

Standard of care today includes minimally invasive surgery in the management of EC. Additional training and experience are required for successful completion of these procedures, just as they are with open procedures. The demonstration of comparable surgical end points (similar numbers of nodes removed, similar frequency of positive nodes, recurrence rates, and survival) along with shortened hospital stays, quicker recovery, and better quality-of-life indicators compared to open procedures suggest that appropriate patients should be counseled regarding this option. Challenges remain on how to increase the minimally invasive training of gynecologic oncologists in practice and fellows in training programs. As with open procedures, defining populations that should be considered for nodal assessment and for postoperative therapies continues to be an important research focus.

Surgical Management of Intraperitoneal Disease

The management of patients with bulky stage III or stage IV disease depends on the ability to resect disease. In patients with distant metastasis, there may be a limited role for surgery such as to provide control of vaginal bleeding. In patients with intraperitoneal disease, options include resecting easily removable disease (uterus, adnexa, omentum) versus a more extensive cytoreductive effort. The value of extensive cytoreductive surgery in EC has not been as well studied as it has in ovarian cancer. Historically, limitations in postoperative therapies (lack of enthusiasm for whole abdominal radiation, marginally effective CT regimens, reliance on hormonal therapy) perhaps reduced interest. Several retrospective reports suggest that survival correlates with volume of residual disease (252–254). Shih et al. (255) reported on 58 patients with stage IV endometrioid disease treated from 1977 to 2003, of whom 9 had no gross residual, 11 had <1 cm residual, and 32 had residual >1 cm. The median survival for the entire population group was 19 months; however, median survival was 42 months for patients with no gross residual disease. In a multivariate analysis of the data, residual disease and the use of postoperative adjuvant CT were independently associated with survival. Bristow et al. (254) demonstrated that optimal cytoreduction (<1 cm) could be obtained in 55% of stage IV patients and required omentectomy (93%), peritoneal stripping (65%), and bowel resection (29%) to do it. In patients with serous histology, similar survival improvements were seen with optimal debulking of intraperitoneal disease (256).

Surgical Recommendations

The contemporary management of EC has significantly changed. We believe that patients must be appropriately counseled with regard to the presumed benefits of lymphadenectomy as well as the potential risks. Data for the ASTEC and Italian lymphadenectomy trials cast doubt as to the benefit of resecting negative nodes, but both studies clearly demonstrate that nodal disease cannot be found unless one searches for it. The clinician is challenged with finding the "needle in the haystack" in a disease where the baseline rate of nodal metastasis in ~9%. The marginal benefit achieved by lymphadenectomy and the downstream costs associated with or without its use in terms of adjuvant therapy, outcomes, and quality of life need to be better defined so that patients and physicians can make choices based on good information. Clinical pathologic models that define low-risk populations for whom lymphadenectomy may be safely omitted appear promising, but must be validated prospectively in large series. In the future, biomarker-based testing or sentinel nodal assessment may serve as an alternative to lymphadenectomy, but cannot be routinely recommended at this point because the data is immature. Increasing the proportion of patients who undergo minimally invasive surgery to manage EC is an important goal and driven by the data. Patients who *a priori* are deemed not to be candidates for staging should be considered for vaginal or minimally invasive hysterectomies. Surgical therapy for EC removes the disease and defines populations at risk for recurrence and death. Surgical staging, or the lack of it, defines patient groups as surgically staged node-positive or -negative, or unstaged. Comprehensive staging most accurately assigns stage and associated prognosis, although the magnitude of the risk assignment is tempered by the frequency of positive nodes, uterine risk factors, and use of adjuvant therapy. Staging also allows for a more tailored approach to the use of adjuvant therapies. For patients with resectable intraperitoneal disease, cytoreductive surgery can result in optimal volumes of residual disease, and perhaps improved outcomes.

PATHOLOGY

Hyperplasia

The current classification of endometrial hyperplasia accepted by both the International Society of Gynecologic Pathologists (ISGP) and the World Health Organization (WHO) is based on the schema of Kurman and Norris (257), which divides hyperplasia on the basis of architectural features into simple or complex and on the basis of cytologic features into typical or atypical (**Table 21.12**). The resulting classification has four categories as follows: *simple hyperplasia* (SH), *complex hyperplasia* (CH), *simple atypical hyperplasia* (SAH), and *complex atypical hyperplasia* (CAH). Simple hyperplasia is defined as an increase in the number of endometrial glands, which may be dilated with little crowding or have an irregular outline and exhibit crowding. Complex hyperplasia is characterized by glands with irregular outlines, marked structural complexity, and back-to-back crowding. The designation "atypical hyperplasia" is used to denote a proliferation of glands exhibiting cytologic atypia, recognized as nuclear enlargement, the presence of nucleoli, or a change from an elongated to a more ovoid or round nucleus. The chromatin may be either evenly or irregularly dispersed. The justification for this classification system rests on three retrospective studies that demonstrate a higher rate of progression of CAH to adenocarcinoma (257–259). It is sometimes difficult to apply this system, which requires one to

TABLE 21.12. Classification of Endometrial Hyperplasia

Types of Hyperplasia	Progressing to Cancer (%)
Simple (cystic without atypia)	1
Complex (adenomatous without atypia)	3
Atypical	
Simple (cystic with atypia)	8
Complex (adenomatous with atypia)	29

make a distinction between cytologically atypical nuclei and those without atypical nuclei, because a spectrum of nuclear variability actually exists. As noted by Kendall et al. (260), the definitions of architectural complexity and nuclear atypia potentially rest on a multitude of criteria, and some but not all criteria may be fully developed in any given case.

Several reports have addressed the reproducibility of diagnoses of hyperplasia (260–262). Intra-observer reproducibility was generally found to be moderate to good, whereas interobserver reproducibility was poor to moderate for various diagnostic categories. These studies probably overestimate the interobserver reproducibility because they used expert gynecologic pathologists and specified the classification to be used. In a prospective study by the GOG, neither community-based nor expert panel diagnosis of atypical hyperplasia was highly accurate (72). The current classification of hyperplasia relies on a combination of multiple architectural and cytologic criteria. It is hardly surprising that interobserver reproducibility is relatively low when multiple criteria are used to classify a lesion, because each pathologist must assign a relative value or weight to each potentially conflicting criterion. Other factors contributing to low reproducibility include (a) the fragmentary nature of curettings, (b) the presence of borderline lesions, (c) uncertainty about the significance of focal hyperplasia, (d) the inadequacy of published descriptions and understanding of terms used to define architectural or cytologic atypia, and (e) the difficulty associated with the translation of verbal descriptions into light microscopic interobserver reproducibility for images.

The gross manifestations of endometrial hyperplasia are highly varied. The endometrium is often of diffusely increased thickness (5 mm to 10 mm or greater), vaguely nodular, tan, and soft without hemorrhage or necrosis. However, hyperplasia may be focal or multifocal in a background of polyps or cycling endometrium, or occasionally associated with a diffusely thin endometrial lining. Part of the variability may reflect a reduction in the ET because of prior endometrial sampling. Coexistent adenocarcinoma is present in 1% to 40% of hysterectomies performed to treat hyperplasia, with the latter number reflecting the frequent co-occurrence of carcinoma with atypical CH.

Endometrial Intraepithelial Neoplasia

On the basis of a combination of morphologic, molecular, and morphometric information, Mutter et al. have proposed an alternative classification scheme to replace the current WHO hyperplasia terminology (263–266). They have presented data that endometrial intraepithelial neoplasia (EIN) is the histopathologic presentation of a monoclonal endometrial preinvasive glandular proliferation that is the immediate pathologic precursor of endometrioid endometrial adenocarcinoma. Monoclonality and forward carryover of EIN mutations into subsequent carcinoma were the original molecular standards used for EIN diagnosis. Computer-assisted morphometric analysis of more than 20 features was carried out initially and the three features seen in molecularly defined precancers enabled an objective delineation of histologic diagnostic criteria (the D-score). The principal components assessed included a reduction in the volume of stroma, an increased variability in nuclear shape gland contour. Several of these features have been translated to characteristics that can be assessed subjectively by the surgical pathologist (**Fig. 21.3**). These features include the following: (a) the area of the glands exceeds that of stroma; (b) nuclear and cytoplasmic features of the affected glandular cells differ from those of the background glands, and may include loss of nuclear polarity or increased nuclear pleomorphism; in the absence of any background glands, a highly abnormal cytology is sufficient; (c) the maximum diameter exceeds 1 mm; (d) benign conditions including disordered proliferation, polyps, and repair are excluded; and (e) the cribriform or maze-like pattern of carcinoma is excluded. There is a high degree of concordance between EIN diagnoses rendered by computer and those made subjectively by pathologists, and either has superior cancer predictive value when compared to the 14-fold increased cancer risk conferred by the presence of atypia compared to lack thereof in the WHO hyperplasia schema. Clinical outcome studies have shown that almost 40% of women with an EIN diagnosis will be diagnosed with EC within 1 year and, and for those who do not develop cancer within 12 months, a 45-fold increased risk of future EC exists. Correspondingly, absence of an EIN lesion in an initial representative biopsy, including those with only benign hyperplasia, confers very high (99%) negative predictive value for concomitant or future adenocarcinoma.

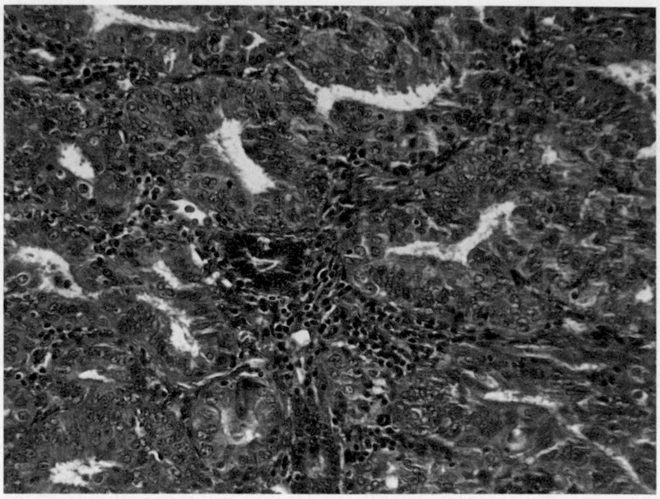

Figure 21.3. A lesion that could be classified in two different systems as either EIN or CAH based on gland crowding and cytologic atypia. Note the presence of a residual inactive endometrial gland that may be used as a reference for estimating cytologic atypia.

Although EIN shares many features with atypical CH, the two entities are not entirely overlapping. The concept of EIN is appealing because there appears to be a strong biologic basis, with EIN representing a clonal process, whereas disordered proliferation and hyperplasia remain as diffuse endometrial physiologic responses to an abnormal stimulus (unopposed estrogen stimulation).

Simple Hyperplasia

In SH, the endometrium is thicker than usual, with dilated glands that have outpouchings and invaginations, producing an irregular outline to the enlarged glands. The glands are crowded, the stroma is more densely cellular than usual, and some foam cells may exist within the stroma. Follow-up of patients with this condition reveals little or no progression to carcinoma.

Complex Hyperplasia

The endometrium is increased in thickness by back-to-back glands in cases of CH. Most glands have irregular outlines. The two main features differentiating this from SH is the high ratio of glands to stroma, with some back-to-back glands that have very little intervening stroma. Epithelial stratification is a frequent finding, producing an appearance of two to four cell layers. Mitotic activity is highly variable, but may range to up to 10 mitotic figures per 10 high-power fields.

Atypical Hyperplasia

Atypical hyperplasia is characterized by cytologic atypia of the glands, which may vary unpredictably according to vagaries of histologic preparation. The architecture may reflect simple or CH, although it is usually complex. The cells lining the glands display nuclear hyperchromatism and nuclear enlargement, and have an increased nucleus–cytoplasm ratio. Nuclei are irregular in size and shape and have a thickened nuclear membrane, inconspicuous to prominent nucleoli, and a coarse chromatin texture. At times, the nuclei may appear clear with scattered, coarse chromatin clumps.

Progression from Hyperplasia to Cancer

The natural history of endometrial hyperplasia is difficult to define for a variety of reasons, four of which follow: (a) pathologic criteria—criteria and terminology for the various forms of hyperplasia have changed repeatedly; (b) initial sampling—the method of initial diagnosis is often curettage, which removes part or all of the lesion to be studied; (c) coexisting lesions—other lesions such as adenocarcinoma may coexist at the time of diagnosis without our knowledge, since the curettage or biopsy samples only a minority of the endometrium; and (d) subsequent intervention—hormonal or surgical intervention usually interrupts observations of the natural history of the hyperplasia. Nevertheless, there are reasonably good data to support the following assertions: (a) endometrial hyperplasia is commonly a consequence of unopposed prolonged estrogen stimulation; (b) some hyperplasias may regress if the estrogenic stimulus is removed or in response to progestational or antiestrogenic treatment; (c) some hyperplasias coexist with, or progress to, invasive adenocarcinoma; and (d) the probability of progression to adenocarcinoma is related to the degree of architectural or cytologic atypia. Progression from hyperplasia to carcinoma occurs in only 1% of patients with SH and in 3% of patients with CH (71). Progression from atypical hyperplasia is much higher; 8% of patients with SAH and 29% of those with CAH develop carcinoma (**Table 21.12**) (71,257). Glandular complexity superimposed on atypia probably places the patient at greater risk than does cytologic atypia alone, but the point is unsettled.

Pathologic Diagnosis

The ISGP and the WHO last revised the classification of uterine tumors in 2003 (267), and the portion pertaining to carcinomas of the endometrium is presented in **Table 21.13**. This relatively simple classification scheme accommodates the vast majority of ECs and distinguishes among neoplasms of significantly different prognosis. Mixed carcinomas with two distinctive cell types are relatively common, and are defined as those carcinomas in which the secondary component constitutes at least 10% of the neoplasm.

In most endometrial samples, the distinction of adenocarcinoma from hyperplasia is straightforward. However, a small fraction of problematic cases with complex proliferations truly tax the abilities of experts as well as novices to classify them correctly. The diagnosis of a well-differentiated adenocarcinoma is made in the presence of any of the following criteria: (a) irregular infiltration of glands in an altered fibroblastic stroma, (b) a confluent glandular pattern that results in either a cribriform arrangement or confluent interconnected glands, or (c) extensive papillary growth of epithelium and stroma into glandular lumina (257).

Histologic Grade

The differentiation of a carcinoma is expressed as its grade. Grade 1 lesions are well differentiated and are generally associated with a good prognosis. Grade 2 tumors (**Fig. 21.4**) are moderately well-differentiated and have an intermediate prognosis, and grade 3 reflects poorly differentiated lesions, which frequently have a poor prognosis. Both architectural criteria and nuclear grade are used in the FIGO and ISGP–WHO committee (268) classification of tumors and are applied to endometrioid cell types including variants and mucinous carcinomas (**Table 21.13**). In contrast, serous, clear cell, and undifferentiated carcinomas are considered high-grade by definition, and are not graded numerically. The architectural grade is determined as follows: grade 1—an adenocarcinoma in which less than 5% of the tumor growth is in solid sheets; grade 2—an adenocarcinoma in which 6% to 50% of the neoplasm is arranged in solid sheets of neoplastic cells; grade 3—an adenocarcinoma in which greater than 50% of the neoplastic cells are in solid masses. Regions of squamous differentiation are excluded from this assessment. The FIGO rules for grading state that notable nuclear atypia, inappropriate for architectural grade, raises the grade of a grade 1 or grade 2 tumor by one. However, FIGO did not define notable nuclear atypia. Justification and clarification for this modification based on extreme nuclear pleomorphism were provided in a recent GOG study. For 715 women with nonserous ECs, three nuclear grades were defined as follows: grade 1—round-to-oval nuclei with even distribution of chromatin and inconspicuous nucleoli; grade 2—irregular, oval nuclei with chromatin clumping and moderate-size nucleoli; and grade 3—large, pleomorphic nuclei with coarse chromatin and large, irregular nucleoli. Patients with tumors of architectural grade 1 or 2, but with a majority of cells having nuclei of grade 3, had a significantly worse behavior, justifying an upgrading by one grade (269).

Taylor et al. (270) proposed a two-tiered system for grading endometrial carcinoma based on a study of 85 patients with stage I and II EC. They divided tumors at 10% intervals based on the percentage of solid tumor growth, and found that tumor recurrences were confined

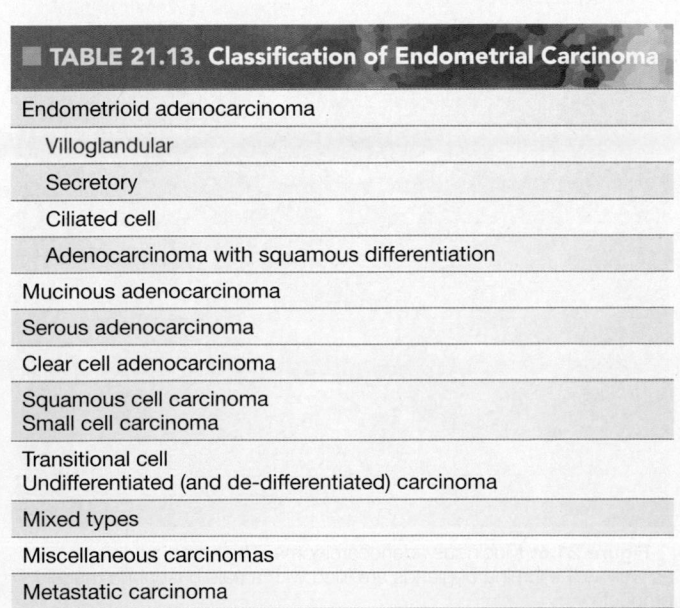

TABLE 21.13. Classification of Endometrial Carcinoma

Endometrioid adenocarcinoma
Villoglandular
Secretory
Ciliated cell
Adenocarcinoma with squamous differentiation
Mucinous adenocarcinoma
Serous adenocarcinoma
Clear cell adenocarcinoma
Squamous cell carcinoma Small cell carcinoma
Transitional cell Undifferentiated (and de-differentiated) carcinoma
Mixed types
Miscellaneous carcinomas
Metastatic carcinoma

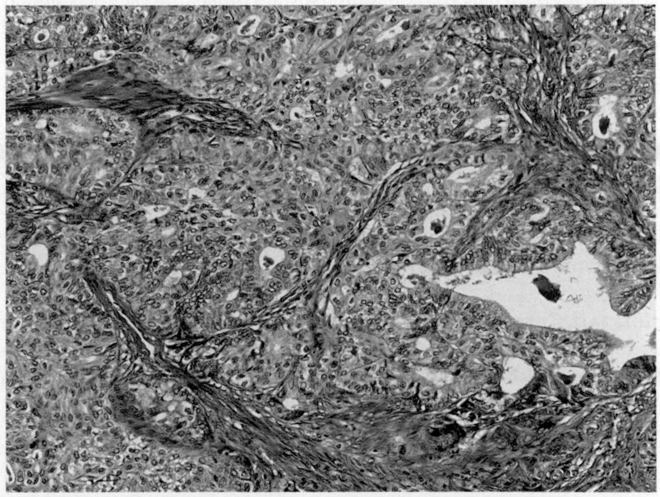

Figure 21.4. Endometrioid adenocarcinoma, grade 2. The glandular component is a caricature of proliferative phase glands, with stratification and a shared luminal border to the neoplastic cells. In grade 2 carcinomas, regions of solid neoplastic growth occupy between 5% and 50% of the surface area of the carcinoma.

to the subset with greater than 20% solid tumor. They also found that this binary division yielded a higher degree of interobserver agreement than three architectural grades. Lax et al. (271) have presented preliminary data on a binary architectural grading system based on the presence of greater than 50% solid growth, a diffusely infiltrative growth pattern, and tumor cell necrosis. These methods will have to be replicated in a larger patient population before an assessment of their prognostic utility can be made.

Cell Types

Endometrioid Adenocarcinoma. Endometrioid adenocarcinoma is the most common form of carcinoma of the endometrium, comprising 75% to 80% of the cases (59,272). It varies from well differentiated to undifferentiated. Characteristically, the glands of endometrioid adenocarcinoma are formed of tall columnar cells that share a common apical border, resulting in a smoothly delineated, round or oval luminal contour. With decreasing differentiation, there is a preponderance of solid growth rather than gland formation, and the cells lining glandular lumina become more numerous but not necessarily clearly stratified. Stromal invasion manifested by a desmoplastic host response or vascular invasion is often not evident in the biopsy or curettage specimen.

Villoglandular Carcinoma. There has been considerable confusion about the definition and significance of papillary carcinoma of the endometrium. A variety of cell types of endometrial adenocarcinoma with differing biologic behavior, including serous, clear cell, mucinous, and villoglandular carcinoma, may grow in a papillary fashion. Thus, the adjective *papillary* does not represent a cell type but rather an architectural pattern (272,273).

Villoglandular carcinoma is a relatively common subtype of endometrioid adenocarcinoma characterized by neoplastic columnar cells covering delicate fibrovascular cores. The apical cytoplasmic borders are straight, the nuclei are usually low-grade, and the tumor cells architecturally resemble those of other endometrioid adenocarcinomas, with which they are often admixed. In the largest study to date, villoglandular carcinomas were better differentiated than ECs, but the age at diagnosis, depth of myometrial invasion, nodal spread, and survival were similar to those of ECs, justifying their classification as a subtype of endometrioid adenocarcinoma (274).

Secretory Carcinoma. Secretory carcinoma is a variant of EC, but it is unusual and represents no more than 2% of the cases (275,276). It is identified by its well-differentiated glandular pattern, consisting of columnar epithelial cells containing intracytoplasmic vacuoles similar to secretory endometrium. It is usually grade 1 architecturally and by nuclear features. There is minimal cellular atypia, stratification, and pleomorphism. The intracellular secretions are not mucin but glycogen. The cellular features of secretory carcinoma differentiate it from clear cell carcinoma, which is more papillary with more pleomorphic nuclei. By its lack of mucin, secretory carcinoma may be differentiated from mucinous carcinoma. Recognition of secretory carcinoma is important because it has a less virulent clinical course (276,277), although the clinical profile of patients is similar to that of patients with adenocarcinoma.

Ciliated Carcinoma. Ciliated carcinoma is rare. Ciliated cells are more commonly identified in endometrial hyperplasia and in benign metaplasia (tubal metaplasia), but they may occur in ECs. Associated with prior exogenous estrogen use, this cell type is reported to have a good prognosis (278).

Adenocarcinoma with Squamous Differentiation. Foci of squamous differentiation are found in about 10% to 25% of endometrial adenocarcinomas (**Fig. 21.5**). Historically, the tumors were sometimes separated into adenoacanthoma or adenosquamous carcinoma based on whether the squamous component appeared histologically benign or malignant (279–283). However, in about 30% of cases, the squamous component is not clearly benign or malignant. In a GOG study of early-stage disease, it was noted that these tumors with squamous regions behave in a fashion similar to ECs without squamous differentiation (284). The squamous areas usually mirror the degree of differentiation, which, coupled with assessment of histologic grade and other conventional prognostic factors, is thus more useful for prognostication and determination of adjuvant therapy than the historic terms *adenoacanthoma* and *adenosquamous carcinoma*, which are confusing and should be abandoned.

Mucinous Adenocarcinoma. Mucinous adenocarcinoma is rare in the endometrium, in contrast to its high frequency in the endocervix. It has been reported to represent between 1% and 9% of endometrial adenocarcinomas (285–287), but the former figure is probably more accurate. If present as the major cellular component of an EC, this tumor resembles mucinous carcinoma seen in the ovary and endocervix. Two patterns occur: In one, the cells are columnar with basally oriented nuclei; in the other, the cells are more pseudostratified, as in an adenocarcinoma of the colon or mucinous carcinoma of the ovary (**Fig. 21.6**). The characteristic cellular pattern

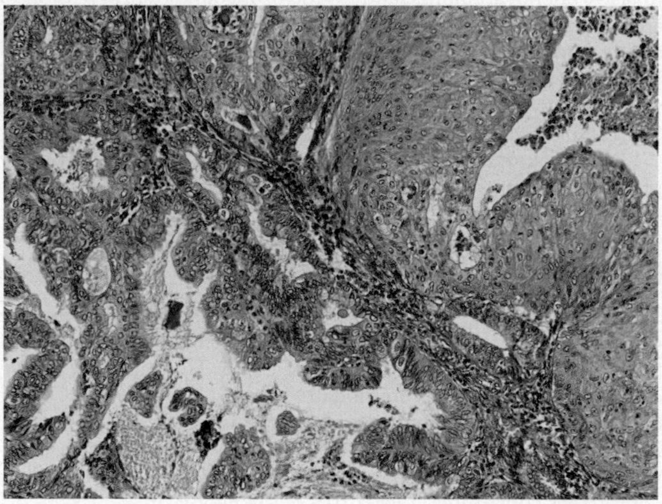

Figure 21.5. Endometrioid adenocarcinoma with squamous differentiation. The squamous component may form keratin pearls, but more often simply is characterized by acquisition of more abundant, deeply eosinophilic cytoplasm and distinct cell borders (upper right of figure). The squamous component may appear histologically benign or malignant.

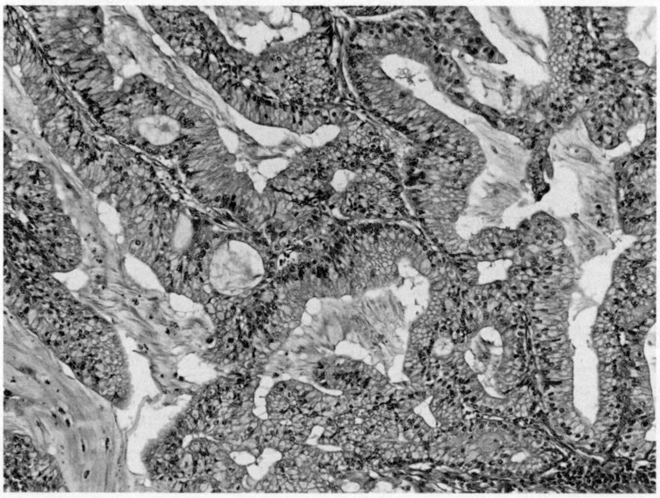

Figure 21.6. Mucinous adenocarcinoma. The apical cytoplasm cells as well as the lumina of glands are filled with a pale basophilic mucoid product.

should represent over 50% of the entire tumor. Typically, there are either papillary processes or cystically dilated glands lined by columnar or pseudostratified columnar epithelium. The cytoplasm is positive for carcinoembryonic antigen (CEA), mucicarmine, and periodic acid–Schiff stain, but it is diastase resistant (287). This tumor differs from clear cell carcinoma and secretory endometrium by having more mucin and less glycogen. The glandular architecture is usually well maintained, and most are well-differentiated (285). To establish the origin in the endometrium, exclusion of a primary endocervical tumor may be required. If the endocervical sample demonstrates the same neoplasm, the site of origin must be carefully established because this cell type is common in the endocervix (288). Neither the pattern, the type of mucin staining, nor the presence of CEA can reliably distinguish mucinous adenocarcinoma of the endometrium from its more common counterpart in the endocervix (289,290). Mucinous carcinoma of the endometrium has the same prognosis as common EC (286).

Serous Carcinoma. Serous carcinoma of the endometrium closely resembles serous carcinoma of the ovary and fallopian tube because its papillary growth and cellular features are similar (**Figs. 21.7** and **21.8**). It is usually found in an advanced stage in older women (291). Fibrous papillary fronds are lined by epithelial cells, which are almost devoid of cytoplasm, but which manifest stratification, atypism, pleomorphism, mitotic figures, and bizarre forms. These fronds often detach or demonstrate a terminal growth of tiny papillary excrescences and individual cells, which detach easily (**Fig. 21.7**). A second pattern of irregular gaping glands lined by cuboidal cells with scalloped, apical borders may be present, particularly in the deeper aspect of the tumor (**Fig. 21.8**). Lymphatic invasion is commonplace in the myometrium. Distinction from clear cell carcinoma may be difficult but can usually be accomplished on the basis of a greater degree of papillary processes, greater nuclear atypia, and less cytoplasm in papillary serous carcinoma. Psammoma bodies are frequently observed in serous carcinoma, but solid growth is more common in clear cell carcinoma.

Serous carcinoma represents approximately 10% of ECs, which is fortunate because it is an aggressive tumor. The tumors often deeply invade the myometrium, and unlike typical endometrioid adenocarcinoma, there is a propensity for peritoneal spread. Unfortunately, advanced-stage disease or recurrence is common even when serous carcinomas are apparently only minimally invasive or when confined to the endometrium in polyps (171,292,293). Because the metastatic disease is often identified only microscopically, about 60% of patients are upstaged following complete surgical staging (171,291,294). A report by Wheeler et al. (295) stressed the prognostic importance

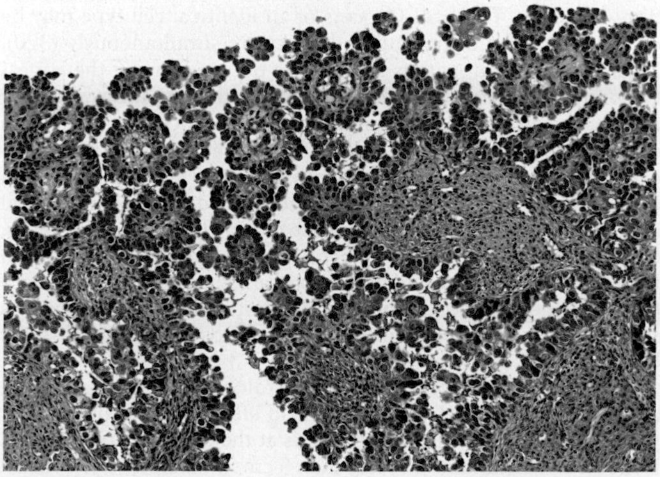

Figure 21.7. Serous carcinoma often arises in endometrium of older women, and superficially, portions usually have a highly papillary architecture.

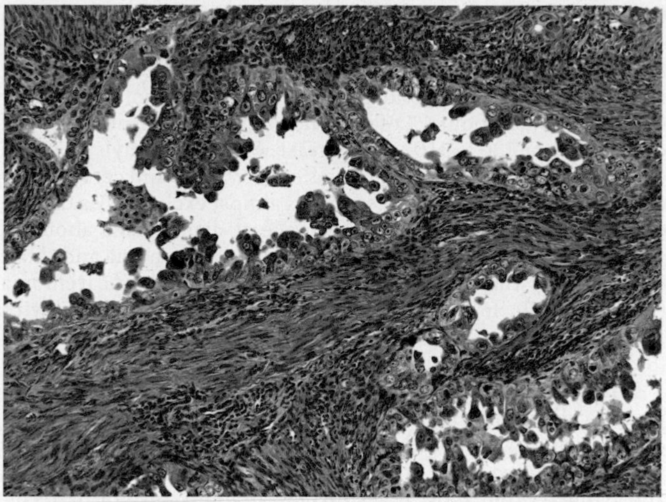

Figure 21.8. Serous carcinoma is characterized by high-grade cytologic atypia in cells that do not share a common apical border. The papillary architecture may be replaced by gaping glands at the interface with the myometrium.

of meticulous surgicopathologic staging. They and others found that serous carcinoma truly confined to the uterus had an overall excellent prognosis, whereas patients with extrauterine disease, even if only microscopic in size, almost always suffered recurrence and death from tumor (296,297).

EIC is a histologically distinctive lesion that is specifically associated with serous carcinoma of the endometrium (298–302). Serous carcinomas most often arise from a background of atrophy or polyps rather than hyperplasia (298,299,301), and they are not epidemiologically related to unopposed estrogen stimulation. EIC has been proposed to represent a form of intraepithelial tumor characteristic of serous carcinoma, and it is the precursor to invasive serous carcinoma. Mutations in *p53* that can be detected immunohistochemically as overexpression of the antigen are found in most cases, and the mutation is shared with that found in the invasive serous carcinoma (**Fig. 21.9**). EIC is usually found in the endometrium harboring a serious carcinoma (299), but occasionally occurs in the absence of any invasive carcinoma. In such cases, it may be associated with synchronous serous carcinoma in the peritoneum (300).

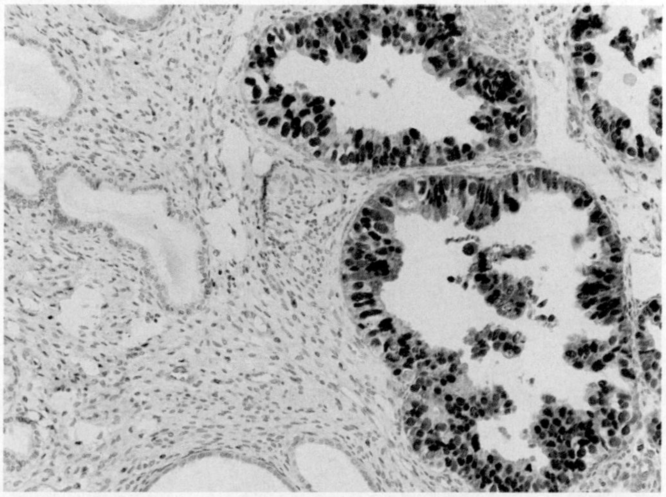

Figure 21.9. Endometrial intraepithelial carcinoma is the precursor lesion of invasive serous carcinoma. It shares histologic and immunohistochemical features with serous carcinoma, including frequent overexpression of p53. In this case, there is nuclear localization of stain in EIC *(right)*, but no staining of the benign glands or stroma of the polyp in which it has arisen *(left)*.

Clear Cell Carcinoma. Clear cell adenocarcinoma of the endometrium is generally recognized and defined on the basis of the distinctive clearing of the cytoplasm of neoplastic cells growing in any combination of solid, glandular, tubulocystic, or papillary configurations. About 4% of endometrial adenocarcinomas are of clear cell type (303–310). In contrast with the diethylstilbestrol (DES)-related clear cell carcinomas of the vagina and cervix, clear cell carcinoma of the endometrium is almost exclusively a disease of menopausal women. The mean age at diagnosis is about 68 years, which is similar to that of serous adenocarcinoma and about 6 years older than that of typical endometrial adenocarcinoma (303,306,310). It is a biologically aggressive neoplasm, with a 5-year survival rate varying from only about 20% to 65% (5,303,306,308,310).

The hallmark of clear cell carcinoma is the presence of neoplastic cells with optically clear cytoplasm, reflecting an abundance of glycogen. Four basic architectural patterns of clear cell adenocarcinoma exist, including solid, glandular, tubulocystic, and papillary, but most cases display an admixture of patterns. The solid pattern consists of masses of large neoplastic cells of polygonal shape with clear to faintly eosinophilic cytoplasm and distinct cell membranes. The glandular pattern is reminiscent of the tubular glands of endometrioid adenocarcinoma, whereas the tubulocystic pattern is formed of dilated spherical-appearing glands. The papillary pattern is architecturally identical to that of serous carcinoma, with generally short, branching fibrovascular cores, often hyalinized, covered by neoplastic cells. The latter three patterns often have lining cells with a hobnail appearance, resulting from the scalloped apex of individual neoplastic cells that project along the surface (**Fig. 21.10**).

Squamous Carcinoma. Although focal squamous differentiation is common in endometrial adenocarcinoma, pure squamous carcinoma of the endometrium is extremely rare, representing less than 1% of EC, and with only about 60 reported cases (311–315). Most patients are postmenopausal, and the average age at diagnosis is about 65 years (311,313). Squamous carcinoma of the endometrium is established as primary in the endometrium after a cervical origin is ruled out. There must be no connection with or spread from benign or malignant cervical squamous epithelium. It is often associated with cervical stenosis, pyometra, and chronic inflammation. About 60% of the cases have been confined to the uterus, and the prognosis for these patients has been relatively good (311). In contrast, less than 15% of women with advanced-stage disease have survived 2 years after diagnosis. Histologic grade does not appear to correlate with the probability of survival.

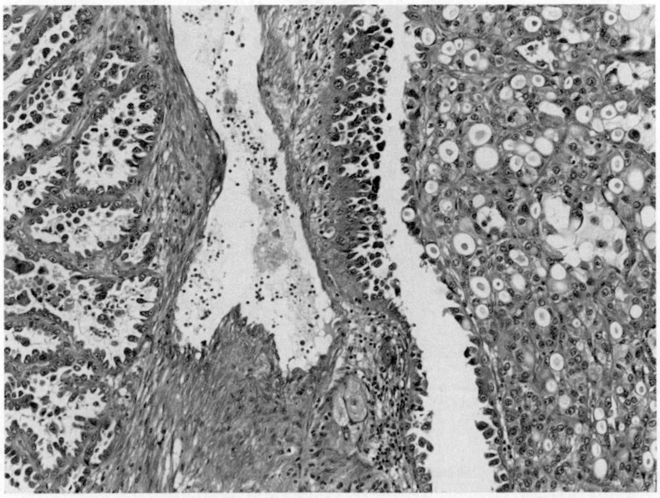

Figure 21.10. Clear cell carcinoma. In this tumor, a tubulocystic pattern with a lining of hobnail cells is present on the left, while a solid pattern is present on the right. Any mixture of solid, tubulocystic, papillary, or glandular architecture may occur.

Undifferentiated Carcinoma. Undifferentiated carcinoma of the endometrium has been described as a distinct tumor type. These neoplasms are composed of a monotonous proliferation of medium-sized, round, or polygonal cells growing in sheets with no specific pattern. Mitotic figures are numerous. No glandular, squamous, or sarcomatous differentiation is detected in routinely stained sections. Keratins and epithelial membrane antigen are detected by immunohistochemistry in fewer than 20% of the cells in most cases, in contrast to diffuse staining in most high-grade endometrioid carcinomas. Selected cases may contain neurosecretory granules in a minority of the cells as demonstrated by immunohistochemical stains. Neurosecretory products are apparently not released into the patient's circulation or are not in an active form because no affected women have manifested symptoms. Most patients present with tumors of advanced stage, and the behavior is usually aggressive. A *glassy cell carcinoma* has also been described, which comprises less than 1% of ECs. It is characterized by cytoplasm that has a ground-glass appearance, as in the cervix. Although few cases have been reported, such as serous and clear cell carcinomas, glassy cell carcinoma appears to be aggressive (316,317).

Mixed Cell Type. If an EC manifests two or more different cell types, each representing at least 10% or more of the tumor, the term *mixed cell type* is appropriate.

Metastatic Carcinoma to the Endometrium. Malignancies in other organs may metastasize to the endometrium. The most common extragenital sites are breast, stomach, colon, pancreas, and kidney, although any disseminated tumor could involve the endometrium. The ovaries are the most likely genital sources of metastasis. Metastatic carcinoma presents as abnormal vaginal bleeding, and the initial specimen for evaluation is usually a biopsy or curetting. Although the metastatic disease may appear as a large focus, individual and small groups of malignant cells may subtly intermingle with normal endometrium or myometrium. Lymphatics are usually involved. Special stains for mucin, CEA, or melanin may suggest that the cells are not of endometrial origin. In some instances, unusual cell types, such as signet ring cells, may be present, suggesting a metastasis from the gastrointestinal (GI) tract. It is uncommon but not exceptional for the endometrial sample to be the first indication of an occult primary lesion (318,319).

Simultaneous Tumors. Cancers of an identical cell type may be discovered in the ovary and endometrium simultaneously (320). Usually, the primary site is assigned to the area having the largest tumor mass and most advanced stage. In certain situations, primary malignancies in the endometrium and ovary may coexist. This "field effect" of the "extended Müllerian system" may occur in 15% to 20% of endometrioid carcinomas of the ovary (321,322). In a review of a GOG study of 74 patients with simultaneously detected endometrial and ovarian carcinomas with disease grossly limited to the pelvis, only 16% of women suffered a recurrence of disease, with a median follow-up of 80 months. This group of patients was atypical, with 86% having endometrioid histology in both sites. Recurrence was statistically related to the presence of microscopic metastases or high histologic grade (323).

Carcinomas of more advanced histologic grade and cell type are more difficult to assign to the field effect because of a higher probability of invasion and metastasis at the time of surgery (277). If the endometrial tumor is less than 5 cm in diameter, the ovarian lesion is unilateral, invasion is less than the middle third, vessels are not involved, and the EC is well-differentiated, metastasis to the ovary is unlikely (324).

Pathologic Factors of Prognostic Significance

Pathologic information has been used to estimate risk of nodal metastasis and to define prognosis (recurrence, survival) in EC. Prognostic factors have been identified within each stage of EC, and the discussion of prognostic factors is probably best served by discussing factors within comparably staged groups, more so than as isolated factors. For example, in GOG 99, which compared observation to pelvic RT in patients with stage I–II EC and pathologically negative LN, a model based on combinations of patient age and tumor grade, depth of invasion, and lymphovascular space invasion (LVI) could predict patients at highest risk for recurrence (144). Similarly, PORTEC identified a combination of two of three factors—age >60, grade 3 tumor, and depth of invasion > 50%—that defined patients at high risk for local-regional failure when managed by surgery alone (325). Increasingly, risk models are used to counsel patients as to the marginal benefit of postoperative therapies.

Predicting Nodal Disease

On the basis of pathologic information available at the time of surgery, the risk for nodal metastasis may be estimated. Physicians who selectively perform nodal dissections frequently do so based on the presence of uterine risk factors that suggest the potential for nodal disease. In patients who did not undergo a nodal dissection at the time of hysterectomy, decisions to offer RT are commonly based on the estimation of risk for nodal disease based on uterine risk factors. In the surgical pathologic study GOG 33, pelvic and para-aortic nodal disease was more frequent with increasing grade (percentage of pelvic nodal metastases: 3% grade 1, 9% grade 2, 18% grade 3), depth of invasion (1% endometrium only, 5% inner one-third, 6% middle one-third, 25% outer one-third myometrial invasion), and LVI (27% with LVI, 7% without LVI) (59). Pelvic and para-aortic nodal metastases were also more common with cervical involvement, when peritoneal cytology was positive, and when extra-nodal (adnexal, intraperitoneal sites) disease was found. In a multivariate model, grade, depth of invasion, and intraperitoneal disease were independent predictors of pelvic nodal disease. In a further analysis of patients participating in GOG 33, 47 of 48 patients with para-aortic nodal disease had one or more factors of palpably enlarged para-aortic nodes, grossly positive pelvic nodes, gross adnexal disease, or outer one-third invasion (61). Despite the use of pathology to help predict nodal disease, many believe that LN assessment is superior as it provides actual information on nodal status, as opposed to an estimate, which can then be used to tailor therapy. As previously discussed, patients at very low risk for nodal involvement may also be specified by uterine risk factors (size, grade, depth of invasion) (172–176).

Prognostic Factors

FIGO Stage

Prognostic factors may be used to categorize patients into high- and low-risk groups and to guide the use of adjuvant therapies. Understanding these factors also allows for the development of novel strategies to reduce risk of recurrence or alter patterns of disease failure. Overall, the patients at highest risk for recurrence and death have spread of disease outside of the uterus, which is reflected by FIGO stage (61). The prognostic utility of surgicopathologic stage has been confirmed in multiple studies of large numbers of patients, using both univariate and multivariate analysis (59,303,326–331). FIGO surgical stage is often the single strongest predictor of outcome for women with endometrial adenocarcinoma in studies using multivariate analyses (303). Although the FIGO clinical staging system of 1971 was generally useful, retrospective comparison of the two methods demonstrated the clear superiority of surgicopathologic staging over clinical staging in predicting outcome.

Patients with intraperitoneal or distant metastases (stage IV) have the poorest prognosis with 5-year survival ranging from 20% to 25% (5). In GOG 122, comparing whole abdominal RT to doxorubicin/cisplatin CT as primary therapy for EC patients with <2-cm residual disease stage III–IV, stage IV (compared to stage III) disease was an independent predictor of shorter PFS (HR 2.2.9) and survival (HR 1.9) (332). Gross intraperitoneal spread frequently indicates the presence of larger tumor burden as many patients with intraperitoneal disease also have adnexal and nodal disease. In GOG 33, 51% of patients with gross intraperitoneal spread had positive pelvic nodes, whereas only 7% without spread had positive pelvic nodes (59). Prognosis may be modified by the volume of residual disease after cytoreductive surgery (252–255).

Patients with nodal metastases (stage IIIC disease) also have poorer prognosis compared to node-negative populations. FIGO data shows 5-year survival to be 57% in stage IIIC patients compared to 74% to 91% when nodes are negative (stage I-II) (5). Patients with positive pelvic but negative para-aortic nodes have a better prognosis compared to those with para-aortic disease (61,333,334). For example, Hoekstra and colleagues reported a series of 85 patients with stage IIIC disease who had a 5-year survival of 61% (334). Patients with positive pelvic nodes had a 5-year survival of 70% compared to 49% when para-aortic disease was present. In 2009, FIGO staging was revised for patients with positive pelvic nodes/negative para-aortic nodes who were reclassified as stage IIIC1, and patients with any positive para-aortic node were classified as Stage IIIC2 (89). This change has been validated in two recent reviews (335,336). Two retrospective series have also suggested that patients with nodal disease in addition to positive cytology, adnexa, or serosa have poorer PFS or survival compared to those patients with positive nodes alone (164,333). Lymphadenectomy (142,163,193), complete surgical resection of bulky nodes (337), and use of CT (194,332,335,338) have been suggested to improve outcomes in patients and modify the prognostic effect of nodal disease.

Patients with FIGO 1988 stage IIIA disease represent a heterogeneous population having adnexal, peritoneal cytology, and/or serosal involvement, but with negative LN. Positive peritoneal cytology as the sole upstaging factor was dropped in the 2009 FIGO staging revisions as a stage defining characteristic (89). In the GOG 33 study, 12% of all patients had positive cytology, and of these, 25% had positive pelvic nodes and 19% had metastases to para-aortic LN (59). Six percent of clinical stage I–II patients have spread of tumor to the adnexa, and of these, 32% have pelvic node metastases compared with 8% pelvic node positivity if adnexal involvement is not present (59). Twenty percent have positive para-aortic node metastases, which is four times greater than if adnexal metastases were not present.

For patients who are completely staged and found to have no extrauterine disease, 4% to 6% of patients have positive cytology as an isolated finding (59,216,339). Published opinions are mixed about the significance of this finding (340–345). In a review of the literature, Wethington categorized patients into groups based on low-risk uterine features (grade 1 to 2, <50% depth of invasion, no LVI) with positive peritoneal cytology. In this group, positive cytology occurred in 11% of cases, and had a recurrence rate of 4%. Patients with higher risk features plus positive cytology had a 32% risk of recurrence (346). Saga reported that positive peritoneal cytology alone in staged patients (n = 32) was associated with a 5-year survival of 87%; however, this was worse than the 97% survival seen in cytology-negative patients (347). In a series of 57 patients with FIGO stage IIIA (1988) disease, cytology appears to carry the same significance as adnexal involvement and was an independent predictor of prognosis (348).

Histologic Cell Types

The histologic classification of endometrial adenocarcinoma is important not only because it facilitates the recognition of lesions as carcinoma, but also because the cell type has consistently been recognized as being important in predicting the biologic behavior and probability of survival. Endometrioid adenocarcinoma accounts for the majority of tumors in the uterine corpus and carries a relatively favorable prognosis. Consequently, the virulence of other cell types is usually related to endometrioid adenocarcinoma.

Adenocarcinoma with squamous differentiation is similar to typical endometrioid adenocarcinoma with respect to the distribution by age and frequency of nodal metastasis, and is associated with a slightly increased probability of survival. *Villoglandular carcinoma* has a biologic behavior similar to that of endometrioid adenocarcinoma (274,349). *Serous carcinoma* has been considered an aggressive histologic type, with OS rates varying from 40% to 60% at 5 years (5,292,294,350–353). *Clear cell carcinoma* also has a highly aggressive behavior, with 5-year survival rates of 30% to 75% (354–357). One of the problems with using histology as a marker for prognosis is that serous cancers are more likely to have spread at presentation than endometrioid tumors. Patients with serous or clear cell tumors present with stage III–IV disease in 41% and 33%, respectively, compared to 14% with endometrioid type (5). Studies suggest that 40% to 70% of serous tumors will have extra-uterine spread at presentation; therefore, complete surgical staging is warranted in this tumor type (171). Given this level of disease spread, it is not surprising that unstaged/clinical stage I serous patients appear to have similar prognosis to stage III–IV endometrioid types. Once patients with serous or clear cell tumors are appropriately allocated into the correct stage, the importance of histology appears to be less (358–361). For example, Creasman et al. evaluated FIGO data and showed that patients with stage I serous tumors had comparable outcomes to those with stage I, grade 3 endometrioid tumors. Five-year survival for stage IB and IC serous tumors was 81% and 55% compared to 84% and 66% for grade 3 tumors (361). In advanced and recurrent EC patients participating in phase 3 GOG CT trials, response rate (RR) to CT was not associated with histologic type, and serous tumor type was not independently associated with PFS (17).

Grade

The degree of histologic differentiation has been considered to be an indicator of tumor spread. The GOG and other studies have confirmed that as grade becomes less differentiated, there is a greater tendency for deep myometrial invasion and, subsequently, higher rates of pelvic and para-aortic LN involvement (59,362–364). Survival has also been consistently related to histologic grade, and in a GOG study of more than 600 women with clinical stage I or occult stage II endometrioid adenocarcinoma, the 5-year relative survival was as follows: grade 1% to 94%; grade 2% to 84%; grade 3% to 72% (61). In patients with early-stage EC participating in the PORTEC trial, the risk of cancer-related death for patients with grade 3 tumors was 4.9 compared to grade 1 to 2 tumors (151).

Myometrial Invasion

Deep myometrial invasion is one of the more important factors correlated with a higher probability of extrauterine tumor spread, treatment failure, and recurrence, and with diminished probability of survival (**Fig. 21.11**) (144,326,365). In a GOG study of over 400 women with clinical stage I and occult stage II endometrioid adenocarcinoma, the 5-year relative survival was 94% when the tumor was confined to the endometrium, 91% when the tumor involved the inner third of the myometrium, 84% when the tumor extended into the middle third, and 59% when the tumor invaded into the outer third of the myometrium (61). Even in node-negative patients, deep myometrial invasion retains prognostic information. For example, Mariani et al. (366) reported that for stage I (node-negative) patients, deep invasion (>66% myometrial invasion) was an independent predictor for recurrence and distant site of failure.

Lymphovascular Space Invasion

Several studies have suggested that LVI is a strong predictor of recurrence and death, and is independent of depth of myometrial invasion or histologic differentiation (**Fig. 21.12**) (303,367,368). In a retrospective series of 628 surgically staged patients, the presence of high-intermediate risk (HIR) uterine characteristics and LVI were associated with nodal metastases (367). The OR for nodal disease was 4.4 with HIR factors, and 11 for LVI. In this series, the LVI and HIR features were independently associated with PFS and survival. Zaino et al. (331) found that LVI was a statistically significant indicator of death from tumor in early clinical stage but not early surgical stage endometrial adenocarcinoma. This suggests that lymphatic invasion helps to identify patients likely to have spread to LN or distant sites, but that its importance is diminished for those in whom thorough sampling of nodes has failed to identify metastasis. Vascular space invasion or capillary-like space (CLS) involvement with tumor exists in approximately 15% of uteri containing adenocarcinoma (59,368,369). Pelvic LN are positive in 27% of cases, which is four times more often if malignant cells are found in the CLS than if absent. The risk of para-aortic node metastases when LVI was present was 19%, which is a sixfold increase over negative CLS involvement (59). Lymphovascular invasion is identified in 35% to 95% of serous carcinomas of the endometrium, where it has generally been associated with an elevated risk of tumor recurrence or death from disease (294,350,352).

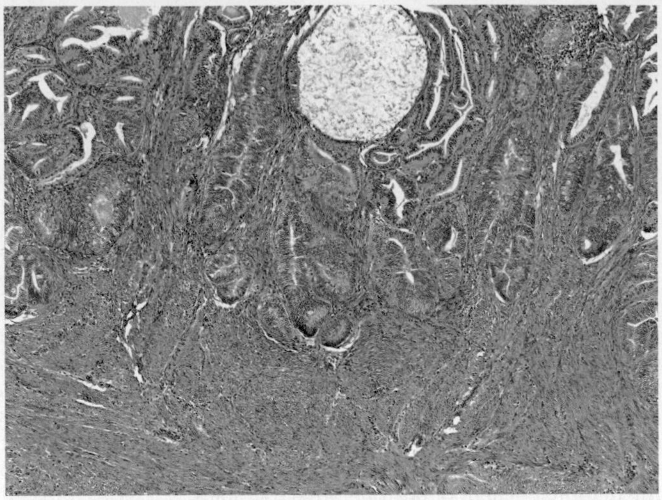

Figure 21.11. Myometrial invasion by endometrial adenocarcinoma may be accompanied by a desmoplastic reaction, but often no such reaction is present, as in this case.

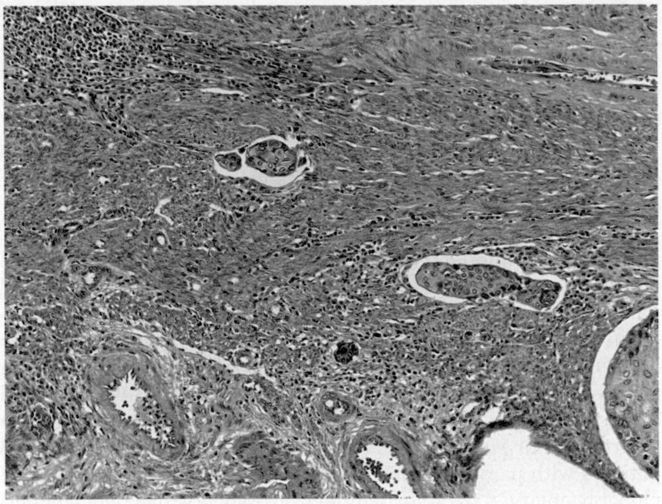

Figure 21.12. Lymphatic invasion by endometrial adenocarcinoma. Nests of neoplastic cells occupy the lumen of an endothelial-lined space. Since artifactual retraction of stroma around tumor may simulate lymphatic spaces, true lymphatic invasion is best assessed in the myometrium adjacent to the tumor.

Patterns of Failure

Another way to approach pathologic information is to understand the pathologic relationships that predict particular patterns of failure. For example, in patients with pathologic negative-node, stage I EC, pelvic sidewall recurrences are rare, and failures occur most frequently at the vaginal cuff or at distant sites (144,370,371). High-risk stage I patients who do not undergo nodal dissections have both pelvic sidewall and distant sites of failure, even with routine use of RT (162). Patients with node-positive disease frequently have recurrences at distant sites, with rare intra-abdominal failures (164,165,334). Patients with stage IV/intraperitoneal disease most commonly fail in the peritoneal cavity. The implications of patterns of failure data are that we may choose our postoperative therapies better by defining patterns of failure for a particular stage distribution or based on the presence of risk factors. The Mayo Clinic group has advocated this approach following a review of patterns of failure data from their group (366,372–375). For example, these investigators suggested that hematogenous, lymphatic, and peritoneal failures could be predicted based on pathologic factors, and that therapy should be directed to reduce failures at these sites depending on pathologic information (60). Whether their finding can be validated in a prospective manner, or if existing therapies effectively control disease at particular sites, needs to be evaluated.

GENERAL MANAGEMENT

Results of Standard Therapy and Their Sequelae

Early uncontrolled trials suggested that progestin therapy after surgery or irradiation was associated with a decreased risk of recurrence in patients with disease confined to the uterus (376). However, large prospective, randomized trials failed to show a survival advantage (377–379). RT has been and remains the standard adjuvant treatment modality for most patients at risk for recurrence. This standard continues to evolve, however. An older, poorly designed study of adjuvant cytotoxic CT showed no benefit for patients treated with single-agent doxorubicin and arrested interest in adjuvant CT for many years (380). By 2006, two prospective trials comparing RT to CT demonstrated similar outcomes for patients treated with CT or RT (379,380). Adjuvant CT improved PFS and survival in patients with advanced-stage disease compared to whole abdominal RT, suggesting an important role for first-line therapy that includes CT (332). Current research focuses on whether outcomes may be improved by adding CT either sequentially or concomitantly with radiation.

ADJUVANT RADIATION THERAPY

RT continues to play an important role in the management of EC, although its role is evolving. It is used adjuvantly, as definitive treatment for patients who are medically inoperable, for local recurrence, and for palliation. Historically, patients were treated with preoperative intracavitary brachytherapy with or without external beam RT followed by hysterectomy. This approach has not been completely abandoned but is used infrequently and usually only in patients with gross cervical or parametrial involvement. Today, most patients undergo primary surgery; then, depending on final pathologic review, the need for RT is determined. Radiation can be delivered with external beam irradiation, brachytherapy, or a combination of both. Brachytherapy is most frequently delivered by an intracavitary technique, where an applicator is inserted into an anatomic cavity, such as a tandem positioned in the uterus or cylinder in the vagina. Brachytherapy can also be performed by interstitial application, where needles are placed into the tissues at risk under general anesthesia, most commonly in the setting of vaginal recurrence following hysterectomy. Brachytherapy dose may be delivered with low dose rate ^{137}Cs sources (low dose rate [LDR]), an ^{192}Ir source (LDR or pulsed dose rate [PDR]), or a high dose rate ^{192}Ir source (high dose rate [HDR]). With LDR, the patient is admitted to the hospital for the applicator insertion and brachytherapy delivery, and usually requires bed rest for several days. This method exposes other personnel to irradiation, is often costlier, and places the patient at risk for deep venous thrombosis and other medical complications. HDR is typically performed over multiple fractions in the outpatient setting, avoids radiation exposure to personnel, and allows for greater flexibility in the dose distribution by use of a stepping source and remote afterloader. PDR also allows for dose optimization with use of a stepping source and is considered gentler on normal tissues as a low dose of radiation is given every hour over several days. PDR also requires hospital admission but personnel radiation exposure is limited.

Early-Stage Disease

Most of the data on adjuvant radiation in EC pertains to patients with early-stage (I–II) disease, as this is the most common presentation and the focus of several randomized trials. The use of radiation in this group of patients, however, has been undergoing significant changes in practice over the last 10 years. The questions yet to be resolved are clarifying which patients will be best served by adjuvant RT and determining the most appropriate radiation modality, either pelvic radiation, vaginal brachytherapy, or a combination.

Benefit of Adjuvant Radiation

Two prospective, randomized trials compared surgery alone to surgery and postoperative external beam radiation. The first trial was conducted by the GOG (study 99) where 392 patients with stage IB–IIB EC who underwent total abdominal hysterectomy/bilateral salpingo-oophorectomy (TAH/BSO) and pelvic/para-aortic LN sampling were randomized to observation (n = 202) or postoperative pelvic radiation (n = 190) to a total dose of 50.4 Gy in 28 fractions (144). The study was designed to allow for an 80% chance of detecting a 58% decrease in the recurrence hazard rate and a 56% decrease in the death hazard rate. Recurrence-free interval (RFI) was the primary end point with all-cause survival as well as recurrence-free survival (RFS) as secondary end points. With a median follow-up of 68 months, the 4-year survival rate was 92% in the radiation arm compared with 86% in the observation arm (Relative hazard: 0.86; $p = 0.557$). The estimated 2-year cumulative incidence of recurrence was 3% versus 12% in favor of the irradiation arm (RH: 0.42; $p = 0.007$), indicating that radiation decreased the hazard rate of recurrence by the required 58%. Specifically, the rate of vaginal recurrence, the most frequent area of recurrence, was 6.4% (13 out of 202) in the surgery-alone arm compared to 1.05% (2 out of 190) in the radiation arm. Of interest, the two patients in the surgery arm that recurred were randomized to radiation but refused adjuvant treatment. In addition, the estimated risk of death from any cause was 14% less in the RT arm, but was not statistically significant. More than half of the deaths were from causes other than treatment or EC, and the paper points out that it was therefore not adequately powered to detect an OS difference, a point often not appreciated by many physicians. This GOG study further identified a subgroup of patients termed HIR, who accounted for two-thirds of the cancer-related deaths and recurrences, and has become a population of interest for further study in currently open trials. The definition of HIR by GOG is determined by the combination of age and intrauterine risk factors including grades 2 or 3, outer one-third myometrial invasion, and LVI. Patients are considered to fall into the HIR category if they are age ≥70 years with one risk factor, age ≥50 years with at least two risk factors, or age ≥ 18 years with all three risk factors. In this HIR patient population, the 4-year cumulative recurrence was 27% without irradiation compared to 13% with irradiation, an absolute benefit of 19%. In contrast, for the low-risk population, there was a 6% versus 2% recurrence rate in unirradiated compared to the irradiated enrollees. The GOG trial 0249 was designed to further refine the roles of CT and RT in the HIR population, and randomized women to adjuvant VCB followed by three cycles of carboplatin and paclitaxel versus pelvic irradiation with either 3D conformal therapy or intensity-modulated radiation therapy (IMRT) to 4,500 to 5,040 cGy in 25 to 28 fractions with an optional brachytherapy boost. Publication of GOG 249 is pending, however, there appeared to be no difference in relapse-free or OS between the two adjuvant treatments.

The second trial was the PORTEC study where 714 patients with stage IB grade 2, 3 and IC grade 1, 2 were randomized after TAH/BSO without LN sampling to observation (n = 360) or pelvic radiation (n = 354) to a total dose of 46 Gy in 23 fractions (151). With a median follow-up of 52 months, the 5-year vaginal/pelvic recurrence rate was 4% in the radiation arm compared to 14% in the observation arm ($p < 0.001$). The corresponding 5-year survival rates were 81% and 85%, respectively ($p = 0.37$). In patients with HIR features by the PORTEC definition (where intermediate-risk factors were outer-half invasion, grade 3 or >60 years old, but excluded deeply invasive high-grade tumors; patients were deemed HIR with two of the three factors), the recurrence risk was reduced from 23% to 5% with adjuvant irradiation. It should be noted here that this is different from the GOG HIR definition, and likely a much lower risk population. An update with a median follow-up of 13.3 years has been recently published (381). The actuarial 15-year locoregional recurrence was statistically different at 6% versus 15% for those with adjuvant irradiation compared to observation with no statistical difference in OS or failure-free survival, distant metastases, or secondary cancers. Most recurrences in the observation arm were vaginal (11% of the 15%).

An additional trial, PORTEC II, was completed as a follow-up study (152). The study population was a HIR population based on the PORTEC definition. As in PORTEC I, the patients underwent a TAH/BSO without LN dissection and were randomized to 46 Gy in 23 fractions of external beam irradiation or vaginal brachytherapy alone, with either 21 Gy in three fractions of high-dose rate therapy or 30 Gy in one LDR fraction. Four hundred twenty-seven patients were enrolled in this noninferiority trial designed with the primary end point of vaginal recurrence. The research question was whether vaginal brachytherapy was as effective at controlling vaginal recurrence as external beam radiation, with fewer toxic effects and improved quality of life. Secondary end points were locoregional recurrence, distant metastases, overall and DFS, and quality of life. At a median follow-up of 45 months, the estimated 5-year vaginal recurrence rates were 1.8% for brachytherapy alone and 1.6% for external irradiation. The nodal failure rate was significantly different at 3.8% for the brachytherapy-alone arm and 0.5% for external beam irradiation, although this difference was not felt to be clinically meaningful. Distant metastases, DFS, and OS were similar in both arms. Eighty percent of the patients had deeply invasive disease, and over 90% had grades 1 or 2 disease. In fact, with central pathologic review, 48% of the patients that were enrolled with grade 1 disease increased to 78.6% of the study population. Final pathology reviewed revealed that 14% of the patients did not fit pathologic eligibility for the trial, although the outcome was unchanged with these patients excluded on reanalysis. It should not be unexpected that pelvic external beam radiation resulted in a similar vaginal recurrence rate to vaginal brachytherapy. In addition, with this lower risk subgroup compared to the GOG 99 HIR population, it should be noted that the pelvic failure rate was quite low, even in the brachytherapy-only arm. Furthermore, GI toxicity and quality of life were significantly improved in the vaginal brachytherapy arm compared to the external beam arm (382,383). The currently enrolling PORTEC 3 trial randomizes high-risk and advanced-stage patients between external irradiation alone and external irradiation with concurrent and adjuvant CT. The patients eligible for PORTEC 3 include those with stage IB if the disease is grade 3 and paired with LVI, IC if grade 3, and Stages IIIA-C or uterine serous or clear cell carcinoma stages IB-III.

The ASTEC/EN.5 trial was actually two trials with separate randomizations combined as one intergroup trial between the United Kingdom Medical Research Council and the National Cancer Institute of Canada (204). This trial examined women with IA grade 3 disease and all grades of IB, and Stages I or II uterine serous or clear cell carcinoma. A LN dissection was not required, and positive cytology was not an exclusion criteria. Positive pelvic nodes were allowed in the ASTEC trial. Patients were randomized to external beam radiation or observation, although vaginal brachytherapy was at the institution's choice, even in the observation arm. The primary outcome measure was OS, and 905 women were enrolled from 112 centers and 7 countries. With a median follow-up of 58 months, no statistical survival difference was noted between the two arms, and the site of the first failure was distant in both arms, that is, approximately 7%. The vaginal and pelvic failure rates were 3.7% versus 1.5% and 2.6% versus 1.1% for observation (with 53% receiving VCB) and pelvic irradiation, respectively (204).

Despite the fact that adjuvant radiation consistently and significantly improved locoregional control in these trials, most of the adjuvant treatment debate focuses on the lack of improvement in OS. The end point of OS is the gold standard for any randomized therapeutic trial in cancer, although when considering early-stage EC, the data should be interpreted with caution. First, in GOG 99, the primary end point was not OS but rather PFS, which was significantly better in the radiation arm (144). Second, because of the relatively high incidence of other comorbidities such as hypertension, DM, and obesity as well as other cancers, the chance of dying from an intercurrent illness is as high if not higher than dying from EC. In the RT arm of the PORTEC trial (151), the 8-year mortality rate from EC was 9.6% compared to 14.4% from other causes and 5.3% from other cancers. In the observation arm, the corresponding rates were 7.5%, 10.6%, and 5.3%. Similar data emerged from GOG 99, which reported that approximately half of the deaths were due to causes other than EC or treatment. This led the authors of GOG 99 to state the following: "With this number of intercurrent deaths in both arms, even if RT reduces the risk of EC-related deaths, the size of this trial is not adequate to reliably detect an OS difference." Thus, it is clear that the competing causes of death in this group of patients having a low cancer-related mortality rate make OS a very elusive end point to attain. Third, even in patients who die from EC, the most common cause is distant rather than local relapse. In the PORTEC trial, the 8-year mortality rate from local versus distant relapse was 1.1% and 7.9%, respectively, in the RT group, and 2% and 5.2%, respectively, in the surgery-alone group (151). Furthermore, women in the observation arm who experienced vaginal relapse received salvage RT with 5-year survival rates of 70%. In the PORTEC 2 trial, vaginal control was the primary end point compared to OS in the ASTEC/EN.5 trial (152,204). In the PORTEC 2 study, 62% and 48% died from intercurrent disease in the external beam and brachytherapy arms, respectively, and 38% versus 52% died of endometrial carcinoma in the irradiation arm and brachytherapy arm, respectively. In the ASTEC/EN.5 trial, 36% of the deaths were observed to be unrelated to disease or treatment. Therefore, it is unrealistic to expect a local treatment modality such as radiation to alter this pattern of relapse. It is also notable that in the GOG 99 and PORTEC I trials, most of the patients did not have poor prognostic features, thus making it difficult to demonstrate any survival advantage to adjuvant radiation. In PORTEC 2, most (80%) of the patients had deeply invasive carcinoma, although those with grade 3 deeply invasive tumors were excluded from the trial. In the ASTEC/EN.5 trial, 75% were deeply invasive but 65% were grades 1 or 2. When the impact of adjuvant radiation in GOG 99 was assessed in the subset of patients with high-risk features (based on age, grade, depth of myometrial invasion, and presence of lymphovascular invasion), the death rate was nonsignificantly lower in the radiation arm (RH: 0.73; 90% CI, 0.43 to 1.26). The PORTEC 2 study included higher risk patients than PORTEC 1 but was powered as a noninferiority study examining the utility of vaginal brachytherapy to prevent local recurrence. Lee et al. in their analysis of the SEER data showed an OS advantage to pelvic radiation for patients with IC grade 1 and grade 3/4 ($p < 0.001$) EC over those treated with surgery alone in their examination of over 21,000 patients. This survival advantage of adjuvant pelvic radiation was significant even in patients who had surgical LN staging (384). All of these issues need to be considered when assessing the benefit of adjuvant radiation. Such debate is not new in the field of oncology, but it is important to note that other oncologists treating cancers of the breast or rectum, when faced with similar results from prospective, randomized trials, have recognized the importance of a multimodality approach in achieving local-regional control as well as survival.

Type of Radiation

There are two types of radiation (intravaginal brachytherapy or pelvic external beam radiation) that could be used either alone or in combination for early-stage EC. Over the last 3 decades, the debate about the appropriate radiation modality has undergone a full circle. In the 1970s and mid-1980s, there was a shift from intravaginal brachytherapy alone to pelvic radiation plus intravaginal brachytherapy. Then, in the late 1980s and early 1990s, there was a shift toward pelvic radiation alone. More recently, and with the increase in surgical LN staging, there has been resurgence in the use of intravaginal brachytherapy alone. A recent article by Patel et al. (385) documented this by probing the SEER database examining the treatment of FIGO stage I and II EC over the years 1995 to 2005. They examined the treatment of 9,815 patients and found that the proportion of those receiving vaginal brachytherapy alone increased from 12.9% to 32.8% as the use of external beam alone decreased from 56.1% to 45.7% over the same time period. The use of both modalities together also decreased from 31% to 21.4% as well.

Intravaginal Brachytherapy Alone or Combined with Pelvic Radiation. In a historically important trial, Aalders et al. (386) reported on 540 patients with stage IB–IC EC who underwent TAH/BSO without LN sampling and postoperative intravaginal brachytherapy to 60 Gy to the vaginal mucosa. The patients then were randomized to observation ($n = 277$) or to supplemental pelvic radiation to 40 Gy ($n = 263$). A significant reduction in local recurrence rates was seen with the addition of pelvic radiation (1.9% vs. 6.9%; $p < 0.01$). With regard to OS, there was no significant difference between the two arms of the study, but in the subset of patients with grade 3 disease and deep myometrial penetration, there was a survival advantage (cause-specific survival) of 18% versus 7% in favor of the pelvic radiation arm (386). The data from this trial contributed to the shift in treatment policy from intravaginal brachytherapy alone to external beam pelvic radiation with or without a brachytherapy boost. As outlined above, in the ASTEC/EN.5 trial, over 50% of the observation arm received vaginal brachytherapy as well. Because the vagina is the most common site of pelvic failure, this paradigm has become more common. Greven et al. (387) reviewed the experience of two institutions to compare the outcome of the two approaches. In that study, there were 270 patients with stage I–II EC: 173 were treated with postoperative pelvic radiation alone, and 97 were treated with a combination of intravaginal and pelvic radiation (387). The corresponding 5-year pelvic control and DFS rates were 96% versus 93% ($p = 0.32$) and 88% versus 83% ($p = 0.41$), respectively. This study as well as others called into question whether the addition of vaginal radiation is needed, particularly when vaginal control rates are excellent with pelvic radiation alone in early-stage disease (388,389). Furthermore, some studies have suggested increased toxicity with the combined approach (388). An examination of the SEER database reviewed 3,395 node-negative EC patients with stages IA, IB, and II disease. Most patients (62.7%) received external beam alone and 37.3% received both external beam and brachytherapy. It was noted that the addition of brachytherapy did not statistically improve survival. A number of other reports (390,391), however, suggest that vaginal vault radiation can be added to pelvic radiation with minimal morbidity and very low rates of recurrence. Some institutions choose to treat to a lower external beam dose of 45 Gy plus a vaginal brachytherapy boost, whereas others prescribe 50.4 Gy to the pelvis without a boost unless higher risk features are present, such as close or positive vaginal margins, extensive LVI, or cervical involvement. As CT becomes an increasingly common part of the treatment paradigm, the former regimen may spare more bone marrow and bowel. In all randomized studies thus reported (GOG 99, PORTEC 1 and 2, and ASTEC/EN.5), the vaginal recurrence rate following adjuvant pelvic irradiation ranges between 1% to 2%, and therefore, any study to examine whether brachytherapy should be added to external beam RT as a boost would require a very large number of patients and more resources than the question warrants.

Intravaginal Brachytherapy Alone. With the increase in surgical LN staging, the use of postoperative intravaginal brachytherapy alone regained its appeal, the rationale being that full surgical LN staging could potentially eliminate the need for pelvic radiation, whereas vaginal brachytherapy could still address the risk of vaginal cuff recurrence, as demonstrated in PORTEC 2. Several additional reports in the past 10 years also demonstrated a very low rate of recurrence either in the vagina or in the pelvis with such an approach (139,206,392–395).

From the above discussion, it is clear that the options available for patients with early-stage endometrioid EC are numerous. Perhaps it is better to consider different options based on the following factors identified as risk factors for recurrence – age, grade, depth of invasion, LVI, histology, and whether a nodal dissection was accomplished.

Cancer Limited to the Mucosa (Formerly Stage IA, grades 1 and 2).

The risk of pelvic LN positivity (57) is ≤3% and the 5-year PFS rate in this group is of the order of 95% to 98%. It is unlikely that postoperative pelvic external beam radiation would add anything to the final outcome (390,396). The role of intravaginal radiation in these patients is also of questionable benefit because of an almost negligible risk of vaginal recurrence with surgery alone. Straughn et al. (370) reported no vaginal recurrence in 103 patients with stage IA grade 1, 2 treated with surgery alone. This is no longer a discreet stage in the 2010 FIGO staging system.

Cancer Limited to the Mucosa, Grade 3

In GOG 33, there were only eight patients with stage IA grade 3 disease, making it difficult to draw any meaningful conclusion (59). There were no relapses in the three patients receiving postoperative radiation as compared with one failure in the five patients who received no postoperative therapy. The risk of LN metastasis in this group of patients is negligible. Straughn et al. (370) reported on eight patients with stage IA grade 3 disease treated with surgery alone, with two of the patients developing isolated vaginal recurrence. Again this subgroup is not formally staged in the new FIGO staging system.

Low-Risk Stage I A, B Grades 1, 2. Straughn et al. (370) reported on 296 patients with IB grade 1, 2 and found only nine (3%) vaginal recurrences and one (0.3%) pelvic recurrence. Horowitz et al. reported on 62 patients who had surgical LN staging and received adjuvant intravaginal brachytherapy. There was one (1.6%) vaginal recurrence and no pelvic recurrence (392). In comparison, data published by Alektiar et al. (397) reported that 233 patients with IB grade 1, 2 showed a vaginal recurrence rate of only 1% and pelvic recurrence of 2% using postoperative intravaginal brachytherapy alone without routine surgical LN staging. In addition, Sorbe et al. (398) reported on 110 patients without retroperitoneal LN sampling with IB grade 1, 2 who were part of a prospective, randomized trial evaluating two different intravaginal brachytherapy doses; the rate of vaginal recurrence was 0.9% and pelvic recurrence 1.8%. These patients also often fit the GOG 99, PORTEC 1, and PORTEC 2 trials, with or without lymphadenectomy. Thus, it seems reasonable to suggest that either observation or intravaginal brachytherapy (irrespective of surgical staging) is a reasonable option. But when deciding on whether adjuvant radiation is needed, it is important to address three issues. First, older patients tend to have higher rates of relapse. In the study by Straughn et al., (370) 8 of the 10 vaginal/pelvic recurrences were in patients ≥60 years old, which was confirmed in the randomized trials. Second, patients with lymphovascular invasion (LVI) have a higher chance of vaginal recurrence as demonstrated by Mariani et al. (373) who reported on 508 patients with stage I EC treated with surgery alone (152 out of 508 were stage IA). The presence of LVI increased the vaginal relapse rate from 3% to 7% ($p = 0.02$) as was confirmed by the GOG 99 trial among others. Recent publications of high-intermediate and high-risk stage I–III endometrial carcinoma patients suggest LVI to be an independent prognostic factor for relapse and survival. (367,399). Third, often the indications for adjuvant radiation are rather arbitrarily based on the amount of myometrial invasion defined in thirds and on whether the tumor is grade 1 versus 2. Yet the amount of myometrial invasion in this group of patients and whether an EC is assigned as grade 1 or 2 do not appear to be significant predictors of outcome (400,401). It is reasonable to offer patients younger than 60 years of age with stage IA grades 1 and 2 disease without LVI observation, whereas those patients ≥60 years or those with LVI are offered adjuvant brachytherapy. It is worth noting that the most common site of recurrence is the vaginal vault and adjuvant brachytherapy is a low-morbidity treatment. When undecided whether to offer brachytherapy, it should be considered that it is a far less intensive treatment than salvage radiation for recurrent disease.

Intermediate to High-Intermediate Risk Stage IB Grade 3 to IC Grades 1,2, 3, Stage II.

Up until the last 10 years, most data in the literature on this group of patients were based on pelvic radiation either alone or in combination with intravaginal brachytherapy (389,390,402,403). Since 1988 and with the increase in surgical LN staging in the United States, a shift occurred with regard to the role of radiation for stage IB grade 3 and even in stage IC disease. For some time, the treatment decision between whole pelvis RT and VCB alone was primarily based on whether the patient had surgical LN staging. If the decision is made that nodal assessment is necessary, which has been called into question for all early-stage patients, an adequate LN sampling/dissection should, at a minimum, meet the GOG guidelines of sampling the obturator, external iliacs, internal iliacs, common iliacs, and para-aortic LN stations, and the minimum number of nodes sampled should be ≥10.

Surgically Staged Patients. For patients with IB grade 3 disease, the retrospective data on intravaginal brachytherapy alone after surgical staging was encouraging (**Table 21.14**). The average rate of vaginal recurrence and pelvic recurrence was reported as 1.3% for both. This compares favorably with the data from the PORTEC I trial where the 5-year rates for vaginal and pelvic recurrence, in the subset of patients with IB grade 3 disease treated with pelvic radiation ($n = 35$), were 0% and 3%, respectively. A multi-institutional review of 220 patients with stage IC EC by Straughn et al. (371) compared adjuvant radiation to no radiation in patients with negative nodes on surgical staging. The investigators concluded that adjuvant radiation is not needed although the 5-year DFS was 74.5% for those treated with surgery alone compared to 92.5% for those treated with adjuvant radiation ($p = 0.0134$). It is unlikely that observation alone, even in those patients with full surgical staging, will be the best approach when VCB carries low morbidity and can greatly decrease the 18% statistically significant difference in DFS from a retrospective study in which it is inferred that patients with the worst prognostic features were the ones who received radiation.

Several investigators have shown the feasibility of such an approach with an average vaginal recurrence rate of 1.6% and pelvic control rate of 2.1% (**Table 21.15**). Thus, intravaginal brachytherapy alone after surgical staging in patients with IB grade 3 and IC EC seems to provide better local/regional control than surgery alone and in a properly selected patient population with very few pelvic failures (144,392,404–407). As described previously, the GOG 0249 trial randomized the HIR population to VCB followed by CT (carboplatin/paclitaxel for three cycles) or pelvic RT (IMRT or 3D conformal) plus an optional cuff brachytherapy boost for high-risk features, and appeared to show equivalence. Note that LN dissection was optional in this trial. In addition, while LN dissection is not allowed, further information may be gained by the PORTEC 3/EN.7 trial that randomizes patients with (1988 FIGO) Stage IB grade 3 with LVI, Stage IC or IIA grade 3, Stage IIB, Stage IIIA or IIIC, or stages IB–III serous or clear cell EC between pelvic RT alone to 48.6 Gy and the same pelvic RT with two cycles of concurrent cisplatin plus four adjuvant cycles of carboplatin/paclitaxel. In the PORTEC 3 trial, the vaginal cuff boost is given in patients with cervical invasion. In the absence of robust evidence, the risk of pelvic failure must be gauged on an individual patient basis to determine whether the risk is sufficient to warrant pelvic radiation versus VCB alone. In the PORTEC trial, 99 patients with Stage IC grade 3 tumors were not randomized but were followed prospectively, and all received pelvic irradiation in the absence of LN evaluation. The locoregional recurrence rate in this high-risk group of patients without a node dissection was 12% (5% vaginal), despite adjuvant irradiation. Note that patients with uterine serous and clear cell carcinoma were not identified separately in this trial, so the percentage of these high-risk pathologies is not known, and given the very high distant failure rate, of 31%, this is noted to be a very high-risk subgroup of patients (162).

With the publication of the two randomized trials, ASTEC and CONSORT, questioning the benefit for lymphadenectomy, many gynecologic oncologists in the United States have chosen to evaluate the nodes only in those patients most at risk for metastatic disease—those with deeply invasive tumors, high-grade disease, high-risk histology, older patients, and those with LVI or a combination of

TABLE 21.14. Outcome for IB Grade 3 EC after Surgical LN Staging and Intravaginal Radiation Therapy (IVRT) Alone

Author	Year	No. of Patients	Median F/U	Vaginal Rec	Pelvic Rec
Fanning	2001	21	52 months	0%	0%
Horowitz	2002	31	65 months	0%	0%
Alektiar	2007	21	46 months	4.8% (1/21)	4.8% (1/21)
Total	—	73	—	1.3% (1/73)	1.3% (1/73)

EC, endometrial cancer; F/U, follow-up; LN, lymph node.

TABLE 21.15. Outcome for IC Endometrial Cancer Grade 1–3 after Surgical LN Staging and IVRT Alone

Author	Year	No. of Patients	Median F/U	Vaginal Rec	Pelvic Rec
Horowitz	2002	50	65 months	2% (1/50)	4% (2/50)
Rittenberg	2003	53	32 months	0%	1.8% (1/53)
Solheim	2005	40	23 months	0%	0%
Alektiar	2007	40	46 months	5% (2/40)	2.5% (1/40)
Total	—	183	—	1.6% (3/183)	2.1% (4/183)

F/U, follow-up; IVRT, Intravaginal Radiation Therapy; LN, lymph node; rec, recurrence.

factors. Examining the trials where routine lymphadenectomy is performed demonstrates the risk for all Stage I patients to be approximately 10% (59,155,156), but selecting the patients at highest risk for disease, while it may not change survival, can certainly guide further treatment paradigms.

No Surgical Lymph Node Staging. In those patients with a combination of high-risk features such as grade 3 tumor, high-risk histologies, LVI, advanced age, or deep myometrial invasion, intravaginal brachytherapy may not be adequate treatment. In the Aalders et al. (386) randomized trial, the rate of local recurrence in the subset of patients with IB grade 3 to IC was 9.3% (13 of 137) for those treated with brachytherapy alone compared to 1.3% (2 of 146) for those treated with brachytherapy and external radiation. This finding is not unexpected as no LN assessment was performed in that trial. Weiss et al. reported on 61 patients with stage IC EC who were treated with postoperative pelvic radiation alone. With a median follow-up of 69.5 months, there was only one recurrence in the pelvis (1.6%). Their review of the published data from the literature for patients with stage IC disease showed a pelvic recurrence of 1.04% in 240 patients treated with pelvic radiation alone compared to 0.97% in 301 patients treated with pelvic and intravaginal radiation. The authors concluded that pelvic radiation alone is sufficient for local-regional control, and clinical efforts should focus on reducing the risk of distant relapse in this subgroup of patients (408). The results of the PORTEC 3 trial may help further stratify patients who may be appropriate candidates for observation or VCB alone, or those at sufficiently high risk who benefit from intensification of therapy, including a combination of adjuvant irradiation and chemotherapy.

Stage II. It is important to recognize the distinction between gross and occult cervical involvement in EC. Gross cervical involvement increases the risk of parametrial extension as well as spread to pelvic LN in a fashion similar to primary cervical cancer. Patients with gross cervical involvement from EC could undergo radical hysterectomy and pelvic LN dissection or preoperative radiation including pelvic radiation and intracavitary brachytherapy followed by simple hysterectomy. For occult cervical involvement, the treatment often consists of simple hysterectomy with or without LN surgical staging and adjuvant radiation. The type of radiation most often utilized is pelvic radiation and intravaginal brachytherapy. Pitson et al. (409) reported on 120 patients treated with such a combination. The 5-year DFS rate was 68% and the rate of pelvic relapse was 5.8% (7 of 120).

There are also emerging data on the role of intravaginal brachytherapy alone in patients with occult cervical involvement who also had surgical LN staging. The rate of pelvic recurrence in four such series ranged from 0% to 6%, but a larger number of patients and longer follow-ups will be necessary in order to confirm this data. (392,394,410,411). Stage II EC is now defined by cervical stromal invasion. The new staging system now only encompasses the latter with true cervical stromal invasion into Stage II (89). Intravaginal brachytherapy alone could be used for surgically staged patients with mucosal involvement alone (392,412), whereas those with disease invading into the stroma, with close margins or with a significant amount of cervical disease, should be treated with pelvic radiation with or without intravaginal brachytherapy boost until trial results demonstrate a better option.

Advanced-Stage Disease

Radiation

The outcome of patients with isolated adnexal involvement (stage IIIA) treated with pelvic radiation is fairly good, although the studied patient numbers are small. Connell et al. (413) reported on 12 patients treated with postoperative pelvic radiation with a 5-year DFS of 70.9%. The weighted average of 5-year DFS and OS rates from literature review in that study were 78.6% and 67.1%, respectively. Patients with isolated serosal involvement (stage IIIA) have a worse prognosis than those with isolated adnexal involvement. Ashman et al. (414) reported on 15 patients with isolated serosal involvement who were treated with pelvic radiation. The 5-year DFS was only 41.5%. If pelvic node involvement (IIIC1) is the only major risk factor, treatment with postoperative pelvic RT can yield a 60% to 72% long-term survival rate (165,415,416), although distant failure is a problem that new trials evaluating CT will hopefully change. Patients with stage IIIC2 disease, by virtue of para-aortic node involvement, represent a particularly high-risk group. Following surgery, these patients are generally treated with extended field radiation to encompass the pelvis and the para-aortic regions. With this aggressive approach, several investigators have reported 30% to 40% survival rates in small patient populations (417–419). The question of whether it is safe to omit radiation even after adequate surgical LN staging in patients with IIIC2 EC was addressed in a study from the Mayo Clinic. Mariani et al. reported on 122 patients with node-positive disease; at 5 years, the risk of pelvic recurrence was 57% after inadequate LN dissection and/or no RT compared to 10% with adequate LN dissection (>10 pelvic nodes and ≥5 para-aortic nodes) and radiation. This difference was statistically significant on univariate ($p < 0.001$) and multivariate analysis ($p = 0.03$), indicating the need for postoperative radiation even after adequate surgical staging (142). The recognition that a significant number of patients with stage III disease fail in the abdomen (373,415) has prompted a number of investigators to evaluate whole abdominal RT in these patients (420,421) and after a small GOG trial a randomized trial was undertaken (422).

Chemoradiation

In the GOG 122 trial, 396 patients with stage III and optimally debulked stage IV disease were randomized to whole abdomen radiation (n = 202) or to doxorubicin–cisplatin chemotherapy (n = 194). With a median follow-up of 74 months, there was significant improvement in both PFS (50% vs. 38%; $p = 0.007$) as well as OS (55% vs. 42%; $p = 0.004$), respectively, in favor of CT (332). To elucidate the right approach for these patients, however, a closer look at this data is warranted. First, the overall absolute rate of relapse was 54% in the radiation arm compared to 50% in the CT arm, a small difference if any, yet the corresponding 5-year PFS rates were 38% and 50% ($p = 0.007$), respectively. Why the discrepancy? The answer is that the 5-year PFS rate for the radiation arm was 38%, whereas the CT arm has two separate 5-year rates. The first one, called unadjusted, was 42%, which is not that significantly different from the 38% rate with radiation, and the second, called "adjusted for stage," was 50%, which was significantly different from the radiation arm. This led us to the second issue: Was the adjustment for stage warranted? The answer is no. Numerically, there were more patients with lymph node involvement in the CT than the radiation arm, but having positive LN was not an independent predictor of poor outcome in this study. Therefore, the adjustment was not warranted, and if any adjustment was needed it should have gone to the radiation arm since there were more patients with positive cytology in this arm, a factor with an HR of 1.8 (95% CI, 0.89 to 1.55) in predicting poor outcome. Third, what should be made of the significant difference in OS? There were 15 deaths unrelated to EC or protocol treatment in the radiation arm compared to only 6 in the chemotherapy arm, raising a question about whether the two arms of the study were truly balanced. Finally, the pelvic recurrence rate was lower in the RT arm which indicates that perhaps both modalities could be used for the advantages they provide—locoregional control for irradiation and distant control for chemotherapy. Another randomized trial comparing adjuvant radiation to CT (doxorubicin–cisplatin–cyclophosphamide) in patients with stage I–III was recently reported and showed no difference in outcome between the two arms (423). With a median follow-up of 95.5 months, the 5-year DFS was 63% in both arms ($p = 0.44$), and the 5-year OS rates were 69% in the radiation arm compared to 66% in the CT arm ($p = 0.77$). What these two trials show is that CT at a minimum is equivalent to radiation in this group of patients and ought to be used, not alone, but rather in combination with radiation. Greven et al. reported the results of Radiation Therapy Oncology Group (RTOG) 9708 on 44 patients with stage I–III EC who were treated with pelvic radiation and intravaginal brachytherapy given concurrently with cisplatin 50 mg/m^2 on days 1 and 28 of radiation, followed by four cycles of cisplatin (50 mg/m^2) and paclitaxel (Taxol) (175 mg/m^2). The 4-year DFS and OS rates for those with stage III disease (66% of patients) were 72% and 77%, respectively (424).

As the follow-up study to GOG 122, GOG 184 was launched. The combination of irradiation and CT was used to control disease and was done in a sequential fashion to limit toxicity. Five hundred fifty-two Stage III and IV patients were enrolled (after 66 patients were enrolled, those with upper abdominal disease were excluded) and received tumor volume-directed irradiation (51% received 5,040 cGy pelvis irradiation alone and 49% received 4,320 to 4,350 cGy of extended field for positive para-aortic disease, or undissected para-aortics) and were then randomized to cisplatin/adriamycin or cisplatin/adriamycin/paclitaxel (425). Growth factors were allowed, and 80% of the patients were able to complete the assigned CT regimen following full-dose RT. The locoregional recurrence rate (any failure in the pelvis, vagina, or para-aortics as first failure) was 10%, which compares favorably with GOG 122 (isolated failures 13% in the whole abdominal irradiation (WAI) arm and 18% in CT arm); Greven's (168) study of 105 irradiated patients with IIIC disease with a pelvic failure rate of 21%; and Mundt's two series, one described 30 patients with stage IIIC treated with postoperative pelvic irradiation with an infield failure rate of 23% and the second, trial of 43 high-risk stage I–IV EC patients treated with CT alone who experienced a 21% actuarial rate of pelvic recurrence as their first or only site of recurrence (426,427). The distant failure rate in these trials was unacceptably high ranging from 26% to 55%. The PORTEC 3 trial described above and the open GOG 0258 address treatment in this advanced population. In the GOG 0258 trial, Stages III or IVA are randomized between volume-directed postoperative irradiation with concurrent cisplatin, followed by four cycles of carboplatin/taxol or six cycles of carboplatin/taxol alone.

SPECIAL SITUATIONS

Positive Cytology Without Adnexal or Serosal Involvement

In this subset of patients, the presence of other adverse features such as aggressive histologies or deep myometrial invasion should be determined first as this is noted but no longer part of the official staging system. The argument to remove it from the staging is that without other factors cytology alone has unclear prognostic value (428). The literature regarding the benefits of treatment in this setting is mixed; even if treatment is beneficial, the appropriate modality still has to be defined. On the basis of the concept that the entire peritoneal cavity is at risk, intraperitoneal radioactive colloidal ^{32}P had been used by some with results that were better than in historic controls (429) but carried significant toxicity. Eltabbakh et al. reported on 27 patients with FIGO grade 1, 2 and <50% myometrial invasion who were treated with intravaginal brachytherapy and megestrol acetate (Megace). None of the patients relapsed or died from their disease. Megace was given for 1 year, and at the end of therapy, 24 patients underwent second-look laparoscopy and peritoneal cytology. In 23 patients, the cytology was negative, and the remaining patients with persistent positive cytology received an additional year of Megace after which cytology was confirmed to be negative (430). Given this, as an isolated risk factor, vaginal brachytherapy with Megace is likely the only adjuvant regimen that may be appropriate in some of these patients.

Definitive Radiation for Inoperable Disease

Patients with medically inoperable stage I–II uterine cancer are usually treated in a fashion similar to those with cervical cancer by using intracavitary applicators with or without pelvic radiation. For patients with clinical stage I grade 1 or 2 and no or minimal evidence of myometrial invasion or LN metastasis on MRI, intracavitary brachytherapy alone may be sufficient provided the uterus is a size and shape that it can be fully covered with the brachytherapy irradiation. There are several applicator choices with one or two tandems (depending on uterus size) and either a cylinder or ovoids. The American Brachytherapy Society Guidelines have recommended either dosing in the uterus 2 cm from the tandem, and treating the upper several centimeters of vagina, or, in the age of image guidance, dosing to the uterine serosa (431). When pelvic radiation is added to brachytherapy, the dose is usually 45 to 50 Gy supplemented with intracavitary brachytherapy. Rouanet et al. (432) treated 250 patients with EC using LDR brachytherapy, which yielded a 5-year DSS of 76.5%. An alternative brachytherapy approach would be to use the Hymen or Simon afterloading system, which consists of multiple Teflon tubes that are inserted into the uterine cavity. With such a treatment approach, Grigsby et al. (433) reported that the 5-year PFS rate of patients with clinical stage I disease treated with a combination of external and intracavitary RT was 94% for grade 1 disease, 92% for grade 2 disease, and 78% for grade 3 disease. High-dose-rate brachytherapy is increasingly used and demonstrates equivalent control (434,435). Nguyen (435) and Niazi (436) reported on patients with clinical stage I–II disease treated with HDR alone or with external irradiation and the disease-specific survival at 8 years was 76% and 91% at 15 years, respectively. Note that many of these patients, by virtue of being medically inoperable, will die of other causes than their early-stage uterine carcinoma. Intriguingly, Fishman published a study comparing the operable with the inoperable and found that those inoperable patients that did not die of intercurrent disease had a similar median 5-year survival (437). Kucera et. al. studied a larger population of 228 and using HDR alone found a DSS at 5 years of 85% and 10 years of 75% (438). For several of these studies, image guidance was not available and the expectation is that dosing the radiation in the appropriate area will increase control and DSS. Although uncommonly seen, IIIB patients are definitively treated with irradiation including external beam and intracavitary/interstitial brachytherapy as they are not surgical candidates (439).

RADIATION THERAPY TECHNIQUES

Intravaginal Brachytherapy

Intracavitary vaginal brachytherapy is designed to deliver dose to the vaginal surface and underlying lymphatic channels at risk of harboring residual disease. Choo and colleagues demonstrated that 95% of vaginal lymphatic channels lie within 5 mm of the vaginal mucosa and therefore this modality is well-suited to deliver this dose effectively, and more safely, than with external beam irradiation. Intravaginal brachytherapy can be delivered using LDR to 60 Gy prescribed to the vaginal mucosa or 30 to 35 Gy prescribed to 0.5-cm depth from the vaginal mucosa using either ovoids for the upper several centimeters of vagina or a cylinder, which allows the length treated to be tailored to the clinical situation. Less commonly, the whole length of the vagina needs to be treated, and should be considered for those with close or positive margins, extensive LVI, or high-risk histologies. HDR brachytherapy guidelines have been established and published for dose and fractionation, although the most common is 700 cGy for three fractions treated at 5-mm depth according to a survey published by Small et. al (440,441). PORTEC-4 is a randomized study that will compare the most common HDR fractionation schemes, including 2,100 cGy versus 1,500 cGy delivered in three fractions.

External Beam Radiation

Pelvic Radiation

Most patients are treated in the postoperative setting. At the time of simulation, the small bowel may be opacified using oral contrast given 60 minutes prior to CT. Vaginal markers are now discouraged as they may displace the vaginal cuff. Patients may be placed in the prone position to displace the small intestines from the radiation field. Prone treatment board allows the abdominal wall and contents to be displaced anteriorly through a hole in the board, to allow displacement of bowel from the pelvis (442). The target volumes are the obturator, external, internal, and lower common iliac nodes, and the proximal two-thirds of the vagina. The presacral and common iliac nodes are encompassed fully in the setting of cervical involvement or pathologic nodal involvement. High-energy linear accelerators (15 MV) are preferred because of their sparing of the skin and subcutaneous tissue when the treatment is a four-field box or when three-dimensional conformal therapy (3DCF) is used, particularly in patients with large tissue separations. The ideal beam arrangement with the conventional four-field pelvic-box technique places the superior border at L5-S1, the inferior border at the bottom of the obturator foramina or at least 3 to 4 cm below the vaginal apex, and the lateral border 1 to 2 cm beyond the widest point of bony pelvis. For the lateral fields, the anterior border is in front of the pubis symphysis to allow external iliac coverage and the posterior border covers S1/S2. The superior and inferior borders are the same for the anterior and posterior fields. All fields are treated daily to a dose of 1.8 Gy. A total dose of 50.4 Gy is given to sterilize microscopic disease, or 45 Gy when combined with intravaginal brachytherapy. 3DCF therapy uses the same beam arrangement, but a planning CT scan is used to outline both tissues at risk and normal tissues. Blocks are placed based on the contours, which allows more accurate targeting and sparing of more normal tissues. Recent evidence suggests decreased acute and late toxicity to the bowel when IMRT is used. Mundt et al. demonstrated a significant reduction in acute and chronic GI toxicity when IMRT was compared to historical controls treated with conventional radiation (443–446). IMRT, compared to the four-field box or 3DCF therapy, uses an inverse planning technique to shape the radiation dose to tissues at risk of harboring microscopic disease and to minimize normal tissue dose. Both 3DCF therapy and IMRT use small collimator "leaves" to finely shape the beam. These "leaves" are mobile and block portions of the generated x-rays. If the collimator "leaves" move while the radiation beam is on and vary the beam intensity, areas of tumor and normal tissue can receive a spectrum of doses; hence the term "intensity modulated." Papers have been published on the use of IMRT in postoperative uterine and cervical carcinoma, vulvar carcinoma, whole abdominal RT, vaginal carcinoma, and intact cervical carcinoma. However, because of the daily variation in bladder and rectal filling and the resultant mobility of the upper vagina, the use of IMRT should be undertaken with caution, and experience with contouring, planning, and delivery is essential (447,448). The introduction of new technology such as tomotherapy (a linear accelerator linked to an online CT scanner), cyberknife (a linear accelerator capable of fiducial imaging to target radiation), and cone beam CT (CT scan mounted to the linear accelerator) for image-guided RT assists in daily target and normal tissue localization. Randomized, prospective data comparing this to traditional therapy is lacking but ongoing trials are evaluating risks, effectiveness, and cost. The NRG TIME-C trial has completed accrual of 1,200 patients and will evaluate patient-reported quality of life, specifically diarrhea at 5 weeks, for patients randomized to 3C versus IMRT.

Extended Field

This technique is mainly used for patients with documented positive para-aortic nodes or patients at risk of disease but without surgical evaluation. Either 3DCF irradiation or IMRT can be utilized (449), although IMRT may significantly reduce the risk of acute and chronic GI toxicity. When para-aortic fields are utilized, attention should be made to the dose delivered to the kidney, especially with increased use of chemotherapy in these patients, and when metrics are well known. The lower border is the same as in pelvic radiation, but the upper border is extended in some patients as high as the T12-L1 interspace. The typical dose is 45 Gy at 1.8 Gy per fraction or 1.5 Gy per fraction if patients develop acute GI toxicity.

Whole Abdomen Radiation Therapy

Whole abdominal radiation therapy (WART) is uncommonly used since the publication of GOG 122. The standard approach is AP/PA open fields with five half-value layer kidney blocks placed over the PA field only (if patient is lying supine) from the start of the treatment. The dose is usually 30.0 Gy at 1.5 Gy per fraction, followed by a 19.8-Gy boost to the pelvis at 1.8 Gy per fraction. The upper border is usually placed 1 cm above the diaphragm, and the lateral borders should extend beyond the peritoneal reflections. The lower border is usually at the bottom of the obturator foramen.

Complications of Radiation

Pelvic Radiation

In GOG 99, the risk of Grade 3 or 4 complications was 14% with RT versus 6% without. In the PORTEC I randomized trial (144), the overall (grades 1 to 4) rate of late complications was 26% in the RT group compared to 4% in the observation group ($p < 0.0001$). Most of the late complications in the RT group, however, were grades 1, 2 (22%), and only 3% were grades 3, 4. It is also important to note that many patients in this trial were treated with AP/PA fields in which the overall rate of complications was 30% compared to 21% for those treated with the four-field box ($p = 0.06$), and even lower for IMRT. The recent 15-year update notes that second malignancies were diagnosed in 16% of the observation patients and 22% of the irradiation patients, a difference that was insignificant. In PORTEC II grades 1 and 2, GI side effects were significantly higher with external beam (delivered using CT planning and with multi-field or 3DCF techniques) than with vaginal brachytherapy (53.8% vs. 12.6%), but grades 3 and 4 were not reported, which is curious, suggesting it was very low and likely not significantly different between the arms. Late grade 3 GI effects were reported in 2% of those receiving EBRT versus <1% of those with VBT. Alternatively, grade 3 atrophy (marked atrophy with or without narrowing or shortening) was reported in <1% of those with EBRT and 2% with VBT. There were no grade 4 or 5 toxicities in either arm. In more advanced disease trials, we see a similar pattern. In GOG 122, those with at least one grade 3 and 4 hematologic toxicity between the arms of WART or CT were 14% versus 88%, respectively. Grade 3 or 4 acute GI toxicity was 13% versus 20% in the WART and CT arms, respectively. Late grades 3 or 4 GI or genitourinary toxicity between the arms were 13% and <1% for WART and 20% and 3% for CT, respectively. Many investigators were surprised that the CT arm had increased acute and late GI effects when compared to WART. Statistical analyses of these results were not reported (332). In GOG 184, where everyone received whole pelvis radiation and 49% pelvis and para-aortic irradiation, the late grade 3 or higher treatment-related GI events were only 5% (425). Acutely pelvic irradiation can cause fatigue, cystitis, diarrhea, skin erythema and breakdown, and vaginitis. Adding a para-aortic field can add nausea and gastritis to the list. VCB is very well tolerated, and complaints during treatment are rare other than discomfort with placement of the device. Late toxicities include intra-abdominal scarring, chronic cystitis or enteritis, bowel obstruction requiring surgery, rectal telangiectasias, and more unusually bone weakening with fracture, fistula formation, kidney or spinal cord damage, second malignancies, menopause if the ovaries are in the field, and with WART liver toxicity. With vaginal brachytherapy, vaginal atrophy, narrowing, dryness, and agglutination are possible.

Radiation Therapy for Local Recurrence

RT can be curative in a select group of patients with small vaginal recurrences who have not received prior radiation. The 5-year local control rate ranges from 42% to 65%, and the 5-year OS rate from 31% to 53% (450–452). Creutzberg et al. (453) reported on survival after relapse from the PORTEC randomized trial. In patients who were initially randomized to surgery alone (n = 46 out of 360), the 5-year survival after vaginal relapse was 65%. But before adopting salvage radiation as a treatment policy for all early-stage EC, a few aspects of this trial need to be addressed. First, the 5-year survival rate from the PORTEC trial is much higher than what is reported in the literature. Most likely, the vaginal recurrences in this trial were detected very early, unlike patients in the community. The extent and size of local recurrence in EC are very significant predictors of outcome (452). Second, this high rate of salvage pertains only to isolated vaginal recurrence. The rate of survival at 3 years for pelvic recurrence in the PORTEC trial was 0%. Third, although the trial does not mention any data on complications, it is not unrealistic to expect a higher complication rate than what is normally seen with adjuvant radiation. With salvage radiation, external beam RT and brachytherapy are often combined and the doses of radiation required are much higher than those used with adjuvant radiation. A study from the M. D. Anderson Cancer Center by Jhingran et al. (454) clearly highlights these issues. They reported on 91 patients who were treated with definitive radiation for isolated vaginal recurrence. The 5-year local control and OS rates were 75% and 43%, respectively. The median dose of radiation was 75 Gy, which often included external radiation and brachytherapy. The rate of grade 4 complications (requiring surgery) was 9%. Thus, when talking with a patient about adjuvant radiation versus radiation reserved for salvage, these issues need to be addressed and compared to the excellent local control and low morbidity obtained with adjuvant irradiation. The currently open GOG 0238 trial randomizes patients with recurrence of endometrial carcinoma limited to the pelvis and vagina to concurrent cisplatin/irradiation versus standard irradiation alone.

SYSTEMIC THERAPIES

Endocrine Therapy

Hormonal agents have proven to be valuable, particularly in the patient with recurrent disease, and reviews of their use have been extensively published. Response rates to endocrine agents including progestins, antiestrogens, and aromatase inhibitors vary (455–462). The overall response to progestins is approximately 25%. However, some trials demonstrate lower RRs, usually in the range of 15% to 20%. These studies generally used more rigorous response criteria and had multi-institutional participation. A higher dose of progestin does not appear to increase the RR. In one randomized trial of 200 mg/d versus 1,000 mg/d of MPA, the overall RR was actually 25% versus 15% favoring the low-dose arm (463). The time to treatment failure and median OS of the low- versus high-dose regimen, respectively, were 3.2 versus 2.5 months and 11.1 versus 7.0 months, all showing no advantage for an increased dose. Prognostic factors related to response were performance status, grade, and progesterone receptor level. The RR was only 8% in poorly differentiated tumors. A phase 2 trial of high-dose megestrol (800 mg orally daily) in 63 patients was associated with a RR of 24% overall, which is similar to lower dose regimens with doses of 40 mg po q.i.d (464). As in the majority of studies with hormonal agents, RRs were statistically higher in patients with grade 1 or 2 lesions (37%) versus grade 3 lesions (8%); $p = 0.02$. In addition to grade, a long disease-free interval (exceeding 2 or 3 years) and positive estrogen or progesterone receptor status have all been associated with an increased frequency of response (455,458,463,464). Age, location of metastatic disease, number of metastatic sites, prior therapy, and weight have also been analyzed by several investigators, but they have not been convincingly linked with response.

Tamoxifen has been investigated in patients with recurrent disease in several studies (461–465). Results have varied, but in general, RRs have been modest in untreated patients. A GOG study evaluated 68 patients with advanced or recurrent disease receiving tamoxifen at 20 mg po b.i.d and showed an overall RR of 10% (90% CI, 5.7 to 17.9) (461). The median progression-free interval was short at 1.9 months (90% CI, 1.7 to 3.2 months) and the OS was 8.8 months (90% CI, 7.0 to 10.1 months). One small randomized phase 2 study comparing megestrol acetate to megestrol acetate with tamoxifen showed no advantage in RR for the combination, with RRs of 20% versus 19%, respectively (466). The lack of synergistic response is supported by observations of EC treated in a nude mouse model. Tumors treated with medroxyprogesterone or tamoxifen plus medroxyprogesterone were devoid of progesterone receptor during the growth inhibitory and regrowth phase of the tumor resulting from receptor downregulation (467). The possibility of alternating tamoxifen with megestrol acetate to exploit the recruitment of progesterone receptors by tamoxifen is an interesting strategy. The GOG performed a phase 2 study with 56 patients with advanced or recurrent EC who had not previously received CT or hormonal manipulation (468). Patients were treated with megestrol acetate at 160 mg/d for 3 weeks alternating with tamoxifen 40 mg po q.i.d for 3 weeks. An overall RR of 27% (90% CI, 17.3 to 38.4) with a 21.4% CR rate was seen, with the duration of response exceeding 20 months in 8 of 15 responders. The RR was 38% for patients with grade 1 disease and 22% for those with grade 3 disease. In another phase 2 GOG study, a similar patient population was treated with tamoxifen 40 mg po daily plus alternating weekly cycles of MPA 200 mg po daily (469). Of the 58 evaluable patients, the RR was 33% (6 complete, 13 partial). Although these phase 2 results are intriguing, a randomized study would be required to determine if alternating hormones is superior to single-hormone approaches. Positive receptor status has been associated with improved disease-free and OS rates (470,471). These data indicate that the receptor status provides important biologic information and that receptor-positive tumors tend to be better differentiated and slower growing than are their receptor-negative counterparts. CT had no effect on hormone receptor capacity in a nude mouse model of xenografted EC (472). Other factors, such as changes in vaginal cytology during treatment (473), and results in the subrenal capsule chemosensitivity assay (474) and in the nude mouse model (475) may help predict response to progestins.

Several studies have evaluated gonadotropin-releasing hormone analogs in patients with metastatic EC. Gallagher et al. (476) noted one complete and five partial responses (PRs) to leuprolide or goserelin in 17 patients (35% response; 95% CI, 13% to 58%) with metastatic disease. Of note, the duration of remission ranged from 7 to 30 months, and 14 of the 17 patients had been previously treated with progestins. Another report described four responses in seven postmenopausal patients with EC treated with goserelin (477). *In vitro* studies in human EC cell lines have suggested that such growth inhibition may have been due to apoptosis (478). The GOG studied goserelin at 3.6-mg subcutaneously monthly in 40 patients with advanced or recurrent disease. Seventy-one percent of patients had received prior RT. There were two complete (5%) and three partial (7%) responses, with an overall RR of 11% (95% CI, 4% to 27%). Goserelin is observed to have limited activity in this patient population, and no additional single-agent studies are planned (456).

Investigation is under way in patients with uterine cancer to evaluate the activity of SERMs. These agents have ER-antagonist activity in breast and uterine tissues and ER-agonist activity in bone. The first reported study to date is from the GOG and fvevaluated anastrozole at 1-mg po daily orally in 23 unselected patients (i.e., 9 patients had grade 2 tumors and 14 patients had grade 3 tumors). A PR rate of 9% was seen (90% CI, 3% to 23%). It is noted that the PR rate of 9% in this study is similar to the 8% reported in grade 3 patients treated with standard progestins (464,470). Another study evaluated the investigational SERM arzoxifene in 37 patients. Twenty-six patients were ER-positive and 22 were progesterone receptor (PR) positive. A RR of 31% (95% CI, 25% to 51%) was seen in this selected patient population with a median duration of response of 13.9 months (457). Additional study of these agents in patients with well-differentiated tumors is warranted (479).

Endometrial Cancer and Cytotoxic Chemotherapy

Recent data illustrating the utility of CT has expanded the role of CT to include not only metastatic disease but also surgically staged advanced disease. The role of CT in the management of high-risk early-stage disease remains investigational.

Early-Stage High-Risk Uterine Cancer

Despite the ability for surgical staging to define a low-risk patient population for most patients with negative pelvic and para-aortic LN, certain subgroups of patients with Stage I–II EC have been shown to have a higher risk of recurrence. These patients may benefit from postoperative adjuvant therapy, either RT alone or in combination with CT. Defining patients that require therapy remains a challenge.

Hogberg et al. (480) reported the results of two randomized studies (NSGO-EC-9501/EORTC -55991 and MaNGO-ILIADE-III) examining the role of sequential adjuvant CT and RT. The two randomized clinical trials included patients with Stage I–III EC with no residual tumor and prognostic factors consistent with high-risk disease. These patients were randomly assigned to either adjuvant RT with or without sequential CT. The authors reported that in the NSGO/EORTC study, the combined modality treatment was associated with a 36% reduction in the risk for relapse or death (HR, 0.064; 95% CI, 0.41 to 0.99; $p = 0.04$). A similar HR was reported in the MaNGO study (HR of 0.61), but no significant significance was appreciated. In the combined analysis of these two trials, the estimate of risk for relapse or death was similar with an HR: 0.69 (CI, 0.46 to 1.03; $p = 0.07$). Careful examination of the two independent studies reveals that the majority of patients in the NSGO- EC-9501/EORTC -55991 trial had stage I disease, whereas patients in the MaNGO-ILIADE-III had predominantly stage IIB–IIIC disease. Overall, these results should be interpreted with caution given the heterogeneity of the population studied.

The role of RT alone or in combination with CT was investigated in the GOG 249, a phase III clinical trial that compared the outcomes of pelvic irradiation versus VCB followed by paclitaxel/carboplatin in patients with high-risk early-stage EC. In the GOG 249 study, there was no PFS benefit of adjuvant CT over the standard EBRT (481).

The results of RTOG 0921, a phase II trial of postoperative IMRT with concurrent cisplatin and bevacizumab followed by four cycles of platinum and taxane, were recently reported. Eligible patients included those who had the following high-risk factors, namely, grade 3 carcinoma with >50% myometrial invasion, grade 2 or 3 disease with any cervical stromal invasion or known extrauterine extension confined to the pelvis. A total of 30 patients were eligible for treatment. The 2-year OS was 96.7% while the disease-free rate was 79.1%. Grade 3 toxicities occurring within the first 90 days included headache, fatigue, syncope, thromboembolic events, hyponatremia, hyperglycemia, vaginal infection, liver function tests elevation, febrile neutropenia, and fatigue. The authors noted that no patient developed an infield pelvic failure. The role of bevacizumab in this patient population continues to be explored (482).

Adjuvant and Advanced Disease

CT for adjuvant and advanced disease has been evaluated in multiple clinical trials. Trials have compared CT to RT as well as to other chemotherapeutic regimens.

The initial combinations to be explored included the use of cyclophosphamide with doxorubicin (483–485), followed by the addition of cyclophosphamide and doxorubicin to cisplatin (CAP) (486–489) and doxorubicin to cisplatin (AP) (490–494). Given the lack of additional benefit with a three-drug combination, the AP regimen became the “standard” to which more contemporary approaches were compared. It is important to note that the majority of these trials enrolled a heterogeneous patient population. Despite the lack of prospective data tailored to individual disease stage, these trials have provided constructive insights to the management of patients with advanced disease.

Chemotherapy versus Radiation Therapy

GOG 122 compared WART to eight cycles of doxorubicin/cisplatin CT in patients with *Stage III–IV disease who underwent surgical assessment and had a maximum of 2 cm of disease postoperatively* (332). The results demonstrated an improved PFS) and OS in patients with CT, with the reduction in recurrences largely due to reduced abdominal and distant sites of disease. The event rates were high in both arms. The Japanese GOG 2033 trial (495) randomized 385 women with *stages IC–III endometrioid adenocarcinomas* to WPR therapy versus CT using the regimen cisplatin, doxorubicin, and paclitaxel. PFS at 5 years was 83.5% versus 81.8% for whole pelvic RT and CT, respectively. However, in a subgroup analysis of patients with Stage IC over the age of 70 years with grade 3 endometrioid tumors or stage II or IIIA, CT was associated with improvement over pelvic RT both in terms of PFS (83.8% vs. 66.2% respectively, $p = 0.024$) and OS (89.7% vs. 73.6%, respectively, $p = 0.006$). GOG 184 (425) randomized 552 women with *stage III disease debulked to a maximum residual of 2 cm or less*, followed by volume-directed RT to doxorubicin and cisplatin (AP) or doxorubicin /cisplatin and paclitaxel (TAP). At 3 years, the proportion of patients alive and free from recurrence was similar (62% AP vs. 64% TAP). The overall hazard for recurrence or death of TAP compared to AP was 0.9 (95% CI, 0.69 to 1.17). In women with gross residual disease at the time of enrollment, TAP was associated with a 50% reduction in the risk of relapse or death (HR 0.50; 95% CI, 0.26 to 0.92).

GOG 258, a randomized phase III trial of cisplatin and tumor volume–directed irradiation followed by carboplatin and paclitaxel for optimally debulked advanced EC for stage III–IV EC was recently completed. Results are pending at this time.

Chemotherapy

Given the phase II activity of single-agent taxanes (496–498), the GOG conducted a randomized trial (GOG 163) (499) *for patients with primary stage III and IV or recurrent EC with* ***measurable disease*** comparing doxorubicin and cisplatin to doxorubicin with 24-hour paclitaxel and granulocyte-colony stimulating factor (G-CSF). There were no significant differences in RR (40% vs. 43%), PFS (median 7.2 vs. 6 months), or OS (median 12.6 vs. 13.6 months) for arm 1 and 2, respectively. The disadvantage of GOG 163 was the lack of platinum in the taxane-containing arm. The addition of a taxane was subsequently studied in GOG 177 (500) (*patients with primary stage III and IV or recurrent EC with* ***measurable disease***). GOG 177 utilized doxorubicin (60 mg/m^2 or 45 mg/m^2 in patients with prior RT) with cisplatin (50 mg/m^2) as the standard arm versus paclitaxel (160 mg/m^2) with doxorubicin (45 mg/m^2) and cisplatin (50 mg/m^2) and G-CSF as the investigational regimen. The primary objective was to determine if the addition of paclitaxel improved RR and PFS and OS. Two hundred seventy-three patients were enrolled, and the study was balanced for history of prior RT (50% vs. 46%), serous carcinoma (15% vs. 19%), stage, grade, and body surface area. Grade 3 and 4 platelet toxicity was higher in the three-drug arm (21% vs. 2%), but other hematologic toxicity was ameliorated with G-CSF: absolute neutrophil count 36% versus 50% and neutropenic fever 3% versus 2%. Non-hematologic grade 3, 4 toxicity was higher in the three-drug arm: GI 59% versus 39% and metabolic 25% versus

13%. Response rates were better with the triplet: CR 22% versus 7%, PR 36% versus 27%, and overall RR 57% versus 34%. Median PFS was 8.3 months versus 5.3 months ($p < 0.0005$), and median OS was 15.3 months versus 12.1 months ($p = 0024$). Responses were similar in serous (48%) versus nonserous histology (45%). Overall, paclitaxel, doxorubicin, cisplatin (TAP) chemotherapy increased 12-month survival to 59% compared to 50% with AP with an HR of 0.75 (0.56 to 0.998). Although the TAP regimen produced an improvement in RR and PFS, survival was minimally increased, and was associated with greater toxicity. The combination of paclitaxel and carboplatin as a doublet has also been evaluated in a variety of phase 2 trials and retrospective studies with RRs in the 43% to 80% range (501,502).

GOG 209, a randomized trial comparing doxorubicin, cisplatin, and paclitaxel (TAP) with carboplatin and paclitaxel (TC) (*stage III, IV or recurrent disease*), was recently reported. TC was not inferior to TAP in terms of PFS (median PFS of TAP vs. TP: 13.5 months vs. 13.3 months: HR 1.03) and OS (40.3 months vs. 36.5 months; HR: 1.05) based on interim analysis results. Overall, the toxicity profile favored TC with less sensory neuropathy (sensory neuropathy > Grade 1: 26% vs. 19%, $p < .01$) (503).

Sequence of Therapeutic Modalities

With the current data in mind, the sequence of therapy in patients with advanced surgically resected disease remains in question. Various approaches have been delineated. An RTOG phase II study (RTOG 9708) (424) was conducted to assess the feasibility, safety, toxicity, and patterns of recurrence and survival when CT was combined with adjuvant radiation for patients with high-risk EC. Pathologic requirements included grade 2 or 3 endometrial adenocarcinoma with either >50% myometrial invasion, cervical stromal invasion, or pelvic-confined extrauterine disease. Radiation included 45 Gy in 25 fractions to the pelvis along with cisplatin (50 mg/m^2) on days 1 and 28. Vaginal brachytherapy was performed after the external beam radiation. Four courses of cisplatin (50 mg/m^2) and paclitaxel (175 mg/m^2) were given at 4-week intervals following completion of RT. Forty-six patients were accrued to the study. Median follow-up was a median of 4.3 years. At 4 years, pelvic, regional, and distant recurrence rates were 2%, 2%, and 19%, respectively. OS and DFS rates at 4 years were 85% and 81%, respectively. Four-year rates for survival and DFS for Stage III patients were 77% and 72%, respectively. There were no recurrences for patients with stage IC, IIA, or IIB. Local-regional control was reported to be excellent following combined modality treatment in all patients suggesting additive effects of CT and radiation. Distant metastases continued to occur in more advanced-staged patients.

Secord and colleagues (504) reported a multicenter evaluation of sequential multimodality therapy and clinical outcome for the treatment of advanced EC. A multicenter retrospective analysis of patients with surgical stages III and IV EC from 1993 to 2007 was conducted. Inclusion criteria included a comprehensive staging procedure including hysterectomy, BSO, +/− selective pelvic/aortic lymphadenectomy, and treatment with adjuvant CT and radiation. One hundred and nine patients with advanced-stage EC were identified who received postoperative adjuvant therapies; 41% (n = 45) CT followed by radiation and then further CT (CRC), 17% (n = 18) radiation followed by CT (RC), and 42% (n = 46) CT followed by radiation (CR). There was no difference in the frequency of adverse effects due to either CT ($p = 0.35$) or RT ($p = 0.14$), dose modifications ($p = 0.055$), or delays ($p = 0.80$) between the various sequencing modalities. There was a significant difference between adjuvant treatment groups for both OS (log rank $p = 0.011$) and PFS (log rank $p = 0.025$), with those receiving CRC having a superior 3-year OS (88%) and PFS (69%) compared to RC (54% and 47%) or CR (57% and 52%). After adjusting for stage, age, grade, race, histology, and cytoreduction status, the OS HR for therapy was 5.74 (95% CI, 1.96 to 16.77) for RC and 2.6 (95% CI, 1.01 to 6.71) for CR, compared to CRC, $p = 0.003$. When the analysis was restricted to optimally cytoreduced patients, those who were treated with RC were at higher risk for disease progression (HR = 3.53 [95% CI, 1.29 to 9.71]), $p = 0.024$, and death (HR = 7.24 [95% CI, 2.25 to 23.37]), $p = 0.001$, than patients who received sequential CRC. The authors reported that sequential CRC was associated with improved survival in women with advanced-stage disease compared to other sequencing modalities with a similar adverse effect profile.

Metastatic/Recurrent Disease

The role of CT in the recurrent/metastatic setting remains palliative and minimizing side effects is of equal importance when selecting a regimen. Previously discussed were the trials enrolling patients with metastatic disease, namely GOG 163, 177, and GOG 209 (499,500,504) As the role of CT in the postoperative setting has expanded, the choices in the recurrent/metastatic setting have shifted and in some cases narrowed. Options and choices are dependent on prior treatment, and in some cases, disease-free interval. The most commonly used single agents today based on RRs of at least 20% include cisplatin, carboplatin, doxorubicin, epirubicin, ifosfamide, docetaxel, paclitaxel, and topotecan.

The RR to **cisplatin** dosages of 50 to 60 mg/m^2 given every 3 weeks was similar in patients with prior (25%) (483,505) and no prior CT (21%) (506–508). **Carboplatin** given in dosages of 300 to 400 mg/m^2 every 4 weeks has been associated with RRs of 29% (509–511), which is similar to cisplatin. **Doxorubicin** in dosages of 55 to 60 mg/m^2 has been associated with an overall RR of 26% (483,512,513) and **epirubicin** with a RR of 26% (514). **Liposomal doxorubicin** was reported in a GOG study of 46 patients receiving 50 mg/m^2 every 4 weeks with an overall RR of 9.5% (95% CI, 2.7% to 26%) (515). It is important to note that 32 patients had received prior doxorubicin therapy. A second study evaluated its efficacy in 19 patients without prior CT and resulted in a 21% RR (516). Of the antimetabolites, **5-fluorouracil** was given in dosages of 15 mg/kg for five consecutive days and then every other day until dose-limiting toxicity occurred. It has displayed a 21% RR in 34 patients, whereas **methotrexate** (517) and **mercaptopurine** (518) have been inactive. **Vincristine** given on a weekly schedule was associated with a RR of 18% in 33 untreated patients (519), but dose-limiting neurotoxicity was substantial. In a phase 2 trial of **paclitaxel** conducted by the GOG (496), 28 patients with recurrent or advanced EC received a dose of 250 mg/m^2 every 21 days. Patients who had received prior pelvic irradiation were treated at an initial dose of 200 mg/m^2. CRs were noted in four patients (14%) and PRs in six (21%) for an overall RR of 36%. A more contemporary GOG study evaluated paclitaxel at 200 mg/m^2 (175 mg/m^2 with prior RT) every 3 weeks in pretreated patients showing an overall RR of 27.3% (95% CI, 15% to 42.8%). The median duration of response was 4.2 months, with an OS of 10.3 months (498). A similar study showed a RR of 43% (95% CI, 6% to 80%) in patients who had all previously been treated with platinum-based therapy (520). A multicenter trial recently reported showed a RR of 21% with PFS of 12 weeks and OS of 43 weeks in 35 patients receiving weekly **docetaxel** at 35 mg/m^2 (497). **Topotecan** was evaluated in a phase 2 trial of untreated advanced or recurrent EC administered initially at 1.5 mg/m^2 every day for 5 days every 3 weeks. The trial was suspended for toxicity, but reopened and completed at 1 mg/m^2 q day for 5 days (or 0.8 mg/m^2/d for patients with prior RT). An overall RR of 20% was seen, with median duration of response of 8 months and OS of 6.5 months (521). A subsequent smaller study by Traina et al. using weekly topotecan dosing of 2.5 to 4.0 mg/m^2 on 2 of 3 weeks' schedule followed by 1 week off showed one PR for 54 weeks with two patients having stable disease (SD) for 15 weeks each. Only two patients required dose reduction for toxicity using the weekly schedule (522).

Epothilones are a novel class of nontaxane microtubule-stabilizing agents that are currently approved for the management of advanced breast cancer. Ixabepilone was recently reported to have an objective

RR of 12%, with a PFS of 2.9 months and a SD in for at least 8 weeks in 60% of patients (523).

Regardless of the available choices, responses to each successive line of therapy are short-lived. As such, focus has centered on the molecular basis of EC and potential targeted agents.

GENETIC CHANGES IN EC AND TARGETED THERAPY

The molecular background of EC provides a platform that lends itself to targeted therapeutics in patients with advanced recurrent or metastatic disease. Historically, ECs have been classified into two types: Type I and Type II cancers. Although our current practice is at this time guided by this classification, it is important to note that The Cancer Genome Atlas Research Network that has reclassified ECs into four molecular groups: (1) POLE (ultra-, mutated), (2) microsatellite unstable tumors, (3) copy-number high tumors with TP53 mutations, and (4) other tumors without these molecular alterations (524).

Biologic agents targeting molecular components are currently under development in numerous clinical trials. Focus has centered on specific histologic subtype- and/or biomarker-driven patient stratification. Evidence suggests that not only are type I and II endometrial tumors distinct entities with diversified genotypic and phenotypic profile (**Table 21.16**), but patients within each subtype may also differ molecularly. Hence, efforts have focused on the application of personalized therapies by utilizing biomarkers able to discriminate patients' dominant profile (11,525).

The PI3K/AKT/ mammalian target of rapamycin (mTOR) pathway represents a major signaling pathway downstream of several growth factor receptor kinases (e.g., epidermal growth factor receptor (EGFR), platelet-derived growth factor receptor (PDGFR), fibroblast growth factor receptor (FGFR), and insulin growth factor receptor and is well known to have a pivotal role in cell survival and growth (526,527). The PI3K/AKT/PTEN pathway is the most commonly altered pathway in type I EC (528). Activation of PI3K leads to the phosphorylation of a secondary messenger to form PIP3 (phosphatidylinositol 3, 4, 5-triphosphate). This process is regulated by PTEN, which dephosphorylates PIP3 to PIP2. Activation of PI3K, resulting in PIP3 subsequently leads to AKT activation. AKT promotes cell growth, proliferation, reduces apoptosis, and increases angiogenesis. Two important regulators of the process include the mammalian target of rapamycin complexes mTORC 1 and 2.

The most common mechanisms of PI3K activation are loss of the phosphatase and tensin homologue (PTEN) tumor suppressor protein function and activating mutations in catalytic PI3K subunit, p110α, which is encoded by the *PIK3CA* gene. Cells that are deficient in PTEN may have a resulting activation of the PI3K pathway. The function of the tumor suppressor gene *PTEN* includes inhibition of cell migration, spreading, and adhesion (529–533). The *PTEN* gene is located on chromosome 10q23, and about 40% of endometrial

TABLE 21.16. Molecular Aberrations of EC by Type

Molecular Aberration	Type I (Endometrioid) EC (%)	Type II (Nonendometrioid) EC (%)	Aberrant Pathway
PTEN loss	80–83	5	PI3K/AKT/mTOR pathway
PIK3CA			
mutation	24–40	20	PI3K/AKT/mTOR pathway
amplification	2–14	46	
PIK3R1 mutation	43	12	PI3K/AKT/mTOR pathway
AKT mutation	3	0	PI3K/AKT/mTOR pathway
K-RAS mutation	10–30	0–10	Ras-Raf-Mek-Erk pathway
MSI	15–45	0–5	–
β-catenin (CTNNB1) mutation	14–50	0	Wnt/β-catenin/LEF-1 pathway
E-cadherin loss	5–50	60–90	Wnt/β-catenin/LEF-1 pathway
TP53 mutation	10–20	90	Tumor suppression
p16 loss	8	45	Cyclin D/CDK4-CDK6/RB
HER2			
over expression	3–10	32–43	Cell surface receptor
amplification	1	17–29	
FGFR-2 mutation	12–16	1	Cell surface receptor
EGFR			
over expression	46	34	
mutation	Unknown	0	
IGFIR over expression	78	unknown	cell surface receptor
Chromosomal Instability STK15, BUB1, CCNB2 LOH at multiple loci			–
EphA2 overexpression	48	unknown	transmembrane protein
EpCAM overexpression	Unknown	96	transmembrane protein
HIF1a overexpression	25%	80%	gene transcription nuclear protein
ARID1A mutation	29–40	18–26	transcription-regulating process

EC, Endometrial Cancer.

carcinomas display loss of heterozygosity of chromosome 10q23, which suggests the involvement of *PTEN* in this disease (529–534). *PTEN* mutations in 30% to 50% of EC tumors make this the most frequent genetic alteration known in this disease (533–535). Genes for the catalytic subunit of PI3K (PI3KCA) are frequently amplified (2% to 14% type I ECs, 46% type II) or mutated (30% type I–II) in EC, leading to constitutive activation (11).

mTOR is a conserved serine/threonine kinase that lies downstream of the phosphatidylinositol 3 kinase/PTEN/AKT pathway and is composed of two subunits, mTORC1 and mTORC2. Activated AKT phosphorylates mTOR directly or indirectly by phosphorylating TSC2 (Tuberous sclerosis complex 2), which in turn stimulates mTORC1. Subsequently, mTORC1 phosphorylates several transcription factors, namely, S6K-1 (ribosomal S6 kinase-1) and 4E-BP1 eukaryote translation initiation factor (4E-binding protein-1 [4EBP1]), thereby leading to the synthesis of proteins involved in proliferation and survival. The second subunit mTORC2 is well less defined, but may mediate activation of AKT in response to mTORC1 inhibitors (527,536,537).

Genomic aberrations in the PI3K pathway in EC has made this an attractive target for biologic agents (538). PI3K/AKT/mTOR pathway inhibitors undergoing active clinical investigation in EC have been investigated by Hennessy et al and Engelman (527,539). Of all the available inhibitors, the rapalogs temsirolimus (CCI-779; Wyeth), ridaforolimus (deforolimus; AP23573, MK-8669; Merck), and everolimus (RAD001; Novartis), which specifically inhibit mTORC-1, are the compounds more extensively tested in EC clinical trials thus far (540).

Preliminary results of a phase II trial (541) of **temsirolimus** in recurrent or metastatic EC (CT naïve, with up to one prior line of hormonal therapy) demonstrated encouraging results with five confirmed PRs (26%) out of 19 evaluable patients. Three of the PRs were in patients with papillary serous tumors. Evaluation of a second cohort, women who must have had treatment with one prior regimen of cytotoxic CT, revealed an RR of 7% (2/27). Overall, temsirolimus activity was seen in all histologic subgroups and grades, regardless of PTEN loss. The most frequent drug-related toxicities were fatigue, mucocutaneous irritation (acne-like maculopapular rashes, mucositis, stomatitis, and diarrhea), and pneumonitis. Grade 3 toxic effects were rare and included lymphopenia, neutropenia, thrombocytopenia, hyperglycemia, and hyperlipidemia. Temsirolimus has also been studied in combination with paclitaxel/carboplatin and has demonstrated good tolerability in a phase I trial (542), prompting the initiation of a phase II study. A recently reported GOG study combining temsirolimus with alternating hormones, megestrol acetate, and tamoxifen, was closed secondary to high levels of venous thrombosis and insufficient additional activity to warrant further study (543). Temsirolimus is currently being explored in combination with other cytotoxic and biologic agents, such as carboplatin/paclitaxel, pegylated liposomal doxorubicin, bevacizumab, AMG386, and AZD2171.

Two phase 2 clinical trials (544,545) have demonstrated clinical responses to intravenous **ridaforolimus** (12.5 mg/d for 5 days every other week) in CT-treated patients (544). A PR rate of 7.7% and an SD rate of 58% to oral ridaforolimus in chemotherapy-naïve patients (545) was also noted. In one study (546), patients with unresectable stage III or IVA or metastatic disease were randomized to oral ridaforolimus (40 mg for 5 d/wk) versus medroxyprogesterone (200 mg/d) or megestrol (60 mg/d). Interim analysis of the first 114 patients demonstrated a median PFS of 36 months for ridaforolimus and 1.9 months for progestin therapy (HR 0.53, $p = 0.008$) with grade 3/4 toxicities of hyperglycemia (19%) and anemia (9%). A trial investigating the combination of ridaforolimus with carboplatin/paclitaxel is underway. In a recent phase II trial (547), 35 heavily pretreated patients with recurrent endometrioid EC received oral **everolimus** at a dose of 10 mg daily. Results were encouraging with 43% and 21% of patients achieving SD at 8 and 16 weeks, respectively. Most common drug-related toxicities included abdominal pain (28%), nausea and vomiting (21%), fatigue, anemia, and lymphopenia. An attempt to correlate response to the molecular status of the primary tumor failed to reveal any significant predictive marker although a trend for K-RAS mutation correlation with therapy resistance was noticed (548).

Recently reported was a study of everolimus and letrozole (549). Everolimus was administered orally at 10 mg daily and letrozole was administered orally at 2.5 mg daily. The primary end point was the clinical benefit rate (CBR). Thirty-five patients were evaluable for response. The CBR was 40% (14 of 35 patients). The confirmed objective RR was 32% (Nine patients had CR while two patients had PR). None of the patients discontinued treatment as a result of toxicity. Currently, GOG 3007 is investigating the combination of everolimus and letrozole or hormonal therapy in advanced EC.

Microsatellite instability (MSI) is found in 20% to 45% of type I tumors (0% to 5% type II tumors), and is caused by inactivation of DNA repair genes such as MLH1, MSH2, MSH6, and PMS2 (550–552). Tumors with MSI have instability (insertions and deletions) in the simple repeated sequences found in coding and noncoding elements of many genes. Resulting frame shift mutations may inactivate some genes including *PTEN*. MSI was first described in HNPCC. One of the most common extracolonic tumors associated with this disease is EC, and MSI has been demonstrated in both hereditary and sporadic tumors (553). MSI in EC has been reported to be between 9% and 43% (546,554–558). In 71% to 92% of sporadic EC, MSI has been found to be associated with hypermethylation of the *hMLH1* promoter region, whereas it seems to be less common in the promoter region of *hMSH2* (376,559). It is likely that methylation of the promoter region is an important mechanism of *hMLH1* gene inactivation in EC (560–562) and a precursor to MSI. Too few studies have been done to reach any conclusion regarding the importance of MSI as a prognostic factor in EC, although defects in MMR systems may alter responsiveness to CT or radiation (563,564) Deletions or mutations of the *PTEN* gene, and MSI due to hypermethylation of the promoter for the mismatch repair gene, *hMLH1*, are both relatively common and early events in the development of a significant proportion of type I endometrioid adenocarcinomas. In contrast, these molecular alterations do not appear to be critical in the pathogenesis of serous or clear cell carcinoma. However, mutations in the *p53* gene are found with high frequency not only in invasive serous carcinoma but also in EIC (302,565), the noninvasive precursor of serous carcinoma, suggesting that a different pathway is followed in the development of the second type of endometrial adenocarcinoma.

TP53 is a tumor suppressor gene, the product of which is a protein involved in the regulation of the cell cycle at the G_1 checkpoint, permitting replication of cells that have acquired various mutations. Mutations of the *p53* gene often result in a protein with a longer half-life, which accumulates in the cell. Upregulation of wild-type (i.e., nonmutated) *p53* may occur after DNA damage and also results in overexpression that is detectable by immunohistochemistry. This appears to be an early event in the development of serous carcinoma, but it is a late event in ECs for which it serves as an indicator of poor prognosis. In addition to the very frequent overexpression of p53 protein in serous carcinoma (566), it has also been related to a higher FIGO stage, clear cell histology, higher histologic grade, and increased depth of myometrial invasion (566–569). Lundgren et al. (570) studied p53 in relation to clinicopathologic variables in 376 consecutive patients with EC stages I-IV. p53 overexpression was found to be a strong significant factor with regard to relapse-free survival in univariate analysis, but it failed to retain its significance when submitted to multivariate analysis.

In contrast, p53 mutations are not often found in type I, low-grade endometrioid tumors (560). This suggests that different subgroups of ECs have different genetic pathways. Much more work is needed to understand the genetic mechanics at play and to translate this into use within the clinical and therapeutic field (561).

The EFGR/Her/ErbB family is composed of four structurally similar tyrosine kinase–functioning receptors: EGFR (, Her1),

ErbB2 (Her2/neu), ErbB3 (Her3), and ErbB4 (Her4). Their activation triggers a cascade of events ultimately leading to cell proliferation and survival (562). This molecular family has garnered a great deal of interest given that it activates important downstream pathways including vascular endothelial growth factor (VEGF), PI3K/AKT, and Ras/Raf/MEK (571). EGFR family-directed therapies include both small molecule tyrosine kinase inhibitors (e.g., erlotinib, gefitinib, and lapatinib) and anti-EGFR monoclonal antibodies (e.g., cetuximab and trastuzumab). Yet, despite EGFR overexpression in both EC subtypes (572), and favorable preclinical studies using EGF receptor antagonists (573,574), clinical trials in unselected EC population have shown little promise. For historical purposes, Erlotinib (Tarceva, Genentech) (150 mg/d orally) was evaluated in 32 assessable women with CT-naive, recurrent, or metastatic EC 615 (575). One prior line of hormonal therapy was permitted. The overall RR was 13% (12.5% with confirmed PR lasting 2 to 36 months, and 47% with SD with a median duration of 3.7 months). A phase 2 trial was performed to evaluate the efficacy and safety of gefitinib (Iressa, AstraZeneca) in patients with persistent/recurrent EC. Women were treated with 500-mg oral gefitinib daily with PFS at 6 months as the primary end point. Four patients experienced PFS ≥6 months, and one had a CR that was not associated with an EGFR mutation. This treatment regimen was tolerable but lacked sufficient efficacy to warrant further evaluation in this setting (576). Lapatinib (Tykerb) was evaluated in GOG 229 D. The second stage accrual was not opened likely due to low activity.

HER2/neu is a proto-oncogene, the product of which is a transmembrane growth factor receptor, p185erb-2, which shares some homology with the EGFR. It is normally expressed at low levels in the cycling endometrium. HER-2/neu is frequently overexpressed or amplified in 10% to 30% of type I and 40% to 80% of type II ECs (577), and has been associated with advanced-stage (578), decreased differentiation, aggressive cell types, particularly including the clear cell type (579), and deep myometrial invasion. The significance of HER2/neu amplification or overexpression as a predictor of survival is somewhat unclear, with no apparent association of overexpression to outcome being identified in several studies (566,579–589), but a statistically significant relationship in most others even after adjusting for other known risk factors. In addition to its potential utility as an indicator of poor prognosis, systemic therapy using antibodies directed against the HER2/neu protein has been investigated for patients with tumors that express the protein at high levels. **Trastuzumab** (Herceptin, Genentech) monotherapy failed to demonstrate significant activity in the recent GOG 181-B study (590). No responses were achieved, although 12 of 34 women experienced stabilization. Given the higher rates of HER-2 overexpression seen in type II tumors, assessment of trastuzumab combined with carboplatin/paclitaxel in serous papillary tumors is underway.

Afatinib, an oral ErbB family blocker that covalently binds and irreversibly blocks all kinase-competent ErbB family members, demonstrated activity against HER 2 amplified uterine serous EC *in vitro* and *in vivo*. Afatinib resulted in inhibition of HER2/neu phosphorylation and inhibited the growth of HER2 neu amplified tumor xenografts (591). A phase II evaluation of Afatinib in patients with persistent or recurrent HER 2 positive uterine serous carcinoma (NCT02491099) is currently in progress.

The **RAS/RAF/MEK pathway** is involved in several crucial cellular functions including angiogenesis, cell cycle regulation, proliferation, and survival. The activation of *RAS* proto-oncogenes through either point mutations or gene amplification has been identified in various malignant tumors. Mutations in the K-*ras* oncogene have been reported in EC and also in endometrial hyperplasia, suggesting that K-*ras* activation may be an early event in the development of endometrioid malignancy. In most studies, the presence of K-*ras* mutations has not been related to stage, grade, depth of invasion, or survival (592–595). K-*ras* mutations may activate the PI3K pathway independent of traditional signaling (596,597). This pathway is under the direct control of upstream cell surface growth receptors that are often affected in EC. Besides the relatively high prevalence of K-*ras* mutations identified in EC (**Table 21.16**), recent data has also illustrated an interesting negative feedback loop involving pS6K. Ramjaun and colleagues recently reported that this pathway is activated in the presence of AKT blockade (598). MEK inhibitors and RAF kinase small molecule inhibitors are currently being investigated. The GOG has explored a single-agent phase II trial of the oral MEK inhibitor ***selumetinib*** (AZD6244) in patients pre-treated with recurrent or persistent EC. Although adequate RRs were achieved, frequent and severe side effects have halted this trial. Clinical trials under development have now focused on the simultaneous blockade of components of both Ras/Raf/MEK and PI3K/AKT/mTOR pathways (598–601).

Angiogenesis mediates the growth of several solid tumors including that of EC. Overexpression of VEGF has been associated with poor prognostic factors in EC such as deep myometrial invasion and LN metastasis (602–604). VEGF expression seems highly variable depending on histologic subtype and disease stage, with early-stage well-differentiated lesions expressing the highest levels (605). To date, treatment of recurrent EC with antiangiogenic agents has revealed mixed results.

The most significant developments in this class of agents have centered on suppressing the vascular endothelial growth factor receptor (VEGFR) ligand. **Bevacizumab** (Avastin, Roche) (15 mg IV every 3 weeks) was investigated in GOG 229E, a study in patients with recurrent or persistent measurable EC after receiving one or two prior cytotoxic regimens (606). Of 52 evaluable patients, 13.5% had objective response (one CR and six PRs) while 40.4% of patients survived progression-free for at least 6 months. Median PFS and OS were 4.2 and 10.5 months, respectively. Although no GI perforations or fistulas occurred, two episodes of grades 3–4 hemorrhage and thromboembolism were reported.

Recently reported were the results of two randomized phase 2 trials evaluating the addition of bevacizumab to carboplatin and paclitaxel in advance or recurrent EC. GOG-86 P was a three-arm trial that evaluated the addition of bevacizumab, temsirolimus, or ixabepilone to carboplatin and paclitaxel in 349 patients. There was no difference in PFS when compared to carboplatin and paclitaxel (607). In contrast, there was an improvement in median OS in the carboplatin/paclitaxel/bevacizumab arm when compared to the historical control, namely, GOG 209 (34 months vs. 22.7 months, $p < 0.039$). The MITO END-2 trial was a randomized phase 2 trial of 108 patients with advanced or recurrent EC. Patients were randomized to carboplatin and paclitaxel +/− bevacizumab. Bevacizumab was continued as maintenance therapy. There was a statistically significant improvement in the median PFS (12 vs. 8.7 months, $p = 0.036$). Although OS was not mature, there was a numerical increase in median OS of 23.5 vs. 18 months, $p = 0.24$) (608).

Recently reported was a two-stage phase 2 study of the combination of temsirolimus and bevacizumab in patients with recurrent or persistent EC. Treatment included bevacizumab 10 mg/kg every other week and temsirolimus 25 mg IV weekly. Forty-nine patients were evaluable. The regimen was associated with significant toxicity, namely, two GI–vaginal fistulas, one grade 3 epistaxis, two intestinal perforations, and one grade 4 thrombosis/embolism was reported. Twelve patients (24.5%) experienced clinical responses (1 complete and 11 PRs), and 23 patients (46.9%) survived progression free for at least 6 months. Median PFS and OS were 5.6 and 16.9 months, respectively (609).

Tyrosine kinase receptor inhibitors are among the various targeted therapeutics under investigation. These agents target several receptors allowing for the pharmacological disruption of several independent pathways. **Sunitinib malate** (Sutent, Pfizer) is an oral small molecule, multitargeted tyrosine kinase inhibitor that targets several receptor tyrosine kinases. In one study (610), 20 evaluable patients with recurrent or metastatic EC, previously treated with at most one CT regimen, received 50 mg sunitinib daily for 4 consecutive weeks followed by 2 weeks off. Three patients (15%) achieved PR and five (25%) stabilization of the disease, four of which were for more than 6 months. Median time to progression and OS were 2.5 and 19 months respectively.

Unfortunately, the antiangiogenic and antiproliferative properties of **sorafenib** (Nexavar, Bayer) (611) and **thalidomide** (Thalomid, Celgene) (612) did not lead to significant objective responses in the corresponding phase 2 clinical trials and were deemed to no further investigation.

New antiangiogenic agents recently studied in EC include the angiokinase inhibitors brivanib, cediranib, BIBF1120, and the VEGF-Trap aflibercept (GOG 229-F).

Powell and colleagues (613) reported a phase 2 trial of brivanib in recurrent or persistent EC. Eligible patients received up to two prior cytotoxic agents, had measurable disease and had a performance status of <2. Treatment consisted of brivanib 800 mg daily. Primary end points included PFS at 6 months and objective tumor response. Forty-three patients were eligible. Eight patients (18.6%) had responses (one CR and seven PRs) and 13 patients (30.2%) had a PFS at 6 months. The median PFS and OS was 3.3 and 10.7 months, respectively. Bender and colleagues (614) evaluated a phase 2 trial of cediranib in the treatment of persistent EC. Cediranib was administered at 30 mg daily. Forty-eight patients were evaluable for efficacy and toxicity. A PR was observed in 12.5% of patients. Fourteen patients (29%) had a 6-month event-free survival. Median PFS was 3.65 months and median OS was 12.5 months. Vascular disorders accounted for the majority of grade 3 toxicities that included hypertension and pulmonary embolus. Diarrhea and fatigue were also reported. One patient sustained a colonic perforation. BIBF-1120 (615) (Nintedanib), a potent small molecule triple receptor tyrosine kinase inhibitor of PDGFR alpha and beta, FGFR, and VEGFR were also recently reported. Patients were treated with single-agent Nintedanib at 200 mg daily. This agent failed to show sufficient activity. Coleman et al. (616) evaluated aflibercept in a similar patient population. Aflibercept, which targets VEGF and placental growth factor, was administered at 4 mg/kg IV q 14 days (q 28-day cycle). The PFS at 6 months was 41%; median PFS and OS were 2.9 months and 14.6 months, respectively. The agent was associated with significant grade 3 to 4 toxicities including cardiovascular, constitutional, hemorrhage, and metabolic toxicities.

Metformin is a biguanide drug that is widely used for the treatment of type II diabetes. Several studies have suggested that this agent can reduce cancer incidence among hyperglycemic patients. Since the first case report describing metformin-induced regression of AEH in one patient nonrespondent to progestogen therapy, a continuously growing body of evidence has brought metformin to the foreground of therapies against EC. Not only does this antidiabetic agent improve the negatively associated EC metabolic profile (insulin resistance, obesity, estrogen excess) (617,618) but it also exhibits activity against EC cells through antiproliferative, proapoptotic, antiangiogenic, and antimetastatic properties (619–625). Metformin is commonly thought of as an insulin sensitizer resulting in an improvement in insulin resistance, followed by a reduction in circulating insulin levels. Metformin inhibits complex I activity in the mitochondria (622), leading to the activation of its downstream target, AMPK, which regulates multiple signaling pathways controlling cellular proliferation, including inhibition of the mTOR pathway (623). Given the interrelationship between these two pathways, metformin is thought to behave as a novel mTOR inhibitor and has been shown to dramatically decrease proliferation in a number of different human cancer cell lines *in vitro* (624–627) Hanna et al. (628) demonstrated a synergistic relationship between paclitaxel and metformin against human EC cell lines (629). A prospective trial is currently conducted evaluating metformin effect in patients with EC.

The Poly (adenosine diphosphate ribose) polymerase (PARP) is a family of nuclear, multifunctional enzymes that mediates the recruitment of the DNA repair machinery through the base-excision repair pathway (630). The antineoplastic effect of PARP inhibitors stems from their ability to enhance the genomic instability of tumor cells by simultaneously targeting DNA repair pathways and exploiting their intrinsic deficiencies in the homologous recombination (HR) pathway through the phenomenon of synthetic lethality (630). PTEN loss is considered a component of BRCA-ness phenotype. It impedes repair of DNA double-strand breaks via HR, thereby creating cellular susceptibility to PARP inhibition (631). Preclinical data have shown a correlation between *in vitro* sensitivity to PARP inhibition and mutated PTEN status in EC cell lines (632), providing a strong rationale for testing PARP inhibitors in EC, especially type I, which harbors PTEN functional loss in 80% of cases. There is a variety of PARP inhibitors in clinical development, including olaparib, veliparib, and iniparib. A phase I study evaluating olaparib observed a dramatic clinical response in one BRCA mutation–negative patient with metastatic EC. After 6 weeks of treatment, complete resolution of symptoms as well as radiologic response of visceral metastases was noted (629).

Iniparib (BSI-201) was studied in the treatment of recurrent carcinosarcoma of the uterus in combination with carboplatin and paclitaxel.

Patients received paclitaxel 175 mg/m^2 IV over 3 hours, followed by carboplatin (AUC 6) plus iniparib 4 mg/kg IV twice weekly beginning on day one. Seventeen patients were evaluable for analysis. The observed proportion responding was 23.5% (4/17 patients). Iniparib plus paclitaxel and carboplatin did not show significant activity to warrant further study (633).

The Role of Immunotherapy in the Management of Patients with Uterine Cancer

Circumventing the multiple mechanisms of malignancy-induced immune suppression has recently dominated the field of oncology. Checkpoint inhibitors have demonstrated significant success in multiple disciplines. Recently, a phase 2 trial of pembrolizumab, a humanized monoclonal antibody to the PD-1 receptor, was conducted in patients with mismatch repair (MMR)–deficient tumors to address whether MMR-deficient tumors were more responsive to PD-1 blockade than MMR-proficient tumors. The authors reported that MMR-deficient cancers had higher objective RRs and improved PFS (634). In another study, Howitt et al. (635) reported that polymerase e-mutated and MSI ECs were associated with a high neoantigen load and a high number of tumor-infiltrating lymphocytes, which was counterbalanced by overexpression of PD-1 and PD-L1 (635). Multiple studies addressing the role of immunotherapy in EC are planned.

Management of Patients with Serous, Clear Cell Histologies

Serous cancer and, to a lesser extent, clear cell ECs tend to spread in a fashion similar to ovarian cancer with a high propensity for upper abdominal relapse. Therefore, whole abdomen radiation has been extensively studied historically in this group of patients (422). Given the mixed results with whole abdomen RT, the recognized patterns of disease spread and failure, and the findings of GOG 122 (332) supporting an increased role for CT, CT has increasingly been used to treat these high-risk histologies. On the basis of the RRs of paclitaxel and carboplatin in other tumors of serous histology, trials investigating paclitaxel and carboplatin in UPSCs have reported RRs of 60% to 70% (636,637). No randomized, prospective trials evaluating multimodality therapy specifically for early- or late-stage uterine serous carcinomas have been reported. A single-institution phase 2 trial for advanced-stage uterine papillary serous histology administered paclitaxel and platinum-based CT for three cycles followed by volume-directed

RT. Patients then received an additional three cycles of CT. The most common toxicity was hematologic and occurred during CT following RT. The PFS for the nine women treated is 46.4 months (638). A similar study administered four cycles of platinum with paclitaxel or epirubicin followed by whole pelvic and vaginal brachytherapy. The 5-year OS for this group was 58.9% (639). Currently, the role of trastuzumab is being explored in patients with uterine serous carcinoma.

With regard to stage I disease, the available data for designing a treatment plan is retrospective. A study of 74 stage I patients with UPSC between 1987 and 2004 who underwent complete staging at Yale University was reported (640). Patients were divided into those who had no residual cancer in the hysterectomy specimen versus those who did. Stage IA patients who had residual in the hysterectomy specimen and who were treated with platinum-based CT had no recurrences (n = 7) versus 6 of 14 (43%) who did not receive treatment. Of 15 patients with stage IB disease, there were no recurrences in the treated group but 10 of 13 nontreated patients (77%) recurred. Platinum-based CT was associated with improved PFS ($p < 0.01$) and OS ($p < 0.05$). Furthermore, no patient who received radiation to the vaginal cuff recurred at the cuff versus 6 of 31 (19%) of those who did not receive vaginal cuff irradiation (641). Recognizing the limits of retrospective studies, these data support the potential benefit of a regimen of platinum-based CT with cuff irradiation in patients with UPSC. Randomized, prospective data is needed to accurately define the best approach in these patients.

In 2009, the SGO produced a review of the management of women with serous EC (641). It was noted that as extrauterine spread was common, even in the setting of minimally invasive/noninvasive disease, surgical staging should be routinely performed. In addition, platinum-based CT should be considered in both early-staged and advanced-staged patients. In addition, the SGO also sponsored a review of clear cell carcinoma of the uterus that supported routine staging, and consideration of postoperative CT (642). The rarity of these tumor types has made histology-based clinical trial difficult to perform. It is hoped that as a better understanding of the molecular pathways evolve in EC, treatment based on histology may become more common. At the present time, using standard CT regimens, there is no data to support different therapies based on histology alone (17).

FUTURE DIRECTIONS

Over a decade ago, the National Cancer Institute convened an expert panel to develop research priorities in gynecologic cancers. The resulting report, Priorities of the Gynecologic Cancer PRG, specified that understanding tumor biology was the central key toward controlling gynecologic cancers. Now nearly a decade later, some hope for a better understanding of EC at a genetic and molecular level is being realized. The GOG 210 study, a prospective surgical pathologic study that created an annotated tissue repository from over 6,000 patients with more than 36,000 specimens serves as a resource for discovery and validation of predictive and prognostic biomarkers. In addition, the Genome Atlas Project has nearly completed an analysis of 500 ECs (endometrioid and serous types) with array-based analyses and second-generation sequencing that will provide information on genome copy number, gene expression profiles, methylation status, whole exome sequencing, and will completely sequence 10% of all cases. It is expected that the knowledge from these datasets will drive clinical research and patient care for the next decade. Increasingly, we can expect that therapies offered to our patients will be based on a more complete understanding of pathways, and that therapies may be matched to address specific genetic changes.

SUMMARY

EC is the most common gynecologic malignancy, and an understanding of presentation, surgical management, and treatment options is required for gynecologic oncologists. Surgical therapy is a mainstay of EC with lymphadenectomy and laparoscopy increasingly integrated. A thorough knowledge of the relationships between uterine factors and extrauterine disease spread is essential. Surgical staging defines extent of disease and largely defines risk of recurrence. Pelvic radiation is associated with better local control, but no improvement in survival for patients with stage I–II EC in randomized trials. CT is increasingly integrated into up-front management of advanced-stage EC, and may have a role in early-stage disease. Combination RT and CT is under evaluation. Targeted agents hold promise; however, a better understanding of molecular and genetic changes is required to improve efficacy.

INTERNATIONAL PERSPECTIVES

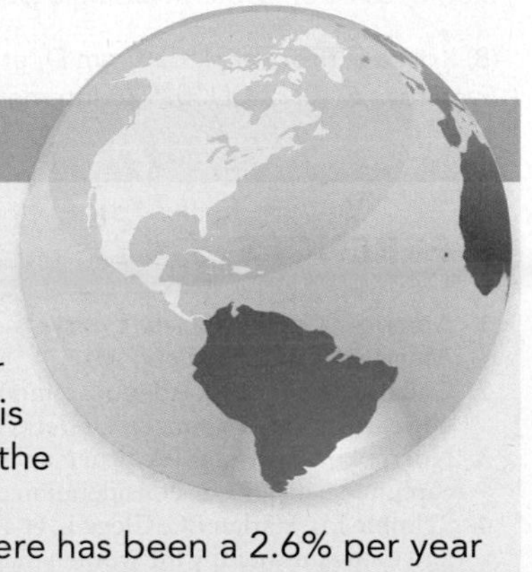

Endometrial Cancer in Canada

Helen MacKay, MD

The presentation, diagnosis, and management of EC as presented in the chapter by McMeekin et al. is applicable in the Canadian context. While the same data is used for decision making, the funding model and some choices are different than the American model of care.

As in the United States, the incidence of EC has been increasing. Since 2004 there has been a 2.6% per year increase in EC among Canadian women. Furthermore, while overall age-standardized mortality rates for cancer declined by 1.2% per year for females in Canada, there was a 2.8% increase in mortality rate associated with EC (2005–2010) (1). These trends are expected to continue. Factors contributing to this rise include the rise in obesity, aging population, the widespread decrease in the use of hormone replacement therapy, population level delays in childbearing, the decreasing rates of hysterectomy for benign disease, and the increasing prevalence of diabetes (2,3). As in other jurisdictions the Canadian Government recognizes that addressing the underlying causes, especially the rise in obesity, are essential if we are to reduce the incidence of this and other cancers.

(*continued*)

INTERNATIONAL PERSPECTIVES (*continued*)

Efforts are being made to optimize the management of EC in some Canadian jurisdictions. Cancer care Ontario (CCO) is developing an Endometrial Cancer Pathway working with multidisciplinary/multi-stakeholder groups utilizing guidelines developed by CCO's Program in Evidence-Based Care and considering multiple sources of evidence-based practice from several jurisdictions. In Canada, for most stages of EC and all cases where fertility-sparing options are being pursued, a fully trained gynecologic oncologist will be involved in the patients' care. The exception is in the management of those diagnosed with stage 1, grade 1 endometrioid EC where a general gynecologist could be involved. Review of all malignant cases by a pathologist who has a specialist interest in gynecologic malignancy is strongly encouraged. Referral to a genetic counselor where Lynch syndrome is suspected is standard of care. Recently, there has been a move toward some centers reporting mismatch repair protein status on all endometrioid ECs.

Canadian investigators recognize the limitations of the dualistic model of EC and the limitations of the current risk stratification systems. Among others, they are seeking to develop practical pared down classifiers of the TCGA subgroups (4), which may ultimately lead to a clinically relevant tool to better define prognostic groups (5,6). Most recognize the need for the development of better validated risk stratification models to select the optimal therapeutic approach for women.

There are no biologic agents approved for the treatment of EC in Canada. Women with metastatic or recurrent EC are managed by multidisciplinary teams. Standard of care systemic therapy for EC based on GOG 209 (6) and earlier studies is carboplatin paclitaxel or a platinum anthracycline combination. Endocrine therapy is considered for those with lower grade ER or PR-positive tumors (7). Referral for clinical trials is strongly encouraged given the limited therapeutic option for the patient with metastatic or recurrent disease.

(1) Canadian Cancer Statistics 2015: Special topic predictions of the future burden of cancer in Canada. http://www.cancer.ca

(2) http://www.statcan.gc.ca

(3) Crosbie EJ, Zwahlen M, Kitchener HC, et al. Body mass index, hormone replacement therapy, and endometrial cancer risk: a meta-analysis. *Cancer Epidemiol Biomark Prev.* 2010;19(12):3119–3130.

(4) Cancer Genome Atlas Research N, Kandoth C, Schultz N, et al. Integrated genomic characterization of endometrial carcinoma. *Nature.* 2013;497(7447):67–73.

(5) Stelloo E, Bosse T, Nout RA, et al. Refining prognosis and identifying targetable pathways for high-risk endometrial cancer; a TransPORTEC initiative. *Modern Pathol.* 2015;28(6):836–844.

(6) Talhouk A, McConechy MK, Leung S, et al. A clinically applicable molecular-based classification for endometrial cancers. *Br J Cancer.* 2015;113(2):299–310.

(7) Miller D, Filiaci V, Fleming G, et al. Randomized phase III noninferiority trial of first line chemotherapy for metastatic or recurrent endometrial carcinoma: a Gynecologic Oncology Group study. *Gynecol Oncol.* 2012;125:771.

(8) Kokka F, Brockbank E, Oram D, et al. Hormonal therapy in advanced or recurrent endometrial cancer [serial online]. *Cochrane Database Syst Rev.* 2010;12:CD007926.International Perspectives

REFERENCES

1. American Cancer Society. *Cancer Facts and Figures 2016*. Atlanta, GA: American cancer Society; 2016.
2. Gallup DG, Stock RJ. Adenocarcinoma of the endometrium in women 40 years of age or younger. *Obstet Gynecol.* 1984;64:417–420.
3. Norris HJ, Tavassoli FA, Kurman RJ. Endometrial hyperplasia and carcinoma, diagnostic consideration. *Am J Surg Pathol.* 1988;7:839–847.
4. Trimble EL, Harlan LC, Clegg L, et al. Pre-operative imaging, surgery, and adjuvant therapy for women diagnosed with cancer of the corpus uteri in community practice in the US. *Gynecol Oncol.* 2005;96:741–748.
5. Creasman W, Odicino F, Maisonneuve P, et al. Carcinoma of the corpus uteri. *Int J Gynecol Obstet.* 2006;95(Suppl 1):S105–S143.
6. Kitchener H, Trimble EL. Endometrial cancer state of the science meeting. *Int J Gynecol Cancer.* 2009;19:134–140.
7. Curtin J, Clarke-Pearson DL. *Pathways to Progress in Women's Cancer. A Research Agenda Proposed by the Society of Gynecologic Oncology*. Chicago, IL: The Society of Gynecologic Oncology; 2012.
8. Naumann RW, Coleman R. The use of adjuvant radiation therapy in early endometrial cancer by members of the Society of Gynecologic Oncologists in 2005. *Gynecol Oncol.* 2007;105:7–12.
9. Singh M, Zaino R, Filiaci V, et al. Relationship of estrogen and progesterone receptors to clinical outcome in metastatic endometrial carcinoma: a Gynecologic Oncology Group study. *Gynecol Oncol.* 2007;106(2):325–333.
10. Engelsen I, Akslen LA, Salverson HB. Biologic markers in endometrial cancer treatment. *APMIS.* 2009;117:693–707.
11. Dedes K, Wetterskog D, Ashworth A, et al. Emerging therapeutic targets in endometrial cancer. *Nat Rev Clin Oncol.* 2011;8:261–271.
12. Plentl AA, Friedman EA. *Lymphatic System of the Female Genitalia: The Morphologic Basis of Oncologic Diagnosis and Therapy.* Philadelphia, PA: WB Saunders; 1971:116.
13. Ries LAG, Eisner CL, Kosary, et al. *SEER Cancer Statistics Review, 1973–1997.* Bethesda, MD: National Cancer Institute; 2000:171–181.
14. Parkin DM, Whelan SL, Ferlay J, et al. *Cancer Incidence in Five Continents*, Vol. 7. IARC Sci. Pub. No. 143. Lyon: IARC; 1997.
15. Yap S, Matthews R. Racial and ethnic disparities in cancer of the uterine corpus. *J Nat Med Assoc.* 2006;98:1930–1933.
16. Maxwell GL, Tian C, Risinger J, et al. Racial disparity in survival among patients with advanced/recurrent endometrial adenocarcinoma: a Gynecologic Oncology Group study. *Cancer.* 2006;107:2197–2205.
17. McMeekin DS, Filiaci V, Thigpen JT, et al. Importance of histology in advanced and recurrent endometrial cancer patients participating in

first-line chemotherapy trials: a Gynecologic Oncology Group study. *Gynecol Oncol.* 2007;106:16–22.
18. Ferguson S, Olshen A, Levine D, et al. Molecular profiling of endometrial cancers from African American and Caucasian women. *Gynecol Oncol.* 2006;101:209–213.
19. Watson P, Lynch H. Extracolonic cancer in hereditary nonpolyposis colorectal cancer. *Cancer.* 1993;71:677–685.
20. Lu K, Dinh M, Kohlman W, et al. Gynecologic cancer as a "sentinel cancer" for women with hereditary nonpolyposis colorectal cancer syndrome. *Obstet Gynecol.* 2005;105:569–574.
21. Berends M, Wu Y, Sijmons R, et al. Toward new strategies to select young endometrial cancer patients for mismatch repair gene mutation analysis. *J Clin Oncol.* 2003;23:4364–4370.
22. Schmeler K, Lynch H, Chen L, et al. Prophylactic surgery to reduce the risk of gynecologic cancers in the Lynch syndrome. *N Engl J Med.* 2006;354:261–269.
23. Hornreich G, Beller U, Lavie O, et al. Is uterine serous papillary carcinoma a *BRCA1*-related disease? Case report and review of the literature. *Gynecol Oncol.* 1999;75:300–304.
24. Levine D, Lin O, Barakat R, et al. Risk of endometrial cancer associated with BRCA mutation. *Gynecol Oncol.* 2001;80:395–398.
25. Beiner M, Fich A, Rosen B, et al. The risk of endometrial cancer in women with *BRCA1* and *BRCA2* mutations. A prospective study. *Gynecol Oncol.* 2007;104:7–10.
26. Barak F, Milgrom R, Laitman Y, et al. The rate of predominant Jewish mutations in the BRCA1, BRCA2, MSH2, MSH6 genes in unselected Jewish endometrial cancer patients. *Gynecol Oncol.* 2010;119:511–515.
27. Bokhman JV. Two pathologenic types of endometrial carcinoma. *Gynecol Oncol.* 1983;10:237–246.
28. Kovalev S, Marchenko ND, Gugliotta BG, et al. Loss of p53 function in uterine papillary serous carcinoma. *Hum Pathol.* 1998;29:613–619.
29. Cao QJ, Belbin T, Socci N, et al. Distinctive gene expression profiles by cDNA microarrays in endometrioid and serous carcinomas of the endometrium. *Int J Gynecol Pathol.* 2004;23:321–329.
30. Akhmedkhanov A, Zeleniuch-Jaquotte A, Toniolo P. Role of exogenous and endogenous hormones in endometrial cancer. *Ann NY Acad Sci.* 2001;943:296–315.
31. Key TJA, Pike MC. The dose effect relationship between unopposed estrogens and endometrial mitotic rate: its central role in explaining and predicting endometrial cancer risk. *Br J Cancer.* 1998;57:205–212.
32. Henderson BE, Feigelson HS. Hormonal carcinogenesis. *Carcinogenesis.* 2000;21:427–433.
33. McDonald TW, Malkasian GD, Gaffey TA. Endometrial cancer associated with feminizing ovarian tumor and polycystic ovarian disease. *Obstet Gynecol.* 1977;49:654–658.
34. Smith DC, Prentice R, Thompson DJ, et al. Association of exogenous estrogen and endometrial carcinoma. *N Engl J Med.* 1975;293:1164–1167.
35. Ziel HK, Finkle WD. Increased risk of endometrial carcinoma among users of conjugated estrogens. *N Engl J Med.* 1975;293:1167–1170.
36. Schottenfeld D. Epidemology of endometrial neoplasia. *J Cell Biochem Suppl.* 1995;23:151–159.
37. MacDonald PC, Edman CD, Hemsell DL, et al. Effect of obesity on conversion of plasma androstenedione to estrone in postmenopausal women with and without endometrial cancer. *Am J Obstet Gynecol.* 1978;130:448–455.
38. Judd HL, Lucas WE, Yen SS. Serum 17 beta-estradiol and estrone levels in postmenopausal women with and without endometrial cancer. *J Clin Endocrinol Metab.* 1976;43:272–278.
39. Grodin, JM, Siiteri PK, MacDonald PC. Source of estrogen production in postmenopausal women. *J Clin Endocrinol Metab.* 1973;36:207–214.
40. Weiss J, Saltzman B, Doherty J, et al. Risk factors for the incidence of endometrial cancer according to the aggressiveness of disease. *Am J Epidemiol.* 2006;164:56–62.
41. Elwood JM, Cole P, Rothman KJ, et al. Epidemiology of endometrial cancer. *J Natl Cancer Inst.* 1977;59:1055–1060.
42. O'Mara BA, Byers T, Schoenfeld E. Diabetes mellitus and cancer risk: a multisite case-control study. *J Chronic Dis.* 1985;38:435–441.
43. Parazzini F, La Vecchia C, Negri E, et al. Diabetes and endometrial cancer: an Italian case-control study. *Int J Cancer.* 1999;81:539–542.
44. Kazer RR. Insulin resistance, insulin-like growth factor I and breast cancer: a hypothesis. *Int J Cancer.* 1995;62:403–406.
45. Rutanen EM. Insulin-like growth factors in endometrial function. *Gynecol Endocrinol.* 1998;12:399–406.
46. Nagamani M, Stuart CA. Specific binding and growth-promoting activity of insulin in endometrial cancer cells in culture. *Am J Obstet Gynecol.* 1998;179:6–12.
47. Killackey MA, Hakes TB, Pierce VK. Endometrial adenocarcinoma in breast cancer patients receiving antiestrogens. *Cancer Treat Rep.* 1985;69:237–238.
48. Fornander T, Cedermark B, Mattsson A, et al. Adjuvant tamoxifen in early breast cancer: occurrence of new primary cancers. *Lancet.* 1989;21:117–120.
49. Fisher B, Costantino JP, Redmond CK, et al. Endometrial cancer in tamoxifen-treated breast cancer patients: findings from the National Surgical Adjuvant Breast and Bowel Project (NSABP) B-14. *J Natl Cancer Inst.* 1994;86:527–537.
50. Magriples U, Naftolin F, Schwartz PE, et al. High-grade endometrial carcinoma in tamoxifen-treated breast cancer patients. *J Clin Oncol.* 1993;11:485–490.
51. Barakat RR, Wong G, Curtin JP, et al. Tamoxifen use in breast cancer patients who subsequently develop corpus cancer is not associated with a higher incidence of adverse histologic features. *Gynecol Oncol.* 1994;55:164–168.
52. van Leeuwen FE, Bernadette J, Coebergh JW, et al. Risk of endometrial cancer after tamoxifen treatment of breast cancer. *Lancet.* 1994;343:448–452.
53. Fornander T, Hellstrom A-C, Moberger B. Descriptive clinicopathologic study of 17 patients with endometrial cancer during or after adjuvant tamoxifen in early breast cancer. *J Natl Cancer Inst.* 1993;85:1850–1855.
54. DeMichele A, Troxel A, Berlin J, et al. Impact of raloxifiene or tamoxifen use on endometrial cancer risk: a population based case-control study. *J Clin Oncol.* 2008:26:4151–4159.
55. Perez E. Appraising adjuvant aromatase inhibitor therapy. *Oncologist.* 2006;11:1058–1069.
56. The Writing Group for the PEPI Trial. Effects of hormone replacement therapy on endometrial histology in postmenopausal women: the postmenopausal estrogen/progestin interventions trial. *JAMA.* 1996;275:370–375.
57. Maxwell GL, Schildkraut J, Calingaert B, et al. Progestin and estrogen potency of combination oral contraceptives and endometrial cancer risk. *Gynecol Oncol.* 2006;103:535–540.
58. Stanford JL, Brinton LA, Berman ML, et al. Oral contraceptives and endometrial cancer: do other risk factors modify the association. *Int J Cancer.* 1993;54:243–248.
59. Creasman WT, Morrow CP, Bundy BN, et al. Surgical pathologic spread patterns of endometrial cancer: a Gynecologic Oncology Group study. *Cancer.* 1987;60:2035–2041.
60. Mariani A, Dowdy S, Keeney G, et al. High-risk endometrial cancer subgroups: candidates for target based adjuvant therapy. *Gynecol Oncol.* 2004;95:120–126.
61. Morrow CP, Bundy BN, Kumar RJ, et al. Relationship between surgical-pathological risk factors and outcome in clinical stages I and II carcinoma of the endometrium. A Gynecologic Oncology Group study. *Gynecol Oncol.* 1991;40:55.
62. Rabban JT, Zaloudek CJ. Minimal uterine serous carcinoma: current concepts in diagnosis and prognosis. *Pathology.* 2007;39:125–133.
63. Wheeler DT, Bell KA, Kurman RJ, et al. Minimal uterine serous carcinoma: diagnosis and clinicopathologic correlation. *Am J Surg Pathol.* 2000;24:797–806.
64. Nakagawa-Okamura C, Sato S, Tsuji I, et al. Effectiveness of mass screening for endometrial cancer. *Acta Cytol.* 2002;46:277–283.
65. Vuento MH, Maatela JI, Tyrkko JE, et al. A longitudinal study of screening for endometrial cancer by endometrial biopsy in diabetic females. *Int J Gynecol Cancer.* 1995;5:390–395.
66. ACOG Committee Opinion. Routine cancer screening. *Obstet Gynecol.* 2006;108:1611–1613.
67. Society of Gynecologic Oncologists. Practice guidelines: uterine corpus-endometrial cancer. *Oncology.* 1998;12:122–126.
68. Gambrell RD Jr, Massey FM, Castenada TA, et al. Use of the progesterone challenge test to reduce the risk of endometrial cancer. *Obstet Gynecol.* 1980;55:732–738.
69. Gorodeski IG, Geier A, Lunenfeld B, et al. Progesterone challenge test in postmenopausal women with pathological endometrium. *Cancer Invest.* 1988;6:481–485.
70. Hunter JE, Tritz DE, Howell MG, et al. The prognostic and therapeutic implications of cytologic atypia in patients with endometrial hyperplasia. *Gynecol Oncol.* 1994;55:66–71.
71. Kurman R, Kaminski P, Norris H. The behavior of endometrial hyperplasia. A long-term study of "untreated" hyperplasia in 170 patients. *Cancer.* 1985;56:403–411.
72. Trimble CL, Kauderer J, Zaino R, et al. Concurrent endometrial carcinoma in women with a biopsy diagnosis of atypical endometrial hyperplasia: a Gynecologic Oncology Group study. *Cancer.* 2006;106:812–819.

73. King A, Seraj IM, Wagner RJ. Stromal invasion in endometrial adenocarcinoma. *Am J Obstet Gynecol.* 1984;149:10–14.
74. Tavassoli F, Kraus FT. Endometrial lesions in uteri resected for atypical endometrial hyperplasia. *Am J Clin Pathol.* 1978;70:770.
75. Randal TC, Kurman RJ. Progestin treatment of atypical hyperplasia and well-differentiated carcinoma of the endometrium under age 40. *Obstet Gynecol.* 1997;90:434–440.
76. Ushijima K, Yahata H, Yoshikawa H, et al. Multicenter phase II study of fertility-sparing treatment with medroxyprogesterone acetate for endometrial carcinoma and atypical hyperplasia in young women. *J Clin Oncol.* 2007;25:2798–2803.
77. Leitao M, Chi D. Fertility sparing options for patients with gynecologic malignancies. *Oncologist.* 2005;10:613–622.
78. Runowicz CD. Gynecologic surveillance of women on tamoxifen: first do no harm. *J Clin Oncol.* 2000;18:3457–3458.
79. ACOG Committee Opinion. Tamoxifen and uterine cancer. *Obstet Gynecol.* 2006;107:1475–1478.
80. Gredmark T, Kvint S, Harvel G, et al. Histopathologic findings in women with post-menopausal bleeding. *Br J Obstet Gynaecol.* 1995;102:133–136.
81. Feldman S, Cook F, Harlow B, et al. Predicting endometrial cancer among women who present with abnormal vaginal bleeding. *Gynecol Oncol.* 1995;56:376–381.
82. Clark TJ, Mann CH, Shah N, et al. Accuracy of outpatient endometrial biopsy in the diagnosis of endometrial cancer: a systematic quantitative review. *Br J Obstet Gynaecol.* 2002;109:313–321.
83. Dijkhuizen FP, Mol B, Brolmann H, et al. The accuracy of endometrial sampling in the diagnosis of patients with endometrial carcinoma and hyperplasia: a meta-analysis. *Cancer.* 2000;89:1765–1772.
84. Iossa A, Cianferoni L, Ciatto S, et al. Hysteroscopy and endometrial cancer diagnosis: a review of 2007 consecutive examinations in self-referred patients. *Tumori.* 1991;77:479–483.
85. Ben-Yehuda O, Kim Y, Leuchter R. Does hysteroscopy improve upon the sensitivity of dilatation and curettage in the diagnosis of endometrial hyperplasia or carcinoma? *Gynecol Oncol.* 1998;68:4–7.
86. Clark TJ, Voit D, Gupta J, et al. Accuracy of hysteroscopy in the diagnosis of endometrial cancer and hyperplasia. A systematic quantitative review. *JAMA.* 2002;288:1610–1621.
87. Bradley WH, Boente MP, Brooker D, et al. Hysteroscopy and cytology in endometrial cancer. *Obstet Gynecol.* 2004;104:1030–1033.
88. Revel A, Tsafrir A, Anteby SO, et al. Does hysteroscopy produce intraperitoneal spread of endometrial cancer cells? *Obstet Gynecol Surv.* 2004;59:280–284.
89. Pecorelli S. Revised FIGO staging for carcinoma of the vulva, cervix, and endometrium. *Int J Gynecol Obstet.* 2009;105:109–110.
90. Tabor A, Watt H, Wald N. Endometrial thickness as a test for endometrial cancer in women with post-menopausal vaginal bleeding. *Obstet Gynecol.* 2002;99:663–670.
91. Smith-Bindman R, Kerlikowske K, Feldstein K, et al. Endovaginal ultrasound to exclude endometrial cancer and other endometrial abnormalities. *JAMA.* 1998;280:1510–1517.
92. Conoscenti G, Mier YJ, Fischer-Tamaro L, et al. Endometrial assessment by transvaginal sonography and histological findings after D&C in women with post-menopausal bleeding. *Ultrasound Obstet Gynecol.* 1995;6:108–115.
93. Tongsong T, Pongnarisorn C, Mahanuphap P. Use of vaginosongraphic measurements of endometrial thickness in the identification of abnormal endometrium in pari- and post-menopausal bleeding. *J Clin Ultrasound.* 1994;22:479–482.
94. Goldstein R, Bree R, Benson C, et al. Evaluation of the woman with post-menopausal bleeding. Society of Radiologists in Ultrasound—consensus conference statement. *J Ultrasound Med.* 2001;20:1025–1036.
95. deKroon CD, deBrock GH, Dieben SW, et al. Saline contrast hysterosonography in abnormal uterine bleeding: a systematic review and meta-analysis. *Br J Obstet Gynaecol.* 2003;110:938–947.
96. Marziale P, Atlante G, Pozzi M, et al. 426 cases of stage I endometrial carcinoma: a clinicopathological analysis. *Gynecol Oncol.* 1989;32:278.
97. Ozalp S, Yalcin OT, Polay S, et al. Diagnostic efficacy of the preoperative lymphoscintigraphy, Ga-67 scintigraphy, and computed tomography for the detection of lymph node metastasis in cases of ovarian or endometrial cancer. *Acta Obstet Gynaecol Scand.* 1999;78:155–159.
98. Zerbe M, Bristow R, Grumbine F, et al. Inability of preoperative computed tomography scans to accurately predict the extent of myometrial invasion and extracorporal spread in endometrial cancer. *Gynecol Oncol.* 2000;78:67–70.
99. Signorelli M, Guerra L, Buda A, et al. Role of integrated FDG PET/CT in the surgical management of patients with high risk clinical early stage endometrial cancer: detection of pelvic nodal metastases. *Gynecol Oncol.* 2009;115:231–235.
100. Savelli L, Testa A, Mabrouk M, et al. A prospective comparison of the accuracy of transvaginal sonography and frozen section assessment of myometrial invasion in endometrial cancer. *Gynecol Oncol.* 2012;124:549–552.
101. Gordon AN, Fleischer AC, Dudley BS, et al. Preoperative assessment of myometrial invasion of endometrial adenocarcinoma by sonography (US) and magnetic resonance imaging (MRI). *Gynecol Oncol.* 1989;34:175–179.
102. Rockall AG, Sohaib SS, Harisinghani MG, et al. Diagnostic performance of nanoparticle enhanced magnetic resonance imaging in the diagnosis of lymph node metastases in patients with endometrial and cervical cancer. *J Clin Oncol.* 2005;23:2813–2821.
103. Messiou C, Spencer JA, Swift SE. MR staging of endometrial cancer. *Clin Radiol.* 2006;61:822–832.
104. Hardesty LA, Sumkin JH, Hakim C, et al. The ability of helical CT to preoperatively stage endometrial carcinoma. *Am J Roentgenol.* 2001;176:603–606.
105. Chung HH, Kang SB, Cho JY, et al. Accuracy of MR imaging for the prediction of myometrial invasion of endometrial cancer. *Gynecol Oncol.* 2007;104:654–659.
106. Rockall AG, Meroni R, Sohaib SA, et al. Evaluation of endometrial carcinoma on magnetic resonance imagining. *Int J Gynecol Cancer.* 2007;17:188–196.
107. Todo Y, Okamoto K, Hayashi M, et al. A validation study of a scoring system to estimate the risk of lymph node metastasis for patients with endometrial cancer for tailoring the indication of lymphadenectomy. *Gynecol Oncol.* 2007;104:623–628.
108. Kalogera E, Scholler N, Powless C, et al. Correlation of serum HE4 with tumor size and myometrial invasion in endometrial cancer. *Gynecol Oncol.* 2011;124(2):270–275.
109. Farias-Eisener R, Su F, Robbins T, et al. Validation of serum biomarkers for detection of early and late stage endometrial cancer. *Am J Obstet Gynecol.* 2010;202:73.e1–e5.
110. Niloff JM, Klug TL, Schaetzl E, et al. Elevation of serum CA 125 in carcinomas of the fallopian tube, endometrium, and endocervix. *Am J Obstet Gynecol.* 1984;148:1057.
111. Hsieh CH, ChangChien CC, Lin H, et al. Can a preoperative CA 125 level be a criterion for full pelvic lymphadenectomy in surgical staging of endometrial cancer? *Gynecol Oncol.* 2002;86:28–33.
112. Rose PG, Sommers RM, Reale FR, et al. Serial serum CA-125 measurements for evaluation of recurrence in patients with endometrial carcinoma. *Obstet Gynecol.* 1994;84:12–16.
113. Nicklin J, Janda M, Gebski V, et al. The utility of serum CA-125 in predicting extra-uterine disease in apparent early-stage endometrial cancer. *Int J Cancer.* 2012;131(4):885–890. doi:10.1002/ijc.26433.
114. Heyman J. The so-called Stockholm Method and the results of treatment of uterine cancer at the Radiumhemmet. *Acta Radiol.* 1935;16:129.
115. Arneson AN, Stanbro WW, Nolan JF. The use of multiple sources of radium within the uterus in the treatment of endometrial cancer. *Am J Obstet Gynecol.* 1948;55:64–78.
116. Asbury RF, Blessing JA, McGuire WP, et al. Aminothiadiazole (NSC 4728) in patients with advanced carcinoma of the endometrium. A phase II study of the Gynecologic Oncology Group. *Am J Clin Oncol.* 1990;13:39–41.
117. Nolan J, Arneson A. An instrument for inserting multiple capsules of radium within the uterus in the treatment of corpus cancers. *Am J Roentgenol.* 1943;49:504.
118. Lewis GC Jr, Slack NH, Mortel R, et al. Adjuvant progestogen therapy in the primary definitive treatment of endometrial cancer. *Gynecol Oncol.* 1974;2:368–376.
119. Dobbie BMW, Taylor C, Waterhouse J. Study of carcinoma of the endometrium. *J Obstet Gynaecol Br Commonw.* 1973;114:106–109.
120. Gray LA. Lymph node excision in treatment of gynecologic malignancies. *Am J Surg.* 1964;108:660–663.
121. Lewis GC, Bundy B. Surgery for endometrial cancer. *Cancer.* 1981;48:568–574.
122. Barakat RR, Lev G, Hummer A, et al. Twelve-year experience in the management of endometrial cancer: a change in surgical and postoperative radiation approaches. *Gynecol Oncol.* 2007;105:150–156.
123. Morrow CP. Curtin JP. *Surgery for Ovarian Neoplasia in Gynecologic Cancer Surgery.* New York, NY: Churchill Livingstone Inc.; 1996:627–716.
124. Morrow CP. Curtin JP. *Surgery for Cervical Neoplasia in Gynecologic Cancer Surgery.* New York, NY: Churchill Livingstone Inc.; 1996:451–568.

125. Soliman P, Frumovitz M, Spannuth W, et al. Lymphadenectomy during endometrial cancer staging: practice patterns among gynecologic oncologists. *Gynecol Oncol.* 2010;119:291–294.
126. Jadoul P, Donnez J. Conservative treatment may be beneficial for young women with atypical endometrial hyperplasia or endometrial adenocarcinoma. *Fert Steril.* 2003;80:1315–1324.
127. International Federation of Gynecology and Obstetrics: classification and staging of malignant tumors in the female pelvis. *Int J Gynaecol Obstet.* 1971;9:172.
128. Tillmanns T, Kamelle S, Abudayyeh I, et al. Panniculectomy with simultaneous gynecologic oncology surgery. *Gynecol Oncol.* 2001;83:518–522.
129. Wright J, Powell M, Herzog T, et al. Panniculectomy: improving lymph node yield in morbidly obese patients with endometrial neoplasms. *Gynecol Oncol.* 2004;94:436–441.
130. Ramirez P, Frumovitz M, Bodurka D, et al. Hormonal therapy for the management of grade 1 endometrial adenocarcinoma: a literature review. *Gynecol Oncol.* 2004;95:133–138.
131. Soliman PT, Oh J, Schmeler K, et al. Risk factors for young premenopausal women with endometrial cancer. *Obstet Gynecol.* 2005;105:575–580.
132. Baker J, Obermair A, Gebski V, et al. Efficacy of oral or intrauterine device-delivered progestin in patients with complex endometrial hyperplasia with atypia or early endometrial adenocarcinoma: a meta-analysis and systematic review of the literature. *Gynecol Oncol.* 2012;125:263–270.
133. Penner K, Dorigo O, Aoyama C, et al. Predictors of resolution of complex atypical hyperplasia or grade 1 endometrial adenocarcinoma in premenopausal women treated with progestin therapy. *Gynecol Oncol.* 2012;124:542–548.
134. Candiani GB, Belloni C, Maggi R, et al. Evaluation of different surgical approach in the treatment of endometrial cancer at FIGO stage I. *Gynecol Oncol.* 1990;37:6–8.
135. Massi G, Savino L, Susini T. Vaginal hysterectomy versus abdominal hysterectomy for treatment of stage I endometrial adenocarcinoma. *Am J Obstet Gynecol.* 1996;174:1320–1326.
136. Scarselli G, Savino L, Ceccherini R, et al. Role of vaginal surgery in the 1st stage endometrial cancer. Experience of the Florence School. *Eur J Gynaecol Oncol.* 1992;13:15–19.
137. Bloss JD, Berman ML, Bloss LP, et al. Use of vaginal hysterectomy for the management of stage I endometrial cancer in the medically compromised patient. *Gynecol Oncol.* 1991;40:74–77.
138. Pitkin RM. Vaginal hysterectomy in obese women. *Obstet Gynecol.* 1977;49:567–569.
139. Orr JW, Holimon J, Orr P. Stage I corpus cancer: is teletherapy necessary. *Am J Obstet Gynecol.* 1997;176:777–789.
140. Homesley HD, Kadar N, Barrett RJ, et al. Selective pelvic and periaortic lymphadenectomy does not increase morbidity in surgical staging of endometrial carcinoma. *Am J Obstet Gynecol.* 1992;167:1225–1230.
141. Abu-Rustum N, Alektiar K, Iasonos A, et al. The incidence of symptomatic lower-extremity lymphedema following treatment of uterine corpus malignancies: a 12-year experience at Memorial Sloan-Kettering Cancer Center. *Gynecol Oncol.* 2006;103:714–718.
142. Mariani A, Dowdy S, Cliby W, et al. Efficacy of systematic lymphadenectomy and adjuvant radiotherapy in node-positive endometrial cancer patients. *Gynecol Oncol.* 2006;101:200–208.
143. Lewandowski G, Torrisi J, Potkul R, et al. Hysterectomy with extended surgical staging and radiotherapy versus hysterectomy alone and radiotherapy in stage I endometrial cancer: a comparison of complication rates. *Gynecol Oncol.* 1990;36:401–404.
144. Keys HM, Roberts JA, Brunetto VL, et al. A phase III trial of surgery with or without adjunctive external pelvic radiation therapy in intermediate risk endometrial adenocarcinoma: a Gynecologic Oncology Group study. *Gynecol Oncol.* 2004;92:744–751.
145. Goudge C, Bernhard S, Cloven N, et al. The impact of complete surgical staging on adjuvant treatment decisions in endometrial cancer. *Gynecol Oncol.* 2004;93:536–539.
146. Sharma C, Deeutsch I, Lewin S, et al. Lymphadenectomy influences the utilization of adjuvant radiation treatment for endometrial cancer. *Am J Obstet Gynecol.* 2011;205:562.e1–562.e9.
147. Partridge EE, Shingleton H, Menck H. The National Cancer Data Base report on endometrial cancer. *J Surg Oncol.* 1996;61:111–123.
148. MacDonald OK, Sause W, Lee J, et al. Does oncologic specialization influence outcomes following surgery in early stage adenocarcinoma of the endometrium. *Gynecol Oncol.* 2005;99:730–735.
149. Roland PY, Kelly FJ, Kulwicki C, et al. The benefits of a gynecologic oncologist: a pattern of care study for endometrial cancer treatment. *Gynecol Oncol.* 2004;93:125–130.
150. Aalders JG, Thomas G. Endometrial cancer—revisiting the importance of pelvic and para-aortic lymph nodes. *Gynecol Oncol.* 2007;104:222–231.
151. Creutzberg CL, van Putten WL, Koper PC, et al. Surgery and postoperative radiotherapy versus surgery alone for patients with stage-1 endometrial carcinoma: multicentre randomised trial. PORTEC Study Group. Post Operative Radiation Therapy in Endometrial Carcinoma. *Lancet.* 2000;355:1404–1411.
152. Nout RA, Smit VT, Putter H, et al. Vaginal brachytherapy versus pelvic external radiotherapy for patients with endometrial cancer of high-intermediate risk (PORTEC 2): an open lable, non inferiority, randomized trial. *Lancet.* 2010, 375:816–823.
153. Trimble E, Kosary C, Park R. Lymph node sampling and survival in endometrial cancer. *Gynecol Oncol.* 1998;71:340–343.
154. COSA-NZ-UK Endometrial Cancer Study Groups. Pelvic lymphadenectomy in high-risk endometrial cancer. *Int J Gynecol Cancer.* 1996;6:102–107.
155. ASTEC Study Group. Efficacy of systematic pelvic lymphadenectomy in endometrial cancer (MRC ASTEC trial): a randomized study. *Lancet.* 2009;373:125–136.
156. Benedetti Panici P, Basile S, Maneschi F, et al. Systematic pelvic lymphadenectomy versus no lymphadenectomy in early-stage endometrial carcinoma: Randomized clinical trial. *J Natl Cancer Inst.* 2008;100:1707–1716.
157. Creasman WT, Mutch DE, Herzog TJ. ATEC lymphadenectomy and radiation therapy: are conclusions valid. *Gynecol Oncol.* 2010;116:293–294.
158. Seamon LG, Fowler JM, Cohn DE. Lymphadenectomy for endometrial cancer: The controversy. *Gynecol Oncol.* 2010;117:6–8.
159. Lee TS, Kim JW, Seong S, et al. Benefit of lymphadenectomy in endometrial cancer: can truth be obtained by randomized controlled trial after ASTEC? *Int J Gynecol Cancer.* 2009;19(8):1467.
160. Nugent EK, Bishop EA, Mathews CA, et al. Do uterine risk factors or lymph node metastasis more significantly affect recurrence in patients with endometrioid adenocarcinoma. *Gynecol Oncol.* 2012;125:94–98.
161. Kwon J, Qiu F, Saski R, et al. Are uterine risk factors more important than nodal status in predicting survival. *Obstet Gynecol.* 2009;114:736–743.
162. Creutzberg C, van Putten W, Warlam-Rodenhuis C, et al. Outcome of high-risk stage IC, grade 3 compared with stage I endometrial carcinoma patients: the postoperative radiation therapy in endometrial carcinoma trial. *J Clin Oncol.* 2004;22:1234–1241.
163. Onda T, Yoshikawa H, Mizutani K, et al. Treatment of node positive endometrial cancer with complete node dissection, chemotherapy and radiation therapy. *Br J Cancer.* 1997;75:1836–1841.
164. McMeekin DS, Lashbrook D, Gold M, et al. Analysis of FIGO stage IIIc endometrial cancer patients. *Gynecol Oncol.* 2001;81:273–278.
165. Nelson G, Randall M, Sutton G, et al. FIGO stage IIIC endometrial carcinoma with metastases confined to pelvic lymph nodes: analysis of treatment outcomes, prognostic variables, and failure patterns following adjuvant radiation therapy. *Gynecol Oncol.* 1999;75:211–214.
166. Arango HA. Hoffman MS, Roberts WS, et al. Accuracy of lymph node palpation to determine need for lymphadenectomy in gynecologic malignancies. *Obstet Gynecol.* 2000;95:553–556.
167. Franchi M, Ghezzi F, Melpigano M, et al. Clinical value of intraoperative gross examination in endometrial cancer. *Gynecol Oncol.* 2000;76:357–361.
168. Janda M, Gebski V, Brand A, et al. Quality of life after total laparoscopic hysterectomy for stage I endometrial cancer (LACE): a randomized trial. *Lancet.* 2010;11(8);772–780.
169. Kim Y, Niloff J. Endometrial carcinoma: analysis of recurrence in patients treated with a strategy minimizing lymph node sampling and radiation therapy. *Obstet Gynecol.* 1993;82:175–180.
170. Faught W, Krepart G, Loctocki R, et al. Should selective para-aortic lymphadenectomy be part of surgical staging for endometrial cancer. *Gynecol Oncol.* 1994;55:51–55.
171. Goff B, Kato D, Schmidt R, et al. Uterine papillary serous carcinoma: patterns of metastatic spread. *Gynecol Oncol.* 1994;54:264–268.
172. Podratz KC, Mariani A, Webb MJ. Staging and therapeutic value of lymph-adenenctomy in endometrial cancer. *Gynecol Oncol.* 1998;70(2):163–164.
173. Mariani A, Webb MJ, Keeney GI, et al. Low risk corpus cancer: is lymphadenectomy or radiotherapy necessary. *Am J Obstet Gynecol.* 2000;182:1506–1519.
174. Mariani A, Dowdy SC, Cliby WA, et al. Prospective assessment of lymphatic dissemination in endometrial cancer: a paradigm shift in surgical staging. *Gynecol Oncol.* 2008;109:11–28.
175. Convery PA, Cantrell LA, DiSanto N, et al. Retrospective review of an intraoperative algorithm to predict lymph node metastasis in low grade endometrial cancer. *Gynecol Oncol.* 2011;123:65–70.
176. Milam M, Java J, Walker JL, et al. Nodal metastasis risk in endometrioid endometrial cancer. *Obstet Gynecol.* 2012;119:286–292.

177. Kang S, Kang WD, Chung HH, et al. Preoperative identification of Low-risk group for lymph node metastasis in endometrial cancer: a Korean GOG study. *J Clin Oncol.* 2012;30:1329–1334.
178. Bernardini M, May T, Khalifa M, et al. Evaluation of two management strategies for preoperative grade 1 endometrial cancer. *Obstet Gynecol.* 2009;114:7–15.
179. Doering DL, Barnhill DR, Weiser EB, et al. Intraopertive evaluation of depth of myometrial invasion in stage I endometrial adenocarcinoma. *Obstet Gynecol.* 1989;74:930–933.
180. Goff BA, Riche LW. Assessment of depth of myometrial invasion in endometrial adenocarcinoma. *Gynecol Oncol.* 1990;38:46–48.
181. Creasman WT, Zaino R, Major FL, et al. Early invasive carcinoma of the cervix (3–5 mm invasion): risk factors and prognosis: a Gynecologic Oncology Group study. *Am J Obstet Gynecol.* 1998;178:62–65.
182. Leblanc E, Querleu D, Narducci F, et al. Surgical staging of early invasive epithelial ovarian tumors. *Semin Surg Oncol.* 2000;19:36–41.
183. Case AS, Rocconi RP, Straughn JM, et al. A prospective blinded evaluation of the accuracy of frozen section for the surgical management of endometrial cancer. *Obstet Gynecol.* 2006;108:1375–1379.
184. Frumovitz M, Slomovitz BM, Singh DK, et al. Frozen section analyses as predictors of lymphatic spread in patients with early-stage uterine cancer. *J Am Coll Surg.* 2004;199:388–393.
185. Frumovitz M, Singh DK, Meyer L, et al. Predictors of final histology in patients with endometrial cancer. *Gynecol Oncol.* 2004;95:463–468.
186. Cohn D, Huh D, Fowler J, et al. Cost-effectiveness analysis of strategies for the surgical management of grade 1 endometrial cancer. *Obstet Gynecol.* 2007;109:1388–1395.
187. Barnes MN, Roland P, Straughn M, et al. Comparison of treatment strategies for endometrial adenocarcinoma: analysis of financial impact. *Gynecol Oncol.* 1999;74:443–447.
188. Mariani A, Webb M, Galli L, et al. Potential therapeutic role of para-aortic lymphadenectomy in node positive endometrial cancer. *Gynecol Oncol.* 2000;76:348–356.
189. McMeekin DS, Lashbrook D, Gold M, et al. Nodal distribution and its significance in FIGO stage III endometrial cancer. *Gynecol Oncol.* 2001;82:375–379.
190. Flanigan C, Mannel R, Walker J, et al. Incidence and location of para-aortic lymph node metastases in gynecologic malignancies. *J Am Coll Surg.* 1995;181:72–74.
191. Abu-Rustum NR, Gomez J, Alektiar KM, et al. The incidence of isolated para-aortic nodal metastasis in surgically staged endometrial cancer patients with negative pelvic lymph nodes. *Gynecol Oncol.* 2009;115:236–238.
192. Chiang AJ, Yu KJ, Chao KC, et al. The incidence of isolated para-aortic nodal metastasis in completely staged endometrial cancer. *Gynecol Oncol.* 2011;121:122–125.
193. Chuang L, Burke T, Tornos C, et al. staging laparotomy for endometrial carcinoma: assessment of retroperitoneal lymph nodes. *Gynecol Oncol.* 1995;58:189–193.
194. Todo Y, Kato H, Kaneuchi M, et al. Survival effect of para-aortic lymphadenectomy in endometrial cancer (SEPAL study): a retrospective cohort analysis. *Lancet.* 2010;375:1165–1172.
195. Hirahatake K, Hareyama H, Sakuragi N, et al. A clinical and pathologic study on para-aortic lymph node metastasis in endometrial carcinoma. *J Surg Oncol.* 1997;65:82–87.
196. Kohler C, Tozzi R, Klemm P, et al. Laparoscopic para-aortic left-sided transperitoneal infrarenal lymphadenectomy in patients with gynecologic malignancies: techniques and results. *Gynecol Oncol.* 2003;91:139–148.
197. Dowdy S, Aletti G, Cliby W. Extra-peritoneal laparoscopic para-aortic lymphadenectomy. A prospective cohort study of 293 patients with endometrial cancer. *Gynecol Oncol.* 2008;111:418–424.
198. Kilgore L, Partridge E, Alvarez R, et al. Adenocarcinoma of the endometrium: survival comparisons of patients with and without pelvic node sampling. *Gynecol Oncol.* 1995;56:29–33.
199. Girardi F, Petru E, Heydarfadai M, et al. Pelvic lymphadenectomy in the surgical treatment of endometrial cancer. *Gynecol Oncol.* 1993;49:177–180.
200. Cragan J, Havrilesky L, Calingaert B, et al. Retrospective analysis of selective lymphadenectomy in apparent early-stage endometrial cancer. *J Clin Oncol.* 2005;23:3668–3675.
201. Chan J, Cheung M, Huh W, et al. Therapeutic role of lymph node resection in endometrioid corpus cancer: a study of 12,333 patients. *Cancer.* 2006;107:1823–1830.
202. Havrilseky LJ, Cragun J, Calingaert B, et al. Resection of lymph node metastases influences survival in stage IIIC endometrial cancer. *Gynecol Oncol.* 2005;99(3):689–695.
203. Bristow RE, Zahurak ML, Alexander CJ, et al. FIGO stage IIIC endometrial carcinoma: Resection of macroscopic nodal disease and other determinants of survival. *Int J Gynecol Cancer.* 2003;13:664–672.
204. ASTEC/EN.5 Study Group, Blake P, Swart AM, Orton J, et al. Adjuvant external beam radiotherapy in the treatment of endometrial cancer (MRC ASTEC and NCIC CTG EN.5 randomized trials): pooled trial results, systematic review, and meta-analysis. *Lancet.* 2009;373:137–146.
205. Fanning J, Nanavati P, Hilgers R. Surgical staging and high dose rate brachytherapy for endometrial cancer: limiting external radiotherapy to node positive tumors. *Obstet Gynecol.* 1996;87:1041–1044.
206. Mohan D, Samuels M, Selim M, et al. Long term outcomes of therapeutic pelvic lymphadenectomy for stage I endometrial adenocarcinoma. *Gynecol Oncol.* 1998;70:165–171.
207. Khoury-Collado F, Abu-Rustum NR. Lymphatic mapping in endometrial cancer: a literature review of current techniques *Int J Gynecol Cancer.* 2008;18:1163–1168.
208. Altgassen C, Muller N, Hornemann A, et al. Immunohistochemical workup of sentinel nodes in endometrial cancer improves diagnostic accuracy. *Gynecol Oncol.* 2009;114:284–287.
209. Nihura H, Okamoto S, Yoshinaga K, et al. Detection of micrometastases in the sentinel lymph nodes of patients with endometrial cancer. *Gynecol Oncol.* 2007;105:683–686.
210. Khoury-Collado F, Murray MP, Hensley ML, et al. Sentinel lymph node mapping for endometrial cancer improves the detection of metastatic disease to regional lymph nodes. *Gynecol Oncol.* 2011;122:251–254.
211. Kang S, Yoo HJ, Hwang JH, et al. Sentinel lymph node biopsy in endometrial cancer: Meta-analysis of 26 studies. *Gynecol Oncol.* 2011;123:522–527.
212. Childers JM, Brzechffa P, Hatch K, et al. Laparoscopically assisted surgical staging of endometrial cancer. *Gynecol Oncol.* 1993;51:33–38.
213. Childers JM, Surwit EA. Combined laparoscopic and vaginal surgery for the management of two cases of stage I endometrial cancer. *Gynecol Oncol.* 1992;45:46–51.
214. Boike G, Lurain J, Bruke J. A comparison of laparoscopic management of endometrial cancer with a traditional laparotomy. *Obstet Gynecol.* 1994;52:105.
215. Magrina JF, Mutone NF, Weaver AL, et al. Laparoscopic lymphadenectomy and vaginal or laparoscopic hysterectomy with bilateral salpingo-oophorectomy for endometrial cancer: morbidity and survival. *Am J Obstet Gynecol.* 1999;181:376–381.
216. Homesley HD, Boike G, Spiegel G. Feasibility of laparoscopic management of presumed stage I endometrial carcinoma and assessment of accuracy of myoinvasion estimates by frozen section: a Gynecologic Oncology Group study. *Int J Gynecol Cancer.* 2004;14:341–347.
217. Malur S, Possover M, Michels W, et al. Laparoscopic assisted vaginal hysterectomy versus abdominal surgery in patients with endometrial cancer—a prospective randomized trial. *Gynecol Oncol.* 2001;80:239–244.
218. Gemignani ML, Curtin J, Zelmanovich J, et al. Laparoscopic assisted vaginal hysterectomy for endometrial cancer: clinical outcomes and hospital charges. *Gynecol Oncol.* 1999;73:5–11.
219. Spirtos NM, Schlaerth J, Gross G, et al. Cost and quality of life analyses of surgery for early endometrial cancer: laparotomy versus laparoscopy. *Am J Obstet Gynecol.* 1996;174(6):1795–1799.
220. Walker J, Piedmonte M, Spirtos N, et al. Recurrence and survival after random assignment to laparoscopy versus laparotomy for comprehensive staging of uterine cancer: GOG LAP2 study. *J Clin Oncol.* 2012;30:695–700.
221. Querleu D, Leblanc E, Castelain B. Laparoscopic pelvic lymphadenectomy in the staging of early carcinoma of the cervix. *Am J Obstet Gynecol.* 1991;164:579–581.
222. Nezhat CR, Burrell MO, Nezhat FR, et al. Laparoscopic radical hysterectomy with para-aortic and pelvic node dissection. *Am J Obstet Gynecol.* 1992;166:864–865.
223. Spirtos N, Schlaerth J, Spirtos T, et al. Laparoscopic bilateral pelvic and para-aortic lymph node sampling: an evolving technique. *Am J Obstet Gynecol.* 1995;172:105–111.
224. Childers JM, Hatch KD, Tran A, et al. Laparoscopic para-aortic lymphadenectomy in gynecologic malignancies. *Obstet Gynecol.* 1993;82:741–747.
225. Scribner D, Walker J, Johnson G, et al. Laparoscopic pelvic and para-aortic lymph node dissection: analysis of first 100 cases. *Gynecol Oncol.* 2001;82:498–503.
226. Fowler JM, Carter JR, Carlson JW, et al. Lymph node yield from laparoscopic lymphadenectomy in cervical cancer: a comparative study. *Gynecol Oncol.* 1993;51:187–192.
227. Eltabbakh G. Effect of surgeon's experience on the surgical outcome of laparoscopic surgery for women with endometrial cancer. *Gynecol Oncol.* 2000;78:58–61.
228. Harkki-Siren P, Kurki T. A nationwide analysis of laparoscopic complications. *Obstet Gynecol.* 1997;89:108–112.

229. Harkki-Siren P, Sjoberg J. Evaluation and the learning curve of the first one hundred laparoscopic hysterectomies. *Acta Obstet Gynecol Scand.* 1995;74:638–641.
230. Tozzi R, Malur S, Koehler C, et al. Laparoscopy versus laparotomy in endometrial cancer: first analysis of survival of a randomized prospective study. *J Minim Invasive Gynecol.* 2005;12:130–136.
231. Walker JL, Piedmonte MR, Spirtos NM, et al. Recurrence and survival after random assignment to laparoscopy versus laparotomy for comprehensive surgical staging of uterine cancer: Gynecologic Oncology Group LAP2 study. *J Clin Oncol.* 2012;30:695–700.
232. Scribner D, Walker J, Johnson G, et al. Surgical management of early stage endometrial cancer in the elderly: is laparoscopy feasible? *Gynecol Oncol.* 2001;83:563–568.
233. Scribner D, Walker J, Johnson G, et al. Laparoscopic pelvic and para-aortic lymph node dissection in the obese. *Gynecol Oncol.* 2002;84:426–430.
234. Eltabbakh G, Shamonki M, Moody J, et al. Hysterectomy for obese women with endometrial cancer: laparoscopy or laparotomy. *Gynecol Oncol.* 2000;78:329–335.
235. O'Hanlan K, Dibble S, Fisher D. Total laparoscopic hysterectomy for uterine pathology: impact of body mass index on outcomes. *Gynecol Oncol.* 2006;103:938–941.
236. Boggess JF, Gehrig PA, Cantrell L, et al. A comparative study of 3 surgical methods for hysterectomy with staging for endometrial cancer: robotic assistance, laparoscopy, laparotomy. *Am J Obstet Gynecol.* 2008;199:360–369.
237. DeNardis SA, Holloway RW, Bigsby GE, et al. Robotically assisted laparoscopic hysterectomy versus total abdominal hysterectomy and lymphadenectomy for endometrial cancer. *Gynecol Oncol.* 2008;111:412–417.
238. Veljovich DS, Paley PJ, Drescher CW, et al. Robotic surgery in gynecologic oncology: program initiation and outcomes after the first year with comparison with laparotomy for endometrial cancer staging. *Am J Obstet Gynecol.* 2008;198:679.e1–e679.e10.
239. Holloway RW, Ahmad S, DeNardis SA, et al. Robotic-assisted laparoscopic hysterectomy and lymphadenectomy for endometrial cancer: Analysis of surgical performance. *Gynecol Oncol.* 2009;115:447–452.
240. Seamon LG, Fowler JM, Richardson DL, et al. A detailed analysis of the learning curve: Robotic hysterectomy and pelvic-aortic lymphadenectomy for endometrial cancer. *Gynecol Oncol.* 2009;114:162–167.
241. Lowe MP, Johnson PR, Kamelle SA, et al. A multi-institutional experience with robotic-assisted hysterectomy with staging for endometrial cancer. *Obstet Gynecol.* 2009;114:236–243.
242. Lim PC, Kang E, Park DH. Learning curve and surgical outcome for robotic-assisted hysterectomy with lymphadenectomy: case-matched controlled comparison with laparoscopy and laparotomy for treatment of endometrial cancer. *J Min Invas Gynecol.* 2010;17:739–748.
243. Seamon L, Cohn D, Richardson D, et al. Robotic Hysterectomy and pelvic-aortic lymphadenectomy for endometrial cancer. *Obstet Gynecol.* 2008;112:1207–1213.
244. Seamon LG, Bryant SA, Rheaume PS, et al. Comprehensive surgical staging for endometrial cancer in obese patients-comparing robotics and laparotomy. *Obstet Gynecol.* 2009;114:16–21.
245. Subramaniam A, Kim K, Bryant S, et al. A cohort study evaluating robotic versus laparotomy surgical outcomes of obese women with endometrial cancer. *Gynecol Oncol.* 2011;122:604–607.
246. Massi G, Savino L, Susini T. Vaginal hysterectomy versus abdominal hysterectomy for the treatment of stage I endometrial adenocarcinoma. *Am J Obstet Gynecol.* 1996;174:1320–1326.
247. Kornblith A, Huang H, Walker J, et al. Quality of life of patients with endometrial cancer undergoing laparoscopic FIGO staging compared with laparotomy: A GOG study. *J Clin Oncol.* 2009;27:5337–5342.
248. Scribner D, Walker J, Johnson G, et al. Laparoscopic pelvic and para-aortic lymph node dissection: analysis of the first 100 cases. *Gynecol Oncol.* 2001;82:498–503.
249. Possover M, Krause N, Plaul K, et al. Laparoscopic para-aortic and pelvic lymphadenectomy: experience with 150 patients and review of literature. *Gynecol Oncol.* 1998;71:19–28.
250. Querleu D, Lebanc E, Cartron G, et al. Audit of preoperative and early complications of laparoscopic lymph node dissection in 1000 cancer patients. *Am J Obstet Gynecol.* 2006;195:1287–1292.
251. Childers JM, Spirtos N, Brainard P, et al. Laparoscopic staging of the patient with incompletely staged early adenocarcinoma of the endometrium. *Obstet Gynecol.* 1994;83:597–600.
252. Goff BA, Goodman A, Muntz HG, et al. Surgical stage IV endometrial carcinoma: a study of 47 cases. *Gynecol Oncol.* 1994;52:237–240.
253. Chi DS, Welshinger M, Venkatraman ES, et al. The role of surgical cytoreductive surgery in stage IV endometrial carcinoma. *Gynecol Oncol.* 1997;67(1):56–60.
254. Bristow RE, Zerbe MJ, Rosenshein N, et al. Stage IVb endometrial carcinoma: the role of cytoreductive surgery and determinants of survival. *Gynecol Oncol.* 2000;78:85–91.
255. Shih KK, Gardner G, Barakat R, et al. Surgical cytoreduction in stage IV endometrioid endometrial carcinoma. *Gynecol Oncol.* 2011;122:608–611.
256. Bristow R, Duska L, Montz F. The role of cytoreductive surgery in the management of stage IV uterine papillary serous carcinoma. *Gynecol Oncol.* 2001;81:92–99.
257. Kurman R, Norris H. Evaluation of criteria for distinguishing atypical endometrial hyperplasia from well-differentiated carcinoma. *Cancer.* 1982;49:2547–2559.
258. Huang S, Amparo E, Fu Y. Endometrial hyperplasia: histologic classification and behavior. *Surg Pathol.* 1988;1:215–225.
259. Hunter JE, Tritz DE, Howell MG, et al. The prognostic and therapeutic implications of cytologic atypia in patients with endometrial hyperplasia. *Gynecol Oncol.* 1994;55:66–71.
260. Kendall BS, Ronnett BM, Isacson C, et al. Reproducibility of the diagnosis of endometrial hyperplasia, atypical hyperplasia, and well-differentiated carcinoma. *Am J Surg Pathol.* 1998;22:1012–1019.
261. Bergeron C, Nogales F, Masseroli M, et al. A multicentric European study testing the reproducibility of the WHO classification of endometrial hyperplasia with a proposal of a simplified working classification for biopsy and curettage specimens. *Am J Surg Pathol.* 1999;23:1102–1108.
262. Skov BG, Broholm H, Engel U, et al. Comparison of the reproducibility of the WHO classifications of 1975 and 1994 of endometrial hyperplasia. *Int J Gynecol Pathol.* 1997;16:33–37.
263. Mutter GL. The Endometrial Collaborative Group. Endometrial intraepithelial neoplasia (EIN): will it bring order to chaos? *Gynecol Oncol.* 2000;76:287–290.
264. Baak JP, Mutter GL. EIN and WHO94. *J Clin Pathol.* 2005;58:1–6.
265. Baak JP, Mutter G, Robboy S, et al. The molecular genetics and morphometry-based endometrial intraepithelial neoplasia classification system predicts disease progression in endometrial hyperplasia more accurately than the 1994 World Health Organization classification system. *Cancer.* 2005;103:2304–2312.
266. Mutter GL, Zaino R, Baak J, et al. Benign endometrial hyperplasia sequence and endometrial intraepithelial neoplasia. *Int J Gynecol Pathol.* 2007;26:103–114.
267. Silverberg S, Kurman R. *Tumors of the Uterine Corpus and Gestational Trophoblastic Disease.* Vol 3. Washington, DC: Armed Forces Institute of Pathology; 1992.
268. Zaino RJ, Silverberg SG, Norris HJ, et al. The prognostic value of nuclear versus architectural grading in endometrial adenocarcinoma: a Gynecologic Oncology Group study. *Int J Gynecol Pathol.* 1994;13:29–36.
269. Zaino RJ, Kurman RJ, Diana KL, et al. The utility of the revised International Federation of Gynecology and Obstetrics histologic grading of endometrial adenocarcinoma using a defined nuclear grading system. *Cancer.* 1995;75:81–86.
270. Taylor R, Zeller J, Lieberman R, et al. An analysis of two versus three grades for endometrial carcinoma. *Gynecol Oncol.* 1999;74:3–6.
271. Lax S, Ronntet B, Pizer E, et al. A binary grading system for uterine endometrioid carcinoma is comparable to FIGO grading for predicting prognosis and has superior interobserver reproducibility. *Mod Pathol.* 1999;12:118A.
272. Fanning J, Evans MC, Peters AJ, et al. Endometrial adenocarcinoma histologic subtypes: clinical and pathologic profile. *Gynecol Oncol.* 1989;32:288–291.
273. Sutton GP, Brill L, Michael H, et al. Malignant papillary lesions of the endometrium. *Gynecol Oncol.* 1987;27:294–304.
274. Zaino FJ, Kurman RJ, Brunetto VL, et al. Villoglandular adenocarcinoma of the endometrium: a clinicopathologic study of 61 cases. *Am J Surg Pathol.* 1998;22:1379.
275. Kusuyama J, Yoshida M, Imai H, et al. Secretory carcinoma of the endometrium. *Acta Cytol.* 1989;33:127.
276. Toban H, Watkins GJ. Secretory adenocarcinoma of the endometrium. *Int J Gynecol Pathol.* 1985;4:328.
277. Christopherson WM, Alberhasky RC, Connelly PF. Carcinoma of the endometrium. I. A clinicopathologic study of clear-cell carcinoma and secretory carcinoma. *Cancer.* 1982;49:1511.
278. Hendrickson MR, Kempson RL. Ciliated carcinoma—a variant of endometrial adenocarcinoma. A report of 10 cases. *Int J Gynecol Pathol.* 1983;2:1–12.
279. Alberhasky RC, Connelly PJ, Christopherson WM. Carcinoma of the endometrium. IV. Mixed adenosquamous carcinoma. A clinical-pathological study of 68 cases with long-term follow-up. *Am J Clin Pathol.* 1982;77:655–664.

280. Julian CG, Daikoku NH, Gillespie A. Adenoepidermoid and adenosquamous carcinoma of the uterus. A clinicopathologic study of 118 cases. *Am J Obstet Gynecol.* 1977;128:106–116.
281. Ng AB, Reagan JW, Storaasli JP, et al. Mixed adenosquamous carcinoma of the endometrium. *Am J Clin Pathol.* 1973;59:765–781.
282. Salazar OM, DePapp EW, Bonfiglio T, et al. Adenosquamous carcinoma of the endometrium. An entity with an inherently poor prognosis? *Cancer.* 1977;40:119–130.
283. Silverberg SG, Bolin MG, DeGiorgi LS. Adenoacanthoma and mixed adenosquamous carcinoma of the endometrium. A clinicopathologic study. *Cancer.* 1972;30:1307–1314.
284. Zaino R, Kurman R, Herbold D, et al. The significance of squamous differentiation in endometrial carcinoma. *Cancer.* 1991;68:2293–2302.
285. Melhem MF, Tobon H. Mucinous adenocarcinoma of the endometrium: a clinicopathological review of 18 cases. *Int J Gynecol Pathol.* 1987;6:347.
286. Ross J, Eifel P, Cox R, et al. Primary mucinous adenocarcinoma of the endometrium. *Am J Surg Pathol.* 1983;7:715–729.
287. Tiltman A. Mucinous carcinoma of the endometrium. *Obstet Gynecol.* 1980;55:244–247.
288. Maier RC, Norris HJ. Coexistence of cervical intraepithelial neoplasia with primary adenocarcinoma of the endocervix. *Obstet Gynecol.* 1980;56:361.
289. Maes G, Fleuren GJ, Bara J, et al. The distribution of mucins, carcinoembryonic antigen, and mucus-associated antigens in endocervical and endometrial adenocarcinomas. *Int J Gynecol Pathol.* 1988;7:112–122.
290. McCluggage WG, Roberts N, Bharucha H. Enteric differentiation in endometrial adenocarcinomas: a mucin histochemical study. *Int J Gynecol Pathol.* 1995;14:250–254.
291. Wilson TO, Podratz KC, Gaffey TA, et al. Evaluation of unfavorable histologic subtypes in endometrial adenocarcinoma. *Am J Obstet Gynecol.* 1990;162:418–423.
292. Carcangiu ML, Chambers JT. Uterine papillary serous carcinoma: a study on 108 cases with emphasis on the prognostic significance of associated endometrioid carcinoma, absence of invasion, and concomitant ovarian carcinoma. *Gynecol Oncol.* 1992;47:298–305.
293. Chan JK, Loizzi V, Youssef M, et al. Significance of comprehensive surgical staging in noninvasive papillary serous carcinoma of the endometrium. *Gynecol Oncol.* 2003;90:181–185.
294. Chambers JT, Merino M, Kohorn EI, et al. Uterine papillary serous carcinoma. *Obstet Gynecol.* 1987;69:109–113.
295. Wheeler D, Bell K, Kurman R, et al. Minimal uterine serous carcinoma: diagnostic and clinicopathologic correlation. *Am J Surg Pathol.* 2000;24:797–806.
296. Huh W, Powell M, Leath C, et al. Uterine papillary serous carcinoma: comparisons of outcomes in surgical stage I patients with and without adjuvant therapy. *Gynecol Oncol.* 2003;91:470–475.
297. Havrilesky L, Alvarez Secord A, Bae-Jump V, et al. Outcomes in surgical stage I uterine papillary serous carcinoma. *Gynecol Oncol.* 2007;105:677–682.
298. Ambros RA, Sherman ME, Zahn CM, et al. Endometrial intraepithelial carcinoma: a distinctive lesion specifically associated with tumors displaying serous differentiation. *Hum Pathol.* 1995;26:1260–1267.
299. Sherman ME, Bitterman P, Rosenshein NB, et al. Uterine serous carcinoma. A morphologically diverse neoplasm with unifying clinicopathologic features. *Am J Surg Pathol.* 1992;16:600–610.
300. Soslow R, Pirong E, Isacson C. Endometrial intraepithelial carcinoma with associated peritoneal carcinomatosis. *Am J Surg Pathol.* 2000;24:726–732.
301. Spiegel G. Endometrial carcinoma *in situ* in postmenopausal women. *Am J Surg Pathol.* 1995;19:417–431.
302. Zheng W, Khurana R, Farahmand S, et al. p53 immunostaining as a significant adjunct diagnostic method for uterine serous carcinoma. *Am J Surg Pathol.* 1998;22:1463–1473.
303. Abeler V, Kjørdstad K, Berle E. Carcinoma of the endometrium in Norway: a histopathological and prognostic survey of a total population. *Int J Gynecol Cancer.* 1992;2:9–22.
304. Abeler VM, Kjorstad KE. Clear cell carcinoma of the endometrium: a histopathological and clinical study of 97 cases. *Gynecol Oncol.* 1991;40:207–217.
305. Abeler VM, Vergote IB, Kjorstad KE, et al. Clear cell carcinoma of the endometrium. Prognosis and metastatic pattern. *Cancer.* 1996;78:1740–1747.
306. Christopherson W, Alberhasky R, Connelly P. Carcinoma of the endometrium. II. Papillary adenocarcinoma: a clinicopathological study of 46 cases. *Am J Clin Pathol.* 1982;77:534–540.
307. Kurman RJ, Scully RE. Clear cell carcinoma of the endometrium. An analysis of 21 cases. *Cancer.* 1976;37:872–882.
308. Lax SF, Pizer ES, Ronnett BM, et al. Clear cell carcinoma of the endometrium is characterized by a distinctive profile of p53, Ki-67, estrogen, and progesterone receptor expression. *Hum Pathol.* 1998;29:551–558.
309. Miller B, Umpierre S, Tornos C, et al. Histologic characterization of uterine papillary serous adenocarcinoma. *Gynecol Oncol.* 1995;56:425–429.
310. Webb GA, Lagios MD. Clear cell carcinoma of the endometrium. *Am J Obstet Gynecol.* 1987;156:1486–149.
311. Goodman A, Zukerberg LR, Rice LW, et al. Squamous cell carcinoma of the endometrium: a report of eight cases and a review of the literature. *Gynecol Oncol.* 1996;61:54–60.
312. Melin JR, Wanner L, Schulz, DM, et al. Primary squamous cell carcinoma of the endometrium. *Obstet Gynecol.* 1979;53:115.
313. Simon A, Kopolovic J, Beyth Y. Primary squamous cell carcinoma of the endometrium. *Gynecol Oncol.* 1988;31:454–461.
314. Tagsjo EB, Rosenberg P, Simonsen E. Primary squamous cell carcinoma of the endometrium. Case report. *Eur J Gynaecol Oncol.* 1993;14:308–310.
315. Yamashina M, Kobara TY. Primary squamous cell carcinoma with its spindle cell variant in the endometrium. A case report and review of literature. *Cancer.* 1986;57:340–345.
316. Christopherson WM, Alberhasky PC, Connelly PJ. Glassy cell carcinoma of the endometrium. *Hum Pathol.* 1982;13:418–421.
317. Hachisuga T, Sugimori H, Kaku T, et al. Glassy cell carcinoma of the endometrium. *Gynecol Oncol.* 1990;36:134–138.
318. Kumar NB, Hart WR. Metastases to the uterine corpus from extravaginal cancers. A clinicopathologic study of 63 cases. *Cancer.* 1982;50:2163.
319. Kumar NB, Schneider V. Metastases to the uterus from extra pelvic primary tumors. *Int J Gynecol Pathol.* 1983;2:134.
320. Piura B, Glezerman M. Synchronous carcinomas of endometrium and ovary. *Gynecol Oncol.* 1989;33:261–264.
321. Eifel P, Hendrickson M, Ross J, et al. Simultaneous presentation of carcinoma involving the ovary and uterine corpus. *Cancer.* 1982;50:163–170.
322. Scully RE. *Tumors of the Ovary and Maldeveloped Gonad.* AFIP Pamphlet No. 16. Washington, DC: Armed Forces Institute of Pathology; 1982:92.
323. Zaino RJ, Whitney C, Brady MF. Simultaneously detected endometrial and ovarian carcinomas: a clinicopathologic study of 74 cases. *Mod Pathol.* 1998;11:118.
324. Ulbright T, Roth L. Metastatic and independent cancers of the endometrium and ovary. A clinicopathologic study of 34 cases. *Hum Pathol.* 1985;16:28–34.
325. Scholten A, van Putten WL, Beerman H, et al. Postoperative radiotherapy for stage I endometrial carcinoma: long term outcome of the randomized PORTEC trial with central pathology review. *Int J Radiation Oncol Biol Phys.* 2005;63:834–838.
326. Boronow R, Morrow C, Creasman W, et al. Surgical staging in endometrial cancer: clinical-pathologic findings of a prospective study. *Obstet Gynecol.* 1984;63:825–832.
327. Gal D, Recio FO, Zamurovic D. The new International Federation of Gynecology and Obstetrics surgical staging and survival rates in early endometrial carcinoma. *Cancer.* 1992;69:200–202.
328. Homesly H, Zaino R. Endometrial cancer: prognostic factors. *Semin Oncol.* 1994;21:71–78.
329. Kosary CL. FIGO stage, histology, histologic grade, age and race as prognostic factors in determining survival for cancers of the female gynecological system: an analysis of 1973–87 SEER cases of cancers of the endometrium, cervix, ovary, vulva, and vagina. *Semin Surg Oncol.* 1994;10:31–46.
330. Wolfson A, Sightler S, Markoe A, et al. The prognostic significance of surgical staging for carcinoma of the endometrium. *Gynecol Oncol.* 1992;45:142–146.
331. Zaino RJ, Kurman RJ, Diana KL, et al. Pathologic models to predict outcome for women with endometrial adenocarcinoma. *Cancer.* 1996;77:1115–1121.
332. Randall M, Filiaci V, Muss H, et al. Randomized phase III trial of WART versus doxorubicin and cisplatin chemotherapy in advanced endometrial carcinoma: A GOG study. *J Clin Oncol.* 2006;24:36–44.
333. Mariani A, Webb M, Keeney G, et al. Stage IIIC endometrioid corpus cancer includes distinct subgroups. *Gynecol Oncol.* 2002;87:112–117.
334. Hoekstra AV, Kim RJ, Small W, et al. FIGO stage IIIC endometrial carcinoma: prognsostic factors and outcomes. *Gynecol Oncol.* 2008;114:273–278.
335. Todo Y, Kato H, Minobe S, et al. A validation study of the new revised FIGO staging system to estimate prognosis for patients with stage IIIC endometrial cancer. *Gynecol Oncol.* 2011:121:126–130.
336. Werner HMJ, Trovik J, Marcickiewicz J, et al. Revison of FIGO surgical staging in 2009 for endometrial cancer validates to improve risk stratification. *Gynecol Oncol.* 2012;125:103–108.
337. Havrilesky LJ, Cragun J, Calingaert B, et al. Resection of lymph node metastases influences survival in stage IIIc endometrial cancer. *Gynecol Oncol.* 2005;99:689–695.
338. Takeshima N, Umayahara K, Fujiwara K, et al. Effectiveness of postoperative chemotherapy for para-aortic lymph node metastasis of endometrial cancer. *Gynecol Oncol.* 2006;102:214–217.

339. Kennedy A, Peterson G, Becker S, et al. Experience with pelvic washings in stage I and II endometrial carcinoma. *Gynecol Oncol.* 1987;28:50–60.
340. Yazigi R, Piver M, Blumenson I. Malignant peritoneal cytology as an indicator in stage I endometrial cancer. *Obstet Gynecol.* 1983;62:359–362.
341. Grimshaw R, Tupper W, Fraser R, et al. Prognostic value of peritoneal cytology in endometrial carcinoma. *Gynecol Oncol.* 1990;36:97–100.
342. Sutton GP. The significance of positive peritoneal cytology in endometrial cancer. *Oncology.* 1990;4:21–26.
343. Konski A, Poulter C, Keys H, et al. Absence of prognostic significance, peritoneal dissemination and treatment advantage in endometrial cancer patients with positive peritoneal cytology. *Int J Radiat Oncol Biol Phys.* 1988;14:49–55.
344. Turner D, Gershenson D, Atkinson N, et al. The prognostic significance of peritoneal cytology for stage I endometrial cancer. *Obstet Gynecol.* 1989;74:775–780.
345. Kadar N, Homesley H, Malfetano J. Positive peritoneal cytology is an adverse risk factor in endometrial carcinoma only if there is other evidence of extrauterine disease. *Gynecol Oncol.* 1992;46:145–149.
346. Wethington S, Medel NIB, Wright JD, et al. Prognostic significance and treatment implications of positive peritoneal cytology in endometrial adenocarcinoma: unraveling a mystery. *Gynecol Oncol.* 2009;115:18–25.
347. Saga Y, Imai M, Joba T, et al. Is peritoneal cytology a prognostic factor of endometrial cancer confined to the uterus. *Gynecol Oncol.* 2006;103:277–280.
348. Havrilesky L, Cragun J, Calingaert B, et al. The prognostic significance of positive peritoneal cytology and adnexal/serosal metastasis in stage IIIa endometrial cancer. *Gynecol Oncol.* 2007;104:401–405.
349. Esteller M, Garcia A, Martinez-Palones JM, et al. Clinicopathologic features and genetic alterations in endometrioid carcinoma of the uterus with villoglandular differentiation. *Am J Clin Pathol.* 1999;111:336–342.
350. Abeler VM, Kjorstad KE. Serous papillary carcinoma of the endometrium: a histopathological study of 22 cases. *Gynecol Oncol.* 1990;39:266–271.
351. Chen J, Trost D, Wilkinson E. Endometrial papillary adenocarcinomas: two clinicopathologic types. *Int J Gynecol Pathol.* 1985;4:279–288.
352. Hendrickson M, Martinez A, Ross J, et al. Uterine papillary serous carcinoma: a highly malignant form of endometrial adenocarcinoma. *Am J Surg Pathol.* 1982;6:93–108.
353. Ward BG, Wright RG, Free K. Papillary carcinomas of the endometrium. *Gynecol Oncol.* 1990;39:347–351.
354. Aquino-Parsons C, Lim P, Wong F, et al. Papillary serous and clear cell carcinoma limited to endometrial curettings in FIGO stage 1a and 1b endometrial adenocarcinoma: treatment implications. *Gynecol Oncol.* 1998;71:83–86.
355. Carcangiu ML, Chambers JT. Early pathologic stage clear cell carcinoma and uterine papillary serous carcinoma of the endometrium: comparison of clinicopathologic features and survival. *Int J Gynecol Pathol.* 1995;14:30–38.
356. Kanbour-Shakir A, Tobon H. Primary clear cell carcinoma of the endometrium: a clinicopathologic study of 20 cases. *Int J Gynecol Pathol.* 1991;10:67–78.
357. Malpica A, Tornos C, Burke TW, et al. Low-stage clear-cell carcinoma of the endometrium. *Am J Surg Pathol.* 1995;19:769–774.
358. Havrilesky L, Alvarez Secord A, Bae-Jump V, et al. Outcomes in surgical stage I uterine papillary serous carcinoma. *Gynecol Oncol.* 2007;105:677–682.
359. Alektiar A, McKee A, Lin O, et al. Is there a difference in outcome between stage I-II endometrial cancer of papillary serous/clear cell and endometrioid FIGO grade 3 cancer? *Int J Radiat Oncol Biol Phys.* 2002;54:79–85.
360. Huh W, Powell M, Leath C, et al. Uterine papillary serous carcinoma: comparisons of outcomes in surgical stage I patients with and without adjuvant therapy. *Gynecol Oncol.* 2003;91:470–475.
361. Creasman WT, Kohler M, Odicino F, et al. Prognosis of papillary serous, clear cell, and grade 3 stage I carcinoma of the uterus. *Gynecol Oncol.* 2004;95:593–596.
362. Chambers SK, Kapp DS, Peschel RE, et al. Prognostic factors and sites of failure in FIGO stage I, grade 3 endometrial carcinoma. *Gynecol Oncol.* 1987;27:180–188.
363. Sutton GP, Geiser HE, Stehman FB, et al. Features associated with survival and disease-free survival in early endometrial cancer. *Am J Obstet Gynecol.* 1989;160:1385–1393.
364. Wharton JT, Mikuta JJ, Mettlin C, et al. Risk factors and current management in carcinoma of the endometrium. *Surg Gynecol Obstet.* 1986;162:515–520.
365. Bucy GS, Mendenhall WM, Morgan LS, et al. Clinical stage I and II endometrial carcinoma treated with surgery and/or radiation therapy: analysis of prognostic and treatment-related factors. *Gynecol Oncol.* 1989;33:290.
366. Mariani A, Webb M, Keeney G, et al. Surgical stage I endometrial cancer: predictors of distant failure and death. *Gynecol Oncol.* 2002;87:274–280.
367. Guntupalli S, Zigheloim I, Kizer N, et al. Lymphovascular space invasion is an independent risk factor for nodal disease and poor outcomes in endometrioid endometrial cancer. *Gynecol Oncol.* 2012;124:31–35.
368. Sivridis E, Buckley CH, Fox H. The prognostic significance of lymphatic vascular space invasion in endometrial adenocarcinoma. *Br J Obstet Gynaecol.* 1987;94:991–994.
369. Hanson M, van Nagell J, Powell D. The prognostic significance of lymph-vascular space invasion in stage I endometrial cancer. *Cancer.* 1985;55:1753–1757.
370. Straughn JM, Huh W, Kelly J, et al. Conservative management of stage I endometrial carcinoma after surgical staging. *Gynecol Oncol.* 2002;84:194–200.
371. Straughn JM, Huh W, Orr J, et al. Stage IC adenocarcinoma of the endometrium: survival comparisons of surgically staged patients with and without adjuvant therapy. *Gynecol Oncol.* 2003;89:295–300.
372. Mariani A, Dowdy S, Keeney G, et al. Predictors of vaginal relapse in stage I endometrial cancer. *Gynecol Oncol.* 2005;97:820–827.
373. Mariani A, Webb M, Kenney G, et al. Endometrial cancer: predictors of peritoneal failure. *Gynecol Oncol.* 2003;89:236–242.
374. Mariani A, Webb M, Keeney G, et al. Predictors of lymphatic failure in endometrial cancer. *Gynecol Oncol.* 2002;84:437–442.
375. Mariani A, Webb M, Rao S, et al. Significance of pathologic patterns of pelvic lymph node metastases in endometrial cancer. *Gynecol Oncol.* 2001;80:113–120.
376. Kauppila A, Kujansuu E, Vihko R. Cytosol estrogen and progestin receptors in endometrial carcinoma of patients treated with surgery, radiotherapy, and progestin. Clinical correlates. *Cancer.* 1982;50(10):2157–2162.
377. Macdonald RR, Thorogood J, Mason MK. A randomized trial of progestogens in the primary treatment of endometrial carcinoma. *Br J Obstet Gynaecol.* 1988;95:166–174.
378. Vergote I, Kjorstad K, Abeler V, et al. A randomized trial of adjuvant progestogen in early endometrial cancer. *Cancer.* 1989;64:1011.
379. von Minckwitz G, Loibl S, Brunnert K, et al. Adjuvant endocrine treatment with medroxyprogesterone acetate or tamoxifen in stage I and II endometrial cancer—a multicentre, open, controlled, prospectively randomised trial. *Eur J Cancer.* 2002;38:2265–2271.
380. Morrow C, Bundy B, Homesley H, et al. Doxorubicin as an adjuvant following surgery and radiation therapy in patients with high-risk endometrial carcinoma, stage I and occult stage II: a Gynecologic Oncology Group study. *Gynecol Oncol.* 1990;36:166–171.
381. Creutzberg CL, Nout RA, Marnix L, et al. Fifteen year radiotherapy outcomes for the randomized PORTEC-1 trial for endometrial cancer. *Int J Rad Oncol Biol Phys.* 2011;81:631–638.
382. Nout RA, Putter H, Jürgenliemk-Schulz IM, et al. Quality of life after pelvic radiotherapy or vaginal brachytherapy for endometrial cancer: first results of the randomized PORTEC-2 trial. *J Clin Oncol.* 2009;27:3547–3556.
383. Nout RA, Putter H, Jürgenliemk-Schulz IM, et al. Five year quality of life of endometrial cancer patients treated in the randomized PORTEC 2 trial and comparison with norm data. *Eur J Cancer.* 2012;48(11):1638–1648.
384. Lee CM, Szabo A, Shrieve DC, et al. Frequency and effect of adjuvant radiation therapy among women with stage I endometrial adenocarcinoma. *JAMA.* 2006;295(4):389–397.
385. Patel MK, Cote ML, Ali-Fehmi R, et al. Trends in the utilization of adjuvant vaginal cuff brachytherapy and/or external beam radiation treatment in stage I and II endometrial cancer: a surveillance, epidemiology, and end-results study. *Int J Radiat Oncol Biol Phys.* 2012;83(1):178–184.
386. Aalders J, Abeler V, Kolstad P, et al. Postoperative external irradiation and prognostic parameters in stage I endometrial carcinoma: clinical and histopathologic study of 540 patients. *Obstet Gynecol.* 1980;56:419–427.
387. Greven KM, D'Agostino RB Jr, Lanciano RM, et al. Is there a role for a brachytherapy vaginal cuff boost in the adjuvant management of patients with uterine-confined endometrial cancer? *Int J Radiat Oncol Biol Phys.* 1998;42:101–104.
388. Randall ME, Wilder J, Greven K, et al. Role of intracavitary cuff boost after adjuvant external irradiation in early endometrial carcinoma. *Int J Radiat Oncol Biol Phys.* 1990;19:49–54.
389. Rush S, Gal D, Potters L, et al. Pelvic control following external beam radiation for surgical stage I endometrial adenocarcinoma. *Int J Radiat Oncol Biol Phys.* 1995;33:851–854.
390. Kucera H, Vaura N, Weghoupt K. Benefit of external irradiation in pathologic stage I endometrial carcinoma: a prospective clinical trial of 605 patients who received postoperative vaginal irradiation and additional pelvic irradiation in the presence of unfavorable prognostic factors. *Gynecol Oncol.* 1990;38:99–104.

391. Nori D, Merimsky O, Batata M, et al. Postoperative high dose-rate intravaginal brachytherapy combined with external irradiation for early stage endometrial cancer: a long-term follow-up. *Int J Radiat Oncol Biol Phys.* 1994;30:831–837.
392. Horowitz NS, Peters WA III, Smith MR, et al. Adjuvant high dose rate vaginal brachytherapy as treatment of stage I and II endometrial carcinoma. *Obstet Gynecol.* 2002;99:235–240.
393. Anderson JM, Stea B, Hallum AV, et al. High-dose-rate postoperative vaginal cuff irradiation alone for stage IB and IC endometrial cancer. *Int J Radiat Oncol Biol Phys.* 2000;46:417–425.
394. MacLeod C, Fowler A, Duval P, et al. High-dose-rate brachytherapy alone post-hysterectomy for endometrial cancer. *Int J Radiat Oncol Biol Phys.* 1998;42:1033–1039.
395. Petereit DG, Tannehill SP, Grosen EA, et al. Outpatient vaginal cuff brachytherapy for endometrial cancer. *Int J Gynecol Cancer.* 1999;9:456–462.
396. Elliot P, Green D. The efficacy of postoperative vaginal irradiation in preventing vaginal recurrence in endometrial cancer. *Int J Gynecol Cancer.* 1994;4:84.
397. Alektiar KM, McKee A, Venkatraman E, et al. Intravaginal high-dose-rate brachytherapy for stage IB (FIGO grade 1, 2) endometrial cancer. *Int J Radiat Oncol Biol Phys.* 2002;53:707–713.
398. Sorbe B, Staumits A, Karlsson L. Intravaginal high-dose-rate brachytherapy for stage I endometrial cancer: a randomized study of two dose-per-fraction levels. *Int J Radiat Oncol Biol Phys.* 2005;62(5):1385–1389.
399. Narayan K, Khaw P, Bernshaw D, et al. Prognostic significance of lymphovascular space invasion and nodal involvement in intermediate- and high-risk endometrial cancer patients treated with curative intent using surgery and adjuvant radiotherapy. *Int J Gynecol Cancer.* 2012;22:260–266.
400. Alektiar KM, McKee A, Lin O, et al. The significance of the amount of myometrial invasion in patients with stage IB endometrial carcinoma. *Cancer.* 2002;95:316–321.
401. Scholten AN, Creutzberg CL, Noordijk EM, et al. Long-term outcome in endometrial carcinoma favors a two—instead of a three—tiered grading system. *Int J Radiat Oncol Biol Phys.* 2002;52:1067–1074.
402. Irwin C, Levin W, Fyles A, et al. The role of adjuvant radiotherapy in carcinoma of the endometrium—results in 550 patients with pathologic stage I disease. *Gynecol Oncol.* 1998;70:247–254.
403. Piver M, Hempling R. A prospective trial of post-operative vaginal radium/cesium for grade 1–2 less than 50% myometrial invasion and pelvic radiation therapy for grade 3 or deep myometrial invasion in surgical stage I endometrial adenocarcinoma. *Cancer.* 1990;66:133.
404. Chadha M, Nanavati PJ, Liu P, et al. Patterns of failure in endometrial carcinoma stage IB grade 3 and IC patients treated with postoperative vaginal vault brachytherapy. *Gynecol Oncol.* 1999;75:103–107.
405. Alektiar KM, Chi D, Barakat RR. Risk stratification of death from endometrial cancer in patients with early stage disease. *Int J Radiat Oncol Biol Phys.* 2007;69(3):S387–S388.
406. Solhjem MC, Petersen IA, Haddock MG. Vaginal brachytherapy alone is sufficient adjuvant treatment of surgical stage I endometrial cancer. *Int J Radiat Oncol Biol Phys.* 2005;62(5):1379–1384.
407. Rittenberg PVC, Lotocki RJ, Heywood MS, et al. High-risk surgical stage 1 endometrial cancer: outcomes with vault brachytherapy alone. *Gynecol Oncol.* 2003;89(2):288–294.
408. Weiss MF, Connell PP, Waggoner S, et al. External pelvic radiation therapy in stage IC endometrial carcinoma. *Obstet Gynecol.* 1999;93:599–602.
409. Pitson G, Colgan T, Levin W, et al. Stage II endometrial carcinoma: prognostic factors and risk classification in 170 patients. *Int J Radiat Oncol Biol Phys.* 2002;53:862–867.
410. Fanning J. Long-term survival of intermediate risk endometrial cancer (stage IG3, IC, II) treated with full lymphadenectomy and brachytherapy without teletherapy. *Gynecol Oncol.* 2001;82:371–374.
411. Ng TY, Nicklin JL, Perrin LC, et al. Postoperative vaginal vault brachytherapy for node-negative stage II (occult) endometrial carcinoma. *Gynecol Oncol.* 2001;81:193–195.
412. Rittenberg PVC, Lotocki RJ, Heywood MS, et al. Stage II endometrial carcinoma: limiting post-operative radiotherapy to the vaginal vault in node-negative tumors. *Gynecol Oncol.* 2005;98(3):434–438.
413. Connell PP, Rotmensch J, Waggoner S, et al. The significance of adnexal involvement in endometrial carcinoma. *Gynecol Oncol.* 1999;74:74–79.
414. Ashman JB, Connell PP, Yamada D, et al. Outcome of endometrial carcinoma patients with involvement of the uterine serosa. *Gynecol Oncol.* 2001;82:338–343.
415. Greven K, Corn B, Lanciano RM. Pathologic stage III endometrial carcinoma. *Cancer.* 1993;71:3697.
416. Mariani A, Webb MJ, Keeney GL, et al. Stage IIIC endometrioid corpus cancer includes distinct subgroups. *Gynecol Oncol.* 2002;87:12–17.
417. Corn BW, Lanciano RM, Greven KM, et al. Endometrial carcinoma with para-aortic lymphadenopathy: patterns of failure and opportunity for cure. *Int J Radiat Oncol Biol Phys.* 1992;24:223.
418. Hicks ML, Piver S, Jeffrey LP, et al. Survival in patients with para-aortic lymph node metastases from endometrial adenocarcinoma clinically limited to the uterus. *Int J Radiat Oncol Biol Phys.* 1993;26:607.
419. Rose PG, Cha SD, Tak WK, et al. Radiation therapy for surgically proven para-aortic node metastasis in endometrial carcinoma. *Int J Radiat Oncol Biol Phys.* 1992;24:229–233.
420. Gibbons S, Martinez A, Schary M, et al. Adjuvant whole abdominopelvic irradiation for high-risk endometrial carcinoma. *Int J Radiat Oncol Biol Phys.* 1991;21:1019–1025.
421. Martinez A, Podratz K. Results of whole abdomino-pelvic radiation with nodal boost for patients with endometrial cancer at high risk of failure in the peritoneal cavity. *Hematol Oncol Clin North Am.* 1988;2:431.
422. Sutton G, Axelrod J, Bundy B, et al. Whole abdominal radiotherapy in the adjuvant treatment of patients with stage III and IV endometrial cancer: a Gynecologic Oncology Group study. *Gynecol Oncol.* 2005;97(3):755–763.
423. Maggi R, Lissoni A, Spina F, et al. Adjuvant chemotherapy vs. radiotherapy in high-risk endometrial carcinoma: results of a randomised trial. *Br J Cancer.* 2006;95(3):266–271.
424. Greven K, Winter K, Underhill K, et al. Final analysis of RTOG 9708: adjuvant postoperative irradiation combined with cisplatin/paclitaxel chemotherapy following surgery for patients with high-risk endometrial cancer. *Gynecol Oncol.* 2006;103(1):155–159.
425. Homesley HD, Filiaci V, Gibbons SK, et al. A randomized phase III trial in advanced endometrial carcinoma of surgery and volume directed radiation followed by cisplatin and doxorubicin with or without paclitaxel: A Gynecologic Oncology Group study. *Gynecol Oncol.* 2009;112:543–552.
426. Mundt AJ, Murphy KT, Rotmensch J, et al. Surgery and postoperative radiation therapy in FIFO stage IIIC endometrial carcinoma. *Int J Radiat Oncol Biol Phys.* 2001;50:1154–1160.
427. Mundt AJ, McBride R, Rotmensch J, et al. Significant pelvic recurrence in high risk pathologic stage I-IV endometrial carcinoma patients after chemotherapy alone: implications for adjuvant radiation therapy. *Int J Radiat Oncol Biol Phys.* 2001;50:1145–1153.
428. Milosevic MF, Dembo AJ, Thomas GM. The clinical significance of malignant peritoneal cytology in stage I endometrial carcinoma. *Int J Gynecol Cancer.* 1992;2:225–235.
429. Soper JT, Creasman WT, Clarke-Pearson DL, et al. Intraperitoneal chromic phosphate ^{32}P suspension therapy of malignant peritoneal cytology in endometrial carcinoma. *Am J Obstet Gynecol.* 1985;153:191–196.
430. Eltabbakh GH, Piver MS, Hempling RE, et al. Excellent long-term survival and absence of vaginal recurrences in 332 patients with low-risk stage I endometrial adenocarcinoma treated with hysterectomy and vaginal brachytherapy without formal staging lymph node sampling: report of a prospective trial. *Int J Radiat Oncol Biol Phys.* 1997;38:373–380.
431. Nag S, Erickson B, Parikh S, et al. The American Brachytherapy Society recommendations for high-dose-rate brachytherapy for carcinoma of the endometrium. *Int J Radiat Oncol Biol Phys.* 2000;48:779–790.
432. Rouanet P, Dubois JB, Gely S, et al. Exclusive radiation therapy in endometrial carcinoma. *Int J Radiat Oncol Biol Phys.* 1993;26:223–228.
433. Grigsby P, Kuske R, Perez CA, et al. Medically inoperable stage I adenocarcinoma of the endometrium treated with radiotherapy alone. *Int J Radiat Oncol Biol Phys.* 1986;13:483.
434. Knocke TH, Kucera H, Weidinger B, et al. Primary treatment of endometrial carcinoma with high-dose-rate brachytherapy: results of 12 years of experience with 280 patients. *Int J Radiat Oncol Biol Phys.* 1997;37:359–365.
435. Nguyen TV, Petereit DG. High-dose-rate brachytherapy for medically inoperable stage I endometrial cancer. *Gynecol Oncol.* 1995;59:370–375.
436. Niazi TM, Souhami L, Portelance L, et al. Long term results of high dose rate brachytherapy in the primary treatment of medically inoperable stage I-II endometrial carcinoma. *Int J Radiat Oncol Biol Phys.* 2005;63:1108–1113.
437. Fishman DA, Roberts KB, Chambers JT, et al. Radiation therapy as exclusive treatment for medically inoperable patients with stage I and II endometrioid carcinoma with endometrium. *Gynecol Oncol.* 1996 May;61(2):189–196.
438. Kucera H, Knocke TH, Kucera E, et al. Treatment of endometrial carcinoma with high-dose-rate brachytherapy alone in medically inoperable stage I patients. *Acta Obstet Gynecol Scand.* 1998;77:1008–1012.
439. Nicklin JL, Petersen RW. Stage 3B adenocarcinoma of the endometrium: a clinicopathologic study. *Gynecol Oncol.* 2000;78:203–207.

440. Small W Jr, Beriwal S, Demanes DJ, et al. American Brachytherapy Society consensus guidelines for adjuvant vaginal cuff brachytherapy after hysterectomy. *Brachytherapy.* 2012;1:58–67.
441. Small W Jr, Erickson B, Kwakwa F. American Brachytherapy Society survey regarding practice patterns of postoperative irradiation for endometrial cancer: current status of vaginal brachytherapy. *Int J Radiat Oncol Biol Phys.* 2005;63:1502–1507.
442. Ghosh K, Padilla LA, Murray KP, et al. Using a belly board device to reduce the small bowel volume within pelvic radiation fields in women with postoperatively treated cervical carcinoma. *Gynecol Oncol.* 2001;83:271–275.
443. Mundt AJ, Lujan AE, Rotmensch J, et al. Intensity-modulated whole pelvic radiotherapy in women with gynecologic malignancies. *Int J Radiat Oncol Biol Phys.* 2002;52(5):1330–1337.
444. Mundt AJ, Mell LK, Roeske JC. Preliminary analysis of chronic gastrointestinal toxicity in gynecology patients treated with intensity-modulated whole pelvic radiation therapy. *Int J Radiat Oncol Biol Phys.* 2003;56(5):1354–1360.
445. Roeske JC, Lujan A, Rotmensch J, et al. Intensity-modulated whole pelvic radiation therapy in patients with gynecologic malignancies. *Int J Radiat Oncol Biol Phys.* 2000;48:1613–1621.
446. Lujan AE, Mundt AJ, Roeske JC, et al. Intensity-modulated radiotherapy as a means of reducing dose to bone marrow in gynecologic patients receiving whole pelvic radiotherapy. *Int J Radiat Oncol Biol Phys.* 2003;57:516–521.
447. Buchali A, Koswig S, Dinges S, et al. Impact of the filling status of the bladder and rectum on their integral dose distribution and the movement of the uterus in the treatment planning of gynaecological cancer. *Radiother Oncol.* 1999;52:29–34.
448. Huh, SJ, Park W, Han Y. Interfractional variation in position of the uterus during radical radiotherapy for cervical cancer. *Radiother Oncol.* 2004;71:73–79.
449. Salama JK, Mundt AJ, Roeske J, et al. Preliminary outcome and toxicity report of extended-field, intensity-modulated radiation therapy for gynecologic malignancies. *Int J Radiat Oncol Biol Phys.* 2006;65:1170–1176.
450. Curran WJ, Whittington R, Peters AJ, et al. Vaginal recurrences of endometrial carcinoma: the prognostic value of staging by a primary vaginal carcinoma system. *Int J Radiat Oncol Biol Phys.* 1988;15:803–808.
451. Sears J, Greven K. Prognostic factors and treatment outcome for patients with locally recurrent endometrial cancer. *Cancer.* 1994;74:1303–1308.
452. Wylie J, Irwin C, Pintilie M, et al. Results of radical radiotherapy for recurrent endometrial cancer. *Gynecol Oncol.* 2000;77:66–72.
453. Creutzberg CL, van Putten WL, Koper PC, et al. PORTEC Study Group. Survival after relapse in patients with endometrial cancer: results from a randomized trial. *Gynecol Oncol.* 2003;89:201–209.
454. Jhingran A, Burke TW, Eifel PJ, et al. Definitive radiotherapy for patients with isolated vaginal recurrence of endometrial carcinoma after hysterectomy. *Int J Radiat Oncol Biol Phys.* 2003;56:1366–1372.
455. Podratz KC, O'Brien PC, Malkasian GD Jr, et al. Effects of progestational agents in treatment of endometrial carcinoma. *Obstet Gynecol.* 1985;66:106–110.
456. Asbury RF, Brunetto VL, Lee RB, et al. Goserelin acetate as treatment for recurrent endometrial carcinoma: a Gynecologic Oncology Group study. *Am J Clin Oncol.* 2002;25:557–560.
457. McMeekin DS, Gordon A, Fowler J, et al. A phase II trial of arzoxifene, a selective estrogen response modulator, in patients with recurrent or advanced endometrial cancer. *Gynecol Oncol.* 2003;90:64–69.
458. Piver MS, Barlow JJ, Lurain JR, et al. Medroxyprogesterone acetate (Depo-Provera) vs. hydroxyprogesterone caproate (Delalutin) in women with metastatic endometrial adenocarcinoma. *Cancer.* 1980;45:268–272.
459. Quinn MA, Cauchi M, Fortune D. Endometrial carcinoma: steroid receptors and response to medroxyprogesterone acetate. *Gynecol Oncol.* 1985;21:314–319.
460. Rose PG, Brunetto VL, et al. A phase II trial of anastrozole in advanced recurrent or persistent endometrial carcinoma: a Gynecologic Oncology Group study. *Gynecol Oncol.* 2000;78(2):212–216.
461. Slavik M, Petty WM, Blessing JA, et al. Phase II clinical study of tamoxifen in advanced endometrial adenocarcinoma: a Gynecologic Oncology Group study. *Cancer Treat Rep.* 1984;68:809–811.
462. Thigpen T, Brady MF, Homesley HD, et al. Tamoxifen in the treatment of advanced or recurrent endometrial carcinoma: a Gynecologic Oncology Group study. *J Clin Oncol.* 2001;19:364–367.
463. Thigpen JT, Brady MF, Alvarez RD, et al. Oral medroxyprogesterone acetate in the treatment of advanced or recurrent endometrial carcinoma: a dose-response study by the Gynecologic Oncology Group. *J Clin Oncol.* 1999;17:1736–1744.
464. Lentz SS, Brady MF, Major FJ, et al. High-dose megestrol acetate in advanced or recurrent endometrial carcinoma: a Gynecologic Oncology Group Study. *J Clin Oncol.* 1996;14:357–361.
465. Quinn MA, Campbell JJ, Murray R, et al. Tamoxifen and aminoglutethimide in the management of patients with advanced endometrial carcinoma not responsive to medroxyprogesterone. *Aust N Z J Obstet Gynaecol.* 1981;21:226–229.
466. Pandya KJ, Yeap BY, Weiner LM, et al. Megestrol and tamoxifen in patients with advanced endometrial cancer: an Eastern Cooperative Oncology Group study (E4882). *Am J Clin Oncol.* 2001;24:43–46.
467. Satyaswaroop PG, Clarke CL, Zaino RJ, et al. Apparent resistance in human endometrial carcinoma during combination treatment with tamoxifen and progestin may result from desensitization following down-regulation of tumor progesterone receptor. *Cancer Lett.* 1992;62:107–114.
468. Fiorica JV, Brunetto VL, Hanjani P, et al. Phase II trial of alternating courses of megestrol acetate and tamoxifen in advanced endometrial carcinoma: a Gynecologic Oncology Group study. *Gynecol Oncol.* 2004;92:10–14.
469. Whitney C, Brunetto V, Zaino R, et al. Phase II study of medroxyprogesterone acetate plus tamoxifen in advanced endometrial carcinoma: a Gynecologic Oncology Group study. *Gynecol Oncol.* 2004;92:4–9.
470. Geisinger K, Homesely H, Morgan T, et al. Endometrial adenocarcinoma. A multiparameter clinicopathologic analysis including the DNA profile and the sex steroid hormone receptors. *Cancer.* 1986;58:1518–1525.
471. Kauppila A. Oestrogen and progestin receptors as prognostic indicators in endometrial cancer. A review of the literature. *Acta Oncol.* 1989;28:561–566.
472. Vering A, Michel RT, Mitze M, et al. Influence of chemotherapy on hormone receptor concentration in a xenotransplanted endometrial cancer. *Eur J Obstet Gynecol Reprod Biol.* 1992;45:131–138.
473. Bonte J, Decoster JM, Ide P. Vaginal cytologic evaluation as a practical link between hormone blood levels and tumor hormone dependency in exclusive medroxyprogesterone treatment of recurrent or metastatic endometrial adenocarcinoma. *Acta Cytol.* 1977;21:218–224.
474. Stratton JA, Mannel RS, Rettenmaier MA, et al. Treatment of advanced and recurrent endometrial carcinoma: correlation of patient response to hormonal and cytotoxic chemotherapy and the response predicted by the subrenal capsule chemo sensitivity assay. *Gynecol Oncol.* 1989;32:55–59.
475. Zaino RJ, Satyaswaroop PG, Mortel R. Hormonal therapy of human endometrial adenocarcinoma in a nude mouse model. *Cancer Res.* 1985;45:539–541.
476. Gallagher CJ, Oliver RT, Oram DH, et al. A new treatment for endometrial cancer with gonadotrophin releasing-hormone analogue. *Br J Obstet Gynaecol.* 1991;98:1037.
477. De Vriese G, Bonte J. Possible role of goserelin, an LH-RH agonist, in the treatment of gynaecological cancers. *Eur J Gynaecol Oncol.* 1993;14:187–191.
478. Kleinman D, Douvdevani A, Schally AV, et al. Direct growth inhibition of human endometrial cancer cells by the gonadotropin-releasing hormone antagonist SB-75: role of apoptosis. *Am J Obstet Gynecol.* 1994;170:96–102.
479. Chan S. A review of selective estrogen receptor modulators in the treatment of breast and endometrial cancer. *Semin Oncol.* 2002;29(3 suppl 11):129–133.
480. Hogberg T, Signorelli M, de Oliveira CF, et al. Sequential adjuvant chemotherapy and radiotherapy in endometrial cancer-results from two randomised studies. *Eur J Cancer.* 2010;46(13):2422–2431.
481. McMeekin DS, Filiacib VL, Aghajanianc C, et al. A randomized phase III trial ofpelvic radiation therapy (PXRT) versus vaginal cuff brachytherapy followed by paclitaxel/carboplatin chemotherpay (VCB/C) in patients with high risk (HR), early stage endometrial cancer (EC): A Gynecologic Oncology Group Trial. *Gynecol Oncol.* 2014;134(2):438.
482. Viswananthan AN, Moughan J, Miller BE, et al. NRG Oncology/RTOG 0921: a phase 2 study of postoperative intensity modulated radiotherapy with concurrent cisplatin and bevacizuman followed by carboplatin and paclitaxel for patietns with endometrial cancer. *Cancer.* 2015;121:2156–2163.
483. Campora E, Vidali A, Mammoliti S, et al. Treatment of advanced or recurrent adenocarcinoma of the endometrium with doxorubicin and cyclophosphamide. *Eur J Gynaecol Oncol.* 1990;11(3):181–183.
484. Muggia FM, Chia G, Reed LJ, et al. Doxorubicin-cyclophosphamide: effective chemotherapy for advanced endometrial adenocarcinoma. *Am J Obstet Gynecol.* 1977;128(3):314–319.
485. Seski JC, Edwards CL, Gershenson DM, et al. Doxorubicin and cyclophosphamide chemotherapy for disseminated endometrial cancer. *Obstet Gynecol.* 1981;58(1):88–91.

486. Edmonson JH, Krook JE, Hilton JF, et al. Randomized phase II studies of cisplatin and a combination of cyclophosphamide-doxorubicin-cisplatin (CAP) in patients with progestin-refractory advanced endometrial carcinoma. *Gynecol Oncol.* 1987;28(1):20–24.
487. Burke TW, Stringer CA, Morris M, et al. Prospective treatment of advanced or recurrent endometrial carcinoma with cisplatin, doxorubicin, and cyclophosphamide. *Gynecol Oncol.* 1991;40(3):264–267.
488. Dunton CJ, Pfeifer SM, Braitman LE, et al. Treatment of advanced and recurrent endometrial cancer with cisplatin, doxorubicin, and cyclophosphamide. *Gynecol Oncol.* 1991;41(2):113–116.
489. Hancock KC, Freedman RS, Edwards CL, et al. Use of cisplatin, doxorubicin, and cyclophosphamide to treat advanced and recurrent adenocarcinoma of the endometrium. *Cancer Treat Rep.* 1986;70(6):789–791.
490. Barrett RJ, Blessing JA, Homesley HD, et al., Circadian-timed combination doxorubicin-cisplatin chemotherapy for advanced endometrial carcinoma. A phase II study of the Gynecologic Oncology Group. *Am J Clin Oncol.* 1993;16(6):494–496.
491. Pasmantier MW, Coleman M, Silver RT, et al. Treatment of advanced endometrial carcinoma with doxorubicin and cisplatin: effects on both untreated and previously treated patients. *Cancer Treat Rep.* 1985;69(5):539–542.
492. Seltzer V, Vogl SE, Kaplan BH. Adriamycin and cis-diamminedichloroplatinum in the treatment of metastatic endometrial adenocarcinoma. *Gynecol Oncol.* 1984;19(3):308–313.
493. Thigpen JT, Brady MF, Homesley HD, et al. Phase III trial of doxorubicin with or without cisplatin in advanced endometrial carcinoma: a gynecologic oncology group study. *J Clin Oncol.* 2004;22(19):3902–3908.
494. Trope C, Johnsson JE, Simonsen E, et al. Treatment of recurrent endometrial adenocarcinoma with a combination of doxorubicin and cisplatin. *Am J Obstet Gynecol.* 1984;149(4):379–381.
495. Susumu N, Sagae S, Udagawa Y, et al. Randomized phase III trial of pelvic radiotherapy vs cisplatin-based combined chemotherapy in patients with intermediate and high-risk endometrial cancer: a JGOG study. *Gynecol Oncol.* 2008;108:236–233.
496. Ball HG, Blessing JA, Lentz SS, et al. A phase II trial of paclitaxel in patients with advanced or recurrent adenocarcinoma of the endometrium: a Gynecologic Oncology Group study. *Gynecol Oncol.* 1996;62(2):278–281.
497. Gunthert AR, Ackermann S, Beckmann MW, et al. Phase II study of weekly docetaxel in patients with recurrent or metastatic endometrial cancer: AGO Uterus-4. *Gynecol Oncol.* 2007;104(1):86–90.
498. Lincoln S, Blessing JA, Lee RB, et al. Activity of paclitaxel as second-line chemotherapy in endometrial carcinoma: a Gynecologic Oncology Group study. *Gynecol Oncol.* 2003;88(3):277–281.
499. Fleming GF, Filiaci VL, Bentley RC, et al. Phase III randomized trial of doxorubicin + cisplatin versus doxorubicin + 24-h paclitaxel + filgrastim in endometrial carcinoma: a Gynecologic Oncology Group study. *Ann Oncol.* 2004;15(8):1173–1178.
500. Fleming GF, Brunetto VL, Cella D, et al. Phase III trial of doxorubicin plus cisplatin with or without paclitaxel plus filgrastim in advanced endometrial carcinoma: a Gynecologic Oncology Group Study. *J Clin Oncol.* 2004;22(11):2159–2166.
501. Hoskins PJ, Swenerton KD, Pike JA, et al. Paclitaxel and carboplatin, alone or with irradiation, in advanced or recurrent endometrial cancer: a phase II study. *J Clin Oncol.* 2001;19(20):4048–4053.
502. Sovak MA, Dupont J, Hensley ML, et al. Paclitaxel and carboplatin in the treatment of advanced or recurrent endometrial cancer: a large retrospective study. *Int J Gynecol Cancer.* 2007;17(1):197–203.
503. Miller D, Filiaci V, Fleming G, et al. Randomized phase III noninferiority trial of first line chemotherapy for metastatic recurrent endometrial carcinoma: a Gynecologic Oncology Group study. 2012 Annual Meeting on Women's Cancer (SGO): late breaking abstract 1. *Gynecol Oncol.* 2012;125:771–773.
504. Secord AA, Havrilesky LJ, O'Malley DM, et al. A multicenter evaluation of sequential multimodality therapy and clinical outcome for the treatment of advanced endometrial cancer. *Gynecol Oncol.* 2009;114(3):442–447.
505. Thigpen JT, Blessing JA, Lagasse LD, et al. Phase II trial of cisplatin as second-line chemotherapy in patients with advanced or recurrent endometrial carcinoma. A Gynecologic Oncology Group study. *Am J Clin Oncol.* 1984;7(3):253–256.
506. Deppe G, Cohen CJ, Bruckner HW. Treatment of advanced endometrial adenocarcinoma with cis-dichlorodiammine platinum (II) after intensive prior therapy. *Gynecol Oncol.* 1980;10(1):51–54.
507. Seski JC, Edwards CL, Herson J, et al. Cisplatin chemotherapy for disseminated endometrial cancer. *Obstet Gynecol.* 1982;59(2):225–228.
508. Thigpen JT, Blessing JA, Homesley H, et al. Phase II trial of cisplatin as first-line chemotherapy in patients with advanced or recurrent endometrial carcinoma: a Gynecologic Oncology Group Study. *Gynecol Oncol.* 1989;33(1):68–70.
509. Burke TW, Munkarah A, Kavanagh JJ, et al. Treatment of advanced or recurrent endometrial carcinoma with single-agent carboplatin. *Gynecol Oncol.* 1993;51(3):397–400.
510. Green JB III, Green S, Alberts DS, et al. Carboplatin therapy in advanced endometrial cancer. *Obstet Gynecol.* 1990;75(4):696–700.
511. Long HJ, Pfeifle DM, Wieand HS, et al. Phase II evaluation of carboplatin in advanced endometrial carcinoma. *J Natl Cancer Inst.* 1988;80(4):276–278.
512. Horton J, Begg CB, Arseneault J, et al. Comparison of adriamycin with cyclophosphamide in patients with advanced endometrial cancer. *Cancer Treat Rep.* 1978;62(1):159–161.
513. Thigpen JT, Buchsbaum HJ, Mangan C, et al. Phase II trial of adriamycin in the treatment of advanced or recurrent endometrial carcinoma: a Gynecologic Oncology Group study. *Cancer Treat Rep.* 1979;63(1):21–27.
514. Calero F, Asins-Codoñer E, Jimeno J, et al. Epirubicin in advanced endometrial adenocarcinoma: a phase II study of the Grupo Ginecologico Espanol para el Tratamiento Oncologico (GGETO). *Eur J Cancer.* 1991;27(7):864–866.
515. Muggia FM, Blessing JA, Sorosky J, et al. Phase II trial of the pegylated liposomal doxorubicin in previously treated metastatic endometrial cancer: a Gynecologic Oncology Group study. *J Clin Oncol.* 2002;20(9):2360–2364.
516. Escobar PF, Markman M, Zanotti K, et al. Phase 2 trial of pegylated liposomal doxorubicin in advanced endometrial cancer. *J Cancer Res Clin Oncol.* 2003;129(11):651–654.
517. Muss HB, Blessing JA, Hatch KD, et al. Methotrexate in advanced endometrial carcinoma. A phase II trial of the Gynecologic Oncology Group. *Am J Clin Oncol.* 1990;13(1):61–63.
518. Dvorak O. Cytembena treatment of advanced gynaecological carcinomas. *Neoplasma.* 1971;18(5):461–464.
519. Broun GO, Blessing JA, Eddy GL, et al. A phase II trial of vincristine in advanced or recurrent endometrial carcinoma. A Gynecologic Oncology Group Study. *Am J Clin Oncol.* 1993;16(1):18–21.
520. Woo HL, Swenerton KD, Hoskins PJ. Taxol is active in platinum-resistant endometrial adenocarcinoma. *Am J Clin Oncol.* 1996;19(3):290–291.
521. Wadler S, Levy DE, Lincoln ST, et al. Topotecan is an active agent in the first-line treatment of metastatic or recurrent endometrial carcinoma: Eastern Cooperative Oncology Group Study E3E93. *J Clin Oncol.* 2003;21(11):2110–2114.
522. Traina TA, Sabbatini P, Aghajanian C, et al. Weekly topotecan for recurrent endometrial cancer: a case series and review of the literature. *Gynecol Oncol.* 2004;95(1):235–241.
523. Dizon DS, Blessing JA, McMeekin DS, et al. Phase II trial of ixabepilone as second-line treatment in advanced endometrial cancer: gynecologic oncology group trial 129-P. *J Clin Oncol.* 2009;27(19):3104–3108.
524. The Cancer Genome Atlas Research Network. Integrated genomic characterization of endometrial cancer. *Nature.* 2013;497:67–72.
525. Westin SN, Broaddus RR. Personalized therapy in endometrial cancer: challenges and opportunities. *Cancer Biol Ther.* 2012;13(1):1–13.
526. Yeramian A, Moreno-Bueno G, Dolcet X, et al. Endometrial carcinoma: molecular alterations involved in tumor development and progression. *Oncogene.* 2013;32(4):403–413.
527. Hennessy BT, Smith DL, Ram PT, et al. Exploiting the PI3K/AKT pathway for cancer drug discovery. *Nat Rev Drug Discov.* 2005;4(12):988–1004.
528. Naumann RW. The role of the phosphatidylinositol 3-kinase (PI3K) pathway in the development and treatment of uterine cancer. *Gynecol Oncol.* 2011;123(2):411–420.
529. Sansal I, Sellers W. The biology and clinical relevance of the *PTEN* tumor suppressor pathway. *J Clin Oncol.* 2004;22:2954–2963.
530. Lee JO, Yang H, Georgescu MM, et al. Crystal structure of the *PTEN* tumor suppressor: implications for its phosphoinositide phosphatase activity and membrane association. *Cell.* 1999;99:323–334.
531. Li J, Yen C, Liaw D, et al. *PTEN*, a putative protein tyrosine phosphatase gene mutated in human brain, breast, and prostate cancer. *Science.* 1997;275:1943–1947.
532. Maxwell GL, Risinger JI, Gumbs C, et al. Mutation of the *PTEN* tumor suppressor gene in endometrial hyperplasias. *Cancer Res.* 1998;58(12):2500–2503.
533. Tamura M, Gu J, Matsumoto K, et al. Inhibition of cell migration, spreading, and focal adhesions by tumour suppressor *PTEN*. *Science.* 1998;280:1614–1617.
534. Peiffer SL, Herzog TJ, Tribune DJ, et al. Allelic loss of sequences from the long arm of chromosome 10 and replication errors in endometrial cancers. *Cancer Res.* 1995;55:1922–1926.
535. Kong D, Suzuki A, Zou TT, et al. *PTEN1* is frequently mutated in primary endometrial carcinomas. *Nat Genet.* 1997;17:143–144.

536. Meric-Bernstam F, Gonzalez-Angulo AM. Targeting the mTOR signaling network for cancer therapy. *J Clin Oncol.* 2009;27(13):2278–2287.
537. Cantley LC. The phosphoinositide 3-kinase pathway. *Science.* 2002; 296(5573):1655–1657.
538. Slomovitz BM, Wu W, Broaddus RR, et al. mTOR inhibition is a rational target for the treatment of endometrial cancer. *Proc Am Soc Clin Oncol.* 2004;22:abstract 5076.
539. Engelman JA. Targeting PI3K signalling in cancer: opportunities, challenges and limitations. *Nat Rev Cancer.* 2009;9(8):550–562.
540. Dancey JE. Clinical development of mammalian target of rapamycin inhibitors. *Hematol Oncol Clin North Am.* 2002;16(5):1101–1114.
541. Oza AM, Elit L, Tsao MS, et al. Phase II study of temsirolimus in women with recurrent or metastatic endometrial cancer: a trial of the NCIC Clinical Trials Group. *J Clin Oncol.* 2011;29(24):3278–3285.
542. Kollmannsberger C, Hirte H, Siu LL, et al. Temsirolimus in combination with carboplatin and paclitaxel in patients with advanced solid tumors: a NCIC-CTG, phase I, open-label dose-escalation study (IND 179). *Ann Oncol.* 2012;23(1):238–244.
543. Fleming GF, Filiaci VL, Hanjani P, et al. Hormone therapy plus temsirolimus for endometrial carcinoma (EC): gynecologic oncologic group trial #248. *J Clin Oncol.* 2011;29 suppl: abstract 5014.
544. Colombo N, McMeekin DS, Schwartz PE, et al. A phase II trial of the mTOR inhibitor AP23573 as a single agent in advanced endometrial cancer. *Proc Am Soc Clin Oncol.* 2007;25: abstract 5516.
545. Mackay H, Welch S, Tsao MS, et al. Phase II study of oral ridaforolimus in patients with metastatic and/or locally advanced recurrent endometrial cancer: NCIC CTG IND 192. *J Clin Oncol.* 2011;29 suppl: abstract 5013.
546. Peltomäki P. Role of DNA mismatch repair defects in the pathogenesis of human cancer. *J Clin Oncol.* 2003;21:1174–1179.
547. Slomovitz BM, Lu KH, Johnston T, et al. A phase 2 study of the oral mammalian target of rapamycin inhibitor, everolimus, in patients with recurrent endometrial carcinoma. *Cancer.* 2010;116(23):5415–5419.
548. Meyer PN, Slomovitz BM, Djordjevic B, et al. The search continues: looking for predictive biomarkers for response mTOR inhibition in endometrial cancer. *J Clin Oncol.* 2011;29 suppl: abstract 5016.
549. Slomovitz BM, Brown J, Johnston TA, et al. A phase II study of everolimus and letrozole in patients with recurrent endometrial cancer. *J Clin Oncol.* 2011;29 suppl: abstract 5012.
550. Jiricny J. The multifaceted mismatch repair system. *Nat Rev Mol Cell Biol.* 2006;7:335–346.
551. MacDonald ND, Salvesen HB, Ryan A, et al. Frequency and prognostic impact of microsatellite instability in a large population based study of endometrial carcinomas. *Can Res.* 2000;60:1750–1752.
552. Basil JB, Goodfellow PJ, Rader JS, et al. Clinical significance of microsatellite instability in endometrial carcinoma. *Cancer.* 2000;89:1758–1764.
553. Dunlop MG, Farrington SM, Carothers AD, et al. Cancer risk associated with germline DNA mismatch repair gene mutations. *Hum Mol Genet.* 1977;6:105–110.
554. Black D, Soslow R, Levine D, et al. Clinicopathologic significance of defective DNA mismatch repair in endometrial carcinoma. *J Clin Oncol.* 2006;24:1745–1753.
555. Caduff RF, Johnston CM, Svoboda-Newman SM, et al. Clinical and pathological significance of microsatellite instability in sporadic endometrial carcinoma. *Am J Pathol.* 1996;148:1671–1678.
556. Duggan BD, Felix JC, Muderspach LI, et al. Microsatellite instability in sporadic endometrial carcinoma. *J Natl Cancer Inst.* 1994;86:1216–1221.
557. Helland A, Børresen-Dale AL, Peltomäki P, et al. Microsatellite instability in cervical endometrial carcinomas. *Int J Cancer.* 1997;70:499–501.
558. Risinger JI, Berchuck A, Kohler MF, et al. Genetic instability of microsatellite in endometrial carcinoma. *Cancer Res.* 1993;53:5100–5103.
559. Esteller M, Levine R, Baylin SB, et al. *MLH1* promoter hypermethylation is associated with the microsatellite instability phenotype in sporadic carcinomas. *Oncogene.* 1998;17:2413–2417.
560. Lax SF, Kendall B, Tashiro H, et al. The frequency of p53, K-ras mutation and microsatellite instability differs in uterine endometrioid and serous carcinoma. *Cancer.* 2000;88:814–824.
561. Lalloo F, Evans G. Molecular genetics and endometrial cancer. *Best Pract Res Clin Gynaecol.* 2001;15:355–363.
562. De Luca A, Carotenuto A, Rachiglio A, et al. The role of the EGFR signaling in tumor microenvironment. *J Cell Physiol.* 2008;214(3):559–567.
563. Bilbao C, Lara P, Ramirez R, et al. Microsatellite instability predicts clinical outcome in radiation treated endometrioid endometrial cancer. *Int J Radiation Oncol Biol Phys.* 2010;76:9–13.
564. Resnick K, Frankel W, Morrison C, et al. Mismatch repair status and outcomes after adjuvant therapy in patients with surgically staged endometrial cancer. *Gynecol Oncol.* 2010;117:234–238.
565. Moll UM, Chalas E, Auguste M, et al. Uterine papillary serous carcinoma evolves via a p53 driven pathway. *Hum Pathol.* 1996;27:1295–1300.
566. Tahiro H, Isacson C, Levine R, et al. p53 mutations are common in uterine serous carcinoma and occur as an early event in their pathogenesis. *Am J Pathol.* 1997;150:177–185.
567. Lukes AS, Kohler MF, Pieper CF, et al. Multivariable analysis of DNA ploidy, p53, and HER-2/neu as prognostic factors in endometrial cancer. *Cancer.* 1994;73:2380–2385.
568. Kihana T, Hamada K, Inoue Y, et al. Mutation and allelic loss of the p53 gene in endometrial carcinoma. Incidence and outcome in 92 surgical patients. *Cancer.* 1995;76(1):72–78.
569. Tashiro H, Isacson C, Levine R, et al. p53 gene mutations are common in uterine serous carcinoma and occur early in their pathogenesis. *Am J Pathol.* 1997;150:177–185.
570. Lundgren C, Auer G, Frankendal B, et al. Nuclear DNA content, proliferative activity, and p53 expression related to clinical and histopathologic features in endometrial carcinoma. *Int J Gynecol Cancer.* 2002;12:110–118.
571. Mendelsohn J. Targeting the epidermal growth factor receptor for cancer therapy. *J Clin Oncol.* 2002;20(18 suppl):1S–13S.
572. Khalifa MA, Mannel RS, Haraway SD, et al. Expression of EGFR, HER-2/neu, p53, and PCNA in endometrioid, serous papillary, and clear cell endometrial adenocarcinomas. *Gynecol Oncol.* 1994;53:84–92.
573. Takahashi K, Saga Y, Mizukami H, et al. Cetuximab inhibits growth, peritoneal dissemination, and lymph node and lung metastasis of endometrial cancer, and prolongs host survival. *Int J Oncol.* 2009;35(4):725–729.
574. Gaikwad A, Wolf JK, Brown J, et al. In vitro evaluation of the effects of gefitinib on the cytotoxic activity of selected anticancer agents in a panel of human endometrial cancer cell lines. *J Oncol Pharm Pract.* 2009;15(1):35–44.
575. Oza AM, Eisenhauer EA, Elit L, et al. Phase II study of erlotinib in recurrent or metastatic endometrial cancer: NCIC IND-148. *J Clin Oncol.* 2008;26(26):4319–4325.
576. Leslie KK, Sill MW, Darcy KM, et al. Efficacy and safety of gefitinib and potential prognostic value of soluble EGFR, EGFR mutations, and tumor markers in Gynecologic Oncology Group phase II trial of persistent of recurrent endometrial cancer. *J Clin Oncol.* 2009;27(suppl 15S):A-e16542.
577. Samarnthai N, Hall K, Yeh IT. Molecular profiling of endometrial malignancies. *Obstet Gynecol Int.* 2010;2010:162363.
578. Berchuck A, Rodriguez G, Kinney R, et al. Overexpression of HER-2/neu in endometrial cancer is associated with advanced stage disease. *Am J Obstet Gynecol.* 1991;164:15–21.
579. Reinartz JJ, George E, Lindgren BR, et al. Expression of p53, transforming growth factor alpha, epidermal growth factor receptor, and c-erbB-2 in endometrial carcinoma and correlation with survival and known predictors of survival. *Hum Pathol.* 1994;25:1075–1083.
580. Rolitsky C, Theil K, McGaughy V, et al. HER-2/neu amplification and over expression in endometrial carcinoma. *Int J Gynecol Pathol.* 1999;18:138–143.
581. Santin A, Bellone S, Van Stedum S, et al. Determination of HER2/neu status in uterine serous papillary carcinoma: Comparative analysis of immunohistochemistry and fluorescence *in situ* hybridization. *Gynecol Oncol.* 2005;98:24–30.
582. Slomovitz B, Broaddus RR, Burke TW, et al. Her-2/neu over expression and amplification in uterine papillary serous carcinoma. *J Clin Oncol.* 2004;22:3126–3132.
583. Kohler MF, Carney P, Dodge R, et al. p53 over expression in advanced-stage endometrial adenocarcinoma. *Am J Obstet Gynecol.* 1996;175:1246–1252.
584. Backe J, Gassel AM, Krebs S, et al. Immunohistochemically detected HER-2/neu—expression and prognosis in endometrial carcinoma. *Arch Gynecol Obstet.* 1997;259:189–195.
585. Pisani AL, Barbuto DA, Chen D, et al. HER-2/neu, p53, and DNA analyses as prognosticators for survival in endometrial carcinoma. *Obstet Gynecol.* 1995;85:729–734.
586. Hetzel DJ, Wilson TO, Keeney GL, et al. HER-2/neu expression: a major prognostic factor in endometrial cancer. *Gynecol Oncol.* 1992;47:179–185.
587. Nazeer T, Ballouk F, Malfetano JH, et al. Multivariate survival analysis of clinicopathologic features in surgical stage I endometrioid carcinoma including analysis of HER-2/neu expression. *Am J Obstet Gynecol.* 1995;173:1829–1834.
588. Saffari B, Jones L, el-Naggar A, et al. Amplification and over expression of HER-2/neu (c-erbB-2) in endometrial cancers: correlation with overall survival. *Cancer Res.* 1995;55:5693–5698.
589. Morrison C, Fanagolo V, Ramirez N, et al. HER-2 is an independent prognostic factor in endometrial cancer: association with outcome in a large cohort of surgically staged patients. *J Clin Oncol.* 2006;24:2376–2385.

590. Fleming GF, Sill MW, Darcy KM, et al. Phase II trial of trastuzumab in women with advanced or recurrent, HER2-positive endometrial carcinoma: a Gynecologic Oncology Group study. *Gynecol Oncol.* 2010;116(1):15–20.
591. Schwab CL, Bellone S, English DP, et al. Afatinib demonstrates remarkable acitivty against HER 2 amplified uterine serous endometrial cancer in vitor and in vivo. *Br J Cancer.* 2014;111:1750–1756.
592. Caduff RF, Johnston CM, Frank TS. Mutations of the K-ras oncogene in carcinoma of the endometrium. *Am J Pathol.* 1995;146:182–188.
593. Esteller M, Garcia A, Martinez-Palones JM, et al. The clinicopathological significance of K-RAS point mutation and gene amplification in endometrial cancer. *Eur J Cancer.* 1997;33:1572–1577.
594. Ito K, Watanabe K, Nasik S, et al. K-ras point mutations in endometrial carcinoma: effect on outcome is dependent on age of patient. *Gynecol Oncol.* 1996;63:238–246.
595. Semczuk A, Berbec H, Kostuch M, et al. K-ras gene point mutations in human endometrial carcinomas: correlation with clinicopathological features and patients' outcome. *J Cancer Res Clin Oncol.* 1998;124:695–700.
596. Courteny KD, Cocoran RB, Engleman JA. The PI3K pathway as a drug target in human cancer. *J Clin Oncol.* 2010;28:1075–1083.
597. Yuan TL, Cantley LC. PI3K pathway alterations in cancer: variations on a theme. *Oncogene.* 2008;27:5497–5510.
598. De Luca A, Maiello MR, D'Alessio A, et al. The RAS/RAF/MEK/ERK and the PI3K/AKT signalling pathways: role in cancer pathogenesis and implications for therapeutic approaches. *Expert Opin Ther Targets.* 2012;16(S2):S17–S27.
599. Wang LE, Ma H, Hale KS, et al. Roles of genetic variants in the PI3K and RAS/RAF pathways in susceptibility to endometrial cancer and clinical outcomes. *J Cancer Res Clin Oncol.* 2012;138(3):377–385.
600. Semczuk A, Berbeć H, Kostuch M, et al. K-ras gene point mutations in human endometrial carcinomas: correlation with clinicopathological features and patients' outcome. *J Cancer Res Clin Oncol.* 1998;124(12): 695–700.
601. Ramjaun AR, Downward J. Ras and phosphoinositide 3-kinase: partners in development and tumorigenesis. *Cell Cycle.* 2007;6(23):2902–2905.
602. Stefansson IM, Salvesen HB, Akslen LA. Vascular proliferation is important for clinical progress of endometrial cancer. *Cancer Res.* 2006;66(6):3303–3309.
603. Salvesen HB, Iversen OE, Akslen LA. Prognostic significance of angiogenesis and Ki-67, p53, and p21 expression: a population-based endometrial carcinoma study. *J Clin Oncol.* 1999;17(5):1382–1390.
604. Kamat AA, Merritt WM, Coffey D, et al. Clinical and biological significance of vascular endothelial growth factor in endometrial cancer. *Clin Cancer Res.* 2007;13(24):7487–7495.
605. Gehrig PA, Bae-Jump VL. Promising novel therapies for the treatment of endometrial cancer. *Gynecol Oncol.* 2010;116(2):187–194.
606. Aghajanian C, Sill MW, Darcy KM, et al. Phase II trial of bevacizumab in recurrent or persistent endometrial cancer: a Gynecologic Oncology Group study. *J Clin Oncol.* 2011;29(16):2259–2265.
607. Aghajanian C, Filiaci VL, Dizon DS, et al. A randomized phase II study of paclitaxel/carboplatin/bevacizumab, paclitaxel/carboplatin/temsirolimus and ixabepilone/carboplatin/bevacizumab as initial therapy for measurable stage III or IVA, stage IVB or recurrent endometrial cancer, GOG86P. *J Clin Oncol.* 2015;33 suppl: abstract 5500.
608. Lorusso D, Ferrandina G, Colombo N, et al. Randomized phase II trial of carboplatin-paclitaxel (CP) compared to carboplatin-paclitaxel-bevacizumab (CPBin advanced (stage III-IV) or recurrent endometrial cancer: the MITO END-2. *J Clin Oncol.* 2015;33 suppl: abstract 5502.
609. Alvarez EA. A Phase II trial of combination bevacizumab and temsirolimus in the treatment of recurrent or persistent endometrial carcinoma: A Gynecologic Group Study. *Gynecol Oncol.* 2013;129(1):22–27.
610. Correa R, Mackay H, Hirte HW, et al. A phase II study of sunitinib in recurrent or metastatic endometrial carcinoma: a trial of the Princess Margaret Hospital, The University of Chicago, and California Cancer Phase II Consortia. *J Clin Oncol.* 2010;28(15 suppl): abstract 5038.
611. Nimeiri HS, Oza AM, Morgan RJ, et al. A phase II study of sorafenib in advanced uterine carcinoma/carcinosarcoma: a trial of the Chicago, PMH, and California Phase II Consortia. *Gynecol Oncol.* 2010;117(1):37–40.
612. McMeekin DS, Sill MW, Benbrook D, et al. A phase II trial of thalidomide in patients with refractory endometrial cancer and correlation with angiogenesis biomarkers: a Gynecologic Oncology Group study. *Gynecol Oncol.* 2007;105(2):508–516.
613. Powell MA, Sill MW, Goodfellow PJ, et al. A phase II trial of brivanib in Recurrent or persistent endometrial cancer: An NRG Oncology / Gynecologic Oncology Group Study. *Gynecol Oncol.* 2014;135(1):38–43.
614. Bender DB, Sill MW, Lankes HA, et al. A phase II evaluation of cediranib in the treatemnt of recurrent of persistent endometrial cancer: An NRG Oncology/Gynecologic Oncology Study Group. *Gynecol Oncol.* 2015;138:507–512.
615. Dizon DS, Sill MW, Schilder JM, et al. A phase II evaluation of Nintedanib (BIBF-1120) in the treatment of recurrent or persistent endometrial cancer: An NRG Oncology/Gynecologic Oncology Study Group. *Gynecol Oncol.* 2014;135(3):441–445.
616. Coleman RL, Sill MW, Lankes HA, et al. A phase II evaluation of Aflibercept in the treatment of recurrent or persistent endometrial cancer: a Gynecologic Oncology Group Study. *Gynecol Oncol.* 2012;127(3):538–543.
617. Soliman PT, Wu D, Tortolero-Luna G, et al. Association between adiponectin, insulin resistance, and endometrial cancer. *Cancer.* 2006;106(11):2376–2381.
618. Chia VM, Newcomb PA, Trentham-Dietz A, et al. Obesity, diabetes, and other factors in relation to survival after endometrial cancer diagnosis. *Int J Gynecol Cancer.* 2007;17(2):441–446.
619. Cantrell LA, Zhou C, Mendivil A, et al. Metformin is a potent inhibitor of endometrial cancer cell proliferation—implications for a novel treatment strategy. *Gynecol Oncol.* 2010;116(1):92–98.
620. Evans JM, Donnelly LA, Emslie-Smith AM, et al. Metformin and reduced risk of cancer in diabetic patients. *BMJ.* 2005;330(7503):1304–1305.
621. Tan BK, Adya R, Chen J, et al. Metformin treatment exerts antiinvasive and antimetastatic effects in human endometrial carcinoma cells. *J Clin Endocrinol Metab.* 2011;96(3):808–816.
622. Brunmair B, Staniek K, Gras F, et al. Thiazolidinediones, like metformin, inhibit respiratory complex I: a common mechanism contributing to their antidiabetic actions? *Diabetes.* 2004;53(4):1052–1059.
623. Hadad SM, Fleming S, Thompson AM. Targeting AMPK: A new therapeutic opportunity in breast cancer. *Crit Rev Oncol Hematol.* 2008;67(1):1–7.
624. Cantrell LA, Zhou C, Mendivil A, et al. Metformin is a potent inhibitor of endometrial cancer cell proliferation—implications for a novel treatment strategy. *Gynecol Oncol.* 2008;116(1):92–98.
625. Gotlieb WH, Saumet J, Beauchamp MC, et al. In vitro metformin anti-neoplastic activity in epithelial ovarian cancer. *Gynecol Oncol.* 2008;110(2):246–250.
626. Zakikhani M, Dowling R, Fantus IG, et al. Metformin is an AMP kinase-dependent growth inhibitor for breast cancer cells. *Cancer Res.* 2006;66(21):10269–10273.
627. Zakikhani M, Dowling RJ, Sonenberg N, et al. The effects of adiponectin and metformin on prostate and colon neoplasia involve activation of AMP-activated protein kinase. *Cancer Prev Res (Phila Pa).* 2008;1(5):369–375.
628. Hanna RK, Zhou C, Malloy KM, et al. Metformin potentiates the effects of paclitaxel in endometrial cancer cells through inhibition of cell proliferation and modulation of the mTOR pathway. *Gynecol Oncol.* 2012;125(2):458–469.
629. Forster MD, Dedes KJ, Sandhu S, et al. Treatment with olaparib in a patient with PTEN-deficient endometrioid endometrial cancer. *Nat Rev Clin Oncol.* 2011;8(5):302–306.
630. Javle M, Curtin NJ. The role of PARP in DNA repair and its therapeutic exploitation. *Br J Cancer.* 2011;105(8):1114–1122.
631. Mendes-Pereira AM, Martin SA, Brough R, et al. Synthetic lethal targeting of PTEN mutant cells with PARP inhibitors. *EMBO Mol Med.* 2009;1(6–7):315–322.
632. Dedes KJ, Wetterskog D, Mendes-Pereira AM, et al. PTEN deficiency in endometrioid endometrial adenocarcinomas predicts sensitivity to PARP inhibitors. *Sci Transl Med.* 2010;2(53):53ra75.
633. Aghajanian C, Sill MW, Secord AA, et al. Iniparib plus paclitaxel and carboplatin as initial treatment of advanced or recurrent uerine carcinosarcoma: a Gynecologic Oncology Group Study. *Gynecol Oncol.* 2012;126(3):424–427.
634. Le DT, Uram JN, Wang H, et al. PD-1 Blockade in Tumors with Mismatch-Repair Deficiency. *N Engl J Med.* 2015;372(26):2509–2520.
635. Howitt BE, Shukla SA, Sholl LM, et al. Association of Polymerase e-mutated and microsatellite-instable endometrial cancers with neoantigen load, number of tumor- infiltrating lymphocytes, and expression of PD-1 and PD-L1. *JAMA Oncol.* 2015;1(9):1319–1323.
636. Zanotti KM, Belinson JL, Kennedy AW, et al. The use of paclitaxel and platinum-based chemotherapy in uterine papillary serous carcinoma. *Gynecol Oncol.* 1999;74:272–277.

637. Ramondetta L, Burke TW, Levenback C, et al. Treatment of uterine papillary serous carcinoma with paclitaxel. *Gynecol Oncol.* 2001;82:156–161.
638. Gehrig PA. Uterine papillary serous carcinoma: a review. *Expert Opin Pharmacother.* 2007;8:809–816.
639. Low JS, Wong EH, Tan HS, et al. Adjuvant sequential chemotherapy and radiotherapy in uterine papillary serous carcinoma. *Gynecol Oncol.* 2005;97:171–177.
640. Kelly MG, O'Malley DM, Hui P, et al. Improved survival in surgical stage I patients with uterine papillary serous carcinoma (UPSC) treated with adjuvant platinum-based chemotherapy. *Gynecol Oncol.* 2005;98(3):353–359.
641. Boruta DM, Gehrig PA, Nickles Fader A, et al. Management of women with uterine serous cancer: A Society of Gynecologic Oncology review. *Gynecol Oncol.* 2009;115:142–153.
642. Olawaiye AB, Boruta DM. Management of women with clear cell endomtrial cancer; A Society of Gynecologic Oncology review. *Gynecol Oncol.* 2009;113:277–283.

CHAPTER 22

Corpus: Mesenchymal Tumors

Mario M. Leitao Jr, Carmen Tornos, Aaron H. Wolfson, and Roisin O'Cearbhaill

INTRODUCTION

Mesenchymal tumors of the uterine corpus are rare, accounting for approximately 7% to 8% of all uterine cancers (1). The outcomes of many of these tumors seem to be less favorable than in many of the more common uterine carcinomas. However, outcomes do vary significantly based on specific histology. These tumors are believed to arise from the mesenchymatous portion of the uterine corpus, and are often considered to be uterine "sarcomas." The World Health Organization (WHO) classification of mesenchymal uterine corpus tumors is summarized in **Table 22.1** (2). Uterine carcinosarcomas (CS) may not be best classified as sarcomas or mesenchymal tumors any longer, but rather as metaplastic carcinomas of the uterus (3). Nevertheless, this group of malignancies will be described as "uterine CS" in this chapter. A key concept is that uterine sarcomas are truly heterogeneous tumors with vastly different clinical presentations, responses to therapy, and outcomes. Until recently, much of the available literature has been extremely limited, as most studies have combined all uterine sarcomas into a single cohort.

TABLE 22.1. WHO Classification of Mesenchymal Tumors of the Uterine Corpus

Mesenchymal Tumors
Endometrial stromal and related tumors
Endometrial stromal sarcoma, low grade
Endometrial stromal nodule
Undifferentiated endometrial sarcoma
Smooth muscle tumors
LMS
Epithelioid variant
Myxoid variant
Smooth muscle tumor of uncertain malignant potential
Leiomyoma, NOS
Histologic variants
Mitotically active variant
Cellular variant
Hemorrhagic cellular variant
Epithelioid variant
Myxoid
Atypical variant
Lipoleiomyoma variant
Growth pattern variants
Diffuse leiomyomatosis
Dissecting leiomyoma
Intravenous leiomyomatosis
Metastasizing leiomyoma
Miscellaneous mesenchymal tumors
Mixed endometrial stromal and smooth muscle tumor
Perivascular epithelioid cell tumor
Adenomatoid tumor
Other malignant mesenchymal tumors
Other benign mesenchymal tumors Mixed Epithelial and Mesenchymal Tumors
Carcinosarcoma (malignant Mullërian mixed tumor; metaplastic carcinoma)
Adenosarcoma
Carcinofibroma
Adenofibroma
Adenomyoma
Atypical polypoid variant

Source: Tumors of the uterine corpus. In: Tavassoli FA, Devilee P, eds. *World Health Organization Classification of Tumours. Pathology and genetics of Tumours of the Breast and Female Genital Organs*. Lyons, France: IARC Press; 2003:217–258, with permission.

EPIDEMIOLOGY AND RISK FACTORS

Histologic Distribution

The histopathologic criteria for uterine sarcomas have evolved significantly over the last few years. Therefore, histologic distribution may have shifted. Many series do not include or specify sarcoma subtypes, and many of these studies report on very small patient cohorts. By combining series with at least 100 cases, including CS, we see that the most common uterine sarcomas are leiomyosarcoma (LMS) and CS (4–9) **(Fig. 22.1A)**. LMS accounts for over two-thirds of uterine sarcomas (4–10) **(Fig. 22.1B)**. Endometrial stromal sarcomas (ESS) account for approximately 25% of true uterine sarcomas; all other subtypes are exceedingly rare, comprising <10% (4–10) **(Fig. 22.1B)**. ESS has traditionally been considered a low-grade tumor. Undifferentiated uterine sarcoma is now the preferred terminology for what was previously described as high-grade ESS.

However, the description of high-grade ESS has been redefined (11). Most recently, Abeler and colleagues (10) reported the largest series of uterine sarcomas ($n = 419$) from the Norwegian Cancer Registry (which describes histologic subtype distribution). This series excluded CS altogether. Of the 419 included sarcomas, 62% were LMS, 20% were ESS, and 18% were various other subtypes including undifferentiated sarcomas (6%), adenosarcomas (5.5%), sarcoma not otherwise specified (NOS) (4.5%), rhabdomyosarcoma (<1%), giant cell sarcoma (<1%), and perivascular epithelioid cell tumors (PEComa; <1%) (10).

Age Distribution

Patients with CS and adenosarcomas (AS) tend to be older at the time of diagnosis compared to those with LMS and ESS. The mean/median ages reported in the published series range from 42 to 51 years for

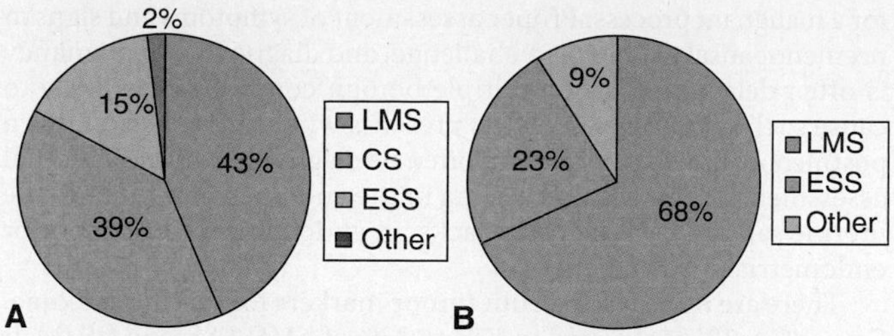

Figure 22.1. Histologic distribution of uterine sarcomas in series with at least 100 cases, **(A)** including CS and **(B)** excluding CS. ESS, endometrial stromal sarcoma; CS, carcinosarcoma; LMS, leiomyosarcoma; AS, adenosarcoma.

ESS (4,5,9,10–16), 48 to 57 years for LMS (4,5,9,10,17–19), 57 to 67 years for CS (4,5,9,20,21), 58 to 66 years for AS (10,22), and 46 years for undifferentiated sarcomas (12). Thus, many patients with CS are postmenopausal at the time of diagnosis, whereas patients with LMS, ESS, or undifferentiated sarcomas may be pre- or perimenopausal at diagnosis. The mean age for patients diagnosed with smooth muscle tumors of uncertain malignant potential (STUMP) is 43 years, and many of these patients are likely to be premenopausal (23). This has potential implications in terms of patient fertility. The other tumor subtypes are so rare that it is difficult to discern a particular pattern of age distribution among them.

Racial Distribution

Zelmanowicz et al. (24) noted that women with CS are more likely to be of African American descent (among 453 patients and controls, 28% vs. 4% other, $p = 0.001$) than those with endometrial adenocarcinomas. In reviews by Mortel et al. and Norris et al. (25,26), 33% and 24% of patients with CS were non-Caucasian, respectively. Brooks et al. (27) reported that the age-adjusted incidence of uterine sarcomas in African American women was twice that of controls. The age-adjusted incidences of LMS for Black and White women, respectively, were 1.5 and 0.9 per 100,000. Those for CS in African American and Caucasian women, respectively, were 4.3 and 1.7 per 100,000. Felix and colleagues (28) noted that African American race was more prevalent among 82 LMS cases (20.7%) compared to 98 EMS cases (6.1%).

Risk Factors

Prior Radiation Exposure

Prior exposure to pelvic radiotherapy (RT) is thought to increase the risk of developing a subsequent uterine sarcoma, primarily CS and undifferentiated sarcoma. However, prior pelvic RT is not thought to increase the risk for uterine LMS or STUMP. In a large series from the Mayo Clinic, only 1 (0.6%) of 208 patients with LMS had received prior pelvic RT (29). In a study from MD Anderson Cancer Center, none of 41 patients with STUMP had a history of pelvic RT (23). In a study by Christopherson et al. (30) only 2 of 33 patients with uterine LMS had a history of RT.

In the series of CS reported by Norris et al. in 1966 (26), 9 of 31 (29%) patients had received pelvic RT 7 to 26 years prior to diagnosis. In a 1986 report by Meredith et al. (31) on 1,208 uterine malignancies, only 30 (2.4%) patients had received prior pelvic RT. Interestingly, only 8 patients had received RT for a gynecologic malignancy; others had pelvic RT for a benign diagnosis. Of irradiated patients, 5 (17%) developed CS, with a crude association of 11%. The risk of endometrial adenocarcinoma after radiation was much less than 2%. It has been suggested that postirradiation CS occur at a younger average age than those arising *de novo* (32). Latency to diagnosis of malignancy is generally shorter in older patients (31). Pothuri et al. (33) compared the clinicopathologic characteristics of 23 cases of uterine cancers occurring in patients with prior history of cervical cancer treated with pelvic RT, to 527 cases of uterine cancers in patients with no history of pelvic RT. CS and undifferentiated sarcomas accounted for 9 (39%) of the 23 radiation-associated malignancies, compared to 33 (8%) of the sporadic cases (33). It appears that radiation-associated malignancies tend to have a worse outcome, possibly due to lack of early symptomatology. In the setting of other, very rare uterine sarcoma subtypes, definitive assessment is precluded.

Hormone Exposure and Obesity

It has been suggested that exposure to hormonal medications, including tamoxifen, may increase the risk of uterine sarcomas. The association of estradiol–progestin therapy was assessed by Jaakkola et al. (34) using data from the Finnish Cancer Registry (which captures nearly 100% of all cancers in Finland) and the Reimbursement Registry of the Social Insurance Institution of Finland. Uterine sarcomas occurred in 76 of the 243,857 women identified as having used estradiol–progestin therapy for more than 6 months. Carcinosarcomas were not included in this analysis. Use of estradiol–progestin therapy was associated with a 60% elevation in risk for any uterine sarcoma (standardized incidence ratio [SIR], 1.6; 95% confidence interval [CI], 1.2–1.9). It was mostly associated with LMS (SIR, 1.8; 95% CI, 1.3–2.4); no statistically significant association with ESS was identified (SIR, 1.4; 95% CI, 0.9–2.1). Additionally, the elevated risk was noted only in women who had used estradiol–progestin therapy for 5 years or more.

The Epidemiology of Endometrial Cancer Consortium (E2C2) recently published a pooled analysis of 15 cohort and case–control observational studies (28). This is the largest series to date assessing risk factors for uterine sarcoma (n = 229) and CS (n = 244) versus endometrioid endometrial carcinomas (n = 7,623) and normal controls (n = 28,829). Uterine sarcomas included all sarcomas of the uterus, with 98 ESS and 82 LMS. Oral contraceptive use, postmenopausal estrogen (ER)-alone use, and postmenopausal ER–progesterone (PR) use were not associated with uterine sarcoma or CS. No association was found when LMS and ESS were analyzed separately. Thus, it seems that the association of hormonal use with risk of uterine sarcoma or CS is not strong. As the risk is exceedingly low, these data should not dissuade use of hormones in appropriate cases.

Interestingly, the E2C2 analyses suggested an association of obesity (BMI $\geq$30 kg/m^2) with uterine sarcoma (OR = 1.73 [95% CI, 1.22–2.46]) and CS (OR = 2.25 [95% CI, 1.60–3.15]). Obesity was also associated with ESS (OR = 1.74 [95% CI, 1.03–2.93]), but not LMS (OR = 1.56 [95% CI, 0.88–2.77]). As ESS is known to be ER-driven, the association with obesity is understandable. However, the association of obesity with CS in this analysis requires further study and validation.

Tamoxifen Use

Tamoxifen use among breast cancer patients may also increase the risk of uterine malignancies, including sarcomas. Using data from the National Israeli Cancer Registry, Lavie and colleagues (35) reported on 1,507 cases of women with breast cancer diagnosed from 1987 to 1988. They noted that uterine cancers developed in 17 of 886 (1.9%) women treated with tamoxifen, compared to only 4 of 621 (0.6%) women who did not receive tamoxifen (OR, 3.1; 95% CI, 1–9.1). The risk of uterine cancer was associated with increased duration of tamoxifen use. A significant association was seen with more than 4 years of tamoxifen use (OR, 6.6; 95% CI, 2.0–21.1), whereas use of tamoxifen for 2 years or less was not associated with an increased risk (OR, 2.1; 95% CI, 0.4–11.6). Uterine sarcomas developed in only four patients in the entire cohort; these included two CS and two rhabdomyosarcomas. All four occurred in patients who received tamoxifen, suggesting a possible association of tamoxifen use and risk of uterine sarcoma. Hoogendoorn and colleagues (36) reported that among patients diagnosed with uterine cancer, CS accounted for a much larger proportion of cases in those who had received prior tamoxifen therapy compared to those who had not (15% vs. 4%, respectively).

Hereditary Predisposition

Hereditary predisposition to certain uterine sarcomas has also been suggested, but this remains to be elucidated. Using the Danish Hereditary Nonpolyposis Colorectal Cancer (HNPCC) Registry, Nilbert et al. (37) identified 164 HNPCC families with predisposing mutations; sarcomas of various sites represented only 1% ($n = 14$) of 1,570 malignant diagnoses. Three sarcomas were uterine: one was a CS in a 44-year-old with loss of MSH2 and MSH6 expression; another CS was seen in a 55-year-old with loss of MSH6 expression; another was an LMS in a 44-year-old with loss of MSH2 and MSH6 expression. Recently, it has been suggested that the prevalence of uterine LMS is increased in women with hereditary retinoblastoma (38). Although the overall risk of uterine sarcoma is low in these hereditary syndromes, it is nevertheless of interest. Because of the high risk of endometrial sarcoma, prophylactic hysterectomy is strongly recommended in women from HNPCC kindreds after childbearing is complete. No such recommendation exists for women with hereditary retinoblastoma, as the potential risk was only recently described. However, we believe that it is reasonable to consider prophylactic total hysterectomy, with retention of ovaries, in women with a history of retinoblastoma who have completed childbearing.

CLINICAL PRESENTATION AND DIAGNOSIS

Presenting Symptoms and Signs

The most common presenting symptom of uterine sarcoma is abnormal vaginal bleeding (4,12,14,22,27,38) (**Table 22.2**). Patients with LMS often present with an abdominopelvic mass, or a mass that is palpable on physical examination (4,27). LMS and ESS are often incidentally diagnosed after surgery for presumed uterine fibroids. ESS was an incidental finding in 42% of cases reported by Memorial Sloan Kettering Cancer Center (16). Therefore, it is quite likely that the vast majority of patients ultimately diagnosed with LMS or ESS would have some abnormal enlargement of the uterus, discovered after presentation with abnormal vaginal bleeding. Vaginal bleeding in a postmenopausal female should be evaluated appropriately, with endometrial sampling and possibly an intravaginal ultrasound (US). An enlarging pelvic mass in a postmenopausal female is suspicious for a malignant process. Proper assessment of symptoms and signs in premenopausal patients is a challenge, and diagnosis of malignancy is often delayed because multiple benign conditions are likely to cause such symptoms. CS often presents with vaginal bleeding in a postmenopausal female and can often be diagnosed with endometrial assessment, as it is a lesion arising in the endometrium (unlike true uterine sarcoma, which often lacks an endometrial component or endometrial involvement).

There are no reliable serum tumor markers for uterine sarcoma. Serum CA-125 is elevated in 17% to 33% of LMS, ESS, and CS (4). It should not be routinely used in the evaluation and diagnosis of these tumors. Preoperative endometrial assessment with office pipelle or dilation and curettage under anesthesia are of limited accuracy. However, endometrial assessments should be performed in all women who present with abnormal vaginal bleeding. Bansal et al. (39) reported that invasive tumor was diagnosed in 86% of uterine sarcoma cases through preoperative endometrial sampling. The correct histology was noted in only 64% of the cases ultimately diagnosed as uterine sarcoma (39). However, a majority of sarcomas in this series (32/46; 70%) were correctly diagnosed as CS on final pathology, as well as four LMS, two ESS, and eight other sarcomas (39).

TABLE 22.2. Common Presenting Symptoms in Patients with Uterine Sarcomas (Percentage of Cases Describing the Symptoms)

Symptom	ESS (%) (4,12,14)	CS (%) (4)	LMS (%) (4,27)	AS (%) (22,38)
Asymptomatic	14	7	11	12
Abnormal vaginal bleeding	68	68	53	61
Abdominopelvic mass	14	16	48	—
Abdominopelvic pain	18	9	23	20
Uterine enlargement	64	—	—	—
Uterine cavity lesion	21	—	—	—
Vaginal discharge	4	—	—	—
Abdominal distention	—	—	—	2

AS, adenosarcoma; CS, carcinosarcoma; ESS, endometrial stromal sarcoma; LMS, leiomyosarcoma.

Preoperative Imaging

Preoperative imaging is of limited accuracy in differentiating benign from malignant uterine lesions, especially in the absence of obvious extrauterine disease; nevertheless, it is often utilized as part of the initial evaluation of these patients. While CS are more often diagnosed via endometrial sampling, preoperative imaging may be valuable in determining the presence of extrauterine disease. Small single-institution retrospective series have suggested that pelvic magnetic resonance imaging (MRI) may be of value in identifying uterine sarcomas and distinguishing them from benign uterine lesions. Namimto et al. (40) reported 100% sensitivity and specificity using diffusion-weighted imaging (DWI) and T2-weighted MRI in distinguishing uterine sarcomas from benign lesions, compared to DWI alone. This seems promising, but it is unlikely to be utilized in clinical practice and its accuracy may not be reliably reproducible. For example, Cornfeld and colleagues (41), using various objective MRI criteria, reported that MRI showed very poor accuracy in distinguishing leiomyomas with atypical imaging features from malignant uterine mesenchymal tumors. Using various MRI-specific criteria, the sensitivity of this imaging modality in identifying uterine sarcoma ranged from only 17% to 56%; however, specificity was 80% to 100% (41).

Serum LDH and MRI

Serum lactate dehydrogenase (LDH) may be an interesting additive to imaging in the evaluation of uterine lesions concerning for LMS (**Table 22.3**). In a prospective trial, Goto and colleagues (42) reported an accuracy of 99.3% in predicting uterine LMS when serum LDH was combined with dynamic MRI. The positive predictive value (PPV) was 91% using the combined assessment, compared to 39% for LDH alone and 71% for MRI (dynamic or not). These results are impressive and require further validation, but it is simple enough to obtain a serum LDH in patients with concerning lesions of the uterus. Another important point is that the series by Goto et al., as well as other series, report a high specificity and nearly 100% negative predictive value (NPV) for MRI, with or without LDH. This may be useful for patients who do not wish to undergo surgery, especially those desiring fertility. It may also help in deciding upon the surgical approach for patients with presumed benign leiomyomas as well as suspicious lesions.

Uterine Morcellation

Laparoscopy has become the standard, preferred approach in the management of women with benign and malignant gynecologic conditions. Morcellation of the uterus, either for removal of the specimen during minimally invasive procedures, for myomectomy

■ TABLE 22.3. Test Characteristics Using Dynamic MRI and Serum LDH in Predicting Uterine LMS from Degenerating Leiomyomas

Test	Sensitivity (%)	Specificity (%)	Accuracy (%)	PPV (%)	NPV (%)
Total serum LDH	100	87.7	86.6	38.5	100
MRI	100	96.9	97.1	71.4	100
Dynamic MRI	100	87.5	90.5	71.4	100
LDH . . . dynamic MRI	100	99.2	99.3	90.9	100

NPV, negative predictive value; PPV, positive predictive value.

Source: Adapted from Goto A, Takeuchi S, Sugimura K, et al. Usefulness of Gd-DTPA contrast-enhanced dynamic MRi and serum determination of LDH and its isozymes in the differential diagnosis of leiomyosarcoma from degenerated leiomyoma of the uterus. *Int J Gynecol Cancer*. 2002;12:354–361, with permission (Lippincott Williams & Wilkins).

for fertility preservation, or for supracervical hysterectomy, has been commonplace for many years. Morcellation is often not done in the setting of CS because these patients tend to be older and the diagnosis of malignancy is known preoperatively. However, it is not unusual that an LMS or ESS is incidentally diagnosed after some form of morcellation, or less-than-total hysterectomy. Morcellation of a uterine LMS is associated with worse outcome. Perri et al. (43) reported a significantly higher rate of recurrence and lower overall survival (OS) in women who had undergone something less than a total abdominal hysterectomy (TAH) and were subsequently diagnosed with uterine LMS. The hazard ratios (HR) for recurrence and survival in TAH compared to other types of resection (myomectomy, morcellation, or supracervical hysterectomy) were 0.39 and 0.36, respectively. Park et al. (44) reported a series in which the 5-year disease-free survival (DFS) was 40% in women who underwent tumor morcellation and were subsequently diagnosed with LMS, compared to 65% in patients with LMS who did not undergo morcellation ($p = 0.04$). Similarly, the 5-year OS was 46% after morcellation, compared to 73% in patients who were not morcellated ($p = 0.04$) (44). Morcellation also appears to have a negative impact on risk of recurrence in ESS, but no adverse impact on OS (45).

The true impact of morcellation of uterine LMS is difficult to fully understand because of the very small cohorts and overall poor quality of published reports. Bogani and colleagues (46) reported the results of an extensive meta-analysis on the impact of morcellation and outcomes in patients with unsuspected uterine LMS. Following an exhaustive review of the available medical literature databases, they identified 60 potential studies. After applying rigorous inclusion material, only four studies remained in the meta-analysis. These included 202 patients (75 morcellated, 127 non-morcellated); all were analyzed retrospectively. The 75 morcellated cases included patients who had undergone open, vaginal, laparoscopic, or hysteroscopic morcellation. Significantly higher rates of overall recurrence, intra-abdominal recurrence, and death were noted in the morcellated cohort. The combined death rate for morcellated versus non-morcellated was 48% and 29%, respectively (OR = 2.42 [95% CI, 1.19–4.92]; $p = 0.01$). The rate of extra-abdominal recurrence was not significantly different. The authors clearly noted a high risk of bias in all four studies.

The higher risk of recurrence and death may be a consequence of disseminated, unrecognized sarcoma during morcellation. The difference in intra-abdominal recurrence rates noted by Bogani and colleagues is very similar to that reported by Oduyebo et al. (47) in a small (but the largest available) series of cases of disseminated disease identified at the time of re-exploration, immediately after morcellation, from an unrecognized LMS. Disseminated sarcomatosis was noted in two out of seven patients (28.6%) with uterine LMS who underwent immediate re-exploration prior to noted recurrence. All seven were presumed to be stage I at the time of initial surgery. Both patients recurred and one died; the other had only 8 months of follow-up. In the five cases without disease at re-exploration, four (80%) have not recurred and are alive without evidence of disease at a median follow-up of 23.4 months (range, 3.5–48.2 months). The true value of re-exploration cannot be definitively stated based on such a small series. Additionally, one cannot comment on whether immediate re-exploration and possible debulking would alter the outcomes. However, immediate re-exploration and possible debulking are reasonable considerations. Re-exploration may provide information to help guide decisions regarding additional therapies. At a minimum, it provides prognostic information and a clearer understanding of the patient's current disease state.

Despite the potential adverse impact of morcellation on outcomes in patients ultimately diagnosed with LMS and ESS, we cannot definitively conclude that morcellation or myomectomy are entirely inappropriate in the management of patients with presumed benign leiomyomas. The risk of LMS and ESS in patients undergoing surgery for presumed benign leiomyoma is quite low. In a combined series of four studies with a total of 4,981 patients, the risk of LMS and ESS after surgery for presumed benign leiomyoma was only 0.24% and 0.06%, respectively (48–51). This risk is no greater in those undergoing surgery for an indication of rapidly enlarging leiomyoma (49).

The risk of unexpected malignancy is associated with age. In two large public database analyses, the risk of any uterine cancer was exceedingly low in women less than 40 years of age, but increased significantly with increasing patient age (52,53). Neither study specifically assessed the prevalence or risk of uterine sarcoma.

In April 2014, the U.S. Food and Drug Administration (FDA) issued a safety communication regarding uterine power morcellation (54). This communication was not an outright ban. It encouraged thoughtful decision-making when considering morcellation, but strongly discouraged it. The FDA communication also specified a need for careful patient counseling regarding the risks of power morcellation before consenting patients for surgery. While the FDA communication comments only on power morcellation, similar concerns remain with respect to myomectomy and supracervical (subtotal) hysterectomy that, as stated previously, are not morcellated. Additionally, little has been mentioned regarding uterine artery embolization of presumed uterine fibroids. In response to the FDA communication, many institutions decided to ban the use of power morcellation altogether. Patient safety is always the prime consideration in surgery. However, when morcellation is completely abandoned, there are many other consequences that must be taken into account. Barron and colleagues (55) reported a decrease in minimally invasive hysterectomies and myomectomies following the FDA announcement. Similarly, Harris et al. (56) reported a decrease in minimally invasive hysterectomy. An increase in surgical complications and readmissions were also noted. It is reasonable to obtain preoperative pelvic MRI when a less-than-total hysterectomy for presumed benign leiomyoma is planned. Appropriate imaging will help localize the tumors, and provides an excellent NPV. Serum LDH may also be useful in determining when morcellation may be less than optimal. However, a patient with a normal serum LDH and/or non-suspicious MRI may reasonably undergo morcellation, with little concern for uterine sarcoma. Morcellation should be avoided in patients with highly suspicious MRI and elevated serum LDH, and in postmenopausal patients with enlarging uterine masses, new uterine masses, or newly symptomatic uterine masses. (As it is unusual for postmenopausal women to experience sudden symptoms from either long-standing benign fibroids or new ones, these cases are highly suspicious for malignancy, and morcellation should be ruled out.) Proper and thoughtful patient selection is likely much more important in surgical decision-making than is the complete abandonment of a particular surgical tool. In December 2013, the Society of Gynecologic Oncology issued a position statement on morcellation, recommending that patients be counseled regarding the risk of occult malignancy prior to undergoing this procedure. They asserted that morcellation is generally contraindicated in the presence of known or suspected malignancy, and may be inadvisable in the treatment of premalignant conditions or risk-reducing surgeries (57).

STAGING AND PROGNOSIS

Staging Systems

The American Joint Committee on Cancer (AJCC) has presented a staging system for soft tissue sarcomas, but there are limitations in applying this to uterine sarcomas. The International Federation of Gynecology and Obstetrics (FIGO) presented a sarcoma-specific system only recently. A modified staging system based on the staging system for endometrial carcinomas was most commonly used (19). In a study at Memorial Sloan Kettering Cancer Center, Zivanovic and colleagues (19) demonstrated that neither the modified FIGO system nor the AJCC staging system was adequate. **Figure 22.2** depicts PFS and OS based on staging, using the modified FIGO and AJCC systems (19). The concordance indices for PFS using the FIGO or AJCC systems were 0.6 and 0.596, respectively, and for OS 0.62 and 0.633, respectively. These are not ideal; in more accurate systems they are usually > 0.7. The prognostic inadequacy of both the modified FIGO and AJCC systems was further confirmed by investigators at Brigham and Women's Hospital (58).

In 2009, FIGO devised a uterine sarcoma-specific staging system for LMS, ESS, and adenosarcoma (3) **(Tables 22.4 and 22.5)**. Carcinosarcomas are staged using the system for endometrial carcinomas (3). There are no clear guidelines with respect to staging other less common uterine sarcomas. However, the 2009 FIGO systems have not yet been validated. Garg and colleagues reported that the 2009 FIGO system did not demonstrate a more accurate prognostic capability compared to the 1988 system for endometrial carcinomas (which was used to stage sarcomas prior to 2009) (21). **Figure 22.3** depicts the stage distribution for newly diagnosed uterine sarcomas using older staging criteria—which essentially stages any disease beyond the uterine corpus and/or cervix as stage III or IV. On presentation, the majority of ESS, LMS, and adenosarcomas appear confined to the uterus and/or cervix (59,60). Carcinosarcomas and undifferentiated sarcomas have a much greater propensity for metastatic spread at time of presentation. The value of preoperative imaging to assess for extrauterine spread has been questioned (61). However, it is reasonable to use imaging preoperatively in patients with newly diagnosed uterine sarcomas to assess for extrauterine spread, as there is at minimum an approximately 25% or greater chance of extrauterine disease **(Fig. 22.3)**, (except in the setting of adenosarcoma). On the basis of very small case reports and series, rarer subtypes are usually confined to the uterus on presentation.

Uterine sarcomas confined to the uterine body (typically stage I) tend to have a worse prognosis than the more common endometrial carcinomas (except for ESS). The 5-year OS for patients with stage I ESS is approximately 97% (62). OS is excellent for patients with ESS, irrespective of stage; including all stages at presentation, OS is approximately 92% (15). This contrasts sharply with the outcomes seen in other uterine sarcomas. The 5-year OS for adenosarcomas confined to the endometrium is 84% (3); this drops to approximately 65% if there is any myoinvasion (5). The 5-year OS for LMS, CS, and undifferentiated sarcoma confined to the uterine corpus is 57%, 62%, and 52%, respectively (19,59,62). Patients diagnosed with STUMP were previously considered to have low-grade LMS. These patients have an outstanding prognosis, which may have biased previous reports on outcomes in LMS.

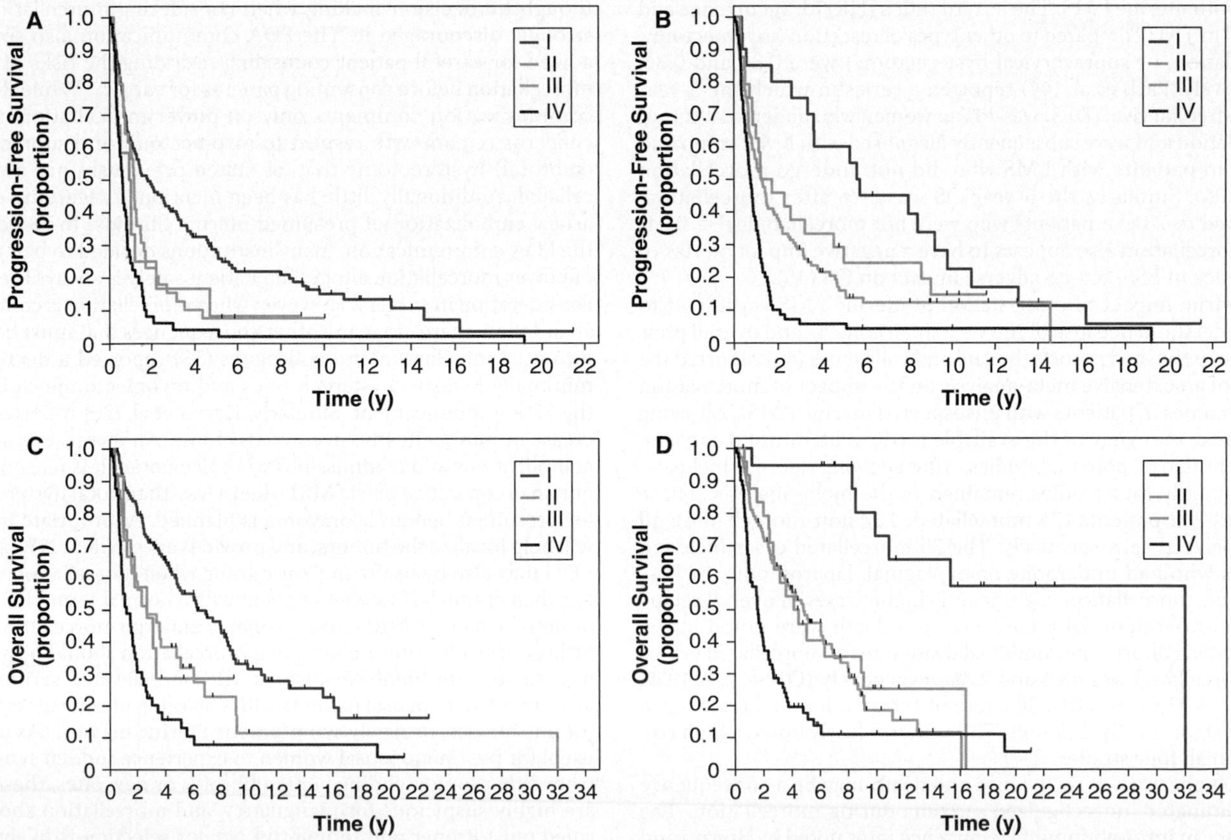

Figure 22.2. Progression-free survival by **(A)** FIGO stage and **(B)** AJCC Staging. OS by **(C)** FIGO stage and **(D)** AJCC stage.

Source: From Zivanovic O, Leitao MM, Iasonos A, et al. Stage-specific outcomes of patients with uterine leiomyosarcoma: a comparison of the International Federation of Gynecology and Obstetrics and American Joint Committee on Cancer Staging systems. *J Clin Oncol*. 2009;27:2066–2072, with permission.

TABLE 22.4. 2009 FIGO Staging System for Uterine LMS and ESS

Stage	Definition
I	Tumor limited to uterus
IA	Less than or equal to 5 cm
IB	More than 5 cm
II	Tumor extends beyond the uterus, within the pelvis
IIA	Adnexal involvement
IIB	Involvement of other pelvic tissues
III	Tumor invades abdominal tissues (not just protruding into the abdomen)
IIIA	One site
IIIB	More than one site
IIIC	Metastasis to pelvic and/or para-aortic lymph nodes
IV	
IVA	Tumor invades bladder and/or rectum
IVB	Distant metastasis

Source: From D'Angelo E, Prat J. Uterine sarcomas: a review. *Gynecol Oncol.* 2010;116:131–139, with permission (Elsevier).

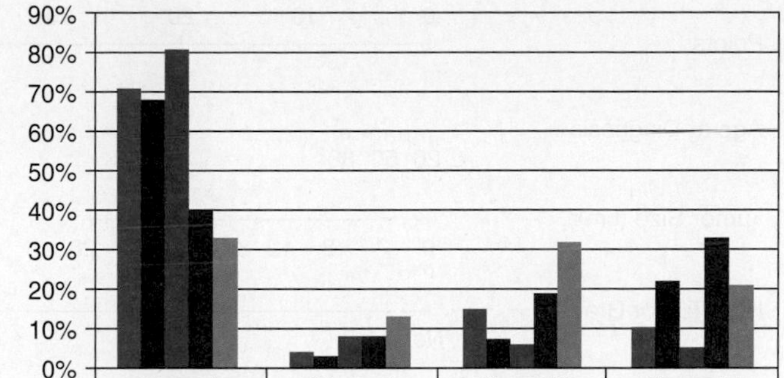

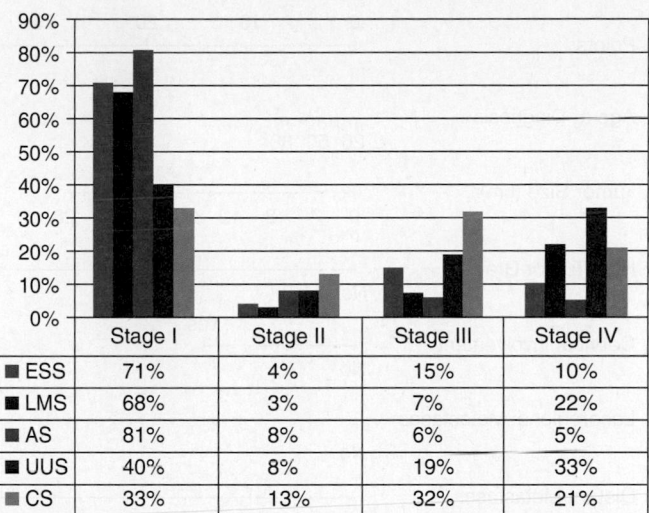

	Stage I	Stage II	Stage III	Stage IV
ESS	71%	4%	15%	10%
LMS	68%	3%	7%	22%
AS	81%	8%	6%	5%
UUS	40%	8%	19%	33%
CS	33%	13%	32%	21%

Figure 22.3. Stage distribution of the more common uterine sarcomas. ESS, endometrial stromal sarcoma; LMS, leiomyosarcoma; AS, adenosarcoma; UUS, undifferentiated uterine sarcoma; CS, carcinosarcoma.

TABLE 22.5. 2009 FIGO Staging System for Uterine Adenosarcomas

Stage	Definition
I	Tumor limited to uterus
IA	Tumor limited to endometrium/endocervix with no myometrial invasion
IB	Less than or equal to half myometrial invasion
IC	More than half myometrial invasion
II	Tumor extends beyond the uterus, within the pelvis
IIA	Adnexal involvement
IIB	Involvement of other pelvic tissues
III	Tumor invades abdominal tissues (not just protruding into the abdomen)
IIIA	One site
IIIB	More than one site
IIIC	Metastasis to pelvic and/or para-aortic lymph nodes
IV	
IVA	Tumor invades bladder and/or rectum
IVB	Distant metastasis

Source: From D'Angelo E, Prat J. Uterine sarcomas: a review. *Gynecol Oncol.* 2010;116:131–139, with permission (Elsevier).

Nomograms

Improved prognostic systems and methods are needed for uterine sarcomas. Nomograms to provide prognostic and predictive information are being used more commonly. A nomogram designed to predict 5-year OS in patients with uterine LMS was developed by investigators at Memorial Sloan Kettering Cancer Center (63) (**Fig. 22.4**). In this nomogram, a total point score is obtained by adding up the various listed clinicopathologic criteria. The score is then plotted against the 5-year OS (line at the bottom) to determine an estimated survival. This nomogram is available online at http://www.mskcc.org/cancer-care/adult/endometrial-other-uterine/leiomyosarcoma/prediction-tools (64). The bootstrap-validated concordance probability (CP) for this nomogram was 0.65. It was externally validated using independent cohorts from two other sarcoma centers (65). The CP in this external validation was 0.67. Although more accurate than the current FIGO or AJCC systems, it is not ideal and requires further development and validation.

Molecular Prognostics

A possible reason for the limited prognostic capabilities of current staging systems and nomograms is that they rely on anatomic, clinical, and pathologic criteria that have not been consistently associated with outcome. A better molecular understanding of these tumors is urgently needed, and may possibly provide more accurate prognostication. Leitao and colleagues (66) have reported that ER and PR receptor expression in uterine LMS is associated with outcome. In their evaluation of cases presenting with extrauterine disease, including cervical extension alone, they found that ER/PR expression was not prognostic; however, it *was* prognostic in patients with disease confined to the uterine body. Most notably, of the 10 PR-overexpressing cases, only 1 patient recurred and died, compared to the 10 PR-non-expressing cases in which 9/10 recurred and 5 died (66). Ioffe and colleagues (67) also reported a possible association with hormone receptor expression and outcome in uterine sarcomas. Subtyping hormone receptors may further improve prognostication (68). Koivisto-Korander and colleagues (69) assessed the immunohistochemical association of various proteins (Ki-67, p53, CD10, CD44, desmin, SMA, ERa, and PR-A) with survival outcomes in patients with CS and LMS. They found that none of the expression patterns of any of these proteins was associated with survival in patients with CS (69). However, in patients with LMS, only E-RA and PR-A overexpression was associated with survival (69).

Expression patterns of other proteins have reportedly been associated with outcome. β-catenin expression has been associated with crude survival in patients with LMS, but not in those with ESS, adenosarcoma, or undifferentiated sarcoma (70). Cyclooxygenase-2 (COX-2) expression has been independently associated with outcome in patients with LMS (71). COX-2 was not prognostic in patients with uterine CS (72). In a series reported by D'Angelo and colleagues (73), P53, p16, Ki67, and bcl-2 expression patterns were found to be associated with outcome in patients with LMS, but only bcl-2 was prognostic in undifferentiated LMS and ESS. CD10 and PTEN expression were not found to be prognostic (73). These are all

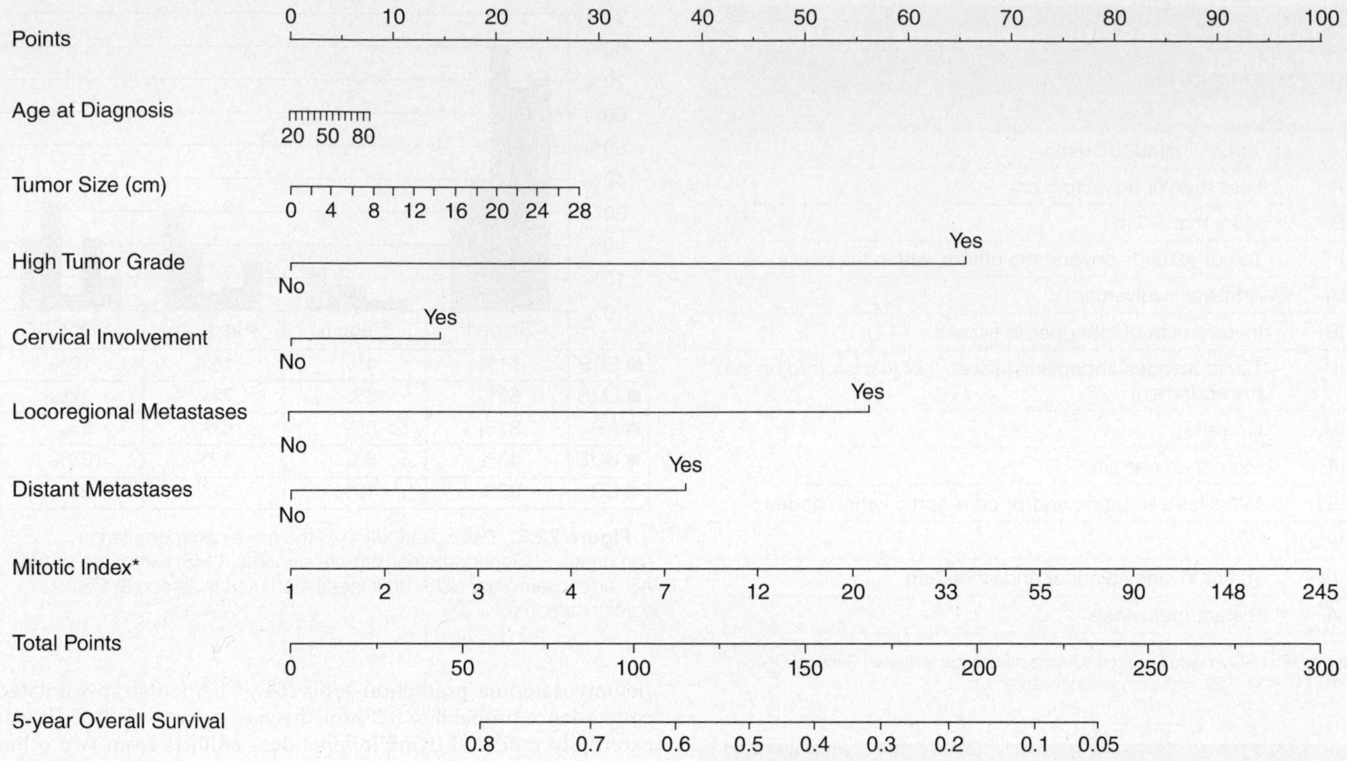

Figure 22.4. Nomogram for 5-year OS for uterine LMS. This is the uterine LMS nomogram for 5-year overall survival. The mitotic index (*asterisk*) was modeled using log transformation; for display purposes, values were converted back to original scale (exponential; CP, 0.671; bootstrap-validated CP, 0.651).

Source: Zivanovic O, Jacks LM, Iasonos A, et al. A nomogram to predict postresection 5-year overall survival for patients with uterine leiomyosarcoma. *Cancer.* 2012;118:660–669, with permission.

interesting, hypothesis-generating reports. As we begin to unravel the molecular biology of these rare tumors, all of the existing studies will require further validation and investigation before we begin to incorporate them into clinically useful prognostic tools. However, improved prognostication will likely come from molecular-based analyses and possibly from protein and/or gene expression profiling. Unfortunately, uterine LMS appears to be hypermutated, making analysis and understanding of these tumors very challenging (74,75). Microarray analyses have revealed that these tumors harbor nearly 4,000 differentially expressed genes, compared to normal myometrium, at a false discovery rate of 0.0001 (76).

Patterns of Recurrence

Patterns of first recurrence are described in **Table 22.6**. The median PFS (i.e., time to recurrence) is greater than 100 months (8.3 years) in patients with ESS, based on the current criteria for diagnosis (12,14,77,78). Previous studies reported median PFS of 15 to 23 months for ESS (5,9). However, this probably reflects the inclusion of tumors now considered to be undifferentiated sarcomas, and not truly ESS. Few data exist on patterns of recurrence for undifferentiated sarcomas, but they are likely to reflect the patterns observed in other sarcomas or in those previously reported for ESS. The median time to recurrence for AS is approximately 40 months (22). LMS and CS have a very short median PFS of 12 to 19 months and 11 to 14 months, respectively (5,9,19,21,75,79). Extrapelvic recurrences are common; 82% of CS involve an extrapelvic site. The most common site of extrapelvic recurrence in ESS and LMS is the lung (80). The abdomen is the most common site of extrapelvic recurrence in adenosarcomas and CS. STUMP tumors have an exceedingly low risk of recurrence and nearly 100% OS. In a report from MD Anderson Cancer Center, only 3 of 41 STUMP cases recurred (1 each at 13, 47, and 68 months) (23). All patients were alive and without evidence of disease at the time of publication (23). The rarity of other uterine sarcomas precludes definitive comments on patterns of recurrence, but most tend to recur locally.

TABLE 22.6. Patterns of First Recurrence in Patients with Select Uterine Sarcomas

	ESS (12,14,78,79)	AS (22)	LMS (5,9,19,21,80,81)	CS (5,9,77,80)
Median PFS (months)	101–130	41	12–19	11–14
Pelvic-only first recurrence[a]	43%	62%	41%	18%
Extrapelvic first recurrence[b]	57%	38%	59%	82%
Most common extrapelvic site	Lung	Abdomen	Lung	Abdomen

AS, adenosarcoma; CS, carcinosarcoma; ESS, endometrial stromal sarcoma (only includes true "low-grade" cases); LMS, leiomyosarcoma; PFS, progression-free survival.

[a]Includes vaginal ± other pelvic recurrence.

[b]Some cases also with concurrent pelvic recurrence.

Molecular Biology and Genetics

The association with expression patterns of certain proteins and outcome is described above. These data are limited and mostly non-validated. The key to improved prognostic and predictive tools, as well as therapeutics, in patients with uterine sarcomas will only be achieved when we attain a significant understanding of the inherent molecular biology of these tumors; at this time, our understanding is limited. Below, we describe some recent molecular studies of particular interest. Many more are in publication, and we expect additional data to be forthcoming. (Further description is provided in the **Pathology** section of this chapter.)

Gene rearrangements have been described and validated in patients with ESS, with at least 75% of tumors demonstrating gene rearrangement (81). The t(7;17) translocation resulting in the *JAZF1-SUZ12* gene fusion is the most common translocation, found in approximately 35% to 50% of ESS (81). Other noted gene fusions are *JAZF1-PHF1, EPC1-PHF1, JAZF1* only, and *PHF1* only (81).

Undifferentiated endometrial sarcomas (previously referred to as high-grade ESS) lack these *JAFZ1*-based rearrangements, and instead frequently harbor the *YWHAE-FAM22A/B* genetic fusion (11,82). The *YWHAE-FAM22A/B* fusion has been proposed as a possible oncogene in the development of undifferentiated (i.e., high-grade) ESS, because of the transforming properties of the YWHAE-FAM22 protein expressed by this gene fusion (11,82). Additionally, the *YWHAE-FAM22A/B* fusion appears to be specific to these tumors, as it was not detected in 827 other cases representing 55 tumor types (11).

LMP2 is an important immuno-protease subunit that is induced by IFN-g, and may be involved in various cell events—possibly including the suppression of tumor cell growth (83). Mice lacking LMP2 spontaneously develop uterine LMS, with an incidence of about 40% at 14 months of age (83). LMP2 expression appears to be absent in human LMS, but is retained in human leiomyomata (83). LMP2 may be involved in the sarcoma-genesis of uterine LMS, and this requires continuous investigation. LMS does not appear to harbor somatic mutations in *EGFR, CDKN2A, MET, KIT, RAS, BRAF, PI3KCA, HER-2,* or *PDGFR-α,* for which targeted therapies are available (84,85).

Growdon and colleagues (85) analyzed uterine CS for the presence of somatic mutations. The rate of mutations identified for each gene analyzed was *PIK3CA* (56%), *KRAS* (44%), *TP53* (33%), *CTNNB1* (6%), and *NRAS* (6%). *TP53* mutation was the only mutational event that retained an independent association with survival. The Akt/β-catenin pathway and alterations in Rb expression may be involved in the development of CS of the uterus (86). This is believed to be modified through transactivation of the *Slug* gene. Cimbaluk et al. (87) assessed immunohistochemical expression of potential therapeutic targets. They found that expression was low in both the epithelial and mesenchymal components for HER-2 (6% and 0%, respectively) and c-Kit (0%, both). EGFR expression in the epithelial and mesenchymal components was 30% and 67%, respectively. COX-2 was expressed in 70% of the epithelial component, but in only 16% of the mesenchymal component. VEGF was highly expressed in both the epithelial and mesenchymal components (100% and 93%, respectively).

Pathology

Malignant mesenchymal tumors can be classified as either pure mesenchymal tumors or tumors with mixed epithelial and mesenchymal components. In the first group, the most common is LMS, followed by ESS, and (rarely) other tumors including rhabdomyosarcoma, liposarcoma, angiosarcoma, chondrosarcoma, osteosarcoma, and alveolar soft-part sarcoma. Mixed epithelial and mesenchymal tumors include CS and AS. In addition, there are three rare mesenchymal tumors that occur in the uterus: uterine tumors resembling ovarian sex cord tumors (UTROSCTs), perivascular epithelioid cell tumors (PEComas), and inflammatory myofibroblastic tumor (88). These entities are usually benign, but may impede the differential diagnosis of malignant lesions.

LMS and Other Smooth Muscle Tumors

LMS are malignant smooth muscle tumors that usually arise *de novo*. Recent studies have shown that some of these tumors have areas of benign morphology, suggesting progression from leiomyoma to LMS (89,90); however, clonality studies support this progression in only a small percentage of cellular or symplastic leiomyomas (90,91). LMS is usually a solitary, poorly circumscribed mass with a soft and fleshy consistency. The cut surface is variegated, with gray areas intermixed with yellow areas of necrosis, and sometimes hemorrhagic areas. The epicenter of the tumor is the myometrium. Most LMS tumors are intramural. Occasionally, they extend into the cervix or beyond the uterus through the serosa (**Figs. 22.5–22.7**).

Microscopically, most LMS are overtly malignant with hypercellularity, coagulative tumor cell necrosis (TCN), abundant mitoses, atypical mitoses, marked cytologic atypia, and infiltrative borders (**Fig. 22.8**). Some lack one or more of these features, and occasionally the differential diagnosis between a benign and a malignant lesion is controversial. The three most important criteria are coagulative TCN, high mitotic rate, and significant cytologic atypia. In conventional LMS (spindle cell type), the diagnosis of malignancy is rendered when any two of the following three criteria are present: TCN, diffuse moderate-to-severe cytologic atypia, and 10 or more mitoses per 10 high-power fields (HPF) (92). TCN is characterized by an abrupt transition from viable to necrotic tissue (**Fig. 22.9**). In contrast, hyaline necrosis, which is seen in some leiomyomas, has an area of hyalinized tissue between the necrotic and viable tumor.

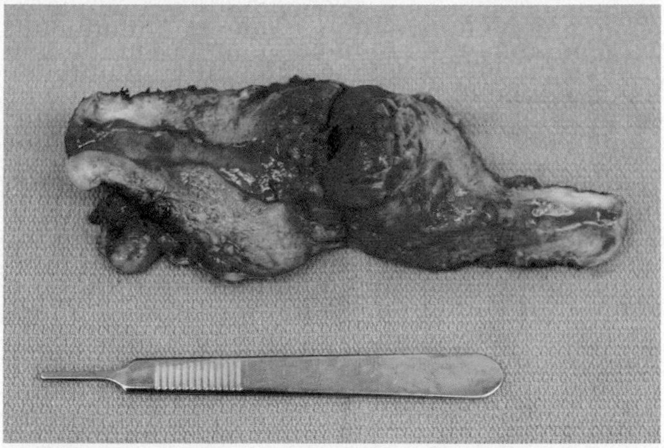

Figure 22.5. LMS, gross.

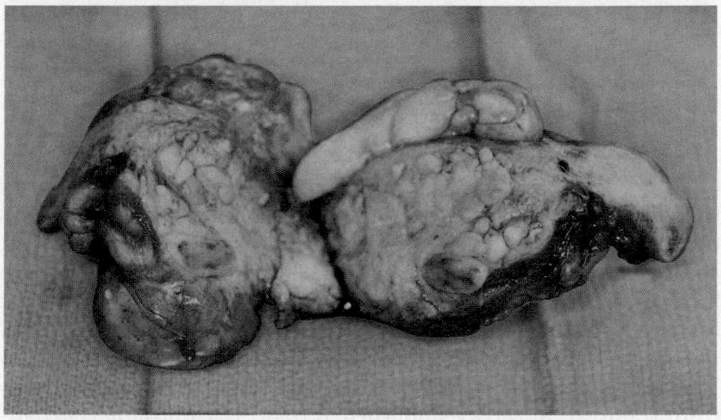

Figure 22.6. LMS, gross, showing heterogenous appearance.

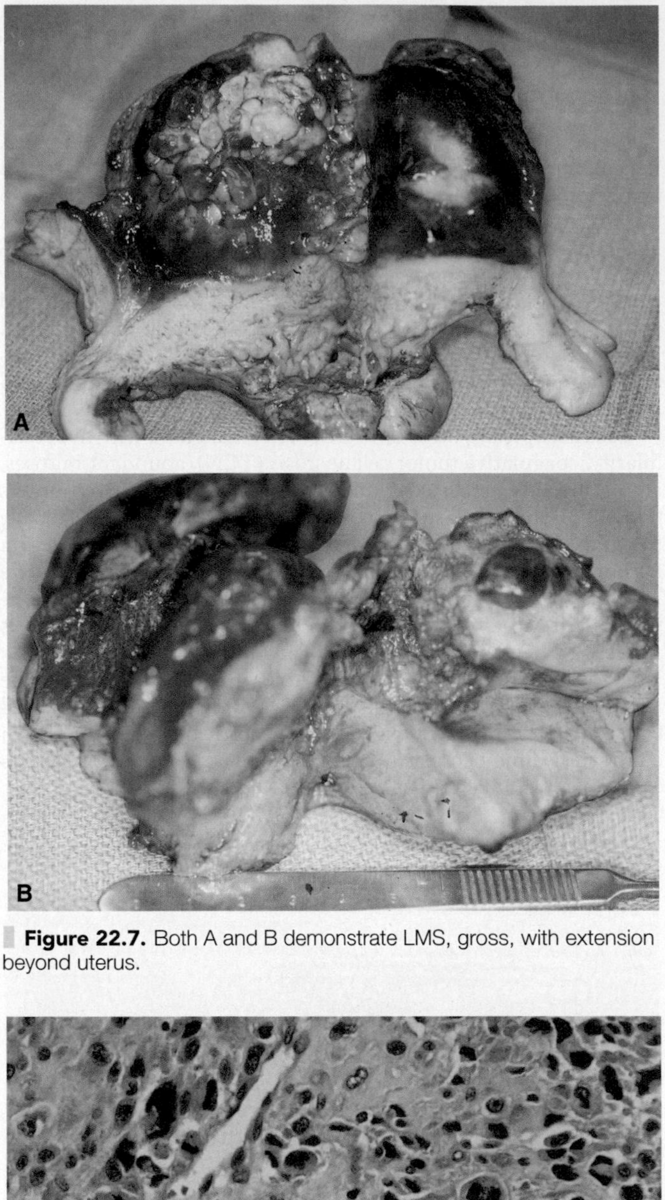

Figure 22.7. Both A and B demonstrate LMS, gross, with extension beyond uterus.

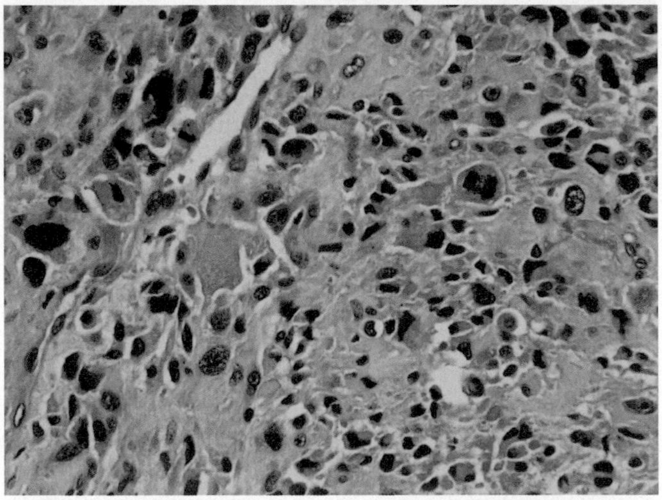

Figure 22.8. LMS, microscopic.

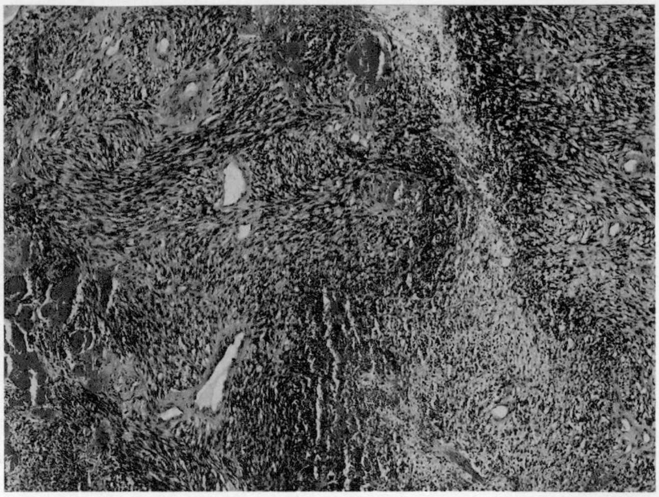

Figure 22.9. LMS, microscopic, with abrupt transition from viable to necrotic tissue.

Some smooth muscle tumors demonstrate histologic features that are not worrisome enough to render an unequivocal diagnosis of sarcoma. These lesions can be classified as atypical leiomyomas, smooth muscle tumors with low malignant potential (low probability of an unfavorable outcome), or STUMP, depending on the histologic features. **Figure 22.10** summarizes the classification of uterine smooth muscle tumors based on histologic characteristics. This classification is largely based upon a large retrospective study from Stanford University, published in 1994 (92)—the largest to date. Tumors that clinically and pathologically appear to be leiomyomas, but have up to 15 mitoses per 10 HPF, behave in a benign fashion, and are classified as mitotically active leiomyomas (92,93). Leiomyomas are more likely to have a high mitotic count if they are excised during the secretory phase of the menstrual cycle, during pregnancy, or while patients are receiving exogenous PR therapy.

Five studies in the literature have addressed the diagnosis and clinical behavior of borderline smooth muscle tumors classified as atypical leiomyomas, tumors with low malignant potential, and tumors of uncertain malignant potential (23,94–97). The overall recurrence rate, based on these studies, is 8.6%. Most tumors recurred as STUMP, although one recurred as LMS (23). Most patients were alive and free of disease when these studies were published; one study reported three disease-specific deaths, all occurring more than 6 years after initial diagnosis (94). There are tumors that lack one of the three major diagnostic criteria (mitoses, atypia, necrosis) but show other worrisome features such as infiltrative borders, lymphovascular invasion, or atypical mitoses. Classification of these tumors is always problematic. It is recommended that any unusual cases be reviewed by a gynecologic pathologist. Two recent studies of atypical leiomyomas or leiomyomas with bizarre nuclei have shown a favorable outcome in the majority of cases (110 cases, including both studies). Only one patient (originally treated with hysterectomy) recurred as an atypical leiomyoma in the retroperitoneum at 87.5 months. All other patients were NED, that is, had no evidence of disease, including the 34 patients treated with myomectomy alone.

Infarcted necrosis of benign leiomyomas is sometimes seen during pregnancy, after uterine artery embolization, thermal balloon endometrial ablation, therapy with tranexamic acid, or therapy with high-dose progestins. In addition, pedunculated submucosal leiomyomas may undergo spontaneous torsion and infarction, even protruding through the cervix. Infarcted leiomyomas should not be confused with LMS. As noted before, infarcted necrosis is not TCN. In addition, infarcted leiomyomas are not associated with significant cytologic atypia, high mitotic rate, atypical mitoses, or invasive borders. An accurate clinical history may be useful in many of these cases.

Several recent studies support the use of immunostains for p16, p53, and Ki67 (proliferative activity marker) in the differential diagnosis of problematic smooth muscle tumors. p16 is overexpressed in uterine LMS compared with leiomyomas and STUMP, suggesting that p16 may be implicated in pathogenesis. In addition, LMS is characterized by higher *p53* expression and higher proliferative activity (Ki67) than other uterine smooth muscle tumors. The combination of high p16, p53, and Ki67 expression supports a diagnosis of LMS, if used in combination with H&E features, gross appearance of the tumor, and clinical features (98–103).

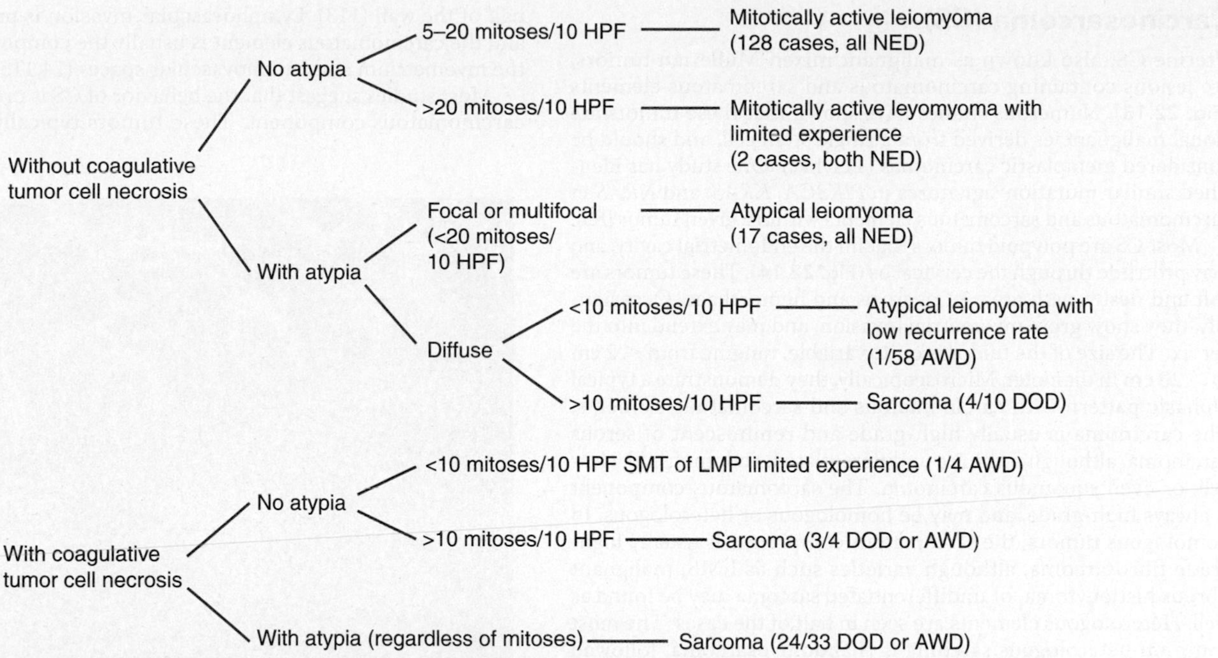

Figure 22.10. Uterine smooth muscle tumors (excluding epithelioid and myxoid types and cervical tumors). AWD, alive with disease; DOD, dead of disease; HPF, high-power fields; LMP, low malignant potential; NED, no evidence of disease; SMT, smooth muscle tumor.

The classification criteria of smooth muscle tumors with either myxoid or epithelioid features differ from the criteria used for spindle cell tumors. Epithelioid tumors have cells that are round rather than spindle-shaped, with round nuclei mimicking epithelial cells (hence the term "epithelioid") (**Fig. 22.11**). Epithelioid LMS have significant cytologic atypia of at least 3 mitoses per 10 HPF, and TCN is demonstrated in 50% of cases (104). A previous study suggests that epithelioid tumors may behave more aggressively than spindle cell tumors, with a higher tendency to metastasize (105). Myxoid LMS is rare, and may be histologically deceiving because of the lack of TCN, minimal atypia, and a low mitotic rate. The most reliable histologic criteria of malignancy are infiltrative borders and lymphovascular invasion (106) (**Fig. 22.12**). Myxoid LMS portends a long-term survival similar to that of other LMS tumors, but at least one study reported better 5-year survival (73%) compared to ordinary LMS (49%) (10).

The histologic parameters of LMS that have been associated with poor prognosis include mitotic rate (107,108), lymphovascular invasion (107), size (108), diffuse high-grade cytologic atypia (109), and negative ER and PR (66). However, many of these characteristics have not been associated with outcome; therefore, they are not entirely validated.

Benign Metastasizing Leiomyoma

Benign metastasizing leiomyoma (BML) is characterized by the presence of a uterine leiomyoma associated with one or more extrauterine smooth muscle tumors that are histologically benign. The most common site of metastasis is the lung, although metastases have also been described in the retroperitoneum, mediastinal lymph nodes, soft tissue, and bone. Before rendering a diagnosis of BML, the pathologist should sample tissue extensively to rule out any aggressive components. The pathogenesis of these tumors is unclear. Some animal experiments suggest that BML may be secondary to lymphatic and hematologic spread, coelomic metaplasia, and intraperitoneal seeding (a pathogenesis similar to that of endometriosis) (110).

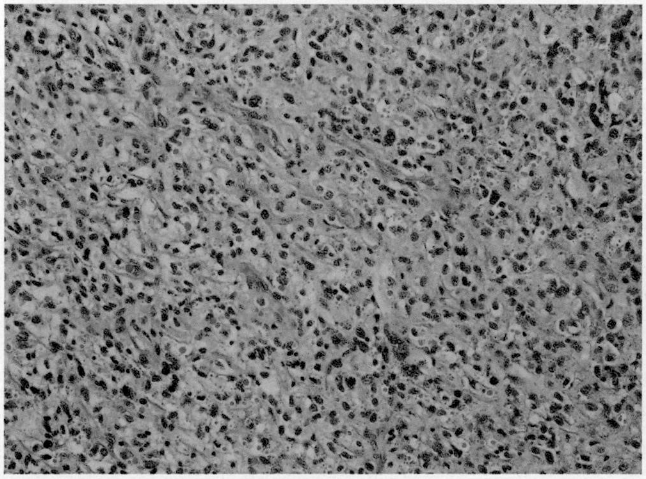

Figure 22.11. Epithelioid LMS, microscopic appearance.

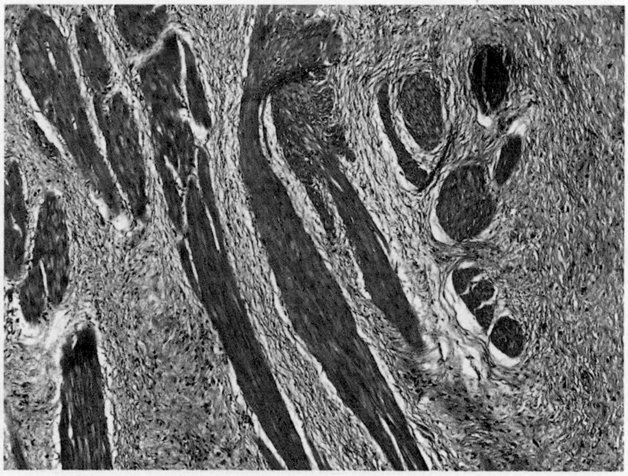

Figure 22.12. Myxoid LMS, microscopic appearance.

Carcinosarcoma (CS)

Uterine CS, also known as malignant mixed Müllerian tumors, are lesions containing carcinomatous and sarcomatous elements **(Fig. 22.13)**. Numerous studies have shown that these tumors are clonal malignancies derived from a single stem cell, and should be considered metaplastic carcinomas (111,112). One study has identified similar mutation signatures in *PIK3CA*, *KRAS*, and *NRAS* in carcinomatous and sarcomatous elements within a given tumor (85).

Most CS are polypoid tumors that fill the endometrial cavity, and may protrude through the cervical os **(Fig. 22.14)**. These tumors are soft and fleshy, with areas of necrosis and hemorrhage. Occasionally, they show gross myometrial invasion, and may extend into the cervix. The size of the tumor is quite variable, ranging from < 2 cm to > 20 cm in diameter. Microscopically, they demonstrate a typical biphasic pattern with carcinomatous and sarcomatous elements. The carcinoma is usually high-grade and reminiscent of serous carcinoma, although some are undifferentiated, endometrioid, clear cell, or even squamous carcinoma. The sarcomatous component is always high-grade, and may be homologous or heterologous. In homologous tumors, the sarcomatous component is usually high-grade fibrosarcoma, although varieties such as LMS, malignant fibrous histiocytoma, or undifferentiated sarcoma may be found as well. Heterologous elements are seen in half of the cases. The most common heterologous sarcoma is rhabdomyosarcoma, followed by chondrosarcoma, and, less often, osteosarcoma or liposarcoma (113). Most CS have myometrial invasion, commonly into less than half of the wall (113). Lymphovascular invasion is present in 60%, and the carcinomatous element is usually the component invading the myometrium and lymphovascular spaces (74,113).

Most studies suggest that the behavior of CS is predicted by the carcinomatous component. These tumors typically metastasize

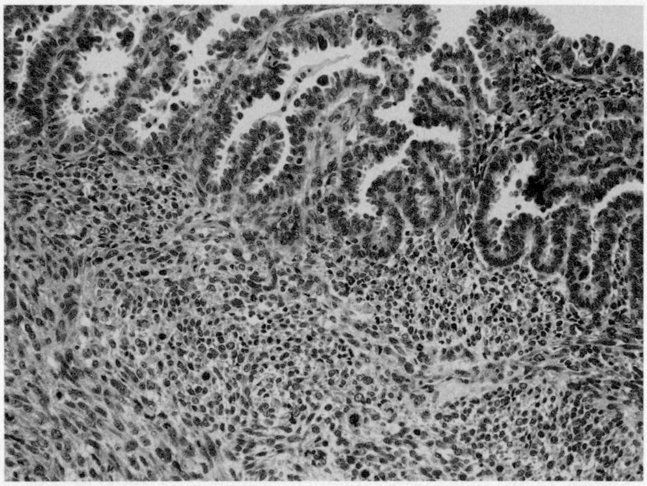

Figure 22.13. CS, microscopic appearance.

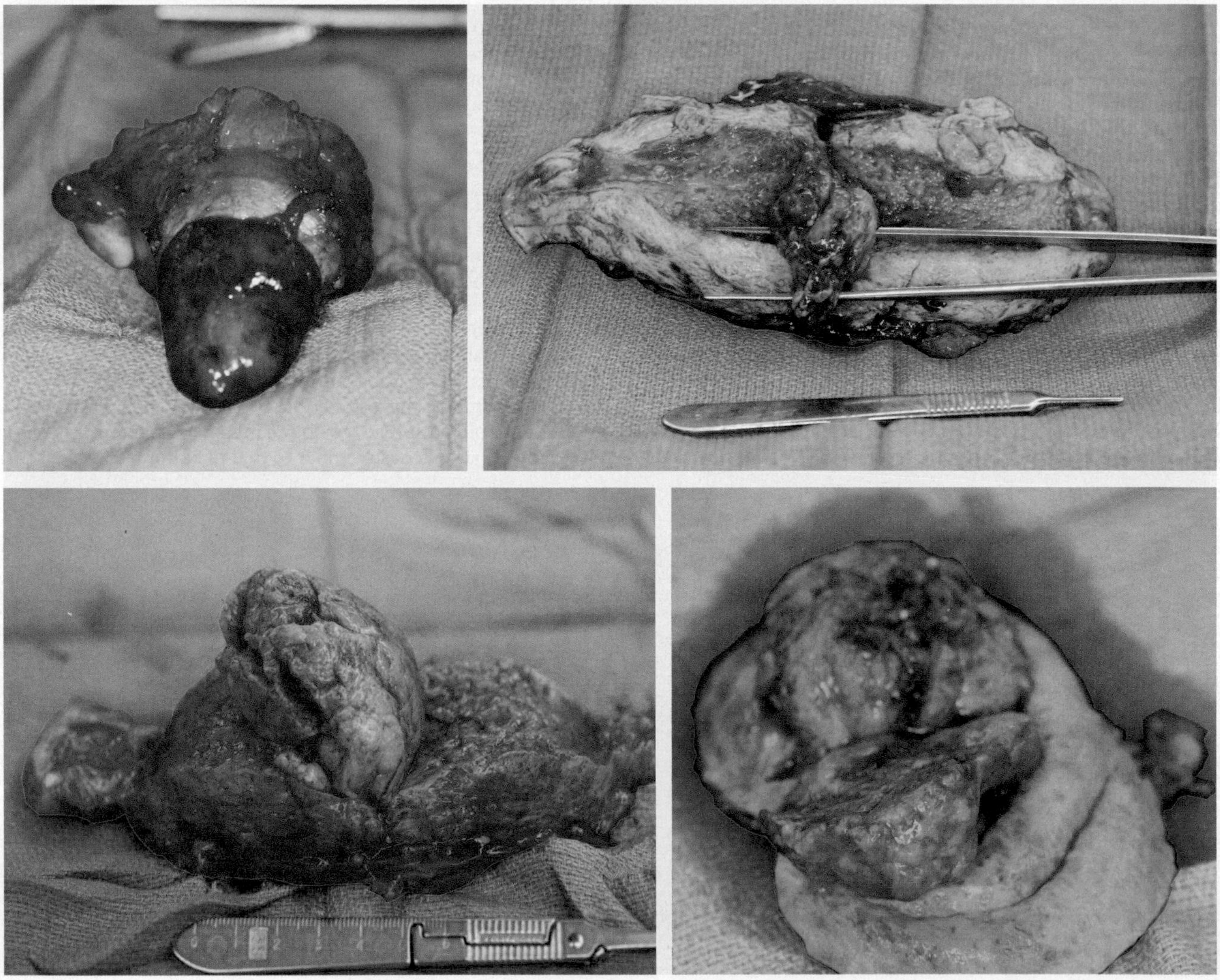

Figure 22.14. CS, gross photographs of four cases demonstrating polypoid nature of lesions.

through lymphatic channels, similar to endometrial carcinomas. Most metastases and recurrences consist of pure carcinoma (29,30). Histopathologic adverse prognostic factors include heterologous elements (in stage I tumors), a high percentage of sarcomatous components in the main tumor and in the recurrences, and deep myometrial invasion (29–31).

Müllerian CS may arise in extrauterine–extraovarian sites. Most have been reported in the peritoneum or retroperitoneum. Some occur at the site of previous RT, and some arise in areas of endometriosis (114–119).

Endometrial Stromal Neoplasms

In the most recent (2014) WHO publication, endometrial stromal tumors are classified as endometrial stromal nodules, low-grade ESS, high-grade ESS, or undifferentiated uterine sarcoma (120). Both endometrial stromal nodules and low-grade ESS are composed of cells identical to those found in the stroma of proliferative endometrium, whereas high-grade ESS and undifferentiated sarcomas are composed of cells with cytologic atypia. The differential diagnosis between an endometrial stromal nodule and an ESS is important, because the nodules are always benign. Differential diagnosis is based upon the presence of infiltrating margins with or without angioinvasion in ESS. These two features are not seen in stromal nodules, which are always well-circumscribed, with pushing (well-defined) margins (121).

Stromal Nodule

Stromal nodules are the least common of the pure endometrial stromal neoplasms. They are usually solitary masses, with diameters ranging from 1.2 to 22 cm, with an average of 7.1 cm (122). On cut section, endometrial stromal nodules are fleshy and often tan-yellow in color. Microscopically they are composed of uniformly bland, small cells resembling normal endometrial stromal cells, with fusiform nuclei and scant cytoplasm. Abundant arterioles, reminiscent of the spiral arterioles of the normal endometrium, are also present. The mitotic rate is low, with most tumors having fewer than 5 mitoses per 10 HPF. Most endometrial stromal nodules are cellular; some have variable amounts of intercellular collagen, which occasionally forms dense collagen bands or nodules (**Fig. 22.15**). Another common finding is the presence of clusters of foamy histiocytes within the tumor. The borders between the tumor and the adjacent myometrium are microscopically pushing. Occasionally, they demonstrate more irregular borders with minimal areas of tumor extending into the adjacent myometrium, usually within 3 mm of the main tumor mass (121). Endometrial stromal nodules lack any associated lymphovascular invasion. Other changes seen in endometrial stromal nodules include smooth muscle metaplasia, cystic degeneration, sex cord–like areas, and necrosis.

Endometrial stromal nodules are sometimes confused with cellular leiomyomas. As both tumors are benign, the misdiagnosis of one for the other is probably of no clinical consequence in a hysterectomy specimen. In a curettage specimen, however, the differential diagnosis is more important. Some histologic features favor a leiomyoma: blood vessels with thick muscular walls, cleft-like spaces, and merging with adjacent myometrium. A battery of IHC stains may be useful. CD10 is usually present in endometrial stromal cells, and smooth muscle tumors stain positively for desmin and h-caldesmon.

Low-Grade ESS

Low-grade ESS is characterized by uniformly bland cells resembling endometrial stromal cells. On gross examination, some comprise a single visible mass, whereas others have multiple masses or diffuse myometrial infiltration by worm-like masses (**Fig. 22.16**). Typically, these tumors permeate the myometrial wall, in some cases, up to the serosa (**Fig. 22.17**). Most have fewer than 10 mitoses per 10 HPF. Some ESS tumors have unusual histologic features that may confound the diagnosis. These include myxoid changes, fibroblastic and/or smooth muscle differentiation, epithelioid changes, and extensive endometrioid glandular differentiation (123–126).

Low-grade ESS is usually positive for ER, PR, and CD10, and approximately 50% have cytogenetic abnormalities involving rearrangements of chromosomes 6, 7, and 17. The most characteristic translocation of these tumors, t(T7;17) (Tp15;q21), generates a fusion of the *JAZF1* and *JJAZ1* genes. The presence of this chromosomal abnormality may be useful in diagnosing difficult cases or recurrent tumors (127).

Low-grade ESS may occur in extrauterine sites including ovary, fallopian tube, cervix, vagina, vulva, pelvis, abdomen, retroperitoneum, placenta, sciatic nerve, or round ligament (128–133). Some are associated with endometriosis. Histologically, they are similar to uterine ESS, and a uterine tumor must be excluded before defining the lesion as a primary extrauterine ESS. The relapse rate for extrauterine ESS is 62%, similar to that of advanced low-grade uterine ESS.

High-grade ESS

The newly described entity of "high-grade ESS" is an infiltrative tumor showing confluent destructive growth, often invading deeply into the myometrial wall. These tumors have areas of high-grade cytology with a brisk mitotic count of >10 mitoses per 10 HPF, necrosis, and often lymphovascular invasion. Approximately 50% have an admixed low-grade component, which is usually fibroblastic. These tumors may demonstrate the same histologic variants seen in other endometrial stromal tumors, including rosettes, glandular, and sex cord–like patterns. High-grade ESS typically harbors the

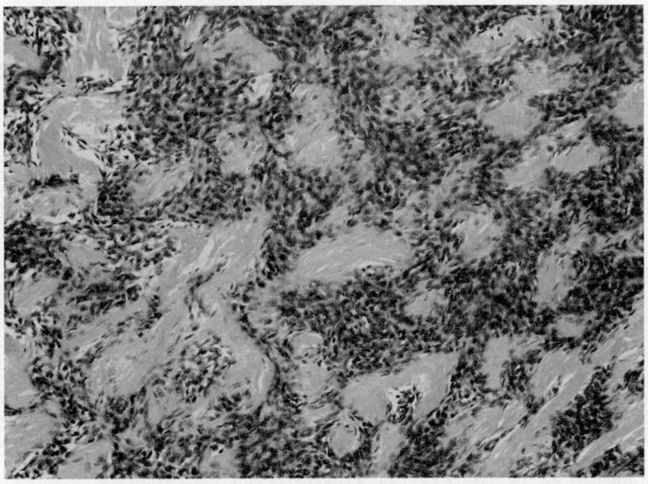

Figure 22.15. Endometrial stromal nodule, microscopic appearance.

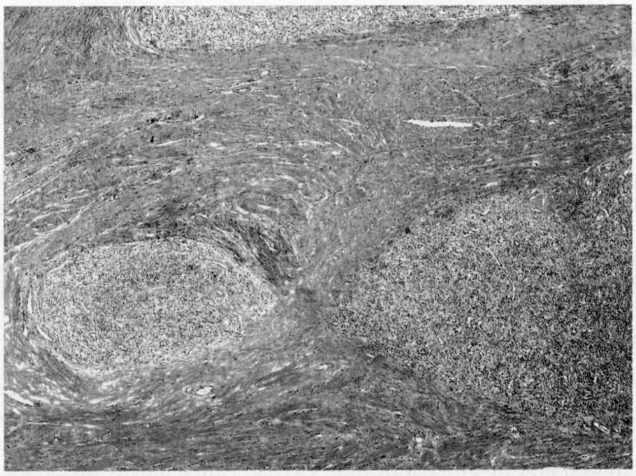

Figure 22.16. Endometrial stromal sarcoma, low-grade, microscopic appearance.

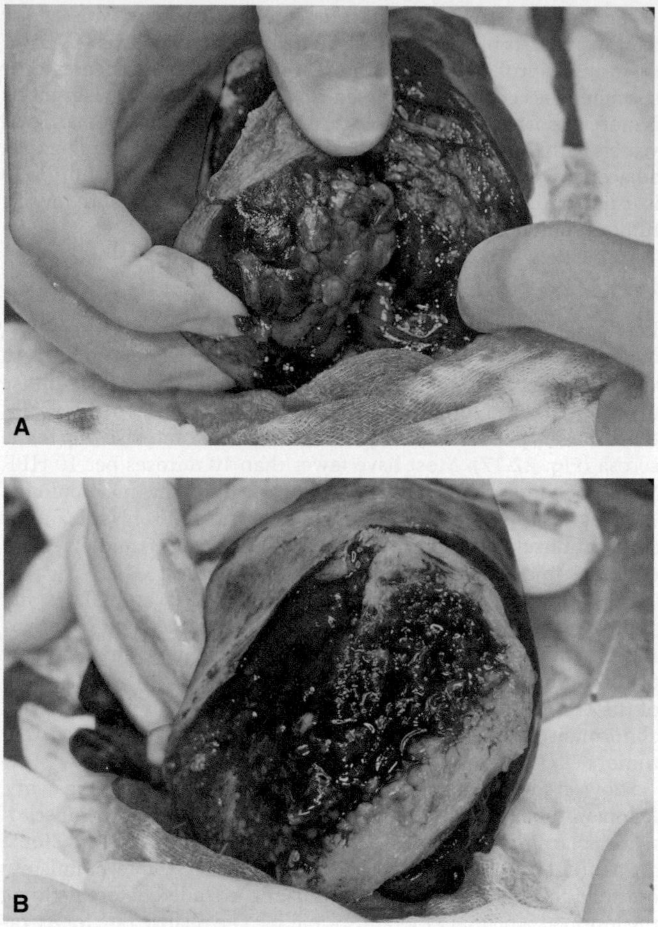

Figure 22.17. Both A and B demonstrate the gross appearance of endometrial stromal sarcoma, low-grade, gross appearance.

TWHAE-FAM22 genetic fusion as a result of t(10;17) (q22;p13). In comparison with low-grade ESS, patients with high-grade ESS have more recurrences and are more likely to die of disease (134). The high-grade component of these tumors is usually negative for CD10, ER, and PR, but positive for cyclin D1 (135). It is usually positive for c-kit, but lacks KIT hotspot mutations (136).

Undifferentiated Uterine Sarcomas

Undifferentiated uterine sarcomas are rare and account for only 6% of all uterine sarcomas (10). They demonstrate cytologic atypia to the extent that they cannot be recognized as arising from endometrial stroma. Morphologically, these high-grade lesions resemble undifferentiated mesenchymal tumors and behave as high-grade sarcomas (10,73,137). It is advisable to describe these entities as "high-grade sarcoma," "undifferentiated sarcoma," or "poorly differentiated uterine sarcoma" (137) rather than as ESS, as this last term may inaccurately suggest an indolent tumor. Undifferentiated uterine sarcomas are usually seen in patients older than 50 years. They have a recurrence rate of over 85%, and are usually fatal (10,73,137). Cheng-Han and Nucci recently authored an excellent review comparing the histology and clinical features of all ESS tumors (138).

Müllerian Adenosarcoma

Müllerian adenosarcomas are mixed Müllerian tumors composed of malignant stroma and benign epithelium. Most adenosarcomas arise in the endometrium; and, rarely, in the endocervix, lower uterine segment, and myometrium (22). Grossly, the majority are solitary polypoid masses with a spongy appearance, secondary to the presence of small cysts. Occasionally, these tumors appear as multiple polyps or masses, and may be multicentric. Their size varies from 1 to 17 cm (mean, 5 cm).

Microscopically, Müllerian AS have a benign epithelial component usually covering the surface of the polyps, and in the form of benign glands uniformly distributed throughout the tumor. The mesenchymal component is usually a low-grade sarcoma that resembles endometrial stroma. The presence of hypercellular stroma around the glands is common, and some tumors have a leaflike papillary growth pattern (**Fig. 22.18**). It may be difficult to arrive at a diagnosis of adenosarcoma because of the very low-grade nature of this tumor. Minimal criteria were described by Clement and Scully in a review of 100 cases of adenosarcoma published in 1990 (22). They include at least one of the following: two or more stromal mitoses per 10 HPF, marked stromal hypercellularity, and significant stromal cell atypia. Even with these criteria, some cases are deceivingly bland, and several have been seen in which the diagnosis was only possible after the review of multiple recurrences of uterine polyps (139). A minority of cases have sarcomatous overgrowth, in which more than 25% of the tumor is composed of pure sarcoma. In these cases, the sarcoma is typically high-grade and the lesions are aggressive (140) (**Fig. 22.19**). Recent studies confirm that histologic parameters associated with increased risk of recurrence include stromal overgrowth, lymphovascular invasion, and myometrial invasion (141,142).

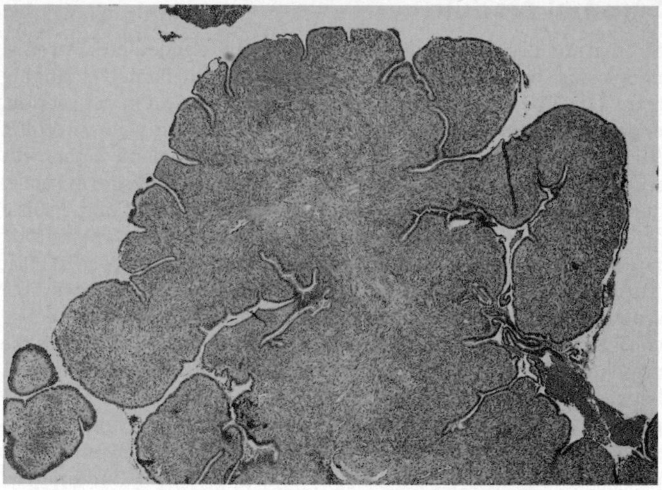

Figure 22.18. Müllerian adenosarcoma, microscopic appearance.

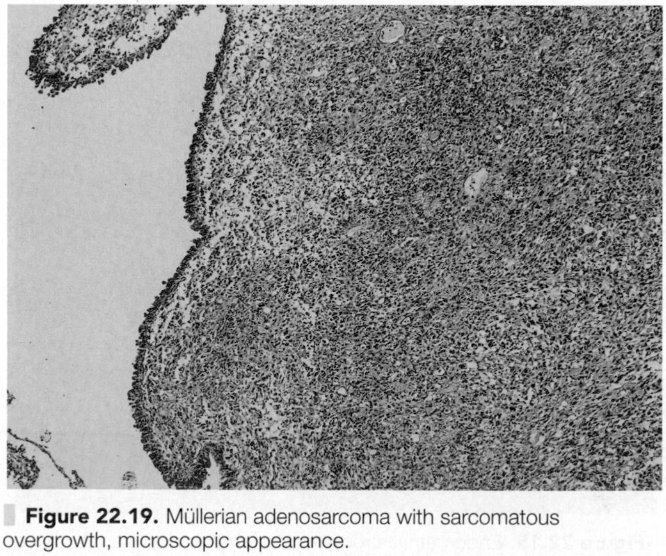

Figure 22.19. Müllerian adenosarcoma with sarcomatous overgrowth, microscopic appearance.

Most AS without stromal overgrowth express ER and PR receptors in the sarcomatous component, which may be used for therapeutic purposes. However, hormonal receptors are negative in AS with stromal overgrowth (139,143). Besides stromal overgrowth, the only other histopathologic features associated with decreased survival are myometrial invasion (22,59,139,140) and the presence of lymphovascular invasion (142). Müllerian AS have been described in extrauterine sites, including the ovary, and in areas of endometriosis in the vagina, rectovaginal septum, gastrointestinal tract, urinary bladder, pouch of Douglas, peritoneum, and liver (144–152).

Uterine Tumor Resembling Ovarian Sex Cord Tumor

In 1976, Clement and Scully (153) coined the term "uterine tumors resembling ovarian sex cord tumors (UTROSCT)" to describe a series of uterine neoplasms with sex cord–like pattern. Since then, sex cord–like patterns have been demonstrated in endometrial stromal neoplasms, smooth muscle neoplasms, and in cases lacking clear endometrial stroma and smooth muscle differentiation. The term UTROSCT should be reserved for this last category. UTROSCTs are tumors of uncertain histogenesis/lineage. Immunohistochemically, these tumors co-express epithelial, myoid, and sex cord markers (154,155). This immuno-profile can also be seen in ESS with sex cord–like areas. However, UTROSCT lacks the typical *JAZF1-JJAZ1* translocation frequently seen in endometrial stromal tumors (156). UTROSCTs are rare, usually submucosal, and well circumscribed, with a yellow cut surface. Histologically, they are composed of sertoliform tubules with low mitotic activity and little nuclear atypia (153–155) (**Fig. 22.20**). Most behave in a benign fashion, although there is at least one reported case of a small bowel metastasis (157).

Perivascular Epithelioid Cell Tumors (PEComas)

(PEComas are rare neoplasms presumably derived from perivascular epithelioid cells that co-express melanocytic and smooth muscle markers. Other tumors belonging to the same family include angiomyolipoma, clear cell/sugar tumor of the lung, lymphangioleiomyomatosis, and myomelanocytic tumor of the ligamentum teres/falciform ligament. PEComas have been described in a variety of locations including visceral organs, soft tissues, skin, oral mucosa, orbit, and base of skull (158). The uterus and gastrointestinal tract are the most common locations for visceral PEComas. About 8% of PEComas occur in patients with the tuberous sclerosis complex. Most of these tumors co-express melanocytic (HMB45, Melan-A,

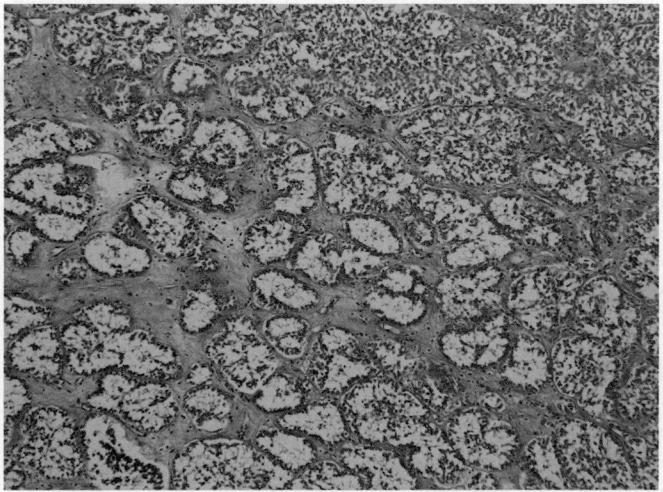

Figure 22.20. UTROSCT, microscopic appearance.

microphthalmia transcription factor, S-100 protein) and smooth muscle markers (desmin, SMA, H-caldesmon). Most uterine PEComas are histologically and clinically benign. They can appear as either grossly well-circumscribed or focally infiltrative masses. Histologically, they are composed of epithelioid cells with abundant clear or eosinophilic cytoplasm, sometimes associated with spindle cells, and a prominent vasculature (158,159). Approximately 25% of reported cases develop metastases and/or recurrences. Most malignant tumors have more than one of these histologic features: size >5 cm, high-grade nuclear features, infiltration of surrounding tissue, necrosis, mitoses >2 per 50 HPF, and lymphovascular invasion. However, there is not a single reliable prognostic indicator other than the presence of lymphovascular invasion (158–161).

A distinct subset including some uterine PEComas harbor *TFE3* gene fusions, and show immunoreactivity for TFE3 protein (162,163). These tumors tend to have distinctive nested/alveolar morphology. In the past, *TFE3* gene fusions were described only in alveolar soft-part sarcomas and in some renal cell carcinomas. PEComas with *TFE3* gene fusions seem to occur in younger people without tuberous sclerosis.

Inflammatory Myofibroblastic Tumor

Inflammatory myofibroblastic tumors (IMT) are rare mesenchymal lesions considered to be of intermediate biologic potential. The most common sites for these tumors include lung, mesentery, omentum, and retroperitoneum. A few cases have been reported in the uterus (164,165), where they present as polypoid masses in the lower uterine segment, or bulky myometrial masses. IMTs range in size from 1 to 12 cm. They are composed of spindle and epithelioid myofibroblastic cells admixed with lymphoplasmacytic infiltrate in variably myxoid stroma cells. IHC expression of ALK is characteristic of all IMTs, and can be used in the differential diagnosis with other uterine spindle cell tumors that are negative (including smooth muscle tumors, ESS, and CS) (164). Most IMTs behave indolently. However, a recent series reported three cases with aggressive behavior including local recurrence, extrauterine spread, or distant metastases. The aggressive tumors were reportedly larger and characterized by a higher percentage of myxoid stroma, higher mitotic count, and necrosis, compared to indolent tumors (166). Given the positive ALK expression, patients with IMT may benefit from targeted therapy.

Other Rare Uterine Sarcomas

Rarely, other sarcomas may be found in the uterine corpus. Rhabdomyosarcomas, although more commonly arising in the cervix of children, have also been encountered in the corpus in adults. These tumors may be of embryonal or pleomorphic histology. They are aggressive, with a 5-year disease-specific survival of only 29%. Patients with pleomorphic rhabdomyosarcoma have a worse prognosis than those with embryonal histology (10,167,168).

Uterine liposarcomas are rare tumors. Some arise in uterine lipoleiomyomas (169), others are associated with smooth muscle tumors, and may represent LMS with cyst-divergent differentiation (168,170).

Other rare sarcomas described in the uterus include angiosarcoma, Ewing sarcoma, alveolar soft-part sarcoma, osteosarcoma, chondrosarcoma, fibrosarcoma, and malignant fibrous histiocytoma (168).

SURGERY

Surgery is a cornerstone in the treatment of a majority of soft tissue sarcomas, including uterine sarcomas. Many women with uterine sarcomas are premenopausal at the time of initial diagnosis; therefore, concerns about fertility and premature menopause should be considered. Surgery to remove the primary tumor—myomectomy, or most often hysterectomy—and inspection of the peritoneal cavity are central to the initial management of these patients. In this section, we will discuss the necessity of performing nodal evaluation, nodal dissection, and removal of the ovaries. The role of cytoreductive procedures for extrauterine disease at the time of diagnosis, and at recurrence, will also be discussed. Fertility-preserving options are extremely limited, but are possible in a few highly select cases (in the setting of less-aggressive mesenchymal tumors).

Uterine Preservation

Myomectomy, or tumor resection with preservation of the uterus, is an option in younger women diagnosed with STUMP or other atypical leiomyomata of the uterus who wish to preserve fertility. Unfortunately, a total hysterectomy (never supracervical) must be performed in a majority of malignant mesenchymal tumors of the uterus. There is no clear option for preserving the uterus in patients diagnosed with LMS, undifferentiated (or high-grade) ESS, or carcinosarcoma. Uterine preservation has been described in eight women diagnosed with "leiomyosarcoma," and successful pregnancies were reported (171). However, it is unclear from this report whether these were all truly high-grade LMS, or whether some, or all, were STUMPs or other tumors of less malignant histologies (171). Until further conclusive investigation is conducted and reported, TAH must still be recommended.

The management of endometrial stromal tumors is somewhat challenging. A confirmed endometrial stromal nodule does not require completion hysterectomy, as it is a benign lesion. However, it may be difficult to confirm whether such a tumor is an endometrial stromal nodule or an ESS without a significant amount of normal myometrium around it, and to state with confidence that there are no infiltrating margins with or without angioinvasion (120). Therefore, a TAH should be recommended in postmenopausal women and in women who have completed childbearing. However, TAH may also be necessary in women who wish to have children. Uterine preservation in the setting of ESS has been reported in a very young (16-year-old) girl (172) and in a 25-year-old who went on to carry a successful pregnancy (173).

Role of Nodal Evaluation or Lymphadenectomy

Two important questions to ask when deciding whether to perform a procedure—in particular, nodal dissections of non-enlarged lymph nodes and removal of ovaries in premenopausal women—are as follows: (1) What is the risk of microscopic disease in those organs? (2) Is there a benefit to removing those organs? Lymph node metastasis in adult soft tissue sarcomas is <3%, with some variation among histologic subtypes (174). Routine regional lymphadenectomy is not recommended for patients with adult soft tissue sarcomas, but resection of bulky isolated metastases can be considered (174).

The risk of lymph metastasis in LMS overall is approximately 7% (4,5,29,60,175–177) (**Table 22.7**). However, the rate of occult lymph node metastasis is less than 3% (175–178). There is no clear benefit to routine lymphadenectomy in patients who present with uterine LMS confined to the uterus and/or clinically normal lymph nodes (4,17,29,60,175). Carcinosarcomas have a higher rate of overall (27%) and occult (20%) lymph node metastasis (4,5,20,59,74,176) (**Table 22.8**).

Undifferentiated endometrial sarcomas are believed to behave similarly, but clear data are lacking. The role of lymphadenectomy beyond debulking of enlarged lymph nodes is still to be determined. Nemani and colleagues (179) suggested that there is a benefit to lymphadenectomy, irrespective of the use of RT. However, the current standard is that all patients, regardless of stage, receive adjuvant systemic chemotherapy (CT). It is quite possible that the therapeutic benefit of lymphadenectomy, if any, in patients with CS may be tempered by this. Nodal dissection in this setting is reasonable and is considered to be standard treatment. The rate of overall and occult lymph node metastasis in ESS is 16% and 6%, respectively (4,5,14–16,180–182) (**Table 22.9**). Deep myometrial invasion and extensive lymph–vascular space invasion (LVSI) further increase the risk of occult metastasis (16). These features are often not obvious at the time of hysterectomy. There is no clear known survival advantage

TABLE 22.7. Lymph Node and Ovarian Metastases in Uterine LMS

	Lymph Node Metastasis		Ovarian Metastasis	
Series	All Cases	Occult Metastasis[a]	All Cases	Occult Metastasis[a]
Ayhan (175)	3/34 (8.8%)	1/27 (3.7%)	—	—
Major (176)	—	2/57 (3.5%)	—	2/59 (3.4%)
Leitao (177)	3/37 (8%)	1/27 (3.7%)	—	—
Goff (178)	—	0/9 (0%)	—	—
Gadducci (179)	—	0/4 (0%)	—	—
Giuntoli (29)	4/36 (11%)	—	—	—
Park (4)	0/11 (0%)	—	—	—
Koivisto (5)	0/15 (0%)	—	—	—
Kapp (60)	23/357 (6.4%)	—	—	—
Total	33/490 (6.7%)	3/124 (2.4%)	4/108 (3.7%)	4/130 (3.1%)

[a]Occult metastasis means nodal metastasis in clinically normal lymph nodes, and disease clinically confined to the uterine corpus and/or cervix.

TABLE 22.8. Lymph Node and Ovarian Metastases in Uterine Carcinosarcoma

	Lymph Node Metastasis		Ovarian Metastasis	
Series	All Cases	Occult Metastasis[a]	All Cases	Occult Metastasis[a]
Major (176)	—	51/287 (18%)	—	36/300 (12%)
Park (20)	—	13/41 (32%)	—	—
Park (4)	8/37 (22%)	—	—	—
Koivisto (5)	6/24 (25%)	—	—	—
Arend (59)	726/2709 (14%)	—	—	—
Galaal (74)	19/34 (56%)	—	—	—
Total	759/2804 (27.1%)	64/328 (19.5%)	—	36/300 (12%)

[a]Occult metastasis means nodal metastasis in clinically normal lymph nodes, and disease clinically confined to the uterine corpus and/or cervix.

to routine lymphadenectomy in these patients (15). Nevertheless, it may be reasonable to consider lymphadenectomy at the time of hysterectomy, recognizing that the therapeutic, prognostic, or predictive value of this in ESS is unknown. Reoperation to complete a lymphadenectomy is not likely to be of any benefit in ESS that does not exhibit deep stromal invasion or extensive LVSI. The rate of lymph node metastasis in adenosarcomas is approximately 3% (59). On the basis of very limited information, lymphadenectomy in patients with disease clinically confined to the uterus may not offer much benefit.

Role of Oophorectomy

The risk of ovarian metastasis is very low in LMS (176,177) (**Table 22.7**). Routine oophorectomy, especially in premenopausal patients, provides no benefit. A SEER analysis actually suggested worse survival in patients undergoing bilateral salpingo-oophorectomy (BSO) (17). It is not entirely clear why removal of the ovaries would lead to a

TABLE 22.9. Lymph Node and Ovarian Metastases in ESS (Low Grade)

	Lymph Node Metastasis		Ovarian Metastasis	
Series	All Cases	Occult Metastasis[a]	All Cases	Occult Metastasis[a]
Park (4)	2/17 (12%)	—	—	—
Koivisto (5)	1/13 (8%)	—	—	—
Dos Santos (16)	7/36 (19%)	2/20 (10%)	11/87 (13%)	0/62 (0%)
Goff (178)	—	0/7 (0%)	—	—
Gadducci (179)	—	0/2 (0%)	—	—
Riopel (180)	3/8 (38%)	1/6 (17%)	—	—
Cheng (14)	4/18 (22%)	—	—	—
Shah (15)	7/100 (7%)	—	—	—
Signorelli (181)	3/19 (16%)	1/16 (6.3%)	—	—
Total	27/211 (12.8%)	4/51 (7.8%)	11/87 (13%)	0/62 (0%)

[a]Occult metastasis means nodal metastasis in clinically normal lymph nodes, and disease clinically confined to the uterine corpus and/or cervix.

worse prognosis, but at the very least these data support retention of the ovaries in premenopausal women who want to retain ovarian function. Occult ovarian metastasis can be seen in approximately 12% of CS (176) (**Table 22.8**). BSO should be recommended for these patients; fortunately, many are postmenopausal. Occult ovarian metastasis in ESS is rare (16) (**Table 22.9**). Ovarian preservation appears to be associated with a higher risk of recurrence; however, this has no impact on OS, and these patients do very well in general (12,15,62). BSO is recommended to reduce the risk of recurrence, but this should be carefully discussed with young premenopausal women. The risk of ovarian metastasis and therapeutic benefit is difficult to discern, because of a lack of large series addressing it in this and other rare uterine sarcomas.

Cytoreductive Surgery for Patients with Extrauterine Disease at Initial Diagnosis

Cytoreductive surgery (CRS) in patients presenting with uterine sarcoma has not been well-described. The only information available describes patients presenting with uterine LMS and extrauterine metastasis (183). The median PFS in patients undergoing a complete gross resection was 14.2 months, compared to 6.8 months for those who had surgery and visible residual disease ($p = 0.002$) (183). OS was 31.9 months compared to 20.2 months, respectively ($p = 0.04$) (183). On multivariate analysis, complete CRS maintained an independent association with PFS, but not with OS. The lack of independent statistical association with OS may be explained by the relatively small number of cases studied. CRS may be a reasonable consideration in highly select cases, in which complete resection of tumor is believed to be feasible without the need for extensive procedures such as exenteration. The potential benefit of surgery should be weighed against the potential risks, and these cases must be individually managed.

Surgery for Recurrent Disease

Data are limited with respect to CRS of recurrent uterine sarcomas. However, CRS may be considered in many of these cases, especially if the patient has had a relatively long disease-free interval and the sites of recurrence appear amenable to a complete surgical resection. Surgery is often considered for recurrent ESS because of the relative indolence of these tumors, long disease-free intervals, and lack of other effective treatments. Currently, the approach to carcinosarcoma is often extrapolated from data for endometrial carcinomas. Resection of recurrent LMS has been described. Surgery for other sarcomas is often considered, but there is no data regarding these very rare uterine sarcomas.

Khoury-Collado et al. (184) described an updated series of 21 patients (from 1997 to 2011) with uterine cancers who developed recurrence in the pelvis after prior RT and underwent pelvic exenteration. The cases included: uterine sarcomas ($n = 6$), CS ($n = 2$), adenosarcomas ($n = 2$), LMS ($n = 1$), and ESS ($n = 1$). In the two carcinosarcoma cases, there was a short time between prior therapy and exenteration, and the median survival after exenteration was only 6 months. The median survival after exenteration for the four other sarcomas was not reached, and the 5-year OS was 66%. Pelvic exenteration may also be a reasonable consideration for patients with isolated pelvic recurrences after prior RT. However, it must be recognized that these operations are quite morbid, and the reported outcomes are based on very small numbers of highly selected patients with uterine sarcomas.

Resection of pulmonary metastases at the time of initial diagnosis and the time of recurrence is often considered for patients with soft tissue sarcomas, and is associated with a favorable survival benefit (185). Specifically, in recurrent uterine sarcomas without other extrathoracic disease, resection of pulmonary metastases is associated with a survival benefit (186). Levenback and colleagues (186) reported a 5-year survival rate of 43% after resection of pulmonary metastases in a group of 45 uterine sarcomas including 38 LMS, 4 ESS, and 3 CS. Unilateral pulmonary recurrence was associated with better survival after metastasectomy than bilateral recurrence (mean survival 39 months vs. 27 months, respectively [$p = 0.02$]). Tumor size, histologic type, use of adjuvant therapy after resection, patient age, and time from hysterectomy to first pulmonary resection were not statistically associated with survival after metastasectomy.

Surgical cytoreduction of recurrent uterine LMS, with or without pulmonary recurrence, has also been reported to provide a possible survival benefit. Leitao and colleagues (80) reported a survival benefit with optimal resection (defined as largest residual tumor mass ≤ 1 cm in diameter) of pulmonary and extrapulmonary first recurrences of uterine LMS. Median survival was 3.9 years after an optimal resection compared to only 0.7 years after suboptimal resection ($p = 0.002$). The only other prognostic factor was time to first recurrence. Median survival was 5.1 years in cases with a time to first recurrence >12 months, compared to 1.5 years in cases with a time to recurrence of ≤ 12 months ($p = 0.005$). Tumor grade, thoracic versus non-thoracic procedures, sites of first recurrence, and use of adjuvant therapy after resection, were not associated with survival. In a larger series by Giuntoli et al. (187), secondary cytoreduction in patients with recurrent uterine LMS was also associated with a survival benefit. Secondary cytoreduction to no gross residual was independently associated with survival after adjusting for site of recurrence, use of CT, RT, combined surgery and CT, and recurrence time (187). Similar to the findings of Leitao et al., a longer time to recurrence was also prognostic of outcome but with 6 months used for the cutoff (187).

RADIATION THERAPY

As the use of RT for patients with uterine sarcomas has been almost exclusively delivered in the postoperative setting (188), the role of preoperative, primary, or palliative RT will not be presented in this section, nor will we offer a detailed discussion of the techniques and complications of adjuvant RT. This has been more fully discussed in Chapter 21 on Corpus: Epithelial Tumors.

Uterine Sarcomas

There is only one published phase III randomized trial comparing observation versus postoperative radiation therapy (PORT) in surgically staged patients with stages I and II uterine sarcomas. This study opened in July 1988 and closed to patient accrual in July 2001. Eligible patients underwent an initial surgical resection that involved mandatory TAH–BSO. Retroperitoneal lymph node dissection was optional (approximately 25% underwent lymph node sampling). The 1988 FIGO staging classification for endometrial carcinoma was applied to these patients (189). Because of the time period of this trial's inception, there were no recommendations regarding either collection of peritoneal washings or omentectomy. The study enrolled 224 patients for randomization from 36 institutions. Patient histologies included the following: 99 LMS, 92 CS, 30 ESS, 1 myxoid LMS, and 2 unclassified cell types. It must be noted that there was a central pathology review of tumor samples; however, no distinction was made regarding low-grade EES, and high-grade undifferentiated uterine sarcomas (UUS). Eligible study patients were randomized to undergo either observation or PORT, consisting of a total dose of approximately 50.4 Gy in 28 daily 1.8-Gy fractions, over 5 to 6 weeks. Two-dimensional (2-D) treatment planning techniques involving bony landmarks were employed to treat the whole pelvis as follows: (a) cranially, the superior aspect of the 5th lumbar vertebra; (b) caudally, the inferior aspect of the obturator foramen; (c) anteriorly, the upper margin of the symphysis pubis; and (d) posteriorly, the level separating the 2nd and 3rd sacral vertebrae. Treatment field arrangements varied from 3 fields, 4-field box (55%), or parallel opposed pair (40%) beams. CT was not administered to any of the study patients (190).

The primary objective of this European Organisation for Research and Treatment of Cancer (EORTC) Gynecological Cancer Group (GCG) trial was to determine whether patients receiving adjuvant pelvic PORT had reduced rates of local (vaginal) and/or regional (pelvic) relapse versus patients receiving no adjuvant therapy, and to assess whether or not improvement in locoregional (LR) control translated into a significant reduction in distant metastases. Secondary objectives of the EORTC-GCG 55874 focused on the impact of PORT on improved OS and PFS without significant increase in toxicity, compared to the observational group (190).

EORTC-GCG 55874 was originally planned to accrue 75 patients per year for 3 years to obtain the projected 77 LR failures necessary for statistical analyses. However, owing to slow accrual of patients, two unplanned interim analyses—the first in April 1995 and the second in December 2001—were required to assess the feasibility of completing the study objectives. Thus, it required 13 years (median follow-up 6.8 years) for patient accrual to record 68 out of the originally planned 77 LR relapses required for adequate statistical evaluation. Of the 224 enrolled patients, adequate follow-up data was available for analysis in 219 patients (due to insufficient follow-up data in two cases in the observational cohort and three cases in the PORT group) (188).

Crude relapse rates for all cell types in EORTC-GCG 55874 were 47% (52/110) in the PORT cohort and 50% (54/109) in the observational arm. There was a significant reduction in overall LR relapse in the PORT group: 24 (21%) compared to 44 (40%) in the observational arm ($p = 0.004$). Furthermore, there was a reduction in isolated LR relapse of 3% in the PORT group versus 18% in the nonirradiated arm. Distant metastases occurred as a component of failure in 49 (46%) patients in the PORT versus 35 (32%) in the observational cohorts. There was a higher rate of isolated distant metastasis in the adjuvant group versus the nonirradiated cohort (25.5% versus 10%, respectively). The primary cause of death was malignant disease in 81% (39/48) of PORT patients and 93% (43/46) of observational patients. There was no significant difference in OS or PFS and no difference in toxicity identified between the two groups (192) **(Figs. 22.21 and 22.22)**.

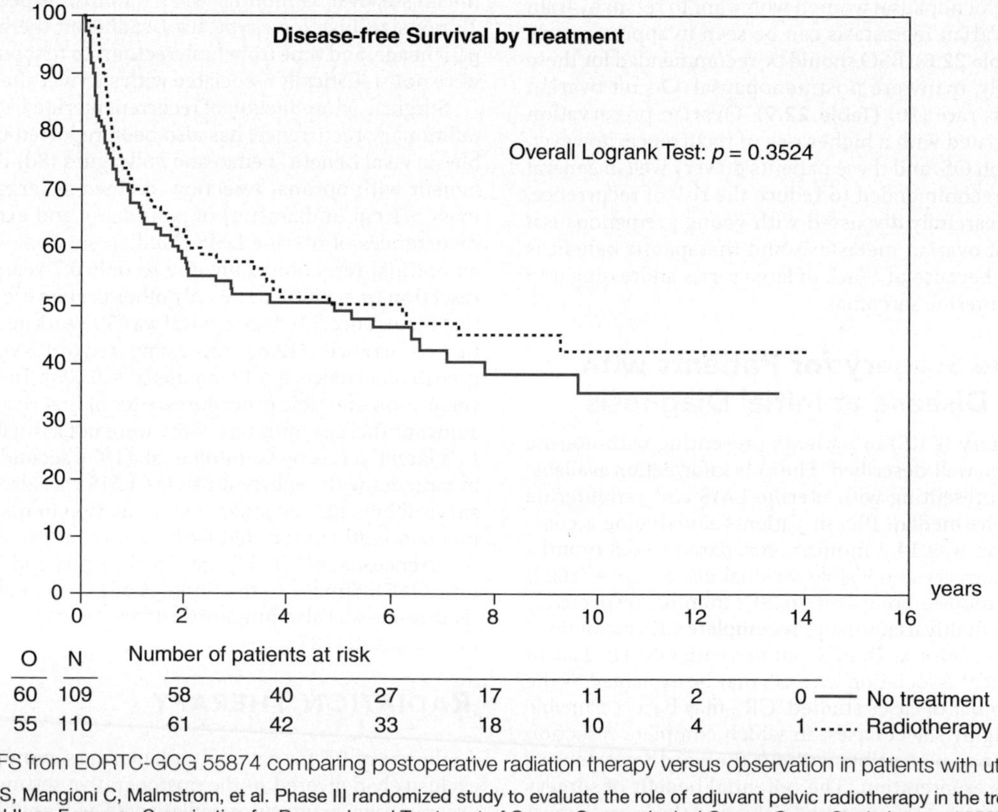

Figure 22.21. DFS from EORTC-GCG 55874 comparing postoperative radiation therapy versus observation in patients with uterine sarcoma.

Source: From Reed NS, Mangioni C, Malmstrom, et al. Phase III randomized study to evaluate the role of adjuvant pelvic radiotherapy in the treatment of uterine sarcomas stages I and II: an European Organisation for Research and Treatment of Cancer Gynaecological Cancer Group Study (protocol 55874). *Eur J Cancer*. 2008;44:808–818, with permission (Elsevier).

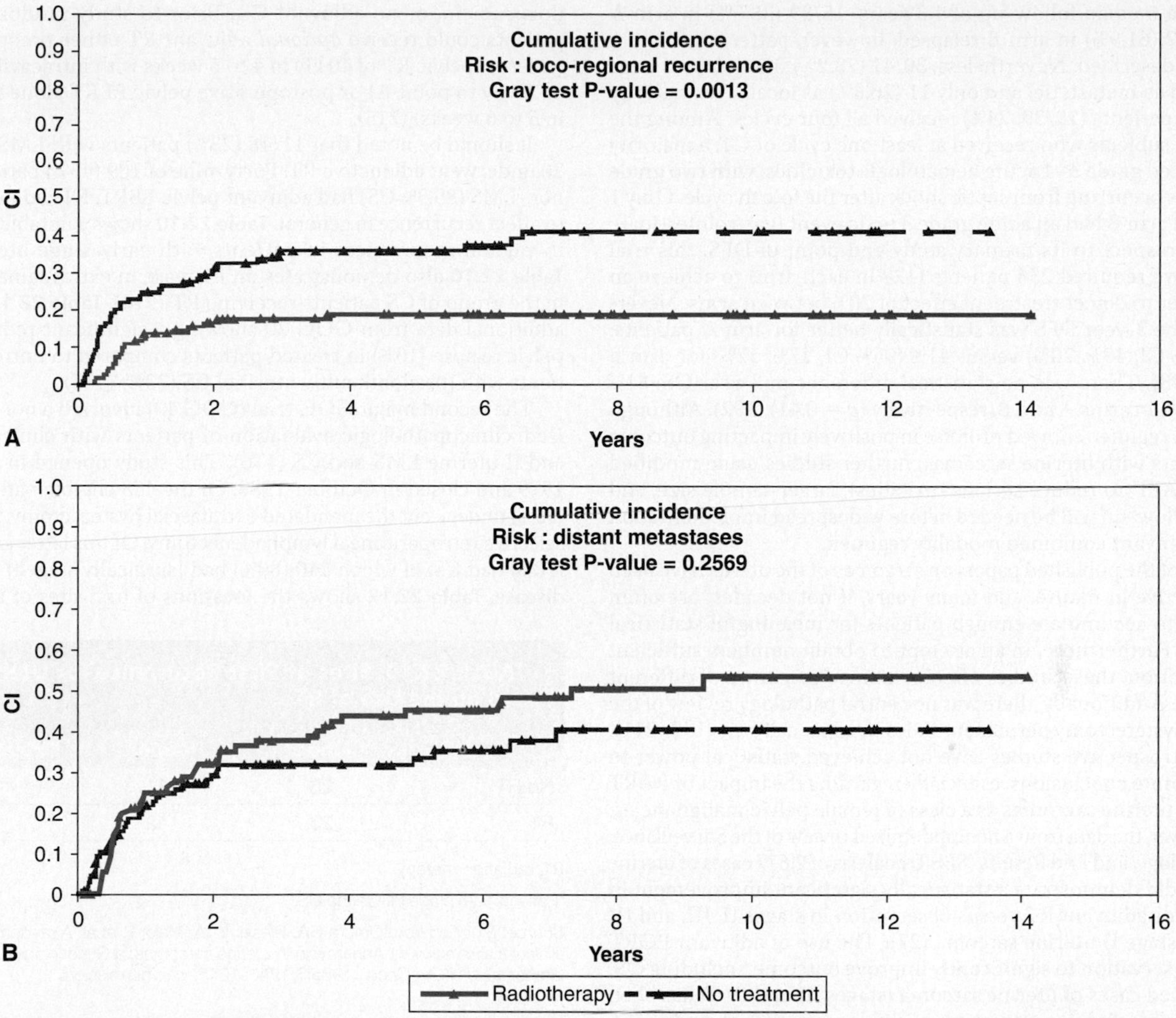

Figure 22.22. Cumulative incidence of **(A)** LR recurrence and **(B)** distant metastases of postoperative adjuvant radiation therapy versus observation in patients with uterine sarcoma.

Source: From Reed NS, Mangioni C, Malmstrom, et al. Phase III randomized study to evaluate the role of adjuvant pelvic radiotherapy in the treatment of uterine sarcomas stages I and II: an European Organisation for Research and Treatment of Cancer Gynaecological Cancer Group Study (protocol 55874). *Eur J Cancer.* 2008;44:808–818, with permission (Elsevier).

With respect to patients with uterine CS in EORTC-GCG 55874, PORT did reduce LR failures from 47% (observational cohort) to 24% (PORT cohort) ($p < 0.05$), while not significantly decreasing the overall rate of distant metastasis (29% observational vs. 35% PORT cohort). This improvement in LR control with adjuvant pelvic PORT was further noted in the evaluation of patients with isolated LR failures (24% observational versus 4% PORT). However, there were more isolated distant failures in the adjuvantly irradiated subset of patients with CS (7% observational versus 15% PORT) (190). This latter finding is similar to that shown for patients with endometrial carcinomas randomized to adjuvant pelvic external beam radiation therapy (EBRT) compared to patients not treated with EBRT (191). Nevertheless, the findings of EORTC-GCG 55874 suggest that pelvic PORT should be considered as adjuvant therapy to improve LR control in patients with stage I and II uterine CS. More importantly, PORT was associated with benefit in patient OS, compared to patients receiving no adjuvant RT (HR, 1.58; 95% CI, 0.83, 3.01) (190).

Concerning patients with stage I and II uterine LMS, LR relapse in the observational group (24%) was comparable to that of the adjuvantly irradiated cohort (20%). The overall rate of distant failure in the observational cohort (33%) was less than that in the PORT cohort (54%). However, isolated LR failures were 14% in the observational cohort and 2% in the PORT cohort. With respect to isolated distant failures, there were 14% in the observational cohort versus 36% in the PORT cohort (190). The findings of EORTC-GCG 55874 may be used to defer adjuvant PORT for patients with stage I and II uterine LMS. Because of the observed impact on improving isolated LR control in this patient subset, one could make an argument for employing pelvic PORT as a salvage or palliative therapy in selected patients with early-stage uterine LMS. Finally, EORTC-GCG 55874 showed a negative impact of PORT on OS in the LMS cohort of early-stage patients (HR, 0.64; 95% CI, 0.36, 1.14) (188).

One reported phase 3 multi-institutional, prospectively randomized clinical trial for stages I, II, and III uterine sarcomas (1988 FIGO criteria) compared experimental adjuvant chemoradiation (arm A) versus standard adjuvant pelvic PORT (arm B) for patients with CS (19 patients), LMS (53 patients), UUS (9 patients) (192). Arm A involved four planned cycles of intravenous (IV) doxorubicin ["A"] (50 mg/m^2) on day 1, cisplatin ["P"] (75 mg/m^2) on day 3, and ifosfamide ["I"] (3 g/m^2/day) with mesna (3 g/m^2/day) on days 1 and 2 every 3 weeks. One month following completion of this "API" CT, arm B patients received pelvic PORT to a total dose of 45 Gy over 5 weeks, with optional vaginal brachytherapy (VBT). The control cohort of patients began pelvic PORT within 8 weeks of surgery, with or without VBT. Of note, this study accrued only 81 of a planned total of 256 subjects (39 and 42 in arms A and B, respectively) from October 2001 through July 2009.

With a median follow-up of 4.3 years, 15/39 (38.5%) in arm A and 26/42 (61.9%) in arm B relapsed; however, patterns of failure were not described. Nevertheless, 30/41 (73.2%) first relapses were described as metastatic, and only 11 (26.8%) as local. The majority of arm A patients (29/39, 74%) received all four cycles. Among the 38 arm A subjects who received at least one cycle of CT, a majority experienced grade 3–4 acute hematologic toxicities, with two grade 5 fatalities occurring from septic shock after the fourth cycle. Only 1 patient in arm B had an acute grade 3 toxic event (gastrointestinal).

With respect to its primary study end point of DFS, this trial would have required 256 patients (128 in each arm) to achieve an 80% power to detect treatment effect of 20% between arms. Nevertheless, the 3-year DFS was statistically better for arm A patients: 55% (95% CI, 40%, 70%) versus 41% (95% CI, 27%, 57%) for arm B ($p = 0.048$). There was no statistical difference in 3-year OS: 81% versus 69% in arms A and B, respectively ($p = 0.41$) (192). Although this novel regimen showed promise in positively impacting outcome for patients with uterine sarcomas, further studies using modified doses of API (to reduce serious toxicities), larger sample size, and longer follow-up will be needed before widespread implementation of this adjuvant combined modality regimen.

Most of the published papers on sarcomas of the uterus have been retrospective in nature, and many years, if not decades, are often required to accumulate enough patients for meaningful statistical analyses. Furthermore, in an attempt to obtain numbers sufficient for evaluation, these studies often combined sarcomas of different cell types. Additionally, there was no central pathology review of the original hysterectomy permanent slides to verify cell type (193–211). These retrospective studies have not achieved statistical power to reach definite conclusions, especially regarding the impact of PORT on OS in uterine sarcomas as a class of female pelvic malignancies.

However, the data from a nonrandomized review of the Surveillance, Epidemiology, and End Results (SEER) analysis of 2,677 cases of uterine sarcoma did demonstrate a statistically significant improvement in survival for adjuvant RT versus observation in stages II, III, and IV (but not stage I) uterine sarcoma (27). The use of adjuvant PORT versus observation to significantly improve outcome, including OS, in advanced cases of uterine sarcoma (stages III and IVA) has been further supported in a retrospective single institutional study of 76 evaluable cases of uterine sarcomas (206). However, another SEER analysis of 1,819 patients with stage I/II uterine CS, and 1,088 with stage I/II uterine LMS, showed improved survival for the subset of patients with CS who did not have any nodal sampling. There was no observed significant survival benefit for CS patients undergoing a node dissection, or for any subset of patients with LMS (212).

Recently, Sampath et al. (213) published a retrospective review—the largest to date—of patients with uterine sarcoma. The investigators conducted a query of the National Oncology Database (Impac Medical Systems, Sunnyvale, CA), identifying 3,650 evaluable patients with a diagnosis of uterine sarcoma. Of this initial group, 2,206 had definitive surgery; of these, 1,128 had CS, 529 had LMS, and 361 had EES, comprising stages I through IV (with unknown stage, however, in approximately one-third of patients). Statistical analyses showed no significant impact on OS for patients receiving predominantly pelvic PORT (with or without VBT) compared to those receiving no adjuvant therapy. However, a significant reduction in LR relapse was noted in the adjuvantly irradiated cohort compared to the observational cohort: 53% at 5 years ($p < 0.001$). In addition, this LR control benefit conferred by adjuvant RT versus observation was preserved on subset analyses of patients with uterine CS ($p < 0.001$), LMS ($p < 0.01$), and ESS ($p < 0.05$) (213). This latter study may be cited as evidence for future trials to prospectively evaluate the incorporation of adjuvant volume-directed RT into the range of potential therapeutic modalities for uterine sarcomas.

The GOG previously conducted two prospective clinical trials of selected patients with uterine sarcomas. The earliest study (GOG 20) reported on 156 evaluable patients with [surgically staged] stage I or II sarcomas of the uterus (214). Patients were enrolled from 1973 to 1982 and randomized to receive at least one cycle of adjuvant doxorubicin, or no adjuvant CT. Prior to study randomization, patients could receive *optional* adjuvant RT either preoperatively (external pelvic RT of 40 Gy in 4 to 5 weeks with intracavitary VBT of 20 Gy to point A) or postoperative pelvic EBRT alone (to 50 Gy in 5 to 6 weeks) (215).

It should be noted that 11/48 (23%) patients with LMS in GOG 20 underwent adjunctive RT. Forty-nine of 109 (45%) patients with non-LMS (85.3% CS) had adjuvant pelvic EBRT. RT did not appear to affect recurrence in general. **Table 22.10** shows a notable decrease in vaginal recurrences in patients with early-stage uterine CS. **Table 22.10** also demonstrates an increase in extravaginal failures in the group of CS patients receiving RT (214). **Table 22.11** depicts additional data from GOG 20 showing a significant reduction in pelvic relapse (10%) in treated patients compared to untreated patients with [predominantly uterine] CS (23%) (215).

The second major GOG trial (GOG 40) involved a nonrandomized, clinicopathologic evaluation of patients with clinical stage I and II uterine LMS and CS (176). This study opened in February 1979 and closed in October 1988. Of the 453 eligible patients, 430 (95%) underwent the mandated extrafascial hysterectomy, BSO, and selective retroperitoneal lymphadenectomy. Of this latter group, 301 (70%) had CS, of which 240 (80%) had [surgically staged] stage I/II disease. **Table 22.12** shows the locations of first sites of relapse(s)

TABLE 22.10. Sites of First Recurrence for Uterine CS[a] Based on the Use of RT

	None	Vaginal	Extravaginal
No RT	28	11	10
RT	23	2	19

RT, radiation therapy.

[a]Patients with stage I/II uterine CS.

Source: Modified from Omura GA, Blessing JA, Major F, et al. A randomized clinical trial of adjuvant Adriamycin in uterine sarcomas: a Gynecologic Oncology Group study. *J Clin Oncol*. 1985;3:1240–1245, with permission.

TABLE 22.11. Sites of First Recurrence for Uterine CS[a] Based on the Use of RT

	Pelvic	Extra-Pelvic
No RT	14/60 (23%)	12/60 (20%)
Pelvic RT	5/49 (10%)	17/49 (35%)

RT, radiation therapy.

[a]85% of this group (93 patients) with non-leiomyosarcomas of the uterus was stage I/II uterine CS.

Source: Modified from Hornback NB, Omura G, Major FJ. Observations on the uterine sarcomas of adjuvant radiation therapy in patients with stage I and II uterine sarcoma. *Int J Radiat Oncol Biol Phys*. 1986;12:2127–2130, with permission (Elsevier).

TABLE 22.12. Sites of First Recurrence for Uterine CS[a] Based on Use of Radiotherapy

	No RT	Pelvic RT
Pelvis	43	20
Abdomen	43	19
Distant	38	31
None	83	59

[a]For patients with uterine CS who may have had more than one relapse.

Source: Modified from Major FJ, Blessing JA, Silverberg SG, et al. Prognostic factors in early-stage uterine sarcoma: a Gynecology Oncology Group study. *Cancer*. 1993;71:1702–1709, with permission (Wiley).

in this subset. Although adjuvant pelvic EBRT was not mandated, it again appears possible that postoperative pelvic PORT plays a role in reducing LR relapses in patients with early-stage uterine CS.

However, in the French pilot study that led to the previously described SARCGYN study (192), 18 patients with optimally debulked surgical stage I, II, and III uterine sarcomas (13/18 with uterine LMS) received three cycles of adjuvant doxorubicin, cisplatin, and ifosfamide, followed by sequential pelvic EBRT to a total dose of approximately 45 Gy in 5 weeks, with or without VBT (209). The investigators then performed a matched case–control study of 18 patients; 16 underwent pelvic RT alone and 2 received no adjuvant treatment. With a median follow-up of 43 months (range, 23 to 56 months), they found that only 5 patients (27.8%) had suffered recurrences. All of these patients failed in extrapelvic sites only. Moreover, neither median survival nor DFS had been reached at the last follow-up. There remains much uncertainty regarding the role of pelvic EBRT for patients with uterine LMS, especially with respect to reserving volume-directed RT in combination with CT as adjunctive treatment, or even as a component of salvage and/or palliative therapeutic intervention (209).

Uterine CS

The most common types of uterine sarcoma histologies currently reported in the literature are referred to as metaplastic carcinoma (111), mixed epithelial and stromal tumors of the uterus (2), historically known as uterine CS, or some variant of mixed Müllerian uterine tumors (195,216–225). There has been one randomized phase 3 prospective trial of adjuvant RT in CS (GOG 150). This study compared whole-abdominal irradiation to three cycles of cisplatin/ifosfamide CT with respect to recurrence rates, DFS, and OS. Also evaluated were therapeutic toxicities. Eligible patients had CS confined to the abdomen and had undergone optimal surgical debulking with no postsurgical residual disease >1 cm. Patients randomized to RT received a total dose of 30 Gy to the whole abdomen using EBRT, followed by a pelvic boost, to a cumulative pelvic dose of approximately 50 Gy.

The first published report on the two treatment cohorts was based on an analysis performed in December 2005 (226). Of the 224 patients enrolled, 206 were evaluable. Of these 206 patients, 105 received adjuvant RT and 101 received CT. The estimated death rate for patients receiving CT was 32.8% lower than those receiving RT ($p = 0.042$). A subsequently published update of GOG 150 based on a May 2006 analysis demonstrated that this reduction in estimated death rate by CT was 31%, relative to RT ($p = 0.046$) (227).

The final analysis of the GOG 150 data was conducted in November 2006 (228). At that time, the median duration of follow-up for patients who were alive at last contact was 63 months. The breakdown of surgical stages for patients in the RT versus CT cohorts is as follows: stage I—35/105 (33.3%) versus 29/101 (28.7%); stage II—11/105 (10.5%) versus 15/101 (14.9%); stage III—45/105 (42.9%) versus 47/101 (46.5%); stage IV—14/105 (13.3%) versus 10/101 (9.9%). The estimated crude probability of relapse within 5 years was nonsignificant: 58% versus 52% for the RT and CT groups, respectively. The sites of first failure are presented in **Table 22.13**. Although not statistically significant, there were fewer vaginal and more abdominal relapses in the adjuvant RT cohort compared to the CT cohort. **Table 22.14** demonstrates an estimated 5-year survival of approximately 35% for patients randomized to adjuvant RT versus 45% in the CT group. After adjusting for stage and age at diagnosis, there was a trend toward reduction of the death rate for those receiving CT (29%) compared to RT (HR, 0.712; 95% CI, 0.484–1.048; $p = 0.085$; 2-tail test). Of interest, patients who received adjuvant RT had more late complications, mainly gastrointestinal, than those undergoing cytotoxic therapy ($p < 0.001$). Two patients undergoing RT died as a direct result of radiation-induced hepatitis (228).

One retrospective single-institutional study from a major academic medical center attempted to further verify the results of GOG 150 by evaluating 49 patients with optimally debulked stage I–IV uterine CS who received either adjuvant RT alone (pelvic or whole abdominal irradiation ± VBT) or predominantly paclitaxel/carboplatin CT (± whole abdominal or pelvic irradiation ± VBT). Although the findings were not statistically significant owing to small sample size, this report did show a reduction in upper abdominal relapses (24% vs. 35%) and extravaginal/pelvic failures in the group receiving combined modality adjuvant therapy compared to the cohort receiving adjuvant RT alone (45% vs. 91%, respectively) (229).

A large single institutional retrospective study of 121 patients with surgically staged I–IV uterine CS (2009 FIGO staging criteria) with central pathologic confirmation of cell type found that the use of any type of adjuvant RT seemed to prevent vaginal failures in all stages. Of note, the use of external beam PORT to the pelvis did impact survival.

TABLE 22.13. Patterns of Failure for Uterine CS

Sites of Recurrence[a]	WAI ($n=105$), Number of Cases	Chemotherapy ($n=101$), Number of Cases
Vagina	4	10
Pelvis	14	14
Abdomen	29	19
Distant	27	24

n, total number of cases in each arm; WAI, whole abdominal irradiation.

[a]Some patients had multiple sites of relapse.

Source: Modified from Wolfson AH, Brady MF, Rocereto T, et al. A Gynecologic Oncology Group randomized phase III trial of whole abdominal irradiation (WAI) vs. cisplatin-ifosfamide and mesna (CIM) as postsurgical therapy in stage I–IV carcinosarcoma (CS) of the uterus. *Gynecol Oncol*. 2007;107:177–185, with permission (Elsevier).

TABLE 22.14. Patterns of Failure in Patients with Surgically Staged Uterine LMS Managed by Surgery with or without External Beam Pelvic Irradiation (+/− Vaginal Brachytherapy +/− Chemotherapy)

Reference	Stage	Vagina	Pelvis	Extrapelvic	Abdomen	Distant	Adjuvant Treatment
178	I, II, III, IV	Not stated	0/13	Not stated	1/13	7/13	Yes[a]
178	I, II, III, IV	Not stated	8/50	Not stated	9/50	17/50	No[a]
241	I, II	Not stated	4/26	10/26	Not stated	Not stated	Mainly yes[a]
29	I, II, III	Not stated	4/23	9/23	Not stated	Not stated	Yes[a]
29	I, II	Not stated	14/69	23/69	Not stated	Not stated	No[a]
Subtotals	—	—	30/181 (16.6%)	42/118 (35.6%)	10/63 (15.9%)	24/63 (38.1%)	—
Totals	—	—	30/181 (16.6%)	76/181 (42.0%)	—	—	—

[a]Nonrandomized.

A more recent population-based retrospective review of 1,581 patients with [surgically staged] stage I and II uterine CS, using FIGO 1988 criteria, found that the use of VBT rose from 4.5% between 1988 and 1999 to 12.5% between 2005 and 2010. Of the total patient sample, 803 (50.8%) had no RT, 636 (40.2%) had PORT with EBRT, and 142 (9.0%) had adjuvant VBT alone. On multivariable analyses, the type of RT did not impact survival; however, VBT was statistically associated with improved OS compared to no adjuvant RT (HR 0.67, 95% CI, 0.47, 0.95) ($p = 0.024$). This latter report and GOG 150 suggest that there may be a role for adjuvant VBT in patients with uterine CS, especially in the setting of early-stage disease.

Results from other retrospective institutional and population-based series focusing solely on uterine CS are inconsistent concerning the impact of adjuvant therapy on outcome. Some demonstrate no survival benefit for postoperative RT (195,219,221,222,224), whereas others show a significant impact of pelvic PORT on survival (216,218,223,225). One of the above studies involved a review of the nonrandomized SEER database of 2,461 women with CS (1973 to 2003) (225). In this dataset, 890 patients received adjuvant RT. The overall 5-year survival of those receiving RT versus no-RT was 41.5% and 33.2%, respectively ($p < 0.001$); furthermore, a significant improvement in survival was observed in all stages of disease, including stage IV.

Finally, there have been several published retrospective reports suggesting that combined adjuvant CT followed by RT to address the high rate of extrapelvic sites of metastases may impart even longer survival, especially in stage I and II disease (179,217,220,230–233). Nevertheless, the role of adjuvant RT in the management of patients with uterine CS remains inconclusive. As there were more vaginal failures in the CT arm of GOG 150, and other sites of relapse (abdominal recurrences) were similar or less common in frequency than those in the RT arm, it may be reasonable to consider postoperative VBT (either high- or low-dose-rate) with CT (of greater than three cycles) for any patient with optimally debulked CS in future trials.

Uterine LMS

There are no existing randomized phase 3 trials that demonstrate any impact of adjuvant RT on LR relapse or survival in this patient population. **Table 22.15** presents data from several retrospective series in which overall pelvic/extrapelvic relapse rates were reportedly 16.6% and 42.0%, respectively, for patients with uterine LMS.

There is still a paucity of information distinguishing upper-abdominal from extra-abdominal distant sites of tumor involvement. The pelvic and extrapelvic percentages were 18.5% (22/119), and 41.2% (49/119) for the nonirradiated patients, respectively, and 12.9% (8/62),

TABLE 22.15. Chemotherapy in LMS of the Uterus

Drug	n	Prior Therapy	Schedule	Overall Response (%)	Reference
Single-agent chemotherapy					
Primary chemotherapy					
Liposomal doxorubicin	32	11 RT	50 mg/m^2 q 4 wk	16	275
Topotecan	36	8 RT	1.5 mg/m^2 × 5 d q 3 wk	11	276
Paclitaxel	33	8 RT	175 mg/m^2 q 3 wk	9	277
Ifosfamide	35	15 RT	1.5 g/m^2 × 5 d q 4 wk (1.2 g/m^2 if prior RT)	17	278
Etoposide	28	7 RT	100 mg/m^2 × 3 d q 3 wk	0	279
Cisplatin	33	8 RT	50 mg/m^2 q 3 wk	3	280
Doxorubicin	28	N/A	60 mg/m^2 q 3 wk	25	281
Piperazinedione	19	N/A	9 mg/m^2 q 3 wk	5[a]	282
Aminothiadiazole	20	N/A	125 mg/m^2 q 1 wk	0	283
Diaziquone	24	N/A	22.5 mg/m^2 q 3 wk	0	284
Trabectedin	20	7 RT	1.5 mg/m^2 over 24 h q3 wk	10	302
Nonprimary chemotherapy					
Gemcitabine	44	11 RT, 35 CT	1,000 mg/m^2 weekly × 3 q 4 wk	21	285
	31	31 CT	1,250 mg/m^2 weekly × 2 q 3 wk	3.2[b]	286
	29	15 RT, 19 CT	1,250 mg/m^2 weekly × 3 q 4 wk	3[b]	287
	56	N/A	1,000 mg/m^2 weekly × 3 q 4 wk	18[b]	288
	22	16 RT, 21 CT	1,000 mg/m^2 weekly × 3 q 4 wk (fixed-dose rate)	19	301
Paclitaxel	48	15 RT, 33 CT	175 mg/m^2 q 3 wk (135 mg/m^2 if prior RT)	8.4	289
Trabectedin	54	54 CT	1.5 mg/m^2 over 24 h q 3 wk	4[b]	290
	49	49 CT	1–1.8 mg/m^2 over 1-3 h q 3 wk	4.1[b]	291
	35	21 RT, 4 CT	1.5mg/m^2 over 24 h q 3 wk	17[b]	303
Trimetrexate	23	7 RT, 10 CT	5 mg/m^2 orally × 5 days q 2 wk	4.3	293
Etoposide	29	6 RT, 27 CT	50 mg/m^2 orally × 21 days q 4 wk	6.9	294
	28	7 RT, 27 CT	100 mg/m^2 days 1, 3, 5 q 4 wk	11	295

TABLE 22.15. Chemotherapy in LMS of the Uterus (*continued*)

Drug	n	Prior Therapy	Schedule	Overall Response (%)	Reference
Amonafide	26	8 RT, 25 CT	300 mg/m^2 × 5 days q 3 wk	4	296
Mitoxantrone	12	12 CT	12 mg/m^2 q 3 wk	0	297
Cisplatin	19	19 CT	50 mg/m^2 q 3 wk	5	298
Temozolomide	11	N/A	180 mg/m^2 orally × 5 days q 4 wk	18[c]	300
Vinorelbine	16	16 CT	30 mg/m^2 weekly × 8	6[c]	299
Combination chemotherapy					
Doxorubicin *plus*	20	N/A	60 mg/m^2 q 3 wk	30	281
Dacarbazine			250 mg/m^2 × 5 d q 3 wk		
Dacarbazine *plus*	18	7 RT	750 mg/m^2 q 4 wk	28	307
Mitomycin			6 mg/m^2 q 4 wk		
Doxorubicin			40 mg/m^2 q 4 wk		
Cisplatin			60 mg/m^2 q 4 wk		
Dacarbazine *plus*	10	10 No CT	750 mg/m^2 q 4 wk	80	308
Mitomycin			6 mg/m^2 q 4 wk		
Doxorubicin			40 mg/m^2 q 4 wk		
Cisplatin			60 mg/m^2 q 4 wk		
Mitomycin *plus*	35	8 RT	8 mg/m^2 q 3 wk	23	309
Doxorubicin			40 mg/m^2 q 3 wk		
Cisplatin			60 mg/m^2 q 3 wk		
Hydroxyurea *plus*	38	11 RT	2 g orally × 1 day q 4 wk	18	310
Dacarbazine			700 mg/m^2 q 4 wk		
Etoposide			300 mg/m^2 × 2 days q 4 wk		
Ifosfamide *plus*	33	9 RT,33 No CT	5 mg/m^2 q 3 wk	30	311
Doxorubicin			50 mg/m^2 q 3 wk		
Gemcitabine *plus*	34	14 RT, 16 CT	900 mg/m^2 days 1, 8 q 3 wk (675 mg/m^2 if prior RT)	53[c]	312
Docetaxel			100 mg/m^2 day 8 q 3 wk (75 mg/m^2 if prior RT)		
Gemcitabine *plus*	42	42 No CT	900 mg/m^2 days 1, 8	36	265
Docetaxel			100 mg/m^2 day 8 q 3 wk		
Gemcitabine *plus*	48	17 RT, 48 CT	900 mg/m^2 days 1, 8 (675 mg/m^2 if prior RT)	27	264
Docetaxel			100 mg/m^2 day 8 q 3 wk (75 mg/m^2 if prior RT)		
Gemcitabine *plus*	24	12 RT, 18 CT	900 mg/m^2 days 1, 8 (675 mg/m^2 if prior RT)	24	301
Docetaxel			100 mg/m^2 day 8 q 3 wk (75 mg/m^2 if prior RT)		
Gemcitabine *plus*	8	No RT, 4 CT	900 mg/m^2 days 1, 8	38	304
Docetaxel			70 mg/m^2 day 8 q 3 wk		
Gemcitabine *plus*	54	11 RT, No CT	900 mg/m^2 days 1, 8 (675 mg/m^2 if prior RT)	32	398
Docetaxel			75 mg/m^2 day 8 q 3 wk (60 mg/m^2 if prior RT)		
Doxorubicin *plus*	38	38 No CT	60 mg/m^2 q 3 wk	19[a]	313
Cyclophosphamide			500 mg/m^2 q 3 wk		
Gemcitabine *plus*	9	N/A	800 mg/m^2 days 1, 8	22	314
Vinorelbine			25 mg/m^2 days 1, 8 q 3 wk		
Temozolomide *plus*	11	10 CT	150 mg/m^2 orally days 1–7 q 2 wk	9.1	316
Thalidomide			200 mg orally daily		

(*continued*)

■ **TABLE 22.15. Chemotherapy in LMS of the Uterus (*continued*)**

Drug	n	Prior Therapy	Schedule	Overall Response (%)	Reference
Doxorubicin *plus*	47	17 RT, No CT	60 mg/m² q 3 wk	60	320
Trabectedin			1.1 mg/m² 3-hr q 3 wk		
Biologic and targeted agents					
Thalidomide	9	14 RT, 29 CT	200–1,000 mg orally daily	0	384
Sorafenib	37	N/A	400 mg orally twice daily	3[c]	385
Sunitinib	23	23 CT	50 mg orally daily × 4 of 6 wk	8.7	381
Aflibercept	41	14 RT, 20 CT	4 mg/kg day 1 q2 wk	0	386
Ridaforolimus	57	57 CT	12.5 mg × 5 days q2 wk	0[c]	393
Ixabepilone	23	6 RT, 23 CT	40 mg/m² q3 wk	0	335
Bevacizumab *plus* Doxorubicin	7	N/A	15 mg/kg q3 wk75 mg/m²	28	390

Note: All chemotherapy agents were given intravenously unless specified.

CT, chemotherapy; N/A, not available; RT, radiation therapy.

[a]Uterine sarcoma.

[b]Adult soft tissue sarcoma.

[c]Adult Leiomyosarcoma.

respectively and 43.5% (27/62) for the radiated patients, (176,180,234). It does not appear that postoperative RT has any significant effect on reducing recurrence in patients with uterine LMS. However, two series combined yielded a pelvic relapse rate of 11.1% (4/36) with RT versus 61.1% (22/36) without adjuvant RT (178,181). One recently reported retrospective series of 69 patients with all stages of uterine LMS (staged as per the 2009 staging criteria), of which 46.4% (32/69) underwent PORT with or without adjuvant CT, found, on multivariable analyses, that PORT significantly reduced pelvic failures (HR, 0.28, 95% CI, 0.11, 0.69; $p = 0.006$) and increased OS (HR, 0.44, 95% CI, 0.23, 0.85; $p = 0.014$), independent of other clinicopathologic factors (235). The major problem is that, despite achieving local control, the majority of these patients have distant extra-abdominal metastases in organs such as the lung. There is a need to develop more effective systemic therapies to improve patient outcome (176,179,236,237).

A retrospective case–control, single-institution study of patients with uterine LMS demonstrated a trend toward improved survival in 31 patients who received adjuvant pelvic irradiation, compared with 31 controls who did not receive adjuvant RT (29,238,239). A recent retrospective study from a consortium of institutions involving 143 patients with surgical stage I–IV uterine LMS reported on 24 patients (17%) who received pelvic PORT and 63 (44%) who had adjuvant and/or palliative CT. This latter study found that the rate of pelvic relapse was significantly reduced ($p = 0.02$) for patients who received RT (18%) versus those who did not (49%). Although not maintained at 90 months of follow-up, this study also showed that the 5-year survival of patients receiving adjuvant RT (70%) was greater than the survival of those who did not (35%) (240). A large single-institutional series of 182 patients with uterine sarcomas, of whom 79 (43.4%) had LMS, recently demonstrated that patients receiving PORT had significantly improved 5-year OS compared to those who did not (71.8% vs. 40.2%, respectively; $p = 0.018$) (241–243). However, the role of adjuvant RT in the management of patients with uterine LMS remains undefined.

ESS

To date, no randomized phase III trials have shown any significant impact of adjuvant RT on outcomes in patients with uterine EES. These tumors can be subdivided into a low-grade category (ESS) or a high-grade category (UUS) of sarcoma. Gadducci and colleagues (244) reported no abdominal or distant recurrences independent of the administration of adjuvant irradiation in all stages of low-grade ESS. Yet, there was a 33.3% (6/18) pelvic recurrence rate, of which the majority did not undergo any RT. This latter finding suggests that postoperative external pelvic RT should at least be considered for the subset of patients with low-grade stage I and II ESS. This has been supported by other retrospective studies (208).

One retrospective report reviewed 28 cases of ESS, of which 19 were low-grade and 9 high-grade (245,246). Fifty percent of the patients in this series underwent adjuvant pelvic RT, with no difference in survival. In addition, almost 30% of patients receiving adjuvant RT relapsed within the treatment field (247). With respect to undifferentiated ESS, another study documented multiple sites of recurrence, including abdominal (34.8% [11/32]), distant (34.8% [11/32]), and pelvic (40.6% [13/32]) sites of relapse (248). However, a more recent small series of 13 patients with all stages of uterine EES reported that the 10 patients who received pelvic PORT (+/− vaginal boost) had an 89% rate of LR control, compared to 50% for the 3 patients who did not (249). Another small retrospective series of 10 patients with stage I/II UUS (as per 2009 FIGO criteria), of whom 8 were treated with PORT, reported that none experienced pelvic failure (250). With the exception of one single-institution, retrospective series (251), no direct survival benefit has been associated with the use of PORT in either EES or UUS (252–254). Thus, the role of RT for patients with uterine EES remains uncertain.

CHEMOTHERAPY

Uterine sarcomas, although far less common than endometrial carcinomas, exhibit two features that suggest a need for systemic therapy: a recurrence rate of at least 50%, even in early-stage disease; and a high propensity for distant failure. The comparatively low incidence of uterine sarcomas has made randomized, controlled trials difficult. Despite this, cooperative group studies have provided data from phase II and III trials supporting the rational selection of systemic CT.

When utilizing CT in the treatment of uterine sarcomas, it is crucial to understand that these neoplasms are heterogeneous. Uterine CS (malignant mixed Müllerian tumors) and LMS constitute 90% of cases entered into clinical trials. These two histologic subtypes are usually the only uterine sarcomas presenting in sufficient numbers to allow meaningful phase 3 studies; however, as each of these two histologic subtypes appears to respond differently to CT, they should be studied separately.

Limited Disease

Uterine sarcoma is associated with a high rate of distant metastasis, even in the absence of intraperitoneal or lymph node metastasis. It has been concluded that this is due to the high rate of hematogenous and lymphatic dissemination (255). Therefore, the role of adjuvant systemic CT is under investigation in patients with apparently limited disease that has been fully resected. A meta-analysis of almost 2,000 patients with localized, resectable soft tissue sarcomas (including uterine sarcomas) in small randomized trials of adjuvant anthracycline-based CT showed improved outcomes with CT compared to local treatment alone. Absolute risk reduction of 12% in recurrence and 11% in death were associated with doxorubicin-based CT combined with ifosfamide (256). Application of these data to uterine sarcoma is somewhat stymied, however, by the range of tumor sites and the heterogeneity of sarcoma subtypes included in this meta-analysis.

The largest randomized trial to date (a phase III GOG trial of 156 evaluable patients) concluded that there was no significant difference between adjuvant CT versus no further therapy in patients with uterine sarcoma. The recurrence rate and median survival of patients treated with doxorubicin compared to no therapy were 41% versus 53% and 73 months versus 55 months, respectively. However, this trial did not segregate different histologic subtypes (214). Adjuvant pelvic RT was optional, and was not balanced between the arms. The fact that there was no protocol-specified schedule of imaging for recurrence may also have affected the results. As is common with advanced disease, more recent trials have segregated histologic subtypes. Previous studies reported that a CT regimen consisting of a combination of cyclophosphamide, vincristine, doxorubicin, and dacarbazine yielded a 68% to 89% 5-year survival in the setting of stage I uterine sarcomas (257–260).

Uterine CS

A nonrandomized study using adjuvant combination CT including etoposide, cisplatin, and doxorubicin demonstrated a 2-year survival of 92% in 23 patients with surgical stage I and stage II uterine CS. However, the fact that 7 patients also received RT makes interpretation of these results difficult (261). A pilot study of 38 patients with surgical stage I and stage II uterine CS concluded that multimodality treatment with CT, including epirubicin and cisplatin, as well as RT yielded 74% OS at a median follow-up of 55 months (230). However, high patient dropouts made these conclusions controversial. A phase 3 GOG study by Sutton et al. (262) of 65 patients with completely resected stage I and II uterine CS treated with adjuvant ifosfamide and cisplatin reported 2- and 5-year survival of 82% and 62%, respectively. As more than half of the recurrences involved the pelvis, the study suggested that a combined sequential approach including CT and RT might be beneficial in this group of patients. This conclusion will require verification in a randomized phase 3 study.

GOG 150, a phase 3 randomized study of patients with stage I–IV uterine CS (44% stage I or II) undergoing maximal resection of all gross diseases, compared whole abdominal RT to three cycles of cisplatin and ifosfamide as adjuvant therapy. Although not statistically significant, there was a trend toward improved outcome in the CT group; the rates of recurrence and estimated death were 21% and 29% lower, respectively, compared to the RT group (228). A small retrospective study of 49 patients with completely resected stage I–IV uterine CS reported superior outcomes in patients treated with adjuvant carboplatin and paclitaxel, with or without RT, compared to patients receiving adjuvant RT alone (263).

Uterine LMS

The role of adjuvant CT following complete resection of early-stage uterine LMS is still under investigation, but the preliminary results of studies of adjuvant systemic CT are promising. Two factors continue to limit the study of adjuvant therapy in the setting of uterine LMS: the relatively low frequency of the disease, which makes it difficult to complete randomized trials in a reasonable period of time; and the lack of highly active therapeutic agents.

The demonstrated activity of gemcitabine plus docetaxel in metastatic uterine LMS led to the investigation of this combination in the adjuvant setting (264,265). A phase 2, single-institution trial of four cycles of fixed-dose-rate gemcitabine and docetaxel following complete resection of stage I–IV disease has been reported (79). Among the 18 patients with early-stage disease, 59% remained disease-free at 2 years, and median OS had not been reached at 5-year follow-up. The Sarcoma Alliance for Research through Collaboration subsequently conducted a phase 2, multicenter study of four cycles of adjuvant fixed-dose-rate gemcitabine plus docetaxel followed by four cycles of doxorubicin in 47 patients with uterus-limited LMS (266). Although 78% of the patients remained progression-free at 2 years, the percentage dropped to 50% at 3-year follow-up (266–268). Of note, age, menopausal status, hormone receptor status, grade, mitotic rate, or FIGO stage were not significantly associated with PFS. An ongoing phase 3 multicenter, randomized trial (GOG 277) is comparing four cycles of gemcitabine plus docetaxel followed by four cycles of doxorubicin to the current standard of observational approach, to determine if adjuvant CT improves outcomes for patients with uterus-limited high-grade LMS (NCT01533207) (269).

Low-Grade ESS

There are no data to support the use of adjuvant CT in patients who have had complete resection of low-grade ESS confined to the uterus. The standard approach in this setting is observation alone. The role of adjuvant hormonal therapy for these patients has not been evaluated prospectively. Given the hormone-sensitive nature of these tumors, it is believed that ER replacement therapy may be detrimental in patients with low-grade ESS (270).

AS

Because of the rarity of these tumors, there are no prospective data on the role of adjuvant systemic therapy for patients with completely resected adenosarcoma. Patients without sarcomatous overgrowth are often treated similarly to patients with ESS. The presence of sarcomatous overgrowth is associated with an increased propensity for disease spread and recurrence (168,271). In a retrospective single-institution review of uterine adenosarcoma, only 1 (20%) of 5 patients with sarcomatous overgrowth was progression-free at 2 years, whereas 14 patients without sarcomatous overgrowth remained progression-free at 2 years (272). Management of patients with sarcomatous overgrowth is often extrapolated from data regarding high-grade soft tissue sarcoma. Patients with soft tissue sarcoma should be encouraged to participate in clinical trials.

Rhabdomyosarcomas

Given the rarity of uterine rhabdomyosarcoma in adults, adjuvant therapy is extrapolated from data on conventional pediatric rhabdomyosarcoma treatment paradigms (273). However, a modified every-3-week schedule consisting of vincristine, actinomycin D, and cyclophosphamide is proposed, as weekly vincristine causes significant neurotoxicity in adults.

Advanced and Recurrent Disease

Neoadjuvant Chemotherapy

To date, there have been no prospective studies evaluating the role of neoadjuvant CT in the treatment of uterine sarcoma. The theoretical appeal of neoadjuvant therapy is that it might potentially facilitate improved surgical outcomes through tumor shrinkage, and also permit *in vivo* assessment of chemosensitivity to first-line drug therapy. The role of PET as an intermediate end point biomarker to assess early treatment response in patients with soft tissue sarcomas undergoing neoadjuvant CT is under investigation (274).

Chemotherapy for Advanced/Recurrent Disease

LMS

Numerous single agents have been and continue to be tested in patients with LMS (**Table 22.15**). Unfortunately, the results have been unimpressive (275–301). Doxorubicin and ifosfamide as primary single-agent CT are the most active in recurrent and advanced uterine LMS. In 1983, the GOG demonstrated seven responses among 28 patients (25%) treated every 3 weeks with single-agent doxorubicin (281). Doxorubicin is considered the most active single agent. The GOG subsequently reported that treatment with liposomal doxorubicin yielded one complete (3.2%) and four partial (13%) responses, but conferred no advantage compared to historical results using doxorubicin alone (275). However, given the lower risk of cardiotoxicity, liposomal doxorubicin may be considered for certain patients in whom doxorubicin therapy is precluded. The GOG demonstrated that ifosfamide had moderate activity, with six partial responses among 35 patients (17%) (278).

As in other types of soft tissue sarcoma, gemcitabine has demonstrated activity, with one (2.3%) complete response and eight (18%) partial responses in cases of persistent or recurrent uterine LMS (285). The median duration of response was only 4.8 months. A similar response rate (19%, based on five partial responses) was found by Pautier et al., who reported a median PFS of 5.5 months. In a small phase II study of temozolomide in advanced soft tissue sarcoma, a partial response was seen in 2 (18%) of 11 patients with LMS (300). Single-agent paclitaxel demonstrated limited activity, with a 9% overall response in 33 patients (277). Intravenous single-agent etoposide demonstrated an overall response of 11% in 28 patients (295), whereas prolonged oral etoposide yielded an overall response of 6.9% in 29 patients (294). However, no complete or partial responses were observed in another GOG phase 2 study of single-agent IV etoposide (100 mg/m^2 daily for 3 days every 3 weeks) (279). Topotecan was tested in 36 patients, with complete response in 1 (3%), partial response in 3 (8%), stable disease in 12 (33%), and tumor progression in 20 patients (56%) (276).

A phase 2 study of the marine-derived drug trabectedin, with a 24-hour infusion schedule in 20 CT-naïve patients who had advanced or recurrent uterine LMS, demonstrated a partial response rate of 10%, and 50% of the patients remained progression-free for at least 6 months (302). A phase 3 study of trabectedin versus dacarbazine led to the FDA approval of trabectedin for patients with LMS and liposarcoma, who previously received anthracycline-based therapy. A total of 212 of the 518 patients on this study had uterine LMS. Patients were randomized 2:1 to trabectedin 1.5 mg/m^2 with a 24-hour IV infusion, or to dacarbazine. The response rate was 9.9%, with a median PFS of 4 months in the trabectedin arm versus 6.9% and 1.5-month PFS in the dacarbazine arm (303).

A small phase II trial of vinorelbine in patients who had failed prior to doxorubicin-based CT demonstrated a partial response in 1 (6%) of 16 patients with LMS (299). Single-agent cisplatin also yielded a poor overall response in phase II trials: 3% to 5% (280,298). In a small study published in 2002, the antifolate compound trimetrexate was associated with an overall response of 4.3% in 28 patients who had received prior treatment (293). Mitoxantrone (297), diaziquone (284), amonafide (296), aminothiadiazole (283), piperazinedione (282), and ixabepilone (304) were inactive as single agents. A phase II trial comparing doxorubicin and docetaxel for advanced soft tissue sarcoma demonstrated no objective responses in the docetaxel group (305). In a phase 2 study of LMS, eribulin, a fully synthetic analog of the marine sponge product halichondrin B, showed some promise (306). However, in the phase 3 study that led to FDA approval of eribulin for treatment of liposarcoma, no apparent advantage was conferred by eribulin, compared to the significantly less expensive dacarbazine, in the uterine LMS subgroup.

Combination CT yields greater response rates (**Table 22.15**) (15,264,265,281,307–314). In 1983, the GOG demonstrated that the combination of doxorubicin and dacarbazine resulted in an overall response rate of 30%. Two years later, the same group demonstrated a 19% response rate using the combination of doxorubicin and cyclophosphamide (313). Both of the phase III trials were too small to draw any definite conclusions. However, as noted above, these trials did enable researchers to observe that LMS had a different chemotherapeutic response profile compared to uterine CS. This resulted in the separation of the two different histologic entities in subsequent trials.

In 1996, the GOG demonstrated an 18% overall response in patients treated with a combination of dacarbazine, etoposide, and hydroxyurea (310). In the same year, using a combination of ifosfamide and doxorubicin, the GOG demonstrated an overall response rate of 30% in patients with advanced LMS and no history of prior treatment (311). A later GOG study showed that treatment with mitomycin, doxorubicin, and cisplatin produced an overall response rate of 23% in 35 patients. Pulmonary toxicity was appreciable, however (309). On the basis of this study, the GOG conducted a phase II trial of dacarbazine, doxorubicin, mitomycin, and cisplatin (DAMP), which produced a 28% response rate. However, the complexity and toxicity of this regimen precluded further investigation, and the study was closed after the first stage of accrual (307).

Fixed-dose-rate gemcitabine plus docetaxel has proved highly active and tolerable (40% overall response rate) in both treated and untreated patients with uterine LMS (315). As initial therapy for metastatic uterine LMS, this combination CT yielded a 36% response rate (2 complete and 13 partial responses) among 42 patients. The response rate for the doublet was 27% in the second-line setting, with a median PFS of greater than 5.6 months. In a more recent French study, the response rate for the doublet as second-line therapy for uterine LMS was 24% (5 partial responses among 22 patients, with a median PFS of 4.7 months). An ongoing phase 2 study (NCT02249702) is comparing the doublet to trabectedin in patients previously treated for uterine LMS.

A phase II trial of gemcitabine plus dacarbazine reported a 19% response rate for the doublet, compared to 13% for dacarbazine alone, in 32 previously treated patients with LMS. A phase II trial of fixed-dose-rate gemcitabine and vinorelbine in patients with advanced soft tissue sarcoma yielded a response rate of 22% in 9 uterine LMS patients, but conferred no advantage over the historical results achieved with single-agent gemcitabine (314). A combination of temozolomide and thalidomide in advanced LMS yielded a partial response in 2 (10%) cases, with no complete response (316).

Pautier et al. reported an impressive response rate of 60% (28 CR) and a median PFS of 8.2 months among 47 uterine LMS patients enrolled in a non-randomized phase II trial of doxorubicin plus 3-hour trabectedin as first-line treatment for advanced LMS (317). An additional 28% (13 patients) had stable disease. Conversely, another randomized phase II study of 3-hour trabectedin plus doxorubicin versus doxorubicin alone as first-line therapy for soft tissue sarcoma was stopped early due to futility, with a reported 13% response rate for the combination regimen and 20% rate for doxorubicin alone (318). The caveat to this cross-trial comparison is that the sequence of CT administration was different in the two trials; additionally, the latter trial was conducted in a population of patients with heterogenous soft tissue sarcoma. Given the significant toxicity associated with the combination regimen, including elevated transaminases, myelosuppression, and febrile neutropenia, further validation is required before this combination could be recommended.

The efforts in LMS treatment continues to focus on identifying active drugs and combination regimens in phase II trials. A pooled analysis of phase 2 studies (undertaken in 2005) compared the response rates of single-agent versus combination therapy. It showed that patients who received first- or second-line CT for treatment of metastatic LMS had a higher response rate with combination CT than with single-agent CT (319). The European GeDDiS trial, a phase 3 comparison of single-agent doxorubicin versus gemcitabine plus docetaxel as first-line treatment in 257 patients with locally advanced or metastatic soft tissue sarcoma, failed to show any difference in

OS between the two regimens. In fact, the hazard ratio favored the superiority of doxorubicin (HR, 1,28, $p = 0.07$) (320). This also held true in the subgroup analysis of the 72 patients with uterine LMS. Although a higher incidence of oral mucositis and febrile neutropenia was associated with doxorubicin, in general it was better tolerated. Only 1 patient (2%) in the doxorubicin arm withdrew from treatment early because of unacceptable toxicity, whereas 13 patients (16%) in the gemcitabine + docetaxel arm experienced significant grade 3 or 4 fatigue and diarrhea. Nevertheless, the higher objective response rates associated with combination therapy may be crucial for select patients with imminent life-threatening organ compromise.

CS

Several drugs have been studied as single agents in the treatment of CS. (**Table 22.16**) (280,281,397,307,321–334). However, only three have demonstrated clear-cut activity: ifosfamide, cisplatin, and paclitaxel (280,321–324,328,333,334). On a 5-day schedule, ifosfamide produced 25 CRs and 12 PRs (overall response rate, 36%) in 102 CT-naïve patients (209). In patients with prior CT, cisplatin produced an 18% response in 28 patients (333). A repeat trial in a larger group of CT-naïve patients documented essentially the same response rate (19%) (280). In both trials, cisplatin was used at 50 mg/m^2 every 3 weeks. Investigators at M.D. Anderson Cancer Center used a higher dose, ranging from 75 mg/m^2 to 100 mg/m^2 every 3 weeks. Only 12 patients with measurable disease were entered into the trial, but 1 CR and 4 PRs were observed (overall response, 42%) (334). However, the lack of randomization and the small number of cases in this trial preclude conclusions about the merits of a higher dose. In another study, treatment with paclitaxel as a single agent was associated with a response rate of 21% in a group of 33 patients with uterine sarcoma who had prior CT; there was an 8.2% response rate in patients who failed appropriate local therapy (328).

Doxorubicin, generally regarded as the most active agent for soft tissue sarcomas, has unfortunately demonstrated inconsistent activity in three trials of patients with uterine carcinosarcoma. The first two studies constituted one arm of each of two randomized trials. In the first, four responses among 41 patients (10%) with uterine CS (281) were observed. The second study demonstrated a 19% response rate utilizing a dose of 60 mg/m^2 every 3 weeks for patients with recurrent or advanced uterine sarcomas (313). The third study employed a range of doses—from 50 mg/m^2 to 90 mg/m^2 every 3 weeks—but this resulted in no response among 9 patients with measurable disease (325). Topotecan 1.5 mg/m^2 daily for 5 days demonstrated unimpressive activity (10% response rate) in patients with advanced or recurrent uterine CS previously treated with CT (326). In phase II studies, etoposide (332), mitoxantrone (297), piperazinedione (287), diaziquone (331), amonafide (329), trimetrexate (327), aminothiadiazole (330), and ixabepilone (335) demonstrated negligible activity.

In general, combination CT regimens usually result in a higher response rate than single-agent regimens. However, not all combination regimens have impacted survival. This is clearly seen in the treatment of uterine CS. There have been numerous reports on combination CT for the treatment of uterine CS (**Table 22.16**) (261,262,281,313,323,327,336–338). A combination of cyclophosphamide, vincristine, doxorubicin, and dacarbazine reportedly yielded a 23% overall response rate (337). A combination of etoposide, hydroxyurea, and dacarbazine yielded a response of 15% in 32 patients (336). Subsequently, an EORTC trial reported on 48 patients with unresectable or recurrent CS who were treated with a combination of cisplatin, doxorubicin, and ifosfamide. The overall response rate was an impressive 56%. Unfortunately, this regimen was also associated with a high incidence of nephrologic and hematologic toxicities (338).

A phase 2 study of carboplatin and paclitaxel as first-line CT for women with advanced uterine CS reported an overall response rate of 54% (13% CR), with a favorable toxicity profile (339). Another smaller study reported a 62% response rate for 13 patients with measurable disease treated with the doublet (340). The addition of the PARP inhibitor iniparib to carboplatin and paclitaxel was associated with a lower-than-expected response rate (24%) and greater toxicity (341).

The first randomized study in 1983 by the GOG, which combined uterine CS with other sarcomas, was too small for subset analysis (281). Nonetheless, combination doxorubicin plus dacarbazine resulted in an overall response of 23% and a trend toward greater response, compared to single-agent doxorubicin (10%). A significant improvement in PFS and OS could not be demonstrated, but two conclusions may be drawn from this trial. First, a greater response to CT was significantly associated with an increase in OS and DFS. Second, uterine CS had a different response profile compared to LMS. Two years later, the GOG compared cyclophosphamide plus doxorubicin to single-agent doxorubicin. A response rate of 25%

TABLE 22.16. Chemotherapy in CS of the Uterus

Drug	n	Prior Therapy	Schedule	Overall Response (%)	Reference
Single-agent chemotherapy					
Primary chemotherapy					
Cisplatin	63	28 RT	50 mg/m^2 q 3 wk	19	379
Ifosfamide	91	34 RT	2 g/m^2 × 3 days q 3 wk	29	322
	102	27 RT	1.5 g/m^2 × 5 days q 3 wk	36	323
	28	8 RT	1.5 g/m^2 × 5 days q 4 wk	32	324
Doxorubicin	21	21 No CT	60 mg/m^2 q 3 wk	19[a]	313
	9	6 No CT	50–90 mg/m^2 q 3 wk	0	325
Piperazinedione	19	19 No CT	9 mg/m^2 q 3 wk	5.3	282
Nonprimary chemotherapy					
Doxorubicin	41	N/A	60 mg/m^2 q 3 wk	10	281
Topotecan	48	16 RT, 44 CT	1.5 mg/m^2 × 5 days q 3 wk	10	326
Trimetrexate	21	N/A	5 mg/m^2 orally × 5 days q 2 wk	4.8	327
Paclitaxel	44	15 RT, 33 CT	170 mg/m^2 q 3 wk	18	328
Amonafide	16	5 RT, 14 CT	300 mg/m^2 × 5 days q 3 wk	6	329

(continued)

■ TABLE 22.16. Chemotherapy in CS of the Uterus (*continued*)

Drug	n	Prior Therapy	Schedule	Overall Response (%)	Reference
Aminothiadiazole	22	10 RT, 18 CT	125 mg/m^2 q 1 wk	5	330
Diaziquone	23	11 RT, 18 CT	22.5 mg/m^2 q 3 wk	4	331
Mitoxantrone	17	17 CT	12 mg/m^2 q 3 wk	0	297
Etoposide	31	14 RT, 29 CT	100 mg/m^2 days 1, 3, 5 q 4 wk	6.5	332
Cisplatin	28	28 CT	50 mg/m^2 q 3 wk	18	333
	12	7 CT	75–100 mg/m^2 q 3 wk	42	333
Combination chemotherapy					
Doxorubicin *plus*	31	N/A	60 mg/m^2 q 3 wk	23	281
Dacarbazine			250 mg/m^2 × 5 days q 3 wk		
Doxorubicin *plus*	30	30 No CT	60 mg/m^2 q 3 wk	19[a]	313
Cyclophosphamide			500 mg/m^2 q 3 wk		
Ifosfamide *plus*	92	25 RT	1.5 g/m^2 × 5 days q 3 wk	54	323
Cisplatin			20 mg/m^2 × 5 days q 3 wk		
Ifosfamide *plus*	88	26 RT	1.6 g/m^2 × 3 days q 3 wk	45	322
Paclitaxel			135 mg/m^2 q 3 wk		
Ifosfamide *plus*	65	65 No CT	1.5 g/m^2 × 5 days q 3 wk	N/A	262
Cisplatin			20 mg/m^2 × 5 days q 3 wk		
Hydroxyurea *plus*	32	11 RT	2 g orally q 4 wk	15	336
Dacarbazine			700 mg/m^2 q 4 wk		
Etoposide			100 mg/m^2 × 3 days q 4 wk		
Etoposide *plus*	4	N/A	100 mg/m^2 × 2 days q 4 wk	100	261
Cisplatin			50 mg/m^2 q 4 wk		
Doxorubicin			50 mg/m^2 q 4 wk		
Cyclophosphamide *plus*	26	14 CT	400 mg/m^2 day 2 q 4 wk	23	337
Vincristine			1 mg/m^2 days 1, 5 q 4 wk		
Doxorubicin			40 mg/m^2 day 2 q 4 wk		
Dacarbazine			200 mg/m^2 × 5 days q 4 wk		
Cisplatin *plus*	32	32 No CT	50 mg/m^2 q 3 wk	56[b]	338
Doxorubicin			45 mg/m^2 q 3 wk		
Ifosfamide			5 g/m^2 q 3 wk		
Gemcitabine *plus*	24	9 RT, 24 CT	600 mg/m^2 days 1, 8, 15	8	343
Docetaxel			35 mg/m^2 days 1, 8, 15		
Paclitaxel *plus*	46	15 RT, 46 No CT	175 mg/m^2 q 3 wk	54	339
Carboplatin			AUC 6 q 3 wk		
Paclitaxel *plus*	13	9 RT, 2 CT	175 mg/m^2 q 3 wk	62	399
Carboplatin			AUC 5 q 3 wk		
Biologic and targeted therapy					
Imatinib	23	23	600 mg orally daily	0	380
Thalidomide	5	NA	200 mg orally daily	0	383
Aflibercept	19	19 CT	4 mg/kg day 1 q 2 wk	0	386
Pazopanib	19	9 RT, 19 CT	800 mg orally daily	0	400
Iniparib *plus*	17	4 RT, 17 No CT	4 mg/kg days 1, 4, 8, 11, 15, 18	24	401
Paclitaxel			175 mg/m^2 q 3 wk		
Carboplatin			AUC 6 q 3 wk		

Note: All chemotherapy agents were given intravenously unless specified.

CT, chemotherapy; N/A, not available; RT, radiation therapy.

[a]Uterine sarcoma.

[b]Female genital tract.

was observed in CS; again, however, numbers were inadequate to determine any significant benefit to the doublet versus single-agent doxorubicin. The trial was closed early because of failure to reach statistical significance (313).

In recognition of the different responses to therapy between CS and LMS, randomized trials began to segregate these two major histologic subtypes into separate patient populations. Unfortunately, this increased the time needed to complete clinical trials. Nonetheless, a large randomized trial was performed and reported in 2000. The GOG evaluated the addition of cisplatin to ifosfamide in 194 eligible patients with CS, and found that this combination regimen improved the overall response rate (from 36% to 54%) and prolonged the median progression-free interval by an absolute 2 months. However, this advantage was not associated with a significant gain in OS, and six treatment-related deaths occurred (323).

On the basis of the finding that paclitaxel showed moderate activity (18% response rate) in advanced uterine carcinoma (328), the GOG carried out a phase III trial of 3-day ifosfamide with or without paclitaxel for advanced disease. The group found that adding paclitaxel produced a 45% response rate, compared to 29% in the ifosfamide single-agent arm. OS was significantly improved. There was a significant decrease in the hazard of death and progression, but, as expected, more sensory neuropathy (322). A meta-analysis supports the use of combination CT in advanced or recurrent uterine CS because of the associated reduction in the risk of death and disease progression compared to single-agent therapy (342). The results of the non-inferiority phase III trial, GOG 261, comparing paclitaxel plus carboplatin and paclitaxel plus ifosfamide as first-line CT for patients with uterine or ovarian carcinosarcoma, are awaited (NCT00954174). Of note, patients on these studies who had had prior RT were eligible to enroll.

Data regarding second-line CT doublets are limited. A phase II trial of weekly gemcitabine and docetaxel in the treatment of recurrent uterine CS reported an 8.3% overall response rate, with a median PFS of only 1.8 months (343). Combination regimens that confer significant improvements in survival are still needed (**Table 22.17**).

ESS

In recurrent ESS, reports support hormonal therapy for patients in the low-grade subgroup (14), and CT for patients with high-grade tumors (344). As noted above, current definitions of ESS do not include high-grade lesions as a component. In a retrospective review of 74 patients with low-grade stromal sarcoma, none of the 10 patients who received CT responded to treatment, compared to 27% of patients treated with hormonal therapy (14). Randomized phase III trials of stromal sarcomas are limited because of the rarity of this disease. Two randomized trials compared single-agent and combination CT in advanced uterine sarcoma, but did not report the response rate of stromal sarcomas separately. The GOG reported a phase 2 study of ifosfamide treatment in 21 cases of recurrent or metastatic ESS. Three patients attained CRs and four had PRs, for an overall response rate of 33.3% (345). Another noncontrolled study showed a 50% response rate to doxorubicin therapy in 10 patients with recurrent ESS (346). Much of the other literature consists of case reports and retrospective studies involving a small number of cases. Published CT regimens include carboplatin plus paclitaxel (347); doxorubicin, cisplatin, and ifosfamide (348); doxorubicin plus ifosfamide (349); doxorubicin, vincristine, and cyclophosphamide (350); and prolonged oral etoposide (351).

AS

In a small retrospective series of AS, three of the five patients treated with doxorubicin- and/or ifosfamide-containing salvage CT showed a brief PR (352). Similar response rates were reported in another retrospective series of patients with recurrent disease treated with doxorubicin plus ifosfamide (353). Patients with soft tissue sarcomas should be encouraged to participate in clinical trials.

High-Grade Undifferentiated Endometrial Sarcoma

There are no prospective trials of CT specifically for high-grade undifferentiated endometrial sarcoma. Case reports of response to ifosfamide- and doxorubicin-based regimens have been documented in the literature (348,354). Gemcitabine plus docetaxel may also have activity in high-grade undifferentiated endometrial sarcoma, as evidenced by a small retrospective case series reporting a 75% response rate among six patients treated with that combination. In that series, the response rate of five patients treated with doxorubicin was 40%. All responses were of short duration. The response rate to second-line CT was only 19%, and no patient responded to re-treatment with a regimen that they had previously responded to. A phase II trial of first-line CT for recurrent or metastatic ESS reported a 33% response rate, but did not segregate high- versus low-grade tumors (355). Owing to the paucity of data available to guide systemic treatment, patients with these tumors should be encouraged to participate in clinical trials.

PEComa

There are no prospective data on systemic CT for PEComa. A case report of a 9-year-old girl with uterine PEComa reported radiographic response following two cycles of neoadjuvant vincristine, ifosfamide, and doxorubicin, but analysis of the surgical specimen did not show any tumor response. Case reports of tamoxifen or anthracycline-based CT following surgical resection of gynecologic PEComa do not suggest any benefit from adjuvant therapy (202). In the metastatic or recurrent setting, CT does not appear to be effective (356). Sirolimus, a mammalian target of rapamycin (mTOR) inhibitor that targets TORC1, shows activity in non-uterine PEComas; however, it has not demonstrated response in uterine PEComa (357). Patients with uterine PEComa should be encouraged to participate in clinical trials.

Rhabdomyosarcoma

Because of the rarity of uterine rhabdomyosarcoma, there are no prospective data to guide optimal therapy (203). In a case series of pediatric patients with rhabdomyosarcoma of the genital tract, complete responses have been reported with the administration of neoadjuvant ifosfamide, vincristine, and actinomycin D combination CT (204). Referral to experienced tertiary cancer centers for multimodality treatment planning and risk stratification is recommended for patients with non-pleomorphic uterine rhabdomyosarcoma (including the alveolar and embryonal subtypes).

Liposarcoma

Uterine liposarcoma is another rare tumor. In contemplating treatment, we must extrapolate from the management of non-uterine liposarcomas, for which agents such as doxorubicin, ifosfamide, trabectedin, and dacarbazine are reportedly active for. The FDA recently approved eribulin, a synthetic analog of halichondrin B, for unresectable or metastatic liposarcoma previously treated with anthracycline-based therapy (358).

Toxicity of Systemic Therapies

The most common toxicities of CT are hematologic and gastrointestinal toxicities. The grade 3–4 adverse effects of CT with overall response rate higher than 5% in LMS and CS are listed in **Tables 22.18** and **22.19**. Combination CT is associated with a much higher incidence of grade 3–4 toxicities compared with the single-agent regimens. In the GOG study, the overall response rate of combination

TABLE 22.17. Phase III Clinical Trials in Uterine Sarcomas

Drug	n	Prior Therapy	Schedule	Overall Response (%)	Median PFS (mos)	Median OS (mos)	Leukopenia (%)	Neutropenia (%)	Thrombocytopenia (%)	Anemia (%)	GI (%)	Neuropathy (%)	Reference
Doxorubicin	41 CS/28 LMS	N/A	60 mg/m² q 3 wk	10/25	3.5[a]	7.7[a]	16	N/A	4	N/A	2	N/A	182
Doxorubicin *plus*	31 CS/20LMS	N/A	60 mg/m² q 3 wk	23/30	5.5[a]	7.3[a]	35	N/A	13	N/A	9	N/A	
Dacarbazine			250 mg/m² × 5 days q 3 wk										
Doxorubicin	21 CS/21LMS	8 RT	60 mg/m² q 3 wk	19[a]	5.1[a]	11.6[a]	10	N/A	0	N/A	N/A	N/A	212
Doxorubicin *plus*	30 CS/17LMS	9 RT	60 mg/m² q 3 wk	19[a]	4.9[a]	10.9[a]	35	N/A	0	N/A	N/A	N/A	
Cyclophosphamide			500 mg/m² q 3 wk										
Ifosfamide	102 CS		1.5 g/m² × 5 days q 3 wk	36	4	7.6	59	36	5	8	5	20	209
Ifosfamide *plus* Cisplatin	92 CS	25 RT	1.5 g/m² × 5 days q 3 wk	54	6	9.4	97	67	64	19	18	29	
			20 mg/m² × 5 days q 3 wk										
Ifosfamide	91 CS		2 g/m² × 3 days q 3 wk	29	3.6	8.4	42	53	3	9	7	0	215
Ifosfamide	88CS	26 RT	1.6 g/m² × 3 days q 3 wk	45	5.8	13.5	36	44	3	15	8	3	
Paclitaxel			135 mg/m² q 3 wk										

Note: All chemotherapy agents were given intravenously.

CS, carcinosarcoma; GI, gastrointestinal; LMS, leiomyosarcoma system; N/A, not available; PFS, progression-free survival; RT, radiation therapy.

[a]Uterine sarcoma.

TABLE 22.18. Grade 3–4 Adverse Effects of Chemotherapy in Leiomyosarcoma LMS (Overall response Rate >5%)

Drug	n	Prior Therapy	Schedule	Overall Response (%)	Leukopenia (%)	Neutropenia (%)	Thrombocytopenia (%)	Anemia (%)	GI (%)	Others	Reference
Liposomal doxorubicin	32	11 RT	50 mg/m^2 q 4 wk	16	13	16	N/A	23	19	Dermatotoxicity 6.5%	275
Topotecan	36	8 RT	1.5 mg/m^2 × 5 days q 3 wk	11	33	90	13	16	17		276
Paclitaxel	33	8 RT	175 mg/m^2 q 3 wk	9	9	33	3	3	0	No neurotoxicity	277
	48	15 RT, 33 CT	175 mg/m^2 q 3 wk	8.4	6.3	17	0	17	42		289
Ifosfamide	35	15 RT	1.5 g/m^2 × 5 days q 4 wk	17	34	N/A	0	0	3	Neurotoxicity 3%, granulocytopenia 11%, dermatotoxicity 14%	278
Doxorubicin	28	N/A	60 mg/m^2 q 3 wk	25	16	N/A	4	N/A	2		281
	29	6 RT, 27 CT	50 mg/m^2 orally × 21 days q 4 wk	6.9	24	35	18	12	6	Neurotoxicity 6%	283
Gemcitabine	44	11 RT, 35 CT	1,000 mg/m^2 weekly × 3 q 4 wk	21	27	34	11.4	6.8	14		285
	22	16 RT, 21 CT	1,000 mg/m^2 weekly × 3 q 4 wk	19	37	32	11	1	0		301
Trabectedin	20	7RT	1.5 mg/m^2 over 24 h q 3 wk	10	55	80	15	5	0	Hepatotoxicity 10%	302
	134	134CT	1.5 mg/m^2 over 24 h q 3 wk	10	N/A	37	17	14	15	Hepatotoxicity 26% Rhabdomyolysis 1%	303
Trabectedin *plus* doxorubicin	47	17RT, No CT	1.1mg/m^2 over 3 h q 3 wk	60	76	78	37	27	19	Hepatotoxicity 39%	320
Dacarbazine	78	78 CT	1g/ m^2 q 3 wk	7	N/A	21	18	12	4		303
Temozolomide	11	N/A	180 mg/m^2 orally × 5 days q 4 wk	18*c*	0	0	0	4	4	Fatigue 4%	300
Vinorelbine	16	16 CT	30 mg/m^2 weekly × 8	6*c*	N/A	N/A	N/A	N/A	N/A	Grade 3 toxicity 67%	299
Doxorubicin *plus* Dacarbazine	20	N/A	60 mg/m^2 q 3 wk	30	35	N/A	13	N/A	9		281
			250 mg/m^2 × 5 days q 3 wk								
Dacarbazine *plus* Mitomycin *plus* Doxorubicin *plus* Cisplatin	18	7 RT	750 mg/m^2 q 4 wk	28	67	78	94	61	44		307
			6 mg/m^2 q 4 wk								
			40 mg/m^2 q 4 wk								

(*continued*)

TABLE 22.18. Grade 3–4 Adverse Effects of Chemotherapy in Leiomyosarcoma LMS (Overall response Rate >5%) (*continued*)

Drug	n	Prior Therapy	Schedule	Overall Response (%)	Leukopenia (%)	Neutropenia (%)	Thrombo-cytopenia (%)	Anemia (%)	GI (%)	Others	Reference
			60 mg/m² q 4 wk								
Mitomycin *plus* Doxorubicin *plus* Cisplatin	35	8 RT	8 mg/m² q 3 wk	23	N/A	N/A	N/A	N/A	N/A	Pulmonary toxicity 8%	309
			40 mg/m² q 3 wk								
			60 mg/m² q 3 wk								
Hydroxyurea *plus* Dacarbazine *plus* Etoposide	38	11 RT	2 g orally × 1 day q 4 wk	18	29	N/A	3	N/A	N/A		310
			700 mg/m² q 4 wk								
			300 mg/m² × 2 days q 4 wk								
Ifosfamide *plus* Doxorubicin	33	9 RT	5 mg/m² /24h q 3 wk	30	0	49	0	0	0	Cardiac toxicity 3%	311
			50 mg/m² q 3 wk								
Gemcitabine *plus* Docetaxel	34	14 RT, 16 CT	900 mg/m² days 1, 8 q 3 wk	53	N/A	21	29	15	12	Dyspnea 21%, fatigue 21%	312
			100 mg/m² day 8 q 3 wk								
	42	42 No CT	As above	36	17	14	14	24	14		264
	48	17 RT, 48 CT	As above	27	23	21	40	25	6.3	Fluid retention syndrome 19%	265
	24	12 RT, 18 CT	As above	24	11	14	26	8	0		301
	54	11 RT, No CT	900 mg/m² days 1, 8 q 3 wk	32	NA	23	28	33	25		398
			75 mg/m² day 8 q 3 wk								
Gemcitabine *plus* Vinorelbine	9	N/A	800 mg/m² days 1, 8	22	28	40	10	5	10		314
			25 mg/m² days 1,8 q3 wk								
Temozolomide *plus* Thalidomide	11	10 CT	150 mg/m² orally × 7 q 2 wk	9.1	N/A	4	4	4	8	Neurotoxicity 12%	316
			200 mg orally daily								
Sunitinib	23	23 CT	50 mg orally daily × 4 of 6 wk	8.7	13	17	13	17	30		381
Bevacizumab *plus* Doxorubicin	7	N/A	15 mg/kg q 3 wk 75 mg/m²	28	N/A	N/A	18	6	0	Alopecia 100% Cardiotoxicity gr ≥2 35%	390

Note: All chemotherapy agents were given intravenously unless specified.

CT, chemotherapy; GI, gastrointestinal system; N/A, not available; RT, radiation therapy.

TABLE 22.19. Grade 3–4 Adverse Effects of Chemotherapy in Uterine Carcinosarcoma (Overall Response Rate >5%)

Drug	n	Prior Therapy	Schedule	Overall Response (%)	Leukopenia (%)	Neutropenia (%)	Thrombo-cytopenia (%)	Anemia (%)	GI (%)	Others	Reference
Doxorubicin	41	N/A	60 mg/m^2 q 3 wk	10	16	N/A	4	N/A	2		281
	21	21 No CT	60 mg/m^2 q 3 wk	19[a]	10	N/A	0	N/A	0		313
Cisplatin	63	28 RT	50 mg/m^2 q 3 wk	19	2	N/A	0	N/A	N/A		280
	28	28 CT	50 mg/m^2 q 3 wk	18	0	N/A	0	N/A	4.2	Nephrotoxicity 22.2%	333
Ifosfamide	91	34 RT	2 g/m^2 × 3 days q 3 wk	29	42	53	3	9	7		322
	102	27 RT	1.5 g/m^2 × 5 days q 3 wk	36	59	36	5	8	5	Neuropathy 20%	323
	28	8 RT	1.5 g/m^2 × 5 days q 4 wk	32	45	24	7	0	0	Dermatotoxicity 35%	324
Topotecan	48	16 RT, 44 CT	1.5 mg/m^2 × 5 days q 3 wk	10	83.3	85.4	39.6	25	8.3		326
Paclitaxel	44	15 RT, 33 CT	170 mg/m^2 q 3 wk	18.2	30	43	7	9	2	Neurotoxicity 7%	328
Doxorubicin *plus*	31	N/A	60 mg/m^2 q 3 wk	23	35	N/A	13	N/A	9		281
Dacarbazine			250 mg/m^2 × 5 days q 3 wk								
Doxorubicin *plus*	30	30 No CT	60 mg/m^2 q 3 wk	19[a]	35	N/A	0	N/A	N/A		313
Cyclophosphamide			500 mg/m^2 q 3 wk								
Ifosfamide *plus*	92	25 RT	1.5 g/m^2 × 5 days q 3 wk	54	97	67	64	19	18	Neuropathy 29%	323
Cisplatin			20 mg/m^2 × 5 days q 3 wk								
Ifosfamide *plus* Cisplatin	65	65 No CT	1.5 g/m^2 × 5 days q 3 wk 20 mg/m^2 × 5 days q 3 wk	N/A	70.8	26.2	63.1	7.7	10.8	Cardiotoxicity 4.6%, neurotoxicity 4.6%, nephrotoxicity 3.1%	262
Ifosfamide *plus*	88	26 RT	1.6 g/m^2 × 3 days q 3 wk	45	36	44	3	15	8	Neuropathy 3%	322
Paclitaxel			135 mg/m^2 q 3 wk								
Hydroxyurea *plus*	32	11 RT	2 g orally q 4 wk	15	24	N/A	6	3	3	Dermatotoxicity 33%, fever 3%	336
Dacarbazine *plus*			700 mg/m^2 q 4 wk								

(*continued*)

ABLE 22.19. Grade 3–4 Adverse Effects of Chemotherapy in Uterine Carcinosarcoma (Overall Response Rate >5%) (*continued*)

Drug	n	Prior Therapy	Schedule	Overall Response (%)	Leukopenia (%)	Neutropenia (%)	Thrombo-cytopenia (%)	Anemia (%)	GI (%)	Others	Reference
Etoposide			100 mg/m^2 × 3 days q 4 wk								
Etoposide *plus*	4	N/A	100 mg/m^2 × 2 days q 4 wk	100	9.5	N/A	N/A	N/A	21.4	Alopecia 100%	261
Cisplatin *plus*			50 mg/m^2 q 4 wk								
Doxorubicin			50 mg/m^2 q 4 wk								
Cyclophosphamide *plus*	26	14 CT	400 mg/m^2 day 2 q 4 wk	23	34.6	N/A	15.4	N/A	N/A	Septicemia 15.4%, neurotoxicity 7.7%	337
Vincristine *plus*			1 mg/m^2 days 1, 5 q 4 wk								
Doxorubicin *plus*			40 mg/m^2 day 2 q 4 wk								
Dacarbazine			200 mg/m^2 × 5 days q 4 wk								
Cisplatin *plus*	32	32 No CT	50 mg/m^2 q 3 wk	56[a]	94.6	84.8	64.8	43.2	53.8	Neurotoxicity 15%, alopecia 64%	338
Doxorubicin *plus*			45 mg/m^2 q 3 wk								
Ifosfamide			5 g/m^2 q 3 wk								
Gemcitabine *plus* Docetaxel	24	9 RT, 24 CT	600 mg/m^2 days 1,8,1535 mg/m^2 days 1,8,15	8	50	46	13	13	13		343
Paclitaxel *plus* Carboplatin	46	15 RT, 46 No CT	175 mg/m^2 q 3 wk AUC 6 q 3 wk	54	43	85	11	11	4.3	Neurotoxicity 11%	339

Note: All chemotherapy agents were given intravenously unless otherwise specified.

CT, chemotherapy; N/A, not available; RT, radiation therapy.

[a]Uterine sarcoma.

ifosfamide plus cisplatin was 54%; however, the rate of grade 3–4 of leukopenia was 97%, and six deaths occurred before the first dose reduction of ifosfamide (323). The more recent GOG phase III trial with ifosfamide plus paclitaxel reported a 45% overall response rate, with tolerable toxicities (322); this seems to be a relatively effective and safe regimen. Ifosfamide should be used with caution in elderly patients, however, because of the risk of encephalopathy. Consideration of reduced-dose regimens may still be reasonable in older patients with good performance status. Among other phase 2 trials of different CT regimens, liposomal doxorubicin plus paclitaxel, doxorubicin, cisplatin, and etoposide plus cisplatin plus doxorubicin, were reported to have less toxicity, with moderate effect. Despite the routine use of growth factor support with gemcitabine and docetaxel, myelosuppression—particularly in previously treated patients—is still the predominant toxicity encountered with this combination (264,265). Lower limb edema is also more common in the second-line setting. Trabectedin requires central venous access, and is associated with fatigue, myelosuppression, transaminitis, and vomiting (290). Steroid premedication is required to reduce hepatotoxicity.

Newer agents such as palifosfamide-tris may have a more tolerable toxicity profile compared to standard CT drugs. Palifosfamide-tris is a stabilized active metabolite of ifosfamide, with less potential for bladder toxicity. A phase 3 randomized study of doxorubicin plus palifosfamide/placebo as first-line CT for patients with metastatic soft tissue sarcoma (NCT01168791) is currently ongoing.

Hormonal Therapy

Although the role of hormonal therapy is clear in breast and endometrial cancers, it has not been extensively evaluated in the setting of mesenchymal uterine tumors. Few uterine sarcomas contain sufficient ER- or PR-receptor protein to influence therapy, the only exception being low-grade ESS or stromal nodules. ER and PR receptors have been identified in 55.5% and 55.8%, respectively, of samples from patients with various types of uterine sarcomas, but the median concentrations are substantially lower than those observed in breast or endometrial cancers. ESS tumors reportedly have higher receptor levels (359). Uniquely, low-grade ESS is hormonally responsive in roughly two-thirds of cases, and long-term maintenance therapy should be beneficial. Several papers have reported that long-term use of tamoxifen for the treatment of breast cancer is related to the development of uterine sarcoma (360,361). This is likely secondary to the stimulatory estrogenic effects of tamoxifen on the uterus. It is therefore reasonable to avoid ER replacement therapy for these patients.

ESS

Progestins, gonadotropin-releasing hormone (GnRH) analogs (362), or aromatase inhibitors (344,363) have been used in the treatment of patients with advanced or recurrent ESS, and several case reports are associated with gain in long-term stability. A retrospective study of patients with low-grade ESS reported a response rate of 27% (5 CRs and 3 PRs), stable disease in 53% (16 patients), and a median time to progression of 24 months in a subgroup of patients receiving hormonal therapy (14). A significant majority received megestrol acetate.

Lantta et al. (364) reported two cases of patients with extensive intraperitoneal low-grade ESS, associated with high levels of PR receptors, who achieved CR on hormonal therapy. Three cases with high levels of PR receptors were reported by Baker et al. (365), all of which achieved PRs or stabilization of disease on oral megestrol acetate. In a collaborative survey of endolymphatic stromal myosis, Piver et al. (366) recorded CRs or PRs to hormonal therapy in 6 of 13 patients (46%) treated with progestational agents. Scribner and Walker (367) reported on 1 patient with extensive ESS of the uterus whose tumor was reduced to resectable size by administration of leuprolide acetate and megestrol acetate. Low-grade ESS has also been reported to express srp27, an ER-induced 24-DK protein suggesting hormone responsiveness (368). Medroxyprogesterone acetate has induced major responses in ESS pulmonary metastatic lesions (369,370). GnRH analogs reportedly controlled tumor progression in one case of recurrent low-grade ESS with moderate ER and PR receptor positivity (362). Medroxyprogesterone acetate and aromatase inhibitors, such as letrozole, were reportedly highly effective and conferred sustained progression control in 6 of 10 cases of low-grade stromal sarcomas (371). Spano et al. presented two cases of ESS with lung metastases treated with aminoglutethimide; both patients achieved CRs and remained disease-free for 14 and 7 years, respectively (344). In a phase 2 trial of mifepristone, a selective PR receptor modulator, in recurrent uterine cancer, no responses (0%) were seen in two patients with low-grade ESS (372).

Other Uterine Sarcomas

There are anecdotal reports of responses to hormonal therapy in adenosarcomas and low-grade LMS (373). A retrospective study of an aromatase inhibitor in selected patients with advanced, predominantly low-volume, disease reported PRs in three patients (9%). Patients whose tumors did not express ER or PR receptors derived no benefit (374). No objective responses were seen in a phase 2 study of letrozole in 27 previously treated patients with advanced ER- or PR-positive uterine LMS (375). The best response was stable disease in 14 (54%) patients. All three patients who received letrozole for >24 weeks had tumors expressing ER and PR in >90% of tumor cells. Another prospective ongoing study is comparing letrozole to observation-alone for newly diagnosed uterine LMS (NCT00414076). One case of letrozole therapy in high-grade uterine carcinosarcoma with marked tumor control was reported, but this has not been well studied (376).

Biologic and Targeted Therapy

In light of the high rates of recurrence and poor response to RT and CT, biologic therapy may hold more promise in the treatment of uterine sarcoma and other types of soft tissue sarcoma. Recent advances in understanding the biology of uterine sarcoma, with respect to probable treatment targets, have concentrated on tyrosine kinase receptors, vascular endothelial growth factor (VEGF), and the phosphatidyl 3-kinase (PI3K)/Akt pathway.

Since the discovery that high proto-oncogene *c-kit* expression in gastrointestinal stromal tumors (GIST) may be amenable to control with tyrosine kinase inhibitors such as imatinib mesylate and sunitinib, there has been some interest in this treatment for uterine sarcomas (377). However, the expression of *c-kit* in uterine sarcomas varies considerably in different studies (378–380). Given the great progress made in the treatment of GIST with imatinib mesylate, a GOG phase 2 evaluation of this drug was conducted in patients with recurrent or persistent carcinosarcoma of the uterus who had previously received other treatment (380). No activity was seen. The GOG investigated sunitinib maleate as a second- or third-line therapy for LMS of the uterus. The trial was reported as negative, with only two PRs (9%) noted among 23 patients (381).

Emoto et al. (382) demonstrated inhibition of a VEGF-expressing malignant mixed tumor cell line by TNP-470, an angiogenesis inhibitor. Another angiogenesis inhibitor, thalidomide, failed to demonstrate any activity in recurrent or persistent uterine CS (383) or uterine LMS (384). A phase 2 study of sorafenib, a small-molecule B-raf and VEGF receptor inhibitor, was also negative, and only one (3%) PR was seen among 37 patients with adult LMS (385). No responses were observed in a phase 2 trial of aflibercept in recurrent or metastatic gynecologic CS or uterine LMS (386).

In a GOG phase 2 study of patients with previously treated uterine CS, no responses were seen with use of pazopanib, an oral multi-target kinase inhibitor. Only 3 (16%) among 19 evaluable patients remained progression-free at 6 months (387). In another phase 2 study of pazopanib, only one PR (2.4%) was reported among 41 patients in the LMS cohort (388). In a phase 3 trial of pazopanib versus placebo as second-line therapy for metastatic soft tissue sarcoma (46% LMS), the response rate in the pazopanib group was 6%. There was a 3-month increase in PFS. Although this did not translate into significant improvement in OS, pazopanib is now FDA-approved for patients with advanced soft tissue sarcoma who previously received CT (389). As there is a potential for life-threatening hepatotoxicity with this drug, patients' liver function should be carefully monitored. Pazopanib is currently being studied in combination with gemcitabine as second-line therapy for LMS (NCT01442662).

A phase 2 study of doxorubicin with bevacizumab in 17 CT-naïve patients with soft tissue sarcoma reported a lower-than-anticipated response rate of 12%, with significant cardiotoxicity (≥ grade 2 in 35% of patients) (390). Among the 7 patients with uterine LMS, there were two (28%) PRs. The addition of bevacizumab to fixed-dose-rate gemcitabine plus docetaxel failed to improve overall response rate, PFS, or OS in a GOG phase 3 trial. A total of 107 CT-naïve patients with advanced or recurrent uterine LMS were accrued to the placebo-controlled trial of gemcitabine plus docetaxel, with or without bevacizumab. The trial was closed early after the planned interim analysis failed to show superiority in the experimental arm. In fact, median PFS was observed to be shorter in the bevacizumab-containing arm versus the control arm: 4.2 and 6.2 months, respectively (391).

Loss of PTEN function results in upregulation of the PI3K/Akt signaling pathway, and has been associated with high-grade and recurrent LMS (392). mTOR is a central regulator of this pathway. Ridaforolimus (formerly deforolimus), an mTOR inhibitor, demonstrated no response in the 56 LMS patients, but 36% had disease stabilization at 16 weeks (393). In a phase 2 study of ridaforolimus in endometrial cancer, no responses were seen in the CS patients (394). A phase 3 study of ridaforolimus as maintenance strategy in patients with metastatic sarcoma who derived benefit from CT reported a disappointing 3-week increase in PFS (395). Although there are published case reports on the activity of sirolimus in non-uterine PEComas, the mTOR inhibitor does not appear to be active in this setting (357).

Aberrant activity of epigenetic enzymes, such as histone deacetylases (HDACs), has been linked to tumorigenesis. HDAC inhibitors appear to exert greater apoptotic effects in tumor cells compared to normal, healthy cells. It is hypothesized that the enhanced sensitivity of tumor cells to HDAC inhibitors is due to the altered expression of apoptotic genes, as a result of alterations in the cancer epigenome (396). The activity of the HDAC inhibitor mocetinostat in combination with gemcitabine, in the treatment of LMS, is currently being explored (NCT02303262).

Tumor genomic profiling may help identify novel therapies for uterine sarcomas. However, our ability to translate these results into effective therapeutic strategies is still in its infancy. An example of this is a negative clinical trial of alisertib, a highly selective small molecule inhibitor of Aurora A kinase (397). Genome-wide transcriptional profiling of uterine LMS demonstrated frequent overexpression of gene products of the mitotic spindle apparatus, including Aurora A kinase; preclinical models in uterine LMS have shown activity for alisertib; disappointingly, however, no clinically meaningful activity was seen in the phase 2 study. Further advances in our understanding of the biology of uterine sarcomas are needed to provide more treatment targets and make long-term disease control possible.

Systemic Therapy: Summary

The current role of CT in the management of uterine sarcomas involves palliative-intent therapy for patients with advanced or recurrent disease. In LMS, the active drugs are doxorubicin, ifosfamide, gemcitabine, and docetaxel. In uterine CS, the drugs of choice are ifosfamide, cisplatin/carboplatin, and paclitaxel. Hormonal therapy, including progestational agents, GnRH analogs, and aromatase inhibitors, has a role in the treatment of advanced or recurrent low-grade ESS. The use of hormonal agents in the treatment of other histologic subtypes has not been well studied. Efforts to identify additional active agents continue.

INTERNATIONAL PERSPECTIVES

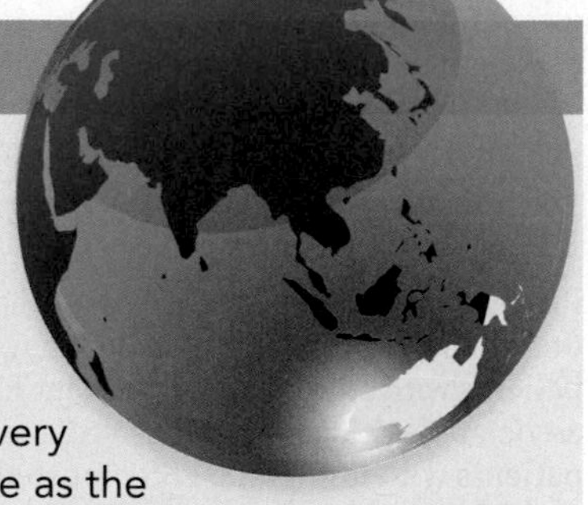

Corpus: Mesenchymal Tumors in Australia

Michael Friedlander, MD

This is a very comprehensive and up-to-date review of uterine mesenchymal tumors by Mataio et al. The general approach to management of patients with uterine sarcomas in the United States, which is outlined in detail in this chapter, is very similar to that in Australia and other countries. These are difficult tumors to manage as the literature is sparse and patchy, the trials have included a heterogeneous group of tumors, there is limited level 1 evidence to support treatment recommendations, the pathologic classifications have changed over time, and many of the studies included a large number of patients with CS. It is now well recognized and widely accepted that uterine CS are high-grade metaplastic epithelial tumors and that the principles of management are the same as in high-grade endometrial carcinomas. It is unfortunate that for so many years, patients with CS have been included in clinical trials as well as in registries together with other uterine sarcomas, which has led to much confusion and has resulted in data that is difficult to interpret. This is a very good example of how a misleading "name" influenced patient management for decades and denied patients with uterine CS inclusion into endometrial cancer clinical trials. Arguably, if they had been included and possibly stratified separately, we would have much more data to base our treatment recommendations on for patients with uterine CS. Fortunately, this has changed recently and these patients are now being included in clinical trials in EC.

There are a number of important points that come through loud and clear in this chapter. First, the importance of expert pathology review is essential to make the correct diagnosis, and all patients should ideally have their diagnosis made by an expert gynecological pathologist or at least reviewed by one and the diagnosis be

INTERNATIONAL PERSPECTIVES (*continued*)

confirmed before making any treatment decisions or recommendations, as these are rare tumors. The other critically important point is that international collaboration and cooperation is essential if progress is to be made. There already is a concerted effort to run randomized trials in these rare tumors that have been subject to expert pathologic review. It is essential that these trials are supported by translational research. Apart from randomized phase II and III clinical trials, there is also a place for single-arm basket trials such as the PARAGON trial, which is being led by ANZGOG, which includes separate phase II trials of patients with ESS as well as other ER-/PR-positive uterine sarcomas who are treated with anastrozole. The basket trial design has made it possible to open this study in Australia and New Zealand, the United Kingdom and Belgium, and it has accrued well and will close in June 2016. There is a translational component and this will be critical in identifying the subset of patients who respond to hormonal therapy.

(1) Conklin CM, Longacre TA. Endometrial stromal tumors: the new WHO classification. *Adv Anat Pathol*. 2014;21(6):383–393.
(2) Mileshkin LR, Edmondson RJ, O'Connell R, et al. Phase II study of anastrozole in recurrent estrogen (ER) / progesterone (PR) positive endometrial cancer: the PARAGON trial--ANZGOG 0903. 2016 ASCO Annual Meeting A(abstract 5520). *J Clin Oncol*. 2016;34(suppl): abstr 5520.

INTERNATIONAL PERSPECTIVES

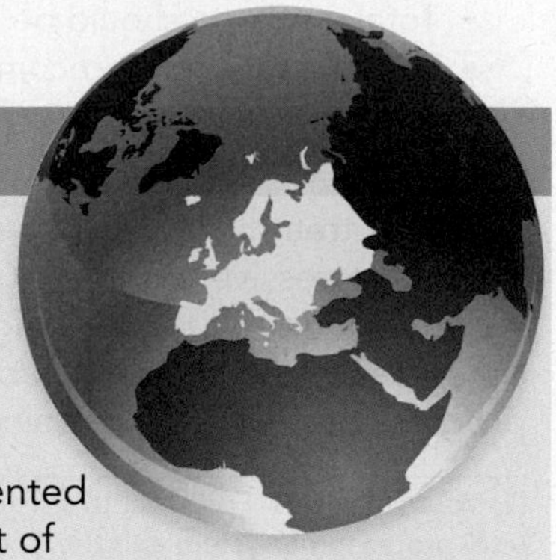

Uterine Mesenchymal Tumors in Poland

Paweł Knapp, MD

Mesenchymal tumors of the uterus are a heterogeneous group of disorders varying in incidence rates, clinical course, and morphologic presentation. Histopathologic examination aimed at determining the type of sarcoma, supplemented by the analysis of the immunophenotype of the tumor, is crucial for the assessment of prognosis and the planning of cancer treatment (1–4).

The RARCARE report, published in 2013 by Stiller et al., analyzed the incidence rates of rare tumors (sarcomas) in 27 countries of the European Union, and demonstrated beyond any doubt that these tumors present a noticeable epidemiologic problem. From 1995 to 2002, a total of 45,568 cases of sarcoma-type tumors were recorded in the databases of 76 European cancer registers. Of those, mesenchymal tumors of the uterus accounted for 4,011 cases, and sarcomas of the remaining soft tissues comprising the urogenital system accounted for another 1,919 cases. Uterine sarcomas belong to a relatively rare group of malignancies, as they account for about 3% to 8% of all uterine tumors. According to Stiller et al., the raw annual incidence rate is approximately 0.6 per 100,000 females (SE $<$ 0.1). As also demonstrated in the RARECARE report, the estimated number of uterine mesenchymal tumors would increase to 2,466 cases recorded each year (5).

Current European trends in the surgical management of uterine mesenchymal tumors depend on the histologic type and the clinical stage of the tumor. Consequently, the type and scope of primary surgical treatment differs depending on the type of the sarcoma; this, however, is not manifested in any significant differences in the surgical procedures described in this chapter. The suggestions of recommendations of European societies regarding the surgical management of the three most common histologic types of the mesenchymal tumors of the uterus are as follows (5,6):

1. CS:
   - The treatment of choice involves simple (or, less commonly, radical) hysterectomy with pelvic lymphadenectomy;
   - The role of para-aortic lymphadenectomy has not been fully elucidated;
   - In case of extrapelvic spread, the principle of total macroscopic resection of tumor is to be followed;
   - Adnexal conservation and fertility-sparing procedures are not recommended;
   - Because of the scope of primary surgery, the pattern of the disease spread, and its sensitivity to chemo- and radiotherapy, surgical approach is of no great importance in the treatment of disease recurrences.
2. LMS:
   - The treatment of choice in FIGO grade I and II LMS patients consists of a simple hysterectomy with adnexectomy and without pelvic lymphadenectomy;
   - The sparing of the ovaries in early stages of the disease has no impact on OS;

(*continued*)

INTERNATIONAL PERSPECTIVES (*continued*)

- Pelvic and para-aortic lymphadenectomy is not recommended in stage I and II tumors;
- Fertility-sparing treatment may be used only in cases of tumors removed, including healthy tissue margins, and in patients motivated in maintaining fertility. The safety of this approach has not been examined thus far;
- Advanced LMS requires total macroscopic cytoreduction, with the importance of systematic lymphadenectomy remaining unclear;
- Because of the radio- and chemoresistance of LMS, surgical management has documented applicability in the treatment of local recurrences and metastases of uterine LMS;
- Non-radical sparing procedures or LMS morcellation significantly worsen the prognoses, regardless of subsequent total procedures.

3. ESS:
   - In low-grade ESS, the treatment of choice consists of a simple hysterectomy;
   - Adnexectomy is recommended in selected cases of low-grade ESS, whereas adnexal conservation is possible in stage I and II tumors;
   - The safety of fertility-sparing treatment has not been elucidated to date;
   - Systematic pelvic and para-aortic lymphadenectomy should be performed in advanced stages of the disease;
   - Total resection should be attempted in advanced or locally recurrent disease;
   - To date, no explicit recommendations were formulated regarding the surgical treatment of high-grade ESS—recommended treatment involves simple hysterectomy and adnexectomy along with resection of all visible neoplastic foci.

Adjuvant treatment of uterine mesenchymal tumors is complementary, as described in this chapter.

The aggressive biology of mesenchymal tumors of the uterus is still the subject of numerous research studies. Elucidation of their biology may be one of the elements facilitating the use of targeted gene therapies or other treatments leading to better and longer control of the disease, thus directly translating into overall and progression-free survival gains.

(1) Voutsadakis IA. Epithelial to mesenchymal transition in the pathogenesis of uterine malignant mixed Mullerian tumors: the role of ubiquitin proteasome system and therapeutic opportunities. *Clin Transl Oncol.* 2012;14(4):243–253.

(2) Seidman MA, Oduyebo T, Muto MG, et al. Peritoneal dissemination complicating morcellation of uterine mesenchymal neoplasms. *PLoS One.* 2012;7(11):e50058.

(3) Kowalewska M, Bakula-Zalewska E, Chechlinska M, et al. microRNAs in uterine sarcomas and mixed epithelial-mesenchymal uterine tumors: a preliminary report. *Tumour Biol.* 2013;34(4):2153–2160.

(4) Zhao Z, Yoshida Y, Kurokawa T, et al. 18F-FES and 18F-FDG PET for differential diagnosis and quantitative evaluation of mesenchymal uterine tumors: correlation with immunohistochemical analysis. *J Nucl Med.* 2013;54(4):499–506.

(5) Stiller CA, Trama A, Serraino D, et al. Descriptive epidemiology of sarcomas in Europe: report from the RARECARE project. *Eur J Cancer.* 2012;49(3):684–695.

(6) Lax S. Mesenchymal uterine tumors. Stromal tumors and other rare mesenchymal neoplasms. *Pathologe.* 2009;30(4):284–291.

INTERNATIONAL PERSPECTIVES

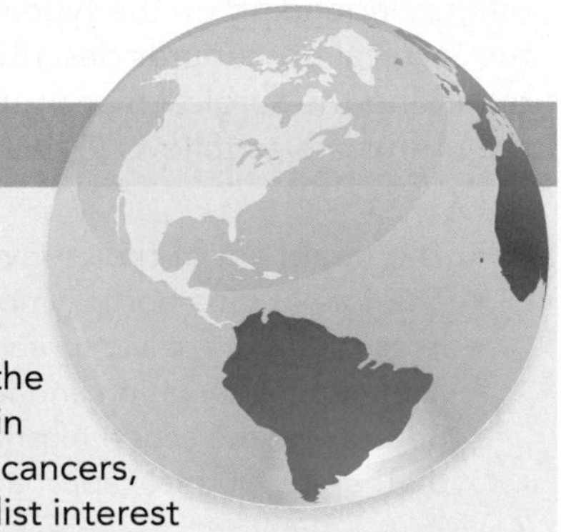

Mesenchymal Tumors in Canada

Helen MacKay, MD

Mesenchymal tumors of the uterine corpus are rare, and randomized data for the management of the individual subtypes are limited, which poses challenges in establishing standard-of-care approaches to treatment. Like all rare gynecologic cancers, involvement of multidisciplinary teams and review by a pathologist with a specialist interest in gynecologic cancers are essential to optimize care. In our jurisdiction, review of uterine sarcoma cases can also include involvement of general sarcoma teams to ensure all options have been considered for the patient.

Given the need for high-quality data, the Gynecologic Cancer Intergroup has advocated for cross-border participation and collaboration in clinical trials. For those tumors, such as uterine adenosarcomas, which occur

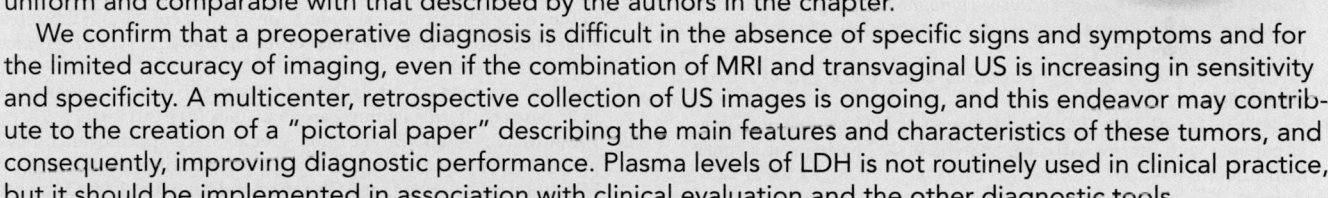

INTERNATIONAL PERSPECTIVES (*continued*)

at very low frequency, development of prospective cancer registries to enable greater understanding and potentially overcome reporting bias has been proposed (1).

Uterine CS were traditionally included in the sarcoma category, but with the emergence of molecular data, they are now considered to be dedifferentiated carcinomas, which explains their aggressive behavior (2). Multimodality treatment should be considered even for early-stage disease (3). Participation in clinical trials, when available, is essential if we are to improve the outcome for women diagnosed with uterine CS. Inclusion of correlative studies and tissue collection as part of study protocols will be key to learning more about the biology of this disease and in identifying potential therapeutic targets. Again, cross-group and international collaboration and participation in protocols is desirable to accelerate the pace of discovery.

---

(1) Friedlander ML, Covens A, Glasspool RM, et al. Gynecologic Cancer InterGroup (GCIG) consensus review for mullerian adenosarcoma of the female genital tract. *Int J Gynecol Cancer*. 2014;24(9 Suppl 3):S78–S82.

(2) McCluggage WG. Uterine carcinosarcomas (malignant mixed Mullerian tumors) are metaplastic carcinomas. *Int J Gynecol Cancer*. 12(6):687–690.

(3) Cantrell LA, Blank SV, Duska LR. Uterine carcinosarcoma: a review of the literature. *Gynecol Oncol*. 2015;137(3):581–588.

INTERNATIONAL PERSPECTIVES

Management of Mesenchymal Tumors in Italy

Angelo Maggioni, MD

Management of uterine mesenchymal tumors is often debated for the rarity of these tumors and the lack of available, large randomized clinical trials. Nevertheless, treatment of mesenchymal tumors in Italian referral centers is mostly uniform and comparable with that described by the authors in the chapter.

We confirm that a preoperative diagnosis is difficult in the absence of specific signs and symptoms and for the limited accuracy of imaging, even if the combination of MRI and transvaginal US is increasing in sensitivity and specificity. A multicenter, retrospective collection of US images is ongoing, and this endeavor may contribute to the creation of a "pictorial paper" describing the main features and characteristics of these tumors, and consequently, improving diagnostic performance. Plasma levels of LDH is not routinely used in clinical practice, but it should be implemented in association with clinical evaluation and the other diagnostic tools.

Removal of the uterus is necessary in almost all cases, and inspection of the peritoneal cavity is frequently practiced, whereas nodal assessment (lymph node assessment; LNA) and removal of the ovaries (BSO) are limited to specific cases. The variability depends on the different histologies: In young premenopausal patients with LMS, neither BSO nor LNA are usually performed; in the same way, nodal dissection is not required for adenosarcoma. Because of the rarity of nodal metastases in LMS, LNA is not part of surgical staging, unless nodes at preoperative or intraoperative evaluation are suspicious. Fertility-preserving surgery is not an option, even for young patients, when the diagnosis of LMS is confirmed, given the extremely poor prognosis of these neoplasms.

After a case in which a woman developed disseminated LMS after an "undiagnosed sarcoma" was treated with laparoscopy and power morcellation, the FDA discouraged the use of power morcellation devices for uterine myomas. This statement had a strong effect on clinical practice in Italy, and morcellation for presumed benign uterine leiomyomas is undergoing a slow decline. Strong data have been recently published on dissemination and worsening of outcome in case of intra-abdominal morcellation of myomas with an unexpected final diagnosis of LMS. Some surgical alternatives are ongoing to maintain the minimally invasive approach to uterine fibroids, especially in cases with very low risk of malignancy, using devices as new intra-abdominal baskets or performing extra-abdominal morcellation (vaginally or abdominally, by doing this procedure inside safe bags).

Removal of gross macroscopic disease at initial diagnosis, when the tumor is spread outside of the uterus, is recommended, when performance status is good and the surgical procedures are considered safe for the patient.

(*continued*)

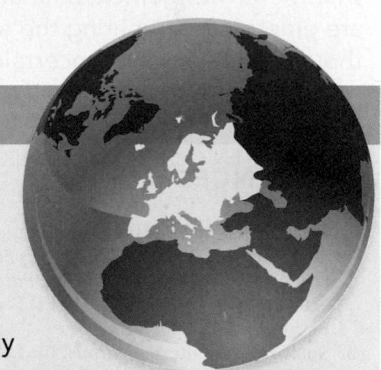

INTERNATIONAL PERSPECTIVES (*continued*)

Surgery for recurrent disease is an option when disease is limited to a single site or confined to limited areas, where the tumor can be radically removed. The disease-free interval plays a role in the decision-making process, even if standardized guidelines are not available. The final strategy is usually personalized according to the patient; however, surgery maintains an important role, especially given the lack of good alternatives.

Adjuvant RT is limited to uterine CS, when the risk for local recurrence is considered high, while its use in the palliative setting is frequent, above all for hemostatic or analgesic purposes.

The need for adjuvant CT is still debated; even if we lack clear evidence of benefit from CT, in terms of OS and DFS, in uterine LMS stage I or II, CT is usually offered to young patients with good performance status and no medical contraindications. The regimens usually used in the first-line setting, both for adjuvant and for metastatic disease, for LMS, CS, and undifferentiated sarcoma are universally accepted by the different Italian referral centers. Uterine LMS is treated upfront with gemcitabine and docetaxel, irrespective of the initial stage of presentation; in the recurrent setting, trabectedin is usually chosen as a second-line option, followed by doxorubicin and dacarbazine, and by ifosfamide. CS is generally treated with carboplatin and paclitaxel in the frontline setting, and with doxorubicin in the second line. In undifferentiated sarcoma, ifosfamide and doxorubicin are frequently used, and gemcitabine alone or in combination with docetaxel can be considered. Hormonal therapy is frequently prescribed for ESS.

Interesting results are expected from the randomized clinical trial on uterine LMS stage I or II, comparing treatment with gemcitabine and docetaxel, followed by doxorubicin versus observation. In Italy, new studies are emerging comparing the association of trabectedin and dacarbazine with actual standard treatment, even though there is some uncertainty about tolerability with this doublet.

REFERENCES

1. Kosary CL. Cancer of the corpus uteri. In: Ries LAG, Young JL, Keel GE, et al., eds. *SEER Survival Monograph: Cancer Survival Among Adults: U.S. SEER Program, 1988-2001, Patient and Tumor Characteristics*. National Cancer Institute, SEER Program, NIH pub. No. 07-6215. Bethesda, MD, 2007:123–132.
2. Tumors of the uterine corpus. In: Tavassoli FA, Devilee P, eds. *World Health Organization Classification of Tumours. Pathology and Genetics of Tumours of the Breast and Female Genital Organs*. Lyons, France: IARC Press; 2003:217–258.
3. D'Angelo E, Prat J. Uterine sarcomas: a review. *Gynecol Oncol*. 2010;116:131–139.
4. Park J, Kim D, Suh D, et al. Prognostic factors and treatment outcomes of patients with uterine sarcoma: analysis of 127 patients at a single institution, 1989–2007. *J Cancer Res Clin Oncol*. 2008;134:1277–1287.
5. Koivisto-Korander R, Butzow R, Koivisto A, et al. Clinical outcome and prognostic factors in 100 cases of uterine sarcoma: experience in Helsinki University Central Hospital 1990–2001. *Gynecol Oncol*. 2008;111:74–81.
6. Kahanpaa K, Wahlstrom T, Grohn P, et al. Sarcomas of the uterus: a clinicopathologic study of 119 patients. *Obstet Gynecol*. 1986;67:417–424.
7. George M, Pejovic MH, Kramar A. Uterine sarcomas: prognostic factors and treatment modalities—study on 209 patients. *Gynecol Oncol*. 1986;24:58–67.
8. Olah KS, Gee H, Blunt S, et al. Retrospective analysis of 318 cases of uterine sarcoma. *Eur J Cancer*. 1991;27:1095–1099.
9. Pautier P, Genestie C, Rey A, et al. Analysis of clinicopathologic prognostic factors for 157 uterine sarcomas and evaluation of grading score validated for soft tissue sarcoma. *Cancer*. 2000;88:1425–1431.
10. Abeler VM, Royne O, Thorensen S, et al. Uterine sarcomas in Norway. A histopathological and prognostic survey of a total population from 1970 to 2000 including 419 patients. *Histopathology*. 2009;54:355–364.
11. Lee CH, Mariño-Enriquez A, Ou W, et al. The clinicopathologic features of YWHAE-FAM22 endometrial stromal sarcomas: a histologically high-grade and clinically aggressive tumor. *Am J Surg Pathol*. 2012;36:641–653.
12. Jin Y, Pan L, Wang X, et al. Clinical characteristics of endometrial stromal sarcoma from and academic medical hospital in China. *Int J Gynecol Cancer*. 2010;20:1535–1539.
13. Vera AAL, Guadarrama MBR. Endometrial stromal sarcoma: clinicopathologic and immunophenotype study of 18 cases. *Ann Diag Pathol*. 2011;15:312–317.
14. Cheng X, Yang G, Schmeler KM, et al. Recurrence patterns and prognosis of endometrial stromal sarcoma and the potential of tyrosine kinase-inhibiting therapy. *Gynecol Oncol*. 2011;121:323–327.
15. Shah LP, Bryant CS, Kumar S, et al. Lymphadenectomy and ovarian preservation in low-grade endometrial stromal sarcoma. *Obstet Gynecol*. 2008;112:1102–1108.
16. dos Santos LA, Garg K, Diaz JP, et al. Incidence of lymph node and adnexal metastasis in endometrial stromal sarcoma. *Gynecol Oncol*. 2011;121:319–322.
17. Garg G, Shah JP, Liu R, et al. Validation of tumor size as staging variable in the revised International Federation of Gynecology and Obstetrics stage I leiomyosarcoma: a population-based study. *Int J Gynecol Cancer*. 2010;20:1201–1206.
18. Loizzi V, Cormio G, Nestola D, et al. Prognostic factors and outcomes in 28 cases of uterine leiomyosarcoma. *Oncology*. 2011;81:91–97.
19. Zivanovic O, Leitao MM, Iasonos A, et al. Stage-specific outcomes of patients with uterine leiomyosarcoma: a comparison of the International Federation of Gynecology and Obstetrics and American Joint Committee on Cancer staging systems. *J Clin Oncol*. 2009;27:2066–2072.
20. Park J, Kim D, Kim J, et al. The role of pelvic and/or para-aortic lymphadenectomy in surgical management of apparently early carcinosarcoma of uterus. *Ann Surg Oncol*. 2010;17:861–868.
21. Pradhan TA, Stevens EE, Ablavsky M, et al. FIGO staging for carcinosarcoma: can the revised staging system predict overall survival? *Gynecol Oncol*. 2011;123:221–224.
22. Clement PB, Scully RE. Mullerian adenosarcoma of the uterus: a clinicopathologic analysis of 100 cases with a review of the literature. *Hum Pathol*. 1990;21:363–381.
23. Guntupalli SR, Ramirez PT, Anderson ML, et al. Uterine smooth muscle tumor of uncertain malignant potential: a retrospective analysis. *Gynecol Oncol*. 2009;113:324–326.
24. Zelmanowicz A, Hildesheim A, Sherman MA, et al. Evidence for a common etiology for endometrial carcinomas and malignant mixed müllerian tumors. *Gynecol Oncol*. 1998;69:253–257.
25. Mortel R, Nedwich A, Lewis GC, et al. Malignant mixed müllerian tumors of the uterine corpus. *Obstet Gynecol*. 1970;35:469–480.
26. Norris HJ, Roth E, Taylor HB. Mesenchymal tumors of the uterus. *Obstet Gynecol*. 1966;28:57–63.
27. Brooks SE, Zhan M, Cote T, et al. Survival epidemiology and end results analysis of 267 cases of uterine sarcomas, 1989–1999. *Gynecol Oncol*. 2004;93:204–208.
28. Felix AS, Cook LS, Gaudet MM, et al. The etiology of uterine sarcomas: a pooled analysis of the epidemiology of endometrial cancer consortium. *Br J Cancer*. 2013;108:727–734.

29. Giuntoli RL, Metzinger DS, DiMarco CS, et al. Retrospective review of 208 patients with leiomyosarcoma of the uterus: prognostic indicators, surgical management, and adjuvant therapy. *Gynecol Oncol.* 2003;89:460–469.
30. Christopherson WM, Williamson EO, Gray LA. Leiomyosarcoma of the uterus. *Cancer.* 1972;29:1512–1517.
31. Meredith RJ, Eisert DR, Kaka Z, et al. An excess of uterine sarcomas after pelvic irradiation. *Cancer.* 1986;58:2003–2007.
32. Varala-Duran J, Nochomovitz LE, Prem KA, et al. Post irradiation mixed Müllerian tumors of the uterus. *Cancer.* 1980;45:1625–1631.
33. Pothuri B, Ramondetta L, Eifel P, et al. Radiation-associated endometrial cancers are prognostically unfavorable tumors: a clinicopathologic comparison with 527 sporadic endometrial cancers. *Gynecol Oncol.* 2006;103:948–951.
34. Jaakkola S, Lyytinen HK, Pukkala E, et al. Use of estradiol-progestin therapy associates with increased risk for uterine sarcomas. *Gynecol Oncol.* 2011;122:260–263.
35. Lavie O, Barnett-Griness O, Narod SA, et al. The risk of developing uterine sarcoma after tamoxifen use. *Int J Gynecol Cancer.* 2008;18:352–356.
36. Hoogendoorn WE, Hollema H, van Boven HH, et al. Prognosis of uterine corpus cancer after tamoxifen treatment for breast cancer. *Breast Cancer Res Treat.* 2008;112:99–108.
37. Nilbert M, Therkildsen C, Nissen A, et al. Sarcomas associated with hereditary nonpolyposis colorectal cancer: broad anatomical and morphological spectrum. *Familial Cancer.* 2009;8:209–213.
38. Francis JH, Kleinerman RA, Seddon J, et al. Increased risk of secondary uterine leiomyosarcoma in hereditary retinoblastoma. *Gynecol Oncol.* 2012;124:254–259.
39. Bansal N, Herzog TJ, Burke W, et al. The utility of preoperative endometrial sampling for the detection of uterine sarcomas. *Gynecol Oncol.* 2008;110:43–48.
40. Namimoto T, Yamashita Y, Awai K, et al. Combined use of T2-weighted and diffusion-weighted 3-T MR imaging for differentiating uterine sarcomas from benign leiomyomas. *Eur Radiol.* 2009;19:2756–2764.
41. Cornfeld D, Israel G, Martel M, et al. MRI appearance of mesenchymal tumors of the uterus. *Eur J Radiol.* 2010;74:241–249.
42. Goto A, Takeuchi S, Sugimura K, et al. Usefulness of Gd-DTPA contrast-enhanced dynamic MRI and serum determination of LDH and its isozymes in the differential diagnosis of leiomyosarcoma from degenerated leiomyoma of the uterus. *Int J Gynecol Cancer.* 2002;12:354–361.
43. Perri T, Korach J, Sadetzki S, et al. Uterine leiomyosarcoma: does the primary surgical procedure matter? *Int J Gynecol Cancer.* 2009;19:257–260.
44. Park J, Park S, Kim D, et al. The impact of tumor morcellation during surgery on the prognosis of patients with apparently early uterine leiomyosarcoma. *Gynecol Oncol.* 2011;122:255–259.
45. Park J, Kim D, Kim J, et al. The impact of tumor morcellation during surgery on the outcomes of patients with apparently early low-grade endometrial stromal sarcoma of the uterus. *Ann Surg Oncol.* 2011;18:3453–3461.
46. Bogani G, Cliby WA, Aletti GD. Impact of morcellation on survival outcomes of patients with unexpected uterine leiomyosarcoma: a systematic review and meta-analysis. *Gynecol Oncol.* 2015;137:167–172.
47. Oduyebo T, Rauh-Hain AJ, Meserve EE, et al. The value of re-exploration in patients with inadvertently morcellated uterine sarcoma. *Gynecol Oncol.* 2014;132:360–365.
48. Leibsohn S, D'Ablaing G, Mishell DR Jr, et al. Leiomyosarcoma in a series of hysterectomies performed for presumed uterine leiomyomas. *Am J Obstet Gynecol.* 1990;162:968–976.
49. Parker WH, Fu YS, Berek JS. Uterine sarcoma in patients operated on for presumed leiomyoma and rapidly growing leiomyoma. *Obstet Gynecol.* 1994;83:414–418.
50. Takamizawa S, Minakami H, Usui R, et al. Risk of complications and uterine malignancies in women undergoing hysterectomy for presumed benign leiomyomas. *Gynecol Obstet Invest.* 1999;48:193–196.
51. Leung F, Terzibachian JJ, Gay C, et al. Hysterectomies performed for presumed leiomyomas: should the fear of leiomyosarcoma make us apprehend non laparotomic surgical routes?. *Gynecol Obstet Fertil.* 2009;37:109–114.
52. Wright JD, Tergas AI, Cui R, et al. Use of electric power morcellation and prevalence of underlying cancer in women who undergo myomectomy. *JAMA Oncol.* 2015;1:69–77.
53. Perkins RB, Handal-Orefice R, Hanchate AD, et al. Risk of undetected cancer at the time of laparoscopic supracervical hysterectomy and laparoscopic myomectomy: implications for the use of power morcellation. *Womens Health Issues.* 2016;26(1):21–26.
54. U.S. Food & Drug Administration. FDA discourages use of laparoscopic power morcellation for removal of uterus or uterine fibroids. http://www.fda.gov/NewsEvents/Newsroom/PressAnnouncements/ucm393689.htm. Accessed January 31, 2016.
55. Barron KI, Richard T, Robinson PS, et al. Association of the U.S. Food and Drug Administration morcellation warning with rates of minimally invasive hysterectomy and myomectomy. *Obstet Gynecol.* 2015;126:1174–1180.
56. Harris JA, Swenson CW, Uppal S, et al. Practice patterns and postoperative complications before and after US Food and Drug Administration safety communication on power morcellation. *Am J Obstet Gynecol.* 2016;214:98.e1–98.e13.
57. Society of Gynecologic Oncology. Morcellation Updates: https://www.sgo.org. Accessed April 18, 2014.
58. Raut CP, Nucci MR, Wang Q, et al. Predictive value of FIGO and AJCC staging systems in patients with uterine leiomyosarcoma. *Eur J Cancer.* 2009;45:2818–2824.
59. Arend R, Bagaria M, Lewin SN, et al. Long- term outcome and natural history of uterine adenosarcomas. *Gynecol Oncol.* 2010;119:305–308.
60. Kapp DS, Shin JY, Chan JK. Prognostic factors and survival in 1396 patients with uterine leiomyosarcomas: emphasis on impact of lymphadenectomy and oophorectomy. *Cancer.* 2008;112:820–830.
61. Nugent EK, Zighelboim I, Case AS, et al. The value of perioperative imaging in patients with uterine sarcomas. *Gynecol Oncol.* 2009;115:37–40.
62. Li N, Wu L, Zhang H, et al. Treatment options in stage I endometrial stromal sarcoma: a retrospective analysis of 53 cases. *Gynecol Oncol.* 2008;108:306–311.
63. Zivanovic O, Jacks LM, Iasonos A, et al. A nomogram to predict postresection 5-year overall survival for patients with uterine leiomyosarcoma. *Cancer.* 2012;118:660–669.
64. Memorial Sloan Kettering Cancer Center. Uterine leiomyosarcoma nomogram. https://www.mskc.org/cancer-care/types/uterine-sarcoma/prediction-tools. Accessed April 18, 2016.
65. Iasonos A, Keung EZ, Zivanovic O, et al. External validation of a prognostic nomogram for overall survival in women with uterine leiomyosarcoma. *Cancer.* 2013;119:1816–1822.
66. Leitao MM Jr, Hensley M, Barakat RR, et al. Immunohistochemical expression of estrogen and progesterone receptors and outcomes in patients with newly diagnosed uterine leiomyosarcoma. *Gynecol Oncol.* 2012;124:558–562.
67. Ioffe YJ, Li AJ, Walsh CS, et al. Hormone receptor expression in uterine sarcomas: prognostic and therapeutic roles. *Gyencol Oncol.* 2009;115:466–471.
68. Rodriguez Y, Baez D, de Oca FM, et al. Comparative analysis of the ERa/ERb ratio and neurotensin and its high-affinity receptor in the myometrium, uterine leiomyoma, atypical leiomyoma, and leiomyosarcoma. *Int J Gynecol Pathol.* 2011;30:354–363.
69. Koivisto-Korander R, Butzow R, Koivisto A, et al. Immunohistochemical studies on uterine carcinosarcoma, leiomyosarcoma, and endometrial stromal sarcoma: expression and prognostic importance of ten different markers. *Tumor Biol.* 2011;32:451–459.
70. Kildal W, Pradhan M, Abeler VM, et al. β-catenin expression in uterine sarcomas and its relation to clinicopathologic parameters. *Eur J Cancer.* 2009;45:2412–2417.
71. Lee CH, Roh J, Choi J, et al. Cyclooxygenase-2 is an independent predictor of poor prognosis in uterine leiomyosarcomas. *Int J Gynecol Cancer.* 2011;21:668–672.
72. Menczer J, Schreiber L, Sukmanov O, et al. COX-2 expression in uterine carcinosarcoma. *Acta Obstet Gynecol.* 2010;89:120–125.
73. D'Angelo E, Spagnoli LG, Prat J. Comparative clinicopathologic and immunohistochemical analysis of uterine sarcomas diagnosed using the World Health Organization classification system. *Hum Pathol.* 2009;40:1571–1585.
74. Galaal K, Kew FM, Tam KF, et al. Evaluation of prognostic factors and treatment outcomes in uterine carcinosarcoma. *Eur J Obstet Gynecol Reprod Biol.* 2009;143:88–92.
75. Leath CA 3rd, Numnum TM, Kendrick JE 4th, et al. Patterns of failure for conservatively managed surgical stage I uterine carcinosarcoma: implications for adjuvant therapy. *Int J Gynecol Cancer.* 2009;19:888–891.
76. Barlin JN, Zhou QC, Leitao MM, et al. Molecular subtypes of uterine leiomyosarcoma and correlation with clinical outcome. *Neoplasia.* 2015;17:183–189.
77. Beck TL, Singhal PK, Ehrenberg HM, et al. Endometrial stromal sarcoma: analysis of recurrence following adjuvant treatment. *Gynecol Oncol.* 2012;125:141–144.
78. Kim WY, Lee JW, Choi CH, et al. Low-grade endometrial stromal sarcoma: a single center's experience with 22 cases. *Int J Cancer.* 2008;18:1084–1089.
79. Hensley ML, Ishill N, Soslow R, et al. Adjuvant gemcitabine plus docetaxel for completely resected stages I-IV high grade uterine leiomyosarcoma: results of a prospective study. *Gynecol Oncol.* 2009;112:563–567.

80. Leitao MM, Brennan MF, Hensley M, et al. Surgical resection of pulmonary and extrapulmonary recurrences of uterine leiomyosarcoma. *Gynecol Oncol.* 2002;87:287–294.
81. Chiang S, Ali R, Melnyk N, et al. Frequency of known gene rearrangements in endometrial stromal tumors. *Am J Surg Pathol.* 2011;35:1364–1372.
82. Lee C, Ou W, Marino-Enriquez A, et al. 14-3-3 fusion oncogenes in high-grade endometrial stromal sarcoma. *Proc Natl Acad Sci USA.* 2012;109:929–934.
83. Hayashi T, Horiuchi A, Sano K, et al. Mice lacking LMP2, immuno-proteasome subunit, as and animal model of spontaneous uterine leiomyosarcoma. *Protein Cell.* 2010;1:711–717.
84. Murray S, Linardou H, Mountzios G, et al. Low frequency of somatic mutations in uterine sarcomas: a molecular analysis and review of the literature. *Mutation Res.* 2010;686:68–73.
85. Growdon WB, Roussel BN, Scialabba VL, et al. Tissue-specific signatures of activating PIK3CA and RAS mutations in carcinosarcomas of gynecologic origin. *Gynecol Oncol.* 2011;121:212–217.
86. Saegusa M, Hashimura M, Kuwata T, et al. Requirement of the Akt/β-catenin pathway for uterine carcinosarcoma genesis, modulating E-cadherin expression through the transactivation of Slug. *Am J Pathol.* 2009;174:2107–2115.
87. Cimbaluk D, Rotmensch J, Scudiere J, et al. Uterine carcinosarcoma: immunohistochemical studies on tissue microarrays with focus on potential therapeutic targets. *Gynecol Oncol.* 2007;105:138–144.
88. Folpe AL, Kwiatkowski DJ. Perivascular epithelioid cell neoplasms: pathology and pathogenesis. *Hum Pathol.* 2010;41:1–15.
89. Mittal K, Joutovsky A. Areas with benign morphologic and immunohistochemical features are associated with some uterine leiomyosarcomas. *Gynecolo Oncol.* 2007;104:362–365.
90. Mittal KR, Chan F, Wei JJ, et al. Molecular and immunohistochemical evidence for the origin of uterine leiomyosarcomas from associated leiomyoma and symplastic leiomyoma-like areas. *Modern Pathol.* 2009;22:1303–1311.
91. Zhang P, Zhang C, Hao J, et al. Use of X chromosome inactivation pattern to determine clonal origins of uterine leiomyoma and leiomyosarcoma. *Hum Pathol.* 2006;37:1350–1356.
92. Bell SW, Kempson RL, Hendrickson MR. Problematic uterine isthmus muscle neoplasms. A clinicopathologic study of 213 cases. *Am J Surg Pathol.* 1994;18:535–558.
93. Perrone T, Dehner LP. Prognostically favorable "mitotically active" the smooth muscle tumors of the uterus. A clinicopathologic study of 10 cases. *Am J Surg Pathol.* 1988;12:1–8.
94. Giuntoli RL, Gostout BS, Di Marco CS, et al. Diagnostic criteria for uterine smooth muscle tumors: Leiomyoma variants associated with malignant behavior. *J Reprod Med.* 2007;52:1001–1010.
95. Ip PP, Cheung AN, Clement PB. Uterine smooth muscle tumors of uncertain malignant potential (STUMP): a clinicopathologic analysis of 16 cases. *Am J Surg Pathol.* 2009;33:992–1005.
96. Ng JS, Chew SH, Low J. A clinicopathologic study of uterine smooth muscle tumors of uncertain malignant potential (STUMP). *Ann Acad Med Singapore.* 2010;39:625–628.
97. Veras E, Zivanovic O, Jacks L, et al. "Low grade leiomyosarcoma" and late recurring smooth muscle tumors of the uterus: a heterogeneous collection of frequently misdiagnosed tumors associated with an overall favorable prognosis relative to conventional uterine leiomyosarcomas. *Am J Surg Pathol.* 2011;35:1626–1637.
98. O'Neill CJ, McBride HA, Connolly LE, et al. Uterine leiomyosarcomas are characterized by high p16, p53, and MIB1 expression in comparison with usual leiomyomas, leiomyoma variants and smooth muscle tumors of unertain malignant potential. *Histopathology.* 2007;50:851–858.
99. Ly A, Mills AM, McKenney JK, et al. Atypical leiomyomas of the uterus: a clinicopathologc study of 51 cases focusing on long-term follow up. *Am J Surg Pathol.* 2013;37:643–649.
100. Croce S, Young RH, Oliva E. Uterine leiomyomas with bizarre nuclei: a clinicopathologic study of 59 cases. *Am J Surg Pathol.* 2014;38:1330–1339.
101. Chen L, Yang B. Immunohistochemical analysis of p16, p53, and Ki67 expression in uterine smooth muscle tumors. *Int J Gynecol Pathol.* 2008;27:326–332.
102. Atkins KA, Arronte N, Darus CJ, et al. The use of p16 in enhancing the histologic classification of uterine smooth muscle tumors. *Am J Surg Pathol.* 2008;32:98–102.
103. Gannon BR, Manduch M, Childs TJ. Differential immunoreactivity of p16 in leiomyosarcomas and leiomyoma variants. *Int J Gynecol Pathol.* 2008;27:68–73.
104. Prayson RA, Goldblum JR, Hart WR. Epithelioid smooth muscle tumors of the uterus: a clinicopathologic study of 18 patients. *Am J Surg Pathol.* 1997;21:383–391.
105. Jones MW, Norris HJ. Clinicopathologic study of 28 uterine leiomyosarcomas with metastases. *Int J Gynecol Pathol.* 1995;14:243–249.
106. Burch DM, Tavassoli FA. Myxoid leiomyosarcoma of the uterus. *Histopathology.* 2011;59:1144–1155.
107. Pelmus M, Penault-Llorca F, Guillou L, et al. Prognostic factors in early stage leiomyosarcoma of the uterus. *Int J Gynecol Pathol.* 2009;19:385–390.
108. D'Angelo E, Espinosa I, Ali R, et al. Uterine leiomyosarcomas: tumor size, mitotic index, and biomarkers Ki67, and Bcl-2 identify 2 groups with different prognosis. *Gynecol Oncol.* 2011;121:328–333.
109. Wang WL, Soslow R, Hensley M, et al. Histopathologic prognostic factors in stage I leiomyosarcoma of the uterus: a detailed analysis of 27 cases. *Am J Surg Pathol.* 2011;35:522–529.
110. Awonuga AO, Shavell VI, Imudia AN, et al. Pathogenesis of benign metastasizing leiomyoma: a review. *Obstet Gynecol Surv.* 2010;65:189–195.
111. McCluggage WG. Malignant biphasic uterine tumors: carcinosarcomas or metaplastic carcinomas? *J Clin Pathol.* 2002;55:321–325.
112. Taylor NP, Zighelboim I, Huettner PC, et al. DNA mismatch repair and TP53 defects are early events in uterine carcinosarcoma tumorigenesis. *Modern Pathol.* 2006;19:1333–1338.
113. Ferguson SE, Tornos C, Hummer A, et al. Prognostic features of surgical stage I uterine carcinosarcoma. *Am J Surg Pathol.* 2007;31:1653–1661.
114. Garamvoelgyii E, Guillou L, Gebhard S, et al. Primary malignant mixed Müllerian tumor of the female peritoneum. A clinical, pathologic, and immunohistochemical study of 3 pieces and review of the literature. *Cancer.* 1994;74:854–860.
115. Rose PG, Rodriguez M, Abdul-Karim FW. Malignant mixed Müllerian tumor of the female peritoneum: treatment and outcome of 3 cases. *Gynecol Oncol.* 1997;65:523–525.
116. Sumathi VP, Murnaghan M, Dobbs SP, et al. Extragenital Müllerian carcinosarcoma arising from the peritoneum: report of 2 cases. *Int J Gynecol Cancer.* 2002;12:764–767.
117. Ko ML, Huang SH, Shen J, et al. Primary peritoneal carcinosarcoma report of a case with 5 year disease free survival after surgery and chemoradiation and review of the literature. *Acta Oncol.* 2005;44:756–760.
118. Shintaku M, Matsumoto T. Primary Müllerian carcinosarcoma of the retroperitoneum: report of a case. *Int J Gynecol Pathol.* 2001;20:191–195.
119. Booth C, Zahn CM, McBroom J, et al. Retroperitoneal Müllerian carcinosarcoma associated with endometriosis: a case report. *Gynecol Oncol.* 2004;93:546–549.
120. Dionigi A, Oliva E, Clement PB, et al. Endometrial stromal nodules and endometrial stromal tumors with limited infiltration: a clinicopathologic study of 50 cases. *Am J Surg Pathol.* 2002;26:567–581.
121. Conklin CM, Longacre TA. Endometrial stromal tumors: The New WHO classification. *Adv Anat Pathol.* 2014;21:383–93.
122. Chang KL, Crabtree GS, Kim Lim-Tan S, et al. Primary uterine endometrial stromal neoplasms: a clinicopathologic study of 117 cases. *Am J Surg Pathol.* 1990;14:415–438.
123. Oliva E, Young RH, Clement PB. Myxoid and fibrous endometrial stromal tumors of the uterus: a report of 10 cases. *Int J gynecol Pathol.* 1999;18:310–319.
124. Yilmaz A, Rush DS, Soslow RA. Endometrial stromal sarcomas with unusual histologic features. A report of 24 primary and metastatic tumors emphasizing fibroblastic and smooth muscle differentiation. *Am J Surg Pathol.* 2002;26:1142–1150.
125. Oliva E, Clement PB, Young RH. Epithelioid endometrial and endometrioid stromal tumors: a report of 4 pieces emphasizing their distinction from epithelioid smooth muscle tumors and other oxyphilic uterine and extrauterine tumors. *Int J Gynecol Pathol.* 2002;21:48–55.
126. Clement PB, Scully RE. Endometrial stromal sarcomas of the uterus with extensive endometrioid glandular differentiation: a report of 3 cases that caused problems in the differential diagnosis. *Int J Gynecol Pathol.* 1992;11:163–173.
127. Nucci MR, Harburger D, Koontz J, et al. Molecular analyses of the JAZF1-JjAZ1 gene fusion by RT-CPR and fluorescence in situ hybridization in endometrial stromal neoplasms. *Am J Surg Pathol.* 2007;31:65–70.
128. Chang KL, Crabtree GS, Soo Kim LT, et al. Primary extrauterine endometrial stromal neoplasms: a clinicopathologic study of 20 cases and a review of the literature. *Int J Gynecol Pathol.* 1993;12:282–296.
129. Irvin W, Pelkey T, Rice L, et al. Endometrial stromal sarcoma of the vulva arising in extraovarian endometriosis: a case report and literature review. *Gynecol Oncol.* 1998;71:313–316.
130. Kondi-Paphitis A, Smyrniotis B, Liapis A, et al. Stromal sarcoma arising in endometriosis. A clinicopathologic and immunohistochemical study of 4 cases. *Eur J Gynaecol Oncol.* 1998;19:588–590.

131. Lacroix-Triki M, Beyris L, Martel P, et al. Low grade endometrial stromal sarcoma arising from sciatic nerve endometriosis. *Obstet Gynecol.* 2004;104:1147–1149.
132. Androulaki A, Papathomas TG, Alexandrou P, et al. Metastatic low grade endometrial stromal sarcoma of clitoris: report of a case. *Int J Gynecol Cancer.* 2007;17:290–293.
133. Sato K, Ueda Y, Sugaya J, et al. Extrauterine endometrial stromal sarcoma with JAZF1/JjAZ1 fusion confirm with RT-PCR and interphase FISH presenting as an inguinal tumor. *Virchows Arch.* 2007;450:349–353.
134. Lee CH, Mariño-Enriquez A, Ou W, et al. The clinicopathologic features of YWHAE-FAM22 endometrial stromal sarcomas: a histologically high-grade and clinically aggressive tumor. *Am J Surg Pathol.* 2012;36:641–653.
135. Lee CH, Ali RH, Rouzbahman M, et al. Cyclin-D1as a diagnostic immunomarker for endometrial stromal sarcoma with YWHAE-FAM22 rearrangement. *Am J Surg Pathol.* 2012;36:1562–1570.
136. Lee CH, Hoang LN, Yip S, et al. Frequent expression of KIT in endometrial stromal sarcoma with YWHAER genetic rearrangement. *Mod Pathol.* 2014;27:751–757.
137. Evans HL, Endometrial stromal sarcoma and poorly differentiated endometrial sarcoma. *Cancer.* 1982;50:2170–2182.
138. Cheng-Han L, Nucci MR. Endometrial stromal sarcoma—the new genetic paradigm. *Histopathology.* 2015;67:1–19.
139. Gallardo A, Prat J. Mullerian adenosarcoma: a clinicopathologic and immunohistochemical study of 55 cases challenging the existence of adenofibroma. *Am J Surg Pathol.* 2009;33:278–288.
140. Clement PB. Mullerian adenosarcoma of the uterus with sarcomatous overgrowth. A clinicopathologic analysis of 10 cases. *Am J Surg Pathol.* 1989;13:28–38.
141. Bernard B, Clarke BA, Malowany JI, et al. Uterine adenosarcomas: a dual-institution update on staging, prognosis and survival. *Gynecol Oncol.* 2013;131:634–639.
142. Carroll A, Ramirez PT, Westin SN, et al. Uterine adenosarcoma: an analysis on management, oucomes and risk factors for recurrence. *Gynecol Oncol.* 2014;135:455–461.
143. Soslow RA, Ali A, Oliva E. Mullerian adenosarcomas: an immunophenotypic analysis of 35 cases. *Am J Surg Pathol.* 2008;32:1013–1021.
144. Anderson J, Behbakht K, De Geest K, et al. Adenosarcoma in a patient with vaginal endometriosis. *Obstet Gynecol.* 2001;98:964–966.
145. Liu L, Davidosmon S, Singh M. Mullerian adenosarcoma of vagina arising in persistent endometriosis: report of a case and review of the literature. *Gynecol Oncol.* 2003;90:486–490.
146. Raffaeli R, Piazzola E, Zanconato G, et al. A rare case of extrauterine adenosarcoma arising in endometriosis of the rectovaginal septum. *Fertil Steril.* 2004;81:1142–1144.
147. Yantiss RK, Clement PB, Young RH. Neoplastic and pre-neoplastic changes in gastrointestinal endometriosis: a study of 17 cases. *Am J Surg Pathol.* 2000;24:513–524.
148. Vata AR, Ruzis EP, Moussabeck O, et al. Endometrioid adenosarcoma of the bladder arising from endometriosis. *J Urol.* 1990;143:813–815.
149. Murugasu A, Miller J, Proietto A, et al. Extragenital Mullerian adenosarcoma with sarcomatous overgrowth arising in an endometriotic cyst in the pouch of Douglas. *Int J Gynecol Pathol.* 2003;13:371–375.
150. Dincer AD, Timmins P, Pietrocola D, et al. Primary peritoneal adenosarcoma with sarcomatous overgrowth associated with endometriosis. *Int J Gynecol Pathol.* 2002;21:65–68.
151. N'Senda P, Wendum D, Balladur P, et al. Adenosarcoma arising in hepatic endometriosis. *Eur Radiol.* 2000;10:1287–1289.
152. Huang GS, Arend RC, Sakaris A, et al. Extragenital adenosarcoma: a case report, review of the literature and management discussion. *Gynecol Oncol.* 2009;115:472–475.
153. Clement PB, Scully RE. Uterine tumors resembling ovarian sex cord tumors. A clinicopathologic analysis of 14 cases. *Am J Clin Pathol.* 1976;66:512–525.
154. Hurrell DP, McCluggage WG. Uterine tumors resembling ovarian sex cord tumor is an immunohistochemically polyphenotypic neoplasm which exhibits coexpression of epithelial, myoid and sec cord markers. *J Clin Pathol.* 2007;60:1148–1154.
155. De leval L, Lim GS, Waltregny D, et al. Diverse phenotypic profile of uterine tumors resembling ovarian sex cord tumors: on immunohistochemical study of 12 cases. *Am J Surg Pathol.* 2010;34:1749–1761.
156. Staats PN, Garcia JJ, Dias-Santagata DC, et al. Uterine tumors resembling ovarian sex cord tumors (UTROSCT) lack the JAZF1-JJAZ1 translocation frequently seen in endometrial stromal tumors. *Am J Surg Pathol.* 2009;33:1206–1212.
157. Biermann K, Heukamp LC, Buttner R, et al. Uterine tumor resembling an ovarian sex cord tumor associated with metastasis. *Int J Gynecol Pathol.* 2008;27:58–60.
158. Folpe AL, Mentzel T, Lehr H, et al. Perivascular epithelioid neoplasms of soft tissue and gynecologic origin. *Am J Surg Pathol.* 2005;29:1558–1575.
159. Vang R, Kempson RL. Perivascular epithelioid cell tumor (PEComa) of the uterus. A subset of HMB45 epithelioid mesenchymal neoplasms with an uncertain relationship to pure smooth muscle tumors. *Am J Surg Pathol.* 2002;26:1–13.
160. Fadare O. Perivascular epithelioid cell tumor (PEComa) of the uterus: on outcome-based clinicopathologic analysis of 41 reported cases. *Adv Anat Pathol.* 2008;15:63–75.
161. Schoolmeester JK, Howitt BE, Hirsch MS, et al. Perivascular epithelioid cell neoplasm (PEComa) of the gynecologic tract: clinicopathologic and immunohistochemical characterization of 16 cases. *Am J Surg Pathol.* 2014;38:176–188.
162. Argani P, Aulmann S, Illei PB, et al. Adistinct subset of PEComas harbor TFE3 fusions. *Am J Surg Pathol.* 2010;34:1395–1406.
163. Agaram NP, Sung YS, Zhang L, et al. Dichotomy of genetic abnormalities in PEComas with therapeutic implications. *Am J Surg Pathol.* 2015;39:813–25.
164. Rabban JT, Zaloudek CJ, Shekitka KM, et al. Inflammatory myofibroblastic tumor of the uterus: a clinicopathologic study of 6 cases emphasizing distinction from aggressive mesenchymal tumors. *Am J Surg Pathol.* 2005;29:1348–1355.
165. Gupta N, Mittal S, Misra R. Inflammatory pseudotumor of the uterus: an unusual pelvic mass. *Eur J Obstet Gynecol Reprod Biol.* 2011;156:118–119.
166. Parra-Herran C, Quick CM, Howitt BE, et al. Inflammatory myofibroblastic tumor of the uterus: clinical and pathologic review of 10 cases including a subset with aggressive clinical course. *Am J Surg Pathol.* 2015;39:157–168.
167. Ferguson SE, Gerald W, Barakat RR, et al. Clinicopathologic features of rhabdomyosarcoma of gynecologic origin in adults. *Am J Surg Pathol.* 2007;31:382–389.
168. Fadare O. Heterologous and rare homologous sarcomas of the uterine corpus: a clinicopathologic review. *Adv Anat Pathol.* 2011;18:60–74.
169. McDonald AG, Dal Chin P, Gangully A, et al. Liposarcoma arising in uterine lipoleiomyoma: a report of the cases and review of the literature. *Am J Surg Pathol.* 2011;35:221–227.
170. Fadare O. Pleomorphic liposarcoma of the uterine corpus with focal smooth muscle differentiation. *Int J Gynecol Pathol.* 2011;30:282–287.
171. Lissoni A, Cormio G, Bonazzi C, et al. Fertility-sparing surgery in uterine leiomyosarcoma. *Gynecol Oncol.* 1998;70:348–350.
172. Stadsvold JL, Molpus KL, Baker JJ, et al. Conservative management of a myxoid endometrial stromal sarcoma in a 16-year-old nulliparous woman. *Gynecol Oncol.* 2005;99:243–245.
173. Yan L, Tian Y, Fu Y, et al. Successful pregnancy after fertility-preserving surgery for endometrial stromal sarcoma. *Fertil Steril.* 2010;93:269.e1–269.e3.
174. Fong Y, Coit DG, Woodruff JM, et al. Lymph node metastasis from soft tissue sarcoma in adults: analysis of data from a prospective database of 1772 sarcoma patients. *Ann Surg.* 1993;217:72–77.
175. Ayhan A, Aksan G, Gultekin M, et al. Prognosticators and the role of lymphadenectomy in uterine leiomyosarcomas. *Arch Gynecol Obstet.* 2009;280:79–85.
176. Major FJ, Blessing JA, Silverberg SG, et al. Prognostic factors in early-stage uterine sarcoma: a Gynecologic Oncology Group study. *Cancer.* 1993;71:1702–1709.
177. Leitao MM, Sonoda Y, Brennan MF, et al. Incidence of lymph node and ovarian metestases in leiomyosarcoma of the uterus. *Gynecol Oncol.* 2003;91:209–212.
178. Goff BA, Rice LW, Fleischhacker D, et al. Uterine leiomyosarcoma and endometrial stromal sarcoma: lymph node metastases and sites of recurrence. *Gynecol Oncol.* 1993;50:105–109.
179. Nemani D, Mitra N, Guo M, et al. Assessing the effects of lymphadenectomy and radiation therapy in patients with uterine carcinosarcoma: a SEER analysis. *Gynecol Oncol.* 2008;111:82–88.
180. Gadducci A, Landoni F, Sartori E, et al. Uterine leiomyosarcoma: analysis of treatment failures and survival. *Gynecol Oncol.* 1996;62:25–32.
181. Riopel J, Plante M, Renaud MC, et al. Lymph node metastases in low-grade endometrial stromal sarcoma. *Gynecol Oncol.* 2005;96:402–406.
182. Signorelli M, Fruscio R, Dell'Anna T, et al. Lymphadenectomy in uterine low-grade endometrial stromal sarcoma: an analysis of 19 cases and a literature review. *Int J Gynecol Cancer.* 2010;20:1363–1366.
183. Leitao MM Jr, Zivanovic O, Chi DS, et al. Surgical cytoreduction in patients with metastatic uterine leiomyosarcoma at the time of initial diagnosis. *Gynecol Oncol.* 2012;125:409–413.

184. Khoury-Collado F, Einstein MH, Bochner BH, et al. Pelvic exenteration with curative intent for uterine malignancies. *Gynecol Oncol.* 2012;124:42–47.
185. Burt BM, Ocejo S, Mery CM, et al. Repeated and aggressive pulmonary resections for leiomyosarcoma metastases extends survival. *Ann Thorac Surg.* 2011;92:1202–1207.
186. Levenback C, Rubin SC, McCormack PM, et al. Resection of pulmonary metastases from uterine sarcomas. *Gynecol Oncol.* 1992;45:202–205.
187. Giuntoli RL 2nd, Garrett-Mayer E, Bristow RE, et al. Secondary cytoreduction in the management of recurrent uterine leiomyosarcoma. *Gynecol Oncol.* 2007;106:82–88.
188. Sutton G, Kavanagh J, Wolfson A, et al. Corpus: mensenchymal tumors. In: Barakat RR, Markman M, Randall ME, eds. *Principles and Practice of Gynecologic Oncology*. 5th ed. Philadelphia, PA: Lippincott, Williams & Wilkins; 2009:733–761.
189. Makker V, Abu-Rustum NR, Alektiar KM, et al. A retrospective assessment of outcomes of chemotherapy-based versus radiation-only adjuvant treatment for completely resected stage I–IV uterine carcinosarcoma. *Gynecol Oncol.* 2008;111(2):249–254.
190. Reed NS, Mangioni C, Malmstrom H, et al. Phase III randomized study to evaluate the role of adjuvant pelvic radiotherapy in the treatment of uterine sarcomas stages I and II: an European Organisation for Research and Treatment of Cancer Gynaecological Cancer Group Study (protocol 55874). *Eur J Cancer.* 2008;44:808–818.
191. Aalders J, Abeler V, Kolstad P, et al. Postoperative external irradiation and prognostic parameters in stage I endometrial carcinoma: clinical and histopathologic study of 540 patients. *Obstet Gynecol.* 1980;56:419–427.
192. Pautier P, Floquet A, Gladieff L, et al. A randomized clinical trial of adjuvant chemotherapy with doxorubicin, ifosfamide, and cisplatin followed by radiotherapy versus radiotherapy alone in patients with localized uterine sarcomas (SARCGYN study). A study of the French Sarcoma Group. *Ann Oncol.* 2013;24:1099–1104.
193. Vongtama V, Karlen JR, Piver SM, et al. Treatment, results and prognostic factors in stage I and II sarcomas of the corpus uteri. *Am J Obstet Gynecol.* 1976;126:139–147.
194. Salazar OM, Bonfiglio TA, Patten SF, et al. Uterine sarcomas: natural history, treatment and prognosis. *Cancer.* 1978;42:1152–1160.
195. Perez CA, Askin F, Baglan RJ, et al. Effects of irradiation on mixed Müllerian tumors of the uterine sarcomas. *Cancer.* 1979;43:1274–1284.
196. Hoffmann W, Schmandt S, Koradiotherapymann RD, et al. Radiotherapy in the treatment of uterine sarcomas: a retrospective analysis of 54 cases. *Gynecol Obstet Invest.* 1996;42:49–57.
197. Knocke TH, Kucera H, Dorfler D, et al. Results of postoperative radiotherapy in the treatment of sarcomas of the corpus uteri. *Cancer.* 1998;83:1972–1979.
198. Ferrer F, Sabater S, Farruterine B, et al. Impact of radiotherapy on local control and survival in uterine sarcomas: a retrospective study from the GRUP Oncologic Catala-Occita. *Int J Radiat Oncol Biol Phys.* 1999;44:47–52.
199. Chauveinc L, Deniaud E, Plancher C, et al. Uterine sarcomas: the Curie Institute experience. Prognostic factors and adjuvant treatments. *Gynecol Oncol.* 1999;72:232–237.
200. Soumarova R, Horova H, Seneklova Z, et al. Treatment of uterine sarcoma: a survey of 49 patients. *Arch Gynecol Obstet.* 2002;266:92–95.
201. Livi L, Paiar F, Shah N, et al. Uterine sarcoma: twenty-seven years of experience. *Int J Radiat Oncol Biol Phys.* 2003;57:1366–1373.
202. Dusenbery KE, Potish RA, Agenta PA, et al. On the apparent failure of adjuvant pelvic radiotherapy to improve survival for women with uterine sarcomas confined to the uterus. *Am J Clin Oncol.* 2005;28:295–300.
203. Dusenberry KE, Potish RA, Judson P. Limitations of adjuvant radiotherapy for uterine sarcomas spread beyond the uterus. *Gynecol Oncol.* 2004;94:191–196.
204. Sorbe B, Johansson B. Prophylactic pelvic irradiation as part of primary therapy in uterine sarcomas. *Int J Oncol.* 2008;32:1111–1117.
205. Sahinler I, Atalar B, Tecer GM, et al. Postoperative radiotherapy in the treatment of uterine sarcomas: long-term results and analysis of prognostic factors. *J BUON.* 2010;15:480–488.
206. Rovirosa A, Ascaso C, Ordi J, et al. How to deal with prognostic factors and radiotherapy results in uterine neoplasms with a sarcomatous component? *Clin Transl Oncol.* 2009;11:681–687.
207. Magnuson WJ, Petereit DG, Anderson BM, et al. Impact of adjuvant pelvic radiotherapy in stage I uterine sarcoma. *Anticancer Res.* 2015;35: 365–370.
208. Hou HL, Meng MB, Chen XL, et al. The prognosis of adjuvant radiation therapy after surgery in uterine sarcomas. *Onco Targets Ther.* 2015;8:2339–2344.
209. Pautier P, Rey A, Haie-Meder C, et al. Adjuvant chemotherapy with cisplatin, ifosfamide, and doxorubicin followed by radiotherapy in localized uterine sarcomas: Results of a case-control study with radiotherapy alone. *Int J Gynecol Cancer.* 2004;14:1112–1117.
210. Denschlag D, Masoud G, Gilbert L. Prognostic factors and outcome in women with uterine sarcoma. *Eur J Surg Oncol.* 2006;33:91–95.
211. Yoney A, Eren B, Eskici S, et al. Retrospective analysis of 105 cases with uterine sarcoma. *Bull Cancer.* 2008;95:E10–E17.
212. Wright JD, Venkatraman ES, Shah M, et al. The role of radiation in improving survival for early-stage carcinosarcomas and leiomyosarcomas. *Am J Obstet Gynecol.* 2008;199:536.e1–536.e8.
213. Sampath S, Schultheiss TE, Ryu JK, et al. The role of adjuvant radiation in uterine sarcomas. *Int J Radiat Oncol Biol Phys.* 2010;76:728–734.
214. Omura GA, Blessing JA, Major F, et al. A randomized clinical trial of adjuvant Adriamycin in uterine sarcomas: a Gynecologic Oncology Group study. *J Clin Oncol.* 1985;3:1240–1245.
215. Hornback NB, Omura G, Major FJ. Observations on the uterine sarcomas of adjuvant radiation therapy in patients with stage I and II uterine sarcoma. *Int J Radiat Oncol Biol Phys.* 1986;12:2127–2130.
216. Gerszten K, Faul C, Kounelis S, et al. The impact of adjuvant radiotherapy on carcinosarcoma of the uterus. *Gynecol Oncol.* 1998;68:8–13.
217. Wong L, See HT, Khoo-Tan HS, et al. Combined adjuvant cisplatin and ifosfamide chemotherapy and radiotherapy for malignant mixed Müllerian tumors of the uterine sarcomas. *Int J Gynecol Cancer.* 2006;16:1364–1369.
218. Molpus KL, Redline-Frazzier S, Reed G, et al. Postoperative pelvic irradiation in early stage uterine mixed Müllerian tumors. *Eur J Gynaecol Oncol.* 1998;19:541–546.
219. Le T. Adjuvant pelvic radiotherapy for uterine carcinosarcoma in a high risk population. *Eur J Surg Oncol.* 2001;27:282–285.
220. Menczer J, Levy T, Piura B, et al. A comparison between different postoperative treatment modalities of uterine carcinosarcoma. *Gynecol Oncol.* 2005;97:166–170.
221. Chi DS, Mychalczak B, Saigo PE, et al. The role of whole-pelvic irradiation in the treatment of early-stage uterine carcinosarcoma. *Gynecol Oncol.* 1997;65:493–498.
222. Callister M, Ramondetta LM, Jhingran A, et al. Malignant mixed Müllerian tumors of the uterus: analysis of patterns of failure, prognostic factors, and treatment outcome. *Int J Radiat Oncol Biol Phys.* 2004;58:786–796.
223. Knocke TH, Weitmann HD, Kucera H, et al. Results of primary and adjuvant radiotherapy in the treatment of mixed Müllerian tumors of the corpus uteri. *Gynecol Oncol.* 1999;73:389–395.
224. Sartori E, Bazzurini L, Gadducci A, et al. Carcinosarcoma of the uterine sarcomas: a clinicopathological multicenter CTF study. *Gynecol Oncol.* 1997;67:70–75.
225. Smith DC, MacDonald OK, Gaffney DK. The impact of adjuvant radiation therapy on survival in women with uterine carcinosarcoma. *Int J Gynecol Cancer.* 2008;18(2):255–261.
226. Wolfson AH, Brady MF, Rocereto TF, et al. A Gynecologic Oncology Group randomized trial of whole abdominal irradiation (WWAI) vs. cisplatin-ifosfamide + mesna (WCIM) in optimally debulked stage I–IV carcinosarcoma (WCS) of the uterine sarcomas. *J Clin Oncol.* 2006;24:256.
227. Wolfson AH, Brady MF, Rocereto TF, et al. A Gynecologic Oncology Group randomized trial of whole abdominal irradiation versus chemotherapy in optimally debulked carcinosarcomas of the uterus. *Int J Gynecol Cancer.* 2006;16:45.
228. Wolfson AH, Brady MF, Rocereto T, et al. A Gynecologic Oncology Group randomized phase III trial of whole abdominal irradiation (WAI) vs. cisplatin-ifosfamide and mesna (CIM) as postsurgical therapy in stage I–IV carcinosarcoma (CS) of the uterus. *Gynecol Oncol.* 2007;107: 177–185.
229. Makker V, Abu-Rustum NR, Alektiar KM, et al. A retrospective assessment of outcomes of chemotherapy-based versus radiation-only adjuvant treatment for completely resected stage I–IV uterine carcinosarcomas. *Gynecol Oncol.* 2008;11:249–254.
230. Manolitsas T, Wain GV, Williams KE, et al. Multimodality therapy for patients with clinical stage I and II malignant mixed müllerian tumors of the uterus. *Cancer.* 2001;91:1437–43.
231. Prat J. FIGO staging for uterine sarcomas. *Int J Gynaecol Obstet.* 2009;104:179.
232. Gonzalez Bosquet J, Terstriep SA, Cliby WA et al. The impact of multi-modal therapy on survival for uterine carcinosarcomas. *Gynecol Oncol.* 2010;116:419–423.
233. Patel N, Hegarty SE, Cantrell LA, et al. Evaluation of brachytherapy and external beam radiation therapy for early stage, node-negative uterine CS. *Brachytherapy.* 2015;14:606–612.
234. Gadducci A, Fabrini MG, Bonuccelli A, et al. Analysis of treatment failures in patients with early-stage uterine leiomyosarcoma. *Anticancer Res.* 1995;15:485–488.

235. Cantrell LA, Havrilesky L, Moore DT, et al. A multi-institutional cohort study of adjuvant therapy in stage I-II uterine carcinosarcoma. *Gynecol Oncol.* 2012;127:22–26.
236. Sorbe B, Paulsson G, Andersson S, et al. A population-based series of uterine carcinosarcomas with long-term follow-up. *Acta Oncologica.* 2013;52:759–766.
237. Gungorduk K, Ozdemir A, Ertas IE, et al. Adjuvant treatment modalities, prognostic predictors and outcomes of uterine carcinosarcomas. *Cancer Res Treat.* 2015;47:282–289.
238. Rovirosa A, Ascaso C, Arenas M, et al. Pathologic prognostic fators in stage I-III uterine carcinosarcoma treated with postoperative radiotherapy. *Arch Gynecol Obstet.* 2014;290:329–334.
239. Einstein MH, Klobocista M, Hou JY, et al. Phase II trial of adjuvant pelvic radiation "sandwiched" between ifosfamide or ifosfamide plus cisplatin in women with uterine carcinosarcoma. *Gynecol Oncol.* 2013;124:26–30.
240. Mahdavi A, Monk BJ, Ragazzo J, et al. Pelvic radiation improves local control after hysterectomy for uterine leiomyosarcomas: a 20-year experience. *Int J Gynecol Cancer.* 2009;19:1080–1084.
241. Wong P, Han K, Sykes J, et al. Postoperative radiotherapy improves local control and survival in patients with uterine leiomyosarcoma. *Radiat Oncol.* 2013;8:128.
242. Mancari R, Signorelli M, Gadducci A, et al. Adjuvant chemotherapy in stage I-II uterine leiomyosarcoma: A multicentric retrospective study of 140 patients. *Gynecol Oncol.* 2014;133:531–536.
243. Ricci S, Giuntoli RL, Eisenhauer E, et al. Does adjuvant chemotherapy improve survival for women with early-stge uterine leiomyosarcoma? *Gynecol Oncol.* 2013;131:629–633.
244. Gadducci A, Sartori E, Landoni F, et al. Endometrial stromal sarcoma: analysis of treatment failure and survival. *Gynecol Oncol.* 1996;63:247–253.
245. Bodner K, Bodner-Adler B, Obermair A, et al. Prognostic parameters in endometrial stromal sarcoma: a clinicopathologic study in 31 patients. *Gynecol Oncol.* 2001;81(2):160–165.
246. Tanz R, Mahfound T, Bazine A, et al. Endometrial stromal sarcoma: prognostic factors and impact of adjuvant therapy in early stages. *Hematol Oncol Stem Cell Ther.* 2012;5:31–35.
247. Malouf GG, Duclos J, Rey A, et al. Impact of adjuvant treatment modalities on the management of patients with stage I-II endometrial sarcoma. *Ann Oncol.* 2010:21:2102–2106.
248. Geller MA, Argenta P, Bradley W, et al. Treatment and recurrence patterns in endometrial stromal sarcomas and the relation to c-kit. *Gynecol Oncol.* 2004;95:632–636.
249. Valduvieco I, Rovirosa A, Colomo L, et al. Endometrial stromal sarcoma. Is there a place for radiotherapy? *Clin Transl Oncol.* 2010;12:226–230.
250. Rios I, Rovirosa A, Morales J, et al. Undifferentiated uterine sarcoma: A rare, not well known aggressive disease: Report of 13 cases. *Arch Gynecol Obstet* 2014; 290:993–997.
251. Weitmann HD, Knocke TH, Kucera H et al. Radiation therapy in the treatment of endometrial stromal sarcoma. *Int J Radiat Oncol Biol Phys* 2001; 49:739–748.
252. Barney B, Tward JD, Skidmore T, et al. Does radiotherapy or lymphadenectomy improve survival in endometrial stromal sarcoma? Int *J Gynecol Cancer* 2009; 19:1232–1238.
253. Leath CA, Huh WK, Hyde Jr, A multi-institutional review of outcomes of endometrial stromal sarcoma. *Gynecol Oncol* 2007; 105:630–634.
254. Chan JK, Kawar NM, Shin JY, et al. Endometrial stromal sarcoma: A population-based analysis. *Br J Cancer* 2008: 99:1210–1215.
255. Rose PG, Piver MS, Tsukada Y, et al. Patterns of metastasis in uterine sarcoma: an autopsy study. *Cancer.* 1989;63:935–938.
256. Pervaiz N, Colterjohn N, Farrokhyar F, et al. A systematic meta-analysis of randomized controlled trials of adjuvant chemotherapy for localized resectable soft-tissue sarcoma. *Cancer.* 2008;113:573–581.
257. Odunsi K, Moneke V, Tammela J, et al. Efficacy of adjuvant CYVADIC chemotherapy in early-stage uterine sarcomas: results of long-term follow-up. *Int J Gynecol Cancer.* 2004;14:659–664.
258. Piver MS, Lele SB, Marchetti DL, et al. Effect of adjuvant chemotherapy on time to recurrence and survival of stage I uterine sarcomas. *J Surg Oncol.* 1988;38:233–239.
259. Hempling RE, Piver MS, Baker TR. Impact on progression-free survival of adjuvant cyclophosphamide, vincristine, doxorubicin (Adriamycin), and dacarbazine (CYVADIC) chemotherapy for stage I uterine sarcoma. A prospective trial. *Am J Clin Oncol.* 1995;18:282–286.
260. Wong C, Lele SB, Natarajan N. Effect of adjuvant chemotherapy on long-term survival of stage I uterine sarcoma. *Proc Am Soc Clin Oncol.* 1999;18:386 (abstract 1492).
261. Resnik E, Chambers SK, Carcangiu ML, et al. A phase II study of etoposide, cisplatin, and doxorubicin chemotherapy in mixed Müllerian tumors (MMT) of the uterus. *Gynecol Oncol.* 1995;56:370–375.
262. Sutton G, Kauderer J, Carson LF, et al. Adjuvant ifosfamide and cisplatin in patients with completely resected stage I or II carcinosarcomas (mixed mesodermal tumors) of the uterus: a Gynecologic Oncology Group study. *Gynecol Oncol.* 2005;96:630–634.
263. Makker V, Abu-Rustum NR, Alektiar KM, et al. A retrospective assessment of outcomes of chemotherapy-based versus radiation-only adjuvant treatment for completely resected stage I–IV uterine carcinosarcoma. *Gynecol Oncol.* 2008;111(2):249–254.
264. Hensley ML, Blessing JA, Degeest K, et al. Fixed-dose rate gemcitabine plus docetaxel as second-line therapy for metastatic uterine leiomyosarcoma: a Gynecologic Oncology Group phase II study. *Gynecol Oncol.* 2008;109:323–328.
265. Hensley ML, Blessing JA, Mannel R, et al. Fixed-dose rate gemcitabine plus docetaxel as first-line therapy for metastatic uterine leiomyosarcoma: a Gynecologic Oncology Group phase II trial. *Gynecol Oncol.* 2008;109:329–334.
266. Hensley ML, Wathen K, et al. Adjuvant treatment of high-risk primary uterine leiomyosarcoma with gemcitabine/docetaxel (GT), followed by doxorubicin (D): results of phase II multicenter trial SARC005.ASCO meeting abstracts. *J Clin Oncol.* 2010;28(Suppl 15):10021.
267. Hensley ML, Wathen JK, Maki RG, et al. Adjuvant therapy for high-grade, uterus-limited leiomyosarcoma: results of a phase 2 trial (SARC 005). *Cancer.* 2013;119:1555–1561.
268. Hensley ML, Wathen JK, Maki RG, et al. Adjuvant therapy for high-grade, uterus-limited leiomyosarcoma: results of a phase 2 trial (SARC 005). *Cancer.* 2013;119(8):1555–1561.
269. Hensley ML. Phase III randomized study of adjuvant chemotherapy comprising gemcitabine hydrochloride and docetaxel followed by doxorubicin hydrochloride versus observation in patients with uterus-limited, high-grade uterine leiomyosarcoma. https://clinicaltrials.gov/ct2/show/NCT01533207
270. Chu MC, Mor G, Lim C, et al. Low-grade endometrial stromal sarcoma: hormonal aspects. *Gynecol Oncol.* 2003;90:170–176.
271. Shi Y, Liu Z, Peng Z, et al. The diagnosis and treatment of Mullerian adenosarcoma of the uterus. *Aust N Z J Obstet Gynaecol.* 2008;48:596–600.
272. Tanner EJ, Toussaint T, Leitao MM Jr, et al. Management of uterine adenosarcomas with and without sarcomatous overgrowth. *Gynecol Oncol.* 2013;129:140–144.
273. Crist WM, Anderson JR, Meza JL, et al. Intergroup Rhabdomyosarcoma Study-IV: results for patients with nonmetastatic disease. *J Clin Oncol* 2001;19:3091–3102.
274. Herrmann K. 18F-FDG-PET/CT Imaging as an early survival predictor in patients with primary high-grade soft tissue sarcomas undergoing neoadjuvant therapy. *Clin Cancer Res.* 2012;18:2024–2031.
275. Sutton G, Blessing J, Hanjani P, et al. Phase II evaluation of liposomal doxorubicin (Doxil) in recurrent or advanced leiomyosarcoma of the uterus: a Gynecologic Oncology Group study. *Gynecol Oncol.* 2005;96:749–752.
276. Miller DS, Blessing JA, Ball H, et al. Phase II trial of topotecan in patients with advanced, persistent, or recurrent uterine leiomyosarcomas: a Gynecologic Oncology Group study. *Am J Clin Oncol.* 2000;23:355–357.
277. Sutton G, Blessing JA, Ball H. Phase II trial of paclitaxel in leiomyosarcoma of the uterus: a Gynecologic Oncology Group study. *Gynecol Oncol.* 1999;74:346–349.
278. Sutton G, Blessing JA, Barrett RJ, et al. Phase II trial of ifosfamide and mesna in leiomyosarcoma of the uterus: a Gynecologic Oncology Group study. *Am J Obstet Gynecol.* 1992;166:556–559.
279. Thigpen T, Blessing JA, Yordan E, et al. Phase II trial of etoposide in leiomyosarcoma of the uterus: a Gynecologic Oncology group study. *Gynecol Oncol.* 1996;63:120–122.
280. Thigpen T, Blessing JA, Beecham J, et al. Phase II trial of cisplatin as first-line chemotherapy in patients with advanced or recurrent uterine sarcomas: a Gynecologic Oncology Group study. *J Clin Oncol.* 1991;9:1962–1966.
281. Omura GA, Major FJ, Blessing JA, et al. A randomized study of Adriamycin with and without dimethyl triazenoimidazole carboxamide in advanced uterine sarcomas. *Cancer.* 1983;52:626–632.
282. Thigpen JT, Blessing JA, Homesley HD, et al. Phase II trial of piperazinedione in patients with advanced or recurrent uterine sarcoma. A Gynecologic Oncology Group study. *Am J Clin Oncol.* 1985;8:350–352.
283. Asbury R, Blessing JA, Smith DM, et al. Aminothiadiazole in the treatment of advanced leiomyosarcoma of the uterine corpus. A Gynecologic Oncology Group study. *Am J Clin Oncol.* 1995;18:397–399.
284. Slayton RE, Blessing JA, Look K, et al. A phase II clinical trial of diaziquone (AZQ) in the treatment of patients with recurrent leiomyosarcoma of

the uterus, a Gynecologic Oncology Group study. *Invest New Drugs.* 1991;9:207–208.
285. Look K, Sandler A, Blessing JA, et al. Phase II trial of gemcitabine as second-line chemotherapy of uterine leiomyosarcoma: a Gynecologic Oncology Group study. *Gynecol Oncol.* 2004;92:644–647.
286. Svancarova L, Blay JY, Judson IR, et al. Gemcitabine in advanced adult soft-tissue sarcomas. A phase II study of the EORTC Soft Tissue and Bone Sarcoma Group. *Eur J Cancer.* 2002;38:556–559.
287. Okuno S, Edmonson J, Mahoney M, et al. Phase II trial of gemcitabine in advanced sarcomas. *Cancer.* 2002;94:3225–3229.
288. Patel SR, Gandhi V, Jenkins J, et al. Phase II clinical investigation of gemcitabine in advanced soft tissue sarcomas and window evaluation of dose rate on gemcitabine triphosphate accumulation. *J Clin Oncol.* 2001;19:3483–3489.
289. Gallup DG, Blessing JA, Andersen W, et al. Evaluation of paclitaxel in previously treated leiomyosarcoma of the uterus: a Gynecologic Oncology Group study. *Gynecol Oncol.* 2003;89:48–51.
290. Yovine A, Riofrio M, Blay JY, et al. Phase II study of ecteinascidin-743 in advanced pretreated soft tissue sarcoma patients. *J Clin Oncol.* 2004;22:890–899.
291. Twelves C, Hoekman K, Bowman A, et al. Phase I and pharmacokinetic study of YondelisTM (Ecteinascidin-743; ET-743) administered as an infusion over 1 h or 3 h every 21 days in patients with solid tumours. *Eur J Cancer.* 2003;339:1842–1851.
292. Garcia-Carbonero R, Supko JG, Maki RG, et al. Ecteinascidin-743 (ET-743) for chemotherapy-naïve patients with advanced soft tissue sarcomas: multicenter phase II and pharmacokinetic study. *J Clin Oncol.* 2005;23:5484–5492.
293. Smith HO, Blessing JA, Vaccarello L. Trimetrexate in the treatment of recurrent or advanced leiomyosarcoma of the uterus: a phase II study of the Gynecologic Oncology Group. *Gynecol Oncol.* 2002;84:140–144.
294. Rose PG, Blessing JA, Soper JT, et al. Prolonged oral etoposide in recurrent or advanced leiomyosarcoma of the uterus: a Gynecologic Oncology Group study. *Gynecol Oncol.* 1998;70:267–271.
295. Slayton RE, Blessing JA, Angel C, et al. Phase II trial of etoposide in the management of advanced and recurrent leiomyosarcoma of the uterus: a Gynecologic Oncology Group study. *Cancer Treat Rep.* 1987;71:1303–1304.
296. Asbury R, Blessing JA, Buller R, et al. Amonafide in patients with leiomyosarcoma of the uterus: a phase II gynecologic oncology group study. *Am J Clin Oncol.* 1998;21:145–146.
297. Muss HB, Bundy BN, Adcock L, et al. Mitoxantrone in the treatment of advanced uterine sarcoma. A phase II trial of the Gynecologic Oncology Group. *Am J Clin Oncol.* 1990;13:32–34.
298. Thigpen JT, Blessing JA, Wilbanks GD. Cisplatin as second-line chemotherapy in the treatment of advanced or recurrent leiomyosarcoma of the uterus. A phase II trial of the Gynecologic Oncology Group. *Am J Clin Oncol.* 1986;9:18–20.
299. Fidias P, Demetri G, Harmon DC, et al. Navelbine shows activity in previously treated sarcoma patients: phase II results from MGH/Dana Farber/Partner's Cancer Care Study. *Proc Am Soc Clin Oncol.* 1998;abstract 1977.
300. Talbot SM, Keohan ML, et al. A phase II trial of temozolomide in patients with unresectable or metastatic soft tissue sarcoma. *Cancer.* 2003;98:1942–1946.
301. Pautier P, Floquet A, Penel N, et al. Randomized multicenter and stratified phase II study of gemcitabine alone versus gemcitabine and docetaxel in patients with metastatic or relapsed leiomyosarcomas: a Federation Nationale des Centres de Lutte Contre le Cancer (FNCLCC) French Sarcoma Group Study (TAXOGEM study). *Oncologist.* 2012;17:1213–1220.
302. Monk BJ, Blessing JA, Street DG, et al. A phase II evaluation of trabectedin in the treatment of advanced, persistent, or recurrent uterine leiomyosarcoma: a Gynecologic Oncology Group study. *Gynecol Oncol.* 2012;124:48–52.
303. Demetri GD, von Mehren M, Jones RL, et al. Efficacy and safety of trabectedin or dacarbazine for metastatic liposarcoma or leiomyosarcoma after failure of conventional chemotherapy: results of a phase III randomized multicenter clinical trial. *J Clin Oncol.* 2016;34:786–793.
304. Takano T, Niikura H, Ito K, et al. Feasibility study of gemcitabine plus docetaxel in advanced or recurrent uterine leiomyosarcoma and undifferentiated endometrial sarcoma in Japan. *Int J Clin Oncol.* 2014;19(5):897–905.
305. Verweij J, Lee SM, et al. Randomized phase II study of docetaxel versus doxorubicin in first- and second-line chemotherapy for locally advanced or metastatic soft tissue sarcomas in adults: a study of the European Organization for Research and Treatment of Cancer Soft Tissue and Bone Sarcoma Group. *J Clin Oncol.* 2000;18:2081–2086.
306. Schoffski P, Ray-Coquard IL, et al. Activity of eribulin mesylate in patients with soft-tissue sarcoma: a phase 2 study in four independent histological subtypes. *Lancet Oncol.* 2011;12:1045–1052.
307. Long H 3rd, Blessing JA, Sorosky J. Phase II trial of dacarbazine, mitomycin, doxorubicin, and cisplatin with sargramostim in uterine leiomyosarcoma: a Gynecologic Oncology Group study. *Gynecol Oncol.* 2005;99:339–342.
308. Edmonson JH, Marks RS, Buckner JC, et al. Contrast of response to dacarbazine, mitomycin, doxorubicin, and cisplatin (DMAP) plus GM-CSF between patients with advanced malignant gastrointestinal stromal tumors and patients with other advanced leiomyosarcomas. *Cancer Invest.* 2002;20:605–612.
309. Edmonson JH, Blessing JA, Cosin JA, et al. Phase II study of mitomycin, doxorubicin and cisplatin in the treatment of advanced uterine leiomyosarcoma: a Gynecologic Oncology Group study. *Gynecol Oncol.* 2002;85:507–510.
310. Currie J, Blessing JA, Muss HB, et al. Combination chemotherapy with hydroxyurea, dacarbazine (DTIC), and etoposide in the treatment of uterine leiomyosarcoma: a Gynecologic Oncology Group study. *Gynecol Oncol.* 1996;61:27–30.
311. Sutton G, Blessing JA, Malfetano JH. Ifosfamide and doxorubicin in the treatment of advanced leiomyosarcoma of the uterus: a Gynecologic Oncology Group study. *Gynecol Oncol.* 1996;62:226–229.
312. Hensley ML, Maki R, Venkatraman E, et al. Gemcitabine and docetaxel in patients with unresectable leiomyosarcoma: results of a phase II trial. *J Clin Oncol.* 2002;20:2824–2831.
313. Muss HB, Bundy B, DiSaia PJ, et al. Treatment of recurrent or advanced uterine sarcoma. A randomized trial of doxorubicin versus doxorubicin and cyclophosphamide (a phase III trial of the Gynecologic Oncology Group). *Cancer.* 1985;15:1648–1653.
314. Dileo P, Morgan JA, Zahrieh D, et al. Gemcitabine and vinorelbine combination chemotherapy for patients with advanced soft tissue sarcomas: results of a phase II trial. *Cancer.* 2007;109:1863–1869.
315. Hensley ML, Anderson S, et al. Activity of gemcitabine plus docetaxel in leiomyosarcoma (LMS) and other histologies: report of an expanded phase II trial [Meeting Abstracts]. *J Clin Oncol.* 2004;22:9010.
316. Boyar MS, Hesdorffer M, Keohan ML, et al. Phase II study of temozolomide and thalidomide in patients with unresectable or metastatic leiomyosarcoma. *Sarcoma.* 2008;2008:412–503.
317. Garcia-Del-Muro X, Lopez-Pousa A, Maurel J, et al. Randomized phase II study comparing gemcitabine plus dacarbazine versus dacarbazine alone in patients with previously treated soft tissue sarcoma: a Spanish Group for Research on Sarcomas Study. *J Clin Oncol.* 2011;29:2528–2533.
318. Campos SM, Brady WE, Moxley KM, et al. A phase II evaluation of pazopanib in the treatment of recurrent or persistent carcinosarcoma of the uterus: a gynecologic oncology study group. *Gynecol Oncol* 2014;133:537–541.
319. Kanjeekal S, Chambers A, Fung MF, et al. Systemic therapy for advanced uterine sarcoma: a systemic review of the literature. *Gynecol Oncol.* 2005;97:624–637.
320. Pautier P, Floquet A, Chevreau C, et al. Trabectedin in combination with doxorubicin for first-line treatment of advanced uterine or soft-tissue leiomyosarcoma (LMS-02): a non-randomised, multicentre, phase 2 trial. *Lancet Oncol.* 2015;16:457–464.
321. Seddon BM, Whelan J, Strauss SJ, et al. GeDDiS: A prospective randomised controlled phase III trial of gemcitabine and docetaxel compared with doxorubicin as first-line treatment in previously untreated advanced unresectable or metastatic soft tissue sarcomas (EudraCT 2009-014907-29). *J Clin Oncol.* 2015;33 Suppl:abstract 10500.
322. Homesley HD, Filiaci V, Markman M, et al. Phase III trial of ifosfamide with or without paclitaxel in advanced uterine carcinosarcomas: a Gynecologic Oncology Group study. *J Clin Oncol.* 2007;25:526–531.
323. Sutton G, Brunetto VL, Kilgore L, et al. A phase III trial of ifosfamide with or without cisplatin in carcinosarcomas of the uterus: a Gynecologic Oncology Group study. *Gynecol Oncol.* 2000;79:147–153.
324. Sutton G, Blessing JA, Rosenshein N, et al. Phase II trial of ifosfamide and mesna in mixed mesodermal tumors of the uterus: a Gynecologic Oncology Group study. *Am J Obstet Gynecol.* 1989;161:309–312.
325. Gershenson DM, Kavanagh JJ, Copeland LJ, et al. High-dose doxorubicin infusion therapy for disseminated mixed mesodermal sarcoma of the uterus. *Cancer.* 1987;59:1264–1267.
326. Miller DS, Blessing JA, Schilder J, et al. Phase II evaluation of topotecan in carcinosarcomas of the uterus: a Gynecologic Oncology Group study. *Gynecol Oncol.* 2005;98:217–221.
327. Fowler JM, Blessing JA, Burger RA, et al. Phase II evaluation of oral trimetrexate in mixed mesodermal tumors of the uterus: a Gynecologic Oncology Group study. *Gynecol Oncol.* 2002;85:311–314.

328. Curtin JP, Blessing JA, Soper JT, et al. Paclitaxel in the treatment of carcinosarcoma of the uterus: a Gynecologic Oncology Group study. *Gynecol Oncol.* 2001;83:268–270.
329. Asbury R, Blessing JA, Podczaski E, et al. A phase II trial of amonafide in patients with mixed mesodermal tumors of the uterus: a Gynecologic Oncology Group study. *Am J Clin Oncol.* 1998;21:306–307.
330. Asbury R, Blessing JA, Moore D. A phase II trial of aminothiadiazole in patients with mixed mesodermal tumors of the uterine corpus: a Gynecologic Oncology Group study. *Am J Clin Oncol.* 1996;19:400–402.
331. Slayton RE, Blessing JA, Clarke-Pearson D. A phase II trial of diaziquone (AZQ) in mixed mesodermal sarcomas of the uterus. *Invest New Drugs.* 1991;9:93–94.
332. Slayton RE, Blessing JA, DiSaia PJ, et al. Phase II trial of etoposide in the management of advanced or recurrent mixed mesodermal sarcomas of the uterus: a Gynecologic Oncology Group study. *Cancer Treat Rep.* 1987;71:661–662.
333. Thigpen JT, Blessing JA, Orr JW Jr, et al. Phase II trial of cisplatin in the treatment of patients with advanced or recurrent mixed mesodermal sarcomas of the uterus: a Gynecologic Oncology Group study. *Cancer Treat Rep.* 1986;70:271–274.
334. Gershenson DM, Kavanagh JJ, Copeland LJ, et al. Cisplatin therapy for disseminated mixed mesodermal sarcoma of the uterus. *J Clin Oncol.* 1987;5:618–621.
335. Duska LR, Blessing JA, Rotmensch J, et al. A Phase II evaluation of ixabepilone (IND #59699, NSC #710428) in the treatment of recurrent or persistent leiomyosarcoma of the uterus: an NRG Oncology/Gynecologic Oncology Group Study. *Gynecol Oncol.* 2014;135:44–48.
336. Currie J, Blessing JA, McGehee R, et al. Phase II trial of hydroxyurea, dacarbazine (DTIC), and etoposide (VP-16) in mixed mesodermal tumors of the uterus: a Gynecologic Oncology Group study. *Gynecol Oncol.* 1996;61:94–96.
337. Piver MS, DeEulis TG, Lele SB, et al. Cyclophosphamide, vincristine, Adriamycin, and dimethyl-triazeno imidazole carboxamide (CYVADIC) for sarcomas of the female genital tract. *Gynecol Oncol.* 1982;14:319–323.
338. van Rijswijk RE, Vermorken JB, Reed N, et al. Cisplatin, doxorubicin and ifosfamide in carcinosarcomas of the female genital tract. A phase II study of the European Organization for Research and Treatment of Cancer Gynaecological Cancer Group (EORTC 55923). *Eur J Cancer.* 2003;39:481–487.
339. Powell MA, Filiaci VL, Rose PG, et al. Phase II evaluation of paclitaxel and carboplatin in the treatment of carcinosarcoma of the uterus: A Gynecologic Oncology Group Study. *J Clin Oncol.* 2010;28:2727–2731.
340. Lacour RA, Euscher E, Atkinson EN, et al. A phase II trial of paclitaxel and carboplatin in women with advanced or recurrent uterine carcinosarcoma. *Int J Gynecol Cancer.* 2011;21:517–522.
341. Aghajanian C, Sill MW, Secord AA, et al. Iniparib plus paclitaxel and carboplatin as initial treatment of advanced or recurrent uterine carcinosarcoma: a Gynecologic Oncology Group Study. *Gynecol Oncol.* 2012;126:424–427.
342. Galaal K, Godfrey K, Naik R, et al. Adjuvant radiotherapy and/or chemotherapy after surgery for uterine carcinosarcoma. *Cochrane Database Syst Rev.* 2011;(1):CD006812.
343. Miller BE, Blessing JA, Stehman FB, et al. A phase II evaluation of weekly gemcitabine and docetaxel for second-line treatment of recurrent carcinosarcoma of the uterus: a gynecologic oncology group study. *Gynecol Oncol.* 2010;118:139–144.
344. Spano JP, Soria JC, Kambouchner M, et al. Long-term survival of patients given hormonal therapy for metastatic endometrial stromal sarcoma. *Med Oncol.* 2003;20:87–93.
345. Sutton G, Blessing JA, Park R, et al. Ifosfamide treatment of recurrent or metastatic endometrial stromal sarcomas previously unexposed to chemotherapy: a study of the Gynecologic Oncology Group. *Obstet Gynecol.* 1996;87:747–750.
346. Berchuck A, Rubin SC, Hoskins WJ, et al. Treatment of endometrial stromal tumors. *Gynecol Oncol.* 1990;36:60–65.
347. Szlosarek PW, Lofts FJ, Pettengell R, et al. Effective treatment of a patient with a high-grade endometrial stromal sarcoma with an accelerated regimen of carboplatin and paclitaxel. *Anticancer Drugs.* 2000;11:275–278.
348. Yamawaki T, Shimizu Y, Hasumi K. Treatment of stage IV "high-grade" endometrial stromal sarcoma with ifosfamide, Adriamycin, and cisplatin. *Gynecol Oncol.* 1997;64:265–269.
349. Ihnen M, Mahner S, Janicke F, et al. Current treatment options in uterine endometrial stromal sarcoma: report of a case and review of the literature. *Int J Gynecol Cancer.* 2007;17:957–963.
350. Lehner LM, Miles PA, Enck RE. Complete remission of widely metastatic endometrial stromal sarcoma following combination chemotherapy. *Cancer.* 1979;433:1189–1194.
351. Lin YC, Kudelka AP, Tresukosol D, et al. Prolonged stabilization of progressive endometrial stromal sarcoma with prolonged oral etoposide therapy. *Gynecol Oncol.* 1995;58:262–265.
352. Tanner EJ Toussaint T, Leitao MM Jr, et al. Management of uterine adenosarcomas with and without sarcomatous overgrowth. *Gynecol Oncol.* 2013;129(1):140–144.
353. Carroll A, Ramirez PT, Westin SN, et al. Uterine adenosarcoma: an analysis on management, outcomes, and risk factors for recurrence. *Gynecol Oncol.* 2014;135:455–461.
354. Thomas MB, Keeney GL, Podratz KC, et al. Endometrial stromal sarcoma: treatment and patterns of recurrence. *Int J Gynecol Cancer.* 2009;19:253–256.
355. Sutton G, Blessing JA, Park R, et al. Ifosfamide treatment of recurrent or metastatic endometrial stromal sarcomas previously unexposed to chemotherapy: a study of the Gynecologic Oncology Group. *Obstet Gynecol.* 1996;87:747–750.
356. Bleeker JS, Quevedo JF, Folpe AL, et al. "Malignant" perivascular epithelioid cell neoplasm: risk stratification and treatment strategies. *Sarcoma.* 2012;2012:541626.
357. Wagner AJ, Malinowska-Kolodziej I, Morgan JA, et al. Clinical activity of mTOR inhibition with sirolimus in malignant perivascular epithelioid cell tumors: targeting the pathogenic activation of mTORC1 in tumors. *J Clin Oncol.* 2010;28:835–840.
358. Schoffski P, Maki RG, Italiano A, et al. Randomized, open-label multicenter, phase III study of eribulin versus dacarbazine in patients (pts) with leiomyosarcoma (LMS) and adipocytic sarcoma (ADI). *J Clin Oncol.* 2015;33 Suppl:abstract LBA10502.
359. Sutton GP, Stehman FB, Michael H, et al. Estrogen and progesterone receptors in uterine sarcomas. *Obstet Gynecol.* 1986;68:709–714.
360. McCluggage WG, Abdulkader M, Price JH, et al. Uterine carcinosarcomas in patients receiving tamoxifen. A report of 19 cases. *Int J Gynecol Cancer.* 2000;10:280–284.
361. Kloos I, Delaloge S, Pautier P, et al. Tamoxifen-related carcinosarcomas occur under/after prolonged treatment: report of five cases and review of the literature. *Int J Gynecol Cancer.* 2002;12:496–500.
362. Burke C, Hickey K. Treatment of endometrial stromal sarcoma with a gonadotropin-releasing hormone analogue. *Obstet Gynecol.* 2004;104:1182–1184.
363. Maluf FC, Sabbatini P, Schwartz L, et al. Endometrial stromal sarcoma: objective response to letrozole. *Gynecol Oncol.* 2001;82:384–388.
364. Lantta M, Kahanpaa K, Karkkainen J, et al. Estradiol and progesterone receptors in two cases of endometrial stromal sarcoma. *Gynecol Oncol.* 1984;18:233–239.
365. Baker TR, Piver MS, Lele SB, et al. Stage I uterine adenosarcoma: a report of six cases. *J Surg Oncol.* 1988;37:128–132.
366. Piver MS, Rutledge FN, Copeland L, et al. Uterine endolymphatic stromal myosis. *Obstet Gynecol.* 1984;63:725–745.
367. Scribner DR Jr, Walker JL. Low-grade endometrial stromal sarcoma: preoperative treatment with depo-lupron and megace. *Gynecol Oncol.* 1998;71:458–460.
368. Navarro D, Cabrera JJ, Leon L, et al. Endometrial stromal sarcoma expression of estrogen receptors, progesterone receptors and estrogen-induced srp27 (24K) suggests hormone responsiveness. *J Steroid Biochem Mol Biol.* 1992;41:589–596.
369. Mansi JL, Ramachandra S, Wiltshaw E, et al. Endometrial stromal sarcomas. *Gynecol Oncol.* 1990;36:113–118.
370. O'Brien AA, O'Briain DS, Daly PA. Aggressive endometrial stromal sarcoma responding to medroxyprogesterone following failure of tamoxifen and combination chemotherapy. Case report. *Br J Obstet Gynaecol.* 1985;92:862–866.
371. Pink D, Lindner T, Mrozek A, et al. Harm or benefit of hormonal treatment in metastatic low-grade endometrial stromal sarcoma: single center experience with 10 cases and review of the literature. *Gynecol Oncol.* 2006;101:464–469.
372. Ramondetta LM, Johnson AJ, Sun CC, et al. Phase 2 trial of mifepristone (RU-486) in advanced or recurrent endometrioid adenocarcinoma or low-grade endometrial stromal sarcoma. *Cancer.* 2009;115:1867–1874.
373. Krumholz BA, Lobovsky FY, Halitsky V. Endolymphatic stromal myosis with pulmonary metastases. Remission with progestin therapy: report of a case. *J Reprod Med.* 1973;10:85–89.
374. O'Cearbhaill R, Zhou Q, Iasonos A, et al. Treatment of advanced uterine leiomyosarcoma with aromatase inhibitors. *Gynecol Oncol.* 2010;116:424–429.
375. George S, Feng Y, Manola J, et al. Phase 2 trial of aromatase inhibition with letrozole in patients with uterina leiomyosarcomas expressing estrogen and/or progesterone receptors. Cancer. 2014;120:738–743.
376. Wang X, Tangjitgamol S, Liu J, et al. Response of recurrent uterine high-grade malignant mixed Müllerian tumor to letrozole. *Int J Gynecol Cancer.* 2005;15:1243–1248.

377. Maki RG. Recent advances in therapy for gastrointestinal stromal tumors. *Curr Oncol Rep.* 2007;9:165–169.
378. Rushing RS, Shajahan S, Chendil D, et al. Uterine sarcomas express KIT protein but lack mutation(s) in exon 11 or 17 of c-KIT. *Gynecol Oncol.* 2003;91:9–14.
379. Winter WE 3rd, Seidman JD, Krivak TC, et al. Clinicopathological analysis of c-kit expression in carcinosarcomas and leiomyosarcomas of the uterine corpus. *Gynecol Oncol.* 2003;91:3–8.
380. Huh WK, Sill MW, Darcy KM, et al. Efficacy and safety of imatinib mesylate (Gleevec) and immunohistochemical expression of c-Kit and PDGFR-beta in a Gynecologic Oncology Group Phase II Trial in women with recurrent or persistent carcinosarcomas of the uterus. *Gynecol Oncol.* 2010;117:248–254.
381. Hensley ML, Sill MW, Scribner DR, et al. Sunitinib malate in the treatment of recurrent or persistent uterine leiomyosarcoma: a Gynecologic Oncology Group phase II study. *Gynecol Oncol.* 2009;115:460–465.
382. Emoto M, Ishiguro M, Iwasaki H, et al. Effect of angiogenesis inhibitor TNP-470 on the growth, blood flow, and microvessel density in xenografts of human uterine carcinosarcoma in nude mice. *Gynecol Oncol.* 2003;89:88–94.
383. Yi-Shin Kuo D, Timmins P, Blank SV, et al. Phase II trial of thalidomide for advanced and recurrent gynecologic sarcoma: a brief communication from the New York Phase II consortium. *Gynecol Oncol.* 2006;100:160–165.
384. McMeekin DS, Sill MW, Darcy KM, et al. A phase II trial of thalidomide in patients with refractory leiomyosarcoma of the uterus and correlation with biomarkers of angiogenesis: a gynecologic oncology group study. *Gynecol Oncol.* 2007;106:596–603.
385. Maki RG, D'Adamo DR, Keohan ML, et al. Phase II study of Sorafenib in patients with metastatic or recurrent sarcomas. *J Clin Oncol.* 2009;27:3133–3140.
386. Mackay HJ, Buckanovich RJ, Hirte H, et al. A phase II study single agent of aflibercept (VEGF Trap) in patients with recurrent or metastatic gynecologic carcinosarcomas and uterine leiomyosarcoma. A trial of the Princess Margaret Hospital, Chicago and California Cancer Phase II Consortia. *Gynecol Oncol.* 2012;125:136–140.
387. Campos SM, Brady WE, Moxley KM, et al. A phase II evaluation of pazopanib in the treatment of recurrent or persistent carcinosarcoma of the uterus: a gynecologic oncology group study. *Gynecol Oncol.* 2014;133:537–541.
388. Sleijfer S, Ray-Coquard I, Papai Z, et al. Pazopanib, a multikinase angiogenesis inhibitor, in patients with relapsed or refractory advanced soft tissue sarcoma: a phase II study from the European organisation for research and treatment of cancer-soft tissue and bone sarcoma group (EORTC study 62043). *J Clin Oncol.* 2009;27:3126–3132.
389. van der Graaf WT, Blay JY, Chawla SP, et al. Pazopanib for metastatic soft-tissue sarcoma (PALETTE): a randomised, double-blind, placebo-controlled phase 3 trial. *Lancet.* 2012;379:1879–1886.
390. D'Adamo DR, Anderson SE, Albritton K, et al. Phase II study of doxorubicin and bevacizumab for patients with metastatic soft-tissue sarcomas. *J Clin Oncol.* 2005;23:7135–7142.
391. Hensley ML, Miller A, O'Malley DM, et al. Randomized phase III trial of gemcitabine plus docetaxel plus bevacizumab or placebo as first-line treatment for metastatic uterine leiomyosarcoma: an NRG Oncology/Gynecologic Oncology Group study. J Clin Oncol. 2015;33:1180–1185.
392. Hu J, Khanna V, Jones M, et al. Genomic alterations in uterine leiomyosarcomas: potential markers for clinical diagnosis and prognosis. *Genes Chromosomes Cancer.* 2001;31:117–124.
393. Chawla SP, Staddon AP, Baker LH, et al. Phase II study of the mammalian target of rapamycin inhibitor ridaforolimus in patients with advanced bone and soft tissue sarcomas. *J Clin Oncol.* 2012;30:78–84.
394. Colombo N, McMeekin DS, Schwartz PE, et al. Ridaforolimus as a single agent in advanced endometrial cancer: results of a single arm, phase 2 trial. *Br J Cancer.* 2013;108:1021–1026.
395. Blay J, Chawla SP, Ray-Coquard, et al. Phase III, placebo-controlled trial (SUCCEED) evaluating ridaforolimus as maintenance therapy in advanced sarcoma patients following clinical benefit from prior standard cytotoxic chemotherapy: long-term (>= 24 months) overall survival results. ASCO meeting abstracts. *J Clin Oncol.* 2012;30(15 Suppl): 10010.
396. Bolden JE, Shi W, Jankowski K, et al. HDAC inhibitors induce tumor-cell-selective pro-apoptotic transcriptional responses. *Cell Death Dis.* 2013;4:e519.
397. Hyman DM, Sill M, Cho JK, et al. A phase II study of alisertib (MLN8237) in recurrent or persistent uterine leiomyosarcoma: an NRG Oncology/Gynecologic Oncology Group Study (GOG-0231D). *J Clin Oncol.* 2015;33 Suppl:abstr e16512.
398. Hensley ML, Miller A, O'Malley DM, et al. Randomized phase III trial of gemcitabine plus docetaxel plus bevacizumab or placebo as first-line treatment for metastatic uterine leiomyosarcoma: an NRG Oncology/Gynecologic Oncology Group study. *J Clin Oncol.* 2015;33(10): 1180–1185.
399. Lacour RA, Euscher E, Atkinson EN, et al. A phase II trial of paclitaxel and carboplatin in women with advanced or recurrent uterine carcinosarcoma. *Int J Gynecol Cancer.* 2011;21:517–522.
400. Campos SM, Brady WE, Moxley KM, et al. A phase II evaluation of pazopanib in the treatment of recurrent or persistent carcinosarcoma of the uterus: a Gynecologic Oncology Group Study. *Gynecol Oncol.* 2014;133:537–541.
401. Aghajanian C, Sill MW, Secord AA, et al. Iniparib plus paclitaxel and carboplatin as initial treatment of advanced or recurrent uterine carcinosarcoma: a Gynecologic Oncology Group Study. *Gynecol Oncol.* 2012;126:424–427.

CHAPTER 23

Epithelial Ovarian Cancer

Gini F. Fleming, Jeffrey D. Seidman, Anna Yemelyanova, and Ernst Lengyel

EPIDEMIOLOGY AND RISK FACTORS

In this chapter "ovarian cancer" will generally refer to a Müllerian cancer arising in the peritoneum, fallopian tube, or ovary. Established risk factors for ovarian cancer include genetic factors, including a known genetic predisposition (e.g., BRCA1/2 and hereditary nonpolyposis colorectal cancer [HNPCC]), and a strong family history for breast and ovarian cancer. Hormonal and reproductive factors include parity, breast-feeding, early menarche, late menopause, menopausal hormonal treatment, oral contraceptive (OCP) use, and endometriosis. The relative risks (RRs) associated with endocrinologic factors are small, though important because they are potentially subject to modulation. The most important risk factor, after having a first-degree relative with the disease, is age. Women younger than 40 years without a positive family history rarely have ovarian cancer. Fifty percent of all cases of ovarian cancer in the United States occur in women over the age of 65. A large meta-analysis including more than 1.3 million women showed clearly that most risk factors show heterogeneity across ovarian cancer histologic subtypes. Of 14 established risk factors including the 10 mentioned above, nine risk factors applied only to certain histologies. In general, reproductive and hormonal risk factors are more strongly associated with clear cell and endometrioid ovarian cancers (1). This suggests that there is no unifying etiology for "ovarian cancer" and that the different histologic subtypes must be considered separately to understand the specific risk profile, biology, and clinical behavior.

Epidemiology

Epithelial ovarian cancer is the leading cause of death from gynecologic cancer in the United States and Europe. Surveillance, Epidemiology, and End Results (SEER) data show that 22,280 new cases of ovarian cancer and 14,240 deaths from ovarian cancer are expected in the United States in 2016 (2). It is estimated that in the United States, 1 in 70 women will develop ovarian cancer, and 1 in 100 women will die of the disease. In Europe, the International Agency for Research on Cancer in Lyon estimated that there will be 44,100 new patients with ovarian cancer and 29,800 deaths in the 27 European reporting countries (3). In both the United States and Europe, ovarian cancer is the fifth most common cause of all cancer deaths in women. Estimates for the global ovarian cancer burden, which includes borderline cancers (the US and European numbers exclude them), are that 225,500 patients will develop epithelial ovarian cancer and about 140,200 will succumb to the disease per year.

Ovarian cancer rates vary between different countries and appear to be linked to socioeconomic status and reproductive patterns. North America and most of the industrialized countries of Europe have high incidence rates, whereas the disease is rare in Asia and Africa. The lowest rates of ovarian cancer are in sub-Saharan Africa (**Fig. 23.1**). Although the reasons for this difference are not well understood, countries with a high incidence rate are generally characterized by smaller family sizes, high-fat diets, higher socioeconomic status, older age, and a predominantly Caucasian population. Once a woman moves from a country with a low incidence of ovarian cancer to one with a high incidence, her risk for the disease tends to approach that of her adopted country rather than that of her country of origin. The fatality rate of ovarian cancer is high (70%), and 80% of deaths occur within 5 years of diagnosis. The age-adjusted mortality in the United States declined by 23% from 9.8/100,000/year to 7.5/100,000/year from 1975 to 2011. It has been hypothesized that this decline in mortality was largely caused by an earlier decline in ovarian cancer incidence, due, for the most part, to the known protective effect of

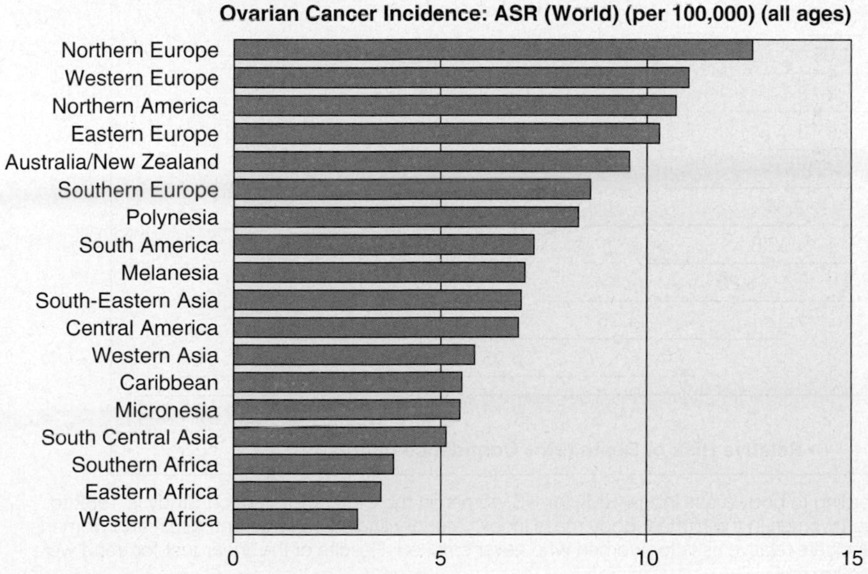

Figure 23.1. Age-standardized incidence rate (ASR) of ovarian cancer in the world.

Source: From Ferlay J, Bray F, Pisani P, et al. *GLOBOCAN 2000: Cancer Incidence, Mortality and Prevalence Worldwide, Version 1.0*. IARC Cancer Base No. 5. Lyon, France: IARC, with permission.

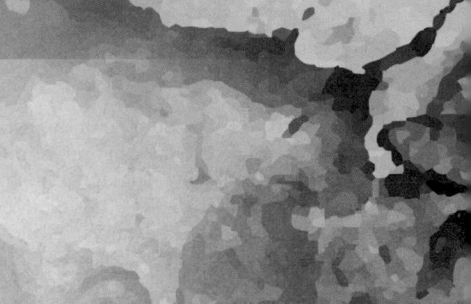

OCP, which were introduced in the 1960s. Today, 80% to 85% of US women have taken OCP at some point in their life. Paralleling the reduction in mortality, the age-adjusted ovarian cancer incidence fell by 26% from 16.3/100,000 women to 12.1/100,000 women (26%). The decline in incidence was then followed by a decline in mortality supporting the hypothesis that OCP contributed to this effect. Still, despite the widespread use of OCP, it is estimated that, because of the expanding and aging US population, the annual number of ovarian cancer cases will increase from 21,000 to 28,591 in the years from 2010 to 2030 (4).

Weight/Body Mass Index

Many epidemiologic studies have reported that height and weight are relevant to the risk of developing ovarian cancer, although the findings of these studies have been inconsistent. In a prospective cohort study that followed 495,477 women for 6 years, body mass index (BMI) and ovarian cancer mortality had a significant association (**Fig. 23.2**). For women with a BMI of 35 to 39, the RR of developing ovarian cancer was 1.5 (CI, 1.1–2), whereas the RR of developing endometrial cancer was 6.3 (CI, 3.8–10.4). In 2012, a meta-analysis that summarized 47 studies involving 25,157 women with ovarian cancer and 81,311 women without the disease found a small but significant increase in RR (1.07) of ovarian cancer per 5-cm increase in height. The RR for ovarian cancer per 5 kg/m^2 increase in BMI was 1.1 in women who did not take hormone replacement therapy (HRT) but only 0.95 in women on HRT (5). High BMI was associated with increased risk for borderline serous (recent BMI, OR, 1.24 per 5 kg/m^2; CI, 1.18–1.3), invasive endometrioid (OR, 1.17; CI, 1.11–1.23), and invasive mucinous (OR, 1.19; CI, 1.06–1.32) tumors. Low-grade serous invasive tumors (RR, 1.13; CI, 1.03–1.25), and high-grade serous invasive cancers in premenopausal women (RR, 1.11; CI, 1.04–1.18) were also associated with an increased BMI, but high-grade serous cancers were not (6). However, an analysis from the Ovarian Cancer Cohort Consortium including over 5,000 women with ovarian cancer did not show any significant association of BMI with ovarian cancer or with any subtype (1). Because obesity does not increase the risk of high-grade serous cancers, reducing BMI is unlikely to prevent most ovarian cancers. Given that the association of obesity and ovarian cancer is either weak or absent, it is possible that it can be attributed to confounding factors, such as type 2 diabetes, high-fat diet, or other factors that are currently unknown (7).

Reproductive Factors: Pregnancy and Breast-feeding

A number of epidemiologic studies have indicated that early menarche and late menopause increase the risk of ovarian cancer, although increased parity, breast-feeding, and use of OCP reduce that risk. Adding to this evidence are several case–control studies showing that pregnancy lowers ovarian cancer risk and that the risk reduction is greater with each additional pregnancy. The unifying feature of these reproductive factors is an increase or decrease in the number of ovulations that a woman experiences throughout her lifetime. However, a pregnancy after age 35 is more protective against ovarian cancer than a pregnancy in a woman 25 years or younger, regardless of the number of times she has given birth, suggesting that pregnancy at older ages involves mechanisms of risk reduction other than cessation of ovulation (8). There is no relationship between the timing of the last pregnancy and ovarian cancer survival. Women who breast-feed for longer than 12 months have a substantial reduction in the risk of ovarian cancer in addition to the risk reduction derived from childbirth, and this is likely to be related to suppression of ovulation (9). However, breast-feeding probably reduces ovarian cancer incidence through several additional mechanisms, including reduced serum concentrations of estradiol and luteinizing hormone (LH) and elevated levels of follicle-stimulating hormone (FSH).

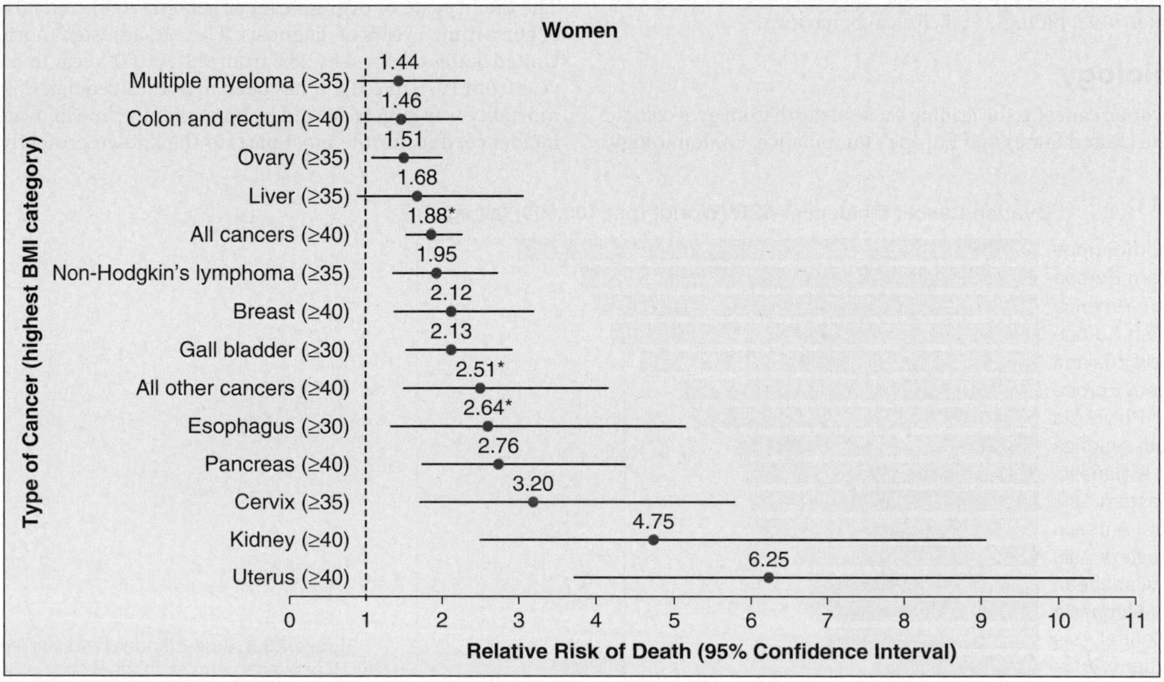

Figure 23.2. Summary of mortality from cancer according to body mass index (BMI) for US women in the Cancer Prevention Study II, 1982 to 1998. For each relative risk, the comparison was between women in the highest body mass index category (indicated in parentheses) and women in the reference category (BMI, 18.5 to 24.9). *Asterisks* indicate relative risks for women who never smoked. Results of the linear test for trend were significant ($p \leq 0.05$) for all cancer sites.

Source: Printed with permission from Calle EE, Rodriguez C, Walker-Thurmond K, et al. Overweight, obesity, and mortality from cancer in a prospectively studied cohort of U.S. adults. *N Engl J Med*. 2003;348:1625–1638.

Oral Contraceptives

Women who use OCP for at least 5 years reduce their risk of ovarian cancer by an average of 50%, with a concomitant decrease in mortality (10–12) (**Fig. 23.3**). Protection against ovarian cancer is probably the most important non-contraceptive benefit of OCP. The largest pooled analysis, a meta-analysis reanalyzing data from 45 epidemiologic studies, which included 23,257 women with ovarian cancer and 87,303 controls, showed that the use of OCP in high-income countries reduced ovarian cancer incidence from 1.2 to 0.8 and mortality from 0.7 to 0.5 per 100 users (10). The data also showed a solid duration–response relationship between ovarian cancer incidence and OCP use, because the level of protection conferred clearly increased with duration of use (12) (**Fig. 23.4**). In addition, the data confirmed that the protective effect continues for decades after OCPs are discontinued and suggested that the earlier a woman begins using OCP, the greater the reduction in her risk for developing ovarian cancer (12). An analysis stratifying the effects of OCP by histologic subtypes showed that a 5-year increase in OCP duration reduced the risk of serous, endometrioid, and clear cell cancer by 14% to 15% (1). However, it is unclear which is more important for a protective effect, the age at which women begin taking OCP or the duration of use. Interestingly, OCP had little effect on risk for mucinous ovarian cancers, which is consistent with the distinct biology of these tumors (13).

The mechanisms underlying the profound and long-lasting protection against ovarian cancer provided by OCP use are not well understood. The protective effects may be mediated by suppression of ovulation, reduction of gonadotropin levels, and/or induction of apoptosis (11). Moreover, OCPs suppress levels of FSH, LH, and estradiol, all of which can promote tumor cell proliferation. In view of the protective effects of parity and breast-feeding, however, a primary mechanism of protection may well involve suppression of ovulation, which reduces the number of lifetime ovulatory cycles and the associated injury to the epithelial cells on the surface of the ovary. According to an older hypothesis (the "incessant ovulation" hypothesis) (14), ovarian cancer develops from an aberration in the repair process of the surface epithelium, which is ruptured and repaired during each ovulatory cycle. In support of this theory, it is well known that domestic egg-laying hens, which are forced to ovulate incessantly, have a high incidence of lesions believed to be ovarian-derived tumors with peritoneal carcinomatosis (15). Alternative hypotheses center on the ability of OCP to treat endometriosis and reduce the risk of acquiring pelvic inflammatory disease (PID), two conditions known to be associated with ovarian cancer (see below). However, these hypotheses are at odds with an origin of ovarian cancer in the fallopian tube (see Pathology section). A case–control study has shown that progestin-only contraceptive users have a reduced risk (0.39) for developing ovarian cancer (16). Moreover, the increase in progestin levels seen during pregnancy suggests that the protective effect of pregnancy may involve progestins as well as the reduction in the number of lifetime ovulations (12). Recent studies in primates indicate that the progestin component of OCPs has a chemopreventive effect by inducing apoptosis of ovarian surface cells that have undergone genetic damage (17). This is supported by the fact that women who use a long-acting progestin-only contraceptive (depot medroxyprogesterone acetate—Depo Provera), which does not completely suppress ovulation, experience a protective effect similar to that observed with OCPs, which completely suppress ovulation (11).

Hormone Replacement Therapy

Currently, the primary indications for the prescription of HRT are severe postmenopausal symptoms and not the prevention of chronic disease. Several prospective cohort studies examined the relationship of postmenopausal estrogen or estrogen/progestin HRT to the risk of developing ovarian cancer. In a prospective, double-blind study, over 8,000 women who had not had a hysterectomy were randomized to either placebo or 0.625 mg conjugated equine estrogen with 2.5 mg medroxyprogesterone acetate (Women's Health Initiative [WHI]) (18). After an average of 5.6 years of follow-up, 20 women in the estrogen/progestin group were diagnosed with an invasive ovarian cancer versus 12 in the placebo group, which was not a significant difference (HR, 1.64; CI, 0.78–3.45). The observational "Million Women Study" (19) showed an increased risk with estrogen-only

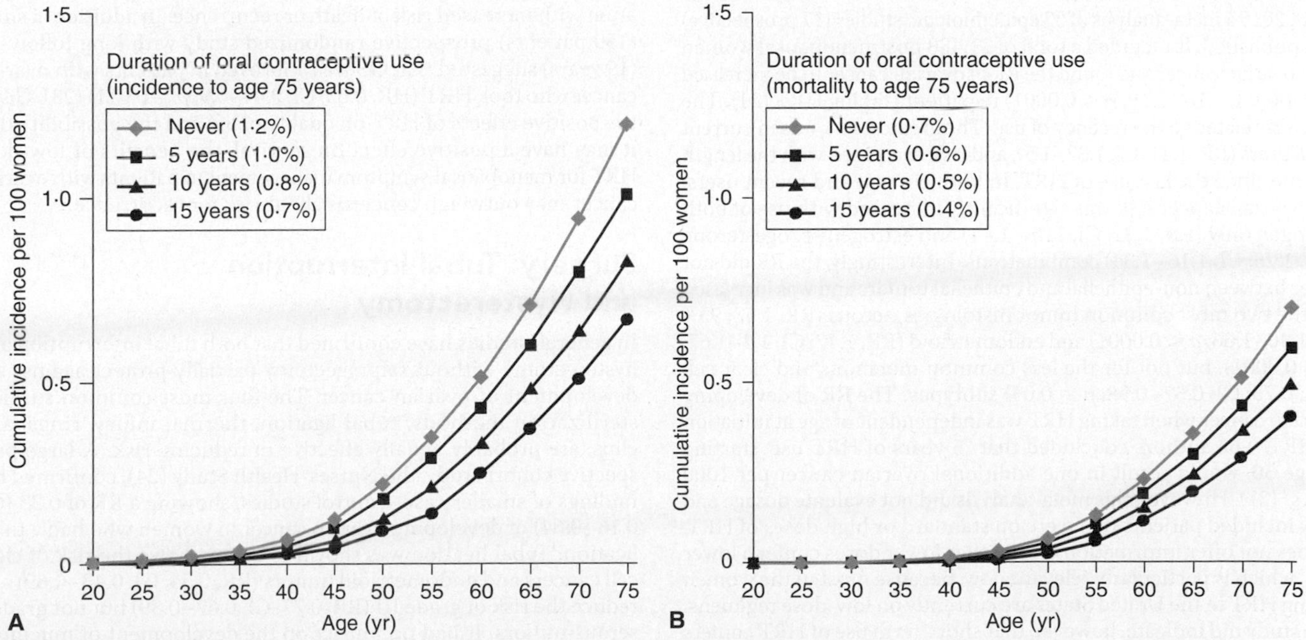

Figure 23.3. Absolute risk of ovarian cancer for women in high-income countries, by duration of use of oral contraceptives. **A:** Cumulative incidence of ovarian cancer per 100 women. **B:** Cumulative mortality from ovarian cancer per 100 women.

Source: From Beral V, Doll R, Hermon C, et al. Ovarian cancer and oral contraceptives: Collaborative reanalysis of data from 45 epidemiological studies including 23,257 women with ovarian cancer and 87,303 controls. *Lancet*. 2008;371:303–314.

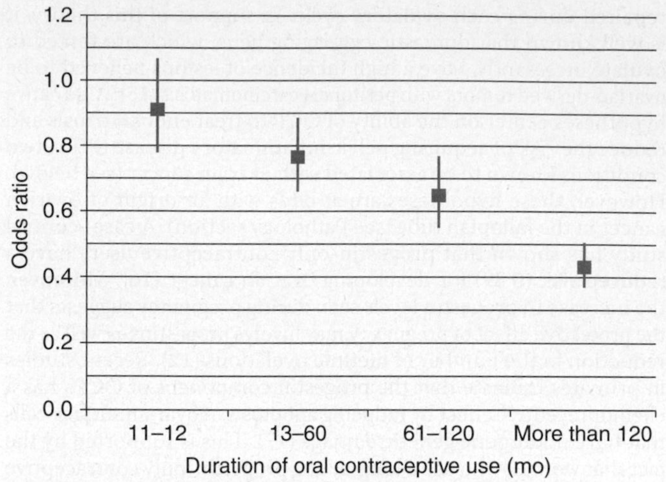

Figure 23.4. Relationship between duration of oral contraceptive pill use and ovarian cancer incidence. There is no evidence of heterogeneity. The estimated value of sigma (σ) is 0.15.

Source: Fig. 3 from Havrilesky LJ, Moorman PG, Lowery WJ, et al. Oral contraceptive pills as primary prevention for ovarian cancer: a systematic review and meta-analysis. *Obstet Gynecol*. 2013;122:139.

HRT (RR, 1.49; CI, 1.2–1.81) and, like the Breast Cancer Detection Demonstration Project, showed a lower risk with estrogen/progestin combination therapy (RR, 1.15; CI, 1–1.33). This study also reviewed the cumulative incidence of gynecologic cancers, including ovarian, endometrial, and breast cancer in women taking HRT. The gynecologic cancer incidence per 1,000 women over 5 years increased from 19 per 1,000 in "never-users" to 26 per 1,000 in current users of estrogen-only HRT, and to 35 per 1,000 in current users of estrogen/progestin combinations (**Fig. 23.5**). The strength of this study, which followed nearly 1 million women, was that the results were adjusted for age at menopause, OCP use, BMI, smoking, and physical activity. HRT was found to be unrelated to the risk of mucinous ovarian cancer. Other data indicate that regular use of vaginal and transdermal estrogen may carry a slightly increased risk of ovarian cancer (19,20).

In 2015 a meta-analysis of 52 epidemiologic studies (17 prospective) was published. It included a total of 21,488 postmenopausal women with ovarian cancer and found the RR of ovarian cancer to be increased by 1.14 (CI, 1.10–1.19, $p < 0.0001$) in patients taking HRT (21). The risk was related to the recency of use. The greatest risk was in current HRT users (RR, 1.41; CI, 1.32–1.5), and risk decreased with the length of time since the last use of HRT. In both current and recent users, the ovarian cancer risk was significantly increased with use of both estrogen only (RR, 1.32; CI, 1.23–1.41) and estrogen–progesterone (RR, 1.25; CI, 1.16–1.34) combinations. Interestingly, the RR did not differ between non-epithelial and epithelial tumors and was increased for the two most common tumor histologies, serous (RR, 1.53; 95% CI, 1.40–1.66; $p < 0.0001$) and endometrioid (RR, 1.42; CI, 1.2–1.67; $p < 0.0001$), but not for the less common mucinous and clear cell (RR, 0.75; CI, 0.57–0.98; $p = 0.04$) subtypes. The RR of developing ovarian cancer when taking HRT was independent of age at initiation of HRT. The authors concluded that "5 years of HRT use, starting at age 50, would result in one additional ovarian cancer per 1000 users" (21). However, this meta-analysis did not evaluate dosage and only included patients that were on standard or high doses of HRT. It does not offer information on whether lower doses confer a lower risk, which is particularly relevant now, because most of the women taking HRT in the United States are currently on low-dose regimens. The study did indicate, however, that short-term use of HRT confers less risk. Although an increased risk for ovarian cancer was found in all current users, it did not persist in those who had used HRT less than 5 years and stopped. Therefore, the judicious use of HRT is not necessarily contraindicated by these data. Current clinical practice is

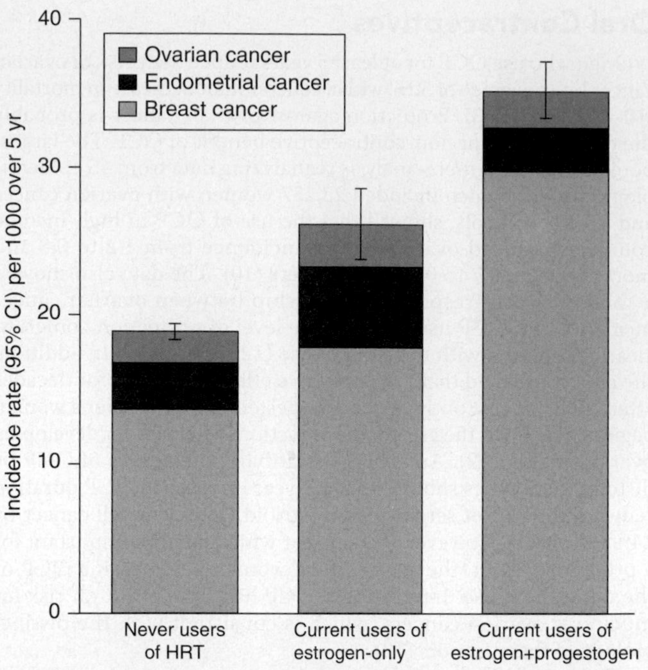

Figure 23.5. Standardized incidence rate (95% CI) for ovarian, endometrial, and breast cancer per 100 women in the study cohort over a 5-year period, for current users of various types of HRT and for never users. Incidence rates are standardized by age, region of residence, socioeconomic status, time since menopause, parity, use of oral contraceptives, body mass index, and alcohol consumption. Rates apply to women with a uterus and ovaries.

Source: Reprinted with permission from Beral V, Million Women Study Collaborators, Bull D, et al. Ovarian cancer and hormone replacement therapy in the Million Women Study. *Lancet*. 2007;369(9574):1703–1710.

to prescribe HRT to patients with severe postmenopausal symptoms and to administer it at the lowest effective dose for less than 5 years.

Interestingly, a meta-analysis (22) of HRT use by women with a history of epithelial ovarian cancer did not show a significant association with increased risk of death or recurrence. In addition, a small (150 patients) prospective randomized study with long follow-up (19 years) suggested that OS was improved in patients with ovarian cancer who took HRT (HR, 0.63; CI, 0.44–0.9; $p = 0.011$) (23). Given the positive effects of HRT on quality of life and the possibility that it may have a positive effect on survival, the benefits of low-dose HRT for menopausal symptom management in patients with ovarian cancer may outweigh concerns about risk for recurrence.

Surgery: Tubal Interruption and Hysterectomy

In general, studies have confirmed that both tubal interruption and hysterectomy without salpingectomy partially protect against the development of ovarian cancer. The four most common surgical sterilization methods, tubal ligation, thermal injury, rings, and clips, are probably equally effective in reducing risk. A large prospective cohort study, the Nurses' Health Study (24), confirmed the findings of smaller case–control studies, showing a RR of 0.33 (CI, 0.16–0.64) of developing ovarian cancer in women who had a tubal ligation. Tubal ligation was shown to almost halve the risk of clear cell cancers and endometrioid tumors (RR, 0.54; CI, 0.43–0.69) and reduce the risk of grade III (RR, 0.77; CI, 0.67–0.89) but not grade 1 serous tumors. It had no impact on the development of mucinous ovarian cancer (25). The same study also reported a weak inverse relationship between hysterectomy and ovarian cancer (RR, 0.67; CI, 0.45–1) and found that the effect of hysterectomy was greater when the surgery was performed at an earlier age (24), a finding that was not confirmed in a later study (25). In the recent analysis by the Ovarian Cancer Cohort Consortium, tubal ligation was associated with reduced risk of endometrioid (RR, 0.6; CI, 0.41–0.88) and clear cell (RR, 0.35; CI, 0.18–0.69) cancers but not with a reduced risk of serous tumors, and hysterectomy was associated with a reduced risk only for clear cell cancers (1).

A retrospective case–control study evaluated the effect of tubal ligation in patients with *BRCA1* mutations (26). Like women unselected for genetic risk, BRCA1 mutation carriers who had undergone a tubal ligation had a considerably reduced risk of developing ovarian cancer (OR, 0.39; CI, 0.22-–0.7). Those who both had a tubal ligation and had used OCP in the past had an even lower odds ratio of developing ovarian cancer (OR, 0.28; CI, 0.15–0.52). Possible explanations for the protective effect of tubal interruption against ovarian cancer include (a) an impaired blood supply to the ovaries/distal fallopian tube through the superior branch of the uterine artery, which causes most women to enter menopause earlier and experience fewer lifetime ovulations; (b) an occlusion of the tube that blocks the upward flow of carcinogens and endometrial tissue from the uterus and reduces pelvic infection rates; and (c) the reduced presence and decreased proliferation of progenitor cells in the fimbriated end of the fallopian tube (27).

Inflammation: PID and Endometriosis

PID is a generalized infection of the female genital tract. Several small case–control studies have suggested that PID is associated with ovarian cancer. However, this association only gained wide acceptance with the publication of a large study (28) comparing the ovarian cancer incidence of 68,000 women who had experienced PID versus 136,000 who had not. In this well-designed study, the hazard ratio for ovarian cancer in patients with a history of PID (adjusted appropriately for confounding factors) was twice as high (HR, 1.92) as that of controls and was even higher (HR, 2.46) in women who had at least five episodes of PID. Such indications of a dose–response effect add credibility to epidemiologic findings.

Endometriosis, characterized by the ectopic growth of endometrial glands in the ovary and the abdominal cavity, affects 10% of women of reproductive age. In smaller case–control studies and one large meta-analysis (1), a history of endometriosis has been consistently shown to be associated with clear cell and endometrioid ovarian carcinoma, with an odds ratio of approximately 2. In many endometrioid and clear cell ovarian cancers, endometriosis is detected histologically adjacent to the carcinoma. Combining data from 13 ovarian cancer case–control studies (7,900 patients with ovarian cancer), the Ovarian Cancer Association Consortium (OCAC) published a definitive report that self-reported endometriosis increased the risk of clear cell (OR, 3.05; CI, 2.4–3.8) and endometrioid ovarian cancer (OR, 2.04; CI, 1.7–2.5) (29). In this report endometriosis was also associated, for the first time, with low-grade serous cancers (OR, 2.11; CI, 1.4–3.2), suggesting that these cancers, which are generally believed to arise from serous borderline tumors (SBTs), can also arise from endometriotic implants. Adjusted for histology and International Federation of Gynecology and Obstetrics (FIGO) stage, women with endometriosis-associated ovarian cancer have similar survival to women with non-endometriosis-associated ovarian cancer (30).

There are two pathologic subtypes of endometriosis: displaced benign ectopic endometrial glands and atypical endometriosis. Endometriosis with cytologic atypia and complex hyperplasia ("atypical endometriosis"), present in 2% to 3% of all patients who undergo surgery for endometriosis, is most likely a direct precursor for type I/low-grade ovarian cancers (31). This hypothesis was supported by a study in which *ARID1A* gene mutations were detected in 30% of endometrioid and 46% of clear cell cancers, as well as in areas of atypical endometriosis that were adjacent to the cancers (32). Many genes expressed in endometriosis are also detected in endometrioid ovarian cancer, but do not overlap with genes expressed in high-grade serous cancers (33). In summary, endometriosis is associated with three histologic subtypes of ovarian cancer: endometrioid, clear cell, and low-grade serous (30). The risk of low-grade serous cancers is 3.77 times higher (CI, 1.24–11.48) in patients with endometriosis, but the risk of high-grade serous cancer is not increased (see also Pathology section) (1).

A common mechanism linking endometriosis and PID to ovarian cancer risk may involve the intensive release of cytokines and the infiltration of immune cells (macrophages) that accompanies inflammation. Some (34), but not all (35), epidemiologic data suggest that the use of anti-inflammatory agents, including aspirin and nonsteroidal anti-inflammatory drugs, protects against ovarian cancer. In the largest meta-analysis to date, aspirin was associated with a 20% reduction in ovarian cancer risk (OR, 0.91; CI, 0.84–0.99), which was most consistent for serous histologies. This beneficial effect was observed with low-dose aspirin (100 mg/d), the dose used for cardiovascular protection. Interestingly, nonaspirin NSAIDs were not significantly associated with a reduction of ovarian cancer risk (36).

Other Risk Factors: Diet, Smoking, Exercise

For the most part, studies that have investigated whether diet affects ovarian cancer risk have had inconsistent and conflicting results. Any association between diet and cancer risk is likely to be difficult to decipher given the inaccuracy of food frequency questionnaires and seasonal differences in the supply of fresh food. Several studies have tried to determine whether vitamin A and β-carotene consumption affects ovarian cancer risk; but although some studies suggested a risk reduction, others could not confirm it. The prospective California Teachers Study, which had almost 100,000 participants, concluded that dietary factors are unlikely to play a major role in ovarian cancer development. In this cohort study, a RR reduction was only found with increased intake of isoflavones, the phytoestrogens found in soy-based foods, some of which have antiestrogenic effects (RR, 0.6; CI, 0.33–1) (37,38). The Women's Health Initiative Dietary Modification Trial was a randomized controlled trial in 48,835 postmenopausal women that prospectively evaluated the effects of reducing fat intake by at least 20% and increasing consumption of vegetables, fruits, and grains on ovarian cancer incidence (39). The overall ovarian cancer HR was not statistically different between the two groups; however, it decreased with the increasing duration of the intervention: for the first 4 years, the risk for ovarian cancer was similar in the intervention and control groups; but over the next 4 years, the risk was lower in the intervention group [0.38 cases per 1,000 person-years in the intervention group vs. 0.64 per 1,000 person-years in the comparison group (HR, 0.6; CI, 0.38–0.96)]. A meta-analysis analyzing 20 epidemiologic studies showed no association between dietary fat intake and epithelial ovarian cancer risk (40). Indirect evidence for the effect of diet on the risk of ovarian cancer is provided by the observations that women from geographic areas with a low incidence of ovarian cancer who relocate to a high-incidence region (North America, Europe) acquire the same risk as women who were born in that region and that ovarian cancer incidence has increased over time in Japan, which is transitioning to a more Westernized eating pattern (41).

Smoking is not generally considered a risk factor for ovarian cancer (42). However, current smoking seems to be associated with an increased risk of developing a mucinous ovarian cancer (OR, 1.78; CI, 1.01–3.15) (43). Smoking cessation reduces this risk back to baseline over 20 years. A large meta-analysis encompassing 28,114 patients concluded that current smoking was associated with a small albeit clinically insignificant increase in ovarian cancer (RR, 1.06; CI, 1.01–1.11). The increased risk was driven by mucinous cancers that are more common in smokers (RR, 1.79; CI, 1.6–2). Interestingly smoking reduced the risk of endometrioid (RR, 0.81; CI, 0.72–0.92) and clear cell (RR, 0.8; CI, 0.65–0.97) and had no association with serous ovarian cancer (44).

Currently, there is no convincing association between physical exercise and ovarian cancer risk and survival (45). A Gynecologic Oncology Group (GOG) trial that recently completed accrual is testing the effect of regular exercise, a low-fat diet, and high intake of vegetables after primary treatment for ovarian cancer on progression-free survival (PFS) (GOG#225: "Can diet and exercise modulate ovarian, fallopian tube, and peritoneal cancer progression-free survival?").

In summary, factors that decrease the number of lifetime ovulations reduce the risk of developing ovarian cancer, whereas hereditary factors increase the risk. From a practical, clinical standpoint, only a positive family history will raise the suspicion of a predisposition to ovarian cancer in an asymptomatic woman.

HEREDITARY OVARIAN CANCER: BRCA AND HNPCC

The study of familial breast and ovarian cancer began in 1866 when the French physician and pathologist Paul Broca noted a much larger than expected incidence of cancer in his wife's family. Over four generations, 10 out of the 24 women in her family died from breast cancer, whereas several more individuals of both sexes developed other malignancies. He concluded that this excess of cancers could not reasonably be attributed to chance. We now estimate that approximately 18% to 24% of invasive epithelial ovarian cancers have an autosomal dominant germ line mutation. *BRCA1* or *BRCA2* is the most common identified genetic mutation in ovarian cancer patients (14% to 18%) followed by mutations in genes linked to Lynch syndrome (*MLH1, MSH2, MSH6, PMS2*); however, of this writing (April 2016), 12 suspected hereditary ovarian cancer genes have been identified (**Table 23.1**) (46–49). These hereditary mutations are the strongest known risk factors for the development of ovarian cancer. They may also provide targets for therapy, as is the case with *BRCA1/2* mutations and poly-ADP-ribose polymerase (PARP) inhibitors.

Biology of BRCA-Associated Ovarian Cancer

The *BRCA* genes are inherited in an autosomal dominant fashion, which means that every first-degree relative of a mutation carrier has a 50% chance of carrying a mutation. The *BRCA* genes function as classic tumor suppressors, with loss of function of both alleles required for cancer formation. Carriers are initially heterozygous for the *BRCA* gene mutation(s) in all cells and then the sporadic loss of the wild-type allele in epithelial breast or fallopian/ovarian cells results in a predisposition to cancer. The BRCA 1/2 proteins regulate cell cycle checkpoints and gene expression. Their most important function is participation in a specific DNA repair pathway, homologous recombination, which is used for the high-fidelity repair of double-strand DNA breaks. Because cells with *BRCA1/2* mutations lack the ability to repair double-strand breaks, they have increased genomic instability and a predisposition to malignant transformation. The ability of cells with *BRCA* mutations to repair DNA cross-links induced by platinum salts is impaired, which is hypothesized to explain the increased platinum sensitivity of patients with *BRCA* mutations (see below). BRCA1 and 2 are components of the Fanconi anemia DNA repair pathway. Several other genes identified to be mutated in ovarian cancer (*BRIP1, PALB2, RAD51C*) are also part of this pathway. The *PALB2* gene, which is part of this pathway, binds *BRCA1/2* at sites of DNA damage.

TABLE 23.1. Multiplex Testing of Hereditary Ovarian Cancer

Mismatch repair/Lynch-HNPCC	*MLH1, MSH2, MSH6, PMS2, EPCAM*
Tumor suppressor	*TP53, PTEN*
Double-strand DNA break repair genes	*BRCA1, BRCA2*, ATM, CHEK2, NBN
Fanconi anemia pathway	*BRIP1*, BARD1, *PALB2*, MRE11A, RAD50, *RAD51C, RAD51D*, FANCP

Currently there are 12 genes (*italicized*) associated with hereditary breast/ovarian cancer syndromes (46–49).

The prevalence of *BRCA1* or *BRCA2* mutations (over 1,000 have been identified) in the general population is about 1:300 to 1:800. However, specific ethnic populations founded by small ancestral groups, such as French Canadians, Icelanders, Mexicans, and Ashkenazi Jews, have a higher mutation rate arising from spontaneous "founder mutations." For example, 2% to 3% of all Jewish women of Eastern European descent have one of three founder mutations (two in *BRCA1* 187delAG and 5382insC; one in *BRCA2* 6174 delT). The cumulative lifetime risk of developing ovarian cancer for women with a *BRCA1* mutation has been estimated at up to 40% by age 70 and for women with a *BRCA2* mutation up to 18%. The number of *BRCA2*-associated ovarian cancers is smaller overall and the age of onset is later than with *BRCA1*. In comparison, the lifetime risk for ovarian cancer for women in the general population is 1.4% (50). Of note, borderline tumors are not associated with *BRCA1/2* mutations. The age of a *BRCA1/2* mutation carrier, however, is very relevant to her absolute risk of ovarian or breast cancer. The highest incidence of ovarian cancer is between ages 50 and 59 for *BRCA1* mutation carriers and between 60 and 69 years for *BRCA2* mutation carriers and then the risks lower with age but always significantly exceed the risk in the general population (51). There are several online tools for calculating the probability of a *BRCA1/2* mutation and for calculating cancer risk regardless of gene status. One is the Breast and Ovarian Analysis of Disease Incidence and Carrier Estimation Algorithm (BOADICEA), which is used to calculate the risk of breast and ovarian cancer based on family history (52).

Clinical Features of *BRCA*-Associated Ovarian Cancer

In general, *BRCA* mutation carriers who develop ovarian cancer have a younger age at diagnosis, are more likely to have cancers of high-grade serous histology originating in the fallopian tube, are less likely to have borderline or mucinous tumors, and have, in the short term, a better prognosis than matched controls with sporadic ovarian cancer (46,53). A breast cancer precedes the ovarian cancer diagnosis in 37% of *BRCA1*-associated cases and 37% of *BRCA2*-associated cases (54).

In 1996, Rubin and colleagues reported results of a retrospective analysis suggesting that there are distinct clinical and pathologic features of *BRCA1*-associated ovarian cancer (52). Among 53 patients with germ line *BRCA1* mutations, the average age at diagnosis was only 48, and the vast majority of cancers were serous adenocarcinomas. Cancers associated with *BRCA1* mutations had a relatively favorable prognosis, with an actuarial median survival of 77 months compared with 29 months for matched controls (**Fig. 23.6**). However, larger studies have shown that although *BRCA1*-related cancers have a better initial prognosis, this advantage decreases over time and eventually reverses at 8 years (47,55). The 5- and 10-year survival rates for noncarriers are 42/30%, for *BRCA1* mutation carriers 45/25%, and for *BRCA2* carriers 54/35%, respectively (55).

Historically, series have reported that *BRCA*-associated cancers are usually of high-grade serous histology; however, recent studies show that *BRCA1*- and *BRCA2*-associated tumors are similar in histology and grade to sporadic cancers (47). In one study of 1,119 *BRCA1/2*-associated ovarian cancers (53), the subtypes included 67% serous, 12% endometrioid, 2% clear cell, and 1% mucinous cancers. The important clinical implication of these findings is that women with endometrioid and clear cell carcinomas should still be considered for *BRCA* mutation testing. In another series of *BRCA*-associated ovarian cancers with centralized pathology review (56), cancers in *BRCA* carriers were compared with those in noncarriers. Mutation-associated tumors were of significantly higher grade

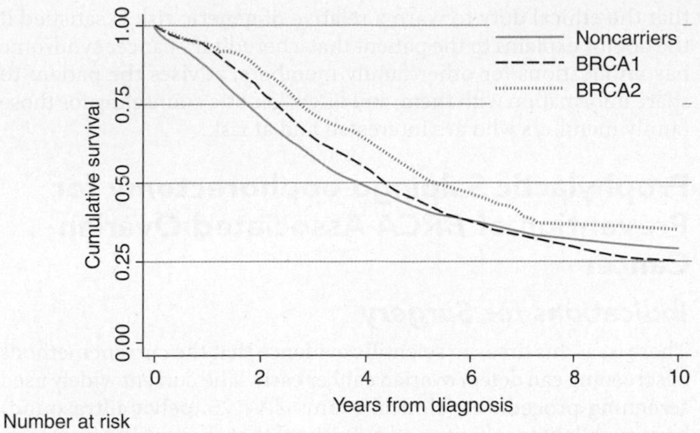

Number at risk						
Noncarriers	1924	2914	2295	1657	1120	812
Carriers						
BRCA1	404	676	499	323	198	118
BRCA2	162	278	239	152	86	58

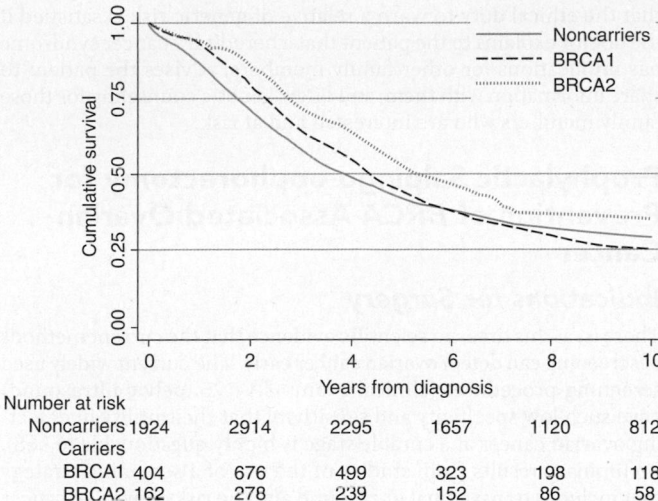

Figure 23.6. Kaplan–Meier estimates of cumulative survival according to BRCA1/2 mutation status.

Source: Fig. 1 from Candido-dos-Reis FJ, Song H, Goode EL, et al. Germline mutation in BRCA1 or BRCA2 and ten-year survival for women diagnosed with epithelial ovarian cancer. *Clin Cancer Res*. 2015;21:652–657.

and stage and less often mucinous than non-mutation-associated tumors. No mucinous and no borderline tumors were found in the mutation-associated group. Primary peritoneal carcinoma occurred rarely in both groups. Restricting genetic testing to women with ovarian cancer who have a family history of hereditary cancers, as ascertained by risk factors, will miss half of the patients with a mutation. Therefore, genetic testing solely based on family history alone can no longer be recommended and all ovarian cancer patients with non-mucinous histology should consider testing to evaluate if they have a hereditary ovarian cancer. A large study, which screened 1,342 unselected patients from the province of Ontario diagnosed with epithelial ovarian cancer, reported a *BRCA1/2* mutation frequency of 13.4% (57). Although this study used multiplex ligation-dependent probe amplification and therefore detected the large deletions that normally elude general sequencing, the current standard method to detect genomic abnormalities is next-generation sequencing. Women with ovarian cancer in their fourth life decade had the highest mutation rate (24%), as did women of Italian (43%), Jewish (30%), or Indo-Pakistani (29%) origin. Importantly, 8% of the mutation carriers detected by the screening had no first-degree relative with ovarian or breast cancer. Among Ashkenazi Jewish women with ovarian cancer, there is an estimated 29% to 40% chance that the disease is related to a *BRCA1* or *BRCA2* mutation (58).

Ovarian cancer in a *BRCA1/2* mutation carrier has specific clinical characteristics when compared with sporadic ovarian cancer. It is probable that the improved 5-year survival of women with *BRCA*-associated ovarian cancers is related to the fact that loss of function of *BRCA* proteins, which participate in DNA damage repair, initially results in a more favorable response to platinum-based chemotherapy. Women with *BRCA1/2*-associated ovarian cancers are less likely to have platinum-resistant disease (14.9%) than those with sporadic ovarian cancer (31.7%), and when these patients recur, they tend to have a higher response to second-line platinum-based chemotherapy, even in the setting of initially platinum-resistant disease (4). Platinum salts induce DNA cross-links, which are recognized by DNA damage repair pathways and are repaired by nucleotide excision repair and homologous recombination (59). It may be because *BRCA1/2*-associated high-grade serous cancers harbor defects in homologous recombination that platinum compounds are more efficient in these cancers. A decrease in *BRCA1* mRNA levels (PCR-based measurement) was associated with a significantly longer survival in 57 unselected ovarian cancer patients (60).

Gene Panel-Testing/Counseling

During the 1990s, clinical testing for hereditary ovarian cancer was limited to *BRCA1/2*; however, with the advent of inexpensive next-generation sequencing, we can now test for a wide variety of genes. While *BRCA* and Lynch syndrome are most commonly associated with ovarian cancer, recent findings suggest that 12 other genes confer an increased risk of ovarian cancer, although their biologic role in tumorigenesis is still being investigated (**Table 23.1**).

Based on three pivotal studies (47–49), most centers perform multiplex testing. Although the specific panels used may vary slightly, most commercial and academic panels include around 20 to 30 genes associated with germ line mutations/insertions/deletions in ovarian cancer. In a cohort of 1,915 ovarian cancer patients identified from GOG protocols 218 and 262 and the Washington University gynecologic tissue bank, 18% were found to have a pathogenic germ line mutation. Approximately 15% had mutations in *BRCA1* (9.5%) or *BRCA2* (5.1%), whereas 3% had mutations in the Fanconi anemia pathway. DNA MMR genes were altered in 0.4% of cases (47). *BRIP1*, a Fanconi anemia pathway gene, is the third most frequent germ line mutation in ovarian cancer patients (0.9–1.6%), conferring a RR of ovarian cancer of about 3.4 (lifetime risk 5.8%) (47). Although *PALB2* increases breast cancer risk, its contribution to ovarian cancer risk is still under investigation. In all these studies, if patients had been selected based solely on clinical criteria (young age, family history, and serous tumor type) a significant proportion of patients with mutations would have been missed. It is estimated that about one-third of patients found to have a non-*BRCA1/2* mutation will experience a change in clinical management (e.g., risk-reducing salpingo-oophorectomy [RRSO], colorectal screening, additional family testing) (48). However, some controversy over the use of panel-testing remains. It should be realized that we do not understand the significance of germ line variants, including copy number variations or mosaicism, for most of the genes in **Table 23.1**, and at this point the presence of variants not clearly associated with increased risk should not guide medical decision making.

It is particularly important to offer genetic testing to patients who have already developed ovarian cancer. The identification of a *BRCA* mutation may impact their treatment, because it might indicate an increased sensitivity to PARP inhibitors as well as to platinum compounds both in the first- and second-line setting (46). Although the up-front treatment (carboplatin/paclitaxel) for *BRCA* mutation-associated ovarian cancers is currently the same as treatment for sporadic ovarian cancers, the treatment of recurrent cancer may include PARP inhibitors in *BRCA1/2* mutation carriers. Also, the unaffected first-degree female relatives of *BRCA* mutation carriers have a 50% probability of carrying the same mutation and can be specifically tested for it. Those first-degree relatives who are found to be *BRCA* negative can be informed that they are not at a significantly greater risk of developing ovarian cancer than the general population, whereas those who carry the mutation can be counseled on risk-reducing strategies. Given that a salpingo-oophorectomy reduces the risk of developing ovarian and fallopian tube cancer by about 80%, it is clinically meaningful to be aware that a woman carries a *BRCA* mutation. Negative findings in multigene testing in a patient with ovarian cancer may reassure the unaffected relatives that there is not a known cancer gene in the family; however, the unaffected first-degree relative's ovarian cancer risk would still be slightly elevated (3–7%) compared to the population risk of 1.4%.

Therefore, a negative test provides useful clinical information that will assist with her care and inform screening recommendations. We believe genetic testing should therefore be routinely offered to all women with non-mucinous high-grade epithelial ovarian cancer, regardless of family history.

Considerable expertise and time is needed to counsel women at risk for hereditary cancer. This is of particular importance when testing using cancer gene panels where interpretation of results and management decisions can be complicated. Specifically, although cancer risk estimates are highly reliable for patients with *BRCA1* and *2* mutations, the level of risk associated with other genes is less clear as are recommendations for cancer risk management (61). A genetic counselor or physician with expertise in treating hereditary cancers in women can provide the patient not only appropriate medical information, but also skilled consideration for her concerns and emotional support. *BRCA*- and Lynch syndrome–directed genetic counseling is important for the effective assessment of risk for the patient and her family and for decision making regarding preventive strategies and therapies. However, most women who undergo genetic testing do not receive in-person genetic counseling (62), and at this time there may not be sufficient genetic counseling resources to allow in-person counseling of all patients. Newer genetic counseling models, including phone counseling and the guided use of Internet resources, are currently being explored.

Until a woman with a *BRCA1/2* mutation chooses to have prophylactic surgery, most practitioners will follow her with pelvic exams, CA-125 testing, and pelvic ultrasound, but there is no evidence that these screening strategies improve ovarian cancer survival. Patients should also have regular breast examinations as well as annual mammograms and breast magnetic resonance imaging (MRI). The evidence for use of tamoxifen for primary prevention of breast cancer in BRCA1 and 2 carriers is very limited. In contrast, several studies have shown that removal of the ovaries before menopause reduces breast cancer risk by about 50% (63). Prophylactic bilateral mastectomy should also be discussed with *BRCA* mutation carriers, and patients should be informed of the techniques available for removing and reconstructing the breast, and the expected psychosocial and sexual effects. Counseling about RRSO should balance the risks and symptoms associated with surgical menopause with the morbidity and high mortality of advanced serous ovarian cancer (51).

Most studies have shown that the reproductive and hormonal factors that affect ovarian cancer risk in the general population also affect risk for women who carry *BRCA1* and *BRCA2* mutations. Narod et al., from Toronto, reported results from a large database, which included 670 women with a history of *BRCA1*-associated ovarian cancer, 124 with a history of *BRCA2*-associated ovarian cancer, and 2,424 mutation carriers with no history of ovarian cancer (64). Use of OCPs reduced the risk of ovarian cancer in women with *BRCA1* mutations (OR 0.56) and *BRCA2* mutations (OR 0.39). The six studies that addressed this question were analyzed together in a meta-analysis (65), showing that the odds ratio (OR) for developing ovarian cancer was 0.65 (CI, 0.47–0.66) in *BRCA1* mutation carriers using OCPs, 0.65 (CI, 0.34–1.24) for *BRCA2* mutation carriers, and 0.58 (CI, 0.46–0.73) for the combined BRCA1/2 group. In summary, OCP use is inversely associated with ovarian cancer risk, whereas a modest but not statistically significant increased risk was observed for breast cancer (65).

Breast-feeding was also found to be protective for carriers of a *BRCA1* mutation (OR 0.74). An effect of similar magnitude was seen for breast-feeding in *BRCA2* mutation carriers, but it was not statistically significant (OR 0.72). Although the Toronto group had previously reported that tubal ligation was protective against ovarian cancer in mutation carriers as well as noncarriers, the association in this expanded cohort was not significant for carriers of either a *BRCA1* (OR 0.8) or a *BRCA2* mutation (OR 0.63). Pregnancy, which had previously been reported to be protective for women carrying a *BRCA* mutation (58), was found to be protective for carriers of *BRCA1* mutations (OR 0.67), but was associated with increased risk for carriers of *BRCA2* mutations (OR 2.74). The reasons for this are not clear.

Finally, it is important to be aware of legislation that addresses issues of discrimination and privacy that are raised by the prospect of increasingly comprehensive genetic information on each patient. The Genetic Information Nondiscrimination Act (GINA) (2008) prohibits health insurers and employers from discriminating on the basis of genetic information (66). Rules governing patient privacy and confidentiality prevent a physician from disclosing genetic test results to a relative without permission from the patient. The American Society of Clinical Oncology (ASCO) guidelines suggest that the ethical duty to warn a relative of genetic risk is satisfied if the doctor explains to the patient that a hereditary cancer syndrome has implications for other family members, advises the patient to share information with them, and offers genetic counseling for those family members who are interested and at risk.

Prophylactic Salpingo-oophorectomy for Prevention of *BRCA*-Associated Ovarian Cancer

Indications for Surgery

There is, at this time, no scientific evidence that the current methods of screening can detect ovarian cancer early. The current widely used screening procedures (clinical exam, CA-125, pelvic ultrasound) have such low specificity and sensitivity that their utility in detecting ovarian cancer at a curable stage is highly questionable (67,68). Preliminary results from studies of the use of a screening strategy that includes transvaginal ultrasound and the risk of ovarian cancer algorithm (ROCA), which detects a significant change in CA-125, have not been promising even in postmenopausal women (68). Such screening is even less efficient in young premenopausal women because ovulating women may have functional cysts, endometriosis, or a hemorrhagic corpus luteum, which can be mistaken for a suspicious mass (**Table 23.4**). The ovarian cancer screening studies have not focused exclusively on high-risk women; however, the US Preventative Task Force indicates that there is no reason to believe that high-risk women will benefit from screening (69). The National Comprehensive Cancer Network (NCCN) guidelines do not support ovarian cancer screening, but state that it can be considered at the clinician's discretion starting at age 30 to 35 years.

In contrast, the evidence does strongly support the efficacy of RRSO in reducing mortality through early detection of ovarian cancer and prevention in unaffected women (**Table 23.2**). In 2002, two large prospective series clearly demonstrated that RRSO reduced the risk of developing Müllerian carcinoma (ovarian, fallopian tube, and peritoneal cancer) in patients with *BRCA1/2* mutations (70,71). Kauff and colleagues from Memorial Sloan-Kettering prospectively studied 170 women with either *BRCA1* or *BRCA2* mutations for 6 years (**Fig. 23.7**). Ninety-eight women who underwent RRSO were compared with 72 women who elected surveillance. Three large prospective studies showed that the RRSO group had significantly fewer *BRCA*-related gynecologic and breast cancers than the surveillance group (51,71,72).

Another larger prospective study reported on the effects of RRSO in *BRCA1* and *BRCA2* germ line mutation carriers separately. Among 1,079 patients, RRSO reduced ovarian cancer risk in women with *BRCA1* mutations by 85% and reduced breast cancer risk in women with *BRCA2* mutations by 72%. There was also a 39% reduction in breast cancer risk in women with *BRCA1* mutations and a reduction in ovarian cancers in women with *BRCA2* mutations, but these were not statistically significant. The absence of a significant reduction in ovarian cancer in *BRCA2* mutation carriers may have been partially attributable to the fact that most women with *BRCA2*-associated ovarian cancer are over 60 years old, whereas the median age of the women in the study was 46 years (57). In another large study coordinated by the Toronto group, 5,783 known carriers of a *BRCA1* or *BRCA2* mutation were identified from an international registry of 32 centers. The overall reduction in risk of Müllerian cancers with RRSO was 80%; the estimated cumulative incidence of peritoneal cancer at 20 years after RRSO was 3.9% for BRCA1 and 1.9% for BRCA2, with most cases occurring less than 5 years after RRSO (73).

Given the strong evidence that RRSO reduces all-cause, breast cancer-specific, and ovarian cancer-specific mortality, the NCCN, the American College of Obstetrics and Gynecology (ACOG), and the Society of Gynecologic Oncology (SGO) (74) have all recommended that prophylactic salpingo-oophorectomy be considered in women with hereditary ovarian cancer syndromes between age 35 and 40 years or after childbearing is completed. Because *BRCA2* mutation

TABLE 23.2. Prospective Observational Studies of Risk-Reducing Salpingo-oophorectomy in Patients with BRCA1/2 Mutations

Author, Journal, Yr	Study Period	RRSO	Surveillance	Mean Follow-Up (yr)	Ovarian Cancer RRSO vs. No RRSO	Hazard Ratio	Comment	Reference
Kauff, NEJM, 2002	1995–2001	98	72	2.1	1 vs. 5	0.15 (0.02–1.31)		(71)
Domcheck, JAMA, 2010	1974–2008	465	1092	3.7	10 vs. 98	0.28 (0.12–0.69	No breast cancer in 247 women with RRM	(72)
Finch, JCO, 2014	1995–2011	3513	2270	5.6	32 vs. 108	0.2 (0.13–0.3)	46 women had an occult cancer at RRSO	(51)

RRM, risk-reducing mastectomy; RRSO, risk-reducing salpingo-oophorectomy.

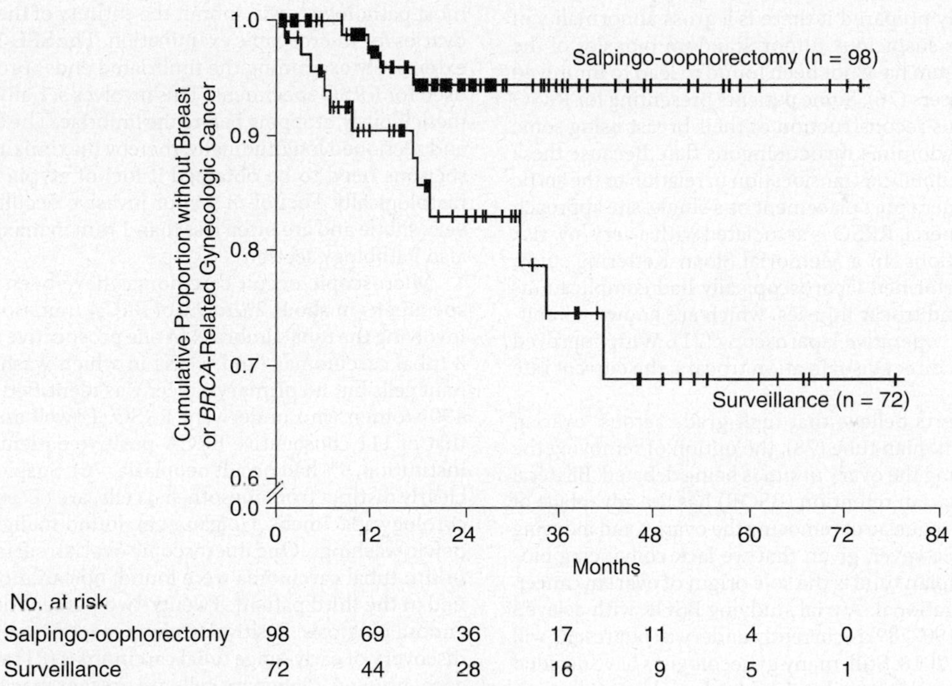

Figure 23.7. Kaplan–Meier estimates of the time to breast cancer or BRCA-related gynecologic cancer among women electing risk-reducing salpingo-oophorectomy and women electing surveillance for ovarian cancer.

p = 0.006 by the log-rank test for the comparison between the actuarial mean times to cancer. A Cox proportional-hazards model for multiple end points, which took into account the different proportions of women in the 2 groups who had breast tissue at risk, yielded a hazard ratio for subsequent breast cancer or *BRCA*-related gynecologic cancer after risk-reducing salpingo-oophorectomy of 0.25 (95% confidence interval, 0.08 to 0.74).
Source: From Kauff ND, Stagopan JM, Robson ME, et al. Risk-reducing salping-oophorectomy in women with a *BRCA1* or *BRCA2* mutation. *N Engl J Med*. 2002;346:1609–1615, with permission.

carriers will develop ovarian cancer at an average age of 58, and only 2% to 3% of them will develop ovarian cancer by age 50 as compared with 10% to 21% of women with *BRCA1* mutations, delaying RRSO in *BRCA2* mutation carriers until age 50 could be considered (72). However, women with *BRCA2* mutations have a 26% to 34% risk of developing breast cancer by the age of 50, and the evidence suggests that the breast cancer risk reduction conferred by RRSO is greater when the ovaries are removed earlier (47). In one study, RRSO *after* a primary diagnosis of breast cancer significantly reduced breast cancer-specific mortality in *BRCA1* mutation carriers (HR, 0.38; CI, 0.19–0.77) (75). The number of BRCA2 carriers was much smaller and a benefit of RRSO not seen. RRSO mostly benefited patients with ER-negative breast cancer. The data also suggest that oophorectomy is most beneficial during the first year of treatment.

Surgery

Because RRSO substantially decreases ovarian cancer risk by about 80% and reduces breast cancer risk by 48% (51,72), the benefits of prophylactic surgery clearly outweigh the associated risks. Some risk (up to 3.9%) of primary peritoneal cancer remains after RRSO, and that risk could arise from an ovarian remnant, an incompletely removed fallopian tube, or a microscopically metastasized occult cancer that could not be recognized at the time of surgery.

The informed consent discussion for RRSO surgery should include not only information about the general risks of surgery and the risk of occult or subsequent cancer, but also information about the likely side effects of surgical menopause. Permission to perform a full staging or debulking procedure if cancer is found may also be obtained. The rate of occult cancer detected with RRSO (which requires an additional surgical procedure) can be up to 10% in a tertiary referral center (76), although in a population-based study of *BRCA1/2* mutation carriers (5,782 patients) undergoing RRSO it was only 4.2% (51). Hysterectomies are not performed routinely, because there are no reports indicating that the intrauterine portion of the fallopian tube gives rise to a fallopian tube cancer and the data associating mutations in *BRCA* and uterine cancer are very limited (77). However, hysterectomy may be indicated to reduce endometrial cancer risk for patients with Lynch syndrome who are also at risk for endometrial cancer (see below), if there is other uterine pathology (e.g., fibroids, incontinence, menorrhagia), or to simplify HRT.

It is usually possible to perform RRSO laparoscopically as an outpatient procedure. Occasionally a laparotomy will be necessary because of extensive intra-abdominal/pelvic adhesions. After a thorough surveillance of the entire abdominal cavity, including the upper abdomen, peritoneal washings are performed and abnormal areas biopsied. The ureter is visualized and the infundibulopelvic vessels are transected about 2 cm superior to the ovary to assure that the entire ovary has been removed. The tube and the superior branch of the uterine artery are transected very close to the uterine cornua. A frozen section is only prepared if there is a gross abnormality of the ovary or any other suspicious tumor. Random biopsies of the omentum and peritoneum have not been found to lead to improved detection of occult cancers (76). Some patients presenting for RRSO will have had a previous reconstruction of their breast using some variation of a rectus abdominis myocutaneous flap. Because these procedures can lead to umbilical translocation in relation to the aortic bifurcation, higher camera port placement or a single-site approach may be required. In general, RRSO is associated with a very low risk of operative complications. In a Memorial Sloan-Kettering study, 4 out of 80 RRSOs performed laparoscopically had complications caused by adhesions and trocar injuries, which are known complications associated with operative laparoscopy (71). With improved optical equipment and direct visualization trocars, the current rate may be lower.

Because many experts believe that high-grade serous "ovarian cancer" arises in the fallopian tube (78), the option of removing the fallopian tube and leaving the ovary *in situ* is being debated. Bilateral salpingectomy with ovarian retention (BSOR) has the advantage of avoiding the long-term sequelae of removing the ovaries and inducing surgical menopause. However, given that we lack convincing biologic data that the fallopian tube is the sole origin of ovarian cancer, BSOR remains investigational. A trial studying BSOR with delayed oophorectomy (NCT01907789) is currently underway but results will not be available before 2018. Still, many gynecologists have decided not to wait for the outcome of randomized trials and have begun to remove the fallopian tube at the time of hysterectomy for noncancer indications, as the surgical risk is small. Since 2010, investigators in British Columbia have educated gynecologists about the potential benefits of salpingectomy, suggesting that they remove the tubes at the time of hysterectomy for benign disease and for sterilization in lieu of a tubal ligation (79).

Postoperative Results

Women who have chosen to undergo RRSO generally report a good overall quality of life. The operation is often accompanied by a significant decrease in perceived risk and therefore a decrease in anxiety. Acute surgical menopause, however, can have a significant negative effect on quality of life (80). Menopause affects bone health and can cause a decrease in sexual desire along with vaginal atrophy and dyspareunia, which affect sexual functioning, leading to a further decrease in sexual desire, discomfort, and avoidance of intimacy. Many patients suffer from vasomotor symptoms, such as hot flashes and night sweats, which lead to sleep disturbances. These symptoms can be alleviated, but not completely eliminated, by HRT. Eisen et al. reported that HRT after RRSO is not associated with an increase in breast cancer risk in *BRCA* mutation carriers and those who received short-term HRT (approximately 3 years duration) after RRSO preserved the reduction in breast cancer risk offered by the surgery (HR, 0.38 vs. 0.37) (81). Still, decision making regarding menopausal therapies in women with *BRCA* mutations who are at increased risk of breast cancer is challenging because of the theoretical risk that HRT will promote growth of occult breast tumors. In addition, results from the WHI have influenced women and physicians to avoid use of cyclic estrogen/progestin HRT. Alternative treatments for vasomotor symptoms, such as venlafaxine and gabapentin, which are less effective than HRT, should be discussed in counseling. None of the "natural" treatments for hot flashes have been shown to be more effective than placebo.

The Pathologic Examination of Risk-Reducing Salpingo-oophorectomy Specimens

A family history of ovarian cancer and/or *BRCA* or other cancer gene mutation should be shared with the pathologist, as only one slide from the fallopian tube and ovary of patients with benign gynecologic disease is normally reviewed (4). In the setting of a known history of genetic predisposition to breast and ovarian cancer, most pathologists will submit the entirety of the fallopian tubes and ovaries for microscopic examination. The SEE-FIM (sectioning and extensively examining the fimbriated ends) protocol is now widely used for RRSO specimens. This involves serially sectioning the tube meticulously, stopping before the fimbriae. The fimbria is amputated and sectioned longitudinally, thereby maximizing exposure. Deeper sections need to be obtained if foci of atypia are to be identified histologically. Foci of *in situ* or invasive occult carcinoma may be very subtle and are often less than 1 mm in maximum diameter (see also Pathology section).

Microscopic occult carcinomas have been identified in RRSO specimens in about 2% to 9% of *BRCA* mutation carriers, generally involving the tubal fimbriae. In one prospective series, 7 ovarian and 3 tubal carcinomas (and 1 case in which washings showed malignant cells but no primary cancer was identified) were found among 490 women who underwent RRSO. Powell and colleagues report that of 111 consecutive BRCA-positive patients treated at a single institution, 9% had occult neoplasia (76). Suspicious epithelial cells, clearly distinct from mesothelial cells, are occasionally identified in cytology specimens. Colgan et al. found malignant cells in 3 of 35 pelvic washings. One microscopic ovarian surface carcinoma and 1 *in situ* tubal carcinoma were found; no carcinoma could be identified in the third patient. Twenty-two percent of specimens showed endosalpingiosis. Positive cytology specimens only rarely lead to the discovery of early-stage tubal carcinomas (81) although sometimes, as mentioned, malignant cells are present in washings at RRSO and there is no identifiable carcinoma by histology (73). Identification of a STIC but no other evidence of disseminated disease generally does not require additional surgery.

Lynch Syndrome—Hereditary Nonpolyposis Colorectal Cancer Syndrome

Epithelial ovarian cancer is also a component of HNPCC syndrome, which refers to patients who fulfill the Amsterdam criteria for Lynch syndrome II. Dr. Henry Lynch, who gave his name to the syndrome, characterized it as autosomal dominant cancer susceptibility syndrome. In addition to a predisposition to develop colorectal and endometrial cancer, women with this syndrome have a 10% to 13% lifetime risk for developing ovarian cancer (82,83) (27% to 71% risk of developing endometrial cancer). These patients develop ovarian cancer at a younger age and present at an earlier stage (83). They also have a higher percentage of low-grade tumors than the general population (84). In a cohort of women with HNPCC and at least two primary cancers, more than half were initially diagnosed with a gynecologic cancer, which preceded the development of a colorectal cancer. Fourteen percent of these women had synchronous cancers; a colorectal and a gynecologic cancer were found simultaneously

(82). Women at risk for Lynch syndrome are identified using either the Amsterdam II or the revised Bethesda criteria, which have been enriched for patients who are likely to have a hereditary origin of their cancer. However, even though the Bethesda criteria have been revised to improve identification, they may still miss as many as 28% of patients with Lynch syndrome.

Lynch syndrome describes patients and families with a germ line mutation in *MLH1, MSH2, MSH6, PMS2*, or *EPCAM*. Lynch syndrome-related tumors exhibit a lengthening or shortening of DNA repeat sequences, which leads to microsatellite instability (MSI), caused by an inability to repair DNA replication errors. The germ line mutations that characterize the syndrome are in genes involved in the DNA mismatch repair pathway, especially *MSH2* and *MLH1*, which account for about 90% of the mutations detected in families with Lynch syndrome. *MSH2* is particularly associated with an excess of endometrial and ovarian carcinomas. Other genes in the MMR family, including *MSH6, PMS1*, and *PMS2*, account for 10% of HNPCC-related cancers (83). To identify patients with HNPCC using tissue specimens, two approaches are used: for MSI analysis, DNA is extracted from macrodissected tumors using paraffin sections and short tandem repeats are amplified. Immunohistochemical stains are performed for *MSH2, MSH6, MLH1*, and *PMS2*. If a MMR protein is absent, despite appropriate controls, confirmatory germ line testing is performed. MSI can be owing to epigenetic changes as well as to Lynch syndrome. If tissue analysis is suggestive of HNPCC the diagnosis should be confirmed through germ line testing for Lynch syndrome-related genes.

A French multicenter study reviewed the cancer incidence in 537 families with Lynch syndrome (85). For women in the study, the cumulative risk for Lynch syndrome-associated cancers was 19% by age 50 and 54% by age 70. The age-specific cumulative risk for ovarian cancer by age 70 was 20% for *MLH1* mutation carriers, 24% for *MSH2* mutation carriers, and 1% for those with *MSH6* mutations (**Fig. 23.8**). The authors found that *MSH6* mutation carriers have much lower cancer risks than those with *MLH1* and *MSH2* mutations. These findings raise the question of whether women with a *MSH6* mutation really need prophylactic surgery, especially if no other family member has been affected by cancer. However, a smaller cohort study did not confirm this low ovarian cancer risk in women affected by *MSH6* mutations (86). This study from the combined Swedish/Danish cancer registry found that the distribution of ovarian cancer histologic subtypes in patients with Lynch syndrome differed considerably from the sporadic ovarian cancer population. They reported that 35% of the ovarian cancers associated with Lynch syndrome were endometrioid and 17% were clear cell, both much higher percentages than are seen in sporadic cases. *PMS2* mutations are associated with a small increased risk of ovarian cancer.

As with *BRCA1/2* patients, RRSO is a very effective method for the prevention of ovarian cancer in patients with a Lynch syndrome mutation. Preoperatively, patients should have a colonoscopy to search for polyps and colon cancer, an endometrial biopsy to exclude an occult endometrial cancer, and a vaginal ultrasound to detect any ovarian masses that will affect the surgical approach (minimally invasive vs. open surgery). In a large study combining all Lynch syndrome patients followed at MD Anderson, UCSF, and Creighton University, none of 61 patients who underwent RRSO and a hysterectomy developed ovarian or uterine cancer. However, 12 (5.5%) of the 223 patients who chose surveillance developed ovarian cancer and 33% developed endometrial cancer (87). Consistent with the French study (85), half of the patients who developed ovarian cancer had a *MLH1* mutation and the other half a *MSH2* mutation, whereas none had a *MSH6* mutation. Clearly RRSO and hysterectomy are effective in preventing gynecologic cancers in women affected by HNPCC. Women with Lynch syndrome and ovarian cancer have a better prognosis with a 5-year survival of 88%.

A critical question for patients with Lynch syndrome is at what age a hysterectomy/BSO should be performed. Two studies reported that the median age for endometrial and ovarian cancer in these patients is 46 to 48 years and 42 to 48 years, respectively. Moreover, a significant number of the women in one study (21% to 42%) developed ovarian cancer before age 40 (86,87). However, the French study found that the risk of developing ovarian cancer for all Lynch syndrome mutation carriers by age 40 does not exceed 2% to 3%. Still, a prudent approach is to perform the hysterectomy and RRSO after the age of 35, or once childbearing is completed. Obviously, such an early intervention requires extensive counseling, balancing the consequences of surgical menopause treated with HRT with the benefits of avoiding ovarian and endometrial cancer.

For patients with Lynch syndrome who prefer not to undergo prophylactic surgery there is no scientifically proven ovarian cancer screening option. According to the NCCN guidelines and most experts, transvaginal ultrasound and CA-125 are acceptable exams in patients with mutations, if the patient is fully aware that these interventions will not necessarily diagnose ovarian cancer early and might even be harmful, because of possible complications of surgical follow-up for a false-positive result (67). However, given that two-thirds of HNPCC-associated ovarian cancers are diagnosed during stages I and II because of their endometrioid and clear cell histology (86,87), a vaginal ultrasound is a reasonable choice for surveillance in a woman who declines prophylactic surgery. Although it has not been thoroughly studied, chemoprevention with OCP together with screening for ovarian and endometrial cancer is currently used in women who want to delay surgery.

	Cumulative Risk, % (95% Confidence Interval)											
	Colorectal Cancer				Endometrial Cancer				Ovarian Cancer			
		Carriers				Carriers				Carriers		
Age, y	All	*MLH1*	*MSH2*	*MSH6*	All	*MLH1*	*MSH2*	*MSH6*	All	*MLH1*	*MSH2*	*MSH6*
20	0 (0–1)	0 (0–1)	0 (0–1)	0	0	0	0	0	0	0	0	0
30	2 (1–3)	1 (0–3)	2 (1–5)	0 (0–1)	0 (0–1)	0 (0–1)	0 (0–1)	0	0	0	0 (0–1)	0
40	5 (3–8)	6 (3–11)	8 (4–13)	1 (0–3)	2 (1–4)	1 (0–4)	2 (0–7)	1 (0–2)	1 (0–1)	0 (0–2)	1 (0–3)	0
50	13 (9–19)	14 (8–27)	20 (13–30)	3 (2–6)	8 (4–15)	9 (3–19)	8 (3–21)	3 (1–8)	3 (1–5)	4 (0–11)	4 (1–9)	0 (0–1)
60	24 (17–35)	28 (16–49)	36 (23–54)	6 (4–12)	23 (12–38)	32 (12–55)	18 (8–53)	9 (5–19)	7 (2–21)	15 (1–45)	11 (2–28)	1 (0–2)
70	35 (25–49)	41 (25–70)	48 (30–77)	12 (8–22)	34 (16–58)	54 (20–80)	21 (8–77)	16 (8–32)	8 (2–37)	20 (1–65)	24 (3–52)	1 (0–3)
80	42 (30–60)	49 (29–85)	52 (31–90)	18 (13–30)	35 (17–60)	57 (22–82)	21 (9–82)	17 (8–47)	8 (2–39)	20 (1–66)	38 (3–81)	1 (0–3)

[a]See eTable 3 (available at http:www.jama.com) for the number of affected individuals and the number of family members contributing to the likelihood for risk estimation.

Figure 23.8. Age-specific cumulative risks of colorectal cancer, endometrial cancer, and ovarian cancer according to gene for mismatch repair mutation carriers.

Source: From Bonadona V, Bonaiti B, Olschwang S, et al. Cancer risk associated with germline mutations in MLH1, MSH2, and MSH6 genes in Lynch syndrome. *JAMA*. 2011;305:2304–2310, with permission.

NAURAL HISTORY OF THE DISEASE: PATTERNS OF SPREAD

Mucinous and Endometrioid Ovarian Cancer

Mucinous neoplasms are the largest of all known ovarian tumors. They can reach diameters of 30 to 40 cm, often compressing adjacent organs (**Fig. 23.9**). Intact removal of these tumors may be challenging because of their weight, the large veins that drain from them, and difficulties visualizing the ureter during the procedure. However, mucinous tumors, especially the largest, tend to be benign. Indeed, 80% of these tumors are benign mucinous cystadenomas, and when malignant, most mucinous tumors are low grade. Although high-grade invasive mucinous cancers are very aggressive and resistant to chemotherapy, they are rare. Only 0.5% to 1.5% of advanced ovarian cancers have a mucinous histology. One large study found that 71% of invasive mucinous tumors found in the ovary were metastases from the gastrointestinal tract (colon, pancreas, and appendix), and only 29% were truly primary mucinous ovarian cancers (88,89). These primary invasive mucinous tumors are often confined to the ovary without surface involvement and are unilateral (metastases are more often bilateral) and of a significant size (≥13 cm) (88). Often patients with mucinous tumors have an elevated level of one of two tumor markers, CEA or CA19-9.

Pseudomyxoma peritonei (PMP) is a condition caused by the production of mucin by glandular cells in the peritoneal cavity. These cells have a benign glandular histology, but their behavior is biologically malignant, as the mucin-producing cells implant diffusely on the abdominal and pelvic peritoneum. The cells then produce thick mucin that encases the bowel and pelvic organs, leading to tumor cachexia and bowel obstruction. The most common origins of PMP are currently thought to be appendiceal neoplasms or ruptured benign mucoceles of the appendix with secondary involvement of the ovary. Patients with PMP can progress for months or years without symptoms. Although their disease often has an indolent course, it cannot be cured (10-year survival is 50% to 60%) (90,91). Currently, it is generally recommended that patients receive aggressive cytoreductive surgery with complete peritonectomy and hyperthermic intraperitoneal chemotherapy (HIPEC) in a specialized center, although there are no randomized data to support this strategy (91).

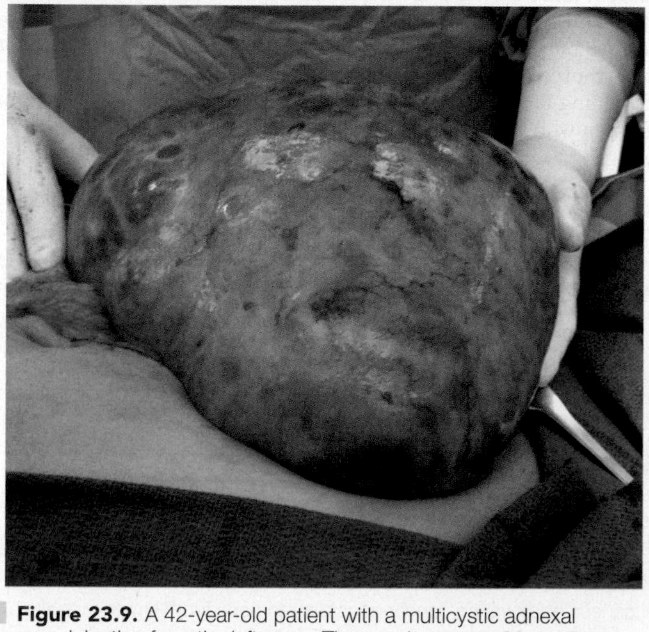

Figure 23.9. A 42-year-old patient with a multicystic adnexal mass originating from the left ovary. The specimen was 20 × 15 cm and weighed 5 pounds. The frozen section returned as a mucinous borderline tumor.

Invasive endometrioid ovarian cancer accounts for about 10% of all ovarian carcinomas and occurs most often in perimenopausal patients. These cancers are often associated with endometriosis (29). Up to 25% of patients of reproductive age with an endometrioid endometrial cancer have a synchronous early-stage endometrioid ovarian cancer (92). Molecularly, these tumors are often clonally related, representing metastatic disease from either the uterus or the ovary (93).

Because of the large size of the primary tumor, both mucinous and endometrioid ovarian cancers are likely to be discovered at an early stage (FIGO I/II). They do not have the pattern of transcoelomic spread along peritoneal surfaces seen with serous cancers and, unlike high-grade serous ovarian cancer, they do not respect anatomic intraperitoneal planes. Locally, they are characterized by thick adhesions to the pelvis and can invade adjacent pelvic organs including the muscularis of the colon and the pelvic sidewall. Advanced metastatic endometrioid and mucinous tumors (FIGO III/IV) implant into the abdominal wall and metastasize to the parenchyma of intra-abdominal organs such as the liver and spleen (88).

Serous Ovarian Cancer

Serous carcinomas originating from Müllerian epithelium, which include ovarian, peritoneal, and fallopian tube cancers, are characterized by transcoelomic spread (13,94). Recently, there have been new insights into the origin of serous "ovarian" cancer, and a putative precursor lesion in the fallopian tube, serous tubal intraepithelial carcinoma (STIC), has been identified. It is now believed that most serous "ovarian" cancer originates in the fallopian tube as STIC (76,95). A small tumor can be easily assigned to a particular anatomic site, but if the tumor is widely disseminated, it is not possible to clearly identify where a serous tumor originated. In the absence of a STIC, serous tumors will default to ovarian. However, this is not very important from a clinical standpoint, because the dissemination patterns of serous ovarian, fallopian tube, and peritoneal cancer are clinically indistinguishable by virtue of their propensity to exfoliate malignant cells into the peritoneal cavity, and patient survival is very similar. A study (96), as well as clinical experience, suggests that all three tumor subtypes grow quickly and disseminate on mesothelial cell-covered body cavities, including the peritoneal cavity or pleural space. Once the cancer cells detach from the ovarian or fallopian tube tumor, they float in the ascites as single cells or as multicellular spheroids (13). The cells follow the normal clockwise circulation of peritoneal fluid up the right paracolic gutter and to the undersurface of the right hemi-diaphragm, where they may implant and grow as surface nodules. All intraperitoneal mesothelium-covered surfaces are at risk, with frequent involvement of the peritoneum, diaphragm, omentum, to a lesser degree the hepatic flexure and splenic hilum, bowel and bowel mesentery, and appendix (94,97).

The most common sites involved in locoregional metastasis are the contralateral ovary, the peritoneum of the cul-de-sac, and the rectosigmoid colon serosa and its mesentery. Colonization of the cul-de-sac with cancer cells often results in obliteration of the rectouterine space. In patients with extensive pelvic disease (**Fig. 23.10**), the uterus, bladder dome, side wall peritoneum overlying the ureter, sigmoid colon, ovarian tumor masses, and appendix become a conglomerate pelvic tumor, and it is very difficult to identify the individual organs or any anatomic borders (98,99). If the tumor is predominantly on the patient's right side, a large tumor mass develops in the right lower quadrant involving the ileocecum, appendix, and right ovary. If the tumor is predominantly on the left side, the conglomerate tumor includes the left ovary, the rectosigmoid and its mesentery, and the left side of the uterus.

The most frequent site of distant metastasis is the omentum. Other than metastases to the contralateral ovary, an omental metastasis is often the largest tumor in the abdominal cavity. Serous cancers initially transform the infracolic omentum, but as the cancer progresses the entire omentum is replaced by tumors (94), reaching from the hepatic to the splenic flexure (**Fig. 23.11**). Because the omentum reaches the

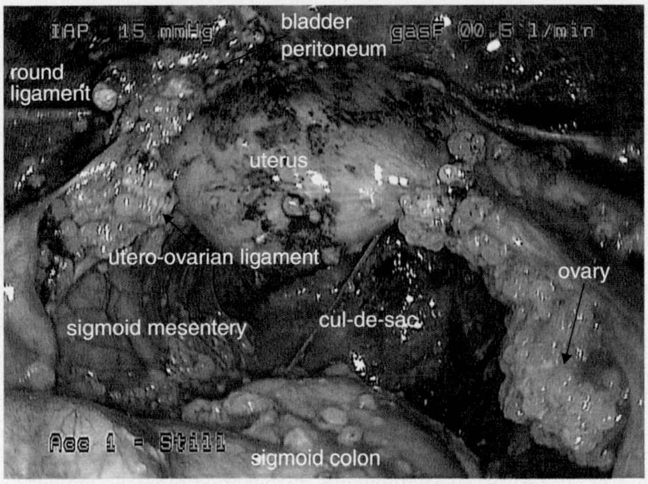

Figure 23.10. Laparoscopic intraoperative image of the pelvis of a patient with disseminated high-volume disease suggestive of ovarian cancer on CT scan. Tumor implants on the sigmoid colon, sigmoid mesentery, pelvic sidewall, ovary, utero-ovarian ligament, and bladder peritoneum.

spleen in the left upper quadrant, there is often a solid tumor at the lower pole of the spleen and at the splenic hilum directly adjacent to the distal pancreas, sometimes requiring an en bloc resection of the distal pancreas and the spleen in order to completely clear the left upper abdomen (100,101). In patients affected by extensive disease, the lesser omentum, which is attached to the lesser curvature of the stomach, is also involved. Despite extensive involvement of the omentum by a serous carcinoma, there is almost never invasion of the gastric or transverse colon muscularis as the tumor is only invading the serosa. It is almost always possible to develop a plane between the tumor and the muscularis and remove the tumor nodules and plaques without a colon or gastric resection. Also, there is rarely tumor in the retroperitoneal, lesser sac, because serous tumors metastasize on mesothelial cell-covered surfaces. Extensive surface involvement of the abdominal or pleural cavity will cause ascites and a pleural effusion, respectively. Patients with extensive intra-abdominal tumor involvement sometimes have extensive involvement of the small

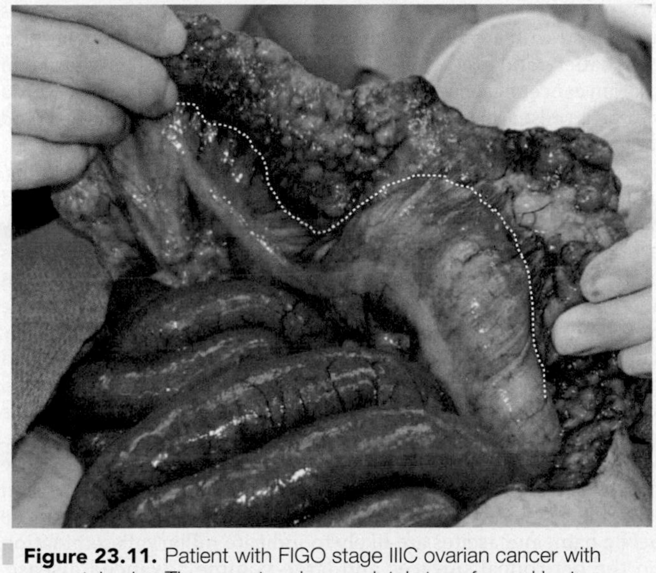

Figure 23.11. Patient with FIGO stage IIIC ovarian cancer with an omental cake. The omentum is completely transformed by tumor nodules. The omentum is lifted superiorly, toward the patient's head. The omental tumor can almost always be dissected off the transverse colon along an avascular plane (***white dotted line***), allowing entry into the lesser sac.

bowel mesentery. A condition described owing to its appearance as "rose budding" will occur when tumor constricts the blood supply to the bowel and limits bowel mobility because of the short mesenteric root. Often these tumors are unresectable because they compromise all blood supply to the small bowel from the superior mesenteric artery and impair venous return through the superior mesenteric vein. In very advanced disease, serous cancers tend to agglutinate the loops of small bowel and cause a high-grade bowel obstruction at many levels (jejunum, ileum).

Women with advanced serous ovarian cancer, who have disseminated miliary disease covering the entire peritoneal surface, including the diaphragms, often have large-volume ascites (102). The ascitic fluid generally contains mesothelial, inflammatory, and tumor cells (13). Rarely, serous tumors will metastasize to the mesothelial cell-covered pericardium, causing a pericardial effusion.

Because FIGO stage IV serous ovarian cancer is defined by several anatomic locations in the upper abdomen and/or a malignant pleural effusion, patients with stage IV disease are a very heterogeneous group. Peritoneal–pleural lymphatic communication through the diaphragm allows trans-diaphragmatic spread of tumor into the mesothelium-covered pleural space, causing a malignant pleural effusion. Because serous cancers have a preference for implantation on the right diaphragm, most patients with FIGO 2013 stage IV disease have a right-sided malignant pleural effusion (37% to 48%) (103,104). Other metastasis patterns that define FIGO stage IVB disease include parenchymal liver metastases, supraclavicular/axillary lymphadenopathy, parenchymal lung metastases, mediastinal adenopathy, and distal vaginal or perineal metastases (103,104). Although serous ovarian cancer disseminates extensively within the abdominal cavity, intra-pulmonary metastasis, or other intra-parenchymal involvement, for example, intrahepatic, spleen, or kidney tumors, are rare. If these are found, the differential diagnosis should be expanded to include a different ovarian cancer histotype (clear cell, mucinous, or carcinosarcoma) or a different tumor origin (gastrointestinal, breast cancer).

Advanced invasive low-grade serous cancers, which represent about 9% of all epithelial ovarian cancers (105,106), have a tumor distribution pattern that is very similar to that of high-grade serous cancers, with metastasis to the omentum (83%), fallopian tube (63%), pelvic peritoneum (49%), and uterine serosa (46%) (107).

Lymph Node Metastasis

Exfoliation followed by implantation is one of two primary modes of ovarian cancer dissemination. The other is via the retroperitoneal lymphatics draining the ovary. This path follows the superior ovarian blood supply in the infundibulopelvic ligament, which contains the ovarian artery and vein as well as extensive lymphatics which terminate in lymph nodes lining the aorta and vena cava up to the level of the renal vessels. The next lymph node stations are at the celiac trunk, from which tumor cells may continue up to the mediastinal and supraclavicular lymph nodes. Lymph channels also pass laterally through the broad ligament and parametrial channels to terminate in the pelvic sidewall lymphatics, including the external iliac, obturator, and hypogastric chains (108). Spread may also occur along the course of the round ligament, resulting in involvement of the inguinal lymphatics (the disease of these patients is now categorized as FIGO IVB). The principal lymphatic drainage of the ovary and fallopian tube appears to be via the para-aortic lymph nodes. Lymph node metastases are correlated with the extent of intra-abdominal disease involvement. Retroperitoneal node involvement has been found in the majority of advanced ovarian cancer cases (109–111).

The initial spread of ovarian cancer, by both the intraperitoneal and lymphatic routes, is clinically occult. As many as 20% of women with the appearance of FIGO stage I/II ovarian cancer have widespread disease (112). Histologic type (serous), grade (III), and CA-125 (high) at diagnosis are risk factors for lymph node metastasis. The true extent of disease can be detected only by histologic examination of visually normal tissues sampled during careful surgical staging

■ **TABLE 23.3. Subclinical Metastases in Apparent Early Ovarian Cancer**

Site	No. of Patients with Involvement	Total Patients	% Involved
Diaphragm	17	223	7.6
Omentum	21	294	7.1
Cytology	13	69	18.8
Peritoneal	6	61	9.8
Pelvic modes	18	202	8.9
Para-aortic modes	35	285	12.3

Source: Modified with permission from Moore DH. Primary management of early epithelial ovarian carcinoma. In: Rubin SC, Sutton GP, eds. *Ovarian Cancer*. New York, NY: McGraw-Hill; 1993:241–254.

(113). Approximately 10% of patients with cancer that appears to be confined to the ovaries will have metastases to the para-aortic nodes. Many patients with apparently localized disease will also have occult disease found in peritoneal washings or in biopsies of the diaphragm and omentum (**Table 23.3**). However, it should be noted that the data in **Table 23.3** predate advanced imaging modalities (e.g., high-resolution computed tomography (CT) scans).

Recurrent Ovarian Cancer

The majority (80%) of patients with advanced ovarian cancer who undergo a combination of platinum- and taxane-based chemotherapy will have a recurrence, although many will have initial complete response to primary treatment (103,114). Of all patients with ovarian cancer, 75% have an intra-abdominal recurrence; the remainder have extra-peritoneal/intrahepatic or distant metastasis with or without intra-abdominal recurrence (115). Twenty-two percent of recurrences occur outside the peritoneal cavity. The locations of intra-abdominal recurrences include the remnants of the omentum, especially at the splenic flexures, the small and large bowel mesentery, and the epiploic appendices, which are peritoneal pouches filled with fat and located along the colon and intraperitoneal rectum. The majority of deaths occur in the first 2 years (53%) and only 46.2% of all patients survive 5 years (SEER data, accessed April 2016).

Following the increased use of intraperitoneal chemotherapy with the publication of GOG#172 (116), several retrospective studies reported a change in the pattern of recurrence. Women treated with intraperitoneal, rather than intravenous, chemotherapy were found to have a higher rate of extra-abdominal recurrences, including brain metastasis, pleural effusions, and mediastinal disease. Robinson et al. found that women with recurrent ovarian cancer treated with intraperitoneal chemotherapy had a 26% risk of extra-abdominal metastasis, whereas women treated with only intravenous chemotherapy had a 7% risk (117). Two other retrospective studies reported even higher extra-peritoneal recurrence rates of 41% to 45% after intraperitoneal chemotherapy (118). It has also been reported that when intraperitoneal chemotherapy is combined with bevacizumab, more patients present with recurrent disease in the central nervous system or the skin (117). Regardless of its combination with intraperitoneal therapy, more pleural and parenchymal metastases are observed after bevacizumab treatment (119).

Clinical Presentation and Diagnostic Work-Up

The diagnosis and treatment of patients with ovarian masses is difficult because of the diversity of clinical presentation, the plethora of differential diagnoses, and the wide range of therapeutic options (**Table 23.4**).

Clinical Presentation of Patients with a Benign Adnexal Mass or Early-Stage Ovarian Cancer

Almost all patients with small adnexal tumors are asymptomatic; the mass is usually discovered incidentally during a work-up for other conditions (**Fig. 23.12**). With increasing size, adnexal masses cause pelvic pressure and pain by compressing surrounding structures. A larger pelvic tumor can cause genitourinary symptoms, including urinary urgency, urinary frequency, and dyspareunia. Posteriorly, a fixed pelvic tumor can compress the sigmoid colon, causing severe constipation and pain. These symptoms can occur in both benign disease and early ovarian cancer. It is impossible to differentiate a benign from a malignant ovarian mass by clinical examination alone. Borderline ovarian tumors, nonserous malignant epithelial ovarian cancer (endometrioid, clear cell, mucinous), and non-epithelial (germ cell, stromal cell) malignant tumors frequently present as large adnexal masses at an early stage without any further abdominal dissemination.

An ovarian mass becomes a surgical emergency if a patient has a sudden onset of abdominal pain. The differential diagnosis in this situation includes rupture, torsion, and possible infarction of the ovarian mass. In addition, severe abdominal pain can also be caused by a hemorrhage inside a cyst, which distends it, or by the rupture of a blood-filled cyst, causing hemoperitoneum. Sudden abdominal pain associated with an adnexal mass is often accompanied by malaise, nausea and vomiting, low-grade fever, an elevated white blood cell count, and elevated C-reactive protein levels, which are all caused by peritoneal irritation. In the presence of acute pain, peritoneal signs, rigidity, and rebound tenderness, urgent expert surgical evaluation should be considered. Evaluation is most often performed laparoscopically. Delaying surgery can result in infarction, hemorrhage, peritonitis, and sepsis. Vaginal bleeding in a patient with an adnexal mass could be an indication of synchronous endometrial and ovarian cancers (92) or a granulosa cell tumor that produces estrogen, causing abnormal bleeding. Sertoli–Leydig cell tumors, which can cause bleeding, can also lead to virilization.

Clinical Presentation of Patients with Advanced Ovarian Cancer

The clinical presentation of advanced ovarian cancer is varied. Treating physicians are often surprised by how few symptoms women with advanced ovarian cancer may experience. Nonspecific symptoms associated with advanced ovarian cancer include anorexia, fatigue, early satiety, and loss of appetite. Although weight loss is unusual in ovarian cancer because of diffuse ascites production, tumor cachexia can be a presenting sign in patients with high-volume disease and long-standing partial bowel obstruction.

Often patients have nonspecific pelvic and abdominal symptoms, including bloating and diffuse, dull, constant abdominal pain caused by the infiltration of the peritoneum and the bowel mesentery or by extensive ascites. Involvement of the small bowel can cause changes in the frequency of bowel movements, with alternating constipation and diarrhea. If the tumor has metastasized to the omentum, there may be upper abdominal discomfort with nausea, belching, early satiety, and fullness. The abdominal cavity may also be distended by several liters of ascites, which can cause a significant increase in abdominal circumference leading to marked discomfort. Extensive ascites can cause significant fatigue, anorexia, pain, nausea/vomiting, and incontinence. In addition, ascites can cause dyspnea, because the lower lung lobes are compressed by the abdominal distension (102). Signs of bowel obstruction, severe urinary symptoms, intense pelvic pain, and ascites are likely to indicate miliary dissemination on the peritoneal surfaces and large-volume advanced disease. Moreover, patients with advanced ovarian cancer sometimes present with deep venous thrombosis (DVT) from large tumors pressing on pelvic veins or as part of the hypercoagulopathy associated with advanced-stage cancer (120).

TABLE 23.4. Differential Diagnosis of an Adnexal Mass

Definition	Description	Mean Age	Clinical Presentation	Imaging	Therapy	Comments
Ectopic pregnancy	Tubal pregnancy, most common in the fimbriated end	Reproductive age women	Positive pregnancy test. History of PID, tubal surgery, fertility treatment, or previous ectopic pregnancies. Pelvic pain, anemia	Pelvic ultrasound	Methotrexate or laparoscopy with salpingectomy or salpingostomy, laparotomy if hemodynamically unstable	Clinical emergency. 10%–15% recurrence risk
Physiologic, functional cysts	Follicular cyst—preovulatory cyst Corpus luteum cyst—postovulatory cyst caused by hemorrhage or cyst formation. Theca lutein cysts are caused by hCG stimulation of the ovary. “Other”: paratubal cysts, hydrosalpinx	Reproductive age women	Depending on size, lower abdominal pain, dyspareunia, signs of latent torsion. On exam freely mobile and unilateral. May present as an acute abdomen when ruptured, torsed, or infarcted: unilateral intermittent, acutely worsening pelvic pain	Pelvic ultrasound. Often > 7cm	Persists for weeks. Oral contraceptives might cause involution/resolution and help with the diagnosis. If a cyst does not resolve within 8 weeks, laparoscopy should be considered	Most frequent benign masses in reproductive age women. A bleeding corpus luteum can cause an acute abdomen, anemia, and hemoperitoneum. Hydrosalpinx is a cystic dilatation of the fallopian tube caused by PID, ectopic pregnancy, endometriosis, or fallopian tube cancer
Polycystic ovaries	Endocrine disorder. Multiple follicle cysts enlarging the ovaries to 2–5 times their normal size	Reproductive age women	Irregular menstrual cycles, anovulation, amenorrhea, acne, hirsutism, subfertility, metabolic syndrome	Pelvic ultrasound, hormonal tests (DHEAS, androstenedione, testosterone, FSH). Glucose tolerance test	Oral contraceptives, metformin, glitazones, weight loss, clomiphene, spironolactone	Often associated with peripheral insulin resistance. Higher risk of endometrial hyperplasia and endometrial cancer
Serous and mucinous cystadenomas	Serous—cystic: thin walled, unilocular. Mucinous—cystic thin walled but may be multicystic		Serous 5–20 cm, mucinous up to 40 cm	Pelvic/abdominal ultrasound	Laparoscopic drainage and removal or laparoscopic cystectomy	May present with torsion or rupture. Cystadenofibroma is a mixed tumor
Germ cell tumors	Benign: teratomas/dermoids. Malignant: immature teratoma/dysgerminoma	Young reproductive age patients	Bilateral in 20%. Elevated β-hCG, AFP, LDH, (CA-125)	Ultrasound. Might show calcifications on X-ray or CT. Solid, partially cystic	Laparoscopic cystectomy removing the entire capsule. If malignant salpingo-oophorectomy, staging	
Sex cord stromal cell tumors	Benign: fibromas, thecomas, Brenner cell tumors Malignant: granulosa cell tumor, Sertoli–Leydig cell tumor	30-menopause, but also postmenopausal patients	Solid, firm tumors resembling fibroids. May produce hormones: estradiol, inhibin. May cause irregular bleeding, uterine hyperplasia	Ultrasound/CT. Solid homogeneous tumors. Granulosa cell tumors are heterogeneous and often rupture	Laparoscopic or laparotomy for ovarian cystectomy or oophorectomy depending on size	In postmenopausal patients benign stromal cell tumors are preoperatively often interpreted as being malignant. Often the CA-125 is normal or not too high

(continued)

TABLE 23.4. Differential Diagnosis of an Adnexal Mass (*continued*)

Definition	Description	Mean Age	Clinical Presentation	Imaging	Therapy	Comments
Peritoneal inclusion cysts	Cystic	Any age	History of multiple pelvic/abdominal surgeries or recurrent pelvic infections or peritoneal dialysis	Ultrasound: multiple thin walled cysts, CT, MRI can often help to establish a diagnosis	Observation vs. ultrasound or CT-guided aspiration with cytology. Surgical intervention for severe symptoms or hydronephrosis. High perioperative morbidity (bowel, ureter injury)	
Fibroids	Benign. Broad ligament or pedunculated fibroids misdiagnosed	30–55 yr	Often asymptomatic. Degeneration or infarction can occur and cause acute pain	Ultrasound, rarely CT or MRI	Observation vs. surgical intervention with myomectomy or hysterectomy	Common in African-American women. Often pedunculated fibroids are mistaken for an adnexal mass
Endometriosis	1–10 cm endometriotic cysts filled with blood, adherent to surrounding organs. Often bilateral. Endometriotic implants occur in the pelvic peritoneum including the cul-de-sac and bladder peritoneum. Nodularity of the uterosacral ligaments	30–45 yr	Pelvic pain. Dyspareunia. May have cyclical pain with menses, infertility, and dyspareunia. May present with acute pain from rupture, rarely torsion. CA-125 100–300 U/mL	Pelvic/abdominal ultrasound. Diagnostic laparoscopy	Conservative treatment. Anti-inflammatory drugs, OCP, GnRH analogues. Laparoscopy with removal of endometriomas and coagulation of endometriotic nodules. Extent of surgery depends on symptoms and desire for future fertility	Common in white nulliparous women. Ovarian endometrioma is also called a "chocolate cyst"
PID/salpingitis	Tubo-ovarian abscess complicates PID in 15% of all women	Young sexually active patients	History of PID, pelvic pain, malaise, vaginal discharge (GO, chlamydia), cervical motion tenderness. Fever, chills, leukocytosis, CRP ↑, Platelets ↑. CA-125: 100–500 U/mL. Coagulopathy if septic	Ultrasound showing one or more masses that are homogenous, cystic, possibly with air fluid levels and septations	Combination antibiotic treatment, CT-guided abscess drainage. Laparoscopy or laparotomy if abscess cannot be drained or if the patient has signs and symptoms of sepsis	High recurrence risk
Appendicitis and appendiceal abscess	Appendicitis, right-sided tenderness, rebound	Younger patients	Fever, guarding, rebound tenderness. Malaise, RLQ pain, nausea, vomiting, absence of vaginal discharge. Pain migration, leukocytosis, CRP ↑, Platelets ↑, CA-125~100-200 U/mL	Ultrasound and CT imaging with contrast. No distinct mass. Features consistent with abscess: enhancement, irregular borders	Laparoscopic surgery	Difficult differential in children and young women. Consider PID and pregnancy
Diverticulitis and diverticular abscess	Diverticulitis mostly in the sigmoid colon causing left-sided pain	Elderly patients	Fever, guarding, rebound tenderness. Malaise, LLQ pain, nausea, vomiting. Pain, leukocytosis, CRP ↑, Platelets ↑, CA-125~100–200 U/mL	Ultrasound and CT imaging with contrast. No distinct mass. Features consistent with abscess: enhancement, irregular borders	Combination antibiotic treatment, CT-guided abscess drainage. Surgery if patient has signs and symptoms of sepsis and for definitive treatment	Presentation in very old patients might be subtle. High recurrence risk

Colon cancer			Anemia, irregular stools. Induration and irregularity. Family history	Sigmoidoscopy/ colonoscopy		60%–70% occur on the left side but cecal cancer can present as right adnexal mass
Early invasive epithelial ovarian cancer	Early serous ovarian cancer, endometrioid or clear cell ovarian cancer		CA-125 ↑ only in 50%	Papillary surface excrescences, areas of necrosis, internal solid elements	Surgical intervention: Consider starting with a laparoscopy to establish a diagnosis. Referral to gynecologic oncologist for full staging	Differential of ovarian malignancy: invasive serous cancer, endometrioid, clear cell cancer. Borderline tumors
Advanced invasive epithelial ovarian cancer	Serous carcinoma with ascites and metastasis to upper abdomen	Postmenopausal women	Persistent bloating, general abdominal pain, early satiety. Vaginal bleeding. CA-125 ↑ in 80%. Platelets ↑	Suspicious adnexal mass and ascites, upper abdominal disease	Exploratory laparotomy, staging, tumor debulking. Referral to gynecologic oncologist	Differentiate between high- and low-volume disease. High-volume disease often requires upper abdominal procedures and bowel surgery
Metastasis	Gastric, colon, breast, and uterine cancer		CA-125 can be elevated. Other tumor markers might be helpful (CEA, CA19-9, CA15-3)	Bilateral solid complex masses in patients with prior cancer history	Excision can be considered for symptomatic relief or if it is the only site of metastatic disease	Poor prognosis compared to ovarian cancer
Rare differential diagnoses	– Pelvic kidney – Disseminated abdominal tuberculosis: Young women unlikely to have ovarian cancer from endemic areas, populations at risk, ascites, CA-125 ↑, absence of a dominant adnexal mass					

AFP, alpha-fetoprotein; CA-125, cancer antigen 125; CRP, C-reactive protein; DHEAS, dehydroepiandrosterone sulfate; FSH, follicle-stimulating hormone; GnRH, gonadotropin-releasing hormone; GO, gonorrhea; hCG, human chorionic gonadotropin; LDH, lactic dehydrogenase; LLQ, left lower quadrant; OCP, oral contraceptive pill; PID, pelvic inflammatory disease; RLQ, right lower quadrant.

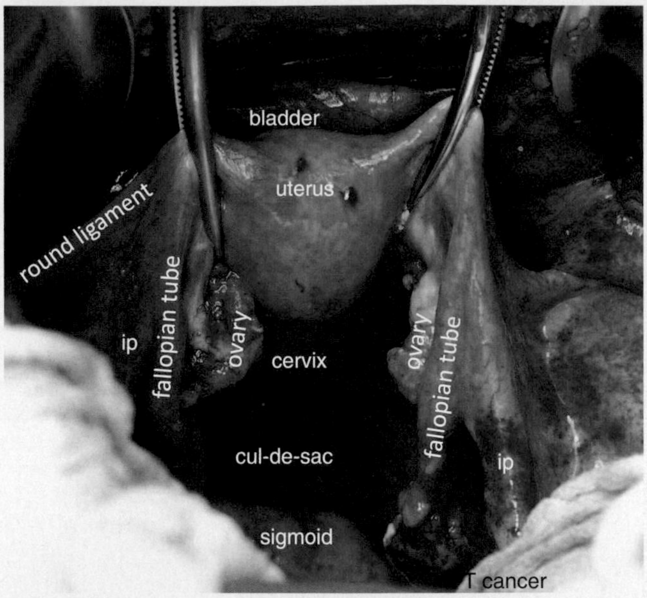

Figure 23.12. Patient with left fallopian tube cancer hanging off the left tubal fimbriae. Fallopian tube (FT), infundibulopelvic (ip) artery and vein.

Because symptoms often develop late, when the cancer is already advanced, ovarian cancer has been called the "silent killer" or "the cancer that whispers." There are no specific symptoms that assist in diagnosing ovarian cancer early. However, a careful review of symptoms in women with ovarian cancer has shown that many have abdominal symptoms, urinary frequency, and pain for 3 months or longer before diagnosis (121). One study suggested that ovarian cancer patients tend to have a combination of symptoms (e.g., increased abdominal size/bloating, early satiety, pelvic/abdominal pain, urinary urge, incontinence), which are more severe, more frequent, and of more recent onset than those symptoms reported by patients without cancer who present to a primary care clinic (121). These symptoms are nonspecific and overlap with several common disorders like irritable bowel syndrome, dyspepsia, and menopause. There is no evidence that screening for any of these symptom clusters can aid in recognizing ovarian cancer earlier or improve on the use of CA-125 and ultrasound (122). Several studies have concluded that the appraisal of symptoms alone is not likely to lead to an earlier diagnosis (123,124).

American College of Obstetrics and Gynecology (ACOG) and SGO (125) consensus guidelines recommend referral to a gynecologic oncologist for postmenopausal women with elevated CA-125, ascites, a nodular/fixed pelvic mass, or evidence of abdominal/distant metastasis. In premenopausal women, a very elevated CA-125, ascites, or evidence of abdominal or distant metastasis should also trigger a referral. These guidelines have a positive predictive value of 39.6% for premenopausal women and 64.6% for postmenopausal women. A benign condition that can closely mimic the constellation of symptoms described in the consensus guidelines is Meigs syndrome (126). This syndrome is characterized by a cytologically benign pleural effusion and ascites, which resolve upon removal of a concomitant ovarian tumor, usually an ovarian fibroma or thecoma.

Diagnosis of Ovarian Cancer

The correct clinical diagnosis of an ovarian mass is difficult and requires considerable experience and clinical judgment (**Table 23.4**). Age is a very important factor in assessing an adnexal mass, as many ovarian tumors have a predilection for a particular age group. In premenarchal girls, an adnexal mass is often germ cell in origin, whereas young women in their reproductive years are most likely to have benign disease. In postmenopausal patients, a complex adnexal mass is particularly concerning for an epithelial cancer, as a normal postmenopausal ovary is atrophic and small ($1.5 \times 1 \times 0.5$ cm) (**Table 23.5**). On average, the volume of a normal ovary is 10 cm^3 in postmenopausal and 20 cm^3 in premenopausal women (127).

An adnexal mass in a woman of reproductive age is a significant diagnostic challenge, because most of these tumors in premenopausal women are benign. However, it is critical that no malignant tumors are missed. The differential diagnosis of an adnexal mass/cyst is described in **Table 23.4**. There are several categories of benign masses, including functional cysts, adenomas, nonmalignant germ cell tumors (mature teratomas/dermoids), nonmalignant sex cord stromal tumors (fibromas), and endometriosis. The most common benign solid ovarian tumors are ovarian fibromas (fibroma/fibrothecoma/cystadenofibroma). Another common solid tumor is a pedunculated fibroid, which may be interpreted on imaging as an adnexal mass. Infectious conditions that may present with similar signs and symptoms include PID, appendicitis, and diverticulitis. For women in their reproductive years, the decision to pursue surgery will depend on the degree of clinical suspicion based on the factors detailed above and their desire for future fertility.

In some patients there is no distinct adnexal mass but a conglomerate tumor in the lower abdomen. The differential diagnosis for this includes an advanced ovarian cancer, an advanced endometrial cancer/sarcoma, colon or appendiceal cancer, and retroperitoneal tumors. A metastatic breast, colon, or lung cancer tumor should be considered in the presence of an atypical pattern of metastasis or abnormal mammogram or chest X-ray (**Table 23.4**) (128,129). It should be remembered, however, that although ovarian cancer is much more prevalent in postmenopausal women than premenopausal

TABLE 23.5. Differential Diagnosis of an Adnexal Mass by Age

History	Age	Differential Diagnosis
Age Pregnancy Menopausal status Family history	Premenarchal	Germ cell tumors, mature teratomas, rhabdomyosarcomas
	Young reproductive age (15–25 years)	Functional cysts, ectopic pregnancy, pelvic inflammatory disease (PID)/salpingitis/tuboovarian abscess (TOA), mature teratomas (dermoid), appendicitis/appendiceal abscess, polycystic ovaries, juvenile granulosa cell tumor, dysgerminoma, endodermal sinus tumor, tuberculosis
	Middle reproductive age (25–35 years)	Endometriosis, functional cysts, polycystic ovaries, serous/mucinous cystadenomas, PID/salpingitis/TOA, mature teratomas (dermoid), Sertoli–Leydig cell tumor
	Advanced reproductive age (35–45 years)	Stromal cell tumors (fibroma/fibrothecoma/cystadenofibroma), pedunculated fibroids, peritoneal cysts, adult granulosa cell tumor
	Perimenopausal (46–52 years)	Functional cysts, fibroids, ovarian cancer, endometrial cancer
	Postmenopausal (<52 years)	Serous/mucinous cystadenomas, ovarian cancer, colon cancer, benign stromal cell tumors, diverticulitis/diverticular abscess, fibroids

women, the most common cause of an adnexal mass in a postmenopausal patient is still a benign cyst. Either this is caused by hormonal imbalances that can exist during perimenopause or this develops postmenopausally, driven by hormones secreted by the postmenopausal ovary. In postmenopausal women, simple unilocular cysts can be monitored, but women with solid or complex masses should be offered surgery. Depending on the level of suspicion for cancer, surgery may begin with a minimally invasive approach that can be converted to an open procedure if the frozen section suggests a borderline tumor or malignancy.

When formulating a diagnosis, the most important factors to consider are the patient's age, menopausal status, family history, clinical exam, and the results of serum (CA-125, HE-4), and imaging studies (ultrasound/CT/MRI) (**Tables 23.4** and **23.5**). Because of the lethality of ovarian cancer, it is considered advisable to "err on the side of caution." The fear of not detecting a malignancy, which could delay diagnosis or lead to inadequate surgery, has shaped the clinical response to adnexal masses for decades. The current treatment paradigm is that every postmenopausal woman with a solid adnexal mass should have a surgical exploration to determine histology. Given that early-stage ovarian cancer has a much better prognosis than advanced-stage disease, many operations are performed with the goal of "catching" a cancer early. Because only histology can exclude the presence of an ovarian cancer, about 5% to 10% of all women will, at some point, undergo surgery to rule out an ovarian cancer, despite the fact that most adnexal masses are benign (130).

Clinical Exam

A focused clinical exam should begin with an assessment of supraclavicular lymph nodes, a breast exam, and percussion of the lungs to detect a pleural effusion. The abdomen should also be evaluated for the presence of an umbilical hernia. The involvement of the umbilicus by an ovarian cancer is colloquially called "*Sister Mary Joseph nodule*," named after an assistant to Dr. William Mayo, who identified the lesion as a sign of advanced malignancy. The abdomen should also be inspected for surgical scars and visible veins ("*caput medusae*") caused by impaired central venous return from extensive intra-abdominal disease. The size and mobility of the adnexal mass should be assessed and the abdomen examined for the presence of ascites, costovertebral angle tenderness from hydronephrosis, and enlarged inguinal lymph nodes. In a patient with extensive ascites, the bowel floats on top of the ascites leading to central tympany on exam, whereas in patients with a large tumor, the tympany is lateral.

On gynecologic exam, a prominent cystocele can be indicative of ascites. The bimanual and rectovaginal exam should attempt to evaluate and characterize the adnexal mass in respect to size, borders (smooth/irregular), mobility (fixed/mobile), and location. Invasive ovarian cancers often have irregular borders and are often fixed to the pelvic sidewall and fill the cul-de-sac. Pelvic examination findings may also include involvement of the parametrium by tumor, or nodularity of the rectovaginal septum. It may not be possible to differentiate the uterus from the tumor and the cervix is sometimes dislocated anteriorly behind the pubic symphysis. Some ovarian tumors are behind the uterus and can be best palpated with a rectovaginal exam after the bladder is emptied. Still, despite best efforts and experience, the pelvic examination is less accurate than ultrasound and CT in detecting and characterizing an adnexal mass, especially if the patient is obese or if the uterus is significantly enlarged.

Laboratory Tests

The laboratory work-up for patients with suspected ovarian cancer generally includes a complete blood count. Patients with ovarian cancer are often hemoconcentrated, whereas patients with gastrointestinal malignancies are frequently anemic. Patients with ovarian cancer often have thrombocytosis (a poor prognostic marker) (120) and may have a low albumin level, which is indicative of tumor cachexia and malnutrition and is associated with higher peri- and postoperative morbidity. A pregnancy test should be part of the work-up for all premenopausal women, as uterine/adnexal enlargement can be because of pregnancy. The current biomarkers used clinically to asses if an adnexal mass is malignant are CA-125, HE-4, and OVA1.

The CA-125 tumor marker (normal <35 U/mL), initially described by Dr. Robert Bast (131), is the most thoroughly investigated serum marker. It is expressed both on Müllerian (tubal, endometrial, endocervical) and coelemic (pericardium, pleura, peritoneum, ovarian surface) epithelium. Only 50% of stage I disease is associated with an elevated serum CA-125, which is one reason that CA-125 is not a good screening method for early-stage ovarian cancer (132) and even in advanced-stage cancers the marker has a 20% to 25% false-negative rate (133). However, 80% of patients with ovarian cancer of any stage who are over 50 years have an elevated CA-125 (133). A meta-analysis by Myers et al. studied the performance of CA-125 as a serum marker to distinguish between benign and malignant adnexal masses (134). In premenopausal women with an adnexal mass, an increased CA-125 predicts a malignancy with the following statistical performance: sensitivity, 50% to 74%; specificity, 26% to 92%; and positive predictive value, 5% to 67%. For postmenopausal women the performance is much better: sensitivity, 69% to 87%; specificity, 81% to 100%; and positive predictive value, 73% to 100%. The CA-125 is highest in serous and lowest in mucinous ovarian cancers. Clear cell and endometrioid ovarian cancer often have lower CA-125 values, around 200 U/mL or normal values (127,133).

A number of gynecologic conditions can falsely elevate CA-125 levels: In premenopausal women, the differential of an elevated CA-125 includes many diseases associated with acute or chronic inflammation, to the extent that CA-125 can be regarded as an acute phase reactant. CA-125 can be elevated in patients with PID, peritoneal tuberculosis, endometriosis, fibroids, pregnancy, cirrhosis of the liver, systemic lupus erythematosus, and inflammatory bowel disease. Moreover, CA-125 is not specific to ovarian cancer, as it is increased, albeit modestly, in most metastatic solid tumors, including gastrointestinal, breast, and endometrial cancer. Patients with mucinous ovarian cancer often have elevated CEA values, but this tumor marker is also nonspecific and is increased in patients with gastrointestinal malignancies, especially colon and gastric cancer. A ratio of CA-125/CEA > 25 is used clinically to exclude a gastrointestinal malignancy (135).

In summary, CA-125 is most useful in distinguishing between a benign and malignant mass when used in conjunction with clinical history (age, menopausal status, imaging). Accompanied by other factors, it may help triage women with an adnexal mass for surgery or observation. Moreover, although a single-threshold CA-125 should not be used for screening an asymptomatic woman, serial measurements can have utility (see below). CA-125 is also helpful in the evaluation of response to therapy in patients with an established diagnosis of ovarian cancer and can assist in the diagnosis of recurrence. However, the early treatment of relapse based on an increase in serum CA-125 levels has not been found to influence patient survival when compared with treatment based on clinical evidence or the appearance of symptoms (136).

Human epididymis (HE) 4 is a secreted glycoprotein expressed on human ovarian cancer cells (137). A meta-analysis by Lin showed that HE4 assays had a pooled sensitivity of 74% (CI, 0.72–0.76) and specificity of 87% (0.85–0.89) in the differentiation of benign and malignant adnexal masses. When the authors compared HE4 with CA-125, the HE4 serum levels demonstrated higher specificity, probably because CA-125 is overexpressed in many common nonmalignant disorders (see above). A combination of HE4 and CA-125 enhances both sensitivity (90% CI, 0.87–0.92) and specificity (85% CI, 0.82–0.87) compared with either test used alone (138).

OVA1 is a test combining five different serum proteins, including CA-125, pre-albumin, apolipoprotein A1, β2-microglobulin, and transferrin. This test was approved by the FDA to aid in the triage of patients with an adnexal mass. It uses an algorithm to generate a score between 0 and 10; patients stratified as high risk have OVA1 scores ≥ 4.4 (postmenopausal) or ≥ 5 (premenopausal). In a summary analysis of two studies with 1,016 patients, OVA1 had a sensitivity of 92.2% (CI, 88.2–94.9) and a specificity of 49.4% (CI, 45.9–53). In contrast, CA-125 had a sensitivity of 70.6% (CI, 64.7–75.8) and a specificity of 89.6% (CI, 87.2–91.6). OVA1 had a negative predictive value of 94.9% (CI, 92.3–96.7) and a positive predictive value of 37.9% (CI34.2–41.8), whereas CA-125 had a negative predictive value of 90.1% (CI, 87.8–92) and a positive predictive value of 69.5% (CI, 63.6–74.8) (139). The study was criticized because of the high prevalence of cancer (9.1%) in the study population, making it difficult to generalize the findings to practices where ovarian cancer is less prevalent. Use in a different clinical setting reduces the test's positive predictive value and increases its negative predictive value. Until the OVA1 test is studied in nonacademic clinical environments, it is difficult to assess its future use in the evaluation of ovarian masses.

Imaging of Adnexal Masses and Early Ovarian Cancer: Ultrasound and MRI

In patients with adnexal masses, a pelvic ultrasound, as well as a complete history, physical examination, and a CA-125, is generally needed to provide the information necessary to determine if surgery is required. Because the patient history and the clinical exam alone cannot reliably differentiate between benign and malignant masses, imaging is commonly performed to help establish a diagnosis and treatment plan.

Ultrasound can detect and characterize ovarian size and morphology. Although vaginal ultrasound provides high-resolution imaging of the ovary, for large ovarian masses, an abdominal ultrasound will complement the vaginal scan. Defined ultrasound criteria help diagnose functional cysts, dermoids, and endometriomas with a high degree of certainty, allowing the choice of conservative, nonoperative treatment. Benign tumors often appear on ultrasound as unilateral with smooth walls, a few smooth cysts, no solid elements or papillary projections, and an absence of ascites. Functional cysts have thin walls and are fluid filled. In general, most benign tumors are cystic and mobile. The risk of malignancy in unilocular cystic tumors (even if they are >10 cm) and septated cystic ovarian tumors is extremely low. In the absence of solid areas or papillary projections, these cysts are never malignant and 38% to 80% resolve within 1 year (130). Dermoids are often cystic with hyper-echoic areas (teeth, hair). Endometriomas have low-level, layered echos (blood) and thick walls. In contrast, malignant tumors are partially solid and cystic, often bilateral, irregular, fixed, and often accompanied by ascites. Patients with tumors that display these features require surgical exploration. Homogenous solid tumors also require surgical exploration, but the most common finding is an ovarian fibroma or a pedunculated fibroid (**Table 23.4**). In summary, ultrasound is excellent for predicting a benign ovarian mass, but is less accurate in the prediction of malignancy or the detection of early-stage ovarian cancer (140).

Several sonography-based predictive models have been developed to differentiate between benign and malignant tumors. Sassone developed a model that integrates inner wall structure, wall thickness, septa, and echogenicity as sonographic markers of malignancy and determined that, in premenopausal women, cysts greater than 6 cm should be further investigated for malignancy (141). Indeed, malignant tumors often present as complex masses with partially solid and partially cystic components. In a pooled estimate of 18 cohort studies of the Sassone model, it was calculated that its sensitivity and specificity in differentiating between a benign and malignant ovarian mass are 84% and 80%, respectively (142). Ueland published the most accurate morphology index based on ovarian volume and morphologic complexity (**Fig. 23.13**) (133,143). The risk of malignancy was related to structural complexity, tumor volume, and a total morphology index score. There was only one malignancy found in 315 tumors with a morphology index <5, indicating that the score is very useful in identifying low-risk tumors. Among 127 patients with a morphology index ≥5 there were 52 invasive or borderline tumors. A group of investigators from Kentucky expanded this finding by adding serial exams to determine if a change in the morphology index over time could aid in deciding if a patient with an adnexal mass needed surgery (144). Adnexal masses that were found to be malignant showed an increase of 1.6 points per month in the morphology index, whereas the scores of benign ovarian tumors only increased 0.3 per month.

The studies described above considered ultrasound in a binary model to differentiate benign from malignant adnexal masses. The International Ovarian Tumour Analysis (IOTA) group expanded this approach using the Assessment of Different Neoplasias in the adneXa (ADNEX) model to differentiate between benign, borderline, primary ovarian cancer, and metastatic cancer (145). This large prospective study of 5,909 patients evaluated in 24 primarily European centers used four clinical variables (age, CA-125, family history, referral center) and six ultrasound variables (lesion diameter, proportion of solid tissue, <10 cysts, number of papillary projections, acoustic shadow, ascites). The area under the receiver operating curve (AUC), differentiating

Size	>4–6 cm
Ovarian volume	Length x width x height x 0.523. Premenopausal > 20 cm^3. Postmenopausal > 10 cm^3.
Morphology	Thick septations > 3 mm (differentiate from a papillary projection) Complex solid and cystic (multi–locular) Solid enhancing nodules Papillary projections
Vascularization	Pulsatility index (PI) > 1. Resistive Index (RI) >0.4. Central intramural blood flow
Other findings	Ascites (60 mL or greater) Uterine invasion Peritoneal thickening, carcinomatosis

A

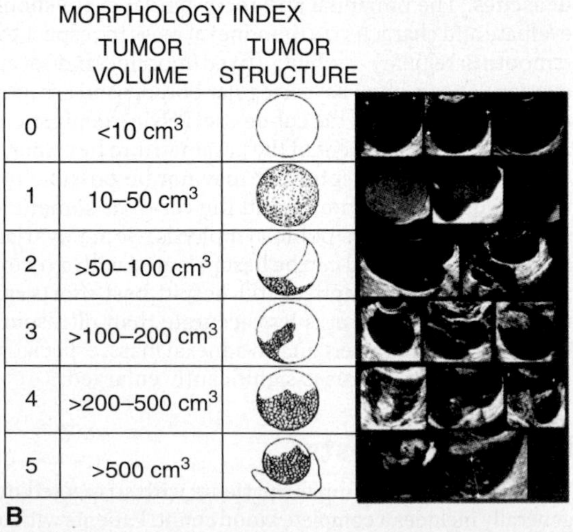

B

Figure 23.13. Imaging characteristics of a malignant adnexal mass. **A:** Criteria for malignancy. **B:** Morphology index with sonographic examples.
Source: **(A)** Adapted from van Nagell JR Jr, Miller RW. Evaluation and management of ultrasonographically detected ovarian tumors in asymptomatic women. *Obstet Gynecol*. 2016;127:848–858; Forstner R, Meissnitzer M, Cunha TM. Update on imaging of ovarian cancer. *Curr Radiol Rep*. 2016;4:31. Miller RW, Ueland FR. Risk of malignancy in sonographically confirmed ovarian tumors. *Clin Obstet Gynecol*. 2012;55:52–64. **(B)** From Elder JW, Pavlik EJ, Long A, et al. Serial ultrasonographic evaluation of ovarian abnormalities with a morphology index. *Gynecol Oncol*. 2014;135:8–12.

between benign and malignant masses, was 0.94, indicating that the model discriminated very well between the two. The model also differentiated well between benign, borderline, primary ovarian cancer, and metastatic cancer with an AUC of 0.85 to 0.99 (145).

Sometimes color flow Doppler is used to aid in distinguishing benign from malignant tumors. The neovascularization of malignant tumors is characterized by an absence of tunica media in tumor blood vessels, leading to reduced flow resistance which can be detected by Doppler. Resistance to blood flow is measured by calculating the pulsatility index (PI) and resistive index (RI). However, these indices, as independent variables, are unreliable for predicting ovarian cancer because the location of tumor vessels is variable (130).

Often ovarian masses are indeterminate on gray-scale ultrasound and, although they provide an insufficient rationale to proceed to surgery, are sufficiently concerning that a second imaging test is ordered for further characterization. Contrast-enhanced MRI is the preferred advanced modality for an ultrasound-indeterminate adnexal lesion because of its high specificity. MRI can differentiate between simple fluid, atypical fluid (mucinous), fresh blood, old hematoma, solid tissue, stromal tissue, and fat (146,147). As with ultrasound, several criteria have been established to differentiate a benign from a malignant mass, including the presence of septations, solid elements, and papillary projections, and solid tissue intensity on T2-weighted MRI. Injection of gadolinium contrast agents adds further information, because solid malignant components within a mass take up the contrast. This also allows a better differentiation of cystic from solid lesions, especially endometriomas, stromal cell tumors, and teratomas. The pretest probability of detecting a borderline or malignant tumor increased from 32% to 77% (95% CI, 69%–85%), with a positive result for malignancy with MRI, and decreased to 4.8% (95% CI, 3%–6%), with a negative result (148). Given this sensitivity and specificity, MRI is a very good (if expensive) test for predicting whether a mass is benign or malignant. However, it is not able to differentiate between borderline and invasive tumors. A meta-analysis found that the average sensitivity and specificity of MRI in distinguishing a borderline or malignant tumor from a benign tumor were 92% (95% CI, 89%–94%) and 85% (95% CI, 82%–87%), respectively. Although this sensitivity is similar to that reported by ultrasound, the specificity of MRI is superior. A comparison of color Doppler, CT scans, and MRI showed that of all three modalities, contrast-enhanced MRI is most helpful in further characterizing an adnexal mass that is indeterminate on ultrasound (146). In a premenopausal woman with an indeterminate ultrasound and a negative contrast-enhanced MRI, the risk of malignancy is 2%, whereas a positive MRI increases the risk of malignancy in the same patient to 80%. Given the high *a priori* probability that a mass in a premenopausal patient is benign, a reasonable approach is to further characterize an ultrasound-indeterminate adnexal lesion by MRI (146–148). If the MRI is reassuring, the patient can be followed with a combination of clinical exam, serial ultrasounds, and CA-125 every 3 to 6 months to capture a malignant adnexal tumor not detected during the initial work-up (140,147). If the mass is stable, the follow-up interval can be extended.

Computed tomography allows the detection and characterization of an adnexal mass, but performs less well than MRI as a secondary imaging modality following gray-scale ultrasound. Even when intravenous contrast is given, CT offers lower soft tissue contrast than MRI (146). CT has a sensitivity of 87% but a low specificity of 16% in differentiating a benign from a malignant ovarian mass (149).

Although the approaches described above are extremely useful in the evaluation of an adnexal mass, other factors will affect the final decision to perform surgery, including the patient's age, clinical symptoms, fertility preferences, medical comorbidities, and the number and extent of previous surgeries. It is important to stress to the patient that although imaging and clinical judgment can be used to characterize many ovarian masses, only histologic examination can confirm the diagnosis. If a patient has a strong family history of cancer, an elevated CA-125, free fluid/ascites, as well as a large mass (>10 cm), there is sufficient reason to perform surgery.

Imaging of Advanced Ovarian Cancer: Computed Tomography, Positron Emission Tomography Scan, and MRI

Because of its reasonable cost and wide availability, CT scanning is currently the preoperative imaging modality most often used in patients with a high clinical suspicion for ovarian cancer. Frequently, patients are found to have an adnexal mass or advanced disease after a CT scan of the abdomen and pelvis ordered for nonspecific clinical symptoms. A CT scan of the pelvis is able to characterize the adnexal mass and discern any involvement of the surrounding organs (bladder, sigmoid, ureter, and pelvic sidewall). In the upper abdomen, retroperitoneal adenopathy, omental and mesenteric involvement, and intrahepatic liver involvement can be detected reliably by CT scans with intravenous contrast (150). Often the CT scan of the abdomen and pelvis is extended to the chest, which allows detection of intra-pulmonary metastasis, pleural effusion, and pleural disease. These findings predict a lower chance of optimal cytoreduction (151).

Preoperative CT scans can identify the presence of disease in anatomic regions that are difficult or technically impossible to resect (e.g., stomach, lesser sac, liver, small bowel mesentery, and adenopathy above the renal vessels). Bristow and colleagues identified 13 diagnostic features and devised a score to predict the chances of optimal cytoreduction in patients with advanced ovarian cancer (152). The 13 factors included in the score were peritoneal thickening; peritoneal implants greater than 2 cm; small and large bowel mesenteric disease greater than 2 cm; omental extension to stomach, spleen, or lesser sac; extension of the tumor to the pelvic sidewall/parametria/hydroureter; large-volume ascites; supra- and infrarenal lymphadenopathy; diaphragm involvement; inguinal canal disease; liver lesions greater than 2 cm; and porta hepatis/gall bladder disease. Using this model, the authors were able to predict surgical outcomes at their own institution with 93% accuracy (152). However, a multi-institutional validation study showed an accuracy of only 34% to 46% (153). This validation study identified disease on the diaphragm and large bowel mesentery implants as the only statistically significant predictors of suboptimal cytoreduction, and even when the score was limited to these two factors there was a 33% false-positive rate (153).

In a joint prospective study at Memorial Sloan-Kettering and MD Anderson Cancer Center involving 350 patients, Suidan and colleagues sought to determine if a CT of the abdomen and pelvis could predict the likelihood of suboptimal debulking. Three clinical (age≥60 years, CA-125≥500 U/mL, ASA 3/4) and six radiologic criteria were significantly associated with suboptimal debulking to more than 1 cm residual tumor size (154). The radiologic criteria included supra-renal retroperitoneal lymph nodes>1cm, diffuse small bowel adhesions/thickening, tumors>1cm in the small bowel mesentery, root of the SMA, perisplenic area, and lesser sac. Forty-eight patients receiving neo-adjuvant chemotherapy (NACT) during the study period were excluded. This prognostic model was found to have a predictive accuracy of 0.758 (154).

Because surgical outcome depends on so many factors other than anatomical disease distribution (comorbidities, surgeon philosophy, advanced surgical techniques), preoperative CT scanning poorly predicts surgical resectability. Therefore, for most patients surgical evaluation of the peritoneal cavity, which often includes a diagnostic laparoscopy, is required to evaluate the resectability of disease (155–157). Still, a patient whose CT scan clearly indicates high-volume ovarian disease should be evaluated carefully before a decision is made to proceed with primary debulking and serious consideration should be given to NACT (135,158).

Positron emission tomography (PET) has been integrated with CT scan for the diagnosis of ovarian cancer and the evaluation of disease recurrence (150,159). CT/PET combines the high anatomic resolution afforded by CT scan with a functional study of tumor fluoro-deoxy glucose (FDG) uptake. Although PET scans have very high sensitivity, they have low specificity because of increased FDG uptake in benign metabolically active tissues and inflammatory changes. In a single-institution prospective study of 101 patients, the combined CT/PET scan had a sensitivity of 100% and specificity of 92% in the correct diagnosis of tumors that were suspicious on ultrasound (160). CT/PET scans seem to be especially useful in further characterizing a suspected recurrence. In a retrospective study, PET/CT showed a sensitivity of 82% and a specificity of 87% in correctly identifying recurrent disease, which was superior to CA-125 or CT/MRI scans used alone (159). CT/PET scans were also found to be particularly effective in the diagnosis of retroperitoneal lymph nodes (161).

Although CT provides good spatial resolution, MRI is a nonradioactive imaging modality that provides excellent soft tissue contrast resolution. In addition to its utility in the diagnosis of an indeterminate ovarian mass (140,146,147) as described above, MRI is also an excellent modality for the characterization of nonadnexal pelvic pathology (e.g., diverticulitis) and for the further characterization of the extent of ovarian cancer in the upper abdomen. The T1-weighted MRI images, after administration of contrast (gadolinium), allow the detection of peritoneal metastases and bowel implants. They also can determine whether the bowel mesentery or diaphragm is involved by cancer and whether a liver tumor is benign or malignant, or is on the surface of the liver or intrahepatic. MRI is better than CT or ultrasound in the diagnosis of small peritoneal metastases, but CT imaging is superior in identifying the involvement of the omentum by ovarian cancer (149).

In recurrent cancer, MRI is especially useful for differentiating postsurgical changes from a recurrence on the vaginal dome, small bowel mesentery, splenic hilum, liver surface, or diaphragm. The reported sensitivity of MRI for recurrent ovarian cancer ranges from 62% to 91% and the specificity from 40% to 100%, depending primarily on tumor size (150).

Screening

No current screening modalities (CA-125, pelvic ultrasound, pelvic examinations), either individually or in combination, have been shown to decrease the risk of death from ovarian cancer. Because ovarian cancer has such a low prevalence (1 case/2,500 women per year), screening low-risk asymptomatic women requires a test or combination of tests with very high sensitivity and specificity, and high positive and negative predictive values. Several studies have shown that, if asymptomatic women were screened for ovarian cancer, between 5 and 33 operations would be required to find one invasive ovarian cancer (65,122,162). This situation is primarily caused by the high false-positive rates of ultrasound and CA-125 in benign disease.

Three large prospective randomized studies from Japan (162), the United States (65), and the United Kingdom (66) have compared women screened for ovarian cancer with CA-125 and/or ultrasound with women who were not screened.

The Shizuoka Cohort Study of Ovarian Cancer Screening ran between 1985 and 1999 and screened 82,487 postmenopausal women using fixed cutoff CA-125 values (<35 U/mL) and pelvic ultrasound (162). Ovarian cancer was detected in 32 patients in the control group and 27 patients in the screening group, suggesting that screening does not detect more ovarian cancers. Among these women, the proportion of stage I cancers was 63% in the screened group and 38% in the observation group ($p = 0.22$) indicating that screening did not lead to a significant stage-shift, which signifies earlier detection. However, the group only reported on ovarian cancer detection and no survival data have been published.

The Prostate, Lung, Colorectal, and Ovarian (PLCO) Cancer Screening Trial (1993–2001) randomized 78,216 postmenopausal women to either annual screening with a fixed cutoff value for CA-125 (<35 U/mL) and ultrasound or to usual medical care (65). Ultrasounds were done yearly for three consecutive years and CA-125 yearly for 5 years. Borderline tumors were considered false positive and were not considered malignant neoplasms. The results showed that screening does not improve mortality from ovarian cancer. False-positive screening results were returned in 3,285 patients, 1,080 (32.9%) underwent surgery and of these 15% (163 women) experienced 222 major complications (20.6 complication rate/100 surgeries). The number of patients diagnosed in late stage ovarian cancer was similar in the screening and observation groups, suggesting that screening does not detect ovarian cancer at an earlier stage.

The UK Collaborative Trial of Ovarian Cancer Screening (UKCTOCS), which ran between 2001 and 2005, assessed the effect of screening on disease mortality in more than 200,000 postmenopausal women (66). Two screening strategies were tested: primary ultrasound screening versus multimodality screening (CA-125 followed by ultrasound). They then annually measured CA-125 and used the ROCA for an interpretation of rises in CA-125 over time (163). ROCA is a computer-based algorithm devised to increase the sensitivity and specificity of CA-125 by looking at the changes in levels of CA-125 over time for an individual, instead of using a single cutoff value as the basis for deciding whether additional tests are needed. Using ROCA, the investigators triaged women to annual screening versus repeat CA-125 versus repeat CA-125 and transvaginal ultrasound. The primary outcome was ovarian cancer death; however, the group did not find a significant reduction in mortality. The mortality reduction with multimodality screening, CA-125, and ultrasound was 15% (CI: 3–30%, $p = 0.21$), and the reduction with ultrasound alone was 11% (CI –7–27, $p = 0.21$). The results suggest that most of the disease detected with multimodality screening was low volume (FIGO I, II, IIIA made up 39% of cancers vs. 26% in patients who did not undergo screening). In a *post hoc* analysis there was evidence of a significant mortality reduction (28%) in the patients who had multimodality screening after 7 years, but given the primary analysis did not identify a significant reduction in mortality, this finding is essentially hypothesis-generating. No stage-shift was observed in patients screened with ultrasound alone; 641 patients needed to be screened to prevent one cancer death. Criticisms of the study included the exclusion of primary peritoneal cancers from the main analysis, the exclusion of prevalent cancers, the persistence of high mortality from ovarian cancer despite screening (53% of patients died within 2.3 years of diagnosis), and the potential of lead-time bias associated with early detection. The study results will be reanalyzed in 3 years, which should give us data that could help us assess the value of the screening approaches.

Even women who are at high risk of developing ovarian cancer because of a *BRCA1* or *BRCA2* mutation have not been shown to significantly benefit from annual pelvic exams, CA-125, and ultrasound (73) because of low sensitivities and very low positive predictive values of the three different screening modalities (164). The inability to detect early ovarian cancer using a yearly screening approach is probably because of the very fast growth rate of high-grade serous carcinoma (HGSC) once it is fully transformed, which reduces the time during which screening can detect preinvasive or early invasive ovarian cancer (96). Another reason that screening tends to be ineffective may be the extent of ovarian cancer disease heterogeneity. In summary, pelvic exams, CA-125, and ultrasound have not been conclusively shown to significantly decrease mortality from ovarian cancer in either low- or high-risk populations. If a woman wants to reduce her risk, tubal ligation/removal, OCP, or a prophylactic salpingo-oophorectomy may currently be the best strategy for primary prevention.

Differential Diagnosis of Ovarian Cancer

The most common cause of malignant ascites in women is ovarian cancer, but patients with metastatic breast, pancreatic, and gastric cancer, which usually has concomitant intrahepatic metastasis, can also present with ascites. Therefore, other cancers should be considered in patients with extensive ascites and CA-125 values around 200 U/mL. Reviewing patients with ascites who presented to an oncology clinic, Ayantunde (102) found diagnoses to be ovarian cancer (37%), pancreaticobiliary cancer (21%), gastric cancer (18%), colon cancer

(4%), and breast cancer (3%). Nonmalignant causes of ascites include pancreatitis, tuberculosis, hepatitis, systemic lupus erythematosus, cirrhosis, ovarian torsion, and Meigs syndrome. Tuberculotic granulomas on the peritoneum combined with ascites are clinically indistinguishable from serous ovarian cancer. A paracentesis will both establish a diagnosis of malignancy and improve the dyspnea, pain, nausea, and vomiting that the patient may be experiencing as a result of large-volume ascites.

Although serous ovarian cancer disseminates extensively within the abdominal cavity or to retroperitoneal lymph nodes, it will only rarely have metastasized elsewhere at the time of initial presentation. Imaging studies that suggest intra-pulmonary metastasis or intra-parenchymal metastases in the liver, spleen, or kidney, especially in the absence of significant intraperitoneal disease or the absence of a significant ovarian tumor, should broaden the differential diagnosis to include a less common ovarian cancer histotype (clear cell, mucinous, or carcinosarcoma) or a different tumor origin (gastrointestinal: colon/gastric/appendiceal or breast cancer). Younger age and bilateral ovarian tumors may also be a sign that the ovarian tumors are of metastatic origin.

Gastric cancers tend to cause drop metastases to the ovary, referred to as Krukenberg tumors, after Friedrich Krukenberg, a German gynecologist and pathologist. Because gastrointestinal malignancies are apt to metastasize to the ovary because of its extensive blood supply, these cancers are important differential diagnoses for women presenting with disseminated intra-abdominal disease on imaging. Indeed, 9% of all patients with colon cancers have metastases to the ovary, and the ovarian tumor is often bigger than the primary colonic tumor; 1% to 3% of all patients operated on for a presumed ovarian cancer are found to have an extragenital cancer (128). Patients who present with predominantly gastrointestinal symptoms, anemia, a high CEA, low CA-125, and a positive hemoccult test should undergo an esophagogastroduodenoscopy (EGD) and a colonoscopy with biopsies. A CA-125/CEA serum ratio greater than 25 has high discriminative power to differentiate between ovarian and colon cancer, but might not be able to exclude a mucinous tumor (135). The median survival for patients who present with peritoneal and ovarian metastasis from colon cancer is only 10 months.

Breast cancer can also metastasize to the ovary and is the most frequent (84%) primary cause of ovarian metastasis of non-GI origin. Metastasis of breast cancer to the ovary was found at autopsy in 23% to 39% patients who died of breast cancer. The median survival after diagnosis of breast cancer metastasized to the ovary is 26 to 54 months (128,129,165). To determine if an ovarian mass is a breast cancer metastasis or a new ovarian cancer in patient with a history of breast cancer, the stage and histology and other prognostic factors (ER/PR, HER2/neu, proliferation) of the previous breast disease should be considered. Patients with stage IV breast disease are much more likely to have distant metastasis than patients with early-stage tumors, and lobular breast cancer metastasizes more often to the ovary than invasive ductal cancer. Most patients with ovarian metastasis from breast cancer are premenopausal (77%) and present with abdominal distension in the absence of ascites. Often these patients have bilateral ovarian involvement (64%), a high CA15-3, and a low CA-125. However, patients with breast cancer and abdominal carcinomatosis can have a high CA-125, which makes the differentiation from ovarian cancer challenging. On pelvic ultrasound, breast cancer metastases to the ovary tend to be more solid appearing than a primary ovarian cancer, which is often multicystic. The benefit of surgery in the treatment of breast cancer metastatic to the ovaries has not been proven and may be limited to the palliation of symptoms by removing a single mass. Retrospective studies have suggested a possible survival benefit for surgery in patients with no residual disease after the operation, but found no benefit in the setting of widely metastatic disease (129). The 5-year survival for women with ovarian metastasis from breast cancer is 26%, which is much higher than that for those with ovarian metastasis from colorectal and gastric cancer (8% and 1%, respectively), but lower than the median survival for primary ovarian cancer (128). Ovarian cancer is the most common non-breast secondary malignancy after treatment for breast cancer. Indeed, a history of breast cancer is associated with a two- to fourfold increase in the risk of developing ovarian cancer and this rate is higher in patients with hereditary breast and ovarian cancer syndrome.

SURGERY

Introduction and Definitions

Surgery plays an important role at every phase of ovarian cancer treatment. Patients newly diagnosed with ovarian cancer usually undergo surgery for the purpose of pathologic diagnosis, cytoreduction, symptom relief, and staging. Indeed, both the old and new FIGO staging systems (**Table 23.6**) require that surgery be performed to confirm the histologic diagnosis and to determine the true extent of the disease. In the recurrent disease setting, surgical biopsy can confirm a diagnosis and also provide therapeutic benefit, as the removal of an isolated mass may render a patient macroscopically tumor-free. In patients with recurrent disease involving extensive tumor dissemination, removal of tumor masses ("debulking" or "cytoreduction") accomplishes significant symptom relief and, in select patients, limited surgery may result in the palliation of bowel obstruction. Clinically there is a distinction between "low-volume advanced-stage disease" and "high-volume advanced disease" because the lower the volume at presentation, the greater the possibility that surgery will result in an absence of residual disease.

The most important prognostic factors predicting long-term survival from ovarian cancer are the FIGO stage and the amount of disease remaining after debulking surgery. Patients with ovarian cancer will benefit from treatment by a gynecologic oncologist or physicians familiar with the disease and skilled in its surgical management.

The widely used 1988 FIGO staging system for ovarian cancer was replaced in 2014 by a new staging system approved by FIGO and published in 2014 which is (166) presented in **Table 23.6**.

The terms for common surgical procedures, as they are used in this chapter, are defined in **Table 23.7**.

Early-Stage Ovarian Cancer

Optimal staging in early ovarian cancer includes careful inspection, palpation, and biopsies of peritoneal surfaces (diaphragm, paracolic gutters, bladder, and cul-de-sac peritoneum), pelvic and diaphragmatic washings, removal of the affected ovary, an infracolic or infragastric omentectomy, and a systematic pelvic and para-aortic lymph node dissection (167). An appendectomy can, though rarely, change the final staging. Preserving the contralateral ovary and the uterus in young patients desiring fertility is considered acceptable in appropriately selected cases of early-stage epithelial invasive and borderline ovarian cancer. Every effort should be made to remove an ovarian mass intact, although it is not clear whether intraoperative rupture affects prognosis. Rupture of an ovarian mass is associated with thick/dense adhesions. If these adhesions contain tumor cells, tumors which otherwise appear to be FIGO stage I should be upstaged to stage II (**Table 23.6**).

Thorough surgical staging of early ovarian cancer is important for establishing the correct FIGO stage in order to determine prognosis and choice of therapy (chemotherapy vs. observation). In a study of 86 patients with ovarian cancer grossly confined to the ovary, approximately 30% of the patients who underwent completion surgery were upstaged. Sixty percent of these patients were upstaged because of microscopic disease in biopsy specimens from adhesions or omentum, whereas the others had either uterine or fallopian tube metastases or positive lymph nodes. Occult metastases were associated with increasing tumor grade and the presence of ascites (168). Other predictors of unappreciated residual disease after primary surgery include a high preoperative CA-125 level and positive cytology from pelvic or diaphragmatic washings (165).

TABLE 23.6. FIGO Ovarian Cancer Staging

Surgical FIGO – Ovarian Cancer Staging 1988		Surgical FIGO – Ovarian Cancer Staging 2014	
I	Tumors limited to one or both ovaries	I	Tumor confined to ovaries or fallopian tubes
IA	Tumor limited to one ovary; capsule intact; no tumor on ovarian surface; no malignant cells in ascites/ peritoneal washings	IA	Tumor limited to one ovary, capsule intact or fallopian tube, no tumor on ovarian or fallopian tube surface, no malignant cells in ascites or peritoneal washings
IB	Tumor limited to both ovaries; capsule intact; no tumor on ovarian surface; no malignant cells in ascites/ peritoneal washings	IB	Tumor involves both ovaries; capsule intact or fallopian tubes, no malignant cells in ascites or peritoneal washings
IC	Tumor limited to ovaries with any of the following: capsule ruptured, tumor on ovarian surface, positive washings/ascites	IC1-3	Tumor limited to one or both ovaries/fallopian tubes IC1: Surgical spill intraoperatively IC2: Capsule rupture before surgery or tumor on ovarian or fallopian tube surface IC3: Malignant cells in the ascites or peritoneal washings
II	Tumor involves one or both ovaries with pelvic extension or implants	II	Tumor involves one or both ovaries or fallopian tube with pelvic extension (below the pelvic brim) or primary peritoneal cancer
IIA	Extension and/or implants on uterus or fallopian tube; negative washings/ascites	IIA	Extension and/or implants on uterus and/or fallopian tubes
IIB	Extension or implants onto other pelvic structures; negative washings/ascites	IIB	Extension to other pelvic intraperitoneal tissues
IIC	Pelvic extension (IIA or IIB) or implants with positive peritoneal washings/ascites		
III	Microscopic peritoneal implants outside of the pelvis; or limited to the pelvis with extension to the small bowel or omentum	III	Tumor involves one or both ovaries or fallopian tubes, or primary peritoneal cancer, with cytologically or histologically confirmed spread to the peritoneum outside the pelvis and/or metastasis to the retroperitoneal lymph nodes
IIIA	Microscopic peritoneal metastases beyond pelvis	IIIA	IIIA1: Positive retroperitoneal lymph nodes only IIIA1(i): Metastasis $\leq$ 10 mm IIIA1(ii): Metastasis $>$ 10 mm IIIA2: Microscopic, extrapelvic (above the pelvic brim) peritoneal involvement $\pm$ positive retroperitoneal lymph nodes
IIIB	Macroscopic peritoneal metastases beyond pelvis $<$ 2 cm in size	IIIB	Macroscopic, extrapelvic, peritoneal metastasis $\leq$ 2 cm $\pm$ positive retroperitoneal lymph nodes. Includes extension to capsule of liver/spleen.
IIIC	Macroscopic peritoneal metastases beyond pelvis $>$ 2 cm and/or positive retroperitoneal or inguinal lymph nodes (pT3B N1 or pT3C)	IIIC	Macroscopic, extrapelvic, peritoneal metastasis $>$ 2 cm $\pm$ positive retroperitoneal lymph nodes. Includes extension to capsule of liver/spleen (no parenchymal involvement).
IV	Distant metastasis including pleural effusion with positive cytology. Distant metastases outside the peritoneal cavity. Parenchymal liver/splenic metastasis.	IV	Distant metastasis excluding peritoneal metastasis
		IVA	Pleural effusion with positive cytology/biopsy
		IVB	Hepatic and/or splenic parenchymal metastasis, metastasis to extra-abdominal organs (including inguinal lymph nodes and lymph nodes outside of the abdominal cavity) Bowel infiltration – transmural with mucosal involvement and umbilical deposit

Comments on FIGO 2014 (166): There is no stage I primary peritoneal cancer. Dense adhesions containing tumor cells justify upgrading apparent stage I tumors to stage II. Rectum invasion is stage IIB. Positive para-aortic lymph node metastases are considered regional lymph nodes (FIGO 2014 IIIA1(ii)). Involvement of retroperitoneal lymph nodes must be proven cytologically or histologically. Examples of metastatic sites which upstage tumors to FIGO 2014 IVB: Transmural bowel infiltration, subcutaneous/umbilicus/abdominal wall, extra-abdominal lymph nodes (inguinal, axillary), and umbilical metastasis.

Complete staging in early disease may obviate the need for cytotoxic chemotherapy. A retrospective subset analysis of patients with FIGO stage I–IIA disease enrolled in the ACTION trial (112,169) found that complete surgical staging was statistically significantly associated with better outcomes, presumably because the unstaged group included patients with occult stage III disease. In this trial, patients were randomly assigned to adjuvant chemotherapy or observation after they had undergone either complete or incomplete staging surgery. Although the trial was not designed to compare different surgical staging procedures (and extent of surgical staging was not randomized), a subgroup analysis of patients with a poorly differentiated tumor found that the optimally surgically staged group ($n = 78$) had a significantly longer ($p < 0.009$) 10-year cancer-specific survival of 85% compared with 56% in patients who were not completely staged ($n = 78$). This improved outcome was independent of age, presumed stage, histology, and whether or not chemotherapy was given (169,170). Moreover, the benefit of adjuvant chemotherapy was seen only in patients with incomplete surgical staging. Incompletely staged patients with a poorly differentiated grade III tumor were found to derive the greatest benefit from adjuvant chemotherapy. However, the role of chemotherapy in relation to staging remains uncertain. The ICON1 trial suggested that both incompletely and completely staged patients with early-stage disease may benefit from adjuvant chemotherapy (171,172).

TABLE 23.7. Terms for Common Surgical Procedures as Used in This Chapter

Procedure	Definition
Paracentesis	Drainage of presumed malignant fluid/ascites in a patient with intra-abdominal tumor masses to establish a diagnosis before initiation of chemotherapy with cytology or to provide symptomatic relief
Biopsy	Biopsy of disseminated disease or an adnexal mass to establish a pathologic diagnosis before initiation of chemotherapy
Primary cytoreductive surgery	Initial laparotomy to establish a diagnosis, stage, and attempt maximal tumor debulking to microscopic disease before the initiation of first-line chemotherapy. Also called by some physicians as "primary debulking"
Interval cytoreduction or interval debulking	Cytoreductive surgery after a biopsy only or a primary suboptimal debulking or a limited surgery (e.g., hysterectomy/BSO) followed by induction chemotherapy
Second look surgery	Surgery performed at the completion of primary chemotherapy in patients who do not have evidence of disease by CT scan or CA-125 to determine if there is residual disease in order to plan for additional chemotherapy. Currently rarely performed
Secondary cytoreductive surgery	Surgery in a patient with recurrent disease who has completed primary treatment, including primary debulking and/or chemotherapy and had been without evidence of disease for 6 months. The procedure is most commonly performed for platinum-sensitive patients with oligometastatic disease. Also called "secondary debulking" by some physicians
Palliative surgery	Surgery performed to relieve symptoms, most commonly performed for a malignant bowel obstruction with the goal to remove the obstruction or perform a diversion. Not primarily intended to remove tumors
Staging surgery	Surgery to evaluate extent of disease guiding treatment decisions (chemotherapy: yes/no) for early stage disease
Posterior pelvic exenteration	*En bloc* resection of bladder serosa, uterus, sigmoid colon, and proximal rectum, as well as ovarian/fallopian tube masses, cul-de-sac tumors with complete parietal pelvic peritonectomy to encompass all pan-pelvic disease (98)
Surgery: complete debulking	
Result: no macroscopic disease	Complete resection (541): cytoreduction of all tumors independent of preoperative tumor load to microscopic residual disease at the completion of surgery—no gross residual tumors left. R0 resection
Surgery: optimal debulking	
Result: macroscopic disease up to 1 cm	Minimal residual (541): macroscopic disease up to 1 cm in diameter after primary surgery. Also called by some physicians as "optimal cytoreduction." R1 resection
Surgery: suboptimal debulking.	
Result: macroscopic disease > 1 cm	Gross residual (541): primary cytoreduction resulting in macroscopic disease larger than 1 cm in size at the end of surgery. R2 resection

The surgical approach to the staging of presumed early-stage ovarian cancer will depend on patient comorbidities and number of previous abdominal operations, as well as on how skilled the surgeon is at minimally invasive surgery. Retrospective studies suggest that both a minimally invasive approach and an open laparotomy allow for comprehensive surgical staging. Concerns regarding the minimally invasive approaches include limited visibility of both diaphragms, the inability to palpate tissue, and the longer operating time. Lymph node counts and the size of the omental specimen obtained are similar for both procedures. Given that bulky disease is only rarely detected in early-stage ovarian cancer patients, a minimally invasive surgical approach may be preferable, as it involves less blood loss, a shorter hospital stay, and faster recovery with less pain and allows patients to start chemotherapy earlier. However, specialized surgical training is necessary (173). Another concern with the laparoscopic approach is the possibility of port site metastasis, although this risk seems to be small (1.18%) and such metastases are often a sign of disseminated intra-abdominal disease (174). In early ovarian cancer, restaging involves multiple biopsies of the diaphragmatic, abdominal, gutter, and pelvic/bladder peritoneum, as well as, at the least, a unilateral salpingo-oophorectomy, omentectomy, pelvic and para-aortic lymph node dissection, and pelvic and diaphragmatic washings for cytology. Patients who do not want to preserve fertility will also have a hysterectomy and removal of the contralateral ovary and tubes.

In most cases, unstaged patients with presumed early-stage invasive ovarian cancer should be staged or given adjuvant chemotherapy if staging is not feasible.

Role of Lymph Node Dissection in Early Ovarian Cancer

When treating both early and advanced ovarian cancer, a surgeon should make two decisions: (a) whether to perform a lymph node sampling, and (b) whether to remove only enlarged or palpably suspicious lymph nodes or to perform a systematic lymph node dissection, removing all visible pelvic and para-aortic lymph nodes within defined anatomic borders. Dye studies have shown that the lymphatic drainage of the ovaries originates under the ovarian surface. Lymph fluid predominantly drains superiorly, along both ovarian vascular pedicles (175). On the left side, the lymphatics follow the infundibulopelvic vein until it drains into the left renal vein. The high left infrarenal, para-aortic lymph nodes often harbor lymph node metastasis and are a known site of (isolated) recurrence. The right infundibulopelvic vein and its accompanying lymphatics reach the inferior vena cava about 1 cm below the right renal vein. Cancer cells are then able to continue traveling along a net of lymphatic vessels covering the inferior vena cava and the interaortocaval space to lymph nodes at the base of the celiac axis, and then through the caval opening in the diaphragm into the chest, reaching thoracic, mediastinal, or prescalene lymph nodes. Secondary lymph drainage routes are along lymphatics draining inferiorly through the utero-ovarian ligament to lymph nodes in the broad ligament and along the external iliac artery to the round ligament and then to inguinal lymph nodes. This spread pattern explains why inguinal lymph node metastasis is sometimes detected in patients with ovarian cancer. There is also minor lymph drainage to lymphatics along the internal iliac artery or lymph nodes in the obturator fossa (176). Ovarian lymph drainage does not reach the uterus, explaining why intrauterine or cervical metastases are rare in serous ovarian cancer.

It is recommended that both the pelvic and high, infrarenal para-aortic lymph nodes should be removed when a systematic lymph node dissection is performed in patients with early ovarian cancer (171,172) (**Fig. 23.14**). However, given the lymphatic drainage of the ovaries, the removal of high para-aortic lymph nodes is the most important (110). The anatomic borders of a pelvic lymph node dissection are laterally, the external iliac artery and the genitofemoral nerve that travels on the psoas muscle; superiorly, the bifurcation of the external and internal iliac artery to the inguinal ligament; and medially, the anterior division of the hypogastric artery and the ureter (**Fig. 23.15**). By slightly elevating and lateralizing the external iliac vein, the surgeon exposes the obturator fossa and the obturator nerve and then clears the lymph nodes superior to the nerve. To enable right para-aortic lymph node dissection, the descending colon and terminal ileum are mobilized by incising the peritoneum around the cecum to expose the inferior vena cava and interaortocaval space. The cecum is reflected medially and the dissection is begun on the right common iliac artery. The precaval fatty tissue containing lymph nodes is removed from the common iliac artery up to the right renal vein, with care taken not to injure the ureter, renal vessels, or the third/horizontal part of the duodenum. Of note, the superior mesenteric artery/vein is anterior to the third part of the duodenum. To remove the left para-aortic lymph nodes, the fat/lymph node containing tissue lateral to the aorta between the bifurcation of the left common iliac artery and the left renal vein is removed. Although it is rarely necessary, the inferior mesenteric artery can be ligated to accomplish a high para-aortic dissection. Because the lymph nodes rest on top of the lumbar vertebral bodies, great care must be taken not to injure the lumbar veins. A systematic lymph node dissection is associated with increased operating time, blood loss, and blood transfusions. Acute complications of the surgery include, rarely, bowel injury (duodenum), venous vascular injuries (IVC, external iliac, hypogastric vein), and ureteral injuries. Long-term complications include lower extremity lymphedema, adhesive disease, and formation of lymphoceles which can become chronic and sometimes infected, requiring drainage, obliteration, or surgery. The rate of positive lymph nodes is very low in mucinous ovarian cancer, and lymph node dissection probably can be omitted in this histologic subtype (109,177).

Several retrospective studies have indicated that the rate of positive lymph nodes in patients of all FIGO stages who undergo a systematic pelvic and para-aortic lymph node dissection is 25% to 53%, with most of the positive lymph nodes found in the high para-aortic and interaortocaval regions (109–111). Because imaging and intraoperative palpation of lymph node beds have a low sensitivity and specificity for the detection of lymph node metastasis, several studies have investigated the role of a systematic pelvic and para-aortic lymph node dissection. In a prospective trial, Maggioni and colleagues randomized 310 patients diagnosed with early FIGO stage I and II ovarian cancer, who had undergone optimal surgical debulking, to receive either a systematic lymph node dissection or lymph node sampling (113). Patients with all major histologic subtypes were represented in the study: serous (39%), endometrioid (21%), mucinous (13%), and clear cell tumors (13%). Positive lymph nodes (which upstage a patient to FIGO 1988 stage IIIC or FIGO 2013 stage IIIA1) were found in 9% of patients in the sampling group and in 22% of the systematic lymph node dissection group ($p < 0.05$), suggesting that 13% were upstaged because of the lymph node dissection. Of those with negative lymph nodes, 66% of the patients in the control arm and 51% in the systematic lymphadenectomy arm received chemotherapy ($p < 0.03$), suggesting that, in an unstaged patient, physicians tend to err on the side of overtreatment. The patients in the systematic lymph node dissection arm spent an average of 90 minutes longer in surgery, lost 300 mL more blood, and significantly received more blood transfusions (22% vs. 36%, $p < 0.05$). Both groups had similar rates of postoperative complications. There was no difference in PFS or overall survival (OS) between the two groups, but the study was underpowered for the detection of a small benefit.

The FIGO 1988 staging categorized patients with lymph node metastasis or intraperitoneal metastasis as FIGO IIIC. Patients with an ovarian cancer limited to the pelvis with positive retroperitoneal lymph nodes have a much better 5-year PFS and OS than patients with a pelvic tumor and intraperitoneal disease. Therefore, the new FIGO staging subclassified patients with "only" retroperitoneal lymph node metastasis as stage IIIA1. A review of the large GOG#182 trial analyzed patients who underwent cytoreduction to microscopic residual disease. The median PFS was 21 months for patients with positive lymph nodes and intraperitoneal disease greater than 2 cm before surgery, 29 months with negative lymph nodes and disease greater than 2 cm, and 48 months for patients who had positive lymph nodes but preoperative intraperitoneal disease less than 2 cm (178).

In summary, systematic lymph node dissection provides important prognostic and staging information for patients with suspected early-stage ovarian cancer, which assists with assigning the correct pathologic stage and enables informed decisions concerning the need for adjuvant chemotherapy.

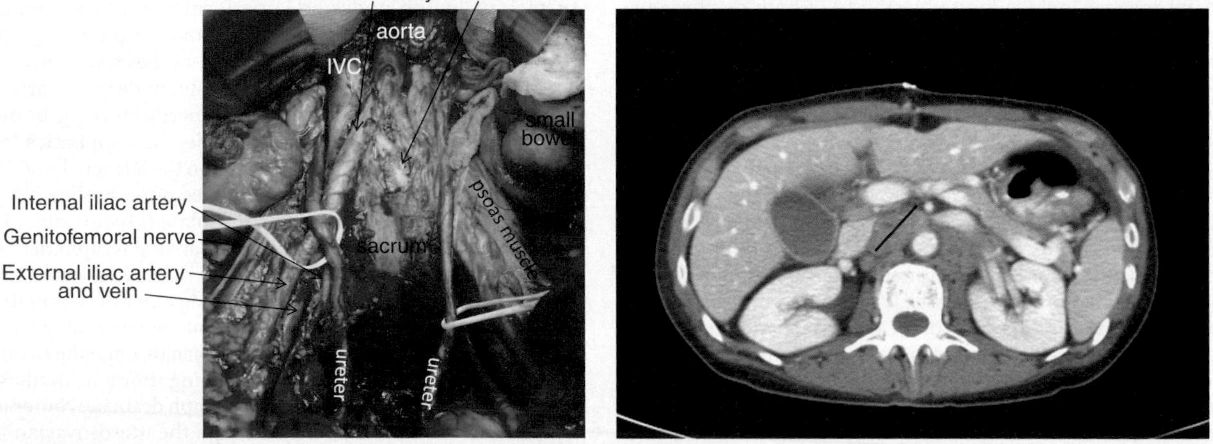

Figure 23.14. Pelvic and high para-aortic lymph node dissection in a patient with FIGO IIIC serous ovarian cancer and bulky para-aortic (see CT scan) and pelvic lymph node metastasis which were surgically removed. Before the lymph node dissection, a posterior exenteration was performed—the next step was to perform an end-to-end anastomosis of the descending colon with the rectum (not shown). The patient was optimally debulked (microscopic disease).

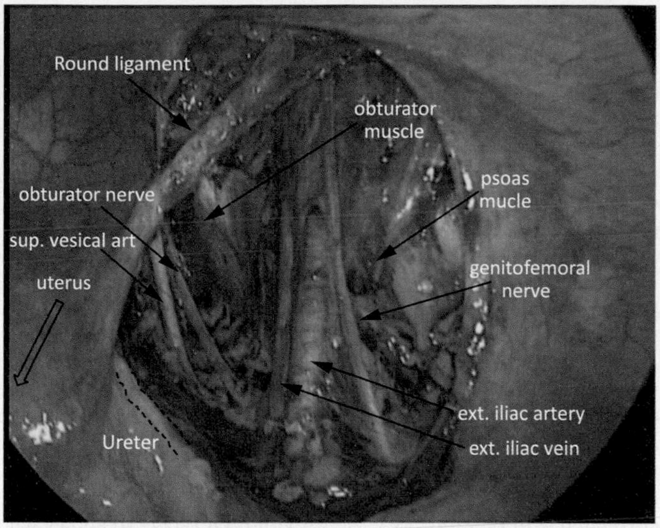

Figure 23.15. Right laparoscopic lymph node dissection in a patient with early ovarian cancer.

Advanced Epithelial Ovarian Cancer

Rationale for Surgical Debulking

Surgical debulking is central to the initial management of advanced FIGO stage III/IV ovarian cancer, and the extent of residual disease after surgery is the only prognostic factor under the control of the operating surgeon. The concept of removing widely disseminated tumors within the abdominal cavity is specific to epithelial ovarian/fallopian/peritoneal, and appendiceal cancers. It is unusual to attempt primary tumor debulking in patients with widely metastatic colon, breast, or gastric cancer. One reason surgical debulking of ovarian cancer is technically feasible is that serous ovarian cancer is usually confined within the peritoneal borders of the abdominal cavity. It spreads along the peritoneal, diaphragmatic surfaces without deep invasion (13) into abdominal organs, and this allows dissection along a surgical plane between an organ and the attached tumor. For example, although the omental tumor is very large and often densely attached to the transverse colon, it is rarely necessary to perform a transverse colon resection and it is almost always possible to sharply dissect the tumor off without injuring the colon muscularis (**Fig. 23.11**). The omental tumor often reaches the splenic hilum and distal pancreas, but rarely invades the parenchyma of these organs. Although ovarian tumors can occlude the pelvis completely and transform the pelvic peritoneum into thick tumor plaques, the pelvis can usually be completely cleared of tumors with a modified posterior exenteration (98). Serous ovarian cancer tumors never extend via direct invasion beyond the lining of the peritoneal surfaces, and a retroperitoneal dissection allows the entire tumor-covered peritoneal reflection to be removed (**Fig. 23.16**) (98). In contrast, uterine sarcomas and colon and breast cancers often grow retroperitoneally, making a complete resection much more challenging.

Several theories have been put forward to explain the strong association of surgical debulking to a state of no visible residual disease with patient survival ("microscopic disease"). One factor could be that the ability to surgically remove all disease correlates with other biologic factors that predispose to better outcomes. However, large bulky tumors may contain necrotic or hypoxic areas that have a low growth fraction and are resistant to chemotherapy. Optimal debulking could then, theoretically, drive remaining microscopic tumor cells into the cell cycle, rendering them more susceptible to cytotoxic chemotherapy.

In advanced "high tumor volume" ovarian cancer, staging traditionally takes place as part of the initial debulking surgery, with the goal of removing all visible disease and, possibly, implanting a port for intraperitoneal chemotherapy (116). In patients with extensive

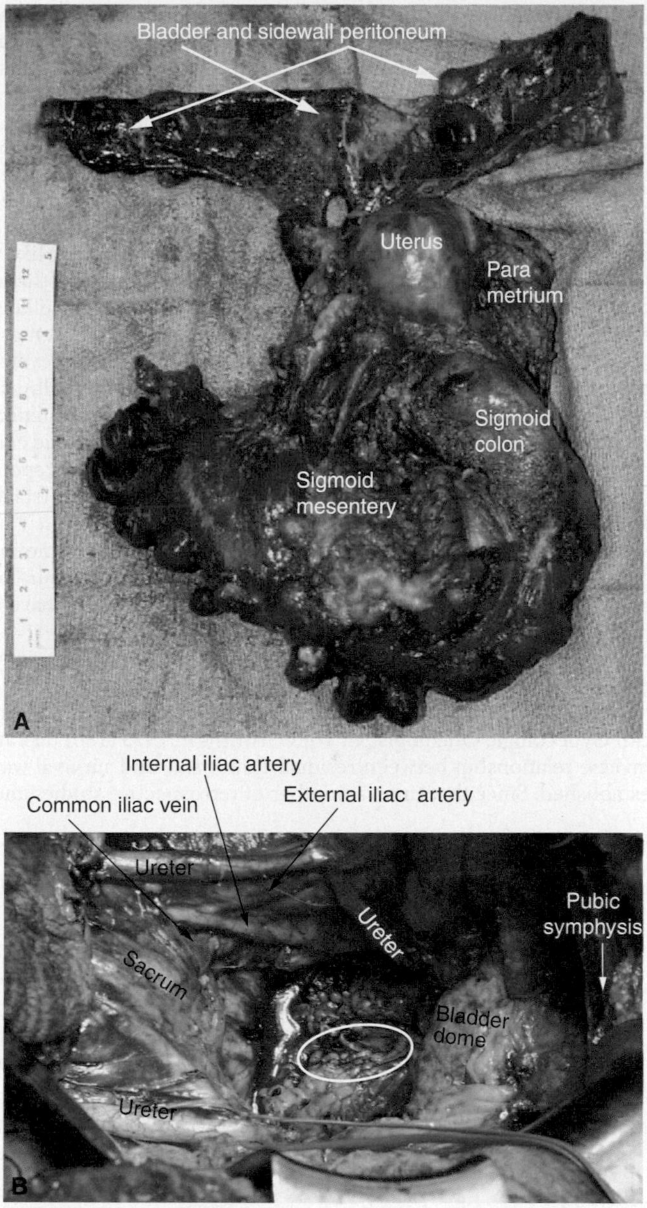

Figure 23.16. Specimen from a modified posterior pelvic exenteration. *En bloc* resection of sigmoid colon and its mesentery, uterus, parametrium, and tumor-covered pelvic peritoneum (cul-de-sac, pelvic sidewall, bladder).

tumor dissemination combined with a chronic bowel obstruction, the cancer leads to tumor-associated cachexia with a catabolic metabolic status, limiting the patient's ability to maintain reasonable nutritional status. Removal of tumor masses ("debulking") produces significant symptom relief from tumors externally pressing on organs in the pelvis or the upper abdomen. Surgical tumor debulking can also reduce ascites production and improve the nutritional and functional status of the patient, resulting in a higher quality of life.

Overall, there is no uniform surgical approach to the treatment of advanced ovarian cancer. Patient (age, nutritional status, comorbidities) and intraoperative factors (disease location, adhesions from previous surgeries, intraoperative stability/anesthesia, blood loss) and the surgical skills of the physician will determine the extent of surgical resection in the individual patient. It requires significant surgical training and experience to successfully remove pelvic and upper abdominal disease with a low complication rate. In Europe, a gynecologist generally collaborates closely with a general surgeon, who usually performs the bowel resections and upper abdominal debulking (e.g., diaphragm stripping, splenectomy). In North America, the majority of debulking, including gastro-intestinal procedures, is performed by a gynecologic oncologist with the consultation of a hepatobiliary surgeon should extensive mobilization of the liver or a liver resection be necessary. Although the comparative efficacy of these two approaches has never been studied, studies on both sides of the Atlantic have shown that high-volume centers have a higher rate of optimal surgical debulking in advanced ovarian cancer. The resectability of extensive disease with acceptable morbidity is likely to reflect a combination of surgical experience, technique, anesthesia care, critical and postoperative care, and nursing. Optimal debulking rates of up to 70% to 80% have been reported in various centers (101,179), but 50% is an accepted quality measure (167). Several centers have shown that a dedicated surgical team and a multidisciplinary effort can improve complete and optimal cytoreduction rates over time. Size and tumor distribution at the beginning and end of surgery should be carefully documented in the operative report in order to define the two most important prognostic factors (stage and residual disease).

The characterization of surgical outcome based on the amount of residual disease at the end of surgery is an accepted measure of surgical success, with the caveat that tumor measurements have a high degree of interobserver variability.

Although many surgeons had previously recommended a maximal debulking effort for patients with advanced ovarian cancer (e.g., Joe V. Meigs 1934), it was not until a retrospective study by the American Gynecologic Oncologist C. Tom Griffiths in 1975 (180) that an inverse relationship between residual tumor size and survival was established. Since that time, a number of retrospective studies and meta-analyses have reported the prognostic value of residual disease for both PFS and OS (89,103,104,179,181–183). In 1992, Hoskins and colleagues (184,185) reviewed survival and surgical results in two GOG studies that enrolled patients with FIGO stage III and IV disease (GOG#52, 97). Defining three different groups (microscopic vs. <2 cm vs. >2 cm residual disease), the authors found that survival is inversely related to the volume of residual disease at the end of surgery. Notably, they also found that, in patients with residual disease greater than 2 cm, increments in the size of residual disease did not appreciably affect survival. Later, Chi and colleagues from Memorial Sloan-Kettering showed that the introduction of radical pelvic dissection and upper abdominal debulking surgery increased the number of patients who could be optimally debulked (101).

In the largest (4,312 women) phase III ovarian cancer trial performed to date (GOG#182), the Gynecological Cancer InterGroup studied the addition of a third chemotherapy group to the standard carboplatin and paclitaxel regimen in women with stage III/IV ovarian cancer (89). Although the addition of a third drug did not show any benefit, the extent of cytoreductive surgery was shown to be significantly correlated with PFS and OS. Patients with FIGO stage III and IV who had no macroscopic disease at the end of surgery, minimal residual disease (<1 cm), or gross residual disease had a median PFS of 29, 16, and 13 months, respectively, and a median OS of 68, 44, and 30 months, respectively. Breakdown by stage is shown in **Figure 23.17**. A meta-analysis of 81 studies by Bristow and colleagues (179) also showed that survival is associated with the amount of residual disease, with a median OS of 22.7 months for patient cohorts in which 25% or fewer were maximally cytoreduced (≤ 3cm residual tumor) and a median OS of 33.9 months for patient cohorts with 75% or greater rates of maximal cytoreduction. Each 10% increase in the proportion

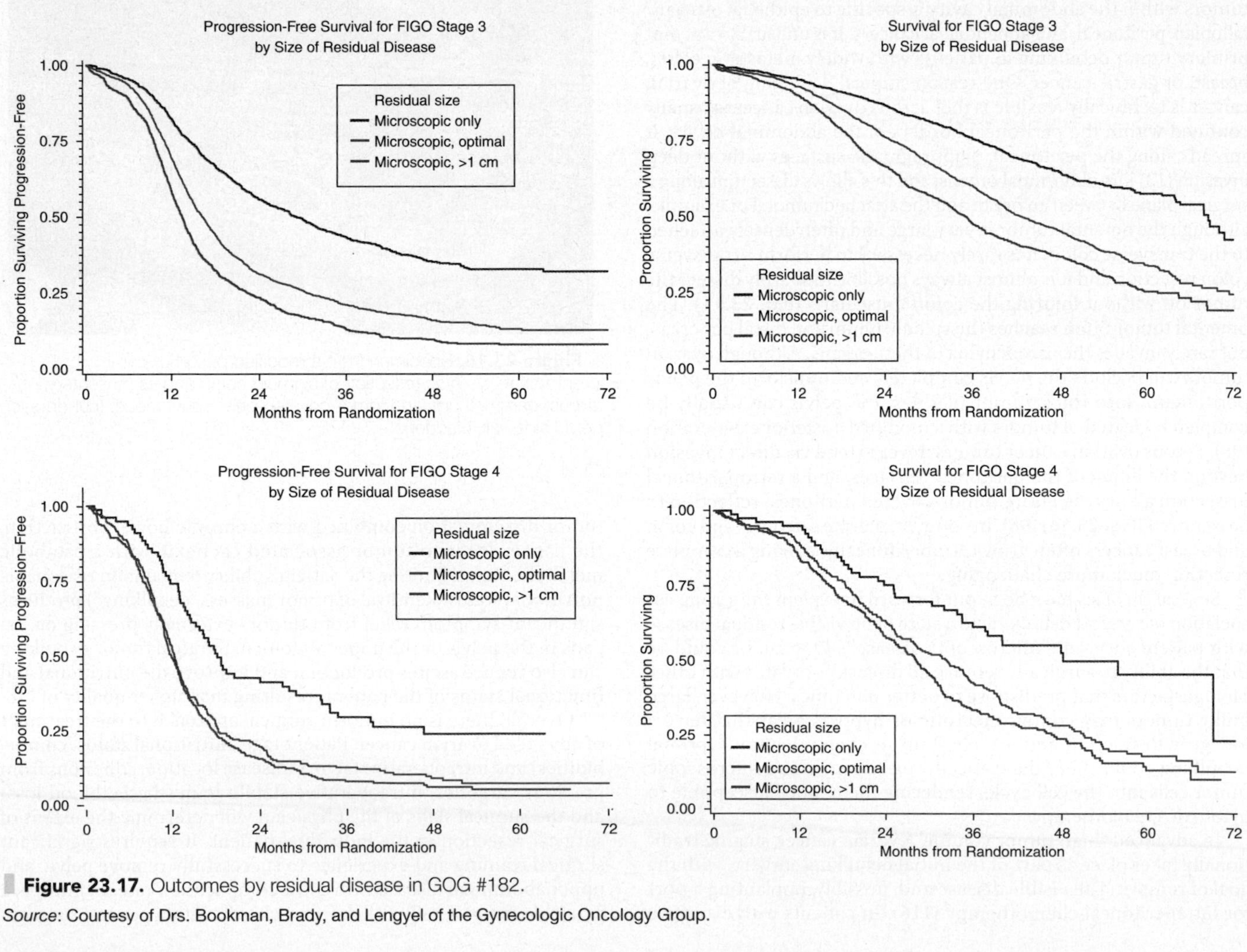

Figure 23.17. Outcomes by residual disease in GOG #182.
Source: Courtesy of Drs. Bookman, Brady, and Lengyel of the Gynecologic Oncology Group.

of patients who were maximally cytoreduced was associated with a 5.5% increase in median cohort survival time.

Improved survival with complete tumor resection is also seen in patients with FIGO stage IV disease. Winter et al., reviewing the experience of GOG#111, #132, #152, and #162, showed that patients with residual disease greater than 5 cm, multiple stage IV defining sites of metastasis (parenchymal liver disease, pleural effusion), and clear cell/mucinous ovarian cancer had a significantly worse survival (103). The median PFS and OS for stage IV patients whose tumor was reduced to microscopic disease were better than those for patients with any amount of visible residual cancer. Patients with residual disease where the single largest lesion is 0.1 to 1.0 cm and 1.1 to 5.0 cm had comparable survival and patients with residual tumor bigger than 5 cm had the worst prognosis. These data have been interpreted to suggest that, even in patients with FIGO stage IV disease, cytoreduction to microscopic disease should be the primary goal at initial surgery. A positive association of stage IV disease optimally debulked to microscopic residual disease with longer survival was also confirmed by review of three prospective phase III Arbeitsgemeinschaft Gynäkologische Onkologie (AGO) trials (AGO-OVAR #3, #5, #7) (104).

Pre-surgical high metastatic tumor load plays an important role in prognosis (184). An important question is whether every patient benefits from surgical debulking, independent of the extent of disease at the beginning of surgery. In GOG#52, patients with large-volume disease at the beginning of surgery, who were optimally debulked using an aggressive upper abdominal procedure, still had shorter survival than patients who initially had low-volume disease, even if the surgical outcome was similar (184). Du Bois and colleagues, summarizing the AGO experience from three prospective phase III trials (3,126 patients from AGO-OVAR #3, #5, #7) with identical inclusion criteria, concluded that complete surgical debulking is associated with improved prognosis in any FIGO substage, but cannot completely overcome the prognostic impact of preoperative disease load (182). Resection to microscopic disease was associated with a longer median OS (microscopic disease: 99.1 months CI, 83.5–not reached; residual <1 cm: 29.6 months CI, 27.4–32.2; residual > 1 cm: 29.6 months CI, 27.4–32). Extending these studies, Horowitz analyzed the impact of preoperative disease burden on survival by studying the impact of aggressive surgery on patients with high- and low-volume disease from GOG#182. Of 1,636 patients with large volume disease preoperatively (upper abdominal disease—diaphragm/spleen/liver/pancreas), 199 (12%) were reduced to microscopic disease, but these patients still had a worse PFS and OS compared with patients with preoperative low-volume disease (186) (**Fig. 23.18**). Therefore, both the preoperative tumor burden, including the extent of upper abdominal disease, and the extent of surgical resection (postoperative tumor burden) influence the PFS and OS of patients with advanced ovarian cancer.

In summary, surgical debulking plays a very important role in the management of advanced ovarian cancer. However, patients with very extensive carcinomatosis and extensive upper abdominal disease and/or mesenteric involvement tend to obtain limited benefit from primary debulking procedures, as many will be suboptimally debulked (186). Surgery alone is never curative in advanced disease and therefore should only be attempted as part of a treatment plan including postoperative chemotherapy. As discussed below, it is not possible to predict with accuracy which patients can be optimally debulked, because neither CT nor PET has sufficient specificity (153,154,187). Sometimes only the direct visualization of tumor distribution by laparoscopy provides the necessary information. The overall goal of cytoreductive surgery for patients with advanced-stage FIGO III/IV ovarian cancer should be, whenever feasible, the complete cytoreduction of all visible disease. The reports of improved outcomes with radical debulking suggest that patients should be counseled about this option. However, it is important to remember that, although

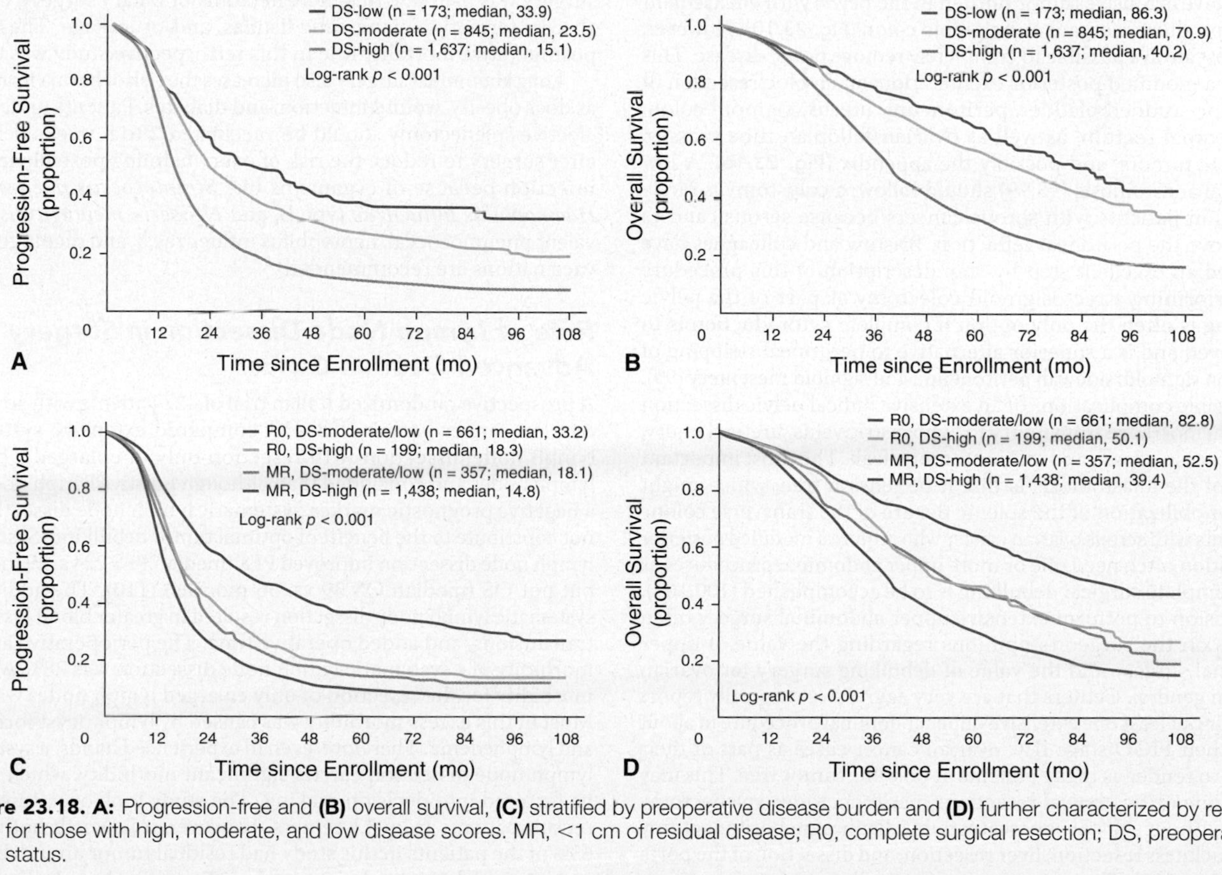

Figure 23.18. A: Progression-free and **(B)** overall survival, **(C)** stratified by preoperative disease burden and **(D)** further characterized by residual disease for those with high, moderate, and low disease scores. MR, <1 cm of residual disease; R0, complete surgical resection; DS, preoperative disease status.

Source: From Horowitz NS, Miller A, Rungruang B, et al. Does aggressive surgery improve outcomes? Interaction between preoperative disease burden and complex surgery in patients with advanced-stage ovarian cancer: an analysis of GOG 182. *J Clin Oncol*. 2015;33(8):937–943.

we justify surgical debulking because it provides symptom relief and it has been shown, in numerous retrospective reviews, to be associated with improved survival, the clinical benefits of radical surgery in ovarian cancer have never been studied in a prospective randomized trial. Heroic attempts to remove unresectable tumors will not benefit patients. In general, complex surgical procedures should be judiciously used in patients with resectable disease, when removal of all visible tumors can be achieved.

Surgical Debulking—Pelvic and Upper Abdominal Procedures

Surgery for patients with advanced ovarian cancer should start with a vertical midline incision extending from the pubic symphysis to above the umbilicus. This allows visualization of the entire abdominal cavity, including the diaphragms, and permits the safe evaluation and resection of upper abdominal disease. Pelvic and diaphragmatic washings and biopsies of suspicious peritoneal surfaces (e.g., paracolic gutters) should be performed. With a careful exploration of the abdominal cavity, the surgeon will be able to evaluate the extent of the disease and plan the surgical approach. Particular attention should be paid to the upper abdomen, as the disease distribution in that region will often determine whether a patient can be optimally debulked. It is helpful to stratify patients with advanced cancer as having either low- and high-volume disease intraoperatively because different surgical strategies are associated with each classification (186,188,189).

Patients with advanced ovarian cancer but low-volume disease should have comprehensive staging, including a total abdominal hysterectomy, bilateral salpingo-oophorectomy, and infragastric omentectomy between the hepatic flexure and the splenic hilum. If the patient can be rendered macroscopically disease free, a pelvic and high para-aortic lymph node dissection is reasonable (110).

Patients with advanced ovarian cancer and high-volume disease usually have extensive tumor burden in the pelvis with encasement of the reproductive organs and sigmoid colon (**Fig. 23.10**). However, it is almost always possible to completely remove pelvic disease. This requires a modified posterior exenteration, an en bloc resection of the tumor-studded bladder, peritoneum, uterus, sigmoid colon, and proximal rectum, as well as ovarian/fallopian tube masses, cul-de-sac tumors, and possibly the appendix (**Fig. 23.16**). A low colorectal anastomosis (98,99) should follow; a colostomy is rarely required in patients with serous cancers because serous cancers grow above the peritoneal reflection. Bristow and colleagues have published an excellent step-by-step description of this procedure (98). Performing a rectosigmoid colectomy as part of the pelvic debulking is often the only option if complete cytoreduction is to be achieved and is a superior alternative to peritoneal stripping of disease on sigmoid, sidewall peritoneum, and sigmoid mesentery (99). The possible complications of an extensive radical pelvic dissection include hemorrhage from injury to hypogastric veins, ureteral injury, pelvic abscess, sepsis, and an anastomotic leak. The most important feature of the anastomosis is that it be tension free, which might require mobilization of the splenic flexure of the transverse colon.

Patients with serous ovarian cancer who require a modified posterior exenteration often need one or more upper abdominal procedures as well if complete surgical debulking is to be accomplished (100,101). The decision to perform extensive upper abdominal surgery often depends on the surgeon's opinions regarding the value of upper abdominal surgery and the value of debulking surgery for ovarian cancer in general. Centers that are very aggressive surgically report performing at least one extensive upper abdominal procedure in about 50% of their FIGO stage IIIC ovarian cancer cases as part of their attempt to render as many patients as possible tumor free. This may include one or two bowel resections, peritonectomy, splenectomy with or without a distal pancreatectomy, diaphragm peritonectomy or full thickness resection, liver resection, and dissection of the porta hepatis (100,101). The most common upper abdominal procedure is diaphragm stripping or resection. Two excellent descriptions of liver mobilization and diaphragm stripping and resection were published by Grimm et al. (190) and Eisenhauer et al. (191). A review (183) of GOG#182 (89), limited to patients with FIGO stage III or IV disease who were optimally debulked (<1 cm), showed that 18% (482 of 2,655 patients) had undergone upper abdominal procedures. The most common procedure was diaphragm surgery (13%), followed by splenectomy and liver surgery (4% each), pancreatectomy (0.5%), and porta hepatis surgery (0.2%) (183). An excellent description of en bloc resection of extensive left upper quadrant disease has been published by Hoffman et al. (192). By using upper abdominal procedures, the authors were able to achieve complete cytoreduction in a high percentage of patients, and OS of patients with upper abdominal disease who were completely cytoreduced was superior to OS of patients with upper abdominal disease who were not completely cytoreduced. However, the preoperative tumor load continues to largely define PFS and OS. Even when aggressive upper abdominal surgery is used to reduce the tumor to microscopic disease, the survival of patients who present with high-volume disease is worse than that of patients who present with low-volume disease (186). As a word of caution, extensive involvement of the upper abdomen with disease may preclude an optimal debulking; aggressive upper abdominal surgery should be performed only when the entire disease can be removed with acceptable morbidity.

Magtibay and colleagues reported on 112 patients at the Mayo Clinic who underwent a splenectomy as part of ovarian cancer debulking (193). The most common indications were metastatic parenchymal involvement (46%), perisplenic involvement from an omental tumor that reached the splenic hilum (42%), and intraoperative trauma (13%). Complications included wound infections (6%), postoperative pneumonitis (4.5%), thromboembolic events (8%), and sepsis (4.5%). The overall perioperative mortality was 5%. A similar complication rate was reported recently; out of 121 patients, 38% had a complication, but severe complications were observed only in 19% (188). Complications were most often observed when ovarian debulking surgery was paired with pancreatectomy or biliary surgery, causing abscess formation, pancreatic fistulas, and/or leakage. The 90-day postoperative mortality rate in this retrospective study was 0.9%.

Long abdominal surgery also increases the risk of hernia formation, as does obesity, wound infection, and diabetes. Patients undergoing elective splenectomy should be vaccinated 2 to 3 weeks before or after surgery to reduce the risk of overwhelming postsplenectomy infection because of organisms like *Streptococcus pneumoniae*, *Haemophilus influenzae* type B, and *Neisseria meningitidis*. Polyvalent pneumococcal, hemophilus influenzae b, and meningococcal vaccinations are recommended.

Role of Lymph Node Dissection in Surgery for Advanced Ovarian Cancer

A prospective randomized Italian trial of 427 patients with advanced ovarian cancer (stages IIIB–IV) compared extensive systematic lymph node dissection with resection only of enlarged ("bulky") lymph nodes and concluded that, although positive lymph nodes are a negative prognostic marker, systematic lymph node dissection did not contribute to the benefit of optimal tumor debulking. Systematic lymph node dissection improved PFS (median PFS 22 vs. 29 months), but not OS (median OS 59 vs. 56 months) (110). The addition of systematic lymph node dissection resulted in greater blood loss, more transfusions, and added operative time. The perioperative and late morbidity of a systematic lymph node dissection was 28%, whereas morbidity for the resection of only enlarged lymph nodes was 18%. Most of this excess morbidity was caused by lymphocyst formation and lymphedema. Therefore, even in experienced hands, a systematic lymph node dissection carries significant morbidity, which should be factored into decision making. The study took over 12 years to recruit patients from 13 centers. However, it is worth noting that 63% of the patients in this study had residual tumor after debulking surgery, which might obviate any benefit of lymph node dissection. The German AGO retrospectively reviewed data from three large phase III trials (AGO-OVAR# 3, 5, 7) of chemotherapy in advanced epithelial ovarian cancer. They found that in the subgroup of patients with no residual disease and no enlarged lymph nodes, a systematic lymph node dissection was associated with a small statistically significant survival benefit (median OS, 108 vs. 83 months) (111).

In summary, the current practice in advanced ovarian cancer is to remove enlarged/suspicious lymph nodes as part of tumor debulking, and one retrospective review suggests systematic pelvic and para-aortic lymph node dissection might therapeutically benefit patients who have been optimally debulked to microscopic residual disease. A large international phase III trial that randomizes patients with advanced ovarian cancer who are debulked to microscopic disease to either systematic lymph node dissection or nodal sampling only is now underway (LION trial: lymphadenectomy in ovarian neoplasms).

Neo-adjuvant Chemotherapy

The European Organization for Research and Treatment of Cancer (EORTC)-GCG and NCIC performed a phase III trial (EORTC#55971) randomizing 718 patients with FIGO (1988) stage IIIC or IV ovarian cancer to either neo-adjuvant platinum-containing chemotherapy followed by interval debulking or to primary debulking surgery followed by platinum-based chemotherapy (135). The largest residual tumor after surgery was less than 1 cm in 80% of patients treated with the neo-adjuvant approach, whereas this was only accomplished in 42% of all patients who underwent up-front debulking. There was a trend toward less blood loss, fewer postoperative infections, and fewer thromboembolic complications in the neo-adjuvant treatment group, as well as a shorter operative time. Most importantly, there was no significant difference in PFS (12 months in both groups) or OS (29/30 months) between the two groups, and this was independent of the rate of optimal debulking accomplished in a specific center (**Fig. 23.19**). The study was criticized for its low PFS and OS results, but most patients had adverse prognostic factors to begin with: 74% had tumors larger than 5 cm (61% >10 cm) in size at baseline, indicating that study participants had very advanced disease. Another, related, criticism of the study was the low rate of optimal debulking. In the primary debulking group 19.4% of all patients were reduced to microscopic disease, whereas the rate was 51.2% for the neo-adjuvant group. In the United States the optimal debulking rate is 40% to 80%.

A second phase III trial (CHORUS) (158), which randomly assigned 552 women to either primary surgery or NACT (three cycles pre- and three cycles postoperatively) also found no significant difference in OS between the two groups (PFS 10.7 vs. 12 months, OS 22.6 vs. 24.1 months). There were fewer complications in the neo-adjuvant group, and more patients in the neo-adjuvant group had an improvement in global quality of life.

Fourteen patients (6%) died in the primary surgery group, which is a much higher mortality rate than has been previously reported in phase III trials of advanced ovarian cancer and may be related to the advanced stage or poor performance status of the patients entered on the study. The median operative time in both groups was short, at 120 minutes, and debulking to microscopic disease was accomplished in only 17% of the women who had primary surgery compared with 39% of those who had primary chemotherapy ($p = 0.0001$). In the primary surgery group 27% did not have a BSO, 24% did not have a hysterectomy, and only 20% had upper abdominal surgery.

Results of these studies started a heated discussion on the role of NACT and the best timing of radical debulking in the front-line treatment of ovarian cancer. This discussion is still ongoing. There are no preoperative factors or imaging studies (153) that can be used to predict the success of interval cytoreduction surgery. For patients with FIGO (1988/2013), stage I–IIIB disease, primary surgery is currently the standard treatment. An exploratory analysis of the EORTC study (194) showed that women with less extensive metastatic disease did better with primary surgery whereas patients with metastatic tumors that are larger than 4.5 cm and patients with FIGO (1988) stage IV did better with NACT. Physicians who feel a primary surgical approach is preferable even in women with large tumor volume note results such as those from a retrospective analysis of patients treated at Memorial Sloan-Kettering Cancer Center during the time of EORTC trial who underwent very aggressive surgery (including upper abdominal surgery), with high rates of optimal debulking, and reported that these patients experienced results that appear superior to those seen in the CHORUS and EORTC trials, with a PFS and OS of 17 months and 50 months, respectively (195).

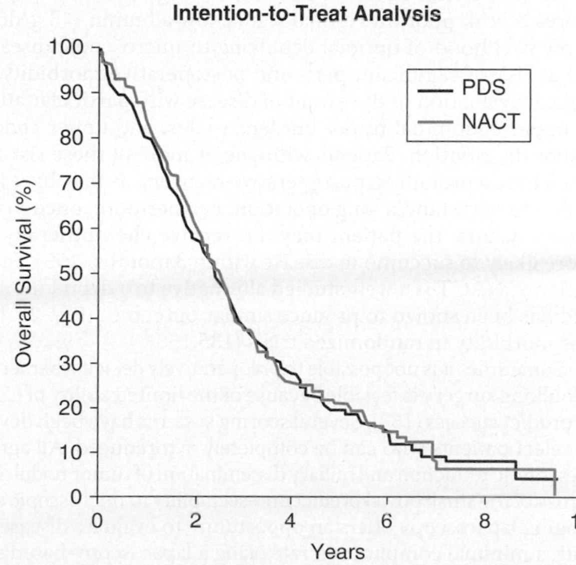

	No. of Events	No. of Patients at Risk				
Primary Debulking Surgery (PDS)	253	336	189	62	14	2
Neoadjuvant Chemotherapy (NACT)	245	334	195	46	13	2

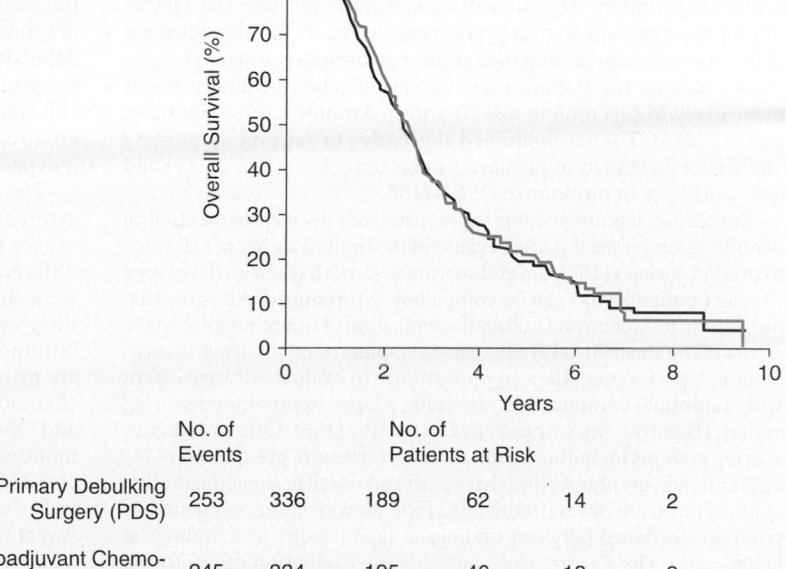

Figure 23.19. Neo-adjuvant chemotherapy versus upfront debulking.

Source: Reprinted with permission from Vergote I, Troupe CG, Amant F, et al. Neoadjuvant chemotherapy or primary surgery in stage IIIC or IV ovarian cancer. N Engl J Med. 2010;363:943–953.

In patients with extensive tumor burden (ascites, poor performance status and several comorbidities, obesity, and older age), NACT is a very reasonable choice. The current standard for a healthier, younger patient with disease that appears resectable is initial aggressive surgery with the goal of accomplishing a complete tumor debulking with no visible residual disease.

Summary of Primary Debulking Surgery for Ovarian Cancer

Many factors contribute to how long a patient with advanced ovarian cancer survives. Inherent genetic characteristics of the tumor may play a more important role in OS than stage or cytoreductive surgical debulking. However, the study of genetic factors in relation to surgical treatment is in its infancy. At present, the degree of surgical debulking is the only prognostic factor that can be influenced by the surgeon. We know that among patients with advanced-stage III/V ovarian cancer, those who undergo a complete debulking have the most favorable prognosis. Whether a complete resection is performed is, at least in part, determined by the surgeon's skill and willingness to engage in a maximal surgical effort. Once the decision has been made to proceed, the goal of every operation in patients with advanced-stage III/IV ovarian cancer should be a complete resection of all visible tumors to microscopic disease (157).

However, ultraradical surgery, involving the addition of upper abdominal procedures to pelvic tumor debulking, will increase morbidity and not every patient is a good candidate for such an aggressive approach (196). Large-volume involvement of the upper abdomen, extended small and large bowel surface and mesentery involvement or multiple liver metastases, may preclude an optimal debulking. Wright and colleagues, reviewing a large administrative database with over 28,000 patients, showed that the complication rate of extensive ovarian cancer debulking (e.g., surgical site, medical, infectious complications) increases with age. Women younger than 50 years, 70 to 80 years, and those older than 80 years have a 17.1%, 29.7%, and 31.5% complication rate, respectively (196).

Two groups of factors should contribute to the decision whether to take a patient to surgery and perform a radical debulking procedure (155): (a) A careful preoperative evaluation of patient-related risk factors: Patients with significant comorbidities and low performance status (American Society of Anesthesiology [ASA] preoperative scores 3 or 4, poor nutritional status, low albumin <3 g/dL) have a low likelihood of optimal debulking to microscopic disease and are at risk of significant peri- and postoperative morbidity; (b) A critical evaluation of the extent of disease with particular attention to upper abdominal tumor burden, ascites, and upper abdominal tumor distribution. Patients with one or more of these risk factors often have a prolonged postoperative recovery, as they have limited ability to withstand a long operation. Furthermore, once a complication occurs, the patient may not receive chemotherapy and is more likely to succumb to disease within 3 months (155). For these patients, NACT is a well-studied alternative to a debulking surgery and has been shown to produce similar outcomes (**Fig. 23.19**) and less morbidity in randomized trials (135,158).

Sometimes it is not possible to preoperatively decide whether radical debulking surgery is feasible because of the limited ability of CT scans to predict success (153). Several scoring systems have been developed to select patients who can be completely cytoreduced. All agree that mesenteric retraction and miliary dissemination of tumor nodules on the serosa of the small bowel predict unresectability to microscopic disease. Staging laparoscopy offers an opportunity to evaluate disease extent with a minimal complication rate using a laparoscopy-based scoring system (Fagotti score or predictive index (PI) (156). Other predictive scoring systems including serum markers (albumin, preoperative CA-125) and radiographic features have performed well in single-institution studies, but were not reproducible (153). However, there is generally good concordance between findings at laparoscopy and findings at laparotomy. The Fagotti score includes the evaluation of peritoneal and diaphragmatic carcinomatosis, omental caking, need for a large/small bowel resection (excluding sigmoid resection), involvement of the stomach, lesser sac, or spleen, and liver surface lesions, assigning a score of 2 for each feature present. A score >10 predicts that it will be impossible to completely cytoreduce a tumor to microscopic disease. At MD Anderson the Fagotti score is used to standardize care. Patients with scores < 8 receive initial cytoreductive surgery, whereas those with scores ≥ 8 receive NACT (157). A prospective trial "SCORPION" conducted at MD Anderson is now testing primary debulking surgery versus NACT in patients with scores from 8 to 12 (157).

Second-look laparotomy was often performed in the 1980s after primary surgery and adjuvant cisplatin-based therapy for prognostic information and to determine the need for further treatment. Chemotherapy was generally continued for those found to have residual small volume disease. Second-look surgery is no longer generally performed, because no therapy instituted as a result of disease found during these procedures altered prognosis. Reoperation following chemotherapy also introduces unnecessary morbidity. About one-third of patients with advanced ovarian cancer were found to be free of disease at a second-look laparotomy, yet over half of these patients eventually experienced a recurrence.

In summary, the extent of primary surgical cytoreduction in patients with advanced ovarian cancer and multiple comorbidities should be determined for every patient individually. If there is doubt, until more data become available, it is reasonable to treat these patients with NACT followed by debulking surgery.

Interval Debulking for Suboptimally Debulked Patients

In this section, the term *interval debulking surgery* refers to a surgical procedure in a patient with persistent abdominal disease after an initial surgical debulking effort and three to four cycles of chemotherapy (**Table 23.7**).

There is conflicting evidence from two large prospective, randomized trials regarding whether interval debulking surgery can improve survival in patients for whom an initial surgical effort did not achieve optimal results (197,198). In a multicenter trial conducted by the EORTC (197), patients with suboptimal (>1 cm) disease remaining after primary cytoreduction were treated with three cycles of cyclophosphamide and cisplatin. Those without progression were randomized to interval debulking surgery and additional chemotherapy versus additional chemotherapy alone. With approximately 140 patients randomized to each arm, patients undergoing interval debulking showed a statistically significant improvement in both progression-free interval and median survival (**Fig. 23.20**). The survival of patients with residual lesions of more than 1 cm after the interval debulking surgery was similar to that of patients who did not undergo the surgery. None of the patients in the interval debulking group died and morbidity was minimal. The long-term results from this study showed that after 5 years PFS and OS were still significantly better for the patients in the interval debulking group and that being randomized to interval debulking remained an independent prognostic factor for improved survival (199).

The GOG prospective, randomized trial of interval secondary cytoreduction in patients with advanced FIGO stage III/IV ovarian cancer with suboptimal (> 1 cm) residual disease, however, had different results (GOG#152) (198). Five hundred fifty patients were enrolled in GOG#152 within 6 weeks of initial surgery. After three cycles of paclitaxel and cisplatin, patients without evidence of tumor progression were randomized to receive either secondary cytoreduction and three additional cycles of chemotherapy or chemotherapy alone. At the time of the report (2004), median PFS and OS (**Fig. 23.21**) for the interval cytoreduction group were 10.5 months and 33.9 months, respectively, compared with 10.7 months and 33.7 months for the chemotherapy-alone group. A consistent lack of effect was seen in all patients regardless of the residual tumor size at the end of the interval debulking surgery.

Several theories have been advanced to explain the difference in outcomes between the GOG and European studies. One point

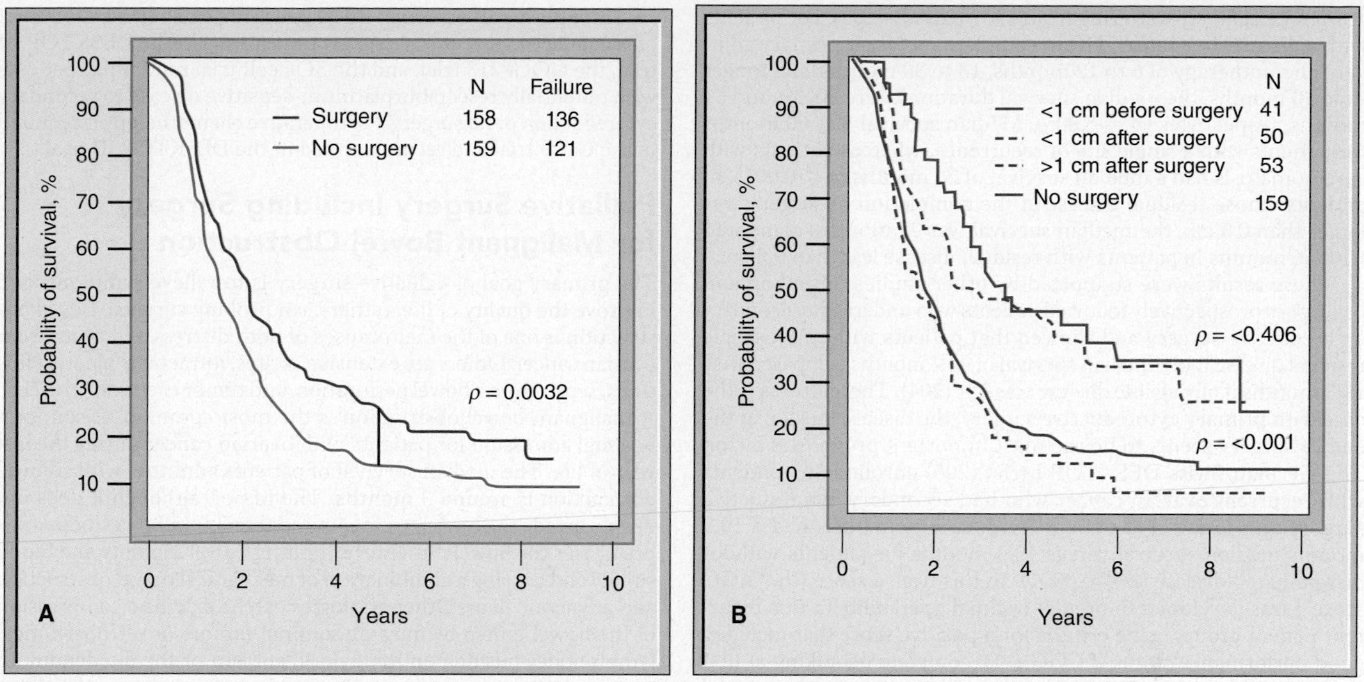

Figure 23.20. A: Survival of patients who underwent interval cytoreductive surgery and no interval surgery. **B:** Survival of patients who underwent interval cytoreductive surgery according to size of tumor lesions versus patients without interval surgery.

Source: From van der Burg ME. Advanced ovarian cancer. *Curr Treat Options Oncol*. 2001;2(2):109–118.

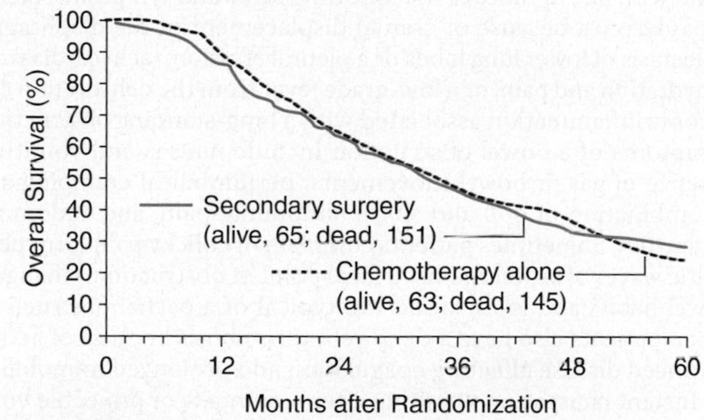

No. at Risk

Secondary surgery	216	187	129	83	49	31
Chemotherapy alone	208	185	124	81	56	22

$p = 0.92$ for the comparison between the groups by the log-rank test

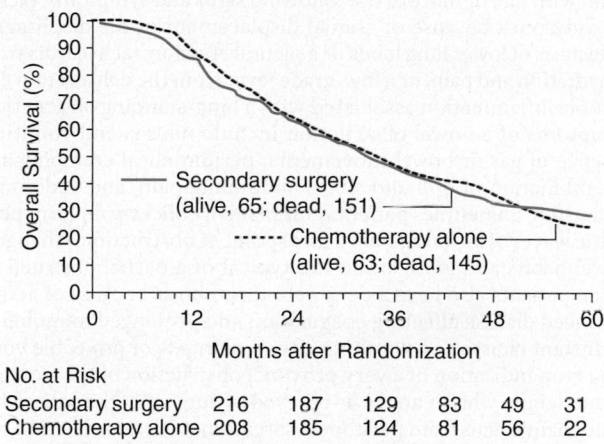

Figure 23.21. Overall survival of patients with advanced ovarian cancer who underwent interval debulking surgery compared with treatment with chemotherapy-only GOG trial.

Source: Rose PG, Nerenstone S, Brady M, et al. A phase III randomized study of interval secondary cytoreduction in patients with advanced-stage ovarian carcinoma with suboptimal residual disease: a Gynecologic Oncology Group study. *Proc Am Soc Clin Oncol*. 2002;21;201A, with permission.

raised is that there were differences in the extent of the initial cytoreduction surgery. In the GOG trial, both the initial and interval cytoreductive operations were clearly defined and were performed almost exclusively by trained gynecologic oncologists, whereas in the EORTC trial the extent of the initial surgery was not clearly defined and surgery was most often performed by general gynecologists. As a result, residual disease following primary surgery measured less than 5 cm in about two-thirds of the GOG patients, compared with one-third of the patients in the EORTC trial. Following chemotherapy, residual disease greater than 1 cm was found in 56% of the GOG patients versus 65% of the European patients. In addition, the chemotherapeutic regimen used in the GOG trial, paclitaxel and platinum, may have been more effective than the platinum and cyclophosphamide combination used by the EORTC. Less effective chemotherapy would increase the benefit of interval cytoreduction in the EORTC trial, which found conversion from suboptimal to optimal residual tumor in 45% of patients as compared with 36% in the GOG trial. Differences in outcomes may also be related to different posttreatment surveillance and to the availability of more effective second-line therapies, because the EORTC trial completed accrual in May 1993 before paclitaxel was introduced into clinical care. It is of interest to note that the similar median and OS in both arms of the GOG trial were substantially longer than those reported in the best (interval cytoreduction) arm of the EORTC trial. We can conclude that patients who had an initial maximal effort at cytoreduction resulting in suboptimal debulking are unlikely to benefit from interval cytoreduction (198). However, patients with advanced ovarian cancer who previously only had a biopsy, removal of the ovary, partial removal of ovarian tumors, or, in general, a limited surgical attempt, may benefit from a second surgery that involves maximal debulking (197).

Secondary Cytoreductive Surgery for Recurrent Disease

Despite modest improvements in adjuvant chemotherapy for ovarian cancer (intraperitoneal chemotherapy (116), dose-intense chemotherapy [200,201], and aggressive primary debulking surgery including upper abdominal procedures) (155,183,186,188–190,192,193,202), the majority (70%) of patients with advanced epithelial ovarian cancer will have a recurrence (89). As there is currently no chemotherapy that can cure recurrent ovarian cancer, surgical resection of recurrent disease is an option for a select group of patients.

In 1992 a retrospective study of secondary cytoreduction for recurrent disease from investigators in Munich showed an OS of 29 months for patients cytoreduced to microscopic residual disease, whereas patients with any visible disease after surgery had a median survival of only 9 months (202). Later, Chi and colleagues reviewed outcomes of 157 patients who had undergone secondary cytoreduction at Memorial Sloan-Kettering from 1987 to 2001 (203). For patients with a disease-free interval from completion of their primary adjuvant chemotherapy of 6 to 12 months, 13 to 30 months, and longer than 30 months, the median survival durations were 30, 39, and 51 months, respectively ($p = 0.005$). Median survival was 60 months for patients with a single site of recurrence, whereas patients with carcinomatosis had a median survival of 28 months ($p < 0.001$). In patients whose residual disease at the completion of surgery was larger than 0.5 cm, the median survival was 27 months, compared with 56 months in patients with residual disease less than 0.5 cm.

These results were supported by other studies. Eisenkop and colleagues prospectively followed patients who underwent secondary cytoreductive surgery and showed that patients with microscopic residual disease had a median survival of 44.4 months compared with 19.3 months if any visible disease was left (204). Therefore, as is the case with primary cytoreductive surgery, the disease burden at the end of surgery seems to be the most important prognostic factor. The German/Swiss DESKTOP I trial (205) enrolled 267 patients with recurrent ovarian cancer who had secondary cytoreductive surgery and found that patients with carcinomatosis had a 19.9 months median survival versus 45.3 months for patients without disseminated disease ($p < 0.0001$). In this trial, a score (the "AGO score") was developed to predict optimal operability in this recurrent patient group, using criteria for a positive score that included good performance status (ECOG ≤ 1), complete debulking at first surgery, and less than 500 cc of ascites. The score was then tested in the DESKTOP II prospectively: 76% of the patients who fulfilled all three criteria had an optimal debulking to no residual disease (206). One-third of the patients that had surgery suffered at least one minor or major complication. However, the AGO score was found to have no independent prognostic value. A retrospective study from the Mayo Clinic that applied the AGO score to 192 women who had secondary cytoreductive surgery between 1998 and 2013 found that a positive AGO score predicted a R0 resection in 84.3% of cases. Thus, a positive AGO score does indicate that secondary debulking surgery for recurrent ovarian cancer is likely to be successful. However, 64.4% patients with a negative score also achieved a R0 resection. The median disease-free interval for the entire group was 1.9 years (207). Overall survival was longer for patients with complete (5.4 years) than with optimal (2.4 years) or suboptimal cytoreduction (1.3 years).

A small subset of patients (4% to 5%) will present with isolated recurrences in retroperitoneal lymph nodes. Several small retrospective studies found that complete resection of lymph nodes limited to one anatomic region (60% are high para-aortic) is associated with significantly improved survival (178). This finding is consistent with the better prognosis of patients who present with localized disease in the pelvis and retroperitoneal lymph node metastasis.

All studies reporting on secondary cytoreductive surgery are retrospective or prospective nonrandomized studies, which have an inherent selection bias for patients in a prognostic group judged suitable for surgical interventions. However, based on the consistent findings of these studies, the following selection criteria for secondary debulking seem reasonable: Patients with (a) a disease-free interval longer than 12 months, (b) platinum-sensitive disease with additional chemotherapy options, (c) oligometastatic or localized intra- or retroperitoneal disease with the absence of ascites and carcinomatosis, and (d) a good performance status (208). For all other patients, the potential morbidity and limited benefit associated with suboptimal secondary cytoreduction should be carefully weighed against the possible benefit of surgery. In cases where radiologic studies do not provide a clear preoperative picture of disease extent, a diagnostic laparoscopy to assess resectability may assist with the decision. In appropriately selected patients secondary cytoreduction is associated with an improved patient outcome, with the largest benefit in patients from whom all visible disease is removed (206). Very rarely is surgery indicated in platinum-resistant recurrences. It should be performed only if a PET/CT shows only one or two lesions and there is no ascites (209).

Three prospective randomized trials will hopefully clarify the impact of secondary cytoreductive surgery on survival. The DESKTOP III trial, the GOG#213 trial, and the SOCceR trial randomize patients with potentially resectable platinum-sensitive disease to secondary cytoreduction or no surgery. Postoperative chemotherapy is required in the GOG trial and recommended in the DESKTOP III trial.

Palliative Surgery Including Surgery for Malignant Bowel Obstruction

The primary goal of palliative surgery is to relieve symptoms and improve the quality of life, rather than prolong survival. Bowel obstruction is one of the main causes of both distress and death from ovarian cancer. Others are extensive ascites, intractable pleural effusions, sepsis from a bowel perforation, and tumor cachexia (210,211). A malignant bowel obstruction is the most common reason for a hospital admission for patients with ovarian cancer during the last year of life. The median survival of patients admitted with a bowel obstruction is around 3 months. The tumor, although it does not deeply invade the bowel, connects and then kinks bowel loops and/or encases the bowel mesentery, limiting bowel mobility and blood supply and causing a combination of mechanical bowel obstruction and adynamic ileus. Other etiologies can be extrinsic compression of the bowel lumen by intra-abdominal tumors or retroperitoneal lymph nodes pushing on the pyloric antrum or the duodenum. In patients without a recurrence, who underwent an extensive debulking procedure or received previous i.p. chemotherapy, adhesions, an old hematoma, or a new incisional hernia may also be the cause of a bowel obstruction.

Patients with advanced disease tend to present to the emergency room with one or more of the following signs and symptoms: tachypnea/dyspnea because of cranial displacement of the diaphragm/atelectasis of lower lung lobes or a pleural effusion, tachycardia from dehydration and pain, or a low-grade fever from the dehydration and chronic inflammation associated with a long-standing obstruction. Symptoms of a bowel obstruction include nausea and vomiting, absence of gas or bowel movements, periumbilical cramping and a combination of dull and sharp abdominal pain, and abdominal distension. Sometimes patients complain of colicky pain from peristaltic waves of bowel against a focal point of obstruction. Changing bowel habits and loose stools are typical of a partial obstruction. Often patients also have a deep vein thrombosis because of active, advanced disease affecting coagulation and prolonged immobility.

Instant nausea and vomiting after oral intake or projectile vomiting is an indication of a very proximal obstruction of the stomach or duodenum which cannot be relieved by surgery. If the patient has an adynamic ileus from peritoneal carcinomatosis, auscultation will show an absence of bowel sounds, but if there is a complete bowel obstruction bowel sounds will be high pitched. Proximal bowel obstruction may be caused either by an extensive upper abdominal tumor load or by enlarged high para-aortic lymph nodes causing extrinsic compression of the duodenum or jejunum. The abdomen of patients with a proximal bowel obstruction is often not distended, which can give the mistaken impression that the problem is limited, although the patients suffer from severe nausea and bilious emesis. Laboratory analysis often shows hemoconcentration, thrombocytosis, low albumin, and hypokalemic, hypochloremic metabolic alkalosis, which is a sign of repeated vomiting and/or long-standing nasogastric tube drainage. Patients with a volvulus or chronic bowel ischemia may have metabolic acidosis, leukocytosis, and an increase in lactate. Although bowel obstruction is a clinical diagnosis, a supine and upright abdominal X-ray ("GI obstruction series") will show air-fluid levels. A chest X-ray may reveal free air. A CT scan of the abdomen and pelvis with oral and intravenous contrast or a small bowel follow-through will permit the evaluation of the small/large bowel over its entire length and will help determine whether there is partial or complete bowel obstruction and whether there are multiple sites of obstruction or a single transition point. The bowel is often dilated proximal to the transition point and collapsed distally.

Treatment options at this point include palliative care with symptom control, a percutaneous endoscopic gastrostomy (PEG) tube, parenteral nutrition, palliative chemotherapy, stents for gastric outlet obstruction or single-site colonic obstruction, and as last resort palliative surgery. Initial treatment for a malignant bowel obstruction should be conservative and may include bowel rest and hydration to correct metabolic abnormalities, which are signs of a long-standing obstruction. Additional supportive measures include treatment with octreotide to reduce secretions, anti-emetics, corticosteroids to reduce inflammation and act as anti-emetics, and narcotics for adequate pain management. In selected patients it is possible to accomplish a temporary surgical correction and relieve the blockage by either removing the tumors obstructing the bowel or by performing a diversion that may involve a colostomy, ileostomy, or a limited bowel resection with intestinal bypass. Preoperative contraindications to an attempted surgical correction of a malignant bowel obstruction include an adynamic ileus caused by carcinomatosis or extensive ascites, diffusely metastatic cancer with bowel obstructions on multiple levels, and involvement of the proximal ileum, duodenum, or stomach. Relative contraindications to palliative surgery for a malignant bowel obstruction are a long-standing obstruction, significant deconditioning and tumor cachexia (low serum albumin), multiple previous abdominal surgeries, and rapidly progressing, chemotherapy-resistant disease (212). Before surgery, consideration should be given to a large bowel stent if the obstruction is in the distal colon.

Because the purpose of palliative surgery is to improve the quality of life, the procedure must be short and limited, with the lowest possible complication rate. A review of patients with ovarian cancer at a single institution who underwent palliative surgery for bowel obstruction found that, in experienced hands and with appropriately selected patients, a surgical correction was possible in 84% of all patients and successful palliation, defined as the ability to tolerate oral intake for at least 60 days after surgery, was achieved in 71% of patients (213). In 16% of patients, a gastrostomy tube was placed and most of the other patients received an ileostomy, a colostomy, or the obstructed area was bypassed. The rate of major surgical complications was 22% and included enterocutaneous fistula formation, abscess formation, bacterial peritonitis, thromboembolic events, and death. The median survival for patients who were able to receive chemotherapy (70%) was 9.7 months, whereas it was 2.4 months for those not treated with chemotherapy (213). A low preoperative albumin ($<$2.5 mg/dL), ascites ($<$2 L), and carcinomatosis were found to be relative contraindications (212). Other studies have shown similar results. Palliative surgery for bowel obstruction in ovarian cancer patients is associated with significant mortality (15% to 25%), whether it is an elective or an emergency procedure. Successful palliation (adequate oral intake $>$ 60 days) is achieved in 53% to 71% of patients and the inoperability rate is around 20% (212–214). These results highlight the importance of discussing possible outcomes with patients, fostering realistic expectations, and learning how the patient defines successful palliation.

Excessive ascites production is also often encountered in patients with progressive disease. Ultrasound-guided intraperitoneal catheter placement is safe and can be performed intermittently as an outpatient procedure. Visceral injury followed by peritonitis is very rare with this procedure, but with repeated paracentesis the ascites may become loculated and drainage incomplete. Often repeated paracenteses are necessary, and in this case, a permanent indwelling abdominal catheter can be placed and the patient or her family instructed on how to drain the ascites. Antiangiogenic therapy may also reduce ascites production.

PATHOLOGY

Classification

The 2014 WHO classification of ovarian epithelial tumors is summarized in **Table 23.8**. Epithelial tumors comprise about half of all ovarian tumors and account for 40% of benign tumors and over

TABLE 23.8. 2014 WHO Histologic Classification of Common Epithelial Tumors of the Ovary

Serous tumors
Benign
Serous cystadenoma
Serous surface papilloma
Serous adenofibroma
Borderline
Serous borderline tumor/atypical proliferative serous tumor
Serous borderline tumor—micropapillary variant/noninvasive low-grade serous carcinoma
Malignant
Low-grade serous carcinoma
High-grade serous carcinoma
Mucinous tumors
Benign
Mucinous cystadenoma
Mucinous adenofibroma
Borderline tumor
Mucinous borderline tumor/atypical proliferative mucinous tumor
Malignant
Mucinous carcinoma
Endometrioid tumors
Benign
Endometriotic cyst
Endometrioid cystadenoma
Endometrioid adenofibroma
Borderline
Endometrioid borderline tumor/atypical proliferative endometrioid tumor
Malignant
Endometrioid carcinoma
Clear cell tumors
Benign
Clear cell cystadenoma
Clear cell adenofibroma
Borderline
Clear cell borderline tumor/atypical proliferative clear cell tumor
Malignant
Clear cell carcinoma
Brenner tumors
Benign
Brenner tumor
Borderline
Borderline Brenner tumor/atypical proliferative Brenner tumor
Malignant
Malignant Brenner tumor
Seromucinous tumors
Benign
Seromucinous cystadenoma
Seromucinous adenofibroma
Borderline
Seromucinous borderline tumor/atypical proliferative seromucinous tumor
Malignant
Seromucinous carcinoma
Undifferentiated carcinoma

Source: Kurman RJ, Carcangiu ML, Herrington CS, et al. *WHO Classification of Tumours of Female Reproductive Organs*. Lyon, France: IARC; 2014:12–13.

95% of malignant tumors. Over 1,200 consecutive ovarian surface epithelial tumors over a 13-year period were recently reviewed at a large US community hospital using uniform pathologic review with current criteria (**Table 23.9**) (215). Although not population based, these data on carcinomas are very similar to population-based data from Canada (216) and Sweden (217).

The apparent cell-type distribution of ovarian cancer has changed significantly in the past two decades as metastatic mucinous carcinomas have been recognized and properly categorized (218). Primary invasive mucinous carcinoma now appears to be quite uncommon, comprising only 3% of ovarian carcinomas and less than 1% of advanced-stage carcinomas (**Table 23.10**) (219). Carcinosarcoma (malignant mixed Müllerian tumor), previously regarded as a rare primary ovarian tumor, now appears to comprise 6% of ovarian carcinomas in the United States. This apparent increase in frequency may be because of more thorough sampling with the identification of small sarcomatous components in otherwise typical HGSCs. There are global geographic differences in the incidence of the different cell types (220). For example, clear cell carcinomas are more common in Japan as compared with North America. The extent to which these differences may reflect variation in diagnostic criteria or other aspects of pathology practice is currently unknown. **Table 23.11** defines the abbreviations used in this section.

Pathogenesis

Dualistic Model of Ovarian Cancer Pathogenesis

Advances in molecular biology correlated with morphologic studies have shed new light on the pathogenesis of ovarian carcinoma and have challenged many of the time-honored concepts of ovarian neoplasia. These studies have led to the proposal of a new model of carcinogenesis (221). Concomitantly, recent studies have provided evidence that the origin of ovarian carcinoma, previously regarded to be the ovarian surface epithelium, may be the fallopian tube in many or possibly even most cases (222,223). The view that ovarian cancer begins in the ovary and spreads systematically to the pelvis, abdomen, and then distant sites is now less favored and the dated

TABLE 23.9. Distribution of 1,247 Ovarian Epithelial Tumors by Cell Type, Washington Hospital Center, 1999 to 2011

	Benign (%)	Atypical Proliferative/ Borderline (%)	Malignant (%)	Total (%)
Serous	48.6	1.8	17.8	68.2
Endometrioid	0.8	0.2	1.9	2.9
Clear cell	0	0.2	2.2	2.4
Mucinous	7.6	1.0	0.8	9.4
Seromucinous	1.8	0.3	0.2	2.3
Transitional	9.9	0.2	0.3	10.4
Mixed	0.6	0	0.7	1.3
Undifferentiated	–	–	0.1	0.1
Carcinosarcoma	–	–	1.6	1.6
Squamous	1.3	–	0.1	1.4
Total	70.6	3.7	25.7	100

Source: Fleming G, Seidman J, Lengyel E. Epithelial ovarian cancer. In: Barakat RR, Berchuck A, Markman M, et al, eds. *Principles and Practice of Gynecologic Oncology*. 6th ed. Philadelphia, PA: Wolters Kluwer/Lippincott Williams & Wilkins: 2013:757–847.

TABLE 23.10. Distribution of 562 Invasive Ovarian Carcinomas by Cell Type, Washington Hospital Center, 1991 to 2013

	Stage I	Stage II	Stage III	Stage IV	Total (%)
High-grade serous	11	18	248	94	371 (66.0)
Low-grade serous	2	0	22	5	29 (5.2)
Endometrioid	21	8	10	2	41 (7.3)
Clear cell	24	8	10	3	45 (8.0)
Mucinous	13	1	1	0	15 (2.7)
Transitional	6	0	0	0	6 (1.1)
Carcinosarcoma	1	5	21	7	34 (6.0)
Seromucinous	4	1	0	0	5 (0.9)
Mixed	4	3	4	2	13 (2.3)
Undifferentiated	0	1	1	0	2 (0.4)
Squamous	0	0	0	1	1 (0.2)
Total (%)	86 (15.3)	45 (8.0)	317 (56.4)	114 (20.3)	562

High-grade serous includes those of peritoneal and tubal origin. Transitional cell carcinomas (other than malignant Brenner tumors) are classified as high-grade serous carcinoma (see text).

Source: Seidman JD, Vang R, Ronnett BM, et al. Distribution and case-fatality ratios by cell type for ovarian carcinomas: a 22 year series of 562 patients with uniform, current histological classification. *Gynecol Oncol*. 2015;136:336–340.

TABLE 23.11. Abbreviations Used in the Pathology Section

AGUS Atypical glandular cells of undetermined significance	
APCCT Atypical proliferative clear cell tumor	
APET Atypical proliferative endometrioid tumor	
APMT Atypical proliferative mucinous tumor	
APST Atypical proliferative serous tumor	
DPAM Disseminated peritoneal adenomucinosis	
ESS Endometrioid stromal sarcoma	
FNA Fine-needle aspiration	
HGSC High-grade serous carcinoma	
HR Homologous recombination	
LGSC Low-grade serous carcinoma	
MBT Mucinous borderline tumor	
MMMT Malignant mixed mesodermal tumor	
MPSC Micropapillary serous carcinoma	
NAC Neo-adjuvant chemotherapy	
PMP Pseudomyxoma peritonei	
SBT Serous borderline tumor	
SEE-FIM Sectioning and extensively examining the fimbriated end	
STIC Serous tubal intraepithelial carcinoma	
TCC Transitional cell carcinoma	
WHO World Health Organization	

concept that ovarian carcinoma, over time, progresses from well to poorly differentiated also appears to be incorrect for the vast majority of cases.

Accumulating clinicopathologic and molecular genetic data have led to the proposal of a new model of ovarian carcinogenesis that reconciles the differing relationships of borderline and malignant tumors among the different cell types. This model divides surface epithelial tumors into two categories, type I and type II, based on their clinicopathologic features and characteristic molecular genetic changes (221).

Type I tumors are low-grade, relatively indolent neoplasms that arise from well-characterized precursor lesions (atypical proliferative [borderline] tumors and endometriosis) and usually present as large stage I neoplasms. This group includes low-grade serous carcinoma (LGSC, invasive micropapillary serous carcinoma [MPSC]), low-grade endometrioid, mucinous, and probably clear cell carcinomas. Clear cell carcinoma, although it exhibits most of the features of type I tumors such as association with a well-established precursor (endometriosis) and frequent large size and presentation in stage I, is typically high grade unlike the other type I tumors. Nonetheless, preliminary molecular genetic data show a greater similarity of clear cell carcinoma to type I as compared with type II tumors.

Type I tumors often harbor mutations in genes encoding protein kinases including *KRAS*, *BRAF*, *PIK3CA*, and *ERBB2*, as well as other signaling molecules including *PTEN* and *CTNNB1* (β-catenin). Borderline (atypical proliferative) serous and mucinous tumors appear to develop from cystadenomas, whereas borderline endometrioid and clear cell tumors arise from endometriosis. Type I carcinomas are heterogeneous and often display areas identical to their benign and atypical proliferative precursors/counterparts. Similar mutations have been identified in the different components of each tumor cell type, providing supportive evidence of the neoplastic sequence of benign to borderline to carcinoma for these cell types.

In contrast, type II tumors, of which the vast majority are HGSC and its variants, are aggressive, high-grade neoplasms from the outset; in the past they have been said to arise *de novo*. Accumulating data support the new paradigm that HGSCs arise from intraepithelial carcinomas, the majority of which have been detected in the tubal mucosa, usually the fimbriae (STIC). It is currently not clear what proportion of HGSC arises from the tube. The vast majority of type II carcinomas have *TP53* mutations, and evidence suggests that essentially all typical HGSCs have *TP53* mutations (224). *TP53* mutations have been found in tubal intraepithelial carcinomas and in a recently described putative precursor lesion of tubal intraepithelial carcinoma designated "p53 signature." This latter lesion appears morphologically normal but overexpresses p53 and can harbor a *TP53* mutation. These findings highlight the role of *TP53* mutation in the early development of HGSC (221) although the importance of the p53 signature and whether it is a bona fide precursor are unclear (225). The dualistic model is supported by findings from many investigators (226).

Development of a type II tumor in a background of a type I tumor (type I to type II progression and/or co-occurrence) is quite uncommon, but does occasionally occur. Histologically this may be seen as HGSC arising within a LGSC or endometriosis, or a mucinous carcinoma with a mural nodule of anaplastic carcinoma. There is a mouse model that appears to replicate this type of progression (227).

The anatomical progression of ovarian carcinoma is becoming better understood. It had generally been assumed that carcinoma originates in the ovary, is confined to the ovary for a period of time, and then disseminates to the pelvis, followed by the abdominal cavity before spreading to distant sites. This view underlies the basis of the FIGO staging system (**Table 23.6**) in which tumors confined to the ovary are stage I, those involving the pelvic organs stage II, with involvement of abdominal organs stage III, and distant sites stage IV. This view also has been used to justify the attempts to develop a screening test. There are, however, significant problems with this assumption. It has been known for many years that HGSC is found disseminated through the peritoneum very early in its course, a finding that led to the now disproven idea of multifocal origin. Further, clinicopathologic comparison of stage I with stage III carcinomas shows that stage I tumors are predominantly type I and nonserous whereas stage III tumors are predominantly type II and most often HGSC. Accordingly, descriptions of progression of ovarian cancer from stage I to advanced stage are in most cases invalid because they describe different tumor types. Furthermore, progression from stage I to advanced stage, a fundamental tenet of the argument for development of a screening test for ovarian cancer, is accordingly flawed. The failure of all screening trials to reduce ovarian cancer mortality is therefore not surprising (67,68).

It is important to appreciate that type II ovarian carcinomas account for the vast majority of ovarian cancer deaths (85% in a recent large series) (219). Most type II tumors are HGSC and at the time of diagnosis, nearly all are widely disseminated throughout the peritoneum with the largest volume of tumor outside the ovaries. Serous carcinoma and its variants (peritoneal serous carcinoma, carcinosarcoma, undifferentiated carcinoma, and mixed carcinomas with a high-grade serous component) account for nearly 90% of cases of peritoneal carcinomatosis from ovarian carcinoma (**Table 23.10**) and accordingly the vast majority of ovarian cancer deaths. These data that analyze stage distribution by histologic type suggest that early- and advanced-stage tumors are fundamentally different diseases and provide further support for the dualistic model (228).

Putative Histopathologic Precursor Lesions

The study of precursors of ovarian carcinoma is very difficult because the ovaries are not readily accessible for screening, and ovarian carcinomas typically present in advanced stage, obliterating or rendering unrecognizable any possible precursor lesions. Furthermore, identification of a putative precursor lesion is based on microscopic examination of a complete oophorectomy specimen, and therefore the natural history of the lesion cannot be observed. Studies on ovaries removed prophylactically from high-risk women, benign tissue adjacent to ovarian carcinomas, normal-appearing ovaries contralateral to stage I carcinomas, and normal ovaries in women with tumors that meet the standard criteria for primary peritoneal serous carcinoma have generated conflicting data.

Surface Epithelial Dysplasia. Historically, investigators have studied ovarian surface epithelium in the vicinity of carcinomas in an attempt to define the putative entity of "ovarian dysplasia" and have reported atypical cellular and nuclear features that appear more frequently in ovarian surface epithelium near or contralateral to carcinomas in comparison to control ovaries. These findings, however, have not been corroborated.

Surface Epithelial Inclusions. The superficial ovarian cortex often contains simple glands and cysts lined by a single layer of flat, cuboidal epithelium or ciliated tubal-type epithelium (**Fig. 23.22**). These are termed surface epithelial or cortical (formerly "germinal") inclusions, and their presence directly correlates with age. Historically, they have been considered to arise after postovulatory repair of the damaged ovarian surface; however, the evidence for this is weak. It has recently been suggested that the origin of inclusions could be the fimbrial epithelium, which is in close apposition with the ovarian surface epithelium (229). In this model, ovulatory disruption of the ovarian surface allows fimbrial epithelium access to the superficial cortical stroma. At present, this is the most compelling hypothesis as it explains the tubal morphology of inclusions and their age distribution, but the evidence is largely circumstantial; furthermore, the role of ovulatory surface disruption does not explain the presence of such inclusions in women who do not ovulate such as those with PCOS. Nonetheless, there is no more than circumstantial evidence for the time-honored surface epithelial origin of these inclusions. Furthermore, the ovarian surface epithelium is not Müllerian in origin; it is mesothelial, and metaplasia of the peritoneal mesothelium to tubal-type epithelium, though widely believed to occur, is another widely held assumption that has not been convincingly demonstrated.

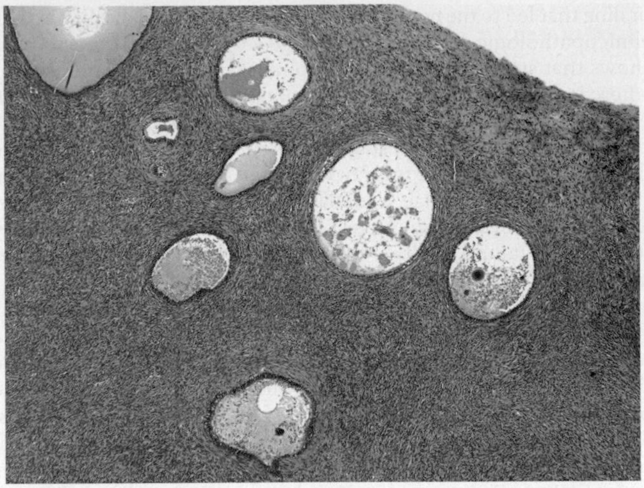

Figure 23.22. Cortical inclusions are lined by ciliated columnar tubal-type epithelium within the ovarian cortical stroma. The ovarian surface is seen at the top right.

Some studies on prophylactic oophorectomy specimens in high-risk women and normal-appearing ovaries contralateral to stage I carcinomas have shown a higher number of these cortical inclusions in comparison to controls, but others have not confirmed these findings. These studies have also evaluated a variety of other features including cortical invaginations (clefts) and surface papillomatosis and some have found the latter two to be more common in cancer-prone ovaries than in controls, but these findings have not been confirmed by other investigators either (230).

Endometriosis. Endometriosis is a well-documented and easily recognized precursor lesion because carcinomas arising in endometriosis are type I tumors, grow slowly, and therefore allow a greater window of opportunity for discovery prior to obliteration of the precursor lesion by the carcinoma. Endometriosis is common and found in about 10% of reproductive-age women, but the risk of malignant transformation in an individual patient is very low. Nonetheless, endometriosis is associated with up to about 20% of ovarian cancers and is acknowledged to be the precursor of most or nearly all endometrioid and clear cell carcinomas and an occasional mucinous carcinoma. Serous carcinomas may be found coincidentally in women with endometriosis but do not appear to be histogenetically related. A pooled analysis of 13 case–control studies with 7,911 ovarian cancer patients and 13,226 controls showed that self-reported endometriosis is associated with an increased risk of endometrioid, clear cell and low-grade serous carcinomas, whereas there was no association with HGSC and mucinous carcinoma (29).

The plausibility of endometriosis as an ovarian cancer precursor is supported by our understanding of endometrial cancer precursors. Atypical endometrial hyperplasia in the uterus is a well-defined precursor of endometrial adenocarcinoma, and changes similar to this lesion are occasionally observed in endometriosis. In addition, atypical changes are also seen in endometriosis in the vicinity of endometrioid adenocarcinomas of the ovary and even more frequently in association with clear cell carcinoma. On occasion, the full morphologic spectrum from endometriosis with hyperplasia to atypical hyperplasia and well-differentiated endometrioid adenocarcinoma can be observed.

Molecular studies of endometriosis have demonstrated molecular alterations including LOH in the *PTEN* gene and MSI, as well as chromosomal aberrations including trisomies and monosomies, all indicative of a neoplastic process. A recent study analyzing the mutation patterns of *ARID1A* and *PIK3CA* in endometriotic lesions and associated carcinomas found evidence that multifocal benign endometriotic lesions are clonally related (231). The revised WHO classification (**Table 23.8**) now includes endometriotic cysts in the category of benign endometrioid tumors.

It has been estimated that carcinoma develops in 0.3% to 3% of cases of endometriosis, but this is likely an overestimate because a large number of cases of endometriosis never come to biopsy. The true figure is probably closer to 0.3%. Ovarian endometriosis is significantly more likely to undergo malignant transformation as compared with extraovarian endometriosis (232).

Further evidence that endometriosis is a precursor of ovarian carcinoma is provided by large studies from Sweden and Japan. In a Swedish study of over 20,000 women hospitalized with endometriosis, after a mean follow-up of 11.4 years, the RR of ovarian cancer in comparison to the control population was 1.9. Patients with a long-standing history of endometriosis (10 years or longer) had a RR of 4.2 (233). In a study in Japan of 6,398 women with endometriosis, the standardized incidence ratio was 9.0 after 17 years of follow-up, with a risk of 13.2 in women diagnosed after age 50 (234). In the latter study, the mean age at diagnosis of ovarian carcinoma was 51, a reflection of the significantly younger age of women with endometriosis-associated cancers.

Benign and Borderline (Atypical Proliferative) Neoplasms. Although the natural history of benign ovarian tumors cannot be directly observed as they must be completely removed for accurate diagnosis, the observation of morphologically benign areas within carcinomas and recent molecular data strongly suggest that borderline tumors are precursors of low-grade serous, endometrioid, and mucinous carcinomas (type I tumors in the dualistic model). Invasive LGSCs (invasive MPSCs) usually display large areas of SBT. Similarly, mucinous borderline tumors (MBTs) are heterogeneous and usually display large areas of mucinous cystadenoma as well as morphologically intermediate forms, which include mucinous cystadenoma with focal atypia and MBT with intraepithelial carcinoma (235). The progression of SBT to LGSC and MBT to mucinous carcinoma is supported by similar molecular changes in the separate components of these neoplasms.

Tubal Intraepithelial Carcinoma. There is an ongoing paradigm shift in our understanding of precursors of HGSC. It has recently been proposed that the origin of most serous carcinomas is the tubal fimbriae (221,223). The typical fallopian tube carcinoma is a HGSC and, until recently, a grossly obvious papillary luminal tumorous mass has generally been required to assign the primary site to the fallopian tube (236). However, a fimbrial carcinoma seems unlikely to cause luminal dilatation except possibly in a short distal segment and could be misinterpreted as ovarian in origin, particularly because the fimbriae normally reside on the ovarian surface. Until relatively recent recognition of the fallopian tube as a potential primary site of pelvic serous carcinogenesis, fallopian tube tissue had not routinely been microscopically examined in its entirety. In fact, only one or two sections of the mid-portion of the tube were often submitted. This led to the underappreciation of small grossly inapparent lesions. The SEE-FIM protocol for pathologic evaluation of the fallopian tubes is becoming increasingly used, particularly in high-risk patients, and led to the description of microscopic lesions. Tubal epithelial atypia, STIC, and small high-grade serous tubal carcinomas have been found in prophylactic specimens from women with *BRCA* mutations (236). In addition, it is frequently impossible to clearly separate the ovary and tube for evaluation in serous carcinoma. All of these observations suggest the possibility that many apparent ovarian cancers are in fact tubal in origin (221,223). Carcinoma involving the tubal mucosa has generally been regarded as secondary when there is also tumor in the ovary, peritoneum, and/or endometrium; however, this is an assumption. Many of the dominant tumorous adnexal masses appear to be paraovarian and/or extensively involve the fallopian tube in a manner consistent with peritoneal or tubal origin. The identification of *TP53* mutations in STICs as well as in HGSCs, in most cases with identical mutations in both, (95,237) provide further support for the tubal origin of many HGSCs.

Meticulous examination of RRSO specimens has disclosed occult invasive carcinomas in about 3% of cases: 53% ovarian, 39% tubal, and 8% peritoneal (229), and it has been suggested that some apparent primary peritoneal carcinomas after RRSO reflect undetected microscopic ovarian carcinomas. It has also been suggested that some apparent peritoneal carcinomas in women who have undergone oophorectomy but not salpingectomy may reflect metastases from primary tubal carcinomas. Foci of STIC and atypical hyperplasia have been reported in RRSO specimens and the tubal fimbria is by far the most common site (76,223,237–239). As noted earlier, the reported frequency of occult invasive carcinomas in prophylactic specimens from high-risk women is 3% but varies widely: 0% to 12% in a compilation of 16 series, which included 1,750 patients (229). In an additional 1%, STIC has been identified, making intraepithelial or invasive tubal carcinoma the majority of occult carcinomas. GOG199, a prospective study of 966 high-risk women, found STIC or invasive carcinoma in 2.6% (240). The wide range among studies could reflect differing thresholds for the diagnosis of tubal carcinoma, particularly intraepithelial carcinoma. In addition, there are several potential sources of bias in these types of studies (241). The interobserver reproducibility of the diagnosis of STIC has not been optimal, but recent data suggest that using p53 and Ki-67 immunostaining in conjunction with morphology markedly improves reproducibility (242). Data on the clinical outcome of isolated STIC are very limited. A recent review showed that 3 of 78 patients (4.5%) developed serous carcinomatosis after relatively limited follow-up (4 years or less) (243).

STICs have been identified in association with a high proportion of HGSCs. STICs contain *TP53* mutations and are cytologically malignant but are confined to the tubal epithelium. More recently, it has been found that there are small foci of morphologically normal tubal epithelium that are immunohistochemically positive for p53 and that have a Ki-67 proliferation index higher than normal tubal epithelium but lower than that found in STICs. A minimum of 12 tubal secretory epithelial cells that are p53 positive has been proposed as a definition for a "p53 signature" that is a candidate for a STIC precursor (244). Such p53 signatures have been associated with STICs as well as apparent ovarian serous carcinoma, but are also not uncommonly found in the general population. *TP53* mutations have been found in a majority of p53 signatures. These findings have led to the proposal that the p53 signature is the long sought precursor of a subset of ovarian HGSCs. These data await confirmation in larger series and by other investigators.

In and around the fimbriae, there is a junction between the tubal epithelium and the mesothelium which has been designated the tubal–peritoneal junction (**Figs. 23.23** and **23.24**). This is a highly tortuous zone and had escaped notice until a recent comprehensive characterization (245). Because junctions between different types of epithelium, such as the gastroesophageal junction and the cervical transformation zone, are often hot spots for carcinogenesis, this region is now of great interest. We recently reported STIC within 1 to 2 mm of this junction, and on occasion STIC can be found precisely at this junction (245).

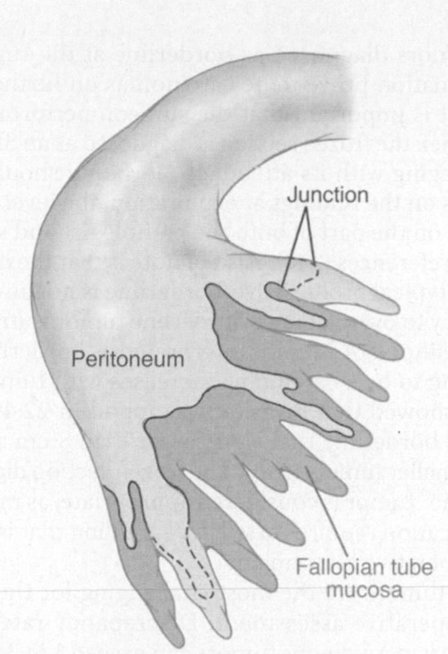

Figure 23.23. Schematic diagram of the fimbrial region showing the tubal–peritoneal junction as a tortuous blue line in and around the fimbriae.

Source: Reproduced from Seidman JD, Yemelyanova A, Zaino RJ, et al. The fallopian tube-peritoneal junction: a potential site of carcinogenesis. *Int J Gynecol Pathol*. 2011;30:304–311, with permission.

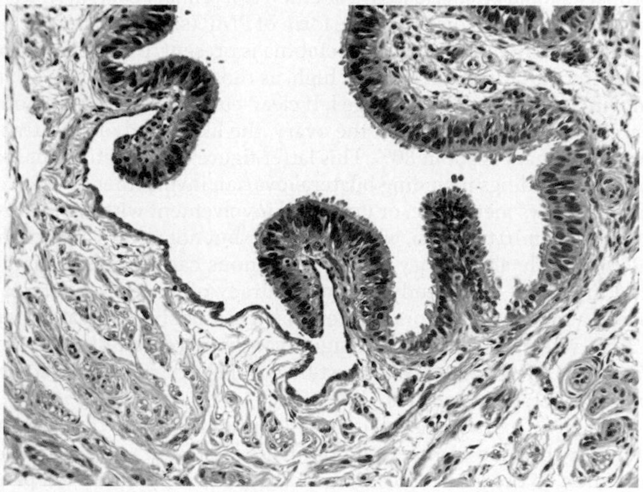

Figure 23.24. Histology of the tubal–peritoneal junction showing a flattened mesothelial lining at bottom left and the columnar tubal epithelium at right and top left.

Intraoperative Consultation (Frozen Section)

Getting the most out of a frozen section requires open lines of communication between the surgeon and the pathologist. The value of clinical information and operative findings to the pathologist should not be underestimated. A frozen section should be requested only when information is needed to determine what surgical procedure will be performed. Unnecessary frozen sections waste valuable resources and introduce opportunities for error (246).

The main purpose of intraoperative consultation for an ovarian mass is to determine whether a malignancy is present so that staging can proceed. However, a simple diagnosis of "malignant" is not enough because metastatic neoplasms to the ovary are not infrequent and may present prior to the diagnosis of the primary lesion. Because 5% to 10% of malignant ovarian masses are metastases from extraovarian primaries, the pathologist should attempt to make as specific a diagnosis as can reasonably be rendered given the limitations of frozen section. The benign versus malignant distinction in most cases is easily made, and the accuracy in most hospitals is over 95% (247). More difficult and hence less accurate is the distinction of a primary from a metastatic tumor, a distinction which will affect the surgical approach. It is somewhat less important to distinguish borderline tumor from carcinoma intraoperatively, as full abdominal exploration is done for both, although full staging is generally done for borderline tumors only when there is a high index of suspicion based on clinical or intraoperative findings (see below). Borderline (atypical proliferative) tumors present a unique intraoperative problem. Low-grade serous neoplasms are heterogeneous, and LGSCs nearly always have benign appearing areas resembling a cystadenoma or an SBT. The amount of tissue that can be examined intraoperatively is limited. Consequently, approximately 20% to 30%

of ovarian tumors diagnosed as borderline at the time of frozen section examination prove to be carcinomas on further sampling. Accordingly, it is important that the surgeon perform a thorough exploration when the frozen section is diagnosed as an SBT. Whether a complete staging with its attendant morbidity should be undertaken depends on the findings at exploration, the level of suspicion for carcinoma on the part of both the pathologist and surgeon, and the patient's preferences (246). Also of note is that the distinction of benign from atypical proliferative/borderline is not always reliable, with a tendency to overdiagnose borderline tumors intraoperatively (247). The likelihood of a tumor interpreted as borderline at frozen section proving to be a carcinoma increases with tumor size. One recent study showed that invasion was found in 22.4% of tumors interpreted as borderline that were larger than 8 cm as compared with 3.2% of smaller tumors (248). The frozen section diagnosis of "at least borderline" tumor is considered appropriate, as more accurate tumor classification requires extensive sampling that is not feasible during intraoperative assessment.

Mucinous tumors are the most challenging for the pathologist during intraoperative assessment. Discrepancy rates for frozen sections of ovarian mucinous tumors can exceed 1 in 3 (249). When a mucinous tumor is diagnosed intraoperatively, it is important for the surgeon to do a complete abdominal exploration. The likelihood of a mucinous tumor being an extraovarian primary increases with the degree of atypia, gross and microscopic complexity, and the presence of extraovarian disease. Simple unilocular mucinous cysts or cystadenomas are nearly always benign primary ovarian tumors. Once any degree of atypia is present, even if mild, an extraovarian primary should be considered in addition to a primary ovarian APMT/MBT. If peritoneal disease in the form of PMP (see PMP later in this chapter) or metastatic adenocarcinoma is present, the likelihood of an extraovarian primary is very high, as most true primary ovarian mucinous carcinomas are stage I. If clear-cut evidence of mucinous carcinoma is present within the ovary, the likelihood of an extraovarian primary is about 80%. This latter figure can be refined based on other findings including bilateral ovarian involvement, which is nearly always metastatic, or unilateral involvement with tumor size smaller than 10 to 13 cm, which is usually but not always metastatic (250). Nearly all primary ovarian mucinous carcinomas are large and unilateral. One study on the accuracy of frozen sections for ovarian mucinous tumors showed that a tumor size of greater than 13 cm was associated with a significantly increased discrepancy rate (251). Accordingly, size must be considered with other factors in intraoperative decisions.

When an extraovarian primary is considered likely, the surgeon should perform a complete abdominal exploration with particular attention to the gastrointestinal and hepatobiliary tracts and pancreas, as most metastatic mucinous carcinomas to the ovaries arise in these sites. The appendix should be removed even if it appears normal, as small appendiceal neoplasms can disseminate.

CAP, WHO, and ICCR Guidelines

The College of American Pathologists (CAP) has issued guidelines for the reporting of ovarian cancer, which were updated in 2016 (252). Support for the 2014 WHO classification of tumors is indicated. Complete reporting with the CAP cancer checklist requires assessment of ovarian surface involvement and tumor rupture. It is therefore important that the pathologist communicate with the surgeon or review the operative report to provide these data. For advanced-stage disease, the size of the largest peritoneal nodule needs to be assessed, and although this is often evident from the gross pathologic examination, input from the surgeon may be required as the tumor may be incompletely resected. In apparent stage III disease, clinical or pathologic information may be needed to determine whether distant metastases have been diagnosed (stage IV). Other required elements of the checklist include specimen type, procedure, specimen integrity, primary site, tumor size, histologic type, lymph node numbers and status, extent of involvement of other organs, status of peritoneal and pleural fluid specimens, and pTNM stage (seventh edition). Grade is required for mucinous and endometrioid carcinomas (HGSC, LGSC, and clear cell carcinoma contain the grade in their definitions); endometrioid carcinomas should be graded using the FIGO system. FIGO stage is recommended but not required. There is an optional chemotherapy response score for patients who have received NACT.

CAP recognizes that LGSC and HGSC are separate tumor types and includes a category of mixed carcinomas. A likely tubal origin of many HGSCs is recognized, as is the unified entity of HGSC of the ovary/fallopian tube/peritoneum. Support for a recent proposal for primary site designation is indicated (222). CAP also recognizes that "invasive implants" are invasive LGSCs.

The 2014 WHO Classification (253), updated from 2003, contains several notable changes from the 2003 edition. First, the fallopian tube is recognized as the likely source of a large majority of HGSCs. Second, HGSC and LGSC are recognized as distinctive tumor types rather than different grades of the same tumor. Invasive peritoneal implants associated with SBT/APST are equated with invasive LGSC. The micropapillary variant of SBT is equated with noninvasive LGSC. WHO does not recommend a category of mixed carcinomas. Finally, seromucinous tumors are placed in their own category, separate from the majority of mucinous tumors which are intestinal type.

The ICCR (International Collaboration on Cancer Reporting) recommendations for data reporting are generally in line with the CAP recommendations. ICCR is also aligned with WHO and CAP in recognition of a likely tubal origin and equating invasive implants with invasive LGSC. They also accept the "atypical proliferative" and "noninvasive LGSC" terminology. None of the three organizations recommends the "low malignant potential" terminology.

Like CAP, ICCR also supports a recent proposal for primary site designation (222), the use of which results in the fallopian tube being considered the primary site in the vast majority of HGSCs.

All three organizations cite the SEE-FIM protocol for complete sampling of the fallopian tubes (237). CAP recommends submitting the fimbriae in total only for patients with HGSC with no gross tubal involvement. All three also accept the FIGO grading system for endometrioid carcinoma and accept all clear cell carcinomas (as well as undifferentiated carcinoma and carcinosarcoma) as high grade.

Cytopathology

There are two types of cytopathologic specimens typically used in evaluation of ovarian epithelial neoplasms: fine-needle aspirates (FNA) of ovarian cysts and peritoneal fluids (obtained by peritoneal washing or by aspiration of ascitic fluid). FNA specimens or effusions from sites of distant metastasis may also be examined. Rarely, the presence of psammoma bodies in a Pap smear will be the first sign of primary or recurrent ovarian or peritoneal serous carcinoma, more commonly when associated with atypical glandular cells of undetermined significance (AGUS) or in older women with symptoms and signs suggesting malignancy. In a review of over 200,000 Pap smears, psammoma bodies were found in 6 patients, 2 of whom proved to have ovarian carcinoma. In a review of 138 cases of AGUS, 5 (3.6%) proved to have ovarian cancers (254).

FNA may be useful in patients who appear to have inoperable ovarian cancer or who cannot undergo surgery for other reasons. Unsatisfactory specimens from ovarian cyst aspirates are common and limit the usefulness of the procedure. FNA specimens from most ovarian carcinomas are cellular and contain cytologically malignant cells, but accurate subclassification is often difficult and may be impossible based solely on cytologic material. FNA of an operable ovarian mass is generally discouraged as the procedure risks conversion of a stage IA carcinoma into stage IC.

Cytologic samples of peritoneal fluid and diaphragmatic scrapings are routinely obtained during staging procedures for ovarian cancer. Cytologic findings are important in substaging FIGO stage I ovarian cancer; malignant cells in peritoneal washings or ascites warrants assignment of tumors to stage IC. Malignant cells are more often present in ascites than in washings, and their presence correlates positively with volume of ascites, serous histology, stage, and positive lymph nodes (255). The cytologic features of tumor cells generally resemble those in FNA specimens but may be more degenerate.

Peritoneal lavage is often performed at the time of RRSO in high-risk women. Occult carcinomas can be identified in these cytology specimens. Colgan and associates found malignant cells in 3 of 35 such specimens in the absence of other evidence of malignancy. Endosalpingiosis, manifested by morphologically benign tubal-type epithelium, was found in 22% (239). Malignant cells reported in washings at RRSO rarely leads to the discovery of early-stage tubal carcinomas (256).

Atypical epithelial cells resembling the ovarian tumor can occasionally be found in peritoneal cytology specimens associated with borderline tumors. This finding has not been associated with adverse outcome and can be ignored except in the small proportion of patients who have bona fide carcinomas (patients with invasive LGSCs or SBTs with invasive implants), who can be substaged based on the presence or absence of epithelial cells resembling the primary ovarian tumor in the cytology specimens. This situation is rarely encountered as most LGSCs or SBTs with invasive implants are stage III.

Endometriosis and endosalpingiosis involving peritoneal surfaces may shed epithelial fragments into peritoneal washings or ascites. In addition, benign fallopian tube epithelium (particularly if salpingitis is present) and benign eutopic endometrial tissue may also be shed into the fluid via expulsion through the fallopian tubes. If the cells in the fluid are not obviously malignant, comparison of the cytologic features of the epithelium in the fluid with those of the tissue sections is essential. Cytologic abnormalities mimicking malignancy may be caused by chemotherapy as well as radiation; accordingly it is important to provide this history to the pathologist.

Borderline Tumors

The borderline category of ovarian epithelial tumors was introduced in the early 1970s in order to describe a group of tumors that did not display invasion, but that occasionally appeared to behave in a malignant fashion. Their behavior appeared to be intermediate between benign cystadenomas and frank serous carcinomas. The classification was intended as provisional, but with its continued use over the past three decades, the borderline category has become entrenched. Recent studies have documented a wide histologic spectrum encompassed by the borderline category, which correlates with behavior. Some experts believe that the borderline group has been sufficiently resolved into benign and malignant types such that the category is no longer needed. However, most prefer to retain the borderline category with some modifications in terminology.

Serous Borderline Tumors

Table 23.12 outlines the terminology, invasion, and behavior of proliferating serous tumors. Tumors at the lower end of the morphologic spectrum of proliferating serous tumors behave in a benign fashion and display a papillary architecture in which papillae have a hierarchical branching pattern. These tumors are termed SBTs or APSTs. Tumors at the upper end of the morphologic spectrum behave like low-grade carcinomas and display a more complex nonhierarchical branching pattern characterized by delicate micropapillae and are classified as SBT with micropapillary features, noninvasive micropapillary (low-grade) serous carcinomas (noninvasive MPSC/noninvasive LGSC). SBTs comprise about 50% of borderline ovarian tumors of all histologic types (**Table 23.9**). The atypical proliferative terminology has been accepted as synonymous with "borderline" whereas "low malignant potential" is currently not favored (257).

The most confusing aspect of SBTs is their association with peritoneal implants in the absence of invasive disease. There are two types of "peritoneal implants": noninvasive and invasive. It is now clear, however, that patients with noninvasive implants have a survival that approaches 100%, whereas those with invasive implants have a prognosis similar to that of patients with invasive LGSC, with 5- and 10-year survival rates of approximately 70% and 40%, respectively (257). Invasive implants are therefore believed to represent metastatic LGSCs. The finding of invasive implants with SBT is very unusual and warrants further sampling of the ovarian tumor to identify occult areas of noninvasive LGSC or invasion. However, invasive implants may be seen in association with ovarian SBT more commonly with and occasionally without micropapillary features and may reflect tumor progression in the peritoneum even in the absence of LGSC in the ovary. The nature of noninvasive implants is unclear. Although there are conflicting data as to whether they arise from the ovarian tumor or are independent peritoneal proliferations, a recent molecular analysis of 62 SBT primary tumor-implant pairs, which included both noninvasive and invasive implants, demonstrated identical *KRAS* or *BRAF* mutations in 59 cases (95%), supporting the origin of the implants from the primary ovarian tumor (258). The prognosis with noninvasive implants is excellent and no therapy is needed, although patients may develop complications because of adhesions. Nonetheless, clinical follow-up may be of value as long-term data now indicate that a small but significant proportion with noninvasive implants will progress to invasive LGSC. Uzan and associates followed 168 women with advanced-stage SBT. Seven (4%) recurred with invasive disease, and among 20 with noninvasive recurrences, 4 (20%) recurred with invasive disease after a mean of 7 years after the noninvasive recurrence (259).

Microinvasion and associated lymph node lesions are found in a minority of cases. Although their origin and significance are not

TABLE 23.12. Terminology, Invasion, and Behavior of Proliferating Serous Tumors

Synonyms	Invasion	Behavior
Serous borderline tumor (SBT)/atypical proliferative serous tumor (APST) without implants	Absent	Benign
SBT/APST with noninvasive implants	Absent	Usually benign, but 4% risk of developing invasive low-grade serous carcinoma, and 5-/10-year survival rates of 95%/90%
Micropapillary SBT/noninvasive micropapillary serous carcinoma/noninvasive low-grade serous carcinoma	Absent, but often associated with invasive peritoneal implants (invasive low-grade serous carcinoma)	Same as invasive low-grade serous carcinoma when invasive implants are present
Low-grade serous carcinoma/well-differentiated serous carcinoma/invasive low-grade serous carcinoma/invasive micropapillary serous carcinoma	Present	5-/10-year survival rates approximately 70%–85%/40%–60%
Invasive implants/invasive low-grade serous carcinoma	Present	5-/10-year survival rates approximately 70%–85%/40%–60%

entirely clear, the survival with microinvasion and/or lymph node lesions in the absence of MPSC or invasive implants is virtually 100%.

To summarize, SBTs can now be subclassified into those for which survival is close to 100% and those with a malignant, though indolent, behavior. SBTs with or without microinvasion, with or without lymph node lesions, and with or without noninvasive implants can, for practical purposes, be considered benign, although, as noted, there is a small long-term risk of developing invasive serous carcinoma when noninvasive implants are present. Serous tumors with invasive implants, in contrast, have recurrence and mortality rates similar to those of LGSC.

Nonserous Borderline Tumors

The vast majority of nonserous borderline tumors are of the mucinous type. Endometrioid, clear cell, and transitional cell types are rare and have never been convincingly demonstrated to be anything but completely benign.

MBTs are not associated with peritoneal implants, and, like SBTs, have virtually 100% survival. Microinvasion (less than 5 mm) is occasionally seen and is not an adverse prognostic factor (235). Intraepithelial carcinoma may also occur in APMTs and although this is usually benign, there are occasional reports of malignant behavior (260). As mucinous tumors are usually very large, malignant behavior may be a manifestation of occult undetected invasion. Aggressive behavior of MBTs in the older literature is virtually always confined to patients with PMP, and it is now clear that nearly all cases of PMP are of gastrointestinal origin (see below).

Primary versus Metastatic Ovarian Carcinomas

Metastatic carcinomas involving the ovaries often have unusual and deceptive features. The ovarian metastases may be the first manifestation of malignancy and may be much larger than the associated primary tumor. They are often cystic and accordingly grossly mimic primary ovarian carcinomas. They occasionally present prior to the identification of the primary tumor. The most common and problematic type of carcinoma metastatic to the ovary is mucinous carcinoma. Metastatic carcinomas are typically bilateral and small (typically less than 10–12 cm) and display ovarian surface and superficial cortical involvement, a nodular pattern of ovarian involvement, and a haphazard infiltrative pattern of stromal invasion. However, some metastatic carcinomas, especially mucinous carcinomas derived from the colorectum, pancreaticobiliary tract, appendix, and endocervix, can exhibit gross and microscopic features simulating a primary ovarian mucinous or endometrioid tumor. In particular, metastases can be large, unilateral, and multicystic and can display deceptive patterns of ovarian involvement. If these patterns are not recognized, these metastatic carcinomas can be misinterpreted as primary ovarian MBTs with intraepithelial carcinoma or well-differentiated mucinous or endometrioid carcinoma. Not infrequently, some of these metastases display highly differentiated areas adjacent to invasive areas, simulating benign and MBT precursor lesions. Intraepithelial and invasive carcinoma in the fallopian tube may also be mimicked by metastatic carcinoma (261,262).

When mucinous carcinomas in the ovaries are rigorously classified based on refined criteria and awareness of deceptive patterns, metastatic mucinous carcinomas are much more commonly encountered than primary ovarian mucinous carcinomas. In general, the presence of a mucinous carcinoma in the ovary, particularly if extraovarian disease is present, should always prompt the pathologist and surgeon to consider the possibility of metastatic mucinous carcinoma. Immunohistochemical analysis can be useful for identifying some metastatic mucinous carcinomas that simulate primary ovarian mucinous tumors; however, the value of currently available markers is limited because of overlapping immunoprofiles of primary tumors and certain metastases (see Metastatic mucinous carcinoma, later in this chapter). Clinical evaluation is usually required to exclude metastatic mucinous carcinoma in the ovary derived from a clinically occult extraovarian source. Many investigators find it a safe and useful practice to consider mucinous carcinoma in the ovary metastatic until proven otherwise (229).

Ovarian Cancer Genetics and Genomics

High-grade serous carcinoma is characterized by nearly ubiquitous presence of *TP53* mutations (263). Missense or nonsense mutations of *TP53* are considered the earliest molecular event in high-grade serous carcinogenesis.

It has been long recognized that approximately 12% to 15% of HGSCs occur in patients with germ line mutations in *BRCA1* and *BRCA2* genes. Recent studies showed that up to 50% of HGSCs are related to inactivation of *BRCA1/2* genes by either germ line or somatic mutation, or through epigenetic mechanisms. The term BRCAness is applied to these tumors that share deficient homologous recombination (HR) DNA repair pathway leading to marked genomic instability. The cases with high levels of genomic aberrations have been shown to have improved survival (264). The impaired HR is thought to be responsible for superior sensitivity to platinum-based chemotherapy. Additionally, some of the cases of acquired platinum resistance have demonstrated secondary reversal of mutations in *BRCA1/2*. A majority of alterations of *BRCA1/2* genes are truncating mutations; however, a small proportion of missense mutations have been described in cases with somatic mutations (265). The data regarding favorable outcome in BRCA-deficient patients are somewhat conflicting as some studies have shown that *BRCA2*, but not *BRCA1* deficiency is associated with improved survival and chemotherapy response (266). Some studies also suggest that the survival benefits seen early are no longer seen 10 to 15 years after diagnosis (54).

Point mutations in oncogenes and tumor suppressor genes other than *TP53*, *BRCA1*, and *BRCA2* are relatively uncommon in HGSCs (263). However, structural variations (gains and losses) are frequent, resulting in a chromosomally unstable or C-class malignancy (dominated by copy number changes) (267). A large study of the gene expression patterns in a cohort of ovarian carcinomas by Tothill et al. that included HGSCs, endometrioid carcinoma, as well as a group of borderline tumors described six groups (C1–C6) with distinct expression profiles (268). All borderline tumors clustered into the C3 subtype. Group C6 was composed almost exclusively of endometrioid carcinomas of low and intermediate grades. HGSCs along with some high- and intermediate-grade endometrioid carcinomas were distributed over four groups (C1, C2, C4, and C5). The Cancer Genome Atlas initiative validated these findings and termed the expression profile-based subtypes of HGSC as Immunoreactive, Differentiated, Proliferative, and Mesenchymal (263).

The mesenchymal subtype (C1) is characterized by extensive stromal desmoplasia and immune cell infiltrate in the stroma. Markers of activated myofibroblasts, vascular endothelial cells, pericytes, extracellular matrix production, cell adhesion, and angiogenesis are overexpressed. High expression of HOX, FAP, and ANGPTL1/2 is observed. This subtype has the worst survival relative to other three.

The immunoreactive subtype (C2) has prominent intratumoral immune cell infiltrates. It is defined by markers of adaptive immune response, particularly those involved in T-cell activation and trafficking. The gene expression signature shows overexpression of T-cell chemokine ligands CXCL11 and CXCL10 and receptor CXCR3. This subtype along with C4 demonstrates improved survival.

The differentiated subtype (C4) also shows intratumoral immune cell infiltrates. Its gene expression pattern is dominated by high expression of MUC1 and MUC16 and expression of SLPI.

The proliferative subtype (C5) demonstrates overexpression of developmental transcription factors including Homeobox genes, high-motility group members, WNT/β-catenin and cadherin signaling pathways, and extracellular marker-related genes. The defining gene expression signature consists of high expression of HMGA2, SOX11, MCM2, and PCN and low expression of MUC1 and MUC16.

Borderline tumors are characterized by a distinct gene expression profile (C3 subtype), low expression of proliferation markers (MKI67,

TOP2A, CCNB1, CDC2, and KIF11), and relative overexpression of MAPK pathway genes (DUSP4, DUSP6, SERPIN5A, MAP3K5, and SPRY2) likely related to mutations in *KRAS* and *BRAF*.

The gene expression pattern of low-grade endometrioid tumors clusters into a distinct C6 subtype and is characterized by low expression of proliferation markers (MKI67, TOP2A, CCNB1, CDC2, and KIF11) and overexpression of transcriptional targets of the β-catenin complex correlating with the presence of β-catenin mutations and reflecting deregulation of the WNT signaling pathway (268).

Ovarian clear cell carcinomas have recurrent *PIK3CA* and *ARID1A* mutations and relatively infrequent *TP53* mutations (32,269,270). Frequent loss of *ARID1A* has also been shown in endometriosis in cases associated with clear cell carcinoma supporting the classification of endometriosis as the precursor lesion.

Endometrioid carcinomas have prevalent *CTNNB1*, *ARID1A*, and *PIK3CA* mutations (32,270). Endometriosis-associated endometrioid carcinomas have frequent loss of *ARID1A*. This alteration has also been shown in the precursor lesion, that is, endometriosis (32).

The data on molecular genetic profiles of mucinous carcinomas are relatively limited. Some studies have demonstrated *KRAS* mutations in more than half of MBT and mucinous carcinomas (271,272). Anglesio et al. demonstrated HER2/neu (*ERBB2*) amplification in 18% of mucinous carcinomas and smaller proportion (6%) of MBT with anecdotal responses to trastuzumab (272,273).

LGSC has been classically associated with *RAS/RAF* and *ERBB2* mutations that are shared with their precursor, SBT (274). *KRAS* and *BRAF* mutations appear mutually exclusive. One study demonstrates that recurrent LGSCs harbor *KRAS*, but not *BRAF*, mutations (275). Additionally, *NRAS* mutations were identified in invasive LGSC but not in SBT (276). Mutations in *USP9X* and *EIF1AX* associated with the mTOR pathway are found in LGSCs and may represent drivers of progression from SBT to carcinoma. Compared with SBTs, LGSCs appear enriched in copy number alterations, particularly loss of 9p and homozygous deletion of the *CDKN2A/2B* locus and hemizygous deletion of 1p36 (277). These copy number changes have been suggested as another potential mechanism of progression.

Serous Tumors

Serous Cystadenoma and Adenofibroma

Benign serous tumors including cystadenomas and adenofibromas are common and account for two-thirds of benign ovarian epithelial tumors and the majority of ovarian serous tumors. Benign serous tumors are equally distributed among unilocular cysts, multilocular cysts, and cystadenofibromas. The vast majority of lesions classified as serous cystadenoma display a serous epithelial lining lacking proliferation, suggesting that this tumor is not neoplastic. In support of this concept is the finding of polyclonality in the epithelium of most serous cystadenomas (278). Furthermore, another study confirmed these findings and found genetic abnormalities in the stroma of serous cystadenofibromas (279). Accordingly, not only are most serous cystadenomas probably not true epithelial neoplasms, the epithelium reflecting cystically dilated inclusions, but also the stroma may be the only neoplastic component. Surprisingly, these may in fact, turn out to be benign stromal tumors, a finding which will eventually lead to reassessment of the place of serous cystadenomas, if any, in the serous neoplastic sequence.

Cystadenomas are lined by pseudostratified, tubal-type epithelium, with the characteristic elongated (secretory cell) and rounded (ciliated cell) nuclei. A single layer of flattened to cuboidal cells with uniform basal nuclei is also common. Mitoses and atypia are generally absent. Psammoma bodies are present in the stroma in 15% of cystadenomas. There is a broad spectrum of epithelial proliferation in benign serous tumors, which is manifested by variation in the prominence and complexity of the papillae, from a simple, single layer and blunt papillae to focal epithelial stratification and detachment of cell clusters approaching the degree of proliferation seen in SBT. Identification of these features in 10% of the tumor separates serous cystadenoma from SBT. If these features are focal (<10%), a diagnosis of serous cystadenoma with focal atypia, or serous cystadenoma with focal epithelial proliferation, is used (257).

SBT/Atypical Proliferative Serous Tumor

The conceptual and practical issues regarding the borderline category are discussed earlier in this chapter. The terminology and behavior of proliferating serous tumors are listed in **Table 23.12**.

Clinical and Operative Findings. The clinical features of patients with SBTs are similar to those for serous cystadenomas; the mean age at diagnosis is 42 years. The risk factors are similar to those for ovarian cancer with notable exceptions of a higher frequency of infertility and a lower frequency of *BRCA* mutations.

SBTs are bilateral in 37% of cases in the older literature; the recent Stanford series showed a 55% bilaterality rate (280). This difference probably reflects more diligent examination of normal-sized ovaries with the identification of small serous proliferations contralateral to obviously tumorous ovaries. Exophytic papillae reflecting ovarian surface involvement are common and are more often found in patients who also have peritoneal implants. Tumors with an exophytic component are associated with implants in up to two-thirds of cases as compared with 10% to 20% of tumors that are completely intracystic.

Gross Findings. SBTs have fine, friable, and exuberant papillary projections in contrast to the smooth-walled cysts of serous cystadenoma. Papillae are nearly always present on the internal surfaces of the cyst and are present on the external surfaces in up to 70% of cases.

Peritoneal endosalpingiosis in patients with SBT is grossly inconspicuous. Noninvasive desmoplastic implants are firm and fibrotic and are covered by an inflammatory exudate in 20% of cases. Invasive implants (metastatic LGSC) resemble typical serous carcinoma but are often less bulky and more calcified.

Thorough sampling of the primary tumor for histologic examination is needed to rule out invasion. Previous recommendations of 1 section per cm of maximum tumor diameter (257) will not identify invasion in a significant minority of cases in which invasion is actually present. Recent data suggest that at least 2 sections per cm are needed to confidently exclude invasion (281) (see below Microinvasion).

Microscopic Findings. SBTs display extensive epithelial stratification, tufting (budding), and detachment of individual cells and cell clusters in addition to hierarchical branching with successively smaller papillae emanating from the larger, more centrally located papillae. Stratification and budding in at least 10% of the tumor warrants a diagnosis of SBT (**Fig. 23.25**). Focal areas of fusion of the epithelial buds may create a Roman bridge or cribriform pattern. Similarly, foci of nonhierarchical branching with fine elongated micropapillae emanating directly from large central papillae are seen not infrequently. When cribriform and/or micropapillary patterns constitute either a 5 mm or greater confluent area, or 10% or greater proportion, the tumor warrants classification as noninvasive LGSC (see below). Ciliated cells resembling fallopian tube epithelium are present in about one-third of tumors. The nuclei of SBTs resemble those in cystadenomas but tend to display slightly more atypia. Nuclei tend to be ovoid or rounded and nucleoli may be prominent. Mitoses are not common. Psammoma bodies are present in up to half of SBTs.

Microinvasion. Two distinct types of lesions have been designated "microinvasion" in SBTs. In most published reports, the two types have not been specifically distinguished or correlated with outcome. The usual type of microinvasion (eosinophilic type) accounts for the vast majority of reported cases. It is characterized by isolated cells and small cell clusters with abundant eosinophilic cytoplasm that appear to be budding from the epithelium into the superficial stromal cores of the papillae (**Fig. 23.26**). The lesion must be smaller than 5 mm and can be multiple. When carefully sought, 10% of reported

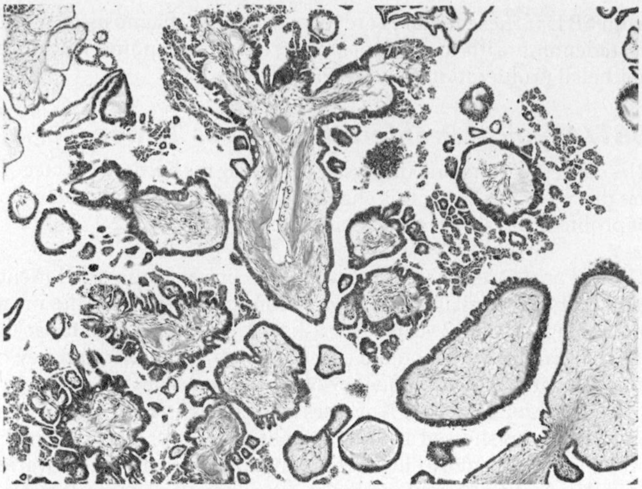

Figure 23.25. Atypical proliferative serous tumor (serous borderline tumor) displaying a complex papillary pattern with detachment of atypical cell clusters at the tips of the papillae.

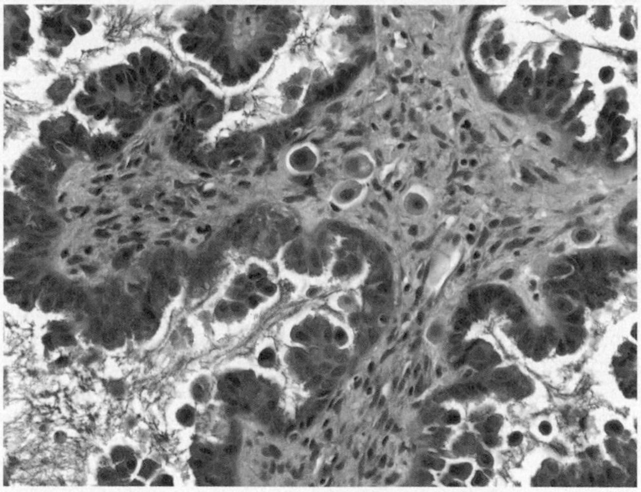

Figure 23.26. Microinvasion in an atypical proliferative serous tumor. The individual cells in the center with abundant eosinophilic cytoplasm reflect the more common type of microinvasion.

APSTs contain microinvasion; however, microinvasion was specifically noted in only 1.3% of reported APSTs up to 1999 (282). More recent series suggest that microinvasion is quite common and may be found in 25% or more of APSTs (283). A recent study evaluating these eosinophilic cells showed loss of expression of several markers, a lower proliferation index, and other findings suggesting that these are not neoplastic, but rather, are terminally differentiated cells, some of which are undergoing apoptosis (284).

The second type of microinvasion occurs less commonly and is characterized by a haphazard infiltrative pattern of small solid nests of cells and micropapillae, often surrounded by a clear space and associated with an identifiable stromal response. This second pattern of invasion closely resembles primary ovarian invasive LGSC (invasive LGSC) as well as "invasive implants" and is often referred to as "microinvasive carcinoma," because the evidence, albeit limited, indicates that it is a manifestation of true invasive carcinoma. To qualify as microinvasive carcinoma, the lesion must be smaller than 5 mm. Multiple foci are permitted.

Microinvasion has been associated with a higher frequency of bilaterality, exophytic growth, and peritoneal implants. Recent evidence suggests that the identification of microinvasion or microinvasive carcinoma is a clue that further sampling might disclose more extensive invasion. A minimum of 2 sections per cm of maximum tumor diameter are needed to maximize detection of occult invasion (281).

A review of 94 patients with microinvasion reported up to 1999, the vast majority of which were not associated with peritoneal implants, showed 100% survival (282). More recently, the Stanford group found that microinvasion was a significant predictor of survival on univariate but not multivariate analysis (285). Although more data are needed, from the standpoint of prognosis and management, microinvasion does not appear to have immediate clinical relevance. Whether or not staging is needed for a woman with microinvasive carcinoma is unclear. There are no data at present suggesting that follow-up or any treatment will influence recurrence or survival.

Associated Peritoneal Lesions: Endosalpingiosis and "Implants". SBTs are often associated with serous lesions involving the peritoneum. Endosalpingiosis, or benign glandular inclusions, are found in 40% of patients. At present, 40% of reported APSTs are associated with peritoneal implants in contrast to 25% in the pre-1980 literature (282). In the Stanford series, 59% had implants (280). However, in population-based and hospital-based material, the figure is in the 10% to 20% range, indicating a significant referral bias to large specialized centers in favor of tumors with implants. A recent population-based series in Denmark reported 14% of patients with implants (286), and a large multi-institutional study in Germany reported that 21.7% of SBTs had implants (287). Among those with implants in these two series, 83% were noninvasive and 17% were invasive.

Endosalpingiosis, or benign glandular inclusions, may involve the peritoneal surfaces in patients with or without benign or malignant serous ovarian tumors. These glands typically are lined by simple columnar epithelium, which displays tubal differentiation. The epithelium may display minor degrees of atypia and form simple papillary structures; psammoma bodies are often present and may persist after degeneration of the epithelium.

About 78% to 83% of all SBT patients with implants have peritoneal epithelial lesions that display a degree of proliferation beyond that usually seen in endosalpingiosis, but that lack features of invasion. These have been designated "noninvasive implants" and have two morphologic forms: epithelial and desmoplastic.

Noninvasive epithelial implants are papillary and resemble the ovarian SBT to some extent (**Fig. 23.27**). The cores of the papillae have fibrovascular support, and the epithelial cells resemble those in endosalpingiosis. Thus, mild atypia is often present, but mitoses are usually absent. Calcification in the form of psammoma bodies is common and may be extensive.

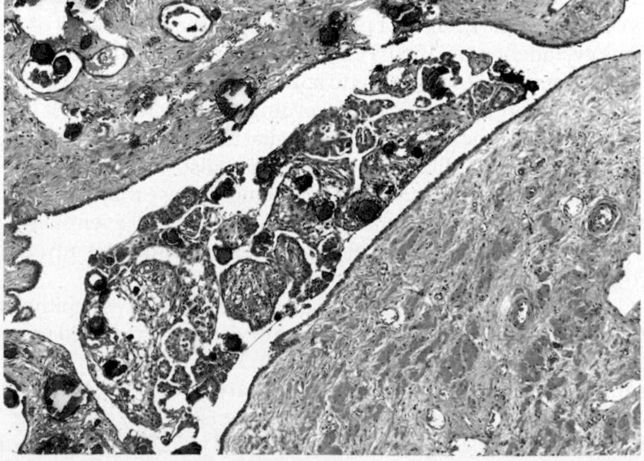

Figure 23.27. Noninvasive epithelial peritoneal implant associated with atypical proliferative serous tumor/serous borderline tumor. The implant displays a papillary architecture with psammomatous calcification. Note there is no invasion of adjacent peritoneum at top left and bottom right.

The desmoplastic noninvasive implant is a plaque-like thickening overlying peritoneal surfaces and may extend into the septae that separate omental lobules creating a low-power appearance that suggests invasion (**Fig. 23.28**). These implants display an exuberant fibroblastic proliferation in which gland-like or papillary structures lined by epithelial cells are present. Psammoma bodies are usually present. The epithelium typically shows minimal cytologic atypia (**Fig. 23.28**). The fibroblastic proliferation often has a granulation tissue-like appearance characterized by edematous fascicles of plump fibroblasts, often with interspersed small vascular channels. Mitotic figures are usually absent, and psammoma bodies are present in over 90% of cases. This type of implant can be very difficult to interpret for pathologists who may be unfamiliar with these rare lesions. As the invasiveness of the implant is the determinant of benign versus malignant behavior in these tumors (see below), expert pathology consultation should be obtained if there is doubt about the diagnosis.

Among patients with SBT or noninvasive LGSC, 17% to 22% of those with implants have invasive implants. About three-fourths of patients with invasive implants have noninvasive LGSC; the finding of invasive implants with SBT is very unusual and warrants further sampling of the ovarian tumor to identify occult areas of noninvasive LGSC or invasion.

The characteristic architectural feature of an invasive implant is a haphazard infiltrative growth pattern (**Fig. 23.29**). A confluent or cribriform glandular pattern may be present. An exophytic pattern is not uncommon and usually displays a micropapillary pattern. Typically, micropapillae are haphazardly arranged and small solid nests of cells embedded in fibrous stroma and surrounded by a clear space or cleft are present (**Fig. 23.29**) (288). Invasive implants often display only mild cytologic atypia, but occasionally atypia is moderate. If severe atypia is present, HGSC should be diagnosed.

Bona fide invasive implants most likely reflect peritoneal metastases of LGSCs (some with undetected occult invasion); less likely, these may be independent lesions which may have progressed from endosalpingiosis or noninvasive implants. As LGSCs are often exophytic, malignant cells can theoretically be shed from the surface of the tumor and implant on peritoneal surfaces even when the primary tumor is not invasive. Invasive implants are associated with a poor prognosis and are considered invasive carcinomas (253).

Lymph Nodes. Nodal endosalpingiosis, or benign glandular inclusions, are found in 45% of patients with SBT/noninvasive LGSC in whom lymph nodes are examined, in comparison to about 10% of women who have nodes removed for other reasons. Up to 42% of these patients have nodes containing serous lesions with proliferative features beyond endosalpingiosis. There is a strong association with invasive peritoneal implants and micropapillary architecture. In the Stanford series, 42% of patients with SBT and lymph node resection had lymph node lesions, but this is likely an overestimate because of consultation bias and may also be related to a higher frequency of node sampling in patients with peritoneal implants (289).

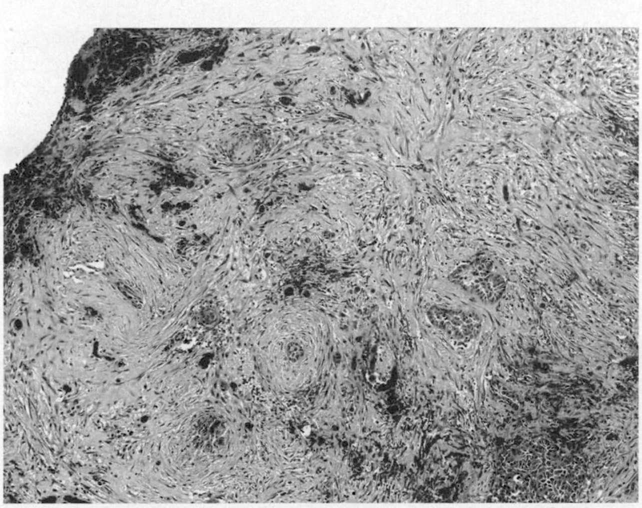

Figure 23.28. Noninvasive desmoplastic peritoneal implant displays an abundant granulation tissue-like spindle cell stroma with rare scattered glands lined by minimally atypical epithelium.

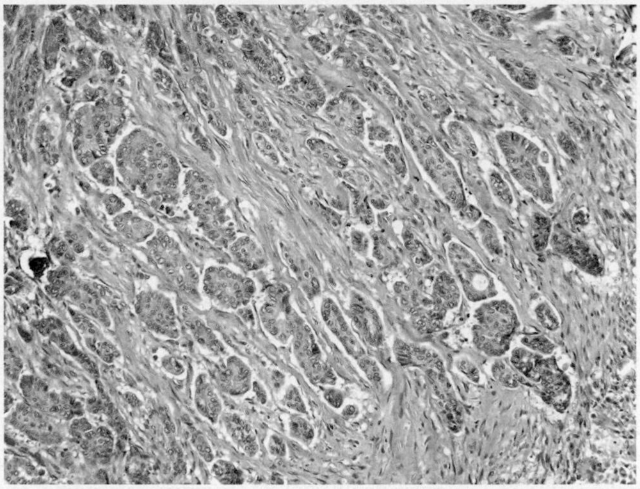

Figure 23.29. Invasive low-grade serous carcinoma/invasive peritoneal implant, characterized by small papillae lined by epithelium with mild atypia and surrounded by clear spaces.

Proliferative serous lesions in lymph nodes have been reported in over 100 cases of SBT. Although these lesions have been referred to as "metastases," it is preferable to refer to them as "associated serous lesions in lymph nodes" or "lymph node involvement" as they may or may not be related to the ovarian tumor.

Lymph node lesions apart from endosalpingiosis can be divided into two types. One is characterized by individual cells and clusters of cells with abundant eosinophilic cytoplasm in the sinuses, predominantly subcapsular sinuses. The nature of these cells is unclear. They resemble the eosinophilic cells seen in "microinvasion," which may be terminally differentiated cells undergoing apoptosis (see above, Microinvasion). They may reflect detached cells from an exophytic tumor surface which are transported to nodes via lymphatic drainage of the peritoneal cavity (284).

The second type of lymph node lesion is characterized by glandular inclusions and papillary serous structures, usually within or just beneath the capsule of the lymph node, that resemble the ovarian SBT. The majority of these papillary serous lesions are also associated with endosalpingiosis in the same lymph node. Cytologic atypia is mild or moderate and mitotic figures are rarely seen. The observation of papillary proliferations arising within endosalpingiosis and the rare reports of SBTs and carcinomas arising within lymph nodes from endosalpingiosis suggest an independent origin of this second type of lymph node lesion.

In the 2006 Stanford series, 8 of 31 patients (26%) with lymph node involvement had invasive peritoneal implants. Among 22 patients with follow-up, 4 were alive with disease and there were 2 deaths, 1 in a patient with indeterminate peritoneal implants (289).

Clinical Behavior. In six prospective randomized trials including 373 patients with SBTs followed for a mean of 6.7 years, the survival was 100% (282). Large studies, some population-based, in the United States, Korea, and Sweden show a 10-year survival of 96% to 100% (290–292). In stage I, the survival does not differ from the expected survival of the general population according to a population-based Denmark study (286). If patients with invasive implants (carcinoma) or indeterminate implants are excluded, then the OS for patients with lymph node lesions other than endosalpingiosis is 98% to 99%. The survival for patients with microinvasion or microinvasive carcinoma unassociated with invasive implants is also nearly100%.

The behavior of SBTs with extraovarian lesions is clearly based on the type of implants that are present. Among patients with noninvasive peritoneal implants, the outcome is less favorable, with a 10-year survival of 90% in a population-based study from Denmark (286). As noted earlier, about 4% of those with noninvasive implants eventually develop invasive carcinoma.

Based on a literature review of 467 noninvasive serous tumors, which included both invasive and noninvasive implants, the survival rate for patients with invasive implants was 66% after a mean follow-up of 7.4 years, compared with 95% for patients with noninvasive implants ($p < 0.0001$) (282). The survival rate for patients with invasive implants is similar to that for patients with invasive low-grade (micropapillary) serous carcinoma (see below) (107), and as noted earlier, invasive implants are equated with invasive LGSC.

Low-Grade Malignant Serous Tumors

This section discusses LGSC; MPSC, invasive and noninvasive types; noninvasive LGSC; micropapillary SBT; psammocarcinoma; and SBT with invasive implants.

Low-grade serous carcinoma is synonymous with invasive MPSC and is a distinctive invasive carcinoma that is currently believed to arise from SBTs (see Pathogenesis, earlier in this chapter). It is not simply a low-grade version of the usual serous carcinoma, as accumulating evidence strongly indicates that this is a distinctively different cell type of ovarian carcinoma. It therefore should not be lumped with HGSC, the usual fatal type of ovarian cancer.

The characteristic micropapillary and cribriform pattern in SBTs has been associated with invasive implants and accordingly with a worse prognosis than typical SBTs (229). Despite the lack of demonstrable invasion, these tumors behave like low-grade carcinomas in contrast to the other tumors in this group (APSTs) which have nearly 100% survival. It was therefore proposed that they be designated noninvasive MPSCs. Others have preferred the term "SBT, micropapillary variant" and "noninvasive low-grade serous carcinoma"; the latter two terms are used synonymously in the current WHO classification (253).

Unfortunately, the term MPSC has been used for two morphologically distinct, albeit related, entities and this has caused some confusion. The noninvasive form of MPSC is a variant of SBT and is also referred to as noninvasive LGSC. The invasive form of MPSC is classified as invasive LGSC, LGSC, or well-differentiated serous carcinoma. It is likely that noninvasive MPSC is a form of *in situ* or intraepithelial carcinoma. Noninvasive LGSCs comprise 14% of SBTs in consultation-based material and 8% in population-based data (286). Invasive LGSCs are quite uncommon and comprise only 5% of ovarian carcinomas and 7% of serous carcinomas (**Table 23.10**).

Clinical and Operative Findings. The mean age of patients with the noninvasive form of LGSC is 42 years; the invasive form, 45 years; and the psammomatous variant (psammocarcinoma), 54 years. For noninvasive LGSC, two-thirds are bilateral as compared with only one-third with SBT. Half of patients are stage I and the remainder are stages II and III. For invasive LGSC, 80% to 90% are bilateral and 93% are advanced stage. Bilateral tumors and those with an exophytic component are more likely to be associated with advanced-stage disease.

Gross Findings. The mean tumor size for the noninvasive form is about 8 cm, and for the invasive form, about 11 cm. Surface involvement is present in 54% of cases. As these tumors are very well differentiated, they tend to have a more papillary and cystic gross appearance like SBTs, and little if any necrosis, in contrast to many typical HGSCs that often have solid areas and extensive necrosis. Bilaterality, exophytic growth, and peritoneal implants are more common with noninvasive LGSC as compared with SBT.

Microscopic Findings. Noninvasive LGSC is a proliferating serous neoplasm, which displays a high degree of epithelial proliferation and complexity but is noninvasive. The tumor displays a characteristic pattern of papillary branching. The distal papillary branches are thin and delicate with minimal fibrovascular support and emanate abruptly from thick, more centrally located papillae without intervening branches of successive intermediate sizes, unlike the hierarchical branching pattern of SBTs. When the papillae fuse, a cribriform pattern or a Roman bridge-like pattern results on the surfaces of the large papillae (**Fig. 23.30**). Both micropapillary and cribriform patterns may be present. A 5 mm in diameter area of a confluent micropapillary pattern or 10% of the tumor occupied by the micropapillary pattern is required for the diagnosis. The majority of noninvasive LGSCs have areas of typical SBT, in contrast to only 2% of HGSCs. In some cases associated with metastases (invasive implants), invasion has been found in the primary tumor after exhaustive histologic sampling (281).

Noninvasive LGSC displays no invasion of the stromal cores of the papillae. Invasion in LGSC is recognized by haphazard infiltrative growth composed of solid nests or complex gland-like structures displaying micropapillae (**Fig. 23.29**). The nests and gland-like structures are often surrounded by a clear space or cleft. Psammoma bodies are common. The psammomatous variant of invasive LGSC, so-called "psammocarcinoma," is characterized by a myriad of psammoma bodies occupying greater than 75% of the papillae.

LGSCs with or without invasion display similar cytologic features. Cells tend to be rounded with scant cytoplasm, and there is mild or moderate nuclear atypia, often with prominent small nucleoli. The cells in SBTs tend to be columnar, are often ciliated, and have less nuclear atypia. Mitotic activity tends to be low. Severe nuclear atypia warrants a designation of HGSC even in the absence of overt invasion. This latter situation reflects HGSC with an architectural pattern simulating SBT, which is quite uncommon; further histologic sampling of the tumor in such cases is likely to identify invasion.

The peritoneal implants associated with noninvasive LGSC are frequently invasive (i.e., carcinoma). Among 157 reported cases of advanced-stage noninvasive LGSC, 45% of the implants were invasive, in comparison to 7% of the implants associated with APSTs ($p < 0.0001$). Noninvasive LGSCs also are more likely to be associated with serous lesions in lymph nodes that replace the node parenchyma, supporting the view that these are either *in situ* or invasive carcinomas with metastatic potential.

Clinical Behavior. Despite the absence of obvious invasion in the noninvasive variant of LGSC, the data indicate that it behaves as a LGSC. Stage I noninvasive LGSC has virtually 100% survival. In contrast to noninvasive LGSCs, invasive LGSCs are rarely stage I. The 5- and 10-year survival rates for patients with advanced-stage noninvasive LGSC are approximately 70% to 85% and 40% to 60%, respectively. After recurrence as invasive carcinoma, the outcome of noninvasive LGSC is similar to that of invasive LGSC, with a PFS of about 2 years and a median survival of 6 to 7 years (107,293,294).

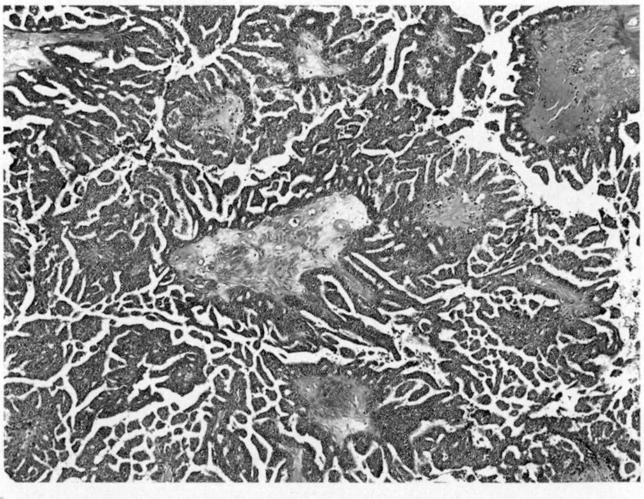

Figure 23.30. Noninvasive micropapillary serous carcinoma/micropapillary serous borderline tumor displays a delicate micropapillary architecture at the surfaces of large papillae, without invasion of underlying stroma.

Although the patterns of spread are similar to ordinary HGSC, LGSC has a significantly better prognosis (295). Stage III LGSC is more likely to be stage IIIA as compared with HGSC, which is nearly always stage IIIC. The natural history of LGSC is characterized by indolent growth that is resistant to chemotherapy and recurrences that maintain the well-differentiated histologic appearance of the primary tumor, even decades later. Rare exceptions show transformation to HGSC.

High-Grade Serous Carcinoma of Ovarian, Tubal, and Peritoneal Origin

High-grade serous carcinoma is the most common type of ovarian cancer and accounts for the majority of ovarian carcinomas. If the clinically and pathologically identical peritoneal and tubal serous carcinomas are included, in addition to carcinosarcoma and undifferentiated carcinoma which are variants, the frequency is over 72% (**Table 23.10**). In over one-third of women with advanced-stage HGSC, the ovaries are small and display predominantly surface involvement. In the past, these findings have justified a diagnosis of primary peritoneal serous carcinoma.

It has been suggested recently that many or even most serous carcinomas classified as ovarian or peritoneal may actually be tubal carcinomas of fimbrial origin. This is discussed further earlier in this chapter (see Pathogenesis). For practical purposes, the clinical and pathologic features of tubal, ovarian, and peritoneal HGSCs are identical as described below.

Clinical and Operative Findings. HGSC most often occurs in the sixth and seventh decades, and the mean age is 63 years for advanced-stage tumors. Nearly all comprehensively staged patients present in advanced stage with tumor usually disseminated throughout the abdominal and pelvic cavities. Although most advanced-stage cases involve both ovaries microscopically, grossly the ovaries are of normal size in one-third to one-half of cases (includes those cases formerly classified as of peritoneal origin). The vast majority of advanced-stage ovarian carcinomas involve peritoneal surfaces, including the pelvic peritoneum and the surfaces of the bowel and other abdominal organs. Both pelvic and abdominal spread can be by direct extension or metastasis. For example, direct extension to the bowel, broad ligament, or uterus can occur by contiguous growth or by metastasis when exfoliation of malignant cells results in seeding of the peritoneal surfaces.

Gross Findings. Serous carcinomas range from microscopic to about 20 cm in greatest dimension. The dominant tumorous mass is typically multilocular, cystic, and solid, with soft, friable papillae filling the cyst cavities; occasionally it is completely solid. The cysts contain serous, turbid, or bloody fluid. The external surfaces often display papillae. Solid areas on cut surface are pink to gray. Hemorrhage and necrosis are often present.

When the ovaries are normal in size, the ovarian surfaces often display papillary excrescences of variable size. The appearance of the fallopian tubes is variable. Sometimes they appear normal and may be adherent to the ovarian tumor. Sometimes they cannot be clearly identified. When the fimbriae are identified and carefully examined, they may appear hyperplastic and splayed over the ovarian or tumor surface. In occasional cases, a tumorous papillary outgrowth of the fimbriae constitutes the largest pelvic tumor. Rarely, the fallopian tube is dilated and filled with tumor; in the past, these were the only cases classified as being of tubal origin.

Omental and other peritoneal metastases are characterized by firm nodules with white or gray cut surfaces, which may coalesce to form an omental cake or large masses adherent to bowel and other structures. A grossly normal omentum contains microscopic tumor in 22% of cases.

Microscopic Findings. HGSCs display complex papillary and solid patterns and marked cytologic atypia (**Fig. 23.31**). Frequently they display a lace-like or labyrinthine pattern characterized by extensive bridging and coalescence of papillae resulting in slit-like spaces. Areas of solid growth and glandular and cribriform patterns are common (**Fig. 23.31**). Cytoplasmic clear cell change may occur, but characteristic architectural patterns of clear cell carcinoma are not present. Nearly all cases display areas of large, pleomorphic nuclei. Multinucleated tumor giant cells may be present (**Fig. 23.31**). Bizarre nuclei greater than 50 μm in diameter are characteristic and occur in 86% of advanced-stage tumors (**Fig. 23.31**). Mitoses, including abnormal mitoses, are numerous and necrosis is often pronounced. Psammoma bodies are present in a majority of cases. Rarely, a completely solid carcinoma without any evidence of glands, papillae, or other recognizable patterns occurs; this is probably a variant of HGSC but is designated undifferentiated carcinoma (see below, Undifferentiated Carcinoma).

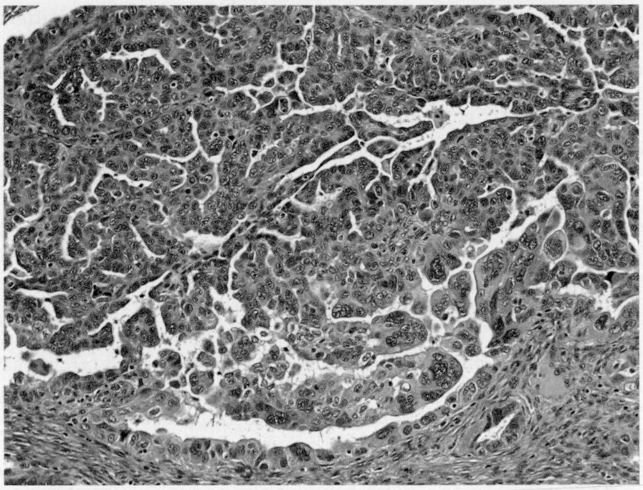

Figure 23.31. High grade serous carcinoma displays papillary growth and severe cytologic atypia with bizarre forms.

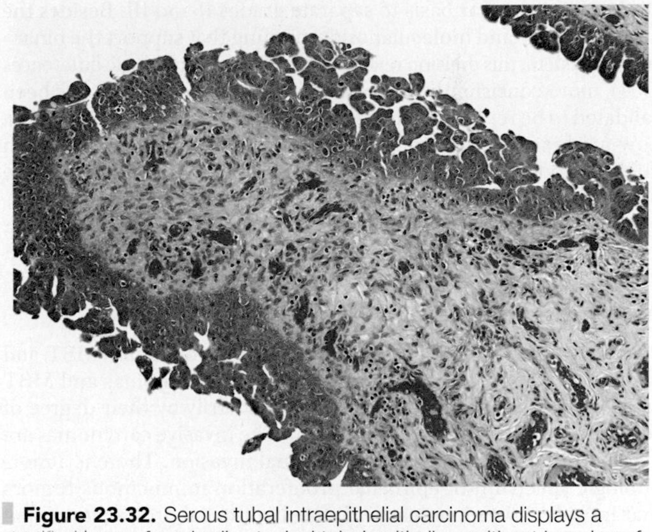

Figure 23.32. Serous tubal intraepithelial carcinoma displays a stratified layer of markedly atypical tubal epithelium without invasion of the underlying lamina propria of the fallopian tube mucosa.

The fallopian tube mucosa displays STIC in a substantial proportion of cases (**Fig. 23.32**). Depending on both interobserver diagnostic reproducibility and on whether the fallopian tubes were entirely embedded for examination, reports of STIC associated with HGSC vary from 19% to 53% in tumors classified as ovarian and from 29% to 56% in tumors classified as peritoneal (237,296–298). As these are typically very small lesions, on the order of 1 to 3 mm or even smaller (245), they may be easily overlooked. STIC is usually, but not always, confined to the fimbriae. Complete embedding of the tube increases the yield of STIC. Accordingly, the fallopian tubes should be meticulously examined and entirely embedded for microscopic examination in all high-grade extrauterine serous carcinomas. As noted earlier, the SEE-FIM protocol is a commonly used guideline for tube sectioning.

Metastatic foci of HGSC may display a variety of patterns. A recent study showed that tumors with germ line or somatic BRCA1 or

BRCA2 abnormalities were more likely to display a pushing pattern or infiltrative micropapillary metastases, whereas those without such abnormalities showed infiltrative metastases with papillary, glandular, and rarely cribriform and micropapillary features (299). These metastatic features appeared more reliable than features of the primary tumor for predicting BRCA mutations.

Foci of serous carcinoma that remain after NACT often display extensive fibrosis, psammomatous calcification with scant carcinomatous epithelium, and even more extreme bizarre nuclear features. Histiocytic response and single-cell invasion are seen in a majority of cases (300). A recently validated chemotherapy response score has been reported (301). STIC may persist after NACT (302).

Grade. There is a bimodal distribution that separates serous carcinomas into a small group of low-grade carcinomas and a much larger group of HGSCs (303). These findings along with the distinctly different molecular genetic profile that distinguish low- from HGSC support that these are two distinct types of carcinoma and also support the use of a two-tier grading system instead of the traditional three-tier systems of well, moderate, and poorly differentiated serous carcinomas. Unlike the two-tier system proposed by Malpica and colleagues from MD Anderson (MDACC), the three-tier system does not have a clinical or molecular basis to separate grades II and III. Besides the morphometric and molecular underpinning that support the binary grading system, this division reveals distinctive epidemiologic differences (304), more consistently separates prognostic groups, and has been validated to be reproducible among generalists and specialists (305). Low-grade serous carcinoma is characterized by uniform cells with mild to moderate nuclear atypia, whereas high-grade tumors have pleomorphic cells with marked nuclear atypia. Low-grade tumors have a mitotic index less than 12 per 10 HPF, and usually much lower, whereas high-grade tumors usually display greater than 12 per 10 HPF.

Mucinous Tumors

Primary ovarian mucinous tumors include cystadenomas, MBT, and carcinomas (intraepithelial and invasive). Cystadenomas and MBT are noninvasive and are distinguished primarily by their degree of complexity and epithelial proliferation. The invasive carcinomas are distinguished by the presence of stromal invasion. There is a morphologic spectrum of epithelial proliferation in mucinous tumors that includes cystadenomas with focal epithelial proliferation, and MBT with intraepithelial carcinoma and/or microinvasion, providing evidence that these tumors constitute a biologic spectrum with individual types representing successive steps in the sequence of ovarian mucinous carcinogenesis. A relatively small proportion of ovarian mucinous tumors arise in a mature cystic teratoma (306), and accordingly are germ cell tumors.

The other types of mucinous tumors seen in the ovary include metastatic mucinous carcinomas, most commonly from the gastrointestinal tract, and low-grade mucinous tumors of appendiceal origin secondarily involving the ovary in association with the clinical syndrome of PMP. Both metastatic mucinous carcinomas and low-grade mucinous tumors of appendiceal origin can simulate primary ovarian mucinous tumors, usually MBT and primary ovarian mucinous carcinoma (235). It is now clear that primary ovarian mucinous carcinomas are much less common than previously believed. Furthermore, most mucinous carcinomas within the ovary prove to be metastatic (218).

Benign Mucinous Tumors, Intestinal and Müllerian (Seromucinous, Endocervical-Like) Types

Mucinous cystadenomas (including the Müllerian type; see below) comprise 15% of benign ovarian epithelial neoplasms (**Table 23.9**). About 80% are of the intestinal type. The mean patient age is about 50 years. Intestinal-type mucinous cystadenomas are unilocular or multilocular tumors of variable size, ranging from a few centimeters to over 30 cm, with a mean of about 10 cm. They are typically unilateral (>95%). The capsule is typically thick and white with a smooth outer surface. The cysts contain thick gelatinous material. They are composed of glands and cysts lined by simple nonstratified mucinous epithelium (**Fig. 23.33**). When epithelial atypia or proliferation resembling MBT is present, this feature must be limited. Tumors composed predominantly of cystadenoma with less than 10% of MBT are diagnosed as mucinous cystadenoma with focal proliferation or focal atypia (235). Up to 18% of mucinous cystadenomas contain transitional cell nests, also referred to as a Brenner tumor component, often in a discrete nodule, which is usually interpreted as a concurrent Brenner tumor (**Fig. 23.34**). Occasionally, cystadenomas have endocervical-type mucinous epithelium. These are referred to as Müllerian-type mucinous, endocervical-like mucinous, or seromucinous cystadenoma. They usually have a papillary architecture in contrast to the pure glandular pattern of the intestinal type.

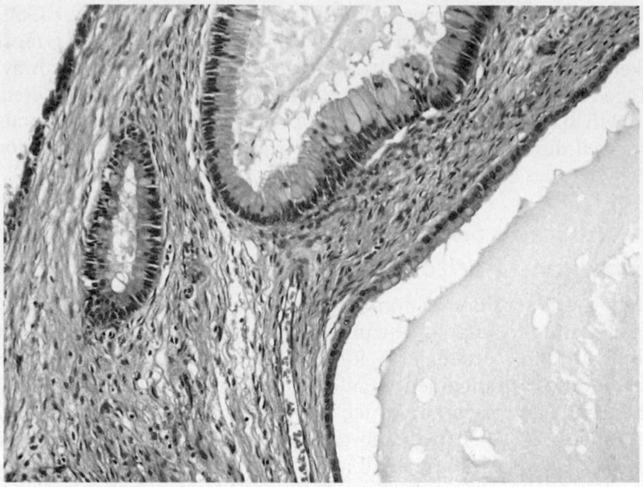

Figure 23.33. Mucinous cystadenoma shows a single layer of columnar epithelium with small basal nuclei and abundant mucin-rich cytoplasm.

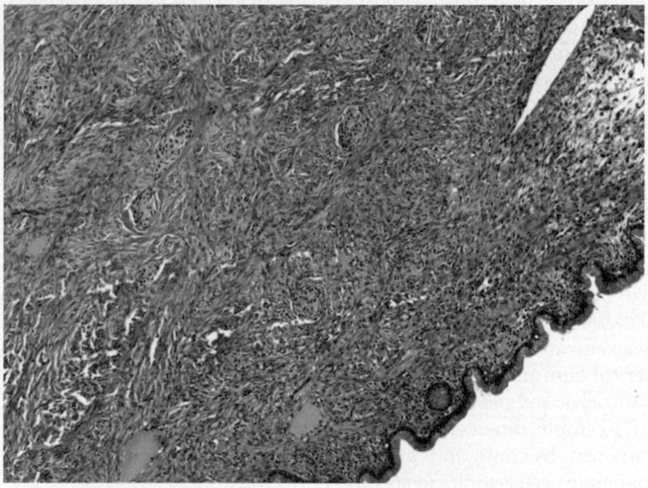

Figure 23.34. Mixed mucinous–Brenner tumor with several Brenner-type (transitional) nests within the stroma toward the top left and a single layer of mucinous epithelium at bottom right.

Mucinous Borderline Tumor, Intestinal Type (Atypical Proliferative Mucinous Tumor)

Although the borderline category was intended mainly for serous tumors, the concept was also extended to mucinous tumors as they also appeared to have intermediate forms. These were most often characterized by PMP and were felt to be analogous to SBTs with peritoneal implants. There are two types of MBT corresponding to

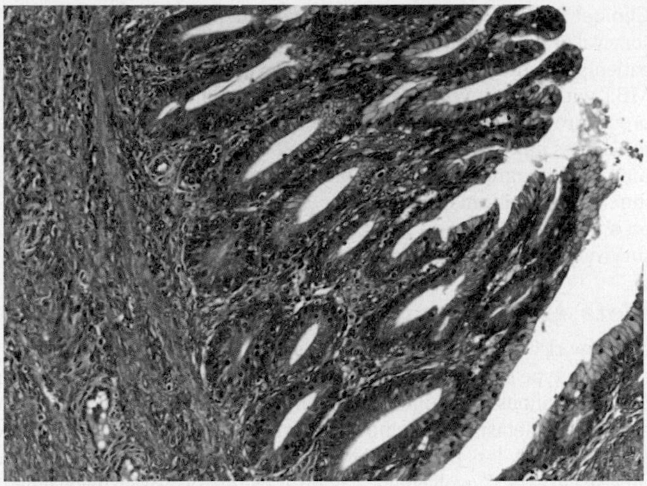

Figure 23.35. Atypical proliferative mucinous tumor shows glandular proliferation, cellular stratification, and mild cytologic atypia.

the two types of mucinous cystadenoma: the gastrointestinal type and the endocervical-like (Müllerian or seromucinous) type. The gastrointestinal type of MBT is typically a large, multicystic tumor with a smooth capsule and is usually unilateral (>95%) with median size of about 20 to 22 cm (235,307). The locules of the tumor are usually filled with mucinous material and the lining appears smooth, without grossly evident papillations. Microscopically, the cysts are lined by stratified, proliferative gastrointestinal-type mucinous epithelium exhibiting tufted and villoglandular or papillary intraglandular growth and displaying mild to moderate nuclear atypia; stromal invasion is absent (**Fig. 23.35**).

Review of the literature on tumors meeting the diagnostic criteria for MBT, gastrointestinal type, reveals a benign behavior. Over 600 stage I tumors have been reported and fewer than 1% of patients have died of the disease. Rare reports of recurrence of well-sampled tumors diagnosed by experts are generally attributed to incomplete resection because of adhesions and/or cystectomy (308). Most fatal tumors had an unknown degree of sampling and are reported in the older literature; most recent studies report 100% survival (235). Approximately 100 "advanced-stage MBTs" have been reported, with nearly 50% mortality. Of these, about 85% have been associated with PMP. More recent studies have established that virtually all cases of PMP are of gastrointestinal (usually appendiceal), not ovarian, origin (see PMP below) (235). The remaining 15% of advanced-stage MBTs reported are probably metastatic mucinous carcinomas that masquerade as MBTs. Therefore, there is no documentation of peritoneal implants associated with true primary ovarian MBT and for practical purposes, advanced-stage MBT does not exist. When these latter tumors are removed from the MBT category, the remainder consist of stage I tumors with benign behavior.

Mucinous Borderline Tumor, Seromucinous (Endocervical-Like or Müllerian) Type (Seromucinous Borderline Tumor (SMBT); Atypical Proliferative Seromucinous Tumor)

The seromucinous type of MBT (SMBT) is grossly, microscopically, and immunophenotypically distinct from the gastrointestinal-type tumor. The seromucinous tumors are much less common, smaller, more frequently bilateral, architecturally resemble SBT, and are much more often associated with endometriosis (over one-third of cases). In addition, they frequently display acute inflammation of the stroma and a combination of endocervical mucinous and serous (ciliated) type epithelium, often admixed with minor components (<10%) of other cell types. Based on a small number of studies, these tumors appear to exhibit benign behavior (235).

Mucinous Borderline Tumors with Intraepithelial Carcinoma

Noninvasive mucinous tumors with marked nuclear atypia are classified as MBT with intraepithelial carcinoma. Intraepithelial carcinomas confined to the ovaries have an excellent prognosis (about 95% survival, with most recent studies reporting 100% survival). A small number of so-called "advanced-stage intraepithelial mucinous carcinomas" have been reported, with a few tumor deaths. In view of the ability of metastatic mucinous carcinomas to simulate MBT with intraepithelial carcinoma, it is likely that some of these apparent advanced-stage intraepithelial carcinomas with adverse outcomes represent metastases from occult extraovarian primary tumors. It is also possible that some of these represent true primary ovarian mucinous carcinomas with foci of destructive invasion in unsampled tissue.

Mucinous Borderline Tumors with Microinvasion

Microinvasion in MBT has been defined as either small foci of stromal invasion characterized by single cells, glands, or small clusters or nests of mucinous epithelial cells within the stroma, or as small foci of confluent glandular or cribriform growth within the stroma. The size criterion for each focus has varied from 2 to 5 mm, with no requirement regarding the number of foci allowed. Some tumors with microinvasion also have intraepithelial carcinoma. Based on the relatively small number of microinvasive tumors with follow-up that have been reported, no well-documented recurrences or deaths owing to the disease have been reported.

Mucinous Tumors Associated with PMP

PMP has historically referred to the presence of mucinous ascites or mucoid nodules adherent to peritoneal surfaces and has not had a consistently applied histopathologic definition. Recent studies have clarified that PMP is a clinicopathologic syndrome in which mucoid peritoneal nodules and/or mucinous ascites are accompanied by low-grade neoplastic mucinous epithelium associated with pools of extracellular mucin. Morphologic, immunohistochemical, and molecular genetic studies have provided compelling evidence that virtually all cases of PMP are derived from low-grade mucinous adenomas, usually of the appendix, and that the ovarian involvement is secondary (235). When intraoperative consultation with frozen section leads to a diagnosis of a mucinous ovarian tumor in the setting of PMP, appendectomy and thorough examination of the gastrointestinal and pancreaticobiliary tracts should be performed. The pathologist should examine the entire appendix microscopically in permanent sections. The rare exception to the gastrointestinal origin of PMP is the occurrence of mucinous tumors arising in ovarian mature cystic teratomas associated with mucinous ascites (309). The terms "disseminated peritoneal adenomucinosis" (DPAM) and "involvement by low-grade appendiceal mucinous neoplasm" are now preferred as specific pathologic diagnostic terms for these low-grade peritoneal and ovarian mucinous tumors, respectively.

Invasive Mucinous Carcinomas

Clinical and Operative Findings. Mucinous carcinomas of the intestinal type are rare and comprise 3% of ovarian carcinomas (**Table 23.10**). Primary ovarian mucinous carcinomas, like MBT, most often present as large unilateral ovarian masses without evidence of ovarian surface involvement or extraovarian disease. The vast majority, generally over 90%, present in FIGO stage I.

Gross Findings. The gross findings are similar to MBTs in that the tumors are typically large, unilateral, multicystic mucus-containing tumors with smooth white capsules and have mean and median sizes of 18 to 22 cm. They may contain solid areas and foci of necrosis and hemorrhage.

Microscopic Findings. Mucinous carcinomas of intestinal type typically are architecturally well differentiated and display a variety of glandular patterns, with most tumors containing areas of MBT

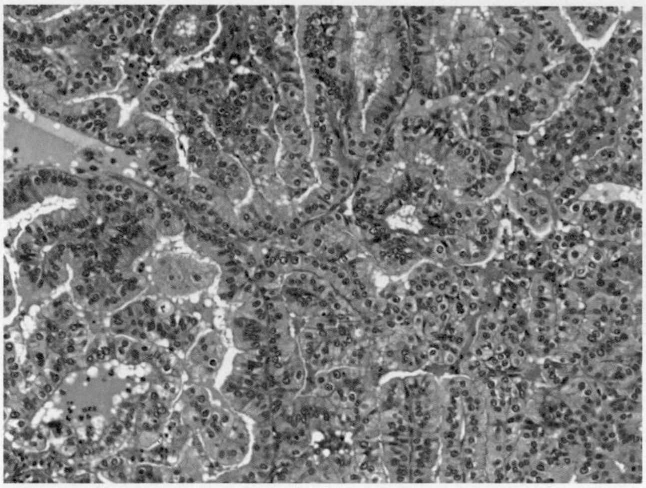

Figure 23.36. Mucinous carcinoma with confluent glandular pattern of invasion manifested by complex and interconnected epithelial proliferation lacking stroma.

adjacent to areas of carcinoma. In addition to destructive stromal invasion, there is a second pattern of invasion termed the "confluent glandular" or "expansile" pattern. In this pattern, the glandular epithelium is markedly crowded and interconnected with little intervening stroma (310) (**Fig. 23.36**). Primary ovarian mucinous carcinomas commonly exhibit this pattern of invasion, and the presence of an infiltrative pattern of stromal invasion should raise concern for metastatic mucinous carcinoma. For tumors composed predominantly of MBTs, the foci of confluent growth should measure more than the upper size limit allowed for microinvasion (5 mm) to qualify for the diagnosis of invasive carcinoma. Mucinous carcinomas of the seromucinous (Müllerian or endocervical-like) type are quite uncommon (311). They are clinically and grossly similar to the borderline tumors of this type. Microscopically, they also resemble MBTs but exhibit destructive stromal invasion or sufficient complex or confluent growth to be classified as carcinoma. Like their noninvasive counterparts, they have a strong association with endometriosis.

As discussed above, it is critical when evaluating a mucinous carcinoma involving the ovary to consider the possibility of an extraovarian primary. Metastatic mucinous carcinomas are usually readily recognized as such when the ovarian tumors exhibit at least two of the following features: bilaterality, smaller size (typically less than 10–12 cm), ovarian surface involvement, a nodular pattern of ovarian involvement, and a haphazard infiltrative pattern of stromal invasion. Immunohistochemistry can be of great value in this distinction. In general, primary ovarian mucinous tumors are positive for CK7 and variably positive for CK20. Most gastrointestinal carcinomas are negative for CK7 and positive for CK20. Molecular tests for HPV and p16 stains are positive in cervical carcinomas and can be of value. Mammaglobin and GCDFP-15 are positive in most breast carcinomas and negative in ovarian mucinous tumors. DPC4 is positive in ovarian mucinous carcinoma and often negative in pancreatic carcinoma. ER and PR are generally not helpful markers as they are usually negative in primary ovarian mucinous tumors. An algorithm has been proposed to assist in the distinction of primary versus metastatic mucinous carcinoma, particularly at the time of intraoperative evaluation when only limited histologic material can be examined. As originally proposed, bilateral mucinous carcinomas and unilateral ones smaller than 10 cm are metastatic, and unilateral ones larger than 10 cm are primary (218). As originally reported, this algorithm correctly classified 90% of mucinous carcinomas. Subsequent studies confirmed and refined the algorithm, also with close to 90% accuracy, and suggest that 13 cm is a better cutoff than 10 cm (250). Because these size measurements are often not extremely precise and may be taken after the tumor has been partially deflated and emptied of its mucinous contents, the 10 to 15 cm size range is of lesser predictive value (312).

Clinical Behavior. Patients with stage I mucinous carcinomas have a survival of about 90%, similar to comprehensively staged FIGO stage I patients with the other cell types of ovarian carcinoma. For patients with MBT with microinvasion and/or intraepithelial carcinoma, a staging procedure is unlikely to yield positive findings, but no data are available to address its value. The extent of the infiltrative pattern of invasion may have prognostic significance (313). Bona fide advanced-stage mucinous carcinomas have a poor prognosis, and limited data based on a recent GOG study and a GCIG meta-analysis suggest that the survival is significantly worse than that for serous carcinomas (88,314).

Metastatic Mucinous Carcinomas

It is now clear that the historical canon that mucinous carcinoma is a common type of primary ovarian cancer is incorrect. As noted earlier, 80% of mucinous carcinomas that involve the ovaries are metastatic from other sites. Metastatic mucinous carcinomas are typically bilateral and small (typically less than 10–12 cm), and display ovarian surface and superficial cortical involvement, a nodular pattern of ovarian involvement, and a haphazard infiltrative pattern of stromal invasion. However, some metastatic mucinous carcinomas can exhibit gross and microscopic features simulating a primary ovarian mucinous tumor. In particular, metastases can be large, unilateral (thus misclassified by the algorithm discussed earlier), and multicystic and can display deceptive patterns of ovarian involvement. Recognizing metastases is especially problematic when the ovarian tumor is the initial manifestation of disease and an extraovarian primary mucinous carcinoma is occult. When mucinous carcinomas in the ovaries are rigorously classified based on refined criteria and awareness of the deceptive patterns, metastatic mucinous carcinomas are much more commonly encountered than primary ovarian mucinous carcinomas (218). In general, the presence of a mucinous carcinoma in the ovary, particularly if extraovarian disease is present, should always prompt the surgeon and pathologist to consider the possibility of metastatic mucinous carcinoma. Immunohistochemical analysis can be useful for identifying some metastatic mucinous carcinomas, but clinical evaluation is essential to exclude a clinically occult extraovarian source. The most common sources of ovarian metastases are colon, endometrium, breast, appendix, and stomach (315).

Endometrioid Tumors

The vast majority of endometrioid ovarian neoplasms are carcinomas. Endometrioid adenofibromas and endometrioid borderline tumors (atypical proliferative endometrioid tumors, APET) are quite uncommon. However, endometriosis is quite common and now regarded as neoplastic. Consequently, endometriomas and endometriotic cysts constitute the majority of true benign endometrioid ovarian neoplasms, notwithstanding the likelihood that their ultimate origin is from the endometrium via tubal reflux. Molecular biologic studies have shown that endometrioid ovarian carcinomas have similarities with and differences from their uterine counterparts.

Endometrioid Adenofibromas

Endometrioid adenofibromas are uncommon benign tumors that comprise less than 1% of ovarian epithelial neoplasms, and 83% are unilateral. The median age is 57 years. The mean diameter is about 10 cm. The external surface is smooth and the cut surface is densely fibrous, often with intermixed cystic areas creating a honeycomb appearance. Microscopically, the dominant pattern is that of an adenofibroma or cystadenofibroma. The epithelial elements are arranged in branching tubular glands and cysts and usually resemble those of proliferative or mildly hyperplastic endometrium. Endometrioid adenofibromas are frequently associated with endometriosis.

Endometrioid Borderline Tumors (EBT) (Atypical Proliferative Endometrioid Tumors [APET])

There is a spectrum of epithelial proliferation, glandular crowding, and cytologic atypia in benign endometrioid neoplasms ranging from mild atypia, mild glandular crowding, and epithelial stratification slightly beyond that seen in endometrioid adenofibromas, to confluent epithelial proliferation lacking stromal support in areas up to 5 mm in diameter resembling atypical hyperplasia and well-differentiated adenocarcinoma of the endometrium. A variety of terms have been employed for these tumors, including proliferating or proliferative endometrioid tumor, atypical endometrioid adenofibroma, endometrioid tumor of low malignant potential, endometrioid borderline tumor, and APET. APET with microinvasion (<5 mm), which is very rare, constitutes the upper end of this spectrum; with invasion >5 mm, a diagnosis of low-grade endometrioid carcinoma is warranted. The behavior of all of the tumors up to and including those with microinvasion has been benign.

Clinical and Operative Findings. EBT comprise only 0.2% of ovarian epithelial neoplasms. Among five series, there were 134 patients with a mean age of about 51 years. Six patients (4%) had bilateral tumors, and all but two were confined to the ovaries. The mean tumor size was about 9 cm. The characteristic gross appearance is cystic in two-thirds and solid and cystic in the rest; the cyst fluid is usually hemorrhagic, brown, or green. Many patients have had endometriosis and some have also had endometrial hyperplasia.

Microscopic Findings. The two characteristic microscopic architectural appearances of EBT are adenofibromatous and glandular/papillary. The glandular/papillary proliferation can show varying degrees of glandular complexity and crowding. When the glandular proliferation becomes confluent, this is considered evidence of invasion and is classified as microinvasion if the confluent area is less than 5 mm. Some investigators prefer to classify these as EBT with intraepithelial carcinoma. A confluent epithelial proliferation or invasion that exceeds 5 mm in diameter warrants a diagnosis of carcinoma (310). The glands show crowding, mild or moderate cytologic atypia, epithelial stratification, and often display tufting and bridging. Severe cytologic atypia warrants a diagnosis of intraepithelial carcinoma, but this is quite rare and should prompt further searching for invasion. Among 134 reported APETs, all of those with clinical follow-up have had a benign behavior after a mean of approximately 5 years (229,316). Rarely, an endometriotic cyst is lined by markedly atypical epithelial cells that have cytologic features of malignancy. If the lesion is well-sampled and invasion is not found, a designation of EBT with intraepithelial carcinoma should be used. Rarely, a cytologically malignant lining of an endometriotic cyst displays clear cell features (see Clear Cell Borderline Tumors below).

Endometrioid Adenocarcinoma

In the older literature, about 15% to 20% of reported ovarian carcinomas have been classified as endometrioid, up to 25% in some reports (317), but when strict criteria are applied, the figure is lower and probably in the range of 10% to 15%. When very strict criteria are used, requiring a readily recognized resemblance to uterine endometrioid carcinoma and classifying nonspecific high-grade adenocarcinomas as serous carcinoma as is currently preferred (318,319), the figure is about 7.2% (**Table 23.10**). Clear cell and endometrioid ovarian cancers are overrepresented in women with Lynch syndrome (320,321).

Clinical and Operative Findings. These tumors are most common in the fifth and sixth decades, and the mean patient age at diagnosis is 55 to 58 years. Tumor size ranges from 12 to 20 cm with a mean of about 15 cm. The stage distribution differs significantly from serous carcinoma. A high proportion of endometrioid carcinomas are diagnosed in stage I: 43% in a review of 874 cases from 19 series, and 53% in our series (**Table 23.10**). About 13% of early-stage (FIGO I–II) cases are bilateral. Endometriosis, which may be extraovarian, in the ipsilateral or contralateral ovary or within the tumor itself, is found in at least 15% to 20% of patients.

Gross Findings. Endometrioid carcinomas have a smooth outer surface. On cut section, they are solid and cystic, with the cysts containing friable soft masses and bloody fluid. Cysts occasionally contain mucus or greenish fluid. Less commonly, the tumor is solid with extensive hemorrhage and necrosis. Tumors arising in endometriosis may display gross findings of an endometriotic cyst containing chocolate-colored fluid, with one or more solid nodules or papillary excrescences protruding from the wall and containing carcinoma.

Microscopic Findings. Destructive infiltrative growth characterizes one pattern of endometrioid carcinoma. This pattern is characterized by angulated glands with an infiltrative pattern, jagged irregularly spaced and unevenly shaped nests, and solid sheets with jagged edges. More commonly, a confluent glandular epithelial proliferation exceeding 5 mm (the limit for microinvasion) is present. This pattern is characterized by extensive glandular branching, budding, true cribriform architecture, and highly complex papillary proliferations (**Fig. 23.37**). Confluent or expansile invasion is the predominant pattern in most endometrioid carcinomas (310).

Architecturally well-differentiated endometrioid adenocarcinoma accounts for the majority of cases and is characterized by a confluent or cribriform proliferation of glands lined by tall, stratified columnar epithelium with sharp luminal margins (**Fig. 23.38**). A villoglandular

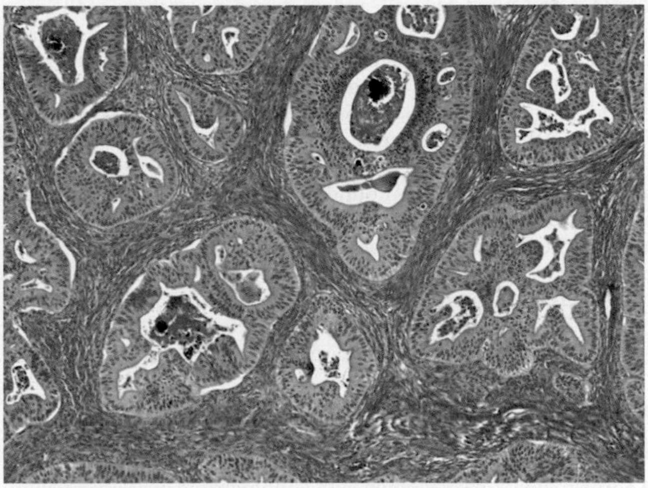

Figure 23.37. Endometrioid adenocarcinoma displaying an infiltrative pattern of cellular islands containing endometrioid-type epithelium with a cribriform pattern.

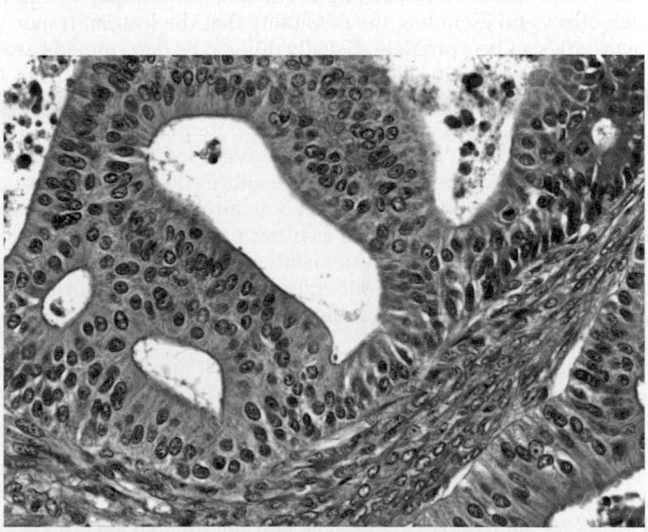

Figure 23.38. Endometrioid adenocarcinoma, high magnification (same case as **Fig. 23.37**) showing tall columnar epithelium with sharply punched out glandular spaces and mild to moderate cytologic atypia.

growth pattern also occurs. Despite the low-grade architecture, high-grade nuclear features are often present. Mitotic figures are common. Squamous differentiation is present in up to 50% of cases. Focal secretory changes are seen in up to a third of cases. In the majority of cases, a component of endometriosis, endometrioid adenofibroma or EBT, can be identified.

Moderately and poorly differentiated endometrioid carcinomas show solid growth, complex glandular and microglandular patterns with marked nuclear pleomorphism and mitotic activity; however, the majority of high-grade carcinomas with these features are usually classified as serous. It has been suggested that solid areas in some endometrioid adenocarcinomas may reflect an undifferentiated component (322).

At present, clinicopathologic and molecular data indicate that it is important to be strict about classifying an adenocarcinoma as endometrioid type. Most predominantly glandular non-clear cell, non-mucinous high-grade ovarian carcinomas are serous carcinomas. Glandular, cribriform, and solid patterns are common in serous carcinoma (318,319). A bona fide endometrioid adenocarcinoma should closely resemble eutopic endometrial carcinomas with tall columnar epithelium and sharp gland lumenal margins. Foci of squamous differentiation, secretory change, endometriosis, or endometrioid adenofibroma can be of value in supporting the diagnosis of endometrioid carcinoma.

Clinical Behavior. Overall, endometrioid carcinomas of the ovary have a better prognosis than typical serous carcinomas because of the high proportion of stage I cases. The favorable prognosis may also result, in part, from the younger age of women diagnosed with endometrioid carcinoma, as young age is an established prognostic factor, and the high frequency of low-grade tumors. However, data on the influence of grade on prognosis are less clear because grade and stage are mutually confounding factors (see below, Prognostic factors). One recent large prospective series found that in stages II and III, the prognosis was significantly better for endometrioid as compared with serous carcinoma. In that series, however, endometrioid carcinomas were significantly more likely to be optimally debulked as compared with serous carcinomas and occurred in younger women. In addition, neither substage nor grade was considered (317).

Endometrioid Carcinoma Associated with Uterine Endometrial Carcinoma

Approximately 14% of women with endometrioid ovarian carcinoma also have endometrial cancer of the uterine corpus. Endometrial hyperplasia is also commonly present. As both tumors are usually well-differentiated endometrioid adenocarcinomas, they resemble each other, and excluding the possibility that the ovarian tumor is metastatic can be a problem. Usually this can be determined based on a careful evaluation of the clinicopathologic features (323). If the uterine endometrial tumor is low grade with no or only inner half myometrial invasion, its metastatic potential is very low and the ovarian tumor can confidently be regarded as independent. If the endometrial tumor is high grade and/or deeply myoinvasive, the features of the ovarian tumors come into play. Bilaterality and a multinodular pattern, as well as other patterns characteristic of metastatic disease indicate metastatic tumor. Close association of the ovarian tumors with either an underlying adenofibroma or endometriosis, if present, can provide evidence that the ovarian tumor is independent.

The median age of women who present with simultaneous uterine and endometrioid ovarian cancer is about 50 years, significantly lower than that the median age of presentation for HGSCs (about 63 years), and close to that for all women with endometrioid carcinomas (55 to 58 years). The median ovarian tumor size is about 9 cm. The majority of tumors in both sites are well differentiated. The 5-year survival is 70% to 92%, and the median survival is 10 years or longer (324), suggesting that a large proportion of these tumors are independent.

Over the last few years, investigators have employed several different molecular strategies to assess the likelihood that simultaneously detected endometrioid adenocarcinomas in the ovary and endometrium represent a single versus two independent primaries. Most of these have relied upon the presence or absence of shared genetic alterations in the ovarian and endometrial adenocarcinomas. The difficulty of correctly classifying some of these cases is highlighted by the fact that virtually every published series of synchronous ovarian and uterine endometrioid adenocarcinomas includes cases that, after being diagnosed using standard histologic criteria, would be reclassified based on molecular analysis (325).

Endometrioid Carcinoma Arising in Endometriosis

On average, 15% to 20% of endometrioid carcinomas of the ovary are associated with endometriosis which may occur within the tumor, the ipsilateral or contralateral ovary, or elsewhere. The frequency can be as high as 42%. It is likely that when strict criteria are applied to diagnose endometrioid carcinoma (see above), some cases would be reclassified as HGSCs and therefore the percentage of endometrioid carcinomas associated with endometriosis would be higher. The majority of bona fide endometrioid carcinomas can be shown to be associated with endometriosis when extensive histologic sampling and meticulous searching for the histologic features of endometriosis are performed, and strict diagnostic criteria are used. In only a minority of cases, however, can direct continuity from endometriosis to atypical hyperplasia to carcinoma be demonstrated. This is most commonly seen in the lining of an endometriotic cyst, which may display a thickening of the cyst wall, papillary excrescences, or a nodule protruding into the cyst. The mean age of women with endometrioid carcinoma associated with endometriosis is 5 to 10 years younger than for women whose endometrioid tumors are unassociated with endometriosis. Tumors associated with endometriosis, and particularly those arising in an endometriotic cyst, are usually architecturally well differentiated and stage I, and therefore the prognosis is excellent. On rare occasions, a limited atypical epithelial proliferation in an endometriotic cyst will raise the differential diagnosis of atypical hyperplasia similar to the type seen in the uterine corpus, versus well-differentiated endometrioid adenocarcinoma. In such cases, criteria for this distinction used in the uterine corpus have been applied with minor modifications. In some of these cases, a diagnosis of EBT may be justified.

The identification of genetic alterations in endometriotic lesions and the observation of a morphologic transition from endometriosis to carcinoma in over one-third of cases indicates that endometriosis is a precursor of endometrioid carcinoma. Progression from endometriosis to benign endometrioid neoplasm to well-differentiated endometrioid carcinoma is analogous to that proposed for progression of LGSC from SBT. Hence, low-grade (well-differentiated) endometrioid carcinomas are classified as type I tumors in the dualistic model of ovarian cancer pathogenesis (see Pathogenesis, earlier in this chapter). Classification of high-grade endometrioid carcinomas is less clear. Overlap of both morphologic and molecular features between high-grade endometrioid and high-grade serous carcinomas has led most authorities to classify the vast majority of gland forming or near-solid cytologically high-grade ovarian carcinomas to the serous category, to the degree that true high-grade endometrioid carcinomas are considered to be very uncommon (318,319).

Clear Cell Tumors

The vast majority of clear cell neoplasms of the ovaries are carcinomas and they comprise 8.0% of ovarian carcinomas (**Table 23.10**). Clear cell adenofibromas and clear cell borderline tumors are vanishingly rare (**Table 23.9**).

Clear Cell Adenofibromas

These are among the rarest of the ovarian epithelial tumors; no cases were found among 1,247 consecutive epithelial tumors in a large community hospital (**Table 23.9**), and only 4 cases were found among 472 clear cell neoplasms from the AFIP consultation service (326). Among 16 reported cases of benign clear cell tumors, the mean age was 49 years. One tumor was bilateral. The median diameter was about 10 cm. Microscopically, the tumor is characterized by tubular glands lined by one or two layers of peg-like or hobnail cells that may bulge into the lumen or are flattened. The cytoplasm is either scanty, often in the hobnail cells, or abundant clear, granular, or eosinophilic in the large polyhedral cells. Nuclear atypia and mitotic activity are minimal. The clinical behavior is said to be benign, although data are very limited. Many experts hesitate to ever make a diagnosis of clear cell adenofibroma, as the likelihood of its representing an inadequately sampled, unusual, or subtle clear cell carcinoma is believed to be very high.

Clear Cell Borderline Tumors (CCBT) (Atypical Proliferative Clear Cell Tumors, APCCT)

CCBT comprise 0.2% of ovarian epithelial tumors (**Table 23.9**). Among approximately 71 cases of CCBT (clear cell adenofibroma of borderline malignancy) in the literature, the mean age is 60 to 70 years. The mean tumor diameter is about 10 to 12 cm. In contrast to the gross appearance of clear cell adenofibroma, a majority are mixed solid and cystic, and there are softer and fleshier areas. Microscopically, the architecture is similar to the clear cell adenofibroma, but glands are more crowded. The tumor has greater epithelial proliferation and atypia than adenofibromas and lacks stromal invasion. The cell types lining the glands and cystic spaces are similar to those in benign tumors but display significant nuclear atypia with coarse chromatin clumping, prominent nucleoli, and mitotic activity up to 3 per 10 HPF. The epithelium may display stratification and budding; true papillary structures are uncommon. Small solid nests of clear cells, significant gland crowding, or papillary growth should raise the suspicion of stromal invasion. Endometriosis is seen in 20% of patients. Distinction of a CCBT from clear cell carcinoma is one of the most difficult distinctions in gynecologic pathology. Some clear cell carcinomas lack an obviously infiltrative pattern and are characterized solely by crowded glands.

Occasionally, an endometriotic cyst is lined by atypical epithelial cells with clear cytoplasm and/or hobnail features characteristic of clear cell neoplasms. This has been designated "atypical endometriosis." Rarely, cytologic features of malignancy are present in this setting. If the lesion is well sampled and invasion is not found, the lesion is classified as CCBT with intraepithelial carcinoma. In our experience in a non-consultative setting, this is the most common appearance of CCBT. Microinvasion should be diagnosed if invasive areas measure less than 5 mm, but this finding should prompt additional sampling to look for diagnostic features of overt carcinoma. There are virtually no published data on clear cell tumors with microinvasion or intraepithelial carcinoma, both of which are exceedingly rare. Peritoneal "implants" have not been described associated with these tumors. Among the limited reported CCBTs, there is one reported recurrence and no tumor deaths.

Clear Cell Carcinomas

Recent data indicate that HGSCs can have areas of clear cells and that such tumors have the other pathologic and immunohistochemical features of HGSC, lack typical patterns of CCC, and should be diagnosed as serous (327). In addition, endometrioid carcinomas may have clear cells reflecting secretory or squamous differentiation (328). Old literature on clear cell carcinomas may therefore be inaccurate because of this classification problem. There is some evidence that clear cell carcinoma is more common in Asia, particularly Japan, and in Asian Americans as compared with Caucasians (329). Clear cell and endometrioid ovarian cancers are overrepresented in women with Lynch syndrome (320,321).

Clinical and Operative Findings. The mean age of patients with clear cell carcinoma is 50 to 56 years. Symptoms usually relate to a pelvic or abdominal mass. Clear cell carcinoma is the most common epithelial ovarian neoplasm to be associated with vascular thrombotic events (18% to 46% of patients) and paraneoplastic hypercalcemia (2% to 10%).

The relationship with endometriosis is strongest for clear cell carcinoma among all cell types of ovarian carcinoma. Accordingly, endometriotic implants are commonly present in close proximity to the tumor or elsewhere in the pelvis or abdomen. About 45% to 60% of clear cell carcinomas present in FIGO stage I, and 10% to 20% in stage II (330) (**Table 23.10**). Seven percent are bilateral; 4% of stage I cases are bilateral (331). Several recent studies have shown that stage I clear cell carcinoma is more likely to be stage IC (50% to 74%) as compared with the other cell types (332,333). This seems to be correlated with a higher risk of tumor rupture, likely because of the extent and inherent difficulty in dissecting adhesions owing to endometriosis (334).

Gross Findings. Tumors range up to 30 cm with a mean diameter of about 12 to 15 cm. Although they may be solid and fibrous with a honeycomb cut surface resembling benign and borderline clear cell tumors, more commonly the cut surfaces reveal a thick-walled unilocular cyst with multiple yellow-beige fleshy nodules protruding into the lumen or a multiloculated cystic mass with cysts containing watery or mucinous fluid. Most tumors arise in endometriosis and often display features of an endometriotic cyst that typically contains chocolate-brown fluid, and a thickened, polypoid, or nodular area in the wall, or a larger solid area reflecting the focus of malignant transformation.

Microscopic Findings. Clear cell carcinomas display several different patterns, which often occur together (**Figs. 23.39–23.41**). These include papillary, tubulocystic, and solid. In a minority of cases, there is a prominent adenofibromatous component. Recently, some investigators have subdivided clear cell carcinomas into those arising in a cyst and those that are more solid and adenofibromatous. The cystic tumors are more frequently papillary, whereas the tubulocystic pattern (**Fig. 23.39**) tends to dominate in the adenofibromatous tumors. The cystic variant appears to be more frequently associated with endometriosis. Some have suggested that the two variants arise along different pathways (326,330).

The solid pattern of clear cell carcinoma is characterized by sheets of polyhedral cells with abundant, clear cytoplasm separated by delicate fibrovascular septae or dense fibrotic stroma. The

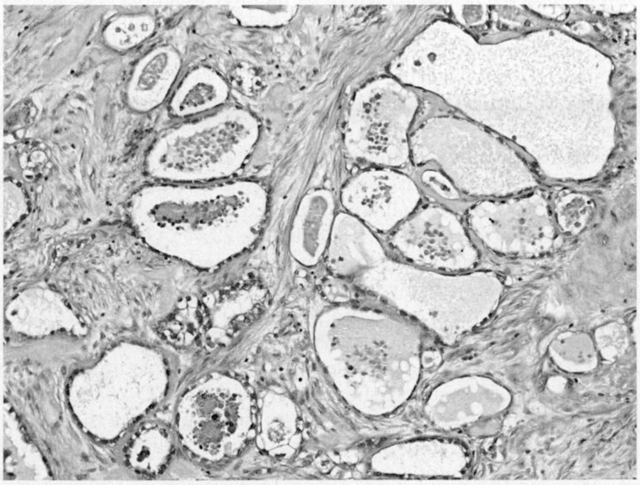

Figure 23.39. Clear cell carcinoma, tubulocystic pattern. This pattern is deceptively benign appearing, characterized by cystic and glandular spaces lined by flattened to low cuboidal epithelium, often with only minimal cytologic atypia.

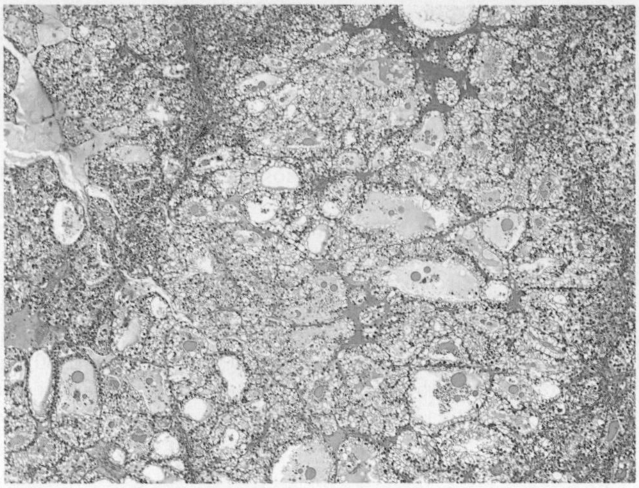

Figure 23.40. Clear cell carcinoma, glandular and solid pattern with an infiltrative pattern of small and medium sized glands lined by cells with abundant clear cytoplasm.

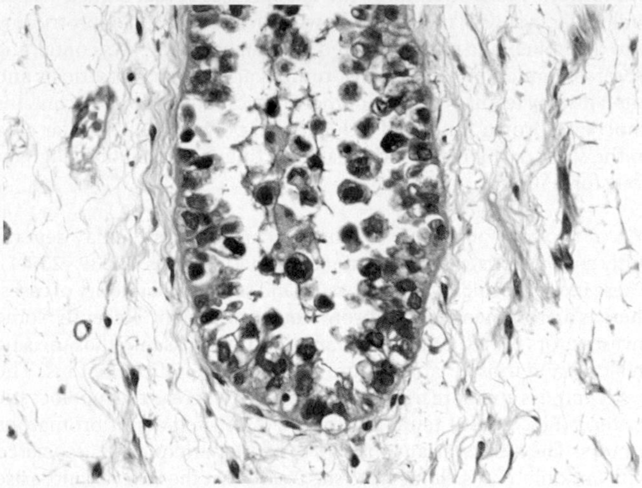

Figure 23.41. Clear cell carcinoma, hobnail pattern, displaying epithelial stratification of markedly atypical cells with clear cytoplasm and snouts protruding into the gland lumen.

papillary pattern is characterized by papillae that are either fibrotic or, more often, hyalinized. In fact, the hyalinized papillary cores are a very characteristic feature of this tumor. The tubulocystic pattern is characterized by varying size tubules and cysts (**Fig. 23.39**). The majority of tumors display combinations of all of these patterns. Despite its name, many of the cells comprising clear cell carcinoma contain eosinophilic cytoplasm with only limited foci of cells with clear cytoplasm. The cells with clear cytoplasm contain glycogen. The nuclei vary from small and rounded and angular to large and pleomorphic with prominent nucleoli (**Fig. 23.41**). Often, the nuclear grade within a tumor varies from mild to markedly atypical. However, at least focally the nuclear grade is nearly always high. Mitotic activity tends to be low, exceeding 10 per 10 HPF in only one-fourth of cases. In the tubulocystic and papillary patterns, the cells often have a hobnail appearance with the nucleus protruding from the papillae, tubule, or cyst, into the lumen (**Fig. 23.41**). Occasionally, the epithelium lining the tubules and cysts is flattened and the nuclear grade is low in these areas, but careful scrutiny will reveal cells with high-grade nuclei elsewhere. Several grading systems have been tested, but none has had consistent and reproducible correlations with prognosis independent of stage. Clear cell carcinoma is considered high-grade in all cases. The distinction of clear cell carcinoma from HGSC and endometrioid carcinoma is occasionally problematic. HNF1β and Napsin A are new immunohistochemical markers that have proved useful in this distinction (328).

Clear cell carcinomas arising in endometriosis are usually cystic and may display atypia of the lining of an endometriotic cyst with either a gradual or abrupt transition to cytologic features of malignancy and invasive clear cell carcinoma. This can be seen in one-third of clear cell carcinomas. If cytologic atypia is marked and invasion is absent, a diagnosis of CCBT with intraepithelial carcinoma is warranted. Cystic clear cell carcinomas are significantly more likely to be associated with endometriosis and atypical endometriosis as compared with the adenofibromatous type (330).

About one-third of reported ovarian clear cell carcinomas are associated with endometriosis either in the involved ovary or elsewhere in the pelvis or abdomen. These figures vary widely and many recent studies have observed 50% or greater associated with endometriosis (229,335). One recent large study found endometriosis to be present in about 90% of cystic clear cell carcinomas, whereas the association of endometriosis with adenofibromatous clear cell carcinomas was only 44% (330). In our experience nearly all ovarian clear cell carcinomas are associated with endometriosis when it is carefully sought, and at least one-third of cases can be demonstrated to have arisen within endometriosis, usually an endometriotic cyst.

Clinical Behavior. There are conflicting data on the behavior of clear cell carcinoma. In some studies, the prognosis appears similar to that for other ovarian carcinomas, but in others, the prognosis is said to be worse. Comprehensively staged ovarian carcinoma (of all histologic types) in FIGO stage I has a 90% or better 5-year survival, and several recent studies have shown comparable survival rates for clear cell carcinoma (335). Evidence that clear cell histology is an adverse prognostic factor in advanced stage is somewhat more convincing. However, recent refinements in the criteria for cell-type assignment suggest that clear cell carcinoma has been overdiagnosed, as a small but significant minority of HGSCs contain clear cells. This misclassification, by removing some HGSCs from the serous group, improves the apparent survival of serous carcinomas by increasing the proportion of the more indolent LGSC (295). The improved survival of serous carcinoma may then appear better than that for clear cell carcinoma, fallaciously supporting the conventional wisdom that the prognosis for clear cell carcinoma is worse than the other cell types (295). The prognostic impact of rupture is controversial. Several studies, including a recent series of 193 patients with stage I clear cell carcinoma in which intraoperative tumor rupture occurred in 36%, have not demonstrated a negative survival impact (334).

Brenner (Transitional Cell) Tumors

Transitional cell tumors comprise 10% of ovarian epithelial tumors. Nearly all of these are benign Brenner tumors; atypical proliferative and malignant forms are very uncommon. The transitional epithelial cell type, characterized by a relatively uniform population of stratified cells with ovoid nuclei displaying nuclear grooves, is named because of its resemblance to urothelium. Evidence suggests that Brenner tumors have some true urothelial differentiation and derive from Walthard nests (336), whereas transitional cell carcinoma (TCC) (unassociated with a benign Brenner component) is a variant of HGSC.

Brenner (Benign Transitional Cell) Tumors

The mean patient age at diagnosis is 56 years. These are common incidental findings and are often microscopic in size. Most tumors are 2 cm or smaller. Multiple microscopic tumors are seen in 17% of patients. Occasionally they are large and may exceed 10 cm. Most tumors are well-circumscribed, firm, and rubbery, with a smooth or slightly bosselated serosal surface. The cut surfaces are typically solid and fibrous, usually gray, white, or yellow, and may be whorled or lobulated; occasionally a cystic component is present.

Microscopically, the characteristic feature is sharply demarcated epithelial nests in a dense fibrous stroma (**Fig. 23.42**). The epithelial

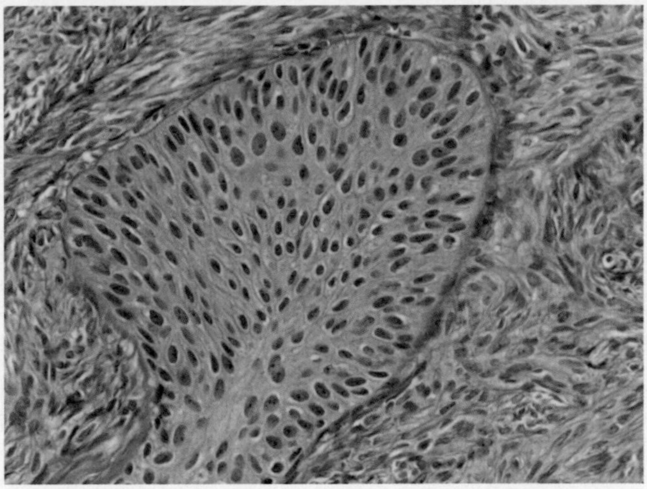

Figure 23.42. Brenner tumor. The transitional cell type is characterized by ovoid to spindled nuclei with prominent nuclear grooves, which resembles urothelium.

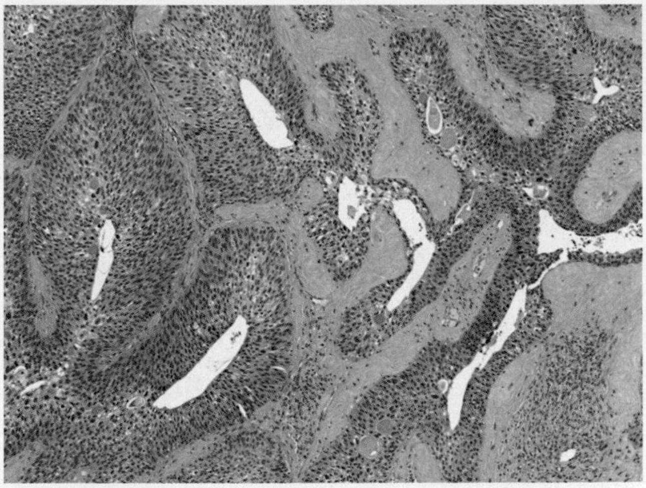

Figure 23.43. Atypical proliferative transitional cell (Brenner) tumor with expansile proliferation of transitional-type epithelium displaying mild to moderate cytologic atypia.

cells are uniform in size with prominent cell borders and pale to eosinophilic cytoplasm. The nuclei are oval and longitudinal grooves are usually present. Atypia and mitotic activity are generally not present. A metaplastic mucinous component may occasionally form the dominant part of the tumor and accounts for the association of Brenner tumors with mucinous cystadenomas. It has been suggested that the majority of nonteratomatous mucinous tumors arise in Brenner tumors as an overgrowth of the mucinous component (337) (see below, Mixed Brenner–mucinous tumors). The stroma varies from closely resembling ovarian cortical stroma to densely fibrous. Hyalinized areas are common, and dystrophic, spiculated calcification is present in about half of the cases. The clinical behavior is benign.

Mixed Brenner–Mucinous Tumors

Tumors containing both Brenner and mucinous components are more common than previously appreciated (**Fig. 23.34**). These are believed to be variants of Brenner tumor and can be classified as metaplastic Brenner tumor or mixed Brenner–mucinous tumor. One-fourth of benign ovarian epithelial tumors that have a mucinous component also contain a Brenner component. Conversely, 16% of tumors with a Brenner component contain a mucinous component. These patients are significantly older than those with pure mucinous or pure Brenner tumor, with a mean age of 68 years. They are unilateral and most often have discrete Brenner and mucinous components, but in 30% the components are admixed. The other clinical and pathologic features are similar to their pure counterparts (337). A recent study showed that the mucinous and Brenner components of the mixed tumors are monoclonal (338).

Atypical Proliferative Brenner (Transitional Cell) Tumors

These rare neoplasms, also termed "atypical proliferative" or "borderline" transitional cell or Brenner tumor, or transitional cell or Brenner tumor "of low malignant potential," present in patients whose mean age is 59 years. They are always unilateral and confined to the ovary. They are much larger than their benign counterparts, are usually cystic, and measure 10 to 28 cm with a mean diameter of 18 cm. Papillary or polypoid masses project into the cyst lumens, and there is usually a benign Brenner component present with a solid and fibrous cut surface. Microscopically, the intracystic papillary component is composed of transitional-type epithelium resembling low-grade noninvasive papillary transitional cell neoplasms of the urinary tract. Mucinous metaplasia may be present in the epithelium lining the papillae. Underneath the papillae and within the wall there may be solid areas of transitional epithelium with little intervening stroma (**Fig. 23.43**). Nearly all cases display areas of benign transitional cell neoplasm. The cytologic features are similar to those in benign transitional cell tumors, but occasionally significant atypia and mitotic activity are present. Among over 50 reported cases of atypical proliferative transitional cell tumors, there has been one local recurrence and no convincing evidence of malignant behavior. Accordingly, the term, "atypical proliferative transitional cell (Brenner) tumor" is preferred.

Malignant Transitional Cell Tumors (Malignant Brenner Tumors and High-Grade Serous Carcinomas with Transitional-Like Features (Transitional-Like Variant of HGSC [TV-HGSC])

High-grade serous carcinomas may have focal areas that display features resembling TCC. Nearly all tumors that have historically been classified as ovarian TCCs are now regarded as HGSCs with transitional-like features by most experts (339). Only about 3% of advanced-stage serous carcinoma were classifiable as TCC based on the predominant pattern. Accordingly, the only true malignant transitional cell tumors of the ovary are malignant Brenner tumors, in which a benign or atypical proliferative Brenner component is identified.

Clinical and Operative Findings. Malignant Brenner tumors comprise 1% of ovarian carcinomas and occur at a mean age of 63 years. The size of malignant Brenner tumors ranges up to 25 cm with a mean diameter of 14 cm. Among stage I tumors, 16% are bilateral. The stage distribution is as follows: stage I, 64%; stage II, 12%; stage III 18%; stage IV, 6%.

Gross Findings. In the malignant Brenner tumor, the benign Brenner component may be identifiable as a solid fibrous nodule within a cyst wall. Sometimes malignant Brenner tumor is completely solid. TV-HGSCs have the gross features of HGSC.

Microscopic Findings. A diagnosis of malignant Brenner tumor is only warranted when a benign or atypical proliferative Brenner component is identified within or is contiguous with the tumor. The characteristic microscopic feature of MBT is thick, blunt, and often elongated papillary folds with fibrovascular cores, lined by transitional-type epithelium resembling urothelium. The papillae often appear to arise from a cyst wall with a similar lining of stratified and atypical transitional cells. A solid pattern is present in about half the cases. Stromal invasion is present and characterized by haphazard infiltrative growth of epithelium at the base of the papillae into the cyst

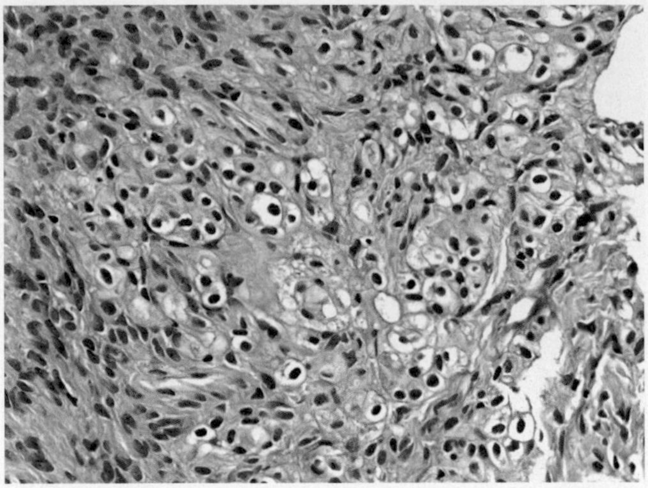

Figure 23.44. Malignant Brenner tumor characterized by small variably sized nests of transitional-type cells with an infiltrative pattern.

wall or extensive areas of solid epithelial proliferation with scant or no fibrovascular support. Another architectural pattern of malignant Brenner tumor is characterized by a solid tumor resembling benign Brenner tumor but the epithelial nests are more angulated and have a disorderly growth pattern which appears invasive (**Fig. 23.44**). In our experience, this latter pattern is the most common pattern of malignant Brenner tumor.

In TV-HGSC, cytologic atypia is prominent. High-grade pleomorphic nuclear features and bizarre giant cells occur in about one-third. MBTs, like their benign counterparts, often have prominent stromal calcification which is usually spiculated, in contrast to TV-HGSC in which calcification is less common and more often psammomatous as in serous carcinomas.

Clinical Behavior. TV-HGSC is clinically different from malignant Brenner tumor. TV-HGSC presents in advanced stage, whereas most malignant Brenner tumors present in stage I. TV-HGSC is a variant of HGSC and thus is a type II tumor. This is supported by similar clinical and pathologic features between these two types of ovarian carcinoma and an immunophenotype that more closely resembles serous carcinoma rather than TCC of the urinary tract. In contrast, malignant Brenner tumor has features of a type I tumor (see Pathogenesis, earlier in this chapter).

Squamous Tumors

Epidermoid cysts comprise 1.4% of ovarian epithelial tumors. They are lined by squamous epithelium and lack teratomatous elements. Pure invasive squamous cell carcinoma is very rare, comprising 0.4% of ovarian carcinomas. In a series of 18 cases, endometriosis was found in 7 cases, and no underlying lesion was found in 11 cases. Invasive squamous cell carcinoma in the ovary is most commonly because of malignant transformation of a mature cystic teratoma; in such cases, the tumor is classified as a germ cell tumor with malignant transformation. Rarely, metastatic disease from the uterine cervix is the source of squamous cell carcinoma in the ovary.

The majority of patients with primary ovarian squamous cell carcinoma present with advanced-stage disease and die within 1 year. Although data are limited, this entity appears to confer a significantly worse prognosis than either HGSC or squamous cell carcinoma arising in a mature cystic teratoma.

Mixed Epithelial Tumors

The presence of two epithelial cell types in an ovarian epithelial neoplasm, each comprising at least 10% of the tumor, warrants a designation of a mixed epithelial tumor. Nonetheless, many experts prefer to ignore the minor components and classify tumors based solely on the predominant component, unless the minor component is invasive/malignant in an otherwise benign tumor or is of a higher grade than the remainder of the tumor. Poorly differentiated serous and endometrioid carcinomas often display overlapping features, and at times, assignment to one or the other group is arbitrary and varies among observers. As discussed earlier, it is believed that there is no clinical or molecular basis for separating high-grade serous and endometrioid carcinomas. Experts believe that most of these tumors are preferably classified as serous, reserving the endometrioid designation for those tumors that display easily recognizable and characteristic features of eutopic endometrioid adenocarcinomas. Similarly, endometrioid and clear cell differentiation are not infrequently mixed. A mucinous component is often observed in benign transitional cell neoplasms (see above, mixed transitional cell-mucinous tumors). When carefully reviewed and classified based on current criteria, bona fide mixed cell types of ovarian carcinomas comprise less than 1% of cases (340).

Undifferentiated Carcinoma

Undifferentiated carcinomas show no readily identifiable features of any of the cell types of ovarian surface epithelial neoplasms. Therefore, any element of glands, papillae, or psammoma bodies removes a tumor from this category. Solid carcinomas with rare foci of glands or papillae are preferably classified as serous, although a few experts include such tumors in the undifferentiated category.

There are four types of primary ovarian undifferentiated carcinoma, referred to as follows: undifferentiated carcinoma not otherwise specified (NOS), non-small-cell neuroendocrine carcinoma, the hypercalcemic type of small cell carcinoma, and the pulmonary type of small cell carcinoma. When strict pathologic criteria are employed for these diagnoses, all types are very rare, together comprising less than 1% of invasive carcinomas. In our series of 562 carcinomas (**Table 23.10**), there were two cases (0.4%) of undifferentiated small cell carcinoma. In all cases when a diagnosis of undifferentiated carcinoma is considered, it is very important to exclude metastatic tumor, particularly from the lungs.

Although data are limited, undifferentiated carcinoma NOS appears to be more common than the other three types. The usual type of undifferentiated carcinoma NOS shares most clinical and pathologic features with HGSC and therefore is probably a variant of this type. The mean age at presentation is 60 years and nearly all present in stages III and IV. Tumors are composed of solid sheets of large pleomorphic cells with high-grade nuclear features, and usually with abundant cytoplasm that is often eosinophilic. Overall, 22% survive 5 years, but only 14% of patients with stage III and IV disease survive 5 years. Although OS appears somewhat worse than that for serous carcinoma, data on this rare tumor are quite limited and when stratified by stage, patients with undifferentiated carcinoma do not have a significantly worse prognosis that those with HGSC.

Non-small-cell neuroendocrine carcinoma is usually associated with another cell type of surface epithelial carcinoma, most often mucinous carcinoma, and therefore is best classified according to the better-differentiated component. Undifferentiated small cell carcinoma associated with hypercalcemia, which is also referred to as malignant rhabdoid tumor of the ovary, is a distinctive neoplasm occurring in young women with a mean age of 23. The characteristic microscopic pattern displays sheets of small cells with interspersed follicle-like spaces. It is associated with a poor prognosis. Genomically, it is characterized by deleterious germ line or somatic mutations in a single gene, *SMARCA4*, in almost all cases (341).

Malignant Mixed Mesodermal Tumor (Carcinosarcoma)

Although previously thought to be rare, carcinosarcomas comprise about 6% of ovarian carcinomas in the United States (**Table 23.10**) and 2.5% in Thailand (342). The mean age at diagnosis, 66 years, is slightly higher than that for HGSC. These tumors are typically large, ranging from 15 to 20 cm in diameter. The stage distribution is identical to that of HGSC. The morphology is similar to its uterine counterpart. The characteristic microscopic feature is an intimate admixture of malignant epithelial and stromal elements. The malignant epithelial element is most commonly a HGSC, but can be of any of the surface epithelial cell types of ovarian tumors. The stromal component usually contains sheets of hyperchromatic rounded to spindled cells with marked nuclear atypia and a high mitotic index. Heterologous elements, most commonly cartilage, osteoid, and rhabdomyoblasts, are commonly found and, as in the uterine counterpart, their frequency depends on the diligence with which they are sought. Occasionally, a tumor that is otherwise a typical carcinoma has a small focus of malignant stroma. Although there are few published data on such tumors, they are classified as MMMTs. Immunohistochemical stains for epithelial markers are often positive in the sarcomatous component, and their behavior and patterns of spread are similar to HGSCs. Like endometrial carcinosarcomas, the majority have been demonstrated to be monoclonal. These observations indicate that these tumors should be classified as metaplastic carcinomas like their uterine counterparts, and accordingly represent a type II tumor (see Pathogenesis, earlier in this chapter). In the older literature, MMMTs were considered aggressive, rapidly fatal tumors with a median survival of approximately 1 year, but more recent data suggest that with cisplatin and either a taxane or ifosfamide therapy, survival rates approaching those for serous carcinoma can be achieved (343). When stratified by stage, some studies, including a large SEER analysis have shown that the disease-specific survival is worse than that for HGSC (344). In the latter study, the 5-year survival for stage III was 24% as compared with 39% for HGSC. Most but not all studies have shown that, like their uterine counterpart, the presence of heterologous elements does not influence prognosis.

Sarcomas

Although primary pure or mixed sarcomas of the ovary are very uncommon, they constitute a heterogeneous group with four different types of neoplasms: endometrioid stromal sarcoma, adenosarcoma, sarcoma arising in a mature teratoma, and miscellaneous soft tissue sarcomas. Most carcinosarcomas are no longer considered sarcomas (see Malignant mixed mesodermal tumors, above). All of these tumors are extremely rare. Sarcomas arising in teratomas are classified as germ cell tumors with secondary malignant transformation.

Endometrial Stromal Sarcoma

Endometrioid stromal sarcoma (ESS; comprising the group of tumors formerly known as low-grade endometrial sarcoma) is an extremely rare primary ovarian neoplasm that is morphologically identical to its uterine counterpart. Among approximately 27 reported cases, 63% have been closely associated with endometriosis from which the tumor probably arises. The mean patient age is 52 years. The mean tumor size is 10 cm. Over 70% present in advanced-stage (FIGO II–III). As primary uterine ESS is often slow growing and prone to late recurrence, it is important to consider the possibility of metastatic tumor from a uterine primary, even if the patient has had a hysterectomy in the remote past. The behavior appears to parallel that of advanced-stage uterine ESS, although data are limited.

Müllerian Adenosarcoma and "Aggressive Endometriosis"

Müllerian adenosarcoma of the ovary is very rare. It is morphologically similar to its uterine counterpart. Nearly 60 cases have been reported (345). The mean age is 54 years and the mean tumor size is 14 cm. Sixty-five percent present in FIGO stage I. Nearly all cases are unilateral. Grossly, the majority are predominantly solid with some cystic areas, and 10% are predominantly cystic. The characteristic microscopic feature is periglandular stromal condensation with atypia and mitotic activity in these hypercellular areas of stroma. Leaflike processes of stroma covered by a single layer of benign epithelium is another characteristic pattern. About 30% have sarcomatous overgrowth. In the largest series (345), among 40 cases, 9 tumors were considered high-grade (moderate or severe atypia and/or 10 or more mitoses per 10 HPF in the most active areas) and 31 were low-grade. Sixty-three percent of stage I tumors recurred. The 5-year recurrence-free survival was 45% for women with low-grade stage I disease and 25% for women with high-grade stage I disease. The overall 5-year survival is about 65%.

Rarely, histologically benign endometriosis appears infiltrative to the surgeon and/or displays perineural and vascular invasion. The stroma can be cellular but there is no atypia and mitotic activity is very low. It can prove difficult to resect and consequently may display low-grade malignant behavior. This may be a form of low-grade adenosarcoma and has been referred to as "aggressive endometriosis." It has also been suggested that these are low-grade endometrial stromal sarcomas with endometrioid glandular differentiation. There are no large series of this entity and it is therefore poorly understood.

Tumors of the Fallopian Tubes

Benign Tumors

The most common benign tumor of the fallopian tube is adenomatoid tumor, also referred to as benign mesothelioma because of its histogenesis which is now known to be mesothelial. These are nearly always incidental findings, typically 1 to 2 cm and often microscopic, and within the myosalpinx. They are firm and yellowish on cut section. Microscopically they display interanastomosing tubules and glands with no atypia or mitotic activity. The cytoplasm is eosinophilic and vacuolated. Of note, a small biopsy of a diffuse malignant mesothelioma can have an identical histologic appearance. This is of little practical concern, as peritoneal mesotheliomas in women are exceedingly rare; we diagnosed 2 malignant peritoneal mesotheliomas during the same period as our consecutive series of 562 ovarian carcinomas over a 22-year period.

The tubal mucosa rarely gives rise to benign papillomas, SBTs, and so-called metaplastic papillary tumor of pregnancy. The myosalpinx, as it is composed of smooth muscle, occasionally gives rise to leiomyomas. Occasional examples of tubal adenomyomas probably represent endometriosis with prominent smooth muscle proliferation. The peritoneal-lined serosal surface, in addition to adenomatoid tumor (see above), also may produce mesothelial/peritoneal cysts. When a mesothelial cyst is multiloculated, the pathologist may consider the possibility of so-called multicystic mesothelioma. However, this latter entity is exceedingly rare and probably not truly neoplastic. A diagnosis of cystic adhesions or multiloculated mesothelial/peritoneal cyst is most appropriate.

Female adnexal tumor of probable Wolffian origin (FATWO) is a rare epithelial neoplasm that is usually found within the broad ligament and probably arises paratubally from mesonephric remnants. It is generally benign; however, it may recur. Several late recurrences and rare fatalities have been reported.

Malignant Tumors

High-Grade Serous Carcinoma. The most common tubal malignancy is HGSC, which is clinically and pathologically identical to HGSC of the ovary and peritoneum. Until recently, carcinoma of the fallopian tube was thought to be rare, comprising less than 1% of gynecologic malignancies. Over the past decade, evidence has been accumulating that a significant proportion of apparent ovarian and peritoneal HGSCs are associated with STIC. Serous tubal intraepithelial carcinoma (STIC) is usually fimbrial and is now felt by most experts to be the source of a majority of these tumors. This is discussed in greater detail earlier in this chapter (see Pathogenesis; and High-grade serous carcinoma).

There are very rare reports of clear cell and endometrioid carcinomas of the fallopian tube. Because these tumors, when ovarian, arise in endometriosis, tubal examples presumably arise in endometriosis as well. Several studies have shown that STIC is specifically associated with serous carcinomas (296,346), so that a tubal epithelial origin of clear cell or endometrioid carcinoma is unlikely.

Tubal carcinosarcomas (malignant mixed Müllerian tumors) rarely occur and are classified as variants of HGSC like their ovarian counterparts. Other types of sarcoma are exceedingly rare.

PROGNOSTIC FACTORS

Universally accepted prognostic factors for patients with ovarian cancer are stage, which reflects a combination of tumor size and disease distribution, and, in patients with stage III and IV disease, volume of residual disease after surgical cytoreduction.

Tumor Stage

The ovarian cancer staging system (**Table 23.6**) was updated in 2014. There will remain variability in survival for patients with the same stage, reflecting both the variability in completeness of staging (particularly for early-stage disease) and the variable biology of different histologic subtypes of ovarian cancer. SEER data from 1999 to 2007 show a 5-year relative survival of 89% for patients with stage I disease, 70% for those with stage II disease, 36% for those with stage III disease, and 17% for those with stage IV disease. Ten-year relative survival rates decrease to 84%, 59%, 23%, and 8%, respectively (347) (**Fig. 23.45**).

Age

Older women have a much worse prognosis. For example, SEER data show that women over the age of 75 with stage III disease have a 5-year relative survival of 21% versus 41% for those aged 50 to 64 years. This is in part because they have an increased incidence of high-stage and high-grade disease at the time of diagnosis (**Table 23.13**) (348). Moreover they may be less able to tolerate aggressive therapy. However, in an analysis of the SEER database, age remained a poor prognostic factor even when results were adjusted for stage, grade, histologic cell type, race, and surgical treatment. A German study found that during the period 1979 to 2003 there was a strong trend of improving survival for all ovarian cancer patients except those aged 75 years and older (349).

Prognostic Variables in Early-Stage Disease

About one-quarter of patients present with stage I or II epithelial ovarian cancer (**Table 23.10**) Prognostic factors are particularly important in stage I disease because chemotherapy can be withheld for the subsets with best prognosis (**Fig. 23.46**). A multivariable analysis of prognostic factors for recurrence in two GOG chemotherapy trials of surgically staged women with "high-risk early-stage" disease (IA/B grade 3, stage IC or II any grade, stage I or II clear cell), GOG #95 and GOG #157, identified four independent predictors of worse prognosis: age > 60 years (HR, 1.57), stage II (HR, 2.7 vs. stage IA or IB), grade 2 (HR, 1.84 vs. grade 1) or grade 3 (HR, 2.47 vs. grade 1), and positive cytology (HR, 1.72) (350).

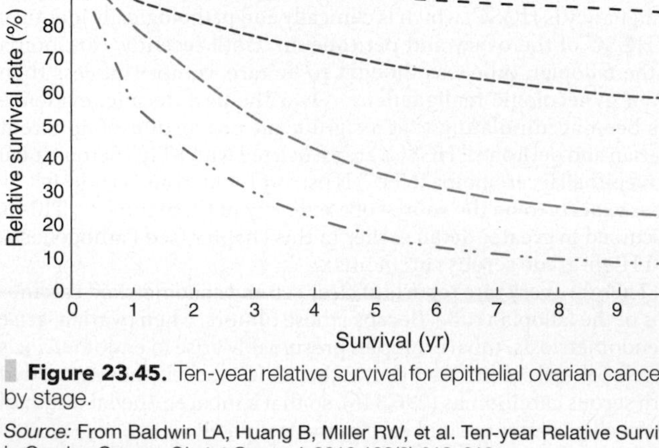

Figure 23.45. Ten-year relative survival for epithelial ovarian cancer by stage.

Source: From Baldwin LA, Huang B, Miller RW, et al. Ten-year Relative Survival in Ovarian Cancer. *Obstet Gynecol.* 2012;120(3):612–618.

TABLE 23.13. SEER Data 1975 to 2001

Incidence of Stage by Age Group				
Age group (*n*)		**n Stage I (%)**	**n Stage II (%)**	**n Stage III–IV (%)**
<20	(628)	388 (62)	46 (7)	194 (31)
20–49	(10,243)	4,340 (42)	773 (8)	5,130 (50)
50–59	(10,788)	2,830 (26)	833 (8)	7, 125 (66)
60–69	(12,201)	2,162 (18)	767(6)	9,272 (76)
70–79	(10,259)	1,409 (14)	636 (6)	8,214 (80)
80+	(3,813)	707 (12)	389 (69)	4,717 (81)
Total	47,932	11,836 (24.6)	3,444 (7.2)	34,652 (72.3)
5-year relative survival by age group and stage				
20–49		0.93	0.87	0.38
50–59		0.91	0.68	0.31
60–69		0.94	0.61	0.23
70–79		0.77	0.51	0.14
80+		0.69	0.11	0.03

Source: Adapted from Wright JD, Chen L, Tergas AI, et al. Trends in Relative Survival for Ovarian Cancer from 1975 to 2011. *Obstet Gynecol.* 2015;125(6):1345–1352.

Histologic Subtype

The distribution of cell types in early-stage disease is very different from the distribution in advanced-stage disease. Most advanced-stage cancers are of high-grade serous histology, whereas less than a quarter of early-stage cancers are serous. Endometrioid and clear cell cancers tend to present at an early stage. (**Table 23.10**) Serous histology has been reported to be a poor prognostic factor in stage I disease, especially in patients who have not been comprehensively staged (351). From 4% to 25% of patients with apparent stage I ovarian cancer will have nodal involvement when lymph nodes are pathologically examined; the risk for lymph node involvement correlates with histology (high risk with high-grade serous and clear cell tumors) and grade (higher risk with higher grade).

Stage I clear cell carcinoma was historically believed to be associated with a worse outcome than other stage I cell types. However, several large series have not confirmed this (331,350,351). Advanced-stage clear cell carcinoma, as discussed below, does have a poor prognosis. Although patients with advanced-stage mucinous tumors also fare poorly, stage I mucinous tumors are generally low grade and have a good prognosis.

In reading older series regarding the importance of tumor histology it should be remembered that diagnostic criteria for the major cell types of ovarian carcinoma have undergone significant shifts over the past two decades. Serous carcinomas have been more clearly distinguished from endometrioid and clear cell carcinomas with which they have often been confused and serous carcinoma has been divided into two distinct groups, the more common high grade and the less common low grade, which are no longer considered different grades of the same tumor, but rather biologically different cell types.

Grade

Analyzing tumor grade as a prognostic factor in general in stage I disease is problematic because of the interplay between histologic subtype and grade and because of issues with reproducibility of grade. Three of the five types of carcinomas, HGSC, LGSC, and clear cell carcinoma, already have a designated grade by definition. In studies

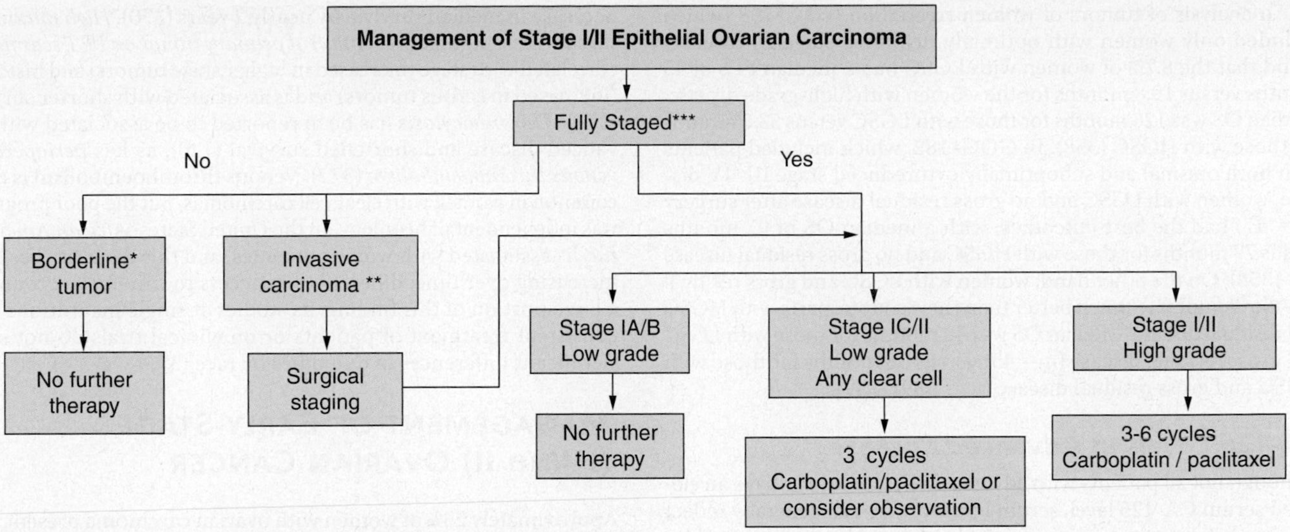

Figure 23.46. Management of stage I/II epithelial ovarian carcinoma.

*For unstaged borderline tumors that have intraepithelial carcinoma, micropapillary architecture > 5 mm, or microinvasion, may consider staging using a mimally invasive approach.

**Some data suggest that the risk of nodal metastatses in grade 1 mucinous tumors is low enough that further staging is not warranted; in some situations, uterus and contralateral ovary may be preserved.

***Full staging includes removal of the affected ovary and tube, omentectomy, LND, possible appendectomy.

that do not separately analyze tumors by cell type, grade is associated not only with the likelihood of lymph node involvement in apparent stage I disease, but with the likelihood of recurrence in fully staged patients with stage I disease. Once cell type is determined, grade adds information primarily for endometrioid and mucinous cell types. From FIGO data for surgically staged stage I disease (352) the overall 5-year survivals are 92%, 85%, and 79% for grade 1, 2, and 3 tumors, respectively. Stage IA and IB grade 1 carcinomas have disease-specific survival rates as high as 97% in the absence of any adjuvant therapy.

Surgical Prognostic Factors in Early-Stage Disease

Malignant ascites is associated with worse outcomes and is incorporated into stage. Although capsular rupture should be avoided where possible, the data on the prognostic significance of capsular rupture are conflicting, likely because there are several confounding variables including time of rupture (preoperative vs. intraoperative) and cause of rupture (spontaneous vs. iatrogenic). The new staging system separates out these categories, which were previously all lumped together as stage IC. Tumor size is not prognostic in stage I disease; low-grade early-stage tumors may be very large. Uncertainty remains regarding adhesions. No problem regarding staging exists when the surgeon encounters discrete implants separate from the primary tumor or when solid tumor is found invading adjacent structures. However, more often there is apparently benign adherence of an ovarian tumor to adjacent structures in the absence of metastatic implants or obvious direct tumor extension. Older literature suggests that such "benign" adhesions, when dense, are associated with a relapse risk equivalent to stage II (353). Adherence is judged to be dense when so described by the surgeon, when sharp dissection was required to mobilize the tumor, when a raw area was left in the place of adherence, or when cyst rupture resulted from dissecting the adhesions free. However, a review of more recent data (354) failed to identify dense adhesions as an independent prognostic factor.

CA-125 Levels in Early-Stage Disease

A report analyzing data from 600 surgically staged (including lymphadenectomy) FIGO stage I epithelial ovarian cancer patients found preoperative serum CA-125 ≥30 U/mL to be an independent predictor of decreased survival (HR, 2.7). Clear cell and mucinous tumors had somewhat lower preoperative CA-125 levels. The only independent predictive factor other than CA-125 was age greater than 70 years (HR, 2.6) (355).

Prognostic Variables in Stage III/IV Disease

Volume of Residual Disease after Surgery

As discussed more extensively in above in the section on Surgery, the volume of residual disease following cytoreduction surgery is consistently and directly correlated with survival for both stage III and stage IV disease (**Fig. 23.18**). Most series have focused on the size of the largest residual mass, and not the total number of lesions, but the number of residual masses may be an important prognostic factor as well. There is, of course, a correlation between volume of disease before surgery and residual disease remaining after surgery. Although patients with stage IIIC disease who are without residual disease after surgery do better than patients with stage IIIC disease that have macroscopic residual disease, they still have a significantly worse prognosis than patients with stage IIIA disease (who are more likely to have low-grade tumors).

Histologic Subtype and Grade in Advanced Disease

In advanced-stage disease, mucinous and clear cell histologies are associated with a significantly worse prognosis, likely because of chemotherapy resistance. Advanced-stage endometrioid tumors are associated with a better prognosis than advanced-stage serous tumors. One retrospective series which included patients with stages IIC–IV disease treated with paclitaxel/platinum following cytoreduction surgery showed a median OS of 121 months for low-grade serous tumors, 64 months for endometrioid tumors, 29 months for clear cell tumors, 15 months for mucinous tumors, and 45 months for a category including high-grade serous, unspecified, and undifferentiated carcinomas (356). The prognostic importance of histology holds even in stage IV disease: A study from Japan reported that women with serous or endometrioid tumors had a median OS of 3.1 years versus 0.9 years for those with clear cell or mucinous tumors (357).

It must be remembered that grade, cell type, and stage are confounded: As noted earlier, the grade is contained in the definition of three of the five cell types of ovarian carcinoma. LGSC is more likely to be stage IIIA or IIIB as compared with HGSC, which nearly always presents as stage IIIC disease. In addition, low-grade serous tumors occur in younger women who tend to have less comorbidity (295).

An analysis of tumors of women treated on GOG#158 (which included only women with optimally debulked stage III disease) found that the 8.7% of women with LGSC had a median PFS of 45 months versus 19.8 months for the women with high-grade disease. Median OS was 126 months for those with LGSC versus 53.8 months for those with HGSC (358). In GOG#182, which included patients with both optimal and suboptimally cytoreduced stage III–IV disease, women with LGSC and no gross residual disease after surgery ($n = 47$) had the best outcomes, with a median OS of 97 months versus 77 months for those with HGSC and no gross residual disease ($n = 358$). On the other hand, women with LGSC and gross residual disease did not fare much better than their counterparts with HGSC and residual disease. Median OS was 42 months for those with LGSC and gross residual disease ($n = 45$) versus 38 months for those with HGSC and gross residual disease ($n = 539$) (359).

CA-125 Levels in Advanced Disease

Although not all patients with advanced ovarian cancer have an elevated serum CA-125 level, serum levels of CA-125 generally reflect volume of disease in women with initially elevated levels. Postoperative (pre-chemotherapy) CA-125 levels have prognostic significance. Decline of CA-125 with chemotherapy is also prognostic. In one study, normalization of CA-125 (level less than 35 U/mL) after the third cycle of treatment was associated with a median OS of 42 months compared with a median survival of 22 months for those whose CA-125 did not normalize. This association held true even within the subgroup of optimal microscopically debulked patients (360).

Genomic Prognostic Factors

BRCA1 and *BRCA2* mutations are associated with both a higher response rate to platinum-based therapies and improved PFS. *BRCA2* mutation carriers appear to have longer survival than *BRCA1* mutation carriers. Some recent analyses suggest that although short-term outcomes are better for mutation carriers, long-term outcomes (10-year) may not be better than average, perhaps reflecting early chemotherapy sensitivity and high rates of eventual recurrence (55,266,361). It is not only *BRCA* mutation carriers whose tumors are more sensitive to platinum agents (and PARP inhibitors); approximately 50% of ovarian cancers have defective homologous DNA repair, and there is widespread ongoing effort to develop a robust biomarker that captures this "BRCAness" and can be used on formalin-fixed paraffin-embedded (FFPE) tissue (362). *BRCA1/2* mutated ovarian cancers harbor significantly increased CD3+ and CD8+ tumor-infiltrating lymphocytes (TILS), and *number of TILS* is independently associated with good outcome (363). Interestingly, tumors with epigenetic silencing of *BRCA1* through promoter hypermethylation do not appear to have any survival advantage. *Somatic mutations in the ADAMTS gene family* (found in 10% of high-grade serous cases) have been found to be significantly associated with a higher genomic-wide mutation rate, better response rate to chemotherapy, and longer PFS and OS (364). *CCNE1 amplification* has been associated with primary chemotherapy-resistant disease and poor outcomes (365). Multiple *genomic expression profiles* with prognostic significance are being developed, but none have yet come into clinical use (263). For example, one publication identified three prognostic groups among high-grade tumors treated with platinum/taxane therapy: The two poor prognostic groups were characterized by increased hypermethylation and stroma-related genes (366).

Other Prognostic Factors

Poor performance status and an increased number of patient-reported symptoms, particularly lower extremity edema, are associated with worse outcomes (367). Increased BMI at the time of diagnosis has not been associated with increased mortality in most studies (368), but a *prediagnosis history of vigorous exercise* was shown in the WHI to be associated with a 26% lower risk of ovarian cancer-specific mortality (369). *Perioperative infection* has been reported to be an independent risk factor for poor outcomes, with an associated decrease in median survival by nearly 2 years (370). *High maximum standardized uptake (SUVmax) of primary tumor on PET scanning* is correlated with stage (increased in higher stage tumors) and histology (increased in serous tumors) and is associated with shorter survival (371). *Thrombocytosis* has been reported to be associated with advanced disease and shortened survival (120), as has *perioperative venous thromboembolism* (372). Venous thromboembolism is more common in women with clear cell carcinomas, but the poor prognosis was independent of histology. In the United States, *African American race* is associated with worse outcomes, and this disparity has been increasing over time; differences in access to care may account for a large portion of this finding, as studies at single institutions with consistent treatment of patients or on clinical trials do not show significant differences in outcomes by race (373).

MANAGEMENT OF EARLY-STAGE (I AND II) OVARIAN CANCER

Approximately 25% of women with ovarian carcinoma present with stage I or II disease. An algorithm for standard management of early-stage disease is shown in **Figure 23.46**. Unlike advanced-stage ovarian cancers, which are usually HGSC, early-stage tumors are more often of mucinous, clear cell, or endometrioid histology (**Table 23.10**).

Surgical Therapy for Early-Stage Ovarian Carcinoma

Surgery will be curative for most patients with stage I ovarian cancer. The optimal surgical procedure for most epithelial ovarian carcinomas is removal of the uterus along with both fallopian tubes and ovaries and complete surgical staging. This is discussed in more detail in the section on Surgery. There are situations in which full staging is not possible or not always needed, such as incompletely staged borderline ovarian carcinomas, grade 1 mucinous tumors, and patients who desire fertility preservation (374). The general advantage of surgical staging in early ovarian cancer is that chemotherapy can sometimes be omitted in a fully staged patient with stage IA or IB disease.

Fertility Preservation

In the younger patient who wishes to retain her childbearing potential and who appears to have a curable cancer (particularly a localized tumor with mucinous, endometrioid, or low-grade serous histology), it is appropriate to preserve the uterus and the contralateral ovary. Any abnormalities in the remaining ovary should be biopsied during surgery and sent for expert frozen section. If the frozen section is ambiguous as to whether the tumor is benign, borderline, or malignant, or if there is doubt about the extent of the disease, final pathology should be awaited and a two-step surgical approach employed. If both ovaries contain invasive tumor on frozen section ovarian preservation is usually not indicated. In rare cases a small implant can be removed using a wedge resection.

Recommendations **(375):**
Stage IA, GI + II, serous, mucinous, endometrioid → Fertility sparing surgery
FIGO IA, clear cell cancer → Consider fertility sparing surgery
FIGO IC, GI + II, serous, mucinous, endometrioid → Consider fertility sparing surgery
FIGO IC, clear cell cancer → No fertility sparing surgery
FIGO IA + IC, GIII→ No fertility sparing surgery

Postoperative Therapy for Stage I Ovarian Carcinoma

Patients with stage IA and IB grade 1 carcinomas have disease-specific survival rates as high as 97% in the absence of any postoperative therapy. Early GOG trials showed that overall patients with stage IA or IB and grade 1 or 2 disease had a 5-year disease-free survival rate (DFS) of 91% and a 5-year OS rate of 94% with surgery alone (376).

Other patients with early-stage disease are considered to have a risk of recurrence high enough to warrant adjuvant therapy. However, the benefit of such treatment has been difficult to prove because the number of patients with higher grade early-stage disease is small (so trials are difficult to complete) and the overall risk of recurrence is not that great (so large trials are needed). Published trials have included multiple histologic types with very different biology and variable staging and generally have lacked the power to show interactions between treatment and grade or histologic subtype. In addition, treatment at recurrence may be curative for a small number of patients who did not receive initial adjuvant treatment.

Radiotherapy for Early-Stage Ovarian Cancer

External Beam Therapy

In the past radiation therapy was used extensively for curative and adjuvant management of low stage and low residual volume ovarian carcinoma of all tumor subtypes. This treatment was largely abandoned in the 1980s with the advent of cisplatin-based therapies. It has been suggested that this should be reconsidered, particularly for nonserous histologies (377). Swenerton et al. performed a population-based non-randomized retrospective cohort review of 703 women from Canada with no macroscopic residual disease after surgery who underwent platinum-based chemotherapy with or without sequential abdominopelvic radiotherapy. Among women with stage I or stage II clear cell, endometrioid, or mucinous histology, the addition of radiotherapy was associated with a 43% decrease in overall mortality (378). No benefit was seen for those with stage III disease or tumors of serous histology. The most common late side effect was chronic GI toxicity, with 41/351 women having chronic grade 2 or higher GI toxicity. A subsequent analysis from the same group looked only at clear cell carcinomas and suggested a benefit specifically for stage IC and stage II disease (379). Given that clear cell carcinomas are often confined to the pelvis, it seems possible that similar benefit and less toxicity could be seen with pelvic radiotherapy alone rather than abdominopelvic radiotherapy for this histologic subgroup, and hopefully future trials will address this issue.

Radiocolloid Therapy

As transcoelomic spread is the main route of dissemination of ovarian cancer, the intraperitoneal instillation of radiocolloids, which deliver high doses of radiation to the peritoneal surfaces, was historically used for early-stage disease. Intraperitoneal ^{32}P, which penetrates only 2 to 3 mm, was the isotope most commonly administered. Therapy was abandoned when randomized data suggested better results with chemotherapy. In addition, a randomized comparison of ^{32}P versus observation did not show any decrease in the risk of relapse or improve survival in patients with more advanced-stage disease who had a surgically confirmed complete remission (380).

Chemotherapy for Early-Stage Ovarian Cancer

As shown in **Figure 23.46**, postoperative chemotherapy is usually recommended for patients with high-grade stage IA or IB tumors and most tumors of stage IC or higher. But it must be appreciated that we do not have good evidence that such treatment improves OS. Randomized trials including platinum-based chemotherapy in early-stage ovarian cancer are summarized in **Table 23.14**. Most are

TABLE 23.14. Randomized Trials of Platinum-Based Chemotherapy in Early-Stage Ovarian Carcinoma

Author (Year)	N	Eligibility	Arms	Outcome
Vergote (1992)	347	Stage I, II, III without residual disease	^{32}P vs. cisplatin	No difference in OS or DFS
Chiara (1994)	70	Stage IA/B Gr 3, any IC, II	WAR vs. cisplatin/cyclophosphamide	5-year OS 53% vs. 71% RFS 50% vs. 74% p = NS
				Only 67% of patients completed WAR
Bolis (1995)	83	Stage IA/B Gr 2/3	Observation vs. cisplatin	5-year DFS 65% vs. 83%
				5-year OS 82% vs. 88%
Bolis (1995)	152	Stage IC	^{32}P vs. cisplatin	5-year DFS 65% vs. 85%
				5-year OS 79% vs. 81%
Trope (2000)	162	Stage I Gr 2/3 or Gr 1 aneuploid/clear cell	Observation vs. carboplatin	5-year DFS 80% vs. 85%
				5-year OS 70% vs. 71% p = NS
Young (2003)	251	Stage IA/B Gr 3 or clear cell IC, II	^{32}P vs. cisplatin/cyclophosphamide	10-year RFS 65% vs. 72% 10-year OS: HR chemo 0.83 p = NS
ICON1 (2003)	477	Physician uncertain about need for chemotherapy	Observation vs. platinum-based chemotherapy	5-year RFS 62% vs. 73% $p = 0.01$ 5-year OS 70% vs. 79% $p = 0.03$
ACTION (2003)	448	Stage IA/B Gr 2–3 All IC, IIA, and clear cell	Observation vs. platinum-based chemotherapy	5-year RFS 68% vs. 76% $p = 0.02$ 5-year OS 78% vs. 85% p = NS
Bell (2006)	427	Stage IA/B Gr 3 or clear cell All IC, II	Carboplatin/paclitaxel three cycles vs. six cycles	HR RFS 0.761 p = NS 5-year OS no difference
Mannel (2011)	542	Stage IA/B Gr 3 or clear cell, IC, II	Carboplatin/paclitaxel three cycles followed by observation vs. followed by weekly paclitaxel × 26	5-year RFS 77% vs. 80% p = NS

DFS, disease free survival; Gr, grade; HR, hazard ratio; NS, not significant; OS, overall survival; RFS, relapse-free survival; WAR, whole abdominal radiotherapy.

Source: From Fleming G, Seidman JD, Lengyel E. Epithelial ovarian cancer. In: Barakat RR, Berchuck A, Markmann M, et al, eds. *Principles and Practic of Gynecologic Oncology.* 6th ed. Philadelphia, PA: Lippincott Williams & Wilkins; 2013:757–847.

older, have variably staged patients, and included multiple different histologic subtypes. Although individual trial results vary somewhat, as a group they have shown fairly consistent improvement in disease-free survival for postoperative chemotherapy versus observation or radiotherapy. However, the only clear demonstration of an OS benefit in the treatment of early-stage ovarian cancer comes from a joint analysis of two large European trials (the ACTION and ICON1 trials), which together randomized 923 patients with early-stage disease (over 90% stage I) to receive either platinum-based chemotherapy or no initial adjuvant treatment. Results of a preplanned combined analysis indicated a statistically significant improvement in both disease-free survival (HR, 0.64) and OS (HR, 0.67) with adjuvant platinum-based therapy (170,381). Yet, even these results are not considered definitive proof of a benefit from chemotherapy in early-stage disease because comprehensive surgical staging (particularly lymph node dissection) was not required for entry into these trials. In a retrospective subset analysis of the ACTION trial, the patients with optimal staging had no benefit from chemotherapy, suggesting that the overall positive results reflected the benefit of chemotherapy in women with low-volume stage III disease. However, only 151 patients (of variable histology) were optimally staged, which is too few to provide statistical power for firm conclusions about the benefit of chemotherapy in this subgroup (**Fig. 23.47**).

It has been suggested that the discrepancy between the benefit in disease-free survival and lack of benefit in OS seen in several of the randomized early-stage chemotherapy trials resulted from increased salvage rates for chemotherapy in patients who recur after observation. However, most patients whose cancer recurs will die of their disease. Investigators at the Royal Marsden Hospital examined the salvage rate after relapse in their series of prospective observation for patients with stage I disease (complete staging not required) (382). Sixty-one (31%) of 194 patients relapsed at a median of 17 months (range 6 months to 15.7 years), and 55 of them received platinum-based chemotherapy at the time of relapse. Progression-free survival at 5 years after relapse was only 24%.

Duration of Chemotherapy for Early-Stage Disease

The GOG 157 trial randomized 427 eligible patients with early-stage disease and unfavorable prognostic markers (stage IA or IB grade 3, clear cell, stage IC, and completely resected stage II) to receive either three or six cycles of carboplatin (area under the curve [AUC] 7.5)/paclitaxel (175 mg/m^2) chemotherapy. Surgical staging was required, although 29% of patients had surgical procedures that were considered inadequate or inadequately documented. Overall 5-year survival did not differ by treatment arm (HR, 1.02). Adjusting for initial FIGO stage and tumor grade, the recurrence rate was 24% lower for patients getting six cycles, but this difference was not statistically significant (relative hazard 0.761; 95% CI, 0.512–1.13, $p = 0.18$) (383). There was a slightly lower estimated benefit of six cycles of chemotherapy in the completely staged group (HR, 0.66 for incompletely staged vs. 0.796 for completely staged patients), but there was no significant evidence of heterogeneity in treatment effect. Toxicity was increased with six cycles; in particular the rate of grade III and IV neurotoxicity was 11% versus only 2% with three cycles. A subsequent exploratory analysis showed that for the 97 women with serous tumors the risk of recurrence was significantly lower after six versus three cycles of chemotherapy; 83% versus 60% (HR, 0.33; CI, 0.14–0.77; $p = 0.04$), whereas for those with nonserous tumors, including clear cell carcinomas, no benefit was seen. The 5-year OS for women with serous carcinomas was 86% for those receiving six cycles of therapy and 73% for those receiving three cycles of therapy; this difference did not reach statistical significance (384). The GOG conducted a subsequent trial (GOG #175) in the same patient population randomizing 542 eligible women to either three cycles of carboplatin (AUC 6)/paclitaxel (175 mg/m^2) or three cycles of the same regimen followed by maintenance therapy with weekly paclitaxel 40 mg/m^2 for 24 weeks. No significant difference in recurrence-free interval (HR, 0.807) or OS was seen. Only 29% of subjects had serous histology, and their results did not differ from those of the overall population (HR, 0.822) (385).

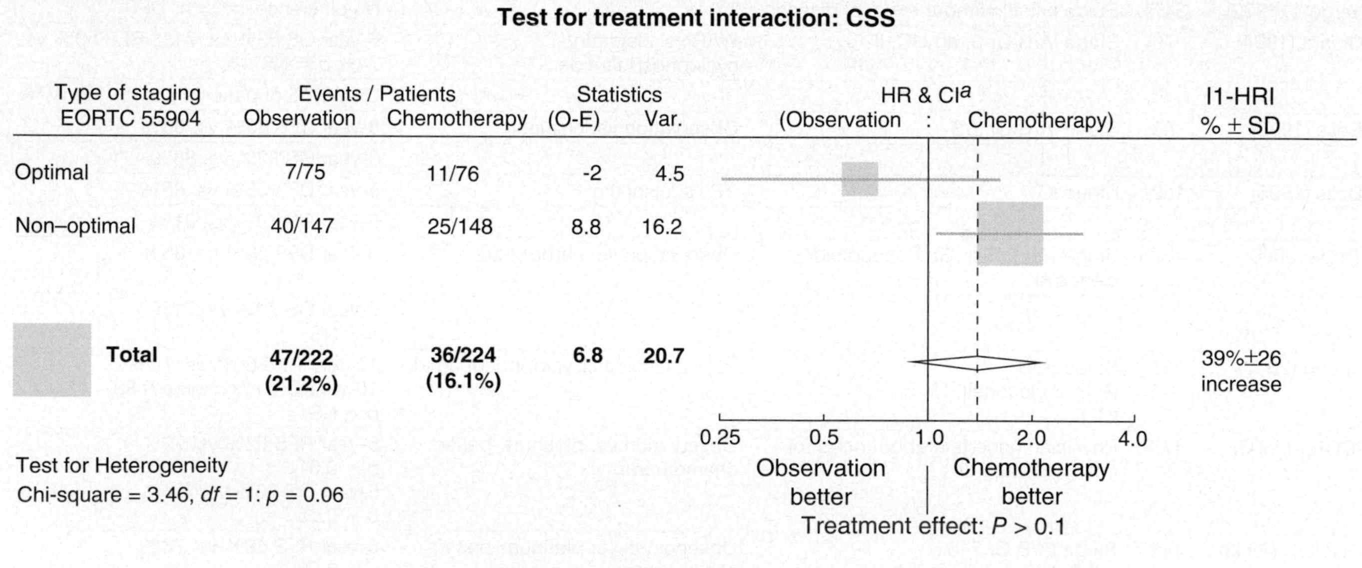

Test for treatment interaction: CSS
Type of staging EORTC 55904
Events / Patients
Observation
Chemotherapy
Statistics
(O-E)
Var.
HR & CI[a]
(Observation : Chemotherapy)
I1-HRI
% ± SD
Optimal
7/75
11/76
-2
4.5
Non–optimal
40/147
25/148
8.8
16.2
Total
47/222 (21.2%)
36/224 (16.1%)
6.8
20.7
39%±26 increase
0.25
0.5
1.0
2.0
4.0
Observation better
Chemotherapy better
Treatment effect: P > 0.1
Test for Heterogeneity
Chi-square = 3.46, df = 1: p = 0.06

[a]95%CI everywhere

Figure 23.47. Forest plots of the interaction between the two staging categories (optimal and nonoptimal) versus treatment effect (adjuvant chemotherapy better vs. observation better) for cancer-specific survival (CSS).

Solid squares = hazard ratios (HRs) for cancer-specific survival (with the area of the square being proportional to the variance of the estimated effect); **length of the horizontal line through the square** = 95% confidence interval (CI); **open diamond** = HR (middle of the diamond); **horizontal points of the diamond** = 95% CI for the combined data. CSS, cancer-specific survival; EORTC, European Organization of Research and Treatment of Cancer; O – E, number of events observed minus number of events expected under the null hypothesis; SD, standard deviation; Var., variance of 1 divided by the logarithm of the HR. Linear trends and heterogeneity of the HRs to detect differences in relative size of treatment effect were assessed by a χ^2 test for interaction. All statistical tests were two-sided.

Source: From Trimbos B, Timmers P, Pecorelli S, et al. Surgical Staging and Treatment of Early ovarian cancer: long-term analysis from a randomized trial. *J Natl Cancer Inst*. 2010;102(13):982–987.

At this time it is recommended that patients with comprehensively staged stage IA or IB low-grade epithelial ovarian cancer receive no postoperative chemotherapy (see **Fig. 23.46**). Patients with grade III or stage IC disease have a relapse risk of at least 20%, and this may be reduced with platinum-based chemotherapy, particularly for those with high-grade serous tumors. Paclitaxel/carboplatin for three to six cycles is the usual treatment for early-stage high-risk disease. It is hoped that future data will better address which women with early-stage ovarian cancers actually derive benefit from therapy and that therapy may be better targeted to different histologic subtypes.

Early-Stage Clear Cell Carcinoma

Seven to 11% of patients with apparent early-stage ovarian clear cell tumors will have retroperitoneal lymph node involvement (386), compared with 28% for early-stage serous carcinomas (387). In general, clear cell carcinomas of the ovary are not graded; they are all considered high grade and have traditionally all been treated with adjuvant chemotherapy. One single-institution experience including 110 stage I clear cell cancers found that 60/110 (56%) were stage IA, 31/110 (28%) were stage IC on basis of rupture-only, and 19/110 (17.3%) were stage IC based on surface involvement and/or positive cytology. Three-year progression-free survival rates for the subgroups were 93%, 90%, and 56% (**Fig. 23.48**) (388). Although the vast majority of patients in this series received chemotherapy, advanced-stage clear cell carcinoma tends to be chemotherapy resistant, and it is not clear that chemotherapy contributed to the good prognosis for those with IA and disease or IC based on rupture only. Future studies should explore whether chemotherapy benefits patients with these subsets of clear cell ovarian cancer.

As described above, retrospective reviews have shown that prognosis in stage IC and II clear cell carcinoma might be improved by the addition of radiotherapy, and hopefully future trials will also address this issue.

Early-Stage Fallopian Tube Carcinomas

Given the current hypothesis that many serous ovarian cancers actually arise in the fallopian tubes, the staging systems for ovarian cancer and fallopian tube cancer have been combined in the new 2014 FIGO staging. A small number of patients present with obvious early-stage disease in the fallopian tubes. This is frequently incidentally detected after surgery for non-oncologic indications such as incontinence or after prophylactic salpingo-oophorectomy performed for cancer prevention in women with a *BRCA* mutation. These patients should be fully surgically staged. Most fallopian tube carcinomas are of high-grade serous histology. Prognosis has been reported to be dependent on depth of invasion of the tumor into the fallopian tube. When controlled for stage and grade, early-stage fallopian tube cancers appear to have a prognosis similar to that of early-stage cancers appearing to arise from the ovary (389); older FIGO data suggest that patients with stage I fallopian tube cancers have a 5-year OS of 81% (390). Adjuvant chemotherapy will be indicated in most situations. There is considerable uncertainty regarding treatment of isolated STIC (serous tubal intraepithelial lesions). One recent review reported that of 78 patients with STIC lesions cytology was obtained in 66 patients and was positive in 7 (10.6%). A variety of surgical operations were performed, but no patient had evidence of disease in the uterus, omentum, or lymph nodes. Three of 67 (4.5%) *BRCA* mutation carriers with STIC lesions were diagnosed with primary peritoneal cancer during follow-up (243). We lack data to support full staging in patients with STIC lesions, data regarding prognostic importance of isolated positive washings in patients with STIC lesions, and data regarding benefit of chemotherapy in these situations.

MANAGEMENT OF BORDERLINE TUMORS

Borderline (sometimes referred to as low malignant potential; LMP) tumors comprise 10% to 20% of ovarian malignancies, and most are serous or mucinous. They were first described by Taylor in 1929 and recognized by FIGO in 1971 as a distinct histologic subtype. Their histology is reviewed in detail in the section on Pathology. In general, patients with borderline tumors present at a younger age (on average 10 years younger) and have earlier-stage disease than women with invasive ovarian carcinomas; over 75% of borderline ovarian tumors are stage I at the time of diagnosis (287).

Current hypotheses suggest that borderline tumors are precursors to type I invasive tumors, SBTs are precursors to low-grade serous tumors, and MBTs are precursors to invasive mucinous tumors. SBTs are more common than MBTs in the United States; in Asia, the rate of MBTs has been reported to be similar or higher than that of SBT (391). Approximately 75% to 80% of borderline tumors are stage I at the time of diagnosis. Nearly all MBTs are stage I at the time of diagnosis. Even when SBTs present with more advanced-stage disease, survival is prolonged. A recent Danish series found women with stage I SBT had a survival similar to that of the general population, whereas among women with advanced-stage disease the 10-year relative survival was 90% for those with noninvasive implants and 60% for those with invasive implants (286). The very long natural history makes accurate collection of outcomes and performing clinical trials challenging. Because these tumors are particularly likely to affect young women, decisions regarding fertility-sparing, egg retrieval, and surgical menopause in the treatment of early-stage disease are often pertinent.

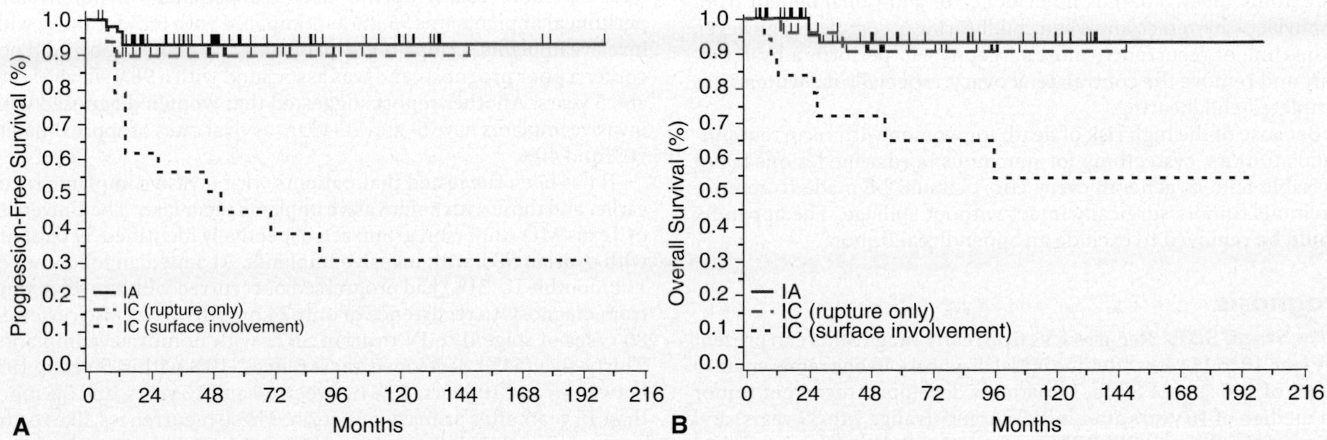

Figure 23.48. Kaplan–Meier survival analysis for ovarian clear cell carcinoma stratified by stage I breakdown—PFS **(A)** and OS **(B)**.

Source: From Shu CA, Zhou Q, Jotwani AR, et al. Ovarian clear cell carcinoma, outcomes by stage: the MSK experience. *Gynecol Oncol*. 2015;139(2):236–241.

Early-Stage Borderline Tumors

Surgery

Surgery is the cornerstone of treatment for early-stage borderline ovarian tumors. It is often not known preoperatively whether an ovarian mass will prove to be a borderline tumor, and the accuracy of frozen section in the diagnosis of ovarian tumors has been reported to be low; 20% to 30% of ovarian tumors diagnosed as borderline at the time of frozen section examination prove to be invasive carcinomas on further sampling (392). Issues of surgical management of an ovarian mass, including borderline tumors, are covered in the section "Surgery." Most often this will involve an initial minimally invasive surgical approach.

A full staging of borderline tumors along with salpingo-oophorectomy and omentectomy has historically been recommended, and the recent large (950 patient) prospective ROBOT study reported that incomplete staging was an independent risk factor for recurrence (287). However, as lymph node involvement in SBTs does not appear to affect prognosis, and as current guidelines recommend no systemic adjuvant therapy for women with implants, even invasive implants (393), upstaging would not have therapeutic implications, and the inferior prognosis for unstaged patients may simply be a result of stage shift.

Therefore, the role of restaging borderline tumors not fully staged at the time of initial surgery remains controversial. In one retrospective multicenter study the rate of upstaging was 14.8% for serous tumors; it is very low for mucinous tumors (394). The most relevant situation for restaging appears to be in women with apparent stage I SBT with microinvasion or micropapillary histology, which has the highest risk of invasive implants. The majority of patients can be followed without additional surgery after obtaining a baseline abdominopelvic CT scan and CA-125 (serous) or CEA (mucinous) tumor marker (391). The ROBOT study reported that elevated CA-125 was associated with peritoneal implants of any type, but was not independently predictive of future relapse (395).

As many women with borderline tumors are in their childbearing years, the efficacy and safety of conservative surgery for early-stage disease are important. There is no evidence that fertility-sparing surgery has an adverse effect on OS in patients with stage I borderline tumors, but it does increase recurrence rates. A meta-analysis of 39 studies including 5,105 women concluded that for women with unilateral tumors recurrence rates were 25.3% for women undergoing cystectomy versus 12.5% for those undergoing unilateral salpingo-oophorectomy; survival was not different. For women with bilateral tumors the recurrence rate was 25.6% for bilateral cystectomy and 26.1% for unilateral salpingo-oophorectomy plus contralateral cystectomy. The cumulative pregnancy rate was 45.4% for unilateral salpingo-oophorectomy and 40.3% for unilateral cystectomy (394). There is no evidence of additional benefit from prophylactic hysterectomy when childbearing is completed; however, at the time of recurrence, most surgeons will perform a hysterectomy and remove the contralateral ovary, especially if a woman has completed childbearing.

Because of the high risk of death for women with recurrent mucinous tumors, cystectomy for mucinous borderline lesions is not advisable and, in general, every effort should be made to remove mucinous tumors surgically intact without spillage. The appendix should be removed to exclude an appendiceal tumor.

Prognosis

Early-Stage SBTs. Recurrences from early-stage SBTs can present very late, 10 to 15 years after the initial diagnosis. In one representative report of 160 stage I SBTs, 11 patients developed recurrent tumor at a median of 16 years after initial surgery (range 7 to 39 years) and 8 died of the disease (396). The prospective ROBOT trial reported that neither microinvasion nor micropapillary growth pattern had an impact on recurrence rate. Similarly, a meta-analysis of 42 studies suggested that lethal recurrence rates were 18.3% for early-stage typical SBTs, 16.8% for micropapillary serous tumors, and 10.7% for borderline tumors with microinvasion (397). Recurrences may still be borderline tumors or may have transformed into invasive cancers. These invasive cancers are more often, but not always, of low grade and carry a significantly worse prognosis than borderline recurrences (**Fig. 23.49**).

Early-Stage Mucinous Borderline Tumors. MBTs tend to be large, and areas of microinvasion can easily be missed if they are not sampled thoroughly. However, the clinical relevance of this is unclear, as microinvasion does not have clear prognostic significance. A review of eight series including 116 patients with mucinous ovarian tumors and stromal microinvasion reported that none developed an invasive recurrence. However, median follow-up in a number of these series was under 5 years. Intraepithelial cancer may also occur in MBTs, and although this is usually benign, there are occasional reports of malignant behavior. In general, although the overall prognosis of early-stage MBTs is excellent, they can occasionally recur and may recur late. Uzan et al. reported that although MBTs relapsed less often than SBTs, the recurrences are much more likely to be invasive (398). Patients with invasive recurrences, like those with other advanced-stage mucinous tumors, do poorly.

Systemic Therapy

Chemotherapy is not indicated for stage I or II borderline tumors, regardless of histology or microinvasion.

Advanced-Stage SBTs

Surgery

Chemotherapy does not appear to have a role in the treatment of borderline tumors; hence surgery is the primary treatment. Retrospective studies suggest that the proportion of patients achieving optimal cytoreduction is stage-for-stage higher for patients with serous low malignant potential tumors and low-grade serous cancers than for those with high-grade serous epithelial ovarian cancer. Residual disease is an important prognostic factor for both recurrence-free and OS.

Prognosis

Residual disease after surgery, the presence of advanced disease prior to surgery, and invasive implants showing clear stromal invasion are poor prognostic factors. Seidman and Kurman reported on a review of 97 publications including 4,129 patients and noted that after 7.4 years of follow-up, the survival of patients with noninvasive peritoneal implants was 95.3% as compared with 66% for those with invasive implants. Lymph node involvement, as noted above, did not confer a poor prognosis and was associated with a 98% survival rate at 6.5 years. Another report suggested that women diagnosed with invasive implants have 5- and 10-year survival rates of approximately 70% and 40%.

It has been suggested that patients with invasive implants recur earlier and those with noninvasive implants recur later. The University of Texas MD Anderson group retrospectively identified 39 patients with ovarian SBT with invasive implants. At a median follow-up of 111 months, 12 (31%) had progressed or recurred with a median time from diagnosis to recurrence of only 24 months. They also reviewed 80 cases of stage II to IV ovarian SBTs with noninvasive implants. Thirty-five (44%) developed recurrences, 10% within 5 years, 19% between 5 and 10 years, 10% between 10 and 15 years, and 5% more than 15 years after primary resection. These recurrences, like recurrences from stage I disease, may be noninvasive, low-grade serous tumors or, occasionally, high-grade serous tumors.

Adjuvant Systemic Therapy

Meta-analysis has shown no benefit of adjuvant systemic therapy for any subset of advanced-stage borderline tumors, including those with invasive implants. Adjuvant therapy is therefore not recommended (393).

Therapy for Advanced-Stage LGSC and Invasive Recurrences of SBTs

As shown in **Figure 23.49**, noninvasive recurrences of borderline tumors continue to have a relatively good prognosis and should be treated with surgical resection. Invasive recurrences have a prognosis similar to that of *de novo* LGSC. Shvartzman et al. identified 112 patients with *de novo* LGSCs and 41 with invasive recurrences of borderline tumors. There were no statistically significant differences between the two groups in median age (42.7 vs. 45.4 years [at relapse]), PFS (19.5 vs. 25 months), or OS (81.8 vs. 82.8 months) (293). Age less than 35 years has been reported to be a poor prognostic factor among patients with advanced-stage LGSC (399).

At this time the recommendation for newly diagnosed LGSC remains surgical removal of all tumor followed by standard chemotherapy. However, this warrants further study. LGSC is a relatively chemotherapy-resistant disease. In a combined analysis of four front-line chemotherapy trials, the Arbeitsgemeinschaft Gynäkologische Onkologie (AGO) reported that the response rate for LGSC was only 23.1% versus 90.1% for HGSC (400). Even lower response rates to neo-adjuvant therapy have been reported, and use of neo-adjuvant therapy for LGSC

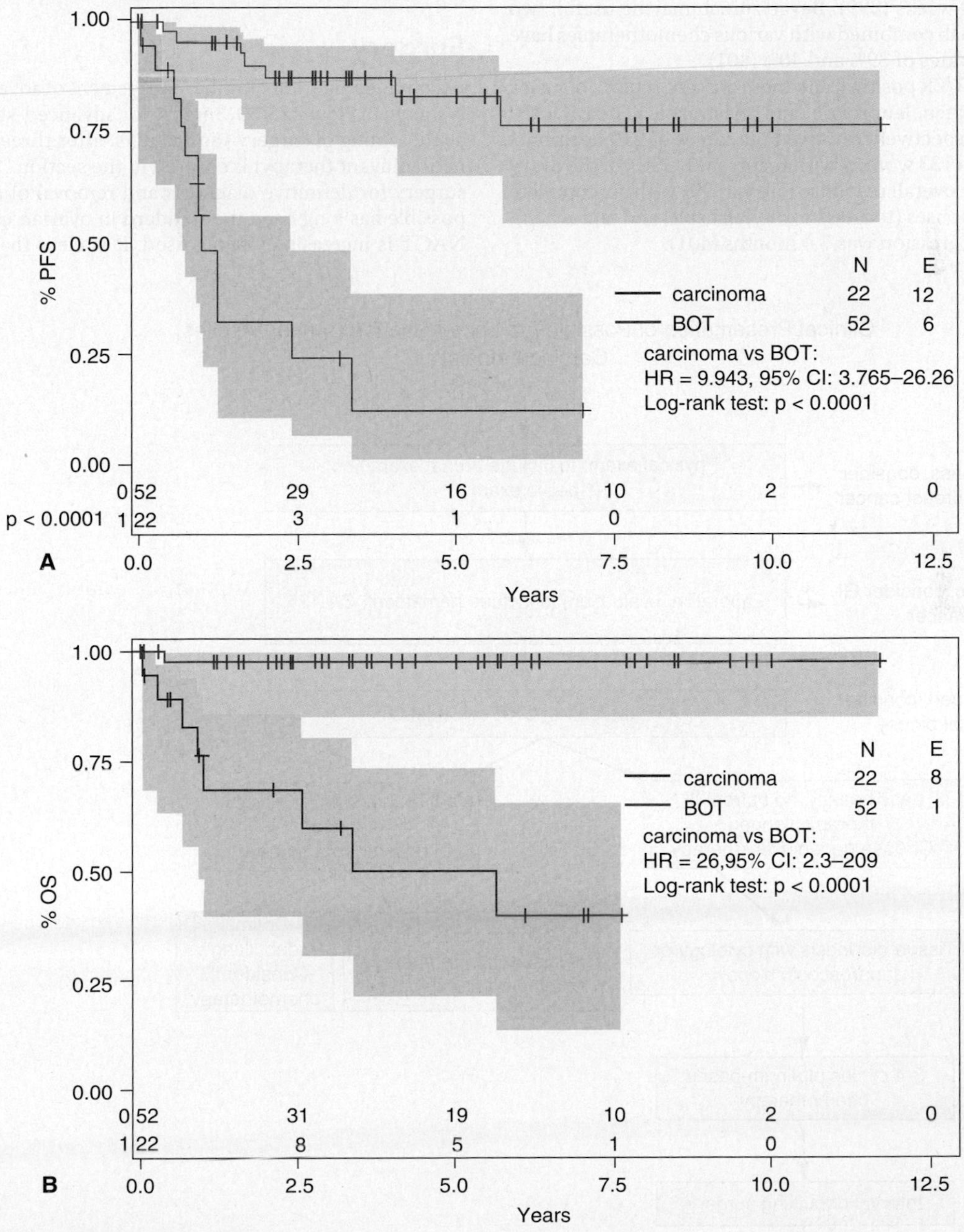

Figure 23.49. A: Progression-free survival (PFS) and **B:** overall survival (OS) after relapse of a borderline ovarian tumor—relapse as invasive carcinoma versus relapse as borderline ovarian tumor (BOT).

Source: From du Bois, Ewald-Riegler N, de Gregorio N, et al. Borderline tumours of the ovary: a cohort study of the Arbeitsgemeinschaft Gynäkologische Onkologie (AGO) Study Group. *Eur J Cancer*. 2013;49(8):1905–1914.)

is not advised (401). A recent abstract presented results of a very small retrospective series of women with advanced-stage LGCS treated with cytoreductive surgery followed by adjuvant hormonal therapy (mostly aromatase inhibitors) and no chemotherapy. When compared with a control group of patients treated with chemotherapy, there was no difference in PFS (402). However CA-125 measurements have been shown to decline with adjuvant chemotherapy for advanced-stage LGSC with normalization of CA-125 after one of first three cycles being associated with better outcomes, suggesting some degree of chemotherapy sensitivity (403). Prospective data regarding the best up-front systemic therapy for this disease are badly needed.

Treatment of progressive unresectable LGSC is problematic. Gershenson et al. reported on a retrospective review of 108 chemotherapy regimens administered to 58 patients with low-grade serous ovarian tumors. There was an overall response rate of 3.7%, with one complete and three partial responses. The median time to progression was 29 weeks (399). Bevacizumab may be useful; two series of bevacizumab combined with various chemotherapies have reported response rates of 39% and 40% (401).

Most LGSC is ER/PR positive, and there are case reports of major responses to tamoxifen, leuprolide, and anastrazole. The MD Anderson group retrospectively reviewed outcomes of 219 hormonal therapy regimens in 133 women with recurrent LGSCs of the ovary or peritoneum. The overall response rate was 9%, with six complete and two partial responses (to anastrazole, letrozole, and tamoxifen). Median time to progression was 7.4 months (401).

As initial reports suggested a high frequency of *KRAS* and *BRAF* mutations in LGSCs, a trial was undertaken with AZD6244 (selumetinib), which inhibits MEK-1/2 (downstream signaling effectors of KRAS/BRAF activating mitogenic signaling) in women with LGSCs. The majority had at least three prior cytotoxic regimens. There was a 15% response rate with a median PFS of 11 months. Of patients for whom sufficient tumor material was available, 6% had *BRAF* mutations and 41% had *KRAS* mutations. No correlation between response and mutation status was observed (404). Other data also suggest that *BRAF* mutations, although common in early-stage borderline tumors, are rare in advanced-stage LGSCs, and therefore agents targeting BRAF may not be useful in the treatment of recurrent disease.

MANAGEMENT OF ADVANCED-STAGE (III AND IV) OVARIAN CANCER

Surgery

A simplified algorithm for the management of advanced-stage disease is shown in **Figure 23.50**. Surgery for advanced-stage disease as well as the timing of surgery (up-front vs. after three or more cycles of neo-adjuvant therapy) is covered in the section "Surgery." Up-front surgery for definitive diagnosis and removal of as much tumor as possible has long been the standard in ovarian cancer therapy, but NACT is increasingly being used. It is clear that women who are

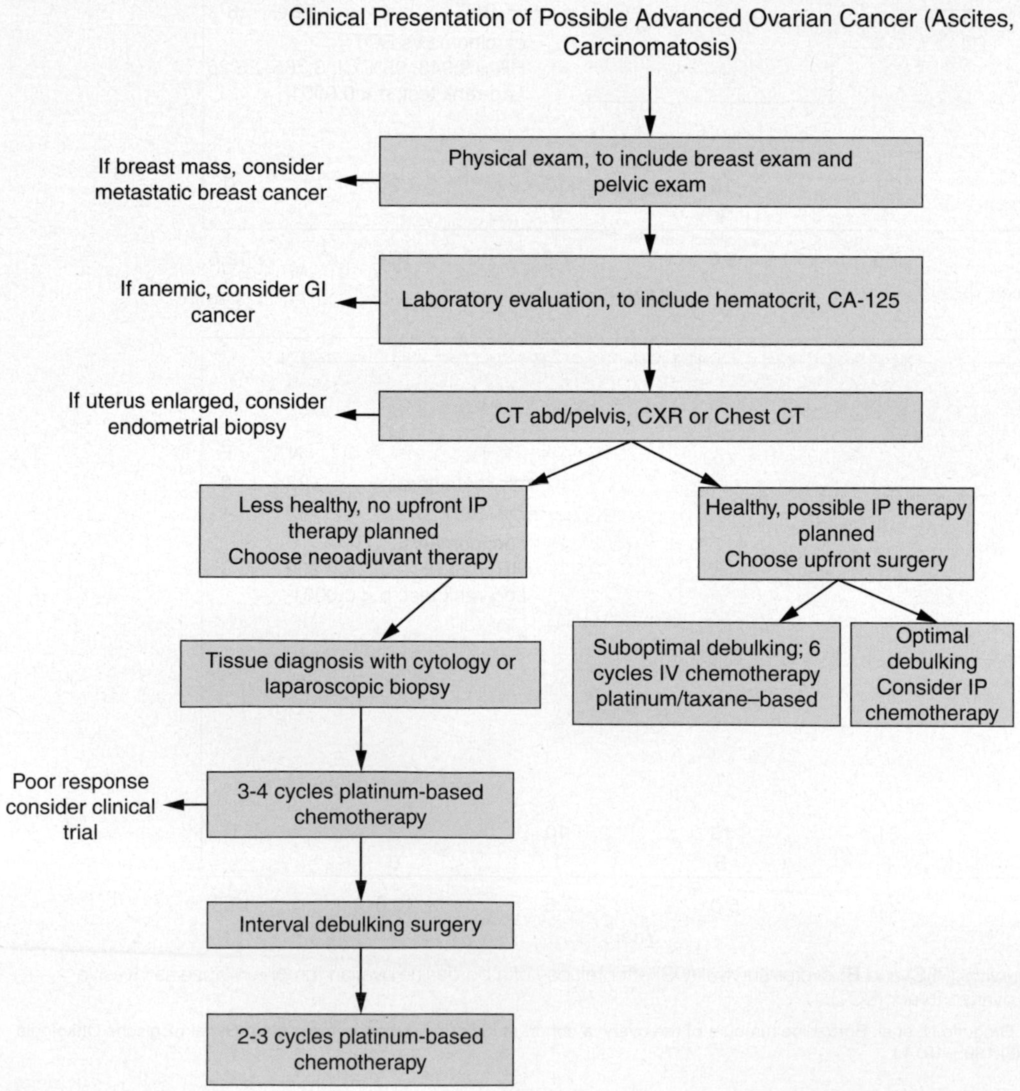

Figure 23.50. Management of advanced-stage ovarian cancer.

successfully surgically debulked to minimal or no residual disease have an improved survival, although how much of this is a direct result of the surgical effort and how much reflects unknown biologic/genetic, social, or health factors in patients who have debulkable disease remain unclear.

Chemotherapy

Treatment is rarely curative for women with advanced-stage ovarian carcinoma, even when there is no residual disease. Whereas the 5-year case fatality rate for women with ovarian cancer overall fell by 7.5% from 1973 to 1999, corresponding to the introduction of platinum and paclitaxel in clinical practice, the 12-year case fatality rate over the same time period declined by only 1.2%, suggesting that in most cases chemotherapy may delay, rather than prevent, death from ovarian cancer (4).

The majority of women with advanced-stage ovarian cancer have HGSC, and they have made up the vast majority of patients in the trials of advanced disease. Hence the trials discussed in this section may be assumed to apply primarily to HGSC. Approximately 50% to 70% of patients with measurable disease after surgery will have a complete or partial response to platinum-based first-line postoperative therapy (405). In trials including optimally and suboptimally debulked patients, at least half will generally have a complete clinical response to platinum-based regimens, with disappearance of all disease on imaging and normalization of CA-125. Unfortunately, even of those with complete clinical remission, the majority eventually develop recurrent disease.

The most common front-line therapy in the United States is currently six cycles of intravenous paclitaxel/carboplatin. Some physicians administer eight or nine cycles of therapy, particularly when interval debulking is performed. However, three small randomized trials that investigated the benefit of prolonging the duration of treatment beyond six cycles all showed an increase in toxicity but no improvement in outcomes (181,406,407). The use of weekly paclitaxel regimens is popular, based on the results of the JGOG 3016 trial discussed below. The benefits of intraperitoneal therapy for patients with optimally debulked tumors are uncertain. Neither addition of a third cytotoxic agent nor maintenance therapy after attaining remission has been shown to improve survival.

Platinum Use

Platinum agents are the most active group of chemotherapy drugs in the treatment of ovarian cancer. This may partially be accounted for by the fact that defects in homologous DNA repair (including BRCA mutations) are common in ovarian cancers and appear to be associated with response to platinum therapy. A variety of different platinum agents have activity. A small ($n = 177$) randomized trial comparing oxaliplatin/cyclophosphamide with cisplatin/cyclophosphamide as first-line therapy showed no difference in PFS or OS between the two treatment groups (408). Multiple randomized trials have confirmed that carboplatin is as active as cisplatin when both are given intravenously (409), and because carboplatin produces substantially less neurotoxicity, nausea, and ototoxicity, it has become the standard for intravenous use. There is some uncertainty as to how high a dose of platinum is needed for optimal efficacy. An older meta-analysis of over 60 published trials showed a correlation between dose intensity of cisplatin and observed response rate, but the correlation held only over a range of doses lower than those used in clinical practice today (410). Multiple trials of varying design have tested higher versus lower doses of platinum agents, including trials using doses of carboplatin requiring stem cell support, but no good evidence supports the use of doses of cisplatin above 50 mg to 100 mg/m^2 every 3 weeks or doses of carboplatin over AUC 5 to 7.5 every 3 weeks. It should be recognized when comparing carboplatin dosing across trials that there may be variation in dosing for a given AUC depending, among other things, on how GFR is calculated. AUC 6 is the most common dose used for first-line therapy in the United States.

Addition of Paclitaxel to Platinum Chemotherapy

In the 1980s, a great deal of excitement was generated by the demonstration that single-agent paclitaxel had substantial activity against platinum-resistant ovarian cancer. A number of randomized trials were rapidly launched comparing platinum-based regimens with and without taxane in the first-line treatment of ovarian cancer.

The results of the first two of these trials (GOG111 and OV-10) clearly demonstrated that combination chemotherapy with paclitaxel and cisplatin prolonged both PFS and OS as compared with cyclophosphamide/cisplatin (411–413). In GOG111, which included 386 women with suboptimally debulked or stage IV disease, the median OS was 37 months for those treated with paclitaxel (135 mg/m^2 over 24 hours) and cisplatin as compared with 25 months for those receiving cyclophosphamide and cisplatin. Similar results were found in the more inclusive (stages IIB–IV) European OV-10 trial, which reported a median OS of 36 months for the paclitaxel-containing arm (175 mg/m^2 over 3 hours) versus 26 months for the cyclophosphamide-containing arm.

The other two trials did not as clearly support the addition of paclitaxel to front-line therapy. The three arms of GOG132 were single-agent paclitaxel (200 mg/m^2 over 24 hours), single-agent cisplatin (100 mg/mg^2), and the combination of cisplatin 75 mg/m^2 plus paclitaxel 135 mg/m^2 over 24 hours (372). A total of 614 women with suboptimally debulked or stage IV disease were treated. The response rate to single-agent paclitaxel in patients with measurable disease was significantly lower than to either of the platinum-containing regimens (42% vs. 67%, $p < 0.01$). However, the difference in median OS (30.2, 25.9, and 26.3 months for patients randomized to cisplatin, paclitaxel, or the combination, respectively) was not statistically significant. The investigators speculated that the lack of benefit for the combination arm related to the fact that almost 50% of patients on the single-agent arms began subsequent treatment (frequently with the therapy of the alternate arm, that is, cisplatin for women who were randomized to paclitaxel and paclitaxel for women who were randomized to cisplatin) prior to overt clinical progression, presumably on the basis of a rising CA-125. By way of contrast, paclitaxel was seldom used as salvage therapy in GOG111 because of its limited availability at the time, and whereas 48% of patients in the cisplatin/cyclophosphamide arm of OV-10 crossed over to paclitaxel as first salvage treatment, it appears that they did so after overt clinical progression. ICON3, a large ($n = 2{,}075$) multinational trial which randomized women with stage I–IV disease to carboplatin AUC 6/paclitaxel chemotherapy versus single-agent carboplatin AUC 6 or CAP (cisplatin/doxorubicin/cyclophosphamide) chemotherapy, found no superiority for the taxane-containing combination in either PFS or OS (hazard ratio for OS 0.98; 95% CI, 0.87–1.10). About a third of patients on carboplatin in the control group went on to receive a taxane at some stage, mostly after the disease had progressed. The results of this trial also appear to contradict those of OV-10 and GOG111, and the explanation remains unclear. However, given that carboplatin plus paclitaxel combination therapy is certainly at least as active as single-agent carboplatin, and that the doublet is both relatively well tolerated in general and platelet-sparing relative to single-agent carboplatin, the combination became standard. Single-agent carboplatin is sometimes used for frail older patients.

Alternate Paclitaxel Dosing. The standard dose of paclitaxel in front-line therapy was 135 mg/m^2 when it was used as a 24-hour infusion and is currently 175 mg/m^2 as a 3-hour infusion every 3 weeks or 80 mg/m^2 as a 1-hour infusion weekly. Neither increasing the every-3-week dose nor using prolonged infusions has been associated with improved outcomes. **Table 23.15** shows some trials testing different taxane regimens. Paclitaxel was historically administered as a 24-hour infusion to minimize hypersensitivity reactions and to diminish neurotoxicity when it was administered in combination with cisplatin. Because an early randomized phase II trial in recurrent disease had suggested slightly better disease-related outcomes with

■ TABLE 23.15. Selected Trials Testing Taxane Variations in Front-Line Therapy

Trial Name	N Stages	ARMS	Median PFS	Median OS
SCOTROC (418)	1077 IC–IV	Carbo AUC 5 + paclitaxel 175 mg/m^2 q3wk	14.8 months	2 years 69%
		Carbo AUC 5 + docetaxel 75 mg/m^2 q3wk	15 months	2 years 64%
Bolis (415)	502 IIB–IV	Carbo AUC 6 + paclitaxel 175 mg/m^2	4 years PFS 41.5%	4 years OS 46.2%
		Carbo AUC 6 + paclitaxel 225 mg/m^2	4 years PFS 39.2%	4 years OS 47.3%
GOG162 (414)	324 III or IV suboptimal	Cisplatin 75 mg/m^2 + paclitaxel 135 mg/m^2/24hr	1.03 years	2.49 years
		Cisplatin 75 mg/m^2 + paclitaxel 135 mg/m^2/96hr	1.05 years	2.54 years
JGOG 3016 (416)	637 II–IV	Carbo AUC 6 q3wk + paclitaxel 180 mg/m^2 q3wk	17.5 months	62.2 months
		Carbo AUC 6 q3wk + paclitaxel 80mg/m^2/wk	28.2 months	100.5 months
GOG262 (200)	692 III–IV (580 w/ bev 112 w/o bev	Carbo AUC 6 q3wk + paclitaxel 175 mg/m^2 q3wk	No Bev 10.3 months Bev 14.7 months	No OS difference between arms
		Carbo AUC 6 q3wk + paclitaxel 80 mg/m^2/wk	No Bev 14.2 months Bev 14.9 months	
MITO-7 (417)	822 IC–IV	Carbo AUC 6 q3wk + Paclitaxel 175 mg/m^2 q3wk	17.3 months	2 years OS 78.9%
		Carbo AUC 2 q1wk + Paclitaxel 60mg /m^2/wk	18.3 months	2 years OS 77.3%
ICON8	IC–IV	Carbo AUC 5 q3wk + Paclitaxel 175 mg/m^2 q3wk	Ongoing	
		Carbo AUC 5 q3wk + Paclitaxel 80 mg/m^2/wk		
		Carbo AUC 2 q1wk + Paclitaxel 80 mg/m^2/wk		

a 24-hour versus a 3-hour paclitaxel infusion, GOG162 randomized women with ovarian cancer to cisplatin 75 mg/m^2 plus paclitaxel 135 mg/m^2, with the paclitaxel administered as either a 24- or a 96-hour infusion. There was no difference in OS or PFS between the two durations of infusion (414). Attempts at escalating the every-3-week paclitaxel dose have also been made. A prospective, randomized trial in previously untreated advanced ovarian cancer patients compared two different doses of paclitaxel (175 vs. 225 mg/m^2), with all patients receiving carboplatin at an AUC of 5. No improvement in survival was reported for the higher dose regimen (415).

More recently, based on data in women with metastatic breast cancer that weekly paclitaxel was superior to every-3-week paclitaxel in terms of response and survival, the Japanese Gynecologic Oncology Group (JGOG) randomly assigned 637 women with stages II to IV ovarian cancer, primary peritoneal cancer, or fallopian tube cancer to 6 cycles of either standard therapy with carboplatin AUC 6 plus paclitaxel 180 mg/m^2 over 3 hours every 21 days or dose-dense therapy with carboplatin AUC 6 every 21 days plus paclitaxel 80 mg/m^2 on days 1, 8, and 15 of a 21-day cycle. Patients with measurable disease who had a major response received three additional cycles of chemotherapy. Interval or secondary debulking surgery was permitted. The dose-dense regimen was superior in terms of both median PFS (28.2 vs. 17.5 months; HR, 0.76; 95% CI, 0.62–0.91) and median OS (100.5 vs. 62.2 months; HR, 0.79, 95% CI, 0.63–0.90) (416). All subgroups (age, stage, residual disease) appeared to benefit, except for women with clear cell or mucinous tumors. The dose-dense regimen was more myelotoxic than standard therapy, and required an increased number of dose delays and reductions. The GOG performed a confirmatory trial (GOG262) using carboplatin AUC 6 with weekly paclitaxel 80 mg/m^2 compared with carboplatin AUC 6 with every-3-week paclitaxel 175 mg/m^2. Bevacizumab 15 mg/kg every 3 weeks, given with chemotherapy and then until progression, was optional, but was selected by 84% ($n = 580$) of patients. Overall, there was no difference between the arms for PFS (14.7 vs. 14.0 months, $p = 0.18$), but in the subset ($n = 112$) that did not receive bevacizumab, PFS was significantly improved (14.2 vs. 10.3 months, $p = 0.03$). Anemia and neuropathy were increased on the weekly paclitaxel arm (200). The mechanism by which bevacizumab might potentially obscure a benefit of weekly paclitaxel remains uncertain. The Multicenter Italian Trials in ovarian cancer (MITO)-7 trial used a regimen of weekly paclitaxel at a somewhat lower dose than the JGOG trial, 60 mg/m^2, and combined it with weekly carboplatin AUC 2. The control arm was every-3-week paclitaxel 175 mg/m^2 plus carboplatin AUC 6 given every 3 weeks. There was no difference in PFS between the arms (18.3 months for weekly and 17.3 months for every 3 weeks), but there was decreased toxicity, including febrile neutropenia, thrombocytopenia, renal toxicity, and neuropathy, as well as significantly better QOL in the weekly arm (417). The fact that this weekly regimen did not outperform the every-3-week regimen when the total cumulative doses of taxane were similar suggests that weekly paclitaxel might be superior to every-3-week paclitaxel only when there is a higher total cumulative dose (and this is supported by an older trial in which weekly paclitaxel used in recurrent ovarian cancer was not superior to every-3-week paclitaxel when total dose was fixed).

ICON8 is an ongoing three-arm trial testing standard therapy with carboplatin every 3 weeks plus paclitaxel every 3 weeks, a regimen of carboplatin every 3 weeks plus weekly paclitaxel, and a regimen in which both carboplatin and paclitaxel are given weekly. No bevacizumab is used. Hopefully the results of this trial will clarify the benefits of weekly paclitaxel administration.

Alternate Taxanes. The Scottish Gynaecological Cancer Trials Group tested the incorporation of docetaxel into front-line therapy (418). A total of 1,077 women with stage IC to IV ovarian or primary peritoneal carcinoma were randomized to six cycles of carboplatin AUC 5 and either docetaxel 75 mg/m^2 or paclitaxel 175 mg/m^2. At a median follow-up of 23 months, there was no difference in PFS (15 months for docetaxel, 14.8 months for paclitaxel) or OS (2-year OS 64% for docetaxel and 69% for paclitaxel). This was confirmed in a subsequent report with longer follow-up. Docetaxel was associated with less neurotoxicity (11% vs. 30% grade ≥ 2 neurosensory toxicity) and more myelotoxicity (11 patients vs. 3 patients with neutropenic fever). Docetaxel represents an option for patients with or at risk for neurotoxicity.

Albumin-bound paclitaxel has been shown to have activity in ovarian cancer, but has not been compared with paclitaxel. Paclitaxel polyglumex (Xyotax; CTI 2103), a microparticle-bound paclitaxel, is being tested by the GOG in a randomized trial (GOG212) as consolidation therapy compared with paclitaxel or no further therapy; accrual completed January 2014, but results are not yet available.

Addition of a Third Cytotoxic Agent to Front-Line Chemotherapy

There are no data that addition of any third cytotoxic agent to front-line chemotherapy of ovarian cancer improves outcomes, despite an immense amount of investigation of this strategy. Multiple randomized phase III trials testing the addition of doxorubicin, epirubicin, gemcitabine, and topotecan to a platinum/taxane backbone either sequentially or all at the same time have all been negative. In addition, an international multiarm randomized study was led by the GOG (GOG182-ICON5) to definitively answer whether triplet cytotoxic chemotherapy improves survival (89). A total of 4,312 advanced-staged ovarian cancer patients were randomized to carboplatin/paclitaxel or carboplatin/paclitaxel combined with either gemcitabine, liposomal doxorubicin, or topotecan. PFS ranged from 15.4 to 17.5 months across the four treatment arms, with an HR of 0.94 to 1.07, which was not statistically different among any of the combination regimens studied.

Substitution of an Alternate Cytotoxic Agent for Paclitaxel

A randomized phase III trial substituting gemcitabine for paclitaxel as front-line therapy showed inferior OS for women on the gemcitabine-containing arm (419). Results with liposomal doxorubicin have been more interesting. The phase III MITO-2 trial randomly assigned 820 chemotherapy-naïve patients with stage IC to IV ovarian cancer to carboplatin AUC 5 plus paclitaxel 175 mg/m^2 or to carboplatin AUC 5 plus PLD 30 mg/m^2, every 3 weeks for six cycles. The primary end point was PFS. Median PFS was 19.0 and 16.8 months with carboplatin/PLD and carboplatin/paclitaxel, respectively (HR, 0.95; 95% CI, 0.81–1.13; $p = 0.58$). Median OS times were 61.6 and 53.2 months with carboplatin/PLD and carboplatin/paclitaxel, respectively (HR, 0.89; 95% CI, 0.72–1.12; $p = 0.32$). Carboplatin/PLD produced less neurotoxicity and alopecia but more hematologic adverse effects. There was no relevant difference in global quality of life after three and six cycles (420). This regimen has not been widely adopted for front-line therapy, partly because the usual dose of carboplatin in the United States is AUC 6, and there are concerns about hematologic toxicity if this dose were added to PLD, partly because of data about possible superiority of weekly paclitaxel and partly because paclitaxel has been relatively easy to combine with other non-neurotoxic agents, and PLD can be more problematic in this regard. Nonetheless, the regimen appears at least as effective as standard dose every-3-week paclitaxel/carboplatin and may be an option for patients with severe neuropathy or taxane allergies.

Addition of Bevacizumab to Primary Chemotherapy

Bevacizumab is a humanized monoclonal antibody targeting vascular endothelial growth factor (VEGF). Elevated VEGF (or VEGF-A) expression occurs in all stages of ovarian cancer and is associated with poor prognosis, including shorter survival. Bevacizumab as a single agent produced response rates in the range of 15% to 20% in the setting of recurrent ovarian cancer (421), which are higher than the response rates seen for other solid tumors. There was therefore great enthusiasm for the addition of bevacizumab to up-front chemotherapy, and two large randomized trials have been performed in this setting, both showing an improvement in PFS, but no improvement in OS (**Table 23.16**).

GOG218 was a placebo-controlled three-arm study in women with stage III (incompletely resected) and stage IV disease (421). This trial compared a control group receiving carboplatin AUC 6/paclitaxel 175 mg/m^2 with carboplatin/paclitaxel with concomitant bevacizumab (15 mg/kg every 3 weeks) and with carboplatin/paclitaxel with concomitant bevacizumab followed by maintenance bevacizumab for an additional 16 doses (once every 3 weeks). In groups receiving bevacizumab, it was not started until cycle 2, to avoid postoperative wound healing problems. Median PFS for the three arms was 10.3, 11.2, and 14.1 months, respectively, but there were no significant differences in OS between the groups. The experimental regimen was tolerable; bowel perforation or fistula requiring medical intervention occurred in 1.2% of patients in the control arm, 2.8% of patients in the concomitant-only bevacizumab arm, and 2.6% of patients in the concomitant plus maintenance bevacizumab arm. Because the primary end point of the study was PFS, the blind was not maintained after progression, and the authors noted that the end point of OS could have been contaminated by the effect of post-progression therapy. Because blocking VEGF inhibits the formation of ascites in preclinical studies, a retrospective subset analysis of GOG218 examined whether the presence of ascites

TABLE 23.16. Randomized Trials with or without Bevacizumab

Trial Name	Population	Arms	Results Median PFS/OS[a]	
GOG218 (Burger, 2011) (421)	Stage III–IV first-line	Bev + Carbo + Paclitaxel →Bev Bev + Carbo + Paclitaxel →Placebo Placebo + Carbo + Paclitaxel →Placebo	14.1 months/39.7 months 11.2 months/38.7 months 10.3 months/39.3 months	
ICON7 (Perren, 2011) (405)	Stage IIB–IV first-line Stage I–IIA if gr3 or clear cell	Bev + Carbo + Paclitaxel →Bev Carbo + Paclitaxel	19 months/HR death 0.85 17.3 months/(0.69–1.04)	
OCEANS (Aghajanian, 2011) (503,542)	Platinum-sensitive first recurrence	Gem + Carbo + Bev→Bev Gem + Carbo + placebo→Placebo	12.4 months/33.6 months 8.4 months/32.9 months	RR = 78% RR = 57%
AURELIA (Pujade-Lauraine, 2012) (488)	Platinum-resistant, 1–2 prior regimens	Chemotherapy + Bev→Bev Chemotherapy (× over at progression) Chemotherapy = PLD, topotecan, or weekly paclitaxel	6.7 months/NA 3.4 months/NA	31% 13%
GOG213 (Coleman, 2016) (480)	Platinum-sensitive first recurrence	Paclitaxel + Carbo+Bev→Bev Paclitaxel + Carbo	13.8 months/42.2 months 10.4 months/37.3 months	$p < 0.0001$ for PFS; $p = 0.056$ for OS

[a]For most studies, OS reported as immature.

might affect the benefit from bevacizumab. Patients with no ascites ($n = 221$) had no improvement with bevacizumab in either PFS (adjusted hazard ratio [AHR] 0.81) or OS (AHR, 0.94), whereas those with ascites had significant improvement in both PFS (AHR, 0.71) and OS (AHR, 0.82). These data require validation before clinical application (422).

A second trial, ICON7, was led by European investigators. This study had only two arms: carboplatin/paclitaxel and carboplatin/paclitaxel with concomitant and 12 additional cycles of consolidation every-3-week bevacizumab). There was no placebo; the bevacizumab dose used was 7.5 mg/kg every 3 weeks rather than the 15 mg/kg used in the GOG218 trial; and women with both high-risk early-stage and with more advanced disease were eligible to participate. The restricted mean PFS for the control group and the group receiving bevacizumab was similar at 20.3 versus 21.8 months; restricted mean OS times were also not different at 44.6 versus 45.5 months. Restricted means were used for analysis because there was evidence of nonproportional hazards. In an exploratory analysis of a predefined subgroup of 502 patients with poor prognosis disease (stage IV or stage III with over 1.0 cm residual disease; similar to the population of GOG218 as a whole), a significant restricted mean OS difference was observed: 34.5 months for standard therapy versus 39.3 months with bevacizumab (423). The most important increase in toxicity was a risk of grade 2 or higher hypertension (18% with bevacizumab and 2% with standard therapy) and the risk for grade 3 or higher thromboembolic events (7% with bevacizumab vs. 3% with standard therapy). The primary quality of life end point in the ICON7 trial was global QoL as assessed by the European Organization for the Research and Treatment of Cancer (EORTC) quality of life questionnaire-core 30 at week 54. At week 54 (approximately just at the end of bevacizumab therapy) the mean score was 6.4 points lower in the bevacizumab arm ($p < 0.0001$) (424). By week 76 global QoL was not significantly different between the arms.

Based on the results of GOG218 and ICON7, the European Medicines Agency approved the use of bevacizumab in combination with paclitaxel plus carboplatin for the front-line treatment of advanced ovarian cancer with at least stage IIIB disease in the European Union. Bevacizumab is not FDA-approved in the United States for front-line use in ovarian cancer, and the National Institute for Health and Care Excellent (NICE) in the UK guidance statement stated that use of bevacizumab for first-line treatment of ovarian cancer is not a cost-effective use of resources (425). Issues discussed have included the lack of OS benefit seen with bevacizumab in either study as a whole and the high cost of the drug.

The appropriate duration of bevacizumab therapy has also been an issue. Because the PFS curves for both GOG218 and ICON7, which administered bevacizumab only for a fixed period of time after completion of chemotherapy, appear to converge at some point after discontinuation of bevacizumab (nonproportional hazards), it has been hypothesized that the bevacizumab benefit is dependent on continued administration. The ongoing MITO-16/MANGO2b trial *Multicenter Phase III Randomized Study with Second-Line Chemotherapy Plus or Minus Bevacizumab in Patients with Platinum-Sensitive Epithelial Ovarian Cancer Recurrence After a Bevacizumab/Chemotherapy First Line* is testing the benefit of bevacizumab in patients already treated with bevacizumab.

It may be that some subsets of patients benefit more from bevacizumab than others. Preliminary data presented at the ASCO in 2014 using a subset of 284 high-grade serous tumors from the ICON7 trial identified a molecular signature ("immune subgroup") in which antiangiogenic therapy might actually confer a worse PFS (HR, 1.73; 95% CI, 1.12–2.68) and OS (HR, 2.00; 95% CI, 1.11–3.61) when compared with chemotherapy alone (426). At the same meeting Winterhoff et al. used a different subset of 380 tumors from the same trial and analyzed response by the molecular classification described by The Cancer Genome Atlas (TCGA) project. They found that the carcinomas of mesenchymal subtype appeared to benefit most from bevacizumab with a median PFS improvement of 9.5 months; the differentiated, immunoreactive, and proliferative subtypes demonstrated median PFS improvements of 5.8, 3.4, and 3.2 months, respectively (427). In an analysis of the predictive power of CD31 expression in patients from GOG 218, the median OS with bevacizumab was found to be 45.6 months compared with 35.9 months with placebo in patients with CD31 high expression (HR, 0.68; 95% CI, 0.52–0.89; $p = 0.0155$). In the CD31 low group, the HR was 1.13 (428). No validations of any of these analyses have been published to date.

Newer antiangiogenic agents have also been tested in the front-line setting. The oral VEGF receptor antagonist, nintedanib (200 mg twice daily), was added to first-line standard therapy in the phase III placebo-controlled AGO-OVAR12 trial and was continued up to 120 weeks. Median PFS was minimally but statistically significantly improved from 16.6 to 17.2 months; grade 3 diarrhea increased from 2% to 21% (429). The phase III AGO-OVAR16 trial compared pazopanib as maintenance treatment after first-line therapy; treatment with pazopanib extended PFS by 5.6 months compared with placebo. Preliminary OS data did not suggest benefit (430).

At this time antiangiogenic therapy is not standard in the United States for front-line therapy of ovarian cancer.

Intraperitoneal Chemotherapy

Intraperitoneal (IP) chemotherapy is a form of dose escalation; it provides a means by which high concentrations of drugs and long durations of tissue exposure can be attained at the peritoneal surface. Because IP progression of disease remains the major source of morbidity and mortality in ovarian cancer, it is a theoretically attractive approach in the treatment of this disease. Many chemotherapeutic agents, including those used for the treatment of ovarian cancer such as cisplatin, carboplatin, topotecan, and paclitaxel, have been tested for feasibility with IP administration. Larger or less water-soluble molecules will stay longer in the peritoneal cavity and have a higher peritoneal cavity-to-plasma concentration ratio (sometimes referred to as "pharmacologic advantage"), but may not get into the bloodstream. The direct penetration of chemotherapy agents into tumor masses is limited to 1 to 2 mm from the tumor surface. Early work by Los et al., using a rat intraperitoneal tumor model, found that the concentration of cisplatin at the periphery of tumor nodules was higher after IP administration of cisplatin, but the concentration at the center of the nodules was identical after IP and IV administration (431). Hence (a) the theoretical benefit is only for very small tumor volumes and (b) agents that do not reach therapeutic systemic levels when given by the IP route need to be administered intravenously (IV) as well. Cisplatin has a 10- to 20-fold pharmacologic advantage when given intraperitoneally. For a given dose of cisplatin, peak concentrations are higher with IV cisplatin, and this has resulted in somewhat decreased toxicity in a randomized comparison of the same doses of cisplatin given IP versus IV, including less hearing loss and neuromuscular toxicity. However, the amount of cisplatin recovered in the urine, reflecting total systemic exposure, is similar regardless of whether the administration is IV or IP. Similarly, carboplatin given IP at an AUC of 6 has been shown to produce an AUC in the peritoneal cavity about 17 times higher than that of carboplatin given intravenously while producing a very similar serum AUC (432). Paclitaxel, on the other hand, has a pharmacologic advantage of about 1,000, and significant levels persist in the peritoneal cavity 1 week after drug administration. However, the dose that can be given is limited by abdominal pain, and serum paclitaxel concentrations detected in patients treated with IP paclitaxel at feasible doses are low (433). It should be recognized that administration of IP chemotherapy can be technically challenging, and catheter-related issues are common.

Clinical Use of Intraperitoneal Therapy for Ovarian Cancer

In January 2006, the NCI issued a clinical alert supporting the use of IP cisplatin chemotherapy in women with optimally surgically debulked ovarian cancer. A meta-analysis of eight trials comparing IP with IV platinum-based chemotherapy (all but one used cisplatin) showed an average 21.6% decrease in the risk of death (HR, 0.79; 95% CI, 0.70–0.89) with IP therapy. Because the expected median duration of survival for women with optimally debulked ovarian cancer receiving standard treatment is approximately 4 years, this size reduction in the death rate was estimated to translate into about a 12-month increase in overall median survival. The power of this analysis was based primarily on the survival benefits for IP chemotherapy observed in the first three randomized trials summarized in **Table 23.17** (116,434,435). However, none of these trials used a modern carboplatin/weekly paclitaxel IV arm, and all

TABLE 23.17. Selected Randomized Trials of Intraperitoneal versus Intravenous Chemotherapy in Optimally Debulked Ovarian Cancer

Author (Year)	N	Regimens	Median PFS	Median OS	Comments
Alberts (1996) (434)	546	IV cyclophosphamide 600 mg/m^2 + IP cisplatin 100 mg/m^2 × 6	N/A	49 months	<2 cm residual disease permitted; 58% of patients in both groups completed 6 cycles of cisplatin
		vs.		vs.	
		IV cyclophosphamide 600 mg/m^2 + IV cisplatin 100 mg/m^2 × 6		41 months $p = 0.02$	
Markman (2001) (435)	462	IV carboplatin AUC 9 × 2 followed by IV paclitaxel 135 mg/m^2/24 h + IP cisplatin 100 mg/m^2 × 6	28 months	63 months	18% of patients on IP arm received ≤2 cycles of IP therapy
		vs.	vs.	vs.	
		IV paclitaxel 135 mg/m^2/24 h + IV cisplatin 75 mg/m^2 × 6	22 months $p = 0.01$	52 months $p = 0.05$	
Armstrong (2006) (116)	416	D1 IV paclitaxel 135 mg/m^2/24 h + D2 IP cisplatin 100 mg/m^2 + D8 IP paclitaxel 60 mg/m^2	24 months	67 months	49% of patients received ≤3 cycles of IP therapy
		vs.	vs.	vs.	
		D1 IV cisplatin 75 mg/m^2 + D1 IV paclitaxel 135 mg/m^2/24 h	19 months	50 months	
Walker (2016) (436)	1,560	D1 IV carboplatin AUC 6 +D1,8,15 IV paclitaxel 80 mg/m^2	24.9 months	N/A	Bevacizumab 15 mg/kg IV D1 given on all arms
		vs.			
		D1 IP carboplatin AUC 6 +D1,8,15 IV paclitaxel 80 mg/m^2	27.3 months		
		vs.			
		D1 IV paclitaxel 135 mg/m^2/3hr +D2 IP cisplatin 75 mg/m^2 +D8 IP paclitaxel 60 mg/m^2	26.0 months		

IP, intraperitoneal; IV, intravenous; OS, overall survival; PFS, progression-free survival.

of them used IP cisplatin at 100 mg/m^2 which has been deemed unacceptably toxic. This is largely because of the cisplatin dose; in the SWOG trial which used a control arm that included cisplatin 100 mg/m^2 IV, the IP arm was actually less toxic. In GOG172, only 42% of patients on the IP arm received the six planned cycles of intraperitoneal therapy because of either cisplatin-related toxicities or catheter problems.

Significant effort was therefore put into developing a more tolerable IP regimen, primarily either reducing the dose of cisplatin or substituting IP carboplatin for IP cisplatin. IP carboplatin can be safely used and appears to have favorable pharmacokinetics (pharmacologic advantage combined with good systemic drug exposure), but there is no evidence yet that it will provide the same survival benefit as IP cisplatin. These less toxic regimens were compared with an IV weekly paclitaxel/every-3-week carboplatin regimen in GOG252. The three arms of GOG252 included the all IV carboplatin plus dose-dense paclitaxel regimen published by the JGOG, the identical regimen with the carboplatin administered IP instead of IV, and a modification of the regimen used in GOG172 with paclitaxel 135 mg/m^2 IV over 3 hours on day 1, cisplatin 75 mg/m^2 IP on day 2, and paclitaxel 60 mg/m^2 IP on day 8. All three arms were combined with bevacizumab, which was administered every 3 weeks and continued for 22 cycles. Results of this trial were reported at the 2016 meeting of the SGO and showed no difference between the three arms, with a median PFS of 26.8 months for the all IV arm, 28.7 months for the IP carboplatin arm, and 27.8 months for the IP cisplatin arm. Toxicity was worst in the IP cisplatin arm, with 11.2% of patients experiencing grade 3 or greater nausea or vomiting compared with 5.1% in the all IV arm and 4.7% in the IP carboplatin arm (436). It is not clear if the negative results of this trial are because of the specific regimens chosen, as the cisplatin dose in the IP arm was lower than the IP cisplatin dose used in previous trials, and the weekly paclitaxel in the control arm may have been advantageous. Alternatively, the use of bevacizumab may in some way have obscured the benefits of IP therapy, as it is postulated to have obscured the benefits of weekly paclitaxel in GOG262.

Ongoing Trials with IP Therapy

Ongoing trials, including iPOCC and OV-21, should provide some additional information regarding the benefits of IP therapy. In the iPOCC trial (GOTIC-001/JGOG 3019), the route of carboplatin administration is the only variable that differs between the two arms: dose-dense weekly paclitaxel at 80 mg/m^2 IV is administered in combination with either IV or IP carboplatin AUC 6 every 3 weeks. Patients with stages II to IV disease are eligible; hence this study will explore the potential of IP chemotherapy in suboptimally debulked disease. It is certainly possible that intraperitoneal therapy might benefit women other than those with initially optimally debulked cancer. For example, some patients might be "chemically debulked" by their first few cycles of chemotherapy. The SWOG 8501 trial (Alberts, **Table 23.17**), perhaps the cleanest of the previous IP therapy trials in that all variables were the same in both arms except the route of cisplatin administration, permitted accrual of women with up to 2 cm of residual disease. Benefit of therapy was not influenced by the extent of residual disease ($p = 0.93$ for interaction of treatment and residual disease, microscopic vs. $\leq$0.5 cm vs. $>$0.5–2 cm). The OV-21/GCIG study incorporates IP therapy after neo-adjuvant treatment. Responders to neo-adjuvant therapy receive interval debulking surgery, and if the residual disease after surgery is less than 1 cm, they are randomized to one of three arms. The control arm is the combination of IV paclitaxel at 135 mg/m^2 followed by IV carboplatin AUC 5 on day 1, and then IV paclitaxel at 60 mg/m^2 on day 8. The second arm is same as the control arm except that carboplatin and day 8 paclitaxel are given by the IP route. The third arm is the same as the second arm, except that IP cisplatin 75 mg/m^2 is substituted for IP carboplatin.

Although it appears that at equal doses, IP cisplatin may be more effective than IV cisplatin, it is not clear that the IP regimens in use today are more effective than an all-IV weekly paclitaxel/every-3-week carboplatin regimen, but they are clearly more toxic. Therefore for many experts, the future role of IP therapy remains uncertain.

Consolidation/Maintenance

Many women with ovarian cancer have an excellent response to first-line chemotherapy, but most will nonetheless relapse and die of their disease. Approximately two-thirds of patients with advanced ovarian cancer will achieve a clinical complete remission following chemotherapy; that is, they will have no evidence of disease on physical examination or in radiographic studies together with a serum CA-125 in the normal range. In the days when second-look laparotomy was used, about one-third of all patients with advanced ovarian cancer were free of disease at a second-look laparotomy following primary cisplatin-based therapy. Such operations, whose purpose was prognostic, are no longer generally performed, because no therapy instituted as a result of disease found at second-look surgery was found to alter prognosis, and over half of those patients who initially presented with stage III or IV disease will recur after a negative second-look operation.

Further therapy after a clinical complete remission would clearly be warranted for many women if an effective treatment could be found. However, despite extensive investigation, no trials of consolidation or maintenance therapy have produced any survival benefit to date. The most promising strategies tested have been maintenance paclitaxel and maintenance bevacizumab, both of which appear to delay progression without improving OS.

Consolidation with Intraperitoneal Chemotherapy

The EORTC randomized women with a pathologic complete remission to front-line platinum-based therapy to no further therapy versus four cycles of intraperitoneal cisplatin at 100 mg/m^2. The trial closed early with less than half of its planned accrual. After a median follow-up of 8 years, the HRs for PFS and OS were 0.89 (95% CI, 0.59–1.33) and 0.82 (95% CI, 0.52–1.29). These results were felt to be suggestive of a treatment benefit, but insufficient to change practice (437).

Consolidative Radiotherapy

A randomized trial of intraperitoneal ^{32}P versus observation after pathologic complete response to primary therapy was negative (380). Whole abdominal radiotherapy after chemotherapy is problematic because of complications including myelosuppression, radiation enteritis, and bowel obstruction. Using conventional techniques, WAR is not able to deliver adequate radiation doses to the upper abdomen, because of limiting toxicities to organs such as liver and kidneys. Several very small randomized trials have been conducted with contradictory results. Nonetheless, some of the results have been intriguing. For example, the Swedish-Norwegian Ovarian Cancer Study Group randomly assigned 98 patients with stage III ovarian cancer who had a pathologic complete response (CR) at second-look surgery after 4 courses of cisplatin/anthracycline chemotherapy to no further therapy, continued chemotherapy with cisplatin/anthracycline to 10 courses total, or whole abdominal radiotherapy. PFS was significantly better (5-year PFS: WAR = 56%, chemotherapy = 36%, control = 35%, $p = 0.032$) and OS trended toward better in the group receiving WAR (438). As discussed above in the section "Early-Stage Disease," there may be a role for radiation in early-stage clear cell carcinomas, and in this situation pelvic radiotherapy might be able to produce the same benefit as whole abdominal radiotherapy.

Consolidative/Maintenance Chemotherapy

As is the case for use of a third cytotoxic agent in front-line combination therapy, use of a third cytotoxic agent such as topotecan or epirubicin for consolidation/maintenance therapy has failed to improve outcomes (439–441). Two small prospective trials of consolidation with high-dose chemotherapy with hematopoietic stem cell support have both been negative (442,443).

Paclitaxel Maintenance Therapy. The most promising trial of maintenance therapy to date has been a Southwest Oncology Group (SWOG)/GOG trial randomizing women in clinical complete remission to either 3 or 12 cycles of IV paclitaxel 175 mg/m^2 every 4 weeks (444). The trial was halted by its data and safety monitoring board after a planned interim efficacy analysis, at a point when there was a statistically significant improvement in time to progression but no difference in OS between the treatment arms (PFS 28 vs. 21 months, one-sided $p = 0.0035$). Because insufficient patients to detect a survival difference had been randomized at the time the study was stopped ($n = 262$) and because patients receiving 3 cycles of therapy were allowed the option of crossing over to 12 cycles, a survival comparison was not possible. The neurotoxicity observed was substantial, even though patients with higher than grade 1 neurotoxicity were excluded from the trial, and the dose of paclitaxel was decreased during the study conduct to 135 mg/m^2 every 4 weeks. However, not very many patients had accrued to the lower dose at the time of study closure, and they were not included in the analysis, so the effect of this dose reduction on therapy efficacy is uncertain. An unplanned retrospective subgroup analysis suggested a trend toward survival benefit in the group of patients who started maintenance therapy with a CA-125 level of less than 10 (445).

A subsequent Italian study group randomized 200 patients with stages IIb to IV disease who were in clinical or pathologic complete response after six courses of paclitaxel/platinum-based chemotherapy to either observation or six consolidation courses of paclitaxel 175 mg/m^2 every 3 weeks. Grade 2 or greater sensory neurotoxicity was reported in 28.0% of the paclitaxel-arm patients. Two-year PFS rates were 54% and 59% (p = not significant) in the control and maintenance arms, respectively. Corresponding 2-year OS rates were 90% and 87% (p = not significant), respectively (446). As mentioned above, GOG212 randomized women in clinical complete remission after primary therapy for stage III or IV disease to maintenance paclitaxel polyglumex, maintenance paclitaxel, or observation, and results are pending. This trial has OS as the end point.

Maintenance with Noncytotoxic Agents. Noncytotoxic agents such as interferon, a monoclonal antibody targeting CA-125 (oregovomab), erlotinib, radioimmunoconjugates including intraperitoneal administration of a 90Y-conjugated antimucin antibody, and matrix metalloproteinase inhibitors have all been tested in phase III trials with no improvement in survival. As discussed above, trials of antiangiogenic agents in the consolidation/maintenance setting have shown some promise, but none are currently approved for this indication.

Specifics of Epithelial Ovarian Cancer with Clear Cell and Mucinous Histology, Including Advanced Disease

Historically, clinical trials for epithelial ovarian cancer included all histologic subtypes together. It has become obvious that this is not appropriate and that the different histologic subtypes are both biologically and clinically distinct. Because high-grade serous tumors make up about two-thirds of advanced-stage disease (see **Table 23.10**), there has been little power to draw conclusions about the relative benefit of the treatment under study to less common subtypes. However, it has become obvious that advanced-stage clear cell and mucinous tumors have a worse prognosis than advanced-stage serous tumors, which may be related to lower sensitivity to standard cytotoxic chemotherapy.

Clear Cell Carcinomas

Clear cell carcinoma accounts for 1% to 12% of epithelial ovarian carcinomas in the United States, but 15% to 25% of epithelial ovarian cancers in Japan. Asian women in the United States who get ovarian cancer are twice as likely to have a clear cell cancer as White women. In Japan, as in Western countries, clear cell carcinoma tends to present at an early stage; in one review, 39% of clear cell cancers were stage I, 13% stage II, 30% stage III, and 6% stage IV (332). Histologic diagnosis may be challenging (see the section "Pathology"), because some HGSCs have a clear cell component and may be misclassified as clear cell carcinomas. There is a high frequency of capsule rupture during surgery for clear cell carcinoma. In the EORTC-ACTION trial, capsule rupture was reported in 44% of clear cell carcinomas versus 19% of serous tumors. The vast majority was because of intraoperative rupture. A review of early-stage clear cell ovarian cancer in British Columbia found that 5-year disease survival for all patients with FIGO stage IC clear cell disease was 67% versus 84% for those stage IA/B clear cell tumors. However, patients with IC disease based on capsule rupture alone, with no positive cytology or surface involvement, had a prognosis similar to those with stage IA disease (379). As discussed above, the benefits of chemotherapy in early-stage clear cell carcinoma are uncertain.

Molecular studies suggest a distinct profile for clear cell carcinomas. Unlike high-grade serous cancers, they are mostly (85%) *p53* wild-type, and they have a lower frequency of *BRCA1* and *2* germ line mutations than high-grade serous tumors. They have low levels of chromosomal instability and a high frequency (up to 40%) of phosphoinositide 3-kinase catalytic alpha (*PIK3CA*) mutations. AT-rich interactive domain-containing protein 1A (*ARID1A*), a tumor suppressor gene, appears to have an inactivating mutation in almost half of clear cell carcinomas (36). Another characteristic feature is the overexpression of the proinflammatory cytokine IL-6. Gene expression profiling suggests some similarities between clear cell carcinomas of the ovary, endometrium, and kidney. Both uterine and ovarian clear cell carcinomas are pathophysiologically linked to malignant transformation of endometriosis, and some current clinical trials allow enrollment of patients with clear cell carcinoma of either the uterus or the ovary.

As discussed above (see "prognosis"), advanced-stage clear cell carcinomas do not respond as well to platinum-based chemotherapy as do high-grade serous tumors (HGSC). Response rates to front-line carboplatin and paclitaxel therapy range from 22% to 56% compared with 70% in HGSC (447). Survival for women with advanced-stage clear cell disease is also inferior to that of women with HGSC. A 2010 meta-analysis which included data from over 8,000 patients on seven international front-line trials using platinum-based regimens identified 221 women with stage III/IV clear cell carcinoma. These women had a median OS of 21.3 months versus 40.8 months for women with serous carcinomas (448). Similar results were seen in a review of data from 544 stage I–IV patients with ovarian clear cell carcinoma who participated in 12 randomized GOG protocols using platinum-based chemotherapy. Although there was no significant difference in PFS or OS for early-stage clear cell carcinoma compared with early stage HGSC, late stage patients with clear cell carcinoma had poorer outcomes compared with those with last stage HGSC, with HR for OS being 1.66. This held true for both optimally debulked (HR, 1.34, $p = 0.003$) and suboptimally debulked (HR, 3.18, $p < 0.001$) disease (448).

Most studies of therapy for recurrent clear cell carcinoma have found low response rates. Investigators from MD Anderson published a retrospective review of 51 patients treated at their institution for recurrent clear cell carcinoma. Among those with platinum-sensitive disease, only 2 (9%) of 22 patients had a partial response to retreatment with carboplatin and paclitaxel; none of the 29 patients given second-line therapy for platinum-resistant disease responded (449). In a study of 75 Japanese women with at least two lines of prior systemic therapy, those whose tumors recurred more than 6 months after completion of chemotherapy had a response rate of 8%, which was similar to the response rate of 6% observed for those whose tumors progressed within 6 months of completing primary chemotherapy (386). This may be because most recurrences occur in women who presented with completely resected stage I disease, and hence there is no way of knowing if the tumor actually shrank in response to chemotherapy, making the term "platinum sensitive" a misnomer. However, the MITO-9 project identified 72 patients with recurrent clear cell carcinoma and found somewhat more optimistic results to second-line therapy, with an overall response rate to platinum of 80% in platinum-sensitive disease. However, there was no central pathology review; in about half of patients the histology was "mixed," and only 28% were stage I at diagnosis, raising the possibility that a number of these tumors might not be considered clear cell with current pathology standards (450).

There are few reports of therapies effective specifically for clear cell carcinomas. The Japanese Gynecologic Oncology Group (JGOG 3017) performed a randomized phase III study comparing paclitaxel plus carboplatin with cisplatin plus irinotecan for the front-line therapy of clear cell carcinoma, and results showed no differences in OS or PFS between the arms (451). Among the nonplatinum agents used in primary and secondary resistant cases in the MITO-9 analysis, gemcitabine appeared to have better activity [response rate (RR) 66%] than topotecan (RR 33%) or liposomal doxorubicin (RR 10%).

There has been interest in the use of mTOR inhibitors (which have activity in the therapy of clear cell kidney cancer) and agents targeting the Akt/PI3K pathway; a report of weekly temsirolimus in five evaluable patients with heavily pretreated clear cell carcinoma of the ovary noted one partial response of 14 months duration (452). Although the response rate in the GOG phase II trial of temsirolimus in women with epithelial ovarian cancer unselected for histology was disappointing at 9.3%, one of the three patients with clear cell histology did have a partial response lasting 4 months (453). A front-line single-arm phase II trial (GOG268; NCT01196429), testing the combination of carboplatin, paclitaxel, and temsirolimus followed by consolidation temsirolimus in the treatment of stage III/IV clear cell carcinoma of the ovary, has fully accrued; results should be available soon. Antiangiogenic agents, which like mTOR inhibitors have activity in the treatment of renal cell carcinoma, are also actively being explored. GY001 is an ongoing phase II trial of cabozantanib in recurrent clear cell carcinoma of the ovary. Cabozantanib inhibits multiple receptor tyrosine kinases including VEGFr and c-Met, which have been shown to be amplified and overexpressed in clear cell adenocarcinomas. A phase II trial of rilotumumab (AMG 102), a monoclonal antibody targeting hepatocyte growth factor (HGF; ligand for cMET), was performed in women with pretreated ovarian cancer unselected for cMET status or histology. One of 31 patients had a complete response, and she had a tumor of endometrioid/clear cell histology (454). The ongoing European NiCCC trial is comparing nintedanib, which targets multiple receptor tyrosine kinases including VEGF, PDGF, and FGF, with chemotherapy (investigator choice of three different agents) in the treatment of recurrent clear cell carcinoma of ovary or endometrium.

Multiple reports suggest that women with clear cell carcinomas are more likely to have a thromboembolic event. In one retrospective study 42% of patients with clear cell carcinoma had a venous thromboembolic event versus only 22% of patients with other histologies. Half of the events occurred postoperatively (455). Venous thromboembolism during primary therapy of ovarian clear cell carcinoma is associated with shorter PFS and OS, and this increase in mortality is not attributable to mortality from the thrombotic event (456). Hypercalcemia related to paraneoplastic expression of parathyroid hormone-related peptide has also been reported to be more common in clear cell carcinoma of the ovary than in other subtypes (457). Bone metastases and brain metastases may occur.

Mucinous Tumors

When gene expression arrays are performed, mucinous tumors group separately from serous, endometrioid, and clear cell ovarian carcinomas. They are not associated with *BRCA* mutations, and often have *KRAS* mutations. *HER2* is amplified in about 20% of mucinous tumors (458). Unlike colorectal adenocarcinomas, they are often immunoreactive for CK7; unlike other ovarian cancers they are frequently immunoreactive for CK20 and CDX2 (which are usually diffusely and strongly reactive in colorectal adenocarcinomas), though the staining is often weak and focal. Early-stage mucinous tumors tend to be low grade and have a good prognosis. They are unlikely to have metastasized to lymph nodes, and as discussed above (see section "Early-Stage Disease"), lymph node dissection is generally not needed in stage IA mucinous tumors. Advanced-stage mucinous tumors, which are uncommon, respond poorly to chemotherapy and are associated with a short survival. MacKay et al. found the median disease-free survival for women with stage III/IV mucinous tumors to be only 14.6 months, even shorter than that for women with clear cell disease (314). It is now known that many tumors thought initially to be advanced-stage mucinous tumors in older studies actually represent metastatic disease from another site, so it is difficult to interpret published results. In a recent international front-line trial for stage III/IV disease that tested five different regimens of cytotoxic chemotherapy in 4,000 women, 44 cases were classified as mucinous adenocarcinoma. Only about one-third of these was judged to be primary mucinous carcinomas by the three central reviewers; the remainder were thought to represent metastatic disease from another site. Interestingly, the median survival did not differ significantly between the groups considered primary ovarian cancers or metastatic tumors from another site, and survival for both groups was significantly shorter than the survival for women with serous carcinoma (14 vs. 42 months, $p < 0.001$) (88).

Based on similarities of mucinous ovarian cancers to colorectal carcinomas, an international trial was launched to compare carboplatin/paclitaxel with or without bevacizumab, with capecitabine/oxaliplatin with or without bevacizumab in the front-line therapy of stage II–IV or recurrent mucinous carcinomas. Unfortunately this trial was closed because of poor enrollment. Of the 16 patients accrued, only 5 were deemed to have correct stage and histology on central pathology review, illustrating some of the difficulties in both clinically identifying and studying advanced mucinous ovarian cancer (459).

CARCINOSARCOMA

Ovarian carcinosarcomas tend to present with advanced disease, and early-stage tumors are unusual. Stage III ovarian carcinosarcoma appears to be more common than either stage III mucinous ovarian cancer or stage III clear cell cancer (**Table 23.10**). Ovarian carcinosarcoma occurs at a slightly older age and has a worse prognosis overall than epithelial ovarian cancer without sarcomatous differentiation, with a median OS in the range of 9 to 24 months. A SEER database review found a 5-year survival of 65.2% for stage I ovarian carcinosarcoma (vs. 80.6% for stage I serous tumors) and of 18.2% for stage III ovarian carcinosarcoma (vs. 33.3% for stage III serous ovarian cancer) (460). The presence of homologous versus heterologous elements has not been found to have any clear influence on outcomes, but the presence of more than 25% sarcomatous histology has been linked to a worse prognosis. Optimal cytoreduction is associated with improved outcomes, and it is generally recommended that operative management of these tumors resembles that of epithelial ovarian cancer. Adjuvant chemotherapy is also generally recommended, although randomized trials showing benefit do not exist. Prospective GOG trials reported response rates of 10% for single-agent doxorubicin, 18% for ifosfamide, and 20% for cisplatin. Retrospective series have suggested that platinum-containing regimens produce higher response rates than nonplatinum-containing regimens, but the optimal regimen remains unknown, and it is unknown whether the percentage of sarcomatous histology in the tumor should influence choice of regimen. One series suggested improved outcomes with cisplatin/ifosfamide versus carboplatin/paclitaxel; another suggested superior outcomes with carboplatin/paclitaxel versus other regimens (461). A case–control series of 50 cases of carcinosarcoma of the ovary treated with first-line platinum–taxane-based therapy and 100 cases of papillary serous ovarian cancer matched by age, stage, and year of diagnosis showed response rates to chemotherapy of 62% for carcinosarcomas and 83% for epithelial ovarian cancers, with median PFS of 11 versus 16 months and median OS of 24 versus 41 months (462). Some trials allow patients with carcinosarcoma of the ovary to participate in trials for carcinosarcoma of the uterus, and in GOG261, women with stage I–IV disease are randomized to front-line therapy with either paclitaxel plus carboplatin or ifosfamide plus paclitaxel. Accrual is complete but results are not yet available.

Follow-Up of Patients Who are Clinically Without Evidence of Disease – Survivorship Issues

There are relatively few studies of long-term effects of therapy for ovarian cancer. A recent systematic review of studies examining QOL in patients who survived ovarian cancer after treatment found that QOL is generally good compared with healthy women, but fear of recurrence, sexual problems, and treatment sequelae, particularly neuropathy, persist (463).

In premenopausal women with ovarian cancer, the removal of the ovaries results in premature menopause. Consequently, they have symptoms including hot flashes and vaginal dryness, and those who achieve long-term survival are at increased risk for osteoporosis. There has historically been some concern about prescribing HRT to ovarian cancer survivors because (1) epidemiologic evidence suggests that estrogen replacement therapy slightly increases the risk of developing ovarian cancer *de novo* and (2) most ovarian cancers express estrogen receptors, and antiestrogens, such as tamoxifen, may produce tumor shrinkage in a small subset of women with advanced ovarian cancer. However, long-term results of the small randomized AHT (Adjuvant Hormone Therapy) trial ($n = 150$) have supported the hypothesis that HRT is safe for ovarian cancer survivors. Women with any stage ovarian cancer were randomized to HRT or no HRT, where HRT selection was according to treating physician preference. At a median follow-up of 19 years for living patients, OS was significantly improved in patients receiving HRT (HR, 0.63; $p = 0.011$). No statistically significant difference in adverse events was seen between groups (23).

Neuropathy is a symptom flagged in most surveys of ovarian cancer survivors. An Italian retrospective review (MITO-4) queried 120 women who received carboplatin AUC 5 plus paclitaxel 175 mg/m^2 every 3 weeks for six cycles and remained in clinical remission. Fifty-four percent had some neurologic toxicity during chemotherapy (42% grade 1, 11% grade 2, and 1% grade 3). The probability of residual neurotoxicity was 15% at 6 months after the end of chemotherapy and 11% at 2 years after the end of chemotherapy (464). Rates of neuropathy are higher with dose-dense weekly paclitaxel regimens and with cisplatin-containing regimens. Whereas there are agents, such as duloxetine, that can provide some symptomatic alleviation for neuropathy, it is best prevented. Patients should be questioned about numbness and tingling in their hands and feet at each visit during treatment, and agent substitution (e.g., docetaxel for paclitaxel, carboplatin for cisplatin) or dose modification should be considered before neuropathy becomes severe, particularly in patients whose life might be affected by neuropathy (e.g., piano player). Neuropathy is more common in older patients and in African Americans.

Risks of second primaries, particularly for patients with a *BRCA* mutation or Lynch syndrome, should be kept in mind. Patients may have been too overwhelmed at the time of diagnosis to consider genetic counseling, and other family members may develop cancers as time goes by, so the issue should be reconsidered during follow-up visits.

Follow-Up of Patients in Remission

National Comprehensive Cancer Network (NCCN) Guidelines (version 2.2015) (465) for follow-up of patients with ovarian cancer who enter a clinical complete remission include a history and clinical exam every 2 to 4 months for 2 years, then 3 to 6 months for 3 years, then annually after 5 years, with CA-125 or other tumor markers at every visit if initially elevated, and imaging only as clinically indicated. Pelvic exam should be performed periodically. A rise in CA-125 in patients with a history of high-grade serous cancer is fairly specific for recurrence, particularly if the pretreatment CA-125 was significantly elevated and a second confirmatory CA-125 shows that the titer is continuing to rise. The CA-125 may rise prior to any evidence of disease on imaging, and, in about a third of all women, over 6 months will elapse between the initial CA-125 rise and the time they develop symptoms. Recurrent ovarian cancer is not curable, and it is not clear that earlier detection can improve either survival or QOL. The Medical Research Council (OV-05) and the European Organization for the Research and Treatment of Cancer (EORTC 55955) conducted a phase 3 trial in which 1,442 women with a clinical complete remission after first-line platinum-containing therapy were followed with serial CA-125 levels, followed by randomization to either initiate treatment at the time of biochemical recurrence (defined as a CA-125 exceeding twice the upper limit of normal) versus waiting until the time of clinical evidence of recurrence. A total of 529 women were randomized. Twenty percent of women had a rise in CA-125 within 6 months of completing primary chemotherapy, 33% between 6 and 12 months, and 45% after 12 or more months. Treatment at the time of CA-125 rise resulted in starting chemotherapy 4.8 months earlier compared with patients treated at the time of clinical recurrence. However, survival (defined as survival from the time of CA-125 rise) did not differ between the two groups, at 25.7 months for women assigned to early treatment and 27.1 months for those assigned to delayed treatment. Most importantly, women receiving early treatment had a worse QOL as measured by a shorter time to deterioration of the global health score on the EORTC QLQ-C30 questionnaire (136). Issues concerning the use of CA-125 as part of follow-up should be discussed with patients. Detection of disease while it is not symptomatic may allow patients more opportunity to participate in trials of new agents, but it cannot be claimed to improve survival, and some women may opt for less aggressive monitoring.

Uses of CA-125 in Ovarian Cancer Treatment

Tumor markers are discussed in the section on Clinical Presentation and Diagnostic Work-Up. As discussed above (see "Screening"), the current usefulness of CA-125 for screening of asymptomatic women is limited, in part because many stage I ovarian cancers are not associated with an elevated serum level of CA-125, and a variety of nonmalignant conditions (endometriosis, tuberculosis, abdominal infections, hepatitis) can elevate CA-125, particularly in premenopausal women. Some more recent large-scale screening trials have used multimodal strategies including CA-125 algorithm (ROCA), which establishes a CA-125 baseline for each woman and evaluates for changes in slope (66). CA-125 is also widely used to monitor for cancer recurrence in patients with complete remission after front-line therapy, but as described above, this has not been shown to improve survival. For women with a high CA-125 at baseline, the marker correlates with volume of disease and is often checked with each cycle of chemotherapy. Multiple studies have shown that the rapidity of CA-125 normalization and depth of CA-125 nadir after completion of primary therapy have prognostic value. For example, one group found median PFS and OS for women with stage III or IV ovarian cancer who achieved a value of less than 35 U/mL after third cycle to be 18 and 42 months, respectively, compared with 9 and 22 months for patients whose tumor marker did not normalize ($p < 0.001$) (360). The authors suggested that in future trials, women whose CA-125 does not normalize after the third cycle should be switched to an alternate regimen. However, at this time there are no clinical interventions known to improve outcomes for those women who do not show the desired decline in CA-125.

CA-125 may be useful for monitoring the effectiveness of second-line chemotherapy, decreasing the need for frequent imaging. A number of CA-125 response definitions, such as 50% or 75% decline, have been developed. Herzog et al. reported that in a large phase III ovarian cancer trial of salvage chemotherapy (OVA301, pegylated liposomal doxorubicin plus trabectedin vs. pegylated liposomal doxorubicin alone), the concordance between CA-125 using modified Rustin criteria (which define a CA-125 response as ≥ 50% reduction in CA-125 levels from pretreatment values, maintained at least 28 days) (466) and that using RECIST (Response Evaluation Criteria in Solid Tumors 1.0) criteria was 79%. The negative predictive value of CA-125 was 89% to 90%, indicating that in most cases, lack of CA-125 response predicts lack of radiologic response. However, the positive predictive value of CA-125 was only 59% to 68%, indicating that response by CA-125 does not always predict a RECIST response. Changes in CA-125 tended to occur first: radiologic response was preceded by a CA-125 decrease in a high proportion of patients, and CA-125 progression preceded RECIST progression in 35% of patients, with a median lead time of 8.4 weeks (467).

Caution should be used when relying on CA-125 to assess response to therapy, particularly in women with heavily pretreated disease. It can occasionally happen that major discordance develops, and the cancer progresses whereas the CA-125 value declines. In addition, there may be a "marker flare" after the first cycle of chemotherapy. Sabbatini et al. reported that only half of the patients who eventually had a CA-125 decline with liposomal doxorubicin therapy had a decline prior to the second cycle of therapy (468). Questions have also been raised as to whether CA-125 response criteria are valid in the setting of anti-VEGF-targeted therapy, because it has been noted that patients on maintenance bevacizumab were noted to sometimes have clinically stable disease for a prolonged period after a rise in CA-125 that would have qualified as progression. It is unclear if the issue is unreliability of CA-125 or the ability of the targeted agent to provide continued benefit even in the setting of slight tumor growth. Removal of ascites will affect CA-125 levels; renal dysfunction does not.

TREATMENT OF PERSISTENT/RECURRENT DISEASE

Ovarian cancer that is resistant to primary chemotherapy or recurs at some point after primary chemotherapy is generally not curable. Nonetheless, some women with recurrent disease will have prolonged survival. Of the women who are not cured by their primary therapy, about 10% will progress on primary platinum treatment and are described as having disease that is "platinum-refractory"; about 15% will progress 0 to 6 months after completion of primary therapy and are said to have "platinum-resistant" disease; and 75% have disease that recurs more than 6 months after primary therapy, which is termed "platinum-sensitive." Sometimes the group of women recurrent between 6 and 12 months after surgery is referred to as "partially platinum-sensitive."

A recent European retrospective review of women receiving antitumor therapy at first recurrence showed median OS to be 43 months for women with platinum-sensitive disease, 20.5 months for partially platinum-sensitive disease, 12.7 months for platinum-resistant disease, and 9.8 months for platinum-refractory disease. Among women with partially platinum-sensitive disease, there was no difference in survival for those who received platinum and non-platinum-based therapy (469).

Secondary Cytoreductive Surgery

Surgery in the treatment of recurrent ovarian cancer is covered in the section "Surgery." It is generally considered indicated when the cancer recurs a prolonged time after primary therapy and/or in a limited site. Two current randomized trials, GOG #213 and the DESKTOP III trial, are addressing whether surgery plus chemotherapy improves survival over chemotherapy alone in women with platinum-sensitive recurrent disease.

Second-Line Chemotherapy

In 1991 Markman et al. published an influential retrospective review of 72 patients who had responded to initial platinum-based therapy and were subsequently re-treated with a platinum- based regimen (470). The response rates were 27% for women with a "platinum-free interval" of 5 to 12 months, 33% for those with a platinum-free interval of 13 to 24 months, and 59% for those with a platinum-free interval of over 24 months.

Platinum-resistant disease is more resistant to most systemic therapies, not just platinum therapy. In women with platinum-resistant disease, response rates to standard chemotherapeutic agents range from 10% to 25%, and duration of response is typically less than 6 months. On comparison, response rates are usually over 30% and duration of response over 8 months for women with platinum-sensitive disease. This appears to be true for noncytotoxic agents as well as cytotoxic agents. A recent trial of single-agent treatment with the antiangiogenic tyrosine kinase inhibitor, cediranib, yielded 26% response rate in platinum-sensitive disease versus no responders in the platinum-resistant cohort (471).

Whereas categories of platinum sensitivity are useful shorthand predictors of the likelihood of response to further treatment, they have primarily been created for use in clinical trials and must be used with clinical judgment when selecting therapy in individual cases. For example, a woman with stage I clear cell carcinoma that recurs with diffuse disease 7 months after completion of adjuvant chemotherapy probably had no response to treatment at all, and her cancer will likely be refractory to further chemotherapy. On the other hand, a woman with suboptimally debulked stage IV serous carcinoma that has responded completely to primary chemotherapy and who has a rise in CA-125 after 5 months probably has chemotherapy-sensitive disease and is very likely to have at least some tumor shrinkage with a second line of platinum-based treatment.

Time since most recent platinum therapy is not the only means of predicting benefit from future treatment. Eisenhauer et al. analyzed the results for 704 patients who had recurrence or persistent disease after primary platinum-based therapy and were treated on a variety of second-line chemotherapy trials (472). Independent predictors of a positive response to second-line therapy were a largest tumor diameter of less than 5 cm, fewer sites of disease, and serous histology. Time to recurrence since primary therapy, when analyzed as a continuous variable, was not independently prognostic and was closely correlated with tumor size. Lee et al. published a nomogram for predicting PFS in women with platinum-sensitive recurrent ovarian cancer. The most important factor contributing to shorter PFS was size of the largest tumor; other descriptors remaining significant in multivariable analysis were platinum-free interval, CA-125 (higher values being worse), number of organ sites of metastasis, and white blood count (higher being worse) (473). The effects of prolonged consolidation therapy on future sensitivity of the tumor to treatment have not been well studied and are likely to vary with the agent used.

Patients with a complete response to second-line platinum therapy will usually have a shorter time to recurrence after the second treatment regimen than after the first (474), and recurrent ovarian cancers eventually become resistant to platinum and all other chemotherapy agents. Hoskins et al. developed a statistic for estimating benefit from further therapy in patients who had received multiple regimens. Women with a time from first to third (or second to fourth, third to fifth, etc.) relapse or progression of 6 months or less had a median survival of under 3 months. In other words, women with minimal or no benefit (with prolonged disease stabilization considered a benefit) from two different therapies in a row have a very poor prognosis (475).

Platinum-Sensitive Disease

Single-Agent Cytotoxic Therapy in Platinum-Sensitive Disease. Platinum agents are the most active front-line drugs for the treatment of ovarian cancer and are generally considered to be the most active agents in women with platinum-sensitive relapsed disease, particularly for women who relapse more than 12 months after completing primary therapy. However, there are few randomized data directly comparing single-agent platinum compounds with other single agents in women with platinum-sensitive disease. The EORTC randomized 86 women to either single-agent paclitaxel or single-agent oxaliplatin. Responses among the 63 platinum-resistant patients were 5 out of 31 (16%) for paclitaxel and 2 out of 32 (6%) for oxaliplatin. Responses among the platinum-sensitive patients were 2 out of 10 (20%) for paclitaxel and 5 out of 13 (38%) for oxaliplatin (476).

Platinum-Based Combination Cytotoxic Therapy in Platinum-Sensitive Disease. There have been several randomized trials comparing platinum-based combination cytotoxic therapy with single-agent platinum therapy in women with platinum-sensitive recurrent ovarian cancer (**Table 23.18**). In general, these show superior response rates and superior PFS with combination therapy. Only one trial has shown an OS benefit with combination therapy. ICON4/AGO-OVAR-2.2, a combined analysis of two parallel trials comparing paclitaxel plus platinum with "conventional platinum-based chemotherapy" (71% received single-agent carboplatin, 17% cisplatin/doxorubicin/cyclophosphamide, and 12% other nontaxane platinum-based regimens), reported an absolute improvement in OS of 5 months with taxane combination therapy (from 24 to 29 months) (477). Only about 40% of the patients in this analysis had received prior taxane therapy, and this has raised concern about the generalizability of the results although there was no significant statistical interaction between survival benefit and prior taxane therapy. Only 31% of patients in the nontaxane arm received taxane therapy at the time of progression. Other trials have not shown a survival benefit to combination chemotherapy in women with platinum-sensitive disease. The GCIG trial randomizing women to carboplatin and to carboplatin plus gemcitabine was not powered to show an OS difference; however, despite a superior response rate (complete response was achieved in only 6% of women on single-agent therapy vs. 15% of women on the combination regimen) and a longer progression-free interval with combination treatment, there was no evidence even of a trend to survival benefit (478). There were no differences in QOL scores between the two arms; the primary difference in toxicities was increased hematologic toxicity of the combination regimen, with 27% vs. 8% grade 3/4 anemia, 70% vs. 12%

TABLE 23.18. Combination Cytotoxic Therapy in Platinum-Sensitive Recurrent Ovarian Cancer

Author (Year)	n	Regimen	RR	Median PFS	Median OS
Bolis (2001) (543)	190	Carboplatin	56%	3 years 12%	3 years 29%
		Carboplatin + Epidoxorubicin	62% p = NS	3 years 25%	3 years 42% p = NS
Cantu (2002) (544)	97	Paclitaxel	45%	9 months	26 months
		CAP	55% p = NS	16 months	35 months
Parmar (ICON4/AGO-OVAR 2.2)	802	Platinum[a]	54%	10 months	24 months
(2003) (477)		Platinum + Paclitaxel	66% $p = 0.06$	13 months	29 months
Pfisterer (2006) (478)	356	Carboplatin	31%	5.8 months	17.3 months
		Carboplatin + Gemcitabine	47% $p = 0.0016$	8.6 months $p = 0.0031$	18 months
Alberts (2008) (545)	61	Carboplatin	32%	8 months	18 months
		Carboplatin + Liposomal doxorubicin	67% $p = 0.02$	12 months $p = 0.06$	26 months $p = 0.02$
Monk (2012) (487)	218[b]	PLD	22.6%	7.5 months	24.1 months (PFI>12 months) 16.4 months (PFI 6–12 months)
		PLD + Trabectedin	35.3%	9.2 months	27 months (PFI > 12 months) 22.4 months (PFI 6–12 months)
Wagner (2012) (481)	466	Carboplatin + PLD	N/A	11.3 months	30.7 months
		Carboplatin + paclitaxel		9.2 months	33 months

CAP, cisplatin/doxorubicin/cyclophosphamide; NS, not significant; OS, overall survival; PFI, platinum-free interval; PFS, progression-free survival; PLD, pegylated liposomal doxorubicin; RR, response rate.

[a]Control arm in CAP or single-agent carboplatin.

[b]Subset of a larger trial.

grade 3/4 neutropenia, and 35% vs. 11% grade 3/4 thrombocytopenia. Addition of bevacizumab to carboplatin/gemcitabine for women with platinum-sensitive recurrence has been shown to improve PFS, but not OS (479,480).

Despite the lack of any OS benefit and the generally increased toxicity with combination therapy, platinum-based combination regimens have become usual treatment for women with disease recurring over 12 months after completion of primary chemotherapy. Combination therapy consistently increases complete response rates, which can allow a second period of time off therapy with no evidence of disease.

Several trials in women with platinum-sensitive disease have compared platinum-based combinations with each other. Most notably the CALYPSO trial compared carboplatin AUC 5 plus pegylated liposomal doxorubicin (PLD) 30 mg/m^2 every 4 weeks with carboplatin AUC 5 plus paclitaxel 175 mg/m^2 every 3 weeks and showed superior PFS for the PLD regimen but no difference in OS between regimens. Again, toxicities differed: The PLD regimen produced less alopecia and neuropathy, but more nausea, mucositis, and hand–foot syndrome (481). The HECTOR trial, which has been reported only in abstract form, compared carboplatin AUC 5 plus topotecan 0.75 mg/m^2 on days 1, 2, and 3 every 3 weeks, with standard therapy consisting of physician/patient choice of either carboplatin plus paclitaxel, carboplatin plus gemcitabine, or carboplatin plus pegylated liposomal doxorubicin. In the standard therapy group, 78% of patients chose gemcitabine plus carboplatin. There was no significant difference in response rate, PFS, or OS between the two arms (482).

Platinum-Resistant Disease

In general, tumors resistant to platinum are more resistant to any cytotoxic agent. A number of phase 3 randomized trials including paclitaxel (483), topotecan (484), pegylated liposomal doxorubicin (483), and gemcitabine (483) as single agents have been informative in guiding our treatment of platinum-resistant disease. They show that response rates to conventional single-agent therapy in this group of women are about 10%, median PFS is about 3 to 4 months, and median OS is 9 to 12 months. Significant differences in terms of response rate or survival between various agents in platinum-resistant disease are not usually seen.

Combinations of cytotoxic agents have not been shown to be superior to single-agent therapy in women with platinum-resistant disease. A small trial randomized 234 women whose disease had recurred within 12 months of initial platinum-based therapy (median: 3 months) to single-agent paclitaxel versus epidoxorubicin plus paclitaxel (485). The response rate was 37% for the combination and 47% for single-agent paclitaxel; median survivals were 12 and 14 months, respectively. A small randomized phase II GINECO (Groupe D'Investigaters Nationaux pour l'Etude des Cancers Ovariens) trial comparing single-agent weekly paclitaxel with weekly paclitaxel plus carboplatin or weekly paclitaxel plus weekly topotecan in patients with platinum- resistant ovarian cancer showed no improvement in response rate or PFS with combination therapy (470,486). A randomized trial of trabectedin plus pegylated liposomal doxorubicin versus pegylated liposomal doxorubicin alone showed that in women with platinum-sensitive disease, both disease response rates and PFS were improved (35% vs. 23%; 9.2 vs. 7.5 months), whereas in women with platinum-resistant disease they were not (12% vs. 13%; 3.7 vs. 4.0 months). There was no difference in OS for either group (487).

Combinations of chemotherapy with antiangiogenic therapy appear to be more promising than combination cytotoxic therapy in the setting of resistant disease. The addition of bevacizumab to standard single-agent therapy (investigator choice of weekly paclitaxel, liposomal doxorubicin, or topotecan) in the open-label phase III AURELIA trial significantly improved PFS (HR, 0.48; $p < 0.001$) and response rate (27.3% vs. 11.8%) in women with platinum-resistant disease, although the OS trend was not significant (488). Bevacizumab is now US FDA-approved for use in combination with weekly paclitaxel, liposomal doxorubicin, or topotecan for women with platinum-resistant disease. The MITO-11 randomized phase II trial combining one of the oral antiangiogenic agents, pazopanib, with paclitaxel compared with paclitaxel alone also showed a significant improvement in PFS for women with platinum-resistant disease (6.35 vs. 3.49 months, $p = 0.0002$) (489).

In summary, platinum-based combinations improve response rates and PFS and have become the usual treatment in the United States as the first salvage regimen for women who relapse more than 12 months after the completion of primary therapy, with single-agent therapy usual in women who have an initial treatment-free interval of less than 6 months, and individualized decisions in those with a 6- to 12-month treatment-free interval. Treatment is not curative, and there are situations in which a patient with late relapse may choose single agent or nonplatinum therapy; it is unlikely that survival is significantly compromised by such a choice. Single-cytotoxic therapy is standard for women with platinum-resistant disease, and combination with bevacizumab improves response rate and PFS in this setting.

Drugs Useful in Treatment of Recurrent Ovarian Cancer

Taxanes, liposomal doxorubicin, topotecan, and gemcitabine have been studied in randomized trials, as discussed above. A number of other agents are occasionally useful. Hexamethamelamine (altretamine) is an older alkylating agent with the advantages (patient convenience) and disadvantages (inappropriate for patients with episodic or partial small bowel obstruction, limited availability for patients without good insurance coverage for outpatient medication) of an oral therapy. It is rarely used, as it produces significant amounts of neuropathy, nausea, and vomiting. A GOG phase 2 trial of single-agent hexamethamelamine in women with platinum-resistant ovarian cancer demonstrated a 10% response rate and a 21% rate of grade 3 emesis (490). Oral etoposide, a topoisomerase II inhibitor, is better tolerated and may be slightly more active. It produces cytopenias and is leukemogenic, which has limited enthusiasm for attempts to incorporate it into front-line therapy, but it remains an occasionally useful salvage agent. Interestingly, intravenous etoposide appears to have minimal activity in women with pretreated ovarian cancer. Ifosfamide has produced response rates of 10% to 20%, but the toxicities, hematologic and neurologic, are excessive compared with those of other available agents, and it is rarely used. Irinotecan has activity, but is associated with substantial diarrhea and nausea, which can be particularly troublesome in ovarian cancer patients with some preexisting level of bowel dysfunction. 5-Fluorouracil has produced response rates of 10% to 33% in older studies. A more recent retrospective review of ovarian cancer patients with a median of four prior chemotherapy regimens treated with 5-FU at 600 mg/m^2 weekly plus leucovorin for 6 weeks of an 8-week cycle reported a response rate of 25%. However, responses were generally short-lived (491). Vinorelbine, capecitabine, and pemetrexed (492) may sometimes be useful; none of them are FDA-approved for use in ovarian cancer.

Taxanes. Although in most parts of the world taxane therapy is now part of front-line treatment for ovarian cancer, taxanes remain very useful in treating recurrent disease. Both weekly paclitaxel (493,494) and docetaxel (495) have shown response rates of 20% to 30% in women who recurred within 6 months of primary platinum–taxane-based combination therapy. Weekly paclitaxel is particularly useful, as it tends to be less myelotoxic than many other regimens. Nab-paclitaxel has the advantage that it does not require steroid premedication to avoid hypersensitivity reactions. Nab-paclitaxel on a schedule of 100 mg/m^2 on days 1, 8, and 15 of a 28-day schedule produced a response rate of 23% in women with platinum/paclitaxel-resistant ovarian cancer (496).

Topotecan. Topotecan is a topoisomerase I inhibitor approved by the FDA for the treatment of recurrent ovarian cancer. A phase III trial compared topotecan on the FDA-approved schedule of 1.5 mg/m^2 for 5 consecutive days repeated every 21 days to liposomal doxorubicin 50 mg/m^2 every 28 days. Response rate was 17% overall for topotecan: 28.8% for platinum-sensitive disease and 6.5% for platinum-resistant disease (483). However, the daily × 5 regimen is not convenient and has proved more myelosuppressive than most treating physicians deem reasonable in the palliative setting. Lower starting doses of 1.0 to 1.25 mg/m^2 are better tolerated, although their efficacy is not as well documented. Individuals at increased risk for myelotoxicity include those with impaired renal function, older age, extensive prior therapy, or prior pelvic irradiation.

Weekly bolus topotecan has been shown to have some activity in a number of small trials and has come into common use because the schedule is more convenient and produces less myelosuppression. The maximum tolerated dose (MTD) in phase 1 studies was 4 mg/m^2, with dose-limiting toxicities of anemia, chronic fatigue, and gastrointestinal distress. A randomized phase 2 trial of topotecan 4 mg/m^2 given 3 weeks out of 4 versus topotecan 1.25 mg/m^2 daily × 5 in 194 women with platinum-resistant ovarian cancer showed a numerically lower response rate for the weekly schedule (2 of 28 vs. 5 of 21 for the daily × 5 regimen) as well as a nonsignificantly decreased PFS (3.0 vs. 4.4 months). Overall survival was similar (9.6 vs. 9.3 months) (497). It is possible that differences between the two schedules would be more evident in patients with platinum-sensitive disease. The GOG attempted to randomize women with platinum-sensitive disease to a weekly versus daily regimen, but enrollment was slow, and the trial was changed to a single-arm phase II trial of weekly topotecan. The response rate for the 15 patients receiving the daily × 5 regimen was 27%, but the confidence intervals around this response rate were very wide given the small number of patients; response rate for the 65 women receiving the weekly regimen was 12% (498).

Liposomal Doxorubicin. Liposomal doxorubicin is also FDA-approved for the treatment of recurrent ovarian cancer. The every-4-week schedule of administration is convenient, and the lack of alopecia is attractive to patients. In the randomized trial comparing liposomal doxorubicin 50 mg/m^2 every 4 weeks with daily × 4 topotecan, the overall response rate was 19.7% (28.4% for women with platinum-sensitive disease and 12.3% for women with platinum-resistant disease). However, there is a high incidence of palmar–plantar erythrodysesthesia using the approved dose of 50 mg/m^2. Markman et al. published a non-randomized phase 2 trial suggesting that there was only a 12% incidence of grade 2 and no grade 3 palmar–plantar erythrodysesthesia when the starting dose was lowered from 50 to 40 mg/m^2. The response rate was 9%; all patients were platinum/paclitaxel resistant, with a median of two prior regimens (483,499). It is not known if doxorubicin or epirubicin would have similar activity; these drugs have well-documented activity in ovarian cancer, mostly in the front-line setting, but a very different side effect profile with more alopecia, nausea, and vomiting. One small phase II trial reported a response rate of 18% to epirubicin at a dose of 150 mg/m^2 in women with platinum-resistant ovarian cancer (472).

Gemcitabine. Single-agent gemcitabine has modest activity in the treatment of recurrent ovarian cancer. Based on experimental models, it was hypothesized that combining gemcitabine with cisplatin might reverse platinum resistance. Cisplatin-resistant cells upregulate nucleotide excision repair complexes, which are thought to be inhibited by gemcitabine. Preclinical models suggested synergy between cisplatin and gemcitabine in platinum-resistant cell lines. A multicenter GOG trial of the combination as second-line therapy in women with platinum-resistant ovarian cancer reported a response rate of 16% (500).

Bevacizumab

Elevated vascular endothelial growth factor (VEGF or VEGF-A) expression occurs in all stages of ovarian cancer and is associated with poor prognosis, including shorter survival. In addition, VEGF (which is also known as vascular permeability factor) overexpression is directly associated with the production of ascitic fluid.

Bevacizumab is a humanized anti-VEGF monoclonal antibody. Prospective trials have reported activity of single-agent bevacizumab against pretreated ovarian cancer to be in the range of 15% to 20%. It is generally well tolerated; however, notable toxicities include hypertension, proteinuria, excess venous thrombosis, and bowel perforation and fistulization. Patients with evidence of bowel obstruction or bowel invasion by tumor should not receive bevacizumab. A phase II trial evaluated the combination of bevacizumab and metronomic (daily low-dose) oral cyclophosphamide in 70 women who had been treated with up to three prior chemotherapy regimens. At 6 months, 56% patients were progression-free and the overall response rate was 24% (501). The response rate for women with platinum-sensitive disease was higher than the response rate for women with platinum-resistant disease (33% vs. 12%) although the difference was not statistically significant. The cyclophosphamide in this regimen was postulated to have an antiangiogenic effect. Interestingly, a subsequent study in women with heavily pretreated ovarian cancer (a median of four prior regimens) and known *BRCA* mutations reported a response rate to single-agent oral cyclophosphamide of 13% (502).

Subsequent interest focused on combinations of bevacizumab and cytotoxic agents (**Table 23.16**). Trials in both platinum-sensitive and platinum-resistant disease have shown improvements in response rate and PFS when bevacizumab is combined with standard therapy. The OCEANS trial was a randomized, double-blind placebo-controlled trial comparing the combination of gemcitabine plus carboplatin plus bevacizumab with the combination of gemcitabine plus carboplatin plus placebo in women with platinum-sensitive recurrent ovarian cancer. Chemotherapy was continued for a planned 6 cycles or up to 10 cycles in patients with continued response. After completion of chemotherapy, bevacizumab or placebo was continued until progression. Overall response rate and median PFS were both significantly improved with the addition of bevacizumab (78%; 12.3 months vs. 57%; 8.6 months) (479). There was no difference in median OS: 33.6 months for the bevacizumab arm and 32.9 months for the placebo arm. Thirty-eight percent of patients in the placebo arm received subsequent bevacizumab (503). Bevacizumab is not FDA-approved for use in platinum-sensitive disease in the United States, and the UK NICE guidelines in 2013 concluded that use in the platinum-sensitive setting was not a cost-effective use of resources (504). The AURELIA trial was conducted in platinum-resistant patients. A total of 361 women with platinum-resistant (but not refractory) ovarian cancer and one or two prior regimens were randomized to standard therapy, consisting of investigators' choice of pegylated liposomal doxorubicin, topotecan, or weekly paclitaxel, with or without bevacizumab. Patients in the chemotherapy arm were permitted to cross over to bevacizumab monotherapy at the time of progression. Overall response rate was significantly improved from 11.8% to 27.3%, and median PFS was improved from 3.4 to 6.7 months by the addition of bevacizumab. Median OS was not significantly different between the arms (13.3 vs. 16.6 months). Of note, 40% of patients on the standard therapy arm crossed over to bevacizumab monotherapy, as permitted by the protocol (488). Patient-reported outcomes were significantly improved for patients getting bevacizumab; the proportion of patients achieving a 15% improvement on the QLQ-OV28 abdominal/GI symptom subscale at week 8/9 increased from 9.3% to 21%, and the percentage of patients having over 15% improvement on the Functional Assessment of Cancer Therapy-Ovarian Cancer Symptom Index (FOSI) at week 8/9 increased from 3.1% to 12.2% (505). On November 14, 2014, the US FDA approved bevacizumab in combination with chemotherapy for the treatment of women with platinum-resistant, recurrent ovarian cancer.

Other antiangiogenics have also been tested in combination with chemotherapy for women with recurrent ovarian cancer. Of particular note are the preliminary results of ICON6, which randomly assigned 456 women with platinum-sensitive relapsed ovarian cancer to chemotherapy with placebo, with concomitant cediranib, or with concomitant cediranib followed by maintenance cediranib for up to 18 months. Time to progression was increased by 3.2 months, and OS was also significantly improved by 2.7 months. Cediranib caused more hypertension, diarrhea, hypothyroidism, hoarseness, bleeding, proteinuria, and fatigue (506).

VEGF increases permeability, leading to ascites formation, and preclinical studies show that VEGF inhibition can suppress ascites. A randomized placebo-controlled phase II ($n = 55$) study with the anti-VEGF decoy receptor, aflibercept, was therefore performed in subjects with ascites and treatment-resistant ovarian cancer. Aflibercept significantly extended time to ascitic drainage compared with placebo (55.1 vs. 23.3 days, respectively; $p = 0.0019$). There was no effect on OS. Aflibercept was associated with more grade 3/4 toxicities, including three fatal GI adverse effects (intestinal perforations) versus one in the placebo group (intestinal fistula) (507). The current Australia and New Zealand Gynaecological Oncology Group (ANZGOG) REZOLVE study is testing intraperitoneal bevacizumab to decrease ascites formation.

PARP Inhibitors

PARP-1 is an enzyme that plays a critical role in the repair of DNA single-strand breaks. In cells that are deficient in double-strand break repair because of defects in homologous recombination (HR), inhibition of PARP produces synthetic lethality. A number of PARP inhibitors have demonstrated activity in the treatment of ovarian cancer.

Olaparib® is an oral PARP inhibitor that received accelerated approval by the US FDA in 2014 for the treatment of ovarian cancer patients with a germ line BRCA mutation who have received at least three prior treatment regimens. A pooled analysis of 205 patients in six trials of olaparib monotherapy showed that among women with a germ line BRCA mutation and three or more lines of prior chemotherapy, the response rate was 36% and the median duration of response was 7.4 months. Forty-two percent of women with platinum-sensitive disease responded versus 26% of those with platinum-resistant disease (508).

The Cancer Genomic Atlas (TCGA) project demonstrated that up to 50% of high-grade serous ovarian cancers (HGSOC) have some defect in the HR pathway, and other reports have shown that the rate of HR mutations is similar between HGSOC and ovarian cancers of clear cell, endometrioid, and carcinosarcoma histologies (509). It is therefore unsurprising that PARP inhibitors also have activity in ovarian cancer patients who do not carry a germ line BRCA mutation. Gelmon et al. treated 64 women with measurable high-grade serous or undifferentiated ovarian cancer with single-agent olaparib at a dose of 400 mg orally twice a day. Confirmed objective responses were observed in 41% of patients with *BRCA1* or *BRCA2* mutations and 24% of women without mutations. Among women with platinum-sensitive disease, responses were seen in 60% (3 of 5) *BRCA1* or *BRCA2* mutation carriers and in 50% (10 of 20) who did not carry a germ line mutation; among women with platinum-resistant disease, responses were seen in 33% (4 of 12) *BRCA1* or *BRCA2* mutation carriers but in only 4% (1 of 26) women who did not carry a germ line mutation (**Fig. 23.51**) (510). There have been challenges in identifying a biomarker that will suggest the presence of HR deficiency. One approach is based on evidence that homologous-repair deficient cancers exhibit global DNA alterations termed "genomic scarring" that are consistent with their reliance on the error-prone nonhomologous end joining (NHEJ) DNA repair pathway. Ongoing trials are testing PARP inhibition in women without a germ line BRCA mutation, hoping to validate tumor assays designed to identify which ovarian cancers in women without a germ line BRCA mutation are likely to respond.

PARP inhibitors are a convenient oral single-agent option for treatment of BRCA mutation carriers, but they are not proven superior to other treatments in this setting. A randomized phase II trial of the oral PARP inhibitor olaparib (high or low dose) versus pegylated liposomal doxorubicin (PLD) in ovarian cancer patients with a germ line *BRCA1* or *BRCA2* mutation who had recurred within 12 months of their most recent platinum-based regimen showed a similar median PFS of 8.8 months for the high-dose olaparib arm (400 mg twice a day; current FDA-approved dosage), 6.5 months for the lower-dose olaparib arm (200 mg twice daily), and 7.1 months for

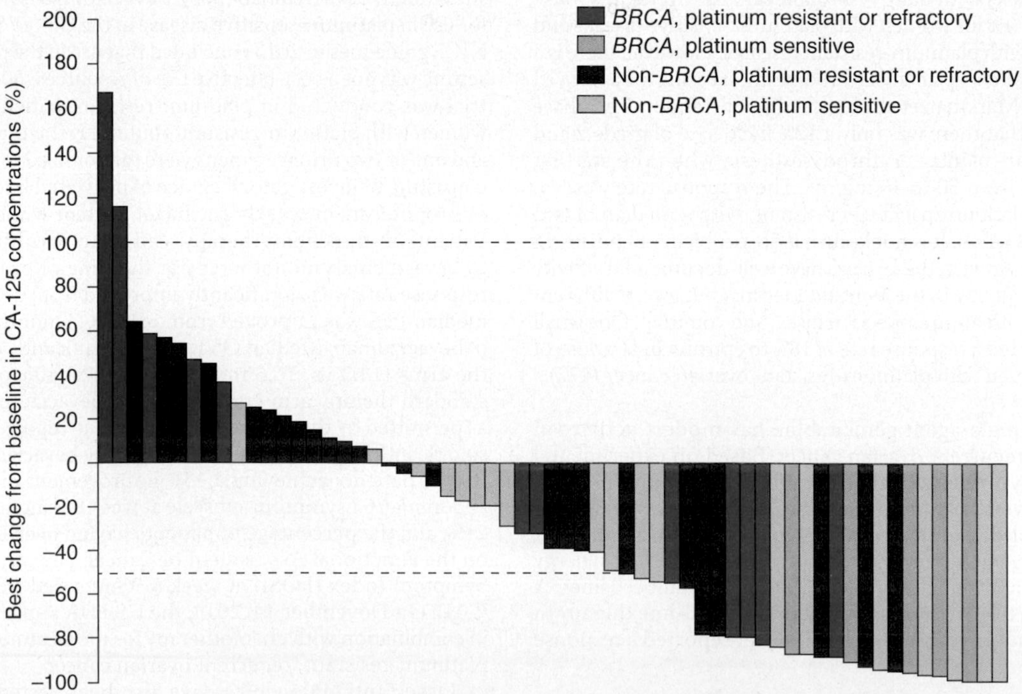

Figure 23.51. Single-agent olaparib therapy in ovarian cancer. Best percentage change from baseline CA-125 concentrations, by platinum sensitivity and resistance and germ line BRCA status.

Source: From Gelmon KA, Tischkowitz M, Mackay H, et al. Olaparib in patients with recurrent high-grade serous or poorly differentiated ovarian carcinoma or triple-negative breast cancer: a phase 2, multicenter, open-label, nonrandomized study. *Lancet Oncol*. 2011;12(9):852–861.

the PLD group. The RECIST response rate was 31% in the high-dose olaparib arm and 18% in the PLD arm. The PFS of 7.1 months seen with PLD exceeded that seen in a previous large randomized trial of patients with unknown BRCA status and similar proportions of patients with platinum-resistant and platinum-sensitive disease (4 months); it has been hypothesized that patients with germ line *BRCA1/2* mutations derive more benefit from PLD treatment than women with nonhereditary ovarian cancers (511).

The most common grade 3 or higher adverse events seen with olaparib have been vomiting and anemia. In the olaparib versus liposomal doxorubicin trial, one heavily pretreated patient receiving low-dose olaparib died of myelodysplastic syndrome, and the US Package Insert for Lynparza® (olaparib) contains the following warning for the development of MDS/AML: *MDS/AML have been confirmed in 6 out of 298 (2%) patients enrolled in a single arm trial of Lynparza monotherapy, in patients with deleterious or suspected deleterious germ line BRCA-mutated advanced cancers.* It is not yet clear how much additional risk for secondary MDS/AML is conferred by use of PARP inhibitors.

Resistance to single-agent therapy PARP inhibitor therapy usually develops in less than a year. Cancers in women with a germ line *BRCA1* or *BRCA2* mutation can develop secondary genetic changes that restore the reading frame of the BRCA protein. Such secondary mutations are associated with the development of platinum resistance, and some similar mutation likely allows development of resistance to PARP inhibitors.

In Europe the European Medicines Agency (EMA) has approved olaparib in a different setting: as maintenance therapy for women with BRCA-mutated ovarian cancer in platinum-sensitive recurrence following response to platinum therapy.

A randomized placebo-controlled phase II trial tested olaparib 400 mg bid versus placebo in 265 women with platinum-sensitive relapsed high-grade serous ovarian carcinomas who were in partial or complete response following their last platinum-containing regimen. Median PFS was significantly longer with olaparib than with placebo (8.4 vs. 4.8 months, $p < 0.001$); this was more pronounced in the group with a germ line or tumor BRCA mutation (11.2 vs. 4.3 months, $p < 0.0001$). Overall survival data at 58% maturity showed no difference between the groups [HR, 0.88 (0.64–1.21)] (512). It has been suggested that post-progression PARP inhibitor therapy may have had a confounding effect on the OS analysis. Several ongoing or completed large, randomized trials are examining the role of maintenance PARP inhibition in ovarian cancer patients both with and without a germ line BRCA mutation, and results should be available soon.

Platinum Hypersensitivity

Repeated courses of carboplatin therapy place patients at risk for hypersensitivity reactions. Such reactions rarely occur with the first treatment; rather, they are associated with cumulative dose and have been reported to occur in up to 27% of women receiving more than seven cycles of carboplatin. These reactions usually occur during drug infusion and are associated with flushing, nausea, and hypertension. They may be severe and/or fatal. Atypical hypersensitivity reactions, occurring after drug infusion, have also been described. A number of desensitization protocols have been published and appear to be generally effective; they often involve premedication with steroids and antihistamines, and starting dilute infusions very slowly then gradually increasing the concentration and rate over 4 to 24 hours (513). Not all patients allergic to carboplatin will be allergic to cisplatin. Hypersensitivity reactions have been reported to be lower with some second-line combinations than others. For example, the CALYPSO trial reported rates of hypersensitivity to be lower with the combination of liposomal doxorubicin plus platinum (15.5%, with 2.4% > grade 2) than with the combination of paclitaxel plus carboplatin (33.1%, with 8.8% > grade 2) (514). Elderly patients in this study had a significantly decreased risk for hypersensitivity reactions. Weekly carboplatin may be associated with an increased risk for hypersensitivity reactions. The role of skin testing in the clinical setting is controversial, and it is not widely used; it has a fairly high negative predictive value, but is not perfectly predictive, and performing the test requires prior experience and use of a control. Routine use of diphenhydramine premedication has been reported to produce a nonsignificant decrease in the rate of these reactions (515).

Hormonal Therapy

Epithelial ovarian cancers frequently express estrogen (ER) and progesterone receptors (PR), and higher levels of PR expression have been associated with improved survival in several analyses (516). However, one recent analysis of androgen receptor (AR), PR, and ER alpha/beta in 196 patients enrolled on a prospective randomized trial of front-line therapy with carboplatin/docetaxel +/– celecoxib found that it was the subgroup with hormone receptor negative disease that had the best prognosis. ER beta nuclear staining was significantly associated with poor prognosis, and AR, which was expressed in 10% of cancers, was associated with a trend toward worse prognosis (517).

Multiple attempts have been made to treat ovarian carcinoma with hormonal therapy, including progestins and antiestrogens. The response rates generally have been quite low, in the range of 10%. Most of the trials were small, many were conducted in patients with platinum-resistant disease, and many were performed decades ago, before steroid receptor analysis was available (516). The GOG completed a randomized trial comparing tamoxifen with thalidomide for the therapy of women who have CA-125 marker elevation but no measurable recurrence of disease. Women treated with thalidomide had a median PFS of 3.2 versus 4.5 months for those treated with tamoxifen, which was not significantly different (518). There is an ongoing trial (NCT01974765) using the AR inhibitor enzalutamide in the therapy of AR-positive ovarian cancer.

Gonadotropin-releasing hormone (GnRH) receptors may also be expressed on ovarian cancers. A few small trials of GnRH analogs have demonstrated low response rates. Attempts have been made to target cytotoxic agents by linking them to a GnRH analog, and a phase II trial of AEZS-108, an LHRH analog linked to doxorubicin, was reported to produce a 14.3% partial response rate in women with platinum-resistant disease (519).

Over 90% of serous borderline ovarian tumors are estrogen-receptor positive (520), and there are case reports of responses to tamoxifen, leuprolide, and anastrozole. The MD Anderson group retrospectively reviewed outcomes to various hormonal therapy regimens in 133 women with recurrent LGSCs and found a 9% response rate (521).

NEW THERAPEUTICS

Treatments Directed at Less Common Histologies

Current trials for low-grade serous cancers are building on the 15% response rate observed with the MEK1/2 inhibitor, selumetinib. GOG281 randomizes women with LGSC and at least one prior chemotherapy regimen to either standard therapy (choice of letrozole, tamoxifen, paclitaxel, liposomal doxorubicin, or topotecan) or the MEK1/2 inhibitor, trametinib. Similarly the phase III MILO trial, which recently completed accrual, is testing the MEK inhibitor MEK162 against standard therapy in recurrent LGSC.

In clear cell carcinoma, interest has focused on the high incidence of *ARID1A* mutations. In a functional profiling of endometriosis-associated clear cell carcinomas presented at the ASCO 2012 meeting, an siRNA kinome screen identified colony stimulating factor-1 receptor (CSF1R) as a synthetically lethal target of *ARID1A*-deficient but not *ARID1A*-intact endometriosis-associated clear cell carcinoma cell lines (522). Dasatinib, a small-molecule inhibitor of BCR-ABL, is also able to inhibit CSF1, and an ongoing NRG/GOG trial, GOG283, is testing dasatinib in the therapy of pretreated ovarian or uterine clear cell carcinomas. Tumors are stratified by expression of BAF250a, the gene encoded by *ARID1A*. More recently, inhibition of the EZH2 methyltransferase has been shown to act in a synthetic lethal manner in *ARID1A*-mutated ovarian cancer cells and *in vivo* models of ARID1A-mutated ovarian tumors (523). A number of EZH2 inhibitors are in development, and this is a promising direction for this group of cancers.

Targeted Therapies in High-Grade Serous Ovarian Cancer

High-frequency "druggable" mutations that would be analogous to the *BCR-ABL* gene in CML do not appear to exist in high-grade serous ovarian cancer. TCGA project analyzed messenger RNA expression, microRNA expression, promoter methylation, and DNA copy number in 489 high-grade serous ovarian adenocarcinomas and the DNA sequences of exons from coding genes in 316 of these tumors. High-grade serous ovarian cancer is characterized by multiple mutations, with an average of 61.9 per tumor. Almost all tumors (96%) have *TP53* mutations, but there were no other high-prevalence mutations found. A few low-prevalence but statistically recurrent somatic mutations in genes including *NF1*, *BRCA1/2*, *RB1*, and *CDK12* were described (263).

Detectable expression of EGFR has been reported in 19% to 92% of ovarian cancers, with studies suggesting that EGFR dysregulation is associated with worse survival. However, no anti-EGFR therapies, including monoclonal antibodies such as cetuximab and matuzumab and small molecule inhibitors such as gefitinib and erlotinib, have been shown to be effective. An EORTC/GCIG randomized phase 3 trial of erlotinib for 2 years versus observation in women with responding or stable disease after first-line platinum-based therapy did not show any benefit to erlotinib therapy (524).

A role for therapy targeting HER2 in ovarian cancer has also been explored. The GOG found that 11.2% of women with progressive or recurrent ovarian cancer had tumors that stained 2+ or 3+ for HER2. However, the response rate to the anti-HER2 monoclonal antibody trastuzumab in the group of women with 2+ or 3+ expression by immunohistochemical evaluation was only 7.3% (525). Gene amplification was not assessed in this study, and it is possible that therapy would be more effective in *HER2*-amplified disease. *HER2* amplification is found in about 20% of mucinous ovarian carcinomas, and there is one report of a dramatic response to the combination of trastuzumab plus carboplatin in this usually chemotherapy-resistant subtype (273). Pertuzumab is a monoclonal antibody that binds to an epitope on HER2 distinct from the trastuzumab-binding site and prevents dimerization of HER2 with other receptors. It has been approved by the US FDA for treatment of HER2-positive metastatic breast cancer in combination with trastuzumab. A subsequent trial that randomized women with platinum-resistant ovarian cancer to gemcitabine or gemcitabine plus pertuzumab showed a 5% response rate for gemcitabine versus 14% for the combination (526).

Volasertib is an intravenously administered small molecule cell-cycle inhibitor that targets Polo-like kinase. A recent randomized phase II trial of patients with platinum-resistant or refractory ovarian cancer compared volasertib with investigator's choice of single-agent nonplatinum cytotoxic chemotherapy. Twenty-four-week disease control rates for volasertib and chemotherapy were 30.6% and 43.1%; 11% of patients receiving volasertib had PFS for more than 1 year versus no patients with chemotherapy. However, there is no biomarker identifying which patients might benefit from volasertib (527).

Agents Targeting Angiogenesis

Antiangiogenic therapy consistently produces a measurable response rate in ovarian cancer, but survival benefits have been difficult to demonstrate. Bevacizumab, a monoclonal antibody targeting VEGF, is the most extensively tested antiangiogenic agent for ovarian cancer, and results of trials of bevacizumab as well as results of numerous trials of small molecule inhibitors of VEGF tyrosine kinase are discussed above. Numerous other antiangiogenic agents continue to be evaluated in women with ovarian cancer, and many of them target different or multiple components of the angiogenic pathway. Ramucirumab (IMC1121B), a monoclonal antibody to VEGFR2, produced a 5% PR rate (3 of 60) among a heavily pretreated group of patients: 75% had platinum-resistant or refractory disease (528). Trebananib (AMG 386) is a peptide-Fc fusion protein that neutralizes the interaction between the Tie2 receptor and angiopoietin-1/2. It has the unusual toxicity profile of inducing peripheral edema and ascites. A randomized phase III trial (Trinova I) of weekly paclitaxel versus weekly paclitaxel plus trebananib in women with recurrent disease and a platinum-free interval of less than 3 months increased PFS from 5.4 to 7.2 months ($p < 0.001$), but interim OS analysis showed no difference between the arms (17.3 vs. 19 months) (529).

Combinations of antiangiogenic therapy with PARP inhibitors are of interest; downregulation of homologous recombination repair genes occurs with hypoxia, with enhancement of PARP inhibitor sensitivity in the hypoxic setting. A multi-institutional randomized phase II study compared the activity of olaparib plus the oral antiangiogenic tyrosine kinase inhibitor, cediranib, with olaparib alone in women with recurrent platinum-sensitive ovarian cancer. The combination significantly extended both response rate and PFS with a median PFS of 9.0 months for olaparib alone and 17.7 months for the combination. A *post hoc* subset analysis by *BRCA* mutation status (carrier vs. noncarrier/unknown) showed that there appeared to be more benefit to the addition of cediranib in patients with wild-type or unknown *BRCA* status in whom there was an increase in PFS from 5.8 months with olaparib alone to 16.6 months with combination therapy (530). Whether these PFS benefits will translate into OS benefits or, as the case with multiple bevacizumab trials, produce improvement in PFS but not OS remains to be seen. The NRG has recently opened NRG-GY005, which will compare standard nonplatinum-based chemotherapy, single-agent cediranib, single-agent olaparib, and the combination of cediranib plus olaparib in platinum-resistant ovarian cancer, and NRG-GY004, which will compare olaparib alone, the combination of cediranib plus olaparib, and standard platinum-based chemotherapy in women with platinum-sensitive disease.

Targeting Homologous Recombination Deficiency

TCGA pathway analyses suggested that homologous recombination is defective in about half of the high-grade serous ovarian tumors analyzed. As discussed above, a large number of PARP inhibitors are being aggressively pursued in this space, as single agents, in maintenance, and in combination with chemotherapy. Combinations with chemotherapy have been problematic because of increased cytopenias. One open-label phase II trial randomized 162 women with platinum-sensitive recurrent disease, unselected for *BRCA1/2* mutation status, to carboplatin AUC 6/paclitaxel 175 mg/m^2 chemotherapy for six cycles followed by no further therapy versus the combination of olaparib plus carboplatin AUC 4/paclitaxel 175 mg/m^2 chemotherapy followed by olaparib maintenance. A lower carboplatin dose had to be used in the combination regimen because of hematologic toxicity. Results have been reported in abstract form. Response rates were not different between the arms; PFS was significantly improved at 12.2 versus 9.6 months. OS did not differ between groups in either the overall patient population or in the patients with BRCA mutations (531).

Other approaches are also being developed to target HR-deficient tumors. For example, HR-deficient tumors are expected to be more sensitive to combinations of checkpoint inhibitors with DNA-damaging chemotherapy. Several approaches to inhibit the ATR-CHK1-WEE1 pathway, including ATR inhibitors such as VX-970 and AZD 6738, WEE1 inhibitors such as AZD1775, and CHK1 inhibitors such as GDC-0452 and LY 2606368, are currently in early clinical trial evaluation in ovarian cancers. AZD1775 has already demonstrated clinical activity as monotherapy in *BRCA*-mutated tumors (362).

Immunologic Therapies

In 2003 Zhang et al. made the observation that among patients in clinical complete remission the presence of intratumoral T cells was a strongly favorable prognostic factor (532). However, no immunotherapy has been approved for the therapy of ovarian cancer.

There remains interest in vaccine-type therapies, which have used a variety of antigens, including MUC 1 carbohydrate epitope, p53 peptide, HER2/neu peptides, and the cancer-testis antigen NY-ESO-1, which are sometimes directly injected, sometimes loaded onto dendritic cells, and sometimes expressed in recombinant viral vectors. However, there have been no randomized trials published showing clinical benefit.

Immunomodulation with novel immune checkpoint inhibitors such as CTLA-4 inhibitors (ipilumimab), PD-1 inhibitors, and PDL-1 inhibitors has produced a great deal of excitement in recent years, and some of these agents have been approved in a number of solid tumors including melanoma, kidney cancer, and lung cancer. A small trial of nivolumab in 20 patients with platinum-resistant ovarian cancer demonstrated an overall response rate of 15%. Two of these responders had complete responses that lasted 17 and 14 months (nivolumab was given only for a year); one of these had a clear cell carcinoma (533). The prolonged duration of the responses achieved has generated substantial excitement, and multiple trials are attempting to determine which ovarian cancer patients will benefit from such immunotherapies.

Other New Directions

The folate receptor is highly overexpressed in ovarian cancer, and a number of therapies have attempted to take advantage of this. Farletuzumab is an antifolate receptor antibody that had appeared promising, but phase III trials adding farletuzumab to standard chemotherapy in both the platinum-resistant and platinum-sensitive setting failed to significantly improve PFS. A prespecified subgroup analysis did demonstrate that patients with farletuzumab exposure above the median had superior PFS and OS compared with placebo, and continued study is planned (534). Vintafolid (EC145) is a conjugate of folic acid and desacetylvinblastine that binds to the folate receptor with high affinity. Phase II results were promising, but a phase III double-blind study (PROCEED) was stopped early by its Data Safety Monitoring Board (DSMB) for futility (535). IMGN853 (mirvetuximab soravtansine) is a folate receptor alpha-targeting antibody drug conjugate that comprises a folate receptor alpha-binding antibody conjugated with the potent maytansinoid, DM4. It is associated with some ocular toxicity. A preliminary report showed an extremely promising objective response rate of 4/10 heavily pretreated platinum-resistant patients, and further studies are planned (536).

Other antibody–drug conjugates have also had promising preliminary results in the therapy of ovarian cancer, but remain early in development. DMOT4039A is an antibody–drug conjugate targeting mesothelin. Three of 10 ovarian cancer patients with platinum-resistant ovarian cancer and a mesothelin IHC score of 3+ treated on the q3 week schedule at the recommended phase 2 dose level had a confirmed partial response (537). NaPi2b is a multitransmembrane sodium-dependent phosphate transporter expressed in human lung, ovarian, and thyroid cancers. DNIB0600A is an antibody–drug conjugate consisting of a monoclonal antibody conjugated to the antimitotic agent monomethyl auristatin E. At the recommended phase 2 dose 41% of patients whose tumor had an IHC score of 2 or 3 for NaPi2b had a confirmed partial response (538).

Aberrant DNA methylation is a frequent epigenetic event in ovarian cancer and represents an additional source of potential molecular markers. Four promoter methylation subtypes significantly associated with survival were identified in high-grade serous tumors by the TCGA project. Wei et al. investigated CpG island hypermethylation across stages III and intravenous ovarian tumors (539). Hierarchical clustering revealed two tumor groups with distinctly different methylation profiles. The duration of PFS after chemotherapy was significantly shorter for patients whose tumors contained high levels of concurrent methylation compared with patients whose tumors had lower tumor methylation levels. Hypomethylating agents and histone deacetylase inhibitors are currently being studied in combination with standard chemotherapies. Matei et al. tested low-dose decitabine administered before carboplatin in 17 patients with heavily pretreated and platinum-resistant ovarian cancer. The regimen induced a 35% objective RR and a PFS of 10.2 months, with 9 patients (53%) free of progression at 6 months. Demethylation of *MLH1*, *RASSF1A*, *HOXA10*, and *HOXA11* in tumor biopsies after treatment positively correlated with PFS, suggesting that low-dose decitabine altered DNA methylation of genes, restoring sensitivity to carboplatin (540). A phase I/II randomized trial of carboplatin with or without SGI-110, a small molecule DNA hypomethylating agent, in patients with platinum-resistant disease has been completed, and results should be available shortly.

REFERENCES

1. Wentzensen N, Poole EM, Trabert B, et al. Ovarian cancer risk factors by histologic subtype: an analysis from the Ovarian Cancer Cohort Consortium. *J Clin Oncol.* 2016;34(24):2888–2898.
2. Siegel RL, Miller KD, Jemal A. Cancer statistics, 2016. *CA Cancer J Clin.* 2016;66:7–30.
3. De Angelis R, Sant M, Coleman MP, et al. Cancer survival in Europe 1999–2007 by country and age: results of EUROCARE—5-a population-based study. *Lancet Oncol.* 2014;15:23–34.
4. Sopik V, Iqbal J, Rosen B, et al. Why have ovarian cancer mortality rates declined? Part II. Case-fatality. *Gynecol Oncol.* 2015;138:750–756.
5. Collaborative Group on Epidemiological Studies of Ovarian Cancer. Ovarian cancer and body size: individual participant meta-analysis including 25,157 women with ovarian cancer from 47 epidemiologic studies. *PLoS Med.* 2012;9:e1001200.
6. Olsen CM, Nagle CM, Whiteman DC, et al. Obesity and risk of ovarian cancer subtypes: evidence from the Ovarian Cancer Association Consortium. *Endocr Relat Cancer.* 2013;20:251–262.
7. Taubes G. Epidemiology faces its limits. *Science.* 1995;269:164–169.
8. Whiteman D, Siskind V, Purdie D, et al. Timing of pregnancy and the risk of epithelial ovarian cancer. *Cancer Epidemiol Biomarkers Prev.* 2003;12:42–46.
9. Jordan S, Siskind V, Green AC, et al. Breastfeeding and risk of epithelial ovarian cancer. *Cancer Causes Control.* 2010;21:109–116.
10. Beral V, Doll R, Hermon C, et al. Ovarian cancer and oral contraceptives: collaborative reanalysis of data from 45 epidemiological studies including 23257 women with ovarian cancer and 87303 controls. *Lancet.* 2008;371:303–314.
11. Schildkraut JM, Calingaert B, Marchbanks PA, et al. Impact of progestin and estrogen potency in oral contraceptives on ovarian cancer risk. *J Natl Cancer Inst.* 2002;94:32–38.
12. Havrilesky LJ, Moorman PG, Lowery WJ, et al. Oral contraceptive pills as primary prevention for ovarian cancer: a systematic review and meta-analysis. *Obstet Gynecol.* 2013;122:139–147.
13. Lengyel E. Ovarian cancer development and metastasis. *Am J Pathol.* 2010;177:1053–1064.
14. Casagrande JT, Louie E, Pike MC, et al. "Incessant ovulation" and ovarian cancer. *Lancet.* 1979;2:170–173.
15. Trevino LS, Buckles EL, Johnson PA. Oral contraceptives decrease the prevalence of ovarian cancer in the hen. *Cancer Prev Res.* 2012;5:343–349.
16. Risch HA. Hormonal etiology of epithelial ovarian cancer, with a hypothesis concerning the role of androgens and progesterone. *J Natl Cancer Inst.* 1998;90:1774–1786.
17. Rodriguez GC, Nagarsheth NP, Lee KL, et al. Progestin-induced apoptosis in the macaque ovarian epithelium: differential regulation of transforming growth factor-β. *J Natl Cancer Inst.* 2002;94:50–60.
18. Anderson GL, Judd HL, Kaunitz AM, et al. Effects of estrogen plus progestin on gynecologic cancers and associated diagnostic procedres. *JAMA.* 2003;290:1739–1748.
19. Beral V, Bull D, Green J, et al. Ovarian cancer and hormone replacement therapy in the million women study. *Lancet.* 2007;369:1703–1710.
20. Morch LS, Lokkegaard E, Andreasen AH, et al. Hormone therapy and ovarian cancer. *JAMA.* 2009;302:298–305.
21. Collaborative Group on Epidemiological Studies of Ovarian Cancer, Beral V, Gaitskell K, et al. Menopausal hormone use and ovarian cancer risk: individual participant meta-analysis of 52 epidemiological studies. *Lancet.* 2015;385:1835–1842.

22. Li D, Ding CY, Qiu LH. Postoperative hormone replacement therapy for epithelial ovarian cancer patients: a systematic review and meta-analysis. *Gynecol Oncol.* 2015;139:355–362.
23. Eeles R, Morden JP, Gore M, et al. Adjuvant hormone therapy may improve survival in epithelial ovarian cancer: results of the AHT Randomized Trial. *J Clin Oncol.* 2015;33(35):4138–4144.
24. Hankinson SE, Hunter DJ, Colditz GA, et al. Tubal ligation, hysterectomy, and risk of ovarian cancer. *JAMA.* 1993;270:2813–2818.
25. Gaitskell K, Green J, Pirie K, et al. Tubal ligation and ovarian cancer risk in a large cohort: substantial variation by histological type. *Int J Cancer.* 2016;138:1076–1084.
26. Narod SA, Sun P, Ghadirian P, et al. Tubal ligation and risk of ovarian cancer in carriers of BRCA1 or BRCA2 mutations: a case-control study. *Lancet.* 2001;357:1467–1470.
27. Tiourin E, Velasco VS, Rosales MA, et al. Tubal ligation induces quiescence in the epithelia of the fallopian tube fimbria. *Reprod Sci.* 2015;22(10):1262–1271.
28. Lin HW, Tu YY, Lin SY, et al. Risk of ovarian cancer in women with pelvic inflammatory disease: a population-based study. *Lancet Oncol.* 2011;12:900–904.
29. Pearce CL, Templeman C, Rossing MA, et al. Association between endometriosis and risk of histological subtypes of ovarian cancer: a pooled analysis of case-control studies. *Lancet Oncol.* 2012;13:385–394.
30. Kim HS, Kim TH, Chung HH, et al. Risk and prognosis of ovarian cancer in women with endometriosis: a meta-analysis. *Br J Cancer.* 2014;110:1878–1890.
31. Vecellini P, Somigliana E, Buggio L, et al. Endometriosis and ovarian cancer. *Lancet Oncol.* 2012;13:188–189.
32. Wiegand KC, Shah S, Al-Agha OM, et al. ARID1A mutations in endometriosis associated ovarian carcinomas. *N Eng J Med.* 2010;363:1532–1543.
33. Banz C, Ungethuem U, Kuban RJ, et al. The molecular signature of endometriosis-associated endometroid ovarian cancer differs significantly from endometriosis-independent endometroid ovarian cancer. *Fertil Steril.* 2009;94:1212–1217.
34. Schildkraut JM, Moorman PG, Halabi S, et al. Analgesic drug use and risk of ovarian cancer. *Epidemiology.* 2006;17:104–107.
35. Bonovas S, Filioussi K, Sitaras NM. Do nonsteroidal anti-inflammatory drugs affect the risk of developing ovarian cancer? a meta-analysis. *Br J Clin Pharmacol.* 2005;60:194–203.
36. Trabert B, Ness RB, Lo-Ciganic WH, et al. Aspirin, nonaspirin nonsteroidal anti-inflammatory drug, and acetaminophen use and risk of invasive epithelial ovarian cancer: a pooled analysis in the Ovarian Cancer Association Consortium. *J Natl Cancer Inst.* 2014;106:djt431.
37. Chiang ET, Lee VS, Canchola AJ, et al. Diet and risk of ovarian cancer in the california teachers study cohort. *Am J Epidemiol.* 2007;165:802–813.
38. Chang ET, Lee VS, Canchola AJ, et al. Dietary patterns and risk of ovarian cancer in the california teachers study cohort. *Nutr Cancer.* 2008;60:285–291.
39. Prentice RL, Thompson CA, Caan B, et al. Low-fat dietary pattern and cancer incidence in the women's health initiative dietary modification randomized controlled trial. *J Natl Cancer Inst.* 2007;99:1534–1543.
40. Hou R, Wu QJ, Gong TT, et al. Dietary fat and fatty acid intake and epithelial ovarian cancer risk: evidence from epidemiological studies. Oncotarget. 2015;6:43099–43119.
41. Li XM, Ganmaa D, Sato A. The experience of Japan as a clue to the etiology of breast and ovarian cancers: relationship between death from both malignancies and dietary practices. *Med Hypotheses.* 2003;60:268–275.
42. Tworoger SS, Gertig DM, Gates MA, et al. Caffeine, alcohol, smoking, and the risk of incident epithelial ovarian cancer. *Cancer.* 2007;112:1169–1177.
43. Soegaard M, Jensen A, Hogdall E, et al. Different risk factor profiles for mucinous and nonmucinous ovarian cancer: results from the danish MALOVA study. *Cancer Epidemiol Biomarkers Prev.* 2007;16:1160–1166.
44. Collaborative Group on Epidemiological Studies of Ovarian Cancer, Beral V, Gaitskell K, et al. Ovarian cancer and smoking: individual participant meta-analysis including 28,114 women with ovarian cancer from 51 epidemiological studies. *Lancet Oncol.* 2012;13:946–956.
45. Moorman PG, Jones LW, Akushevich L, et al. Recreational physical activity and ovarian cancer risk and survival. *Annu Epidemiol.* 2011;21:178–187.
46. Alsop K, Fereday S, Meldrum C, et al. BRCA mutation frequency and patterns of treatment response in BRCA mutation-positive women with ovarian cancer: a report from the australian ovarian cancer study group. *J Clin Oncol.* 2012;30(21):2654–2663.
47. Norquist BM, Harrell MI, Brady MF, et al. Inherited mutations in women with ovarian carcinoma. *JAMA Oncol.* 2016;2(4):482–490.
48. Desmond A, Kurian AW, Gabree M, et al. Clinical actionability of multigene panel testing for hereditary breast and ovarian cancer risk assessment. *JAMA Oncol.* 2015;1:943–951.
49. Walsh T, Casadei S, Lee MK, et al. Mutations in 12 genes for inherited ovarian, fallopian tube and peritoneal carcinoma identified by massively parallel sequencing. *Proc Natl Acad Sci U S A.* 2011;108:18032–18037.
50. Chen S, Parmigiani G. Meta-analysis of BRCA1 and BRCA2 penetrance. *J Clin Oncol.* 2007;25:1329–1333.
51. Finch AP, Lubinski J, Moller P, et al. Impact of oophorectomy on cancer incidence and mortality in women with a BRCA1 or BRCA2 mutation. *J Clin Oncol.* 2014;32(15):1547–1553.
52. Epidemiology CfCG. BOADICEA. University of Cambridge; 2016. http://ccge.medschl.cam.ac.uk/boadicea/
53. Rubin SC, Benjamin I, Behbakht K, et al. Clinical and pathological features of ovarian cancer in women with germ-line mutations of BRCA1. *N Eng J Med.* 1996;335:1413–1416.
54. Mavaddat N, Barrowdale D, Andrulis IL, et al. Pathology of breast and ovarian cancers among BRCA1 and BRCA2 mutation carriers: results from the consortium of investigators and modifiers for BRCA1/2 (CIMBA). *Cancer Epidemiol Biomarkers Prev.* 2012;2:134–147.
55. Candido-dos-Reis FJ, Song H, Goode EL, et al. Germline mutation in BRCA1 or BRCA2 and ten-year survival for women diagnosed with epithelial ovarian cancer. *Clin Cancer Res.* 2015;21:652–657.
56. Werness BA, Ramus SJ, DiCioccio RA, et al. Histopathology, FIGO stage, and BRCA mutation status of ovarian cancers from the gilda radner familial ovarian cancer registry. *Int J Gynecol Pathol.* 2004;23:29–34.
57. Zhang Z, Royer R, Li S, et al. Frequencies of BRCA1 and BRCA2 mutations among 1342 patients with invasive ovarian cancer. *Gynecol Oncol.* 2011;121:353–357.
58. Modan B, Hartge P, Hirsch-Yechezel G. Oral contraceptives and the risk of ovarian cancer among carriers and noncarriers of a BRCA1 and BRCA2 mutation. *N Eng J Med.* 2001;345:235–240.
59. Lord CJ, Ashworth A. The DNA damage response and cancer therapy. *Nature.* 2012;481:287–292.
60. Quinn JE, James CR, Stewart GE. BRCA1 mRNA expression levels predict for overall survival an ovarian cancer after chemotherapy. *Clin Cancer Res.* 2007;13:7413–7420.
61. Easton DF, Pharoah PD, Antoniou AC, et al. Gene-panel sequencing and the prediction of breast-cancer risk. *N Engl J Med.* 2015;372:2243–2257.
62. Armstrong J, Toscano M, Kotchko N, et al. Utilization and outcomes of BRCA genetic testing and counseling in a national commercially insured population: the ABOUT Study. *JAMA Oncol.* 2015;1(9):1251–1260.
63. Hartmann LC, Lindor NM. The role of risk-reducing surgery in hereditary breast and ovarian cancer. *N Engl J Med.* 2016;374:454–468.
64. McLaughlin JR, Risch HA, Lubinski J, et al. Reproductive risk factors for ovarian cancer in carriers of BRCA1 and BRCA2 mutations: a case-control study. *Lancet Oncol.* 2007;8:34.
65. Moorman PG, Havrilesky LJ, Gierisch JM, et al. Oral contraceptives and risk of ovarian cancer and breast cancer among high-risk women: a systematic review and meta-analysis. *J Clin Oncol.* 2013;31:4188–4198.
66. Leib JR, Hoodfar E, Haidle JL, et al. The new genetic privacy law. *Community Oncol.* 2008;5:351–354.
67. Buys S, Partridge E, Black A, et al. Effect of screening on ovarian cancer mortality: the Prostate, Lung, Colorectal and Ovarian (PLCO) Cancer Screening Randomized Controlled Trial. *JAMA.* 2011;305:2295–2303.
68. Jacobs IJ, Menon U, Ryan A, et al. Ovarian cancer screening and mortality in the UK Collaborative Trial of Ovarian Cancer Screening (UKCTOCS): a randomised controlled trial. *Lancet.* 2016;387:945–956.
69. Moyer VA, Force USPST. Screening for ovarian cancer: U.S. Preventive Services Task Force reaffirmation recommendation statement. *Ann Intern Med.* 2012;157:900–904.
70. Rebbeck TR, Lynch HT, Neuhausen SL, et al. Prophylactic oophorectomy in carriers of BRCA1 or BRCA2 mutations. *N Eng J Med.* 2002;346:1616–1622.
71. Kauff ND, Stagopan JM, Robson ME, et al. Risk-reducing salpingo-oophorectomy in women with a BRCA1 or BRCA2 mutation. *N Eng J Med.* 2002;346:1609–1615.
72. Domchek SM, Friebel TM, Singer CF, et al. Association of risk-reducing surgery in BRCA1 or BRCA2 mutation carriers with cancer risk and mortality. *JAMA.* 2010;304:967–975.
73. Finch A, Beiner M, Lubinski J, et al. Salpingo-oophorectomy and the risk of ovarian, fallopian tube, and peritoneal cancers in women with a BRCA1 or BRCA2 mutation. *JAMA.* 2006;296:185–192.
74. Lancaster JM, Powell CB, Chen LM, et al. Society of gynecologic oncology statement on risk assessment for inherited gynecologic cancer predispositions. *Gynecol Oncol.* 2015;136:3–7.
75. Metcalfe K, Lynch HT, Foulkes WD, et al. Effect of oophorectomy on survival after breast cancer in BRCA1 and BRCA2 mutation carriers. *JAMA Oncol.* 2015;1:306–313.

76. Powell BC, Chen LM, McLennan J, et al. Risk-reducing salpingo-oophorectomy (RRSO) in BRCA mutation carriers. *Int J Gynecol Cancer.* 2011;21:846–851.
77. Shu CA, Pike MC, Jotwani AR, et al. Uterine cancer after risk-reducing salpingo-oophorectomy without hysterectomy in women with BRCA mutations. *JAMA Oncol.* 2016. doi:10.1001/jamaoncol.2016.1820.
78. Bowtell DD, Bohm S, Ahmed AA, et al. Rethinking ovarian cancer II: reducing mortality from high-grade serous ovarian cancer. *Nat Rev Cancer.* 2015;15:668–679.
79. McAlpine JN, Hanley GE, Woo MM, et al. Opportunistic salpingectomy: uptake, risks, and complications of a regional initiative for ovarian cancer prevention. *Am J Obstet Gynecol.* 2014;210:471.e1–471.e11.
80. Finch A, Metcalfe KA, Chiang JK, et al. The impact of prophylactic salpingo-ophorectomy on menopausal symptoms and sexual function in women who carry a BRCA mutation. *Gynecol Oncol.* 2011;121:163–168.
81. Eisen A, Lubinski J, Gronwald J, et al. Hormone therapy and the risk of breast cancer in BRCA1 mutation carriers. *J Natl Cancer Inst.* 2008;100:1361–1362.
82. Lu KH, Dinh M, Kohlmann W, et al. Gynecologic cancer as a "sentinel cancer" for women with hereditary nonpolyposis colorectal cancer syndrome. *Obstet Gynecol.* 2005;105:569–574.
83. Lynch HT, Chapelle A. Hereditary colorectal cancer. *N Eng J Med.* 2003;348:919–932.
84. Watson P, Butzow R, Lynch HT, et al. The clinical features of ovarian cancer in hereditary nonpolyposis colorectal cancer. *Gynecol Oncol.* 2001;82:223–228.
85. Bonadona V, Bonaïti B, Olschwang S, et al. Cancer risk associated with germline mutations in MLH1, MSH2, and MSH6 genes in lynch syndrome. *JAMA.* 2011;305:2304–2310.
86. Ketabi Z, Bartuma K, Bernstein I, et al. Ovarian cancer linked to lynch syndrome typically presents as early-onset, non-serous epithelial tumors. *Gynecol Oncol.* 2011;121:462–465.
87. Schmeler KM, Lynch HT, Chen LM, et al. Prophylactic surgery to reduce the risk of gynecologic cancers in the lynch syndrome. *N Eng J Med.* 2006;354:261–269.
88. Zaino R, Brady MF, Lele S, et al. Advanced stage mucinous adenocarcinoma of the ovary is both rare and highly lethal. *Cancer.* 2011;117:554–562.
89. Bookman MA, Brady MF, McGuire WP, et al. Evaluation of new platinum-based treatment regimens in advanced-stage ovarian cancer: a phase III trial of the Gynecologic Cancer Intergroup. *J Clin Oncol.* 2009;27:1419–1425.
90. Sugerbaker PH. New standard of care for appendiceal epithelial neoplasms and pseudomyxoma peritoneii. *Lancet Oncol.* 2006;7:69–76.
91. Passot G, Vaudoyer D, Villeneuve L, et al. What made hyperthermic intraperitoneal chemotherapy an effective curative treatment for peritoneal surface malignancy: a 25-year experience with 1,125 procedures. *J Surg Oncol.* 2016;113:796–803.
92. Walsh C, Holschneider C, Hoang Y, et al. Coexisting ovarian malignancy in young women with endometrial cancer. *Obstet Gynecol.* 2005;106:693–699.
93. Dizon DS, Birrer MJ. Making a difference: distinguishing two primaries from metastasis in synchronous tumors of the ovary and uterus. *J Natl Cancer Inst.* 2016;108(6):djv442.
94. Sehouli J, Senyuva F, Fotopoulou C, et al. Intra-abdominal tumor dissemination pattern and surgical outcome in 214 patients with primary ovarian cancer. *J Surg Oncol.* 2009;99:424–427.
95. Kuhn E, Kurman RJ, Vang R, et al. TP53 mutations in serous tubal intraepithelial carcinoma and concurrent pelvic high-grade serous carcinoma-evidence supporting the clonal relationship of the two lesions. *J Pathol.* 2012;226:421–426.
96. Brown PO, Palmer C. The preclinical natural history of serous ovarian cancer: defining the target for early detection. *PLoS Med.* 2009;6:1–11.
97. Dauplat J, Hacker NF, Nieberg R, et al. Distant metastases in epithelial ovarian carcinoma. *Cancer.* 1987;60:1561–1566.
98. Bristow RE, del Carmen M, Kaufman H, et al. Radical oophorectomy with primary stapled colorectal anastomosis for resection of locally advanced epithelial ovarian cancer. *J Am Coll Surg.* 2003;197:565–574.
99. Aletti GD, Podratz KC, Jones MB, et al. Role of rectosigmoidectomy and stripping of pelvic peritoneum in outcomes of patients with advanced ovarian cancer. *J Am Coll Surg.* 2006;203:521–526.
100. Kehoe SM, Eisenhauer EL, Chi DS. Upper abdominal surgical procedures: liver mobilization and diaphragm peritonectomy/resection, spenectomy, and distal pancreatectomy. *Gynecol Oncol.* 2008;111:S51–S55.
101. Chi DS, Eisenhauer EL, Zivanovic O, et al. Improved progression-free and overall survival in advanced ovarian cancer as a result of a change in surgical paradigm. *Gynecol Oncol.* 2009;114:26–31.
102. Ayantunde A, Parsons S. Pattern and prognostic factors in patients with malignant ascites: a retrospective study. *Ann Oncol.* 2007;18:945–949.
103. Winter WE, Maxwell GL, Tian C, et al. Tumor residual after surgical cytoreduction in prediction of clinical outcome in stage IV epithelial ovarian cancer: a Gynecological Oncology Group study. *J Clin Oncol.* 2008;26:83–89.
104. Wimberger P, Wehling M, Lehmann N, et al. Influence of residual tumor on outcome in ovarian cancer patients with FIGO stage IV disease. *Ann Surg Oncol.* 2010;17:1642–1648.
105. McGuire WP, Hoskins WJ, Brady MF, et al. Taxol and cisplatin improves outcome in advanced ovarian cancer as compared to cytoxan and cisplatin. *N Eng J Med.* 1996;334:1–6.
106. Ozols RF, Bundy B, Greer BE, et al. Phase III trial of carboplatin and paclitaxel compared with cisplatin and paclitaxel in patients with optimally resected stage III ovarian cancer: a Gynecologic Oncology Group study. *J Clin Oncol.* 2003;21:3194–3200.
107. Gershenson D, Sun CC, Lu K, et al. Clinical behavior of stage II-IV low-grade serous carcinoma of the ovary. *ObstetGynecol.* 2006;108: 361–368.
108. Mangan CE, Rubin SC, Rabin DS, et al. Lymph node nomenclature in gynecologic oncology. *Gynecol Oncol.* 1986;23:222–226.
109. Morice P, Joulie F, Camatte S, et al. Lymph node involvement in epithelial ovarian cancer: analysis of 276 pelvic and paraaortic lymphadenectomies and surgical implications. *J Am Coll Surg.* 2003;197:198–205.
110. Benedetti P, Maggioni A, Hacker NF, et al. Systematic aortic and pelvic lymphadenectomy versus resection of bulky nodes only in opitmally debulked advanced ovarian cancer: a randomized clinical trial. *J Natl Cancer Inst.* 2005;97:560–566.
111. Du Bois A, Reuss A, Harter P, et al. Potential role of lymphadenectomy in advanced ovarian cancer: a combined exploratory analysis of three propectively randomized phase III multicenter trials. *J Clin Oncol.* 2010;28:1733–1739.
112. Timmers PJ, Zwinderman AH, Coens C, et al. Understanding the problem of inadequately staging early ovarian cancer. *Eur J Cancer.* 2010;46:880–884.
113. Maggioni A, Benedetti Panici P, Dell'Anna T, et al. Randomised study of systematic lymphadenectomy in patients with epithelial ovarian cancer macroscopically confined to the pelvis. *Br J Cancer.* 2006;95:699–704.
114. Winter WE, Maxwell L, Tian C, et al. Prognostic factors for stage III epithelial ovarian cancer: a Gynecologic Oncology Group study. *J Clin Oncol.* 2007;25:3621–3627.
115. Cormio G, Rossi C, Cazzolla A, et al. Distant metastases in ovarian carcinoma. *Int J Gynecol Cancer.* 2003;13:125–129.
116. Armstrong DK, Bundy B, Wenzel L, et al. Intraperitoneal cisplatin and paclitaxel in ovarian cancer. *N Engl J Med.* 2006;353:34–43.
117. Robinson W, Beyer J, Griffin S, et al. Extraperitoneal metastases from recurrent ovarian cancer. *Int J Gynecol Cancer.* 2012;22:43–46.
118. Esselen K, Rodriguez N, Growdon W, et al. Patterns of recurrence in advanced epithelial ovarian, fallopian tube and peritoneal cancers treated with intraperitoneal chemotherapy. *Gynecol Oncol.* 2012;127:51–54.
119. Petrillo M, Amadio G, Salutari V, et al. Impact of bevacizumab containing first line chemotherapy on recurrent disease in epithelial ovarian cancer: a case-control study. *Gynecol Oncol.* 2016;142(2):231–236.
120. Stone RL, Nick AM, McNeish IA, et al. Paraneoplastic thrombocytosis in ovarian cancer. *N Engl J Med.* 2012;366:610–618.
121. Goff BA, Mandel LS, Melancon CH, et al. Frequency of symptoms of ovarian cancer in women presenting to primary care clinics. *JAMA.* 2004;291:2705–2712.
122. Pavlik EJ, Saunders BA, Doran S, et al. The search for meaning - symptoms and transvaginal sonography screening for ovarian cancer. *Cancer.* 2012;115:3689–3698.
123. Rossing MA, Wicklund KG, Cushing-Haugen KL, et al. Predictive value of symptoms for early detection of ovarian cancer. *J Natl Cancer Inst.* 2010;102:222–229.
124. Lim AWW, Mesher D, Gentry-Maharaj A, et al. Predictive value of symptoms for ovarian cancer: comparison of symptoms reported by questionaire, interview, and general practitioner notes. *J Natl Cancer Inst.* 2012;104:114–124.
125. Committee on Gynecologic Practice. The role of the obstetrician-gynecologist in the early detection of epithelial ovarian cancer. *Obstet Gynecol.* 2011;117:742–746.
126. Ray A, Masch WR, Saukkonen K, et al. Case records of the Massachusetts General Hospital: case 18-2016. A 52-year-old woman with a pleural effusion. *N Engl J Med.* 2016;374:2378–2387.
127. van Nagell JR Jr, Miller RW, DeSimone CP, et al. Long-term survival of women with epithelial ovarian cancer detected by ultrasonographic screening. *Obstet Gynecol.* 2011;118:1212–1221.
128. Skirnisdottir I, Garmo H, Holmberg L. Non-genital tract metastases to the ovaries presented as ovarian tumors in Sweden 1990–2003:

occurence, origin and survival compared to ovarian cancer. *Gynecol Oncol.* 2007;105:166–171.
129. Ayhan A, Guvenal T, Salman MC, et al. The role of cytoreductive surgery in nongenital cancers metastatic to the ovaries. *Gynecol Oncol.* 2005;98:235–241.
130. van Nagell JR Jr, Miller RW. Evaluation and management of ultrasonographically detected ovarian tumors in asymptomatic women. *Obstet Gynecol.* 2016;127:848–858.
131. Bast RC, Feeney M, Lazarus H, et al. Reactivity of a monoclonal antibody with human ovarian carcinoma. *J Clin Invest.* 1981;68:1331–1337.
132. Mann W, Patsner B, Coher H, et al. Preoperative serum CA-125 levels in patients with with surgical stage I invasive ovarian adenocarcinoma. *J Natl Cancer Inst.* 1998;80:208–213.
133. Miller RW, Ueland FR. Risk of malignancy in sonographically confirmed ovarian tumors. *Clin Obstet Gynecol.* 2012;55:52–64.
134. Myers ER, Bastian LA, Havrilesky LJ, et al. Management of adnexal mass. *Evid Rep Technol Assess (Full Rep).* 2006;130:1–145.
135. Vergote I, Troupe CG, Amant F, et al. Neoadjuvant chemotherapy or primary surgery in stage IIIC or IV ovarian cancer. *N Eng J Med.* 2010;363:943–953.
136. Rustin GJ, van der Burg ME, Griffin CL, et al. Early versus delayed treatment of relapsed ovarian cancer (MRC OVO5/EORTC 55955) a randomised trial. *Lancet.* 2010;376:1155–1163.
137. Rauh-Hain JA, Melamed A, Buskwofie A, et al. Adnexal mass in the postmenopausal patient. *Clin Obstet Gynecol.* 2015;58:53–65.
138. Zhen S, Bian LH, Chang LL, et al. Comparison of serum human epididymis protein 4 and carbohydrate antigen 125 as markers in ovarian cancer: a meta-analysis. *Mol Clin Oncol.* 2014;2:559–566.
139. Longoria TC, Ueland FR, Zhang Z, et al. Clinical performance of a multivariate index assay for detecting early-stage ovarian cancer. *Am J Obstet Gynecol.* 2014;210:78 e71–e79.
140. Liu J, Xu Y, Wang J. Ultrasonography, computed tomography and magnetic resonance imaging for diagnosis of ovarian carcinoma. *Eur J Radiol.* 2007;62:328–334.
141. Sassone A, Timor-Tritsch I, Artner A, et al. Transvaginal sonographic characterization of ovarin disease: evaluation of a new scoring system to predict ovarian malignancy. *Obstet Gynecol.* 1991;78:70–76.
142. Geomini P, Kruitwagen R, Bremer GL, et al. The accuracy of risk scores in predicting ovarian malignancy. *Obstet Gynecol.* 2009;113:384–394.
143. Ueland FR, DePriest PD, Pavlik EJ, et al. Preoperative differentiation of malignant from benign ovarian tumors: the efficacy of morphology indexing and Doppler flow sonography. *Gynecol Oncol.* 2003;91:46–50.
144. Elder JW, Pavlik EJ, Long A, et al. Serial ultrasonographic evaluation of ovarian abnormalities with a morphology index. *Gynecol Oncol.* 2014;135:8–12.
145. Van Calster B, Van Hoorde K, Valentin L, et al. Evaluating the risk of ovarian cancer before surgery using the ADNEX model to differentiate between benign, borderline, early and advanced stage invasive, and secondary metastatic tumours: prospective multicentre diagnostic study. *BMJ.* 2014;349:g5920.
146. Kinkel K, Lu Y, Mehdizade A, et al. Indeterminate ovarian mass at US: incremental value of second imaging test for characterizatoin: meta-analysis and Bayesian analysis. *Radiology.* 2005;236:85–94.
147. Anthoulakis C, Nikoloudis N. Pelvic MRI as the "gold standard" in the subsequent evaluation of ultrasound-indeterminate adnexal lesions: a systematic review. *Gynecol Oncol.* 2014;132:661–668.
148. Medeiros L, Fretas L, Rosa D, et al. Accuracy of magnetic resonance imaging in ovarian tumor: a systematic quantitative review. *Am J Obstet Gynecol.* 2011;204:e1–e10.
149. Balan P. Ultrasonography, computed tomography and magnetic resonance imaging in the assessment of pelvic pathology. *Eur J Radiol.* 2006;58:147–155.
150. Gadducci A, Cosio S. Surveillance of patients after initial treatment of ovarian cancer. *Crit Rev Oncol Hematol.* 2009;71:43–52.
151. Borley J, Wilhelm-Benartzi C, Yazbek J, et al. Radiological predictors of cytoreductive outcomes in patients with advanced ovarian cancer. *BJOG.* 2015;122:843–849.
152. Bristow RE, Duska L, Lambrou N, et al. A model for predicting surgical outcome in patients with advanced ovarian carcinoma using computed tomography. *Cancer.* 2000;89:1532–1540.
153. Axtell A, Lee MH, Bristow RE, et al. Multi-institutional reciprocal validation study of computed tomography predictors of suboptimal primary cytorecuction in patients with advanced ovarian cancer. *J Clin Oncol.* 2007;25:384–389.
154. Suidan RS, Ramirez PT, Sarasohn DM, et al. A multicenter prospective trial evaluating the ability of preoperative computed tomography scan and serum CA-125 to predict suboptimal cytoreduction at primary debulking surgery for advanced ovarian, fallopian tube, and peritoneal cancer. *Gynecol Oncol.* 2014;134:455–461.
155. Aletti GD, Eisenhauer E, Santillan A, et al. Identification of patient groups at highest risk from traditional approach to ovarian cancer treatment. *Gynecol Oncol.* 2011;120:23–28.
156. Petrillo M, Vizzielli G, Fanfani F, et al. Definition of a dynamic laparoscopic model for the prediction of incomplete cytoreduction in advanced epithelial ovarian cancer: proof of a concept. *Gynecol Oncol.* 2015;139:5–9.
157. Nick AM, Coleman RL, Ramirez PT, et al. A framework for a personalized surgical approach to ovarian cancer. *Nat Rev Clin Oncol.* 2015;12(4):239–245.
158. Kehoe S, Hook J, Nankivell M, et al. Primary chemotherapy versus primary surgery for newly diagnosed advanced ovarian cancer (CHORUS): an open-label, randomised, controlled, non-inferiority trial. *Lancet.* 2015;386:249–257.
159. Antunovic L, Cimitan M, Borsatti E, et al. Revisiting the clinical value of 18 F-FDG PET/CT in detection of recurrent epithelial ovarian carcinomas. *Clin Nucl Med.* 2012;37:e184–e188.
160. Risum S, Hogdall C, Loft A, et al. The diagnostic value of PET/CT for ovarian cancer: a prospective study. *Gynecol Oncol.* 2007;105:145–149.
161. Dauwen H, Van Calster B, Deroose CM, et al. PET/CT in the staging of patients with a pelvic mass suspicious for ovarian cancer. *Gynecol Oncol.* 2013;131:694–700.
162. Kobayashi H, Yamada Y, Sado T, et al. A randomized study of screening for ovarian cancer: a multicenter study in Japan. *Int J Gynecol Cancer.* 2008;18:414–420.
163. Skates SJ, Menon U, MacDonald N, et al. Calculation of the risk of ovarian cancer from serial CA-125 values for preclinical detection in postmenopausal women. *J Clin Oncol.* 2003;21:206s–210s.
164. Van der Velde N, Mourits M, Arts HJG, et al. Time to stop ovarian cancer screening in BRCA1/2 mutation carriers? *Int J Cancer.* 2009;124:919–923.
165. Ayhan A, Gultekin M, Celik NY, et al. Occult metastasis in early ovarian cancers: risk factors and associated prognosis. *Am J Obstet Gynecol.* 2007;196:81.e1–e6.
166. Prat J, FIGO Committee on Gynecologic Oncology. Staging classification for cancer of the ovary, fallopian tube, and peritoneum. *Int J Gynaecol Obstet.* 2014;124:1–5.
167. Verleye L, Ottevanger PB, van der Graaf W, et al. EORTC-GCG process indicators for ovarian cancer surgery. *Eur J Cancer.* 2009;45:517–526.
168. Garcia-Soto AE, Boren T, Wingo SN, et al. Is comprehensive surgical staging needed for thorough evaluation of early-stage ovarian carcinoma? *Am J Obstet Gynecol.* 2012;206:242.e1–242.e5.
169. Trimbos JB, Vergote I, Bolis G, et al. Impact of adjuvant chemotherapy and surgical staging in early-stage ovarian carcinoma: European Organisation for Research and Treatment of Cancer: adjuvant chemotherapy in ovarian neoplasm trial. *J Natl Cancer Inst.* 2003;95:113–125.
170. Trimbos B, Timmers P, Pecorelli S, et al. Surgical staging and treatment of early ovarian cancer: long-term analysis from a randomized trial. *J Natl Cancer Inst.* 2010;102:982–987.
171. Colombo N, Guthrie D, Chiari S, et al. International Collaborative Ovarian Neoplasm trial 1: a randomized trial of adjuvant chemotherapy in women with early-stage ovarian cancer. *J Natl Cancer Inst.* 2003;95:125–132.
172. Collinson F, Qian W, Fossati R, et al. Optimal treatment of early-stage ovarian cancer. *Ann Oncol.* 2014;25:1165–1171.
173. Chi DS, Abu-Rustum NR, Sonoda Y, et al. The safety and efficacy of laparoscopic surgical staging of apparent stage I ovarian and fallopian tube cancers. *Am J Obstet Gynecol.* 2005;192:1614–1619.
174. Zivanovic O, Sonoda Y, Diaz JP, et al. The rate of port-site metastases after 2251 laparoscopic procedures in women with underlying malignant disease. *Gynecol Oncol.* 2008;111:431–437.
175. DiRe F, Fontanelli R, Raspagliesi F, et al. Pelvic and para-aortic lymphadenetomy in cancer of the ovary. *Balliere's Clin Obstet Gynaecol.* 1989;3:131–138.
176. Eichner E, Bove ER. In vivo studies on the lymphatic drainage of the human ovary. *Obstet Gynecol.* 1954;3:287–297.
177. Schmeler KM, Frumovitz M, Deavers M, et al. Prevalence of lymph node metastasis in primary mucinous carcinoma of the ovary. *Obstet Gynecol.* 2010;116:269–273.
178. Rungruang B, Miller A, Richard SD, et al. Should stage IIIC ovarian cancer be further stratified by intraperitoneal vs. retroperitoneal only disease?: a gynecologic oncology group study. *Gynecol Oncol.* 2012;124:53–58.
179. Bristow RE, Tomacruz RS, Armstrong DK, et al. Survival effect of maximal cytoreductive surgery for advanced ovarian carcinoma during the platinum era: a meta-analysis. *J Clin Oncol.* 2002;20:1248–1259.

180. Griffiths CT. Surgical resection of tumor bulk in the primary treatment of ovarian carcinoma. *Natl Cancer Inst Monogr.* 1975;42:101–104.
181. Hakes TB, Chalas E, Hoskins WJ, et al. Randomized prospective trial of 5 versus 10 cycles of cyclophosphamide, doxorubicin, and cisplatin in advanced ovarian carcinoma. *Gynecol Oncol.* 1992;45:284–289.
182. Du Bois A, Reuss A, Pujade-Lauraine E, et al. Role of surgical outcome as prognostic factor in advanced epithelial ovarian cancer: a combined exploratory analysis of prospectively randomized phase 3 multicenter trials. *Cancer.* 2009;115:1234–1244.
183. Rodriguez N, Miller A, Richard SD, et al. Upper abdominal procedures in advanced stage ovarian or primary peritoneal carcinoma patients with minimal or no gross residual disease: an analysis of Gynecologic Oncology Group (GOG) 182. *Gynecol Oncol.* 2013;130:487–492.
184. Hoskins WJ, Bundy BN, Thigpen JT, et al. The influence of cytoreductive surgery on recurrence-free interval and survival in small-volume stage III epithelial ovarian cancer: a gynecologic oncology group study. *Gynecol Oncol.* 1992;47:159–166.
185. Hoskins WJ, McGuire WP, Brady MF, et al. The effect of diameter of largest risidual disease on survival after primary cytoreductive surgery in patients with suboptimal residual epithelial ovarian carcinoma. *Am J Obstet Gynecol.* 1994;170:974–979.
186. Horowitz NS, Miller A, Rungruang B, et al. Does aggressive surgery improve outcomes? Interaction between preoperative disease burden and complex surgery in patients with advanced-stage ovarian cancer: an analysis of GOG 182. *J Clin Oncol.* 2015;33(8):937–943.
187. Boj SF, Hwang CI, Baker LA, et al. Organoid models of human and mouse ductal pancreatic cancer. *Cell.* 2015;160:324–338.
188. Benedetti Panici P, Di Donato V, Fischetti M, et al. Predictors of post-operative morbidity after cytoreduction for advanced ovarian cancer: analysis and management of complications in upper abdominal surgery. *Gynecol Oncol.* 2015;137:406–411.
189. Greggi S, Falcone F, Carputo R, et al. Primary surgical cytoreduction in advanced ovarian cancer: an outcome analysis within the MITO (Multicentre Italian Trials in Ovarian Cancer and Gynecologic Malignancies) Group. *Gynecol Oncol.* 2016;140:425–429.
190. Grimm C, Harter P, Heitz F, et al. The sandwich technique of diaphragmatic stripping or full-thickness resection for advanced ovarian cancer: how to keep it short and simple. *Int J Gynecol Cancer.* 2015;25:131–134.
191. Eisenhauer EL, Chi DS. Liver mobilization and diaphragm peritonectomy/resection. *Gynecol Oncol.* 2007;104:25–28.
192. Hoffman MS, Tebes SJ, Sayer RA, et al. Extended cytoreduction of intraabdominal metastatic ovarian cancer in the left upper quadrant utilizing en bloc resection. *Am J Obstet Gynecol.* 2007;197:209.e1–e209.e4; discussion 209.e4–209.e5.
193. Magtibay PM, Adams PB, Silverman MB, et al. Splenectomy as part of cytoreductive surgery in ovarian cancer. *Gynecol Oncol.* 2006;102:369–374.
194. van Meurs HS, Tajik P, Hof MH, et al. Which patients benefit most from primary surgery or neoadjuvant chemotherapy in stage IIIC or IV ovarian cancer? An exploratory analysis of the European Organisation for Research and Treatment of Cancer 55971 randomised trial. *Eur J Cancer.* 2013;49:3191–3201.
195. Chi DS, Musa F, Dao F, et al. An analysis of patients with bulky advanced stage ovarian, tubal, and peritoneal carcinoma treated with primary debulking surgery (PDS) during an identical time period as the randomized EORTC-NCIC trial of PDS vs neoadjuvant chemotherapy (NACT). *Gynecol Oncol.* 2012;124:10–14.
196. Wright J, Lewin SN, Deutsch I, et al. Defining the limits of radical cytoreductive surgery for ovarian cancer. *Gynecol Oncol.* 2011;123:467–473.
197. Van Der Burg MEL, Van Lent M, Buyse M, et al. The effect of debulking surgery after induction chemotherapy on the prognosis in advanced epithelial ovarian cancer. *N Eng J Med.* 1995;332:629–634.
198. Rose PG, Nerenstone S, Brady MF, et al. Secondary surgical cytoreduction for advanced ovarian carcinoma. *N Eng J Med.* 2004;351:2489–2497.
199. van der Burg ME. Advanced ovarian cancer. *Curr Treat Options Oncol.* 2001;2:109–118.
200. Chan JK, Brady MF, Penson RT, et al. Weekly vs. every-3-week paclitaxel and carboplatin for ovarian cancer. *N Eng J Med.* 2016;374:738–748.
201. Katsumata N, Yasuda M, Takahasi F, et al. Dose-dense paclitaxel once a week in combination with carboplatin every 3 weeks for advanced ovarian cancer: a phase3, open-label, randomised controlled trial. *Lancet.* 2009;9698:1331–1338.
202. Jänicke F, Hölscher M, Kuhn W, et al. Radical surgical procedure improves survival time in patients with recurrent ovarian cancer. *Cancer.* 1992;70:2129–2136.
203. Chi DS, McCaughty K, Diaz JP, et al. Guidelines and selection criteria for secondary cytoreductive surgery in patients with recurrent, platinum-senstive epithelial ovarian carcinoma. *Cancer.* 2006;106:1933–1939.
204. Eisenkop SM, Friedman RL, Spirtos NM. The role of secondary cytoreductive surgery in the treatment of patients with recurrent epithelial ovarian carcinoma. *Cancer.* 2000;88:144–153.
205. Harter P, Hahmann M, Lueck HJ, et al. Surgery for recurrent ovarian cancer: role of peritoneal carcinomatosis. Exploratory analysis of the DESKTOP I trial about risk factors, surgical implications, and prognostic value of peritoneal carcinomatosis. *Ann Surg Oncol.* 2009;13:1702–1710.
206. Harter P, Sehouli J, Reuss A, et al. Propective validation study of a predictive score for operability of recurrent ovarian cancer. *Int J Gynecol Cancer.* 2011;21:289–295.
207. Janco JM, Kumar A, Weaver AL, et al. Performance of AGO score for secondary cytoreduction in a high-volume U.S. center. *Gynecol Oncol.* 2016;141:140–147.
208. Díaz-Montes TP, Bristow RE. Secondary cytoreduction for patients with recurrent ovarian cancer. *Curr Oncol Rep.* 2012;7:451–458.
209. Musella A, Marchetti C, Palaia I, et al. Secondary cytoreduction in platinum-resistant recurrent ovarian cancer: a single-institution experience. *Ann Surg Oncol.* 2015;22:4211–4216.
210. Radwany SM, von Gruenigen VE. Palliative and end-of-life care for patients with ovarian cancer. *Clin Obstet Gynecol.* 2012;55:173–184.
211. Hope JM, Pothuri B. The role of palliative surgery in gynecologic cancer cases. *Oncologist.* 2013;18:73–79.
212. Perri T, Korach J, Ben-Baruch G, et al. Bowel obstruction in recurrent gynecologic malignancies: defining who will benefit from surgical intervention. *Eur J Surg Oncol.* 2014;40:899–904.
213. Pothuri B, Vaidya A, Aghajanian C, et al. Palliative surgery for bowel obstruction in recurrent ovarian cancer: an updated series. *Gynecol Oncol.* 2003;89:306–313.
214. Kolomainen DF, Daponte A, Barton DP, et al. Outcomes of surgical management of bowel obstruction in relapsed epithelial ovarian cancer (EOC). *Gynecol Oncol.* 2012;125:31–36.
215. Fleming G, Seidman JD, Lengyel E. Epithelial ovarian cancer. In: Barakat RR, Berchuck A, Markmann M, et al, eds. *Principles and Practic of Gynecologic Oncology.* 6th ed. Philadelphia, PA: Lippincott Williams & Wilkins; 2013:755–845.
216. Kobel M, Kalloger SE, Huntsman DG, et al. Differences in tumor type in low-stage versus high-stage ovarian carcinomas. *Int J Gynecol Pathol.* 2010;29:203–211.
217. Akeson M, Jakobsen AM, Zetterqvist BM, et al. A population-based 5-year cohort study including all cases of epithelial ovarian cancer in western Sweden: 10-year survival and prognostic factors. *Int J Gynecol Cancer.* 2009;19:116–123.
218. Seidman JD, Kurman RJ, Ronnett BM. Primary and metastatic mucinous adenocarcinomas in the ovaries: incidence in routine practice with a new approach to improve intraoperative diagnosis. *Am J Surg Pathol.* 2003;27:985–993.
219. Seidman JD, Vang R, Ronnett BM, et al. Distribution and case-fatality ratios by cell-type for ovarian carcinomas: a 22-year series of 562 patients with uniform current histological classification. *Gynecol Oncol.* 2015;136:336–340.
220. Sung PL, Chang YH, Chao KC, et al. Global distribution pattern of histological subtypes of epithelial ovarian cancer: a database analysis and systematic review. *Gynecol Oncol.* 2014;133:147–154.
221. Kurman RJ, Shih IeM. Molecular pathogenesis and extraovarian origin of epithelial ovarian cancer—shifting the paradigm. *Hum Pathol.* 2011;42:918–931.
222. Singh N, Gilks CB, Wilkinson N, et al. Assignment of primary site in high-grade serous tubal, ovarian and peritoneal carcinoma: a proposal. *Histopathology.* 2014;65:149–154.
223. Salvador S, Gilks B, Kobel M, et al. The fallopian tube: primary site of most pelvic high-grade serous carcinomas. *Int J Gynecol Cancer.* 2009;19:58–64.
224. Vang R, Levine DA, Soslow RA, et al. Molecular alterations of TP53 are a defining feature of ovarian high-grade serous carcinoma: a rereview of cases lacking TP53 mutations in The Cancer Genome Atlas Ovarian Study. *Int J Gynecol Pathol.* 2016;35:48–55.
225. Cass I, Walts AE, Barbuto D, et al. A cautious view of putative precursors of serous carcinomas in the fallopian tubes of BRCA mutation carriers. *Gynecol Oncol.* 2014;134:492–497.
226. Steffensen KD, Waldstrom M, Grove A, et al. Improved classification of epithelial ovarian cancer: results of 3 danish cohorts. *Int J Gynecol Cancer.* 2011;21:1592–1600.

227. Wu R, Baker SJ, Hu TC, et al. Type I to type II ovarian carcinoma progression: mutant Trp53 or Pik3ca confers a more aggressive tumor phenotype in a mouse model of ovarian cancer. *Am J Pathol.* 2013;182:1391–1399.
228. Yemelyanova AV, Cosin JA, Bidus MA, et al. Pathology of stage I versus stage III ovarian carcinoma with implications for pathogenesis and screening. *Int J Gynecol Cancer.* 2008;18:465–469.
229. Seidman JD, Cho KR, Ronnett BM. Surface epithelial tumors of the ovary. In: Kurman RJ, Ellenson LH, Ronnett BM, eds. *Blaustein's Pathology of the Female Genital Tract.* 6th ed. New York, NY: Springer-Verlag; 2011:679–784.
230. Seidman JD, Wang BG. Evaluation of normal-sized ovaries associated with primary peritoneal serous carcinoma for possible precursors of ovarian serous carcinoma. *Gynecol Oncol.* 2007;106:201–206.
231. Anglesio MS, Bashashati A, Wang YK, et al. Multifocal endometriotic lesions associated with cancer are clonal and carry a high mutation burden. *J Pathol.* 2015;236:201–209.
232. Stern RC, Dash R, Bentley RC, et al. Malignancy in endometriosis: frequency and comparison of ovarian and extraovarian types. *Int J Gynecol Pathol.* 2001;20:133–139.
233. Brinton LA, Gridley G, Persson I, et al. Cancer risk after a hospital discharge diagnosis of endometriosis. *Am J Obstet Gynecol.* 1997;176:572–579.
234. Kobayashi H, Sumimoto K, Moniwa N, et al. Risk of developing ovarian cancer among women with ovarian endometrioma: a cohort study in Shizuoka, Japan. *Int J Gynecol Cancer.* 2007;17:37–43.
235. Ronnett BM, Kajdacsy-Balla A, Gilks CB, et al. Mucinous borderline ovarian tumors: points of general agreement and persistent controversies regarding nomenclature, diagnostic criteria, and behavior. *Hum Pathol.* 2004;35:949–960.
236. Vang R, Wheeler JE. Diseases of the Fallopian tube and paratubal region. In: Kurman RJ, Ellenson LK, Ronnett BM, eds. *Blaustein's Pathology of the Female Genital Tract.* 6th ed. New York: Springer-Verlag; 2011:529–578.
237. Kindelberger DW, Lee Y, Miron A, et al. Intraepithelial carcinoma of the fimbria and pelvic serous carcinoma: evidence for a causal relationship. *Am J Surg Pathol.* 2007;31:161–169.
238. Domchek SM, Friebel TM, Garber JE, et al. Occult ovarian cancers identified at risk-reducing salpingo-oophorectomy in a prospective cohort of BRCA1/2 mutation carriers. *Breast Cancer Res Treat.* 2010;124:195–203.
239. Colgan TJ, Murphy J, Cole DE, et al. Occult carcinoma in prophylactic oophorectomy specimens: prevalence and association with BRCA germline mutation status. *Am J Surg Pathol.* 2001;25:1283–1289.
240. Sherman ME, Piedmonte M, Mai PL, et al. Pathologic findings at risk-reducing salpingo-oophorectomy: primary results from Gynecologic Oncology Group Trial GOG-0199. *J Clin Oncol.* 2014;32:3275–3283.
241. Klaren HM, van't Veer LJ, van Leeuwen FE, et al. Potential for bias in studies on efficacy of prophylactic surgery for BRCA1 and BRCA2 mutation. *J Natl Cancer Inst.* 2003;95:941–947.
242. Visvanathan K, Vang R, Shaw P, et al. Diagnosis of serous tubal intraepithelial carcinoma based on morphologic and immunohistochemical features: a reproducibility study. *Am J Surg Pathol.* 2011;35:1766–1775.
243. Patrono MG, Iniesta MD, Malpica A, et al. Clinical outcomes in patients with isolated serous tubal intraepithelial carcinoma (STIC): a comprehensive review. *Gynecol Oncol.* 2015;139:568–572.
244. Lee Y, Medeiros F, Kindelberger D, et al. Advances in the recognition of tubal intraepithelial carcinoma: applications to cancer screening and the pathogenesis of ovarian cancer. *Adv Anat Pathol.* 2006;13:1–7.
245. Seidman JD. Serous tubal intraepithelial carcinoma localizes to the tubal-peritoneal junction: a pivotal clue to the site of origin of extrauterine high-grade serous carcinoma (ovarian cancer). *Int J Gynecol Pathol.* 2015;34:112–120.
246. Tornos C, Soslow R. Frozen section of ovarian lesions. In: Soslow RA, Tornos C, eds. *Diagnostic Pathology of Ovarian Tumors.* New York, NY: Springer; 2011:111–115.
247. Heatley MK. A systematic review of papers examining the use of intraoperative frozen section in predicting the final diagnosis of ovarian lesions. *Int J Gynecol Pathol.* 2012;31:111–115.
248. Shih KK, Garg K, Soslow RA, et al. Accuracy of frozen section diagnosis of ovarian borderline tumor. *Gynecol Oncol.* 2011;123:517–521.
249. Storms AA, Sukumvanich P, Monaco SE, et al. Mucinous tumors of the ovary: diagnostic challenges at frozen section and clinical implications. *Gynecol Oncol.* 2012;125:75–79.
250. Yemelyanova AV, Vang R, Judson K, et al. Distinction of primary and metastatic mucinous tumors involving the ovary: analysis of size and laterality data by primary site with reevaluation of an algorithm for tumor classification. *Am J Surg Pathol.* 2008;32:128–138.
251. Pongsuvareeyakul T, Khunamornpong S, Settakorn J, et al. Accuracy of frozen-section diagnosis of ovarian mucinous tumors. *Int J Gynecol Cancer.* 2012;22:400–406.
252. Gilks CB, Movahedi-Lankarani S, Baker PM, et al. *Protocol for the Examination of Specimens from Patients with Primay Tumors of the Ovary or Fallopian Tube.* College of American Pathologists; 2016. Also available at www.cap.org
253. Kurman RJ, Carcangiu ML, Herrington CS, et al. *WHO Classification of Tumours of Femal Reproductive Organs.* Lyon, France: IARC Press; 2014.
254. Tam KF, Cheung AN, Liu KL, et al. A retrospective review on atypical glandular cells of undetermined significance (AGUS) using the Bethesda 2001 classification. *Gynecol Oncol.* 2003;91:603–607.
255. Ayhan A, Gultekin M, Taskiran C, et al. Ascites and epithelial ovarian cancers: a reappraisal with respect to different aspects. *Int J Gynecol Cancer.* 2007;17:68–75.
256. Agoff SN, Mendelin JE, Grieco VS, et al. Unexpected gynecologic neoplasms in patients with proven or suspected BRCA-1 or -2 mutations: implications for gross examination, cytology, and clinical follow-up. *Am J Surg Pathol.* 2002;26:171–178.
257. Seidman JD, Soslow RA, Vang R, et al. Borderline ovarian tumors: diverse contemporary viewpoints on terminology and diagnostic criteria with illustrative images. *Hum Pathol.* 2004;35:918–933.
258. Ardighieri L, Zeppernick F, Hannibal CG, et al. Mutational analysis of BRAF and KRAS in ovarian serous borderline (atypical proliferative) tumours and associated peritoneal implants. *J Pathol.* 2014;232:16–22.
259. Uzan C, Zanini-Grandon AS, Bentivegna E, et al. Outcome of patients with advanced-stage borderline ovarian tumors after a first peritoneal noninvasive recurrence: impact on further management. *Int J Gynecol Cancer.* 2015;25:830–836.
260. Khunamornpong S, Settakorn J, Sukpan K, et al. Mucinous tumor of low malignant potential ("borderline" or "atypical proliferative" tumor) of the ovary: a study of 171 cases with the assessment of intraepithelial carcinoma and microinvasion. *Int J Gynecol Pathol.* 2011;30:218–230.
261. Rabban JT, Vohra P, Zaloudek CJ. Nongynecologic metastases to fallopian tube mucosa: a potential mimic of tubal high-grade serous carcinoma and benign tubal mucinous metaplasia or nonmucinous hyperplasia. *Am J Surg Pathol.* 2015;39:35–51.
262. Stewart CJ, Leung YC, Whitehouse A. Fallopian tube metastases of non-gynaecological origin: a series of 20 cases emphasizing patterns of involvement including intra-epithelial spread. *Histopathology.* 2012;60:E106–E114.
263. Cancer Genome Atlas Research Network. Integrated genomic analyses of ovarian carcinoma. *Nature.* 2011;474:609–615.
264. Baumbusch LO, Helland A, Wang Y, et al. High levels of genomic aberrations in serous ovarian cancers are associated with better survival. *PLoS One.* 2013;8:e54356.
265. Birkbak NJ, Kochupurakkal B, Izarzugaza JM, et al. Tumor mutation burden forecasts outcome in ovarian cancer with BRCA1 or BRCA2 mutations. *PLoS One.* 2013;8:e80023.
266. Yang D, Khan S, Sun Y, et al. Association of BRCA1 and BRCA2 mutations with survival, chemotherapy sensitivity, and gene mutator phenotype in patients with ovarian cancer. *JAMA.* 2011;306:1557–1565.
267. Ciriello G, Miller ML, Aksoy BA, et al. Emerging landscape of oncogenic signatures across human cancers. *Nat Genet.* 2013;45:1127–1133.
268. Tothill RW, Tinker AV, George J, et al. Novel molecular subtypes of serous and endometrioid ovarian cancer linked to clinical outcome. *Clin Cancer Res.* 2008;14:5198–5208.
269. Ho ES, Lai CR, Hsieh YT, et al. p53 mutation is infrequent in clear cell carcinoma of the ovary. *Gynecol Oncol.* 2001;80:189–193.
270. Kuo KT, Mao TL, Jones S, et al. Frequent activating mutations of PIK3CA in ovarian clear cell carcinoma. *Am J Pathol.* 2009;174:1597–1601.
271. Cuatrecasas M, Villanueva A, Matias-Guiu X, et al. K-ras mutations in mucinous ovarian tumors: a clinicopathologic and molecular study of 95 cases. *Cancer.* 1997;79:1581–1586.
272. Vereczkey I, Serester O, Dobos J, et al. Molecular characterization of 103 ovarian serous and mucinous tumors. *Pathol Oncol Res.* 2011;17:551–559.
273. McAlpine JN, Wiegand KC, Vang R, et al. HER2 overexpression and amplification is present in a subset of ovarian mucinous carcinomas and can be targeted with trastuzumab therapy. *BMC Cancer.* 2009;9:433.
274. Anglesio MS, Arnold JM, George J, et al. Mutation of ERBB2 provides a novel alternative mechanism for the ubiquitous activation of RAS-MAPK in ovarian serous low malignant potential tumors. *Mol Cancer Res.* 2008;6:1678–1690.
275. Tsang YT, Deavers MT, Sun CC, et al. KRAS (but not BRAF) mutations in ovarian serous borderline tumour are associated with recurrent low-grade serous carcinoma. *J Pathol.* 2013;231:449–456.
276. Emmanuel C, Chiew YE, George J, et al. Genomic classification of serous ovarian cancer with adjacent borderline differentiates RAS pathway and TP53-mutant tumors and identifies NRAS as an oncogenic driver. *Clin Cancer Res.* 2014;20:6618–6630.

277. Kuo KT, Guan B, Feng Y, et al. Analysis of DNA copy number alterations in ovarian serous tumors identifies new molecular genetic changes in low-grade and high-grade carcinomas. *Cancer Res*. 2009;69:4036–4042.
278. Cheng EJ, Kurman RJ, Wang M, et al. Molecular genetic analysis of ovarian serous cystadenomas. *Lab Invest*. 2004;84:778–784.
279. Hunter SM, Anglesio MS, Sharma R, et al. Copy number aberrations in benign serous ovarian tumors: a case for reclassification? *Clin Cancer Res*. 2011;17:7273–7282.
280. Longacre TA, McKenney JK, Tazelaar HD, et al. Ovarian serous tumors of low malignant potential (borderline tumors): outcome-based study of 276 patients with long-term (> or =5-year) follow-up. *Am J Surg Pathol*. 2005;29:707–723.
281. Seidman JD, Kraus JA, Yemelyanova A, et al. Ovarian low grade serous neoplasms: evaluation of sampling recommendations based on tumors expected to have invasion (those with peritoneal invasive low grade serous carcinoma (invasive implants)) [abstract]. *Modern Pathol*. 2009;22(suppl 1):236A.
282. Seidman JD, Kurman RJ. Ovarian serous borderline tumors: a critical review of the literature with emphasis on prognostic indicators. *Hum Pathol*. 2000;31:539–557.
283. Kraus JA, Seidman JD. The relationship between papillary infarction and microinvasion in ovarian atypical proliferative ("borderline") serous and seromucinous tumors. *Int J Gynecol Pathol*. 2010;29:303–309.
284. Maniar KP, Wang Y, Visvanathan K, et al. Evaluation of microinvasion and lymph node involvement in ovarian serous borderline/atypical proliferative serous tumors: a morphologic and immunohistochemical analysis of 37 cases. *Am J Surg Pathol*. 2014;38:743–755.
285. McKenney JK, Balzer BL, Longacre TA. Patterns of stromal invasion in ovarian serous tumors of low malignant potential (borderline tumors): a reevaluation of the concept of stromal microinvasion. *Am J Surg Pathol*. 2006;30:1209–1221.
286. Hannibal CG, Vang R, Junge J, et al. A nationwide study of serous "borderline" ovarian tumors in Denmark 1978–2002: centralized pathology review and overall survival compared with the general population. *Gynecol Oncol*. 2014;134:267–273.
287. du Bois A, Ewald-Riegler N, de Gregorio N, et al. Borderline tumours of the ovary: a cohort study of the Arbeitsgmeinschaft Gynakologische Onkologie (AGO) Study Group. *Eur J Cancer*. 2013;49:1905–1914.
288. Bell KA, Smith Sehdev AE, Kurman RJ. Refined diagnostic criteria for implants associated with ovarian atypical proliferative serous tumors (borderline) and micropapillary serous carcinomas. *Am J Surg Pathol*. 2001;25:419–432.
289. McKenney JK, Balzer BL, Longacre TA. Lymph node involvement in ovarian serous tumors of low malignant potential (borderline tumors): pathology, prognosis, and proposed classification. *Am J Surg Pathol*. 2006;30:614–624.
290. Sherman ME, Mink PJ, Curtis R, et al. Survival among women with borderline ovarian tumors and ovarian carcinoma: a population-based analysis. *Cancer*. 2004;100:1045–1052.
291. Akeson M, Zetterqvist BM, Dahllof K, et al. Population-based cohort follow-up study of all patients operated for borderline ovarian tumor in western Sweden during an 11-year period. *Int J Gynecol Cancer*. 2008;18:453–459.
292. Park JY, Kim DY, Kim JH, et al. Surgical management of borderline ovarian tumors: the role of fertility-sparing surgery. *Gynecol Oncol*. 2009;113:75–82.
293. Shvartsman HS, Sun CC, Bodurka DC, et al. Comparison of the clinical behavior of newly diagnosed stages II-IV low-grade serous carcinoma of the ovary with that of serous ovarian tumors of low malignant potential that recur as low-grade serous carcinoma. *Gynecol Oncol*. 2007;105:625–629.
294. Smith Sehdev AE, Sehdev PS, Kurman RJ. Noninvasive and invasive micropapillary (low-grade) serous carcinoma of the ovary: a clinicopathologic analysis of 135 cases. *Am J Surg Pathol*. 2003;27:725–736.
295. Seidman JD, Yemelyanova A, Cosin JA, et al. Survival rates for international federation of gynecology and obstetrics stage III ovarian carcinoma by cell type: a study of 262 unselected patients with uniform pathologic review. *Int J Gynecol Cancer*. 2012;22:367–371.
296. Tang S, Onuma K, Deb P, et al. Frequency of serous tubal intraepithelial carcinoma in various gynecologic malignancies: a study of 300 consecutive cases. *Int J Gynecol Pathol*. 2012;31:103–110.
297. Seidman JD, Zhao P, Yemelyanova A. "Primary peritoneal" high-grade serous carcinoma is very likely metastatic from serous tubal intraepithelial carcinoma: assessing the new paradigm of ovarian and pelvic serous carcinogenesis and its implications for screening for ovarian cancer. *Gynecol Oncol*. 2011;120:470–473.
298. Leonhardt K, Einenkel J, Sohr S, et al. p53 signature and serous tubal in-situ carcinoma in cases of primary tubal and peritoneal carcinomas and serous borderline tumors of the ovary. *Int J Gynecol Pathol*. 2011;30:417–424.
299. Reyes MC, Arnold AG, Kauff ND, et al. Invasion patterns of metastatic high-grade serous carcinoma of ovary or fallopian tube associated with BRCA deficiency. *Mod Pathol*. 2014;27:1405–1411.
300. Bromley AB, Altman AD, Chu P, et al. Architectural patterns of ovarian/pelvic high-grade serous carcinoma. *Int J Gynecol Pathol*. 2012;31:397–404.
301. Bohm S, Faruqi A, Said I, et al. Chemotherapy response score: development and validation of a system to quantify histopathologic response to neoadjuvant chemotherapy in tubo-ovarian high-grade serous carcinoma. *J Clin Oncol*. 2015;33:2457–2463.
302. Colon E, Carlson JW. Evaluation of the fallopian tubes after neoadjuvant chemotherapy: persistence of serous tubal intraepithelial carcinoma. *Int J Gynecol Pathol*. 2014;33:463–469.
303. Malpica A, Deavers MT, Lu K, et al. Grading ovarian serous carcinoma using a two-tier system. *Am J Surg Pathol*. 2004;28:496–504.
304. Plaxe SC. Epidemiology of low-grade serous ovarian cancer. *Am J Obstet Gynecol*. 2008;198:459 e451–e458; discussion 459 e458–e459.
305. Malpica A, Deavers MT, Tornos C, et al. Interobserver and intraobserver variability of a two-tier system for grading ovarian serous carcinoma. *Am J Surg Pathol*. 2007;31:1168–1174.
306. Kerr SE, Flotte AB, McFalls MJ, et al. Matching maternal isodisomy in mucinous carcinomas and associated ovarian teratomas provides evidence of germ cell derivation for some mucinous ovarian tumors. *Am J Surg Pathol*. 2013;37:1229–1235.
307. Riopel MA, Ronnett BM, Kurman RJ. Evaluation of diagnostic criteria and behavior of ovarian intestinal-type mucinous tumors: atypical proliferative (borderline) tumors and intraepithelial, microinvasive, invasive, and metastatic carcinomas. *Am J Surg Pathol*. 1999;23:617–635.
308. Irving JA, Clement PB. Recurrent intestinal mucinous borderline tumors of the ovary: a report of 5 cases causing problems in diagnosis, including distinction from mucinous carcinoma. *Int J Gynecol Pathol*. 2014;33:156–165.
309. McKenney JK, Soslow RA, Longacre TA. Ovarian mature teratomas with mucinous epithelial neoplasms: morphologic heterogeneity and association with pseudomyxoma peritonei. *Am J Surg Pathol*. 2008;32:645–655.
310. Chen S, Leitao MM, Tornos C, et al. Invasion patterns in stage I endometrioid and mucinous ovarian carcinomas: a clinicopathologic analysis emphasizing favorable outcomes in carcinomas without destructive stromal invasion and the occasional malignant course of carcinomas with limited destructive stromal invasion. *Mod Pathol*. 2005;18:903–911.
311. Taylor J, McCluggage WG. Ovarian seromucinous carcinoma: report of a series of a newly categorized and uncommon neoplasm. *Am J Surg Pathol*. 2015;39:983–992.
312. Yemelyanova A, Seidman JD. Metastatic tumors. In: Soslow RA, Tornos C, eds. *Diagnostic Pathology of Ovarian Tumors*. New York, NY: Springer; 2011:133–144.
313. Khunamornpong S, Settakorn J, Sukpan K, et al. Primary ovarian mucinous adenocarcinoma of intestinal type: a clinicopathologic study of 46 cases. *Int J Gynecol Pathol*. 2014;33:176–185.
314. Mackay HJ, Brady MF, Oza AM, et al. Prognostic relevance of uncommon ovarian histology in women with stage III/IV epithelial ovarian cancer. *Int J Gynecol Cancer*. 2010;20:945–952.
315. Bruls J, Simons M, Overbeek LI, et al. A national population-based study provides insight in the origin of malignancies metastatic to the ovary. *Virchows Arch*. 2015;467:79–86.
316. Roth LM, Emerson RE, Ulbright TM. Ovarian endometrioid tumors of low malignant potential: a clinicopathologic study of 30 cases with comparison to well-differentiated endometrioid adenocarcinoma. *Am J Surg Pathol*. 2003;27:1253–1259.
317. Storey DJ, Rush R, Stewart M, et al. Endometrioid epithelial ovarian cancer: 20 years of prospectively collected data from a single center. *Cancer*. 2008;112:2211–2220.
318. Soslow RA. Histologic subtypes of ovarian carcinoma: an overview. *Int J Gynecol Pathol*. 2008;27:161–174.
319. McCluggage WG. My approach to and thoughts on the typing of ovarian carcinomas. *J Clin Pathol*. 2008;61:152–163.
320. Chui MH, Gilks CB, Cooper K, et al. Identifying Lynch syndrome in patients with ovarian carcinoma: the significance of tumor subtype. *Adv Anat Pathol*. 2013;20:378–386.
321. Vierkoetter KR, Ayabe AR, VanDrunen M, et al. Lynch Syndrome in patients with clear cell and endometrioid cancers of the ovary. *Gynecol Oncol*. 2014;135:81–84.
322. Silva EG, Deavers MT, Bodurka DC, et al. Association of low-grade endometrioid carcinoma of the uterus and ovary with undifferentiated

carcinoma: a new type of dedifferentiated carcinoma? *Int J Gynecol Pathol.* 2006;25:52–58.
323. Murray MP, Park KJ. Pathology of endometrioid tumors. In: Soslow RA, Tornos C, eds. *Diagnostic Pathology of Ovarian Tumors.* New York, NY: Springer; 2011:75–90.
324. Zaino R, Whitney C, Brady MF, et al. Simultaneously detected endometrial and ovarian carcinomas—a prospective clinicopathologic study of 74 cases: a gynecologic oncology group study. *Gynecol Oncol.* 2001;83:355–362.
325. Cho KR, Shih Ie M. Ovarian cancer. *Annu Rev Pathol.* 2009;4:287–313.
326. Zhao C, Wu LS, Barner R. Pathogenesis of ovarian clear cell adenofibroma, atypical proliferative (borderline) tumor, and carcinoma: clinicopathologic features of tumors with endometriosis or adenofibromatous components support two related pathways of tumor development. *J Cancer.* 2011;2:94–106.
327. Han G, Gilks CB, Leung S, et al. Mixed ovarian epithelial carcinomas with clear cell and serous components are variants of high-grade serous carcinoma: an interobserver correlative and immunohistochemical study of 32 cases. *Am J Surg Pathol.* 2008;32:955–964.
328. Lim D, Ip PP, Cheung AN, et al. Immunohistochemical comparison of ovarian and uterine endometrioid carcinoma, endometrioid carcinoma with clear cell change, and clear cell carcinoma. *Am J Surg Pathol.* 2015;39:1061–1069.
329. Fuh KC, Shin JY, Kapp DS, et al. Survival differences of Asian and Caucasian epithelial ovarian cancer patients in the United States. *Gynecol Oncol.* 2015;136:491–497.
330. Veras E, Mao TL, Ayhan A, et al. Cystic and adenofibromatous clear cell carcinomas of the ovary: distinctive tumors that differ in their pathogenesis and behavior: a clinicopathologic analysis of 122 cases. *Am J Surg Pathol.* 2009;33:844–853.
331. Timmers PJ, Zwinderman AH, Teodorovic I, et al. Clear cell carcinoma compared to serous carcinoma in early ovarian cancer: same prognosis in a large randomized trial. *Int J Gynecol Cancer.* 2009;19:88–93.
332. Takano M, Kikuchi Y, Yaegashi N, et al. Clear cell carcinoma of the ovary: a retrospective multicentre experience of 254 patients with complete surgical staging. *Br J Cancer.* 2006;94:1369–1374.
333. Magazzino F, Katsaros D, Ottaiano A, et al. Surgical and medical treatment of clear cell ovarian cancer: results from the multicenter Italian Trials in Ovarian Cancer (MITO) 9 retrospective study. *Int J Gynecol Cancer.* 2011;21:1063–1070.
334. Suh DH, Park JY, Lee JY, et al. The clinical value of surgeons' efforts of preventing intraoperative tumor rupture in stage I clear cell carcinoma of the ovary: a Korean Multicenter Study. *Gynecol Oncol.* 2015;137:412–417.
335. Bennett JA, Dong F, Young RH, et al. Clear cell carcinoma of the ovary: evaluation of prognostic parameters based on a clinicopathological analysis of 100 cases. *Histopathology.* 2015;66:808–815.
336. Roma AA, Masand RP. Ovarian Brenner tumors and Walthard nests: a histologic and immunohistochemical study. *Hum Pathol.* 2014;45:2417–2422.
337. Seidman JD, Khedmati F. Exploring the histogenesis of ovarian mucinous and transitional cell (Brenner) neoplasms and their relationship with Walthard cell nests: a study of 120 tumors. *Arch Pathol Lab Med.* 2008;132:1753–1760.
338. Wang Y, Wu RC, Shwartz LE, et al. Clonality analysis of combined Brenner and mucinous tumours of the ovary reveals their monoclonal origin. *J Pathol.* 2015;237:146–151.
339. Ali RH, Seidman JD, Luk M, et al. Transitional cell carcinoma of the ovary is related to high-grade serous carcinoma and is distinct from malignant brenner tumor. *Int J Gynecol Pathol.* 2012;31:499–506.
340. Mackenzie R, Talhouk A, Eshragh S, et al. Morphologic and molecular characteristics of mixed epithelial ovarian cancers. *Am J Surg Pathol.* 2015;39:1548–1557.
341. Witkowski L, Goudie C, Foulkes WD, et al. Small-cell carcinoma of the ovary of hypercalcemic type (malignant rhabdoid tumor of the ovary): a review with recent developments on pathogenesis. *Surg Pathol Clin.* 2016;9:215–226.
342. Khunamornpong S, Suprasert P, Chiangmai WN, et al. Metastatic tumors to the ovaries: a study of 170 cases in northern Thailand. *Int J Gynecol Cancer.* 2006;16(suppl 1):132–138.
343. Leiser AL, Chi DS, Ishill NM, et al. Carcinosarcoma of the ovary treated with platinum and taxane: the memorial Sloan-Kettering Cancer Center experience. *Gynecol Oncol.* 2007;105:657–661.
344. Rauh-Hain JA, Diver EJ, Clemmer JT, et al. Carcinosarcoma of the ovary compared to papillary serous ovarian carcinoma: a SEER analysis. *Gynecol Oncol.* 2013;131:46–51.
345. Eichhorn JH, Young RH, Clement PB, et al. Mesodermal (mullerian) adenosarcoma of the ovary: a clinicopathologic analysis of 40 cases and a review of the literature. *Am J Surg Pathol.* 2002;26:1243–1258.
346. Maeda D, Ota S, Takazawa Y, et al. Mucosal carcinoma of the fallopian tube coexists with ovarian cancer of serous subtype only: a study of Japanese cases. *Virchows Arch.* 2010;457:597–608.
347. Baldwin LA, Huang B, Miller RW, et al. Ten-year relative survival for epithelial ovarian cancer. *Obstet Gynecol.* 2012;120:612–618.
348. Wright JD, Chen L, Tergas AI, et al. Trends in relative survival for ovarian cancer from 1975 to 2011. *Obstet Gynecol.* 2015;125:1345–1352.
349. Gondos A, Holleczek B, Arndt V, et al. Trends in population-based cancer survival in Germany: to what extent does progress reach older patients? *Ann Oncol.* 2007;18:1253–1259.
350. Chan JK, Tian C, Monk BJ, et al. Prognostic factors for high-risk early-stage epithelial ovarian cancer: a Gynecologic Oncology Group study. *Cancer.* 2008;112:2202–2210.
351. Seidman JD, Yemelyanova AV, Khedmati F, et al. Prognostic factors for stage I ovarian carcinoma. *Int J Gynecol Pathol.* 2010;29:1–7.
352. Heintz AP, Odicino F, Maisonneuve P, et al. Carcinoma of the ovary. FIGO 26th Annual Report on the Results of Treatment in Gynecological Cancer. *Int J Gynaecol Obstet.* 2006;95(suppl 1):S161–S192.
353. Dembo AJ, Davy M, Stenwig AE, et al. Prognostic factors in patients with stage I epithelial ovarian cancer. *Obstet Gynecol.* 1990;75:263–273.
354. Seidman JD, Cosin JA, Wang BG, et al. Upstaging pathologic stage I ovarian carcinoma based on dense adhesions is not warranted: a clinicopathologic study of 84 patients originally classified as FIGO stage II. *Gynecol Oncol.* 2010;119:250–254.
355. Obermair A, Fuller A, Lopez-Varela E, et al. A new prognostic model for FIGO stage 1 epithelial ovarian cancer. *Gynecol Oncol.* 2007;104:607–611.
356. Bamias A, Sotiropoulou M, Zagouri F, et al. Prognostic evaluation of tumour type and other histopathological characteristics in advanced epithelial ovarian cancer, treated with surgery and paclitaxel/carboplatin chemotherapy: cell type is the most useful prognostic factor. *Eur J Cancer.* 2012;48:1476–1483.
357. Mizuno M, Kajiyama H, Shibata K, et al. Prognostic value of histological type in stage IV ovarian carcinoma: a retrospective analysis of 223 patients. *Br J Cancer.* 2015;112:1376–1383.
358. Bodurka DC, Deavers MT, Tian C, et al. Reclassification of serous ovarian carcinoma by a 2-tier system: a Gynecologic Oncology Group Study. *Cancer.* 2012;118:3087–3094.
359. Fader AN, Java J, Ueda S, et al. Survival in women with grade 1 serous ovarian carcinoma. *Obstet Gynecol.* 2013;122:225–232.
360. Skaznik-Wikiel ME, Sukumvanich P, Beriwal S, et al. Possible use of CA-125 level normalization after the third chemotherapy cycle in deciding on chemotherapy regimen in patients with epithelial ovarian cancer: brief report. *Int J Gynecol Cancer.* 2011;21:1013–1017.
361. Kotsopoulos J, Rosen B, Fan I, et al. Ten-year survival after epithelial ovarian cancer is not associated with BRCA mutation status. *Gynecol Oncol.* 2016;140:42–47.
362. Konstantinopoulos PA, Ceccaldi R, Shapiro GI, et al. Homologous recombination deficiency: exploiting the fundamental vulnerability of ovarian cancer. *Cancer Discov.* 2015;5:1137–1154.
363. Strickland KC, Howitt BE, Shukla SA, et al. Association and prognostic significance of BRCA1/2-mutation status with neoantigen load, number of tumor-infiltrating lymphocytes and expression of PD-1/PD-L1 in high grade serous ovarian cancer. *Oncotarget.* 2016;7(12):13587–13598.
364. Liu Y, Yasukawa M, Chen K, et al. Association of somatic mutations of ADAMTS genes with chemotherapy sensitivity and survival in high-grade serous ovarian carcinoma. *JAMA Oncol.* 2015;1:486–494.
365. Patch AM, Christie EL, Etemadmoghadam D, et al. Whole-genome characterization of chemoresistant ovarian cancer. *Nature.* 2015;521:489–494.
366. Chen P, Huhtinen K, Kaipio K, et al. Identification of prognostic groups in high-grade serous ovarian cancer treated with platinum-taxane chemotherapy. *Cancer Res.* 2015;75:2987–2998.
367. Matsuo K, Ahn EH, Prather CP, et al. Patient-reported symptoms and survival in ovarian cancer. *Int J Gynecol Cancer.* 2011;21:1555–1565.
368. Yang HS, Yoon C, Myung SK, et al. Effect of obesity on survival of women with epithelial ovarian cancer: a systematic review and meta-analysis of observational studies. *Int J Gynecol Cancer.* 2011;21:1525–1532.
369. Zhou Y, Chlebowski R, LaMonte MJ, et al. Body mass index, physical activity, and mortality in women diagnosed with ovarian cancer: results from the Women's Health Initiative. *Gynecol Oncol.* 2014;133:4–10.
370. Matsuo K, Prather CP, Ahn EH, et al. Significance of perioperative infection in survival of patients with ovarian cancer. *Int J Gynecol Cancer.* 2012;22:245–253.
371. Nakamura K, Hongo A, Kodama J, et al. The pretreatment of maximum standardized uptake values (SUVmax) of the primary tumor is predictor for poor prognosis for patients with epithelial ovarian cancer. *Acta Med Okayama.* 2012;66:53–60.

372. Gunderson CC, Thomas ED, Slaughter KN, et al. The survival detriment of venous thromboembolism with epithelial ovarian cancer. *Gynecol Oncol.* 2014;134:73–77.
373. Terplan M, Schluterman N, McNamara EJ, et al. Have racial disparities in ovarian cancer increased over time? An analysis of SEER data. *Gynecol Oncol.* 2012;125:19–24.
374. Kleppe M, Wang T, Van Gorp T, et al. Lymph node metastasis in stages I and II ovarian cancer: a review. *Gynecol Oncol.* 2011;123:610–614.
375. Satoh T, Hatae M, Watanabe Y, et al. Outcomes of fertility-sparing surgery for stage I epithelial ovarian cancer: a proposal for patient selection. *J Clin Oncol.* 2010;28:1727–1732.
376. Young RC, Walton LA, Ellenberg SS, et al. Adjuvant therapy in stage I and stage II epithelial ovarian cancer. Results of two prospective randomized trials. *N Engl J Med.* 1990;322:1021–1027.
377. Thomas G. Revisiting the role of radiation treatment for non-serous subtypes of epithelial ovarian cancer. *Am Soc Clin Oncol Educ Book.* 2013. doi:10.1200/EdBook_AM.2013.33.e205.
378. Swenerton KD, Santos JL, Gilks CB, et al. Histotype predicts the curative potential of radiotherapy: the example of ovarian cancers. *Ann Oncol.* 2011;22:341–347.
379. Hoskins PJ, Le N, Gilks B, et al. Low-stage ovarian clear cell carcinoma: population-based outcomes in British Columbia, Canada, with evidence for a survival benefit as a result of irradiation. *J Clin Oncol.* 2012;30:1656–1662.
380. Varia MA, Stehman FB, Bundy BN, et al. Intraperitoneal radioactive phosphorus (32P) versus observation after negative second-look laparotomy for stage III ovarian carcinoma: a randomized trial of the Gynecologic Oncology Group. *J Clin Oncol.* 2003;21:2849–2855.
381. Trimbos JB, Parmar M, Vergote I, et al. International collaborative ovarian neoplasm trial 1 and adjuvant chemotherapy in ovarian neoplasm trial: two parallel randomized phase III trials of adjuvant chemotherapy in patients with early-stage ovarian carcinoma. *J Natl Cancer Inst.* 2003;95:105–112.
382. Ahmed FY, Wiltshaw E, A'Hern RP, et al. Natural history and prognosis of untreated stage I epithelial ovarian carcinoma. *J Clin Oncol.* 1996;14:2968–2975.
383. Bell J, Brady MF, Young RC, et al. Randomized phase III trial of three versus six cycles of adjuvant carboplatin and paclitaxel in early stage epithelial ovarian carcinoma: a Gynecologic Oncology Group study. *Gynecol Oncol.* 2006;102:432–439.
384. Chan JK, Tian C, Fleming GF, et al. The potential benefit of 6 vs. 3 cycles of chemotherapy in subsets of women with early-stage high-risk epithelial ovarian cancer: an exploratory analysis of a Gynecologic Oncology Group study. *Gynecol Oncol.* 2010;116:301–306.
385. Mannel RS, Brady MF, Kohn EC, et al. A randomized phase III trial of IV carboplatin and paclitaxel x 3 courses followed by observation versus weekly maintenance low-dose paclitaxel in patients with early-stage ovarian carcinoma: a Gynecologic Oncology Group Study. *Gynecol Oncol.* 2011;122:89–94.
386. del Carmen MG, Birrer M, Schorge JO. Clear cell carcinoma of the ovary: a review of the literature. *Gynecol Oncol.* 2012;126:481–490.
387. Ditto A, Martinelli F, Reato C, et al. Systematic para-aortic and pelvic lymphadenectomy in early stage epithelial ovarian cancer: a prospective study. *Ann Surg Oncol.* 2012;19:3849–3855.
388. Shu CA, Zhou Q, Jotwani AR, et al. Ovarian clear cell carcinoma, outcomes by stage: the MSK experience. *Gynecol Oncol.* 2015;139:236–241.
389. Vaysse C, Touboul C, Filleron T, et al. Early stage (IA-IB) primary carcinoma of the fallopian tube: case-control comparison to adenocarcinoma of the ovary. *J Gynecol Oncol.* 2011;22:9–17.
390. Heintz AP, Odicino F, Maisonneuve P, et al. Carcinoma of the fallopian tube. FIGO 26th Annual Report on the Results of Treatment in Gynecological Cancer. *Int J Gynaecol Obstet.* 2006;95(suppl 1):S145–S160.
391. Morice P, Uzan C, Fauvet R, et al. Borderline ovarian tumour: pathological diagnostic dilemma and risk factors for invasive or lethal recurrence. *Lancet Oncol.* 2012;13:e103–e115.
392. Song T, Choi CH, Kim HJ, et al. Accuracy of frozen section diagnosis of borderline ovarian tumors. *Gynecol Oncol.* 2011;122:127–131.
393. Harter P, Gershenson D, Lhomme C, et al. Gynecologic Cancer InterGroup (GCIG) consensus review for ovarian tumors of low malignant potential (borderline ovarian tumors). *Int J Gynecol Cancer.* 2014;24:S5–S8.
394. Vasconcelos I, de Sousa Mendes M. Conservative surgery in ovarian borderline tumours: a meta-analysis with emphasis on recurrence risk. *Eur J Cancer.* 2015;51:620–631.
395. Fotopoulou C, Sehouli J, Ewald-Riegler N, et al. The value of Serum CA125 in the diagnosis of borderline tumors of the ovary: a subanalysis of the prospective multicenter ROBOT Study. *Int J Gynecol Cancer.* 2015;25:1248–1252.
396. Silva EG, Tornos C, Zhuang Z, et al. Tumor recurrence in stage I ovarian serous neoplasms of low malignant potential. *Int J Gynecol Pathol.* 1998;17:1–6.
397. Vasconcelos I, Darb-Esfahani S, Sehouli J. Serous and mucinous borderline ovarian tumours: differences in clinical presentation, high-risk histopathological features, and lethal recurrence rates. *BJOG.* 2016;123:498–508.
398. Uzan C, Nikpayam M, Ribassin-Majed L, et al. Influence of histological subtypes on the risk of an invasive recurrence in a large series of stage I borderline ovarian tumor including 191 conservative treatments. *Ann Oncol.* 2014;25:1312–1319.
399. Gershenson DM, Bodurka DC, Lu KH, et al. Impact of age and primary disease site on outcome in women with low-grade serous carcinoma of the ovary or peritoneum: results of a Large Single-Institution Registry of a Rare Tumor. *J Clin Oncol.* 2015;33:2675–2682.
400. Grabowski JP, Harter P, Heitz F, et al. Operability and chemotherapy responsiveness in advanced low-grade serous ovarian cancer. An analysis of the AGO Study Group metadatabase. *Gynecol Oncol.* 2016;140:457–462.
401. Della Pepa C, Tonini G, Santini D, et al. Low grade serous ovarian carcinoma: from the molecular characterization to the best therapeutic strategy. *Cancer Treat Rev.* 2015;41:136–143.
402. Fader AN, Jernigan AM, Bergstrom J, et al. Primary cytoreductive surgery and adjuvant hormone therapy in women with advanced low-grade serous carcinoma: reducing overtreatment without compromising survival? Presented at SGO Annual Meeting on Women's Cancer, San Diego, March 22, 2016; abstract 68.
403. Fader AN, Java J, Krivak TC, et al. The prognostic significance of pre- and post-treatment CA-125 in grade 1 serous ovarian carcinoma: a gynecologic Oncology Group study. *Gynecol Oncol.* 2014;132:560–565.
404. Farley J, Brady WE, Vathipadiekal V, et al. Selumetinib in women with recurrent low-grade serous carcinoma of the ovary or peritoneum: an open-label, single-arm, phase 2 study. *Lancet Oncol.* 2013;14:134–140.
405. Perren TJ, Swart AM, Pfisterer J, et al. A phase 3 trial of bevacizumab in ovarian cancer. *N Engl J Med.* 2011;365:2484–2496.
406. Bertelsen K, Jakobsen A, Stroyer J, et al. A prospective randomized comparison of 6 and 12 cycles of cyclophosphamide, adriamycin, and cisplatin in advanced epithelial ovarian cancer: a Danish Ovarian Study Group trial (DACOVA). *Gynecol Oncol.* 1993;49:30–36.
407. Lambert HE, Rustin GJ, Gregory WM, et al. A randomized trial of five versus eight courses of cisplatin or carboplatin in advanced epithelial ovarian carcinoma. A North Thames Ovary Group Study. *Ann Oncol.* 1997;8:327–333.
408. Misset JL, Vennin P, Chollet PH, et al. Multicenter phase II-III study of oxaliplatin plus cyclophosphamide vs. cisplatin plus cyclophosphamide in chemonaive advanced ovarian cancer patients. *Ann Oncol.* 2001;12:1411–1415.
409. Aabo K, Adams M, Adnitt P, et al. Chemotherapy in advanced ovarian cancer: four systematic meta-analyses of individual patient data from 37 randomized trials. Advanced Ovarian Cancer Trialists' Group. *Br J Cancer.* 1998;78:1479–1487.
410. Levin L, Hryniuk WM. Dose intensity analysis of chemotherapy regimens in ovarian carcinoma. *J Clin Oncol.* 1987;5:756–767.
411. Muggia FM, Braly PS, Brady MF, et al. Phase III randomized study of cisplatin versus paclitaxel versus cisplatin and paclitaxel in patients with suboptimal stage III or IV ovarian cancer: a gynecologic oncology group study. *J Clin Oncol.* 2000;18:106–115.
412. McGuire WP, Hoskins WJ, Brady MF, et al. Cyclophosphamide and cisplatin compared with paclitaxel and cisplatin in patients with stage III and stage IV ovarian cancer. *N Engl J Med.* 1996;334:1–6.
413. Piccart MJ, Bertelsen K, James K, et al. Randomized intergroup trial of cisplatin-paclitaxel versus cisplatin-cyclophosphamide in women with advanced epithelial ovarian cancer: three-year results. *J Natl Cancer Inst.* 2000;92:699–708.
414. Spriggs DR, Brady MF, Vaccarello L, et al. Phase III randomized trial of intravenous cisplatin plus a 24- or 96-hour infusion of paclitaxel in epithelial ovarian cancer: a Gynecologic Oncology Group Study. *J Clin Oncol.* 2007;25:4466–4471.
415. Bolis G, Scarfone G, Polverino G, et al. Paclitaxel 175 or 225 mg per meters squared with carboplatin in advanced ovarian cancer: a randomized trial. *J Clin Oncol.* 2004;22:686–690.
416. Katsumata N, Yasuda M, Isonishi S, et al. Long-term results of dose-dense paclitaxel and carboplatin versus conventional paclitaxel and carboplatin for treatment of advanced epithelial ovarian, fallopian tube, or primary peritoneal cancer (JGOG 3016): a randomised, controlled, open-label trial. *Lancet Oncol.* 2013;14:1020–1026.
417. Pignata S, Scambia G, Katsaros D, et al. Carboplatin plus paclitaxel once a week versus every 3 weeks in patients with advanced ovarian

cancer (MITO-7): a randomised, multicentre, open-label, phase 3 trial. *Lancet Oncol.* 2014;15:396–405.

418. Vasey PA, Jayson GC, Gordon A, et al. Phase III randomized trial of docetaxel-carboplatin versus paclitaxel-carboplatin as first-line chemotherapy for ovarian carcinoma. *J Natl Cancer Inst.* 2004;96:1682–1691.
419. Gordon AN, Teneriello M, Janicek MF, et al. Phase III trial of induction gemcitabine or paclitaxel plus carboplatin followed by paclitaxel consolidation in ovarian cancer. *Gynecol Oncol.* 2011;123:479–485.
420. Pignata S, Scambia G, Ferrandina G, et al. Carboplatin plus paclitaxel versus carboplatin plus pegylated liposomal doxorubicin as first-line treatment for patients with ovarian cancer: the MITO-2 randomized phase III trial. *J Clin Oncol.* 2011;29:3628–3635.
421. Burger RA, Brady MF, Bookman MA, et al. Incorporation of bevacizumab in the primary treatment of ovarian cancer. *N Engl J Med.* 2011;365:2473–2483.
422. Ferriss JS, Java JJ, Bookman MA, et al. Ascites predicts treatment benefit of bevacizumab in front-line therapy of advanced epithelial ovarian, fallopian tube and peritoneal cancers: an NRG Oncology/GOG study. *Gynecol Oncol.* 2015;139:17–22.
423. Oza AM, Cook AD, Pfisterer J, et al. Standard chemotherapy with or without bevacizumab for women with newly diagnosed ovarian cancer (ICON7): overall survival results of a phase 3 randomised trial. *Lancet Oncol.* 2015;16:928–936.
424. Stark D, Nankivell M, Pujade-Lauraine E, et al. Standard chemotherapy with or without bevacizumab in advanced ovarian cancer: quality-of-life outcomes from the International Collaboration on Ovarian Neoplasms (ICON7) phase 3 randomised trial. *Lancet Oncol.* 2013;14:236–243.
425. Dyer M, Richardson J, Robertson J, et al. NICE guidance on bevacizumab in combination with paclitaxel and carboplatin for the first-line treatment of advanced ovarian cancer. *Lancet Oncol.* 2013;14:689–690.
426. Gourley C, McCavigan A, Perren T, et al. Molecular subgroup of high-grade serous ovarin cancer (HGSOC) as a predictor of outcome following bevacizumab. *J Clin Oncol.* 2014;32:abstract 5502.
427. Winterhoff B, Kommoss S, Oberg A, et al. Bevacizumab and improvement of progression-free survival (PFS) for patients with the mesenchymal subtype of ovarian cancer. *J Clin Oncol.* 2014;32:abstract 5509.
428. Birrer M, Choi Y, Brady MF, et al. Retrospective analysis of candidate predictive tumor biomarkers (BMs) for efficacy in the GOG-0218 trial evaluating front-line carboplatin-paclitaxel (CP) +/- bevacizumab (BEV) for epithelial ovarian cacner (EOC). *J Clin Oncol.* 2015;33:abstract 5505.
429. du Bois A, Kristensen G, Ray-Coquard I, et al. Standard first-line chemotherapy with or without nintedanib for advanced ovarian cancer (AGO-OVAR 12): a randomised, double-blind, placebo-controlled phase 3 trial. *Lancet Oncol.* 2016;17:78–89.
430. du Bois A, Floquet A, Kim JW, et al. Incorporation of pazopanib in maintenance therapy of ovarian cancer. *J Clin Oncol.* 2014;32:3374–3382.
431. Los G, Mutsaers PH, van der Vijgh WJ, et al. Direct diffusion of cis-diamminedichloroplatinum(II) in intraperitoneal rat tumors after intraperitoneal chemotherapy: a comparison with systemic chemotherapy. *Cancer Res.* 1989;49:3380–3384.
432. Miyagi Y, Fujiwara K, Kigawa J, et al. Intraperitoneal carboplatin infusion may be a pharmacologically more reasonable route than intravenous administration as a systemic chemotherapy. A comparative pharmacokinetic analysis of platinum using a new mathematical model after intraperitoneal vs. intravenous infusion of carboplatin—a Sankai Gynecology Study Group (SGSG) study. *Gynecol Oncol.* 2005;99:591–596.
433. Fujiwara K, Armstrong D, Morgan M, et al. Principles and practice of intraperitoneal chemotherapy for ovarian cancer. *Int J Gynecol Cancer.* 2007;17:1–20.
434. Alberts DS, Liu PY, Hannigan EV, et al. Intraperitoneal cisplatin plus intravenous cyclophosphamide versus intravenous cisplatin plus intravenous cyclophosphamide for stage III ovarian cancer. *N Engl J Med.* 1996;335:1950–1955.
435. Markman M, Bundy BN, Alberts DS, et al. Phase III trial of standard-dose intravenous cisplatin plus paclitaxel versus moderately high-dose carboplatin followed by intravenous paclitaxel and intraperitoneal cisplatin in small-volume stage III ovarian carcinoma: an intergroup study of the Gynecologic Oncology Group, Southwestern Oncology Group, and Eastern Cooperative Oncology Group. *J Clin Oncol.* 2001;19:1001–1007.
436. Walker JL, Brady MF, Wenzel L. A phase II trial of bevacizumab with IV versus IP chemotherapy for ovarian, fallopian tube, and peritoneal carcinoma: an NRG Oncology Study. *Gynecol Oncol.* Presented at SGO Annual Meeting on Women's Cancer, San Diego, March 22, 2016;Late Breaking Abstract 6.
437. Piccart MJ, Floquet A, Scarfone G, et al. Intraperitoneal cisplatin versus no further treatment: 8-year results of EORTC 55875, a randomized phase III study in ovarian cancer patients with a pathologically complete remission after platinum-based intravenous chemotherapy. *Int J Gynecol Cancer.* 2003;13(suppl 2):196–203.
438. Sorbe B, Swedish-Norgewian Ovarian Cancer Study G. Consolidation treatment of advanced (FIGO stage III) ovarian carcinoma in complete surgical remission after induction chemotherapy: a randomized, controlled, clinical trial comparing whole abdominal radiotherapy, chemotherapy, and no further treatment. *Int J Gynecol Cancer.* 2003;13:278–286.
439. Pfisterer J, Weber B, Reuss A, et al. Randomized phase III trial of topotecan following carboplatin and paclitaxel in first-line treatment of advanced ovarian cancer: a gynecologic cancer intergroup trial of the AGO-OVAR and GINECO. *J Natl Cancer Inst.* 2006;98:1036–1045.
440. De Placido S, Scambia G, Di Vagno G, et al. Topotecan compared with no therapy after response to surgery and carboplatin/paclitaxel in patients with ovarian cancer: Multicenter Italian Trials in Ovarian Cancer (MITO-1) randomized study. *J Clin Oncol.* 2004;22:2635–2642.
441. Bolis G, Danese S, Tateo S, et al. Epidoxorubicin versus no treatment as consolidation therapy in advanced ovarian cancer: results from a phase II study. *Int J Gynecol Cancer.* 2006;16(suppl 1):74–78.
442. Papadimitriou C, Dafni U, Anagnostopoulos A, et al. High-dose melphalan and autologous stem cell transplantation as consolidation treatment in patients with chemosensitive ovarian cancer: results of a single-institution randomized trial. *Bone Marrow Transplant.* 2008;41:547–554.
443. Pujade-Lauraine E, Cure H, Battista C, et al. High dose chemotherapy in ovarian cancer. *Int J Gynecol Cancer.* 2001;11(suppl 1):64–67.
444. Markman M, Liu PY, Wilczynski S, et al. Phase III randomized trial of 12 versus 3 months of maintenance paclitaxel in patients with advanced ovarian cancer after complete response to platinum and paclitaxel-based chemotherapy: a Southwest Oncology Group and Gynecologic Oncology Group trial. *J Clin Oncol.* 2003;21:2460–2465.
445. Markman M, Liu PY, Moon J, et al. Impact on survival of 12 versus 3 monthly cycles of paclitaxel (175 mg/m^2) administered to patients with advanced ovarian cancer who attained a complete response to primary platinum-paclitaxel: follow-up of a Southwest Oncology Group and Gynecologic Oncology Group phase 3 trial. *Gynecol Oncol.* 2009;114:195–198.
446. Pecorelli S, Favalli G, Gadducci A, et al. Phase III trial of observation versus six courses of paclitaxel in patients with advanced epithelial ovarian cancer in complete response after six courses of paclitaxel/platinum-based chemotherapy: final results of the After-6 protocol 1. *J Clin Oncol.* 2009;27:4642–4648.
447. Jain A, Seiden MV. Rare epithelial tumors arising in or near the ovary: a review of the risk factors, presentation, and future treatment direction for ovarian clear cell and mucinous carcinoma. *Am Soc Clin Oncol Educ Book.* 2013. doi:10.1200/EdBook_AM.2013.33.e200.
448. Farley J, Brady WE, Birrer M, et al. An evaluation of survival of ovarian cancer patients with clear cell carcinoma versus serous carcinoma treated with platinum therapy: a Gynecologic Oncolopgy Group experience. *J Clin Oncol.* 2013;31:abstract 5534.
449. Crotzer DR, Sun CC, Coleman RL, et al. Lack of effective systemic therapy for recurrent clear cell carcinoma of the ovary. *Gynecol Oncol.* 2007;105:404–408.
450. Esposito F, Cecere SC, Magazzino F, et al. Second-line chemotherapy in recurrent clear cell ovarian cancer: results from the multicenter italian trials in ovarian cancer (MITO-9). *Oncology.* 2014;86:351–358.
451. Sugiyama T, Okamoto A, Enomoto T, et al. Randomized phase III trial of irinotecan plus cisplatin compared with paclitaxel plus carboplatin as first-line chemotherapy for ovarian clear cell carcinoma: JGOG3017/GCIG Trial. *J Clin Oncol.* 2016;34(24):2881–2887.
452. Takano M, Kikuchi Y, Kudoh K, et al. Weekly administration of temsirolimus for heavily pretreated patients with clear cell carcinoma of the ovary: a report of six cases. *Int J Clin Oncol.* 2011;16:605–609.
453. Behbakht K, Sill MW, Darcy KM, et al. Phase II trial of the mTOR inhibitor, temsirolimus and evaluation of circulating tumor cells and tumor biomarkers in persistent and recurrent epithelial ovarian and primary peritoneal malignancies: a Gynecologic Oncology Group study. *Gynecol Oncol.* 2011;123:19–26.
454. Martin LP, Sill M, Shahin MS, et al. A phase II evaluation of AMG 102 (rilotumumab) in the treatment of persistent or recurrent epithelial ovarian, fallopian tube or primary peritoneal carcinoma: a Gynecologic Oncology Group study. *Gynecol Oncol.* 2014;132:526–530.
455. Duska LR, Garrett L, Henretta M, et al. When 'never-events' occur despite adherence to clinical guidelines: the case of venous thromboembolism in clear cell cancer of the ovary compared with other epithelial histologic subtypes. *Gynecol Oncol.* 2010;116:374–377.
456. Diaz ES, Walts AE, Karlan BY, et al. Venous thromboembolism during primary treatment of ovarian clear cell carcinoma is associated with decreased survival. *Gynecol Oncol.* 2013;131:541–545.

457. Savvari P, Peitsidis P, Alevizaki M, et al. Paraneoplastic humorally mediated hypercalcemia induced by parathyroid hormone-related protein in gynecologic malignancies: a systematic review. *Onkologie*. 2009;32:517–523.
458. Chao WR, Lee MY, Ruan A, et al. Assessment of HER2 Status Using Immunohistochemistry (IHC) and Fluorescence In Situ Hybridization (FISH) techniques in mucinous epithelial ovarian cancer: a comprehensive comparison between ToGA biopsy method and ToGA surgical specimen method. *PLoS One*. 2015;10:e0142135.
459. Brown J. Rare tumors review. SGO presentation, San Diego, March 22, 2016.
460. George EM, Herzog TJ, Neugut AI, et al. Carcinosarcoma of the ovary: natural history, patterns of treatment, and outcome. *Gynecol Oncol*. 2013;131:42–45.
461. del Carmen MG, Birrer M, Schorge JO. Carcinosarcoma of the ovary: a review of the literature. *Gynecol Oncol*. 2012;125:271–277.
462. Rauh-Hain JA, Growdon WB, Rodriguez N, et al. Carcinosarcoma of the ovary: a case-control study. *Gynecol Oncol*. 2011;121:477–481.
463. Ahmed-Lecheheb D, Joly F. Ovarian cancer survivors' quality of life: a systematic review. *J Cancer Surviv*. 2016;10(5):789–801.
464. Pignata S, De Placido S, Biamonte R, et al. Residual neurotoxicity in ovarian cancer patients in clinical remission after first-line chemotherapy with carboplatin and paclitaxel: the Multicenter Italian Trial in Ovarian cancer (MITO-4) retrospective study. *BMC Cancer*. 2006;6:5.
465. National Comprehensive Cancer Network. NCCN version 2.2015. http://www.NCCN.org. Accessed April 24, 2016.
466. Rustin GJ, Vergote I, Eisenhauer E, et al. Definitions for response and progression in ovarian cancer clinical trials incorporating RECIST 1.1 and CA 125 agreed by the Gynecological Cancer Intergroup (GCIG). *Int J Gynecol Cancer*. 2011;21:419–423.
467. Herzog TJ, Vermorken JB, Pujade-Lauraine E, et al. Correlation between CA-125 serum level and response by RECIST in a phase III recurrent ovarian cancer study. *Gynecol Oncol*. 2011;122:350–355.
468. Sabbatini P, Mooney D, Iasonos A, et al. Early CA-125 fluctuations in patients with recurrent ovarian cancer receiving chemotherapy. *Int J Gynecol Cancer*. 2007;17:589–594.
469. Freyer G, Ray-Coquard I, Fischer D, et al. Routine clinical practice for patients with recurrent ovarian carcinoma: results from the TRO-CADERO Study. *Int J Gynecol Cancer*. 2016;26:240–247.
470. Markman M, Rothman R, Hakes T, et al. Second-line platinum therapy in patients with ovarian cancer previously treated with cisplatin. *J Clin Oncol*. 1991;9:389–393.
471. Hirte H, Lheureux S, Fleming GF, et al. A phase 2 study of cediranib in recurrent or persistent ovarian, peritoneal or fallopian tube cancer: a trial of the Princess Margaret, Chicago and California Phase II Consortia. *Gynecol Oncol*. 2015;138:55–61.
472. Eisenhauer EA, Vermorken JB, van Glabbeke M. Predictors of response to subsequent chemotherapy in platinum pretreated ovarian cancer: a multivariate analysis of 704 patients [see comments]. *Ann Oncol*. 1997;8:963–968.
473. Lee CK, Simes RJ, Brown C, et al. Prognostic nomogram to predict progression-free survival in patients with platinum-sensitive recurrent ovarian cancer. *Br J Cancer*. 2011;105:1144–1150.
474. Markman M, Markman J, Webster K, et al. Duration of response to second-line, platinum-based chemotherapy for ovarian cancer: implications for patient management and clinical trial design. *J Clin Oncol*. 2004;22:3120–3125.
475. Hoskins PJ, Le N. Identifying patients unlikely to benefit from further chemotherapy: a descriptive study of outcome at each relapse in ovarian cancer. *Gynecol Oncol*. 2005;97:862–869.
476. Piccart MJ, Green JA, Lacave AJ, et al. Oxaliplatin or paclitaxel in patients with platinum-pretreated advanced ovarian cancer: a randomized phase II study of the European Organization for Research and Treatment of Cancer Gynecology Group. *J Clin Oncol*. 2000;18:1193–1202.
477. Parmar MK, Ledermann JA, Colombo N, et al. Paclitaxel plus platinum-based chemotherapy versus conventional platinum-based chemotherapy in women with relapsed ovarian cancer: the ICON4/AGO-OVAR-2.2 trial. *Lancet*. 2003;361:2099–2106.
478. Pfisterer J, Plante M, Vergote I, et al. Gemcitabine plus carboplatin compared with carboplatin in patients with platinum-sensitive recurrent ovarian cancer: an intergroup trial of the AGO-OVAR, the NCIC CTG, and the EORTC GCG. *J Clin Oncol*. 2006;24:4699–4707.
479. Aghajanian C, Blank SV, Goff BA, et al. OCEANS: a randomized, double-blind, placebo-controlled phase III trial of chemotherapy with or without bevacizumab in patients with platinum-sensitive recurrent epithelial ovarian, primary peritoneal, or fallopian tube cancer. *J Clin Oncol*. 2012;30:2039–2045.
480. Coleman R, Brady MF, Herzog TJ, et al. A phase III randomized controlled clinical trial of carboplatin and paclitaxel alone or in combination with bevacizumab followede by bevacizumab and secondary cytoreductive surgery in platinum-sensitive, recurrent ovarian, peritoneal primary and fallopian tube cancer (Gynecologic Oncology Group 0213). *Gynecol Oncol*. 2015;137:abstract 3.
481. Wagner U, Marth C, Largillier R, et al. Final overall survival results of phase III GCIG CALYPSO trial of pegylated liposomal doxorubicin and carboplatin vs paclitaxel and carboplatin in platinum-sensitive ovarian cancer patients. *Br J Cancer*. 2012;107:588–591.
482. Sehouli J, Meier W, Wimberger P, et al. Topotecan plus carboplatin versus standard therapy with paclitaxel plus carboplatin (PC) or gemcitabine plus carboplatin (GC) or carboplatin plus pegylated dosorubicin (PLDC): a randomized phase III trial of the NOGGO-AGO-Germaine-AGO Austria and GEICO-GCIG intergroupd study (HECTOR). *J Clin Oncol*. 2012;abstract 5031.
483. Gordon AN, Fleagle JT, Guthrie D, et al. Recurrent epithelial ovarian carcinoma: a randomized phase III study of pegylated liposomal doxorubicin versus topotecan. *J Clin Oncol*. 2001;19:3312–3322.
484. ten Bokkel Huinink W, Gore M, Carmichael J, et al. Topotecan versus paclitaxel for the treatment of recurrent epithelial ovarian cancer. *J Clin Oncol*. 1997;15:2183–2193.
485. Buda A, Floriani I, Rossi R, et al. Randomised controlled trial comparing single agent paclitaxel vs epidoxorubicin plus paclitaxel in patients with advanced ovarian cancer in early progression after platinum-based chemotherapy: an Italian Collaborative Study from the Mario Negri Institute, Milan, G.O.N.O. (Gruppo Oncologico Nord Ovest) group and I.O.R. (Istituto Oncologico Romagnolo) group. *Br J Cancer*. 2004;90:2112–2117.
486. Lortholary A, Largillier R, Weber B, et al. Weekly paclitaxel as a single agent or in combination with carboplatin or weekly topotecan in patients with resistant ovarian cancer: the CARTAXHY randomized phase II trial from Groupe d'Investigateurs Nationaux pour l'Etude des Cancers Ovariens (GINECO). *Ann Oncol*. 2012;23:346–352.
487. Monk BJ, Herzog TJ, Kaye SB, et al. Trabectedin plus pegylated liposomal doxorubicin (PLD) versus PLD in recurrent ovarian cancer: overall survival analysis. *Eur J Cancer*. 2012;48:2361–2368.
488. Pujade-Lauraine E, Hilpert F, Weber B, et al. Bevacizumab combined with chemotherapy for platinum-resistant recurrent ovarian cancer: the AURELIA open-label randomized phase III trial. *J Clin Oncol*. 2014;32:1302–1308.
489. Pignata S, Lorusso D, Scambia G, et al. Pazopanib plus weekly paclitaxel versus weekly paclitaxel alone for platinum-resistant or platinum-refractory advanced ovarian cancer (MITO 11): a randomised, open-label, phase 2 trial. *Lancet Oncol*. 2015;16:561–568.
490. Markman M, Blessing JA, Moore D, et al. Altretamine (hexamethylmelamine) in platinum-resistant and platinum-refractory ovarian cancer: a Gynecologic Oncology Group phase II trial. *Gynecol Oncol*. 1998;69:226–229.
491. Peled Y, Levavi H, Krissi H, et al. The use of Fluorouracil (5-FU) and leucovorin in women with heavily pretreated advanced ovarian carcinoma. *Am J Clin Oncol*. 2013;36:472–474.
492. Miller DS, Blessing JA, Krasner CN, et al. Phase II evaluation of pemetrexed in the treatment of recurrent or persistent platinum-resistant ovarian or primary peritoneal carcinoma: a study of the Gynecologic Oncology Group. *J Clin Oncol*. 2009;27:2686–2691.
493. Kaern J, Baekelandt M, Trope CG. A phase II study of weekly paclitaxel in platinum and paclitaxel-resistant ovarian cancer patients. *Eur J Gynaecol Oncol*. 2002;23:383–389.
494. Markman M, Hall J, Spitz D, et al. Phase II trial of weekly single-agent paclitaxel in platinum/paclitaxel-refractory ovarian cancer. *J Clin Oncol*. 2002;20:2365–2369.
495. Markman M, Zanotti K, Webster K, et al. Phase 2 trial of single agent docetaxel in platinum and paclitaxel-refractory ovarian cancer, fallopian tube cancer, and primary carcinoma of the peritoneum. *Gynecol Oncol*. 2003;91:573–576.
496. Coleman RL, Brady WE, McMeekin DS, et al. A phase II evaluation of nanoparticle, albumin-bound (nab) paclitaxel in the treatment of recurrent or persistent platinum-resistant ovarian, fallopian tube, or primary peritoneal cancer: a Gynecologic Oncology Group study. *Gynecol Oncol*. 2011;122:111–115.
497. Sehouli J, Stengel D, Harter P, et al. Topotecan weekly versus conventional 5-day schedule in patients with platinum-resistant ovarian cancer: a randomized multicenter phase II trial of the North-Eastern German Society of Gynecological Oncology Ovarian Cancer Study Group. *J Clin Oncol*. 2011;29:242–248.
498. Herzog TJ, Sill MW, Walker JL, et al. A phase II study of two topotecan regimens evaluated in recurrent platinum-sensitive ovarian, fallopian tube or primary peritoneal cancer: a Gynecologic Oncology Group Study (GOG 146Q). *Gynecol Oncol*. 2011;120:454–458.

499. Markman M, Kennedy A, Webster K, et al. Phase 2 trial of liposomal doxorubicin (40 mg/m^2) in platinum/paclitaxel-refractory ovarian and fallopian tube cancers and primary carcinoma of the peritoneum. *Gynecol Oncol.* 2000;78:369–372.
500. Brewer CA, Blessing JA, Nagourney RA, et al. Cisplatin plus gemcitabine in platinum-refractory ovarian or primary peritoneal cancer: a phase II study of the Gynecologic Oncology Group. *Gynecol Oncol.* 2006;103:446–450.
501. Garcia AA, Hirte H, Fleming G, et al. Phase II clinical trial of bevacizumab and low-dose metronomic oral cyclophosphamide in recurrent ovarian cancer: a trial of the California, Chicago, and Princess Margaret Hospital phase II consortia. *J Clin Oncol.* 2008;26:76–82.
502. Kummar S, Oza AM, Fleming GF, et al. Randomized trial of oral cyclophosphamide and veliparib in high-grade serous ovarian, primary peritoneal, or fallopian tube cancers, or BRCA-mutant ovarian cancer. *Clin Cancer Res.* 2015;21:1574–1582.
503. Aghajanian C, Goff B, Nycum LR, et al. Final overall survival and safety analysis of OCEANS, a phase 3 trial of chemotherapy with or without bevacizumab in patients with platinum-sensitive recurrent ovarian cancer. *Gynecol Oncol.* 2015;139:10–16.
504. Pinilla-Dominguez P, Richardson J, Robertson J, et al. NICE guidance on bevacizumab in combination with gemcitabine and carboplatin for treating the first recurrence of platinum-sensitive advanced ovarian cancer. *Lancet Oncol.* 2013;14:691–692.
505. Stockler MR, Hilpert F, Friedlander M, et al. Patient-reported outcome results from the open-label phase III AURELIA trial evaluating bevacizumab-containing therapy for platinum-resistant ovarian cancer. *J Clin Oncol.* 2014;32:1309–1316.
506. Ledermann JA, Embleton AC, Raja F, et al. Cediranib in patients with relapsed platinum-sensitive ovarian cancer (ICON6): a randomised double-blind,placebo-controlled phase I trial. *Lancet.* 2016;387:1066–1074.
507. Gotlieb WH, Amant F, Advani S, et al. Intravenous aflibercept for treatment of recurrent symptomatic malignant ascites in patients with advanced ovarian cancer: a phase 2, randomised, double-blind, placebo-controlled study. *Lancet Oncol.* 2012;13:154–162.
508. Matulonis UA, Penson RT, Domchek SM, et al. Olaparib monotherapy in patients with advanced relapsed ovarian cancer and a germline BRCA1/2 mutation: a multi-study analysis of response rates and safety. *Ann Oncol.* 2016.
509. Pennington KP, Walsh T, Harrell MI, et al. Germline and somatic mutations in homologous recombination genes predict platinum response and survival in ovarian, fallopian tube, and peritoneal carcinomas. *Clin Cancer Res.* 2014;20:764–775.
510. Gelmon KA, Tischkowitz M, Mackay H, et al. Olaparib in patients with recurrent high-grade serous or poorly differentiated ovarian carcinoma or triple-negative breast cancer: a phase 2, multicentre, open-label, non-randomised study. *Lancet Oncol.* 2011;12:852–861.
511. Kaye SB, Lubinski J, Matulonis U, et al. Phase II, open-label, randomized, multicenter study comparing the efficacy and safety of olaparib, a poly (ADP-ribose) polymerase inhibitor, and pegylated liposomal doxorubicin in patients with BRCA1 or BRCA2 mutations and recurrent ovarian cancer. *J Clin Oncol.* 2012;30:372–379.
512. Ledermann J, Harter P, Gourley C, et al. Olaparib maintenance therapy in patients with platinum-sensitive relapsed serous ovarian cancer: a preplanned retrospective analysis of outcomes by BRCA status in a randomised phase 2 trial. *Lancet Oncol.* 2014;15:852–861.
513. Makrilia N, Syrigou E, Kaklamanos I, et al. Hypersensitivity reactions associated with platinum antineoplastic agents: a systematic review. *Met Based Drugs.* 2010;2010. doi:10.1155/2010/207084.
514. Joly F, Ray-Coquard I, Fabbro M, et al. Decreased hypersensitivity reactions with carboplatin-pegylated liposomal doxorubicin compared to carboplatin-paclitaxel combination: analysis from the GCIG CALYPSO relapsing ovarian cancer trial. *Gynecol Oncol.* 2011;122:226–232.
515. Mach CM, Lapp EA, Weddle KJ, et al. Adjunct histamine blockers as premedications to prevent carboplatin hypersensitivity reactions. *Pharmacotherapy.* 2016;36(5):482–487.
516. Voutsadakis IA. Hormone receptors in serous ovarian carcinoma: prognosis, pathogenesis, and treatment considerations. *Clin Med Insights Oncol.* 2016;10:17–25.
517. van Kruchten M, van der Marel P, de Munck L, et al. Hormone receptors as a marker of poor survival in epithelial ovarian cancer. *Gynecol Oncol.* 2015;138:634–639.
518. Hurteau JA, Brady MF, Darcy KM, et al. Randomized phase III trial of tamoxifen versus thalidomide in women with biochemical-recurrent-only epithelial ovarian, fallopian tube or primary peritoneal carcinoma after a complete response to first-line platinum/taxane chemotherapy with an evaluation of serum vascular endothelial growth factor (VEGF): a Gynecologic Oncology Group Study. *Gynecol Oncol.* 2010;119:444–450.
519. Emons G, Gorchev G, Sehouli J, et al. Efficacy and safety of AEZS-108 (INN: zoptarelin doxorubicin acetate) an LHRH agonist linked to doxorubicin in women with platinum refractory or resistant ovarian cancer expressing LHRH receptors: a multicenter phase II trial of the ago-study group (AGO GYN 5). *Gynecol Oncol.* 2014;133:427–432.
520. Abu-Jawdeh GM, Jacobs TW, Niloff J, et al. Estrogen receptor expression is a common feature of ovarian borderline tumors. *Gynecol Oncol.* 1996;60:301–307.
521. Gershenson DM, Sun CC, Iyer RB, et al. Hormonal therapy for recurrent low-grade serous carcinoma of the ovary or peritoneum. *Gynecol Oncol.* 2012;125:661–666.
522. Miller RW, Brough R, Bajrami I, et al. Functional profiling of clear cell ovarian cancer. *J Clin Oncol.* 2012;20:abstract 5035.
523. Bitler BG, Aird KM, Garipov A, et al. Synthetic lethality by targeting EZH2 methyltransferase activity in ARID1A-mutated cancers. *Nat Med.* 2015;21:231–238.
524. Vergote IB, Jimeno A, Joly F, et al. Randomized phase III study of erlotinib versus observation in patients with no evidence of disease progression after first-line platin-based chemotherapy for ovarian carcinoma: a European Organisation for Research and Treatment of Cancer-Gynaecological Cancer Group, and Gynecologic Cancer Intergroup study. *J Clin Oncol.* 2014;32:320–326.
525. Bookman MA, Darcy KM, Clarke-Pearson D, et al. Evaluation of monoclonal humanized anti-HER2 antibody, trastuzumab, in patients with recurrent or refractory ovarian or primary peritoneal carcinoma with overexpression of HER2: a phase II trial of the Gynecologic Oncology Group. *J Clin Oncol.* 2003;21:283–290.
526. Makhija S, Amler LC, Glenn D, et al. Clinical activity of gemcitabine plus pertuzumab in platinum-resistant ovarian cancer, fallopian tube cancer, or primary peritoneal cancer. *J Clin Oncol.* 2010;28:1215–1223.
527. Pujade-Lauraine E, Selle F, Weber B, et al. Volasertib versus chemotherapy in platinum-resistant or -refractory ovarian cancer: a randomized phase II Groupe des Investigateurs Nationaux pour l'Etude des Cancers de l'Ovaire Study. *J Clin Oncol.* 2016;34:706–713.
528. Penson RT, Moore KM, Fleming GF, et al. A phase II study of ramucirumab (IMC-1121B) in the treatment of persistent or recurrent epithelial ovarian, fallopian tube or primary peritoneal carcinoma. *Gynecol Oncol.* 2014;134:478–485.
529. Monk BJ, Poveda A, Vergote I, et al. Anti-angiopoietin therapy with trebananib for recurrent ovarian cancer (TRINOVA-1): a randomised, multicentre, double-blind, placebo-controlled phase 3 trial. *Lancet Oncol.* 2014;15:799–808.
530. Liu JF, Barry WT, Birrer M, et al. Combination cediranib and olaparib versus olaparib alone for women with recurrent platinum-sensitive ovarian cancer: a randomised phase 2 study. *Lancet Oncol.* 2014;15:1207–1214.
531. Oza AM, Cibula D, Benzaquen AO, et al. Olaparib combined with chemotherapy for recurrent platinum-sensitive ovarian cancer: a randomised phase 2 trial. *Lancet Oncol.* 2015;16:87–97.
532. Zhang L, Conejo-Garcia JR, Katsaros D, et al. Intratumoral T cells, recurrence, and survival in epithelial ovarian cancer. *N Engl J Med.* 2003;348:203–213.
533. Hamanishi J, Mandai M, Ikeda T, et al. Safety and antitumor activity of anti-PD-1 antibody, nivolumab, in patients with platinum-resistant ovarian cancer. *J Clin Oncol.* 2015;33:4015–4022.
534. Vergote I, Armstrong D, Scambia G, et al. A randomized, double-blind, placebo-controlled, phase iii study to assess efficacy and safety of weekly farletuzumab in combination with carboplatin and taxane in patients with ovarian cancer in first platinum-sensitive relapse. *J Clin Oncol.* 2016:34(19):2271–2278.
535. Ledermann JA, Canevari S, Thigpen T. Targeting the folate receptor: diagnostic and therapeutic approaches to personalize cancer treatments. *Ann Oncol.* 2015;26:2034–2043.
536. Moore KM, Martin LP, Seward SM, et al. Preliminary single agent activity of IMGN853, a folate receptor alpha (FRalpha)-targeting antibody-drug conjegate (ADC), in platinum-resistant epithelial ovarian cacner (IEOC) patients (pts): phase I trial. *J Clin Oncol.* 2015;33:5518.
537. Weekes CD, Lamberts LE, Borad MJ, et al. Phase I study of DMOT4039A, an antibody-drug conjugate targeting mesothelin, in patients with unresectable pancreatic or platinum-resistant ovarian cancer. *Mol Cancer Ther.* 2016;15:439–447.
538. Burris HA, Gordon MS, Gerber DE, et al. A phase I study of DNIB0600A, an antibody-drug conjugate (ADC) targeting NaPi2b in patients (pts)

with non-small cell lung cancer (NSCLC) or platinum-resistnat ovarian cacner (OC). *J Clin Oncol.* 2015;32:5s.
539. Wei SH, Chen CM, Strathdee G, et al. Methylation microarray analysis of late-stage ovarian carcinomas distinguishes progression-free survival in patients and identifies candidate epigenetic markers. *Clin Cancer Res.* 2002;8:2246–2252.
540. Matei D, Fang F, Shen C, et al. Epigenetic resensitization to platinum in ovarian cancer. *Cancer Res.* 2012;72:2197–2205.
541. Zapardiel I, Morrow CP. New terminnology for cytoreduction in advanced ovarian cancer. *Lancet.* 2011;12:214.
542. Aghajanian C, Sill MW, Darcy KM, et al. Phase II trial of bevacizumab in recurrent or persistent endometrial cancer: a Gynecologic Oncology Group study. *J Clin Oncol.* 2011;29:2259–2265.
543. Bolis G, Scarfone G, Giardina G, et al. Carboplatin alone vs carboplatin plus epidoxorubicin as second-line therapy for cisplatin- or carboplatin-sensitive ovarian cancer. *Gynecol Oncol.* 2001;81:3–9.
544. Cantu MG, Buda A, Parma G, et al. Randomized controlled trial of single-agent paclitaxel versus cyclophosphamide, doxorubicin, and cisplatin in patients with recurrent ovarian cancer who responded to first-line platinum-based regimens. *J Clin Oncol.* 2002;20:1232–1237.
545. Alberts DS, Liu PY, Wilczynski SP, et al. Randomized trial of pegylated liposomal doxorubicin (PLD) plus carboplatin versus carboplatin in platinum-sensitive (PS) patients with recurrent epithelial ovarian or peritoneal carcinoma after failure of initial platinum-based chemotherapy (Southwest Oncology Group Protocol S0200). *Gynecol Oncol.* 2008;108:90–94.

CHAPTER 24

Ovarian Germ Cell Tumors

Daniela Matei, Robert E. Emerson, and Jubilee Brown

INTRODUCTION

Significant improvement in the management of ovarian germ cell tumors (OGCTs) has been achieved during the past three decades. The development of more effective chemotherapy (CT) regimens is the leading cause for improved outcome in this rare group of patients. Other advancements in the field include the development of a more precise surgical staging system, improved radiographic imaging, more sophisticated pathology techniques, and improved supportive care and symptom control that has enabled safe delivery of treatment. A substantial number of patients with OGCT are long-term survivors and suffer minimal morbidity from treatment. Fertility-sparing surgical procedures enable young women with OGCT to preserve their reproductive potential. These positive results in clinical outcome reflect the ability to build on the treatment success in testicular cancer, as well as a collaborative effort among multiple specialties (gynecologic oncology, medical oncology, pathology, and radiology).

PATHOLOGY

The 2014 World Health Organization classification of OGCTs includes dysgerminoma, yolk sac tumor, embryonal carcinoma, nongestational choriocarcinoma, mixed germ cell tumors, and teratomas (immature teratoma (IT), mature teratoma, and various types of monodermal teratoma) (1,2). Although mature teratomas are relatively common, representing approximately 20% of ovarian tumors, the malignant germ cell tumors are less common and account for 2% to 3% of all ovarian cancers. Both mature teratomas and malignant germ cell tumors usually occur in young women, with a peak age of incidence in the late teens to early twenties. The age range is, however, broad, with rare cases of OGCTs being diagnosed in postmenopausal women.

Dysgerminoma

Dysgerminoma is the most common malignant OGCT, but it represents only 1% to 2% of ovarian malignant tumors overall (1). The mean patient age at presentation is approximately 22 years (1). A small percentage of these tumors are associated with disorders of sexual development with a Y chromosome–containing karyotype, and in this situation the tumor may be associated with gonadoblastoma. Most dysgerminomas, however, occur in normal females who present with abdominal enlargement, a growing mass, or pain. About 10% of dysgerminomas are bilateral on gross examination and another 10% have microscopic involvement of the contralateral ovary. Association with gonadoblastoma increases the risk of bilateral involvement by dysgerminoma.

On gross examination, dysgerminomas are usually large, white to gray, lobulated masses that have no more than very focal hemorrhage or necrosis. Prominent hemorrhage, necrosis, or cystic changes are not expected and, if present, suggest a mixed germ cell tumor. Microscopically, dysgerminomas are composed of nests and cords of primitive germ cells, with clear to pale eosinophilic cytoplasm and prominent cytoplasmic borders (**Fig. 24.1**). Nuclei are enlarged but are relatively uniform in size. The nuclei may be rounded or have flat sides. The nests of tumor cells are separated by bands of fibrous tissue with lymphocytes. Occasionally, noncaseating granulomas may be present. Small cysts or pseudoglandular spaces may sometimes be seen, often representing inadequate specimen fixation. Syncytiotrophoblast cells are present in about 3% of dysgerminomas and do not, in the absence of cytotrophoblast cells, indicate a mixed germ cell tumor. These tumors have been designated dysgerminoma with syncytiotrophoblastic giant cells, but have the same prognosis as dysgerminomas (2).

Dysgerminomas contain cytoplasmic glycogen that can be visualized using the periodic acid Schiff (PAS) stain. Membranous immunoreactivity for placenta-like alkaline phosphatase (PLAP), c-kit (CD117), and podoplanin (D2-40) is also commonly observed. The most helpful immunohistochemical stain is probably the nuclear transcription factor OCT 3/4, which is highly sensitive and specific for dysgerminoma and embryonal carcinoma as a group (3). Dysgerminomas stain negatively for CD30, whereas embryonal carcinomas are positive for CD30. In contrast to yolk sac tumor, dysgerminoma is negative for α-fetoprotein (AFP). Syncytiotrophoblast cells, if present, will display human chorionic gonadotropin (hCG) staining.

Dysgerminoma is the only OGCT that commonly displays c-kit staining. Approximately 25% to 50% of dysgerminomas harbor c-kit mutations, but the mutations do not necessarily indicate imatinib sensitivity (4–6).

Yolk Sac Tumor

Yolk sac tumors (formerly also known as endodermal sinus tumors) are the second most common malignant OGCTs, accounting for

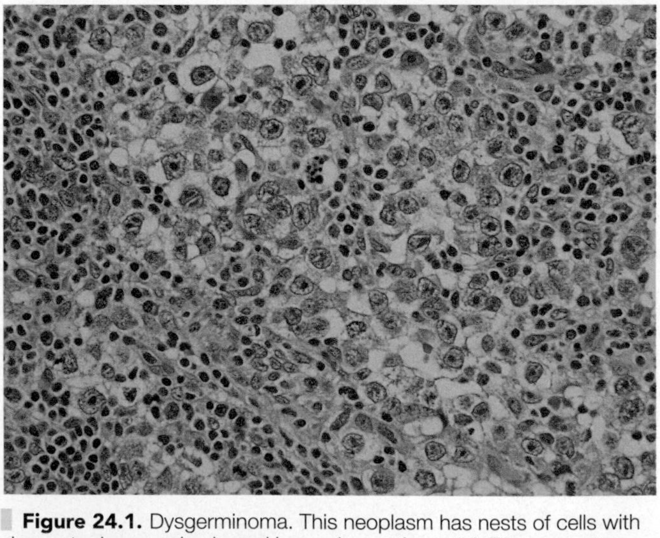

Figure 24.1. Dysgerminoma. This neoplasm has nests of cells with clear cytoplasm and enlarged hyperchromatic nuclei. Fibrous septae containing lymphocytes separate nests of tumor.

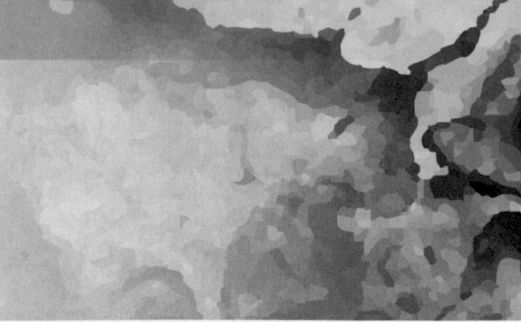

about 20% of cases. Recently, a proposal to rename the tumor as "primitive endodermal tumor" has been made (2), but although this may more accurately represent the range of differentiation seen in these tumors, this name has not yet gained significant usage. The peak incidence of this tumor is at approximately 19 years of age, and they occur very rarely beyond age 40.

Ovarian yolk sac tumors are typically large and unilateral, although metastasis to the opposite ovary may occur. These tumors have a smooth external surface unless rupture or invasion into surrounding structures has occurred. On sectioning, these neoplasms are solid and cystic and tan to gray in color, commonly with hemorrhage and necrosis. The cut surface may appear mucoid or gelatinous. Yolk sac tumors may have many different histologic patterns. The most common microscopic pattern in primary ovarian tumors is the reticular or microcystic pattern (**Fig. 24.2**). The tumor has a mesh-like pattern, and it displays a network of flattened or cuboidal epithelial cells with varying degrees of atypia. The endodermal sinus (festoon) pattern contains Schiller–Duval bodies (**Fig. 24.3**) that have a central capillary surrounded by connective tissue and a peripheral layer of columnar cells. These structures are situated in cavities lined by yolk sac tumor cells. When present, Schiller–Duval bodies may be a helpful diagnostic feature, but they are not present in all yolk sac tumors (7).

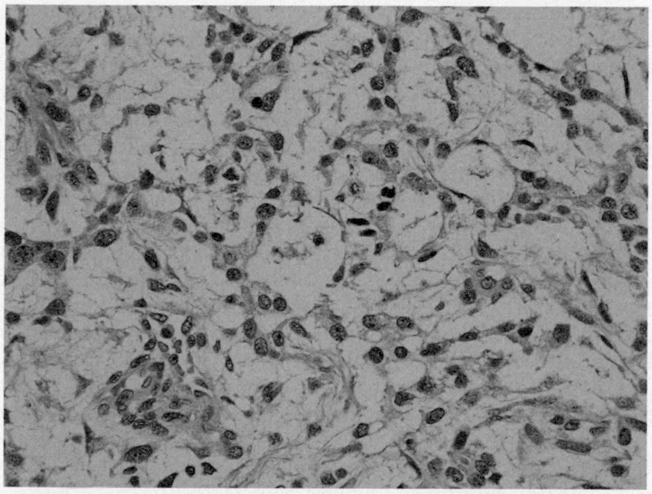

Figure 24.2. Reticular pattern of yolk sac tumor. There is a mesh-like arrangement of cuboidal tumor cells.

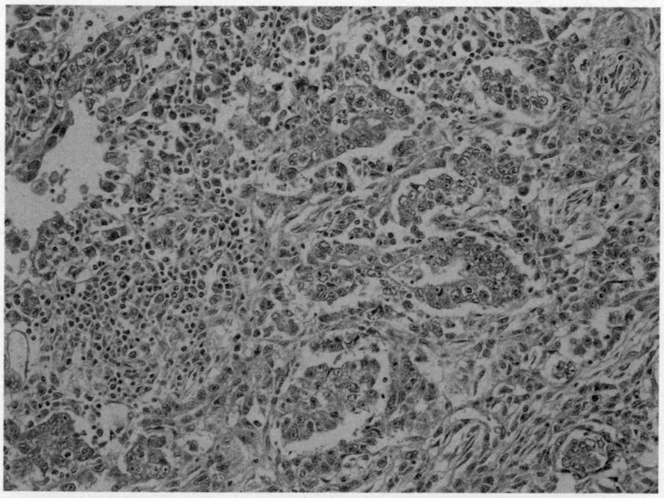

Figure 24.3. Schiller–Duval bodies, papillary structures with central blood vessels, are seen in the endodermal sinus pattern of yolk sac tumor.

Other less common patterns of yolk sac tumor include polyvesicular vitelline, enteric, solid, parietal, glandular, endometrioid-like, hepatoid, and mesenchymal patterns (8). Most patterns of yolk sac tumor may contain eosinophilic hyaline globules that are PAS positive and diastase resistant. These globules may be seen in non–germ cell tumors, and they are not specific for yolk sac tumor. They do not contain AFP. Yolk sac tumors usually show cytoplasmic staining for keratin and AFP, although the parietal pattern of yolk sac tumor typically does not contain AFP. AFP-negative parietal pattern yolk sac tumor may be seen following CT (9). Some types of yolk sac tumor, particularly glandular pattern yolk sac tumor, may closely resemble endometrioid, clear cell, or other adenocarcinomas. Age is an important and distinctive factor, because OGCTs usually occur in younger patients than epithelial ovarian tumors. Lack of staining for keratin 7 and epithelial membrane antigen supports a diagnosis of yolk sac tumor. Glypican-3 is more sensitive as a yolk sac tumor marker, but it is not entirely specific as staining is seen in embryonal carcinoma, hepatocellular carcinoma, and some other tumors. The pluripotency marker SALL4 may, because of the limited sensitivity of the AFP immunohistochemical stain, be useful in some cases, but is also expressed in other germ cell tumors and, rarely, in other tumors. Clear cell carcinoma is, perhaps, the tumor most likely to be mistaken for yolk sac tumor; these tumors were combined as "mesonephroma ovarii" prior to the 1940s (10). Very rarely, yolk sac tumor components have been seen in association with other tumors, usually ovarian endometrioid carcinomas, in older adult women, and these tumors may be less responsive to CT (10).

Embryonal Carcinoma

Embryonal carcinoma is rare in the ovary, either as pure embryonal carcinoma or as a component of a mixed germ cell tumor, in contrast to its frequent presence in testicular mixed germ cell tumors (11). When it is present, ovarian embryonal carcinoma is usually associated with yolk sac tumor in a mixed germ cell tumor. The diagnosis of ovarian embryonal carcinoma can prompt consideration of performing chromosomal analysis, because some tumors may be associated with Y chromosome–containing gonadal dysgenesis (2). On gross examination, embryonal carcinoma characteristically displays areas of hemorrhage and necrosis. Microscopically, this tumor is composed of very crowded, high nucleus-to-cytoplasm ratio cells with enlarged, pleomorphic nuclei and with prominent nucleoli. Glandular, solid, and papillary patterns may be seen. Vascular invasion is common. Embryonal carcinoma stains for PLAP, keratin AE1/AE3, CD30, and OCT3/4 (11). In contrast to dysgerminoma, embryonal carcinoma seldom stains for c-kit. Syncytiotrophoblast cells may be present, but, if not accompanied by cytotrophoblast cells, do not indicate the presence of a choriocarcinoma component.

Choriocarcinoma

Primary nongestational ovarian choriocarcinoma is rare, either as pure choriocarcinoma or as a component of a mixed OGCT. Choriocarcinomas display abundant hemorrhage and necrosis on gross examination (**Fig. 24.4**). Microscopically, these neoplasms show a plexiform pattern composed of an admixture of syncytiotrophoblast and cytotrophoblast cells (**Fig. 24.5**). Syncytiotrophoblastic giant cells have abundant eosinophilic to amphophilic cytoplasm that contains multiple atypical, hyperchromatic nuclei. Cytotrophoblast cells are round and often have well-defined cell borders, clear to lightly eosinophilic cytoplasm, and single nuclei that are usually less darkly staining than the syncytiotrophoblast cells. Blood vessel invasion is commonly seen. Cytotrophoblast cells do not produce hCG. Syncytiotrophoblast cells are formed from cytotrophoblast cells and do produce hCG. Choriocarcinoma may also stain for cytokeratin, α-inhibin, and glypican-3. Intermediate trophoblast cells within the tumor will stain for human placental lactogen (12,13). Nongestational choriocarcinoma must be distinguished from gestational choriocarcinoma because the former has a worse prognosis and requires more aggressive therapy.

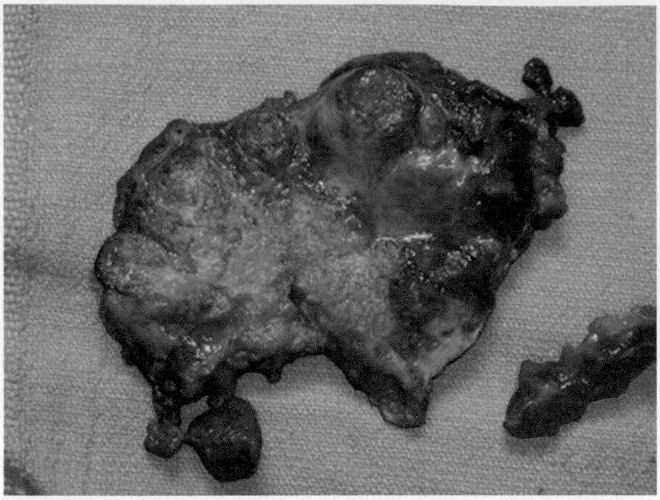

Figure 24.4. Choriocarcinoma. This ovarian neoplasm is extremely hemorrhagic.

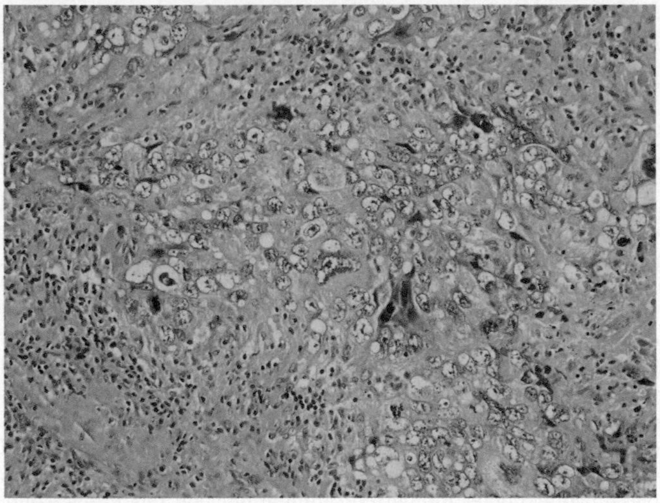

Figure 24.5. Choriocarcinoma. Syncytiotrophoblast cells have dark cytoplasm and multiple atypical nuclei. Cytotrophoblast cells have lighter cytoplasm and single atypical nuclei. Both cell types are admixed in choriocarcinoma. Areas of hemorrhage and necrosis are common.

Mixed Germ Cell Tumors

Mixed germ cell tumors of the ovary contain two or more different types of germ cell neoplasm. They are much less common in the ovary than in the testis. Malignant mixed germ cell tumors are large, unilateral neoplasms, but the gross appearance on the cut surface depends on the types of germ cell tumors present. The most common germ cell tumor element in the Armed Forces Institute of Pathology series was dysgerminoma (80%), followed by yolk sac tumor (70%), teratoma (53%), choriocarcinoma (20%), and embryonal carcinoma (13%) (2). The most frequent combination has been dysgerminoma and yolk sac tumor. Syncytiotrophoblast may occur either as a component of choriocarcinoma or as isolated cells in other germ cell tumor elements. The diagnosis and determination of prognosis of malignant mixed germ cell tumors depend on adequate tumor sampling to detect small areas of different types of germ cell tumor.

Polyembryoma was formerly considered a distinct category of germ cell tumor, but may also be considered a variant of mixed germ cell tumor in which layers of embryonal carcinoma and yolk sac tumor are closely arranged in a pattern that mimics early embryonic development. The microscopic appearance of the resulting embryoid bodies includes an embryonic disc separating a ventral space resembling yolk sac cavity and a dorsal space resembling amniotic cavity. Teratoma is also present in most cases.

Teratomas

Ovarian teratomas are germ cell tumors that typically contain tissue derived from two or three embryonic layers; however, monodermal teratomas with tissue of only one type, such as thyroid (struma ovarii), carcinoid tumor, or primitive neuroectodermal tumor, also exist. Teratomas represent approximately 95% of OGCT. Teratomas are subclassified according to whether immature neuroectodermal tissue is present (IT) or absent (mature teratoma). In contrast to other OGCT types, ovarian pure teratomas (both mature and immature) do not contain 12p amplification (14). Ovarian teratomas that are part of a mixed germ cell tumor do, in contrast, have 12p amplification and may have isochromosome 12p, suggesting that these tumors have a different pathogenesis than pure ovarian teratomas (14,15). The pure ovarian teratomas may arise from a benign germ cell tumor in a parthenogenetic-like process (similar to pediatric testicular teratoma), whereas teratomas coexisting with a malignant OGCT component derive from malignant germ cells (similar to postpubertal testicular teratoma).

Most teratomas are mature cystic teratomas that contain differentiated tissue components such as skin, glandular epithelium, glial tissue, cartilage, and bone. Any tissue type present in adults may be represented in teratomas. The widest variety of tissue types is characteristically identified in a nodule in the wall of the cystic neoplasms. Mature cystic teratomas are benign neoplasms; however, rare examples may contain a somatic malignancy such as squamous cell carcinoma, papillary thyroid carcinoma, sarcoma, or other non–germ cell tumor. Such malignant transformation is seen in 0.2% to 1.4% of mature teratomas. A rare, recently described unusual clinical manifestation of ovarian mature teratomas is autoimmune encephalitis associated with antibodies to the *N*-methyl-D-aspartate receptor (16). The encephalitis may present with psychiatric symptoms and is typically responsive to surgical removal of the teratoma.

ITs in adult women, in contrast to mature cystic teratomas, are uncommon tumors. They represent about 3% of all ovarian teratomas, but ITs are the third most common form of malignant OGCTs. Most immature ovarian teratomas are unilateral neoplasms. ITs are predominantly solid tumors, but they may contain some cystic areas. The cut surface of ITs is soft and fleshy or encephaloid in appearance (**Fig. 24.6**). Areas of hemorrhage and necrosis are common. Microscopically, these tumors contain a variety of mature and immature tissue components. The immature elements almost always consist of immature neural tissue in the form of small round blue cells focally organized into rosettes and tubules (**Fig. 24.7**).

There is a correlation between disease prognosis and the degree of immaturity in the teratoma. The three-tiered grading system is still most often used (1). Grade 1 ITs display some immaturity, but

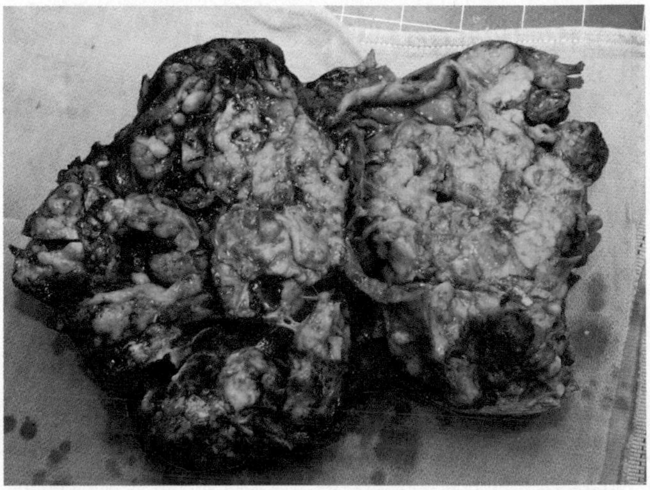

Figure 24.6. Ovarian immature teratoma. The neoplasm is predominantly solid and has a soft, encephaloid appearance.

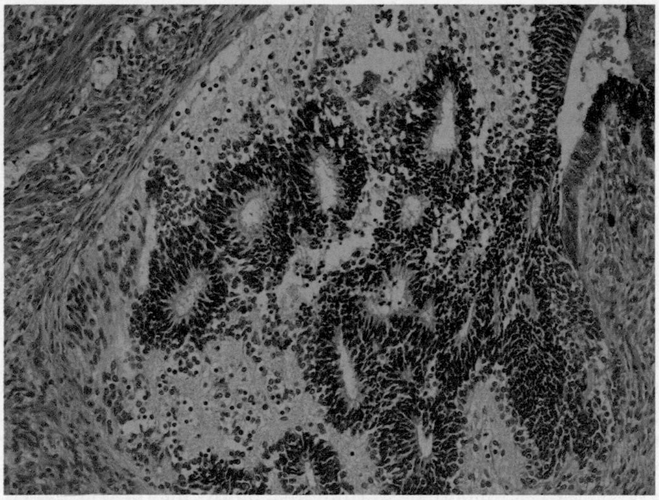

Figure 24.7. Ovarian immature teratoma. Immature neural tissue forms tubules.

the immature neural tissue does not exceed, in aggregate, the area of one low-power field (40× total magnification) in any slide. Grade 2 ITs contain immature neural tissue in one to three low-power fields in any slide. Grade 3 ITs contain immature neural tissue in greater than three low-power fields in at least one slide. Some authors prefer classifying ITs as either low (grade 1)- or high (grades 2 and 3)-grade teratomas. Overgrowth of immature neuroectodermal tissue in an extensive, confluent mass represents primitive neuroectodermal tumor that has a poor prognosis. In patients whose neoplasm has disseminated beyond the ovary, the grade of the tumor metastasis is important in predicting survival and determining treatment.

Occasionally, patients may have peritoneal implants that contain only mature glial tissue (gliomatosis peritonei), but genetic data suggest that these mature glial implants may represent a metaplastic phenomenon rather than actual tumor implants (2). The behavior of gliomatosis peritonei is typically benign, although they may rarely progress to a high grade glioma. It is extremely important to sample peritoneal disease thoroughly in order to identify foci of IT.

Molecular Characteristics

Biologically, OGCTs, like testis cancer, are derived from primordial germ cells, which undergo defective meiosis. Karyotypic abnormalities are common and include aneuploidy or chromosomal rearrangements (17). In contrast, benign teratomas commonly have a normal karyotype. One report notes chromosomal abnormalities in 7% of mature teratomas (14,15). Analysis of centromeric heteromorphism suggests that 65% to 70% of benign teratomas result from a post–meiosis I type error (homozygotes), whereas the remaining 30% to 35% are caused by defective meiosis I, as demonstrated by heterozygosity of centromeric markers (14). Among malignant OGCTs, aneuploidy and chromosomal translocations or truncations similar to those encountered in testicular carcinoma have been widely reported (17,18). The presence of an isochromosome 12p (i12p) has been noted in ovarian tumors (19), albeit less commonly than in testis cancer. Gains of 12p material may be present in 77% of dysgerminomas and lower percentages of other malignant OGCTs. Other chromosomal aberrations such as loss or gain in chromosomes 1, 11, 12, 16, and X can be identified (20). The association between dysgerminoma and dysgenetic gonads is well recognized and should be managed accordingly, as will be discussed. MicroRNAs from the *miR-371-373* and *miR-302* clusters are overexpressed in all germ cell tumors, anecdotally correlate with disease burden, and are promising candidate biomarkers for disease monitoring and diagnosis (21). Additionally, *KIT* gene mutations appear to be amplified in dysgerminomas and may represent a potential therapeutic target (6). Other mutations in dysgerminomas have been occasionally identified including *DICER1*, *TP53*, and *KRAS* (4). Protein expression and gene mutation studies of OGCT have recently been reviewed, and overexpression of *POU5F1*, *KIT*, *NANOG*, *PDPN*, and *SOX2* is notable among the frequently overexpressed genes (4).

Clinical Features

Malignant germ cell tumors of the ovary occur mainly in girls and young women. In the clinical series reported from the M.D. Anderson Cancer Center (MDACC), the age of the patients ranged from 6 to 40 years, with a median age of 16 to 20 years, depending on the histologic type (22). A recent evaluation of the National Cancer Institute's Surveillance, Epidemiology, and End Results (SEER) database shows a median age at diagnosis of 22 years (range: 0 to 93 years), with 91% of patients being less than 40 years at diagnosis (23). There are ethnic and racial differences in the incidence of germ cell tumors, with increased incidence of OGCTs among pediatric black females compared with black males and among Hispanic girls aged 10 to 19 years, as compared with non-Hispanics (24). Interestingly, a case–cohort study from the Children Oncology Group, including 274 cases (195 OGCTs and 79 testicular cancers), showed that a family history of cancer was inversely correlated with the risk of developing germ cell tumors (25).

Signs and symptoms in these patients are rather consistent. The combination of abdominal pain associated with a palpable pelvic-abdominal mass is present in approximately 85% of patients (26–28). Ten percent of patients present with acute abdominal pain, usually caused by cyst/tumor rupture, hemorrhage, or ovarian torsion. This finding is somewhat more common in patients with endodermal sinus tumor or mixed germ cell tumors and is frequently misdiagnosed as acute appendicitis. Less common signs and symptoms include abdominal distention (35%), fever (10%), and vaginal bleeding (10%). A few patients exhibit isosexual precocity, because of hCG production by tumor cells.

In a small percentage of cases, OGCTs occur during pregnancy or in the immediate postpartum period (27). In the series reported by Gordon (29), 20 of 158 patients with dysgerminoma were diagnosed during pregnancy or after delivery. Nondysgerminomatous ovarian tumors occur less frequently during pregnancy, but rare cases have been reported (30–33). Marked increase in AFP heralds the presence of a germ cell tumor with yolk sac component. By and large, patients with OGCTs diagnosed during pregnancy can be treated successfully, without compromising the health of the fetus. Surgical resection of tumors and CT have been performed safely in mid- and third trimesters. However, rapid disease progression and/or pregnancy termination/miscarriage have been recorded, especially for nondysgerminomatous tumors (34).

Many germ cell tumors possess the unique property of producing biologic markers that are detectable in serum. The development of specific and sensitive radioimmunoassay techniques to measure hCG and AFP led to dramatic improvements in patient monitoring. Serial measurements of serum markers aid the diagnosis and, more importantly, are useful for monitoring response to treatment and detection of subclinical recurrences. **Table 24.1** illustrates typical findings in the sera of patients with various tumor histologic types. Endodermal sinus tumor and choriocarcinoma are prototypes for AFP and hCG production, respectively. Embryonal carcinoma can secrete both hCG and AFP, but most commonly produces hCG. Mixed tumors may produce either, both, or none of the markers, depending on the type and quantity of elements present. Dysgerminoma is commonly devoid of hormonal production, although a small percentage of tumors produce low levels of hCG, if multinucleated syncytiotrophoblastic giant cells are present. An elevated level of AFP or high level of hCG (>100 units/mL) denotes the presence of tumor elements other than dysgerminoma. Therapy should be adjusted accordingly (see Dysgerminoma section). Although ITs are associated with negative markers, a few tumors can produce AFP. A third tumor marker is lactic dehydrogenase (LDH), which

■ **TABLE 24.1. Serum Tumor Markers in Malignant Germ Cell Tumors of the Ovary**

Histology	AFP	hCG
Dysgerminoma	–	±
Endodermal sinus tumor	+	–
Immature teratoma	±	–
Mixed germ cell tumor	±	±
Choriocarcinoma	–	+
Embryonal carcinoma	±	+

AFP, α-fetoprotein; hCG, human chorionic gonadotropin.

is frequently and nonspecifically elevated in patients with OGCTs. Unfortunately, it is less specific than hCG or AFP, which limits its usefulness. CA-125 also can be nonspecifically elevated in patients with OGCTs (35). Age over 40 to 45 years, stage greater than I, yolk sac tumor histology, and treatment outside a referral center have been identified as prognostic factors that affect survival (23,36).

SURGERY

Operative Findings

Malignant germ cell tumors of the ovary tend to be quite large. In the MDACC series, these tumors ranged in size from 7 to 40 cm, with a median size of 16 cm (26). Predominance of right-sided over left-sided involvement was noted. Bilaterality of tumor involvement (especially true stage IB disease) is exceedingly rare, except for dysgerminoma. Bilateral involvement occurs in 10% to 15% of dysgerminoma patients (29,37–40). For nondysgerminomatous tumors, bilateral involvement signifies either advanced disease with metastatic spread to the contralateral ovary or the presence of a mixed germ cell tumor with prominent dysgerminoma component. Ascites may be noted in approximately 20% of cases. Rupture of tumors, either preoperatively or intraoperatively, occurs in approximately 20% of cases. Torsion of the ovarian pedicle was documented in 5% of patients in the MDACC series.

Benign cystic teratoma is associated with malignant germ cell tumors in 5% to 10% of cases. These coexistent teratomas may occur in the ipsilateral ovary, in the contralateral ovary, or bilaterally. Likewise, a preexisting gonadoblastoma may be noted in association with dysgerminoma and dysgenetic gonads related to a 46XY karyotype (20,41–43). Malignant germ cell tumors generally spread along the peritoneal surface or through lymphatic dissemination. Although the relative frequency of these two principal mechanisms of dissemination is difficult to discern, it is generally accepted that these neoplasms more commonly metastasize to lymph nodes than epithelial tumors. The high prevalence of inadequate staging procedures makes the true incidence of lymph node involvement uncertain. It is our impression that although still uncommon, malignant OGCTs have a somewhat greater predilection than epithelial tumors to metastasize hematogenously to the parenchyma of the liver or lung. The stage distribution is also very different from that of epithelial tumors. In most large series, approximately 60% to 70% of tumors will be stage I (29). The next most common stage is stage III, accounting for 25% to 30% of tumors. Stages II and IV are relatively uncommon.

Extent of Primary Surgery

The initial treatment approach for a patient suspected of having a malignant OGCT is surgery, both for diagnosis and for therapy. The route of surgery, whether through a vertical midline incision or through a minimally invasive approach, should be determined based on surgical experience with the intent to avoid tumor rupture (NCCN guidelines). A thorough determination of the disease extent by inspection and palpation should be made. If the disease appears confined to one or both ovaries, comprehensive staging biopsies should be performed in adult patients.

The type of primary operative procedure depends on the surgical findings. Because many of these patients are young women, for whom preservation of fertility is a priority, minimizing the surgical resection while ensuring removal of tumor bulk must be thoughtfully balanced. As noted previously, bilateral ovarian involvement is rare, except for the case of pure dysgerminoma. Bilateral involvement may be found in cases of advanced disease (stages II to IV), in which there is metastasis from one ovary to the opposite gonad, or in cases of mixed germ cell tumors with a dysgerminoma component. Therefore, fertility-sparing unilateral salpingo-oophorectomy with preservation of the contralateral ovary and of the uterus can be performed in most patients. Ovarian cystectomy as the sole treatment is not recommended (44–46). If the contralateral ovary appears grossly normal on careful inspection, it should be left undisturbed. However, in the case of pure dysgerminoma, biopsy may be considered, because occult or microscopic tumor involvement occurs in a small percentage of patients. Unnecessary biopsy, however, may result in future infertility because of peritoneal adhesions or ovarian failure. If the contralateral ovary appears abnormally enlarged, a biopsy or ovarian cystectomy should be performed. If frozen examination reveals a dysgenetic gonad or if there are clinical indications suggesting a hermaphrodite phenotype, then bilateral salpingo-oophorectomy is indicated. However, it is difficult to establish this diagnosis on frozen section. This determination should preferably be made by finding the karyotype preoperatively. If benign cystic teratoma is found in the contralateral ovary, an event that can occur in 5% to 10% of patients, then contralateral ovarian cystectomy with preservation of remaining normal ovarian tissue is recommended.

An important problem, albeit rare, is bilateral gonadal involvement in a patient who desires to preserve fertility and who is a candidate for postoperative CT. There are no data regarding the ability of CT to eradicate a primary ovarian tumor. In testis cancer, there are presumptive data suggesting that tumor may persist after CT in the gonad and that the testis may be a drug sanctuary. In exceptional situations, it may be reasonable to preserve an involved ovary in a patient who will be receiving CT. However, it is conceivable that ovarian preservation could increase the risk for recurrence in these selected cases. The decision to preserve an involved ovary is difficult and must be made carefully considering patients' wishes.

The advent of *in vitro* fertilization technology also has an impact on operative management (47). Convention has dictated that if a bilateral salpingo-oophorectomy is necessary, a hysterectomy should also be performed. However, with current assisted reproduction technologies (ARTs) involving donor oocyte and hormonal support, a woman without ovaries could potentially sustain a normal intrauterine pregnancy. Similarly, if the uterus and one ovary are resected because of tumor involvement, current techniques provide the opportunity for oocyte retrieval from the remaining ovary, *in vitro* fertilization with sperm from her male partner, and embryo implantation into a surrogate's uterus. As the field of ART is evolving, traditional guidelines concerning surgical treatment in young patients with gynecologic tumors have to be thoughtfully adapted to individual circumstances.

Surgical Staging

Surgical staging remains the standard of care in adult patients to determine the extent of disease, provide prognostic information, and guide postoperative management. A meticulous approach is important for every patient, but it is of critical importance for those patients with early clinical disease to detect the presence of occult or microscopic metastases and provide CT in those situations. Staging of OGCTs follows the same principles applicable to epithelial ovarian tumors, as described by the International Federation of

Gynecologists and Obstetricians (see **Table 24.2**). Proper staging procedures consist of the following:

1. Although a transverse incision is cosmetically superior, a vertical midline incision is usually necessary for adequate exposure, appropriate staging biopsies, and resection of large pelvic tumors or metastatic disease in the upper abdomen. Minimally invasive surgical approaches for gynecologic cancer staging have become widely accepted, and although trials specific to this approach for malignant OGCTs have not been performed, this approach is considered preferable to open surgery when the same surgical outcomes can be obtained.
2. Ascites, if present, should be evacuated and submitted for cytologic analysis. If no peritoneal fluid is noted, cytologic washings of the pelvis and bilateral paracolic gutters should be performed prior to manipulation of the intraperitoneal contents.
3. The entire peritoneal cavity and its structures should be carefully inspected and palpated in a methodical manner. We generally prefer to start with the subphrenic spaces and move caudad toward the pelvis. The subdiaphragmatic areas, omentum, colon, all peritoneal surfaces, the entire retroperitoneum, and small intestinal serosa and mesentery should be evaluated. Any suspicious areas should be submitted for biopsy or excised.
4. Next, the primary ovarian tumor and pelvis should be examined. Both ovaries should be carefully assessed for size, presence of obvious tumor involvement, capsular rupture, external excrescences, or adherence to surrounding structures.
5. If the disease seems to be limited to the ovary or localized to the pelvis, then random staging biopsies of structures at risk should be performed. These sites should include the omentum (with generous biopsies from multiple areas) and the peritoneal surfaces of the following sites: bilateral paracolic gutters, cul-de-sac, lateral pelvic walls, vesicouterine reflection, and subdiaphragmatic areas. Any adhesions should also be generously sampled.
6. The paraaortic and bilateral pelvic lymph node–bearing areas should be carefully palpated. Any suspicious nodes should be excised or sampled. If no suspicious areas are detected, these areas should be sampled. There is no evidence that a complete paraaortic and/or pelvic lymphadenectomy is advantageous.
7. If obvious gross metastatic disease is present, it should be excised if feasible, or at least sampled to document disease extent. The concept of cytoreductive surgery is discussed below. There are insufficient data at present to support the use of minimally invasive surgery in the setting of metastatic disease.

TABLE 24.2. FIGO Staging of Ovarian Germ Cell Tumors

Stage	Description
I	Tumor limited to ovaries
IA	Tumor limited to one ovary, no ascites, intact capsule
IB	Tumor limited to both ovaries, no ascites, intact capsule
IC	Tumor either stage IA or IB, but with ascites present containing malignant cells or with ovarian capsule involvement or rupture or with positive peritoneal washings
II	Tumor involving one or both ovaries with extension to the pelvis
IIA	Extension to uterus or tubes
IIB	Involvement of both ovaries with pelvic extension
IIC	Tumor either stage IIA or IIB, but with ascites present containing malignant cells or with ovarian capsule involvement or rupture or with positive peritoneal washings
III	Tumor involving one or both ovaries with tumor implants outside the pelvis or with positive retroperitoneal or inguinal lymph nodes. Superficial liver metastases qualify as stage III
IIIA	Tumor limited to the pelvis with negative nodes but with microscopic seeding of the abdominal peritoneal surface
IIIB	Negative nodes, tumor implants in the abdominal cavity <2 cm
IIIC	Positive nodes or tumor implants in the abdominal cavity >2 cm
IV	Distant metastases present

FIGO, International Federation of Gynecologists and Obstetricians.

Most patients receive initial surgery without the care of a gynecologic oncologist and do not undergo comprehensive staging. On referral of such a patient to a university or a tertiary care center, the oncologist is faced with the dilemma of inadequate staging information. In such cases, postoperative studies including CT scan of the abdomen are recommended. If histopathologic and available information from the first surgery clearly indicates the use of systemic CT, reexploration for obtaining staging information is inadvisable. Reoperation for comprehensive staging may be appropriate for patients who would undergo surveillance and forego CT in the event of negative comprehensive staging. This is an area of current debate, because some patients may be candidates for surveillance, using salvage CT in the event of recurrent disease.

Cytoreductive Surgery

If widely spread tumor is encountered at initial surgery, it is recommended that the same principles concerning cytoreductive surgery applied in the surgical management of advanced epithelial ovarian cancer be followed. Specifically, as much tumor as is technically feasible and safe should be resected. However, because of their rarity, there is scant information in the literature on the impact of cytoreductive surgery of malignant germ cell tumors. In a study of the Gynecologic Oncology Group (GOG), Slayton et al. (48) found that 15 of 54 (28%) patients with completely resected disease at primary surgery failed CT with a combination of vincristine, dactinomycin, and cyclophosphamide (VAC), as opposed to 15 of 22 (68%) patients with incompletely resected disease treated with the same regimen. Furthermore, a higher percentage of patients with bulky postoperative residual disease (82%) failed CT compared with those with minimal residual disease (55%). In a subsequent GOG study reported by Williams, patients received the combination regimen of cisplatin, vinblastine, and bleomycin (PVB). In this study, patients with nondysgerminomatous tumors and clinically nonmeasurable disease after surgery had a greater likelihood of remaining progression free than those with measurable disease (65% vs. 34%) (49). In addition, patients who had been surgically debulked to optimal disease had an outcome intermediate between patients with suboptimal disease and those with optimal disease without debulking.

Even with epithelial tumors, the relative influence of tumor biology, surgical skill, and aggressiveness remains uncertain. Germ cell tumors, especially dysgerminomas, are generally much more chemosensitive than epithelial ovarian tumors. Therefore, aggressive resection of metastatic disease in these cases, especially resection of bulky retroperitoneal nodes, is questionable. The surgeon must exercise thoughtful and mature intraoperative judgment when encountering such situations, carefully weighing the risks of cytoreductive maneuvers in the setting of chemosensitive tumors. There is no substitute for surgical experience and a clear understanding of the biologic behavior of these neoplasms. Even in the face of extensive metastatic disease, it is possible to perform a fertility-sparing procedure with preservation of a normal contralateral ovary, though outcomes data are lacking.

The value of secondary cytoreductive surgery in the management of OGCTs is even less clear than that of primary cytoreductive surgery. Although secondary cytoreduction is of questionable benefit for patients with refractory epithelial ovarian cancer

(50,51), germ cell tumors are relatively more chemosensitive than epithelial tumors and are more likely to respond to second-line therapy. Therefore, if a patient has an isolated focus of persistent tumor after first-line CT in an area such as the lung, liver, retroperitoneum, or brain, then surgical extirpation should be considered before changing CT regimens. Although this clinical situation is extremely rare, it has been encountered in other situations involving chemosensitive tumors, such as gestational trophoblastic disease and testicular cancer.

Unlike testicular cancer, the finding of a residual mass after completion of CT is less common in patients with OGCTs because these women are likely to have considerable tumor debulking at the time of the diagnostic surgical procedure and thus enter CT with significantly less tumor burden. At completion of CT, men with nonseminomatous tumors or seminoma may have persistent mature teratoma or desmoplastic fibrosis. In patients with bulky dysgerminoma, residual masses after CT are very likely to represent desmoplastic fibrosis. Although a number of patients with pure ovarian ITs or mixed germ cell tumors have persistent mature teratoma at the completion of CT, as documented by second-look laparotomy (52), the majority is left with multiple small peritoneal implants rather than with a dominant mass. However, it is now recognized that occasional patients who have received CT for ITs or mixed germ cell tumors containing teratoma will have bulky residual teratoma after CT. The natural history or biologic implications of these findings are not clear. In testicular cancer, patients with bulky residual teratoma may experience slow progression of tumor (53) or may develop overtly malignant tumors over time (54–57). There are similar anecdotal reports of progressive mature teratoma in OGCT patients after CT (58–60). Considering this information, it seems appropriate to resect persistent masses in patients with negative markers after CT for germ cell tumors containing IT. If viable neoplasm is found, additional CT should be considered. However, if only mature teratoma is resected, observation is generally recommended.

Second-Look Laparotomy

Since 1960, second-look laparotomy was included in the routine management of patients with epithelial ovarian cancer to assess disease status after a fixed interval of CT. This approach was extrapolated to the management of patients with OGCTs. In a review of the MDACC experience with second-look laparotomy, findings were negative in 52 of 53 patients (61). The one patient with positive findings at second-look laparotomy had an elevated AFP level prior to surgery, which accurately predicted residual disease. This patient received subsequent CT with PVB, entering prolonged remission. Of the patients with negative findings, one woman relapsed 9 months after the negative second-look surgery and subsequently died. Thirteen patients in this series had biopsy-proven evidence of residual mature teratoma (so-called "chemotherapeutic retroconversion") at second-look laparotomy; treatment was discontinued in all patients and none developed recurrence. Thus, in this series, second-look surgery did not add prognostic information or alter the therapeutic management of patients. The role of second-look surgery is further obscured in the setting of advancement in imaging techniques (CT scanning, positron emission tomography (PET), and MRI) and in an era where tumor marker measurements are part of routine care of patients with germ cell tumors.

The GOG experience with second-look laparotomy in OGCTs has been reviewed (52). One hundred and seventeen patients who were enrolled prospectively on GOG protocols using cisplatin-based CT after initial surgical staging and cytoreduction (GOG protocols #45, 78, and 90) underwent second-look surgical procedures. Of these, 45 surgical procedures were performed in patients who received three courses of cisplatin, etoposide, and bleomycin (BEP) after complete tumor resection. In this subgroup, 38 patients had negative findings, 2 patients had IT, and 5 patients had mature teratoma. One of the patients with residual IT received further CT and one did not. Both women with residual IT and the rest of the patients remained disease free. One patient with negative second-look surgery findings subsequently relapsed and succumbed to disease. Hence, in the subgroup of patients with completely resected primary OGCTs, the benefit of second-look surgery is nil. In contrast, 72 patients in this series treated with similar CT had advanced incompletely resected tumors before beginning adjuvant treatment. In this subgroup, 48 patients did not have teratoma elements in their primary tumor. At second-look surgery, 45 patients had no residual tumor and 3 patients displayed persistent endodermal sinus tumor or embryonal carcinoma. All three of the latter patients died despite further treatment. Five patients with negative second laparotomies recurred, of which only one was salvaged with CT. Thus, the value of second-look surgery in patients with incompletely resected germ cell tumors, not containing teratoma, is arguably minimal. However, in the subgroup of patients with incompletely resected tumors containing teratoma elements (total of 24 patients), second-look surgery had an impact on subsequent management. Of these patients, 16 were found to have mature teratoma at second look, which was bulky or progressive in 7 cases. Four additional patients were found to have residual IT. Fourteen of the total 16 patients with teratoma and 6 of the 7 women with bulky residual tumor remained disease free after surgical resection. Therefore, although second-look laparotomy is not necessary in patients with tumor completely resected primarily or in those patients with initially incompletely resected tumor not containing teratoma, clinical benefit can be derived in those patients with incompletely resected primary tumor that contains elements of teratoma (see **Table 24.3**).

Advances in imaging technology, including the advent of positron emission tomography (PET) scanning, may further obviate the need for surgical reexploration. Although PET scan is sensitive for detecting active (malignant) tumor, its usefulness in evaluating residual mature teratoma is more limited (62–65). A positive PET scan in the setting of a residual mass after treatment is highly indicative of viable tumor and, when used in conjunction with traditional radiographic techniques (CT scan, MRI) and tumor marker determinations, can predict relapses with accuracy (66). A recent series demonstrates that in patients with residual masses after treatment for seminoma, a positive PET scan represents strong evidence that the residual mass contains persistent tumor. In contrast, if the PET scan is negative, residual masses are unlikely to contain active tumor. The specificity of the PET scan in this situation was 100%, the sensitivity was 80%,

TABLE 24.3. Results of Second-Look Surgery in Patients Enrolled on GOG Protocols

Primary Surgery	Total Number	Positive Second Look: Progression-Free/Total Number	Negative Second Look: Progression-Free/Total Number
Completely resected tumor	45	7/7[a]	37/38
Incompletely resected tumor	24	16/20[b]	4/4
Teratoma present/teratoma absent	48	0/3[c]	41/45

[a]Five mature teratomas and two immature teratomas.

[b]Sixteen mature teratomas and four immature teratomas.

[c]Three embryonal carcinoma and yolk sac tumors.

Source: Reprinted with permission from Williams SD, Blessing JA, DiSaia PJ, et al. Second-look laparotomy in ovarian germ cell tumors: the Gynecologic Oncology Group experience. *Gynecol Oncol*. 1994;52(3):287–291.

and the positive and negative predictive values were 100% and 95%, respectively (67). Although studies using PET scanning in OGCT are scant (68,69), the concepts are very similar and can be extrapolated from the testis cancer literature.

CHEMOTHERAPY FOR OGCTS

Chemotherapy: From VAC to PEB

One of the great triumphs of cancer treatment in the 1970s and 1980s has been the development of effective CT for testicular cancer (70,71). The lessons learned from prospective, randomized trials in testicular cancer were subsequently applied to OGCTs. Presently, the overwhelming majority of patients with OGCTs survive their disease with the judicious use of surgery and cisplatin-based combination CT. There are many similarities, but a few important differences between testicular cancer and OGCTs.

Historically, the first regimens used successfully for women with OGCTs were *VAC* or VAC-type regimens. Such treatments had curative potential, especially for early-stage disease. However, among patients with advanced disease, the number of long-term survivors after VAC therapy remained under 50%. In the series reported from the MDACC, although 86% of patients with stage I tumors were cured with VAC, the efficacy of the regimen was significantly lower for patients with advanced disease (22). Only 57% of stage II patients and 50% of stage III patients achieved long-term control. The two patients with stage IV tumors in this series succumbed to the disease. Similarly, in a GOG study, only 7 out of 22 patients with incompletely resected OGCTs achieved long-term disease control after VAC, as compared with 39 of 54 patients with completely resected tumors (72). In that report, 11 of 15 patients with stage III and both patients with stage IV disease progressed within 12 months. These data suggest that VAC CT was insufficient for the treatment of advanced stage and/or incompletely resected OGCTs.

Because of the experience gained from the treatment of testicular tumors demonstrating the superiority of cisplatin-based regimens, new platinum-based regimens were tested in patients with OGCTs. Gershenson reported the efficacy of PVB in a small series of patients treated at the MDACC (73). Among 15 patients, 7 received PVB in the adjuvant setting and 8 received the combination at the time of recurrence. Six of seven patients treated with PVB upfront became long-term survivors. Among them, three women had optimally debulked stage III disease.

Subsequently, the PVB combination was evaluated prospectively in GOG protocol #45 (49). In this study, 47 of 89 patients with nondysgerminomatous ovarian tumors (53%) were disease free, with a median follow-up of 52 months. The latest treatment failure occurred at 28 months. Eight other patients had durable remissions with second-line therapy and a few other patients had nonprogressive or slowly progressive IT. Thus, the 4-year overall survival (OS) was approximately 70%. Of note, 29% of patients enrolled in this trial had received prior radiation or CT, which might have negatively affected the overall outcome. As discussed previously, patients who were debulked to optimal disease fared better than those who were not. Histologic type and marker elevation before treatment were not associated with adverse outcome. However, even among patients with nonmeasurable and presumably small volume disease, and without prior treatment, 8 of 30 patients treated with PVB ultimately failed.

In testicular cancer, subsequent experience has documented that etoposide is at least equivalent to vinblastine and produces improved survival in patients with high tumor volume (71). Furthermore, the use of etoposide in place of vinblastine led to reduced neurologic toxicity, abdominal pain, and constipation. The latter two adverse effects are particularly important for patients with OGCTs, because many would have had recent abdominal surgery. These observations led to the evaluation of the combination of BEP (**Table 24.4**) in patients with OGCTs. In a series from the MDACC, long-term remissions were recorded in 25 of 26 patients treated with BEP (74). The only patient who succumbed to disease had been noncompliant with treatment, monitoring, and follow-up. In this series, four patients with measurable disease after surgery had complete remissions after BEP treatment. This led to a prospective GOG study evaluating BEP in patients with OGCTs (75). The regimen was highly effective, 91 of 93 enrolled patients being free of disease at follow-up. On the basis of these data, although BEP and VAC have not been prospectively compared, BEP emerged as the preferred regimen for patients with OGCTs. The inclusion of cisplatin in the treatment of ovarian tumors resulted indisputably in an improvement in survival and disease control, as shown by the results of GOG studies, as well as by other clinical series (76–78). These results of therapy are summarized in **Table 24.5**.

TABLE 24.4. The BEP Regimen[a]

Cisplatin	20 mg/m^2 days 1–5
Etoposide (VP-16)	100 mg/m^2 days 1–5
Bleomycin	30 units IV weekly

BEP, bleomycin, etoposide, and cisplatin.

TABLE 24.5. Adjuvant Chemotherapy

Institution	Regimen	Progression Free/ Total (%)
GOG (75)	BEP	89/93 (94)
Australia (77)	Multiple	9/10 (88)
Hospital 12 de Octubre (76)	PVB or BEP	9/9 (98)
M.D. Anderson (73)	PVB	4/4 (98)
M.D. Anderson (74)	BEP	20/20 (98)

BEP, cisplatin, etoposide, bleomycin; GOG, Gynecologic Oncology Group; PVB, cisplatin, vinblastine, bleomycin.

Differences in Outcome for Patients with Completely Resected Tumors versus Advanced Stage Disease

It is clear that several prognostic factors impact the outcome of patients with OGCTs and that there are important differences between testicular cancer and OGCTs. Debulking surgery plays a central role in the management of ovarian tumors, but has a less important role in testicular cancer. In the hands of an experienced surgeon, the majority of women with ovarian tumors are debulked to minimal and often clinically undetectable disease before starting CT. Therefore, unlike patients with testicular cancer, most women who are candidates for CT have minimal or no residual disease. However, even in this circumstance, there seems to be little doubt that adjuvant therapy is appropriate in the majority of cases. The anticipated risk of relapse with surgery alone in patients with advanced disease is as high as 75% to 80%. Particularly, patients with embryonal carcinoma, endodermal sinus tumors, and mixed tumors containing these elements are considered to be at very high risk of recurrence without postoperative therapy. This risk can be minimized by the use of adjuvant CT. In GOG protocol #78, 50 of 51 patients with completely resected OGCTs remained free of disease when three cycles of BEP were given adjuvantly. Other studies using cisplatin-based therapy have given similar results (**Table 24.6**). The recommended treatment for most patients (with the exception of patients with grade 1 IT, or stage IA dysgerminoma) is adjuvant CT with three courses of BEP. Virtually all patients with early-stage or

TABLE 24.6. Chemotherapy of Advanced Disease

Institution	Regimen	Progression Free/ Total (%)
GOG (49)	PVB	47/89 (52)
Australia (77)	Multiple	42/46 (89)
Hospital 12 de Octubre (76)	PVB or BEP	15/19 (78)
M.D. Anderson (73)	PVB	7/11 (63)
M.D. Anderson (74)	BEP	5/6 (82)

BEP, bleomycin, etoposide, and cisplatin; GOG, Gynecologic Oncology Group; PVB, cisplatin, vinblastine, bleomycin.

completely resected disease will survive after careful surgical staging and cisplatin-based adjuvant CT. More recently, clinical series and observations are beginning to suggest that surveillance with careful follow-up after surgery may be an acceptable alternative for carefully selected patients, as discussed below. Given the fact that surgery followed by CT is curative for most patients, this course of action should be taken only after very careful consideration. Further studies are needed in this area.

In contrast, most clinical series have shown worse clinical outcome for patients with metastatic disease or with incompletely resected tumors (see **Table 24.7**). Current clinical trials in testicular cancer separate patients with small tumor volume and a resultant excellent prognosis from those with bulky tumor or liver and brain involvement (79). Patients in the former group are usually complete responders to CT and long-term survivors, whereas only about 50% to 60% of the latter patients are cured. Hence, clinical trials for patients with good prognostic factors investigate shorter or less toxic CT aimed at minimizing toxicity (80), while preserving efficacy. In contrast, clinical trials for patients with high-risk disease have evaluated more intensive CT regimens with the goal of improving the likelihood of cure (81,82). For instance, high-dose chemotherapy (HDCT) with stem cell rescue was tested for patients with high-risk testicular cancer in a multi-institutional clinical protocol (ECOG protocol 3894). Patients considered to have high risk for relapse were randomized to receive four cycles of BEP (control arm) versus two cycles of BEP followed by HDCT with autologous stem cell rescue in the form of two (tandem) courses using carboplatin, etoposide, and cyclophosphamide as a conditioning regimen (experimental arm). The 1-year durable complete response rate was 52% after BEP + HDCT and 48% after BEP alone ($p = 0.53$) (83). The results of the trial disproved the concept that more aggressive CT in the first-line setting improves outcome of high-risk testicular cancer patients when compared with standard-dose BEP (84).

Dependable risk stratification, similar to the one used for testicular tumors, is not currently in use for OGCTs. The only clinical prognosticators for outcome of OGCTs remain stage at diagnosis and increase in tumor marker levels (85). Whether this reflects an inherent biologic difference between OGCTs and testis cancer or merely an underestimation of tumor volume because of intraperitoneal spread is not clear. In summary, with the exception of patients with grade 1 IT or stage IA dysgerminoma, the available evidence supports that women with OGCT should receive three to four cycles of BEP CT after cytoreductive surgery. Therapy courses longer than four cycles are not supported, regardless of tumor volume.

TABLE 24.7. A Typical Antiemetic Regimen

Granisetron 1 mg IV 30 minutes prior to cisplatin daily for 5 days
Or
Ondansetron 0.15 mg/kg IV 30 minutes prior and 4 hours after cisplatin daily for 5 days
Plus
Dexamethasone 20 mg IV 30 minutes prior to cisplatin on days 1 and 2
Plus
Aprepitant 125 mg PO on day 1 and 80 mg PO on days 2 and 3, prior to cisplatin infusion

PO, by mouth.

Management of Residual or Recurrent Disease

The large majority of patients with OGCTs are cured with surgery and platinum-based CT. However, a small percentage of patients have persistent or progressive disease during treatment or recur after completion of treatment. Like in testicular cancer, these treatment failures are categorized as platinum resistant (progression during or within 4 to 6 weeks of completing treatment) or platinum sensitive (recurrence beyond 6 weeks from platinum-based therapy).

Most recurrences occur within 24 months from primary treatment, and nearly all cause specific deaths within 5 years of diagnosis (23). In a series from the MDACC, 42 treatment failures were identified among 160 patients with OGCTs treated between 1970 and 1990 (86). Treatment failure in these patients was attributed to inadequate surgery in 14 patients, inadequate radiation in 5 patients, inadequate CT in 16 patients (underdosing and noncompliance), treatment-related toxicity in 1 patient, and unidentifiable causes in 6 patients. A significant number of patients included in this series had received VAC-based CT, which accounted for the higher than expected rate of recurrence.

Given the high curability rate of OGCTs with primary treatment, the management of recurrent disease represents a complex and often difficult issue, and preferably should be performed in a specialized center. Data to guide the management of patients with recurrent OGCTs are scant and largely extrapolated from the clinical experience with testicular cancer. The single most important prognostic factor in patients with testicular cancer is whether or not they are refractory to cisplatin. The likelihood of cure with high-dose salvage therapy in patients who relapse from a complete remission after initial therapy is as high as 60% or more. On the other hand, in patients who are truly cisplatin refractory, the likelihood of long-term survival and cure is significantly less. However, up to 30% to 40% of these patients can become long-term survivors. Approximately 30% of patients with recurrent platinum-sensitive testicular cancer can be salvaged with second-line CT (vinblastine, ifosfamide, platinum) (81). High-dose therapy with carboplatin, etoposide with or without cyclophosphamide or ifosfamide, and stem cell rescue has been shown to be highly active in this setting (87,88). Generally, in patients who are not cisplatin refractory, one course of standard-dose therapy, usually cisplatin, vinblastine, and ifosfamide, is given. If an initial response is seen, then two subsequent courses of HDCT (carboplatin and etoposide) with stem cell rescue are undertaken (89). A report from the Indiana University describes this approach among 184 patients with recurrent testicular cancer. At a median follow-up of 48 months, 116 patients were in complete remission. Remarkably, of the subgroup of 40 patients who were platinum refractory, 18 became disease free after HDCT (90). Although this approach has not been prospectively tested in women with recurrent platinum-sensitive OGCTs, because of the rarity of such patients, the concepts are very similar and support the use of high-dose therapy in this setting. A recent retrospective analysis on the use of HDCT for recurrent OGCTs at Indiana University revealed that patients with recurrent OGCTs tend to be referred late and have worse outcomes compared with their male counterparts (91). Of 13 women treated with HDCT for recurrent OGCTs, 11 had yolk sac tumors and 8 were platinum refractory. In this series, four achieved long-term survival; however, only five received HDCT as second-line therapy, the rest being referred late in the course of their disease (91). It is, therefore, important to consider early referral to a specialized center for management of recurrent disease to maximize chances of cure. An ongoing Alliance phase III clinical trial (NCT02375204) is comparing standard-dose salvage CT with paclitaxel, ifosfamide, and cisplatin versus a high-dose regimen with paclitaxel and ifosfamide followed by high-dose carboplatin and etoposide, with stem cell rescue as first salvage regimen for relapsed germ cell tumors. The results of the study will set the definitive approach for the management of recurrent germ cell tumors.

Active agents in the setting of recurrence after HDCT include ifosfamide, taxanes, gemcitabine, and oxaliplatin (92–94). In a phase II trial from the Indiana University, the combination of gemcitabine and paclitaxel induced objective responses in 10 of 31 patients who had recurred after HDCT. Of those, five patients were free of disease 2 years after treatment (94). The combination of gemcitabine and oxaliplatin induced a 46% response rate in a group of 31 patients with recurrent germ cell tumors. Over 60% of these patients were platinum resistant or refractory (95). A new class of agents with promising clinical activity includes the cyclin-dependent kinase (CDK) inhibitors. In a clinical trial including 29 patients with recurrent germ cell tumors treated with the CDK4/6 inhibitor palbociclib, the 6-month progression-free survival (PFS) was 28%, suggesting promising activity (96). Referral for treatment with investigational agents for recurrent, refractory OGCTs is appropriate.

Immediate Toxicity of Chemotherapy

Acute adverse effects of CT can be substantial, and these patients should be treated by physicians experienced in their management. About 25% of patients develop febrile neutropenic episodes during CT and require hospitalization and broad-spectrum antibiotics. Cisplatin can be associated with nephrotoxicity. This can be avoided by ensuring adequate hydration during and immediately after CT and by avoidance of aminoglycoside antibiotics. Bleomycin can cause pulmonary fibrosis. Pulmonary function testing is frequently used to follow these patients. However, the value of carbon monoxide diffusion capacity to predict early lung disease has been challenged (97). The most effective method for monitoring patients with germ cell tumors is careful physical examination of the chest. Findings of early bleomycin lung disease are a lag or diminished expansion of one hemithorax or fine bibasilar rales that do not clear with cough. These findings can be very subtle, but if present immediate discontinuation of bleomycin should be mandated. It is important to note that randomized trials in good prognosis testicular cancer have suggested that bleomycin is an important component of the treatment regimen, particularly if only three courses of therapy are given (98,99). Other randomized trials have shown that carboplatin is inferior to cisplatin and cannot be substituted for cisplatin without worsening therapeutic outcome (100,101).

Patients with advanced OGCTs should receive three to four courses of treatment given in full dose and on schedule. There is presumptive evidence in testicular cancer that the timeliness of CT may be associated with outcome. Thus, treatment is given regardless of hematologic parameters on the scheduled day of treatment. Because most patients will not develop neutropenic fever or infection, hematopoietic growth factors are not routinely necessary (102). It is reasonable to use hematopoietic growth factors to avoid dose reductions for patients with previous episodes of neutropenic fever or in unusually ill patients who are at a higher risk of myelosuppressive complications or those who received prior radiotherapy. Modern antiemetic therapy, an example of which is shown in **Table 24.7**, has greatly lessened CT-induced emesis. By following these guidelines and providing supportive care as indicated, virtually all patients can be treated on schedule, in full or nearly full dose. CT-related mortality should be less than 1%. In GOG protocol #78, there were no toxic deaths among 93 patients treated. Late effects of CT are discussed below.

Immature Teratoma

The situation of patients with IT is more complex. ITs are categorized as grade 1, 2, or 3 depending on the amount of immature neuroepithelium in the tumor, based on Thurlbeck and Scully's system, which was modified by Norris (2). Our current treatment strategy for adults with ITs is based on a retrospective analysis of 58 patients, in which higher grade correlated with prognosis. Specifically, only 1 of 14 patients with grade 1 IT recurred, but there was an 18% recurrence rate for grade 2 tumors and a 70% recurrence rate for grade 3 tumors (3). These data were further informed by a report of 41 patients with IT by Gershenson et al. (103) in which 94% of patients treated with surgery only recurred, compared with 14% of patients treated with surgery and CT. These studies set the current standard of care for women with IT, which is surveillance for stage I grade 1 IT and adjuvant CT with three courses of BEP for all other patients (4). This recommendation has come into question based on the probable underestimation of tumor stage in the Norris report and multiple studies in the pediatric and adult population that suggest observation may be a viable approach in a subset of these patients. Although surgery followed by adjuvant therapy cures virtually all patients with localized high-grade teratoma, it is possible that the risk of relapse is sufficiently low in a defined population of well-staged patients, to warrant clinical observation with careful follow-up, such that relapsing patients would be diagnosed with small volume tumor and cured with subsequent salvage CT.

Studies supporting surgery without CT in the pediatric population include the Pediatric Oncology Group/Children's Cancer Group Intergroup Study (INT) 0106, which reported on 44 girls with completely resected ovarian IT who were observed closely without adjuvant CT. In this series, 26 patients had grade 2 or 3 IT, and 13 patients had microscopic foci of yolk sac tumor. At 4 years, the event-free survival (EFS) was 97.7% with only one recurrence, which was salvaged with BEP; the OS rate was thus 100%. The authors concluded that surgery alone is curative for children with completely resected ovarian IT (104,105). Additionally, investigators at Mount Vernon and Charing Cross Hospitals in England have observed 15 patients with stage IA tumors after initial surgical treatment (106). Of these, nine patients had grade 2 or 3 IT and six had elements of endodermal sinus tumor. There were three recurrences in this series, one of nine in the pure IT group and two of six in the mixed histology group. Two of these patients were salvaged with CT, and one patient died of pulmonary embolus. Of note is that the patient who died became pregnant 4 months after diagnosis and could not be followed adequately because of her pregnancy. Investigators at the University of Milan have also reported the clinical outcomes of 32 patients with pure ovarian IT followed prospectively (107). In this group, nine patients had grade 2 and 3 stage IA ITs and were treated with surgery and intensive surveillance. Only two recurrences were noted in this group. They consisted of one case of mature teratoma and one case of gliosis. The mature teratoma was resected, and the patient with gliosis was followed without treatment. Both patients are alive and well, and never received CT. Furthermore, among four patients with stage IC tumors treated with surgical resection and surveillance, there was one case of gliosis and one recurrence with mature tissue, which was resected (no CT). All patients are currently free of disease. Subsequently, Mann et al. (108) reported on the outcomes of 54 pediatric patients in the United Kingdom with ovarian IT after complete surgical resection and no adjuvant CT. The EFS and OS rates were 85.9% and 95.1%, respectively, also supporting primary surgical treatment for completely resected ovarian ITs in pediatric patients.

Most recently, the Malignant Germ Cell International Collaborative and the GOG published outcomes on pediatric and adult patients with ovarian ITs to establish a uniform treatment approach across all age groups (109). Of 179 patients included (98 pediatric, 81 adult), 90 pediatric patients had surgery alone, whereas all adult patients had adjuvant CT. The 5-year EFS and OS rates were 91% and 99% among pediatric patients, and were 87% and 93% among adults, respectively. Grade was the most important risk factor for relapse, suggesting that surgery alone was sufficient for patients with grade 1 tumors across all ages and all stages. Because postoperative CT did not decrease relapses in the pediatric cohort, the authors suggest that high-grade recurrent disease in the pediatric patient is not chemosensitive. Adult patients with higher grade tumors may do well with observation alone, using CT or second surgery in the event of relapse. Although this concept is supported by evidence derived from the pediatric literature and limited information in adults, this hypothesis has not been tested prospectively and should be approached with caution until future trials inform best practice for adults.

DYSGERMINOMA

Dysgerminoma is the female equivalent of seminoma. This disease differs from its nondysgerminomatous counterparts in several respects. First, it is more likely to be localized to the ovary at the time of diagnosis (stage I). Bilateral involvement is more common, as is its spread to retroperitoneal lymph nodes. Although less relevant now than before the era of modern CT, dysgerminoma is very sensitive to radiation (29,39,110).

Observation for Stage I Tumors

Approximately 75% to 80% of dysgerminoma patients are stage I at diagnosis (38,111). In a previous era, clinical observation was deemed appropriate for women with tumors less than 10 cm and without contralateral ovarian involvement, whereas adjuvant radiotherapy (RT) was recommended for larger tumors (112). The size-based distinction was subsequently called into question (111,113), and currently observation is considered appropriate for the majority of patients with stage IA disease. In a series reported by LaPolla et al. (111), seven of nine patients with stage IA dysgerminoma followed without postoperative RT remained disease free. All but one patient had tumors greater than 10 cm. In another report, among 14 patients with stage IA dysgerminoma treated with surveillance, 5 recurred. Of those, four patients were salvaged with radiation and one was salvaged with radiation followed by CT. All stage IA patients are alive, free of disease (110). Similarly, Gordon (29) reported that the 5-year survival among 72 patients with stage IA pure dysgerminoma treated conservatively was 95%. The recurrence rate in this case series was 17%, with four deaths attributable to disease. However, in this series, salvage CT was offered to only one patient, which may explain the unfavorable outcomes. A report from Mount Vernon and the Charing Cross Hospitals quoted two relapses among nine patients with stage IA dysgerminoma treated with observation. Both were cured with salvage CT (114). A partial summary of reports' observation after surgery in stage I dysgerminoma is presented in **Table 24.8**.

TABLE 24.8. Results of Clinical Surveillance after Surgery in Patients with Stage IA Dysgerminoma

Institution	Period	Progression Free/Total Number (%)	Overall Survival/Total Number (%)
AFIP (27)	Before 1968	46/57 (79)	52/57 (89)
Hopkins (29)	1930–1981	58/72 (79)	67/72 (92)
Mayo Clinic (110)	1950–1984	9/14 (63)	14/14 (98)
Iowa Hospitals (111)	1935–1985	7/7 (98)	7/7 (98)
M.D. Anderson (112)	1947–1974	5/5 (98)	5/5 (98)
Mount Vernon Hospital (106)	1973–1995	6/9 (65)	9/9 (98)

AFIP, Armed Forces Institute of Pathology.

Currently, patients with stage IA dysgerminoma are observed after unilateral salpingo-oophorectomy, regardless of the size of the primary tumor. Careful follow-up is required, because as many as 15% to 25% of patients will experience a recurrence. However, because of the tumor's chemosensitivity, virtually all patients can be salvaged successfully at the time of recurrence, if adequate early detection of recurrent tumors is achieved.

Radiation Therapy

In the past, many stage I patients and all patients with higher stage tumors received RT (38). Radiation was delivered to the ipsilateral hemipelvis (with shielding of the contralateral ovary and the head of the femur) and to the paraaortic nodes. A single field with the upper limit at T10–T11 and the lower limit at L4–L5 level was used. For stage III retroperitoneal disease, curative RT used an additional field for mediastinum and supraclavicular nodes. In the presence of peritoneal involvement, the whole abdomen and pelvis, mediastinum, and supraclavicular nodes were irradiated. Typically, 30 Gy (7.5 to 9 Gy/week) was given as prophylactic irradiation for stage I tumors. For curative irradiation of stage III disease, 35 to 40 Gy total dose was given to the pelvis, and a boost (10 Gy) was delivered to the involved nodes. When irradiating above the diaphragm, DePalo gave 30 additional Gy 3 to 6 weeks after completion of irradiation below the diaphragm. When irradiating the entire abdominal cavity, the fields were similar to those used for epithelial tumors (112,115–117). The results of RT were excellent. DePalo et al. (38) reported that all 13 stage I patients (12 stage IA and 1 with stage IB) treated with RT were alive and free of disease, with a median follow-up of 77 months. The 5-year relapse-free survival (RFS) for 12 stage III patients was 61.4%, and the OS was 89.5%. Lawson and Adler (115) reported that 10 of 14 stage I–III patients were alive, with a median follow-up of 54 months. In this small series, there was no correlation between survival and the stage of disease or the size of the primary tumor. Others reported similar results, with overall progression-free rates varying between 70% and 90% (see **Table 24.9**) (39,40). However, despite the remarkable radiosensitivity of dysgerminoma, RT is rarely performed nowadays, because CT is equally or more effective, less toxic, and less likely to compromise gonadal function. Given that most patients are cured with surgery alone or surgery and CT, and the young age at the time of diagnosis, consideration should also be given to the delayed carcinogenic effects of intermediate dose radiation. Review of the SEER database shows that 10 of 70 patients (13%) who received RT for a malignant OGCT developed a second cancer, significantly higher than patients who did not receive RT (23).

Chemotherapy

Dysgerminoma is very responsive to cisplatin-based CT (74,118). Since 1984, patients with advanced dysgerminoma were eligible for GOG protocols. Patients enrolled on these studies received three to four courses of PVB or BEP. In a combined analysis, 20 patients were evaluated (119). All had stage III or IV disease and most of them had suboptimal (greater than 2 cm) residual tumor. With a median follow-up of 26 months, 19 of the 20 women were disease free. Among 11 patients with clinically measurable tumor, 10 had complete responses to CT. Fourteen patients who underwent second-look laparotomy had completely negative results. Thus, it appears that nearly all patients with advanced dysgerminoma treated with chemotherapy will be durable complete responders.

Considering that patients with stage III dysgerminoma would require extensive radiation and still carry a risk of failure and that such patients probably fare worse with subsequent CT, it is clear that these patients should be treated primarily with CT. For most,

TABLE 24.9. Effects of Radiotherapy in Women with Pure Dysgerminoma

Institution	Period	Stage	Progression Free/Total Number of Patients (%)
AFIP (27)	Before 1968	I–III	12/14 (84)
Mayo Clinic (110)	1950–1984	I–IV	16/20 (79)
M.D. Anderson (112)	1947–1974	I–III	26/31 (83)
Florence (40)	1960–1983	IC–III	21/26 (79)
NCI Milan (38)	1970–1982	I–III	21/25 (83)
Iowa Hospitals (111)	1935–1985	I–III	12/13 (90)
Sweden (39)	1927–1984	I–IV	49/60 (82)
Egypt (147)	1978–1989	II–III	10/15 (65)
Prince of Whales Hospital (115)	1969–1983	II–III	10/14 (71)

AFIP, Armed Forces Institute of Pathology.

the preferred adjuvant therapy is BEP. This regimen almost invariably prevents recurrence in nondysgerminomatous tumors and certainly will do so in dysgerminoma. Most patients treated with BEP will retain fertility. An alternative regimen tested by the GOG consists of a 3-day regimen with carboplatin and etoposide. On this protocol, all 39 patients with pure dysgerminoma remained free of disease at a median follow-up of 7.8 years (120). Although highly active, this regimen is not recommended for routine use because of significantly less experience accumulated with its use and the concern that this regimen is not as effective in tumors containing nondysgerminomatous elements.

The implications of elevated hCG or AFP levels in patients with dysgerminoma should be emphasized. These tumor markers are usually increased in patients with nondysgerminomatous tumors. Therefore, AFP elevation denotes the presence of elements other than dysgerminoma, and treatment should be tailored accordingly. An elevated hCG level can be occasionally seen in pure dysgerminoma. This finding should not alter therapy, but it should prompt reexamination of the tumor specimen to determine whether syncytiotrophoblastic cells are present or if the tumor contains nondysgerminomatous elements.

In summary, the majority of dysgerminoma patients have stage I disease at diagnosis. These patients can be treated with unilateral salpingo-oophorectomy and can be observed carefully with regular pelvic examinations, abdominopelvic CT, and tumor markers including LDH. Fifteen to 25% of patients observed will experience recurrence and will require CT. In patients with more advanced disease, the risk of recurrence is significant enough to warrant adjuvant treatment. The majority of patients receive three cycles of BEP CT. Radiation might be considered as initial treatment only in unusual circumstances, such as in older patients or in those with serious concomitant illness that preclude the use of systemic CT.

Late Effects of Treatment

As the prognosis of patients with OGCTs has dramatically improved with the evolution of modern combination CT, attention is focused on the late effects of therapy. There is a considerable body of literature on the late effects of treatment in testicular cancer patients, yet the information available for women with OGCTs remains limited. However, many analogies can be drawn.

Sequelae of Surgery

Fertility-sparing surgery is the accepted standard for most patients with malignant OGCT, because most patients are of reproductive age or younger when diagnosed (NCCN guidelines [121]). Young patients with OGCTs undergo at least one, if not multiple, surgical procedures. Although there is no available information on the long-term effects of surgery on these patients, future infertility related to pelvic surgery with subsequent peritoneal and tubal adhesions is well described. Therefore, meticulous surgical technique and avoidance of unnecessary operative maneuvers (e.g., biopsy of a normal contralateral ovary) are required for preventing future complications (44,122,123). Another cause of infertility in this population is unnecessary bilateral salpingo-oophorectomy and hysterectomy, because fertility-sparing surgery is possible in nearly all patients with malignant OGCT, and long-term outcomes including pregnancy are excellent. In a series from Milan, among 55 patients treated with fertility-sparing surgery, without further CT, 12 out of 12 patients who attempted conception became pregnant and 12 normal deliveries were recorded (124). Two additional pregnancies occurred in this group and resulted in termination, one of which was because of in-uterus detection of fetal malformation. Recently, Gershenson reported the findings of GOG protocol 9901 (124). Among 132 survivors of OGCTs treated with surgery and platinum-based CT, 71 patients had fertility-sparing procedures. Of those fertile survivors, 62 (87.3%) maintained menstrual periods and 24 survivors reported 37 successful pregnancies. Although the survivors reported increased incidence of gynecologic problems and diminished sexual pleasure, they also tended to have stronger, more positive relationships with their significant others (125).

The extent of upfront surgical staging required for optimal outcomes is under scrutiny. Pediatric patients with malignant OGCTs typically undergo collection of ascites or cytologic washings and examination of the peritoneal surfaces and retroperitoneal lymph nodes with sampling or excision of abnormal areas, without lymphadenectomy, peritoneal biopsies, or omentectomy (126). Because surveillance may be an acceptable strategy for a growing number of patients, and treatment with CT may be successful in the small percentage of patients who relapse, future investigations may support limiting surgical staging, but this remains the standard of care in adult patients at present. When a patient presents to the gynecologic oncologist after initial surgery with incomplete staging, restaging may not be uniformly indicated, and surveillance may instead be considered (127).

As with any group of patients with a history of pelvic surgery, patients with OGCTs may develop functional cysts in the residual ovary. Muram et al. (127) reported his experience with 27 patients with OGCTs who underwent unilateral salpingo-oophorectomy and were followed for 12 to 215 months after completion of therapy. Of the 18 patients who maintained ovarian function, 13 (72%) developed functional cysts during follow-up. A trial of oral contraceptives and serial ovarian surveillance with sonography is helpful is distinguishing functional cysts from tumor recurrence.

Sequelae of Radiation Therapy

There is limited information about the late effects of RT in dysgerminoma patients. In a review of the late effects of RT in patients receiving abdominal therapy for ovarian dysgerminoma at the MDACC, there was a small increase in reported dyspareunia and the number of bowel movements (128). Somewhat surprisingly, at a median follow-up of 12 years, none of the 43 patients treated with RT developed small bowel obstruction. No other significant intestinal or bladder problems were recorded. As expected, none of the patients treated with radiation conceived (129). A recent review of the SEER database indicates an increased risk of secondary malignancy in patients who received radiation for a malignant OGCT. In this study, 10 of 70 patients (10%) who received RT for a malignant OGCT developed a second cancer, significantly higher than in patients who did not receive RT (23). In practice, RT is rarely administered, because CT is effective and preservation of ovarian function is preferred (37,130).

Sequelae of Chemotherapy

The evolutionary development and refinement of combination CT have resulted in the cure of a high percentage of patients with chemosensitive tumors, such as lymphomas, testicular cancer, gestational trophoblastic disease, and malignant OGCTs. Within the last few years, several reports have described the long-term effects of CT in cancer survivors. As expected, most reports refer to the more common lymphomas and testicular cancers.

A recently recognized effect of CT used for the treatment of germ cell tumors is the risk of secondary malignancies. The epipodophyllotoxins teniposide and etoposide are associated with the development of acute myelogenous leukemia (AML) with certain morphologic and cytogenetic features (131–135). This treatment complication appears to be dose-(131,132) and schedule-dependent (134). Of 348 male germ cell tumor patients receiving three to four courses of BEP as first-line therapy at Indiana University, two developed etoposide-related leukemia. None of the 67 patients who received only three courses developed AML (131). Similarly, in the study reported by Pedersen-Bjergaard et al. (131) 5 out of 212 patients developed acute leukemia or myelodysplastic syndrome after etoposide therapy. However, all patients who developed AML received more than 2,000 mg/m^2 of etoposide. None of the 130 patients who received less than this dose developed AML. Morphologically, these leukemias are monocytic or myelomonocytic (M4 or M5). Characteristic chromosomal translocations (mostly involving the 11q23 region) are frequently, but not always, present. Leukemia after etoposide treatment occurs within 2 to 3 years compared with alkylating agent–induced AML, which has a longer latency period. Late occurrence of chronic myelogenous leukemia after treatment of testicular cancer was reported (136). In the GOG protocol testing the efficacy of BEP in women with OGCTs, 1 case of AML was recorded among 91 patients treated (75). An additional case of lymphoma was diagnosed during follow-up in this series, yet a correlation between CT and lymphoproliferative disorders has not been reported to date. Taking these issues into account, most clinicians consider BEP as the CT regimen of choice. The incidence of second neoplasms is quite low, particularly in patients receiving low cumulative etoposide doses. The continued use of etoposide over vinblastine is based on its superior efficacy demonstrated in testis cancer (71). Furthermore, vinblastine-induced abdominal pain and ileus are troublesome for some patients, particularly for those who underwent abdominal surgery, such as women with OGCTs. The risk/benefit ratio continues to favor etoposide over vinblastine.

There also continues to be considerable focus on the long-term effects of CT on gonadal function. Studies of patients with a variety of cancers suggest that, although ovarian dysfunction or failure is a risk of CT, the majority of survivors can anticipate normal menstrual and reproductive function (137–139). Factors such as old age at initiation of therapy, greater cumulative drug dose (140), and longer duration of therapy (139) have an adverse effect on future gonadal function. Successful pregnancies after treatment with combination CT have been well documented in other types of malignancies, including Hodgkin's disease, non-Hodgkin's lymphomas, and leukemia. There are similar reports in patients with malignant OGCTs (124,141–143). In a review of the MDACC series (141), 27 (68%) of 40 patients who had retained a normal contralateral ovary and uterus maintained regular menses consistently after completion of CT, and 33 (83%) were having regular menses at the time of follow-up. Of 16 patients who had attempted to become pregnant, 12 were successful. One patient underwent an elective first-trimester abortion, and the other 11 patients bore 22 healthy infants over time, none of which had a major birth defect. In a series from Milan, among 169 patients with OGCTs, 138 underwent fertility-sparing surgery, and of those, 81 underwent adjuvant CT (123). After treatment, all but one woman recovered menstrual function, and 55 conceptions were recorded. Forty normal full-term babies were delivered. There were four babies with congenital malformations, one in a patient who did not receive CT and three in women who had received CT (the difference was not statistically significant).

The GOG evaluated the quality of life and psychosocial characteristics of survivors of OGCTs compared with matched controls. In this analysis, the survivors appeared to be well adjusted, were able to develop strong relationships, and were free of significant depression (144). The impact on fertility was modest or none in patients undergoing fertility-sparing surgeries (125). OGCT survivors appeared to be free of any major physical illnesses at a median follow-up of 10 years, as compared with matched controls. The only differences were higher rates of reported hypertension (17% vs. 8%, $p = 0.02$), hypercholesterolemia (9.8% vs. 4.4%, $p = 0.09$), and hearing loss (5.3% vs. 1.5%, $p = 0.09$) compared with controls (145). Among chronic functional problems, numbness, tinnitus, nausea elicited by reminders of CT (vs. general nausea triggers for controls), and Raynaud's symptoms were reported more frequently by survivors. Interestingly, late effects of treatment are more pronounced among children receiving treatment for germ cell tumors (146). Specifically, neurotoxicity, growth abnormalities, pulmonary toxicity, and gastrointestinal toxicity have been reported in a higher proportion than in adult patients. Despite persistence of a few sequelae of treatment, in general, OGCT survivors enjoy a healthy life comparable to that of controls, justifying administration of curative treatment in full and timely dosing.

SUMMARY

Virtually all patients with early-stage, completely resected OGCTs survive after careful surgical staging and three courses of adjuvant BEP. Furthermore, up to 80% of patients with incompletely resected or advanced tumors are expected to be long-term survivors. Acute toxicity of treatment is relatively modest. An important, but fortunately unusual late complication of treatment is etoposide-induced leukemia. However, patients receiving the usually administered cumulative dose of etoposide are at low risk for developing AML. Otherwise, late consequences of CT are limited. Efforts should concentrate on fertility preservation for patients who desire subsequent pregnancies.

The majority of dysgerminoma patients have stage I disease at diagnosis. These patients usually can be treated with unilateral salpingo-oophorectomy and careful postoperative observation without adjuvant treatment. CT is offered at the time of recurrence. In patients with more advanced but resected disease, the risk of recurrence is significant enough to warrant upfront adjuvant treatment, which for most patients is CT because of its near universal effectiveness and limited impact on fertility. In patients with incompletely resected tumor or for patients who recur after previous radiation, CT similar to that given for tumors other than dysgerminoma is appropriate.

Surgery continues to have a pivotal role in the management of all patients with OGCTs. Initial careful surgical staging is important in selecting appropriate subsequent therapy (although this is currently a matter of some debate). Second-look laparotomy is not necessary in patients who have no residual tumor after their initial surgical procedure and who receive adjuvant CT. This procedure also does not seem warranted in patients with advanced tumors without elements of teratoma. The judicious use of surgery followed by CT will cure the majority of patients with OGCTs at the expense of minimal and predictable immediate and late toxicities. The role of surveillance in low-risk patients is expanding. In most circumstances, fertility can be preserved.

INTERNATIONAL PERSPECTIVES

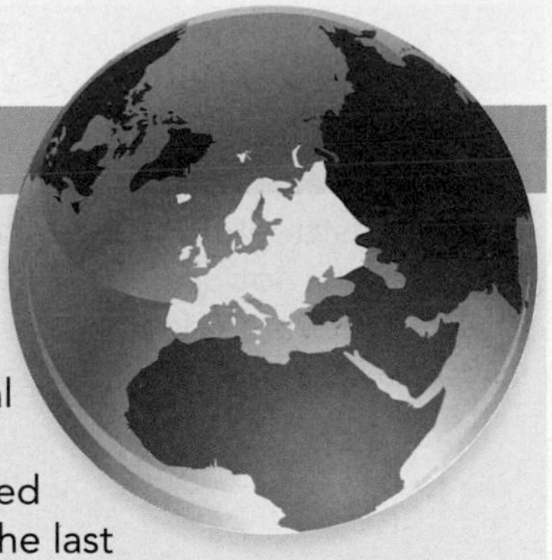

Ovarian Germ Cell Tumors: The Spanish View

Luis M. Chiva, MD, PhD

Germ cell tumors of the ovary, which are relatively uncommon, exemplify a special group of female tumors that are associated with an excellent prognosis after adequate surgical and adjuvant therapy. This excellent prognosis has been attributed to the tumors' biologic characteristics, as well as improvements in treatment over the last few decades.

Specific features of these tumors make their management unique. For example, early age at onset calls for a physician/patient shared decision-making process for the consideration of fertility-sparing options. Even adjuvant therapy with platinum-based CT does not preclude future pregnancies. Furthermore, the elevation of specific tumor-associated markers at the time of diagnosis and relapse gives us the opportunity to offer timely therapeutic interventions.

In Spain, germ cell tumors are rare, and patients who develop these tumors are typically managed as in the United States. In many cases, the diagnosis is made after an unexpected finding during a laparoscopic procedure undertaken to assess a pelvic mass in a young woman. After referral to a gynecologic oncologist, laparotomy and comprehensive surgical staging are usually performed. A fertility-sparing procedure can be offered to young patients. Adjuvant therapy (usually BEP) is given in most cases, except to patients with stage IA or IB pure dysgerminoma or stage IA pure IT, grade 1.

Follow-up is carried out similar to that of patients with epithelial tumors, including the assessment of specific tumor markers. CT scan is the basic imaging tool for ruling out recurrence and subsequently PET/CT scan if any suspicious findings are identified.

Unfortunately in Spain, as in other countries, there are still unanswered questions in the management of these tumors, such as whether thorough surgical staging is needed, the definitive indications for adjuvant CT, the best chemotherapeutic combinations in recurrent disease, and the most efficient surveillance schedule. Furthermore, there are poorly understood differences in treatment approaches between pediatric oncologists and gynecologic oncologists that should be explored and clarified. International collaborative trials among specialties investigating these rare tumors, even though challenging, are one of the safest ways to address some of the unknown aspects of this disease.

INTERNATIONAL PERSPECTIVES

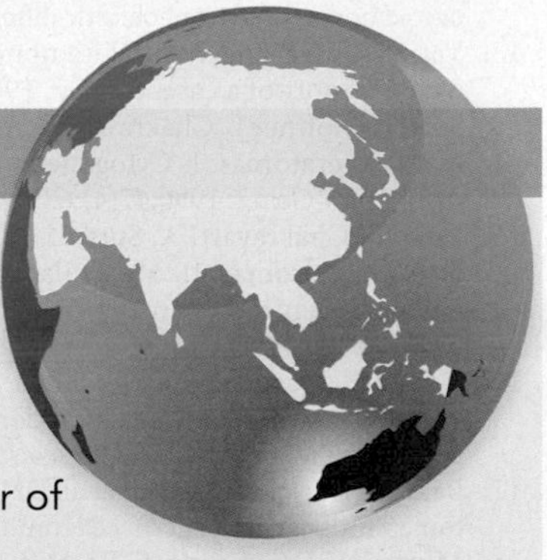

Ovarian Germ Cell Tumors (Korea)

Sang-Yoon Park, MD, PhD

In South Korea, the incidence of OGCTs has not changed significantly over the past decade, with 127 cases reported in 1999 and 122 cases reported in 2011. In contrast, there has been a slightly increased incidence of epithelial ovarian cancer of 1.5% annually.

As in other parts of the world, OGCTs, compared with epithelial ovarian cancer, are typically diagnosed at a young age. Issues of concern in the management of these tumors include fertility preservation and the late effects of cancer and its treatment. Fortunately, high cure rates can be expected. In general, we consider fertility preservation even in cases involving the ovaries, uterus, and brain. Therefore, multidisciplinary team care is strongly advocated in our institution and in our country. Because OGCTs are chemosensitive in most cases, cure is our primary treatment endpoint. Therefore, timely initiation of CT without delay is stressed.

With the exception of stage IA dysgerminoma or grade I IT, in which surveillance is appropriate, we recommend adjuvant CT for all patients. Our standard regimen consists of four cycles of combination BEP, and we

(*continued*)

INTERNATIONAL PERSPECTIVES (*continued*)

expect greater than 90% of patients to be rendered disease-free. Alternative regimens include PVB or carboplatin and etoposide. For patients with recurrent germ cell tumors, we generally use taxanes and gemcitabine.

For posttreatment surveillance, we follow appropriate tumor markers, such as AFP and/or hCG. If tumor markers are not useful in a particular patient's germ cell tumor type, sonography and MRI scans are preferred over CT scans to decrease radiation exposure. Our patients are educated on the long-term morbidities of specific CT regimens, and they are followed accordingly.

REFERENCES

1. Tavassoli FA, Devilee P, eds. *World Health Organization Classification of Tumors: Pathology and Genetics of Tumours of the Breast and Female Genital Organs*. Lyon, France: IARC Press; 2003.
2. Kurman RJ, Norris HJ. Malignant germ cell tumors of the ovary. *Hum Pathol*. 1977;8(5):551–564.
3. Cheng L, Thomas A, Roth LM, et al. OCT4: a novel biomarker for dysgerminoma of the ovary. *Am J Surg Pathol*. 2004;28(10):1341–1346.
4. Sever M, Jones TD, Roth LM, et al. Expression of CD117 (c-kit) receptor in dysgerminoma of the ovary: diagnostic and therapeutic implications. *Mod Pathol*. 2005;18(11):1411–1416.
5. Hoei-Hansen CE, Kraggerud SM, Abeler VM, et al. Ovarian dysgerminomas are characterised by frequent KIT mutations and abundant expression of pluripotency markers. *Mol Cancer*. 2007;6:12.
6. Cheng L, Roth LM, Zhang S, et al. KIT gene mutation and amplification in dysgerminoma of the ovary. *Cancer*. 2011;117(10):2096–2103.
7. Kurman RJ, Norris HJ. Endodermal sinus tumor of the ovary: a clinical and pathologic analysis of 71 cases. *Cancer*. 1976;38(6):2404–2419.
8. Roth LM. Variants of yolk sac tumor. *Pathol Case Rev*. 2004;10:186–192.
9. Damjanov I, Amenta PS, Zarghami F. Transformation of an AFP-positive yolk sac carcinoma into an AFP-negative neoplasm. Evidence for in vivo cloning of the human parietal yolk sac carcinoma. *Cancer*. 1984;53:1902–1907.
10. Ramalingam P, Malpica A, Silva EG, et al. The use of cytokeratin 7 and EMA in differentiating ovarian yolk sac tumors from endometrioid and clear cell carcinomas. *Am J Surg Pathol*. 2004;28(11):1499–1505.
11. Kurman RJ, Norris HJ. Embryonal carcinoma of the ovary: a clinicopathologic entity distinct from endodermal sinus tumor resembling embryonal carcinoma of the adult testis. *Cancer*. 1976;38:2420–2433.
12. Beck JS, Fulmer HF, Lee ST. Solid malignant ovarian teratoma with "embryoid bodies" and trophoblastic differentiation. *J Pathol*. 1969;99(1):67–73.
13. Vance RP, Geisinger KR. Pure nongestational choriocarcinoma of the ovary. Report of a case. *Cancer*. 1985;56(9):2321–2325.
14. Surti U, Hoffner L, Chakravarti A, et al. Genetics and biology of human ovarian teratomas. I. Cytogenetic analysis and mechanism of origin. *Am J Hum Genet*. 1990;47(4):635–643.
15. Deka R, Chakravarti A, Surti U, et al. Genetics and biology of human ovarian teratomas. II. Molecular analysis of origin of nondisjunction and gene-centromere mapping of chromosome I markers. *Am J Hum Genet*. 1990;47(4):644–655.
16. Tabata E, Masuda M, Eriguchi M, et al. Immunopathological significance of ovarian teratoma in patients with anti-N-methyl-d-aspartate receptor encephalitis. *Eur Neurol*. 2014;71(1–2):42–48
17. Baker BA, Frickey L, Yu IT, et al. DNA content of ovarian immature teratomas and malignant germ cell tumors. *Gynecol Oncol*. 1998;71(1):14–18.
18. Murty VV, Dmitrovsky E, Bosl GJ, et al. Nonrandom chromosome abnormalities in testicular and ovarian germ cell tumor cell lines. *Cancer Genet Cytogenet*. 1990;50(1):67–73.
19. Speleman F, De Potter C, Dal Cin P, et al. i(12p) in a malignant ovarian tumor. *Cancer Genet Cytogenet*. 1990;45(1):49–53.
20. Shen DH, Khoo US, Zhang Y, et al. Cytogenetic study of malignant ovarian germ cell tumors by chromosome in situ hybridization. *Int J Gynecol Cancer*. 1998;8:222–232.
21. Murray MJ, Halsall DJ, Hook CE, et al. Identification of microRNAs from the miR-371-373 and miR-302 clusters as potential serum biomarkers of malignant germ cell tumors. *Am J Clin Pathol*. 2011;135:119–125.
22. Gershenson DM, Copeland LJ, Kavanagh JJ, et al. Treatment of malignant nondysgerminomatous germ cell tumors of the ovary with vincristine, dactinomycin, and cyclophosphamide. *Cancer*. 1985;56(12):2756–2761.
23. Solheim O, Gershenson DM, Trope CG, et al. Prognostic factors in malignant ovarian germ cell tumors (The Surveillance, Epidemiology, and End Results experience 1978-2010). *Eur J Cancer*. 2014;50:1942–1950.
24. Poynter JN, Amatruda JF, Ross JA. Trends in incidence and survival of pediatric and adolescent patients with germ cell tumors in the United States, 1975 to 2006. *Cancer*. 2010;116(20): 4882–4891.
25. Poynter JN, Radzom AH, Spector LG, et al. Family history of cancer and malignant germ cell tumors in children: a report from the Children's Oncology Group. *Cancer Causes Control*. 2010;21(2):181–189.
26. Gershenson DM, Del Junco G, Copeland LJ, et al. Mixed germ cell tumors of the ovary. *Obstet Gynecol*. 1984;64(2):200–206.
27. Asadourian LA, Taylor HB. Dysgerminoma. An analysis of 105 cases. *Obstet Gynecol*. 1969;33(3):370–379.
28. De Backer A, Madern GC, Oosterhuis JW, et al. Ovarian germ cell tumors in children: a clinical study of 66 patients. *Pediatr Blood Cancer*. 2006;46(4):459–464.
29. Gordon A, Lipton D, Woodruff JD. Dysgerminoma: a review of 158 cases from the Emil Novak Ovarian Tumor Registry. *Obstet Gynecol*. 1981;58(4):497–504.
30. Christman JE, Teng NN, Lebovic GS, et al. Delivery of a normal infant following cisplatin, vinblastine, and bleomycin (PVB) chemotherapy for malignant teratoma of the ovary during pregnancy. *Gynecol Oncol*. 1990;37(2):292–295.
31. Farahmand SM, Marchetti DL, Asirwatham JE, et al. Ovarian endodermal sinus tumor associated with pregnancy: review of the literature. *Gynecol Oncol*. 1991;41:156–160.
32. Horbelt D, Delmore J, Meisel R, et al. Mixed germ cell malignancy of the ovary concurrent with pregnancy. *Obstet Gynecol*. 1994;84(4 pt 2):662–664.
33. Rajendran S, Hollingworth J, Scudamore I. Endodermal sinus tumour of the ovary in pregnancy. *Eur J Gynaecol Oncol*. 1999;20(4):272–274.
34. Bakri YN, Ezzat A, Akhtar, et al. Malignant germ cell tumors of the ovary. Pregnancy considerations. *Eur J Obstet Gynecol Reprod Biol*. 2000;90(1):87–91.
35. Sekiya S, Seki K, Nagai Y. Rise of serum CA 125 in patients with pure ovarian yolk sac tumors. *Int J Gynaecol Obstet*. 1997;58(3):323–324.
36. Mangili G, Sigismondi C, Gadducci A, et al. Outcome and risk factors for recurrence in malignant ovarian germ cell tumors: a MITO-9 retrospective study. *Int J Gynecol Cancer*. 2011;21(8):1414–1421.
37. Ayhan A, Bildirici I, Gunalp S, et al. Pure dysgerminoma of the ovary: a review of 45 well staged cases. *Eur J Gynaecol Oncol*. 2000;21(1):98–101.
38. De Palo G, Lattuada A, Kenda R, et al. Germ cell tumors of the ovary: the experience of the National Cancer Institute of Milan. I. Dysgerminoma. *Int J Radiat Oncol Biol Phys*. 1987;13(6):853–860.
39. Bjorkholm E, Lundell M, Gyftodimos A, et al. Dysgerminoma. The Radiumhemmet series 1927–1984. *Cancer*. 1990;65(1):38–44.
40. Santoni R, Cionini L, D'Elia F, et al. Dysgerminoma of the ovary: a report on 29 patients. *Clin Radiol*. 1987;38(2):203–206.
41. Berg FD, Kurzl R, Hinrichsen MJ, et al. Familial 46, XY pure gonadal dysgenesis and gonadoblastoma/dysgerminoma: case report. *Gynecol Oncol*. 1989;32(2):261–267.
42. Fisher RA, Salm R, Spencer RW. Bilateral gonadoblastoma/dysgerminoma in a 46 XY individual: case report with hormonal studies. *J Clin Pathol*. 1982;35(4):420–424.
43. Kingsbury AC, Frost F, Cookson WO. Dysgerminoma, gonadoblastoma, and testicular germ cell neoplasia in phenotypically female and male siblings with 46 XY genotype. Cancer. 1987;59(2):288–291.
44. Schwartz PE. Surgery of germ cell tumours of the ovary. Forum (Genova). 2000;10(4):355–365.

45. Peccatori F, Bonazzi C, Chiari S, et al. Surgical management of malignant ovarian germ-cell tumors: 10 years' experience of 129 patients. *Obstet Gynecol.* 1995;86(3):367–372.
46. Gershenson DM. Fertility-sparing surgery for malignancies in women. *J Natl Cancer Inst Monogr.* 2005;34(1):43–47.
47. Saunders DM, Ferrier AJ, Ryan J. Fertility preservation in female oncology patients. *Int J Gynecol Cancer.* 1996;6:161–167.
48. Slayton RE, Hreshchyshyn MM, Silverberg SC, et al. Treatment of malignant ovarian germ cell tumors: response to vincristine, dactinomycin, and cyclophosphamide (preliminary report). *Cancer.* 1978;42(2):390–398.
49. Williams SD, Blessing JA, Moore DH, et al. Cisplatin, vinblastine, and bleomycin in advanced and recurrent ovarian germ-cell tumors. A trial of the Gynecologic Oncology Group. *Ann Intern Med.* 1989;111(1):22–27.
50. Scarabelli C, Gallo A, Carbone A. Secondary cytoreductive surgery for patients with recurrent epithelial ovarian carcinoma. *Gynecol Oncol.* 2001;83(3):504–512.
51. Parazzini F, Raspagliesi F, Guarnerio P, et al. Role of secondary surgery in relapsed ovarian cancer. *Crit Rev Oncol Hematol.* 2001;37(2):121–125.
52. Williams SD, Blessing JA, DiSaia PJ, et al. Second-look laparotomy in ovarian germ cell tumors: the gynecologic oncology group experience. *Gynecol Oncol.* 1994;52(3):287–291.
53. Andre F, Fizazi K, Culine S, et al. The growing teratoma syndrome: results of therapy and long-term follow-up of 33 patients. *Eur J Cancer.* 2000;36(11):1389–1394.
54. Chen RJ, Huang PT, Lin MC, et al. Advanced stage squamous cell carcinoma arising from mature cystic teratoma of the ovary. *Acta Obstet Gynecol Scand.* 2001;80(1):84–86.
55. Ronnett BM, Seidman JD. Mucinous tumors arising in ovarian mature cystic teratomas: relationship to the clinical syndrome of pseudomyxoma peritonei. *Am J Surg Pathol.* 2003;27(5):650–657.
56. Vartanian RK, McRae B, Hessler RB. Sebaceous carcinoma arising in a mature cystic teratoma of the ovary. *Int J Gynecol Pathol.* 2002;21(4):418–421.
57. Shen DH, Khoo US, Xue WC, et al. Ovarian mature cystic teratoma with malignant transformation. An interphase cytogenetic study. *Int J Gynecol Pathol.* 1998;17(4):351–357.
58. Geisler JP, Goulet R, Foster RS, et al. Growing teratoma syndrome after chemotherapy for germ cell tumors of the ovary. *Obstet Gynecol.* 1994;84 (4 pt 2):719–721.
59. Itani Y, Kawa M, Toyoda S, et al. Growing teratoma syndrome after chemotherapy for a mixed germ cell tumor of the ovary. *J Obstet Gynaecol Res.* 2002;28(3):166–171.
60. Kattan J, Droz JP, Culine S, et al. The growing teratoma syndrome: a woman with nonseminomatous germ cell tumor of the ovary. *Gynecol Oncol.* 1993;49(3):395–399.
61. Gershenson DM, Copeland LJ, del Junco G, et al. Second-look laparotomy in the management of malignant germ cell tumors of the ovary. *Obstet Gynecol.* 1986;67(6):789–793.
62. Albers P, Bender H, Yilmaz H, et al. Positron emission tomography in the clinical staging of patients with Stage I and II testicular germ cell tumors. *Urology.* 1999;53(4):808–811.
63. Hain SF, O'Doherty MJ, Timothy AR, et al. Fluorodeoxyglucose positron emission tomography in the evaluation of germ cell tumours at relapse. *Br J Cancer.* 2000;83(7):863–869.
64. Kollmannsberger C, Oechsle K, Dohmen BM, et al. Prospective comparison of [18F]fluorodeoxyglucose positron emission tomography with conventional assessment by computed tomography scans and serum tumor markers for the evaluation of residual masses in patients with nonseminomatous germ cell carcinoma. *Cancer.* 2002;94(9):2353–2362.
65. Sanchez D, Zudaire JJ, Fernandez JM, et al. 18F-fluoro-2-deoxyglucose-positron emission tomography in the evaluation of nonseminomatous germ cell tumours at relapse. *BJU Int.* 2002;89(9):912–916.
66. Sugawara Y, Zasadny KR, Grossman HB, et al. Germ cell tumor: differentiation of viable tumor, mature teratoma, and necrotic tissue with FDG PET and kinetic modeling. *Radiology.* 1999;211(1):249–256.
67. Becherer A, De Santis M, Karanikas G, et al. FDG-PET is superior to CT in the prediction of viable tumour in post-chemotherapy seminoma residuals. *Eur J Radiol.* 2005;54(2):284–288.
68. Murphy JJ, Tawfeeq M, Chang B, et al. Early experience with PET/CT scan in the evaluation of pediatric abdominal neoplasms. *J Pediatr Surg.* 2008;43(12):2186–2192.
69. Basu S, Rubello D. PET imaging in the management of tumors of testis and ovary: current thinking and future directions. *Minerva Endocrinol.* 2008;33(3):229–256.
70. Einhorn LH, Donohue J. Cis-diamminedichloroplatinum, vinblastine, and bleomycin combination chemotherapy in disseminated testicular cancer. *Ann Intern Med.* 1977;87(3):293–298.
71. Williams SD, Birch R, Einhorn LH, et al. Treatment of disseminated germ-cell tumors with cisplatin, bleomycin, and either vinblastine or etoposide. *N Engl J Med.* 1987;316(23):1435–1440.
72. Slayton RE, Park RC, Silverberg SG, et al. Vincristine, dactinomycin, and cyclophosphamide in the treatment of malignant germ cell tumors of the ovary. A Gynecologic Oncology Group Study (a final report). *Cancer.* 1985;56(2):243–248.
73. Gershenson DM, Kavanagh JJ, Copeland LJ, et al. Treatment of malignant nondysgerminomatous germ cell tumors of the ovary with vinblastine, bleomycin, and cisplatin. *Cancer.* 1986;57(9):1731–1737.
74. Gershenson DM, Morris M, Cangir A, et al. Treatment of malignant germ cell tumors of the ovary with bleomycin, etoposide, and cisplatin. *J Clin Oncol.* 1990;8(4):715–720.
75. Williams S, Blessing JA, Liao SY, et al. Adjuvant therapy of ovarian germ cell tumors with cisplatin, etoposide, and bleomycin: a trial of the Gynecologic Oncology Group. *J Clin Oncol.* 1994;12(4):701–706.
76. Culine S, Lhomme C, Kattan J, et al. Cisplatin-based chemotherapy in the management of germ cell tumors of the ovary: The Institut Gustave Roussy Experience. *Gynecol Oncol.* 1997;64(1):160–165.
77. Segelov E, Campbell J, Ng M, et al. Cisplatin-based chemotherapy for ovarian germ cell malignancies: the Australian experience. *J Clin Oncol.* 1994;12(2):378–384.
78. Dimopoulos MA, Papadopoulou M, Andreopoulou E, et al. Favorable outcome of ovarian germ cell malignancies treated with cisplatin or carboplatin-based chemotherapy: a Hellenic Cooperative Oncology Group study. *Gynecol Oncol.* 1998;70(1):70–74.
79. Einhorn LH. Curing metastatic testicular cancer. *Proc Natl Acad Sci USA.* 2002;99(7):4592–4595.
80. Einhorn LH, Williams SD, Loehrer PJ, et al. Evaluation of optimal duration of chemotherapy in favorable-prognosis disseminated germ cell tumors: a Southeastern Cancer Study Group protocol. *J Clin Oncol.* 1989;7(3):387–391.
81. Einhorn LH. Salvage therapy for germ cell tumors. *Semin Oncol.* 1994;21(4 suppl 7):47–51.
82. Bokemeyer C, Kollmannsberger C, Meisner C, et al. First-line high-dose chemotherapy compared with standard-dose PEB/VIP chemotherapy in patients with advanced germ cell tumors: a multivariate and matched-pair analysis. *J Clin Oncol.* 1999;17(11):3450–3456.
83. Motzer RJ, Nichols CJ, Margolin KA, et al. Phase III randomized trial of conventional-dose chemotherapy with or without high-dose chemotherapy and autologous hematopoietic stem-cell rescue as first-line treatment for patients with poor-prognosis metastatic germ cell tumors. *J Clin Oncol.* 2007;25(3):247–256.
84. Daugaard G, Skoneczna I, Aass N, et al. A randomized phase III study comparing standard dose BEP with sequential high-dose cisplatin, etoposide, and ifosfamide (VIP) plus stem-cell support in males with poor-prognosis germ-cell cancer. An intergroup study of EORTC, GTCSG, and Grupo Germinal (EORTC 30974). *Ann Oncol.* 2011;22:1054–1061.
85. Murugaesu N, Schmid P, Dancey G, et al. Malignant ovarian germ cell tumors: identification of novel prognostic markers and long-term outcome after multimodality treatment. *J Clin Oncol.* 2006;24(30):4862–4866.
86. Messing MJ, Gershenson DM, Morris M, et al. Primary treatment failure in patients with malignant ovarian germ cell neoplasms. *Int J Gynecol Cancer.* 1992;2(6):295–300.
87. Broun ER, Nichols CR, Turns M, et al. Early salvage therapy for germ cell cancer using high dose chemotherapy with autologous bone marrow support. *Cancer.* 1994;73(6):1716–1720.
88. Broun ER, Nichols CR, Gize G, et al. Tandem high dose chemotherapy with autologous bone marrow transplantation for initial relapse of testicular germ cell cancer. *Cancer.* 1997;79(8):1605–1610.
89. Lotz JP, Andre T, Donsimoni R, et al. High dose chemotherapy with ifosfamide, carboplatin, and etoposide combined with autologous bone marrow transplantation for the treatment of poor-prognosis germ cell tumors and metastatic trophoblastic disease in adults. *Cancer.* 1995;75(3):874–885.
90. Einhorn LH, Williams SD, Chamness A, et al. High dose chemotherapy and stem cell rescue for metastatic germ cell rumors. *N Engl J Med.* 2007;357(4):340–348.
91. Ammakkanavar NR, Matei D, Abonour R, et al. High-dose chemotherapy for recurrent ovarian germ cell tumors. *J Clin Oncol.* 2015;33(2):226–227.

92. Loehrer PJ, Gonin R, Nichols CR, et al. Vinblastine plus ifosfamide plus cisplatin as initial salvage therapy in recurrent germ cell tumor. *J Clin Oncol.* 1998;16(7):2500–2504.
93. Hinton S, Catalano P, Einhorn LH, et al. Phase II study of paclitaxel plus gemcitabine in refractory germ cell tumors (E9897): a trial of the Eastern Cooperative Oncology Group. *J Clin Oncol.* 2002;20(7):1859–1863.
94. Einhorn LH, Brames MJ, Juliar B, et al. Phase II study of paclitaxel plus gemcitabine salvage chemotherapy for germ cell tumors after progression following high-dose chemotherapy with tandem transplant. *J Clin Oncol.* 2007;25(5):513–516.
95. Kollmannsberger C, Beyer J, Liersch R, et al. Combination chemotherapy with gemcitabine plus oxaliplatin in patients with intensively pretreated or refractory germ cell cancer: a study of the German Testicular Cancer Study Group. *J Clin Oncol.* 2004;22(1):108–114.
96. Vaughn DJ, Hwang WT, Lal P, et al. Phase 2 trial of the cyclin-dependent kinase 4/6 inhibitor palbociclib in patients with retinoblastoma protein-expressing germ cell tumors. *Cancer.* 2015;121(9):1463–1468.
97. McKeage MJ, Evans BD, Atkinson C, et al. Carbon monoxide diffusing capacity is a poor predictor of clinically significant bleomycin lung. New Zealand Clinical Oncology Group. *J Clin Oncol.* 1990;8(5):779–783.
98. Loehrer PJ, Johnson D, Elson P, et al. Importance of bleomycin in favorable-prognosis disseminated germ cell tumors: an Eastern Cooperative Oncology Group trial. *J Clin Oncol.* 1995;13(2):470–476.
99. de Wit R, Stoter G, Kaye SB, et al. Importance of bleomycin in combination chemotherapy for good-prognosis testicular nonseminoma: a randomized study of the European Organization for Research and Treatment of Cancer Genitourinary Tract Cancer Cooperative Group. *J Clin Oncol.* 1997;15:1837–1843.
100. Bajorin DF, Sarosdy MF, Pfister DG, et al. Randomized trial of etoposide and cisplatin versus etoposide and carboplatin in patients with good-risk germ cell tumors: a multiinstitutional study. *J Clin Oncol.* 1993;11(4):598–606.
101. Horwich A, Sleijfer DT, Fossa SD, et al. Randomized trial of bleomycin, etoposide, and cisplatin compared with bleomycin, etoposide, and carboplatin in good-prognosis metastatic nonseminomatous germ cell cancer: a Multiinstitutional Medical Research Council/European Organization for Research and Treatment of Cancer Trial. *J Clin Oncol.* 1997;15:1844–1852.
102. American Society of Clinical Oncology. Recommendations for the use of hematopoietic colony-stimulating factors: evidence-based, clinical practice guidelines. *J Clin Oncol.* 1994;12(11):2471–2508.
103. Gershenson DM, del Junco G, Silva EG, et al. Immature teratoma of ovary. *Obstet Gynecol.* 1986;68:624–629.
104. Cushing B, Giller R, Ablin A, et al. Surgical resection alone is effective treatment for ovarian immature teratoma in children and adolescents: a report of the pediatric oncology group and the children's cancer group. *Am J Obstet Gynecol.* 1999;181(2):353–358.
105. Marina NM, Cushing B, Giller R, et al. Complete surgical excision is effective treatment for children with immature teratomas with or without malignant elements: a Pediatric Oncology Group/Children's Cancer Group Intergroup Study. *J Clin Oncol.* 1999;17(7):2137–2143.
106. Dark GG, Bower M, Newlands ES, et al. Surveillance policy for stage I ovarian germ cell tumors. *J Clin Oncol.* 1997;15(2):620–624.
107. Bonazzi C, Peccatori F, Colombo N, et al. Pure ovarian immature teratoma, a unique and curable disease: 10 years' experience of 32 prospectively treated patients. *Obstet Gynecol.* 1994;84(4):598–604.
108. Mann JR, Gray ES, Thornton C, et al. Mature and immature extracranial teratomas in children: the UK Children's Cancer Study Group experience. *J Clin Oncol.* 2008;26:3590–3597.
109. Pashankar F, Hale JP, Dang H, et al. Is adjuvant chemotherapy indicated in ovarian immature teratomas? A combined data analysis from the Malignant Germ Cell Tumor International Collaborative. *Cancer.* 2016;122(2):230–237.
110. Buskirk SJ, Schray MF, Podratz KC, et al. Ovarian dysgerminoma: a retrospective analysis of results of treatment, sites of treatment failure, and radiosensitivity. *Mayo Clin Proc.* 1987;62(12):1149–1157.
111. LaPolla JP, Benda J, Vigliotti AP, et al. Dysgerminoma of the ovary. *Obstet Gynecol.* 1987;69(6):859–864.
112. Krepart G, Smith JP, Rutledge F, et al. The treatment for dysgerminoma of the ovary. *Cancer.* 1978;41(3):986–990.
113. Thomas GM, Dembo AJ, Hacker NF, et al. Current therapy for dysgerminoma of the ovary. *Obstet Gynecol.* 1987;70(2):268–275.
114. Patterson DM, Murugaesu N, Holden L, et al. A review of the close surveillance policy for stage I female germ cell tumors of the ovary and other sites. *Int J Gynecol Cancer.* 2008;18(1): 43–50.
115. Lawson AP, Adler GF. Radiotherapy in the treatment of ovarian dysgerminomas. *Int J Radiat Oncol Biol Phys.* 1988;14(3):431–434.
116. Freed JH, Cassir JF, Pierce VK, et al. Dysgerminoma of the ovary. *Cancer.* 1979;43(3):798–805.
117. Marks RD, Underwood PB, Othersen HB, et al. Dysgerminoma—100% control with combined therapy in six consecutive patients with advanced disease. *Int J Radiat Oncol Biol Phys.* 1978;4(5–6):453–456.
118. Culine S, Lhomme C, Kattan J, et al. Cisplatin-based chemotherapy in dysgerminoma of the ovary: thirteen-year experience at the Institut Gustave Roussy. *Gynecol Oncol.* 1995;58(3):344–348.
119. Williams SD, Blessing JA, Hatch KD, et al. Chemotherapy of advanced dysgerminoma: trials of the Gynecologic Oncology Group. *J Clin Oncol.* 1991;9(11):1950–1955.
120. Williams SD, Kauderer J, Burnett AF, et al. Adjuvant therapy of completely resected dysgerminoma with carboplatin and etoposide: a trial of the Gynecologic Oncology Group. *Gynecol Oncol.* 2004;95(3):496–499.
121. http://www.nccn.org/professionals/physician_gls/pdf/aya.pdf
122. Kanazawa K, Suzuki T, Sakumoto K. Treatment of malignant ovarian germ cell tumors with preservation of fertility: reproductive performance after persistent remission. *Am J Clin Oncol.* 2000;23(3):244–248.
123. Zanetta G, Bonazzi C, Cantu M, et al. Survival and reproductive function after treatment of malignant germ cell ovarian tumors. *J Clin Oncol.* 2001;19(4):1015–1020.
124. Gershenson DM, Miller AM, Champion VL, et al. Reproductive and sexual function after platinum-based chemotherapy in long-term ovarian germ cell tumor survivors: a Gynecologic Oncology Group Study. *J Clin Oncol.* 2007;25(19):2792–2797.
125. Billmore D, Vinocur C, Rescorla F, et al. Outcome and staging evaluation in malignant germ cell tumors of the ovary in children and adolescents: an intergroup study. *Int J Gynecol Cancer.* 2011;21:1414–1421.
126. Gershenson DM. Current advances in the management of malignant germ cell and stromal tumors of the ovary. *Gynecol Oncol.* 2012;125:515–517.
127. Muram D, Gale CL, Thompson E. Functional ovarian cysts in patients cured of ovarian neoplasms. *Obstet Gynecol.* 1990;75(4):680–683.
128. Howell S, Shalet S. Gonadal damage from chemotherapy and radiotherapy. *Endocrinol Metab Clin North Am.* 1998;27(4):927–943.
129. Casey AC, Bhodauria S, Shapter A, et al. Dysgerminoma: the role of conservative surgery. *Gynecol Oncol.* 1996;63(3):352–357.
130. Nichols CR, Breeden ES, Loehrer PJ, et al. Secondary leukemia associated with a conventional dose of etoposide: review of serial germ cell tumor protocols. *J Natl Cancer Inst.* 1993;85(1):36–40.
131. Pedersen-Bjergaard J, Daugaard G, Hansen SW, et al. Increased risk of myelodysplasia and leukaemia after etoposide, cisplatin, and bleomycin for germ-cell tumours. *Lancet.* 1991;338(8763):359–363.
132. Pui CH. Epipodophyllotoxin-related acute myeloid leukaemia. *Lancet.* 1991;338(8780):1468.
133. Pui CH, Ribeiro RC, Hancock ML, et al. Acute myeloid leukemia in children treated with epipodophyllotoxins for acute lymphoblastic leukemia. *N Engl J Med.* 1991;325(24):1682–1687.
134. Ratain MJ, Kaminer LS, Bitran JD, et al. Acute nonlymphocytic leukemia following etoposide and cisplatin combination chemotherapy for advanced non-small-cell carcinoma of the lung. *Blood.* 1987;70(5):1412–1417.
135. Pedersen-Bjergaard J, Brondum-Nielsen K, Karle H, et al. Chemotherapy-related - late occurring – Philadelphia chromosome in AML, ALL and CML. Similar events related to treatment with DNA topoisomerase II inhibitors? *Leukemia.* 1997;11(9):1571–1574.
136. Horning SJ, Hoppe RT, Kaplan HS, et al. Female reproductive potential after treatment for Hodgkin's disease. *N Engl J Med.* 1981;304(23): 1377–1382.
137. Byrne J, Mulvihill JJ, Myers MH, et al. Effects of treatment on fertility in long-term survivors of childhood or adolescent cancer. *N Engl J Med.* 1987;317(21):1315–1321.
138. Siris ES, Leventhal BG, Vaitukaitis JL. Effects of childhood leukemia and chemotherapy on puberty and reproductive function in girls. *N Engl J Med.* 1976;294(21):1143–1146.
139. Nicosia SV, Matus-Ridley M, Meadows AT. Gonadal effects of cancer therapy in girls. *Cancer.* 1985;55(10):2364–2372.
140. Gershenson DM. Menstrual and reproductive function after treatment with combination chemotherapy for malignant ovarian germ cell tumors. *J Clin Oncol.* 1988;6(2):270–275.
141. Brewer M, Gershenson DM, Herzog CE, et al. Outcome and reproductive function after chemotherapy for ovarian dysgerminoma. *J Clin Oncol.* 1999;17(9):2670–2675.
142. Pektasides D, Rustin GJ, Newlands ES, et al. Fertility after chemotherapy for ovarian germ cell tumours. *Br J Obstet Gynaecol.* 1987;94(5):477–479.

143. Rustin GJ, Pektasides D, Bagshawe KD, et al. Fertility after chemotherapy for male and female germ cell tumours. *Int J Androl.* 1987;10(1):389–392.
144. Champion V, Williams SD, Miller A, et al. Quality of life in long-term survivors of ovarian germ cell tumors: a Gynecologic Oncology Group Study. *Gynecol Oncol.* 2007;105(3):687–694.
145. Matei D, Miller AM, Monahan P, et al. Chronic physical effects and health care utilization in long-term ovarian germ cell tumor survivors: a Gynecologic Oncology Group study. *J Clin Oncol.* 2009;27(25):4142–4149.
146. Hale GA, Marina NM, Jones-Wallace D, et al. Late effects of treatment for germ cell tumors during childhood and adolescence. *J Pediatr Hematol Oncol.* 1999;21(2):115–122.
147. Zaghloul MS, Khattab TY. Dysgerminoma of the ovary: good prognosis even in advanced stages. *Int J Radiat Oncol Biol Phys.* 1992;24(1):161–165.

CHAPTER 25

Ovarian Sex Cord–Stromal Tumors

David M. Gershenson, Sean C. Dowdy, and Robert H. Young

INTRODUCTION

The intraovarian matrix that supports the germ cells and is covered by the surface epithelium consists of cells originating from the sex cords and mesenchyme of the embryonic gonad. Granulosa cells and Sertoli cells, generally considered to be homologous, are derived from the sex cord cells, whereas the pluripotent mesenchymal cells are the precursors of theca cells, Leydig cells, and fibroblasts. Neoplastic transformation of these cellular constituents, either singly or in various combinations collectively, results in neoplasms that are termed sex cord–stromal tumors (SCSTs). The classification of the SCSTs provides the template from which this chapter endeavors to stratify and define these tumor entities according to their morphologic characteristics (**Table 25.1**).

The SCSTs are estimated to account for approximately 7% of all malignant ovarian neoplasms (1). Although SCSTs account for a decreasing proportion of all ovarian malignancies with advancing age, the annual age-related incidence continues to increase through the seventh decade of life (2). Overall, the majority of these tumors are benign or of low malignant potential and are associated with a favorable long-term prognosis. In addition, a significant proportion of SCSTs are diagnosed in patients younger than age 40 years and have the potential to produce a variety of steroid hormones. Hence, adequate knowledge of the natural history of each of these tumors is imperative in diagnosing and individualizing definitive surgical and adjuvant therapy.

SCSTs account for nearly 90% of all functioning ovarian neoplasms (3). With the exception of fibromas, the clinical presentation of patients with SCSTs is frequently governed by the clinical manifestations resulting from the endocrinologic abnormalities. Excessive estrogen production, whether from increased tumor synthesis or peripheral conversion of androgens, influences end-organ responses, which are usually age dependent and can range from isosexual precocious puberty to menometrorrhagia to postmenopausal bleeding. In addition, the associated risks for endometrial cancer and possibly breast cancer must be recognized (4–6). Conversely, the rapid onset of signs ranging from early defeminization to frank virilization heralds a hyperandrogenic state. Elevated circulating levels of testosterone and/or androstenedione provide strong evidence for the presence of an SCST. Although granulosa cell, theca cell, and Sertoli cell tumors are generally considered to be estrogenic, and Sertoli–Leydig cell tumors (SLCTs) and steroid cell tumors (SCTs) are predominantly androgenic, the functional endocrinologic capacities of these tumors are impossible to predict based on their morphologic features. It should also be noted that miscellaneous ovarian tumors, both primary and metastatic, that are not in the SCST family may be androgenic or estrogenic if their stroma is stimulated to undergo luteinization.

TABLE 25.1. Classification of Sex Cord–Stromal Tumors

Granulosa stromal cell tumors
Granulosa cell tumor
Adult type
Juvenile type
Tumors in the thecoma–fibroma group
Thecoma (including subset associated with sclerosing peritonitis)
Fibroma (including cellular form)–fibrosarcoma
Sclerosing stromal tumor
Microcystic stromal tumor
Sertoli stromal cell tumors
Sertoli cell tumor
Sertoli–Leydig cell tumor
Well differentiated
Of intermediate differentiation
Poorly differentiated
With heterologous elements
Retiform
Sex cord tumor with annular tubules
Unclassified sex cord–stromal tumors
Gynandroblastoma
Steroid cell tumors
Leydig cell tumors
Steroid cell tumor not otherwise specified

GRANULOSA CELL TUMORS

Although granulosa cell tumors (GCTs) of the ovary were initially described by Rokitansky (7) in 1859, the pathogenesis of these neoplasms remains ill defined. At least in part, this is a reflection of the low incidence of GCTs, and hence the limited number of cases managed at any single institution. Although molecular aberrations crucial to the pathogenesis of GCTs have been elucidated recently, to our knowledge there are no recognized risk factors for their development (4,8). Reproductive factors, including the use of fertility-promoting agents and oral contraceptives, do not appear to increase the risk of disease. Unkila-Kallio et al. (9) studied a possible link between fertility-promoting agents and GCTs using the nationwide Finnish Cancer Registry. They analyzed the occurrence of GCTs in Finland from 1965 to 1994 against sales statistics for ovulation inducers. The incidence of GCTs declined by nearly 40% from 1965–1969 to 1985–1994 despite a 13-fold increase in the use of clomiphene citrate and a 200-fold increase in human menopausal gonadotropin use; oral contraceptive use increased fivefold. In another series of 240 GCTs, prior use of oral contraceptives and a history of infertility were associated with improved survival on univariable, but not multivariable analysis (10). No hereditary predisposition for any of the SCSTs has been identified (11), although a case report described the occurrence of adult GCTs in two first-degree relatives (12).

GCTs comprise 5% of all ovarian malignancies, but account for approximately 70% of malignant SCSTs (4–6,13–20). The annual incidence of GCTs in the United States and other developed countries varies from 0.4 to 1.7 cases per 100,000 women (5,6,8,19,21,22). Quirk and Natarajan reported histology-specific age-adjusted ovarian cancer incidence rates that were standardized to the recently adopted year 2000 U.S. standard population utilizing data from the Surveillance, Epidemiology, and End Results (SEER) program (23). Out of a total of 23,484 microscopically confirmed cases of primary ovarian cancer, 293 (1.2%) were of sex cord–stromal origin. Although GCTs have been diagnosed from infancy through the tenth decade of life, the average age at the time of diagnosis in over 750 cases was 52 years (4–6,14,16–19). Considering that GCTs occurring after the third decade of life appear to be histologically distinct, in most instances, from those occurring in children and younger adults, the clinical and pathologic characteristics for the juvenile and adult GCTs will be addressed separately.

GCTs: Adult Type

Adult-type granulosa cell tumors (AGCTs), histologically described below, account for 95% of all GCTs. The majority of patients will present with one or a combination of the following clinical symptoms: abnormal vaginal bleeding, abdominal distention, and abdominal pain (5,6,16–19,24). The latter symptoms are most frequently attributable to the gross size of the tumor at the time of diagnosis, with the majority exceeding 10 cm in diameter and many exceeding 15 cm (5,17,19). In one series, 12% had ascites at diagnosis (24). In many series, menometrorrhagia, oligomenorrhea, or amenorrhea in premenopausal women or bleeding in postmenopausal women are the most common reasons for seeking medical assistance. These and other clinical manifestations such as breast tenderness, uterine myohypertrophy, and endometrial hyperplasia are caused by hyperestrogenism associated with GCT.

The endocrine function of AGCTs, specifically the production of estrogens, has been repeatedly demonstrated. In a detailed retrospective analysis of endometrial specimens from 69 patients with GCTs, Gusberg and Kardon (25) observed histologic features consistent with unopposed estrogen, including atypical adenomatous hyperplasia in 42% of the evaluated cohort, adenocarcinoma *in situ* (4) in 5%, and invasive adenocarcinoma in 22%. Similarly, Evans et al. (4) noted endometrial hyperplasia in 55% and adenocarcinoma in 13% of their GCT study population. Other investigators have corroborated the high prevalence of glandular hyperplasia and have reported adenocarcinoma frequencies ranging from 3% to 27% (5,6,14,16–19,26,27). Selective ovarian venous catheterizations during surgery have documented hormonal production, including the secretion of large quantities of estrogen from the ovary harboring the GCT. The return of serum estrogen to physiologic levels after surgical resection has also been demonstrated. Occasionally, patients with GCTs present with endometrial changes (decidual reaction of the stroma or secretory characteristics of the glands) consistent with tumor production of progesterone (28). Rarely, virilizing changes such as oligomenorrhea, hirsutism, and other masculinizing signs may accompany GCTs (29–31).

Pathology

AGCTs have an average diameter of approximately 12 cm, but a subset, 10% to 15% of the cases, are small and not appreciated on pelvic examination (32). Most characteristically, they are predominantly cystic, with numerous locules filled with fluid or clotted blood and separated by solid tissue (**Fig. 25.1**), or they are solid, with large areas of hemorrhage. The solid tissue may be gray-white or yellow and soft or firm. A rare tumor is cystic, usually thin walled, but occasionally thick walled, and multilocular or unilocular (30).

Microscopic examination reveals an almost exclusive population of granulosa cells or, more often, an additional component of theca cells, fibroblasts, or both. The granulosa cells grow in a wide variety of patterns. The better differentiated tumors usually have microfollicular, macrofollicular, insular, or trabecular patterns. The microfollicular pattern is characterized by numerous small cavities (Call–Exner bodies) (**Fig. 25.2**) that may contain eosinophilic fluid, one or a few degenerating nuclei, hyalinized basement membrane material, or, rarely, basophilic fluid. The microfollicles are typically separated by well-differentiated granulosa cells that contain scanty cytoplasm and pale, angular, or oval, often grooved nuclei arranged haphazardly in relation to one another and to the follicles. The uncommon macrofollicular pattern is characterized by cysts lined by well-differentiated granulosa cells beneath which theca cells are present. The trabecular and insular forms of GCTs are characterized by bands and islands of granulosa cells separated by fibromatous or thecomatous stroma. The less well-differentiated forms of the AGCT typically have a water silk (moire silk), gyriform, or diffuse (sarcomatoid) pattern alone or in combination. The first two patterns are manifested by parallel undulating or zigzag rows of granulosa cells, generally in single file, whereas the diffuse form is characterized by

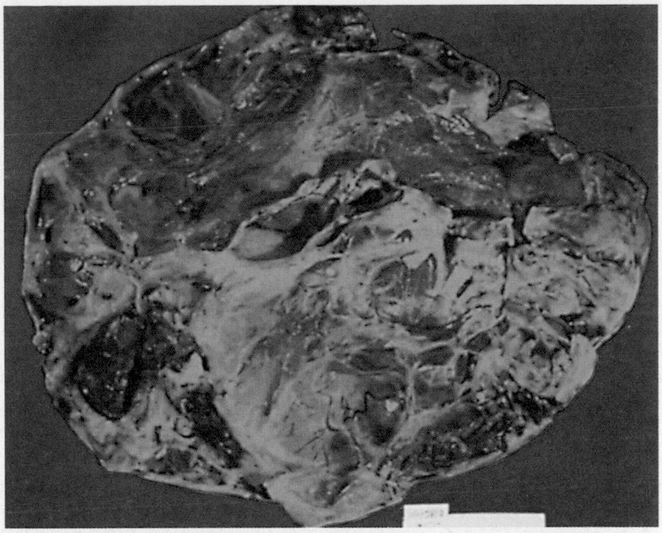

Figure 25.1. Granulosa cell tumor. The sectioned surface is composed predominantly of multiple cysts filled with blood.

Source: Reprinted with permission from Case Records of the Massachusetts General Hospital, Case 89–1961. *N Engl J Med*. 1961;265:1210–1214.

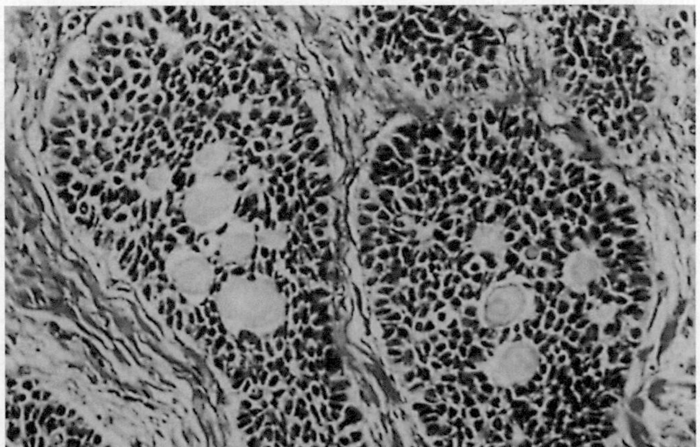

Figure 25.2. Granulosa cell tumor, adult type, microfollicular pattern. Several nests of granulosa cells with small oval and angular nuclei enclose multiple Call–Exner bodies.

a monotonous, patternless cellular growth. In some AGCTs, the neoplastic cells have moderate to abundant quantities of dense or vacuolated cytoplasms; the term *luteinized granulosa cell tumor* is appropriate when such cells predominate (28). The cells in GCTs usually have round to oval, pale, and often grooved nuclei (**Fig. 25.2**), but rarely the cells are spindle-shaped, resembling a cellular fibroma or low-grade fibrosarcoma; mitotic figures (MFs) may be numerous, but are rarely atypical. There is usually only mild nuclear atypia, but approximately 2% of tumors contain mononucleate and multinucleate cells with large, bizarre, hyperchromatic nuclei, the presence of which does not appear to worsen the prognosis (33).

Natural History

AGCTs are low-grade malignancies with a propensity to remain localized and indolent. Ninety percent are stage I at diagnosis (27). The 10-year survival rate for stage I disease ranges from 86% to 96%; for disease that is more advanced at diagnosis, the 10-year survival rate ranges from 26% to 49% (27). Bilaterality occurs in less than 10% (24). Tumor rupture occurred in 22% of a series of 97 cases (24). A unique feature of GCTs is that they recur at extended time intervals from primary therapy, suggesting the presence of persistent occult disease with a very indolent growth rate. For patients who recur, the median time to recurrence is 6 years and median survival after recurrence is 5.6 years (4,14). In a series of 160 stage I GCTs, median time to recurrence was 12 years and median overall survival (OS) was similar between patients with and without recurrence (34).

Prognostic Factors

The staging system for GCTs is the same as that used for epithelial ovarian cancer. It was revised in 2014 (International Federation of Gynecology and Obstetrics [FIGO]). Whereas surgical stage has been recognized as the most important prognostic factor for GCTs, the impact of tumor size, rupture, histologic subtype, nuclear atypia, and mitotic activity on outcome is less clear; larger, well-characterized series are necessary to clarify existing discrepancies (8,35,36). As noted above, GCTs are large and therefore prone to rupture. Rupture appears to adversely impact survival in stage I patients, justifying stratification as stage IC (14,34). In a series of 240 patients, treatment prior to 1984, age greater than 60 years, tumor size greater than 10 cm, advanced stage, residual tumor, and use of hormonal therapy were associated with GCT-related death. However, only stage was associated with recurrence on multivariate analysis (10). Tumor size has been variably associated with risk of death (5,15,19,21,37). Increasing degrees of nuclear atypia and increasing mitotic frequency per 10 high-power fields (HPFs) have been correlated inversely with prognosis. Specimens from patients with more advanced disease tend to demonstrate higher grade of atypia and/or more MFs (5,14,15,19). Despite its somewhat subjective assessment, nuclear grade has reportedly been a reliable prognostic indicator in stage I cases (14,19). The significance of histologic subtypes has been debated, and they appear to be of minimal value. Several investigative groups (4,5,13–15,19) have failed to confirm Kottmeier's (38) report of the prognostic importance of histologic patterns alone in GCTs. Similarly, the results of investigations utilizing flow cytometric analysis of DNA content have been inconsistent. Klemi et al. (39) reported a significant survival advantage for patients with tumors demonstrating normal ploidy and/or an S-phase fraction (SPF) of less than 6%. However, other investigators have suggested that nondiploid GCTs are infrequently encountered (40,41). Another investigation of 20 GCTs found that the degree of nuclear atypia, mitotic count, Ki-67 index, and DNA aneuploidy were not predictive of tumor recurrence (34). Chadha et al. (40) reported that three of five aneuploid tumors from a total population of 43 pathologically diagnosed GCTs were vimentin-negative but positive for cytokeratin and epithelial membrane antigen, and therefore cautioned that such highly aneuploid tumors may represent undifferentiated carcinomas. Indeed, it is clear that some series of GCTs in the literature include undifferentiated carcinomas not otherwise specified, or recently recognized entities such as the large-cell carcinoma of hypercalcemic type. Therefore, series with unusually large numbers of late-stage or poor-prognosis cases should be evaluated cautiously.

Investigators have analyzed several potential molecular markers, including p53 status, telomerase, Ki-67, c-myc, HER2/neu, and vascular endothelial growth factor (VEGF) in GCTs (42–48). To date, no molecular marker provides prognostic information for GCTs beyond what is known from stage and histopathologic parameters.

Ala-Fossi et al. (49) stained 30 GCTs for the inhibin subunit. All 24 stage I and II tumors were positive, whereas four of six stage II–IV tumors were negative. Those that were negative were poorly differentiated and exhibited rapid disease progression. Whether other observers would have accepted these tumors as valid GCTs is a concern. Stage was the sole independent prognostic factor.

Serum Markers

The majority of patients presenting with advanced GCTs will recur. Therefore, the identification of a specific serum tumor marker(s) would facilitate early detection of recurrent disease and monitoring of treatment effectiveness (4,5,17,19). As noted above, serum estrogens are generally produced by GCTs and have been utilized as an indicator of disease status (50). Unfortunately, serum estradiol levels are occasionally normal, and more frequently are only marginally increased, making them less than ideal for monitoring in a significant number of patients. Several proteins derived from granulosa cells, including inhibin, follicle-regulating protein, and Müllerian-inhibiting substance (MIS), are useful markers (51–59). In a prospective evaluation of 27 patients with GCTs, Jobling et al. (53) demonstrated that serum inhibin levels are typically elevated sevenfold above normal follicular phase levels prior to primary surgical management. In a comparative investigation of serum inhibin B and anti-Müllerian hormone, elevations in both were noted in 123 patients with primary and recurrent GCTs. The area under the curve of each was >0.90, and somewhat higher when used in combination (59a). Mom et al. (60) showed that inhibin B was the predominant form of inhibin secreted by these tumors, with a sensitivity and specificity of 89% and 100%, respectively, compared with 67% and 100% for inhibin A. Elevations in inhibin B were present in 85% of recurrences, and predated clinical evidence of recurrence by a median of 11 months. Both inhibin and calretinin have become useful immunohistochemical markers to assist in the diagnosis of GCTs and other SCSTs (61).

GCTs: Juvenile Type

Ovarian neoplasms are relatively rare in childhood and adolescence. When encountered, the majority are of germ cell origin, with only 5% to 7% being SCSTs. The latter are predominantly of the granulosa cell type in this age group, and demonstrate a distinct tumor morphology and to a degree biology from the typical AGCT considered above (62). Approximately 90% of the GCTs diagnosed in prepubertal girls and in most women less than 30 years of age will be of the juvenile type (JGCT). In a clinicopathologic analysis of 125 cases of JGCT, 44% occurred prior to age 10 and only 3% after the third decade of life (63). The majority of prepubertal patients present with clinical evidence of isosexual precocious pseudopuberty, which may include breast enlargement, development of pubic hair, increased vaginal secretions, advanced somatic development, and other secondary sex characteristics (63–67). Serum estradiol levels were reported as elevated in 17 of 17 cases of JGCTs with pseudopuberty (65). In addition, elevated levels of serum progesterone (6 of 10) and testosterone (6 of 8) were likewise observed, as well as suppressed levels of luteinizing hormone and follicle-stimulating hormone (FSH). The occasional patient will harbor an androgen-secreting JGCT accompanied by virilization (63,65,66). Although the signs of either precocious pseudopuberty or virilization are dramatic, the most consistent clinical sign at presentation in patients with JGCTs is increasing abdominal girth. Young et al. (63) indicated that in only 2 of 113 nonpregnant patients with JGCTs was the treating physician unable to palpate a mass on abdominal, pelvic, and/or rectal examination. Abdominal pain, dysuria, and constipation may coexist. Infrequently, a surgical emergency is encountered following spontaneous rupture or torsion of the enlarged ovary. JGCTs may occur in infants, who appear to have a more favorable prognosis than older individuals (68). Hasiakos et al. (69) described a case of JGCT associated with pregnancy, and reviewed the literature.

The frequency of bilaterality for JGCTs is estimated to be 5%, similar to that for AGCTs (70). When stage was assigned based on surgical and histologic parameters, 88% were stage IA, 2% stage IB, 8% stage IC, and 3% stage II. As noted, extraovarian spread is infrequently encountered at exploration, whereas rupture of the tumor is noted in approximately 10% of cases. Ascites contributes to the abdominal distention in 10% to 36% of cases (63,65).

JGCTs have been reported in association with enchondromatosis alone (Ollier's disease) or concomitantly with hemangiomas (Maffucci's syndrome) (65,71–73). Individuals with these relatively uncommon mesodermal dysplasias generally present prior to puberty and frequently develop secondary neoplasms, most commonly sarcomas, after the second decade of life. JGCTs are the next most frequent tumor associated with these disorders and become evident during the first and second decades of life. These observations appear to imply more than coincidental occurrences and suggest a generalized mesodermal dysplasia, perhaps contributing to the pathogenesis of these neoplastic processes. In addition, congenital bilateral JGCTs of the ovary have been reported in leprechaunism, a disease characterized by insulin resistance resulting from an insulin receptor defect (74).

Pathology

The appearances of JGCTs are similar to the adult form; a solid and cystic neoplasm, in which the cysts contain hemorrhagic fluid, is common (63,64,67). Uniformly solid and uniformly cystic neoplasms are also encountered; the latter may be multilocular or, in rare instances, unilocular. The solid component is typically yellow-tan or gray and occasionally exhibits extensive necrosis, hemorrhage, or both.

Microscopic examination typically reveals a predominantly solid cellular tumor with focal follicle formation, but occasionally, a uniformly solid or a uniformly follicular pattern is seen. In the solid areas, the neoplastic cells may be arranged diffusely or as multiple nodules of various sizes. The follicles typically vary in size and shape; Call–Exner bodies are rarely encountered, and the follicles rarely reach the large size of those in the macrofollicular AGCT. The follicular lumens in the juvenile tumor contain eosinophilic or basophilic fluid, which stains with mucicarmine in approximately two of three cases.

The two characteristic cytologic features of the neoplastic juvenile granulosa cells that distinguish them from those of AGCT are their generally rounded, hyperchromatic nuclei, which almost always lack grooves, and their almost invariable moderate to abundant eosinophilic or vacuolated (luteinized) cytoplasm (**Fig. 25.3**). Nuclear atypia in JGCTs varies from minimal to marked; in approximately 13% of the cases, severe degrees are present. The mitotic rate also varies greatly, but is generally higher than that seen in AGCTs, often being five or more per 10 HPF (63,64).

Natural History

In the initial series by Young et al. (63), 98% of 125 patients with JGCTs were less than 35 years of age, and 78% were 20 years or less. Notwithstanding the customary presenting complaint of increased abdominal girth and the clinical documentation of a large mass (64% >10 cm), 90% of the JGCTs analyzed by Young et al. (63) were stage IA or IB. The corresponding survival rate for these patients, with an average follow-up of 3.5 years, was 97%. Included were nine stage IA2 patients with rupture of the tumor, all of whom were alive and free of disease. Patients presenting with associated isosexual pseudoprecocious puberty may have a more favorable prognosis. Assessing 80 such cases from 212 reported JGCTs, only two cancer-related deaths (2.5%) were observed. Presumably, the clinical manifestations lead to early diagnosis and excellent outcomes (63,65–67).

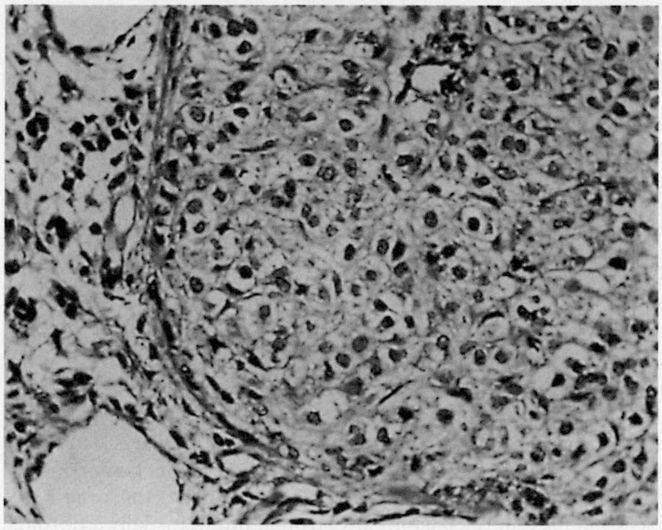

Figure 25.3. Granulosa cell tumor, juvenile type. A nodule of tumor is composed of large cells with abundant cytoplasm and slightly pleomorphic, hyperchromatic nuclei.

Although the presentation of early symptoms and localized disease is similar to that of AGCTs, the natural history of JGCTs differs notably in several respects. Although the adult form frequently includes a latency period with recurrences remote from initial diagnosis, the juvenile counterpart is characteristically aggressive in advanced stages, and the time to relapse is generally within 3 years of the initial diagnosis (63,65,67). Thirteen cases of stage II, III, or IV disease were abstracted from three analyses, with a combined sample size of 180 patients (63,65,66). Of these 13 patients, only three (23%) were alive when reported; notably, the recurrences and deaths occurred within a relatively brief interval.

Prognostic Factors

Young et al. (63) noted that surgical stage represented the most reliable prognostic indicator. Tumor size, mitotic activity, and nuclear atypia were significant predictors only when analyzed without regard to stage. In that series, rupture did not correlate with outcome. Schneider et al. (75) reported on a group of 54 SCSTs in children and adolescents from Germany (45 JGCTs and 9 others). They addressed the outcome of patients with "accidental" stage IC disease, defined as violation of the tumor capsule during surgery, versus "natural" stage IC tumors, with preoperative rupture or malignant ascites. Among 12 patients with accidental stage IC disease, there were no recurrences. In contrast, five of the nine patients with natural stage IC disease recurred ($p = 0.001$). Assessment of DNA content via flow cytometry in JGCTs demonstrated nondiploid patterns in nearly half (76,77). However, Jacoby et al. (76) were unable to correlate DNA ploidy or SPF with either stage of disease or prognosis in patients with localized disease. In the series by Schneider et al. (75), mitotic activity correlated with prognosis. There were no relapses in 35 patients whose tumors exhibited low or moderate mitotic activity. Among those with high mitotic activity (>19 mitoses per 10 HPFs), approximately half recurred.

Serum Markers

Although information specific to JGCTs is limited, the various tumor markers discussed above for AGCTs would appear to be applicable to JGCTs for monitoring of recurrent disease.

Tumors in the Thecoma–Fibroma Group

As the ovarian stromal cell is the precursor of both fibroblasts and theca cells, pure thecomas and pure fibromas represent extremes along a continuum, with a significant percentage of the tumors having admixtures of theca cells and collagen-producing spindle cells. Nonetheless, the majority of tumors in the thecoma–fibroma group are readily subcategorized based on relatively distinct histologic characteristics. The major subcategories include thecoma, fibroma–fibrosarcoma, sclerosing stromal cell tumor (SST) and microcystic stromal tumor. The latter neoplasm is currently placed in the stromal category, although it has differing features from other pure stromal neoplasms, and in time may lead to a separate categorization. Another recently described entity is the so-called "luteinized thecoma associated with sclerosing peritonitis," which is also placed in this grouping tentatively (see below, section on Thecoma). Finally, the literature contains the designation "luteinized thecoma." This has been used in the past for any stromal tumor, usually a fibroma, containing lutein cells. However, recognizing that lutein cells may be seen in many neoplasms, the category "luteinized thecoma" as such does not merit its own designation. The presence of many luteinized stromal cells in a stromal tumor may merit notice, as it may explain the presence of androgenic clinical manifestations.

Thecoma

Thecomas (**Fig. 25.4**) are almost invariably clinically benign (4,78,79). They account for less than 1% of ovarian neoplasms and occur at an older age than other SCSTs. The majority of patients are in their sixth and seventh decades at the time of diagnosis (4,78). Combining two large series totaling over 140 patients, less than 10% presented prior to age 30. Based on a compendium of nearly 300 cases, bilaterality occurs with a frequency of approximately 2% and extraovarian spread occurs rarely, if at all (4,78–,80).

The primary presenting signs and symptoms in patients with thecomas are abnormal vaginal bleeding and/or an abdominal/pelvic mass (78–80). The former promotes initiation of medical intervention in the majority of postmenopausal patients, whereas increasing abdominal girth or a palpable mass is more frequently the main presenting complaint in premenopausal patients. Lesion size has been reported to vary from less than 1 to 40 cm in diameter (78,79,80). They are, on average, smaller than GCTs.

Thecomas are considered to be among the most hormonally active of the SCSTs. The abnormal bleeding encountered in 60% of patients is presumably attributable to excess estrogen production (78,79). In the series reported by Evans et al. (4), endometrial hyperplasia was observed in 37% of the evaluable patients, and adenocarcinoma consistent with an unopposed estrogen effect was documented in an additional 27%. All the uterine cancers were well-differentiated and minimally invasive, but two patients subsequently died of endometrial carcinoma. Other coexisting uterine pathologic findings potentially influenced by elevated circulating estrogen levels included leiomyomata, myohypertrophy, and endometrial polyps.

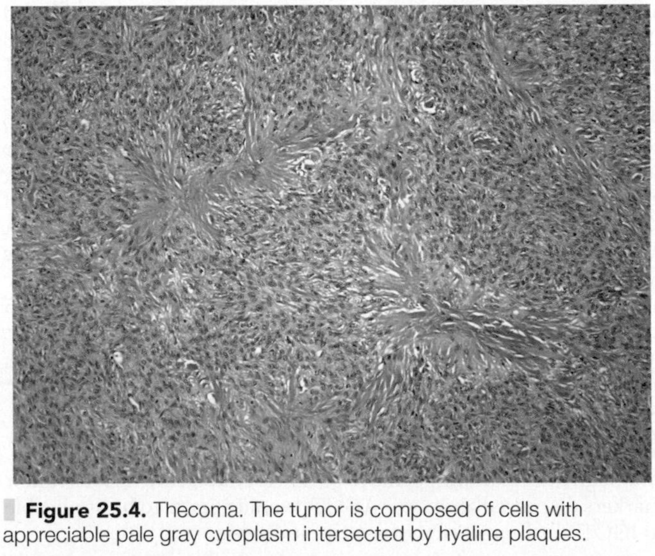

Figure 25.4. Thecoma. The tumor is composed of cells with appreciable pale gray cytoplasm intersected by hyaline plaques.

An enigmatic tumor that has been considered a variant of luteinized thecoma has been associated with sclerosing peritonitis (81). These tumors are often bilateral and frequently have a brisk mitotic rate, but have not demonstrated metastatic potential. Sclerosing peritonitis has, however, been fatal owing to pursuant complications. Schonman et al. (82) presented a case of luteinized thecoma associated with sclerosing peritonitis treated with ovarian wedge resection. Despite recurrent bowel obstruction, the was successfully treated with high-dose steroids. She achieved pregnancy and was free of symptoms 18 months following treatment.

Fibroma–Fibrosarcoma

Fibromas are the most commonly encountered SCST, accounting for approximately 4% of all ovarian neoplasms. These typically endocrine-inert tumors are seldom bilateral, and vary in size from microscopic to extremely large masses. Although infrequently diagnosed prior to age 30, fibromas can occur at any age; the average age of diagnosis is the latter half of the fifth decade of life (83). As their size increases, fibromas tend to become more edematous, leading to the escape of increasing quantities of fluid from the tumor surfaces. Ascites is detected in association with 10% to 15% of ovarian fibromas that exceed a diameter of 10 cm (84). Furthermore, 1% of patients develop a hydrothorax in addition to the hydroperitoneum (Meigs syndrome) (85). Gorlin's syndrome is associated with an inherited predisposition to the development of ovarian fibromas along with several other abnormalities, the most frequent of which is the appearance of basal cell nevi at an early age (86).

Approximately 10% of ovarian fibromatous tumors demonstrate increased cellularity and varying degrees of mitotic activity. These tumors are designated cellular fibromas and are considered to be tumors of low malignant potential, particularly if ruptured or associated with adhesions (87). Fibrosarcomas are distinguished by their greater cellular density and, most notably, moderate to marked pleomorphism and even greater mitotic activity (88). Few cases have been reported, but their diagnosis may be facilitated by the presence of elevated inhibin levels, supporting a sex cord origin (89).

Sclerosing Stromal Cell Tumors

SSTs were initially described by Chalvardjian and Scully (90) in 1973 as a distinct subgroup within the thecoma–fibroma family of ovarian tumors. This relatively rare tumor characteristically differentiates itself histologically and clinically from both thecomas and fibromas (91,92). The tumors are on average the same size as fibromas and thecomas, but have a more variegated sectioned surface, which is often at least focally edematous. Histologically, the presence of pseudolobulation of cellular areas separated by edematous to sclerotic connective tissue and prominent vascularity are distinguishing features. Clinically, SSTs commonly manifest during the second and third decades of life, with 80% being diagnosed prior to age 30. This is unique among ovarian stromal tumors (93). They are often associated with other stromal tumors, including thecomas (94). The signs and symptoms that most commonly prompt medical evaluation include menstrual irregularities and/or pelvic pain (95). Ascites is seldom encountered; this further distinguishes SSTs from fibromas (95). In contrast to thecomas, SSTs are usually inactive endocrinologically (90). However, in a limited number of cases steroidogenic activity has been demonstrated, even including androgenic manifestations, particularly if the patient is pregnant (95–99). To date, all SSTs have been clinically benign, and with one exception (100), all have been unilateral. One report noted an elevated CA-125 level (101), but this is unusual.

Microcystic Stromal Tumor

This rare neoplasm (102) typically is unassociated with endocrine manifestations. There are no distinctive gross features. The tumors are often initially believed to be thecomas until the peculiar microcystic formations, which result in the entity being named as it is, are observed. Relatively frequent cytologic atypia may lead to an erroneous diagnosis of a neoplasm with an aggressive nature, but the follow-up information to date indicates a benign outcome in the vast majority of cases. Although these tumors, as noted earlier, are tentatively placed in the stromal category, they differ from most stromal tumors in that they fail to stain for inhibin and calretinin. They also typically show nuclear beta-catenin positivity (103). According to the prominence of the microcysts, a variety of erroneous diagnoses may result, some of them significant, such as potential misclassification as yolk sac tumor, especially if the tumor occurs in the younger female as they sometimes do.

Natural History

Stromal tumors with rare exceptions are benign neoplasms, and any associated morbidity or mortality is generally attributable to side effects of treatment or concurrent disease (4,78,80,83,104). Examples of the latter include deaths from endometrial carcinoma resulting from the unopposed estrogen produced by the thecomas (4). Although cases of "malignant thecomas" have been reported, critical reappraisal of such tumors invariably results in histologic reassignment to sarcomas or diffuse GCTs (105). DNA ploidy analyses of thecomas and fibromas demonstrate aneuploid patterns in the majority, most commonly trisomy and/or tetrasomy 12, which offer a clue to their pathogenesis (106,107).

Prognostic Factors

The prognosis for patients diagnosed with cellular fibromas is generally favorable. Recurrences of these tumors of low malignant potential are generally correlated with adherent disease, rupture, or incomplete removal at the time of primary cytoreduction (87). In contrast, fibrosarcomas have a higher likelihood of recurrence, but fortunately are rare.

SERTOLI STROMAL CELL TUMORS

This category includes pure Sertoli cell tumors and SLCTs. Nomenclature-wise, it could also include Leydig cell tumors; however, Leydig cell tumors have been traditionally been classified in the steroid cell category because they share with those tumors a uniform population of cells of endocrine secreting type (with either eosinophilic or pale lipid-rich cytoplasm) and lack an epithelial element.

Neoplasms arising in the ovary, exhibiting morphologic characteristics similar to those of the testes during various stages of gonadogenesis, were recognized and elegantly described by Meyer (108,109). He reasoned that the origin of these tumors was the male blastema and coined the term *arrhenoblastoma*. Considering the functional nature of these male homologs and the varying degrees of associated defeminization and/or masculinization, the term *androblastoma* was also adopted. However, Morris and Scully (110), in 1958, contended that both designations implied masculinization, which is frequently absent; furthermore, a variety of unrelated androgen-producing ovarian tumors exist. Therefore, they recommended the adoption of the morphologic designation SLCT, a nomenclature based on morphology rather than clinical manifestations.

Sertoli Cell Tumors

Sertoli cell tumors are rare, accounting for less than 5% of all Sertoli stromal cell tumors (93). The average age at presentation is about 30 years, but this lesion can occur at any age. Evidence of estrogen production has been observed in approximately two-thirds of the reported cases. Consistent with excess estrogen production, isosexual precocious puberty has been witnessed during the first decade of life, menstrual disorders during the reproductive decades, and postmenopausal bleeding in the decades after the climacteric. Reflecting tumor size (average 9 cm), capsular distention, and/or adnexal torsion, and abdominal distention and/or pain are frequent complaints. Pelvic examination generally confirms the presence of tumor under these circumstances. The frequency of excessive renin production in association with Sertoli cells appears to exceed mere chance (111–113). Evaluation of refractory hypertension and hypokalemia has, rarely, resulted in the discovery of a Sertoli cell tumor as the origin of the excess renin. An occasional Sertoli cell tumor has arisen in a patient with Peutz–Jeghers syndrome (PJS) (114,115).

Pathology

On gross examination, these rare tumors are typically solid, lobulated, and yellow (93,116). Microscopic examination shows hollow or solid tubules lined by cells that usually exhibit relatively bland cytologic features, but rare tumors exhibit moderate to severe nuclear atypia. In most of these tumors, a tubular pattern predominates, but occasionally a diffuse pattern is conspicuous.

Prognosis

The great majority of these rare tumors have been unilateral stage I lesions. The greater majority of Sertoli cell tumors are well differentiated, and are rarely malignant (93). Excision of the tumor results in prompt resolution of the hyperestrogenic state.

Sertoli–Leydig Cell Tumors

SLCTs are extremely uncommon, accounting for less than 0.2% of all ovarian tumors. As implied by their designation, the tumors contain both Sertoli and Leydig cell elements. The clinical characteristics, specifically endocrine, are related to the degree of histologic differentiation and the presence of a retiform pattern and/or heterologous elements ((described below, in section on Pathology of Sertoli-Leydig Cell Tumors), the latter two variants being less often androgenic. The average patient age at diagnosis is approximately 25 years, with the majority (70% to 75%) of the tumors becoming clinically manifest during the second and third decades of life. Less than 10% occur either prior to menarche or after the climacterium. Patients harboring well-differentiated tumors present at an average age of 35 years, or 10 years later than patients with intermediate or poorly differentiated lesions. Conversely, tumors with retiform patterns are generally detected 10 years earlier than the intermediate and poorly differentiated tumors (117–119). Based on the compiled data from three reported series totaling over 300 patients, the frequency of extraovarian spread of disease at the time of diagnosis is approximately 2.5%. The likelihood of encountering bilateral tumors is even less (117–119).

The most frequent complaints at the time of presentation of, in these generally healthy adolescents and young adults, are menstrual disorders, virilization, and nonspecific symptoms resulting from an abdominal mass. Nearly one-half of the patients experience sufficient abdominal pain or discomfort or note abdominal distention, or palpate a mass on self-examination, prompting them to seek professional assessment. Whereas capsular distention and/or intralesional hemorrhage or necrosis of the tumor and/or adjacent visceral compression by the tumor account for the associated chronic or intermittent pain, acute abdominal pain necessitating emergency intervention invariably reflects vascular compromise from torsion. Although lesion size varies according to histologic differentiation (approximately 5 cm for well-differentiated tumors to >15 cm for poorly differentiated tumors), abdominal, vaginal, and/or rectal examination readily identifies an adnexal mass in approximately 95% of symptomatic patients. The most common premonitory symptoms, namely, menstrual disorders and subtle androgenic manifestations, predate by several months, and sometimes years, the recognition of the overt clinical signs or symptoms. Irregular bleeding, oligomenorrhea, and postmenopausal bleeding, retrospectively, have been attributed to either excess androgens or estrogens. The etiology of the latter is presumably the peripheral conversion of androgens to estrogens or, rarely, from an estrogen-secreting SLCT. Frank virilization occurs in 35% of the patients with SLCTs, and another 10% to 15% have some clinical manifestations consistent with androgen excess. The most frequent androgenic symptom complex encountered includes amenorrhea, voice deepening, and hirsutism. In addition, breast atrophy, clitorimegaly, loss of female contour, and temporal hair recession, for example, are signs of masculinization witnessed in patients with SLCTs (117–119). The prevalence of androgenic manifestations appears to be independent of the degree of histologic differentiation, but is observed less frequently in heterologous SLCTs and only occasionally in patients harboring retiform lesions (118,120–123). Although the preoperative diagnosis of SLCT in the absence of androgenic excess may be impossible, this neoplastic entity should constitute the primary preoperative diagnosis in patients with androgenic manifestations presenting during the second through the fourth decades of life with a unilaterally palpable adnexal mass.

Uncommonly, estrogen manifestations are witnessed in the context of presumed end-organ estrogenic responses, including postmenopausal bleeding and endometrial polyp formation, hyperplasia, and adenocarcinoma. Cautious interpretation of such observations is required, realizing that peripheral conversion of androgens to estrogens may be as plausible as a primary estrogen-secreting SLCT. As expected from the clinical findings, most patients demonstrating signs of defeminization or virilization have elevated plasma testosterone levels (117–119). Whereas plasma androstenedione may occasionally be elevated, the urinary 17-ketosteroids, including dehydroepiandrosterone, are usually normal, with the occasional patient presenting with a slightly elevated level. An elevated testosterone/androstenedione ratio generally suggests the presence of an androgen-secreting ovarian tumor, most likely an SLCT. Recognizing that certain gonadotropin-releasing hormone (GnRH) agonists modulate androgen production by downregulating gonadotropin levels and through a direct effect on the ovary, Pascale et al. (124) demonstrated successful suppression of testosterone and androstenedione in five virilized women with the administration of GnRH agonists. Their data suggest that androgen-secreting tumors of the ovary appear to be less autonomous than such tumors originating in the adrenal gland. Surgical excision of the SLCTs results in a precipitous drop in androgen levels and, over time, partial to complete resolution of the clinical manifestations associated with androgen excess is observed.

The coexistence of other diseases with SLCTs has been chronicled. The frequency with which thyroid disease is observed in these patients appears to exceed mere chance. Furthermore, several cases of other mesenchymal tumors have occurred in patients with SLCTs, including sarcoma botryoides of the cervix as well as Ollier's disease (118,125). The latter is a rare disease, but it is associated with other SCSTs, specifically JGCTs, as noted above. Finally, there appears to be a tendency toward familial occurrence (118).

Pathology

Gross Features. SLCTs vary in size from small to huge masses, but most are between 5 and 15 cm in diameter. The majority are solid, often yellow, and lobulated (**Fig. 25.5**), but many are solid and cystic. Pure cystic tumors are exceptionally rare, in contrast to GCTs. Poorly differentiated tumors tend to be larger than more differentiated tumors, and more frequently contain areas of hemorrhage and necrosis (118). Tumors with heterologous or retiform components are more often cystic than other tumors in this category (120,121,123,126). The heterologous tumors occasionally simulate mucinous cystic tumors on gross examination, and retiform tumors may contain large edematous intracystic papillae, resembling serous papillary tumors, or may be soft and spongy, with varying degrees of cystification (123).

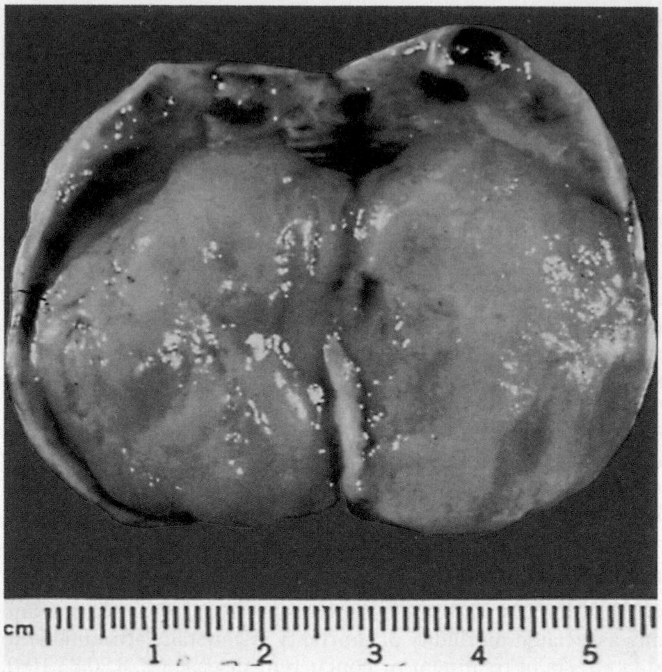

Figure 25.5. Sertoli–Leydig cell tumor. The sectioned surface of the tumor is focally lobulated and was yellow in the fresh state.

Microscopic Features. Well-differentiated SLCTs are characterized by a predominantly tubular pattern (127). On low-power examination, a nodular architecture is often conspicuous, with fibrous bands intersecting lobules composed of small, round, hollow, or, less often, solid tubules lined by well-differentiated cells and separated by variable numbers of Leydig cells. Rarely the tubules appear pseudoendometrioid (128).

SLCTs of intermediate and poor differentiation form a continuum characterized by a variety of patterns and combinations of cell types (117–119). Some tumors exhibit intermediate differentiation in some areas and poor differentiation in others; less commonly, tumors of intermediate differentiation contain well-differentiated foci. Both the Sertoli cells and the Leydig cells may exhibit varying degrees of immaturity. In tumors of intermediate differentiation, immature Sertoli cells have small, round, oval, or angular nuclei, generally scanty cytoplasm, and are arranged typically in ill-defined masses, often creating a lobulated appearance on low power; solid and hollow tubules, nests, broad columns of Sertoli cells, and, most characteristically, thin cords resembling the sex cords of the embryonic testis are often present (**Fig. 25.6**). These structures are separated by stroma, which ranges from fibromatous to densely cellular to edematous, and typically contains clusters of well-differentiated Leydig cells (**Fig. 25.6**). Cysts containing eosinophilic secretion may be present, creating a thyroid-like appearance, and follicle-like spaces are encountered rarely. The Sertoli cell and Leydig cell elements, singly or in combination, may contain varying and sometimes large amounts of lipid, in the form of small or large droplets. When a significant amount of the stromal component comprises immature cellular mesenchymal tissue with high mitotic activity resembling a nonspecific sarcoma, the tumor is poorly differentiated.

Fifteen percent of SLCTs have a substantial retiform component, and are so designated because they are composed of a network of elongated tubules and cysts, both of which may contain papillae, resembling the rete testis (33). This pattern is usually accompanied by other patterns of SLCTs, but sometimes an entire tumor has a retiform pattern.

Heterologous elements occur in approximately 20% of Sertoli cell tumors (124,129). In a series of these tumors, 18% contain glands and cysts lined by moderately to well-differentiated intestinal-type epithelium (124). Mesenchymal heterologous elements, encountered

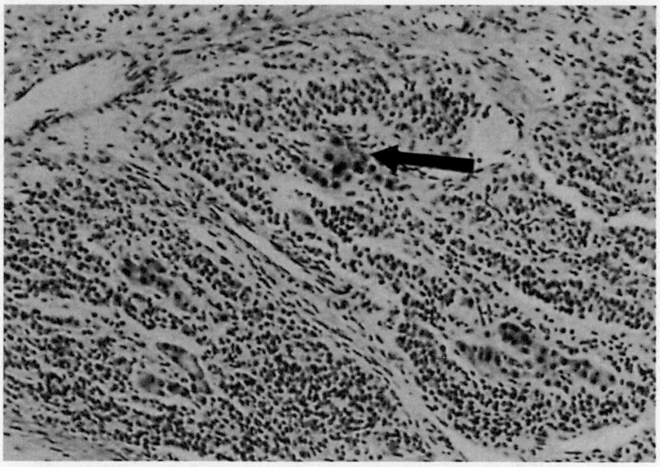

Figure 25.6. Sertoli–Leydig cell tumor, intermediate differentiation. Nests of large Leydig cells *(arrow)* lie among bands of immature Sertoli cells.

Source: Reprinted with permission from Morris JM, Scully RE. *Endocrine Pathology of the Ovary*. St. Louis, MO: Mosby; 1958;82–96.

in 5% of Sertoli cell tumors, include islands of cartilage arising on a sarcomatous background, areas of embryonal rhabdomyosarcoma, or both (129).

Natural History

SLCTs display characteristics that differ markedly from their epithelial counterparts, notably in regard to their malignant potential. Despite an average size of approximately 16 cm, only 2% to 3% of SLCTs have demonstrable extraovarian spread at the time of detection. Furthermore, Young et al. (63) identified only 29 clinically malignant cases in their series of 220 SLCTs observed at varying intervals, and they noted an 18% malignancy rate among 164 patients with adequate follow-up. At least in part, the more favorable prognosis reflects the abrupt onset of androgenic manifestations and the early detection of nonspecific symptoms, which promote prompt medical assessment. Nevertheless, the natural history of the malignant variant includes early recurrences, with approximately two-thirds becoming evident within 1 year of treatment and only 6% to 7% recurring after 5 years. The abdominal cavity (including the pelvis) and the retroperitoneal nodes are the most frequent sites for recurrences. In addition, the contralateral ovary, lungs, liver, and bone are other reported sites of recurrent metastatic disease. The collective salvage rates in patients with clinically malignant disease are low, with extrapolated estimates being less than 20%.

Prognostic Factors

Stage is the most important predictor of outcome in SLCTs. Fortunately, 97% of SLCTs are reportedly stage I at diagnosis, and less than 20% of these localized tumors become clinically malignant. The most cogent phenotypic prognostic determinant for stage I SLCTs is the degree of histologic differentiation (117–119). Approximately one-half of the reported SLCTs are of intermediate differentiation, 10% are well differentiated, 20% are heterologous, and the remainder are poorly differentiated. No extraovarian spread or subsequent recurrences were encountered by Young and Scully (127) among 23 well-differentiated SLCTs. However, approximately 10% of intermediate and 60% of poorly differentiated tumors, as well as 20% of heterologous tumors, demonstrated clinically malignant behavior (118). The heterologous tumors contain either endodermal elements such as gastrointestinal epithelium and carcinoids or mesenchymal elements including skeletal muscles and/or cartilage. The endodermal elements are typically associated with intermediately differentiated homologous elements and represent 75% of the heterologous SLCTs. Their corresponding prognosis parallels that of the intermediately differentiated homologous tumors. In contrast, heterologous tumors containing mesenchymal elements account for 5% of all SLCTs and invariably coexist with a poorly differentiated homologous component. The clinically aggressive malignant behavior of poorly differentiated heterologous tumors is evidence by the extremely low rates of survival (118).

Retiform patterns, tumor size, mitotic activity, and tumor rupture appear to increase in frequency because the degree of tumor differentiation decreases (117–119). Approximately 10% of neoplasms express histologic patterns resembling the rete testis. They are more commonly observed in younger patients (average age, 15 years) and are generally larger, possibly secondary to the less frequent association of androgenic manifestations and, hence, a later clinical presentation (120–123). SLCTs harboring a retiform pattern are associated with a 20% rate of malignancy, significantly higher than the 12% rate in nonretiform SLCTs. Young and Scully (123) noted that 14 of 25 retiform cases were of intermediate differentiation, with 1 demonstrating poorly differentiated homologous histology and 10 exhibiting heterologous elements (3 intermediate and 7 poorly differentiated). Arguably, the less favorable prognosis reflects the frequency of associated heterologous and/or poorly differentiated homologous lesions. This concept is supported by the finding that the majority of the metastatic lesions do not contain retiform patterns (123). However, the adverse characteristics of the retiform component are during examination of tumors of intermediate differentiation. Although only 4 of over 100 reported intermediately differentiated SLCTs were clinically malignant, 3 of the 4 contained retiform patterns (118).

Tumor size, mitotic activity, and rupture have been reported to influence prognosis (117,118). The size, mitotic index, and rupture frequency appear to increase because histologic dedifferentiation increases. Notwithstanding these associations, substratification of intermediate and poorly differentiated lesions according to these parameters identifies significant prognostic differences.

The frequency of androgen excess has been addressed above, with 50% or more of patients diagnosed with SLCTs either directly or indirectly displaying clinical manifestations of hyperandrogenism. Serum testosterone levels are invariably elevated when virilization is present, and selective venous catheterization has documented the ovary as the site of origin (130,131). In addition, immunostaining was positive for testosterone in eight SLCTs analyzed, including a limited number of tumors from patients without clinical signs or symptoms of androgen excess (2,132). The Leydig cells, as anticipated, were shown to be the cell of origin for the synthesis of testosterone. Following cytoreductive surgery, serum testosterone levels are rapidly cleared from the circulation and have been reported on occasion to increase again due to the burden of recurrent metastatic disease.

Other unique secretory products, namely, inhibin and alpha fetoprotein (AFP), have been reported in a limited number of SLCTs and are proteins generally equated with GCTs and germ cell tumors, respectively (121,123,131–133). In addition to GCTs, the Sertoli and Leydig cells have been shown to produce inhibin in testicular tissues, and presumably these same cell types are the site of origin in the SLCTs. Motoyama et al. (133) summarized the literature and reported the 14th case of an elevated serum AFP accompanying SLCTs. A clinically malignant course was appreciated in 43% of the described population, which had a mean age of 16 years. In addition, the majority (57%) was described as having a retiform component, a frequency substantially higher than the 10% usually seen in larger SLCT samples. Preferential AFP sampling may account for a portion of this seemingly unusually high frequency in that, histologically, the retiform pattern may be confused with a yolk sac tumor, particularly in the absence of clinical androgenic manifestations. The Sertoli and Leydig cells appear to be the cells of origin for AFP within the tumor. Employing immunostaining, Gagnon et al. (132) confirmed that Leydig cells appear to be the predominant site for AFP synthesis, but Sertoli cells are also capable of producing this oncoprotein. Testing four retiform and four nonretiform SLCTs, they demonstrated a 50% positivity rate in both histologic subtypes. The precise frequency of both inhibin and AFP positivity and their correlation with disease activity await larger confirmatory assessments.

Ovarian Sex Cord Tumor with Annular Tubules

In 1970, Scully (70) described a limited series of unique ovarian tumors characterized by either simple or complex ring-shaped tubules, and proposed the morphologic designation ovarian sex cord tumor with annular tubules (SCTATs). The distinctive cellular elements of these neoplasms were judged to be histologically representative of an intermediate between Sertoli cell and GCTs. Shen et al. (134) reported that SCTATs accounted for 6% of the sex cord tumors treated at their institution. An association with PJS was recognized by Scully, and in a subsequent report of 74 cases of SCTAT, Young et al. (135) noted that approximately 1 in 3 SCTATs occurred in patients with PJS. Ovarian sex cord tumors with annular tubules occurring in association with PJS are typically small (many microscopic), multifocal, calcified, and bilateral. The average age of presentation is the early to mid-portion of the fourth decade of life (135,136). The non-PJS tumors are considerably larger, seldom multifocal or calcified, and invariably unilateral. The average age of these patients is the mid- to latter portion of the third decade of life.

Abnormal vaginal bleeding is the most common presenting complaint, including menstrual irregularities during the reproductive era and postmenopausal bleeding during the mature years. Menometrorrhagia followed by prolonged episodes of amenorrhea is common in non-PJS patients. Abdominal pain or discomfort is less frequently encountered, but generally accompanies grossly involved adnexa or other incidental pelvic pathology. In addition, the signs and symptoms accompanying intussusception secondary to colonic polyp formation may be manifested in PJS-associated patients. The majority of PJS-associated SCTATs are not detectable via clinical examination and are appreciated unexpectedly during surgical or pathologic assessment. In contrast, the majority of non-PJS SCTATs are palpable on abdominal and/or vaginal examination. Although these tumors are seldom encountered during the first decade of life, isosexual precocity is invariably witnessed when SCTATs are diagnosed in affected children (135–138).

Considering the rarity of both PJS, an autosomal dominant disorder, and SCTAT, the frequent concurrency of these two processes suggests a potential linkage in their pathogenesis. Approximately 36% of SCTATs are observed in patients with PJS. In addition, 15% of PJS-associated SCTATs also develop adenoma malignum of the cervix (AMC), a neoplasm that defies early diagnosis and is associated with a relatively high mortality rate (135,139–141). A recent report of 34 patients with PJS demonstrated a significantly elevated risk (relative risk = 20.3) of breast and gynecologic malignancies in women (142); one patient had a Sertoli–Leydig tumor and three had sex cord tumors with annular tubules. The PJS gene was mapped to chromosome 19p13.3 (143) and was later identified as a novel serine–threonine kinase, STK11 (144). Because of the wide variety of malignancies occurring in individuals with PJS, STK11 is believed to function as a general tumor-suppressor gene.

Contingent on the patient's age, precocious puberty, menstrual irregularities, or postmenopausal bleeding are clinical manifestations of SCTATs, indirectly attesting to their endocrine activity (135–139,141,145,146). These signs of hyperestrogenism and the corresponding effects on the endometrium were readily recognized in the initial description of these unique tumors (62). Numerous reports have confirmed the presence of endometrial hyperplasia and/or polyp formation, particularly in PJS-associated SCTATs. Although similar signs in endometrial histology can be observed in non-PJS SCTATs, clinical histories of menorrhagia followed by episodes of amenorrhea are more frequent (134–137,145,146). Endometrial sampling in a limited population of such patients has demonstrated a spectrum from atrophic glandular to secretory or decidualized endometrium, suggestive of significant levels of progesterone production (134,136,146). Assessment of circulating steroid levels has confirmed the presence of excessive estrogen in essentially all SCTAT cases (134,145–147). However, normal progesterone levels have been observed in PJS-associated tumors, but elevated quantities of progesterone have been documented in non-PJS patients (134,145–147). Shen et al. (134) demonstrated elevated estrogen and progesterone levels (and normal testosterone levels) in two SCTAT patients without PJS, documenting glandular atrophy and decidual stromal changes. Utilizing selective ovarian venous sampling, Crain (146) demonstrated a significant progesterone gradient between peripheral and ovarian venous serum in a non-PJS patient with pseudodecidual changes of the endometrium. Complete resolution of the manifestations attributed to these hormonal imbalances is routinely observed, with surgical extirpation of the ovarian neoplasm.

Pathology

Grossly, the PJS-associated tumors are small, solid and yellow. The non-PJS-associated neoplasms, which are almost always grossly visible, may be similar, but in some cases are solid and cystic or mostly cystic. This tumor is characterized microscopically by the presence of simple and complex annular tubules (**Fig. 25.7**). The simple tubules have the shape of a ring, with the nuclei oriented around the periphery and around a central hyalinized body composed of basement membrane material; an intervening anuclear cytoplasmic zone forms the major component of the ring. The more numerous complex tubules are rounded structures comprising intercommunicating rings revolving around multiple hyaline bodies. In patients with PJS, the tumors are typically multifocal and exhibit calcification.

Prognostic Factors

Notwithstanding their histologic similarities, the differences in the natural history and long-term prognosis for SCTATs associated with PJS and SCTATs independent of PJS are readily apparent. Those detected in women with PJS are benign. Important in the management of this entity, however, is the recognition that approximately 15% of these patients will harbor an AMC. In addition, there are almost always exceptions to the rule. Barker et al. (148) reported a 54-year-old woman with SCTAT and PJS demonstrating aggressive malignant behavior, with multiple recurrences. In their review of the literature, the authors identified two previous such patients. Because of delayed declaration of symptoms, the diagnosis of AMC is frequently made following examination of the hysterectomy specimen. In a recent

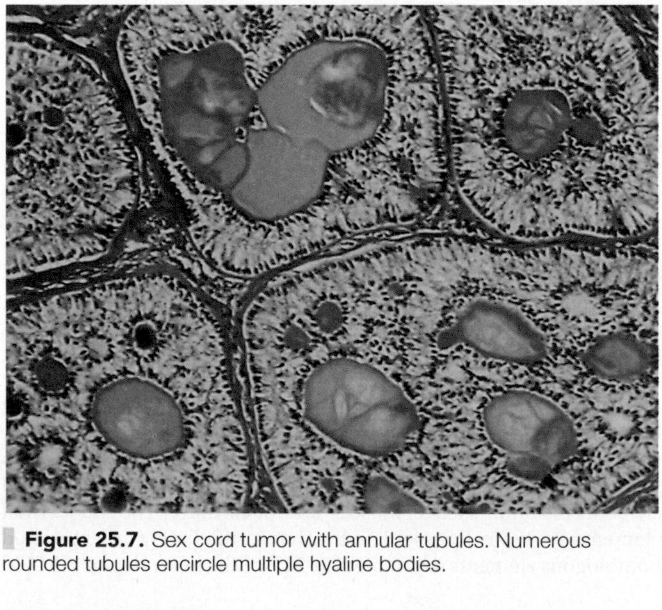

Figure 25.7. Sex cord tumor with annular tubules. Numerous rounded tubules encircle multiple hyaline bodies.

review by Srivatsa et al. (141), the prognosis for PJS patients with SCTAT and AMC is ominous, reflecting high AMC recurrence rates and refraction to treatment.

Based on the compiled data from four reported series including 63 patients with SCTATs and without clinically apparent PJS, the rate of malignancy was approximately 20% (134–137). Primary extraovarian extension and/or frequency of recurrence has been correlated with the original tumor size and mitotic activity. The tumor characteristically has a relatively long doubling time, a propensity for lymphatic dissemination, and is apt to remain lateralized. Because the primary ovarian lesion is invariably unilateral, the lymphatic metastases are invariably ipsilateral, extending within the confines from the paraaortic region to the supraclavicular area. The nature of the retroperitoneal metastases generally facilitates surgical resection and repeat cytoreduction. This tumor's indolent growth pattern, coupled with the relative ease of resection, affords patients extended palliation.

Because SCTATs possess characteristics of both granulosa cells and Sertoli cells, tumor markers elicited by either or both cell types indicate that diagnosis and surveillance of these tumors may be utilized, as well. The increased serum estrogen levels and corresponding clinical manifestations recognized in SCTATs suggest that monitoring hormone levels may be useful. Unfortunately, serum estradiol lacks adequate sensitivity, particularly when the residual tumor volume is limited. However, recent reports demonstrate the potential value and sensitivity of two unique secretory proteins as tumor markers for SCTATs. Gustafson et al. (147) illustrated the applicability of monitoring serum inhibin and MIS in the management of a patient with advanced, recurrent SCTAT. More recently, Puls et al. (149) reported an excellent correlation between serum inhibin and MIS levels and the clinical status of a patient with SCTAT during administration of chemotherapy (CT). The ultimate utility of these tumor markers awaits a study achieving accrual of sufficient numbers of patients with SCTATs to address adequately sensitivity and specificity issues.

SCSTs, Unclassified

This ill-defined group of tumors, which accounts for less than 10% of tumors in the sex cord–stromal category, comprises those in which a predominant pattern of testicular or ovarian differentiation is not clearly recognizable. Talerman et al. (150) have recently segregated proposed the designation "diffuse nonlobular androblastoma" for this group of tumors. The six ovarian tumors they reported were mostly estrogenic and had a predominant diffuse proliferation of cells resembling theca cells, granulosa cells, or both, but five of the six cases also contained steroid-type cells and tubules typical of Sertoli cell neoplasia.

SCSTs may be particularly difficult to subclassify when they occur in pregnant patients because of alterations in their usual clinical and pathologic features (151). Their nature is rarely suggested clinically because, during pregnancy, estrogenic manifestations are not recognizable and androgenic manifestations are rare. In one study, 17% of 36 SCSTs that were removed during pregnancy were placed in the unclassified group, and many of those classified in the granulosa cell or Sertoli–Leydig cell category had large areas with an indifferent appearance (151).

Gynandroblastoma

Gynandroblastoma is an extremely rare SCST (if strict morphologic criteria are followed to establish the diagnosis). Microscopically, these tumors must demonstrate readily identifiable (at least 10%) granulosa cells and tubules of Sertoli cells. Not surprisingly, the corresponding stromal cells, namely, theca and/or Leydig cells, may also be present in varying degrees. In a recent review of the world literature, Martin-Jimenez et al. (152) were able to identify only 17 authenticated cases of gynandroblastoma. Patients presented at an average age of 29.5 years (range, 16 to 65 years), with primary symptoms of menstrual disturbances consistent with the predominant functional status of the tumor. Commonly, a hyperandrogenic clinical profile is elicited, but signs and symptoms of excessive estrogens or no endocrine manifestations can be encountered. Amenorrhea, hirsutism, and clitorimegaly are frequently noted in association with elevated testosterone levels. Conversely, the common end-organ responses to hyperestrogenism include menometrorrhagia, postmenopausal bleeding, and endometrial hyperplasia. Although the unilateral masses are typically small, 75% are palpable prior to surgical exploration and are characterized by well-differentiated ovarian and testicular constituent elements. Regardless of the associated hormonal activity, gynandroblastomas are considered to be of low malignant potential. To date, only a single case was reported to be clinically malignant resulting in the death of the patient (153). A gynandroblastoma in pregnancy has also been reported (154).

Steroid Cell Tumors

SCTs constitute only 0.1% of all ovarian neoplasms. The predominant components of these tumors are steroid hormone–secreting cells, including lutein cells, Leydig cells, and adrenocortical cells. Until recently, the term *lipid cell tumors* was applied to these neoplasms, but Hayes and Scully (155) noted that 25% of such designated tumors did not contain appreciable intracellular fat. Hence, the functional designation SCT was suggested and stratified into three subclasses: stromal luteoma, Leydig cell tumor, and SCTs not otherwise specified (SCTNOT). The stromal luteoma category was introduced in 1964 to describe small neoplasms in the steroid cell family that were almost certainly of stromal origin. However, it is now felt that they are best considered, simply, small SCTs and do not have sufficiently unique aspects to merit separate classification. Leydig cell tumors, are, however, sufficiently distinctive as to merit classification from the larger body of overall SCTs placed in the group of SCTNOT.

Leydig Cell Tumors

Leydig cell tumors are rare. By combining two reviews (156,157) that summarize the English-language literature prior to and after 1966, 38 Reinke-positive cases affording adequate abstraction were identified. These invariably unilateral tumors are typically small, ranging in size from 0.7 to 15 cm, with a mean of 2.7 cm, and are therefore frequently not detectable via clinical examination or pelvic imaging. The average age at diagnosis is 58 years (range, 37 to 86 years), with only a small percentage occurring prior to the climacterium. The initial clinical manifestations are usually consistent with a hyperandrogenic state. Overt signs of virilization are observed in greater than 80% of the patients. These include one or more of the following: hirsutism, acne, deepening of the voice, breast atrophy, clitorimegaly, and male pattern baldness. In contrast to the frequently dramatic onset and progression of virilization witnessed with SLCTs, ovarian Leydig cell tumors are generally characterized by a more indolent course. Paraskevas and Scully (156) reported an interval of 7 years between recognized onset of signs and symptoms of androgen excess and diagnosis. Analysis of serum androgens demonstrated that testosterone was consistently elevated when urinary 17-ketosteroids were normal or marginally increased. These observations suggest minimal production of androstenedione or dehydroepiandrosterone. Conversely, estrogenic manifestations are occasionally witnessed, such as irregular menses or postmenopausal bleeding (156,157). Pathologic assessment of the uterus may reveal endometrial hyperplasia, polyp formation, and/or carcinoma in the presence or absence of leiomyomata and/or myohypertrophy. Whether the hyperestrogenic features are a result of tumor secretion of estrogens, or peripheral conversion of androgens to estrogens, remains to be ascertained.

Pathology. Histologically, Leydig cell tumors are typically composed of a monotonous proliferation of cells with abundant eosinophilic cytoplasm, and they less often have pale foamy lipid-rich cells than SCTNOT. The cells are predominantly cytologically bland, but bizarre nuclear atypia may be encountered this is almost always unassociated with mitotic activity, and should not lead to concern for malignancy. Roth and Sternberg (158) subdivided these tumors according to location and possibly the cell of origin, namely, Leydig cell tumors of hilar type versus nonhilar type. Whereas the latter presumably arise from ovarian stromal cells and are extremely rare, the former tumors are located in the hilus of the ovary and encroach on or extend into the ovarian stroma to varying degrees. Other features of Leydig cell tumors (including location in the ovarian hilus or adjacent to nonmedullated nerve fibers, association with hilar cell hyperplasia, fibrinoid vascular changes in the tumor, and clustering of cells around vessels) indicate that tumors lacking crystals of Reinke should likely be considered Leydig cell tumors (156).

Prognostic Factors. In a review of the English literature through 1988, 38 Reinke-positive cases were accrued and only a single case of a clinically malignant lesion was identified (156,157). Based on tumor size (15 cm) alone, this sole example might be considered an outlier. Hence, similar to stromal luteomas, ovarian Leydig cell tumors are essentially benign neoplasms with primary postsurgical concerns consisting of regression of the androgen-induced alterations. Generally speaking, significant regression is witnessed, but significant residual sequelae are appreciated in approximately one-half of the patients.

Steroid Cell Tumors, Not Otherwise Specified

Neoplasms identified as SCTs but lacking the specific characteristics of Leydig cell tumors are collectively classified as SCTNOS. The average age at presentation of patients harboring SCTNOS is 43 (10 to 15 years earlier than Leydig cell tumors); the tumors have been diagnosed from early childhood to the ninth decade of life (159). These generally solid yellow tumors are usually larger than Leydig cell tumors. The average size at diagnosis is approximately 8.5 cm. Furthermore, a higher frequency of bilaterality (5%) in advanced disease is encountered with these neoplasms. In their review of 63 collated cases, Hayes and Scully (159) reported that 81% of cases were localized (stage I), 6% were stage II, and 13% were stage III or IV. Curiously, they noted that the average age (54 years) of patients with advanced disease was 10 years older than the group as a whole. At least in part, these findings reflect the absence of documented advanced malignancies during the first two decades of life.

Clinical signs and/or symptoms of androgen excess ranging from heterosexual precocity in prepubertal girls to amenorrhea, hirsutism, and/or virilization during the reproductive and/or postmenopausal age prompt the majority of patients to seek medical advice (159,160). Not infrequently, these androgenic changes may have been present for many years (161). Additional concerns at presentation include increasing abdominal girth, reflecting tumor size and, rarely, ascites, abdominal pain, Cushingoid symptoms, and irregular uterine bleeding. The latter may represent clinical manifestations of estrogen excess (159,162), which has been suggested to occur at a frequency of 6% to 23%. Whether the source of estrogen is *de novo* synthesis by the tumor or from peripheral conversion of androgens remains to be determined. Isosexual precocious pseudopuberty has been detected in young girls harboring SCTNOS (159,163,164). An additional 10% to 15% of patients are asymptomatic, with tumors detected incidentally during routine pelvic examination or at the time of hysterectomy or other surgical interventions.

The steroid hormone–secreting capacities of SCTNOS are more diverse than those of most SCSTs. Whereas approximately one in four patients does not demonstrate clinical manifestations of hormonal imbalances, the majority of patients with SCTNOS show evidence of androgen excess (10% to 15% estrogen excess), and a lesser percentage show evidence of cortisol excess. These excesses are demonstrable via assessment of end-organ responses and serum/plasma steroid levels. Whereas elevated plasma levels of corticosteroids are typically observed in conjunction with SCTNOS, the number of overt presentations with Cushing's syndrome is limited (163,165–167). However, 17% of the clinically malignant tumors reported by Hayes and Scully (159) were associated with Cushing's syndrome. The serum testosterone and androstenedione levels are invariably elevated, as are urinary 17-ketosteroids; presumably, the latter reflect the level of excess androstenedione production.

Pathology.

Gross Features. These tumors are typically solid, well-circumscribed, occasionally lobulated (**Fig. 25.8**), and on average measure 8.4 cm in diameter (159). Approximately 5% are bilateral. They are typically yellow or orange but are occasionally red, dark brown, or black. Necrosis, hemorrhage, and cystic degeneration are occasionally observed.

Microscopic Features. On microscopic examination, the tumor cells are typically arranged diffusely but occasionally grow in nests, irregular clusters, thin cords, and columns. The polygonal to rounded tumor cells have distinct cell borders, central nuclei, and moderate to abundant amounts of cytoplasm varying from eosinophilic and granular to vacuolated and spongy (**Fig. 25.9**). In approximately 60% of the cases, nuclear atypia is absent or minimal and mitotic activity

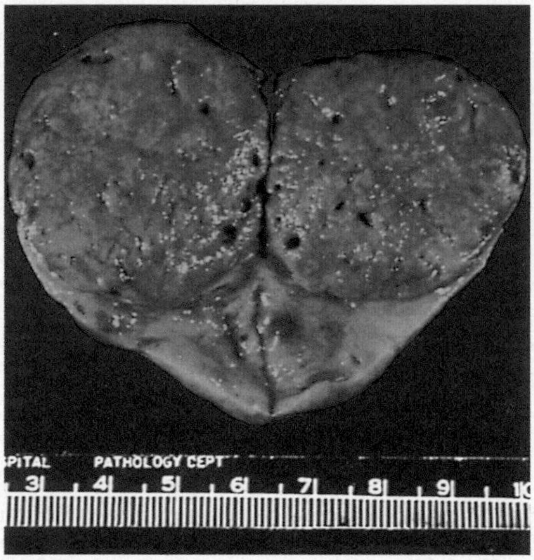

Figure 25.8. Steroid cell tumor, unclassified. The sectioned surface of the tumor is lobulated and was yellow-orange in the fresh state. This tumor was from a 9-year-old virilized girl.

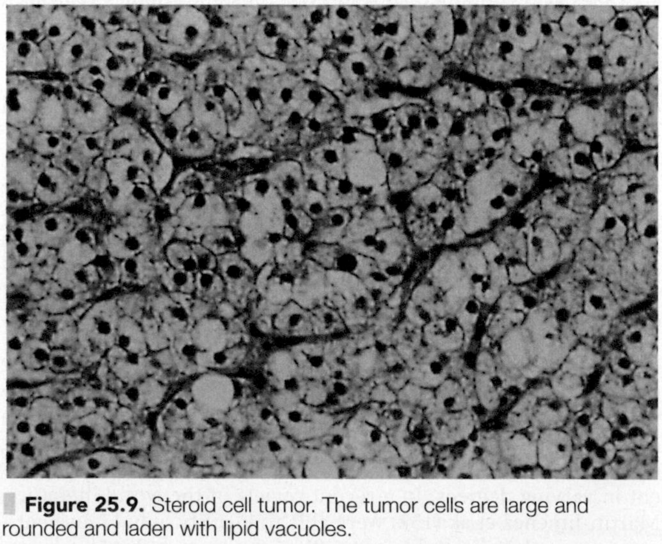

Figure 25.9. Steroid cell tumor. The tumor cells are large and rounded and laden with lipid vacuoles.

Source: Reprinted with permission from Hayes MC, Scully RE. Ovarian steroid cell tumors not otherwise specified [lipid cell tumors]: a clinicopathologic analysis of 63 cases. *Am J Surg Pathol*. 1987;11:835–845.

is low (less than 2 MFs per 10 HPFs). In the remaining cases, grades 1 to 3 nuclear atypia (**Fig. 25.3**) is present, usually associated with an increase in mitotic activity (up to 15 MFs per 10 HPFs). Occasional small SCTs (formally placed in the stromal luteoma category) are associated with hyperthecosis, which may contribute to the androgenic manifestations in such cases.

Prognosis. In contrast to the benign natural history of Leydig cell tumors, SCTNOS are associated with an appreciable rate of clinical malignancy (although there may be a reporting bias). In the largest series in the literature, 43% of patients with follow-up of 3 or more years demonstrated extraovarian disease, either at primary surgery or during subsequent follow-up (168). Unfortunately, to date, salvage therapy has been abysmal. Multiple factors appear to correlate with the frequency of disseminated disease including age, stage, tumor size, mitotic activity, tumor necrosis, hemorrhage, and symptoms of Cushing's syndrome. The average age of patients with clinical malignancies is 16 years older than patients without metastatic disease and 3 or more years of observation. No clinically malignant cases have been reported to date in patients younger than 20 years of age. All malignant SCTNOS were reported to measure 7 cm or more in greatest diameter (159). In fact, 78% of all tumors 7 cm or larger were malignant, whereas only 21% of all benign tumors exceeded this dimension. The most cogent determinant correlating with malignant potential was mitotic activity, with 92% of malignant tumors displaying 2 or more MFs per 10 HPFs. Similarly, in the presence of necrosis, 86% were malignant; if hemorrhage was present, 77% were malignant. In addition, three of four patients (17% of all malignant cases) with recognizable Cushing's syndrome harbored clinically malignant disease (159).

Although the majority of recurrences become clinically manifest within 3 years of diagnosis, Hayes and Scully (159) reported that 22% of recurrences occurred after 3 years and that, in fact, all of these cases occurred after 5 years; the longest interval was 19 years. Therefore, the duration of posttreatment surveillance should be adjusted accordingly. The only currently available utilizable markers for SCTNOS include the steroid hormones that were elevated prior to definitive treatment.

TREATMENT

The definitive management of SCSTs is dependent on one or more of the following: surgical stage, histologic subtype, patient's age and desire for fertility preservation, and various prognostic factors. Surgical resection alone is sufficient for SCSTs lacking malignant potential. Postoperative adjunctive therapy should be considered for patients with advanced disease and SLCTs with poor differentiation or mesenchymal heterologous elements (169).

Operative Management

Surgery remains the cornerstone of treatment for patients with SCSTs. Following sampling of peritoneal washings for cytologic assessment, inspection and palpation of the viscera are conducted to detect macroscopic disease. Resection of the ovarian tumor constitutes sufficient therapy for the essentially benign neoplasms, including thecomas, fibromas, gynandroblastomas, stromal luteomas, Leydig cell, sclerosing stromal, Sertoli cell, and well-differentiated SLCTs. Furthermore, sex cord tumors with annular tubules associated with PJS are also considered benign and can be similarly managed, but it is imperative that the endocervix be evaluated and subsequently monitored for the potential development of an AMC.

Upon histologic confirmation of GCTs, intermediate or poorly differentiated SLCTs, SCSTs with annular tubules independent of PJS, and SCTNOTs, surgical staging is required. This includes multiple peritoneal biopsies, omentectomy, and resection of grossly suspicious pelvic or paraaortic lymph nodes. Careful inspection of the peritoneum is critical because residual disease is strongly correlated with recurrence. However, there appears to be little benefit to performing routine lymphadenectomy in the absence of grossly suspicious lymph nodes. In three series totaling 180 patients with GCTs and SLCTs, no lymph node metastases were found among those who underwent pelvic and/or paraaortic lymphadenectomy (170–174). Furthermore, isolated retroperitoneal recurrences are rare. In 34 patients with recurrent GCTs, 2 recurred in the retroperitoneum only; 2 in the pelvis and retroperitoneum; and 1 in the pelvis, abdomen, and retroperitoneum (170). In another series of 87 patients, only 2 of 18 recurrences were isolated to the retroperitoneum (171). Overall, approximately 10% to 15% of first recurrences involve the retroperitoneum. Following careful surgical staging, in the absence of extraovarian disease, conservation of the uterus and contralateral ovary is reasonable in patients wishing preservation of fertility. In a review of the 1988 to 2001 SEER database, Zhang et al. (175) identified 376 patients with ovarian SCST. The survival for the group of 110 patients with stage I–II disease who underwent conservative surgery without hysterectomy was similar to that of patients who underwent standard surgery. For older patients or those with advanced-stage disease or bilateral ovarian involvement, abdominal hysterectomy and bilateral salpingo-oophorectomy are usually indicated. Others have reported conservative management for patients with advanced JGCTs treated with cytoreduction and CT, leading to prolonged disease-free intervals and multiple pregnancies (172). However, if the uterus is preserved, a thorough curettage must be performed in all patients with estrogen-producing tumors whether they are considered to be benign or potentially malignant (173). If maintenance of fertility is not a concern, a hysterectomy and residual salpingo-oophorectomy should be performed. Although no randomized evidence exists pertaining to the efficacy of cytoreduction in SCSTs, based on the benefits observed with their epithelial counterparts, we endorse an aggressive maximum effort at primary surgery if metastatic disease is encountered. In a recent multivariate analysis of 176 patients with GCTs, only residual disease after primary surgery and tumor size were predictive of recurrence (37). The value of secondary cytoreduction continues to be controversial, but appears to be meritorious for the more indolent tumor types such as GCTs and SCTATs not associated with PJS. Repeat cytoreduction frequently affords these patients extended palliation, and should be considered the cornerstone for treatment of recurrent disease.

Postoperative Management and Management of Recurrent Disease

Granulosa Cell Tumors (Adult)

The vast majority of women with stage I disease have an excellent prognosis after surgery alone, and do not require adjuvant therapy. For those with stage IC disease, consideration can be given to adjuvant therapy on an individualized basis. However, the management of stage IC GCT remains controversial. Recently, in a study of 104 women with stage I GCTs, Wilson et al. (34) observed higher relapse rates (43% vs. 24%; $p = 0.02$) and shorter time to relapse (10.2 vs. 16.2 years; $p = 0.007$) in patients with stage IC versus stage IA disease. Most women presenting with stages II–IV disease would be advised to have postoperative therapy, depending on their individual characteristics. However, in some centers in the United States and Europe, patients with metastatic disease are initially treated with surgery alone and only receive CT at the time of relapse.

Whereas some investigators have reported improved outcomes in patients treated with adjuvant radiation therapy (RT), other investigators have found no clear value to the use of adjuvant RT (4,6,17,176). Because of the rarity of GCT, it is difficult to conduct prospective trials in these patients. Two retrospective reports provide some data on the use of RT. Savage et al. (177) reviewed the courses of 62 women treated for adult GCTs at the Royal Marsden Hospital from 1969 to 1995. Thirty-eight (61%) had stage I disease. Eleven of the stage I patients had adjuvant pelvic radiation. The 10-year disease-free survival of these patients was 77% versus 78% for stage I patients treated with surgery alone. Unfortunately, neither complete surgical staging information nor the features that led to the selection of patients for adjuvant radiation was provided. For eight patients with inoperable disease (or residual disease postoperatively), radiation resulted in complete responses in four (50%) that lasted 16 months to 5 years.

Wolf et al. (176) reported on 34 patients with GCTs treated with radiation at the M.D. Anderson Cancer Center, 14 of whom had measurable disease. Six of the 14 (43%) had a clinical complete response. Three of the responders were alive without evidence of disease 10 to 21 years after radiation.

The Gynecologic Oncology Group (GOG) has reported the largest series of women with ovarian SCSTs treated with CT. They used four cycles of cisplatin, bleomycin, and etoposide (BEP) (178). Eligible patients had incompletely resected stage II to IV or recurrent disease. Seventy-five patients entered, but 18 were ineligible because of incorrect histology or disease status. Of the 57 eligible patients, 41 had recurrent disease and 16 had primary disease. Thirty-nine had gross residual disease following surgery. Forty-eight had GCTs, seven had SLCTs, one had a malignant thecoma, and one had an unclassified SCST. This CT combination was considered to be active, with 11 of 16 primary-disease patients and 21 of 41 recurrent-disease patients remaining progression-free at a median follow-up of 3 years. Recognizing the prolonged natural history of these tumors, longer follow-up of this cohort will be important. The regimen was fairly toxic, with two bleomycin-related fatalities among the first six patients treated with the initial bleomycin dose of 20 U/m^2 (maximum 30 U) weekly for 9 weeks. The bleomycin dose was then reduced (20 U/m^2 every 3 weeks × 4 cycles), with no further toxicity. Grade 4 myelotoxicity occurred in 61% of the patients. The value of bleomycin in the treatment of this tumor type remains in question (179).

Gershenson et al. (180) also reported on the use of BEP in a group of nine women with poor prognosis of SCSTs of the ovary with poor prognosis (seven had metastatic disease). The median PFS was 14 months, with a median survival time of 28 months. In the same report, these investigators describe activity with paclitaxel in patients with GCTs who failed platinum-based therapies. In an earlier series, Gershenson et al. (168) found that cisplatin, doxorubicin, and cyclophosphamide showed activity in the treatment of metastatic ovarian stromal tumors, including two SLCTs. The overall response rate was 63% in this series.

The management of patients with recurrent disease must be individualized. The majority of relapses occur in the pelvis or abdomen, but liver, lung, or bone recurrences are also observed. Given the characteristic indolent growth pattern of GCTs, with long disease-free intervals, surgical resection of disease recurrence is often the initial step in the management of appropriate patients. Pecorelli et al. (181) treated 38 patients with advanced ($n = 7$) or recurrent ($n = 31$) GCTs with cisplatin, vinblastine, and bleomycin (PVB) in a prospective trial through the European Organization for Research and Treatment of Cancer. Of the seven women who presented with advanced disease (stages II to IV), one was alive and disease-free at 81 months. Five died between 4 and 12 months after the start of PVB, and another was alive with disease at 2 months. Among the 31 women with recurrent disease, 7 were alive without further evidence of disease 24 to 81 months from the start of PVB. Consistent with the indolent course observed with GCTs in some women, another 11 patients were alive with disease at a mean of 45 months from the start of PVB (median, 39 months).

The wisdom of using a germ cell–like regimen for stromal tumors is questionable. Uygun et al. (182) reported on a small series of 11 women with recurrent GCTs. Most had cyclophosphamide, Adriamycin (doxorubicin), and cisplatin in the adjuvant setting. Four were treated with cyclophosphamide and cisplatin for recurrence and survived 35 to 73 months after recurrence.

Taxanes have also been reportedly active in SCSTs. A case report documented a dramatic response to paclitaxel in a patient with a GCT 2 years following cessation of platinum-based therapy (183). Subsequently, Brown et al. (184) reported a retrospective review of the M.D. Anderson Cancer Center experience with taxane therapy in 44 patients with newly diagnosed or recurrent SCSTs. Eleven patients received paclitaxel and a platinum drug for newly diagnosed SCSTs; all were alive at the time of the study, with a median follow-up of 52 months. Of 37 patients treated with a taxane for recurrent SCST, 7 had no measurable disease after secondary cytoreductive surgery, and 30 had measurable disease. The response rate in the latter cohort was 42%. In a follow-up study, Brown et al. (185) retrospectively compared the efficacy and side effects of taxanes, with or without platinum, with the combination of BEP. The outcomes of the two groups were similar, but the side effects associated with the BEP regimen appeared to be greater. The authors concluded that taxane and platinum CT warrants further investigation in SCSTs. The GOG recently completed accrual on a phase 2 trial of paclitaxel in women with stromal tumors with measurable disease (GOG protocol 187)—either previously untreated or recurrent. Results are pending. In addition, a GOG randomized phase 2 study of paclitaxel and carboplatin versus BEP in patients with SCSTs is ongoing.

Given the overall experience with cytotoxic CT for SCSTs over the past 3+ decades, it appears that these neoplasms are only moderately chemosensitive. Two recent studies have further elucidated this perspective. In a report of 27 patients with GCTs who received CT, nine patients had measurable disease and were evaluable for response (186). One (11%) of these patients had a complete response, and one (11%) had a partial response, for an overall response rate of 22%. The authors also evaluated 15 studies including 224 patients with measurable disease who received CT, and noted a response rate of 50%. However, they emphasized the lack of standardized response criteria, making a valid comparison very difficult.

Meisel et al. (187) reported a retrospective cohort study of 118 patients with GCTs, 10 (8%) of whom received adjuvant CT. Thirty-two patients experienced at least one relapse. The authors were unable to discern any definite benefit of treatment with CT for relapse compared with other strategies—surgery alone, hormonal therapy, RT, etc. However, the numbers were quite small. They concluded that adjuvant therapy did not appear to improve time to first relapse.

Considerable rationale exists for the utilization of hormone-based approaches in GCTs. A proportion of these tumors express steroid hormone receptors (188). Responses of GCTs, occasionally long-term, to medroxyprogesterone acetate and to GnRH antagonists have been reported (189–193). Fishman et al. (194) treated six patients with recurrent or persistent GCTs with monthly intramuscular injections of leuprolide acetate. Four patients had received prior cisplatinum-based CT. Five patients had evaluable disease: two had partial responses and three had stable disease. The leuprolide was well tolerated.

Aromatase inhibitors have also been used in GCTs. Three reports have documented remissions in seven women who received aromatase inhibitors for recurrent GCTs (195–197).

In a systematic review of 415 potentially relevant studies, van Meurs et al. (198) identified 19 eligible studies that included 31 patients with GCTs treated with 38 evaluable hormonal therapies. Overall, the authors reported a 25.8% complete response rate and a 45.2% partial response rate. Four patients had stable disease, and five had disease progression. Median PFS was 18 (range 0 to 60) months.

Antiangiogenesis drugs have also demonstrated activity in SCSTs. Farkkila et al. (48) found that VEGF and VEGF-2 were highly expressed in primary and recurrent GCTs. In addition, although VEGF protein expression was not predictive of tumor recurrence in this series, high levels of circulating VEGF were found in the serum of women with primary GCTs. Tao et al. (199) reported on eight patients with recurrent GCTs (seven adults and one juvenile) who were treated with bevacizumab. One patient had a complete response and two had a partial response. The GOG conducted a phase 2 trial of bevacizumab in 36 women with recurrent sex cord–stromal ovarian tumors (200). The majority (32 patients) had GCTs, and four had unclassified SCSTs. These 36 patients received a total of 491 cycles of bevacizumab, with a median of 9 treatment cycles per patient. Six (16.7%) patients had a partial response, and 28 (77.8%) had stable disease. The median PFS was 9.3 months. There is also an ongoing French randomized phase 2 trial comparing bevacizumab plus weekly paclitaxel followed by bevacizumab maintenance therapy, versus weekly paclitaxel followed by observation, in patients with recurrent ovarian SCSTs.

Garcia-Donas et al. (201) have also suggested that ketoconazole (a CYP17 inhibitor) may have benefit in metastatic GCTs, reporting on a patient with recurrent GCT who remained progression-free for 10 months while on the drug.

Granulosa Cell Tumors (Juvenile)

Calaminus et al. (202) reported the outcome of 33 patients with JGCTs—24 treated with surgery alone and 9 with surgery and cisplatin-based CT. There have been 6 relapses, with 60 months median follow-up: 2 of 20 stage IA, 2 of 8 stage IC, and 2 of 5 stage IIC to IIIC. Three patients with stage IIC to IIIC disease treated with adjuvant cisplatinum-based therapy remained disease-free at 46 to 66 months after diagnosis. Furthermore, Powell and Otis (203) reported short-term disease control in two teenagers with stage III JGCTs following surgery and cisplatin-based CT.

German investigators published their 15-year experience (1985 to 2000) with 54 SCSTs in children and adolescents (75). Forty-five were JGCTs. Twelve received adjuvant CT for stages IC to IIIC disease. BEP and cisplatin, etoposide, and ifosfamide (PEI) were the most commonly used regimens. Six patients remained in remission after adjuvant CT 15 to 106 months later. A seventh developed a contralateral JGCT 10 years after her initial primary tumor. Five of the 12 have recurred, 3 of whom died 16 to 28 months from diagnosis.

Powell et al. (204) reported a patient with long-term disease-free survival (DFS) following salvage CT for recurrent JGCT. The patient had presented with stage IIIC disease, initially treated by resection of all gross disease followed by carboplatin and etoposide for 6 cycles. She recurred 13 months later with limited disease in the liver and a mass at the inferior aspect of the spleen. She underwent gross total resection followed by six cycles of bleomycin and paclitaxel. The patient was disease-free 44 months later, delivering a normal baby at Caesarian section.

Recently, Benesch et al. (205) reported a case of a 4 1/2-year-old patient diagnosed with a stage IA JGCT. One year after diagnosis, the patient developed a recurrent in a paraaortic lymph node, which was treated with surgery, RT, and conventional treatment followed by high-dose CT. Seven months later, she was diagnosed with a second relapse in a paratracheal lymph node treated with surgery and RT followed by a 2-year course of a combination of bevacizumab, paclitaxel, thalidomide, and pegylated interferon. At the time of the report, the patient was in complete remission 6 years after the second relapse.

Auguste et al. (206) sequenced the transcriptome of four JGCTs and compared them with control transcriptomes. They detected in-frame duplications within the oncogene AKT1 in >60% of the tumor specimens studied. These observations may hold promise for the future use of targeted therapeutics in this tumor type.

Sertoli–Leydig Cell Tumors

Therapy for those few individuals presenting with high-stage SLCTs, as well as for individuals with recurrent disease, must be individualized. The effectiveness of RT is unknown (119). Reports exist of responses to vincristine, actinomycin D, and cyclophosphamide and cisplatin, doxorubicin, and cyclophosphamide (168,207). Schneider et al. (75) reported on three patients with SLCTs who were treated with platinum-based CT. One patient with stage IC disease with intermediate differentiation received two cycles of the combination of cisplatin and etoposide and was disease-free at 47 months. Two other patients, both of whom had stage IC poorly differentiated SLCTs, were dead of tumor at 7 and 19 months, respectively, after receiving either BEP or PEI. Given the functional hormonal nature of many of these neoplasms, consideration could also be given to some form of hormonal manipulation, such as luteinizing hormone–releasing agonists or antagonists (208).

Recently, the Italian cooperative group, Multicentre Italian Trials in Ovarian Cancer, reported their experience with 21 patients with SLCTs (209). Five patients received adjuvant CT—platinum-based CT in four (BEP in two and paclitaxel/carboplatin in two), and one received the combination of methotrexate, 5-fluorouracil, and cyclophosphamide. Three of the five patients subsequently died of disease. Seven patients (one stage IAG1, three stage IAG2, one stage ICG2, and two stage IIICG3) relapsed, four of whom had stage IA disease and did not receive adjuvant CT. Five of these patients were treated with surgery plus CT, one received CT alone, and one received palliation only. All six patients who received CT were treated with platinum-based regimens—either BEP or paxlitaxel/carboplatin. At the time of the report, two patients—one with stage IAG1 and one with stage IAG2—were clinically disease-free, and the other five died of disease.

Gui et al. (210) reported 40 cases of stage IA or IC ovarian SLCTs seen at Peking Union Medical College Hospital in Beijing, China, between 1966 and 2009. Of 34 cases with intermediate or poor differentiation, 23 received adjuvant CT (platinum-based CT, 17; nonplatinum-based CT, 6) following surgery. None of the 23 patients relapsed, whereas 2 of 11 patients who did not receive adjuvant CT relapsed.

Sex Cord Tumor with Annular Tubules

Given the rarity of this tumor, the collective experience with systemic therapy for SCTATs is scant. Their endocrine activities suggest that the tumors may retain responsiveness to perturbation of gonadotropin levels. A case report documents a complete response to etoposide, bleomycin, and cisplatin in a patient with recurrent SCTAT (149). A more recent Chinese report of 13 patients with SCTAT noted that six (46.2%) patients experienced 14 recurrences (211). Two of these patients achieved a complete response without further recurrence after secondary cytoreductive surgery and CT with platinum, etoposide, and bleomycin or platinum, vinblastine, and bleomycin. Three patients achieved a partial response and were alive with disease at the time of the report after surgery and/or RT.

MOLECULAR PATHOGENESIS

Our current knowledge regarding various autocrine and endocrine regulatory mechanisms influencing ovarian function, the overexpression of inhibin in several SCSTs, the alterations in ovarian steroidogenesis, and the changes in circulating gonadotropin levels in SCSTs provides clues regarding the pathogenesis of these tumors. Investigations to date exploring the interactive regulatory mechanisms of inhibin, activin, follistatin, and FSH have predominantly included the more common GCTs. FSH provides a fundamental regulatory role in the differentiation processes of granulosa cells during the early stages of follicle development. Specifically, FSH stimulates cell proliferation (mitosis), increases the availability of cell-surface prolactin and luteinizing hormone receptors, and induces aromatase activity, resulting in increased estradiol production. Other growth regulatory factors such as insulin-like growth factor (IGF) and epidermal growth factor modulate these actions, including the enhancement of the mitogenic effects of FSH. In addition, FSH secretion from the anterior pituitary is modulated in part by the serum levels of inhibin, activin, estrogens, and/or androgens.

Inhibin, a heterodimeric glycoprotein hormone composed of an α-subunit and one of two β-subunits, is secreted by the granulosa cells of the ovary (212). Inhibin A consists of αA and βA; inhibin B consists of αB and βB. Petraglia et al. (213) demonstrated that serum inhibin B was dramatically increased in eight of nine patients with GCTs, whereas inhibin A was slightly increased in all patients. Its major physiologic function is to inhibit the secretion of FSH by the anterior pituitary gland (214). Inhibin is expressed in excessive quantities by GCTs. Although it maintains its regulatory function pertaining to FSH suppression, it appears to be ineffective in controlling estrogen production and cell proliferation within the gonad. Robertson et al. (215) reviewed the various serum-based assays for inhibin.

Activin, also a peptide hormone of ovarian granulosa cell origin, is composed of two β-subunits that are identical to those of inhibin. In contrast to inhibin, activin stimulates the secretion of FSH, induces the production of estradiol when having a negative impact on progesterone production, and promotes granulosa cell differentiation (214).

Lin et al. (216) performed comparative genomic hybridization of a set of 37 adult-type GCTs (36 primaries, 1 recurrence) obtained from five hospitals in Taiwan. All patients had stage I disease except for one stage III patient with limited disease at initial diagnosis. Twenty-two (61%) of the 36 primary tumors had chromosomal imbalances. The nonrandom changes included loss of 22q in 31% of tumors, gain of chromosome 14 in 25% of tumors, and gain of chromosome 12 in 14% of tumors. Monosomy 22 frequently coexisted with trisomy 14. High-level amplification, as can be seen in many aggressive carcinomas, was not detected in any of these GCTs. Similar findings have been reported elsewhere (217,218). As a sole abnormality, trisomy 12 has also been found in fibromas and fibroepitheliomas, in addition to GCTs (219,220). Menczer et al. (221) looked for HER2/neu expression in 12 GCTs and saw no immunohistochemical (IHC) staining. An Austrian group examined the IHC expression of the HER family of receptors—HER1 (EGFR), HER2, HER3, and HER4—in 38 adult GCTs and 2 of the juvenile type (222). Thirty-one cases (77.5%) were positive for at least one of the receptors (EGFR, HER3, or HER4). None of the 40 cases showed a positive reaction for HER2. Twenty-six of 40 (65%) showed reactivity for EGFR. HER3 and HER4 expression was observed in 18 (45%) and 23 (57.5%) tumors, respectively. Kusamura et al. (223) investigated HER2 expression in 18 GCTs: all cases were negative. They also showed a markedly low likelihood of IHC staining for p53 and low proliferative indices in these tumors. Richards et al. (224) used a mouse model to investigate granulosa cell tumorigenesis. They showed that formation of GCTs by stable activation of β-catenin (CTNNB1) in granulosa cells is accelerated by concomitant *Kras* activation or PTEN loss. It has yet to be confirmed if these are crucial pathways in the development of GCTs in humans.

Shah and colleagues (225) performed whole-transcriptome paired-end RNA sequencing on four GCTs. They discovered a point mutation, missense point mutation, 402C→G (C134W), in *FOXL2*, a member of the forkhead–winged helix family of transcription factors. This gene is known to be involved in ovarian differentiation, is required for the normal development of granulosa cells, and may alter cell cycle progression and apoptosis (226,227). They and others have demonstrated that FOXL2 mutations are present in over 95% of GCTs, but a small minority of JGCTs (228,229). These results support a molecular basis for the disparate clinical course observed between JGCTs and AGCTs, provide a means to improve diagnosis in difficult cases, and suggest that *FOXL2* is a key driver of GCT pathogenesis. Molecular studies of JGCTs are limited, but in one investigation AKT1 duplication was identified in >60% of JGCTs tested. These findings may lead to useful therapeutic targets in the future (206,230).

Another major finding has been that of *DICER1* mutations in ovarian SCSTs (231–233). Schultz et al. (231) reported that, among 296 kindreds including 325 children with pleuropulmonary blastoma (PPB), 3 children had both PPB and SLCT. Among family members of PPB patients, they identified six ovarian SCSTs. Germline *DICER1* mutations were identified in four of six patients with SCSTs from PPB kindreds and in two of three children with ovarian SCSTs and no personal or family history of PPB. In another report, Heravi-Moussavi et al. (232) found somatic *DICER1* mutations in the RNAse IIIb domain in 26/43 (60%) SLCTs, including 4 tumors with additional germline *DICER1* mutations. Thus far, discovery of these mutations has translated into a therapeutic target.

Chu et al. (234) examined the estrogen receptor (ER) isoform gene expression in a small series of GCTs and serous cystoadenocarcinomas of the ovary (four of each). They demonstrated widespread expression of ER-α in both tumor types but at relatively low levels, similar to or less than what is seen in the endometrium. ER-β expression in the GCTs, however, was severalfold higher than that of ER-α. Fuller and Chu (235) have provided an informative review of various signaling pathways that are important in the regulation of growth, differentiation, and apoptosis of normal granulosa cells, which may contribute to the molecular pathogenesis of GCTs. Because of the important role of the IGF system in development of the dominant follicle, and its contribution to epithelial ovarian cancer, Alexiadis et al. (236) characterized the expression of several components of the IGF system in a series of nine GCTs. Interestingly, pregnancy-associated plasma protein-A (PAPP-A) expression was highest in the GCTs. PAPP-A is a metalloproteinase synthesized by granulosa cells, the activity of which leads to increased IGF bioavailability. Anttonen et al. (237) studied samples from a cohort of 80 GCT patients from the University of Helsinki and examined several growth regulatory factors known to be important in normal granulosa cell function, including anti-Müllerian hormone, inhibin-α, and GATA transcription factors. They found a correlation between high GATA4 expression and higher likelihood of recurrence. Interestingly, GATA4 and SMAD3 appear to cooperate to reduce GCT cell apoptosis and may contribute to the oncogenic phenotype observed with FOXL2 mutations (238).

The natural history of SCSTs is uniquely different from that of their epithelial counterparts and provides an intriguing tumor model. The vast majority of these neoplasms are characteristically of low malignant potential. They are typically unilateral and remain localized, retain hormone-secreting functions consistent with their well-differentiated appearance, and recurrences, when encountered, are usually delayed. In contrast, a small percentage of otherwise phenotypically similar tumors demonstrate a more virulent course and are generally refractory to therapy. The SCST subtypes display a bimodal age distribution, notably with JGCTs, SSCTs, SLCTs, and SCTATs, occurring predominantly during the first three decades of life. The association of these tumors with several uncommon congenital disease entities, such as enchondromatosis, leprechaunism, and PJS, provides clues to their underlying genetic etiologies. Uniquely, several of these functioning neoplasms, including AGCTs, JGCTs, SLCTs, and SCTATs, overexpress growth-regulatory substances including inhibin, MIS, and follicle-regulating protein. Given the limited number of ovarian SCSTs available for study, our current understanding of the mechanism of oncogenesis in these tumors is understandably limited.

SUMMARY

The principal problem related to the study of SCSTs and the development of effective therapy is their rarity. Although this interesting group of tumors has been studied extensively from a histologic standpoint, there are surprisingly few features that distinguish tumors more likely to recur or have aggressive behavior, and much of the information is conflicting.

Surgery remains the cornerstone of treatment for patients with SCSTs. Furthermore, for young patients desirous of fertility preservation, fertility-sparing surgery is possible in a large proportion of cases because these tumors tend to be unilateral and nonmetastatic. Patients who appear to have a worse prognosis, and for whom postoperative therapy would appear to be indicated, include those with metastatic SCSTs of any histotype and those with stage I poorly differentiated SLCTs. For patients with SCSTs confined to the ovary, postoperative therapy is not recommended. For those with stage IC disease, the issue of postoperative therapy is unresolved.

Standard postoperative treatment consists of platinum-based CT. The BEP regimen is currently the most popular combination. However, this is a relatively toxic regimen, hence the interest in

INTERNATIONAL PERSPECTIVES

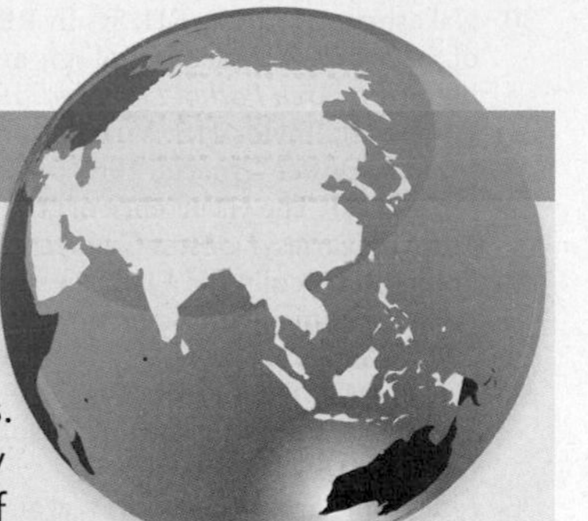

Ovarian Sex Cord–Stromal Tumors in Israel

Uzi Beller, MD

This is an excellent chapter discussing tumors not often seen in our daily practices. Although they are rare, it is of utmost importance to manage them appropriately because they commonly occur in young women of reproductive age. The authors of this chapter have been "global consultants" on the management of ovarian sex cord–stromal tumors for the past four decades, providing their colleagues with guidance on the conservative management of these tumors and the preservation of fertility in these young women.

The thorough understanding of the biology and, most importantly, the natural history of these rare tumors is mutual to all parts of the world, and one finds minimal deviation between continents or countries in this respect.

This chapter is a solid reference for practitioners for managing their patients and for medical students and trainees for learning about these tumors and how to treat them. With today's knowledge and understanding of sex cord–stromal tumors of the ovary, young women can be safely treated with preservation of fertility following the guidelines presented in this comprehensive chapter.

alternative combinations, such as taxane/platinum chemotherapy. However, more study of this latter combination is warranted. An ongoing GOG study should help resolve the issue. In general, available experience with CT to date suggests that any regimen may be only moderately effective, and of those who do benefit, only about 50% enjoy a durable remission.

Beyond platinum-based CT, there is no consensus concerning recommended second-line or salvage therapy. Hormonal medications clearly have some degree of activity in GCTs. Antiangiogenesis agents hold promise. In addition, there is probably a limited role for radiation. This gap in our armamentarium underscores the need for novel target-based therapeutics developed through the study of the genes and pathways involved in the pathogenesis of these neoplasms. Thus far, the association of GCTs with FOXL2 mutations, the association of JGCTs with AKT1 mutations, and the association of some SLTs with DICER1 mutations have not translated into targeted therapies. However, the future appears bright for identification of novel therapies for this group of rare ovarian tumors.

REFERENCES

1. Koonings PP, Campbell K, Mishell DR Jr, et al. Relative frequency of primary ovarian neoplasms: a 10-year review. *Obstet Gynecol.* 1989;74(6):921–926.
2. Cramer DW, Devesa SS, Welch WR. Trends in the incidence of endometrioid and clear cell cancers of the ovary in the United States. *Am J Epidemiol.* 1981;114(2):201–208.
3. Tavassoli FA. Ovarian tumors with functioning manifestations. *Endocrinol Pathol.* 1994;5(3):137–148.
4. Evans AT, Gaffey TA, Malkasian GD Jr, et al. Clinicopathologic review of 118 granulosa and 82 theca cell tumors. *Obstet Gynecol.* 1980;55(2):231–238.
5. Malmstrom H, Hogberg T, Risberg B, et al. Granulosa cell tumors of the ovary: prognostic factors and outcome. *Gynecol Oncol.* 1994;52(1): 50–55.
6. Ohel G, Kaneti H, Schenker JG. Granulosa cell tumors in Israel: a study of 172 cases. *Gynecol Oncol.* 1983;15(2):278–286.
7. Rokitansky CV. Über abnormalities des corpus luteum. *Allg Wien Med Z.* 1859;4:253–254.
8. Schumer ST, Cannistra SA. Granulosa cell tumor of the ovary. *J Clin Oncol.* 2003;21(6):1180–1189.
9. Unkila-Kallio L, Leminen A, Tiitinen A, et al. Nationwide data on falling incidence of ovarian granulosa cell tumours concomitant with increasing use of ovulation inducers. *Hum Reprod.* 1998;13(10):2828–2830.
10. Bryk S, Färkkilä A, Bützow R, et al. Clinical characteristics and survival of patients with an adult-type ovarian granulosa cell tumor: a 56-year single-center experience. *Int J Gynecol Cancer.* 2015;25(1):33–41.
11. Werness BA, Ramus SJ, Whittemore AS, et al. Histopathology of familial ovarian tumors in women from families with and without germline BRCA1 mutations. *Hum Pathol.* 2000;31(11):1420–1424.
12. Stevens TA, Brown J, Zander DS, et al. Adult granulosa cell tumors of the ovary in two first-degree relatives. *Gynecol Oncol.* 2005;98(3):502–505.
13. Bjorkholm E. Granulosa cell tumors: a comparison of survival in patients and matched controls. *Am J Obstet Gynecol.* 1980;138(3):329–331.
14. Bjorkholm E, Silfversward C. Prognostic factors in granulosa-cell tumors. *Gynecol Oncol.* 1981;11(3):261 274.
15. Fox H, Agrawal K, Langley FA. A clinicopathologic study of 92 cases of granulosa cell tumor of the ovary with special reference to the factors influencing prognosis. *Cancer.* 1975;35(1):231–241.
16. Pankratz E, Boyes DA, White GW, et al. Granulosa cell tumors. A clinical review of 61 cases. *Obstet Gynecol.* 1978;52(6):718–723.
17. Piura B, Nemet D, Yanai-Inbar I, et al. Granulosa cell tumor of the ovary: a study of 18 cases. *J Surg Oncol.* 1994;55(2):71–77.
18. Schweppe KW, Beller FK. Clinical data of granulosa cell tumors. *J Cancer Res Clin Oncol.* 1982;104(1–2):161–169.
19. Stenwig JT, Hazekamp JT, Beecham JB. Granulosa cell tumors of the ovary. A clinicopathological study of 118 cases with long-term follow-up. *Gynecol Oncol.* 1979;7(2):136–152.
20. Young RH, Scully RE. Ovarian sex cord–stromal tumours: recent advances and current status. *Clin Obstet Gynaecol.* 1984;11(1):93–134.
21. Bjorkholm E, Silfversward C. Granulosa- and theca-cell tumors. Incidence and occurrence of second primary tumors. *Acta Radiol Oncol.* 1980;19(3):161–167.
22. Muir CS, Waterhouse JAH, Mack TM, et al. *Cancer Incidence in Five Continents* (IARC Scientific Publication No. 88). Vol V. Lyon, France: International Agency for Research on Cancer; 1987.
23. Quirk JT, Natarajan N. Ovarian cancer incidence in the United States, 1992–1999. *Gynecol Oncol.* 2005;97(2):519–523.
24. Cronje HS, Niemand I, Bam RH, et al. Review of the granulosa-theca cell tumors from the Emil Novak ovarian tumor registry. *Am J Obstet Gynecol.* 1999;180(2 pt 1):323–327.
25. Gusberg SB, Kardon P. Proliferative endometrial response to theca-granulosa cell tumors. *Am J Obstet Gynecol.* 1971;111(5):633–643.
26. Stuart GC, Dawson LM. Update on granulosa cell tumours of the ovary. *Curr Opin Obstet Gynecol.* 2003;15(1):33–37.
27. Chen VW, Ruiz B, Killeen J, et al. Pathology and classification of ovarian tumors. *Cancer.* 2003;97(suppl 10):2631–2642.
28. Young RH, Oliva E, Scully RE. Luteinized adult granulosa cell tumors of the ovary: a report of four cases. *Int J Gynecol Pathol.* 1994;13(4):302–310.
29. Zanagnolo V, Pasinetti B, Sartori E. Clinical review of 63 cases of sex cord stromal tumors. *Eur J Gynaecol Oncol.* 2004;25(4):431–438.

30. Nakashima N, Young RH, Scully RE. Androgenic granulosa cell tumors of the ovary. A clinicopathologic analysis of 17 cases and review of the literature. *Arch Pathol Lab Med.* 1984;108(10):786–791.
31. Norris HJ, Taylor HB. Virilization associated with cystic granulosa tumors. *Obstet Gynecol.* 1969;34(5):629–635.
32. Fathalla MF. The occurrence of granulosa and theca tumours in clinically normal ovaries. *J Obstet Gynaecol Br Commonw.* 1967;74(2):279–282.
33. Young RH, Scully RE. Ovarian sex cord–stromal tumors with bizarre nuclei: a clinicopathologic analysis of 17 cases. *Int J Gynecol Pathol.* 1983;1(4):325–335.
34. Wilson MK, Fong P, Mesnage S, et al. Stage I granulosa cell tumours: a management conundrum? Results of long-term follow up. *Gynecol Oncol.* 2015;138(2):285–291.
35. Miller BE, Barron BA, Wan JY, et al. Prognostic factors in adult granulosa cell tumor of the ovary. *Cancer.* 1997;79(10):1951–1955.
36. Fujimoto T, Sakuragi N, Okuyama K, et al. Histopathological prognostic factors of adult granulosa cell tumors of the ovary. *Acta Obstet Gynecol Scand.* 2001;80(11):1069–1074.
37. Sun HD, Lin H, Jao MS, et al. A long-term follow-up study of 176 cases with adult-type ovarian granulosa cell tumors. *Gynecol Oncol.* 2012;124(2):244–249.
38. Kottmeier HL. *Carcinoma of the Female Genitalia.* Baltimore, MD: Williams & Wilkins; 1953.
39. Klemi PJ, Joensuu H, Salmi T. Prognostic value of flow cytometric DNA content analysis in granulosa cell tumor of the ovary. *Cancer.* 1990;65(5):1189–1193.
40. Chadha S, Cornelisse CJ, Schaberg A. Flow cytometric DNA ploidy analysis of ovarian granulosa cell tumors. *Gynecol Oncol.* 1990;36(2):240–245.
41. Evans MP, Webb MJ, Gaffey TA, et al. DNA ploidy of ovarian granulosa cell tumors. Lack of correlation between DNA index or proliferative index and outcome in 40 patients. *Cancer.* 1995;75(9):2295–2298.
42. Ala-Fossi SL, Maenpaa J, Aine R, et al. Prognostic significance of p53 expression in ovarian granulosa cell tumors. *Gynecol Oncol.* 1997;66(3):475–479.
43. Kappes S, Milde-Langosch K, Kressin P, et al. p53 mutations in ovarian tumors, detected by temperature-gradient gel electrophoresis, direct sequencing and immunohistochemistry. *Int J Cancer.* 1995;64(1):52–59.
44. Villella J, Herrmann FR, Kaul S, et al. Clinical and pathological predictive factors in women with adult-type granulosa cell tumor of the ovary. *Int J Gynecol Pathol.* 2007;26(2):154–159.
45. King LA, Okagaki T, Gallup DG, et al. Mitotic count, nuclear atypia, and immunohistochemical determination of Ki-67, c-myc, p21-ras, c-erbB2, and p53 expression in granulosa cell tumors of the ovary: mitotic count and Ki-67 are indicators of poor prognosis. *Gynecol Oncol.* 1996;61(2):227–232.
46. Liu FS, Ho ES, Lai CR, et al. Overexpression of p53 is not a feature of ovarian granulosa cell tumors. *Gynecol Oncol.* 1996;61(1):50–53.
47. Dowdy SC, O'Kane DJ, Keeney GL, et al. Telomerase activity in sex cord–stromal tumors of the ovary. *Gynecol Oncol.* 2001;82(2):257–260.
48. Färkkilä A, Anttonen M, Pociuviene J, et al. Vascular endothelial growth factor (VEGF) and its receptor VEGFR-2 are highly expressed in ovarian granulosa cell tumors. *Eur J Endocrinol.* 2011;164(1):115–122.
49. Ala-Fossi SL, Aine R, Punnonen R, et al. Is potential to produce inhibins related to prognosis in ovarian granulosa cell tumors? *Eur J Gynaecol Oncol.* 2000;21(2):187–189.
50. Kaye SB, Davies E. Cyclophosphamide, Adriamycin, and cis-platinum for the treatment of advanced granulosa cell tumor, using serum estradiol as a tumor marker. *Gynecol Oncol.* 1986;24(2):261–264.
51. Boggess JF, Soules MR, Goff BA, et al. Serum inhibin and disease status in women with ovarian granulosa cell tumors. *Gynecol Oncol.* 1997;64(1):64–69.
52. Gustafson ML, Lee MM, Asmundson L, et al. Müllerian inhibiting substance in the diagnosis and management of intersex and gonadal abnormalities. *J Pediatr Surg.* 1993;28(3):439–444.
53. Jobling T, Mamers P, Healy DL, et al. A prospective study of inhibin in granulosa cell tumors of the ovary. *Gynecol Oncol.* 1994;55(2):285–289.
54. Lane AH, Lee MM, Fuller AF Jr, et al. Diagnostic utility of müllerian inhibiting substance determination in patients with primary and recurrent granulosa cell tumors. *Gynecol Oncol.* 1999;73(1):51–55.
55. Lappohn RE, Burger HG, Bouma J, et al. Inhibin as a marker for granulosa cell tumor. *Acta Obstet Gynecol Scand Suppl.* 1992;7(suppl 155):61–65.
56. Lappohn RE, Burger HG, Bouma J, et al. Inhibin as a marker for granulosa cell tumors. *N Engl J Med.* 1989;321(12):790–793.
57. Rey RA, L'homme C, Marcillac I, et al. Antimüllerian hormone as a serum marker of granulosa cell tumors of the ovary: comparative study with serum alpha-inhibin and estradiol. *Am J Obstet Gynecol.* 1996;174(3):958–965.
58. Rodgers KE, Marks JF, Ellefson DD, et al. Follicle regulatory protein: a novel marker for granulosa cell cancer patients. *Gynecol Oncol.* 1990;37(3):381–387.
59. Sluijmer AV, Heineman MJ, Evers JL, et al. Peripheral vein, ovarian vein and ovarian tissue levels of inhibin in a postmenopausal patient with a granulosa cell tumour. *Acta Endocrinol (Copenh).* 1993;129(4):311–324.
59a. Färkkilä A, Koskela S, Bryk S, et al. The clinical utility of serum anti-Müllerian hormone in the follow-up of ovarian adult-type granulosa cell tumors: a comparative study with inhibin B. Int J Cancer. 2015;137(7):1661–1671.
60. Mom CH, Engelen MJA, Willemse PHB, et al. Granulosa cell tumors of the ovary: the clinical value of serum inhibin A and B levels in a large single center cohort. *Gynecol Oncol.* 2007;105(2):365–372.
61. McCluggage WG, Young R. Immunohistochemistry as a diagnostic aid in the evaluation of ovarian tumors. *Semin Diagn Pathol.* 2005;22(1):3–32.
62. Scully RE. Stromal luteoma of the ovary: a distinctive type of lipoid-cell tumor. *Cancer.* 1964;17(6):769–778.
63. Young RH, Dickersin GR, Scully RE. Juvenile granulosa cell tumor of the ovary. A clinicopathological analysis of 125 cases. *Am J Surg Pathol.* 1984;8(8):575–596.
64. Lack EE, Perez-Atayde AR, Murthy AS, et al. Granulosa theca cell tumors in premenarchal girls: a clinical and pathologic study of ten cases. *Cancer.* 1981;48(8):1846–1854.
65. Plantaz D, Flamant F, Vassal G, et al. Granulosa cell tumors of the ovary in children and adolescents. Multicenter retrospective study in 40 patients aged 7 months to 22 years. *Arch Fr Pediatr.* 1992;49(9):793–798.
66. Vassal G, Flamant F, Caillaud JM, et al. Juvenile granulosa cell tumor of the ovary in children: a clinical study of 15 cases. *J Clin Oncol.* 1988;6(6):990–995.
67. Zaloudek C, Norris HJ. Granulosa tumors of the ovary in children: a clinical and pathologic study of 32 cases. *Am J Surg Pathol.* 1982;6(6):513–522.
68. Bouffet E, Basset T, Chetail N, et al. Juvenile granulosa cell tumor of the ovary in infants: a clinicopathologic study of three cases and review of the literature. *J Pediatr Surg.* 1997;32(5):762–765.
69. Hasiakos D, Papakonstantinou K, Goula K, et al. Juvenile granulosa cell tumor associated with pregnancy: report of a case and review of the literature. *Gynecol Oncol.* 2006;100(2):426–429.
70. Scully RE. Sex cord tumor with annular tubules: a distinctive ovarian tumor of the Peutz-Jeghers syndrome. *Cancer.* 1970;25(5):1107–1121.
71. Asirvatham R, Rooney RJ, Watts HG. Ollier's disease with secondary chondrosarcoma associated with ovarian tumour. A case report. *Int Orthop.* 1991;15(4):393–395.
72. Tamimi HK, Bolen JW. Enchondromatosis (Ollier's disease) and ovarian juvenile granulosa cell tumor. *Cancer.* 1984;53(7):1605–1608.
73. Tanaka Y, Sasaki Y, Nishihira H, et al. Ovarian juvenile granulosa cell tumor associated with Maffucci's syndrome. *Am J Clin Pathol.* 1992;97(4):523–527.
74. Brisigotti M, Fabbretti G, Pesce F, et al. Congenital bilateral juvenile granulosa cell tumor of the ovary in leprechaunism: a case report. *Pediatr Pathol.* 1993;13(5):549–558.
75. Schneider DT, Calaminus G, Wessalowski R, et al. Ovarian sex cord–stromal tumors in children and adolescents. *J Clin Oncol.* 2003;21(12):2357–2363.
76. Jacoby AF, Young RH, Colvin RB, et al. DNA content in juvenile granulosa cell tumors of the ovary: a study of early- and advanced-stage disease. *Gynecol Oncol.* 1992;46(1):97–103.
77. Swanson SA, Norris HJ, Kelsten ML, et al. DNA content of juvenile granulosa tumors determined by flow cytometry. *Int J Gynecol Pathol.* 1990;9(2):101–109.
78. Bjorkholm E, Silfversward C. Theca-cell tumors. Clinical features and prognosis. *Acta Radiol Oncol.* 1980;19(4):241–244.
79. Burandt E, Young RH. Thecoma of the ovary: a report of 70 cases emphasizing aspects of its histopathology different from those often portrayed and its differential diagnosis. *Am J Surg Pathol.* 2014;38(8):1023–1032.
80. Barrenetxea G, Schneider J, Centeno MM, et al. Pure theca cell tumors. A clinicopathologic study of 29 cases. *Eur J Gynaecol Oncol.* 1990;11(6):429–432.
81. Staats PN, McCluggage WG, Clement PB, et al. Luteinized thecomas (thecomatosis) of the type typically associated with sclerosing peritonitis: a clinical, histopathologic, and immunohistochemical analysis of 27 cases. *Am J Surg Pathol.* 2008;32(9):1273–1290.
82. Schonman R, Klein Z, Edelstein E, et al. Luteinized thecoma associated with sclerosing peritonitis—conservative surgical approach followed by corticosteroid and GnRH agonist treatment—a case report. *Gynecol Oncol.* 2008;111(3):540–543.
83. Dockerty MB, Mason JC. Ovarian fibromas: clinical and pathologic study of 283 cases. *Am J Obstet Gynecol.* 1944;47:741–752.

84. Samanth KK, Black WC. Benign ovarian stromal tumors associated with free peritoneal fluid. *Am J Obstet Gynecol.* 1970;107(4):538–545.
85. Meigs JV. Fibroma of the ovary with ascites and hydrothorax: Meigs' syndrome. *Am J Obstet Gynecol.* 1954;67(5):962–987.
86. Raggio M, Kaplan AL, Harberg JF. Recurrent ovarian fibromas with basal cell nevus syndrome (Gorlin syndrome). *Obstet Gynecol.* 1983;61(suppl 3):95S–96S.
87. Prat J, Scully RE. Cellular fibromas of the ovary: a comparative clinicopathologic analysis of seventeen cases. *Cancer.* 1981;47(11):2663–2670.
88. Irving JA, Alkushi A, Young RH, et al. Cellular fibromas of the ovary: a study of 75 cases including 40 mitotically active tumors emphasizing their distinction from fibrosarcoma. *Am J Surg Pathol.* 2006;30(8):929–938.
89. Wang J, Papanastasopoulos P, Savage P, et al. A unique case of extraovarian sex-cord stromal fibrosarcoma, with subsequent relapse of differentiated sex-cord tumor. *Int J Gynecol Pathol.* 2015;34(4):363–368.
90. Chalvardjian A, Scully RE. Sclerosing stromal tumors of the ovary. *Cancer.* 1973;31(3):664–670.
91. Gee DC, Russell P. Sclerosing stromal tumours of the ovary. *Histopathology.* 1979;3(5):367–376.
92. Lam RM, Geittmann P. Sclerosing stromal tumor of the ovary. A light, electron microscopic and enzyme histochemical study. *Int J Gynecol Pathol.* 1988;7(3):280–290.
93. Oliva E, Alvarez T, Young RH. Sertoli cell tumors of the ovary. A clinicopathologic and immunohistochemical study of 54 cases. *Am J Surg Pathol.* 2005;29(2):143–156.
94. Roth LM, Gaba AR, Cheng L. On the pathogenesis of sclerosing stromal tumor of the ovary: a neoplasm in transition. *Int J Gynecol Pathol.* 2014;33(5):449–462.
95. Suit PF, Hart WR. Sclerosing stromal tumor of the ovary. An ultrastructural study and review of the literature to evaluate hormonal function. *Cleve Clin J Med.* 1988;55(2):189–194.
96. Cashell AW, Cohen ML. Masculinizing sclerosing stromal tumor of the ovary during pregnancy. *Gynecol Oncol.* 1991;43(3):281–285.
97. Ismail SM, Walker SM. Bilateral virilizing sclerosing stromal tumours of the ovary in a pregnant woman with Gorlin's syndrome: implications for pathogenesis of ovarian stromal neoplasms. *Histopathology.* 1990;17(2):159–163.
98. Katsube Y, Iwaoki Y, Silverberg SG, et al. Sclerosing stromal tumor of the ovary associated with endometrial adenocarcinoma: a case report. *Gynecol Oncol.* 1988;29(3):392–398.
99. Bennett JA, Oliva E, Young RH. Sclerosing stromal tumors with prominent luteinization during pregnancy: a report of 8 cases emphasizing diagnostic problems. *Int J Gynecol Path.* 2015;34(4):357–362.
100. Healy DL, Burger HG, Mamers P, et al. Elevated serum inhibin concentrations in postmenopausal women with ovarian tumors. *N Engl J Med.* 1993;329(21):1539–1542.
101. van Winter JT, Podratz KC, Gaffey TA. Sclerosing stromal tumor of the ovary in a 13-year-old girl. *Adolesc Pediatr Gynecol.* 1993;6:164–165.
102. Irving JA, Young RH. Microcystic stromal tumor of the ovary: report of 16 cases of a hitherto uncharacterized distinctive ovarian neoplasm. *Am J surg Pathol.* 2009;33(3):367–375.
103. Irving JA, Lee CH, Yup S, et al. Microcystic stromal tumor. A distinctive ovarian sex cord-stromal neoplasm characterized by FOXL2, SF-1, cyclin D1, and β-catenin nuclear expression and CTNNB1 mutations. *Am J Surg Pathol.* 2015;39(10):1420–1426.
104. Mancuso A, Grosso M, D'Anna R, et al. Anatomo-clinical considerations on the ovarian fibroma. *Clin Exp Obstet Gynecol.* 1995;22(2):115–119.
105. Waxman M, Vuletin JC, Urcuyo R, et al. Ovarian low-grade stromal sarcoma with thecomatous features: a critical reappraisal of the so-called "malignant thecoma." *Cancer.* 1979;44(6):2206–2217.
106. Micci F, Haugom L, Abeler VM. Consistent numerical chromosome aberrations in thecofibromas of the ovary. *Virchows Arch.* 2008;452(3):269–276.
107. Lage JM, Weinberg DS, Huettner PC, et al. Flow cytometric analysis of nuclear DNA content in ovarian tumors. Association of ploidy with tumor type, histologic grade, and clinical stage. *Cancer.* 1992;69(11):2668–2675.
108. Meyer R. Pathology of some special ovarian tumors and their relation to sex characteristics. *Am J Obstet Gynecol.* 1931;22:697–713.
109. Novak E. Life and works of Robert Meyer. *Am J Obstet Gynecol.* 1947;53(1):50–64.
110. Morris M, Scully RE. *Endocrine Pathology of the Ovary.* St. Louis, MO: Mosby; 1958:82–96.
111. Aiba M, Hirayama A, Sukurada M, et al. Spironolactone body-like structure in rennin-producing Sertoli-cell tumors of the ovary. *Surg Pathol.* 1990;3:143–149.
112. Ehrlich EN, Dominguez OV, Samuels LT, et al. Aldosteronism and precocious puberty due to an ovarian androblastoma (Sertoli cell tumor). *J Clin Endocrinol Metab.* 1963;23:358–367.
113. Korzets A, Nouriel H, Steiner Z, et al. Resistant hypertension associated with a rennin-producing ovarian Sertoli cell tumor. *Am J Clin Pathol.* 1986;85(2):242–247.
114. Ferry JA, Young RH, Engel G, et al. Oxyphilic Sertoli cell tumor of the ovary: a report of three cases, two in patients with the Peutz-Jeghers syndrome. *Int J Gynecol Pathol.* 1994;13(3):259–266.
115. Ravishankar S, Mangray S, Kurkchubasche A, et al. Unusual Sertoli cell tumor associated with sex cord tumor with annular tubules in Peutz-Jeghers syndrome: report of a case and review of the literature on ovarian tumors in Peutz-Jeghers syndrome. *Int J Surg Path.* 2016;24(3):269–73.
116. Tavassoli FA, Norris HJ. Sertoli tumors of the ovary. A clinicopathologic study of 28 cases with ultrastructural observations. *Cancer.* 1980;46(10):2281–2297.
117. Roth LM, Anderson MC, Govan AD, et al. Sertoli-Leydig cell tumors: a clinicopathologic study of 34 cases. *Cancer.* 1981;48(1):187–197.
118. Young RH, Scully RE. Ovarian Sertoli-Leydig cell tumors with a retiform pattern: a problem in histopathologic diagnosis. A report of 25 cases. *Am J Surg Pathol.* 1983;7(8):755–771.
119. Zaloudek C, Norris HJ. Sertoli-Leydig tumors of the ovary. A clinicopathologic study of 64 intermediate and poorly differentiated neoplasms. *Am J Surg Pathol.* 1984;8(6):405–418.
120. Roth LM, Slayton RE, Brady LW, et al. Retiform differentiation in ovarian Sertoli-Leydig cell tumors. A clinicopathologic study of six cases from a Gynecologic Oncology Group study. *Cancer.* 1985;55(5):1093–1098.
121. Talerman A. Ovarian Sertoli-Leydig cell tumor (androblastoma) with retiform pattern. A clinicopathologic study. *Cancer.* 1987;60(12):3056–3964.
122. Young RH. Sertoli-Leydig cell tumors of the ovary: review with emphasis on historical aspects and unusual variants. *Int J Gynecol Pathol.* 1993;12(2):141–147.
123. Young RH, Scully RE. Ovarian Sertoli-Leydig cell tumors. A clinicopathological analysis of 207 cases. *Am J Surg Pathol.* 1985;9(8):543–569.
124. Pascale MM, Pugeat M, Roberts M, et al. Androgen suppressive effect of GnRH agonist in ovarian hyperthecosis and virilizing tumours. *Clin Endocrinol(Oxf).* 1994;41(5):571–576.
125. Weyl-Ben Arush M, Oslander L. Ollier's disease associated with ovarian Sertoli-Leydig cell tumor and breast adenoma. *Am J Pediatr Hematol Oncol.* 1991;13(1):49–51.
126. Young RH, Prat J, Scully RE. Ovarian Sertoli-Leydig cell tumors with heterologous elements. I. Gastrointestinal epithelium and carcinoid: a clinicopathologic analysis of thirty-six cases. *Cancer.* 1982;50:2448–2456.
127. Young RH, Scully RE. Well-differentiated ovarian Sertoli-Leydig cell tumors: a clinicopathological analysis of 23 cases. *Int J Gynecol Pathol.* 1984;3(3):277–290.
128. McCluggage WG, Young RH. Ovarian Sertoli-Leydig cell tumors with pseudoendometrioid tubules (pseudoendometrioid Sertoli-Leydig cell tumors). *Am J Surg Pathol.* 2007;31(4):592–597.
129. Prat J, Young RH, Scully RE. Ovarian Sertoli-Leydig cell tumors with heterologous elements. II. Cartilage and skeletal muscle: a clinicopathologic analysis of twelve cases. *Cancer.* 1982;50(11):2465–2475.
130. Cohen I, Shapira M, Cuperman S, et al. Direct in-vivo detection of atypical hormonal expression of a Sertoli-Leydig cell tumour following stimulation with human chorionic gonadotrophin. *Clin Endocrinol(Oxf).* 1993;39(4):491–495.
131. Ohashi M, Hasegawa Y, Haji M, et al. Production of immunoreactive inhibin by a virilizing ovarian tumour (Sertoli-Leydig tumour). *Clin Endocrinol(Oxf).* 1990;33(5):613–618.
132. Gagnon S, Tetu B, Silva EG, et al. Frequency of alpha-fetoprotein production by Sertoli-Leydig cell tumors of the ovary: an immunohistochemical study of eight cases. *Mod Pathol.* 1989;2(1):63–67.
133. Motoyama I, Watanabe H, Gotoh A, et al. Ovarian Sertoli-Leydig cell tumor with elevated serum alpha-fetoprotein. *Cancer.* 1989;63(10):2047–2053.
134. Shen K, Wu PC, Lang JH, et al. Ovarian sex cord tumor with annular tubules: a report of six cases. *Gynecol Oncol.* 1993;48(2):180–184.
135. Young RH, Welch WR, Dickersin GR, et al. Ovarian sex cord tumor with annular tubules: review of 74 cases including 27 with Peutz-Jeghers syndrome and four with adenoma malignum of the cervix. *Cancer.* 1982;50(7):1384–1402.
136. Hart WR, Kumar N, Crissman JD. Ovarian neoplasms resembling sex cord tumors with annular tubules. *Cancer.* 1980;45(9):2352–2363.
137. Ahn GH, Chi JG, Lee SK. Ovarian sex cord tumor with annular tubules. *Cancer.* 1986;57:1066–1073.
138. Solh HM, Azoury RS, Najjar SS. Peutz-Jeghers syndrome associated with precocious puberty. *J Pediatr.* 1983;103(4):593–595.
139. Nomura K, Furusato M, Nikaido T, et al. Ovarian sex cord tumor with annular tubules. Report of a case. *Acta Pathol Jpn.* 1991;41:701–706.

140. Podczaski E, Kaminski PF, Pees RC, et al. Peutz-Jeghers syndrome with ovarian sex cord tumor with annular tubules and cervical adenoma malignum. *Gynecol Oncol.* 1991;42(1):74–78.
141. Srivatsa PJ, Keeney GL, Podratz KC. Disseminated cervical adenoma malignum and bilateral ovarian sex cord tumors with annular tubules associated with Peutz-Jeghers syndrome. *Gynecol Oncol.* 1994;53(2):256–264.
142. Boardman LA, Thibodeau SN, Schaid DJ, et al. Increased risk for cancer in patients with the Peutz-Jeghers syndrome. *Ann Intern Med.* 1998;128(11):896–899.
143. Hemminki A, Tomlinson I, Markie D, et al. Localization of a susceptibility locus for Peutz-Jeghers syndrome to 19p using comparative genomic hybridization and targeted linkage analysis. *Nat Genet.* 1997;15(1):87–90.
144. Jenne DE, Reimann H, Nezu J, et al. Peutz-Jeghers syndrome is caused by mutations in a novel serine threonine kinase. *Nat Genet.* 1998;18(1):38–43.
145. Benagiano G, Bigotti G, Buzzi M, et al. Endocrine and morphological study of a case of ovarian sex-cord tumor with annular tubules in a woman with Peutz-Jeghers syndrome. *Int J Gynaecol Obstet.* 1988;26(3):441–452.
146. Crain JL. Ovarian sex cord tumor with annular tubules: steroid profile. *Obstet Gynecol.* 1986;68(suppl 3):75S–79S.
147. Gustafson ML, Lee MM, Scully RE, et al. Müllerian inhibiting substance as a marker for ovarian sex-cord tumor. *N Engl J Med.* 1992;326(7):466–471.
148. Barker D, Sharma R, McIndoe A, et al. An unusual case of sex cord tumor with annular tubules with malignant transformation in a patient with Peutz-Jeghers syndrome. *Int J Gynecol Pathol.* 2009;29(1):27–32.
149. Puls LE, Hamous J, Morrow MS, et al. Recurrent ovarian sex cord tumor with annular tubules: tumor marker and chemotherapy experience. *Gynecol Oncol.* 1994;54(3):396–401.
150. Talerman A, Hughesdon PE, Anderson MC. Diffuse nonlobular ovarian androblastoma usually associated with feminization. *Int J Gynecol Pathol.* 1982;1(2):155–171.
151. Young RH, Dudley AG, Scully RE. Granulosa cell, Sertoli-Leydig cell, and unclassified sex cord–stromal tumors associated with pregnancy: a clinicopathological analysis of thirty-six cases. *Gynecol Oncol.* 1984;18(2):181–205.
152. Martin-Jimenez A, Condor-Munro E, Valls-Porcel M, et al. Gynandroblastoma of the ovary. Review of the literature. *J Gynecol Obstet Biol Reprod.* 1994;23(4):391–394.
153. Novak ER. Gynandroblastoma of the ovary: review of 8 cases from the Ovarian Tumor Registry. *Obstet Gynecol.* 1967;30(5):709–715.
154. Kalir T, Friedman F Jr. Gynandroblastoma in pregnancy: case report and review of literature. *Mt Sinai J Med.* 1998;65(4):292–295.
155. Hayes MC, Scully RE. Stromal luteoma of the ovary: a clinicopathological analysis of 25 cases. *Int J Gynecol Pathol.* 1987;6(4):313–321.
156. Paraskevas M, Scully RE. Hilus cell tumor of the ovary. A clinicopathological analysis of 12 Reinke crystal-positive and nine crystal-negative cases. *Int J Gynecol Pathol.* 1989;8(4):299–310.
157. Dunnihoo DR, Grieme DL, Woolf RB. Hilar-cell tumors of the ovary. Report of 2 new cases and a review of the world literature. *Obstet Gynecol.* 1966;27(5):703–713.
158. Roth LM, Sternberg WH. Ovarian stromal tumors containing Leydig cells. II. Pure Leydig cell tumor, non-hilar type. *Cancer.* 1973;32(4):952–960.
159. Hayes MC, Scully RE. Ovarian steroid cell tumors (not otherwise specified). A clinicopathological analysis of 63 cases. *Am J Surg Pathol.* 1987;11(11):835–845.
160. Harris AC, Wakely PE Jr, Kaplowitz PB, et al. Steroid cell tumor of the ovary in a child. *Arch Pathol Lab Med.* 1991;115(2):150–154.
161. Davidson BJ, Waisman J, Judd HL. Long-standing virilism in a woman with hyperplasia and neoplasia of ovarian lipidic cells. *Obstet Gynecol.* 1981;58(6):753–759.
162. Taylor HB, Norris HJ. Lipid cell tumors of the ovary. *Cancer.* 1967;20(11):1953–1962.
163. Adeyemi SD, Grange AO, Giwa-Osagie OF, et al. Adrenal rest tumour of the ovary associated with isosexual precocious pseudopuberty and cushingoid features. *Eur J Pediatr.* 1986;145(3):236–238.
164. Dengg K, Fink FM, Heitger A, et al. Precocious puberty due to a lipid-cell tumour of the ovary. *Eur J Pediatr.* 1993;152(1):12–14.
165. Clement PB, Young RH, Scully RE. Clinical syndromes associated with tumors of the female genital tract. *Semin Diagn Pathol.* 1991;8(4):204–233.
166. Donovan JT, Otis CN, Powell JL, et al. Cushing's syndrome secondary to malignant lipoid cell tumor of the ovary. *Gynecol Oncol.* 1993;50(2):249–253.
167. Young RH, Scully RE. Ovarian steroid cell tumors associated with Cushing's syndrome: a report of three cases. *Int J Gynecol Pathol.* 1987;6(1):40–48.
168. Gershenson DM, Copeland LJ, Kavanagh JJ, et al. Treatment of metastatic stromal tumors of the ovary with cisplatin, doxorubicin, and cyclophosphamide. *Obstet Gynecol.* 1987;70(5):765–769.
169. Gershenson DM. Chemotherapy of ovarian germ cell tumors and sex cord stromal tumors. *Semin Surg Oncol.* 1994;10(4):290–298.
170. Abu-Rustum N, Restivo A, Ivy J, et al. Retroperitoneal nodal metastasis in primary and recurrent granulosa cell tumors of the ovary. *Gynecol Oncol.* 2006;103(1):31–34.
171. Thrall MM, Paley P, Pizer E, et al. Patterns of spread and recurrence of sex cord-stromal tumors of the ovary. *Gynecol Oncol.* 2011;122(2):242–245.
172. Powell JL, Kotwall CA, Shiro BC. Fertility-sparing surgery for advanced juvenile granulosa cell tumor of the ovary. *J Pediatr Adolesc Gynecol.* 2014;27(4):e89–e92.
173. Ottolina J, Ferrandina G, Gadducci A, et al. Is the endometrial evaluation routinely required in patients with adult granulosa cell tumors of the ovary? *Gynecol Oncol.* 2015;136(2):230–234.
174. Park JY, Jin KL, Kim DY, et al. Surgical staging and adjuvant chemotherapy in the management of patients with adult granulosa cell tumors of the ovary. *Gynecol Oncol.* 2012;125(1):80–86.
175. Zhang M, Cheung MK, Shin JY, et al. Prognostic factors responsible for survival in sex cord stromal tumors of the ovary—an analysis of 376 women. *Gynecol Oncol.* 2007;104(2):396–400.
176. Wolf JK, Mullen J, Eifel PJ, et al. Radiation treatment of advanced or recurrent granulosa cell tumor of the ovary. *Gynecol Oncol.* 1999;73(1):35–41.
177. Savage P, Constenla D, Fisher C, et al. Granulosa cell tumours of the ovary: demographics, survival and the management of advanced disease. *Clin Oncol.* 1998;10(4):242–245.
178. Homesley HD, Bundy BN, Hurteau JA, et al. Bleomycin, etoposide, and cisplatin combination therapy of ovarian granulosa cell tumors and other stromal malignancies: a Gynecologic Oncology Group study. *Gynecol Oncol.* 1999;72(2):131–137.
179. Colombo N, Parma G, Franchi D. An active chemotherapy regimen for advanced ovarian sex cord–stromal tumors. *Gynecol Oncol.* 1999;72(2):129–130.
180. Gershenson DM, Morris M, Burke TW, et al. Treatment of poor-prognosis sex cord–stromal tumors of the ovary with the combination of bleomycin, etoposide, and cisplatin. *Obstet Gynecol.* 1996;87(4):527–531.
181. Pecorelli S, Wagenaar HC, Vergote IB, et al. Cisplatin (P), vinblastine (V) and bleomycin (B) combination chemotherapy in recurrent or advanced granulosa (-theca) cell tumours of the ovary. An EORTC Gynaecological Cancer Cooperative Group Study. *Eur J Cancer.* 1999;35(9):1331–1337.
182. Uygun K, Aydiner A, Saip P, et al. Clinical parameters and treatment results in recurrent granulosa cell tumor of the ovary. *Gynecol Oncol.* 2003;88(3):400–403.
183. Tresukosol D, Kudelka AP, Edwards CL, et al. Recurrent ovarian granulosa cell tumor: a case report of a dramatic response to Taxol. *Int J Gynecol Cancer.* 1995;5(2):156–159.
184. Brown J, Shvartsman HS, Deavers MT, et al. The activity of taxanes in the treatment of sex cord-stromal ovarian tumors. *J Clin Oncol.* 2004;22(17):3517–3523.
185. Brown J, Shvartsman HS, Deavers MT, et al. The activity of taxanes compared with bleomycin, etoposide, and cisplatin in the treatment of sex cord-stromal ovarian tumors. *Gynecol Oncol.* 2005;97(2):489–496.
186. van Meurs HS, Buist MR, Westermann AM, et al. Effectiveness of chemotherapy in measurable granulosa cell tumors. *Int J Gynecol Cancer.* 2014;24(3):496–505.
187. Meisel JL, Hyman DM, Jotwani A, et al. The role of systemic chemotherapy in the management of granulosa cell tumors. *Gynecol Oncol.* 2015;136(3):505–511.
188. Chadha S, Rao BR, Slotman BJ, et al. An immunohistochemical evaluation of androgen and progesterone receptors in ovarian tumors. *Hum Pathol.* 1993;24(1):90–95.
189. Fishman A, Kudelka A, Edwards C, et al. GnRH agonist (Depot-Lupron) in the treatment of refractory or persistent ovarian granulosa cell tumor (GCT). *Proc Am Soc Clin Oncol.* 1994;13:236(abst).
190. Isaacs R, Forgeson G, Allan S. Progestogens for granulosa cell tumours of the ovary [Letter]. *Br J Cancer.* 1992;65:140. doi:10.1038/bjc.1992.28.
191. Malik ST, Slevin ML. Medroxyprogesterone acetate (MPA) in advanced granulosa cell tumours of the ovary—a new therapeutic approach? *Br J Cancer.* 1991;63:410–411. doi:10.1038/bjc.1991.94.
192. Martikainen H, Penttinen J, Huhtaniemi I, et al. Gonadotropin-releasing hormone agonist analog therapy effective in ovarian granulosa cell malignancy. *Gynecol Oncol.* 1989;35:406–408. doi:10.1016/0090-8258(89)90089-9.
193. Hardy RD, Bell JG, Nicely CJ, et al. Hormonal treatment of a recurrent granulosa cell tumor of the ovary: case report and review of the literature. *Gynecol Oncol.* 2005;96:865–869. doi:10.1016/j.ygyno.2004.10.042.
194. Fishman A, Kudelka AP, Tresukosol D, et al. Leuprolide acetate for treating refractory or persistent ovarian granulosa cell tumor. *J Reprod Med.* 1996;41(6):393–396.

195. Freeman SA, Modesitt SC. Anastrozole therapy in recurrent ovarian adult granulosa cell tumors: a report of 2 cases. *Gynecol Oncol.* 2006;103:755–758. doi:10.1016/j.ygyno.2006.06.022.
196. Korach J, Perri T, Beiner M, et al. Promising effect of aromatase inhibitors on recurrent granulosa cell tumors. *Int J Gynecol Cancer.* 2009;19:830–833. doi:10.1111/IGC.0b013e3181a261d7.
197. AlHilli MM, Long HJ, Podratz KC, et al. Aromatase inhibitors in the treatment of recurrent ovarian granulosa cell tumors: brief report and review of the literature. *J Gynecol Obstet Res.* 2012;38(1):340–344.
198. van Meurs HS, van Lonkhuijzen LRCW, Limpens J, et al. Hormone therapy in ovarian granulosa cell tumors: a systematic review. *Gynecol Oncol.* 2014;134(1):196–205.
199. Tao X, Sood AK, Deavers MT, et al. Anti-angiogenesis therapy with bevacizumab for patients with ovarian granulosa cell tumors. *Gynecol Oncol.* 2009;114(3):431–436.
200. Brown J, Brady WE, Schink J, et al. Efficacy and safety of bevacizumab in recurrent sex cord-stromal ovarian tumors: results of a phase 2 trial of the Gynecologic Oncology Group. *Cancer.* 2014;120(3):334–351.
201. Garcia-Donas J, Hurtado A, Garcia-Casado Z, et al. Cytochrome P17 inhibition with ketoconazole as treatment for advanced granulosa cell ovarian tumor. *J Clin Oncol.* 2013;31(10):e165–e166.
202. Calaminus G, Wessalowski R, Harms D, et al. Juvenile granulosa cell tumors of the ovary in children and adolescents: results from 33 patients registered in a prospective cooperative study. *Gynecol Oncol.* 1997;65(3):447–452.
203. Powell JL, Otis CN. Management of advanced juvenile granulosa cell tumor of the ovary. *Gynecol Oncol.* 1997;64(2):282–284.
204. Powell JL, Connor GP, Henderson GS. Management of recurrent juvenile granulosa cell tumor of the ovary. *Gynecol Oncol.* 2001;81(1):113–116.
205. Benesch M, Lackner H, Pilhatsch A, et al. Long-term remission in a female with multiple relapsed juvenile granulosa cell tumor. *J Pediatr Hematol Oncol.* 2015;37(8):e486–e489.
206. Auguste A, Bessiere L, Todeschini AL, et al. Molecular analyses of juvenile granulosa cell tumors bearing AKT1 mutations provide insights into tumor biology and therapeutic leads. *Hum Mol Genetics.* 2015;24(23):6687–6698.
207. Schwartz PE, Smith JP. Treatment of ovarian stromal tumors. *Am J Obstet Gynecol.* 1976;125(3):402–411.
208. Emons G, Schally AV. The use of luteinizing hormone releasing hormone agonists and antagonists in gynaecological cancers. *Hum Reprod.* 1994;9(7):1364–1379.
209. Sigismondi C, Gadducci A, Lorusso D, et al. Ovarian Sertoli-Leydig cell tumors. A retrospective MITO study. *Gynecol Oncol.* 2012;125(3):673–676.
210. Gui T, Cao D, Shen K, et al. A clinicopathological analysis of 40 cases of ovarian Sertoli-Leydig cell tumors. *Gynecol Oncol.* 2012;127(2):384–389.
211. Qian Q, You Y, Yang J, et al. Management and prognosis of patients with ovarian sex cord tumor with annular tublules: a retrospective study. *BMC Cancer.* 2015;15:270–277. doi:10.1186/s12885-015-1277-y.
212. Burger HG. Inhibin. *Reprod Med Rev.* 1992;1:1–20.
213. Petraglia F, Luisi S, Pautier P, et al. Inhibin B is the major form of inhibin/activin family secreted by granulosa cell tumors. *J Clin Endocrinol Metab.* 1998;83(3):1029–1032.
214. Ying SY. Inhibins, activins, and follistatins: gonadal proteins modulating the secretion of follicle-stimulating hormone. *Endocr Rev.* 1988;9(2):267–293.
215. Robertson DM, Stephenson T, Pruysers E, et al. Characterization of inhibin forms and their measurement by an inhibin alpha-subunit ELISA in serum from postmenopausal women with ovarian cancer. *J Clin Endocrinol Metab.* 2002;87(2):816–824.
216. Lin YS, Eng HL, Jan YJ, et al. Molecular cytogenetics of ovarian granulosa cell tumors by comparative genomic hybridization. *Gynecol Oncol.* 2005;97(1):68–73.
217. Mayr D, Kaltz-Wittmer C, Arbogast S, et al. Characteristic pattern of genetic aberrations in ovarian granulosa cell tumors. *Mod Pathol.* 2002;15(9):951–957.
218. Caburet S, Anttonen M, Todeschini AL, et al. Combined comparative genomic hybridization and transcriptomic analyses of ovarian granulosa cell tumors point to novel candidate driver genes. *BMC Cancer.* 2015;15:251. doi:10.1186/s12885-015-1283-0.
219. Fletcher JA, Gibas Z, Donovan K, et al. Ovarian granulosa stromal cell tumors are characterized by trisomy 12. *Am J Pathol.* 1991;138(3): 515–520.
220. Halperin D, Visscher DW, Wallis T, et al. Evaluation of chromosome 12 copy number in ovarian granulosa cell tumors using interphase cytogenetics. *Int J Gynecol Pathol.* 1995;14(4):319–323.
221. Menczer J, Schreiber L, Czernobilsky B, et al. Is Her-2/neu expressed in nonepithelial ovarian malignancies? *Am J Obstet Gynecol.* 2007;196(1):79e1–79e4.
222. Leibl S, Bodo K, Gogg-Kammerer M, et al. Ovarian granulosa cell tumors frequently express EGFR (Her-1), Her-3, and Her-4: an immunohistochemical study. *Gynecol Oncol.* 2006;101(1):18–23.
223. Kusamura S, Derchain S, Alvarenga M, et al. Expression of p53, c-erbB-2, Ki-67, and CD34 in granulosa cell tumor of the ovary. *Int J Gynecol Cancer.* 2003;13(4):450–457.
224. Richards JS, Fan H-Y, Liu Z, et al. Either Kras activation or Pten loss similarly enhance the dominant-stable CTNNB1-induced genetic program to promote granulosa cell tumor development in the ovary and testis. *Oncogene.* 2012;31(12):1504–1520.
225. Shah SP, Köbel M, Senz J, et al. Mutation of FOXL2 in granulosa-cell tumors of the ovary. *N Engl J Med.* 2009;360(26):2719–2729.
226. Cocquet J, Pailhoux E, Jaubert F, et al. Evolution expression of FOXL2. *J Med Genet.* 2002;39(12):916–922.
227. Schmidt D, Ovitt CE, Anlag K, et al. The murine winged-helix transcription factor FOXL2 is required for granulosa cell differentiation and ovary maintenance. *Development.* 2004;131(4):933–942.
228. Goulvent T, Ray-Coquard I, Borel S, et al. DICER1 and FOXL2 mutations in ovarian sex cord-stromal tumours: a GINECO Group study. *Histopathology.* 2016;68(2):279–285.
229. Al-Aha O, Huwalt HF, Chow C, et al. FOXL2 is a sensitive and specific marker for sex cord-stromal tumors of the ovary. *Am J Surg Pathol.* 2011;3(4):484–494.
230. Bessière L, Todeschini AL, Auguste A, et al. A hot-spot of in-frame duplications activates the oncoprotein AKT1 in juvenile granulosa cell tumors. *EBioMedicine.* 2015;2(5):421–431.
231. Schultz KA, Pacheco MC, Yang J, et al. Ovarian sex cord-stromal tumors, pleuropulmonary blastoma and DICER1 mutations: a report from the International Pleuropulmonary Blastoma Registry. *Gynecol Oncol.* 2011;122(2):246–250.
232. Heravi-Moussavi A, Anglesio MS, Cheng SW, et al. Recurrent somatic DICER1 mutations in nonepithelial ovarian cancers. *N Eng J Med.* 2012;366(3):234–242.
233. Rio Frio T, Bahubeshi A, Kanellopoulou A, et al. DICER1 mutations in familial multinodular goiter with and without ovarian Sertoli-Leydig cell tumors. *JAMA.* 2011;305(1):68–77.
234. Chu S, Mamers P, Burger HG, et al. Estrogen receptor isoform gene expression in ovarian stromal and epithelial tumors. *J Clin Endocrinol Metab.* 2000;85(3):1200–1205.
235. Fuller PJ, Chu S. Signalling pathways in the molecular pathogenesis of ovarian granulosa cell tumours. *Trends Endocrinol Metab.* 2004;15(3):122–128.
236. Alexiadis M, Mamers P, Chu S, et al. Insulin-like growth factor, insulin-like growth factor-binding protein-4, and pregnancy-associated plasma protein-A gene expression in human granulosa cell tumors. *Int J Gynecol Cancer.* 2006;16(6):1973–1979.
237. Anttonen M, Unkila-Kallio L, Leminen A, et al. High GATA-4 expression associates with aggressive behavior, whereas low anti-müllerian hormone expression associates with growth potential of ovarian granulosa cell tumors. *J Clin Endocrinol Metab.* 2005;90(12):6529–6535.
238. Anttonen M, Pihlajoki M, Andersson N, et al. 23. FOXL2, GATA4, and SMAD3 co-operatively modulate gene expression, cell viability and apoptosis in ovarian granulosa cell tumor cells. *PLoS One.* 2014;9(1):e85545.

CHAPTER 26

Gestational Trophoblastic Disease: Molar Pregnancy and Gestational Trophoblastic Neoplasia

Julian C. Schink and John R. Lurain

INTRODUCTION

Gestational trophoblastic disease (GTD) describes a continuum of interrelated lesions that arise from abnormal proliferation of placental trophoblasts, ranging from benign hydatidiform mole to invasive mole, malignant choriocarcinoma (CCA), placental site trophoblastic tumor (PSTT), and epithelioid trophoblastic tumor (ETT) (**Table 26.1**). Hydatidiform moles, both complete and partial, are benign lesions that resolve following uterine evacuation in the vast majority of cases. Persistent GTD refers to disease that does not resolve after molar evacuation or that becomes malignant and requires active management. Invasive moles, CCA, PSTT, and ETT, are collectively referred to as gestational trophoblastic neoplasia (GTN), with varying degrees of malignant potential. GTN most commonly arises after a molar pregnancy, though it can develop after any pregnancy. Historically, GTD was associated with high rates of morbidity and mortality. Hydatidiform mole was associated with serious medical and surgical complications, and the mortality rate for invasive mole approached 15%. The mortality rate for CCA was near 100% if metastatic disease was present and 60% for nonmetastatic disease even if hysterectomy was performed. Earlier detection with ultrasonography, the use of human chorionic gonadotropin (hCG) as a disease-specific biomarker, advances in uterine evacuation, and the introduction of chemotherapy (CT) into the management of GTN have significantly decreased the risk of death associated with GTD and have allowed many women to preserve their fertility after treatment. This chapter will describe the epidemiology and pathology of molar pregnancy and GTN and will discuss the changes in diagnosis and management that have transformed GTN from one of the most deadly to one of the most curable solid tumors in women, with cure rates higher than 90% even in the presence of metastasis (1–3).

EPIDEMIOLOGY

Epidemiologic data for GTD are unreliable, primarily because of inconsistent case definitions, no centralized databases, and the rarity of certain forms of the disease. Similarly, defining the risk factors that contribute to the development of GTD has been challenging, with an inability to adequately identify at-risk populations and a lack of control groups (4). Based on available data, hydatidiform mole develops in women during their reproductive years, with an incidence that varies widely across different geographic regions. In North America, Australia, New Zealand, and Europe, the incidence of molar pregnancy has been reported as 0.6 to 1.1 per 1,000 pregnancies, but it is two- to three-fold higher in Southeast Asia and Japan (2.0 per 1,000 pregnancies) (5–8). In Taiwan, hydatidiform mole occurs in 1 of 125 pregnancies, whereas the incidence in the United States is approximately 1 in 1,500 pregnancies. In a study from Ireland, the incidence of complete and partial mole was reported as 1 in 1,945 and 1 in 695 pregnancies, respectively (9).

Despite this geographic variation, the risk of hydatidiform mole has not been linked to any specific ethnic or racial differences, cultural factors, or differences in reporting of hospital-based and population-based data (10–12). However, several studies have reported a link between molar pregnancy and socioeconomic and dietary factors, specifically that the risk of complete molar pregnancy increases with decreased consumption of vitamin A (carotene) and animal fat (13,14). Regions with a higher incidence of vitamin A deficiency also have a higher incidence of molar pregnancy. A history of infertility is also associated with increased risk of complete and partial mole (15), and a history of spontaneous abortion increases the risk of both complete and partial moles two- to three-fold compared with women without a history of miscarriage (15–17).

The two strongest risk factors for complete hydatidiform mole are maternal age and prior molar pregnancy (17). Both very young women and women over the age of 40 have a higher risk of complete molar pregnancy, with older women having a 5- to 10-fold higher risk (18,19). In women over the age of 50, one in every three pregnancies is molar (4). These observations suggest that the ova of older women are predisposed to the abnormal fertilization events that lead to hydatidiform mole. The risk of a second complete molar pregnancy is 1%, approximately 10- to 20-fold higher than the risk of molar pregnancy in the general population (20,21), and the risk of a third mole is 15% to 20% (22,23), regardless of a change in partner (24).

Familial repetitive hydatidiform mole (17) has been linked to a missense mutation in the *NLRP7* locus (25,26) on chromosome 19 (27); in one report, this mutation was present in 60% of patients who had two molar pregnancies (28). The mutated gene is involved in maternal imprinting (29) and is seen in familial clusters of complete moles of biparental origin rather than androgenetic origin (26,30).

There is less information regarding the epidemiology of partial molar pregnancy, though it is clear that it differs from that of complete molar pregnancy (18,19). Partial mole does not appear to be linked to vitamin A deficiency (31) or advanced maternal age (17), but is associated with a history of irregular menstruation and use of high estrogen–containing oral contraceptives (31).

Locally invasive GTN develops in approximately 15% of patients after molar evacuation. CCA occurs in 1 in 50,000 pregnancies (including term, miscarriage, abortion, or ectopic) (32). CCA is 1,000 times more likely to develop after a complete molar pregnancy than after other pregnancy events, with half of all CCA cases arising

TABLE 26.1. National Institutes of Health Clinical Classification of Gestational Trophoblastic Disease

I. Benign GTD
    A. Complete hydatidiform mole
    B. Partial hydatidiform mole

II. Malignant GTD
    A. Nonmetastatic (invasive mole or CCA)
    B. Metastatic
        1. CCA
        2. PSTT
        3. ETT

CCA, choriocarcinoma; ETT, epithelioid trophoblastic tumor; GTD, gestational trophoblastic disease; PSTT, placental site trophoblastic tumor.

from molar pregnancies. The risk of CCA increases in women with advanced maternal age and prior hydatidiform mole, and is higher in women of Asian, American Indian, and African American descent (12). Menarche after age 12, light menstrual flow, and long-term use of oral contraceptives are also associated with a higher risk of CCA (33), though the association between postmolar GTN and oral contraceptive use is not entirely clear (34,35). Women with type A blood also have an increased risk of CCA (7,36).

PSTT and ETT are extremely rare forms of malignant GTN, and there are insufficient data to characterize the epidemiology or risk factors. Approximately 95% of PSTT and ETT lesions develop after a term pregnancy or nonmolar abortion (37), often several months or even years later.

Pathology and Chromosomal Features

Trophoblastic Differentiation and GTD

Molar pregnancies and GTN originate from the placental trophoblast, which is derived from the outermost layer of the blastocyst, called the trophectoderm (38). The trophoblast is composed of cytotrophoblast, syncytiotrophoblast, and intermediate trophoblast. Syncytiotrophoblast invades the endometrial stroma upon implantation of the blastocyst and secretes hCG and other proteins to regulate the implantation site microenvironment. Cytotrophoblast fuses with syncytiotrophoblast to form the chorionic villi that cover the chorionic sac. Nonvillous cytotrophoblast differentiates into intermediate trophoblast, categorized as either implantation site or chorion type. Implantation site intermediate trophoblast loses the ability to proliferate but invades the maternal decidua and myometrium in a highly controlled manner, migrating to the maternal spiral arteries to facilitate oxygen and waste transfer between the fetus and the mother (**Fig. 26.1**).

Invasion of healthy trophoblast into the maternal endometrium is a normal, tightly regulated event in pregnancy that is required for the vascular connection between the fetus and the mother. When regulatory mechanisms are impaired, invasive and vascular tumors arise. For example, TGF-β and a proteoglycan, decorin, have an inhibitory effect on nonvillous trophoblast cell growth, migration, and invasion, and this negative regulation is lost in trophoblast lesions (39,40).

Most GTD lesions (except partial mole) derive from the fetus and not from the mother and, therefore, contain only paternal genetic material (38). A large body of work on the immunobiology of GTD has suggested that a maternal immunologic response is activated by paternal antigens in the trophoblastic cells of GTD lesions, thereby promoting their regression and sensitizing them to CT; conversely, women with persistent GTD or aggressive disease may have greater histocompatibility such that the paternal antigens do not elicit a strong immune response from the mother (41).

All three types of trophoblast can proliferate to produce GTD lesions (42), and each type expresses different antigens that have been useful in the immunohistochemical analysis and differential diagnosis of trophoblastic lesions (43); they may also provide insight into the pathogenic mechanisms underlying GTN (**Table 26.2**). Expression of Ki-67, proliferating cell nuclear antigen, and p53 is significantly higher in GTD compared with normal tissues and can differentiate between GTD and spontaneous abortion (44). p63 isoforms are differentially expressed in cytotrophoblast and intermediate trophoblast (45) and may be useful in differentiating between PSTT (p63 negative) and ETT (p63 positive). Human leukocyte antigen G is also expressed in intermediate trophoblasts, but not in villous cytotrophoblasts or syncytiotrophoblasts, and may be useful in the diagnosis of various GTD lesions (46). Several growth factors and oncogenes are abnormally expressed in molar tissues and CCA (15,47,48). Both complete mole and CCA overexpress c-myc, c-erb2, and bcl-2. Epidermal growth factor (EGF) receptor was found to be more highly expressed in CCA and complete moles compared with normal placenta and partial moles, suggesting that EGF family members may be involved in GTN pathogenesis (49). In addition, there is increased expression of matrix metalloproteinase (MMP-1

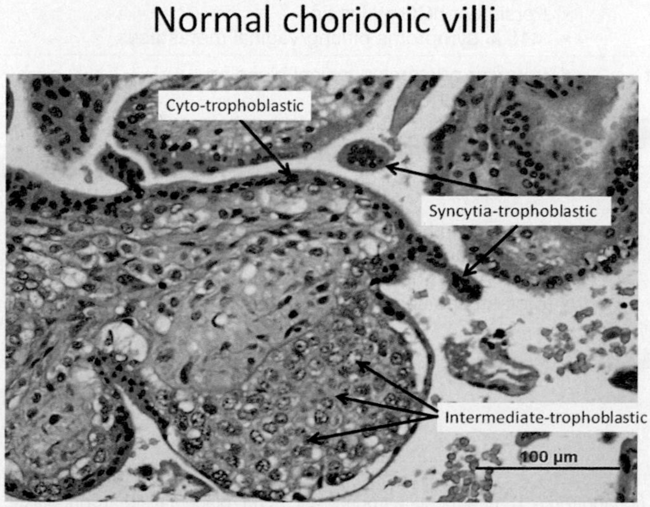

Figure 26.1. Normal trophoblast differentiation. Cytotrophoblast, syncytiotrophoblast, and intermediate trophoblast are labeled in this photomicrograph.

TABLE 26.2. Immunohistochemical Markers for Differential Diagnosis of GTD

Marker	Application
Ki-67, PCNA, p53	Spontaneous abortion (negative)
	GTD (positive)
	CCA (diffusely positive in 50% cells)
	PSTT (>10% labeling index)
p63	PSTT (negative)
	ETT (positive)
HLA-G	Nonvillous IT (positive)
	PSTT (implantation site IT positive)
	ETT (chorionic-type IT positive)
β-hCG	CCA (syncytiotrophoblast positive)
Inhibin α	CCA (trophoblast and IT positive)
	PSTT (diffusely positive)
	ETT (diffusely positive)
hPL	CCA (IT positive)
	PSTT (diffusely positive)
Mel-CAM	PSTT (diffusely positive)
Cytokeratin	CCA (all cells positive)
	PSTT (diffusely positive)
	ETT (diffusely positive)
p57kip2	Complete mole (negative)
	Partial mole (positive)
Cyclin E	ETT (relatively greater staining than placental site nodule)

CCA, choriocarcinoma; ETT, epithelioid trophoblastic tumor; GTD, gestational trophoblastic disease; IT, intermediate trophoblast; PCNA, proliferating cell nuclear antigen; PSTT, placental site trophoblastic tumor.

and MMP-2) and decreased expression of tissue inhibitor of metalloproteinase 1 in CCA compared with either hydatidiform mole or normal placenta, implicating the dysregulation of extracellular matrix (ECM) in the invasion and metastasis of CCA (50). Characterizing the molecular pathogenesis of GTD is an active area of research that may reveal new diagnostic and prognostic markers, as well as lead to targeted therapies.

Hydatidiform Mole

Molar pregnancies arise from the proliferation of villous cytotrophoblast and syncytiotrophoblast, which produces lesions on the maternal decidua (51,52). A comparison of the characteristics and cytogenetics of complete and partial moles is provided in **Table 26.3**. Complete hydatidiform moles show early uniform enlargement of villi with hyperplastic and atypical trophoblast, and do not contain a fetus/embryo or villous capillaries (**Fig. 26.2**). Most complete moles (approximately 90%) are 46,XX and arise from the fertilization of an "empty" anucleated egg—missing the pronucleus and maternal chromosomes—by a single sperm followed by duplication of paternal haploid chromosomes (**Fig. 26.3**) (53,54). The other 10% of complete moles are either 46,XY or 46,XX and are produced by dispermic fertilization of an anucleated egg. Some complete moles can also arise from the loss of maternal chromosomes during the first cleavage. Regardless of monospermic or dispermic fertilization, complete moles contain only paternal chromosomes (androgenetic), though maternal DNA is present in the mitochondria of the egg (55). The presence of excess paternal material leads to trophoblastic hyperplasia, with no formation of a fetus because of the absence of maternal chromosomal DNA. Loss of maternally imprinted genes and extra paternally imprinted genes may also inhibit embryo formation (56).

In contrast, partial hydatidiform moles contain fetal/embryonic tissue, and the chorionic villi show varying degrees of focal enlargement and edema, predominantly syncytiotrophoblast hyperplasia, scalloping of the villous outline, prominent stromal inclusions, and functional villous circulation (**Fig. 26.4**) (57). Like complete moles, the trophoblast is hyperplastic, but shows only mild atypia. In later stages of partial molar pregnancy, the fetus shows congenital abnormalities, such as syndactyly of the fingers and toes (57). The majority of partial moles are triploid, most often 69,XXY, with two sets of paternal chromosomes because of either dispermic fertilization of a normal egg or duplication of chromosomes in a single sperm after fertilization of a normal egg (**Fig. 26.3**) (51,56,58).

Invasive Mole

Invasive mole is a condition in which hydatidiform mole, with hydropic villi and proliferating trophoblast, has invaded the myometrium through the tissue or veins (**Fig. 26.5**). Molar villi may be observed on the uterine serosa, and extrauterine tubal and ovarian moles can occur (59). Invasive moles are less hydropic, and trophoblastic proliferation is easily seen (**Table 26.3**) (57).

Choriocarcinoma

Approximately 2% of women with complete moles may develop CCA, characterized by a mixture of cytotrophoblast and syncytiotrophoblast hyperplasia, hemorrhage, necrosis, and the absence of chorionic villi (**Fig. 26.6**) (57). Direct invasion of the myometrium and vasculature is also present, which permits metastasis to the lungs, brain, liver, pelvis and vagina, kidney, intestines, and spleen. Immunohistochemical markers can confirm a histologic diagnosis

TABLE 26.3. Clinicopathologic Features of Gestational Trophoblastic Diseases

Disease	Pathologic Features	Clinical Features
Complete mole	• Diploid (46,XX and some 46,XY) • No fetus or embryo • Diffuse swelling of villi • Diffuse trophoblastic hyperplasia	• Vaginal bleeding • Large for date uterine size • Bilateral theca lutein cysts • hCG can be >100,000 mIU/mL
Partial mole	• Triploid (69,XXY; 69,XYY; 69,XXX) • Abnormal fetus or embryo • Focal swelling of villi • Focal trophoblastic hyperplasia with mild atypia	• Symptoms of incomplete or missed abortion • Vaginal bleeding • hCG rarely elevated >100,000 mIU/mL
Invasive mole	• Trophoblastic hyperplasia • Swollen villi • Myometrial invasion	• Irregular postmolar vaginal bleeding • Persistent hCG elevation • <15% symptoms of lung/vaginal metastases
Choriocarcinoma	• Mixture of cytotrophoblast and syncytiotrophoblast hyperplasia • No villi • Myometrial invasion and metastatic potential • Hemorrhage • Necrosis	• Irregular postmolar vaginal bleeding • Persistent hCG elevation • Metastases and associated symptoms
PSTT	• Diploid • IT hyperplasia • No villi • Less hemorrhage and necrosis • High potential for lymphatic invasion and metastasis • Focal hCG production	• Low serum hCG • Enlarged uterus • hCG levels normal to 1,000 mIU/mL • Metastases and associated symptoms
ETT	• IT nodules surrounded by hyalinized ECM • Extensive necrotic tissue • Preserved blood vessel structure • Hemorrhage and metastases rare	

ECM, extracellular matrix; ETT, epithelioid trophoblastic tumor; hCG, human chorionic gonadotropin; IT, intermediate trophoblast; PSTT, placental site trophoblastic tumor.

Source: Adapted from Lurain JR. Gestational trophoblastic disease I: epidemiology, pathology, clinical presentation and diagnosis of gestational trophoblastic disease, and management of hydatidiform mole. *Am J Obstet Gynecol.* 2010;203(6):531–539, with permission.

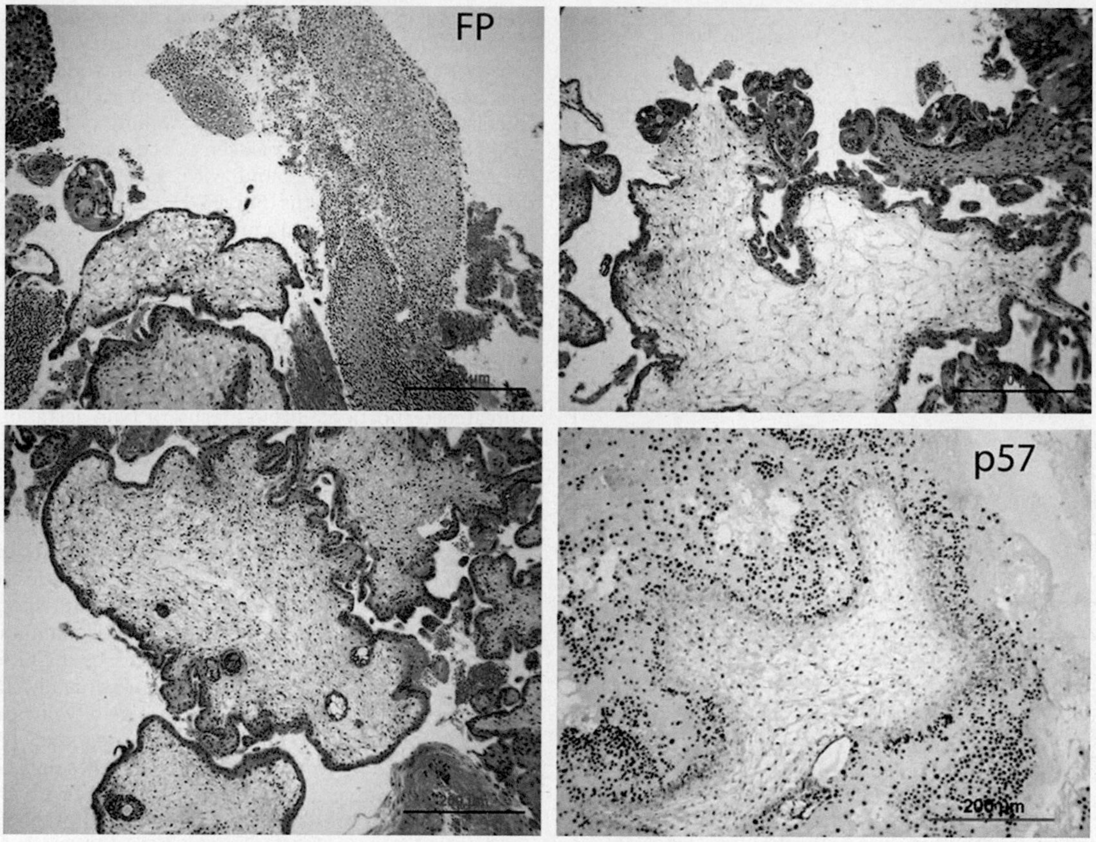

Figure 26.2. Partial hydatidiform mole. **Upper left:** large chorionic villi and fetal parts (FP); **Upper right:** large irregular contour and trophoblastic proliferation; **Lower left:** large irregular contour with pseudoinclusion cysts; **Lower right:** chorionic villous stromal cells stain positive for p57.

of CCA, with tumors staining strongly for hCG and inhibin α in the trophoblast, human placental lactogen (hPL), and inhibin α in the intermediate trophoblast, and cytokeratin in all trophoblast cells (**Tables 26.2** and **26.3**) (60). Ki-67 is diffusely expressed in approximately half of the cells (61).

Placental Site Trophoblastic Tumor

PSTT lesions are usually diploid and monomorphic, developing from the placental implantation site intermediate trophoblast after a normal or aborted uterine pregnancy (62). PSTT lesions contain primarily mononuclear intermediate trophoblast without chorionic villi that infiltrates the uterine wall in sheets or cords between myometrial fibers (**Fig. 26.7**). Compared with CCA, there is less hemorrhage, necrosis, and vascular invasion, but there is a higher risk of lymphatic metastasis. hCG production is focal, leading to relatively lower serum levels (**Table 26.3**). These tumors may be diagnosed immunohistochemically and may contain diffuse cytokeratin and hPL (63), as well as inhibin α (60) and Mel-CAM (**Table 26.2**) (61). The Ki-67 labeling index is also usually elevated (>10%) in a neoplastic lesion of nonvillous trophoblast (61).

Epithelioid Trophoblastic Tumor

ETT is a rare malignant tumor that arises from neoplastic transformation of chorion-type intermediate trophoblast (62). These lesions appear as nodules of mononuclear intermediate trophoblast, surrounded by hyalinized ECM within extensive necrotic tissue and with preserved blood vessel structure (**Fig. 26.8** and **Table 26.3**). Intratumor hemorrhage and metastases are rarely observed. ETT tumor cells show diffuse expression of immunohistologic markers, including cytokeratin and inhibin α (**Table 26.2**) (64). Cyclin E staining is higher in ETT than in placental site nodule and can help in differentiating between the two (64–66).

MANAGEMENT OF MOLAR PREGNANCY

Clinical Presentation

Approximately 80% to 90% of women with complete hydatidiform mole present with vaginal bleeding, occurring at 6 to 16 weeks' gestation. Women may also present with larger uterine size than expected for gestational date, toxemia, hyperemesis, and hyperthyroidism in the first or second trimester. However, the widespread use of ultrasonography in developed countries and accurate hCG tests to evaluate vaginal bleeding have led to earlier diagnosis of molar pregnancy, and other clinical signs and symptoms are seen less often (**Table 26.4**) (67). hCG levels can be greater than 100,000 mIU/mL in a complete molar pregnancy, and there are no fetal heart tones (**Table 26.3**); however, hCG levels vary widely in individual patients, and with earlier ultrasound detection, patients may not present with extremely elevated hCG. It should also be emphasized that a high hCG level alone is not sufficient for a diagnosis of hydatidiform mole, and a confirmatory ultrasound should be performed. In approximately 15% of women with complete hydatidiform mole, ultrasound imaging reveals the presence of bilateral theca lutein cyst enlargement of the ovaries (5,67–70).

Partial hydatidiform mole presents quite differently from complete mole. The vast majority of patients—greater than 90%—present with symptoms of incomplete or missed abortion. Vaginal bleeding occurs in 75% of patients with a partial molar pregnancy, and uterine enlargement, hyperemesis, hypertension, hyperthyroidism, and theca lutein cysts are not often seen. Presenting hCG levels are higher than 100,000 mIU/mL in only 10% of patients (70–73).

Diagnosis

Ultrasonography is the primary means of preoperative diagnosis of molar pregnancy, and its introduction has made diagnosis at much

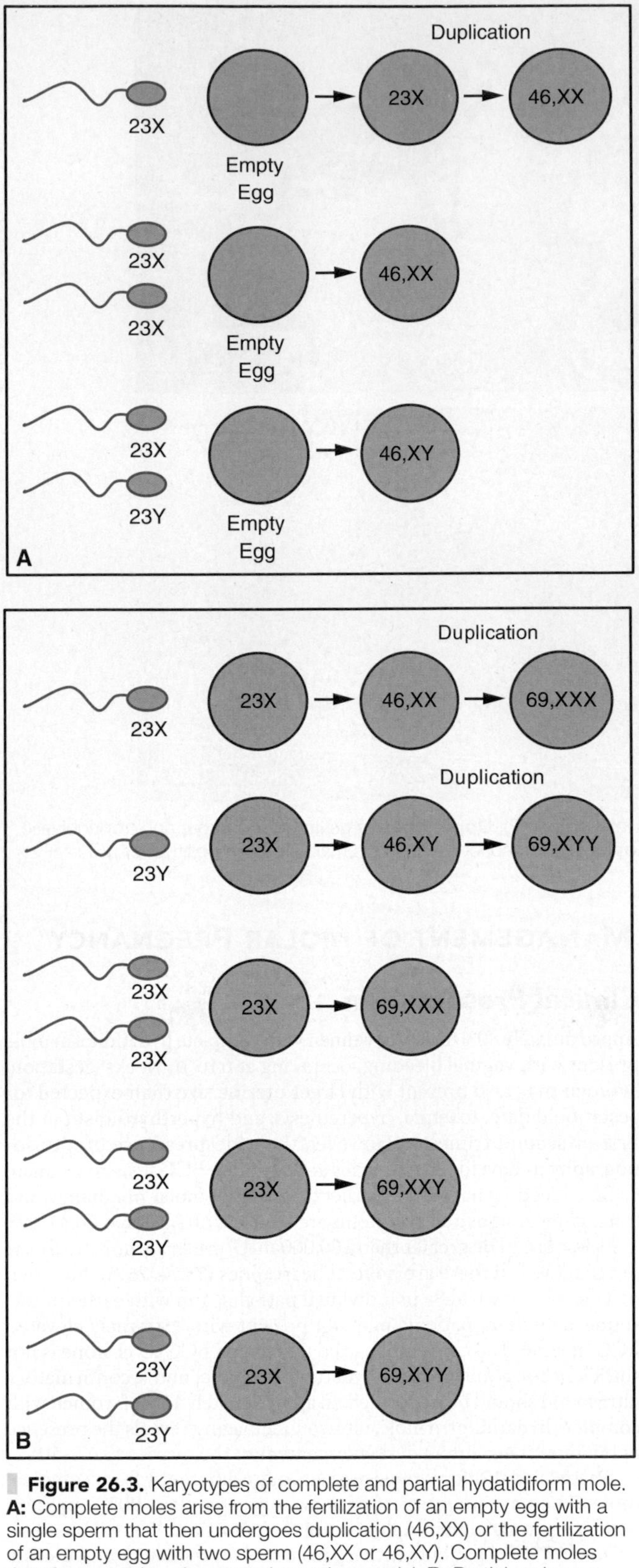

Figure 26.3. Karyotypes of complete and partial hydatidiform mole. **A:** Complete moles arise from the fertilization of an empty egg with a single sperm that then undergoes duplication (46,XX) or the fertilization of an empty egg with two sperm (46,XX or 46,XY). Complete moles therefore contain only paternal genetic material. **B:** Partial moles are triploid (69,XXY; 69XYY; or 69XXX) and arise from either dispermic fertilization of a normal egg or duplication of chromosomes in a single sperm after fertilization of a normal egg.

earlier stages possible (69,74–76). Ultrasound not only provides information on the type of molar pregnancy, but also determines involvement of the endometrial cavity or myometrium, assesses the risk of uterine perforation, and detects theca lutein cysts and vaginal metastases. The diffuse hydropic swelling of the chorionic villi in complete molar pregnancy is seen as a characteristic vesicular "snowstorm" pattern on ultrasound, with many holes within the placenta and the absence of a fetus (**Fig. 26.9**). However, because this pattern is also seen in women with missed abortion, hematometra, or uterine fibroids, ultrasound diagnosis alone is not very specific. When ultrasound diagnosis is combined with elevated hCG and the absence of fetal heartbeat, molar pregnancy is the most likely diagnosis. For partial moles, ultrasonography can detect focal cystic spaces in the placental and the enlarged gestational sac (76). Ultrasound may show the snowstorm pattern and a viable fetus, which may also indicate threatened abortion, fibroid uterus, or twin gestation with a single missed abortion and a complete mole. Partial mole can be confirmed with chorionic villus sampling that shows triploidy.

The most accurate disease-specific marker of GTD is hCG, which is produced by hydatidiform moles and CCA and can be measured quantitatively in the blood and urine. Placental hCG is a glycoprotein of two subunits, a common α subunit that is similar to the α subunit of pituitary hCG and a placenta-specific β subunit. In a normal pregnancy, hCG is essential for maintaining placental vascular supply. As pregnancy progresses, hCG is secreted by syncytiotrophoblasts, increasing to approximately 60,000 mIU/mL at 10 weeks and then declining to a range of values around 12,000 mIU/mL through the remainder of the pregnancy (77). hCG molecules secreted by trophoblast-derived moles and GTN are more heterogeneous than in a normal pregnancy, with transformation of the trophoblast resulting in fragmentation of the hCG molecule, and several forms of hCG are present, including hyperglycosylated, nicked, C-terminal truncated β subunit, free β subunit, nicked free β subunit, and free α subunit (78). Normally, hyperglycosylated hCG is produced by cytotrophoblasts early in gestation and acts as an autocrine regulator of trophoblast invasion of the implantation site and establishment of the fetomaternal circulation. Hyperglycosylated β subunit is produced by GTN lesions and promotes the growth and invasion of the malignant trophoblasts (79).

It is, therefore, essential that quantitative assays used to diagnose or follow-up GTD detect all forms of the hCG protein and its degradation products. In one study, Cole et al. (80) compared several commercially available hCG tests and found significant variations in assay results related to differences in recognition of hCG variants. The most common hCG assay is a monoclonal antibody sandwich assay (81). Complete hydatidiform moles present with markedly elevated hCG, with half of the patients having levels greater than 100,000 mIU/mL (82,83). Because hCG levels in a normal pregnancy are highest at the end of the first trimester, hCG measurements need to be taken at several times to differentiate a complete molar pregnancy from a normal gestation, multiple gestation, or pregnancy complicated by diseases that are associated with an enlarged placenta. By contrast, hCG levels greater than 100,000 mIU/mL are seen in only 10% of patients with partial moles (71,72).

Diagnosis of complete and partial moles may also include pathologic examination of curettage tissue; however, with the diagnosis of hydatidiform mole occurring earlier in gestation, histologic analysis can be challenging (84,85). Cytogenetic analysis can differentiate between complete mole (androgenetic diploidy), partial mole (diandric triploidy), and hydropic abortus (biparental diploidy). A hydropic abortus can contain enlarged villi, but lacks proliferating trophoblast (57). Immunohistochemical analysis may also help to confirm a diagnosis of molar pregnancy; specifically, p57kip2 expression can differentiate between complete and partial hydatidiform moles (**Table 26.2**) (86–90). This protein is paternally imprinted and maternally expressed; therefore, the villous cytotrophoblast cells in complete moles, which lack maternal chromosomes, will stain negative for p57kip2, whereas partial moles and hydropic abortus will stain positive. Fluorescence *in situ* hybridization can be used

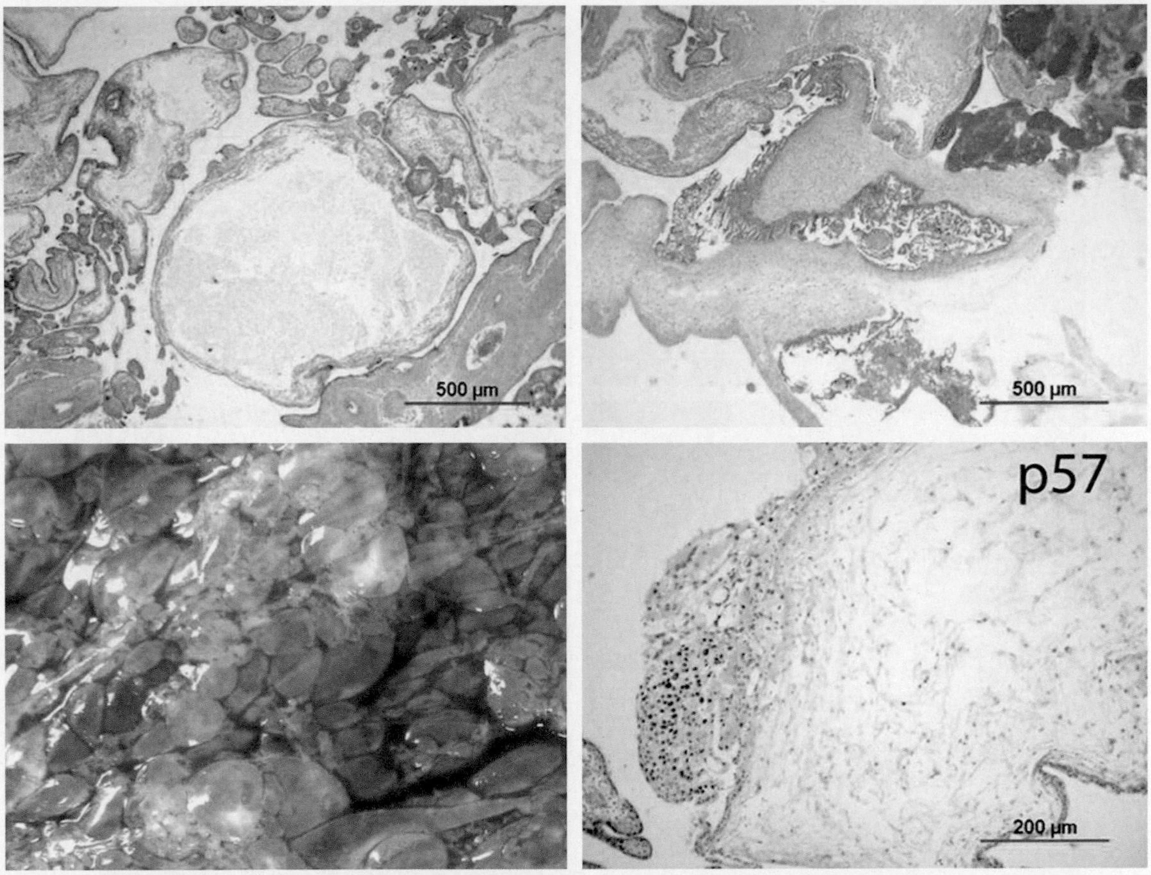

Figure 26.4. Complete hydatidiform mole. **Upper left:** large round chorionic villi with cistern formation; **Upper right:** large irregular contour with extensive trophoblastic proliferation; **Lower left:** gross morphology of large cystic chorionic villi; **Lower right:** chorionic villous stromal cells stain negative for p57.

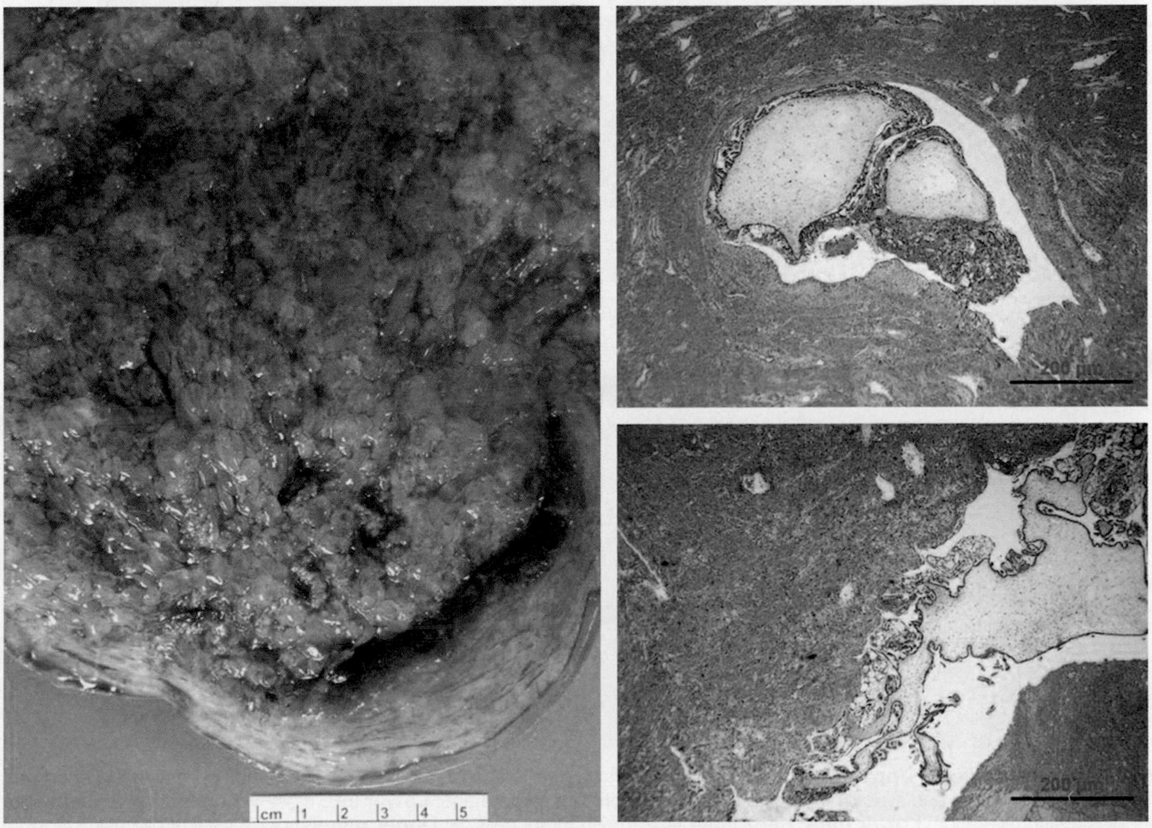

Figure 26.5. Invasive mole. Macrophotograph of molar product of conception that occupies the entire endometrial cavity and invades the myometrium (*left panel*). Photomicrographs show molar chorionic villi infiltrating into the myometrium (*right panels*).

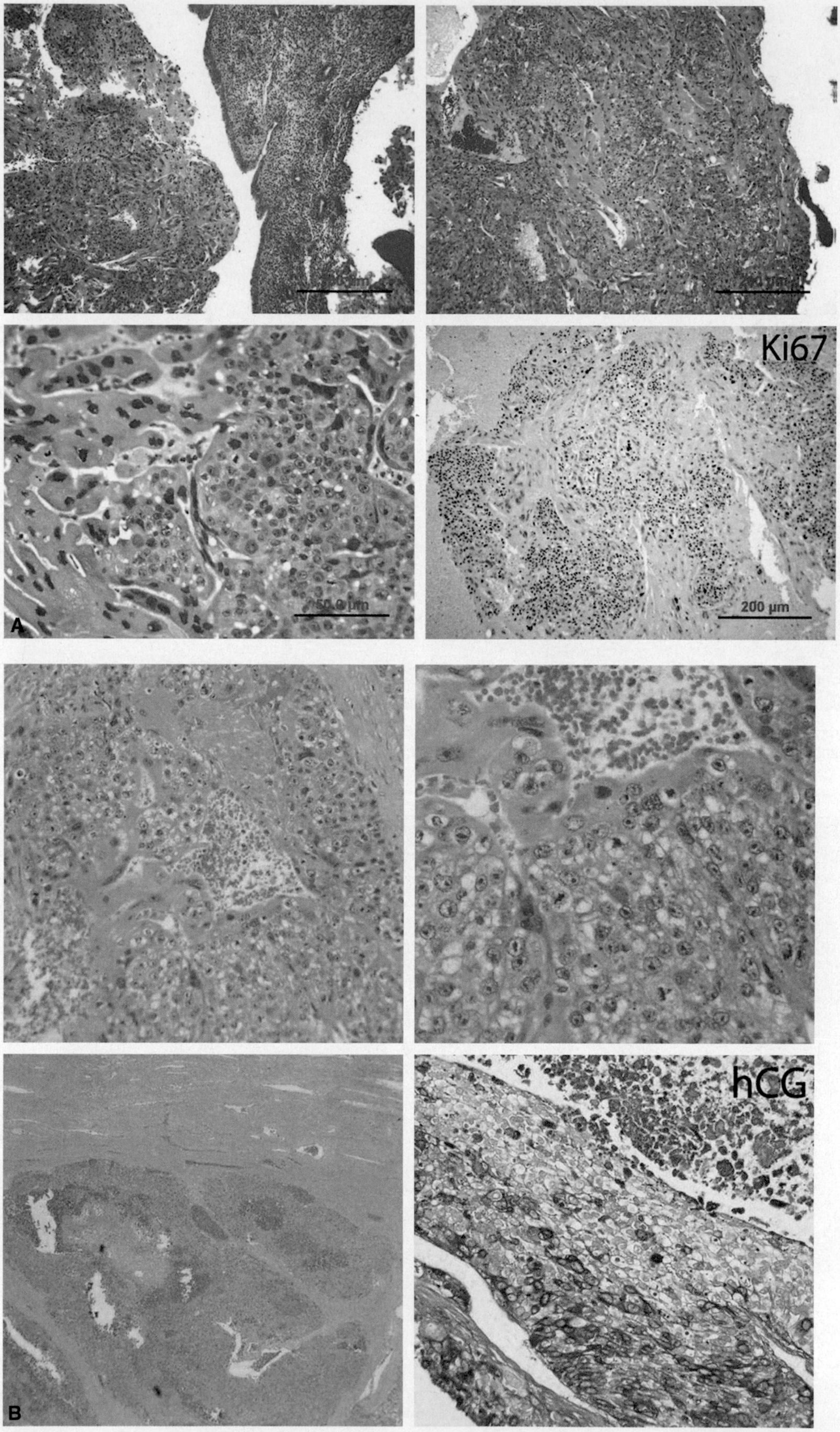

Figure 26.6. Choriocarcinoma. **A: Upper left:** fragment of trophoblastic proliferation in the background of normal-appearing endometrium; **Upper right:** sheath of cytotrophoblastic and syncytiotrophoblastic proliferation with hemorrhage; **Lower left:** close view of biphasic cytotrophoblastic and syncytiotrophoblast cell proliferation; **Lower right:** Ki-67 index is >50% in tumor cells. **B: Upper panels:** close view of biphasic cytotrophoblastic and syncytiotrophoblastic proliferation; **Lower left:** tumor invasion into myometrium with characteristic hemorrhage; **Lower right:** immunostain for hCG is positive in most syncytiotrophoblast cells.

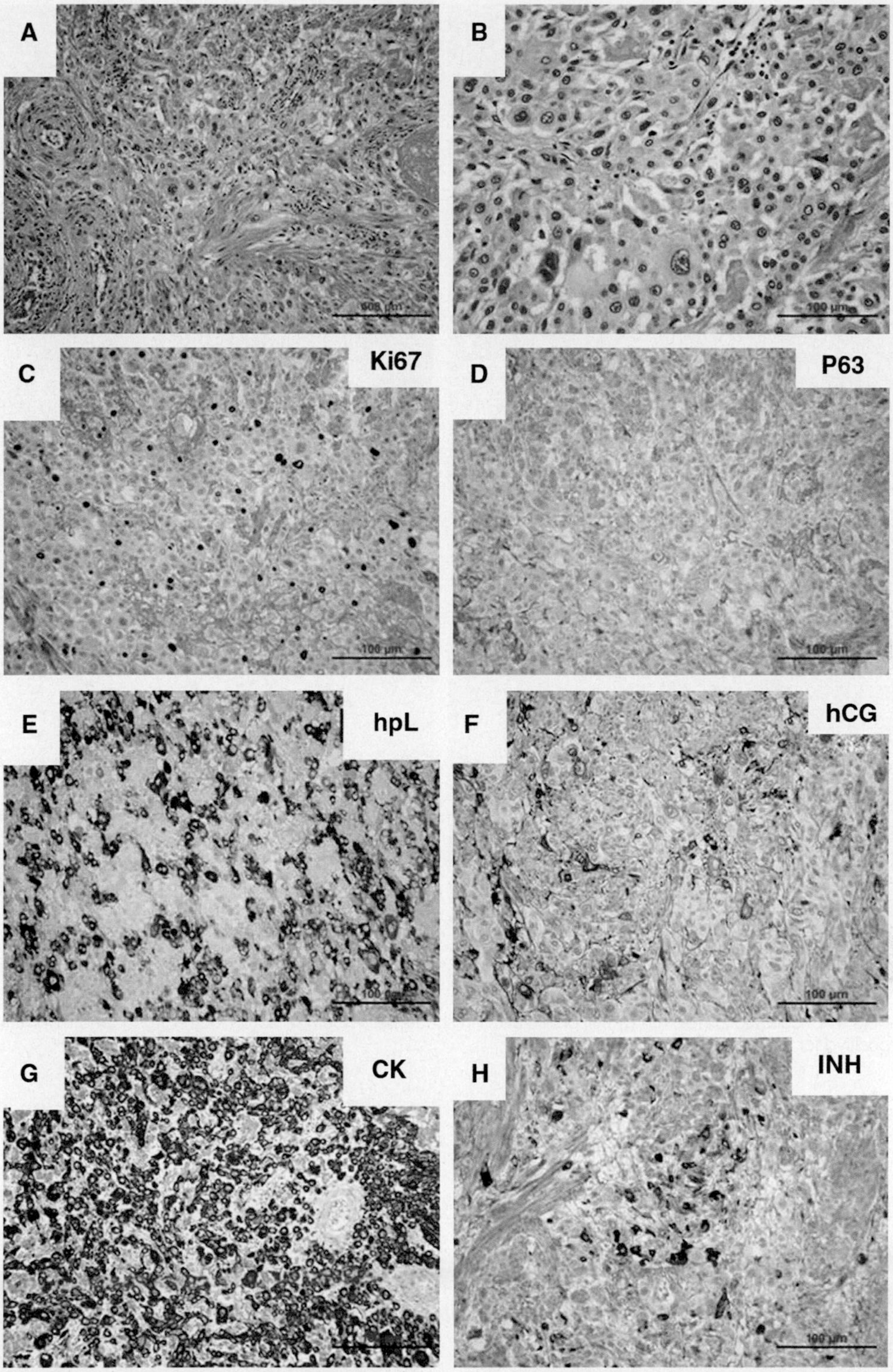

Figure 26.7. Placental site trophoblastic tumor (PSTT). **A, B:** Histology shows mostly intermediate placental site trophoblastic cell proliferation and infiltration into the myometrium. **C:** Tumor cells show moderate cytologic atypia and have an increased Ki-67 index (>20%). Tumor cells are also negative for p63 **(D)**, which excludes a diagnosis of epithelioid trophoblastic tumor; are strongly and diffusely positive for human placental lactogen **(E)** and pan-cytokeratin **(G)**; and are diffusely positive for hCG **(F)** and inhibin **(H)**. CK, cytokeratin; hPL, human placental lactogen; INH, inhibin.

to distinguish between p57kip2-positive partial moles (triploid) and hydropic abortus (diploid) (91). *PHLDA2* is another maternally imprinted gene that can be used to identify partial moles (92).

False-Positive and False-Negative hCG Tests

hCG measurements are a critical diagnostic tool for GTD, but some assays may produce false-positive or "phantom" hCG results (93). False-positive hCG tests, some as high as 800 mIU/mL, can lead to unnecessary surgery and CT in healthy patients (94). These false-positive results are due to the presence of nonspecific heterophilic antibodies that mimic hCG and can interfere with the hCG sandwich assay. These antibodies are present in 3% to 4% of healthy people. Because the large antibody does not pass through the glomerulus into the urine, false-positive hCG test results can be identified by determining hCG levels in the urine. In addition, serial dilution of the serum sample would not show a decrease in the detected antibody.

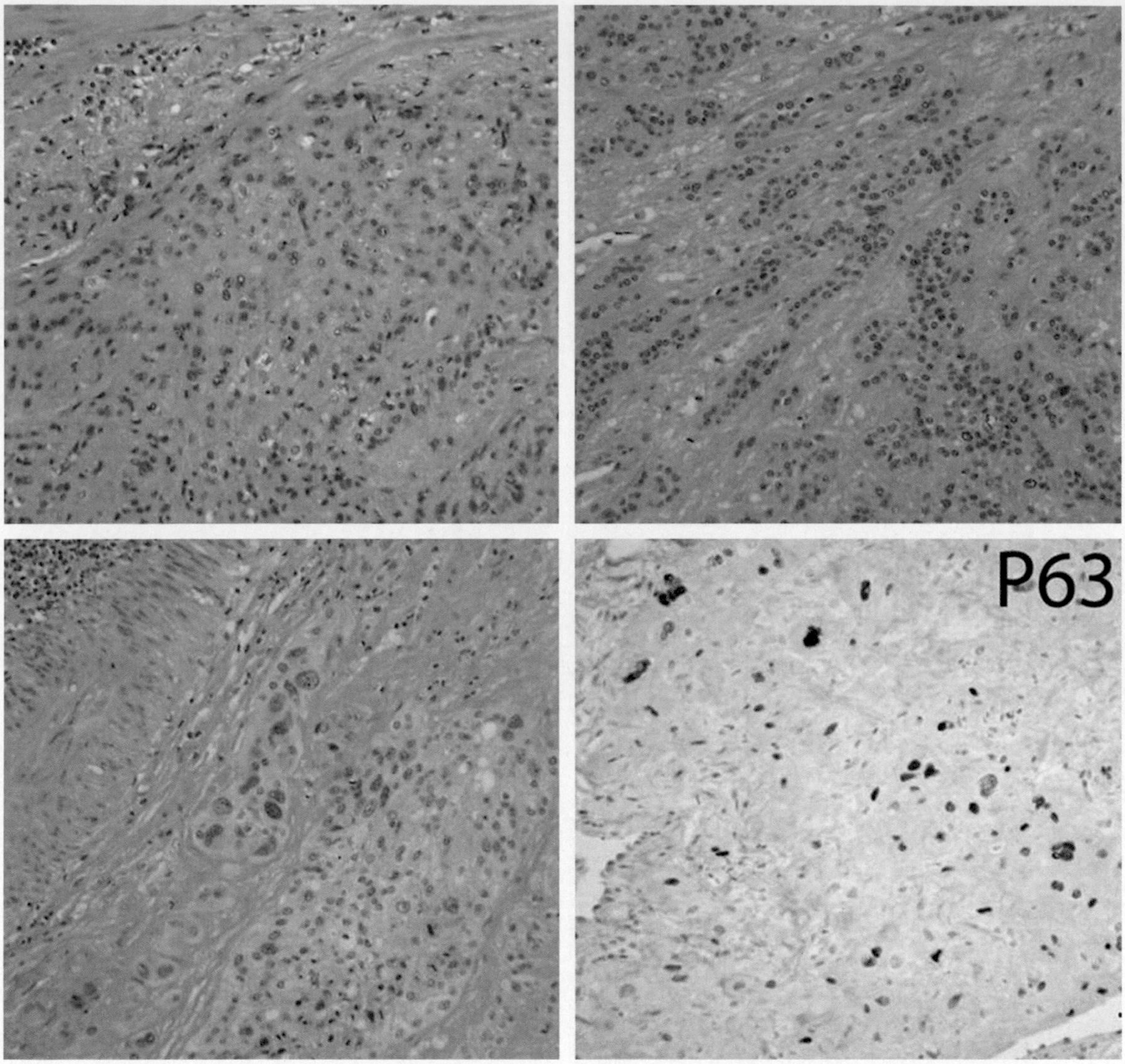

■ **Figure 26.8.** Epithelioid trophoblastic tumor. Tumor cell proliferation in sheets (*upper left*) or cords (*upper right*), and myometrial invasion (*lower left*). Tumor cells stain positive for p63.

■ **TABLE 26.4. The Changing Clinical Signs of Molar Pregnancy**

	Incidence (%)	
Clinical Sign	**1970s**	**2010s**
Vaginal bleeding	100	90
Uterine enlargement	54	28
Toxemia	22	1
Hyperemesis	28	8
Hyperthyroidism	10	<1
Trophoblastic emboli	2	<1
Bilaterally enlarged ovaries	15	15
Absence of fetal heart sounds	100	100

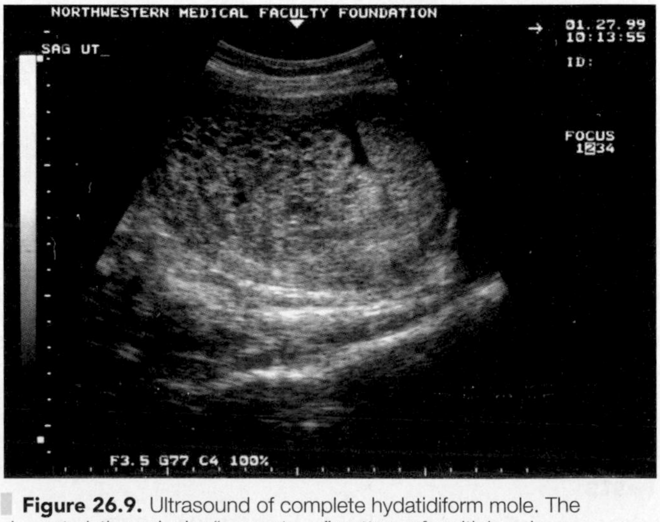

■ **Figure 26.9.** Ultrasound of complete hydatidiform mole. The characteristic vesicular "snowstorm" pattern of multiple echoes, appearing as holes within the placenta. No fetus is present.

Luteinizing hormone (LH) can also cross-react with hCG assays, leading to falsely elevated hCG in women with elevated pituitary follicle-stimulating hormone, LH, or hCG. hCG normally increases with age, and perimenopausal and postmenopausal women may have low-level hCG test results. To determine whether the hCG detected in the serum is from the pituitary, women may be given oral contraceptive to suppress LH, followed by simultancous measurement of LH and hCG (95,96).

Serum hCG may be incorrectly measured by enzyme-linked immunosorbent assay when levels are extremely high because of the "hook effect." These falsely low or negative results are caused by oversaturation of the signaling antibodies used to detect hCG by the assay equipment, and can be avoided by diluting the serum in cases where very high levels are suspected or anticipated (97).

Treatment

Suction evacuation and curettage is the preferred treatment for hydatidiform mole in patients who wish to preserve their fertility (**Table 26.5**) (98,99). Patients should undergo a preoperative evaluation including vital signs, laboratory tests, and electrocardiogram to identify any medical complications, such as anemia, preeclampsia, and hyperthyroidism. The patient's blood type and hCG levels should also be measured preoperatively. If the patient is hemodynamically stable, the type of molar evacuation procedure can be selected (100,101). If the uterus is greater than 12-week size, ultrasound monitoring should be used to prevent uterine perforation and ensure complete removal of the molar tissue. Suction evacuation and curettage is performed under conscious sedation or anesthesia, and the cervix is dilated to allow passage of a 12- to 14-mm suction cannula into the lower uterine segment. The cannula is rotated to remove the intrauterine contents. Intravenous oxytocin should be started at the onset of the procedure and continued postoperatively for several hours to enhance uterine contraction. Rh-negative patients will also need to receive Rh immunoglobulin during evacuation because the Rh D factor is expressed by trophoblastic cells (100,101). Gentle sharp curettage should be applied after suction evacuation. At least 2 units of blood should be available because of the risk of bleeding, which increases with uterine size. Postoperative respiratory distress may occur because of trophoblastic embolization, excessive fluid resuscitation, or massive oxytocin infusion. Attention to blood and crystalloid replacement reduces the risk of pulmonary complications, although all patients should be monitored with a pulse oximeter for at least 2 hours after surgery. Patient outcomes can be improved with the judicious use of equipment, ready access to blood products, careful monitoring during the procedure, and anticipation and treatment of complications.

TABLE 26.5. Evacuation of Hydatidiform Mole

Preoperative evaluation and preparation 1. Chest X-ray 2. Complete blood count 3. Electrolytes 4. Baseline oxygen saturation 5. Type and cross 2 units of blood 6. Set up Rho (D) immunoglobulin (RhoGAM) if patient is Rh-negative
Surgical procedure (with ultrasound guidance if uterus is >12 weeks size) 1. Premedication and paracervical anesthesia 2. Dilatation 3. Suction curettage—leave cannula at lower uterine segment until majority of molar tissue has been removed 4. Begin intravenous oxytocin infusion 5. Gentle sharp curettage
Postevacuation 1. Monitor respiratory status and uterine bleeding for at least 2 hours 2. Give RhoGAM if Rh-negative 3. Prescribe contraceptive 4. Follow hCG levels every 2 weeks until 2 consecutive normal results, then every month for 6 months and every 3 months twice

hCG, human chorionic gonadotropin.

For patients who have completed childbearing and do not wish to preserve their fertility, hysterectomy may be performed as an alternative to suction evacuation and curettage (**Fig. 26.10**). Hysterectomy removes the risk of local myometrial invasion, and focal disease can be ruled out in patients with persistent GTD. The high cost of this procedure and the risk of complications should limit the use of hysterectomy to those patients at high risk of postmolar GTD, including women over the age of 40, greater than gestational date uterine size, theca lutein cysts greater than 6 cm, hCG greater than 100,000 mIU/mL, and medical complications of pregnancy. However, metastatic disease may still be present after hysterectomy, with a 3% to 5% risk of postmolar GTN, and patients should be followed up with serial hCG testing (98).

Medical induction of labor and hysterotomy are not recommended, because of the increased risk of maternal morbidity, including blood loss, incomplete evacuation requiring surgical intervention, and the need for Cesarean delivery in subsequent pregnancies. This approach also increases the risk of trophoblastic dissemination and development of postmolar GTN requiring CT (99).

Use of prophylactic CT—either methotrexate or actinomycin D—at the time of evacuation or immediately afterward can reduce

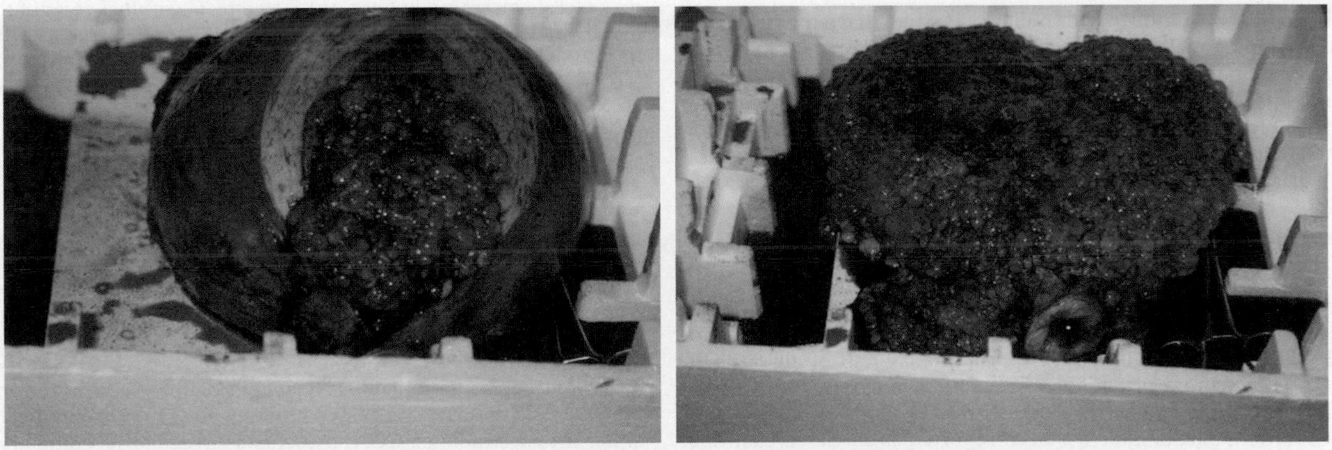

Figure 26.10. In selected patients, hysterectomy may decrease the likelihood of postmolar GTN. This photograph shows a 16-week uterus filled with complete hydatidiform mole.

the risk of postmolar GTN from 15%–20% to 3%–8%. However, this approach exposes patients to chemotherapeutic toxicity, but benefits only a small number of patients. Because all patients who are found to have persistent postmolar GTN with serial hCG testing can be cured with CT, in general, prophylactic CT is not recommended. Its use should be limited to those patients who have a greater than normal risk of postmolar GTN, or who are less likely to comply with serial hCG testing during follow-up (102–104).

Molar Pregnancy and Coexisting Fetus

Twin pregnancies of a complete mole and normal fetus occur approximately once in every 22,000 to 100,000 pregnancies and may be difficult to distinguish from partial mole. Ultrasound can usually differentiate between these two scenarios, though cytogenetics may help distinguish a normal viable fetus from a triploid nonviable fetus in a partial mole. Patients with a twin normal/complete mole pregnancy are at higher risk of hemorrhage, preterm delivery, and other complications, as well as a higher risk of persistent GTN. Although suction evacuation and curettage are often recommended to terminate the pregnancy, 40% of these pregnancies will result in a normal viable fetus if left untreated (105–107). Our approach to this very rare situation is to carefully counsel the patient about this risk of life-threatening hemorrhage, pregnancy loss, and prematurity, in support of shared decision-making.

Follow-Up

Clinical findings of successful evacuation include prompt uterine involution, ovarian cyst regression, and cessation of bleeding. Definitive follow-up after molar evacuation requires serial serum quantitative hCG measurements every 1 to 2 weeks until three consecutive normal tests, and then every 3 months for 6 months to 1 year after normalization. More than 50% of patients will achieve a normal hCG within 2 months of evacuation. Women should be counseled to avoid pregnancy after GTD; contraception is recommended for 6 months after the first normal hCG result so that any postmolar elevation in hCG that is detected can be distinguished from the hCG rise that occurs in a normal pregnancy. Oral contraceptives are preferred because they suppress LH and remove any interference with hCG assay measurements. Studies have shown that oral contraceptives do not increase the risk of postmolar GTN (108–110). Fertility preservation is achieved in over 80% of women with hydatidiform mole. High-risk postmolar disease is more often seen in patients who are not compliant with serial hCG measurements or are lost to follow-up (3). There is a 1% to 2% increased risk of developing a second complete molar pregnancy and a much lower risk of a second partial molar pregnancy (111).

Pregnancy after Hydatidiform Mole

All women with a history of molar pregnancy have a higher risk of developing malignant disease in a subsequent pregnancy (111). After molar evacuation, women should be counseled to wait at least 6 months from the time of hCG normalization to become pregnant. For all future pregnancies, pathologic examination of the placenta and other products of conception and measurement of hCG 6 weeks postpartum are recommended.

Persistent GTD/Postmolar GTN

Postmolar invasive mole or CCA occurs after 15% to 20% of complete and 1% to 5% of partial molar pregnancies, and invasive mole is seen more frequently (85% to 90%) than CCA (10% to 15%) (51,52,58,100,112–117). Approximately half of all cases of CCA arise from a prior molar pregnancy, but only 2% to 3% of all hydatidiform moles will progress to CCA (118). A diagnosis of CCA after a partial mole has been reported as single cases in the literature (51,52,58,119–125). Of women with invasive mole, 15% will have metastatic disease to the lungs or vagina. Most PSTTs and ETTs arise after nonmolar pregnancies, sometimes years after the pregnancy event (64,124,125).

The likelihood of persistent GTD after a molar pregnancy is higher in women who initially presented with marked trophoblastic growth, as indicated by hCG levels greater than 100,000 mIU/mL, excessive uterine size (>20 weeks), and theca lutein cysts greater than 6 cm in diameter. Women who have at least one of these risk factors have a 40% chance of developing postmolar GTN, compared with a 4% risk in those with none of these factors. Other risk factors for postmolar GTN include age greater than 40 years, repeat molar pregnancy, aneuploidy mole, and medical complications of molar pregnancy, such as toxemia, hyperthyroidism, and trophoblastic embolization (100).

At the molecular level, studies have found that women who will develop postmolar disease are more likely to show telomerase activity (126). Conversely, apoptotic activity measured by various techniques is higher in hydatidiform moles that spontaneously regress versus those that go on to develop postmolar GTN (127,128). Other studies have found that hydatidiform moles that are more likely to progress to malignant disease have lower expression of the antiapoptotic gene Mcl-1 (129), ferritin light polypeptide, and insulin-like growth factor–binding protein 1 (130).

For women with persistent GTD, a second curettage can be considered if their WHO score is low (<5). This approach was considered controversial in the past, because retrospective studies showed a variety of results from no benefit and significant perforation risk to significant response (131–134). The recently published results of the prospective clinical trial, Gynecologic Oncology Group study (GOG 242), clearly support the option of second curettage rather than CT for this low risk group of women with post molar GTN. In this study, of 60 women with postmolar GTN, WHO score 0–6, 24 (40%) were able to avoid CT. Grade 3–4 toxicity was limited to one patient with uterine perforation and one patient with hemorrhage requiring transfusion. None of the six women with WHO score of 5 or 6 responded completely to second curettage; therefore it is recommended that this treatment option be limited to patients with a WHO score of 0–4 (135).

Quiescent GTD

Some women with a history of GTD or spontaneous abortion may have a consistently low level of hCG (<200 mIU/mL for at least 3 months) but no detectable disease. In such situations, there is usually no evidence of hyperglycosylated hCG, a finding that, if present, is indicative of cytotrophoblastic invasion. This "quiescent GTD" does not respond to either surgery or CT. It is believed that the hCG being detected in these patients is produced by dispersed foci or individual slow-growing syncytiotrophoblast cells, with no invasive potential in the absence of cytotrophoblast or intermediate trophoblast.

Approximately one-quarter of patients with quiescent GTD go on to develop active GTN, with detectable increases in both hCG and hyperglycosylated hCG levels (112,113,136,137). These patients may secrete increased hyperglycosylated hCG within 5 years of the initial pregnancy event, weeks to months before a detectable rise in hCG or clinical evidence of GTN (138). To diagnose quiescent GTD, false-positive hCG testing should be ruled out and the patient examined for any evidence of disease. Patients should be monitored closely with periodic hCG testing and should avoid pregnancy (95). CT and surgery should be avoided unless a diagnosis of GTN can be made, based on either a sustained rise in hCG or the appearance of disease.

GESTATIONAL TROPHOBLASTIC NEOPLASIA

Clinical Presentation

The clinical presentation of GTN depends on the pregnancy event, the extent of disease, and histopathology (1–3). Postmolar GTN, either invasive mole or CCA, presents as irregular bleeding after evacuation of a hydatidiform mole (usually a complete mole). Invasive mole is diagnosed clinically rather than pathologically, with persistent hCG elevation after molar evacuation. CCA occurs in association with any pregnancy event, with approximately 25% of cases occurring after abortion or tubal pregnancy, 25% after term or preterm gestation, and 50% after a molar pregnancy. Sometimes, a metastatic vaginal lesion may be disrupted during pelvic examination, which can lead to uncontrolled vaginal bleeding. Women with postmolar GTN may also present with an enlarged, irregular uterus and bilateral ovarian enlargement. There are no signs or symptoms that differentiate between postmolar GTN and GTN arising after a nonmolar pregnancy event, because these symptoms are related to the invasion and metastasis of the tumor. GTN should be considered in patients who present with postpartum bleeding and uterine subinvolution, although other causes include endomyometritis, tumors in other organ systems, or another pregnancy. Uterine perforation and metastases can cause abdominal pain, hemoptysis, melena, or increased intracranial pressure that leads to headaches, seizures, or hemiplegia. Symptoms suggesting pulmonary involvement include dyspnea, cough, and chest pain, and early respiratory failure requiring mechanical ventilation may develop. A diagnosis of GTN should be considered for any woman of reproductive age who presents with pulmonary symptoms (121). Symptoms of brain metastases include vomiting, seizures, headache, hemiparesis, and speech and visual disturbances (139). Liver and gastrointestinal metastases are rare and usually are seen with simultaneous lung or brain involvement; these patients have the lowest survival rate (140). PSTT and ETT often present with irregular vaginal bleeding and an enlarged uterus, with hCG levels from normal to 1,000 mIU/mL, sometimes years after a previous pregnancy. PSTT may also present with liver, lung, or brain metastases, or complications such as neoplastic nephrotic syndrome (124,125).

Diagnosis

The International Federation of Gynecology and Obstetrics (FIGO) defined a set of criteria for diagnosing persistent GTD in 2002 (**Table 26.6**) (141). Postmolar GTN is usually diagnosed when hCG levels plateau or rise during follow-up after molar evacuation, without histologic diagnosis. An hCG plateau is defined as a less than 10% decline in four measurements taken over 3 weeks. A rise is defined as a greater than 20% increase in three measurements taken over 2 weeks. The presence of elevated hCG in addition to metastases usually indicates CCA, whereas with PSTT and ETT, serum hCG levels are only slightly elevated, making differential diagnosis particularly challenging (64,124,125). The free hCG β subunit may be the best biomarker for diagnosing PSTT and the β core fragment for ETT (38,77). Although a diagnosis of GTN can be confirmed pathologically by examination of curettage or hysterectomy specimens, the placenta, or biopsy of metastatic lesions, the risk of hemorrhage is too high, and biopsy of vaginal lesions should be avoided (142).

For any patient with suspected or established GTN, a metastatic workup and evaluation of risk factors is performed (2,3,143) A complete history, physical examination, and laboratory tests (including complete blood cell count, coagulation study, serum chemistries, blood type and antibody screening, and quantitative serum hCG level) should be taken. Radiologic studies should start with a chest X-ray; if abnormal, a CT or MRI of the chest should be performed to detect pulmonary metastases. If the physical examination and the chest X-ray are normal and there are no symptoms of metastasis, other sites of metastasis are rarely present.

In general, we reserve further evaluation for metastatic disease only in the presence of lung metastases. The vast majority of patients with brain involvement (94%) have associated lung metastases; conversely, 20% of patients with lung metastases also have brain metastases. Brain metastases tend to appear in the parietal lobe and on the right side of the brain (**Fig. 26.11**). To detect central nervous system (CNS) lesions and brain involvement, MRI is significantly more sensitive than CT scan. Cerebrospinal fluid (CSF) hCG testing was a valuable tool prior to the development of CT scan and MRI scanning, but is rarely indicated in practice. If performed, a serum/CSF hCG ratio of less than 60:1 is a sensitive marker of CNS metastasis (143), although false positives can occur if measurements are taken when hCG levels are falling. CT scan of the abdomen, pelvic ultrasound, and MRI may be useful to detect extensive uterine disease and, specifically, to identify patients who may benefit from hysterectomy. Biopsy of metastases is not recommended, because the associated risks of biopsy outweigh the benefits of confirming a diagnosis of metastatic disease.

Staging and Risk Scoring

In 2002, FIGO adopted a combined anatomic staging system and a modified version of the WHO risk factor scoring system for GTN (**Tables 26.7** and **26.8**) (144). The FIGO stage is designated by a Roman numeral and is followed by the modified WHO score designated by an Arabic numeral, separated by a colon. The risk score takes into account eight criteria, each of which is given a score from 0 to 4. Treatment of GTN is based on the classification of patients into risk groups defined by the stage and risk factor scoring system (145). The FIGO system is essential for selecting initial therapy for patients with GTN that will ensure the best possible outcomes with the fewest side effects. A recent study found that most patients classified as low risk but who have an initial level of hCG greater than 400,000 mIU/mL will fail initial CT, suggesting that perhaps these patients would benefit from multiagent CT (146). Patients with hCG levels between 100,000 and 400,000 mIU/mL will either respond to a single-agent regimen or require a change in regimen to achieve cure. Note that this staging and risk factor scoring system do not apply to either PSTT or ETT.

TABLE 26.6. FIGO 2000 Criteria for Diagnosis of Persistent GTD/Postmolar GTN

hCG plateau lasting for four measurements over a period of at least 3 weeks (days 1, 7, 14, and 21)
Rise in hCG of 10% or more for three measurements over at least 2 weeks (days 1, 7, and 14)
Persistence of elevated hCG 6 months after mole evacuation
Presence of a histologic diagnosis of CCA

CCA, choriocarcinoma; hCG, human chorionic gonadotropin.

Source: From FIGO Oncology Committee. FIGO staging for gestational trophoblastic neoplasia 2000. FIGO Oncology Committee. *Int J Gynaecol Obstet*. 2002;77(3):285–287, with permission.

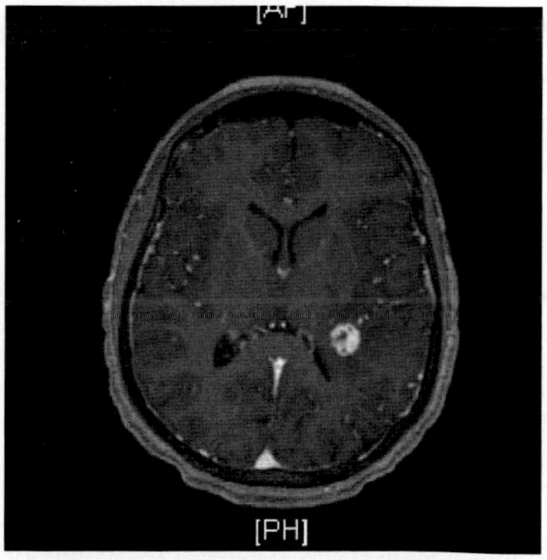

Figure 26.11. MRI of the brain. MRI showing right parietal lobe lesion with central hemorrhage.

■ TABLE 26.7. FIGO 2000 Staging for Gestational Trophoblastic Neoplasiav

Stage	Description
I	Disease confined to uterus
II	Disease extends outside uterus but is limited to genital structures (adnexa, vagina, broad ligament)
III	Disease extends to lungs with or without genital tract involvement
IV	Disease involves other metastatic sites

Source: From FIGO Oncology Committee. FIGO staging for gestational trophoblastic neoplasia 2000. FIGO Oncology Committee. *Int J Gynaecol Obstet*. 2002;77(3):285–287, with permission.

■ TABLE 26.8. FIGO 2000 Risk Scoring System for Gestational Trophoblastic Neoplasia

	Score			
Risk Factor	0	1	2	4
Age, years	≤39	>39	–	–
Antecedent pregnancy	Mole	Abortion	Term	
Pregnancy event to treatment interval, months	<4	4–6	7–12	>12
Pretreatment hCG, mIU/mL	$<10^3$	10^3–10^4	10^4–10^5	$>10^5$
Largest tumor mass, including uterus, cm	<3	3–4	≥5	–
Site of metastases	–	Spleen, kidney	GI tract	Brain, liver
No. of metastases	–	1–4	5–8	>8
Previous failed chemotherapy	–	–	Single drug	≥2 drugs

Source: From FIGO Oncology Committee. FIGO staging for gestational trophoblastic neoplasia 2000. FIGO Oncology Committee. *Int J Gynaecol Obstet*. 2002;77(3):285–287, with permission.

■ TABLE 26.9. Chemotherapy for Low-Risk Gestational Trophoblastic Neoplasia

Regimen	Primary Remission Rate (%)
MTX 0.4 mg/kg (max 25 mg)/day IV or IM for 5 days; repeat every 2 weeks	87–93
MTX 30–50 mg/m² IM weekly	49–74
MTX 1 mg/kg IM days 1, 3, 5, and 7; folinic acid 0.1 mg/kg IM days 2, 4, 6, and 8; repeat every 15–18 days or as needed	74–90
MTX 100 mg/m² IVP, then 200 mg/m² in 500 mL D5W over 12 hours; folinic acid 15 mg IM or PO every 12 hours for 4 doses beginning 24 hours after start of MTX; repeat every 18 days or as needed	69–90
Act D 10–13 mcg/kg IV (with a max daily dose of 0.5 mg) every day for 5 days; repeat every 2 weeks	77–94
Act D 1.25 mg/m² IV every 2 weeks (max 2 mg/day)	69–90
Alternating MTX 0.4 mg/kg (max 25 mg)/day IV daily for 5 days alternating every two weeks with Act D 10–13 mcg/kg (with a max daily dose of 0.5 mg) IV daily for 5 days	100

Act D, actinomycin D; D5W, dextrose 5% in water; IM, intramuscular; IV, intravenous; IVP, intravenous push; MTX, methotrexate; PO, by mouth.

Management

The cure rate for high-risk GTN—most commonly CCA—is currently greater than 90%, and for low-risk disease it approaches 100%, primarily because of the inherent sensitivity of trophoblastic neoplasms to CT, the effective use of hCG as a marker of early disease, the referral of patients to specialized centers, the identification of predictive factors of treatment response that has permitted individualization of therapy, and the use of combined surgery, radiation, and CT in the highest risk patients. Management of PSTT and ETT is more challenging because these neoplasms are often resistant to CT, and hCG level is not a strong marker of these diseases (2,3,147).

Low-Risk GTN

Patients in the low-risk group are those with Stage I disease (nonmetastatic) or Stage II and III disease (metastatic) with a risk score of less than 7. Stage I patients with a WHO score of 0–4 may benefit from a second curettage. When CT is indicated, these patients should undergo single-agent treatment with either methotrexate or actinomycin D (148,149), which has achieved survival rates approaching 100%. There are several different CT protocols for low-risk nonmetastatic GTN that have produced comparable results in nonrandomized, retrospective studies (**Table 26.9**). Taken together, these studies suggest that the 5-day methotrexate or the 8-day methotrexate–folinic acid protocol and the 5-day actinomycin D protocols or the biweekly single-dose actinomycin D protocols are significantly more effective than weekly intramuscular (IM) methotrexate. An ongoing phase III randomized international multi-institutional GOG study (GOG 275) is testing biweekly actinomycin D versus multiday (either 5- or 8-day) methotrexate. Remission rates with each of these protocols vary because of differences in drug doses, schedules, routes of administration, and patient factors. These studies also found that initial resistance to CT is associated with older age, higher hCG, nonmolar antecedent pregnancy, histopathologic diagnosis of CCA, presence of metastases, and higher FIGO score. Common side effects of these regimens are stomatitis, mucositis of the gastrointestinal tract, pleuritis, conjunctivitis, and skin rash.

CT is continued until hCG values have returned to normal, and at least one course is administered after the first normal hCG level is achieved. A recent retrospective study compared relapse rates in women from the UK and the Netherlands with low-risk disease who were treated with methotrexate alternating with folinic acid (150). A greater number of patients relapsed with only two consolidation courses than those who received three consolidation courses after reaching the institutional normal hCG value of less than 5 mIU/mL. If hCG levels plateau at a point above normal during treatment, or if toxicity limits the ability to administer the chosen regimen, CT is changed to an alternative single-agent regimen. Multiagent CT is indicated in the event of a significant elevation in hCG, development of metastases, or resistance to sequential single-agent CT. Although there are differences in primary remission rates with each of the CT protocols, the cure rate remains high and most patients are able to preserve their fertility.

The John I. Brewer Trophoblastic Disease Center reviewed 30 years of experience treating low-risk nonmetastatic GTN to determine the most effective therapy, evaluate toxicity, and identify the factors associated with treatment resistance (**Table 26.10**) (151). Of 253 patients who received initial therapy of single-agent methotrexate (0.4 mg/kg, maximum 25 mg) as an IV push for 5 days every 2 weeks, only 5 required subsequent multiagent CT (90% complete response), and all patients achieved permanent remission. Only 12 patients experienced significant side effects with methotrexate, most commonly stomatitis, leading to a change in therapy to another

TABLE 26.10. Treatment of Low-Risk GTN at the Brewer Trophoblastic Disease Center

Regimens: MTX 0.4 mg/kg (max 25 mg)/day IV for 5 days, repeat every 2 weeks; Act D 10–13 mcg/kg IV every day for 5 days, repeat every 2 weeks

	Complete Remission Rate to Initial Single-Agent MTX	Required Multiagent Chemotherapy or Surgery (%)	Cured (%)
Lurain and Elfstrand (1995) (1962–1990) (151)	89.3% (226/253 nonmetastatic, low-risk GTN)	2	100
Roberts and Lurain (1996) (1962–1992) (183)	65.6% (40/61 metastatic, low-risk GTN)	3	100
Chapman-Davis et al. (2009) (1979–2009) (184)	81% (291/360 FIGO low-risk GTN[a])	6	100

[a]Stage I disease (nonmetastatic) and Stage II and III disease (metastatic), risk score <7.

agent, and no life-threatening toxicities were noted. Resistance to the initial single-agent methotrexate regimen was associated with high pretreatment hCG, nonmolar antecedent pregnancy, and clinicopathologic diagnosis of CCA. These findings are consistent with those of other centers and suggest that the most effective treatment protocol for low-risk nonmetastatic GTN is methotrexate 0.4 mg/kg (maximum total dose 25 mg) IM or IV push given once daily for 5 days every other week (151–168).

Two retrospective case studies compared 5-day IM methotrexate and 8-day methotrexate–folinic acid protocols in patients with low-risk nonmetastatic GTN; one study found that there was no difference in remission rates (76%) (157), and the other reported lower remission rates in patients receiving methotrexate–folinic acid (72%) than in patients receiving methotrexate alone (92%) (167). Gleeson et al. (168) subsequently reported a 69% primary remission rate in patients with nonmetastatic postmolar GTN treated with weekly methotrexate alone and a 75% remission rate with methotrexate–folinic acid.

As an alternative to methotrexate, actinomycin D may be given as an IV push of 10 to 12 μg/kg daily for 5 days every other week or as a single 1.25 mg/m^2 (max dose 2.0 mg/m^2) IV dose every other week (169–173). The primary remission rate for patients with nonmetastatic postmolar GTN was 88% for 5-day actinomycin D and 78% for pulsed actinomycin D (174). However, actinomycin D is more often used as a second-line therapy in patients with methotrexate resistance or with contraindications to methotrexate, because it is associated with higher perceived toxicity, particularly alopecia, and produces local tissue injury in cases of IV extraversion (175).

Several studies have compared weekly methotrexate and biweekly actinomycin D regimens for treatment of low-risk, nonmetastatic GTN. Across three randomized clinical trials, IM methotrexate was associated with lower primary complete response rates (49% to 53%) than pulsed actinomycin D (69% to 90%) (176–178). In the phase 3 GOG study (178), there was a higher complete response for biweekly IV actinomycin D than for weekly IM methotrexate (70% vs. 53%, $p = 0.01$), and in patients with lower risk scores (<5), the response rate was 73% and 58%, respectively ($p = 0.03$). Both regimens were less effective in patients with risk scores of 5 or 6 or if the diagnosis was CCA (complete response: 42% and 9%, respectively). Actinomycin D was associated with a high incidence of grade 1 alopecia and grade 1 nausea. In another randomized study of patients with stage I nonmetastatic GTN, complete remission was achieved in 74% of women who received methotrexate–folinic acid and in 100% of women who received 5-day actinomycin D (179). In a retrospective study of patients with low-risk, mostly nonmetastatic GTN, Abrao et al. (180) reported no significant difference in the complete remission rates with 5-day regimens of methotrexate or actinomycin D or combination therapy (69%, 61%, and 79%, respectively); however, the incidence of side effects was much higher in patients receiving the combination therapy than either single-agent regimen.

For patients with low-risk metastatic GTN (Stage II or III, score <7), single-agent CT with multiday dosing of either methotrexate or actinomycin D is appropriate; however, the biweekly actinomycin D protocols used for nonmetastatic disease should not be used in these patients (**Table 26.9**). Three specialized trophoblastic disease centers in the United States have reported remission rates of 48% to 67% in patients with low-risk, metastatic GTN with single-agent CT, with 1% to 14% of patients requiring multiagent therapy after failure of single-agent therapy with or without surgery (**Table 26.10**) (181–183). In this group of patients, resistance to single-agent therapy was associated with pretreatment hCG levels >100,000 mIU/mL, age older than 35 years, a FIGO score >4, and the presence of large vaginal metastases.

At the Brewer Trophoblastic Disease Center, we examined risk factors for developing resistance to initial methotrexate therapy in 358 patients with low-risk GTN treated between 1979 and 2009 (**Table 26.10**) (184). Patients initially received methotrexate 0.4 mg/kg (max 25 mg) IV push daily for 5 days every 14 days. Actinomycin D 0.5 mg IV push daily for 5 days every 14 days was used in 64 patients who developed resistance or toxicity to initial methotrexate CT, and multiagent regimens were used in 20 patients for whom either single-agent CT failed. The complete response rate to initial methotrexate was 81%, and the complete response rate to actinomycin D as secondary therapy was 75% (94% overall complete response rate to sequential single-agent CT). The remaining patients achieved permanent remission with multiagent CT with or without surgery. Resistance to initial methotrexate CT was associated with increasing FIGO score ($p < 0.0001$), clinicopathologic diagnosis of CCA ($p = 0.028$), higher pretreatment hCG ($p = 0.001$), and presence of metastatic disease ($p = 0.018$).

In general, primary treatment failure occurs in 10% to 30% of patients with low-risk GTN and in 30% to 50% of patients with low-risk, metastatic disease. Most patients who are resistant to the initial CT will be placed into remission after changing to another single-agent CT. Patients with low-risk nonmetastatic disease will rarely require multiagent CT, and approximately 15% of patients with low-risk, metastatic GTN will require multiagent CT with or without surgery. The higher rate of failure of initial single-agent therapy in patients with higher FIGO scores has led some to propose an intermediate risk group of patients who have metastatic disease with scores of 5 or 6. Ideally, treatment failure should be identified as early as possible to limit patient exposure to ineffective CT cycles. Several groups have tried to determine an hCG cutoff value that can predict treatment resistance, in order to allow prompt changes in treatment (185–187). One group found that a cutoff value of 737 mIU/mL was able to predict resistance to 8-day methotrexate with a specificity of 97.5% (188). If treatment change is necessary, the risk score is recalculated to determine the most appropriate second-line regimen.

In patients with low-risk GTN who do not wish to preserve their fertility, adjuvant hysterectomy may be performed with the initiation of CT to reduce the length of treatment required to achieve remission (189). Other indications for hysterectomy in low-risk GTN include persistent, CT-resistant disease in the uterus or to treat uterine tumor hemorrhage.

High-Risk GTN

Chemotherapy. Patients in the high-risk group have metastatic GTN, either stage IV disease or stage II and III disease with a risk factor score greater than 6. These patients are treated more aggressively with multiagent CT, with or without adjuvant radiation or surgery (**Table 26.11**). With this approach, cure rates have

■ TABLE 26.11. EMA-CO Chemotherapy for High-Risk Gestational Trophoblastic Neoplasia

Treatment Day	Regimen	
1	Etoposide	100 mg/m² IV over 30 minutes
	Act D	0.5 mg IVP
	MTX	100 mg/m² IVP, then 200 mg/m² in 500 mL D5W over 12 hours
2	Etoposide	100 mg/m² IV over 30 minutes
	Act D	0.5 mg IVP
	Folinic acid	15 mg IM or PO every 12 hours for 4 doses starting 24 hours after start of MTX (on day 1)
8	Cyclophosphamide	600 mg/m² IV
	Vincristine	1.0 mg/m² IVP

Cycle repeats every 2 weeks (i.e., days 15, 16, and 22).

Act D, actinomycin D; D5W, dextrose 5% in water; IM, intramuscular; IV, intravenous; IVP, intravenous push; MTX, methotrexate; PO, by mouth.

reached 80% to 90%. Treatment delay or dose reduction because of side effects increases the likelihood of tumor resistance and treatment failure (2,3,147). Historically, a combination treatment of methotrexate, actinomycin D, and cyclophosphamide or chlorambucil (MAC) was used as first-line therapy for high-risk, metastatic GTN and achieved cure in 63% to 71% of patients (**Table 26.12**) (190,191). Over time, the regimen of choice shifted to a combination of cyclophosphamide, hydroxyurea, actinomycin D, methotrexate with folinic acid, vincristine, and doxorubicin (CHAMOCA) (**Fig. 26.12**). The primary remission rate in high-risk, metastatic GTN was reported to be 82% with this regimen (192). However, a subsequent randomized trial comparing MAC and CHAMOCA found that the primary remission rate and the cure rate were inferior for CHAMOCA, which also had a more toxic side-effect profile (193). The addition of etoposide to a regimen containing high-dose methotrexate with folinic acid, actinomycin D, and vincristine (EMA-CO) improved both primary remission and

■ TABLE 26.12. Treatment of High-Risk GTN at Brewer Trophoblastic Disease Center

Brewer et al. (1968) (190)	MTX and/or Act D followed by MAC: 39% survival
	Initial MAC: 65% survival
Lurain and Brewer (1985) (1968–1982) (191)	MAC: 63% (29/46) complete remission
Schink et al. (1992) (1986–1991) (195)	EMA-CO: 83% (10/12) complete remission
Escobar et al. (2003) (1986–2001) (200)	EMA-CO: 76% (19/25) complete response rate
	92% (23/25) survival
Lurain et al. (2006) (201)	EMA-CO: 66.7% (20/30) complete response rate
	93.3% (28/30) survival
Lurain et al. (2010) (1986–2009, FIGO high-risk only[a]) (204)	EMA-CO: 54% (14/26) complete response rate
	92% (24/26) survival

[a]Stage II and III disease, risk score ≥7 and Stage IV disease.

survival rates in patients with high-risk GTN (**Table 26.12**) (194,195). The EMA-CO regimen for high-risk GTN has reportedly complete response rates of 71% to 78% and long-term survival rates of 85% to 94% (196–204). The survival rates exceed the complete response rates because GTN is a unique malignancy where secondary therapies often result in cure. In our study series (200,201,204), we reported complete response rates of 76%, 67%, and 54% and overall survival rates of 92%, 93%, and 92% with EMA-CO treatment, respectively. Deaths occurred only in patients with FIGO stage IV disease with scores greater than 12, and no treatment-related deaths or severe toxicities were seen. Neutropenia was rare, although alopecia and anemia were common, and mild paresthesia and stomatitis occurred in 20% of patients.

Patients with widely metastatic disease as evidenced by a very high WHO/FIGO score (>12) are at significant risk for pulmonary, intraperitoneal, or intracranial hemorrhage, this risk may be mitigated by starting treatment with low dose induction chemotherapy. The use of induction low-dose etoposide 100 mg/m² and cisplatin 20 mg/m² (EP); days 1 and 2, every 7 days has been used at Charing Cross since 1995 to reduce early deaths before commencing EMA-CO. EP induction was given to 23.1% of 140 high-risk patients (33 of 140 patients) with a large disease burden for one to four cycles, and the early death rate was reduced to only 0.7%, compared with 7.2% in the pre-1995 cohort (205).

Though aggressive multiagent therapy is associated with high levels of toxicity, single-agent therapy is not appropriate for high-risk patients, because the success rate of secondary CT after failure of single-agent therapy is only 20% to 50%. Based on current evidence, EMA-CO is the initial treatment of choice for patients with high-risk, metastatic GTN. The regimen has high complete response rates and survival rates, as well as low toxicity that improves patient adherence to treatment and thus reduces the risk of drug resistance. CT is continued for at least two to three courses after the first normal hCG level is achieved.

Radiation

For patients who present with brain metastases, whole brain radiation (3,000 cGy in 200 cGy fractions) or, in selected patients, surgical excision with stereotactic radiation is indicated and is usually performed at the start of CT to lower the risk of hemorrhage (140,206–208). In these patients, the EMA-CO regimen is modified such that methotrexate is increased to 1 g/m² with 30 mg of folinic acid every 12 hours for 3 days starting 32 hours after the start of infusion (209). Intrathecal and high-dose methotrexate may also be used in some centers (209,210). Patients are also treated with dexamethasone to decrease edema and phenytoin sodium to prevent seizure. During therapy, patients undergo serial CT scans or MRIs to monitor the lesions. Once a complete response has been achieved, hCG levels in the CSF should be measured, ideally by radioimmunoassay to detect low levels of protein. The plasma to CSF ratio of hCG should be less than 60 (144). Patients with brain metastases have a cure rate of 50% to 80% depending on symptoms and the number, size, and location of brain lesions.

Surgery

Approximately 50% of patients with high-risk, metastatic GTN will require adjuvant surgical procedures, usually hysterectomy and pulmonary resection, for CT-resistant disease or to control hemorrhage and sepsis (211–219). Selected patients with focal disease may be candidates for partial lung, liver, or brain resection. Imaging with fluorodeoxyglucose positron emission tomography (PET), with CT scan for anatomic localization, may help with targeted surgery (220). For women with excessive vaginal bleeding, selective arterial embolization may be beneficial (221,222). We reviewed a series of 50 patients with high-risk GTN who were treated at the Brewer Trophoblastic Disease Center from 1986 through 2005 with EMA-CO as primary or secondary therapy. Twenty-four patients (48%) underwent 28 adjuvant surgical procedures, and 21 (87.5%) were cured. Fifteen of 17 patients who underwent hysterectomy;

Disease		1960s	1970s	1980s	1990s	2000–present
Low-Risk GTN		Methotrexate x 5d IV		→	→	→
High Risk GTN	1st Line	MTX	MAC →	CHAMOCA → EMACO	→	→
	2nd			MAC → BEP	EMA-EP	→
	3rd				BEP	→
	4th					VIP → ICE
	5th					TP/TE
PSTT	1st			EMA-EP →	→	
	2nd					TP/TE

Figure 26.12. Evolution of chemotherapy for GTN at the John I. Brewer Trophoblastic Disease Center. Chemotherapy regimens are shown for low-risk disease, as well as the first-line therapy and subsequent regimens for recurrent or resistant high-risk disease. For PSTT, chemotherapy may be used in patients with metastatic disease and in patients with nonmetastatic disease and poor prognostic factors.

4 of 5 patients who had resistant foci of CCA in the lung resected; all 4 patients who had suturing of the uterus, uterine artery embolization, small bowel resection, and salpingectomy for bleeding; and 1 patient who had uterine wedge resection for resistant CCA survived (213).

Second-Line/Salvage Therapy

Despite the use of multimodal primary therapy, approximately 30% of patients with high-risk GTN will have an incomplete response or will relapse from remission and will require secondary CT (223–230). Risk factors for relapse include the presence of multiple metastases to sites other than the lung and vagina and inadequate first-line CT. Salvage CT with the EMA-EP regimen, in which etoposide and cisplatin have been substituted for cyclophosphamide and vincristine in the EMA-CO regimen, is the most appropriate for patients who have not responded (plateaued low hCG levels) or experienced a relapse (reelevation of hCG after a complete response) to first-line EMA-CO. This regimen is highly toxic and usually requires granulocyte colony-stimulating factor support by the third cycle. Salvage CT combined with surgical excision of persistent tumor will result in cure for most of these high-risk patients (228–230). In patients who have developed resistance to methotrexate-containing protocols, drug combinations containing etoposide and platinum with bleomycin, ifosfamide, or paclitaxel have also been effective (224,231). At the Brewer Trophoblastic Disease Center, we reported on 26 patients with persistent or relapsed high-risk GTN who received secondary platinum-based salvage CT. The overall survival was 61.5% (16/26). Of the 16 patients for whom primary therapy with methotrexate/actinomycin D–based CT without etoposide failed, 10 (63%) had complete clinical responses to bleomycin, etoposide, and cisplatin; etoposide, ifosfamide, and cisplatin; and ifosfamide, carboplatin, and etoposide; and 10 (63%) were cured. Of the 10 patients for whom primary therapy with EMA-CO failed, 9 (90%) had complete clinical responses to EMA-EP or bleomycin, etoposide, cisplatin, but only 6 (60%) subsequently achieved a lasting remission (223). Most recently, we reviewed the effect of etoposide/platinum-based salvage therapy in 49 women (20 of whom were treated secondarily at our center) with high-risk GTN treated between 1986 and 2010 for whom initial multiagent therapy with EMA-CO had failed (**Table 26.13**) (230). Salvage therapy included etoposide and a platinum agent with methotrexate and actinomycin D (EMA-EP), bleomycin (BEP), ifosfamide (VIP, ICE), or paclitaxel (TP/TE). Of the 28 patients who developed resistance to EMA-CO, 82% achieved lasting complete responses to salvage therapy. Three of four patients who received RT for brain metastases survived, and 82% of patients who required surgical procedures to remove metastases survived. High hCG level at the start of salvage therapy ($p < 0.001$), a higher number of metastatic sites ($p < 0.02$), and metastases to sites other than the lung and vagina ($p < 0.05$) were associated with lower survival in these patients. Patients with metastases in the brain, liver, and gastrointestinal tract have a 75%, 73%, and 50% survival rate, respectively (229).

TABLE 26.13. Secondary Treatment of EMA-CO–Resistant, High-Risk GTN

Regimen	Patients	Complete Response, No. (%)	Survival, No. (%)
EMA-EP	19	11 (58)	9 (47)
BEP	16	11 (69)	9 (56)
VIP	2	1 (50)	1 (50)
ICE	6	4 (67)	3 (30)
TP/TE	3	2 (67)	1 (33)
Totals	46	29 (63)	23 (82)

BEP, bleomycin, etoposide, platinum agent; EMA-CO, etoposide, methotrexate, actinomycin D, cyclophosphamide, vincristine; EMA-EP, etoposide, methotrexate, actinomycin D, platinum agent; TP/TE, paclitaxel, platinum agent/paclitaxel, etoposide; VIP and ICE, etoposide, platinum agent, ifosfamide.

Source: Adapted from Lurain JR, Schink JC. Importance of salvage therapy in the management of high-risk gestational trophoblastic neoplasia. *J Reprod Med.* 2012;57(5–6):219–224, with permission.

PSTT and ETT

Because of the relative resistance of PSTT and ETT to CT and the high risk of lymphatic spread, hysterectomy with lymph node dissection is the recommended treatment. Prior to surgery, histologic diagnosis of PSTT with endometrial biopsy or curettage specimen should be confirmed with immunohistochemical staining for the presence of hPL and the absence of hCG. CT should be used in patients with metastatic disease and in patients with nonmetastatic disease and poor prognostic factors, including a long interval between last pregnancy and diagnosis (>2 years), deep myometrial invasion, tumor necrosis, and mitotic count greater than 5/10 high-power fields (232,233). Though we do not know the optimal CT regimen for PSTT and ETT, the current treatment of choice is a platinum-containing regimen, such as EMA-EP or a paclitaxel/cisplatin–paclitaxel/etoposide (TP/TE) doublet. With hysterectomy and CT, the survival rate is approximately 100% for nonmetastatic disease and 50% to 60% for metastatic disease (234–236).

Reasons for Treatment Failure

We identified patients who were transferred to the Brewer Trophoblastic Disease Center after treatment failure elsewhere, in order to determine the causes of treatment failure. We also compared our second-line treatment results from 1979 to 2006 with previous reports from 1962 to 1978 (**Table 26.14**) (237). The most common reasons for treatment failure for GTN were (1) use of single-agent CT for patients with high-risk disease and (2) inappropriate use of weekly IM methotrexate CT for treatment of patients with metastatic disease, FIGO scores ≥7, and/or nonpostmolar CCA. Successful secondary GTN treatment in these patients improved from 59% during 1962 through 1978 to 93% during 1979 through 2006, most likely as a result of center experience and the use of more effective CT regimens. It is recommended that clinicians request advice from or referral for treatment to centers with expertise in management of GTN for patients who fail single-agent therapy for low-risk disease and for any patient with high-risk disease (238).

Follow-Up of GTN

After hCG has returned to normal levels and treatment has been completed, serum quantitative hCG levels should be obtained at 1-month intervals for 12 months. The risk of relapse is approximately 3% in the first year after completing therapy and drops to less than 1% thereafter. Physical examinations are performed at intervals of 6 to 12 months, and other testing is rarely indicated.

Pregnancy after GTN

Successful treatment of GTN with CT has allowed most women to preserve their fertility, despite exposure to drugs that are toxic to the ovary. Most women resume normal ovarian function after CT and exhibit no increase in infertility, however, menopause may occur earlier. Contraception should be maintained during treatment and for 1 year after completion of CT, preferably using oral contraceptives, to allow for uninterrupted hCG follow-up and to permit the ovulation of eggs that may have been damaged by exposure to cytotoxic drugs.

Successful pregnancies have been reported after GTN, without an increased rate of abortion, stillbirth, congenital anomalies, prematurity, or major obstetric complications (22,239,240). There is no evidence for reactivation of disease with subsequent pregnancies, although patients who have had one trophoblastic disease episode have a 1% to 2% risk of a second GTD event, independent of previous CT (4). Therefore, pelvic ultrasound is recommended in the first trimester of any post-GTN pregnancy to confirm a normal gestation. The products of contraception or placentas from future pregnancies should also be carefully examined histopathologically, and a serum quantitative hCG level should be determined 6 weeks after any pregnancy.

Risk of Secondary Malignancies

Because of the relatively short exposure of patients with GTN to intermittent schedules of methotrexate and actinomycin D and the infrequent use of alkylating agents, there are concerns of increased susceptibility to the development of other malignancies. A retrospective study in 1996 from Charing Cross demonstrated an increased use of etoposide-containing drug combinations for treatment of GTN that has led to an increased risk of secondary malignancies, including acute myelogenous leukemia, colon cancer, melanoma, and breast cancer (241). Because of this, and an association with alopecia and severe nausea, the use of etoposide-containing regimens is limited to patients with high-risk disease. A follow-up study from Charing Cross, in 2015, looked back at the original cohort and extending it to include 1903 women treated between 1958 and 2000, with follow-up beginning in 2006. They found: "Subsequent cancer risks for patients cured of gestational trophoblastic tumors with modern chemotherapy appear similar to those of the normal population with no overall increased risk of malignancy after MTX-FA or EMA-CO. However, there was evidence of an increased risk of leukemia after EMA-CO and some evidence of other site-specific increased risks based on small patient numbers. All major treatments except MTX-FA increased the risk of early menopause."(242).

TABLE 26.14. Overall Results of Treatment of GTN at the Brewer Center 1962–2006

Treatment Site/Dates	Number	Survival
Primarily at Brewer Center	740	702 (95%)[a]
1962–1978	359	329 (92%)
1979–2006	381	373 (98%)
Secondarily at Brewer Center	64	47 (73%)[a]
1962–1978	37	22 (59%)[b]
1979–2006	27	25 (93%)[b]
Total	804	749 (93%)

[a] $p < 0.05$.

[b] $p < 0.005$.

Source: Adapted from Lurain JR, Hoekstra AV, Schink JC. Results of treatment of patients with gestational trophoblastic neoplasia referred to the Brewer Trophoblastic Disease Center after failure of treatment elsewhere (1979–2006). *J Reprod Med*. 2008;53(7):535–540, with permission.

CONCLUSIONS

The more widespread use of ultrasound to evaluate patients who present with vaginal bleeding has led to earlier diagnosis of hydatidiform mole. Although hCG is a disease-specific marker for complete molar pregnancy, levels vary widely in individual patients, and those who are diagnosed with earlier-stage disease may not show highly elevated hCG. The majority of patients with molar pregnancy are successfully treated with suction evacuation and curettage, and the risk of a second molar pregnancy or development of postmolar neoplasia is low (1).

Cure rates for both nonmetastatic and low-risk, metastatic GTN should approach 100% with the judicious use of second curettage or initial single-agent methotrexate or actinomycin D. Approximately 20% of low-risk patients will develop resistance to the initial chemotherapeutic agent, but 90% will be cured by the use of sequential single-agent treatment. Eventually, approximately 10% of patients will require multiagent CT, with or without surgery, to achieve remission. With aggressive, multimodality therapy—EMA-CO with adjuvant RT or surgery as indicated—cure rates for high-risk GTN have reached 80% to 90%. Though one-third of high-risk patients fail first-line therapy or experience a relapse from remission, salvage therapy with platinum-containing drug regimens, with or without surgery, will cure most patients with resistant GTN (147).

REFERENCES

1. Lurain JR. Gestational trophoblastic disease. I. Epidemiology, pathology, clinical presentation and diagnosis of gestational trophoblastic disease, and management of hydatidiform mole. *Am J Obstet Gynecol.* 2010;203:531–539.
2. Seckl MJ, Sebire NJ, Berkowitz RS. Gestational trophoblastic disease. *Lancet.* 2010;376:717–729.
3. Berkowitz RS, Goldstein DP. Current management of gestational trophoblastic diseases. *Gynecol Oncol.* 2009;112:654–662.
4. Strohl AE, Lurain JR. Clinical epidemiology of gestational trophoblastic disease. *Curr Obstet Gynecol Rep.* 2013;3(1):40–43. doi:10.1007/s13669-013-0070-7
5. Bracken MB. Incidence and aetiology of hydatidiform mole: an epidemiological review. *Br J Obstet Gynaecol.* 1987;94(12):1123–1135.
6. Atrash HK, Hogue CJ, Grimes DA. Epidemiology of hydatidiform mole during early gestation. *Am J Obstet Gynecol.* 1986;154(4):906–909.
7. Palmer JR. Advances in the epidemiology of gestational trophoblastic disease. *J Reprod Med.* 1994;39(3):155–162.
8. Fukunaga M, Ushigome S, Endo Y. Incidence of hydatidiform mole in a Tokyo hospital: a 5-year (1989 to 1993) prospective, morphological, and flow cytometric study. *Hum Pathol.* 1995;26(7):758–764.
9. Jeffers MD, O'Dwyer P, Curran B, et al. Partial hydatidiform mole: a common but underdiagnosed condition. A 3-year retrospective clinicopathological and DNA flow cytometric analysis. *Int J Gynecol Pathol.* 1993;12(4):315–323.
10. Bagshawe KD, Dent J, Webb J. Hydatidiform mole in England and Wales 1973–1983. *Lancet.* 1986;2(8508):673–677.
11. Takeuchi S. Incidence of gestational trophoblastic disease by regional registration in Japan. *Hum Reprod.* 1987;2(8):729–734.
12. Smith HO, Qualls CR, Prairie BA, et al. Trends in gestational choriocarcinoma: a 27-year perspective. *Obstet Gynecol.* 2003;102(5 Pt 1):978–987.
13. Berkowitz RS, Cramer DW, Bernstein MR, et al. Risk factors for complete molar pregnancy from a case-control study. *Am J Obstet Gynecol.* 1985;152(8):1016–1020.
14. Parazzini F, La Vecchia C, Mangili G, et al. Dietary factors and risk of trophoblastic disease. *Am J Obstet Gynecol.* 1988;158(1):93–99.
15. Fulop V, Mok SC, Berkowitz RS. Molecular biology of gestational trophoblastic neoplasia: a review. *J Reprod Med.* 2004;49(6):415–422.
16. Acaia B, Parazzini F, La Vecchia C, et al. Increased frequency of complete hydatidiform mole in women with repeated abortion. *Gynecol Oncol.* 1988;31(2):310–314.
17. Parazzini F, Mangili G, La Vecchia C, et al. Risk factors for gestational trophoblastic disease: a separate analysis of complete and partial hydatidiform moles. *Obstet Gynecol.* 1991;78(6):1039–1045.
18. Parazzini F, La Vecchia C, Pampallona S. Parental age and risk of complete and partial hydatidiform mole. *Br J Obstet Gynaecol.* 1986;93(6):582–585.
19. Sebire NJ, Foskett M, Fisher RA, et al. Risk of partial and complete hydatidiform molar pregnancy in relation to maternal age. *BJOG.* 2002;109(1):99–102.
20. Sand PK, Lurain JR, Brewer JI. Repeat gestational trophoblastic disease. *Obstet Gynecol.* 1984;63(2):140–144.
21. Berkowitz RS, Im SS, Bernstein MR, et al. Gestational trophoblastic disease: subsequent pregnancy outcome, including repeat molar pregnancy. *J Reprod Med.* 1998;43(1):81–86.
22. Garrett LA, Garner EI, Feltmate CM, et al. Subsequent pregnancy outcomes in patients with molar pregnancy and persistent gestational trophoblastic neoplasia. *J Reprod Med.* 2008;53(7):481–486.
23. Sebire NJ, Fisher RA, Foskett M, et al. Risk of recurrent hydatidiform mole and subsequent pregnancy outcome following complete or partial hydatidiform molar pregnancy. *BJOG.* 2003;110(1):22–26.
24. Tuncer ZS, Bernstein MR, Wang J, et al. Repetitive hydatidiform mole with different male partners. *Gynecol Oncol.* 1999;75(2):224–226.
25. Kou YC, Shao L, Peng HH, et al. A recurrent intragenic genomic duplication, other novel mutations in NLRP7 and imprinting defects in recurrent biparental hydatidiform moles. *Mol Hum Reprod.* 2008;14(1):33–40.
26. Wang CM, Dixon PH, Decordova S, et al. Identification of 13 novel NLRP7 mutations in 20 families with recurrent hydatidiform mole; missense mutations cluster in the leucine-rich region. *J Med Genet.* 2009;46(8):569–575.
27. Moglabey YB, Kircheisen R, Seoud M, et al. Genetic mapping of a maternal locus responsible for familial hydatidiform moles. *Hum Mol Genet.* 1999;8(4):667–671.
28. Messaed C, Chebaro W, Di Roberto RB, et al. NLRP7 in the spectrum of reproductive wastage: rare non-synonymous variants confer genetic susceptibility to recurrent reproductive wastage. *J Med Genet.* 2011;48(8):540–548.
29. Murdoch S, Djuric U, Mazhar B, et al. Mutations in NALP7 cause recurrent hydatidiform moles and reproductive wastage in humans. *Nat Genet.* 2006;38(3):300–302.
30. Fisher RA, Hodges MD, Newlands ES. Familial recurrent hydatidiform mole: a review. *J Reprod Med.* 2004;49(8):595–601.
31. Berkowitz RS, Bernstein MR, Harlow BL, et al. Case-control study of risk factors for partial molar pregnancy. *Am J Obstet Gynecol.* 1995;173(3 Pt 1):788–794.
32. Ngan S, Seckl MJ. Gestational trophoblastic neoplasia management: an update. *Curr Opin Oncol.* 2007;19(5):486–491.
33. Buckley JD, Henderson BE, Morrow CP, et al. Case-control study of gestational choriocarcinoma. *Cancer Res.* 1988;48(4):1004–1010.
34. Stone M, Dent J, Kardana A, et al. Relationship of oral contraception to development of trophoblastic tumour after evacuation of a hydatidiform mole. *Br J Obstet Gynaecol.* 1976;83(12):913–916.
35. Costa HL, Doyle P. Influence of oral contraceptives in the development of post-molar trophoblastic neoplasia—a systematic review. *Gynecol Oncol.* 2006;100(3):579–585.
36. Palmer JR, Driscoll SG, Rosenberg L, et al. Oral contraceptive use and risk of gestational trophoblastic tumors. *J Natl Cancer Inst.* 1999;91(7):635–640.
37. Osborne R, Dodge J. Gestational trophoblastic neoplasia. *Obstet Gynecol Clin North Am.* 2012;39(2):195–212.
38. Shih IM, Kurman RJ. The pathology of intermediate trophoblastic tumors and tumor-like lesions. *Int J Gynecol Pathol.* 2001;20(1):31–47.
39. Xu G, Guimond MJ, Chakraborty C, et al. Control of proliferation, migration, and invasiveness of human extravillous trophoblast by decorin, a decidual product. *Biol Reprod.* 2002;67(2):681–689.
40. Xu G, Chakraborty C, Lala PK. Expression of TGF-beta signaling genes in the normal, premalignant, and malignant human trophoblast: loss of smad3 in choriocarcinoma cells. *Biochem Biophys Res Commun.* 2001;287(1):47–55.
41. Berkowitz RS, Goldstein DP. Recent advances in gestational trophoblastic disease. *Curr Opin Obstet Gynecol.* 1998;10(1):61–64.
42. Bentley RC. Pathology of gestational trophoblastic disease. *Clin Obstet Gynecol.* 2003;46(3):513–522.
43. Shih I-M. Trophogram, an immunohistochemistry-based algorithmic approach, in the differential diagnosis of trophoblastic tumors and tumorlike lesions. *Ann Diagn Pathol.* 2007;11(3):228–234.
44. Kale A, Soylemez F, Ensari A. Expressions of proliferation markers (Ki-67, proliferating cell nuclear antigen, and silver-staining nucleolar organizer regions) and of p53 tumor protein in gestational trophoblastic disease. *Am J Obstet Gynecol.* 2001;184(4):567–574.
45. Shih IM, Kurman RJ. p63 expression is useful in the distinction of epithelioid trophoblastic and placental site trophoblastic tumors by profiling trophoblastic subpopulations. *Am J Surg Pathol.* 2004;28(9):1177–1183.
46. Singer G, Kurman RJ, McMaster MT, et al. HLA-G immunoreactivity is specific for intermediate trophoblast in gestational trophoblastic disease and can serve as a useful marker in differential diagnosis. *Am J Surg Pathol.* 2002;26(7):914–920.
47. Fulop V, Mok SC, Genest DR, et al. p53, p21, Rb and mdm2 oncoproteins: expression in normal placenta, partial and complete mole, and choriocarcinoma. *J Reprod Med.* 1998;43(2):119–127.
48. Fulop V, Mok SC, Genest DR, et al. c-myc, c-erbB-2, c-fms and bcl-2 oncoproteins: expression in normal placenta, partial and complete mole, and choriocarcinoma. *J Reprod Med.* 1998;43(2):101–110.
49. Hussein MR. Analysis of p53, BCL-2 and epidermal growth factor receptor protein expression in the partial and complete hydatidiform moles. *Exp Mol Pathol.* 2009;87(1):63–69.
50. Petignat P, Laurini R, Goffin F, et al. Expression of matrix metalloproteinase-2 and mutant p53 is increased in hydatidiform mole as compared with normal placenta. *Int J Gynecol Cancer.* 2006;16(4):1679–1684.
51. Szulman AE, Surti U. The syndromes of hydatidiform mole. I. Cytogenetic and morphologic correlations. *Am J Obstet Gynecol.* 1978;131(6):665–671.
52. Szulman AE, Surti U. The syndromes of hydatidiform mole. II. Morphologic evolution of the complete and partial mole. *Am J Obstet Gynecol.* 1978;132(1):20–27.
53. Kajii T, Ohama K. Androgenetic origin of hydatidiform mole. *Nature.* 1977;268(5621):633–634.
54. Fisher RA, Newlands ES. Gestational trophoblastic disease. Molecular and genetic studies. *J Reprod Med.* 1998;43(1):87–97.

55. Azuma C, Saji F, Tokugawa Y, et al. Application of gene amplification by polymerase chain reaction to genetic analysis of molar mitochondrial DNA: the detection of anuclear empty ovum as the cause of complete mole. *Gynecol Oncol.* 1991;40(1):29–33.
56. Lawler SD, Fisher RA, Dent J. A prospective genetic study of complete and partial hydatidiform moles. *Am J Obstet Gynecol.* 1991;164(5 Pt 1):1270–1277.
57. Lage JM. Gestational trophoblastic diseases. In: Robboy SJ, Anderson MC, Russell P, eds. *Pathology of the Female Reproductive Tract.* Edinburgh, UK: Churchill Livingstone; 2001:759–781.
58. Lage JM, Mark SD, Roberts DJ, et al. A flow cytometric study of 137 fresh hydropic placentas: correlation between types of hydatidiform moles and nuclear DNA ploidy. *Obstet Gynecol.* 1992;79(3):403–410.
59. Gaber LW, Redline RW, Mostoufi-Zadeh M, et al. Invasive partial mole. *Am J Clin Pathol.* 1986;85(6):722–724.
60. Shih IM, Kurman RJ. Immunohistochemical localization of inhibin-alpha in the placenta and gestational trophoblastic lesions. *Int J Gynecol Pathol.* 1999;18(2):144–150.
61. Shih IM, Kurman RJ. Ki-67 labeling index in the differential diagnosis of exaggerated placental site, placental site trophoblastic tumor, and choriocarcinoma: a double immunohistochemical staining technique using Ki-67 and Mel-CAM antibodies. *Hum Pathol.* 1998;29(1):27–33.
62. Oldt RJ 3rd, Kurman RJ, Shih IeM. Molecular genetic analysis of placental site trophoblastic tumors and epithelioid trophoblastic tumors confirms their trophoblastic origin. *Am J Pathol.* 2002;161(3):1033–1037.
63. Rhoton-Vlasak A, Wagner JM, Rutgers JL, et al. Placental site trophoblastic tumor: human placental lactogen and pregnancy-associated major basic protein as immunohistologic markers. *Hum Pathol.* 1998;29(3):280–288.
64. Shih IM, Kurman RJ. Epithelioid trophoblastic tumor: a neoplasm distinct from choriocarcinoma and placental site trophoblastic tumor simulating carcinoma. *Am J Surg Pathol.* 1998;22(11):1393–1403.
65. Mao TL, Seidman JD, Kurman RJ, et al. Cyclin E and p16 immunoreactivity in epithelioid trophoblastic tumor—an aid in differential diagnosis. *Am J Surg Pathol.* 2006;30(9):1105–1110.
66. Bamberger AM, Aupers S, Milde-Langosch K, et al. Expression pattern of the cell cycle promoter cyclin e in benign extravillous trophoblast and gestational trophoblastic lesions: correlation with expression of Ki-67. *Int J Gynecol Pathol.* 2003;22(2):156–161.
67. Curry SL, Hammond CB, Tyrey L, et al. Hydatidiform mole: diagnosis, management, and long-term followup of 347 patients. *Obstet Gynecol.* 1975;45(1):1–8.
68. Kohorn EI. Molar pregnancy: presentation and diagnosis. *Clin Obstet Gynecol.* 1984;27(1):181–191.
69. Soto-Wright V, Bernstein M, Goldstein DP, et al. The changing clinical presentation of complete molar pregnancy. *Obstet Gynecol.* 1995;86(5):775–779.
70. Hou JL, Wan XR, Xiang Y, et al. Changes of clinical features in hydatidiform mole: analysis of 113 cases. *J Reprod Med.* 2008;53(8):629–633.
71. Szulman AE, Surti U. The clinicopathologic profile of the partial hydatidiform mole. *Obstet Gynecol.* 1982;59(5):597–602.
72. Czernobilsky B, Barash A, Lancet M. Partial moles: a clinicopathologic study of 25 cases. *Obstet Gynecol.* 1982;59(1):75–77.
73. Berkowitz RS, Goldstein DP, Bernstein MR. Natural history of partial molar pregnancy. *Obstet Gynecol.* 1985;66(5):677–681.
74. Santos-Ramos R, Forney JP, Schwarz BE. Sonographic findings and clinical correlations in molar pregnancy. *Obstet Gynecol.* 1980;56(2):186–192.
75. Benson CB, Genest DR, Bernstein MR, et al. Sonographic appearance of first trimester complete hydatidiform moles. *Ultrasound Obstet Gynecol.* 2000;16(2):188–191.
76. Fine C, Bundy AL, Berkowitz RS, et al. Sonographic diagnosis of partial hydatidiform mole. *Obstet Gynecol.* 1989;73(3 Pt 1):414–418.
77. Cole LA. Human chorionic gonadotropin and associated molecules. *Expert Rev Mol Diagn.* 2009;9(1):51–73.
78. Ozturk M, Berkowitz R, Goldstein D, et al. Differential production of human chorionic gonadotropin and free subunits in gestational trophoblastic disease. *Am J Obstet Gynecol.* 1988;158(1):193–198.
79. Cole LA, Khanlian SA. Hyperglycosylated hCG: a variant with separate biological functions to regular hCG. *Mol Cell Endocrinol.* 2007;260–262:228–236.
80. Cole LA, Shahabi S, Butler SA, et al. Utility of commonly used commercial human chorionic gonadotropin immunoassays in the diagnosis and management of trophoblastic diseases. *Clin Chem.* 2001;47(2):308–315.
81. Cole LA. hCG, its free subunits and its metabolites. Roles in pregnancy and trophoblastic disease. *J Reprod Med.* 1998;43(1):3–10.
82. Berkowitz R, Ozturk M, Goldstein D, et al. Human chorionic gonadotropin and free subunits' serum levels in patients with partial and complete hydatidiform moles. *Obstet Gynecol.* 1989;74(2):212–216.
83. Menczer J, Modan M, Serr DM. Prospective follow-up of patients with hydatidiform mole. *Obstet Gynecol.* 1980;55(3):346–349.
84. Fowler DJ, Lindsay I, Seckl MJ, et al. Histomorphometric features of hydatidiform moles in early pregnancy: relationship to detectability by ultrasound examination. *Ultrasound Obstet Gynecol.* 2007;29(1):76–80.
85. Sebire NJ, Rees H, Paradinas F, et al. The diagnostic implications of routine ultrasound examination in histologically confirmed early molar pregnancies. *Ultrasound Obstet Gynecol.* 2001;18(6):662–665.
86. Sarmadi S, Izadi-Mood N, Abbasi A, et al. p57KIP2 immunohistochemical expression: a useful diagnostic tool in discrimination between complete hydatidiform mole and its mimics. *Arch Gynecol Obstet.* 2011;283(4):743–748.
87. Castrillon DH, Sun D, Weremowicz S, et al. Discrimination of complete hydatidiform mole from its mimics by immunohistochemistry of the paternally imprinted gene product p57KIP2. *Am J Surg Pathol.* 2001;25(10):1225–1230.
88. Fisher RA, Hodges MD, Rees HC, et al. The maternally transcribed gene p57(KIP2) (CDNK1C) is abnormally expressed in both androgenetic and biparental complete hydatidiform moles. *Hum Mol Genet.* 2002;11(26):3267–3272.
89. Thaker HM, Berlin A, Tycko B, et al. Immunohistochemistry for the imprinted gene product IPL/PHLDA2 for facilitating the differential diagnosis of complete hydatidiform mole. *J Reprod Med.* 2004;49(8):630–636.
90. McConnell TG, Murphy KM, Hafez M, et al. Diagnosis and subclassification of hydatidiform moles using p57 immunohistochemistry and molecular genotyping: validation and prospective analysis in routine and consultation practice settings with development of an algorithmic approach. *Am J Surg Pathol.* 2009;33(6):805–817.
91. Chiang S, Fazlollahi L, Nguyen A, et al. Diagnosis of hydatidiform moles by polymorphic deletion probe fluorescence in situ hybridization. *J Mol Diagn.* 2011;13(4):406–415.
92. Genest DR, Dorfman DM, Castrillon DH. Ploidy and imprinting in hydatidiform moles. Complementary use of flow cytometry and immunohistochemistry of the imprinted gene product p57KIP2 to assist molar classification. *J Reprod Med.* 2002;47(5):342–346.
93. Palmieri C, Dhillon T, Fisher RA, et al. Management and outcome of healthy women with a persistently elevated beta-hCG. *Gynecol Oncol.* 2007;106(1):35–43.
94. Rotmensch S, Cole LA. False diagnosis and needless therapy of presumed malignant disease in women with false-positive human chorionic gonadotropin concentrations. *Lancet.* 2000;355(9205):712–715.
95. Hancock BW. hCG measurement in gestational trophoblastic neoplasia: a critical appraisal. *J Reprod Med.* 2006;51(11):859–860.
96. Papapetrou PD, Anagnostopoulos NI. A gonadotropin and alpha-subunit suppression test for the assessment of the ectopic production of human chorionic gonadotropin and its subunits after the menopause. *J Clin Endocrinol Metab.* 1985;60(6):1187–1195.
97. Grenache DG, Dighe AS, Fantz CR, et al. Falsely decreased human chorionic gonadotropin (hCG) results due to increased concentrations of the free β subunit and the β core fragments in quantitative hCG assays. *Clin Chem.* 2010;56:1839–1844.
98. Soper JT. Surgical therapy for gestational trophoblastic disease. *J Reprod Med.* 1994;39(3):168–174.
99. Tidy JA, Gillespie AM, Bright N, et al. Gestational trophoblastic disease: a study of mode of evacuation and subsequent need for treatment with chemotherapy. *Gynecol Oncol.* 2000;78(3 Pt 1):309–312.
100. Berkowitz RS, Goldstein DP. Clinical practice. Molar pregnancy. *N Engl J Med.* 2009;360(16):1639–1645.
101. Hancock BW, Tidy JA. Current management of molar pregnancy. *J Reprod Med.* 2002;47(5):347–354.
102. Kashimura Y, Kashimura M, Sugimori H, et al. Prophylactic chemotherapy for hydatidiform mole. Five to 15 years follow-up. *Cancer.* 1986;58(3):624–629.
103. Kim DS, Moon H, Kim KT, et al. Effects of prophylactic chemotherapy for persistent trophoblastic disease in patients with complete hydatidiform mole. *Obstet Gynecol.* 1986;67(5):690–694.
104. Limpongsanurak S. Prophylactic actinomycin D for high-risk complete hydatidiform mole. *J Reprod Med.* 2001;46(2):110–116.
105. Steller MA, Genest DR, Bernstein MR, et al. Clinical features of multiple conception with partial or complete molar pregnancy and coexisting fetuses. *J Reprod Med.* 1994;39(3):147–154.

106. Fishman DA, Padilla LA, Keh P, et al. Management of twin pregnancies consisting of a complete hydatidiform mole and normal fetus. *Obstet Gynecol.* 1998;91(4):546–550.
107. Sebire NJ, Foskett M, Paradinas FJ, et al. Outcome of twin pregnancies with complete hydatidiform mole and healthy co-twin. *Lancet.* 2002;359(9324):2165–2166.
108. Berkowitz RS, Goldstein DP, Marean AR, et al. Oral contraceptives and postmolar trophoblastic disease. *Obstet Gynecol.* 1981;58(4): 474–477.
109. Curry SL, Schlaerth JB, Kohorn EI, et al. Hormonal contraception and trophoblastic sequelae after hydatidiform mole (a Gynecologic Oncology Group Study). *Am J Obstet Gynecol.* 1989;160(4):805–809; discussion 809–811.
110. Deicas RE, Miller DS, Rademaker AW, et al. The role of contraception in the development of postmolar gestational trophoblastic tumor. *Obstet Gynecol.* 1991;78(2):221–226.
111. Rice LW, Lage JM, Berkowitz RS, et al. Repetitive complete and partial hydatidiform mole. *Obstet Gynecol.* 1989;74(2):217–219.
112. Lurain JR, Brewer JI, Torok EE, et al. Natural history of hydatidiform mole after primary evacuation. *Am J Obstet Gynecol.* 1983;145(5):591–595.
113. Feltmate CM, Batorfi J, Fulop V, et al. Human chorionic gonadotropin follow-up in patients with molar pregnancy: a time for reevaluation. *Obstet Gynecol.* 2003;101(4):732–736.
114. Hancock BW, Nazir K, Everard JE. Persistent gestational trophoblastic neoplasia after partial hydatidiform mole incidence and outcome. *J Reprod Med.* 2006;51(10):764–766.
115. Feltmate CM, Growdon WB, Wolfberg AJ, et al. Clinical characteristics of persistent gestational trophoblastic neoplasia after partial hydatidiform molar pregnancy. *J Reprod Med.* 2006;51(11):902–906.
116. Berkowitz RS, Goldstein DP, Bernstein MR. Evolving concepts of molar pregnancy. *J Reprod Med.* 1991;36(1):40–44.
117. Mosher R, Goldstein DP, Berkowitz R, et al. Complete hydatidiform mole: comparison of clinicopathologic features, current and past. *J Reprod Med.* 1998;43(1):21–27.
118. Lurain JR. Gestational trophoblastic tumors. *Semin Surg Oncol.* 1990;6(6):347–353.
119. Paradinas FJ, Browne P, Fisher RA, et al. A clinical, histopathological and flow cytometric study of 149 complete moles, 146 partial moles and 107 non-molar hydropic abortions. *Histopathology.* 1996;28(2):101–110.
120. Sebire NJ, Fisher RA, Rees HC. Histopathological diagnosis of partial and complete hydatidiform mole in the first trimester of pregnancy. *Pediatr Dev Pathol.* 2003;6(1):69–77.
121. Heifetz SA, Czaja J. In situ choriocarcinoma arising in partial hydatidiform mole: implications for the risk of persistent trophoblastic disease. *Pediatr Pathol.* 1992;12(4):601–611.
122. Menczer J, Girtler O, Zajdel L, et al. Metastatic trophoblastic disease following partial hydatidiform mole: case report and literature review. *Gynecol Oncol.* 1999;74(2):304–307.
123. Gardner HA, Lage JM. Choriocarcinoma following a partial hydatidiform mole: a case report. *Hum Pathol.* 1992;23(4):468–471.
124. Allison KH, Love JE, Garcia RL. Epithelioid trophoblastic tumor: review of a rare neoplasm of the chorionic-type intermediate trophoblast. *Arch Pathol Lab Med.* 2006;130(12):1875–1877.
125. Baergen RN, Rutgers JL, Young RH, et al. Placental site trophoblastic tumor: a study of 55 cases and review of the literature emphasizing factors of prognostic significance. *Gynecol Oncol.* 2006;100(3):511–520.
126. Cheung AN, Zhang DK, Liu Y, et al. Telomerase activity in gestational trophoblastic disease. *J Clin Pathol.* 1999;52(8):588–592.
127. Wong SY, Ngan HY, Chan CC, et al. Apoptosis in gestational trophoblastic disease is correlated with clinical outcome and Bcl-2 expression but not Bax expression. *Mod Pathol.* 1999;12(11):1025–1033.
128. Chiu PM, Ngan YS, Khoo US, et al. Apoptotic activity in gestational trophoblastic disease correlates with clinical outcome: assessment by the caspase-related M30 CytoDeath antibody. *Histopathology.* 2001;38(3):243–249.
129. Fong PY, Xue WC, Ngan HY, et al. Mcl-1 expression in gestational trophoblastic disease correlates with clinical outcome: a differential expression study. *Cancer.* 2005;103(2):268–276.
130. Feng HC, Tsao SW, Ngan HY, et al. Differential expression of insulin-like growth factor binding protein 1 and ferritin light polypeptide in gestational trophoblastic neoplasia: combined cDNA suppression subtractive hybridization and microarray study. *Cancer.* 2005;104(11):2409–2416.
131. van Trommel NE, Massuger LF, Verheijen RH, et al. The curative effect of a second curettage in persistent trophoblastic disease: a retrospective cohort survey. *Gynecol Oncol.* 2005;99(1):6–13.
132. Schlaerth JB, Morrow CP, Rodriguez M. Diagnostic and therapeutic curettage in gestational trophoblastic disease. *Am J Obstet Gynecol.* 1990;162(6):1465–1470; discussion 1470–1471.
133. Pezeshki M, Hancock BW, Silcocks P, et al. The role of repeat uterine evacuation in the management of persistent gestational trophoblastic disease. *Gynecol Oncol.* 2004;95(3):423–429.
134. Garner EI, Feltmate CM, Goldstein DP, et al. The curative effect of a second curettage in persistent trophoblastic disease: a retrospective cohort survey. *Gynecol Oncol.* 2005;99(1):3–5.
135. Osborne RJ, Filiaci VL, Schink JC, et al. Second curettage for low-risk nonmetastatic gestation trophoblastic neoplasia. *Obstet Gynecol.* 2016;128:1–9.
136. Cole LA, Butler SA, Khanlian SA, et al. Gestational trophoblastic diseases: 2. Hyperglycosylated hCG as a reliable marker of active neoplasia. *Gynecol Oncol.* 2006;102(2):151–159.
137. Khanlian SA, Cole LA. Management of gestational trophoblastic disease and other cases with low serum levels of human chorionic gonadotropin. *J Reprod Med.* 2006;51(10):812–818.
138. Cole LA, Khanlian SA. Inappropriate management of women with persistent low hCG results. *J Reprod Med.* 2004;49(6):423–432.
139. Neubauer NL, Latif N, Kalakota K, et al. Brain metastasis in gestational trophoblastic neoplasia: an update. *J Reprod Med.* 2012;57(7–8):288–292.
140. Barber EL, Schink JC, Lurain JR. Hepatic metastasis in gestational trophoblastic neoplasia: patient characteristics, prognostic factors, and outcomes. *J Reprod Med.* 2014;59(5–6):199–203.
141. FIGO Oncology Committee. FIGO staging for gestational trophoblastic neoplasia 2000. FIGO Oncology Committee. *Int J Gynaecol Obstet.* 2002;77(3):285–287.
142. Berry E, Hagopian GS, Lurain JR. Vaginal metastases in gestational trophoblastic neoplasia. *J Reprod Med.* 2008;53(7):487–492.
143. Lurain JR, Casanova LA, Miller DS, et al. Prognostic factors in gestational trophoblastic tumors: a proposed new scoring system based on multivariate analysis. *Am J Obstet Gynecol.* 1991;164(2):611–616.
144. Athanassiou A, Begent RH, Newlands ES, et al. Central nervous system metastases of choriocarcinoma: 23 years' experience at Charing Cross Hospital. *Cancer.* 1983;52(9):1728–1735.
145. Ngan HY, Bender H, Benedet JL, et al. Gestational trophoblastic neoplasia, FIGO 2000 staging and classification. *Int J Gynaecol Obstet.* 2003;83(Suppl 1):175–177.
146. McGrath S, Short D, Harvey R, et al. The management and outcome of women with post-hydatidiform mole 'low-risk' gestational trophoblastic neoplasia, but hCG levels in excess of 100 000 IUl(−1). *Br J Cancer.* 2010;102(5):810–814.
147. Lurain JR. Gestational trophoblastic disease. II. Classification and management of gestational trophoblastic neoplasia. *Am J Obstet Gynecol.* 2011;204:11–18.
148. Lurain JR. Pharmacotherapy of gestational trophoblastic disease. *Expert Opin Pharmacother.* 2003;4(11):2005–2017.
149. Alazzam M, Tidy J, Hancock BW, et al. First line chemotherapy in low risk gestational trophoblastic neoplasia. *Cochrane Database Syst Rev.* 2009;(1):CD007102.
150. Lybol C, Sweep FC, Harvey R, et al. Relapse rates after two versus three consolidation courses of methotrexate in the treatment of low-risk gestational trophoblastic neoplasia. *Gynecol Oncol.* 2012;125(3):576–579.
151. Lurain JR, Elfstrand EP. Single-agent methotrexate chemotherapy for the treatment of nonmetastatic gestational trophoblastic tumors. *Am J Obstet Gynecol.* 1995;172(2 Pt 1):574–579.
152. Hammond CB, Borchert LG, Tyrey L, et al. Treatment of metastatic trophoblastic disease: good and poor prognosis. *Am J Obstet Gynecol.* 1973;115(4):451–457.
153. Hammond CB, Hertz R, Ross GT, et al. Primary chemotherapy for nonmetastatic gestational trophoblastic neoplasms. *Am J Obstet Gynecol.* 1967;98(1):71–78.
154. Bagshawe KD, Dent J, Newlands ES, et al. The role of low-dose methotrexate and folinic acid in gestational trophoblastic tumours (GTT). *Br J Obstet Gynaecol.* 1989;96(7):795–802.
155. Garrett AP, Garner EO, Goldstein DP, et al. Methotrexate infusion and folinic acid as primary therapy for nonmetastatic and low-risk metastatic gestational trophoblastic tumors: 15 years of experience. *J Reprod Med.* 2002;47(5):355–362.
156. Berkowitz RS, Goldstein DP, Bernstein MR. Ten year's experience with methotrexate and folinic acid as primary therapy for gestational trophoblastic disease. *Gynecol Oncol.* 1986;23(1):111–118.
157. Wong LC, Choo YC, Ma HK. Methotrexate with citrovorum factor rescue in gestational trophoblastic disease. *Am J Obstet Gynecol.* 1985;152(1):59–62.
158. McNeish IA, Strickland S, Holden L, et al. Low-risk persistent gestational trophoblastic disease: outcome after initial treatment with low-dose methotrexate and folinic acid from 1992 to 2000. *J Clin Oncol.* 2002;20(7):1838–1844.

159. Khan F, Everard J, Ahmed S, et al. Low-risk persistent gestational trophoblastic disease treated with low-dose methotrexate: efficacy, acute and long-term effects. *Br J Cancer*. 2003;89(12):2197–2201.
160. Growdon WB, Wolfberg AJ, Goldstein DP, et al. Evaluating methotrexate treatment in patients with low-risk postmolar gestational trophoblastic neoplasia. *Gynecol Oncol*. 2009;112(2):353–357.
161. Wong LC, Ngan HY, Cheng DK, et al. Methotrexate infusion in low-risk gestational trophoblastic disease. *Am J Obstet Gynecol*. 2000;183(6):1579–1582.
162. Berkowitz RS, Goldstein DP, Bernstein MR. Methotrexate infusion and folinic acid in the primary therapy of nonmetastatic gestational trophoblastic tumors. *Gynecol Oncol*. 1990;36(1):56–59.
163. Elit L, Covens A, Osborne R, et al. High-dose methotrexate for gestational trophoblastic disease. *Gynecol Oncol*. 1994;54(3):282–287.
164. Hoffman MS, Fiorica JV, Gleeson NC, et al. A single institution experience with weekly intramuscular methotrexate for nonmetastatic gestational trophoblastic disease. *Gynecol Oncol*. 1996;60(2):292–294.
165. Homesley HD, Blessing JA, Rettenmaier M, et al. Weekly intramuscular methotrexate for nonmetastatic gestational trophoblastic disease. *Obstet Gynecol*. 1988;72(3 Pt 1):413–418.
166. Homesley HD, Blessing JA, Schlaerth J, et al. Rapid escalation of weekly intramuscular methotrexate for nonmetastatic gestational trophoblastic disease: a Gynecologic Oncology Group study. *Gynecol Oncol*. 1990;39(3):305–308.
167. Smith EB, Weed JC Jr, Tyrey L, et al. Treatment of nonmetastatic gestational trophoblastic disease: results of methotrexate alone versus methotrexate—folinic acid. *Am J Obstet Gynecol*. 1982;144(1):88–92.
168. Gleeson NC, Finan MA, Fiorica JV, et al. Nonmetastatic gestational trophoblastic disease: weekly methotrexate compared with 8-day methotrexate-folinic acid. *Eur J Gynaecol Oncol*. 1993;14(6):461–465.
169. Osathanondh R, Goldstein DP, Pastorfide GB. Actinomycin D as the primary agent for gestational trophoblastic disease. *Cancer*. 1975;36(3):863–866.
170. Petrilli ES, Morrow CP. Actinomycin D toxicity in the treatment of trophoblastic disease: a comparison of the five-day course to single-dose administration. *Gynecol Oncol*. 1980;9(1):18–22.
171. Twiggs LB. Pulse actinomycin D scheduling in nonmetastatic gestational trophoblastic neoplasia: cost-effective chemotherapy. *Gynecol Oncol*. 1983;16(2):190–195.
172. Schlaerth JB, Morrow CP, Nalick RH, et al. Single-dose actinomycin D in the treatment of postmolar trophoblastic disease. *Gynecol Oncol*. 1984;19(1):53–56.
173. Petrilli ES, Twiggs LB, Blessing JA, et al. Single-dose actinomycin-D treatment for nonmetastatic gestational trophoblastic disease: a prospective phase II trial of the Gynecologic Oncology Group. *Cancer*. 1987;60(9):2173–2176.
174. Kohorn EI. Decision making for chemotherapy administration in patients with low-risk gestational trophoblastic neoplasia. *Int J Gynecol Cancer*. 1996;6:279–285.
175. Kohorn EI. Is lack of response to single-agent chemotherapy in gestational trophoblastic disease associated with dose scheduling or chemotherapy resistance? *Gynecol Oncol*. 2002;85(1):36–39.
176. Gilani MM, Yarandi F, Eftekhar Z, et al. Comparison of pulse methotrexate and pulse dactinomycin in the treatment of low-risk gestational trophoblastic neoplasia. *Aust N Z J Obstet Gynaecol*. 2005;45(2):161–164.
177. Yarandi F, Eftekhar Z, Shojaei H, et al. Pulse methotrexate versus pulse actinomycin D in the treatment of low-risk gestational trophoblastic neoplasia. *Int J Gynaecol Obstet*. 2008;103(1):33–37.
178. Osborne RJ, Filiaci V, Schink JC, et al. Phase III trial of weekly methotrexate or pulsed actinomycin for low-risk gestational trophoblastic neoplasia: a Gynecologic Oncology Group study. *J Clin Oncol*. 2011;29(7):825–831.
179. Lertkhachonsuk AA, Israngura N, Wilailak S, et al. Actinomycin d versus methotrexate-folinic acid as the treatment of stage I, low-risk gestational trophoblastic neoplasia: a randomized controlled trial. *Int J Gynecol Cancer*. 2009;19(5):985–988.
180. Abrao RA, de Andrade JM, Tiezzi DG, et al. Treatment for low-risk gestational trophoblastic disease: comparison of single-agent methotrexate, dactinomycin and combination regimens. *Gynecol Oncol*. 2008;108(1):149–153.
181. DuBeshter B, Berkowitz RS, Goldstein DP, et al. Management of low-risk metastatic gestational trophoblastic tumors. *J Reprod Med*. 1991;36(1):36–39.
182. Soper JT, Clarke-Pearson DL, Berchuck A, et al. 5-day methotrexate for women with metastatic gestational trophoblastic disease. *Gynecol Oncol*. 1994;54(1):76–79.
183. Roberts JP, Lurain JR. Treatment of low-risk metastatic gestational trophoblastic tumors with single-agent chemotherapy. *Am J Obstet Gynecol*. 1996;174(6):1917–1923; discussion 1923–1914.
184. Chapman-Davis E, Hoekstra AV, Rademaker AW, et al. Treatment of nonmetastatic and metastatic low-risk gestational trophoblastic neoplasia: factors associated with resistance to single-agent methotrexate chemotherapy. *Gynecol Oncol*. 2012;125(3):572–575.
185. Shigematsu T, Hirakawa T, Yahata H, et al. Identification of chemotherapeutic refractory cases based on human chorionic gonadotropin values among patients with low-risk persistent trophoblastic disease treated with 8-day methotrexate-folinic acid. *Eur J Gynaecol Oncol*. 2003;24(2):113–116.
186. Rotmensch J, Rosenshein NB, Block BS. Comparison of human chorionic gonadotropin regression in molar pregnancies and post-molar nonmetastatic gestational trophoblastic neoplasia. *Gynecol Oncol*. 1988;29(1):82–86.
187. van Trommel NE, Massuger LF, Schijf CP, et al. Early identification of resistance to first-line single-agent methotrexate in patients with persistent trophoblastic disease. *J Clin Oncol*. 2006;24(1):52–58.
188. Kerkmeijer LG, Thomas CM, Harvey R, et al. External validation of serum hCG cutoff levels for prediction of resistance to single-agent chemotherapy in patients with persistent trophoblastic disease. *Br J Cancer*. 2009;100(6):979–984.
189. Clark RM, Nevadunsky NS, Ghosh S, et al. The evolving role of hysterectomy in gestational trophoblastic neoplasia at the New England Trophoblastic Disease Center. *J Reprod Med*. 2010;55(5–6):194–198.
190. Brewer JI, Torok EE, Webster A, et al. Hydatidiform mole: a follow-up regimen for identification of invasive mole and choriocarcinoma and for selection of patients for treatment. *Am J Obstet Gynecol*. 1968;101(4):557–563.
191. Lurain JR, Brewer JI. Treatment of high-risk gestational trophoblastic disease with methotrexate, actinomycin D, and cyclophosphamide chemotherapy. *Obstet Gynecol*. 1985;65(6):830–836.
192. Begent RH, Bagshawe KD. The management of high-risk choriocarcinoma. *Semin Oncol*. 1982;9(2):198–203.
193. Curry SL, Blessing JA, DiSaia PJ, et al. A prospective randomized comparison of methotrexate, dactinomycin, and chlorambucil versus methotrexate, dactinomycin, cyclophosphamide, doxorubicin, melphalan, hydroxyurea, and vincristine in "poor prognosis" metastatic gestational trophoblastic disease: a Gynecologic Oncology Group study. *Obstet Gynecol*. 1989;73(3 Pt 1):357–362.
194. Newlands ES, Bagshawe KD, Begent RH, et al. Results with the EMA/CO (etoposide, methotrexate, actinomycin D, cyclophosphamide, vincristine) regimen in high risk gestational trophoblastic tumours, 1979 to 1989. *Br J Obstet Gynaecol*. 1991;98(6):550–557.
195. Schink JC, Singh DK, Rademaker AW, et al. Etoposide, methotrexate, actinomycin D, cyclophosphamide, and vincristine for the treatment of metastatic, high-risk gestational trophoblastic disease. *Obstet Gynecol*. 1992;80(5):817–820.
196. Bolis G, Bonazzi C, Landoni F, et al. EMA/CO regimen in high-risk gestational trophoblastic tumor (GTT). *Gynecol Oncol*. 1988;31(3):439–444.
197. Bower M, Newlands ES, Holden L, et al. EMA/CO for high-risk gestational trophoblastic tumors: results from a cohort of 272 patients. *J Clin Oncol*. 1997;15(7):2636–2643.
198. Kim SJ, Bae SN, Kim JH, et al. Risk factors for the prediction of treatment failure in gestational trophoblastic tumors treated with EMA/CO regimen. *Gynecol Oncol*. 1998;71(2):247–253.
199. Matsui H, Suzuka K, Iitsuka Y, et al. Combination chemotherapy with methotrexate, etoposide, and actinomycin D for high-risk gestational trophoblastic tumors. *Gynecol Oncol*. 2000;78(1):28–31.
200. Escobar PF, Lurain JR, Singh DK, et al. Treatment of high-risk gestational trophoblastic neoplasia with etoposide, methotrexate, actinomycin D, cyclophosphamide, and vincristine chemotherapy. *Gynecol Oncol*. 2003;91(3):552–557.
201. Lurain JR, Singh DK, Schink JC. Primary treatment of metastatic high-risk gestational trophoblastic neoplasia with EMA-CO chemotherapy. *J Reprod Med*. 2006;51(10):767–772.
202. Turan T, Karacay O, Tulunay G, et al. Results with EMA/CO (etoposide, methotrexate, actinomycin D, cyclophosphamide, vincristine) chemotherapy in gestational trophoblastic neoplasia. *Int J Gynecol Cancer*. 2006;16(3):1432–1438.
203. Lu WG, Ye F, Shen YM, et al. EMA-CO chemotherapy for high-risk gestational trophoblastic neoplasia: a clinical analysis of 54 patients. *Int J Gynecol Cancer*. 2008;18(2):357–362.
204. Lurain JR, Singh DK, Schink JC. Management of metastatic high-risk gestational trophoblastic neoplasia: FIGO stages II–IV: risk factor score > or = 7. *J Reprod Med*. 2010;55(5–6):199–207.
205. Alifrangis C, Agarwal R, Short D, et al. EMA/CO for high-risk gestational trophoblastic neoplasia: good outcomes with induction low-dose etoposide-cisplatin and genetic analysis. *J Clin Oncol*. 2013;31(2):280–286.

206. Evans AC Jr, Soper JT, Clarke-Pearson DL, et al. Gestational trophoblastic disease metastatic to the central nervous system. *Gynecol Oncol.* 1995;59(2):226–230.
207. Small W Jr, Lurain JR, Shetty RM, et al. Gestational trophoblastic disease metastatic to the brain. *Radiology.* 1996;200(1):277–280.
208. Bakri Y, Berkowitz RS, Goldstein DP, et al. Brain metastases of gestational trophoblastic tumor. *J Reprod Med.* 1994;39(3):179–184.
209. Rustin GJ, Newlands ES, Begent RH, et al. Weekly alternating etoposide, methotrexate, and actinomycin/vincristine and cyclophosphamide chemotherapy for the treatment of CNS metastases of choriocarcinoma. *J Clin Oncol.* 1989;7(7):900–903.
210. Newlands ES, Holden L, Seckl MJ, et al. Management of brain metastases in patients with high-risk gestational trophoblastic tumors. *J Reprod Med.* 2002;47(6):465–471.
211. Mutch DG, Soper JT, Babcock CJ, et al. Recurrent gestational trophoblastic disease: experience of the Southeastern Regional Trophoblastic Disease Center. *Cancer.* 1990;66(5): 978–982.
212. Newlands ES, Bower M, Holden L, et al. Management of resistant gestational trophoblastic tumors. *J Reprod Med.* 1998;43(2):111–118.
213. Lurain JR, Singh DK, Schink JC. Role of surgery in the management of high-risk gestational trophoblastic neoplasia. *J Reprod Med.* 2006;51(10):773–776.
214. Alazzam M, Hancock BW, Tidy J. Role of hysterectomy in managing persistent gestational trophoblastic disease. *J Reprod Med.* 2008;53(7):519–524.
215. Pisal N, North C, Tidy J, et al. Role of hysterectomy in management of gestational trophoblastic disease. *Gynecol Oncol.* 2002;87(2):190–192.
216. Tomoda Y, Arii Y, Kaseki S, et al. Surgical indications for resection in pulmonary metastasis of choriocarcinoma. *Cancer.* 1980;46(12):2723–2730.
217. Xu LT, Sun CF, Wang YE, et al. Resection of pulmonary metastatic choriocarcinoma in 43 drug-resistant patients. *Ann Thorac Surg.* 1985;39(3):257–259.
218. Fleming EL, Garrett L, Growdon WB, et al. The changing role of thoracotomy in gestational trophoblastic neoplasia at the New England Trophoblastic Disease Center. *J Reprod Med.* 2008;53(7):493–498.
219. Kanis MJ, Lurain JR. Pulmonary resection in the management of high-risk gestational trophoblastic neoplasia. *Int J Gynecol Cancer.* 2016;26(4):796–800.
220. Dhillon T, Palmieri C, Sebire NJ, et al. Value of whole body 18FDG-PET to identify the active site of gestational trophoblastic neoplasia. *J Reprod Med.* 2006;51(11):879–887.
221. Vogelzang RL, Nemcek AA Jr, Skrtic Z, et al. Uterine arteriovenous malformations: primary treatment with therapeutic embolization. *J Vasc Interv Radiol.* 1991;2(4):517–522.
222. Lim AK, Agarwal R, Seckl MJ, et al. Embolization of bleeding residual uterine vascular malformations in patients with treated gestational trophoblastic tumors. *Radiology.* 2002;222(3):640–644.
223. Lurain JR, Nejad B. Secondary chemotherapy for high-risk gestational trophoblastic neoplasia. *Gynecol Oncol.* 2005;97(2):618–623.
224. Yang J, Xiang Y, Wan X, et al. Recurrent gestational trophoblastic tumor: management and risk factors for recurrence. *Gynecol Oncol.* 2006;103(2):587–590.
225. Ngan HY, Tam KF, Lam KW, et al. Relapsed gestational trophoblastic neoplasia: a 20-year experience. *J Reprod Med.* 2006;51(10):829–834.
226. Powles T, Savage PM, Stebbing J, et al. A comparison of patients with relapsed and chemo-refractory gestational trophoblastic neoplasia. *Br J Cancer.* 2007;96(5):732–737.
227. Mao Y, Wan X, Lv W, et al. Relapsed or refractory gestational trophoblastic neoplasia treated with the etoposide and cisplatin/etoposide, methotrexate, and actinomycin D (EP-EMA) regimen. *Int J Gynaecol Obstet.* 2007;98(1):44–47.
228. Newlands ES, Mulholland PJ, Holden L, et al. Etoposide and cisplatin/etoposide, methotrexate, and actinomycin D (EMA) chemotherapy for patients with high-risk gestational trophoblastic tumors refractory to EMA/cyclophosphamide and vincristine chemotherapy and patients presenting with metastatic placental site trophoblastic tumors. *J Clin Oncol.* 2000;18(4):854–859.
229. Lurain JR, Schink JC. Importance of salvage therapy in the management of high-risk gestational trophoblastic neoplasia. *J Reprod Med.* 2012;57(5–6):219–224.
230. Wang J, Short D, Sebire NJ, et al. Salvage chemotherapy of relapsed or high-risk gestational trophoblastic neoplasia (GTN) with paclitaxel/cisplatin alternating with paclitaxel/etoposide (TP/TE). *Ann Oncol.* 2008;19(9):1578–1583.
231. Hoekstra AV, Lurain JR, Rademaker AW, et al. Gestational trophoblastic neoplasia: treatment outcomes. *Obstet Gynecol.* 2008;112(2 Pt 1):251–258.
232. Bower M, Paradinas FJ, Fisher RA, et al. Placental site trophoblastic tumor: molecular analysis and clinical experience. *Clin Cancer Res.* 1996;2(5):897–902.
233. Chang YL, Chang TC, Hsueh S, et al. Prognostic factors and treatment for placental site trophoblastic tumor-report of 3 cases and analysis of 88 cases. *Gynecol Oncol.* 1999;73(2):216–222.
234. Papadopoulos AJ, Foskett M, Seckl MJ, et al. Twenty-five years' clinical experience with placental site trophoblastic tumors. *J Reprod Med.* 2002;47(6):460–464.
235. Hassadia A, Gillespie A, Tidy J, et al. Placental site trophoblastic tumour: clinical features and management. *Gynecol Oncol.* 2005;99(3):603–607.
236. Schmid P, Nagai Y, Agarwal R, et al. Prognostic markers and long-term outcome of placental-site trophoblastic tumours: a retrospective observational study. *Lancet.* 2009;374(9683):48–55.
237. Lurain JR, Hoekstra AV, Schink JC. Results of treatment of patients with gestational trophoblastic neoplasia referred to the Brewer Trophoblastic Disease Center after failure of treatment elsewhere (1979–2006). *J Reprod Med.* 2008;53(7):535–540.
238. Kohorn E. Regional centers for trophoblastic disease. *Am J Obstet Gynecol.* 2007;196(2):95–96.
239. Woolas RP, Bower M, Newlands ES, et al. Influence of chemotherapy for gestational trophoblastic disease on subsequent pregnancy outcome. *Br J Obstet Gynaecol.* 1998;105(9):1032–1035.
240. Matsui H, Iitsuka Y, Suzuka K, et al. Early pregnancy outcomes after chemotherapy for gestational trophoblastic tumor. *J Reprod Med.* 2004;49(7):531–534.
241. Rustin GJ, Newlands ES, Lutz JM, et al. Combination but not single-agent methotrexate chemotherapy for gestational trophoblastic tumors increases the incidence of second tumors. *J Clin Oncol.* 1996;14(10):2769–2773.
242. Savage P, Cooke R, O'Nions J, et al. Effects of single-agent and combination chemotherapy for gestational trophoblastic tumors on risks of second malignancy and early menopause. *J Clin Oncol.* 2015;33(5):572–578.

CHAPTER 27

Breast Cancer

David A. Edmonson, Tina Rizack, Margaret M. Steinhoff, C. James Sung, Hanan I. Khalil, Jarslow T. Hepel, Sonali V. Pandya, Robert D. Legare, and Don S. Dizon

INTRODUCTION

Breast cancer is the most common cancer in women, diagnosed in 1.2 million women worldwide each year. Treatment paradigms require an understanding of the natural history of the disease, including the various patterns of metastases and recurrence, and both the prognostic and predictive factors that may influence both response to treatment and overall survival (OS). In addition, the complexities that govern medical and surgical decisions make the management of breast cancer far more complicated than that of other disease sites. This chapter will provide the essential information regarding breast cancer, with an emphasis on recent developments. It stresses an interdisciplinary view of disease management by providing the foundational aspects of breast disease and treatment.

EPIDEMIOLOGY

Each year, more than 200,000 women and more than 2,000 men are diagnosed with breast cancer in the United States. It is estimated that one in eight women will be diagnosed with breast cancer in their lifetime. Fortunately, mortality from breast cancer has been steadily declining since 1990, at a rate of 3.1% per year in women under 50 years of age and 2.1% per year in older women (1). Still, more than 40,000 women succumb to breast cancer each year, making it the second most lethal malignancy behind lung cancer.

RISK FACTORS

Risk factors for breast cancer have been well characterized (**Table 27.1**). In general, factors associated with increased exposure to estrogen are well established. This includes female gender, early menarche, late menopause, later age at first pregnancy, and nulliparity. The use of combined estrogen and progesterone hormone therapy is a risk factor, although the Women's Health Initiative demonstrated that estrogen-only preparations (only indicated for women without an intact uterus) resulted in a lower risk of breast cancer (2). Of note, there is no evidence that oral contraceptive use increases risk (3), and a 2015 meta-analysis of women undergoing hormonal treatment for infertility came to similar conclusions (4). Among modifiable risk factors, obesity, weight gain in later life, and the consumption of alcohol have been identified in prospective observational studies (5). Race is a risk factor as well, though some data suggest it may be tumor-type specific. For example, Warner et al. (6) showed that Black women had a 21% higher risk of breast cancer–specific death, but this appeared limited to hormone receptor–positive tumors; there were no differences in survival among women with triple-negative or human epidermal growth factor-2 (HER2)–positive tumors. Family history is also a strong epidemiologic risk factor, and clinical models, such as the Tyrer–Cuzick, Gail, and Claus models, can assist in the prediction of breast cancer risk (7). Beyond classification of risk based on family history (familial risk), familial risk attributed to genetic mutations have been characterized. Among the best characterized are mutations involving BRCA1, localized to chromosome 17q21, and BRCA2, on chromosome 13q12-13, both of which confer a risk for breast cancer as high as 80% among carriers (8,9). However, genetic mutations beyond BRCA1 have also been characterized that carry an increased risk of breast cancer, including Li–Fraumeni syndrome (TP53), hereditary diffuse gastric cancer (CDH1), CHEK2, a member of the Fanconi Anemia–BRCA pathway involved in checkpoint function, and DNA repair mediated by BRCA1 and p53, and PALB2, another gene in the same pathway (7).

Environmental risks include prior radiation exposure, chemical exposure, and work/lifestyle factors. Work evaluating the long-term effects of environmental factors has established prior radiation exposure as an additional risk factor. The therapeutic use of mantle-field radiation in women with lymphoma and the sequelae of the atomic bombing of Japan in World War II identified the heightened risks of breast cancer, particularly in young women. This was shown in a study by Hancock et al. (10), which noted that radiation exposure in women with Hodgkin disease had an elevated risk of breast cancer compared to normal women, which increased by 6 to 15 fold, beginning approximately 10 years after completion of therapy.

TABLE 27.1. Risk Factors for Breast Cancer

Increased Estrogen Exposure	Female gender Early menarche Late menopause Use of postmenopausal estrogen/progesterone hormone therapy
Parity	Late age at first pregnancy Nulliparity
Lifestyle Factors	Obesity Weight gain later in life Alcohol consumption
Race	Black race
Family History	Breast cancer in first-degree relatives Male breast cancer
Genetic Mutations	BRCA1/2 TP53 CDH1 CHECK2 PALB2
Environmental	Prior radiation exposure Night shift work Polycyclic aromatic hydrocarbon exposure
Breast Findings	Benign breast lesions Dense breast tissue

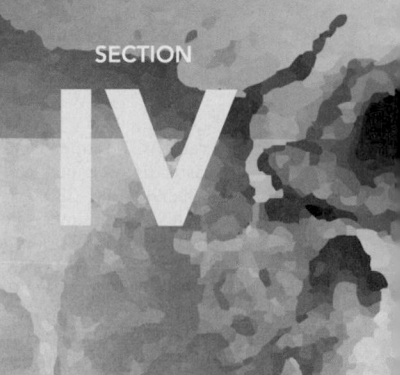

Chemical exposure is of increasing interest as a possible risk factor for the development of breast cancer. Several observances seem to suggest that there is some type of cause–effect relationship. In several regions of the country, there are unusually high incidences of breast cancer. In the 1990s, NIEHS and the National Cancer Institute cofunded the Long Island Breast Cancer Study Project (11,12). This was one of the largest and most comprehensive studies conducted exploring the possible link between breast cancer and environmental exposures, which evaluated three widespread pollutants, organochlorine pesticides (DDT), its metabolite DDE, polychlorinated biphenyls, and polycyclic aromatic hydrocarbons (PAHs), all of which were common within the Long Island area. The study showed that there was a modest increased risk of breast cancer with PAH exposure; however, no other definitive relationship between chemicals and breast cancer risk could otherwise be identified.

Multiple studies have looked at the relationship between night shift work and increased risk of breast cancer. A 2013 meta-analysis of 10 studies by Wang et al. (13) showed a pooled adjusted relative risk (RR) of 1.19 for those "ever exposed to night shift work and breast cancer". A dose–response relationship was also suggested, with a 3% increase in risk for every 5 years exposed to night shift work. More alarming is that their work suggested that an increase of 500 night shifts would result in a 13% increase in breast cancer risk.

The theoretical association appears to involve disruption of normal circadian rhythms, which may result in the suppression of melatonin output, with disruptions in pathways associated with melatonin, including angiogenesis, oxidation, and immune regulation. Lower levels of melatonin may also result in continuous production of estrogen as well as altering the estrogen receptor (ER), thus, increasing the risk of breast cancer (13–15).

Multiple studies have identified an association between breast cancer and breast findings, including the presence of benign breast lesions and increased density of breast tissue. For example, in a study by Hartmann et al. (16), the RR for breast cancer ranged from 1.27 for nonproliferative lesions to 1.88 for proliferative lesions without atypia to 4.24 in lesions with atypia, and this risk persisted for as long as 25 years after biopsy. Boyd and colleagues (17) reported on the association between risk and breast density (measured in percentage of the total breast). Using 1,112 matched case–control pairs they determined the association between risk and reported that women with density of 75% or greater had a significantly increased risk of breast cancer (odds ratio [OR] 4.7, 95% CI 3.0 to 7.4), with younger women notably at greatest risk.

ANATOMY

The breast is a modified sweat gland composed of two components: the large ducts and the terminal duct-lobular unit (TDLU), surrounded by adipose and fibrous tissue, lymphatics, nerves, and blood vessels. The surface of the breast is attached to the underlying fibrous tissue *via* Cooper ligaments, and the mammary gland lies over the pectoralis major muscle extending vertically along the second to sixth ribs and horizontally from the sternum to the anterior midaxillary line. The axillary tail comprises mammary tissue as well and extends laterally from the chest wall into the axilla. The large duct system of subsegmental, segmental, and lactiferous ducts converge and empty onto the nipple. The TDLU is the most distal part of this branching ductal system, and is felt to be the site of origin of most pathologic entities of the breast, including fibrocystic changes, ductal hyperplasias, and the majority of carcinomas (18). It is connected to the subsegmental ducts and represents the secretory unit of the gland.

Mobility of the breast tissue over the chest wall is through the retromammary bursa, which lies between the superficial and deep fascia. The vast lymphatic system of the breast is composed of a network over the entire surface of the chest, neck, and abdomen, with increased density under the axilla. There are three main lymphatic pathways of the breast: the axillary pathway, which drains the upper and lower halves of the breast into the lateral axillary nodal chain; the transpectoral pathway, which drains into the supraclavicular nodes; and the internal mammary (IM) pathway, draining the inner halves of the breast into the nodes of the IM chain.

NATURAL HISTORY OF BREAST CANCER

Breast cancers can have predictable features. For example, breast cancer is more likely to be diagnosed in the central or outer quadrants of the breast than in the inner regions (19), and some studies suggest that more cancers occur in the left rather than the right breast (20). Within the breast, cancer travels along ducts (intraductal carcinoma), and the process of invasion begins when the tumor erodes through the basement membrane. Continued growth results as the tumor spreads along adjacent lobules, breast lymphatics, perineural routes, and vascular spaces. When it involves the dermal lymphatics, the overlying dermis becomes edematous and red with the classic appearance of peau d'orange. Continued growth of the primary tumor can result in the involvement of the pectoralis and intercostal muscles, ribs, and the clavicle.

While less frequently encountered, locally advanced or metastatic disease at diagnosis is sometimes seen in clinical practice. Tumor spread can occur locally by direct extension, lymphatically, or *via* intravascular means. Lymphatic spread of tumor from the breast travels to the locoregional nodes of the chest: the axillary, intramammary, and supraclavicular nodal basins, and increasing tumor size is a well-known predictor of nodal involvement. A medial or central lesion of the breast is more likely to metastasize to the IM nodes than outer quadrant lesions, and this has been theorized to explain their worse prognosis compared to upper outer breast tumors (19). Vascular invasion can be observed, even with small tumors.

Metastatic disease from breast cancer can occur in any organ site. Lee (21) reviewed the published autopsy series in a 1983 report that included more than 2,000 women who had died of breast cancer. The most commonly involved organs were the lungs, bones, nodes, and liver. The pleural space, adrenal glands, and brain represented the next most commonly involved sites. Bloom (22) compared a group of women with untreated breast cancer with a cohort of patients treated with radical or modified radical mastectomy, with or without irradiation, and reported overall 10-year survival rates of 3.6% in the untreated cohort versus 34% in the treated group.

CLINICAL PRESENTATION OF BREAST CANCER

In countries where mammographic screening is established, women will often present with an abnormal mammogram. However, presentation with a clinical breast mass or even advanced disease still occurs in resource-rich countries, though it is more common in resource-poor settings. For women in their childbearing years, a delay in diagnosis may be attributed to benign causes such as recent trauma, changes with pregnancy, or due to breast-feeding. For women presenting with a mass, signs and symptoms of disease include breast tenderness, skin changes, bloody nipple discharge, or changes in the shape and size of the breast, with or without axillary adenopathy. Rarely do women present only with axillary adenopathy without evidence of a breast primary (occult breast carcinoma). Lastly, inflammatory breast cancer (IBC) presents as a tender, red, and swollen breast, often mistaken for mastitis. A crusting rash emanating from the nipple is sine qua non for Paget disease of the breast, which is almost uniformly associated with an underlying malignancy. Rarely will women present with metastatic breast cancer (MBC), a phenomenon more likely in resource-poor areas.

BREAST IMAGING

Breast imaging can be performed as a screening tool in asymptomatic women to detect early cancer, in high-risk women, or as a diagnostic examination in women suspected of having breast cancer or previously treated for breast cancer. Mammography remains the most widely used technique for screening, and it is the only modality proven to decrease mortality. Computer-aided detection (CAD), a tool designed to help the radiologist improve the detection of breast cancer, is frequently used by interpreting radiologists; the benefits and consequences will be reviewed.

Modalities such as ultrasound (US) and magnetic resonance imaging (MRI) serve as adjunct tools in the diagnostic setting or high-risk screening. In addition, breast tomosynthesis is used in some centers as an additional technique.

Mammography

The efficacy of mammography has been widely established by multiple randomized controlled trials demonstrating absolute mortality reduction, achieved by mammography's ability to detect both ductal carcinoma in situ (DCIS) and invasive breast cancer at a smaller size and earlier stage than in unscreened women. However, the value of mammography has also been called into question recently. A 2012 meta-analysis performed by the Independent United Kingdom Panel on Breast Cancer Screening that included 11 randomized trials confirmed that mammography is associated with a 20% reduction in breast cancer mortality (23), and other studies suggest that women between 40 and 69 years stand to benefit the most, particularly if implemented for at least 10 years (24). In 2014, long-term follow-up data from the Canadian National Breast Screening study were reported (25). Pooled results for women aged 40 to 49 years and 50 to 59 years showed no decrease in breast cancer mortality associated with screening. The cumulative breast cancer mortality was unchanged regardless of screening mammography (hazard ratio [HR] 0.99, 95% CI 0.88 to 1.12). Whether this points to flaws in trial design or is due to improvements in systemic management for newly diagnosed breast cancer are points that remain controversial.

In 2009, the United States Preventive Services Task Force reported modified recommendations for screening that include: biennial screening mammography for women aged 50 to 74 years and recommendations against routine screening mammography in women aged 40 to 49 years (26). In lieu of routine screening in younger women, the task force favored an individualized approach based on the goals and preferences of patients balanced with careful consideration of the risks and benefits of mammography in this particular population. Since then, the American Cancer Society has released guidelines as well and recommends routine screening starting at 45 years, at which point annual mammography should be conducted until age 54, after which they can transition to biennial screening (27). However, other organizations, including the American College of Radiology (ACR) (28) and the American College of Obstetrics and Gynecology (29), still recommend routine mammographic screening starting at age 40.

It is important to recognize that not all cancers will be found by mammography (30,31). For example, Esserman et al. (30) evaluated 866 patients to evaluate the impact of screening mammography and reported that 15% and 30% of women have either mammographically occult disease or will present with an interval breast cancer (i.e., cancer presenting in between mammograms), respectively. In a screening population, up to 10% of patients will be "recalled" for additional imaging, either additional mammographic views, spot compression views to determine if the area represents superimposed tissue versus a true mass or magnification views to better characterize calcifications, or US evaluation to determine the solid or cystic nature of a mass. Of all positive screening examinations, approximately 5% to 10% will have a diagnosis of cancer. Of all recommended biopsies, 25% to 40% will be positive for cancer. It is anticipated that the addition of tomosynthesis to two-dimensional conventional mammography will effectively decrease the "recall" rate and positive screening rate, and decrease the anxiety caused to patients. It is also expected to increase the sensitivity of mammography.

Mammography Regulations and Reporting

The Breast Imaging Reporting and Data System (BIRADS), first published in 1993, is a lexicon developed by the ACR to standardize terminology used in reporting findings on mammograms (32). It includes terms for describing features of masses (shapes and margins) and calcifications (morphology and distribution). It defines final assessment categories to describe the radiologist's level of suspicion about a mammographic abnormality to comply with the federally mandated Mammography Quality Standards Act (MQSA) regulations. All mammograms must be assessed, with a final BIRADS category of 0 to 6 (**Table 27.2**).

The report must include the date of comparison films, the indication for the examination (screening, recall, clinical finding, or follow-up), an assessment of overall breast composition to indicate the relative possibility that a lesion may be hidden by normal tissue, limiting the sensitivity of the examination, a description of any significant findings, and an overall summary impression.

Diagnostic Mammography

Diagnostic mammography is reserved for women with clinical signs or symptoms that suggest breast cancer (palpable mass, skin thickening, nipple retraction, or nipple discharge); recalls for further mammographic evaluation due to abnormal screening examination; or personal history of breast cancer. Patients with breast augmentation may be considered diagnostic because of more effort and time involved with obtaining necessary views, but should be audited in the screening group.

TABLE 27.2. BIRADS Assessment Categories

BIRADS 0	Examination is not complete. Often means additional workup is needed (e.g., spot compression, US)
BIRADS 1	No change in examination from prior; no abnormal findings appreciated
BIRADS 2	Benign finding, detected at routine screening. This includes breast cyst, fibroadenoma, fatty densities, surgical scar, scattered microcalcifications, and the presence of breast implants
BIRADS 3	*Probably* benign finding; typically, a 6-month follow-up will be needed. Findings included are tiny clusters of calcifications, focal asymmetric areas of nonpalpable fibroglandular densities, focal findings such as a dilated duct, generalized distribution of lesions, such as calcifications
BIRADS 4 **4A** **4B** **4C**	Suspicious or indeterminate findings identified. A biopsy should be performed. Finding associated with a **low** suspicion of breast cancer Finding associated with an **intermediate** suspicion of breast cancer Finding of **moderate** concern of being cancer
BIRADS 5	Very high probability of breast cancer, which requires immediate action
BIRADS 6	Imaging of a known cancer, proven by biopsy
Categorization of Breast Density	
Almost entirely fatty	
Few areas of fibroglandular density identified	
Heterogenous density, which may obscure a small mass	
Extreme density, associated with a lower sensitivity of mammography	

Film versus Digital Mammography

Film mammography is extremely effective and has been widely accepted as a screening modality for the past 20 to 30 years. With this technique, the mammography images are recorded as hard copy on film and developed by the technologist, then presented to the radiologist for review. Digital mammography uses a digital detector to replace the screen-film of conventional mammography. Radiation transmitted through the breast is absorbed by an electronic detector, with a response faithful over a wide range of intensities. The recorded information can be displayed using computer image–processing techniques to allow arbitrary settings of image brightness and contrast without need for further exposure to patients. The lower system noise would be expected to enhance the visibility of subtle contrast differences between tumors and normal background tissue. The processes of image acquisition, storage, and display are separated, allowing optimization of each. The average patient dose of radiation is slightly lower than that of film mammography. Examination time for each patient is shorter, permitting increased patient throughput. Images are more easily archived and accessed in Picture Archiving Communication Systems (PACS).

The Digital Mammographic Imaging Screening Trial reported a benefit of digital over screen-film mammography in certain groups of women (33). In this study, 49,528 asymptomatic women presenting for screening mammography at 33 sites in the United States and Canada underwent both digital and film mammography, with the examinations interpreted independently by two radiologists. While in the entire population the diagnostic accuracy of digital and film mammography was similar, the accuracy of digital mammography was significantly higher than that of film mammography in the following groups: women under the age of 50 years, women with heterogeneously dense or extremely dense breasts on mammography, and premenopausal or perimenopausal women. The results are understandable, because the technical advantages of digital mammography permit x-ray transmission manipulation to enhance visualization of subtle changes in tissue over the entire breast. It is known that the major limitation of mammography is that cancer can be hidden by adjacent breast tissue; with digital mammography, the visibility of a mass or cancer present in an image can be increased if contrast is adjusted.

The effect of transition to digital mammography from film screen was evaluated in a separate study that audited practice data from baseline year of film screen, year 1 digital, year 2 digital, and year 3 digital (34). In this practice, there was an increase in the recall rate with digital mammography (6.05 recall rate with film screen to 7.1% to 8.5% with digital technique), which persisted as a higher rate even at year 3. However, the cancer detection rate also increased for at least 2 years after the transition to digital, suggesting that cancers that may have been obscured with film screen mammography were more likely to be visible by digital technique. Overall, calcifications were significantly better seen by digital technique, an important point because calcifications often mark earlier, more treatable, disease.

Computer-Aided Detection

CAD allows for the identification of suspicious findings on mammograms to assist the radiologist's interpretation. A 2008 meta-analysis reported that CAD demonstrated no significant impact on the cancer detection rate (OR 1.04, 95% CI 0.96 to 1.13) and was associated with an increased rate of recall (OR 1.10, 95% CI 1.08 to 1.12) (35). However, the quality of the data was comprised due to significant heterogeneity in the studies included.

A prospective trial sought to evaluate the impact of double reading versus single reading plus CAD (36). There was no significant difference in the double reading regimen versus the single reading with CAD regimen for identification of masses or microcalcifications. However, more parenchymal deformities were detected in the double reading regimen, while more asymmetric densities were found by single reading plus CAD. In addition, there was a significant trend for improved cancer detection in women with dense breasts with double reading. Despite overall equivalence, double reading is costlier and more time consuming compared to single reading with the aid of CAD. As a result, CAD is likely to continue to be more widely used.

Ultrasound

Ultrasonography is a valuable adjunct to mammography, largely due to being widely available and relatively inexpensive. It is typically indicated for targeted examination, most often to determine the cystic versus solid nature of a mass, and is often used to characterize lesions as more likely to be benign or malignant. Prevalence-screening studies in women with radiographically dense breasts, especially younger women, have shown that targeted breast US may be useful. In one experience that included more than 800 women 30 years or younger presenting with a focal breast sign or symptom, targeted US had 100% sensitivity and negative predictive value (37). However, the limitations of breast US as a screening tool are well-known, as it requires a skilled operator, is labor intensive, and lacks standardized examination technique and interpretation criteria. Moreover, it does not detect microcalcifications, which can signal the earliest forms of cancer, the in situ disease.

Tomosynthesis

Tomosynthesis is a three-dimensional mammographic technique allowing better visualization of breast lesions by minimizing effects of overlapping tissue. The acquisition of images mimics conventional mammography with breast positioning and compression. Multiple low-dose images are obtained at different angles during a sweep of the x-ray tube, resulting in a digital data set which can be reconstructed into tomographic sections through the breast. Digital breast tomosynthesis was approved for clinical use in February 2011.

There are no prospective studies of tomosynthesis versus routine mammography, despite its availability. However, retrospective studies suggest it can be useful as a single test or in combination with digital mammography. For example, the largest retrospective study compared digital mammography alone ($n = 281,187$) or in combination with tomosynthesis ($n = 173,663$) (38). The addition of tomosynthesis resulted in a higher positive predictive value for recall from 4% to 6% and for biopsy from 24% to 29%. This resulted in 16/1,000 fewer recalls and 1.2/1,000 more cancers detected.

Tomosynthesis has been implemented in larger imaging centers across the United States. It is expected that within a few years there will be more data available to better determine the utility of tomosynthesis. It is unknown whether there will be additional cost or reimbursement for the procedure. The technique as of now is being reimbursed as for two-dimensional digital mammography. However, the equipment is expensive and the reading time for the radiologist is increased, with multiple more images to be interpreted. As more breast imagers become adept at the technology, a clearer sense of the increased reading time will be available.

Given its ability to minimize the effects of overlapping tissue, tomosynthesis is expected to be more beneficial in women with dense breasts, and may not yield more information in women with fatty breast tissue, in whom lesions are less likely to be obscured by overlapping tissue. However, more large scale trials will need to be performed to evaluate who will best benefit from the examination.

Breast MRI

MRI of the breast has evolved over the past 2.5 decades from a research tool to the most sensitive imaging modality in the detection of breast cancer, particularly for women deemed at high risk for breast cancer. Contrast-enhanced breast MRI is the most accurate modality in the clinical evaluation and staging of breast cancer. For breast lesion detection, intravenous injection of gadolinium-based contrast enhancement allows visualization of breast cancer against the background of glandular tissue. This distinction relies on the determination that tumor angiogenesis and surrounding tissue permeability allow contrast uptake within cancer. That is, a significant number of invasive tumors demonstrate rapid wash-in of contrast by 2 minutes and washout with time. Significant overlap between the enhancement pattern of benign and malignant processes exists, which must be recognized, and which lowers the specificity of breast MRI.

Technical standards for breast MRI are set by the ACR for proper imaging, interpretation, and accreditation (39). MRI of the breast should be performed with a dedicated breast coil, using at least a 1.5 Tesla magnet, and imaging parameters should be instituted to optimize high spatial and temporal resolution. MRI with a 3 Tesla magnet is evolving and slowly spreading; however, its advantage over the more commonly used 1.5 Tesla magnets is not known yet.

Ample data support the superiority of MRI over all other breast screening modalities, including mammography, US, and scintigraphy. MR sensitivity for the detection of invasive breast cancer ranges between 71% and 100%, though specificity is low at approximately 65%, likely due to overlap in the enhancement patterns between benign and malignant lesions (40,41). In general, the estimated negative predictive value of MRI is high, ranging between 90% and 95%. Although previous studies in DCIS showed low and variable sensitivities, with improved techniques, contemporary studies suggest it is more accurate than even mammography. For example, in one study of 79 women with pathologically proven DCIS, the detection rate for mammogram and MRI was 91% and 85%, respectively. However, when compared by the size of disease, MRI was significantly more accurate, especially in women under 50 years (42).

Breast MR reporting is standardized based on the ACR BI-RADS MR lexicon, which incorporates terminology and specific descriptors of breast MRI findings, in addition to assigning a final BIRADS category in the assessment, similar to mammography. The fifth edition of BIRADS introduced some changes to the prior MR BIRADS lexicon. By definition, an enhancing focus is less than 5 mm, and any space-occupying lesion 5 mm or larger constitutes a mass. Masses are evaluated based on shape, margin characteristics, internal enhancement, and kinetic analysis. To mention some descriptors of malignancy, an irregular mass, spiculated margins, heterogeneous/rim enhancement, and rapid wash-in and washout kinetics are characteristic of malignancy. Nonmass enhancement (NME) can be focal, linear, segmental, regional, or diffuse. The typical MR appearance of DCIS is NME in a linear or segmental distribution. As such, analysis of breast MR–enhancing lesions involves analyzing both lesion morphology and kinetics of enhancement to provide the most specificity in lesion characterization.

Screening Breast MRI

For women at high risk for breast cancer, breast MRI is a validated screening modality in addition to mammography. Studies have demonstrated that MRI is much more sensitive than even mammography or US in these patients. As an example, Kuhl et al. (43) conducted a surveillance study that included more than 500 women at high risk for breast cancer, defined by family history and/or genetic mutational analysis. With a median follow-up of 5.3 years, MRI was found to be far more sensitive than either mammogram or US (91% vs. 33% and 40%, respectively). Among women deemed at "higher" risk, the sensitivity favored MRI over mammogram (100% vs. 25%), although specificity was equivalent (96% to 97%). Additional work showed that MRI can detect a tumor in approximately 4% of high-risk women with mammographically occult breast cancer (44). In another study of high-risk women screened with all three modalities, 33% of cancers were visible by MR only, compared to 11% by mammography only, and 3% by US only (45). These data were validated by two recent review studies that evaluated more than 4,000 women and found that breast MR sensitivity alone ranges from 71% to 100%, mammography from 25% to 50%, mammography with US from 48% to 67%, all modalities together from 80% to 100%, and MR specificity from 93% to 98% (46,47).

In 2007, the American Cancer Society published new guidelines for high-risk screening with MRI based on scientific evidence and expert opinion (**Table 27.3**) (48). According to these new guidelines, high risk is defined as a lifetime risk of 20% to 25% or greater, being a, BRCA gene mutation carrier or first-degree relative of a BRCA carrier, women treated at an early age with chest radiation, and hereditary syndromes that place women at high risk for breast cancer. Currently, there are not enough data to support for or against annual breast MRI in women with a personal history of breast cancer or with high-risk lesions, and these patients are to be assessed on a case-to-case basis.

TABLE 27.3. Criteria for Use of an Annual MRI as an Adjunct to Mammography as a Screening Test for Breast Cancer

Known BRCA mutation
First-degree relative of a known BRCA mutation carrier (but otherwise not tested)
Personal risk of breast cancer exceeds 20% (using risk prediction models)
Prior radiation to the chest before the age of 30
Known familial genetic syndrome with an increased risk of breast cancer (e.g., Li–Fraumeni)

Breast MRI also serves to screen the contralateral breast in women with recently diagnosed breast cancer. A recent multicenter prospective trial evaluating contralateral breast cancer in women with recently proven breast cancer found clinically and mammographically occult breast cancer in 3.1% of 969 women, with a sensitivity of 91% and a negative predictive value of 99% (49).

Preoperative Evaluation of Breast Cancer

There are several clinical scenarios in which breast MRI is useful in addition to mammography, with the most common indication being preoperative staging of a newly diagnosed invasive cancer or DCIS. Breast MRI can delineate clinically and mammographically occult additional disease, including in situ disease associated with invasive cancer, and can detect noncalcified DCIS. In that regard, MRI is superior to mammography or US in defining local extent of the disease and can identify additional sites of disease. As an example, Liberman et al. (50) found that 48% of women who underwent preoperative MRI of the breast had additional foci of disease unsuspected by mammography. In a separate study by Girardi et al. (51), additional mammographically occult cancer was detected in 9% of patients staged with MRI preoperatively. As such, the addition of breast MRI can aid in surgical planning, including decisions regarding the role of mastectomy or the consideration for neoadjuvant chemotherapy (NACT).

However, the use of preoperative breast MRI is not without controversy. Braun et al. (52) evaluated the influence of preoperative MRI on surgical management in a retrospective study that included 160 patients with operable breast cancer and reported that it changed the clinical management in 27.5% of patients. This included findings of more widespread disease than otherwise suspected in 19% of cases. However, they also noted that 14 cases (9%) required additional surgical procedures for what was ultimately found to be benign pathology. Further fueling the controversy are the results of the comparative effectiveness of MRI in breast cancer (COMICE) trial, which included more than 1,600 patients randomly assigned to a preoperative MRI or not (53). This trial showed that MRI did not decrease surgical negative margins and was associated with a higher rate of mastectomy. However, more recent data suggest a more positive role of preoperative MRI, whereby Obdeijin et al. (54) and Sung et al. (55) found significantly lower reexcision rates of 18.9% and 29%, respectively, in patients staged with preoperative MRI as opposed to reexcision rates of 37.4% and 45% with no MRI. Another study by Fortune–Greeley et al. (56) in 2014 demonstrated that there is a 40% reduction in the rate of reexcision of invasive lobular cancer with MR, without increasing the mastectomy rate. The effect of MRI staging on patient mortality outcome is still unknown. On the basis of these findings, we support a thoughtful approach to the role of preoperative MRI and feel it is a reasonable test for women with dense breasts, especially if they have a histologic diagnosis of invasive lobular cancer.

Breast MRI: Other Roles

Recurrence following breast conservation therapy is better detected by MRI than mammography or US, with high specificity and negative predictive value (57). In addition, MRI has a role in determining the response to NACT, and it is more reliable than mammography or US in that respect. However, while MRI may not show residual enhancement following chemotherapy, it is not 100% accurate in the detection of residual disease. In at least one report, MRI was associated with a 23% risk of underestimation (58). For women presenting with suspicious clinical findings for breast cancer and negative conventional imaging tests, MRI of the breast has an added value. These instances include a woman with a palpable suspicious mass, women with metastatic axillary lymph nodes but no mammographically defined breast primary cancer, and those with pathologic unilateral nipple discharge or Paget disease and a negative mammogram and US. MRI use to workup mammographic calcifications or other mammographic abnormality is discouraged, and suspicious findings should undergo core biopsy. A helpful role of MRI in such clinical scenarios would be to delineate the extent of disease and to rule out an underlying occult invasive component.

BREAST PATHOLOGY

Fibrocystic Changes

The breast ducts and lobules can show a wide range of benign nonproliferative and proliferative epithelial lesions. Nonproliferative lesions include cysts (macroscopic and microscopic), duct ectasia, fibrosis, and apocrine metaplasia. Proliferative lesions were first separated into different risk categories based on the work of Dupont and Page (59). Compared to normal breast (**Figs. 27.1** and **27.2**), patterns associated with a mildly increased risk (~two-fold) of subsequent breast carcinoma are considered proliferative changes, and include usual ductal epithelial hyperplasia (**Fig. 27.3**), lobular hyperplasia, sclerosing adenosis, radial scars, and intraductal papillomas (60). Both sclerosing adenosis and radial scars (**Figs. 27.4 and 27.5**) show distortion of normal breast architecture, and this irregular gland pattern may mimic an invasive carcinoma. These benign proliferations maintain a normal myoepithelial cell layer, which can be highlighted by immunohistochemical (IHC) stains. Intraductal papillomas have fibrovascular cores lined by myoepithelial cells and one or more layers of epithelial cells (**Fig. 27.6**). Papillomas involving large ducts near the nipple may cause a bloody nipple discharge.

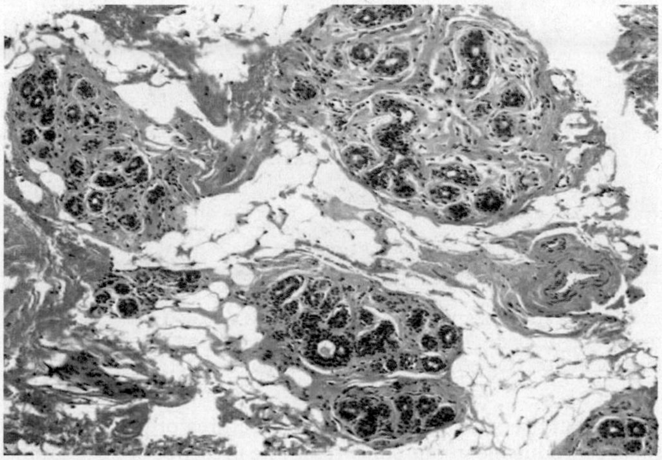

Figure 27.1. Normal breast lobules. Three TDLUs are surrounded by adipose and fibrous tissue.

Atypical ductal hyperplasia (ADH) and atypical lobular hyperplasia (ALH) are associated with an approximately fivefold higher increased risk of subsequent breast cancer (60). ADH is characterized by architectural patterns approaching that of in situ carcinoma, while ALH shows expansion of the lobule by a loose, monomorphic cell

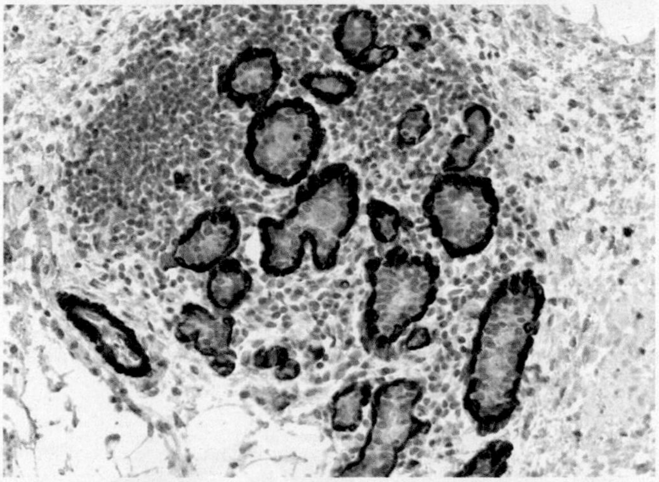

Figure 27.2. Normal breast lobule. Presence of myoepithelial cells is illustrated by positive staining for smooth muscle myosin heavy chain.

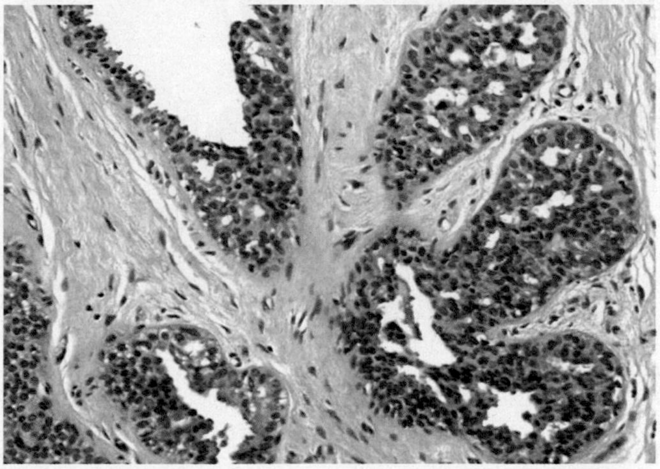

Figure 27.3. Usual ductal hyperplasia. Slightly expanded ducts are filled with hyperplastic ductal epithelial cells and myoepithelial cells in an irregular fenestrated growth pattern.

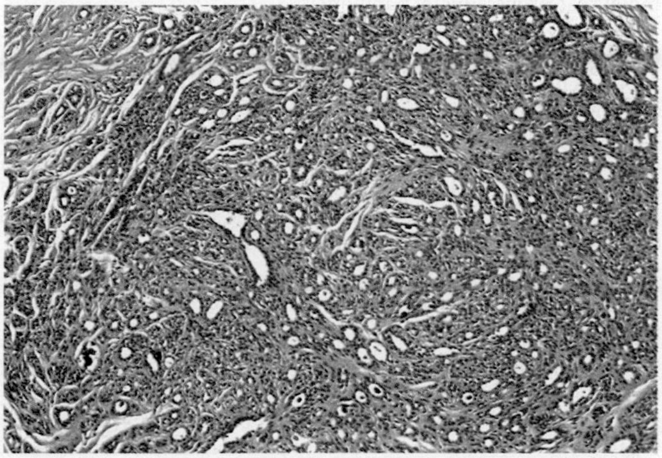

Figure 27.4. Sclerosing adenosis. A well-developed lobulocentric distribution of dilated ducts and overgrowth of spindly myoepithelial cells may be mistaken as malignancy in core biopsy or frozen section.

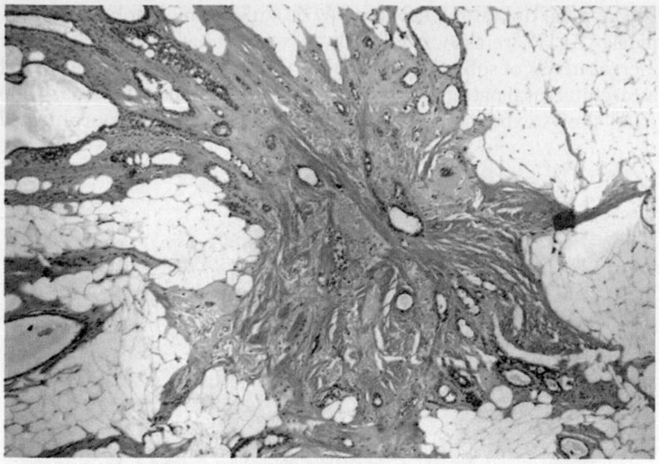

Figure 27.5. Radial scar. A stellate lesion with irregular ducts radiating from the elastotic center, the entrapped glands may mimic an invasive ductal carcinoma.

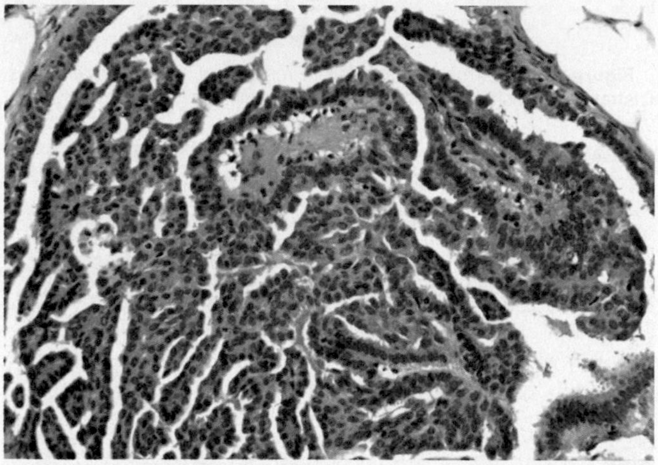

Figure 27.6. Intraductal papilloma. A well-circumscribed papillary proliferation fills a dilated duct. The presence of fibrovascular core of the papillae indicates benignity.

population (**Figs. 27.7 and 27.8**). Reproducibility of the diagnosis of ADH is still problematic, but more uniform criteria are now used by most pathologists (61). There is still controversy as to whether size criteria should be used to separate ADH from low-grade DCIS (two completely involved ducts or 2 mm). ADH can also involve a radial scar or intraductal papilloma.

A newly appreciated group of lesions are columnar cell change, columnar cell hyperplasia, and flat epithelial atypia (**Figs. 27.9 and 27.10**). These lesions were originally described by Azzopardi (62), and their significance has been reappraised due to their frequent association with mammographically detected microcalcifications (63). More recently, it has been noted that flat epithelial atypia (**Fig. 27.11**) has a high association with low-grade DCIS (64) and invasive tubular carcinoma (65). Molecular studies may be able to further characterize these lesions and their role in breast carcinogenesis.

Ductal Carcinoma In Situ

DCIS or intraductal carcinoma is a heterogenous group of lesions with the proliferation of malignant cells confined within the ductal system. Traditionally, DCIS was classified on the basis of its architectural pattern, often dichotomized as comedo and noncomedo types. Noncomedo patterns include solid, cribriform, micropapillary, clinging, and papillary types. Combinations of these patterns are not uncommon in a biopsy. Several grading schemes incorporating both architectural and nuclear features have been proposed, but the Holland version, in which nuclear features predominate, was most reproducible in one study (66). The presence of intraluminal necrosis and calcifications is usually noted, along with the nuclear grade and pattern(s).

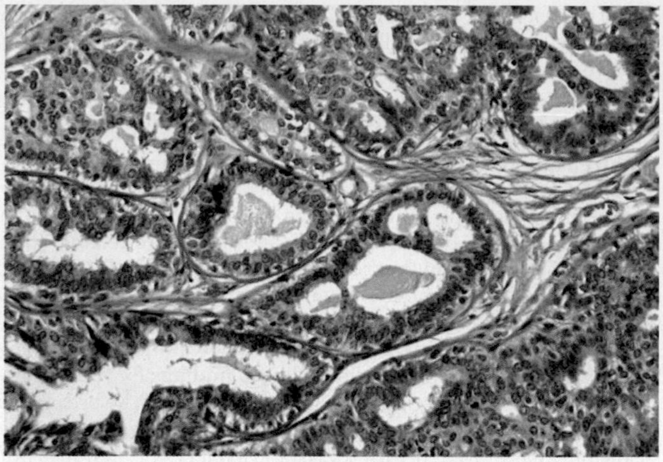

Figure 27.7. ADH. The proliferation has a cribriform growth pattern approaching that of a DCIS, but the microlumens are more irregular in sizes and shapes.

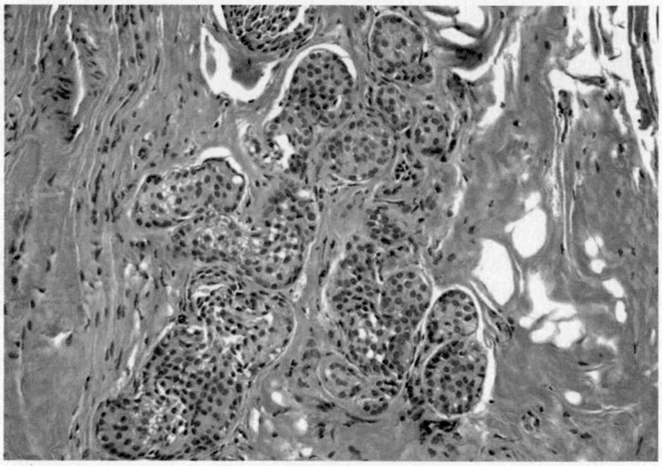

Figure 27.8. ALH. The lobular glands are somewhat expanded with a loose monomorphic cell population.

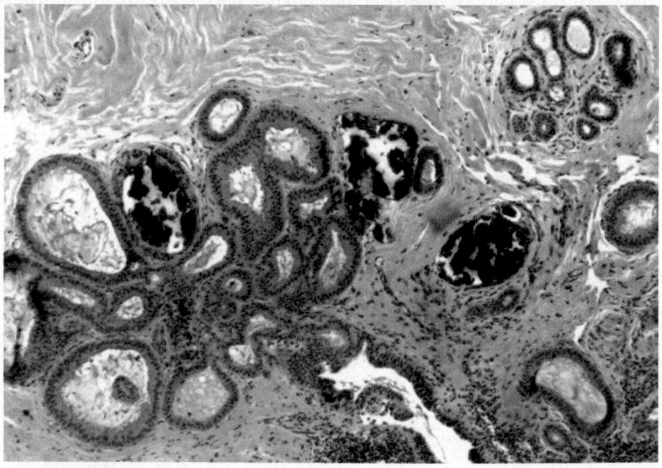

Figure 27.9. Columnar cell change. Variably dilated acini with microcystic change lined by columnar cells, frequently associated with luminal secretions and/or microcalcifications.

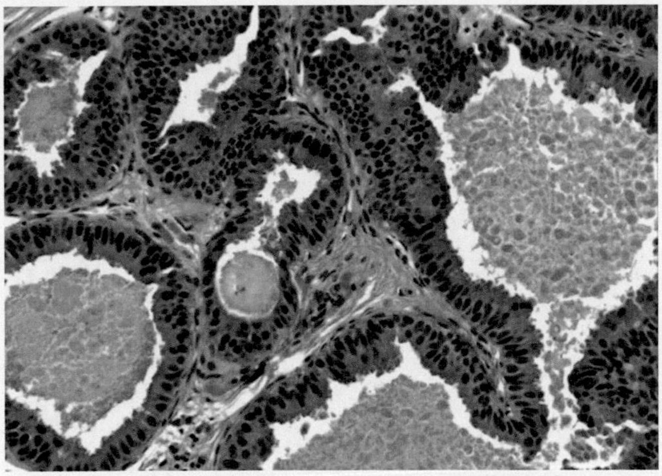

Figure 27.10. Columnar cell hyperplasia. Columnar cell change with piling up of several layers or stratification associated with luminal secretions.

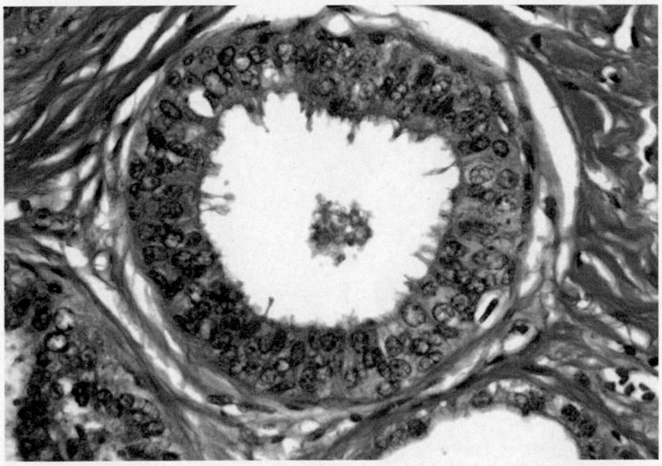

Figure 27.11. Flat epithelial hyperplasia. This is a columnar lesion characterized by mildly atypical epithelial cells, which may represent a precursor of or the earliest morphologically recognizable form of low-grade DCIS.

Comedo-type DCIS (comedocarcinoma) shows a solid proliferation of large, pleomorphic nuclear grade 3 epithelial cells with numerous mitoses and central necrosis containing cellular debris, so-called "comedo-necrosis" (Fig. 27.12). The necrotic material often becomes calcified, and these coarse calcifications have a distinctive mammographic appearance outlining the ductal system ("casting calcifications"). Periductal fibrosis and inflammation is common in comedo-type DCIS and can be a diagnostic problem, as microinvasion is a feature more frequently associated with comedo-type DCIS than other patterns (67). Extension of the large pleomorphic cells into the distal lobular unit is a pattern known as "cancerization of lobules."

The solid, cribriform, papillary, and micropapillary patterns of noncomedo DCIS are usually composed of uniform low-grade or intermediate-grade nuclei. Cribriform patterns show smooth, rounded, "punched-out" spaces (Fig. 27.13). The micropapillary subtype does not contain fibrovascular cores, whereas papillary DCIS does (Fig. 27.14). The "clinging" or "flat" type of DCIS may have either low- or high-grade nuclei. Microcalcifications may be associated with these noncomedo patterns and may be detected by mammography. Their pattern of distribution is less specific than that of the comedo DCIS and may be similar to that seen in benign conditions. Lesion size is often problematic by pathologic evaluation, as most DCIS is not grossly evident. It is not practical to submit all tissue from an excisional biopsy for microscopic evaluation, so sectioning

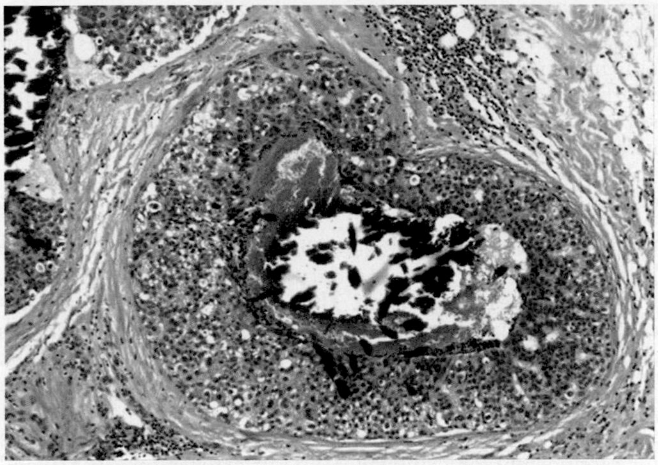

Figure 27.12. Comedo-type DCIS. Markedly expanded ducts are filled with high-grade neoplastic ductal cells with central necrosis and calcifications.

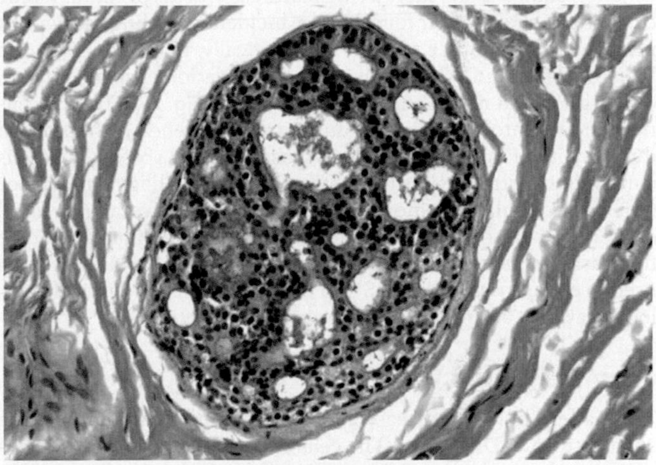

Figure 27.13. Cribriform DCIS. Expanded duct is filled with low-to-intermediate-grade neoplastic cells forming secondary rigid cribriform microlumens resembling "punched out" spaces.

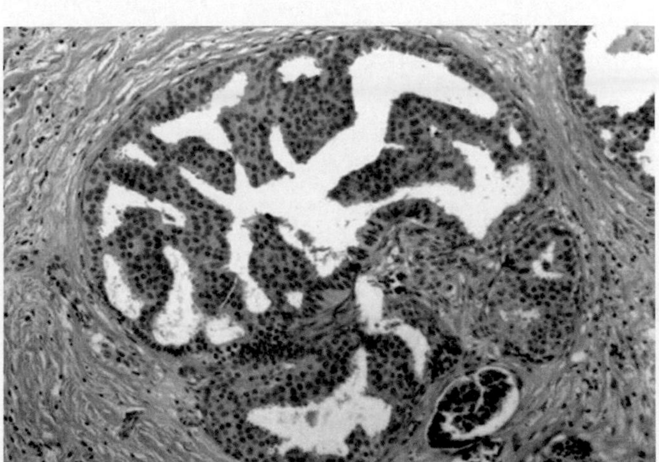

Figure 27.14. Micropapillary DCIS. Low-grade neoplastic ductal cells form papillary fronds in an expanded duct. The papillary fronds lack fibrovascular core.

is guided by the type of lesion and radiographic findings. Mammography can often give a more accurate size of the lesion, but only in tumors that are entirely marked by calcifications. Margin width is most easily measured microscopically in perpendicular sections, which requires the presence of colored inks for unique identification of each margin.

Paget Disease of the Nipple

Paget disease of the nipple reflects direct extension of DCIS, usually high grade, into the lactiferous ducts and adjacent skin. Clinically, the nipple appears excoriated. The DCIS may or may not be accompanied by invasive carcinoma. Histologically, the Paget cells are large round cells with prominent nucleoli and pale cytoplasm. They occur singly within the layers of the epidermis, or may form groups at the dermal–epidermal junction, mimicking malignant melanoma (**Fig. 27.15**). Lesional cells of Paget disease are positive for carcinoembryonic antigen (CEA) or cytokeratin 7 (CK7) and negative for Melan-A and HMB-45 (**Fig. 27.16**).

Lobular Carcinoma In Situ

Lobular carcinoma in situ (LCIS) was first described by Foote and Stewart in 1941 and has been an enigma ever since. It is a multicentric lesion, with no identifying features on gross or radiographic evaluation, and is often found as an incidental finding in biopsies performed for another reason. Histologically, in classic LCIS, the lobule is distended by a monomorphic population of small uniform cells with round nuclei and scant cytoplasm (**Fig. 27.17**). The cells may extend into the adjacent duct, growing beneath the normal ductal epithelium, a pattern known as "pagetoid spread." There is continuing controversy as to whether LCIS is an obligate precursor of invasive lobular carcinoma or just a marker of overall increased cancer risk in either breast. Certainly, LCIS is often found adjacent to invasive lobular carcinoma. The term "lobular neoplasia" is often used to encompass both LCIS and ALH, which have identical cytologic features, but minor differences in architecture.

Pleomorphic LCIS

This pattern of in situ disease involves larger ducts and mimics the solid pattern of DCIS (68). The cells are evenly spaced, slightly dyscohesive, and may have visible intracytoplasmic lumina (**Fig. 27.18**). Immunohistochemistry for E-cadherin demonstrates loss of this membrane protein (**Fig. 27.19**). Treatment should be similar to DCIS, as this pattern of LCIS is considered a precursor lesion of invasive carcinoma rather than just a risk factor for subsequent disease (69).

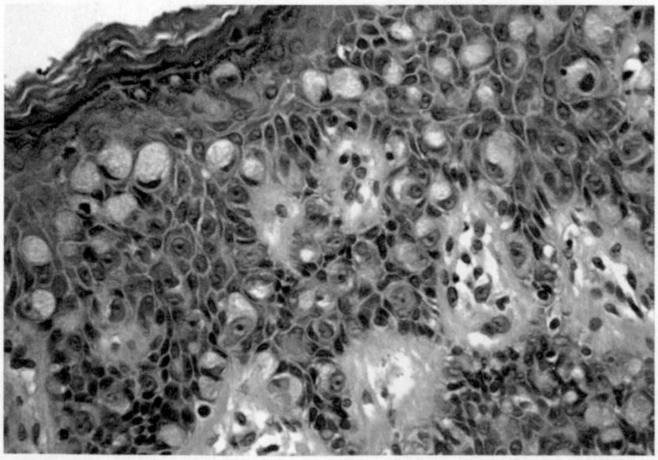

Figure 27.15. Paget disease. Large, round, pale neoplastic cells occur singly within the epidermis, mimicking malignant melanoma.

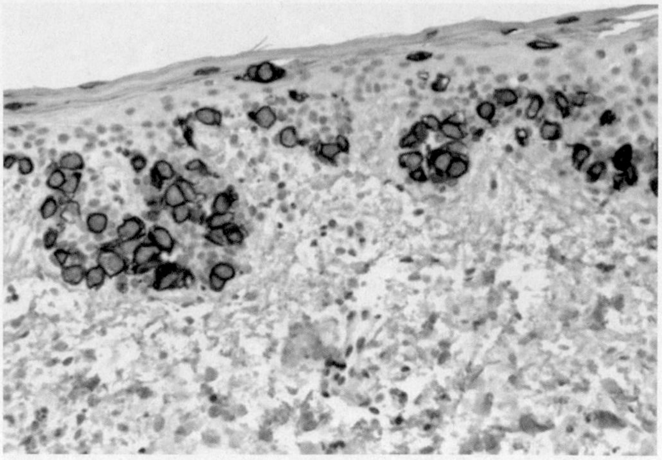

Figure 27.16. Paget disease. Paget disease cells are positive for CEA or CK7 and negative for Melan-A and HMB-45, which are positive in malignancy melanoma.

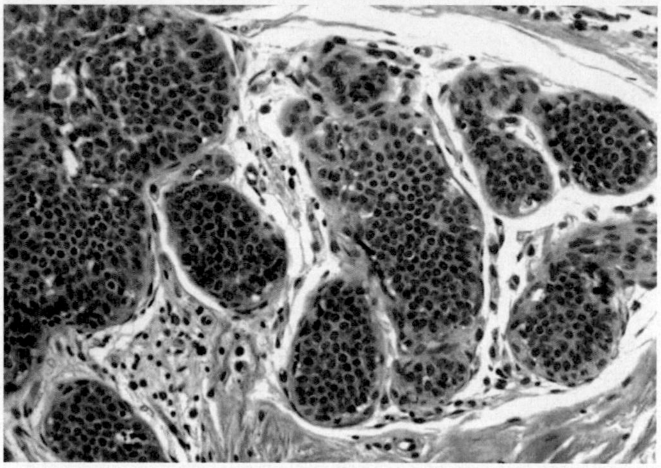

Figure 27.17. LCIS. An expanded lobule is markedly distended by a monomorphic population of small uniform cells. The underlying lobular architecture is still recognizable.

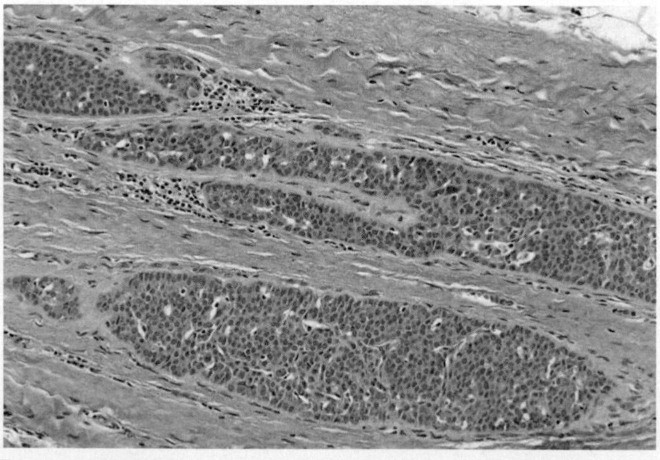

Figure 27.18. Pleomorphic LCIS. This pattern of LCIS involves larger ducts with evenly spaced and slightly dyscohesive tumor cells, mimicking solid pattern of DCIS.

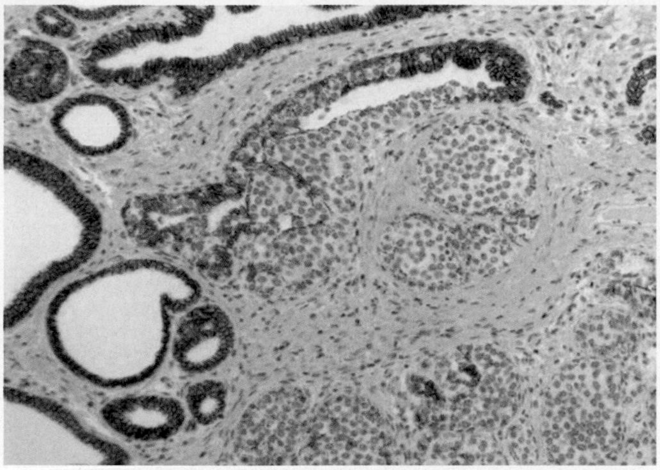

Figure 27.19. LCIS. Loss of membranous e-Cadherin staining of LCIS in contrast with adjacent normal ducts with positive staining.

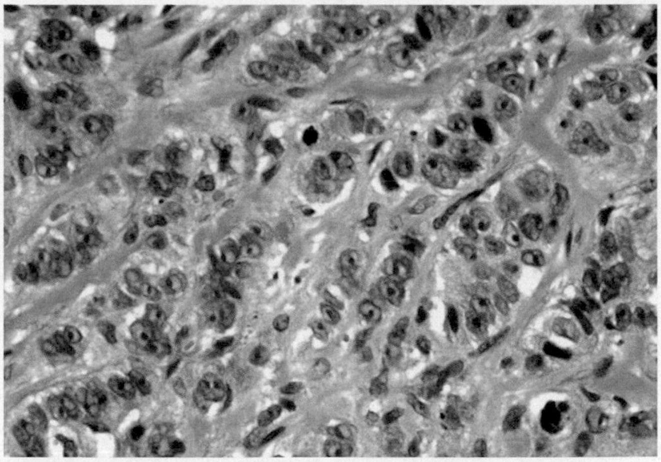

Figure 27.20. Invasive ductal carcinoma. Small solid cords of neoplastic cells with moderate-to-severe cytologic atypia are surrounded by a fibrous stroma.

Invasive Carcinoma

Invasive carcinoma of the breast is defined by the presence of stromal invasion, usually manifest by a fibrotic, desmoplastic stromal reaction around the invading cells. Tumor may be microinvasive (<1 mm) within an area of DCIS or may form an obvious tumor mass, clinically or radiographically. Tumors are classified by the pattern of growth into ductal and lobular forms. Breast carcinoma is surgically staged using the AJCC staging system based on the size of the invasive component. Synoptic checklist reporting using templates devised by the College of American Pathologists (CAP) aids in ensuring that all important pathologic features are documented. DCIS may be focally present adjacent to the invasive component or intermixed with invasive tumor. The term "EIC" denotes a tumor with an extensive in situ component, defined as at least 25% of the tumor mass.

Invasive Ductal Carcinoma

The majority of invasive tumors of the breast are ductal and have varying morphologic patterns that have led to several subclassifications. Most of the special types listed below are distinguished because they have an extremely good prognosis. The majority of tumors (~75%) have no specific features and are designated carcinoma not otherwise specified or carcinoma of no special type. These tumors may be composed of small glands, tubules, solid cords, or nests of cells with varying degrees of cytologic atypia surrounded by a reactive (desmoplastic) fibrous stroma (**Fig. 27.20**). The recommended grading system is the Nottingham modification, which is based on adding scores for architectural pattern, nuclear pleomorphism, and mitotic count (**Table 27.4**) (70). Grade 1 tumors (well differentiated) have 3 to 5 points, Grade 2 tumors (moderately differentiated) have 6 to 7 points, and Grade 3 tumors (poorly differentiated) have 8 to 9 points. While initially applied only to invasive ductal carcinoma, this system can also be applied to invasive lobular carcinomas and has been validated in numerous studies (71).

TABLE 27.4. Modified Nottingham Histologic Scoring System for Invasive Breast Tumor Grade

Glandular (acinar)/tubular differentiation	
1 point	>75% of tumor area forming glandular/tubular structures
2 points	10% to 75% of tumor area forming glandular/tubular structures
3 points	<10% of tumor area forming glandular/tubular structures
Nuclear pleomorphism	
1 point	Nuclei are small with little increase in size compared to normal breast epithelial cells, regular outlines, uniform nuclear chromatin, and little variation in size
2 points	Cells are larger than normal with open vesicular nuclei, visible nucleoli, and moderate variability in both size and shape
3 points	Cells have vesicular nuclei, often with prominent nucleoli, exhibiting marked variation in size and shape, occasionally with very large and bizarre forms
Mitotic count	
1 point	≤7 mitoses per 10 high-power fields
2 points	8–14 mitoses per 10 high-power fields
3 points	≥15 mitoses per 10 high-power fields

Overall grade: Grade 1: 3 to 5 points; Grade 2: 6 to 7 points; Grade 3: 8 to 9 points.

Special Types

Mucinous Carcinoma

Mucinous (or colloid) carcinoma usually occurs in postmenopausal women. The tumor is well circumscribed and may have a gelatinous gross appearance. Microscopically, nests of uniform small cells are surrounded by pools of mucin (**Fig. 27.21**). The in situ component is minimal, but may also show intraductal mucin production. Pure mucinous tumors are low grade and have an excellent prognosis, with a low risk of lymph node metastasis (72). This is not true, however, of mixed carcinomas with a prominent nonmucinous, usual invasive ductal carcinoma component.

Tubular Carcinoma

Tubular carcinoma is a well-differentiated invasive carcinoma composed of small glands or tubules that can be difficult to distinguish from some benign lesions, especially radial scars. The tubules are arranged haphazardly, often with a surrounding cellular stroma. They are somewhat angular with open lumens and are lined by a single layer of monomorphic epithelial cells (**Fig. 27.22**). Myoepithelial cells are absent, and IHC for myoepithelial markers (smooth muscle myosin heavy chain, calponin, p63, and/or CD10) is helpful in confirming the diagnosis on needle biopsy. Within this group, tumors with at least 75% tubules and grade 1 nuclei have an excellent prognosis (73). Invasive tubular carcinoma is often associated with a low-grade micropapillary or cribriform DCIS or adjacent atypical columnar cell lesions (65). Tubular carcinomas are small, usually less than 1 cm, and are frequently detected by screening

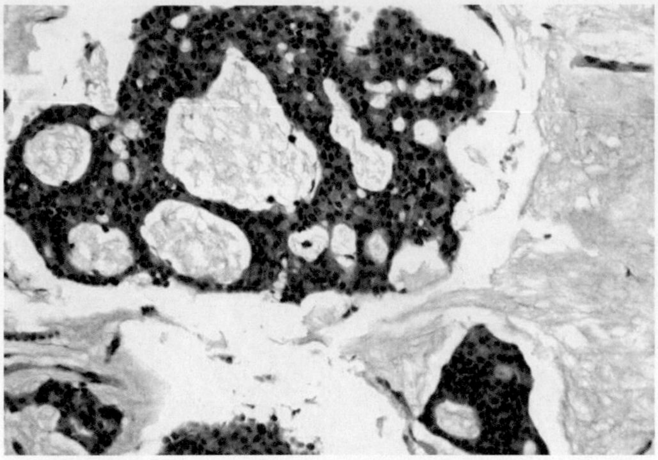

Figure 27.21. Mucinous carcinoma. Nests of low-grade neoplastic cells in a cribriform pattern are surrounded by a large pool of mucin, rendering a gelatinous gross appearance.

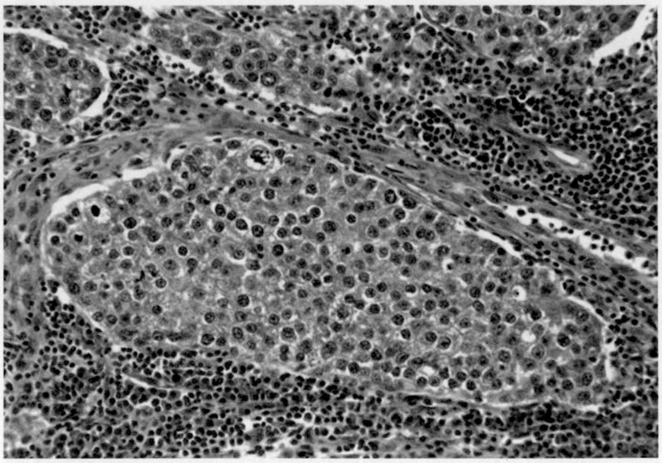

Figure 27.23. Medullary carcinoma. Highly pleomorphic neoplastic cells in a syncytial sheet pattern are surrounded by a diffuse lymphocytic infiltrate.

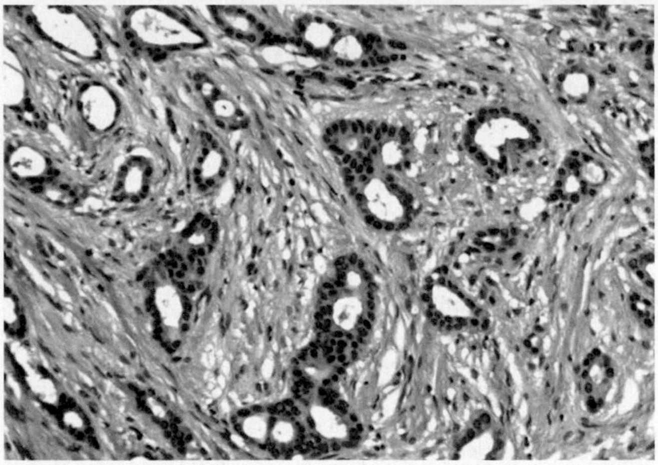

Figure 27.22. Tubular carcinoma. Well-formed angular, oval, and tubular glands with a single layer of neoplastic ductal cells diffusely infiltrate a desmoplastic fibrous stroma. Myoepithelial cells are absent from these tubules.

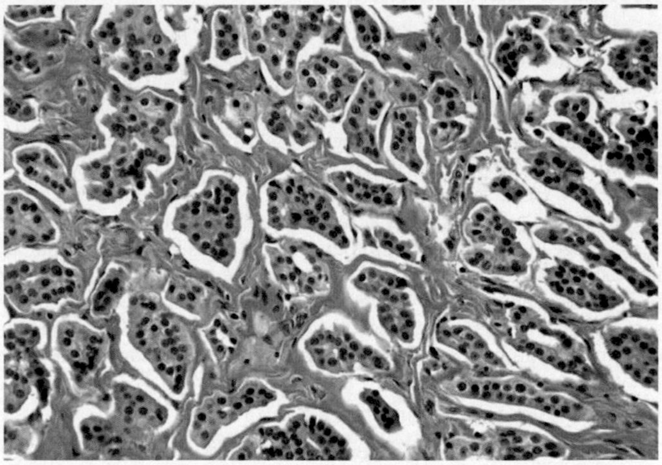

Figure 27.24. Invasive micropapillary carcinoma. Small clusters of intermediate-grade neoplastic cells lie within small clear spaces of a fibrocollagenous stroma mimicking tumor cells in angiolymphatic spaces. The tumor cells display reversed polarity, whereby the E-Cadherin negative luminal (apical) edge of the tumor cells is at the periphery of the tumor clusters.

mammography. Tumors with a component of usual invasive ductal carcinoma should not be included in this category. Invasive cribriform carcinoma, which also has a good prognosis, may be mixed with tubular carcinoma.

Medullary Carcinoma

Medullary carcinomas occur more commonly in women under 50 and have a higher frequency in BRCA1 mutation carriers. Clinically, the tumor is well circumscribed and may mimic a fibroadenoma. Microscopically, the tumor is composed of solid syncytial sheets of large anaplastic cells with pleomorphic nuclei, prominent nucleoli, and abundant mitotics (**Fig. 27.23**). Gland formation is absent. The tumor has a pushing border and is surrounded by a dense lymphoplasmacytic infiltrate. Only tumors with this strict morphology and no component of typical invasive ductal carcinoma have a good prognosis.

Micropapillary Carcinoma

Micropapillary carcinoma is a recently described entity with a characteristic morphology, high incidence of positive nodes at presentation despite small tumor size, and poor OS (74). The tumor is composed of small clusters of malignant cells floating within small clear spaces resembling lymphatic channels (**Fig. 27.24**). Most tumors have high nuclear grade and true lymphatic space invasion. A component of usual invasive ductal carcinoma may be present.

Papillary Carcinoma

Papillary carcinoma is a rare subtype. Several different entities are encompassed within this terminology. Solid papillary carcinoma and encapsulated (intracystic or encysted) papillary carcinoma have indolent behavior like a DCIS, although they lack surrounding myoepithelial cells (**Fig. 27.25**) (75). Encapsulated papillary carcinoma forms a well-circumscribed mass and may have DCIS present in adjacent ducts. Invasive papillary carcinomas have evidence of destructive stromal invasion adjacent to larger solid nests.

Inflammatory Carcinoma

The term "inflammatory carcinoma" originated as a clinical term to describe a patient presenting with a reddened edematous breast suggesting mastitis. Skin biopsies from such patients often show tumor thrombi in dermal lymphatic channels (**Fig. 27.26**), but this is not true in every case.

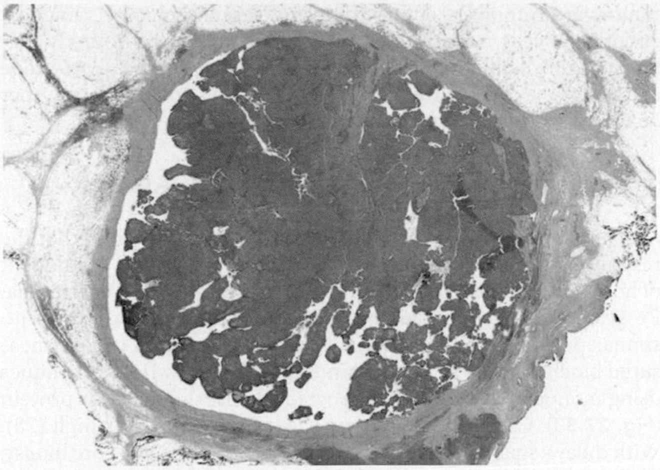

Figure 27.25. Solid or encapsulated (intracystic) papillary carcinoma. Low power shows a well-circumscribed tumor with branching network of fibrovascular stroma. A cystic formation is not necessary for the diagnosis.

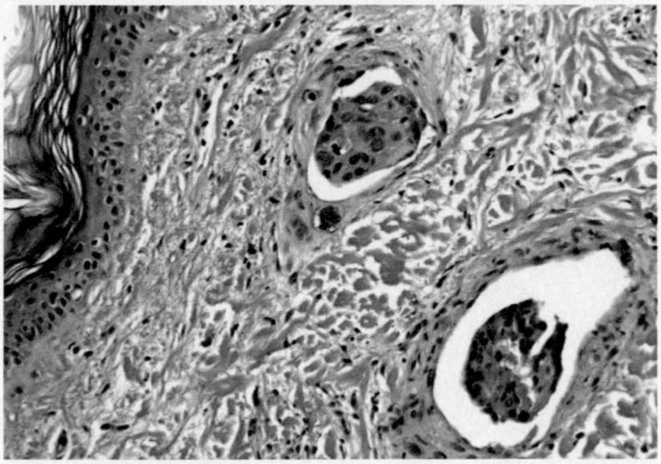

Figure 27.26. Inflammatory carcinoma. Carcinomatous emboli are present in dilated dermal lymphatics.

Invasive Lobular Carcinoma

Invasive lobular carcinoma comprises approximately 10% of all breast cancers. The classic form of invasive lobular carcinoma is composed of small monotonous tumor cells with scant cytoplasm growing in linear columns ("Indian file") or in concentric ("targetoid") patterns around normal ducts and lobules (**Figs. 27.27** and **27.28**). A mild stromal desmoplastic reaction may be present around the tumor cells, but many invasive lobular carcinomas do not form a discrete tumor mass. This diffuse growth pattern can be a problem when attempting conservative surgical excision, and tumors are frequently upstaged after surgery (76).

Variant forms of invasive lobular carcinoma include alveolar, solid, and trabecular patterns and are composed of the same monomorphic small cells. Signet ring cell carcinoma (**Fig. 27.29**), in which the cells contain prominent intracytoplasmic vacuoles, is considered a variant of invasive lobular carcinoma due to its similar growth patterns. Another variant is pleomorphic lobular carcinoma, in which the columns of cells show marked nuclear atypia.

Stage for stage, the prognosis of patients with invasive lobular carcinoma is no different from invasive ductal carcinoma. However, the patterns of metastatic disease are different, with lobular carcinomas having a propensity to metastasize to the meninges and peritoneal and pleural surfaces. Invasive lobular carcinomas and mixed lobular and ductal invasive carcinomas appear to be more

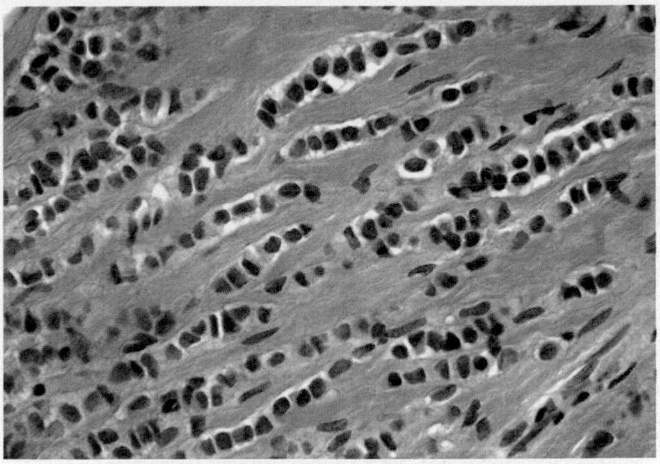

Figure 27.27. Invasive lobular carcinoma. Small monotonous tumor cells invade in linear "Indian file" pattern.

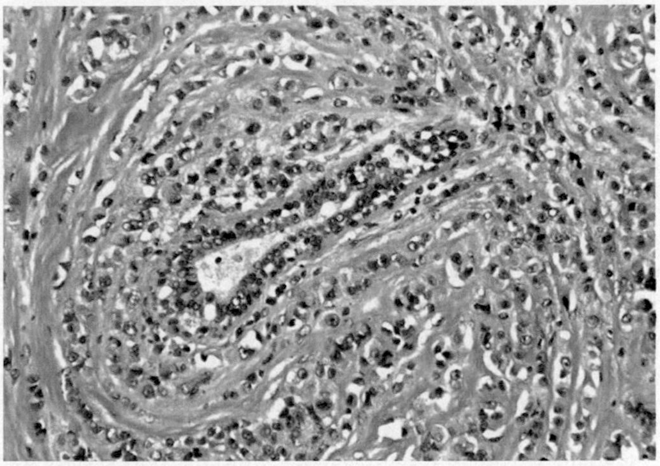

Figure 27.28. Invasive lobular carcinoma. Tumor cells infiltrate in a concentric pattern around a normal duct.

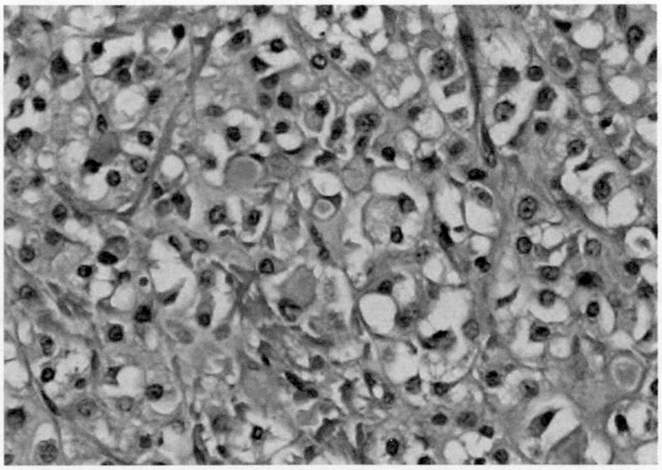

Figure 27.29. Signet ring cell carcinoma. Tumor cells contain a large amount of intracytoplasmic mucin, which pushes the nuclei to the cell periphery, thus resembling signet rings.

frequent in postmenopausal women taking combination hormone replacement therapy (77).

Tubulolobular Carcinoma

This tumor shows a mixture of invasive lobular and tubular carcinoma growth patterns with low-grade nuclei. The mixed architectural pattern parallels the expression of markers of ductal and lobular differentiation, and these tumors appear to have a good prognosis.

Other Tumors

Metaplastic Carcinoma

The term "metaplastic carcinoma" is used to describe tumors with prominent morphologic patterns different from usual ductal and lobular patterns. The term encompasses epithelial tumors (carcinomas) showing squamous cell differentiation, monophasic spindle cell carcinoma, and biphasic tumors with both epithelial and mesenchymal elements (**Fig. 27.30**). Spindle cell (sarcomatoid) carcinomas express epithelial markers (cytokeratins) despite their spindle cell morphology and are aggressive tumors with a high rate of extranodal metastases. Biphasic tumors (biphasic sarcomatoid carcinoma or carcinosarcoma) may contain heterologous elements, such as malignant cartilage or bone (**Fig. 27.31**).

Phyllodes Tumors

Phyllodes tumors, formerly known as "cystosarcoma phyllodes" are biphasic tumors similar to fibroadenomas with a spectrum of morphology and biologic behavior. The median age at diagnosis is 45, which is several decades longer than that of fibroadenoma. These tumors are grossly well circumscribed but are infiltrative on microscopic examination. They are composed of benign glandular elements with a prominent stromal component showing varying degrees of hypercellularity, nuclear atypia, and mitotic activity (**Fig. 27.32**). The older term "cystosarcoma phyllodes" refers to the leaflike architectural pattern with intervening cystic spaces. While features such as size, mitotic activity, and cellular atypia correlate with clinical behavior, attempts to reliably divide these tumors into benign and malignant forms are not always successful. The lower grade tumors tend to recur, especially if incompletely excised due to the subtle infiltrative margin. Overall, lymph node metastases are uncommon and surgery is the primary treatment.

Angiosarcoma

Angiosarcoma is the most common primary sarcoma of the breast and may be associated with previous radiation therapy (RT). The tumors are composed of anastomosing vascular channels lined by endothelial cells, which range from mildly atypical to frankly malignant. The distinction between a benign angioma and a low-grade angiosarcoma can be difficult to determine on a small biopsy. Other histologic patterns of primary breast sarcoma also occur.

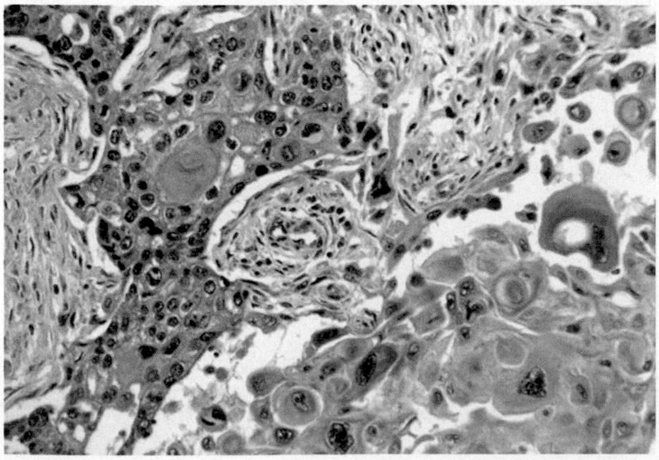

Figure 27.30. Metaplastic carcinoma. The area to the right of this poorly differentiated invasive breast carcinoma shows squamous differentiation.

REQUIRED TESTS ON BREAST CANCER

Measurement of ER in breast cancers is performed to predict the response of an invasive tumor to endocrine therapy or the benefit of hormonal therapy for risk reduction in cases of in situ carcinoma. Progesterone receptor (PR) is an ER-regulated gene product with similar prognostic implications. Hormone receptors can be measured biochemically by ligand-binding assays or by IHC techniques using monoclonal antibodies directed against the receptor protein (**Fig. 27.33**). Correlation between the two techniques is high (78). With today's smaller tumors usually diagnosed by needle core biopsy, IHC is the preferred method of analysis. This method also allows for the distinction between invasive tumor, in situ tumor, and nontumor elements. The American Society of Clinical Oncology (ASCO) and CAP published a joint guideline containing an algorithm for testing, interpretation, and reporting, as well as requirements for standardization and validation of testing techniques (79). Both the

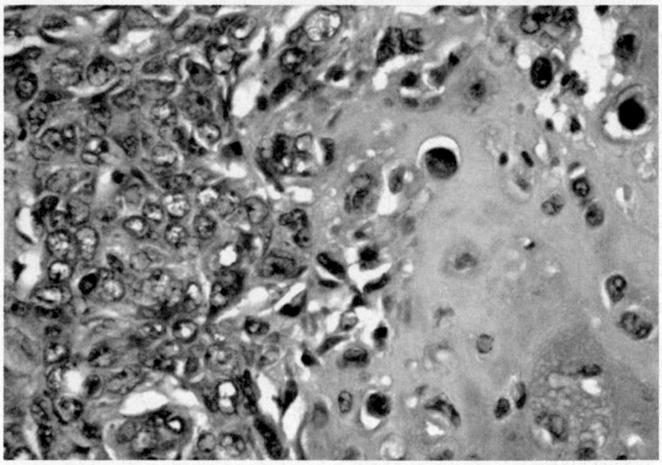

Figure 27.31. Metaplastic carcinoma. A well-developed cartilaginous focus is seen in this poorly differentiated invasive carcinoma with chondroid differentiation.

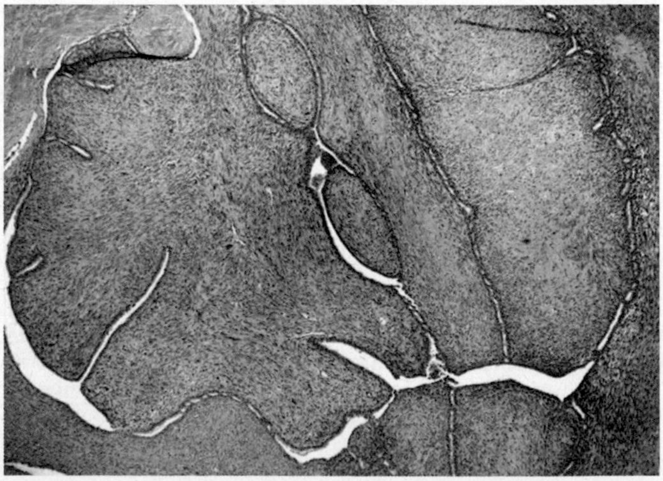

Figure 27.32. Phyllodes tumor. Phyllodes tumors have leaflike architectural pattern with intervening cystic spaces. They are composed of benign glandular elements with a prominent stroma showing varying degrees of hypercellularity, nuclear atypia, and mitotic activity.

percentage of cells stained and the intensity of the staining should be reported. A positive result is defined as greater that 1% of cell nuclei staining positive.

HER-2/neu

HER-2/neu, or c-erbB2, is an oncogene whose protein product is a membrane receptor tyrosine kinase. Overexpression of HER2 is associated in most, if not all, cases with the presence of additional copies of the gene that codes for the HER2 protein on chromosome 17. While the cause of this HER2 gene amplification, which is found only in the patient's breast cancer cells, is not understood, its biologic implications are clear—increased density of HER2 on the surface of the malignant cells leads to the formation of both homo- (HER2:HER2) and heterodimers with other members of the HER receptor family (HER1, HER3, and HER4), triggering activation of tyrosine kinases associated with the intracellular portions of the receptors, which in turn trigger a number of signaling pathways that enhance cancer cell growth and proliferation, resistance to apoptosis, and metastatic potential.

Amplification of HER-2/neu is seen in most cases of comedo-type DCIS and in approximately 20% to 30% of invasive ductal carcinomas, usually of high grade. It can be detected by IHC for the protein product or by gene amplification techniques, such as fluorescence in situ hybridization (FISH) or chromogenic in situ hybridization. Increased copy number is closely associated with elevated protein expression. Amplification of HER-2/neu identifies a subset of patients with a poor prognosis who benefit from treatment with trastuzumab, a monoclonal antibody directed against the HER-2/neu receptor.

The ASCO and the CAP defined criteria for HER2-positive (HER2+) breast cancer (80). These guidelines were revised in 2013 as follows: 1) at least 10% of the tumor's cells exhibit uniform intense membrane staining (3+) for HER2 by IHC stain (**Fig. 27.34**); or 2) their tumor cells display either an average of six or greater HER2 signals per cell; or 3) a ratio of HER2 to chromosome 17 (using a centromeric probe) (HER2/CEP17) signals by in situ hybridization (ISH) of ≥2 (regardless of HER2 copy number); or 4) HER2/CEP17 ratio <2 with an average HER2 copy number ≥6 per cell (**Fig. 27.35**).

Other Markers

Proliferation rate measured by flow cytometry (S-phase fraction), DNA image cytometry, or IHC (Ki67 MIB-1 antibody) has a relation to clinical outcome (81). However, these and other markers suffer from problems with standardization of results between laboratories (82).

Genomic Studies and Breast Cancer Subtypes

Molecular techniques have shown that breast cancer is a heterogeneous disease. Perou et al. (83) were the first to use gene expression profiling to classify breast cancers into distinct molecular groups based on the expression of distinct "intrinsic" genes. Luminal A tumors show high expression of ER and related genes, with low proliferation. Luminal B tumors also show expression of ER but have high proliferation and show variable expression of PR and HER2. The HER2-enriched group of tumors express the HER2 oncoprotein and related genes, with variable expression of hormone receptors. Basal-like tumors express basal (myoepithelial) markers like cytokeratin 5/6 and epidermal growth factor (EGFR), and typically lack expression of ER, PR, and HER2 (triple-negative tumors). This subgroup of tumors is the most frequent type found in BRCA1-associated breast cancer. The molecular subtyping of breast cancers has begun to identify unique therapeutic options for the different tumor types, and this remains an important area of therapeutic research (84).

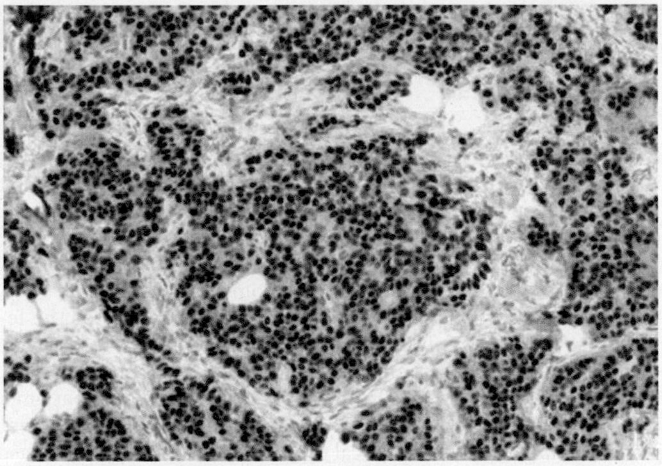

Figure 27.33. Positive ER. Greater than 90% of tumor cells of this invasive ductal carcinoma are strongly positive for ER.

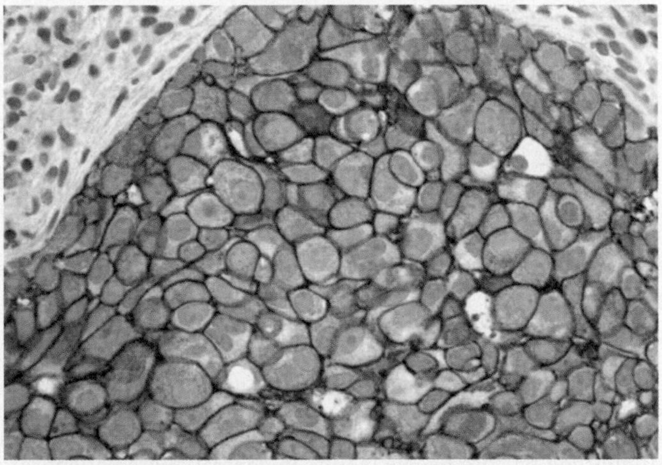

Figure 27.34. Positive HER-2/neu. Strong (3+) Her-2/neu membrane immunoreactivity is seen in this invasive ductal carcinoma.

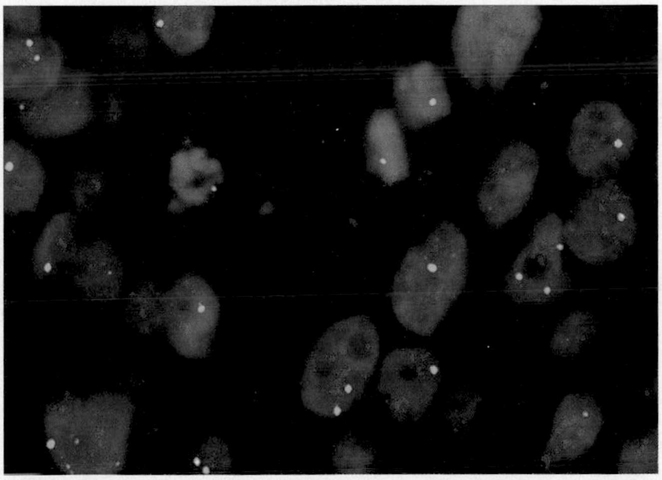

Figure 27.35. Amplification of HER-2/neu gene (*red dots*) by FISH. The centromere of chromosome 17 appears as green signals.

SURGICAL MANAGEMENT

In Situ Disease

In the past, DCIS was managed, like any breast cancer, by mastectomy. This was effective from a cancer point of view and resulted in a local recurrence rate of only 1% (85). However, current treatment mirrors the approach to early invasive breast cancer, and breast conservation therapy is the standard of care for most cases. It should be noted, however, there are no phase III studies comparing breast conservation therapy with total mastectomy in DCIS.

For women with DCIS, margin status and the size of the lesion appear to be significant factors related to risk of recurrence (86,87). Despite the use of breast-conserving treatment (BCT), some women may still require mastectomy, and for these patients, the indications for mastectomy for DCIS include: (1) persistent positive margins after wide local excision; (2) multicentric disease (i.e., DCIS involving more than one quadrant); and (3) a large tumor-to-breast size ratio for which breast-conserving surgery (BCS) would result in a personally defined cosmetically unacceptable result (88). All women who undergo mastectomy should also have a sentinel lymph node biopsy performed to ensure the absence of occult invasive disease.

While sentinel node biopsy is standard for women with DCIS undergoing mastectomy, it is not entirely clear if it plays a role in BCT. In the largest series looking at this issue, nodal involvement was seen in only 5% of cases; however, 70% of these metastases were detected only by IHC staining (89). In general, we typically consider lymphatic mapping for women with a span of DCIS greater than 4 cm or those who present with a mass on mammography. Other considerations include women with palpable DCIS, high-grade DCIS on core biopsy, and the presence (or question of) microinvasion.

Early Invasive Disease

Early invasive breast cancer, defined as tumors less than 2 cm in size, is almost uniformly diagnosed by imaging modalities (e.g., mammogram and/or breast US or MRI). The diagnosis is often established by core needle biopsy. In general, these patients are treated with wide local excision as part of BCT. Contraindications to this include multicentricity, a poor breast–tumor volume ratio, and women in whom RT is contraindicated (e.g., serious connective tissue disorders, pregnancy, or prior irradiation). Particular attention to the location of the tumor, its palpability, fixation to the skin or underlying chest wall, cutaneous changes, nipple irregularities, and regional nodal assessment are paramount.

The aim of BCS is to resect the primary tumor with clear margins. This can be achieved either with the needle localization technique or one of the other many techniques that have been described in the literature to localize the lesion, such as intraoperative US localization (90) or radioisotope-guided resection (91).

For women undergoing wide local excision, the ideal margin for breast cancer in a wide local excision continues to be a controversial topic. However, a consensus statement supported by both the Society of Surgical Oncology (SSO) and American Society of Therapeutic Radiation Oncology (ASTRO) and based on a meta-analysis of 33 studies, including more than 28,000 patients was released in 2014 (92). The report concluded that positive margins are associated with a two-fold increased risk in in-breast tumor recurrence (IBTR) rates, compared to negative margins. The risk is not altered by differences in biology, endocrine therapy, or a radiation boost. However, wider surgical margins do not significantly reduce the risk of IBTR, regardless of patient age, less favorable biology, or extensive intraductal component. Given these results, the consensus statement adopts an adequate margin when there is pathologically no evidence of invasive tumor at the surgically inked margin.

In 2015, Chagpar et al. (93) reported the results of a randomized trial evaluating the role of resecting additional tissue circumferentially around the tumor cavity (called cavity shaved margins) on outcomes in more than 200 women undergoing BCS (i.e., partial mastectomy) for stage 0 to III breast cancer. The median age of the patients was 61 years (range, 33 to 94). Of those enrolled, 23%, 19%, and 53% had invasive cancer, DCIS alone, or both, respectively. Compared to those who did not undergo shaved margins, shave margins resulted in a significantly lower rate of positive margins (19% vs. 34%, $p = 0.01$) and were subjected to less second surgical procedures (10% vs. 21%, $p = 0.02$).

Locally Advanced Breast Cancer

Locally advanced breast cancer (LABC) is variously defined, though reasonable definitions include patients with a primary tumor size greater than 3 to 5 cm, involvement of the chest wall, skin ulceration or satellitosis, and/or positive axillary nodes. For these patients, the evolving standard is to offer neoadjuvant therapy prior to any planned surgical treatment. From a surgical standpoint, neoadjuvant treatment is associated with a higher rate of breast conservation, without a reduction in either disease-free survival (DFS) or OS, without an increase in the complication rate of surgery, and without delay in onset of further postoperative treatment (94). The use of NACT does result in a 30% to 40% decrease in the incidence of axillary nodal involvement and up to a 20% complete response rate in responding patients (95–97).

Approximately 25% of patients who are not candidates for breast conservation before treatment will be candidates for BCT after the administration of NACT. All patients considered for NACT should undergo an axillary evaluation to help establish the nodal stage. For women with clinically evident nodal disease, a needle biopsy can be performed, with either axillary US with needle biopsy, or sentinel node biopsy in nonpalpable disease. For women with clinically negative axillary examination, further workup is necessary, because clinical examination is associated with a false-negative rate in excess of 20%. US with fine needle aspiration cytology of suspicious nodes has a reported sensitivity and specificity of 36% to 92% and 69% to 100%, respectively (98,99).

For women with no evidence of axillary node involvement prior to NACT, sentinel node biopsy is often used in this population, although the timing remains controversial. Mamounas (100) reviewed the experience of the National Surgical Adjuvant Breast and Bowel Project (NSABP) B-27 clinical trial and reported that a sentinel lymph node can be identified in 85% and is falsely negative in 11%, confirming that sentinel node biopsy after NACT is both feasible and accurate. Of interest, they also reported that 30% to 40% of patients with a positive sentinel node biopsy before neoadjuvant therapy are downstaged after treatment and may not require axillary dissection.

For patients treated with neoadjuvant therapy, clinical and radiologic assessment should be performed following the completion of 2 to 3 cycles (**Fig. 27.36**). For those patients who are candidates or otherwise opt to proceed with surgery, a decision to proceed with mastectomy or BCS depends on clinical factors. The contraindications for breast conservation in this setting are similar to those for primary BCT and include residual tumor >5 cm, skin edema or involvement, chest wall fixation, diffuse calcifications on mammogram (obtained posttreatment), multicentric disease, and contraindications to RT.

Early consultations with both plastic surgery and radiation oncology should be performed in patients undergoing mastectomy who express an interest in immediate reconstruction, preferably before any surgery takes place. Immediate reconstruction can be associated with a slightly higher rate of complications, which may result in a delay in postoperative treatment. In addition, those who undergo RT may experience issues with cosmesis.

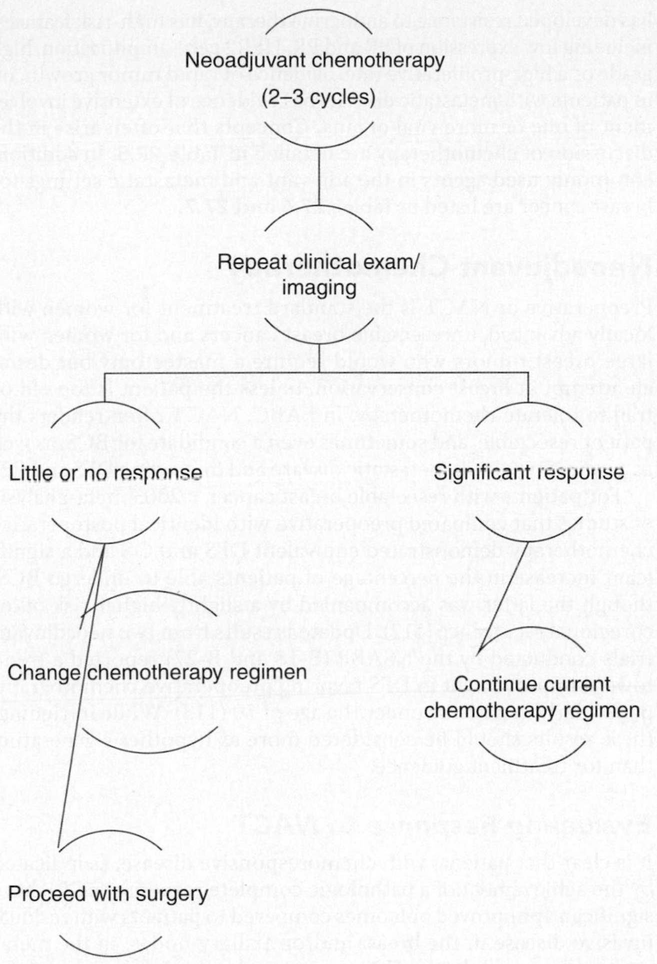

Figure 27.36. Neoadjuvant treatment of breast cancer: an algorithm.

Management of the Axilla

Women without clinical evidence of axillary involvement from invasive breast cancer are managed with a sentinel node biopsy to stage the axilla. In contrast, a complete axillary lymph node dissection (ALND) is indicated in the following situations: node-positive disease at presentation; IBC; clinical stage T4 breast cancer; failed sentinel node mapping during surgery; and axillary recurrence after prior breast cancer treatment. The NSABP B-32 trial evaluated the impact of sentinel node biopsy with or without ALND in more than 5,600 women, almost 4,000 of whom had pathologically node-negative disease (101). Compared to women who underwent both procedures, there was no difference in OS in those undergoing sentinel node biopsy alone (HR 1.20, 95% CI 96 to 1.5), and 8-year OS rate estimates were 90% and 92% in the sentinel node–only group and the combined procedure group, respectively. There was also no difference in DFS or regional node recurrences as first events (14 vs. 8, respectively).

Traditionally, all patients with a positive sentinel node biopsy underwent an ALND. However, contemporary clinical trials have challenged this paradigm. The American College of Surgeons Oncology Group Z-0011 study (Z11 study) was designed to determine whether ALND was necessary for survival or local control in the setting of BCS with whole breast irradiation and adjuvant systemic therapy in patients with SLN metastases, specifically with one to two positive sentinel nodes (102). This phase 3 study prospectively enrolled 891 patients with T1-2 tumors and a clinically negative axilla undergoing BCT with whole breast radiation. In this group, patients with one to two positive sentinel nodes identified at surgery were randomized to undergo ALND or no further treatment. With a median follow-up of 6.3 years, the OS rate was 91.8% in the ALND group versus 92.5% in the sentinel node biopsy group alone. The rate of nodal recurrence in the sentinel node-only arm was 0.4% and 0.9%, respectively. There was no significant difference in OS or locoregional recurrence between the two groups, despite a 27% rate of pathologic node involvement among the group who underwent ALND. Of note, all patients received whole breast radiation (third field nodal irradiation was not allowed), and the overwhelming majority received adjuvant systemic therapy (96% in ALND arm and 97% in sentinel node biopsy arm). In addition, the study did not include patients who received NACT or underwent mastectomy.

The International Breast Cancer Study Group (IBCSG) 23-01 evaluated 931 patients, of whom 464 underwent ALND and 467 did not (103). Ninety-one percent of patients in both groups underwent BCS and 9% underwent mastectomy. The purpose of the multicenter randomized controlled trial was to identify whether ALND might be overtreatment in patients who have micrometastases only in the sentinel node. The enrollment eligibility criteria was broadened to include tumors ≤5 cm and one or more micrometastases (<2 mm) in the sentinel nodes, multifocal or multicentric tumors. At median follow-up of 5 years, there was no difference in DFS or OS between the arms, despite a 13% pathologic finding of positive nonsentinel nodes in those who underwent ALND. The rate of regional recurrence in the no-ALND arm was <1%, comparable to findings of other studies.

Lastly, the EORTC 10981–22023 AMAROS (After mapping of the Axilla: Radiotherapy or Surgery) trial was a randomized, multicenter, open-label phase 3, noninferiority trial that evaluated radiotherapy versus surgery of the axilla after positive sentinel node biopsy (104). In this analysis, 17% underwent mastectomy in the ALND group and 18% underwent mastectomy in the axillary radiotherapy group. Eighty-two percent underwent BCS in both groups. A median of two sentinel nodes was excised in both groups, and a median of one sentinel node was positive, of which 59% had macrometastasis in the ALND group and 62% had macrometastasis in the axillary radiotherapy arm. The results showed no significant difference between the two groups (ALND vs. axillary radiotherapy) in 5-year axillary recurrence, DFS, and OS. There was a higher incidence of lymphedema and more severe symptoms of lymphedema in the dissected group.

Technique of Axillary Lymph Node Dissection

In the United States, standard practice for ALND requires removal of level I and level II lymph nodes. Level I is defined as nodal tissue lateral to the pectoralis minor muscle, and level II is defined as nodal tissue posterior to the pectoralis minor muscle. Level III nodes (nodal tissue medial to the pectoralis minor muscle) are generally not included in the dissection due to increased morbidity. Retrieval of level III nodes requires transection of the pectoralis minor muscle. Interpectoral nodes (Rotter nodes) should be removed if suspicious. At minimum, 10 nodes should be retrieved during the procedure. The axilla is bounded by the axillary vein superiorly, the serratus anterior muscle medially, the latissimus dorsi muscle laterally, the subscapularis muscle posteriorly, and the clavipectoral fascia anteriorly. The thoracodorsal nerve to the latissimus muscle and the long thoracic nerve to the serratus anterior muscle is preserved. If possible, the main trunk of the intercostobrachial nerve is also preserved to decrease the risk of arm paresthesias. The risk of lymphedema with this procedure is quoted at 6% to 50% (105,106).

Sentinel Lymph Node Biopsy

The sentinel lymph node biopsy is performed using radioactive colloid material (technetium 99), blue dye (methylene blue or lymphazurin blue), or a combination of both. Using both the radioactive colloid and the blue dye increases the identification rate to 95%. The sentinel lymph node identification rate with a periareolar/subareolar injection of the radiocolloid and blue dye injection is higher than that with a peritumoral injection. The radioactive colloid is typically injected in the Nuclear Medicine department, and a lymphoscintigram, which shows the lymphatic drainage pattern of the tumor, is obtained. The vast majority of drainage is in the ipsilateral axilla. Additionally, blue dye is injected prior to surgery. During the surgery, a separate axillary incision is made to perform the procedure. Dissection includes incising the clavipectoral fascia to enter the axilla. The axilla is interrogated with a handheld gamma probe to identify sentinel node(s). The sentinel node can be "hot," "blue," or "hot and blue." The radiotracer facilitates identification by emitting high activity sound ("hot node"), and the blue dye stains the node, assisting in the visualization of the sentinel node ("blue node"). The node is carefully dissected from the surrounding tissue. Each sentinel node is excised and counted over 10 seconds. For sentinel lymph node identification with radioactivity, the node with counts greater than the 10% of the most radioactive node is excised. If blue dye is used, any blue node or node with an adjacent blue-stained lymphatic is a sentinel node. Before completion of the procedure, the axilla is palpated for any grossly abnormal nodes, as false negativity is common with nodes replaced by tumor.

An anatomical description by Clough divided the axilla into four zones, separated by the lateral thoracic vein and the second intercostal brachial nerve. In this scheme, in 242 stageI/II breast cancer patients, the sentinel node was identified medial to the vein 98.2% of the time, usually below the nerve (86.8%.) The upper lateral zone, adjacent to the lymphatic drainage of the arm, never contained the sentinel node (107). The lower axilla is the most common location of the sentinel node(s). While lymphatic mapping to the IM chain has been performed, its impact on outcome remains unclear.

Intraoperative assessment of sentinel lymph nodes using touch imprints and routine IHC staining is used by some to enable an immediate therapeutic lymphadenectomy if the nodes are positive, thus sparing the patient from a second procedure. However, intraoperative assessment may have unacceptable rates of false-negative results, ranging from 36% to 71% (108).

Oncoplastic Surgery

Immediate reconstruction after mastectomy is safe from an oncologic perspective and beneficial to a patient's well-being. A more ideal technique of complete resection of the breast with preservation of the unaffected structures was primarily championed by Simmons et al. (109). They compared recurrence patterns in women treated by skin-sparing mastectomy (SSM) versus non-SSM and demonstrated local recurrence rates of 3.90% and 3.25%, respectively, with an equivalent distant recurrence rate of 3.9% at 5 years. A subsequent 2010 meta-analysis of SSM/nipple areolar sparing mastectomy (NSM) versus non-SSM confirmed these findings, reporting equivalent local recurrence rates (6.2% vs. 4.0%) regardless of technique, with a follow-up of 37.5 to 101 months (110). This technique has been extended to patients with more advanced disease treated with NACT.

While the reconstructed breast has proved to appear more natural, the desire for improved breast conservation remains paramount, with a goal of providing not only the greatest assurance of nipple-areolar function, but to a lesser extent, minimizing the sense of loss by the patient. Adopting techniques from breast reduction, breast surgeons have now expanded their armamentarium in achieving cosmetically desirable lumpectomy. Incorporation of breast reduction or mastopexy with lumpectomy has yielded successful results that translate into improved cosmetic outcome for patients with either macromastia or ptotic breasts. More recently, an array of techniques has been developed that utilize simple reshaping or local tissue transfer to diminish skin retraction post lumpectomy (111). The essential goal of oncoplastic surgery is greater attainment of clear margins, reduced reexcision and mastectomy, and ultimately, improved patient satisfaction and well-being.

SYSTEMIC THERAPY

Cytotoxic chemotherapy and biologic agents against HER2 are commonly given to patients with early- and advanced-stage breast cancer whose disease is either hormone-insensitive (ER- and PR-negative), has developed resistance to endocrine therapy, has high-risk features, including low expression of ER and PR, HER2 gene amplification, high grade or a high proliferative rate, evidence of rapid tumor growth, or, in patients with metastatic disease, has evidence of extensive involvement of one or more vital organs. Concepts that often arise in the discussion of chemotherapy are detailed in **Table 27.5**. In addition, commonly used agents in the adjuvant and metastatic settings for breast cancer are listed in **Tables 27.6 and 27.7**.

Neoadjuvant Chemotherapy

Preoperative or NACT is the standard treatment for women with locally advanced, unresectable breast cancers and for women with large breast tumors who would require a mastectomy but desire an attempt at breast conservation, unless the patient is too old or frail to tolerate chemotherapy. In LABC, NACT often renders the patient resectable, and sometimes even a candidate for BCS, as well as eradicating occult metastatic disease and improving DFS and OS.

For patients with resectable breast cancer, a 2005 meta-analysis of studies that compared preoperative with identical postoperative chemotherapy demonstrated equivalent DFS and OS and a significant increase in the percentage of patients able to undergo BCS, though the latter was accompanied by a slightly higher risk of locoregional recurrence (112). Updated results from two neoadjuvant trials conducted by the NSABP (B-18 and B-27) reported a trend toward improvement in DFS favoring preoperative chemotherapy, particularly in patients under the age of 50 (113). While intriguing, these results should be considered more as hypothesis generating than for treatment guidance.

Evaluating Response to NACT

It is clear that patients with chemoresponsive disease, as indicated by the achievement of a pathologic complete response (pCR), have significantly improved outcomes compared to patients with residual invasive disease in the breast and/or axillary nodes; in the meta-analysis discussed above, pCR was associated with 52% improvements in both DFS and OS (112). However, the optimal method to assess response to NACT is controversial.

■ TABLE 27.5. Concepts around Chemotherapy for Breast Cancer

Dose intensity	For many chemotherapeutic agents, higher drug concentrations result in increased killing of cancer cells in vitro (or a dose–response curve). However, it is not entirely clear that increasing dose improves outcomes in breast cancer. For example, high-dose therapy with autologous hematopoietic stem cell transplantation appeared promising in early trials, but this was not borne out in randomized trials and has since been abandoned.
Dose density	The administration of similar or lower doses of one or more agents more frequently. This often allows administration of a higher overall dose of a drug with less toxicity, and also may increase the drug's cytotoxic effects by increasing the likelihood of catching a higher proportion of cancer cells in the most vulnerable phases of their cell cycle.
Non–cross-resistant drug combinations	Using agents, either concurrently or sequentially, with different mechanisms of action, different mechanisms of drug resistance, and, when possible, nonoverlapping toxicities. Switching to a non–cross-resistant drug or regimen may improve response, even when the patient is responding to the initial regimen.

TABLE 27.6. Agents Used in the Treatment of Breast Cancer

Adjuvant or Neoadjuvant Setting	Metastatic Setting
Anthracyclines • Doxorubicin + Cyclophosphamide (AC) • Epirubicin + Cyclophosphamide (EC)	Anthracyclines • Doxorubicin or Epirubicin • Liposomal Doxorubicin
Taxanes • Paclitaxel (weekly, every 2 weeks) • Docetaxel (every 3 weeks)	Taxanes and other Microtubulin Targeted agents • Paclitaxel • Docetaxel • nAb-paclitaxel • Ixabepilone • Eribulin • Vinorelbine
Cyclophosphamide (IV)	Cyclophosphamide (Oral)
Fluoropyrimidines • 5-FU in combination with Cyclophosphamide and Methotrexate (CMF)	Fluoropyrimidines • 5FU • Capecitabine
Platinum agents • Carboplatin	Platinum agents • Carboplatin • Cisplatin
HER2-directed agents • Trastuzumab • Pertuzumab	HER2-directed agents • Trastuzumab • Pertuzumab • Ado-Trastuzumab Emtansine • Lapatinib
Endocrine therapy • Tamoxifen • Aromatase inhibitors • GnRH Analogs	Endocrine therapy • Tamoxifen • Aromatase inhibitors • Fulvestrant • GnRH Analogs
	CDK Inhibitors • Palbociclib + Letrozole
	mTOR Inhibitors • Everolimus + Exemestane
	Gemcitabine Etoposide

TABLE 27.7. Acceptable Regimens for Breast Cancer[a]

Doxorubicin + Cyclophosphamide (AC, every 2 weeks)	AC→Paclitaxel (weekly × 12)
AC→Docetaxel (every 3 weeks)	Docetaxel + Cyclophosphamide (TC)
Cyclophosphamide, Methotrexate, 5-Fluorouracil (CMF)	Carboplatin + Docetaxel[b]

[a]All regimens can be combined with trastuzumab for HER2-positive breast cancer treatment.

[b]Typically reserved for HER2-positive breast cancers, in combination with Trastuzumab.

In patients with visible or palpable disease, response (or lack thereof) can often be assessed on physical examination. Sequential imaging studies (discussed earlier) can usually indicate whether a patient is responding or not, though occasionally clinically "stable" tumors will prove to be largely or totally replaced with fibrous tissue. However, imaging can be relatively insensitive for assessing the breast and axilla for microscopic disease following resolution of any visible tumor mass or abnormal nodes.

The NSABP utilized a definition of pCR that required the absence of invasive disease in the breast, irrespective of the presence of any residual disease in the axillary nodes (113). In addition, others have reported that the presence of residual DCIS in the breast, in the absence of residual invasive disease, had no impact on survival outcomes (114). Despite these reports, it has become clear that persistent disease in the axillary nodes is associated with higher recurrence rates, while conversion from node-positive to node-negative disease with NACT indicates a good prognosis (115). On the basis of these findings, most contemporary US studies use the absence of invasive disease in the breast **and** axilla (ypT0/isN0) as their definition of pCR.

However, one analysis suggests that breast cancer subtype matters when employing a definition of pCR (116). Using a more stringent definition of pCR that included the absence of either invasive or in situ disease in the breast and negative lymph nodes, pCR was found to correlate with prognosis (measured by both DFS and OS) only in patients with more aggressive cancers (e.g., TNBC, ER-/HER2 positive, and atypical ER-positive tumors), but not in those ER-positive (luminal A) breast cancers. Despite the finding that patients with less aggressive cancers were also less likely to obtain a pCR, they had similar outcomes whether or not they achieved one.

Other investigators suggest that extent of residual disease after NACT may be prognostic in the absence of a pCR. European investigators have used a number of scoring systems, the best known of which is the Miller/Payne grading system, to assess post-NACT pathologic specimens for both residual disease and chemotherapy response, and the results of which have been shown to correlate with DFS and OS (117). In the United States, Symmans and colleagues (118) reported that the size and cellularity of residual invasive disease in the breast and number and size of metastatic deposits in the axillary nodes predicted distant recurrence. These variables are incorporated into a formula called the patient's Residual Cancer Burden (RCB). Of interest, patients with minimal residual disease (RCB-I) appear to be at no greater risk of distant disease recurrence than patients with a pCR (RCB-0), while patients with more extensive residual disease (RCB-II and -III) are at much greater risk of recurrence, especially if their tumor is hormone receptor-negative. RCB analyses have been incorporated into a number of NACT studies, both to stratify non-pCR responses and to validate this methodology.

NACT Regimens

A general principle regarding NACT regimens is that chemotherapeutic agents that have proven effectiveness in the adjuvant setting should have similar efficacy against disease in the breast and axillary nodes as well as occult metastatic disease in the neoadjuvant setting. Thus, there is no reason to use different regimens based on when the chemotherapy is given with respect to surgery. The choice of specific chemotherapy drugs and regimens should be based on our understanding of therapy response as related to tumor biology and patient subsets and is similar to the considerations on the approach to adjuvant treatment.

What to do for patients who are not responding to NACT is unknown. In one trial, patients not responding after four cycles of the anthracycline-based regimen were switched to docetaxel, and while 55% had a clinical response to the taxane, their pCR rate was only 2%, and their 3-year survival was markedly inferior to the responsive patients (119). In the GeparTrio trial, patients who did not respond with at least a 50% reduction in tumor size after two cycles of TAC were randomly assigned to either four more cycles of TAC or four cycles of vinorelbine and capecitabine (NX) every 21 days (120). While both groups of patients had similar clinical response (51%) and pCR (5% to 6%) rates, a recent update of the trial reported that patients switched to NX demonstrated significant (41%) improvement in DFS compared to patients who continued on TAC. Meanwhile, patients responding after two cycles of TAC were randomized to four or six more cycles of the same regimen, and while the longer treatment duration had only a modest impact on the pCR rate (24% vs. 21%), it did result in significant improvement in DFS.

Treatment for patients who go to surgery after NACT and are found to have significant residual disease is based on their tumor type. Patients with ER-positive tumors typically receive adjuvant endocrine therapy, while patients with HER2+ cancers receive trastuzumab. For all others, there is no evidence that administration of additional chemotherapy, sometimes referred to as "adjuvant after neoadjuvant," in a patient who has received both an anthracycline and a taxane in the preoperative setting will reduce recurrences. As such, adjuvant treatment in these patients is usually not recommended.

HER2-Positive Disease

Given the rapid growth kinetics of HER2+ breast cancers, it is not surprising that a significant percentage of patients with these cancers present with large tumors or locally advanced disease, making them good candidates for neoadjuvant therapy. While the percentage of patients with HER2+ cancers who achieve a pCR with NACT alone, especially those with hormone receptor-negative/HER2+ disease, is relatively high, blocking HER2 signaling clearly enhances the chemosensitivity of HER2+ breast cancers. An analysis of two randomized trials demonstrated significant improvements in pCR rates with the addition of trastuzumab to chemotherapy versus chemotherapy alone (RR 2.07, 95% CI 1.41 to 3.03) (121). Combining trastuzumab with chemotherapy was also associated with a reduction in the relapse rate (26% vs. 39%, 95% CI 0.48 to 0.94) and a trend toward improvement in the risk of death (13% vs. 20% mortality rate).

Given concerns about the risk of cardiac dysfunction associated with concomitant administration of an anthracycline and trastuzumab, combining these agents is typically avoided until further data on the safety of that approach becomes available. Our standard neoadjuvant regimen for a HER2+ patient includes four cycles of doxorubicin and cyclophosphamide (AC) administered every 2 or 3 weeks followed by 12 weeks of weekly paclitaxel plus trastuzumab. It is important to remember that following surgery, all patients should then continue on single-agent trastuzumab to complete a full year of the biologic treatment. Other appropriate neoadjuvant regimens for patients with HER2+ cancers include those used in the adjuvant treatment setting (**Table 27.6**).

There is continued interest in the administration of dual HER2-targeted treatments together with NACT to overcome potential trastuzumab resistance. The NeoAdjuvant Lapatinib and/or Trastuzumab Treatment Optimization (Neo-ALTTO) trial randomly assigned 453 women with stage II–III HER2+ breast cancers to lapatinib 1,500 mg daily, trastuzumab, or the combination of trastuzumab and lapatinib 1,000 mg daily (122). Patients received 6 weeks of HER2-targeted therapy alone, followed by 12 weeks of weekly paclitaxel (80 mg/m^2) along with their assigned HER2-targeted treatment, then underwent surgery. Compared to those patients treated with trastuzumab or lapatanib alone, those who were treated with both drugs experienced a significantly higher clinical response rate at the end of treatment (67% vs. 30% and 52%, respectively), which was confirmed at the time of surgery (80% vs. 71% and 74%). In addition, these patients had a higher pCR rate (51% vs. 30% and 25%), although it was not reflected by the proportion of patients treated with BCS (41% vs. 39% and 43%).

The NeoSPHERE trial was an open-label randomized phase II trial that enrolled 417 women with operable, locally advanced, or inflammatory HER2+ breast cancer and randomly assigned them to 12 weeks of treatment using one of four regimens: docetaxel (100 mg/m^2 every 3 weeks for four cycles) plus trastuzumab (group A), docetaxel plus trastuzumab and pertuzumab (group B), pertuzumab plus trastuzumab alone (group C), or docetaxel plus pertuzumab (group D) (123). After surgery, patients on the docetaxel arms received three cycles of 5-fluorouracil, epirubicin, and cyclophosphamide (FEC) and completed a year of trastuzumab, while patients in group C received both docetaxel and FEC followed by trastuzumab. The pCR rates were 29%, 46%, 17%, and 24% in groups A, B, C, and D, respectively. Compared to women with hormone-receptor–positive disease, the pCR rates were generally higher in women with hormone-receptor–negative tumors. Serious (grade 3/4) adverse events in patients treated with docetaxel (groups A, B, and D) included neutropenia, febrile neutropenia, and diarrhea. The addition of pertuzumab to the docetaxel plus trastuzumab combination did not appear to increase toxicity, including cardiac adverse events. These results are fascinating not only because of the higher pCR rate seen on the chemotherapy plus trastuzumab and pertuzumab arm, but also because of the frequency of pCRs associated with dual HER2-targeted therapy alone, raising the intriguing possibility that there may be a subset of HER2+ patients who can be effectively treated without the toxic effects of chemotherapy.

Adjuvant Chemotherapy

The Early Breast Cancer Trialists' Collaborative Group (EBCTCG) published an update on the role of adjuvant chemotherapy in early-stage breast cancer in 2012, and for the first time added an analysis of the benefits of the addition of a taxane (paclitaxel or docetaxel), concurrently or sequentially, to anthracycline-based adjuvant chemotherapy (124). In older trials that included a no-chemotherapy arm, administration of anthracycline-based adjuvant chemotherapy reduced breast cancer recurrences by 27%, resulting in an absolute improvement in the 10-year recurrence rate of 8% (39.4% vs. 47.4%), a 6.5% reduction in breast cancer–related mortality, and a 5% improvement in overall mortality. Chemotherapy regimens that included six cycles of cyclophosphamide with standard doses of either doxorubicin or epirubicin and 5-fluorouracil (CAF or CEF) resulted in larger relative improvements in OS (36%) than regimens in which patients received just four cycles of standard-dose doxorubicin or epirubicin with cyclophosphamide (AC or EC) (22%). Compared to nonchemotherapy controls, administration of cyclophosphamide, methotrexate, 5-fluorouracil (CMF) was associated with a 30% relative reduction in breast cancer recurrence (29.6% vs. 39.8%), which resulted in a 6.2% improvement in breast cancer mortality and a 4.7% improvement in overall mortality. All of these results were highly statistically significant due to the large numbers of women involved (8,575 women in the anthracycline-based trials, 5,253 in the CMF trials). The difference in the outcomes for the control groups likely reflects different patient populations, with only 18% of patients treated on the anthracycline-based trials having node-negative cancers compared to 66% on the CMF trials. Benefits from chemotherapy were essentially equivalent across multiple patient subgroups, including age, node status, hormone receptor status, and tumor grade, and administration of adjuvant endocrine therapy (tamoxifen) did not reduce the benefit of receiving adjuvant chemotherapy.

A number of studies have compared anthracycline-based regimens with standard or near-standard CMF. Studies on which patients (9,527 women, of whom 53% were node-positive) received higher cumulative doses of anthracycline (such as six cycles of CAF or CEF) demonstrated superiority of anthracycline-based therapy, with a relative 11% reduction in breast cancer recurrences, corresponding to a 2.6% absolute benefit, a 20% reduction in breast cancer mortality (4.1% absolute), and a 16% reduction in overall mortality (3.9% absolute). In contrast, studies that compared briefer anthracycline-based regimens, such as four cycles of AC or EC to CMF (5,122 women, of whom 61% were node-positive), failed to show improvement in outcomes.

With regard to the benefits of adding a taxane to anthracycline-based adjuvant chemotherapy, the recent meta-analysis identified an overall relative reduction rate in breast cancer recurrence of 14%, breast cancer mortality of 13%, and overall mortality of 11%. Studies in which the taxane was added to an anthracycline regimen of standard duration demonstrated the greatest benefit for the new class of agents, including a 16% reduction in recurrences (4.6% absolute), 14% improvement in breast cancer mortality (2.8% absolute), and 14% improvement in overall mortality (3.2% absolute), while studies in which patients on the nontaxane arm continued on their anthracycline-based regimen to match the duration of treatment of patients assigned to receive the taxane failed to show significant improvements in outcomes. The aggregate results were consistent across age groups, nodal status, and hormone receptor status. In the majority of studies included in the 2012 meta-analysis, the taxane (whether paclitaxel or docetaxel) was administered q3weeks, thus potentially underestimating the benefits of dose-dense q2week or weekly paclitaxel.

A meta-analysis of 10 trials that compared standard versus dose-dense adjuvant chemotherapy reported that dose-dense treatment was associated with relative improvements in DFS (17% to 19%) and OS (15% to 16%), whether the dose-dense regimen used similar or modified chemotherapy doses compared to the control regimen. However, this difference was seen only in patients with ER-negative cancers (in whom the DFS benefit was 29%), not in patients with ER-positive cancers (8% benefit, which did not reach statistical significance).

HER2-Negative Disease

For patients with hormone receptor-negative (or triple-negative) breast cancer, adjuvant chemotherapy is often indicated, especially if the tumor size is greater than 10 mm, and regardless of nodal status.

However, for patients with hormone receptor-positive disease, the role of chemotherapy should be individualized, taking into account the substantial risk reduction expected from adjuvant endocrine therapy. Genomic tools are now available to identify patients likely to do well with adjuvant endocrine therapy alone from those who would be expected to receive greater relative benefit from the addition of chemotherapy. Of those available, perhaps the one most widely used in the United States is the Onco*type* DX assay, which is a PCR-based array that measures gene expression by mRNA for a total of 16 cancer-related genes, some of which reflect its level of estrogen stimulation (and thus likely sensitivity to endocrine therapies) and some of which correlate with cell proliferation and metastasis (associated with relative insensitivity to endocrine therapies and potential greater benefit from chemotherapy), relative to five "housekeeping" genes. Paik and colleagues (125) demonstrated that the recurrence score (RS) derived from the levels of expression of these genes is both prognostic for risk of recurrence in untreated patients and predictive of degree of risk reduction achieved with endocrine therapy (specifically tamoxifen) and CMF chemotherapy.

The prognostic significance of a low score among patients with node-negative breast cancer was recently shown in a prospective trial in which more than 1,600 patients with a low RS (≤10) were directed toward observation (126). At 5 years, the rate of survival from invasive breast cancer was 94% and greater than 99% remained free from breast cancer recurrence. OS in this population at 4 years was 98%. Further results from this trial will inform the benefits of adjuvant chemotherapy among women with higher RS. More limited data support its use in patients with a limited number (1 to 3) of involved axillary nodes (127), and this is being tested in an ongoing trial, RxPONDER (SWOG 1007, NCT01272037).

MammaPrint is a microarray-based gene expression assay that measures mRNA levels for 70 genes that reflect tumor proliferation, invasion, and angiogenesis. The score derived from this assay has been shown to be prognostic of risk of recurrence in patients with ER-positive, node-negative cancers (128), but it has not yet demonstrated the ability to predict benefit from the addition of adjuvant chemotherapy to endocrine therapy. This assay is also being studied in a prospective clinical trial called MINDACT (Microarray in Node-Negative Disease May Avoid Chemotherapy, NCT00433589), which is designed to determine if patients with ER-positive disease with 0 to 3 involved lymph nodes considered higher risk by clinical features but low risk by MammaPrint can be spared chemotherapy.

Several contemporary clinical trials have broadened the options for adjuvant chemotherapy in women deemed to be at sufficient risk of recurrence. The U.S. Oncology Trial 9735 enrolled more than 1,000 women (greater than 50% with node-positive disease and greater than 70% with ER-positive disease) and randomly assigned treatment with AC or docetaxel and cyclophosphamide (TC) every 3 weeks for four cycles (129). At a median of 7 years' follow-up, TC remained superior to AC, with a 26% improvement in DFS, which translated into a 6% absolute increase, and a 31% rise in OS (5% absolute benefit). The DFS benefit was apparent independent of age, nodal status, and hormone receptor status (though not statistically significant in the subgroups). Short-term toxicities were comparable across the two arms of the study, but four patients on the AC arm have died of possible late complications of treatment, one with congestive heart failure and three with leukemia or myelodysplasia. Though of relatively modest size, this study has had a major impact on the treatment of patients with low- to intermediate-risk disease in the United States, presumably due to the appeal of avoiding exposure to an anthracycline without (apparently) sacrificing efficacy. In the NSABP B-38 trial, almost 5,000 women with node-positive, early-stage breast cancer were randomly assigned to one of three regimens: dose-dense AC followed by dose-dense paclitaxel (AC-T), dose-dense AC followed by paclitaxel plus gemcitabine (AC-TG), or a three-drug combination of docetaxel plus AC (TAC) (130). There were no significant differences in either DFS or OS at 5 years between any of the regimens. However, TAC was associated with significantly higher rates of febrile neutropenia (9% vs. 3% with AC-T and AC-TG). The regimens with paclitaxel, on the other hand, were associated with higher rates of neuropathy.

HER2-Positive Disease

The goal of HER2-directed therapy is to block this activation, which also has the effect of enhancing sensitivity to other antitumor treatments. It is now widely indicated in the adjuvant context based on seminal results from three randomized trials that consistently demonstrated substantial improvements in DFS and OS with the addition of trastuzumab during or after standard adjuvant chemotherapy (**Table 27.8**) (131–135).

For HER2+ patients in whom chemotherapy is recommended, and provided they have no contraindication to administration of an anthracycline (no characteristics suggesting an increased risk of significant cardiotoxicity), we administer doxorubicin plus cyclophosphamide for four cycles (AC) followed by weekly paclitaxel for 12 weeks. We administer trastuzumab weekly with paclitaxel, but once completed, trastuzumab is administered every 3 weeks to complete 1 year. For patients with any contraindication to treatment with an anthracycline, or for those who, after discussing treatment alternatives, opt not to receive an anthracycline, combining trastuzumab with a nonanthracycline regimen, such as docetaxel plus carboplatin (TC) is an option.

Given concerns about the incidence of cardiotoxicity seen in patients with HER2+ MBC who received both an anthracycline and trastuzumab, and the demonstrated synergy between trastuzumab and a variety of chemotherapeutic agents in vitro, the Breast Cancer International Research Group (BCIRG) 006 trial was designed to test the efficacy and toxicity of a nonanthracycline–based chemotherapy regimen plus trastuzumab against a standard anthracycline-based chemotherapy regimen with or without trastuzumab (**Table 27.8**) (131). The use of carboplatin alongside docetaxel and trastuzumab (TCH) was associated with a lower rate of congestive heart failure (0.4%) compared to arms containing doxorubicin (0.4% vs. 0.7% and 2% with AC→D or AC→DTr, respectively), and was also associated with a lower likelihood of a sustained drop in left ventricular ejection fraction (9.4% vs. 11.2% and 18.6%, respectively). In addition to reducing cardiac toxicity, dropping the anthracycline reduced vomiting and mucositis, and appeared to markedly reduce, if not eliminate, the small but real risk (0.33% in patients on AC-T or AC-TH) of developing a treatment-related leukemia.

As with patients treated with anthracyclines, all patients receiving trastuzumab should have cardiac function evaluated prior to starting chemotherapy and prior to starting trastuzumab, after which cardiac monitoring should be individualized based on patient age, baseline ejection fraction, and risk factors for developing cardiac dysfunction. At our institution, we utilize echocardiograms for this purpose. Guidelines from the National Comprehensive Cancer

■ TABLE 27.8. Adjuvant Trials in HER2-Positive Breast Cancer

Trial	Regimens	N	DFS (vs. Control)	OS
NCCTG 9831 NSABP B-31	Chemotherapy[a] + Tr vs. Chemotherapy alone	4,045[b]	HR = 0.69 (95% CI, 0.57–0.85)	HR = 0.67 (95% CI, 0.48–0.93)
HERA	Chemotherapy[c] followed by Tr[d] (1 year) vs. Chemotherapy alone	5,090	HR = 0.76 (95% CI, 0.43–0.67)	HR = 0.76 (95% CI, 0.47–1.23)[e]
BCIRG 006[f]	AC→D Tr vs. Carboplatin + D + Tr vs. AC→D	3,222	HR = 0.61 (95% CI, 0.48–0.76) HR = 0.67 (95% CI, 0.54–0.83)	HR = 0.59 (95% CI, 0.42–0.85) HR = 0.66 (95% CI, 0.47–0.93)

BCIRG, Breast Cancer International Research Group; D, Docetaxel; HERA, Herceptin Adjuvant trial; NCCTG, North Central Clinical Trials Group; NSABP, National Surgical Breast and Bowel Project; Tr, Trastuzumab.

[a]In both studies, treatment was administered for 52 weeks. All patients received four cycles of doxorubicin 60 mg/m2 and cyclophosphamide 600 mg/m2 (AC) every 3 weeks followed by paclitaxel (T), administered at 80 mg/m2 weekly for 12 weeks (NCCTG), or either 80 mg/m2 weekly for 12 weeks or 175 mg/m2 every 3 weeks for four cycles (NSABP). All patients on NSABP B-31 started Tr **concurrent** with paclitaxel; one-third of patients on NCCTG study started trastuzumab concurrent with paclitaxel; the rest started it **sequentially**, after completing paclitaxel.

[b]The results were reported as a joint analysis of both studies.

[c]In HERA, less than 25% received both an anthracycline and a taxane.

[d]Patients randomly assigned to Tr were further randomly assigned to 1 versus 2 years of therapy. There was no difference between 1 or 2 years of trastuzumab therapy.

[e]Results are reported with Tr for 1 year. They are confounded by cross-over; 52% of patients on observation ultimately were treated with Tr.

[f]Results of the second interim analysis are presented.

Center Network can be used to modify or hold treatment based on changes to cardiac function (136).

Whether patients with a small HER2+ breast cancer (i.e., less than 1 cm) require treatment (especially 1 year of trastuzumab) is not clear, and there are no randomized data to inform this. The best data come from a single-arm trial that enrolled more than 400 patients with HER2+ tumors (48% of whom had a tumor less than 10 mm in size) treated with single agent paclitaxel weekly for 12 weeks plus trastuzumab (for a 1-year treatment duration) (137). With 4 years of follow-up, the 3-year rates of overall and recurrence-free survival were excellent at 99% for each end point. When evaluated by tumor size (using 10 mm as a cutoff) they did not find a difference in outcomes. While these data do not definitively indicate that patients with small tumors should receive treatment, it does offer support for it in patients who desire adjuvant therapy.

Metastatic Disease

HER-2 Negative Disease

As noted previously, chemotherapy is appropriate treatment for patients with MBC that is hormone-insensitive (ER- and PR-negative) or refractory (having progressed on one or more endocrine therapies), displays aggressive biology (rapid disease progression or early recurrence following adjuvant or neoadjuvant therapy), or is associated with significant symptoms or evidence of extensive or rapidly progressive involvement of vital organs (most often the liver or lungs), which is referred to as visceral crisis. Choice of chemotherapeutic agent or combination of agents depends upon the extent and biology of the patient's disease, her age, performance status and comorbid medical conditions, timing and extent of prior treatment, and her doctor's willingness to accept the risks of various toxicities as a tradeoff for antitumor efficacy, with the understanding that her condition is not curable and that differences in survival with various approaches are modest at best. Common agents used in MBC are listed in **Table 27.6**.

A 2013 meta-analysis compared combination versus single-agent chemotherapy in this setting and found that there was no difference in OS associated with either approach, even when analyzed by line of chemotherapy, schema of treatment, and dose intensity (138). Interestingly, in an analysis for progression-free survival (PFS; 8 trials, 866 women), combination therapy was significantly associated with a higher risk of progression compared to single-agent treatment (HR 1.16, $p = 0.01$). Combination therapy resulted in significantly higher overall response rates (RR 1.13, $p = 0.008$), but at the expense of a higher rate of febrile neutropenia (RR 1.32, $p = 0.01$).

HER-2 Positive Disease

For women with HER2+ MBC, the optimal first-line regimen is not known, as few have been tested in randomized trials. While taxane-based regimens remain commonly administered, some doctors and patients will opt for regimens not usually associated with hair loss, such as vinorelbine-, gemcitabine-, capecitabine-, or liposomal doxorubicin-trastuzumab. Combinations of chemotherapeutic agents given with trastuzumab may (paclitaxel and carboplatin vs. single agent paclitaxel) or may not (docetaxel and carboplatin vs. single agent docetaxel) produce higher RR and improved time to progression (TTP), but have not been shown to improve OS (139,140).

When a patient has achieved maximal benefit from a chemotherapy-trastuzumab combination or starts to develop cumulative toxicities, she is often switched to single-agent trastuzumab "maintenance" therapy, a logical strategy given the level of activity of single-agent trastuzumab, but this approach has not been tested in a randomized trial. What is clear is that HER2+ patients progressing on treatment retain sensitivity to HER2-targeted therapies. For example, in one study that included patients who had progressed on trastuzumab and randomly assigned to capecitabine with continuation of trastuzumab versus capecitabine alone, combination treatment resulted in a superior TTP (8.2 vs. 5.6 months) and OS (25.5 vs. 20.4 months) (141). Even before these results became available, it had been routine practice in patients with HER2+ MBC who were progressing on one chemotherapy-trastuzumab combination to change the cytotoxic agent but continue trastuzumab.

In addition to trastuzumab, lapatinib has modest single-agent activity in patients with HER2+ MBC who have progressed on trastuzumab; however, in patients previously treated with an anthracycline, taxane, and trastuzumab, the combination of capecitabine and lapatinib bested single-agent capecitabine in terms of TTP (6.2 vs. 4.3 months) and OS (75.0 vs. 56.4 weeks) (142).

For these patients, dual HER2-directed agents may also play a role. In one trial, women with HER2+ MBC who had progressed on one or more trastuzumab-containing regimens were assigned to treatment with single-agent lapatinib versus lapatinib and trastuzumab (143). Patients on the combination arm had a superior clinical benefit rate (24.7% vs. 12%), improved TTP (12 vs. 8 weeks), and a nonsignificant improvement in OS (52 vs. 39 weeks). In the CLEOPATRA trial, 808 HER2+ patients with treatment-naïve MBC received docetaxel plus trastuzumab and were also randomly assigned to pertuzumab or placebo (144). Patients assigned to the dual targeted agents had improved RR (80% vs. 69%), PFS (19 vs. 12 months), and a trend toward improved OS. The addition of pertuzumab was associated with higher rates of diarrhea, mucositis, rash, and febrile neutropenia (14% vs. 8%), but no increase in cardiac toxicity.

Duration of Treatment

The optimal duration of treatment with chemotherapy in MBC is unknown. In general, studies of more prolonged administration of chemotherapy have demonstrated prolongation of TTP but little or no improvement in OS, often associated with increased toxicity and inferior quality of life. A meta-analysis of 11 trials, which compared fixed duration chemotherapy with treatment to disease progression, confirmed prolongation of PFS, with a modest increase in OS. In practice, treatment is often administered until a response plateau is reached (based on imaging studies or tumor marker), development of bothersome cumulative toxicities, or the patient requests a treatment break. In patients with hormone receptor–positive disease, an effort to delay disease progression by initiating some novel (to the patient) form of endocrine therapy is reasonable, though this is not supported by any objective data. Whether to resume chemotherapy as soon as there is evidence of disease progression or to wait until the patient begins to have symptoms is not known, and best left to a joint decision between the patient and her physician.

ENDOCRINE THERAPY

The role of endocrine therapy has grown significantly over the past several years as both our understanding of breast cancer has matured and as new therapeutic options have developed. It has become increasingly clear that endocrine therapy is the backbone of treatment for hormonally responsive breast cancer, independent of stage.

Adjuvant Setting for Hormone Receptor–Positive Disease

Perhaps no data set has been more instructive in helping to define the benefit of adjuvant hormonal therapy than the meta-analysis generated by the Early Breast Cancer Trialists' Collaborative Group (145). One of the principles appreciated through this overview analysis is that the proportional benefit of a given treatment is constant through risk groups (e.g., stage) and that the absolute benefit changes based on the estimated risk of systemic recurrence. For instance, if hormonal therapy decreases the risk of cancer recurrence by 30% in a given individual, the absolute benefit would be 3% if the 10-year risk of relapse were 10%, but 18% if the 10-year risk of relapse were 60%. This concept of proportional and absolute benefit from adjuvant therapy is a guiding principle when women are counseled regarding treatment options in the adjuvant setting.

Tamoxifen was the first hormonal agent used in the adjuvant setting for breast cancer (146,147). As a selective estrogen receptor modulator (SERM), tamoxifen has differential effects on various tissues. While tamoxifen may achieve its beneficial effect in the treatment of breast cancer through multiple means, the principle mode of action appears to be through competitive binding to the ER. By preventing estrogen binding, translocation and nuclear binding of the ER is inhibited, altering transcriptional and posttranscriptional events mediated by the receptor. The antagonistic properties of tamoxifen toward breast cancer are contrasted against its agonistic effects on other tissues, such as the bone and uterus. Tamoxifen, like estrogen, improves bone mineral density in postmenopausal women and is a risk factor for endometrial cancer. Tamoxifen may negatively affect bone density in premenopausal women. The risk of endometrial cancer with the use of tamoxifen is estimated at two- to three-fold over the general population risk, though the risk is likely lower in premenopausal women and perhaps close to the general population. It is recommended that women on tamoxifen follow general guidelines for gynecologic screening and follow-up, but importantly, report any menstrual changes, dysfunctional uterine bleeding, or other symptoms to their gynecologist. Women should discuss the use of tamoxifen with their gynecologist to ensure that they are being properly evaluated.

Another important risk associated with tamoxifen is that of venous thrombosis. While perhaps less so in premenopausal women, as demonstrated by the NSABP P-1 trial, tamoxifen carries an approximate two-fold increased risk for deep venous thrombosis compared to the general population (148). This risk is sometimes described as similar to that associated with the use of oral contraceptives and may influence choice of hormonal therapy in the postmenopausal setting.

Other potential side effects of tamoxifen include hot flashes, weight gain, mood changes, increased vaginal discharge, cataracts, and rarely retinal abnormalities. Several studies have suggested an increase in risk of stroke with tamoxifen. Tamoxifen can increase fertility by increasing ovarian stimulation and is a teratogen and is therefore contraindicated during pregnancy. Moreover, premenopausal women on tamoxifen need to ensure appropriate contraception, as it is possible to become pregnant while on this medication.

The benefits of adjuvant tamoxifen have been demonstrated in multiple clinical trials (**Tables 27.9** and **27.10**); most notably, the EBCTCG showed a trend toward improved recurrence-free survival with higher doses of tamoxifen taken in the adjuvant setting, though without any benefit in mortality (158). Thus, 20 mg/day is the recommended dose.

The duration of treatment for women taking tamoxifen has changed recently. Historically, a 5-year course of tamoxifen was standard. Newer clinical trials have, however, have suggested a benefit to extended tamoxifen administration. Specifically, two large clinical trials, the Adjuvant Tamoxifen: Longer versus Shorter (ATLAS) (156) and the Adjuvant Tamoxifen: To offer more (aTTom) (157) trials, showed an approximate further 3% to 4% reduction in the risk of recurrence for 10 versus 5 years of tamoxifen. As well, in the ATLAS trial, 10 years of therapy was associated with an approximate 2% benefit in survival. The principal benefit of extended duration of tamoxifen was appreciated after the 10 years of treatment (156).

Aromatase inhibitors block estrogen production by preventing conversion of androgens produced by the adrenal gland, such as androstenedione to estrogens, such as estrone, which is later converted to estradiol. This block occurs in the breast as well as in peripheral tissues such as adipose tissue. The resulting decrease in circulating estrogen has been demonstrated through multiple clinical trials to be effective treatment for receptor-positive breast cancer. Of the three commercially available aromatase inhibitors, anastrozole and letrozole are nonsteroidal and exemestane is. There are currently no demonstrable differences in efficacy or toxicity between these three products. Toxicities of aromatase inhibitors commonly include hot flashes and joint or muscle aches.

Unlike tamoxifen, aromatase inhibitors can contribute to osteopenia and osteoporosis, with an increased incidence of fractures, and therefore bone density should be followed carefully in women receiving these medicines. Other possible side effects include hypertension, gastrointestinal disturbance, depression, urovaginal symptoms, and possibly cardiac events. Aromatase inhibitors are not associated with an increased risk of endometrial cancer and have a lower risk for deep venous thrombosis compared to tamoxifen (159).

Several studies have demonstrated the efficacy of aromatase inhibitors in the adjuvant setting and have defined their superiority compared with tamoxifen (**Tables 27.9** and **27.10**). On the basis of these trials, it is recommended that all postmenopausal women receiving adjuvant hormonal therapy receive at least 2 to 3 years of an aromatase inhibitor unless contraindicated. Five years of an aromatase inhibitor, tamoxifen followed by an aromatase inhibitor, or an aromatase inhibitor followed by tamoxifen are all options. Decisions regarding extending adjuvant endocrine therapy beyond 5 years are made on an individualized basis, in part based on prognostics and patient preference. However, treatment with an aromatase inhibitor alone beyond 5 years is the subject of current investigation.

■ TABLE 27.9. Seminal Trials of Endocrine Therapy in the Adjuvant Setting: 5 Years of Therapy

Trial	N	Arms	Disease-Free Survival	*p*-Value	Overall Survival	*p*-Value	Follow-up (years)
Scottish Tamoxifen Trial (147)	1,312[a]	T P	76.2% 61.6%	$p < 0.0001$	83.6% 76.8%	$p = >0.002$	2.5–8
NSABP B-14 (149)	2,644[b]	T P	83% 77%	$p < 0.0001$	93% 92%	$p = 0.3$	4
ATAC (150)	6,241[c]	A T	80.3% 76%	$p = 0.04$	23.5% 24%	$p = 0.09$	10
Intergroup Exemestane Study (151)	4,599[d]	T→ E T→	77% 73%	$p < 0.0001$	84.7% 82.4%	$p = 0.04$	7.6
Team (152)	9,700[e]	E T→E	86% 85%	$p = 0.60$	90% 90%	–	5.1
BIG 1-98 (153)	8,010[f]	L First T First	84% 81.4%	$p = 0.003$	96% 95.2%	–	2
		L L→T T→L	87.9% 87.6% 86.2%	NS	–	–	6

A, Anastrozole; E, Exemestane; ER, Estrogen Receptor; L, Letrozole; P, Placebo; T, Tamoxifen.

[a]included pre and postmenopausal node-negative and postmenopausal node-positive, and ER status unknown.

[b]included pre- and postmenopausal node-negative.

[c]included postmenopausal, 84% know to be ER-positive.

[d]included postmenopausal, ER-positive or unknown, node-positive and -negative. Patients receiving exemestane would have received Tamoxifen for 2 to 3 years prior.

[e]postmenopausal, ER-positive, node-positive and -negative.

[f]adjusted for cross-over.

■ TABLE 27.10. Seminal Trials of Endocrine Therapy in the Adjuvant Setting: 10 Years of Therapy

Trial	N	Arms	Disease-Free Survival	*p*-Value	Overall Survival	*p*-Value	Follow-up (years)
MA 17 (154,155)[a]	5,169[b]	T→L T→P	93% 87% HR = 0.52	$p \leq 0.001$ $p \leq 0.001$	96% 93.6% HR = 0.61	$p = 0.25$ $p \leq 0.001$	5.3
ATLAS (156)	6,846[c]	T × 5 years T × 10 years	79% 82%	$p = 0.002$	79% 81%	$p = 0.01$	7.5
aTTom (157)	6,953[d]	T × 5 years T × 10 years	81% 83%	$p = 0.003$	73.9% 75.5%	$p = 0.1$	4.2

[a]adjusted for cross-over.

[b]postmenopausal, ER-positive, node-positive and -negative.

[c]premenopausal, ER-positive, node-positive and -negative.

[d]pre- and postmenopausal, ER-positive and unknown, node-positive and -negative.

The degree of benefit and choice of hormonal therapy may be further influenced by primary tumor characteristics. The level of expression and potentially the relative expression of ER and PR positivity in breast cancer cells may be predictive of the responsiveness of the tumor to hormonal manipulation (151). It is therefore important to incorporate the degree of ER and PR positivity into adjuvant therapy decisions. Going against the conventional understanding of how the ER and PR expression predicts for benefit from endocrine therapy, the recent EBCTCG report on tamoxifen has shown uniform benefit in ER-positive tumors regardless of the level of expression and no benefit in ER-negative tumors independent of PR expression (145). This remains an area of active investigation. The differential benefit to tamoxifen and aromatase inhibitors in the postmenopausal ER+/HER2+ setting also requires further study.

Ovarian Ablation or Suppression

Ovarian ablation (OA) has long been explored as a therapeutic option for premenopausal women with breast cancer. As the ovaries are the major source for estrogen, silencing the ovaries *via* surgical oophorectomy, radiotherapy, or the use of GnRH analogs may provide a benefit, although controversy continues as to its role in modern breast cancer management. The EBCTG overview on OA included 12 trials that compared OA by surgery or radiation to control and encompassed 2012 women with early breast cancer (158). The meta-analysis concluded that OA was associated with both disease-free and OS advantages compared to observation. At 15 years, 52% of those who underwent OA were alive compared with 46% of those who did not undergo OA ($p = 0.001$); furthermore, 45% and 39%, respectively, remained disease free ($p = 0.0007$). When trials using

OA versus chemotherapy following breast surgery were analyzed, however, the benefits of OA were more modest and did not achieve statistical significance. Despite these findings, OA cannot be considered equivalent to chemotherapy, as these trials compared OA to chemotherapy that is considered inferior to modern adjuvant chemotherapy. Still, among premenopausal women who do not receive chemotherapy, OA may play a significant role in management.

Since the meta-analysis, several results have been published in this area. The combined analysis of the Suppression of Ovarian Function Trial (SOFT) and the Tamoxifen and Exemestane Trial, with a median follow-up of 68 months, noted a 4% improvement in DFS with the use of exemestane versus tamoxifen and ovarian suppression (91.1% vs. 87.3% with HR 0.72, $p < 0.001$) (160). This benefit was seen both in women who did and did not receive adjuvant chemotherapy. While the SOFT trial demonstrated no overall benefit for tamoxifen and ovarian suppression over tamoxifen alone, there did appear to be a benefit in women whose risk was high enough to include the use of adjuvant chemotherapy and in women who were less than 35 years of age (161).

Endocrine Therapy in MBC

Hormonal therapy is optimal initial therapy in the setting of stage IV hormone receptor–positive, HER2-negative breast cancer, unless aggressive recurrence mandates chemotherapy to maximize time to response to avert impending organ failure (e.g., significant hepatic metastasis). Options in the premenopausal setting include ovarian suppression with or without the addition of tamoxifen or an aromatase inhibitor, or even tamoxifen alone. In the postmenopausal setting, tamoxifen or aromatase inhibitors are effective options; however, more recent data have demonstrated improved outcome when fulvestrant is used as initial therapy as opposed to an aromatase inhibitor. Fulvestrant is a pure anti-estrogen approved for use in the postmenopausal setting and is given by monthly intramuscular injection. Data from the FIRST trial demonstrated a significantly improved time to progression when 205 women were randomized to first-line fulvestrant versus anastrozole (23.4 vs. 13.1 months), and both treatments were well tolerated (162). Aromatase inhibitors remain a good option for first-line therapy and have been clearly shown to be superior to tamoxifen. A meta-analysis of more than 8,500 patients treated with either first-line aromatase inhibitors or tamoxifen showed a significant survival benefit with aromatase inhibitors (163).

Hormonal resistance eventually evolves over time, necessitating the use of chemotherapy for cancer control. The mechanisms behind the evolution of hormonal resistance and strategies to reinduce hormonal sensitivity in stage IV breast cancer continue to be actively investigated. A recently published study looking at reversing hormonal resistance with the addition of everolimus, an mTOR inhibitor, or placebo to second-line endocrine therapy with exemestane demonstrated a significant improvement in PFS from 3 to 7 months in favor of everolimus (164). This regimen has been challenging to administer, in part due to significant stomatitis associated with everolimus.

Dysregulation of the cell cycle by the acquisition of genetic mutations is a common feature of cancer cells, providing a selective growth advantage. As cyclin-dependent kinases have a critical role in regulating cell cycle kinetics, they are a relevant target for clinical investigation. The Paloma-1 trial demonstrated that the cyclin-dependent kinase 4 and 6 inhibitor palbociclib in combination with letrozole in the first-line metastatic setting of ER+, HER2-negative breast cancer in postmenopausal women was associated with an increase in response rate and a doubling of median PFS from 10.2 months with letrozole alone to 20.2 months with the combination of letrozole and palbociclib (165). Palbociclib was approved in this setting in May 2015. On the basis of these results, palbociclib was evaluated in postmenopausal women with metastatic disease who had progressed on an aromatase inhibitor in the adjuvant setting or after one or more lines of therapy (including one prior line of chemotherapy combination) in the Paloma-3 trial (166). Compared to fulvestrant alone, the addition of palbociclib resulted in a significant improvement in PFS (9.2 vs. 3.8 months; HR 0.42, 95% CI 0.32 to 0.56). Palbociclib is associated with neutropenia, but rarely febrile neutropenia, and appears to be well tolerated, making it a practical addition to endocrine therapy in this setting.

Patients with HER2+, hormone receptor–positive MBC may not require first-line treatment with chemotherapy (and anti-HER2 treatment). Instead, the combination of an aromatase inhibitor with anti-HER2–targeted therapy has improved PFS compared to endocrine therapy alone (167,168).

Neoadjuvant Endocrine Therapy

As in the adjuvant and metastatic setting, hormonal therapy can also be beneficial for women presenting with LABC. If chemotherapy is not being employed, neoadjuvant (preoperative) hormonal therapy in the hormonally positive setting can be effective in increasing the ability to completely surgically resect the primary tumor in locally advanced disease, as well as in increasing the chances for BCS. Studies suggest that neoadjuvant aromatase inhibitors can be equally as effective as chemotherapy, with comparable response rates and rates of breast conservation (169,170). In postmenopausal women, aromatase inhibitors appear to be superior to tamoxifen (169).

Endocrine Therapy for Risk Reduction

The use of tamoxifen in early adjuvant trials appeared to have the benefit of decreasing the risk of second primary breast tumors. Also, tamoxifen in the NSABP B-24 trial demonstrated a decreased risk of invasive and in situ disease in women with a history of DCIS (170). On the basis of these findings, evaluations of tamoxifen for prevention have been published, which support their use in this setting (**Table 27.11**). A meta-analysis of four prevention trials utilizing tamoxifen in normal or higher risk women showed a 38% reduction in the incidence of invasive breast cancer (174). Only the rate of ER-positive breast cancer was reduced. The risk of endometrial cancer was increased by a factor of 2.4, and the risk of thromboembolic events was increased by 1.9. Importantly, there was no detectable improvement in overall mortality or breast cancer–specific mortality rates.

Tamoxifen was compared directly to another SERM, raloxifene, as prevention for high-risk postmenopausal women. Initially published in 2006, raloxifene appeared similar to tamoxifen in decreasing the risk of invasive breast cancer but was less effective in decreasing the risk of DCIS (172). However, with longer follow-up, raloxifene was inferior to tamoxifen in the prevention of invasive breast cancer (RR 1.24, CI 1.05 to 1.47), and the difference in rates of DCIS was no longer statistically significant (RR 1.22, CI 0.95 to 1.59). Raloxefine was associated with a reduced incidence of endometrial cancer (RR 0.55, CI 0.36 to 0.83) and thromboembolic events (RR 0.75, CI 0.6 to 0.93) compared to tamoxifen. Overall, there was no difference in mortality.

Several data sets also demonstrate the efficacy of aromatase inhibitors for prevention in postmenopausal women with increased risk of breast cancer (154) (**Table 27.11**). Also, anastrozole was similar to tamoxifen in risk reduction in the setting of DCIS (175).

On the basis of these trials, raloxifene, tamoxifen, and aromatase inhibitors are reasonable options to reduce one's risk of breast cancer. While tamoxifen can be used in both pre- and postmenopausal women, raloxifene and aromatase inhibitors are reserved as risk-reducing agents only in postmenopausal women. Aromatase inhibitors have been defined as a reasonable alternative to tamoxifen in the setting of DCIS.

Radiation Therapy

RT is an important and well-established treatment modality for women with breast cancer. RT has been shown to reduce the risk of local and regional recurrence and to prevent the need for salvage mastectomy in women undergoing BCS, as well as to improve local and regional control in women following mastectomy who have

TABLE 27.11. Seminal Trials of Endocrine Therapy for Risk Reduction

Trial	N	Arms	Cumulative Rate of Invasive Breast Cancer (per 1,000)	p-Value	Cumulative Rate of Noninvasive Breast Cancer (per 1,000)	p-Value	Follow-up (years)
NSABP P-1 (170)	13,207	T P	24.8 42.5	$p < 0.001$	10.2 15.8	$p = 0.008$	7
IBIS I (171)	7,154	T P	61.8 80.9	$p < 0.0001$	10.1 16.1	$p = 0.047$	16
MAP.3 (172)	4,560	E P	4.8 14.1	$p = 0.002$	3.9 6.2	$p = 0.31$	2.9
IBIS II (173)	3,864	A P	16.7 32.9	$p = 0.001$	3.1 10.3	$p = 0.009$	5

A, Anastrozole; E, Exemestane; P, Placebo; T, Tamoxifen.

high-risk disease. Importantly, this reduction in local failure has been shown to translate into improved OS with long-term follow-up (176).

Breast-Conserving Therapy

As discussed above, BCT consisting of adjuvant radiation following BCS is the standard approach for women with localized, operable breast cancer. However, not all women will be candidates for BCT due to relative contraindications to RT, including some connective tissue disorders (e.g., scleroderma and lupus) and prior breast irradiation.

Although one of the earliest trials evaluating BCT showed inferior results compared with mastectomy, this trial used insufficient radiation doses by modern standards. Subsequent trials conducted in both Europe and North America have all shown equivalent DFS and OS between BCT and mastectomy. The largest of these was NSABP B06, which randomly assigned 1,843 patients to one of three arms: total mastectomy, lumpectomy alone, or lumpectomy with radiation. With 20 years, follow-up results, there were no survival differences between women treated with total mastectomy or lumpectomy with radiation (DFS rates, 36% and 35% [$p = 0.26$], respectively, and OS rates of 47% and 46% [$p = 0.57$], respectively) (177). Local disease control was also similar: 90% and 86%, respectively.

For women undergoing BCT, RT results in a two-thirds reduction in locoregional recurrence. Again, this was best demonstrated in NSABP B06, in which, with 20-year follow-up, lumpectomy and radiation more than halved the rate of local recurrence compared to lumpectomy alone (14% vs. 39%), which again is the largest of the studies addressing this question, randomizing 1,262 patients to lumpectomy verses lumpectomy and radiation. Twenty-year follow-up results showed a local failure rate of 39% with lumpectomy alone and 14% with lumpectomy and radiation (177). The impact of RT on survival was addressed in the EBCTCG meta-analysis that included the individual patient data from more than 10,000 patients treated on 1 of 17 randomized trials (178). They reported that the addition of RT to surgery significantly reduced the risk of a first recurrence (local or distant) at 10 years from 35% to 19% ($p < 0.0001$). More importantly, this translated into an OS benefit seen at 15-years' follow-up, with an absolute reduction in overall mortality of 3.8% ($p = 0.0005$).

While the benefits of RT have been effectively established, ongoing work is aiming to better elucidate who may *not* benefit from RT, thus sparing them from the potential toxicities of treatment. In 1989, the NSABP initiated the B-21 trial, evaluating over 1,000 women with low-risk disease undergoing BCS (179). Women of all ages with tumors less than or equal to 1 cm and ER-positive, lymph node-negative disease were included. Patients were randomly assigned to adjuvant treatment with tamoxifen alone versus RT alone versus both RT and tamoxifen. The primary end points were IBTR and incidence of contralateral breast cancer. As reported, tamoxifen was not as effective in preventing IBTR as RT alone, but both were less effective than the combination of RT and tamoxifen. The incidence of IBTR at 8 years on tamoxifen alone, RT alone, and the combination was 16.5%, 9.3%, and 2.8%, respectively. Another subgroup felt to be at lower risk of recurrence is older patients, as they tend to have more indolent tumor biology. A trial by the CALGB evaluated the additional benefit of RT in women 70 years of age or older treated by lumpectomy and tamoxifen (180,181). These women had tumors less than 2 cm in size and were ER-positive and lymph node-negative. The rate of IBTR was 4% versus 1% at 5 years ($p < 0.001$) and 10% versus 2% at 10 years ($p < 0.001$) for women treated with endocrine therapy alone versus those receiving RT, respectively. While the rate of local recurrence was again higher among women who did not receive radiation, the absolute benefit of radiation was small, suggesting that it may be reasonable for older women with small tumors to forego RT, provided they are candidates for endocrine therapy (182).

Postmastectomy Radiation Therapy

For women who undergo a mastectomy and are deemed to be at moderate to high risk for local recurrence, RT to the chest wall and regional lymphatics is indicated. The criteria that define "moderate" and "high" risk have evolved over time and continues to do so as our understanding of the important factors related to local–regional recurrence grows.

Early trials of postmastectomy RT showed a decrease in local recurrence but no apparent benefit in OS (176). However, the trials varied greatly in radiation technique and dose, and some included patients who did not receive systemic therapy. However, there have been three modern era trials that have evaluated the benefit of postmastectomy RT. The Danish Breast Cancer Cooperative group (DBCCG) conducted one trial that included 1,708 premenopausal women with pathologic stage II or III breast cancer who were treated with CMF chemotherapy and randomly assigned to observation or to treatment with RT of the chest wall and regional nodes (183). RT was associated with a significant reduction in locoregional recurrence (alone or with evidence of distant disease) compared to chemotherapy alone (9% vs. 32%, respectively, $p < 0.001$). It was also associated with a significant survival benefit at 10 years (54% of those who received RT were alive vs. 45% of those who received CMF only, $p < 0.001$). A second DBCCG trial included more than 1,300 postmenopausal women with stage II–III breast cancer who were treated with tamoxifen (30 mg/day for 1 year) and randomly assigned to treatment with RT or no RT (184). With a median follow-up of over 10 years, RT was associated with a significant reduction in locoregional recurrence compared to tamoxifen (8% vs. 35%, respectively, $p < 0.001$) and a significant improvement in OS (45% and 36%, respectively, $p = 0.03$). Despite these results, the

DBCCG trials have been criticized for the low number of axillary lymph nodes removed on axillary dissection and higher than expected axillary recurrent rates in the control groups.

Another trial conducted in British Columbia also addressed the question of postmastectomy RT by randomizing more than 300 women to CMF chemotherapy with or without RT (185). This trial also showed a local–regional control benefit and OS benefit to RT, yet unlike the Danish trials, the median number of axillary lymph nodes removed on axillary dissection was 11. At 20-years' follow-up, isolated recurrence was 10% versus 26% and OS was 47% versus 37% in favor of postmastectomy RT. The relative magnitude of benefit from RT was similar in women with 1 to 3 positive nodes (HR 0.76, 95% CI 0.50 to 1.15) compared to those with ≥4 positive nodes (HR 0.70, 95% CI 0.46 to 1.06).

The Early Breast Cancer Trialists' Collaborative Group also performed a meta-analysis of individual patient data from randomized trials of postmastectomy RT (176). This analysis included 8,500 women, and for those with any involved axillary nodes, RT resulted in a 17% absolute reduction in 5-year local recurrence (6% vs. 23%) and a 4.4% absolute improvement in 15-year OS (40.2% vs. 35.8%). An update of this analysis showed that the reduction in locoregional recurrence and breast cancer mortality is evident not only in patients with four or more involved axillary lymph nodes but also in those with one to three involved axillary nodes (186). In women treated with mastectomy and axillary dissection, the addition of RT reduced the risks of locoregional recurrence from 20.3% to 3.8% at 10 years, any recurrence (local or distant) from 45.7% to 34.2% at 10 years, and breast cancer mortality from 47.0% to 37.9% at 15 years.

Postmastectomy RT, therefore, should be administered to all patients with locally advanced disease (T4 or ≥4 positive nodes). However, RT should be *offered* to patients with 1 to 3 positive nodes or involved surgical margins, as these patients are also at moderate to high risk for local recurrence. Furthermore, a subset of patients with node-negative disease is at risk for recurrence and may benefit from postmastectomy RT. A combination of some of the following risk factors defines this latter group: young age, T2 or greater disease, lymphovascular space invasion, close margins, and triple-negative disease (187,188).

Radiation Therapy to the Regional Lymph Nodes

RT not only improves the likelihood of tumor control in the breast or along the chest wall, but also improves regional control in the draining lymph node basins for patients at risk for harboring micrometastatic disease at these sites. The role of RT in axillary management has been looked at in several important clinical trials, such as the ACOSOG Z0011 trial (discussed above), which suggested that RT to the axillary may not be necessary, particularly for those felt to be at low risk for recurrence (102). However, it should be noted that all patients in this trial received breast irradiation and there was no central review of the radiation fields, which is important for quality control. The importance of the latter point was shown in a retrospective review of the radiation fields used in this trial, which revealed that 19% of patients were treated with regional nodal irradiation (RNI) targeting the axilla and supraclavicular fossa (SCF), and an additional 50% of patient were treated with "high" tangents targeting the level I/II axilla (189). The EORTC's AMAROS trial also evaluated a similar question, and is discussed above.

The management of lymph nodes beyond the low axilla was evaluated in two additional trials. In both trials, all patients had breast surgery and ALND and then were randomly assigned to undergo RNI, including the high axillary, supraclavicular, and IM lymph nodes versus breast or chest wall RT alone. In the NCIC MA.20 trial, 1,832 women with node-positive or high-risk node-negative disease were included (190). At 10 years, RNI resulted in significant improvements of all end points, including DFS (HR 0.76, $p = 0.01$), isolated locoregional DFS (HR 0.59, $p = 0.0009$), and distant DFS (HR 0.76, $p = 0.03$). However, there was no corresponding statistically significant difference in OS. In the EORTC 22922/10925 trial, 4,004 women with node-positive or centrally and medially located node-negative disease were enrolled (191). As before, there were significant improvements in all end points at 10 years, including DFS (HR 0.89, $p = 0.04$) and distant DFS (HR 0.86, $p = 0.02$). In addition, there was a significant reduction in breast cancer mortality (HR 0.82, $p = 0.02$), although only a trend was noted toward improvement in OS (HR 0.82, $p = 0.06$). These trials demonstrate that for high-risk patients, RNI improves not only regional disease control but also impacts risk of metastatic disease and breast cancer mortality.

The inclusion of the IM nodes in RNI has been controversial. Classic surgical data have shown that the risk of IM node involvement can be as high as 20% to 40%, particularly for patients who have medial tumors and involved axillary lymph nodes (192,193). In addition, retrospective data suggest that RT to the IM chain may confer a survival benefit (194,195). However, clinical relapse in the IM chain even in these patients is uncommon, with estimates placing this at less than 1% (196). To further add to the controversy, regarding increased cardiac dose and resulting risk for cardiac mortality when the IM nodes are treated on the left side.

To evaluate the benefits of IM nodal irradiation, Hennequin et al. (197) randomized women with positive axillary lymph nodes or those with centrally/medically located tumors irrespective of nodal status to breast and supraclavicular irradiation with or without IM nodal irradiation. At 10 years, there was no difference in primary end point of OS. Despite these results, some have criticized the trial because it included patients that may have been at a relatively low risk of recurrence, and as a result, it was underpowered for the primary end point.

Radiation Therapy for In Situ Breast Disease

Approximately 20% to 30% of patients treated with local excision alone for DCIS have a recurrence, with about half of these recurrences being invasive cancer. As a result, radiation is often delivered as a means of risk reduction. To date, four randomized trials have compared excision alone with excision followed by whole breast RT, and all have demonstrated that RT reduces the risk of a subsequent breast event by 38% to 62% (198).

In addition, an EBCTCG meta-analysis suggested that the same proportional benefit was seen across risk groups, with the largest absolute benefits seen in patients with high risk factors; size >2 cm, high grade, presence of comedonecrosis, and positive resection margins. However, even in women with small, low-grade tumors resected with negative margins, the absolute reduction in IBTR with RT at 10 years was still 18%. However, there is no significant difference in breast cancer–specific mortality or overall mortality with or without RT for DCIS.

Attempts at identifying subgroups of patients at low risk for recurrence following excision alone have met with limited success. Wong et al. (199) prospectively evaluated a series of patients treated with wide resection margins of at least 1 cm and still reported a 5-year recurrence rate of 12%. A prospective trial run by ECOG evaluated patients with low-grade tumors less than 2.5 cm and high-grade tumors less than 1 cm (200). Five-year IBTR was 6.1% in the low-grade group and 15.3% in the high-grade group despite a mean tumor size of only 6 and 5 mm, respectively. The RTOG also led a study that compared observation to RT in more than 600 women with low-risk DCIS (201). Compared to observation, RT resulted in a significantly lower rate of IBTR at 7 years (0.9% vs. 6.7%, respectively, $p < 0.001$).

Partial Breast Irradiation

Standard RT consists of irradiating the whole breast; however, for select patients, partial breast RT may be an option. The concept of partial breast RT arose out of the realization that the majority of tumor recurrences occur at or near the region of the lumpectomy site (202,203). Thus, for well-selected patients, only the breast tissue surrounding the tumor bed needs radiation treatment.

Limiting RT to a smaller portion of the breast results in two major advantages. First, there is a reduction in the volume of irradiated tissue, thereby preserving these tissues from potential deleterious radiation effects. This includes minimal-to-no dose exposure to the heart and lung. Second, by reducing the volume of treatment, the overall treatment time can be safely accelerated to deliver the entire course of radiation within a week or less. This approach is referred to as accelerated partial breast irradiation (APBI), and is generally defined as radiotherapy delivered to less than the whole breast employing fractions higher than 1.8 to 2.0 Gy/day over a period of less than 5 to 6 weeks. Multiple techniques have been developed and are being developed for the delivery of APBI. In North America, the most commonly used techniques are multi-catheter interstitial brachytherapy, intracavitary brachytherapy, and 3D conformal external beam RT. Multiple single-institutional as well as multi-institutional trials, some with follow-up beyond 10 years, have demonstrated results comparable to those of whole breast irradiation (204). Phase III randomized trials comparing whole breast RT and APBI have been completed. One trial, conducted by the Groupe Européen de Curiethérapie of European Society for Radiotherapy and Oncology (GEC-ESTRO) (205), enrolled 1,184 women with early-stage breast cancer treated with BCS and randomly assigned them to treatment using standard whole breast RT or APBI (using an interstitial multi-catheter technique). At 5 years' follow-up, there was no statistically significant difference in IBTR (1.4% vs. 0.9%), DFS, OS, or late toxicity.

At this time, the American Brachytherapy Society (ABS), American Society of Breast Surgeons (ASBS), and ASTRO have published guidelines for appropriate patient selection for APBI (**Table 27.12**) (206,207).

TABLE 27.12. Guidelines for Appropriate Patient Selection for APBI

ASTRO "Suitable" Criteria:
Patient factors
Age ≥60 years
BRCA1/2 mutation not present
Pathologic factors:
Tumor size ≤2 cm
T stage: T1
Margins negative by at least 2 mm
Any Grade
No LVSI
ER Positive
Unicentric and Unifocal
Histology
Invasive ductal or other favorable subtypes
Pure DCIS or EIC not allowed
Associated LCIS is allowed
Nodal factors
N stage: pN0 (i–, i+)
Nodal surgery: Sentinel node biopsy or axillary node dissection
Treatment factors
Neoadjuvant therapy not allowed
ABS:
Age ≥50 years
Invasive carcinoma (any histology) or DCIS
Tumor size ≤3 cm
Margins negative (no tumor at inked margin)
ER positive or negative
No LVSI
Lymph node-negative (pN0)
ASBS (Updated 2008)
Age ≥45 years
Invasive ductal carcinoma or DCIS
Tumor size ≤3 cm
Margins negative by at least 2 mm
Lymph node-negative (pN0)

Radiation Therapy: Other Indications

For patients who experience locally recurrent breast cancer, local therapy with surgery and/or radiation may be an option. For some, cure can be achieved, and in most, RT can help reduce the risk of significant morbidity of uncontrolled, local disease.

Oligometastatic disease is a transitional state between localized disease and widespread systemic disease, where the volume and number of metastatic deposits is limited, and local therapy (with or without systemic therapy) is an option. Although only a small percentage of these patients can have long-term DFS, this is in distinct contrast to patients with widespread metastatic disease in whom cure is not possible. While such tumor biology is considered quite rare in breast cancer, aggressive local therapy with radiation and/or surgery should be considered for select patients. Stereotactic body RT or stereotactic radiosurgery is an ideal method of RT for these patients. With this method, high ablative doses of radiation are delivered in a highly conformal manor with extreme precision. This is typically done in just one to five treatments or fractions and can be applied not just to the brain but almost any part of the body. The large radiation doses result in a high probability of local disease control, and the conformality and precision allows for a low risk of side effects and complications (208,209).

For patients with widespread metastatic disease, RT can be used effectively for palliation of lesions involving the chest wall, regional lymphatics, bone, brain, lung, and liver, among other areas. Indication for radiation in this setting include palliation of symptomatic lesions not responding or unlikely to respond to systemic therapy and prevention of complications of local disease progression such as impending pathologic fracture from bone metastasis, impingement of the spinal cord or nerve roots from spine metastasis, or neurologic sequelae from brain metastases. Palliative radiation courses usually last from a one-time 8 Gy 1-day treatment to a 2- to 3-week course of 2.5 to 3 Gy per fraction for a total dose of 30 to 37.5 Gy.

Radiation Therapy Techniques

Radiation treatment planning and delivery has dramatically evolved since the inception of BCT; from low-energy Cobalt units using indiscriminant en face treatment fields, to high-energy linear accelerators with rudimentary 2D planning, and now to modern computed tomography (CT)–based, 3D treatment planning with sophisticated dose modulation. This is important to understand, as we have come a long way in our ability to spare normal tissues, and this needs to be considered when evaluating long-term toxicity data from obsolete techniques that are clearly inferior and posed substantial higher risk to underlying organs compared to modern methods.

For modern radiation treatment planning, the process begins with the "simulation." This is a session at which the patient position for treatment is established. For breast cancer, this is typically in the supine position with the ipsilateral arm up, although other treatment positions are sometimes used to optimize target and normal tissue geometry. Appropriate immobilization devices are used to ensure the stability and reproducibility of the patient position during daily treatments. Tattoos are placed to allow for precise positioning with aid of in-room targeting lasers. A CT scan is obtained in the established treatment position. This data set is used to design treatment portals and to perform dose calculations. This allows for tailoring the treatment fields to the specific anatomy of the patient and allows for optimization of target doses and normal tissue sparing. Once an appropriate treatment plan is generated, the virtual plan is verified on the patient *via* imaging through the treatment portals. The whole process undergoes rigorous quality assurance procedures to ensure the utmost accuracy in all facets of treatment delivery.

Intact Breast

Following BCS, the entire residual breast tissue is included in the irradiated volume with or without regional lymph node groups depending on the risk of subclinical disease spread to these regions. Treatment portals are oriented tangential to the breast to avoid lung and heart irradiation. Photon energies of 4 to 6 MV are preferred to treat the breast. Energies greater than 6 MV may underdose superficial tissue beneath the skin surface, but may be helpful in decreasing hot spots for patients with large breasts. Dose modulation with wedges, tissue compensators, electronic compensation (field-in-field techniques), or intensity-modulated radiation therapy (IMRT) is used to optimize dose distribution and dose homogeneity across the target volumes. The prescription dose used is 45 to 50.4 Gy in 1.8 to 2.0 Gy per fraction over 25 to 28 treatments given 5 days/week over 5 to 6 weeks. This is followed by a boost to the tumor bed consisting of 10 to 16 Gy in 1.8 to 2.0 Gy per fraction to at total dose of 60 to 66 Gy over 6 to 7 weeks of treatment.

The tumor bed has the highest risk of harboring subclinical or microscopic disease, and clinical evidence has shown that it is the site at highest risk for recurrence. The value of adding a tumor bed boost was evaluated by two randomized trials. The EORTC 22881–10882 trial involved more than 5,300 women with stage I or II breast cancer who were randomly assigned to whole breast treatment with or without a tumor bed boost of 16 Gy (210). With a median follow-up of 17 years, there was no difference in 20-year OS between the boost and the no-boost group (60% vs. 61%, respectively, HR 1.05, 95% CI 0.92 to 1.19). However, the rate of IBTR favored those who underwent a boost (9% vs. 13%, HR 0.65, 99% CI 0.52 to 0.81). A separate randomized trial from Lyon, France also showed a reduction in local relapse with a 10 Gy boost (211). The boost targets the lumpectomy cavity with an appropriate margin. Planning should be performed using CT-based simulation to ensure appropriate target coverage and can be delivered using one of several techniques including *en face* electrons, three-dimensional conformal RT (3D-CRT), IMRT, Accuboost, or other brachytherapy techniques (212,213).

Long-term data have now emerged demonstrating that hypofractionated whole breast RT is an appropriate option for many patients. This allows for the shortening of overall treatment time to 3 to 4 weeks from 5 to 7 weeks with standard fractionation. Whelan et al. (214) reported an update of the Canadian study that randomized more than 1,200 women to either standard whole breast irradiation (50 Gy in 25 fractions) or to a hypofractionated regime (42.5 Gy in 16 fractions). The IBTR rate at 10 years was similar: 6.7% for standard fractionation and 6.2% for hypofractionation. Good-to-excellent cosmetic outcome was also similar: 71.3% and 69.8%, respectively. Long-term outcomes from the United Kingdom Standardization of Breast Radiotherapy (START) trials have also been recently published (215). START-B enrolled 2,215 women and randomized them to receive either 50 Gy in 25 fractions or 40 Gy in 15 fractions. At 10 years, the local-regional recurrence rate was not statistically different, 5.5% versus 4.3%, for standard- and hypofractionation, respectively. The side effects of RT, including breast shrinkage, telangiectasia, and breast edema, were notably less common with hypofractionation, and cosmetic outcomes were not different between the two treatment schedules.

These trials provided robust, level 1 evidence that hypofractionation is safe and equally effective. Although there are some limitations to hypofractionation whole breast irradiation, many women can now be offered this more convenient treatment option.

Chest Wall

For women at high risk for local or regional recurrence following mastectomy, RT is delivered to the chest wall and regional lymphatics. Similar to intact breast treatment, a 3D-CRT technique using tangentially oriented beams is used. Tissue-equivalent bolus material is used on the chest wall surface, for at least a portion of the treatment, to increase dose build-up in superficial chest wall tissues. Other techniques such as *en face* electrons fields, mixed electron and photon fields, and IMRT can also be used to target the tissues at risk. The typical prescription dose is 45 to 50.4 Gy in 1.8 to 2.0 Gy per fraction over 25 to 28 treatments over 5 to 6 weeks. This can be followed by a boost to the mastectomy scar/operative bed to a total dose of 60 to 66 Gy.

For patients undergoing mastectomy, reconstructive options are an important consideration for most women. The plastic surgeon should be involved early in the multidisciplinary management of these patients, as many factors can have significant implications on the ultimate cosmetic outcome. Among these factors are the type of reconstruction used and sequencing of reconstruction and postmastectomy radiation.

Regional Lymphatics

From a radiation oncology perspective, the regional lymphatics are divided into four anatomical groups: low axilla (level I and lower lever II), high axilla (high level II and level III), SCF, and IM chain. Each of these regions can be targeted based on risk of subclinical disease involvement. The low axilla is inadvertently included in most tangential whole breast radiation fields. This typically includes the first echelon lymph nodes, as most sentinel nodes are found in these regions.

For patients with node-negative disease, the risk of a recurrence in the axilla or SCF is uncommon, and inclusion of these nodal regions is not necessary. For patients with involved axillary lymph nodes, and particularly those with four or more involved nodes, the SCF is at risk and should be treated. The SCF is typically treated with a single anterior oblique field that is matched to the tangential breast fields. The matching technique is crucial to prevent beam overlap and thus significant dose hot spots at the beam junctions. For women with involved axillary lymph nodes who undergo a completion axillary dissection, treatment of the high axilla is generally not necessary, as the risk of failure after an *en bloc* resection is not common.

Avoiding irradiation of the high axilla in these patients is desirable, as irradiation increases the risk of arm lymphedema following axillary dissection. Thus, treatment of the high axilla is typically reserved for patients at high risk of subsequent axillary failure. This includes patients who do not undergo axillary evaluation but are at risk for axillary lymph node involvement, patients with positive sentinel lymph nodes who do not undergo a completion dissection, and patients with involved axillary lymph nodes who undergo dissection but have high risk factors. The high axilla is typically treated by extending the oblique SCF field laterally. Often a posterior field, posterior axillary boost, or PAB, is added to supplement dose to the posterior portion of the axilla. The IM nodes are located in the first five intercostal spaces adjacent to the IM vessels, just lateral to the sternum. The first three intercostal spaces are typically targeted for treatment as these represent the highest risk region. Several techniques can be used to treat the IM nodes. The most common methods are either a matched *en face* or oblique electron field or a modification of the whole breast tangential beams. Regional lymph nodes are treated to a total dose of 45 to 50.4 Gy in 1.8 to 2.0 Gy per fraction.

Accelerated Partial Breast Irradiation

Numerous techniques for the delivery of APBI have been employed involving both external beam and brachytherapy techniques. The most common techniques used in North America are interstitial multi-catheter brachytherapy (IMB), intracavitary balloon brachytherapy (IBB), and 3D-CRT. IMB is characterized by the percutaneous placement of multiple catheters into and surrounding the lumpectomy cavity in such a fashion as to deliver the prescription dose to the tumor bed with a margin of 1.0 to 1.5 cm. This technique is versatile and can conform to the most complex tumor bed geometry. IBB was developed as a simplification of the IMB technique. IBB involves the percutaneous placement of a single catheter applicator into the lumpectomy cavity. This is performed either at the time of surgery under direct visualization with an open cavity or postoperatively under US and/or CT guidance. Once the end of the applicator is positioned within the lumpectomy cavity, the balloon at the end of the applicator is inflated to conform to the cavity. Dose is prescribed to a 1-cm distance from the balloon surface to encompass the tumor bed with an appropriate margin. Several balloon and balloon-like catheters are commercially available, including Mammosite, Contura, and SAVI. APBI using 3D-CRT is an external beam technique that employs four to five noncoplanar, tangential oriented beams targeted to the lumpectomy cavity. To account for breast motion, respiratory motion, patient motion, and setup error, a larger margin of 2.5 cm is used with this technique. A prescription dose of 34.0 Gy in 10 fractions given twice daily is used for IMB and IBB, and a dose of 38.5 Gy in 10 fractions is used for APBI using 3D-CRT.

Pregnancy-Associated Breast Cancer

Pregnancy-associated breast cancer (PABC) is defined as cancer diagnosed either during pregnancy or up to 12 months postpartum, and breast cancer is among the most commonly diagnosed cancers encountered in pregnant women. The incidence of PABC ranges from 0.02% to 0.1%, and 17 to 100 per 100,000 pregnancies may be affected (216). With the increasing trend of delaying childbearing to an older age, the incidence of PABC is reportedly increasing in some countries. For example, data from Sweden showed that between 1963 and 2002, the incidence increased from 16 to 37.4 per 100,000 deliveries, with an additional increase in breast cancer seen between the first and second year after delivery, from 10.6 to 15 per 100,000 deliveries (217). Deciding on the best treatment of PABC is challenging due to potential conflicts between maternal and fetal well-being.

Most women diagnosed with PABC present with a painless breast mass, though this cannot be presumed to be malignant; the majority of palpable masses identified during pregnancy are benign, including lactating adenomas, fibroadenomas, and galactoceles. However, further evaluation is warranted if palpable findings persist. Unfortunately, given the physiologic changes associated with pregnancy, diagnostic delays are common and are believed to contribute to the advanced stages at diagnosis among pregnant women.

Typically, breast US is the first diagnostic study used to evaluate a palpable breast and/or axillary mass during pregnancy given its safety and high sensitivity and specificity (218). However, mammography may be helpful, especially to rule out multicentric, multifocal, and/or bilateral breast cancer. MRI has also been used during pregnancy; however, as gadolinium crosses the placenta and has been associated with fetal abnormalities in rats, contrast-enhanced breast MRI is not recommended (219).

Although the usefulness of mammography during pregnancy has been questioned, recent studies have reported on both the safety and relative efficacy of mammography during pregnancy. With proper abdominal shielding, the irradiation dose to the fetus from a standard two-view mammogram is <50 mrad (0.5 μGy). It is within the limits considered acceptable during pregnancy and well below the threshold exposure of 10 rad (100 mGy), at which point the estimated risk of fetal malformations and central nervous system problems is 1% (220).

The use of other imaging modalities should be limited to those required for treatment planning. If a workup for metastatic disease is necessary, acceptable evaluations during pregnancy include chest radiographs, abdominal/liver US and noncontrast skeletal MRI (221). US guided core biopsies can be performed safely, and as in the nonpregnant patient, these are the preferred methods for diagnosis.

Historically, PABC carried a dismal prognosis, with survival rates of less than 20% at 5 years. However, it is likely the prognosis is not directly attributable to the onset of cancer in pregnancy. Rather it reflects poor prognostic features of breast cancer when diagnosed in pregnant women compared to age-matched nonpregnant counterparts, including larger tumors that are more often node-positive (222). These cancers are more often infiltrating ductal adenocarcinomas, often high grade, hormone receptor-negative, and HER2/neu positive, with associated lymphovascular invasion (223,224).

Available data on the overall prognosis of women with PABC are conflicting. A meta-analysis of 30 papers (3,628 cases and 37,100 controls) showed PABC was associated with a poorer OS, especially in women diagnosed in the postpartum period (225). It is important to note that the meta-analysis included articles dating back to 1965, when less effective treatment options were available, and included postpartum patients, though poorer outcomes in PABC diagnosed in the postpartum period have been corroborated by other studies (226).

Treatment Approach to PABC

Treatment strategies are determined by tumor biology, stage, gestational age, and patient/family wishes, and guidelines for pregnant women essentially follow those set forth for nonpregnant women, with the exception of RT. Pregnancy termination is rarely indicated for the treatment of PABC and should be reserved for aggressive tumors diagnosed early in the first trimester in which an aggressive treatment strategy is recommended, or in situations where the woman desires this prior to treatment. A multidisciplinary approach is essential to providing optimal care, allowing for cooperation between medical, surgical and radiation oncology, radiology, obstetrics, and neonatology.

Surgery

The safety of surgical intervention at any stage in the pregnancy is well established, and a modified radical mastectomy has traditionally been considered the standard of care. This approach virtually eliminates the need for irradiation and allows optimal control of disease within the axilla. However, given that most women with PABC will receive adjuvant or NACT, resulting in a delay of radiotherapy until after delivery, BCS is increasingly seen as a reasonable alternative for pregnant women, particularly if the diagnosis is made in the latter second and third trimester.

Lymph node staging remains the most important predictor of systemic recurrence, and accurate nodal staging is crucial to determining appropriate systemic therapy. As in nonpregnant patients, axillary US and image-guided FNA of suspicious nodes may be helpful in diagnosing those patients with locally advanced disease. This is of particular relevance to patients for whom neoadjuvant therapy is being considered. Although the sensitivity and specificity of sentinel lymph node biopsy in pregnancy has not been systematically evaluated, this technique has been used successfully in pregnant patients, and expert panels feel this can be considered after an informed discussion. The majority of data are with regard to the use of Tc-99 colloid, which is considered safe in pregnancy (227). The lower radioactive dose associated with the 1-day protocol is preferred. Sentinel lymph node biopsy is considered safe and accurate from a maternal perspective, with only one unsuccessful mapping and one recurrence among 97 patients with PABC (227). While methylene blue dye might be used (228), isosulfan dye alone is not recommended because of the low (1%) but potentially harmful risk of anaphylactic maternal reaction (229).

Radiotherapy

Therapeutic RT during pregnancy is contraindicated, and if indicated, it is typically delayed until the postpartum period. However, this has been challenged by some who feel that the risks of radiation to the fetus are overestimated and exposure can be reduced sufficiently by proper shielding, resulting in fetal exposure doses that fall below accepted threshold levels (230). The lack of prospective data and the option of mastectomy for patients with PABC, however, continue to make the use of RT during PABC contraindicated.

Systemic Therapy

As in nonpregnant women, chemotherapy often plays a crucial role in both the adjuvant and neoadjuvant treatment in women with PABC. The effects of chemotherapy on fetal development and growth vary depending on gestational age at the time of exposure. When administered during the first trimester, chemotherapy effects are characterized as "all-or-nothing" and may result in high rates of miscarriages and congenital malformations (216). As a result, chemotherapy should be avoided during the first trimester. Outside of the first trimester, chemotherapy has proven to be relatively safe. The second and third trimesters of pregnancy are characterized primarily by fetal growth and maturation, as organogenesis is complete. For example, the prevalence of fetal transformations declines from 14% in the first trimester to 3% in the second and third trimesters, comparable to the baseline US major malformation risk in the general population of 3% (216). While chemotherapy delivered after the first trimester is not associated with fetal anomalies, increased rates of growth restriction, intrauterine and neonatal death, prematurity, and hemopoietic suppression have been reported (216).

When chemotherapy is administered (as neoadjuvant or adjuvant therapy), it is generally recommended that doses be adjusted to increasing weight. While prospective case series have reported on the use of anthracycline-based chemotherapy administered every 3 to 4 weeks during the second and third trimesters, there are few prospective trials. Among the largest prospectively recorded series, Hahn and colleagues (231) reported that among 57 women treated with FAC in the second and third trimesters, there were no stillbirths, miscarriages, or perinatal deaths. The median gestational age at delivery was 37 weeks (range 29 to 42 weeks), and the most common neonatal complication was respiratory distress, 10% of which required ventilator support. These findings have been replicated in other reports. Most data show that anthracyclines are safe, with preference for doxorubicin rather than epirubicin, with which more fetal cardiac toxicities have been reported (232).

Taxanes used in other malignancies, such as ovarian cancer, have shown similar results. A review of 8 articles included 11 pregnancies from women who received taxanes (majority with paclitaxel). There were 12 newborns recorded, resulting in 92.31% cases of a healthy child with 20 months of follow-up (233). As paclitaxel has been shown to have less placental transport, its use is favored over docetaxel (221).

Although HER2-directed therapy is an integral part of the treatment of HER2-positive breast cancers, trastuzumab is associated with adverse effects on pregnancy and should not be administered. In a recent review of 18 reports of trastuzumab use in the literature, oligohydramnios and anhydramnios was found in 1/3 of cases (234). In addition, most pregnancies resulted in premature delivery, and four of the newborns died of complications related to prematurity, particularly respiratory failure. This contraindication extends to other HER2-directed agents, such as lapatinib, TDM-1, and pertuzumab, especially since we do not have enough data to inform benefits versus risks. In response to the lack of data, the US MotHER registry was created in 2008 to prospectively gather data on HER2-directed therapy in pregnancy (235).

For women diagnosed with hormone receptor–positive breast cancer, the use of endocrine manipulation has been less extensively studied in the context of pregnancy. As a result, there are no long-term data available on children following exposure to tamoxifen or an aromatase inhibitor in utero. However, animal and preclinical data suggest that tamoxifen at least is teratogenic, and as such, it (and by extrapolation, aromatase inhibitors) is best reserved until completion of the pregnancy.

The developmental impact of chemotherapy on children has also been evaluated. Most recently, Amant and colleagues (236) documented the outcomes of 129 children exposed to chemotherapy during pregnancy, matched to 129 controls consisting of children whose mothers were not exposed during pregnancy. There were no differences among the groups in regard to cognitive, cardiac, or general development of children during early childhood. However, kids exposed to chemotherapy in utero were more frequently born premature. While prematurity was associated with cognitive impairment in this study, the association was independent of whether or not their mothers received cancer treatment. This stresses the importance of avoiding iatrogenic premature delivery whenever possible and to deliver patients as near full-term whenever possible.

Pregnancy after Breast Cancer Treatment

For women who become pregnant after breast cancer treatment, there appears to be no negative impact on survival outcomes. A study by Azim et al. (237), which included 333 patients with 686 matched nonpregnant controls, showed that pregnancy after breast cancer was not detrimental to their risk of recurrence. This is sometimes used to support a notion of the "healthy-mother effect," which is, that only healthy women give birth, and those who are sick in relation to their breast cancer will not (238).

For women treated with BCT, breast feeding may still be an option. For example, Higgins and Haffty (239) reported on 11 patients who subsequently experienced 13 pregnancies. Following delivery, lactation was possible in the treated breast in four instances but not in six others. In three women, lactation was pharmacologically suppressed. In the majority of cases, lactation was possible in the untreated breast. The time interval from initial treatment did not appear to impact successful lactation; however, in four instances where lactation was not successful, a circumareolar incision was performed, suggesting that lactation may be less likely to occur in the case of centrally located lesions where the anatomy of central ducts may be altered.

There are no strict guidelines to inform the best time to attempt pregnancy after breast cancer. While it may seem helpful to wait a period of time prior to attempting pregnancy, there are no available data to inform whether prognosis is impacted based on the extent of time from treatment to pregnancy. Furthermore, women with a risk of breast cancer may develop recurrent disease many years after, such that a waiting period of 2 years may not be as reassuring as it seems.

In this regard, fertility must be discussed with patients, preferably prior to adjuvant treatment. This is in keeping with clinical practice guidelines published by ASCO for fertility preservation in patients diagnosed with cancer (240).

Breast Cancer in the Elderly Patient

Age is a well-documented risk factor for the development of breast cancer, and decisions regarding effective therapy can be complicated by a real or perceived limited life expectancy, multiple competing comorbidities and limited data gleaned from randomized trials. Furthermore, defining the "elderly population" is problematic. Much of the literature defines "elderly" broadly and includes women as young as 65 years of age and may even exclude women older than 80 years of age.

Despite the high prevalence of breast cancer in older women, they are less likely to receive standard care and may have worse outcomes as a result. In a study of more than 120,000 women, increasing age was associated with lower surgical rates, less frequent use of radiation, and increased use of primary endocrine therapy (241). We advocate that decisions on treatment be based on a careful, individualized assessment of physiologic age, estimated life expectancy, risks, benefits, treatment tolerance, patient preference, and potential treatment barriers.

While there is currently no standard method of geriatric assessment, tools have attempted to estimate the relative benefit of treatment, taking into account both tumor biologic characteristics as well as a patient's life expectancy. Other potentially useful scales for evaluating chemotherapy toxicity have undergone prospective evaluation and include using low nutritional status (as evaluated using the Mini-Nutritional Assessment) and decreased mobility (evaluated using the timed Up and Go test) to predict increased toxicity to chemotherapy (242); the Cancer and Aging Research Group (CARG) risk score (243); and Chemotherapy Risk Assessment Scale for High-Age Patients (CRASH) score (244). However, these scales need further validation before being used routinely.

Compared to younger women, older women are more likely to have breast cancers that are ER- and PR-positive and HER2-negative, well- or moderately differentiated with a low proliferation index. In contrast, tumor size and nodal involvement have been shown to increase with age, and one analysis of SEER registry data shows older women are diagnosed with metastatic disease more frequently than younger women.

Surgery

Despite earlier studies suggesting that primary medical treatment with tamoxifen was as effective as surgery for the treatment of operable breast cancer in elderly patients, more recent randomized studies have demonstrated a more favorable outcome following surgical management of these patients. A recent Cochrane review also concluded that primary endocrine therapy alone is inferior to surgery for local control of operable breast cancer in older women, and suggests that the option of endocrine therapy alone should be limited to those women whose competing comorbidities preclude them from proceeding to surgery or women who refuse surgery at all (245).

Standard of care for operable breast cancer in older women is similar to those in their younger counterparts. Older patients tolerate surgery as well as their younger counterparts, and the operative mortality of patients who are in reasonable health with a reasonable functional status is negligible (246). Careful evaluation of significant comorbidities will identify the small group of women who would suffer significant morbidity and/or mortality from surgery. Furthermore, the widespread adoption and acceptance of axillary sentinel node biopsy has served to decrease further the risk associated with operative management of breast cancer. In support of this, the IBCSG compared the outcome of axillary clearance versus no clearance in women older than 60 years (median age, 74 years) with clinically negative, operable breast cancer (247). All women with endocrine-responsive breast cancer received 5 years of tamoxifen. Although axillary relapse was not the primary end point, the results were reassuring in this subgroup, showing a relapse rate of ~2% after 5 years of follow-up. Avoiding axillary clearance was associated with an improvement in early quality-of-life measures. These data, in combination with the results of the ACOSOG Z0011 trial discussed earlier, support a limited role of ALND in older women.

Radiotherapy

While the role of postoperative RT in general has been well established, recent retrospective and prospective trials have specifically looked at the role of RT in older women. These data show that while there may be a group of women whose margin of therapeutic benefit for postoperative RT is small enough that radiation can be safely omitted, currently, breast RT remains the standard of care when indicated.

The CALGB 9343 trial randomly assigned women 70 years or older with a clinical stage 1, ER+ breast cancer to lumpectomy plus tamoxifen with or without whole breast RT (180). At completion of a 12.6-year median follow-up, the locoregional recurrence was 2% among patients receiving whole breast RT compared to 10% for those who did not receive whole breast RT. No OS difference was noted. Despite a lower beneficial therapeutic margin, the subset of patients who underwent RT still had a 3% lower risk of breast recurrences favoring radiation in medically fit patients. The PRIME II trial also evaluated the effect of whole breast RT omission following BCS and endocrine therapy in more than 1,300 patients (≥65 years) with T1-2 (≤3 cm), node-negative disease on outcomes (248). IBTR rates were 1.2% and 4.1% with versus without RT, respectively, and again, no differences were found between the two groups in regional recurrence, distant metastases, contralateral breast cancers, or new breast cancers.

The decision to forego RT must take into account the best prognostic estimates and balance carefully a patient's life expectancy with the risk of serious adverse events from RT. Current trials evaluating intraoperative RT, APBI, such as the NSABP B-39 trial, may help to define better the options of postoperative RT for elderly patients.

Systemic Therapy

The benefit of adjuvant hormonal therapy for endocrine-responsive breast cancers is of particular relevance to elderly patients, given that approximately 80% older women have ER+ cancers. Despite this, tamoxifen does carry risks, including rare cases of endometrial cancers and an increased rate of thromboembolic events. With this in mind, it is notable that patients with small (<1 cm), node-negative tumors with other serious comorbid conditions and a life expectancy of less than 10 years are unlikely to benefit significantly from endocrine manipulation.

For women in whom an aromatase inhibitor is being considered, two analyses specifically reported on the outcomes following treatment with aromatase inhibitors among older women. The MA.17 trial evaluated the additional advantage of extended letrozole after 5 years of tamoxifen and did not find an interaction between age and treatment, suggesting that letrozole would be of benefit to older patients as it is for younger women (249). This was consistent with the findings from the Breast International Group (BIG) I-98 trial, which compared letrozole with tamoxifen and showed a significant benefit in favor of letrozole (153). Thus, in regards to elderly women who are at increased risk of bone loss and cardiovascular complications, the long-term risks of aromatase inhibitors may be significant and must be taken into account when recommending adjuvant endocrine therapy.

Despite an overall favorable biologic profile in breast cancer in the elderly, older women deemed to be at a substantial risk of recurrence should be offered chemotherapy. Retrospective analyses of the SEER database have reported a statistically significant reduction in all-cause mortality of 15% to 28% among elderly women with ER-negative cancers treated with chemotherapy, particularly node-positive patients (250,251). Still, most experts suggest limiting chemotherapy to elderly women with hormone receptor-negative tumors that are considered high risk and whose life expectancy exceeds 5 years.

Few women with node-negative, hormone receptor–positive breast cancers are likely to benefit from chemotherapy. Gene-based risk assessment tools, such as the 21-gene recurrence assay, may help to distinguish those women with node-negative tumors and possibly 1 to 3 positive nodes whose risk is sufficiently high enough to warrant chemotherapy. To date, the optimal chemotherapy regimen, dose, and schedule for elderly patients remain undefined. Therefore, treatment approach recommendations regarding regimen should mirror those used in younger women and individualized based on the patient's comorbidities. For example, patients with a history of heart failure may be best treated using a nonanthracycline–based regimen such as docetaxel and cyclophosphamide (252). All women with a HER2-positive cancer and who are otherwise offered systemic chemotherapy should be offered trastuzumab.

INTERNATIONAL PERSPECTIVES

Lynette Denny, MBChB, MMED, PhD, FCOG (SA), South Africa

Early detection and the appropriate treatment of women with breast cancer have resulted in a significant decline in mortality from this disease, possibly exceeding the impact of screening mammography. Clinical breast examination and self-examination may reduce morbidity but are unlikely to have a significant impact on mortality. From the perspective of women with breast cancer in low- and middle-income countries (LMICs), mortality from breast cancer is much higher than in high-income countries (HICs). The main reasons for these disparities are related to (1) late presentation, (2) poor access to quality health services, (3) lack of modern treatment facilities and options, and (4) lack of adequate training of health care professionals in the care of women with breast cancer.

Providing services for women in LMICs requires de novo recognition of cancer as a significant health problem for people living in these countries, and in fact, breast cancer has become the commonest cancer in women in many developing countries, including Africa. Yet, there is a paucity of access to surgical oncology, chemotherapy, hormone therapy, pathology, and radiation. Furthermore, palliative care is hardly practised, and as an example, only approximately 11 countries in Africa provide oral morphine. Where radiation facilities do exist, they are unable to meet the needs of the cancer community; for instance, there are two radiation machines in Ethiopia, a country of 80 million inhabitants. It is important, as we work toward greater equity in the provision of cancer care, to understand the complex nature of interventions required and the absolute necessity for multidisciplinarity. Many countries have one or two pathologists, and even obtaining estrogen or progestogen receptors is impossible. In some settings, surgery is performed without any histology to guide adjuvant therapy, and in other settings, surgery is inappropriately performed, leaving women with disfigurement and great suffering.

Much work is necessary to improve the survival and quality-of-life outcomes for women with breast cancer worldwide. It will take a strong, international, and collaborative commitment to meet the multiple needs already identified and delivered in a socially appropriate manner, cognizant of the differences in infrastructure and affordability across LMICs and HICs.

INTERNATIONAL PERSPECTIVES

Helen MacKay, MBChB, BSc., MRCP, and MD
and Maureen Trudeau, MD, FRCPC, Canada

The presentation, diagnosis, and management of breast cancer as presented in the chapter by Edmonson et al. are applicable in the Canadian context. While the same data are used for decision making, the funding model and some choices of therapy are different from the American model of care. The key points relating to technological advances, screening mammography, surgical resection, radiotherapy, and systemic treatment apply. Cancer Care Ontario guidelines have recently been published (1), and parts of those guidelines have been adopted as ASCO guidelines, reflecting the similarity of Canadian and American practice recommendations (2,3).

The availability of specific drugs in the adjuvant or metastatic setting differs across jurisdictions depending on the interpretation and strength of the evidence and criteria for funding (e.g., pertuzumab is not currently funded publicly in the neoadjuvant setting, and ixabepilone is not funded for metastatic disease). Specific regimens in the adjuvant setting include the use of FEC-D (5 fluorouracil, epirubicin, cyclophosphamide followed by docetaxel) as a standard anthracycline–taxane regimen along with variations of AC-paclitaxel and AC-docetaxel regimens. The most widely used genomic tool for prediction of benefit from hormonal therapy only or of the addition of chemotherapy for early, node-negative (including micromets), ER+, HER2-disease is Oncotype DX; although other assays are being considered. The evidence summaries of pregnancy-associated breast cancer

(*continued*)

INTERNATIONAL PERSPECTIVES (continued)

(PABC) and breast cancer in the elderly are welcome additions to the outline of evidence and complex issues faced in clinical practice. The outline of PABC is similar to Canadian recommendations recently published as well (4).

(1) Eisen A, Fletcher GG, Gandhi S, et al. Optimal systemic therapy for early breast cancer in women: a clinical practice guideline. *Curr Oncol.* 2015;22(Suppl 1):S67–S81.

(2) Denduluri N, Somerfield MR, Eisen A, et al. Selection of optimal adjuvant chemotherapy regimens for early breast cancer and adjuvant targeted therapy for human epidermal growth factor receptor 2-positive breast cancers: an American Society of Clinical Oncology Guideline Adaptation of the Cancer Care Ontario Clinical Practice Guideline [published online April 18, 2016]. *J Clin Oncol.* 2016.

(3) Henry NL, Somerfield MR, Abramson VG, et al. Role of patient and disease factors in adjuvant systemic therapy decision making for early-stage, operable breast cancer: American Society of Clinical Oncology Endorsement of Cancer Care Ontario Guideline Recommendations [published online July 1, 2016]. *J Clin Oncol.* 2016.

(4) Raphael J, Trudeau ME, Chan K. Outcome of patients with pregnancy during or after breast cancer: a review of the recent literature. *Curr Oncol.* 2015;22(Suppl 1):S8–S18.

KEY POINTS

1. Technological advances have improved our ability to classify breast cancers, going from histopathologic characterization of a tumor into the genomic signature that the tumor carries. Luminal, basaloid, and HER2 overamplified breast cancers are a part of this new classification, which may yet help determine the best way to individualize treatments.
2. The mammogram remains the key screening test for women. Ultrasound is useful in distinguishing a benign versus malignant lesion or in the evaluation of a nonmammographically apparent mass. Breast MRI is indicated in selected populations as a screening tool and as an adjunct to mammography for treatment planning purposes.
3. Mastectomy and breast conservation surgeries achieve equivalent outcomes, the latter of which is possible with the use of adjuvant RT. Sentinel node biopsy is the standard of care in the surgical management of the new patient with breast cancer, with a clinically negative axillary examination. Completion axillary dissection in those patients with a positive sentinel node remains standard of care, though considerable controversy exists as to whether this standard must be applied uniformly.
4. The adjuvant treatment of breast cancer must be individualized. While chemotherapy plays an important role in the adjuvant setting, we are recognizing the variable response and benefits that can be achieved, particularly in those women who are ER+, and even in those women who are HER2/neu negative. Patients with high-risk node-negative (1 cm or more if ER-negative, 2 cm or more if ER+) or node-positive breast cancer who are HER2/neu positive, warrant treatment with an anthracycline, taxane treatment, and adjuvant trastuzumab therapy.
5. Endocrine therapy remains the most potent agents for women with ER+ breast cancer.
6. Radiotherapy achieves a reduction in local recurrence when used as an adjuvant modality. This becomes important, as evidence indicates that local recurrence is a predictor of mortality from breast cancer.

The treatment of breast cancer calls for a coordinated multimodality approach that ensures all aspects of the disease are being expeditiously and appropriately addressed.

REFERENCES

1. Siegel RL, Miller KD, Jemal A. Cancer statistics, 2015. *CA Cancer J Clin.* 2015;65:5–29.
2. Chlebowski RT, Hendrix SL, Langer RD, et al. Influence of estrogen plus progestin on breast cancer and mammography in healthy postmenopausal women: the Women's Health Initiative Randomized Trial. *JAMA.* 2003;289:3243–3253.
3. Marchbanks PA, Curtis KM, Mandel MG, et al. Oral contraceptive formulation and risk of breast cancer. *Contraception.* 2012;85:342–350.
4. Gennari A, Costa M, Puntoni M, et al. Breast cancer incidence after hormonal treatments for infertility: systematic review and meta-analysis of population-based studies. *Breast Cancer Res Treat.* 2015;150:405–413.
5. Michels KB, Mohllajee AP, Roset-Bahmanyar E, et al. Diet and breast cancer: a review of the prospective observational studies. *Cancer.* 2007;109:2712–2749.
6. Warner ET, Tamimi RM, Hughes ME, et al. Racial and ethnic differences in breast cancer survival: mediating effect of tumor characteristics and sociodemographic and treatment factors. *J Clin Oncol.* 2015;33:2254–2261.
7. Scalia-Wilbur J, Colins BL, Penson RT, et al. Breast cancer risk assessment: moving beyond BRCA 1 and 2. *Semin Radiat Oncol.* 2016;26:3–8.
8. Miki Y, Swensen J, Shattuck-Eidens D, et al. A strong candidate for the breast and ovarian cancer susceptibility gene BRCA1. *Science.* 1994;266:66–71.
9. Wooster R, Neuhausen SL, Mangion J, et al. Localization of a breast cancer susceptibility gene, BRCA2, to chromosome 13q12-13. *Science.* 1994;265:2088–2090.
10. Hancock SL, Tucker MA, Hoppe RT. Breast cancer after treatment of Hodgkin's disease. *J Natl Cancer Inst.* 1993;85:25–31.
11. Gammon MD, Santella RM, Neugut AI, et al. Environmental toxins and breast cancer on Long Island. I. Polycyclic aromatic hydrocarbon DNA adducts. *Cancer Epidemiol Biomarkers Prev.* 2002;11(8):677–685.
12. Schoenfeld ER, O'Leary ES, Henderson K, et al. Electromagnetic fields and breast cancer on Long Island: a case–control study. *Am J Epidemiol.* 2003;158:47–58.

13. Wang F, Yeung KL, Chan WC, et al. A meta-analysis on dose–response relationship between night shift work and the risk of breast cancer. *Ann Oncol.* 2013;24:2724–2732.
14. Koppes LLJ, Geuskens GA, Pronk A, et al. Night work and breast cancer risk in a general population prospective cohort study in The Netherlands. *Eur J Epidemiol.* 2014;29:577–584.
15. Schernhammer ES, Kroenke CH, Laden F, et al. Night work and risk of breast cancer. *Epidemiol Camb Mass.* 2006;17:108–111.
16. Hartmann LC, Sellers TA, Frost MH, et al. Benign breast disease and the risk of breast cancer. *N Engl J Med.* 2005;353:229–237.
17. Boyd NF, Guo H, Martin LJ, et al. Mammographic density and the risk and detection of breast cancer. *N Engl J Med.* 2007;356:227–236.
18. Wellings SR, Jensen HM, Marcum RG. An atlas of subgross pathology of the human breast with special reference to possible precancerous lesions. *J Natl Cancer Inst.* 1975;55:231–273.
19. Gaffney DK, Tsodikov A, Wiggins CL. Diminished survival in patients with inner versus outer quadrant breast cancers. *J Clin Oncol.* 2003;21:467–472.
20. Tulinius H, Sigvaldason H, Olafsdóttir G. Left and right sided breast cancer. *Pathol Res Pract.* 1990;186:92–94.
21. Lee YT. Breast carcinoma: pattern of metastasis at autopsy. *J Surg Oncol.* 1983;23:175–180.
22. Bloom HJ. The influence of delay on the natural history and prognosis of breast cancer: a study of cases followed for five to twenty years. *Br J Cancer.* 1965;19:228–262.
23. Independent UK Panel on Breast Cancer Screening. The benefits and harms of breast cancer screening: an independent review. *Lancet.* 2012;380:1778–1786.
24. Schopper D, de Wolf C. How effective are breast cancer screening programmes by mammography? Review of the current evidence. *Eur J Cancer.* 2009;45:1916–1923.
25. Miller AB, Wall C, Baines CJ, et al. Twenty five year follow-up for breast cancer incidence and mortality of the Canadian National Breast Screening Study: randomised screening trial. *BMJ.* 2014;348:g366.
26. US Preventive Services Task Force. Screening for breast cancer: U.S. Preventive Services Task Force recommendation statement. *Ann Intern Med.* 2009;151:716–726, W-236.
27. Oeffinger KC, Fontham ET, Etzioni R, et al. Breast cancer screening for women at average risk: 2015 guideline update from the American Cancer Society. *JAMA.* 2015;314:1599–1614.
28. Mainiero MB, Lourenco A, Mahoney MC, et al. ACR appropriateness criteria breast cancer screening. *J Am Coll Radiol.* 2013;10:11–14.
29. American College of Obstetricians-Gynecologists. Practice bulletin no. 122: breast cancer screening. *Obstet Gynecol.* 2011;118:372–382.
30. Esserman LJ, Shieh Y, Rutgers EJ, et al. Impact of mammographic screening on the detection of good and poor prognosis breast cancers. *Breast Cancer Res Treat.* 2011;130(3):725–734.
31. Shaw CM, Flanagan FL, Fenlon HM, et al. Consensus review of discordant findings maximizes cancer detection rate in double-reader screening mammography: Irish National Breast Screening Program experience. *Radiology.* 2009;250:354–362.
32. American College of Radiology. *American College of Radiology Breast Imaging Reporting and Data System BI-RADS.* 5th Ed. In: D'Orsi CJ, Sickles EA, Mendelson EB, et al., eds. Reston, VA: American College of Radiology; 2013.
33. Pisano ED, Gatsonis C, Hendrick E, et al. Diagnostic performance of digital versus film mammography for breast-cancer screening. *N Engl J Med.* 2005;353:1773–1783.
34. Glynn CG, Farria DM, Monsees BS, et al. Effect of transition to digital mammography on clinical outcomes. *Radiology.* 2011;260:664–670.
35. Taylor P, Potts HWW. Computer aids and human second reading as interventions in screening mammography: two systematic reviews to compare effects on cancer detection and recall rate. *Eur J Cancer.* 2008;44:798–807.
36. Gilbert FJ, Astley SM, Gillan MG, et al. Single reading with computer-aided detection for screening mammography. *N Engl J Med.* 2008;359:1675–1684.
37. Loving VA, DeMartini WB, Eby PR, et al. Targeted ultrasound in women younger than 30 years with focal breast signs or symptoms: outcomes analyses and management implications. *AJR Am J Roentgenol.* 2010;195:1472–1477.
38. Friedewald SM, Rafferty EA, Rose SL, et al. Breast cancer screening using tomosynthesis in combination with digital mammography. *JAMA.* 2014;311:2499–2507.
39. DeMartini WB, Rahbar H. Breast magnetic resonance imaging technique at 1.5 T and 3 T: requirements for quality imaging and American College of Radiology accreditation. *Magn Reson Imaging Clin N Am.* 2013;21:475–482.
40. DeMartini W, Lehman C. A review of current evidence-based clinical applications for breast magnetic resonance imaging. *Top Magn Reson Imaging.* 2008;19:143–150.
41. Seely JM, Nguyen ET, Jaffey J. Breast MRI in the evaluation of locally recurrent or new breast cancer in the postoperative patient: correlation of morphology and enhancement features with the BI-RADS category. *Acta Radiol.* 2007;48:838–845.
42. Proulx F, Correa JA, Ferré R, et al. Value of pre-operative breast MRI for the size assessment of ductal carcinoma in situ. *Br J Radiol.* 2016;89:20150543. doi:10.1259/bjr.20150543.
43. Kuhl CK, Schrading S, Leutner CC, et al. Mammography, breast ultrasound, and magnetic resonance imaging for surveillance of women at high familial risk for breast cancer. *J Clin Oncol.* 2005;23:8469–8476.
44. Morris EA, Liberman L, Ballon DJ, et al. MRI of occult breast carcinoma in a high-risk population. *AJR Am J Roentgenol.* 2003;181:619–626.
45. Riedl CC, Ponhold L, Flöry D, et al. Magnetic resonance imaging of the breast improves detection of invasive cancer, preinvasive cancer, and premalignant lesions during surveillance of women at high risk for breast cancer. *Clin Cancer Res.* 2007;13:6144–6152.
46. Medeiros LR, Duarte CS, Rosa DD, et al. Accuracy of magnetic resonance in suspicious breast lesions: a systematic quantitative review and meta-analysis. *Breast Cancer Res Treat.* 2011;126:273–285.
47. Peters NH, Borel Rinkes IH, Zuithoff NP, et al. Meta-analysis of MR imaging in the diagnosis of breast lesions. *Radiology.* 2008;246:116–124.
48. Saslow D, Boetes C, Burke W, et al. American Cancer Society guidelines for breast screening with MRI as an adjunct to mammography. *CA Cancer J Clin.* 2007;57:75–89.
49. Lehman CD, Gatsonis C, Kuhl CK, et al. MRI evaluation of the contralateral breast in women with recently diagnosed breast cancer. *N Engl J Med.* 2007;356:1295–1303.
50. Liberman L, Morris EA, Dershaw DD, et al. MR imaging of the ipsilateral breast in women with percutaneously proven breast cancer. *AJR Am J Roentgenol.* 2003;180:901–910.
51. Girardi V, Carbognin G, Camera L, et al. Multifocal, multicentric and contralateral breast cancers: breast MR imaging in the preoperative evaluation of patients with newly diagnosed breast cancer. *Radiol Med.* 2011;116:1226–1238.
52. Braun M, Pölcher M, Schrading S, et al. Influence of preoperative MRI on the surgical management of patients with operable breast cancer. *Breast Cancer Res Treat.* 2008;111:179–187.
53. Turnbull L, Brown S, Harvey I, et al. Comparative effectiveness of MRI in breast cancer (COMICE) trial: a randomised controlled trial. *Lancet.* 2010;375:563–571.
54. Obdeijn IM, Tilanus-Linthorst MM, Spronk S, et al. Preoperative breast MRI can reduce the rate of tumor-positive resection margins and reoperations in patients undergoing breast-conserving surgery. *AJR Am J Roentgenol.* 2013;200:304–310.
55. Sung JS, Li J, Da Costa G, et al. Preoperative breast MRI for early-stage breast cancer: effect on surgical and long-term outcomes. *AJR Am J Roentgenol.* 2014;202:1376–1382.
56. Fortune-Greeley AK, Wheeler SB, Meyer AM, et al. Preoperative breast MRI and surgical outcomes in elderly women with invasive ductal and lobular carcinoma: a population-based study. *Breast Cancer Res Treat.* 2014;143:203–212.
57. Belli P, Costantini M, Romani M, et al. Magnetic resonance imaging in breast cancer recurrence. *Breast Cancer Res Treat.* 2002;73:223–235.
58. Chen JH, Bahri S, Mehta RS, et al. Impact of factors affecting the residual tumor size diagnosed by MRI following neoadjuvant chemotherapy in comparison to pathology. *J Surg Oncol.* 2014;109:158–167.
59. Dupont WD, Page DL. Risk factors for breast cancer in women with proliferative breast disease. *N Engl J Med.* 1985;312:146–151.
60. Santen RJ, Mansel R. Benign breast disorders. *N Engl J Med.* 2005;353:275–285.
61. Schnitt SJ, Connolly JL, Tavassoli FA, et al. Interobserver reproducibility in the diagnosis of ductal proliferative breast lesions using standardized criteria. *Am J Surg Pathol.* 1992;16:1133–1143.
62. Azzopardi JG. Benign and malignant proliferative epithelial lesions of the breast; a review. *Eur J Cancer Clin Oncol.* 1983;19:1717–1720.
63. Fraser JL, Raza S, Chorny K, et al. Columnar alteration with prominent apical snouts and secretions: a spectrum of changes frequently present in breast biopsies performed for microcalcifications. *Am J Surg Pathol.* 1998;22:1521–1527.
64. Collins LC, Achacoso NA, Nekhlyudov L, et al. Clinical and pathologic features of ductal carcinoma in situ associated with the presence of flat epithelial atypia: an analysis of 543 patients. *Mod Pathol.* 2007;20:1149–1155.
65. Fernández-Aguilar S, Simon P, Buxant F, et al. Tubular carcinoma of the breast and associated intra-epithelial lesions: a comparative study

with invasive low-grade ductal carcinomas. *Virchows Arch Int J Pathol.* 2005;447:683–687.
66. Wells WA, Carney PA, Eliassen MS, et al. Pathologists' agreement with experts and reproducibility of breast ductal carcinoma-in-situ classification schemes. *Am J Surg Pathol.* 2000;24:651–659.
67. de Mascarel I, MacGrogan G, Mathoulin-Pélissier S, et al. Breast ductal carcinoma in situ with microinvasion: a definition supported by a long-term study of 1248 serially sectioned ductal carcinomas. *Cancer.* 2002;94:2134–2142.
68. Sullivan ME, Khan SA, Sullu Y, et al. Lobular carcinoma in situ variants in breast cores: potential for misdiagnosis, upgrade rates at surgical excision, and practical implications. *Arch Pathol Lab Med.* 2010;134:1024–1028.
69. O'Malley FP. Lobular neoplasia: morphology, biological potential and management in core biopsies. *Mod Pathol.* 2010;23(Suppl 2):S14–S25.
70. Elston CW, Ellis IO. Pathological prognostic factors in breast cancer. I. The value of histological grade in breast cancer: experience from a large study with long-term follow-up. C. W. Elston & I. O. Ellis. Histopathology. 1991; 19; 403–410. *Histopathology.* 2002;41:151–152, discussion 152–153.
71. Bane AL, Tjan S, Parkes RK, et al. Invasive lobular carcinoma: to grade or not to grade. *Mod Pathol.* 2005;18:621–628.
72. Diab SG, Clark GM, Osborne CK, et al. Tumor characteristics and clinical outcome of tubular and mucinous breast carcinomas. *J Clin Oncol.* 1999;17(5):1442–1448.
73. Goldstein NS, Kestin LL, Vicini FA. Refined morphologic criteria for tubular carcinoma to retain its favorable outcome status in contemporary breast carcinoma patients. *Am J Clin Pathol.* 2004;122:728–739.
74. Pettinato G, Manivel CJ, Panico L, et al. Invasive micropapillary carcinoma of the breast: clinicopathologic study of 62 cases of a poorly recognized variant with highly aggressive behavior. *Am J Clin Pathol.* 2004;121:857–866.
75. Collins LC, Carlo VP, Hwang H, et al. Intracystic papillary carcinomas of the breast: a reevaluation using a panel of myoepithelial cell markers. *Am J Surg Pathol.* 2006;30:1002–1007.
76. Moatamed NA, Apple SK. Extensive sampling changes T-staging of infiltrating lobular carcinoma of breast: a comparative study of gross versus microscopic tumor sizes. *Breast J.* 2006;12:511–517.
77. Daling JR, Malone KE, Doody DR, et al. Relation of regimens of combined hormone replacement therapy to lobular, ductal, and other histologic types of breast carcinoma. *Cancer.* 2002;95:2455–2464.
78. Allred DC. The utility of conventional and molecular pathology in managing breast cancer. *Breast Cancer Res.* 2008;10(Suppl 4):S4.
79. Hammond ME, Hayes DF, Dowsett M, et al. American Society of Clinical Oncology/College of American Pathologists guideline recommendations for immunohistochemical testing of estrogen and progesterone receptors in breast cancer (unabridged version). *Arch Pathol Lab Med.* 2010;134:e48–e72.
80. Wolff AC, Hammond ME, Hicks DG, et al. Recommendations for human epidermal growth factor receptor 2 testing in breast cancer: American Society of Clinical Oncology/College of American Pathologists clinical practice guideline update. *Arch Pathol Lab Med.* 2014;138:241–256.
81. Daidone MG, Silvestrini R. Prognostic and predictive role of proliferation indices in adjuvant therapy of breast cancer. *J Natl Cancer Inst Monogr.* 2001;(30):27–35.
82. Dowsett M, Nielsen TO, A'Hern R, et al. Assessment of Ki67 in breast cancer: recommendations from the International Ki67 in Breast Cancer working group. *J Natl Cancer Inst.* 2011;103:1656–1664.
83. Perou CM, Sørlie T, Eisen MB, et al. Molecular portraits of human breast tumours. *Nature.* 2000;406:747–752.
84. Cadoo KA, Traina TA, King TA. Advances in molecular and clinical subtyping of breast cancer and their implications for therapy. *Surg Oncol Clin N Am.* 2013;22:823–840.
85. Boyages J, Delaney G, Taylor R. Predictors of local recurrence after treatment of ductal carcinoma in situ: a meta-analysis. *Cancer.* 1999;85:616–628.
86. Douglas-Jones AG, Logan J, Morgan JM, et al. Effect of margins of excision on recurrence after local excision of ductal carcinoma in situ of the breast. *J Clin Pathol.* 2002;55:581–586.
87. Neuschatz AC, DiPetrillo T, Steinhoff M, et al. The value of breast lumpectomy margin assessment as a predictor of residual tumor burden in ductal carcinoma in situ of the breast. *Cancer.* 2002;94(7):1917–1924.
88. Patani N, Cutuli B, Mokbel K. Current management of DCIS: a review. *Breast Cancer Res Treat.* 2008;111:1–10.
89. Wilkie C, White L, Dupont E, et al. An update of sentinel lymph node mapping in patients with ductal carcinoma in situ. *Am J Surg.* 2005;190:563–566.
90. Haid A, Knauer M, Dunzinger S, et al. Intra-operative sonography: a valuable aid during breast-conserving surgery for occult breast cancer. *Ann Surg Oncol.* 2007;14:3090–3101.
91. Duarte GM, Cabello C, Torresan RZ, et al. Radioguided Intraoperative Margins Evaluation (RIME): preliminary results of a new technique to aid breast cancer resection. *Eur J Surg Oncol.* 2007;33:1150–1157.
92. Moran MS, Schnitt SJ, Giuliano AE, et al. Society of Surgical Oncology-American Society for Radiation Oncology consensus guideline on margins for breast-conserving surgery with whole-breast irradiation in stages I and II invasive breast cancer. *Int J Radiat Oncol Biol Phys.* 2014;88:553–564.
93. Chagpar AB, Killelea BK, Tsangaris TN, et al. A randomized, controlled trial of cavity shave margins in breast cancer. *N Engl J Med.* 2015;373(6):503–510.
94. Fisher B, Brown A, Mamounas E, et al. Effect of preoperative chemotherapy on local-regional disease in women with operable breast cancer: findings from National Surgical Adjuvant Breast and Bowel Project B-18. *J Clin Oncol.* 1997;15:2483–2493.
95. Khan A, Sabel MS, Nees A, et al. Comprehensive axillary evaluation in neoadjuvant chemotherapy patients with ultrasonography and sentinel lymph node biopsy. *Ann Surg Oncol.* 2005;12:697–704.
96. Kuerer HM, Sahin AA, Hunt KK, et al. Incidence and impact of documented eradication of breast cancer axillary lymph node metastases before surgery in patients treated with neoadjuvant chemotherapy. *Ann Surg.* 1999;230:72–78.
97. Mansour EG, Gray R, Shatila AH, et al. Survival advantage of adjuvant chemotherapy in high-risk node-negative breast cancer: ten-year analysis—an intergroup study. *J Clin Oncol.* 1998;16:3486–3492.
98. Mainiero MB. Regional lymph node staging in breast cancer: the increasing role of imaging and ultrasound-guided axillary lymph node fine needle aspiration. *Radiol Clin North Am.* 2010;48:989–997.
99. Somasundar P, Gass J, Steinhoff M, et al. Role of ultrasound-guided axillary fine-needle aspiration in the management of invasive breast cancer. *Am J Surg.* 2006;192:458–461.
100. Mamounas EP. Impact of neoadjuvant chemotherapy on locoregional surgical treatment of breast cancer. *Ann Surg Oncol.* 2015;22:1425–1433.
101. Krag DN, Anderson SJ, Julian TB, et al. Sentinel-lymph-node resection compared with conventional axillary-lymph-node dissection in clinically node-negative patients with breast cancer: overall survival findings from the NSABP B-32 randomised phase 3 trial. *Lancet Oncol.* 2010;11:927–933.
102. Giuliano AE, Hunt KK, Ballman KV, et al. Axillary dissection vs no axillary dissection in women with invasive breast cancer and sentinel node metastasis: a randomized clinical trial. *JAMA.* 2011;305:569–575.
103. Galimberti V, Cole BF, Zurrida S, et al. Axillary dissection versus no axillary dissection in patients with sentinel-node micrometastases (IBCSG 23-01): a phase 3 randomised controlled trial. *Lancet Oncol.* 2013;14:297–305.
104. Donker M, van Tienhoven G, Straver ME, et al. Radiotherapy or surgery of the axilla after a positive sentinel node in breast cancer (EORTC 10981-22023 AMAROS): a randomised, multicentre, open-label, phase 3 non-inferiority trial. *Lancet Oncol.* 2014;15:1303–1310.
105. Petrek JA, Heelan MC. Incidence of breast carcinoma-related lymphedema. *Cancer.* 1998;83:2776–2781.
106. Petrek JA, Senie RT, Peters M, et al. Lymphedema in a cohort of breast carcinoma survivors 20 years after diagnosis. *Cancer.* 2001;92:1368–1377.
107. Clough KB, Nasr R, Nos C, et al. New anatomical classification of the axilla with implications for sentinel node biopsy. *Br J Surg.* 2010;97:1659–1665.
108. Van Diest PJ, Torrenga H, Borgstein PJ, et al. Reliability of intraoperative frozen section and imprint cytological investigation of sentinel lymph nodes in breast cancer. *Histopathology.* 1999;35:14–18.
109. Simmons RM, Fish SK, Gayle L, et al. Local and distant recurrence rates in skin-sparing mastectomies compared with non-skin-sparing mastectomies. *Ann Surg Oncol.* 1999;6:676–681.
110. Lanitis S, Tekkis PP, Sgourakis G, et al. Comparison of skin-sparing mastectomy versus non-skin-sparing mastectomy for breast cancer: a meta-analysis of observational studies. *Ann Surg.* 2010;251:632–639.
111. Chen CY, Calhoun KE, Masetti R, et al. Oncoplastic breast conserving surgery: a renaissance of anatomically-based surgical technique. *Minerva Chir.* 2006;61:421–434.
112. Mauri D, Pavlidis N, Ioannidis JP. Neoadjuvant versus adjuvant systemic treatment in breast cancer: a meta-analysis. *J Natl Cancer Inst.* 2005;97:188–194.
113. Rastogi P, Anderson SJ, Bear HD, et al. Preoperative chemotherapy: updates of National Surgical Adjuvant Breast and Bowel Project Protocols B-18 and B-27. *J Clin Oncol.* 2008;26:778–785.

114. Mazouni C, Peintinger F, Wan-Kau S, et al. Residual ductal carcinoma in situ in patients with complete eradication of invasive breast cancer after neoadjuvant chemotherapy does not adversely affect patient outcome. *J Clin Oncol.* 2007;25:2650–2655.
115. Rouzier R, Extra JM, Klijanienko J, et al. Incidence and prognostic significance of complete axillary downstaging after primary chemotherapy in breast cancer patients with T1 to T3 tumors and cytologically proven axillary metastatic lymph nodes. *J Clin Oncol.* 2002;20:1304–1310.
116. von Minckwitz G, Untch M, Blohmer JU, et al. Definition and impact of pathologic complete response on prognosis after neoadjuvant chemotherapy in various intrinsic breast cancer subtypes. *J Clin Oncol.* 2012;30:1796–1804.
117. Ogston KN, Miller ID, Payne S, et al. A new histological grading system to assess response of breast cancers to primary chemotherapy: prognostic significance and survival. *Breast.* 2003;12:320–327.
118. Symmans WF, Peintinger F, Hatzis C, et al. Measurement of residual breast cancer burden to predict survival after neoadjuvant chemotherapy. *J Clin Oncol.* 2007;25:4414–4422.
119. Heys SD, Hutcheon AW, Sarkar TK, et al. Neoadjuvant docetaxel in breast cancer: 3-year survival results from the Aberdeen trial. *Clin Breast Cancer.* 2002;3(Suppl 2):S69–S74.
120. Huober J, von Minckwitz G, Denkert C, et al. Effect of neoadjuvant anthracycline-taxane-based chemotherapy in different biological breast cancer phenotypes: overall results from the GeparTrio study. *Breast Cancer Res Treat.* 2010;124:133–140.
121. Petrelli F, Borgonovo K, Cabiddu M, et al. Neoadjuvant chemotherapy and concomitant trastuzumab in breast cancer: a pooled analysis of two randomized trials. *Anticancer Drugs.* 2011;22:128–135.
122. Baselga J, Bradbury I, Eidtmann H, et al. Lapatinib with trastuzumab for HER2-positive early breast cancer (NeoALTTO): a randomised, open-label, multicentre, phase 3 trial. *Lancet.* 2012;379:633–640.
123. Gianni L, Pienkowski T, Im YH, et al. Efficacy and safety of neoadjuvant pertuzumab and trastuzumab in women with locally advanced, inflammatory, or early HER2-positive breast cancer (NeoSphere): a randomised multicentre, open-label, phase 2 trial. *Lancet Oncol.* 2012;13:25–32.
124. Early Breast Cancer Trialists' Collaborative Group (EBCTCG), Peto R, Davies C, et al. Comparisons between different polychemotherapy regimens for early breast cancer: meta-analyses of long-term outcome among 100,000 women in 123 randomised trials. *Lancet.* 2012;379:432–444.
125. Paik S, Shak S, Tang G, et al. A multigene assay to predict recurrence of tamoxifen-treated, node-negative breast cancer. *N Engl J Med.* 2004;351:2817–2826.
126. Sparano JA, Gray RJ, Makower DF, et al. Prospective validation of a 21-gene expression assay in breast cancer. *N Engl J Med.* 2015;373:2005–2014.
127. Albain KS, Barlow WE, Shak S, et al. Prognostic and predictive value of the 21-gene recurrence score assay in postmenopausal women with node-positive, oestrogen-receptor-positive breast cancer on chemotherapy: a retrospective analysis of a randomised trial. *Lancet Oncol.* 2010;11:55–65.
128. van de Vijver MJ, He YD, van't Veer LJ, et al. A gene-expression signature as a predictor of survival in breast cancer. *N Engl J Med.* 2002;347:1999–2009.
129. Jones S, Holmes FA, O'Shaughnessy J, et al. Docetaxel with cyclophosphamide is associated with an overall survival benefit compared with doxorubicin and cyclophosphamide: 7-year follow-up of US oncology research trial 9735. *J Clin Oncol.* 2009;27:1177–1183.
130. Swain SM, Tang G, Geyer CE Jr, et al. Definitive results of a phase III adjuvant trial comparing three chemotherapy regimens in women with operable, node-positive breast cancer: the NSABP B-38 trial. *J Clin Oncol.* 2013;31:3197–3204.
131. Slamon D, Eiermann W, Robert N, et al. Adjuvant trastuzumab in HER2-positive breast cancer. *N Engl J Med.* 2011;365:1273–1283.
132. Goldhirsch A, Gelber RD, Piccart-Gebhart MJ, et al. 2 years versus 1 year of adjuvant trastuzumab for HER2-positive breast cancer (HERA): an open-label, randomised controlled trial. *Lancet.* 2013;382:1021–1028.
133. Gianni L, Dafni U, Gelber RD, et al. Treatment with trastuzumab for 1 year after adjuvant chemotherapy in patients with HER2-positive early breast cancer: a 4-year follow-up of a randomised controlled trial. *Lancet Oncol.* 2011;12:236–244.
134. Perez EA, Romond EH, Suman VJ, et al. Four-year follow-up of trastuzumab plus adjuvant chemotherapy for operable human epidermal growth factor receptor 2-positive breast cancer: joint analysis of data from NCCTG N9831 and NSABP B-31. *J Clin Oncol.* 2011;29:3366–3373.
135. Romond EH, Perez EA, Bryant J, et al. Trastuzumab plus adjuvant chemotherapy for operable HER2-positive breast cancer. *N Engl J Med.* 2005;353:1673–1684.
136. NCCN Clinical Practice Guidelines in Oncology: Survivorship (V 2.2015). http://www.nccn.org/professionals/physician_gls/f_guidelines.asp#survivorship.
137. Tolaney SM, Barry WT, Dang CT, et al. Adjuvant paclitaxel and trastuzumab for node-negative, HER2-positive breast cancer. *N Engl J Med.* 2015;372:134–141.
138. Dear RF, McGeechan K, Jenkins MC, et al. Combination versus sequential single agent chemotherapy for metastatic breast cancer. *Cochrane Database Syst Rev.* 2013;(12):CD008792.
139. Robert N, Leyland-Jones B, Asmar L, et al. Randomized phase III study of trastuzumab, paclitaxel, and carboplatin compared with trastuzumab and paclitaxel in women with HER-2-overexpressing metastatic breast cancer. *J Clin Oncol.* 2006;24:2786–2792.
140. Valero V, Forbes J, Pegram MD, et al. Multicenter phase III randomized trial comparing docetaxel and trastuzumab with docetaxel, carboplatin, and trastuzumab as first-line chemotherapy for patients with HER2-gene-amplified metastatic breast cancer (BCIRG 007 study): two highly active therapeutic regimens. *J Clin Oncol.* 2011;29:149–156.
141. von Minckwitz G, du Bois A, Schmidt M, et al. Trastuzumab beyond progression in human epidermal growth factor receptor 2-positive advanced breast cancer: a German Breast Group 26/Breast International Group 03-05 study. *J Clin Oncol.* 2009;27:1999–2006.
142. Cameron D, Casey M, Press M, et al. A phase III randomized comparison of lapatinib plus capecitabine versus capecitabine alone in women with advanced breast cancer that has progressed on trastuzumab: updated efficacy and biomarker analyses. *Breast Cancer Res Treat.* 2008;112:533–543.
143. Blackwell KL, Burstein HJ, Storniolo AM, et al. Randomized study of Lapatinib alone or in combination with trastuzumab in women with ErbB2-positive, trastuzumab-refractory metastatic breast cancer. *J Clin Oncol.* 2010;28:1124–1130.
144. Baselga J, Cortés J, Kim SB, et al. Pertuzumab plus trastuzumab plus docetaxel for metastatic breast cancer. *N Engl J Med.* 2012;366:109–119.
145. Early Breast Cancer Trialists' Collaborative Group (EBCTCG). Effects of chemotherapy and hormonal therapy for early breast cancer on recurrence and 15-year survival: an overview of the randomised trials. *Lancet.* 2005;365:1687–1717.
146. Fisher B, Costantino J, Redmond C, et al. A randomized clinical trial evaluating tamoxifen in the treatment of patients with node-negative breast cancer who have estrogen-receptor-positive tumors. *N Engl J Med.* 1989;320:479–484.
147. Adjuvant tamoxifen in the management of operable breast cancer: the Scottish Trial. Report from the Breast Cancer Trials Committee, Scottish Cancer Trials Office (MRC), Edinburgh. *Lancet.* 1987;2:171–175.
148. Fisher B, Costantino JP, Wickerham DL, et al. Tamoxifen for prevention of breast cancer: report of the National Surgical Adjuvant Breast and Bowel Project P-1 Study. *J Natl Cancer Inst.* 1998;90:1371–1388.
149. Benson JR. Re: Five versus more than five years of tamoxifen for lymph node-negative breast cancer: updated findings from the National Surgical Adjuvant Breast and Bowel Project B-14 Randomized Trial. *J Natl Cancer Inst.* 2001;93(19): 1493–1494.
150. Sestak I, Distler W, Forbes JF, et al. Effect of body mass index on recurrences in tamoxifen and anastrozole treated women: an exploratory analysis from the ATAC trial. *J Clin Oncol.* 2010;28(21):3411–3415.
151. Coombes RC, Kilburn LS, Snowdon CF, et al. Survival and safety of exemestane versus tamoxifen after 2–3 years' tamoxifen treatment (Intergroup Exemestane Study): a randomised controlled trial. *Lancet.* 2007;369:559–570.
152. Bliss JM, Kilburn LS, Coleman RE, et al. Disease-related outcomes with long-term follow-up: an updated analysis of the intergroup exemestane study. *J Clin Oncol.* 2012;30(7):709–717.
153. Breast International Group (BIG) 1-98 Collaborative Group, Thürlimann B, Keshaviah A, et al. A comparison of letrozole and tamoxifen in postmenopausal women with early breast cancer. *N Engl J Med.* 2005;353:2747–2757.
154. Goss PE, Ingle JN, Alés-Martínez JE, et al. Exemestane for breast-cancer prevention in postmenopausal women. *N Engl J Med.* 2011; 364(25):2381–2391.
155. Jin H, Tu D, Zhao N, et al. Longer-term outcomes of letrozole versus placebo after 5 years of tamoxifen in the NCIC CTG MA.17 trial: analyses adjusting for treatment crossover. *J Clin Oncol.* 2012;30(7):718–721.
156. Davies C, Pan H, Godwin J, et al. Long-term effects of continuing adjuvant tamoxifen to 10 years versus stopping at 5 years after diagnosis of oestrogen receptor-positive breast cancer: ATLAS, a randomised trial. *Lancet.* 2013;381:805–816.
157. Gray RG, Rea D, Handley K, et al. aTTom: Long-term effects of continuing adjuvant tamoxifen to 10 years versus stopping at 5 years in 6,953

women with early breast cancer. *J Clin Oncol.* 2013;31(Suppl; abstr 5). http://meetinglibrary.asco.org/content/112995-132.

158. Early Breast Cancer Trialists' Collaborative Group (EBCTCG), Davies C, Godwin J, et al. Relevance of breast cancer hormone receptors and other factors to the efficacy of adjuvant tamoxifen: patient-level meta-analysis of randomised trials. *Lancet.* 2011;378:771–784.
159. Amir E, Seruga B, Niraula S, et al. Toxicity of adjuvant endocrine therapy in postmenopausal breast cancer patients: a systematic review and meta-analysis. *J Natl Cancer Inst.* 2011;103(17):1299–1309.
160. Pagani O, Regan MM, Francis PA; TEXT and SOFT Investigators & International Breast Cancer Study Group. Exemestane with ovarian suppression in premenopausal breast cancer. *N Engl J Med.* 2014;371:1358–1359.
161. Francis PA, Regan MM, Fleming GF. Adjuvant ovarian suppression in premenopausal breast cancer. *N Engl J Med.* 2015;372:436–446.
162. Robertson JF, Llombart-Cussac A, Rolski J, et al. Activity of fulvestrant 500 mg versus anastrozole 1 mg as first-line treatment for advanced breast cancer: results from the FIRST study. *J Clin Oncol.* 2009;27:4530–4535.
163. Mauri D, Pavlidis N, Polyzos NP, et al. Survival with aromatase inhibitors and inactivators versus standard hormonal therapy in advanced breast cancer: meta-analysis. *J Natl Cancer Inst.* 2006;98:1285–1291.
164. Baselga J, Campone M, Piccart M, et al. Everolimus in postmenopausal hormone-receptor-positive advanced breast cancer. *N Engl J Med.* 2012;366:520–529.
165. Finn RS, Crown JP, Lang I, et al. The cyclin-dependent kinase 4/6 inhibitor palbociclib in combination with letrozole versus letrozole alone as first-line treatment of oestrogen receptor-positive, HER2-negative, advanced breast cancer (PALOMA-1/TRIO-18): a randomised phase 2 study. *Lancet Oncol.* 2015;16:25–35.
166. Turner NC, Huang Bartlett C, Cristofanilli M. Palbociclib in hormone-receptor-positive advanced breast cancer. *N Engl J Med.* 2015;373:209–219.
167. Johnston S, Pippen J Jr, Pivot X, et al. Lapatinib combined with letrozole versus letrozole and placebo as first-line therapy for postmenopausal hormone receptor-positive metastatic breast cancer. *J Clin Oncol.* 2009;27:5538–5546.
168. Kaufman B, Mackey JR, Clemens MR, et al. Trastuzumab plus anastrozole versus anastrozole alone for the treatment of postmenopausal women with human epidermal growth factor receptor 2-positive, hormone receptor-positive metastatic breast cancer: results from the randomized phase III TAnDEM study. *J Clin Oncol.* 2009;27:5529–5537.
169. Ellis MJ, Ma C. Letrozole in the neoadjuvant setting: the P024 trial. *Breast Cancer Res Treat.* 2007;105(Suppl 1):33–43.
170. Fisher B, Land S, Mamounas E, et al. Prevention of invasive breast cancer in women with ductal carcinoma in situ: an update of the National Surgical Adjuvant Breast and Bowel Project experience. *Semin Oncol.* 2001;28:400–418.
171. Cuzick J, Sestak I, Cawthorn S, et al. Tamoxifen for prevention of breast cancer: extended long-term follow-up of the IBIS-I breast cancer prevention trial. *Lancet Oncol.* 2015;16(1):67–75.
172. Vogel VG, Costantino JP, Wickerham DL, et al. Update of the National Surgical Adjuvant Breast and Bowel Project Study of Tamoxifen and Raloxifene (STAR) P-2 trial: preventing breast cancer. *Cancer Prev Res.* 2010;3:696–706.
173. Cuzick J, Sestak I, Forbes JF, et al. Anastrozole for prevention of breast cancer in high-risk postmenopausal women (IBIS-II): an international, double-blind, randomised placebo-controlled trial. *Lancet.* 2014;383(9922):1041–1048.
174. Cuzick J, Powles T, Veronesi U, et al. Overview of the main outcomes in breast-cancer prevention trials. *Lancet.* 2003;361:296–300.
175. Forbes JF, Sestak I, Howell A, et al. Anastrozole versus tamoxifen for the prevention of locoregional and contralateral breast cancer in postmenopausal women with locally excised ductal carcinoma in situ (IBIS-II DCIS): a double-blind, randomised controlled trial. *Lancet.* 2016;387(10021):866–873. doi:10.1016/S0140-6736(15)01129-0.
176. Clarke M, Collins R, Darby S, et al. Effects of radiotherapy and of differences in the extent of surgery for early breast cancer on local recurrence and 15-year survival: an overview of the randomised trials. *Lancet.* 2005;366:2087–2106.
177. Fisher B, Jeong JH, Anderson S, et al. Twenty-five-year follow-up of a randomized trial comparing radical mastectomy, total mastectomy, and total mastectomy followed by irradiation. *N Engl J Med.* 2002;347:567–575.
178. Early Breast Cancer Trialists' Collaborative Group (EBCTCG), Darby S, McGale P, et al. Effect of radiotherapy after breast-conserving surgery on 10-year recurrence and 15-year breast cancer death: meta-analysis of individual patient data for 10,801 women in 17 randomised trials. *Lancet.* 2011;378:1707–1716.
179. Fisher B, Bryant J, Dignam JJ, et al. Tamoxifen, radiation therapy, or both for prevention of ipsilateral breast tumor recurrence after lumpectomy in women with invasive breast cancers of one centimeter or less. *J Clin Oncol.* 2002;20:4141–4149.
180. Hughes KS, Schnaper LA, Bellon JR, et al. Lumpectomy plus tamoxifen with or without irradiation in women age 70 years or older with early breast cancer: long-term follow-up of CALGB 9343. *J Clin Oncol.* 2013;31:2382–2387.
181. Hughes KS, Schnaper LA, Berry D, et al. Lumpectomy plus tamoxifen with or without irradiation in women 70 years of age or older with early breast cancer. *N Engl J Med.* 2004;351:971–977.
182. Hepel JT, Wazer DE. Should a woman age 70 to 80 years receive radiation after breast-conserving surgery? *J Clin Oncol.* 2013;31:2377–2381.
183. Overgaard M, Christensen JJ, Johansen H, et al. Evaluation of radiotherapy in high-risk breast cancer patients: report from the Danish Breast Cancer Cooperative Group (DBCG 82) Trial. *Int J Radiat Oncol Biol Phys.* 1990;19:1121–1124.
184. Overgaard M, Jensen MB, Overgaard J, et al. Postoperative radiotherapy in high-risk postmenopausal breast-cancer patients given adjuvant tamoxifen: Danish Breast Cancer Cooperative Group DBCG 82c randomised trial. *Lancet.* 1999;353:1641–1648.
185. Ragaz J, Olivotto IA, Spinelli JJ, et al. Locoregional radiation therapy in patients with high-risk breast cancer receiving adjuvant chemotherapy: 20-year results of the British Columbia randomized trial. *J Natl Cancer Inst.* 2005;97:116–126.
186. EBCTCG (Early Breast Cancer Trialists' Collaborative Group), McGale P, Taylor C, et al. Effect of radiotherapy after mastectomy and axillary surgery on 10-year recurrence and 20-year breast cancer mortality: meta-analysis of individual patient data for 8135 women in 22 randomised trials. *Lancet.* 2014;383:2127–2135.
187. Jagsi R, Raad RA, Goldberg S, et al. Locoregional recurrence rates and prognostic factors for failure in node-negative patients treated with mastectomy: implications for postmastectomy radiation. *Int J Radiat Oncol Biol Phys.* 2005;62:1035–1039.
188. Wang J, Shi M, Ling R, et al. Adjuvant chemotherapy and radiotherapy in triple-negative breast carcinoma: a prospective randomized controlled multi-center trial. *Radiother Oncol.* 2011;100:200–204.
189. Jagsi R, Chadha M, Moni J, et al. Radiation field design in the ACOSOG Z0011 (Alliance) Trial. *J Clin Oncol.* 2014;32:3600–3606.
190. Whelan TJ, Olivotto IA, Levine MN. Regional nodal irradiation in early-stage breast cancer. *N Engl J Med.* 2015;373:1878–1879.
191. Poortmans PM, Collette S, Kirkove C, et al. Internal mammary and medial supraclavicular irradiation in breast cancer. *N Engl J Med.* 2015;373:317–327.
192. Morrow M, Foster RS. Staging of breast cancer: a new rationale for internal mammary node biopsy. *Arch Surg.* 1981;116:748–751.
193. Veronesi U, Cascinelli N, Bufalino R, et al. Risk of internal mammary lymph node metastases and its relevance on prognosis of breast cancer patients. *Ann Surg.* 1983;198:681–684.
194. Chang JS, Park W, Kim YB, et al. Long-term survival outcomes following internal mammary node irradiation in stage II–III breast cancer: results of a large retrospective study with 12-year follow-up. *Int J Radiat Oncol Biol Phys.* 2013;86:867–872.
195. Thorsen LB, Offersen BV, Danø H, et al. DBCG-IMN: a population-based cohort study on the effect of internal mammary node irradiation in early node-positive breast cancer. *J Clin Oncol Off J Am Soc Clin Oncol.* 2016;34(4):314–320. doi:10.1200/JCO.2015.63.6456.
196. Freedman GM, Fowble BL, Nicolaou N, et al. Should internal mammary lymph nodes in breast cancer be a target for the radiation oncologist? *Int J Radiat Oncol Biol Phys.* 2000;46:805–814.
197. Hennequin C, Bossard N, Servagi-Vernat S, et al. Ten-year survival results of a randomized trial of irradiation of internal mammary nodes after mastectomy. *Int J Radiat Oncol Biol Phys.* 2013;86:860–866.
198. Early Breast Cancer Trialists' Collaborative Group (EBCTCG), Correa C, McGale P, et al. Overview of the randomized trials of radiotherapy in ductal carcinoma in situ of the breast. *J Natl Cancer Inst Monogr.* 2010;2010:162–177.
199. Wong JS, Kaelin CM, Troyan SL, et al. Prospective study of wide excision alone for ductal carcinoma in situ of the breast. *J Clin Oncol.* 2006;24:1031–1036.
200. Hughes LL, Wang M, Page DL, et al. Local excision alone without irradiation for ductal carcinoma in situ of the breast: a trial of the Eastern Cooperative Oncology Group. *J Clin Oncol.* 2009;27:5319–5324.
201. McCormick B, Winter K, Hudis C, et al. RTOG 9804: a prospective randomized trial for good-risk ductal carcinoma in situ comparing radiotherapy with observation. *J Clin Oncol.* 2015;33:709–715.
202. Veronesi U, Marubini E, Mariani L, et al. Radiotherapy after breast-conserving surgery in small breast carcinoma: long-term results of a randomized trial. *Ann Oncol.* 2001;12:997–1003.

203. Vicini FA, Kestin LL, Goldstein NS. Defining the clinical target volume for patients with early-stage breast cancer treated with lumpectomy and accelerated partial breast irradiation: a pathologic analysis. *Int J Radiat Oncol Biol Phys.* 2004;60:722–730.
204. Hepel JT, Wazer DE. A comparison of brachytherapy techniques for partial breast irradiation. *Brachytherapy.* 2012;11:163–175.
205. Strnad V, Ott OJ, Hildebrandt G, et al. 5-year results of accelerated partial breast irradiation using sole interstitial multicatheter brachytherapy versus whole-breast irradiation with boost after breast-conserving surgery for low-risk invasive and in-situ carcinoma of the female breast: a randomised, phase 3, non-inferiority trial. *Lancet.* 2016;387(10015):229–238. doi:10.1016/S0140-6736(15)00471-7.
206. Shah C, Vicini F, Wazer DE, et al. The American Brachytherapy Society consensus statement for accelerated partial breast irradiation. *Brachytherapy.* 2013;12:267–277.
207. Consensus Statement for Accelerated Partial Breast Irradiation (APBI). https://www.breastsurgeons.org/new_layout/about/statements/PDF_Statements/APBI.pdf.
208. Rusthoven KE, Kavanagh BD, Cardenes H, et al. Multi-institutional phase I/II trial of stereotactic body radiation therapy for liver metastases. *J Clin Oncol.* 2009;27:1572–1578.
209. Wang XS, Rhines LD, Shiu AS, et al. Stereotactic body radiation therapy for management of spinal metastases in patients without spinal cord compression: a phase 1–2 trial. *Lancet Oncol.* 2012;13:395–402.
210. Bartelink H, Maingon P, Poortmans P, et al. Whole-breast irradiation with or without a boost for patients treated with breast-conserving surgery for early breast cancer: 20-year follow-up of a randomised phase 3 trial. *Lancet Oncol.* 2015;16:47–56.
211. Romestaing P, Lehingue Y, Carrie C, et al. Role of a 10-Gy boost in the conservative treatment of early breast cancer: results of a randomized clinical trial in Lyon, France. *J Clin Oncol.* 1997;15:963–968.
212. Hepel JT, Evans SB, Hiatt JR, et al. Planning the breast boost: comparison of three techniques and evolution of tumor bed during treatment. *Int J Radiat Oncol Biol Phys.* 2009;74:458–463.
213. Leonard KL, Hepel JT, Styczynski JR, et al. Breast boost using noninvasive image-guided breast brachytherapy vs. external beam: a 2:1 matched-pair analysis. *Clin Breast Cancer.* 2013;13:455–459.
214. Whelan TJ, Pignol JP, Levine MN, et al. Long-term results of hypofractionated radiation therapy for breast cancer. *N Engl J Med.* 2010;362:513–520.
215. Haviland JS, Owen JR, Dewar JA, et al. The UK Standardisation of Breast Radiotherapy (START) trials of radiotherapy hypofractionation for treatment of early breast cancer: 10-year follow-up results of two randomised controlled trials. *Lancet Oncol.* 2013;14:1086–1094.
216. National Toxicology Program. NTP monograph: developmental effects and pregnancy outcomes associated with cancer chemotherapy use during pregnancy. *NTP Monogr.* 2013;(2):i–214.
217. Andersson TM, Johansson AL, Hsieh CC, et al. Increasing incidence of pregnancy-associated breast cancer in Sweden. Obstet Gynecol. 2009;114(3):568–572.
218. Navrozoglou I, Vrekoussis T, Kontostolis E, et al. Breast cancer during pregnancy: a mini-review. *Eur J Surg Oncol.* 2008;34:837–843.
219. Oto A, Ernst R, Jesse MK, et al. Magnetic resonance imaging of the chest, abdomen, and pelvis in the evaluation of pregnant patients with neoplasms. *Am J Perinatol.* 2007;24:243–250.
220. Streffer C, Shore R, Konermann G, et al. Biological effects after prenatal irradiation (embryo and fetus). A report of the International Commission on Radiological Protection. *Ann ICRP.* 2003;33:5–206.
221. Amant F, Loibl S, Neven P, et al. Breast cancer in pregnancy. *Lancet.* 2012;379:570–579.
222. Middleton LP, Chen V, Perkins GH, et al. Histopathology of breast cancer among African-American women. *Cancer.* 2003;97(1 Suppl):253–257.
223. Amant F, von Minckwitz G, Han SN, et al. Prognosis of women with primary breast cancer diagnosed during pregnancy: results from an international collaborative study. *J Clin Oncol.* 2013;31:2532–2539.
224. Murphy CG, Mallam D, Stein S, et al. Current or recent pregnancy is associated with adverse pathologic features but not impaired survival in early breast cancer. *Cancer.* 2012;118:3254–3259.
225. Azim HA Jr, Santoro L, Russell-Edu W, et al. Prognosis of pregnancy-associated breast cancer: a meta-analysis of 30 studies. *Cancer Treat Rev.* 2012;38:834–842.
226. Callihan EB, Gao D, Jindal S, et al. Postpartum diagnosis demonstrates a high risk for metastasis and merits an expanded definition of pregnancy-associated breast cancer. *Breast Cancer Res Treat.* 2013;138:549–559.
227. Gropper AB, Calvillo KZ, Dominici L, et al. Sentinel lymph node biopsy in pregnant women with breast cancer. *Ann Surg Oncol.* 2014;21:2506–2511.
228. Pruthi S, Haakenson C, Brost BC, et al. Pharmacokinetics of methylene blue dye for lymphatic mapping in breast cancer-implications for use in pregnancy. *Am J Surg.* 2011;201:70–75.
229. Raut CP, Daley MD, Hunt KK, et al. Anaphylactoid reactions to isosulfan blue dye during breast cancer lymphatic mapping in patients given preoperative prophylaxis. *J Clin Oncol.* 2004;22:567–568.
230. Kal HB, Struikmans H. Radiotherapy during pregnancy: fact and fiction. *Lancet Oncol.* 2005;6:328–333.
231. Hahn KM, Johnson PH, Gordon N, et al. Treatment of pregnant breast cancer patients and outcomes of children exposed to chemotherapy in utero. *Cancer.* 2006;107:1219–1226.
232. Framarino-Dei-Malatesta M, Perrone G, Giancotti A, et al. Epirubicin: a new entry in the list of fetal cardiotoxic drugs? Intrauterine death of one fetus in a twin pregnancy. Case report and review of literature. *BMC Cancer.* 2015;15:951.
233. Zagouri F, Sergentanis TN, Chrysikos D, et al. Taxanes for ovarian cancer during pregnancy: a systematic review. *Oncology.* 2012;83:234–238.
234. Zagouri F, Sergentanis TN, Chrysikos D, et al. Trastuzumab administration during pregnancy: a systematic review and meta-analysis. *Breast Cancer Res Treat.* 2013;137:349–357.
235. The MotHER Pregnancy Registry. http://www.motherpregnancyregistry.com/.
236. Amant F, Vandenbroucke T, Verheecke M, et al. Pediatric outcome after maternal cancer diagnosed during pregnancy. *N Engl J Med.* 2015;373:1824–1834.
237. Azim HA Jr, Kroman N, Paesmans M, et al. Prognostic impact of pregnancy after breast cancer according to estrogen receptor status: a multicenter retrospective study. *J Clin Oncol.* 2013;31:73–79.
238. Sankila R, Heinävaara S, Hakulinen T. Survival of breast cancer patients after subsequent term pregnancy: 'healthy mother effect.' *Am J Obstet Gynecol.* 1994;170:818–823.
239. Higgins S, Haffty BG. Pregnancy and lactation after breast-conserving therapy for early stage breast cancer. *Cancer.* 1994;73:2175–2180.
240. Loren AW, Mangu PB, Beck LN, et al. Fertility preservation for patients with cancer: American Society of Clinical Oncology clinical practice guideline update. *J Clin Oncol.* 2013;31:2500–2510.
241. Lavelle K, Sowerbutts AM, Bundred N, et al. Is lack of surgery for older breast cancer patients in the UK explained by patient choice or poor health? A prospective cohort study. *Br J Cancer.* 2014;110:573–583.
242. Soubeyran P, Fonck M, Blanc-Bisson C, et al. Predictors of early death risk in older patients treated with first-line chemotherapy for cancer. *J Clin Oncol.* 2012;30:1829–1834.
243. Hurria A, Togawa K, Mohile SG, et al. Predicting chemotherapy toxicity in older adults with cancer: a prospective multicenter study. *J Clin Oncol.* 2011;29:3457–3465.
244. Extermann M, Boler I, Reich RR, et al. Predicting the risk of chemotherapy toxicity in older patients: the Chemotherapy Risk Assessment Scale for High-Age Patients (CRASH) score. *Cancer.* 2012;118:3377–3386.
245. Hind D, Wyld L, Reed MW. Surgery, with or without tamoxifen, vs tamoxifen alone for older women with operable breast cancer: cochrane review. *Br J Cancer.* 2007;96:1025–1029.
246. Audisio RA, Bozzetti F, Gennari R, et al. The surgical management of elderly cancer patients; recommendations of the SIOG surgical task force. *Eur J Cancer.* 2004;40:926–938.
247. International Breast Cancer Study Group, Rudenstam CM, Zahrieh D, et al. Randomized trial comparing axillary clearance versus no axillary clearance in older patients with breast cancer: first results of International Breast Cancer Study Group Trial 10-93. *J Clin Oncol.* 2006;24:337–344.
248. Kunkler IH, Williams LJ, Jack WJ, et al. Breast-conserving surgery with or without irradiation in women aged 65 years or older with early breast cancer (PRIME II): a randomised controlled trial. *Lancet Oncol.* 2015;16:266–273.
249. Muss HB, Tu D, Ingle JN, et al. Efficacy, toxicity, and quality of life in older women with early-stage breast cancer treated with letrozole or placebo after 5 years of tamoxifen: NCIC CTG intergroup trial MA.17. *J Clin Oncol.* 2008;26:1956–1964.
250. Elkin EB, Hurria A, Mitra N, et al. Adjuvant chemotherapy and survival in older women with hormone receptor-negative breast cancer: assessing outcome in a population-based, observational cohort. *J Clin Oncol.* 2006;24:2757–2764.
251. Giordano SH, Duan Z, Kuo YF, et al. Use and outcomes of adjuvant chemotherapy in older women with breast cancer. *J Clin Oncol.* 2006;24:2750–2756.
252. Freyer G, Campone M, Peron J, et al. Adjuvant docetaxel/cyclophosphamide in breast cancer patients over the age of 70: results of an observational study. *Crit Rev Oncol Hematol.* 2011;80:466–473.

CHAPTER 28

Management of Infections in Patients with Gynecologic Malignancy

Amar Safdar, Kenneth Rolston, and Donald Armstrong

Patients with gynecologic cancer are susceptible to infections. The risk of developing an infection can arise from a number of factors that may be related to the neoplasm and antineoplastic therapy, or both. Tumor encroachment and invasion of adjacent structures, necrosis of expanding tumor mass, surgical tumor excision and removal of internal organs including lymph nodes, and diversion procedures that disrupt protective barriers in the lower and upper female reproductive tract are some of the factors. Patients with these malignancies may also be susceptible to a host of infections due to the presence of drug- or radiation-induced mucositis, severe neutropenia, long-term sequelae of prior abdominopelvic radiation therapy, and the presence of indwelling foreign devices (1,2).

The wide spectrum of causative microorganisms most frequently arise from endogenous vaginal, urethral, and intestinal tract colonization with bacteria and Candida species. The normal aerobic and anaerobic vaginal bacterial flora may be altered in patients undergoing antimicrobial and antineoplastic therapy. Among factors that influence changes in colonization are hormonal dysfunction, alteration in the composition of mucosal secretions including innate immune functions, frequent exposure to broad-spectrum antimicrobial agents, antineoplastic drug and radiation therapy, instrumentation, and prolonged, often multiple hospitalizations. In a recent report, however, patients receiving external-beam radiotherapy for gynecologic malignancy did not experience changes in aerobic microflora in the vagina, cervix, or rectum (3,4). Whereas significant growth in vaginal yeast species occurred during the first 2 weeks after radiation therapy commenced, *Candida albicans* and *Candida tropicalis* were most prominent. The increase of vaginal growth in *Candida* species returned to preradiation levels after 4 weeks (5). Exposure to health care facilities, especially centers that care for immunocompromised oncology patients, has been recognized as a major influence, albeit transient in most instances, in promoting changes in cutaneous, orointestinal, and genitourinary microflora. The changes in vaginal and lower urinary tract microflora occur less commonly, even following repeat exposure to the hospital environment, and are often limited to patients who undergo instrumentation. The health care–associated microorganisms are frequently less susceptible to commonly prescribed antibiotics, and optimum selection of antimicrobial drugs poses a daunting challenge. It is, however, important to appreciate that changes in a host's microflora are in most cases transient, and restitution of normal intestinal and vaginal flora occurs once factors promoting the change have been removed.

The female genital tract is rich in anaerobic microflora. Peptococcaceae are prominent in the normal vaginal bacterial flora. Quantitative vaginal cultures in recent studies showed that anaerobic bacteria outnumbered aerobic bacteria by nearly 10:1; peptococci, *Lactobacillus, Corynebacterium, Eubacterium*, and *Bacteroides* species are frequently isolated (6). *Escherichia coli, Klebsiella* species, and *Enterobacter* species are the aerobic gram negatives, and streptococci, enterococci, and coagulase-negative staphylococcus are gram-positive bacteria isolated from the lower female genital tract. These organisms provide an important reference to local and invasive infections seen in patients undergoing treatment for gynecologic malignancy.

This chapter provides an overview of infections encountered in patients receiving treatment for cancers involving the female reproductive system. A detailed review of specific diseases such as postsurgical abdominopelvic infections, febrile neutropenia, and bacteremia is presented. A focused discussion regarding the changing epidemiology of causative organisms, the increasing rate of infection due to drug-resistant organisms, and an update on new antimicrobial agents is briefly provided.

PATIENTS WITH FEVER

The factors that increase the risk of infection are shown in **Table 28.1**. Knowledge of underlying predisposing factor(s) is necessary in the selection of appropriate empiric therapy. Antibiotic prophylaxis and/or recent treatment with broad-spectrum antimicrobial drugs have been associated with the risk of infection(s) due to nondrug-susceptible microorganisms, including systemic candidiasis. Awareness of specific cancer and cancer therapy–associated risks, and the host's underlying immune dysfunction, may allow for proper selection of empiric antibiotic therapy in critically ill patients prior to the results of diagnostic microbiologic and radiographic studies being known. It is important to note that patients with gynecologic cancer may have a high risk of polymicrobial infections due to the presence of physiologic microflora resulting from anatomic proximity to the lower intestinal and urinary tracts. In certain infections, such as deep tissue abscess, cellulitis in patients with chronic fistula tract, presence of large necrotic tumor, and history of multiple recent instrumentations, the probability of polymicrobial infection remains high (7). Furthermore, in patients with a known anaerobic bloodstream infection, concurrent bacteremia due to aerobic organism(s) is not uncommon (7). Patients with advanced cancer, history of radiation therapy, and extensive pelvic surgery may develop obstruction to the pelvic venous and lymphatic flow. The aberration in physiologic/anatomic defenses and stagnation heightens the risk of cellulitis, abscess formation, and septic thrombophlebitis. Furthermore, these factors also unfavorably influence response to antimicrobial therapy. Several comprehensive cancer centers and other institutions that care for large numbers of patients with cancer have developed infectious disease consultative services with a special interest and expertise in infections seen in this high-risk patient population. **Table 28.2** provides a breakdown of the various infectious and noninfectious causes prompting infectious disease consultation requests from the gynecologic oncology clinical service at the MD Anderson Cancer Center.

TUMOR-RELATED INFECTIONS

Tumor-associated infections are dependent on the anatomic site, type, and extent of tumor involvement. In patients with an early stage of locally involved cancer such as stage I cervical cancer, most infections remain localized to the vagina, whereas in patients with

TABLE 28.1. Predisposing Risk Factors and Infections in Patients with Gynecologic Tumors

Tumor related
Obstruction of gastrointestinal or urinary tract
Erosion into bowel, urinary tract, peritoneum, or retroperitoneal space
Necrosis of rapidly growing cancer promotes abscess formation
Lymphatic obstruction
Surgery
Aspiration pneumonia
Hospital-acquired pneumonia, including ventilator-associated pneumonia
Wound infection; skin, and skin structure infection
Tissue necrosis due to disruption of blood supply
Infected hematoma
Fistula tract communication between intestinal and urinary tracts
Complicated peritonitis
Septic deep thrombophlebitis
Fasciitis, myositis, and gas gangrene are rare complications
Chemotherapy
Febrile neutropenia
Pneumonia
Neutropenic enterocolitis
Radiation therapy
Enteritis
Urinary tract infection
Poor wound healing
Catheter and implantable devices
Device infection
Peritonitis
Bloodstream infection
Urinary tract infection

advanced cervical cancer, infections may involve the uterus, fallopian tubes, ovaries, and other deep pelvic structures and retroperitoneum. Infections may present as tubo-ovarian or deep pelvic abscess, endometritis, and less frequently pyometra (**Figs. 28.1–28.3**). Extension of these infections to adjacent structures may present as ascending pyelonephritis, rectal abscess, and complicated peritonitis. These are often serious, requiring surgical debridement or intervention by invasive radiology (8,9). It is also important to note that an infection may be the primary presentation of an undiagnosed malignancy involving the female reproductive tract. In a study of postmenopausal women who presented with tubo-ovarian abscess, nearly half of these patients were subsequently diagnosed with a gynecologic malignancy (10). Therefore, a thorough investigation of possible underlying cancer should be considered in postmenopausal women or those without sexually transmitted diseases who present with tubo-ovarian abscess or pyometra.

In a large study conducted at the M. D. Anderson Cancer Center in the 1970s, septicemia, pneumonia, and peritonitis in patients with gynecologic cancer were associated with high infection-associated mortality (11). In the last two decades, in patients at an increased risk for infections, early diagnosis, identification of factors associated with poor treatment outcome, empiric therapy with new-generation broad-spectrum antimicrobial drugs, advances in antineoplastic and target-centered radiation therapy, and improved surgical techniques have substantially improved outcomes. The recent favorable outcomes for serious systemic bacterial and *Candida* species infections are in most part due to the availability of well-tolerated broad-spectrum antimicrobial drugs. The recent emergence and spread of multidrug-resistant (MDR) organisms, however, may mitigate these advances, such that the treatment course of patients with solid-organ cancer with limited immune suppression, life-threatening septicemia, pneumonia, peritonitis, and abdominopelvic infections may mimic those of the antibiotic nascent era (11).

TABLE 28.2. Infectious Diseases Consultations Performed for the Gynecologic Oncology Clinical Service at MD Anderson Cancer Center, Houston, Texas[a]

Reason for Consultation	Number (%)
Intra-abdominal/pelvic abscess	43 (11)
Surgical wound infection	41 (10)
Complicated urinary tract infection	38 (10)
Neutropenic fever	36 (9)
Pneumonia	35 (9)
Unexplained fever (including tumor fever)	35 (9)
Bacteremia	32 (8)
Diarrhea (including *C. difficile* associated)	30 (8)
Nonspecific cutaneous eruption (rash)	21
Leukocytosis/leukemoid reaction	19
Infection with MDR organism[b]	16
Fungemia	11
Varicella-zoster infection	5
Meningitis	2
Miscellaneous[c]	9

[a]Consultations performed by K.R. from January 2001 to December 2011.
[b]MDR—multidrug resistant, defined as resistance to three or more different classes of antimicrobial agents, included cellulitis, wound breakdown/dehiscence.
[c]Included travel and other immunizations.

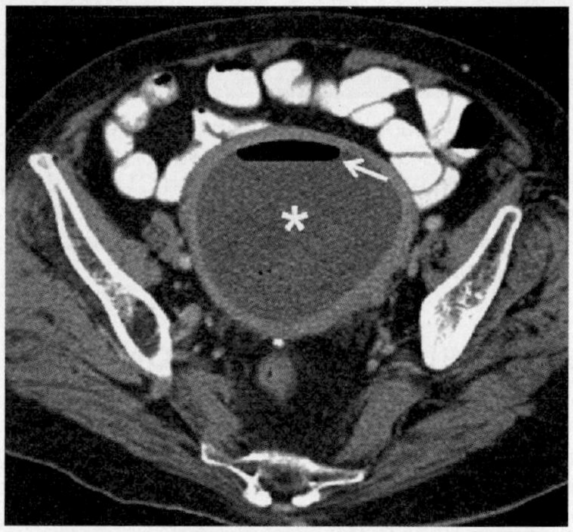

Figure 28.1. A 73-year-old woman with endometrial cancer presented with pelvic pain, fever, and vaginal bleeding. Axial CT scan performed with enteric and IV contrast demonstrates a markedly distended endometrial cavity containing fluid (*asterisk*). Air is also present, with an air–fluid level (*arrow*). In a febrile patient, this is highly suggestive of infection/endometritis. At D&C, blood and pus were drained from the uterine cavity, compatible with pyohematometra.

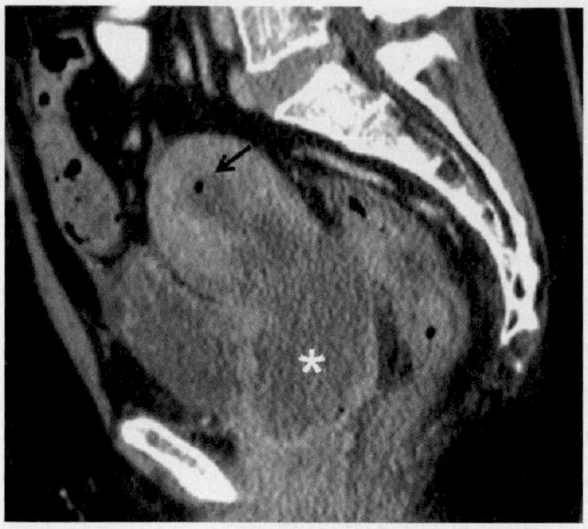

Figure 28.2. A 46-year-old woman with cervical cancer presented with pelvic pain and fever. Sagittal contrast-enhanced CT image demonstrates a large cervical mass (*asterisk*). There is obstruction of the endometrial cavity, which is mildly distended and contains fluid and air (*arrow*), compatible with infection/pyometra.

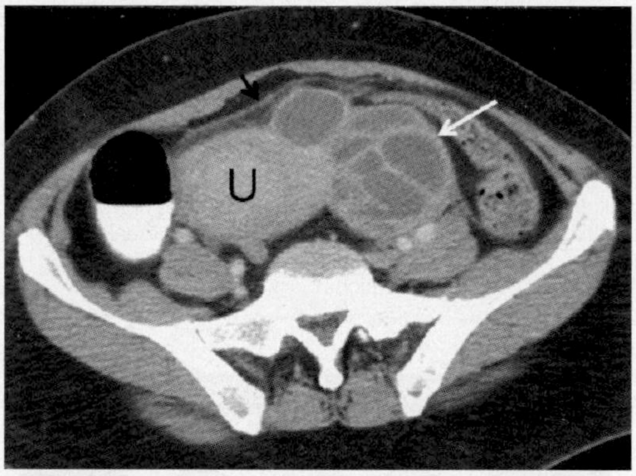

Figure 28.3. A 40-year-old woman with cervical cancer presented with fever and left lower quadrant pain and was diagnosed with tubo-ovarian abscess. Axial contrast-enhanced CT scan demonstrates a complex, multiloculated mass with thick septations (*white arrow*) to the left of the uterine fundus (*u*). There are inflammatory changes in the pelvic fat (*black arrow*).

SURGERY-RELATED INFECTIONS

Patients undergoing surgery for cervical cancer have a higher rate of infectious complications, compared with patients with endometrial cancer who tolerate surgery better and have fewer infections during the early and late postoperative period (12). Pelvic exenteration is performed in patients with advanced and/or treatment-refractory cervical and upper reproductive tract malignancies. Infections remain as serious complications following pelvic exenteration; early post-surgical wound infection and wound dehiscence are not uncommon (13,14). Urinary tract infections frequently occur in patients with urinary fistula and/or in those who develop urethral obstruction. Studies show that greater than 40% of patients undergoing pelvic exenteration for gynecologic and rectal cancer had urinary tract infection, wound dehiscence, or both (13). Late infections such as ascending pyelonephritis may be serious, as they frequently recur and are seen in patients with usually irreparable structural damage to the urinary reservoir such as neobladder, stenosis of urethra, or surgical anastomosis site. Ureterointestinal fistula, stones in the urinary reservoir, and surgical, radiation, or chronic/recurring infection/inflammation-induced narrowing all contribute to increased risk of infections. Unless the anatomical abnormality is corrected, these patients remain at increased risk for recurrent urinary tract infections and complications arising from prolonged systemic antibiotic therapy and repeat hospitalizations.

In a recent large study of over 6,854 patients undergoing surgery for gynecologic cancer at the Cleveland Clinic, the overall frequency of surgical site infection (SSI) was 5.4%. The rate of SSI was 7% in patients undergoing laparotomy, which was three and a half times higher than the rate of SSI following minimally invasive surgery ($p < 0.001$) (15). In those patients who had a laparotomy, independent predictors of SSI included: (a) diagnosis of endometrial cancer, (b) obesity, (c) the presence of ascites, (d) anemia, and (e) perioperative blood transfusion. Furthermore, patients with American Society of Anesthesiologists class ≥3 and those who underwent more complex surgical procedures also had a higher rate of SSI. Significant risk factors for deep tissue or organ SSI were hypoalbuminemia, preoperative weight loss, respiratory comorbidities, complex surgery, and the need for perioperative blood transfusion. Patients who developed SSIs had a significantly longer hospital stay and higher rates of reoperation, development of sepsis, and wound dehiscence. The risk of acute renal failure or 30-day mortality, however, was not adversely impacted by the presence of SSIs in these patients.

In cases of surgically related, suspected infection, empiric therapy includes adequate coverage for possible polymicrobial infection. The choice should include drugs that provide adequate coverage for enteric coliforms, enterococci, including vancomycin-resistant *Enterococcus* species, especially in patients who have known prior intestinal or genitourinary tract colonization due to these drug-resistant bacteria and/or are receiving care at centers with known high prevalence for these pathogens (16). As most infections in this setting may also have an anaerobe as a copathogen, even in patients with negative microbiologic evidence of anaerobic infection, antibiotic selection should entertain unisolated anaerobic bacteria. We recommend secondary suppressive antimicrobial therapy in patients with recurrent deep pelvic infection to reduce morbidity and subsequent hospitalization and surgeries. It is critical to select high-risk patients judiciously so patients are not given prolonged courses of broad-spectrum antibiotics, which is the single most important factor in promoting selection for or less commonly development of *de novo* drug-resistant bacteria and fungi.

Infections remain the main concern in patients following radical vulvar resection and inguinal lymph node dissection. In 67 patients undergoing 112 inguinal lymphadenectomies, early postoperative cellulitis was noted in nearly one-third, and early surgical wound breakdown also occurred in over 20% (17).

Wound Infection

Infected surgical wounds in patients following female genital tract surgery include *Staphylococcus aureus*, including MDR or semisynthetic methicillin-resistant *S. aureus* (MRSA) obtained from health care microflora (health care-associated; HA) or community-acquired (CA) MRSA, which has now become the leading source of MRSA infections in the United States and globally. *Streptococcus* species (group A, B, C, non-Enterococcus D and G) are also common pathogens in this population. Nearly one-third of infections, especially those with involvement of the lower intestinal tract and urinary tract, are less likely to be monomicrobial.

In certain subpopulations of patients who have been receiving systemic corticosteroids for extended periods, patients with morbid obesity, malnutrition, **cancer-related cachexia,** and poorly controlled diabetes mellitus have a higher risk of developing postoperative wound infections. Coagulase-negative *Staphylococcus*, *Streptococcus* species, *S. aureus*, enteric gram-negative bacteria, and *Bacteroides* species are potential pathogens.

Patients who have a complicated hospital course following surgery may develop infections due to organisms acquired from the health care microenvironment. In critically ill patients, infections are treated empirically, and the spectrum of causative organism(s) may not be available at the time of medical decision making. Knowledge of regional and institutional prevalence of drug-resistant organisms is required in prescribing an appropriate treatment regimen. The empiric therapy in patients with prolonged hospitalization and anatomic abnormalities such as enterourethral, entero- or rectovaginal, or enterovesicular fistula increases the probability of recurrent infection due to resistant HA–gram-negative bacteria such as *Pseudomonas* species, extended-spectrum beta-lactamases and carbapenemases producing Enterobacteriaceae, including *E. coli* and *Klebsiella pneumoniae*. Other nonfermentative gram-negative bacteria like nosocomial *Acinetobacter* spp. and *Stenotrophomonas maltophilia* are often resistant to a wide variety of commonly used broad-spectrum antibiotics; successful treatment for MDR bacterial disease remains a consternating task (18,19).

Intra-abdominal and Pelvic Abscess

An infected collection within the peritoneal cavity may develop as a consequence of breach in the physical barriers resulting from tumor progression and tumor necrosis and may also occur in patients undergoing instrumentation, or as a consequence of reconstructive surgery and implantation of prosthetic devices. The secondary seeding of the intraperitoneal tumor mass in patients with bloodstream infection arising from a different primary source, such as the urinary tract, or antineoplastic therapy–induced orointestinal mucositis or indwelling vascular device may also occur. The spectrum of causative organisms includes enteric bacteria such as *E. coli*, *Enterococcus*, *Staphylococcus* species, *Bacteroides*, and other anaerobes. *Candida* species infection is less frequent in non-neutropenic patients, although patients with high yeast counts in multiple body sites referred as high *Candida* colonization index, exposure to prolonged broad-spectrum antibiotics, poorly controlled diabetes mellitus, systemic corticosteroid use, as well as stay in critical care units and presence of foreign devices may increase the risk for tissue-invasive candidiasis.

Hematogenous or direct seeding of the retroperitoneal space may lead to paraspinal and psoas abscess; these infections escape early detection, as patients may not have high-grade fever, and increase in chronic low back pain remains subject to interpretation. In the absence of a direct extension from the intestinal or urinary tract, these retroperitoneal infections are usually monomicrobial; diagnosis requires prompt computed tomography (CT) or magnetic resonance imaging (MRI) scans and aspiration of the infected collection (**Figs. 28.4** and **28.5**). In tuberculosis endemic regions, *Mycobacterium tuberculosis* must be considered in determining the etiology of these infections, especially in patients in whom the vertebral column is involved.

Pelvic abscesses that develop after instrumentation or following surgery are often polymicrobial, and treatment is directed toward normal intestinal tract and cutaneous microflora (20).

Peritoneal infections following bowel perforation, anastomotic leaks, or fistula tracts may present with fever, abdominal pain, and fistula drainage and/or surgical wound dehiscence. Most infections, as expected, are polymicrobial and Enterobacteriaceae, *S. aureus*, *Streptococcus*, and *Enterococcus* species, including vancomycin-resistant strains, are frequently encountered. *Bacteroides fragilis* and *Clostridium* species are common anaerobes; *Fusobacterium*, *Peptostreptococcus*, and *Eubacterium* occur less commonly. Patients with peritoneal infections following surgery involving the nonsterile bowel and lower genitourinary tract may also have an increased risk for *Pseudomonas* species infection involving the deep pelvic and lower abdominal tissue and/or organs.

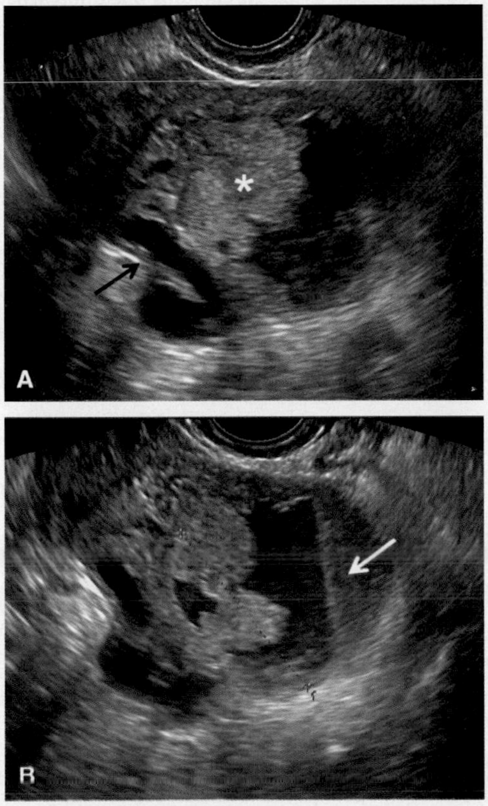

Figure 28.4. A 52-year-old woman with fallopian tube carcinoma initially diagnosed as tubo-ovarian abscess. She presented to the emergency department with left lower quadrant pain and fever. **A:** Transvaginal ultrasound demonstrates a complex left adnexal mass with a tubular configuration of fluid-filled component (*arrow*) and a solid component (*asterisk*). **B:** Additional image demonstrates fluid-debris level within this mass (*arrow*). Initially, this was thought to represent a tubo-ovarian abscess; however, the patient had no risk factors for pelvic inflammatory disease. At surgery, fallopian tube carcinoma was found.

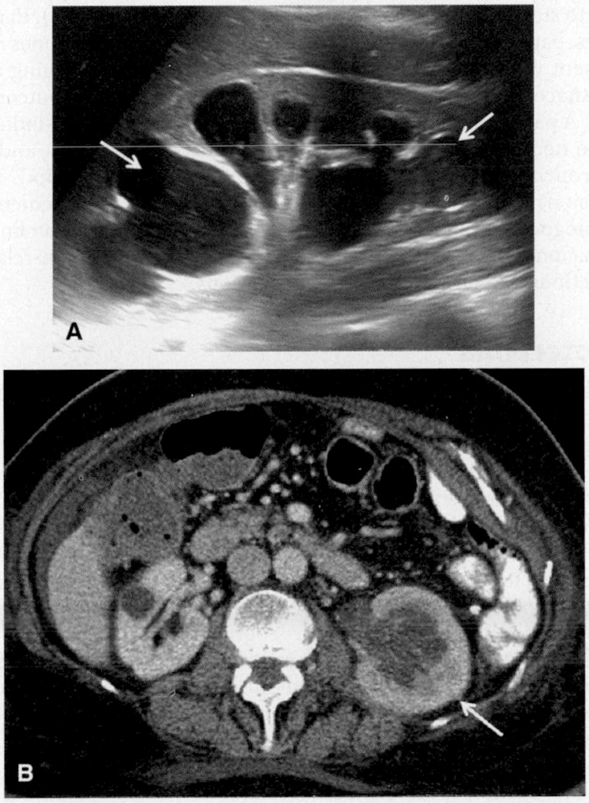

Figure 28.5. A 48-year-old woman with cervical cancer presented with left flank pain and fever. **A:** Sagittal gray-scale ultrasound image of the left kidney demonstrates marked hydronephrosis compatible with ureteral obstruction secondary to the patient's cervical neoplasm. There is echogenic debris present in the dilated collecting system (*arrows*) compatible with pus in the setting of pyonephrosis. **B:** Axial contrast-enhanced CT scan in the same patient demonstrates the enlarged left kidney with hydronephrosis (*arrow*). There is a delayed nephrogram compared with the right, compatible with obstruction. The left nephrogram is also heterogeneous and there is perinephric inflammatory change compatible with pyelonephritis. The right kidney is normal with the exception of a small cyst.

Chemotherapy and Radiation-Related Infections

Patients receiving chemotherapy may have an increased risk of infection; neutropenia for less than a week increases risk of systemic bacterial infections due to *S. aureus*, *Pseudomonas*, *E. coli*, and other coliform bacteria. Patients who remain neutropenic for longer than 5 to 7 days are also at an increased risk for developing tissue-invasive *Candida* species infection (1,2). Disruption of orointestinal and genitourinary tract mucosa compromises an important barrier in the prevention of bacterial and fungal invasion. In patients with severe treatment-induced mucositis, α-hemolytic streptococcal and anaerobic septicemia may lead to devastating consequences including rapidly progressive multiorgan failure, disseminated intravascular coagulation, hemodynamic collapse, and death (21).

Radiation therapy in patients with vulvar, vaginal, and cervical cancer causes microvascular damage to the tissue and may lead to difficult-to-treat intestinal, vaginal, and urologic complications.

Increased doses of radiation for gynecologic cancer have been associated with improved cancer-free survival (22). However, with increased radiation dose, the rate of complications has also risen (23). Noninfectious complications arising from high-dose radiotherapy include damage to the organs in the radiation field, including necrosis of tissue and bone; fistula formation, enteritis, proctitis, aseptic degenerative arthritis of pelvic and sacroiliac joints increase the risk of pathologic fracture. Radiation-induced fibrosis may result in vaginal, rectal, and ureteric stenosis and predisposes to secondary infection due to stagnation and inadequate physiologic drainage (24). In rare cases, patients with radiation-induced necrosis of pelvic bones may present with osteomyelitis; for these patients, a challenging and multifaceted treatment approach is needed for successful outcomes (25). A patient with osteomyelitis in the setting of radiation-induced bone necrosis may need extensive surgical debridement and an appropriate selection of antibiotics for a prolonged period. The excisional defects create additional complexity due to placement of autologous or cadaveric biologic graft prosthetics. A high clinical suspicion remains critical in the timely diagnosis of radiation-related infectious and noninfectious complications.

Bacteremia

Most hematogenous bloodstream infections in adult neutropenic cancer patients are due to coagulase-negative *Staphylococcus*, viridians streptococci, *E. coli*, *Pseudomonas aeruginosa*, and *S. aureus* observed in a prospective case-controlled study (26). In patients with solid-organ cancer, *E. coli* and coagulase-negative *Staphylococcus* account for nearly 40% of bacteremia, whereas *Pseudomonas*, *S. aureus*, and enterococcal bloodstream infections account for 10% or less, each (27). *Klebsiella* species, other Enterobacteriaceae, and *S. maltophilia* are of serious concern and may become prominent bloodstream infections in certain geographic regions.

Cancer patients with bacteremia who present with extensive tissue involvement/infection are significantly less likely to respond to antimicrobial therapy (28). Other factors associated with poor prognosis in bacteremic adult patients with an underlying malignancy include shock, infection due to MDR bacteria, and *Pseudomonas* and *Clostridium* species infection (28).

Bacteroides and *Clostridium* species are the most frequent cause of anaerobic bacteremia, which is most frequently seen in patients with abdominal and pelvic malignancy (28,29). In cancer patients with nonsporulating anaerobes, bacteremia, *B. fragilis*, and *Fusobacterium* are isolated more frequently compared with *Peptostreptococcus* and *Eubacterium* species (30). Polymicrobial infections are more frequent in patients with anaerobic bacteremia compared with aerobic bacterial infections. *E. coli*, *Pseudomonas*, *Klebsiella* species, and among gram-positive cocci *Streptococcus*, *Enterococcus*, and *Staphylococcus epidermidis*, may accompany anaerobic bloodstream infection (30). Concurrent candidemia is uncommon in patients with bacteremia due to anaerobic bacteria, unless patients (a) have a high *Candida* colonization index, (b) have an indwelling intravascular catheter, (c) are receiving care in a critical care unit, (d) have poorly controlled diabetes, (e) have parenteral nutritional support, or (f) have severe and prolonged treatment-induced neutropenia. Over 90% of patients with nonsporulating anaerobic bacteremia may also have a deep tissue abscess (30). The authors suggest that all patients with gynecologic malignancy who present with anaerobic bacteremia be thoroughly evaluated for an infected abdominopelvic or pelvic collection, which may not be clinically apparent at the time of initial presentation.

Hematogenous *Clostridium* species infection is often seen in patients with gastrointestinal or genitourinary cancer, and acute leukemia (31). Nearly one-third of patients with bacteremia with *Clostridium* species alone and nearly half with polymicrobial infections present with septic shock (31). *Clostridium perfringens* is a common species, and *Clostridium septicum* is uncommon, although serious *C. septicum* infections are seen in patients with intra-abdominal neoplasms (31,32). Diffuse, rapidly spreading cellulitis involving the abdominal wall, groin, and upper thigh area, gas gangrene, and acute intravascular hemolysis indicate the possibility of clostridial infection (33). Early appropriate therapy remains critical in improving response and outcome for patients with deep tissue anaerobic infection with or without accompanying bacteremia.

Febrile Neutropenia

The organisms associated with infections in patients with neutropenia are shown in **Table 28.3**. *Pseudomonas* spp. is a well-recognized cause of serious systemic infections in febrile neutropenic patients. The other nonfermentative gram-negative bacteria such as *S. maltophilia* have emerged and present as life-threatening pneumonia, bacteremia, or deep tissue infection; these infections are commonly resistant to standard broad-spectrum antipseudomonal antibiotics, and despite appropriate therapy, response may remain suboptimal (18). Patients with peripheral absolute blood neutrophil counts of less than 500 have significantly higher risk of serious infection, especially if the duration of neutropenia is more than 5 to 7 days (1,2). During the first 5 days of neutropenia, bacterial infections are prominent; if neutropenia

TABLE 28.3. Microorganisms Commonly Associated with Infection in Neutropenic Patients

Gram-negative organisms
Escherichia coli
Klebsiella spp.
Pseudomonas aeruginosa
Stenotrophomonas maltophilia
Enterobacter spp.
Gram-positive organisms
Staphylococcus spp. including vancomycin-tolerant organisms
Staphylococcus aureus
Coagulase-negative *Staphylococcus* such as *S. epidermidis* and *S. saprophyticus*
β-Hemolytic streptococci, group A, B, G
α-Hemolytic streptococci (viridans streptococcus spp.)
Enterococcus spp. including vancomycin-resistant strains
Fungi[a]
Candida spp. including *C. albicans, C. glabrata, C. tropicalis,* and *C. parapsilosis*

[a]Patients receiving multiple courses of fluconazole therapy or prolonged antifungal suppression or prophylaxis are at higher risk for infections due to drug-resistant *C. glabrata* and *C. krusei*.

extends beyond a week, invasive candidiasis becomes a concern; and in patients with greater than 2 weeks of profound neutropenia, invasive mold infections such as aspergillosis may occasionally be encountered. In most patients with gynecologic malignancy, isolation of a mold even from sterile samples does not indicate invasive fungal disease; in patients with no known established predisposing factors (31), these saprophytic molds usually represent colonization or laboratory contamination (34).

Catheter-Related Bloodstream Infection

In patients with solid-organ cancer, nearly 70% of gram-positive bacteremia is associated with an infected indwelling vascular catheter; similarly, 60% of gram-negative bacteremia is also related to an infected catheter, whereas only 19% of gram-negative bacteremia in patients with hematologic cancer is due to an infected catheter (35). Coagulase-negative *Staphylococcus* remains the most commonly isolated microorganism in blood cultures drawn from an indwelling central venous catheter and is frequently regarded as catheter-related bloodstream infection. Similarly, *S. aureus*, including MRSA bacteremia, may result from an infected indwelling catheter, and successful therapy requires selection of antimicrobial agents that penetrate the biofilm and are effective against the sessile nongrowth stationary phase of the bacteria (36). *S. aureus* bloodstream infections are associated with high rates of complications (37). Patients with solid-organ cancer with catheter-related *S. aureus* bacteremia have a fivefold higher probability of developing intravascular complications such as septic thrombosis and, less commonly, infective endocarditis (37).

Patients with gynecologic malignancy have a higher rate of postoperative infection, catheter malfunction, and unplanned catheter removal following external intravascular catheters compared with subcutaneous/implantable venous access devices (38,39). Nearly one-third of all intravascular catheters were associated with delayed complications in this cancer population; bacteremia was significantly more common in patients with nonimplantable (Hickman catheters) compared with implantable indwelling intravenous devices such as infusaport or peripheral access system ports (40).

IMPLANTABLE DEVICE INFECTIONS

Peritoneal, hepatic, and pleural implantable devices for delivering chemotherapy or drainage of recurring malignant effusions have been successfully used in the last two decades. These devices are well tolerated; major complications including bowel perforation are uncommon, and serious infections are seen in less than 5% of cases (41–46). Overall, infections are seen in less than 20% of cases. While serious infections, including pocket infections, are seldom noticed, when these do occur they should be treated aggressively, with prompt removal of the infected reservoir and appropriate systemic antimicrobial therapy (41) (**Fig. 28.6**). Abdominal pain and chemotherapy-related discomfort remain the main problems associated with these chemotherapy infusion devices.

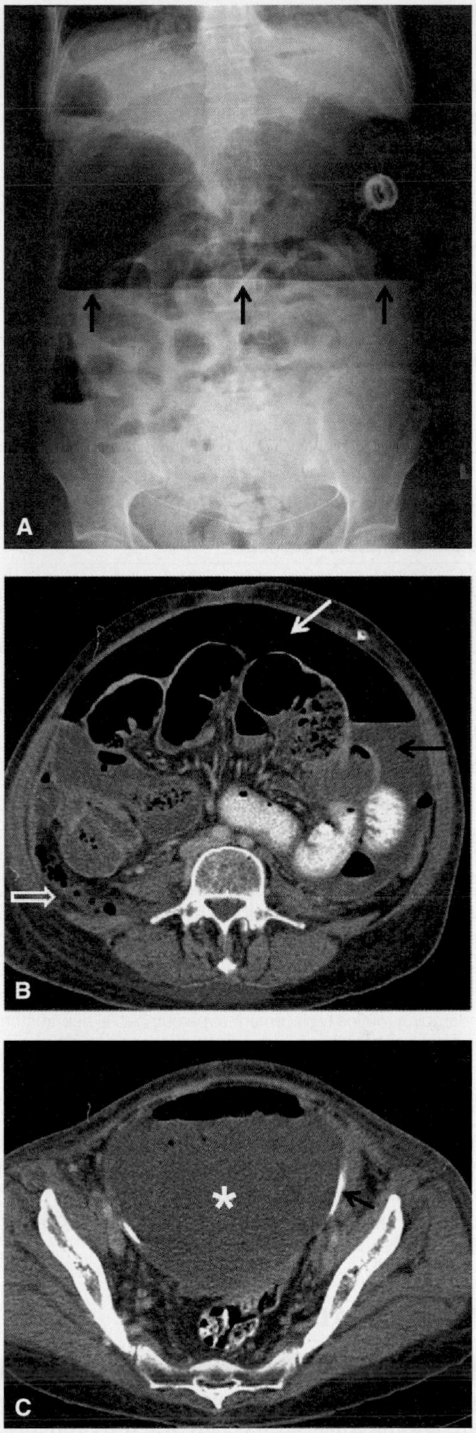

Figure 28.6. A 53-year-old woman with recurrent papillary serous carcinoma of the ovary with serosal bowel implants undergoing intraperitoneal chemotherapy presented with abdominal pain, vomiting, and fever. **A:** Upright abdominal radiograph demonstrates large amounts of free intraperitoneal air with air–fluid level due to the presence of ascites fluid (*arrows*). Multiple dilated air-filled loops of bowel are noted. Intraperitoneal chemotherapy infusion catheter is in place with port in the left upper abdomen. These findings are compatible with perforated viscus. **B:** Axial contrast-enhanced CT scan in the same patient demonstrates a large amount of free intraperitoneal air (*white arrow*) and ascites fluid (*black arrow*). There are multiple dilated loops of bowel. There is a mottled gas collection in the right lower quadrant posterior to the cecum (*open white arrow*). At surgery, perforated cecum was confirmed. **C:** Large loculated fluid and gas-containing collection in the pelvis is compatible with an abscess (*asterisk*). The chemotherapy infusion catheter is visualized at the posterior wall of the abscess (*black arrow*).

Urinary Tract Infection

Patients with gynecologic cancer have an increased risk of urinary tract infection. The factors that promote infections are listed in **Table 28.4**. Nearly one-third of patients, while undergoing pelvic radiotherapy for gynecologic cancer, may have symptoms of urinary tract infection at the onset of therapy or develop infection during the course of radiation therapy (47). Despite appropriate treatment, infections may recur and require several courses of antibiotic therapy (47). Patients who have undergone pelvic exenteration remain at increased risk for ascending urinary tract infection (14); recurrent pyelonephritis in these patients leads to an increased risk of scarring and permanent renal damage. Older patients with advanced gynecologic and urologic malignancies are now being considered for pelvic exenteration surgery (48). In these and other patients with lower renal reserves, a severe episode of pyelonephritis may precipitate

TABLE 28.4. Factors Promoting Urinary Tract Infections

Tumor obstruction
Retrograde urine flow leading to ascending pyelonephritis
Stagnation in patients with outlet obstruction and abscess formation
Instrumentation
Cystoscopy-related introduction of pathogens
Dilatation of strictures
Foreign body
Urethral stent
Percutaneous nephrostomy tube placement/replacement[a]
Surgical drains for extended duration
Radiotherapy
Inflammation of bladder mucosa
Suppression of local innate cellular and acellular immune response
Surgery
Urinary diversions
Organ resection
Lymph node dissection
Anastomotic leak
Chronic surgical wound breakdown
Chemotherapy
Neutropenia
Suppression of local immune surveillance and response to bacterial invasion
Mucosal damage and disruption

[a]Patients undergoing routine replacement of percutaneous nephrostomy tubes may develop transient bacteremia in the event of prior colonization.

irreversible renal failure, prompting prolonged renal replacement therapy. We suggest that in selected high-risk patients, preemptive antimicrobial therapy or even secondary antibiotic prophylaxis be considered after an episode of urinary tract infection, especially pyelonephritis.

ANTIMICROBIAL AGENTS

It is important to refer to the spectrum of local and regional drug resistance among commonly encountered pathogens in selecting appropriate antimicrobials, especially when treatment is initiated empirically, or in patients awaiting microbiologic drug susceptibility results.

SURGICAL ANTIMICROBIAL PROPHYLAXIS

Operative Site

Guidelines for the administration of antibiotics to uninfected patients undergoing pelvic surgical procedures were first proposed by Ledger et al. in 1975 (49). Prophylactic antibiotics are indicated for women undergoing pelvic surgery for malignancy. There have been few studies evaluating this prophylaxis in such cases. Recently, cefazolin was shown to be inferior to cefotetan as a single-dose prophylaxis in women undergoing elective abdominal hysterectomy (50). A placebo-controlled trial showed that using a broad-spectrum cephalosporin plus beta-lactamase inhibitor significantly reduced the risk of major operation-site infection from 27% in patients not given antimicrobial prophylaxis, whereas none of the patients given antibiotic developed operative-site infection (51).

The overall postoperative infection rate has been as high as 46%, and SSI is seen in nearly one-fourth of patients (52). The risk of postoperative infection is adversely affected by prolonged duration of surgery >5 hours, presence of remote infection at the time of surgery, and duration of hospitalization longer than 3 weeks; in patients with all three risk factors, the relative risk of infections increases to 7.3%, compared with 3% in patients who have only one of these risk factors (52). Risk factors that have been associated with an increased incidence of infection in patients undergoing surgery for reproductive tract neoplasms include lower socioeconomic status, preoperative colonization, failure to administer perioperative heparin, obesity, advanced patient age, a longer operative period, and a longer hospital stay prior to surgery (53,54). Extent of surgery plays a central role in predicting probability and severity of postoperative infections (12–14,54). However, these risk factors were not have not been uniformly reported by investigators.

Clinical Investigation

The overall operative-site infection rate after gynecologic surgery ranges from 6.7% to 44%. One study reported that patients with preoperative cervical colonization did not have an increase in postoperative complications such as duration of hospitalization, operative time, or febrile episodes compared with patients in whom no cervical colonization was demonstrated (55). An overall decrease in significant postoperative infections with the utilization of preoperative antimicrobial prophylaxis was reported in retrospective studies among patients undergoing radical hysterectomy (56,57). The benefit, however, was thought to be associated only with reduced local wound infections (58).

Prospective data have not resolved this issue. The numbers of patients in comparative studies have been small, and the data may therefore be inadequate for detecting a statistically significant difference in infection rates. Rosenshein et al. noted no significant difference in overall operative-site infection after preoperative prophylaxis (59), an observation shared by Marsden et al (60). In contrast, significantly lower incidences of infection following preoperative antimicrobial prophylaxis were reported by Sevin et al. (61) and Micha et al. (62). Sevin et al. reported that a short course (three doses) of prophylaxis was as effective as a long course consisting of 12 doses in preventing major infection after radical hysterectomy (63). If separate operative-site data from prospective studies are combined, the overall incidence of pelvic infection and wound infection was significantly reduced by the administration of prophylactic antimicrobials.

A cost–benefit analysis of three doses of cefazolin antimicrobial prophylaxis showed a 29% reduction in infectious morbidity following vaginal hysterectomy, and an 18% reduction in postoperative infections in patients following abdominal hysterectomy (64).

One patient population that has a significant surgical incision breakdown includes women undergoing radical vulvectomy. Anecdotal experience indicates that the principal pathogens are *S. aureus* and *S. epidermidis*. Not unexpectedly, the administration of broad-spectrum medications, such as piperacillin or mezlocillin, failed to significantly reduce the incidence of postoperative wound infection; 8 of 12 women undergoing radical vulvectomy for vulvar carcinoma who were given single-dose piperacillin or mezlocillin developed postoperative infections (65). We recommend a *Staphylococcus* active antimicrobial for women undergoing radical or modified vulvectomy for vulvar carcinoma. Drain sites fall into the same category. The foreign body undoubtedly contributes to the infections; in our opinion, local attention, rather than broad-spectrum parenteral or oral antibiotics, is the appropriate preventive approach.

AGENT ADMINISTRATION

Intravenous administration of antibiotics is recommended to achieve high serum and tissue drug concentration, and should be given before anesthesia. Antibiotics for women undergoing hysterectomy for benign indications are administered by suppository, by spray, and orally, with significant reduction in operative-site infection (66–68). There are no similar data for women undergoing hysterectomy for gynecologic cancer, and these routes of administration are presently not advised.

Timing of Drug Administration

The first dose of an antibiotic should be given intravenously in the operating room. Combination regimens and prolonged administration did not appear to offer superior infection prevention when compared with that provided by a single agent given once. If the interval between the first dose and opening of the vagina exceeds 2.5 to 3 hours, a second intravenous dose should be given 15 to 30 minutes before the anticipated vaginal entry. This conclusion is based on data provided by Shapiro et al. (69). This has not been clinically studied, but administration at longer fixed intervals has not enhanced protection at hysterectomy for benign indications. In cancer patients who are expected to undergo a prolonged surgical procedure (>4 hours), the dose may be repeated after 4 to 6 hours.

Recommendations

Intravenous administration of 2 g cefazolin should be given in the operating room. Cefazolin provides activity against gram-negative and gram-positive aerobic and anaerobic bacteria; it is an uncommon therapeutic agent and is comparatively inexpensive—beneficial attributes for a prophylactic antibiotic. A single dose of a prophylactic agent did not result in the selection of a resistant species, as did three doses of antibiotics at hysterectomy for benign disease (70). A 1-g dose may suffice, but 2 g was superior to 1 g for vaginal hysterectomy, and three 1-g doses over 16 hours were statistically inferior to a single 2-g dose for cesarean delivery (71). A single dose (1 g) of cefotetan was significantly ($p < 0.05$) superior to 1 g of cefazolin in preventing operative-site infection after elective abdominal hysterectomy for benign diagnoses. The high drug acquisition cost was offset by an overall reduction in hospital costs, owing to fewer infections and shorter hospital stays in patients given cefotetan compared with cefazolin (72). Kobamatsu et al. also found superior protection for women undergoing radical hysterectomy when using expanded-spectrum cephalosporins compared with first-generation agents (73). Other alternatives include ampicillin–sulbactam, although there is little evidence to support this practice; similarly, metronidazole as a single agent may be less effective at preventing infection compared with broad-spectrum cephalosporin agents (74). More prospective data are necessary in patients with gynecologic cancer undergoing surgery.

If the patient is allergic to cephalosporins, or has a history of a type I immediate hypersensitivity reaction to a penicillin, and if she is not allergic to a tetracycline, the recommendation is 100 mg doxycycline orally at bedtime the night before surgery, and again on the day of surgery about 3 hours before departure for the operating room. This regimen has been evaluated prospectively in Parkland Memorial Hospital in a nonrandomized study using very few patients and no control regimen. If the woman is allergic to tetracycline, the recommendation is intravenous administration of 900 mg of clindamycin given preoperatively, as for cefazolin. The new generation of fluoroquinolones such as moxifloxacin may be particularly suited for the gynecologic cancer patient scheduled for pelvic surgery because of its aerobic and anaerobic spectrum of antibacterial activity and extended drug half-life. Prospective, controlled studies are needed.

BOWEL PREPARATION

Unobstructed Bowel

In elective gynecologic surgical cases in which no bowel surgery is anticipated, such as a hysterectomy and staging procedure for endometrial cancer, most centers do not utilize a mechanical bowel preparation. However, in more complex cases such as ovarian cancer cytoreduction and pelvic exenteration in which opening or resection of the intestine is likely, the use of mechanical bowel preparation is still used in many centers. There are approximately 10^{11} bacteria in a gram of feces, making sepsis a major hazard if the colon is opened. It is desirable to reduce the patient's normal colonic microflora to diminish the postoperative infection rate in case it is necessary to perform a colonic resection and reanastomosis. Preparation for colonoscopy is a regimen of clear liquids the day before surgery and 3 tablespoons of Fleet Phospho Soda in one-half cup of cool water at 4:00 PM and 6:00 PM the day before surgery. Patients should be cautioned to drink eight to ten 8–fluid ounce glasses of clear liquids the day before surgery. Additional clear fluid is acceptable. Some surgeons prefer to add a Fleet enema 2 hours before surgery. An alternative mechanical preparation is whole gut irrigation with chilled polyethylene glycol and electrolyte therapy or a similar lavage solution given orally at a rate of approximately 1 L/h until the rectal effluent is colorless, but for not more than 4 hours.

A recent large cohort, multicenter, randomized trial has placed routine mechanical bowel preparation practice into serious question; in patients who underwent elective colorectal surgery, no difference in anastomotic leak or other septic complications such as fascia dehiscence were noted in the group of patients who had preoperative bowel preparation versus those who did not (75). Enhanced recovery pathways have been proposed internationally to hasten surgical recovery through the attenuation of the stress response. Nelson and colleagues recently reviewed the literature on "enhanced recovery" pathways (ERPs) in gynecologic oncology to assess its efficacy (76). The Enhanced Recovery After Surgery (ERAS) Society was contacted to identify any unpublished protocols. Seven investigations were identified. Common interventions included allowing oral intake of fluids up to 2 hours before induction of anesthesia, solids up to 6 hours before anesthesia, carbohydrate supplementation, intra- and postoperative euvolemia, aggressive nausea/vomiting prophylaxis, and oral nutrition and ambulation the day of surgery. In addition, mechanical bowel preparations, the nil per os (NPO) after midnight rule, nasogastric tubes, and intravenous opioids were not utilized. While no randomized data are available in gynecologic oncology, significant improvements in patient satisfaction, length of stay, and cost were observed in ERP cohorts compared with historic controls. Morbidity, including infectious morbidity, mortality, and readmission rates were no different between groups. Given the above data, the benefit of mechanical bowel preparation in complex cases, such as ovarian cancer cytoreduction and pelvic exenteration, is becoming more and more controversial.

Preoperative oral antibiotics are still recommended by many authorities. In the antimicrobial approach, 1 g each of erythromycin and neomycin is given orally at 1:00 PM, 2:00 PM, and 11:00 PM the day before surgery. This regimen was initially proposed in 1971 by Nichols and Condon (77). An alternative is 1 g each of metronidazole and neomycin at 2:00 PM and at 11:00 PM the day before surgery. There should be no need to add further antimicrobial prophylaxis to 2 g of cefazolin or other agents.

Obstructed Bowel

There can be no mechanical prophylaxis for preoperative management of the obstructed bowel. Treatment principles include fluid and electrolyte therapy with mechanical decompression of the bowel from above and timed surgical intervention. Women with mechanical intestinal obstruction immediately after surgery may respond to conservative treatment with decompression only. If necessary, surgery should be performed within 24 hours of the mechanical obstruction; these patients have the lowest mortality rate. A dose of intravenous antibiotic should be given in the operating room before the procedure, with a second dose given in the recovery room, and a third dose 8 hours later if it is necessary to enter the bowel lumen. The single-agent or combination regimen should provide broad coverage of both gram-positive and gram-negative aerobic and anaerobic bacterial species with a broader spectrum of antibacterial activity than with cefazolin. Evaluation has produced no evidence for a superior regimen. A single agent usually suffices unless the patient is septic, in which case antibiotic combination is appropriate because therapy, not prophylaxis, is necessary.

BUNDLED INTERVENTIONS

A recently described approach in many surgical subspecialties to decrease SSIs is the use of "bundled" interventions. In this setting, a "bundle" is defined as a set of evidence-based practices performed collectively with the goal of reducing 30-day SSIs. Johnson and colleagues recently reported their outcomes with prospectively implementing a perioperative SSI bundle of sterile closing tray and staff glove change for fascia and skin closure, dressing removal at 24 to 48 hours, dismissal with 4% chlorhexidine gluconate, and follow-up nursing phone call (78). This bundle was added to their prior established (preintervention) elements of patient education, 4% chlorhexidine gluconate shower before surgery, antibiotic administration, 2% chlorhexidine gluconate and 70% isopropyl alcohol coverage of incisional area, and cefazolin redosing 3 to 4 hours after incision. The overall 30-day SSI rate was 38 of 635 (6.0%) among all cases in the preintervention period compared with 2 of 190 (1.1%) in the postintervention period. Overall, the relative risk reduction in SSI was 82.4% ($p = 0.01$). Many, if not all, of the bundled interventions have been incorporated in many centers to minimize SSIs after gynecologic oncology surgery.

CLINICAL SYNDROMES

Peritonitis and Intra-abdominal Abscess

Etiology

Infection in the patient with pelvic cancer most commonly involves the pelvis and abdomen. The potential causes of infection include complications of the primary tumor, surgery, and antineoplastic therapy including radiation and chemotherapy. The tumor can compromise the integrity of the vaginal wall and allow seeding of endogenous vaginal flora into the pelvic and peritoneal cavities. Previous antibiotics, radiation therapy, and the tumor itself may alter the normal genital flora. The tumor can also erode into the bowel and allow entry of fecal material into the peritoneal cavity. Rare cases of several other syndromes arising from untreated pelvic tumor, including spontaneous clostridial gas gangrene and pneumoperitoneum, have been reported (79). Peritonitis, with or without abscess formation, may occur postoperatively after hysterectomy or with bowel injury. Radiation therapy to the pelvis can cause radiation enteritis, leading to a chronic diarrheal syndrome, which may develop years after radiation therapy is completed. These patients are also at higher risk for bowel adhesions and subsequent obstruction, and subclinical perforation may present as late insidious intra-abdominal or deep pelvic abscess. Macro- and micronutrient **malabsorption** in patients with chronic diarrheal state may enhance susceptibility to severe systemic infections and extenuate the healing process.

Signs and Symptoms

In the patient with pelvic cancer, peritonitis may develop at any time, including at initial diagnosis (e.g., tumor infiltration of bowel), immediately postoperatively, or days or weeks after surgery (e.g., tumor infiltration or radiation therapy). The signs are generally dramatic and familiar: abdominal pain, fever, and signs of peritoneal irritation. However, among postoperative patients or patients who have received radiation or corticosteroid therapy, the physical findings may resemble those typical of a routine postoperative patient, making the diagnosis more difficult. To ensure proper diagnosis, frequent physical examinations and CT scan should be obtained early in the course of the disease.

Abscess formation can also occur in several settings. In some patients, a subclinical microperforation of the bowel is successfully walled off by the body's immune system, forming a pericolic or intraperitoneal abscess. This has been shown to occur 7 to 10 days after microperforation (80). Fever or mechanical obstruction may be the only presenting sign. Subphrenic, psoas, or liver abscesses may present as a fever of unknown origin and may require a methodical, diligent evaluation for diagnosis. A fistula, usually caused by tumor but also occurring postoperatively, may form between any two organ systems, including the bladder, vagina, bowel, or skin. Persistent suppuration despite therapy or the presence of a feculent discharge from the skin, bladder, or vagina may suggest the development of a fistula.

Diagnosis

The diagnosis of peritonitis is usually made on clinical grounds. In patients who have clinical evidence of peritonitis but are unable to undergo surgery because of bulky tumor, multiple prior surgeries, or general debility, paracentesis with appropriate cultures may be useful in guiding antibiotic therapy. Radiologic investigation is generally required to diagnose an abscess. Regular plain x-ray films of the abdomen are seldom revealing. A sonogram, CT scan, or MRI of the abdomen may show the collection (**Figs. 28.7 and 28.8**). A gallium scan may also be helpful. In a particularly confusing case in which abnormalities of scans can represent an abscess, metastatic tumor, or postoperative changes, a labeled leukocyte scan may be

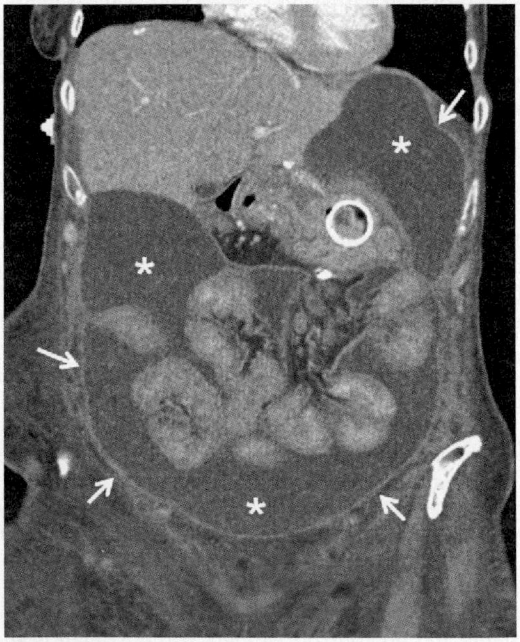

Figure 28.7. A 58-year-old woman with metastatic ovarian cancer presented with fever, abdominal pain, and elevated peripheral white blood cell count. Coronal contrast-enhanced CT scan showed multiple loculated fluid collections in the abdomen and pelvis (*asterisk*) with central displacement of small bowel loops. There is thickening and enhancement of the peritoneal reflection (*arrows*). These findings could be seen with either peritoneal carcinomatosis or peritonitis. Aspiration of the fluid was compatible with infection and peritonitis.

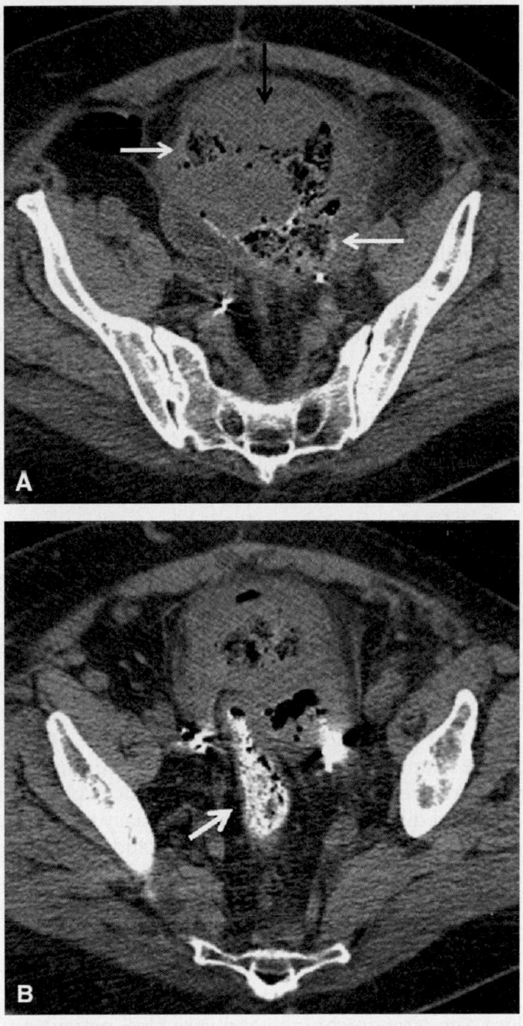

■ **Figure 28.8.** A 65-year-old woman with recurrent cervical cancer and fistula tract with rectum. **A:** Axial CT image performed with enteric contrast shows the large recurrent mass in the midline pelvis (*black arrow*). There are mottled collections of gas and enteric contrast present within this mass (*white arrows*) suggesting fistulization with bowel. **B.** Slightly more inferior image demonstrates the contrast-filled rectum (*arrow*) partially encased by the mass. This was the site of fistulization.

needed to diagnose the abscess with certainty; presently, however, these scans are seldom used due to inconsistent results and the fact that several days are required to complete the process.

The diagnosis of a fistula requires demonstration of abnormal drainage from one organ system to another. This can be shown by intravenous or intravesical injection of dye for fistulae arising from the bladder, oral or rectal instillation of dye for those arising from the gastrointestinal tract, or a fistulogram for a fistula involving the skin (**Fig. 28.9**).

In all cases, laboratory abnormalities, including an elevated leukocyte count, reactive thrombocytosis, an elevated erythrocyte sedimentation rate, C-reactive protein, and abnormal liver function tests, may suggest the diagnosis and direct the workup. The microbiologic diagnosis in each of these syndromes requires culture for aerobes and anaerobes. Blood cultures are only rarely positive. Some patients may have an unexplained bacteremia of enteric aerobic gram-negative rods or anaerobes. This is probably from a microperforation of the bowel. Any patient with pelvic tumor and enteric gram-negative rods or anaerobic bacteremia should be radiologically evaluated for evidence of perforation.

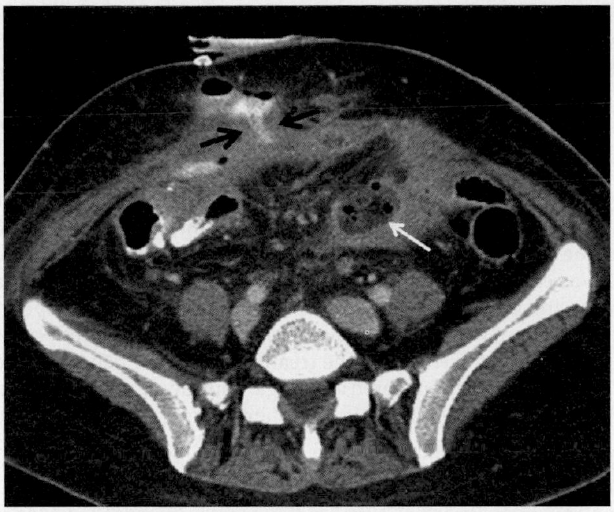

■ **Figure 28.9.** A 61-year-old woman with recurrent fallopian tube carcinoma and carcinomatosis status post exploratory laparotomy, partial small bowel resection presented with draining anterior abdominal wall wound. Axial CT scan performed with enteric and IV contrast demonstrates a loop of small bowel adherent to the anterior abdominal wall with enteric contrast-containing tract within the abdominal wall soft tissues (*black arrows*). There is a contrast-containing collection in the overlying subcutaneous soft tissues. These findings are compatible with enterocutaneous fistula. Additional intraperitoneal abscess is noted (*white arrow*).

Therapy

Acute, generalized peritonitis where gastrointestinal perforation is suspected usually requires urgent surgery to irrigate the peritoneum and repair any perforation. Broad-spectrum antibiotic coverage with agents such as cefoxitin, ticarcillin–clavulanic acid, piperacillin–tazobactam; metronidazole, clindamycin with ampicillin, and an aminoglycoside such as tobramycin or amikacin is generally effective for the polymicrobial infection. Addition of aminoglycosides is particularly important for patients who have been recently or frequently hospitalized or who have had past courses of antibiotics. These situations predispose the patient to the development of resistant organisms.

Effective treatment of an abscess requires drainage. Percutaneous drainage is adequate in many cases, but laparotomy is occasionally required. Large or persistent abscesses may require placement of a suction drain. Patients with fistulae often require resection of the involved tissue.

For intra-abdominal infection, intravenous antibiotics directed at the recovered bacteria should continue for at least 10 to 14 days after drainage. Some patients who have been on antibiotics may have evidence of pus but no growth on cultures. In this situation, broad-spectrum antibiotics directed at enteric gram-negative rods and anaerobes should be administered. Laboratory parameters such as leukocyte counts should be followed to determine the exact duration.

Patients who are inoperable can be treated with chronic suppressive therapy, intravenously or orally. Oral agents such as amoxicillin–clavulanic acid (875 mg bid) or clindamycin (450 mg q 6 to 8 hours) may be effective. Ciprofloxacin, moxifloxacin, or levofloxacin alone should not be used in this situation because they provide limited coverage for *Enterococcus* species.

Patients with infections due to vancomycin-resistant enterococci and/or vancomycin-tolerant (81) *Streptococcus* or *Staphylococcus* species may be treated with daptomycin (6 mg/kg daily) or linezolid (600 mg twice daily), usually in combination with drugs with gram-negative and anaerobic activity. Tigecycline may also be used as an alternative; it has broad-spectrum antimicrobial activity including promising *in vitro* results against MDR bacteria such as extended-spectrum beta-lactamase-positive *E. coli*, MDR *Acinetobacter*, *S. maltophilia*, carbapenemases producing *K. pneumoniae*, vancomycin-resistant enterococci, and MDR *S. aureus*. There are limited clinical data for its use in patients with gynecologic malignancy, and due to poor activity against *Pseudomonas* species it should be used cautiously in neutropenic patients and those with prior invasive pseudomonal invasive disease or known bacterial colonization. Furthermore, emergence of drug-resistant bacteria or selection of less-susceptible organisms remains a concern for widespread use of drugs with broad-spectrum antimicrobial coverage. Similarly, antipseudomonal carbapenems such as imipenem-cilastatin and meropenem should also be reserved for seriously ill patients with polymicrobial infection, as emergence and spread of MDR gram-negative bacteria are increasing in immunosuppressed cancer patients (82). Ertapenem, a carbapenem without antipseudomonal activity, was as effective as piperacillin-tazobactam for the treatment of acute pelvic infection (83) and can be administered as a single daily dose, albeit due to lack of enterococcal coverage, it is important to select patients carefully.

Urinary Tract Infection

Etiology

Many clinical situations predispose a patient to urinary tract infection. Urinary tract infection continues to be the leading cause of infectious morbidity in this population. One study showed that half of the patients with pelvic cancer admitted to the hospital because of infection had a urinary tract infection; *E. coli* was the most common organism isolated (84). Another report found that the frequency of urinary tract infections is increased as much as threefold in patients undergoing pelvic irradiation (22–24). Many patients who undergo pelvic surgery require prolonged bladder catheterization, usually with a Foley catheter. These patients may develop the well-recognized infectious complications of chronic bladder catheterization, the most common of which is recurrent infection. In addition, tumor can cause urinary obstruction and subsequent infection. The role of antiseptic or antibiotic-impregnated urinary catheters has not yet been defined.

Signs and Symptoms

Some patients with gynecologic malignancy and urinary tract infection have the familiar clinical picture of dysuria, fever, flank or suprapubic tenderness, elevated leukocyte count, and abnormal urinalysis. In many others, these signs and symptoms are obscured by the rest of the clinical picture. For instance, a postoperative patient may be expected to have abdominal tenderness, an elevated leukocyte count, and fever. The physician should consider the entire clinical setting before embarking on a course of therapy.

Diagnosis

Diagnosis is generally made on the basis of a urine culture, from a "clean catch" or through a catheter, but the initial urinalysis is extremely helpful. Pyuria is expected in any nongranulocytopenic patient with a urinary tract infection. Gram stain of urinary sediment can direct antibiotic therapy in advance of the culture results. A common problem confronting the physician is when patients, especially those with indwelling catheters or nephrostomy tubes, have positive urine cultures but do not appear to be ill. Differentiating colonization from invasive infection is frequently not simple and requires clinical judgment. Any patient who is not severely neutropenic should also have pyuria along with positive urine cultures. The absence of pyuria in a patient with a positive urine culture suggests the likelihood of simple asymptomatic **bacteriuria.** From a practical standpoint, in a clinically stable patient, it is reasonable to withhold antibiotics pending repeated urinalysis and urine culture. If an organism persists, therapy may be considered.

Therapy

Therapy should be based on the sensitivity pattern of the recovered organism. Intravenous antibiotics are reserved for patients with drug-resistant bacteria and those with systemic infection, ascending infection, or pyelonephritis. Optimum duration of therapy in a patient with a urethral stent or a permanent indwelling catheter is often difficult to determine. It is virtually impossible to eradicate an infection in the presence of a foreign body, and removal of the foreign object is highly desirable; however, removal is not always feasible. A patient with a urinary tract infection and a foreign body in the urinary collecting system should be considered for chronic suppressive therapy if she has recurrent infection. In general, among patients with gram-negative rods, chronic suppressive therapy may include ampicillin, trimethoprim-sulfamethoxazole, doxycycline, or an oral fluoroquinolone such as ciprofloxacin. Patients with a chronic enterococcal infection may benefit from chronic suppressive therapy with amoxicillin–clavulanic acid (Augmentin®) or amoxicillin alone or doxycycline.

In patients with pyuria and fever in whom a urinary tract infection is suspected, empiric antibiotic therapy should be given pending urine culture results. Gram stain of urinary sediment may be helpful in directing treatment. However, for those cases in which Gram stain is not helpful, broad-spectrum coverage should be given. For a patient who has had frequent or prolonged hospitalizations, effective coverage of potentially resistant gram-negative rods dictates that two drugs be given, preferably a beta-lactam and an aminoglycoside. Cefazolin (1 to 2 g IV, q 8 hours) and gentamicin (4 to 5 mg/kg/day IV in three divided doses) is a good empiric combination for many patients. For more debilitated patients or those with prolonged hospitalizations and frequent past courses of antibiotics, advanced generation cephalosporin, such as ceftazidime (1 to 2 g IV, q 8 hours) or cefepime (1 g IV, q 8 hours) should be substituted for cefazolin. After culture results are known, antibiotics can be adjusted and the spectrum narrowed. For any gynecologic cancer patient with an unexplained predisposition to recurrent urinary tract infection, a full investigation should be undertaken to exclude obstruction from tumor as the cause.

Wound Infections

There are important variables that influence the development of wound infection after surgery. These include hospital flora, patient microflora, operative technique and variables, patient nutritional status, and competency of innate and adaptive immune function. Women being treated for reproductive tract cancer may be at risk because of specific problems with immunocompetency, prior chemotherapy or radiotherapy, poor nutritional status, hypoproteinemia, being economically disadvantaged, or suffering from an advanced cancer-associated catabolic state. Additional risk factors for incisional infection include obesity, inadequately controlled diabetes, and systemic corticosteroid use. Surgical variables include operative procedures in excess of 4 hours, breaks in surgical technique, capacious inoculum at the operative site, excessive cautery, passive drains, shaving of the area in which the incision is made immediately before surgery, and placement and types of sutures. Infections may range from a mild cellulitis to a devastating fasciitis, deep infection with myonecrosis, and mixed anaerobic–aerobic synergistic abdominopelvic gangrene (85).

Cellulitis

Etiology

Cellulitis is a relatively frequent occurrence. The presence of a foreign body in a wound is an unavoidable risk factor in many cases, but this variable should be removed or reduced as much as possible. Devitalized tissue, especially fat, can also act as a foreign body. Excess cautery causes thermal injury; the charred tissue may act as a foreign body. The presence of significant amounts of devitalized tissue usually produces a wound defect. A mechanical wound retractor can cause fat necrosis, and there appears to be only minimal ability to resorb these areas during wound healing. These areas should be carefully identified and excised before closing the wound. If drains are used, they should be closed, and drains should be vacuumed. Drains should not exit through the wound but rather through an adjacent puncture site, and they should be removed as early as possible. *S. aureus* is recovered from 50% or more of wound infections. If the operative procedure involves transection of the vagina, the infections may harbor other species of normal flora of the lower reproductive tract, such as gram-positive and gram-negative anaerobes and Enterobacteriaceae. Cellulitis of the leg occurs with increased frequency in patients after vulvectomy (86). The affected leg is not always edematous. Group B beta-hemolytic streptococci are frequently recovered. Prophylactic therapy with oral penicillin may reduce recurrences in some patients (86). Increased prevalence of penicillinases among clinical streptococcal isolates cautions against penicillin preparation without beta-lactamase inhibitor.

Signs and Symptoms

Cellulitis is almost uniformly associated with pain and erythema in the incisional margins, with an increase in local skin and tissue temperature, and many times with fever. Incisions are usually tender at examination. Incisional cellulitis may not become evident until the fourth postoperative day or later.

Diagnosis

The infected surgical incision should be explored. This can frequently be performed at the bedside. Opposing skin edges in such incisions are usually separated without difficulty and may expose underlying purulent material, seromas, hematomas, or any combination of these. The wound should be explored thoroughly, and if the wound shows unusual features, aerobic and anaerobic cultures should be obtained. Foreign bodies such as sutures or drains should be removed, and obviously necrotic areas should adequately be debrided. It is important to document deep fascial integrity. If this cannot be done at the bedside, it should be performed in the operating room.

Therapy

The wound should be packed open with fine-mesh gauze approximated to the incisional margins and changed with each dressing change. The dressing is changed two to four times daily, avoiding harsh chemical and repeat mechanical debridement in the absence of necrotic tissue. Commonly used solutions are hydrogen peroxide, acetic acid, and Dakin's solution (0.25% sodium hypochlorite). In general, these debriding solutions should be removed from the wound with sterile normal saline before packing because they may impede healing. Except in unusual instances, it is unnecessary to administer parenteral antimicrobials. These incisions may be left open to heal by secondary intent, or they may be closed before discharge from the hospital after the margins exhibit healthy viable granulation tissue. The optimal time for secondary closure is about the 4th day after institution of wound therapy. Studies have shown that normal wound healing occurs as long as the hematocrit exceeds 17%, but that a lower level will impede healing (87).

Necrotizing Fasciitis

Necrotizing fasciitis is a potentially life-threatening infection of the soft tissues above deep fascia that can involve the abdominal wall or vulva with extension to the proximal thighs and buttocks (87). There are several descriptive names for this infection, such as beta-hemolytic streptococcal gangrene, hospital gangrene, gram-negative anaerobic cutaneous gangrene, nonclostridial gas gangrene, gangrenous erysipelas, or synergistic necrotizing cellulitis, but the name used by most is that coined by Wilson in 1952, that is, necrotizing fasciitis (88). This significant infection has been reported in patients with endometrial cancer following irradiation and hysterectomy (89–91). It has also been found in endopelvic fascia, in a suprapubic catheter site during chemotherapy, in the vulva in diabetes, and after diagnostic laparoscopy (92–97).

Etiology

Bacteria recovered from necrotizing fasciitis–infected sites include anaerobes, particularly *Peptostreptococcus, Prevotella,* and *Bacteroides* species, as well as *E. faecalis, S. aureus,* and Enterobacteriaceae. These bacteria produce large quantities of proteolytic and other enzymes and toxins that allow rapid spread to contiguous tissues. Superficial vessels are occluded, depriving the affected areas of oxygen, other nutrients, and antibiotics. This deprivation interferes with bacterial eradication. Patients at particularly high risk of developing this infection include women older than 50 years of age and those with arteriosclerotic heart disease, diabetes, or other chronic diseases.

Signs and Symptoms

Early in the course of necrotizing fasciitis, the signs and symptoms are those of any wound cellulitis. Because there is no response to the usual methods of therapy, antibiotic therapy will frequently be initiated. The infection, however, seems to smolder initially, then rapidly progresses to involve the wound and to produce clinical sepsis. Mortality rates for this infection have been as high as 76%. The degree of disease evident on the skin is only a small fraction of the total amount of tissue that is involved because the skin is not the primary area of infection. Hallmarks of this infection include severe pain in contrast to scant physical findings, edema that is unusual for the apparently minimal degree of infection, and superficial tissue crepitus may be present. The skin overlying the affected area becomes blue or brown as the disease progresses, and there may be formation of bullae. Edema progresses, and there may be seepage of grayish fluid from the skin and does not bleed if cut. Lack of familiarity with this infection and failure to recognize its signs may delay diagnosis. Even when recognized and treated early, there is a high mortality rate.

Diagnosis

Diagnostic criteria as first outlined by Fisher et al. include (98) the following:

1. Extensive necrosis of the superficial fascia with widespread undermining of surrounding tissue
2. A moderate to severe systemic toxic reaction
3. Absence of muscle involvement
4. Failure to demonstrate *Clostridium* species in the wound or blood cultures
5. Absence of major vascular occlusion
6. Histologic demonstration of intense leukocytic infiltration, focal necrosis of the superficial fascia and surrounding tissues, and microvascular thrombosis

Early diagnosis followed as soon as possible by appropriate treatment produces the highest cure rate. Radiologic evaluation, particularly with MRI, may confirm the diagnosis rapidly and should be ordered whenever the disease is suspected. The average interval between diagnosis and initiation of treatment is approximately 5 days. If the interval is 4 days or less, survival rates are high, but an interval of 7 days or more is more likely to result in patient death because even intense antimicrobial therapy is rarely successful at this late stage.

Therapy

Although the administration of broad-spectrum antimicrobials is important, wide and often disfiguring surgical debridement is the treatment required for preservation of life. The excision must extend to areas that bleed. Adjunctive therapy with whirlpool baths and perhaps hyperbaric oxygen may be considered early in the course of the disease.

Clostridial Myonecrosis

Clostridial myonecrosis (gas gangrene) was described by Altmeier (99). It is an infection that occurs in muscle and adjacent tissues beneath the deep fascia and is seen most commonly after trauma.

However, it can be seen after intra-abdominal surgery or surgery in an area that has been contaminated by feces. Mortality rates are about 25%, and poor prognostic factors are leukopenia, advanced age, renal failure, and intravascular hemolysis.

Etiology

Clostridial myonecrosis is caused by *C. perfringens* (80% to 95%), *C. novyi* (10% to 40%), or *C. septicum* (5% to 20%). It is usually seen in association with gastrointestinal mucosal ulceration or perforation because *Clostridium* species are normal inhabitants of the gastrointestinal tract. *C. perfringens* may be isolated from as many as 20% of women with upper genital tract infections not involving sexually transmitted diseases. The mere presence of *C. perfringens* in a wound does not mean that the patient will develop gas gangrene; it develops in only 1% to 2% of wounds in which that species can be isolated.

Signs and Symptoms

Early signs and symptoms of clostridial myonecrosis are tense edema in tissue that is extremely tender and pain that rapidly intensifies. If an incision is open, it is not uncommon to see a swollen, herniated muscle. There is frequently a serosanguinous, dirty discharge that has many gram-positive or gram-variable rods but few leukocytes. There may also be gas bubbles, and the secretions have a particularly sweet, offensive odor. The surrounding tissue frequently has crepitus. The skin becomes red to green-purple and then turns yellow before becoming a characteristic bronze color. The usual incubation period is about 2 to 3 days, but it can be as short as 6 hours. With progression of the infection, the patient becomes obviously ill, pale, and sweaty, with increased pulse rate and decreased blood pressure. Temperature is usually elevated, but hypothermia and shock may occur early in the course of the illness.

Diagnosis

A positive wound culture may accompany the characteristic signs and symptoms of clostridial myonecrosis. X-ray films of the affected area frequently show gas deep in the tissues. Blood cultures grow clostridia in approximately 15% of the cases. It is common to find a decrease in hemoglobin and an increase in circulating leukocytes. Involved muscle is pale and edematous, with loss of elasticity, and it does not bleed or contract with stimulation. Histologic findings demonstrate coagulation necrosis of muscle fibers.

Therapy

Clostridial myonecrosis is another infection that requires prompt and extensive debridement in the operating room. Cultures must be performed, and because clostridia may develop plasmid-mediated antibiotic resistance, repeated cultures with sensitivity testing may be required if a patient is slow to respond. In addition to wide debridement, the treatment of choice is penicillin G at a dose of 1 to 2 million units every 2 to 3 hours. Gram stain also may indicate the presence of gram-negative bacteria, in which case coverage should be provided for those bacteria as well. Chloramphenicol is as effective against *Clostridium* species as it is against many gram-negative species, although, seldom used due to potentially life-threatening drug toxicity. Metronidazole, imipenem, or clindamycin, all of which have good *in vitro* activity against *C. perfringens*, may be considered. Other antibiotics with good *in vitro* activity include tetracycline, erythromycin, and rifampin. Hyperbaric oxygen may be adjunctive, but its efficacy is uncertain.

Intraperitoneal Catheter Infections

Etiology

Delivery of chemotherapeutic agents through an intraperitoneal catheter has enabled physicians to deliver high concentrations of drug locally while decreasing systemic side effects (44,100). However, intraperitoneal catheters can become infected at the exit site, along the catheter tunnel, or secondary peritonitis may occur in rare cases. *S. epidermidis* is the most common organism followed by *S. aureus* and *Streptococcus* species. Gram-negative bacilli and anaerobes, presumably from the bowel, are also found, especially in patients with polymicrobial infections. Patients who have been treated for bacterial peritonitis in the past may develop peritonitis due to *Candida* species.

Signs and Symptoms

With exit-site or tunnel infections, patients report discomfort at the site. Patients with peritonitis may complain of diffuse abdominal pain, with or without a change in bowel pattern. Fever may be absent in peritonitis, making the diagnosis more difficult because many patients with pelvic tumor have abdominal pain. On examination, patients with exit-site or tunnel infections have redness and sometimes have discharge where the catheter has been inserted. Patients with peritonitis have tenderness, and frequently have abdominal rebound.

Diagnosis

Diagnosis of exit-site and tunnel infections is made clinically, with support from a Gram stain and culture of any discharge. Patients with suspected peritonitis should have withdrawal of peritoneal fluid for cell count and microbiologic evaluation. A rough guideline, derived from experience among patients receiving continuous ambulatory peritoneal dialysis, is that any leukocyte count in peritoneal fluid >100 cells/mm^3 suggests infection. Gram stain and culture should reveal the specific organism. Chemical peritonitis after instillation of chemotherapy can mimic infectious peritonitis. Peritoneal fluid cultures are often not helpful in distinguishing between infectious and chemical peritonitis, especially in infections due to a fastidious organism. Use of biomarkers such as C-reactive protein or procalcitonin remains uncertain.

Therapy

For patients with peritonitis, systemic therapy is advised according to the recovered organisms. Treatment should be continued 10 days or longer, with serial peritoneal fluid cell counts guiding therapy. The peritoneum provides a large absorptive surface, and antibiotics delivered intraperitoneally readily enter the intravascular space; however, we suggest that intraperitoneal antibiotic therapy should be reserved for patients with serious, treatment-refractory infection. Treatment of fungal peritonitis is a unique problem. Amphotericin B can cause adhesions if delivered intraperitoneally. Echinocandins such as micafungin, caspofungin appear to be the treatment of choice for patients with intra-abdominal and peritoneal candidiasis (101). Fluconazole, which can be administered orally or intravenously, was shown in one study of patients receiving continuous ambulatory peritoneal dialysis to effectively treat *C. albicans* peritonitis and should be avoided in patients with *Candida glabrata* and *Candida krusei* infection (102). Fluconazole may be used for long-term therapy in patients with *Candida* peritonitis who have responded to initial aggressive therapy with micafungin (100 mg IV daily) or caspofungin (70 mg × 1 IV followed by 50 mg IV daily).

Septic Pelvic Thrombophlebitis

Septic pelvic thrombophlebitis, also known as suppurative pelvic thrombophlebitis, is a disorder that has been diagnosed most frequently after antimicrobial therapy for pelvic infection after cesarean section or septic abortion, but it can be seen as a complication of infection after any type of pelvic surgery. The mortality rate observed in 1917 was 52% after surgical therapy (103). Fortunately, this complication of pelvic infection is now very rare. The use of antimicrobial prophylaxis and the enhanced antibacterial activity of current therapeutic regimens are presumed to be paramount in the disappearance of this potentially lethal infection.

Etiology

Septic pelvic thrombophlebitis is clot formation in the pelvic veins as a result of infection. It can be seen after hysterectomy, other pelvic operative procedures including brachytherapy, and in association with pelvic trauma or perirectal abscess. Classically, there is relative venous stasis before phlebitis that develops adjacent to pelvic infection. The intimal lining of the veins is invaded by bacteria, including Enterobacteriaceae, especially *E. coli*, aerobic and anaerobic streptococci, and *Bacteroides*. The veins involved may be the ovarian, hypogastric, or uterine, with essentially equal involvement in the right and left sides. If common iliac veins are involved, clot formation is more frequently seen on the left for unknown reasons. Infected clot may embolize to the lungs, kidneys, liver, brain, and spleen.

Signs and Symptoms

A clinical diagnosis may not be readily evident. Presentation is essentially that of a fever of unknown cause, and the physician must rule out infections such as pyelonephritis, pneumonia, and pelvic or abdominal abscess. The most frequent presentation currently seen is persistence of fever associated with tachycardia after clinical response to antimicrobial therapy for a pelvic infection. Physical examination is normal in most instances, but it may be possible to palpate tender cords in the vaginal fornices. In patients with bacteremia and septic emboli, chills are observed in as many as 67%, pyrexia may be elevated to 41°C, and the variations in temperature may be quite hectic. Dyspnea, tachypnea, pleuritic pain, cough, hemoptysis, restlessness, anxiety, and perhaps angina may all be seen with septic embolization.

Diagnosis

Compatible clinical presentation and CT or MRI scan are used for diagnosis (104). Criteria for diagnosis of venous thrombosis using CT studies include enlargement of the involved vein(s), sharply defined vessel walls enhanced by contrast media, and a low-density intraluminal mass (105). Diagnosis using MRI is based on intense intraluminal signals from clot in involved veins and a lack of signal with normal blood flow in uninvolved vessels; no contrast agent is needed. Blood culture should be performed if there is suspicion of septicemia. Tests for blood gases, a chest radiograph, and IV contrast-enhanced chest CT scan (or in patients with contraindication to IV contrast use, a ventilation-perfusion scan) may be performed to assess pulmonary embolization. A gallium scintiscan may be necessary to identify very small septic embolic foci in the lungs.

Therapy

Early treatment of venous thrombosis was surgical (103). The first to advocate the use of anticoagulants in addition to antibiotics were Schulman and Zatuchni (106). In some cases antibiotics alone may be adequate, and can be used for patients in whom anticoagulation may be detrimental (107). In the largest published study of heparin therapy, the mean time to become afebrile was 2.5 days, and the average duration of heparin therapy was 8 days (108,109). It is unnecessary to initiate warfarin sodium (Coumadin) therapy in patients without evidence of emboli. Thromboembolism during or after treatment with heparin has not been reported. Antibiotic therapy must be continued. If there is significant improvement in the pulse rate and temperature pattern within 12 to 48 hours after the addition of heparin, reassessment is mandatory. Treatment with low-molecular-weight heparin has not been studied or standardized for this condition (110). Heparin therapy is not without complications. Between 2% and 5% of patients may have an allergic reaction; bleeding occurs in 7% to 10% of patients; and the most devastating effect is the development of the "white clot syndrome" (111). This occurs in <1% of patients, but it may be associated with major limb amputation in 20% of those suffering from it, and death has been reported in nearly half of these patients. This phenomenon is a paradoxical arterial platelet aggregation associated with thrombocytopenia, and it should be suspected in patients with decreasing platelet counts or an increasing requirement of heparin to maintain adequate anticoagulation. The only current indications for surgical intervention are embolization during heparin therapy or lack of response. The usual intervention is placement of a vena cava filter, a procedure usually performed by an interventional radiologist.

Neutropenia and Fever

Etiology

Patients with severe neutropenia are at particularly high risk for severe morbidity and mortality unless empiric intravenous antibiotic therapy is instituted at the first evidence of fever or clinical worsening. Most commonly, the febrile neutropenic patient does not have an obvious source of fever. Even in those with bacteremia, the source is rarely clinically evident. Bacteria often enter the bloodstream through the gastrointestinal tract because of the small chemotherapy-induced disruption of the intestinal mucosa and the accompanying neutropenia and thrombocytopenia. Neutropenic patients may also develop a clinically diagnosed group of infections, including pneumonia and cellulitis. Neutropenic patients with these clinically diagnosed infections may progress very rapidly, may have exceedingly subtle clinical signs and symptoms, and always require early, aggressive therapy of their infections to achieve a response.

Signs and Symptoms

Fever is often the only complaint of patients with neutropenia and bacteremia. Patients receiving chemotherapy should be instructed to take their own temperature at home twice a day (more frequently if a subjective feeling of fever develops) and to contact their treating physician for temperatures above 38.0°C or 100.4°F.

Diagnosis

Diagnosis is made by blood culture. Of all febrile, neutropenic patients from whom blood cultures are obtained, only 10% to 20% have an organism isolated. The others probably have enough organisms to cause fever and systemic illness, but an insufficient burden of microorganisms to be cultivated using current standard culture-based techniques. Coagulase-negative *Staphylococcus*, *S. aureus*, streptococci, *E. coli*, *Klebsiella* species, and *Pseudomonas* species are frequently isolated bacteria (112). In a recent report of 2,142 patients with febrile neutropenia, 499 (23%) patients developed bacteremia due to gram-positive bacteria (57%) and gram-negative bacteria (34%), and polymicrobial infection was seen in 10% (113). Mortality rates were lowest (5%) in patients with gram-positive infection, followed by 18% mortality with gram-negative bacteremia, and they 13% in patients diagnosed with polymicrobial bloodstream infection (113). Polymicrobial infections are often underreported, and neutropenic patients with intestinal and genitourinary tract mucosal damage have a higher risk of systemic infection due to multiple microorganisms (7).

Therapy

The Infectious Disease Society of America (IDSA) updates guidelines for management of patients with fever and neutropenia. Full consideration of this complex topic is beyond the scope of this chapter (114). In general, a febrile neutropenic patient should receive antibiotics with activity against *P. aeruginosa*, pending results of blood cultures. Numerous regimens are effective, and their use should be determined according to sensitivity patterns for *P. aeruginosa* at a given hospital. In general, good results have been achieved with a beta-lactam antibiotic plus beta-lactamase inhibitor such as ticarcillin–clavulanic acid, piperacillin–tazobactam, or a third/fourth-generation cephalosporin such as ceftazidime or cefepime, or a carbapenem such as imipenem or meropenem with or without an aminoglycoside. Monitoring peak and trough levels of aminoglycosides is recommended to maintain drug levels in optimum therapeutic range and to mitigate drug-induced ototoxicity and nephrotoxicity. The choice of the specific aminoglycoside (e.g., tobramycin, amikacin) is dictated by the sensitivity patterns in a given hospital. Once-daily dosing of aminoglycosides is not recommended for the neutropenic patient but can be given in other settings. The length of therapy for neutropenic patients is determined by many factors and must be individualized. An infectious disease specialist should follow patients with prolonged neutropenia and fever.

Fungal Infections

Etiology

Patients with pelvic cancer may be at risk for the development of fungal infections, particularly those caused by *Candida* species, including *C. albicans*, *C. tropicalis*, *C. parapsilosis*, and *C. glabrata* (115). Infection may include fungemia, pelvic abscess, or infected urinary stents in patients with extensive pelvic disease and urinary outflow obstruction. Risk factors for the development of invasive candidiasis include prolonged courses (7 to 10 days) of intravenous broad-spectrum antibiotics; an intravenous catheter, particularly a central venous catheter; major abdominal surgery; treatment-induced severe neutropenia for longer than a week; and immunosuppressive therapy, especially with corticosteroids. Patients with enteric or colonic fistula or bowel perforation have an increased risk for tissue-invasive candidiasis (116).

Signs and Symptoms

Patients with the appropriate risk factors who have unexplained fevers may be fungemic. Other than fevers, which can include rigors and hypotension and closely resemble bacteremia, there may be no other symptoms. Blood cultures are positive in only 50% of patients with autopsy-proven disseminated candidiasis. Any blood culture positive for yeast should be considered significant. A full evaluation for a hidden source should be completed, including a thorough reevaluation with history and physical examination, and appropriate laboratory tests that include repeat blood cultures. It is imperative to perform an expert ophthalmoscopic examination for possible *Candida* vitritis, retinitis/retinal abscesses, or endophthalmitis in all patients with presumed, probable, or definite fungemia, since this complication may occur in up to 5% to 15% of patients with fungemia (117).

Presence of multiple body–site *Candida* species colonization proportionally increases the risk of invasive candidiasis, including fungemia and acute disseminated candidiasis (118).

Candida species may cause urinary tract infection in a patient with such indwelling devices as a Foley catheter, internal stents, or percutaneous nephrostomies. Rarely a "fungus ball," consisting of a matted mass of yeast, may cause urinary tract obstruction.

Candida species invasive lung disease is exceedingly rare and may occasionally be seen in critically ill intensive care unit high-risk patients or patients with refractory relapsed acute leukemia and prolonged severe neutropenia. Thus, recovery of any yeast from a respiratory specimen should be considered most likely due to oropharyngeal contamination of lower respiratory tract culture. Unlike patients with leukemia and recipients of allogeneic hematopoietic stem cell transplantation, in patients with gynecologic malignancy invasive mold disease is exceedingly rare. Identification of filamentous fungi, such as *Aspergillus*, should be approached with caution, and mold-active drug therapy reserved for highly immunosuppressed patients with clinical and radiographic features suggestive of invasive aspergillosis (119).

Diagnosis

The diagnosis of a fungal infection is often difficult. The physician must differentiate between invasive disease, which must be treated, and colonization, which does not require systemic antifungal therapy. The recovery of fungi from a urine, sputum, or wound culture does not necessarily mean that the fungus is pathogenic, and clinical judgment must be used to determine if a patient requires therapy. In general, cultures from sterile sites (e.g., blood, cerebrospinal fluid, pleural or peritoneal fluid) should be considered to represent invasive infection until a full evaluation is done. Also, *Candida* recovered from the initial specimen of drainage from an obstructed biliary or urinary tract should be considered to be potentially associated with invasive fungal disease.

With most specimens, however, the distinction between colonization and infection is not so simple. For urine, the presence or absence of pyuria is the simplest and most reliable means of differentiation. Those without pyuria are very likely only colonized and need no therapy. In such patients, a repeat urinalysis and culture may clarify the situation. Recently approved fungal antigen assays including serum beta D glucan and galactomannan have provided much-needed diagnostic sensitivity and specificity in select groups of patients at high risk for invasive fungal disease (120).

Therapy

Treatment options for invasive candidiasis have expanded in recent years. Amphotericin B has the longest record for treatment of invasive fungal infections (115). The optimal duration of therapy for candidemia is not well defined and should be determined by individual responses. However, a 7- to 14-day course of therapy is probably adequate for most episodes (115).

Since the introduction of fluconazole in 1990, the option for invasive candidiasis, severe drug toxicity associated with amphotericin B is observed less and less (115,121). Echinocandins such as caspofungin (70-mg load and then 50 daily IV) showed comparable response in patients with invasive candidiasis versus patients randomized to receive amphotericin B (101). A large prospective trial comparing first two available echinocandins demonstrated 75% efficacy for micafungin compared with 70% in patients treated with caspofungin at the end of antifungal therapy; there were also nonsignificant higher responses among patients with *Candida* peritonitis (67% vs. 40%) and deep tissue abscesses (100% vs. 67%) in the micafungin verses caspofungin groups, respectively (122). These new classes of drugs offer comparable effectiveness but have fewer side effects than the amphotericin B products.

Patients who have *Candida* species consistently cultured from urine but no evidence of systemic fungal infection may benefit from bladder irrigation with amphotericin B, which reduces or eradicates bladder yeast colonization, and may prevent invasive fungal infection. Fluconazole is increasingly being given for this indication and appears to be effective.

Pneumonia

Etiology

Postoperative pneumonia remains a common cause of fever in any surgical patient, including those with gynecologic cancer. Infection may occur from aspiration during intubation or extubation or from hypoaeration due to "splinting" in patients with severe postoperative pain. Postobstructive pneumonia may occur in patients with tumor metastatic to the lungs. In addition, pneumonia may occur in patients with chemotherapy-induced neutropenia.

Signs and Symptoms

The familiar signs and symptoms of pneumonia are cough, fever, chest discomfort, dyspnea, and evidence of pulmonary consolidation on lung examination.

Diagnosis

The diagnosis is usually suggested by the clinical situation and by the findings on physical examination. These are further supported by chest radiographs and sputum examination and culture. Chest radiography may show consolidation. Gram-negative organisms predominate in the mouth flora of hospitalized patients, so an aspiration pneumonia occurring in a hospitalized patient is typically due to gram-negative rods. Although thought by many to be a substantial contributor, anaerobes are seldom isolated in hospitalized patients with aspiration pneumonia.

Therapy

Empiric, rather than pathogen-directed, coverage of patients with clinical pneumonia following a major surgical procedure is usually necessary and varies according to the setting (123). For a patient who has been hospitalized less than 3 days and has had no other recent hospitalizations or recent courses of oral or intravenous antibiotics, single-drug therapy with levofloxacin or moxifloxacin is adequate (123). For the patient who has been hospitalized for a longer period or who has recently received broad-spectrum antibiotics (increasing the likelihood of infection due to multidrug-resistant organisms), *P. aeruginosa* should be covered by the addition of an aminoglycoside such as gentamicin or tobramycin (3 to 5 mg/kg per day in three divided doses), and a beta-lactam should be selected to cover the usual isolates in that hospital. *S. maltophilia* is now increasingly seen in cancer patients without traditional risk factors such as severe neutropenia, prolonged stay in critical care units, or mechanical ventilation (124). Treatment includes high-dose trimethoprim–sulfamethoxazole (15 mg/kg in three to four divided doses) in combination with a second drug to which the bacteria are susceptible (18). Patients with *S. aureus* pulmonary infection may present with rapid clinical deterioration, and necrotizing pneumonia due to MRSA is often seen as a complication following a recent influenza virus–like illness; postviral bacterial infections are especially serious superinfections and require urgent, appropriate antibiotic therapy. Vancomycin (1 g twice daily), or linezolid (600 mg every 12 hours) may be given in patients with lobar or multifocal pneumonia and history of recent influenza-like illness. Therapy for patients with pneumonia should extend up to 10 to 14 days depending on a) clinical response; b) concurrent bacteremia; c) presence of empyema or complicated parapneumonic effusion; or d) secondary hematogenous foci of infection dissemination. Various professional societies have codified recommendations for pneumonia management (125).

Diarrhea Associated with Antibiotics or Chemotherapy

Etiology

Diarrhea is a common finding in patients undergoing treatment of gynecologic malignancy. In a study of 351 hospitalized women with gynecologic cancer in the 1980s, 12% developed diarrhea during the course of their hospital stay; 10% had diarrhea due to *C. difficile* (126). In cancer patients *C. difficile*–associated diarrhea (CDAD) is most commonly a result of exposure to broad-spectrum antibiotics, or in some cases chemotherapy alone (126,127).

Signs and Symptoms

Antibiotic-associated diarrhea can occur at any time during an antibiotic course and for at least a month after discontinuation. Patients typically develop abdominal pain, fever, and frequent watery diarrhea defined as three or more unformed bowel movements in 24 hours lasting for ≥2 days; however, CDAD may sometimes cause abdominal pain and fever without diarrhea.

Diagnosis

Any patient with antibiotic- or chemotherapy-associated diarrhea should have a full evaluation of stool, including routine cultures and antitoxin immunoassays or nucleic acid amplification tests (128). In patients with a highly suspicious clinical presentation but no evidence of *C. difficile* toxin in stool, sigmoidoscopy or colonoscopy may reveal intense mucosal ulceration; inflammation and the pathognomonic pseudomembranes are observed in a small number of cases with advanced disease. One study has suggested that evaluation of stool for *C. difficile* toxin is the only cost-effective test (126). A markedly elevated white blood cell count may also be a clue to diagnosis (129). In a recent retrospective study from a tertiary care cancer center, polymerase chain reaction increased the yield of *C. difficile* cases by twofold compared with that of the standard cytotoxic assay (130). Presently, in most secondary and tertiary care medical centers, nucleic amplification assays have largely replaced the less sensitive immunoassays.

Therapy

Oral therapy with metronidazole (250 mg to 500 mg four times daily for 2 to 4 weeks) is adequate to treat most cases of antibiotic-associated diarrhea (127–129). Because of continued reports of vancomycin-resistant bacteria (131), the use of oral vancomycin is restricted in many hospitals. However, response to metronidazole has been compromised in part with the emergence and spread of hypervirulent North American Pulsed Field type 1 (NAP1) *C. difficile* strains in the United States and Europe (132). Most institutions are currently following IDSA guidelines for moderate and severe CDAD; oral vancomycin should be given only to patients with strong suspicion or proven CDAD and those who have not responded to metronidazole. Some patients may require repeated or prolonged courses of metronidazole or oral vancomycin, particularly if their clinical course necessitates continuation of the provocative agent (i.e., continued antibiotics or chemotherapy). Antidiarrheal compounds such as Lomotil or Imodium should not be given routinely. If, however, diarrhea persists after appropriate tests and cultures, symptomatic therapy should be considered. Nitazoxanide is a nitrothiazolide and effectively treats intestinal infestation of *Cryptosporidium* and *Giardia* species; at low concentrations nitazoxanide also inhibits *C. difficile*. A recent trial showed that nitazoxanide 500 mg twice daily was as effective in eradicating *C. difficile* as metronidazole given 250 mg four times daily (133). Nitazoxanide may be used for patients with metronidazole-refractory or recurrent *C. difficile* colitis, although in our experience the clinical efficacy of nitazoxanide in patients who had failed first-line anti *C. difficile* drugs remains less favorable. In a recent trial fidaxomicin (200 mg twice daily) or vancomycin (125 mg four times daily) orally for 10 days was assessed for clinical response and early relapses (134). The overall response was comparable for both treatment groups; patients treated with fidaxomicin had significantly lower rate of recurrence of *C. difficile* infection associated with non-NAP1 (nonvirulent) strains (134). Currently, this option is being used in patients with relapsed CDAD or those with high risk for relapsed infection.

Noninfectious Causes of Fever

Not all patients with gynecologic malignancy and fever have an infection. Pulmonary embolus, drug-related fever, and tumor-related fever represent the main noninfectious sources of fever; however, other sources such as factitious fever, underlying collagen vascular disorder, autoimmune disorders, and foreign-body-type hypersensitivity reaction, must also be considered. The use of biologic markers such as procalcitonin (PCT) and neopterin levels has been suggested to help distinguish between infectious and noninfectious causes of fever, although further studies are needed to validate these tests prior to routine clinical use (135). Similarly, soluble triggering receptor expressed on myeloid cells-1 (sTREM-1) along with PCT have been suggested to improve recognition of patients with true infection and may help determine whether or not to start empiric antimicrobial therapy (136). Unfortunately, neither PCT nor sTREM-1 by itself has shown consistency in differentiating infectious conditions versus tumor or treatment-related febrile response. It is, however, postulated that a combination of systemic PCT and local and/or systemic sTREM-1 or CRP and/or neopterin may help to distinguish patients with infection from those with noninfectious illness. Results from several randomized intervention studies on PCT-guided antimicrobial therapy in sepsis or pneumonia show PCT may aid in clinical decision-making (136,137). At present, randomized trials to assess the role of select biomarker panels including PCT, neopterin, and sTREM-1 are lacking.

Pulmonary embolus should be considered in a bed-bound or postoperative patient with any combination of fever, chest pain, dyspnea, or an abnormal chest radiograph. Patients with bulky pelvic tumors are also at risk. A high level of suspicion is important, and spiral intravenous contrast-enhanced chest CT scans or ventilation-perfusion scans may establish the diagnosis; in rare instances, a more definite pulmonary angiogram may be performed. Therapy remains anticoagulation with low-molecular-weight heparin. For patients who are unable to tolerate these drugs or who continue to have pulmonary emboli despite therapy, inferior vena caval filters are required.

Many drugs, including antibiotics, may cause fever (138). Patients typically develop fever and a diffuse maculopapular rash after several days of therapy. Eosinophilia, although a helpful sign, is usually lacking. Mild elevations in liver function tests may be present though nonspecific. Atypical presentations of drug fever, including patients without rash or those who develop fever weeks into therapy or after completion of therapy, can also occur. Discontinuing the antibiotic(s) and observing the patient usually make the diagnosis. It is important to remember that some drug fevers may take as long as a week to resolve completely. Supportive measures, such as antipyretics and antipruritics, may decrease symptoms.

The diagnosis of tumor fever can be made only after systematic exclusion of all other potential causes of fever. Most patients with tumor fever have metastatic disease involving the liver or lung. In these patients, the fever may be as high as 40°C, and chills may be absent; when not febrile, these patients often feel relatively well. In patients suspected of having tumor fever, a clinical trial of broad-spectrum antibiotics is given. If the fever does not abate and no other clear infection source is evident, the likelihood of tumor fever increases. Nonsteroidal anti-inflammatory agents such as naprosyn often produce an immediate and sustained response when administered to patients with tumor fever. This should only be done after infectious causes of fever have essentially been excluded, and a trial of broad-spectrum antibiotic therapy has not resulted in defervescence.

REFERENCES

1. Safdar A, Armstrong D. Infections in patients with neoplastic diseases. In: Grenvik M, Ayers SM, Holbrook PR, et al. eds. *Textbook of Critical Care*. 4th ed. Philadelphia, PA: W.B. Saunders; 2000:715–726.
2. Safdar A, Armstrong D. Infectious morbidity in critically ill patients with cancer. *Crit Care Clin.* 2001;17:531–570.
3. Gilstrap LC, Gibbs RS, Michel TJ, et al. Genital aerobic bacterial flora of women receiving radiotherapy for gynecologic malignancy. *Gynecol Oncol.* 1986;23:35–39.
4. Gordon AN, Martens M, LaPread Y, et al. Response of lower genital tract flora to external pelvic irradiation. *Gynecol Oncol.* 1989;35:233–235.
5. Talwar P, Chakrabarti A, Patel F, et al. Yeasts at different mucosal sites in patients with carcinoma cervix before and following radiotherapy. *J Hyg Epidemiol Microbiol Immunol.* 1992;36:311–316.
6. Evaldson G, Heimdahl A, Kager L, et al. The normal human anaerobic microflora. *Scand J Infect Dis.* 1982;35:9–15.
7. Rolston KVI, Bodey GP, Safdar A. Polymicrobial infection in patients with cancer: an underappreciated and underreported entity. *Clin Infect Dis.* 2007;45:228–233.
8. Barton DPJ, Fiorica JV, Hoffman MS, et al. Cervical cancer and tubo-ovarian abscesses: a report of three cases. *J Reprod Med.* 1993;38:561–564.
9. Imachi M, Tanaka S, Ishikawa S, et al. Spontaneous perforation of pyometra presenting as generalized peritonitis in a patient with cervical cancer. *Gynecol Oncol.* 1993;50:384–388.
10. Protopappas AG, Diakomanolis ES, Milingos SD, et al. Tubo-ovarian abscess in postmenopausal women: gynecologic malignancy until proven otherwise. *Eur J Obstet Gynecol Reprod Biol.* 2004;114:203–209.
11. Inagaki J, Rodriguez V, Bodey GP. Causes of death in cancer patients. *Cancer.* 1974;33:568–573.
12. Iatrakis G, Sakellaropoulos G, Georgoulias N, et al. Gynecologic cancer and surgical infectious morbidity. *Clin Exp Obstet Gynecol.* 1998;25:36–37.
13. Chang HK, Lo KY, Chiang HS. Complications of urinary diversion after pelvic exenteration for gynecologic malignancy. *Int Urogynecol J.* 2000;11:358–360.
14. Wydra D, Emerich J, Sawicki S, et al. Major complications following exenteration in cases of pelvic malignancies: a 10-year experience. *World J Gastroenterol.* 2006;12:1115–1119.
15. Mahdi H, Gojayev A, Buechel M, et al. Surgical site infection in women undergoing surgery for gynecologic cancer. *Int J Gynecol Cancer.* 2014;24:779–786.
16. Matar MJ, Safdar A, Rolston KV. Relationship of colonization with vancomycin-resistant enterococci and risk of systemic infection in patients with cancer. *Clin Infect Dis.* 2006;42:1506–1507.
17. Gould N, Kamelle S, Tillmanns T, et al. Predictors of complications after inguinal lymphadenopathy. *Gynecol Oncol.* 2001;82:329–332.
18. Safdar A, Rolston KV. Stenotrophomonas maltophilia: changing spectrum of a serious bacterial pathogen in patients with cancer. *Clin Infect Dis.* 2007;45:1602–1609.
19. Safdar A, Rodriguez GH, Balakrishnan M, et al. Changing trends in etiology of bacteremia in patients with cancer. *Eur J Clin Microbiol Infect Dis.* 2006;25:522–526.
20. McWilliams GD, Hill MJ, Dietrich CS III. Gynecologic emergencies. *Surg Clin North Am.* 2008;88:265–283.
21. Han XY, Kamana M, Rolston KV. Viridans streptococci isolated by culture from blood of cancer patients: clinical and microbiologic analysis of 50 cases. *J Clin Microbiol.* 2006;44:160–165.
22. Green JA, Kirwan JM, Tierney JF. Survival and recurrence after concomitant chemotherapy and radiotherapy for cancer of the uterine cervix. *Lancet.* 2001;385:781–786.
23. Yessaian A, Magistris A, Burger RA, et al. Radical hysterectomy followed by tailored postoperative therapy in the treatment of stage 1B2 cervical cancer: feasibility and indications for adjuvant therapy. *Gynecol Oncol.* 2004;94:61–66.
24. Jurado M, Martinez-Monge R, Garcia-Foncillas J, et al. Pilot study of concurrent cisplatin, 5-fluorouracil, and external beam radiotherapy prior to radical surgery +/− intraoperative electron beam radiotherapy in locally advanced cervical cancer. *Gynecol Oncol.* 1999;74:30–37.
25. Micha JP, Goldstein BH, Rettenmaier MA, et al. Pelvic radiation necrosis and osteomyelitis following chemoradiation for advanced stage vulvar and cervical carcinoma. *Gynecol Oncol.* 2006;101:349–352.
26. Wisplinghoff H, Cornely OA, Moser S, et al. Outcomes of nosocomial bloodstream infections in adult neutropenic patients: a prospective cohort and matched case-control study. *Infect Control Hosp Epidemiol.* 2003;24:905–911.
27. Anatoliotaki A, Valatas V, Mantadakis E, et al. Bloodstream infections in patients with solid tumors: associated factors, microbial spectrum and outcome. *Infection.* 2004;32:65–71.
28. Elting LS, Rubenstein EB, Rolston KV, et al. Outcomes of bacteremia in patients with cancer and neutropenia: observations from two decades of epidemiological and clinical trials. *Clin Infect Dis.* 1997;25:247–259.
29. Zahar JR, Farhat H, Chachaty E, et al. Incidence and clinical significance of anaerobic bacteremia in cancer patients: a 6-year retrospective study. *Clin Microbiol Infect.* 2005;11:724–729.
30. Fainstein V, Elting LS, Bodey GP. Bacteremia caused by non-sporulating anaerobes in cancer patients—a 12-year experience. *Medicine (Baltimore).* 1989;68:151–162.
31. Bodey GP, Rodriguez S, Fainstein V, et al. Clostridial bacteremia in cancer patients—a 12-year experience. *Cancer.* 1991;67:1928–1942.
32. Pelletier JP, Plumbley JA, Rouse EA, et al. The role of *Clostridium septicum* in paraneoplastic sepsis. *Arch Pathol Lab Med.* 2000;124:353–356.
33. Safdar A. Strategies to enhance immune function in hematopoietic transplantation recipients who have fungal infections. *Bone Marrow Transplant.* 2006;38:327–337.
34. Safdar A, Singhal S, Mehta J. Clinical significance of non-*Candida* fungal blood isolation in patients undergoing high-risk allogeneic hematopoietic stem cell transplantation (1993–2001). *Cancer.* 2004;100:2456–2461.
35. Raad I, Hachem R, Hanna H, et al. Sources and outcome of bloodstream infections in cancer patients: the role of central venous catheters. *Eur J Clin Microbiol Infect Dis.* 2007;26:549–556.
36. Raad I, Hanna H, Jiang Y, et al. Comparative activities of daptomycin, Linezolid, and tigecycline against catheter-related methicillin-resistant *Staphylococcus* bacteremic isolates embedded in biofilm. *Antimicrob Agents Chemother.* 2007;51:1656–1660.

37. Ghanem GA, Boktour M, Warneke C, et al. Catheter-related *Staphylococcus aureus* bacteremia in cancer patients: high rate of complications with therapeutic implications. *Medicine (Baltimore).* 2007;86:54–60.
38. Estes JM, Rocconi R, Straughn JM, et al. Complications of indwelling venous access devices in patients with gynecologic malignancies. *Gynecol Oncol.* 2003;91:591–595.
39. Silver DF, Hempling RE, Recio FO, et al. Complications related to indwelling caval catheters on a gynecologic oncology service. *Gynecol Oncol.* 1998;70:329–333.
40. Minassian VA, Sood AK, Lowe P, et al. Long-term central venous access in gynecologic cancer patients. *J Am Coll Surg.* 2000;191:403–409.
41. Roybal JJ, Feliberti EC, Rouse L, et al. Pump removal in infected patients with hepatic chemotherapy pumps: when is it necessary? *Am Surg.* 2006;72:880–884.
42. Strecker EP, Heber R, Boos I, et al. Preliminary experience with locoregional intraarterial chemotherapy of uterine cervical or endometrial cancer using the peripheral implantable port system (PIPS): a feasibility study. *Cardiovasc Intervent Radiol.* 2003;26:118–122.
43. Shoji T, Tanaka F, Yanagihara K, et al. Phase II study of repeated intrapleural chemotherapy using implantable access system for management of malignant pleural effusion. *Chest.* 2002;121:821–824.
44. Sakuragi N, Nakajima A, Nomura E, et al. Complications related to intraperitoneal administration of cisplatin or carboplatin for ovarian carcinoma. *Gynecol Oncol.* 2000;79:420–423.
45. Driesen P, Boutin C, Viallat JR, et al. Implantable access system for prolonged intrapleural immunotherapy. *Eur Respir J.* 1994;7:1889–1892.
46. Adachi S, Noda T, Ito K, et al. Complications associated with CDDP intraperitoneal chemotherapy. *Asia Oceania J Obstet Gynaecol.* 1994;20:7–12.
47. Prasad KN, Pradhan S, Datta NR. Urinary tract infection in patients of gynecologic malignancies undergoing external pelvic radiotherapy. *Gynecol Oncol.* 1995;57:380–382.
48. Roos EJ, Van Eijkeren MA, Boon TA, et al. Pelvic exenteration as treatment of recurrent or advanced gynecologic and urologic cancer. *Int J Gynecol Cancer.* 2005;15:624–629.
49. Ledger WJ, Gee C, Lewis WP. Guidelines for antibiotic prophylaxis in gynecology. *Am J Obstet Gynecol.* 1975;121:1038–1045.
50. Hemsell DL, Johnson ER, Hemsell PG, et al. Cefazolin is inferior to cefotetan as single-dose prophylaxis for women undergoing elective total abdominal hysterectomy. *Clin Infect Dis.* 1995;20:677–684.
51. Hemsell DL, Bernstein SG, Bawdon RE, et al. Preventing major operative site infection after radical abdominal hysterectomy and pelvic lymphadenectomy. *Gynecol Oncol.* 1989;35:55–60.
52. Velasco E, Thuler LC, Martins CA, et al. Risk factors for infectious complications after abdominal surgery for malignant disease. *Am J Infect Control.* 1996;24:1–6.
53. Brooker DC, Savage JE, Twiggs LB, et al. Infectious morbidity in gynecologic cancer. *Am J Obstet Gynecol.* 1987;156:513–520.
54. Morgan LS, Daly JW, Monif GR. Infectious morbidity associated with pelvic exenteration. *Gynecol Oncol.* 1980;10:318–328.
55. Orr JW Jr, Shingleton HM, Hatch KD, et al. Correlation of perioperative morbidity and colonization to radical hysterectomy interval. *Obstet Gynecol.* 1982;59:726–731.
56. Berkeley AS, Orr JW, Cavanagh D, et al. Comparative effectiveness and safety of cefotetan and cefoxitin as prophylactic agents in patients undergoing abdominal or vaginal hysterectomy. *Am J Surg.* 1988;155:81–85.
57. Mann WJ Jr, Orr JW, Shingleton HM, et al. Perioperative influences on infectious morbidity in radical hysterectomy. *Gynecol Oncol.* 1981;11:207–212.
58. Gussman D, Reva J, Carlson JA Jr. Prophylaxis for radical hysterectomy. *Infect Surg.* 1987;6:55.
59. Rosenshein NB, Ruth JC, Villar J, et al. A prospective randomized study of doxycycline as a prophylactic antibiotic in patients undergoing radical hysterectomy. *Gynecol Oncol.* 1983;15:201–206.
60. Marsden DE, Cavanagh D, Wisniewski BJ, et al. Factors affecting the incidence of infectious morbidity after radical hysterectomy. *Am J Obstet Gynecol.* 1985;152:817–821.
61. Sevin BU, Ramos R, Lichtinger M, et al. Antibiotic prevention of infections complicating radical abdominal hysterectomy. *Obstet Gynecol.* 1984;64:539–545.
62. Micha JP, Kucera PR, Birkett JP, et al. Prophylactic mezlocillin in radical hysterectomy. *Obstet Gynecol.* 1987;69:251–254.
63. Sevin BU, Ramos R, Gerhardt RT, et al. Comparative efficacy of short-term versus long-term cefoxitin prophylaxis against postoperative infection after radical hysterectomy: a prospective study. *Obstet Gynecol.* 1991;77:729–734.
64. Shapiro M, Schoenbaum SC, Tager IB, et al. Benefit-cost analysis of antimicrobial prophylaxis in abdominal and vaginal hysterectomy. *JAMA.* 1983;249:1290–1294.
65. van Lindert AC, Giltaij AR, Derksen MD, et al. Single-dose prophylaxis with broad-spectrum penicillins (piperacillin and mezlocillin) in gynecologic oncological surgery, with observation on serum and tissue concentrations. *Eur J Obstet Gynecol Reprod Biol.* 1990;36:137–145.
66. Smith CV, James W Orr, Gibbs RL, et al. Oral doxycycline vs. parenteral cefazolin: prophylaxis for vaginal hysterectomy. *Infect Surg.* 1989;99:64.
67. Turner S. The effect of penicillin vaginal suppositories on morbidity in vaginal hysterectomy and on the vaginal flora. *Am J Obstet Gynecol.* 1950;60:806–812.
68. Wright VC, Lanning MN, Natale R. Use of a topical antibiotic spray in vaginal surgery. *Can Med Assoc J.* 1978;118:1395–1398.
69. Shapiro M, Munoz A, Tager IB, et al. Risk factors for infection at the operative site after abdominal or vaginal hysterectomy. *N Engl J Med.* 1982;307:1661–1666.
70. Hemsell DL, Heard MC, Hemsell PG, et al. Alterations in lower reproductive tract flora after single-dose piperacillin and triple-dose cefoxitin at vaginal and abdominal hysterectomy. *Obstet Gynecol.* 1988;72:875–880.
71. Hemsell DL, Bawdon RE, Hemsell PG, et al. Single-dose cephalosporin for prevention of major pelvic infection after vaginal hysterectomy: cefazolin versus cefoxitin versus cefotaxime. *Am J Obstet Gynecol.* 1987;156:1201–1205.
72. Hemsell DL, Johnson ER, Hemsell PG, et al. Cefazolin inferior to cefotetan for single-dose prophylaxis in women undergoing hysterectomy. *Clin Infect Dis.* 1995;20:677.
73. Kobamatsu Y, Makinoda S, Yamada T, et al. Evaluation of the improvement of cephems on the prophylaxis of pelvic infection after radical hysterectomy. *Gynecol Obstet Invest.* 1991;32:102–106.
74. Bratzler DW, Hunt DR. The surgical infection prevention and surgical care improvement projects: national initiatives to improve outcomes for patients having surgery. *Clin Infect Dis.* 2006;43:322–330.
75. Contant CM, Hop WC, van't Sant HP, et al. Mechanical bowel preparation for elective colorectal surgery: a multicenter randomized trial. *Lancet.* 2008;370:2112–2117.
76. Nelson G, Kalogera E, Dowdy SC. Enhanced recovery pathways in gynecologic oncology. *Gynecol Oncol.* 2014;135(3):586–594.
77. Nichols RL, Condon RE. Preoperative preparation of the colon. *Surg Gynecol Obstet.* 1971;132:323–337.
78. Johnson MP, Kim SJ, Langstraat CL, et al. Using bundled interventions to reduce surgical site infection after major gynecologic cancer surgery. *Obstet Gynecol.* 2016;127(6):1135–1144.
79. Douvier S, Nabholtz JM, Friedman S, et al. Infectious pneumoperitoneum as an uncommon presentation of endometrial carcinoma: report of two cases. *Gynecol Oncol.* 1989;33:392–394.
80. Weinstein WM, Onderdonk AB, Bartlett JG, et al. Experimental intra-abdominal abscesses in rats: development of an experimental model. *Infect Immun.* 1974;10:1250–1255.
81. Safdar A, Rolston KV. Vancomycin tolerance, a potential mechanism for refractory gram-positive bacteremia observational study in patients with cancer. *Cancer.* 2006;106:1815–1820.
82. Ohmagari N, Hanna H, Graviss L, et al. Risk factors for infections with multidrug-resistant *Pseudomonas aeruginosa* in patients with cancer. *Cancer.* 2005;104:205–212.
83. Roy S, Higareda I, Angel-Muller E, et al. Ertapenem once a day versus piperacillin-tazobactam every 6 hours for treatment of acute pelvic infections: a prospective, multicenter, randomized, double-blind study. *Infect Dis Obstet Gynecol.* 2003;11:27–37.
84. McNeeley SG Jr, Hopkins MP, Ehlerova B, et al. Infection on a gynecologic oncology service. *Gynecol Oncol.* 1990;37:183–187.
85. Henderson W. Synergistic bacterial gangrene abdominal hysterectomy. *Obstet Gynecol.* 1977:49(1 suppl):24–27.
86. Bouma J, Dankert J. Recurrent acute leg cellulitis in patients after radical vulvectomy. *Gynecol Oncol.* 1988;29:50–57.
87. Hunt TK, Rabkin J, von Smitten K. Effects of edema and anemia on wound healing and infection. *Curr Stud Hematol Blood Transfus.* 1986;53:101–113.
88. Bahary CM, Joel-Cohen SJ, Neri A. Necrotizing fasciitis. *Obstet Gynecol.* 1977;50:633–637.
89. Wilson B. Necrotizing fasciitis. *Am Surg.* 1952;18:416–431.
90. Daly JW, King CR, Monif GR. Progressive necrotizing wound infections in postirradiated patients. *Obstet Gynecol.* 1978;52 suppl:5S–8S.
91. Husseinzadeh N, Nahhas WA, Manders EK, et al. Spontaneous occurrence of synergistic bacterial gangrene following external pelvic irradiation. *Obstet Gynecol.* 1984;63:859–862.

92. Bearman DM, Livengood CH III, Addison WA. Necrotizing fasciitis arising from a suprapubic catheter site. A case report. *J Reprod Med.* 1988;33:411–413.
93. Hoffman MS, Turnquist D. Necrotizing fasciitis of the vulva during chemotherapy. *Obstet Gynecol.* 1989;74:483–484.
94. Roberts DB. Necrotizing fasciitis of the vulva. *Am J Obstet Gynecol.* 1987;157:568–571.
95. Pruyn SC. Acute necrotizing fasciitis of the endopelvic fascia. *Obstet Gynecol.* 1978;52 suppl:25–45.
96. Sotrel G, Hirsch E, Edelin KC. Necrotizing fasciitis following diagnostic laparoscopy. *Obstet Gynecol.* 1983;62(3 suppl):67S–69S.
97. McNeeley SG Jr, Hendrix SL, Bennett SM, et al. Synthetic graft placement in the treatment of fascial dehiscence with necrosis and infection. *Am J Obstet Gynecol.* 1998;179:1430–1434.
98. Fisher JR, Conway MJ, Takeshita RT, et al. Necrotizing fasciitis. Importance of roentgenographic studies for soft-tissue gas. *JAMA.* 1979;241:803–806.
99. Altmeier WA. Gas gangrene. *Surg Gynecol Obstet.* 1947;84:504.
100. Fujiwara K, Sakuragi N, Suzuki S, et al. First-line intraperitoneal carboplatin-based chemotherapy for 165 patients with epithelial ovarian carcinoma: results of long-term follow-up. *Gynecol Oncol.* 2003;90:637–643.
101. Mora-Duarte J, Betts R, Rotstein C, et al. Comparison of caspofungin and amphotericin B for invasive candidiasis. *N Engl J Med.* 2002;347:2020–2029.
102. Blot SI, Vandewoude KH, Waele JJ. *Candida* peritonitis. *Curr Opin Crit Care.* 2007;13:195–199.
103. Miller C. Ligation or excision of the pelvic veins in the treatment of puerperal pyaemia. *Surg Gynecol Obstet.* 1917;25:431.
104. Twickler DM, Setiawan AT, Evans RS, et al. Imaging of puerperal septic thrombophlebitis: prospective comparison of MR imaging, CT, and sonography. *AJR Am J Roentgenol.* 1997;169:1039–1043.
105. Zerhouni EA, Barth KH, Siegelman SS. Demonstration of venous thrombosis by computed tomography. *AJR Am J Roentgenol.* 1980;134:753–758.
106. Schulman H, Zatuchni G. Pelvic thrombophlebitis in the puerperal and postoperative gynecology patient. Obscure fever as an indication for anticoagulant therapy. *Am J Obstet Gynecol.* 1964;90:1293–1296.
107. Twickler DM, Setiawan AT, Evans RS, et al. Imaging of puerperal septic thrombophlebitis: prospective comparison of MR imaging, CT, and sonography. *AJR Am J Roentgenol.* 1997;169:1039–1043.
108. Josey WE, Staggers SR Jr. Heparin therapy in septic pelvic thrombophlebitis: a study of 46 cases. *Am J Obstet Gynecol.* 1974;120:228–233.
109. Brown CE, Stettler RW, Twickler D, et al. Puerperal septic pelvic thrombophlebitis: incidence and response to heparin therapy. *Am J Obstet Gynecol.* 1999;181:143–148.
110. Lee AY, Levine MN, Baker RI, et al. Low-molecular-weight heparin versus a coumadin for the prevention of recurrent venous thromboembolism in patients with cancer. *N Engl J Med.* 2003;349:146–153.
111. Stanton PE Jr, Evans JR, Lefemine AA, et al. White clot syndrome. *South Med J.* 1988;81:616–620.
112. Raad II, Escalante C, Hachem RY, et al. Treatment of febrile neutropenic patients with cancer who require hospitalization. A prospective randomized study comparing imipenem and cefepime. *Cancer.* 2003;98:1039–1047.
113. Klastersky J, Ameye L, Maertens J, et al. Bacteremia in febrile neutropenic cancer patients. *Int J Antimicrob Agents.* 2007;30(suppl 1):51–59.
114. Freifeld AG, Bow EJ, Sepkowitz KA, et al. Clinical practice guideline for the use of antimicrobial agents in neutropenic patients with cancer: 2010 Update by the Infectious Diseases Society of America. *Clin Infect Dis.* 2011;52:427–431.
115. Rex JH, Walsh TJ, Sobel JD, et al. Practice guidelines for the treatment of candidiasis. Infectious Diseases Society of America. *Clin Infect Dis.* 2000;30:662–678.
116. Marsh PK, Tally FP, Kellum J, et al. Candida infections in surgical patients. *Ann Surg.* 1983;198:42–47.
117. Lamaris GA, Esmaeli B, Chamilos G, et al. Fungal endophthalmitis in a tertiary care cancer center: a review of 23 cases. *Eur J Clin Microbiol Infect Dis.* 2008;27:343–347.
118. Laverdière M, Rotstein C, Bow EJ, et al. Impact of fluconazole prophylaxis on fungal colonization and infection rates in neutropenic patients. The Canadian Fluconazole Study. *J Antimicrob Chemother.* 2000;46:1001–1008.
119. Scott H, Griffin D. Ovarian cancer complicated by invasive pulmonary aspergillus. *Gynecol Oncol.* 2006;100(1):216–217.
120. Eggimann P, Marchetti O. Is (1→3)-β-D-glucan the missing link from bedside assessment to pre-emptive therapy of invasive candidiasis? *Crit Care.* 2011;15:1017.
121. Rex JH, Pappas PG, Karchmer AW, et al. A randomized and blinded multicenter trial of high-dose fluconazole plus placebo versus fluconazole plus amphotericin B as therapy for candidemia and its consequences in nonneutropenic subjects. *Clin Infect Dis.* 2003;36:1221–1228.
122. Pappas PG, Rotstein CM, Betts RF, et al. Micafungin versus caspofungin for treatment of candidemia and other forms of invasive candidiasis. *Clin Infect Dis.* 2007;45:883–893.
123. Marik PE. Aspiration pneumonitis and aspiration pneumonia. *N Engl J Med.* 2001;344:665–671.
124. Aisenberg G, Rolston KV, Dickey BF, et al. *Stenotrophomonas maltophilia* pneumonia in cancer patients without traditional risk factors for infection, 1997–2004. *Eur J Clin Microbiol Infect Dis.* 2007;26:13–20.
125. Mandell LA, Wunderrink RG, Anzueto A, et al. Infectious Diseases Society of America/American Thoracic Society consensus guidelines on the management of community-acquired pneumonia in adults. *Clin Infect Dis.* 2007;44(suppl 2):S27–S72.
126. Cirisano FD, Greenspoon JS, Stenson R, et al. The etiology and management of diarrhea in the gynecologic oncology patient. *Gynecol Oncol.* 1993;50:45–48.
127. Satin AJ, Harrison CR, Hancock KC, et al. Relapsing *Clostridium difficile* toxin-associated colitis in ovarian cancer patients treated with chemotherapy. *Obstet Gynecol.* 1989;74:487–489.
128. Turgeon DK, Novicki TJ, Ouick J, et al. Six rapid tests for direct detection of *Clostridium difficile* and its toxins in fecal samples compared with the fibroblast cytotoxicity assay. *J Clin Microbiol.* 2003;41:667–670.
129. Wanahita A, Goldsmith EA, Marino BJ, et al. *Clostridium difficile* infection in patients with unexplained leukocytosis. *Am J Med.* 2003;115:543–546.
130. Kaltsas A, Simon M, Unruh LH, et al. Clinical and laboratory characteristics of Clostridium difficile infection in patients with discordant diagnostic test results. *J Clin Microbiol.* 2012;50:1303–1307.
131. Low DE, Keller N, Barth A, et al. Clinical prevalence, antimicrobial susceptibility, and geographic resistance patterns of enterococci: results from the SENTRY Antimicrobial Surveillance Program, 1997–1999. *Clin Infect Dis.* 2001;32(suppl 2):S133–S145.
132. Drekonja DM, Butler M, MacDonald R, et al. Comparative effectiveness of Clostridium difficile treatments: a systematic review. *Ann Intern Med.* 2011;155:839–847.
133. Musher DM, Logan N, Hamill RJ, et al. Nitazoxanide for the treatment of *Clostridium difficile* colitis. *Clin Infect Dis.* 2006;43:421–427.
134. Louie TJ, Miller MA, Mullane KM, et al. Fidaxomicin versus vancomycin for Clostridium difficile infection. *N Engl J Med.* 2011;364:422–431.
135. Ruokonen E, Ilkka L, Niskanen M, et al. Procalcitonin and neopterin as indicators of infection in critically ill patients. *Acta Anaesthesiol Scand.* 2002;46:398–404.
136. Schultz MJ, Determann RM. PCT and sTREM-1: the markers of infection in critically ill patients? *Med Sci Monit.* 2008;14:RA241–RA247.
137. Gibot S, Cravoisy A. Soluble form of the triggering receptor expressed on myeloid cells-1 as a marker of microbial infection. *Clin Med Res.* 2004;2:181–187.
138. Hirschmann JV. Fever of unknown origin in adults. *Clin Infect Dis.* 1997;24:291–300; Quiz 301–302.

CHAPTER 29

Management of Surgical Complications of Gynecologic Cancer Treatment

Andreas Obermair, Donal J. Brennan, and Robert E. Bristow

General Complications of Gynecologic Cancer Surgery

Stroke

Stroke is estimated to occur following gynecologic oncology surgery in less than 1% of patients. Risk factors reflect those in the general population: history of previous stroke or transient ischemic attack, atherosclerosis, hypertension, diabetes, and advanced age (1). The etiology of stroke is attributed to hypoperfusion injury, hemorrhage, or embolism. In contrast to cardiac surgery, the majority of noncardiac stroke is due to cerebrovascular thrombosis, rather than embolic events (2). Hypotension (relative to the patient's baseline blood pressure) increases the risk of stroke in patients undergoing noncardiac, non-neurologic surgery (3,4). Despite this, no evidence is available that intraoperative monitoring or regulation of blood pressure reduces the incidence of stroke. Avoidance of severe hyperglycemia and hypoglycemia is recommended, though there is a lack of consensus regarding glucose targets (2).

Cardiac Events

Major noncardiac surgery is associated with major cardiac events (cardiac arrest, myocardial infarction, heart failure, arrhythmias) in 0.5% to 3.0% (3,5). Perioperative myocardial infarction is associated with a 50% to 70% mortality rate and carries a high risk for future cardiac events. More than half of perioperative myocardial infarctions are unrecognized (asymptomatic non-ST elevation), and the incidence peaks during the first 24 hours postoperatively. Recent myocardial infarction, heart failure, ischemic heart disease, diabetes, renal insufficiency, cerebrovascular disease, obesity, sleep apnea, and poor functional status constitute high-risk factors.

Prevention of perioperative cardiac events should focus on evaluation of risk factors, risk stratification, and maximization of patient function. Good evidence supports the continuation of β-blockers and HMG-CoA reductase inhibitors ("statins") throughout the perioperative period for patients already treated with β-blockers. Perioperative measures should focus on maintenance of normothermia and postoperative monitoring of serum troponin levels.

Deep Vein Thrombosis and Pulmonary Embolism

Deep vein thrombosis (DVT) and/or pulmonary embolism comprise the spectrum of complications known as venous thromboembolism (VTE). VTE following surgery is the most common cause of peri- and postoperative death (6). DVT affects 0.1% of patients each year, but the incidence is significantly higher among patients undergoing surgical treatment for gynecologic cancer, occurring in up to 20% of cases (7).

Patients with gynecologic cancer are at high risk for VTE because of their underlying malignancy, increased age, and the extensive nature of treatment. The underlying mechanism of the development of VTE includes increased release of procoagulant factors, cytokine imbalance, and activation of the antifibrinolytic pathways. Clinical risk factors include a history of VTE, obesity, immobility, trauma, prolonged surgical time, radiation therapy, and increasing complexity of surgery. Patients with the highest risk for developing postoperative VTE have two or more of the following: age greater than 60 years, malignancy, and history of VTE (8). Early ambulation, heparin, low-molecular-weight heparin, and sequential compression devices (graduated compression stockings or intermittent pneumatic compression) are effective in reducing the incidence of VTE (9). The incidence of VTE in patients undergoing major gynecologic cancer surgery is decreased with dual, prolonged (4-week) prophylaxis without increasing bleeding complications (10). Current guidelines recommend VTE prophylaxis for at least 4 weeks following surgery in the absence of bleeding or other contraindications.

Bladder and Ureteral Injury

Injuries to the lower urinary tract (laceration, transection, crush injury, ligation, thermal injury, injury through devascularization) are uncommonly diagnosed intraoperatively; the outcomes of patients who are diagnosed late (urinomas, peritonitis, sepsis, fistula) are worse (11). The risk of bladder/ureter injury ranges between 1.1% and 5.3% in patients undergoing a radical hysterectomy and is approximately 1% in standard hysterectomy for uterine cancer (11–14). Bladder injuries recognized at the time of the initial surgical procedure should be repaired immediately, using a standard two-layered closure of delayed absorbable suture. Bladder injuries diagnosed postoperatively (e.g., fistula) may be treated with an indwelling catheter for a period of several weeks. If spontaneous closure does not occur with prolonged drainage, surgical repair is indicated. Ureteral injuries recognized intraoperatively should be repaired by excising the injured segment of ureter, placement of a ureteral stent, and reapproximating the distal urinary tract (ureteroureterostomy, ureteroneocystostomy with psoas hitch, and possibly a Boari flap). Ureteral injuries detected remote from the initial surgical procedure can be managed by attempted placement of a ureteral stent, which can be accomplished either retrograde via cystoscopy or antegrade via a percutaneous nephrostomy tube. If spontaneous closure does not occur after an observation period of 4 to 6 weeks, or if stent placement is not feasible, surgical repair is indicated. Long-term outcomes are generally excellent.

Injury to Small and Large Bowel

Bowel injuries occur in approximately 1% of patients undergoing surgery for gynecologic cancer. Risk factors include previous surgery, adhesions, and previous radiotherapy. Most bowel injuries are recognized at the time of open surgery; however, this is not the case in laparoscopic surgery. A recent systematic review demonstrated that the rate of bowel injury at laparoscopic hysterectomy for malignancy was 1:246 (15). The majority of injuries occur either during establishment of a pneumoperitoneum or with the use of electrosurgical devices. Approximately 40% of laparoscopic bowel injuries are not recognized intraoperatively, and the mortality rate in this group is as high as 3% (15).

Small bowel enterotomies can be closed in one layer using delayed absorbable suture, while large bowel injuries of greater than 2 cm should be closed in two layers. Small or large bowel injuries require primary bowel resection if the blood supply to the bowel is compromised or if injuries occur at multiple levels. The general principles of management of a bowel injury requiring resection are similar to that of any bowel anastomosis (hand-sewn or stapled). After resection of the injured segment of bowel, the anastomosis must be patent, tension-free, and well vascularized. If any of these three conditions are unmet, the risk of leakage is very high.

Nerve Injury

Poor patient position, improper placement of retractor blades, and radical surgical dissection increase the risk of nerve injury (11). *Neurapraxia* is caused by compression leading to changes in intraneural microcirculation, and is fully reversible. *Axonotmesis* (crush injury) will sever axons, and the function will resolve with gradual regeneration of nerve fibers. Transection of nerve fibers causes aberrant regeneration of the axons (misalignment), resulting in permanent functional losses.

The lumbosacral plexus is at risk for injury during gynecologic surgery. The use of short retractor blades or flexible blades with packs placed under the blades instead of self-retainers may reduce the risk of nerve injury intraoperatively (11). Additionally, avoidance of long-term hip extension (femoral nerve) or flexion (sciatic nerve) in lithotomy position will decrease the risk of nerve injuries.

Hemorrhage

Intraoperative hemorrhage is defined as blood loss greater than 1,000 mL, or any requirement for intraoperative blood transfusion. Significant hemorrhage can be expected in 4% to 7.5% of patients undergoing surgery for advanced ovarian cancer (16). Risk factors include anemia prior to surgery, history of prolonged bleeding, blood-thinning medication and herbs/supplements, and intraoperative hypothermia. The principles of management of intraoperative hemorrhage are local and systemic. Local hemostatic control plus the systemic correction of any coagulopathy are the two crucial aspects of managing any significant hemorrhage.

Local measures include tamponade (packs) or the use of an omental autologous transplant (OAT) patch (17); atraumatic grasping, identification and control of all feeding vessels and bleeding sources; identification of sensitive structures (ureters, nerves); the selective use of sutures, clips, diathermy, patches; and the use of topical hemostatic agents. Internal iliac artery ligation should be considered if other measures fail to control pelvic hemorrhage. Finally, "damage control" surgery, with placement of pelvic packing, transfer to the intensive care unit for stabilization, and return to the operating room for pack removal after 24 to 48 hours, may be a last resort.

Postoperative Ileus

Postoperative adynamic ileus is delayed gastrointestinal tract recovery; it may impair wound healing and increase the risk of infections. Gastrointestinal motility is controlled by the enteric autonomous nervous system and influenced by neural reflexes (interfered with by regional anesthesia), inflammation/trauma (tissue handling) and neurohumoral substances (systemic analgesia). Medical illnesses (e.g., diabetes mellitus) or medications may increase the risk of ileus.

Differentiating postoperative ileus from a mechanical small bowel obstruction (SBO) is critical. Bowel sounds are an unreliable indicator and are usually quiet or absent with ileus, but may be high-pitched or absent with SBO. Computed tomography (CT; with oral Gastrografin) or a water-soluble contrast study is recommended to help differentiate ileus from SBO. Failure of contrast to reach the cecum by 4 hours is highly suggestive that surgical intervention will be required and can help differentiate early postoperative SBO from an ileus. Water-soluble contrast may also be therapeutic and may allow a quicker resolution of an adhesive SBO. The treatment of ileus is conservative and nonsurgical, and includes restriction of oral intake, nasogastric tube suction, intravenous fluid and electrolyte replacement, and discontinuation of systemic opioids if possible. Total parenteral nutrition should be considered after 7 to 10 days without satisfactory oral nutrient intake.

Postoperative SBO

Postoperative SBO results from a mechanical blockage of intestinal motility. Possible causes include herniation of bowel (port sites, internal herniation), early adhesions, intussusceptions, and small bowel tumors. The characteristic presentation of SBO is that patients initially recover well (pass flatus, tolerate oral intake), but then develop nausea, vomiting, colicky abdominal discomfort, and pain. CT will show a site of bowel obstruction (transition point), gaseous distension of small bowel, and paucity of air in the rectum. Effective management of SBO requires an expedited diagnosis followed by a short (48 to 72 hours) conservative trial of nasogastric suction and fluid resuscitation in the absence of clinical evidence of strangulation such as peritonism, fever, tachycardia, or leukocytosis. Fluid lost from the nasogastric tube should be replaced with additional crystalloid intravenous fluids and potassium supplementation. There are two indications for surgery for SBO: first, failed conservative management, and second, if there is suspicion of strangulation and loss of bowel vascular perfusion.

Surgical Site Infection

Surgical site infections (SSIs) lead to delayed wound healing, revision surgery, increased use of antibiotics, and increased length of hospital stay (18). On average, a patient with an SSI spends 7 days longer in hospital, is 60% more likely to spend time in the ICU, is five times more likely to be readmitted within 30 days of discharge, and is twice as likely to die (19). The incidence rates vary depending on patient factors and type of surgery, and range from 2% to 10% after laparotomy, while the rate is lower with minimally invasive surgery. Risk factors for SSI include concomitant systemic disease (diabetes, anemia, immunosuppression, immunosuppressive therapy with radiotherapy, chemotherapy, or steroids), obesity, advanced age, preexisting infection, hematoma, damaged tissue, extensive surgery, hypothermia, hemorrhage, and use of drains or catheters (20). Infection control programs reduce the rates of SSI by 35% to 41% (21). Prophylactic antibiotics are most effective when administered 30 to 60 minutes preoperatively. A preoperative Chlorhexidine shower is as effective as bar soap or detergents. Trials on antibacterial sutures are ongoing.

DISEASE SITE–SPECIFIC SURGICAL COMPLICATIONS

Surgery for Ovarian Cancer—Cytoreductive Surgery

Acute Complications

Ovarian cancer cytoreductive surgery has evolved to a contemporary approach designed to achieve complete cytoreduction, with an accepted increase in morbidity balanced against the maximal benefit with respect to long-term survival. A comprehensive approach to advanced-stage ovarian cancer must address disease not only in the pelvis; it also frequently involves surgery on the large and small bowel, diaphragm, liver, spleen, and distal pancreas. Recognition and management of associated perioperative complications is critical. The morbidity of extensive surgical cytoreduction is increased with age, poor nutritional status, and poor functional status (22–26).

Surgical staging for apparent "early" ovarian cancer, including retroperitoneal node dissection, may disrupt the lymphatic system and may cause chylous ascites in the short term. Patients will present with ascites in the early postoperative phase and an injury to the urinary collection system needs to be excluded. The aspiration of chylous is diagnostic.

Spillage of ovarian tumors is more common with minimally invasive surgery than with laparotomy and may upstage ovarian cancer, necessitating adjuvant chemotherapy (27). Meticulous surgical dissection, the use of containment devices (bags), and early conversion to open surgery are strategies to minimize the risk of spillage.

The en bloc resection of locally advanced ovarian cancer (radical oophorectomy or modified posterior exenteration) carries an operative mortality of 0% to 8%, with more contemporary series reporting rates of 4% or lower (28–30). Wound complications are seen in 6% to 34% of patients, particularly with severe hypoalbuminemia (<3.0 ng/dL) and large-volume ascites (31). The estimated blood loss with radical oophorectomy ranges from 800 to 2,900 mL, with as many as 87% of patients receiving blood product transfusion.

Intestinal complications with radical cytoreduction are among the most commonly encountered, with prolonged ileus reported in up to 40% of patients. A large series of 587 patients recently reported an average incidence of postoperative ileus of 30.3% (25.9% without bowel resection, 38.5% with bowel resection) (32). The pattern of spread of ovarian cancer necessitates bowel resection in 19% to 54% of cases (33,34). Colorectal anastomotic leak occurs in fewer than 4% of cases and can lead to abscess, fistula formation, sepsis, and reoperation; the mean time to diagnosis is 19 days (range, 4 to 32 days) (28,29,34–37). Anastomoses below the peritoneal reflection and less than 6 cm from the anal verge are at the highest risk for failure (38). Anastomotic dehiscence can present with insidious symptoms if it is contained, or progressive sepsis with tachycardia, tachypnea, fever, and peritonism if frank fecal peritonitis is present. The investigation of choice to assess a colorectal anastomosis is a CT of the abdomen with rectal contrast.

While there are limited data in gynecologic oncology patient populations, randomized studies on the management of colorectal disorders suggest that mechanical bowel preparation does not lower the risk of anastomotic leak. A recent meta-analysis of 18 randomized controlled trials with over 5,800 patients confirmed that administration of mechanical bowel preparation yielded no difference in anastomotic leak rates (4.4% vs. 4.5%; odds ratio [OR], 0.99 [0.74, 1.13]) or wound complications (9.6% vs. 8.5%; OR, 1.16 [0.95, 1.42]) (39). However, it is sensible to perform a mechanical bowel preparation if a proximal stoma is planned, to prevent a column of stool feeding an anastomotic leak should it occur, or slowing progress following reversal of a loop ileostomy.

Studies of intraperitoneal pelvic drain placement in the setting of a rectal anastomosis similarly suggest no benefit to lowering the risk of anastomotic leak (40). Intestinal diversion has historically been utilized for protection of a rectal anastomosis during primary cytoreductive surgery. Older data suggest that up to 59% of patients requiring rectal anastomosis also underwent protective intestinal diversion with colostomy or ileostomy. Based on more contemporary data, intestinal diversion to "protect" a colorectal anastomosis is not routinely required but may be advisable in patients with very low anastomoses, technically suboptimal anastomoses, or severe hypoalbuminemia (21% leak rate with albumin <3.0 g/dL vs. 3.4% leak rate with albumin >3.0 g/dL) (29,36).

Initial management of anastomotic leak generally requires a laparotomy once the patient has been stabilized. Cardiovascular and respiratory support may be required and broad-spectrum antibiotics should be administered. At laparotomy, great care must be taken not to damage adherent loops of small bowel, and the anastomosis must be exposed and inspected. If a major dehiscence is found, the anastomosis will have to be taken down and a Hartmann's procedure performed with formation of an end colostomy. Care should be taken to seal the distal stump with a linear stapler; as the bowel may be edematous, the staple line should be oversewn with permanent suture that protects the staple line and may make it easier to identify the rectal stump at future surgeries to restore continuity. If the anastomotic leak is small, the anastomosis seems intact, and only minimal soiling is present, the leak can be oversewn, a washout performed, and a protective loop ileostomy fashioned.

Anastomotic dehiscence can very rarely be managed conservatively. Occasionally, if a leak is contained (classically demonstrated on CT by small air-containing abscess around the staple line) and the patient is clinically well, treatment may simply involve antibiotic therapy and bowel rest. A low colorectal dehiscence in a patient with a covering ileostomy may be managed by transanal drainage, which is usually performed at EUA whereby a Foley Catheter can be placed transanally through the staple-line defect to drain the abscess cavity. Once the abscess has drained the anastomosis will often heal spontaneously.

Upper abdominal procedures including splenectomy, distal pancreatectomy, partial hepatectomy, and diaphragmatic peritonectomy or full-thickness resection may be required to render a patient completely free of visible disease. Development of pleural effusions following diaphragmatic peritonectomy or resection occurs in 9% to 64% of patients, although these can be managed with thoracentesis alone in the majority of symptomatic patients. When full-thickness resections are required, perioperative morbidity has been reported in as many as 20% of patients (41,42). A small postoperative pneumothorax will frequently resolve spontaneously and can be monitored with daily chest radiographs. Chest tube placement is occasionally required for major resections of the right hemidiaphragm, large pleural effusions, or worsening pneumothorax.

Acute complications associated with splenectomy include hemorrhage, left lower lobe atelectasis, splenic vein thrombosis, arteriovenous fistula between the splenic artery and vein, and infectious morbidity (43,44). Overwhelming post-splenectomy infection, most commonly due to *Streptococcus pneumoniae*, is a serious complication with a prevalence of 3.2% and a mortality rate as high as 70% (45). Vaccinations for pneumococcus, meningococus, and *Haemophilus influenza* type B are the cornerstones of prevention. Postoperatively, antibiotic prophylaxis is recommended.

Distal pancreatectomy is occasionally indicated to achieve complete disease resection and can result in pancreatic fistula (leak) and pancreatic pseudocyst formation (33,46). Intraoperative placement of a closed suction drain in the left upper quadrant can be useful to monitor for signs of early fistula formation and to prevent pseudocyst formation. Mild enzyme leakage has little clinical impact and can be managed with prolonged drainage and standard oral feeding. Enzyme leakage greater than threefold the upper limit of normal more than 3 days after the operation, or the presence of pain, fever, or leukocytosis requires delay of oral nutrition, administration of antibiotics, somatostatin analogues, and parenteral nutrition.

Chronic Complications

Ovarian cancer patients may experience long-term sequelae related to prior cytoreductive surgery, often exacerbated by the presence of disease recurrence or carcinomatosis. More commonly encountered complications requiring operative intervention are mechanical bowel obstruction or anastomotic stricture. SBO in ovarian cancer patients is best approached with an extended trial of bowel rest and decompression with nutritional supplementation unless bowel dilation is greater than 5 cm, at which point the risk of perforation increases. Carcinomatous ileus can be confused with mechanical bowel obstruction; however, this condition is unlikely to be surgically correctable. If mechanical SBO is refractory to conservative measures, surgical options include resection with reanastomosis, diverting ileostomy, enterocolonic bypass, or palliative percutaneous gastrostomy. Associated complications may include anastomotic failure, blind loop syndrome, or short gut syndrome. Finally, late complications may follow extensive resection of the ileum or a right hemicolectomy; these late complications include chronic diarrhea from impaired absorption of water, fat, and bile salts, and problems related to poor absorption of nutrients, including the fat-soluble vitamins and vitamin B_{12}.

Centralization of Ovarian Cancer Surgery Services

An extensive body of data exists supporting the relationship between surgical volume and mortality; however, the mechanisms underlying this association remain elusive. In ovarian cancer, the relationship between hospital volume and outcome has been controversial; however, recent population-based studies demonstrate an independent relationship between high-volume physicians working in high-volume hospitals and improved disease-free and overall survival (47–49).

The relationship between hospital volume and surgical complications is less clear. Population-based data demonstrate that the 30-day readmission rate following surgery for stage IIIC/IV ovarian cancer is 19% (50), which is consistent with previously published single institution studies (51). The most common reasons for readmission are infection (35%), dehydration (34%), ileus/obstruction (26%), metabolic/electrolyte derangements (23%), and anemia (12%) (92). There does not appear to be a significant relationship between 30-day readmission rates and hospital or physician volume; however, readmission is an independent predictor of reduced overall survival (50).

An analysis of the Agency for Healthcare Research and Quality's Nationwide Inpatient Sample demonstrated that the overall complication rate after surgery for ovarian cancer is 22% (52). Complications are significantly increased in high-volume compared to low-volume hospitals, possibly reflecting a more aggressive approach to cytoreduction. However, patients who experience a complication in a low-volume hospital are almost 50% more likely to die, suggesting that failure to rescue from complications is an important source of the volume-based variation in ovarian cancer outcomes (52).

Although the multifactorial nature of the relationship between volume and outcome in ovarian cancer surgery requires further investigation, it is clear that hospital and physician volume do predict improved survival; this is not due to a reduced complication rate, but may be related to the availability of multidisciplinary teams to manage complications in a timely and appropriate manner.

Surgery for Uterine Cancer

Acute Complications

Until recently, total abdominal hysterectomy was considered the standard surgical approach to hysterectomy for uterine cancer. However, minimally invasive surgical techniques have become increasingly popular due to their favorable outcomes in treatment. To date, three prospective randomized controlled clinical trials are available to compare outcomes from open and laparoscopic surgery for uterine cancer (12–14). The Gynecologic Oncology Group (GOG) **LAP2 Trial (GOG 222)** recruited a total of 2,616 women (12). Patients were eligible if they had clinical stage I to IIA uterine cancer; all histological cell types were allowed; and all patients had to have undergone pelvic and aortic lymph node dissection. The Australian **LACE Trial** enrolled 760 patients. Patients were eligible if they had endometrioid cell type, clinical stage I disease; patients were not eligible if they had a uterine size larger than 10 weeks gestation, had evidence of extrauterine spread (ovarian masses, enlarged lymph nodes), or were unfit for surgery due to medical comorbidities (14). The **Dutch TLH Trial** aimed to compare outcomes in early-stage endometrial cancer treated by laparoscopy or laparotomy. Patients with early-stage endometrial cancer (endometrioid cell type, FIGO grade 1 or 2, clinical stage I disease, negative endocervical curettage) or complex endometrial hyperplasia with atypia were eligible (13). Intraoperative surgical complications were comparable in all three trials.

In the LAP2 trial, postoperative surgical complications were significantly more common in patients who had a laparotomy than in patients who had a laparoscopic procedure (21% vs. 14%). Postoperative ileus (8% vs. 4%) and cardiac arrhythmia (2% vs. 1%) were significantly more common in patients in the open/laparotomy group. In the LACE trial, the open/laparotomy group had a 44% higher incidence of postoperative complications (18.6% in open, 12.9% in laparoscopic) compared to patients in the laparoscopy arm. The incidence of serious adverse events was 74% higher in the open group compared to the laparoscopy group (14.3% for open, 8.2% for laparoscopy). Wound infections or dehiscence were the main contributors to the difference in postoperative complications between laparoscopic (2.0%) and open (8.9%) groups. An open surgical approach (laparotomy), higher Charlson's medical comorbidities score, moderately or poorly differentiated tumors on curetting, lower performance status prior to surgery, obesity, and anemia were independently associated with an increased risk for surgical adverse events (53). Patient's age at surgery was not a risk factor for surgical complications. The Dutch TLH trial recorded comparable postoperative surgical complications in the open and the laparoscopic group (10.6% open/laparotomy; 11.9% laparoscopy). Interestingly, the incidence of postoperative complications was similar among all three trials for patients randomized to the laparoscopic arm (ranging from 11.9% to 14%). In contrast, the incidence of postoperative complications in the open/laparotomy arm was significantly lower in the Dutch TLH trial (10.6%) compared to LACE (18.6%) or LAP2 (21%). In the Dutch TLH trial, no patient required a retroperitoneal node dissection, whereas in the U.S. LAP2 trial, all patients required a pelvic and aortic lymph node dissection. In the Australian LACE trial, approximately half of patients had a retroperitoneal node dissection; however, no differences in the incidence of acute surgical complications were observed between the treatment arms when stratified by nodal dissection status.

Hysterectomy is irrevocably associated with loss of fertility, which should be considered in the context of young women desiring a family. Alternative options currently evaluated in clinical trials include systemic and intrauterine progestin treatment and may result in total pathological responses in up to 50% to 70% of patients (54).

Chronic Complications

Lymphedema and lymphocele are the main chronic complications following surgery for uterine cancer, and the incidence varies depending on the type of surgery and extent of lymph node removal. Overall, lymphedema occurs in 20% of patients following hysterectomy with lymphadenectomy (55). Obesity, the number of lymph nodes removed, the extent of surgery, postoperative infection, radiation therapy, and postoperative DVT increase the risk of developing lymphedema. Lymphoceles are an accumulation of lymphatic fluid in dead space due to postoperative leakage of lymphatic fluid coupled with incomplete lymphatic reabsorption. Most lymphoceles are asymptomatic and found incidentally. The true incidence is therefore unknown (range, 0% to 58.5%) (56–58).

Morcellation

The use of power morcellation in gynecological surgery has come under scrutiny recently following a case of inadvertent dissemination of an unrecognized leiomyosarcoma, which was highlighted by a Food and Drug Administration (FDA) safety notice (59).

First described in 1993 (60), electric power morcellators have become an important adjunct to minimally invasive gynecologic surgery and were used in up to 15% of minimally invasive hysterectomies in the United States up to 2012 (61) resulting in a significant proportion of women avoiding a laparotomy. Compared to a minimally invasive approach, laparotomy is associated with a prolonged hospital stay, more postoperative pain, increased wound complications, venous thromboembolism, and incisional hernias (62).

Increased scrutiny of power morecellation has not only focused on the inadvertent dissemination of unrecognized malignancy but also on other morcellation-related complications. A review of the FDA Manufacturer and User Facility Device Experience database identified 55 complications (11 involving more than 1 organ) including 6 deaths from 1993 through 2013. Bowel injuries (n = 31) were the most commonly reported complications, followed by vascular injuries (n = 27) and injuries to the kidney (n = 3), ureter (n = 3), bladder (n = 1), and diaphragm (n = 1) (61).

Occult uterine malignancies may be present in 9 to 100 per 10,000 women undergoing power morcellation (59,63–65). Multiple studies have demonstrated that patient age is the most important risk factor and morcellation should be avoided in postmenopausal women (66). Given the association between tamoxifen and uterine sarcoma it is advisable to avoid morcellation in these patients, but women are also at risk of inadvertently being diagnosed with endometrial cancers following morcellation of specimens.

While much of the controversy involves the use of electric power morcellation, morcellation can also be used as a surgical technique in vaginal and open surgery with or without the use of power morcellators. The major risk of morcellation is peritoneal seeding of an occult malignancy. Three retrospective cohort studies included patients who underwent exploratory surgery shortly after inadvertent morcellation of a presumed stage 1 uterine sarcoma (64,67,68). Nine of 31 patients (29%) with presumed stage 1 leiomyosarcoma had disseminated peritoneal disease at their second procedure, and five of nine patients (55%) with STUMPS had peritoneal nodules (69). Although some studies suggest that morcellation of stage 1 leiomyosarcoma is associated with a worse outcome, these data should be interpreted with care given the aggressive and unpredictable nature of this disease. Although the numbers are relatively small, this data agrees with previous studies that advocated completion surgery and restaging of uterine malignancy found inadvertently after morcellation for presumed benign disease (68). Data are lacking with respect to the risks associated with inadvertent morcellation of endometrial carcinoma.

Surgery for Cervical Cancer: Radical Hysterectomy and Pelvic Exenteration

Acute Complications

Radical hysterectomy for early-stage cervical cancer is associated with a major complication rate (excessive blood loss, urinary/gastrointestinal tract injury, nerve injury) of 5% to 10%. Vesicovaginal and ureterovaginal fistulas occur in 1% to 3% of cases and typically present within 14 days of surgery with urinary leakage per vagina, commonly associated with pain or fever (70). A CT-Urogram with IV contrast is usually diagnostic for a ureteric fistula. If an injury to the urinary tract is suspected, a cystoscopy with or without a retrograde pyelogram, instillation of methylene blue dye intravenously or via retrograde instillation into the bladder can also help to distinguish a vesicovaginal from ureterovaginal fistula or a combined ureteric plus vesicovaginal fistula.

Small vesicovaginal fistulas can often be managed with prolonged catheterization and continuous decompression of the bladder for 4 to 6 weeks. Ureterovaginal fistulas can often be managed with ureteral stenting or percutaneous nephrostomy.

For nonhealing fistulas, larger fistulas (>1 cm), or complex fistulas involving both ureter and bladder, surgical management with closure is indicated. Typically closure is optimal in a dry environment and can be approached vaginally with a Latzko partial colpocleisis if the defect is small, apical, and not in proximity to the ureter. Bulbocavernosus or Martius fat pad grafts can also be used (71). Trigone involvement or larger complex fistulas are best approached abdominally with re-implantation of the ureter(s) into the bladder or a layered closure with or without an omental flap (72). Urinary retention due to sensory loss and voiding dysfunction are well-recognized complications of radical hysterectomy and result from the denervation of the bladder during the parametrial dissection. Most patients are managed with prolonged bladder decompression for 3 to 7 days with a transurethral or suprapubic catheter. A retrograde voiding trial is recommended to assess for bladder function prior to removal of the catheter, and postvoid residual values of less than 100 mL are generally acceptable.

Minimally invasive approaches to radical hysterectomy, including both traditional laparoscopic and robotically assisted techniques, may offer several health-related benefits including less pain, shorter hospital stay, and more rapid return to full activity than the abdominal approach. However, the incidence of vaginal cuff complications/dehiscence (1.6% to 4.1%) may be higher than that observed with laparotomy (<0.5%); there is also a potential higher risk for nerve injuries (73,74).

Total pelvic exenteration (TPE) is primarily indicated as salvage therapy for cervical cancer patients who have failed radiation therapy or require combined treatment of recurrence in the central pelvis. Acute perioperative morbidity related to TPE is high, with up to 75% of patients experiencing a major complication, and mortality rates of 1% to 5% are typical. Furthermore, reoperation rates to address major complications are high, with rates of 16% to 25.6% reported in the literature (75,76). Morbidity of TPE is attributable to long operative times, compromised healing of the irradiated field, and the complexity of the surgical reconstruction. Significant blood loss, infectious morbidity primarily involving the urinary tract, sepsis, wound complications, fistulas, ileus, and anastomotic leaks of the intestinal or urinary anastomosis are some of the more commonly reported complications. Sepsis, adult respiratory distress syndrome, heart failure, pulmonary embolus, and multiorgan system failure are typical terminal events.

The acute complication rate for both urinary continent and incontinent and urinary diversion ranges from 17% to 20%; these complications include urinary leak, fistula, or anastomotic failure (77). Such problems can be managed conservatively in many cases with prolonged conduit drainage and diversion with percutaneous nephrostomy. Refractory leaks may require surgical revision of the reservoir. Despite the high risk of complications, 5-year survival is in the range of 50% (76,78,79).

Chronic Complications

Urinary retention following radical hysterectomy is usually self-limited; however, long-standing bladder dysfunction may require patient intermittent self-catheterization. Long-term rectal dysfunction is similarly encountered and manifests as constipation or urgency. Nerve-sparing radical hysterectomy, which preserves autonomic and splanchnic innervation to the bladder and rectum, has been reported to decrease bladder and rectal morbidity (70,80). Ureteral strictures are encountered in 1% to 3% of patients and may present with fever and pain, but may be asymptomatic and can lead to loss of renal function. Management is with ureteral stent placement, if possible, or percutaneous nephrostomy placement. Rarely, a ureteric re-implantation may be required. Colonic stomas may be prone to prolapse, hernia, or stricture. However, the most commonly reported intestinal complication is bowel obstruction. Unlike early postoperative bowel obstruction, late obstructions are more likely due to adhesive disease or disease recurrence. Sexual dysfunction is an underreported long-term side effect following radical hysterectomy (81).

Patients undergoing pelvic exenteration are at risk for a number of long-term complications. Urinary diversions are prone to stomal stricture, chronic urinary tract infection, renal dysfunction, nephrolithiasis, metabolic alterations, and difficulty with accessing the reservoir (78,79). Reestablishing intestinal continuity after exenteration has been advocated to minimize the long-term psychosocial and quality-of-life issues surrounding two permanent abdominal stomas but has been associated with a higher risk of reoperation (50% to 60%) and disease recurrence (79). Sexual dysfunction and distorted body image are common problems associated with pelvic exenteration.

Surgery in the Irradiated Field

Radiation induces a complex series of tissue changes including vascular sclerosis and tissue ischemia, the end result of which is fibrosis. Tissue planes are obliterated and healing is compromised. It is estimated that approximately 5% to 7% of patients who undergo radiation therapy for cervical cancer will experience major treatment complications that require surgery (82). The most common sites of intestinal injury in patients who undergo pelvic irradiation are areas that typically lie in the pelvic field. The terminal ileum is the most frequent site of late injury, because of the greater radiosensitivity of the small intestine compared with the colon. The most common indications for reoperative surgery in patients irradiated for cervical or endometrial cancer are intestinal stricture (44%), intestinal fistula or perforation (32%). Radiation damage frequently leads to matted loops of distal ileum densely fixed in the pelvis associated with obstruction or fistula. In the setting of intestinal necrosis, perforation, or abscess formation, resection should be attempted if it can be done without undue risk of damage to adjacent structures. Alternative, more conservative approaches such as intestinal bypass procedures are less morbid, but may lead to the development of blind loop syndrome or result in subsequent spontaneous perforation or fistula formation. In a series of 77 patients who underwent surgery for radiation injury to the small intestine, no difference in short-term complications was noted between patients who underwent resection compared to those who underwent bypass (83).

Urinary tract complications that may lead to surgery in a previously radiated patient include radiation-induced nonhealing or complex ureterovaginal or vesicovaginal fistulas and ureteral strictures, which may compromise renal function. Asymptomatic strictures are more common and underreported in the literature, and may lead to a silent loss of renal function. Most cases of radiation injury to the lower urinary tract can be managed conservatively with ureteric stent placement, percutaneous nephrostomy, or attempts at endoureteral dilation. Recurrent cancer must always be considered, and the appropriate diagnostic biopsies and imaging obtained, prior to consideration for surgical correction or urinary diversion (84).

Surgery for Vulvar Cancer

Acute Complications

Surgical innovation in vulvar cancer evolved as a way to minimize the risk of surgical complications associated with the en bloc radical vulvectomy and bilateral inguinal lymphadenectomy popularized by Stanley Way in the 1950s, rather than from a concern about poor survival outcomes. Vulvar or groin wound breakdown occurs in as many as 50% of patients following radical vulvectomy (85–87). Development of a wound infection is predictive of future wound breakdown and lymphedema (86). Risk factors include increased patient age, obesity, diabetes mellitus, smoking, and prior radiation to the groin. The use of myocutaneous, cutaneous, or skin flaps can reduce tension on suture lines, prevent wound breakdown or infection, and improve cosmetic and functional outcome. A nonrandomized, prospective study showed a reduction in wound breakdown for patients undergoing radical vulvectomy with lymph node dissection and hyperbaric oxygen therapy (88).

Contemporary management of vulvar cancer is tailored to the size and location of the primary tumor, and generally consists of radical partial vulvectomy or wide radical excision combined with ipsilateral or bilateral inguinal lymphadenectomy through separate groin incisions (89). The incidence rates of wound infection, cellulitis, and wound breakdown are 21% to 39%, 21% to 57%, and 17% to 39%, respectively. Optimizing glucose control in patients with diabetes mellitus, using appropriate antibiotic prophylaxis, and sparing the saphenous vein are important prevention strategies (90). Compared to systematic groin node dissection, sentinel lymph node biopsy (SLNB) is associated with a reduction in groin wound breakdown (11.7% vs. 34%) and cellulitis (4.5% vs. 21.3%) (91).

Chronic Complications

Chronic complications from vulvar cancer surgery are often a result of groin node dissection. As many as 50% of patients requiring a groin dissection will experience a long-term complication related to the procedure. Lymphedema occurs in 14% to 48% of patients requiring surgery to the vulva and the groins and in almost 100% of patients requiring postoperative radiation treatment. Lymphedema presents as leg swelling or heaviness of the lower limbs (92). It is regarded as the most debilitating long-lasting side effect from vulvar cancer surgery and results in an inability to perform daily activities, impacts psychological and social well-being, and represents a significant financial burden associated with the treatment (93). Obesity, the number of lymph nodes removed, extent of surgery, postoperative infection, radiation therapy to the groins, and postoperative DVT increase the risk of developing lymphedema after groin dissection (94). SLNB has been associated with a 1.9% incidence rate of lymphedema, compared with 25.2% in patients undergoing systematic groin dissection (91). Lymphocele formation develops in 7% to 19% of patients after inguinal–femoral lymphadenectomy (85).

Over half of women who undergo vulvectomy report sexual dysfunction and psychological issues resulting in dyspareunia, problems with micturition, negative feelings about body image, decreased desire, and inability to orgasm (93). Providing information before and after surgery that details how the treatment may affect sexuality and change anatomy, as well as the provision of methods for how to cope with feelings regarding the illness, may decrease anxiety. The FACT-V questionnaire is a valid and reliable tool that can measure the impact of treatment on QOL and improve standardization or quality-of-life research efforts.

REFERENCES

1. Szeder V, Torbey M. Prevention and treatment of perioperative stroke. *Neurologist*. 2008;14(1):30–36.
2. Ng JLW, Chan MTV, Gelb AW. Perioperative stroke in noncardiac, nonneurosurgical surgery. *Anesthesiology*. 2011;115(4):879–890.
3. Devereaux PJ, Yang H, Yusuf S, et al. Effects of extended-release metoprolol succinate in patients undergoing non-cardiac surgery (POISE trial): a randomised controlled trial. *Lancet*. 2008;371(9627):1839–1847.
4. Bijker JB, Wilton A, Van Klei Y, et al. Intraoperative hypotension and 1-year mortality after noncardiac surgery. *Surv Anesthesiol*. 2011;55(1):40.
5. Poldermans D, Bax J, Boersma E, et al. Guidelines for pre-operative cardiac risk assessment and peri-operative cardiac management in non-cardiac surgery: the Task Force for Pre-operative Cardiac Risk Assessment and Peri-operative Cardiac Management in Non-cardiac Surgery of the European Society of Cardiology (ESC) and endorsed by the European Society of Anaesthesiology (ESA). *Eur Heart J*. 2009;30(22):2769–2812.
6. Agnelli G, Bolis G, Capussotti L, et al. A clinical outcome-based prospective study on venous thromboembolism after cancer surgery. *Ann Surg*. 2006;243(1):89–95.
7. Silverstein MD, Heit JA, Mohr DN, et al. Trends in the incidence of deep vein thrombosis and pulmonary embolism: a 25-year population-based study. *Arch Intern Med*. 1998;158(6):585–593.
8. Clarke-Pearson DL, Dodge RK, Synan I, et al. Venous thromboembolism prophylaxis: patients at high risk to fail intermittent pneumatic compression. *Obstet Gynecol*. 2003;101(1):157–163.
9. Einstein MH, Pritts EA, Hartenbach EM. Venous thromboembolism prevention in gynecologic cancer surgery: a systematic review. *Gynecol Oncol*. 2007;105(3):813–819.
10. Einstein MH, Kushner DM, Connor JP, et al. A protocol of dual prophylaxis for venousthromboembolism prevention in gynecologic cancer patients. *Obstet Gynecol*. 2008;112(5):1091.
11. Mendez LE. Iatrogenic injuries in gynecologic cancer surgery. *Surg Clin North Am*. 2001;81(4):897–923.
12. Walker JL, Piedmonte MR, Spirtos NM, et al. Laparoscopy compared with laparotomy for comprehensive surgical staging of uterine cancer: Gynecologic Oncology Group Study LAP2. *J Clin Oncol*. 2009;27(32):5331–5336.
13. Mourits MJE, Bijen CB, Arts HtJ, et al. Safety of laparoscopy versus laparotomy in early-stage endometrial cancer: a randomised trial. *Lancet Oncol*. 2010;11(8):763–771.
14. Obermair A, Janda M, Baker J, et al. Improved surgical safety after laparoscopic compared to open surgery for apparent early stage endometrial cancer: results from a randomised controlled trial. *Eur J Cancer*. 2012;48(8):1147–1153.
15. Llarena NC, Shah AB, Milad MP. Bowel injury in gynecologic laparoscopy: a systematic review. *Obstet Gynecol*. 2015;125:1407–1417.
16. Vergote I, Tropé CG, Amant F. European Organization for Research and Treatment of Cancer-Gynaecological Cancer Group; NCIC Clinical Trials

Group. Neoadjuvant chemotherapy or primary surgery in stage IIIC or IV ovarian cancer. *N Engl J Med.* 2010;363(10):943–953.
17. Hammond IG, Obermair A, Taylor JD, et al. The control of severe intraoperative bleeding using an overlay autogenous tissue (OAT) patch: case reports. *Gynecol Oncol.* 2004;94(2):564–566.
18. Klevens RM, Edwards JR, Richards CL Jr, et al. Estimating health care-associated infections and deaths in U.S. hospitals, 2002. *Public Health Rep.* 2007;122(2):160–166.
19. Perencevich EN, Sands KE, Cosgrove SE, et al. Health and economic impact of surgical site infections diagnosed after hospital discharge. *Emerg Infect Dis.* 2003;9(2):196–203.
20. Malone DL, Genuit T, Tracy JK, et al. Surgical site infections: reanalysis of risk factors. *J Surg Res.* 2002;103(1):89–95.
21. Stulberg JJ, Delaney CP, Neuhauser DV, et al. Adherence to surgical care improvement project measures and the association with postoperative infections. *JAMA.* 2010;303(24):2479–2485.
22. Winter WE III, Maxwell GL, Tian C, et al. Prognostic factors for stage III epithelial ovarian cancer: a Gynecologic Oncology Group Study. *J Clin Oncol.* 2007;25(24):3621–3627.
23. Winter WE III, Maxwell GL, Tian C, et al. Tumor residual after surgical cytoreduction in prediction of clinical outcome in stage IV epithelial ovarian cancer: a Gynecologic Oncology Group Study. *J Clin Oncol.* 2008;26(1):83–89.
24. Aletti GD, Eisenhauer EL, Santillan A, et al. Identification of patient groups at highest risk from traditional approach to ovarian cancer treatment. *Gynecol Oncol.* 2011;120(1):23–28.
25. Langstraat C, Aletti GD, Cliby WA. Morbidity, mortality and overall survival in elderly women undergoing primary surgical debulking for ovarian cancer: a delicate balance requiring individualization. *Gynecol Oncol.* 2011;123(2):187–191.
26. Thrall MM, Goff BA, Symons RG, et al. Thirty-day mortality after primary cytoreductive surgery for advanced ovarian cancer in the elderly. *Obstet Gynecol.* 2011;118(3):537–547.
27. Cadron I, Leunen K, Van Gorp T, et al. Management of borderline ovarian neoplasms. *J Clin Oncol.* 2007;25(20):2928–2937.
28. Obermair A, Hagenauer S, Tamandl D, et al. Safety and efficacy of low anterior en bloc resection as part of cytoreductive surgery for patients with ovarian cancer. *Gynecol Oncol.* 2001;83(1):115–120.
29. Mourton SM, Temple LK, Abu-Rustum NR, et al. Morbidity of rectosigmoid resection and primary anastomosis in patients undergoing primary cytoreductive surgery for advanced epithelial ovarian cancer. *Gynecol Oncol.* 2005;99(3):608–614.
30. Park JY, Seo SS, Kang S, et al. The benefits of low anterior en bloc resection as part of cytoreductive surgery for advanced primary and recurrent epithelial ovarian cancer patients outweigh morbidity concerns. *Gynecol Oncol.* 2006;103(3):977–984.
31. Nugent EK, Hoff JT, Gao F, et al. Wound complications after gynecologic cancer surgery. *Gynecol Oncol.* 2011;121(2):347–352.
32. Bakkum-Gamez JN, Langstraat CL, Martin JR, et al. Incidence of and risk factors for postoperative ileus in women undergoing primary staging and debulking for epithelial ovarian carcinoma. *Gynecol Oncol.* 2012;125(3):614–620.
33. Chi DS, Zivanovic O, Levinson KL, et al. The incidence of major complications after the performance of extensive upper abdominal surgical procedures during primary cytoreduction of advanced ovarian, tubal, and peritoneal carcinomas. *Gynecol Oncol.* 2010;119(1):38–42.
34. Hoffman MS, Griffin D, Tebes S, et al. Sites of bowel resected to achieve optimal ovarian cancer cytoreduction: implications regarding surgical management. *Am J Obstet Gynecol.* 2005;193(2):582–586.
35. Bristow RE, del Carmen MG, Kaufman HS, et al. Radical oophorectomy with primary stapled colorectal anastomosis for resection of locally advanced epithelial ovarian cancer. *J Am Coll Surg.* 2003;197(4):565–574.
36. Richardson DL, Mariani A, Cliby WA. Risk factors for anastomotic leak after recto-sigmoid resection for ovarian cancer. *Gynecol Oncol.* 2006;103(2):667–672.
37. Peiretti M, Bristow RE, Zapardiel I, et al. Rectosigmoid resection at the time of primary cytoreduction for advanced ovarian cancer. A multi-center analysis of surgical and oncological outcomes. *Gynecol Oncol.* 2012;126(2):220–223.
38. Vignali A, Fazio VW, Lavery IC, et al. Factors associated with the occurrence of leaks in stapled rectal anastomoses: a review of 1,014 patients. *J Am Coll Surg.* 1997;185(2):105–113.
39. Guenaga KF, Matos D, Wille-Jorgensen P. Mechanical bowel preparation for elective colorectal surgery. *Cochrane Database Syst Rev.* 2011;9:CD001544.
40. Jesus EC, Karliczek A, Matos D, et al. Prophylactic anastomotic drainage for colorectal surgery. *Cochrane Database Syst Rev.* 2004;4:CD002100.
41. Cliby W, Dowdy S, Feitoza SS, et al. Diaphragm resection for ovarian cancer: technique and short-term complications. *Gynecol Oncol.* 2004;94(3):655–660.
42. Zapardiel I, Peiretti M, Zanagnolo V, et al. Diaphragmatic surgery during primary cytoreduction for advanced ovarian cancer: peritoneal stripping versus diaphragmatic resection. *Int J Gynecol Cancer.* 2011;21(9):1698–1703.
43. Magtibay PM, Adams PB, Silverman MB, et al. Splenectomy as part of cytoreductive surgery in ovarian cancer. *Gynecol Oncol.* 2006;102(2):369–374.
44. Eisenkop SM, Spirtos NM, Lin WC. Splenectomy in the context of primary cytoreductive operations for advanced epithelial ovarian cancer. *Gynecol Oncol.* 2006;100(2):344–348.
45. Di Sabatino A, Carsetti R, Corazza GR. Post-splenectomy and hyposplenic states. *Lancet.* 2011;378(9785):86–97.
46. Kehoe SM, Eisenhauer EL, Abu-Rustum NR, et al. Incidence and management of pancreatic leaks after splenectomy with distal pancreatectomy performed during primary cytoreductive surgery for advanced ovarian, peritoneal and fallopian tube cancer. *Gynecol Oncol.* 2009;112(3):496–500.
47. Cliby WA, Powell MA, Al-Hammadi N, et al. Ovarian cancer in the United States: contemporary patterns of care associated with improved survival. *Gynecol Oncol.* 2015;136(1):11–17.
48. Bristow RE, Chang J, Ziogas A, et al. Impact of National Cancer Institute Comprehensive Cancer Centers on ovarian cancer treatment and survival. *J Am Coll Surg.* 2015;220(5):940–950.
49. Bristow RE, Chang J, Ziogas A, et al. High-volume ovarian cancer care: survival impact and disparities in access for advanced-stage disease. *Gynecol Oncol.* 2014;132(2):403–410.
50. Eskander RN, Chang J, Ziogas A, et al. Evaluation of 30-day hospital readmission after surgery for advanced-stage ovarian cancer in a medicare population. *J Clin Oncol.* 2014;32(36):4113–4119.
51. Henretta MS, Scalici JM, Engelhard CL, et al. The revolving door: hospital readmissions of gynecologic oncology patients. *Gynecol Oncol.* 2011;122(3):479–483.
52. Wright JD, Herzog TJ, Siddiq Z, et al. Failure to rescue as a source of variation in hospital mortality for ovarian cancer. *J Clin Oncol.* 2012;30(32):3976–3982.
53. Kondalsamy-Chennakesavan S, Janda M, Gebski V, et al. Risk factors to predict the incidence of surgical adverse events following open or laparoscopic surgery for apparent early stage endometrial cancer: results from a randomised controlled trial. *Eur J Cancer.* 2012;48(14):2155–2162.
54. Baker J, Obermair A, Gebski V, et al. Efficacy of oral or intrauterine device-delivered progestin in patients with complex endometrial hyperplasia with atypia or early endometrial adenocarcinoma: a meta-analysis and systematic review of the literature. *Gynecol Oncol.* 2012;125(1):263–270.
55. Ryan M, Stainton MC, Jaconelli C, et al. The experience of lower limb lymphedema for women after treatment for gynecologic cancer. *Oncol Nurs Forum.* 2003;30(3):417–423.
56. Logmans A, Kruyt RH, de Bruin HG, et al. Lymphedema and lymphocysts following lymphadenectomymay be prevented by omentoplasty: a pilot study. *Gynecol Oncol.* 1999;75(3):323–327.
57. Benedetti-Panici P, Maneschi F, Cutillo G, et al. A randomized study comparing retroperitonealdrainage with no drainage after lymphadenectomy in gynecologic malignancies. *Gynecol Oncol.* 1997;65(3):478–482.
58. Achouri A, Huchon C, Bats A-S, et al. Postoperative lymphocysts after lymphadenectomy for gynaecological malignancies: preventive techniques and prospects. *Eur J Obstet Gynecol Reprod Biol.* 2012;161(2):125–129.
59. Food and Drug Administration. *Quantitative Assessment of the Prevalence of Unsuspected Uterine Sarcoma in Women Undergoing Treatment of Uterine Fibroids.* Silver Spring, MD: US FDA; 2014.
60. Steiner RA, Wight E, Tadir Y, et al. Electrical cutting device for laparoscopic removal of tissue from the abdominal cavity. *Obstet Gynecol.* 1993;81(3):471–474.
61. Milad MP, Milad EA. Laparoscopic morcellator-related complications. *J Minim Invasive Gynecol.* 2014;21(3):486–491.
62. Nieboer TE, Johnson N, Lethaby A, et al. Surgical approach to hysterectomy for benign gynaecological disease. *Cochrane Database Syst Rev.* 2009;19(2):CD003677.
63. Hagemann IS, Hagemann AR, LiVolsi VA, et al. Risk of occult malignancy in morcellated hysterectomy: a case series. *Int J Gynecol Pathol.* 2011;30(5):476–483.
64. Seidman MA, Oduyebo T, Muto MG, et al. Peritoneal dissemination complicating morcellation of uterine mesenchymal neoplasms. *PLoS One.* 2012;7(11):e50058.
65. Wright JD, Tergas AI, Burke WM, et al. Uterine pathology in women undergoing minimally invasive hysterectomy using morcellation. *JAMA.* 2014;312(12):1253–1255.

66. Wright JD, Cui RR, Wang A, et al. Economic and survival implications of use of electric power morcellation for hysterectomy for presumed benign gynecologic disease. *J Natl Cancer Inst.* 2015;107(11).
67. Oduyebo T, Rauh-Hain AJ, Meserve EE, et al. The value of re-exploration in patients with inadvertently morcellated uterine sarcoma. *Gynecol Oncol.* 2014;132(2):360–365.
68. Einstein MH, Barakat RR, Chi DS, et al. Management of uterine malignancy found incidentally after supracervical hysterectomy or uterine morcellation for presumed benign disease. *Int J Gynecol Cancer.* 2008;18(5):1065–1070.
69. Liu FW, Galvan-Turner VB, Pfaendler KS, et al. A critical assessment of morcellation and its impact on gynecologic surgery and the limitations of the existing literature. *Am J Obstet Gynecol.* 2015;212(6):717–724.
70. Likic IS, Kadija S, Ladjevic NG, et al. Analysis of urologic complications after radical hysterectomy. *Am J Obstet Gynecol.* 2008;199(6):644. e1–e3.
71. Pushkar DY, Dyakov VV, Kasyan GR. Management of radiation-induced vesicovaginal fistula. *Eur Urol.* 2009;55(1):131–137.
72. Hackethal A, Brennan DJ, Land R, et al. Feasibility and outcomes of uretero-ureterostomy and extravesical ureteroneocystostomy as part of radical surgery for infiltrating gynecologic disease. *Int J Gynecol Cancer.* 2013;23(6):1139–1145.
73. Cronin B, Sung VW, Matteson KA. Vaginal cuff dehiscence: risk factors and management. *Am J Obstet Gynecol.* 2012;206(4):284–288.
74. Kho RM, Akl MN, Cornella JL, et al. Incidence and characteristics of patients with vaginal cuff dehiscence after robotic procedures. *Obstet Gynecol.* 2009;114:231–235.
75. De Wever I. Pelvic exenteration: surgical aspects and analysis of early and late morbidity in a series of 106 patients. *Acta Chir Belg.* 2011;111(5):273–281.
76. Khoury-Collado F, Einstein MH, Bochner BH, et al. Pelvic exenteration with curative intent for recurrent uterine malignancies. *Gynecol Oncol.* 2012;124(1):42–47.
77. Hockel M, Dornhofer N. Pelvic exenteration for gynaecological tumours: achievements and unanswered questions. *Lancet Oncol.* 2006;7(10):837–847.
78. Berek JS, Howe C, Lagasse LD, et al. Pelvic exenteration for recurrent gynecologic malignancy: survival and morbidity analysis of the 45-year experience at UCLA. *Gynecol Oncol.* 2005;99(1):153–159.
79. Goldberg GL, Sukumvanich P, Einstein MH, et al. Total pelvic exenteration: the Albert Einstein College of Medicine/Montefiore Medical Center Experience (1987 to 2003). *Gynecol Oncol.* 2006;101(2):261–268.
80. Jackson KS, Naik R. Pelvic floor dysfunction and radical hysterectomy. *Int J Gynecol Cancer.* 2006;16(1):354–363.
81. Vrzackova P, Weiss P, Cibula D. Sexual morbidity following radical hysterectomy for cervical cancer. *Expert Rev Anticancer Ther.* 2010;10(7):1037–1042.
82. Perez CA, Breaux S, Bedwinek JM, et al. Radiation therapy alone in the treatment of carcinoma of the uterine cervix. II. Analysis of complications. *Cancer.* 1984;54(2):235–246.
83. Smith ST, Seski JC, Copeland LJ, et al. Surgical management of irradiation-induced small bowel damage. *Obstet Gynecol.* 1985;65(5):563–567.
84. Gellrich J, Hakenberg OW, Oehlschlager S, et al. Manifestation, latency and management of late urological complications after curative radiotherapy for cervical carcinoma. *Onkologie.* 2003;26(4):334–340.
85. Hopkins MP, Reid GC, Morley GW. Radical vulvectomy. The decision for the incision. *Cancer.* 1993;72(3):799–803.
86. Leminen A, Forss M, Paavonen J. Wound complications in patients with carcinoma of the vulva: comparison between radical and modified vulvectomies. *Eur J Obstet Gynecol Reprod Biol.* 2000;93(2):193–197.
87. Cavanagh D, Fiorica JV, Hoffman MS, et al. Invasive carcinoma of the vulva - changing trends in surgical management. *Am J Obstet Gynecol.* 1990;163(3):1007–1015.
88. Reedy MB, Capen CV, Baker DP, et al. Hyperbaric oxygen therapy following radical vulvectomy: an adjunctive therapy to improve wound healing. *Gynecol Oncol.* 1994;53(1):13–16.
89. Stehman FB, Bundy BN, Dvoretsky PM, et al. Early stage-I carcinoma of the vulva treated with ipsilateral superficial inguinal lymphadenectomy and modified radical hemivulvectomy - a prospective study of the Gynecologic Oncology Group. *Obstet Gynecol.* 1992;79(4):490–497.
90. Zhang X, Sheng X, Niu J, et al. Sparing of saphenous vein during inguinal lymphadenectomy for vulvar malignancies. *Gynecol Oncol.* 2007;105(3):722–726.
91. Van der Zee AGJ, Oonk MH, De Hullu JA, et al. Sentinel node dissection is safe in the treatment of early-stage vulvar cancer. *J Clin Oncol.* 2008;26(6):884–889.
92. Gould N, Kamelle S, Tillmanns T, et al. Predictors of complications after inguinal lymphadenectomy. *Gynecol Oncol.* 2001;82(2):329–332.
93. Janda M, Obermair A, Cella D, et al. Vulvar cancer patients' quality of life: a qualitative assessment. *Int J Gynecol Cancer.* 2004;14(5):875–881.
94. Cormier JN, Rourke L, Crosby M, et al. A. The surgical treatment of lymphedema: a systematic review of the contemporary literature (2004–2010). *Ann Surg Oncol.* 2012;19(2):642–651.

CHAPTER 30

Management of Pain

Russell K. Portenoy, Ebtesam Ahmed, and Pauline Lesage

The heterogeneous patient population managed by gynecologic oncologists presents a broad range of problems in pain management. Acute pains are highly prevalent, including the rather straightforward incisional pain that follows surgical procedures. Chronic pain occurs in the context of numerous other physical and psychosocial symptoms, often in the population with advanced disease. Gynecologic oncologists have the opportunity to treat pain across all of these contexts, and in so doing, assist patients in maintaining an acceptable quality of life throughout the course of the illness.

Scope of the Problem

Persistent pain is experienced by almost two-thirds of cancer patients with metastatic disease, more than half of those receiving antineoplastic therapy, and about one-third of cancer survivors (1–3). The limited data specific to gynecologic tumors mirror these rates (4,5). For example, a retrospective survey that evaluated 88 women with advanced cervical cancer observed that pain was reported by 81% and was considered to be one of the predominating symptoms by treating clinicians (6). Persistent pain may be related to tissue injury caused by the neoplasm itself, a late effect of an antineoplastic therapy, or a pathology unrelated to the cancer (7–9); most patients with persistent pain have active disease and pain that can be attributed directly to the tumor.

Observational studies suggest that an opioid-based therapeutic regimen can provide satisfactory relief of chronic cancer pain in 70% to 90% of patients (10,11). Undertreatment remains a serious problem, however, despite the availability of well-accepted guidelines for pain management (12–18).

Although the prevalence of severe acute pain in patients with gynecologic cancers has not been determined, and is likely changing with the increasing use of minimally invasive procedures, it is nonetheless presumed to be extremely common. Although acute pain is potentially controllable in a very large majority of cases, some scenarios such as the management of acute postoperative pain after ambulatory surgery pose challenges.

Patients with cancer, and particularly those with advanced disease, also experience numerous symptoms other than pain. Across cancers, the most common of these symptoms are fatigue and psychologic distress (3). Studies suggest that distress is often multifactorial and determined by interactions involving multiple symptoms, physical losses, and psychologic, social, or spiritual concerns (17). Pain may or may not be the predominating source of distress at any point in time. Other symptoms, such as fatigue, may be perceived to be the most distressing symptom adversely affecting quality of life (19). When pain is accompanied by significant fatigue, assessment of the latter symptom and treatment of its causes may become the focus of care (15) in the hope that improved fatigue may enhance the positive impact on quality of life achieved from pain reduction. A therapeutic approach that addresses concomitant symptoms of any type may yield similar benefits.

Assessment of Cancer Pain

The assessment of chronic pain in patients with gynecologic cancer requires an understanding of its phenomenology, pathophysiology, and syndromes. This assessment should also consider the broad range of physical, psychologic, and social disturbances concurrently experienced by these patients. Patients with acute pain, particularly acute postoperative pain, pose less complex management problems, but could still potentially benefit from a comprehensive assessment. The patient's description of the pain, findings on physical examination, objective data from imaging and other tests, and information about the extent of the malignant disease and its treatment are all utilized to assess the likely etiology and underlying pathophysiology of the pain and, if possible, to identify a specific cancer syndrome (20).

National medical organizations have developed guidelines in an effort to more effectively detect and monitor pain. The Joint Commission on Accreditation of Healthcare Organizations developed a standard requiring that pain be assessed initially and periodically in all hospitalized patients. The National Comprehensive Cancer Network Adult Cancer Pain Guidelines require a formal pain assessment, measurement of pain intensity, reassessment of pain intensity at specific intervals, psychosocial support, and specific educational material (15).

Definition of Pain

According to the International Association for the Study of Pain, pain is "an unpleasant sensory and emotional experience associated with actual or potential tissue damage, or described in terms of such damage" (20). This definition underscores the important observation that the pain reported by a patient may be perceived by the clinician to be greater than or less than the observable degree of tissue injury. When pain is acute, and when it is persistent and clearly related to tumor injury, a physical process capable of explaining the pain can usually be identified and is often considered an adequate explanation for the pain. Even in these contexts, however, a careful assessment of psychosocial disturbances is needed to clarify the extent to which pain expression is influenced by factors other than tissue damage.

The definition of pain can be further clarified by the distinctions among nociception, pain, and suffering (**Fig. 30.1**) (21). Nociception is the physiologic process activated by potentially tissue-damaging stimuli. Clinically, nociception is inferred to exist whenever tissue damage is identified. Pain is the perception of nociception and, like other perceptions, can be determined by more than the activity in the sensorineural apparatus alone. Pain that persists after tissue injury heals illustrates the importance of processes other than nociception when pain becomes chronic.

Suffering, or "total pain," can be defined as a more global aversive experience determined by numerous perceptions, one of which may be pain. Among the many other factors that may contribute to suffering are the perception of physical deterioration, the experience of symptoms other than pain, psychologic disturbances (e.g., depression

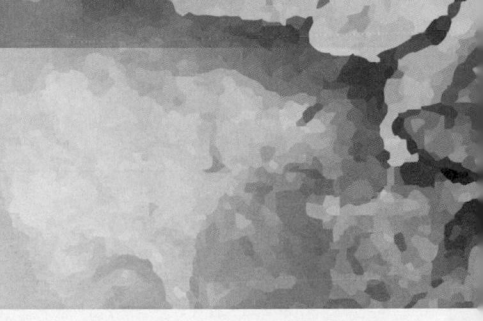

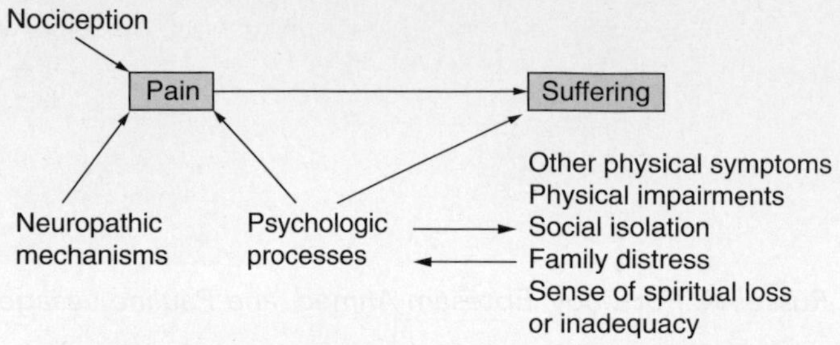

Figure 30.1. Distinctions and interactions between nociception, pain, and suffering.

Source: Reproduced with permission from Portenoy RK. Cancer pain: pathophysiology and syndromes. *Lancet*. 1992:339:1026–1031.

or anxiety), disruption in the family, social isolation, and fear of death. Just as an inordinate focus on nociception, rather than pain, can lead to interventions that reduce tissue damage without alleviating pain, an emphasis on pain management alone in patients with profound suffering determined by other factors can fail to mitigate the burden of illness even if physical comfort is enhanced (22,23).

Evaluation of the Pain Complaint

The comprehensive assessment of pain should include information about temporal characteristics (onset and duration), course (stable or changing since onset, relatively constant, or widely fluctuating), severity (both average and worst), location, quality, and provocative and palliative factors. This evaluation is complemented by information about the patient's extent of disease, related medical and psychosocial conditions, present and past pain management strategies and their outcomes, and the impact of the pain on the patient's daily life and functioning (1,23). Information about the patient's and family's knowledge of, expectations about, and goals for pain management is also salient (24).

Characteristics of Pain

Intensity

The measurement and recording of pain intensity is an essential element in the comprehensive assessment of pain. The most common approaches are a verbal rating scale (none, mild, moderate, severe, excruciating), a numerical scale (where 0 is no pain and 10 is the worst pain imaginable), and a visual analogue scale (VAS) that uses a 10-cm line anchored at one end by the words "no pain" or "least possible pain" and at the other end by "worst possible pain." There are also a variety of scales that use drawings of faces (from smiling to distress) or other types of drawings that may be used for patients who cannot manage other types of tools (e.g., Wong–Baker Pain Rating Scale for children). The choice of scale is less important than consistency in its use over time.

Formal instruments have also been developed that describe pain in multiple dimensions. An example is the Brief Pain Inventory (BPI), a patient self-rating scale that assesses pain intensity and pain interference in various areas of function (25). A short-form version of the BPI (BPI-SF) and translations in multiple languages are available. Examples of older multidimensional pain measurement tools are the McGill Pain Questionnaire (26), which assesses the sensory, affective, and evaluative components of pain, and Memorial Pain Assessment Card, which measures pain intensity, pain relief, and mood on VASs and verbal scales (27). Multidimensional pain scales may be particularly useful in pain research. A consensus has emerged highlighting the importance of multidimensional pain assessment in studies that evaluate pain treatments (28).

Temporal

Acute pain usually has a well-defined onset and a readily identifiable cause (e.g., surgical incision). It may be associated with anxiety, overt pain behaviors (moaning or grimacing), and signs of sympathetic hyperactivity (including tachycardia, hypertension, and diaphoresis).

In contrast, chronic pain is characterized by an ill-defined onset and a prolonged, fluctuating course. Overt pain behaviors and sympathetic hyperactivity are typically absent, and vegetative signs, including lassitude, sleep disturbance, and anorexia, may be present. A clinical depression evolves in some patients. Most patients with chronic cancer pain also experience periodic flares of pain, or "breakthrough pain," an observation with important therapeutic implications. (29–31).

Topographic

The distinctions among focal, multifocal, and generalized pains may influence both the assessment and treatment of the patient. Some therapies, such as nerve blocks, specifically depend on the specific location and extent of the pain.

The distinction between focal and referred pain is similarly important. Focal pains are experienced superficial to the underlying nociceptive lesion, whereas referred pains are experienced at a site distant from the nociceptive lesion. Pain may be referred from a lesion involving any of a large group of structures, including nerve, bone, muscle, or other soft tissue, and viscera (32). Various subtypes can be distinguished: (a) pain referred anywhere along the course of an injured peripheral nerve (such as pain in the thigh or knee from a lumbar plexus lesion); (b) pain referred along a course of the nerve supplied by a damaged nerve root (known as radicular pain); (c) pain referred to the lower part of the body, usually the feet and legs, from a lesion involving the spinal cord (called funicular pain); and (d) pain referred to a site remote from the nociceptive lesion and outside the dermatome affected by the lesion (e.g., shoulder pain from diaphragmatic irritation).

Knowledge of pain referral patterns is needed to target appropriate assessment procedures. For example, a patient with recurrent cervical cancer who reports progressive pain in the inguinal region may require evaluation of numerous structures to identify the underlying pathology responsible for the pain, including the subjacent pelvic bones and hip joint, pelvic sidewall, paraspinal gutter at an upper lumbar spinal level, and intraspinal region at the upper lumbar level.

Etiology

The etiology of acute pain is usually clear-cut. Further evaluation to determine the underlying lesion or pathophysiology of the pain is not indicated unless the course varies from the expected. In contrast, the etiology of chronic pain may be more difficult to characterize. In most cases, pain is due to direct invasion of pain-sensitive structures by the neoplasm (1,3). The structures most often involved are bone and neural tissue, but pain can also occur when there is an obstruction of hollow viscus, distention of organ capsules, distortion or occlusion of blood vessels, and infiltration of soft tissues. The etiology of pain in less than a quarter of patients relates to an antineoplastic treatment, and less than 10% of patients have pain unrelated to the neoplasm or its treatment (33).

Pathophysiology

Clinicians have found it useful to characterize pain according to inferences related to pathophysiology. Although this type of classification greatly simplifies a very complex biology, it has been effectively used to help guide treatment.

Pain is labeled *nociceptive* if it is inferred that the sustaining mechanisms involve ongoing tissue injury involving either somatic or visceral structures. The diagnosis is made based on the finding of tissue injury and the quality of the pain. The quality of somatic nociceptive pain is typically described as aching, stabbing, throbbing, or pressure-like. The quality of visceral nociceptive pain is largely determined by the structures involved. Obstruction of hollow viscus is usually associated with complaints of gnawing or crampy pain, whereas injury to organ capsules or mesentery is associated with an aching or stabbing discomfort.

Pain is labeled *neuropathic* if the evaluation suggests that it is sustained by abnormal somatosensory processing in the peripheral or the central nervous system (CNS) and there is some identifiable neurologic injury. Neuropathic pain represents approximately 40% of cancer pain syndromes and can be disease-related (e.g., tumor invasion of nerve plexus) or treatment-related (chemotherapy-induced painful polyneuropathy) (34). Among those with metastatic disease, neuropathic pain usually results from neoplastic injury to peripheral nerves.

Neuropathic pain is diagnosed on the basis of the patient's verbal description of the pain and evidence of injury to neural tissue. Patients may use any of a variety of verbal descriptors but specific terms, such as "burning," "shock-like," or "electrical," are particularly suggestive of neuropathic pain (35). Areas of abnormal sensations are often found on physical examination. These may include hypesthesia (a numbness or lessening of feeling), paresthesias (abnormal nonpainful sensations such as tingling, cold, or itching), hyperalgesia (increased perception of painful stimuli), hyperpathia (exaggerated pain response), and allodynia (pain induced by nonpainful stimuli such as a light touch or cool air).

Psychogenic pain, a conventional term for some of the disorders labeled in psychiatric parlance as somatoform disorders, reflects the clinical impression that pain results primarily from psychopathologic processes. Although psychologic factors and comorbid psychiatric disorders often influence pain expression, psychogenic pain itself appears to be rare.

Although the diagnosis of psychogenic pain is seldom appropriate, the existence of this condition emphasizes the importance of psychosocial and psychiatric evaluation as part of the pain assessment. The diagnosis of comorbid psychiatric disorders can lead to important therapeutic opportunities. The prevalence of major depression in heterogeneous populations with cancer approaches 10% and may be much higher in various subgroups, including patients who are newly diagnosed (36–38).

If the assessment of the pain does not provide enough information to categorize it using one or more of these labels, it is important to acknowledge this and avoid labeling the patient with a term that may direct care inappropriately. The greatest concern in this regard is the labeling of pain as psychogenic when the assessment does not yield positive evidence of a psychiatric disorder but an alternative answer is lacking. In this case, it is better to label the pain *idiopathic* than to speculate about underlying factors that are not clearly demonstrable from the evaluation.

TABLE 30.1. Cancer Pain Syndromes

I. Pain associated with direct tumor involvement
A. Due to invasion of bone
1. Base of skull
2. Vertebral body
3. Generalized bone pain
B. Due to invasion of nerves
1. Peripheral nerve syndromes
2. Painful polyneuropathy
3. Brachial, lumbar, sacral plexopathies
4. Leptomeningeal metastases
5. Epidural spinal cord compression
C. Due to invasion of viscera
D. Due to invasion of blood vessels
E. Due to invasion of mucous membranes
II. Pain associated with cancer therapy
A. Postoperative pain syndromes
1. Post-thoracotomy syndrome
2. Postmastectomy syndrome
3. Postradical neck dissection
4. Postamputation syndromes
B. Postchemotherapy pain syndromes
1. Painful polyneuropathy
2. Aseptic necrosis of bone
3. Steroid pseudorheumatism
4. Mucositis
C. Postirradiation pain syndromes
1. Radiation fibrosis of brachial or lumbosacral plexus
2. Radiation myelopathy
3. Radiation-induced peripheral nerve tumors
4. Mucositis
III. Pain indirectly related or unrelated to cancer
A. Myofascial pains
B. Postherpetic neuralgia
C. Chronic headache syndromes

Pain Syndromes

Efforts to improve the assessment of cancer pain have been greatly encouraged by the description of numerous pain syndromes, each of which is defined by a cluster of symptoms and signs (39,40). Syndrome identification in patients with gynecologic cancers can help direct the diagnostic evaluation, clarify the prognosis, and target therapeutic interventions (**Tables 30.1** and **30.2**).

TABLE 30.2. Pain Syndromes Commonly Encountered Among Patients with Gynecologic Cancer

Acute pain syndromes
At any stage of disease:
Postoperative pain
Mucositis
In advanced stages of disease:
Recurrent bowel obstruction
Ureteral obstruction
Movement-related pain in brachial/lumbosacral plexopathy
Movement-related pain from bony lesions
Cancer-related chronic pain syndromes
Brachial/lumbosacral plexopathy
Chronic abdominal pain: bowel obstruction, ascites, hepatomegaly
Tenesmoid pain
Bone pain from metastases
Treatment-related chronic pain syndromes
Postmastectomy syndrome
Radiation-induced plexopathy
Chemotherapy-induced peripheral neuropathy (paclitaxel, cisplatin)

MANAGEMENT OF ACUTE PAIN

Although the treatment of patients with acute pain, particularly postoperative pain, is typically less challenging than the long-term management of chronic pain, the outcomes achieved in routine practice settings are often inadequate. Given the potential efficacy of widely used strategies, such as patient-controlled analgesia, less-than-satisfactory outcomes may be more related to systems issues, such as access to a pain service or prolonged pharmacy preparation times, than purely clinical issues. Cancer patients also commonly have concurrent medical problems, psychologic disturbances, and prior and current drug exposures that may increase the heterogeneity of the population and diminish the likelihood that routine measures provide adequate relief of pain. The need for clinicians and administrators to attend to the problem of acute pain and provide the resources and systems for expert management is therefore particularly important in this population.

"Routine" Approach to Postoperative Pain

Despite great variability in the pharmacokinetics and pharmacodynamics of single opioid doses, many patients with severe acute pain respond adequately to a standard opioid regimen consisting of parenteral doses of a short-acting drug administered "as needed." For example, an opioid-naïve patient with acute severe pain may be treated initially using intravenous morphine 5 mg every 3 hours as needed. If the patient has a history of current opioid use for pain, a higher starting dose is needed and a reasonable guideline would be to initiate dosing so that each intravenous dose is calculated to be equivalent to roughly 5% to 10% of the total opioid consumption during the previous 24 hours. This calculation of equivalent doses is based on the information in an equianalgesic dose table. If the starting dose or interval selected initially is not quickly effective, an increase in the dose or shortening of the dosing interval should be considered.

Acute severe pain generally should be treated with a short-acting drug. Many agents other than morphine are available for parenteral therapy, including hydromorphone, oxymorphone, and fentanyl. Meperidine was often used in the past, and although likely to be well tolerated during brief therapy, is generally not preferred because its toxic metabolite, normeperidine, imparts risks that are not shared by other similar drugs.

The intramuscular route was also commonly used in the past. There is no advantage to this, and painful injections have been supplanted by use of the intravenous route.

The proportion of cancer patients with postoperative pain who will be undertreated by an as-needed dosing schedule can be diminished if several factors are recognized. Most important, titration may be needed. The variability in analgesic requirements may require changes in the starting dose, adjustment in the dosing interval during the immediate postoperative period, or both. Some patients require several dose adjustments. Similarly, variability in pain duration after any particular operation is great and the duration of opioid treatment must be flexible, determined solely by patient response. Some patients have concerns about opioid-induced side effects and addiction, which may augment distress and diminish patient compliance with therapy unless strong reassurance is provided by the physician and other staff.

In some populations, the routine approach to postoperative pain management can be enhanced by the use of a nonopioid analgesic, specifically a nonsteroidal anti-inflammatory drug (NSAID). In the United States, ketorolac, ibuprofen, and acetaminophen all have been approved for short-term parenteral use. In opioid-naïve patients, a standard dose of ketorolac can provide analgesia equivalent to a parenteral dose of morphine of 10 mg. The addition of intravenous ketoprofen (not approved in the United States) to intravenous patient-controlled analgesia with tramadol after major gynecologic cancer surgery was shown to significantly reduce opioid consumption (41). At the present time in the United States, patients who are highly predisposed to opioid side effects or toxicity, such as those with severe preexisting lung disease, may benefit from a trial of one of the intravenous nonopioid analgesics, either in lieu of opioid therapy or in combination with an opioid. Ketorolac and ibuprofen should not be used when NSAID treatment is contraindicated.

Patient-Controlled Analgesia

Patient-controlled analgesia (PCA) has achieved great popularity in the management of postoperative pain and there is strong evidence that it improves analgesia, decreases the risk of pulmonary complications, and increases patient satisfaction when compared with conventional opioid analgesia (42). Theoretically, the self-administration of small doses on a frequent basis allows the patient to tailor the dose to the pain and enhance a sense of personal control while achieving a more stable plasma drug concentration. However, not all studies of this modality have been positive. For example, a randomized, controlled trial of 227 gynecologic cancer patients undergoing intra-abdominal surgery found that patients who were switched from parenteral to oral morphine on the first postoperative day experienced the same degree of pain control as those who received parenteral morphine via PCA pump (43). The latter studies suggest that careful attention to dosing rather than the availability of a pump per se is the key factor in achieving adequate pain control.

If PCA is selected, effective analgesia in the opioid-naïve patient is usually attained using morphine at a dose of 1 mg intravenously every 6 minutes as needed, or another opioid at an equivalent dose. Patients already receiving opioid therapy can be treated using higher-dose PCA. Each intravenous dose of the new opioid may be calculated to be roughly equivalent to approximately 5% of the total daily dose of opioid taken during the prior day, and this dose may be initiated with a longer initial dosing interval, such as 10 or 15 minutes.

Other Approaches to Acute Pain Management

Advances in pain research have suggested a variety of other strategies that may be useful as adjunctive therapies for acute cancer-related pain, including postoperative pain. Some strategies require the expertise of pain specialists.

Preemptive Analgesia

The administration of an analgesic prior to surgical tissue injury may reduce postoperative pain and opioid requirements, and possibly have long-term benefits. For example, pretreatment with sustained-release morphine or oxycodone reduced postoperative pain and analgesic requirements (44,45). Although this type of approach is seldom used due to conflicting data in the literature and uncertainty about the specific approach likely to be safe and effective in large groups of patients, it may be worthwhile considering if the acute pain is predictable and likely to be a therapeutic challenge.

Postoperative Combination Therapy

As noted previously, the addition of an NSAID in combination with an opioid can augment analgesia and reduce the use of opioids, potentially leading to reduction of opioid side effects. A recent controlled trial, for example, demonstrated that postoperative celecoxib improved outcomes and was well tolerated in patients undergoing laparoscopic surgery (46). Equally important, there is now substantial data demonstrating that the combination of an opioid and gabapentin, a neuronal calcium channel modulator widely used for the treatment of chronic neuropathic pain, improves a range of outcomes in diverse surgeries, including hysterectomy (47).

Intraspinal Analgesia

Epidural analgesia is now common practice in many hospitals. There is strong evidence favoring this approach over parenteral opioid therapy for some patients (48,49). Pain may be controlled with fewer opioid side effects and at a lower risk of some postoperative complications

(50). Some studies suggest benefits that are prolonged into the recovery phase after surgery, but the extant data are insufficient to judge these benefits adequately (51). Some side effects are more likely with this technique than with conventional systemic opioid therapy, including pruritus and hypotension. Staff with special competencies are needed to implement the approach safely. Given the extant evidence, patients undergoing major gynecologic surgery should be considered for epidural analgesia if the resources exist to provide it. Although there is less clinical experience in the use of subarachnoid opioid administration for postoperative pain, the technique can also provide excellent relief (52).

Regional Anesthetic Techniques

There are numerous regional anesthetic techniques that may be useful for the management of acute pain. The simplest is the application of local anesthetic at the surgical site. Topical anesthetics that are longer acting are in development and may offer substantial benefits in the future.

Neural blockade capable of denervating the painful site is a potential approach in most types of surgery. Catheters that deliver local anesthetic at a dose high enough to produce a sensory block can be placed in the epidural space or along peripheral nerves or plexus. Regional anesthesia can be used during an operation and then continued into the postoperative setting for pain control.

Other Approaches

Transcutaneous electrical nerve stimulation (TENS) has been suggested as a useful modality for incisional pain after abdominal surgery (53). Despite the evident simplicity and safety of the approach, and its obvious potential, it has been used very little in this setting.

Cognitive approaches, including stress reduction, relaxation, hypnosis, and distraction techniques, may also reduce postoperative pain and analgesic requirements (54,55). These techniques are labor intensive and are almost never sufficient as the sole means of analgesia. Nonetheless, studies have established that higher levels of anxiety and depression can negatively influence postoperative pain (56,57), and efforts to reduce anxiety through preoperative education and postoperative psychologic interventions are likely to have salutary effects.

MANAGEMENT OF CHRONIC CANCER PAIN

The successful management of acute postoperative pain is an important concern of the gynecologic oncologist, and optimal pain management should be considered a standard of care. The treatment of chronic pain is a far more challenging problem, however, particularly among those with advanced illness (**Table 30.3**)

TABLE 30.3. Approaches Used in the Management of Chronic Cancer Pain

Primary therapies	
	Radiation therapy
	Chemotherapy
	Surgery
	Antibiotics
Primary analgesic therapies	
	Pharmacologic approaches
	Interventional approaches
	Physiatric approaches
	Neurostimulatory approaches
	Psychologic approaches
	Complementary and alternative medicine approaches

Cancer Pain, Symptom Distress, and Palliative Care

Most cancer patients who experience chronic pain also develop other physical and psychologic symptoms. Pain, fatigue, and psychologic distress are the most prevalent symptoms across cancer populations (58). As described before, the pain assessment should identify and evaluate nonpain symptoms so that concurrent therapy of the most problematic symptoms can be initiated.

Symptom distress, in turn, is only one aspect of the multifaceted problem of suffering (59,60). The assessment of suffering requires an evaluation in multiple domains, including the physical, psychologic, social, and spiritual. Palliative care has emerged as a therapeutic model (61) focused on the assessment and management of problems that relate to these domains and to other domains codified by specialists in the field (62). In the United States, palliative care is a formal medical subspecialty (Hospice and Palliative Medicine); specialist certification is also available for nurses, social workers, and chaplains.

Specialist palliative care is now being provided by institution-based consultation services in most US hospitals. Community-based palliative care for patients with advanced illness and short life expectancy is provided through more than 6,000 hospice agencies in the United States. Community-based, specialist-level palliative care is emerging now, and is likely to become more available in the future.

The broad focus of palliative care on the relief of illness burden experienced by the patient and family may translate into numerous specific interventions, which often include goal setting and advance care planning discussions, symptomatic therapies, treatments to address psychosocial or spiritual distress, concrete services in the home, and efforts to manage caregiver distress and burden. The oncologist is key in providing these interventions during most of the patient's illness. This effort, overall, may be considered early integration of generalist-level palliative care into routine oncologic practice. Referral to specialist services to address complex needs, or provide hospice home care services during the period when death is anticipated relatively soon, is central to the role of the generalist.

In a provisional clinical opinion, the American Society of Clinical Oncology (ASCO) addresses the integration of palliative care into standard oncology care (63).

General Principles of Chronic Pain Management

The development of a successful strategy for pain management must include consideration of the etiology and pathophysiology of pain, the patient's medical status, and the goals of care. Although the main approach for the management of cancer pain is opioid-based pharmacotherapy, other interventions, including disease-oriented treatments (e.g., surgery, chemotherapy, or radiation) or other analgesic techniques, may be appropriate in selected cases.

Role of Primary Therapies

Effective treatment of the pathology underlying the pain can be analgesic. Primary treatment includes antineoplastic therapies and interventions directed at specific structural pathologies (e.g., lysis of adhesions). There is evidence in a limited number of cancers that specific chemotherapy regimens yield analgesic effects and it is a common observation that patients who attain a partial or complete response also experience improved symptoms. In a study of patients with metastatic breast cancer, for example, palliative chemotherapy with doxorubicin with or without vinorelbine resulted in an improvement of pain in 60.4% of the 111 patients who suffered from pain at baseline (64,65); although patients with an objective tumor response were more likely to have an improvement in pain (84.9%), fully 61% of patients with stable disease also benefited. In a small study of patients with advanced ovarian cancer, palliative chemotherapy was associated with improvement in symptom control, emotional well-being, and global quality of life (66).

Radiation therapy commonly is used to manage pain and there is evidence that it can provide effective and durable palliation of pain and other symptoms in chemotherapy-refractory patients with ovarian cancer (67,68). Radiation therapy can also provide analgesia to as many as 80% of those treated for bone metastases (69). Patients with widespread bone metastases or bone pain refractory to local field radiotherapy may benefit from treatment with radiopharmaceuticals, such as strontium 89 or samarium-153 (70). In addition, analgesia may be an expected result when radiation is used to treat epidural disease, tumor ulceration, cerebral metastases, superior vena cava obstruction, and bronchial obstruction.

Unfortunately, many patients with chronic cancer pain have no options for further primary therapy with analgesic intent. The approach to these patients involves a diverse group of analgesic treatments. Several concurrent interventions are often required to manage pain. The benefits of analgesic therapies must be balanced against their risks and the burden of therapy. Repeated assessments are essential in this process and often lead to adjustments in the therapy.

THERAPEUTIC APPROACHES: PHARMACOLOGIC MANAGEMENT

Prospective trials indicate that more than 70% of patients can achieve adequate relief of cancer pain using a pharmacologic approach (12–14). Effective pain management requires expertise in the administration of three groups of analgesic medications: NSAIDs, opioid analgesics, and adjuvant analgesics. The term *adjuvant analgesics* is applied to a diverse group of drugs that also have primary indications other than pain but can be effective analgesics in specific circumstances, such as in the treatment of neuropathic pain.

A model approach to the selection of these drugs, known as the "analgesic ladder," was developed by the World Health Organization (WHO) in the 1980s and remains influential today (**Fig. 30.2**) (71). According to this approach, patients with mild-to-moderate cancer-related pain are first treated with acetaminophen or NSAID. This drug is combined

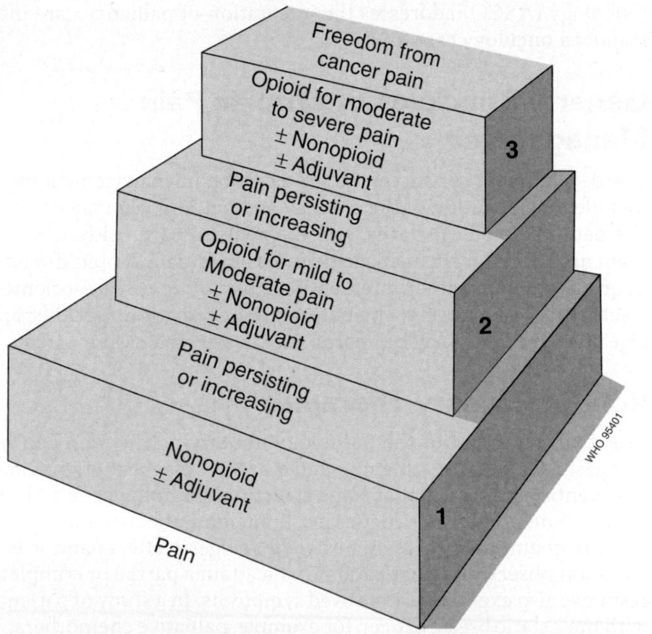

Figure 30.2. The three-step "analgesic ladder" proposed by an expert committee of the Cancer Unit of the World Health Organization.

Source: Reproduced with permission from the World Health Organization. *Cancer Pain Relief*, 2nd Ed. Geneva, Switzerland: World Health Organization; 1996.

with an adjuvant drug that can be selected either to provide additional analgesia (i.e., an adjuvant analgesic) or to treat a side effect of the analgesic or a coexisting symptom. Patients with moderate-to-severe pain, and those with less severe pain that does not respond to a trial of an NSAID, should be treated with an opioid conventionally used to treat moderate pain (sometimes designated a "weak" opioid). This drug may be combined with acetaminophen or an NSAID and an adjuvant drug if there is an indication for one. Those patients with severe pain and those with moderate pain that does not respond to the initial opioid should receive an opioid conventionally used for severe pain (sometimes designated a "strong" opioid), which may be combined with acetaminophen or an NSAID, or with an adjuvant drug, as indicated.

The analgesic ladder is important historically, and is still widely cited in the developing world in an effort to encourage policy makers to expand medical access to opioid drugs. In most developed countries, however, it is not an adequate clinical guideline, given the availability of numerous opioid formulations and other analgesic modalities. Nonetheless, the fundamental concept promoted by the analgesic ladder model—opioid therapy on a long-term basis should be considered the mainstay for the therapy of chronic moderate-to-severe pain related to active cancer—remains widely accepted and a very important message of the original paradigm.

Nonsteroidal Anti-inflammatory Drugs

In the United States, the nonopioid analgesics comprise acetaminophen and the NSAIDs (**Table 30.4**). These drugs have a well-established role in the treatment of cancer pain (72,73). On the basis of clinical observations, NSAIDs appear to be especially useful in patients with bone pain or pain related to grossly inflammatory lesions, and relatively less useful in patients with neuropathic pain. In addition, NSAIDs have an opioid-sparing effect that may be helpful in preventing the occurrence of dose-related side effects (74).

NSAIDs inhibit the enzyme cyclooxygenase (COX) to reduce production of peripheral and central prostaglandins, and this action presumably underlies their analgesic effects. There are multiple forms of COX. COX-1 is relatively more constitutive, physiologically active in many tissues, and COX-2 is relatively inducible, produced as part of the inflammatory cascade. Compounds that are more selective for COX-2 than COX-1 have a lower risk of inducing gastrointestinal adverse effects (75,76), and some drugs that are relatively COX-2 selective have been labeled in this way and promoted for their enhanced gastrointestinal safety. In the United States, the only drug of the latter type now on the market is celecoxib. Rofecoxib and valdecoxib were previously available, but were taken off the market due to concerns related to cardiovascular safety.

The clinical decision to offer an NSAID to a patient with cancer usually hinges on the assessment of drug-related risk. Gastrointestinal toxicity is well recognized, and in recent years, cardiovascular safety has become a prominent concern. Based on numerous studies, it is most reasonable to conclude that all NSAIDs are prothrombotic and pose an increased risk of peripheral vascular disease, myocardial infarction, transient ischemic attacks, and stroke (77–79). Mechanistically, this risk is associated with COX-2 inhibition, whether produced by the nonselective COX-1 and COX-2 inhibitors or by the COX-2 selective drugs. Although the risk varies across drugs, large comparative studies have been retrospective and results have been conflicting. In the United States, all NSAIDs now have a boxed warning in the package insert, which offer cautions about both gastrointestinal and cardiovascular risks. Among all commercially available NSAIDs, naproxen generally is viewed as having the lowest risk of cardiovascular toxicity.

All NSAIDs may also produce varied adverse renal effects. Fluid overload, acute nephritis, and chronic kidney disease are potential problems. All these may cause hepatotoxicity, and a bleeding diathesis is possible with most.

Although all NSAIDs have the potential to produce adverse gastrointestinal effects, ranging from pain or nausea to frank ulceration and hemorrhage, there are important drug-selective differences. The

■ TABLE 30.4. Nonsteroidal Anti-Inflammatory Drugs (NSAIDs)

Class and Generic Name	Approx. Half-Life (h)	Dosing Schedule	Recommended Starting Dose[a]	Comment[b]
P-aminophenol derivatives				
Acetaminophen[c]	3–4	q 4–6 h	650 mg q 4 h (5 doses daily)	Overdosage produces hepatic toxicity. Not anti-inflammatory and therefore not preferred as first-line analgesic or coanalgesic in patients with bone pain. Lack of GI or platelet toxicity; at high doses, liver function tests should be monitored.
Napthylalkanones				
Nabumetone	22–30	q 24 h	500–1,000 mg q 12 h	Appears to have a relatively low risk of GI toxicity; once-daily dosing can be useful.
Salicylates				
Acetylsalicylic acid[c]	3–12[d]	q 4–6 h	650 mg q 4 h (5 doses daily)	Standard for comparison. May not be tolerated as well as some of the newer NSAIDs.
Diflunisal[c]	8–12	q 12 h	1,000 mg × 1, then 500 mg q 12 h	Less GI toxicity than aspirin
Choline magnesium trisalicylate[c]	8–12	q 12 h	500–1,000 mg q 12 h	Choline magnesium trisalicylate and salsalate have minimal GI toxicity and no effect on platelet aggregation despite anti-inflammatory effects. May therefore be particularly useful in some cancer patients.
Salsalate	8–12	q 12 h	500–1,000 mg q 12 h	
Proprionic acids				
Ibuprofen[c]	3–4	q 4–8 h	400–600 mg q 8 h	Available over-the-counter.
Naproxen[c]	13	q 12 h	250–500 mg q 12 h	Available as a suspension.
Naproxen sodium[c]	13	q 12 h	275–550 mg q 12 h	—
Fenoprofen	2–3	q 6 h	200 mg q 6 h	—
Ketoprofen	2–3	q 6–8 h	25–50 mg q 8 h	—
Flurbiprofen[c]	5–6	q 8–12 h	100 mg q 12 h	—
Oxaprozin	40	q 24 h	600 mg q 24 h	Once-daily dosing may be useful.
Acetic acids				
Indomethacin	4–5	q 8–12 h	25 mg q 8 h	Available in sustained-release and rectal formulations. Higher incidence of side effects, particularly GI and CNS, than propionic acids.
Tolmetin	1	q 6–8 h	200 mg q 8 h	
Sulindac	14	q 12 h	150 mg q 12 h	Less renal toxicity than other NSAIDs.
Diclofenac	2	q 6–8 h	25 mg q 8 h	
Ketorolac[c]	4–7	q 4–6 h	30–60 mg load, then 15–30 mg q 6 h (parenteral); 10 mg q 6 h (oral)	Only parenteral formulation available. Approved for postoperative use. Experience too limited to evaluate higher doses.
Oxicams				
Piroxicam	45	q 24 h	20 mg q 24 h	Administration of 40 mg for over 3 weeks is associated with a high incidence of peptic ulcer, particularly in the elderly.
Fenamates				
Mefenamic acid[c]	2	q 6 h	250 mg q 6 h	Not recommended for use longer than 1 week and, therefore, not indicated in cancer pain therapy.
Cox-2 inhibitors				
Celecoxib	11	q 12 h	100–200 mg q 12 h	Fewer GI side effects; no effect on platelet function.

Note: CNS, central nervous system; GI, gastrointestinal.

[a]Starting dose should be one-half to two-thirds of the recommended dose for the elderly, those on multiple drugs, and those with renal insufficiency. Doses must be individualized. Low initial doses should be titrated upward if tolerated and clinical effect is inadequate. Doses can be incremented weekly. Studies of NSAIDs in the cancer population are meager; dosing guidelines are thus empiric.

[b]With all NSAIDs, stool guaiac and liver function tests, BUN, creatinine, and urinalysis should be monitored; frequency of monitoring should be increased for those on relatively high doses.

[c]Pain is approved indication.

[d]Half-life of aspirin increases with dose.

COX-2 selective agents, such as celecoxib, are less likely to cause these effects, as are several of the so-called nonselective agents, such as ibuprofen and diclofenac. Co-administration of a proton pump inhibitor, such as omeprazole, or the prostaglandin analogue misoprostol, should also be considered to reduce the risk of gastrointestinal damage induced by NSAIDs (80,81).

Given their risk profile, NSAIDs should be administered with caution to patients with significant predisposing factors for peptic ulcer disease, cardiovascular disease, renal disease, or bleeding diathesis. If there is no strong contraindication for therapy, patients who are predisposed to ulcer disease should be considered for a trial of celecoxib in the United States and patients who may be at relatively high risk of cardiovascular toxicity should be offered naproxen first (79,82,83).

Other factors may also be important in the selection of an NSAID. First, there is substantial variability in the response of individual patients to different agents, and the response to an NSAID in the past should guide drug selection in the present. Second, it may be useful to consider the drug's duration of effect when selecting an NSAID. The need to improve treatment adherence or provide a simpler dosing regimen encourages the use of a drug that can be administered once daily (e.g., nabumetone) or twice daily (e.g., celecoxib and many others), whereas the desire for as-needed dosing suggests the use of a short-duration drug (e.g., ibuprofen). Finally, drug selection may be influenced by cost, which varies greatly among both drugs and pharmacies.

The toxicities associated with the use of NSAIDs are dose-related and often occult until severe morbidity occurs. Although patients with cancer pain are commonly treated with standard doses, it is reasonable to explore the dose range and seek the minimal effective dose for long-term therapy. Dose escalation in poor responders is limited by dose-related toxicities and a ceiling dose for analgesia above which additional dose increments fail to produce more relief (74). If an increase in dose maintains the therapy in the conventionally accepted safe range and provides more analgesia, it should be continued. The lack of additional pain relief following a dose increase, however, suggests that the ceiling has been reached, and the dose can then be lowered to the previously effective dose or the drug can be discontinued. All patients receiving an NSAID should be evaluated periodically for occult fecal blood, changes in blood pressure, and effects on renal or hepatic function.

Opioid Analgesics

Expertise in the administration of opioid analgesics (**Table 30.5**) is the foundation of cancer pain management. The clinician should have knowledge of opioid pharmacology and a clear grasp of practical guidelines for dosing (15).

TABLE 30.5. Opioid Analgesics

Drug	Dose (mg) Equianalgesic to Morphine 10 mg IM[a] PO	IM	Half-Life (h)	Peak Effect (h)	Duration (h)	Comment[b]
Morphine	20–30	10	2–3	0.5–1.0	3–6	Standard for comparison
Morphine CR	20–30	10	2–3	3–4	8–12	Various formulations are not bioequivalent
Morphine SR	20–30	10	2–3	2–3	12–24	—
Codeine	200	130	2–3	1.5–2.0	3–6	Combined with aspirin or acetaminophen. Usually for moderate pain. Also available without coanalgesic
Hydromorphone	7.5	1.5	2–3	0.5–1.0	2–4	Potency may be greater, i.e., hydromorphone: morphine = 3:1 rather than 6.7:1 during prolonged use
Hydromorphone CR	7.5	—	~ 11	12–16	~ 13	
Oxycodone	20	—	2–3	1	3–4	Combined with aspirin or acetaminophen, for moderate pain; available orally without coanalgesic and useful for severe pain
Oxycodone CR	20	—	2–3	2–3	8–12	—
Oxymorphone	10	1	2–3	1.5–3.0	2–4	—
Oxymorphone CR	20 (oral)		2–3	1.5–3.0	2–4	—
Hydrocodone	30 (oral)	—	3–4	1–2	4–8	
Hydrocodone CR	30 (oral)	—	7–9	5	8–12	
Methadone	20	10	12–190	0.5–1.5	4–12	Although 1:1 ratio with morphine was in single-dose study, there is a change with chronic dosing, and large dose reduction (75%–90%) is needed when switching to methadone. Risk of delayed toxicity
Levorphanol	4	2	12–15	0.5–1	4–6	Usage limited because only 2 mg tablets are available
Fentanyl	—	—	7–12	—	—	Can be administered as a continuous IV infusion or SC infusion; based on clinical experience, 100 μg/h is roughly equianalgesic to morphine 4 mg/h
Fentanyl TTS	—	—	16–24	—	48–72	Based on clinical experience, 100 μg is roughly equianalgesic to morphine 4 mg
Meperidine	300	75	2–3	0.5–1.0	3–4	Not preferred for cancer patients owing to potential toxicity
Tapentadol	—	—	4–5	1	4–6	Mixed mechanism drugs, having both opioid and monoaminergic mechanisms of action; sometimes used for moderate cancer pain.
Tramadol	—	—	6–8	~2	3–6	

[a]Dose that provides analgesia equivalent to 10 mg intramuscular morphine.
[b]All opioids may produce various common side effects, (e.g., constipation, nausea, sedation). Respiratory depression is rare in cancer patients.
IM, intramuscular; IV, intravenous; SC, subcutaneous.

Opioid Classes

Based on receptor interactions, the opioid analgesics can be divided broadly into pure agonists and agonist–antagonists. The pure agonist drugs used in the management of chronic cancer pain are agonists at the μ-receptor subtype. The agonist–antagonist drugs comprise a mixed agonist–antagonist subclass, which includes drugs that are weak antagonists at the μ receptor and agonists at another receptor subtype, and a partial agonist subclass, which includes drugs that are partial agonists at the μ receptor. In the United States, the mixed agonist–antagonist drugs include pentazocine, nalbuphine, dezocine, and butorphanol, and the partial agonists include buprenorphine.

All the agonist–antagonist drugs share properties that together suggest a limited role in the management of chronic cancer pain. These drugs have a ceiling dose for analgesia, and all have the potential to produce an abstinence syndrome in patients already physically dependent on an agonist drug. Some of the mixed agonist–antagonists, particularly pentazocine, are also more likely to produce psychotomimetic effects than the pure agonist drugs. In patients with chronic pain, the lack of oral formulations for all but pentazocine and buprenorphine (sublingual and transdermal formulations) also limits the utility of these drugs. The transdermal buprenorphine patch increases the utility of buprenorphine for chronic pain; it will soon be joined by an intraoral film. The latter drugs have been designed for patients who are opioid-naïve or have very limited opioid exposure, and both this characteristic and its cost presumably will limit its use for cancer pain.

The opioid agonist drugs, the prototype of which is morphine, are preferred in the management of chronic cancer pain. To optimize the administration of these drugs, widely accepted dosing guidelines must be applied systematically.

"Weak" Versus "Strong" Opioids

Unlike the division of the opioids into agonist and agonist–antagonist classes, the distinction between "weak" opioids and "strong" opioids, which was originally incorporated into the WHO analgesic ladder approach (71), is more operational than pharmacologic. None of the "weak" drugs is characterized by a ceiling effect that would limit its use to pain of lesser severity. In the United States, the oral opioids commonly used for chronic, generally moderate pain, include combination products containing acetaminophen plus either codeine, hydrocodone, or oxycodone. Tramadol, a unique centrally acting analgesic with a mechanism of action that is partly opioid, also is generally included with this group, as is tapentadol, a newer analgesic with a mixed mechanism somewhat similar to tramadol. In the United States, the oral opioids used conventionally on the third rung of the analgesic ladder for chronic pain that is generally severe include morphine, hydromorphone, oxycodone, oxymorphone, levorphanol, fentanyl, and methadone.

Although meperidine is sometimes used orally for chronic pain of moderate severity, its risk profile suggests that it should not be selected for the patient with cancer pain. Accumulation of its toxic metabolite, normeperidine, may produce tremulousness, hyperreflexia, myoclonus, and even seizures (84). A similar concern existed with the use of propoxyphene, which is no longer available in the United States.

As suggested by the analgesic ladder, the simplest approach to the management of moderate pain in the cancer patient with limited or no prior exposure to opioids begins with a combination product containing a nonopioid drug and an opioid, usually codeine, oxycodone, or hydrocodone. Codeine is not preferred because genetic variability in its metabolism may be associated with unpredictable relationship between dose and response. After selection of one of these combination drugs, the dose can be increased to maximally safe levels of the coanalgesic; in products containing acetaminophen, this is usually less than 4 g per day. A lower maximal total daily dose—2.6 grams—should be applied in the elderly, patients with any type of hepatic dysfunction, and those who may be unable to comply with the instruction to avoid all over-the-counter medications containing this drug.

Selection of an Opioid for Severe Pain

The selection of an opioid for severe cancer pain is empirical. Traditionally, morphine was considered to be the preferred first-line drug based on worldwide experience, ease of dosing, and the availability of numerous formulations. The intra-individual variability in the response to the different opioids is very substantial, however, and any of the other drugs may yield a better response in the individual patient. This variability also suggests that therapeutic failure with one drug may be followed by remarkable success with another (85).

The predominant metabolic pathway for morphine is glucuronidation to morphine-3-glucuronide (M3G) and morphine-6-glucuronide (M6G), and the accumulation of morphine metabolites may be associated with side effects, such as myoclonus and chronic nausea (86). Renal insufficiency results in accumulation of M3G and M6G (87,88). For this reason, morphine should be administered cautiously to patients with renal insufficiency. Although the supporting data are limited, morphine is often viewed unfavorably when patients have very poor renal function, are on dialysis, or have renal function that is expected to change. In the latter situations, hydromorphone and fentanyl are often preferred (84,89,90).

The selection of an opioid for the treatment of severe cancer pain is also influenced by pharmacokinetic factors, the most salient of which is duration of effect. In an effort to improve adherence and convenience, numerous long-acting modified-release formulations of short half-life opioids have been developed. Oral once-daily or twice-daily formulations of morphine, oxycodone, oxymorphone, hydrocodone, and hydromorphone are available in the United States or other countries. Transdermal fentanyl provides a dosing interval of 2 to 3 days and is preferred by some patients (91).

Although both levorphanol and methadone have relatively long half-lives (**Table 30.6**), patients typically require doses at least every 6 hours to maintain stable effects. Methadone has become an increasingly popular drug for chronic pain, presumably because of its low cost, potential for unexpectedly high potency, and relatively low abuse potential and low likelihood of diversion by individuals with a history of substance use disorder. Clinical experience suggests that rotation to methadone after inadequate treatment with another opioid can indeed produce surprisingly good results, an outcome that has been speculated to be related to the D-isomer in the racemate formulation that is commercially available in most countries; this isomer is not an opioid, but rather blocks another receptor (the *N*-methyl-D-aspartate (NMDA) receptor) that may potentiate analgesia or reverse some degree of opioid tolerance (92,93).

Methadone is a challenging drug to use, however, and clinicians must understand its unique pharmacology in order to administer it in a safe manner. Methadone's half-life ranges between 12 and 190 hours, and substantial delayed toxicity has been observed many days after methadone treatment was begun or altered. Its potential to have an unexpectedly high potency when substituting for another opioid increases the challenge of dose selection when starting the drug. It can prolong the QTc interval (94,95), a risk that suggests the need to obtain a baseline ECG, and periodic ECG monitoring thereafter, in patients who may be predisposed to this phenomenon (96,97). Given the increased potential for serious toxicity and the need for prolonged monitoring with methadone, its administration should be undertaken only by clinicians with the knowledge and experience necessary to ensure safety.

Routes of Administration

The oral and transdermal routes are preferred in the management of chronic cancer pain. Alternative routes may be required, however, and the clinician must recognize their indications and be familiar with the accepted approaches.

Transdermal Delivery

The transdermal route of administration is available for the highly lipophilic opioids buprenorphine and fentanyl. Transdermal fentanyl, which offers a 48-hour to 72-hour dosing interval, is preferred by

TABLE 30.6. Commonly Used Pharmacologic Approaches in the Management of Opioid Side Effects

Opioid Side Effect	Treatment
Constipation	**Approaches for all patients:** Increase fluid intake and dietary fiber Ensure coanalgesic or adjuvant (comfort and convenience, etc.) **Discuss approaches with patient and select one or more:** Daily contact laxative plus stool softener (e.g., senna plus docusate) Daily osmotic laxative Intermittent use of laxative **Consider alternative approaches in refractory cases:** Opioid antagonist—methylnaltrexone or naloxegol Lubiprostone Prokinetic agent (metoclopramide)
Nausea	**Several approaches:** If associated with vertigo or if markedly exacerbated by movement, antivertiginous drug (e.g., scopolamine, meclizine) If associated with early satiety, prokinetic agent (metoclopramide) In other cases, dopamine antagonist drugs (e.g., prochlorperazine, haloperidol, metoclopramide) or 5HT antagonists (ondansetron, granisetron, others)
Somnolence, mental clouding	If analgesia is satisfactory, reduce opioid dose by 25% to 50% If analgesia is satisfactory and the toxicity involves confusion, consider a trial of a neuroleptic (e.g., haloperidol) If analgesia is satisfactory and the toxicity is somnolence, consider a trial of a psychostimulant (e.g., methylphenidate or modafinil) Consider pharmacologic approaches to reduce the opioid requirement (addition of a coanalgesic or adjuvant) Consider trial of an alternative opioid If appropriate, consider nonpharmacologic analgesic approaches

some patients and may be associated with relatively less constipation than oral opioid formulations (98,99). The transdermal route may be very useful for the patient who is unable to swallow or absorb an orally administered opioid. Transdermal fentanyl may not be effective in cachectic patients because the lack of an adequate subcutaneous drug reservoir may result in a relatively higher level of hepatic metabolism. Patients with very low albumin levels and those with frequent infections may be at relatively higher risk for toxicity from transdermal fentanyl because of sudden increases in the free fraction of fentanyl and increased absorption from the reservoir during fever (100–102).

Although buprenorphine is a partial agonist with a ceiling dose, and a capacity to induce abstinence if administered to a patient who is already physically dependent on another opioid, studies suggest that some patients with severe cancer can benefit (103,104). The transdermal formulation of this drug available in the United States provides a relatively low dose range, which may complicate treatment of severe pain.

Rectal

Rectal formulations of oxymorphone, hydromorphone, and morphine are available in the United States. There is also anecdotal experience with rectal administration of controlled-release morphine or oxycodone tablets. The rectal route is usually considered for patients who are relatively opioid nontolerant and become temporarily unable to take oral medications. The potency of opioids administered rectally is believed to approximate oral dosing (105), absorption is variable, and relative potency may be higher or lower than expected; this depends on a variety of factors, including location of the suppository (low in the rectum, where the blood supply is systemic, or high in the rectum, where blood flows through the portal circulation) and contents of the rectum at the time of dosing (106,107).

Oral and Nasal Transmucosal

Absorption through the oral or nasal cavity can potentially occur with any opioid, and those that are lipophilic and relatively potent may be absorbed sufficiently to have clinical use (108). Multiple types of transmucosal formulations of fentanyl have been approved after having been shown to be safe and efficacious when used as a "rescue" dose for the treatment of breakthrough pain in cancer patients receiving a fixed-schedule opioid. These formulations, which are known as *transmucosal immediate-release formulations (TIRFs),* include an intraoral lozenge, an effervescent buccal tablet, a buccal patch, a sublingual tablet, sublingual spray, and a nasal spray. In the United States, all of these products, including generics, have a mandatory shared risk evaluation and mitigation strategy, the purpose of which is to reduce the risk of abuse and unintentional overdose.

All of the TIRFs are efficacious and have an onset of action faster than orally administered drugs (109–112). A few comparative trials suggest that patients with cancer-related breakthrough pain have better outcomes when treated with these drugs instead of an oral opioid. These data have limitations, however, and the appropriate positioning of these drugs against relatively less costly ones in the therapeutic armamentarium for cancer-related breakthrough pain remains uncertain. Patients who demonstrate that a short-acting oral opioid does not satisfactorily address breakthrough pain due to a slow onset of effect, those with very rapid-onset breakthrough pains, and those who have a particularly good response to fentanyl may be considered empirically for a trial of one of these drugs. There are insufficient data to recommend one formulation over another, and this decision will usually be based on availability, cost, and patient preference. Given the perception that rapid-onset formulations address an unmet clinical need, other formulations are in development.

In some clinical situations, a trial of an injectable formulation placed under the tongue is reasonable. Although there is considerable experience in the use of sublingual administration of concentrated oral morphine solution during the care of patients at the end of life, this drug is relatively hydrophilic, and is poorly absorbed by this route; it is likely that most of the effects obtained occur following enteral absorption after swallowing (113).

Intranasal butorphanol is available, but as noted, this opioid is an agonist–antagonist and has characteristics that make it unfavorable for long-term administration to cancer patients. It is rarely used in this setting. As noted, buprenorphine may be useful in some patients with cancer pain, but the sublingual preparations indicated in the United States for the office-based treatment of substance use disorder provide doses that would rarely meet the needs of the cancer patients with pain.

Parenteral Injection

Patients who are unable to swallow or absorb opioid drugs are candidates for long-term parenteral dosing. Repetitive intramuscular or subcutaneous injections are painful and should rarely be considered.

Repetitive intravenous injections may be effective, but these usually require skilled nursing and may be associated with prominent "bolus" effects (toxicity at peak concentration, pain breakthrough at the trough, or both). Repetitive dosing through a "butterfly" needle placed under the skin has been used effectively in end-of-life care, and experience suggests that the needle can be in place for a week without the development of local pain or other problems.

Continuous Infusion

Continuous infusion eliminates the fluctuations in plasma concentration associated with repetitive bolus injections. Any opioid available in an injectable formulation can be used for continuous infusion. The availability of continuous subcutaneous infusion using ambulatory infusion devices has markedly enhanced the clinical utility of infusion techniques, allowing long-term administration of opioids and other drugs in the home environment (114). A diverse group of pumps that range considerably in features, complexity, and cost are now available, and the clinician often has the option of selecting a pump based on the needs and resources of the patient. PCA can be combined with continuous infusion to address episodic pains. In most cities, skilled nursing organizations can assist in the management of therapy at home.

Intraspinal Opioids

The discovery of opioid receptors in the spinal cord provided the foundation for the development of techniques to deliver opioid analgesics intraspinally. Intraspinal administration can provide selective analgesia (i.e., without the sensory or motor blockade produced by local anesthetics) at doses lower than those required systemically. The strongest indication for a trial of intraspinal opioid administration is the occurrence of intolerable somnolence or confusion in patients who are not experiencing adequate analgesia during systemic opioid treatment of pain.

Many methods of intraspinal opioid administration are now in use (115). The most commonly used include a percutaneous epidural catheter, which is usually tunneled to the anterior abdominal wall and there connected to an ambulatory infusion pump; a totally implanted epidural catheter connected to a subcutaneous portal, which in turn is connected to an ambulatory pump; and an intrathecal catheter connected to a totally implanted continuous infusion device. Implantable pump systems, which are refilled percutaneously, are often chosen for patients with life expectancies of three or more months.

A controlled trial that compared neuraxial infusion to comprehensive medical management demonstrated that the spinal opioid treatment improved pain, side effects, quality of life, and even survival (116). Patients with cancer pain that is poorly responsive to systemic therapy should be considered for a neuraxial approach if the resources exist to implement and monitor it.

The preferred drugs for chronic intraspinal infusion are morphine and hydromorphone, but many others are used empirically, and admixtures (e.g., opioid plus local anesthetic or clonidine, or both) are now commonplace. Based on a systematic review of the literature (117), an expert panel created an algorithm for the progressive use of an array of drugs during intrathecal therapy (118). Therapy is initiated with either morphine or hydromorphone. If a second agent is needed, either the local anesthetic bupivacaine or the α_2-adrenergic agonist clonidine may be selected. Clonidine was shown in a controlled trial to be effective in neuraxial analgesia (119). Ziconotide, a unique calcium channel blocker, is also now available in the United States and has been shown to be effective for cancer pain in controlled trials (120). The use of a combination of drugs may help to potentiate analgesia and reduce side effects, such as sensory and motor block, urinary retention, pruritus, and nausea.

Guidelines for the Administration of Opioid Drugs

As noted, all patients who develop moderate-to-severe persistent pain should be considered for an opioid-based regimen. Although the opioid-naïve patient usually is offered a short-acting combination product, it is acceptable to initiate therapy with a long-acting formulation, as long as the dose is appropriate (121). For example, long-acting morphine can be started in the opioid-naïve patient at a dose of 15 mg twice daily, or 20 to 30 mg once daily, depending on the formulation. Long-acting oxycodone or oxymorphone can be started at doses of 10 mg twice daily or 5 mg twice daily, respectively. Transdermal fentanyl can be initiated at 12 μg/hour in opioid-naïve patients. Given the availability of these long-acting formulations in doses appropriate for the opioid-naïve, the decision to start a short-acting or long-acting drug in a patient with new-onset persistent pain is a clinical judgment based on patient preference, convenience, cost and availability, and experience.

If a patient is receiving a short-acting drug, but pain is not controlled, it is conventional practice to switch to a single-entity agonist opioid, typically in a long-acting formulation. Starting doses may be slightly higher if the patient has required regular administration of the short-acting drug. On a daily basis, the milligram dose of a long-acting drug is the same as the short-acting formulation of the same drug.

Following selection of a starting dose, dose adjustment is almost always required. Once a favorable balance between analgesia and side effects is obtained, this is usually maintained for a prolonged time unless there is progression in the pain-producing pathology. Although several large surveys have established that patients with stable disease usually demonstrate stable dosing patterns, most patients with cancer pain do not have stable disease. Recurrent pain or the new occurrence of side effects necessitates another period of dose titration. Inadequate adjustment of the dose is probably the most common reason for unsuccessful long-term management of cancer pain.

In all cases, the dose of an opioid should be increased until acceptable analgesia is produced or intolerable and unmanageable side effects supervene. Ceiling doses for the pure agonist opioids have not been identified clinically, and occasionally doses can become extremely high—equivalent to grams of morphine per day—as upward dose titration proceeds. At relatively high doses, it is important to reassess the nature of the pain, ensure that expressed need for treatment is not related to other factors (e.g., so-called "chemical coping" or the possibility of addiction), and also establish that the benefits of therapy clearly outweigh the side effects and burdens.

Surveys have demonstrated that one-half to two-thirds of patients with cancer pain will experience clinically significant breakthrough pain (122), and it is common to co-administer a short-acting drug—an approach known as "rescue" dosing—to treat it. As described previously, the rapid-onset transmucosal fentanyl formulations have been developed specifically in an effort to improve the management of breakthrough cancer pain.

Treatment of common side effects is an essential element in the successful management of opioid therapy. Patients who experience intolerable toxicity despite treatment should be designated as poorly responsive to the specific drug and route, and an alternative strategy for pain control should be implemented. This may include more sophisticated management of the treatment-limiting side effect, the addition of a pharmacologic or nonpharmacologic analgesic approach that could reduce the opioid requirement, or opioid rotation.

Opioid rotation, or the switching from one drug to another in an effort to improve the outcomes of an opioid regimen, is now widely used, despite guidelines based on experience rather than research (123). Switching requires an appreciation of relative potency, as codified on the equianalgesic dose table (**Table 30.6**). To switch to another opioid drug or route, the equianalgesic dose table is used to calculate a dose of the new drug that would be theoretically equianalgesic with the old drug or route. With few exceptions, the dosing regimen based on this calculated dose should be reduced by 25% to 50% to account for incomplete cross-tolerance between drugs; a larger reduction, 75% to 90%, is prudent if the new drug is methadone (because of a unique pharmacology in this agent). In contrast, no reduction in the equianalgesic dose is needed if the switch is to transdermal fentanyl (because a reduction is already built into the recommended equianalgesic ratios).

Management of Common Opioid Side Effects

Although there is no maximum dose or ceiling dose for the μ-agonist opioids, the appearance of side effects imposes a practical limit on dose escalation. Given the importance of side effects in determining the response to an opioid, the successful management of common adverse side effects is a fundamental aspect of therapy (**Table 30.7**) (124).

Constipation is a highly prevalent side effect of opioid therapy (125). It may contribute to abdominal pain, distension, nausea, and worsening anorexia, and occasionally may progress to obstipation and bowel obstruction. The management of drug-induced constipation should begin with the elimination of nonessential constipating drugs and, if possible, an increase in both fluid and fiber intake. Fiber should not be increased in those with possible partial bowel obstruction or marked debility because of the potential for worsening obstruction.

There is broad consensus that the likelihood of opioid-induced constipation is high enough to warrant prophylactic therapy. There are numerous types of laxatives, including bulk-forming agents, osmotic agents, lubricants, surfactants, contact cathartics, prokinetic drugs, and opioid antagonists (126). The conventional first-line approach is a combination of a stool softener, usually docusate, and a cathartic agent, such as senna. Most patients respond to this therapy. The osmotic agent, propylethylene glycol, in a powdered formulation offers another well-tolerated and usually effective approach. Other osmotic agents, such as lactulose, are often tried in more refractory cases. Lubiprostone, a chloride channel opener approved for opioid-induced constipation in noncancer patients, is available in the United States and may also be considered. Other approaches are rarely tried, including trials of metoclopramide, misoprostol, colchicine, or donepezil.

Opioid antagonist therapy, using a drug that does not cause systemic withdrawal, should be considered when constipation has not responded to routine approaches. A parenteral antagonist, methylnaltrexone, is commercially available in the United States and can be used to manage acute constipation, or with dosing 2 to 3 times weekly (127–129). This drug is a large and polar molecule that does not cross the blood–brain barrier. Another peripherally acting opioid antagonist, alvimopan, is approved for the management of postoperative ileus and has a similar mode of action (130). Oral naloxone has very limited oral bioavailability and is sometimes tried for refractory constipation as well; the starting dose of 0.8 mg twice daily may be doubled every 2 to 3 days until favorable effects occur or side effects are experienced (131,132). A new oral agent, naloxegol, is a polyethylene glycol (PEG)ylated form of naloxone and is classified as a peripherally acting μ-opioid receptor antagonist. This drug is approved for opioid-induced constipation in noncancer patients and may be an important addition to the management of refractory opioid-induced constipation (133).

Nausea or vomiting constitutes a problem for some 10% to 30% of cancer patients receiving opioid therapy (134). Potential contributing etiologies should be evaluated and the treatment adjusted accordingly. If the assessment suggests that factors other than opioids are contributing to the nausea, antiemetic therapy may be combined with specific interventions to reverse or minimize these factors. The usual first-line drugs are the dopamine antagonists, including prochlorperazine, metoclopramide, and haloperidol, and the 5HT antagonists such as ondansetron (135). Patients with refractory nausea may need other pharmacologic approaches, such as a corticosteroid or a commercially available cannabinoid such as tetrahydrocannabinol (THC) or nabilone. Some nauseated patients appear to benefit from empirical treatment with a drug used for vertigo, such as meclizine or scopolamine. In difficult cases, combinations of drugs from unrelated classes are often tried.

Sedation or mental clouding is very common when an opioid regimen is begun or the dose increased. Most patients develop tolerance to this effect relatively quickly, but some do not, and some have other factors that cause cognitive impairment and compound the effect of the opioid. If these side effects are mild, reassurance and education are usually sufficient interventions. When toxicity is severe or persistent enough to compromise the benefits of therapy, other interventions are needed. Treatment of potential etiologies other than the opioid, when feasible and indicated, is the first step in management. If pain is well controlled, it is reasonable to try an opioid dose reduction of 25% to 50%.

Symptomatic therapies for opioid-induced sedation or mental clouding should also be considered (**Table 30.7**). Methylphenidate has been shown to decrease opioid-induced sedation in cancer patients (136,137). The starting dose is 5 mg at breakfast and at lunchtime; dose titration is often needed, while monitoring side effects, including anorexia, jitteriness, anxiety, and insomnia. Other psychostimulants that have been used empirically for this indication include dextroamphetamine, amphetamine, modafinil, and armodafinil (138,139). A role for modafinil in cancer has been suggested by a positive controlled study that demonstrated improvement across cognitive, mood, and fatigue outcome measures, with the maximum benefit at 8 weeks after initiation of treatment. Other drugs that may be considered

TABLE 30.7. Adjuvant Analgesics

Indication	Drugs
Neuropathic pain	Antidepressants
	Tricyclic antidepressants
	Amitriptyline
	Desipramine
	"Newer" antidepressants
	Duloxetine
	Anticonvulsants
	Gabapentin
	Pregabalin
	Sodium channel blockers
	Mexiletine
	α_2-Adrenergic agonists
	Clonidine
	Tizanidine
	NMDA receptor antagonists
	Ketamine
	Cannabinoids
	THC
	Topical anesthetics
	Capsaicin
	Lidocaine
	Miscellaneous
	Baclofen
Bone pain	Bisphosphonates (e.g., pamidronate)
	Denosumab Calcitonin
	Radiopharmaceuticals (e.g., strontium 89 and samarium 153)
Bowel obstruction	Scopolamine
	Glycopyrrolate
	Octreotide
Multipurpose	Corticosteroids
	Dexamethasone Prednisone

in refractory cases include the cholinesterase inhibitor donepezil and other psychostimulants such as caffeine, dexmethylphenidate, and atomoxetine (140,141). A systematic review concluded that the data pertaining to these drugs was insufficient to draw conclusions. Methylphenidate or modafinil are generally considered first.

Tolerance, Physical Dependence, and Addiction

The clinical implications of tolerance, physical dependence, and addiction are commonly misunderstood by patients and clinicians. These misapprehensions may lead to concern about adverse events and, possibly, undertreatment of pain.

Tolerance is a pharmacologic property of opioid drugs defined by the need for escalating doses to maintain effects (142). Patients may have other reasons for declining analgesic effects, however, among which are progressive nociception and increasing psychologic distress. Clinical observations suggest that the most common reason that efficacy declines over time is worsening pain due to progression of a nociceptive lesion. Fear of analgesic tolerance should never delay the implementation of opioid therapy, and tolerance should not be invoked to explain the need for higher opioid doses unless a comprehensive reassessment has failed to identify an alternative explanation.

Physical dependence also is a pharmacologic property of opioid drugs, which is defined by the occurrence of an abstinence syndrome following abrupt dose reduction or administration of an antagonist (142). Neither the dose nor the duration of dosing required to produce physical dependence is known, and it is prudent to assume that all patients who have received an opioid drug for more than a few days have the potential for withdrawal. This implies that dosing should not be discontinued suddenly and that antagonist drugs, including the agonist–antagonist opioids, should be avoided.

Patients who become physically dependent on opioids appear to develop increased sensitivity to the effects of antagonist drugs. Very small doses of naloxone may produce a severe abstinence syndrome. For this reason, the use of naloxone should be limited to patients with symptomatic respiratory depression. When naloxone must be used in patients receiving chronic opioid therapy, only a dilute solution (e.g., 0.4 mg in 10 mL saline) should be administered and incremental doses should be given only until respiration improves. The goal of this intervention is improved respiration and not a return of consciousness, which may be associated with recurrent pain and withdrawal phenomena.

Both tolerance and physical dependence are distinct from addiction. Because the labels applied to patients can determine the attitudes and behaviors of caregivers, it is extremely important that appropriate terms are used to describe these phenomena. Patients who are perceived to have the capacity for withdrawal should be labeled physically dependent and not "addicted."

Addiction is a genetic, psychologic, and behavioral syndrome characterized by craving, loss of control over drug use, compulsive use, and continued use despite harm to the patient or others (143). Although abusable drugs, including opioids, can be shown to have reinforcing effects in animals, the capacity to produce addiction should not be considered an inherent property of the drug. Addiction presumably results from an interaction between the drug and a variety of factors that predispose the individual to develop an addictive pattern of use. These factors probably encompass genetic vulnerability, situational factors, and psychologic disturbances, as well as access to the drug.

Cancer patients who engage in aberrant drug-taking behaviors, such as hoarding or selling, unsanctioned dose escalation, or manipulation of the medical system to obtain additional drugs, may or may not meet criteria for the diagnosis of addiction. If such aberrant behaviors are identified, measures should be taken to eliminate them while a detailed assessment is performed to clarify their meaning (143). In some cases, aberrant drug-related behaviors appear to be driven by uncontrolled pain. This has been termed *pseudoaddiction* and is managed by improved efforts to provide pain relief. Pseudoaddiction can coexist with addiction, however, and care should be taken to ensure that the complaint of pain does not result in a missed diagnosis of addiction. A careful pain history, institution of more controls over prescribing, and monitoring over time should facilitate clarification of these distinctions.

Occasionally, aberrant behaviors are related to a psychiatric disorder other than addiction or to the development of a mild encephalopathy, which leads to confusion about drug taking. Again, these explanations for problematic drug use are not mutually exclusive, and the complexity of the clinical situation requires careful assessment and perhaps referral of the patient to a pain specialist or an addiction medicine specialist (144). The clinician must avoid the stigmatizing label of addiction for patients who have reasonable alternative explanations for aberrant behaviors, but should be willing to render the diagnosis of addiction in those who actually have this disease.

The risk of true iatrogenic addiction is clearly relevant in judging the overall utility of opioid therapy for chronic cancer pain. There is substantial evidence that this risk is extremely low among those with no prior history of abuse or addiction (145). It is now widely accepted that all patients who are being considered for a trial of an opioid should be evaluated for risk factors that may predict aberrant drug-related behavior, such as a history of substance abuse, a family history of substance abuse, and major psychiatric disorder; however, fear of addiction should not be considered a contraindication to opioid therapy of severe cancer pain. Rather, patients should be stratified by risk before therapy begins, and monitored for aberrant drug-related behavior during the course of therapy. Should concerns arise, the clinician may structure therapy so as to reduce risk, or refer appropriately (146,147).

Adjuvant Drugs

Most patients with cancer pain require multiple drugs for symptom management. Some of these adjuvant drugs are used to treat symptoms other than pain, particularly those that occur as side effects of the opioid (**Table 30.7**). Other drugs are used in an effort to provide additive analgesia. The latter drugs comprise acetaminophen, the NSAIDs, and the so-called adjuvant analgesics (148). In recent years, the number of adjuvant analgesics has increased substantially, and several have become approved for primary pain indications due to the abundance of evidence for analgesic efficacy.

The adjuvant analgesics are particularly helpful in the treatment of pain syndromes that are often relatively less responsive to opioids, such as neuropathic pain (**Table 30.7**). In the setting of advanced illness, corticosteroids are commonly used (149); these drugs may also improve anorexia, nausea, and fatigue. Alternatives include specific anticonvulsants and antidepressants. Evidence for analgesic efficacy is best for gabapentin and pregabalin (150–152); for the tricyclic antidepressants, such as amitriptyline and desipramine (153–155); and for the serotonin and norepinephrine reuptake inhibitors, such as duloxetine (156). Gabapentin or pregabalin is usually tried first, given their lack of drug–drug interactions, but sequential trials of various drugs are often required before a well-tolerated and effective adjuvant analgesic is identified.

If the drugs with relatively good evidence of analgesic efficacy in neuropathic pain are not tolerated or are ineffective, trials of other anticonvulsants or antidepressants may be undertaken empirically. Other second-line agents for neuropathic pain include oral sodium channel blockers (e.g., mexiletine) or a brief infusion of lidocaine (157), ketamine (158–161), or a cannabinoid (162,163). At subanesthetic doses, ketamine may be used for treatment of severe refractory pain (158,159). The evidence of benefit is quite limited, however. Cannabinoids are analgesic and a new cannabis derivative, nabiximols (a 1:1 mixture of THC and cannabidiol), is under development specifically for pain related to advanced cancer. There are also several published randomized trials demonstrating at least short-term benefits for smoked (164–166) or vaporized (167,168) cannabis in patients with neuropathic pain, none of which were conducted in patients with cancer-related neuropathic pain. Both the gamma-aminobutyric acid (GABA) agonist, baclofen, and the α_2-adrenergic drugs, tizanidine and clonidine, are sometimes tried in selected patients with refractory neuropathic pain (169,170).

The use of topical agents represents another adjuvant analgesic strategy. A lidocaine patch (171) is available and has shown efficacy in postherpetic neuralgia (172). This formulation is commonly tried for all types of neuropathic and musculoskeletal pains. Topical creams are also used empirically in patients with cancer pain, including compounds containing other local anesthetics, capsaicin, an NSAID, a tricyclic antidepressant, or an opioid (173–175).

Opioid-refractory malignant bone pain is another syndrome for which adjuvant analgesics are often considered. The preferred drugs include bisphosphonates, denosumab (a monoclonal antibody targeting RANK), radiopharmaceuticals, and calcitonin (176–179). Although the bisphosphonates carry the risks of renal insufficiency and osteonecrosis of the jaw, there is evidence that they can improve overall morbidity associated with bone metastases, and a trial of one of these agents is typically considered in the setting of significant bone pain (180).

Adjuvant analgesics are also commonly employed in the setting of bowel obstruction that is not surgically correctable. Aggressive pharmacotherapy, particularly in those with advanced disease, may control symptoms and obviate the need for drainage procedures. Treatment usually involves the combination of anticholinergic drugs (e.g., scopolamine or glycopyrrolate), octreotide, corticosteroids, and opioids (181).

Other Approaches for Chronic Pain Management

Although most patients with cancer pain can achieve adequate relief with pharmacologic approaches alone, a multimodality strategy should always be considered in an effort to optimize the balance between analgesia and side effects, promote better function, or concurrently manage other problems. Multiple therapies are commonly needed to address the broader palliative care concerns of the patient and family, which derive from the complex interaction between pain and suffering.

When the focus is pain control, there are a large number of noninvasive and invasive approaches that may be considered adjunctive to opioid-based pharmacotherapy. Only a small minority of patients will require an invasive analgesic modality if the other therapies are optimally administered.

Interventional Approaches

The interventional strategies include injections, neural blockade, and implant therapies. Trigger point injections may be considered within the purview of all practitioners. Myofascial pains are extremely common in patients with chronic cancer pain, and the use of local anesthetic injections into painful trigger points may be a useful adjunctive approach in these patients.

The advances in neuraxial infusion of opioids and other drugs, as described previously, have largely supplanted the neurodestructive approaches that were employed in the past for pain syndromes refractory to systemic opioid therapy. Nonetheless, some types of neural blockade continue to be widely used (182).

Temporary somatic nerve blocks may be diagnostic, prognostic, or therapeutic. Diagnostic blocks elucidate the afferent pathways involved in the experience of pain. Prognostic blocks are implemented prior to a neurolytic procedure, and although extensive clinical experience indicates that a favorable response does not predict permanent relief following neurolysis, the failure to achieve pain relief with local anesthetic is commonly viewed as a contraindication to a destructive procedure. Repeated therapeutic blocks with local anesthetic are occasionally used in cancer patients who obtain substantial and fairly prolonged relief after such a temporary block. Recently, local anesthetics have been used to provide more prolonged neural blockade through techniques of perineural or epidural infusion.

Neural blockade with neurolytic solutions, usually alcohol or phenol, have been developed to denervate virtually any area of the body (183). Their use is very limited, however, because of the short-term risks associated with the injection of these substances, such as damage to soft tissues and local hemorrhage or infection, and the longer-term risks of neuritis and deafferentation pain. The one generally accepted exception is celiac plexus blockade for the management of epigastric pain due to neoplastic invasion of the celiac axis. The response to neurolytic celiac plexus blockade in pain due to pancreatic cancer has been observed to be so satisfactory that earlier use is warranted whenever the typical pain syndrome occurs (184–186).

Intermittent nitrous oxide inhalation is an anesthetic technique that has proven useful in the management of severe breakthrough pain in patients with advanced cancer (187). Although the availability of masks that reduce ambient leakage of the gas has increased the potential usefulness of this approach, it continues to be applied rarely.

Neurostimulatory Approaches

It has been appreciated for some time that stimulation of afferent neural pathways may result in analgesia. The best-known application of this principle is TENS. Other approaches include percutaneous electrical nerve stimulation, dorsal column stimulation, deep brain stimulation, motor cortex stimulation, and transcranial stimulation. Published experience in the use of these modalities for the management of cancer pain is meager (188,189). Surveys of the techniques that have been used most extensively in noncancer pain (TENS and dorsal column stimulation) suggest that the majority of patients will achieve analgesia soon after the approach is implemented but fewer obtain prolonged relief. A trial of TENS is usually considered in patients with neuropathic pain that has been difficult to manage with opioids.

Physiatric Approaches

Although evidence from clinical trials is lacking, the potential for analgesic effects from physiatric therapies, including the use of orthoses or prostheses, occupational therapy and physical therapy, and modalities such as heat, cold, vibration, and ultrasound, is well accepted. For example, refractory movement–induced pains may be partially relieved by bracing the painful part, such as in patients with back pain due to metastatic lesions of the spine and those with arm pain related to a malignant brachial plexopathy; and a well-fitting prosthesis can reduce stump pain. In addition to the potential for salutary effects on symptoms, physical therapy and occupational therapy can potentially forestall painful complications, such as contractures, and generally increase well-being.

Neurosurgical Approaches

Procedures designed to denervate the painful area surgically have been developed for every level of the nervous system from peripheral nerves to cortex. Historically, the most useful approach has been cordotomy. Like neurolytic blocks, however, these procedures are rarely considered now, largely due to the advent of more sophisticated, nondestructive interventions such as neuraxial infusion.

Psychologic Approaches

Some patients or families who present with severe psychologic distress may benefit from a multidisciplinary approach in which psychologic interventions are emphasized within a program designed to palliate symptoms and provide family support. These goals may be accomplished in some cases through referral to a hospice or palliative care program. Occasionally, patients with psychiatric disorders are identified, indicating the need for further assessment and treatment by an appropriate specialist (190).

Specific cognitive and behavioral approaches have also been applied in the management of pain and related symptoms (191). Cognitive approaches include relaxation training, distraction techniques, hypnosis, and biofeedback, all of which may enhance a patient's sense of personal control and reduce pain. Although experienced personnel are required to implement many of these approaches, the nonspecialist can teach several forms of relaxation training. Cognitive–behavioral therapy, which has achieved wide acceptance in the management of noncancer pain, is occasionally considered in patients with limited disease whose level of functional impairment is perceived to be out of proportion to the effects of the neoplasm.

Complementary and Alternative Medicine Approaches

Therapies that are typically considered to be complementary or alternative have had a growing role in pain management (192). These approaches are often very attractive to patients because they endorse a holistic strategy that is perceived as providing hope and self-control. Some interventions that are termed "complementary" are actually used routinely by specialists in pain medicine or palliative care. These include mind–body therapies (e.g., relaxation, meditation, and others), nutritional support, acupuncture, and massage. Interventions such as homeopathy, naturopathy, and many others, are considered to be far outside the mainstream and are rarely suggested. Healthcare professionals have the difficult task of expressing concerns about some of the latter therapies, while respecting patients' pursuit of complementary treatments that may be beneficial or, at least, pose no significant chance of harm.

CONCLUSION

Pain is highly prevalent among patients with gynecologic tumors. The clinicians involved in the care of these patients have a challenging task in providing state-of-the-art management approaches for both acute and chronic pain. Fortunately, the most effective strategy for both acute and chronic pain, namely, opioid-based pharmacotherapy, is clearly within the purview of all practitioners. The knowledge and skills necessary to optimize this therapy, and integrate it with the broader principles of palliative care, are fundamental to the practice of gynecologic oncology.

REFERENCES

1. Van den Beuken-van Everdingen, de Rijke JM, Kessels AG, et al. Prevalence of pain in patients with cancer: a systematic review of the past 40 years. *Ann Oncol.* 2007;18(9):1437–1449.
2. Van den Beuken-van Everdingen, de Rijke JM, Kessels AG, et al. High prevalence of pain in patients with cancer in a large population-based study in The Netherlands. *Pain.* 2007;132(3):312.
3. Teuissen SC, Wesker W, Kruitwagen C, et al. Symptom prevalence in patients with incurable cancer: a systematic review. *J Pain Symptom Manage.* 2007;34(1):94.
4. Ferrell B, Smith S, Cullinane C, et al. Symptom concerns of women with ovarian cancer. *J Pain Symptom Manage.* 2003;25:528–538.
5. Olson SH, Mignone L, Nakrasieve C, et al. Symptoms of ovarian cancer. *Obstet Gynecol.* 2001;98:212–217.
6. Kim YJ, Munsell MF, Park JC, et al. Retrospective review of symptoms and palliative care interventions in women with advanced cervical cancer. *Gynecol Oncol.* 2015;139(3):553–558.
7. Costantini M, Ripamonti C, Beccaro, et al. Prevalence, distress, management, and relief of pain during the last 3 months of cancer patients' life. Results of an Italian mortality follow-back survey. *Ann Oncol.* 2009;20(4):729–735.
8. Anderson KG, Henrik K. Persistent pain after breast cancer treatment: A critical review of risk factors and strategies for prevention. *J Pain.* 2011;12(7):725–746.
9. Perkins FM, Kehlet H. Chronic pain as an outcome of surgery. *Anesthesiology.* 2000;93:1123–1133.
10. Meuser T, Pietruck C, Radbruch L, et al. Symptoms during cancer pain treatment following WHO-guidelines: a longitudinal follow up study of symptoms prevalence, severity and etiology. *Pain.* 2001;93(3):247–257.
11. Beck SL, Towsley GL, Berry PH, et al. Core aspects of satisfaction with pain management: cancer patients' prespectives. *J Pain Symptom Manage.* 2010;39:100–115.
12. Greco MT, Roberto A, Corli O. Quality of cancer pain management: an update of a systemic review of undertreatment of patients with cancer. *J Clin Oncol.* 2014;32(36):4149–4154.
13. Deandrea S, Montanari M, Moja L, et al. Prevalence of undertreatment in cancer pain. A review of published literature. *Ann Oncol.* 2008;19(12):1985–1991.
14. Foley K. How well is cancer pain treated? *Palliat Med.* 2011;25(5):398–401.
15. National Comprehensive Cancer Network (NCCN). NCCN Clinical practice guidelines in oncology. http://www.nccn.org/professionals/physician_gls/f_guidelines.asp. Accessed January 12, 2016.
16. Ripamonti CI, Bandieri E, Roila F; ESMO Guidelines Working Group. Management of cancer pain: ESMO Clinical Practice Guidelines. *Ann Oncol.* 2011;22 suppl 6:vi69.
17. Newell S, Sanson-Fisher RW, Girgis A, et al. The physical and psychosocial experiences of patients attending an outpatient medical oncology department: a cross-sectional study. *Eur J Cancer Care.* 1999;8:73–82.
18. Fairchild A. Under-treatment of cancer pain. *Curr Opin Support Palliat Care.* 2010;4:11.
19. National Comprehensive Cancer Network Practice Guidelines in Oncology: Cancer-Related Fatigue; 2016. http://www.nccn.org/professionals/physician_gls/pdf/fatigue.pdf. Accessed January 16, 2016.
20. Merskey H, Bogduk N, eds. *Classification of Chronic Pain: Descriptions of Chronic Pain Syndromes and Definitions of Pain Terms.* 2nd Ed. Seattle, WA: IASP Press; 1994.
21. Classification of chronic pain. Descriptions of chronic pain syndromes and definitions of pain terms. Prepared by the International Association for the Study of Pain, Subcommittee on Taxonomy. *Pain Suppl.* 1986;3:S1.
22. Kroenke K, Zhong X, Theobald D, et al. Somatic symptoms in patients with cancer experiencing pain or depression: prevalence, disability, and health care use. *Arch Intern Med.* 2010;170:1686.
23. Zaza C, Baine N. Cancer pain and psychosocial factors: a critical review of the literature. *J Pain Symptom Manage.* 2002;24:526.
24. Redinbaugh EM, Baum A, DeMoss C, et al. Factors associated with the accuracy of family caregiver estimates of patient pain. *J Pain Symptom Manage.* 2002;23:31.
25. Daut RL, Cleeland CS, Flanery RC. Development of the Wisconsin Brief Pain Questionnaire to assess pain in cancer and other diseases. *Pain.* 1983;17:197.
26. Melzack R. The McGill Pain Questionnaire: major properties and scoring methods. *Pain.* 1975;1:277.
27. Fishman B, Pasternak S, Wallenstein SL, et al. The memorial pain assessment card. A valid instrument for the evaluation of cancer pain. *Cancer.* 1987;60:1151.
28. Turk DC, Dworkin RH, Allen RR, et al. Core outcome domains for chronic pain clinical trials: IMMPACT recommendations. *Pain.* 2003;106:337–345.
29. Davies A, Buchanan A, Zeppetella G, et al. Breakthrough cancer pain: an observational study of 1000 European oncology patients. *J Pain Symptom Manage.* 2013;46:619.
30. Deandrea S, Corli O, Consonni D, et al. Prevalence of breakthrough cancer pain: a systematic review and a pooled analysis of published literature. *J Pain Symptom Manage.* 2014;47:57.
31. Davies AN. Breakthrough cancer pain. *Curr Pain Headache Rep.* 2014;18:420.
32. Gerwin RD. Myofascial and visceral pain syndromes: visceral-somatic pain representations. *J Musculoskelet.* 2002;10:165–175.
33. Marcus NJ. Pain in cancer patients unrelated to the cancer or treatment. *Cancer Invest.* 2005;23(1):84–93.
34. Mols F, Beijers T, Vreugdenhil G, et al. Chemotherapy-induced peripheral neuropathy and its association with quality of life: a systematic review. *Support Care Cancer.* 2014;22:2261.
35. Jensen TS, Baron R, Haanpaa M, et al. A new definition of neuropathic pain. *Pain.* 2011;152:2204–2205.
36. Sharpe M, Strong V, Allen K, et al. Major depression in outpatients attending a regional cancer centre: screening and unmet treatment needs. *Br J Cancer.* 2004;90(2):314–320.
37. Prieto JM, Atala J, Blanch J, et al. Role of Depression as a predictor of mortality among cancer patients after stem-cell transplantation. *J Clin Oncol.* 2005;23:6063–6071.
38. Coyne JC, Palmer SC, Shapiro PJ, et al. Distress, psychiatric morbidity, and prescriptions for psychotropic medication in breast cancer waiting room sample. *Gen Hosp Psychiatry.* 2004;26:121–128.

39. Chang VT, Janjan N, Jain S, et al. Update in cancer pain syndromes. *J Palliat Med.* 2006;9(6):1414–1434.
40. Cherny NI. Pain assessment and cancer pain syndromes. In: Hanks G, Cherny NI, Christakis N, et al. eds. *Oxford Text Book of Palliative Medicine.* 4th Ed. Oxford, UK: Oxford University Press; 2010:599–626.
41. Tuncer S, Pirbudak L, Balat O, et al. Adding ketoprofen to intravenous patient-controlled analgesia with tramadol after major gynecologic cancer surgery: a double-blinded, randomized, placebo-controlled clinical trial. *Eur J Gynaecol Oncol.* 2003;24:181–184.
42. Liu SS, Wu CL. The effect of analgesic technique on postoperative patient-reported outcomes including analgesia: a systematic review. *Anesth Analg.* 2007;105(3):789–808.
43. Pearl ML, McCauley DL, Thompson J, et al. A randomized controlled trial of early oral analgesia in gynecologic oncology patients undergoing intra-abdominal surgery. *Obstet Gynecol.* 2002;99:704–708.
44. Bellissant E, Estebe JP, Sebille V, et al. Effect of preoperative oral sustained-release morphine sulfate on postoperative morphine requirements in elective spine surgery. *Fundam Clin Pharmacol.* 2004;18(6):709–714.
45. Reuben SS, Steinberg RB, Maciolek H, et al. Preoperative administration of controlled-release oxycodone for the management of pain after ambulatory laparoscopic tubal ligation surgery. *J Clin Anesth.* 2002;14(3):223–227.
46. White PF, Sacan O, Tufanogullari B, et al. Effect of short-term postoperative celecoxib administration on patient outcome after outpatient laparoscopic surgery. *Can J Anaesth.* 2007;54(5):342–348.
47. Mathiesen O, Moiniche S, Dahl JB. Gabapentin and postoperative pain: a qualitative and quantitative systematic review, with focus on procedure. *BMC Anesthesiol.* 2007;7:6.
48. Marret E, Remy C, Bonnet F; Postoperative Pain Forum Group. Meta-analysis of epidural analgesia versus parenteral opioid analgesia after colorectal surgery. *Br J Surg.* 2007;94(6):665–673.
49. Simon DA, Connor JP, Kushner DM, et al. Epidural analgesia superior to patient-controlled analgesia for postoperative pain relief in gynecologic oncology surgery. *J Pelvic Med Surg.* 2007;13(4):191–196.
50. Fleron MH, Weiskopf RB, Bertrand M, et al. A comparison of intrathecal opioid and intravenous analgesia for the incidence of cardiovascular, respiratory, and renal complications after abdominal aortic surgery. *Anesth Analg.* 2003;97:2–12.
51. Sprung J, Sanders MS, Warner ME, et al. Pain relief and functional status after vaginal hysterectomy: intrathecal versus general anesthesia. *Can J Anaesth.* 2006;53(7):690–700.
52. Ballantyne JC, Carwood CM. Comparative efficacy of epidural, subarachnoid, and intracerebroventricular opioids in patients with pain due to cancer. *Cochrane Database Syst Rev*. 2005;(1):CD005178.
53. Bjordal JM, Johnson MI, Ljunggreen AE. Transcutaneous electrical nerve stimulation (TENS) can reduce postoperative analgesic consumption. A meta-analysis with assessment of optimal treatment parameters for postoperative pain. *Eur J Pain.* 2003;7:181–188.
54. Good M, Anderson GC, Stanton-Hicks M, et al. Relaxation and music reduce pain after gynecologic surgery. *Pain Manag Nurs.* 2002;3:61–70.
55. Watt MC, Stewart SH, Lefaivre MJ, et al. A brief cognitive-behavioral approach to reducing anxiety sensitivity decreases pain-related anxiety. *Cogn Behav Ther*. 2006;35(4):248–256.
56. Ozalp G, Sarioglu R, Tuncel G, et al. Preoperative emotional states in patients with breast cancer and postoperative pain. *Acta Anaesthesiol Scand.* 2003;47:26–29.
57. Vaughn F, Wichowski H, Bosworth G. Does preoperative anxiety level predict postoperative pain? *AORN J.* 2007;85(3):589–604.
58. Cherny NI. The problem of suffering and the principles of assessment in palliative medicine. In: Cherny NI, Fallon MT, Kaasa S, et al. (eds). *Oxford Textbook of Palliative Medicine.* 5th Ed. Oxford, UK: Oxford University Press; 2015:35–48.
59. Homsi J, Walsh D, Rivera N, et al. Symptom evaluation in palliative medicine: patient report vs systematic assessment. *Support Care Cancer.* 2006;14:444.
60. Apolone G, Corli O, Caraceni A, et al. Pattern and quality of care of cancer pain management. Results from the Cancer Pain Outcome Research Study Group. *Br J Cancer*. 2009;100:1566.
61. Yennurajalingam S, Urbauer DL, Casper KL, et al. Impact of a palliative care consultation team on cancer-related symptoms in advanced cancer patients referred to an outpatient supportive care clinic. *J Pain Symptom Manage.* 2011;41:49.
62. The National Consensus Project for Quality Palliative Care. *Clinical Practice Guidelines for Quality Palliative Care.* 3rd Ed. Washington, DC: American Hospital Association; 2013.
63. Smith TJ, Temin S, Alesi ER, Abernethy AP, et al. American Society of Clinical Oncology provisional clinical opinion: the integration of palliative care into standard oncology care. *J Clin Oncol.* 2012;30(8):880–887.
64. Schrijvers D. Disease modifying therapies in advanced cancer. In: Cherny NI, Fallon MT, Kaasa S, et al. (eds). *Oxford Textbook of Palliative Medicine.* 5th Ed. Oxford, UK: Oxford University Press; 2015:765–770.
65. Geels P, Eisenhauer E, Bezjak A, et al. Palliative effect of chemotherapy: objective tumor response is associated with symptom improvement in patients with metastatic breast cancer. *J Clin Oncol.* 2000;18:2395–2405.
66. Doyle C, Crump M, Pintilie M, et al. Does palliative chemotherapy palliate? Evaluation of expectations, outcomes, and costs in women receiving chemotherapy for advanced ovarian cancer. *J Clin Oncol.* 2001;19:1266–1274.
67. Tinger A, Waldron T, Peluso N, et al. Effective palliative radiation therapy in advanced and recurrent ovarian carcinoma. *Int J Radiation Oncology Biol Phys.* 2001;51:1256–1263.
68. Spanos WJ Jr, Pajak TJ, Emami B, et al. Radiation palliation of cervical cancer. *J Natl Cancer Inst Monogr.* 1996;21:127–130.
69. Falkmer U, Jarhult J, Wersall P, et al. A systematic overview of radiation therapy effects in skeletal metastases. *Acta Oncol.* 2003;42:620–633.
70. Hillegonds DJ, Franklin S, Shelton DK, et al. The management of painful bone metastases with an emphasis on radionuclide therapy. *J Natl Med Assoc.* 2007;99(7):785–794.
71. WHO analgesic pain ladder available online. www.who.int/cancer/palliative/painladder/en/. Accessed December 19th, 2015.
72. Mercadante S, Fulfaro F, Casuccio A. A randomised controlled study on the use of anti-inflammatory drugs in patients with cancer pain on morphine therapy: effects of dose-escalation and a pharmacoeconomic analysis. *Eur J Cancer.* 2002;38:1358–1363.
73. Mercadante S. The use of anti-inflammatory drugs in cancer pain. *Cancer Treat Rev.* 2001;27:51–61.
74. Mercadante S, Fulfaro F, Casuccio A. A randomised controlled study on the use of anti-inflammatory drugs in patients with cancer pain on morphine therapy: effects of dose-escalation and a pharmacoeconomic analysis. *Eur J Cancer.* 2002;38:1358–1363.
75. Bombardier C, Laine L, Reicin A, et al. Comparison of upper gastrointestinal toxicity of rofecoxib and naproxen in patients with rheumatoid arthritis. *VIGOR Study Group. N Engl J Med.* 2000;343:1520–1528.
76. Silverstein FE, Faich G, Goldstein JL, et al. Gastrointestinal toxicity with celecoxib vs. nonsteroidal anti-inflammatory drugs for osteoarthritis and rheumatoid arthritis: the CLASS study: a randomized controlled trial. Celecoxib long-term arthritis safety study. *JAMA.* 2000;284:1247–1255.
77. Waksman JC, Brody A, Phillips SD. Nonselective nonsteroidal antiinflammatory drugs and cardiovascular risk: are they safe? *Ann Pharmacother.* 2007;41:1163–1173.
78. Hinz B, Renner B, Brune K. Drug insight: cyclo-oxygenase-2 inhibitors-a critical appraisal. *Nat Clin Pract Rheumatol.* 2007;3:552–560.
79. Trelle S, Reichenbach S, Wandel S, et al. Cardiovascular safety of non-steroidal anti-inflammatory drugs: network meta-analysis. *BMJ.* 2011;342:c7086.
80. Lazzaroni M, Porro GB. Management of NSAID-induced gastrointestinal toxicity: focus on proton pump inhibitors. *Drugs.* 2009;69:51.
81. Lanza FL, Chan FK, Quigley EM; Practice Parameters Committee of the American College of Gastroenterology. Guidelines for prevention of NSAID-related ulcer complications. *Am J Gastroenterol.* 2009;104:728.
82. Schmidt M, Christiansen CF, Mehnert F, et al. Non-steroidal anti-inflammatory drug use and risk of atrial fibrillation or flutter: population based case-control study. *BMJ.* 2011;343:d3450.
83. Antman EM, Bennett JS, Daugherty A, et al. Use of nonsteroidal antiinflammatory drugs: an update for clinicians: a scientific statement from the American Heart Association. *Circulation.* 2007;115:1634.
84. Dean M. Opioids in renal failure and dialysis patients. *J Pain Symptom Manage.* 2004;28(5):497–504.
85. Quigley C. Opioids in people with cancer-related pain. *BMJ Clin Evid.* 2008;2008:2408.
86. Penson RT, Joel SP, Gloyne A, et al. Morphine analgesia in cancer pain: role of the glucuronides. *J Opioid Manag.* 2005;1:83.
87. Quigley C, Joel S, Patel N, et al. Plasma concentrations of morphine, morphine-6-glucuronide and morphine-3-glucuronide and their relationship with analgesia and side effects in patients with cancer-related pain. *Palliat Med.* 2003;17:185.
88. Penson RT, Joel SP, Bakhshi K, et al. Randomized placebo-controlled trial of the activity of the morphine glucuronides. *Clin Pharmacol Ther.* 2000;68:667.
89. Launay-Vacher V, Karie S, Fau JB, et al. Treatment of pain in patients with renal insufficiency: the World Health Organization three-step ladder adapted. *J Pain.* 2005;6:137.
90. Murtagh FE, Chai MO, Donohoe P, et al. The use of opioid analgesia in end-stage renal disease patients managed without dialysis: recommendations for practice. *J Pain Palliat Care Pharmacother.* 2007;21(2):5–16.

91. Hadley G, Derry S, Moore RA, et al. Transdermal fentanyl for cancer pain. *Cochrane Database Syst Rev*. 2013;10:CD010270.
92. BrysonJ, Tamber A, Seccareccia D, et al. Methadone for treatment of cancer pain. *Curr Oncol Rep*. 2006;8:282–288.
93. Leppert W. The role of methadone in cancer pain treatment—a review. *Int J Clin Pract*. 2009;63:1095.
94. Reddy S, Hui D, El Osta B, et al. The effect of oral methadone on the QTc interval in advanced cancer patients: a prospective pilot study. *J Palliat Med*. 2010;13:33.
95. Cruciani RA, Sekine R, Homel P, et al. Measurement of QTc in patients receiving chronic methadone therapy. *J Pain Symptom Manage*. 2005;29:385–391.
96. Krantz MJ, Martin J, Stimmel B, et al. QTc interval screening in methadone treatment. *Ann Intern Med*. 2009;150:387.
97. Chou R, Cruciani RA, Fiellin DA, et al. Methadone safety: a clinical practice guideline from the American Pain Society and College on Problems of Drug Dependence, in collaboration with the Heart Rhythm Society. *J Pain*. 2014;15:321.
98. Van Seventer R, Smit JM, Schipper RM, et al. Comparison of TTS-fentanyl with sustained-release oral morphine in the treatment of patients not using opioids for mild-to-moderate pain. *Curr Med Res Opin*. 2003;19:457.
99. Tassinari D, Sartori S, Tamburini E, et al. Adverse effects of transdermal opiates treating moderate-severe cancer pain in comparison to long-acting morphine: a meta-analysis and systematic review of the literature. *J Palliat Med*. 2008;11:492.
100. Heiskanen T, Mätzke S, Haakana S, et al. Transdermal fentanyl in cachectic cancer patients. *Pain*. 2009;144(1–2):218–222.
101. Ashburn MA, Ogden LL, Zhang J, et al. The pharmacokinetics of transdermal fentanyl delivered with and without controlled heat. *J Pain*. 2003;4:291.
102. Carter KA. Heat-associated increase in transdermal fentanyl absorption. *Am J Health Syst Pharm*. 2003;60:191.
103. Muriel C, Failde I, Micó JA, et al. Effectiveness and tolerability of the buprenorphine transdermal system in patients with moderate to severe chronic pain: a multicenter, open-label, uncontrolled, prospective, observational clinical study. *Clin Ther*. 2005;27:451–462.
104. Naing C, Aung K, Racloz V, et al. Safety and efficacy of transdermal buprenorphine for the relief of cancer pain. *J Cancer Res Clin Oncol*. 2013;139:1963.
105. Wilkinson TJ, Robinson BA, Begg EJ, et al. Pharmacokinetics and efficacy of rectal versus oral sustained-release morphine in cancer patients. *Cancer Chemother Pharmacol*. 1992;31:251.
106. Walsh D, Tropiano PS. Long-term rectal administration of high-dose sustained-release morphine tablets. *Support Care Cancer*. 2002;10:653.
107. Moolenaar F, Meijler WJ, Frijlink HW, et al. Clinical efficacy, safety and pharmacokinetics of a newly developed controlled release morphine sulphate suppository in patients with cancer pain. *Eur J Clin Pharmacol*. 2000;56:219.
108. Weinberg DS, Inturrisi CE, Reidenberg B, et al. Sublingual absorption of selected opioid analgesics. *Clin Pharmacol Ther*. 1988;44:335–342.
109. Rauck R, Reynolds L, Geach J, et al. Efficacy and safety of fentanyl sublingual spray for the treatment of breakthrough cancer pain: a randomized, double-blind, placebo-controlled study. *Curr Med Res Opin*. 2012;28:859.
110. Jandhyala R, Fullarton JR, Bennett MI. Efficacy of rapid-onset oral fentanyl formulations vs. oral morphine for cancer-related breakthrough pain: a meta-analysis of comparative trials. *J Pain Symptom Manage*. 2013;46:573.
111. Portenoy RK, Burton AW, Gabrail N, et al. A multicenter, placebo-controlled, double-blind, multiple-crossover study of Fentanyl Pectin Nasal Spray (FPNS) in the treatment of breakthrough cancer pain. *Pain*. 2010;151:617.
112. Kosugi T, Hamada S, Takigawa C, et al. A randomized, double-blind, placebo-controlled study of fentanyl buccal tablets for breakthrough pain: efficacy and safety in Japanese cancer patients. *J Pain Symptom Manage*. 2014;47:990.
113. Coluzzi PH. Sublingual morphine: efficacy reviewed. *J Pain Symptom Manage*. 1998;16:184–192.
114. Wilcock A, Jacob JK, Charlesworth S, et al. Drugs given by a syringe driver: a prospective multicentre survey of palliative care services in the UK. *Palliat Med*. 2006;20(7):661–664.
115. Swarm RA, Karanikolas M, Cousins MJ. Interventional Approaches for Chronic Pain. In: Cherny NI, Fallon MT, Kaasa S, et al. (eds). *Oxford Textbook of Palliative Medicine*. 5th Ed. Oxford, UK: Oxford University Press; 2015:589–598.
116. Smith TJ, Staats PS, Deer T, et al. Implantable Drug Delivery Systems Study Group. Randomized clinical trial of an implantable drug delivery system compared with comprehensive medical management for refractory cancer pain: impact on pain, drug-related toxicity, and survival. *J Clin Oncol*. 2002;20:4040–4049.
117. Bennett G, Serafini M, Burchiel K, et al. Evidence-based review of the literature on intrathecal delivery of pain medication. *J Pain Symptom Manage*. 2000;20:S12–S36.
118. Hassenbusch SJ, Portenoy RK, Cousins M, et al. Polyanalgesic Consensus Conference 2003: an update on the management of pain by intraspinal drug delivery—report of an expert panel. *J Pain Symptom Manage*. 2004;27:540–563.
119. Eisenach JC, DuPen S, Dubois M, et al. Epidural clonidine analgesia for intractable cancer pain. *Pain*. 1995;61:391–399.
120. Staats PS, Yearwood T, Charapata SG, et al. Intrathecal ziconotide in the treatment of refractory pain in patients with cancer or AIDS: a randomized controlled trial. *JAMA*. 2004;291:63–70.
121. Klepstad P, Kaasa S, Jystad A, et al. Immediate- or sustained-release morphine for dose finding during start of morphine to cancer patients: a randomized, double-blind trial. *Pain*. 2003;101:193.
122. Caraceni A, Martini C, Zecca E, et al. Breakthrough pain characteristics and syndromes in patients with cancer pain. An international survey. *Palliat Med*. 2004;18:177.
123. Reddy A, Yennurajalingam S, Pulivarthi K, et al. Frequency, outcome, and predictors of success within 6 weeks of an opioid rotation among outpatients with cancer receiving strong opioids. *Oncologist*. 2013;18:212.
124. Swegle JM, Logemann C. Management of common opioid-induced adverse effects. *Am Fam Physician*. 2006;74:1347–1354.
125. Kyle G. Constipation and palliative care—where are we now? *Int J Palliat Nurs*. 2007;13(1):6–16.
126. Ford AC, Brenner DM, Schoenfeld PS. Efficacy of pharmacological therapies for the treatment of opioid-induced constipation: systematic review and meta-analysis. *Am J Gastroenterol*. 2013;108:1566.
127. Dutka J, Lowe SS, Michaud M, et al. Long-term use of methylnaltrexone for the management of constipation in advanced cancer. *J Support Oncol*. 2009;7:177.
128. Centeno C, Carranza O, Zuriarrain Y, et al. A prospective study of methylnaltrexone for opioid-induced constipation in advanced illness: should we use it or not? *J Pain Symptom Manage*. 2013;46:e1.
129. Watkins JL, Eckmann KR, Mace ML, et al. Utilization of methylnaltrexone (relistor) for opioid-induced constipation in an oncology hospital. *P T*. 2011;36:33.
130. Jansen JP, Lorch D, Langan J, et al. A randomized, placebo-controlled phase 3 trial (Study SB-767905/012) of alvimopan for opioid-induced bowel dysfunction in patients with non-cancer pain. *J Pain*. 2011;12:185.
131. Liu M, Wittbrodt E. Low-dose oral naloxone reverses opioid-induced constipation and analgesia. *J Pain Symptom Manage*. 2002;23:48.
132. Culpepper-Morgan JA, Inturrisi CE, Portenoy RK, et al. Treatment of opioid-induced constipation with oral naloxone: a pilot study. *Clin Pharmacol*. 1992;52:90–95.
133. Chey WD, Webster L, Sostek M, et al. Naloxegol for opioid-induced constipation in patients with noncancer pain. *N Engl J Med*. 2014;370:2387.
134. Keeley PW. Nausea and vomiting in people with cancer and other chronic diseases. *BMJ Clin Evid*. 2009;2009.
135. Laugsand EA, Kaasa S, Klepstad P. Management of opioid-induced nausea and vomiting in cancer patients: systematic review and evidence-based recommendations. *Palliat Med*. 2011;25:442.
136. Bruera E, Driver L, Barnes E, et al. Patient controlled methylphenidate for cancer related fatigue: a preliminary report. *J Clin Oncol*. 2003;21:4439–4443.
137. Wilwerding MB, Loprinzi CL, Maillard JA, et al. A randomized, crossover evaluation of methylphenidate in cancer patients receiving strong opioids. *Support Care Cancer*. 1995;3:135–138.
138. Cox JM, Pappagallo M. Modafinil: a gift to portmanteau. *Am J Hosp Palliat Care*. 2001;18:408.
139. Webster L, Andrews M, Stoddard G. Modafinil treatment of opioid-induced sedation. *Pain Med*. 2003;4:135.
140. Mercadante S, Serretta R, Casuccio A. Effects of caffeine as an adjuvant to morphine in advanced cancer patients. A randomized, double-blind, placebo-controlled, crossover study. *J Pain Symptom Manage*. 2001;21:369.
141. Stone P, Minton O. European Palliative Care Research collaborative pain guidelines. Central side-effects management: what is the evidence to support best practice in the management of sedation, cognitive impairment and myoclonus? *Palliat Med*. 2011;25:431.
142. Savage SR, Joranson DE, Covington EC, et al. Definitions related to the medical use of opioids: evolution towards universal agreement. *J Pain Symptom Manage*. 2003;26(1):655–667.
143. Portenoy RK. Acute and chronic pain. In: Ruiz P, Strain E, eds. *Lowinson & Ruiz's Substance Abuse: A Comprehensive Textbook*, 5th Ed. Philadelphia, PA: Lippincott, Williams and Wilkins; 2011:695.

144. Katz NP, Adams EH, Benneyan JC, et al. Foundations of opioid risk management. *Clin J Pain*. 2007;23:103.
145. Heit HA. The truth about pain management: the difference between a pain patient and an addicted patient. *Eur J Pain*. 2001;5(suppl A):27–29.
146. Passik SD, Kirsh KL, Donaghy KB, et al. Pain and aberrant drug-related behaviors in medically ill patients with and without histories of substance abuse. *Clin J Pain*. 2006;22:173–181.
147. Miaskowski C. The use of risk-management approaches to protect patients with cancer-related pain and their healthcare providers. *Oncol Nurs Forum*. 2008;35 suppl:20–24.
148. Lussier D, Portenoy RK. Adjuvant analgesics. In: Cherny N, Kaasa S, Fallon M, et al. (eds). *Oxford Textbook of Palliative Medicine*, 5th Edition. Oxford: Oxford University Press; 2015:578–588.
149. Mercadante SL, Berchovich M, Casuccio A, et al. A prospective randomized study of corticosteroids as adjuvant drugs to opioids in advanced cancer patients. *Am J Hosp Palliat Care*. 2007;24:13.
150. Backonja MM, Canafx DM, Cundy KC. Efficacy of Gabapentin enacarbil vs placebo in patients with postherpetic neuralgia and a pharmacokinetic comparison with oral Gabapentin. *Pain Med*. 2011;12:1098–1108.
151. Sandercock D, Cramer M, Wo J, et al. Gabapentin extended release for the treatment of painful diabetic peripheral neuropathy. Efficacy and tolerability in a double-blind, randomized, controlled clinical trial. *Diabetes Care*. 2009;32(2):e20.
152. Gilron I, Flatters SJ. Gabapentin and pregabalin for the treatment of neuropathic pain: a review of laboratory and clinical evidence. *Pain Res Manag*. 2006;11(suppl A):16A–29A.
153. Kalso E, Tasmuth T, Neuvonen PJ. Amitriptyline effectively relieves neuropathic pain following treatment of breast cancer. *Pain*. 1996;64:293–302.
154. Watson CPN. The treatment of neuropathic pain: antidepressants and opioids. *Clin J Pain*. 2000;16:S49–S55.
155. Max MB, Lynch SA, Muir J, et al. Effects of desipramine, amitriptyline, and fluoxetine on pain in diabetic neuropathy. *N Engl J Med*. 1992;326:1250.
156. Wernicke JF, Pritchett YL, D'Souza DN, et al. A randomized controlled trial of duloxetine in diabetic peripheral neuropathic pain. *Neurology*. 2006;67(8):1411–1420.
157. Sloan P, Basta M, Storey P, et al. Mexiletine as an adjuvant analgesic for the management of neuropathic cancer pain. *Anesth Analg*. 1999;89:760–761.
158. Jackson K, Ashby M, Howell D, et al. The effectiveness and adverse effects profile of "burst" ketamine in refractory cancer pain: The VCOG PM 1-00 study. *J Palliat Care*. 2010;26:176.
159. Prommer EE. Ketamine for pain: an update of uses in palliative care. *J Palliat Med*. 2012;15:474.
160. Salas S, Frasca M, Planchet-Barraud B, et al. Ketamine analgesic effect by continuous intravenous infusion in refractory cancer pain: considerations about the clinical research in palliative care. *J Palliat Med*. 2012;15:287.
161. Bell RF, Eccleston C, Kalso EA. Ketamine as an adjuvant to opioids for cancer pain. *Cochrane Database Syst Rev*. 2012;11:CD003351.
162. Burns TL, Ineck JR. Cannabinoid analgesia as a potential new therapeutic option in the treatment of chronic pain. *Ann Pharmacother*. 2006;40:251–260.
163. Iskedjian M, Bereza B, Gordon A, et al. Meta-analysis of cannabis based treatments for neuropathic and multiple sclerosis-related pain. *Curr Med Res Opin*. 2007;23(1):17–24.
164. Wilsey B, Marcotte T, Tsodikov A, et al. A randomized, placebo-controlled, crossover trial of cannabis cigarettes in neuropathic pain. *J Pain*. 2008;9:506.
165. Ellis RJ, Toperoff W, Vaida F, et al. Smoked medicinal cannabis for neuropathic pain in HIV: a randomized, crossover clinical trial. *Neuropsychopharmacology*. 2009;34:672.
166. Ware MA, Wang T, Shapiro S, et al. Smoked cannabis for chronic neuropathic pain: a randomized controlled trial. *CMAJ*. 2010;182:E694.
167. Wilsey B, Marcotte T, Deutsch R, et al. Low-dose vaporized cannabis significantly improves neuropathic pain. *J Pain*. 2013;14:136.
168. Wallace MS, Marcotte TD, Umlauf A, et al. Efficacy of inhaled cannabis on painful diabetic neuropathy. *J Pain*. 2015;16:616.
169. Eisenach JC, DuPen S, Dubois M, et al. Epidural clonidine analgesia for intractable cancer pain. The Epidural Clonidine Study Group. *Pain*. 1995;61:391.
170. Malanga GA, Gwynn MW, Smith R, et al. Tizanidine is effective in the treatment of myofascial pain syndrome. *Pain Physician*. 2002;5:422.
171. Gammaitoni AR, Davis MW. Pharmacokinetics and tolerability of lidocaine patch 5% with extended dosing. *Ann Pharmacother*. 2002;36:236–240.
172. Rowbotham MC, Davies PS, Fields HL. Topical lidocaine gel relieves postherpetic neuralgia. *Ann Neurol*. 1995;37:246.
173. Derry S, Lloyd R, Moore RA, et al. Topical capsaicin for chronic neuropathic pain in adults. *Cochrane Database Syst Rev*. 2009;(4):CD007393.
174. Lin J, Zhang W, Jones A, et al. Efficacy of topical non-steroidal anti-inflammatory drugs in the treatment of osteoarthritis: meta-analysis of randomised controlled trials. *BMJ*. 2004;329:324.
175. Ho KY, Huh BK, White WD, et al. Topical amitriptyline versus lidocaine in the treatment of neuropathic pain. *Clin J Pain*. 2008;24:51.
176. Patrick DL, Cleeland CS, von Moos R, et al. Pain outcomes in patients with bone metastases from advanced cancer: assessment and management with bone-targeting agents. *Support Care Cancer*. 2015;23:1157.
177. Cleeland CS, Body JJ, Stopeck A, et al. Pain outcomes in patients with advanced breast cancer and bone metastases: results from a randomized, double-blind study of denosumab and zoledronic acid. *Cancer*. 2013;119:832.
178. Martin M, Bell R, Bourgeois H, et al. Bone-related complications and quality of life in advanced breast cancer: results from a randomized phase III trial of denosumab versus zoledronic acid. *Clin Cancer Res*. 2012;18:4841.
179. Martinez-Zapata MJ, Roque I, Figuls M, et al. Calcitonin for metastatic bone pain. *Cochrane Database Syst Rev*. 2006;(3):CD003223.
180. Lipton A. Efficacy and safety of intravenous bisphosphonates in patients with bone metastases caused by metastatic breast cancer. *Clin Breast Cancer*. 2007;7(suppl 1):S14–S20.
181. Jervoise H, Andreyev N, Davidson SE, et al. Practice guidance on the management of acute and chronic gastrointestinal problems arising as a result of treatment for cancer. *Gut*. 2012;61(2):179–192.
182. Christo PJ, Mazloomdoost D. Interventional pain treatments for cancer pain. *Ann N Y Acad Sci*. 2008;1138:299–328.
183. Jackson TP, Gaeta R. Neurolytic blocks revisited. *Curr Pain Headache Rep*. 2008;12(1):7–13.
184. Mercadante S, Catala E, Arcuri E, et al. Celiac plexus block for pancreatic cancer pain: factors influencing pain, symptoms and quality of life. *J Pain Symptom Manage*. 2003;26(6):1140–1147.
185. Arcidiacono PG, Calori G, Carrara S, et al. Celiac plexus block for pancreatic cancer pain in adults. *Cochrane Database Syst Rev*. 2011;(3): CD007519.
186. Wyse JM, Carone M, Paquin SC, et al. Randomized, double-blind, controlled trial of early endoscopic ultrasound-guided celiac plexus neurolysis to prevent pain progression in patients with newly diagnosed, painful, inoperable pancreatic cancer. *J Clin Oncol*. 2011;29:3541.
187. Parlow JL, Miline B, Tod DA, et al. Self-administration nitrous oxide for the management of incident pain in terminally ill patients: a blinded case series. *Palliat Med*. 2005;19(1):3–8.
188. Hurlow A, Bennett MI, Robb KA, et al. Transcutaneous electric nerve stimulation (TENS) for cancer pain in adults. *Cochrane Database Syst Rev*. 2012;3:CD006276.
189. Robb K, Oxberry SG, Bennett MI, et al. A cochrane systematic review of transcutaneous electrical nerve stimulation for cancer pain. *J Pain Symptom Manage*. 2009;37:746.
190. Roth AJ, Massie MJ. Psychiatric complications in cancer patients. In: Lenhard RE, Osteen RT, Gansler T, eds. *Textbook of Clinical Oncology*. Atlanta, GA: American Cancer Society; 2001:837–852.
191. Brothers BM, Thornton LM, Anderson B. Cognitive and behavioral interventions. In: Holland JC, ed. *Psychooncology*. New York, NY: Oxford University Press; 2010:415–421.
192. Pan CX, Morrison S, Ness J, et al. Complementary and alternative medicine in the management of pain, dyspnea, and nausea and vomiting near the end of life: a systematic review. *J Pain Symptom Manage*. 2000;20:374–387.

CHAPTER 31

Nutrition Support of Patients with Gynecologic Cancer

Priya Simoes and Mark Schattner

INTRODUCTION

Cachexia and weight loss are common manifestations of cancer and exert major impact on quality of life and survival. Malnutrition is a complex, multifactorial phenomenon that leads to progressive weight loss and deficiency of specific nutrients. Both cancer and its various therapeutic modalities contribute to cachexia. Advances in understanding nutritional requirements and intermediary metabolism, and major technologic progress in the ability to provide nutritional support, have made it possible to feed almost any patient with cancer. Nevertheless, the indications for and the appropriate use of the various modalities of nutritional support are still evolving, and many questions remain unanswered.

Malnutrition in most patients with cancer is usually a manifestation of general calorie and protein deficits that result in progressive weight loss and weakness; however, it is important to recognize that in some patients, specific nutrient deficiencies, such as magnesium deficiency or vitamin B_{12} deficiency, can be present even in the absence of weight loss and can contribute significantly to morbidity and even mortality.

Gynecologic malignancies and their multimodal therapies may be associated with severe malnutrition. Although some nutritional problems occur in patients with cervical and endometrial cancer, they are most commonly seen in those with ovarian cancer, particularly in advanced stages when intra-abdominal metastasis severely impairs gastrointestinal function. Because of the high incidence of malnutrition and its impact on the patient with cancer, nutritional assessment and appropriate therapy should be integral parts of the overall treatment plan.

NUTRITIONAL ASSESSMENT

Nutritional assessment in cancer patients is an ongoing process. It should be a part of the patient's initial evaluation and should be updated periodically. It is especially important to determine the nutritional state prior to therapeutic interventions as well as during and after acute illness, to identify those patients who would benefit from nutritional support. The nutritional assessment method used must be simple, accurate, and inexpensive. Anthropometric parameters, serum protein measurements, and immunologic tests have classically formed the basis of the nutritional evaluation; however, they all have significant deficiencies.

Anthropometric and Biochemical Markers

Anthropometric measurements such as weight, skinfold thickness, mid-arm muscle circumference, and creatinine/height index can all provide useful information but have major limitations. Change in weight is the single most useful measurement of nutritional status when the change does not reflect changes in total body water. The often-present edema, effusions, ascites, and intravenous hydration that often accompany treatment limit the use of weight as a nutritional parameter. In addition, inaccuracies in scales and different clothing can provide misleading information on weight changes. Measurements of skinfold and mid-arm muscle circumference (1) are useful tools in studies but have very limited use in clinical practice. Lumbar skeletal muscle mass, measured by computed tomography (CT), has also been used as a nutritional indicator to determine prognosis and disease recurrence among patients with gynecologic cancers. However, this method requires special imaging software and technical expertise, and its clinical utility is limited (2). A creatinine/height index derived by dividing the patient's 24-hour creatinine excretion by that of a healthy person of the same height offers a sensitive measure of early protein-calorie malnutrition (3) but requires collection of a 24-hour urine specimen and is affected by alterations in renal function, which may not be indicative of the nutritional state.

Low levels of serum proteins such as albumin, prealbumin, transferrin, and retinol-binding protein were classically thought to represent malnutrition. However, in the malnourished sick patient, low levels of these proteins can be nonspecific. They are dependent on intact hepatic synthetic function as well as hydration status. They can be low as a manifestation of severe illness (infection, metastatic cancer, multisystem organ failure) in a normal nutritional state. In addition, they can function as acute-phase reactants and therefore can be normal or elevated in a clinically malnourished patient. Therefore, their role is limited. Similar limitations apply to immunologic parameters such as total lymphocyte count and delayed cutaneous hypersensitivity. In simple starvation, both these measures may be decreased and can return to normal with initiation of nutritional support. However, in the cancer patient undergoing chemotherapy, surgery, or radiotherapy or in the midst of an acute illness, these parameters have little value in the assessment of the nutritional state (4,5).

The above parameters have been combined to create numerous nutritional assessment indices. The most extensively studied is the Prognostic Nutritional Index (PNI), which factors measurements of serum albumin, serum transferrin, triceps skinfold, and delayed cutaneous hypersensitivity (6). Buzby et al. prospectively studied the PNI in patients undergoing gastrointestinal surgery and found that it could accurately stratify patients into high, intermediate, or low risk of developing postoperative complications (7). It must be understood, however, that the index is only as good as the parameters from which it is calculated, and the same limitations outlined above are present in any of these indices.

Subjective Global Assessment

The clinical assessment of the nutritional status has always been used to some extent as part of the general medical history and physical examination. The validity of a formal clinical assessment of the nutritional status was demonstrated in the landmark study by Baker et al., who developed the Subjective Global Assessment (SGA) as a formal clinical assessment of nutritional status (8). The SGA is based on a complete history and physical examination, with emphasis on six areas: change in weight, dietary intake, gastrointestinal symptoms, functional capacity, physiologic stress, and physical signs of nutritional deficiencies. These are used to place the patient into three groups. Group "A" (normal nutritional status) consists of patients without restriction of food intake or absorption, no change in functional status, and stable or increasing weight. Group "B" (mild malnutrition) consists of patients with evidence of decreased food intake and functional status but little or no change in body weight, while those with severe reduction in food intake, functional status, and loss of weight comprise Group "C" (severe malnutrition).

The SGA has consistently been shown to be reproducible and reliable in identifying patients at risk for developing complications associated with malnutrition. In the initial study of 59 patients electively admitted to a general surgical ward, interobserver reproducibility in classification of the nutritional status was 81%, and in a later study of 202 patients, it was found to be 91% accurate (8,9). The initial study by Baker and colleagues showed a significant increase in incidence of infection, use of antibiotics, and length of hospitalization in Group "C" when compared with Group "A" (8). In the follow-up study of 202 patients undergoing gastrointestinal surgery, the rate of septic and nonseptic complications in Group "C" was seven times greater than in Group "A" (9). The SGA provides a simple, reproducible, and accurate method to identify malnourished patients who could benefit from nutritional support. Clinical assessments similar to the SGA have been proved superior to immunologic testing, plasma protein measurements, and bioelectrical impedance in providing a useful evaluation of nutritional status (8–13).

More recently, the SGA has been shown to predict short- and long-term survival and tolerance to chemotherapy among women with ovarian cancer (14,15). It is now considered the preferred method of nutritional assessment for patients with gynecologic cancers (15,16).

Prevalence of Malnutrition

The prevalence of malnutrition depends on the tumor type and stage, the organs involved, and the anticancer therapy. Concurrent nonmalignant conditions such as diabetes and intestinal diseases can be important contributing factors.

The prevalence of weight loss during the 6 months preceding diagnosis of cancer was reported from a multicenter cooperative study of patients with 12 types of cancer (17). The lowest frequency (31% to 40%) and severity of weight loss were found in patients with breast cancer, hematologic cancers, and sarcomas. Intermediate frequency and severity of weight loss was found in patients with colon, prostate, and lung cancer (54% to 64%). Patients with cancer of the pancreas and stomach had the highest frequency (over 80%) and severity of weight loss. However, it is worthwhile noting that approximately 35% of the patients with lung cancer lost more than 5% of their body weight. This underscores the fact that even if the tumor does not involve the gastrointestinal tract directly, there can be significant weight loss because of systemic and metabolic derangements and loss of appetite. Furthermore, the study did not report on patients with gynecologic malignancies, in whom weight loss can also be very frequent and severe. Other studies revealed that over 40% of patients receiving medical treatment for a variety of cancers were malnourished (18,19). Among surgical patients in a Veterans Administration hospital, 39% of those undergoing a major operation for cancer were malnourished, as judged by either a nutrition risk index or a combination of weight loss and low serum proteins (20).

Data on the prevalence and impact of malnutrition in patients with gynecologic tumors mirror the observations in patients with other cancers. In a study of 67 consecutive patients hospitalized with gynecologic cancers at the University of Texas, it was found that 54% were malnourished as determined by the PNI (21). In 1983, Tunca (22) examined the nutritional state of gynecologic oncology patients at time of diagnosis using serum albumin, serum transferrin, immune response, and weight loss. Patients with advanced (stage III or IV) ovarian carcinoma had the highest incidence of severe malnutrition, whereas those with cancer of the cervix, endometrium, or vulva reported weight loss with no indication of malnutrition from serum markers or immune response testing. Orr et al. (23,24) assessed the degree of protein-calorie malnutrition and evidence of vitamin deficiency in 78 patients with untreated cervical cancer. The incidence of protein-calorie malnutrition as assessed by anthropometrics, serum markers, and immune testing was directly related to tumor stage: 4% in stage I, 20% in stage II and III, and 60% in stage IV disease (23). Two-thirds of patients with untreated cervical cancer were found to have reduced blood levels of at least one vitamin. Mean serum levels of folate, β-carotene, and vitamin C at the time of admission were all significantly below control values (24). Similar observations of significant protein-calorie malnutrition were seen in 25 patients with endometrial cancer (25). Using the SGA to study 194 patients with gynecologic cancers, Laky showed that 24% of all patients were malnourished. The prevalence of malnutrition was highest in ovarian cancer (67%) and lowest in endometrial cancer (6%) (16).

Significance of Malnutrition

The impact of malnutrition on the cancer patient was demonstrated in a report by Warren in 1932 (26). Based on data from autopsies, the conclusion was that cachexia was the leading cause of death in a group of 400 patients with various cancers. More recent studies have confirmed the significant impact of malnutrition on the quality of life and prognosis of the cancer patient. In the aforementioned multicenter cooperative study of patients receiving chemotherapy (17), those who presented with weight loss at the time of diagnosis had decreased performance status and survival compared with those who presented without weight loss. In a study of patients with limited, inoperable lung cancer, weight loss was a major predictive factor for survival (18). The negative impact of malnutrition was also demonstrated in surgical patients with malignant and benign diseases. Malnourished patients undergoing a major operation were at greater risk for postoperative morbidity and mortality than were well-nourished patients (20,27).

The impact of malnutrition on patients with a primary gynecologic malignancy is striking. While examining the role of total parenteral nutrition (TPN) in their patients, Terada and colleagues noted that those patients who developed major complications such as a fistula, wound infection, pneumonia, renal failure, respiratory failure, or those who died had significantly more weight loss and lower serum transferrin levels at the time of presentation (28). They concluded that these parameters might be of value in predicting clinical outcome in patients requiring nutritional support. This was confirmed in a study by Geisler, who found that in patients with ovarian cancer, those who were malnourished had increased postoperative complications. This difference could be mitigated if preoperative nutritional support could reverse the malnutrition (29).

Several other studies have confirmed the relationship of malnutrition to poor surgical outcome in patients with primary gynecologic malignancies. Donato et al. reported that of the 104 patients with ovarian carcinoma undergoing intestinal surgery, those considered to be malnourished on the basis of serum protein measurements and weight loss preoperatively had significantly more infectious complications, while other variables including preoperative bowel obstruction, extent of debulking, number of intestinal procedures, or hand versus stapled anastomosis failed to correlate with the rate of infectious complications (30). Poor nutritional status has been shown to be an independent predictor of prolonged postoperative ICU stay in patients with ovarian cancer (31). Hertlein stratified gynecologic cancer patients at risk for malnutrition using a nutritional risk screening (NRS) tool (NRS 2002). The NRS 2002 was calculated using two components: "impaired nutritional status" and "severity of disease," which were each given an individual score from 0 to 4. The sum of the two scores constituted the final NRS (32,33). Those with NRS scores $>$ 3 were at increased risk for perioperative infectious (6.9% vs. 3.2%) and noninfectious complications (15.8% vs. 4.5%). They also had longer hospital stay (10 vs. 6 days). Patients with ovarian cancer had the highest prevalence of malnutrition (33). In another study of gynecologic cancer patients undergoing surgery,

Uppal and colleagues found that patients with preoperative hypoalbuminemia (defined as serum albumin < 3 g/dL) were 6 times more likely to develop a perioperative complication and 10 times more likely to die within 30 days of surgery compared with those with normal albumin levels (34).

In addition to predicting surgical outcome and perioperative complications, malnutrition is associated with increased neutropenic fever following chemotherapy, prolonged hospital stays, decreased quality of life, and reduced overall survival among women with gynecologic cancers (14–16,21,35).

Etiology of Malnutrition

Cancer can induce a wide variety of derangements in nutritional status, ranging from generalized malnutrition with severe weight loss and muscle wasting to a single nutrient deficiency. The etiology of malnutrition in the cancer patient is multifactorial. Nutritionally relevant derangements can be induced by the tumor locally (i.e., gastrointestinal obstruction), by malabsorption, or by humoral factors produced by the tumor itself or by reaction of the immune system to the tumor. All modalities of cancer therapy, surgery, radiation, chemotherapy, immunotherapy, and palliative treatments may be associated with side effects and complications that can impair nutritional status.

Cancer cachexia is defined as an ongoing loss of skeletal muscle mass (with or without loss of fat mass) that cannot fully be reversed by nutritional support and leads to progressive functional impairment. It is diagnosed by the presence of these three criteria: (1) weight loss > 5% over the past 6 months (in absence of simple starvation); (2) BMI < 20 and any degree of weight loss > 2%; or (3) appendicular skeletal muscle index consistent with sarcopenia (males < 7.26 kg/m^2; females < 5.45 kg/m^2) and any degree of weight loss > 2% (36).

The etiologic factors of malnutrition in the cancer patient are generally due to three major factors: decreased food intake, malabsorption, and abnormal metabolism.

Impaired Food Intake and Malabsorption

Both tumor and cancer treatment modalities can lead to decreased food intake through direct effects on the gastrointestinal tract or systemic effects leading to anorexia. Obstruction of the gastrointestinal tract can be caused by any gynecologic malignancy through external compression, or more rarely, by direct invasion. Occasionally, localized obstructions can be relieved surgically or endoscopically; however, obstruction due to peritoneal carcinomatosis seen in advanced ovarian cancer is particularly difficult to manage surgically. Often, draining gastrostomy with parenteral nutrition (when appropriate) is the only option for providing nutrition and symptomatic relief (37,38).

Tumors can induce anorexia without local involvement of the gastrointestinal tract. The pathophysiology of this phenomenon is not well understood. Norton et al. (39) utilized a model of surgically coupled tumor-bearing and normal rats with parabiotic cross-circulation to show that tumor-induced anorexia is mediated by circulating substances. Tumor-induced impairment of smell and taste has been well described (27,40–43), but the mechanism has not been defined. There is growing evidence that glycoproteins, cytokines, and neuropeptides play an important role in the pathogenesis of cancer cachexia. Bernstein et al., (44,45) demonstrated in a rat model that infusion of tumor necrosis factor (TNF) mimics tumor-induced anorexia and these effects are mediated via the area postrema and the caudal medial nucleus of the solitary tract in the central nervous system.

Therapies used for gynecologic malignancies often result in complications that impair nutrient intake and absorption. Surgical interventions can lead to fistulae, short bowel syndrome, infections, and ileus, all of which impair oral intake significantly. In a review of 12 years of colonic surgery in gynecologic oncology patients, the rate for major systemic complications (myocardial infarction, pulmonary embolism, renal failure, sepsis) was 13.7%, and the rate of major bowel complications (abscess, fistulae, hemorrhage, obstruction) was 12.1% (46). Adjuvant radiation and chemotherapy have been shown to increase the incidence of major complications after pelvic exenteration (47).

Radiotherapy can lead to damage of the gastrointestinal tract, most commonly affecting the small bowel, followed by the transverse colon, sigmoid, and rectum. Predisposing risk factors include previous abdominal surgery, pelvic inflammatory disease, thin body habitus, hypertension, and diabetes mellitus (48). In general, a dose of 5,000 rads is the threshold for significant injury. In the acute phase of radiation enteritis, virtually all patients experience anorexia, nausea, and vomiting, which are thought to be mediated by effects of serotonin on the gut (49) and the central nervous system (50). This is followed 2 to 3 weeks later by direct injury to the intestinal mucosa, resulting in diarrhea and mild-to-moderate malabsorption. Most patients will have complete resolution of these acute symptoms. However, a significant minority of patients who received radiotherapy will experience chronic dysfunction of the gastrointestinal tract (51). There is often a latent period of 1 to 2 years, and possibly as long as 20 years, before the symptoms of chronic radiation enteropathy surface (52,53). In a review of 102 patients with radiation enteritis after treatment for cervical or endometrial cancer, the median time to development of severe symptoms such as obstruction or perforation was 18 months (54).

Chronic radiation enteropathy is characterized pathologically by transmural injury leading to submucosal fibrosis, edema, lymphatic ectasia, and obliterative endarteritis, which can induce colicky abdominal pain, diarrhea, steatorrhea, ulceration, perforation, stricture, and fistula formation (48). Yeoh et al. (55) retrospectively studied the effects of pelvic irradiation given for the treatment of cervical cancer in 30 randomly selected women who had undergone radiotherapy 1 to 6 years earlier. Significant dysfunction of the gastrointestinal tract was detected. Nineteen of the patients had frequency of bowel movements, bile acid absorption, and vitamin B_{12} absorption outside of the control range. The authors concluded that abnormal gastrointestinal function is essentially an inevitable long-term complication of pelvic irradiation (55). Huaebye and colleagues (56) prospectively studied the gastrointestinal motility patterns in 41 patients with chronic abdominal complaints after radiotherapy for gynecologic cancer. Impaired fasting motility was found in 29% of patients, and motor response after a meal was attenuated in 24%. Postprandial delay of the migrating motor complex was found to be an independent predictor of malnutrition as assessed by weight loss and serum albumin. Impaired motility of the small bowel, therefore, is a key factor in the symptoms experienced by patients with chronic radiation enteropathy. Chronic radiation enteritis predisposes to numerous secondary complications. Danielsson et al. (57) studied 20 patients with chronic or intermittent diarrhea occurring two or more years after receiving radiotherapy for gynecologic tumors. Bile acid malabsorption was detected in 65% of patients, while evidence of bacterial overgrowth on D-xylose or cholyl-glycine breath tests was found in 45%. Treatment with bile acid binders or antibiotics resulted in a significant decline in the number of daily bowel movements. In 47 patients with gynecologic malignancies who had gastrointestinal complaints lasting more than 4 months after radiotherapy, Kwitko et al (58). found 19 partial small bowel obstructions, 11 cases of malabsorption, and 5 fistulae. The mortality from radiation damage to the small bowel in this report was 32%. More recently, Boland reported on a 25-year experience with post-resection short bowel syndrome secondary to radiation therapy. The majority of the cases were in women who received pelvic radiation for gynecologic cancers. One-third of these patients developed short bowel syndrome within a year after radiation and two-thirds remained dependent on long-term TPN (59). Improved fractionation of radiotherapy and protective shielding of the intestine where possible have reduced these complication rates (60).

Chemotherapy is often associated with decreased food intake. Mucositis and diarrhea are commonly seen during therapy with cytotoxic agents that affect the replicating cells of the intestinal mucosa, such as 5-flourouracil, methotrexate, and bleomycin. The vinca alkaloids can cause ileus and constipation mediated by toxic effects on gastrointestinal neural pathways, while cisplatin and nitrosoureas are highly emetic (61,62). Significant nausea, vomiting, stomatitis, and diarrhea occur in 15% of patients receiving intravenous taxol and in 55% of those receiving the drug orally (63). In addition to direct effects on the GI tract, chemotherapy in women with gynecologic cancers has significant effects on olfactory and gustatory function, leading to reduced appetite and weight loss (64).

The psychological impact of a malignancy and its associated therapies can also lead to decreased nutrient intake. Depression is a frequent cause of anorexia in this population, with up to 58% of cancer patients having depressive symptoms and 38% meeting criteria for major depression (65).

Metabolic Derangements

Even with normal nutrient intake, patients with cancer are at risk for malnutrition due to inefficient nutrient utilization and wasteful metabolic pathways. Cancer cachexia is associated with altered metabolism of carbohydrates, fat, protein, vitamins, and minerals.

Increase in basal energy expenditure (BEE) has been reported in many but not all studies of patients with malignancy (66–68). In patients with newly diagnosed small cell lung cancer, Russel et al. showed a mean increase of 37% in BEE, which fell substantially in those who responded to chemotherapy (69). Similar findings have been reported for gastric cancer and sarcoma (67,70). Elevated BEE will drop after tumor resection (71). There are limited data on the metabolic rate in patients with gynecologic cancers (72). Dickerson et al. used indirect calorimetry to determine the resting energy expenditure in 31 patients with ovarian cancer and 30 patients with cervical cancer. Fifty-five percent of those with ovarian cancer were found to be hypermetabolic (BEE >110% predicted by the Harris–Benedict equation), while only 13% of patients with cervical cancer were hypermetabolic. These differences could not be explained by differences in the extent of disease, nutritional status, body temperature, or nutrient intake (73).

Abnormalities in carbohydrate metabolism in cancer patients include glucose intolerance and peripheral insulin resistance (74–76). These most often become apparent in the patient with advanced metastatic cancer found to have hyperglycemia, which is refractory to high-dose insulin infusion (77,78). In comparison, in simple starvation, patients are most often euglycemic or hypoglycemic. The hyperglycemia seen in cancer patients is exacerbated by increased hepatic gluconeogenesis. Shaw et al. (79) showed that this increase in glucose production is correlated with tumor burden and decreases after tumor resection.

Lipid metabolism may also be abnormal in patients with a malignancy. There is often increased lipolysis with weight loss, and this leads to a decrease in fat mass, which can be out of proportion to the loss of lean body mass (76). In addition, patients with cancer are often hyperlipidemic, and this may be mediated by TNF-α. In contrast to normal homeostasis, cancer patients fail to suppress lipolysis with glucose infusion (79,80). Several causes of increased lipolysis have been proposed, including decreased food intake, stress response to illness with adrenal medullary stimulation and increased circulating catecholamine levels, insulin resistance, and release of lipolytic factors produced by the tumor itself or by myeloid tissue cells (81). One such factor has been well characterized. Lipid mobilizing factor (LMF), a 24-kDa glycoprotein produced by tumors has been shown to stimulate increased lipid mobilization from adipocytes. LMF is thought to act through binding of β-adrenergic receptors and subsequent upregulation of mitochondrial uncoupling proteins (82,83). Animal studies have shown that LMF causes loss of body weight (specifically a loss of body fat), which is independent of caloric food intake (84). The activity of LMF in the urine and serum of cancer patients has been shown to correlate with the degree of weight loss and tumor burden (85,86). In addition to its effect on lipid metabolism, there is preliminary evidence that LMF may protect tumor cells from free radical toxicity and may therefore make tumors less responsive to certain chemotherapeutic agents that induce oxidative damage (87).

High total body protein turnover, with increased synthesis and catabolism, characterizes the alterations of protein metabolism seen in cancer patients. This results in depletion of muscle mass and loss of nitrogen, and contrasts with the adaptive decrease in protein turnover seen in patients with uncomplicated starvation (88). TPN given to patients with cancer will result in gains of weight and body fat, net gains of total body nitrogen, but no suppression of the high protein flux (88,89). The predominant mechanism of muscle protein loss in cancer patients is an ubiquitin-associated pathway (90). In this pathway, polyubiquitin chains are attached to proteins, which are then recognized and degraded by a proteasome complex. This pathway is regulated, in part, by proteolysis-inducing factor (PIF). PIF is a 24-kDa glycoprotein produced by human tumors and was found in the urine of cancer patients who were losing weight, but not in the urine of cancer patients who were maintaining their weight. In fact, PIF expression directly correlates with the severity of weight loss. There are multiple mechanisms by which PIF induces weight loss. PIF has a direct effect on skeletal muscle by decreasing protein synthesis and increasing protein degradation by upregulating the ubiquitin-proteasome dependent pathway. PIF also increases the expression of pro-inflammatory cytokines (i.e., interleukin-6 and -8), which independently cause weight loss, and induces the shedding of syndecans (transmembrane proteoglycans), which has been shown to be related to increased metastases and mortality (91–93). Effective treatment of the underlying cancer has been shown to reverse ubiquitin-dependent proteolysis of skeletal muscle (94). Better understanding of this process holds the promise of improving therapy to attenuate the loss of protein seen in patients with cancer.

Cytokines also play an important role in inducing metabolic derangements. Interleukin 6 and TNF are released during interaction of host cells with tumor, and high serum levels are present in patients with advanced cancer and cachexia (95–97). They mediate increased energy expenditure, whole body protein turnover, rise in serum triglyceride levels, and high glycerol turnover (98). TNF causes protein wasting, depletion of body fat, and anorexia in animal models by activation of an ATP-dependent proteolytic pathway (95,99). Genetic polymorphisms may result in higher levels of circulating cytokines and a greater degree of weight loss in some patients compared with others (100). Interventions to downregulate these cytokines result in improved appetite, body weight, and quality of life (96).

The combined effects of these wasteful and inefficient alterations in metabolism make it difficult to restore nutritional status in the patient with cancer and cachexia despite the use of specialized nutritional support.

NUTRITIONAL THERAPIES

There are four types of nutritional therapies: parenteral nutrition, enteral nutrition, oral dietary therapy, and drug therapy aimed at improving appetite and food intake. Depending on the patient's condition, nutritional support in the cancer patient has two distinct objectives: (1) provision of nutrition during anticancer therapies to counteract their nutritionally related side effects and improve outcome following these therapies and (2) support in patients with long-term or permanent severe impairment of the gastrointestinal tract. In these patients, nutritional support may be required for indefinite periods of time. Results of numerous clinical trials support the use of nutritional support only in limited situations during anticancer therapies. In the group with prolonged gastrointestinal failure, nutritional support may be a lifesaving therapy because patients could die of starvation without TPN or enteral feeding.

Total Parenteral Nutrition

Total parenteral nutrition is an effective method for delivery of nutrients directly into the blood, and thus overcomes the major causes of cancer-induced weight loss, including decreased food intake and dysfunction of the gastrointestinal tract. Survival for more than 20 years in patients nourished exclusively by TPN clearly demonstrates the lifesaving role of this method of nutritional support. Initially, it seemed logical that TPN would be an effective adjuvant therapy for most cancer patients undergoing radiation therapy, surgery, or chemotherapy because of the accompanying cachexia and inability to eat adequately. Randomized studies, however, have shown that TPN only benefits a select subgroup of cancer patients during anticancer therapy.

Efficacy

In patients receiving chemotherapy with or without radiation therapy, TPN can lead to improvements of several nutritional parameters. Both body weight and body fat increase. Deficits of specific vitamins, minerals, and trace elements can be corrected, and hydration status can be improved (88,101). TPN, however, does not alter many of the metabolic derangements encountered in the cancer patient. Increased glucose oxidation and turnover persist as does muscle proteolysis and increased lipolysis (74,79,102,103). Finally, TPN does not stop the overall losses of body nitrogen (104).

The relevant issue for the clinician is the effect of TPN on the morbidity and mortality associated with cancer therapy and whether TPN can allow more intense therapy, as was initially hoped. Numerous randomized trials have examined this issue. Studies of patients undergoing chemotherapy for carcinoma of the ovary (37), lung (105,106), colon (104), testes (107), lymphoma (108), and other tumors (109) have been conducted. However, the patients in these studies were largely unselected. Many were not malnourished and others had adequate oral intake with intact gastrointestinal function, making intravenous nutrition unnecessary, futile, and potentially harmful. Numerous meta-analyses concluded that nondiscriminatory use of TPN in patients undergoing chemotherapy offers no improvement in mortality, response to chemotherapy, or reduction in treatment-associated complications (110–112). This conclusion was echoed in a consensus statement from the National Institutes of Health, the American Society for Parenteral and Enteral Nutrition, and the American Society for Clinical Nutrition (113). The improvement in nutritional parameters afforded by TPN in patients receiving chemotherapy does not necessarily translate into improved clinical outcome. Thus, the routine use of TPN in these patients is not indicated.

There are circumstances, however, in which nutritional support with parenteral nutrition should be considered. These include prevention of the effects of starvation in a patient unable to tolerate oral or enteral feedings for a prolonged period of time (usually more than 7 to 10 days), maximization of performance status in a malnourished patient prior to chemotherapy or surgery, and in patients undergoing bone marrow transplantation (114). TPN may have a stimulatory effect on tumor cell cycle kinetics (115). It was hoped that this effect would induce improved tumor response to cell cycle–specific chemotherapy. Conclusive proof of such a response remains elusive.

A few randomized studies have examined the use of TPN in patients receiving radiotherapy to the abdomen and pelvis (116,117). The role of TPN in the perioperative period has been extensively studied (118–121). At Memorial Sloan Kettering Cancer Center, a prospective study of 117 patients undergoing curative resection for pancreatic cancer randomized to receive TPN or intravenous fluids in the postoperative period showed no benefit from routine use of postoperative TPN (122). The group receiving TPN had a significant increase in postoperative infectious complications. The largest prospective randomized trial investigating the role of TPN in the perioperative setting was the Veterans Administration Cooperative Study. In this study, 395 patients were randomized to receive 7 to 15 days of preoperative and 3 days of postoperative TPN, or oral feeding plus intravenous fluids. TPN did not improve morbidity or 90-day mortality. However, subgroup analysis showed that patients considered to be severely malnourished had fewer infectious complications if they received TPN. The authors concluded that the routine administration of preoperative TPN should be limited to patients who are severely malnourished, unless there are other specific indications (20).

Randomized studies specifically examining the role of perioperative TPN in patients with gynecologic malignancies are lacking. In a report by Terada (28), perioperative parenteral nutritional support was given to 84 of 99 patients. There were no major complications attributed to TPN, but 27% of the patients experienced minor complications: 11% due to central line placement or catheter sepsis, 2% due to fluid overload, and 13% had metabolic complications. There was no report on overall perioperative morbidity or mortality in comparison to patients who did not receive perioperative TPN.

These data and others provided the basis for a consensus statement from the National Institutes of Health, the American Society for Parenteral and Enteral Nutrition, and the American Society for Clinical Nutrition regarding the use of perioperative TPN, which states the following: (a) 7 to 10 days of preoperative TPN in a malnourished patient with gastrointestinal cancer results in a 10% reduction in postoperative complications; (b) routine use of postoperative TPN in malnourished surgical patients who did not receive preoperative TPN results in a 10% increase in complications; (c) if by postoperative day 5 to 10 a patient is unable to tolerate oral or enteral feedings, then TPN is indicated to prevent the adverse effects of starvation. This panel, however, cautioned that in the majority of studies examining perioperative TPN, the amount and type of parenteral nutrition given was not optimal, and patients were often given excess calories. Therefore, the results may differ with the provision of relatively hypocaloric formulas (113). It is reasonable to extend these recommendations to the gynecologic oncology patient undergoing surgery (**Table 31.1**).

Composition of TPN Solution

Once the decision to proceed with parenteral nutritional support is made, access to a large bore central vein should be obtained. This allows the use of calorically dense, hypertonic solutions, which are often necessary in severely ill patients who may have restriction on the amount of intravenous fluids they can receive. The solution must provide the protein and caloric needs, fluid, minerals, trace elements, and vitamins. Estimates of nutrition requirements are based on weight and adjusted for the degree of physiologic stress encountered by the patient, and there are numerous formulas and charts that provide these. Generally, patients require approximately 30 kcal/kg nonprotein calories, 1 g/kg amino acids, and about 2,000 mL of fluid. As illness severity increases and organs' functions change, adjustments may be required. Nonprotein calories can be provided as dextrose or lipid, and the relative amounts of these should also be individualized. Lipids provide 9 kcal/g compared with 3.4 for dextrose

TABLE 31.1. Indications for TPN in Hospitalized Patients with Gynecologic Cancers

Perioperative	• 7–10 days preoperatively in a malnourished patient (who cannot be fed enterally) • Postoperative complications that prevent oral or enteral intake for more than 7–10 days • Enterocutaneous fistula • *No* indication for routine use
During radiation or chemotherapy	• Maximization of performance status prior to therapy in a malnourished patient who cannot be fed enterally • Severe persistent (more than 7–10 days) mucositis, diarrhea, ileus, or emesis • *No* indication for routine use
General	• After 7–10 days of inability to tolerate oral or enteral feeding due to any cause

(in dextrose solutions, glucose is present as glucose monohydrate; hence, a gram contains less than 4 kcal). Lipid calories are particularly useful in patients who have high caloric requirements but cannot tolerate a large fluid load. In addition, lipids are useful in patients with severe pulmonary or hepatic dysfunction as glucose metabolism produces more carbon dioxide, which can add to the burden of the ailing lung and can lead to fatty infiltration of the liver. Up to 60% of caloric requirements can be provided as lipid, but serum triglyceride levels must be monitored closely. Appropriate electrolyte content of TPN solutions is of critical importance. The amounts have to be tailored to the patient's requirements and organ function. Care must be taken to prevent potentially fatal hypokalemia or hypophosphatemia (particularly in the patient with severe weight loss), which can be precipitated by insulin-induced transport of the minerals to the intracellular space when inadequate amounts are given. Other electrolyte disorders, such as cisplatin-induced hypomagnesemia and syndrome of inappropriate antidiuretic hormone secretion (SIADH), are common in the patient with gynecologic malignancy and must be addressed when ordering TPN. The TPN solution must also contain vitamins, minerals, and trace elements. Typically, these are available as standard commercial combination products. However, certain patients require specific modifications. For example, a patient with persistent diarrhea requires zinc supplementation in excess of the amounts present in standard trace element solutions.

Complications

Complications associated with TPN can be classified as catheter related, metabolic, or infectious. Catheter complications most often occur during placement of a central venous catheter and include pneumothorax, hemothorax, arterial injury, and hematoma. These can all be minimized when the procedure is performed by an experienced physician (123). Cobb et al. reported a 3% incidence of pneumothorax, arrhythmia, thrombus, or bleeding during 523 intravenous catheter placements (124). A more recent study of subcutaneous peripheral infusion ports in women with gynecologic malignancies demonstrated a thrombosis rate of 26% during a mean follow-up of 105 days. The authors concluded that other types of vascular access devices may be preferable in this patient population (125). Another study demonstrated a higher rate of catheter-related infections in patients with external central venous catheters compared with subcutaneous infusion ports (126).

Metabolic derangements are frequently encountered during support with TPN, and the prescribing physician must be well versed in the pathophysiology of these disorders. Hyperglycemia is the most common abnormality, and if not corrected, can lead to an osmotic diuresis, dehydration, acidosis, and hyperosmolar coma. One metabolic complication that deserves special mention is the "refeeding syndrome." In chronically ill patients with severe malnutrition, there is often a depletion of total body phosphorus and potassium. The phosphorous deficits may be masked by increased renal phosphorous absorption designed to maintain normal serum levels. When nutritional support is initiated, the infusion of a large glucose load with subsequent surge in insulin leads to increased cellular uptake of phosphorous and potassium, which may induce severe life-threatening hypokalemia and hypophosphatemia (123,127). These disorders cause widespread tissue and organ dysfunction, including muscle weakness, rhabdomyolysis, heart failure, cardiac arrhythmias, and respiratory failure, and may result in death in extreme cases (127,128). Therefore, in patients with evidence of severe undernutrition, nutrition support should be initiated with small amounts of dextrose calories, supplemental phosphorous and potassium, and careful monitoring of serum phosphorous and electrolytes.

TPN has been associated with cholestatic liver disease, as well as fatty infiltration of the liver and glycogen deposition. These abnormalities have been attributed to infusion of excessive glucose calories, imbalance of amino acids, and rarely, fatty acid deficiency (129). Elevation of serum transaminases may occur, but it is generally mild (129,130). Severe liver dysfunction in adult TPN recipients is rare and requires a search for causes other than TPN.

Infections are particularly serious complications in patients with malignancy receiving TPN. In an evaluation of seven studies comparing TPN plus chemotherapy to chemotherapy alone, Klein and Koretz found four studies that showed an increase in infectious complications in patients receiving TPN (117). A meta-analysis by the American College of Nutrition showed a fourfold increase in infections when patients receiving chemotherapy were given TPN (112). In a prospective, randomized study of TPN following pancreatic resection, recipients of TPN had significantly more infectious complications (122). Data from a VA randomized cooperative study showed that patients with mild-to-moderate malnutrition given perioperative TPN had increased rates of infections, while those with severe malnutrition developed significantly fewer infections when supported with TPN (20). Infectious complications are related to both central venous catheters and a variety of sites (wound infection, abscess, and pneumonia).

Home TPN

Long-term TPN in the home can be a lifesaving treatment in an appropriately selected group of patients. It is clear that cancer patients who have had severe gastrointestinal injury, such as massive intestinal resection or severe radiation enteritis, and in whom the cancer has been cured or is well controlled, benefit from long-term TPN at home (131). A study at the Mayo Clinic examined the outcomes of patients with gynecologic malignancies on home TPN. Inoperable bowel obstruction was the indication for TPN in most of these patients. Quality-of-life parameters, including nausea, vomiting, fatigue, comfort, and morale, significantly improved in patients on home TPN compared with pre-TPN status, especially in those with Karnofsky status > 40 (132). Scolapio described 54 patients treated with home TPN after radiation enteritis. The majority had ovarian cancer, and the main causes of intestinal failure were intestinal obstruction from radiation strictures and short bowel syndrome. Approximately half of the patients initiated TPN within 6 months of completing radiation. Over two-thirds of the patients died due to recurrent cancer. However, survival rates and TPN-related complications were comparable to those in patients with benign diseases like Crohn's disease and intestinal necrosis who required home TPN (133). The role of TPN in advanced or end-stage disease is controversial. For patients with inoperable bowel obstruction due to metastatic ovarian cancer, predicting which patients will benefit from home TPN can be difficult (134). In a review of 9,897 days of home TPN administered to 75 patients with various cancers and intestinal obstruction, it was shown that a Karnofsky performance status greater than 50 at the initiation of TPN could accurately predict which patients would have improved quality of life while on home TPN. The authors concluded that home TPN should be avoided if the performance status is below this level (135). In addition, patients with a life expectancy of less than 2 to 3 months will not benefit from home TPN (103,135). In a study from Yale-New Haven Hospital of 17 patients with inoperable bowel obstruction due to malignancy, patients with ovarian cancer had the shortest survival (39 days) compared to patients with colon cancer (90 days) and appendiceal cancer (184 days) (136). A study from the Mayo Clinic in 52 patients with advanced incurable cancer on home TPN found just two patients with ovarian cancer who survived longer than 12 months (132). A recent study from Brown University evaluated 55 patients with terminal ovarian cancer and found the use of TPN conferred a median survival benefit of 4 weeks (137). Patients on TPN were also more likely to receive concurrent chemotherapy (64% vs. 26%). In another study by Diver et al., 115 women with gynecologic malignancies underwent venting gastrostomy tube placement for malignant bowel obstruction. The median survival of patients receiving TPN was 9.6 weeks versus 4.6 weeks in those not receiving TPN (138).

Currently, the best selection criteria for such patients are a fair or better performance status and the potential for further antitumor therapy (**Table 31.2**). Only a highly selected minority of patients with

TABLE 31.2. Indications for Home TPN in Patients with Gynecological Cancers

- Severe chronic radiation enteropathy
- Short bowel syndrome
- Persistent enterocutaneous fistula
- Selected patients with obstruction due to peritoneal carcinomatosis. (Selection based on performance status and potential for further chemotherapy)

end-stage cancer and inoperable bowel obstruction can potentially benefit from home TPN. There are several quality-of-life and ethical issues to be considered among this group of patients, and more data from randomized controlled trials is required.

Recently developed techniques for placing feeding tubes make it possible to hydrate and feed patients enterally, even in the presence of gastrointestinal obstruction, and thus obviate the need for home TPN in patients with upper gastrointestinal tract dysfunction.

Enteral Nutrition

Enteral feeding delivers a liquid-nutrient formula into the gastrointestinal tract through tubes placed into the stomach or small intestine. As in oral feeding, an adequately functioning small intestinal mucosa is required for absorption of nutrients. Enteral feeding can overcome many difficulties encountered in patients with a wide variety of gastrointestinal tract dysfunction. A proximal gastrointestinal obstruction can be bypassed; tubes can be placed distal to obstructions as far as the jejunum, and thus circumvent obstructing lesions of the oral cavity, esophagus, stomach, duodenum, or proximal jejunum (139,140). The liquid-nutrient formula can be delivered as a slow, continuous infusion, thus maximizing absorption by a limited intestinal surface, which can be overwhelmed by the higher volume delivered during oral feeding. Such an approach may be useful in patients with radiation enteritis, short bowel syndrome (with adequate remaining short bowel, usually 3 to 4 ft.), or partial obstruction of the bowel.

Route of Administration and Nutrient Formula

Short-term (<2 weeks) access to the gastrointestinal tract can be obtained through nasogastric or nasoenteric tubes. Patients requiring longer nutritional support should have a gastrostomy or jejunostomy tube placed endoscopically, radiologically, or surgically. In comparison to nasal tubes, gastrostomy or jejunostomy tubes are wider (15 to 24 Fr) and therefore less likely to be obstructed by medications or nutrient solutions. In addition, they are fixed in the stomach or the upper intestine and do not migrate into the esophagus. Thus, the risk of aspiration is considerably decreased (139). These tubes are more comfortable and aesthetically pleasing. These benefits were demonstrated in a randomized study of patients after an acute dysphagic stroke, which showed patients fed with a gastrostomy tube had more optimal provision of nutrients, achieved a better nutritional state, and had less mortality than those fed with nasogastric tubes (141). Patients with gastrostomy tubes have been shown in prospective studies to receive over 90% of prescribed feedings compared to only 55% in patients fed through nasal tubes. These differences are largely attributed to nasogastric tube dislodgment (142). In a randomized study of 33 women with gynecologic malignancies, enteral feedings through a needle catheter jejunostomy maintained postoperative nutrition as measured by serum transferrin levels and was associated with few complications (143). The authors concluded that women with gynecologic cancers should have a jejunostomy placed at the time of operation if it is anticipated that long-term nutritional support will be required.

Endoscopically placed percutaneous gastrostomy tube (PEG) has become the procedure of choice for placement of enteral feeding tubes because of its ease, safety, and the ability to perform it on an outpatient basis. Percutaneous jejunostomy (PEJ) tubes can also be placed endoscopically (140). PEJs allow for continued enteral feeding in patients with gastric resection, gastric outlet obstruction, or gastroparesis. Major complications (bleeding, peritonitis, abdominal wall abscess, colonic perforation, and aspiration) from PEG and PEJ placement are rare, occurring in 0% to 2.5% of patients, while minor complications (wound infection, tube migrations, or leak) are seen in 5% to 15% (70,140,144). More than 100 different enteral feeding formulas are currently commercially available. They are designed to provide complete nutrition, single nutrients, or only fluids and electrolytes. Formulas differ in protein concentration, calories, osmolarity, and percentage of nonprotein calories delivered as carbohydrates or fats. Enteral feeding formulas, which provide 1,500 to 2,000 kcal/day, normally contain all the necessary nutrients including proteins, vitamins, minerals, and trace elements. In addition, there are disease-specific formulations for patients with diabetes or hepatic, renal, or pulmonary dysfunction. The choice of formula should be individualized, and it often helps to minimize problems such as diarrhea, bloating, or hyperglycemia.

Enteral solutions may be administered by either bolus feedings or continuous infusion. Bolus feeding is possible when the tip of the feeding tube is in an intact stomach. Up to 500 mL of a feeding formula can be infused over 10 to 15 minutes by a syringe or gravity into the stomach. The pyloric sphincter regulates flow into the duodenum. All bolus feedings should be done with the patient sitting upright to minimize the risk of aspiration. When the tip of the feeding tube is distal to the pylorus, continuous feeding must be employed to avoid abdominal distention and diarrhea. Rates as high as 150 mL/hour are generally well tolerated (139).

Efficacy

Data from randomized trials examining the efficacy of enteral nutrition given as an adjuvant therapy in patients receiving chemotherapy for a variety of cancers have failed to demonstrate a clear benefit in terms of survival or response to treatment (145–149). The validity of the conclusions of these studies, however, is limited by their small size and poor design. Similar difficulties plague the studies examining the role of standard enteral nutrition in the perioperative period (150–152). Accepted indications for enteral nutrition in cancer patients include (a) obstruction of the upper digestive tract in those in whom enteral access can be safely obtained beyond the site of obstruction, (b) the presence of chronic malnutrition due to inadequate oral intake, and (c) perioperative support of the malnourished patient (153).

Complications

Enteral nutrition is generally safe if careful attention is paid to the following: (a) choice of an appropriate formula, (b) infusion into an appropriate portion of the gastrointestinal tract, (c) use of the correct infusion method, and (d) an ongoing clinical and metabolic monitoring of the patient. The most serious complication of enteral feeding is aspiration, which occurs in 1% to 32% of patients (145). The risk is minimized by keeping patients upright during bolus feedings and using jejuna feedings if there is predisposition for aspiration, gastroparesis, or an impaired gag reflex. Diarrhea is reported in 5% to 30% of patients receiving enteral nutrition (154). While the diarrhea may be related to underlying disorders of the gastrointestinal tract, such as radiation enteritis or short bowel syndrome, a commonly overlooked cause is medications. Patients on enteral feeding often receive magnesium-containing antacids or antibiotics, both of which may induce diarrhea. Metabolic complications include dehydration, azotemia, hyperglycemia, and hyperkalemia. These are usually due to the patient's underlying disease and can be avoided with the choice of the proper formula and careful monitoring.

Home Enteral Nutrition

Home enteral nutrition (HEN) is increasingly being used to provide nutrients and fluids outside the hospital. Cancer is the most common indication for its use and accounts for 42% of all patients receiving HEN (131). It is a safe therapy in patients with cancer, with only a 0.4% annual rate of complications requiring hospitalization (155). The overall 1-year survival for cancer patients on HEN is 30%. However, in patients with cancer of the head and neck who have been successfully treated, HEN has provided good nutrition for periods exceeding 7 years (70,139). Regular medical follow-up is essential to ensure appropriate functioning of the feeding tube and optimization of the nutrition regimen. This form of therapy is useful in patients with gynecologic malignancies with upper gastrointestinal tract obstructions that cannot be treated surgically.

Oral Dietary Therapy

Patients who are able to eat but have impairment of the gastrointestinal tract or have special metabolic requirements may benefit from a specialized oral dietary therapy. Often, this may obviate the need for more costly and complex interventions such as parenteral nutrition. In oral dietary therapy, the regular diet is modified based on the pathophysiologic changes induced by the underlying disorder, with the goal of providing the most optimal nutrition possible. When the main problem is inadequate food consumption, various commercial oral supplements can be used, but usually for only short periods because of taste fatigue. Some preparations provide complete nutrition, while others are intended to supplement deficits of specific nutrients. Problems common in patients with gynecologic malignancies, such as partial small bowel obstruction, chronic radiation enteritis, and short bowel syndrome, may all be amenable to dietary therapies. In partial small bowel obstruction or motility dysfunction, a diet comprised of frequent, small, calorically dense meals with minimal amounts of fiber is indicated. Patients with radiation enteritis should receive a low-fat, low-fiber, and lactose-free diet. Dietary management of short bowel syndrome patients includes frequent small meals; limitation of fiber, lactose, and simple sugars; taking liquids separately from meals; and supplementation of calcium and zinc orally and magnesium and vitamin B_{12} parenterally.

Bye et al. (156) conducted a prospective, randomized trial of a low-fat, low-lactose diet in 143 women with gynecologic malignancies undergoing radiation therapy. The intervention group had significantly less diarrhea. Diarrhea in the control group correlated with increased fatigue and decreased physical function. The authors concluded that diet intervention during radiotherapy reduced the severity of diarrhea, influenced patients' ability to cope with diarrhea, and gave them more control over their situation.

The successful implementation of prescribed diets depends to a large extent on a dietician converting the prescribed diet to a meal plan and working with the patient to implement it. In a prospective, randomized study of 57 patients undergoing chemotherapy for ovarian, breast, or lung cancer, those who received intensive dietary counseling had improved long-term food intake (157). Similar data have been demonstrated in cancer patients undergoing radiotherapy (158) and in patients with acute leukemia undergoing induction chemotherapy (159).

Postoperative Timing of Oral Feeding

Traditionally, concern for postoperative ileus and impaired bowel function have led to delayed feeding after abdominal surgery. In a prospective randomized trial at the University of Indiana, patients undergoing major gynecologic abdominal surgery were randomized into two groups, the first was advanced to a regular diet after return of bowel sounds and passage of flatus, and the second was fed on the first postoperative day with liquids and then advanced to a solid diet. Early feeding was associated with shorter time to tolerance of a solid diet and shorter duration of hospital stay, but a higher incidence of postoperative emesis (160). Subsequent studies in patients with gynecologic malignancies undergoing abdominal surgery have shown similar results, with quicker recovery of intestinal function, reduced postoperative wound complications, improved quality-of-life scores, and shorter duration of hospital stay in those fed early after surgery (161–163).

Postoperative Immunonutrition

Nutrients such as arginine, glutamine, omega-3 fatty acids, and nucleotides are thought to enhance the immune response, modulate inflammation, and improve protein synthesis after surgery. They are added to enteral formulas or oral diets to improve postoperative wound healing and recovery. Two large meta-analyses have examined the benefits of immunonutrition in the perioperative period in patients undergoing major abdominal surgery. The majority of these patients had gastrointestinal malignancies. There was a reduced rate of infectious complications including abdominal abscesses, pneumonia, and wound infections, as well as noninfectious complications, including anastomotic leaks, in the group receiving immunonutrition. No differences in overall mortality were found among the two groups (164). These findings were supported by a recent study in gynecologic oncology patients at UCSF undergoing laparotomy, given an immune-modulated diet in the perioperative period. Patients receiving immune-modulated diets had lower incidence of wound complications (19.6% vs. 33%), leading the authors to conclude that an immune-modulated diet may be protective for the development of surgical site infections (165). A dose of 0.5 to 1 liter/day for 5 to 7 days prior to surgery is recommended (166). A study in patients with colorectal cancer found an increase in tumor infiltrating CD4 and CD 8 cells after they were given immune nutrition. The authors hypothesized that immune nutrients may reduce infections and exert antitumor effects by this mechanism (167). Current ESPEN guidelines recommend perioperative immunonutrition for patients undergoing upper gastrointestinal surgery, but no recommendations exist for patients with gynecologic malignancies. ASPEN guidelines recommend its use even among critically ill postoperative patients (168).

Pharmacologic Agents

Agents that will reverse the wasting seen in advanced cancers have long been sought to complement or replace the provision of nutrients via the oral, enteral, or parenteral route. Hormones, appetite stimulants, and most recently, cytokine antagonists have been examined. Studies of growth hormone IGF-I alone or IGF-I with insulin in cancer-bearing rodent models showed significant attenuation of tumor-induced weight loss. In human clinical trials, these agents provided modest gain in weight but no improvement in quality of life or other benefits (169–171).

Hormones

Ghrelin, a potent orexigenic peptide hormone produced by the stomach, has been shown to increase appetite and caloric intake in normal individuals and in animal models of cancer cachexia. It was therefore hypothesized that ghrelin may be an effective treatment for cancer-induced cachexia. One small randomized study showed that intravenous ghrelin led to a marked increase in energy and caloric intake, with no side effects (172). There was concern that its use would be limited by its promotion of cellular proliferation and invasion of certain types of cancer, but a randomized, placebo-controlled, double-blind, double cross-over study demonstrated that ghrelin was safe and well tolerated. Unfortunately, it did not show any change in nutritional intake (173).

Appetite Stimulants

Anabolic steroids have no proven efficacy in treating cancer cachexia. In a murine model, administration of norandrolone propionate resulted in weight gain, but this was largely due to fluid retention (174). In human trials, steroids produced transient improvement of nutritional parameters and appetite, but continued use is associated with negative nitrogen balance, net calcium loss, glucose intolerance, and immunosuppression (171).

Megestrol acetate is a progestational agent that has been shown to improve appetite and ameliorate weight loss in numerous, but not all, studies of patients with cancer and cachexia (171). Doses in these studies ranged from 160 to 1,200 mg/day, and maximal weight gain was generally seen within 8 weeks. However, the change in weight is largely due to increased adipose tissue and edema (175). Nevertheless, improvement in quality of life has consistently been demonstrated in several large prospective studies in patients with cancer cachexia treated with megestrol acetate (176,177). It is generally well tolerated but can exacerbate underlying diabetes mellitus, increase thrombotic risk, and rarely lead to adrenal suppression. Dronabinol, a marijuana derivative, has shown some promise in small studies, improving appetite and causing weight gain; however, large randomized trials are lacking (171).

Cytokine Inhibitors

Inhibitors of cytokines involved in cancer cachexia and anorexia have the potential to be potent agents in the treatment of malnutrition in cancer. Monoclonal antibodies against TNF lead to improved food intake and diminished loss of protein and fat in murine models of cancer cachexia. Similar data are available for anti-IL-6 (178,179) and anti-IFN-γ. Suramin, a direct IL-6 receptor antagonist, decreased several key parameters of cachexia in tumor-bearing mice (180). In a recent study from Japan, a novel inhibitor of IL-1 and TNF-α showed that direct injection of the drug into tumor did not alter tumor growth but did result in attenuation of loss of body weight and epididymal fat in tumor-bearing mice (181). Human studies utilizing the anticytokine approach are limited. Pentoxifylline and thalidomide have been shown to inhibit TNF-*a*. In two small studies, thalidomide at a dose of 200 mg daily attenuated loss of weight and lean body mass in patients with esophageal and pancreatic cancer (182,183). Interestingly, recent data showed that the clinical anticachexia effects of megestrol acetate are due, at least in part, to the inhibition of cytokines (96) (**Table 31.3**). COX-2 inhibitors like Ibuprofen and celecoxib have been studied for their ability to attenuate the acute-phase response in patients with advanced cancer. However, the data from these studies has remained largely inconclusive (184,185).

In a recent study, Mantovani et al. showed that combination therapy with megestrol acetate, eicosapentaenoic acid, thalidomide, and L-carnitine increased lean body mass and appetite and decreased resting energy expenditure and fatigue in patients with cancer cachexia (186).

Elemental Supplements and Vitamins

A few preclinical and clinical studies have examined the role of elemental supplements, administered in liquid or powder form, in mitigating the gastrointestinal symptoms following pelvic radiation. However, these supplements are poorly tolerated and have not proven to be of benefit so far (187,188). Antioxidant vitamins such as vitamins C and E have proven to be of some benefit in ischemic reperfusion injury (189). In a study by Kennedy, 20 patients with severe symptomatic radiation proctitis were given vitamins C and E for 4 weeks. The group receiving vitamin supplementation had improvement in diarrhea, bleeding, and fecal urgency (190). Some trials have examined the effect of combined omega-3 fatty acids, especially eicosapentaenoic acid, and vitamin E in cancer cachexia. However, there is still insufficient evidence to support their use (191,192).

Drugs to Relieve Symptoms

The use of medications to relieve cancer- or treatment-related symptoms that impair oral intake is an important adjuvant to nutritional support in these patients. For example, optimal antiemetic therapy can now adequately control acute and delayed emesis in 70% to 90% of patients (193). Despite this, the incidence of chemotherapy-induced nausea and emesis is underestimated by oncologists and nurses (194). This highlights the importance of a careful history and review of systems when completing a nutritional evaluation of a cancer patient. Many cancer patients assume that nausea and vomiting are normal during treatment and will not report it as a problem unless specifically asked.

ETHICAL CONSIDERATIONS

Prior to the advent of enteral and parenteral feedings, the inability to receive nutrients through oral intake inevitably led to wasting and death. Therefore, in the majority of patients, the natural history of cancer led to death because of dehydration and starvation. In patients with potentially curable or stable disease, nutritional support, when indicated, is an important and often critical part of the overall treatment plan. On the other hand, the role of nutritional support in the terminally ill is a subject filled with ethical and legal dilemmas. These problems come to light when the wishes of the patient or the patient's representative are not in agreement with the recommendations of the physicians. For example, a patient

TABLE 31.3. Pharmacologic Agents Used for the Treatment of Cancer Cachexia and Anorexia

Class of Agent	Example	Efficacy	Adverse Effects
Hormones	Insulin, IGF, GH	Attenuation of tumor-induced weight loss, *no* improvement in survival or quality of life demonstrated	Hypoglycemia, Hypokalemia
Anabolic steroids	Oxandrolone, nandrolone	Transient improvement in appetite	Fluid retention, Net loss of calcium and nitrogen, Hyperglycemia, Immunosuppression
Progestational agents	Megestrol acetate	Improved appetite, weight, and quality of life	Weight gain is mostly due to fluid retention and adipose tissue, May exacerbate diabetes mellitus, Rare cases of adrenal insufficiency
Cannabinoids	Dronabinol	Improved appetite and weight gain in small studies	CNS effects (slurred speech, nausea, dizziness, sedation)
Cytokine inhibitors	Pentoxifylline, thalidomide, suramin monoclonal antibodies to IL-1, IL-6, and TNF-α	Improved food intake and attenuation of protein and lean body mass loss	Peripheral neuropathy Rash Daytime somnolence

CNS, central nervous system.

may wish to forego nutritional support despite recommendations that such a therapy should be given. Alternatively, patients or their representatives may want to initiate or continue TPN even after all anticancer therapies have failed and the patient is in a terminal state. Two general principles apply: in the first case, autonomy, and in the second, medical futility.

Autonomy is the right of competent patients to make decisions over their care and implies that the physician must solicit these decisions. It was not until the mid-1960s that autonomy began to supersede the Hippocratic tradition with its emphasis on the authoritarian role of the physician. This principle is clearly outlined in a report from the President's Commission for the study of Ethical Problems in Medicine and Biomedical and Behavioral Research, which states: "The voluntary choice of a competent and informed patient should determine whether or not life-sustaining therapy will be undertaken, while health care institutions and professionals should try to enhance patients' abilities to make decisions on their own and to promote understanding of the available options" (195). With regard to most treatments (surgery, chemotherapy, radiation therapy), the patient's knowledge and experience may be very limited, and thus, the physician's recommendations may form the sole basis for the patient's decisions. This is often not the case with nutrition. People understand the role of nutrition in sustaining life, and it is often hard for a lay person to understand why parenteral nutrition may not be indicated or even harmful when the patient has no other source of nourishment.

The principle of medical futility often surfaces in discussion of nutritional support of the cancer patient, especially if the disease is advanced and unresponsive to therapy. There are four aspects to medical futility (196): (1) lack of physiologic rationale for the proposed therapy; (2) failure of the same therapy in a previous attempt; (3) all possible treatments for the underlying disease have failed; (4) the therapy will not improve quality of life or achieve a goal of care (such as living to see a particular life event). In the case of parenteral (and rarely enteral) nutritional support of the cancer patient, aspects 3 and 4 may be specifically applicable.

It should be noted that these principles, autonomy and medical futility, should govern decisions for both initiation and withdrawal of an ongoing therapy.

Religious beliefs often strongly influence decisions regarding nutritional support. Publicly stated opinions on the subject include: (1) a statement from the Archbishop of Canterbury that removal from life support was permitted if it was better to allow the patient to die (197); (2) a papal statement from Pope John Paul II in 2004 concluded that "Artificial nutrition was ordinary and proportionate, and as such morally obligatory" as long as it obtains the goals of "providing nourishment to the patient" and "alleviating suffering." While this statement referred specifically to the provision of artificial nutrition in persistent vegetative states, the same principles may be applied to other end-of-life situations (198), and (3) a review of Orthodox Jewish rabbinical decisions that concluded "the imperative to preserve life supersedes, with a few exceptions, quality of life considerations" (199).

The decision to withhold or withdraw parenteral nutrition should involve an explanation that dying patients experience less hunger and thirst and that dehydration may even alleviate symptoms like choking or drowning sensation from secretions, coughing, nausea, and vomiting (200,201). The potential harmful effects of artificial nutrition support, including electrolyte abnormalities, infection, and fluid overload, should also be discussed. Ultimately, the end decision must remain with the patient or his/her surrogate. The American Dietetic association position paper on artificial nutrition and hydration in the terminally ill states "The patient's expressed desire is the primary guide for determining the extent of nutrition and hydration", emphasizing the principle of autonomy (202).

Legally and ethically, an informed adult with the capacity to make decisions has the right to ask for artificial nutrition support to be withheld, even if such a decision results in death. For the gynecologic oncologist, management of the patient with an inoperable bowel obstruction due to peritoneal carcinomatosis is a difficult and recurrent problem. A recent review attempted to outline the role of parenteral nutrition in this population (134). TPN should be considered in only those patients with a good performance status, and careful attention must be paid to medical and symptomatic outcomes, as well as ethical considerations. It is interesting to note the views of patients on various life-sustaining treatments. In a study from the University of Michigan, 90% of women undergoing treatment for a gynecologic cancer could envision a time when they would refuse ventilator support, but only 37% could foresee a time when they would refuse artificial nutrition (203). It is important for the physician and other members of the health care team to inform the patient and the family that in the terminally ill, provision of food and water by enteral or parenteral routes will not improve comfort (204) and, in fact, may add to discomfort (203–206). At Memorial Sloan Kettering Cancer Center, TPN is used infrequently in patients with gynecologic cancer and bowel obstruction due to malignant carcinomatosis who do not receive any further anticancer therapy. TPN is used under these conditions only when it is judged that it will enhance the quality of life of a patient who is not at imminent risk of dying in spite of widely metastatic disease. When considering the chance of improving quality of life, the burden of TPN administration and monitoring and the risk of complications must be considered.

REFERENCES

1. Trosian MJ. Nutritional assessment. In: Kaminski ME, ed. *Hyperalimentation: A Guide for Clinicians*. New York, NY: Marcel Dekker; 1985:47.
2. Kuroki LM, Mangano M, Allsworth JE, et al. Pre-operative assessment of muscle mass to predict surgical complications and prognosis in patients with endometrial cancer. *Ann Surg Oncol*. 2015;22(3):972–979. doi:10.1245/s10434-014-4040-8.
3. Nixon DW, Heymsfield SB, Cohen AE, et al. Protein-calorie undernutrition in hospitalized cancer patients. *Am J Med*. 1980;68(5):683–690. http://www.ncbi.nlm.nih.gov/pubmed/6769330. Accessed March 6, 2016.
4. Dowd PS, Heatley RV. The influence of undernutrition on immunity. *Clin Sci (Lond)*. 1984;66(3):241–248. http://www.ncbi.nlm.nih.gov/pubmed/6420109. Accessed March 6, 2016.
5. Meakins JL, Christou NV, Shizgal HM, et al. Therapeutic approaches to anergy in surgical patients. Surgery and levamisole. *Ann Surg*. 1979;190(3):286–296. http://www.pubmedcentral.nih.gov/articlerender.fcgi?artid=1344654&tool=pmcentrez&rendertype=abstract. Accessed March 6, 2016.
6. Mullen JL, Buzby GP, Waldman MT, et al. Prediction of operative morbidity and mortality by preoperative nutritional assessment. *Surg Forum*. 1979;30:80–82. http://www.ncbi.nlm.nih.gov/pubmed/538705. Accessed March 6, 2016.
7. Buzby GP, Mullen JL, Matthews DC, et al. Prognostic nutritional index in gastrointestinal surgery. *Am J Surg*. 1980;139(1):160–167. http://www.ncbi.nlm.nih.gov/pubmed/7350839. Accessed March 6, 2016.
8. Baker JP, Detsky AS, Wesson DE, et al. Nutritional assessment: a comparison of clinical judgement and objective measurements. *N Engl J Med*. 1982;306(16):969–972. doi:10.1056/NEJM198204223061606.
9. Detsky AS, Baker JP, O'Rourke K, et al. Predicting nutrition-associated complications for patients undergoing gastrointestinal surgery. *JPEN J Parenter Enteral Nutr*. 1987;11(5):440–446. http://www.ncbi.nlm.nih.gov/pubmed/3656631. Accessed March 6, 2016.
10. Crowe PJ, Snyman AM, Dent DM, et al. Assessing malnutrition in gastric carcinoma: bioelectrical impedance or clinical impression? *Aust N Z J Surg*. 1992;62(5):390–393. http://www.ncbi.nlm.nih.gov/pubmed/1575661. Accessed March 6, 2016.
11. Ottow RT, Bruining HA, Jeekel J. Clinical judgment versus delayed hypersensitivity skin testing for the prediction of postoperative sepsis and mortality. *Surg Gynecol Obstet*. 1984;159(5):475–477. http://www.ncbi.nlm.nih.gov/pubmed/6495145. Accessed March 6, 2016.
12. Pettigrew RA, Hill GL. Indicators of surgical risk and clinical judgement. *Br J Surg*. 1986;73(1):47–51. http://www.ncbi.nlm.nih.gov/pubmed/3947877. Accessed March 6, 2016.
13. Detsky AS, Baker JP, Mendelson RA, et al. Evaluating the accuracy of nutritional assessment techniques applied to hospitalized patients: methodology and comparisons. *JPEN J Parenter Enteral Nutr*. 1984;8(2):153–159. http://www.ncbi.nlm.nih.gov/pubmed/6538911. Accessed March 7, 2016.

14. Gupta D, Lammersfeld CA, Vashi PG, et al. Can subjective global assessment of nutritional status predict survival in ovarian cancer? *J Ovarian Res*. 2008;1(1):5. doi:10.1186/1757-2215-1-5.
15. Phippen NT, Lowery WJ, Barnett JC, et al. Evaluation of the Patient-Generated Subjective Global Assessment (PG-SGA) as a predictor of febrile neutropenia in gynecologic cancer patients receiving combination chemotherapy: a pilot study. *Gynecol Oncol*. 2011;123(2):360–364. doi:10.1016/j.ygyno.2011.07.093.
16. Laky B, Janda M, Cleghorn G, et al. Comparison of different nutritional assessments and body-composition measurements in detecting malnutrition among gynecologic cancer patients. *Am J Clin Nutr*. 2008;87(6):1678–1685. http://www.ncbi.nlm.nih.gov/pubmed/18541556. Accessed March 6, 2016.
17. Dewys WD, Begg C, Lavin PT, et al. Prognostic effect of weight loss prior to chemotherapy in cancer patients. Eastern Cooperative Oncology Group. *Am J Med*. 1980;69(4):491–497. http://www.ncbi.nlm.nih.gov/pubmed/7424938. Accessed March 6, 2016.
18. Lanzotti VJ, Thomas DR, Boyle LE, et al. Survival with inoperable lung cancer: an integration of prognostic variables based on simple clinical criteria. *Cancer*. 1977;39(1):303–313. http://www.ncbi.nlm.nih.gov/pubmed/832246. Accessed March 6, 2016.
19. Ollenschläger G, Viell B, Thomas W, et al. Tumor anorexia: causes, assessment, treatment. *Recent results cancer Res Fortschritte der Krebsforsch Progrès dans les Rech sur le cancer*. 1991;121:249–259. http://www.ncbi.nlm.nih.gov/pubmed/1857862. Accessed March 7, 2016.
20. Perioperative total parenteral nutrition in surgical patients. The veterans affairs total parenteral nutrition cooperative study group. *N Engl J Med*. 1991;325(8):525–532. doi:10.1056/NEJM199108223250801.
21. Santoso JT, Canada T, Latson B, et al. Prognostic nutritional index in relation to hospital stay in women with gynecologic cancer. *Obstet Gynecol*. 2000;95(6 pt 1):844–846. http://www.ncbi.nlm.nih.gov/pubmed/10831978. Accessed March 6, 2016.
22. Tunca JC. Nutritional evaluation of gynecologic cancer patients during initial diagnosis of their disease. *Am J Obstet Gynecol*. 1983;147(8):893–896. http://www.ncbi.nlm.nih.gov/pubmed/6418009. Accessed March 17, 2016.
23. Orr JW, Wilson K, Bodiford C, et al. Nutritional status of patients with untreated cervical cancer. I. Biochemical and immunologic assessment. *Am J Obstet Gynecol*. 1985;151(5):625–631. http://www.ncbi.nlm.nih.gov/pubmed/3919584. Accessed March 6, 2016.
24. Orr JW, Wilson K, Bodiford C, et al. Nutritional status of patients with untreated cervical cancer. II. Vitamin assessment. *Am J Obstet Gynecol*. 1985;151(5):632–635. http://www.ncbi.nlm.nih.gov/pubmed/3919585. Accessed March 6, 2016.
25. Orr JW, Wilson K, Bodiford C, et al. Corpus and cervix cancer: a nutritional comparison. *Am J Obstet Gynecol*. 1985;153(7):775–779. http://www.ncbi.nlm.nih.gov/pubmed/3934976. Accessed March 7, 2016.
26. Warren RS, Starnes HF, Gabrilove JL, et al. The acute metabolic effects of tumor necrosis factor administration in humans. *Arch Surg*. 1987;122(12):1396–1400. http://www.ncbi.nlm.nih.gov/pubmed/3689116. Accessed March 7, 2016.
27. Dempsey DT, Mullen JL, Buzby GP. The link between nutritional status and clinical outcome: can nutritional intervention modify it? *Am J Clin Nutr*. 1988;47(2 suppl):352–356. http://www.ncbi.nlm.nih.gov/pubmed/3124596. Accessed March 7, 2016.
28. Terada KY, Christen C, Roberts JA. Parenteral nutrition in gynecology. *J Reprod Med*. 1988;33(12):957–960. http://www.ncbi.nlm.nih.gov/pubmed/3145977. Accessed March 7, 2016.
29. Geisler JP, Linnemeier GC, Thomas AJ, et al. Nutritional assessment using prealbumin as an objective criterion to determine whom should not undergo primary radical cytoreductive surgery for ovarian cancer. *Gynecol Oncol*. 2007;106(1):128–131. doi:10.1016/j.ygyno.2007.03.008.
30. Donato D, Angelides A, Irani H, et al. Infectious complications after gastrointestinal surgery in patients with ovarian carcinoma and malignant ascites. *Gynecol Oncol*. 1992;44(1):40–47. http://www.ncbi.nlm.nih.gov/pubmed/1730424. Accessed March 28, 2016.
31. Díaz-Montes TP, Zahurak ML, Bristow RE. Predictors of extended intensive care unit resource utilization following surgery for ovarian cancer. *Gynecol Oncol*. 2007;107(3):464–468. doi:10.1016/j.ygyno.2007.07.074.
32. Kondrup J, Rasmussen HH, Hamberg O, et al. Nutritional risk screening (NRS 2002): a new method based on an analysis of controlled clinical trials. *Clin Nutr*. 2003;22(3):321–336. http://www.ncbi.nlm.nih.gov/pubmed/12765673. Accessed December 1, 2015.
33. Hertlein L, Kirschenhofer A, Fürst S, et al. Malnutrition and clinical outcome in gynecologic patients. *Eur J Obstet Gynecol Reprod Biol*. 2014;174:137–140. doi:10.1016/j.ejogrb.2013.12.028.
34. Uppal S, Al-Niaimi A, Rice LW, et al. Preoperative hypoalbuminemia is an independent predictor of poor perioperative outcomes in women undergoing open surgery for gynecologic malignancies. *Gynecol Oncol*. 2013;131(2):416–422. doi:10.1016/j.ygyno.2013.08.011.
35. Gupta D, Lis CG, Vashi PG, et al. Impact of improved nutritional status on survival in ovarian cancer. *Support Care Cancer*. 2010;18(3):373–381. doi:10.1007/s00520-009-0670-y.
36. Fearon K, Strasser F, Anker SD, et al. Definition and classification of cancer cachexia: an international consensus. *Lancet Oncol*. 2011;12(5):489–495. doi:10.1016/S1470-2045(10)70218-7.
37. Abu-Rustum NR, Barakat RR, Venkatraman E, et al. Chemotherapy and total parenteral nutrition for advanced ovarian cancer with bowel obstruction. *Gynecol Oncol*. 1997;64(3):493–495. doi:10.1006/gyno.1996.4605.
38. Jong P, Sturgeon J, Jamieson CG. Benefit of palliative surgery for bowel obstruction in advanced ovarian cancer. *Can J Surg*. 1995;38(5):454–457. http://www.ncbi.nlm.nih.gov/pubmed/7553472. Accessed March 7, 2016.
39. Norton JA, Moley JF, Green MV, et al. Parabiotic transfer of cancer anorexia/cachexia in male rats. *Cancer Res*. 1985;45(11 pt 1):5547–5552. http://www.ncbi.nlm.nih.gov/pubmed/3863707. Accessed March 7, 2016.
40. DeWys WD. Anorexia as a general effect of cancer. *Cancer*. 1979;43(5 suppl):2013–2019. http://www.ncbi.nlm.nih.gov/pubmed/376105. Accessed March 7, 2016.
41. DeWys WD, Walters K. Abnormalities of taste sensation in cancer patients. *Cancer*. 1975;36(5):1888–1896. http://www.ncbi.nlm.nih.gov/pubmed/1192373. Accessed March 7, 2016.
42. Trant AS, Serin J, Douglass HO. Is taste related to anorexia in cancer patients? *Am J Clin Nutr*. 1982;36(1):45–58. http://www.ncbi.nlm.nih.gov/pubmed/6953761. Accessed March 7, 2016.
43. Carson JA, Gormican A. Taste acuity and food attitudes of selected patients with cancer. *J Am Diet Assoc*. 1977;70(4):361–365. http://www.ncbi.nlm.nih.gov/pubmed/845347. Accessed March 7, 2016.
44. Bernstein IL. Neutral mediation of food aversions and anorexia induced by tumor necrosis factor and tumors. *Neurosci Biobehav Rev*. 1996;20(1):177–181. http://www.ncbi.nlm.nih.gov/pubmed/8622825. Accessed March 7, 2016.
45. Bernstein IL, Taylor EM, Bentson KL. TNF-induced anorexia and learned food aversions are attenuated by area postrema lesions. *Am J Physiol*. 1991;260(5 pt 2):R906–R910. http://www.ncbi.nlm.nih.gov/pubmed/2035702. Accessed March 7, 2016.
46. Burnett AF, Potkul RK, Barter JF, et al. Colonic surgery in gynecologic oncology. Risk factor analysis. *J Reprod Med*. 1993;38(2):137–141. http://www.ncbi.nlm.nih.gov/pubmed/8445606. Accessed March 7, 2016.
47. Orr JW, Shingleton HM, Hatch KD, et al. Gastrointestinal complications associated with pelvic exenteration. *Am J Obstet Gynecol*. 1983;145(3):325–332. http://www.ncbi.nlm.nih.gov/pubmed/6824022. Accessed March 7, 2016.
48. Turtel PS, Shike M. Diseases of the small bowel. In: Shils ME, Olsen JA, SM, ed. *Modern Nutrition in Health and Disease*. 9th Ed. Philadelphia, PA: Lippincott Williams & Wilkins.
49. Scarantino CW, Ornitz RD, Hoffman LG, et al. On the mechanism of radiation-induced emesis: the role of serotonin. *Int J Radiat Oncol Biol Phys*. 1994;30(4):825–830. http://www.ncbi.nlm.nih.gov/pubmed/7525517. Accessed March 7, 2016.
50. Bodis S, Alexander E, Kooy H, et al. The prevention of radiosurgery-induced nausea and vomiting by ondansetron: evidence of a direct effect on the central nervous system chemoreceptor trigger zone. *Surg Neurol*. 1994;42(3):249–252. http://www.ncbi.nlm.nih.gov/pubmed/7940114. Accessed March 7, 2016.
51. Sedgwick DM, Howard GC, Ferguson A. Pathogenesis of acute radiation injury to the rectum. A prospective study in patients. *Int J Colorectal Dis*. 1994;9(1):23–30. http://www.ncbi.nlm.nih.gov/pubmed/8027619. Accessed March 7, 2016.
52. Kinsella TJ, Bloomer WD. Tolerance of the intestine to radiation therapy. *Surg Gynecol Obstet*. 1980;151(2):273–284. http://www.ncbi.nlm.nih.gov/pubmed/6996179. Accessed March 7, 2016.
53. Loiudice TA, Lang JA. Treatment of radiation enteritis: a comparison study. *Am J Gastroenterol*. 1983;78(8):481–487. http://www.ncbi.nlm.nih.gov/pubmed/6410908. Accessed March 7, 2016.
54. Libotte F, Autier P, Delmelle M, et al. Survival of patients with radiation enteritis of the small and the large intestine. *Acta Chir Belg*. 1995;95(4 suppl):190–194. http://www.ncbi.nlm.nih.gov/pubmed/8779298. Accessed March 7, 2016.
55. Yeoh E, Horowitz M, Russo A, et al. A retrospective study of the effects of pelvic irradiation for carcinoma of the cervix on gastrointestinal function. *Int J Radiat Oncol Biol Phys*. 1993;26(2):229–237. http://www.ncbi.nlm.nih.gov/pubmed/8491681. Accessed March 7, 2016.
56. Husebye E, Hauer-Jensen M, Kjørstad K, et al. Severe late radiation enteropathy is characterized by impaired motility of proximal small

intestine. *Dig Dis Sci*. 1994;39(11):2341–2349. http://www.ncbi.nlm.nih.gov/pubmed/7956601. Accessed March 7, 2016.

57. Danielsson A, Nyhlin H, Persson H, et al. Chronic diarrhoea after radiotherapy for gynaecological cancer: occurrence and aetiology. *Gut*. 1991;32(10):1180–1187. http://www.pubmedcentral.nih.gov/articlerender.fcgi?artid=1379382&tool=pmcentrez&rendertype=abstract. Accessed March 7, 2016.
58. Kwitko AO, Pieterse AS, Hecker R, et al. Chronic radiation injury to the intestine: a clinico-pathological study. *Aust N Z J Med*. 1982;12(3):272–277. http://www.ncbi.nlm.nih.gov/pubmed/6956295. Accessed March 7, 2016.
59. Boland E, Thompson J, Rochling F, et al. A 25-year experience with postresection short-bowel syndrome secondary to radiation therapy. *Am J Surg*. 2010;200(6):690–693; discussion 693. doi:10.1016/j.amjsurg.2010.07.035.
60. Curran WJ. Radiation-induced toxicities: the role of radioprotectants. *Semin Radiat Oncol*. 1998;8(4 suppl 1):2–4. http://www.ncbi.nlm.nih.gov/pubmed/9794993. Accessed March 7, 2016.
61. Bajorin D, Kelsen D. Toxicity of antineoplastic therapy. In: Turnbull ADM, ed. *Surgical Emergencies in the Cancer Patient*. Chicago, USA: Year Book Medical Publishers; 1987:14.
62. Mitchell EP, Schein PS. Gastrointestinal toxicity of chemotherapeutic agents. *Semin Oncol*. 1982;9(1):52–64. http://www.ncbi.nlm.nih.gov/pubmed/7071609. Accessed March 7, 2016.
63. Calbresi P, Chabner B. Chemotherapy of neoplastic diseases. In: Gilman AG, Rall TW, Nies AS, et al, eds. *The Pharmacologic Basis of Theraputics*. New York, NY: Pergamon Press; 1990:1201.
64. Steinbach S, Hummel T, Böhner C, et al. Qualitative and quantitative assessment of taste and smell changes in patients undergoing chemotherapy for breast cancer or gynecologic malignancies. *J Clin Oncol*. 2009;27(11):1899–1905. doi:10.1200/JCO.2008.19.2690.
65. Massie MJ. Prevalence of depression in patients with cancer. *J Natl Cancer Inst Monogr*. 2004;(32):57–71. doi:10.1093/jncimonographs/lgh014.
66. Arbeit JM, Lees DE, Corsey R, et al. Resting energy expenditure in controls and cancer patients with localized and diffuse disease. *Ann Surg*. 1984;199(3):292–298. http://www.pubmedcentral.nih.gov/articlerender.fcgi?artid=1353395&tool=pmcentrez&rendertype=abstract. Accessed March 7, 2016.
67. Dempsey DT, Feurer ID, Knox LS, et al. Energy expenditure in malnourished gastrointestinal cancer patients. *Cancer*. 1984;53(6):1265–1273. http://www.ncbi.nlm.nih.gov/pubmed/6692317. Accessed March 7, 2016.
68. Hansell DT, Davies JW, Burns HJ. The relationship between resting energy expenditure and weight loss in benign and malignant disease. *Ann Surg*. 1986;203(3):240–245. http://www.pubmedcentral.nih.gov/articlerender.fcgi?artid=1251083&tool=pmcentrez&rendertype=abstract. Accessed March 7, 2016.
69. Russell DM, Shike M, Marliss EB, et al. Effects of total parenteral nutrition and chemotherapy on the metabolic derangements in small cell lung cancer. *Cancer Res*. 1984;44(4):1706–1711. http://www.ncbi.nlm.nih.gov/pubmed/6322985. Accessed March 7, 2016.
70. Shike M, Berner YN, Gerdes H, et al. Percutaneous endoscopic gastrostomy and jejunostomy for long-term feeding in patients with cancer of the head and neck. *Otolaryngol Head Neck Surg*. 1989;101(5):549–554. http://www.ncbi.nlm.nih.gov/pubmed/2512533. Accessed March 7, 2016.
71. Luketich JD, Mullen JL, Feurer ID, et al. Ablation of abnormal energy expenditure by curative tumor resection. *Arch Surg*. 1990;125(3):337–341. http://www.ncbi.nlm.nih.gov/pubmed/1689565. Accessed March 7, 2016.
72. Gadducci A, Cosio S, Fanucchi A, et al. Malnutrition and cachexia in ovarian cancer patients: pathophysiology and management. *Anticancer Res*. 2001;21(4B):2941–2947. http://www.ncbi.nlm.nih.gov/pubmed/11712791. Accessed March 7, 2016.
73. Dickerson RN, White KG, Curcillo PG, et al. Resting energy expenditure of patients with gynecologic malignancies. *J Am Coll Nutr*. 1995;14(5):448–454. http://www.ncbi.nlm.nih.gov/pubmed/8522723. Accessed March 7, 2016.
74. Holroyde CP, Gabuzda TG, Putnam RC, et al. Altered glucose metabolism in metastatic carcinoma. *Cancer Res*. 1975;35(12):3710–3714. http://www.ncbi.nlm.nih.gov/pubmed/1192429. Accessed March 9, 2016.
75. Holroyde CP, Skutches CL, Boden G, et al. Glucose metabolism in cachectic patients with colorectal cancer. *Cancer Res*. 1984;44(12 pt 1):5910–5913. http://www.ncbi.nlm.nih.gov/pubmed/6388829. Accessed March 9, 2016.
76. Kern KA, Norton JA. Cancer cachexia. *JPEN J Parenter Enteral Nutr*. 1988;12(3):286–298. http://www.ncbi.nlm.nih.gov/pubmed/3292798. Accessed March 9, 2016.
77. Lundholm K, Holm G, Scherstén T. Insulin resistance in patients with cancer. *Cancer Res*. 1978;38(12):4665–4670. http://www.ncbi.nlm.nih.gov/pubmed/719645. Accessed March 9, 2016.
78. Cersosimo E, Pisters PW, Pesola G, et al. The effect of graded doses of insulin on peripheral glucose uptake and lactate release in cancer cachexia. *Surgery*. 1991;109(4):459–467. http://www.ncbi.nlm.nih.gov/pubmed/2008651. Accessed March 9, 2016.
79. Shaw JH, Wolfe RR. Fatty acid and glycerol kinetics in septic patients and in patients with gastrointestinal cancer. The response to glucose infusion and parenteral feeding. *Ann Surg*. 1987;205(4):368–376. http://www.pubmedcentral.nih.gov/articlerender.fcgi?artid=1492741&tool=pmcentrez&rendertype=abstract. Accessed March 9, 2016.
80. Beutler B, Cerami A. Cachectin and tumour necrosis factor as two sides of the same biological coin. *Nature*. 1986;320(6063):584–588. doi:10.1038/320584a0.
81. Klein S, Wolfe RR. Whole-body lipolysis and triglyceride-fatty acid cycling in cachectic patients with esophageal cancer. *J Clin Invest*. 1990;86(5):1403–1408. doi:10.1172/JCI114854.
82. Todorov PT, McDevitt TM, Meyer DJ, et al. Purification and characterization of a tumor lipid-mobilizing factor. *Cancer Res*. 1998;58(11):2353–2358. http://www.ncbi.nlm.nih.gov/pubmed/9622074. Accessed March 9, 2016.
83. Bing C, Russell ST, Beckett EE, et al. Expression of uncoupling proteins-1, -2 and -3 mRNA is induced by an adenocarcinoma-derived lipid-mobilizing factor. *Br J Cancer*. 2002;86(4):612–618. doi:10.1038/sj.bjc.6600101.
84. Russell ST, Zimmerman TP, Domin BA, et al. Induction of lipolysis in vitro and loss of body fat in vivo by zinc-alpha2-glycoprotein. *Biochim Biophys Acta*. 2004;1636(1):59–68. doi:10.1016/j.bbalip.2003.12.004.
85. Groundwater P, Beck SA, Barton C, et al. Alteration of serum and urinary lipolytic activity with weight loss in cachectic cancer patients. *Br J Cancer*. 1990;62(5):816–821. http://www.pubmedcentral.nih.gov/articlerender.fcgi?artid=1971511&tool=pmcentrez&rendertype=abstract. Accessed March 9, 2016.
86. Beck SA, Groundwater P, Barton C, et al. Alterations in serum lipolytic activity of cancer patients with response to therapy. *Br J Cancer*. 1990;62(5):822–825. http://www.pubmedcentral.nih.gov/articlerender.fcgi?artid=1971524&tool=pmcentrez&rendertype=abstract. Accessed March 9, 2016.
87. Sanders PM, Tisdale MJ. Role of lipid-mobilising factor (LMF) in protecting tumour cells from oxidative damage. *Br J Cancer*. 2004;90(6):1274–1278. doi:10.1038/sj.bjc.6601669.
88. Shike M, Russel DM, Detsky AS, et al. Changes in body composition in patients with small-cell lung cancer. The effect of total parenteral nutrition as an adjunct to chemotherapy. *Ann Intern Med*. 1984;101(3):303–309. http://www.ncbi.nlm.nih.gov/pubmed/6087702. Accessed March 9, 2016.
89. Burt ME, Stein TP, Schwade JG, et al. Whole-body protein metabolism in cancer-bearing patients. Effect of total parenteral nutrition and associated serum insulin response. *Cancer*. 1984;53(6):1246–1252. http://www.ncbi.nlm.nih.gov/pubmed/6420040. Accessed March 9, 2016.
90. Hasselgren P-O, Wray C, Mammen J. Molecular regulation of muscle cachexia: it may be more than the proteasome. *Biochem Biophys Res Commun*. 2002;290(1):1–10. doi:10.1006/bbrc.2001.5849.
91. Tisdale MJ. Mechanisms of cancer cachexia. *Physiol Rev*. 2009;89(2):381–410. doi:10.1152/physrev.00016.2008.
92. Falconer JS, Fearon KC, Plester CE, et al. Cytokines, the acute-phase response, and resting energy expenditure in cachectic patients with pancreatic cancer. *Ann Surg*. 1994;219(4):325–331. http://www.pubmedcentral.nih.gov/articlerender.fcgi?artid=1243147&tool=pmcentrez&rendertype=abstract. Accessed March 10, 2016.
93. Cabal-Manzano R, Bhargava P, Torres-Duarte A, et al. Proteolysis-inducing factor is expressed in tumours of patients with gastrointestinal cancers and correlates with weight loss. *Br J Cancer*. 2001;84(12):1599–1601. doi:10.1054/bjoc.2001.1830.
94. Tilignac T, Temparis S, Combaret L, et al. Chemotherapy inhibits skeletal muscle ubiquitin-proteasome-dependent proteolysis. *Cancer Res*. 2002;62(10):2771–2777. http://www.ncbi.nlm.nih.gov/pubmed/12019153. Accessed March 9, 2016.
95. Tracey KJ, Wei H, Manogue KR, et al. Cachectin/tumor necrosis factor induces cachexia, anemia, and inflammation. *J Exp Med*. 1988;167(3):1211–1227. http://www.pubmedcentral.nih.gov/articlerender.fcgi?artid=2188883&tool=pmcentrez&rendertype=abstract. Accessed March 9, 2016.
96. Mantovani G, Macciò A, Lai P, et al. Cytokine activity in cancer-related anorexia/cachexia: role of megestrol acetate and medroxyprogesterone acetate. *Semin Oncol*. 1998;25(2 suppl 6):45–52. http://www.ncbi.nlm.nih.gov/pubmed/9625383. Accessed March 9, 2016.
97. Pfitzenmaier J, Vessella R, Higano CS, et al. Elevation of cytokine levels in cachectic patients with prostate carcinoma. *Cancer*. 2003;97(5):1211–1216. doi:10.1002/cncr.11178.
98. Warren RS, Donner DB, Starnes HF, et al. Modulation of endogenous hormone action by recombinant human tumor necrosis factor. *Proc Natl*

Acad Sci U S A. 1987;84(23):8619–8622. http://www.pubmedcentral.nih.gov/articlerender.fcgi?artid=299597&tool=pmcentrez&rendertype=abstract. Accessed March 9, 2016.

99. Llovera M, García-Martínez C, López-Soriano J, et al. Role of TNF receptor 1 in protein turnover during cancer cachexia using gene knockout mice. *Mol Cell Endocrinol*. 1998;142(1–2):183–189. http://www.ncbi.nlm.nih.gov/pubmed/9783914. Accessed March 10, 2016.
100. Deans DAC, Tan BHL, Ross JA, et al. Cancer cachexia is associated with the IL10 -1082 gene promoter polymorphism in patients with gastroesophageal malignancy. *Am J Clin Nutr*. 2009;89(4):1164–1172. doi:10.3945/ajcn.2008.27025.
101. Lowry SF, Smith JC, Brennan MF. Zinc and copper replacement during total parenteral nutrition. *Am J Clin Nutr*. 1981;34(9):1853–1860. http://www.ncbi.nlm.nih.gov/pubmed/6792897. Accessed March 9, 2016.
102. Jeevanandam M, Horowitz GD, Lowry SF, et al. Cancer cachexia and protein metabolism. *Lancet (London, England)*. 1984;1(8392):1423–1426. http://www.ncbi.nlm.nih.gov/pubmed/6145877. Accessed March 10, 2016.
103. Sharp JW, Roncagli T. Home parenteral nutrition in advanced cancer. *Cancer Pract*. 1993;1(2):119–124. http://www.ncbi.nlm.nih.gov/pubmed/8324537. Accessed March 10, 2016.
104. Nixon DW, Moffitt S, Lawson DH, et al. Total parenteral nutrition as an adjunct to chemotherapy of metastatic colorectal cancer. *Cancer Treat Rep*. 1981;65 suppl 5:121–128. http://www.ncbi.nlm.nih.gov/pubmed/6809321. Accessed March 9, 2016.
105. Serrou B, Cupissol D, Plagne R, et al. Parenteral intravenous nutrition (PIVN) as an adjunct to chemotherapy in small cell anaplastic lung carcinoma. *Cancer Treat Rep*. 1981;65 suppl 5:151–155. http://www.ncbi.nlm.nih.gov/pubmed/6286118. Accessed March 10, 2016.
106. Valdivieso M, Bodey GP, Benjamin RS, et al. Role of intravenous hyperalimentation as an adjunct to intensive chemotherapy for small cell bronchogenic carcinoma. *Cancer Treat Rep*. 1981;65 suppl 5:145–150. http://www.ncbi.nlm.nih.gov/pubmed/6809324. Accessed March 9, 2016.
107. Samuels ML, Selig DE, Ogden S, et al. Iv hyperalimentation and chemotherapy for stage III testicular cancer: a randomized study. *Cancer Treat Rep*. 1981;65(7–8):615–627. http://www.ncbi.nlm.nih.gov/pubmed/6166374. Accessed March 14, 2016.
108. Daly JM, Reynolds J, Thom A, et al. Immune and metabolic effects of arginine in the surgical patient. *Ann Surg*. 1988;208(4):512–523. http://www.pubmedcentral.nih.gov/articlerender.fcgi?artid=1493753&tool=pmcentrez&rendertype=abstract. Accessed March 9, 2016.
109. Fletcher JP, Little JM. A comparison of parenteral nutrition and early postoperative enteral feeding on the nitrogen balance after major surgery. *Surgery*. 1986;100(1):21–24. http://www.ncbi.nlm.nih.gov/pubmed/3088751. Accessed March 9, 2016.
110. Klein S, Simes J, Blackburn GL. Total parenteral nutrition and cancer clinical trials. *Cancer*. 1986;58(6):1378–1386. http://www.ncbi.nlm.nih.gov/pubmed/3091243. Accessed March 9, 2016.
111. McGeer AJ, Detsky AS, O'Rourke K. Parenteral nutrition in cancer patients undergoing chemotherapy: a meta-analysis. *Nutrition*. 1990;6(3):233–240. http://www.ncbi.nlm.nih.gov/pubmed/2152097. Accessed March 9, 2016.
112. Parenteral nutrition in patients receiving cancer chemotherapy. American College of Physicians. *Ann Intern Med*. 1989;110(9):734–736. http://www.ncbi.nlm.nih.gov/pubmed/2494922. Accessed March 14, 2016.
113. Klein S, Kinney J, Jeejeebhoy K, et al. Nutrition support in clinical practice: review of published data and recommendations for future research directions. *Clin Nutr*. 1997;16(4):193–218. http://www.ncbi.nlm.nih.gov/pubmed/16844599. Accessed March 14, 2016.
114. Weisdorf SA, Lysne J, Wind D, et al. Positive effect of prophylactic total parenteral nutrition on long-term outcome of bone marrow transplantation. *Transplantation*. 1987;43(6):833–838. http://www.ncbi.nlm.nih.gov/pubmed/3109088. Accessed March 9, 2016.
115. Baron PL, Lawrence W, Chan WM, et al. Effects of parenteral nutrition on cell cycle kinetics of head and neck cancer. *Arch Surg*. 1986;121(11):1282–1286. http://www.ncbi.nlm.nih.gov/pubmed/3096261. Accessed March 9, 2016.
116. Kinsella TJ, Malcolm AW, Bothe A, et al. Prospective study of nutritional support during pelvic irradiation. *Int J Radiat Oncol Biol Phys*. 1981;7(4):543–548. http://www.ncbi.nlm.nih.gov/pubmed/6166598. Accessed March 9, 2016.
117. Klein S, Koretz RL. Nutrition support in patients with cancer: what do the data really show? *Nutr Clin Pract*. 1994;9(3):91–100. http://www.ncbi.nlm.nih.gov/pubmed/8078449. Accessed March 9, 2016.
118. Detsky AS, Baker JP, O'Rourke K, et al. Perioperative parenteral nutrition: a meta-analysis. *Ann Intern Med*. 1987;107(2):195–203. http://www.ncbi.nlm.nih.gov/pubmed/3111322. Accessed March 9, 2016.
119. Fan ST, Lo CM, Lai EC, et al. Perioperative nutritional support in patients undergoing hepatectomy for hepatocellular carcinoma. *N Engl J Med*. 1994;331(23):1547–1552. doi:10.1056/NEJM199412083312303.
120. Holter AR, Fischer JE. The effects of perioperative hyperalimentation on complications in patients with carcinoma and weight loss. *J Surg Res*. 1977;23(1):31–34. http://www.ncbi.nlm.nih.gov/pubmed/406484. Accessed March 9, 2016.
121. Holter AR, Rosen HM, Fischer JE. The effects of hyperalimentation on major surgery in patients with malignant disease: a prospective study. *Acta Chir Scand Suppl*. 1976;466:86–87. http://www.ncbi.nlm.nih.gov/pubmed/828429. Accessed March 9, 2016.
122. Brennan MF, Pisters PW, Posner M, et al. A prospective randomized trial of total parenteral nutrition after major pancreatic resection for malignancy. *Ann Surg*. 1994;220(4):436–441; discussion 441–444. http://www.pubmedcentral.nih.gov/articlerender.fcgi?artid=1234412&tool=pmcentrez&rendertype=abstract. Accessed March 9, 2016.
123. Weinsier RL, Bacon J, Butterworth CE. Central venous alimentation: a prospective study of the frequency of metabolic abnormalities among medical and surgical patients. *JPEN J Parenter Enteral Nutr* 1982;6(5):421–425. http://www.ncbi.nlm.nih.gov/pubmed/6818370. Accessed March 9, 2016.
124. Cobb DK, High KP, Sawyer RG, et al. A controlled trial of scheduled replacement of central venous and pulmonary-artery catheters. *N Engl J Med*. 1992;327(15):1062–1068. doi:10.1056/NEJM199210083271505.
125. Cunningham MJ, Collins MB, Kredentser DC, et al. Peripheral infusion ports for central venous access in patients with gynecologic malignancies. *Gynecol Oncol*. 1996;60(3):397–399. doi:10.1006/gyno.1996.0061.
126. Estes JM, Rocconi R, Straughn JM, et al. Complications of indwelling venous access devices in patients with gynecologic malignancies. *Gynecol Oncol*. 2003;91(3):591–595. http://www.ncbi.nlm.nih.gov/pubmed/14675682. Accessed March 14, 2016.
127. Weinsier RL, Krumdieck CL. Death resulting from overzealous total parenteral nutrition: the refeeding syndrome revisited. *Am J Clin Nutr*. 1981;34(3):393–399. http://www.ncbi.nlm.nih.gov/pubmed/6782855. Accessed March 14, 2016.
128. Solomon SM, Kirby DF. The refeeding syndrome: a review. *JPEN J Parenter Enteral Nutr*. 1990;14(1):90–97. http://www.ncbi.nlm.nih.gov/pubmed/2109122. Accessed March 9, 2016.
129. Sheldon GF, Peterson SR, Sanders R. Hepatic dysfunction during hyperalimentation. *Arch Surg*. 1978;113(4):504–508. http://www.ncbi.nlm.nih.gov/pubmed/416812. Accessed March 9, 2016.
130. Burt ME, Lowry SF, Gorschboth C, et al. Metabolic alterations in a noncachectic animal tumor system. *Cancer*. 1981;47(9):2138–2146. http://www.ncbi.nlm.nih.gov/pubmed/7226107. Accessed March 9, 2016.
131. Howard L, Ament M, Fleming CR, et al. Current use and clinical outcome of home parenteral and enteral nutrition therapies in the United States. *Gastroenterology*. 1995;109(2):355–365. http://www.ncbi.nlm.nih.gov/pubmed/7615183. Accessed March 9, 2016.
132. Hoda D, Jatoi A, Burnes J, et al. Should patients with advanced, incurable cancers ever be sent home with total parenteral nutrition? A single institution's 20-year experience. *Cancer*. 2005;103(4):863–868. doi:10.1002/cncr.20824.
133. Scolapio JS, Ukleja A, Burnes JU, et al. Outcome of patients with radiation enteritis treated with home parenteral nutrition. *Am J Gastroenterol*. 2002;97(3):662–666. doi:10.1111/j.1572-0241.2002.05546.x.
134. Philip J, Depczynski B. The role of total parenteral nutrition for patients with irreversible bowel obstruction secondary to gynecological malignancy. *J Pain Symptom Manage*. 1997;13(2):104–111. http://www.ncbi.nlm.nih.gov/pubmed/9095568. Accessed March 9, 2016.
135. Cozzaglio L, Balzola F, Cosentino F, et al. Outcome of cancer patients receiving home parenteral nutrition. Italian Society of Parenteral and Enteral Nutrition (S.I.N.P.E.). *JPEN J Parenter Enteral Nutr*. 1997;21(6):339–342. http://www.ncbi.nlm.nih.gov/pubmed/9406131. Accessed March 14, 2016.
136. August DA, Thorn D, Fisher RL, et al. Home parenteral nutrition for patients with inoperable malignant bowel obstruction. *JPEN J Parenter Enteral Nutr*. 1991;15(3):323–327. http://www.ncbi.nlm.nih.gov/pubmed/1907683. Accessed March 9, 2016.
137. Brard L, Weitzen S, Strubel-Lagan SL, et al. The effect of total parenteral nutrition on the survival of terminally ill ovarian cancer patients. *Gynecol Oncol*. 2006;103(1):176–180. doi:10.1016/j.ygyno.2006.02.013.
138. Diver E, O'Connor O, Garrett L, et al. Modest benefit of total parenteral nutrition and chemotherapy after venting gastrostomy tube placement. *Gynecol Oncol*. 2013;129(2):332–335. doi:10.1016/j.ygyno.2013.02.002.
139. Shike M. Enteral feeding. In: Shils ME, Olsen JA, Shike M et al, ed. *Modern Nutrition in Health and Disease*. 9th Ed. Philadelphia, PA: Lippincott Williams & Wilkins; 1999:1643.

140. Shike M, Latkany L. Direct percutaneous endoscopic jejunostomy. *Gastrointest Endosc Clin N Am.* 1998;8(3):569–580. http://www.ncbi.nlm.nih.gov/pubmed/9654569. Accessed March 9, 2016.
141. Norton B, Homer-Ward M, Donnelly MT, et al. A randomised prospective comparison of percutaneous endoscopic gastrostomy and nasogastric tube feeding after acute dysphagic stroke. *BMJ.* 1996;312(7022):13–16. http://www.pubmedcentral.nih.gov/articlerender.fcgi?artid=2349687&tool=pmcentrez&rendertype=abstract. Accessed March 9, 2016.
142. Di Lorenzo C, Lachman R, Hyman PE. Intravenous erythromycin for postpyloric intubation. *J Pediatr Gastroenterol Nutr.* 1990;11(1):45–47. http://www.ncbi.nlm.nih.gov/pubmed/2136585. Accessed March 9, 2016.
143. Spirtos NM, Ballon SC. Needle catheter jejunostomy: a controlled, prospective, randomized trial in patients with gynecologic malignancy. *Am J Obstet Gynecol.* 1988;158(6 pt 1):1285–1290. http://www.ncbi.nlm.nih.gov/pubmed/3132853. Accessed March 15, 2016.
144. Safadi BY, Marks JM, Ponsky JL. Percutaneous endoscopic gastrostomy. *Gastrointest Endosc Clin N Am.* 1998;8(3):551–568. http://www.ncbi.nlm.nih.gov/pubmed/9654568. Accessed March 15, 2016.
145. Strong RM, Condon SC, Solinger MR, et al. Equal aspiration rates from postpylorus and intragastric-placed small-bore nasoenteric feeding tubes: a randomized, prospective study. *JPEN J Parenter Enteral Nutr.* 1992;16(1):59–63. http://www.ncbi.nlm.nih.gov/pubmed/1738222. Accessed March 15, 2016.
146. Elkort RJ, Baker FL, Vitale JJ, et al. Long-term nutritional support as an adjunct to chemotherapy for breast cancer. *JPEN J Parenter Enteral Nutr.* 1981;5(5):385–390. http://www.ncbi.nlm.nih.gov/pubmed/6796711. Accessed March 15, 2016.
147. Evans WK, Nixon DW, Daly JM, et al. A randomized study of oral nutritional support versus ad lib nutritional intake during chemotherapy for advanced colorectal and non-small-cell lung cancer. *J Clin Oncol.* 1987;5(1):113–124. http://www.ncbi.nlm.nih.gov/pubmed/3027267. Accessed March 15, 2016.
148. Bozzetti F. Effects of artificial nutrition on the nutritional status of cancer patients. *JPEN J Parenter Enteral Nutr.* 1989;13(4):406–420. http://www.ncbi.nlm.nih.gov/pubmed/2506378. Accessed March 15, 2016.
149. Bounous G, Gentile JM, Hugon J. Elemental diet in the management of the intestinal lesion produced by 5-fluorouracil in man. *Can J Surg.* 1971;14(5):312–324. http://www.ncbi.nlm.nih.gov/pubmed/4107102. Accessed March 15, 2016.
150. Smith RC, Hartemink RJ, Hollinshead JW, et al. Fine bore jejunostomy feeding following major abdominal surgery: a controlled randomized clinical trial. *Br J Surg.* 1985;72(6):458–461. http://www.ncbi.nlm.nih.gov/pubmed/3926036. Accessed March 15, 2016.
151. Ryan JA, Page CP, Babcock L. Early postoperative jejunal feeding of elemental diet in gastrointestinal surgery. *Am Surg.* 1981;47(9):393–403. http://www.ncbi.nlm.nih.gov/pubmed/6792958. Accessed March 15, 2016.
152. Flynn MB, Leightty FF. Preoperative outpatient nutritional support of patients with squamous cancer of the upper aerodigestive tract. *Am J Surg.* 1987;154(4):359–362. http://www.ncbi.nlm.nih.gov/pubmed/3661837. Accessed March 15, 2016.
153. Kirby DF, Teran JC. Enteral feeding in critical care, gastrointestinal diseases, and cancer. *Gastrointest Endosc Clin N Am.* 1998;8(3):623–643. http://www.ncbi.nlm.nih.gov/pubmed/9654573. Accessed March 15, 2016.
154. Bliss DZ, Guenter PA, Settle RG. Defining and reporting diarrhea in tube-fed patients-what a mess! *Am J Clin Nutr.* 1992;55(3):753–759. http://www.ncbi.nlm.nih.gov/pubmed/1550053. Accessed March 15, 2016.
155. Sherry BA, Gelin J, Fong Y, et al. Anticachectin/tumor necrosis factor-alpha antibodies attenuate development of cachexia in tumor models. *FASEB J.* 1989;3(8):1956–1962. http://www.ncbi.nlm.nih.gov/pubmed/2721856. Accessed March 15, 2016.
156. Bye A, Ose T, Kaasa S. Quality of life during pelvic radiotherapy. *Acta Obstet Gynecol Scand.* 1995;74(2):147–152. http://www.ncbi.nlm.nih.gov/pubmed/7900512. Accessed March 15, 2016.
157. Ovesen L, Allingstrup L, Hannibal J, et al. Effect of dietary counseling on food intake, body weight, response rate, survival, and quality of life in cancer patients undergoing chemotherapy: a prospective, randomized study. *J Clin Oncol.* 1993;11(10):2043–2049. http://www.ncbi.nlm.nih.gov/pubmed/8410128. Accessed March 14, 2016.
158. Maciá E, Moran J, Santos J, et al. Nutritional evaluation and dietetic care in cancer patients treated with radiotherapy: prospective study. *Nutrition.* 1991;7(3):205–209. http://www.ncbi.nlm.nih.gov/pubmed/1802209. Accessed March 14, 2016.
159. Ollenschläger G, Thomas W, Konkol K, et al. Nutritional behaviour and quality of life during oncological polychemotherapy: results of a prospective study on the efficacy of oral nutrition therapy in patients with acute leukaemia. *Eur J Clin Invest.* 1992;22(8):546–553. http://www.ncbi.nlm.nih.gov/pubmed/1425861. Accessed March 14, 2016.
160. Schilder JM, Hurteau JA, Look KY, et al. A prospective controlled trial of early postoperative oral intake following major abdominal gynecologic surgery. *Gynecol Oncol.* 1997;67(3):235–240. doi:10.1006/gyno.1997.4860.
161. Minig L, Biffi R, Zanagnolo V, et al. Reduction of postoperative complication rate with the use of early oral feeding in gynecologic oncologic patients undergoing a major surgery: a randomized controlled trial. *Ann Surg Oncol.* 2009;16(11):3101–3110. doi:10.1245/s10434-009-0681-4.
162. Steed HL, Capstick V, Flood C, et al. A randomized controlled trial of early versus "traditional" postoperative oral intake after major abdominal gynecologic surgery. *Am J Obstet Gynecol.* 2002;186(5):861–865. http://www.ncbi.nlm.nih.gov/pubmed/12015496. Accessed March 15, 2016.
163. Charoenkwan K, Matovinovic E. Early versus delayed oral fluids and food for reducing complications after major abdominal gynaecologic surgery. *Cochrane database Syst Rev.* 2014;12:CD004508. doi:10.1002/14651858.CD004508.pub4.
164. Marik PE, Zaloga GP. Immunonutrition in high-risk surgical patients: a systematic review and analysis of the literature. *JPEN J Parenter Enteral Nutr.* 2010;34(4):378–386. doi:10.1177/0148607110362692.
165. Chapman JS, Roddy E, Westhoff G, et al. Post-operative enteral immunonutrition for gynecologic oncology patients undergoing laparotomy decreases wound complications. *Gynecol Oncol.* 2015;137(3):523–528. doi:10.1016/j.ygyno.2015.04.003.
166. Waitzberg DL, Saito H, Plank LD, et al. Postsurgical infections are reduced with specialized nutrition support. *World J Surg.* 2006;30(8):1592–1604. doi:10.1007/s00268-005-0657-x.
167. Caglayan K, Oner I, Gunerhan Y, et al. The impact of preoperative immunonutrition and other nutrition models on tumor infiltrative lymphocytes in colorectal cancer patients. *Am J Surg.* 2012;204(4):416–421. doi:10.1016/j.amjsurg.2011.12.018.
168. McClave SA, Taylor BE, Martindale RG, et al. Guidelines for the provision and assessment of nutrition support therapy in the adult critically ill patient: Society of Critical Care Medicine (SCCM) and American Society for Parenteral and Enteral Nutrition (A.S.P.E.N.). *JPEN J Parenter Enteral Nutr.* 2016;40(2):159–211. doi:10.1177/0148607115621863.
169. Bartlett DL, Stein TP, Torosian MH. Effect of growth hormone and protein intake on tumor growth and host cachexia. *Surgery.* 1995;117(3):260–267. http://www.ncbi.nlm.nih.gov/pubmed/7878530. Accessed March 14, 2016.
170. Tomas FM, Chandler CS, Coyle P, et al. Effects of insulin and insulin-like growth factors on protein and energy metabolism in tumour-bearing rats. *Biochem J.* 1994;301(pt 3):769–775. http://www.pubmedcentral.nih.gov/articlerender.fcgi?artid=1137054&tool=pmcentrez&rendertype=abstract. Accessed March 14, 2016.
171. Ottery FD, Walsh D, Strawford A. Pharmacologic management of anorexia/cachexia. *Semin Oncol.* 1998;25(2 suppl 6):35–44. http://www.ncbi.nlm.nih.gov/pubmed/9625382. Accessed March 15, 2016.
172. Neary NM, Small CJ, Wren AM, et al. Ghrelin increases energy intake in cancer patients with impaired appetite: acute, randomized, placebo-controlled trial. *J Clin Endocrinol Metab.* 2004;89(6):2832–2836. doi:10.1210/jc.2003-031768.
173. Strasser F, Lutz TA, Maeder MT, et al. Safety, tolerability and pharmacokinetics of intravenous ghrelin for cancer-related anorexia/cachexia: a randomised, placebo-controlled, double-blind, double-crossover study. *Br J Cancer.* 2008;98(2):300–308. doi:10.1038/sj.bjc.6604148.
174. Lydén E, Cvetkovska E, Westin T, et al. Effects of nandrolone propionate on experimental tumor growth and cancer cachexia. *Metabolism.* 1995;44(4):445–451. http://www.ncbi.nlm.nih.gov/pubmed/7723666. Accessed March 14, 2016.
175. Strang P. The effect of megestrol acetate on anorexia, weight loss and cachexia in cancer and AIDS patients (review). *Anticancer Res.* 1997;17(1B):657–662. http://www.ncbi.nlm.nih.gov/pubmed/9066597. Accessed March 14, 2016.
176. Beller E, Tattersall M, Lumley T, et al. Improved quality of life with megestrol acetate in patients with endocrine-insensitive advanced cancer: a randomised placebo-controlled trial. Australasian Megestrol Acetate Cooperative Study Group. *Ann Oncol.* 1997;8(3):277–283. http://www.ncbi.nlm.nih.gov/pubmed/9137798. Accessed March 14, 2016.
177. Skarlos DV, Fountzilas G, Pavlidis N, et al. Megestrol acetate in cancer patients with anorexia and weight loss. A Hellenic Co-operative Oncology Group (HeCOG) study. *Acta Oncol.* 1993;32(1):37–41. http://www.ncbi.nlm.nih.gov/pubmed/8466763. Accessed March 14, 2016.
178. Fujimoto-Ouchi K, Tamura S, Mori K, et al. Establishment and characterization of cachexia-inducing and -non-inducing clones of murine colon 26 carcinoma. *Int J cancer.* 1995;61(4):522–528. http://www.ncbi.nlm.nih.gov/pubmed/7759158. Accessed March 14, 2016.
179. Gelin J, Moldawer LL, Lönnroth C, et al. Role of endogenous tumor necrosis factor alpha and interleukin 1 for experimental tumor growth and the development of cancer cachexia. *Cancer Res.* 1991;51(1):415–421. http://www.ncbi.nlm.nih.gov/pubmed/1703040. Accessed March 14, 2016.

180. Strassmann G, Kambayashi T. Inhibition of experimental cancer cachexia by anti-cytokine and anti-cytokine-receptor therapy. *Cytokines Mol Ther.* 1995;1(2):107–113. http://www.ncbi.nlm.nih.gov/pubmed/9384667. Accessed March 14, 2016.
181. Yamamoto N, Kawamura I, Nishigaki F, et al. Effect of FR143430, a novel cytokine suppressive agent, on adenocarcinoma colon26-induced cachexia in mice. *Anticancer Res.* 1998;18(1A):139–144. http://www.ncbi.nlm.nih.gov/pubmed/9568068. Accessed March 14, 2016.
182. Khan ZH, Simpson EJ, Cole AT, et al. Oesophageal cancer and cachexia: the effect of short-term treatment with thalidomide on weight loss and lean body mass. *Aliment Pharmacol Ther.* 2003;17(5):677–682. http://www.ncbi.nlm.nih.gov/pubmed/12641516. Accessed March 14, 2016.
183. Gordon JN, Trebble TM, Ellis RD, et al. Thalidomide in the treatment of cancer cachexia: a randomised placebo controlled trial. *Gut.* 2005;54(4):540–545. doi:10.1136/gut.2004.047563.
184. Lai V, George J, Richey L, et al. Results of a pilot study of the effects of celecoxib on cancer cachexia in patients with cancer of the head, neck, and gastrointestinal tract. *Head Neck.* 2008;30(1):67–74. doi:10.1002/hed.20662.
185. McMillan DC, Wigmore SJ, Fearon KC, et al. A prospective randomized study of megestrol acetate and ibuprofen in gastrointestinal cancer patients with weight loss. *Br J Cancer.* 1999;79(3–4):495–500. doi:10.1038/sj.bjc.6690077.
186. Mantovani G, Macciò A, Madeddu C, et al. Randomized phase III clinical trial of five different arms of treatment in 332 patients with cancer cachexia. *Oncologist.* 2010;15(2):200–211. doi:10.1634/theoncologist.2009-0153.
187. McGough C, Baldwin C, Norman A, et al. Is supplementation with elemental diet feasible in patients undergoing pelvic radiotherapy? *Clin Nutr.* 2006;25(1):109–116. doi:10.1016/j.clnu.2005.09.007.
188. Henson CC, Burden S, Davidson SE, et al. Nutritional interventions for reducing gastrointestinal toxicity in adults undergoing radical pelvic radiotherapy. *Cochrane Database Syst Rev.* 2013;11:CD009896. doi:10.1002/14651858.CD009896.pub2.
189. Borek C. Radiation and chemically induced transformation: free radicals, antioxidants and cancer. *Br J Cancer Suppl.* 1987;8:74–86. http://www.pubmedcentral.nih.gov/articlerender.fcgi?artid=2149458&tool=pmcentrez&rendertype=abstract. Accessed March 17, 2016.
190. Kennedy M, Bruninga K, Mutlu EA, et al. Successful and sustained treatment of chronic radiation proctitis with antioxidant vitamins E and C. *Am J Gastroenterol.* 2001;96(4):1080–1084. doi:10.1111/j.1572-0241.2001.03742.x.
191. Fearon KCH, Von Meyenfeldt MF, Moses AGW, et al. Effect of a protein and energy dense N-3 fatty acid enriched oral supplement on loss of weight and lean tissue in cancer cachexia: a randomised double blind trial. *Gut.* 2003;52(10):1479–1486. http://www.pubmedcentral.nih.gov/articlerender.fcgi?artid=1773823&tool=pmcentrez&rendertype=abstract. Accessed February 22, 2016.
192. Gogos CA, Ginopoulos P, Salsa B, et al. Dietary omega-3 polyunsaturated fatty acids plus vitamin E restore immunodeficiency and prolong survival for severely ill patients with generalized malignancy: a randomized control trial. *Cancer.* 1998;82(2):395–402. http://www.ncbi.nlm.nih.gov/pubmed/9445198. Accessed February 22, 2016.
193. Licitra L, Spinazzé S, Roila F. Antiemetic therapy. *Crit Rev Oncol Hematol.* 2002;43(1):93–101. http://www.ncbi.nlm.nih.gov/pubmed/12098610. Accessed March 17, 2016.
194. Grunberg SM, Deuson RR, Mavros P, et al. Incidence of chemotherapy-induced nausea and emesis after modern antiemetics. *Cancer.* 2004;100(10):2261–2268. doi:10.1002/cncr.20230.
195. Deciding to Forego Life-Sustaining Treatment: A Report on the Ethical, Medical, and Legal Issues in Treatment Decisions. https://repository.library.georgetown.edu/handle/10822/796378. Accessed March 17, 2016.
196. Shils ME. Nutrition and medical ethics: the interplay of medical decisions, patients' rights, and the judicial system. In: Shils ME, Olsen JA, Shike M et al, ed. *Modern Nutrition in Health and Disease.* 9th Ed. Philadelphia, PA: Williams & Wilkins; 1999:1689.
197. Coggan HD. Edwin Stevens Lecture. On dying and dying well. Moral and spiritual aspects. *Proc R Soc Med.* 1977;70(2):75–81. http://www.pubmedcentral.nih.gov/articlerender.fcgi?artid=1542954&tool=pmcentrez&rendertype=abstract. Accessed March 17, 2016.
198. Pope John Paul II. Care for patients in a "permanent" vegetative state. *Origins.* 2004;33(43):737, 739–740. http://www.ncbi.nlm.nih.gov/pubmed/15139351. Accessed March 17, 2016.
199. Schostak RZ. Jewish ethical guidelines for resuscitation and artificial nutrition and hydration of the dying elderly. *J Med Ethics.* 1994;20(2):93–100. http://www.pubmedcentral.nih.gov/articlerender.fcgi?artid=1376434&tool=pmcentrez&rendertype=abstract. Accessed March 17, 2016.
200. Casarett D, Kapo J, Caplan A. Appropriate use of artificial nutrition and hydration-fundamental principles and recommendations. *N Engl J Med.* 2005;353(24):2607–2612. doi:10.1056/NEJMsb052907.
201. Ganzini L, Goy ER, Miller LL, et al. Nurses' experiences with hospice patients who refuse food and fluids to hasten death. *N Engl J Med.* 2003;349(4):359–365. doi:10.1056/NEJMsa035086.
202. Maillet JO, Potter RL, Heller L. Position of the American Dietetic Association: ethical and legal issues in nutrition, hydration, and feeding. *J Am Diet Assoc.* 2002;102(5):716–726. http://www.ncbi.nlm.nih.gov/pubmed/12009001. Accessed March 17, 2016.
203. Brown D, Roberts JA, Elkins TE, et al. Hard choices: the gynecologic cancer patient's end-of-life preferences. *Gynecol Oncol.* 1994;55(3 pt 1):355–362. doi:10.1006/gyno.1994.1306.
204. McCann RM, Hall WJ, Groth-Juncker A. Comfort care for terminally ill patients. The appropriate use of nutrition and hydration. *JAMA.* 1994;272(16):1263–1266. http://www.ncbi.nlm.nih.gov/pubmed/7523740. Accessed March 9, 2016.
205. Zerwekh JV. The dehydration question. *Nursing (Lond).* 1983;13(1):47–51. http://www.ncbi.nlm.nih.gov/pubmed/6549673. Accessed March 28, 2016.
206. Schmitz P. The process of dying with and without feeding and fluids by tube. *Law Med Health Care.* 1991;19(1–2):23–26. http://www.ncbi.nlm.nih.gov/pubmed/1910129. Accessed March 28, 2016.

CHAPTER 32

Palliative and Supportive Care

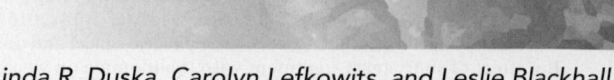

Linda R. Duska, Carolyn Lefkowits, and Leslie Blackhall

INTRODUCTION

Palliative care is a critical element of the comprehensive care of women with gynecologic cancer. The World Health Organization (WHO) defines palliative care as "an approach that improves the quality of life (QOL) of patients and their families facing the problems associated with life threatening illness, through the prevention and relief of suffering by means of early identification and impeccable assessment and treatment of pain and other problems, physical, psychosocial and spiritual (1)." This definition, complemented by similar statements from the American Society of Clinical Oncology (ASCO) (2) and the Society of Gynecologic Oncology (SGO) (3), supports the utilization of palliative care throughout the course of disease for women with gynecologic cancer. Provision of palliative care to patients with cancer has been associated with multiple benefits including both improved clinical outcomes (QOL, symptom control, and patient and caregiver satisfaction) and improved health care utilization outcomes (decreased hospital costs, inpatient and intensive care unit [ICU] admissions) (4).

It is essential to distinguish between palliative care and hospice care or end-of-life care. Unlike hospice care, palliative care may be provided at any point in the disease course and can be offered concurrently with disease-directed therapy, including curative-intent therapy (**Fig. 32.1**). Palliative care focuses on the treatment of symptoms related to both the cancer and cancer therapy, including pain, anxiety, depression, fatigue, and nausea. It also encompasses communication with patients and families about their goals and preferences for care, to ensure that the treatment plan, throughout the disease course, reflects the patient's values and preferences. Patients and their families who are suspicious of the word hospice and reluctant to accept a "hospice consultation" may be willing to accept palliative care if the main purpose is explained accurately: a focus on symptom management with subsequent decrease in suffering. A public opinion survey by the Center to Advance Palliative Care found that the phrase "an extra layer of support" was one that the public found helpful when explaining the role of palliative care (5); this phrase also may be helpful to clinicians when explaining palliative care to patients and families. Another study suggested that the term "supportive care," which is sometimes used synonymously with palliative care, may be more acceptable to referring providers, including oncologists (6). In contrast, hospice care is a specialized end-of-life service, most often covered by the Medicare Hospice Benefit (MHB), which is available to patients with a prognosis of 6 months or less who are no longer pursuing anticancer therapy.

Despite concerns that increased attention to symptom management or advance care planning might hasten death by diminishing the focus on life-prolonging therapies, no study of palliative care has ever shown an association between palliative care and shortened life expectancy. In fact, there is some evidence that early integration of palliative care into standard oncologic care may actually prolong life. In the most well known of the randomized studies in cancer patients, 151 patients with newly diagnosed metastatic non–small cell lung cancer were randomized to integration of outpatient palliative care from the time of cancer diagnosis versus usual oncologic care (7). The early palliative care integration group had significant improvements in QOL and mood, as well as a statistically significantly improved overall survival (11.6 vs. 8.9 months, $p = 0.02$), despite less aggressive intervention at the end of life (7). Other randomized studies in general oncology have shown a similar improvement in QOL with the integration of palliative care into active cancer care (8–14), prompting ASCO to write a Clinical Opinion in 2012 stating that "combined standard oncology care and palliative care should be considered early in the course of illness for any patient with metastatic cancer and/or high symptom burden (15)."

It is therefore imperative that gynecologic oncologists be familiar with the tools and management options of palliative care for their patients. This chapter will focus on the scope of palliative care as it applies to women with gynecologic cancer, with special emphasis on the regulations governing palliative care services in the United States. The importance of this topic cannot be overemphasized: The SGO has concluded that "palliative care significantly improves QOL for patients and their families," and the addition of basic level palliative care is included among the SGO's five Choosing Wisely recommendations (3,16). The SGO's position emphasizes the fundamental importance of palliative care to the delivery of high-quality gynecologic cancer care.

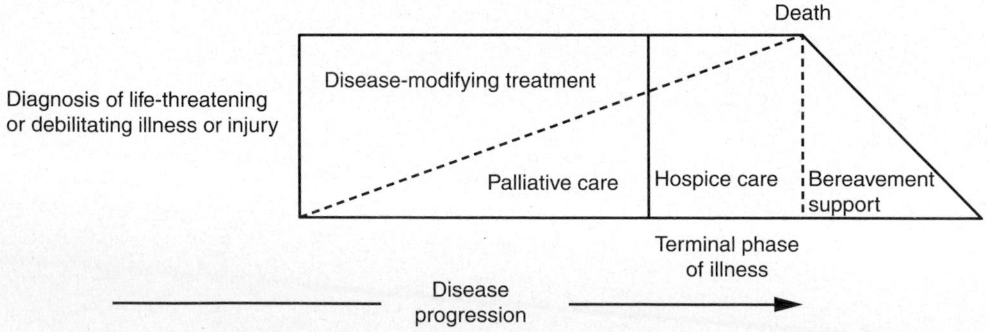

Figure 32.1. The simultaneous care model for palliative care, defined by the Centers for Medicare and Medicaid Services in its proposed Hospice Conditions of Participation and as adapted from the World Health Organization.

Source: From A National Framework and Preferred Practices for Palliative and Hospice Care Quality: A Consensus Report, by the National Quality Forum, Washington, DC. Copyright 2006 by the National Quality Forum. Reproduced with permission.

Systems of Palliative Care Delivery: Specialized Palliative Care, Basic Palliative Care, and Hospice Care

It is important to distinguish between basic and specialty palliative care. Specialty palliative care is provided by an interdisciplinary team with dedicated training in palliative care. In contrast, basic (or primary) palliative care can be provided by any clinician who cares for patients with serious illness; in the case of gynecologic cancer, this may include the gynecologic oncologist, medical oncologist, radiation oncologist, and primary care provider.

Specialty Palliative Care

Core members of the specialty palliative care team include a palliative care–trained physician, nurse or advanced practice provider, a social worker, and a chaplain. Other members may include pharmacists, nutritionists, rehabilitation therapists, and direct care workers. While specialty palliative care is most commonly available as an inpatient hospital consultation service, provision of specialty palliative care is increasing in outpatient clinics (17,18). As of 2010, National Cancer Institute (NCI)-designated cancer centers reported 92% availability of inpatient specialty palliative care consultation teams and 59% availability of outpatient specialty palliative care (compared with 74% and 22%, respectively, for non-NCI cancer centers) (17). In 2006, palliative care (officially called Hospice and Palliative Medicine) was officially recognized by the American Board of Medical Specialties and co-sponsored by multiple other medical boards. Until 2012, clinicians could be "grandfathered in" to board certification in palliative care by documenting a certain number of hours of clinical experience and sitting for written board exams. After 2012, board certification in palliative care requires completion of a 1-year clinical fellowship and written board exams. The data supporting the clinical and economic benefits of early integration of palliative care into standard oncology care are based on trials of specialty palliative care interventions (19).

Basic Palliative Care

Basic palliative care clinical services delivered by non-palliative care specialists is termed "primary palliative care (20)." It is neither feasible, nor desirable, that all palliative care be delivered by specialists. It is not feasible as there are not enough palliative care specialists in the country to care for all patients with serious, life-limiting illnesses. It is not desirable because the inclusion of another set of providers for every woman with gynecologic cancer might cause fragmentation of care, undermining the therapeutic relationship between the patient and her oncologist (20).

Many gynecologic oncologists have been exposed to primary palliative care education during fellowship and feel comfortable caring for their patients' basic needs with respect to symptom management and end-of-life care. A small percentage of gynecologic oncologists are also boarded in palliative care through the efforts of the American Board of Obstetrics and Gynecology; others have completed fellowships in both Gynecologic Oncology and Palliative care. As a result of the growing recognition of the importance of palliative care in this setting, increasing numbers of gynecologic oncologists are becoming boarded in palliative care or becoming familiar with palliative care strategies. Growing interest in palliative care strategies is evidenced by high attendance at SGO courses aimed at teaching symptom management, and interest in the SGO's Palliative Care Network. For gynecologic oncologists, primary palliative care should include core elements of palliative care, such as basic symptom management and aligning treatment choices with patient goals (20). More complex issues, such as existential distress and refractory symptom management, may be better addressed by palliative care specialists (**Table 32.1**).

TABLE 32.1. Representative Skill Sets for Primary and Specialty Palliative Care

Primary palliative care
• Basic management of pain and symptoms
• Basic management of depression and anxiety
• Basic discussions about ○ Prognosis ○ Goals of treatment ○ Suffering ○ Code status
Specialty palliative care
• Management of refractory pain or other symptoms
• Management of more complex depression, anxiety, grief, and existential distress
• Assistance with conflict resolution regarding goals or methods of treatment ○ Within families ○ Between staff and families ○ Among treatment teams
• Assistance in addressing cases of near futility

From Quill TE, Abernethy AP. Generalist plus specialist palliative care—creating a more sustainable model. *N Engl J Med*. 2013;368:1173–1175, © 2013 Massachusetts Medical Society. Reprinted with permission from Massachusetts Medical Society.

Hospice Care

The MHB was first offered in 1983; it is a benefit of Medicare Part A that covers comprehensive end of life (EOL) care (21). To be eligible for the MHB, a patient must be "certified" by two physicians as having a prognosis of 6 months or less. For gynecologic cancer patients, one physician can be the gynecologic oncologist and the other the hospice physician. Eligibility also requires that the patient waive the traditional Medicare parts A and D for care related to the terminal illness, including prescription medications. The hospice benefit applies *only* to care or medications related to the terminal diagnosis; a patient may continue to receive care for coexisting unrelated medical problems covered by Medicare parts A and D and can continue to see her physicians under Medicare Part B coverage. Unlike traditional Medicare benefits, which usually require a 20% co-pay, the MHB coverage is almost 100% for all services including medications (some hospices may require a 5% co-pay).

The hospice benefit is structured as benefit periods (two 90-day periods followed by an unlimited number of 60-day periods). Between benefit periods, the hospice provider must reevaluate and recertify the patient. Patients may revoke the MHB at any time, at which point traditional Medicare coverage is immediately available. There are four levels of hospice care—two outpatient and two inpatient. These include:

- Routine home care—routine palliative care services in the patient's home or nursing facility.
- Continuous home care—intended for crisis management of acute symptoms. It involves intensive home nursing for a minimum of 8 hours during each 24-hour time period.
- General inpatient care—intended for short-term control of acute symptoms that cannot be managed at home. It can be provided by a hospice facility, hospital, or skilled nursing facility (SNF).
- Respite care—intended to give caregivers respite. It is reimbursed for no more than 5 days in each benefit period. Respite care can take place in a hospice facility, hospital, or SNF.

The MHB offers a fixed per diem payment to the hospice program, with rates varying by geographical location. The initial intake of a new patient is particularly time-and resource-intensive and generally costs the hospice far more than the daily per diem; thus it is financially beneficial to the hospice program to have a patient in the program for more than 2 weeks before death. More importantly, late hospice referrals do not give the hospice team enough time to complete the goals of safe and comfortable dying and effective grieving. Data from the National Hospice and Palliative Care Organization show that 34.5% of hospice patients died within 7 days of admission in 2013 (22). Many states offer a Medicaid hospice benefit similar to the MHB. Most private insurers also offer a hospice benefit but these are variable.

The hospice team develops a care plan that meets the individual's needs. The team consists of the patient's physician, the hospice physician (or medical director), nurses, home health aides, social workers, clergy, trained volunteers, and therapists (speech, physical, occupational) if needed. Hospice services are multidimensional. They include pain and symptom management, provision of drugs and medical supplies, assistance with emotional, psychosocial, and spiritual aspects of dying, and support for the family in caring for the patient.

Retrospective data in nongynecologic cancers suggest that hospice care is associated with no decrease in, or in some cases improved, survival. Family members of hospice patients are more likely to report better QOL, lower rates of physical and psychosocial distress, and better quality of death for their loved ones than patients treated in the hospital at the end of life (23–25). One cohort study retrospectively studied 81 patients with gynecologic cancer who died secondary to cancer recurrence and/or progression and who were offered hospice services. Patients who declined hospice when it was recommended were considered not to have utilized hospice whether or not they ultimately received supportive care. Median time for receiving supportive care was longer in the hospice group (8 weeks vs. 1 week) and patients in the nonhospice group were more likely to have an invasive procedure performed or antineoplastic therapy administered within 4 weeks of death. In the subset of patients with recurrent disease (73%), the median overall survival for patients who chose hospice was 17 months, compared with 9 months for the group not utilizing hospice (26). Other studies have confirmed these results in gynecologic cancer patients, and suggest that between 20% and 60% of patients who die of ovarian cancer utilize hospice (27–29).

PRIMARY PALLIATIVE CARE FOR THE GYNECOLOGIC ONCOLOGIST

Symptom Management

Gynecologic cancer patients often experience both disease- and treatment-related symptoms throughout the course of their illness; the high symptom burden in this population has been well documented (30–32). Symptoms may go unrecognized and therefore untreated for a multitude of reasons. Clinicians may assume that patients will initiate discussions about symptoms, while patients expect their physicians to ask about symptoms. Moreover, patients may have a disincentive to report symptoms to their physician due to fears about prompting a change in treatment, though assessment of symptom burden is required to appropriately identify and address symptoms.

Patient-reported outcomes are the gold standard for quantifying patient experience and/or symptoms (33). Several validated scales exist to measure symptom burden, including the Edmonton Symptom Assessment System and the Memorial Symptom Assessment Scale. More recently, investigation has turned to use of routine recording and monitoring of symptoms through the electronic health record; a recent study of 636 gynecologic cancer outpatients found it to be feasible to electronically record patient symptoms and use that data as a basis for referral to psychosocial and supportive care (34). The National Comprehensive Cancer Network (NCCN) guidelines recommend routine screening by the oncology team for uncontrolled symptoms (35). Management of symptoms in gynecologic cancer patients is thoroughly covered in the SGO White Paper on palliative care (36). Basic tenets of symptom management will be reviewed here.

Pain

Pain management is discussed in detail in Chapter 31.

Nausea and Vomiting

Nausea and vomiting are common symptoms in cancer patients, and have special significance in ovarian cancer because of the high incidence of bowel obstruction in this population. We favor an etiology-based approach to patients with this symptom (37), although a protocol-based approach is often more appropriate for those very close to the end of life (38). The etiologic approach relies on a detailed history, including associated symptoms, timing, frequency, and exacerbating and relieving factors. A mnemonic for the differential diagnosis of nausea that categorizes by mechanism is VOMIT—Vestibular apparatus, Obstruction, Motility/Mind, Infection/Inflammation, and Toxins/Tumor. **Table 32.2** summarizes this approach.

Causes of nausea and vomiting in the cancer patient can be roughly divided into those that originate from central nervous system (CNS) sites and those that originate from the gastrointestinal (GI) tract. Chemotherapy and other toxins cause nausea and vomiting via their direct effect on the chemoreceptor trigger zone and vomiting centers. Ondansetron and other 5H3 blockers are very effective in reducing chemotherapy-induced vomiting, and have radically improved the QOL for those receiving highly emetogenic chemotherapy (39). These medications cause less sedation and delirium than phenothiazines, but are extremely constipating; prophylaxis and monitoring for this side effect is imperative. Another targeted agent for chemotherapy-induced nausea and vomiting is the NKI-receptor antagonist class of medications (aprepitant, casopitant, and rolapitant) (40). Phenothiazines are well studied and quite effective but can cause sedation, delirium, and extrapyramidal symptoms. Haloperidol, due to its effects on dopamine, is an effective antiemetic and has minimal side effects when used in low doses (41).

Anticipatory nausea most commonly occurs in the setting of poorly controlled nausea and vomiting caused by chemotherapy, which leads to vomiting in anticipation of chemotherapy. Improved prevention and treatment of the underlying cause of the vomiting is crucial, but may not be sufficient. For patients with severe anticipatory symptoms, behavioral interventions including relaxation techniques, and hypnosis may be used. Benzodiazepine medications (particularly lorazepam) are commonly prescribed for this symptom (42).

Delayed gastric emptying in gynecologic malignancies is due to a variety of causes including chemotherapy-induced gastroparesis, carcinomatosis, ascites, mechanical obstruction, and constipation, is common. Gastric distension, caused by retained food or gastric fluids, activates stretch receptors that feed into the nausea and vomiting centers. Etiologically-based treatment seeks to improve gastric motility through the use of metoclopramide or, less commonly, erythromycin, or to decrease production of gastric fluid through the use of ranitidine, H2 blockers, anticholinergic agents such as scopolamine, or glycopyrrolate (43). Dietary and behavioral interventions are often recommended as well. In selected settings, therapeutic paracentesis can be very effective (44).

The surgical management of malignant bowel obstruction is described below. For the obstructed patient, many of the recommendations above are appropriate, although for the completely obstructed patient, metoclopramide is contraindicated because its use will cause cramping. Octreotide is often recommended for the completely obstructed patient, although recent studies have questioned its efficacy. Steroids are commonly prescribed; however, there is less evidence regarding the efficacy of steroids than of the agents mentioned above (44,45). Pharmacologic management in this setting can be challenging, and attention must be paid to route of administration. Depending on the patient's ability to tolerate oral medications, nonoral options should be considered, including oral dissolving tablets (ondansetron), sublingual preparations (haloperidol), rectal suppositories (prochlorperazine), or intravenous formulations.

TABLE 32.2. Nausea and Vomiting

	Location	Causes	Symptoms	Symptomatic Treatment	
CNS	Vestibular	Metastatic lesions to CNS	Vertigo, movement related nausea	Scopalamine, meclizine	Uncommon
	Cortical	Increased ICP Anxiety, pain Anticipatory	Headache, neurologic signs Vomiting associated with these symptoms Nausea/vomiting "anticipates" noxious stimulus	Steroids Treatment of pain/anxiety Treatment of noxious stimulus, benzodiazepines, haloperidol, Zyprexa, CBT	Uncommon Uncommon Common
	Chemoreceptor trigger zone D2 (dopamine) 5HT3 NK1 vomiting center Achm H1 5HT2	Drugs (chemotherapy) Metabolic (renal failure, liver failure)	Temporal association with medication or toxin	Pretreatment and prophylaxis 5-HT_3 receptor blockers Phenothiazines Metoclopramide NK1 antagonist	Very common
GI	Stomach	Delayed gastric emptying due to: Mechanical obstruction (partial) Gastroparesis (chemotherapy, opioids) Ascites Paraneoplastic syndrome	Early satiety, bloating, reflux, vomiting of undigested food	Metoclopramide Small frequent, calorie dense meals Therapeutic paracentesis where appropriate Ranitidine/H2 blockers	Very common
	Small and large bowel	Mechanical bowel obstruction (partial or complete) paraneoplastic		Metoclopramide (partial obstruction only) Steroids Octreotide Dietary interventions Ranitidine/H2 blockers Anticholinergics	Common (very common in ovarian cancer)

CNS, central nervous system; ICP, intracranial pressure; CBT, cognitive behavioral therapy.

Lymphedema

Lymphedema is a prevalent symptom in women with gynecologic cancer; it is underreported and often untreated. In a large, population-based study, morbidity from lymphedema was experienced by 10% of women after gynecologic cancer treatment, with highest prevalence (36%) among vulvar cancer survivors and lowest (5%) among ovarian cancer survivors (46). Needs relating to managing the symptoms of lymphedema were often unmet. Physical therapy, including lymphatic massage and special exercises, can be helpful for patients with lymphedema, in conjunction with compression bandages and garments. The best way to manage lymphedema is to avoid it if possible: for example, by following algorithms such as the Mayo criteria to avoid unnecessary pelvic node dissection, or by performing sentinel lymph node dissection for vulvar cancer rather than complete groin lymphadenectomy when appropriate. Preoperative preparation is also important, as symptoms may be easier for the patient to manage emotionally if they are not completely unexpected.

Neuropathy

Chemotherapy-induced peripheral neuropathy is one of the most common neurologic complications of cancer treatment; up to 90% of cancer patients treated with chemotherapy will have peripheral neuropathy (47). Neuropathy severity generally increases with treatment dose and duration and decreases after treatment stops. Sensory symptoms (such as tingling, numbness, pain) are more likely to improve over time than motor symptoms (such as difficulty with buttons), but in some patients will persist. Classes of medications used for empiric treatment of peripheral neuropathy include anticonvulsants, antidepressants, opioids, non-opioid analgesics, and topical agents, but quality data is lacking (48,49). First-line therapy usually consists of gabapentin or pregabalin. Gabapentin starting dose is 100 to 300 mg once a day at bedtime, titrated up to 3,600 mg per day in divided doses, if needed. Amitriptyline or nortriptyline can also be used, and have been shown to be efficacious in some studies. One randomized trial showed improvement with use of duloxetine (60 mg/day) over placebo (50).

Constipation

Constipation in the gynecologic oncology patient most commonly arises as a direct effect of disease or as a side effect of medication. Constipating medications commonly used in gynecologic oncology include opioids and selective 5-HT3 antagonists such as ondansetron. Constipation can cause and exacerbate other symptoms including pain and nausea; it must be anticipated and proactively managed. Constipation is a common side effect of opioids, and the only side effect that is not expected to improve or resolve with chronic opioid use. A prophylactic bowel regimen should be considered with every opioid prescription. The percentage of patients treated with an opioid that are offered or prescribed a bowel regimen is considered a quality measure by the Center for Medicare & Medicaid (51). Patients should be counseled regarding constipation at the time of opioid prescription and should be instructed to titrate their bowel regimen to the goal of daily soft bowel movement. Despite widespread use, docusate is not effective as either prophylaxis or treatment. A stimulant laxative such as senna is a good first-line therapy (starting dose 2 tabs q.h.s., max 8 tabs/day, divided b.i.d.). Other pharmacologic options include bisacodyl (PO or PR), or osmotic agents such as polyethylene glycol-3,350 (not a good option for patients with early satiety, as it requires consuming 4 to 8 oz of fluid with every dose), sorbitol, lactulose, and milk of magnesia. Nonpharmacologic options, which can be used to supplement pharmacologic options but are generally not sufficient alone, include increasing activity level and fluid intake. When treating existing constipation, bowel obstruction should be ruled out first, either clinically or with imaging. In addition to the therapies mentioned above, methylnaltrexone, which is a mu-opioid-receptor antagonist, can be used for refractory opioid-induced constipation. Methylnaltrexone is administered 8 to 12 mg SQ q.o.d. because of its limited ability to cross the blood–brain barrier, it does not affect analgesia or precipitate opioid withdrawal (52).

Fatigue

One of the most common and distressing symptoms patients with advanced cancer experience is fatigue (53). Fatigue may be elevated at the time of cancer diagnosis, and typically increases during treatment (54). Prevalence estimates of fatigue during treatment range from 25% to 99% depending on the patient population, type of treatment received, and method of assessment (53). In the majority of studies, 30% to 60% of patients report moderate-to-severe fatigue during treatment, which in some cases may lead to treatment discontinuation. While fatigue usually improves in the year after treatment completion, studies of cancer survivors suggest that approximately one-quarter to one-third experience persistent fatigue for up to 10 years after cancer diagnosis (55,56). Cancer-related fatigue is multidimensional and can cause impairment of QOL by producing a negative impact on other domains of life such as the social and emotional domains. Fatigue is particularly present in women with gynecologic malignancy (57). In one study of ovarian cancer patients, fatigue was reported by 67% of patients in the last year of life, increasing to 93% in the last 3 months (58). More than half of women with cervical cancer have fatigue (59). Unfortunately, treatment options for fatigue are limited and the literature on pharmacologic interventions is very heterogeneous. There is evidence to suggest that methylphenidate may be effective, with a Cochrane meta-analysis showing an estimated superior effect for methylphenidate in cancer-related fatigue (60). Studies in breast cancer have suggested physical exercise and psychosocial interventions may also be helpful in treating cancer-related fatigue (61).

Malignant Bowel Obstruction

In gynecologic cancer, malignant bowel obstruction may occur from either a functional obstruction by tumor or a failure of normal peristalsis due to tumor coating the intestinal serosa (carcinomatous ileus). Nonmalignant causes of bowel obstruction may also occur, due to adhesive disease from radical surgery, radiation damage to normal tissue, or scarring from intraperitoneal chemotherapy. Patients most commonly present with abdominal distension, nausea and vomiting, and pain from the distension of the intestinal wall and interrupted peristalsis. In the end-of-life setting with advanced, incurable disease, conservative measures are recommended, with nasogastric drainage for comfort and intravenous hydration. Gastric tubes can be placed for comfort if the bowel obstruction does not resolve with conservative measures. In rare situations, a palliative surgery may be considered. Palliative surgery should be undertaken with caution, as morbidity is 5% to 49% and mortality 5% to 15% (62). Median survival in recurrent ovarian cancer patients after palliative bowel surgery is approximately 12 months (62).

Anorexia/Cachexia

Anorexia, or loss of appetite, is a common complication of advanced cancer. Cancer cachexia is "a multifactorial syndrome defined by an ongoing loss of skeletal muscle mass (with or without loss of fat mass) that cannot be fully reversed by conventional nutritional support and leads to progressive functional impairment (63)." The syndrome of anorexia and cachexia in advanced cancer is mediated by a complex interplay of metabolic, cytokine, and neuroendocrine-mediated events. The mnemonic ANOREXIA addresses potentially reversible causes of anorexia (Aches and pain, Nausea and GI dysfunction, Oral candidiasis, Reactive [or organic] depression or anxiety, Evacuation problems [constipation, retention], Xerostomia [dry mouth], Iatrogenic [radiation, chemotherapy, drugs], Acid-related problems [gastritis, peptic ulcers]) (64). While potentially reversible causes of anorexia should certainly be evaluated and addressed, it is also important for clinicians, patients, and families to understand that in the absence of identifiable reversible factors, anorexia and cachexia are often part of the natural history of the disease process itself. Given the central role that food and feeding play in caretaking in our culture, anorexia is often very distressing to caregivers. It is important to explain to caregivers that with anorexia/cachexia of advanced cancer, the patient is generally not made uncomfortable by their decreased intake; forcing the patient to eat, while well intentioned, is often far more uncomfortable and traumatic for the patient.

Options for pharmacologic therapies for anorexia include prokinetic agents such as metoclopramide (10 mg PO AC and HS), low-dose steroids such as dexamethasone (regimens vary: 2 to 16 mg/d), and progestational agents such as megestrol acetate (MA; regimens vary: 160 to 1,600 mg/day; starting dose usually 400 mg/d), among others. A randomized study in 2010 examined five different pharmacologic regimens for cancer cachexia (medroxyprogesterone [MPA] or MA, eicosapentaenoic acid [EPA], L-carnitine, thalidomide and a combination of MPA/MA, EPA, L-carnitine, and thalidomide). The combination regimen was found to be most effective with increase in lean body mass; decrease in resting energy expenditure; improvement in fatigue, appetite, and QOL; and improvement in Eastern Cooperative Oncology Group (ECOG) performance status (65).

Dyspnea

Dyspnea is a common and distressing symptom in cancer that is present in more than half of all patients with advanced cancer (66) and approximately 40% of those with gynecologic malignancies (67). Acute dyspnea warrants evaluation for pulmonary embolism or pneumonia depending on the clinical circumstances. Patients with fatigue and deconditioning as a result of their malignancy often report dyspnea with exertion as well. Patients with cancer may also have other causes of dyspnea such as chronic obstructive pulmonary disease and congestive heart failure, putting them at higher risk of dyspnea. Severe dyspnea or air hunger is extremely frightening and can lead to panic attacks, while anxiety can also worsen dyspnea. Treatment of the underlying cause is important but may not be possible or provide complete relief of this symptom. Multiple clinical trials testify to the usefulness and safety of opioids, especially morphine, for the treatment of dyspnea in both cancer and non-cancer settings (68). Immediate-release morphine may be given prior to exertion to increase exercise capacity (69). Benzodiazepines are often recommended for dyspnea when this symptom is associated with significant anxiety, but their use in the ambulatory setting is not currently supported by the literature (66).

Delirium

Delirium is an acute change in mental status that may fluctuate and has several underlying physiological causes. It is characterized by a constellation of features, including acute onset, fluctuating course, altered level of consciousness, inattention, and cognitive impairments (70). It is further characterized based on the level of arousal and psychomotor activity as hyperactive, hypoactive, or mixed. Hypoactive delirium, which is characterized by sedation, lethargy, and psychomotor retardation, can be easily mistaken for fatigue or depression. Delirium in cancer patients is common; prevalence ranges from 10% to 30% in hospitalized patients with cancer and up to 85% in the terminal phase of illness (71). It is associated with significant morbidity, including increased length of hospitalization, functional decline, decreased life expectancy, higher health care costs, and considerable distress for both patients and family members (72). Without a high index of suspicion, it can easily go unnoticed and untreated. Several screening tools for delirium have been validated in patients with cancer, including the Memorial Delirium Assessment Scale, the Delirium Rating Scale-Revised 98, and the Confusion Assessment Method (71). The evaluation of delirium should include a complete history and physical and comprehensive evaluation for reversible etiologies, with the understanding that delirium is often multifactorial (**Table 32.3**).

TABLE 32.3. Contributing Factors to Delirium

Common and treatable
• Medications (anticholinergics, opioids, sedatives, steroids, antidepressants, H2 blockers, metoclopramide, baclofen) • Withdrawal symptoms from abruptly stopping home medications (benzodiazepines, opiates, SSRIs, barbiturates) • Infection • Constipation • Urinary retention • Uncontrolled pain
Less common but treatable
• Electrolyte disturbances • Anemia • Dehydration • Immobilization • Depression, social isolation • Vision or hearing impairment • Emotional distress • Unfamiliar environment
Less common and less treatable
• Cardiac or pulmonary failure with ischemia, hypoxia, or hypercapnia • Renal failure • Hepatic failure with encephalopathy • Neurologic dysfunction due to brain metastases, seizure activity, or stroke

Tucker RO, Nichols AC. *UNIPAC 4. Managing Nonpain Symptoms.* Glenview, IL: American Academy of Hospice & Palliative Medicine; 2012.

Management of delirium begins with addressing reversible underlying etiologies. If symptoms persist, both nonpharmacologic and pharmacologic methods may be utilized. Nonpharmacologic strategies include frequent reorientation, lights on and off at appropriate times, family member presence, optimizing sensory input (hearing aids, glasses when indicated), minimizing noise and disruption at night, and encouraging cognitively stimulating activities. For pharmacologic management, the mainstay of treatment is low-dose Haldol, 0.5 to 2 mg PO or IV q2 to 12 hours. Atypical antipsychotics (including olanzapine, risperidone, quetiapine, ziprasidone, and aripiprazole) have also been used, though they are more expensive and have not been shown to have superior efficacy. Patients receiving antipsychotics should be monitored for side effects including extrapyramidal symptoms and prolonged QT interval. A QTc interval greater than or equal to 500 ms or increase of 60 ms (or 20%) from baseline indicates increased risk of torsades des pointes and should prompt consideration of discontinuation of the antipsychotic and consultation with a cardiologist, taking into account the patient's prognosis and goals of care.

Use of psychostimulants, such as methylphenidate, have been suggested as a possible pharmacologic management for hypoactive delirium. Though no randomized controlled trials have been performed, one small open label prospective trial (73) and several case reports have suggested a benefit. Pharmacotherapy has also been studied to prevent delirium, but a recent review concluded that current evidence is not supportive of use of either cholinesterase inhibitors or antipsychotics for the prevention of delirium (71). Benzodiazepines are occasionally appropriate as an adjunct treatment in patients with agitation refractory to neuroleptics, but for the most part should be avoided given that they can worsen delirium and agitation.

Depression

Depressive symptoms are common among patients with cancer; roughly 45% of patients with solid tumors report depressive symptoms and 15% receive a diagnosis of major depression (74). One study of low-income women with breast or gynecologic cancer found that 17% met criteria for moderate-to-severe depressive disorders. Only 12% of those meeting criteria were receiving medication and only 5% were seeing a counselor or participating in a support group (75). Depressive symptoms in cancer patients have been associated with multiple adverse outcomes including less satisfaction with care, increased use of health services, delayed return to work, reduced QOL, elevated risk of suicide, and increased mortality (74).

Several barriers to the accurate diagnosis of depression are unique to patients with cancer. Standard characterizations of depressive symptoms include both somatic and emotional/cognitive symptoms, but the somatic symptoms (fatigue, weight loss, etc.) are also common symptoms of cancer and its treatment. Additionally, it can be challenging to distinguish between normal and pathological responses to severe illness. Patients with cancer are at risk of both overdiagnosis of depression (if symptoms related to normal grief reaction are over-interpreted as depression) and underdiagnosis (if depressive symptoms in a patient with cancer are believed to be "normal" given the presence of serious illness). The presence of hopelessness, worthlessness, anhedonia, or suicidal ideation can help distinguish clinical depression from grief reaction, as none of these are expected in a normal grief reaction. Temporal variation can also be helpful. Patients experiencing a normal grief reaction will generally have symptoms that wax and wane, whereas patients with depression will have continuous symptoms (76).

While there is no consensus on the single best approach to diagnose depression in patients with cancer, a single screening question such as "are you depressed?" performs reasonably well, with sensitivity of 72%, specificity of 83%, positive predictive value of 44%, and negative predictive value of 94%. The addition of a second question (regarding low interest/pleasure in doing things) improves sensitivity (91%), specificity (86%), positive predictive value (57%), and negative predictive value (98%) (77). These simple screening questions can be used to trigger either a more extensive evaluation or a referral to a mental health or palliative care specialist. Providers must either implement routine depression screening (as recommended by both the NCCN and IOM) or maintain a high index of suspicion to avoid overlooking this common issue and its associated morbidity.

Both psychotherapy and antidepressant medications have shown efficacy in treating depression in patients with cancer. Medication options include tricyclic antidepressants (TCAs), serotonin-specific reuptake inhibitors (SSRIs), and serotonin–norepinephrine reuptake inhibitors (SNRIs). TCAs may be particularly useful if neuropathic pain or insomnia are part of the picture, but their use is often limited by anticholinergic side effects. SSRIs are less sedating than TCAs, but side effects may include headache, nausea, and insomnia. A recent review of antidepressants concluded that there is no evidence to recommend one over another based on efficacy, and so differences in onset of action, side effects, and available routes of administration may drive choice of medication (78). In gynecologic cancer patients who have neuropathy or neuropathic pain related to their disease or its treatment, use of an SNRI such as venlafaxine or duloxetine may also provide some neuropathic pain relief. TCAs, SSRIs, and SNRIs all take several weeks to achieve therapeutic effect. For patients for whom quicker symptom relief is desired or life expectancy is short, use of a psychostimulant such as methylphenidate is another option. Utilization of mental health professionals should be considered, when available, for complex cases.

Anxiety

Transient anxiety is a near-universal reaction to the stressful circumstances surrounding the diagnosis and treatment of cancer. For a significant number of patients, however, anxiety becomes more severe, pervasive, and disabling, and may impact their cancer treatment and QOL (79). The cancer patient with disabling anxiety will often have had a preexisting mood disorder such as panic attacks, generalized anxiety disorder, or depression. Treatment of this symptom includes pharmacologic and nonpharmacologic methods. Cognitive behavioral therapy (CBT), mindfulness-based stress reduction, supportive-expressive psychotherapy, and relaxation training have all shown utility in the treatment or prophylaxis of anxiety in the cancer patient (80–83). Pharmacologic therapy should emphasize antidepressants, with similar recommendations as those noted above. Benzodiazepines, especially short-acting agents such as alprazolam and lorazepam, are not recommended for long-term use due to their addictive potential, as well as their association with sedation, delirium, and falls (84).

Symptom Management in the Last Days of Life

Despite the fact that most cancer patients say they would prefer to die at home, approximately a third of them will spend their final days in a hospital or an ICU (85). Predicting when a patient is in the final days of her life is not always simple. Hui and colleagues have identified the following physical findings as predictive of 3-day mortality: nonreactive pupils, decreased response to verbal and visual stimuli, inability to close eyelids, drooping of nasolabial fold, neck hyperextension, grunting of vocal cords, upper GI tract bleeding, pulselessness of radial artery, decreased urine output, Cheyne–Stokes breathing, respiration with mandibular movement, and the "death rattle" created by uncleared bronchial secretions (86).

Care in the final days of life should focus on optimizing symptom management and minimizing non-beneficial interventions. Involvement of a specialty palliative care team may be appropriate where available. In a gynecologic cancer population, drowsiness, decreased well-being, anorexia, and tiredness were present in more than 70% of patients in the last week of life (87). When the care of a hospitalized patient transitions to being purely focused on comfort, all medications that are not directly related to comfort should be discontinued. The decision about whether any given medication, such as an antiarrhythmic or an anticonvulsant, should be continued to prevent unpleasant symptoms must be individualized to the patient and her ability to take the medication. In the last few days of life as a patient becomes unable to take oral (PO) medications, medications must be transitioned to sublingual, intravenous (IV), subcutaneous (SC), or per rectum (PR). Medications should be ordered and made available as needed for anticipated symptoms including pain, nausea, dyspnea, delirium, and upper airway secretions. Though noise created by uncleared bronchial secretions (sometimes referred to as "death rattle") is not thought to be uncomfortable for the patient, it is often distressing to family members and can be treated with anticholinergic medication. Options include glycopyrrolate 0.1 to 0.2 mg IV or SC q4 hours prn, atropine 0.4 mg SC q 15 minutes prn, or scopolamine patch 1.5 mg. Counseling the family that the symptom is not uncomfortable for the patient may help alleviate distress. Though lab tests and telemetry should be discontinued, consideration should be given to continuing to check temperature and respiratory rate, given that fever creates discomfort and should be treated with Tylenol (IV or PR), and tachypnea creates discomfort and should be treated with opioids even in nonverbal patients.

When rounding on a patient in the last few days of life, vital signs and as-needed (prn) medication use should be reviewed with the nurse caring for the patient. If the nurse is inexperienced in caring for patients in the final days of life, a conversation about why certain vital signs are being followed and what signs should prompt administration of prn medications (restlessness, agitation, brow furrowing, tachypnea) may be helpful. Examination of the patient should include at least a general visual inspection for signs of distress or agitation, with note taken of signs reviewed above that may be predictive of death within 3 days. Touching the patient's hand will reveal fever or cool/mottled extremities, if present. Anticipatory counseling should be offered to the family in terms of what to expect as death approaches, but should only be given if the family expresses interest. Consideration should be given to mentioning signs including waxing and waning consciousness, mottled extremities (not painful to patient) and irregular breathing with periods of apnea (family may observe pauses in breathing and think the patient has passed only to have them breathe again) that are a normal part of the dying process. It may be helpful to mention to families that while we do not know for sure whether unresponsive patients process tactile or auditory sensory input, it may be comforting to both patient and family for them to touch and talk to the patient, even after she no longer responds to them. See **Table 32.4** for a sample order set for a patient receiving comfort-focused care in the last hours to days of life.

TABLE 32.4. Sample Order Set for End of Life for Non-pain Symptoms

Category	Sample Order	Comments
Vital signs	Temperature and respiratory rate q4 hours prn	Fever should be treated because it causes discomfort; tachypnea should be treated with opioids because it may reflect pain or dyspnea
Mouth care	Oral care q2–4 hours	Particularly important for patients who are unconscious and mouth breathing
Oxygen	Oxygen by nasal cannula prn for comfort	Oxygen is not necessary unless patient is alert and complaining of dyspnea relieved by oxygen, otherwise it is preferable to avoid attaching an additional tube to the patient
Anxiety/ Agitation	Lorazepam 0.5–1 mg IV q1 hour prn	In a conscious or semiconscious patient, may consider treating agitation with opioids or Haldol first, as agitation may reflect pain or delirium, and benzodiazepines can worsen delirium and may be sedating
Delirium and/or Nausea	haloperidol 0.5 mg IV q4 hours prn	Important to instruct nursing that haloperidol can be used for nausea
Secretions	Glycopyrrolate 0.2 mg IV q4 hours prn OR Atropine ophthalmic 1% solution 2 drops SL q30 min prn	Sounds related to secretions are not uncomfortable for the patient, but may be treated if they are upsetting to the family
Fever	Acetaminophen 650 mg PO or PR q 4 h prn	In an unconscious patient, fever should be treated with PR Tylenol as fever causes discomfort
Constipation	Dulcolax 10 mg PR daily prn	In patient with life expectancy >24–48 h, consider treating constipation as it can cause discomfort and delirium and a single large bowel movement after suppository will require less frequent moving of the unconscious patient than multiple frequent small bowel movements
Eye Care	Ocular lubricant 1 application both eyes q8 h prn	Particularly important in patients who are unconscious and may not close eyes completely, their eyes may become dry
Nutrition	PO foods and fluids as tolerated for comfort	

Communication

Breaking Bad News

Physicians at all levels of training feel ill-prepared for conversations regarding end-of-life care (88). Although efforts have been made in recent years to improve training in this regard (89), it is estimated that only 5% of practicing oncologists have formal training in breaking bad news or discussing prognosis (90). The literature suggests that patients prefer to have prognostic information, even when the news is worse than expected. Moreover, withholding of bad news may result in a loss of trust between the patient and her physician.

There are several helpful protocols for communication of bad news. One of the best known is the SPIKES protocol, a six-step protocol that incorporates the principles of communication and counseling (91). The SPIKES protocol emphasizes that these conversations should start by clarifying what the patient knows. Information should be provided based on the patient and family members' level of knowledge using clear, nonmedical language; open-ended, empathetic statements; responses to strong emotions; and adequate time for questions. Clinicians should check comprehension frequently and allow moments of silence for processing information.

Prognosis

Talking to patients and their family members about prognosis and end-of-life care is a common and extremely important part of the job of caring for those with life-limiting malignancies. Patients who have a good understanding of their prognosis are less likely to die in the hospital, are more likely to have hospice care at the end of life, and have a better QOL (92). However, many studies continue to document problems with communication. Between a third and three quarters of patients with advanced cancers in recent studies do not understand that their disease is incurable, and most patients have overoptimistic expectations of prognosis (93). Physicians and nurses caring for patients who request aggressive and futile interventions at the end of life based on unrealistic expectations for cure are impacted as well, with several studies documenting moral distress and burnout under these circumstances (94).

Although almost all oncologists agree with the importance of accurate communication regarding prognosis, in practice they tend to avoid or postpone the discussion and instead focus on positive, optimistic formulations about the illness and treatment (95,96). This hesitation to initiate more substantive and realistic discussions of prognosis is often framed in terms of concerns about the impact of such discussions on the patient and, in particular, concerns that such conversations will cause the patient to be depressed, lose hope, and even die more quickly. However, as many have pointed out, physicians who avoid discussing death are also protecting themselves, since talking about this topic causes anxiety, feelings of inadequacy, failure, and loss of control in doctors as well as patients (97).

While there is no evidence that cancer patients who are better informed about their condition have higher rates of depression (95), they do tend to be more satisfied with the communication skills of overly optimistic practitioners (98). This may be because while almost all patients want to be informed of the "truth" in a general way, they also want the truth to be good news and they want their physicians to provide them with hope (99). Almost half of patients with cancer do not want to know their life expectancy even when close to the end of life (100). They "collude" with their physicians in avoiding end-of-life discussions (96). Both patients and family members may misunderstand, discount, or misinterpret negative prognostic information when it is provided (101).

In the face of these serious barriers, it is no wonder that planning for end of life is often lacking in cancer care. The simplistic model in which the oncologist presents full, explicit information regarding prognosis and choices for treatment to the grateful patient who then makes rational choices regarding care by weighing the risks and benefits of treatment disintegrates in the face of the realities of medical practice where prognosis is hard to predict, patients and their family members are distressed and looking for hope, and the oncologist feels internal and external pressure to be optimistic. Several authors have synthesized years of data regarding decisional styles and informational needs of patients and their family members, which may provide a way forward out of the dilemmas outlined above (98,102). One consistent finding is that while many patients do not want to know their prognosis, they do want to know what is going to happen to them: meaning whether or not they can be cured of their cancer and what the treatments can do for them (103). These desires seem contradictory, but in fact may not be so. While patients are often reluctant to hear information about how long they have to live, they are more open to being told that they will, eventually, in some unknown time frame, die of their disease. One way of framing this more qualitative discussion of prognosis is by utilizing the concept of illness trajectory. The illness trajectory of incurable cancer is one of relative stability in functioning until 3 to 6 months prior to death when rapid declines in the ability to perform activities of daily living heralds the onset of terminal stages and is associated with increased risk of harm from systemic treatments (104). Early discussions of the expected course and trajectory of care in these terms can provide the patient and family with a general overview of the goals of treatment, which is to prolong the period of time in which the patient is able to feel well and lead a relatively normal life, while acknowledging that the cancer will eventually be fatal. Describing the clinical signs of progressive disease in terms of functional decline, increasing symptom burden and resistance to disease-specific treatment provides the patient with information that is understandable and useful for advance care planning (ACP) and decision making and gives them a clearer road map for the future. More detailed discussions of life expectancy can be reserved for patients closer to the end of life, when more accurate predictions can be made (105).

This way of framing the discussion avoids the pitfalls of discussing statistical information about length of life. Not only do many patients wish to avoid such discussions, many have a poor understanding of statistics, and struggle to interpret such information. Furthermore, providing accurate prognostic information to an individual patient is very difficult until very close to the end of life since prognosis is a bell curve, and any individual patient can live for much longer or shorter than the average life expectancy of their group. **Table 32.5** presents three different ways of discussing goals of care/prognosis. The purely factual statement, while truthful, seems cold and uncompassionate, and may leave the patient feeling uncared for and in search of hope. The hopeful statement, while true, is ambiguous and many patients hearing this might believe that the treatment they are getting is aimed at cure, because of the emphasis on hopeful new research. The doctor using the second formulation is likely to have higher patient satisfaction, but more poorly informed patients. The illness trajectory formulation is aimed at balancing hope with realism and provides the basis for further discussion.

Finally, it should be noted that these discussions are best carried out in a collaborative and interprofessional manner. Involvement of nursing, social work, and chaplaincy where appropriate can improve the quality of care and may decrease moral distress for all providers.

Advance Care Planning

Advance care planning is a broad paradigm that includes the steps required to enable patients to guide their future health care so that it is consistent with their goals when they are no longer capable of making decisions for themselves. ACP includes discussions about goals for care at the end of life, designation of a health care power of attorney (HPA), and completion of an advance directive (AD) (also called a living will). ACP has been shown to improve compliance with the end-of-life wishes of patients, enhance patient and family satisfaction with care, and reduce family stress, anxiety, and depression.

Code status is just one component of ACP and may be included in an AD. Code status may be a required part of documentation for

TABLE 32.5. Styles of Communication

Style of Discussion	Example
Factual	Your cancer is incurable. This chemotherapy has a 50% chance of prolonging your life. On average, most people with your cancer live for 3 years if they do chemotherapy and 2 years if they do not do the chemotherapy.
Hopeful	Your cancer is incurable; however, we have some really excellent new treatments and every day there is new research into the causes of cancer and new hope that will allow us to fight this disease.
Illness trajectory	Your cancer is incurable; however, there are many treatments that can prolong your life and improve your QOL, and our hope is that we can keep you feeling well and leading a normal life for as long as possible. Over time, we know that this type of cancer will stop responding well to treatment and when it progresses patients become weaker, need more help at home, and have more side effects from chemotherapy. When that happens we will do everything we can to help you feel as well as possible for as long as possible by treating your symptoms and making sure you can continue to enjoy your life.

a hospital admission, but determining code status is not, or should not, be as simple as asking a patient if she wants cardiopulmonary resuscitation (CPR). A code status discussion should take into account an individual patient's chance for recovery and her underlying values and ideally should take place in the context of a broader discussion about goals of care and care preferences. It is also important to keep in mind that a meta-analysis of hospital CPR outcomes for patients with cancer showed that only 6.7% survived to discharge (9.1% with localized disease and 5.6% with metastatic disease) (106). A recent study of patients with advanced cancer found that after viewing an educational video regarding ACP, fewer patients wanted CPR or ventilation; the patients found the video acceptable and would recommend it to others (107). A randomized trial by the same group found that patients with advanced cancer who viewed a video of CPR were less likely to opt for CPR than those who listened to a verbal narrative (108).

While most patients believe that addressing ACP is an important part of their cancer care (109,110), oncology providers often find it difficult to discuss and assume that patients will be hesitant or even unwilling to have the conversation (111). Retrospective studies of deceased cancer patients found that only 19% had a documented AD (112). One study specific to gynecologic cancer patients found that 54% of gynecologic oncologists deferred end-of-life discussions until the patient experienced a major decline in functional status (113). Another study of women with breast and gynecologic cancers found that 50% of women self-reported completing an AD and 48% had named an HPA, but review of medical records documented an AD and HPA for 24% and 14% of women, respectively (114). A meta-analysis of the cancer literature concluded that "all stakeholders are reluctant to initiate ACP early and prefer to delay ACP until the issues raised, particularly those surrounding preferences for end of life care, are more clinically relevant (115)."

The concept of POLST (physician orders for life-sustaining treatment) originated at the Oregon Health and Science University in the 1990s and is meant to complement (not replace) the AD. The POLST form allows the patient's wishes regarding end-of-life treatment to be expressed in an unambiguous medical order with specific treatment instructions. The use of the POLST form communicates the patient's wishes regarding the use of so-called extreme measures (such as ventilators) but also specifies decisions regarding the use of antibiotics, peripheral nutrition, and other medical interventions. It is signed by the physician and by the patient or her surrogate and a copy should be placed in the medical record. The POLST form varies from state to state.

Increasing compliance with ACP is a goal of all cancer providers and their patients. However, the literature suggests that patients expect their physicians to introduce the topic, and that cancer patients prefer that this introduction be made by their primary oncologist (115). It is therefore important for gynecologic oncologists to feel comfortable introducing the topic to their patients. ACP can be a process rather than a single discussion and should not be confused with completion of the AD, which is only a small part of the overall process. Inclusion of nonphysician providers may be important in increasing compliance with completion of AD (114).

Running a Successful Family Meeting

One of the most important tools to facilitate communication with people with advanced disease is the family meeting (116). Family meetings (or conferences) are meetings that include the family caregivers, the patient (where possible), and a multidisciplinary group of health professionals, and are undertaken for multiple purposes including: discussing diagnosis, treatment, prognosis; clarifying the goals of care; developing a plan of care for the patient and caregivers; and discharge planning. Most of the data with respect to the utility of family meetings is derived from the ICU setting, with limited data specific to gynecologic cancer patients.

One study from MD Anderson described family meetings for patients with cancer (117), as follows: A formal meeting with the patient and her family was arranged, also including health care providers, a palliative care physician, a social worker, a chaplain, and a case manager. The meeting began with the social worker introducing the participants. The palliative care physician then discussed the clinical scenario, including cancer history and treatment plan, options for symptom management, prognosis including ADs, and discharge planning. The social worker recorded the meeting, making note of any distress shown by the family or the patient.

Not all family meetings can be run with this sort of multidisciplinary model, but gynecologic oncologists can successfully run a family meeting that attends to all the domains of the patient and her family, even with limited resources. Careful planning is essential. Before the meeting, the physician should decide which issues are to be addressed, which providers will be present, where the meeting will take place, and whether or not the patient will be part of the meeting. The goal of the meeting should be clearly stated to all participants, and time should be allowed for all family members to express their opinions.

Teaching Communication

Numerous studies indicate that patient-oncologist communication is suboptimal, particularly when focusing on issues at the end of life (118). Fortunately, communication skills can be taught, even to busy clinicians, as evidenced by the SCOPE trial, performed with medical, radiation, and gynecologic oncologists in the United States (119). Clinicians were randomly assigned to complete a 1-hour interactive CD-ROM program about responding to patients' negative emotions. Oncologists in the intervention group used more empathetic statements and were more likely to respond to negative emotions empathetically. Perhaps most importantly, patients of intervention oncologists reported greater trust in their oncologists than did patients of control oncologists.

Impact of Communication on Outcomes

Good communication can improve quality of care at the end of life. The group from Duke found that, in a cohort of women with persistent or recurrent ovarian cancer, women who had earlier end-of-life discussions with their health care providers had care that more highly conformed with EOL quality measures (28). Additionally, they were less likely to die in the hospital. The authors stressed that early EOL discussions, preferably conducted more than 30 days from death, increased hospice utilization and were crucial to reducing hospitalizations, ICU admissions, and invasive procedures in the last 30 days of life.

Caregiver Needs

Caregivers, most often family members, are called upon to provide physical care as well as emotional and practical support (120,121). They may experience significant stress in this role, including financial stress if they are unable to continue working while providing care, as well as anxiety about the future. Risk factors for caregiver distress include: other life stresses, poor social support, lower socioeconomic status, younger age, and a closer caregiver–patient relationship (121). Caregivers may be at high risk themselves for health problems resulting from the stress of caring for a gynecologic cancer patient (122). There is therefore a significant need for education of caregivers, who may feel unprepared for their new role, as well as emotional and, where needed, spiritual support (123).

The Australian Ovarian Cancer Study studied the QOL of 99 caregivers of women with ovarian cancer, and reported significantly lower mental and physical QOL for these caregivers when compared to the population norm (121). Mean distress and unmet needs increased over time. Highest unmet needs in the last 6 months of life included managing emotions about prognosis, fear of cancer spread, balancing the caregiver's own needs and the patient's needs, impact of caring on work, and making decisions in the context of uncertainty. Caregiver optimism was associated with improved mental well-being and decreased distress. The authors suggest that caregivers would benefit from early contact with psychosocial staff rather than waiting for post-death referral to bereavement services. Additionally, caregivers having access to providers as well as information resources and support groups may be helpful in fulfilling the need for information that was identified in this study.

QUALITY OF LIFE

There is no common definition for QOL. The WHO defines QOL as an "individual's perception of their position in life in the context of the culture and value systems in which they live and in relation to their goals, expectations, standards and concerns (124)." Health-related QOL, or HRQOL, encompasses symptoms, functioning, psychological well-being, and meaning and fulfillment.

Scales and Measures

Several validated and reliable questionnaires are available for assessment of HRQOL for cancer patients, including the European Organization for Research and Treatment of Cancer (EORTC-QLQ-C30) and the Functional Assessment of Cancer-General version (FACT-G). Domain-specific instruments assess specific domains, such as fatigue or psychological distress. The FACT-G version 4 questionnaire includes the following four subscales: physical well-being, social well-being, emotional well-being, and functional well-being. The subscales can be analyzed separately or together to produce a total HRQOL score. The FACT-G has demonstrated reliability, validity, and responsiveness to change over time (125). The Functional Assessment of Cancer Therapy-Ovarian (FACT-O) is a multidimensional questionnaire developed and validated for use by ovarian cancer patients. There are also specific subscales for cervical cancer (FACT-Cx), endometrial cancer (FACT-En), and vulvar cancer (FACT-V). Higher FACT scores are associated with better HRQOL.

Quality at the End of Life

The National Quality Forum published the following EOL quality performance measures, with a lower occurrence representing better quality of care: admission to ICU within 30 days of death, hospital admission more than 14 days in the last 30 days of life, more than one hospital admission during the last 30 days of life, more than one ED visit during the last 30 days, death in an acute care setting, initiation of a new chemotherapy regimen in the last 30 days, chemotherapy within 14 days of death, and hospice admission less than 3 days before death (126). In women with ovarian cancer, these aggressive care interventions (ACE) at EOL were not associated with improvement in survival for patients with ovarian cancer, and serve as good general quality indicators for gynecologic cancers (27).

Other groups have provided data specific to gynecologic cancer patients regarding ACE. The group from Montefiore reported that timely palliative medicine consultation was associated with lower ACE scores, but only 18% of patients received a "timely" (defined as 30 or more days before death) palliative care consultation (127). Another study from the same group reported the following retrospective data with respect to ACE: median days in hospital during last 6 months of life was 24 days, 30% of patients had an emergency department visit, and 21% were admitted to the ICU. 50% had terminal extubation and 13% had CPR at the EOL. 76% of patients received chemotherapy during the last 6 months of life and 30% in the last 6 weeks (128). 66% of patients were DNR/DNI, 49% enrolled in hospice (median 16 days, range 0 to 149 days), 64% had a family meeting in this study.

QOL as a Clinical Trial Endpoint

HRQOL has evolved into an important albeit secondary endpoint for many cancer clinical trials. In 2014 the ASCO Cancer Research Committee met to discuss "the design of future clinical trials that would produce results that are clinically meaningful to patients." Clinically meaningful was defined as significantly improved survival, significantly improved QOL, or both (129). Recognizing the importance of a patient's specific symptom burden, the ASCO work group suggested that serial assessment of specific cancer-related symptoms using validated instruments constitutes a meaningful clinical outcome. While ovarian cancer patients are willing to undergo significant toxicity in the front-line treatment setting when cure is possible, they are less accepting of toxicities and impairment in daily routine in the recurrent disease treatment setting (130). The study from Havrilesky et al. (131) confirms this finding: 95 women with advanced or recurrent ovarian cancer were willing to accept a shorter progression-free survival (PFS) to avoid severe side effects of treatment: 6.7 months to reduce nausea and vomiting from severe to mild, 5 months to reduce neuropathy from severe to mild, and 3.7 months to reduce abdominal symptoms from severe to moderate. While PFS remained a driver of patient preference, women were willing to trade PFS time for reduction in treatment-related toxicity.

The Gynecology Oncology Group (GOG) has been incorporating HRQOL endpoints into their phase 3 studies for the past decade. In GOG 240, a randomized trial of chemotherapy with or without bevacizumab in patients with advanced or recurrent cervical cancer, the primary QOL endpoint was the score on the Functional Assessment of Cancer Therapy-Cervix Trial Outcome Index (FACT-Cx TOI) (132). Improvements in overall survival and PFS attributed to the incorporation of bevacizumab into the treatment of advanced cervical cancer were not accompanied by any significant deterioration in health-related QOL, allowing the authors to conclude that the addition of bevacizumab achieved a desirable outcome overall. The GOG has also included QOL as a secondary endpoint in several of its recent phase 3 randomized trials in ovarian cancer (133–136). In one of these studies, the GOG showed for the first time that in ovarian cancer patients, baseline QOL scores predicted overall survival (134), and this has been confirmed by others (135).

Other clinical trial groups have also incorporated QOL as clinical trial endpoints. A well-known and practice-changing example is the CALYPSO study, which has changed the standard of care for women with recurrent platinum-sensitive ovarian cancer, run by the

Gynecologic Cancer InterGroup (137). This study was undertaken primarily to identify a treatment regimen for these women that would be non-inferior to traditional therapy and better tolerated from a symptom standpoint. Quality-of-life evaluations (European Organization for Research and Treatment of Cancer Quality of Life Questionnaire C30 version 3.0 and OV-28 version 1.0) were required at 3-month intervals while on treatment, and every 3 months for 1 year from date of enrollment. The primary endpoint was non-inferiority of the less toxic regimen. The study was able to demonstrate that the new regimen was better tolerated than the standard regimen, with improvement in overall QOL, as well as an improvement in overall survival. Progression-free and overall survival remain the primary endpoints of cancer clinical trials, confirmed by the ASCO 2014 workgroup. However, the inclusion of HRQOL as a secondary endpoint allows a more comprehensive interpretation of results and leads to improved clinical decision-making.

BARRIERS TO THE USE OF PALLIATIVE CARE IN GYNECOLOGIC ONCOLOGY

Lack of Specialty Palliative Care Services

Not all facilities have the ability to provide access to specialty palliative care services. Not-for-profit hospitals and public hospitals were, respectively, 4.8 times and 7.1 times more likely to have a palliative care program as compared to for-profit hospitals (138). On a national level in the United States, there are not enough specialty palliative care providers to see all patients who might benefit (20,139,140). The 2015 *State-by-State Report Card* from the Center to Advance Palliative Care and the National Palliative Care Research Center demonstrates that access to palliative care remains inadequate for millions of Americans living with serious illness, despite continuing growth in the number of US hospitals reporting palliative care programs (141). Access to palliative care services depends on geography, with the highest penetration in the New England (88% of hospitals), Pacific (77% of hospitals), and mid-Atlantic (77% of hospitals) states, and lowest in the west south central (43% of hospitals) and east south central (42% of hospitals) states (138). One-third of hospitals in the United States report no palliative care services of any kind, and one-third of states received a grade of C or D. Access to palliative care in community settings such as nursing homes remains limited for people who are not hospice eligible.

Gynecologic oncologists should be able to provide primary palliative care for their own patients, but not all of them feel trained to provide these services. In fact, the majority of gynecologic oncology fellows report insufficient palliative care education during fellowship, with only 11% reporting a palliative care rotation or formal training (142,143). While both fellowship directors and fellows believe that palliative care education is critical, the formal curriculum is not well developed (144). Future development of formal primary palliative care curricula and institution of this curricula into fellowship training programs will be important in training gynecologic oncologists to provide appropriate care.

Poor Reimbursement

Current reimbursement schedules are not structured to support early integration of palliative care into oncology care. Historically, providers were not reimbursed for end-of-life discussions with their patients, or for addressing advanced directives. However, the Centers for Medicare and Medicaid Services (CMS) recently proposed and finalized regulations that will allow Medicare to pay physicians and other qualified health care professionals for providing ACP (145). Specifically, in a proposed regulation released July 8, 2015, CMS introduced two new billing codes for ACP provided to Medicare beneficiaries. On October 30, 2015, CMS finalized these proposed provisions, allowing physicians and other health professionals to bill Medicare for ACP, as a separate service, starting January 1, 2016. Previous Medicare coverage rules only allowed reimbursement for ACP under very limited circumstances. There are currently no plans for improved reimbursement for palliative care services in conjunction with cancer care.

Institutional Limitations

Institutional limitations include the lack of financial support for specialty palliative care, poor reimbursement for palliative care services, and lack of legislation promoting and supporting the integration of palliative care into routine oncology care (17,140,146). Pay-for-performance quality improvement initiatives have shown promise in facilitating the integration of palliative care (147).

Misconceptions about Palliative Care

One of the biggest barriers to the use of palliative care is the misconception, by both patients and providers, that it is synonymous with end-of-life care. A public opinion survey noted that 70% of people self-identified as "not at all knowledgeable" about palliative care (148). Data from providers has shown that many lack knowledge of locally available specialty palliative care services, and mistakenly consider palliative care to be synonymous with end-of-life care and thus incompatible with anticancer therapy (148,149). Due to similar misconceptions, cancer center executives worry that the presence of specialty palliative care could negatively affect their hospital mortality rate and national rating (17). One study found that providers preferred the term "supportive care" to "palliative care" and would be more likely to refer patients to a service named "supportive care (6)." When that institution changed the name of their palliative care service to supportive care, they saw a 40% increase in referrals and a change toward referrals earlier in the disease course (150). The IOM report "Dying in America" concluded that "one of the greatest remaining challenges is the need for better understanding of the role of palliative care among both the public and professionals across the continuum of care so that hospice and palliative care can achieve their full potential for patients and their families (139)."

Misconceptions specific to hospice are also prevalent. There remains a significant lack of education on the part of both providers and patients and family members regarding the benefit of hospice, as well as a suspicion on the part of patients that "hospice means they will kill me faster (151)." Claims of "death panels" remain in the common culture and contribute to reluctance on the part of patients to discuss hospice options. A Kaiser Family Foundation survey from 2013 found that more than one-third (35%) of people ages 65 and over incorrectly believed that a panel was created by the Affordable Care Act to make end-of-life decisions for Medicare beneficiaries (152). Other barriers to timely hospice utilization include overestimation of prognosis, the lack of physician awareness of the demonstrated benefits, and the requirement to forgo anticancer therapy prior to hospice enrollment. Education about the benefits and true nature of hospice will be very important in helping our patients to accept this important benefit at the end of life.

IMPROVING PALLIATIVE CARE FOR WOMEN WITH GYNECOLOGIC CANCERS

Education

Most of the primary palliative care for women with gynecologic cancers will be provided by gynecologic oncologists. Several studies have suggested that fellowship trainees, both medical and gynecologic oncology fellows, do not believe they are adequately trained to address most of the palliative care issues they will face during their careers. Medical oncology fellows have reported inadequate training in symptom management, and little training in giving bad news. Several studies address the issue of palliative care delivery education specifically in gynecologic oncology fellowships. The survey data from Eskander suggest that gynecologic oncology fellows felt the education was lacking, with this result obtained by asking specifically about attending gynecologic oncologists, teaching and direct feedback (rather than about a formal curriculum) (142). A similar survey study from Lefkowits et al. (144) noted that 100% of gynecologic oncology fellowship programs had didactic coverage of palliative topics and 48% had an available palliative care rotation. There was, however, no correlation between the topics that were formally taught and the topics that were considered by the faculty to be the most important. There is clearly room for improving the palliative care curriculum and exposure in gynecologic oncology fellowships. The change of the fellowship governing board to Accreditation Council of Graduate Medical Education expected in 2016–2017 and the associated new Milestones should continue to address this important issue.

Partnering with Specialty Palliative Care

One study of gynecologic cancer patients who were discontinuing chemotherapy found that patients who had seen palliative care prior to the decision to discontinue chemotherapy (compared with those who were referred to palliative care only after the decision to discontinue chemotherapy) had better QOL, emotional functioning and social functioning, less depression, less insomnia, and fewer issues with communication. The patients with earlier palliative care integration also received less chemotherapy within the last 6 weeks of life, and earlier palliative care was an independent predictor of improved overall survival. Another study of patients who had died of gynecologic cancer found that 49% had been referred to palliative care, but only 18% had been referred more than 30 days before their death (127). Among a group of gynecologic cancer patients meeting ASCO recommendations for early palliative care integration, only 53% were referred to palliative care (153). These data, taken together with the robust data in the general oncology literature demonstrating benefits of early specialty palliative care integration (4), suggest that we are likely underutilizing specialty palliative care in women with gynecologic cancer. A cost-effectiveness analysis using clinical benefit data from the Temel trial in lung cancer found routine palliative care referral to be at least cost-effective, possibly even cost-saving, for patients with platinum-resistant ovarian cancer. Gynecologic oncology providers should familiarize themselves with the specialty palliative care resources available at their institutions and utilize them liberally, including early in the disease course for patients with advanced disease or high symptom needs. Palliative care enhances both the quality and the value of gynecologic cancer care.

CONCLUSION

The Center to Advance Palliative Care defines palliative care as "specialized medical care for people living with serious illness. It focuses on providing relief from the symptoms and stress of a serious illness...the goal is to improve QOL for both the patient and the family...Palliative care is appropriate at any age and at any stage in a serious illness and can be provided along with curative treatment." Palliative care involves meticulous evaluation and treatment of the symptoms of cancer and the side effects of cancer therapy. It also involves talking frankly and compassionately with patients and caregivers about the disease and its prognosis, and their goals and expectations; it involves optimizing not just quantity, but also QOL. As providers of both surgical and medical oncology throughout the disease course, gynecologic oncologists have unique longitudinal relationships with their patients and are thus well positioned to provide basic palliative care. The education of gynecologic oncology providers must prepare them for that role. With mounting evidence of the clinical and health systems benefits of specialty palliative care, those services are becoming more and more ubiquitous and should be liberally utilized as "an extra layer of support" for patients with complex needs related to symptom management or navigating goals of care. Gynecologic oncology providers must join the WHO (1), the IOM (139), ASCO (2), and the SGO (3) in recognizing that palliative care is an integral component of high-quality, comprehensive, and individualized care for our patients.

REFERENCES

1. World Health Organization. WHO Definition of Palliative Care. 2002. http://www.who.int/cancer/palliative/definition/en/. Accessed December 24, 2015.
2. Ferris FD, Bruera E, Cherny N, et al. Palliative cancer care a decade later: accomplishments, the need, next steps—from the American Society of Clinical Oncology. *J Clin Oncol.* 2009;27(18):3052–3058.
3. Rimel BJ, Burke WM, Higgins RV, et al. Improving quality and decreasing cost in gynecologic oncology care. Society of Gynecologic Oncology recommendations for clinical practice. *Gynecol Oncol.* 2015;137(2):280–284.
4. Parikh RB, Kirch RA, Smith TJ, et al. Early specialty palliative care-translating data in oncology into practice. *N Engl J Med.* 2013;369(24):2347–2351.
5. McInturff B, Harrington L. Presentation of 2011 Research on Palliative Care. 2011.
6. Fadul N, Elsayem A, Palmer JL, et al. Supportive versus palliative care: what's in a name?: A survey of medical oncologists and midlevel providers at a comprehensive cancer center. *Cancer.* 2009;115(9):2013–2021.
7. Temel JS, Greer JA, Muzikansky A, et al. Early palliative care for patients with metastatic non-small-cell lung cancer. *N Engl J Med.* 2010;363(8):733–742.
8. Bakitas M, Lyons KD, Hegel MT, et al. Effects of a palliative care intervention on clinical outcomes in patients with advanced cancer: the Project ENABLE II randomized controlled trial. *JAMA.* 2009;302(7):741–749.
9. Bakitas MA, Tosteson TD, Li Z, et al. Early versus delayed initiation of concurrent palliative oncology care: patient outcomes in the ENABLE III randomized controlled trial. *J Clin Oncol.* 2015;33(13):1438–1445.
10. Brumley R, Enguidanos S, Jamison P, et al. Increased satisfaction with care and lower costs: results of a randomized trial of in-home palliative care. *J Am Geriatr Soc.* 2007;55(7):993–1000.
11. Gade G, Venohr I, Conner D, et al. Impact of an inpatient palliative care team: a randomized control trial. *J Palliat Med.* 2008;11(2):180–190.
12. Meyers FJ, Carducci M, Loscalzo MJ, et al. Effects of a problem-solving intervention (COPE) on quality of life for patients with advanced cancer on clinical trials and their caregivers: simultaneous care educational intervention (SCEI): linking palliation and clinical trials. *J Palliat Med.* 2011;14(4):465–473.
13. Pantilat SZ, O'Riordan DL, Dibble SL, et al. Hospital-based palliative medicine consultation: a randomized controlled trial. *Arch Intern Med.* 2010;170(22):2038–2040.
14. Rabow MW, Dibble SL, Pantilat SZ, et al. The comprehensive care team: a controlled trial of outpatient palliative medicine consultation. *Arch Intern Med.* 2004;164(1):83–91.
15. Smith TJ, Temin S, Alesi ER, et al. American Society of Clinical Oncology provisional clinical opinion: the integration of palliative care into standard oncology care. *J Clin Oncol.* 2012;30(8):880–887.
16. *Choosing Wisely: an initiative of the ABIM* Foundation. 2015. http://www.choosingwisely.org/. Accessed December 24, 2015.
17. Hui D, Elsayem A, De la Cruz M, et al. Availability and integration of palliative care at US cancer centers. *JAMA.* 2010;303(11):1054–1061.
18. Rabow M, Kvale E, Barbour L, et al. Moving upstream: a review of the evidence of the impact of outpatient palliative care. *J Palliat Med.* 2013;16(12):1540–1549.
19. Parikh RB, Temel JS. Early specialty palliative care. *N Engl J Med.* 2014;370(11):1075–1076.
20. Quill TE, Abernethy AP. Generalist plus specialist palliative care—creating a more sustainable model. *N Engl J Med.* 2013;368(13):1173–1175.
21. Friedman BT, Harwood MK, Shields M. Barriers and enablers to hospice referrals: an expert overview. *J Palliat Med.* 2002;5(1):73–84.
22. NHPCO's Facts and Figures Hospice Care in America 2014 Edition. http://www.nhpco.org/sites/default/files/public/Statistics_Research/2014_Facts_Figures.pdf. Accessed January 31, 2016.
23. Connor SR, Pyenson B, Fitch K, et al. Comparing hospice and nonhospice patient survival among patients who die within a three-year window. *J Pain Symptom Manag.* 2007;33(3):238–246.
24. Wright AA, Keating NL, Balboni TA, et al. Place of death: correlations with quality of life of patients with cancer and predictors of bereaved caregivers' mental health. *J Clin Oncol.* 2010;28(29):4457–4464.
25. Teno JM, Clarridge BR, Casey V, et al. Family perspectives on end-of-life care at the last place of care. *JAMA.* 2004;291(1):88–93.

26. Keyser EA, Reed BG, Lowery WJ, et al. Hospice enrollment for terminally ill patients with gynecologic malignancies: impact on outcomes and interventions. *Gynecol Oncol.* 2010;118(3):274–277.
27. von Gruenigen V, Daly B, Gibbons H, et al. Indicators of survival duration in ovarian cancer and implications for aggressiveness of care. *Cancer.* 2008;112(10):2221–2227.
28. Lopez-Acevedo M, Havrilesky LJ, Broadwater G, et al. Timing of end-of-life care discussion with performance on end-of-life quality indicators in ovarian cancer. *Gynecol Oncol.* 2013;130(1):156–161.
29. Wright AA, Hatfield LA, Earle CC, et al. End-of-life care for older patients with ovarian cancer is intensive despite high rates of hospice use. *J Clin Oncol.* 2014;32(31):3534–3539.
30. Lefkowits C, Teuteberg W, Courtney-Brooks M, et al. Improvement in symptom burden within one day after palliative care consultation in a cohort of gynecologic oncology inpatients. *Gynecol Oncol.* 2015;136(3):424–428.
31. Lefkowits C, Rabow MW, Sherman AE, et al. Predictors of high symptom burden in gynecologic oncology outpatients: who should be referred to outpatient palliative care? *Gynecol Oncol.* 2014;132(3):698–702.
32. Grover S, Hill-Kayser CE, Vachani C, et al. Patient reported late effects of gynecological cancer treatment. *Gynecol Oncol.* 2012;124(3):399–403.
33. Snyder CF, Aaronson NK. Use of patient-reported outcomes in clinical practice. *Lancet.* 2009;374(9687):369–370.
34. Wagner LI, Schink J, Bass M, et al. Bringing PROMIS to practice: brief and precise symptom screening in ambulatory cancer care. *Cancer.* 2015;121(6):927–934.
35. Levy MH, Back A, Benedetti C, et al. NCCN clinical practice guidelines in oncology: palliative care. *J Natl Compr Canc Netw.* 2009;7(4):436–473.
36. Landrum LM, Blank S, Chen LM, et al. Comprehensive care in gynecologic oncology: the importance of palliative care. *Gynecol Oncol.* 2015;137(2):193–202.
37. Stephenson J, Davies A. An assessment of aetiology-based guidelines for the management of nausea and vomiting in patients with advanced cancer. *Support Care Cancer.* 2006;14(4):348–353.
38. Gupta M, Davis M, LeGrand S, et al. Nausea and vomiting in advanced cancer: the Cleveland Clinic protocol. *J Support Oncol.* 2013;11(1):8–13.
39. Naeim A, Dy SM, Lorenz KA, et al. Evidence-based recommendations for cancer nausea and vomiting. *J Clin Oncol.* 2008;26(23):3903–3910.
40. dos Santos LV, Souza FH, Brunetto AT, et al. Neurokinin-1 receptor antagonists for chemotherapy-induced nausea and vomiting: a systematic review. *J Natl Cancer Inst.* 2012;104(17):1280–1292.
41. Hardy JR, O'Shea A, White C, et al. The efficacy of haloperidol in the management of nausea and vomiting in patients with cancer. *J Pain Symptom Manag.* 2010;40(1):111–116.
42. Aapro MS, Molassiotis A, Olver I. Anticipatory nausea and vomiting. *Support Care Cancer.* 2005;13(2):117–121.
43. Davis MP, Hallerberg G; Palliative Medicine Study Group of the Multinational Association of Supportive Care in Cancer. A systematic review of the treatment of nausea and/or vomiting in cancer unrelated to chemotherapy or radiation. *J Pain Symptom Manag.* 2010;39(4):756–767.
44. Smith EM, Jayson GC. The current and future management of malignant ascites. *Clin Oncol.* 2003;15(2):59–72.
45. Ripamonti C, Bruera E. Palliative management of malignant bowel obstruction. *Int J Gynecol Cancer.* 2002;12(2):135–143.
46. Beesley V, Janda M, Eakin E, et al. Lymphedema after gynecological cancer treatment: prevalence, correlates, and supportive care needs. *Cancer.* 2007;109(12):2607–2614.
47. Kim JH, Dougherty PM, Abdi S. Basic science and clinical management of painful and non-painful chemotherapy-related neuropathy. *Gynecol Oncol.* 2015;136(3):453–459.
48. Saif MW, Syrigos K, Kaley K, et al. Role of pregabalin in treatment of oxaliplatin-induced sensory neuropathy. *Anticancer Res.* 2010;30(7):2927–2933.
49. Rao RD, Michalak JC, Sloan JA, et al. Efficacy of gabapentin in the management of chemotherapy-induced peripheral neuropathy: a phase 3 randomized, double-blind, placebo-controlled, crossover trial (N00C3). *Cancer.* 2007;110(9):2110–2118.
50. Smith EM, Pang H, Cirrincione C, et al. Effect of duloxetine on pain, function, and quality of life among patients with chemotherapy-induced painful peripheral neuropathy: a randomized clinical trial. *JAMA.* 2013;309(13):1359–1367.
51. Centers for Medicare and Medicaid Services. http://www.cms.gov/Medicare/Quality-Initiatives-Patient-Assessment-Instruments/Hospice-Quality-Reporting/Current-Measures.html. Accessed January 9, 2016.
52. Thomas J, Karver S, Cooney GA, et al. Methylnaltrexone for opioid-induced constipation in advanced illness. *N Engl J Med.* 2008;358(22):2332–2343.
53. Lawrence DP, Kupelnick B, Miller K, et al. Evidence report on the occurrence, assessment, and treatment of fatigue in cancer patients. *J Natl Cancer Inst Monogr.* 2004(32):40–50.
54. Bower JE. Cancer-related fatigue-mechanisms, risk factors, and treatments. *Nat Rev Clin Oncol.* 2014;11(10):597–609.
55. Bower JE, Ganz PA, Desmond KA, et al. Fatigue in long-term breast carcinoma survivors: a longitudinal investigation. *Cancer.* 2006;106(4):751–758.
56. Servaes P, Gielissen MF, Verhagen S, et al. The course of severe fatigue in disease-free breast cancer patients: a longitudinal study. *Psychooncology.* 2007;16(9):787–795.
57. Wang XS, Woodruff JF. Cancer-related and treatment-related fatigue. *Gynecol Oncol.* 2015;136(3):446–452.
58. Price MA, Bell ML, Sommeijer DW, et al. Physical symptoms, coping styles and quality of life in recurrent ovarian cancer: a prospective population-based study over the last year of life. *Gynecol Oncol.* 2013;130(1):162–168.
59. Kim YJ, Munsell MF, Park JC, et al. Retrospective review of symptoms and palliative care interventions in women with advanced cervical cancer. *Gynecol Oncol.* 2015;139(3):553–558.
60. Mucke M, Mochamat, Cuhls H, et al. Pharmacological treatments for fatigue associated with palliative care. *Cochrane Database Syst Rev.* 2015;5:CD006788.
61. Meneses-Echavez JF, Gonzalez-Jimenez E, Ramirez-Velez R. Effects of supervised multimodal exercise interventions on cancer-related fatigue: systematic review and meta-analysis of randomized controlled trials. *Biomed Res Int.* 2015;2015:328636.
62. Hope JM, Pothuri B. The role of palliative surgery in gynecologic cancer cases. *Oncologist.* 2013;18(1):73–79.
63. Fearon K, Strasser F, Anker SD, et al. Definition and classification of cancer cachexia: an international consensus. *Lancet Oncol.* 2011;12(5):489–495.
64. Tucker RO, Nichols AC. *UNIPAC 4. Managing Nonpain Symptoms.* Glenview, IL: American Academy of Hospice & Palliative Medicine; 2012.
65. Mantovani G, Maccio A, Madeddu C, et al. Randomized phase III clinical trial of five different arms of treatment in 332 patients with cancer cachexia. *Oncologist.* 2010;15(2):200–211.
66. Viola R, Kiteley C, Lloyd NS, et al. The management of dyspnea in cancer patients: a systematic review. *Support Care Cancer.* 2008;16(4):329–337.
67. Dudgeon DJ, Kristjanson L, Sloan JA, et al. Dyspnea in cancer patients: prevalence and associated factors. *J Pain Symptom Manag.* 2001;21(2):95–102.
68. Jennings AL, Davies AN, Higgins JP, et al. A systematic review of the use of opioids in the management of dyspnoea. *Thorax.* 2002;57(11):939–944.
69. Light RW, Muro JR, Sato RI, et al. Effects of oral morphine on breathlessness and exercise tolerance in patients with chronic obstructive pulmonary disease. *Am Rev Respir Dis.* 1989;139(1):126–133.
70. Casarett DJ, Inouye SK; American College of Physicians-American Society of Internal Medicine End-of-Life Care Consensus Panel. Diagnosis and management of delirium near the end of life. *Ann Intern Med.* 2001;135(1):32–40.
71. Breitbart W, Alici Y. Evidence-based treatment of delirium in patients with cancer. *J Clin Oncol.* 2012;30(11):1206–1214.
72. Irwin SA, Pirrello RD, Hirst JM, et al. Clarifying delirium management: practical, evidenced-based, expert recommendations for clinical practice. *J Palliat Med.* 2013;16(4):423–435.
73. Gagnon B, Low G, Schreier G. Methylphenidate hydrochloride improves cognitive function in patients with advanced cancer and hypoactive delirium: a prospective clinical study. *J Psychiatry Neurosci.* 2005;30(2):100–107.
74. Fisch MJ, Zhao F, Manola J, et al. Patterns and predictors of antidepressant use in ambulatory cancer patients with common solid tumors. *Psychooncology.* 2015;24(5):523–532.
75. Ell K, Sanchez K, Vourlekis B, et al. Depression, correlates of depression, and receipt of depression care among low-income women with breast or gynecologic cancer. *J Clin Oncol.* 2005;23(13):3052–3060.
76. Periyakoil VS. Differentiating grief and depression in patients who are seriously ill. *Am Fam Physician.* 2012;86(3):232, 234.
77. Mitchell AJ. Are one or two simple questions sufficient to detect depression in cancer and palliative care? A Bayesian meta-analysis. *Br J Cancer.* 2008;98(12):1934–1943.
78. Gartlehner G, Hansen RA, Morgan LC, et al. Comparative benefits and harms of second-generation antidepressants for treating major depressive disorder: an updated meta-analysis. *Ann Intern Med.* 2011;155(11):772–785.
79. Traeger L, Greer JA, Fernandez-Robles C, et al. Evidence-based treatment of anxiety in patients with cancer. *J Clin Oncol.* 2012;30(11):1197–1205.
80. Leon-Pizarro C, Gich I, Barthe E, et al. A randomized trial of the effect of training in relaxation and guided imagery techniques in improving psychological and quality-of-life indices for gynecologic and breast brachytherapy patients. *Psychooncology.* 2007;16(11):971–979.
81. Petersen RW, Quinlivan JA. Preventing anxiety and depression in gynaecological cancer: a randomised controlled trial. *BJOG.* 2002;109(4):386–394.

82. Moorey S, Cort E, Kapari M, et al. A cluster randomized controlled trial of cognitive behaviour therapy for common mental disorders in patients with advanced cancer. *Psychol Med.* 2009;39(5):713–723.
83. Speca M, Carlson LE, Goodey E, et al. A randomized, wait-list controlled clinical trial: the effect of a mindfulness meditation-based stress reduction program on mood and symptoms of stress in cancer outpatients. *Psychosom Med.* 2000;62(5):613–622.
84. Clegg A, Young JB. Which medications to avoid in people at risk of delirium: a systematic review. *Age Ageing.* 2011;40(1):23–29.
85. Goodman DC, Morden NE, Chang CH, et al. In: Bronner KK, ed. *Trends in Cancer Care Near the End of Life: A Dartmouth Atlas of Health Care Brief.* Lebanon, NH: The Dartmouth Institute for Health Policy & Clinical Practices; 2013. http://www.dartmouthatlas.org/downloads/reports/Cancer_brief_090413.pdf
86. Hui D, Dos Santos R, Chisholm G, et al. Bedside clinical signs associated with impending death in patients with advanced cancer: preliminary findings of a prospective, longitudinal cohort study. *Cancer.* 2015;121(6):960–967.
87. Spoozak L, Seow H, Liu Y, et al. Performance status and symptom scores of women with gynecologic cancer at the end of life. *Int J Gynecol Cancer.* 2013;23(5):971–978.
88. Fallowfield L, Jenkins V. Communicating sad, bad, and difficult news in medicine. *Lancet.* 2004;363(9405):312–319.
89. Back AL, Arnold RM, Tulsky JA, et al. Teaching communication skills to medical oncology fellows. *J Clin Oncol.* 2003;21(12):2433–2436.
90. Baile WF. *Practice Guidelines for Patient/Physician Communication: Breaking Bad News, Version 1.01.* Rockledge, PA: National Comprehensive Cancer Network; 2000.
91. Baile WF, Buckman R, Lenzi R, et al. SPIKES—A six-step protocol for delivering bad news: application to the patient with cancer. *Oncologist.* 2000;5(4):302–311.
92. Wright AA, Zhang B, Ray A, et al. Associations between end-of-life discussions, patient mental health, medical care near death, and caregiver bereavement adjustment. *JAMA.* 2008;300(14):1665–1673.
93. Weeks JC, Catalano PJ, Cronin A, et al. Patients' expectations about effects of chemotherapy for advanced cancer. *N Engl J Med.* 2012;367(17):1616–1625.
94. Curtis JR, Burt RA. Why are critical care clinicians so powerfully distressed by family demands for futile care? *J Crit Care.* 2003;18(1):22–24.
95. Mack JW, Smith TJ. Reasons why physicians do not have discussions about poor prognosis, why it matters, and what can be improved. *J Clin Oncol.* 2012;30(22):2715–2717.
96. The AM, Hak T, Koeter G, et al. Collusion in doctor–patient communication about imminent death: an ethnographic study. *West J Med.* 2001;174(4):247–253.
97. Jackson VA, Mack J, Matsuyama R, et al. A qualitative study of oncologists' approaches to end-of-life care. *J Palliat Med.* 2008;11(6):893–906.
98. Helft PR. Necessary collusion: prognostic communication with advanced cancer patients. *J Clin Oncol.* 2005;23(13):3146–3150.
99. Parker SM, Clayton JM, Hancock K, et al. A systematic review of prognostic/end-of-life communication with adults in the advanced stages of a life-limiting illness: patient/caregiver preferences for the content, style, and timing of information. *J Pain Symptom Manag.* 2007;34(1):81–93.
100. Fried TR, Bradley EH, O'Leary J. Prognosis communication in serious illness: perceptions of older patients, caregivers, and clinicians. *J Am Geriatr Soc.* 2003;51(10):1398–1403.
101. Zier LS, Sottile PD, Hong SY, et al. Surrogate decision makers' interpretation of prognostic information: a mixed-methods study. *Ann Intern Med.* 2012;156(5):360–366.
102. Murray SA, Kendall M, Boyd K, et al. Illness trajectories and palliative care. *BMJ.* 2005;330(7498):1007–1011.
103. Kutner JS, Steiner JF, Corbett KK, et al. Information needs in terminal illness. *Soc Sci Med.* 1999;48(10):1341–1352.
104. Lunney JR, Lynn J, Foley DJ, et al. Patterns of functional decline at the end of life. *JAMA.* 2003;289(18):2387–2392.
105. Enzinger AC, Zhang B, Schrag D, et al. Outcomes of prognostic disclosure: associations with prognostic understanding, distress, and relationship with physician among patients with advanced cancer. *J Clin Oncol.* 2015;33(32):3809–3816.
106. Reisfield GM, Wallace SK, Munsell MF, et al. Survival in cancer patients undergoing in-hospital cardiopulmonary resuscitation: a meta-analysis. *Resuscitation.* 2006;71(2):152–160.
107. Volandes AE, Levin TT, Slovin S, et al. Augmenting advance care planning in poor prognosis cancer with a video decision aid: a preintervention-postintervention study. *Cancer.* 2012;118(17):4331–4338.
108. Volandes AE, Paasche-Orlow MK, Mitchell SL, et al. Randomized controlled trial of a video decision support tool for cardiopulmonary resuscitation decision making in advanced cancer. *J Clin Oncol.* 2013;31(3):380–386.
109. Diaz-Montes TP, Johnson MK, Giuntoli RL II, et al. Importance and timing of end-of-life care discussions among gynecologic oncology patients. *Am J Hosp Palliat Care.* 2013;30(1):59–67.
110. Epstein AS, Shuk E, O'Reilly EM, et al. 'We have to discuss it': cancer patients' advance care planning impressions following educational information about cardiopulmonary resuscitation. *Psychooncology.* 2015;24(12):1767–1773.
111. Ozanne EM, Partridge A, Moy B, et al. Doctor–patient communication about advance directives in metastatic breast cancer. *J Palliat Med.* 2009;12(6):547–553.
112. Sharma RK, Dy SM. Documentation of information and care planning for patients with advanced cancer: associations with patient characteristics and utilization of hospital care. *Am J Hosp Palliat Care.* 2011;28(8):543–549.
113. El-Sahwi KS, Illuzzi J, Varughese J, et al. A survey of gynecologic oncologists regarding the end-of-life discussion: a pilot study. *Gynecol Oncol.* 2012;124(3):471–473.
114. Clark MA, Ott M, Rogers ML, et al. Advance care planning as a shared endeavor: completion of ACP documents in a multidisciplinary cancer program. *Psychooncology.* 2015. Epub October 21, 2015.
115. Johnson S, Butow P, Kerridge I, et al. Advance care planning for cancer patients: a systematic review of perceptions and experiences of patients, families, and healthcare providers. *Psychooncology.* 2016;25(4):362–386.
116. Hudson PL, Girgis A, Mitchell GK, et al. Benefits and resource implications of family meetings for hospitalized palliative care patients: research protocol. *BMC Palliat Care.* 2015;14(1):73.
117. Yennurajalingam S, Dev R, Lockey M, et al. Characteristics of family conferences in a palliative care unit at a comprehensive cancer center. *J Palliat Med.* 2008;11(9):1208–1211.
118. Pollak KI, Arnold RM, Jeffreys AS, et al. Oncologist communication about emotion during visits with patients with advanced cancer. *J Clin Oncol.* 2007;25(36):5748–5752.
119. Tulsky JA, Arnold RM, Alexander SC, et al. Enhancing communication between oncologists and patients with a computer-based training program: a randomized trial. *Ann Intern Med.* 2011;155(9):593–601.
120. Le T, Leis A, Pahwa P, et al. Quality-of-life issues in patients with ovarian cancer and their caregivers: a review. *Obstet Gynecol Survey.* 2003;58(11):749–758.
121. Butow PN, Price MA, Bell ML, et al. Caring for women with ovarian cancer in the last year of life: a longitudinal study of caregiver quality of life, distress and unmet needs. *Gynecol Oncol.* 2014;132(3):690–697.
122. Beesley VL, Price MA, Webb PM, et al. Loss of lifestyle: health behaviour and weight changes after becoming a caregiver of a family member diagnosed with ovarian cancer. *Support Care Cancer.* 2011;19(12):1949–1956.
123. Pitceathly C, Maguire P. The psychological impact of cancer on patients' partners and other key relatives: a review. *Eur J Cancer.* 2003;39(11):1517–1524.
124. WHOQOL Measuring Quality of Life. http://www.who.int/mental_health/media/68.pdf. Accessed January 31, 2016.
125. Cella DF, Tulsky DS, Gray G, et al. The Functional Assessment of Cancer Therapy scale: development and validation of the general measure. *J Clin Oncol.* 1993;11(3):570–579.
126. Earle CC, Park ER, Lai B, et al. Identifying potential indicators of the quality of end-of-life cancer care from administrative data. *J Clin Oncol.* 2003;21(6):1133–1138.
127. Nevadunsky NS, Gordon S, Spoozak L, et al. The role and timing of palliative medicine consultation for women with gynecologic malignancies: association with end of life interventions and direct hospital costs. *Gynecol Oncol.* 2014;132(1):3–7.
128. Nevadunsky NS, Spoozak L, Gordon S, et al. End-of-life care of women with gynecologic malignancies: a pilot study. *Int J Gynecol Cancer.* 2013;23(3):546–552.
129. Ellis LM, Bernstein DS, Voest EE, et al. American Society of Clinical Oncology perspective: raising the bar for clinical trials by defining clinically meaningful outcomes. *J Clin Oncol.* 2014;32(12):1277–1280.
130. Minion LE, Coleman RL, Alvarez RD, et al. Endpoints in clinical trials: what do patients consider important? A survey of the Ovarian Cancer National Alliance. *Gynecol Oncol.* 2016;140(2):193–198.
131. Havrilesky LJ, Alvarez Secord A, Ehrisman JA, et al. Patient preferences in advanced or recurrent ovarian cancer. *Cancer.* 2014;120(23):3651–3659.
132. Penson RT, Huang HQ, Wenzel LB, et al. Bevacizumab for advanced cervical cancer: patient-reported outcomes of a randomised, phase 3 trial (NRG Oncology-Gynecologic Oncology Group protocol 240). *Lancet Oncol.* 2015;16(3):301–311.

133. Armstrong DK, Bundy B, Wenzel L, et al. Intraperitoneal cisplatin and paclitaxel in ovarian cancer. *N Engl J Med.* 2006;354(1):34–43.
134. Wenzel L, Huang HQ, Monk BJ, et al. Quality-of-life comparisons in a randomized trial of interval secondary cytoreduction in advanced ovarian carcinoma: a Gynecologic Oncology Group Study. *J Clin Oncol.* 2005;23(24):5605–5612.
135. Mutch DG, Orlando M, Goss T, et al. Randomized phase III trial of gemcitabine compared with pegylated liposomal doxorubicin in patients with platinum-resistant ovarian cancer. *J Clin Oncol.* 2007;25(19):2811–2818.
136. Wenzel LB, Huang HQ, Armstrong DK, et al. Health-related quality of life during and after intraperitoneal versus intravenous chemotherapy for optimally debulked ovarian cancer: a Gynecologic Oncology Group Study. *J Clin Oncol.* 2007;25(4):437–443.
137. Pujade-Lauraine E, Wagner U, Aavall-Lundqvist E, et al. Pegylated liposomal Doxorubicin and Carboplatin compared with Paclitaxel and Carboplatin for patients with platinum-sensitive ovarian cancer in late relapse. *J Clin Oncol.* 2010;28(20):3323–3329.
138. Dumanovsky T, Augustin R, Rogers M, et al. The growth of palliative care in U.S. hospitals: a status report. *J Palliat Med.* 2016;19(1):8–15.
139. Institute of Medicine. *Dying in America: Improving Quality and Honoring Individual Preferences Near the End of Life.* Washington, DC: National Academies Press; 2014. https://iom.nationalacademies.org/~/media/Files/Report%20Files/2014/EOL/Report%20Brief.pdf. Accessed January 16 2015.
140. Partridge AH, Seah DS, King T, et al. Developing a service model that integrates palliative care throughout cancer care: the time is now. *J Clin Oncol.* 2014;32(29):3330–3336.
141. America's Care of Serious Illness. 2015 state-by-state report card on access to palliative care in our nation's hospitals 2015. https://reportcard.capc.org/wp-content/uploads/2015/08/CAPC-Report-Card-2015.pdf. Accessed December 25, 2015.
142. Eskander RN, Osann K, Dickson E, et al. Assessment of palliative care training in gynecologic oncology: a gynecologic oncology fellow research network study. *Gynecol Oncol.* 2014;134(2):379–384.
143. Lesnock JL, Arnold RM, Meyn LA, et al. Palliative care education in gynecologic oncology: a survey of the fellows. *Gynecol Oncol.* 2013;130(3):431–435.
144. Lefkowits C, Sukumvanich P, Claxton R, et al. Needs assessment of palliative care education in gynecologic oncology fellowship: we're not teaching what we think is most important. *Gynecol Oncol.* 2014;135(2):255–260.
145. 10 FAQs: Medicare's Role in End-of-Life Care. November 5, 2015. http://kff.org/medicare/fact-sheet/10-faqs-medicares-role-in-end-of-life-care/. Accessed December 25, 2015.
146. Lopez-Acevedo M, Lowery WJ, Lowery AW, et al. Palliative and hospice care in gynecologic cancer: a review. *Gynecol Oncol.* 2013;131(1):215–221.
147. Bernacki RE, Ko DN, Higgins P, et al. Improving access to palliative care through an innovative quality improvement initiative: an opportunity for pay-for-performance. *J Palliat Med.* 2012;15(2):192–199.
148. McInturff B, Harrington E. 2011 Public opinion research on palliative care: a report based on research by public opinion strategies. Center to Advance Palliative Care, American Cancer Society and the American Cancer Society Action Network. https://media.capc.org/filer_public/18/ab/18ab708c-f835-4380-921d-fbf729702e36/2011-public-opinion-research-on-palliative-care.pdf. Accessed September 23, 2016.
149. Schenker Y, Crowley-Matoka M, Dohan D, et al. Oncologist factors that influence referrals to subspecialty palliative care clinics. *J Oncol Pract.* 2014;10(2):e37–e44.
150. Dalal S, Palla S, Hui D, et al. Association between a name change from palliative to supportive care and the timing of patient referrals at a comprehensive cancer center. *Oncologist.* 2011;16(1):105–111.
151. Yennurajalingam S, Parsons HA, Duarte ER, et al. Decisional control preferences of Hispanic patients with advanced cancer from the United States and Latin America. *J Pain Symptom Manag.* 2013;46(3):376–385.
152. Kaiser Family Foundation. Kaiser Health Tracking Poll: March 2013. http://kff.org/health-reform/poll-finding/march-2013-tracking-poll. Accessed December 25, 2015.
153. Lefkowits C, Binstock AB, Courtney-Brooks M, et al. Predictors of palliative care consultation on an inpatient gynecologic oncology service: are we following ASCO recommendations? *Gynecol Oncol.* 2014;133(2):319–325.

Index

Note: Page numbers followed by *f* indicate figures; those followed by *t* indicate tables.

B

C

I

M

O

P

Q

R

T